OPERATIVE TECHNIQUES IN ORTHOPAEDIC SURGERY

Third Edition

VOLUME FOUR

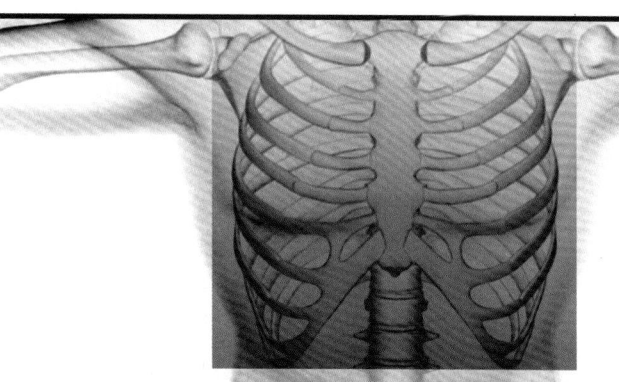

OPERATIVE TECHNIQUES IN ORTHOPAEDIC SURGERY

Third Edition

VOLUME FOUR

EDITORS-IN-CHIEF

Sam W. Wiesel, MD

Chairman and Professor
Department of Orthopaedic Surgery
Georgetown University Medical School
Washington, District of Columbia

Todd J. Albert, MD

Surgeon in Chief Emeritus
Hospital for Special Surgery
Professor of Orthopaedics
Weill Cornell Medical College
New York, New York

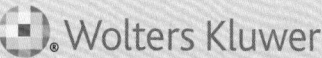

Philadelphia • Baltimore • New York • London
Buenos Aires • Hong Kong • Sydney • Tokyo

Director, Medical Practice: Brian Brown
Senior Development Editor: Stacey Sebring
Marketing Manager: Phyllis Hitner
Production Project Manager: Bridgett Dougherty
Design Coordinator: Steve Druding
Manufacturing Coordinator: Beth Welsh
Prepress Vendor: Absolute Service, Inc.

3rd edition

9 8 7 6 5 4 3 2 1

Printed in China

Library of Congress Cataloging-in-Publication Data

Names: Wiesel, Sam W., editor. | Albert, Todd J., editor.
Title: Operative techniques in orthopaedic surgery / editors in-chief, Sam
   W. Wiesel, Todd J. Albert.
Description: Third edition. | Philadelphia : Wolters Kluwer, 2022. |
   Includes bibliographical references and index.
Identifiers: LCCN 2020057251 | ISBN 9781975145071 hardcover | ISBN
   9781975145088 (epub) | ISBN 9781975145095
Subjects: MESH: Orthopedic Procedures—methods
Classification: LCC RD755 | NLM WE 168 | DDC 617.9—dc23
LC record available at https://lccn.loc.gov/2020057251

EDITORS-IN-CHIEF – DEDICATIONS

We would like to dedicate this Volume to the memory of Richard H. Rothman, MD, PhD whose guidance and mentorship is responsible for our success and that of generations of orthopaedic surgeons. That influence also has led to improvements in the lives of thousands of his patients and those of his orthopaedic offspring.

SAM W. WIESEL, MD AND TODD J. ALBERT, MD

January 5, 2021

DEDICATION

To our wives, Robin, Nancy, Katie, and Vesta, and our children, Mark and Alexis, Chelsea, Alex and Julia, Annie and Sam, and Yara and Noora. We also dedicate this book to Richard H. Rothman and John M Fenlin Jr.—two legends in the field of orthopaedics who had profound influence over our careers and will be missed.

—GRW, MLR, BBW, AND SN

This book is dedicated with enormous love to my extraordinary and inspiring wife, Shelly,
who supported me and raised our four darling children while I did what I did.
My heartfelt wish is that these pages will help to bring at least a small ray of clarity and hope to the reader.

—JB

To my two amazing children, Kai and Lexi, for being so loving, inquisitive, and full of laughter.
You'll always be my inspiration.

—JIH

I dedicate my work on this textbook to all those hardworking surgeons who use these techniques to care for the children.
I would like to thank my wife, Mary, and children, Erin, Colleen, John, and Kelly, for their tolerance of Dad's "homework."
I would also like to thank my orthopaedic mentors for inspiring me to go beyond clinical care and work to contribute to the field through teaching, research, and orthopaedic leadership.

—JMF

For Marcia: thank you for being the most amazing, giving, loving person I know and supporting me through this and every other endeavor. For Julia and James: thank you for growing into the amazing people you are becoming—I could not be more proud. For the Lord Jesus: thank you for these good and perfect gifts.

—JMR

The Sports Medicine section of this wonderful text is dedicated to athletes of all ages, abilities, and levels. It is an honor and a pleasure to treat these special patients. And I encourage all readers to embrace the concept of lifelong learning!

—MDM

To my parents, Dennis and Barbara, who supported my pursuit of a career in orthopaedic surgery; to my wife, Mary, and my children, Ford, Ben, and Charlotte, who tolerated my time spent on this educational endeavor; to all of the contributing foot and ankle educators for sharing their expertise so that providers worldwide may optimize their patient care.

—MEE

To Drs. Kenneth Francis, Ralph Marcove, and William F. Enneking, three great innovators, pioneers, developers, and critical thinkers in the field of orthopaedic oncology. I had the privilege to work with all these great doctors and I dedicate my work on this project to these world class surgeons. Additionally, the love and support of my wife, Jane, and children, Alison and Eric, enabled me to fully pursue, to the highest degree, all these academic and surgical aspirations. Without their support, this compendium would not have been possible.

—MMM

To my mother, Phyllis, who found the best in people, had compassion for all, and whose insight, guidance, and love have always made me believe that anything is possible.

—PT3

I'd like to dedicate this work to my wife Mary, for allowing me the flexibility to maintain an academic career, and to our four daughters training to be future Orthopaedic Surgeons—Lauren, Stephanie, Allison, and Susanne—who will hopefully learn from this text and eventually contribute to making it better in the future for all those that have the privilege of being in the field of Orthopaedics and having the opportunity to give patients their lives back.

—SDB

For my mother: her intelligence, passion for discovery, and goal-directed perfectionism motivated me.
For my father: his love of life, concern for others, and pureness of heart balanced me.
For both: their unending love, pride, and support of me made everything worthwhile.

—TRH

To my parents, Arundhati and Gowri. I know that I don't thank you nearly enough for the herculean effort that it took to raise someone like me. As a father of three now, I have a greater appreciation for the sacrifices that parents make for their children. I love you both and am so grateful for all that you've done for me.

—WNS

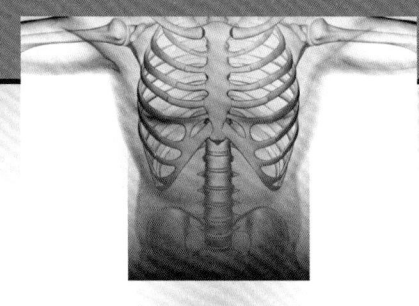

Editorial Board

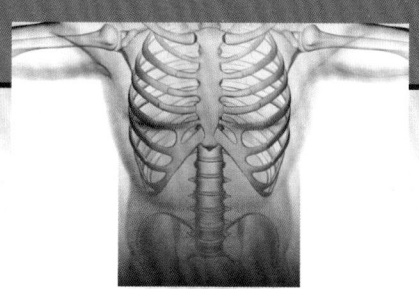

Contents

VOLUME 2

PART 4 PEDIATRICS

SECTION I Trauma

VOLUME 4

PART 8 FOOT AND ANKLE

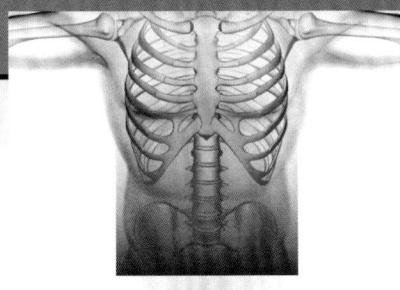

Contributors

PART 8 Foot and Ankle

Jorge I. Acevedo, MD
Director, Foot and Ankle Center of Excellence
Southeast Orthopedic Specialists
Jacksonville, Florida

Samuel B. Adams, MD
Associate Residency Program Director
Director of Foot and Ankle Research
Associate Professor
Department of Orthopaedic Surgery
Duke University Medical Center
Durham, North Carolina

Robert S. Adelaar, MD
Department of Orthopedics
Medical College of Virginia
Virginia Commonwealth University
West Hospital
Richmond, Virginia

Rocco Aicale, MD
Orthopaedic Resident Doctor
Clinica Ortopedica
Università degli Studi di Salerno
Salerno, Italy

Craig C. Akoh, MD
Fellow
Department of Surgery
Duke University Hospital
Durham, North Carolina

Annunziato Amendola, MD
Professor of Orthopaedic Surgery
Chief, Division of Sports Medicine
Duke University
Durham, North Carolina

Kamil M. Amer, MD
Resident
Department of Orthopaedics
Rutgers New Jersey Medical School
Clifton, New Jersey

John G. Anderson, MD
Codirector, Assistant Program Director,
  Associate Professor
Department of Orthopaedic Surgery
Orthopaedic Associates of Michigan
Grand Rapids, Michigan

Robert B. Anderson, MD
Director, Foot and Ankle
Titletown Sports Medicine and Orthopedics
Associate Team Physician, Green Bay Packers
Green Bay, Wisconsin

Michael S. Aronow, MD
Clinical Professor
Department of Orthopaedic Surgery
University of Connecticut School of Medicine
Orthopedic Associates of Hartford
Hartford, Connecticut

Mathieu Assal
Chief, Foot and Ankle Service
Université of Genève
Clinique La Colline
Geneva, Switzerland

Jonathon D. Backus, MD
Assistant Professor
Department of Orthopaedic Surgery
Washington University in Saint Louis
St. Louis, Missouri

Heather Barske, MD, FRCSC
Assistant Professor
Foot and Ankle Surgery
University of Manitoba
Surgeon, Winnipeg Regional Health Authority
Pan Am Clinic
Winnipeg, Manitoba, Canada

Daniel Baumfeld, MD
Adjunct Professor
Department of Orthopedics
Universidade Federal de Minas Gerais
São Paulo, Brazil

Christoph Becher, MD
Assistant Professor of Orthopaedic Surgery
Medizinische Hochschule Hannover
Hannover, Germany

Thomas B. Bemenderfer, MD, MBA
Foot and Ankle Fellow
Orthopaedic Associates of Michigan
Grand Rapids, Michigan

Gregory C. Berlet, MD
Foot and Ankle Surgeon
Orthopedic Foot and Ankle Center
Worthington, Ohio

James L. Beskin, MD
Orthopedic Surgeon
Peachtree Orthopedics
Atlanta, Georgia

Eric M. Bluman, MD
Assistant Professor of Orthopaedic Surgery
Harvard Medical School
Boston, Massachusetts

Donald R. Bohay, MD
Codirector/Associate Professor
Department of Orthopaedic Surgery
Orthopaedic Associates of Michigan
Grand Rapids, Michigan

Michel Bonnin, MD, PhD
Orthopedic Surgeon
Department of Orthopedic Surgery
Centre Orthopédique Santy – Hôpital Privé
  Jean Mermoz
Lyon, France

Jonathan Bourget-Murray, MD
Chief Resident
Department of Surgery
University of Calgary Cumming School of
  Medicine
Foothills Medical Centre
Calgary, Alberta, Canada

Michael E. Brage, MD
Attending Surgeon
Department of Orthopaedics and Sports
  Medicine
University of Washington
Seattle, Washington

Lloyd C. Briggs, Jr., MD
Foot and Ankle Surgeon
Orthopaedic Institute of Ohio
Lima, Ohio

Kimberly K. Broughton, MD
Clinical Fellow in Foot and Ankle Surgery
Department of Orthopaedics
Brigham and Women's Hospital
Jamaica Plain, Massachusetts

John T. Campbell, MD
Director of Research
Department of Orthopaedic Surgery
Institute for Foot and Ankle Reconstruction
Mercy Medical Center
Baltimore, Maryland

Kristin C. Caolo, BA
Research Assistant
Foot and Ankle
Hospital for Special Surgery
New York, New York

Rebecca Cerrato, MD
Orthopedic Surgeon
Institute for Foot and Ankle Reconstruction
Mercy Medical Center
Baltimore, Maryland

Jie Chen, MD, MPH
Clinical Fellow
Department of Orthopaedic Surgery
Duke University Hospital
Chapel Hill, North Carolina

Christopher P. Chiodo, MD
Chief, Foot and Ankle Surgery Service
Department of Orthopaedic Surgery
Brigham and Women's Hospital
Jamaica Plain, Massachusetts

Michael P. Clare, MD
Orthopedic Surgeon
360 Orthopedics
Sarasota, Florida

Thomas O. Clanton, MD
Foot and Ankle Specialist
The Steadman Clinic
Vail, Colorado

J. Chris Coetzee, MD
Orthopedic Surgeon
Twin Cities Orthopedics
Edina, Minnesota

Jean-Alain Colombier, MD
Department of Orthopaedic Surgery
Clinique de L'Union
St. Jean, France

Michael J. Coughlin, MD
Chief, Coughlin Foot and Ankle Clinic
St. Alphonsus Hospital
Boise, Idaho

Justin S. Cummins, MD
Department of Orthopaedics and Sports
  Medicine
Essentia Health
Duluth, Minnesota

Tim Daniels, MD
Professor of Surgery
Department of Orthopaedic Surgery
St. Michael's Hospital
Toronto, Ontario, Canada

Hodges Davis, MD
Professor
Department of Orthopaedic Surgery
OrthoCarolina
Charlotte, North Carolina

Jonathan Day, MS
Orthopedic Surgeon
Hospital for Special Surgery
New York, New York

Richard J. de Asla, MD
Instructor in Orthopaedic Surgery
Department of Orthopaedic Surgery
Massachusetts General Hospital
Boston, Massachusetts

Jonathan T. Deland, MD
Professor
Department of Orthopedic Surgery
Weill Cornell Medical College
Orthopedic Surgeon
Foot and Ankle Service
Hospital for Special Surgery
New York, New York

Bryan D. Den Hartog, MD
Associate Professor of Orthopaedic Surgery
Sanford School of Medicine
University of South Dakota
Rapid City, South Dakota

James K. DeOrio, MD
Professor and Program Chair
Department of Orthopaedic Surgery
Duke University Hospital
Durham, North Carolina

Matthew J. DeOrio, MD
The Orthopaedic Center
Huntsville, Alabama

Benedict F. DiGiovanni, MD
Professor
Department of Orthopaedics and
  Rehabilitation
University of Rochester Medical Center
Rochester, New York

Andrew Dodd, MD, FRCSC
Clinical Lecturer
Department of Surgery
University of Calgary Cumming School of
  Medicine
Foothills Medical Centre
Calgary, Alberta, Canada

Brian Donley, MD
Professor of Surgery
Cleveland Clinic Lerner College of Medicine
Cleveland, Ohio

Mark C. Drakos, MD
Assistant Attending Orthopedic Surgeon
Sports Medicine and Foot and Ankle
Hospital for Special Surgery
New York, New York

Thomas Dreher, MD
Chief of Pediatric Orthopaedics and
  Traumatologie
University Children's Hospital Zurich
Zurich, Switzerland

Mark E. Easley, MD
Chief, Foot and Ankle Division
Department of Orthopaedic Surgery
Duke University Medical Center
Durham, North Carolina

Patrick B. Ebeling, MD
Orthopedic Surgeon
Twin Cities Orthopedics
Burnsville, Minnesota

Andrew J. Elliott, MD
Assistant Professor Orthopedics
Department of Foot and Ankle Surgery
Hospital for Special Surgery
New York, New York

Adolph S. Flemister, Jr., MD
Orthopaedic Foot and Ankle Surgeon
University of Rochester
Rochester, New York

Amanda N. Fletcher, MD, MS
Department of Orthopaedic Surgery
Duke University
Durham, North Carolina

Carol Frey, MD
Co-Director, Sports Medicine Fellowship
Departments of Orthopedic Surgery and
  Family Medicine
Los Angeles County Harbor – UCLA Medical
  Center
Manhattan Beach, California

Taggart T. Gauvain, MD
Assistant Professor
Department of Orthopaedic Surgery
University of Texas John P. and Katherine G.
  McGovern Medical School
Pearland, Texas

Alessio Giai Via, MD
Assistant
Department of Trauma and Orthopaedic
  Surgery
Ospedale Sant'Anna
San Fermo della Battaglia
Como, Italy

Brian D. Giordano, MD
Orthopaedic Surgeon
University of Rochester
Rochester, New York

Mark Glazebrook, MD
Professor of Surgery
Dalhousie University
President, Canadian Orthopedic Association
  2019–2020
Halifax, Nova Scotia, Canada

John S. Gould, MD
Professor of Surgery
Division of Orthopaedic Surgery
Chief, Foot and Ankle
University of Alabama at Birmingham
Birmingham, Alabama

Christopher E. Gross, MD
Associate Professor
Department of Orthopaedic Surgery
Medical University of South Carolina
Charleston, South Carolina

Gregory P. Guyton, MD
Chief, Foot and Ankle Service
Department of Orthopaedic Surgery
MedStar Union Memorial Hospital
Baltimore, Maryland

Kamran Hamid, MD
Assistant Professor
Loyola University Medical Center
Chicago, Illinois

Paul Hamilton, MBBS, FRCS(Tr&Orth)
Consultant Orthopaedic Surgeon
Department of Trauma and Orthopaedics
Epsom and Saint Helier University Hospitals
 NHS Trust
Epsom, United Kingdom

Thomas G. Harris, MD
Faculty
Department of Orthopaedic Surgery
Los Angeles County Harbor – UCLA Medical
 Center
Torrance, California

Paul J. Hecht, MD
Associate Professor of Orthopaedic Surgery
Geisel School of Medicine
Dartmouth College
Hanover, New Hampshire

Beat Hintermann, MD
Chairman, Clinic of Orthopaedics and
 Traumatology
Kantonsspital Baselland
Associate Professor
University of Basel
Basel, Switzerland

Stefan G. Hofstaetter, MD
Department of Orthopaedics
Klinikum Wels-Grieskirchen
Wels, Austria

Amanda M. Holleran, MD
Fellow
Department of Orthopaedics
University of Rochester Medical Center
Rochester, New York

George B. Holmes, Jr., MD
Professor
Department of Orthopaedic Surgery
Rush University Medical Center
Chicago, Illinois

Andrew Hsu, MD
Assistant Clinical Professor
Department of Orthopaedics
UCI Health
Orange, California

Jeannie Huh, MD
San Antonio Military Medical Center
Department of Orthopaedics and
 Rehabilitation
Assistant Professor of Surgery
Uniformed Services University of the Health
 Sciences
San Antonio, Texas

Joshua G. Hunter, MD
Orthopedic Surgeon
Steward Orthopedic and Sports Medicine
 Center
Salt Lake City, Utah

Jason M. Hurst, MD
Associate Partner
Joint Implant Surgeons, Inc.
New Albany, Ohio

James J. Hutson, Jr., MD
Professor Emeritus of Orthopedic Trauma
 Surgery
Miller School of Medicine University of
 Miami
Flat Rock, North Carolina

Christopher F. Hyer, DPM
Foot and Ankle Surgeon
Orthopedic Foot and Ankle Center
Worthington, Ohio

James R. Jastifer, MD
Clinical Assistant Professor
Department of Orthopaedic Surgery
Western Michigan University Homer Stryker
 MD School of Medicine
Kalamazoo, Michigan

A. Holly Johnson, MD
Orthopedic Surgeon
Hospital for Special Surgery
New York, New York

Catherine E. Johnson, MD
Orthopaedic Surgeon
Foot and Ankle Specialists
Baton Rouge Orthopaedic Clinic
Baton Rouge, Louisiana

Jeffrey E. Johnson, MD
Professor
Department of Orthopaedic Surgery
Washington University in Saint Louis
St. Louis, Missouri

Thierry Judet, MD
Chief
Department of Orthopedics
Hôpital Raymond Poincaré
Garches, France

Rishin J. Kadakia, MD
Assistant Professor
Emory University Medical Center
Atlanta, Georgia

Cambre N. Kelly, PhD
Department of Biomedical Engineering
Duke University
Durham, North Carolina

John G. Kennedy, MD
Professor
Department of Orthopedic Surgery
NYU Langone Health
New York, New York

Kevin L. Kirk, DO
Orthopaedic Surgeon
Burkhart Research Institute for Orthopaedics
Department of Orthopaedic Surgery
San Antonio Orthopaedic Group
San Antonio, Texas

Markus Knupp, MD
Head of the Institute
Foot and Ankle Department
Mein Fusszentrum
Basel, Switzerland

Sahil Kooner, MD, FRCSC
Fellow
Department of Orthopaedic Surgery
University of Toronto
Toronto, Ontario, Canada

Sameh A. Labib, MD
Professor
Department of Surgery
Emory University School of Medicine
Atlanta, Georgia

Jeremy M. LaMothe, MD, PhD, FRCSC
Orthopaedic Surgeon
University of Calgary Cumming School of
 Medicine
Calgary, Alberta, Canada

Travis M. Langan, DPM
Surgeon
Orthopedics and Sports Medicine
Carle Foundation Hospital
Champaign, Illinois

Jean Langlois, MD, PhD
Orthopedic Surgeon
Department of Orthopedic Surgery
Centre Orthopédique Santy – Hôpital Privé
 Jean Mermoz
Lyon, France

Johnny T.C. Lau, MD, FRCSC
Assistant Professor
Department of Surgery
University of Toronto
Toronto, Ontario, Canada

Ian L. D. Le, MD, FRCSC
Clinical Assistant Professor
Department of Surgery
University of Calgary Cumming School of
 Medicine
Foothills Medical Centre
Calgary, Alberta, Canada

Simon Lee, MD
Assistant Professor
Department of Orthopaedic Surgery
Rush University Medical Center
Chicago, Illinois

Anna-Kathrin Leucht, MD
Foot and Ankle Fellow
Department of Orthopaedics
University of British Columbia
Footbridge Clinic
Vancouver, British Columbia, Canada

David S. Levine, MD
Orthopedic Surgeon
Hospital for Special Surgery
Assistant Professor of Orthopedic Surgery
Weill Cornell Medical College
New York, New York

Robert B. Lewis, MD
Orthopedic Surgeon
Midcoast Hospital
Brunswick, Maine

Sheldon Lin, MD
Department of Orthopaedics
Rutgers New Jersey Medical School
Newark, New Jersey

Nicola Maffulli, MD, MS, PhD, FRCP, FRCS(Orth)
Professor and Chair
Trauma and Orthopaedic Surgery
Università degli Studi di Salerno
Baronissi, Campania, Italy

Peter Mangone, MD
Orthopaedic Surgeon
Blue Ridge Bone and Joint, Division of
 EmergeOrtho
Co-Director Foot and Ankle Center of
 Excellence
Volunteer Clinical Instructor
MAHEC Residency and Fellowship
 Programs
Asheville, North Carolina

Jared M. Maker, DPM
Orthopedic and Sports Medicine Surgeon
Carle Foundation Hospital
Champaign, Illinois

Jeffrey A. Mann, MD
Private Practice
Oakland, California

Roger A. Mann, MD
Clinical Professor of Orthopaedic Surgery
University of California
Oakland, California

Richard M. Marks, MD
Southeastern Orthopaedics and Sports
 Medicine
West Columbia, South Carolina

Andrew Marsh, MD, MSc, FRCSC
Fellow
Department of Orthopaedic Surgery
University of Toronto
Toronto, Ontario, Canada

William C. McGarvey, MD
Professor
Department of Orthopaedic Surgery
McGovern Medical School
University of Texas Health Science Center
Houston, Texas

Ronan McKeown, MD, FRCSI(Tr&Orth), MFSEM
Lead Clinician Orthopaedic Surgery
Southern Trust
County Armagh, Ireland

Marc Merian-Genast, MD
Praxis für Fuss- und Sprunggelenkschirurgie
Münchenstein, Switzerland

Stuart D. Miller
Assistant Professor
Department of Orthopaedic Surgery
Johns Hopkins University School of Medicine
MedStar Union Memorial Hospital
Baltimore, Maryland

Caio Nery, MD
Head of the Orthopedic Clinic
Orthopedics and Trauma
Universidade Federal de São Paulo
São Paulo, Brazil

Christopher Nicholson, MD
Optim Orthopedics
Savannah, Georgia

Florian Nickisch, MD
Department of Orthopaedic Surgery
University of Utah Orthopaedic Center
Salt Lake City, Utah

James A. Nunley II, MD
Goldner Jones Endowed Professor of
 Orthopaedic Surgery
Duke University Medical Center
Durham, North Carolina

Tahir Ögüt, MD
Professor of Orthopaedic Surgery
Istanbul University Cerrahpasha Medical School
Istanbul, Turkey

Irvin C. Oh, MD
Associate Professor
Department of Orthopaedics and
 Rehabilitation
University of Rochester Medical Center
Rochester, New York

Francesco Oliva, MD, PhD
Associate Professor
Trauma and Orthopaedic Surgery
Departments of Medicine and Surgery
Università degli Studi di Salerno
Baronissi, Italy

Martin J. O'Malley, MD
Associate Professor of Orthopedics
Hospital for Special Surgery
Weil Cornell Medical College
New York, New York

Justin Orr, MD
Foot and Ankle Orthopaedic Surgeon
Director, Orthopaedic Residency Program
William Beaumont Army Medical Center
El Paso, Texas

Cristian Ortiz, MD
Universidad de los Andes
Traumatología y Ortopedia
Santiago, Chile

Fred W. Ortmann, MD
Greensboro Orthopaedics
Greensboro, North Carolina

Thomas G. Padanilam, MD
Partner
Toledo Orthopaedic Surgeons
Toledo, Ohio

Geert I. Pagenstert, MD
Professor of Orthopaedic Surgery
University of Basel
Swiss Olympic Medical Center
Basel, Switzerland

Nikiforos Pandelis Saragas, MBBCh, PhD
Head Foot and Ankle Unit
Department of Orthopaedic Surgery
University of the Witwatersrand
Johannesburg, South Africa

Selene G. Parekh, MD, MBA
Professor
Department of Orthopaedic Surgery
Director of Digital Strategy and Innovation
Partner, North Carolina Orthopaedic Clinic
Adjunct Faculty, Fuqua Business School
Duke University
Durham, North Carolina

Kyle S. Peterson, DPM
Foot and Ankle Surgeon
Suburban Orthopaedics
Bartlett, Illinois

Phinit Phisitkul, MD
Tri-State Specialists
Sioux City, Iowa
Medical Director
Riverview Surgical Center
South Sioux City, Nebraska
Adjunct Assistant Professor
College of Allied Health Professions
University of Nebraska Medical Center
Omaha, Nebraska

Michael S. Pinzur, MD
Professor of Orthopaedic Surgery and
 Rehabilitation
Loyola University Health System
Maywood, Illinois

Gregory C. Pomeroy, MD
Orthopedic Surgeon
St. Mary's Hospital
Portland, Maine

Marcelo Prado
Doctor in Orthopaedic and Traumatology
Foot and Ankle Surgeon
Hospital Israelita Albert Einstein
São Paulo, Brazil

Casey Pyle, MD
Fellow, Orthopaedic Surgery
Los Angeles County Harbor-UCLA Medical
 Center
Torrance, California

George E. Quill, Jr., MD
Assistant Clinical Professor
Department of Orthopedic Surgery
University of Louisville School of Medicine
Director, Foot and Ankle Services
Louisville Orthopedic Clinic and Sports
 Rehabilitation Center
Louisville, Kentucky

Stephen M. Quinnan, MD
Associate Professor of Orthopaedic Surgery
Chief, Orthopaedic Trauma
University of Miami – Jackson
Director of Orthopaedic Surgery
Jackson South
University of Miami Miller School of
  Medicine
Don Soffer Clinical Research Center
Miami, Florida

Mark A. Reiley, MD
Inventor, Board Member, and CMO
Reiley Pharmaceuticals, Inc.
Washington, District of Columbia

David R. Richardson, MD
Associate Professor
Orthopaedic Surgery and Biomedical
  Engineering
University of Tennessee, Campbell Clinic
Memphis, Tennessee

Martinus Richter, MD, PhD
Head, Department of Foot and Ankle Surgery
Krankenhaus Rummelsberg
Schwarzenbruck, Germany

Miranda J. Rogers, MD
Department of Orthopaedic Surgery
University of Utah Hospital
Salt Lake City, Utah

Keir A. Ross, MD
Orthopaedic Surgeon
NYU Langone Health
New York, New York

Roxa Ruiz, MD
Senior Attending Foot and Ankle Surgeon
Center of Excellence for Foot and Ankle
  Surgery
Orthopaedic Clinic
Kantonsspital Baselland
Liestal, Switzerland

Richard W. Rutherford, MD
EmergeOrtho
Durham, North Carolina

Charlie Saltzman, MD
Chairman, Department of Orthopaedic
  Surgery
University of Utah Orthopaedic Center
Salt Lake City, Utah

G. James Sammarco, MD
Clinical Professor
Department of Orthopaedic Surgery
University of Cincinnati Medical Center
Cincinnati, Ohio

V. James Sammarco, MD
Orthopaedic Surgeon
Foot and Ankle
OrthoCincy
Cincinnati, Ohio

Roy W. Sanders, MD
Professor and Chairman
Department of Orthopaedic Surgery
University of South Florida
Director, Orthopaedic Trauma Service
Florida Orthopaedic Institute
Tampa, Florida

Thomas P. San Giovanni, MD
Clinical Professor of Orthopedic Surgery
Florida International University Herbert
  Wertheim College of Medicine
Chief, Foot and Ankle Surgery
UHZ Sports Medicine Institute
Miami, Florida

James Santangelo, MD
Orthopaedic Surgeon
Womack Army Medical Center
Fort Bragg, North Carolina

Robert D. Santrock, MD
Associate Professor
Department of Orthopaedics
Robert C. Byrd Health Sciences Center
West Virginia University
Morgantown, West Virginia

Oliver N. Schipper, MD
Anderson Orthopaedic Clinic
Arlington, Virginia

Lew Schon, MD, FACS, FAAOS
Department of Orthopaedic Surgery
New York University Langone
New York, New York
Director Orthopedic Innovation
Institute of Foot and Ankle Reconstruction
Mercy Medical Center
Baltimore, Maryland

Karl M. Schweitzer, Jr., MD
Foot and Ankle Orthopaedic Surgeon
Duke Orthopaedics
Raleigh, North Carolina

Aaron T. Scott, MD
Associate Professor
Department of Orthopaedic Surgery
Wake Forest University School of Medicine
Winston Salem, North Carolina

Steven L. Shapiro, MD
Savannah Orthopaedic Foot and Ankle
Savannah, Georgia

Akhil Sharma, BS
Research Fellow
Department of Orthopaedic Surgery
Duke University
Durham, North Carolina

Glenn G. Shi, MD
Orthopedic Surgeon
Mayo Clinic
Jacksonville, Florida

Chloe Shields, BS
Research Assistant
University of Miami
Coral Gables, Florida

Yoshiharu Shimozono, MD
Orthopedic Surgeon
NYU Langone Health
New York, New York

Sam Singh, MRCS, FRCS(Orth)
Consultant Orthopaedic Surgeon
Department of Trauma and Orthopaedics
Guy's and Saint Thomas' NHS Foundation
  Trust
London, United Kingdom

Bertil W. Smith, MD
Foot and Ankle Surgeon
Southern California Permanente Medical
  Group
San Marcos, California

Emmanouil D. Stamatis, PhD
Director, Department of Reconstructive Foot
  and Ankle Surgery
Mediterraneo Hospital
Athens, Greece

Michael M. Stephens, FRCSI, MS
Consultant Orthopaedic Surgeon
Department of Orthopaedics
Mater Private Hospital
Dublin, Ireland

J. Jordan Stivers, MD
Resident
Department of Orthopaedic Surgery
Washington University in Saint Louis
St. Louis, Missouri

Karen M. Sutton, MD
Associate Attending Orthopedic Surgeon
Department of Sports Medicine
Hospital for Special Surgery
Stamford, Connecticut

James P. Tasto, MD
Clinical Professor
Department of Orthopaedic Surgery
University of California at San Diego
Founder, San Diego Sports Medicine and
  Orthopaedic Center
San Diego, California

Dean C. Taylor, MD
Professor of Orthopaedic Surgery
Duke University Medical Center
James R. Urbaniak Sports Sciences Institute
Durham, North Carolina

Hajo Thermann
Professor
Medical Specialist for Surgery,
  Trauma Surgery
HKF International Center for Hip,
  Foot and Knee
ATOS Klinik Heidelberg
Heidelberg, Germany

Sandra L. Tomak, MD
Orthopaedic Surgeon
Connecticut Orthopaedic Specialists
Guilford, Connecticut

Joseph Tracey, MS
Medical Student
Department of Orthopaedics
Medical University of South Carolina
Charleston, South Carolina

Hans-Joerg Trnka, MD
Professor
Department of Pediatric Orthopedics and
    Foot Surgery
Orthopädisches Spital Speising Wien
Director, Fusszentrum Wien
Vienna, Austria

H. Robert Tuten, MD
Orthopaedic Surgeon
St. Mary's Hospital
Department of Orthopaedic Surgery
Richmond, Virginia

Victor Valderrabano, MD, PhD
Professor
Department of Orthopaedic Surgery
Swiss Ortho Center
Basel, Switzerland

C. Niek van Dijk, MD
Head, Ankle Unit
FIFA Medical Centre of Excellence
Madrid and Porto, Spain
Emeritus Professor of Orthopaedic Surgery
Academic Medical Centre
University of Amsterdam
Amsterdam, The Netherlands

Emilio Wagner, MD
Foot and Ankle Surgeon
Department of Orthopaedic Surgery
Clínica Alemana de Santiago
Associate Professor
Universidad del Desarrollo
Santiago, Chile

Pablo Wagner, MD
Foot and Ankle Surgeon
Department of Orthopaedic Surgery
Clínica Alemana de Santiago
Universidad del Desarrollo
Santiago, Chile

**Roland Walker, MB ChB, MSc,
FRCS(Tr&Orth)**
Consultant Orthopaedic Surgeon
Department of Trauma and Orthopaedics
Guy's and Saint Thomas' NHS Foundation
    Trust
London, United Kingdom

Raymond J. Walls, MD
Assistant Professor
Department of Orthopaedic Surgery
Yale University School of Medicine
New Haven, Connecticut

Markus Walther, MD, PhD
Medical Director
Department of Foot and Ankle Surgery
Schön Klinik München Harlaching
Munich, Bavaria, Germany

Tibor Warganich, MD
Department of Orthopedic Surgery
Sanford Orthopedics and Sports Medicine
Bemidji, Minnesota

B. Collier Watson, DO
Foot and Ankle Surgeon
Hughston Clinic
Columbus, Georgia

Wolfram Wenz, MD
Foot Surgeon
Experts First
Heidelberg, Germany

Joan R. Williams, MD
Orthopedic Surgeon
Kaiser Permanente Southern California
San Diego, California

Michael G. Wilson, MD, MBA
Orthopaedic Surgeon
Cayuga Orthopaedics
Ithaca, New York

Bryan L. Witt, MD
Foot and Ankle Surgeon
Orthopaedic Associates of Michigan
Grand Rapids, Michigan

Omar Yaldo, MD
Resident
Department of Orthopaedic Surgery
Spectrum Health
Grand Rapids, Michigan

**Alastair Younger, MB, ChB, ChM, MSc,
FRCSC**
Professor
Department of Orthopaedics
The University of British Columbia Faculty
    of Medicine
Footbridge Clinic
Vancouver, British Columbia, Canada

PART 9 Spine

Junyoung Ahn, MD
Orthopaedic Surgeon
Rush University Medical Center
Chicago, Illinois

Todd J. Albert, MD
Surgeon in Chief Emeritus
Hospital for Special Surgery
Professor of Orthopaedics
Weill Cornell Medical College
New York, New York

David Greg Anderson, MD
Professor
Department of Orthopaedic Surgery
Rothman Orthopaedic Institute
Philadelphia, Pennsylvania

Griffin R. Baum, MD
Assistant Professor
Department of Neurosurgery
Donald and Barbara Zucker School of
    Medicine at Hofstra/Northwell
New York, New York

Arianne J. Boylan, MD
Assistant Professor
Department of Neurosurgery
Yale University School of Medicine
New Haven, Connecticut

Rachel Bratescu, MD
Resident
Department of Orthopaedic Surgery
Houston Methodist Hospital
Houston, Texas

Keith H. Bridwell, MD
Professor
Department of Orthopedic Surgery
Washington University in Saint Louis School
    of Medicine
St. Louis, Missouri

Jacob J. Bruckner, MD
Research Fellow
Department of Orthopaedics
University of Maryland School of Medicine
Baltimore, Maryland

Jael E. Camacho, MD
Research Fellow
Department of Orthopaedics
University of Maryland Medical Center
Baltimore, Maryland

Jose A. Canseco, MD, PhD
Rothman Orthopaedic Institute
Spine Surgery Fellow
Department of Orthopaedics
Thomas Jefferson University Hospital
Philadelphia, Pennsylvania

Michael Chang, BA
Research Fellow
Department of Orthopaedic Surgery
Thomas Jefferson University
Philadelphia, Pennsylvania

Saad B. Chaudhary, MD
Assistant Professor
Department of Orthopedics
Icahn School of Medicine at Mount Sinai
New York, New York

Morgan N. Chen, MD
Assistant Clinical Professor of Orthopedic
    Surgery
Mount Sinai Hospital
Clinical Assistant Professor of Surgery
College of Osteopathic Medicine at the New
    York Institute of Technology
New York, New York

Alan H. Daniels, MD
Associate Professor of Orthopaedic Surgery
Brown University Warren Alpert Medical
    School
Providence, Rhode Island

Kevin J. DiSilvestro, MD
Resident
Department of Orthopaedic Surgery
Brown University Warren Alpert Medical School
Providence, Rhode Island

James E. Dowdell, MD
Orthopedic Spine Surgeon
Hospital for Special Surgery
Instructor of Orthopedic Surgery
Weill Cornell Medical College
New York, New York

S. Harrison Farber, MD
Neurosurgery Resident
Barrow Neurological Institute
Phoenix, Arizona

Saifal-Deen Farhan, MD
Assistant Professor
Department of Orthopaedic Surgery
University of California Irvine
Orange, California

Richard G. Fessler, MD, PhD
Professor
Department of Neurosurgery
Rush Medical College
Chicago, Illinois

Michael A. Finn, MD
Assistant Professor
Department of Neurological Surgery
University of Colorado Denver
UCHealth Spine Center
Aurora, Colorado

Steven R. Garfin, MD
Interim Dean
Professor of Orthopaedic Surgery
University of California San Diego School of
  Medicine
San Diego, California

James S. Harrop, MD
Professor
Departments of Neurological and Orthopedic
  Surgery
Director, Division of Spine and Peripheral
  Nerve Surgery
Co-Director, Quality and Safety
Neurosurgery Director of Delaware Valley
  SCI Center
Thomas Jefferson University
Philadelphia, Pennsylvania

Andrew C. Hecht, MD
Chief of Spine Surgery
Department of Orthopedic Surgery
Mount Sinai Health System
New York, New York

John Heflin, MD
Associate Professor of Orthopaedics
University of Utah Health Care
Primary Children's Hospital
Salt Lake City, Utah

John G. Heller, MD
Baur Professor of Orthopaedic Surgery
Spine Fellowship Director
The Emory Spine Center
Department of Orthopaedic Surgery
Emory University School of Medicine
Atlanta, Georgia

George S. Ibrahim, MD
Resident Physician
Department of Orthopaedic Surgery
George Washington University
Washington, District of Columbia

Claude Jarrett, MD
Executive Board Member
Wilmington Health Associates
Orthopaedic Surgeon
New Hanover Regional Medical Center
Wilmington, North Carolina

Nathaniel W. Jenkins, MS
Research Coordinator
Department of Orthopaedic Surgery
Rush University Medical Center
Chicago, Illinois

S. Babak Kalantar, MD
Associate Professor of Orthopaedic Surgery
Chief, Division of Spine Surgery
MedStar Georgetown University Hospital
Washington, District of Columbia

Christopher G. Kalhorn, MD, FACS, FAANS
Associate Professor of Neurosurgery
Department of Neurosurgery
MedStar Georgetown University Hospital
Washington, District of Columbia

Yoshihiro Katsuura, MD
Orthopedic Surgeon
Department of Spine Surgery
Hospital for Special Surgery
New York, New York

Floreana A. Kebaish, MD
Chief Resident
Department of Orthopaedic Surgery
Johns Hopkins University School of Medicine
Baltimore, Maryland

Khaled M. Kebaish, MD
Chief of Spine
Professor of Orthopaedic and Neurosurgery
Johns Hopkins University School of Medicine
Baltimore, Maryland

Michael P. Kelly, MD, MSc
Associate Professor
Department of Orthopedic Surgery
Washington University in Saint Louis School
  of Medicine
St. Louis, Missouri

Christopher K. Kepler, MD, MBA
Assistant Professor
Department of Orthopaedic Surgery
Thomas Jefferson University
Philadelphia, Pennsylvania

James S. Kercher, MD
Orthopedic Surgeon
Peachtree Orthopedics
Atlanta, Georgia

Choll W. Kim, MD, PhD
Director of Minimally Invasive Spine Surgery
Spine Institute of San Diego
San Diego, California

James W. Klunk, MD
Fellow
Department of Orthopaedics
MedStar Union Memorial Hospital
Baltimore, Maryland

Gregory Kuzmik, MD
Resident
Department of Neurosurgery
Yale University School of Medicine
New Haven, Connecticut

Steven K. Leckie, MD
Orthopedic Surgeon
Beth Israel Deaconess Hospital Plymouth
Duxbury, Massachusetts

Yu-Po Lee, MD
Clinical Professor
Department of Orthopaedic Surgery
University of California Irvine
Orange, California

Lawrence G. Lenke, MD
Professor of Orthopedic Surgery
Department of Orthopedic Surgery
Columbia University College of Physicians
  and Surgeons
New York, New York

David J. Love, MD
Spine Fellow
Department of Orthopaedics
University of Maryland School of Medicine
Baltimore, Maryland

Steven C. Ludwig, MD
Professor and Chief of Spine Surgery
Department of Orthopaedics
University of Maryland School of Medicine
Baltimore, Maryland

Keith W. Lyons, MD
Resident
Department of Orthopaedic Surgery
Dartmouth-Hitchcock Medical Center
Lebanon, New Hampshire

Satyajit V. Marawar, MD
Chief of Orthopedic Surgery
VA Medical Center
Associate Professor in Orthopedic Surgery and
  Neurosurgery
Upstate Medical University
Syracuse, New York

Alejandro Marquez-Lara, MD
Orthopaedic Surgery Resident
Rush University Medical Center
Chicago, Illinois

Kevin M. McGrail, MD
Chair, Department of Neurosurgery
MedStar Georgetown University Hospital
Georgetown University School of Medicine
Washington, District of Columbia

Umesh S. Metkar, MD
Orthopedic Spine Surgeon
Beth Israel Deaconess Medical Center
Boston, Massachusetts

Keith W. Michael, MD
Assistant Professor
Department of Orthopedic Surgery
Emory University
Atlanta, Georgia

Christopher M. Mikhail, MD
Resident
Department of Orthopedics
Icahn School of Medicine at Mount Sinai
New York, New York

Brad W. Moatz, MD
Orthopedic Surgeon
MedStar Union Memorial Hospital
Baltimore, Maryland

Sreeharsha V. Nandyala, MD
Resident
Department of Orthopedic Surgery
Massachusetts General Hospital
Boston, Massachusetts

Samuel C. Overley, MD
Orthopaedic Surgeon
UAMS Health
Little Rock, Arkansas

James M. Parrish, MPH
Research Coordinator
Department of Orthopaedic Surgery
Rush University Medical Center
Chicago, Illinois

Shalin Patel, MD
Assistant Professor
Department of Orthopedic Surgery
George Washington University
Washington, District of Columbia

Shyam A. Patel, MD
Resident
Department of Orthopaedic Surgery
Brown University Warren Alpert Medical
  School
Providence, Rhode Island

Adam M. Pearson, MD, MS
Assistant Professor of Orthopaedics
Dartmouth-Hitchcock Medical Center
Lebanon, New Hampshire

Andrew Platt, MD
Neurosurgery Specialist
University of Chicago
Chicago, Illinois

Sheeraz A. Qureshi, MD, MBA
Patty and Jay Baker Endowed Chair
Minimally Invasive Spine Surgery
Hospital for Special Surgery
Associate Professor of Orthopaedic Surgery
Weill Cornell Medical College
New York, New York

Raj Rao, MD
Professor
Department of Orthopedic Surgery
George Washington University
Washington, District of Columbia

Daniel Refai, MD
Assistant Professor
Department of Surgery
Emory University School of Medicine
Atlanta, Georgia

John M. Rhee, MD
Professor
Orthopaedic Surgery
Emory University
Atlanta, Georgia

K. Daniel Riew, MD
Professor
Department of Orthopedic Surgery
Columbia University College of Physicians
  and Surgeons
New York, New York

Jeffrey A. Rihn, MD
Associate Professor of Orthopaedic Surgery
Rothman Orthopaedic Institute
Malvern, Pennsylvania

Gerald E. Rodts, Jr., MD
Professor
Department of Surgery
Emory University School of Medicine
Atlanta, Georgia

Kern Singh, MD
Professor
Department of Orthopaedic Surgery
Rush University Medical Center
Spine Surgeon
Midwest Orthopaedics at Rush
Chicago, Illinois

Laura A. Snyder, MD
Neurosurgeon
Barrow Neurological Institute
Phoenix, Arizona

Selvon St. Clair, MD, PhD
Orthopaedic Surgeon
Orthopaedic Institute of Ohio
Lima, Ohio

Geoffrey Stricsek, MD
Fellow
Department of Medicine
Emory University
Atlanta, Georgia

P. Justin Tortolani, MD
Clinical Professor
Department of Orthopaedic Surgery
University of Maryland School of Medicine
Spine Institute
St. Joseph Medical Center
Baltimore, Maryland

Alexander R. Vaccaro, MD, PhD
Departments of Orthopaedic Surgery and
  Neurological Surgery
Rothman Orthopaedic Institute
Thomas Jefferson University
Philadelphia, Pennsylvania

Bradley K. Weiner, MD
Professor, Vice Chair, and Chief of Spinal
  Surgery
Houston Methodist Hospital
Department of Orthopedic Surgery
Houston, Texas

Andrew P. White, MD
Spine Surgeon
Department of Orthopedics
Beth Israel Deaconess Medical Center
Boston, Massachusetts

Sam W. Wiesel, MD
Chairman and Professor
Department of Orthopaedic Surgery
Georgetown University Medical School
Washington, District of Columbia

Ernest J. Wright, MD
Neurosurgeon
Ascension Saint Thomas Hospital
Nashville, Tennessee

Joon S. Yoo, BA
Research Coordinator
Department of Orthopaedic Surgery
Rush University Medical Center
Chicago, Illinois

S. Tim Yoon, MD, PhD
Professor
Department of Orthopedic Surgery
Emory University
Atlanta, Georgia

Lukas P. Zebala, MD
Associate Professor
Department of Orthopedic Surgery
Washington University in Saint Louis School
  of Medicine
St. Louis, Missouri

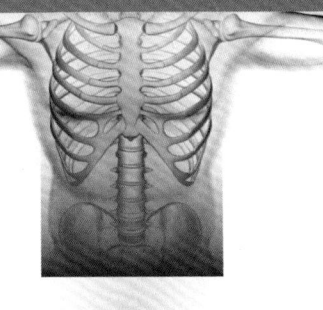

Preface to the Second Edition

The purpose of the second edition of *Operative Techniques in Orthopaedic Surgery* remains the same as the first: to describe in a detailed, step-by-step manner the technical parts of "how to do" the majority of orthopaedic procedures.

It is assumed that the surgeon understands the "why" and the "when," although this information is covered in outline form at the beginning of each procedure.

Each of the nine major sections has been carefully reviewed and updated in both its content and artwork. The second edition has given each section editor the ability to include additional procedures and has also placed more emphasis in creating online content which is easily accessible and fully searchable.

The section editors and chapter authors have done an excellent job. Each has specific expertise and experience in their area and has given their time and effort most generously. It has again been stimulating to interact with these wonderful and talented people, and I am honored to have been able to play a part in this rewarding experience.

I also would like to thank all of the people at Wolters Kluwer. Dave Murphy has been especially helpful and had a great deal of input into this edition, as with the first edition. I would like, as well, to acknowledge Bob Hurley, who was a driving force for the first edition and has been a great resource for this second one as well.

Finally, special thanks goes to Brian Brown, the new acquisitions editor. It has been a wonderful experience to work with Brian who has done an excellent job of bringing this text to completion.

SAM W. WIESEL, MD
Washington, DC
January 2, 2015

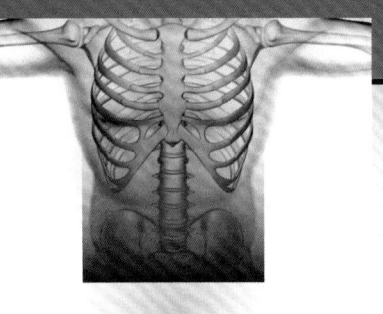

Preface to the First Edition

When a surgeon contemplates performing a procedure, there are three major questions to consider: Why is the surgery being done? When in the course of a disease process should it be performed? And, finally, what are the technical steps involved? The purpose of this text is to describe in a detailed, step-by-step manner the "how to do it" of the vast majority of orthopaedic procedures. The "why" and "when" are covered in outline form at the beginning of each procedure. However, it is assumed that the surgeon understands the basics of "why" and "when," and has made the definitive decision to undertake a specific case. This text is designed to review and make clear the detailed steps of the anticipated operation.

Operative Techniques in Orthopaedic Surgery differs from other books because it is mainly visual. Each procedure is described in a systematic way that makes liberal use of focused, original artwork. It is hoped that the surgeon will be able to visualize each significant step of a procedure as it unfolds during a case.

The text is divided into nine major topics: Adult Reconstruction; Foot and Ankle; Hand, Wrist, and Forearm; Oncology; Pediatrics; Shoulder and Elbow; Sports Medicine; Spine; and Pelvis and Lower Extremity Trauma. Each chapter has been edited by a specialist who has specific expertise and experience in the discipline. It has taken a tremendous amount of work for each editor to enlist talented authors for each procedure and then review the final work. It has been very stimulating to work with all of these wonderful and talented people, and I am honored to have taken part in this rewarding experience.

Finally, I would like to thank everyone who has contributed to the development of this book. Specifically, Grace Caputo at Dovetail Content Solutions, and Dave Murphy and Eileen Wolfberg at Lippincott Williams & Wilkins, who have been very helpful and generous with their input. Special thanks, as well, goes to Bob Hurley at LWW, who has adeptly guided this textbook from original concept to publication.

SWW
January 1, 2010

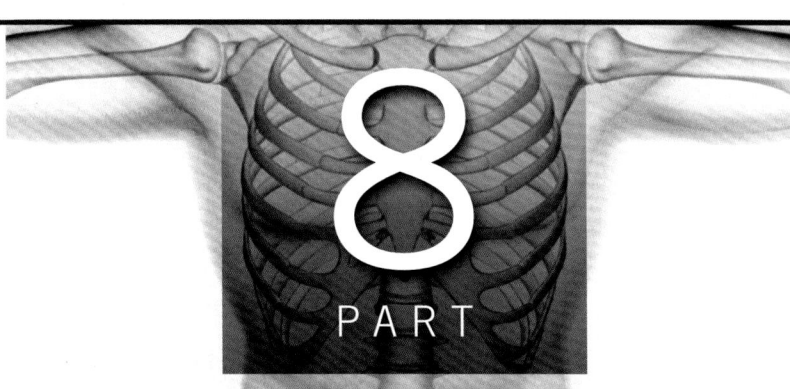

8

PART

Foot and Ankle

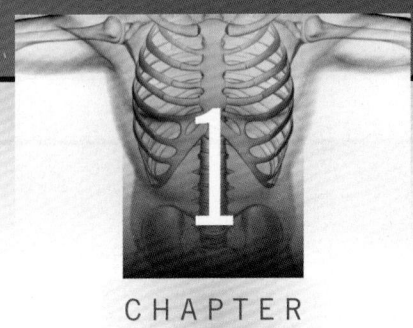

CHAPTER 1

Forefoot
Distal Chevron Osteotomy:
Perspective 1

Hans-Joerg Trnka and Stefan G. Hofstaetter

DEFINITION

- The first reports of a distal metatarsal osteotomy date back to Reverdin, who described in 1881 a subcapital closing wedge osteotomy for the correction of hallux valgus deformity.
- The chevron osteotomy has become widely accepted for correction of mild and moderate hallux valgus deformities. In the initial reports by Austin and Leventen[1] and Miller and Croce,[13] no fixation was mentioned. They suggested that the shape of the osteotomy and impaction of the cancellous capital fragment on the shaft of the first metatarsal provided sufficient stability to forego fixation.
- To increase the indication for this technically simple osteotomy, internal fixation and a lateral soft tissue release have been added.

ANATOMY

- The special situation distinguishing the first metatarsophalangeal (MTP) joint from the lesser MTP joints is the sesamoid mechanism.
  - On the plantar surface of the metatarsal head are two longitudinal cartilage-covered grooves separated by a rounded ridge. The sesamoids run in these grooves.
  - The sesamoid bone is contained in each tendon of the flexor hallucis brevis; they are distally attached by the fibrous plantar plate to the base of the proximal phalanx.
- The head of the first metatarsal is rounded and cartilage-covered and articulates with the smaller concave elliptic base of the proximal phalanx.
- Fan-shaped ligamentous bands originate from the medial and lateral condyles of the metatarsal head and run to the base of the proximal phalanx and the margins of the sesamoids and the plantar plate.
- Tendons and muscles that move the great toe are arranged in four groups:
  - Long and short extensor tendons
  - Long and short flexor tendons
  - Abductor hallucis
  - Adductor hallucis
- Blood supply to the metatarsal head
  - First dorsal metatarsal artery
  - Branches from the first plantar metatarsal artery

PATHOGENESIS

- Extrinsic causes
  - Hallux valgus occurs predominantly in shoe-wearing populations and only occasionally in the unshod individual.
  - Although shoes are an essential factor in the cause of hallux valgus, not all individuals wearing fashionable shoes develop this deformity.
- Intrinsic causes
  - Hardy and Clapham[3] found in a series of 91 patients a positive family history in 63%.
  - Coughlin[2] reported that a bunion was identified in 94% of 31 mothers whose children inherited a hallux valgus deformity.
  - Association of pes planus with the development of a hallux valgus deformity has been controversial.
  - Hohmann[5] was the most definitive that hallux valgus is always combined with pes planus.
  - Coughlin[2] and Kilmartin and Wallace[8] noted no incidence of pes planus in the juvenile patient.
  - Pronation of the foot imposes a longitudinal rotation of the first ray, which places the axis of the MTP joint in an oblique plane relative to the floor. In this position, the foot appears to be less able to withstand the deformity pressures exerted on it by either shoes or weight bearing.
  - The simultaneous occurrence of hallux valgus and metatarsus primus varus has been frequently described. The question of cause and effect continues to be debated.

PATIENT HISTORY AND PHYSICAL FINDINGS

- Patient history often includes the following:
  - Pain in narrow shoes
  - Symptomatic intractable keratoses beneath the second metatarsal head (in 40% of patients)
  - Lateral deviation of the great toe
  - Pronation of the great toe
  - Keratosis medial plantar underneath the interphalangeal joint
  - Bursitis over the medial aspect of the medial condyle of the first metatarsal head
  - Hypermobility of the first metatarsocuneiform joint
- Physical examination for hallux valgus deformity includes the following:
  - Hallux valgus angle: Normal is 15 degrees or less.
  - Intermetatarsal angle: Normal is 9 degrees or less.

- Measurement of the position of the medial sesamoid relative to a longitudinal line bisecting the first metatarsal shaft
  - Grade 0: no displacement of sesamoid relative to the reference line
  - Grade I: overlap of less than 50% of sesamoid relative to the reference line
  - Grade II: overlap of greater than 50% of sesamoid relative to the reference line
  - Grade III: sesamoid completely displaced beyond the reference line
- Joint congruency: measuring the lateral displacement of the articular surface of the proximal phalanx with respect to the corresponding articular surface of the metatarsal head, as seen on a dorsoplantar roentgenogram

IMAGING AND OTHER DIAGNOSTIC STUDIES

- Radiographs of the foot should always be obtained with the patient in the weight-bearing position with anteroposterior (AP) **(FIG 1)**, lateral, and oblique views. The following criteria are examined:
  - Hallux valgus angle
  - Intermetatarsal angle
  - Sesamoid position
  - Joint congruency
  - Distal metatarsal articular angle (DMAA): the relationship between the articular surface of the first metatarsal head and a line bisecting the first metatarsal shaft (normal is 10 degrees or less)
  - Arthrosis of the first MTP joint

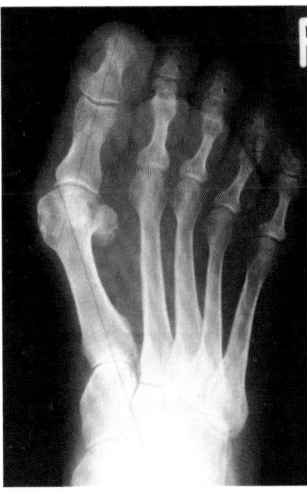

FIG 1 A 72-year-old woman with hallux valgus before surgery.

DIFFERENTIAL DIAGNOSIS

- Ganglion
- Hallux rigidus

NONOPERATIVE MANAGEMENT

- Comfortable wider shoes
- Orthotics
- Spiral dynamics physiotherapy in adolescents

SURGICAL MANAGEMENT

Indications

- Symptomatic hallux valgus deformity with a first intermetatarsal angle of up to 16 degrees
- Stable first metatarsocuneiform joint

Contraindications

- Narrow metatarsal head so that adequate translation is not possible
- Intermetatarsal angle of more than 16 degrees
- Impaired vascular status
- Skeletally immature patient
- Severe osteoarthritic changes

Preoperative Planning

- Standard weight-bearing AP and lateral radiographs are mandatory.
- The hallux valgus and intermetatarsal angles and tibial sesamoid position are measured.
- A preoperative drawing is helpful.
- Clinical examination includes measurement of active and passive range of motion of the first MTP joint as well as inspection of the foot for plantar callus formation indicative of transfer metatarsalgia and stability of the first tarsometatarsal joint.

Positioning

- The foot is prepared in the standard manner.
- The patient is positioned supine.
- An ankle tourniquet is optional.

Approach

- The lateral soft tissue release and the chevron osteotomy are performed through a straight midline incision.

CHEVRON AND TRANSARTICULAR LATERAL SOFT TISSUE RELEASE

Exposure

- The procedure is typically performed under peripheral nerve block.
- A straight medial incision over the metatarsal head is performed **(TECH FIG 1A)**.
- The medial MTP joint capsule is opened with a longitudinal incision **(TECH FIG 1B)**. The joint is inspected for degenerative changes.

- The metatarsal head is now exposed, and Hohmann retractors are placed dorsal and plantar just extra-articular of the first MTP joint.
- The plantar Hohmann retractor protects the plantar artery to the metatarsal head and the dorsal retractor protects the dorsal intra-articular blood supply originating from the capsule.

Lateral Release and Preparation of the Metatarsal Head

- The capsule is released from the plantar and the dorsal aspect of the base of the proximal phalanx **(TECH FIG 2A,B)**.
- While the toe is plantar subluxed **(TECH FIG 2C)**, scissors are placed intra-articular proximal to the sesamoids from medial to lateral **(TECH FIG 2D)**.
- Parallel to this, a beaver knife is inserted and the lateral joint capsule (metatarsosesamoid ligament) is divided immediately superior to the lateral sesamoid **(TECH FIG 2E)**.
- The lateral capsule is fenestrated at the first MTP joint, and a varus stress is applied to the hallux to complete the lateral release **(TECH FIG 2F)**. The medial eminence is now minimally shaved to achieve a plane surface but also to preserve as much metatarsal head width as possible **(TECH FIG 2G)**.

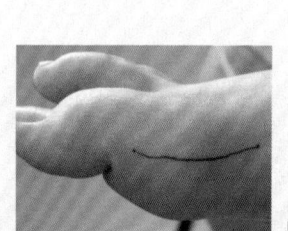
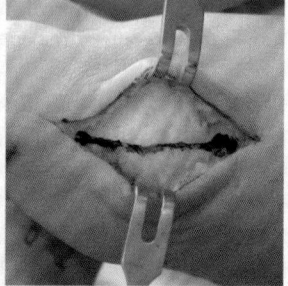

TECH FIG 1 A. Medial skin incision. **B.** Longitudinal capsular incision.

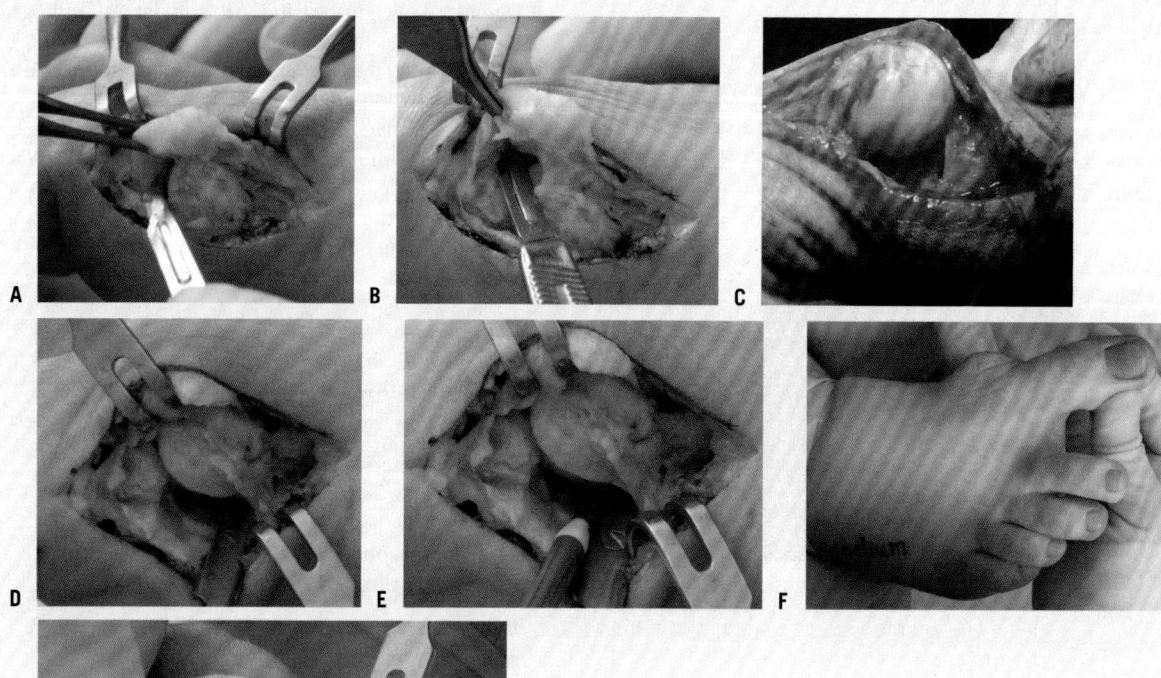

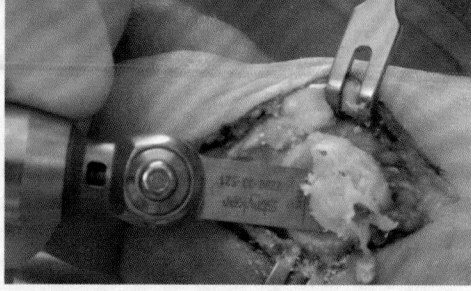

TECH FIG 2 A–C. The capsule is released, and the toe is plantar subluxed. **D.** A scissor is now placed intra-articular proximal to the sesamoids from medial to lateral. **E.** A beaver knife is inserted, and the lateral capsule is incised. **F.** The great toe is brought into 20 degrees of varus to demonstrate the release of the lateral structures. **G.** The medial eminence is minimally resected.

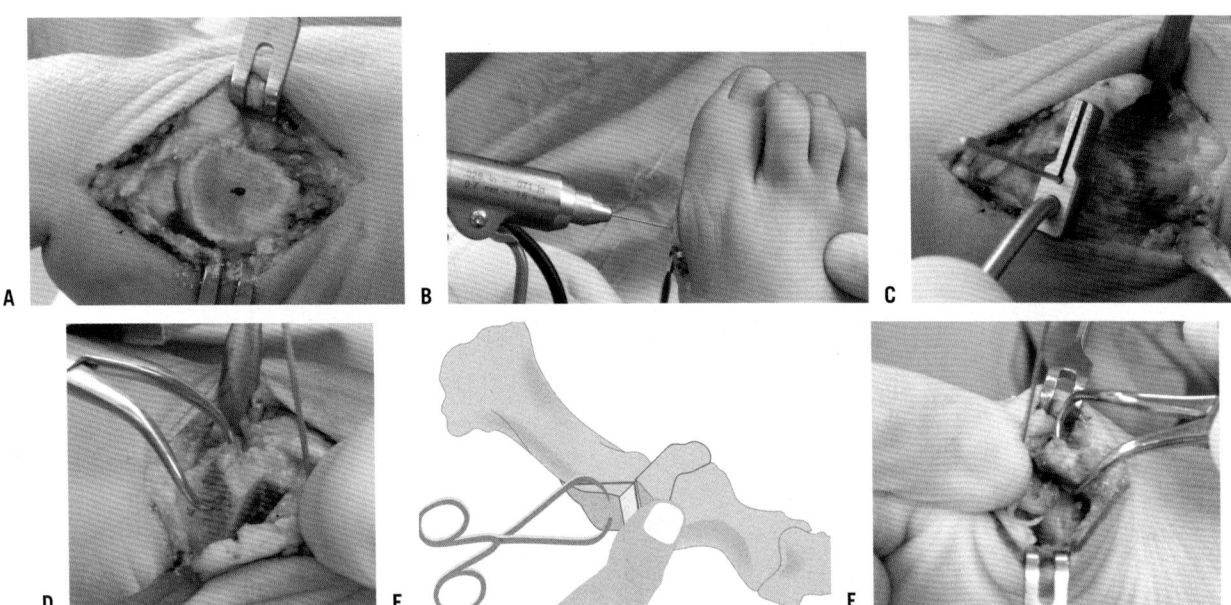

TECH FIG 3 A,B. A guidewire marks the apex of the osteotomy. It should be 20 degrees inclined from medial to lateral and pointing at the head of the fourth metatarsal. **C.** The osteotomy is performed using an osteotomy guide. **D,E.** The metatarsal head is pushed laterally, whereas the metatarsal shaft is pulled medially. **F.** A guidewire used as a joystick may be placed into the distal fragment.

Osteotomy Creation

- A 1.0-mm Kirschner wire is drilled a little bit dorsal to the center of the exposed medial eminence. This wire is generally inclined 20 degrees from medial to lateral, aiming at the head of the fourth metatarsal **(TECH FIG 3A,B)**.
  - In the situation of an elevated position of the first metatarsal, the inclination may be increased.
  - If shortening or lengthening of the first metatarsal is needed, the wire can be aimed to the fifth or third metatarsal head.

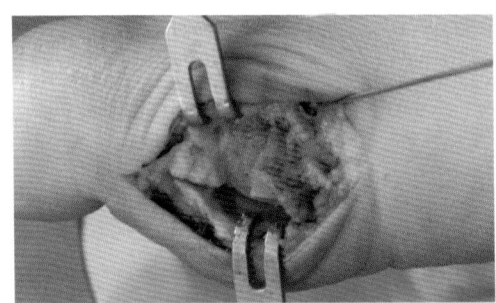

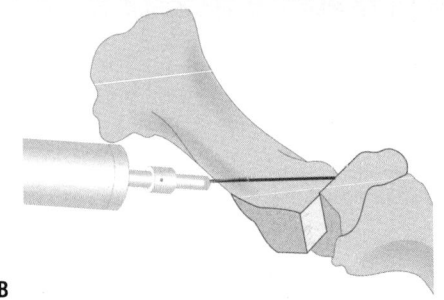

TECH FIG 4 A guidewire for the 2.0 AutoFix screw (Stryker, Kalamazoo, MI) is placed.

- By using a saw guide **(TECH FIG 3C)**, two cuts are then made with an oscillating power saw so that they form an angle of 60 degrees proximal to the drill hole.
- Once the capital fragment is freely mobile, the metatarsal shaft is pulled medially by using a towel clip while pushing the metatarsal head laterally with the help of the thumb of the other hand. A keywire may be inserted into the distal fragment as a "joystick" to facilitate the lateral translation and to avoid tilting of the head **(TECH FIG 3D–F)**.
- In the situation that the DMAA is increased, a wedge from the distal dorsal cut can be excised to place the metatarsal head in a more varus position. If there is only a minor increase of the DMAA, this may also be achieved by impacting the metatarsal head onto the shaft.

Guidewire Placement

- A guidewire for a cannulated AutoFix 2.0 screw (Stryker, Kalamazoo, MI) is inserted from the distal dorsal metatarsal shaft obliquely to lateral plantar of the metatarsal head **(TECH FIG 4)**.
- It is now advised to check the position of the osteotomy and the guidewire with a C-arm or a Fluoroscan.

Screw Insertion and Closure

- The length of the screw is now measured with the cannulated depth gauge **(TECH FIG 5A)**.
- The cannulated head countersink is now used **(TECH FIG 5B)** and the totally self-tapping and self-drilling screw is inserted **(TECH FIG 5C)**.
- Then, the medial eminence is excised in line with the metatarsal shaft, taking care not to excise too much bone off the metatarsal head **(TECH FIG 5D)**.
- While an assistant holds the great toe in a slightly overcorrected position, the medial joint capsule is repaired with U-type sutures **(TECH FIG 5E)**.

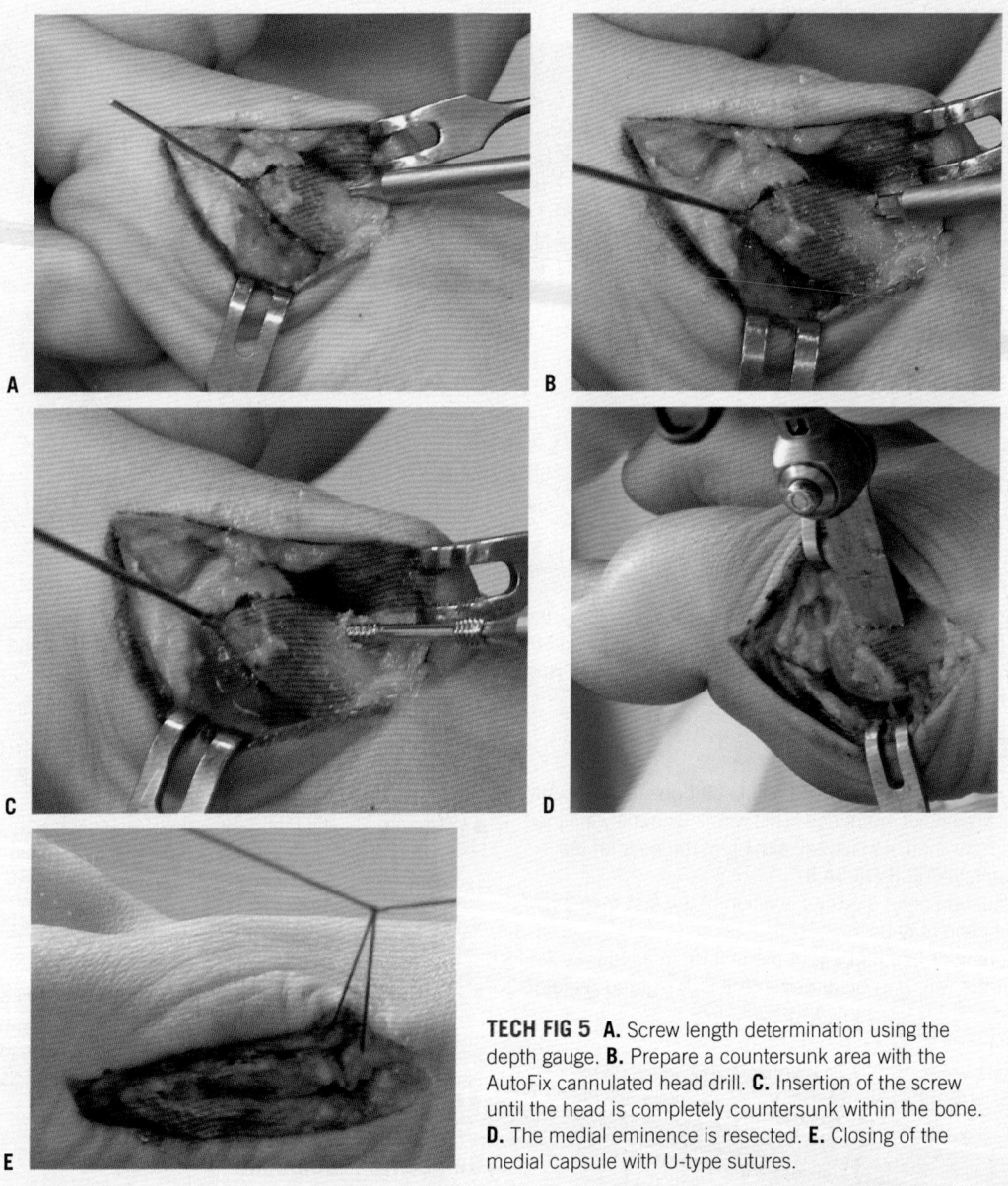

TECH FIG 5 A. Screw length determination using the depth gauge. **B.** Prepare a countersunk area with the AutoFix cannulated head drill. **C.** Insertion of the screw until the head is completely countersunk within the bone. **D.** The medial eminence is resected. **E.** Closing of the medial capsule with U-type sutures.

TECHNIQUES

Pearls and Pitfalls

Lateral Tilt of the Metatarsal Head	• Lateral release to avoid lateral tilting of the head, joystick in the distal fragment, intraoperative Fluoroscan control
Avascular Necrosis	• Careful soft tissue dissection
Intraoperative Fracture of the Metatarsal Head	• A guidewire at the apex of the osteotomy will prevent overpenetration of the distal fragment with the saw blade.

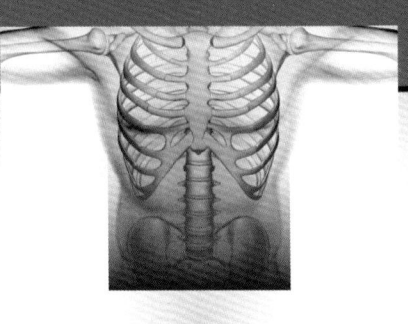

Preface

Techiques in modern Orthopaedic Surgery continue to evolve at a rapid pace. The principles associated with most modern procedures however generally remain rooted in generally sound historical tenets established over the last 150 years.

The goal of the Third Edition of "*Orthopaedic Techniques in Orthopaedic Surgery*" continues to be to describe in a detailed and step by step manner the technical parts of how to do the majority of orthopaedic procedures. The "*why*" and "*when*" are covered in outline form at the beginning of each chapter, but it is assumed that the surgeon understands this information. Each of the nine major topics have been revised to include updated procedures. Additionally, the audio visual part of the text has been increased and continues to evolve. I am very proud of the final text, and very grateful to all the section editors and the authors. I have very much enjoyed working with all of them and it has been a great privilege for me.

I would also like to welcome Dr. Todd Albert as a Co-Editor in Chief for this Edition. I have known Todd since he was a resident at Jefferson under Dr. Richard Rothman. He has had an outstanding career. He is an internationally known academic spine surgeon and has had major administrative roles leading the Rothman Institute in Philadelphia and the Hospital for Special Surgery in New York. Dr. Albert will assume the sole Editor in Chief position for the fourth edition. I am absolutely delighted that he has been able to join us.

Finally, I would like to thank all of the people at Wolters Kluwer for their hardwork. I can still remember when Bob Hurley, in 2000, proposed the first edition of this text. The first time around it took us ten years to get it put together. Brian Brown took over as Production Editor in the middle of the second edition and has been the guiding force for this text since then. I think "*Operative Techniques in Orthopaedic Surgery*" is in good hands as we look to the future.

Sam W. Wiesel, MD
Washington, DC
January 5, 2021

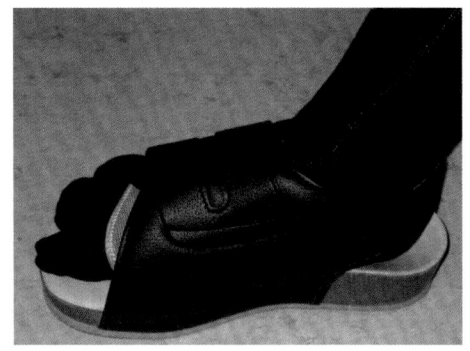
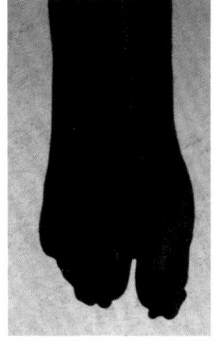

FIG 2 A. Rathgeber postoperative shoe (OFA Rathgeber [Ofa Bamberg, Bamberg, Germany]). **B.** Postoperative hallux valgus compression stocking used after suture removal.

POSTOPERATIVE CARE

- Starting immediately postoperatively, ice application to the foot is helpful to reduce swelling.
- Provided that the bone quality was intraoperatively sufficient, patients are allowed to walk with a postsurgical type shoe (OFA Rathgeber [Ofa Bamberg, Bamberg, Germany]) **(FIG 2A)** on the same day (limited for 4 weeks).
- Weekly changes of the tape dressing are necessary.
- An alternative to weekly dressing changes is the postoperative hallux valgus sock, which also reduces postoperative edema **(FIG 2B)**.
- Radiographs are taken intraoperatively and at 4 weeks of follow-up.
- After radiographic union is achieved, normal dress shoes with a more rigid sole are allowed.
- After 4 weeks, physiotherapy to achieve normal forefoot function is recommended.

OUTCOMES

- In the early years of this technique, it was limited to patients 50 years and younger. This was represented by the study of Johnson et al,[7] which established a contraindication for using a chevron osteotomy in patients older than 50 years. However, Trnka et al[20-22] and Schneider et al[18] have shown that age is not a limiting factor for the chevron osteotomy **(FIG 3)**.
- Another important issue that was stretched out over the years was the combination of a lateral soft tissue release and

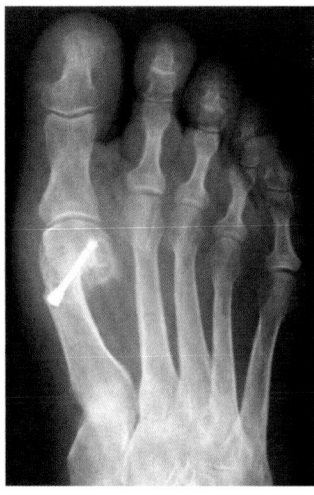

FIG 3 The same patient as in **FIG 1** after surgery.

a distal chevron osteotomy. Earlier reports expressed concern about an increased risk of avascular necrosis if a lateral release is performed in addition to a chevron osteotomy. Jahss,[6] Mann,[9] Mann and Coughlin,[10] Mann and Donato,[11] and Meier and Kenzora[12] have all suggested that avascular necrosis frequently accompanies distal chevron with lateral soft tissue release, citing an incidence of up to 40%. Pochatko et al[15] and Trnka et al[20-22] could not support this in their publications and found no increased risk of avascular necrosis.

- Chevron osteotomy was for many years limited to mild hallux valgus deformities.[17,19] Designed primarily without fixation, the concern was stability and loss of fixation. As it became more obvious that a lateral soft tissue release is important for correction of more severe deformities, this concern gained weight. According to papers by Harper[4] and Sarrafian,[17] lateral displacement is limited up to 50% of metatarsal width.
- Over a period of 14 years, we have modified and developed the chevron osteotomy. By reviewing each step of the development with clinical studies, we now perform a chevron osteotomy with lateral soft tissue release and single screw fixation.
- Trnka et al[21] reported in 2000 a series of 43 patients (57 feet) with 2- and 5-year follow-up. Radiographic evaluation revealed a preoperative average hallux valgus angle of 29 degrees and a preoperative average intermetatarsal angle of 13 degrees. At the 2-year follow-up, those angles averaged 15 and 8 degrees, respectively, and at the 5-year follow-up, they averaged 16 and 9 degrees, respectively. The results at these two follow-up periods proved that the chevron osteotomy is a reliable procedure for mild and moderate hallux valgus deformity and that there are no differences in outcome based on age.
- Schneider et al[18] reported in 2004 a series of 112 feet (73 patients) with a minimum follow-up of 10 years. For 47 feet (30 patients), the results were compared with those from an interim follow-up of 5.6 years. The American Orthopaedic Foot & Ankle Society (AOFAS) score improved from a preoperative mean of 46.5 points to a mean of 88.8 points after a mean of 12.7 years. The first MTP angle showed a mean preoperative value of 27.6 degrees and was improved to 14.0 degrees. The first intermetatarsal angle improved from a preoperative mean of 13.8 to 8.7 degrees. The mean preoperative grade of sesamoid subluxation was 1.7 on a scale of 0 to 3 and improved to 1.2. Measured on a scale of 0 to 3, arthritis of the first MTP joint progressed from a mean of 0.8 to 1.7. The progression of arthritis of the first MTP joint between 5.6 and 12.7 years postoperatively was statistically significant. Excellent clinical results after chevron osteotomy not only proved to be consistent but also showed further

improvement over a longer follow-up period. The mean radiographic angles were constant, without recurrence of the deformity. So far, the statistically significant progression of first MTP joint arthritis has not affected the clinical result, but this needs further observation.

- Sanhudo[16] retrospectively reviewed 50 feet with moderate to severe hallux valgus deformity in 34 patients with a mean follow-up of 30 months. There was a mean AOFAS score improvement of 39.6 (44.5 to 84.1) points. The hallux valgus angle and intermetatarsal angle improved a mean of 22.7 and 10.4 degrees, respectively. He concluded that the chevron osteotomy is also indicated for moderate to severe hallux valgus deformity.

- Park et al[14] performed a level II study to compare chevron osteotomies with dorsolateral approach for lateral release and chevron osteotomies with transarticular lateral release. One hundred and twenty-two female patients (122 feet) who underwent a distal chevron osteotomy as part of a distal soft tissue procedure for the treatment of symptomatic unilateral moderate to severe hallux valgus constituted the study cohort. The 122 feet were randomly divided into two groups: namely, a dorsal first web space approach (group D; 60 feet) and a medial transarticular approach (group M; 62 feet). The clinical and radiographic results of the two groups were compared at a mean follow-up time of 38 months.

- Yammine and Assi[23] demonstrated in a meta-analysis the importance of the lateral soft tissue release for the final outcome of the chevron osteotomy.

- The final clinical and radiographic outcomes between the two approaches for distal soft tissue procedures were comparable and equally successful. Accordingly, the results of this study suggest that the medial transarticular approach is an effective and reliable means of lateral soft tissue release compared with the dorsal first web space approach.

COMPLICATIONS

- Avascular necrosis of the metatarsal head
  - A lateral release does not increase the incidence.[15]
- Hallux varus
- Malpositioning
- Loss of fixation

REFERENCES

1. Austin DW, Leventen EO. A new osteotomy for hallux valgus: a horizontally directed "V" displacement osteotomy of the metatarsal head for hallux valgus and primus varus. Clin Orthop Relat Res 1981;(157):25–30.
2. Coughlin MJ. Roger A. Mann Award. Juvenile hallux valgus: etiology and treatment. Foot Ankle Int 1995;16(11):682–697.
3. Hardy RH, Clapham JC. Observations on hallux valgus based on a controlled series. J Bone Joint Surg Br 1951;33-B(3):376–391.
4. Harper MC. Correction of metatarsus primus varus with the chevron metatarsal osteotomy: an analysis of corrective factors. Clin Orthop Relat Res 1989;(243):180–183.
5. Hohmann G. Hallux valgus. In: Fuss und Bein. Ihre Erkrankungen und deren Behandlung. München, Germany: J.F. Bergmann, 1951: 145–156.
6. Jahss MH. Hallux valgus: further considerations—the first metatarsal head. Foot Ankle 1981;2(1):1–4.
7. Johnson JE, Clanton TO, Baxter DE, et al. Comparison of chevron osteotomy and modified McBride bunionectomy for correction of mild to moderate hallux valgus deformity. Foot Ankle 1991;12(2): 61–68.
8. Kilmartin TE, Wallace WA. The significance of pes planus in juvenile hallux valgus. Foot Ankle 1992;13(2):53–56.
9. Mann RA. Bunion surgery: decision making. Orthopedics 1990;13(9): 951–957.
10. Mann RA, Coughlin MJ. Adult hallux valgus. In: Coughlin MJ, Mann RA, eds. Surgery of the Foot and Ankle. St. Louis: Mosby, 1999: 150–269.
11. Mann RA, Donatto KC. The chevron osteotomy: a clinical and radiographic analysis. Foot Ankle Int 1997;18(5):255–261.
12. Meier PJ, Kenzora JE. The risks and benefits of distal metatarsal osteotomies. Foot Ankle 1985;6(1):7–17.
13. Miller S, Croce WA. The Austin procedure for surgical correction of hallux abductor valgus deformity. J Am Podiatry Assoc 1979;69(2):110–118.
14. Park Y-B, Lee K-B, Kim S-K, et al. Comparison of distal soft-tissue procedures combined with a distal chevron osteotomy for moderate to severe hallux valgus: first web-space versus transarticular approach. J Bone Joint Surg Am 2013;95(21):e158.
15. Pochatko DJ, Schlehr FJ, Murphey MD, et al. Distal chevron osteotomy with lateral release for treatment of hallux valgus deformity. Foot Ankle Int 1994;15(9):457–461.
16. Sanhudo JA. Correction of moderate to severe hallux valgus deformity by a modified chevron shaft osteotomy. Foot Ankle Int 2006;27(8): 581–585.
17. Sarrafian SK. A method of predicting the degree of functional correction of the metatarsus primus varus with a distal lateral displacement osteotomy in hallux valgus. Foot Ankle 1985;5(6):322–326.
18. Schneider W, Aigner N, Pinggera O, et al. Chevron osteotomy in hallux valgus: ten-year results of 112 cases. J Bone Joint Surg Br 2004;86(7): 1016–1020.
19. Shereff MJ, Yang QM, Kummer FJ. Extraosseous and intraosseous arterial supply to the first metatarsal and metatarsophalangeal joint. Foot Ankle 1987;8(2):81–93.
20. Trnka HJ, Hofmann S, Salzer M, et al. Clinical and radiological results after Austin bunionectomy for treatment of hallux valgus. Arch Orthop Trauma Surg 1996;115:171–175.
21. Trnka HJ, Zembsch A, Easley ME, et al. The chevron osteotomy for correction of hallux valgus: comparison of findings after two and five years of follow-up. J Bone Joint Surg Am 2000;82(10): 1373–1378.
22. Trnka HJ, Zembsch A, Wiesauer H, et al. Modified Austin procedure for correction of hallux valgus. Foot Ankle Int 1997;18(3): 119–127.
23. Yammine K, Assi C. A meta-analysis of comparative clinical studies of isolated osteotomy versus osteotomy with lateral soft tissue release in treating hallux valgus. Foot Ankle Surg 2019;25(5):684–690.

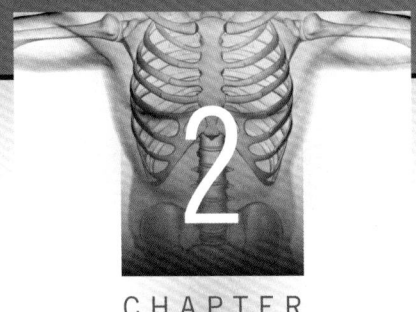

2
CHAPTER

Distal Chevron Osteotomy:
Perspective 2

Paul Hamilton, Sam Singh, and Michael G. Wilson

SURGICAL MANAGEMENT

- The primary indication for a chevron osteotomy is symptomatic hallux valgus deformity with a moderate deformity with an intermetatarsal angle of less than 15 degrees. The first metatarsocuneiform joint should be stable. The osteotomy can also be used to correct an abnormal distal metatarsal articular angle. It is used as a sole procedure in those presenting with minimal transfer symptoms.

Preoperative Planning

- Anteroposterior and lateral weight-bearing radiographs of the foot are evaluated for metatarsal length, intermetatarsal angle, hallux valgus angle, distal metatarsal articular angle, and interphalangeal angle for cases that may require a proximal phalangeal osteotomy to obtain complete correction.
- Congruency of the joint, presence of osteophytes, the size of the bony medial eminence, and the position and condition of the sesamoids are noted.

Positioning

- Surgery is performed on an outpatient basis.
- Prophylactic antibiotics are administered.
- A thigh tourniquet is applied.
- The patient is positioned supine with a sandbag under the ipsilateral buttock, so the big toe points to the ceiling.

CHEVRON OSTEOTOMY

Exposure

- Perform the distal soft tissue release either through a first web space incision or through the medial incision developing the approach over extensor hallucis longus into the first web space. Take care to avoid stripping the lateral metatarsal head soft tissues. We then perform the osteotomy in a step manner as described in the following text.
- Approach the metatarsal through a medial longitudinal incision extending from a point 1 cm proximal to the medial eminence to the medial flare of the proximal phalanx. This can be extended distally if a phalangeal osteotomy is required. Identify the dorsal medial cutaneous nerve, and incise the medial capsule sharply in a single longitudinal direction (TECH FIG 1A).
- Expose the medial eminence and resect it 1 mm medial to the sagittal sulcus (TECH FIG 1B).
- The most important part of the exposure is the identification of the plantar vascular supply (TECH FIG 1C). The osteotomy must be extracapsular. This plantar vascular supply must remain attached to the capital fragment to minimize any risk of avascular necrosis (AVN).

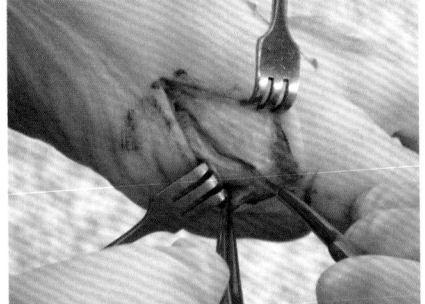 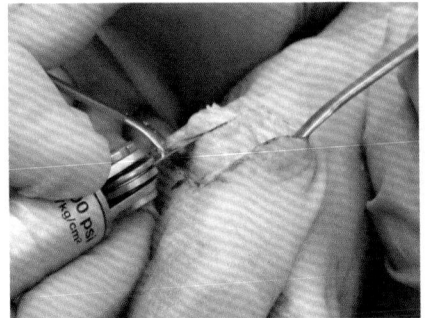 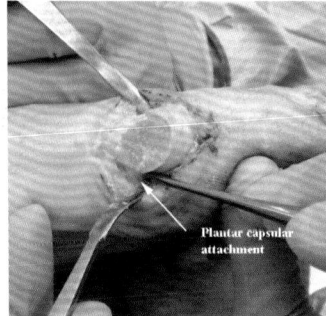

TECH FIG 1 A. After the skin is incised and the dorsal medial nerve is protected, the capsule is incised in a longitudinal fashion. **B.** The medial eminence is resected. **C.** Exposure and preservation of the plantar capsular attachment.

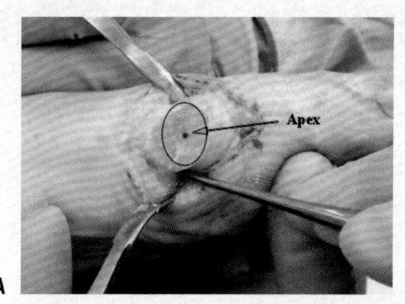
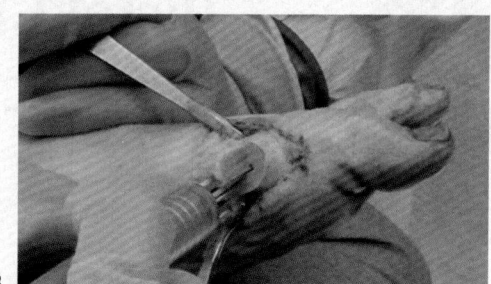
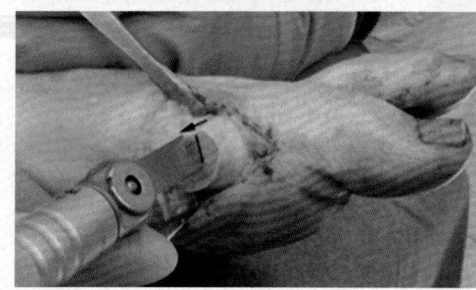

TECH FIG 2 A. An imaginary ellipse based on the articular surface is made, and the center is marked with ink. This is used as the apex of the osteotomy. **B.** The longitudinal cut is performed, ensuring that the proximal limb is extra-articular and the vascular bundle is maintained to the head. **C.** The saw blade is placed at 90 degrees to the longitudinal cut (*black line*) and then angled to produce a chevron osteotomy of between 60 and 80 degrees (*black arrow*).

Osteotomy

- The *apex of the osteotomy* is defined as the center of an imaginary ellipse or circle started by the articular surface of the metatarsal. Mark the apex with ink (**TECH FIG 2A**).
- Create the transverse limb of the osteotomy from the apex to the plantar surface of the metatarsal. The obliquity of this cut varies; the most important factor being that the osteotomy must remain extra-articular and the plantar vascular supply must be maintained to the metatarsal head (**TECH FIG 2B**). Complete the osteotomy through to the lateral side.
- Perform the vertical osteotomy by measuring a 90-degree angle to the plantar cut and then angling the saw blade to reduce this angle by 10 to 20 degrees. The exact angle is not crucial; we find that aiming for the angle to be between 60 and 80 degrees produces a stable osteotomy (**TECH FIG 2C**). Complete this osteotomy to the lateral side to allow displacement of the head fragment. Take care to protect the extensor hallucis longus tendon while performing the vertical osteotomy.

Compression and Fixation

- Use a sharp towel clip to grasp the proximal fragment and use the thumb to apply lateral displacement to the capital fragment (**TECH FIG 3A**). We allow a maximum of 50% displacement.

A McDonald dissector can be used to tease the capital fragment over if required.
- Use in-line force to compress the head fragment onto the shaft, allowing cancellous impaction (**TECH FIG 3B**). This aids in the immediate stability of the osteotomy while fixation is achieved.
- Fixation can be achieved using a 1.6-mm Kirschner wire or a compression screw. We pass the Kirschner wire in a retrograde fashion under direct vision from the plantar head obliquely across to the proximal fragment and through an appropriately placed small skin incision (**TECH FIG 3C**). Back the wire out to leave it a few millimeters deep to cartilage, thus maintaining excellent fixation without penetrating the joint. If a compression screw is used, follow the product guidance and ensure the screw does not penetrate the joint. Shave the redundant neck cortex, approximating to 50% of the protruding portion. Check for stability of the osteotomy.
- Imbricate the medial capsule with a strong absorbable suture while holding the hallux in a neutral or slightly abducted position with the aid of a swab.
- Confirm the reduction in the intermetatarsal angle, screws, and relocation of the sesamoids with image intensification with the foot flat on the image intensifier. Assess the need for a proximal phalangeal osteotomy.
- Close the wound in layers with continuous Monocryl to the skin, and apply a forefoot bandage to maintain the correction.

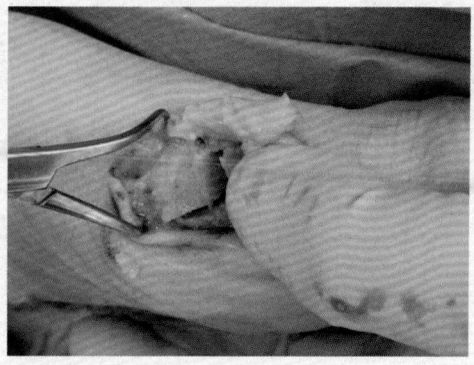
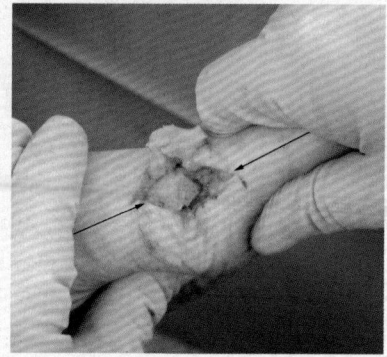

TECH FIG 3 A. The osteotomy is displaced and held with a clip. **B.** In-line compression as indicated by the *black arrows* is performed to impact the cancellous fragments together to increase stability. *(continued)*

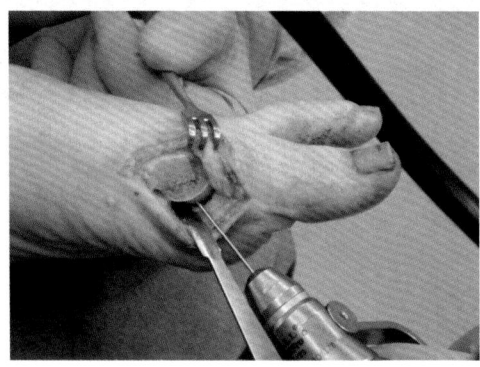

C

TECH FIG 3 *(continued)* **C.** A 1.6-mm Kirschner wire is passed in a retrograde fashion across the osteotomy site.

TECHNIQUES

Pearls and Pitfalls

Exposure	• The most important part of the exposure is that of the plantar vascular bundle. Failure to do so may compromise the blood supply to the metatarsal head.
Osteotomy	• If displacement of the osteotomy is difficult, check that all cuts have been completed. A limited lateral capsulotomy may be performed if needed, restricting the knife cuts to the lateral soft tissues distal to the metatarsal head.
Distal Metatarsal Articular Angle Correction	• To correct an abnormal distal metatarsal articular angle, a small medial wedge from the vertical limb of the osteotomy can be performed. This will make the osteotomy more unstable, and care must be taken to achieve good fixation.

POSTOPERATIVE CARE

- If safe, patients are discharged home on the day of surgery with strict advice to elevate the foot whenever resting for the first 2 weeks.
- In most cases, they are allowed to bear weight on their heel and lateral forefoot in a hard-soled postoperative shoe.
- Cast immobilization is not required.
- The wound is inspected at 2 weeks, at which time, the hallux is restrapped and patients are taught simple passive and active toe flexion–extension exercises.
- At 4 weeks postoperatively, the osteotomy is assessed. The Kirschner wire is removed in the outpatient setting.
- At 6 weeks, the osteotomy is checked radiologically, and if there is consolidation at the line of the osteotomy, the patient is instructed to wear a wide shoe or sneaker and to progress to full weight bearing as tolerated. Strapping of the hallux is discontinued at this time.

OUTCOMES

- The chevron osteotomy is the most commonly performed distal chevron osteotomy for mild hallux valgus in the United States,[4] and outcomes are excellent.[2,5,9]
- AVN with the use of a lateral release remains a concern. Recent reports suggest very low rates of AVN when correcting moderate deformities with the chevron osteotomy with a lateral release.[1,3,5,7] The improved correction that we see with a lateral release means that we perform it in every case.
- Evidence also now suggests that concern that the osteotomy should be reserved for patients younger than 50 years old may not be true, with equivalent results in differing age groups.[6,8]

COMPLICATIONS

- Complications include AVN, stiffness, nerve injury, wound problems, infection, undercorrection, overcorrection, fractures, chronic regional pain disorder, and deep vein thrombosis.
- Delayed union and nonunion are rare complications with the use of fixation.

REFERENCES

1. Kuhn MA, Lippert FG III, Phipps MJ, et al. Blood flow to the metatarsal head after chevron bunionectomy. Foot Ankle Int 2005;26:526–529.
2. Nery C, Barroco R, Réssio C. Biplanar chevron osteotomy. Foot Ankle Int 2002;23:792–798.
3. Peterson DA, Zilberfarb JL, Greene MA, et al. Avascular necrosis of the first metatarsal head: incidence in distal osteotomy combined with lateral soft tissue release. Foot Ankle Int 1994;15:59–63.
4. Pinney S, Song K, Chou L. Surgical treatment of mild hallux valgus deformity: the state of practice among academic foot and ankle surgeons. Foot Ankle Int 2006;27:970–973.
5. Potenza V, Caterini R, Farsetti P, et al. Chevron osteotomy with lateral release and adductor tenotomy for hallux valgus. Foot Ankle Int 2009;30:512–516.
6. Schneider W, Aigner N, Pinggera O, et al. Chevron osteotomy in hallux valgus: ten-year results of 112 cases. J Bone Joint Surg Br 2004;86B:1016–1020.
7. Singh SK, Jayasakera N, Nazir S, et al. Use of a polydioxanone (PDS) suture to stabilize the chevron osteotomy: a review of 30 cases. J Foot Ankle Surg 2004;43:306–310.
8. Trnka HJ, Zembsch A, Easley ME, et al. The chevron osteotomy for correction of hallux valgus: comparison of findings after two and five years of follow-up. J Bone Joint Surg Am 2000;82A:1373–1378.
9. Trnka HJ, Zembsch A, Weisauer H, et al. Modified Austin procedure for correction of hallux valgus. Foot Ankle Int 1997;18:119–127.

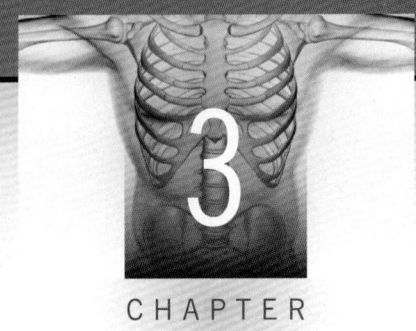

Biplanar Distal Chevron Osteotomy and Rotational Biplanar Chevron Osteotomy

Caio Nery, Marcelo Prado, and Daniel Baumfeld

DEFINITION

- Hallux valgus is a common condition that can affect both adults and adolescents.[2,5] Patients complain of pain and restriction with activities of daily living because of the lateral deviation of the great toe, the medial deviation of the first metatarsal, and the onset of inflammation at the progressively worsening medial eminence of the first metatarsal head. The gender proportion of the hallux valgus deformity is 15 women for every man (15:1).[16]

ANATOMY

- The first metatarsophalangeal (MTP) joint's complex anatomy is directly related to its complex physiology. The concave articular surface of the great toe's proximal phalanx articulates with the convex first metatarsal head. Its physiologic relationship is maintained by the surrounding articular capsule and collateral ligaments.[5] At the plantar aspect of the first MTP joint, the sesamoid complex acts as a rail on which the first metatarsal head glides congruently with the intrinsic and extrinsic tendons, providing power and stability to the joint.[12]

PATHOGENESIS

- Incongruent first MTP joint (physiologic distal metatarsal articular angle [DMAA])
  - The literature suggests that lateral deviation of the great toe is the primary event leading to hallux valgus deformity. This primary deforming force has a reciprocal relationship with metatarsus primus varus; the first and second intermetatarsal angle (IMA) worsens with an increase in the hallux valgus angle (HVA) and vice versa.[12,22] The valgus of the proximal phalanx produces forces whose vectors determine the lateral deviation of the head of the first metatarsal.[4,7,12,14]
- Congruent first MTP joint (increased DMAA)
  - With an increased DMAA, hallux valgus is present despite congruency of the first MTP joint. The articular surface of the first metatarsal head is in a valgus position relative to the first metatarsal shaft axis; therefore, hallux valgus is present even without an imbalance of the muscle forces on the first MTP joint.[14] However, this imbalance leads to a worsening of the deformity. Hallux valgus with an increased DMAA is less common than the incongruent type and typically occurs in men and younger patients (juvenile hallux valgus).[3–7] Recent studies showed that the MTP joint is predominantly congruent in males with the hallux valgus deformity.[16]

- Metatarsal rotation
  - The first metatarsal rotation may be the cause for the metatarsus varus itself, the apparent bunion, the apparent metatarsal head lateral slope, and even sesamoid malposition. The shape of the lateral edge of the metatarsal head, which consistently changes from round to angular when pronation is corrected, has also been implicated as a risk factor for recurrence of hallux valgus and for worse clinical results. Rotational deformity is not associated only with severe deformities, as moderate and even subtle hallux valgus can often require correction of pronation. In CT scans, it has been described that 87% of the individual with hallux valgus have internal rotation deformity, making pronation a serious concern for every surgeon that deals with this deformity.[9,11,23,24]

NATURAL HISTORY

- Shoe wear may contribute to the development of hallux valgus deformity.[2,12,20] A narrow and triangular toe box combined with high heels may force lateral deviation of the great toe, leading to a mechanical disadvantage of the abductor hallucis muscle. In males, the deformity has a clear inheritance pattern and seems to be transmitted by the mother; shoe wear do not play a significant role in the genesis of hallux valgus in men.[16]
- Persistence of these deforming forces may create a relative lateral displacement of the extensor hallucis longus and flexor hallucis longus tendons, which in turn may increase valgus deviation of the great toe. Eventually, the first MTP joint's medial capsule and collateral ligament become attenuated, whereas its lateral soft tissues become contracted.
- The laterally deviated hallux proximal phalanx exerts a varus-producing force to the first metatarsal head, thereby worsening the metatarsus primus varus deformity.[22] Because the sesamoid complex is attached to the proximal phalanx, the sesamoid position typically remains anatomic as the first metatarsal head subluxates medially. Other recent concept is the rotation (pronation) of the metatarsal head relatively to the first metatarsal, with an internal "torsion" of the metatarsal.[9,11] Progression of this displacement often produces the functional deficits and pronation of the great toe.[12]
- Because the first MTP joint is stable and congruent but malaligned with respect to the first metatarsal axis (increased DMAA), juvenile and adolescent hallux valgus deformity should prompt evaluation for potential associated pathology, such as metatarsus adductus, hypermobility, or ligamentous laxity.[16,17]

PATIENT HISTORY AND PHYSICAL FINDINGS

- Patients typically complain of pain over the first metatarsal head's medial eminence, especially while standing and walking in a narrow toe box shoe. Occasionally, patients develop a symptomatic bursitis over the medial eminence. In males with the deformity, there is an early onset of the symptoms.[16]
- Pain plantar to the first metatarsal head suggests a symptomatic and incongruent articulation of the sesamoids with the first metatarsal head. Compensation for this discomfort may lead to transfer metatarsalgia.
- An imbalance of forefoot pressures created by the malalignment of the first ray secondary to hallux valgus may also lead to transfer metatarsalgia.
- We routinely review the patient's general health, activity level, and family history of hallux valgus. We always check for comorbidities that may have a direct impact on the success of corrective bunion surgery, particularly diabetes, arthritis, and neurovascular diseases.[2,12]
- To fully appreciate the degree of hallux valgus deformity, the involved foot must be examined with the patient standing.
- We evaluate the range of motion and alignment of the ankle, hindfoot, midfoot, and forefoot with the patient standing and walking.
- Frontal plane pronation or a valgus position of the hallux is clinically observable and best assessed with the patient standing.[9,11,23]
- The lesser toes are carefully examined for deformities, which can be rigid or supple, requiring different types of treatment.[13]
- Pronation of the great toe must be assessed as well as the presence of callosities under the toes and forefoot associated with metatarsalgia.[1,12]
- Passive correction of hallux valgus is attempted. With the patient standing, pressure is applied over the lateral face of the great toe, trying to correct its valgus deviation. Patients with passive correctable lateral deviation of the great toe will need less invasive or hazardous procedures for the treatment of their hallux valgus deformity, particularly the adductor hallucis release.
- Hypermobility of the first ray can have an influence on the onset of the hallux valgus deformity as well as on its treatment.
- It is easy to differentiate the flexible and rigid forms of hammer or claw toes by applying thumb pressure in the forefoot sole and elevating the metatarsal heads; in the flexible forms, the deformities reduces or disappears completely; in the rigid forms, the maneuver does not change the hammer or claw toes.

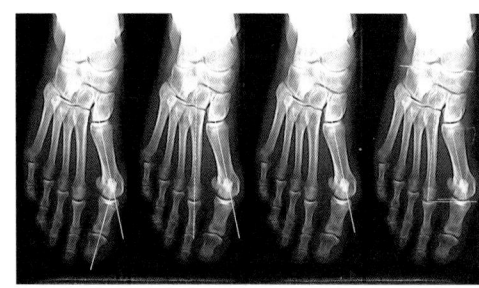

FIG 1 AP radiograph of a patient with hallux valgus. **Left.** HVA (up to 15 degrees). **Second from left.** First IMA (up to 9 degrees). **Second from right.** Sesamoid position. In this patient, the tibial sesamoid is divided into two halves by the diaphyseal axis of the first metatarsal, which means the beginning of a grade 2 sesamoid subluxation (normal is grade 0). **Right.** Relative length of the first and second metatarsals; normal is up to 5 mm.

- A positive MTP joint drawer sign indicates the presence of a capsulitis and instability of the joint due to the lesion of the plantar capsule or collateral ligaments, more commonly the lateral portion of the plantar plate.

IMAGING AND OTHER DIAGNOSTIC STUDIES

- Hallux valgus must be assessed with a minimum of anteroposterior (AP) and lateral weight-bearing radiographs of the foot.
- The HVA is determined by the intersection of the diaphyseal axes of the first metatarsal and the proximal phalanx. Arbitrarily, a normal HVA does not exceed 15 degrees **(FIG 1)**.
- The IMA is the angle between the diaphyseal axes of the first and second metatarsals. Arbitrarily, a normal IMA does not exceed 9 degrees (see **FIG 1**).
- The sesamoid position is determined by its relationship with the first metatarsal diaphyseal axis. Typically, the sesamoids remain in their anatomic position; with progressive hallux valgus deformity, the first metatarsal head progressively subluxates medially in relation to the sesamoids.
  - Normal (grade 0) sesamoid position: The tibial and fibular sesamoids are equidistant from the bisecting line of the first metatarsal.
  - Sesamoid position grades 1 to 3: Grades 1 to 3 signify an increasingly greater lateral position of the tibial sesamoid relative to the bisecting line of the tibial shaft axis, with grade 3 indicating that the tibial sesamoid is positioned completely lateral to the reference line **(FIG 2)**.
  - The interphalangeal angle is measured between the axis of both the proximal and distal phalanx of the great toe; arbitrarily, its normal value is up to 10 degrees.

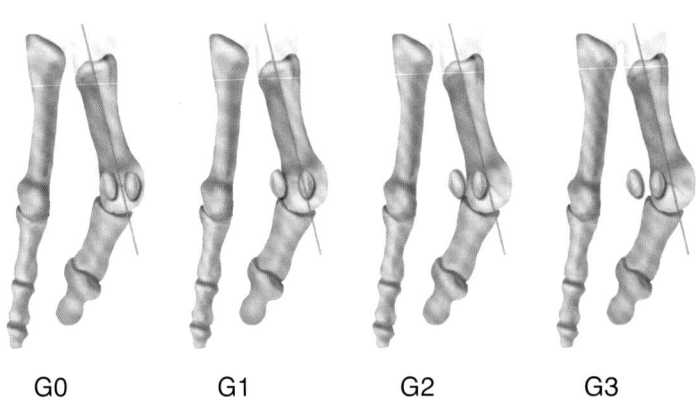

G0   G1   G2   G3

FIG 2 Evaluation of hallucal sesamoid position. Grade 0, no displacement of sesamoids relative to the middle diaphyseal axis of the first metatarsal (normal). Grade 1, overlap of less than 50% of the tibial (medial) sesamoid to the reference line. Grade 2, overlap of more than 50% of the tibial sesamoid to the reference line. Grade 3, tibial sesamoid completely displaced beyond the reference line.

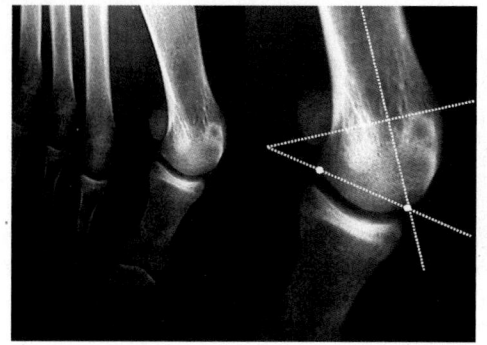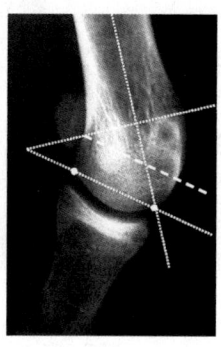

FIG 3 A. AP radiograph from a patient with juvenile hallux valgus in which the absolute congruence of the MTP joint can be noted. The misalignment of the distal articular surface of the metatarsal determines the hallux valgus deformity. **B.** Both edges of the metatarsal head articular surface are marked. The DMAA is measured between the line that connects the articular edges and the perpendicular to the diaphyseal axis of the first metatarsal. The normal value is up to 8 degrees.

- The DMAA is obtained by the intersection of the line that connects the articular edges of the head and the line bisecting the first metatarsal shaft. The DMAA normal value is up to 8 degrees **(FIG 3)**.[15,20] Inter- and intraobserver reliability for measuring the DMAA is poor.
- The proximal phalanx articular angle is measured between the tangent to the proximal articular surface of the proximal phalanx of the great toe and the line bisecting the diaphyseal axis of the same phalanx. It is considered normal up to 10 degrees.
- Relative length of the first and second rays is measured pre- and postoperatively. Most osteotomies lead to shortening of the first metatarsal. In our experience, greater than 5 mm of first metatarsal shortening of the first metatarsal frequently results in transfer metatarsalgia.
- The HVA, DMAA, and IMA are significantly higher in males, indicating that hallux valgus presents as a more severe deformity among males.[16,17]
- Frontal plane pronation or a valgus position of the hallux is also measurable through sesamoid axial views. Pronation observed on axial views can be correlated with the "apparent" sesamoid subluxation on the AP radiographic projection and the lateral shape of the metatarsal head (the round shape of the lateral head is consider a sign of metatarsal rotation) **(FIG 4)**.[11]

DIFFERENTIAL DIAGNOSIS

- Hallux valgus interphalangeus
- Hallux rigidus
- Sesamoiditis

NONOPERATIVE MANAGEMENT

- Patient education
  - Although there is no concrete evidence that shoe wear causes hallux valgus, we believe that wearing shoes with tight toe boxes and high heels contributes to the worsening of deformity.
  - Patients with intrinsic factors contributing to hallux valgus, such as an increased DMAA, should be educated that they are particularly prone to external forces worsening their hallux valgus deformity.[5]
- Orthotic devices and insoles may relieve symptoms but generally do not correct deformity. Moreover, patients already in need of wider toe boxes may need to find shoes with extra depth to accommodate both their foot deformity and the orthotic device. In juvenile hallux valgus (skeletally immature patients), the use of a custom-made night splint could limit the progression but cannot reverse the deformity.[18]
- In skeletally mature patients, intermittent use of a corrective splint does not adequately counterbalance many hours of shoe wear with a narrow toe box and a high heel.

SURGICAL MANAGEMENT

- The primary indication for the biplanar distal chevron osteotomy is moderate hallux valgus deformity with a 1–2 IMA of 14 degrees or less associated with a DMAA greater than 8 degrees.[15]
- The indications for the rotational biplanar chevron osteotomy (RBCO) are mild to moderate hallux valgus deformity associated with hallux pronation related to internal

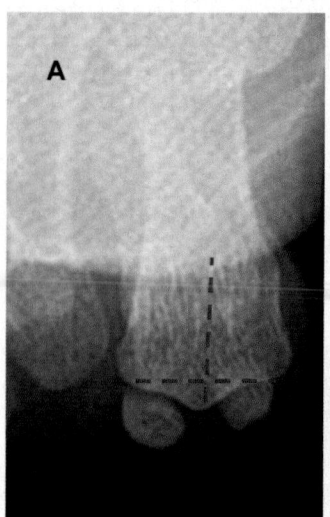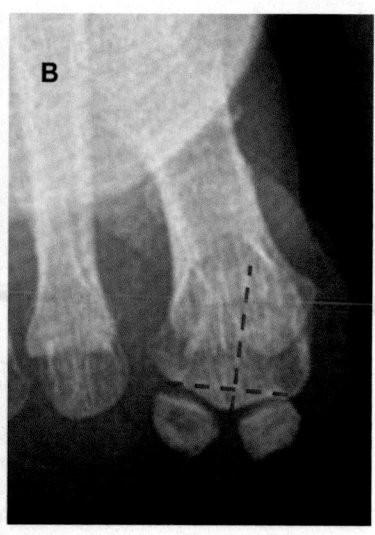

FIG 4 Tangential views of the sesamoids (*broken lines*) during weight-bearing neutral (**A**) pronation (**B**). The degree of longitudinal rotation of the metatarsal is clearly demonstrated by the position of the sesamoids, which still retain a normal relationship to their facets beneath the metatarsal head.

rotation of the first metatarsal bone. This is radiographically observed with the position of first metatarsal head condyles and the laterally subluxated sesamoids on an AP loaded forefoot x-ray.[23]

- Reports of the traditional distal chevron technique over the past two decades suggest that comparable outcomes are achieved for younger and older patients.[10]
- In our hands, contraindications to any distal first metatarsal osteotomy for hallux valgus correction include asymptomatic deformity, a 1–2 IMA exceeding 15 degrees, first MTP joint stiffness or degenerative arthritis, and osteoporosis or osteopenia.
- The biplanar distal chevron and rotational chevron osteotomy can be used as a complementary procedure in the surgical treatment of severe hallux valgus deformities in which the DMAA is abnormal. The combination of two or even three osteotomies in the same ray can be considered safe if the blood supply to the metatarsal head is unharmed.[19]

Preoperative Planning

- Satisfactory neurovascular status
- Is the hallux valgus passively correctible? The surgeon should assess associated lesser toes deformities, including fixed versus flexible deformity, impingement or overlap on the first toe, and presence of plantar calluses.
- Using radiographic measurements from preoperative weight-bearing radiographs of the foot, we always have a preoperative estimation of the required lateral translation of the first metatarsal head and wedge resection to correct the increased DMAA and the presence and amount of rotation.[24]

Positioning

- The patient is positioned supine, with the plantar aspect of the operated foot in line with the end of the operating table.

- We stand on the side of the table immediately adjacent to the operated foot; our assistant stands at the end of the table.
- We routinely use a tourniquet.

Approach

- A 5-cm longitudinal midaxial medial incision is made, centered over the medial eminence (**FIG 5**).
- Careful subcutaneous dissection is performed to protect the dorsal and plantar medial sensory nerves to the hallux.
- Although the distal metatarsal metaphysis must be exposed, periosteal stripping is kept to a minimum, and the lateral vascular supply to the first metatarsal head remains protected.
- In our experience, with the proper indications outlined earlier, we rarely need to perform a risky lateral dissection of the adductor hallucis tendon at the joint line.
  - A routine portion of the exposure, lateral dislocation of the metatarsal head, serves as a physiologic release of the adductor hallucis by bringing its phalangeal insertion closer to its origin.[10,12,15]

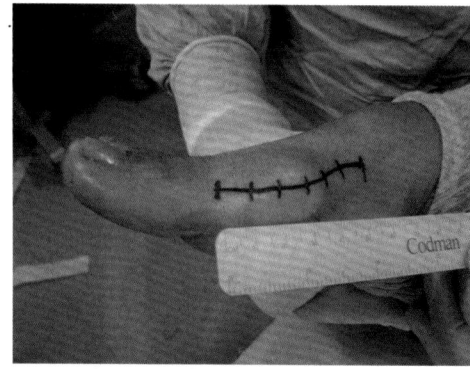

FIG 5 The skin incision is centered over the medial eminence.

CAPSULOTOMY

- We use a Y-shaped incision over the medial face of the MTP joint capsule, creating three distinct flaps that we reapproximate at the completion of the procedure to achieve optimal tensioning (**TECH FIG 1A,B**).
- A short V capsular flap attached to the base of the hallux proximal phalanx may be used as an anchor to correct

the deformity. We always preserve the relatively thin dorsal capsular flap continuous with the lateral capsule to maintain the blood supply to the first metatarsal head. The stout plantar capsular flap attached to the sesamoids serves to reestablish the optimal first metatarsal head–sesamoid position when tensioned after completion of the osteotomy.

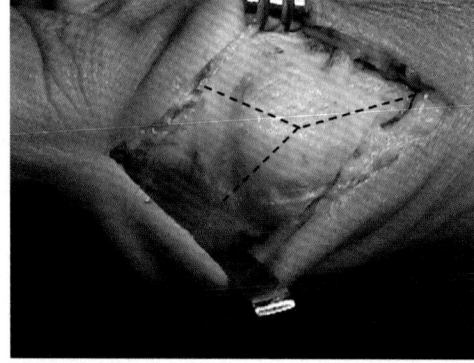

A

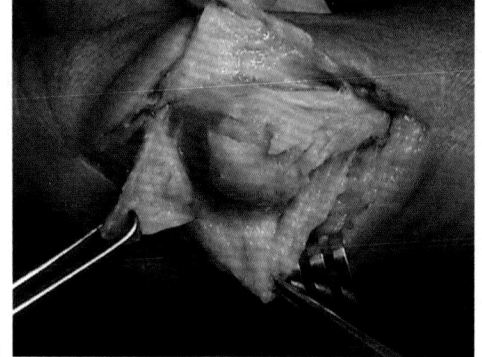

B

TECH FIG 1 A. The Y figure over the medial face of the MTP joint demarcating the capsular flaps. **B.** Following the Y figure, the articular capsule is divided to create the three flaps: a V flap attached to the base of the proximal phalanx, a thin dorsal flap, and a strong plantar flap.

MEDIAL AND DORSAL METATARSAL HEAD EXPOSURE

- After capsulotomy, the first metatarsal head's medial eminence and sagittal groove are exposed.
- Starting at the medial aspect of the sagittal groove, we resect the medial eminence with a small oscillating saw from dorsal to plantar, in line with the medial edge of the foot **(TECH FIG 2A,B)**.
- We make sure to preserve the integrity of the metatarsal head and medial cortex of the metatarsal shaft **(TECH FIG 2C,D)**.

- Occasionally, a "dorsal bunion" is present in the absence of degenerative change. We routinely resect this dorsal eminence in line with the dorsal cortex of the metatarsal shaft to eliminate any chance for impingement and potentially improve cosmesis **(TECH FIG 2E)**.

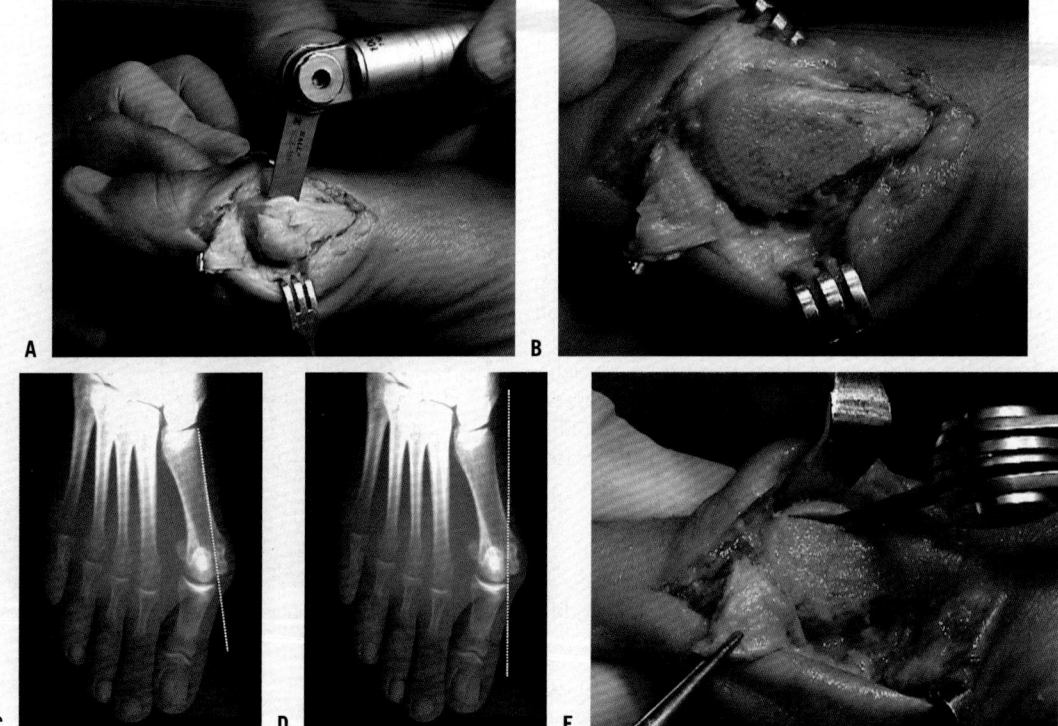

TECH FIG 2 A,B. The beginning of the medial prominence removal. With the sagittal groove used as a guide, the saw is oriented in a dorsoplantar direction. **C.** The medial osteotomy must follow the medial border of the foot to preserve the integrity of the metatarsal head and diaphysis. The wrong way to do this is shown. **D.** The right way to proceed to the prominence resection is shown. **E.** The dorsal prominence of the metatarsal head is resected in line with the dorsal diaphyseal cortex.

BIPLANAR CHEVRON OSTEOTOMY

- As a point of reference, we mark the geometric center of the first metatarsal head with a sharp instrument on the prepared medial surface **(TECH FIG 3A)**. From this point, we draw the segments (arms) of the planned osteotomy.
- We cut the plantar arm of the osteotomy parallel to the inferior surface of the foot **(TECH FIG 3B)**, thereby creating a broad and stable surface area to promote healing between the two osteotomy fragments. If some degree of plantar displacement of the metatarsal head is desirable, one can make the plantar arm cut with the saw oriented in a dorsomedial to plantar–lateral direction. The incline of the cut will determine the amount of plantar displacement of the metatarsal head.[21]
- According to the preoperative radiographic DMAA estimate, we plan a medially based wedge resection as part of the dorsal

limb osteotomy to rotate the capital fragment into a more physiologic relationship with the first metatarsal shaft. Three methods exist to determine the correct size for the medial wedge to be removed[15]:
- A trigonometric formula (wedge width = tan DMAA × first metatarsal head width [in millimeters])
- Drawing the wedge corresponding to the measured DMAA over the AP radiographic image of the first metatarsal
- By direct vision during the operation, make the distal cut parallel to the distal metatarsal articular surface and the proximal cut perpendicular to the long axis of the first metatarsal **(TECH FIG 3C–E)**.
- The saw blade must not violate the inferior portion of the metatarsal head fragment.

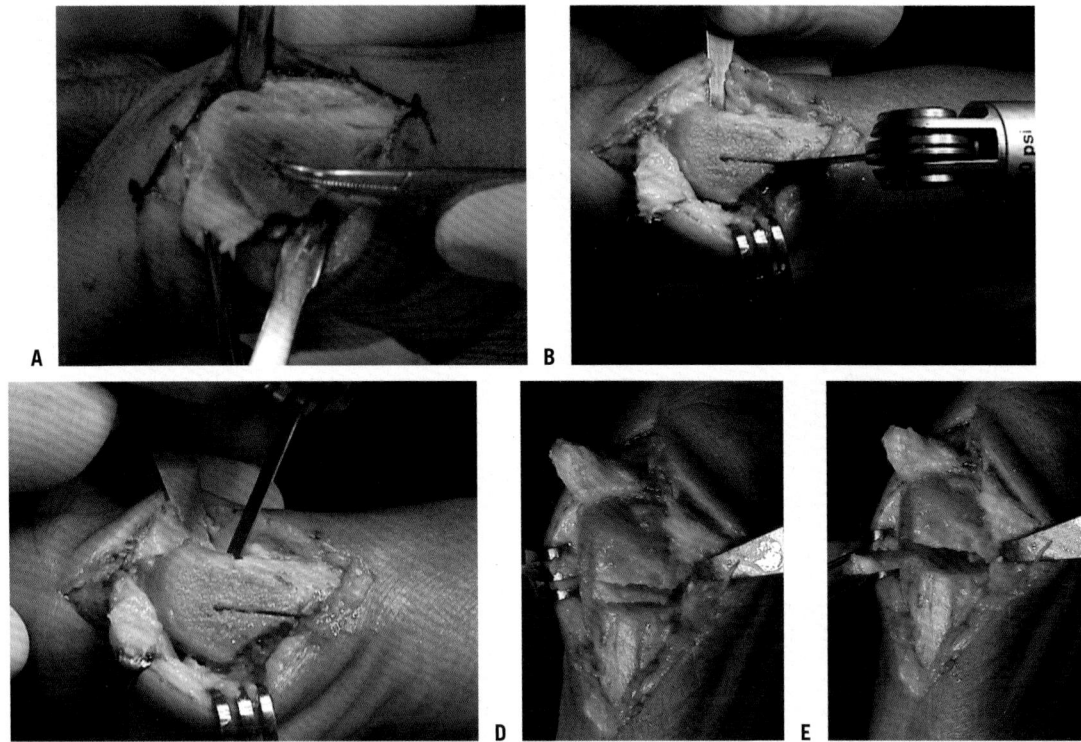

TECH FIG 3 A. Marking the geometric center of the metatarsal head. **B.** The plantar arm of the osteotomy, parallel to the plantar surface of the foot. **C.** The positioning of the saw during the planning of the dorsal arm of the osteotomy. There is a posterior inclination of 10 to 15 degrees to create an acute vertex for the osteotomy. **D.** The dorsal segment of the osteotomy is made using two cuts. The distal one is parallel to the distal articular surface, and the proximal cut is perpendicular to the metatarsal diaphyseal axis so that a medially based wedge is produced. **E.** The metaphyseal bone wedge is removed.

TRANSLATION AND SCREW FIXATION

- In my experience, each millimeter of lateral metatarsal head translation corresponds to 1 degree of 1–2 IMA correction. Using average physiologic dimensions, the metatarsal head may be translated laterally up to 6 mm to create a 9-degree 1–2 IMA without forfeiting osteotomy stability.
- After dorsal wedge resection and simultaneous to lateral translation, rotate the metatarsal head to create a physiologic DMAA and achieve optimal bony apposition at the dorsal aspect of the osteotomy.[10,14]
- Gentle longitudinal traction on the hallux and concomitant pressure with the thumb over the medial capital fragment facilitates lateral displacement **(TECH FIG 4A)**.
- By driving the great toe as a joystick, the capital fragment is rotated under direct vision to correct the DMAA.
- Once the proper positioning of the fragments is obtained, apply gentle pressure on the great toe to coapt the osteotomy site **(TECH FIG 4B)**.
- In our experience, it is not necessary to check the position of the fragments and the amount of correction with fluoroscopy but, for those who think that it is advisable, this is the right moment to do that. You can use a 1.2-mm Kirschner wire to

maintain the fragments temporarily during the fluoroscopic checking.
- We routinely secure the osteotomy with a single screw, either a solid screw placed in lag fashion or a headless cannulated or noncannulated dual-pitch compression screw while maintaining manual reduction of the osteotomy.
  - Screw position: 5 mm proximal to the dorsal arm of the biplanar chevron osteotomy, on the first metatarsal shaft **(TECH FIG 4C)**
  - Screw trajectory: we aim the screw 10 degrees distally and 15 degrees laterally to target the optimal portion of the laterally translated distal fragment, compress the fragments, and limit the risk of penetrating the plantar articular surface.[10]
- Using a 2.7-mm solid screw
  - Initial 2.0-mm drill hole, followed by overdrill of the near cortex with a 2.7-mm drill to create a lag effect
  - Because of the screw trajectory and relatively thin overlying capsule and skin, consider using a countersink.
  - Insertion of the 2.7-mm screw to carefully compress the osteotomy and maintain reduction **(TECH FIG 4D)**

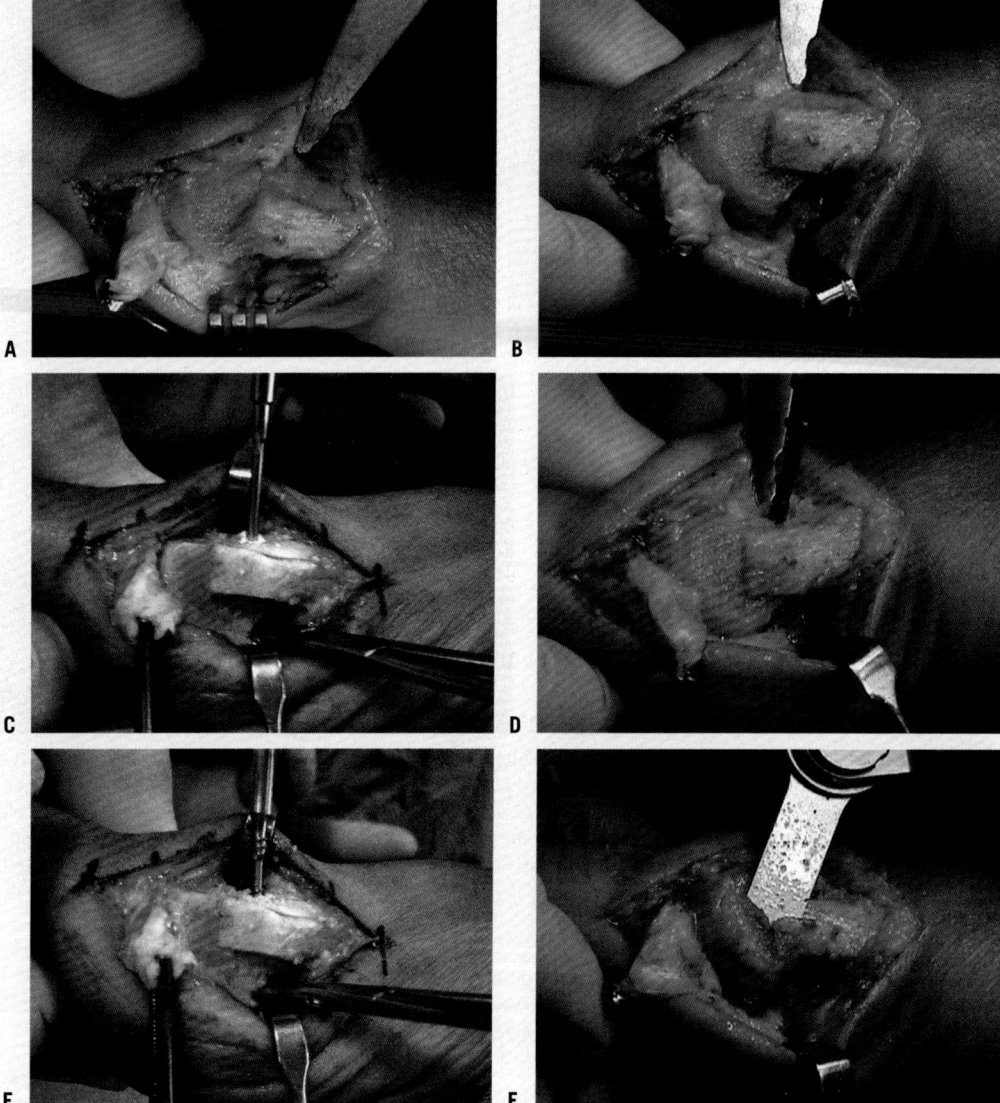

TECH FIG 4 A. With light distraction applied on the great toe, the cephalic fragment is laterally dislocated and internally rotated to reduce both the IMA and the DMAA. **B.** Gentle pressure is applied on the great toe for cooptation the osteotomy site. **C.** Making a drill hole at the dorsal aspect of the metaphysis of the metatarsal. **D.** The introduction of a 2.7-mm screw to achieve the bone fixation. **E.** Bone fixation with a Herbert-type screw. **F.** The metaphyseal remaining portion must be removed from dorsal to plantar to clear the medial border of the metatarsal.

- Using a headless cannulated or noncannulated dual-pitch screw
  - Guide pin (if cannulated)
  - Dual-diameter drill corresponding to the particular screw system
  - Insertion of the screw after proper screw length has been determined, with compression of the fragments and stability created at the osteotomy **(TECH FIG 4E)**

- Carefully resect the residual medial prominence of the proximal fragment with an oscillating saw, directing the saw blade from dorsal to plantar while avoiding any violation of the first metatarsal diaphysis **(TECH FIG 4F).**
- We routinely irrigate the first MTP joint with saline solution to remove undesirable detritus.

ROTATION BIPLANAR CHEVRON OSTEOTOMY (TECH FIG 5)

- As described for the biplanar chevron osteotomy, the geometric center of the first metatarsal head with a sharp instrument on the prepared medial surface from this point, the surgeon can draw the segments (arms) of the planned osteotomy.

- A double limb osteotomy is performed. The dorsal limb starts at the first metatarsal head center and is perpendicular to the long axis of the metatarsal shaft. The inferior limb starts at the same point and is angulated 120 degrees to the first one, thereby

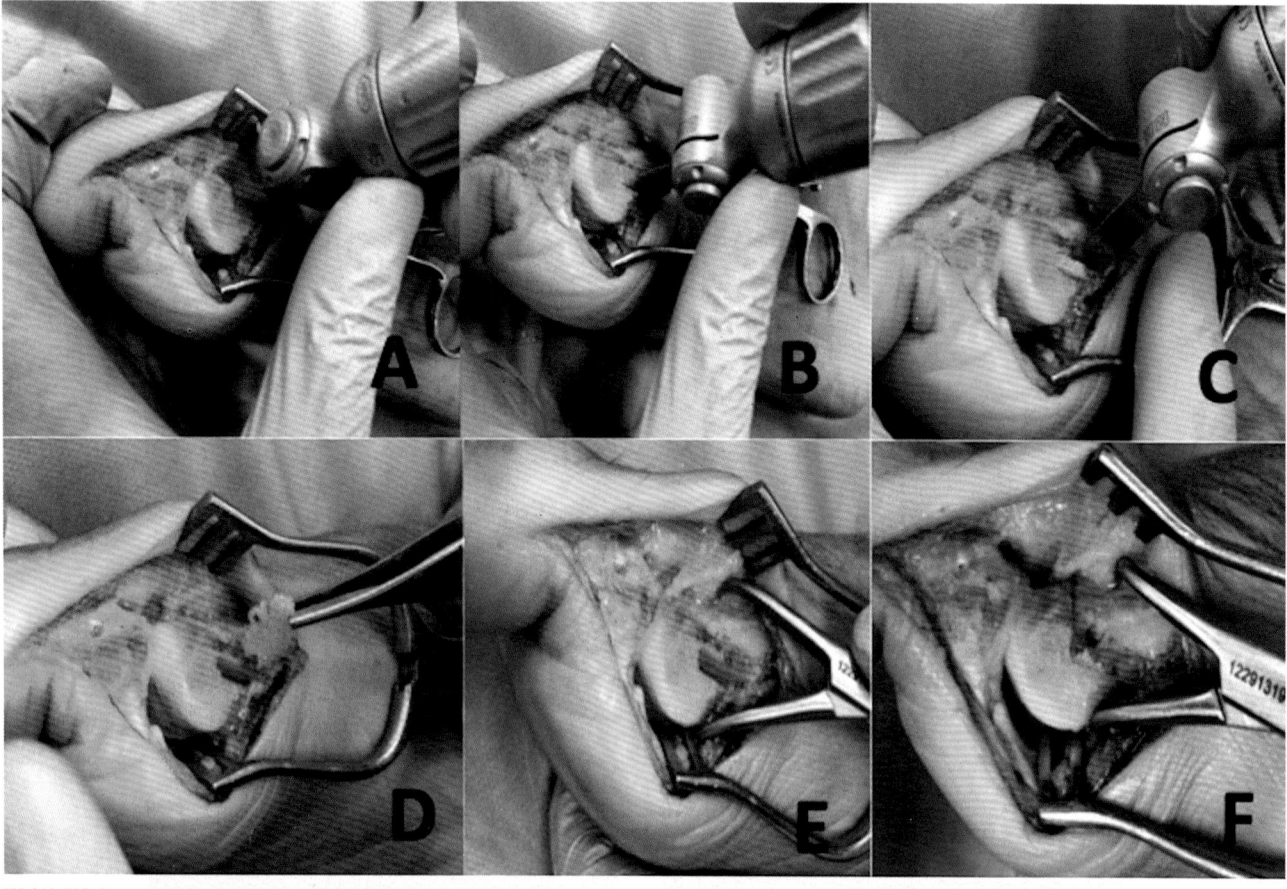

TECH FIG 5 RBCO. **A.** Dorsal cut. **B.** First plantar cut. **C.** Second plantar cut. **D.** Removal of the wedge. **E.** Position of the clamp to close the wedge. **F.** Fragment rotation and wedge closure.

creating a broad and stable surface area to promote healing between the two osteotomy fragments. After that, a medial-based wedge parallel to the plantar limb is performed and removed according to the preoperative radiographic rotation estimated.[23]
- The distal metatarsal fragment is then displaced laterally, just like in the conventional chevron osteotomy.

- After that, correction of the metatarsal rotational deformity is undertaken using the gap left by the medial wedge removal.
- Osteotomy fixation is done by using an almost vertical compression screw, as described for the biplanar chevron osteotomy.

CAPSULORRHAPHY

- We judiciously resect redundant medial capsule. Holding the proximal phalanx in optimal alignment relative to the long axis of the first metatarsal in both the sagittal and transverse planes facilitates determining the overlap of residual medial capsule.
  - In anticipation of some tendency toward recurrence of deformity, we typically hold the hallux in a slight varus and plantarflexion position.
  - In my experience, this optimal position is best maintained by the assistant holding the first metatarsal, the MTP joint, and hallux between the thumb and the second finger of the assistant's hand so that the hallux rests in the space between the assistant's first and second metacarpals **(TECH FIG 6A,B)**.
- With the assistant maintaining the optimal position, we resect the redundant capsular flaps.

- Next, we check the relationship of the medial sesamoid and first metatarsal head, applying greater tension to the plantar flap to reduce the head on the sesamoids if necessary. We place a 2-0 nonabsorbable buried suture at the central corners of both the dorsal and plantar capsular flaps and systematically close the capsulotomy from distal to proximal **(TECH FIG 6C)**.
- Appose the residual V-shaped flap attached to the medial aspect of the proximal phalanx to the previously sutured dorsal and plantar flaps.
- In my experience, removing greater capsular redundancy from the dorsal portion of the phalangeal flap facilitates correction of hallux pronation **(TECH FIG 6D–F)**.

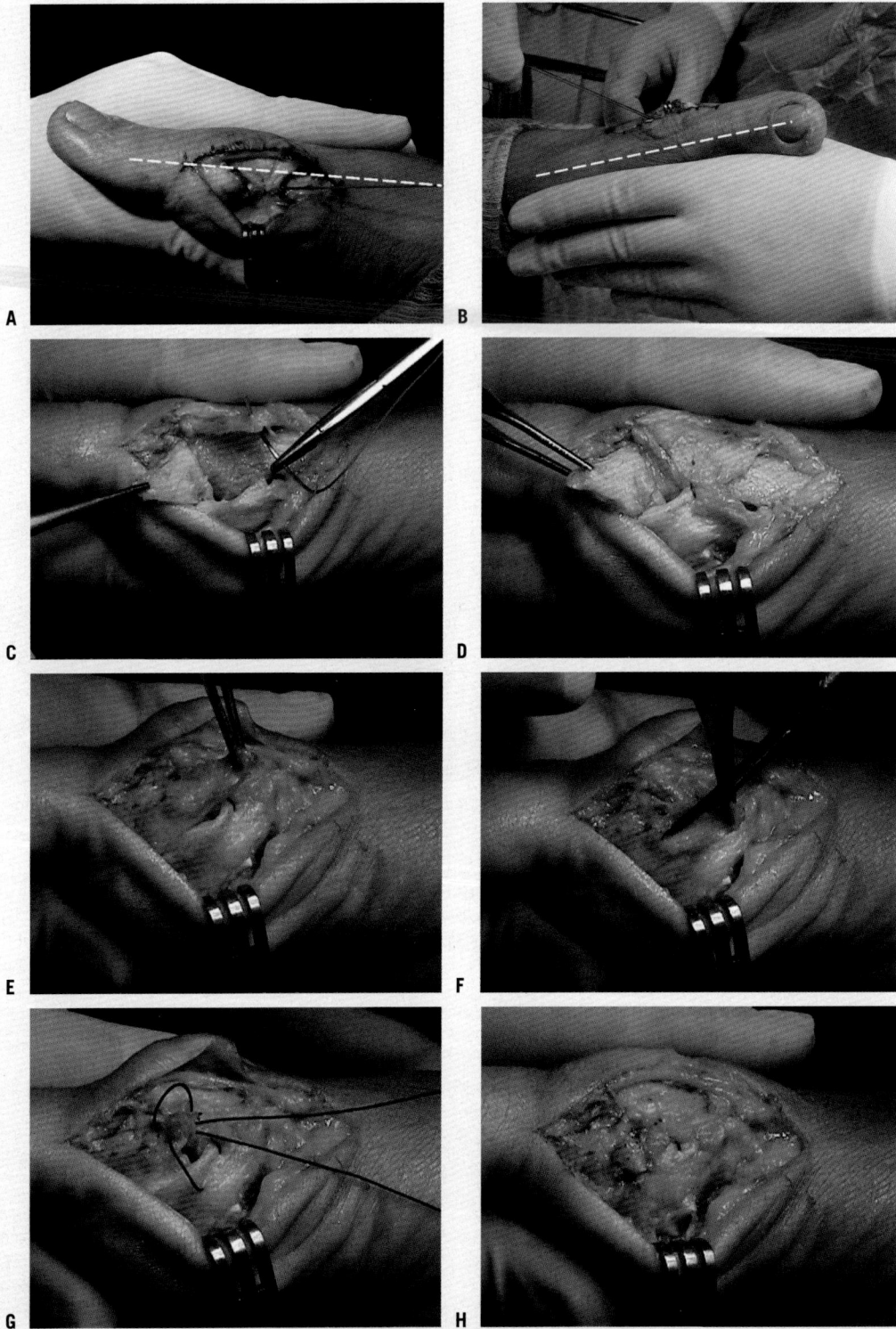

TECH FIG 6 A,B. The best way to keep the hallux in the right position during the capsulorrhaphy. The great toe must be aligned with the first metatarsal in the sagittal and transverse planes (*broken lines*). **C.** After resecting the excess, the dorsal flap is sutured to the plantar capsular flap. **D.** The V-shaped flap attached to the proximal phalanx is apposed to the dorsal and plantar flaps. **E,F.** The excess of the V flap is determined and resected. **G.** A single suture is placed in the vertex of the V-shaped flap. After the toe is released, its adequate position is checked. **H.** While the great toe is kept at the right position, the capsular suture is finished.

- We use a single suture, which is placed at the center of the Y, where the capsular flaps meet **(TECH FIG 6G)**.
  - Once the medial capsulorrhaphy is complete, the assistant releases the toe. Ideally, the hallux should maintain its corrected alignment without external support.
  - Occasionally, we augment the capsulorrhaphy with complementary tensioning sutures to obtain the desired position. Again, the hallux must be held in the corrected position or even slight varus as noted earlier **(TECH FIG 6H)**.

- Close the subcutaneous tissue with interrupted absorbable sutures.
- We favor using absorbable subcuticular sutures and interrupted fine nylon suture in young patients (more favorable skin) and older patients (less favorable skin), respectively. We routinely use a bunion dressing, or H dressing, in the first web space to relieve tension on the medial capsulorrhaphy. We wrap the forefoot with a sterile cotton bandage followed by an adhesive bandage that maintains slight compression on the first metatarsal.

TECHNIQUES

Pearls and Pitfalls

Indications Biplanar Chevron Osteotomy	• Proximal first metatarsal osteotomy with a 1–2 IMA greater than 15 degrees. • In my experience, the power of 1–2 IMA correction is limited by the width of the metatarsal head. • In general, 1 mm of lateral translation equals 1 degree of 1–2 IMA correction. • A biplanar osteotomy is not required, unless the DMAA exceeds 8 degrees.
Indications Rotation Biplanar Chevron Osteotomy	• Mild to moderate hallux valgus deformity associated with hallux pronation related to internal rotation of the first metatarsal bone • Sign of rotation in AP x-rays—position of first metatarsal head condyles, laterally subluxated sesamoids on an AP loaded forefoot, rounded shape of the metatarsal head
Approach	• We routinely perform the skin incision 2 mm dorsal to the medial midaxial line to identify and protect the dorsomedial sensory nerve to the hallux.
Capsular Flaps	• Develop the capsular flaps carefully to allow optimal soft tissue balancing during capsulorrhaphy.
Medial Eminence Resection	• Perform the medial eminence resection in line with the medial foot and not the medial aspect of the first metatarsal. • Less resection is better (limits potential for varus).
Biplanar Chevron Osteotomy	• The plantar arm should be parallel to the plantar plane of the foot. • The apex of the wedge to be resected dorsally should coincide with the lateral cortex of the head to avoid shortening of the metatarsal.
Rotation Biplanar Chevron Osteotomy	• The inferior limb of the osteotomy is angulated 120 degrees to the first one. • The medial-based wedge parallel to the plantar limb is responsible to correct the rotation deformity
Screw Fixation	• Direct the drill and screw laterally to capture the plantar "tongue" of the distal fragment. • Avoid placing a screw that penetrates the plantar cortex at the metatarsal head–sesamoid complex. • Remember to countersink the dorsal metaphyseal cortex when using a 2.7-mm screw.
Capsulorrhaphy	• Be sure that your assistant maintains the great toe at the right position during capsulorrhaphy.
Dressing	• Should maintain the great toe in the optimal position for 3 weeks

POSTOPERATIVE CARE

- Anticipated dried blood may harden the bandage and create pressure-related symptoms postoperatively. This occurs often enough that we routinely change the patient's bandage on postoperative day 3 or 4.[11]
- We allow my patients to bear weight in a Barouk postoperative shoe after the first dressing change. This orthosis concentrates the patient's weight on the rear of the foot while protecting the forefoot. Our patients do not routinely require crutches or assistive devices, but the occasional elderly patient with comorbidities may benefit from temporary use of a walker.

- We routinely change the bandage for my bunion patients at 10-day intervals to confirm that proper great toe alignment is maintained. To confirm that the alignment and reduction are maintained, we obtain a radiograph of the operated foot at 3 weeks after surgery. In our experience, at 1 month postoperatively, patients may transfer to a pair of soft and wide lace-up shoes and initiate hallux range-of-motion exercises.
- In our practice, it takes an average of 3 to 4 months for patients to reach the maximum range of motion and return to regular shoe wear and full activity.

OUTCOMES

- Patient satisfaction rates after distal biplanar chevron osteotomy for moderate hallux valgus deformity approach 90%, depending on appropriate patient expectations and selection.[14]
- In our experience, the procedure reliably and reproducibly corrects the 1–2 IMA, HVA, and increased DMAA (**FIG 6**) and can be useful as a complementary procedure in severe cases (**FIG 7**).
- There is no report in the literature regarding the outcomes of the rotation chevron osteotomy, only technical description.[11,23,24] However, there are some reports about the rotation correction with other types of technique and good results are presented.[9,24]

COMPLICATIONS

- Complications are similar to other distal first metatarsal osteotomies for correction of hallux valgus.

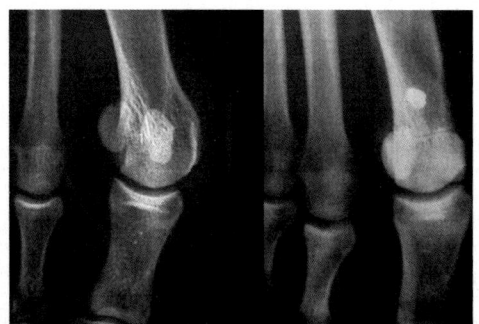
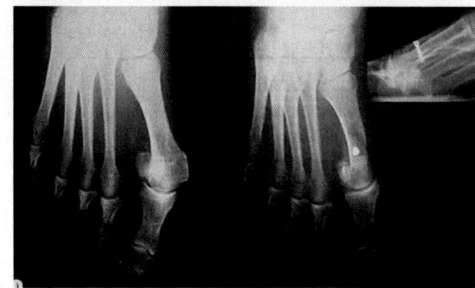
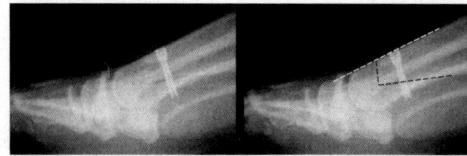

FIG 6 A. Preoperative and postoperative radiographic images of a right foot with hallux valgus with increased DMAA, treated by the biplanar chevron osteotomy. The correction of the DMAA and the sesamoid position is easy to see. The valgus of the great toe was also satisfactorily corrected. **B.** In these images, we can see the correction obtained with the biplanar distal chevron osteotomy. The cephalic fragment was 6 mm laterally dislocated to correct the IMA and the sesamoid position. The DMAA and HVA were corrected to normal values. In the lateral view, we can see the size and position of the screw used in the fragment fixation. **C.** Lateral views of a patient treated by the biplanar distal chevron osteotomy, where we can see both the plantar and dorsal arms of the osteotomy, the position of the screw used in its fixation, and the alignment of the cephalic fragment with the metatarsal diaphysis resulting from the dorsal fragment resection (*broken lines*).

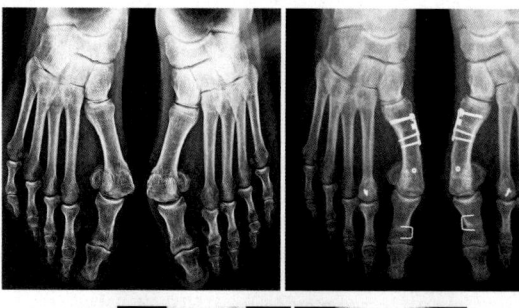
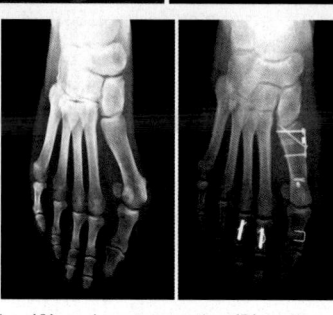

FIG 7 Preoperative (**A**) and postoperative (**B**) radiographic images of a patient with severe hallux valgus deformity with increased DMAA treated by the combination of a proximal opening wedge osteotomy, a distal biplanar chevron osteotomy, and a proximal phalangeal closing wedge "Akin" osteotomy.

- Recurrence or undercorrection
  - Inappropriate preoperative planning
    - Stretching the indications
  - Usually due to inadequate
    - Lateral translation
    - Rotation of the first metatarsal head
    - Soft tissue balancing during the capsulorrhaphy
  - Lack of proper postoperative bunion dressing
- Avascular necrosis of the head of the first metatarsal
  - Overzealous lateral soft tissue stripping
  - Overpenetration of the saw blade into the lateral capsule
  - Although radiographic first metatarsal head changes are frequently observed after distal metatarsal osteotomies, they rarely progress to symptomatic necrosis and collapse of the metatarsal head.[8]
- First MTP joint stiffness
  - In our experience, joint stiffness responds to physical therapy and advancing the weight-bearing status. We maintain that slight overcorrection and some MTP joint stiffness is preferable to undercorrection and full MTP joint motion.
- Hallux varus
  - Overresection of the medial capsule
  - Unnecessary overrelease of the lateral capsule and adductor hallucis tendon

REFERENCES

1. Alexander IJ, ed. Disorders of the first MTP joint. In: The Foot: Examination and Diagnosis, ed 2. New York: Churchill Livingstone, 1997: 69–82.
2. Campbell JT. Hallux valgus: adult and juvenile. In: Richardson EG, ed. OKU, Orthopaedic Knowledge Update: Foot and Ankle, ed 3. Rosemont, IL: American Academy of Orthopaedic Surgery, 2004:3–15.
3. Coughlin MJ. Forefoot disorders. In: Baxter DE, ed. The Foot and Ankle in Sport. St Louis: Mosby, 1994:221–244.

4. Coughlin MJ. Hallux valgus with increased DMAA. In: Nunley JA, Pfeffer GB, Sanders RW, et al, eds. Advanced Reconstruction Foot and Ankle. Rosemont, IL: American Academy of Orthopaedic Surgery, 2004:3–18.

5. Coughlin MJ. Roger A. Mann Award. Juvenile hallux valgus: etiology and treatment. Foot Ankle Int 1995;16:682–697.

6. Coughlin MJ. Second metatarsophalangeal joint instability in the athlete. Foot Ankle 1993;14:309–319.

7. Coughlin MJ, Carlson RE. Treatment of hallux valgus with an increased distal metatarsal articular angle: evaluation of double and triple first ray osteotomies. Foot Ankle Int 1999;20:762–770.

8. Easley ME, Kelly IP. Avascular necrosis of the hallux metatarsal head. Foot Ankle Clin 2000;5:591–608.

9. Hatch DJ, Santrock RD, Smith B, et al. Triplane hallux abducto valgus classification. J Foot Ankle Surg 2018;57(5):972–981.

10. Johnson KA, ed. Chevron osteotomy. In: Master Techniques in Orthopaedic Surgery: The Foot and Ankle. New York: Raven, 1994:31–48.

11. Kim JS, Young KW. Sesamoid position in hallux valgus in relation to the coronal rotation of the first metatarsal. Foot Ankle Clin 2018;23(2):219–230.

12. Myerson MS, ed. Hallux valgus. In: Foot and Ankle Disorders, ed 2. Philadelphia: WB Saunders, 2000:213–288.

13. Nery C. Tornozelo e Pé. In: Barros TEP, Lech O, eds. Exame Físico em Ortopedia. São Paulo, Brazil: Sarvier, 2001:267–300.

14. Nery C, Barrôco R, Maradei S, et al. Osteotomia em chevron biplana: apresentação de técnica. Acta Ortop Brasil 1999;7:47–52.

15. Nery C, Barroco R, Réssio C. Biplanar chevron osteotomy. Foot Ankle Int 2002;23:792–798.

16. Nery C, Coughlin MJ, Baumfeld D, et al. Hallux valgus in males—part 1: demographics, etiology, and comparative radiology. Foot Ankle Int 2013;34(5):629–635.

17. Nery C, Coughlin MJ, Baumfeld D, et al. Hallux valgus in males—part 2: radiographic assessment of surgical treatment. Foot Ankle Int 2013;34(5):636–644.

18. Nery C, Mizusaki J, Magalhães AAC, et al. Tratamiento conservador del hallux valgus juvenil mediante ortesis nocturnas. Rev Española Cir Osteo 1997;187:32–37.

19. Nery C, Réssio C, de Azevedo Santa Cruz G, et al. Proximal opening-wedge osteotomy of the first metatarsal for moderate and severe hallux valgus using low profile plates. Foot Ankle Surg 2013;19:276–282.

20. Nery C, Réssio C, Netto AA, et al. Avaliação radiológica do hálux valgo: estudo populacional de novos parâmetros angulares. Acta Ortop Brasil 2001;9:41–48.

21. Pearce CJ, Sexton SA, Sakellariou A. The triplanar chevron osteotomy. Foot Ankle Surg 2008;14(3):158–160.

22. Piggott H. The natural history of hallux valgus in adolescence and early adult life. J Bone Joint Surg Br 1960;42B:749–760.

23. Prado M, Baumfeld T, Nery C, et al. Rotational biplanar chevron osteotomy. Foot Ankle Surg 2020;26(4):473–476.

24. Smith WB, Dayton P, Santrock RD, et al. Understanding frontal plane correction in hallux valgus repair. Clin Podiatr Med Surg 2018;35(1):27–36.

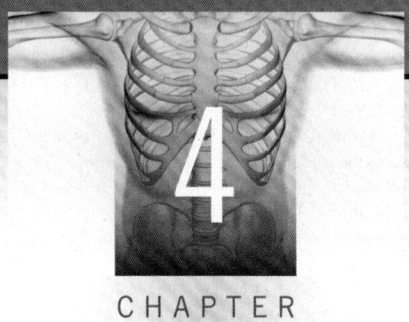

CHAPTER 4

Extending the Indications for the Distal Chevron Osteotomy

James L. Beskin

DEFINITION

- The distal chevron osteotomy has proven to be a reliable, reproducible method of bunion repair for mild to moderate deformity. By altering the location and displacement of the osteotomy, the indications can be expanded to more complex deformities while preserving the straightforward surgical exercise.
- The apex of the chevron osteotomy can be modified to a more proximal location along with a reduced angle to provide a stable healing surface that facilitates maximal lateral translation.
- The proximal location of the osteotomy also reduces the risk of avascular necrosis and permits safe lateral capsule release needed for larger corrections.
- This technique facilitates treatment for moderate to severe bunion deformity with a straightforward surgical method using limited, readily available internal fixation.

ANATOMY

- Factors contributing to a bunion deformity vary among individuals. The diverse anatomic features require scrutiny during surgical planning.
- Pertinent to the corrective factors of a translational osteotomy is the width of the distal metatarsal. The amount of correction may be limited in a small, narrow, or "hourglass"-shaped bone.
- The distal metatarsal articular angle (DMAA) may be altered by varus or valgus rotation during a distal osteotomy. This additional corrective factor should be scrutinized during the surgical planning.
- The sesamoid position is assessed for optimal correction. Station III subluxation usually requires a lateral capsule release to restore normal joint mechanics.
- Hypermobility of the first ray is a potential concern. Correction by lateral translation of the distal metatarsal may be compromised if the cuneiform–metatarsal joint is unstable.

IMAGING AND DIAGNOSTIC STUDIES

- Weight-bearing anteroposterior and lateral radiographs are used to determine bone morphology, associated disease, and deformity parameters used in decision making.
- The ideal correction of the intermetatarsal angle is based on a line drawn along the first metatarsal that is parallel to the second metatarsal shaft and touches the medial base of the first metatarsal or cuneiform (FIG 1). This line crosses the first metatarsal shaft bisector near the ideal location for a corrective osteotomy (*red circle*). It also estimates the amount of translational correction needed and whether there is sufficient bone remaining at the lateral metatarsal to receive the distal metatarsal head. In this example, the osteotomy could be placed slightly distal to the intersecting lines to utilize cancellous bone and still have adequate bone to place the capital fragment (*dotted orange line*).
- The grade of sesamoid subluxation is evaluated to determine whether a lateral capsular release is indicated. The DMAA is assessed to determine if varus or valgus rotational correction is needed at the time of the osteotomy.

SURGICAL MANAGEMENT

Positioning

- The patient is positioned supine. The surgery is usually done under an ankle tourniquet.

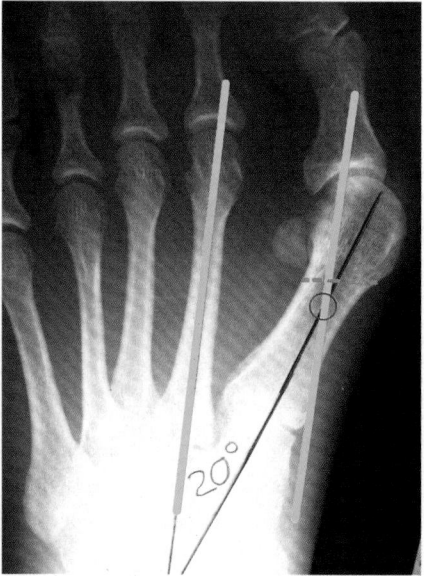

FIG 1 The "ideal correction" is found by drawing a line parallel to the second metatarsal that touches the base of the first metatarsal. The position where this line crosses the first metatarsal bisector helps determine the location and degree of translation possible for the first metatarsal osteotomy.

SOFT TISSUE PREPARATION

- When significant sesamoid subluxation is present (grade II or III), use a dorsal first web incision to expose the lateral capsule.
- A Freer elevator is helpful to probe and identify the dorsal margin of the subluxed lateral sesamoid. Then incise the capsule longitudinally just dorsal to the sesamoid from the phalanx to well proximal to the lateral sesamoid. The adductor tendon is plantar to this incision and is preserved. Leave the intermetatarsal ligament intact. The purpose of this longitudinal cut is to allow medialization of the plantar sesamoid complex at the time of medial capsule repair. Inspect the lateral sesamoid for wear or osteophytes that can be trimmed. Release adhesions and confirm that a Freer elevator can be easily passed from proximal to distal between the metatarsal head and sesamoids.
- Expose the medial joint through a longitudinal incision. Identify and protect the superficial peroneal nerve. Mobilize the tissues to widely expose the capsule from the medial sesamoid inferiorly to the extensor hallucis longus tendon superiorly. The medial plantar digital nerve is also at risk as the dissection nears the medial sesamoid and needs to be protected.
- Cut the capsule longitudinally and slightly plantar to the center of the metatarsal. Reflect the capsule to expose the medial metatarsal eminence and the joint; avoid stripping the dorsal and plantar aspect to minimize risk of vascular insult.

BONE PREPARATION

- Remove the medial eminence with a power saw. The amount of bone is based on radiographic interpretation. Avoid excessive removal to prevent hallux varus. Usually, the cut is 1 to 2 mm medial to the articular margin or the sagittal groove.
- Determine the apex of the osteotomy and mark it with a surgical pen (**TECH FIG 1**). It is typically 15 to 20 mm from the articular surface. Outline the proximal limbs at an angle of about 35 to 45 degrees. If the limbs are too short, there may be instability; if they are too long, there may be difficulty translating or rotating the distal head portion.
- Next, use a Freer elevator to gently strip the periosteum and soft tissue over the area where the osteotomy is anticipated to cut the dorsal and plantar aspects of the metatarsal. Again, leave the tissues distal to the bone cut in place to minimize vascular compromise.
- The osteotomy can be affected by the angle of the saw position with either a dorsal, plantar, proximal, or distal angulation. Generally, a straight or neutral cut is best, although slight proximal angulation and shortening will facilitate translation for a large correction.
- After completing the osteotomy, the distal head fragment should be mobile and ready for translation. Lateral translation is facilitated by applying traction to the toe with one hand and using the other hand to pull with a towel clip on the apex of the proximal metatarsal. Thumb pressure against the head while maintaining traction will allow repositioning of the metatarsal with minimum force (**TECH FIG 2A**). If the head fragment is not readily mobilized, the osteotomy needs to be rechecked and cut. Too much force can break the lateral metatarsal spike.
- Because the osteotomy is often proximal to the metaphyseal bone, the lateral cortex may appear as a spike. The distal head is then perched on this lateral process to maintain length (**TECH FIG 2B**). Up to 90% translation is possible and satisfactorily stabilized with 0.054 Kirschner wires (K-wires). Slight varus or valgus tilt can be applied as indicated by the DMAA.
- Using 0.054 smooth K-wires, direct a pin from the proximal third of the metatarsal medially while also engaging the lateral metatarsal cortex before entering the distal head fragment. These three points of fixation help maximize stability with large corrections (**TECH FIG 3**). Place a second similar pin and check the position with radiographic control. K-wires are typically percutaneous, bent, and left out of the skin but can be cut adjacent to the bone and removed electively. Alternatively, a buried small, 3-mm cannulated screw can be used for one of the K-wires, but a second point of fixation, such as a percutaneous K-wire, is recommended for several weeks for larger, unstable corrections. Place the guide pin for the screw first, usually central at the medial metatarsal and confirm proper distal position. Then insert a percutaneous 0.054 K-wire to supplement stability during screw insertion. If deemed stable, the K-wire can be removed or left in for a few weeks for better fixation. When a screw is used, a headless screw may be preferable due to the potential for symptomatic hardware at the medial metatarsal. Using a screw provides internal fixation for earlier removal of the percutaneous K-wire (3 to 4 weeks) and reduces the risk of osteotomy drift after K-wires are pulled.
- Cut the large prominence of bone left medially after lateral head translation and fixation and contour it in line with the distal head's medial margin. It is important to cut this back proximal enough to avoid a residual bump at the mid-metatarsal area. Note that pins/screws must be proximal enough to allow adequate bone removal (**TECH FIG 4**).

TECH FIG 1 Usual location for the osteotomy.

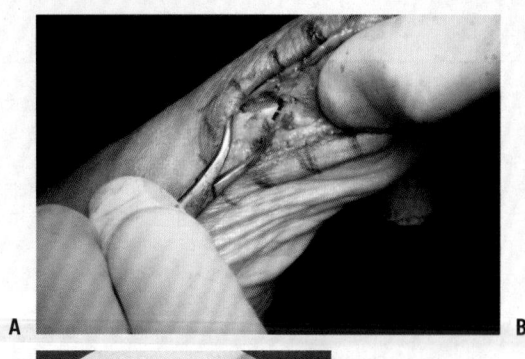

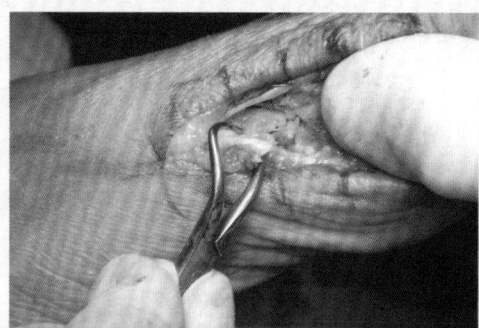

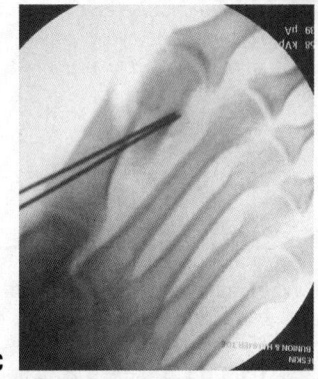

TECH FIG 2 A. The osteotomy is translated laterally with traction and thumb pressure on the distal end while counterpressure is applied with a towel clip to the medial spike of the proximal end. **B.** The lateral cortex of the proximal metatarsal provides a stable spike to perch the distal head fragment. **C.** Radiographic check of pin placement and alignment.

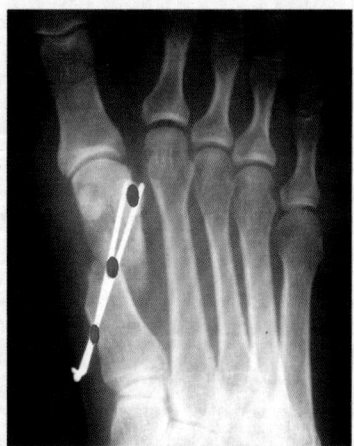

TECH FIG 3 Optimal pin placement. Note contact with the medial and lateral aspect of the proximal metatarsal before entering the distal head fragment.

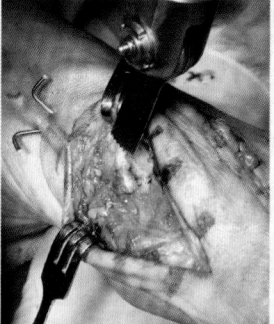
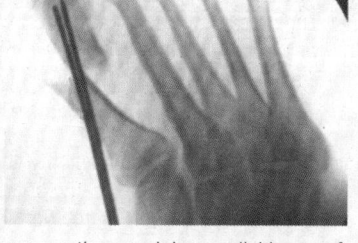

TECH FIG 4 The saw is used to remove the remaining medial bump of the first metatarsal. This needs to be contoured in line with the medial metatarsal head to avoid symptoms at this area postoperatively.

SOFT TISSUE CLOSURE

- Tighten the medial capsule by removing a U-shaped wedge of tissue from the plantar limb of the capsule to near the medial sesamoid. The amount of tissue removed is judged to allow adequate correction of the hallux valgus. Next, close the defect in the plantar capsule with two figure-8 sutures using nonabsorbable 0 or 2-0 suture. A small stout needle facilitates passing suture here. Then perform a "pants-over-vest" closure between the plantar and dorsal capsule to medialize and improve sesamoid position. The goal is to bring the medial sesamoid to the medial margin of the metatarsal head (**TECH FIG 5**). Skin closure and bunion dressings are then applied.

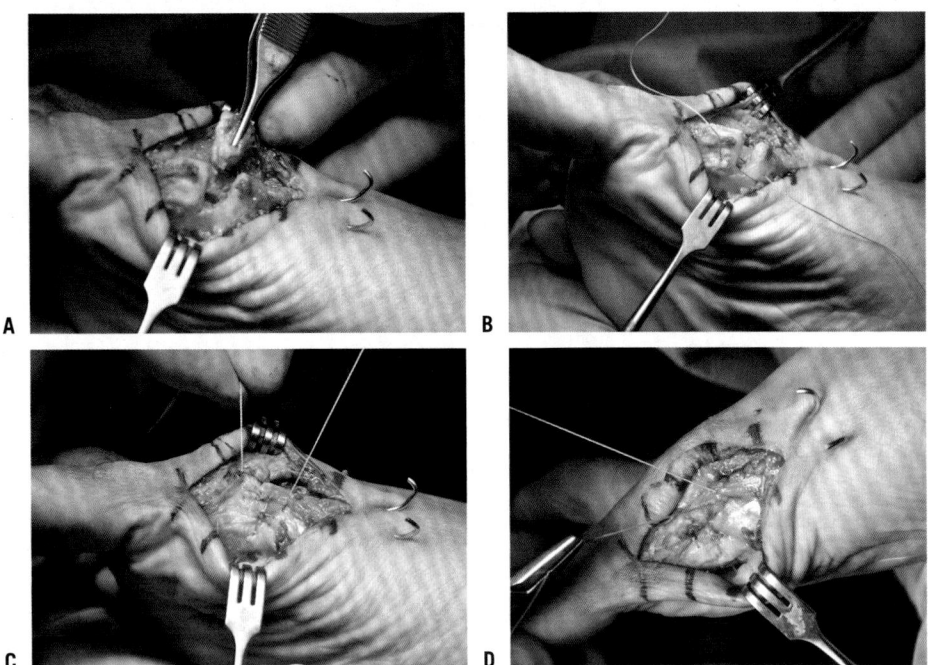

TECH FIG 5 A,B. From the longitudinal capsule incision, a U-shaped wedge of capsule is removed from the plantar limb of the capsule and then sutured to tighten and correct the hallux valgus. **C.** Suture is placed in a pants-over-vest technique to advance the plantar capsule medially and dorsally. **D.** The remaining capsule is closed.

TECHNIQUES

Pearls and Pitfalls

- Avoid routine lateral adductor tendon release to reduce the risk of hallux varus unless specifically indicated by the clinical situation. The increased lateral translation of the osteotomy usually decompresses the lateral structures. The main focus is to realign the sesamoids under the metatarsal head.

- An aggressive contouring of the proximal portion of the metatarsal is necessary to reduce the risk of a residual bony bump near the osteotomy site. This often goes into the medullary canal. The K-wires or screw need to be placed proximal enough to avoid being cut out during this maneuver.

- Two K-wires are recommended to reduce the risk of metatarsal head migration until healing callus has developed. Alternatively, using a headless screw may allow earlier pin removal.

- Other stabilization techniques such as custom plates can be utilized, but too rigid fixation may reduce or delay the callus healing response needed to fill the lateral offset created with this technique.

POSTOPERATIVE CARE

- Patients are instructed to keep the limb elevated the majority of the first 2 weeks postoperatively. They are allowed weight bearing and able to "heel walk" in a postoperative shoe with crutches for balance and offload to comfort.
- At 2 weeks, sutures are removed and another bunion dressing is applied. The patient is instructed to passively dorsiflex and plantarflex the toe.
- At 5 weeks, the pins are removed and the patient is taught to use a compression wrap and toe spacer. Aggressive range-of-motion exercises are initiated. For maximal translation cases, pins are sometimes left in for 6 weeks if no callus is seen on the fifth week x-ray. With adjunctive screw fixation, the pin may be removed at this time.
- Patients are followed on a 3- to 4-week basis to monitor healing and alignment (**FIG 2**).
- With larger osteotomy translation and correction, radiographic healing can take 3 months or more. However, the osteotomy is usually stable for activities of daily living within 2 months. Sports and strenuous activities may require 3 to 5 months of healing.

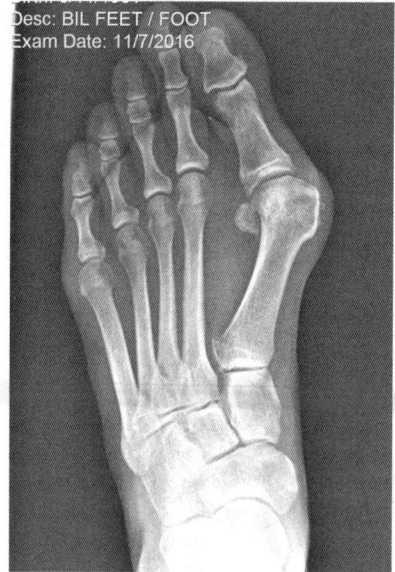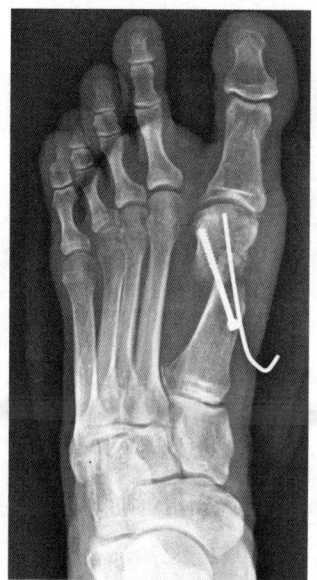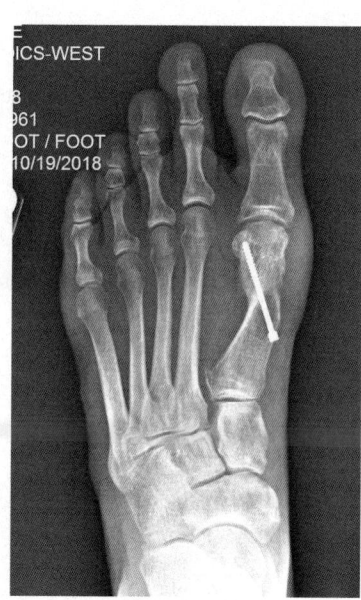

FIG 2 A. Preoperative x-ray. **B.** Postoperative x-ray showing initial combined screw and K-wire technique. Note the proximal placement of hardware allows adequate medial metatarsal resection. **C.** Postoperative 4.5 months with satisfactory bone healing.

OUTCOMES

- We assessed 72 procedures in 62 patients operated on between January 1, 2002, and December 30, 2003. American Orthopaedic Foot and Ankle Society (AOFAS) scores and radiographic assessments were obtained from 39 at an average of 27.6 months after surgery.
- AOFAS scores averaged 93.3, with complete radiographic healing in all patients.
- Hallux valgus angle correction averaged 22.3 degrees, and intermetatarsal angle correction averaged 7.7 degrees.
- This continues to be my primary bunion procedure with similar outcomes over the past 20 years.

COMPLICATIONS

- Complications included symptomatic hallux varus deformities that were due to routine adductor release. This has been revised to a limited lateral capsule release as described here with preservation of the adductor tendon in most cases.
- There were symptomatic medial diaphyseal "bumps" due to inadequate resection of the medial metatarsal after translation. This is now being addressed with more aggressive medial contouring.
- Occasionally, the osteotomy will drift into dorsal or plantar angulation. Plantar angulation is well tolerated unless causing significant toe elevation should not be revised. Dorsal angulation may limit toe dorsiflexion and promote

load transfer to the lesser metatarsals and may require revision.
- No cases of avascular necrosis were identified.

SUGGESTED READINGS

Austin DW, Leventen EO. A new osteotomy for hallux valgus. Clin Orthop Relat Res 1981;(157):25–30.
Harper MC. Correction of metatarsus primus varus with the chevron metatarsal osteotomy. An analysis of corrective factors. Clin Orthop Relat Res 1989;(243):180–183.
Johnson KA, Cofield RH, Morrey BF. Chevron osteotomy for hallux valgus. Clin Orthop Relat Res 1979;(142):44–47.
Murawski D, Beskin JL. Increased displacement maximizes the utility of the distal chevron osteotomy for hallux vagus deformity correction. Foot Ankle Int 2008;29:155–163.
Oh IS, Kim MK, Lee SH. New modified technique of osteotomy for hallux valgus. J Orthop Surg 2004;12:235–238.
Sanhudo JA. Correction of moderate to severe hallux valgus deformity by a modified chevron shaft osteotomy. Foot Ankle Int 2006;27:581–585.
Sarrafian SK. A method of predicting the degree of functional correction of the metatarsus primus varus with a distal lateral displacement osteotomy in hallux valgus. Foot Ankle Int 1985;5:322–326.
Schneider W, Aigner N, Pinggera O, et al. Chevron osteotomy in hallux valgus. Ten-year result of 112 cases. J Bone Joint Surg Br 2004;86(7):1016–1020.
Song JH, Kang C, Hwang DS, et al. Comparison of radiographic and clinical results after extended distal chevron osteotomy with distal soft tissue release with moderate versus severe hallux valgus. Foot Ankle Int 2019;40:297–306.
Stienstra JJ, Lee JA, Nakadate DT. Large displacement distal chevron osteotomy for the correction of hallux valgus deformity. J Foot Ankle Surg 2002;41:213–220.

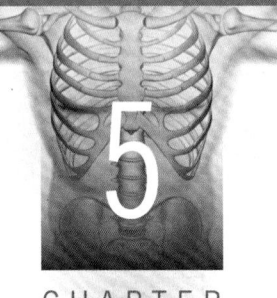

CHAPTER 5

Percutaneous Hallux Valgus Correction

A. Holly Johnson, Jonathan Day, Oliver N. Schipper, Jorge I. Acevedo, Rebecca Cerrato, Alastair Younger, and Peter Mangone

DEFINITION

- Minimally invasive correction of hallux valgus has been described using a technique employing percutaneous chevron and Akin osteotomies.[5,11,12]
- Minimally invasive bunionectomy offers the benefits of smaller incisions and minimal soft tissue disruption while achieving rigid internal fixation (**FIG 1**).
- There is evidence for reduced postoperative pain while maintaining comparable radiographic correction in the hallux valgus angle (HVA) and 1–2 intermetatarsal angle (IMA) compared to traditional open approaches.[5,6,12,13]

ANATOMY

- The hallux (first or great toe) is formed by the first metatarsal, proximal phalanx, and distal phalanx. Additionally, two small plantar bones, the sesamoids, are within the flexor hallucis brevis tendon and articulates with the first metatarsal.
- The hallux has three joints for articulation: the tarsometatarsal joint (formed by the medial cuneiform and metatarsal), the metatarsophalangeal joint (formed by the metatarsal and proximal phalanx), and the interphalangeal joint (formed by the proximal and distal phalanx).
- The function of the sesamoid bones is to dissipate force during weight bearing and also to act as a pulley for the flexor hallucis brevis muscles in flexion of the hallux.[8]
- Hallux valgus (bunion) deformity is characterized by lateral deviation of the great toe at the metatarsophalangeal joint, medial deviation of the first metatarsal, and a consequent valgus deformity at the first metatarsal phalangeal joint.
- In addition, as the first metatarsal phalangeal joint falls into valgus, the sesamoids displace laterally.
- The dorsal medial digital nerve and dorsal lateral digital nerve have been found consistently between 10 and 2 o'clock position in either right and left feet.[7]

PATHOGENESIS

- Hallux valgus is a progressive deformity of the first metatarsophalangeal joint that is initially caused by failure of the medial collateral and sesamoid ligaments.[10]
- Failure of medial support causes the metatarsal head to shift medially and pronate, and the proximal phalanx to drift into a valgus position.
- Pronation and medial subluxation of the metatarsal head causes the lateral shift of the sesamoids, abductor hallucis, adductor hallucis, flexor hallucis longus, and extensor hallucis longus.
- This results in a prominent medial eminence. The bursa overlying the medial eminence becomes thickened due to repetitive extrinsic forces such as footwear.[10]

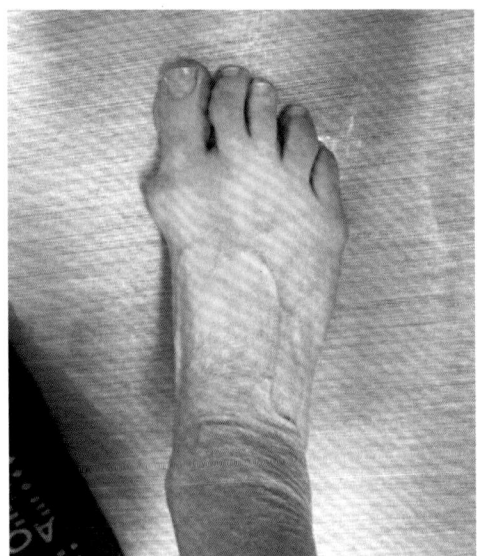
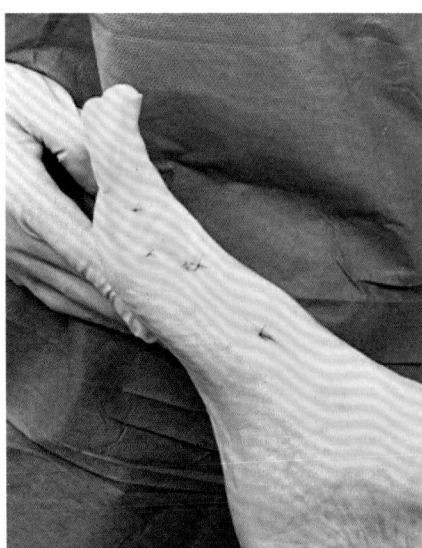
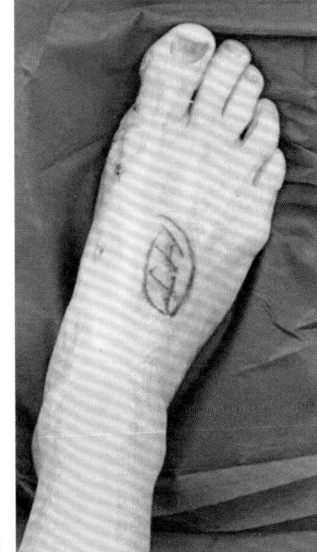

FIG 1 **A.** Preoperative hallux valgus deformity. **B,C.** Postoperative minimally invasive percutaneous chevron and Akin osteotomies.

NATURAL HISTORY

- Hallux valgus deformity is the most common forefoot condition in adults, with approximately 23% of the adult population affected by this condition. It is significantly more prevalent in adult females.[1,9]
- Hallux valgus was first described in the late 1800s by the German surgeon, Carl Hueter,[2] who characterized the deformity as a lateral deviation of the first metatarsophalangeal joint.
- Over a century later, debate continues regarding the contribution of extrinsic and intrinsic factors to the deformity, and the precise etiology is not fully understood.
- Generally, it is accepted that hallux valgus is a progressive deformity of multifactorial etiology, with several predisposing factors. Commonly cited factors include genetic predisposition, restricted footwear, first ray hypermobility, pes planovalgus, and neuromuscular disorders such as cerebral palsy.[1,10]

PATIENT HISTORY AND PHYSICAL FINDINGS

- Patients typically present with a chronic progressive pain of the medial first metatarsophalangeal joint.
- It is often described as sharp or deep pain that is exacerbated by ambulation and certain shoe wear. The frequency and severity of pain usually worsens with time and can be debilitating. Patients often describe an associated increase in size of the deformity.
- The physical exam should include evaluation of the resting position and standing posture of the hallux as well as range of motion. The classical presentation is lateral deviation of the proximal phalanx with medial deviation of the first metatarsal head, resulting in a prominent medial eminence at the first metatarsophalangeal joint. The deformity may be more severe when weight bearing. The prominence is often erythematous and tender to palpation. Patients may exhibit hypermobility of both the metatarsophalangeal and tarsometatarsal joints with increased motion in the transverse plane.[1]

IMAGING AND OTHER DIAGNOSTIC STUDIES

- Radiographic assessment with weight-bearing plain anteroposterior (AP), oblique, and lateral views are the gold standard (FIG 2).
- Severity of hallux valgus can be classified as mild, moderate, or severe based on several validated AP radiographic parameters: the HVA, IMA, and lateral subluxation of the sesamoids (TABLE 1).

DIFFERENTIAL DIAGNOSIS

- Gout
- Hallux rigidus
- Sesamoiditis
- Turf toe

NONOPERATIVE MANAGEMENT

- In general, conservative management includes a trial of wider shoe wear as well as shoe modification including the addition of orthotics and/or additional padding. Toe spacers that prevent the hallux from rubbing against the second toe may be used as well.

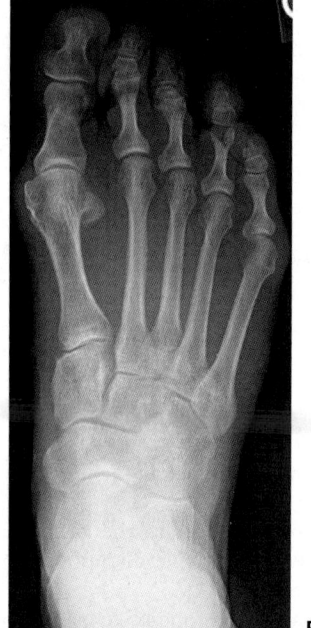 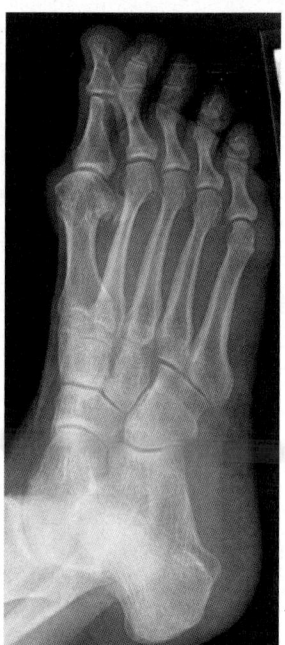
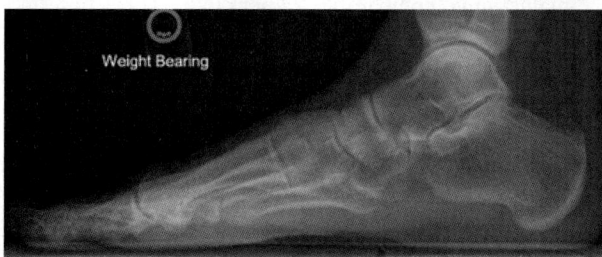

FIG 2 Preoperative weight-bearing plain radiographs. **A.** AP. **B.** Oblique. **C.** Lateral.

SURGICAL MANAGEMENT

Preoperative Planning

- Standard weight-bearing radiographs of the AP, lateral, and oblique views should be reviewed prior to surgery to assess severity of HVA and IMA (see FIG 2). A sesamoid view can be considered to assess for lateral subluxation of the sesamoids.
- Concomitant deformities and abnormalities, such as lesser metatarsophalangeal joint subluxation, hammer toes, degenerative changes in the hallux or midfoot, and so forth should

TABLE 1 Classification of Hallux Valgus Deformity

Classification	HVA	IMA	Lateral Subluxation of Sesamoids
Normal	<15 degrees	<9 degrees	—
Mild	<20 degrees	≤11 degrees	<50%
Moderate	20–40 degrees	<16 degrees	50%–75%
Severe	HVA >40°	≥16 degrees	>75%

HVA, hallux valgus angle; IMA, 1–2 intermetatarsal angle.

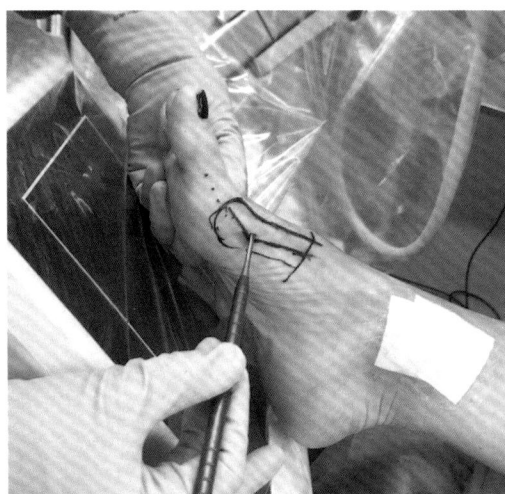

FIG 3 Marker outlines medial portal placement.

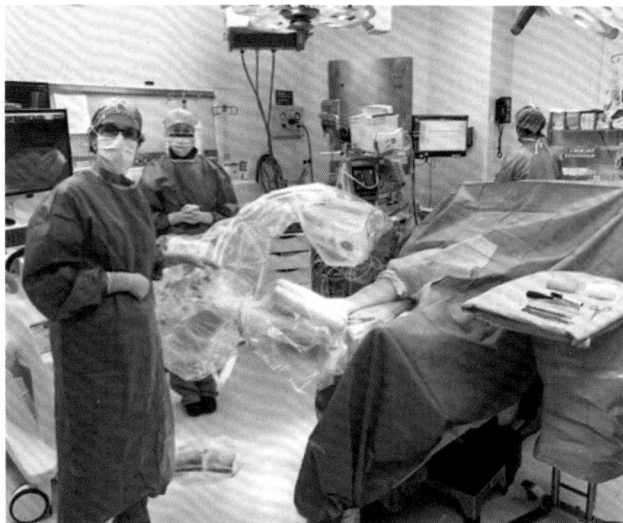

FIG 4 Intraoperative positioning of the patient in supine with the operative foot extended off the operating table distally and in slight eversion to allow room for the mini C-arm.

be assessed. In some cases, these issues may be addressed in the same setting as the hallux valgus correction.

- Bone quality should be considered prior to surgery as well as the presence of any prior hardware in or around the joint.
- The power box for the burr should be capable of delivering high torque at a low speed in order to efficiently cut through bone while minimizing heat production to avoid thermal injury to bone/soft tissue. A 6000 rpms or less is required for the burrs to work efficiently to cut or morselize bone, whereas speeds higher than this, risk thermal injury to the soft tissue and bone.

Positioning

- The patient is placed supine on the operating table with the involved foot extending off the bed distally and in slight external rotation to allow easy access for AP and lateral fluoroscopy of the forefoot (**FIGS 3** and **4**).
- The operative leg is elevated using a bump or blankets, whereas the nonoperative leg may be secured away from the operative field. Frog legging the nonoperative leg may also allow easier access to the operative foot.
- The mini C-arm is positioned next to the patient, ipsilateral to the surgeon's dominant hand. For instance, a right-handed surgeon would position the C-arm on the right side of the patient.
- A tourniquet is generally not indicated as this can increase chances of thermal injury to the soft tissues and bone necrosis.

Approach

- The standard working approach is from the medial portal.
- The medial incision is made directly over the metadiaphyseal junction of the medial first metatarsal just proximal to the flare of the medial eminence (see **FIG 3**). Care should be taken to avoid injuring the dorsomedial sensory nerve branch.
- In severe deformities, an additional dorsal lateral incision may be created over the first metatarsophalangeal joint in order to release lateral ligaments (lateral sesamoid phalangeal

ligament, lateral metatarsosesamoid ligament, adductor hallucis tendon). Care should be taken to avoid releasing the lateral collateral ligament. Any lateral soft tissue release is performed *after* the metatarsal osteotomy is performed, translated, and fixed. Release before this point results in difficulty controlling the position of the metatarsal head during the shift.

- Instruments usually include a 3-mm wedge burr and 2- × 20-mm Shannon burr. The authors prefer to use two 3.0- to 4.0-mm fully threaded cannulated beveled screws for fixation. A 2- × 12-mm Shannon burr is typically used for the Akin osteotomy (**FIG 5**).

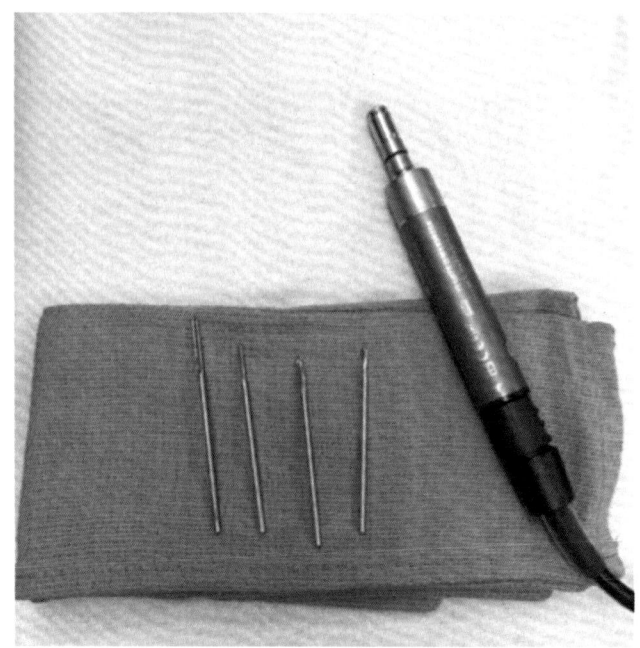

FIG 5 Various sizes of wedge and Shannon burrs.

DISTAL FIRST METATARSAL OSTEOTOMY

- The operative leg is identified and marked preoperatively.
- The patient is placed supine on the operating table with the operative foot extending off the table distally (see **FIG 4**).
- The first metatarsal is identified and traced out with a skin marker.
- Use a guidewire to locate the central axis on lateral fluoroscopic view.
- Under fluoroscopic guidance, a 3- to 5-mm longitudinal incision is made medially over the metadiaphyseal junction of the first metatarsal.
- A hemostat is used to bluntly dissect down to bone to avoid damaging the dorsomedial sensory nerve branch. A periosteal elevator may be used to elevate soft tissue dorsally, but avoid soft tissue stripping plantarly to prevent injury to the vascular supply of the first metatarsal head.
- Resection of the medial eminence may be done before or after the metatarsal osteotomy. Use a small beaver blade to release the plantar edge of the capsule off the eminence. Next, under AP fluoroscopic guidance, insert a 3-mm wedge burr or 2-mm Shannon burr (6000 rpm) directly into the eminence and gently resect bone, rotating the hand plantar and dorsally (**TECH FIG 1**). Take care not to overresect the bone by checking fluoroscopy in multiple planes. Always irrigate the burr and incision to prevent thermal injury to the skin and bone. Express and remove excess bone debris with a rasp and irrigation using a large-bore angiocatheter.
- Under AP fluoroscopic guidance, insert a 2- × 20-mm Shannon burr (6000 rpm) into the incision, just proximal to the medial eminence. This ensures an extracapsular osteotomy. The burr is started slightly more dorsal than plantar. Angle the burr 10 to 20 degrees plantarly and distally to avoid shortening the first metatarsal. If shortening or lengthening of the metatarsal is desired, the trajectory of the burr may be altered to achieve the desired length. After confirming burr direction using AP fluoroscopy, advance the burr through the lateral cortex to create the apex of the osteotomy (**TECH FIG 2**).

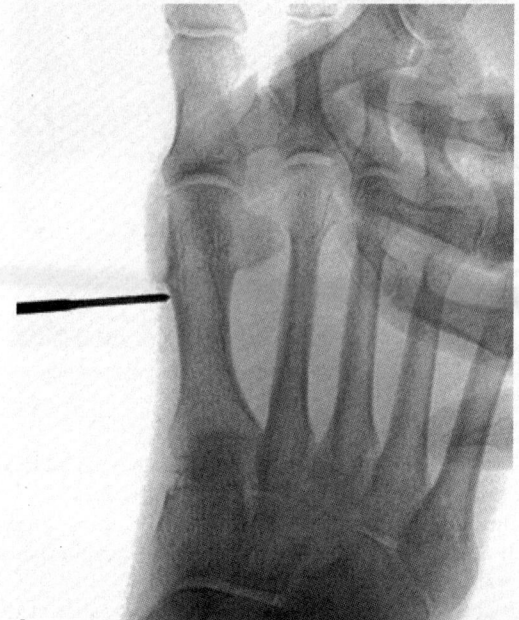

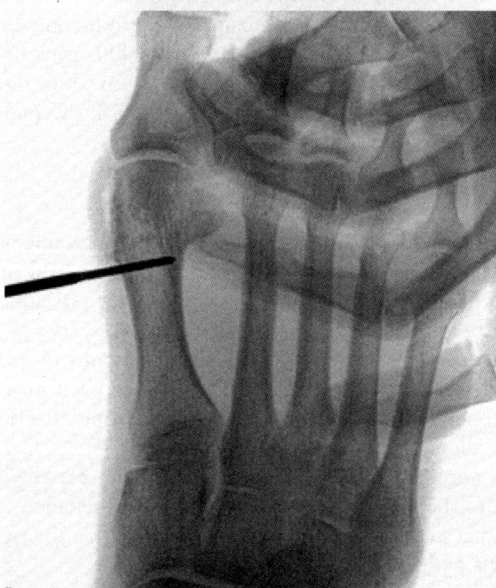

TECH FIG 2 Chevron osteotomy. **A.** Confirming trajectory just proximal to the medial eminence resection. **B.** Advancing the burr to create the chevron osteotomy.

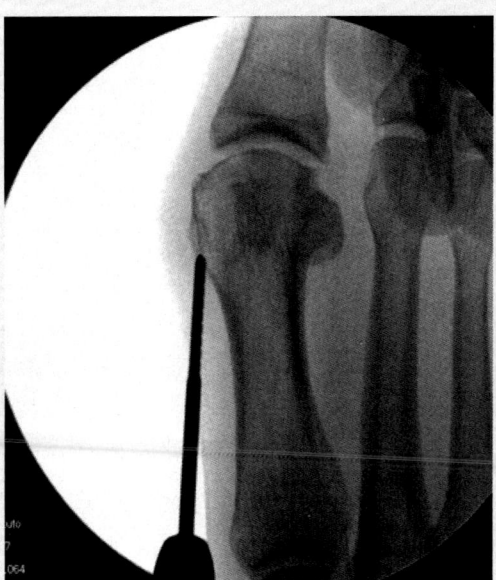

TECH FIG 1 Trajectory of the wedge or Shannon burr for medial eminence resection.

- Complete the dorsal vertical limb of the chevron osteotomy by rotating the hand plantarly and proximally, in a supination motion. Use the medial cortex osteotomy site as the fulcrum of rotation. Gently oscillate the burr in and out to ensure that the cut has reached the distal cortex. Remember to gently irrigate the incision and burr to prevent skin thermal injury.
- Next, complete the plantar limb of the chevron osteotomy by rotating the hand dorsally and distally, using the medial cortex osteotomy site as the fulcrum of rotation. A shorter plantar limb allows for easier rotational correction.

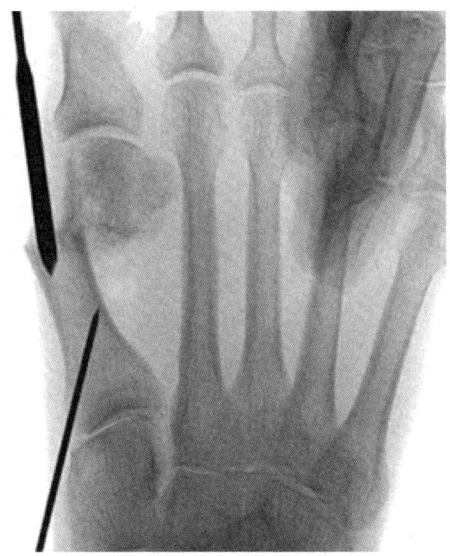

TECH FIG 3 Using the head-shifting tool, the first metatarsal head is shifted laterally relative to the shaft.

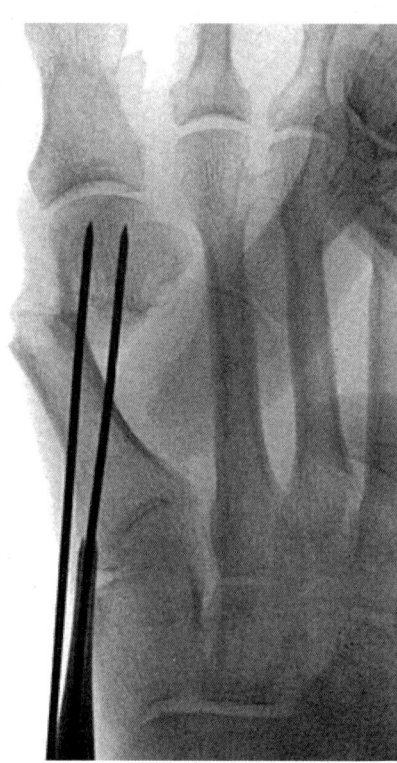

TECH FIG 4 Guidewire fixation of the proximal metatarsal to the distal capital fragment.

- Alternatively, a transverse osteotomy may be performed in lieu of a chevron. In this case, the starting point for the burr and the fulcrum medially are unchanged. The dorsal cut is made vertically by rotating the hand plantarly and the burr dorsally; the plantar cut is then made by rotating the hand dorsally and the burr plantarly.
- Once the capital fragment is mobile, insert a Kirschner wire, elevator, or head-shifting tool through the medial incision and into the first metatarsal shaft.
- Pull traction on the hallux while placing varus stress distally to shift the first metatarsal head laterally relative to the shaft. Placing the hallux in varus stress during lateral translation of the head avoids unwanted angulation of the metatarsal head. Using AP and lateral fluoroscopic views, ensure that proper alignment and rotation of the head relative to the shaft is maintained. If rotational correction is needed, supinate the hallux as well **(TECH FIG 3)**.
- Insert a 1.4-mm guidewire through the proximal medial cortex midaxially at the base of the shaft, angling approximately 1 cm lateral to the first metatarsal head. Place the guidewire through the proximal medial and distal lateral first metatarsal shaft cortices prior to engaging the capital fragment for stability of the construct. The wire should exit the lateral cortex approximately 10 to 15 mm proximal to the osteotomy. Confirm wire trajectory and position on AP and lateral fluoroscopy and then drive the guidewire into the capital fragment.
- Insert a second guidewire distal to the first through the medial proximal first metatarsal cortex and into the capital fragment. Check AP and lateral fluoroscopy views to confirm guidewire position **(TECH FIG 4)**.
- Alternatively, these guidewires may be placed prior to shifting the capital fragment. This avoids having to hold the reduction while placing guidewires.
- Measure each guidewire. Typically, 4 to 6 mm is subtracted from the measurement to ensure the screw is fully buried in the bone and does not breach the metatarsal phalangeal joint. Then, sequentially overdrill and place a 3.0- to 4.0-mm fully threaded cannulated headless beveled screw **(TECH FIG 5)**.

Check AP, internal oblique, and lateral fluoroscopic views to ensure screw heads are not prominent or screw tips are not perforating the metatarsal phalangeal joint space.
- Excise the distal medial step-off of the first metatarsal shaft using the Shannon or wedge burr through the distal screw insertion incision. Either enter the center of the overhanging bone and cut the piece dorsally and plantarly or perform this from a

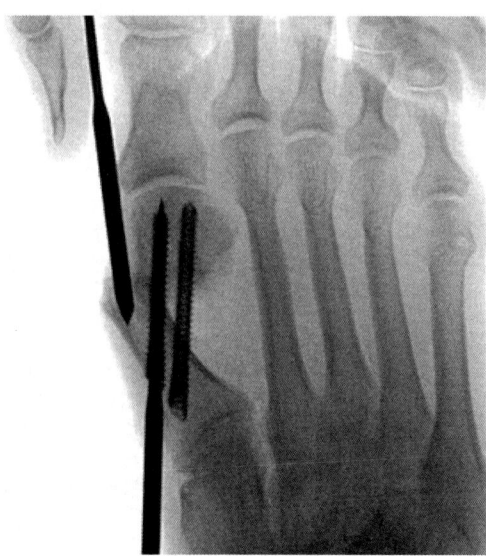

TECH FIG 5 AP fluoroscopic view confirms placement of fully threaded cannulated beveled screws without screw prominence.

plantar to dorsal trajectory to avoid damaging the dorsomedial sensory nerve branch **(TECH FIG 6)**. Remove the free bone fragment or impact it against the osteotomy site to serve as bone graft.

- If a medial eminence resection was not performed at the beginning of the case, a Shannon burr or wedge burr may be used to complete the resection at this point.
- In severe deformities requiring lateral ligament release (lateral sesamoid phalangeal ligament, lateral metatarsosesamoid ligament, adductor hallucis tendon), create an additional dorsal first web space incision at the level of the first metatarsophalangeal joint. Under AP fluoroscopic view, use a beaver blade to cut the ligaments, making sure to avoid severing the lateral collateral ligament. Lateral release should not be performed until after fixation of the osteotomy.

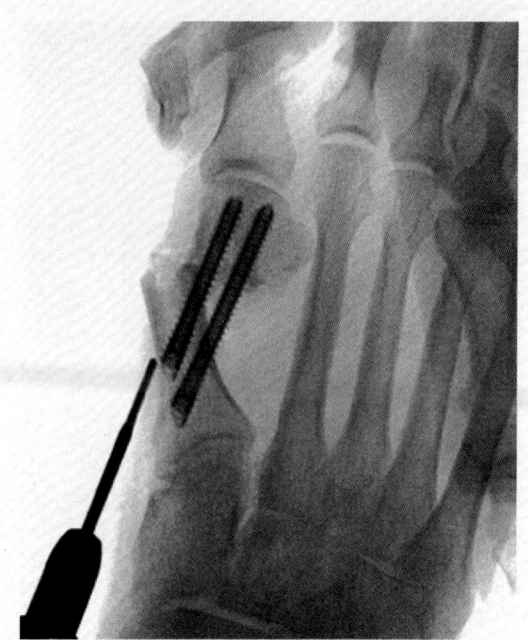

TECH FIG 6 Trajectory of burr for excision of the medial bony step-off after fixation.

AKIN OSTEOTOMY

- If hallux interphalangeus deformity is noted, or if further hallux valgus correction is desired, an Akin osteotomy may be performed. The authors perform an Akin in the vast majority of the time they use the percutaneous chevron for hallux valgus correction.
- Under fluoroscopic guidance, a midaxial medial hallux proximal phalanx incision is made at the junction of the middle and proximal one-third of the bone. Use a periosteal elevator to elevate both dorsal and plantar.
- Insert the 2- × 12-mm Shannon burr midaxially while preserving the lateral cortex **(TECH FIG 7)**.
- Complete the dorsal limb while holding the hallux interphalangeal joint dorsiflexed to prevent damage to the extensor hallucis longus tendon. Complete the plantar limb with the joint flexed to avoid damage to the flexor hallucis longus tendon.
- Place the hallux gently in varus to close down the osteotomy and achieve correction. Place a wire percutaneously across the osteotomy site from the medial base of the proximal phalanx through the distal lateral cortex or retrograde from distal to proximal. After confirming position and correction using AP and lateral fluoroscopy, measure the wire, overdrill, and fix with a 2.0- to 3.0-mm headless screw **(TECH FIG 8)**.
- Close the incisions with a single suture or adhesive strips. Dress with a nonadherent layer and 4- × 4-inch gauze. Place saline-moistened gauze in the first web space and wrap around the medial forefoot to maintain varus stress. Overwrap the gauze and dress as desired to maintain hallux valgus correction.

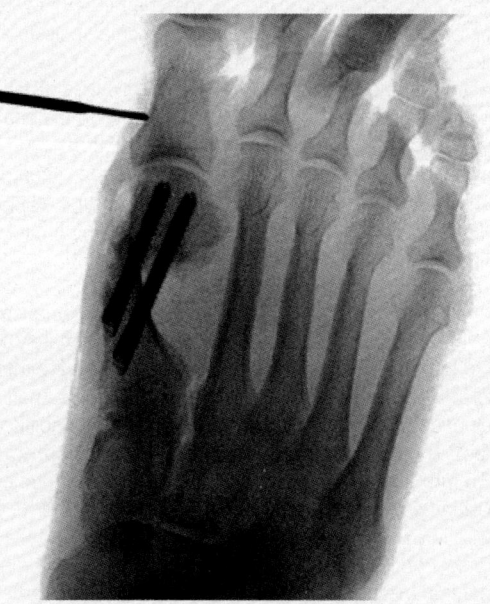

TECH FIG 7 Insertion and trajectory for Akin osteotomy.

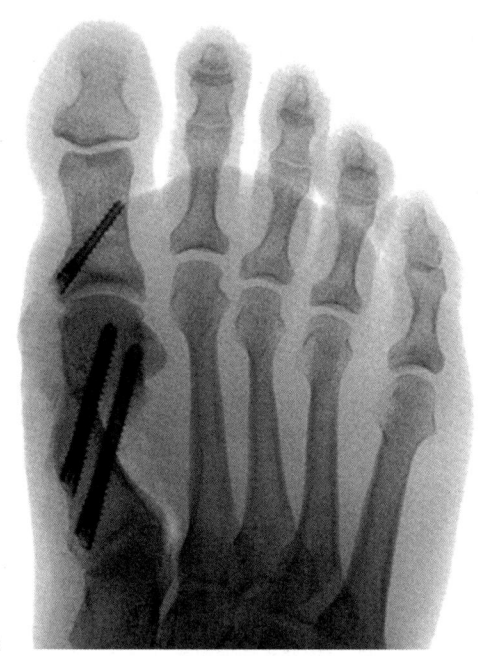 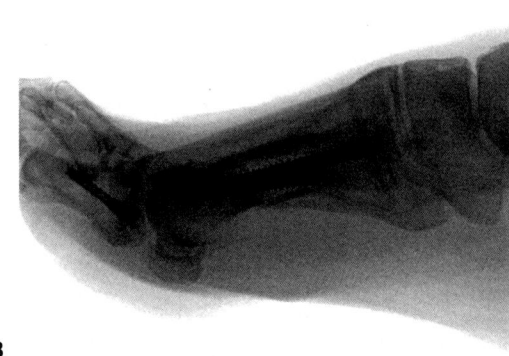

A   B

TECH FIG 8 Final AP (**A**) and lateral (**B**) final fluoroscopic views showing proper screw placement and alignment of minimally invasive percutaneous chevron and Akin osteotomies.

TECHNIQUES

Pearls and Pitfalls

Indications	• Percutaneous correction is indicated in mild to severe deformities without rigid joint arthritis.
Contraindications	• Infection, avascular necrosis, Charcot arthropathy, poor bone stock, rigid hallux valgus
Tourniquet Use	• A tourniquet is not required and may even increase the chance of thermal injury and bone necrosis. Placing the patient in a slight Trendelenburg may reduce bleeding.
Avoiding Neurovascular Damage	• When using the periosteal elevator, care should be made to elevate tissue dorsally rather than plantarly to avoid damaging the blood supply to the first metatarsal head.
Medial Eminence Resection	• If medial eminence resection is needed, the authors recommend resecting the medial eminence prior to distal first metatarsal osteotomy when it is most prominent and stable.
Preventing Thermal Skin Injury	• We recommend copious irrigation whenever using the burr, inserting wires, or overdrilling guidewires to minimize risk of thermal injury to the skin or bone necrosis.
Reducing Risk for Screw Prominence	• Use of beveled screws or recessing nonbeveled screws and subtracting 4–6 mm from guidewire measurement are recommended to reduce risk of prominent hardware.

POSTOPERATIVE CARE

- The surgical dressing is left in place for the first 2 weeks, at which time, a new dressing or soft toe splint may be exchanged at the first postoperative visit.
- Weight bearing in a flat postoperative shoe or boot is allowed as tolerated for the first 4 to 6 weeks, followed by transition into a supportive shoe.
- A soft forefoot compression sleeve may be applied after suture removal to help reduce edema.
- Physical therapy can be initiated after the wounds have healed.

OUTCOMES

- Minimally invasive surgical (MIS) techniques to correct the hallux valgus deformity offers the benefits of small percutaneous incisions while achieving rigid internal fixation for correction.
  - Surgical outcomes have demonstrated comparable patient-reported clinical outcomes when compared with traditional open approaches.[4-6]
  - Some studies suggest greater correction of the HVA with the MIS technique.[5,11]

- Recent studies have suggested the rate of nonunion is less than 1% and that complications usually occur with less surgical experience.[3]
- Several studies have demonstrated the MIS bunionectomy is associated with significantly less pain postoperatively.[5,6]

COMPLICATIONS

- Infection
- Nonunion
- Iatrogenic or postoperative fracture
- Screw prominence
- Shortening of the first metatarsal
- Skin thermal burn

REFERENCES

1. Hecht PJ, Lin TJ. Hallux valgus. Med Clin North Am 2014;98(2): 227–232.
2. Hueter C. Klinik der Gelenkkrankheiten mit Einschluß der Orthopädie, vol 2. Leipzig: Vogel, 1877.
3. Iannò B, Familiari F, De Gori M, et al. Midterm results and complications after minimally invasive distal metatarsal osteotomy for treatment of hallux valgus. Foot Ankle Int 2013;34(7):969–977.
4. Kadakia AR, Smerek JP, Myerson MS. Radiographic results after percutaneous distal metatarsal osteotomy for correction of hallux valgus deformity. Foot Ankle Int 2007;28(3):355–360.
5. Lai MC, Rikhraj IS, Woo YL, et al. Clinical and radiological outcomes comparing percutaneous chevron-Akin osteotomies vs open scarf-Akin osteotomies for hallux valgus. Foot Ankle Int 2018;39(3): 311–317.
6. Lee M, Walsh J, Smith MM, et al. Comparing percutaneous chevron/Akin (PECA) and open scarf/Akin osteotomies. Foot Ankle Int 2017; 38(8):838–846.
7. Malagelada F, Dalmau-Pastor M, Fargues B, et al. Increasing the safety of minimally invasive hallux surgery—an anatomical study introducing the clock method. Foot Ankle Surg 2018;24(1): 40–44.
8. Mann RA, Coughlin MJ. Hallux valgus—etiology, anatomy, treatment and surgical considerations. Clin Orthop Relat Res 1981;(157): 31–41.
9. Nix S, Smith M, Vicenzino B. Prevalence of hallux valgus in the general population: a systematic review and meta-analysis. J Foot Ankle Res 2010;3(1):21.
10. Perera A, Mason L, Stephens M. The pathogenesis of hallux valgus. J Bone Joint Surg Am 2011;93(17):1650–1661.
11. Siddiqui NA, LaPorta G, Walsh AL, et al. Radiographic outcomes of a percutaneous, reproducible distal metatarsal osteotomy for mild and moderate bunions: a multicenter study. J Foot Ankle Surg 2019;58(6):1215–1222.
12. Vernois J, Redfern D. Percutaneous chevron; the union of classic stable fixed approach and percutaneous technique. Fuß Sprunggelenk 2013;11(2):70–75.
13. Vernois J, Redfern DJ. Percutaneous surgery for severe hallux valgus. Foot Ankle Clin 2016;21(3):479–493.

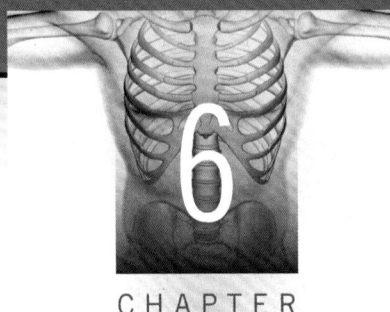

6

CHAPTER

Akin Osteotomy

Paul Hamilton and Sam Singh

SURGICAL MANAGEMENT

- The primary indication for an Akin osteotomy is hallux valgus interphalangeus or in cases in which residual hallux valgus causes pressure on the second toe on the load stimulation test.
- The Akin osteotomy is most commonly used to accompany a scarf or chevron osteotomy.
- An isolated Akin osteotomy is contraindicated in the treatment of hallux valgus.
- We use a proximal medial closing wedge osteotomy that is fixed by a varisation staple (Ortho Solutions, Essex, UK).
- The osteotomy is fashioned within metaphyseal cancellous bone, ensuring excellent cancellous healing. The osteotomy, by being close to the apex of the deformity at the interphalangeal (IP) joint, allows for more powerful correction.

Preoperative Planning

- Surgery is performed on an outpatient basis.
- Anteroposterior (AP) and lateral weight-bearing radiographs of the foot are evaluated for metatarsal length, intermetatarsal angle, hallux valgus angle, distal metatarsal articular angle, and IP angle for cases that may require a proximal phalangeal osteotomy to obtain complete correction.
- Congruency of the joint, presence of osteophytes, the size of the bony medial eminence, and position and condition of the sesamoids are noted.

Preparation and Positioning

- Prophylactic antibiotics are administered.
- A thigh tourniquet is applied.
- The patient is positioned supine with a sandbag under the ipsilateral buttock, so the big toe points to the ceiling.

AKIN OSTEOTOMY

Exposure

- The exposure is performed usually as an extension to the midline longitudinal incision from the metatarsal osteotomy. If performed as an isolated procedure, the exposure must allow visualization of the metatarsophalangeal (MTP) joint proximally and the shaft of the proximal phalanx distally. The exposure of the shaft of the phalanx may require excision of overlying fatty tissue.
- After dissecting directly onto bone, the exposure is completed by periosteal elevation above and below the phalanx. Two small pointed retractors are placed above and below the phalanx to protect the extensor and flexor tendons (TECH FIG 1).

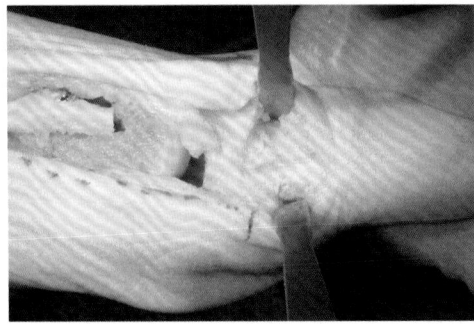

TECH FIG 1 Incision is made directly to bone with subperiosteal dissection above and below the proximal phalanx.

Kirschner Wire Placement

- A 1-mm Kirschner wire is placed in the midportion of the phalanx in the sagittal plane approximately 3 mm distal to the phalangeal flare (TECH FIG 2A).
- Traction on the big toe allows us to visualize the joint to ensure the wire is not intra-articular (TECH FIG 2B).
- The Kirschner wire is removed and the hole marked (TECH FIG 2C).

Osteotomies

- Make the proximal cut parallel to the phalangeal base (TECH FIG 3A).
- To maintain control of the osteotomy, the lateral cortex is scored but not penetrated with the saw blade, thus allowing it to act as a hinge.
- The second osteotomy is created to produce a wafer of bone with the apex laterally (TECH FIG 3B). When removed, it should look like a fine slice of lemon.
- The wedge is closed with direct pressure. This "greensticks" the intact but weakened lateral cortex.

Staple Placement

- The varisation staple (usually 8 mm; 10 mm in larger feet) is selected, and the tip of the distal end is marked with a pen (TECH FIG 4A).

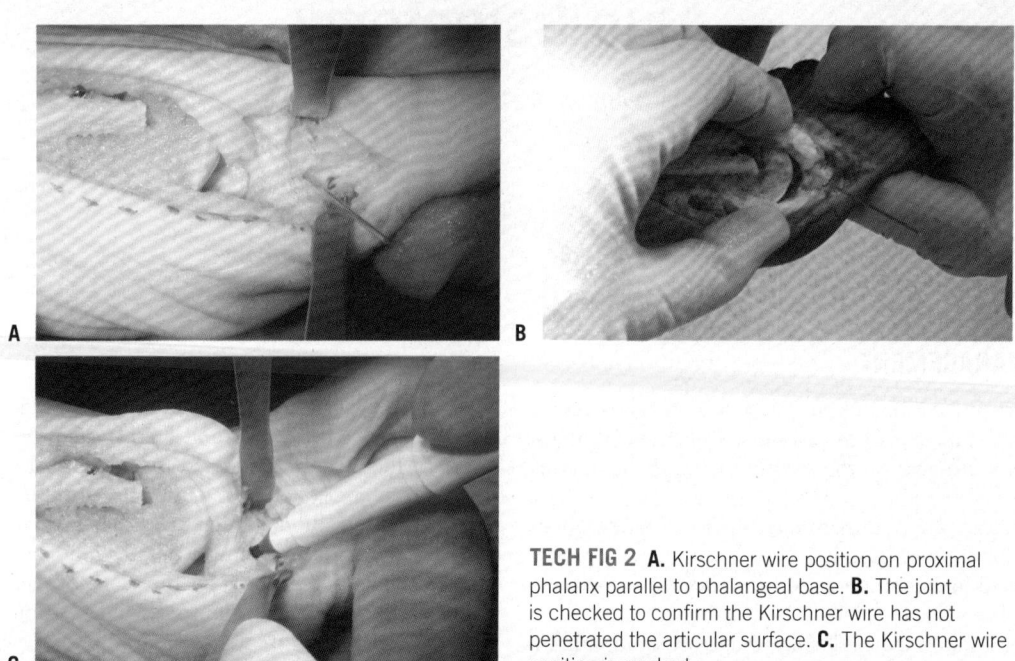

TECH FIG 2 A. Kirschner wire position on proximal phalanx parallel to phalangeal base. **B.** The joint is checked to confirm the Kirschner wire has not penetrated the articular surface. **C.** The Kirschner wire position is marked.

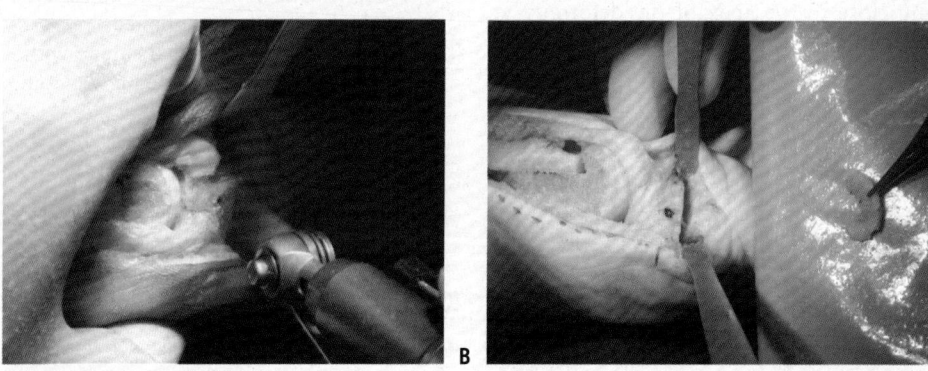

TECH FIG 3 A. The osteotomy is performed parallel to the phalangeal base. **B.** The second cut is performed to produce a small sliver of bone.

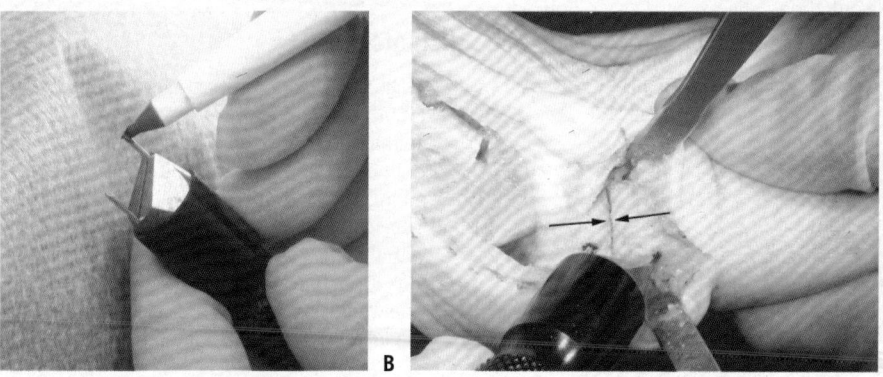

TECH FIG 4 A. The staple is marked with a pen. **B.** The osteotomy is compressed (*arrows*), and the marked staple is placed in the correct position. *(continued)*

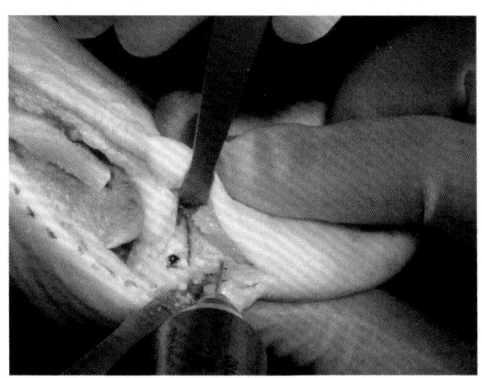 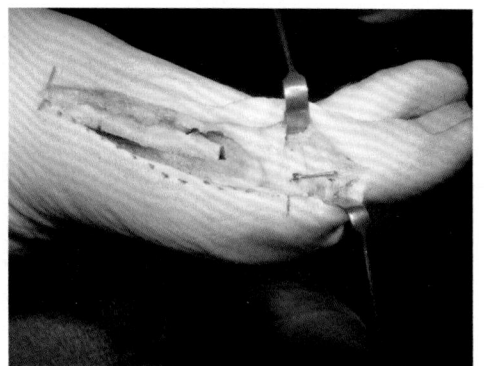

C   D

TECH FIG 4 *(continued)* **C.** The distal mark is then drilled with a Kirschner wire. **D.** The staple is inserted with the osteotomy compressed.

- The staple is placed with the osteotomy compressed.
  - It should be on the midportion of the phalanx in the sagittal plane **(TECH FIG 4B)**.
  - The distal staple leaves an ink mark. This mark is drilled with a 1-mm Kirschner wire **(TECH FIG 4C)**, and then the hole is marked. The position for the staple can then be identified by the two bone marks.
- While maintaining compression, the staple is inserted in the predrilled holes.

- The stability of the fixation is checked **(TECH FIG 4D)**, and axial traction confirms the staple is not in the joint.

Wound Closure

- The wound is closed in layers with continuous Monocryl to skin, and a forefoot bandage is applied to maintain the correction.

CASE EXAMPLE (COURTESY OF MARK E. EASLEY, MD)

Background, Surgical Approach, and Preoperative Planning

- A 30-year-old woman with symptomatic left hallux valgus had increased intermetatarsal and hallux valgus angles.
- Radiograph suggests congruent (symmetric) hallux valgus deformity that may be indicative of an increased distal metatarsal articular angle **(TECH FIG 5A)**.

- Plan for combination biplanar distal chevron and Akin osteotomies.
- Typically a medial midaxial longitudinal approach is used through skin and capsule, extending it more distally than the approach typically used for distal chevron osteotomy alone.
- The dorsomedial sensory cutaneous nerve to the hallux and the extensor hallucis longus tendon must be protected dorsally.

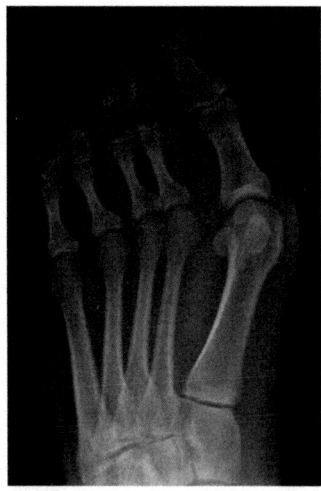 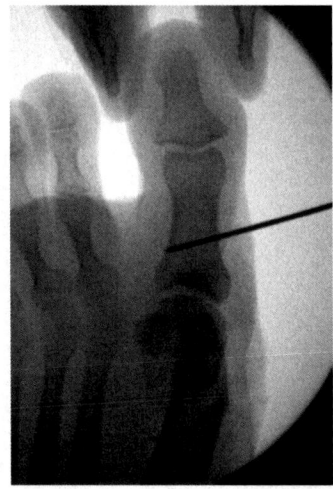

A   B

TECH FIG 5 A. Preoperative radiograph of 30-year-old woman with symptomatic left hallux valgus. Note congruency/symmetry of the MTP joint, suggestive of an increased distal metatarsal articular angle. **B.** Intraoperative fluoroscopy of guide pin for planning oblique proximal phalanx osteotomy.

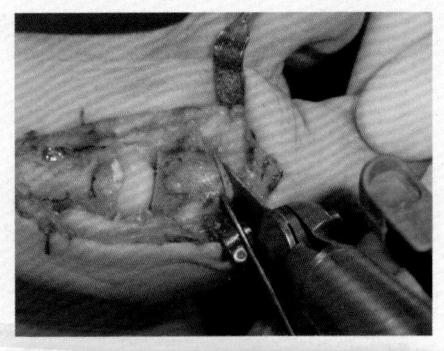

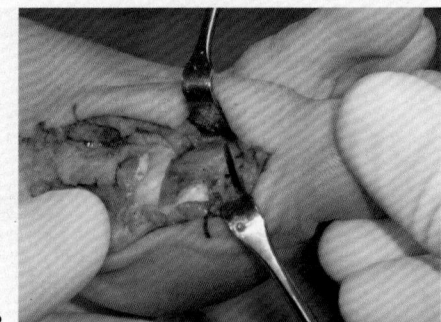

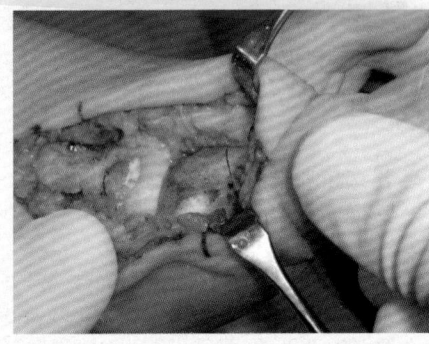

TECH FIG 6 A. Medial wedge resection for Akin osteotomy using the guide pin as a reference. The saw blade is perpendicular to the proximal phalanx shaft axis. **B,C.** Approximating the Akin osteotomy: open (**B**), closed (**C**).

- The plantar medial sensory nerve and flexor hallucis longus tendon need to be protected plantarly, with minimal periosteal stripping.
  - If possible, the plantar medial attachment of the medial capsule/medial collateral ligament on the proximal phalanx should be preserved.
- Intraoperative fluoroscopy is undertaken to plan for medially based closing wedge obliquely oriented osteotomy. A small-diameter Kirschner wire is used to guide the osteotomy **(TECH FIG 5B)**.

Osteotomy Creation

- Medial cortex base wedge resection, using the Kirschner wire as a reference **(TECH FIG 6A)**
- The saw blade is perpendicular to the proximal phalanx shaft axis.
- The lateral cortex is not violated.
- With the wedge of bone removed and lateral cortex intact, the osteotomy is closed **(TECH FIG 6B,C)**.
- Should the osteotomy not completely approximate, with the soft tissues protected, the saw blade may be reinserted into the osteotomy, with the osteotomy held closed as much as possible and run to make the surfaces fully congruent.

Osteotomy Fixation

- With the osteotomy held closed, a cannulated screw guide pin is inserted from the proximal medial aspect of the proximal phalanx without violating the MTP joint **(TECH FIG 7A)**.
- The guide pin should be nearly perpendicular to the oblique osteotomy and not violate the IP joint **(TECH FIG 7B)**.
- A lateral fluoroscopy image can be obtained to confirm that the guide pin is in optimal sagittal plane position.
- After overdrilling the guide pin and with the osteotomy manually compressed and rotation controlled, the cannulated screw is inserted **(TECH FIG 7C,D)**.

Closure and Follow-up

- The periosteum and capsule are closed in concert with the standard medial capsular closure for hallux valgus correction **(TECH FIG 8A)**.
- Follow-up radiographs to confirm satisfactory healing and alignment **(TECH FIG 8B)**.

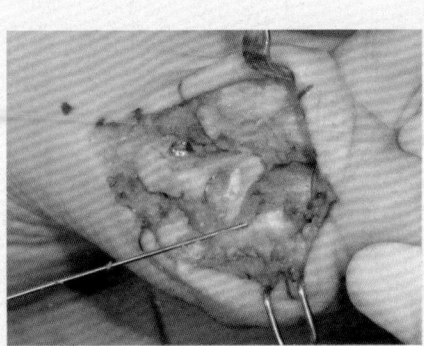

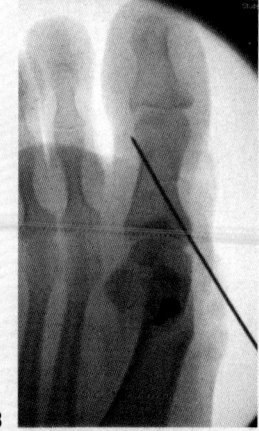

TECH FIG 7 A. Manual compression being maintained across osteotomy during guide pin insertion for cannulated screw fixation. **B.** Intraoperative fluoroscopy shows the guide pin is nearly perpendicular to the osteotomy and does not violate the MTP or IP joints. *(continued)*

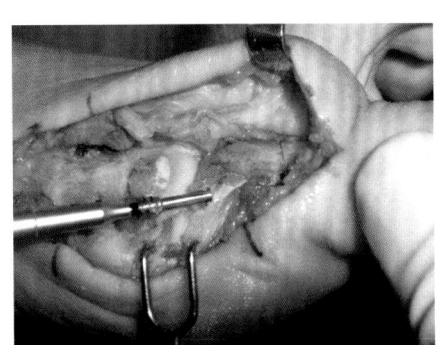

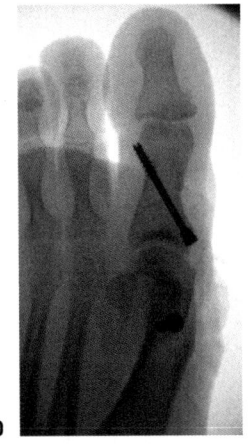

TECH FIG 7 *(continued)* **C.** With manual compression maintained at the osteotomy, the cannulated screw is inserted. **D.** Intraoperative fluoroscopy demonstrates that the screw is maintaining compression at the osteotomy without violating the MTP or IP joints.

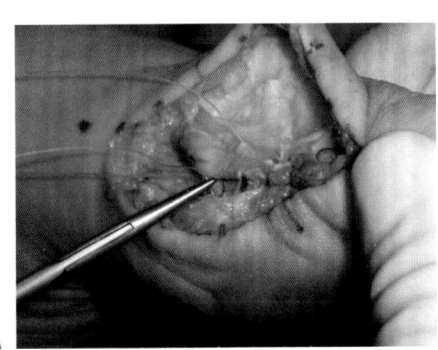

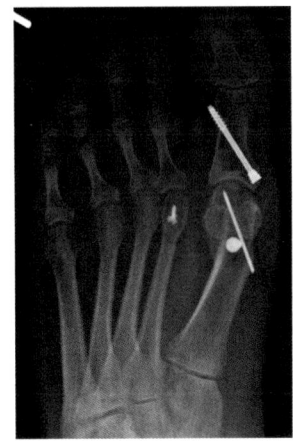

TECH FIG 8 A. Periosteal and capsular closure in concert with routine medial capsular imbrication for hallux valgus correction. **B.** Follow-up AP radiograph.

TECHNIQUES

Pearls and Pitfalls

Exposure	• The orientation of the osteotomy can be difficult if performed in the absence of a metatarsal osteotomy. Avoid the temptation to use a small incision, instead taking care to expose the MTP joint and the shaft of the phalanx.
Staple Insertion	• Resistance may be encountered when inserting the staple due to the hard subchondral bone. Avoid using excess force when inserting the staple, as this may fracture the lateral "greensticked" cortex. Either repeat the Kirschner wire drilling or accept the staple 2–3 mm proud if a good hold is achieved.
Inadvertent Lateral Cortex Fracture	• If the lateral cortex is fractured, then a compression screw is inserted from medial to lateral, spanning the osteotomy.
Overcorrection	• The osteotomy is very powerful, as it is at the apex of the deformity. Aim for a very fine segment of bone; it can be cut again if required.
Unable to Greenstick the Lateral Cortex	• Often, a rectangle of bone as opposed to a wedge has been removed. Forcing it to close will crack the lateral cortex. Instead, use a gentle to-and-fro motion with the running saw while applying gentle compressive force. This thins the lateral cortex until the osteotomy closes without "bouncing back" once pressure is removed.

POSTOPERATIVE CARE

- If safe, patients are discharged home on the day of surgery with strict advice to elevate the foot whenever resting for the first 2 weeks.
- In most cases, they are allowed to bear weight on their heel and lateral forefoot in a hard-soled postoperative shoe.
- Cast immobilization is not required.
- The wound is inspected at 2 weeks, at which time, the hallux is restrapped, and patients are taught simple passive and active toe flexion–extension exercises.
- At 5 weeks postoperatively, the osteotomy is assessed with radiographs.
  - If there is some consolidation at the line of the osteotomy, the patient is instructed to wear a wide shoe or sneaker and to progress to full weight bearing as tolerated.
  - Strapping of the hallux is discontinued at this time.
  - Delayed union or nonunion is rare with this osteotomy.

OUTCOMES

- The most common indication for an Akin osteotomy is in combination with a metatarsal osteotomy for hallux valgus. Outcomes are therefore reported together with satisfaction rates at between 85% and 95%.[2,3,6,7] Very few studies have concentrated solely on the Akin.

COMPLICATIONS

- Complications of this osteotomy are rare[1,4,5,7] but can include nonunion, nerve damage, infection, displacement of the osteotomy, and overcorrection or undercorrection. Failure to recognize propagation of the lateral cortex may increase the risk of subsequent displacement and need for further intervention.

REFERENCES

1. Douthett SM, Plaskey NK, Fallat LM, et al. Restrospective analysis of the Akin osteotomy. J Foot Ankle Surg 2018;57(1):38–43.
2. Frey C, Jahss M, Kummer FJ. The Akin procedure: an analysis of results. Foot Ankle 1991;12:1–6.
3. Garrido IM, Rubio ER, Bosch MN, et al. Scarf and Akin osteotomies for moderate and severe hallux valgus: clinical and radiographic results. Foot Ankle Surg 2008;14:194–203.
4. Hammel E, Abi Chala ML, Wagner T. Complications of first ray osteotomies: a consecutive series of 475 feet with first metatarsal scarf osteotomy and first phalanx osteotomy [in French]. Rev Chir Orthop Reparatrice Appar Mot 2007;93:710–719.
5. Liszka H, Gądek A. Comparison of the type of fixation of Akin osteotomy. Foot Ankle Int 2019;40(4):390–397.
6. Mitchell LA, Baxter DE. A Chevron-Akin double osteotomy for correction of hallux valgus. Foot Ankle 1991;12:7–14.
7. Neumann JA, Reay KD, Bradley KE, et al. Staple fixation for Akin proximal phalangeal osteotomy in the treatment of hallux valgus interphalangeus. Foot Ankle Int 2015;36(4):457–464.

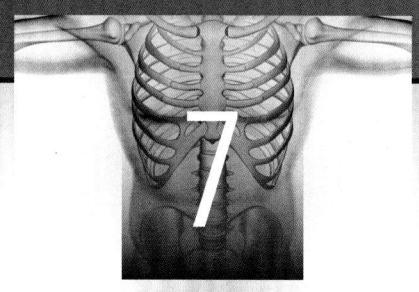

7

CHAPTER

Scarf Osteotomy

Roland Walker, Paul Hamilton, and Sam Singh

SURGICAL MANAGEMENT

- The primary indication for a scarf osteotomy is symptomatic hallux valgus deformity with an intermetatarsal angle of less than 20 degrees. The first tarsometatarsal (metatarsocuneiform) joint should be stable.
- It is a versatile osteotomy that can allow shortening, lengthening, rotation, displacement, or plantarization of the first metatarsal head. Thus, indications include symptomatic hallux valgus with or without mild transfer symptoms, juvenile hallux valgus with an abnormal distal metatarsal articular angle (DMAA), arthritic hallux valgus not severe enough for a fusion, and revision surgery in suitable cases.

Preoperative Planning

- Anteroposterior (AP) and lateral weight-bearing radiographs of the foot are evaluated for metatarsal length, intermetatarsal angle, hallux valgus angle, DMAA, and interphalangeal angle for cases that may require a proximal phalangeal osteotomy to obtain complete correction. Plantar opening and/or dorsal subluxation of the first tarsometatarsal joint suggests instability and a Lapidus fusion should be considered as an alternative.
- Congruency of the joint, presence of osteophytes, the size of the bony medial eminence, and position and condition of the sesamoids are noted.

Positioning

- Surgery is performed on an outpatient basis.
- Prophylactic antibiotics are administered.
- A thigh or ankle tourniquet is applied.
- The patient is positioned supine with a sandbag under the ipsilateral buttock so that the big toe points toward the ceiling.

SOFT TISSUE RELEASE

- Approach the metatarsal through a medial longitudinal incision extending from the proximal metatarsal shaft to the medial flare of the proximal phalanx **(TECH FIG 1A)**. This can be extended distally if a phalangeal osteotomy is required.
  - Identify the dorsal medial cutaneous nerve and incise the medial capsule sharply in a single longitudinal direction, plantar to the nerve.
  - Expose the medial eminence and the metatarsal shaft using subperiosteal sharp dissection, taking care to protect the plantar neck vascular bundle to the metatarsal head **(TECH FIG 1B)**.
  - Create a proximal plantar window by subperiosteal dissection under the midmetatarsal shaft. The proximal plantar exposure can be performed safely without any disruption to the plantar blood supply.
  - Sharp dissect over-the-top of the first metatarsal, into the first web space, taking care not to buttonhole the joint capsule.
  - Put a laminar spreader in the first web space as proximally as possible and gently open it to facilitate the view for the lateral release. A small Langenbeck retractor placed just inside the joint capsule will also improve the view.
  - Use a banana blade to perform the lateral release **(TECH FIG 1C)**. First release the suspensory ligament and the metatarsal attachment of the lateral collateral ligament by carefully dissecting all the soft tissue off the lateral side of the metatarsal head. The fibular sesamoid will then come into view. If it doesn't, there may be osteophyte on the lateral metatarsal head, which can be resected. Take care not to divide the phalangeal attachment of the collateral ligament; otherwise, hallux varus may result. This release is usually sufficient for mild to moderate hallux valgus. The suspensory ligament can also be divided through the joint or through the osteotomy by sweeping a blade above the fibular sesamoid right up to the proximal phalanx. These techniques mean that a separate first web space incision is not routinely needed.
- In moderate to severe hallux valgus, a second stage of the lateral release may be required. This is achieved by pushing the banana blade deep and lateral to the fibular sesamoid, leaving a cuff of tissue (the suspensory ligament) attached to the sesamoid. This maneuver detaches the transverse head of the adductor hallucis tendon and can be extended proximally to also detach the oblique head of this muscle. Deep to the adductor hallucis tendons, there is a fascial layer attaching the fibular sesamoid to the plantar plate of the second metatarsophalangeal joint. This must also be divided for a complete release.

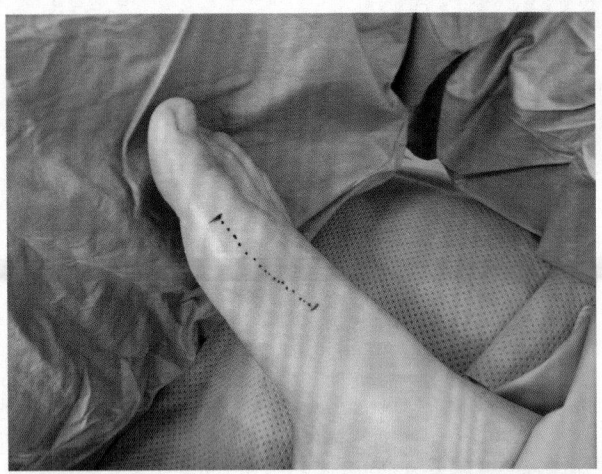

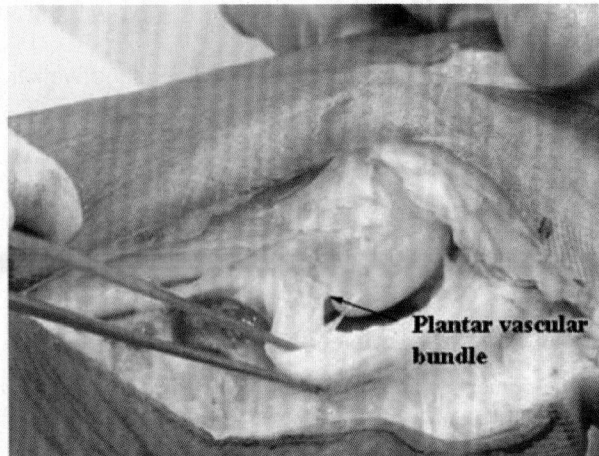

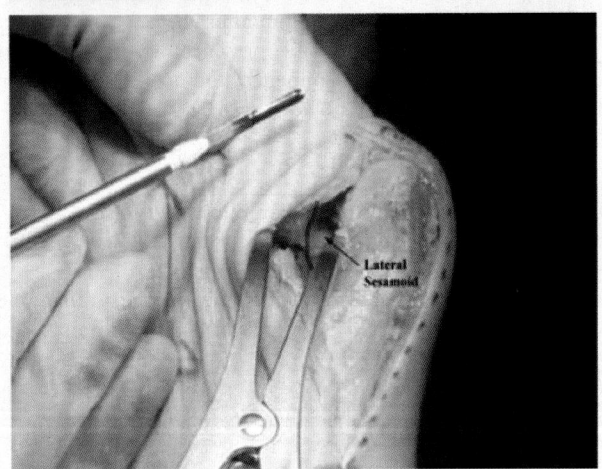

TECH FIG 1 **A.** The incision is made from the tarsometatarsal joint to the proximal metatarsal shaft. **B.** Preserve the plantar blood supply to the capital fragment. **C.** First web space exposure and suspensory ligament release using a banana blade. *Green line* demonstrates plane of adductor release if this is required.

Once again, take care not to divide the phalangeal attachment of the collateral ligament by purposefully exiting the distal part of the release laterally, into the first web space. The surgeon should be able to palpate the plantar fat and skin only through the web space once this full release has been performed.

- Judging the extent of the lateral release is based on surgeon experience, but we have found complete release of the suspensory ligament alone is sufficient in the majority of cases. After adequate release, the hallux valgus must completely passively correct and the sesamoids should also reduce fully.

SHORT SCARF OSTEOTOMY

- For many foot and ankle surgeons, a short scarf osteotomy has become standard. This modification is safe with similar outcomes and has the advantages of a smaller incision and exposure plus single-screw fixation.[2] We use it routinely for nearly all cases, reserving the long scarf for patients with poor bone quality and revision cases. The short scarf can be combined with basal osteotomies for correction of severe hallux valgus with intermetatarsal angle of greater than 20 degrees and also facilitates correction of the DMAA if this is required.
- Begin by performing a minimal resection of the medial eminence (**TECH FIG 2A**). This cut must preserve all of the medial sulcus and creates a small area of cancellous bone for the

medial soft tissues to heal back onto. Orientate this cut perpendicular to the angle of the longitudinal cut.
- Perform the distal transverse cut first and reference from the preoperative x-rays to avoid undue lengthening or shortening of the ray. The cut is dorsal and usually parallel with the articular surface, 2 to 3 mm behind the articular cartilage and angled perpendicular to the second metatarsal shaft, usually toward the third or fourth metatarsophalangeal joint (**TECH FIG 2B**). Slight shortening is acceptable for an arthritic first metatarsophalangeal joint. Lengthening should be avoided except in revision cases if the initial operation has unduly shortened the first ray. When performing the distal cut, elevate the hand to complete the lateral part of the osteotomy.

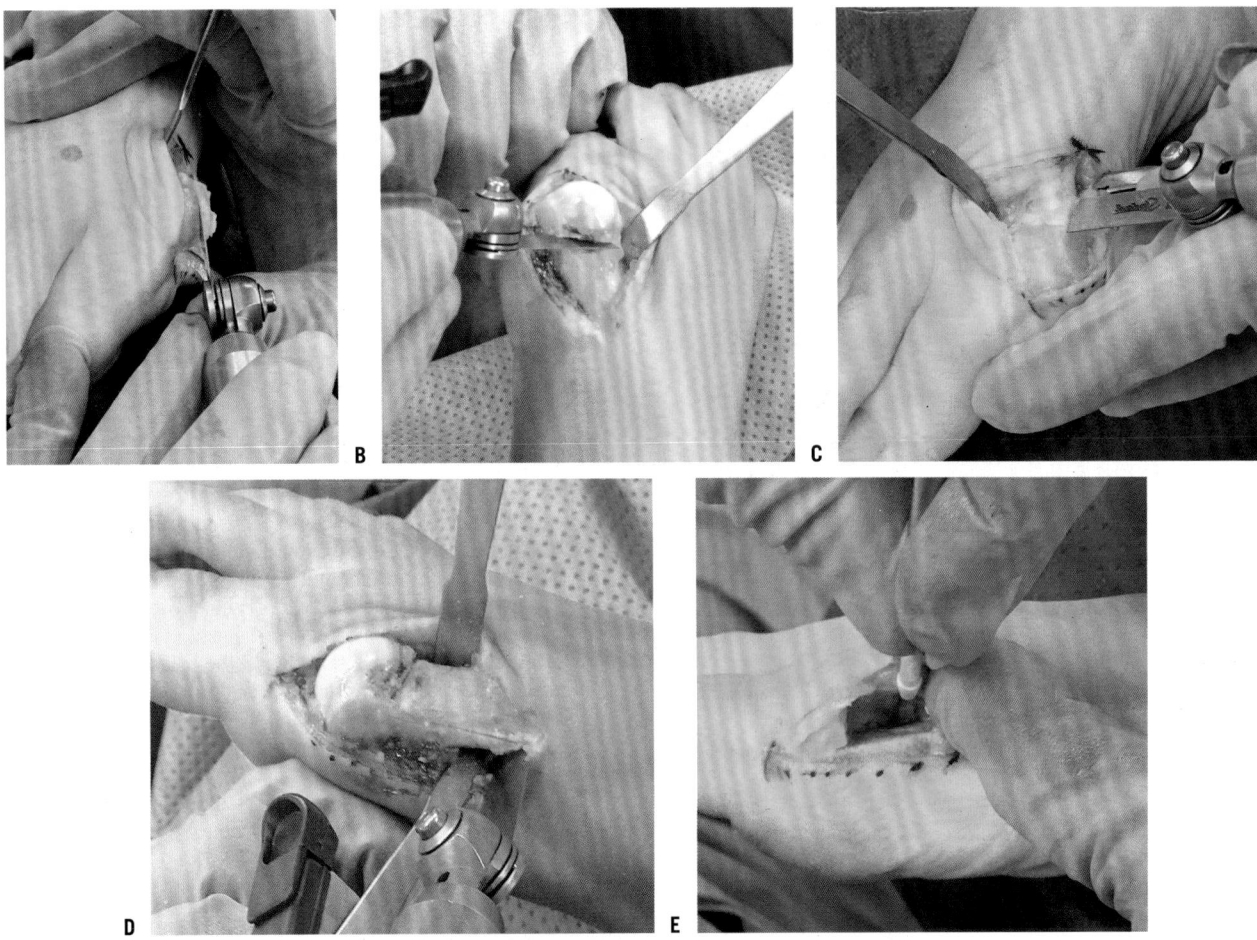

TECH FIG 2 A. Minimal resection of medial eminence preserving the sulcus. **B.** Transverse cuts, avoiding convergence. **C.** Longitudinal cut in the same plane as the plantar metatarsal surface. **D.** Plantar transverse cut is parallel or slightly divergent to the distal transverse cut. **E.** Release of the capsule through the osteotomy.

- Start the longitudinal cut but only go through the medial cortex **(TECH FIG 2C)**. This is begun distally 5 mm from the articular surface and 2 to 3 mm from the dorsal surface of the metatarsal and finishes in the diaphyseal portion of the metatarsal, 2 to 3 mm from the proximal plantar surface of the metatarsal. The osteotomy is usually just over half the length of the metatarsal and must be long enough to allow two screw fixation of this is required.
- Complete the longitudinal cut in the same plane as the plantar orientation of the metatarsal. Also orientate the cut relative to the plantar aspect of forefoot. Slight plantarization of the metatarsal head is optimal.
- The proximal plantar cut must be parallel or slightly divergent from the distal cut to facilitate lateral translation and maximize rotational stability **(TECH FIG 2D)**. Consider using a narrower saw blade for this cut to reduce the risk of notching the metatarsal shaft, which can cause a stress fracture.
- The two transverse cuts should be angled at 60 degrees to the longitudinal cut as chevrons, for maximum stability of the osteotomy.
- The two fragments should separate easily. Avoid levering them apart, which risks metatarsal fracture.

- These steps may need to be repeated if there has been failure to complete all the cuts, but take care to avoid double cutting. This can cause excessive hollowing of the cancellous bone, referred to as *troughing*.
- Release of the capsule and periosteum on the lateral side may be needed if it is preventing displacement. This can often be achieved through the osteotomy, particularly distally **(TECH FIG 2E)**. In our experience, this additional release makes a substantial difference to the mobility of the fragments and allows us to easily dial in the correction.

Displacement

- Perform displacement and/or rotation with guidance from preoperative radiographs by putting traction on the toe to distract the osteotomy and pushing the head fragment laterally. Usually, when traction is released, the two ends of the osteotomy key in and the head fragment will be relatively stable. If it is not, use pointed or curved clamps to hold the displacement **(TECH FIG 3)**.

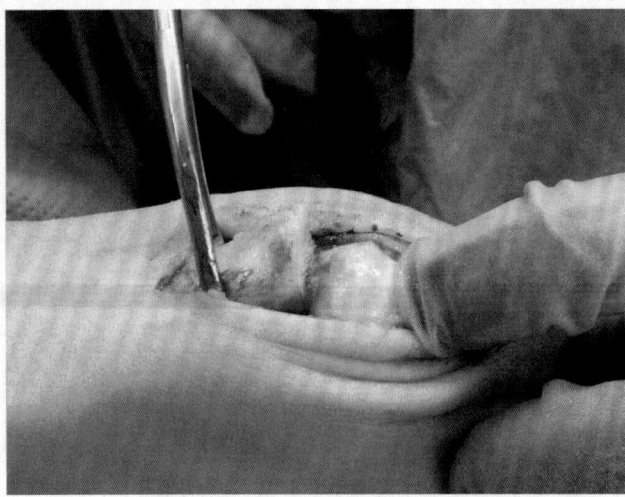

TECH FIG 3 Displacement of the fragment, held with compression clamp.

- Ensure that is no unwanted rotation in the sagittal or frontal planes. Ensure that the osteotomy surfaces are well opposed and keyed in.
- If a correction of the DMAA is required, consider taking extra wedge cuts from the distal metatarsal shaft and the proximal tail of the head fragment to ensure better bone contact and more rotational stability. This takes some thought and planning preoperatively in order to avoid shortening. We recommend using a second screw for fixation if correcting a DMAA abnormality.
- Up to two-thirds of lateral displacement can be obtained while maintaining a strong lateral strut and good bone apposition.

Fixation

- Obtain screw fixation using Barouk screws (DePuy Synthes, Warsaw, IN). These are cannulated, self-tapping screws with a long distal thread and a threaded head to allow compression and burial of the head.
- Place the distal screw first.
  - Pass the guidewire from the proximal fragment into the head fragment as vertically as possible while still maintaining good distal fixation. Typically, the screw is directed toward the tibial sesamoid.
  - Directly visualize the guidewire in the joint (**TECH FIG 4A**), and withdraw it to be flush with the articular surface so that it can be measured (**TECH FIG 4B**). A screw at least 4 mm less than the measured amount is used to avoid intra-articular penetration.
  - During the drilling over the guidewire, ensure that the drill countersink is seated fully to avoid inadvertent fracture during screw placement.
  - Implant the screw carefully ensuring there is good compression across the osteotomy and no rotation of the capital fragment. Ensure the screw head is completely flush with the metatarsal shaft. Typical screw lengths are 14 mm to 20 mm.
  - Directly inspect the joint. If the view is limited, tap the guide wire back into the joint. If you only see a wire, then the screw tip cannot have breached the joint.
- Single-screw fixation is sufficient if the osteotomy is rotationally stable with well keyed-in proximal and distal surfaces. If there is any rotational instability or a DMAA correction is included, add a second screw in the diaphysis:
  - Place the second guidewire for the proximal screw in the midline in an oblique direction to reach the plantar cortex of the distal fragment.
  - Measure it by withdrawing the guidewire so as to be flush with the cortex. This screw length equals the measurement from the wire. Use the long drill as this is a bicortical screw. Retraction of the plantar tissue protects and allows direct visualization of the wire and the drill.
  - Directly visualize the screw to confirm compression and length.

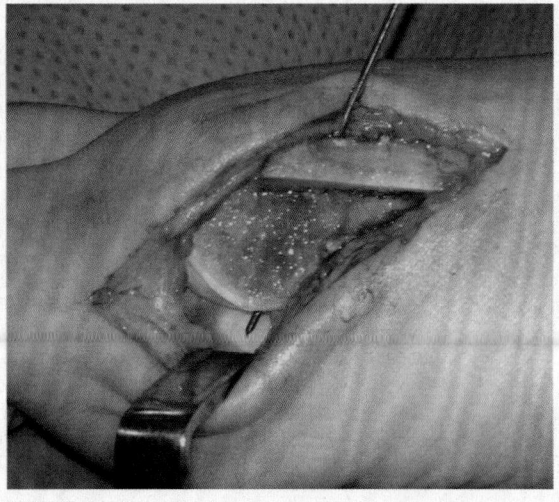
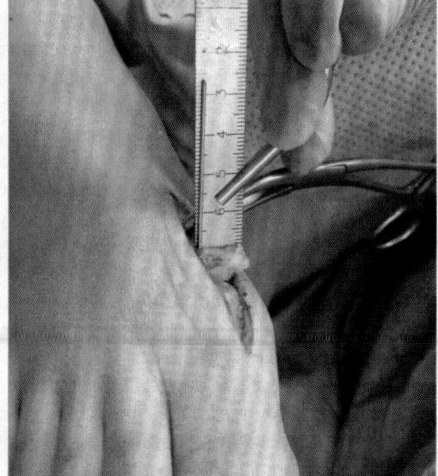

TECH FIG 4 A. Distal wire placement. **B.** Measure the screw length with the wire withdrawn flush to the metatarsal head.

Completion

- Resect the overhanging distal aspect of the dorsal fragment, placing the saw flat on the medial head and cutting toward the medial side of the metatarsal shaft (**TECH FIG 5**). Shape the distal cortical bone, so it is smooth and rounded and check the osteotomy for stability.
- Imbricate the medial capsule with a strong absorbable suture (eg, no. 1 Vicryl) using a box stitch centered on the metatarsal head while your assistant pushes up on the metatarsal head to simulate weight bearing. You can then judge the tension needed in the medial repair to achieve a perfect correction.
- Confirm the reduction of the intermetatarsal angle, screw position, and relocation of the sesamoids with image intensification with the foot flat on the image intensifier to simulate weight bearing. Assess the need for a proximal phalangeal osteotomy.
- Complete the capsular repair with further interrupted sutures and then close the skin with a continuous 3-0 Vicryl Rapide or other absorbable suture. Apply a well-padded forefoot bandage. No strapping should be required to maintain the correction, and the patient should be free to bend the toe.

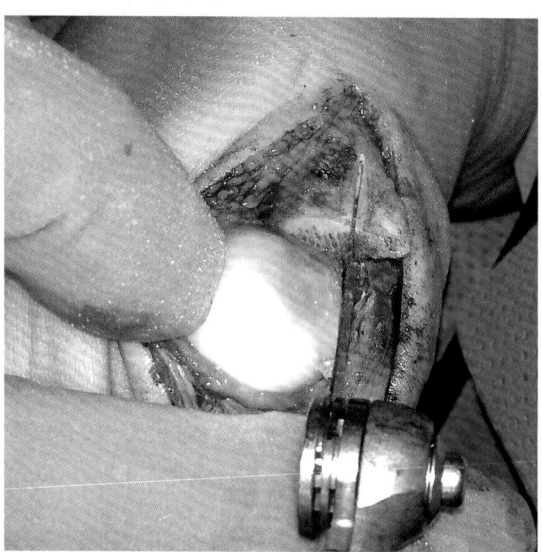

TECH FIG 5 Residual medial bony protuberance excised.

LONG SCARF OSTEOTOMY

- The steps for the long scarf osteotomy are identical to the short scarf. The longitudinal cut, however, is longer and the plantar cut is made in the metaphyseal flare rather than in the diaphysis.
- Care must be taken not to enter the tarsometatarsal joint with the proximal cut.
- Displacement is the same. Occasionally, the proximal lateral corner of the head fragment must be trimmed to avoid impingement with the second metatarsal shaft, in the case of a large displacement.
- Fixation is always with two screws using the technique described earlier.

TECHNIQUES

Pearls and Pitfalls

The osteotomy is complete, but the head fragment will not shift easily.	• After completing the cuts successfully, if displacement is still difficult, then check that the periosteum is not tethering the distal lateral corner of the proximal fragment.
The distal transverse cuts do not key in once the head fragment is shifted.	• The transverse cuts converge, so a second cut of the proximal tail is required.
Rotational Osteotomy to Correct Distal Metatarsal Articular Angle	• If using the scarf osteotomy to correct the DMAA, then additional wedge cuts from the distal metatarsal shaft and the proximal plantar tail are needed to allow for lateral or medial rotation of the metatarsal head as desired.
Longitudinal Cut	• The direction of the longitudinal cut can depress the metatarsal head, depending on the requirements of the patient. Check the angle of the saw blade from the end of the bed before committing to this cut to avoid elevating the head.
Transverse Cut	• Double cutting the transverse cuts can shorten the osteotomy in cases where the joint is very stiff or there is very severe hallux valgus deformity.

Screws	• Direct visualization of the metatarsophalangeal joint is made to avoid joint penetration. Take care to avoid seating the proximal screw too deep into the very thin dorsal cortex, as this may reduce screw hold.
Proximal Plantar Exposure	• This is a safe exposure and does not compromise the blood supply to the metatarsal. It is a vital step: Once completed, it allows orientation of the longitudinal cut parallel to the plantar surface; identification of the flare of the first tarsometatarsal joint ensures the transverse cut is not intra-articular; and a clear view of the lateral plantar surface allows the surgeon to pass the guidewire under direct vision and check the screw length.

POSTOPERATIVE CARE

- If safe, patients are discharged home on the day of surgery with strict advice to elevate the foot whenever resting for the first 2 weeks.
- In most cases, they are allowed to bear weight on their heel and lateral forefoot in a hard-soled postoperative shoe for 5 weeks.
- Cast immobilization is not required.
- The wound is inspected at 2 weeks, and if clean and dry, no further dressings are required. The patient may start to wash the foot and moisturize the scar.
- At 5 weeks postoperatively, the osteotomy is assessed with radiographs (**FIG 1A,B**). If there is some consolidation at the line of the osteotomy, the patient is instructed to wear a wide shoe or sneaker and to progress to full weight bearing as tolerated. Delayed union or nonunion is rare with this osteotomy.

OUTCOMES

- The scarf osteotomy is now a widely used method of correction for hallux valgus; it is particularly popular in Europe.
- Satisfaction rates range from 88% to 92%,[3,4,9,10] equivalent to those of the chevron osteotomy,[5,6] including patients defined as having severe hallux valgus. In a review of five recent publications,[5,7,9–11] the hallux valgus angle was improved on average by 16 degrees (range 11 to 21), the intermetatarsal angle by 6.4 (range 3 to 10), and the American Orthopaedic Foot & Ankle Society score by 45 (range 37 to 55).
- A learning curve for performing the scarf osteotomy has also been noted, with higher complication rates seen in early series.[1]
- Short scarf osteotomy is a safe and effective modification of the traditional technique.[2,12] In a recent series of 166 cases, there were no cases with intra- or postoperative fracture, loss of position, or avascular necrosis (AVN).[12]

COMPLICATIONS

- The main complication seen is stiffness, which occurs in up to 5% of cases.[8] Other complications include wound problems, infection, undercorrection, overcorrection, intraoperative fracture, postoperative metatarsal stress-fracture, dorsomedial nerve damage, chronic regional pain disorder, and deep vein thrombosis.
- Delayed union and AVN are rare complications.
- Fracture risk can be reduced by preserving the lateral strut when placing the proximal screw.

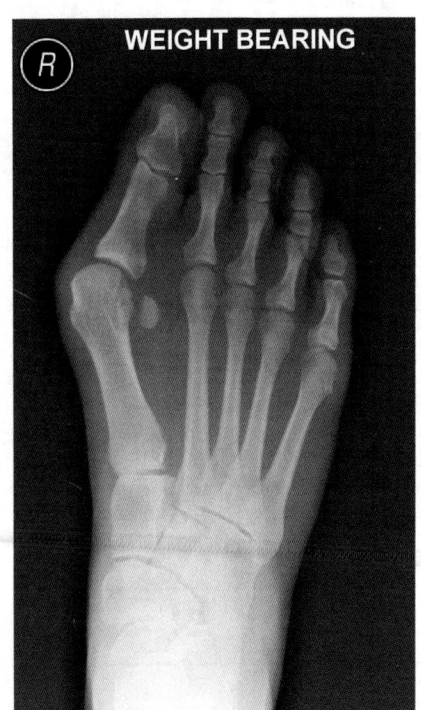
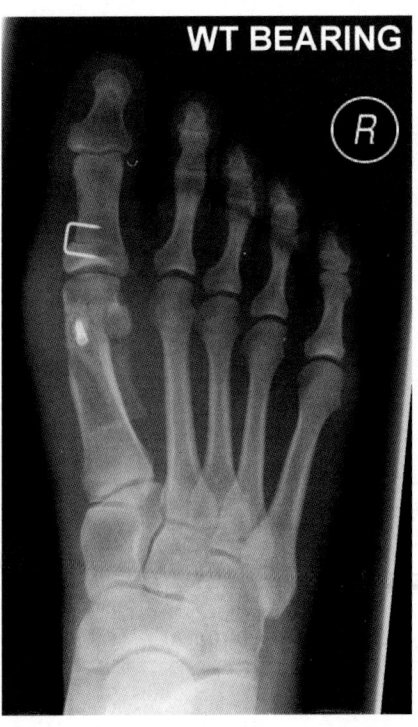

FIG 1 A. Preoperative AP radiograph of a moderate hallux valgus deformity. **B.** Postoperative radiograph after short scarf osteotomy plus Akin osteotomy. Note the proximal end of the osteotomy is in the diaphysis, and the single screw is vertically orientated in the coronal plain, finishing in the medial portion of the head.

REFERENCES

1. Barouk LS, Barouk P. The scarf first metatarsal osteotomy in the correction of hallux valgus deformity. Interact Surg 2007;2:2–11.
2. Barouk P, Vioreanu M, Barouk LS. The short scarf 1st metatarsal osteotomy. In: Bentley G, ed. European Surgical Orthopaedics and Traumatology: The EFFORT Textbook. London: Springer, 2014: 3433–3450.
3. Berg RP, Olsthoorn PG, Pöll RG. Scarf osteotomy in hallux valgus: a review of 72 cases. Acta Orthop Belg 2007;73:219–223.
4. Crevoisier X, Mouhsine E, Ortolano V, et al. The scarf osteotomy for the treatment of hallux valgus deformity: a review of 84 cases. Foot Ankle Int 2001;22:970–976.
5. Deenik AR, Pilot P, Brandt SE, et al. Scarf versus chevron osteotomy in hallux valgus: a randomized controlled trial in 96 patients. Foot Ankle Int 2007;28:537–541.
6. Deenik AR, van Mameren H, de Visser E, et al. Equivalent correction in scarf and chevron osteotomy in moderate and severe hallux valgus: a randomized controlled trial. Foot Ankle Int 2008;29:1209–1215.
7. Garrido IM, Rubio ER, Bosch MN, et al. Scarf and Akin osteotomies for moderate and severe hallux valgus: clinical and radiographic results. Foot Ankle Surg 2008;14:194–203.
8. Hammel E, Abi Chala ML, Wagner T. Complications of first ray osteotomies: a consecutive series of 475 feet with first metatarsal Scarf osteotomy and first phalanx osteotomy [in French]. Rev Chir Orthop Reparatrice Appar Mot 2007;93:710–719.
9. Jones S, Al Hussainy HA, Ali F, et al. Scarf osteotomy for hallux valgus. A prospective clinical and pedobarographic study. J Bone Joint Surg Br 2004;86:830–836.
10. Lipscombe S, Molly A, Sirikonda S, et al. Scarf osteotomy for the correction of hallux valgus: midterm clinical outcome. J Foot Ankle Surg 2008;47:273–277.
11. Perugia D, Basile A, Gensini A, et al. The scarf osteotomy for severe hallux valgus. Int Orthop 2003;27:103–106.
12. Rajeev A, Tumia N. Three-year follow-up results of combined short scarf osteotomy with Akin procedure for hallux valgus. J Foot Ankle Surg 2019;58(5):837–841.

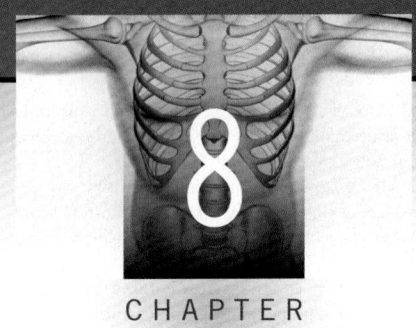

8

CHAPTER

Proximal Crescentic Osteotomy

Roger A. Mann and Jeffrey A. Mann

SURGICAL MANAGEMENT

- The distal soft tissue procedure and proximal metatarsal osteotomy has been widely used for bunion corrections for more than 30 years. It is a reliable, reproducible procedure that can be used to treat a wide range of bunion deformities.
- The procedure is indicated for a hallux valgus deformity with an incongruent metatarsophalangeal joint, an intermetatarsal angle of more than 10 to 12 degrees, and a distal metatarsal articular angle of less than 10 degrees.

- It is carried out in three main steps:
  - Release of the contracted lateral capsular structures: the adductor hallucis tendon, the transverse metatarsal ligament, and the lateral joint capsule
    - By freeing up these three structures, the sesamoid sling can be replaced beneath the first metatarsal head.
  - Preparation of the medial joint structures
    - Exposure and plication of the medial joint capsule
    - Excision of the medial eminence
  - Exposure of the base of the first metatarsal and proximal crescentic metatarsal osteotomy

TECHNIQUES

RELEASE OF THE LATERAL JOINT STRUCTURES

Exposure

- Make a 2.5-cm incision on the dorsal aspect of the first web space between the first and second metatarsal heads.
  - Deepen this incision through the subcutaneous tissue.
- Place a Weitlaner retractor to expose the web space.
  - On the floor of the web space lies the adductor hallucis, which passes obliquely to insert into the lateral sesamoid and the base of the proximal phalanx (TECH FIG 1A,B).
- Identify the capsule between the subluxated fibular sesamoid and the lateral base of the first metatarsal head.
- Use a scalpel to release the capsule. By extending the incision distally in this interval, detach the adductor hallucis tendon from its insertion into the base of the proximal phalanx.
- Detach the adductor tendon from the lateral aspect of the fibular sesamoid, dissecting proximally until the flexor hallucis brevis muscle tissue is noted (TECH FIG 1C).
- Place a Weitlaner retractor between the first and second metatarsal heads, placing the transverse metatarsal ligament under tension (TECH FIG 1B,D).

- Transect the transverse metatarsal ligament.
  - While carrying out this step, it is important that only ligamentous tissue is cut because directly beneath the ligament lies the common nerve to the first web space and the accompanying vessels.

Release the Lateral Joint Capsule

- Make an incision through the dorsal aspect of the joint capsule at the level of the joint line and pass the knife blade to the plantar aspect of the metatarsal (TECH FIG 1E,F).
- With the blade well seated against the bone, pass the scalpel proximally, stripping the origin of the capsule off the metatarsal head over a distance of about 1.5 cm.
- This creates a flap of the lateral joint capsule to be used later in the repair (TECH FIG 1G).
- Bring the hallux into about 25 degrees of varus, which ensures that no lateral contracture remains.

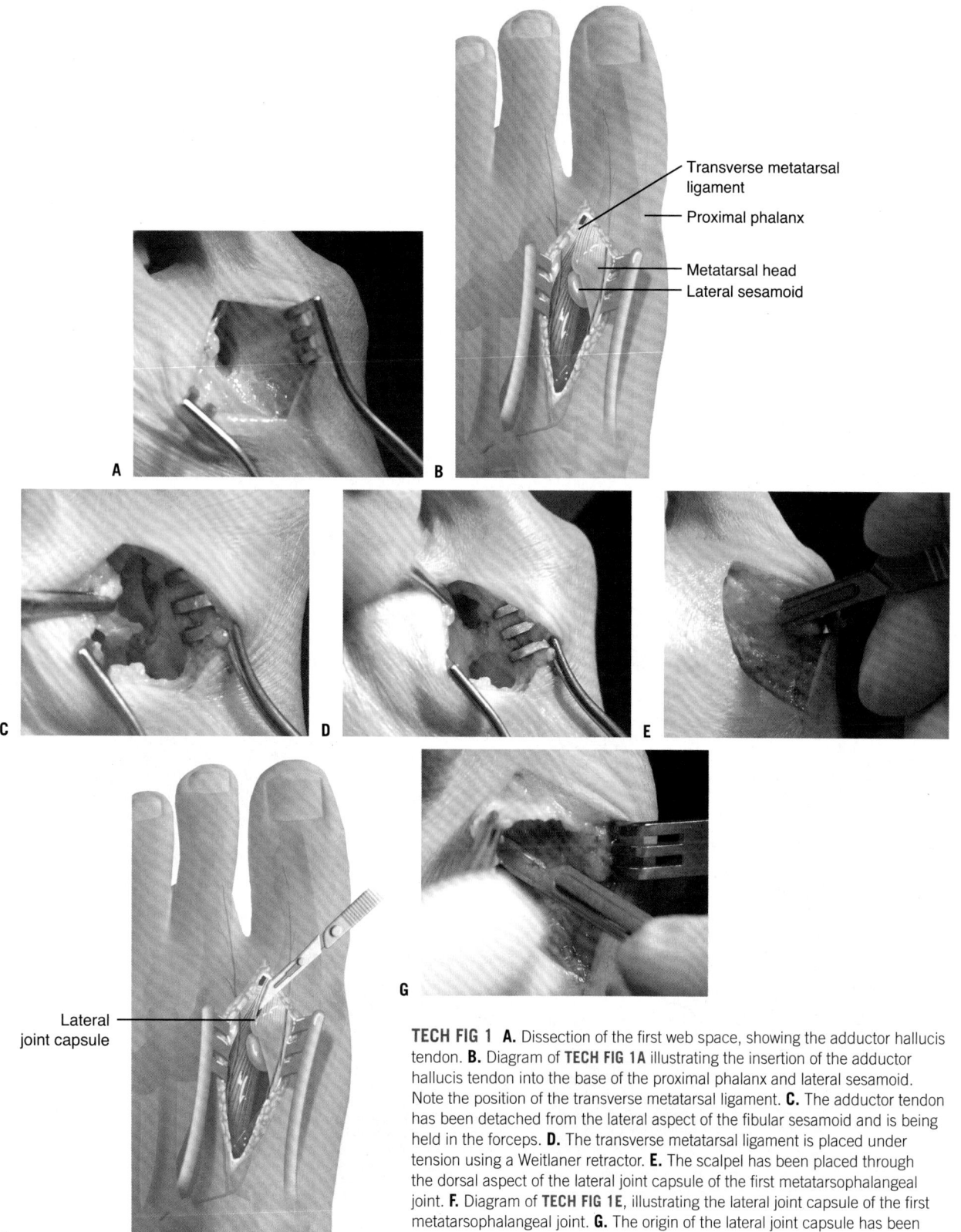

Transverse metatarsal
ligament

Proximal phalanx

Metatarsal head
Lateral sesamoid

Lateral
joint capsule

TECH FIG 1 **A.** Dissection of the first web space, showing the adductor hallucis
tendon. **B.** Diagram of **TECH FIG 1A** illustrating the insertion of the adductor
hallucis tendon into the base of the proximal phalanx and lateral sesamoid.
Note the position of the transverse metatarsal ligament. **C.** The adductor tendon
has been detached from the lateral aspect of the fibular sesamoid and is being
held in the forceps. **D.** The transverse metatarsal ligament is placed under
tension using a Weitlaner retractor. **E.** The scalpel has been placed through
the dorsal aspect of the lateral joint capsule of the first metatarsophalangeal
joint. **F.** Diagram of **TECH FIG 1E**, illustrating the lateral joint capsule of the first
metatarsophalangeal joint. **G.** The origin of the lateral joint capsule has been
stripped off the metatarsal head, creating the flap of tissue held in the forceps.

PREPARATION OF THE MEDIAL JOINT CAPSULE

- Approach the medial joint capsule through a longitudinal incision in the midline starting at the middle of the proximal phalanx and proceeding proximally just past the medial eminence.
- Identify the plane between the subcutaneous tissue and the joint capsule; take care to work along this plane.
  - Dissecting dorsally at first, pull the skin flap away from the capsule to expose the dorsal medial cutaneous nerve, which is then carefully retracted.
- Next, dissect the skin flap off the plantar half of the capsule until the abductor hallucis muscle and tendon are identified.
  - Take care in this area because the plantar medial cutaneous nerve lies just plantar to the abductor tendon.
- The capsulotomy that we prefer starts with a vertical cut in the medial joint capsule, made 2 to 3 mm proximal to the base of the proximal phalanx.
- Make a second, parallel cut 3 to 8 mm proximal to the first cut, depending on the severity of the hallux valgus deformity. A more severe deformity requires more resection of tissue from the medial joint capsule **(TECH FIG 2A)**.
- Bring together these two parallel capsular cuts dorsally through an inverted V-shaped incision.

- On the plantar side, make an upright V-shaped incision through the abductor hallucis tendon that ends at the tibial sesamoid **(TECH FIG 2B)**.
- Remove this capsular tissue **(TECH FIG 2C)**.
- While making the cut through the abductor hallucis tendon, keep the tip of the knife blade inside the joint to avoid damaging the plantar medial cutaneous nerve.
- Make an incision through the joint capsule on the dorsal aspect of the medial eminence.
- Peel the capsular flap proximally and plantarward until the medial eminence is completely exposed **(TECH FIG 2D–F)**.
- Perform an osteotomy to remove the medial eminence.
  - Start the osteotomy 1 to 2 mm medial to the sagittal sulcus; the osteotomy is in line with the medial aspect of the metatarsal shaft **(TECH FIG 2G)**.
  - The medial eminence can be removed with a 16-mm osteotome or with a saw blade. This is strictly the choice of the operating surgeon.
- After performing the osteotomy, inspect the metatarsal to be sure there are no rough edges of bone. Rongeur off any bony prominence.

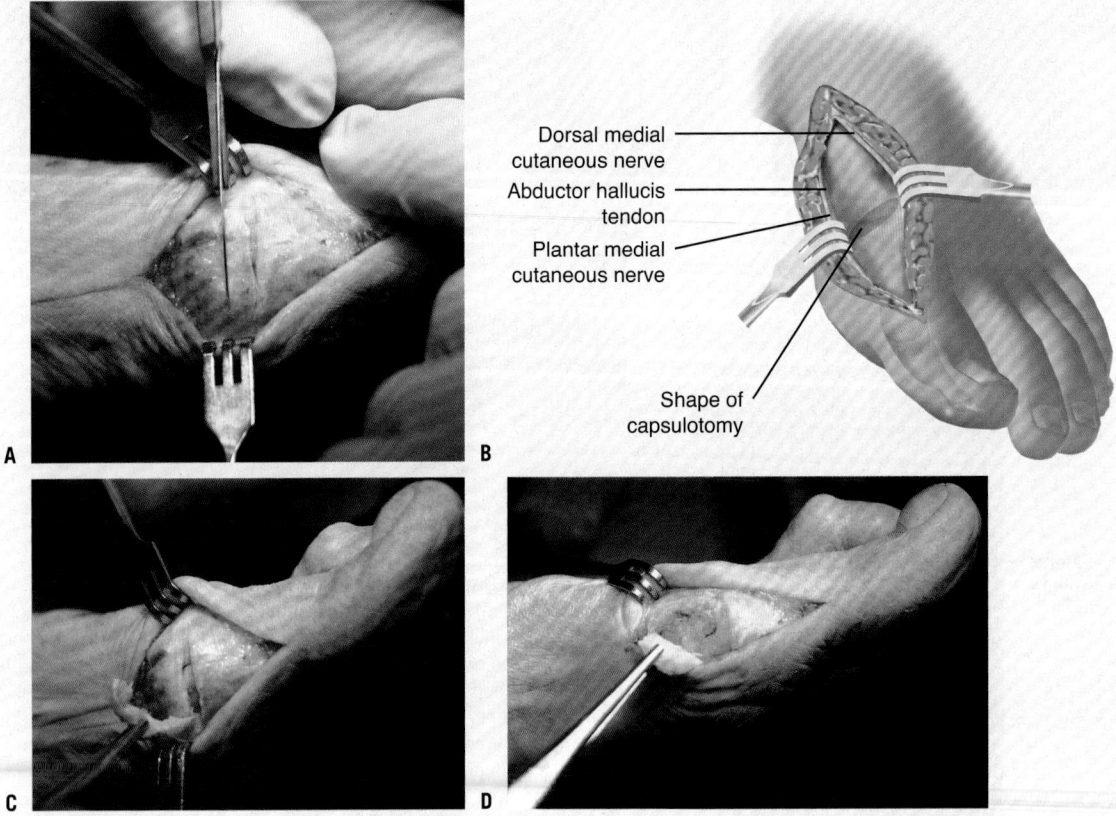

TECH FIG 2 A. Exposure of the medial joint capsule, showing the parallel cuts that represent the vertical limbs of the capsulotomy. **B.** Diagram of **TECH FIG 2C**, demonstrating the shape of the medial joint capsulotomy. **C.** Removing the medial joint capsular tissue. **D.** A dorsal incision is made, and the capsular flap is peeled proximally and plantarward. *(continued)*

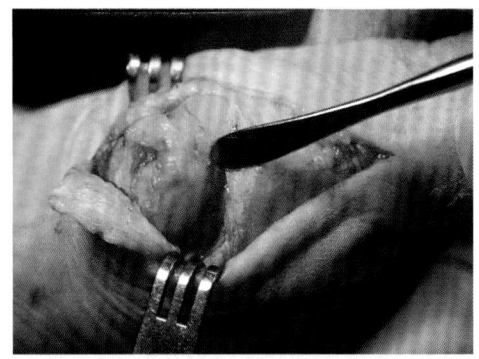

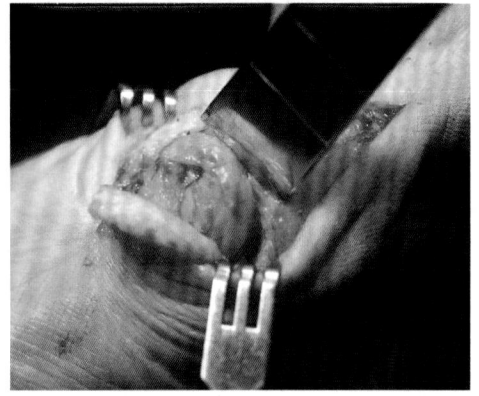

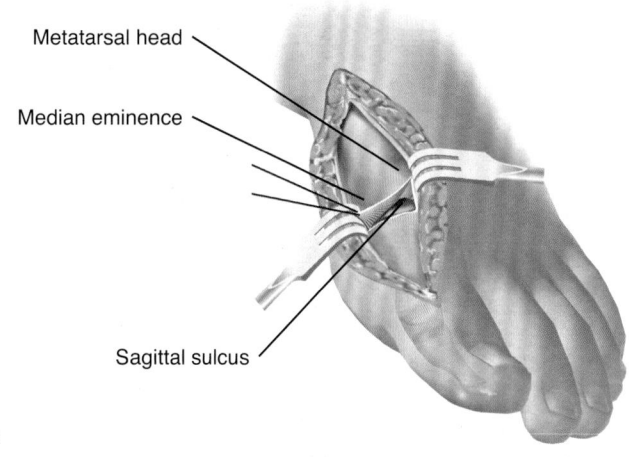

Metatarsal head

Median eminence

Sagittal sulcus

TECH FIG 2 *(continued)* **E.** The medial eminence has been completely exposed. The sagittal sulcus is demonstrated by the Freer elevator. **F.** Diagram of the medial eminence after the capsular flap has been retracted. Note the sagittal sulcus. **G.** The osteotomy—to remove the medial eminence—is started 1 to 2 mm medial to the sagittal sulcus and is performed in line with the medial aspect of the metatarsal shaft.

APPROACH TO THE PROXIMAL CRESCENTIC OSTEOTOMY

- Make an incision directly over the extensor hallucis longus tendon, from just proximal to the metatarsal cuneiform joint distally about 2.5 to 3 cm.
  - Usually, a large vessel crosses this plane; cut or cauterize it when the approach is made.
- Mobilize the extensor tendon and retract it either medially or laterally to expose the metatarsal shaft.
- As the metatarsal shaft is exposed, it is not necessary to be subperiosteal.
  - Working just above the periosteal plane allows the tissues to move easily.
- Identify the metatarsal cuneiform joint.
  - Make a mark on the metatarsal 1 cm distal to the joint; this is where the crescentic osteotomy will be created.
  - Make a second mark on the metatarsal 1 cm distal to the osteotomy site; this is where the screw will be placed that stabilizes the osteotomy (**TECH FIG 3A,B**).
  - To confirm that the osteotomy site is correct, note the flare on the lateral aspect of the metatarsal that marks the junction of the diaphyseal and metaphyseal bone.
    - This is located about 1 cm distal to the metatarsal cuneiform joint.
- Advance a guide pin for the 4.0-mm cannulated screw, a short distance into the metatarsal, beginning at the marked site.
  - The pin should be angled at about 50 degrees to the long axis of the metatarsal in the sagittal plane (see **TECH FIG 3B**). At this angle, the pin and subsequent screw will pass into the plantar aspect of the proximal metatarsal fragment and will not violate the joint.

- Carry out the osteotomy using a crescent-shaped saw blade.
  - This blade comes in two lengths. It is easier to start with a shorter blade and then use the longer blade if necessary to complete the osteotomy (**TECH FIG 3B,C**).
- Positioning of the foot in preparation for the osteotomy is a critical part of this procedure.
  - Sit at the side of the table holding the foot in one hand.
  - Hold the foot in a neutral position in regard to dorsiflexion–plantarflexion and inversion–eversion.
  - Place the saw with the concavity facing proximally toward the heel.
  - The angle of the saw blade should be neither perpendicular to the bottom of the foot nor perpendicular to the metatarsal but about halfway between those positions (see **TECH FIG 3B**).
- Start the osteotomy cut by applying firm pressure to the blade.
  - After making the initial cut into the bone, carefully evaluate the position of the saw blade to be sure that it will cut through the lateral cortex of the metatarsal shaft.
- Sometimes in a wide metatarsal, the blade will not penetrate both cortices.
    - If the medial cortex is not completely cut, it is safe and simple to complete the osteotomy in this area.
    - However, it is difficult and potentially dangerous to complete an osteotomy laterally, as there is a major artery in the space between the first and second metatarsals that could be harmed.

TECHNIQUES

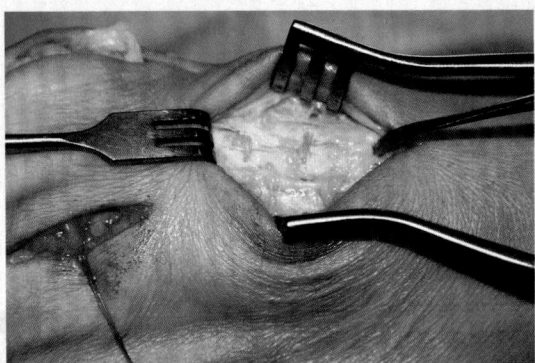

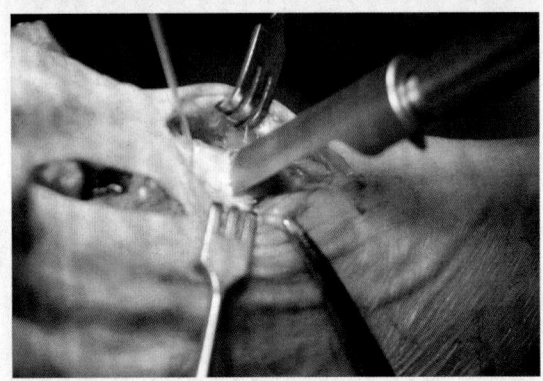

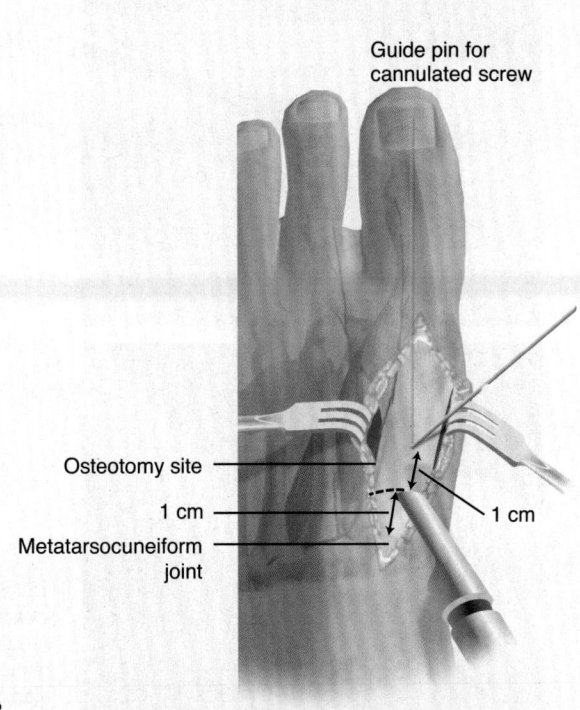

Guide pin for
cannulated screw

Osteotomy site

1 cm

Metatarsocuneiform
joint

1 cm

TECH FIG 3 A. The first metatarsal shaft is exposed. The Freer elevator points to the metatarsocuneiform joint. One centimeter distal to the joint marks the site of the osteotomy, and 1 cm more distally marks the screw insertion site. **B.** Diagram of the first metatarsal shaft demonstrating the metatarsocuneiform joint. Note the osteotomy site and angle of the saw blade. Also note the screw insertion site. **C.** The osteotomy is performed with a crescent-shaped saw blade.

- Make the cut by moving the saw in a medial–lateral direction along the arc of the saw blade.
  - While cutting, apply a little bit of pressure to the blade toward the heel, as this helps to stabilize the blade in the plane of its cut.
  - Once the cut is established, moving the saw blade back and forth without a lot of pressure plantarward will produce a nice smooth cut.
- It is important that the cut passes all the way through the metatarsal so that the distal portion of the bone is totally free and has no bony attachments to the proximal fragment.

- If a medial piece of bone is still present, use a 4- to 6-mm osteotome to cut through the bone.
- Pass a knife blade along the medial side of the cut to be sure that the cut is completely free of any bony or periosteal attachment.
- Return your attention to the first web space.
  - Place a figure-8 suture of 2-0 chromic into the cut end of the adductor hallucis tendon. It is easier to place this stitch before the osteotomy site has been reduced.

CORRECTION OF THE OSTEOTOMY

- Correcting the osteotomy is the most technically demanding part of the bunion procedure.
  - The objective is to stabilize the base of the metatarsal while rotating the distal portion of the metatarsal around the osteotomy site.

Aligning the Metatarsal

- The first step is to push the proximal portion of the cut metatarsal in a medial direction so that it is at the medial excursion of the metatarsal cuneiform joint. This can be accomplished with a Freer elevator **(TECH FIG 4A)**.

- Grasp the metatarsal head firmly with your other hand and rotate the distal aspect of the metatarsal in a lateral direction around the osteotomy site.
  - Examining the osteotomy site demonstrates that the distal fragment rotates no more than 2 to 3 mm around the "crescent" **(TECH FIG 4B)**.
- Hold the osteotomy site in this alignment and drill the previously placed guide pin across the osteotomy site until the plantar cortex is engaged.
  - Once this occurs, the osteotomy site is reasonably stable.
- Measure the guide pin to determine the screw length, which is usually 28 to 30 mm.

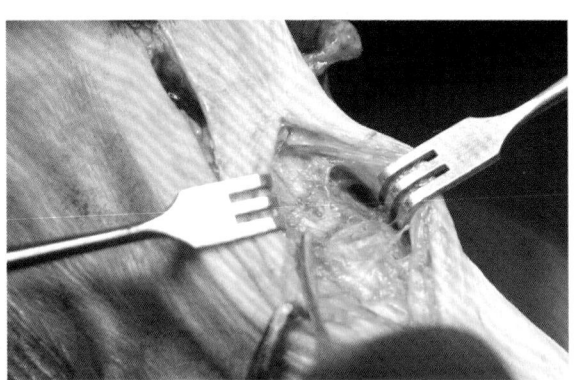

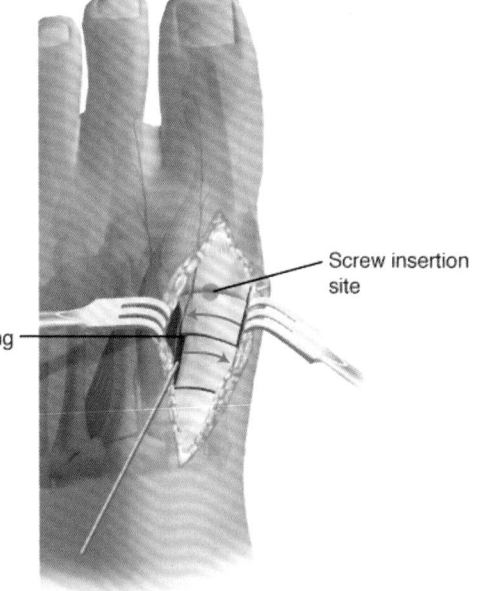

Screw insertion site

2–3 mm overhang

TECH FIG 4 A. The osteotomy is corrected by pushing the proximal portion of the cut metatarsal in a medial direction (note the Freer elevator) while rotating the distal aspect of the metatarsal in a lateral direction around the osteotomy site. **B.** Diagram of the osteotomy site. The surgeon's hand is pushing the metatarsal shaft in a lateral direction. The Freer elevator is pushing the metatarsal base in a medial direction. Note the 2- to 3-mm overhang on the lateral aspect of the osteotomy site.

- When learning to perform this procedure, or if there is a question as to the alignment of the osteotomy, at this point, obtaining a radiograph is warranted.
  - If the guide pin is not providing adequate stability, a second pin or Kirschner wire can be used for supplemental fixation while evaluating the radiograph.
  - If the radiograph shows that the intermetatarsal angle is not sufficiently closed down, remove the guide pin and remanipulate the osteotomy site until the intermetatarsal angle is adequately corrected.

Screw Placement

- While holding the osteotomy site corrected, overdrill the guide pin with the appropriate-sized drill for the cannulated screw set (**TECH FIG 5A**).
  - Usually, it is adequate to advance the drill to a position just past the osteotomy site, so that the guide pin does not back out when the drill is removed.
- Use a countersink, mainly on the distal side of the screw hole, to make the screw head less prominent. However,

excessive countersinking can cause the screw head to be pulled through the screw hole site and produce instability of the osteotomy site.

- Place a partially threaded 4.0-mm cannulated screw across the osteotomy site and carefully tighten it (**TECH FIG 5B**).
  - Be cautious as the screw is tightened because the island of bone is only about 5 or 6 mm and can be cracked if the screw is tightened too firmly.

Verifying Stability

- Check the stability of the osteotomy site by moving the distal fragment in the sagittal plane, looking for any motion at the osteotomy site.
  - Mild instability of the osteotomy can be addressed by carefully tightening the screw or by adding a small-diameter Kirschner wire for supplemental fixation.
  - Occasionally, a small plate may need to be added to the first metatarsal to secure the osteotomy if there is gross instability.

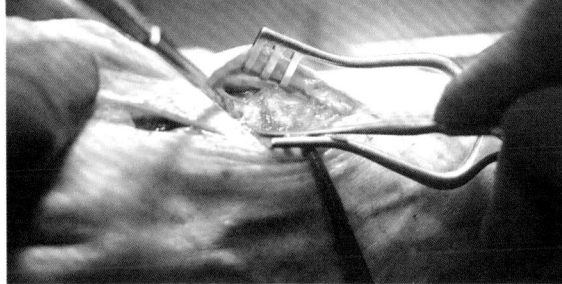

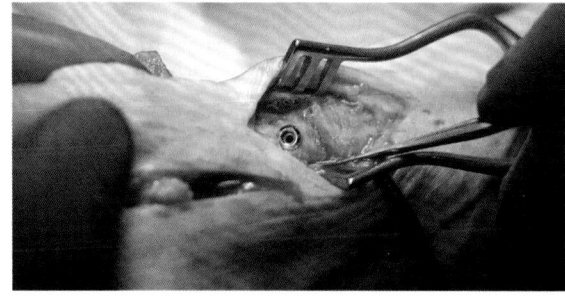

TECH FIG 5 A. The osteotomy site is being held while the cannulated drill is advanced over the guide pin. **B.** The cannulated screw has been placed to stabilize the osteotomy site.

RECONSTRUCTION OF THE MEDIAL JOINT CAPSULE

- The first step in reconstructing the medial joint capsule is to hold the great toe in correct alignment:
  - Neutral dorsiflexion–plantarflexion
  - Zero to 5 degrees of varus
- Rotate the toe to correct pronation, which brings the sesamoids back underneath the metatarsal head.
  - Reduction of the sesamoids has been achieved if they are visible along the plantar aspect of the medial eminence.
- Pull the proximal joint capsule distally to see whether the proximal and distal flaps of the capsule juxtapose one another **(TECH FIG 6A)**.
- If they do, then the capsular flaps are approximated.
- If insufficient capsule has been removed, then more capsular tissue needs to be removed before it is plicated.
  - The capsular flaps should not be overlapped in a pants-over-vest fashion, as this creates too much bulk over the medial eminence.
- To repair the medial capsule, place four to six sutures of 2-0 chromic into the joint capsule with the toe held in correct alignment.

- The first suture is placed as plantar as possible and incorporates the abductor hallucis tendon **(TECH FIG 6B)**.
  - The suture line progresses dorsally **(TECH FIG 6C)**.
- Once the sutures are placed and tied, check the alignment of the toe.
  - The toe should be in neutral position as far as varus and valgus is concerned, or possibly, in a little bit of varus.
  - In general, if the final alignment of the toe is in more than 5 degrees of valgus, extracapsular tissue should be removed.
- Return your attention to the first web space.
  - Sew the adductor hallucis tendon (already tagged with a suture) to the flap of capsule that was stripped off the metatarsal head.
  - If the toe had been positioned in a little too much varus when plicating the medial capsule, tension can be placed on this web space repair to prevent a hallux varus from occurring.
- Thoroughly irrigate the wounds with antibiotic solution and then close them with interrupted silk.
- Apply a sterile compression dressing and then release the tourniquet.

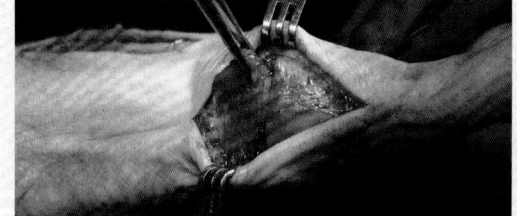 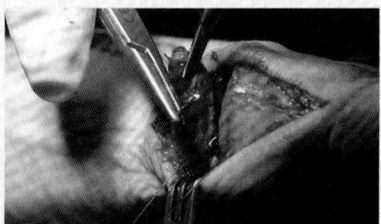 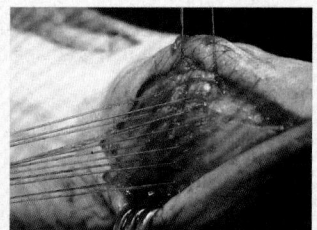

A   B   C

TECH FIG 6 A. With the toe held in neutral position, the medial capsular flaps are checked for proper alignment. **B.** The first suture for repairing the medial joint capsule is placed as plantar as possible; it incorporates the abductor hallucis tendon. **C.** A total of four to six sutures are used to repair the medial joint capsule.

TECHNIQUES

Pearls and Pitfalls

Indications	• Incongruent metatarsophalangeal joint • Intermetatarsal angle of more than 10–12 degrees • Distal metatarsal articular angle of less than 10 degrees
First Web Space Dissection	• Release the entire adductor hallucis tendon off its insertion in the sesamoid and proximal phalanx. • Check adequate release of lateral structures by pulling the toe into maximum varus. • Do not dissect plantar to the transverse metatarsal ligament.
Medial Capsulotomy	• Start with a 3-mm medial capsulotomy for a milder bunion deformity and a larger medial capsulotomy for a more advanced bunion deformity. • Avoid the dorsal and plantar medial cutaneous nerves. • When plicating the medial capsule, do not overlap the capsular flaps in a "pants-over-vest" fashion, as this creates too much bulk over the medial eminence.
Medial Eminence Osteotomy	• The median eminence osteotomy is started 1 to 2 mm medial to the sagittal sulcus and is performed in line with the medial aspect of the metatarsal shaft.

Crescentic Metatarsal Osteotomy	• The crescentic osteotomy is performed 1 cm distal to the metatarsocuneiform joint, at the flare of the base of the proximal phalanx. • The angle of the saw blade for the osteotomy cut should be neither perpendicular to the bottom of the foot nor perpendicular to the metatarsal but about halfway between those positions.
Fixation of Metatarsal Osteotomy	• The guide pin for the cannulated screw should be angled at about 50 degrees to the long axis of the metatarsal. • Leave adequate bone bridge (1 cm) between the cannulated screw and the metatarsal osteotomy. • Avoid penetrating the metatarsal cuneiform joint with the screw fixating the osteotomy site.
Correcting Metatarsal Osteotomy	• Avoid overcorrection or undercorrection of the metatarsal osteotomy. Check the alignment with a Fluoroscan if there is any doubt as to the degree of correction.

POSTOPERATIVE CARE

- The initial postoperative dressing is changed 1 to 2 days after surgery.
  - A dressing incorporating firm gauze and adhesive tape is used to hold the toe in correct alignment.
  - The patient is permitted to ambulate in a postoperative shoe.
- The patient is seen about 8 to 10 days after surgery, at which point the sutures are removed and a radiograph is obtained.
- Based on the alignment of the toe in this radiograph, it is determined how the toe is dressed—namely, into a little more varus or valgus or held in a neutral position.
- The dressings are changed on a weekly basis to ensure that the alignment of the toe remains correct.
- At 3 to 5 weeks after surgery, another radiograph is obtained to confirm the alignment of the toe.
  - If the alignment is not correct, it can still be corrected by pulling the toe into more varus or valgus, depending on what the radiograph dictates.
- After 8 weeks, the dressings are removed and the patient is started on range-of-motion exercises.

OUTCOMES

- Proximal metatarsal osteotomy and distal soft tissue release decreases the bunion deformity to an average of 10 degrees and decreases the intermetatarsal angle to an average of 5 degrees.
- A 90% to 95% rate of patient satisfaction has been reported as well as improvements in pain level and improvements in overall function.

COMPLICATIONS

- Recurrence of hallux valgus deformity
- Hallux varus
- Dorsiflexion of metatarsal osteotomy
- Nonunion of osteotomy site
- Delayed union of osteotomy site

SUGGESTED READINGS

Coughlin MJ, Anderson RB. Hallux valgus. In: Coughlin MJ, Saltzman CL, Anderson RB, eds. Mann's Surgery of the Foot and Ankle, ed 9. Philadelphia: Elsevier, 2014:155–321.

Dreeban S, Mann RA. Advanced hallux valgus deformity: long-term results utilizing the distal soft tissue procedure and proximal metatarsal osteotomy. Foot Ankle Int 1996;17:142–144.

Thordarson DB, Rudicel SA, Ebramzadeh E, et al. Outcome study of hallux valgus surgery—an AOFAS multi-center study. Foot Ankle Int 2001;22:956–959.

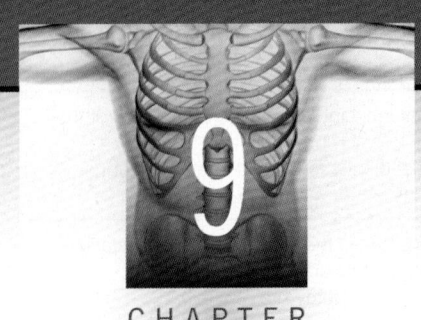

9

CHAPTER

Ludloff Osteotomy

Hans-Joerg Trnka and Stefan G. Hofstaetter

DEFINITION

- Symptomatic hallux valgus associated with a first intermetatarsal angle greater than 15 degrees is typically corrected with a proximal first metatarsal osteotomy and distal soft tissue procedure when nonoperative treatment fails.
- Multiple techniques for the hallux valgus deformity correction have been described.[5]
- In 1918, Ludloff[4] described an oblique osteotomy from the dorsal–proximal to distal–plantar aspects of the first metatarsal, and the procedure was performed without internal fixation.
- The procedure recently gained renewed attention when Chiodo et al[1] and Myerson[6] recommended adding internal fixation and modified several parts of the technique.
- The modified Ludloff osteotomy has been extensively studied with biomechanical and mathematical investigations.

ANATOMY

- The special situation distinguishing the first metatarsophalangeal (MTP) joint from the lesser MTP joints is the sesamoid mechanism.
  - On the plantar surface of the metatarsal head are two longitudinal cartilage-covered grooves separated by a rounded ridge. The sesamoids run in these grooves.
  - The sesamoid bone is contained in each tendon of the flexor hallucis brevis; they are distally attached by the fibrous plantar plate to the base of the proximal phalanx.
- The head of the first metatarsal is rounded and cartilage-covered and articulates with the smaller concave elliptical base of the proximal phalanx.
- Fan-shaped ligamentous bands originate from the medial and lateral condyles of the metatarsal head and run to the base of the proximal phalanx and the margins of the sesamoids and the plantar plate.
- Tendons and muscles that move the great toe are arranged in four groups:
  - Long and short extensor tendons
  - Long and short flexor tendons
  - Abductor hallucis
  - Adductor hallucis
- Blood supply to the metatarsal head
  - First dorsal metatarsal artery
  - Branches from the first plantar metatarsal artery

PATHOGENESIS

- Extrinsic causes
  - Hallux valgus occurs almost exclusively in shoe-wearing populations but only occasionally in the unshod individual.
  - Although shoes are an essential factor in the cause of hallux valgus, not all individuals wearing fashionable shoes develop this deformity.
- Intrinsic causes
  - Hardy and Clapham[2] found, in a series of 91 patients, a positive family history in 63%.
  - Mann and Coughlin[5] reported that a bunion was identified in 94% of 31 mothers whose children inherited a hallux valgus deformity.
  - The association of pes planus with the development of a hallux valgus deformity has been controversial.
  - Hohmann was the most definitive proponent that hallux valgus is always combined with pes planus.
    - Mann and Coughlin[5] and Kilmartin and Wallace[3] noted no incidence of pes planus in the juvenile patient.
    - Pronation of the foot imposes a longitudinal rotation of the first ray that places the axis of the MTP joint in an oblique plane relative to the floor. In this position, the foot appears to be less able to withstand the deformity pressures exerted on it by either shoes or weight bearing.[8]
- The simultaneous occurrence of hallux valgus and metatarsus primus varus has been frequently described. The question of cause and effect continues to be debated.

PATIENT HISTORY AND PHYSICAL FINDINGS

- Physical findings associated with hallux valgus deformity include the following:
  - Pain in narrow shoes
  - Symptomatic intractable keratoses beneath the second metatarsal head (in 40% of patients)
  - Lateral deviation of the great toe
  - Pronation of the great toe
  - Keratosis medial plantar underneath the interphalangeal joint
  - Bursitis over the medial aspect of the medial condyle of the first metatarsal head
  - Hypermobility of the first metatarsocuneiform joint

- Physical examination for hallux valgus deformity should include the following:
  - Hallux valgus angle measurement: Normal is 15 degrees or less.
  - Intermetatarsal angle measurement: Normal is 9 degrees or less.
  - Sesamoid position measurements
  - Joint congruency

IMAGING AND OTHER DIAGNOSTIC STUDIES

- Radiographs of the foot should always be obtained with the patient in the weight-bearing position, with anteroposterior (AP), lateral, and oblique views. The following criteria are examined:
  - Hallux valgus angle
  - Intermetatarsal angle
  - Sesamoid position
  - Joint congruency
  - Distal metatarsal articular angle: the relationship between the articular surface of the first metatarsal head and a line bisecting the first metatarsal shaft (normal is 10 degrees or less)
  - Arthrosis of the first MTP joint

DIFFERENTIAL DIAGNOSIS

- Ganglion
- Hallux rigidus

NONOPERATIVE MANAGEMENT

- Comfortable wider shoes
  - Orthotics
  - Spiral dynamics physiotherapy in adolescents

SURGICAL MANAGEMENT

- Indications
  - Symptomatic hallux valgus deformity with a first inter-metatarsal angle of more than 15 degrees
  - Stable first metatarsal–cuneiform joint
- Contraindications
  - Narrow metatarsal so that adequate rotation of the dorsal fragment is not possible
  - Severe osteoporosis
  - Skeletally immature patient
  - Severe osteoarthritic changes

Preoperative Planning

- Standard weight-bearing AP and lateral radiographs are mandatory.
- The hallux valgus and intermetatarsal angles and tibial sesamoid position are measured.
- A preoperative drawing is helpful.
- Clinical examination includes measurement of active and passive range of motion of the first MTP joint as well as inspection of the foot for plantar callus formation indicative of transfer metatarsalgia and stability of the first tarsometatarsal joint.

Positioning

- The foot is prepared in the standard manner.
- The patient is positioned supine.
- An ankle tourniquet is optional.

Approach

- The lateral soft tissue release and the Ludloff osteotomy are performed through a straight midline incision.

LUDLOFF AND TRANSARTICULAR LATERAL SOFT TISSUE RELEASE

- The procedure is typically performed under the peripheral nerve.
- Make a midaxial skin incision over the medial first MTP joint, extending to the first tarsometatarsal joint (TECH FIG 1A–C).
- Continue deep dissection bluntly.
- The medial MTP joint capsule is opened with a longitudinal incision (TECH FIG 1D,E). The joint is inspected for degenerative changes.

Lateral Release and Preparation of the Metatarsal Head

- The capsule is released from the plantar and the dorsal aspect of the base of the proximal phalanx (TECH FIG 2A,B).
- While the toe is plantar subluxed (TECH FIG 2C), scissors are placed intra-articular proximal to the sesamoids from medial to lateral (TECH FIG 2D).
- Parallel to this, a beaver knife is inserted and the lateral joint capsule (metatarsosesamoid ligament) is divided immediately superior to the lateral sesamoid (TECH FIG 2E).

- The lateral capsule is fenestrated at the first MTP joint, and a varus stress is applied to the hallux to complete the lateral release (TECH FIG 2F).
- The medial eminence is now minimally shaved not only to achieve a plane surface but also to preserve as much metatarsal head width as possible (TECH FIG 2G).
- After careful subcutaneous dissection to avoid damage to the dorsomedial nerve bundle, expose the periosteum of the first metatarsal and insert dorsal–proximal and distal–plantar Hohmann retractors (TECH FIG 2H).

Beginning the Osteotomy

- Plan an oblique first metatarsal osteotomy from the dorsal–proximal first metatarsal (immediately distal to the first tarsometatarsal joint) to the plantar–distal first metatarsal (immediately proximal to the sesamoid complex). First, mark the osteotomy with the electrocautery (TECH FIG 3A).
- The osteotomy is inclined from medial to lateral plantar at an angle of 10 degrees (TECH FIG 3B).

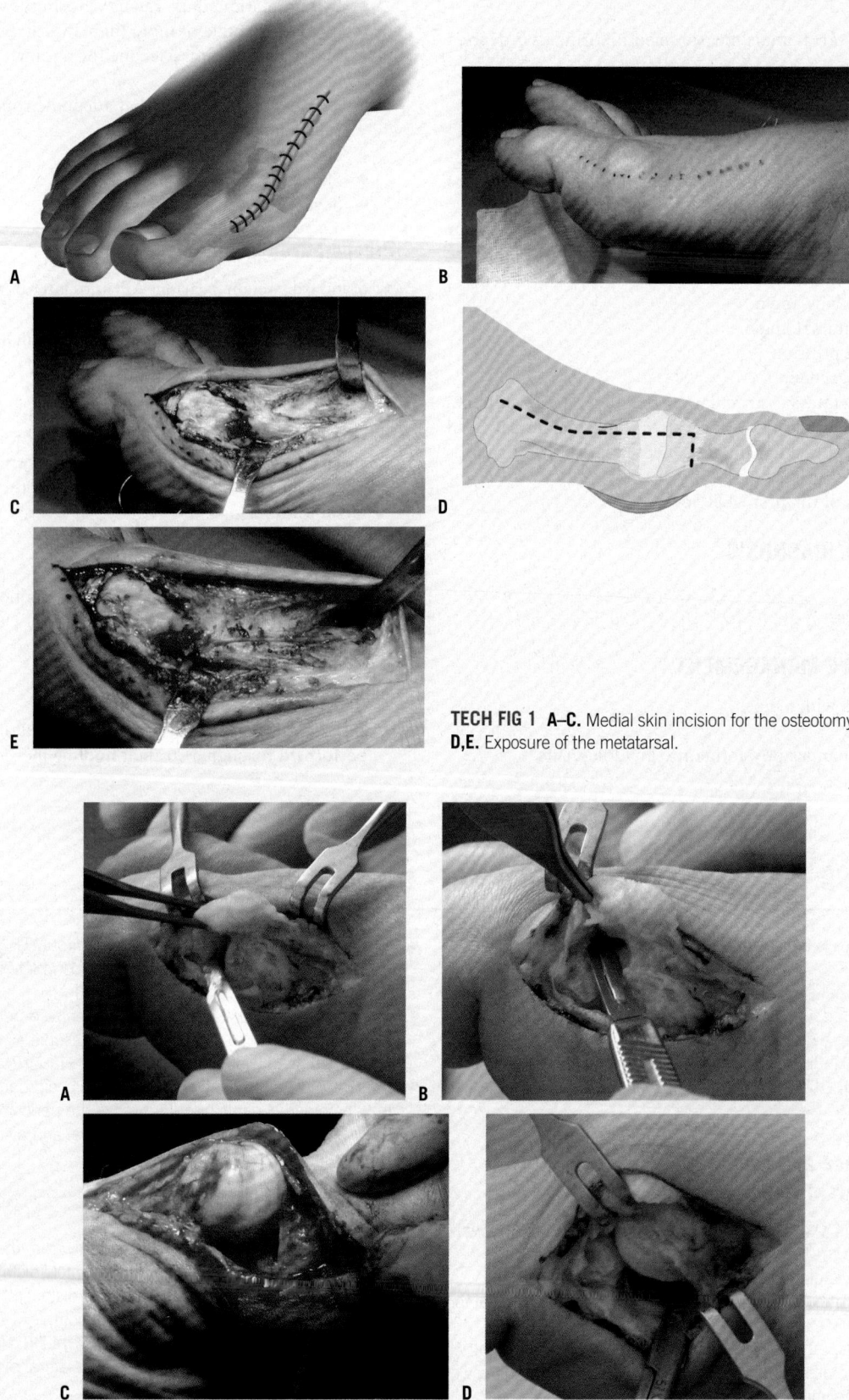

TECH FIG 1 A–C. Medial skin incision for the osteotomy. **D,E.** Exposure of the metatarsal.

TECH FIG 2 A–C. The capsule is released, and the toe is plantar subluxed. **D.** A scissor is now placed intra-articular proximal to the sesamoids from medial to lateral. *(continued)*

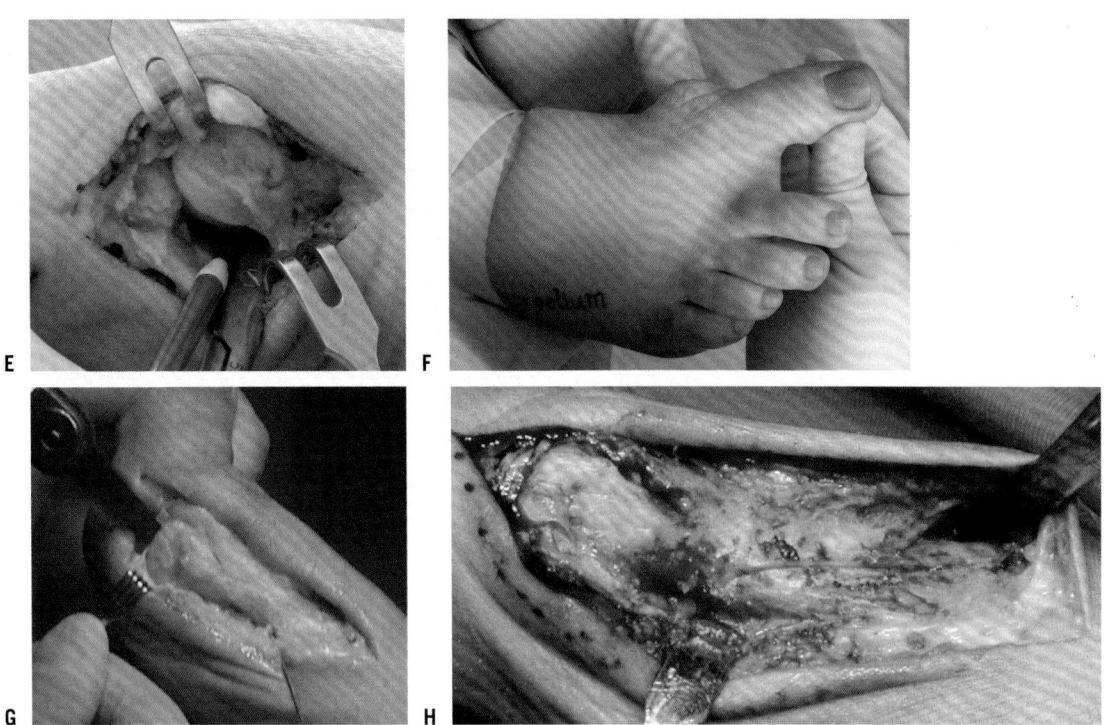

TECH FIG 2 *(continued)* **E.** A beaver knife is inserted, and the lateral capsule is incised. **F.** The great toe is brought into 20 degrees of varus to demonstrate the release of the lateral structures. **G.** The medial eminence is minimally resected. **H.** The metatarsal is exposed using two Hohmann retractors.

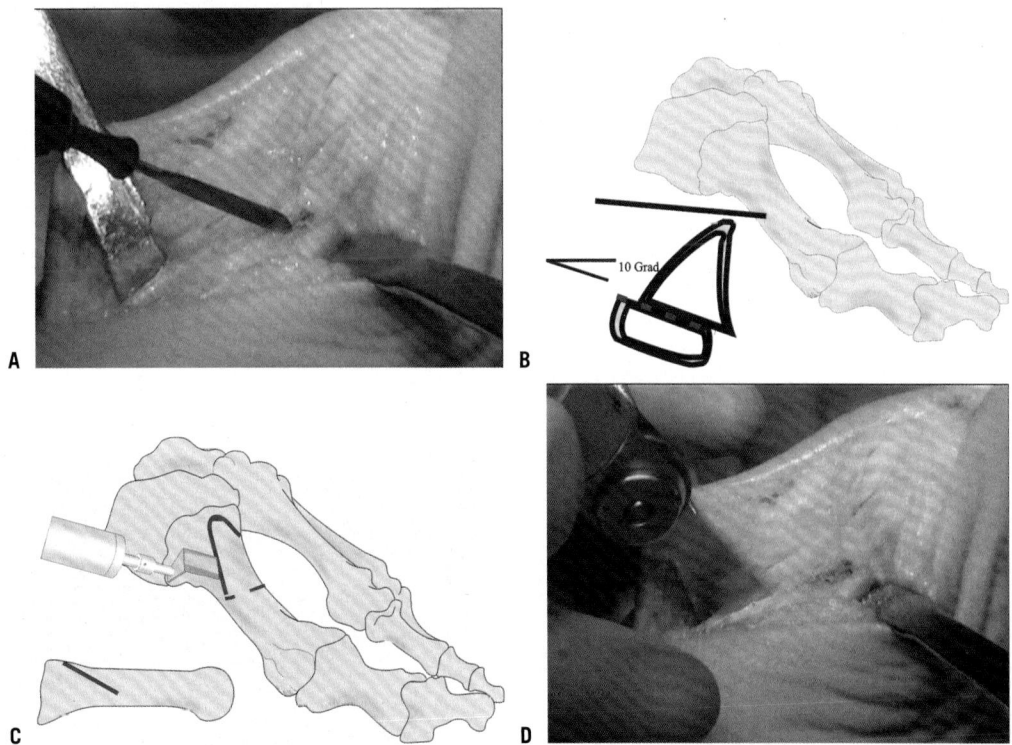

TECH FIG 3 A. The osteotomy is marked. **B.** The osteotomy should be 10 degrees inclined from medial to lateral. **C,D.** The proximal two-thirds of the osteotomy is performed first. *(continued)*

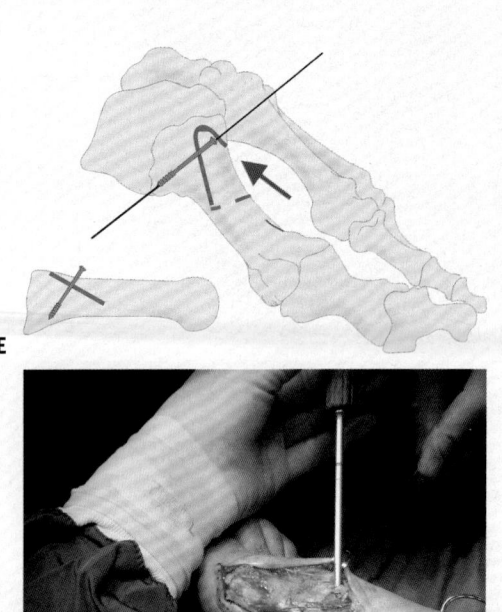

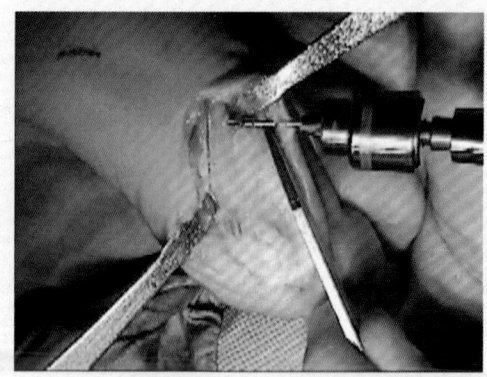

TECH FIG 3 *(continued)* **E–G.** The proximal 3.0-mm cannulated titanium screw is inserted but not tightened.

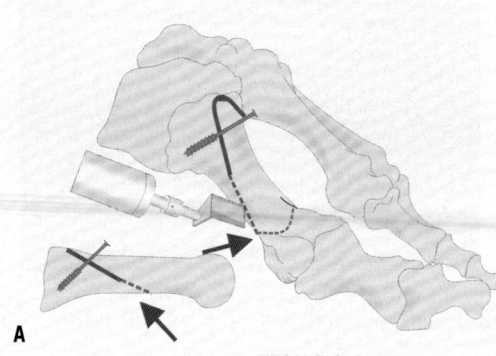

- Perform only the dorsal two-thirds of the osteotomy initially to guarantee a stable situation (**TECH FIG 3C,D**).
- Insert a guidewire for a 3.0- or 4.0-mm cannulated screw (DePuy Synthes, Paoli, PA) or a Charlotte multiuse compression screw (Wright Medical Technology, Arlington, PA) in the proximal aspect of the dorsal fragment perpendicular to the osteotomy (**TECH FIG 3E,F**).
- Insert the first screw without full compression (**TECH FIG 3G**).

Osteotomy Completion and Internal Fixation

- Complete the plantar third of the osteotomy (**TECH FIG 4A,B**).
- Using a towel clip, gently pull the plantar fragment medially and rotate the dorsal fragment laterally with gentle thumb pressure on the first metatarsal head's medial aspect (**TECH FIG 4C,D**).

- After confirming the desired correction fluoroscopically, tighten the first screw to secure the osteotomy.
- Insert a second Charlotte multiuse compression screw from plantar to dorsal across the distal aspect of the osteotomy (**TECH FIG 4E**).

Completion and Closure

- Resect the medial eminence (**TECH FIG 5A**). This is not done before the osteotomy because, otherwise, too much of the metatarsal head might be resected.
- Shave the slight medial bone prominence at the osteotomy smooth with the edge of the saw blade (**TECH FIG 5B**).
- While an assistant holds the great toe in a slightly overcorrected position, repair the medial joint capsule with U-type sutures and tighten the first web space sutures (**TECH FIG 5C**).
- Wrap the foot in a traditional, mildly compressive wet-and-dry bunion dressing.

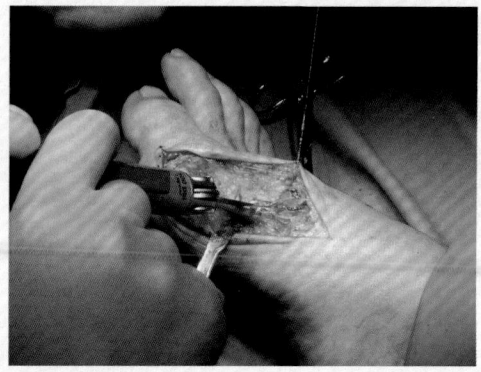

TECH FIG 4 A,B. Osteotomy of the plantar third. *(continued)*

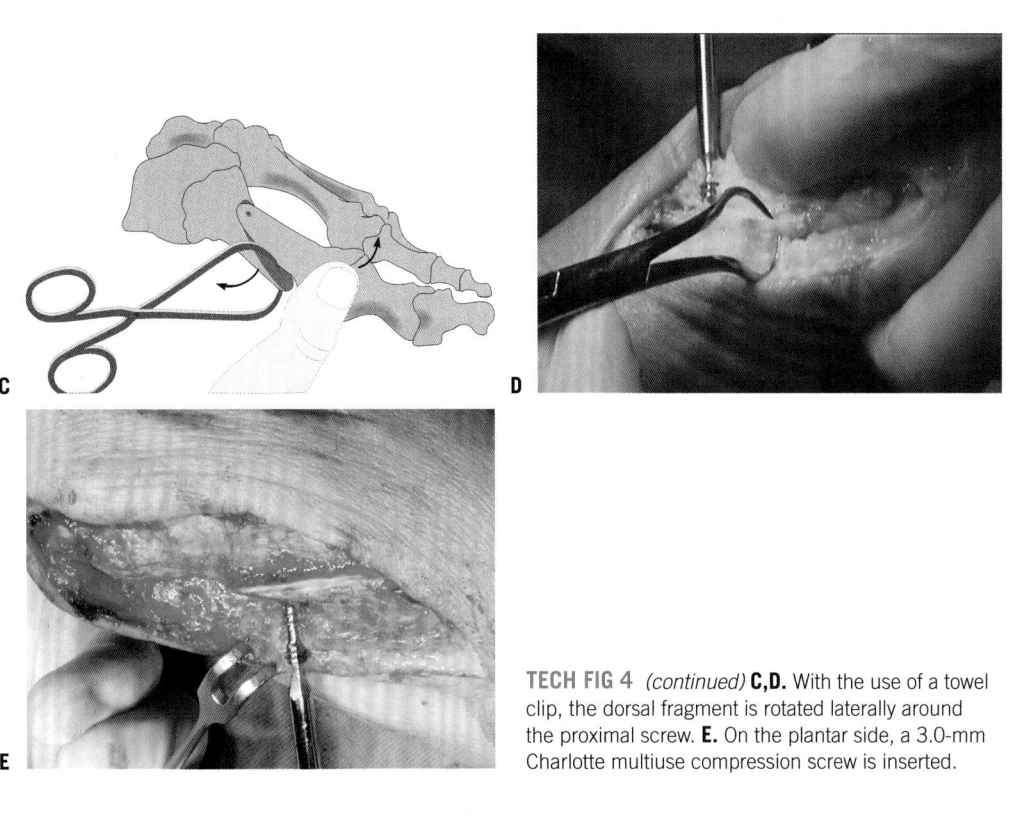

TECH FIG 4 *(continued)* **C,D.** With the use of a towel clip, the dorsal fragment is rotated laterally around the proximal screw. **E.** On the plantar side, a 3.0-mm Charlotte multiuse compression screw is inserted.

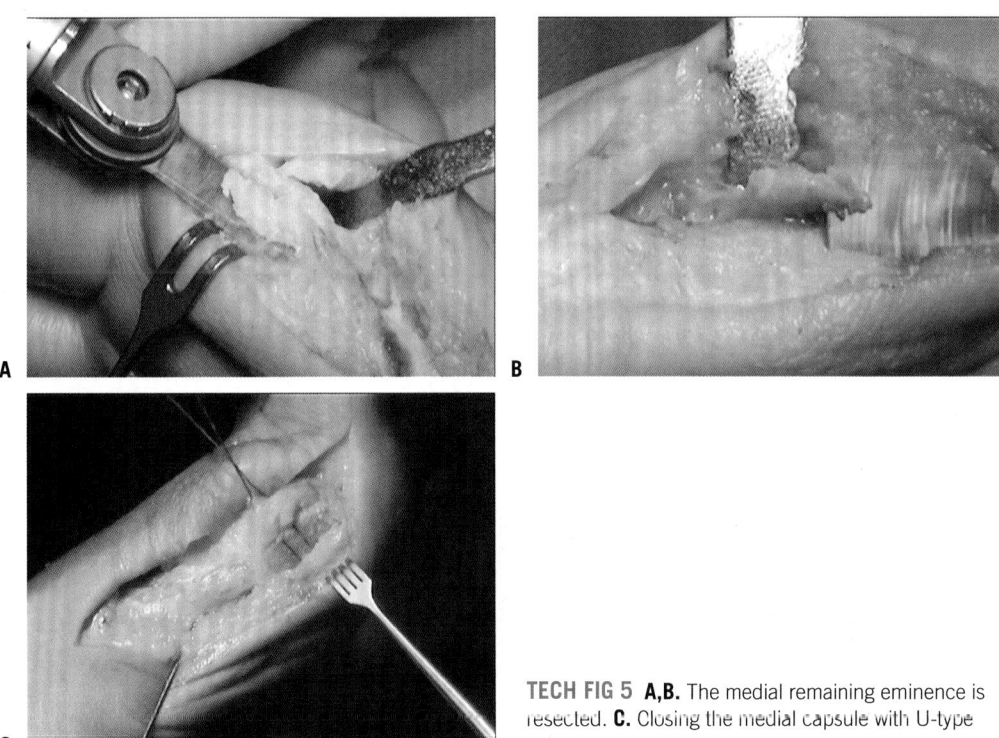

TECH FIG 5 A,B. The medial remaining eminence is resected. **C.** Closing the medial capsule with U-type sutures.

Pearls and Pitfalls

- Avoid short osteotomy because it would create too small of a contact area.

- There should be a long enough distance between the two screws; otherwise, the rotational control is not guaranteed.

- When the screws do not have enough bite, use a cast for postoperative treatment.

POSTOPERATIVE CARE

- Starting immediately postoperatively, ice application to the foot is helpful to reduce swelling.
- Provided that the bone quality was intraoperatively sufficient, patients are allowed to walk with a postsurgical cork-soled shoe (OFA Rathgeber Health Shoes, Ofa Bamberg GmbH, Bamberg, Germany) **(FIG 1A)** on the same day.
- If the bone quality was not sufficient, the patient is put in a walker boot or a short-leg cast.
- Weekly changes of the tape dressing are necessary.
- An alternative to weekly dressing changes is the postoperative hallux valgus compression stocking, which also reduces postoperative edema **(FIG 1B)**.
- Radiographs are taken intraoperatively and at 6 weeks of follow-up **(FIGS 2 and 3)**.
- After radiographic union is achieved, normal dress shoes with a more rigid sole are allowed.
- After 6 weeks, physiotherapy to achieve normal forefoot function is recommended.

OUTCOMES

- Chiodo et al[1] presented their results on 82 consecutive Ludloff cases. Follow-up was possible in 70 cases (85%) at an average of 30 months (range 18 to 42 months). In their series, no symptomatic transfer lesions were found on the second metatarsal. The mean American Orthopaedic Foot and Ankle Society (AOFAS) forefoot score improved from 54 to 91 points. The mean hallux valgus and first intermetatarsal angles before surgery were 31 degrees and 16 degrees, respectively; postoperatively, they averaged 11 and 7 degrees. Complications included prominent hardware requiring removal (7%, 5/70), hallux varus deformity

(6%, 4/70), delayed union (4%, 3/70), superficial infection (4%, 3/70), and neuralgia (4%, 3/70). The average patient age was not mentioned in the study.
- Saxena and McCammon[7] reported the results of 14 procedures in 12 patients with the original technique. The mean hallux valgus angle was corrected from 30.1 to 13.4 degrees and the intermetatarsal angle from 15.9 to 10.8 degrees.
- Weinfeld[10] reported in 2001 a series of 31 patients. The mean hallux valgus angle was corrected from 36.7 to 10.8 degrees and the mean first intermetatarsal angle from 14.8 to 3.9 degrees.
- Trnka et al[9] reviewed the results of 99 patients (111 feet), with an average age of 56 years (range 20 to 78 years), in a multicenter study. The average AOFAS score improved significantly from 46 ± 11 points before surgery to 88 ± 13 points at follow-up. Patients younger than 60 years of age had a significantly higher AOFAS score (90 ± 12 points) than patients older than 60 years of age (82 ± 17 points). The average preoperative hallux valgus angle of 35 ± 7 degrees decreased significantly to 8 ± 9 degrees, and the average intermetatarsal angle decreased significantly from 17 ± 2 degrees to 8 ± 3 degrees. All osteotomies united without dorsiflexion malunion. In the early postoperative period, 17% (18/111) had bony callus formation at the osteotomy site.

COMPLICATIONS

- Potential complications are similar to other proximal osteotomies.
- Hallux varus in 8% and 6%
- Delayed union
- Loss of fixation
- Iatrogenic fracture

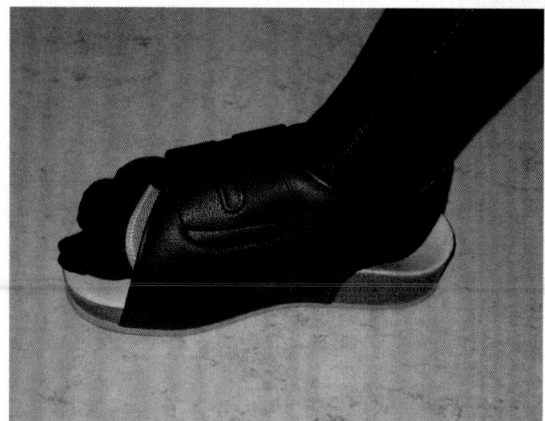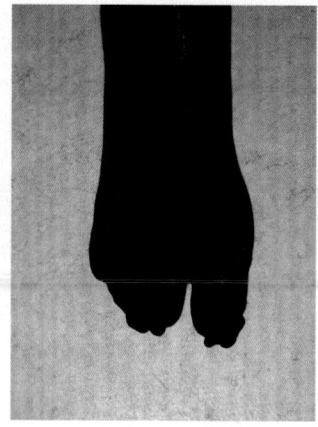

FIG 1 A. Rathgeber postoperative shoe (OFA Rathgeber). **B.** Postoperative hallux valgus compression stocking used after suture removal.

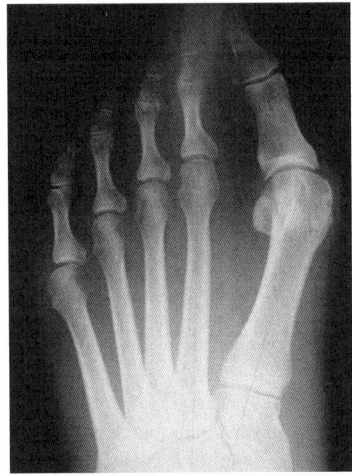

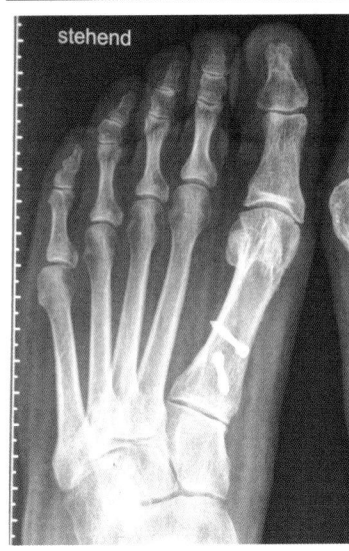

FIG 2 Forty-three-year-old woman before surgery (**A**) and 15 years after the Ludloff osteotomy (**B**).

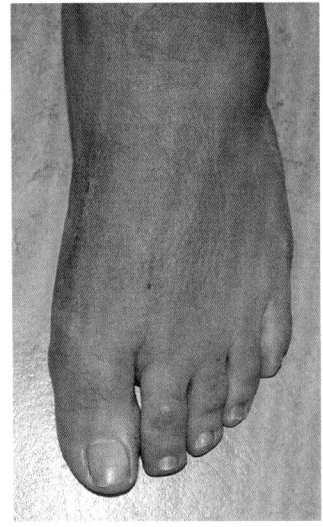

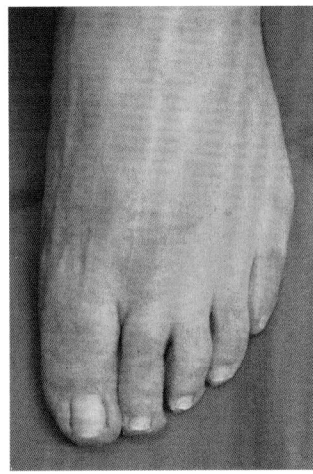

FIG 3 Clinical picture of the same patient 6 weeks (**A**) and 15 years (**B**) after surgery.

REFERENCES

1. Chiodo CP, Schon LC, Myerson MS. Clinical results with the Ludloff osteotomy for correction of adult hallux valgus. Foot Ankle Int 2004;25:532–536.
2. Hardy R, Clapham J. Observations on hallux valgus. J Bone Joint Surg Br 1951;33B:376–391.
3. Kilmartin TE, Wallace WA. The significance of pes planus in juvenile hallux valgus. Foot Ankle 1992;13(2):53–56.
4. Ludloff K. Die Beseitigung des Hallux valgus durch die schräge planta-dorsale Osteotomie des Metatarsus I. Arch Klin Chir 1918;110: 364–387.
5. Mann RA, Coughlin MJ. Adult hallux valgus. In: Coughlin MJ, Mann RA, eds. Surgery of the Foot and Ankle. St Louis: Mosby, 1999:150–269.
6. Myerson MS. Hallux valgus. In: Myerson MS, ed. Foot and Ankle Disorders. Philadelphia: WB Saunders, 2000:213–288.
7. Saxena A, McCammon D. The Ludloff osteotomy: a critical analysis. J Foot Ankle Surg 1997;36:100–105.
8. Trnka H-J, Hofstaetter SG. The Ludloff osteotomy. Techniques Foot Ankle Surg 2005;4:263–268.
9. Trnka H-J, Hofstaetter SG, Hofstaetter JG, et al. Intermediate-term results of the Ludloff osteotomy in 111 feet. J Bone Joint Surg Am 2008;90A:531–539. Erratum in: J Bone Joint Surg Am 2008;90A:1337.
10. Weinfeld SB. The Ludloff osteotomy for correction of hallux valgus: results of 31 cases by one surgeon. Presented at: the 31st Annual Meeting of the American Orthopaedic Foot and Ankle Society, San Francisco, CA, March 3, 2001.

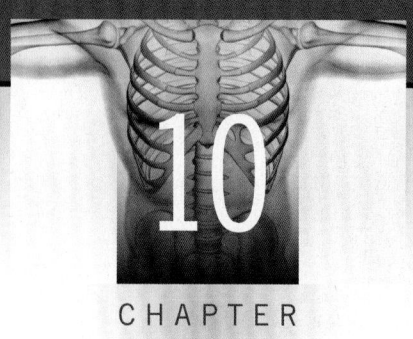

Mau Osteotomy

Kyle S. Peterson, Christopher F. Hyer, and Gregory C. Berlet

DEFINITION

- Hallux valgus is a static subluxation of the first metatarsophalangeal (MTP) joint with medial deviation of the first metatarsal and lateral or valgus rotation of the hallux. A medial or dorsomedial prominence is present and usually called a *bunion*.
- The development of hallux valgus is debated but occurs almost exclusively in shod populations.
  - Other causes that may contribute to a hallux valgus deformity include heredity, pes planus, metatarsus primus varus, systemic arthritis, neuromuscular disorders, excessive roundness of the metatarsal head, and abnormal obliquity of the first metatarsal joint.
  - Hypermobility may also be another causative factor in the formation of a bunion, and a first metatarsal–cuneiform joint fusion may be an appropriate alternative procedure.
- Hallux valgus can lead to painful motion of the joint or difficulty with footwear.
- Surgical correction of bunion deformity is a common procedure.
  - For larger deformities, a proximal osteotomy of the first metatarsal is required.
  - The Mau proximal osteotomy technique is an accepted and proven technique. This osteotomy has the advantage over other proximal osteotomies of being inherently stable, having a reproducible surgical technique, and minimizing the common complications of other proximal osteotomies.

ANATOMY

- The first MTP joint is two joints with a ball-and-socket type of joint between the first metatarsal and proximal phalanx. The second portion is a groove on the plantar first metatarsal that articulates with the dorsal surface of two sesamoids. These joints share a common capsule and interrelated muscles.
- Collateral ligaments are fan-shaped ligaments that originate from the medial and lateral epicondyles of the first metatarsal head. These ligaments run vertical, horizontal, and oblique from the first metatarsal head, proximal phalanx, and sesamoids.
- The sesamoids (medial and lateral) are separated by a rounded ridge (crista) and are connected by the intersesamoidal ligament. The lateral sesamoid is also connected to the plantar plate of the second metatarsal head by the

transverse intermetatarsal (IM) ligament. In addition to collateral ligament attachments, each sesamoid is contained by a separated tendon of the flexor hallucis brevis muscle.
- Intrinsic muscles that insert on the proximal phalanx are the abductor hallucis (plantar medial) and the oblique–transverse head of the adductor hallucis (plantar lateral phalanx). Both of these tendons also blend in with the flexor hallucis brevis to invest each corresponding sesamoid. These intrinsic muscles act to maintain alignment of the hallux and balance the forces of each other.
- Extrinsic muscles include the flexor hallucis longus (FHL) and extensor hallucis longus (EHL). The FHL lies within a groove plantar to the intersesamoidal ligament. It proceeds distally to insert into the base of the distal phalanx. The EHL runs over the dorsal surface of the proximal phalanx and inserts into the base of the distal phalanx. Over the first MTP, the EHL is anchored to the sesamoids by the extensor sling.

PATHOGENESIS

- The development of hallux valgus varies depending on the causative factor.
- The function of the abductor hallucis muscle is to plantarflex, adduct, and invert the proximal phalanx. The reverse is true for the adductor hallucis muscle. When these muscles act together, a straight plantarflexion force is produced and the transverse–frontal plane forces are neutralized.
- When the adductor hallucis muscle gains the mechanical advantage, such as in removing the tibial sesamoid or pronation, a hallux valgus deformity may ensue. The sesamoids are pulled laterally, thus eroding the crista. The metatarsal head is pushed medially, stretching the medial ligaments, and the abductor hallucis slides beneath the metatarsal head, pronating the hallux.
- As the deformity progresses, the EHL and FHL have been shown to become a dynamic deforming force.

NATURAL HISTORY

- The progression of a hallux valgus deformity is usually gradual, but when multiple causative factors are present, progression can be more rapid.
- As the deformity progresses, the hallux drifts laterally and either over or under a stable second digit. Over time, the second MTP joint can dislocate.
- As the hallux drifts laterally, it assumes less weight bearing and a diffuse callus may occur underneath the second metatarsal head.

PATIENT HISTORY AND PHYSICAL FINDINGS

- The chief compliant of a bunion deformity is usually pain. Pain can be located over several areas in a bunion deformity: median eminence, dorsal first MTP joint, medial or lateral sesamoids, or impingement on the second digit.
- A thorough general medical history may include gout, osteoarthritis, rheumatoid arthritis, diabetes, or peripheral vascular disease.
- Other important factors include style of shoes and if any shoe gear modification has been attempted, physical activity of the patient, and occupational demands.
- Patient expectations are also important. Goals of surgery should include increasing activity and decreasing pain. Forewarning the patient of limitations after surgery is necessary, such as the possibility of not returning to tight fashionable shoes.
- The physical examination should start with the patient weight bearing to assess the bunion and lesser toe deformities and compare them to the other foot.
- Evaluation of the vascular status is important. The perfusion is determined by palpating the posterior tibial and dorsal pedis arteries. Perfusion of a digit can be assessed by the capillary refill. Appropriate vascular studies such as transcutaneous oxygen, ankle–brachial index, digital pressures, and segmental pressures are useful when perfusion to the foot is in doubt.
- The first MTP joint range of motion is assessed for crepitus, pain, or impingement if a dorsal spur is present. Motion is also assessed with the hallux in a corrected position to determine the degree of associated contracture of the soft tissues. Normal range of motion is 70 to 90 degrees of dorsiflexion. Joint range of motion is compared to that of the opposite foot.
- Transverse plane mobility is assessed by distracting the hallux while the metatarsal head is pushed laterally to see clinical reduction of the IM angle.
- The median eminence is assessed for its prominence and underlying bursa. Neuritic pain can be elicited from the nearby dorsal or plantar cutaneous nerves.

- The tibial and fibular sesamoids are directly palpated while putting the joint through a range of motion to indicate intra-articular derangement.
- The first tarsometatarsal joint excursion is assessed by grasping proximal to this joint and moving the first metatarsal and comparing it to the opposite foot. Normal range of motion is 10 mm of excursion. A hypermobile first ray is more than 15 mm of excursion.
- Range of motion of the hallux interphalangeal joint is evaluated in the transverse and sagittal plane as well as joint quality.
- Pain may also occur from lesser toe deformities or transfer lesions that may accompany the bunion deformity. A symptomatic intractable plantar keratoma beneath the second metatarsal head is present in most patients. Other associated problems include neuromas, corns, and tailor's bunion.

IMAGING AND OTHER DIAGNOSTIC STUDIES

- The radiologic examination should include weight-bearing lateral, anteroposterior (AP), and oblique views (**FIG 1**).
- Several measurements are obtained using these radiographs to determine the severity of the bunion deformity, including the IM 1–2 angle (IM1–2), hallux valgus angle (HVA), tibial sesamoid position, distal metatarsal articular angle (DMAA), and congruency of the first MTP joint.
  - The IM1–2 angle is determined by measuring the angle subtended by the lines bisecting the longitudinal axis of the first and second metatarsals.
    - Normal is less than 9 degrees (**FIG 2A**).
  - The HVA is determined by measuring the angle subtended by the lines bisecting the first metatarsal and proximal phalanx of the hallux.
    - Normal is 15 degrees or less (**FIG 2B**).
  - Tibial sesamoid position describes the relationship of the tibial sesamoid to the bisection of the first metatarsal.
    - The position of the sesamoid is determined by a numerical sequence of one to seven with increasing deformity.
    - Normal is a position of one to three (**FIG 2C**).

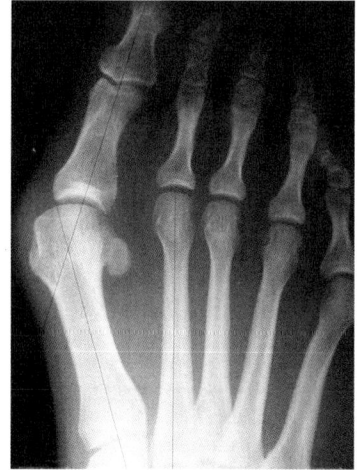
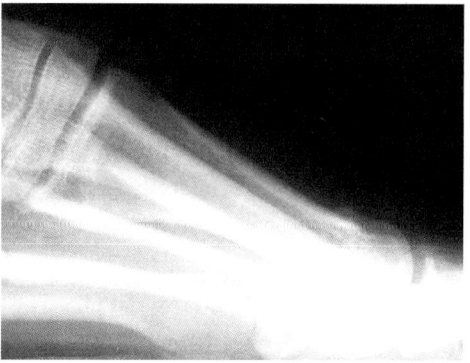

FIG 1 Preoperative weight-bearing AP (**A**) and lateral (**B**) foot radiographs.

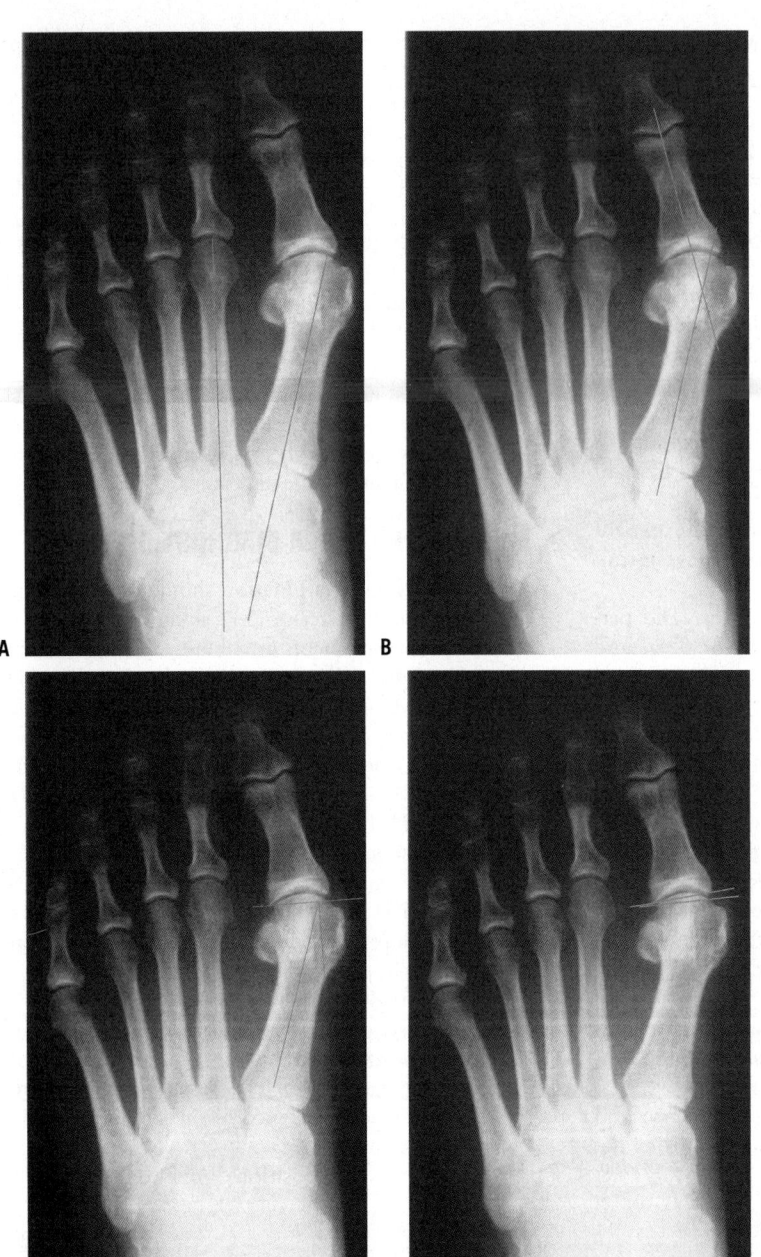

FIG 2 A. The IM angle measures the splay between the first and second. **B.** The HVA measures the angle formed between the proximal phalanx and first metatarsal. **C.** The tibial sesamoid position describes the position of the tibial sesamoid relative to the bisection of the first metatarsal. **D.** The DMAA measures the relationship of the articular surface of the first metatarsal head to the bisection of the first metatarsal. **E.** A deviated joint in which the articular surfaces are not parallel with each other.

- The DMAA is the angle subtended by a line representing the articular cartilage of the first metatarsal head and a perpendicular line to the bisection of the shaft of the first metatarsal.
  - Normal measures less than 8 degrees **(FIG 2D)**.
  - An increase in the DMAA may demonstrate a structural deformity in the head of the metatarsal.
- The first MTP joint may be described as congruent, deviated, or subluxed.
  - A congruent joint is one in which the cartilage surfaces of the first metatarsal head and proximal phalanx are parallel.
  - A deviated joint is one in which the cartilage lines intersect at a point outside of the joint.
  - In a subluxed joint, the cartilage lines intersect within the joint **(FIG 2E)**.
- Degenerative arthritis at the first MTP joint can be evaluated on each weight-bearing radiograph.

DIFFERENTIAL DIAGNOSIS

- Metatarsus primus varus
- Hallux varus
- Gout
- Hallux rigidus

NONOPERATIVE MANAGEMENT

- Conservative treatment options for hallux valgus deformities are limited.
- Shoe wear modifications such as an extra-wide and deep toe box can help accommodate the deformity. Also, a soft upper leather can be stretched over the bunion to provide accommodation.
- Custom-made shoes may help individuals reluctant or unable to undergo a surgical procedure.
- Bunion pads, night splints, and toe spacers tend to be of little use.
- A custom-made orthosis may be beneficial if an associated flatfoot deformity is present. The use of an orthosis has not been demonstrated to prevent a hallux valgus deformity or slow its progression. Others have proposed using orthoses postoperatively to prevent recurrence.

SURGICAL MANAGEMENT

- Bunions can be classified by their severity. This classification is used to facilitate the decision-making process of how to treat the deformity.
  - Mild bunion: HVA less than 20 degrees, congruent joint, IM angle less than 11 degrees. Pain is usually due to a medial eminence.
  - Moderate bunion: HVA 20 to 40 degrees, incongruent joint, IM angle 11 to 18 degrees. The hallux is usually pronated and presses against the second digit.
  - Severe bunion: HVA more than 40 degrees, subluxed joint, IM angle more than 18 degrees. Hallux is often overriding or underlapping the second digit; painful transfer lesion underneath the second metatarsal head; possible arthritic changes to the first MTP joint.
- The indications for hallux valgus surgery using the Mau osteotomy include the following:
  - Painful moderate to severe bunion deformity
  - Deformity unresponsive to conservative treatment
- In addition, the authors frequently use the Mau osteotomy also to correct painful tailor's bunion deformities of the fifth metatarsal. The advantages and technical ease of the osteotomy directly translate to the successful use of the Mau osteotomy for the fifth metatarsal.
  - The indications for tailor's bunion surgery using the Mau osteotomy include the following:
    - Painful, moderate to severe tailor's bunion deformity with an enlarged lateral exostosis and an increased IM 4–5 angle
    - Deformity unresponsive to conservative treatment

Preoperative Planning

- Routine preoperative clearance is obtained via history and physical. This may include an electrocardiogram, chest radiograph, and laboratory workup.
- A prophylactic antibiotic of choice is given 30 minutes before the procedure. Also, one tablet of 200 mg celecoxib (Celebrex) is given.

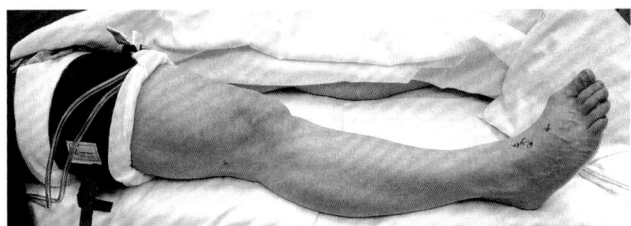

FIG 3 A well-padded thigh tourniquet set to 300 mm Hg.

Positioning

- The patient is placed supine on the operating table with a bump placed under the contralateral hip.
- A well-padded pneumatic thigh tourniquet is used and set to 300 mm Hg (**FIG 3**).

Approach

- Typically, two incisions are used to provide adequate exposure.
  - The first incision is placed over the first web space, and the second is placed on the medial aspect of the first metatarsal (**FIG 4A**).
  - The second incision starts at the first tarsometatarsal joint and courses distal and medially over the first MTP joint for the medial eminence resection and plication of the capsule (**FIG 4B**).

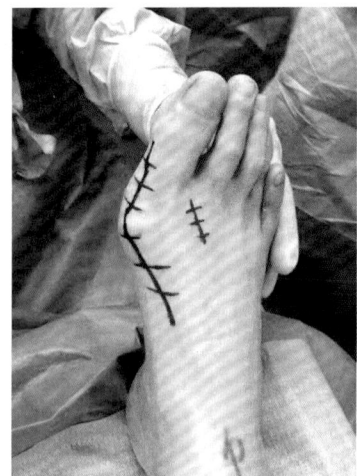

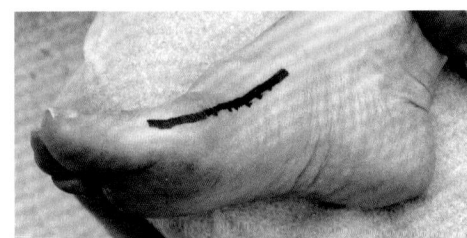

FIG 4 A. Two-incision approach for Mau osteotomy and distal soft tissue procedure. **B.** Medial incision starts at the first tarsometatarsal joint and courses distal and medially for the distal soft tissue procedure.

TECHNIQUES

LATERAL RELEASE OF THE FIRST METATARSOPHALANGEAL JOINT

- Using an incision in the first web space **(TECH FIG 1A)**, perform the lateral release first. Carry dissection through the subcutaneous layer.
- Typically, the first structure incised is the superficial portion of the transverse ligament.
- Use blunt dissection to view the lateral first MTP joint and fibular sesamoid.

- Release the adductor tendon from the plantar–lateral base of the proximal phalanx and fibular sesamoid **(TECH FIG 1B)**.
- Incise the deep portion of the transverse ligament. The lateral capsule of the first MTP joint is "pie crusted," and a varus stress is placed on the joint.

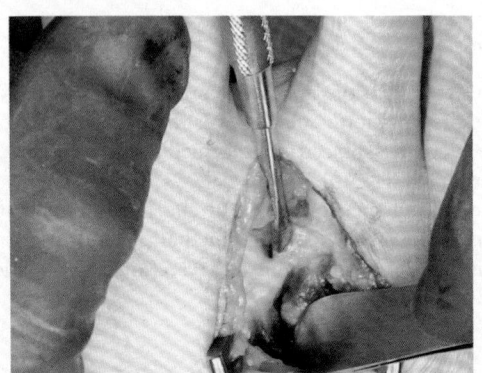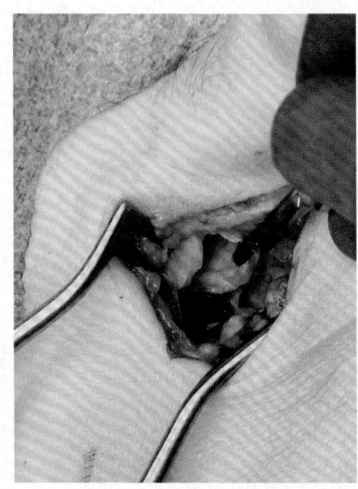

TECH FIG 1 A. The first structure identified in a lateral release is the superficial portion of the deep transverse metatarsal ligament. **B.** Blunt dissection is carried deep to identify and release the adductor hallucis tendon.

MEDIAL CAPSULORRHAPHY

- Using a standard medial approach, perform an inverted-L capsulotomy. The alternative dorsal–medial skin incision, which is placed over the first dorsal metatarsal artery and nerve, can cause nerve irritation and entrapment.
- This allows exposure of the enlarged medial eminence and release of the stretched medial sesamoid suspensory ligament **(TECH FIG 2A)**. Remove the periosteum from the metatarsal head medially and dorsally but keep it intact at the neck plantarly to preserve the nutrient artery.

- Resect the medial eminence using a sagittal saw **(TECH FIG 2B)**.
  - Take the eminence from dorsolateral to plantar–medial. Remove the eminence in this orientation to prevent staking of the metatarsal head and loss of the sagittal groove, which can lead to medial subluxation of the tibial sesamoid and promote hallux varus.

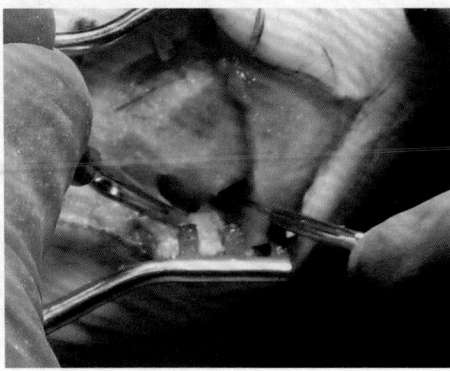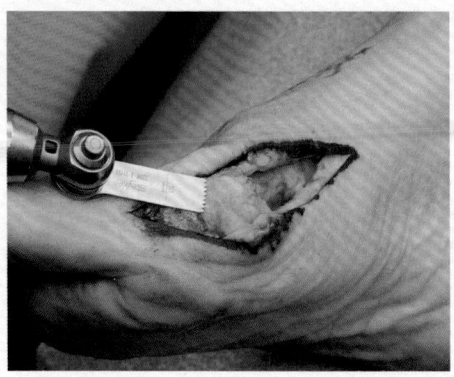

TECH FIG 2 A. Release of the stretched medial sesamoid suspensory ligament. **B.** Minimal exostectomy of the medial eminence.

MAU OSTEOTOMY

Exposure

- Carry the dissection deep to the first metatarsal shaft.
  - The skin incision can be placed slightly plantar to the first metatarsal to avoid surrounding neurovascular structures such as the first dorsal metatarsal artery and nerve. With this incision, a potentially nonpainful scar results as the incision is not placed directly over bone. The EHL tendon is not encountered with this incision and is retracted safely.
  - Identify the first tarsometatarsal joint but do not disturb the capsule. An 18-gauge needle can be placed in the joint for reference.
  - Starting 1 cm from the first tarsometatarsal joint, reflect the periosteum plantar–proximal to dorsal–distal only in line with the osteotomy, thereby preserving the rest of the periosteum (**TECH FIG 3**).
  - Much of the periosteum is retained to promote adequate bone healing.

Osteotomy

- The osteotomy does not incorporate the entire metatarsal shaft as does the traditional Mau osteotomy. The osteotomy ends in the midshaft of the first metatarsal.
- Complete the osteotomy with a sagittal saw parallel to the weight-bearing surface to prevent unwanted dorsal angulation of the first metatarsal.
- The Mau is started proximal–plantar and ends distal–dorsal (**TECH FIG 4**).
- A self-retaining retractor is useful to protect the surrounding neurovascular and tendinous structures.
- Using the straight medial incision avoids tendinous structures and allows excellent visualization of the medial metatarsal shaft to complete the osteotomy.
- To maintain complete control while completing the osteotomy, a smooth guide pin for the selected cannulated screw can be placed perpendicular across the completed proximal portion of the osteotomy. Then the osteotomy can be completed without fear of losing the orientation.

Reduction and Fixation

- After completing the osteotomy, rotate the distal fragment.
  - Optimal rotation of the osteotomy may be facilitated by placing a large reduction bone clamp on the first metatarsal head and neck of the second metatarsal to help reduce the IM1–2 angle (**TECH FIG 5A**).
- Place two temporary Kirschner wires (0.025 inch) from dorsal to plantar perpendicular to the osteotomy site (**TECH FIG 5B**).
- Reduction of the IM1–2 angle is mostly obtained by rotation of the distal fragment. It is acceptable to allow slight lateral translation of the distal fragment relative to the proximal fragment to further correct the IM angle.
- We recommend using intraoperative fluoroscopy to confirm proper position of the first metatarsal head over the tibial sesamoids, congruent joint alignment, and satisfactory orientation of the osteotomy (**TECH FIG 5C,D**).
- We use a towel clip to provisionally advance the capsule into the desired position to assess sesamoid alignment.
- Redundant capsular tissue is excised and optimal correction is obtained with a tibial sesamoid position less than 2 and an IM1–2 angle less than 9 degrees.
  - About 4 mm of redundant capsule is removed from the inverted-L portion of the capsulotomy to help reduce and advance the sesamoids upon closure.
  - With larger deformities, more capsule may need to be removed to reduce the tibial sesamoid position adequately.
- To correct pronation of the hallux, the towel clip can be rotated to correct the deformity and a double simple suture is placed to maintain the correction.
- We use two 2.5- or 3.0-mm headless cannulated screws for final fixation (**TECH FIG 5E**).

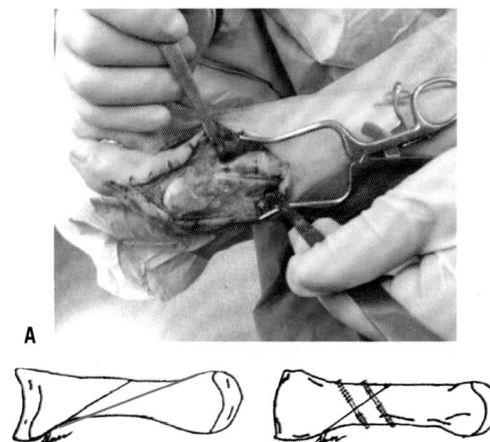

TECH FIG 4 A. The osteotomy is placed parallel to the weight-bearing surface of the foot and the osteotomy is completed from proximal–plantar to distal–dorsal. **B.** The traditional Mau osteotomy (*red line*) and the slight modification (*black line*). The modified Mau does not incorporate the entire metatarsal shaft as does the traditional Mau osteotomy. The modified Mau osteotomy with two-screw fixation.

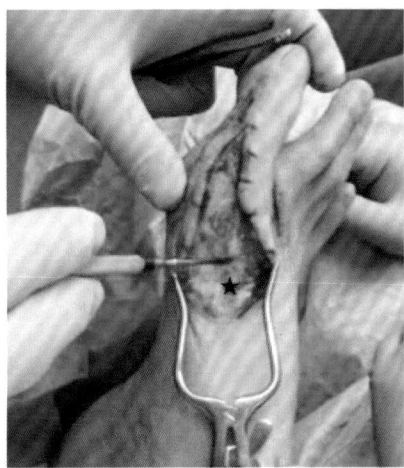

TECH FIG 3 Identification of the first tarsometatarsal joint (star) and starting point of the osteotomy 1 cm distal to the joint (Freer elevator).

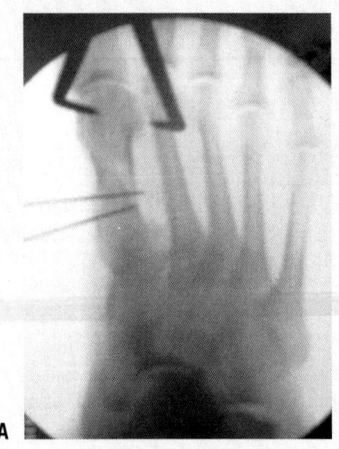

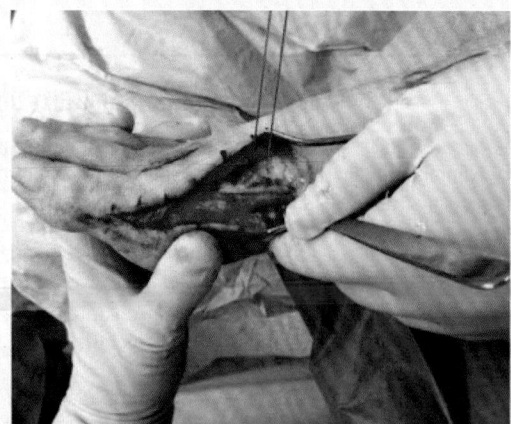

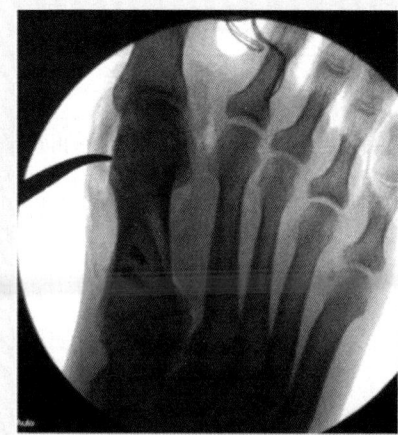

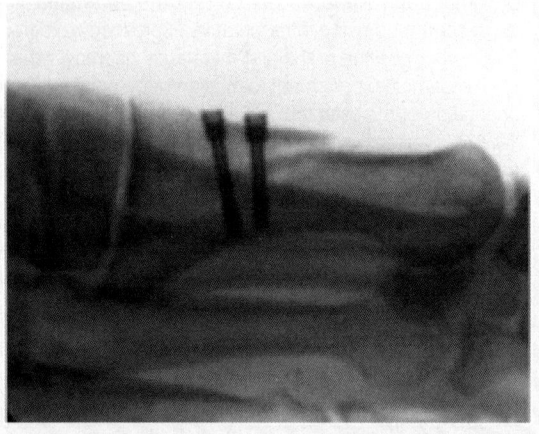

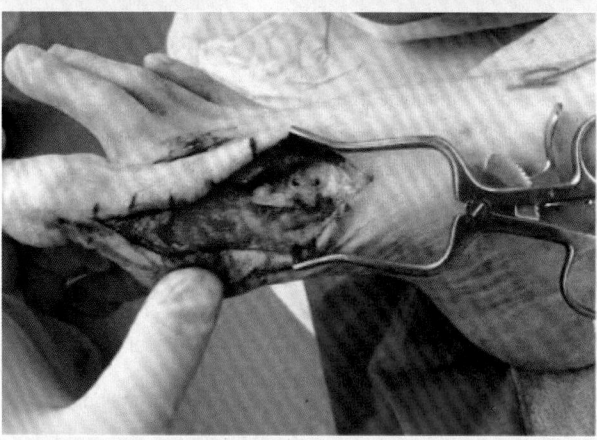

TECH FIG 5 A. Fluoroscopic image showing reduction of IM1–2 angle with large reduction bone clamps. The clamp is placed medially at the first metatarsal head and laterally around the second metatarsal head. **B.** Temporary fixation of the osteotomy with two parallel Kirschner wires from dorsal to plantar. **C.** Intraoperative fluoroscopy of AP foot, showing final fixation and excellent reduction of the IM1–2 angle. **D.** Lateral intraoperative fluoroscopy demonstrating parallel headless screw fixation following Mau osteotomy. **E.** Final fixation of Mau osteotomy with two 3.0-mm cannulated headless screws.

Closure

- To complete the medial capsulorrhaphy, close the capsule using a double simple suture or pants-over-vest technique with 0-0 absorbable suture **(TECH FIG 6A)**.
  - Placing a sponge in the first interspace while closing the capsule will splint the toe in the corrected position.
- Close the subcutaneous layer with 2-0 absorbable suture. The skin is closed based on the surgeon's preference, with either a running subcuticular closure with 3-0 absorbable suture or simple interrupted sutures with 3-0 nylon **(TECH FIG 6B)**.
- Place a soft toe spica dressing by dividing a sponge in thirds and wrapping lateral to medial around the hallux to maintain correction. Use caution to prevent aggressive splinting, which can cause overcorrection and potential hallux varus.

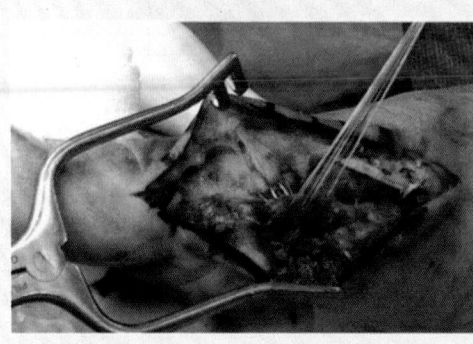

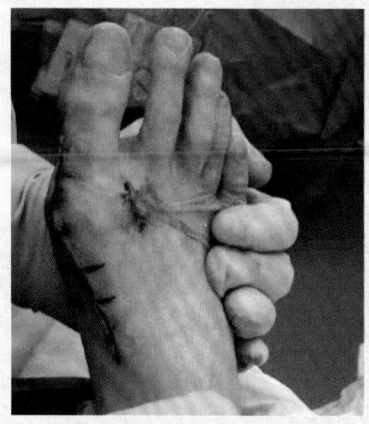

TECH FIG 6 A. Completion of the medial capsulorrhaphy with pants-over-vest technique with 0-0 absorbable suture. **B.** Final skin closure with running subcuticular 3-0 absorbable suture.

MAU OSTEOTOMY FOR CORRECTION OF TAILOR'S BUNION DEFORMITIES OF THE FIFTH METATARSAL

- One incision is used along the lateral aspect of the fifth metatarsal **(TECH FIG 7A)**.
- Dissection is carried through the skin and subcutaneous tissues.
- A longitudinal capsular incision is made, and the periosteal tissues are released around the fifth metatarsal head and the distal third of the fifth metatarsal **(TECH FIG 7B)**.
- The planned osteotomy is directed in a dorsal–distal to proximal–plantar direction starting at the neck of the metatarsal to the mid-diaphysis **(TECH FIG 7C)**.

- The osteotomy is then completed with a microsagittal saw.
- The distal fragment of the osteotomy is then translated medially and temporarily fixated using two guidewires of choice **(TECH FIG 7D)**.
- Final fixation is then achieved with two parallel, 2.5-mm cannulated headless screws **(TECH FIG 7E)**.
- Standard wound closure is performed with absorbable and nonabsorbable sutures.

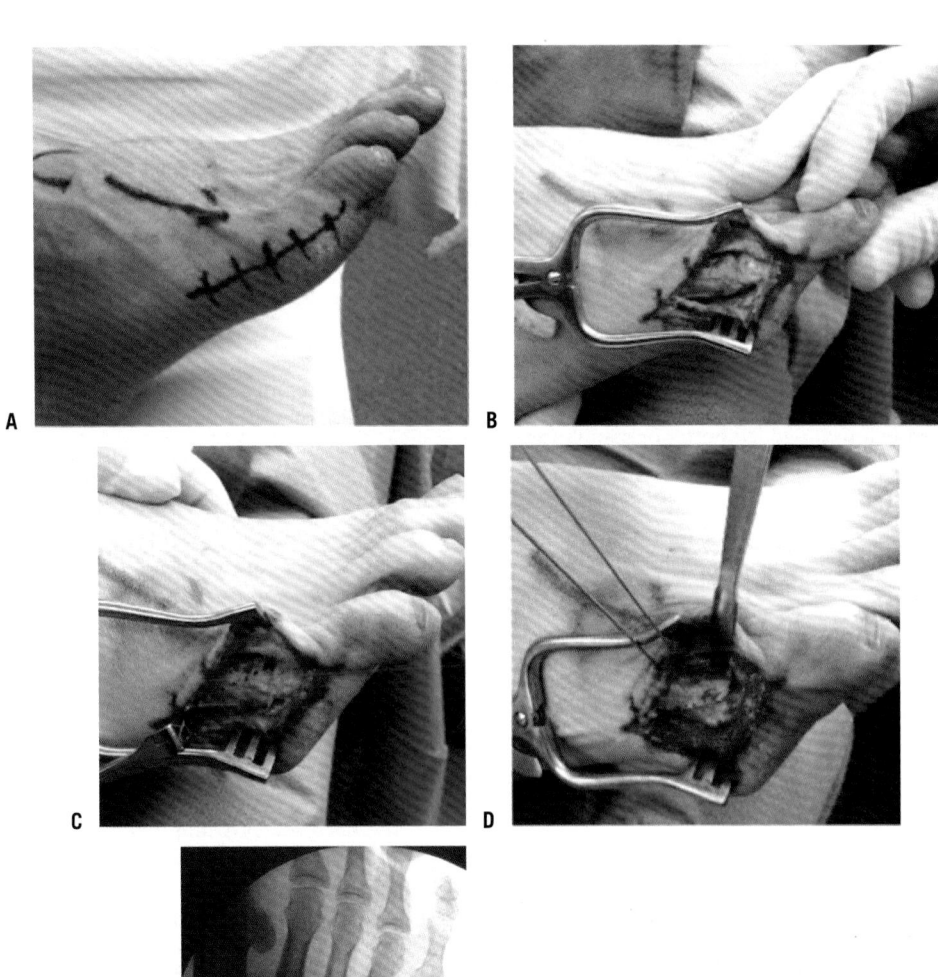

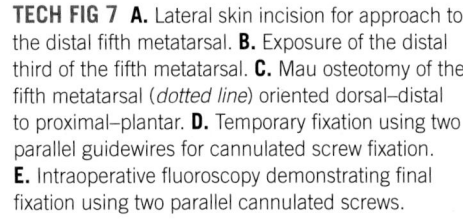

TECH FIG 7 A. Lateral skin incision for approach to the distal fifth metatarsal. **B.** Exposure of the distal third of the fifth metatarsal. **C.** Mau osteotomy of the fifth metatarsal (*dotted line*) oriented dorsal–distal to proximal–plantar. **D.** Temporary fixation using two parallel guidewires for cannulated screw fixation. **E.** Intraoperative fluoroscopy demonstrating final fixation using two parallel cannulated screws.

Pearls and Pitfalls

Incision	• Incision is placed medial to the first metatarsal and slightly plantar to avoid the surrounding neurovascular structures. This allows fast deep dissection.
Medial Capsulorrhaphy	• Placing a varus stress on the hallux will expose redundant capsular tissue that can be incorporated within the L portion of the capsulotomy and can be adequately removed.
Osteotomy	• The periosteum is elevated only in line with the osteotomy. The proximal portion of the osteotomy should be at least 1 cm distal from the first tarsometatarsal joint. This will·also prevent placement of the osteotomy within the first tarsometatarsal joint. • The saw blade is kept parallel to the weight-bearing surface of the foot to prevent unwanted dorsal angulation of the first metatarsal head after completion of the osteotomy. • To maintain complete control of the osteotomy, a guidewire for the cannulated screw can be placed perpendicular in the completed proximal portion of the osteotomy. The osteotomy can be completed dorsodistally without fear of losing the orientation.
IM1–2 Reduction	• Reduction can be achieved with large reduction clamps or by using a Freer elevator on the lateral portion of the proximal fragment and placing counterpressure on the first metatarsal head. Intraoperative fluoroscopy is recommended after placing temporary fixation to achieve an IM angle less than 9 degrees.
Screw Placement	• Placing a screw too distal may cause fracture of the dorsal portion of the osteotomy site. Allow adequate space between the screws and the distal aspect of the osteotomy to prevent fracture.
Unrecognized Hypermobility of the First Tarsometatarsal Joint	• This may result in the inability to effectively reduce the IM1–2 angle after temporary fixation. If encountered, the fist tarsometatarsal joint may be temporarily pinned and permanent fixation placed. The pin across the first tarsometatarsal joint can be removed 4–6 weeks postoperatively.

POSTOPERATIVE CARE

• The patient is placed in a well-padded posterior splint after surgery and instructed to remain non–weight bearing with an assistive device until the first postoperative visit 7 to 10 days after surgery.

• Seven to 10 days after surgery, the sutures are removed and the patient is fully weight bearing in a below-knee immobilizing boot.

• The weight-bearing boot is maintained until bony consolidation occurs typically at 5 to 6 weeks postoperatively.
  • Three weight-bearing radiographs (AP, lateral, oblique) are obtained at each visit until bony healing of the osteotomy site is seen typically between 5 and 6 weeks.

• A removable compression and control strap is prescribed at this point to splint the hallux in a neutral position as the patient transitions to regular shoe gear.

• Physical therapy is instituted at 6 weeks postoperative as the transition from the walking boot to shoes occurs.

• Light activities are permitted until approximately 12 weeks postoperative when full sport may be resumed.

OUTCOMES

• After a proximal osteotomy and distal soft tissue release, 90% to 95% patient satisfaction rates have been reported.[2,3,6]

• One study reviewed retrospective results of the Mau osteotomy and found excellent correction of a moderate to severe bunion deformity in 24 patients.[5]

• A retrospective review of 23 patients found a significant improvement in American Orthopaedic Foot and Ankle Society (AOFAS) scores from 47 preoperatively to 92 postoperative. Additionally, hallux abductovalgus and

IM angles demonstrated a statistically significant improvement. No complications of nonunion or undercorrection were encountered.[8]

• Data has also been shown to advocate the use of a Mau-Reverdin double metatarsal osteotomy for the correction of hallux valgus. A high rate of satisfaction with AOFAS scores and a statistically significant improvement of radiographic angles were shown from preoperative to postoperative.[7]

• Biomechanical studies using sawbones and fresh frozen cadaver models showed superior stability with the Mau osteotomy in terms of fatigue, strength, and stiffness compared to other proximal osteotomies.[1,9]
  • The Mau osteotomy is an inherently stable osteotomy that allows early postoperative weight bearing without the need for cast immobilization as required for other proximal osteotomies due to complications such as dorsal malunion and nonunion.
  • The Mau is a stable osteotomy due to the dorsal shelf to help reduce dorsal displacement forces and broad bony apposition to facilitate two-screw fixation.

• The authors performed a follow-up study comparing the Mau and crescentic osteotomies. Both osteotomies showed comparable correction of the moderate to severe bunion deformity, but significantly more complications were associated with the crescentic osteotomy. Complications included dorsal malunion, placement of screws within the tarsometatarsal joint, and nonunion.[4]

• The Mau osteotomy is technically easier to perform than other proximal osteotomies with fewer complications, as seen in multiple studies, and excellent correction of a bunion deformity **(FIG 5)**.

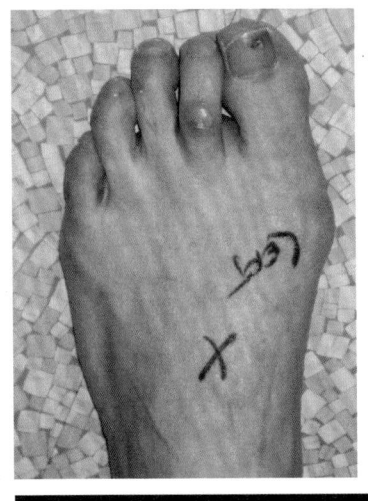 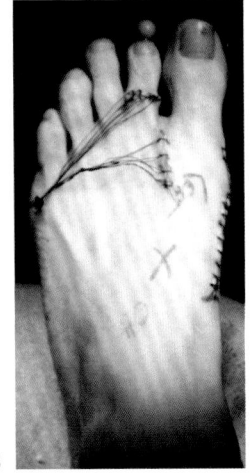 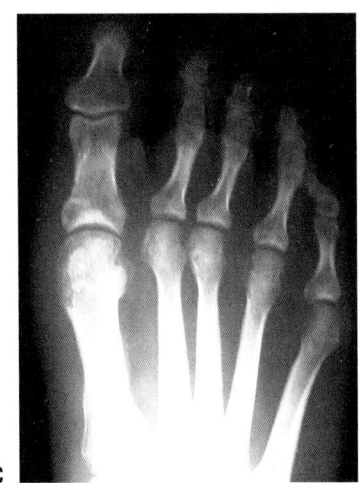

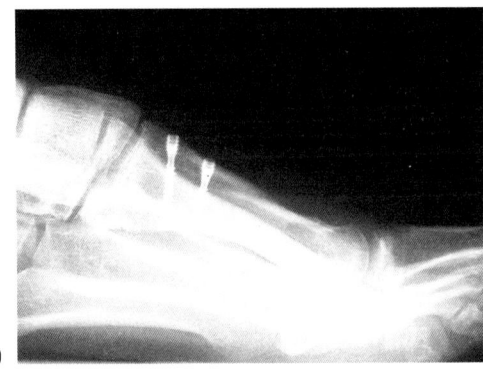

FIG 5 A. Preoperative weight-bearing appearance of the bunion deformity of the patient in **FIG 1**. **B.** Final postoperative appearance closure with 3-0 suture. **C,D.** Postoperative AP and lateral foot radiographs showing excellent reduction of the IM1–2 angle.

COMPLICATIONS

- One of the most common complications after bunion surgery is recurrence. This may be due to selection of the inappropriate procedure to correct the moderate to severe bunion deformity or intraoperative failure to obtain an adequate alignment to correct the deformity.
- Hallux varus is a complication that occurs less often than recurrence. It occurs as a result of overcorrection of the deformity and is much more difficult to correct.
- Other complications include shortening, dorsal malunion, and transfer lesions, which can occur with all proximal osteotomies.

- Although a rare occurrence with the Mau osteotomy, nonunion can become painful and problematic for both the patient and the surgeon.[4,5] The authors recommend revision of a Mau osteotomy nonunion with locking plate fixation and autogenous bone graft supplementation (**FIG 6**).

REFERENCES

1. Acevedo JI, Sammarco VJ, Boucher HR, et al. Mechanical comparison of cyclic loading in five different first metatarsal shaft osteotomies. Foot Ankle Int 2002;23:711–716.
2. Chiodo C, Schon L, Myerson MS, et al. Clinical results with the Ludloff osteotomy for correction of adult hallux valgus. Foot Ankle Int 2004;25:532–536.
3. Easley ME, Kiebzak GM, Davis WH, et al. Prospective, randomized comparison of proximal crescentic and proximal chevron osteotomies for correction of hallux valgus deformity. Foot Ankle Int 1996;17:307–316.
4. Glover JP, Hyer CF, Berlet GC, et al. A comparison of crescentic and Mau osteotomies for correction of hallux valgus. J Foot Ankle Surg 2008;47:103–111.
5. Glover JP, Hyer CF, Berlet GC, et al. Early results of the Mau osteotomy for correction of moderate to severe hallux valgus. J Foot Ankle Surg 2008;47:237–242.
6. Mann RA, Rudicel S, Graves SC, et al. Hallux valgus repair utilizing a distal soft tissue procedure and proximal metatarsal osteotomy: a long-term follow-up. J Bone Joint Surg Am 1992;74A:124–129.
7. Neese DJ, Zelent ME. The modified Mau-Reverding double osteotomy for correction of hallux valgus: a retrospective study. J Foot Ankle Surg 2009;48(1):22–29.
8. Thangarajah T, Ahmed U, Malik S, et al. The early functional outcome of Mau osteotomy for the correction of moderate-severe hallux valgus. Orthop Rev (Pavia) 2013;5(4):e37.
9. Trnka HJ, Parks BG, Ivanic G, et al. Six first metatarsal shaft osteotomies: mechanical and immobilization comparisons. Clin Orthop Relat Res 2000;381:256–265.

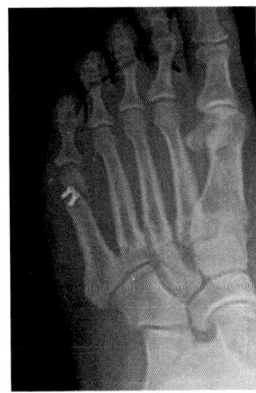 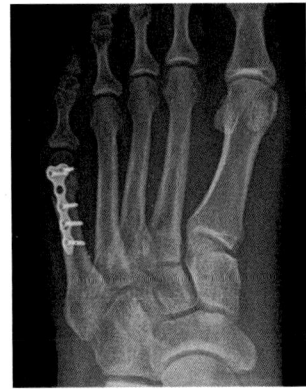

FIG 6 A. Preoperative radiograph demonstrating a nonunion of a fifth metatarsal Mau osteotomy. **B.** Postoperative radiograph demonstrating surgical revision with locking plate fixation and autogenous calcaneal bone graft.

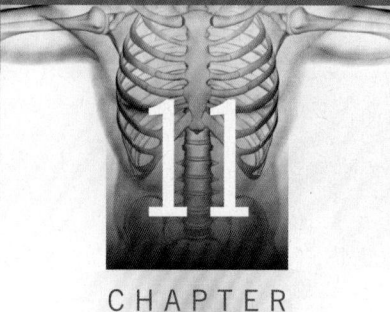

Proximal Chevron Osteotomy with Plate Fixation

Matthew J. DeOrio and James K. DeOrio

DEFINITION

- Correction of major bunion deformities through the proximal portion of the first metatarsal is one method of reducing the angle between the first and second metatarsal.[3–6]
- More than 138 techniques have been described for bunion correction, with widely varied methods of fixation of these osteotomies including pins or screws.
  - Pins provide little inherent stability and have been associated with postoperative infections.
  - Getting excellent fixation of screws can be a problem in cases in which there is poor bone quality.
- Plates, although widely used in all other osteotomies, have not been routinely employed in bunion surgery because of the fear of prominence and irritation of the patient's foot.
- Recently, the use of locking plates and locking screws has been increasing in the orthopaedic world. The locking plates provide essentially a fixed-angle device, which allows for a potentially stronger method of fixation.[4]
  - The advantages of plate fixation for the patient include no external pins, potentially no second procedure to remove hardware, less pain because the osteotomy is stable, and early full or at least partial weight bearing.
- Advantages for the surgeon are that it is possible to do any osteotomy for the first metatarsal and that excellent and secure fixation is obtained.
- Although many different configurations of the osteotomy can be used, the proximal chevron osteotomy permits a greater degree of correction compared with distal osteotomies. It does this through both an angular and translational displacement of the distal portion of the first metatarsal.[2] It does not, however, provide a good correction for rotational deformity increasingly believed to be the main deformity in bunions.

SURGICAL MANAGEMENT

Approach

- The procedure is performed through a single midmedial longitudinal approach to the first metatarsal with the use of an Esmarch tourniquet (**FIG 1**) or pneumatic calf tourniquet.

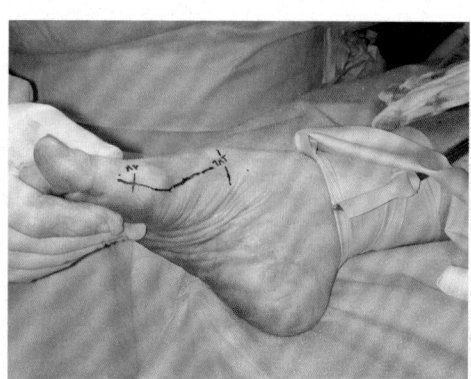
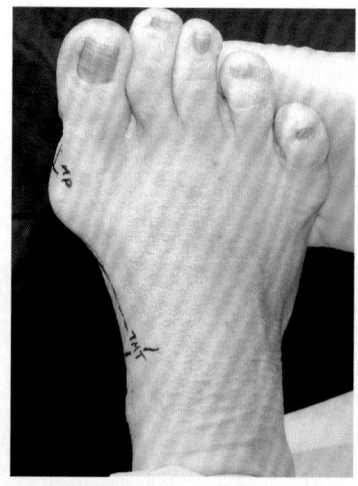

A **B**

FIG 1 A. Simulated weight-bearing view of foot. **B.** A midmedial approach to the first metatarsal is used. The first metatarsophalangeal and first TMT joints are identified.

EXPOSURE

- The skin and subcutaneous tissues are incised sharply to expose the first metatarsophalangeal joint capsule. Care is taken to protect the medial dorsal and plantar cutaneous nerves.
- A vertical capsular resection is performed to remove about 3 to 5 mm of capsule just proximal to the base of the proximal phalanx **(TECH FIG 1)**.
  - A longitudinal incision may also be made in the capsule, excising the midportion.
- A dorsomedial incision is made in the capsule parallel to the first metatarsal, creating a plantarly based capsular flap with exposure of the medial eminence. Similarly, if you make a longitudinal ellipse of the capsule tissue, the medial eminence will likewise be exposed.

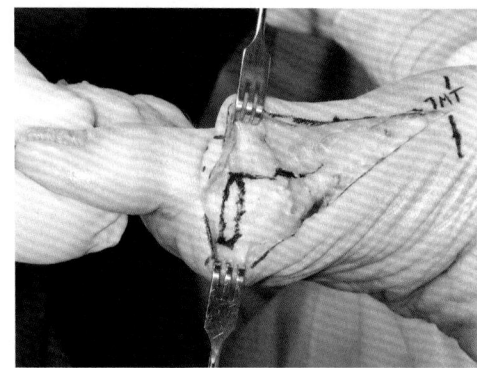

TECH FIG 1 Thick skin flaps are preserved, and a vertical segment of redundant capsule is excised.

RELEASE OF LATERAL JOINT STRUCTURES

- The lateral soft tissues are released from within the metatarsophalangeal joint after distraction of the sesamoids from the first metatarsal with a lamina spreader.
  - First, use a blunt Freer elevator to develop some space and then cut the capsular tissue with a sharp no. 15 blade **(TECH FIG 2)**.
    - The medial approach to the release avoids making a separate 1–2 incision, and the medial incision is just as effective.[1,6] It is no longer necessary to make a separate

incision to release the lateral capsule. And it has been shown that release of the adductor does not significantly improve the ability to correct hallux valgus.[2]

- Complete release can be confirmed when the great toe can be brought into about 15 degrees of varus through the metatarsophalangeal joint.
- The proximal first metatarsal is subsequently exposed both dorsally and plantarly.

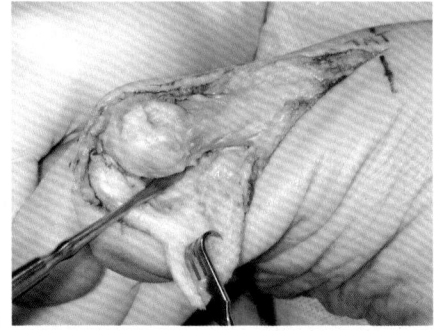
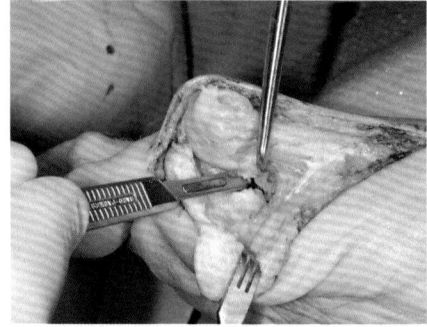

TECH FIG 2 A. A plantarly and proximally based capsular flap is created, and the capsule is released with a Freer elevator. **B.** A no. 15 blade is used to complete the release of the lateral capsular attachment to the lateral sesamoid.

METATARSAL OSTEOTOMY

- The location of the tarsometatarsal (TMT) joint is confirmed, and a point is marked about 20 mm distally from the first TMT joint for the apex of the osteotomy and at the midpoint in the dorsoplantar direction.
- A proximally based chevron osteotomy is created at an angle of about 60 degrees using a microsagittal saw.
- Complete release, both plantarly and dorsally, is confirmed, and care is taken not to fracture either limb of the chevron osteotomy (**TECH FIG 3A,B**).

- The proximal fragment is grasped with a towel clamp and the distal fragment angulated laterally.
  - It also is translated 3 to 5 mm laterally and plantarly enough to coapt the superior portion of the chevron, leaving an opening in the plantar portion of the osteotomy (**TECH FIG 3C**).

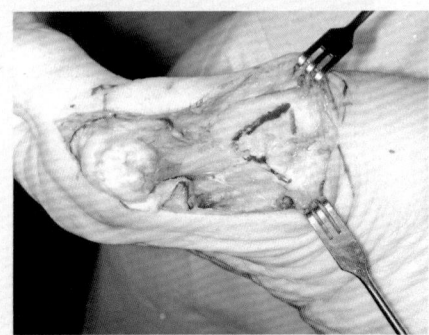
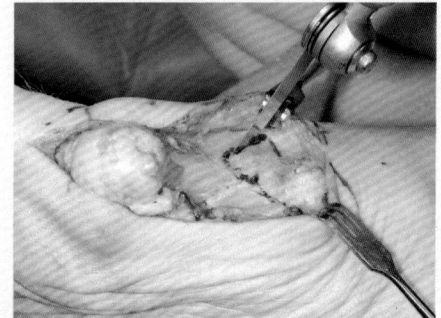
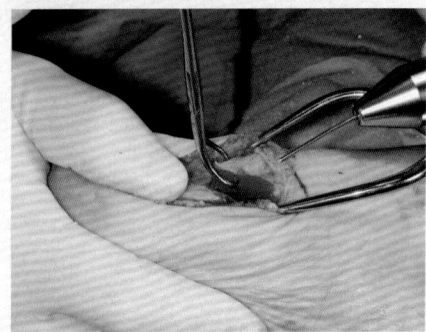

TECH FIG 3 A,B. A microsagittal saw is used to create a 60-degree chevron osteotomy with the apex 20 mm from the TMT joint. **C.** A pointed towel clip is used to hold the proximal metatarsal while the shaft is angulated and translated laterally to decrease the 1–2 intermetatarsal angle and narrow the foot. A K-wire is advanced from the TMT joint into the shaft to hold the correction temporarily.

OSTEOTOMY FIXATION

- The translated position is secured temporarily with a 0.062-inch Kirschner wire (K-wire).
- The prominent proximal fragment is cleaned of periosteum and removed flush with the distal fragment.
- This removed portion is then placed as bone graft between the fragments at the opening created in the chevron osteotomy from the plantar translation (**TECH FIG 4A,B**).

- A four-hole locking plate is used to bridge the osteotomy medially (**TECH FIG 4C**).
  - Care is exercised to avoid penetrating the TMT articulation with screws.
- The medial eminence is removed 1 mm medial to the sagittal sulcus (**TECH FIG 4D**).
- The K-wire is removed, stability is confirmed, and correction and alignment are confirmed with fluoroscopy (**TECH FIG 4E**).

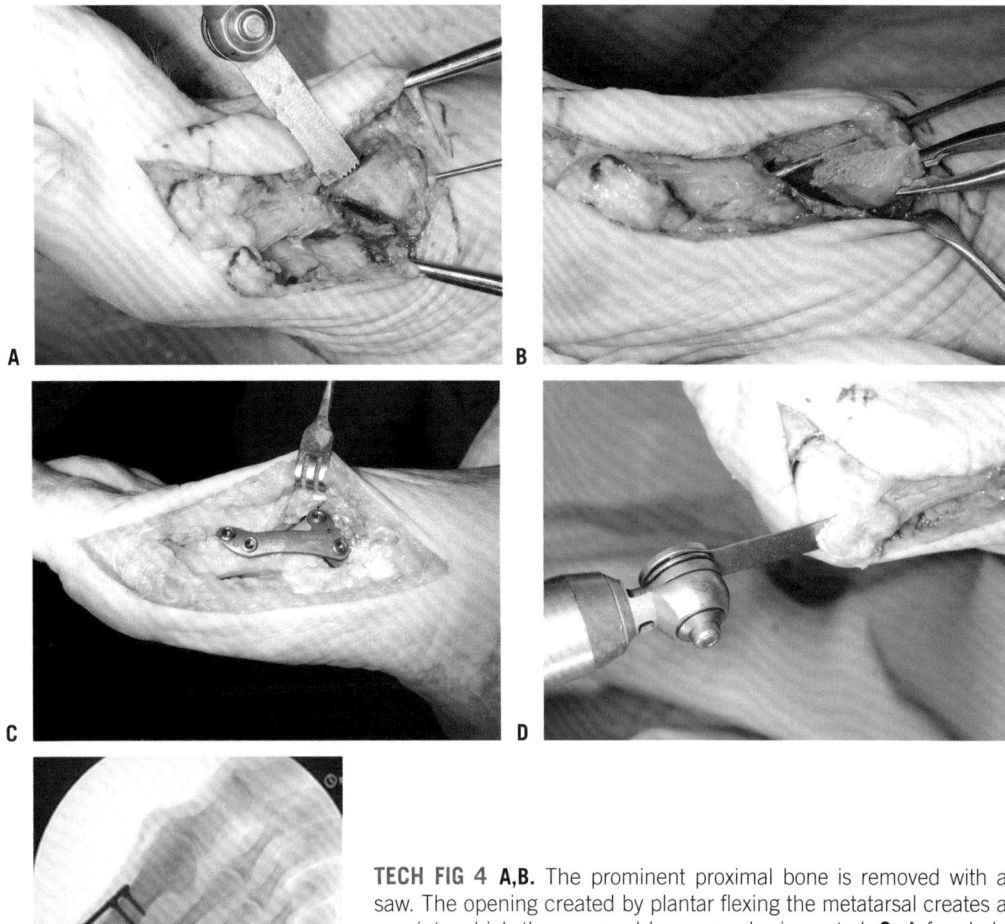

TECH FIG 4 A,B. The prominent proximal bone is removed with a saw. The opening created by plantar flexing the metatarsal creates a gap into which the removed bone may be impacted. **C.** A four-hole locking plate is applied at the osteotomy site. **D.** The prominent medial eminence is removed 1 mm medial to the sagittal sulcus. **E.** Correction of the hallux valgus angle and the 1–2 intermetatarsal angle is confirmed with fluoroscopy.

CAPSULE AND SOFT TISSUE CLOSURE

- Meticulous capsular closure is performed with 2-0 Vicryl sutures, holding the toe in slight varus and supination (**TECH FIG 5A**).

- The deep tissues also are closed over the plate to avoid symptomatic prominent hardware.
- The skin is closed with interrupted vertical mattress 3-0 nylon sutures and a compressive dressing (**TECH FIG 5B**).

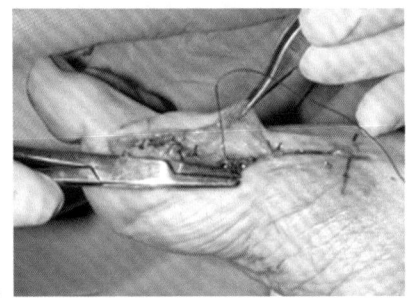

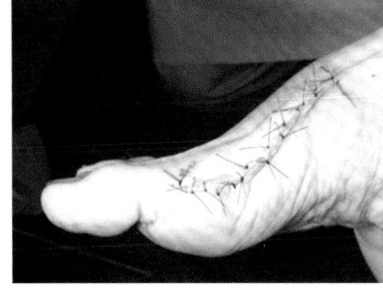

TECH FIG 5 A. The capsular flaps are closed with 2-0 interrupted Vicryl sutures with the hallux held in good position. Soft tissue coverage of the plate also is obtained. **B.** The skin is closed with interrupted 3-0 nylon vertical mattress sutures.

Pearls and Pitfalls

Indications	• Large symptomatic hallux valgus deformity with minimal degenerative change and a 1–2 intermetatarsal angle greater than 15 degrees
Exposure	• During the approach, dissect thick tissue flaps to allow for improved wound healing.
Metatarsal Osteotomy	• Pay particular attention to keeping the saw in the same plane while performing the proximal chevron osteotomy to ensure good bony apposition at the site of fixation. Do not overcorrect the 1–2 metatarsal angle; a negative angle may lead to hallux varus.
Locking Plate Fixation	• If the plate requires contouring for larger intermetatarsal angles, do not bend the plate through the locking holes or the screws will not seat properly in the plate.
Capsular Closure	• By removing redundant medial capsule during the approach, the capsule repair can be accomplished more efficiently at the conclusion of the procedure. The great toe should be positioned in slight varus, about 2 degrees, to allow healing of the capsular tissues in a good position. These tissues will stretch over time. Do not overtighten the capsule because this will overcorrect the toe position and result in varus malalignment. Capsular imbrication also can be used to correct pronation deformity of the hallux.

POSTOPERATIVE CARE

- Bunion dressings are applied at the time of surgery, and sutures are removed 2 to 3 weeks from the date of surgery.
- Heel weight bearing can be allowed immediately postoperatively, with advancement to weight bearing as tolerated in a regular shoe at 6 weeks postoperatively.
- Radiographs are obtained at 6 weeks and 3 months.

REFERENCES

1. Ahn JY, Lee HS, Chun H, et al. Comparison of open lateral release and transarticular lateral release in distal chevron metatarsal osteotomy for hallux valgus correction. Int Orthop 2013;37(9):1781–1787.
2. Augoyard R, Largey A, Munoz MA, et al. Efficacy of first metatarsophalangeal joint lateral release in hallux valgus surgery. Orthop Traumatol Surg Res 2013;99(4):425–431.
3. Easley ME, Kiebzak GM, Davis WH, et al. Prospective, randomized comparison of proximal crescentic and proximal chevron osteotomies for correction of hallux valgus deformity. Foot Ankle Int 1996;17:307–316.
4. Gallentine JW, DeOrio JK, DeOrio MJ. Bunion surgery using locking-plate fixation of proximal metatarsal chevron osteotomies. Foot Ankle Int 2007;28(3):361–368.
5. McCluskey LC, Johnson JE, Wynarsky GT, et al. Comparison of stability of proximal crescentic metatarsal osteotomy and proximal horizontal "V" osteotomy. Foot Ankle Int 1994;15:263–270.
6. Sammarco GJ, Russo-Alesi FG. Bunion correction using proximal chevron osteotomy: a single-incision technique. Foot Ankle Int 1998;19:430–437.

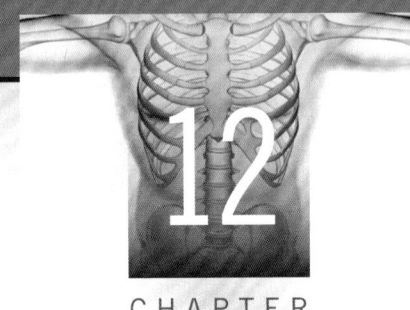

12

CHAPTER

Closing Wedge Proximal Osteotomy

Sam Singh and Michael G. Wilson

SURGICAL MANAGEMENT

- The primary indication for a proximal closing wedge oste-otomy is a symptomatic hallux valgus deformity with a first intermetatarsal angle (IMA) of 14 degrees or greater.
- The first metatarsocuneiform (MC) joint should be sta-ble. We evaluate stability of this joint both by physical examination and radiographs. On physical examination, the cuneiform is stabilized in one hand, whereas the first metatarsal is translated superiorly and inferiorly with the other hand. On weight-bearing radiographs, the MC joint is inspected for incongruency on the anteroposterior (AP) view and plantar widening on the lateral view. We favor a Lapidus-type procedure for hallux valgus associated with first MC joint instability.
- Relative contraindications to this osteotomy include mild osteoarthritic changes in the first metatarsophalangeal (MTP) joint and the presence of an inflammatory arthrop-athy. In the presence of mild osteoarthritic changes, an ac-tive individual who understands the possible future need for a fusion may remain a candidate for a corrective oste-otomy. Similarly, given the improved medical management of inflammatory arthropathy, an informed patient with well-managed rheumatoid arthritis may also be a candidate for reconstructive hallux valgus surgery rather than fusion.
- Absolute contraindications to this osteotomy are advanced osteoarthritis of the first MTP joint or the skeletally im-mature patient, in whom the very proximal nature of this osteotomy can jeopardize the growth plate.

Preoperative Planning

- AP and lateral weight-bearing radiographs of the foot are evaluated for metatarsal length, IMA, and hallux valgus angle. Congruency of the joint, the size of the bony medial eminence, and the position of the sesamoids are noted. We routinely mark the proposed osteotomy on the radiograph (**FIG 1**).

Positioning

- We perform this procedure on an outpatient basis. Prophy-lactic antibiotics are administered. A thigh tourniquet is applied. The patient is positioned supine with a small sand-bag placed under the ipsilateral buttock to ensure the foot points up, allowing for easier osteotomy orientation.

Approach

- We perform the proximal closing wedge osteotomy with a distal soft tissue procedure through two incisions.
  - The first is a dorsal first web space incision extended proximally in a lazy S curve to the dorsal first MC joint. This incision allows access for lateral release and prox-imal osteotomy.
  - The second medial midaxial incision over the first MTP joint is the traditional approach for medial capsulo-tomy, medial eminence resection, and medial capsular plication.

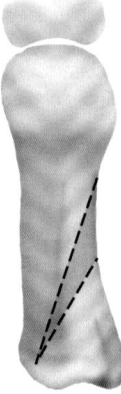

FIG 1 Line diagram showing the closing wedge osteotomy.

SOFT TISSUE RELEASE AND BUNIONECTOMY

- Perform a standard lateral release of the first MTP joint through a dorsal incision centered over the first web space.
- After incising the skin, continue deep dissection bluntly.
- Using sharp dissection, release the tendinous insertion of the adductor hallucis muscle onto the fibular sesamoid and proximal phalanx; we have not found it necessary to reattach this structure proximally (**TECH FIG 1A**).
- Release the suspensory metatarsal–sesamoid ligaments and make multiple sharp perforations in the lateral capsule at the

joint line. Apply a varus force to the hallux, completing the capsular release.
- Approach the medial eminence through a midline longitudinal incision extending from just proximal to the medial eminence to the base of the proximal phalanx. Identify the dorsal medial cutaneous nerve and incise the medial capsule sharply in a longitudinal direction (**TECH FIG 1B**). Expose the medial eminence and resect it 1 mm medial to the sagittal sulcus. Overresection can lead to a postoperative varus deformity.

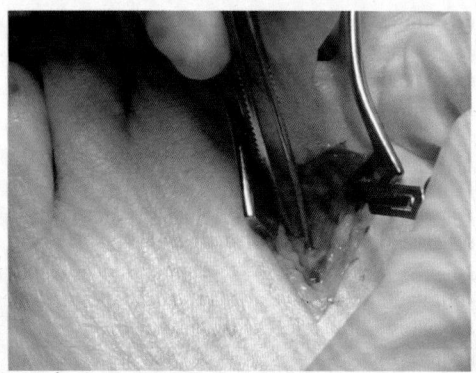
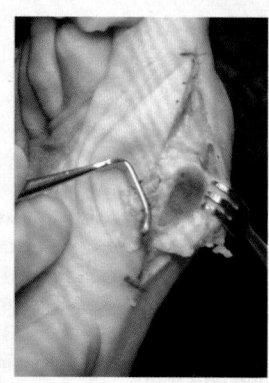

TECH FIG 1 A. The adductor hallucis tendon is released off the proximal phalanx and fibula sesamoid. The suspensory ligaments of the fibula sesamoid are released. **B.** Medial capsulotomy and exostectomy.

OSTEOTOMY

- Extend the first web space incision in an S shape to the first MC joint (**TECH FIG 2A**).
- Approach the dorsal metatarsal shaft through the interval between the extensor hallucis brevis and extensor hallucis longus.
- Retraction with two small pointed retractors facilitates exposure of the metatarsal base.
- The proposed wedge for resection has its apex on the medial cortex about 3 mm from the MC joint. The proposed long oblique osteotomy should leave a large residual proximal fragment for maximal contact area and solid fixation.

- The first cut, the proximal of the two, is perpendicular to the weight-bearing axis of the foot. This is demonstrated during surgery by the simulated weight-bearing test. To maintain control of the osteotomy, the medial cortex is scored but not penetrated with the saw blade (**TECH FIG 2B**).
- After making the second distal cut, excise a lateral wedge-shaped wafer of bone; this leaves a defect, which is compressed with a towel clip. This "greensticks" the intact but weakened medial cortex and the IMA is reduced (**TECH FIG 2C–E**).

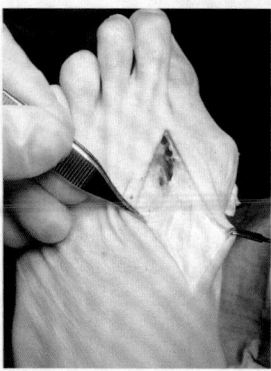
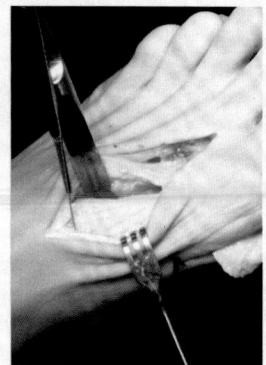
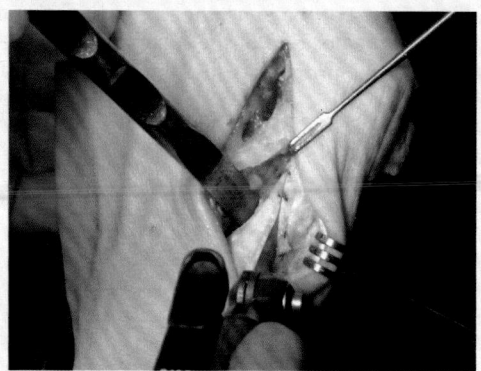

TECH FIG 2 A. The web space incision is extended proximally in a lazy S shape toward the base of the first metatarsal. The extensor hallucis brevis is identified and protected. **B.** The first tarsometatarsal joint is localized to define the limit of the cut. *(continued)*

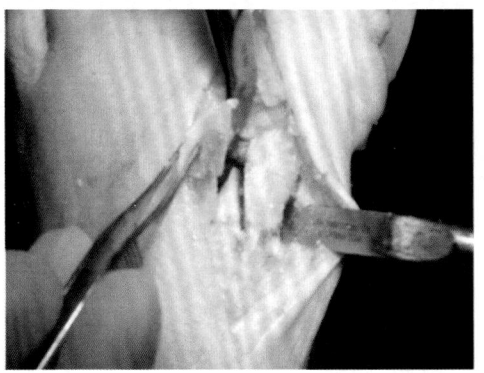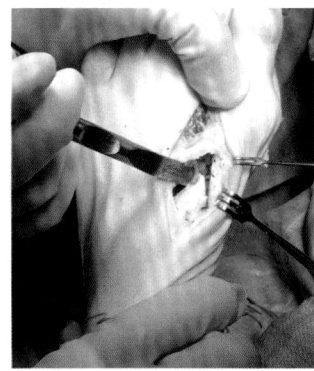

TECH FIG 2 *(continued)* **C–E.** The two osteotomies leave a wedge-shaped segment of bone, which is removed.

REDUCTION, FIXATION, AND CLOSURE

- Insert two 2.7-mm cortical screws (Synthes, Paoli, PA) from the lateral to medial cortex in a lag screw fashion **(TECH FIG 3A,B)**.
  - The small size of the proximal fragment does not allow both screws to be parallel to the osteotomy, but this is not vital, as compression has already been obtained with the reduction forceps.
- Confirm the reduction in the IMA, screws, and relocation of the sesamoids with image intensification.

- Imbricate the medial capsule with a strong absorbable suture while holding the hallux in a neutral or slightly abducted position **(TECH FIG 3C)**.
- Close the wounds in layers with interrupted nylon sutures to the skin and apply a forefoot bandage to maintain the correction **(TECH FIG 3D)**.

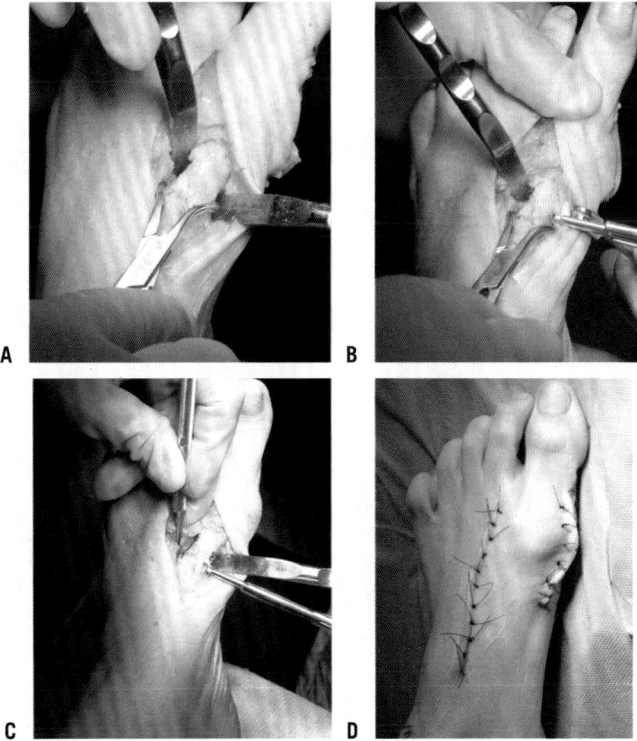

TECH FIG 3 A. Compression with the clamp greensticks the medial cortex. **B,C.** Two screws are inserted in a lag screw fashion. **D.** The capsule is repaired. The skin is closed.

Pearls and Pitfalls

Keep the center of correction proximal.	• The apex of the deformity is the MC joint. To maximize the power of the osteotomy, the center of correction should be as close to the joint as possible, leaving a safe bridge of medial cortex.
Beware the short osteotomy!	• If the osteotomy is too short, it will exit the lateral cortex too proximally, leaving a small proximal fragment. This compromises the contact area and stability of the osteotomy, precludes adequate fixation, and decreases the corrective power of the osteotomy.
Maintain continuous control of the osteotomy.	• By only scoring the medial cortex, complete control of the osteotomy segments is maintained at all times.
Avoid early full weight bearing.	• The excessive sagittal loading can lead to a dorsiflexion malunion.

POSTOPERATIVE CARE

- If safe, patients are discharged home on the day of surgery with strict advice to elevate the foot whenever resting for the first 2 weeks.
- In most cases, patients are allowed to bear weight on their heel and lateral forefoot in a hard-soled postoperative shoe.
- In noncompliant patients, those with poor bone quality or revision cases, we do not hesitate to use cast immobilization from the outset or fixation with three screws (**FIG 2A,B**).
- The wound is inspected, and sutures are removed at 2 weeks, at which time, the hallux is restrapped, and patients are taught simple passive and active toe flexion–extension exercises.
- At 6 weeks postoperatively, the osteotomy is assessed with radiographs (**FIG 3**).
  - If there is some consolidation at the line of the osteotomy, the patient is instructed to wear a wide shoe or sneaker and to progress weight bearing as tolerated.

- Strapping of the hallux is discontinued at this time.
- If there is evidence of a delayed union, the patient is kept non–weight bearing in a hard-soled postoperative shoe.

OUTCOMES

- A review of our first 40 cases with an average age at surgery of 51 years identified one case of transfer metatarsalgia in a patient who had not had it before surgery, one malunion due to loss of fixation, one delayed union requiring prolonged immobilization, and one asymptomatic nonunion. Shortening of the first metatarsal was minimal with this technique, with an average of 0.98 mm (−1 to 3 mm).
- In the subset of 11 patients with a severe deformity and an IMA exceeding 18 degrees (range, 18 to 22 degrees), the average postoperative IMA was 7.8 degrees, with an average 1.8 mm of shortening.

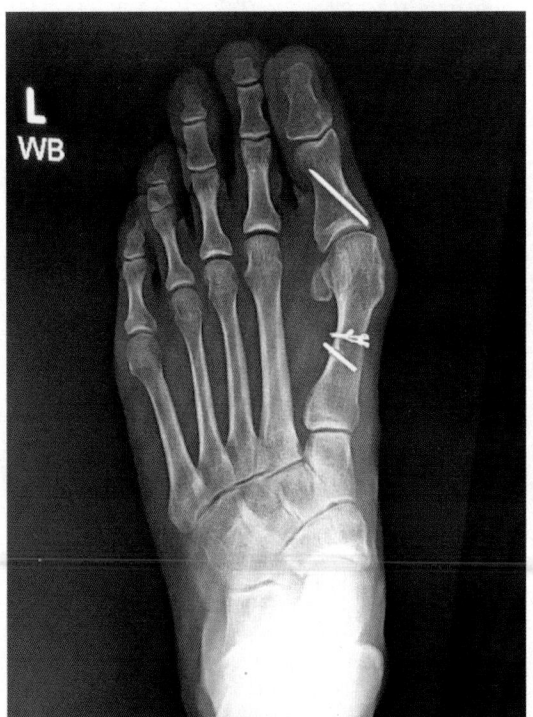 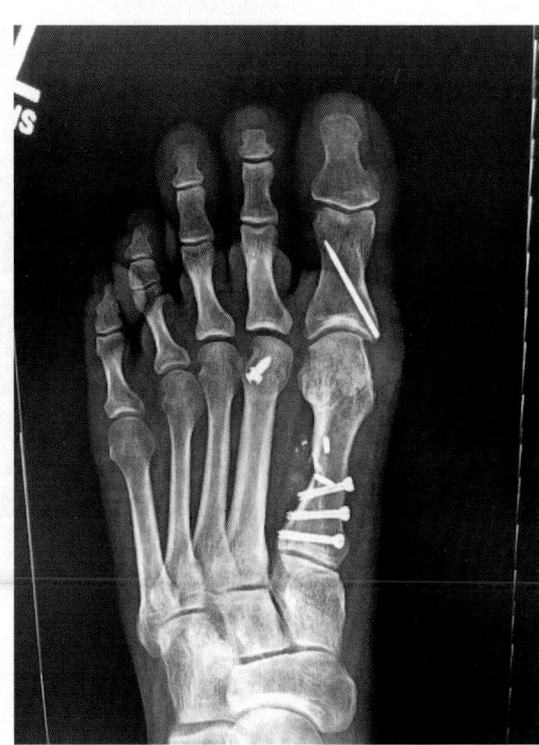

FIG 2 A,B. Preoperative and postoperative radiographs of a revision case; note fixation with three screws.

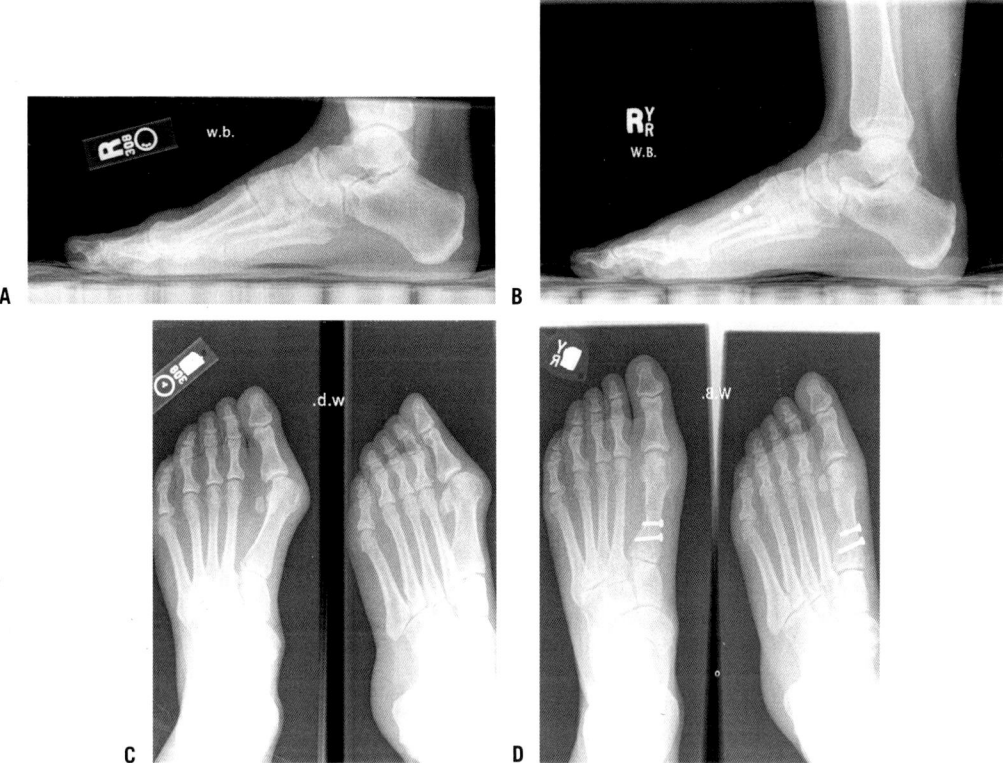

FIG 3 A–D. Preoperative and postoperative radiographs.

- Some studies have reported more shortening (average of 5 mm) with similar osteotomies, but this may be due to two factors:
  - A transverse rather than long oblique closing wedge osteotomy
  - Dorsiflexion malunion, which may make the metatarsal appear shorter on radiographic evaluation
- The stability of this osteotomy is not compromised even when correcting hallux valgus with a large intermetatarsal deformity. This is in contrast to the scarf, Ludloff, and proximal crescentic osteotomies in which bone contact area is substantially reduced.

COMPLICATIONS

- Complications include those of any hallux valgus surgery: iatrogenic fracture, injury to the dorsal medial cutaneous nerve, superficial infection, loss of fixation, and delayed union.

- The risk of iatrogenic fracture can be minimized by using appropriate-diameter screws, leaving a bridge of at least 3 mm between screws, and both drilling and tapping the near cortex (even when using a self-tapping screw).

SUGGESTED READINGS

Mann RA, Rudicel S, Graves SC. Repair of hallux valgus with a distal soft-tissue procedure and proximal metatarsal osteotomy. A long-term follow-up. J Bone Joint Surg Am 1992;74:124–129.

Ruch JA, Banks AS. Proximal osteotomies of the first metatarsal in the correction of hallux abducto valgus. In: McGlamry ED, Banes AS, Downey MS, eds. Comprehensive Textbook of Foot Surgery. Baltimore: Williams & Wilkins, 1987:195–211.

Trnka HJ, Mühlbauer M, Zembsch A, et al. Basal closing wedge osteotomy for correction of hallux valgus and metatarsus primus varus: 10- to 22-year follow-up. Foot Ankle Int 1999;20:171–177.

Trnka HJ, Parks BG, Ivanic G, et al. Six first metatarsal shaft osteotomies: mechanical and immobilization comparisons. Clin Orthop Relat Res 2000;(381):256–265.

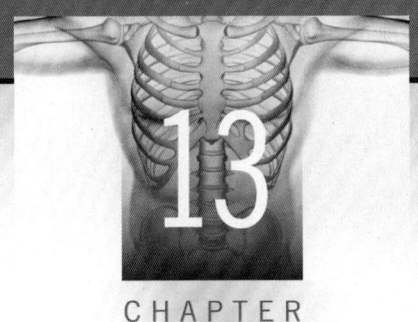

13
CHAPTER

Proximal Opening Wedge Osteotomy for Hallux Valgus Correction

Nikiforos Pandelis Saragas

BACKGROUND

- The proximal opening wedge osteotomy is one of the more than 150 procedures described for the treatment of hallux valgus (HV), indicating the complexity of this deformity.
- It was first described by Trethowan[13] in 1923. Trethowan used no fixation, as he thought that by maintaining an intact lateral cortex and using a well-fitting wedge graft, the osteotomy was relatively stable.
- The procedure was initially performed mainly for adolescent bunions with questionable results. It was also used in the pediatric population with minimal deformity, prophylactically to prevent progression of the deformity.[2,9,12]
- The proximal opening wedge osteotomy fell out of favor in subsequent years due to concerns regarding stability and nonunion at the osteotomy site. More recently, the possibility of arthritis in the first metatarsophalangeal joint (MPJ) due to "jamming" and recurrence of the deformity as a result of the metatarsal lengthening created by the opening wedge was questioned.[3,4,14]
- The earlier concerns have largely been addressed by the advent of more refined surgical techniques, superior internal fixation, and improvement in bone grafting. The addition of a distal closing "chevron-type" wedge osteotomy counteracts the lengthened first metatarsal and negates the increased distal metatarsal articular angle (DMAA), which does occur with the proximal opening wedge osteotomy being a rotational osteotomy.[1,5,11]

SURGICAL MANAGEMENT

- The proximal opening wedge osteotomy is reserved for the correction of moderate to severe (HV angle >30 degrees and 1–2 intermetatarsal [IM] angle >15 degrees) HV deformity.
- The procedure is performed in combination with a lateral distal soft tissue release and a closing distal medial-based wedge osteotomy (chevron-type).

Positioning

- The patient is placed supine on the table with a bolster under the ipsilateral buttock if the lower limb is too externally rotated.
- A thigh tourniquet is used. Although the procedure is done under general anesthetic, a regional block may be given for postoperative pain relief.

TECHNIQUES

EXPOSURE

- The first part of the procedure is the lateral distal soft tissue release while the first web space is still wide.
- A 1- to 1.5-cm incision is made on the dorsum of the first web space.
- The adductor hallucis tendon is identified and is sharply dissected from its insertion on the proximal phalanx of the hallux.
- The dissection is carried proximally, and the sesamoid suspensory ligament (between the lateral hallucal sesamoid and the first metatarsal) is transected. There is no need to release the lateral hallucal sesamoid completely.

CAPSULOTOMY

- A lateral capsulotomy is next performed. At this stage, one should be able to passively push the hallux into ±20 degrees varus.
- A medial incision is made, extending from just distal to the first MPJ proximally along the shaft of the first metatarsal to the first tarsometatarsal (TM) joint.
- The incision is carried down to the medial capsule (identified by the vertical orientation of its fibers). Care should be taken not to injure the medial cutaneous nerve, which should be in the dorsal flap.
  - Inferiorly, the dissection is carried down to the abductor hallucis tendon.

- A vertical capsular incision is made approximately 2 to 3 mm proximal to the articular surface.
- A more proximal incision is made parallel to the first and joined above with an inverted V and inferiorly with a V, thus excising an elliptical piece of capsule.
  - The width of this capsular piece is determined by the size of the medial eminence and the amount of deformity that is to be corrected (**TECH FIG 1**).
- A horizontal capsular incision is now made from the dorsal extent of the vertical incision, proximally to the first TM joint.
- The capsule is then sharply dissected off the medial eminence.
- The medial eminence is cut with a small oscillating saw.
- Care is taken to remain medial to the groove and flush with the medial shaft of the first metatarsal.
- If there is a significant dorsal bunion, this, too, is resected.

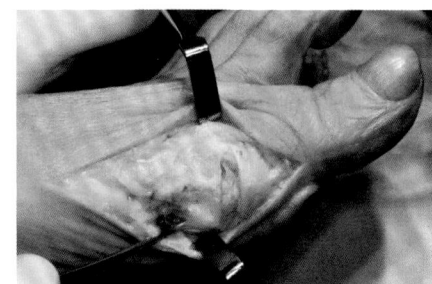

TECH FIG 1 Medial capsulotomy. The abductor hallucis tendon is immediately above the lower retractor.

OSTEOTOMY AND PLATING

- The first TM joint is identified with a needle or under fluoroscopy.
- A transverse proximal osteotomy is performed approximately 1 cm from the TM joint.
- The osteotomy must not be completed, that is, maintain an intact lateral cortex.
- Depending on the set, the osteotomy is carefully prised open with either one or two osteotomes or a small distractor, taking care not to fracture the lateral cortex (**TECH FIG 2A**).
- It is prudent at this stage to use fluoroscopy to determine the amount of opening required to correct the 1–2 IM angle (<8 degrees) and thus deciding on the size wedge plate.

- I found two plates that are particularly good in providing stable fixation for early weight bearing and are low profile (Metatarsal Osteotomy Plate, Arthrex, Inc., Naples, FL, and OrthoLink Medial Wedge Osteotomy Plate, Tornier, Inc., Bloomington, MN) (**TECH FIG 2B**).
- Once the plate is placed, once again the correction is checked under fluoroscopy.
- The holes closest to the osteotomy are filled first.
- Bone obtained from either the excised medial eminence or autologous bone from the medial distal tibial metaphysis is used as bone graft (**TECH FIG 2C**).

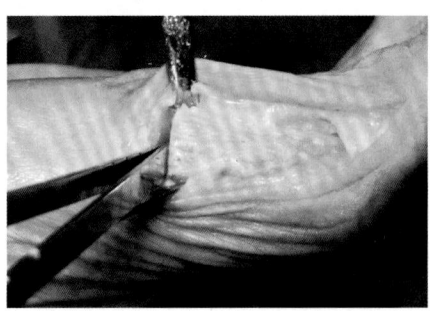

A

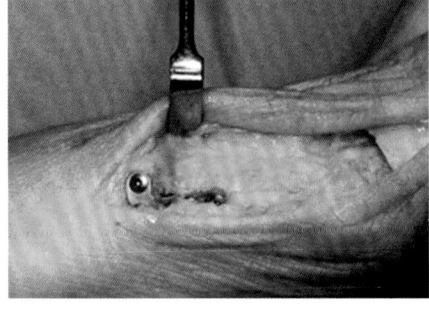

C

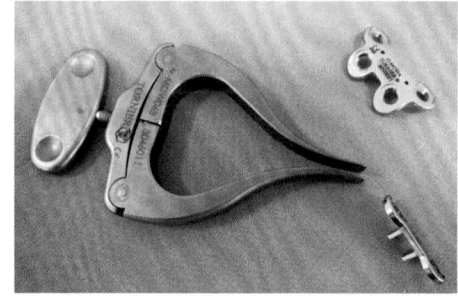

B

TECH FIG 2 A. Opening wedge osteotomy. Maintaining the integrity of the lateral cortex. **B.** OrthoLink Medial Wedge Osteotomy Plate (Tornier) for bunion correction. **C.** Placement of the Arthrex plate and bone graft.

TECHNIQUES

SECURING BONE GRAFT

- A 1-cm longitudinal medial incision is made along the distal tibia approximately 2 cm from the tip of the medial malleolus.
- The dissection is carried down to bone, and a 7-mm trephine needle is used to core out cancellous bone. This can be done several times until enough bone is obtained (**TECH FIG 3A**).
- Once the proximal osteotomy is secured, the distal medial-based closing wedge osteotomy (biplanar chevron) is performed (**TECH FIG 3B,C**). The resected bone wedge can be used as bone graft as well.

- If the DMAA is normal, only a "shortening" chevron is required (**TECH FIG 3D**).
- This osteotomy is secured with a cannulated compression screw.
- The medial capsulorrhaphy is then completed with 2-0 absorbable suture, and the alignment of the hallux is then checked clinically and radiologically (**TECH FIG 3E**).
- Any HV interphalangeus or pronation can be addressed with an Akin osteotomy.

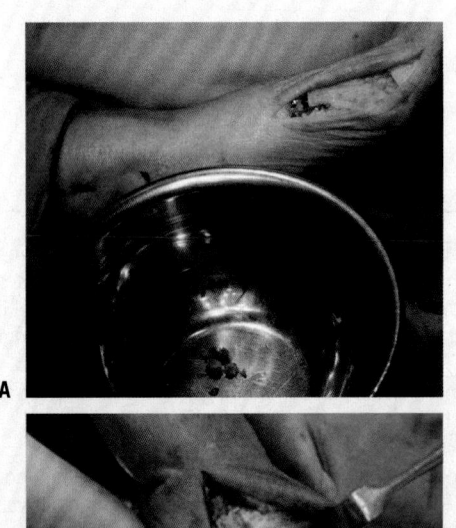
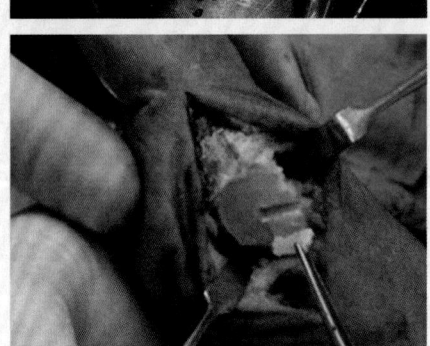
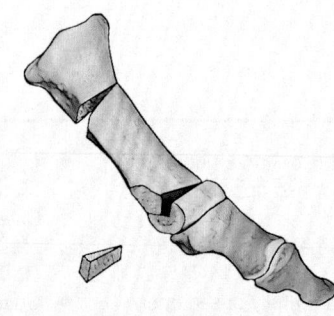
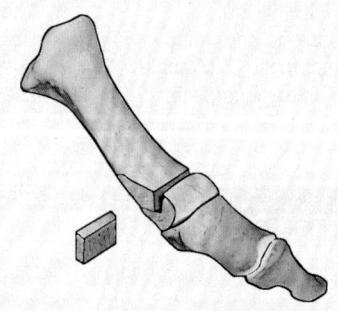
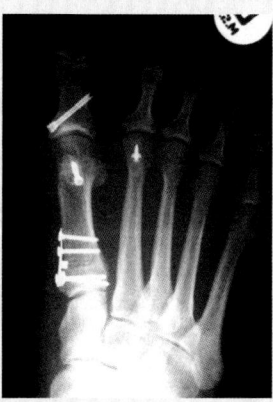

TECH FIG 3 A. A trephine needle is used to obtain cancellous autologous bone graft. **B,C.** Distal medial-based closing wedge osteotomy (biplanar chevron). **D.** Shortening chevron. **E.** Intraoperative fluoroscopy to check alignment after the medial capsulorrhaphy.

COMPLETION

- Skin is closed with absorbable 3-0 subcuticular suture.
- The foot is bandaged with a compression bandage with or without Reston foam spacer in the first web space (**TECH FIG 4**).

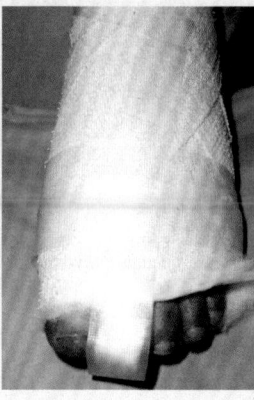

TECH FIG 4 Postoperative dressing with Reston foam.

Pearls and Pitfalls

- The distal lateral soft tissue release should be done through the first web space, as this gives better visualization of the structures and avoids damage to the articular cartilage if the lateral release is attempted through the medial incision.
- A transverse osteotomy is preferable (safer) and is carried out not less than 1 cm distal to the first TM joint.
- The osteotomy is carefully prised open with two flat osteotomes or a special distractor (comes with the Tornier set).
- Be aware of the larger IM angles (>17 degrees). There is a risk of distracting the osteotomy rather than opening it.
- Place the distractor as close to the medial cortex as possible to gain the maximum effect of opening the osteotomy rather than running the risk of distracting.
- Try placing the plate as plantar as possible on the medial surface, as the opening osteotomy tends to plantar flex the first metatarsal.
- Intraoperative fluoroscopy is a must! Use it liberally during all stages of the procedure. Once the medial capsulorrhaphy is complete, the first MPJ congruency is checked with fluoroscopy. Varus complications can be reduced by doing so.
- *Do not* overcorrect the first MPJ, expecting it to lose position later.
- Check the rotation of the hallux.
- Do not panic if the lateral cortex is violated. Trust the plate and bone graft.
- Do not forget the DMAA and/or HV interphalangeus, which will require a distal biplanar chevron and/or Akin osteotomy, respectively.
- The Akin osteotomy does not address the increased DMAA.
- Fifty percent of the success of the procedure is the aftercare. The surgeon must do the follow-up until discharge (6 weeks).
- Use the correct instruments, that is, an appropriate-size oscillating saw/blade. Do not compromise.

POSTOPERATIVE CARE

- The patient remains on strict bed rest with the operated foot elevated overnight.
- The following morning, the patient is mobilized in a wedge-heel postoperative shoe. Weight bearing on the heel as tolerated.
- Mobilization of the hallux begins as soon as is comfortable.
- Weekly checkup/dressings/strapping for first 2 weeks and then 2 weekly for the following 4 weeks
- X-rays are obtained at 6 weeks.
- The postoperative shoe is discontinued at 6 weeks if x-rays show union. Mobilization, footwear, scar care, and activities are explained to the patient.
- A night splint may be used for a further 4 to 6 weeks.

OUTCOMES

- The proximal opening wedge osteotomy is a powerful procedure for the correction of moderate to severe HV deformities, which pretty much meets the requirements for an excellent, if not ideal, proximal osteotomy. It is relatively simple with predictable correction and reproducible and stable enough to allow early weight bearing.
- The results in the literature are uniformly good.
- Wukich et al[15] reviewed 18 of their cases and had an 89% satisfaction rate. The HV angle and 1–2 IM angle improved by 13.5 and 9 degrees, respectively. They found no instances of malunion or nonunion with complete patient satisfaction.[15]
- Cooper et al[3] reported on 23 patients also with complete patient satisfaction. They achieved a mean correction of 15 degrees for the HV angle and 7 degrees for the 1–2 IM angle.[3]
- Shurnas[10] reported the initial experience on 50 patients. He obtained a mean correction of 20 degrees in the HV angle and 12 degrees in the 1–2 IM angle. Mean time to healing was 5 to 8 weeks with no instances of nonunion, malunion, or delayed union. All patients were satisfied with their outcome. The mean increase in the first metatarsal length of 1.9 mm was not significant.[10]

- Shurnas[10] also reported on a retrospective review of more than 90 patients with a minimum 2-year follow-up and found better than 90% good and excellent results.
  - There were five varus overcorrections, one nonunion, one delayed union, and two recurrences.[10]
- Saragas[8] showed an improvement in the American Orthopaedic Foot & Ankle Society (AOFAS) score from 51.3 to 86.8, with over 90% good or excellent results in 46 patients (64 feet). There were 5 cases of hallux varus, of which only 1 was symptomatic. Two developed significant recurrent HV deformity but were asymptomatic. A nonunion developed in 1 case and needed bone grafting.[8]
- Randhawa and Pepper[7] reported on 25 proximal opening wedge osteotomies. The HV angle improved by a mean of 30 degrees and the 1–2 IM angle by 8 degrees. There was an 80% satisfaction rate. They had 1 hallux varus, 1 nonunion, and 1 recurrence.[7]
- Nery et al[6] reported on 41 patients (70 feet). They used two types of fixation plates (Darco BOW or Arthrex LPS plate).
  - A biplanar chevron and/or Akin osteotomy was added as deemed fit depending on the magnitude of the distal angles.
  - The HV angle improved by a mean of 14 degrees and the 1–2 IM angle by 8 degrees. The AOFAS score improved from a mean 50 to 82. Even though both fixation systems were similar regarding correction capacity and stability, the Arthrex system scored significantly higher than Darco in the AOFAS postoperative evaluation, possibly due to the extremely low profile of the Arthrex, avoiding local symptoms.[6]
- The earlier studies have found no adverse effects as a result of violating the lateral cortex or the increased length of the first metatarsal.
- In recent years, several authors have published on the double osteotomy.
- Siekmann et al[11] reported on 32 patients at a mean follow-up period of 59.3 months. The total postoperative AOFAS score was 94.2, and radiographic union was achieved in all cases. Two cases of early avascular necrosis of the first metatarsal head were diagnosed but no late sequelae of arthritis or metatarsal head collapse.[11]

- Forty-five patients (49 feet) were reviewed by Jeyaseelan et al[5] at a mean follow-up of 35.4 months. They, too, reported a high postoperative AOFAS score and a low complication rate of 4.1%. They concluded that the procedure is reliable, safe, and with excellent outcomes.[5]
- In a similar series of 45 patients (47 feet) with a mean follow-up of 45 months, Al-Nammari et al[1] also found that the procedure provides powerful correction. They used the Manchester-Oxford Foot Questionnaire with a mean postoperative score of 12.9.[1]

COMPLICATIONS

- The author of this chapter had five varus overcorrections (prior to obtaining intraoperative fluoroscopy), of which one required arthrodesis.
  - Two developed recurrent HV (asymptomatic).
  - One nonunion requiring bone grafting
- Hardware irritation occurred in two cases and led to removal of the internal fixation.

REFERENCES

1. Al-Nammari SS, Christofi T, Clark C. Double fist metatarsal and Akin osteotomy for severe hallux valgus. Foot Ankle Int 2015;36(10):1215–1222.
2. Bonney G, Macnab I. Hallux valgus and hallux rigidus: a critical surgery of operative results. J Bone Joint Surg Br 1952;34:366–385.
3. Cooper MT, Berlet GC, Shurnas PS, et al. Proximal opening-wedge osteotomy of the first metatarsal for correction of hallux valgus. Surg Technol Int 2007;16:215–219.
4. Hardy MA, Grove JR. Opening wedge osteotomy of the first metatarsal using the Arthrex® Low Profile Plate and Screw System™. Podiatry Internet J 2007;2(4)2.
5. Jeyaseelan L, Chandrashekar D, Mulligan A, et al. Correction of moderate to severe hallux valgus with combined proximal opening wedge and distal chevron osteotomies: a reliable technique. Bone Joint J 2016;98-B(9):1202–1207.
6. Nery C, Réssio C, de Azevedo Santa Cruz G, et al. Proximal opening-wedge osteotomy of the first metatarsal for moderate and severe hallux valgus using low profile plates. Foot Ankle Surg 2013;19:276–282.
7. Randhawa S, Pepper D. Radiographic evaluation of hallux valgus treated with opening wedge osteotomy. Foot Ankle Int 2009;30:427–431.
8. Saragas NP. Proximal opening-wedge osteotomy of the first metatarsal for hallux valgus using a low profile plate. Foot Ankle Int 2009;30:976–980.
9. Scranton PE Jr, Zuckerman JD. Bunion surgery in adolescents: results of surgical treatment. J Pediatr Orthop 1984;4(1):39–43.
10. Shurnas PS. Proximal opening wedge osteotomy of the first metatarsal: biomechanical and clinical evaluation. In: Proceedings from the American Academy of Orthopaedic Surgeons Annual Meeting; March 22–26, 2006; Chicago, IL.
11. Siekmann W, Watson TS, Roggelin M. Correction of moderate to severe hallux valgus with isometric first metatarsal double osteotomy. Foot Ankle Int 2014;35(11):1122–1130.
12. Simmonds FA, Menelaus MB. Hallux valgus in adolescents. J Bone Joint Surg Br 1960;42(4):761–768.
13. Trethowan J. Hallux valgus. In: Choyce CC, ed. A System of Surgery. New York: PB Hoeber, 1923:1046–1049.
14. Watson TS, Shurnas PS. The proximal opening wedge osteotomy for the correction of hallux valgus deformity. Tech Foot Ankle Surg 2008;7:17–24.
15. Wukich DK, Roussel AJ, Dial DM. Correction of metatarsus primus varus with an opening wedge plate: a review of 18 procedures. J Foot Ankle Surg 2009;48(4):420–426.

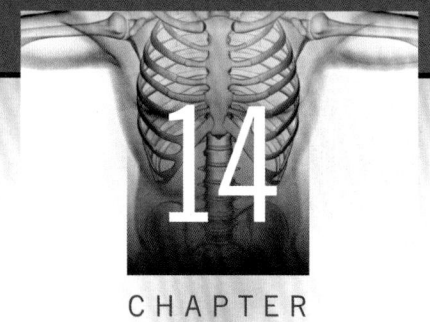

14
CHAPTER

The Proximal Rotational Metatarsal Osteotomy for Hallux Valgus

Pablo Wagner and Emilio Wagner

DEFINITION

- Hallux valgus (HV) is a multiplanar deformity, including metatarsus varus, hallux valgus and first ray pronation.
- A coronal malalignment (metatarsal pronation or external rotation) is present in most HV patients (87%).[7]
- Metatarsal pronation consists of metatarsal rotation in addition to rotation of the whole sesamoid complex and great toe itself.
- Persistent pronation in operated HV patients increases the deformity relapse rate at long term up to 12 times.[8,9]
- The key in determining how to treat HV is to determine which deformities are present in a specific case. If metatarsus varus and pronation exist, both should be corrected to achieve the best possible outcome with the lowest achievable relapse rate.

ANATOMY

- The first metatarsal is approximately 5 cm long. The metatarsophalangeal joint is congruent and allows motion in all three planes. The tarsometatarsal (TMT) joint is a bilobulated joint that participates during the gait cycle as part of the shock absorption mechanism. It distributes the pressure between the whole forefoot on weight bearing, actively unloading the lesser metatarsals.[15,16]
- Soft tissue attachments proximally to the first metatarsal are the TMT capsule, collateral ligaments, peroneus longus tendon, and tibialis anterior tendon. Distally, in addition to the metatarsophalangeal capsule and the medial and lateral collaterals, the abductor tendon spans this joint medially, and the adductor tendon (with two origins) inserts into the proximal phalanx on its lateral edge and to the lateral sesamoid. The metatarsosesamoid ligament is a structure that originates at the lateral sesamoid and inserts laterally at the metatarsal head–neck. The intermetatarsal ligament spans the intermetatarsal 1–2 space and goes from the second metatarsal to the lateral sesamoid.

PATHOGENESIS

- It is not known whether pronation occurs before, after, or simultaneously with the first metatarsal varus.
- When the metatarsal varizes and rotates, the sesamoid complex rotates in conjunction, given their mutual multiple ligamentous attachments. As the sesamoid complex is congruent to sesamoid facets on the metatarsal and continuous with the medial capsule and deep intermetatarsal and metatarsosesamoid ligaments, during the initial pronation, the sesamoid complex rotates following the metatarsal, without dislocating from its facets (FIG 1).
  - In long-standing HV, dislocation of the sesamoid complex from the metatarsal sesamoid facets can occur, given that as metatarsal varus increases, the intermetatarsal ligament and adductor tendon keep their attachments to the lateral sesamoid, a loose medial capsule is present, and there is a constant lateralizing vector pull of the flexor hallucis longus (FHL) tendon that goes in between the sesamoids. All this factors contribute in a dislocation of the sesamoids from the metatarsal sesamoid facets in long standing HV.[6,11,12]
- The FHL traverses between the sesamoids and inserts into the distal phalanx. If the sesamoid complex is pronated-lateralized in an HV patient, the FHL tendon will constantly pull the great toe into valgus, progressively increasing the deformity and/or contributing to HV relapse.
  - The sesamoid lateral displacement is directly correlated with metatarsal pronation.[7]

NATURAL HISTORY

- As shown by some authors, HV surgery relapse rate ranges from 30% to 70% in the long term.[1–4,13]
- As previously said, 87% of patients have medial ray pronation. In patients without HV, pronation can measure up to 14 degrees. On the other hand, in HV patients, the mean is significantly higher (22 degrees).
  - The pronation of the medial ray has been identified by some authors as an important recurrence factor.
  - Shibuya et al[13] identified it as the most important relapse factor. They published a recurrence rate of 51% when the postoperative sesamoid position was above 4 following the Hardy and Clapham classification and 60% if the sesamoid position was above 5.
  - Similarly, Kaufmann et al[5] demonstrated the sesamoid position to be a significant relapse factor.
  - Park and Lee[10] showed that sesamoid position can even be a relapse factor identified in immediate postoperative non–weight-bearing radiographs.
  - The first publications that identified postoperative persistent first ray pronation as an HV relapse factor were two studies by Okuda et al.[8,9] One focused on sesamoid incomplete postoperative reduction and the other on metatarsal bone pronation.
  - As it was presented by Kim and Young,[6] tibial sesamoid position is directly related to metatarsal pronation.

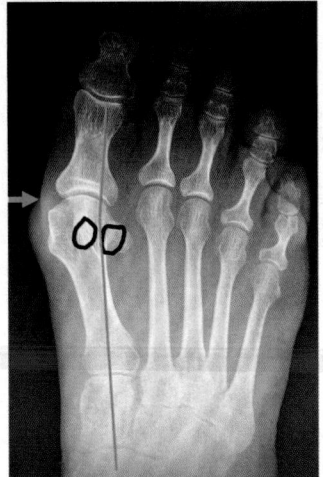 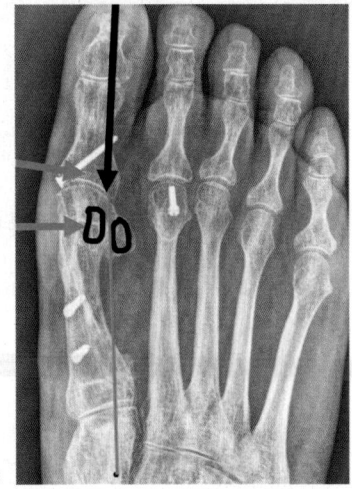 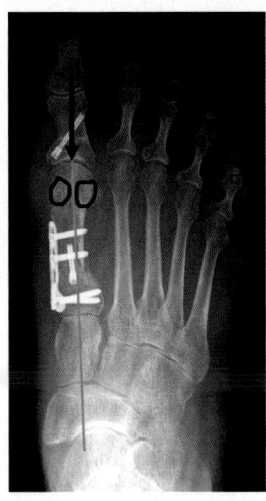

FIG 1 AP weight-bearing foot x-rays. **A.** Laterally displaced sesamoids (*circles*) contribute to further increase HV deformity by having a constant laterally displaced tendon pull (lateral to the metatarsophalangeal joint center; *arrow*). **B.** HV managed with the scarf technique. Sesamoids (*circles*) are still laterally displaced influenced by a persistent metatarsal pronation (round lateral head contour), producing a lateral pull at the metatarsophalangeal joint (*bottom blue arrow*). A laterally displaced FHL pull (*black arrow*) further contributes to the HV deformity (*top blue arrow*). This contributes to a progressive increase–relapse in HV deformity. **C.** HV managed with the PROMO technique. Sesamoids (*circles*) are centrally located below the metatarsal head, with a centered FHL pull (*black arrow*). There is no lateral thrust at the metatarsophalangeal joint. The metatarsal head lateral contour is squared.

PATIENT HISTORY AND PHYSICAL FINDINGS

- Patient history may include the following:
  - Family history of HV
  - Pain over medial bunion eminence and metatarsalgia that improves with wide soft shoes.
  - Unable to wear elegant or narrow shoes. Many patients hide their feet out of sight.
- Patient physical finding may include the following:
  - HV
  - Prominent medial bunion
  - Big toe pronation (as seen looking at the nail bed orientation)
  - Second or third ray metatarsalgia (pain plantarly and/or dorsally)
  - Medial arch flattening (flatfoot)
  - Bunionette
  - Claw toes

IMAGING AND OTHER DIAGNOSTIC STUDIES

- The gold standard for metatarsal pronation and varus measurement is a weight-bearing computed tomography scan.
- The pronation angle is measured between a line through the sesamoid facets (image where the sesamoids are wider) and the floor line. This is a straightforward and fast technique and takes into account the functional axis of the metatarsal (sesamoids facet).
- Another pronation measurement method considers using the anteroposterior (AP) foot weight-bearing view.[14]
  - This method divides pronation in three stages: 10 to 20 degrees, 20 to 30 degrees, and more than 30 degrees.
  - It is based on the metatarsal head lateral round shape. This roundness represents the metatarsal condyles that are visible laterally given the metatarsal rotation (pronation).
    - In stage 1 (10 to 20 degrees), the lateral first metatarsal head shape is rounded, but an acute angle at

the lateral joint corner can be seen before continuing with the condyle (step) **(FIG 2A,B)**.
- For stage 2 (20 to 30 degrees), a continuous line from the joint line to the metatarsal condyles can be seen with no acute angle or step between them, but it does not form a perfectly round circle **(FIG 2C,D)**.
- For stage 3, the metatarsal condyles line is continuous with the first metatarsal metatarsophalangeal joint, forming a perfect round line. A circle can be superimposed on the metatarsal head, and its contour will be congruent with the metatarsal head laterally **(FIG 2E,F)**.

DIFFERENTIAL DIAGNOSIS

- Metatarsus adductus
- Hallux dislocation
- Gout (podagra)
- First metatarsophalangeal synovitis

NONOPERATIVE MANAGEMENT

- Nonoperative treatment can be effective to improve symptoms.
- Most of the time, silicone devices are used to protect the bony prominence from direct shoe pressure.

SURGICAL MANAGEMENT

- The rationale behind proximal rotational metatarsal osteotomy (PROMO) is that it consists of a single oblique osteotomy through which rotation is performed. It offers several advantages:
  - Given the obliquity of the osteotomy, rotation, pronation, and varus correction are all achieved at the same time, without the requirement of wedge resection.
  - No undesired shortening of the metatarsal occurs. (But if desired, shortening is easy to achieve.)

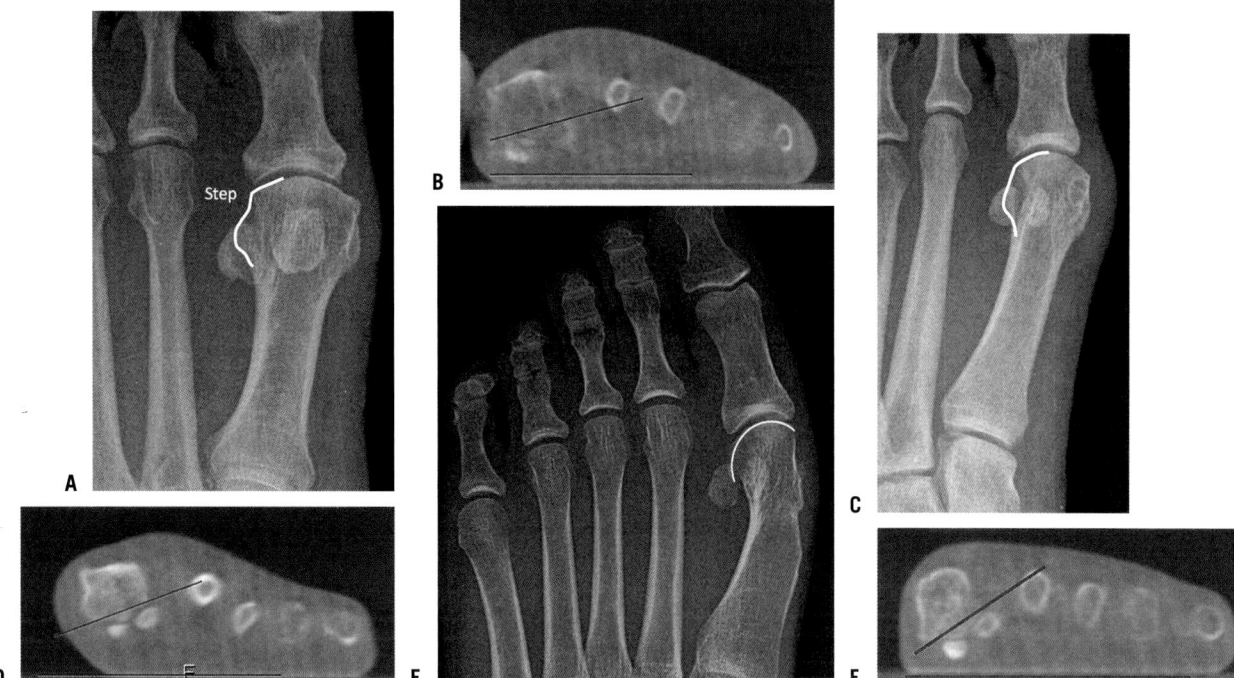

FIG 2 Comparisons of x-rays versus weight-bearing computed tomography (WBCT) scans in three patients. **A,B.** WBCT shows with 15 degrees of first metatarsal pronation (stage 1). The x-ray shows at the lateral corner of the head an acute angle followed by a round shape (condyle) with a straight segment in between (step). **C,D.** WBCT shows 22 degrees of first metatarsal pronation (stage 2). The x-ray shows at the lateral corner of the head a continuum of the distal joint with the lateral round shape. No step is present. **E,F.** WBCT shows 32 degrees of first metatarsal pronation (stage 3). The x-ray shows a completely round head shape laterally with no step.

- The osteotomy angulation is from dorsal distal to plantar proximal, so weight bearing closes the osteotomy, making nonunion extremely rare **(FIG 3A–D).**
- Indications
  - Age younger than 65 years, to avoid poor bone quality that could compromise fixation
  - Mild to moderate HV deformity (HV angle <40 degrees)
  - Stable TMT joint
  - Pronation has to be present.

Preoperative Planning

- To calculate the osteotomy angulation needed to correct the patient's varus and pronation, the intermetatarsal angle (IMA) and pronation angle have to be measured. An AP weight-bearing foot x-ray is needed.

- Metatarsal pronation can be measured on the AP weight-bearing foot x-ray and is classified as stage 1, 2, or 3.
- Using the provided table, choose the osteotomy angulation that corresponds to the IMA and pronation measured **(TABLE 1).**

Positioning

- Patient is positioned supine on the operating table.
- No gluteal bumps are required. Feet should lie comfortably.
- Bone prominences should be protected or padded.
- Regarding equipment, x-ray machine is necessary. Depending on the type available, an x-ray tech is needed or not.

Approach

- A medial minimally invasive or an open approach can be used.

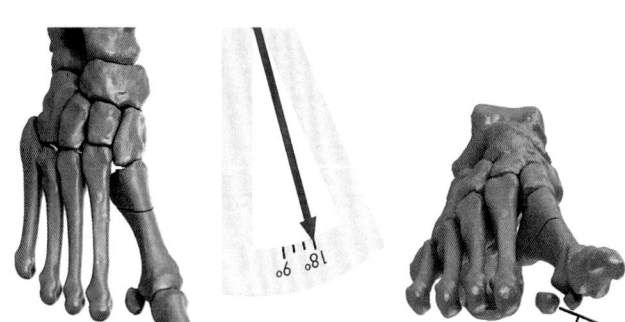

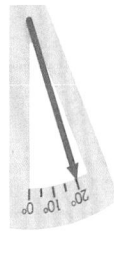

A

FIG 3 Three-dimensional representations of a metatarsus varus with pronation. **A.** IMA of 18 degrees and pronation of 20 degrees are measured at the sesamoid facets. *(continued)*

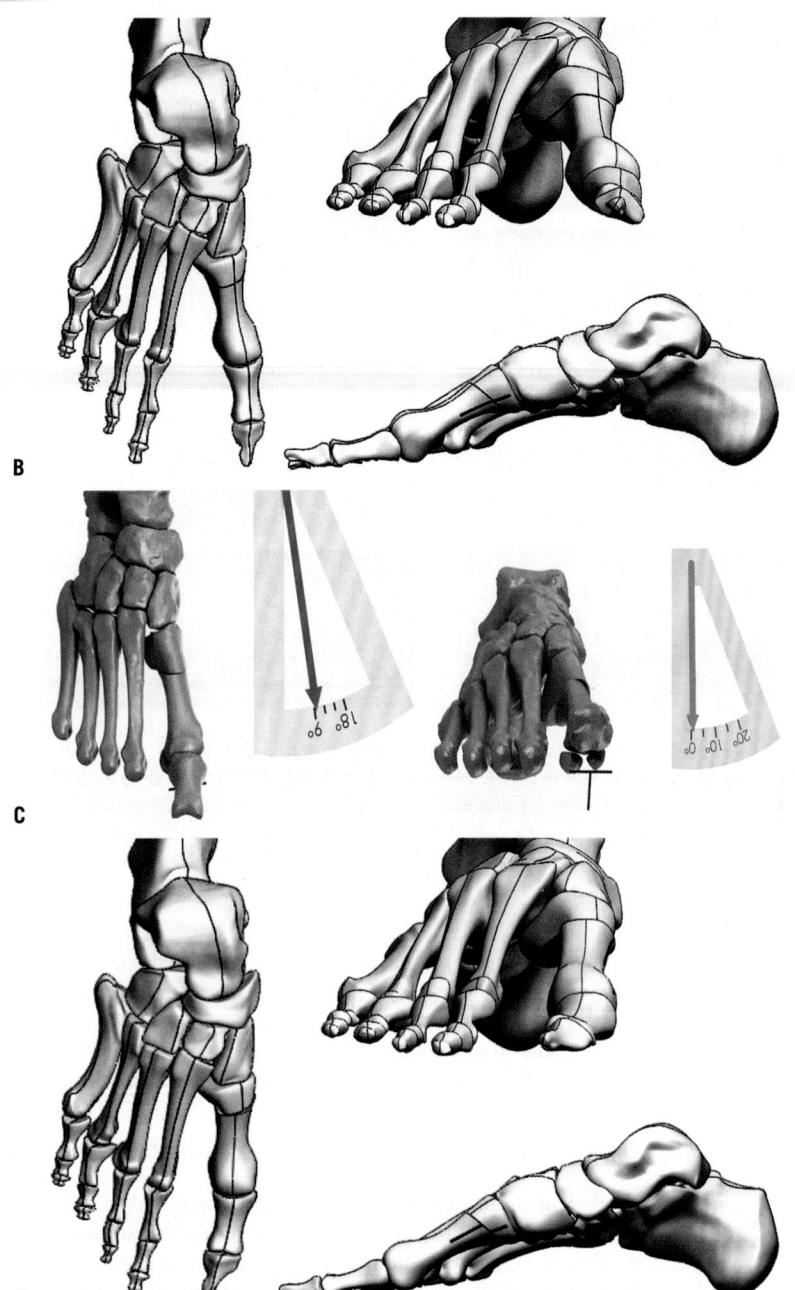

FIG 3 *(continued)* **B.** The PROMO is shown, drawn in three planes. **C,D.** After correction, the varus and pronation are corrected.

B

C

D

IMA (degrees)	10–19	20–29	30–39
8–10	38	28	23
11–12	47	33	28
13–14	55	38	33
15–17	55	42	38
18–20	55	47	42

TABLE 1 Proximal Rotational Metatarsal Osteotomy Angulation Calculation[a]

Pronation Angle (degrees)

[a]To obtain the osteotomy angulation needed to correct a certain deformity, find the value in the table that corresponds to the patient's intermetatarsal angle (IMA) and pronation angle.

EXPOSURE

- For a medial minimally invasive, approach, an incision is made approximately 4 cm long starting at the TMT joint and ending close to the metatarsal neck (identified by palpation) **(TECH FIG 1A)**.
  - Alternatively, an open approach from the TMT joint to the proximal phalanx can be used (same approach as in Scarf osteotomy).

- The soft tissues dorsal and plantar of the metatarsal at the mid-diaphysis are dissected, without violating the TMT joint or the metatarsal neck plantarly **(TECH FIG 1B)**.

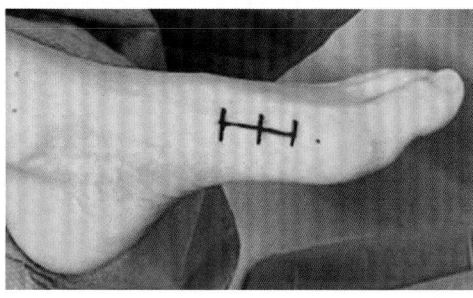 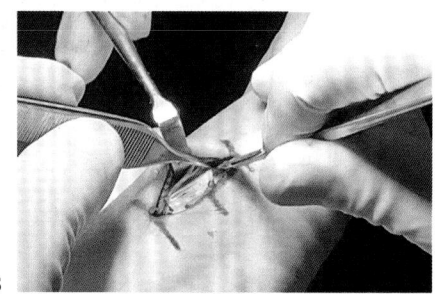

TECH FIG 1 A. The medial minimally invasive approach starts at the TMT joint and extends distally for 3 to 4 cm. If an open approach is chosen, the incision should extend to the metatarsal head. **B.** All dorsal and plantar soft tissue should be dissected off the metatarsal.

PLACEMENT OF GUIDEWIRE AND POSITIONING JIG

- Drive a 1.6-mm Kirschner wire (K-wire) 1 cm distal to the TMT joint at the metatarsal equator. This guidewire should be parallel to the floor and perpendicular to the metatarsal.
  - A tray lid can be used as weight-bearing surface for the foot to help with the parallelism. An assistant should hold the tray lid against the foot sole to simulate weight bearing while the surgeon drives the wire parallel to the lid (weight-bearing surface) **(TECH FIG 2A)**.
  - After this wire is in place, under fluoroscopy (AP foot view), reposition it to leave the wire perpendicular to the metatarsal **(TECH FIG 2B,C)**.

- Double-check with the tray lid that the wire is parallel to the foot sole (weight-bearing surface).
- Slide the positioning jig through the 0-degree hole onto the K-wire aligned with the metatarsal **(TECH FIG 2D)**.
- Add a 1.6-mm K-wire through the jig using the hole that matches the pronation measured in your preoperative planning (eg, 10 to 20 degrees) **(TECH FIG 2E)**.
- Remove the 0-degree wire and positioning jig.

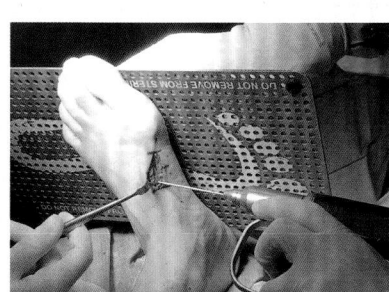 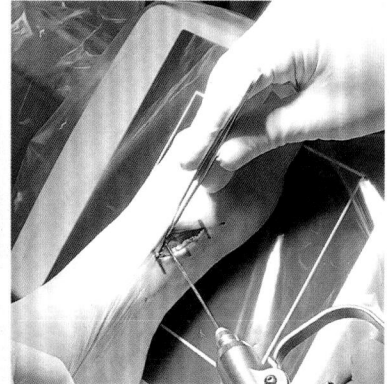 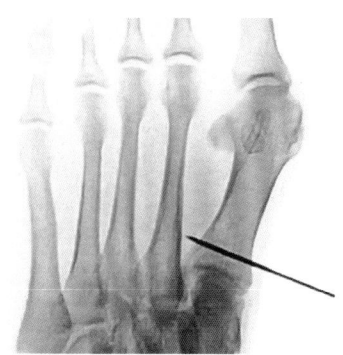

TECH FIG 2 A. The initial guidewire should be driven 1 cm distal to the TMT joint, parallel to the foot sole. It helps to hold a tray lid (or similar) to the patient's foot sole (simulating a weight-bearing surface) and drive the guidewire parallel to the lid. Drive it through only the proximal metatarsal cortex. **B.** Under fluoroscopy, make sure this guidewire is perpendicular to the metatarsal before driving it through the distal metatarsal cortex. **C.** Fluoroscopic AP foot view. It shows the guidewire perpendicular to the metatarsal. *(continued)*

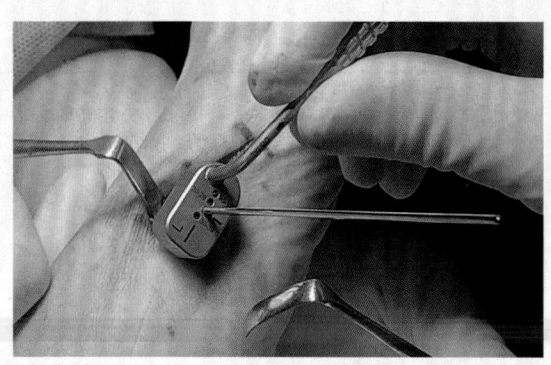 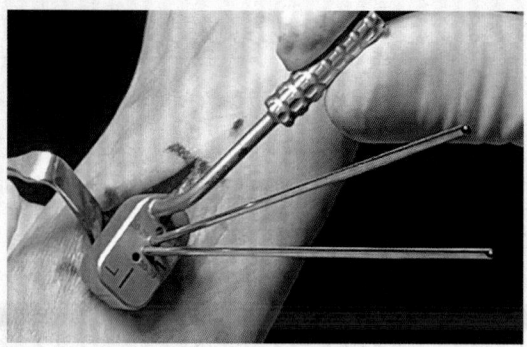

TECH FIG 2 *(continued)* **D.** Slide the positioning jig on its 0-degree hole through the guidewire, holding it aligned with the metatarsal. **E.** Add a 1.6-mm K-wire using the hole labeled with the pronation angle measured (10 to 20, 20 to 30, or more than 30 degrees). Then remove the initial guidewire and the jig.

OSTEOTOMY AND ROTATION JIG

- Slide the osteotomy jig through the K-wire using the hole labeled with the osteotomy angulation previously chosen (eg, 42 degrees). Fix the jig distally at the metatarsal equator **(TECH FIG 3A,B)**.
  - Make sure the jig is distal to the TMT joint and with adequate soft tissue dissection.
- Choose the osteotomy slot on the jig that exits plantarly 1 cm distal to the TMT joint **(TECH FIG 3C)**.
- With the oscillating saw, perform the osteotomy, leaving the lateral metatarsal cortex intact. Remove the osteotomy jig **(TECH FIG 3D)**.

- Apply the rotation jig on the distal wire through its 0-degree hole **(TECH FIG 3E)**.
- Add a second wire using the pronation hole that corresponds to the pronation value previously measured and chosen for the osteotomy calculation (eg, 10 to 20 degrees). Remove the 0-degree wire and the rotation jig **(TECH FIG 3F)**.
- You will have now two wires divergent from each other. This divergence is the pronation that is going to be corrected.

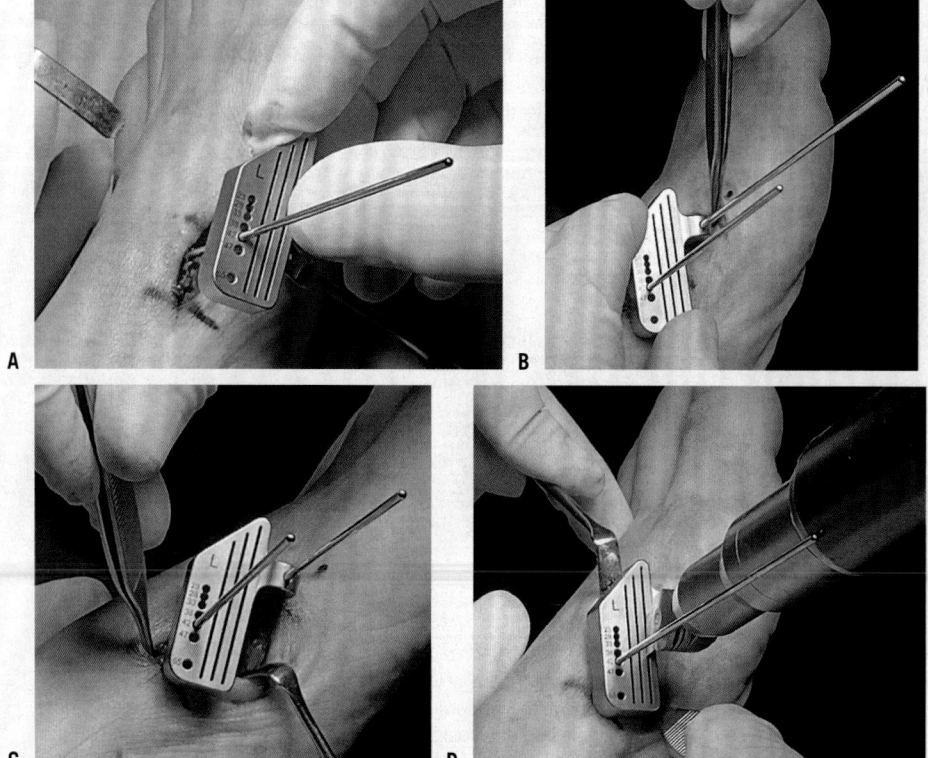

TECH FIG 3 A. Slide the osteotomy jig through the K-wire using the hole labeled with the chosen osteotomy angulation (see **TABLE 1**). **B.** Fix the osteotomy jig distally at the metatarsal equator. **C.** Choose the osteotomy slot that does not violate the TMT joint. **D.** Perform a partial osteotomy (leave lateral metatarsal cortex intact). *(continued)*

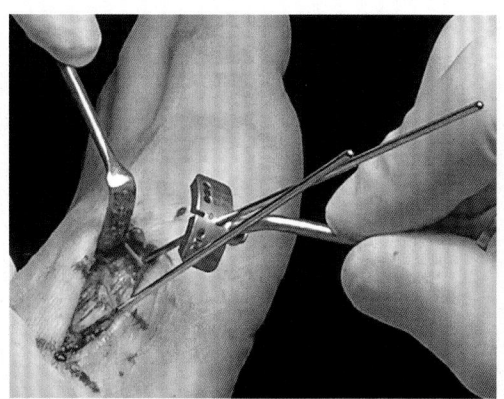
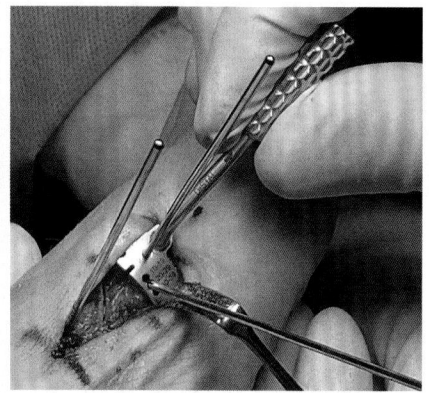

TECH FIG 3 *(continued)* **E.** Slide the rotational jig through the distal K-wire using its 0-degree hole. **F.** While holding the jig aligned with the metatarsal, drive a K-wire through the hole labeled with the pronation measured. Then remove the 0-degree wire and jig.

OSTEOTOMY COMPLETION AND BONE ROTATION

- Using the saw blade, finish the osteotomy (plantar cortex). Once the osteotomy is completed, release the periosteum and peroneus longus fibers that attach laterally to the distal metatarsal segment **(TECH FIG 4A)**.
  - In cases of osteotomies above 42 degrees of angulation, using a rongeur to remove the most plantar proximal spike of the distal segment may be necessary to help loosen up the distal fragment.
  - Move the distal fragment to make sure it easily moves and rotates. Any soft tissue attachment will compromise the adequate correction **(TECH FIG 4B)**.
- Grab the distal metatarsal segment using a Backhaus or towel clamp. Using the clamp, internally rotate (supinate) the distal

metatarsal segment until both medial wires become parallel to each other from a "mediolateral" view **(TECH FIG 4C)**.
- Always overrotate the distal segment slightly, given that some rotation is normally lost during the next steps of the procedure. If you look at the foot in a dorsoplantar view, that is, AP view, the wires have to be divergent from each other **(TECH FIG 4D)**.
- The plantar–medial border of the distal fragment should end up being flush with the medial cortex of the proximal segment **(TECH FIG 4E)**.
  - It is possible to add a 1- to 2-mm distal segment lateral displacement (distal translation–chevron effect) if necessary, depending on the HV severity.

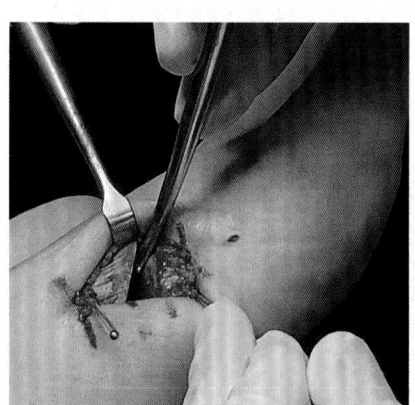
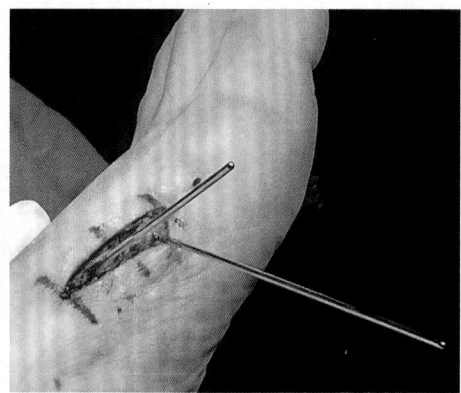
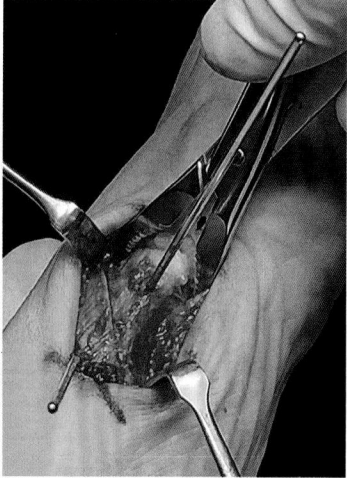

TECH FIG 4 A. Complete the osteotomy using a saw. Release all soft tissues laterally at the osteotomy site. Use a rongeur or elevator to make sure no soft tissue is restraining the osteotomy movement. **B.** Medial view of the foot showing the divergence of the wires. This is the pronation that will be corrected with the PROMO. **C.** Apply a clamp at the distal metatarsal. Rotate the metatarsal until the wires are parallel (a minimum overcorrection is desired) from a mediolateral view. *(continued)*

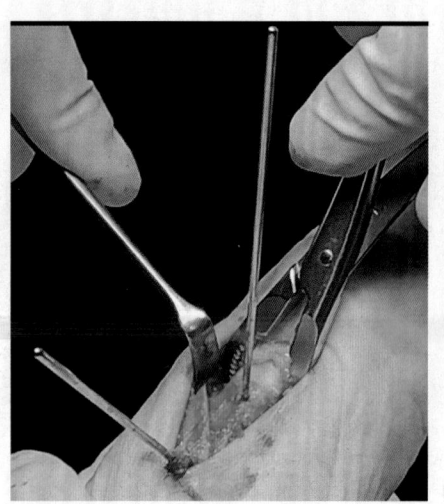
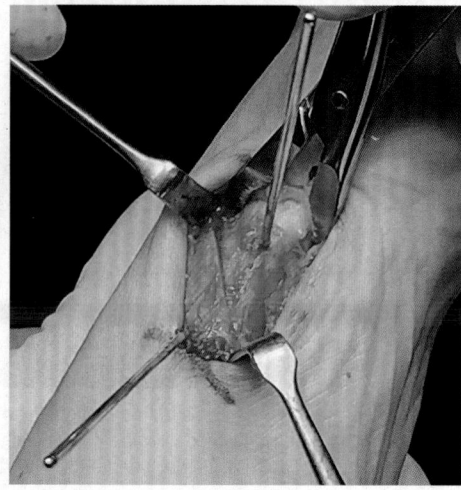

TECH FIG 4 *(continued)* **D.** The wires should diverge in the AP plane (because of the metatarsus varus correction). **E.** The osteotomy should be flush at the plantar medial cortex. Dorsally, a 2-mm step will occur.

PROVISIONAL FIXATION

- Drive two wires perpendicular to the osteotomy for provisional fixation.
  - Start with one wire starting distal plantar on the distal segment and directed dorsal proximal. This wire should start as plantarly as proximal as possible on the distal fragment **(TECH FIG 5A)**.
  - Add a second wire starting proximal dorsal to distal plantar. Start this wire as distal as possible on the proximal segment and aim it parallel to the first wire **(TECH FIG 5B,C)**.
- Check under fluoroscopy that metatarsal correction was achieved **(TECH FIG 5D,E)**.

- The second metatarsal should be parallel to the distal metatarsal segment. The metatarsal head should have changed to a more squared shaped laterally. The sesamoids could be still slightly laterally dislocated given that the great toe is still in valgus and no capsular reefing has been performed.
- The Akin osteotomy aligns the great toe and therefore the FHL tendon and the whole sesamoid complex. In this case, no capsular reefing was performed, but an Akin was performed. In the final postoperative x-rays, a complete sesamoid relocation can be seen.

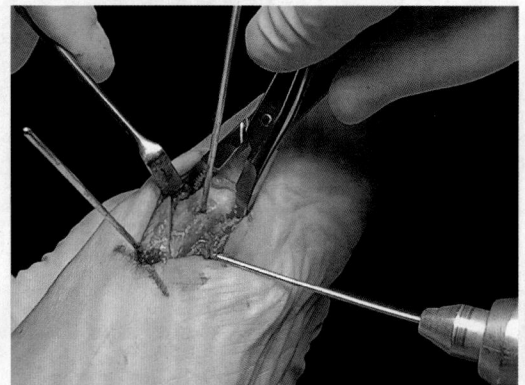
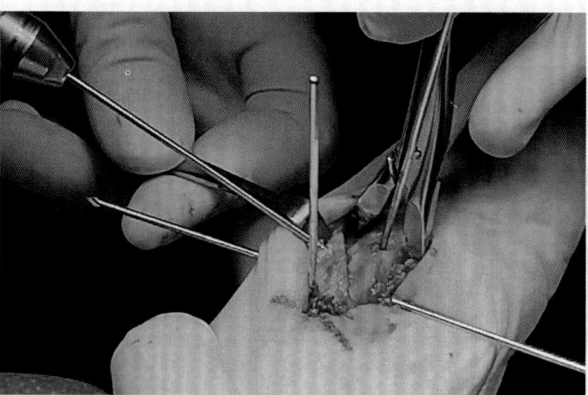

TECH FIG 5 Provisional fixation of the osteotomy. **A.** Drive the first K-wire plantar–dorsal. **B.** Drive a second wire dorsal–plantar, parallel to the first wire. *(continued)*

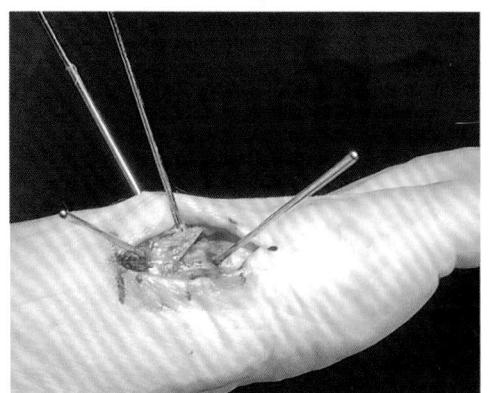

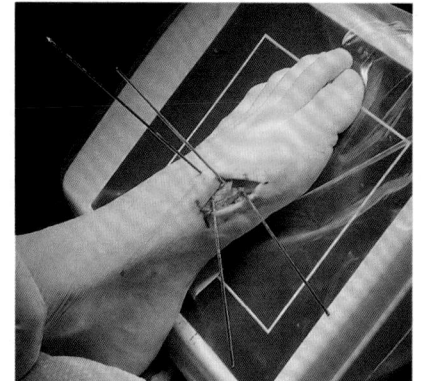

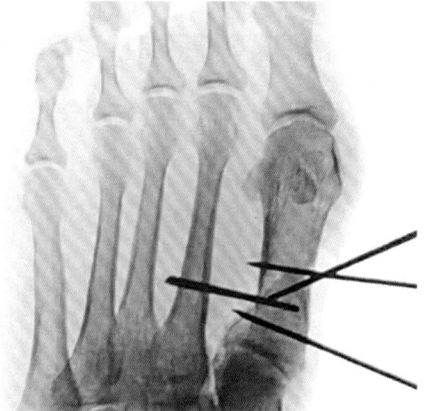

TECH FIG 5 *(continued)* **C.** After transient fixation, make sure the guidewires are still parallel to each other (or slightly overrotated). Leave both osteotomy wires dorsally prominent. **D.** Check the osteotomy correction radiographically. **E.** Fluoroscopic view of the metatarsal correction. The distal metatarsal segment should be parallel to the second metatarsal. No lateral round sign at the head should be seen (pronation corrected).

ADDUCTOR TENDON RELEASE

- Adductor tendon release can be performed before or after the osteotomy completion (**TECH FIG 6A**).
- Place a beaver blade in the intermetatarsal space between the first and second metatarsal heads (**TECH FIG 6B**).
  - Angle your hand 30 degrees proximal and lateral to aim to the lateral aspect of the first metatarsophalangeal joint. Insert the blade in this angulation.

- Enter the metatarsophalangeal capsule and then release the adductor tendon by surrounding the lateral proximal phalangeal corner.
- After the tendon is released, a brighter spot can be seen on x-rays.
- Remove the beaver blade and try applying a varus movement on the great toe to make sure the adductor tendon was completely.

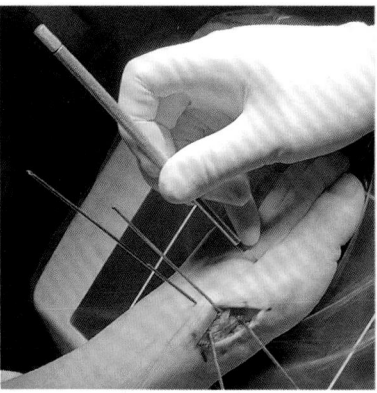

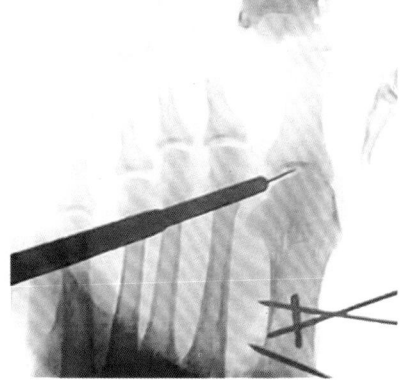

TECH FIG 6 A. Adductor release is performed percutaneously in the metatarsal 1–2 space. **B.** Under x-ray, enter the metatarsophalangeal joint laterally. Do not violate the plantar capsule. Using a beaver blade or similar, section the adductor tendon by surrounding the lateral edge of the proximal phalanx.

DEFINITIVE FIXATION

- Remove any bone steps medially on the metatarsal that could prevent a good bone–plate apposition **(TECH FIG 7A)**.
- Apply a locking plate medially with the precision guide in place. Check that the plate center is at the level of the osteotomy. Make sure that proximally the plate is distal to the TMT joint.
- Fix the plate with three threaded olive wires to the metatarsal. Drive the recommended wire through the precision guide for interfragmentary screw placement **(TECH FIG 7B)**.
  - Measure the screw length using the supplied instruments.

- Drive a 3.0- or 3.5-mm cannulated fully threaded screw across the osteotomy **(TECH FIG 7C)**.
  - Make sure that the screw head is not prominent dorsally to avoid dorsal discomfort.
- After positioning this screw, replace the plate olive wires one by one with 2.5-mm locking screws **(TECH FIG 7D)**.
- Check the correct metatarsal fixation and final position under x-ray.
  - Sometimes, an abnormal distal metatarsal articular angle (DMAA) is present. Do not hesitate to add a distal biplanar chevron if necessary **(TECH FIG 7E,F)**.

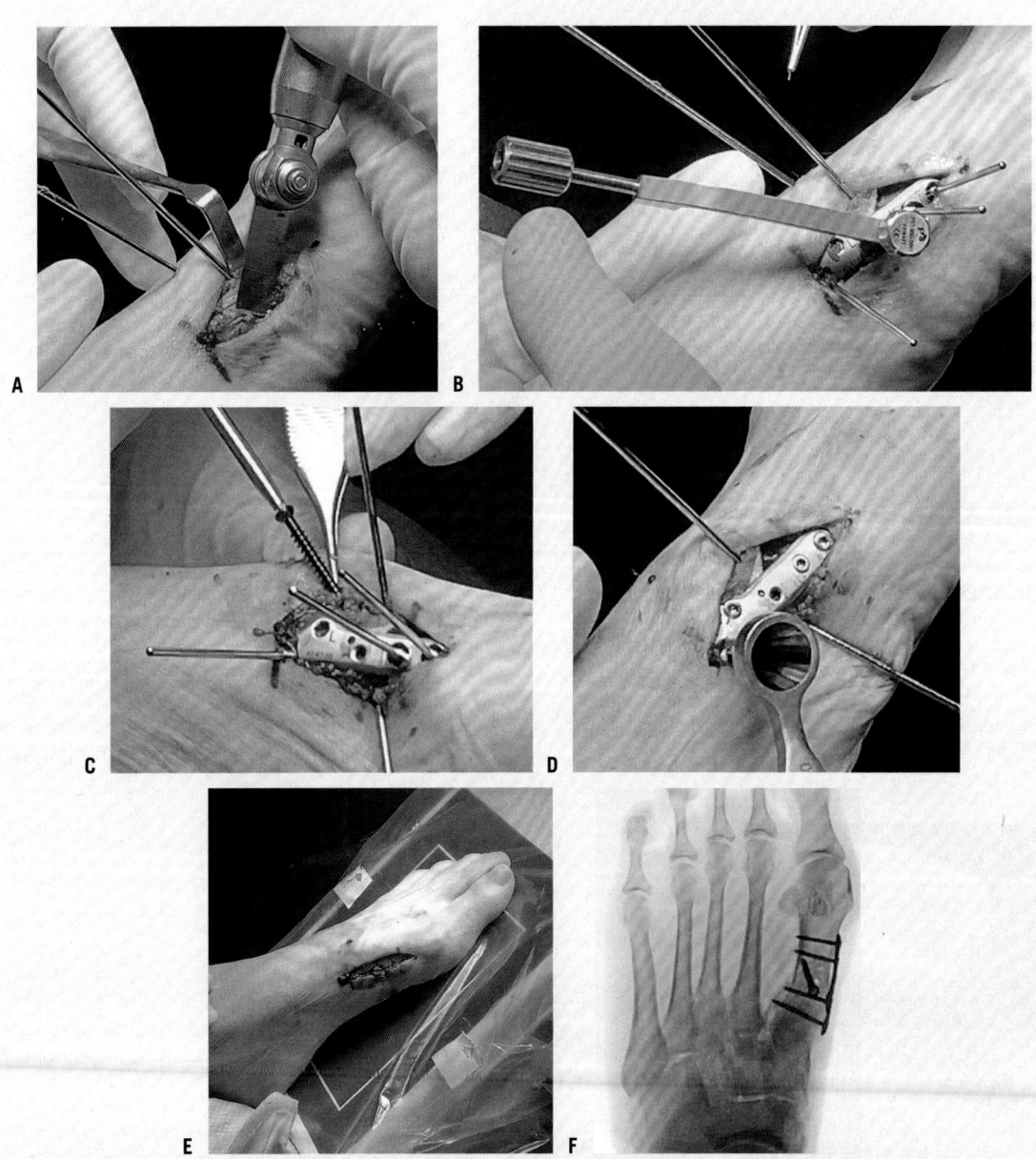

TECH FIG 7 **A.** Remove any bone steps at the osteotomy site to help with plate–bone apposition. Remove the guide-wires. **B.** Fix the plate medially using three olive wires. **C.** Using the precision guide, drive the appropriate wire and subsequent cannulated screw through the osteotomy. **D.** Lock the plate using four 2.5-mm locking screws. **E,F.** Check under x-ray that a satisfactory metatarsal alignment was achieved.

MEDIAL EMINENCE RESECTION AND AKIN OSTEOTOMY

- The Akin osteotomy is optional depending on the foot cosmesis to achieve a straight great toe.
- Using an open or a minimally invasive approach, for example, using a Shannon burr, proceed to remove the medial head eminence (if any) **(TECH FIG 8)**.

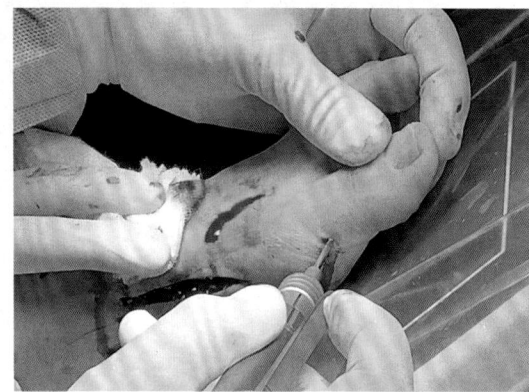

TECH FIG 8 If desired, perform an Akin osteotomy (open or minimally invasive).

CLOSURE

- During surgery, care has to be taken to gently manipulate soft tissues. Skin is never grabbed with pickups.

- Close the subcutaneous layer with resorbable suture (three or four stitches) and proceed with skin closure with intradermal technique.

TECHNIQUES

Pearls and Pitfalls

Osteotomy is rotating but not correcting IMA.	• This is because the osteotomy rotation was performed not keeping the osteotomy closed. It must be kept in mind that while the metatarsal is supinated, a simultaneous valgus deviation occurs. But this will only occur if the osteotomy is kept closed and congruent during rotation. If the metatarsal is exclusively rotated not taking care of correcting the varus, the pronation will be corrected but the varus will not, resulting in an incongruent osteotomy. The surgeon should be conscious, that while rotating the metatarsal, a light valgus push should be applied to the metatarsal to keep a closed osteotomy and achieve an IMA correction.
Osteotomy does not achieve full IMA correction, or desired rotation is not achieved.	• Make sure osteotomy is free of soft tissues. Frequently periosteum and peroneus longus fibers hold the distal fragment preventing an adequate rotation. If rotation was corrected, but there is an undercorrection of the IMA, translate the osteotomy laterally about 2–3 mm. This does not hinder the PROMO stability and improves the IMA correction.
Correction is lost once applying plate.	• Overrotate slightly during transient fixation. Once applying the plate, use olive wires through the plate holes to aid holding correction, before locking the plate. Make sure no bone steps are present medially to avoid the plate to reproduce the deformity (this plate first compresses and then locks)
Great toe is still in valgus after the PROMO procedure.	• Check the metatarsal length; it should not be longer than before. Check the DMAA; it should not be more than 10 degrees. If additional correction is needed although having a satisfactory rotational correction, add a distal chevron (biplanar if DMAA is altered). Performing a PROMO in addition to the chevron does not increase the nonunion risk. If none of the above is present, make sure the adductor tendon was released. Add an Akin osteotomy to improve the HV angle.
Sesamoids are still laterally displaced on the AP foot view after adequate IMA and pronation correction.	• A few millimeters of lateral sesamoids displacement will be self-corrected after medial closure and/or Akin osteotomy. If the head recovered its squared shape, that means pronation was corrected. If sesamoids are evidently dislocated, perform a lateral metatarsosesamoid ligaments release (percutaneous or open) and push the sesamoid complex under the metatarsal head, making sure the IMA is completely corrected. Finally, medially retension the metatarsophalangeal capsule.

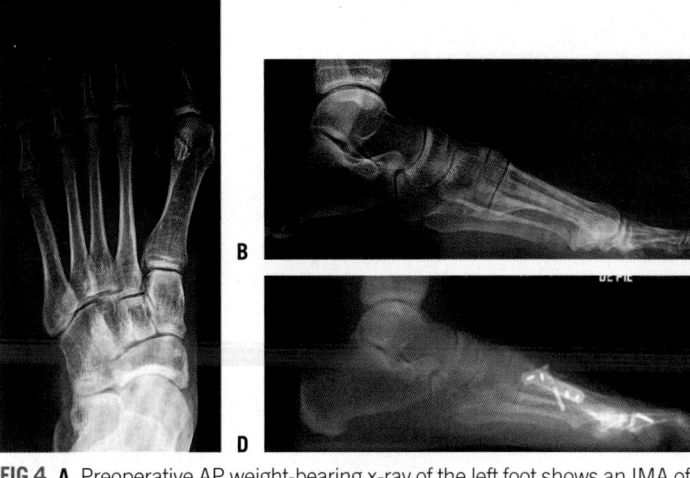
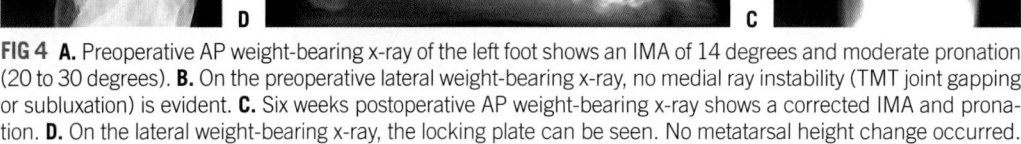

FIG 4 A. Preoperative AP weight-bearing x-ray of the left foot shows an IMA of 14 degrees and moderate pronation (20 to 30 degrees). **B.** On the preoperative lateral weight-bearing x-ray, no medial ray instability (TMT joint gapping or subluxation) is evident. **C.** Six weeks postoperative AP weight-bearing x-ray shows a corrected IMA and pronation. **D.** On the lateral weight-bearing x-ray, the locking plate can be seen. No metatarsal height change occurred.

POSTOPERATIVE CARE

- One month of partial weight bearing (or weight-bearing lateral feet border if bilateral surgery) was performed.
- Rehabilitation is normally performed by the patient with everyday activities. Formal physical therapy is not needed.
- Postoperative medications, 10 days of acetaminophen and anti-inflammatories, are the painkillers of choice. Tramadol drops are prescribed as needed for pain.
- Oral antithrombotic prophylaxis is prescribed for 10 days using dabigatran or rivaroxaban.
- AP and lateral weight-bearing x-rays are taken preoperatively, at 6 weeks, 3 months, and 1 year postoperatively (**FIG 4**).
- During the first month postoperatively, the foot is notably swollen. During the second and third months, swelling rapidly decreases, and the patient is able to fit into smaller and thinner shoes. It can take a year for the swelling to completely disappear.

OUTCOMES

- Functional outcomes significantly improve over time after HV surgery. Lower Extremity Functional Scale scores increase from 53 preoperatively to 73 at 1 year postoperatively.
- Regarding radiologic correction, IMA improves from 15.5 to 5 and HVA from 32 to 5 degrees.
- Recurrence factors for operated HV are severe preoperative HV, incomplete postoperative angular correction, insufficient sesamoid reduction, insufficient pronation reduction, and joint hyperlaxity. References are shown elsewhere.

COMPLICATIONS

- Infection
- Deep venous thrombosis
- Wound dehiscence
- Deformity relapse 4% (in 2 years follow-up according to our latest data)
- Dorsal malunion 1% (This is extremely rare with the PROMO, thanks to the oblique nature of the osteotomy and to the locking plate used.)
- Nonunion 1%

REFERENCES

1. Adam SP, Choung SC, Gu Y, et al. Outcomes after scarf osteotomy for treatment of adult hallux valgus deformity. Clin Orthop Relat Res 2011;469(3):854–859.
2. Bock P, Kluger R, Kristen KH, et al. The Scarf osteotomy with minimally invasive lateral release for treatment of hallux valgus deformity: intermediate and long-term results. J Bone Joint Surg Am 2015;97(15):1238–1245.
3. Deveci A, Firat A, Yilmaz S, et al. Short-term clinical and radiologic results of the scarf osteotomy: what factors contribute to recurrence? J Foot Ankle Surg 2013;52(6):771–775.
4. Jeuken RM, Schotanus MG, Kort NP, et al. Long-term follow-up of a randomized controlled trial comparing scarf to chevron osteotomy in hallux valgus correction. Foot Ankle Int 2016;37(7):687–695.
5. Kaufmann G, Sinz S, Giesinger JM, et al. Loss of correction after chevron osteotomy for hallux valgus as a function of preoperative deformity. Foot Ankle Int 2019;40:287–296.
6. Kim JS, Young KW. Sesamoid position in hallux valgus in relation to the coronal rotation of the first metatarsal. Foot Ankle Clin 2018;23(2):219–230.
7. Kim Y, Kim JS, Young KW, et al. A new measure of tibial sesamoid position in hallux valgus in relation to the coronal rotation of the first metatarsal in CT scans. Foot Ankle Int 2015;36(8):944–952.
8. Okuda R, Kinoshita M, Yasuda T, et al. Postoperative incomplete reduction of the sesamoids as a risk factor for recurrence of hallux valgus. J Bone Joint Surg Am 2009;91(7):1637–1645.
9. Okuda R, Kinoshita M, Yasuda T, et al. The shape of the lateral edge of the first metatarsal head as a risk factor for recurrence of hallux valgus. J Bone Joint Surg Am 2007;89:2163–2172.
10. Park CH, Lee WC. Recurrence of hallux valgus can be predicted from immediate postoperative non-weight bearing radiographs. J Bone Joint Surg Am 2017;99(14):1190–1197.
11. Saltzman CL, Aper RL, Brown TD. Anatomic determinants of first metatarso-phalangeal flexion moments in hallux valgus. Clin Orthop Relat Res 1997;(339):261–269.
12. Scranton PE Jr, Rutkowski R. Anatomic variations in the first ray: part I. Anatomic aspects related to bunion surgery. Clin Orthop Relat Res 1980;(151):244–255.
13. Shibuya N, Kyprios EM, Panchani PN, et al. Factors associated with early loss of hallux valgus correction. J Foot Ankle Surg 2018;57(2):236–240.
14. Wagner P, Wagner E. Is the rotational deformity important in our decision-making process for correction of hallux valgus deformity? Foot Ankle Clin 2018;23(2):205–217.
15. Wang Y, Li Z, Zhang M. Biomechanical study of tarsometatarsal joint fusion using finite element analysis. Med Eng Phys 2014;36:1394–1400.
16. Wong D, Zhang M, Yu J, et al. Biomechanics of first ray hypermobility: an investigation on joint force during walking using finite element analysis. Med Eng Phys 2014;36:1388–1393.

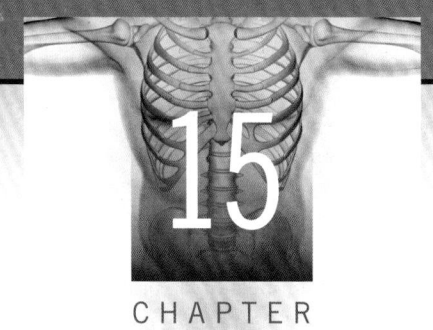

15
CHAPTER

Arthrodesis of the First Metatarsocuneiform Articulation (Lapidus Procedure)

Ian L. D. Le, Jonathan Bourget-Murray, and Andrew Dodd

DEFINITION

- Arthrodesis of the first metatarsal cuneiform joint (ie, Lapidus procedure) is a powerful surgical technique for the correction of hallux valgus deformity. So, in addition to a first metatarsophalangeal (MTP) soft tissue procedure, a Lapidus procedure may be performed.
- This procedure was founded on the premise that hallux valgus was an epiphenomenon to metatarsus primus varus arising from first tarsometatarsal (TMT) hypermobility and a medially oriented first TMT joint.
- The original Lapidus procedure described a capsulorrhaphy of the distal first MTP coupled with an arthrodesis of the first TMT joint. This was done by removing a small wedge of bone from the cuneiform articulation laterally and plantarward to ensure appropriate plantarflexion of the first metatarsal.
- Since originally being described by Albrecht in 1911 and popularized by Paul W. Lapidus in 1934, several modifications have been proposed in an effort to decrease perioperative complications.
- Historically, the postoperative convalescence involved a prolonged period of immobilization and non–weight bearing for several weeks to limit the risks of developing a nonunion or other complications.
- With the advent of improved fixation techniques, early weight bearing is now possible without jeopardizing the deformity correction with outcomes and complication rates comparable to those previous published.

ANATOMY

- The goal of the surgery is to obtain a plantigrade foot with optimal functional biomechanics to allow for (1) an efficacious and painless gait, (2) shock absorption, and (3) assist in maintaining balance and in the distribution of normal forces.
- Weight should be evenly distributed across the "tripod of the foot," which includes the first metatarsal head, the fifth metatarsal head, and the calcaneus.
- The lateral column of the foot is naturally more mobile to accommodate for the flexibility needed when walking on uneven ground.
- The medial column on the other hand is far more rigid, as it carries most of the load while standing and must allow efficient power for push-off.
- The first TMT joint is typically 30 mm in the dorsoplantar plane and 15 mm wide in the mediolateral plane.

PATHOGENESIS

- An equinus contracture is often an underlying feature predisposing the midfoot to increased abnormal stresses. This can lead to eventual instability and ultimately collapse the medial longitudinal arch.
- Debate exists with regard to whether first TMT hypermobility is the primary or a secondary phenomenon responsible for the development of hallux valgus.
- Patients may develop first TMT hypermobility in both the axial and sagittal planes.
  - Axial instability presents as metatarsus primus varus and resultant hallux valgus.
  - Sagittal instability presents as first metatarsal dorsiflexion with predisposition to dorsolateral peritalar subluxation.
- Furthermore, many patients have a medially oriented first TMT joint and tendency toward metatarsus primus varus.

NATURAL HISTORY

- In the face of underlying first TMT hypermobility or an equinus contracture, a hallux valgus deformity will inevitably develop and progress over time—both in symptomatology and in the severity of the deformity.
- Consequently, it is imperative to treat any underlying pathology concomitantly when treating patients with hallux valgus.

PATIENT HISTORY AND PHYSICAL EXAMINATION

- Physical examination:
  - First MTP range of motion (ROM): The examiner assesses flexion and extension of the first MTP in its resting position and reassesses these when the first metatarsal is held in a corrected position (out of varus). A significant loss of ROM in the corrected position is indicative of loss of congruency at the MTP joint. Surgical consideration for a distal metatarsal osteotomy may be needed following the Lapidus procedure.
  - First TMT hypermobility: The examiner rests their index and middle finger of one hand over the dorsal aspect of the patient's first TMT joint while their thumb rests on the plantar surface of the lesser metatarsals. With the other hand, the examiner grasps the first metatarsal and moves it up and down and side to side. Normally, very little motion should be appreciated at the first TMT joint. Excessive motion or translation (>9 mm) is abnormal and indicative of first TMT hypermobility/instability. Occasionally, intercuneiform instability may also be noted.

- Lesser metatarsalgia: With hypermobility of the first TMT joint, the first metatarsal rests relatively elevated to the adjacent lesser metatarsals, resulting in pain and callosities. Callosities are often appreciated beneath the lesser metatarsal heads. Claw toes and extensor recruitment can result in distal migration of the plantar forefoot fat pad, exacerbating the symptoms arising from the lesser metatarsalgia.
- Equinus/Silfverskiöld test: The examiner corrects the hindfoot position to a neutral subtalar position and assesses ankle dorsiflexion ROM both with the knee in full extension and with the knee in >25 degrees of flexion. An inability of dorsiflex the ankle beyond 5 degrees while the knee is fully extended yet improves with knee flexion is indicative of isolated gastrocnemius tightness. Meanwhile, equivalent ankle dorsiflexion, or inability to obtain ≥10 degrees of dorsiflexion, with the knee in extension or flexion is indicative of Achilles tightness (both the soleus and gastrocnemius are involved).

IMAGING AND OTHER DIAGNOSTIC STUDIES

- Plain weight-bearing three-view series of the foot should be obtained: anteroposterior (AP), lateral, and oblique views. Every effort should be made to obtain a true lateral projection, where the domes of the superior aspect of the talus are superimposed.
- Radiographic features of first TMT hypermobility
  - Signs of second and third metatarsal overload (hypertrophied cortical thickening, stress fracture, etc.)
  - Dorsal translation or dorsiflexion of the first metatarsal
  - Plantar widening at the first TMT joint
  - First to third TMT arthrosis
  - First MTP dorsal osteophytes
- Occasionally, plain radiographs of the ankle are needed to rule out adjacent joint involvement.
- Axial sesamoid view can be helpful to assess the extent of metatarsosesamoid arthrosis and degree of sesamoid subluxation.
- Full-length standing radiographs of the lower extremity may be obtained if there is suspicion of concomitant lower extremity malalignment.
- Seldom is a computed tomography scan, magnetic resonance imaging, or other advance imaging modalities needed.

DIFFERENTIAL DIAGNOSIS

- Hallux rigidus
- Metatarsosesamoid arthrosis
- Lesser metatarsalgia
- Interdigital neuroma
- Gout or other inflammatory arthropathy

NONOPERATIVE MANAGEMENT

- Many patients with hallux valgus and hypermobility of the first TMT joint are asymptomatic.
- However, once symptoms develop, progression is inevitable, especially in patients with an underlying equinus contracture.
- Initial management should be directed toward conservative management of local symptoms.
  - Modalities such as nonsteroidal anti-inflammatory drugs, activity modification, rest, weight loss, shoe modifications, and orthotics may be considered.

- In patients with an equinus contracture, a well-directed physiotherapy program focusing at stretching the soleus and gastrocnemius muscles can be helpful.

SURGICAL MANAGEMENT

- Indications:
  - Hallux valgus with associated metatarsus primus varus and first TMT hypermobility
  - Hallux valgus with first TMT arthrosis
  - Revision of failed previous hallux valgus surgery
- Contraindication:
  - Open physeal growth plates

Preoperative Planning

- Radiographs are reviewed to assess the following:
  - Hallux valgus angle (HVA) (normal, <15 degrees)
  - Intermetatarsal angle (IMA) (normal, <9 degrees)
    - Distal metatarsal articular angle (normal, <10 degrees)
  - Proximal phalangeal articular angle (normal, <10 degrees)
- First MTP joint is reviewed to assess the following:
  - Joint congruity
  - Degree of sesamoid subluxation
  - Relative lengths of metatarsal heads (normal, cascade of gradual shortening from second to fifth metatarsal)
- Lateral foot radiographs are reviewed to assess the following:
  - Meary's angle or lateral talar-first metatarsal angle (normal, 0 degrees)
- Based on the aforementioned radiographic parameters, an operative plan is formulated to address the following:
  - Degree of correction needed
  - Need to excise lateral wedge from medial cuneiform
  - Need for concomitant second or third metatarsal shortening osteotomies
- Preoperatively, the surgeon should assess for any underlying equinus contracture and decide if percutaneous Achilles tendon lengthening or a gastrocnemius slide is needed.
- Goals of surgery include correcting the following:
  - The hallux valgus deformity
  - The hypermobility of the first ray
  - Metatarsus primus varus
  - Pronation of the first metatarsal or phalanges
  - Hallux valgus interphalangeus (if present)
  - Medial eminence

Patient Positioning

- The patient is placed supine on a radiolucent table with a padded wedge or bump under the ipsilateral hip to correct for the natural external rotation of the lower extremity.
- The arms are placed on arm boards and any bony prominences along with the ulnar nerve is carefully padded.
- A tourniquet is applied to the thigh.
  - The tourniquet should be placed as proximal as possible to allow access to the proximal tibia should bone graft be needed.
- Once the limb is prepped and draped, a towel bump may be placed under the knee to allow easier access to the dorsum of the foot.
- Exsanguinate the operative limb and inflate the tourniquet (250 to 300 mm Hg).

EXPOSURE

- Make an incision over the dorsomedial aspect of the first metatarsocuneiform joint—between the extensor hallucis longus and brevis tendons. The incision should be long enough to adequately expose and protect the deep peroneal nerve and dorsalis pedis artery (**TECH FIG 1**).

- Identify the first TMT joint by moving the first metatarsal. Expose the joint through a longitudinal incision and careful subperiosteal dissection medially and laterally.

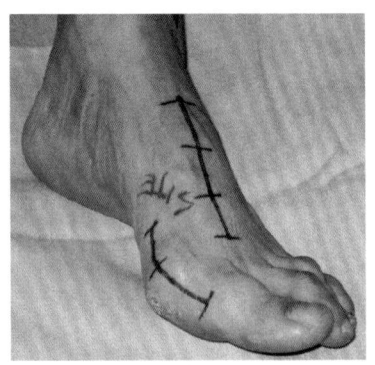 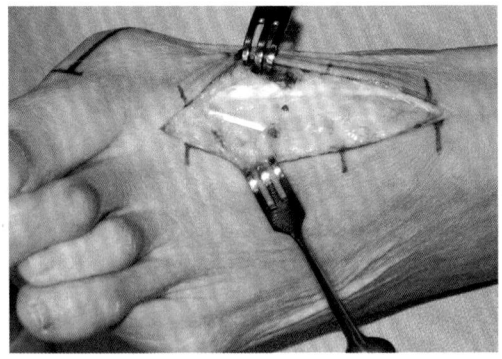

A   B

TECH FIG 1 A. Planned incisions. **B.** Incision between extensor hallucis longus and extensor hallucis brevis.

CORRECTION OF METATARSUS PRIMUS VARUS AND PREPARATION OF THE FIRST TARSOMETATARSAL JOINT

- Using a quarter-inch osteotome, remove any visible osteophytes overlying the first TMT joint.
  - You may wish to save these as they may serve later as bone graft (if needed).
- At this point, the joint is prepared in one of two ways depending if the first TMT joint is medially angled:
  - If there is a need to correct a medially angled first TMT joint:
    - Insert an elevator into the joint to determine the slope of the joint. A depth gauge can be used to assess the depth of the joint. This distance can then be marked on the saw blade with a marking pen for a safer and more accurate cut. By using an oscillating saw, resect a small wedge of bone from the lateral medial cuneiform. The first metatarsal should then plantarflex and abduct. This should be performed by removing as little bone as possible.
    - Use an osteotome to denude the corresponding articular surface of the metatarsal. Maintain the subchondral bone. Avoid excessive metatarsal shortening.
  - If there is no medially angled first TMT joint or if there is an excessively short first metatarsal:
    - Prepare the joint using a series of osteotomes and curettes. Remove only articular cartilage and a small amount of subchondral bone to prevent further shortening. Once complete, there should be two congruent opposing surfaces for arthrodesis.

- Use an oblong curette to ensure there is no residual plantar lip, which may result in excessive dorsiflexion. Meticulous attention is warranted as appropriate plantar resection as this is integral to the success of the surgery.
- Fenestrate the subchondral bone multiple times with a 2.0-mm drill to improve angiogenic and osseous grown to the arthrodesis site (**TECH FIG 2**).

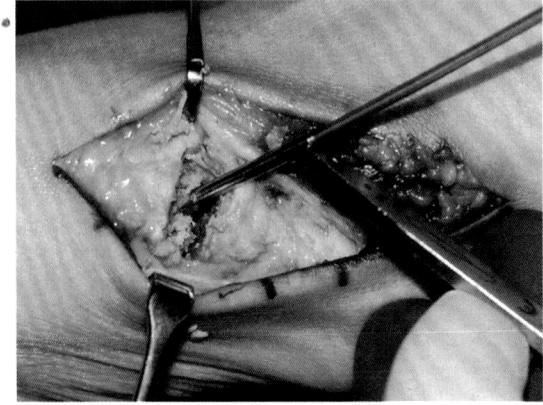

TECH FIG 2 Joint preparation.

DISTAL SOFT TISSUE PROCEDURE

- Extend the dorsal incision down to the first web space, taking care to avoid the digital nerves and the dorsals pedis artery as it divides proximal to the first intermetatarsal space, giving rise to the deep plantar artery.
  - Alternatively, make a second separate incision in the first web space.
- Deep to the attenuated intermetatarsal ligament is the fibular sesamoids and adductor hallucis tendon; leave these intact.
- Protect the fibular sesamoid, identify the first MTP capsule, and incise it longitudinally (**TECH FIG 3**).
- Make a separate medial incision over the first MTP joint, again watching for the crossing dorsal cutaneous nerves.
- Develop a flap superficial to the first MTP capsule, taking care to avoid thinning the capsule itself.
- Sharply incise the capsule full thickness longitudinally and reflect it plantar and dorsal.
- Tease back the capsular reflections to the first metatarsal head proximally to release the adhesions and allow the sesamoids to move independently.
- Grasp the plantar capsule with a Kocher. With gentle pressure, the metatarsal head should be easily reducible over the sesamoids while simultaneously correcting the IMA and closing the gap at the first TMT joint.
- Resect a minimal amount of medial eminence with a rongeur to allow shaping of the medial metatarsal head into a rounded surface.

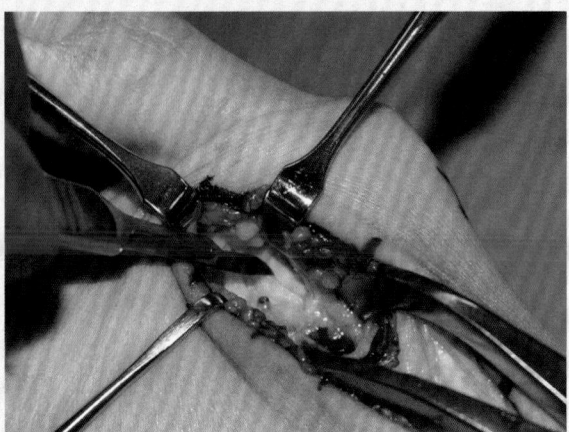

TECH FIG 3 Distal soft tissue release.

STABILIZATION

- Before stabilization, manually reduce the first metatarsal to ensure the foot rests in plantigrade.
  - Placing the foot on a flatfoot plate intraoperatively can help in assessing forefoot and hindfoot position.
- Use Kirschner wires to temporarily maintain your reduction.
- With the metatarsal in the correct position
- Use a burr to create a small trough on the dorsal aspect of the first metatarsal approximately 2 cm from the joint and tapering out distally. This countersinking technique will provide a platform for the head of the screw and insure full contact. Failure to do so causes eccentric loading and lessens the degree of compression achieved with the screw.
- Secure a 4.0-mm lag screw after overdriving the near cortex to the external diameter of the screw (4.0 mm) and a far cortex with a 2.9-mm drill (**TECH FIG 4**).
- Place a second 4.0-mm lag screw from the dorsal surface of the medial cuneiform to the plantar aspect of the first metatarsal. Do so using the same technique described earlier.
- In the past, this construct was further stabilized by placing a third 4.0-mm screw from the first metatarsal into the base of the second metatarsal, but this is now believed to be unnecessary.
- Alternative (and more robust) fixation methods include the use of dorsomedial or plantar locking plate fixation with or without additional lag screw fixation.
- Several recent studies have reported promising data in favor of plate fixation for the modified Lapidus arthrodesis.

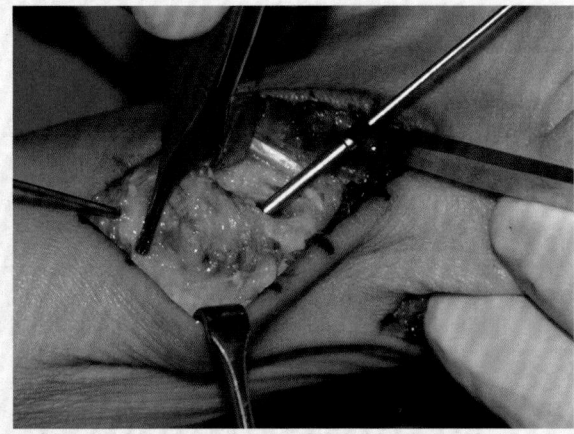

TECH FIG 4 Placement of a 4.0-mm screw after drilling in a lag screw fashion.

BONE GRAFTING

- With improved surgical techniques and more robust fixation methods, the shear strain–relieving bone grafting is now not typically performed.
  - If bone grafting is performed
    - Use a 5.0-mm burr to create two small troughs on the dorsomedial and dorsolateral aspects of the first TMT joint to serve as sites for shear strain–relieving bone graft **(TECH FIG 5A,B)**.

- Also, place bone graft in any gaps at the arthrodesis site.
- Bone graft is obtained from the local procedure or lateral calcaneus bone graft.
- Obtain AP, lateral, and oblique plain film radiographs to ensure appropriate positioning and correction, which is often not seen in detail under C-arm fluoroscopy **(TECH FIG 5C,D)**.

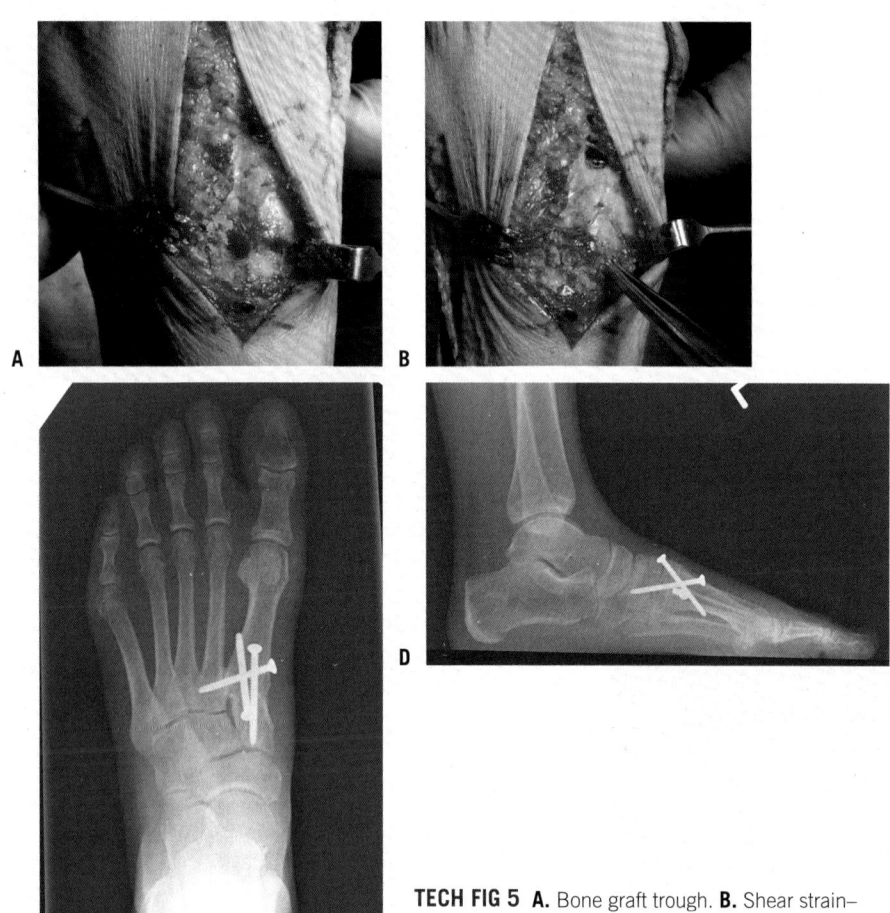

TECH FIG 5 A. Bone graft trough. **B.** Shear strain–relieving bone graft. **C.** Final AP radiograph. **D.** Final lateral radiograph.

WOUND CLOSURE

- Plicate the medial first MTP capsule. Excessive capsule may be excised if redundant.
- It should not be necessary to overtighten the capsule to add additional correction to the hallux valgus.
- Close the remaining incisions in layers.

TECHNIQUES

ADDITIONAL PROCEDURES TO CONSIDER

- Gastrocnemius slide or percutaneous Achilles tendon lengthening
  - Persistent equinus contracture and forefoot overload
- Akin osteotomy
  - Presence of associated hallux valgus interphalangeus
- Second or third metatarsal shortening
  - Loss of metatarsal head parabola
  - Particularly problematic in patients wearing high-heeled shoes

CASE EXAMPLE (COURTESY OF MARK E. EASLEY, MD)

Background and Imaging

- A 75-year-old woman with recurrent/persistent hallux valgus after prior distal procedure
- Symptoms included pain with activity, push-off during gait, and with shoe wear as well as tenderness over the medial eminence.
- Minimal pain and no mechanical symptoms with hallux MTP joint ROM
- Radiographs revealed increased IMA and HVA (**TECH FIG 6A**), incongruent/asymmetric MTP joint, relatively narrow first metatarsal, and no obvious plantar gapping of the first TMT joint (**TECH FIG 6B**).

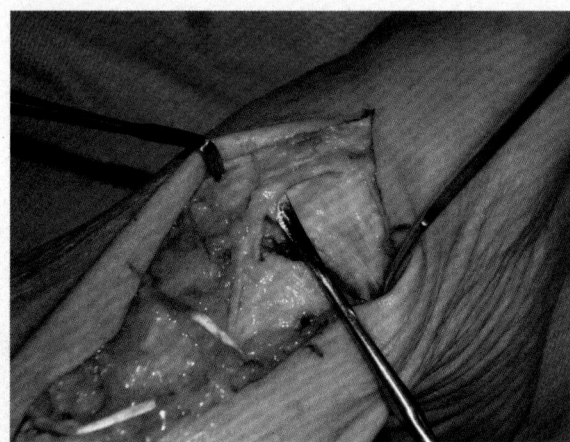

TECH FIG 7 Intraoperative photo of the dorsal incision to the first TMT joint, identifying the deep neurovascular bundle after superficial peroneal nerve branch to dorsomedial hallux, extensor hallucis longus and brevis, and tibialis anterior tendon protected.

Exposure

- A longitudinal dorsal incision is made over the lateral aspect of first TMT joint.
- The superficial peroneal nerve branch to dorsomedial hallux and extensor hallucis longus and brevis is protected.
- On medial aspect of first TMT joint, the tibialis anterior tendon is protected.
- On lateral aspect of TMT joint, the deep neurovascular bundle is protected (**TECH FIG 7**).

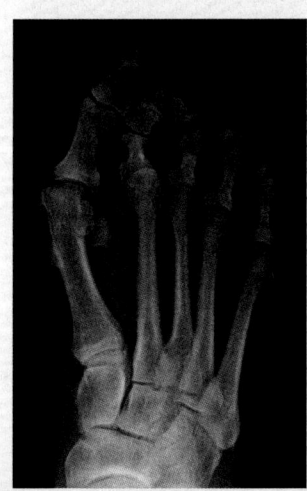

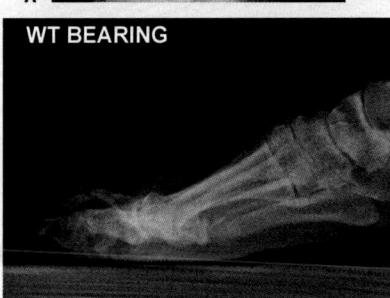

WT BEARING

TECH FIG 6 A 75-year-old woman with recurrent/persistent hallux valgus deformity. **A.** AP view. Note relatively narrow first metatarsal. **B.** Lateral view. In this case, there was no plantar gapping of the first TMT joint to suggest hypermobility.

Tarsometatarsal Joint Preparation

- Initial removal of lateral and plantar cartilage and bone to limit risk of first metatarsal dorsiflexion and correct IMA (**TECH FIG 8A**).
- To limit dorsiflexion, the dorsal rim of cartilage is initially left intact as a reminder to maintain dorsal subchondral bone (**TECH FIG 8B**).
- The first TMT joint is deep, typically 3 cm. The plantar most cartilage and bone must be removed, or it will impinge and promote first metatarsal dorsiflexion that could lead to lesser metatarsal head transfer metatarsalgia (**TECH FIG 8C–E**).
- After cartilage removal, the subchondral bone must be penetrated to promote fusion (**TECH FIG 8F**).

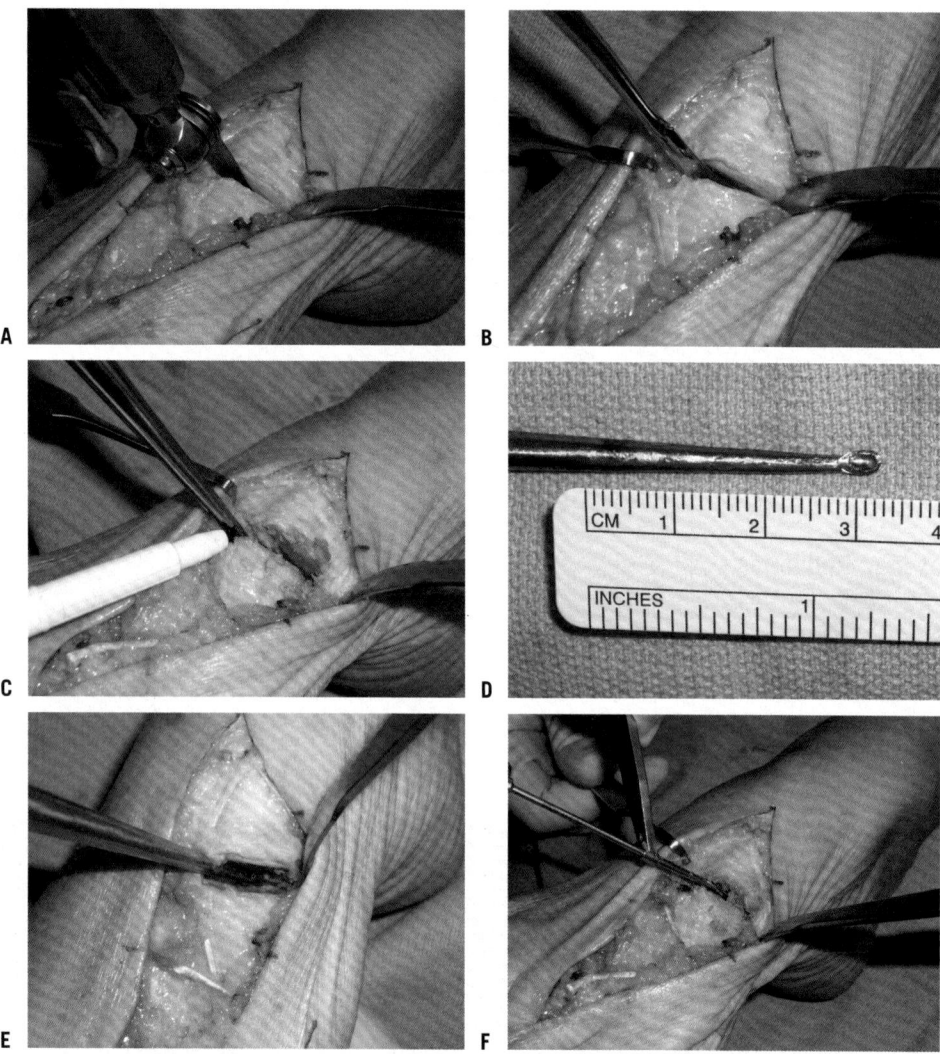

TECH FIG 8 First TMT joint preparation. **A.** Initial removal of lateral and plantar cartilage and bone to limit risk of first metatarsal dorsiflexion and correct IMA. **B.** Dorsal rim of cartilage is initially left intact as a reminder to maintain dorsal subchondral bone. At conclusion of joint preparation, this rim of cartilage is removed. **C.** Curette in the first TMT joint being marked to demonstrate joint depth. **D.** Approximate 3 cm depth noted. **E.** The plantar most cartilage and bone must be removed, or it may impinge and promote first metatarsal dorsiflexion. **F.** After cartilage removal, the subchondral bone must be penetrated to promote fusion.

Distal Soft Tissue Procedure

- In this case, the dorsal longitudinal incision was extended to the first web space and second MTP joint.
- Through the dorsal incision, the lateral release of the suspensory ligament between the lateral capsule and the lateral sesamoid is released to allow the metatarsal head to reduce over the sesamoids.
- Through a medial midaxial incision over the first MTP joint, the medial capsulotomy is performed. In this revision surgery, there was a medial capsular defect that was repaired at the conclusion of the surgery to reconstitute the medial capsule **(TECH FIG 9)**.
- A medial eminence resection was not necessary because it had been performed as part of the index procedure.

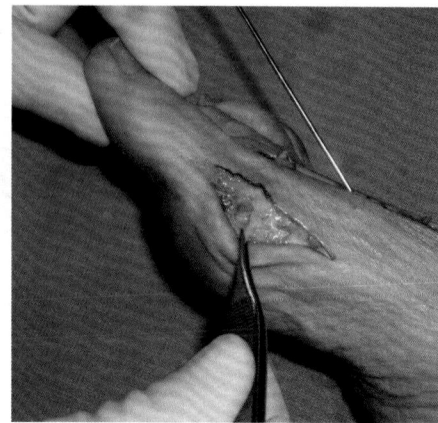

TECH FIG 9 In this revision surgery, a medial capsular defect was identified. To reconstitute the medial capsule, this defect was repaired at the conclusion of the surgery.

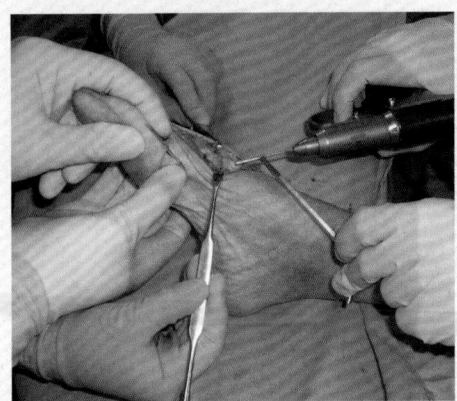
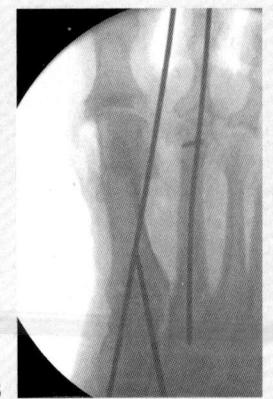
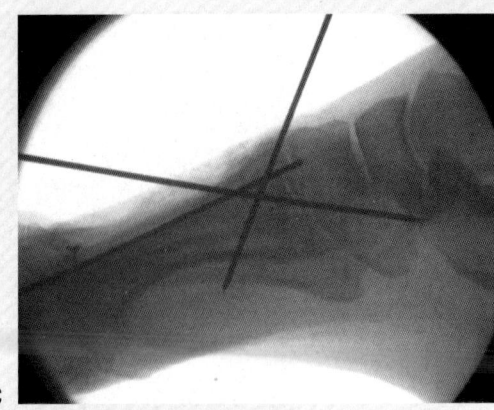

TECH FIG 10 Provisional first TMT joint fixation. **A.** With the first surgeon holding the reduction, the second surgeon places the provisional pins to maintain the reduction. **B.** Intraoperative AP fluoroscopy to confirm satisfactory correction of the IMA. **C.** Intraoperative lateral fluoroscopy demonstrating the first metatarsal dorsiflexion was avoided.

Tarsometatarsal Joint Reduction

- With the first surgeon holding the reduction, the second surgeon places the provisional pins to maintain the reduction **(TECH FIG 10A)**.
- Intraoperative fluoroscopy to confirm satisfactory correction of the IMA and that first metatarsal dorsiflexion has been avoided **(TECH FIG 10B,C)**.

Fixation

- In place of the more lateral proximal to distal guide pin, a compression screw is placed while the reduction is maintained.
- In place of the more medial distal to proximal guide pin, a second compression is placed **(TECH FIG 11A,B)**.
- Intraoperative fluoroscopy is performed to confirm that IMA correction has been maintained **(TECH FIG 11C)**.

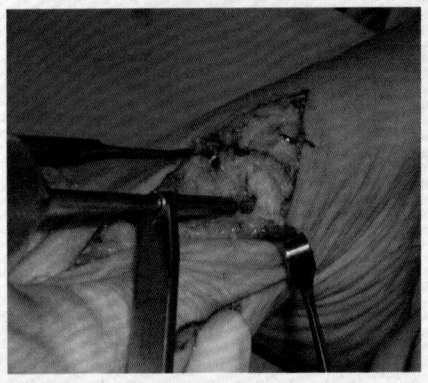
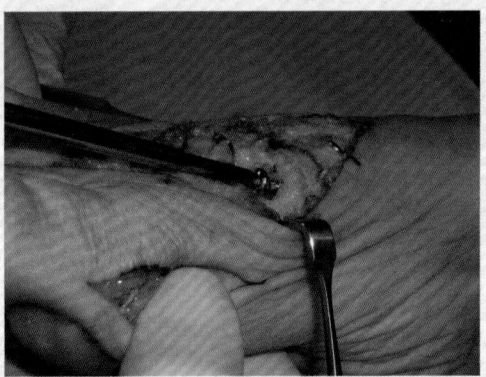
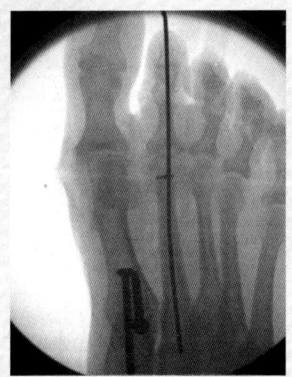

TECH FIG 11 A. Distal guide pin, a compression screw, is placed while the reduction is maintained. **B.** In place of the more medial distal to proximal guide pin, a second compression is placed. **C.** Intraoperative fluoroscopy to confirm that IMA correction has been maintained.

TECHNIQUES

Pearls and Pitfalls

Persistent Dorsiflexed First Metatarsal or Lesser Metatarsalgia	• Failure to resect plantar aspect of the first TMT joint
Nonunion	• Inadequate joint preparation or inadequate fixation, lack of bone graft
Hallux Varus	• Overcorrection of IMA • Release of adductor hallucis tendon

POSTOPERATIVE CARE

- A well-molded posterior plaster splint is applied postoperatively to accommodate postoperative swelling.
- Analgesia is best managed with a single-shot popliteal block supplemented with a saphenous nerve block.
- At 2 weeks, patients are transitioned into a removable boot.
- Patient may mobilize using crutches or a knee scooter.
- The postoperative care for the patient in the example case is as follows:
  - Bunion strapping for 6 to 8 weeks postoperatively
  - Protected weight bearing in a short-leg cast for 4 to 6 weeks followed by transition to a walking boot—provided radiographs suggest satisfactory bridging trabeculation at arthrodesis site.
  - Advance to full weight bearing onto forefoot at 6 to 8 weeks provided radiographs suggest satisfactory bridging trabeculation at arthrodesis site (**FIG 1**).
- Traditionally, a 6- to 12-week period of non–weight-bearing immobilization was recommended before allowing patients to progress to full weight bearing to allow consolidation of the arthrodesis site. Such limitations may be difficult for some patients while imparting patients to potential complications associated with prolonged immobilization.
- Recent studies have demonstrated early weight bearing after a modified Lapidus arthrodesis does not increase the risk of nonunion. Patients should remain strictly non–weight bearing for the first 10 to 14 days, followed by 4 to 6 weeks of protected weight bearing as tolerated in a walking boot.
- Despite recent literature suggesting that early weight bearing does not increase perioperative complications; further research is necessary to support this protocol following different fixation constructs (ie, a locking plate with a compression screw, a compression screw and nonlocking plate, a two-crossed screw construct, or a three-crossed screw construct).

OUTCOMES

- With appropriate surgical indications, surgical technique, and patient compliance, the patient satisfaction rate is beyond 90%.
- Rates of nonunion rates are typically well below 5%.
- Recurrence is rare.

COMPLICATIONS

- See the Pearls and Pitfalls section.

SUGGESTED READINGS

Bendnarz PA, Manoli A II. Modified Lapidus procedure for the treatment of hypermobile hallux valgus. Foot Ankle Int 2000;21:816–821.

Blitz MN, Lee T, Williams K, et al. Early weight bearing after modified Lapidus arthrodesis: a multicenter review of 80 cases. J Foot Ankle Surg 2010;49:357–362.

Coetzee JC, Wickum D. The Lapidus procedure: a prospective cohort outcome. Foot Ankle Int 2004;25:526–531.

Coughlin MJ. Hallux valgus. Instr Course Lect 1997;46:357–391.

Coughlin MJ, Mann R, Saltzman C. Surgery of the Foot and Ankle, ed 8. Philadelphia: Elsevier, 2007.

DeVries JG, Granata JD, Hyer CF. Fixation of first tarsometatarsal arthrodesis: a retrospective comparative cohort of two techniques. Foot Ankle Int 2011;32:158–162.

DiGiovanni CW, Kuo R, Tejwani N, et al. Isolated gastrocnemius tightness. J Bone Joint Surg Am 2002;84:962–970.

Hansen ST. Hallux valgus surgery: Morton and Lapidus were right! Clin Podiatr Med Surg 1996;13:347–354.

Kazzaz S, Singh D. Postoperative cast necessity after a Lapidus arthrodesis. Foot Ankle Int 2009;30:746–751.

Lapidus PW. The author's bunion operation from 1931 to 1959. Clin Orthop 1960;16:119–135.

Mann R. Disorders of the first metatarsophalangeal joint. J Am Acad Orthop Surg 1995;3:34–43.

Morton DJ. Evolution of the longitudinal arch of the human foot. J Bone Joint Surg Am 1924;22:56–90.

Morton DJ. The Human Foot: Its Evolution, Physiology and Functional Disorders. New York: Columbia University Press, 1935.

Patel S, Ford LA, Etcheverry J, et al. Modified Lapidus arthrodesis: rate of nonunion in 227 cases. J Foot Ankle Surg 2004;43:37–42.

Pedowitz W, Kovatis P. Flatfoot in the adult. J Am Acad Orthop Surg 1995;3:293–302.

Prissel MA, Hyer CF, Grambart ST, et al. A multicenter, retrospective study of early weightbearing for modified Lapidus arthrodesis. J Foot Ankle Surg 2016;55:226–229.

Sangeorzan BJ, Hansen ST Jr. Modified Lapidus procedure for hallux valgus. Foot Ankle 1989;9:262–266.

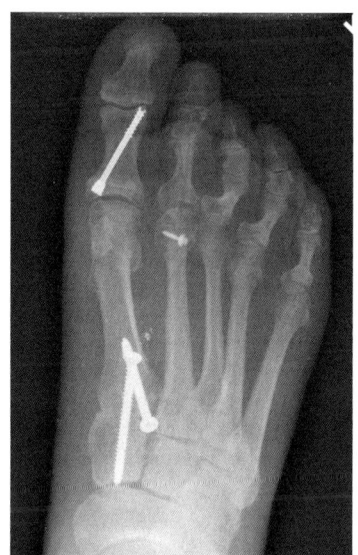

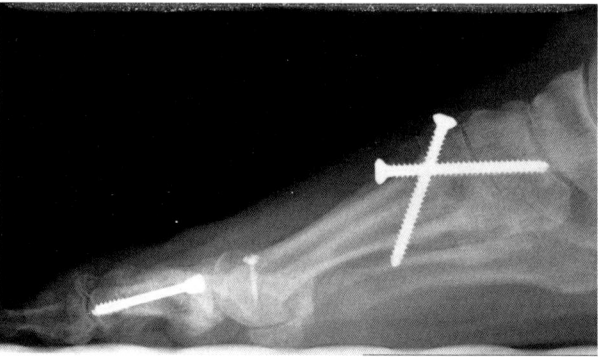

FIG 1 Follow-up weight-bearing radiographs of the patient in **TECH FIGS 6** to **11**. **A.** AP view demonstrating satisfactory hallux metatarsal head on sesamoids and correction of HVA and IMA. Note supplemental Akin osteotomy to optimize correction. **B.** Lateral view demonstrating no dorsiflexion of first metatarsal.

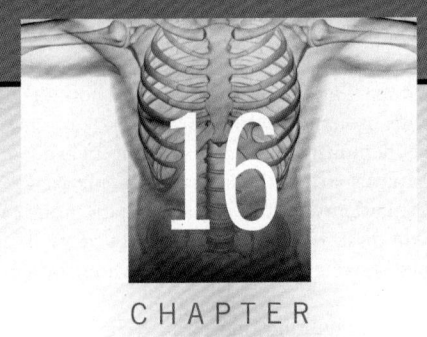

16
CHAPTER

Percutaneous First Tarsal Metatarsal Arthrodesis (Lapidus Procedure) for Hallux Valgus

Amanda N. Fletcher and Alastair Younger

DEFINITION

- The Lapidus procedure, a technique that entails first tarsometatarsal (TMT) joint arthrodesis, was described and popularized as a treatment for hallux valgus deformity by Paul W. Lapidus.[3,4] The Lapidus procedure was described for hallux valgus correction and involved realignment of the metatarsal with a TMT fusion and correction of the hallux valgus angle with a lateral release and medial plication at the first metatarsophalangeal (MTP) joint.
- Because Dr. Lapidus performed his first Lapidus bunion operation in 1931, many technique modifications have been described and the indications broadened.
- The Lapidus procedure is now widely used in treating many forefoot and midfoot pathologies associated with first TMT joint dysfunction including primary hallux valgus, failed or recurrent hallux valgus, hallux varus, metatarsal adductus, lesser metatarsalgia, and inflammatory or posttraumatic arthritis.
- Arthroscopic or minimally invasive surgery (MIS) Lapidus techniques have recently been described,[6,7,9] although reported outcomes are limited given the novelty of the technique. The theorized benefits include smaller incisions, less wound complications, less swelling, less joint stiffness, less pain, and earlier mobilization. Additionally, more precise joint débridement, preparation, and correction may decrease the risk of nonunion and malunion.

ANATOMY

- The motion of the first ray is complex involving the first TMT joint, the cuneiform–navicular joints, and the talonavicular joint.
- The first TMT joint is made up of an articulation between the medial cuneiform and the first metatarsal. This joint relies on osseous, ligamentous, and muscular support to maintain its alignment and stability.
- The dorsal and plantar first cuneometatarsal ligaments provide sagittal stabilization, resisting plantar and dorsal displacement of the first ray, respectively.[14] There is no intermetatarsal ligament between the first and second metatarsal. The peroneus longus and flexor hallucis longus tendons are dynamic stabilizers that serve to minimize dorsal instability.
- The first TMT joint is a partial ball-and-socket joint with triaxial motion including a slight degree of dorsomedial to plantarolateral motion.
  - Greater than 4 degrees of sagittal range of motion and greater than 8 degrees of transverse motion at the first TMT joint constitute excessive range of motion.[10]

- The first ray plays a key role in maintaining the structure of the medial column and provides a stable support for efficient gait and propulsion during push off. In the setting of TMT hypermobility, the medial column is destabilized with an abnormal dorsiflexion motion and resultant medial displacement of the first metatarsal.
- To reinstate a stable medial column construct for propulsion and concurrently treat the hallux valgus deformity, a TMT joint fusion may be indicated.
- The dorsal medial and lateral digital nerves have been found consistently between 10 o'clock and 2 o'clock position at the first MTP joint level.[8]

PATHOGENESIS

- Hallux valgus is a three-dimensional deformity affecting both the soft tissue and bony structures of the first ray. The deformity often includes varus position of the metatarsal, valgus deviation of the phalanx, pronation of the hallux (primarily through the TMT joint), lateral translation or subluxation of the sesamoid complex, and first TMT hypermobility.
- The multifactorial etiology of hallux valgus continues to be debated. There are many anatomic and biomechanical factors, both intrinsic and extrinsic in origin, that are involved and often coexist in the same patient. Remodeling of the bony anatomy likely also contributes particularly in the adolescent patients.
- One theory is that an equinus deformity or tight heel cord drives the midfoot into plantarflexion causing longitudinal collapse and instability. This results in first TMT hypermobility. Axial instability causes metatarsus primus varus and resultant hallux valgus, whereas sagittal instability predisposes to a dorsiflexed first metatarsal. A heel cord lengthening may be merited in some individuals.
- Patients with hallux valgus deformity have a 3.62 mm increase of the first ray sagittal motion,[11] and clinical hypermobility was noted in 96% of patients with recurrent hallux valgus.[2] Hypermobility is present in both the sagittal and transverse planes and is most notable in the dorsomedial direction.[12]
- First TMT joint instability or hypermobility has been described as a main cause of both primary and recurrent hallux valgus. Unaddressed first metatarsal pronation likely leads to failure even in the setting of a corrected intermetatarsal angle.[5]
- The Lapidus procedure stabilizes the medial column and restores the first ray alignment in all three dimensions by derotating the first metatarsal and reducing the subluxed sesamoids.

NATURAL HISTORY

- Although there are many different variations of the natural progression, one commonly recognized is this: equinus → predisposition to medial longitudinal arch collapse and instability → first TMT hypermobility → metatarsus primus varus → hallux valgus → lesser metatarsal overload.
- In general, hallux valgus associated with first TMT hypermobility is a progressive condition in both terms of deformity and symptomatology. Depending on the severity of deformity, nonsurgical measures are typically unsuccessful.
- First TMT hypermobility can cause signs of second and third metatarsal overload including stress fractures or second and third TMT arthrosis. Second metatarsalgia is a common symptom caused by increased loading of the second ray due to a dysfunctional first ray. This may lead to damage to the plantar plate, claw toe deformity, and subluxed or dislocated lesser MTP joints. First TMT hypermobility must be recognized and addressed prior to or concomitantly with these associated conditions.

PATIENT HISTORY AND PHYSICAL FINDINGS

- History: Patients commonly present with a symptomatic hallux valgus deformity and tenderness at the first TMT and MTP joints. Symptomatic hallux valgus often causes difficulty with shoe wear. Given the genetic predisposition of hallux valgus, a family history should be obtained.
- Physical exam: The physical exam should begin with inspection to gauge the severity of the deformity (**FIG 1**), callous formation (particularly beneath the lesser metatarsals), previous surgical incisions, or other foot deformities. Every patient should also undergo an assessment of first TMT range of motion (evaluating for hypermobility in both the sagittal and transverse planes), first MTP range of motion, and the presence of an equinus contracture. The definition of hypermobility remains largely subjective, and quantifying the degree of first TMT hypermobility has been difficult in clinical practice.
- Drawer test for first TMT hypermobility in the sagittal plane
  - Standing at the foot of the patient, the examiner cups the forefoot with both hands placing the fingers on the dorsal aspect and thumb on the plantar aspect of the foot. The index and middle fingers of the medial hand are placed at the dorsal TMT joint and the thumb at the plantar TMT joint. The lateral hand stabilizes the lateral metatarsals. The thumb and fingers of the examining hand are used to test dorsal and plantar translation of the first TMT joint. Alternatively, the index and middle fingers of the lateral hand can rest over the dorsal first TMT joint to monitor motion while the medial hand grasps the first metatarsal between the thumb and fingers. Transverse motion can also be tested here. Minimal motion should be palpated, and excessive motion or translation is indicative of first TMT hypermobility.
- Equinus/Silfverskiöld test for determination of isolated gastrocnemius equinus versus soleus and gastrocnemius equinus
- Subluxation of the lesser toes: Lesser ray instability can be examined by determining if there is MTP subluxation on clinical examination. The lesser toe is subluxed into dorsiflexion and may have increased translation compared to the other toes or the contralateral side secondary to plantar plate deficiency.

IMAGING AND OTHER DIAGNOSTIC STUDIES

- The radiographic assessment should include weight-bearing plain anteroposterior (AP), oblique, lateral, and axial sesamoid views (**FIG 2**). Advanced imaging is infrequently needed.
- The severity of hallux valgus can be classified as mild, moderate, or severe based on several validated AP radiographic parameters: the hallux valgus angle (normal is less than 15 degrees), 1-2 intermetatarsal angle (normal is less than 9 degrees), and lateral subluxation of the sesamoids.
- An increased 1-2 intermetatarsal angle indicates first TMT hypermobility in the transverse plane.

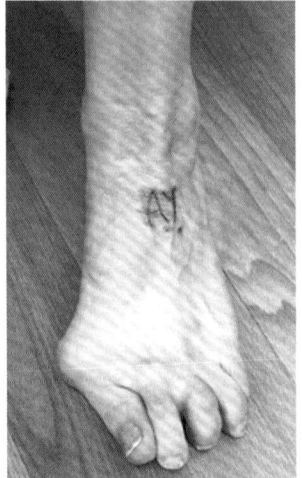

FIG 1 Severe hallux valgus deformity.

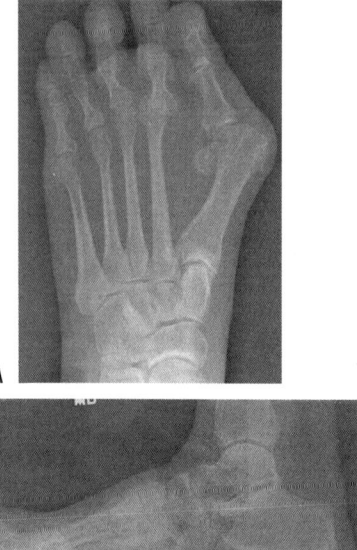

FIG 2 Preoperative AP (**A**) and lateral (**B**) plain radiographs of a patient with severe hallux valgus deformity. First metatarsal pronation and lateral subluxation of the sesamoids are seen on the AP radiograph (**A**).

- The lateral radiographs are reviewed for dorsal translation or dorsiflexion of the first metatarsal with plantar widening at the first TMT joint.
- Additional radiographic evidence indicative of first TMT hypermobility includes signs of second and third metatarsal overload (cortical thickening, stress fractures), arthritis of the Lisfranc joints, and arthritis of the first MTP joint.
- Evaluate for metatarsus adductus as this may make correction of the first ray difficult if the lesser metatarsal heads are not moved laterally.

DIFFERENTIAL DIAGNOSIS

- Hallux rigidus
- Inflammatory arthropathy
- Metatarsosesamoid arthrosis
- Lesser metatarsalgia
- Interdigital neuroma
- Plantar plate tear of the lesser MTP joints

NONOPERATIVE MANAGEMENT

- Nonoperative management for symptomatic hallux valgus should be initiated first. Education and reassurance are helpful as patients may be concerned about the natural history. There is little evidence to determine what may cause progression. Appropriate shoe wear, pads, spacers, taping, and orthotics may be beneficial.
- Nonoperative treatment is warranted in patients with contraindications to first TMT arthrodesis: arthritis of the first MTP joint, skeletal immaturity, generalized ligamentous laxity, short first metatarsal, previous sesamoiditis, infection, avascular necrosis, smoking, poorly controlled diabetes, Charcot arthropathy, and poor bone stock.

SURGICAL MANAGEMENT

- When surgical correction is warranted for symptomatic hallux valgus with hypermobility of the first TMT joint, traditional open Lapidus techniques, or recently described minimally invasive Lapidus techniques may be considered.
- In general, a Lapidus procedure is useful for a more severe hallux valgus deformity and a distal procedure beneficial for a lesser deformity.

Preoperative Planning

- Begin with a thorough history and physical exam to evaluate the primary pathology as well as coexisting deformities and abnormalities to determine if concomitant correction is warranted.

- Consider all prior foot surgeries. A common reason for failed or recurrent hallux valgus after primary correction is unaddressed first metatarsal pronation.[5] Thus, location of previous incisions and presence of hardware should be evaluated to determine if MIS or a traditional open technique is more appropriate.
- Standard weight-bearing radiographs including AP, lateral, oblique, and axial sesamoid views should be obtained and thoroughly reviewed preoperatively.
- Ensure conservative measures have been exhausted prior to surgical planning.
- Anesthesia: The surgery can be performed with a peripheral nerve block, spinal, or general anesthesia. A calf tourniquet, rather than a thigh tourniquet, is required with a peripheral nerve block.
- Equipment:
  - Arthroscopy equipment: 2.9-mm arthroscope
  - Minimally invasive instruments: 3.5-mm shaver, MICA burr, two 12-mm burrs, or a wedge burr
  - Reduction device: Many companies make a compression and distraction device that is useful for reduction of the first to second metatarsal heads.
  - Fixation: cannulated, partially threaded, 3.5-mm cancellous screws (used to hold reduction between the first and second rays), 4-mm headless screws, 3.5- to 4-mm fully threaded cortical screws
  - Other instruments: Scalpels, beaver blades, elevators, and the instruments from the minimally invasive set are useful.

Positioning

- The patient is positioned supine, and bony prominences are padded. The leg should be positioned at the end of the bed. A beanbag or stack of blankets can be used to bump the ipsilateral hip to allow slight internal rotation of the foot. The operative leg should be mobile and free to be moved off of the side of the bed for imaging.
- An arthroscopy tower is placed on the contralateral side of the bed. The scrub nurse and table are also positioned on the opposite side of the bed.
- The C-arm is placed at the foot of the bed on the same side as the operative extremity. The MICA console is also placed on the surgical side of the bed.

Approach

- The procedure is performed through multiple percutaneous dorsal and medial incisions about the first TMT joint.

PERCUTANEOUS FIRST TARSOMETATARSAL ARTHRODESIS (LAPIDUS)

Joint Preparation

- The first MTP joint is localized with examination and intraoperative AP fluoroscopy.
- Using a beaver blade, a 5-mm dorsolateral incision is made at the lateral aspect of the first MTP joint to release the lateral capsule and the lateral metatarsosesamoid ligament.
  - Care should be taken to avoid injuring the dorsolateral sensory nerve branch.
- The blade is passed into the MTP joint by palpation and the position confirmed with the C-arm. The blade is then passed onto the dorsal side of the MTP joint to release the dorsal lateral capsule. The blade is reversed and taken down to the plantar side of the metatarsal head and the plantar lateral capsule released, including the lateral metatarsosesamoid ligament, which is a thickening of the lateral capsule.
- The adductor tendon is also percutaneously released off the lateral side of the sesamoid.
  - The beaver blade is passed in a distal to proximal direction just lateral to the lateral sesamoid to release the tendon.
- A percutaneous 5-mm medial-based incision is made over the first metatarsal head at the level of the medial eminence. Blunt dissection is carried down to the medial eminence.
- The burr is inserted through this incision and is used to remove the medial eminence medial to the level of the sagittal groove. The nondominant hand is used to guide the depth of the burr.
- The exostectomy debulks the medial eminence to allow mobilization of the medial capsule and prevents the medial eminence from blocking the correction. The mobilized bone fragment acts as a soft tissue release and allows the capsule to scar back down in the corrected position after dressings are applied.
  - Care should be taken to avoid injuring the dorsomedial sensory nerve branch by using initial blunt dissection **(TECH FIG 1A)**.

- AP fluoroscopy is then used to identify the first TMT joint. Using a direct medial approach at the level of the TMT joint, a beaver blade is used to penetrate through the medial soft tissues to the level of the joint. An elevator is placed into the joint and the medial capsule released. A small curette can also be used to lever the joint open **(TECH FIG 1B,C)**.
- The 2- × 12-mm burr is placed though the medial TMT incision and the joint cartilage removed. This is performed by dividing the proximal (medial cuneiform) and distal (base of first metatarsal) joint surfaces into four quadrants each, with a total of eight quadrants to sequentially débride **(TECH FIG 1D)**.
  - Proximal: dorsomedial, dorsolateral, plantaromedial, plantarolateral
  - Distal: dorsomedial, dorsolateral, plantaromedial, plantarolateral
  - Care should be taken to avoid penetrating the subchondral bone, especially in older osteoporotic patients. The nondominant hand is used to guide the burr and ensure precise removal. When the burr is intra-articular, the vibratory motion between the two bones can be felt.
  - Care is taken while débriding dorsally not to damage the dorsomedial and dorsolateral neurovascular bundles and laterally not to penetrate the second metatarsal.
- Once adequate intra-articular space has been created, the 2.9-mm scope is inserted and the cartilage removal confirmed. Any residual cartilage is then removed and the cartilage debris flushed out.
  - Dorsomedial, plantaromedial, or dorsolateral 5-mm incisions may be created at the first TMT joint as either a viewing or working portal for further débridement under direct arthroscopic visualization.
  - The 3.5-mm shaver is used to remove debris. Any residual cartilage can be removed using the shaver or the 2- × 12-mm burr.
  - This step is crucial as complete removal of cartilage will provide the best chance of a successful union **(TECH FIG 1E,F)**.

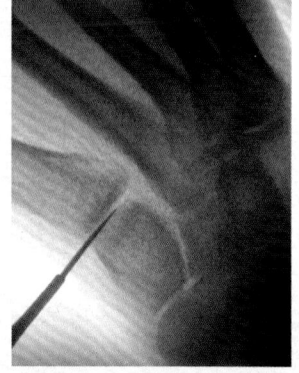

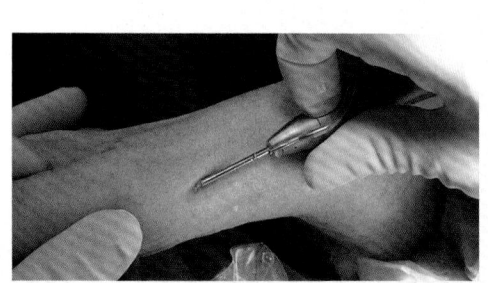

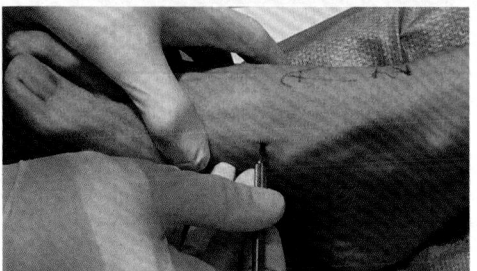

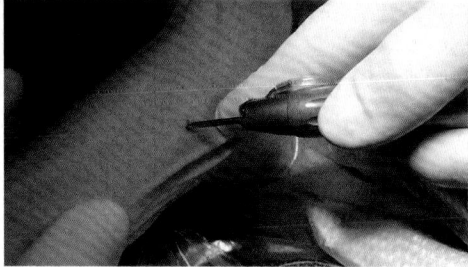

TECH FIG 1 A. Medial eminence resection through a medial-based incision at the level of the first metatarsal head. **B.** Establishing the medial incision at the level of the first TMT joint. **C.** AP fluoroscopic view demonstrating localization of the first TMT joint with an elevator placed in the joint. **D.** Débridement of the first TMT joint with a 2- × 12-mm burr. *(continued)*

A

C

B

D

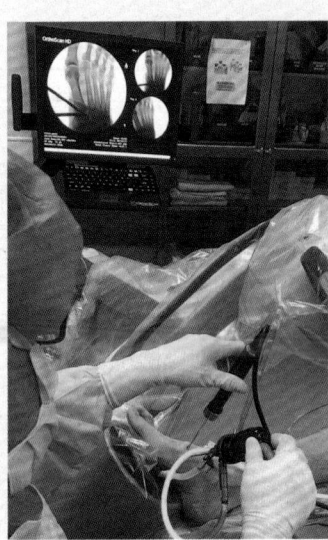

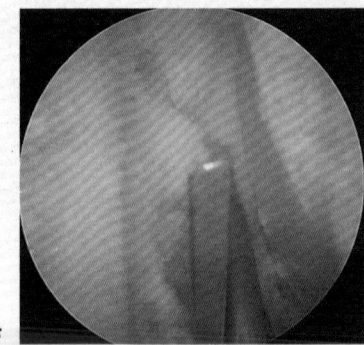

TECH FIG 1 *(continued)* **E.** First TMT joint débridement under arthroscopic visualization. **F.** Arthroscopic view from the dorsomedial portal demonstrating further débridement of the plantar cartilage.

Reduction and Fixation

- The distal end of the first ray is then reduced and derotated. A 2-mm Kirschner wire (K-wire) is placed into the second metatarsal head and another 2-mm K-wire into the first metatarsal head with calculated positioning to allow derotation of the first ray.
  - For example, if 30 degrees of malrotation is to be corrected, the K-wires are positioned 15 degrees of out of plane in each metatarsal head.
- The two K-wires are then rotated into parallel position, and a reduction device is placed over the two K-wires, derotating the first ray.
- The compressor is tightened over the K-wires, closing the first intermetatarsal angle.

- The dorsiflexed first metatarsal is plantarflexed and correctly aligned in the sagittal plane.
- Multiplanar intraoperative fluoroscopic views are used to confirm the reduction and return of the sesamoids to their anatomic position under the first metatarsal head. The reduction can be held by placing a third K-wire from the first to second metatarsal head. Care should be taken with derotation as the first ray can be underreduced or overreduced.
- Through a medial-based incision, a cannulated, partially threaded, cancellous 3.5-mm screw is placed using a guided K-wire between the first and second metatarsals at the meta-diaphyseal junction. The two metatarsals are compressed together, increasing the correction **(TECH FIG 2A)**. The screw is

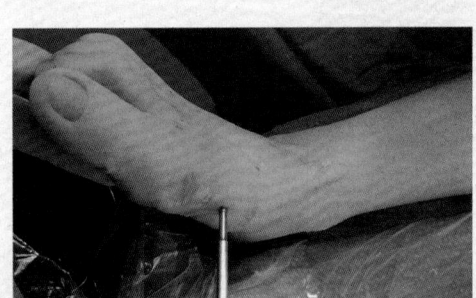

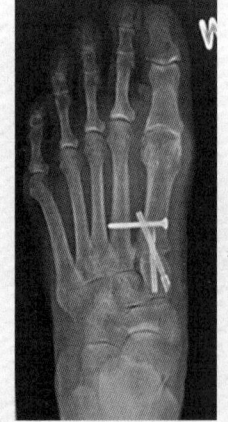

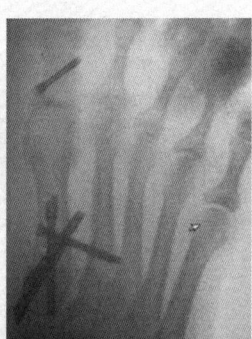

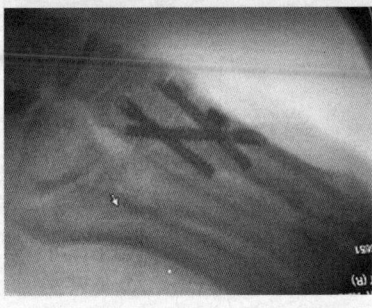

TECH FIG 2 A. Placement of a partial thread cancellous screw between the first and second metatarsal. **B–D.** Variations for fixation across the TMT joint. **B.** AP radiograph of two crossing screws: one anterograde and one retrograde. **C,D.** AP and lateral images showing use of three screws: two anterograde and one retrograde.

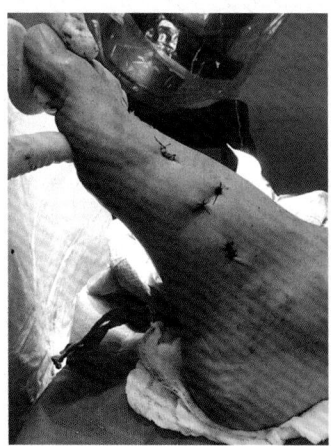
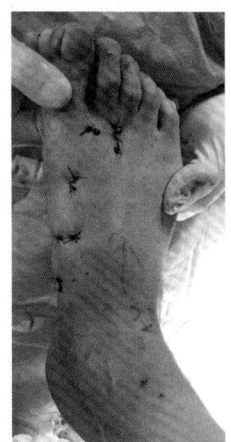
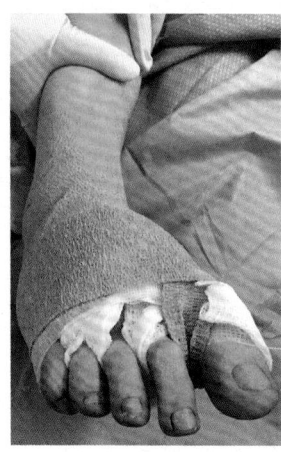

TECH FIG 3 A,B. The closed incisions. **C.** Postoperative wrapping with gauze and cling dressing applied to help maintain the correction.

placed central from plantar to dorsal at the second metatarsal and should be proximal at the metadiaphyseal junction. Stress fractures can occur if the screw is not central or proximal.
  - Alternatively, a lagged, fully threaded 3.5-mm screw can be used for fixation between the first and second rays. However, the authors' techniques have evolved to prefer the former method.
- The compressor/distractor is removed, and the reduction is again reviewed under intraoperative fluoroscopy.
- Starting at the medial eminence, a K-wire from the headless cannulated screw set is placed along the metatarsal shaft toward the medial or middle cuneiform. A cannulated, beveled 4- × 60-mm headless screw is placed retrograde just short of the navicular–middle cuneiform joint.
  - Alternatively, 3.5- to 4-mm fully threaded cortical screws can be used for fixation. Care should be taken to recess nonbeveled screws by subtracting 4 to 6 mm from the guidewire measurement to help reduce the risk of prominent hardware.
- A second and third screw are placed from the dorsal cortex of the first ray retrograde into the medial cuneiform.

- There are multiple variations for fixation across the TMT joint **(TECH FIG 2B–D)**:
  - Two crossing screws: one anterograde, one retrograde
  - Three screws: two anterograde, one retrograde
  - Three screws: two retrograde, one anterograde
  - Three screws: all retrograde
    - The authors' techniques have evolved to prefer three retrograde screws placed distal to proximal from the first metatarsal to the medial cuneiform.

Completion

- Multiplanar fluoroscopic images confirm the correct position of the hardware. Care is taken to ensure there is no unintentional penetration into the navicular cuneiform joints and that hardware prominence is minimized.
- The wounds are irrigated and closed with Monocryl or nylon sutures **(TECH FIG 3A,B)**.
- Sterile dressings and a short walker boot are applied. Gauze and 4-inch cling dressings are applied to maintain correction with the hallux in neutral to slight varus **(TECH FIG 3C)**.

TECHNIQUES

Pearls and Pitfalls

Contraindications	• Arthritis of the first MTP joint, skeletal immaturity, generalized ligamentous laxity, short first metatarsal, previous sesamoiditis, infection, avascular necrosis, Charcot arthropathy, and poor bone stock
Preventing Thermal Skin Injury	• The use of copious irrigation while using the burr, inserting K-wires, or drilling helps minimize the risk of thermal injury to the skin and bone necrosis. Additionally, the burr should be capable of delivering high torque at a low speed in order to efficiently cut through bone while minimizing heat production.
Preventing Hardware Prominence	• The use of beveled screws or recessing nonbeveled screws by subtracting 4–6 mm from the guidewire measurement help reduce the risk of prominent hardware.
Preventing Nonunion and First Metatarsal Shortening	• The joint preparation is critical for the prevention of these two complications. Both intraoperative fluoroscopy and arthroscopy allow precise débridement of the cartilaginous joint surfaces without violating the subchondral bone.
Preoperative Counseling	• It is important to counsel patients preoperatively and set appropriate expectations that, although this is a minimally invasive technique, swelling may take 3–6 months to resolve completely.
Hardware Malposition	• With a percutaneous technique, it is harder to ensure the correct starting point and trajectory of the screws. Screws need to have appropriate fixation in both bones at each side of the joint and not penetrate any other joint.

Undercorrection or Overcorrection of the Deformity	• It may be more challenging to ensure correct reduction of the hallux valgus deformity. The steps outlined should be carefully followed. An additional Akin osteotomy of the proximal phalanx may be required.
Metatarsus Adductus	• Metatarsus adductus may prevent correct realignment of the first metatarsal and leave a residual medial eminence and raised hallux valgus angle. Lesser metatarsal osteotomies may be required to allow correction of the first ray.
Lesser Toe Deformity	• Lesser toes should be corrected at the time of the original surgery including lesser metatarsal osteotomies, MTP joint releases, flexor tendon releases, and phalangeal osteotomies. In some cases, reduction of the MTP joint and K-wire fixation may be required.
A Broad Forefoot	• The wide forefoot can be particularly problematic in some patients. The width of the forefoot is contributed to by both the first and fifth ray deformity. A fifth ray osteotomy may be required at the same time as the first ray surgery.

POSTOPERATIVE CARE

- The patient remains non–weight bearing for the first 2 days postoperatively and then may bear weight as tolerated in a short walker boot.
- Elevation of the operative extremity is important to reduce postoperative swelling.
- The patient is seen in clinic 2 weeks postoperatively for a dressing change and taping or dressing to maintain correction of the first ray and lesser toes **(FIG 3)**.
- Radiographs are obtained at the 6-week follow-up appointment. The patient is transitioned to normal shoe wear at that time.
- Three-month follow-up: The patient is seen again at 3 months postoperatively, and repeat radiographs are obtained. This is typically the last follow-up appointment in the absence of concerns or complications (see **FIG 3C**).

OUTCOMES

- A meta-analysis of 29 studies with a total of 1470 operated feet concluded that the traditional open first TMT arthrodesis had higher corrective power compared with meta-analysis data on proximal, diaphyseal, and distal metatarsal osteotomies.[13]
- MIS Lapidus techniques achieve equivalent correction with rigid internal fixation while maintaining the benefits of small percutaneous incisions.
- Variations of this percutaneous technique have been described[6,7,9] with good radiographic correction and postoperative functional assessment.[9] However, due to the novelty of this procedure, the literature is limited with minimal reported outcomes and no direct comparison of open and MIS Lapidus techniques.
- The theorized advantages of the MIS Lapidus technique include smaller incisions, less wound complications, less swelling, less joint stiffness, and earlier mobilization. Additionally, MIS techniques allow direct visualization of the joint surface and a more thorough preparation of the arthrodesis site with minimal bone removal and better control of the arthrodesis position.[6] Ideally, these advantages limit the risk of nonunion, a shortened first metatarsal, and malunion.

COMPLICATIONS

- Nonunion, malunion, shortening of the first metatarsal, and dorsal elevation of the first metatarsal with subsequent overloading of the lesser metatarsals have been worrisome complications of the Lapidus procedure and its modifications for decades. Other complications include sesamoid pain, decreased motion at the first MTP joint, and loss of correction.
- Results from a recent systematic review analyzing eight studies and 443 traditional open Lapidus arthrodeses with an early postoperative weight-bearing protocol (defined as <2 weeks) demonstrated a nonunion rate of 3.61%.[1]
- Skin thermal burns are a complication unique to MIS procedures. This risk can be minimized with consistent intraoperative irrigation and the proper equipment.

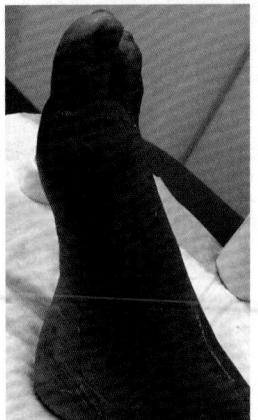 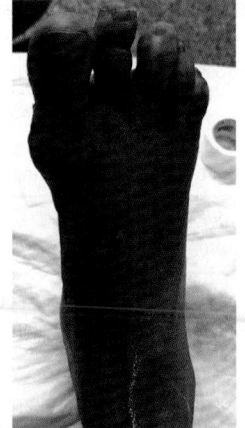 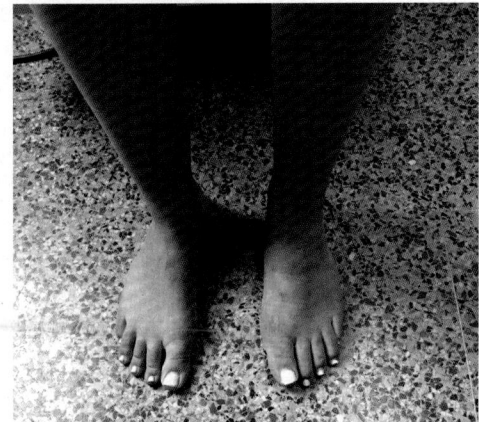

FIG 3 A,B. Two-week postoperative photographs after suture removal. **C.** Three-month postoperative photo of healed incisions.

REFERENCES

1. Crowell A, Van JC, Meyr AJ. Early weightbearing after arthrodesis of the first metatarsal-medial cuneiform joint: a systematic review of the incidence of nonunion. J Foot Ankle Surg 2008;57(6):1204–1206.
2. Ellington JK, Myerson MS, Coetzee JC, et al. The use of the Lapidus procedure for recurrent hallux valgus. Foot Ankle Int 2011;32(7): 674–680.
3. Lapidus PW. A quarter of a century of experience with the operative correction of the metatarsus varus primus in hallux valgus. Bull Hosp Joint Dis 1956;17(2):404–421.
4. Lapidus PW. The author's bunion operation from 1931 to 1959. Clin Orthop 1960;16:119–135.
5. Li S, Myerson MS. Evolution of thinking of the Lapidus procedure and fixation. Foot Ankle Clin 2010;25(1):109–126.
6. Lui TH, Chan KB, Ng S. Arthroscopic Lapidus arthrodesis. Arthroscopy 2005;21(12):1516.
7. Lui TH, Ling SK, Yuen SC. Endoscopic-assisted correction of hallux valgus deformity. Sports Med Arthrosc Rev 2016;24(1):e8–e13.
8. Malagelada F, Dalmau-Pastor M, Sahirad C, et al. Anatomical considerations for minimally invasive osteotomy of the fifth metatarsal for bunionette correction—a pilot study. Foot (Edinb) 2019;36:39–42.
9. Michels F, Guillo S, de Lavigne C, et al. The arthroscopic Lapidus procedure. Foot Ankle Surg 2011;17(1):25–28.
10. Myerson M, Allon S, McGarvey W. Metatarsocuneiform arthrodesis for management of hallux valgus and metatarsus primus varus. Foot Ankle 1992;13(3):107–115.
11. Shibuya N, Roukis TS, Jupiter DC. Mobility of the first ray in patients with or without hallux valgus deformity: systematic review and meta-analysis. J Foot Ankle Surg 2017;56(5):1070–1075.
12. Singh D, Biz C, Corradin M, et al. Comparison of dorsal and dorsomedial displacement in evaluation of first ray hypermobility in feet with and without hallux valgus. Foot Ankle Surg 2016;22(2):120–124.
13. Willegger M, Holinka J, Ristl R, et al. Correction power and complications of first tarsometatarsal joint arthrodesis for hallux valgus deformity. Int Orthop 2015;39(3):467–476.
14. Wukich DK, Donley BG, Sferra JJ. Hypermobility of the first tarsometatarsal joint. Foot Ankle Clin 2005;10(1):157–166.

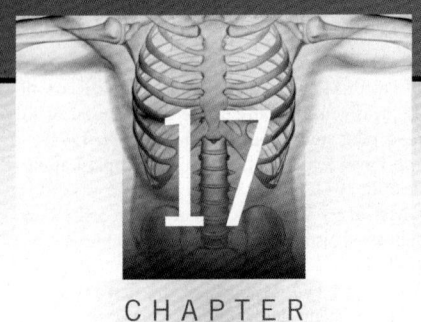

Lapiplasty: Three-Dimensional First Tarsometatarsal Arthrodesis for Hallux Valgus

Robert D. Santrock

DEFINITION

- The Lapiplasty procedure is the third generation of Paul Lapidus's procedure originally described in 1934 for correction of hallux valgus through arthrodesis of the first tarsometatarsal (TMT) joint.[6]
  - The original procedure was a uniplanar correction of the transverse plane and was later modified in 1989 by Sangeorzan and Hansen Jr[11] to be a biplanar correction of the transverse and sagittal planes.
  - The Lapiplasty procedure was developed to additionally incorporate correction of the frontal plane rotation often seen in hallux valgus.[3,5] It is a true triplanar correction of the hallux valgus deformity.
- The Lapiplasty procedure was developed with these principles in mind:
  - The pathogenesis of hallux valgus includes an unstable first TMT joint in most cases.
  - The frontal plane rotation must be corrected in addition to the transverse plane deviation.
  - All correction of deformity must be made before cutting any bone to avoid the need for recutting (which leads to shortening of the first ray); therefore, reproducibility was a must.
  - The procedure should be compatible with rapid (or even immediate) weight bearing to be as minimally disruptive to the patient's lifestyle postoperatively.[2]

ANATOMY

- The pertinent anatomy here includes the entire first ray, from the medial cuneiform to the hallux.
- Both the first TMT joint and the first metatarsophalangeal (MTP) joint are involved with correction of hallux valgus. The first TMT joint has abnormal bony morphology at the first cuneiform in hallux valgus patients.[7] This creates an "unstable" joint and subsequently allows the entire first metatarsal to rotate (pronate) in the frontal plane and deviate in the transverse plane (metatarsal varus). Occasionally, there is elevation of the sagittal plane as well, making the hallux valgus deformity a triplanar deformity.
- Other structures to be aware of while performing this procedure include
  - The insertions of the anterior tibial tendon and the peroneus longus tendon
  - The course of the extensor hallucis longus (EHL) tendon in the foot
  - The terminal branches of the dorsalis pedis artery and the sensory nerves of the medial foot

- The relationships of the structures of the lateral first MTP joint, including the fibular sesamoid and its ligamentous attachments (the accessory suspensory ligament), and the course of the deep peroneal nerve and adductor hallucis in the first web space.

PATHOGENESIS

- The hallux valgus deformity has virtually been redefined in recent years from a singular, transverse plane deformity to a multiplane, three-dimensional (3-D) deformity.
  - Although description of frontal plane rotational contribution to the deformity of hallux valgus dates back to 1956,[8] it was not until the advent of weight-bearing computed tomography that true understanding of the 3-D deformity of hallux valgus could be realized.[5]
  - We now understand that most hallux valgus deformities have rotation (pronation of the metatarsal) in the frontal plane that accompanies the transverse plane deformity of increased intermetatarsal angle (IMA) and hallux valgus angle (HVA).
  - Previously described surgeries failed to routinely address this multiplanar deformity, and subsequently, a high percentage of traditional bunion (metatarsal osteotomy) surgeries resulted in recurrence.
- There is significant evidence that there is distinct morphologic difference in the first TMT joint surfaces in patients with hallux valgus.
  - Mason suggested that hallux valgus patients are more likely to have a unifacet or bifacet first TMT joint.[7] Such shaped joints are perhaps more unstable (especially in frontal plane rotation) and may thus lead to the development of the hallux valgus deformity.

NATURAL HISTORY

- The natural history of hallux valgus deformity is slow progression of great toe deviation laterally. Eventually, impingement upon the second toe and other lesser toes leads to additional deformities such as hammertoes and crossover toe deformities with possible plantar plate rupture and instability of the lesser MTP joints.
- The weight-bearing axis shifts laterally in the foot; this leads to "overload" conditions and may manifest as metatarsalgia or stress fracture.
- The malalignment of the great toe MTP joint and the metatarsal sesamoid joints leads to pain, stiffness, and eventual cartilage damage. This results in symptomatic arthritis of the great toe MTP joint.

PATIENT HISTORY AND PHYSICAL FINDINGS

- A thorough clinical and radiographic exam is required for adequate preparation of any hallux valgus corrective surgery, but the Lapiplasty procedure does not rely on certain angular measurements such as IMA, HVA, or distal metatarsal articular angle.
- The key clinical physical examination findings necessary to understand before performing the Lapiplasty procedure are similar to those of many other hallux valgus corrections.
  - The foot should have an adequate neurovascular exam to predict appropriate healing.
  - There should be the exclusion of equinus contracture and hindfoot malalignment (ie, pathologic flat foot deformity or posterior tibial tendon dysfunction). The first MTP joint should be free of arthritis. This exam does not rely on the presence of first TMT joint arthrosis, pain, or hypermobility.
  - The presence of metatarsus adductus should also be identified. Metatarsus adductus is likely of a different pathogenesis, and as a result, this condition may require addressing the deformities of the lesser metatarsals.

IMAGING AND OTHER DIAGNOSTIC STUDIES

- The radiographic exam requires weight-bearing x-rays of the foot. It is recommended to obtain an anteroposterior, oblique, lateral, and axial sesamoid views.
  - The axial sesamoid view is of utmost importance to gauge the presence of first metatarsal coronal/frontal plane rotation **(FIG 1)**, and this view (along with the anteroposterior x-ray) will help assess the presence of sesamoid subluxation.
  - The identification of metatarsal rotation and sesamoid position are key steps preoperative planning.

DIFFERENTIAL DIAGNOSIS

- Hallux valgus
- Hallux valgus secondary to metatarsus adductus
- Hallux valgus concomitantly with pathologic flat foot deformity
- Hallux valgus concomitantly with equinus contracture
- Degenerative hallux valgus
- Hallux rigidus

NONOPERATIVE MANAGEMENT

- The conservative treatments for hallux valgus are symptomatic treatments only. Therefore, the only reasonable treatments shy of surgery are shoe modifications and activity modifications to reduce pain.
- There are no conservative treatments to correct or adjust the malalignments of hallux valgus.

SURGICAL MANAGEMENT

- The Lapiplasty procedure is indicated for all hallux valgus deformities. However, there are some special considerations as well as some true contraindications.
- Certain findings must be either addressed prior to Lapiplasty or in the same setting as Lapiplasty, including metatarsus adductus, hallux valgus interphalangeus, equinus contracture, hindfoot valgus, and pathologic flatfoot deformity.
- Prior failed hallux valgus surgery is another special consideration. One must evaluate the bone and joint orientations to determine whether reversal of the osteotomies previously deployed can be added to the Lapiplasty procedure to ensure a true triplanar anatomic correction.
- Contraindications to the Lapiplasty procedure include active infection at the surgical site, inadequate vascular exam, end-stage degenerative joint disease of the first MTP joint, significant osteoporosis, and neuropathic disease of the surgical foot.

Preoperative Planning

- The preoperative planning is usually complete with the described physical examination and radiographic analysis described.
- The procedure requires specialized equipment, the Lapiplasty System (Treace Medical Concepts, Ponte Vedra Beach, FL). The devices referred to in the Techniques section are from this kit and manufacturer.

Positioning

- The patient is placed supine on a radiolucent operating room table. It is occasionally necessary to place a hip bump under the operative side if the patient has excessive hip external rotation.

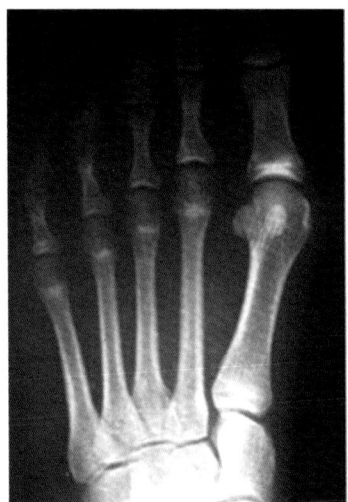

FIG 1 A. Weight-bearing anteroposterior radiograph showing the sesamoids appearing to be subluxated into the first web space but are in fact only pronated with the metatarsal. **B.** Weight-bearing axial sesamoid radiograph showing the sesamoids rotated with the pronated metatarsal.

- A thigh (preferred) or proximal calf tourniquet is applied to the operative limb, and the limb is prepped and draped in the usual fashion to the knees to keep from being limited by the drapes while moving the leg around for fluoroscopic imaging.
  - The leg is exsanguinated and the tourniquet inflated to the appropriate pressure for the entire procedure.
- This procedure is guided by fluoroscopic imaging, so one should be well versed in using image intensification. This procedure is especially suited for the mini C-arm. The mini C-arm should be placed at the foot of the bed, on the operative side.
  - The procedure can be done with a large C-arm as well, but it is a bit more cumbersome.

Approach

- It is essential to keep the incision dorsal with this technique to allow the guidance system to work properly.

FIRST TARSOMETATARSAL JOINT RELEASE

- The initial incision is made over the dorsal aspect of the first TMT joint, just medial to the EHL tendon (TECH FIG 1).
  - The incision is developed until the entire dorsal aspect of the first TMT joint is exposed.
- The entire dorsal and medial aspects of the first TMT joint are subperiosteally dissected.
- This joint release is to allow for rotation of a frontal plane deformity.

- Resection of the plantar lateral flair at the base of the first metatarsal promotes free rotation at the TMT at the time of correction.
  - This is done with an oscillating saw that is used within the first TMT joint.
  - The saw blade is passed dorsal–plantar repeatedly in the lower half of the joint to "plane" the joint surfaces.
- A small elevator is then used to open a soft tissue pocket at the proximal aspect of the 1–2 metatarsal interspace.

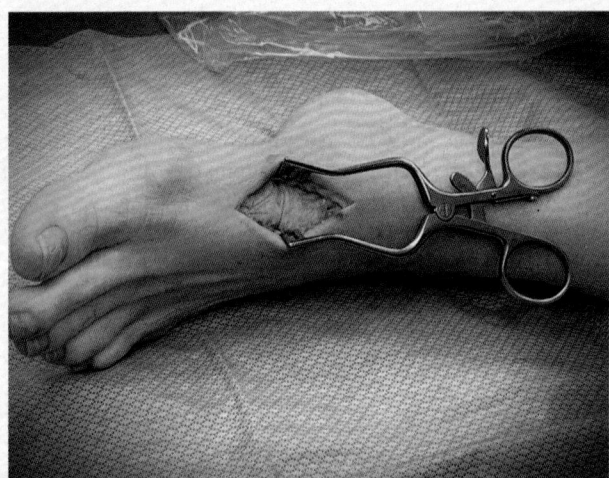

TECH FIG 1 Dorsal incision, adjacent to the EHL tendon, with exposure and release of the first TMT joint.

FIRST METATARSOPHALANGEAL JOINT RELEASE

- The Lapiplasty Fulcrum is placed into this space between the first and second metatarsal bases.
  - The fulcrum is maintained as far proximal as possible, and its proximal edge should be aligned parallel to the first TMT. This position is confirmed on lateral fluoroscopy views.
- It is necessary at this time to increase the mobility of the first MTP joint.
  - A first small webspace incision is made dorsally, and the tight lateral structures are gradually released until the joint

is mobilized. Typically, the lateral joint capsule and the accessory suspensory ligaments of the lateral sesamoid are targeted with this approach. The adductor hallucis tendon is left intact.
- Avoid opening the medial capsule of the first MTP joint at this time because destabilizing the medial structures will not allow the system to properly correct all three planes of the deformity.

PLACEMENT OF THE BONE POSITIONER DEVICE AND CORRECTION OF THE DEFORMITY

- A bone positioner device (Lapiplasty Positioner) is ready to be applied.
- A small stab incision is made over the second metatarsal approximately 1.5 to 2.0 cm distal from the first TMT joint.
  - The positioner is applied distal to the fulcrum and joint **(TECH FIG 2)**.
  - The medial aspect of the positioner should be applied to the plantar medial ridge on the first metatarsal. The lateral portion of the positioner is placed over the lateral cortex of the second metatarsal.
- The correction of the deformity is achieved in all three planes simultaneously by tightening the positioner knob.

- Clinical visualization and fluoroscopy are performed to confirm satisfactory deformity reduction.
  - The goal is to achieve complete correction of the IMA and tibial sesamoid position to normal values before proceeding to the next steps.
  - Care should be taken to ensure normal first ray sagittal plane position prior to proceeding (ie, no dorsiflexion or plantarflexion should be seen on the lateral fluoroscopic image).
- A holding pin is placed through the cannulation in the positioner to temporarily stabilize the corrected position.

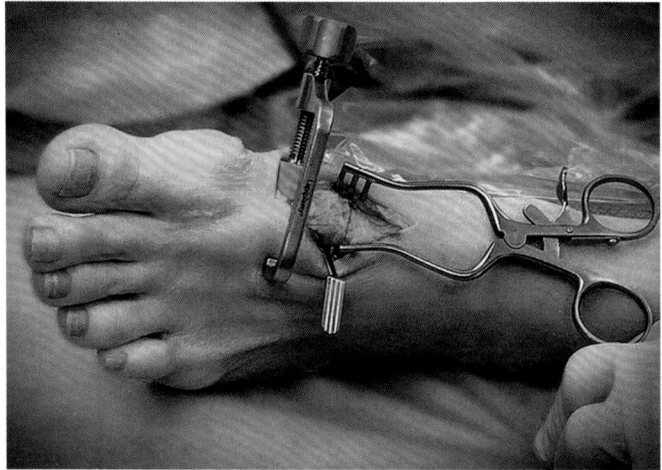
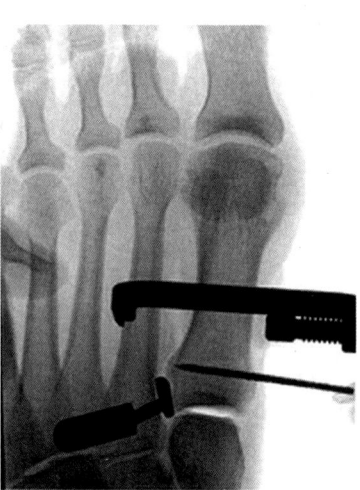

A   **B**

TECH FIG 2 A. Bone positioner and fulcrum being used to make a triplanar correction of hallux valgus deformity. **B.** Radiographic image of bone positioner and fulcrum in place with triplanar correction of hallux valgus deformity.

JOINT RESECTION AND PREPARATION

- The Lapiplasty Joint Seeker is then introduced through the dorsal aspect of the first TMT joint and maintained in the far lateral portion of the joint space.
  - This acts as a placement guide for the Lapiplasty Cut Guide and ensures that the cuts are made correctly in the sagittal plane to prevent dorsiflexion of the first ray at the time of arthrodesis.
- The cutting guide is then placed and aligned to parallel the midline of the first metatarsal and temporarily pinned in place **(TECH FIG 3)**. It is recommended that fluoroscopy be used to confirm the alignment of the cutting guide.
  - Once the position has been confirmed, a final offset pin can be introduced to secure the cutting jig position.

- The joint seeker is then removed, and the cuts on the base of the metatarsal and cuneiform can be completed.
- The fragments from the cuneiform and metatarsal cuts are removed.
  - A drill bit is used to fenestrate the joint surfaces, and the bone chips produced through this process are left to act as bone graft.
  - This joint surface preparation process increases the surface area and promotes rapid arthrodesis of the first TMT joint.

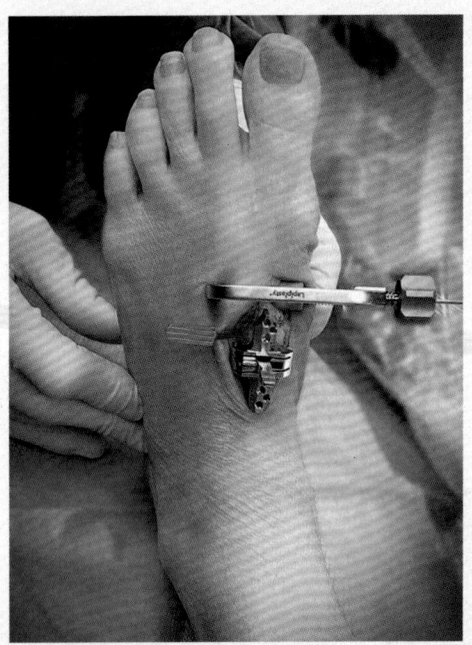
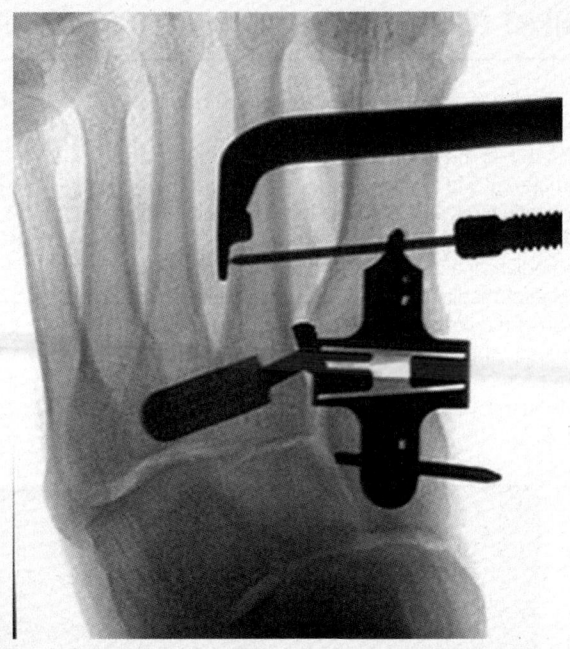

TECH FIG 3 **A.** Cutting guide in place. **B.** Radiographic image of cutting guide placement and the projected joint resection.

JOINT COMPRESSION AND TEMPORARY FIXATION OF ARTHRODESIS SITE

- Once preparation is completed, the first TMT joint is axially compressed with the Lapiplasty Joint Compressor and held in the corrected position with one or two terminally threaded olive wires (**TECH FIG 4**).
  - A smooth wire may also act as a substitute for an olive wire being placed from the medial first metatarsal to the intermediate cuneiform to prevent any derotation.

- The positioner and compressor are removed at this time, and correction is evaluated under fluoroscopy. If the position is satisfactory, the final fixation can be applied.

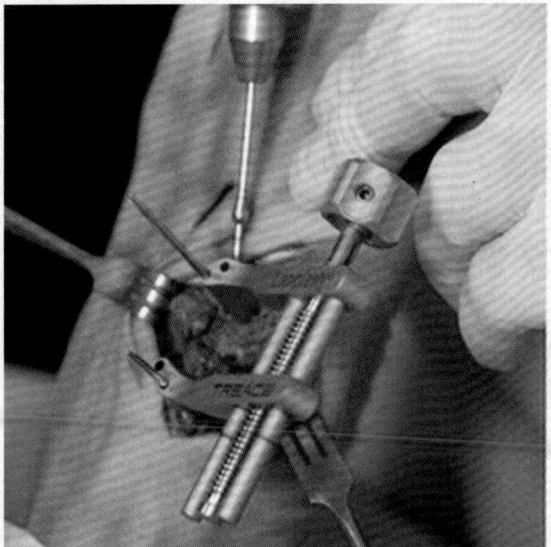
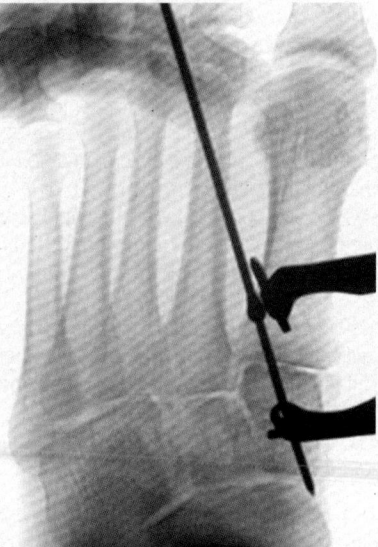

TECH FIG 4 Photograph (**A**) and radiograph (**B**) showing the compressed first TMT joint with a compression olive wire.

BIPLANAR PLATE APPLICATION

- The current technique uses a biplanar fixation construct (Lapiplasty System) that offers improved stability.[2] This construct allows for physiologic micromotion (that is presumed to occur with weight bearing) to promote quick callous bone healing (secondary bone healing) as described by Perren[9] and the AO Foundation (Arbeitsgemeinschaft fur Osteosynthesefragen).
- The initial plate is applied straight dorsal across the first TMT joint as far lateral as possible.
  - Once the plate is positioned, it is temporarily held with plate tacks through the center drill guides.
  - The open guides are drilled in preparation for screw placement.
  - The drill guides are then removed, and the locking screws are placed.

- The plate tacks are removed, the drill guide holes are drilled, the drill guides are removed, and the final two locking screws are applied to the plate.
- A second plate is applied medially across the first TMT joint, 90 degrees to the dorsal plate.
  - This plate is held with two plate tacks and then secured in sequence with four additional locked screws (**TECH FIG 5**).
  - It is important that the medial plate be inferior to the sagittal midline of the first metatarsal.
- Once the biplanar plate construct is complete, a "splay" test should be performed to assess instability between the first and second rays.
  - If the splay test confirms 1–2 intercuneiform joint instability, a transverse screw is used to stabilize the joint.

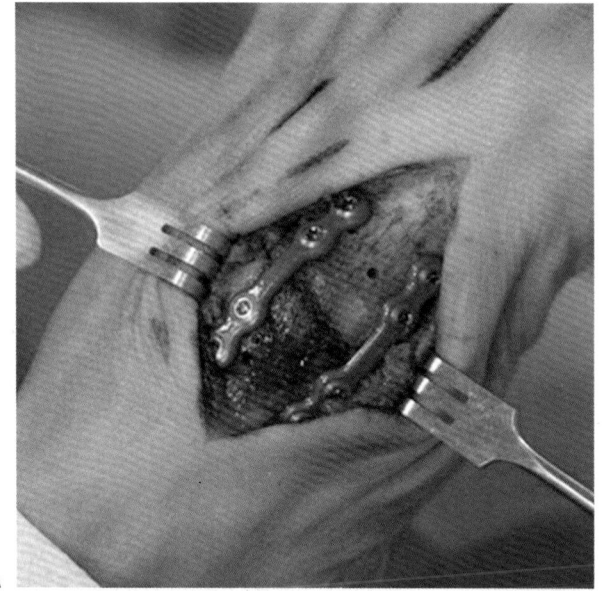

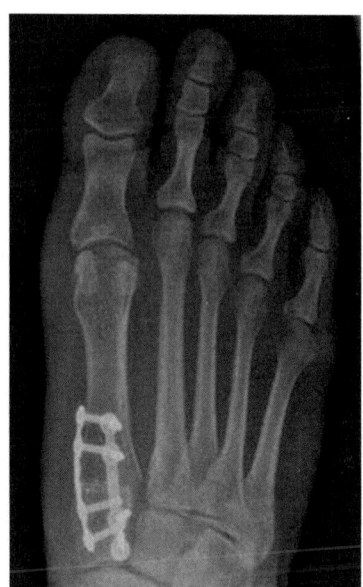

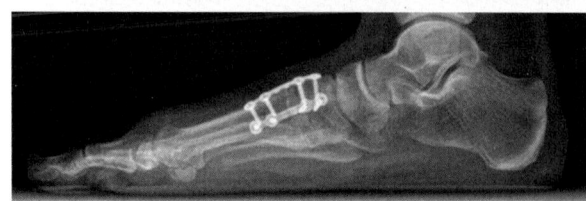

TECH FIG 5 Photograph (**A**) and anteroposterior (**B**) and lateral (**C**) radiographs of the final biplanar Lapiplasty construct.

FINAL TREATMENT FOR THE FIRST METATARSOPHALANGEAL HEAD AND COMPLETION

- Once the first TMT joint has been stabilized, the surgeon can direct their attention to the first MTP joint. If needed, a medial-based incision is used to access the joint.
  - Depending on deformity chronicity, there may be a significant capsular thickening present that may require thinning and a dorsal ridge on the first metatarsal head that may

require removal. Aggressive bone resection at this level is not indicated.
- Once any additional procedures have been completed, the wounds are copiously irrigated and closed in the standard fashion.
- The patient is placed into a sterile dressing and a walking cast boot.

Pearls and Pitfalls

Indications	• Lapiplasty is not recommended for patients with arthritic MTP joints, significant osteoporosis, or dense neuropathy. • Be cautious of concomitant deformities such as equinus, pathologic flatfoot, metatarsus adductus, and hallux valgus interphalangeus.
Positioning	• A mini C-arm is the preferred image intensification.
Incision	• A dorsal approach immediately adjacent to the EHL tendon is preferred.
Release	• Meticulous attention to the full release of the TMT joint is key to obtaining a triplanar correction.
Medial First Metatarsal Head	• Never open the medial capsule until the Lapiplasty is completed.
Biplanar Plating	• Be certain that the dorsal plate is as lateral as possible. • Be certain that the two plates are no less than 90 degrees to one another in the final construct.

POSTOPERATIVE CARE

- The surgery is outpatient, and the system is designed for an accelerated protected weight-bearing program. The walking boot is the preferred immobilization device for the first 6 weeks postoperatively. No strapping of the toe is required or recommended.
- Most patients begin the protected walking in a boot from postoperative days 0 to 7, and self-directed gentle range of motion of the first MTP joint is started early.
- Nonimpact exercise in a boot is permissible immediately.
- X-rays are obtained at 6 weeks, if all is well, the patient is transitioned to a running shoe.
- At 3 months postoperatively, most patients can return to all types of footwear, including fashion shoes.
- At 4 months postoperatively, x-rays are repeated, and if all is well, a return to impact sports (running and jumping) is permitted.
- Most patients do not need physical therapy.
- Some swelling is common for several months (6 to 9 months), and patients should be counseled on this normal occurrence.
- Clinical exams and x-rays are completed at 6 and 12 months postoperatively to ensure continued satisfaction and maintenance of correction.

OUTCOMES

- A study by Ray and colleagues[10] showed a recurrence rate of 3.2% in their cohort undergoing hallux valgus triplane correction with Lapiplasty TMT arthrodesis and a near-immediate weight-bearing protocol over a 13.5-month period.
- Dayton et al[4] published a series of 109 triplanar corrections evaluated at a mean of 17.4 months and reported a 0.9% recurrence rate.
- A multicenter prospective outcome study, ALIGN3D, is under way in hopes of further verifying the long-term benefits of the procedure.[1]
  - The study will enroll up to 200 patients, aged 18 to 55 years, at up to 15 clinical sites in the United States. The postmarket study is designed to evaluate the ability of the Lapiplasty procedure to consistently and reliably correct all three dimensions of the hallux valgus

deformity and maintain the correction following accelerated return to weight bearing.
  - The study's primary end point is radiographic retention of the hallux valgus deformity correction at 24 months of follow-up. Secondary end points include change in 3-D radiographic alignment, clinical radiographic healing, time to start of weight bearing in a boot and in shoes, pain, quality of life, and range of motion of the first MTP joint.

COMPLICATIONS

- Loss of correction or recurrence of deformity is the most common complication following all hallux valgus correction. The rate of radiographic recurrence can range from 30% to 70%. Lapiplasty thus far has exhibited a recurrence rate of only 3.2%.[10]
- Development of nonunion or delayed union is possible. These complications are rare due to the enhancement of "biologic" healing provided by the biplanar plating system.
  - A recent study documented a 97.4% stable union rate in 195 cases of biplanar plating supporting this stable, yet not rigid, biplane fixation concept.[4]
- Shortening of the first ray segment is usually a concern for the original Lapidus procedure and more so, for the modified Lapidus procedure. With the Lapiplasty procedure, it has been frequently observed that the restoration of the length is maintained by the "correct before cut" technique currently described. Minimal bone is removed to allow well coaptation of osseous surfaces.
  - Long-term studies are needed, but, with more than 10,000 procedures performed, the adopters of the Lapiplasty procedure report to a great degree the elimination of transfer metatarsalgia. Thus, to date, shortening has not been of clinical relevance.

REFERENCES

1. Dayton P, Carvalho S, Egdorf R, et al. Comparison of radiographic measurements before and after triplane tarsometatarsal arthrodesis for hallux valgus. J Foot Ankle Surg 2020;59(2):291–297.
2. Dayton P, Ferguson J, Hatch D, et al. Comparison of the mechanical characteristics of a universal small biplane plating technique without compression screw and single anatomic plate with compression screw. J Foot Ankle Surg 2016;55:567–571.

3. Dayton P, Kauwe M, DiDomenico L, et al. Quantitative analysis of the degree of frontal rotation required to anatomically align the first metatarsal phalangeal joint during modified tarsal-metatarsal arthrodesis without capsular balancing. J Foot Ankle Surg 2016; 55(2):220–225.

4. Dayton P, Santrock R, Kauwe M, et al. Progression of healing on serial radiographs following first ray arthrodesis in the foot using a biplanar plating technique without compression. J Foot Ankle Surg 2019;58(3):427–433.

5. Kim Y, Kim JS, Young KW, et al. A new measure of tibial sesamoid position in hallux valgus in relation to coronal rotation of the first metatarsal in CT scans. Foot Ankle Int 2015;36(8):944–952.

6. Lapidus P. Operative correction of the metatarsus varus primus in hallux valgus. Surg Gynecol Obstet 1934;58:183–191.

7. Mason LW, Tanaka H. The first tarsometatarsal joint and its association with hallux valgus. Bone Joint Res 2012;1(6):99–103.

8. Mizuno S, Sima Y, Yamazaki K. Detorsion osteotomy of the first metatarsal bone in hallux valgus. J Jpn Orthop Assoc 1956; 30:813–819.

9. Perren SM. Evolution of the internal fixation of long bone fractures. The scientific basis of biological internal fixation: choosing a new balance between stability and biology. J Bone Joint Surg Br 2002;84:1093–1110.

10. Ray JJ, Koay J, Dayton PD, et al. Multicenter early radiographic outcomes of triplanar tarsometatarsal arthrodesis with early weightbearing. Foot Ankle Int 2019;40(8):955–960.

11. Sangeorzan BJ, Hansen ST Jr. Modified Lapidus procedure for hallux valgus. Foot Ankle 1989;9:262–266.

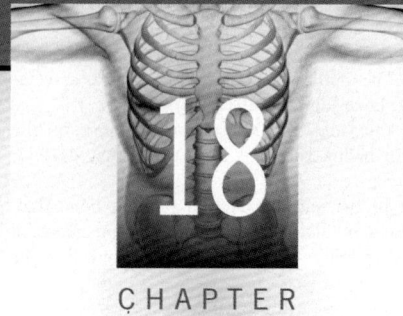

18
CHAPTER

Revision Hallux Valgus Correction

Patrick B. Ebeling and J. Chris Coetzee

DEFINITION

- Recurrent hallux valgus is a partial or complete return of valgus deformity at the first metatarsophalangeal (MTP) joint after surgical correction.
- Metatarsus primus varus is an increase in the 1–2 intermetatarsal angle (1–2 IMA) due to obliquity or hypermobility of the first tarsometatarsal (TMT) joint.

ANATOMY[7]

- The first TMT joint is 27 to 30 mm deep and irregularly shaped (FIG 1).
- The dorsalis pedis artery and deep peroneal nerve are just lateral to the extensor hallucis longus tendon (FIG 2).
- The two heads of the adductor hallucis muscle converge to a single tendon and insert on the lateral sesamoid at the first MTP joint.
- The sesamoids are contained in the capsuloligamentous complex of the MTP joint.
- The dorsal medial cutaneous branch of the superficial peroneal nerve runs along the dorsal medial aspect of the first MTP joint.
- The plantar medial cutaneous branches of the medial plantar nerve run along the plantar aspect of the first MTP joint near the articulations of the sesamoids.
- On the plantar aspect of the first metatarsal head, there are medial and lateral facets for articular with the sesamoids. These facets are separated by a central crista.
- In neutral rotation, the lateral aspect of the first metatarsal head is flat.

PATHOGENESIS

- Recurrence of hallux valgus is most often due to an improperly chosen initial procedure or improper surgical technique.
- Less frequently, factors such as poor bone or tissue quality, infection, patient noncompliance, and instrumentation failure can lead to recurrent hallux valgus.
- Rotational undercorrection and unrecognized metatarsus primus varus are the most common reasons for failure.
- If uncorrected, either rotation of the first metatarsal or metatarsus primus varus will create a valgus moment at the first MTP joint.
- An intact adductor hallucis or a tight lateral joint capsule will exacerbate the valgus moment.

NATURAL HISTORY

- Some partial recurrences of hallux valgus may be tolerable with nonoperative treatment.
- A residual or recurrent medial prominence can result in pain, tenderness, and an overlying bursitis.
- If there is an uncorrected rotational deformity or metatarsus primus varus, the deformity will most likely progress over time.

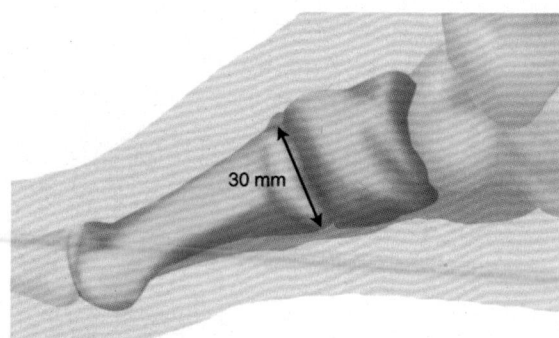

FIG 1 Lateral view of the first TMT joint. The joint is an average of 30 mm deep.

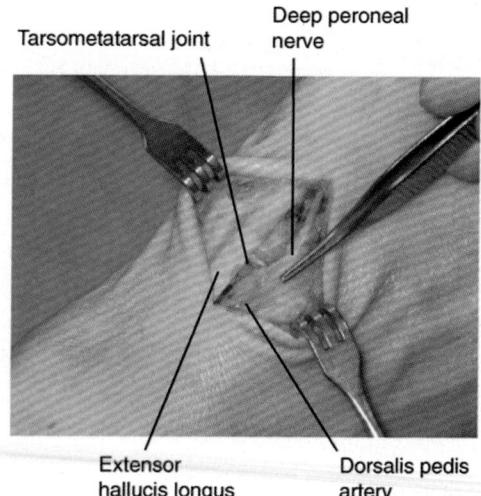

FIG 2 The extensor hallucis longus over the TMT joint. The dorsalis pedis and deep peroneal nerve are just lateral to the tendon.

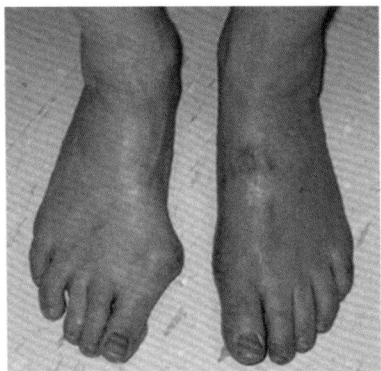

FIG 3 Picture after previous bilateral distal bunion procedures. The *left* side is 6 months after revision with a Lapidus procedure, and the *right* side is preoperative.

- Progressive deformity often leads to second toe overload and, ultimately, to painful deformity of the second toe and/or arthritis at the second TMT joints.
- Lesser metatarsal overload can also occur due to shortening of the first metatarsal, dorsiflexion malunion, or subluxation of the sesamoids.
- Prolonged hallux valgus, especially with an incongruent joint, can lead to degenerative changes at the first MTP joint and/or the sesamoid–first metatarsal articulations.

PATIENT HISTORY AND PHYSICAL FINDINGS

- Patients report valgus deformity at the first MTP joint that is either recurrent or was never fully corrected (**FIG 3**).
- The examiner should evaluate for symptoms associated with metatarsus primus varus:
  - Hypermobility of the first TMT joint[4,5]
    - Mobility of the first TMT joint is tested by holding the lesser metatarsal heads stable with one hand while passively dorsiflexing the first metatarsal head.
    - Hypermobility has been defined as elevation of the first metatarsal head more than 5 to 8 mm above the level of the second metatarsal head (**FIG 4**).
  - Degenerative changes at the first TMT joint
    - Tenderness at the joint line
    - Osteophytes at the dorsal aspect of the joint
  - Lesser toe overload
    - Patients may report feeling as if there is a rock in their shoe.
    - The medial lesser toes should be inspected for claw toe or hammer toe deformity, overlap, large plantar callus, or plantar ulcers (**FIG 5**).
    - The plantar surface of the MTP joints is palpated for tenderness.
    - The proximal phalanx is translated to evaluate for instability of the MTP joint.
- The examiner should evaluate for signs and symptoms associated with first metatarsal rotation:
  - Pronation of the toe is best appreciated clinically with the patient weight bearing.
- The examiner should evaluate for other potential causes of the recurrent deformity:
  - Infection
  - Failure of fixation
  - Generalized ligamentous laxity
  - Osteoporosis

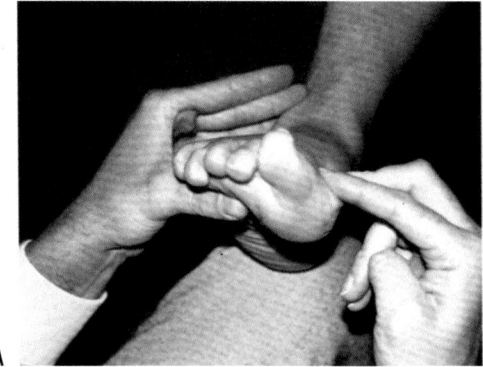

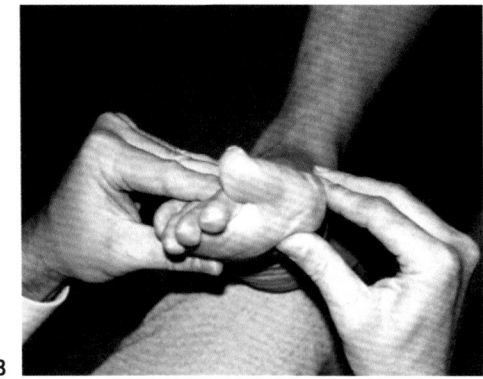

FIG 4 A,B. First TMT hypermobility.

- The examiner should evaluate for first MTP joint arthritis.
  - Advanced radiographic arthritis of the first MTP joint is an indication for arthrodesis.
  - Range of motion of the first MTP joint with the hallux valgus deformity corrected is an indication of expected motion after surgical correction. Severely limited motion may be an indication for arthrodesis.

IMAGING AND OTHER DIAGNOSTIC STUDIES

- Anteroposterior (AP), lateral, and oblique weight-bearing radiographs of the foot should be obtained and evaluated for the following:
  - Surgical changes from the initial surgery, including any retained instrumentation

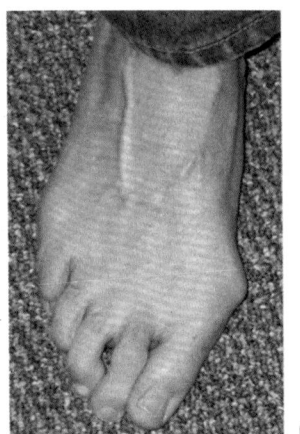
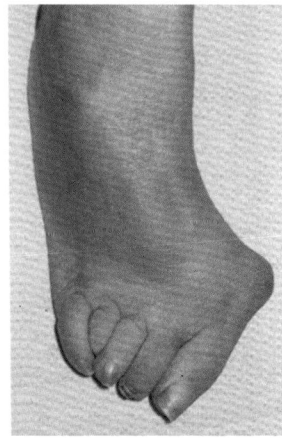

FIG 5 A,B. Claw toe deformity.

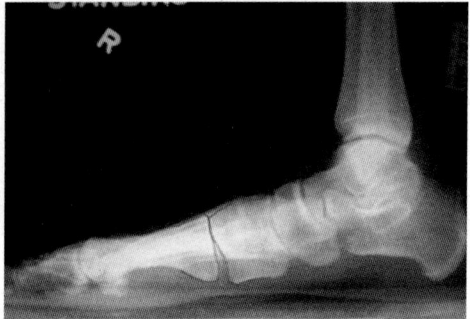

FIG 6 Plantar gapping of the first TMT joint as well as dorsal translation of the first metatarsal on weight-bearing radiographs.

- Congruency of first MTP joint
- Sagittal alignment of the first ray
- Hallux valgus angle (HVA)
  - Angle between long axes of first metatarsal and proximal phalanx
  - Normal is 0 to 15 degrees of valgus.
- 1–2 IMA
  - Angle between long axes of first and second metatarsals
  - Normal angle is less than 9 degrees.
- Distal metatarsal articular angle (DMAA)
  - Angle between long axis of metatarsal shaft and base of distal metatarsal joint surface
  - Normal is less than 15 degrees of valgus.
- Radiologic signs of metatarsus primus varus
  - Increased 1–2 IMA
  - Plantar gap at first TMT joint on weight-bearing lateral image **(FIG 6)**
  - Signs of lesser toe overload such as claw toe or crossover toe deformity
- Radiographic signs of first metatarsal rotation[8,10]
  - Rounded shape of the lateral first metatarsal head on AP view **(FIG 7)**[10]
  - Weight-bearing sesamoid view (modified Bernard view) **(FIG 8)**[8]

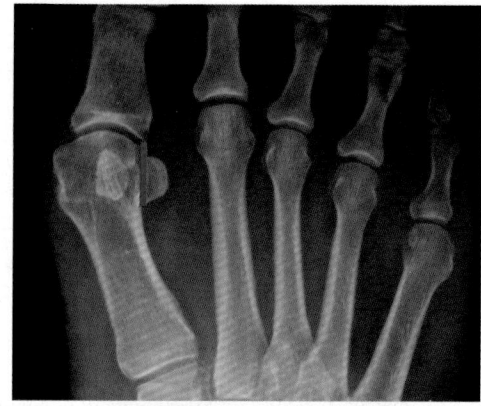

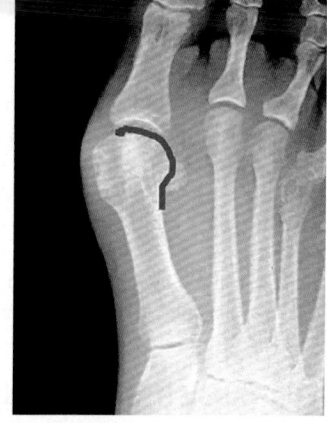

FIG 7 A. AP view of foot demonstrating rotation of first metatarsal with rounded lateral border of first metatarsal head. **B.** AP view of foot without rotational deformity of first metatarsal (*red line*). Note flat lateral border of first metatarsal head.

DIFFERENTIAL DIAGNOSIS

- Undercorrection of hallux valgus deformity
- Unrecognized or misunderstood characteristics of initial deformity
- Loss of fixation

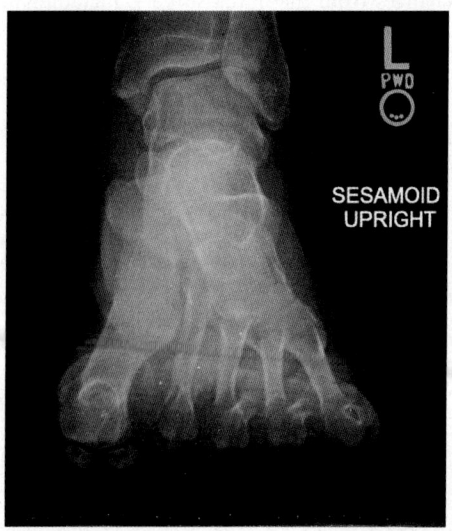

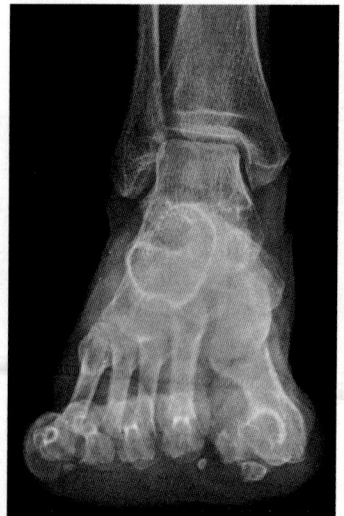

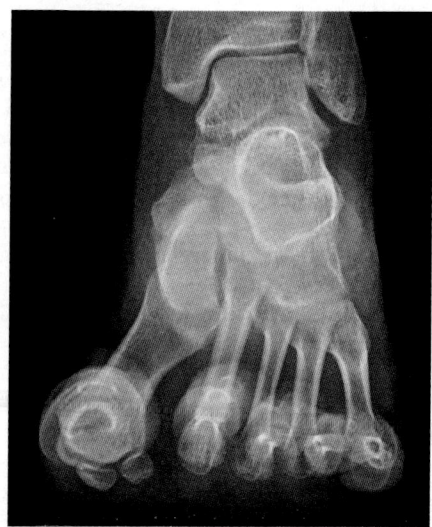

FIG 8 Weight-bearing sesamoid views. **A.** Well-aligned sesamoids. **B.** Lateral displacement of sesamoids. **C.** Reduced sesamoids with first metatarsal rotation.

- Generalized tissue laxity
- Infection
- Arthritis of first MTP joint (7).

NONOPERATIVE MANAGEMENT

- Shoe wear modification
  - Wide toe box
  - Low heels
- Orthotics
  - Medial arch support for associated pes planus
  - Metatarsal pad for associated second toe overload
- Symptomatic treatment
  - Activity modification
  - Over-the-counter medications

SURGICAL MANAGEMENT

- It is important to fully understand the details of the previous procedure.
- Seldom can a failed distal or shaft procedure be revised with another such procedure.

- Most salvage procedures rely on stabilizing the base of the first metatarsal.

Preoperative Planning

- Be prepared to remove any retained instrumentation.
- The age and position of previous incisions must be taken into account.
- The surgeon must evaluate the need for adjunct procedures, including shortening of the lesser metatarsals, correction of lesser toe deformities, and Akin phalangeal osteotomy.

Positioning

- The patient is positioned supine.
- A tourniquet is applied.
- The foot should be positioned to allow access for intraoperative imaging.

Approach

- The approach depends on the procedure to be performed.

LAPIDUS PROCEDURE (FIRST TARSOMETATARSAL JOINT FUSION) (VIDEO)

First Tarsometatarsal Joint Preparation

- Make a 6-cm incision over the dorsum of the first TMT joint.
- Identify the interval between the extensor hallucis longus and the extensor hallucis brevis.
- Incise the capsule of the first TMT joint and release it all around the medial and lateral borders of the joint to allow adequate exposure (**TECH FIG 1A,B**).
- Remove the cartilage from the first TMT joint using small osteotomes and small curettes.
  - Adequate exposure is critical. The plantar aspect of the first TMT joint must be visualized and prepared in order to avoid dorsiflexion malunion.
  - If the first metatarsal is shortened, only the cartilage should be removed.
  - If the first metatarsal is long, a small laterally based wedge can be removed from the medial cuneiform to facilitate reduction of the 1–2 IMA.

- A small plantarly based osteotomy can be performed to plantarflex the first metatarsal, if necessary.
- Use a 2.0-mm drill to perforate the subchondral surfaces of the joint.
- Expose and decorticate the medial aspect of the base of the second metatarsal and the lateral aspect of the base of the first metatarsal (**TECH FIG 1C**).

Distal Soft Tissue Procedure

- Make a direct medial incision over the first MTP joint.
- Capsulotomy
  - We prefer a straight, longitudinal capsulotomy in most revision cases.
  - If there is a redundant capsule, then an elliptical capsulotomy is performed.

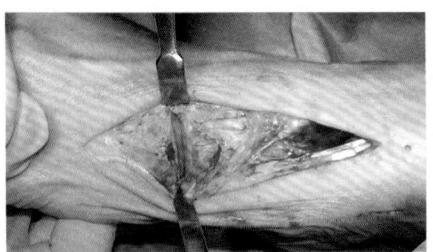 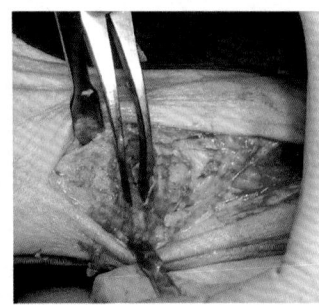 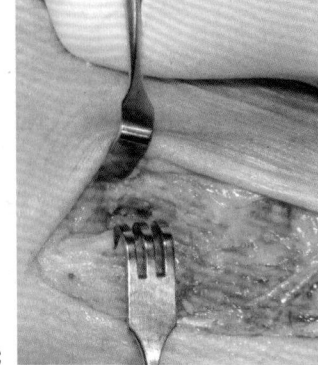

A   B   C

TECH FIG 1 A,B. With the initial exposure, only the dorsal 10 to 15 mm of the TMT joint is visualized. A small lamina spreader or distractor is required to expose the plantar half of the joint. This is a requirement of the procedure to avoid fusing the joint in dorsiflexion. With the distractor in place, the medial aspect of the base of the second metatarsal can be denuded of soft tissue to prepare for intermetatarsal fusion. **C.** Decortication of the lateral aspect of the base of the first metatarsal and the medial aspect of the second metatarsal to allow fusion.

TECHNIQUES

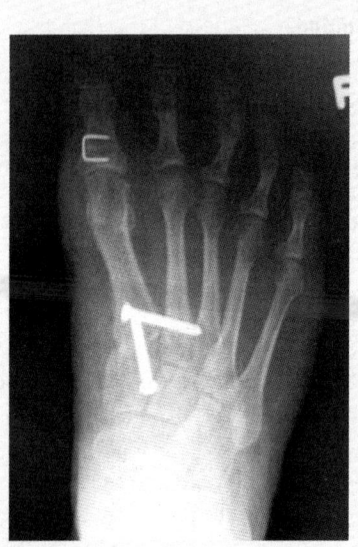 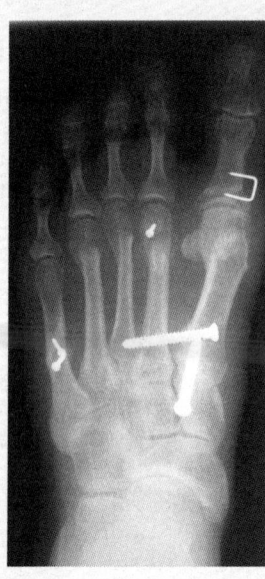

TECH FIG 2 Screw placement for a salvage of a failed distal procedure. **A.** The first metatarsal length was well preserved with the initial procedure. **B.** The first metatarsal length was such that a second metatarsal shortening was indicated to limit second metatarsal overload.

- Medial exostectomy
  - This is often more limited in revision cases.
  - Exposing cancellous bone at the medial eminence may help with healing of the capsule.
- Lateral soft tissue release
  - We prefer a transarticular lateral release.
    - A small lamina spreader facilitates exposure.
    - A beaver blade or no. 15 blade scalpel is passed just dorsal to the fibular sesamoid to release the lateral capsule.
    - Force the MTP joint into varus to complete the lateral release.
  - Lateral release can also be performed through a separate first dorsal web space incision.
    - Make a 2-cm incision in the first web space.
    - Use blunt dissection to identify the adductor hallucis tendon.
      - Identify and protect the terminal branch of the deep peroneal nerve.
    - Incise the adductor hallucis tendon at the lateral aspect of the fibular sesamoid.
    - Incise the lateral capsule longitudinally to allow reduction of the sesamoids.
    - Force the MTP joint into varus to complete the lateral release.
  - The vessels along the plantar lateral aspect of the metatarsal neck, just proximal to the lateral capsule, provide a significant source of blood supply to the metatarsal head and should be avoided.

Fixation of the First Tarsometatarsal Joint

- Reduce the first metatarsal in all three planes.
  - Parallel to the second metatarsal in the coronal plane
  - Neutral rotation in the axial plane
  - Not dorsiflexed in the sagittal plane
- Screw fixation (preferred technique)
  - Place a 3.5-mm cortical screw across the first TMT joint from proximal to distal using a compression technique.
  - Place a second 3.5-mm cortical screw from the medial aspect of the base of the first metatarsal into the base of the second metatarsal.

- Other methods of fixation
  - Plate fixation is useful where bone quality is poor or if a previous proximal procedure was performed.
  - Intramedullary devices specific to the first TMT joint are also available.
- Bone graft obtained from removal of the medial prominence can be placed in the 1–2 intermetatarsal space to augment the intermetatarsal arthrodesis.
- Use intraoperative imaging to confirm the position of the screws and reduction of the deformity **(TECH FIG 2)**.

Akin Osteotomy

- We employ an oblique Akin osteotomy **(TECH FIG 3)**.
  - This provides an abundant surface area for healing.
  - A screw is placed from proximal to distal perpendicular to the osteotomy.
  - It is possible to correct a rotational deformity of the interphalangeal joint through the Akin osteotomy, but this should not serve as a substitute for adequate correction of first metatarsal rotation.

Closure

- Reapproximate the capsule with absorbable suture **(TECH FIG 4A)**.
- The correction of the axial deformity is achieved with bony realignment, not capsular repair **(TECH FIG 4B)**.
  - An AP view prior to capsular closure should confirm reduction of the sesamoids.
  - If this is not the case, ensure that both 1–2 IMA and first metatarsal rotation have been adequately corrected.
- Motion of the first MTP joint should be maintained after capsular closure **(TECH FIG 4C,D)**.
- Close the wounds in layers.
- Obtain final fluoroscopic images to confirm alignment.
  - We strive for a slight overcorrection because the tendency is for recurrence, particularly in a revision procedure **(TECH FIG 4E)**.
- Clinical and radiographic results are presented **(TECH FIG 5)**.

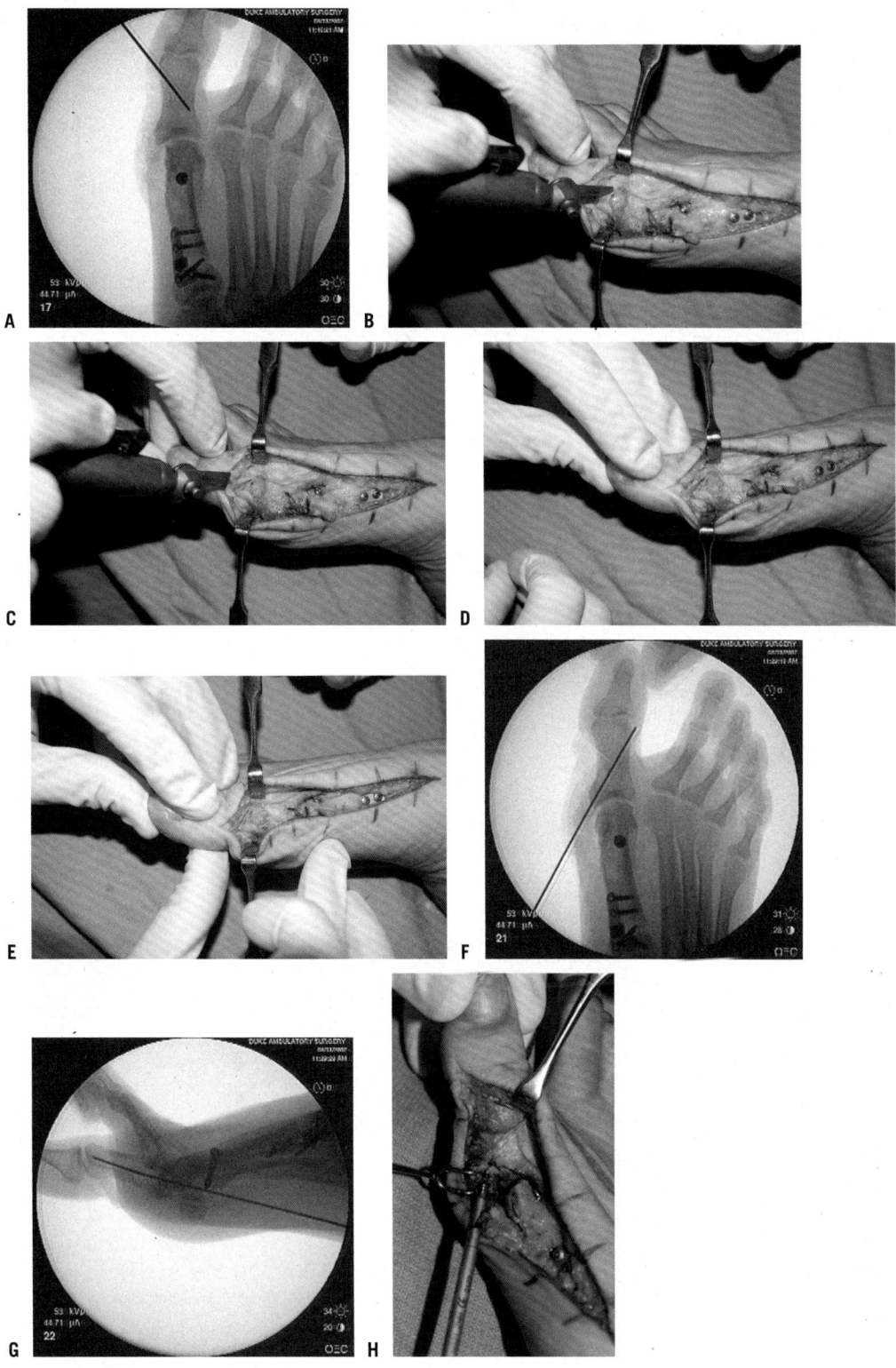

TECH FIG 3 Akin osteotomy (medially based wedge resection of proximal phalanx). **A.** Fluoroscopic view of reference pin to guide saw cut. **B.** Initial cut. **C.** Second cut. **D.** Osteotomy open. **E.** Osteotomy closed. **F.** Fluoroscopic view of guide pin for screw fixation (note that it is perpendicular to the closed osteotomy). **G.** Lateral fluoroscopic view confirming that pin is contained in the proximal phalanx. **H.** Screw insertion with osteotomy reduced.

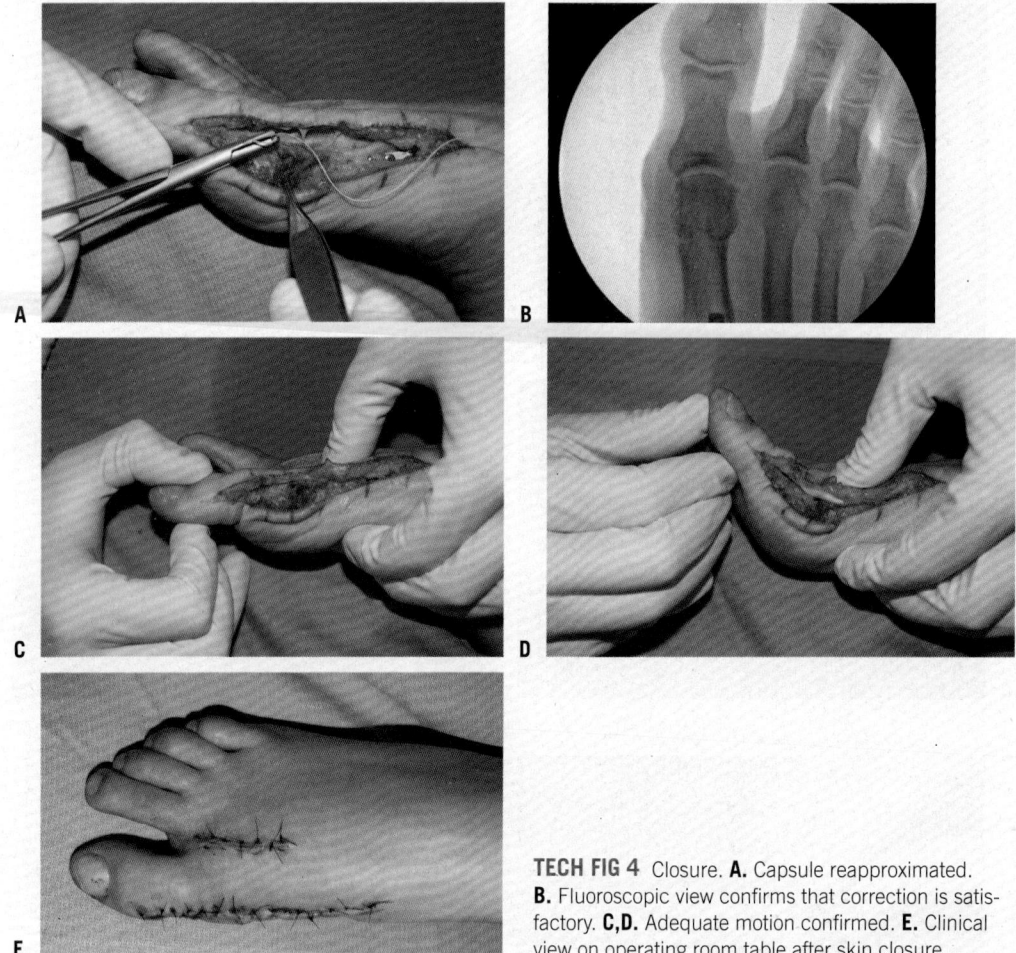

TECH FIG 4 Closure. **A.** Capsule reapproximated. **B.** Fluoroscopic view confirms that correction is satisfactory. **C,D.** Adequate motion confirmed. **E.** Clinical view on operating room table after skin closure.

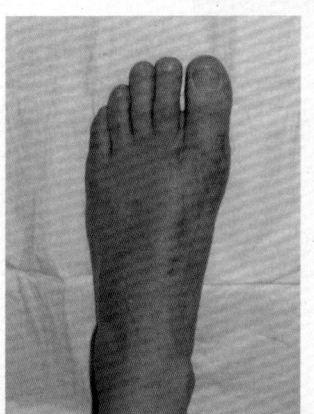
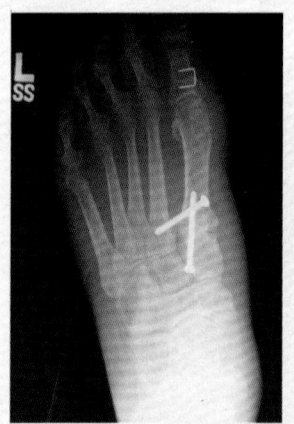
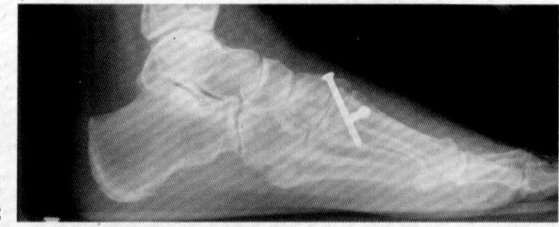

TECH FIG 5 **A.** Early follow-up clinical view. **B.** Weight-bearing AP radiograph. **C.** Lateral radiograph.

CASE EXAMPLE: PROXIMAL OPENING WEDGE OSTEOTOMY

Background

- A 33-year-old woman after distal bunion correction
  - Persistent symptomatic hallux valgus deformity **(TECH FIG 6A)**
  - Has failed appropriate nonoperative management
  - Motion well preserved in first MTP joint
  - Symptoms of second toe overload but no deformity
- Radiographs **(TECH FIG 6B,C)**
  - Prior distal procedure to first metatarsal head
  - Increased 1–2 IMA
  - Increased HVA
  - Questionable increase in the DMAA
  - Relatively short first metatarsal compared to second metatarsal
  - No obvious second toe deformity
  - Flat contour of the lateral first metatarsal head, indicating no significant pronation

Distal Soft Tissue Procedure

- Approach
  - Use previous dorsomedial incision.
  - Extend incision proximally to perform the proximal osteotomy.
- Capsulotomy
  - We prefer a straight, longitudinal capsulotomy in most revision cases.
  - If there is a redundant capsule, then an elliptical capsulotomy is performed.
- Medial exostectomy
  - This is often more limited in revision cases.
  - Exposing cancellous bone at the medial eminence may help with healing of the capsule.
- Lateral release
  - We prefer a transarticular lateral release.
    - A small lamina spreader facilitates exposure.
    - A beaver blade or no. 15 blade scalpel is passed just dorsal to the fibular sesamoid to release the lateral capsule.
    - Force the MTP joint into varus to complete the lateral release.
- Lateral release can also be performed through a separate first dorsal web space incision.
  - This must be performed judiciously to avoid putting the blood supply to the metatarsal head at risk, especially when simultaneous distal osteotomy is performed.
  - Technique
    - Make a 2-cm incision in the first web space.
    - Use blunt dissection to identify the adductor hallucis tendon.
      - Identify and protect the terminal branch of the deep peroneal nerve.
    - Incise the adductor hallucis tendon at the lateral aspect of the fibular sesamoid.
    - Incise the lateral capsule longitudinally to allow reduction of the sesamoids.
    - Force the MTP joint into varus to complete the lateral release.
- The vessels along the plantar lateral aspect of the metatarsal neck, just proximal to the lateral capsule, provide a significant source of blood supply to the metatarsal head and should be avoided.

Proximal Osteotomy

- In this case, a proximal medial opening wedge osteotomy was performed.
  - All traditional osteotomies, when they heal, shorten the first metatarsal slightly.
  - An opening wedge osteotomy may not lengthen the first metatarsal, but the risk of shortening is diminished.
  - The goal in this case was to preserve length, given that the patient was experiencing a second toe overload.
  - Given the osteotomy is performed from the medial side and the lateral cortex is left intact, it may also have less of a tendency to develop a dorsiflexion malunion, which could exacerbate the second toe overload.

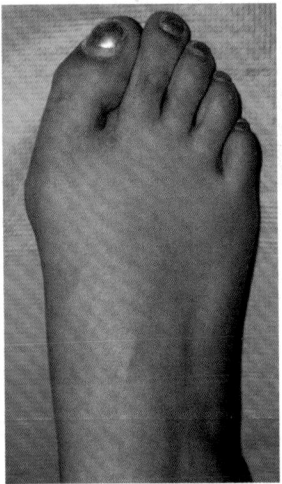
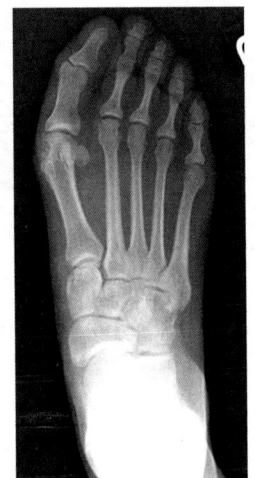
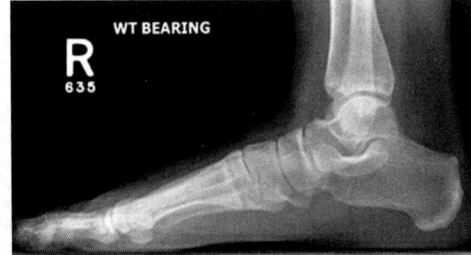

TECH FIG 6 Preoperative evaluation of 33-year-old woman with failed prior bunion correction. **A.** Clinical view. **B.** AP weight-bearing radiograph. **C.** Lateral weight-bearing foot x-ray.

TECHNIQUES

- Fluoroscopy is used to determine the trajectory of the osteotomy and the depth of the saw cut **(TECH FIG 7A)**.
- We make the osteotomy in the oblique plane to increase the surface area and target the more proximal aspect of the lateral metatarsal base where the cortex is wider and the soft tissue support is greater **(TECH FIG 7B)**.
- The saw cut approaches the lateral cortex without violating it.
- The osteotomy is gently opened with a triple osteotome technique **(TECH FIG 7C–E)**.

- The medial plate with spacer is placed and secured with screws **(TECH FIG 7F)**.
  - One of the proximal screws may be placed across the osteotomy to lend further support to the construct **(TECH FIG 7G)**.

Distal Biplanar Chevron Osteotomy

- With exposure, the actual (not radiographic) DMAA can be evaluated **(TECH FIG 8)**.
- The correction of the 1–2 IMA through the proximal osteotomy will increase any greater than physiologic DMAA.

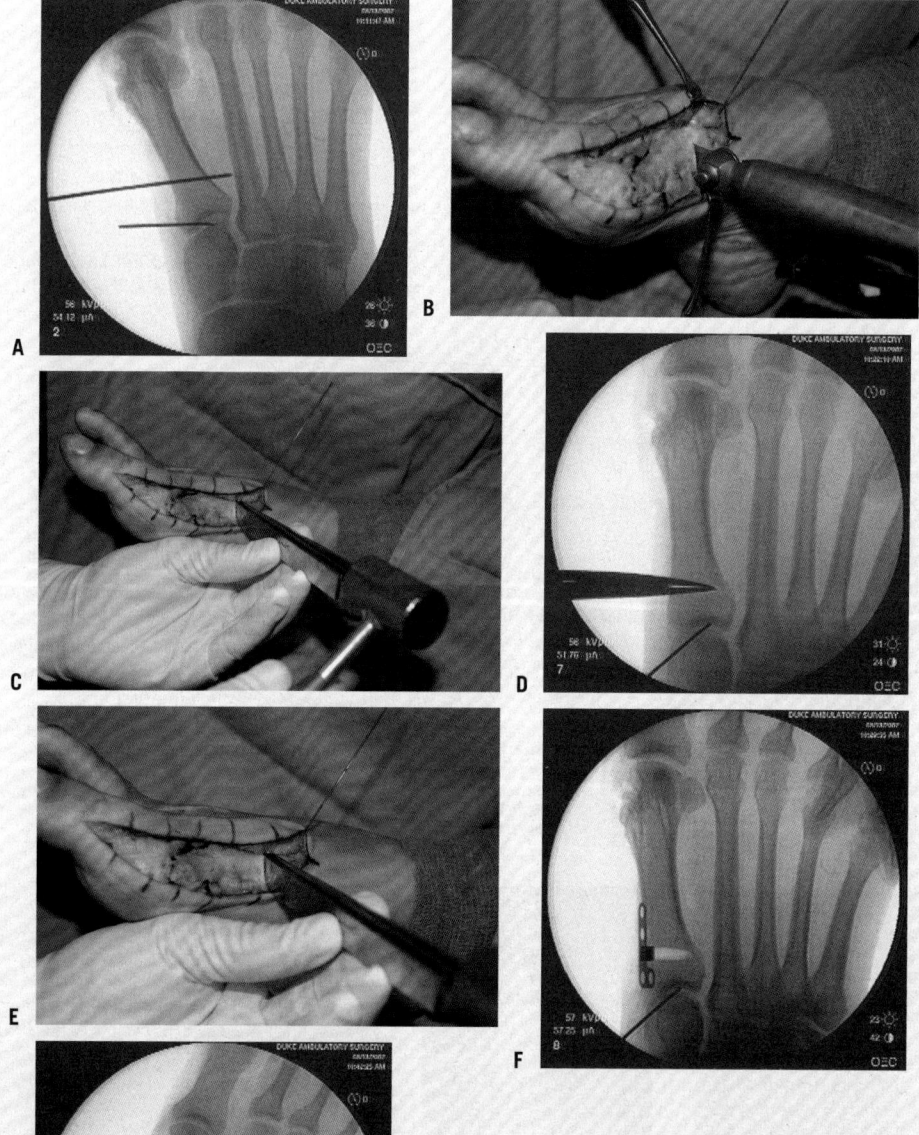

TECH FIG 7 Proximal first metatarsal opening wedge osteotomy. **A.** Fluoroscopic view of reference pin to guide saw blade trajectory. **B.** Microsagittal saw for osteotomy. (Note: Saw blade is perpendicular to metatarsal shaft.) **C.** Triple osteotome technique for opening the osteotomy. **D.** Fluoroscopic view of triple osteotome technique (note lateral cortex intact). **E.** Close-up of triple osteotome technique. **F.** Initial positioning of medial opening wedge plate. **G.** Reference pin to orient osteotomy (note final fixation of proximal osteotomy).

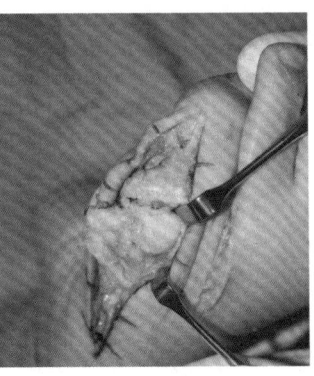

TECH FIG 8 Suggestion of increased DMAA (metatarsal head oriented laterally relative to first metatarsal shaft). Note lateral release performed through a separate dorsal first web space incision.

- A distal biplanar chevron osteotomy (Reverdin-Green osteotomy) affords greater correction, satisfactory stability, and a simple means of correcting the increased DMAA **(TECH FIG 9A)**.
  - We check a pin under fluoroscopic guidance to determine the orientation of the osteotomy (see **TECH FIG 7G**).
  - The osteotomy has a long plantar limb that provides large surface area for healing and excellent contact for screw placement **(TECH FIG 9B)**.
  - A medial closing wedge osteotomy is performed through the short dorsal limb to correct the increased DMAA **(TECH FIG 9C–G)**.
  - We routinely secure this osteotomy with a single screw placed in lag fashion **(TECH FIG 9H)**.
  - The medial prominence is resected **(TECH FIG 9I)**.

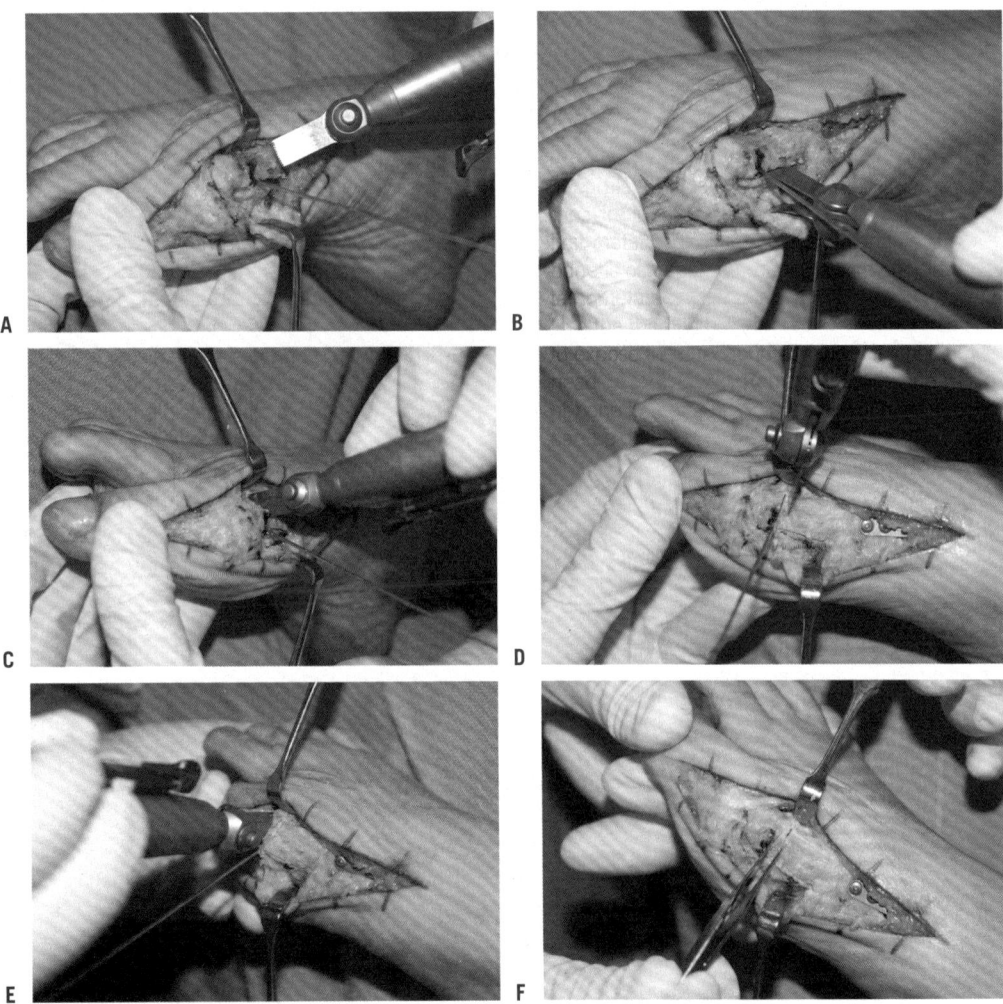

TECH FIG 9 Biplanar distal chevron osteotomy. **A.** Osteotomy marked on metatarsal. **B.** Long plantar limb. **C.** Short dorsal limb. **D–I.** Correcting the increased DMAA using a medially based wedge of dorsal limb. **D.** Initial cut. **E.** Second cut. **F.** Wedge completed. *(continued)*

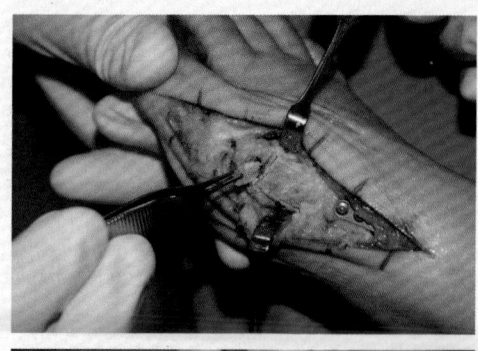

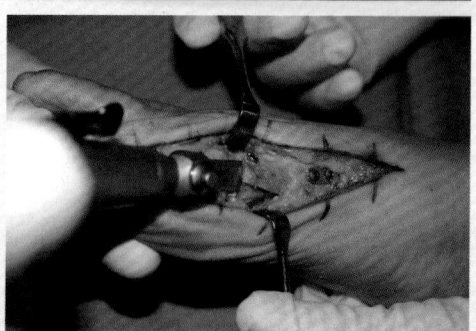

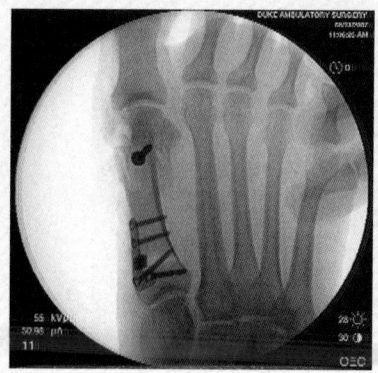

TECH FIG 9 *(continued)* **G.** Wedge extracted. **H.** Distal fragment translated laterally, oriented properly, and secured with a screw to the proximal fragment. **I.** Medial prominence resected.

LUDLOFF METATARSAL OSTEOTOMY

- This procedure could be used instead of a Lapidus procedure in cases where rotational correction is not required.[9]

Indications

- Smokers or patients with other medical issues that place them at risk for delayed or nonunion of a first TMT arthrodesis.
- Patients unable to be non–weight bearing for an extended period (eg, obesity, rheumatoid arthritis, contralateral joint problems, shoulder problems).
- Patients with less severe deformities
  - Expected correction of the 1–2 IMA is 8 to 16 degrees.[9]
  - No rotational correction can be achieved

Technique[1,6]

- Distal soft tissue procedure is as described earlier.
- Make an incision over the medial aspect of the first metatarsal.
- The optimal osteotomy starts on the dorsum, 1 cm from the TMT joint, and extends distal and plantar to a point just proximal to the sesamoid articulation **(TECH FIG 10A)**.
- The osteotomy should be angled from proximal dorsal to distal plantar.
- The axis of rotation should be within 5 mm from the proximal end of the osteotomy.

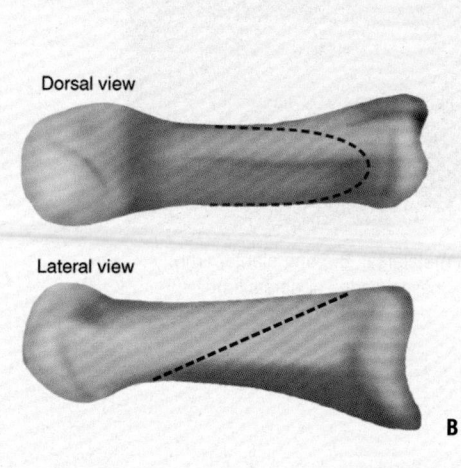

Dorsal view

Lateral view

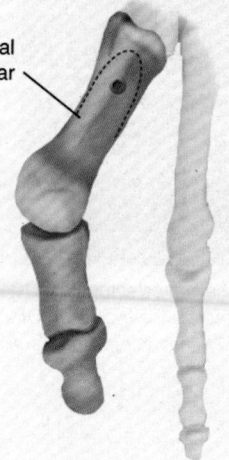

1st screw dorsal to plantar

TECH FIG 10 A–D. Ludloff osteotomy. **A.** A long oblique cut is made from dorsal–proximal to plantar–distal. **B.** After osteotomy and before rotation. The proximal screw is placed first, from dorsal to plantar. *(continued)*

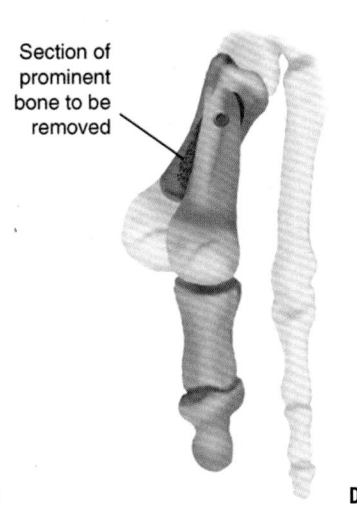

Section of prominent bone to be removed

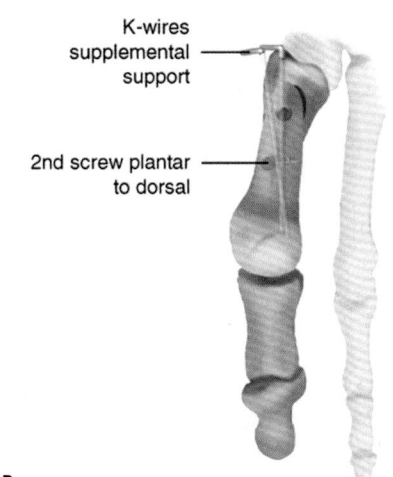

K-wires supplemental support

2nd screw plantar to dorsal

C   **D**

TECH FIG 10 *(continued)* **C.** The distal (capital) portion of the metatarsal is now rotated laterally to correct the intermetatarsal angle before the second screw is added. **D.** This is followed by the second screw, usually from plantar to dorsal, and insertion of a Kirschner wire.

- Complete the proximal part of the osteotomy first and insert the proximal screw from dorsal to plantar.
    - Since this screw will serve as the axis of rotation for the distal capital fragment, it should be slightly longer than the measured length and should not yet be fully tightened.
- Complete the distal part of the osteotomy.

- Rotate the distal capital fragment laterally to obtain the desired amount of correction.
- Insert the second screw and then fully tighten the first screw **(TECH FIG 10B–D)**.
- Remove any prominent medial bone.
- Capsular repair and wound closure are as described earlier.

DORSAL OPENING WEDGE OSTEOTOMY

Indications

- Dorsiflexion malunion of a proximal metatarsal osteotomy
- Dorsal malunion or nonunion of a Lapidus procedure **(TECH FIG 11)**
- No recurrent hallux valgus deformity

Technique

- Make a 6-cm incision over the dorsum of the first metatarsal base.
- Identify the interval between the extensor hallucis longus and the extensor hallucis brevis.
- Perform an osteotomy 1.5 cm distal to the first TMT joint, leaving the plantar cortex intact.
    - For a failed Lapidus procedure with nonunion of the first TMT arthrodesis, the osteotomy is done through the previous fusion site.

- Place a triangular, tricortical bone graft with the wide surface placed dorsally to plantarflex the first metatarsal.
    - Either an allograft or an iliac crest autograft can be used.
    - A small distractor is helpful in distracting and keeping the osteotomy open.
- An intraoperative simulated weight-bearing lateral view radiograph can be helpful to confirm appropriate reduction before final fixation.
- Fix the osteotomy with a small fragment screw from distal to proximal across the bone graft or with a dorsal plate that spans the bone graft **(TECH FIG 11A,B)**.
- Close the wound in layers.

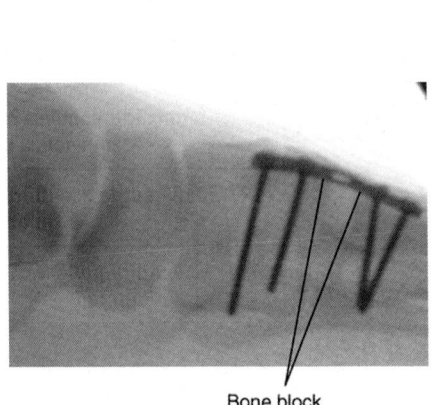

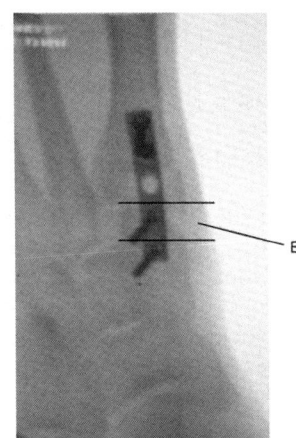

Bone block

A   Bone block   **B**

TECH FIG 11 A. Dorsiflexion malunion of a proximal metatarsal osteotomy. **B.** Dorsal open wedge osteotomy and bone grafting of a malunion of a Lapidus procedure.

GREAT TOE FUSION

Indications

- Severe degenerative changes of the first MTP joint secondary to previous bunion surgery
- Avascular necrosis of the metatarsal head
- Severe recurrence of a hallux valgus in a rheumatoid patient

TECHNIQUES

Pearls and Pitfalls

Indications	• Understand the reason for failure of the first surgery.
	• Obtain adequate imaging to determine the position of the first metatarsal in all three planes: 1–2 IMA, dorsiflexion, and rotation.
	• Evaluate DMAA and the potential need for a distal first metatarsal osteotomy.
	• Identify any existing instrumentation and be prepared to remove it.
	• Determine the age and location of all previous incisions in order to plan the surgical approach.
	• Significant arthritis of the first MTP joint is an indication for arthrodesis.
Medial Exostectomy and Lateral Soft Tissue Release	• Only a minimal medial exostectomy may be needed.
	• Avoid injury to the plantar lateral vessels to minimize the risk of vascular insult to the first metatarsal head.
	• The terminal branch of the deep peroneal nerve is vulnerable to injury in the first web space.
	• Excessive lateral release can lead to a hallux varus deformity.
First TMT Joint Preparation	• Take care not to inadvertently shorten the first metatarsal. Use a saw very sparingly.
	• The first TMT joint is about 25–30 mm deep. Take care to expose and prepare the entire joint surface to avoid fusing the joint in dorsiflexion.
	• A small Inge retractor or a smooth lamina spreader is invaluable in exposing the joint.
	• Careful preparation of the 1–2 intermetatarsal joint is mandatory to minimize the incidence of nonunion.
Positioning of the First Metatarsal	• To avoid dorsiflexion of the first metatarsal, it is helpful to hold the metatarsals in one hand while the screws are placed.
	• An intraoperative simulated weight-bearing lateral x-ray can be helpful in assessing sagittal plane position.
	• Ensure you have corrected first metatarsal rotation. The shape of the lateral aspect of the first metatarsal head on the AP view is a useful indicator.
	• Sesamoid reduction should be accomplished with correction of the first metatarsal position, not the capsular closure.
Shortening of the First Metatarsal	• It is not uncommon to find the first metatarsal shortened with the initial bunion procedure.
	• If this is the case, and if there are signs of significant lesser metatarsal overload, a second and sometimes third metatarsal shortening osteotomy should be done.

POSTOPERATIVE CARE

- Dress the wounds.
- Apply a well-padded slipper great toe spica fiberglass cast in the operating room.
- At 2 weeks, the cast is removed to allow wound check and suture removal.
- Apply either a new slipper cast or a postoperative bunion shoe for an additional 4 weeks.
- Patients are instructed to bear weight on the heel only for 6 weeks.
- X-rays are performed at 6 weeks, and if there is radiographic and clinical evidence of fusion, weight bearing and shoe wear are progressed and physical therapy is begun.

- At 8 weeks, patients can often return to swimming and biking.
- More vigorous physical activity is delayed until 3 months after surgery.

OUTCOMES

- In appropriately chosen patients, revision hallux valgus correction is a reliable option for recurrent hallux valgus.[2–4]
- A prospective cohort study reported an 80% satisfaction rate after the Lapidus procedure for recurrent hallux valgus in carefully selected patients.[2]
- The same prospective cohort study suggested an increased risk of nonunion in smokers.[2]

COMPLICATIONS

- Nonunion of the first TMT arthrodesis
  - Most common complication of a Lapidus procedure (6% to 10%)
  - Increased risk in smokers
- Transfer metatarsalgia
  - Dorsiflexion malunion of the first metatarsal
  - Lesser metatarsal length discrepancy
- Recurrent or persistent deformity
  - Failure to adequately correct first metatarsal rotation
  - Failure to adequately correct 1–2 IMA
  - Inadequate lateral release
- Hallux varus
  - Excessive lateral release
  - Overcorrection of 1–2 IMA
- Painful instrumentation
- Nerve injury
- Infection

REFERENCES

1. Beischer AD, Ammon P, Corniou A, et al. Three-dimensional computer analysis of the modified Ludloff osteotomy. Foot Ankle Int 2005;26(8):627–632.
2. Bock P, Lanz U, Kroner A, et al. The Scarf osteotomy: a salvage procedure for recurrent hallux valgus in selected cases. Clin Orthop Relat Res 2010;468(8):2177–2187.
3. Coetzee JC, Resig SG, Kuskowski M, et al. The Lapidus procedure as salvage after failed surgical treatment of hallux valgus: a prospective cohort study. J Bone Joint Surg Am 2003;85(1):60–65.
4. Ellington JK, Myerson MS, Coetzee JC, et al. The use of the Lapidus procedure for recurrent hallux valgus. Foot Ankle Int 2011;32(7):674–680.
5. King DM, Toolan BC. Associated deformities and hypermobility in hallux valgus: an investigation with weightbearing radiographs. Foot Ankle Int 2004;25(4):251–255.
6. Klaue K, Hansen ST, Masquelet AC. Clinical, quantitative assessment of first tarsometatarsal mobility in the sagittal plane and its relation to hallux valgus deformity. Foot Ankle Int 1994;15(1):9–13.
7. Mann RA. Disorders of the first metatarsophalangeal joint. J Am Acad Orthop Surg 1995;3(1):34–43.
8. Mortier J-P, Bernard J-L, Maestro M. Axial rotation of the first metatarsal head in a normal population and hallux valgus patients. Orthop Traumatol Surg Res 2012;98(6):677–683.
9. Nyska M, Trnka HJ, Parks BG, et al. The Ludloff metatarsal osteotomy: guidelines for optimal correction based on a geometric analysis conduction on a sawbone model. Foot Ankle Int 2003;24(1):34–39.
10. Yamaguchi S, Sasho T, Endo J, et al. Shape of the lateral edge of the first metatarsal head changes depending on the rotation and inclination of the first metatarsal: a study using digitally reconstructed radiographs. J Orthop Sci 2015;20(5):868–874.

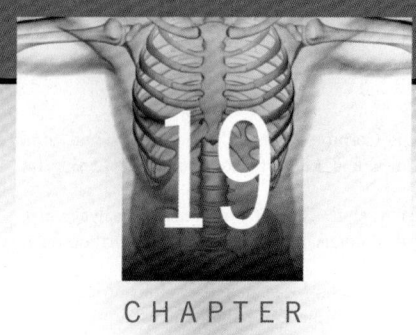

19
CHAPTER

Metatarsal Lengthening in Revision Hallux Valgus Surgery

James A. Nunley II and Jason M. Hurst

DEFINITION

- Shortening of the first metatarsal may occur after first metatarsal osteotomies for hallux valgus correction.[1-3]
- If the first metatarsal is considerably shortened, the patient may develop painful transfer metatarsalgia of the lesser toes.[7]

ANATOMY

- The physiologically normal first metatarsal is generally of similar length to or slightly shorter than the neighboring second metatarsal.
- This length relationship between the first metatarsal and the lesser metatarsals allows for a smooth, progressive weight transfer and optimizes the windlass mechanism during gait.
- The relative plantar position of the first metatarsal head (and sesamoids) also makes the windlass mechanism more effective in transferring weight to the lesser toes and may compensate for a physiologically shorter first metatarsal.

PATHOGENESIS

- Some metatarsal shortening occurs with the majority of all first metatarsal osteotomies performed during hallux valgus correction.[6]
- An iatrogenically shortened first metatarsal can disrupt the normal forefoot weight transfer mechanism and cause a pathologic overload of the adjacent metatarsals.
- Relative dorsiflexion of the metatarsal head can also occur after hallux valgus correction with metatarsal osteotomy, exacerbating the mechanical disadvantage of the shortened metatarsal and further contributing to transfer metatarsalgia.

NATURAL HISTORY

- Transfer metatarsalgia generally does not resolve spontaneously, particularly if coupled with a concomitant forefoot fat pad atrophy.
- Mild transfer metatarsalgia is generally well tolerated, as the patient is able to modify gait, stance, and activity to compensate.
- However, the problem may progress, with painful callus formation developing under the lesser metatarsal heads. Severe, recalcitrant transfer metatarsalgia may cause debilitating forefoot pain that often persists until normal forefoot biomechanics are restored or reasonable footwear accommodation is used.

PATIENT HISTORY AND PHYSICAL FINDINGS

- The great toe usually, but not always, appears shorter than the adjacent metatarsal, especially when compared to the contralateral foot (FIG 1).
- The plantar surface of the forefoot usually, but not always, has calluses under the lesser metatarsal heads.
- The lesser metatarsal heads are tender.
- When examined simultaneously, the first metatarsal head (and sesamoids) may appear elevated and more proximal relative to the second metatarsal head, particularly when compared to the contralateral foot.
- The medial forefoot incisions from prior forefoot surgery must be noted in anticipation of potential revision surgery.
- Hallux metatarsophalangeal (MTP) joint alignment must be examined. A recurrence of hallux valgus deformity after prior surgery will need to be corrected in conjunction with metatarsal lengthening.
- Hallux MTP joint motion must be determined. Stiffness and crepitance may suggest arthrosis that may favor first MTP joint arthrodesis over first metatarsal lengthening (FIG 2).

IMAGING AND OTHER DIAGNOSTIC STUDIES

- Weight-bearing plain radiographs are mandatory; we recommend bilateral radiographs to include the contralateral foot for comparison.

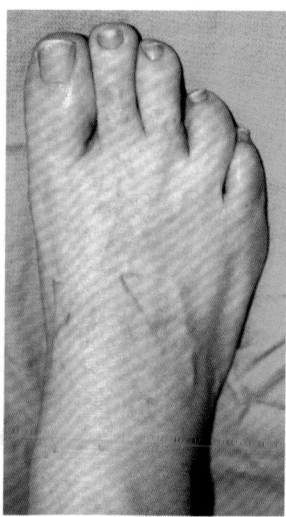

FIG 1 Foot with relatively short first metatarsal after distal first metatarsal osteotomy.

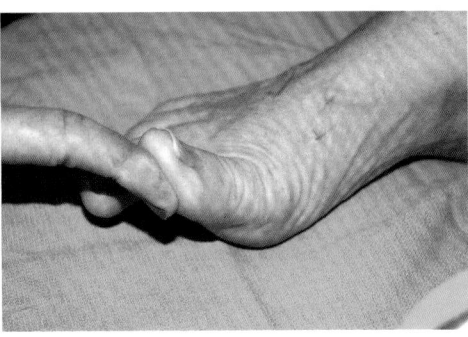

FIG 2 Assessing range of motion of hallux MTP joint before metatarsal lengthening.

- Anteroposterior (AP) radiographs of the symptomatic foot indicate the amount of first metatarsal shortening, the presence of residual deformity (particularly the first metatarsal head–sesamoid relationship), the nature of the prior hallux valgus surgery, and the integrity of the first MTP joint **(FIG 3A)**.
- Lateral radiographs suggest the degree of concomitant elevation of the first metatarsal **(FIG 3B)**.

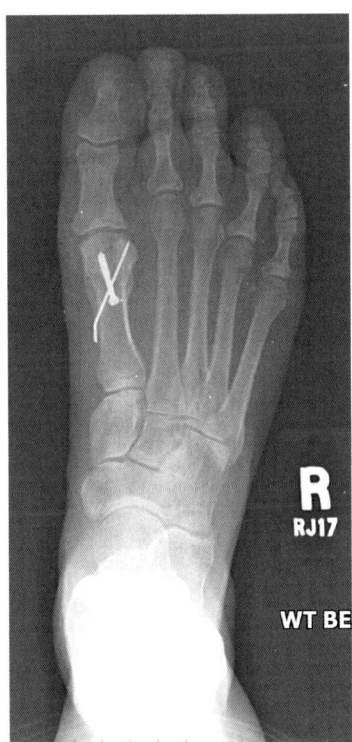

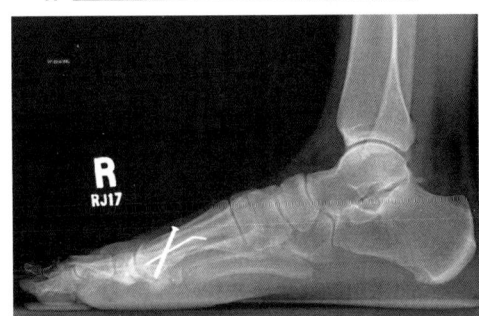

FIG 3 Preoperative radiographs of foot before hardware removal, application of external fixator, and metatarsal corticotomy. **A.** AP view. **B.** Lateral view.

- Contralateral foot radiographs provide some indication of the required lengthening, which is useful in surgical planning.

DIFFERENTIAL DIAGNOSIS

- Recurrence of hallux valgus
- First metatarsal head avascular necrosis
- Dorsiflexed malunion of first metatarsal

NONOPERATIVE MANAGEMENT

- Oral anti-inflammatory medication
- Shoe wear modification (ie, greater stiffness in combination with a rocker sole to unload the forefoot)
- Orthotics with medial posting for the first metatarsal and metatarsal support for the lesser metatarsals

SURGICAL MANAGEMENT

- Surgical management is indicated when nonoperative treatments have failed and other causes are not responsible for the forefoot pain and transfer metatarsalgia.
- Two broad categories may be considered in the surgical management of transfer metatarsalgia secondary to a short first metatarsal: shortening of the lesser metatarsals and lengthening of the first metatarsal.[4,5,8,9]
  - With severe first metatarsal shortening, a combination of these two approaches may need to be considered.
  - First metatarsal lengthening affords the advantage of correcting the problem at its source in lieu of performing surgery on lesser metatarsals that are physiologically normal but subject to an overload phenomenon.

Preoperative Planning

- Weight-bearing plain radiographs are essential to plan the desired lengthening and potential realignment of the metatarsal and MTP joint, determine the need for hardware removal from previous surgery, and identify potential arthritis in the MTP joint.
  - The contralateral first metatarsal, if not previously operated, serves as an ideal template to determine how a more physiologic first metatarsal anatomy may be restored.
  - To account for magnification, relative lengths of the first and second metatarsals may be used as a reference.
- Once the patient is deemed appropriate for metatarsal lengthening, the appropriate position for the external fixator half-pins and corticotomy should be planned radiographically.

Positioning

- The patient should be placed in the supine position on the operating table.
- A bump should not be placed under the ipsilateral hip to allow external rotation of the leg and better access to the medial side of the foot.

Approach

- A four-pin single-plane external fixator will be placed along the medial border of the first metatarsal, and a short, longitudinal dorsal approach to the metatarsal is needed to perform the metatarsal osteotomy **(FIG 4)**.
  - The incision may need to incorporate or be within previous surgical scars to minimize the risk of soft tissue complications.

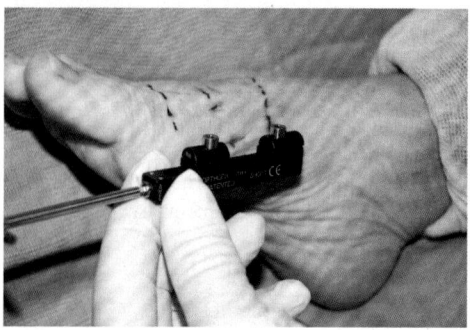

FIG 4 External fixator is held against metatarsal to determine appropriate adjustment of fixator.

- The four drill holes for the external fixator pins are created percutaneously, under fluoroscopic guidance, using a 1.5-mm Kirschner wire or the small-diameter drill corresponding to the particular external fixator set.
- After percutaneous placement of the four external fixator pins, a longitudinal dorsal approach to the metatarsal is used to perform the metatarsal corticotomy.
- Occasionally, a distal soft tissue procedure is necessary, and surgical incisions must be planned carefully. In our experience, this procedure is most effective for a shortened first metatarsal and satisfactory alignment of the first MTP joint.

PLACEMENT OF THE EXTERNAL FIXATOR PINS

- Using a surgical marker, plan the incision for the corticotomy by drawing a 2-cm line along the middle third of the dorsal border of the first metatarsal (see **FIG 4**).
- Using the closed external fixator as a drill guide, create four drill holes (two proximal and two distal) percutaneously along the medial side of the metatarsal using a 1.5-mm Kirschner wire. The external fixator must not be fully distracted when using it as a drill guide; however, it should be slightly distracted in order to apply initial compression after performing the corticotomy.
- With respect to sequence of drill holes, we recommend creating the most distal drill hole first and the most proximal one second, after which these half-pins are secured and the external fixator is attached. This sequence ensures that a monorail external fixator is parallel to the first metatarsal.
  - Alternatively, a hinged external fixator may be employed that can be adjusted to accommodate the pins while still creating longitudinal distraction (**TECH FIGS 1–4**).
  - Place all four pins into the drill holes in a similar percutaneous fashion, and check their position using fluoroscopy (**TECH FIG 5**).
- Some external fixator half-pins are tapered (eg, 2.5-mm tapered threads with 3.0-mm shafts) and thus should not be advanced beyond the lateral cortex of the first metatarsal and then reversed, as they will then lose their stability.

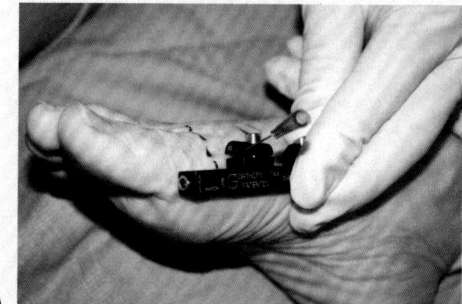

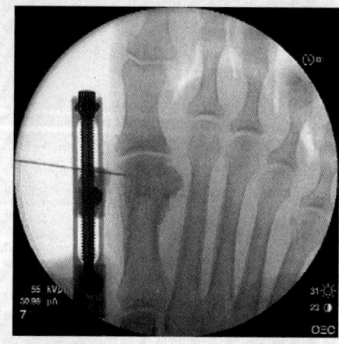

TECH FIG 1 Determining proper location for external fixator, using a needle as a reference. **A.** Clinical view. **B.** Fluoroscopic view.

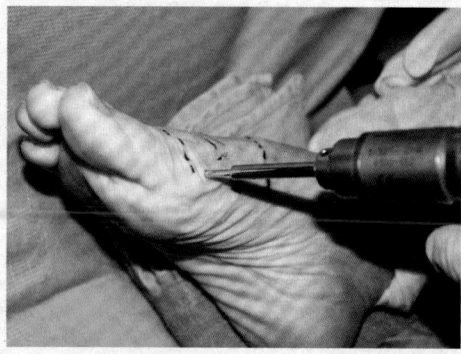

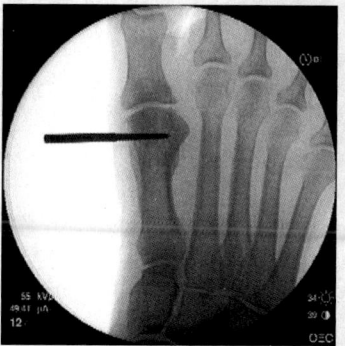

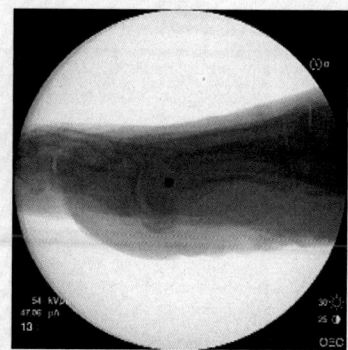

TECH FIG 2 First pin placed in distal first metatarsal. **A.** Clinical view. **B.** AP fluoroscopic view. **C.** Lateral fluoroscopic view.

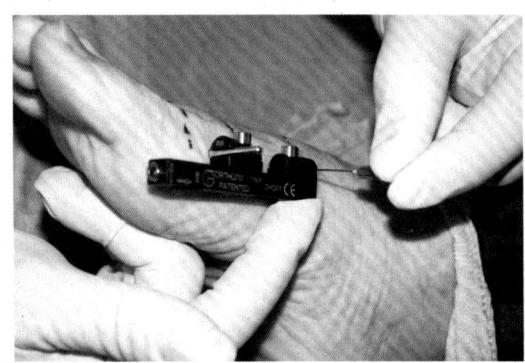
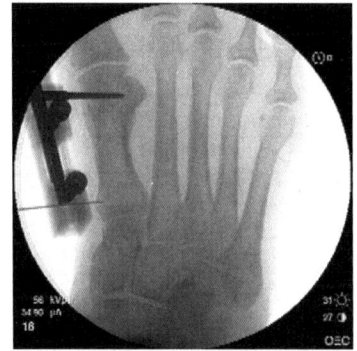

TECH FIG 3 Determining optimal proximal pin position. **A.** Clinical view. **B.** Fluoroscopic view.

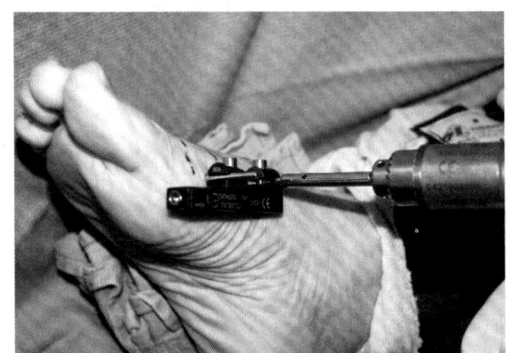
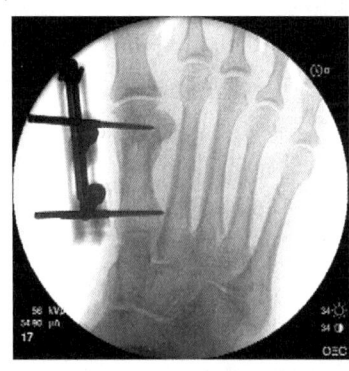
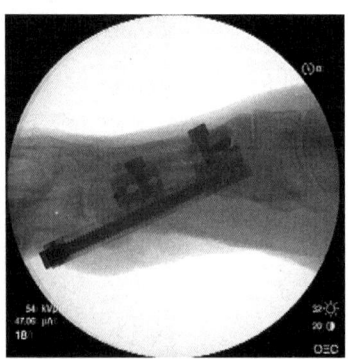

TECH FIG 4 Placing second pin in proximal first metatarsal. **A.** Clinical view. **B.** AP fluoroscopic view. **C.** Lateral fluoroscopic view.

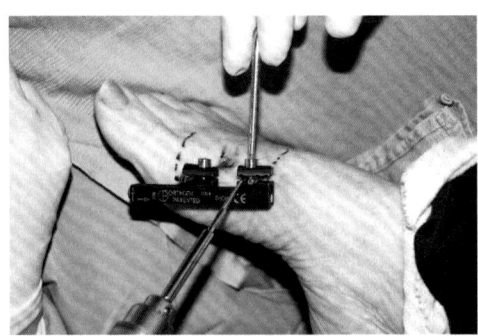
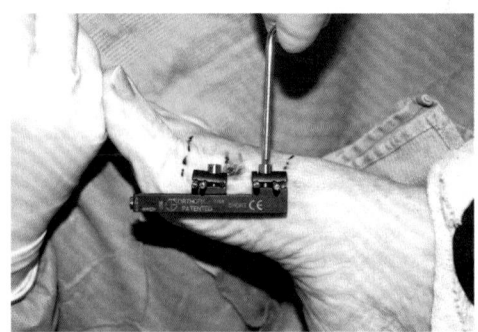
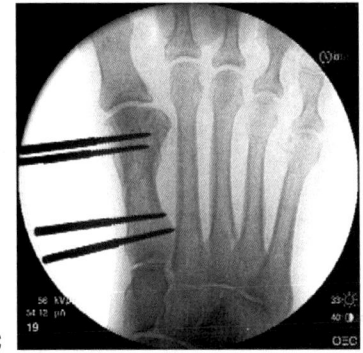

TECH FIG 5 Final two pins placed. **A.** Second most proximal pin being placed. **B.** External fixator tightened. **C.** Fluoroscopic view of all four pins secured. (Note that the external fixator was removed; no further adjustments are made so that the external fixator may be re-positioned on the pins so that the metatarsal maintains its anatomic alignment.)

CREATING THE CORTICOTOMY

- Make a 2-cm incision along the dorsal border of the metatarsal between the central two fixator pins (**TECH FIG 6A**).
- Dissect sharply to bone, and incise the periosteum transversely at the site of the planned corticotomy. Avoid unnecessary periosteal stripping; the periosteum only needs to be elevated directly at the corticotomy site.
- Make a transverse osteotomy using a mini-sagittal saw while simultaneously cooling the blade with iced saline irrigation (**TECH FIG 6B**).

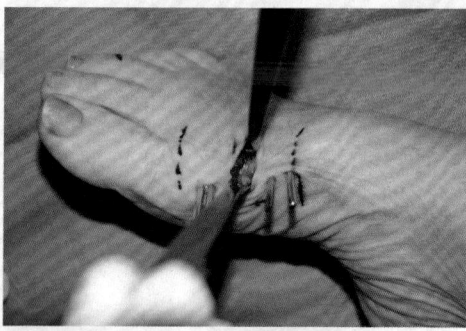
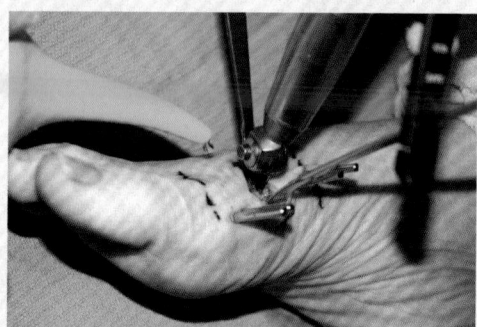

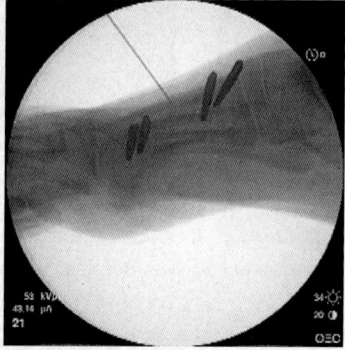

TECH FIG 6 A. Minimally invasive incision for metatarsal corticotomy with minimal periosteal stripping. **B.** Corticotomy being performed (irrigation is being performed to diminish the risk of bone necrosis from the saw). **C.** Before making the corticotomy, the ideal location is confirmed fluoroscopically (the external fixator has been removed to allow for better access during corticotomy).

APPLYING THE EXTERNAL FIXATOR

- After creating the corticotomy, confirm adequacy and distractibility of the distal and proximal first metatarsal segments with careful distraction through the external fixator and fluoroscopic confirmation (**TECH FIG 7A,B**).
- Add dummy pins to increase stability of the fixator (**TECH FIG 7C,D**).
- Compress the corticotomy using the external fixator; little compression is required—essentially the width of the saw blade (**TECH FIG 7E,F**).
- Using fluoroscopic imaging, verify adequate bone-on-bone contact of the two first metatarsal segments and secure the fixator set screws.
- Occasionally, there is slight subluxation of the two first metatarsal segments, and this should be adjusted so that the bony apposition is anatomic.

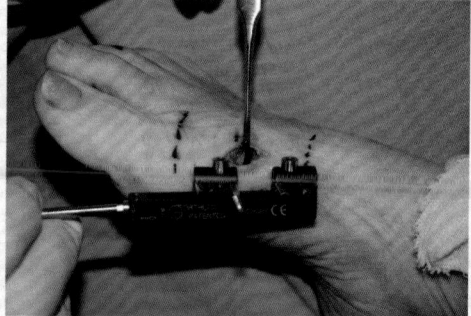
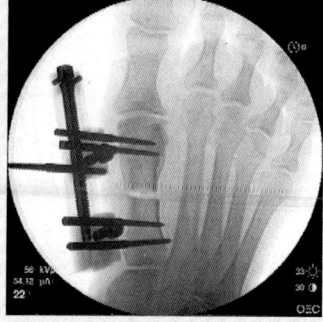

TECH FIG 7 A,B. The external fixator is replaced with the metatarsal in its preoperative position, and the corticotomy is distracted to confirm that it is complete. Additional "dummy" pins are added to the external fixator to afford greater fixator stability. *(continued)*

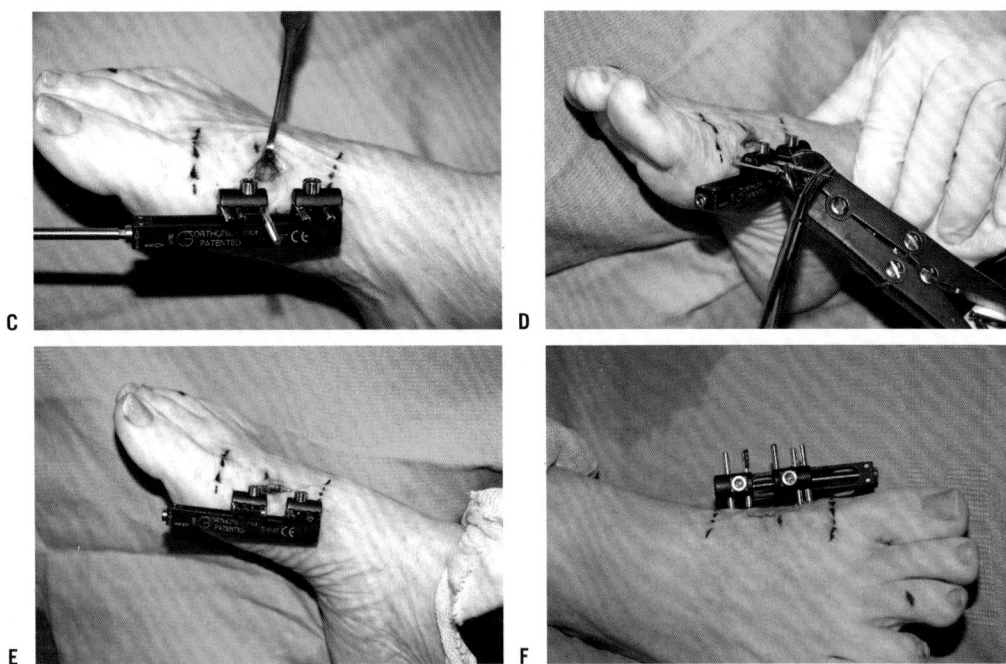

TECH FIG 7 *(continued)* **C.** Adding the pin. **D.** Trimming the pin. **E,F.** The corticotomy is compressed to its anatomic, preoperative position, and the external fixator is tightened.

WOUND CLOSURE

- We approximate the periosteum with 4-0 absorbable polyglactin suture and close the skin with 4-0 nylon suture.

- Apply a soft dressing. The patient can be discharged to home, non–weight bearing the same day of the procedure.

TECHNIQUES

Pearls and Pitfalls

Placement of the External Fixator Pins	• Use the external fixator as a drill guide. • Be sure to place the distal two pins in the plantar half of the distal fragment. This helps impart relative plantarflexion of the distal fragment and metatarsal head, thus limiting the potential for first metatarsal elevation.
Creating the Corticotomy	• Cool the saw blade to limit thermal necrosis of the bone edges.
Applying the External Fixator	• The wound may be reapproximated before placing the fixator, but be sure to verify good bony contact clinically and using fluoroscopic imaging.
Sequence of External Fixator Pins	• Placing the distal- and proximalmost pins first ensures that the external fixator is parallel to the first metatarsal and that no pin will violate the MTP or tarsometatarsal joints.
Stiffness of the First MTP Joint	• In our experience, with gradual distraction, preoperative motion of the first MTP joint is not compromised.
Formation of Bone ("Regenerate")	• Bone or callus does not form immediately with distraction at the corticotomy site; it may lag several weeks behind.

Failure of the Regenerate to Form	• Occasionally, the regenerate will not form despite appropriate distraction technique. Once the full desired distraction has been achieved, alternating quarter-turn distraction and compression may stimulate formation of the regenerate. Use of an external bone stimulator may be considered. As a last resort, the intercalary segment may be bone grafted, and internal fixation may be substituted for the external fixator, albeit only with a history of clean and healthy pin sites (the risk of infection with internal fixation is increased after previous external fixation in close proximity).
Duration of the External Fixator	• Generally, the regenerate becomes adequately stable for external fixator removal by 8–10 weeks, but occasionally, 12–14 weeks is required. We routinely remove the external fixator in the office setting.

POSTOPERATIVE CARE

- The patient is kept non–weight bearing. The first metatarsal needs to be protected until the regenerate has formed at the lengthening site. Weight bearing may compromise the stability of the corticotomy and the external fixator; moreover, weight bearing is not axial at the corticotomy site.
- We routinely see the patient in the clinic about 7 days postoperatively for wound inspection, patient education on distraction, and initiation of first metatarsal lengthening.
- We typically set the distraction rate for 1 mm per day (a quarter-turn of the external fixator every 6 hours).
- The patient should be given instructions in pin care and the number of days to distract the device to yield the desired length.
- We encourage daily first MTP joint range of motion to prevent joint contracture.
- The patient should return to the clinic regularly for radiographs to verify adequate distraction, appropriate position of the distal segment, and passive range of motion of the first MTP joint (**FIG 5A**).
- The lengthening phase is complete once the first metatarsal has reached the desired length, typically the physiologic length based on the first–second metatarsal length ratio from the physiologically normal contralateral foot.

- Partial weight bearing is allowed when there is radiographic evidence of consolidation within the distracted segment so long as it does not impinge on the external fixator. Boot or brace modifications typically allow for weight bearing even with the external fixator in place (**FIG 5B**).
- The fixator is removed once there is satisfactory radiographic consolidation of the regenerate. The patient can resume full weight bearing once the fixator is removed, but we recommend several weeks of protected weight bearing in a surgical shoe or boot to avoid fracture through the half-pin holes, which are potential stress risers (**FIG 5C,D**).
- **FIG 3** shows the radiographic clinical progression throughout the lengthening treatment.

OUTCOMES

- See the 2007 study by Hurst and Nunley.[2]

COMPLICATIONS

- Pin tract infection (inadequate pin care)
- First MTP joint stiffness (failure to perform intermittent first MTP joint range of motion)
- Early consolidation of distracted segment (distraction schedule too slow)

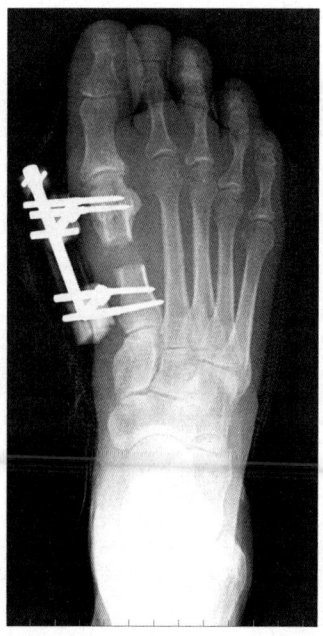

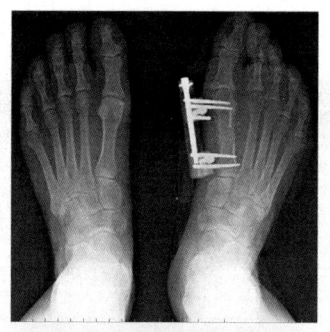

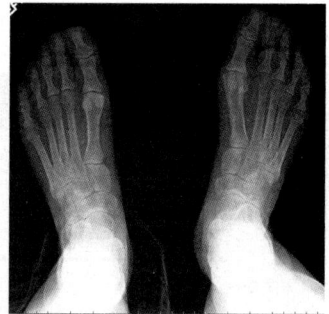

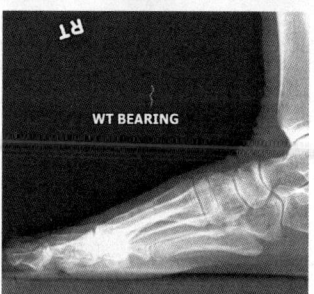

FIG 5 A. Distraction at 3 weeks (regenerate is not yet evident). **B.** Distraction at 10 weeks, regenerate is present but not mature. **C,D.** Radiographic appearance at final 12-month follow-up. First metatarsal consolidation is complete, and adequate lengthening has been obtained.

- Loss of hallux valgus correction (rare, with routine distraction schedule)
- Dorsiflexion of the metatarsal head (poor pin placement or premature removal of external fixator)
- Nonunion (poor fixation or stability of external fixator or premature removal of external fixator)

REFERENCES

1. Holden D, Siff S, Butler J, et al. Shortening of the first metatarsal as a complication of metatarsal osteotomies. J Bone Joint Surg Am 1984;66(4):582–588.
2. Hurst JM, Nunley JA II. Distraction osteogenesis for the shortened metatarsal after hallux valgus surgery. Foot Ankle Int 2007;28:194–198.
3. Jones RO, Harkless LB, Baer MS, et al. Retrospective statistical analysis of factors influencing the formation of long-term complications following hallux abducto valgus surgery. J Foot Surg 1991;30:344–349.
4. Mather R, Hurst J, Easley M, et al. First metatarsal lengthening. Tech Foot Ankle Surg 2008;7:25–30.
5. Nunley JA. The short first metatarsal after hallux valgus surgery. In: Nunley JA, Pfeffer GB, Sanders RW, et al, eds. Advanced Reconstruction: Foot and Ankle. Rosemont, IL: American Academy of Orthopaedic Surgeons, 2004:31–33.
6. Nyska M, Trnka H, Parks BG, et al. Proximal metatarsal osteotomies: a comparative geometric analysis conducted on sawbone models. Foot Ankle Int 2002;23:938–945.
7. Sammarco GJ, Idusuyi OB. Complications after surgery of the hallux. Clin Orthop Relat Res 2001;(391):59–71.
8. Saxby T, Nunley JA. Metatarsal lengthening by distraction osteogenesis: a report of two cases. Foot Ankle 1992;13:536–539.
9. Urbaniak JR, Richardson WJ. Diaphyseal lengthening for shortness of the toe. Foot Ankle 1985;5:251–256.

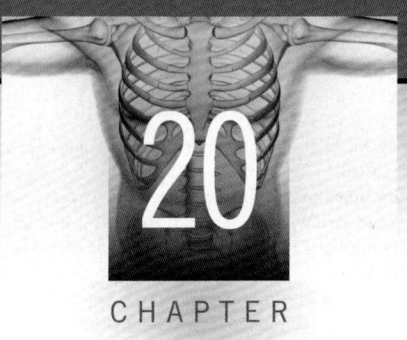

Moberg Osteotomy

Tibor Warganich, Thomas G. Harris, and Casey Pyle

DEFINITION

- Hallux rigidus is a degenerative condition of the first metatarsophalangeal (MTP) joint.
- This leads to a functional limitation of motion of this joint, especially with respect to dorsiflexion.
- Other terms, such as hallux limitus and dorsal bunion, have also been used to describe this condition.
- Hallux rigidus affects about 3% of the adult population.[5]
- This chapter pertains to the surgical procedure of a dorsal closing wedge osteotomy of the proximal phalanx, popularized by Moberg. Although it was initially recommended for young patients (younger than 18 years of age), Moberg[9] extended the indications to include adults.
- It is usually performed in conjunction with a cheilectomy as a joint salvaging procedure, preserving or improving MTP joint motion and allowing for future revision surgery if needed.

ANATOMY

- Usually, dorsiflexion is blocked by a dorsal osteophyte on the metatarsal head. In some cases, there is an osteophyte or ossicle on the dorsum of the base of the proximal phalanx. Dorsiflexion is also limited by contracture of the plantar portion of the MTP joint capsule.
- Articular erosion is characteristically seen on the dorsum of the articular surface of the first metatarsal head and, to a lesser extent, on the dorsum of the base of the proximal phalanx.[8]
- The medial and plantar aspects of the MTP joint are usually spared until later in the disease process (FIG 1).

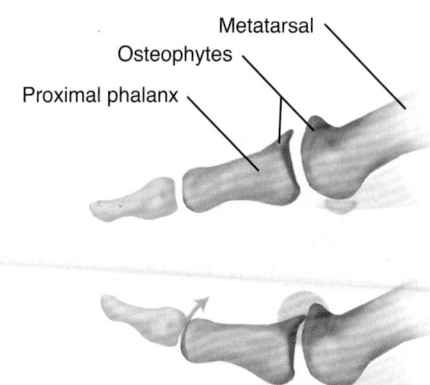

Metatarsal
Osteophytes
Proximal phalanx

FIG 1 Hallux rigidus: Dorsiflexion of proximal phalanx produces painful impingement at the MTP joint.

PATHOGENESIS

- The primary etiology of the hallux rigidus is not known.
- A common cause is trauma, and hallux rigidus may occur after a fracture, sprain, or crush injury. Furthermore, it is thought that microtrauma may injure the articular cartilage over time, leading to degeneration.[4]
- Systemic conditions such as gout and rheumatoid arthritis can also cause degeneration of the first MTP joint, simulating the idiopathic form.

NATURAL HISTORY

- Hallux rigidus is more common in adults than in adolescents.
- Generalized degenerative changes tend to progress with increasing age, but this has not been linked with symptoms.[12]
- Women are affected more often than men and boys, and the condition is often bilateral.

PATIENT HISTORY AND PHYSICAL FINDINGS

- Patients usually describe an insidious onset of activity-related pain at the first MTP joint.
- Swelling and stiffness are common complaints.
- On physical examination in the characteristic case, dorsiflexion motion is measurably limited and plantarflexion motion with force is painful. In some cases, forceful dorsiflexion is also painful but not as painful as forceful plantarflexion.
- Limitation of dorsiflexion usually leads to problems with running, walking on inclines, and wearing high-heeled shoes.
- The increasing dorsal prominence can lead to problems with shoe wear.
- Paresthesias may rarely occur distal to the MTP joint with the compression of the dorsal cutaneous nerves by the dorsal osteophyte and tight-fitting shoes.
- Adaptive gait measures such as a supinated forefoot to unload the painful medial forefoot may lead to lateral foot pain and calluses.[7]
- There is usually generalized enlargement of the joint due to a combination of osteophytes and soft tissue swelling.
- In severe cases with full loss of cartilage and motion, there is sometimes no irritability even with forced flexion. These patients often just have pain because of the osteophytic enlargement causing impingement in the shoe. In these cases, a simple cheilectomy with limited dissection often leads to satisfactory results. These are patients often in their 70s and 80s.
- Interphalangeal joint hyperextension may develop to compensate for restricted MTP joint dorsiflexion, but this is very uncommon.[2]

- Axial loading of the great toe is usually not painful unless severe degeneration or a large osteochondral defect is present.
- Passive plantarflexion of the hallux can also produce pain, as this is thought to bring the inflamed synovium and MTP capsule over the dorsal osteophyte.

IMAGING AND OTHER DIAGNOSTIC STUDIES

- Three weight-bearing views (anteroposterior [AP], lateral, and oblique) of the foot are usually sufficient.
- Weight-bearing views are important because non–weight-bearing views often obscure the dorsal first metatarsal osteophyte. In the non–weight-bearing views, the toes are usually in passive extension, and this may obscure the dorsal osteophyte.
- The AP view is important to assess the amount of medial or lateral joint narrowing.
- The AP view can overestimate the amount of degenerative change as osteophytes may overlie the joint, creating the impression that the joint space is abnormally decreased. Also, a non–weight-bearing AP view can exaggerate the narrowing of the MTP joint space because of the passive extension posturing of the toes at the MTP joint.
- Lateral osteophytes are common and are often early indicators of hallux rigidus. They are also notable at the base of the proximal phalanx.
- Occasionally, a computed tomography scan is useful for detecting osteochondral injuries. Magnetic resonance imaging can be useful as well for detecting chondral damage **(FIG 2)**.

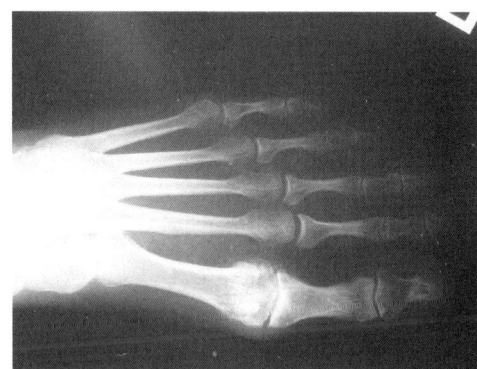

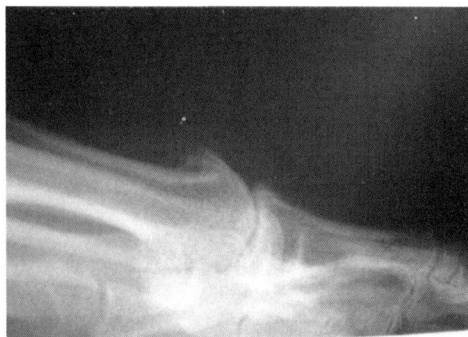

FIG 2 A. AP weight-bearing view of foot showing decreased MTP joint space. The surgeon must be wary not to overestimate joint space loss on the AP view alone because overhanging osteophytes may cause joint space to appear obliterated. **B.** Lateral weight-bearing view of foot showing dorsal osteophytes of metatarsal head and proximal phalanx.

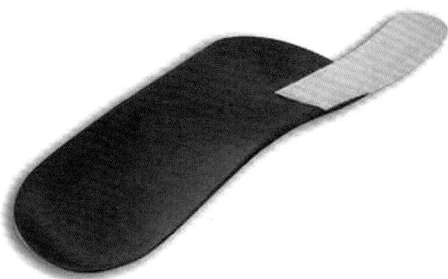

FIG 3 Typical Morton type of extension to an orthotic. This is thought to decrease dorsiflexion at the MTP joint.

DIFFERENTIAL DIAGNOSIS

- MTP synovitis
- Hallux valgus
- Sesamoiditis or sesamoid fracture

NONOPERATIVE MANAGEMENT

- The decision to pursue nonoperative treatment depends on the patient's symptoms and the extent of the degenerative changes. Patients with mild synovitis and minimal complaints can be treated with rest and anti-inflammatory medications.
- The hallux can be taped or braced to limit dorsiflexion, thus resting the joint.
- There are many devices available to increase the rigidity of the medial forefoot. This limits the motion of the MTP joint, thus minimizing the dorsiflexion impingement pain.
  - A Morton extension is an example **(FIG 3)**.
- Steroid injections can be given in the MTP joint. This will help with pain relief temporarily but does not slow the degenerative process.
- Standard shoes with a high toe box are helpful for cases of hallux rigidus. This increases the space for the dorsal osteophytes and reduces pressure on the irritable joint.
- A shoe with a stiff-soled rocker bottom is also helpful and helps with gait smoothness.
- These shoe wear modifications can be effective, but patient compliance and acceptance vary from case to case.
- A study with a minimum follow-up of 14 years showed that the pain associated with hallux rigidus remained the same in 22 of 24 feet.[12]

SURGICAL MANAGEMENT

- We routinely perform a cheilectomy with a proximal phalanx osteotomy. The osteotomy is not a stand-alone procedure but is used to augment the effect of the cheilectomy.[13]
- If the osteotomy is to be combined with a cheilectomy, stable internal fixation is important to secure the osteotomy so that early motion of the MTP joint can be started within 1 to 2 weeks after the surgery.

Preoperative Planning

- All radiographs and other imaging studies should be closely reviewed.
  - Special attention should be directed to the lateral radiograph. This study will show the dorsal osteophytes from the distal metatarsal head and proximal phalanx.

- No specific physical examinations need to be done under anesthesia, but it is important to document the passive range of motion (both dorsiflexion and plantarflexion) before the onset of the procedure.
  - The surgeon should alert the patient that we are "stealing" motion from plantarflexion and giving it to dorsiflexion.

Positioning

- The patient is placed supine on the operating table. A Martin-type tourniquet is applied to the supramalleolar region of the ankle.
- The procedure is usually done under ankle block anesthesia.

- A mini C-arm is also used during the procedure and should be available.
- Antibiotics are given before the procedure.
- Positioning is not as important for this procedure as for other operations.

Approach

- Usually, a dorsomedial approach is used, and the extensor hallucis longus (EHL) is retracted laterally. This will provide good access to both the medial and lateral sides of the MTP joint.
- A directly medial approach to the first MTP joint can be used as well, but this approach can limit access to the lateral side of the joint and is technically more difficult.

TECHNIQUES

EXPOSURE AND CHEILECTOMY

- Make a dorsomedial incision (**TECH FIG 1A**), taking care to identify and protect the dorsomedial cutaneous nerve.
- Retract the EHL laterally (**TECH FIG 1B**).
- Make the MTP capsulotomy in line with the skin incision; the capsule edges can be tagged with a 2-0 Vicryl suture for ease of identification later but is not routinely done.
  - If they are not tagged, carefully identify the dorsal capsule during closure.
  - Retract the capsular edges both plantarly and dorsally.
- Inspect the MTP joint closely.
  - Examine the joint surfaces for osteochondral defects or chondral flaps as well as overall degeneration within the MTP joint.
- Use a reciprocating saw to remove 1 to 2 mm of the medial eminence.
  - This is done to promote healing of the capsule to the bone.

- Perform a dorsal cheilectomy of the metatarsal head, as described elsewhere. Bone is removed flush with the surface of the dorsum of the metatarsal neck (**TECH FIG 1C,D**).
  - We try to limit our resection to only the degenerated area of the metatarsal head but can remove up to a third of the metatarsal head if needed.
- It is important to gain access to and inspect the lateral side of the MTP joint.
  - Increase the lateral exposure as needed.
  - Osteophytes, which can be hard to detect on radiographs, are often evident on the lateral side of the joint. If present, these osteophytes are removed.
- If present, remove osteophytes or ossicles from the proximal phalanx with a rongeur.

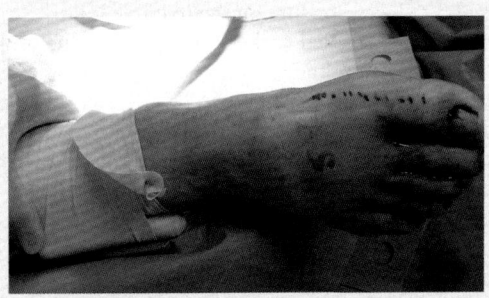 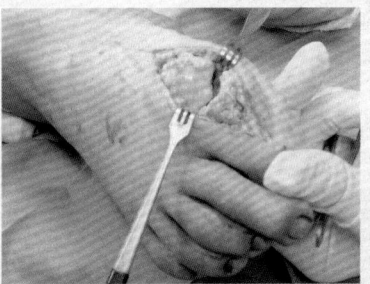 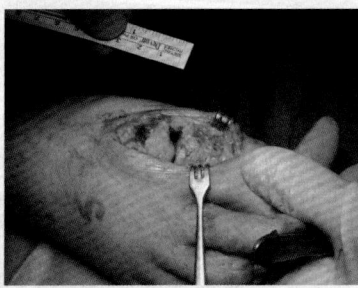

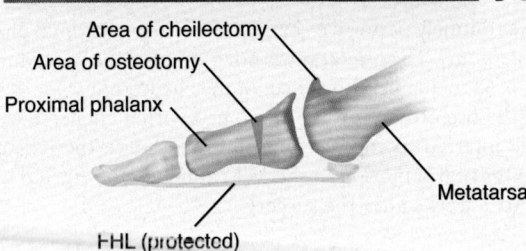

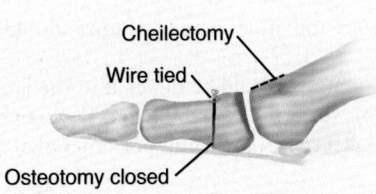

TECH FIG 1 A. Typical line of incision; note tourniquet at supramalleolar region. **B.** The MTP joint widely is exposed. The EHL tendon is retracted laterally. Note exuberant osteophytes on metatarsal head and also osteophytes overhanging from proximal phalanx. **C.** MTP joint after cheilectomy and medial eminence resection. Soft tissue around area of future proximal phalanx osteotomy has been removed. **D.** Cheilectomy and proximal phalanx osteotomy. Shaded areas will be removed. Protection of the flexor hallucis longus (*FHL*) is paramount.

PROXIMAL PHALANX OSTEOTOMY

- Expose the plantar aspect of the proximal phalanx sufficiently to protect the flexor hallucis longus (FHL) tendon.
- During the creation of the osteotomy, be careful to ensure you have enough lateral joint exposure to protect the EHL tendon.
- Place a 0.062-inch smooth Kirschner wire transversely from medial to lateral as a guidewire (**TECH FIG 2A**).
  - It is placed parallel and as close to the articular surface of the proximal phalanx as possible without entering the joint.
  - Use a mini C-arm to verify the proper extra-articular placement of the Kirschner wire (**TECH FIG 2B**). Place the guidewire such that the osteotomy is made just distal to the guide pin. Be wary of what type of internal fixation you are using before making the osteotomy. Try to ensure that the proximal aspect of the osteotomy has enough room to safely accept the internal fixation.
  - Once the placement of the Kirschner wire has been verified, the osteotomy can begin.
- To maximize the amount of dorsiflexion of the tip of the toe, make the osteotomy as close to the articular surface as feasible. However, if the proximal fragment is too small, sometimes it will fragment postoperatively.

- Use an oscillating saw with a 0.5-cm blade width to make the first cut in the phalanx just distal to the surface of the Kirschner wire.
  - The initial cut is incomplete, leaving the plantar cortex intact. (Use irrigation to keep the bone cool during the osteotomy to prevent thermal necrosis.)
  - This protects the FHL and maintains stability in the phalanx in preparation for the second cut.
- Make a second, oblique cut measured 5 mm distal to the first cut (**TECH FIG 2C**).
  - In very mild cases of hallux rigidus, a 3- to 4-mm wedge is used.
  - Keep this cut as parallel as possible to the first cut, looking at the dorsal surface.
  - This width is measured with a sterile ruler.
  - If the two cuts are not parallel, an angular deformity (hallux valgus or varus) can ensue.
  - If there is significant preoperative abductus (lateral angulation), it may help the appearance of the toe to make the medial part of the wedge bigger than the lateral side.
  - As with the first cut, it is important not to finish the osteotomy completely.
- Weaken the remaining plantar cortex with multiple 1.5-mm drill holes. The osteotomy is then completed or "greensticked" (dorsiflexion) manually.

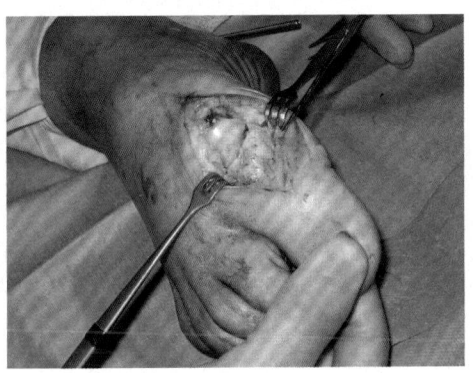

A

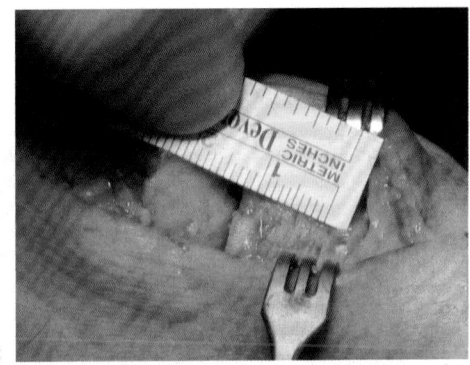

C

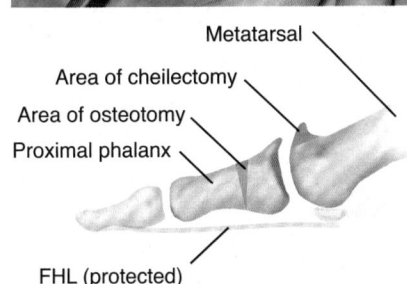

Metatarsal
Area of cheilectomy
Area of osteotomy
Proximal phalanx

FHL (protected)

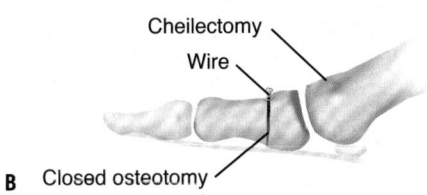

Cheilectomy
Wire

B   Closed osteotomy

TECH FIG 2 A. Placement of Kirschner wire from medial to lateral to ensure extra-articular placement of osteotomy. **B.** Placement of Kirschner wire to ensure extra-articular placement. *FHL,* flexor hallucis longus. **C.** A sterile ruler is used to measure exact dimension of osteotomy.

FIXATION OF THE OSTEOTOMY

- Various options exist for fixation of the fracture site including cerclage wires, minifragment screw fixation (3.0 mm partially threaded), threaded screws alone, multiple percutaneous (0.045 or 0.054 inch) smooth Kirschner wires, or a DynaNite staple (Arthrex, Inc., Naples, FL).

Wire Fixation

- The osteotomy is fixed with 28-gauge wire placed through 1.5-mm drill.
- Make one drill hole at the proximal-dorsomedial aspect of the basal fragment **(TECH FIG 3A)**.
  - Start this hole just adjacent to the articular cartilage at the base of the proximal phalanx and angle it about 45 degrees toward the intramedullary cavity.

- This starting point is about 4 mm from the osteotomy and helps to avoid breakage of a rather fragile tunnel.
- It is helpful to pass the wire from proximal to distal; this places most of the tension on the distal side of the osteotomy when the wire is pulled through the distal segment.
- Start the distal drill hole 3 to 4 mm from the osteotomy and angle it about 45 degrees to the plane of the proximal phalanx **(TECH FIG 3B)**.
- A wire pass instrument can be used to allow the 28-gauge wire passed through the proximal aspect of the osteotomy.
  - As an alternative, a wire passer can be fashioned from the terminal 6 inches of the 28-gauge fixation wire.

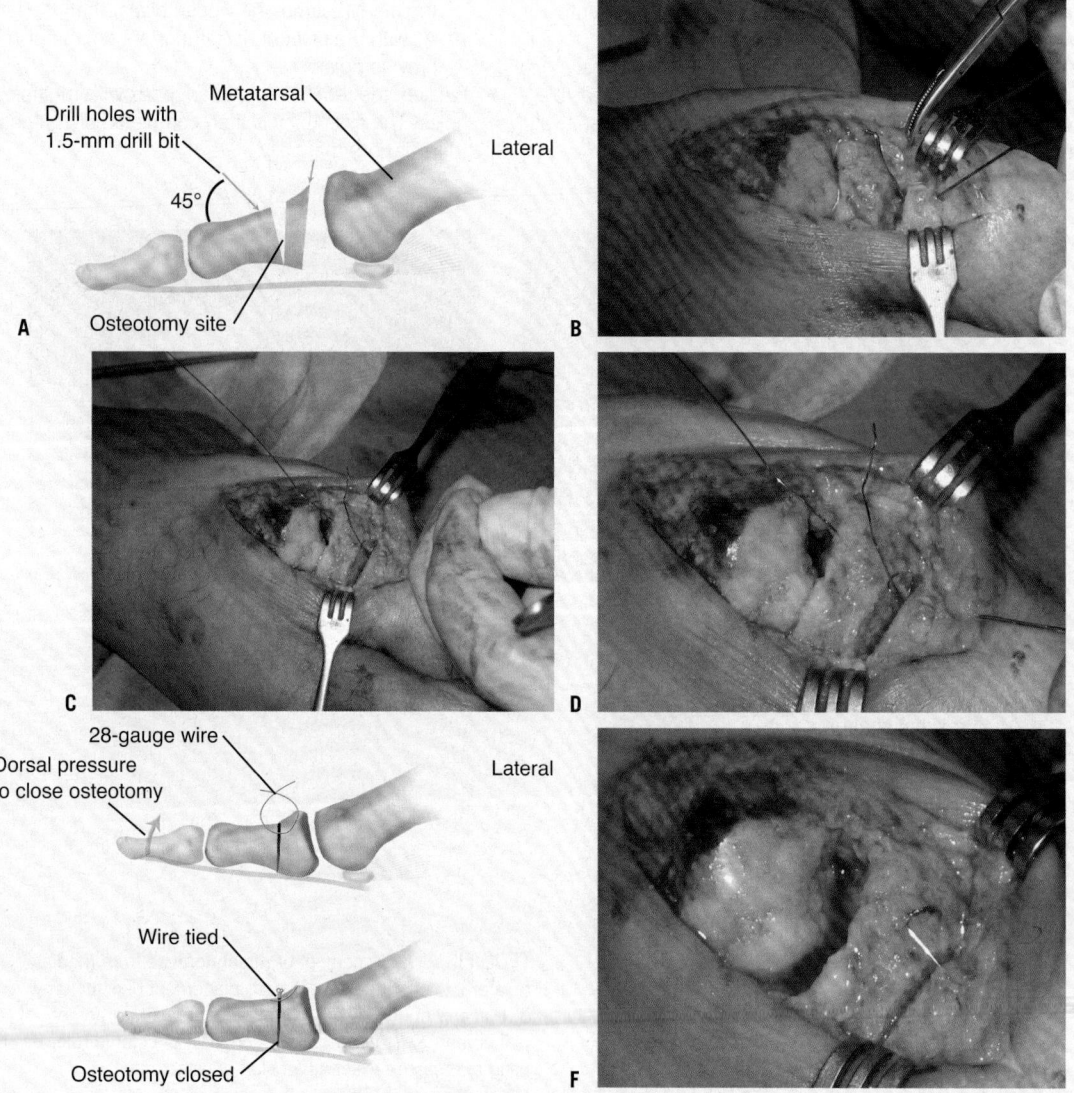

TECH FIG 3 A. Creation of proximal and distal drill holes with 1.5-mm drill. Note that the plantar cortex is intact. **B.** Wire loop going into distal aspect of osteotomy. **C.** Wire going into wire loop from proximal to distal. **D.** Close-up of wire going into loop. **E.** Dorsal pressure is used to close the osteotomy; the wire is tied; the osteotomy is closed. **F.** The wire is tied and placed into soft tissue over osteotomy.

- The other 28-gauge wire is modified in the following ways:
  - A 6-inch piece of 28-gauge wire is folded onto itself to form a small loop.
  - The loop is compressed with a small hemostat to fit through the 1.5-mm hole. We usually fold the wire onto itself and form a small loop with the aid of a small hemostat or mosquito.
  - This loop is then passed into the distal drill hole and into the osteotomy site.
  - Once located within the osteotomy, usually with the assistance of a small hemostat, the created loop is expanded and made larger.
  - This loop is made large enough, so the wire from the proximal osteotomy site can be placed through it **(TECH FIG 3C,D)**.
- Once the proximal wire is placed through the loop, the wire with the loop is pulled distally, pulling the proximal wire with it.
- The assistant places dorsiflexion pressure on the plantar tip of the hallux, closing the wedge osteotomy site as the wire is tightened and twisted **(TECH FIG 3E)**.
  - While the surgeon applies finger tension on the wire, maintaining a closed osteotomy, the wire is twisted about five revolutions.
  - The wire is cut, leaving about 5 mm of residual wire to be bent and placed against the bone **(TECH FIG 3F)**.

DynaNite Fixation

- Alternatively, a Dynanite staple may be used. This is our more recent preferred method of fixation because there is less chance of fracture of the proximal fragment, avoids potential chance of infection with percutaneous Kirschner wires, and allows compressive forces across the osteotomy.
- The staple is oriented with one tine distal to the osteotomy site, and the tine placed proximal in the subchondral bone.

(A 0.054-inch Kirschner wire is placed obliquely across the osteotomy to help hold the position before the staple is placed.) A sizing guide is included to determine which staple will fit best. Typically, a size 9-mm long staple with 7-mm tines is sufficient.
- The system uses a double-barreled drill guide to ensure that guide holes are correctly spaced on the dorsum of the osteotomized phalanx. The double drill guide should be well centered in the bone fragment proximal to the osteotomy in the subchondral bone and the middle of the phalangeal shaft on the distal segment.
- Use a 1.6-mm drill to create a pilot hole to the far cortex at the proposed site of blade entry on the proximal fragment. Then, insert an alignment pin through the guide into the pilot hole to secure the guide in place **(TECH FIG 4A)**.
- This process is then repeated in the distal segment, and a second alignment pin can be placed into the guide in preparation for staple placement **(TECH FIG 4B)**.
- The staple is placed into the delivery device, and the knob is turned clockwise until the tines of the staple are parallel with each other **(TECH FIG 4C)**.
- While holding the drill guide securely in place, the alignment pins are removed, and the staple tines are placed through the windows of the guide into the holes. The guide can then be removed and the staple inserted manually into the bone perpendicular to the osteotomy site **(TECH FIG 4D)**.
- The staple inserted is then removed by turning the knob counterclockwise to release the staple and initiate compression. The provisional Kirschner wire is then removed. The staple is then completely inserted via gentle mallet strikes in the included impactor **(TECH FIG 4E)**.
- Postoperative radiographs demonstrate the placement of staple and alignment of the proximal phalanx. Note the slight dorsiflexion through the proximal phalanx osteotomy on the lateral view **(TECH FIG 4F,G)**.

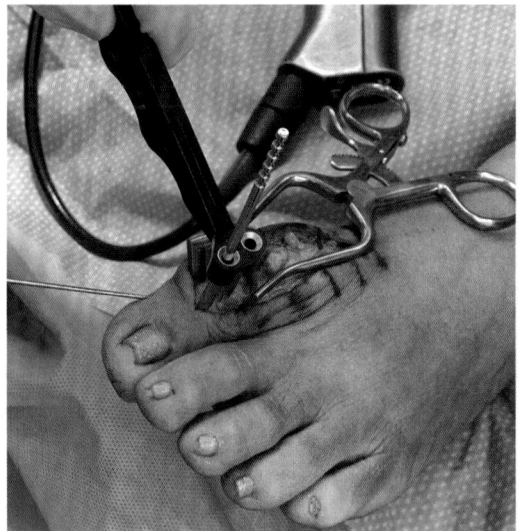 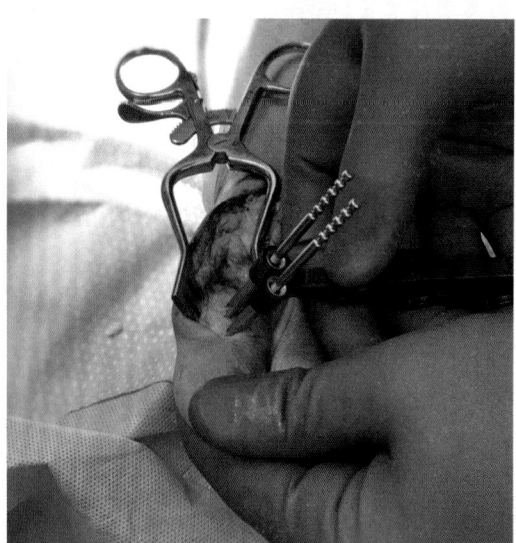

A   B

TECH FIG 4 A. With the reduction held with a Kirschner wire, the drill guide is approximated over the osteotomy site, with attention given to centering the holes over the respective bone fragments. The pilot hole is then made with a 1.6-mm drill bit. **B.** After placing the alignment pin in the proximal hole, the second, distal hole is drilled, and pin is placed to check alignment (inlay). *(continued)*

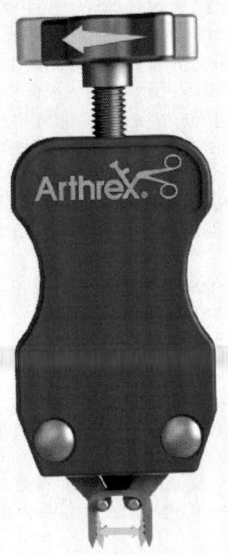

C

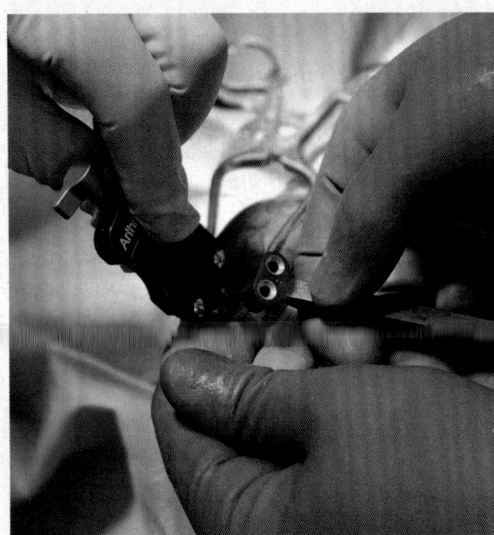

D

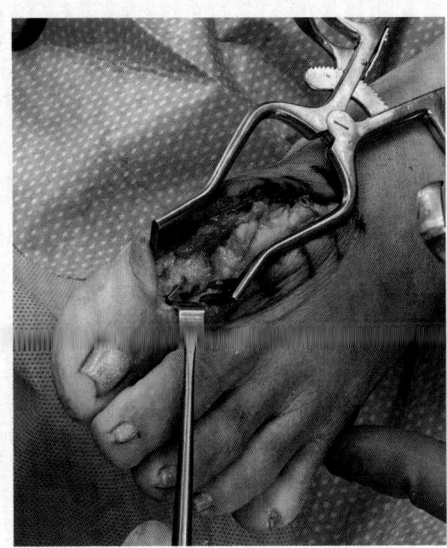

E

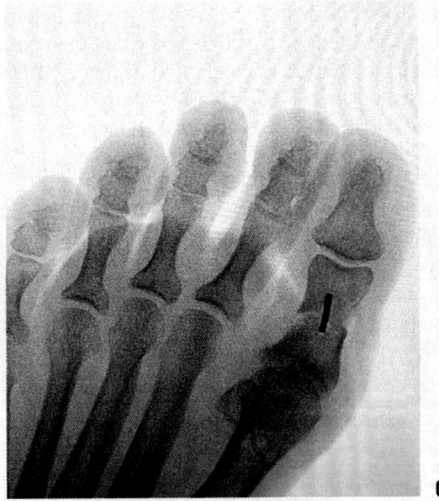

F

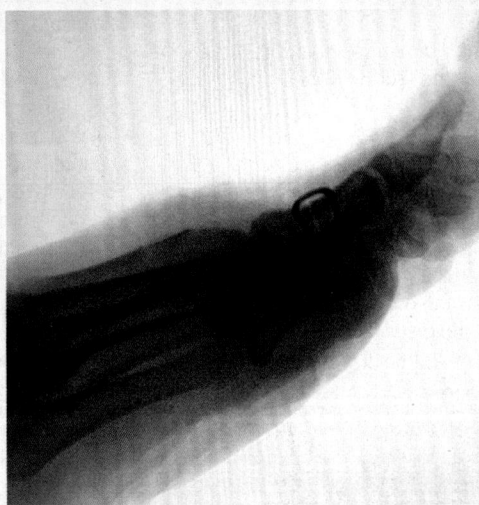

G

TECH FIG 4 *(continued)* **C.** The staple is secured within the inserter, and tines are confirmed to be parallel. **D.** The tines are inserted through the drill guide windows to confirm placement, and the staple is then inserted manually. **E.** The inserter and Kirschner wire are removed, and the impactor is used to mallet the staple securely in place. **F.** Anteroposterior fluoroscopy image demonstrating central placement of the nitinol staple across osteotomy site. **G.** Lateral fluoroscopy image demonstrating the closing-wedge Moberg osteotomy held and compressed by nitinol staple.

CLOSURE

- Close the capsule with nonabsorbable suture, usually 2-0 in diameter.
  - Try to completely cover the osteotomy site with soft tissue. Sometimes, this is not possible, given the limited amount of distal capsule and thin periosteum.

- Close the skin with nylon-type suture in an interrupted fashion.
- Apply a soft dressing consisting of a nonadherent dressing, 4 × 4 gauze, and 4-inch Kling.
- Apply a 2- or 3-inch elastic bandage over this, and the patient is placed in a hard-soled postoperative shoe.

Pearls and Pitfalls

Indications	• If the MTP joint has end-stage degeneration, the patient may have residual postoperative pain and be better served with an arthrodesis.
Intra-articular Osteotomy	• Use of Kirschner wire and a mini C-arm can decrease the incidence of an intra-articular placement of the proximal limb of the osteotomy.
Angular Deformity after Surgery	• Extreme care should be taken to make the second cut of the osteotomy as parallel as possible to the first. "Parallel" is from the perspective of looking at the dorsal surface of the proximal phalanx. • It is important to visualize the medial and lateral aspect of the joint and the proximal phalanx.
Flexor Hallucis Longus Injury	• Careful exposure of the proximal phalanx is essential. • Incomplete plantar osteotomy and "greensticking" the osteotomy after multiple drill holes
Nonunion	• Rare, but bony, apposition is important, as is solid fixation with the wire technique described. • Greensticking of the plantar cortex is also helpful.
Proximal Fragment Fracture	• Creation of 1.5-mm drill hole as close to the proximal articular cartilage as possible • Avoid making the osteotomy too close to the articular surface, let alone cutting into the articular surface. • Pull wire from proximal to distal.

POSTOPERATIVE CARE

- Postoperatively, patients are placed in a hard-soled shoe for 3 to 6 weeks.
- Weight bearing as tolerated is allowed the day after surgery when blood coagulation is complete.
- Patients are initially seen 7 to 10 days after surgery. The patient is instructed to massage the operative site to desensitize the wound beginning 1 week postoperatively.
- Passive dorsiflexion exercises of the MTP joint are begun 1 to 2 weeks after surgery.
- Plantarflexion-type exercises are not started until 4 weeks postoperatively to avoid early tension on the fixation of the osteotomy site. Initially, the patients may complain of decreased ability to plantarflex the toe and having a decreased passive range of motion, especially in reference to the contralateral hallux. This improves with time.
- Less emphasis is placed on plantarflexion unless the resting posture of the hallux is above ground.

OUTCOMES

- The use of a dorsal closing wedge osteotomy increases the space at the dorsal MTP joint (**FIG 4**). In effect, the osteotomy draws the dorsal aspect of the phalanx away from the dorsal aspect of the first metatarsal head. The osteotomy may reduce the joint compression force on the dorsum of the first MTP joint during the toe-off phase of gait.
- In one long-term study, eight women who had 10 toes treated for hallux rigidus by dorsal wedge osteotomy of the proximal phalanx were reviewed after an average follow-up of 22 years (no cheilectomies were done in this study).[1]
  - Five toes were symptom-free, four others did not restrict walking, and only one had required MTP fusion. The authors concluded that dorsal wedge osteotomy afforded long-lasting benefits for hallux rigidus.
- A recent study examined the outcomes of 81 patients with advanced Hattrup and Johnson grade III disease undergoing combination of cheilectomy and proximal phalanx osteotomy with a minimum follow-up period of 2 years (average 4.3 years).
  - An improvement in mean difference in passive dorsiflexion of 27.0 degrees was reported. The mean American Orthopaedic Foot and Ankle Society score improved from 67.2 preoperatively to 88.7 postoperatively with 85.2% patients stating they were satisfied or very satisfied with the procedure.
- Four patients were eventually converted to arthrodesis.

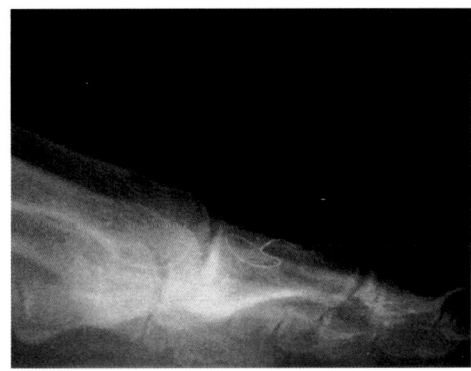

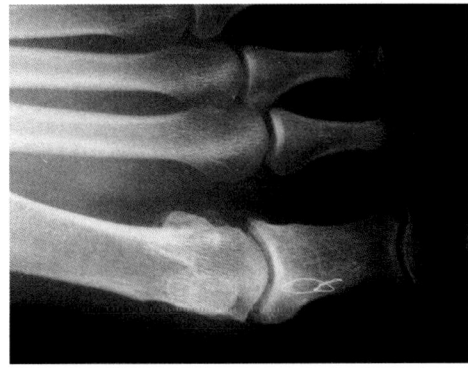

FIG 4 A. Lateral radiograph showing healed osteotomy and area of resection from cheilectomy. **B.** AP radiograph displaying healed osteotomy of proximal phalanx.

- Great results were demonstrated with a combined dorsal closing wedge osteotomy and cheilectomy in patients with advanced disease.[10]
  - The authors have described their experience in comparing patients with both cheilectomies and those with proximal phalanx osteotomies and found the patients with osteotomies had similar satisfaction with the procedure and similar time to wear standard shoes.[14]
- In 2010, Roukis[11] performed a level IV systematic review of 11 studies including a total of 374 instances of hallux rigidus treated with a combination of dorsal cheilectomy and dorsiflexion osteotomy with a minimum follow-up of 12 months (average of 51.1 months).
  - Regarding pain, 149 out of 167 (89.2%) of patients reported that their pain was relieved or improved.
  - Regarding overall outcome, 139 out of 217 (64.1%) of patients reported an "excellent outcome."
  - Five of the studies reported on range of motion with an average gain of 9 degrees of dorsiflexion, from an average of 20.3 degrees preoperatively to 29.3 degrees postoperatively.
  - Reported revision rate was 18 procedures or 4.8%.
- Hunt et al[6] discussed the results of 34 patients (total 35 feet) who underwent a biplanar wedge osteotomy for the combined treatment of hallux rigidus and hallux valgus interphalangeus. This hybrid Moberg-Akin osteotomy is achieved by directing the osteotomy from dorsal-medial to plantar-lateral and removing a wedge from the dorsal-medial cortex. After 6 patients were lost to follow-up, the remaining 29 were followed for a minimum of 6 months (average of 22.5 months).
  - All osteotomies healed, and the interphalangeal angle decreased from 16.1 degrees preoperatively to 11.1 degrees ($P < .01$) postoperatively.
  - Regarding overall outcome, good or excellent results were obtained in 26 of 29 feet, with one patient reporting a poor result due to a nonoperative wound dehiscence.
  - Five of the studies reported on range of motion with an average gain of 9 degrees of dorsiflexion, from an average of 20.3 degrees preoperatively to 29.3 degrees postoperatively.
  - One patient requested hardware removal, but no patients required additional procedures.

COMPLICATIONS

- Intra-articular osteotomy
- FHL injury and laceration
- Angular deformity after surgery
- Fragmentation of the proximal fragment of the proximal phalanx
- Nonunion[3]
- Malunion, including rotational malunion[1]
- Failure to improve
- EHL injury and laceration

REFERENCES

1. Citron N, Neil M. Dorsal wedge osteotomy of the proximal phalanx for hallux rigidus. Long-term results. J Bone Joint Surg Br 1987; 69(5):835–837.
2. Feldman R, Hutter J, Lapow L, et al. Cheilectomy and hallux rigidus. J Foot Surg 1983;22:170–174.
3. Frey CC, Jahss MJ, Kummer FJ. The Akin procedure: an analysis of results. Foot Ankle 1991;12:1–6.
4. Giannestras NJ. Hallux rigidus. Foot Disorders: Medical and Surgical Management, ed 2. Philadelphia: Lea & Febiger, 1973:400.
5. Gould N, Schneider W, Ashikaga T. Epidemiological survey of foot problems in the continental United States: 1978–1979. Foot Ankle 1980;1:8–10.
6. Hunt KJ, Anderson RB. Biplanar proximal phalanx closing wedge osteotomy for hallux rigidus. Foot Ankle Int 2012;33:1043–1050.
7. Mann RA, Clanton TO. Hallux rigidus: treatment by cheilectomy. J Bone Joint Surg Am 1988;70(3):400–406.
8. McMaster MJ. The pathogenesis of hallux rigidus. J Bone Joint Surg Br 1978;60(1):82–87.
9. Moberg E. A simple procedure for hallux rigidus. Clin Orthop Relat Res 1979;(142):55–56.
10. O'Malley MJ, Basran HS, Gu Y, et al. Treatment of advanced stages of hallux rigidus with cheilectomy and phalangeal osteotomy. J Bone Joint Surg Am 2013;95(7):606–610.
11. Roukis TS. Outcomes after cheilectomy with phalangeal dorsiflexory osteotomy for hallux rigidus: a systematic review. J Foot Ankle Surg 2010;49(5):479–487.
12. Smith RW, Katchis SD, Ayson LC. Outcomes in hallux rigidus patients treated nonoperatively: a long-term follow-up study. Foot Ankle Int 2000;21:906–913.
13. Thomas PJ, Smith RW. Proximal phalanx osteotomy for the surgical treatment of hallux rigidus. Foot Ankle Int 1999;20:3–12.
14. Warganich T, Weksler M, Harris T. Functional outcome analysis of hallux rigidus patients undergoing cheilectomy vs. cheilectomy and proximal phalanx osteotomy: a patient's perspective. Orthop Muscul Syst 2014;3:180–185.

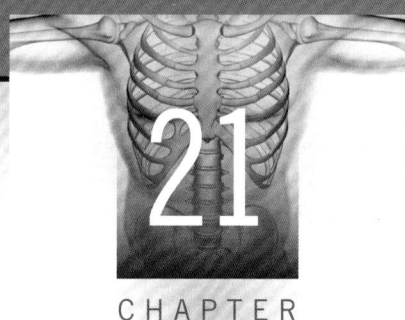

21

Dorsal Cheilectomy for Hallux Rigidus

Richard M. Marks

DEFINITION

- Hallux rigidus refers to limited dorsiflexion of the first meta-tarsophalangeal (MTP) joint as a result of dorsal osteophyte impingement.
- Plantarflexion is typically not limited but may be restricted if a large dorsal osteophyte is present.
- In advanced stages, global arthrosis of the first MTP joint is present.

ANATOMY

- The first MTP joint is supported medially and laterally by collateral ligaments that provide medial–lateral stability (FIG 1A).

- The plantar aspect of the joint consists of the following:
  - The sesamoid complex, including attachments of two slips of the flexor hallucis brevis, which invest the sesamoids (FIG 1B)
  - The plantar plate, a thick fibrous band of tissue that additionally invests and supports the sesamoids. The flexor hallucis longus runs between the sesamoids (FIG 1C).
- The dorsal aspect of the joint includes the capsule, the attachment of the extensor hallucis brevis to the base of the proximal phalanx, and the extensor hallucis longus within the extensor hood.

PATHOGENESIS

- Congenital hallux rigidus (tends to be bilateral)
- Concomitant hallux interphalangus

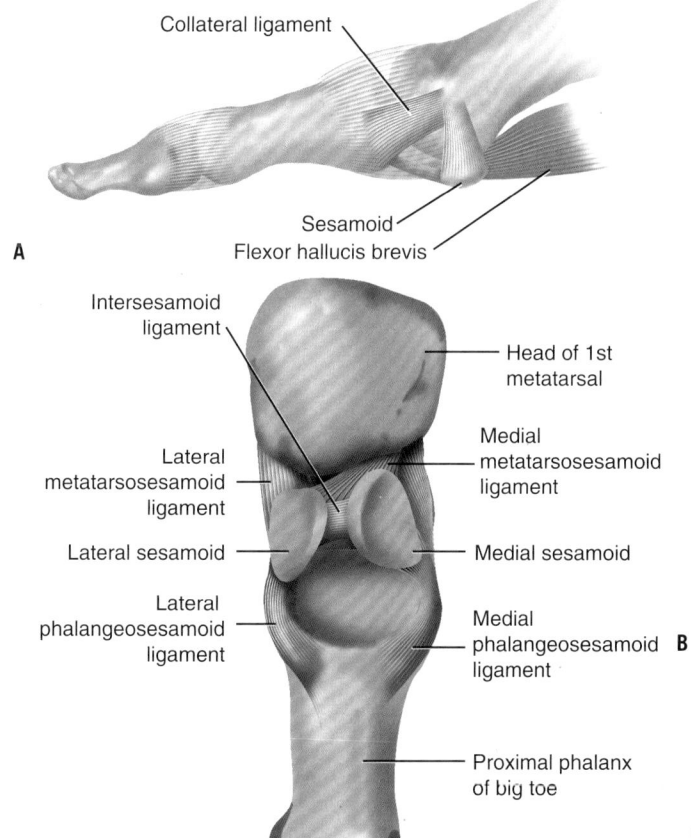

A

Collateral ligament

Sesamoid
Flexor hallucis brevis

C

Intersesamoid ligament

Head of 1st metatarsal

Lateral metatarsosesamoid ligament

Medial metatarsosesamoid ligament

Lateral sesamoid

Medial sesamoid

Lateral phalangeosesamoid ligament

Medial phalangeosesamoid ligament

Proximal phalanx of big toe

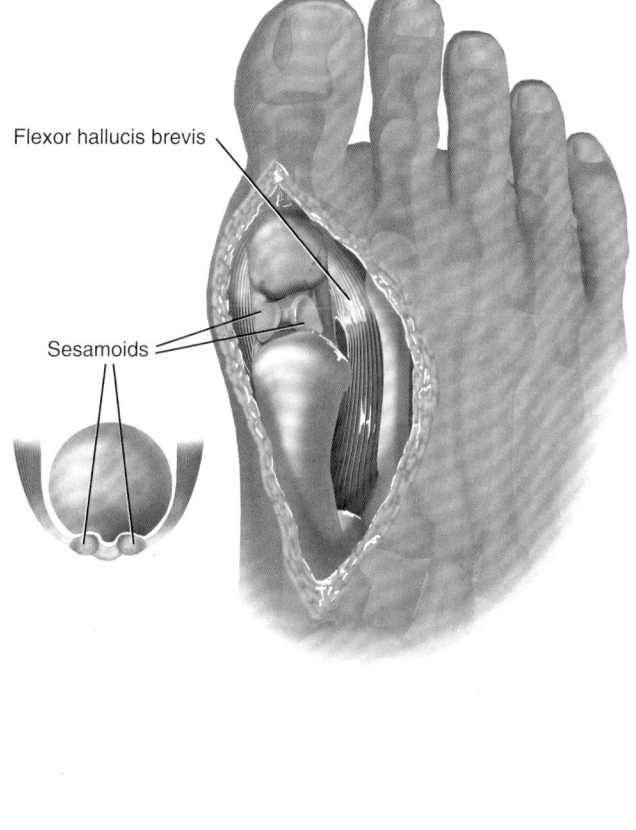

Flexor hallucis brevis

Sesamoids

B

FIG 1 **A.** Medial aspect of first MTP joint anatomy. Collateral ligaments afford medial–lateral stability. **B.** Dorsal aspect of first MTP joint anatomy. **C.** Detail of first MTP joint anatomy with detail of sesamoid complex.

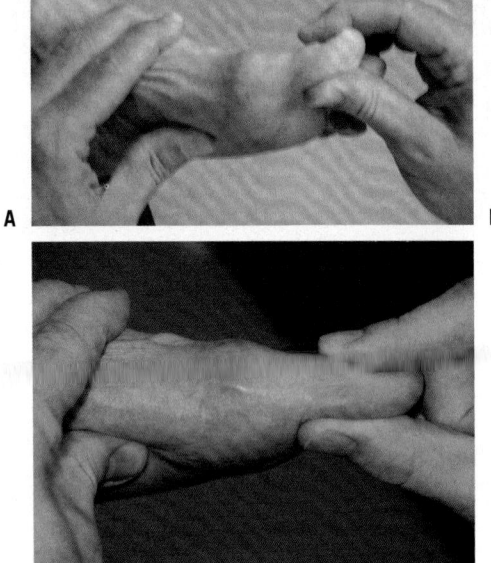

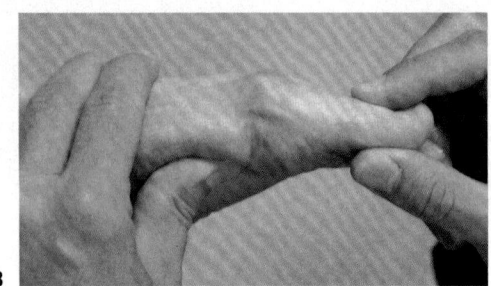

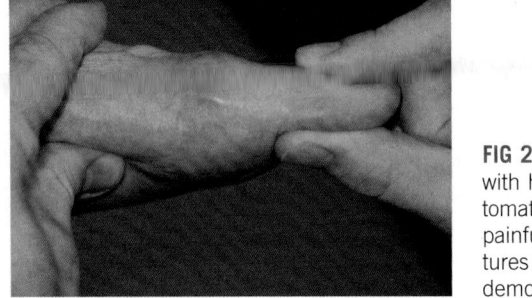

FIG 2 Assessing first MTP joint motion in a patient with hallux rigidus. **A.** Dorsiflexion produces symptomatic impingement. **B.** Often, plantarflexion is also painful, with traction of the dorsal soft tissue structures over the dorsal osteophyte. **C.** Neutral position demonstrating dorsal osteophyte.

- A flat or chevron-shaped MTP joint. This tends to concentrate stresses more centrally.
- Abnormal joint biomechanics
- Trauma to the dorsal articular cartilage, either by a direct blow or repetitive microtrauma
- Cartilage damage secondary to inflammatory reactions from gout or inflammatory arthritis

NATURAL HISTORY

- Abnormal stresses across the MTP joint—through alterations of biomechanics, increased concentration of dorsal cartilage stresses and wear, inflammatory reaction, or direct cartilage injury—result in reactive dorsal osteophyte and marginal osteophytes. If those stresses are not alleviated or corrected, more global arthritic changes may evolve.

PATIENT HISTORY AND PHYSICAL FINDINGS

- Sagittal range of motion is assessed (FIG 2). Pain is typically elicited with extremes of motion, secondary to dorsal impingement, and with plantar motion traction on the dorsal osteophyte.
- A positive grind test indicates more global arthritis, a relative contraindication for cheilectomy.
- Note presence or absence of tenderness with the sesamoid complex examination.

IMAGING AND OTHER DIAGNOSTIC STUDIES

- Standing anteroposterior (AP), lateral, and oblique radiographs are required (FIG 3A,B).
  - The joint space may be obliterated by osteophytes on the AP radiograph, so the oblique radiograph may provide a better view of the retained joint surface.

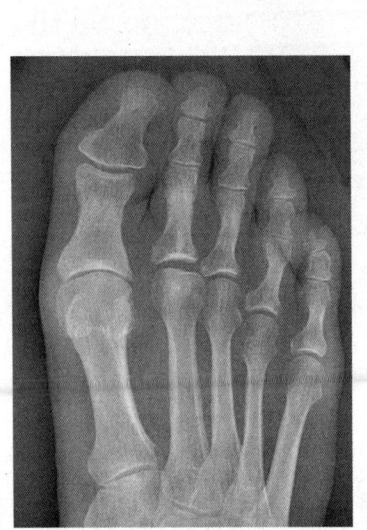

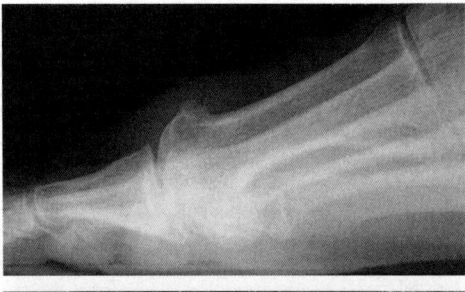

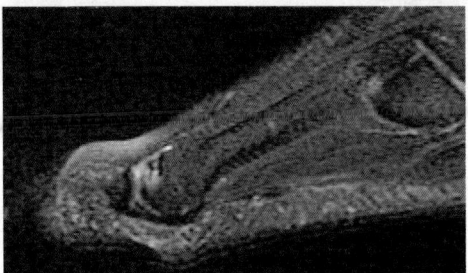

FIG 3 Radiographs of a patient with hallux rigidus. **A.** AP view demonstrating joint space narrowing. **B.** Lateral view with dorsal osteophyte on first metatarsal head. **C.** MRI is not required in the evaluation of hallux rigidus but provides detail if the degree of degenerative change is mild and an osteochondral defect is suspected.

- The AP radiograph is useful to evaluate medial and lateral osteophytes, and the lateral radiograph will reveal the presence of metatarsus elevatus and the extent of the dorsal osteophyte.
- Axial sesamoid view will provide additional information about the sesamoid complex.
- Magnetic resonance imaging (MRI) is helpful if osteochondral defect of the metatarsal head is suspected (**FIG 3C**).

DIFFERENTIAL DIAGNOSIS

- Arthrosis (advanced hallux rigidus)
- Osteochondral defect
- "Turf toe," sesamoid complex injury
- Gout

NONOPERATIVE MANAGEMENT

- Nonoperative treatment consists of the institution of nonsteroidal anti-inflammatory drugs (NSAIDs), accommodative orthotics, and, rarely, physical therapy if gait abnormality is present.
- Accommodative orthotics are designed to restrict sagittal range of motion of the hallux and to redistribute weight-bearing stresses across the first MTP joint with the use of a Morton extension.
- If sesamoid inflammation is present, protective padding is added around the sesamoids and the orthotic is welled out under the sesamoids to provide stress relief.

SURGICAL MANAGEMENT

Preoperative Planning

- Preoperatively, patients are assessed for whether they are appropriate candidates for cheilectomy or for fusion if there are symptoms of more global arthritis of the first MTP joint.
- Cheilectomy is performed for predominantly dorsal arthritic symptoms and for failure to respond to nonoperative means of treatment, as outlined in the previous section.

Positioning

- Preoperatively, patients receive a regional ankle block consisting of a 1:1 mixture of 0.5% bupivacaine and 1% lidocaine, without epinephrine.
- Intravenous antibiotics are administered in the holding area, 30 to 45 minutes before the procedure.
- The patient is placed supine on the operating room table, with the foot at the distal edge of the table to allow for easier fluoroscopic access.
- The foot, ankle, and lower leg are prepped and draped to the lower calf with the use of a leg holder.

Approach

- The first MTP joint is approached dorsally, starting distally from the midportion of the proximal phalanx and extending proximally 3 cm proximal to the joint.

INCISION AND EXPOSURE

- The incision is made medial to the extensor hallucis longus tendon, taking care to preserve the tendon within its sheath (**TECH FIG 1A**).
- Once the tendon is brought laterally and protected, the incision is carried down through the dorsal capsule and distally past the base of the proximal phalanx.
- Loose bodies and proliferative synovium are excised.

- The dorsal aspect of the collateral ligaments is reflected to allow for exposure of the medial and lateral aspects of the joint. Care must be taken to avoid inadvertently destabilizing the joint.
- Hohmann or Senn retractors are placed medially and laterally to protect the soft tissues. Particular attention is paid to protect the extensor hallucis longus tendon distally (**TECH FIG 1B,C**).

TECHNIQUES

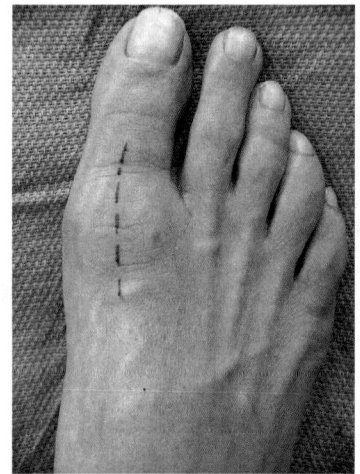 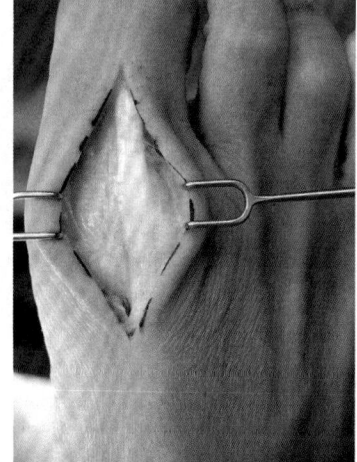 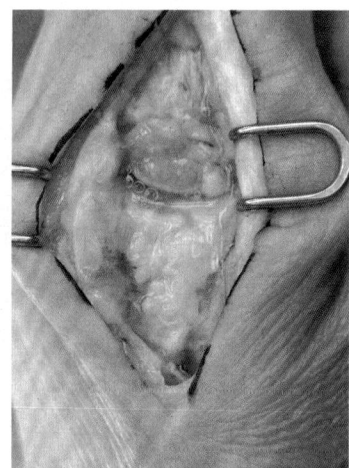

TECH FIG 1 Approach. **A.** Dorsomedial incision. **B.** Identify and protect the dorsomedial sensory nerve to the hallux and the extensor hallucis longus tendon. **C.** Longitudinal capsulotomy after nerve and tendon are retracted.

TECHNIQUES

CHEILECTOMY

- The dorsal osteophyte is resected from the base of the proximal phalanx with a flexible chisel **(TECH FIG 2A,B)**. The hallux is maximally dorsiflexed during this maneuver to protect the central and plantar cartilage of the first metatarsal head.
- The hallux is maximally plantarflexed to allow for examination of the cartilage of the metatarsal head.
- The dorsal 25% to 30% of the metatarsal head articular surface is resected with a flexible chisel **(TECH FIG 2C–F)**, beginning distally and angled proximally to exit at the metaphyseal–diaphyseal junction of the metatarsal.
  - The extent of articular surface resection frequently corresponds to the wear pattern of the cartilage.
  - Avoid exiting too far proximal in the diaphyseal bone, which might weaken the metatarsal.

- Alternatively, a microsagittal saw can be used to resect bone from a proximal to distal direction, but care must be taken to avoid excessive articular cartilage resection. I prefer to start the cartilage resection from the metatarsal head distally.
- Medial and lateral osteophytes are resected, taking care to avoid destabilization of the collateral ligaments.
- The hallux is maximally dorsiflexed and inspected for any residual impingement **(TECH FIG 2G)**. If necessary, additional bone is resected and motion is reevaluated.
- Fluoroscopy can be used to verify adequacy of bone resection, in both the AP and sagittal planes **(TECH FIG 2H,I)**.
- If discrete osteochondral defect is noted, the base of the defect is drilled in multiple directions with a 0.045-inch Kirschner wire to facilitate bleeding into the defect and formation of fibrocartilage.

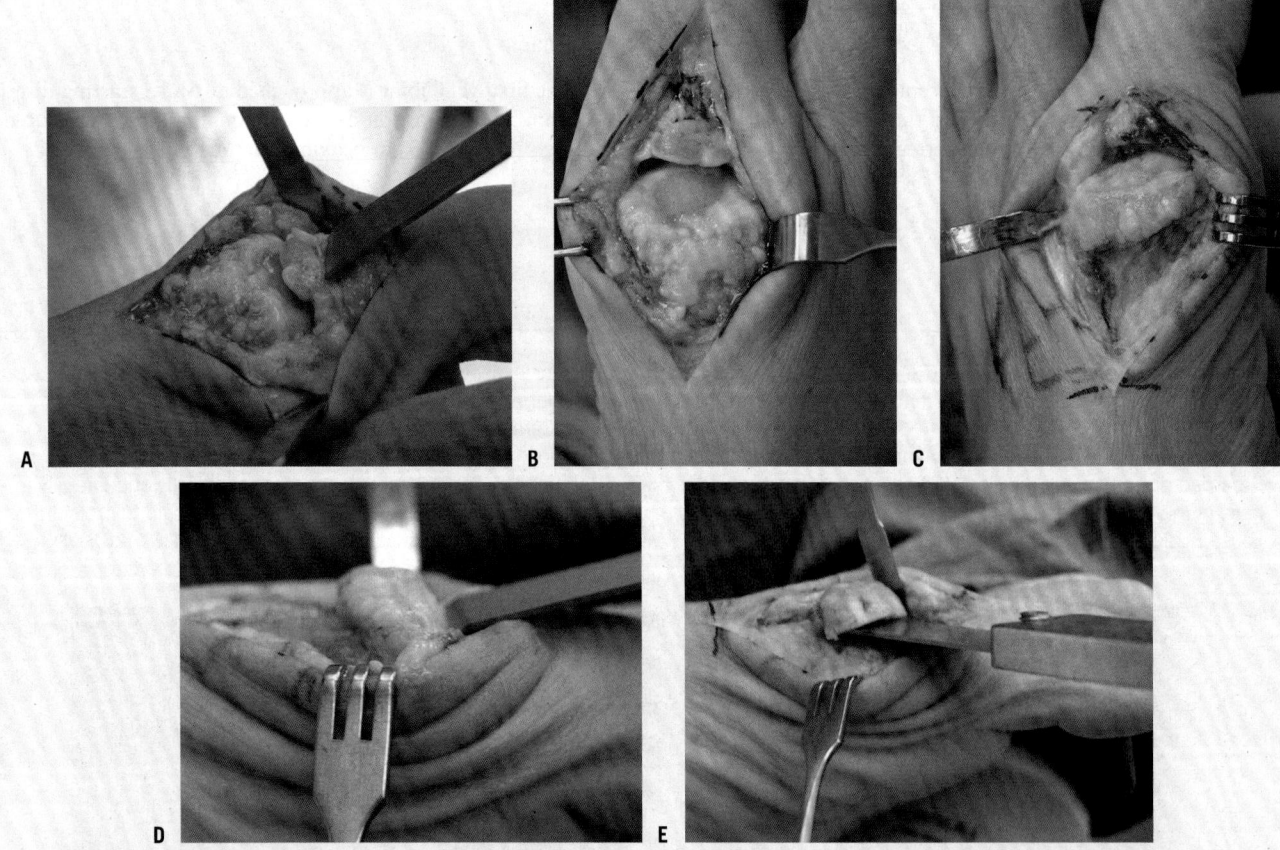

TECH FIG 2 A–F. Resection. **A.** Removing dorsal osteophyte on proximal phalanx. **B.** Joint exposed, demonstrating typical degenerative wear pattern. Note medial and lateral osteophytes. **C.** Dorsal view of dorsal osteophyte. **D.** Sagittal view of large dorsal osteophyte and chisel positioned for resection. **E.** Chisel to resect osteophyte and dorsal one-fourth to one-third of residual articular surface. *(continued)*

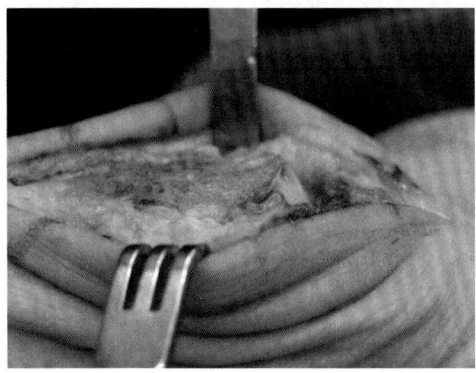
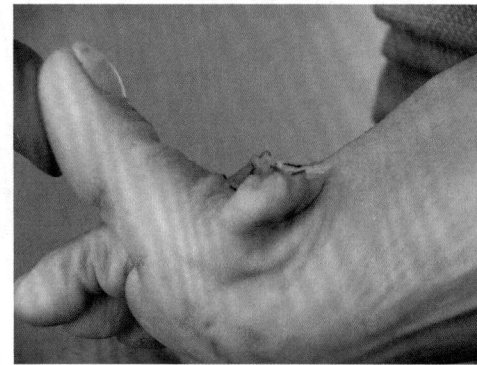

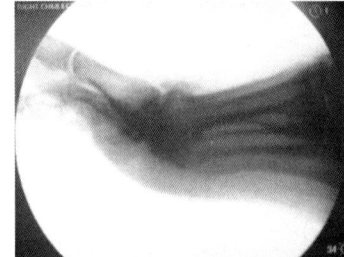
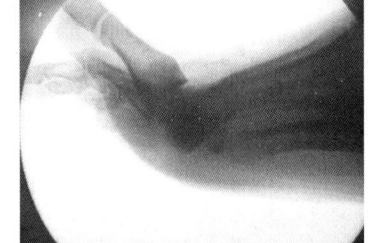

TECH FIG 2 *(continued)* **F.** After osteophyte resection. **G–I.** Checking first the MTP joint range of motion after resection. **G.** Passive dorsiflexion of the toe relative to the metatarsal shaft axis should approach 90 degrees. **H.** Fluoroscopy prior to osteophyte resection. **I.** Fluoroscopy after osteophyte resection.

WOUND CLOSURE

- The wound is irrigated, and a thin film of bone wax is applied to the cancellous bone of the dorsal metatarsal.
- Closure of the capsule is performed with a 2-0 absorbable suture. If necessary, the extensor mechanism is centralized to prevent valgus drift of the hallux postoperatively.
- Subcutaneous closure is performed with either 2-0 or 3-0 absorbable suture, and the skin is closed with simple 4-0 nylon suture. A sterile compressive dressing is applied.

TECHNIQUES

Pearls and Pitfalls

Indications	• Verify that the patient is experiencing symptoms of mechanical dorsal impingement. • Global arthritis with a positive grind test and pain at rest is a contraindication for cheilectomy.
Approach	• Avoid destabilization of the extensor hallucis longus. Medial and lateral exposure should preserve the collateral ligaments. • Avoid injury to the dorsomedial cutaneous branch of the superficial peroneal nerve.
Bone Resection	• To protect the articular surface of the metatarsal, maximally dorsiflex the hallux while performing resection of the dorsal base of the proximal phalanx. • Twenty-five percent to 30% of the articular surface of the metatarsal head needs to be resected to avoid residual impingement. Inadequate bone resection is responsible for most failures.

POSTOPERATIVE CARE

- Patients are instructed to elevate the operative leg for the first 10 days, with heel weight bearing in a postoperative shoe (**FIG 4**).
- At 10 days, sutures are removed and Steri-Strips applied. Postoperative radiographs are obtained at this visit.

- At this point, weight bearing as tolerated is permitted in a postoperative shoe. The patient weans to a sneaker or comfortable shoe over the successive 10 to 14 days.
- Physical therapy is also instituted at 10 days, concentrating on reestablishing range of motion, diminishing edema, and performing scar massage.

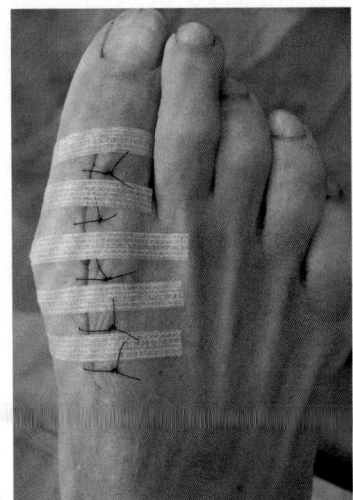

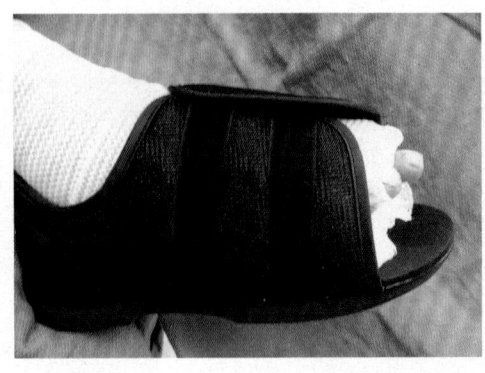

FIG 4 Postoperative management. **A.** Closure. **B.** Immediate weight bearing in a postsurgical shoe.

- Physical activity such as biking, swimming, and elliptical trainer and StairMaster usage is instituted shortly thereafter. Running activities are typically withheld until approximately 3 months after surgery.
- The use of an accommodative orthotic with a Morton extension is occasionally prescribed for a period of time if patients complain of discomfort after activities or continued weight bearing on the lateral aspect of the foot is necessary.

OUTCOMES

- Good to excellent outcomes after cheilectomy range from 72% to 92%.
- Better results are noted with grades I and II.
- Poorer outcomes are reported if there is over 50% loss of articular cartilage at time of surgery.
- No correlation is noted between postoperative radiographic deterioration of joint space and clinical outcome.
- Results do not tend to diminish with time.
- Less than 8% of patients subsequently require fusion.

COMPLICATIONS

- Inadequate bone resection
- Destabilization of the collateral ligaments
- Dorsomedial cutaneous nerve damage
- Progression of arthritis

SUGGESTED READINGS

Coughlin MJ, Shurnas PS. Hallux rigidus: demographics, etiology, and radiographic assessment. Foot Ankle Int 2003;24:731–743.

Coughlin MJ, Shurnas PS. Hallux rigidus. Grading and long-term results of operative treatment. J Bone Joint Surg Am 2003;85-A(11):2072–2088.

Feltham GT, Hanks SE, Marcus RE. Age-based outcomes of cheilectomy for the treatment of hallux rigidus. Foot Ankle Int 2001;22:192–197.

Hattrup SJ, Johnson KA. Subjective results of hallux rigidus following treatment with cheilectomy. Clin Orthop Relat Res 1998;(226):182–191.

Mann RA, Clanton TO. Hallux rigidus: treatment by cheilectomy. J Bone Joint Surg Am 1988;70(3):400–406.

Mulier T, Steenwerckx A, Thienpont E, et al. Results after cheilectomy in athletes with hallux rigidus. Foot Ankle Int 1999;20:232–237.

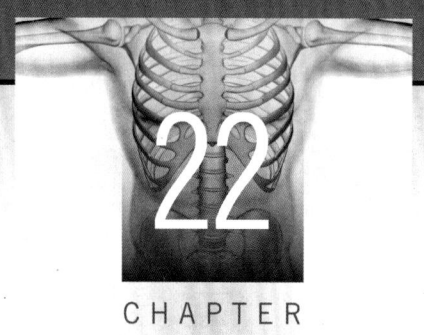

22
CHAPTER

Dorsal Cheilectomy, Extensive Plantar Release, and Microfracture Technique

Hajo Thermann

DEFINITION

- Hallux rigidus, osteoarthrosis of the first metatarsophalangeal (MTP) joint, was first described in 1887.
- Pain and restriction in range of motion (ROM) in the first MTP joint are the major characteristics of hallux rigidus.
- After hallux valgus, hallux rigidus is the second most common deformity of the first MTP joint. The big toe is the location in the foot with the highest incidence of osteoarthrosis; estimates suggest that nearly 10% of the adult population is affected by hallux rigidus.[11,12]
- The incidence of hallux rigidus is higher in women than in men.

ANATOMY

- The first MTP joint is a stable joint formed by the rounded head of the first metatarsal bone fitting into the concave proximal facet of the proximal phalanx.
- The joint is enhanced by the plantar and collateral ligaments. The deep transverse metatarsal ligament is connected to the second ray.
- The sesamoid bones are embedded in the flexor hallucis brevis tendon. They are accommodated at the underside of the first metatarsal in two longitudinally oriented grooves. In a normal relationship, the sesamoids glide distally and proximally within the grooves by a combination of active and passive forces.
- The extensor hallucis longus tendon covers the dorsal side of the first MTP joint and inserts into the base of the distal phalanx.
- The dorsomedial cutaneous nerve is in danger when using a dorsomedial approach to the joint. It is the most medial branch of the superficial peroneal nerve. An anatomic study has shown that the minimum distance from the medial edge of the extensor hallucis longus tendon is 6 mm.[21]

PATHOGENESIS

- The mechanism responsible for developing hallux rigidus remains unclear.
- In theory, damage to the cartilage surface of the first MTP joint, that is, osteochondral fractures or chondral defects, may lead gradually to posttraumatic arthrosis.
- Alternatively, repetitive microtrauma to the first MTP joint, with eccentric overload and stresses that exceed physiologic stresses, may result in hallux rigidus, as seen in football players and ballet dancers.
- The contact distribution shifts dorsally with increasing degrees of extension.[1] This is consistent with the observation

that chondral erosions often initially affect the dorsal aspect of the articular surface of the first metatarsal.
- Various factors, in isolation or in combination, have been suggested as contributing to the development of first MTP joint arthrosis:
  - Hyperextension injury (ie, turf toe injury) to the hallux
  - Metatarsus primus elevates
  - Osteochondral lesions
  - Long first metatarsal
  - Wearing inappropriate shoes
- In 2003, Coughlin and Shurnas[5] evaluated 114 patients treated operatively for hallux rigidus over a 19-year period in a single surgeon's practice for demographics, etiology, and radiographic findings associated with hallux rigidus.
  - The disease was not associated with metatarsus primus elevatus, first ray hypermobility, increased first metatarsal length, Achilles or gastrocnemius tendon tightness, abnormal foot posture, symptomatic hallux valgus, adolescent onset, footwear, or occupation.
  - Hallux rigidus was associated with hallux valgus interphalangeus, female gender, and a positive family history in bilateral cases.
  - In most cases, the problem was bilateral, except when trauma was involved, when the problem was unilateral.
  - Metatarsus adductus was more common in patients with hallux rigidus than in the general population, but no significant correlation was found.
  - A flat or chevron-shaped MTP joint was more common in patients with hallux rigidus.

NATURAL HISTORY

- The natural history of hallux rigidus is similar to that of degenerative arthritis in any joint. Once the process has started, the articular cartilage is more susceptible to injury, resulting from shear and compressive forces. The subchondral bone shares these stresses, which subsequently lead to increased subchondral bone density and formation of periarticular osteophytes. The osteophytes limit first MTP joint motion and further compromise the normal mechanics of this joint. This effect can accelerate the degenerative process.
- The natural history are, at the end point, stiffness and constant pain. The length of time that elapses from initial symptoms to constant pain varies widely. The standard time frame over, which daily or recreational sports activities become painful is about 5 to 10 years, whereas athletes (eg, tennis and basketball players) who experience constant and

repetitive impacts develop constant symptoms in a shorter period of time. In most patients, stiffness is not an issue.

- Outcomes in 22 patients with hallux rigidus representing 24 feet treated nonoperatively at an average follow-up of 14.4 years showed that the pain remained about the same in 22 feet, improved with time in 1 foot, and became worse in 1 foot. There was measurable loss of cartilage space radiographically over time in 16 of 24 feet, and in 8 of the 16 feet, the loss of cartilage space was dramatic.[9]

PATIENT HISTORY AND PHYSICAL FINDINGS

- Hallux rigidus is associated with a positive family history of great toe problems in almost two-thirds of patients.[5]
  - The standard history is a trauma at the MTP joint several years earlier, but more often, we find active persons—mostly former athletes—who are performing high-impact sports such as tennis, golf, or basketball. Starting with "feeling the joint" after exercising, it becomes a progressively limiting factor that prevents them from performing their sport at their normal level.
  - The true etiology of hallux rigidus is often not known.
- In the early stages, the patient complains of pain only on dorsiflexion of the great toe; the ROM is unaffected or only moderately restricted. In the midstage of hallux rigidus, the patient complains of motion-dependent pain. Dorsiflexion of the great toe is restricted. Osteophytes may occur dorsal to the first metatarsal head and may be palpable, the plantar structures become tight, plantar flexion becomes painful at the sesamoid–metatarsal joint (mostly medial), and the ROM also is restricted. A dynamic stress test in dorsiflexion (ie, pressure with the thumb on the medial or lateral sesamoid) can distinguish between sesamoid–metatarsal head pain and MTP pain. Unfortunately, this test is not clear in the presence of ongoing stiffness and arthritic changes of the MTP joint. The late stages present with reduced to complete inhibited dorsiflexion and plantar flexion of the toe, with palpable osteophytes dorsal (medial and lateral) to the metatarsal head and especially around the entire phalangeal base.
- The most striking physical manifestation of hallux rigidus noticed by patients is the bony prominence at the dorsum of the metatarsal head, which is disturbing and painful, especially in firm leather shoes.

- Methods for examining the first MTP joint are as follows:
  - ROM, dorsiflexion, and plantar flexion are checked. In the early stages, restriction of dorsiflexion ("dorsal impingement") is found. In later stages, restriction of plantar flexion and pain at the midrange of the motion arc (indicative of global first MTP joint degenerative joint disease) also are found.
  - Palpation of the first MTP joint. In later stages, palpable and painful osteophytes are present as a symptom of ongoing osteoarthritis.
  - Inspection for clinical changes in form or color of the first MTP joint

IMAGING AND OTHER DIAGNOSTIC STUDIES

- Standard weight-bearing anteroposterior (AP) **(FIG 1A,B)** and lateral radiographs of the foot as well as weight-bearing radiographs of the metatarsals and, in cases of sesamoid pathologies, a sesamoid special radiograph should be performed.
- Coughlin and Shurnas[6] proposed a classification system based on the radiographic system of Hattrup and Johnson[13] that is representative of the natural history. It includes ROM, as well as radiographic and examination findings, as follows:
  - Grade 0: dorsiflexion of 40 to 60 degrees (ie, 20% loss of normal motion), normal radiographic results, and no pain
  - Grade 1: dorsiflexion of 30 to 40 degrees, dorsal osteophytes, and minimal to no other joint changes
  - Grade 2: dorsiflexion of 10 to 30 degrees; mild flattening of the MTP joint; mild to moderate joint narrowing or sclerosis; and dorsal, lateral, or medial osteophytes
  - Grade 3: dorsiflexion of less than 10 degrees, often less than 10 degrees plantar flexion, severe radiographic changes with hypertrophied cysts or erosions or with irregular sesamoids, constant moderate to severe pain, and pain at the extremes of the ROM
  - Grade 4: stiff joint, radiographs showing loose bodies or osteochondritis dissecans, and pain throughout the entire ROM
- Magnetic resonance imaging (MRI) scans are recommended in patients, which have nearly normal radiographs and severe symptoms. In our experience, the majority of these patients undergoing operative management of hallux rigidus

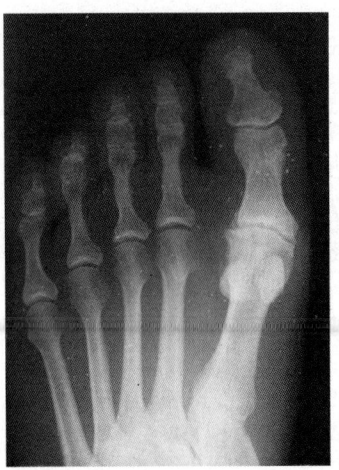 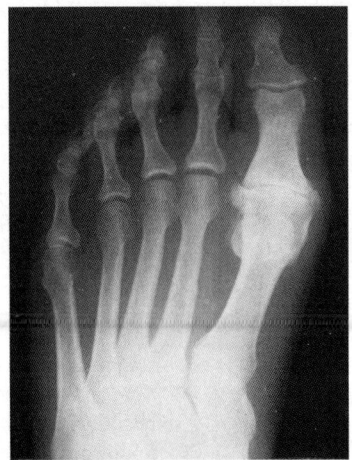 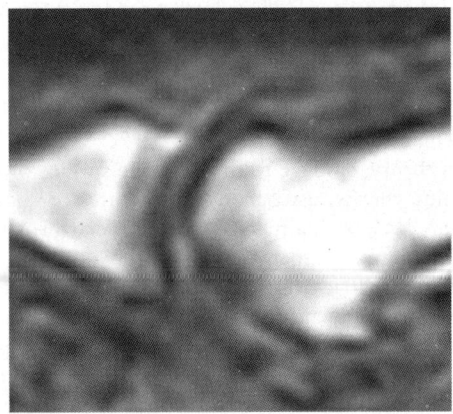

FIG 1 A. Hallux rigidus grade 2 on AP weight-bearing radiograph. **B.** Hallux rigidus grade 3 on AP weight-bearing radiograph. **C.** MRI showing an osteochondral lesion of the metatarsal head.

had an associated osteochondral lesion of the first metatarsal head. Also, arthrosis in the sesamoid–metatarsal joint or osteonecrosis in the sesamoids can be identified on MRI.

- Indication for an MRI is the suspicion of an osteochondral lesion or to identify whether the cartilage lesion is suitable for a joint reconstruction. Massive joint destruction is a contraindication a joint-saving procedure.
- The MRI examination should include sagittal, axial, and coronal views with T1-weighted (repetition time [TR] 35 ms, echo time [TE] 16 ms) and high-resolution gradient echo (TR 1060 ms, TE 16 ms) images **(FIG 1C)**.

DIFFERENTIAL DIAGNOSIS

- Gout
- Rheumatoid arthritis
- Psoriatic arthritis
- Reiter syndrome
- Infectious arthritis
- Sesamoid osteonecrosis

NONOPERATIVE MANAGEMENT

- The primary nonoperative treatments of hallux rigidus are anti-inflammatory therapy and pain relief by orthotic devices.[20]
  - Anti-inflammatory drugs (eg, diclofenac) may be used systemically and locally.
  - Injections in the joint should be restricted to single cases. A single shot of corticosteroids may lead to pain relief.
  - Cooling devices also inhibit the inflammation process.
  - Orthotic devices such as stiff inserts for shoes or rocker bottom soles take pressure from the MTP joint by facilitating the scrolling process. To further alleviate pressure on the joint, a shoe with a roomy toe box should be worn, and high heels should be avoided.
  - Physical therapy helps keep the joint mobile.
- The question is whether immobilizing the joint by orthotics or stiff insoles in early arthritis is a reasonable approach because doing so results in the functional breakdown of the MTP joint.
  - In our practice, we prefer to keep the joint mobile by physical therapy and manual therapy and by having the patient perform exercises for dorsiflexion and plantar flexion daily (eg, aqua jogging on tiptoes).

- Chondroitin and glucosamine sulfate, so-called sympathetic slow-acting drugs in osteoarthritis,[14,19] have comparable success in improving the pain and symptoms of osteoarthritis.
- Additional nonsteroidal anti-inflammatory drugs and ice can be applied to support progress at the beginning of the physical therapy program.

SURGICAL MANAGEMENT

- The goal of surgical treatment is to achieve a pain-free joint.
- Several surgical approaches have been proposed in the literature, including resection arthroplasty, interpositional arthroplasty,[2,12,15] MTP replacement (implant arthroplasty), arthrodesis,[11] and cheilectomy,[11,13,16] which has emerged as the most popular choice for surgical intervention.
  - Indications for performing a cheilectomy are controversial.[6,7] Some authors recommend cheilectomy as a treatment for lower grades only,[10,11,13,17] whereas others have reported successful results even for higher grades of the disease.[7,8]
  - Cheilectomy resects the dorsal obstacle but does not address the plantar pathology, which includes tremendous shortening of the plantar capsular as well as the short flexors and plantar osteophytes of the phalangeal base.
  - Cheilectomy alone without plantar release, in our opinion, cannot be successful.
- A remaining cartilage lesion also may be responsible for persistent symptoms. This observation led to our idea of stimulating fibrocartilage regeneration by microfracturing the subchondral bone with a specially designed awl to open the zone of vascularization.
- Steadman et al[23] has developed a microfracture technique for the knee that creates fibrocartilage in chondral lesions.
  - It has been shown to be effective in comparison to untreated lesions in experimental studies in horses[9] and in clinical studies of the knee[18,22,23] and talus.[4]
- Coughlin and Shurnas[5] types 2 and 3 lesions are indications for the microfracture technique.
  - In type 3 lesions, the patient must be informed that the surgery has only limited success.
- A contraindication for cheilectomy with microfracture is the stiff joint of types 3 and 4 osteoarthritis. In this case, in patients with a low activity level who want good ROM, a resurfacing-type prosthesis (not a "head resection" type) is a good alternative and is being used with increasing frequency **(FIG 2A)**.

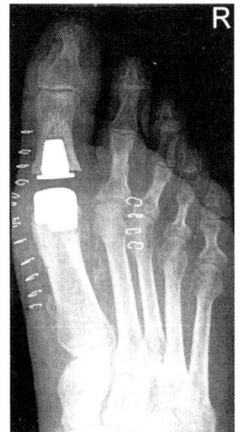 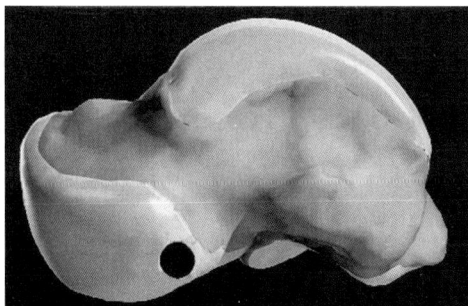 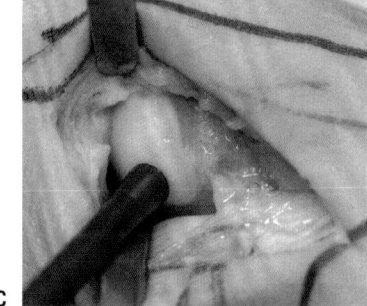

FIG 2 A. Postoperative radiograph of first MTP joint prosthesis. **B,C.** Osteochondral autograft transplantation from the plantar medial talus.

- Patients with isolated, painful osteochondral lesions without degenerative joint disease may be considered in rare cases for microfracture alone (for a small, contained lesion) or for an osteochondral transplantation from the plantar medial talus **(FIG 2B,C)**.

Preoperative Planning

- Standard weight-bearing AP and lateral radiographs as well as, in some cases, MRI evaluation should be performed for grading the patient according to the Coughlin and Shurnas[6] classification, and the cartilage damage should be assessed.

- The clinical examination should include measurement of active and passive ROM and determination of power in extension and plantar flexion, along with a dynamic stress test for evaluation of sesamoid pathology.

Positioning

- The patient is placed supine on the operating table.
- We recommend general anesthesia and Esmarch using a tourniquet placed at the thigh.
  - Lower extremity Esmarch and regional anesthesia or foot block is possible, based on individual preferences.

EXPOSURE

- A 4- to 5-cm incision is made anteromedially **(TECH FIG 1A)**, being careful to protect the dorsal nerve above the first metatarsal head.
- The fatty tissue and the subcutaneous tissue are dissected, and the joint capsule is prepared.

- The extensor hallucis longus tendon is retracted and the joint exposed **(TECH FIG 1B,C)**.
- The joint is then inspected by flexing the great toe in the plantar direction.

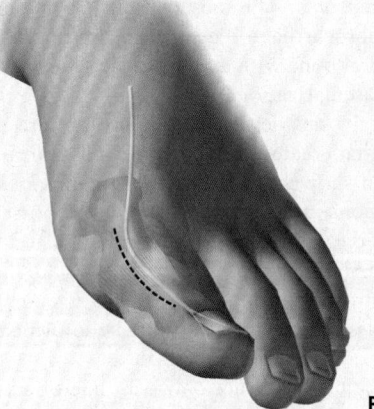 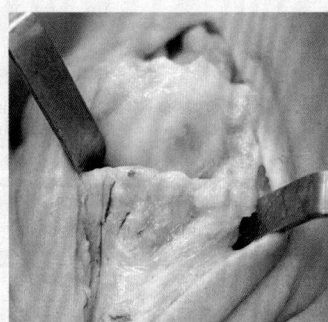 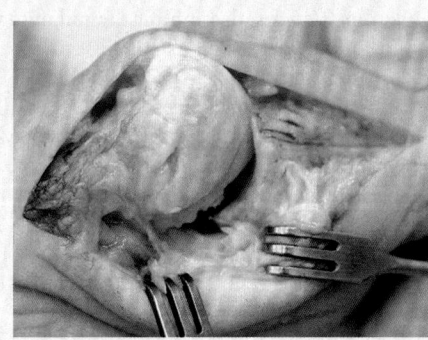

TECH FIG 1 A. Anteromedial approach. **B,C.** Joint exposure from the lateral side showing the restriction in plantar flexion.

CHEILECTOMY

- After inspection of the joint, the dorsal osteophytes on the base of the proximal phalanx are removed.
- Cheilectomy is performed with an oscillating saw.
- The cut is performed in line with the dorsal metatarsal shaft.
  - The resection must not exceed about 15% to 20% of the metatarsal head **(TECH FIG 2A)** because this leads to a jerking motion of the toe.

- Osteophytes remaining on the medial and lateral facet of the joint are removed with a sharp rongeur, plantar flexing the proximal phalanx **(TECH FIG 2B)**.
  - The rims are smoothed with a rasp.
- The final movements in dorsiflexion and plantar flexion have to be smooth without any jerking, as this will be painful without anesthesia.

TECHNIQUES

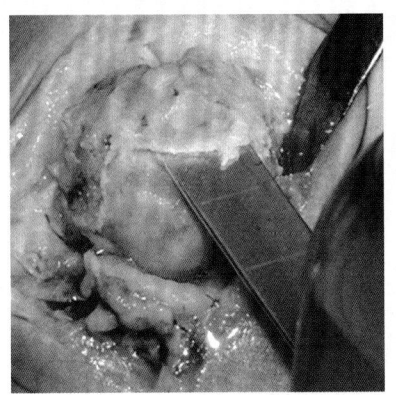

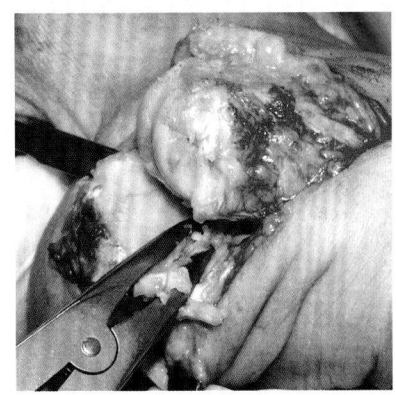

TECH FIG 2 **A.** Cheilectomy. **B.** Resection of remaining osteophytes.

EXTENSIVE PLANTAR RELEASE

- Release of the plantar structures is important for improving the ROM.
  - Because of the inhibition of dorsiflexion in the first MTP joint, contracture of the plantar structures (joint capsule, short toe flexors) has taken place.
- The joint capsule and the short flexors with the sesamoid bones are released subperiosteally using a McGlamry elevator **(TECH FIG 3A,B)**.
- The phalangeal attachment of the plantar capsule and the insertion of the short flexor muscles are released **(TECH FIG 3C)**.
  - This maneuver must be performed cautiously so as not to detach the tendons from their insertion.

- The joint is inspected again for plantar osteophytes of the phalangeal base and unstable cartilage parts, which will be resected.
  - Further resection to the metatarsal head must be avoided to prevent joint instability.
  - The rims are smoothed again with a rasp.
  - Osteophytes at the proximal sesamoid site must be resected because this also is a source for plantar pain and restricted dorsiflexion **(TECH FIG 3D)**.

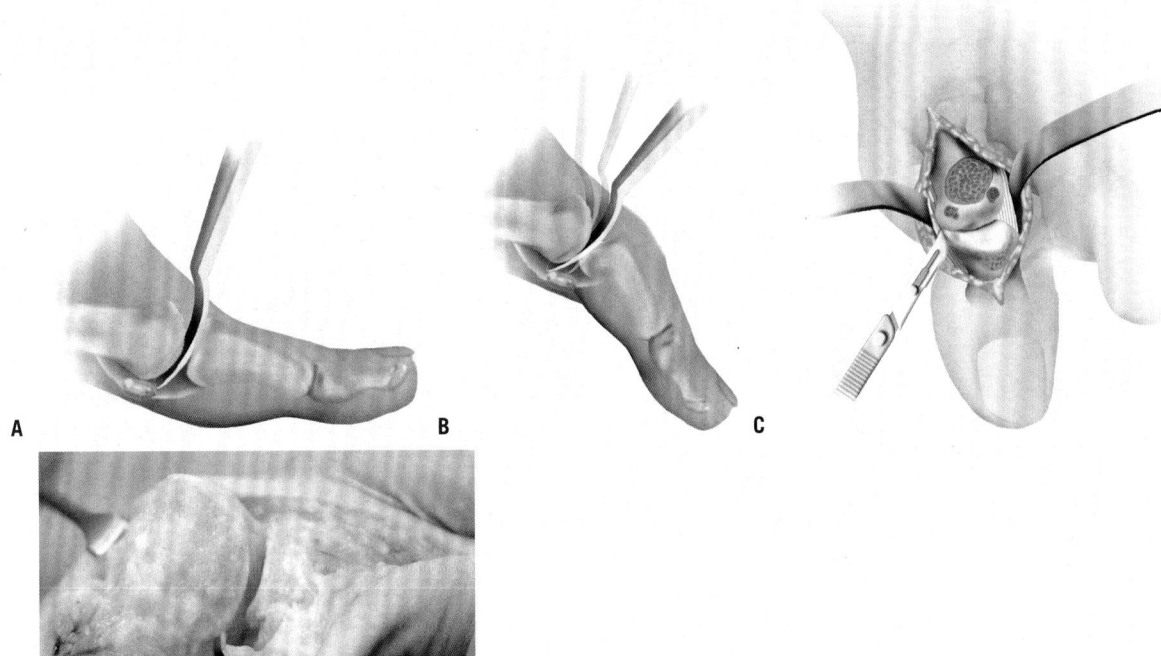

TECH FIG 3 **A,B.** Plantar release using a McGlamry elevator. **C.** Release of the distal capsule and short flexors using a scalpel. **D.** Plantar flexion after plantar release and resection of osteophytes.

TECHNIQUES

MICROFRACTURE

- The remaining cartilage lesions at the first MTP joint or the proximal phalanx must be débrided of all remaining unstable cartilage and fibrous tissue.
  - The calcified cartilage layer must be completely removed.
- Using an awl, the microfractures are placed approximately 1 to 2 mm apart and about 2 to 4 mm deep **(TECH FIG 4)**.

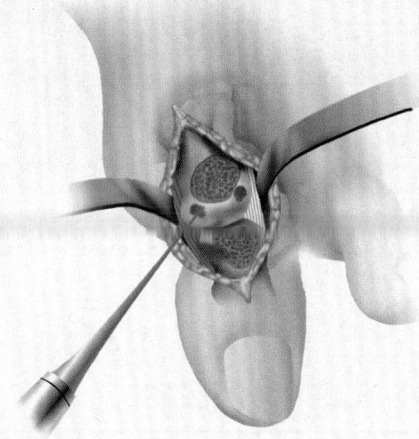

TECH FIG 4 Microfracturing of the metatarsal head.

AUTOLOGOUS MATRIX-INDUCED CHONDROGENESIS (AMIC) PROCEDURE

- In a fourth-degree cartilage lesion the sclerotic subchondral bone plate is débrided by a burr until normal bone is visible.
- Bone marrow aspirate is taken from the iliac crest and spread over the lesion and clotted for several minutes.

- An acellular matrix covers exactly the defect and is fixed by fibrin glue. Additionally, growth factors can be injected over the matrix to enhance biologic activity **(TECH FIG 5)**.

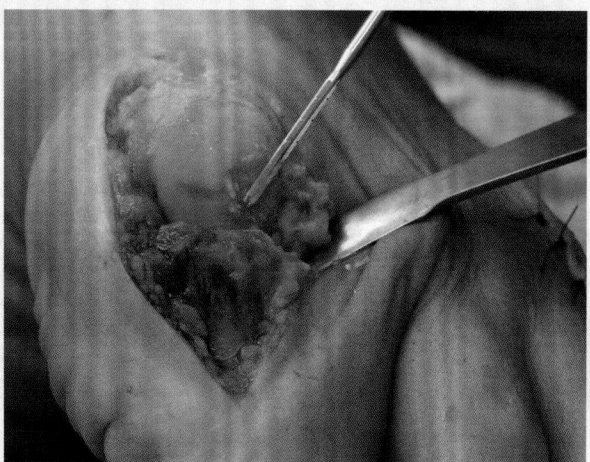
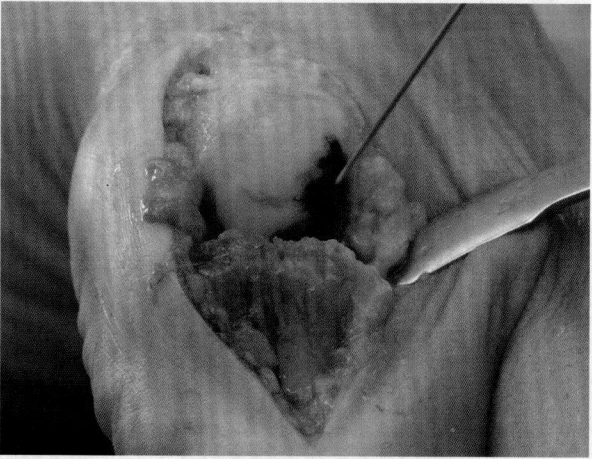

TECH FIG 5 Autologous matrix-induced chondrogenesis (AMIC) procedure of the metatarsal head. **A.** Chondroplasty with a burr. **B.** Injection of bone marrow aspirate. *(continued)*

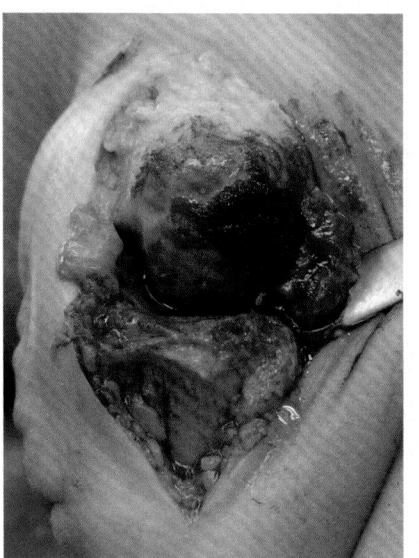
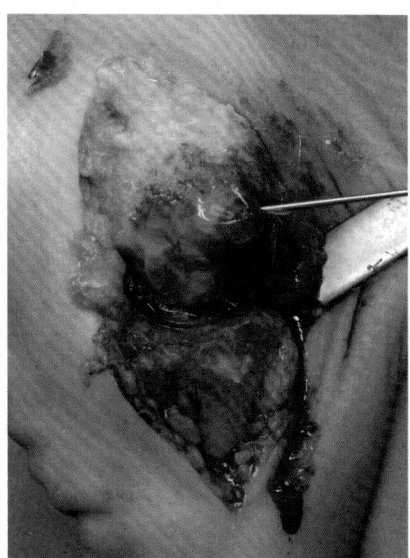
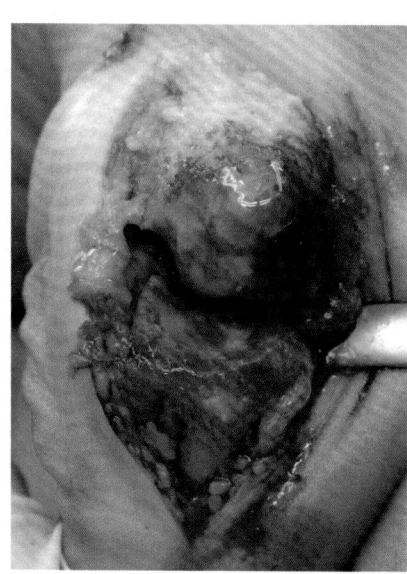

TECH FIG 5 *(continued)* **C.** Implantation of an acellular matrix scaffold. **D,E.** Fixation with fibrin glue.

AKIN OSTEOTOMY

- In cases of valgus deformity of the big toe without hallux valgus deformity is evident, the cartilage lesion is mostly at the lateral condyle of the first metatarsal head is located.
- Cartilage reconstruction without an alignment reconstruction wound lead to a failure of the procedure to unload the lateral

MTP joint a classic closed wedge oblique Akin osteotomy must be performed.
- The closed wedge osteotomy enables furthermore a decompression of the MTP joint **(TECH FIG 6)**.

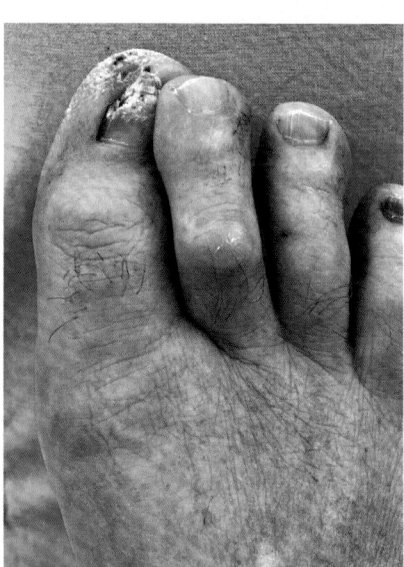
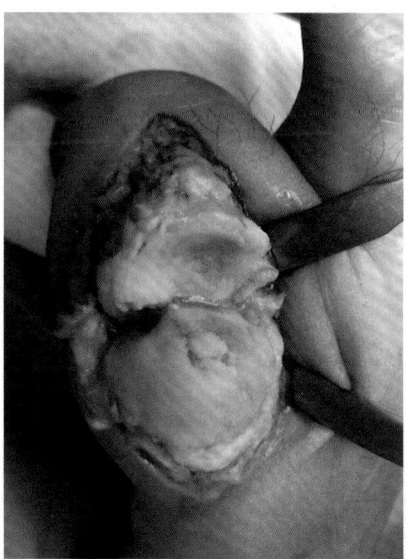
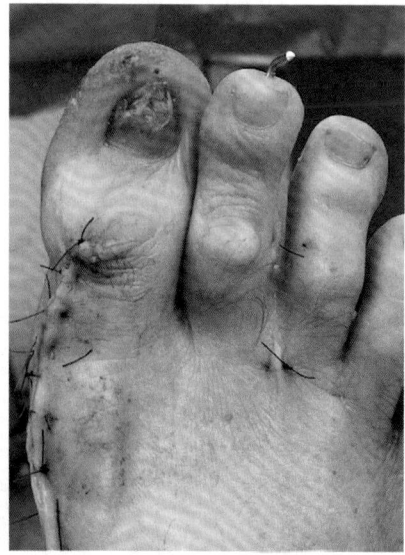

TECH FIG 6 A. Varus deformity of the big toe in a hallux rigidus. **B.** Lateral MTP joint cartilage damage. **C.** Akin osteotomy for alignment correction and unloading of the lateral MTP joint.

WOUND CLOSURE

- The joint capsule is closed with interrupted absorbable sutures, and a 0.8-mm drain is placed between the capsule and the continuous subcutaneous suture.
- The skin is sutured intracutaneously.
- Infiltration of the skin with bupivacaine and morphine decreases pain and need for painkillers after surgery.
- A small splint, which fixes the joint in dorsiflexion, is important to stretch the released shortened plantar structures (TECH FIG 7).

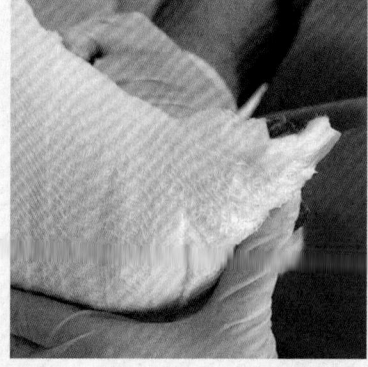

TECH FIG 7 Splint in 40 degrees of dorsiflexion.

TECHNIQUES

Pearls and Pitfalls

Resection of the Metatarsal Head	• Do not exceed 20% of the metatarsal head circumference. • Too much resection may lead to instability of the joint.
Plantar Release of Flexor Tendons	• Rough detachment of the short flexors may result in weak plantar flexion. • Using the McGlamry rasp, a distinct sound must be heard and felt.

POSTOPERATIVE CARE

- After surgery, a gauze-and-tape compression dressing is applied to the wound, and the hallux is fixed in 30 to 40 degrees of dorsiflexion with a plantar cast for 2 days to support plantar release and to improve immediate ROM after surgery.
- A second-generation cephalosporin is given intraoperatively.
- In our practice, from the second day, patients wear a post-surgical shoe with full weight bearing for 2 weeks to reduce loading and its accompanying pain and swelling. This allows the patient to become pain-free more quickly and makes it possible to regain dorsiflexion earlier (FIG 3).
  - The shoe permits good mobility and excellent conditions for decreased swelling and improved wound healing.
- "Aggressive" treatment of pain and swelling is crucial for the success of the surgical procedure because regaining and stabilizing the intraoperatively attained ROM is the postsurgical goal.

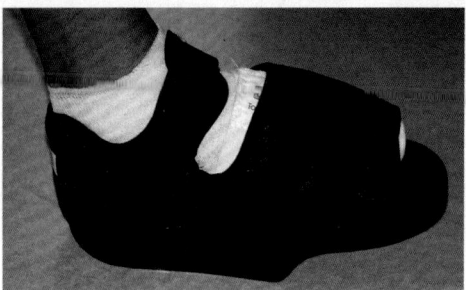

FIG 3 Forefoot postsurgical shoe.

- Passive and active ROM exercises are started from the second day if wound conditions and pain permit.
  - After removal of skin sutures, aggressive stretching is necessary to maintain ROM.
  - At this point, the patient should walk without the postsurgical shoe, focusing on a normal gait.
  - The rehabilitation program also includes isometric and proprioceptive training.
- Cooling, nonsteroidal anti-inflammatory drugs, and physical therapy with joint distraction support the daily self-guided dorsiflexion exercises.
- At 3 to 4 months, the maximum ROM usually has been achieved. The patient must be aware that there is only a limited time frame for achieving good motion.

OUTCOMES

- In a prospective study, 36 patients (26 women and 10 men) with 37 cases of hallux rigidus were operated by the senior author (HT) using the described technique.[3]
  - Patients were examined and interviewed preoperatively as well as 1 year (mean 12 months; 28 cases) and 2 years (mean 23 months; 22 cases) postoperatively and rated using the American Orthopaedic Foot & Ankle Society (AOFAS) hallux MTP–interphalangeal score[17] and by a visual analog scale (VAS; not scaled 10 cm, where 0 is very poor and 10 is excellent).
  - The average age of the 36 patients at the time of surgery was 50 years (range, 31–64 years).
  - Preoperative radiographs following Hattrup and Johnson's[13] classification revealed 25 cases of grade 2 and 12 of grade 3. No patient was classified as grade 1.

- Two patients, both grade 3, refused the follow-up examination.
- Retrospectively, several of these patients would have been classified grade 4 and should not have been considered for cheilectomy. We believe grade 3 is an indication if microfracturing and the plantar release are added for treatment, and the joint is not stiff before surgery.
- According to the AOFAS score, the results revealed a significant improvement from 43 points preoperatively to an average of 78 points (range, 35 to 100 points) after both 1 and 2 years postoperatively.
  - The average outcome on the VAS after 2 years was 7.1 for pain (preoperatively, 2.2; after 1 year, 7.0), 7.1 for function (preoperatively, 2.8; after 1 year, 6.7), and 7.4 for satisfaction (preoperatively, 1.1; after 1 year, 6.6).
  - Clinical examination showed an average improvement in ROM of 22 degrees.[3]

COMPLICATIONS

- In patients with coexisting hallux valgus deformity, correction of the axis with a soft tissue release is essential for a successful result. However, the obligatory immobilization of the osteotomy reduces the options for postoperative management, and results sometimes are less successful in regaining ROM.
- If too much metatarsal head is resected with the cheilectomy, first MTP joint instability may ensue.
- Rough detachment of the short flexors may result in weak plantar flexion.

REFERENCES

1. Ahn TK, Kitaoka HB, Luo ZP, et al. Kinematics and contact characteristics of the first metatarsophalangeal joint. Foot Ankle Int 1997;18:170–174.
2. Barca F. Tendon arthroplasty of the first metatarsophalangeal joint in hallux rigidus: preliminary communication. Foot Ankle Int 1997;18:222–228.
3. Becher C, Kilger R, Thermann H. Results of cheilectomy and additional microfracture technique for the treatment of hallux rigidus. Foot Ankle Surg 2005;3:155–160.
4. Becher C, Thermann H. Results of microfracture in the treatment of articular cartilage defects of the talus. Foot Ankle Int 2005;26: 583–589.
5. Coughlin MJ, Shurnas PS. Hallux rigidus: demographics, etiology, and radiographic assessment. Foot Ankle Int 2003;24:731–743.
6. Coughlin MJ, Shurnas PS. Hallux rigidus. Grading and long-term results of operative treatment. J Bone Joint Surg Am 2003;85(11): 2072–2088.
7. Easley ME, Davis WH, Anderson RB. Intermediate to long-term follow-up of medial-approach dorsal cheilectomy for hallux rigidus. Foot Ankle Int 1999;20:147–152.
8. Feltham GT, Hanks SE, Marcus RE. Age-based outcomes of cheilectomy for the treatment of hallux rigidus. Foot Ankle Int 2001;22: 192–197.
9. Frisbie DD, Trotter GW, Powers BE, et al. Arthroscopic subchondral bone plate microfracture technique augments healing of large chondral defects in the radial carpal bone and medial femoral condyle of horses. Vet Surg 1999;28:242–255.
10. Geldwert JJ, Rock GD, McGrath MP, et al. Cheilectomy: still a useful technique for grade I and grade II hallux limitus/rigidus. J Foot Surg 1992;31:154–159.
11. Gould N. Hallux rigidus: cheilotomy or implant? Foot Ankle 1981;1: 315–320.
12. Hamilton WG, O'Malley MJ, Thompson FM, et al. Roger Mann Award 1995. Capsular interposition arthroplasty for severe hallux rigidus. Foot Ankle Int 1997;18:68–70.
13. Hattrup SJ, Johnson KA. Subjective results of hallux rigidus following treatment with cheilectomy. Clin Orthop Relat Res 1988;(226): 182–191.
14. Hua J, Sakamoto K, Kikukawa T, et al. Evaluation of the suppressive actions of glucosamine on the interleukin-1 beta-mediated activation of synoviocytes. Inflamm Res 2007;56:432–438.
15. Lau JT, Daniels TR. Outcomes following cheilectomy and interpositional arthroplasty in hallux rigidus. Foot Ankle Int 2001;22: 462–470.
16. Mann RA, Clanton TO. Hallux rigidus: treatment by cheilectomy. J Bone Joint Surg Am 1988;70(3):400–406.
17. Mulier T, Steenwerckx A, Thienpont E, et al. Results after cheilectomy in athletes with hallux rigidus. Foot Ankle Int 1999;20:232–237.
18. Pässler HH. Die Technik der Mikrofrakturierung für die Behandlung von Knorpelschäden. Zentralbl Chir 2000;125:500–504.
19. Reginster JY, Deroisy R, Rovati LC, et al. Long-term effects of glucosamine sulphate on osteoarthritis progression: a randomised, placebo-controlled clinical trial. Lancet 2001;357:251–256.
20. Smith RW, Katchis SD, Ayson LC. Outcomes in hallux rigidus patients treated nonoperatively: a long-term follow-up study. Foot Ankle Int 2000;21:906–913.
21. Solan MC, Lemon M, Bendall SP. The surgical anatomy of the dorsomedial cutaneous nerve of the hallux. J Bone Joint Surg Br 2001;83(2):250–252.
22. Steadman JR, Briggs KK, Rodrigo JJ, et al. Outcomes of microfracture for traumatic chondral defects of the knee: average 11-year follow-up. Arthroscopy 2003;19:477–484.
23. Steadman JR, Rodkey WG, Singleton SB, et al. Microfracture technique for full-thickness chondral defects: technique and clinical results. Oper Tech Orthop 1997;7:300–304.

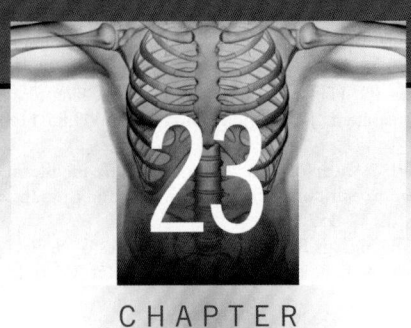

23
CHAPTER

Capsular Interpositional Arthroplasty

Andrew J. Elliott and Martin J. O'Malley

DEFINITION

- Hallux rigidus refers to degenerative arthritis of the first metatarsophalangeal (MTP) joint that is characterized by pain, decreased range of motion (ROM), and proliferative osteophyte formation.

ANATOMY

- The first MTP joint is composed of the dorsal joint capsule, the medial and lateral collateral ligaments, the plantar plate–sesamoid–flexor hallucis brevis (FHB) tendon complex, the first metatarsal head, and the proximal articulating end of the proximal phalanx.
- Pathology is limited primarily to the first MTP joint, with prominent dorsal osteophyte on the metatarsal head.

PATHOGENESIS

- The origin of progressive first MTP joint cartilage degeneration is uncertain. Most attribute hallux rigidus to biomechanical disturbance or local pathology that leads to repetitive stress on articular cartilage and subsequent deterioration of the cartilage surface.
- Trauma
- Inflammatory arthritides (eg, rheumatoid arthritis, gout)
- Primary osteoarthritis
- Associated factors such as long first metatarsal, flat metatarsal head, metatarsus primus elevatus, pronated feet, or hallux valgus interphalangeus are often found in patients with arthritis of the first MTP joint.
- Long first metatarsal may be correlated with development of hallux rigidus.

NATURAL HISTORY

- Initially, pain is localized to the dorsal aspect of the great toe MTP joint. Loss of motion is minimal but can be seen with activities that require maximum dorsiflexion. Over time, generally several years, the degree of involvement and loss of motion increase. Eventually, in the end stage of the process, the first MTP joint will lose nearly all motion. A varus or valgus deformity is usually not associated with this process.
- Pain may or may not progress as osteophytes form to stabilize the joint.
- Progression of osteophytes and joint space narrowing on radiographs may or may not correlate with symptoms.

PATIENT HISTORY AND PHYSICAL FINDINGS

- Typical history is swelling around the first MTP joint. Patients will complain frequently of a progressive increase in the size of the MTP joint and attribute this to a bunion-type deformity.
- Occasionally, avoidance gait can result and cause an increased weight-bearing load on the lateral aspect of the foot.
- Initially, a tender dorsal osteophyte will be noted with MTP joint flexion retrograde elevation and uncovering of the dorsal portion of the articulation. Pain may be associated with local dorsal cutaneous nerve irritation caused by the osteophyte.
- Limited dorsiflexion with abutment of articular surfaces of the phalanx onto the metatarsal head can be seen. Periarticular osteophytes can be noted, particularly laterally.
- Compensatory hyperextension of the hallucal interphalangeal joint can be seen with long-standing disease.
- Axial compression of the MTP joint with pain can often differentiate the level of involvement of the degenerative process.
- Pain is felt with dorsiflexion activities (wearing high-heeled shoes, running, yoga).
- Progressive proliferation of osteophytes about the joint occurs and pain is felt with small toe box shoes.
- Decreased dorsiflexion and plantarflexion motion of the joint is seen, and pain is elicited with attempting these motions.
- Physical examination includes the following:
  - Visualize the dorsal osteophyte to check for swelling.
  - For lesser toe evaluation, examine for hammer toe formation or evidence of a more systemic process: Presence of multiple hammer toe formation with hallux rigidus suggests rheumatoid arthritis.
  - Evaluate ROM for dorsal-based blocking of dorsiflexion.
  - Check axial compression by stabilizing the first metatarsal while compressing the proximal phalanx against the metatarsal head. Increasing levels of pain are associated with more complete joint involvement.
  - Tomassen sign: With the ankle held in neutral, dorsiflexion of the MTP joint is measured. A positive result is suggestive of a stenosing flexor hallucis longus (FHL) tenosynovitis and not a static dorsal osteophyte.
  - Pain at the midrange of the motion arc implies a global first MTP joint arthritis that may not be amenable to dorsal cheilectomy alone but instead is better treated with interpositional arthroplasty or arthrodesis.

IMAGING AND OTHER DIAGNOSTIC STUDIES

- Standard weight-bearing anteroposterior (AP), oblique, and lateral radiographs of the foot
  - Grade I: small lateral spurs with joint space preservation
  - Grade II: metatarsal and phalangeal osteophytes with dorsal joint space narrowing and subchondral sclerosis
  - Grade III: marked osteophyte formation with loss of joint space and subchondral cyst formation **(FIG 1)**
- Laboratory studies if serologic etiology suspected

DIFFERENTIAL DIAGNOSIS

- Trauma
- Primary osteoarthritis
- Degenerative arthritis
- Rheumatoid arthritis
- Seronegative arthropathy
- Gout
- Stenosing FHL tendon[10]

NONOPERATIVE MANAGEMENT

- Low-heeled shoes
- Steel shanks
- Stiff Morton extension orthoses
- Nonsteroidal anti-inflammatory drugs
- Cortisone injection
- Rocker sole shoe or over-the-counter rocker shoe

SURGICAL MANAGEMENT

- Grade I: cheilectomy to address mild osteophyte formation, joint space intact, minimal dorsal spur formation
- Grade II: cheilectomy with Moberg dorsal phalangeal osteotomy to address moderate osteophyte formation, joint space narrowing, subchondral sclerosis, bony proliferation on metatarsal head and phalanx on radiograph, or significant intraoperative joint involvement
- Grade III: interposition arthroplasty or fusion to address marked osteophyte formation, loss of visible joint space, extensive bony proliferation[2,3]

Preoperative Planning

- Standing AP and lateral foot radiographs to anticipate level of intervention
- Consider consent for cheilectomy, Moberg dorsal osteotomy, and interposition arthroplasty. Although arthrodesis could be considered as well, the goal of interpositional arthroplasty is to preserve motion in end-stage first MTP joint arthritis.
- Patients who do well with interpositional arthroplasty typically are moderately but not extremely active athletes who wish for retention of dorsiflexion of the toe for activities of daily living such as sports or use of certain shoe wear.
- Relative contraindications to interpositional arthroplasty include cases in which first MTP joint arthrodesis may be favored.
  - Long second metatarsal (potential risk for development of transfer metatarsalgia) (see **FIG 1A**)
  - Hallux valgus
  - Sesamoid arthritis
  - First tarsometatarsal instability: inflammatory arthritides
  - High-demand patients (athletes, dancers) present a challenge as we believe that they should be discouraged from this procedure yet are also not ideal candidates for first MTP joint arthrodesis.[6]
- Poor vascular status, neuropathy, and infection are absolute contraindications to this procedure.

Positioning

- The patient is placed supine with a bump under the contralateral lumbar region if needed to evert the foot for better exposure.
- The foot is placed at the bottom corner of the bed.
- A bolster is placed under the greater trochanter of the ipsilateral hip to avoid external rotation of the operated extremity.
- A mini C-arm is placed on the ipsilateral side of the bed, about 6 feet past the corner of the operating room table and at a 45-degree angle. In our experience, this positioning affords the best access to the foot and simplifies intraoperative imaging. Blankets or sheets are used to elevate the

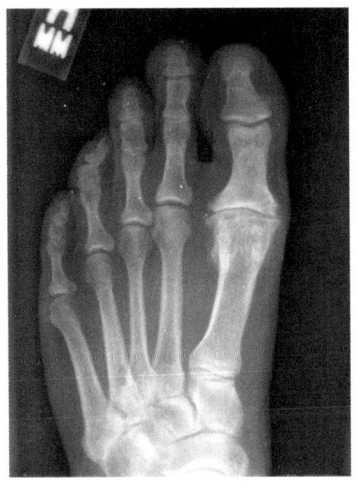
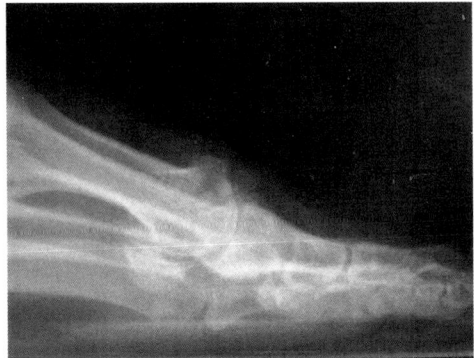

FIG 1 A. AP view of a foot with hallux rigidus with a relatively longer second metatarsal and the suggestion of second metatarsal overload with flattening of the metatarsal head. **B.** Lateral view of the foot demonstrating dorsal osteophytes and joint space narrowing.

operated extremity to facilitate lateral fluoroscopic imaging unobstructed by the contralateral lower extremity.

Approach

- Two approaches are commonly used: dorsal and medial.
- The dorsal approach allows for easier access to the lateral osteophyte. This approach makes suturing the interposition tissue to plantar surface of the joint difficult, however.
- In contrast, the medial incision allows for easier access to the plantar surface and is the approach used by the senior

author (WGH). The capsule is carefully protected, with particular attention given to protecting the plantar nerve (Joplin nerve) as well as the dorsal cutaneous branch.
- Protect the extensor hallucis longus (EHL) tendon and the dorsal and plantar digital nerves. Identify the extensor hallucis brevis (EHB) and the joint capsule.
- Ankle block anesthesia is used, plus an Esmarch ankle tourniquet with three wraps approximating 300 mm Hg, incorporating a full roll of Webril wrapped around the ankle to protect the skin overlying the Achilles tendon.

EXPOSURE AND CAPSULOTOMY

- A longitudinal midaxial medial approach to the first MTP joint is performed (**TECH FIG 1A**).
- The dorsomedial sensory cutaneous nerve to the hallux is identified and protected throughout the procedure.
- A thin layer of adventitial tissue may be mobilized to later be closed over the interpositional arthroplasty to further support the toe.
- The EHL tendon is identified (**TECH FIG 1B**), and the interval between the EHL and the underlying EHB is developed (**TECH FIG 1C**).

- The EHL and FHL tendons are identified and must remain protected throughout the procedure, not only from being transected but also from being tethered by suture.
- A longitudinal medial capsulotomy is performed to expose the arthritic joint.
- The capsule is reflected from the proximal phalanx (**TECH FIG 1D,E**).
- We often use a towel clamp to carefully mobilize the base of the proximal phalanx (**TECH FIG 1F,G**).

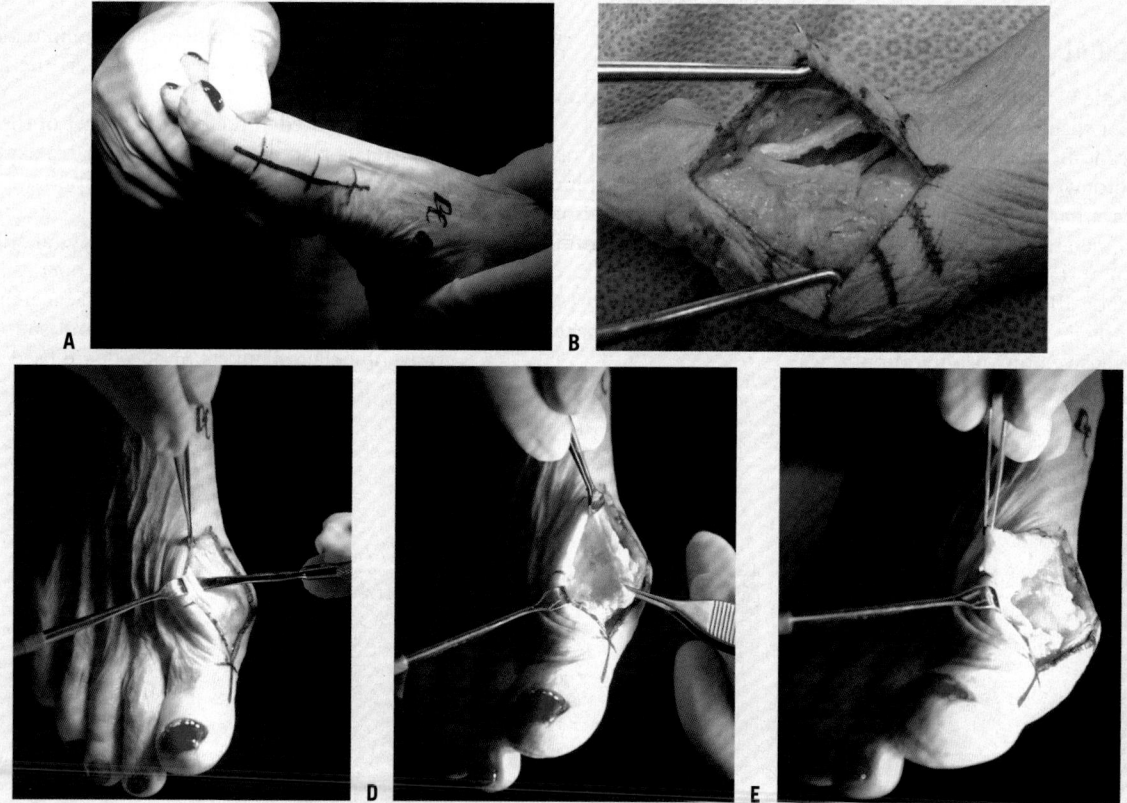

TECH FIG 1 A. Midaxial incision centered over the medial first MTP joint. **B.** Cadaveric specimen demonstrating medial approach with the adventitial tissue over the medial joint capsule exposed and the EHL tendon and dorsomedial sensory cutaneous nerve identified. **C.** First MTP joint capsule being defined while elevating the EHL tendon. **D,E.** Dorsal capsule being reflected off the proximal phalanx. *(continued)*

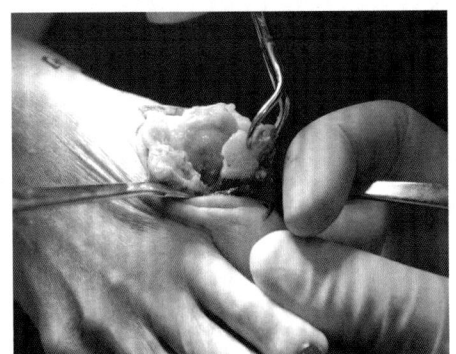 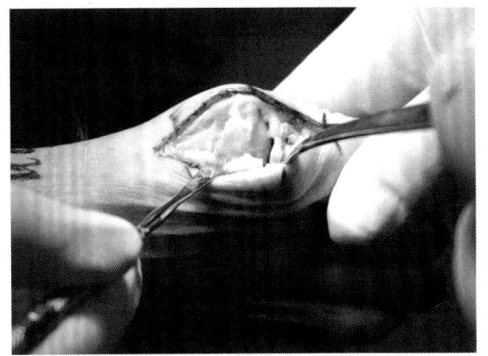

TECH FIG 1 *(continued)* **F,G.** Use of a towel clip to mobilize the proximal phalanx.

CHEILOTOMY AND PHALANGEAL OSTEOTOMY

- Inspect joint and, if over 50% of joint cartilage remains, consider proceeding with cheilectomy with or without dorsal (Moberg) closing wedge osteotomy of the phalanx.[2,3]
- If less than 50% of joint cartilage remains, perform cheilectomy of the dorsal third of the metatarsal head.
- Subperiosteally release the dorsal capsule, the EHB tendon insertion, and the plantar plate–FHB from the proximal phalanx base **(TECH FIG 2A).**

- Resect 25% (roughly 8 mm) of the proximal phalanx with a sagittal saw, protecting the EHL and FHL **(TECH FIG 2B,C).**
- We recommend that no more than this is resected from the proximal phalanx to avoid potential postoperative instability of the residual first MTP joint **(TECH FIG 2D,E).**

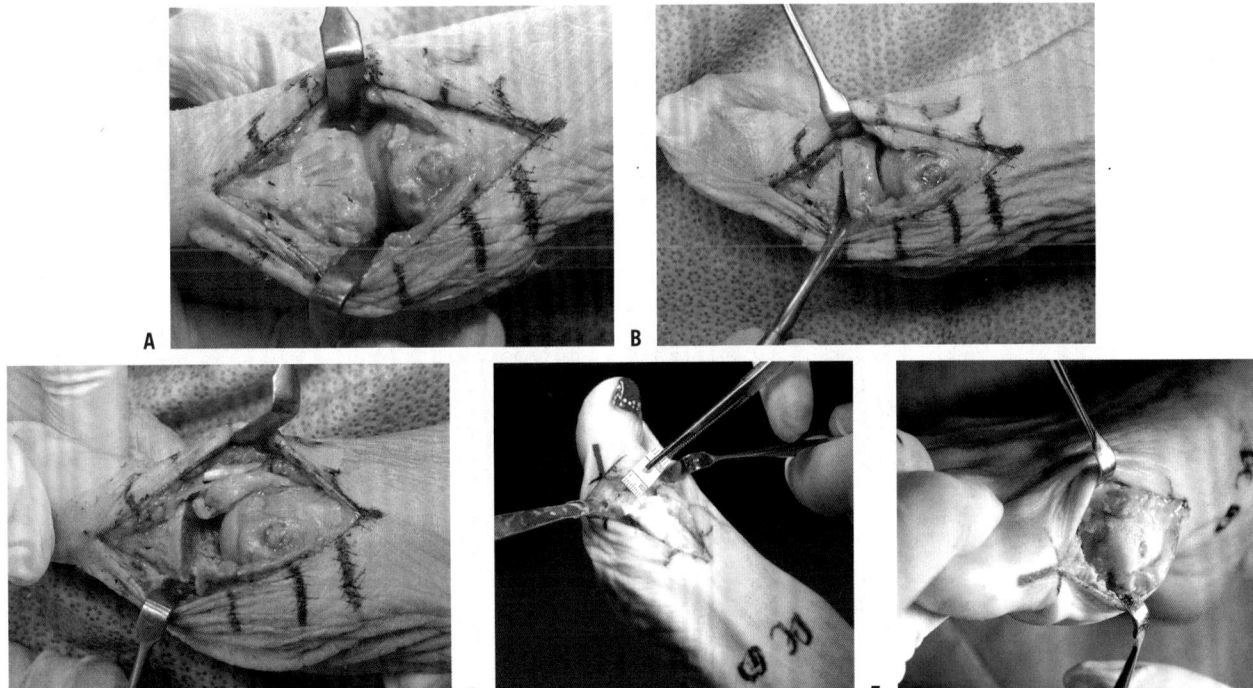

TECH FIG 2 A. Cadaveric specimen with exposed first MTP joint. **B,C.** Cadaveric specimen demonstrating 25% resection of proximal phalanx base. Excessive resection of the proximal phalanx base must be avoided to maintain joint stability. **D.** Measuring planned resection from base of proximal phalanx. **E.** Gap created after dorsal cheilectomy and proximal phalanx resection.

TECHNIQUES

INTERPOSITION ARTHROPLASTY

- Transect EHB tendon approximately 3 cm proximal to the joint. This prevents the capsular tissue from being retracted during gait. Moreover, the EHB tendon may then be used to augment the soft tissue interposition. Mobilize the EHB into the joint space **(TECH FIG 3A,B)**.
- Suture capsular tissue to stumps of the FHB tendon with 0-0 nonabsorbable suture.
  - The dorsal capsule is mobilized into the joint and approximated with the FHB tendon in a balanced fashion.
  - Should the capsule not mobilize adequately, the dorsal cheilectomy may need to be increased.
  - Protect the FHL tendon and the plantar nerves during suturing.
- Typically, there remains a thin layer of adventitial tissue that is superficial to the capsule that can be carefully approximated to further support the toe.

- Evaluate balance and motion of the toe. Dorsiflexion should be uninhibited throughout the motion arc **(TECH FIG 3C,D)**.
- Although originally described, we rarely use a Kirschner wire (K-wire) to support the reconstruction.
- In our experience, the EHL tendon needs to be lengthened in less than 5% of these surgeries, or almost never. However, when necessary, we prefer to perform the lengthening through a horizontal Z pattern.
- The capsule is cut proximally such that it can be rotated down over the top of the metatarsal head. The capsule is mobilized and secured with 2-0 nonabsorbable suture. Repair is done via 2-0 or 3-0 Vicryl.

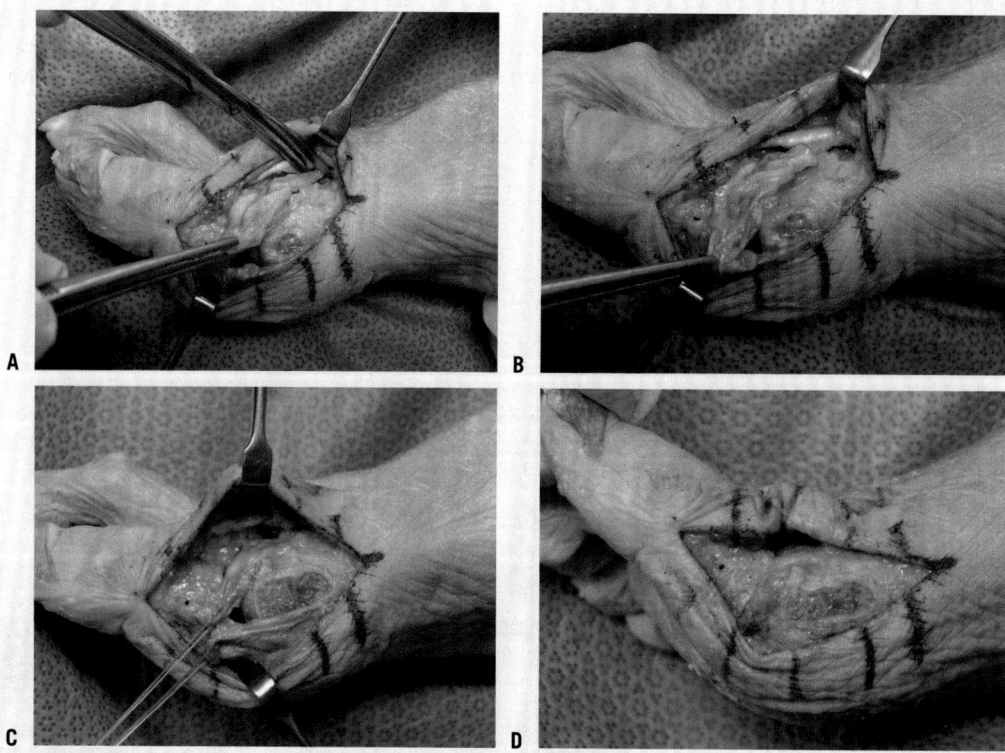

TECH FIG 3 Cadaveric specimen. **A.** Dorsal capsule with EHB. **B.** EHB transected and tendon–capsule complex mobilized into joint. **C.** Capsule sutured to plantar plate. **D.** Toe taken through ROM.

Pearls and Pitfalls

Insufficient Capsular Tissue	• Allograft (gracilis, hamstring, or fascia lata[5]) or autograft (plantaris[1] or hamstring) may be used for insufficient capsule. These can be placed into a cavity prepared by use of MTP joint fusion reamers[4] or a burr[1] instead of proximal phalanx resection.
Push-off Weakness	• Perform oblique osteotomy of the proximal phalanx to decompress the MTP joint but leave the FHB–sesamoid complex attachment intact.[13]
Floppy Toe	• Take care not to resect too much proximal phalanx. • Place a K-wire at resection site, confirm with fluoroscopy, and cut along the wire.
Toe Sits in Dorsiflexion	• Lengthen the EHL if the toe sits in an extended position after reconstruction. • Consider pinning with 0.062-inch K-wire for 3 weeks.
Anatomic Considerations	• Avoid tethering the FHL tendon with the permanent sutures. • Avoid injury to the plantar or dorsomedial digital nerves.
Relative Lengths of the First and Second Metatarsals	• A long second metatarsal may be subject to transfer metatarsalgia with a capsular interpositional arthroplasty. We view a long second metatarsal as a relative contraindication to first MTP joint interpositional arthroplasty. Consider second metatarsal shortening osteotomy for patients with long second metatarsal to prevent transfer metatarsalgia.
Achieving Optimal Soft Tissue Balancing of the First MTP Joint	• Balance the capsule when attaching it to the plantar plate. Then balance the toe relative to the first metatarsal by reapproximating the residual adventitial tissue. Although originally described, pinning should not be necessary.
Suture Placement	• Use of a Hintermann retractor or lamina spreader with a K-wire hole attachment allows for excellent distraction of the joint to facilitate suture placement.

POSTOPERATIVE CARE

• Weight bearing as tolerated in postoperative shoe for 4 to 6 weeks. Begin gentle passive ROM at home.
• Sutures are removed in 10 to 14 days.
• If a pin is used temporarily, it is removed at 3 to 4 weeks.
• Patients should be made aware before surgery that they will have a "floppy" toe for several months until the joint tissues and tendons stabilize with time.

OUTCOMES

• Between 73% and 94% of patients report good to excellent results.[1,4–9,11–13]
• In our experience, transfer metatarsalgia develops to some degree in 30% of patients.[6] These patients can be successfully managed with orthoses, lesser metatarsal shortening osteotomy, or lesser metatarsal plantar condylectomy.

COMPLICATIONS

• Transfer metatarsalgia, particularly with a long second metatarsal
• Resecting too little bone, leading to impingement and pain
• Cock-up deformity
• Hallux valgus or varus
• Floppy toe or stiffness
• Weakness of push-off with the first toe
• Injury to the dorsal and plantar digital nerves
• Tethering of the FHL tendon by the capsular sutures
• Floating great toe (rare and observed when EHL contracture is present and EHL is not lengthened)

ACKNOWLEDGMENT

• The authors would like to thank Timothy Charlton and William G. Hamilton for their outstanding work on the previous edition chapter.

REFERENCES

1. Barca F. Tendon arthroplasty of the first metatarsophalangeal joint in hallux rigidus: preliminary communication. Foot Ankle Int 1997; 18:222–228.
2. Coughlin MJ, Shurnas PS. Hallux rigidus: demographics, etiology, and radiographic assessment. Foot Ankle Int 2003;24:731–743.
3. Coughlin MJ, Shurnas PS. Hallux rigidus: grading and long-term results of operative treatment. J Bone Joint Surg Am 2003;85:2072–2088.
4. Coughlin MJ, Shurnas PS. Soft-tissue arthroplasty for hallux rigidus. Foot Ankle Int 2003;24:661–672.
5. Givissis PK, Symeonidis PD, Kitridis DM, et al. Minimal resection interpositional arthroplasty of the first metatarsophalangeal joint. Foot (Edinb) 2017;32:1–7.
6. Hamilton WG, Hubbard CE. Hallux rigidus. Excisional arthroplasty. Foot Ankle Clin 2000;5:663–671.
7. Hamilton WG, O'Malley MJ, Thompson FM, et al. Roger Mann Award 1995. Capsular interposition arthroplasty for severe hallux rigidus. Foot Ankle Int 1997;18:68–70.
8. Johnson JE, McCormick JJ. Modified oblique Keller capsular interposition arthroplasty (MOKCIA) for treatment of late-stage hallux rigidus. Foot Ankle Int 2014;35:415–422.
9. Kennedy JG, Chow FY, Dines J, et al. Outcomes after interposition arthroplasty for treatment of hallux rigidus. Clin Orthop Rel Res 2006;445:210–215.
10. Kirane YM, Michelson JD, Sharkey NA. Contribution of the flexor hallucis longus to loading of the first metatarsal and first metatarsophalangeal joint. Foot Ankle Int 2008;29:367–377.
11. Lau JTC, Daniels TR. Outcomes following cheilectomy and interpositional arthroplasty in hallux rigidus. Foot Ankle Int 2001;22:462–470.
12. Mafulli N, Papalia R, Palumbo A, et al. Quantitative review of the operative management of hallux rigidus. Br Med Bull 2011;98:75–98.
13. Mroczek KJ, Miller SD. The modified oblique Keller procedure: a technique for dorsal approach interposition arthroplasty sparing the flexor tendons. Foot Ankle Int 2003;24:521–522.

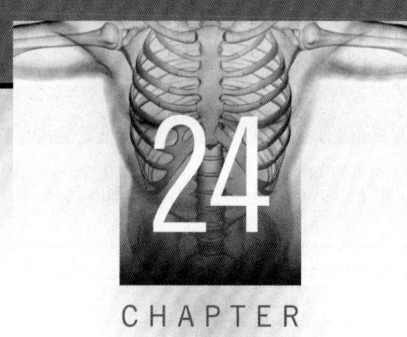

CHAPTER

24

The CARTIVA Procedure

Mark Glazebrook, Tim Daniels, and Rishin J. Kadakia

DEFINITION

- Hallux rigidus, degenerative changes of the first metatarsophalangeal joint (MTPJ), is the most common location for arthritis in the foot. It is reported to affect approximately 3% of adults older than the age of 50 years.[10]
- The incidence of hallux rigidus is higher in females and nearly 50% of cases are bilateral. Hallux rigidus is the second most common pathology associated with the first MTPJ secondary to hallux valgus.[4,5]
- In the majority of patients with hallux rigidus, there is a positive family history of great toe pathology.[6]
- Patients frequently present with pain, stiffness, loss of range of motion (ROM), and osteophyte formation that can cause pain with shoe wear.

ANATOMY

- The first MTPJ consists of the convex head of the first metatarsal bone articulating with the concave base of the proximal phalanx. There are several dynamic and static structures that play integral functions in first MTPJ functioning and stability.
- Varus and valgus static stability is provided by stout lateral and medial collateral ligaments. Dynamic stability in the sagittal plane is also provided by various muscular attachments medially and laterally.
- The plantar capsuloligamentous confluence consists of the thick plantar plate and the sesamoid complex—consisting of the two sesamoid bones invested in the flexor hallucis brevis tendon. The flexor hallucis longus courses between the two sesamoid bones to attach distally.
- The sesamoid complex serves as a fulcrum for the flexor digitorum brevis and allows more power to be generate during plantar flexion.[1]
- The dorsal stability is provided by the dorsal joint capsule and the extensor hood, which also has dynamic stability from the attachment of the extensor hallucis brevis and the EHL passing over.
- The first MTPJ bears approximately 40% to 60% of the body's weight during ambulation and can see up to eight times the regular body weight during high-impact activities.[11,12]

PATHOGENESIS

- The etiology of hallux rigidus can vary depending on the patient case and can frequently be multifactorial.
- Systemic conditions such as rheumatoid arthritis or gout could lead to the development of hallux rigidus, and these cases can be bilateral with multijoint involvement.

- A history of either a traumatic injury or repetitive microtrauma can often lead to the early development of posttraumatic hallux rigidus.
- In most cases, the development of hallux rigidus can be idiopathic with no identifiable cause.
- There is literature supporting certain anatomic factors that may be associated with the development of hallux rigidus such as metatarsus adductus, hallux valgus interphalangeus, and a flat and square-shaped first metatarsal.[6]

NATURAL HISTORY

- Early disease frequently presents with cartilage loss at the dorsal aspect of the joint with dorsal osteophyte formation. In its early stages, ROM is frequently not severely limited, and pain is primarily seen with maximal dorsiflexion.
- As the arthritis progresses, the entire joint becomes involved leading to more diffuse stiffness and pain with all ranges of motion.
- Radiographic changes include a progressive loss of joint space and osteophyte formation as the disease progresses.
- Similar to degenerative changes in other joints, hallux rigidus evolves gradually over time, and progression rates can vary depending on a variety of factors.

PATIENT HISTORY AND PHYSICAL FINDINGS

- Patients typically present with pain and soft tissue swelling surrounding the first MTPJ. Dorsal osteophytes can be palpable and cause pain with shoe wear. Furthermore, large dorsal osteophytes may also cause compression of the dorsomedial cutaneous nerve leading to radiating pain even at rest.
- In early stages, patients complain of dorsal pain and pain with maximal dorsiflexion due to dorsal impingement. Activities such as running or wearing high-heeled shoes may be particularly painful given the degree of first MTPJ dorsiflexion required.
- It is imperative to carefully evaluate ROM of the first MTPJ and to determine exactly which aspects of motion are particularly bothersome. The majority of patients have pain with maximum dorsi-flexion and plantar flexion, with minimal or no midrange pain. If the patient has pain throughout the arc of motion, this indicates a reactive synovitis and influences the surgical options (recommendations). The first clinical sign of mild (early) arthritis of the first MTPJ is pain with forced plantar flexion.
- As the degenerative process progresses, cartilage degeneration usually progresses from the dorsum of the metatarsal head to plantar. Clinically, this is accompanied by a

progressive loss of ROM and radiographic advancement of arthritis with loss of joint space and osteophyte formation.
- Patients may off-load the first ray as symptoms worsen leading to overload of the lateral ray and pain laterally.
- Careful examination of other joints in the foot and body is necessary as multijoint involvement may indicate a systemic process requiring further workup and management.
- Some patients may present with first MTPJ arthritis and an elevated first metatarsal (metatarsus elevatus). If this is present, an improved ROM dorsally is sometimes observed by depressing the first metatarsal while dorsiflexion the first toe.
- It is important to assess the location of the pain and examine the sesamoid first metatarsal articulation. If the patient has plantar medial pain that is exaggerated by direct compression over the tibial sesamoid, then the sesamoid articulation can be considered a pain generator. The presence of sesamoid pain may indicate further workup is required.

IMAGING AND OTHER DIAGNOSTIC STUDIES

- Standard weight-bearing anteroposterior (AP) and lateral radiographs of the foot are most commonly all that is necessary for the diagnosis and management of hallux rigidus (FIG 1).
- Advanced imaging studies are rarely needed except in special cases. Computed tomography scan may be useful in cases with cystic changes or deformity for preoperative planning purposes. Magnetic resonance imaging may be indicated if there is radiographic or clinical concern for osteochondral lesions in the metatarsal head, sesamoid pain, or sesamoid osteonecrosis.
- Patients with midrange pain may have an inflammatory arthritis and should be assessed for seronegative or seropositive arthropathies. A referral to a rheumatologist may be indicated if the clinical findings support this diagnosis (periarticular cysts, symmetric joint space narrowing, other joint involvement, constitutional symptoms).

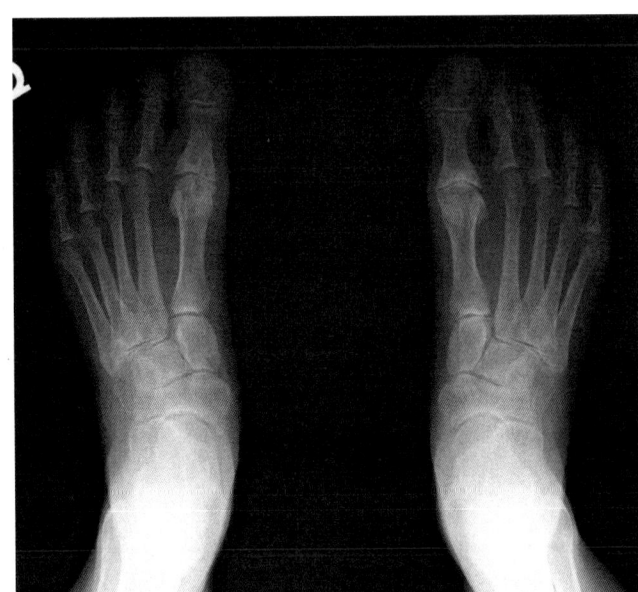

FIG 1 Standing AP radiograph of a patient with bilateral hallux rigidus.

- Coughling and Shurnas[7] developed a classification system summarized in the following text involving both radiographic and clinical factors that is most commonly used for hallux rigidus.
  - Grade 0—no radiographic findings, joint stiffness but no pain, 20% loss of dorsiflexion compared to contralateral
  - Grade 1—dorsal osteophyte formation, mild pain and pain at maximal dorsiflexion, further loss of dorsiflexion to approximately 50% of contralateral
  - Grade 2—more diffuse osteophyte formation, metatarsal head flattening, mild joint spare loss/sclerosis, moderate pain with motion but not at midrange, 75% loss of dorsiflexion compared to contralateral
  - Grade 3—similar radiographic findings but with greater joint space narrowing, involvement of the sesamoids, pain is worse than grade 2 and more constant but still not present at midrange, almost complete loss of dorsiflexion
  - Grade 4—similar radiographic findings and dorsiflexion but now with pain at mid-ROM with passive ROM

DIFFERENTIAL DIAGNOSIS

- Inflammatory arthropathy: rheumatoid arthritis, psoriatic arthritis, etc.
- Gout
- Trauma
- Osteochondral defect
- Infection
- Sesamoid complex injury such as a plantar plate tear
- Sesamoid osteonecrosis
- Sesamoid arthritis

NONOPERATIVE MANAGEMENT

- Nonoperative treatment is the first line of management in patients with hallux rigidus.
- There are a host of treatment options available that depend on the severity of the symptoms and patient limitations.
- Most orthotics aimed at relieving pain from hallux rigidus work by off-loading and decreasing motion of the first MTPJ, primarily dorsiflexion.
  - The Morton extension orthotic is an example of this and provides rigid longitudinal support to the first MTPJ and limits dorsiflexion during push off.
- Wide toe box shoes can prevent pain associated with irritation from dorsal osteophytes.
- Activity modification to avoid sports or activities that cause excessive first MTPJ dorsiflexion can be helpful.
- Oral anti-inflammatories can provide pain relief but must be tolerated by patients, and side effect profiles of long-term use must be considered.
- Intra-articular cortisone injections can provide pain relief for some patients.

SURGICAL MANAGEMENT

- The decision to pursue surgical treatment of hallux rigidus is dependent on the severity of symptoms and lack of response to nonoperative care.
- There are a wide variety of surgical treatment options available, and certain treatment options depends on the stage of arthritic changes and patient factors.

- MTPJ arthrodesis is the most reliable treatment for end-stage arthritis of the first MTPJ as it provides reliable pain relief. However, this sacrifices of ROM, which can impact activities and shoe wear.
- Dorsal cheilectomy is a joint-sparing procedure for early stages of disease that can improve ROM and eliminate mechanical symptoms from dorsal osteophytes and dorsal MT head cartilage degeneration.
- There are a host of other joint-sparing procedures aimed to maintain motion and provide pain relief such as interpositional arthroplasty or partial and total toe replacement with prosthesis. The major challenge to joint-sparing options is reliably providing the patient with pain-free and improved motion while maintaining bone stock if a fusion is required as salvage at a later stage.
- The CARTIVA implant (Wright Medical Group, Memphis, TN) is a synthetic polyvinyl alcohol hydrogel implant that was developed as an alternative joint-sparing procedure and bone-sparing option for the management of hallux rigidus. This implant is placed into the metatarsal head articulating with the base of the proximal phalanx. It aims to provide pain relief while maintaining ROM.
- *Indications*: This synthetic implant is indicated for patients who have failed an appropriate course of nonoperative management of hallux rigidus and desire to maintain some ROM with pain relief.
- *Contraindications*: Active infection of the first MTPJ, documented allergy to the material in the implant, inadequate bone stock to support the implant, avascular necrosis of the metatarsal head, large osteochondral defects or periarticular cysts, active gout, sesamoid arthritis, and systemic processes that lead to bony destruction.

Preoperative Planning

- Clinical history, physical examination, and imaging studies must be reviewed to ensure that the appropriate indications and contraindications are met before proceeding with surgery.
- Radiographs should be reviewed to estimate the size of the metatarsal head. The implant comes in two diameters—8 and 10 mm. Both implants should be available as the final determination is made during the surgery. It is important that at least a 2- to 4-mm circumferential rim of bone is available for implant support.

Positioning

- After either general or regional anesthesia, the patient is placed supine on the operating room table with a bump under the ipsilateral hip so that the foot is pointing directly up to the ceiling. The patient is positioned so that the foot is at the very distal end of the table to allow easy access for fluoroscopy.
- Either a thigh tourniquet or calf tourniquet can be used for the procedure and is up to surgeon preference.
- The foot and ankle is prepped and draped in the standard fashion per surgical protocol.

Approach

- The first MTPJ is approached utilizing a dorsal approach similar to that used for cheilectomy and first MTPJ arthrodesis.

INCISION AND EXPOSURE OF THE FIRST METATARSOPHALANGEAL JOINT

- Approximately, a 6-cm dorsal incision is used along the medial aspect of the extensor hallucis longus (EHL) tendon. Sharp dissection is carried through the skin, and care is taken to protect the EHL tendon within its tendon sheath. The tendon is mobilized laterally to allow access to the first MTPJ. The dorsomedial cutaneous skin nerve will travel medial in the wound, and care must be taken not to injury this medial superficial structure.
- The MTPJ arthrotomy is made longitudinally in line with the skin incision, and the joint capsule is elevated both medially and laterally. Do not completely release the collateral ligaments as this would cause instability of the first MTPJ; however, enough soft tissue release must be performed to visualize the entire metatarsal head for implantation (**TECH FIG 1**).
- At this point, dorsal osteophytes from the proximal phalanx and the metatarsal head can be removed; however, adequate metatarsal head circumference must be maintained to support the implant (at least a 2- to 4-mm cortical rim surrounding the implant is necessary).

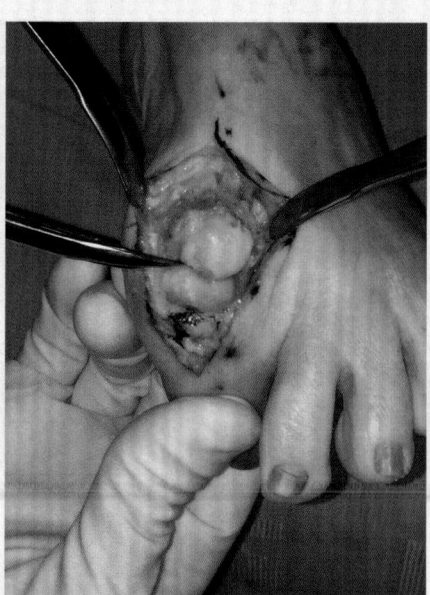

TECH FIG 1 Dorsal exposure with adequate soft tissue release allowing exposure of the first metatarsal head.

APPROPRIATE IMPLANT POSITION AND LOCATION

- The concave end of the guidewire placer (either 8- or 10-mm size) is placed in the center of the metatarsal head in both the sagittal and coronal plane to allow central placement of the guidewire. Ensure that there is at least a 2-mm cortical circumference of bone surrounding the implant. The position of the guidewire can be confirmed using intraoperative fluoroscopy. The guidewire placer is then removed **(TECH FIG 2)**.
- An alternative technique is to asymmetrical place the implant in the location of maximal cartilage wear. In this case, appropriate wire positioning is not checked on fluoroscopy as it will vary depending on the location of cartilage wear. However, it is imperative to ensure that there is still an adequate rim of cortical bone to support the implant if placed in an eccentric position.

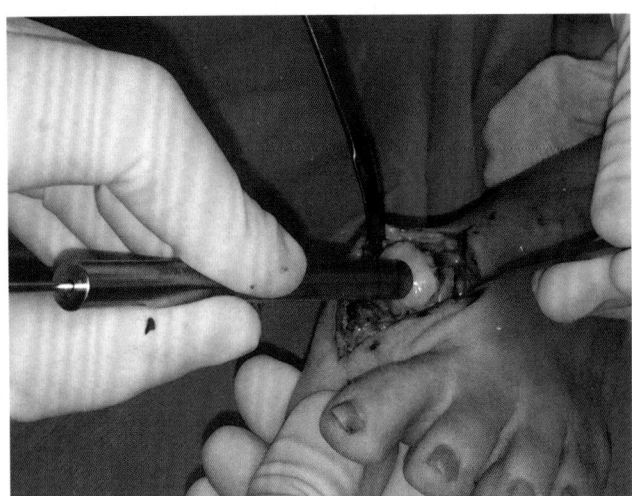

TECH FIG 2 Guidewire placement to ream for the implant.

PREPARING THE METATARSAL HEAD FOR THE IMPLANT

- The appropriately sized reamer is passed over the guidewire, and implantation site is created by reaming. It is important to irrigate the implantation site during reaming to avoid osteonecrosis secondary to overheating. The reamer is started prior to contact with the metatarsal head **(TECH FIG 3)**. Advance the reamer until it is flush with the surrounding metatarsal head surface, but do not compress or apply to much pressure as this will increase the implantation site. Ensure that the drill is in line with the guidewire to ensure that the implant does not sit off axis. The guidewire is then removed, and the implant site is irrigated and cleaned of any soft tissue and bony debris **(TECH FIG 4)**.

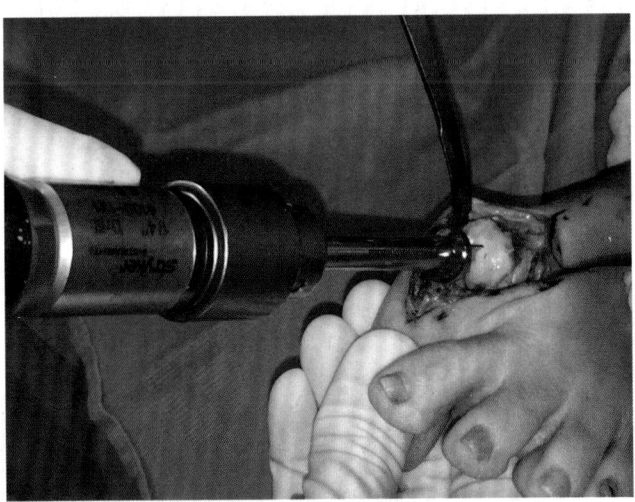

TECH FIG 3 Reaming for implant placement.

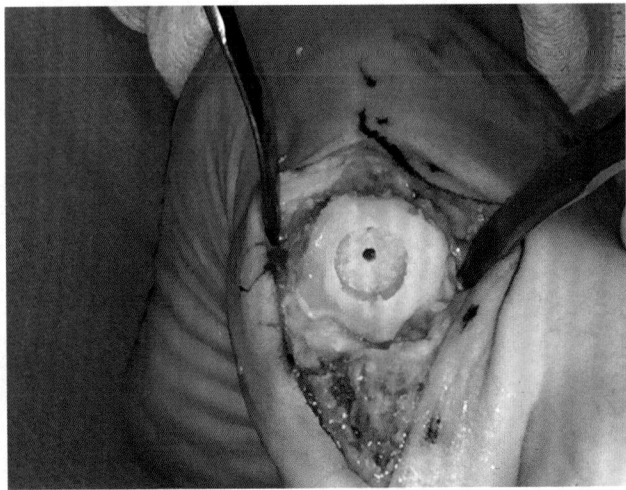

TECH FIG 4 Implant site cleaned of any bony and soft tissue.

TECHNIQUES

IMPLANT PREPARATION

- The appropriately sized synthetic implant is removed from the sterile packing and placed on the back table (**TECH FIG 5**). The introducer device is moistened with sterile saline to allow for easy implant insertion. The implant is then inserted into the introducer in the "round up" position with the curved end of the implant facing upward and the flat end (the end to be placed into the metatarsal head) coming out of the introducer tube (**TECH FIG 6**). The introducer tube is held firmly, and the end of the tube is covered to ensure that the implant does not come out as it is brought into the operative field from the back table.

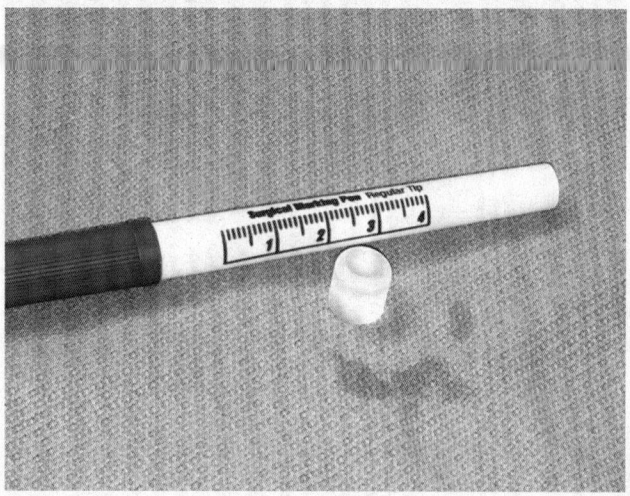

TECH FIG 5 The CARTIVA implant.

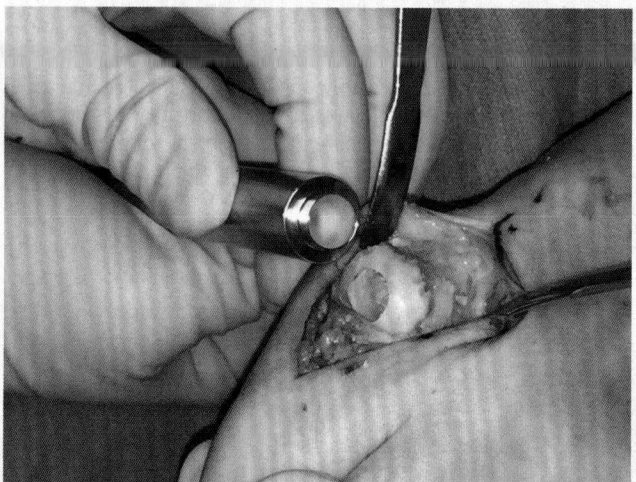

TECH FIG 6 The implant loaded into the introducer tube. Note that the flat end of the implant is facing out of the tube.

INSERTION OF THE IMPLANT

- The distal end of the introducer tube (with the flat end of the implant) is then placed at the implantation site perpendicular to the metatarsal head. The placer is pushed carefully through the introducer tube while maintaining the distal end of the introducer tube at the implantation site. Maintaining the introducer tube is critical as this will allow press-fit of the implant into the implantation site (**TECH FIG 7**).
- After insertion, the implant will be visible and should be slightly proud (minimum of 0.5 to 1.5 mm, preferably 1.5 to 2.5 mm) in relation to the surrounding articular surface.

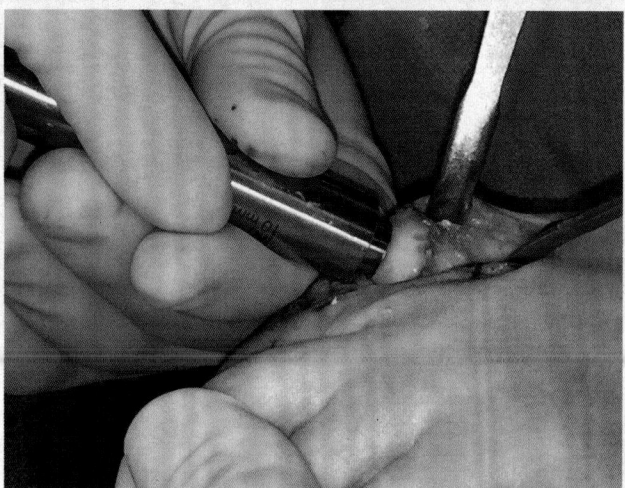
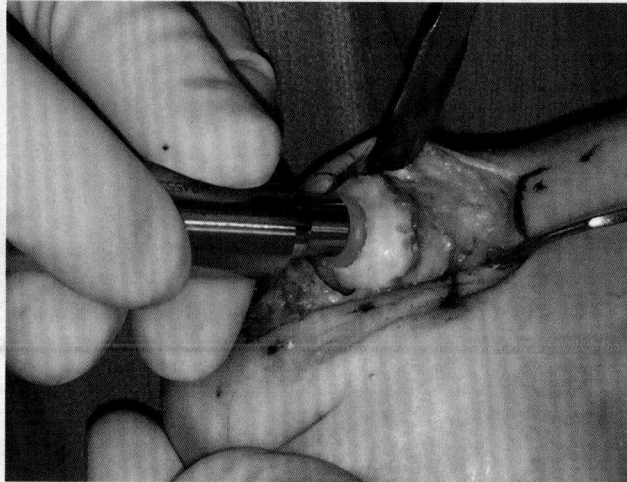

TECH FIG 7 Implant press-fit into the metatarsal head.

RANGE OF MOTION EVALUATION

- After successful implantation, the ROM of the first MTPJ should be clinically evaluated, and the implant should be inspected through ROM to ensure it is well seated and that motion has been achieved with no limitations **(TECH FIG 8)**.

- At this time, any additional synovitis or osteophytes can be removed; again, care must be taken to ensure not to remove too much bone as to compromise implant stability.

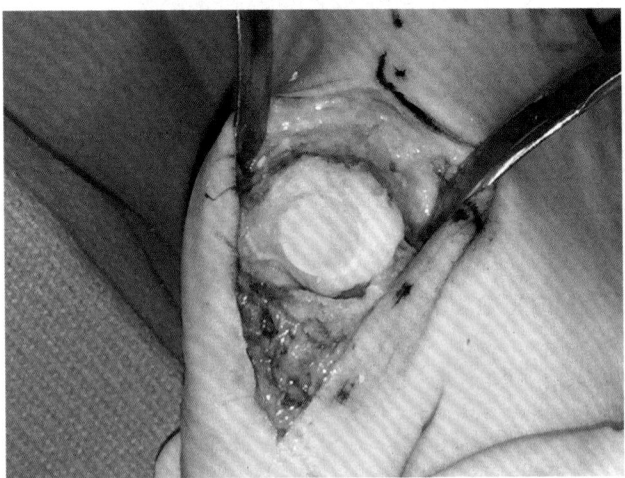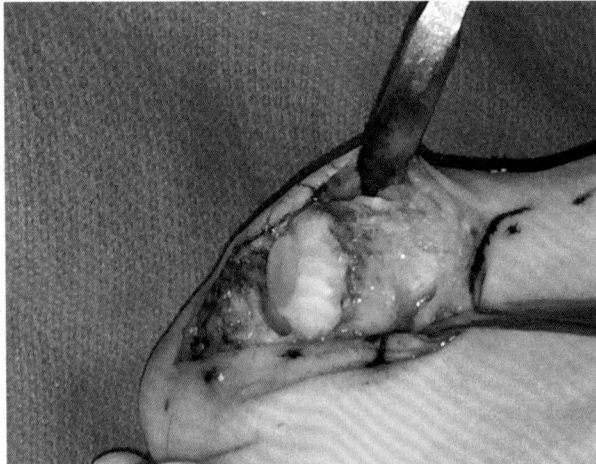

TECH FIG 8 Implant seated in the metatarsal head.

CLOSURE

- The MTPJ and surrounding soft tissues are thoroughly irrigated with sterile normal saline.
- The tourniquet can be released at this time, and adequate hemostasis could be obtained prior to wound closure.

- The capsular layer is closed with 2-0 absorbable suture, and subcutaneous/skin closure is performed per surgeon protocol.
- A sterile dressing is applied, and the patient is placed into a postopcrative shoe.

TECHNIQUES

Pearls and Pitfalls

Surgical Approach	• Avoid injury to the dorsomedial cutaneous branch of the superficial peroneal nerve during the approach. • Excessive release of the collateral ligaments can lead to MTPJ instability.
Implantation Site Preparation	• Prior to drilling the implant site, ensure that there is an adequate rim of cortical bone as inadequate support may lead to a cortical rim fracture sacrificing stability.
Implant Insertion	• Do not over ream as the implant needs to sit slightly proud. If the implant sites flush intraoperatively, the implant may need to be removed and revised with bone grafting.

POSTOPERATIVE CARE

- Patients are placed into a postoperative shoe and kept heel weight bearing in the immediate postoperative period.
- Approximately 2 to 3 weeks postoperatively, the patient returns to clinic to have their sutures removed. At this time, if the incision has healed well, the patient is instructed to begin gentle passive ROM of the first MTPJ.

- Patients remain in the postoperative shoe for 4 to 6 weeks postoperatively and are then transitioned in a regular shoe.
- Low-impact activity such as stationary biking, elliptical, and swimming can resume once the patient has comfortably transitioned to a regular shoe. High-impact activities such as running typically begin about 12 weeks after surgery.
- The patient should curtail or avoid completely any activity that causes pain or swelling at the first MTP joint, such as

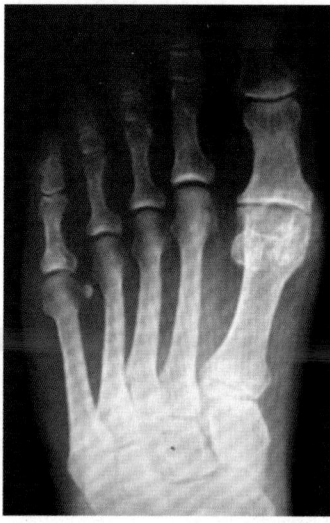 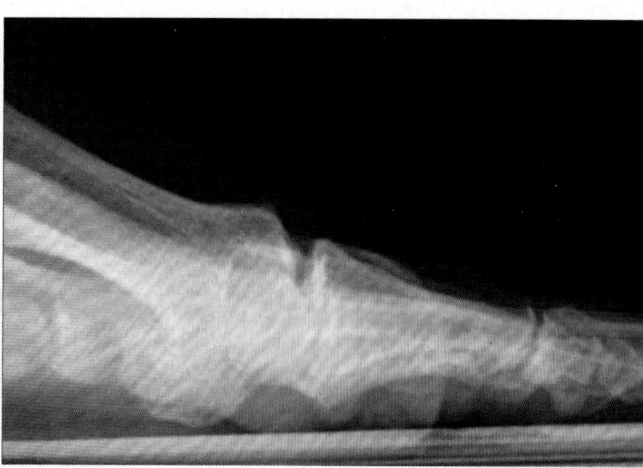

FIG 2 Postoperative weight-bearing AP and lateral radiograph.

running or jumping activities, as well as any direct loading on the toe, such as push-ups or yoga positions, for a minimum of 3 months and sometimes up to 6 months after surgery to avoid an early implant failure. Further revision surgery should not be considered until at least 9 months after surgery if pain or loss of motion is the concern **(FIG 2)**.

• Physical therapy is routinely not needed but can be provided to assist patients with ROM of the first MTPJ and gait training as they transition out of the postoperative shoe.

OUTCOMES

• Baumhauer et al[3] performed a prospective, randomized multicenter study comparing outcomes between first MTPJ arthrodesis and a synthetic cartilage implant for surgical treatment of hallux rigidus. In their study, they looked at the procedure's ability to decrease pain, improve function, and its safety profile. They enrolled 152 patients in the synthetic implant group and 50 patients in the arthrodesis group and followed these patients for 2 years. They found that there was no significant different between the two procedures with regard to safety, pain relief, and function at 2 years. The patients receiving the synthetic implant also demonstrated a 6.2-degree increase in ROM.

• Glazebrook et al[9] followed the earlier cohort of patients who received the synthetic implant 5 years postoperatively and demonstrates that these results were maintained. At 24 months, 9.2% of the patients had undergone implant removal and conversion to arthrodesis. Between 2 and 5 years, 7.6 of the patients underwent implant removal and conversion to arthrodesis. At a mean follow-up of 5.8 years, visual analog scale (VAS), foot and ankle ability measure (FAAM) activities of daily living (ADL), and FAAM Sports scores improved by 57.9, 33.0 and 47.9, respectively. ROM was also maintained. A 93.4% of the patients reported that they would undergo the procedure again.

• There is evidence to suggest that a synthetic cartilage implant may also demonstrate good results in even advanced stages of disease.[8] Baumhauer et al[2] evaluated a cohort of 202 patients and stratified their surgical treatment based on their stage of disease. Even after stratifying by grade, there was no significant different with regard to outcomes between a synthetic cartilage implant and first MTPJ arthrodesis.

COMPLICATIONS

• MTPJ instability
• Progression of hallux rigidus
• Implant subsidence
• Cortical rim fracture
• Painful neuroma secondary to damage to dorsomedial cutaneous nerve
• Infection

REFERENCES

1. Aper RL, Saltzman CL, Brown TD. The effect of hallux sesamoid resection on the effective moment of the flexor hallucis brevis. Foot Ankle Int 1994;15(9):462–470.
2. Baumhauer JF, Singh D, Glazebrook M, et al. Correlation of hallux rigidus grade with motion, VAS pain, intraoperative cartilage loss, and treatment success for first MTP joint arthrodesis and synthetic cartilage implant. Foot Ankle Int 2017;38(11):1175–1182.
3. Baumhauer JF, Singh D, Glazebrook M, et al. Prospective, randomized, multi-centered clinical trial assessing safety and efficacy of a synthetic cartilage implant versus first metatarsophalangeal arthrodesis in advanced hallux rigidus. Foot Ankle Int 2016;37(5):457–469.
4. Bingold AC, Collins DH. Hallux rigidus. J Bone Joint Surg Br 1950;32-B:214–222.
5. Bonney G, Macnab I. Hallux valgus and hallux rigidus; a critical survey of operative results. J Bone Joint Surg Br 1952;34-B:366–385.
6. Coughlin MJ, Shurnas PS. Hallux rigidus: demographics, etiology, and radiographic assessment. Foot Ankle Int 2003;24(10):731–743.
7. Coughlin MJ, Shurnas PS. Hallux rigidus. Grading and long-term results of operative treatment. J Bone Joint Surg Am 2003;85(11):2072–2088.
8. Daniels TR, Younger AS, Penner MJ, et al. Midterm outcomes of polyvinyl alcohol hydrogel hemiarthroplasty of the first metatarsophalangeal joint in advanced hallux rigidus. Foot Ankle Int 2017;38(3):243–247.
9. Glazebrook M, Blundell CM, O'Dowd D, et al. Midterm outcomes of a synthetic cartilage implant for the first metatarsophalangeal joint in advanced hallux rigidus. Foot Ankle Int 2019;40(4):374–383.
10. Hamilton WG, O'Malley MJ, Thompson FM, et al. Roger Mann Award 1995. Capsular interposition arthroplasty for severe hallux rigidus. Foot Ankle Int 1997;18(2):68–70.
11. McCormick JJ, Anderson RB. Rehabilitation following turf toe injury and plantar plate repair. Clin Sports Med 2010;29(2):313–323.
12. Stokes IA, Hutton WC, Stott JR, et al. Forces under the hallux valgus foot before and after surgery. Clin Orthop Relat Res 1979;(142):64–72.

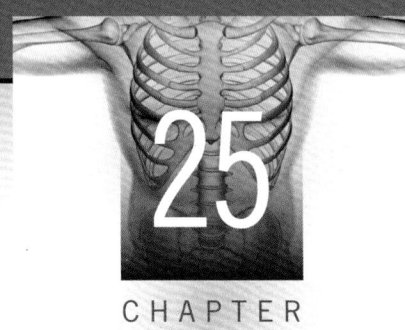

25
CHAPTER

Arthrosurface HemiCAP Resurfacing

Thomas P. San Giovanni

DEFINITION

- Hallux rigidus is an arthritic condition of the first metatarsophalangeal (MTP) joint. It is the most common form of arthritis affecting the foot.
- An estimated 2% to 10% of the general population displays varying grades of hallux rigidus.[3,10,12]

ANATOMY

- Hallux rigidus involves the first MTP joint, which comprises the articulation between the first metatarsal head, the proximal phalangeal base, and the sesamoid complex.
- Although the proximal phalanx is often involved, the predominant disease involves the dorsal aspect of the metatarsal head with articular cartilage loss and dorsal osteophyte formation (FIG 1).

PATHOGENESIS

- The cause of hallux rigidus is controversial and is likely multifactorial.
- Predisposing or associated factors cited in the literature include flat, square-shaped metatarsal head morphology; metatarsus

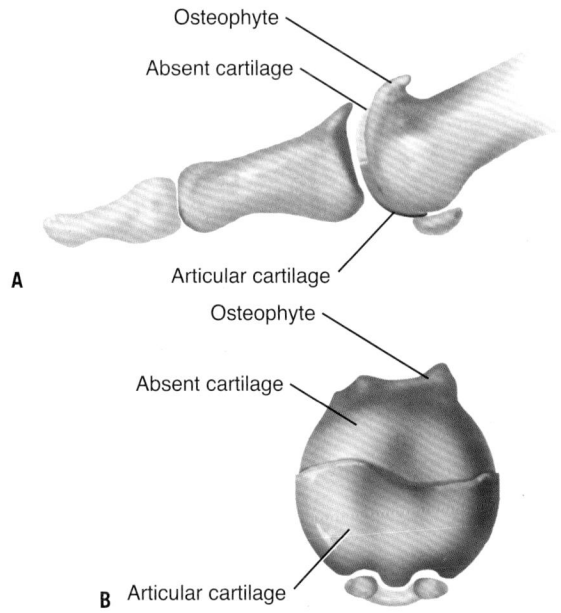

Osteophyte

Absent cartilage

Articular cartilage

A

Osteophyte

Absent cartilage

B Articular cartilage

FIG 1 **A.** Lateral diagram depicting articular cartilage loss and osteophyte along the dorsal aspect of the first MTP joint. **B.** Frontal view showing dorsal articular cartilage loss extending into the central aspect.

adductus; hallux valgus interphalangeus; positive family history with bilateral condition; and trauma.[3,12]
- Isolated or repetitive injury may cause damage to the dorsal aspect of the joint, which leads to altered mechanics (compressive and shear forces increased dorsally). Progressive deterioration of the articular surface, osteophyte formation, and joint contracture ensue.

NATURAL HISTORY

- In its early stages, articular cartilage loss is present along the dorsal aspect of the first metatarsal head. As the condition progresses, articular cartilage loss extends to the central aspects of the metatarsal head and lastly the plantar aspect (FIG 2).
- Although less involved, the proximal phalanx will exhibit varying degrees of articular cartilage loss and dorsal osteophyte formation.
- The natural history of hallux rigidus is one of gradual, progressive worsening.[11]

PATIENT HISTORY AND PHYSICAL FINDINGS

- Patients present with complaints of dull, aching, and, at times, sharp pain along the dorsal aspect of the joint associated with weight-bearing activities.
- Complaints of stiffness and development of a painful dorsal bony prominence are characteristic of the condition.
- The physical examination reveals tenderness overlying the first metatarsal head with a notable dorsal bony prominence, along with limited range of motion of the first MTP joint, particularly dorsiflexion (FIG 3).
- The examiner should assess for pain on midmotion, crepitus, positive first MTP grind test, and plantar tenderness overlying the sesamoids, which represents more extensive disease.

IMAGING AND OTHER DIAGNOSTIC STUDIES

- Weight-bearing anteroposterior (AP), lateral, and oblique views are obtained. The examiner should assess for joint space narrowing, presence of dorsal osteophytes, and joint congruity.
- Computed tomography (CT) and magnetic resonance imaging (MRI) advanced imaging studies are generally not obtained. Evaluation with MRI may occasionally be indicated if the radiographs appear normal but suspicion remains for a central osteochondral defect of the metatarsal head. CT scan is occasionally obtained to assess or confirm the presence of severe metatarsosesamoid involvement, which

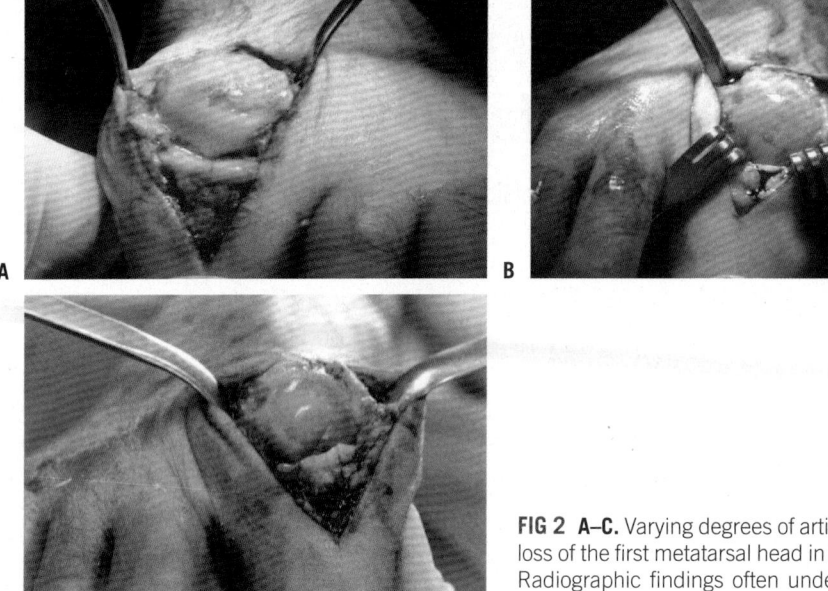

FIG 2 A–C. Varying degrees of articular cartilage loss of the first metatarsal head in hallux rigidus. Radiographic findings often underestimate the extent of disease seen intraoperatively.

can negatively impact outcomes of joint-sparing procedures by affecting the predictability of pain relief. Patients with severe metatarsosesamoid involvement may be more suitable for an arthrodesis; unless in an effort to preserve motion they can accept a scenario where pain may be reduced with a metatarsal head resurfacing, but some degree of residual plantar-based pain may persist.

GRADING SYSTEMS FOR HALLUX RIGIDUS

- Clinical grading system: This system by Coughlin and Shurnas[3] takes into account the subjective and objective findings of pain, motion assessment, and radiographic features.
- Radiographic grading system: The radiographic grading system often used in the literature,[7] grades 1, 2, and 3, signify the percentage of joint space narrowing, the presence or absence of subchondral sclerosis or subchondral cyst, and the degree of osteophyte formation (**TABLE 1; FIG 4**).
- Intraoperative grading system: We have found that the preoperative radiographic grade often underestimates the degree of arthritic involvement of the first MTP joint found at the time of surgery. For this reason, the author (T. P. San Giovanni,

unpublished data) has developed an intraoperative grading system for hallux rigidus for more accurate documentation of the location and extent of full-thickness articular cartilage loss on direct visualization (**FIG 5**). Direct visualization and documentation of the intra-articular hallux rigidus grade provides more accurate and useful information for which to follow clinical outcomes rather than radiographic grades which may be inaccurate due to underestimation of actual extent of cartilage loss. We believe it will serve as a basis for more accurate subject grouping in outcome studies for particular grade-specific procedures. Ultimately, the prognostic value for various procedures can be evaluated on the specific grade actually visualized at surgery and minimizes the interobserver and intraobserver errors typically encountered with other grading systems. This should lead to better evidence-based outcomes research in hallux rigidus surgery and eventually the optimal procedure(s) can be determined and performed based on the specific grade encountered. With well-informed counseling of the patient preoperatively, various surgical options can be provided based on what is encountered intraoperatively. Provided the patient has a solid understanding of the potential

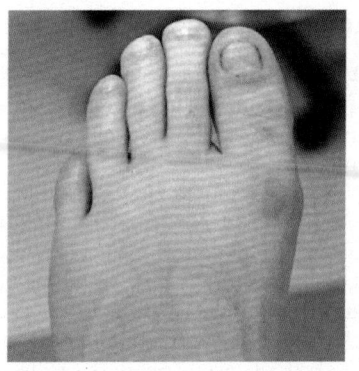 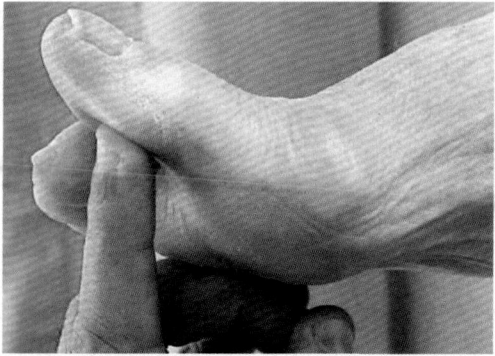

FIG 3 A. Dorsal view of foot in hallux rigidus. Shoe wear may cause irritation over the dorsal bony prominence. **B.** Limited dorsiflexion is noted on the clinical examination.

Table 1 Radiographic Grading System for Hallux Rigidus

Grade	Dorsal Osteophyte	Joint Space	Subchondral Bone
1	Mild to moderate	Space preserved	Normal appearance
2	Moderate	<50% narrowing	Subchondral sclerosis
3	Marked	>50% narrowing	Subchondral sclerosis with or without bone cyst formation

From Hattrup SJ, Johnson KA. Subjective results of hallux rigidus following treatment with cheilectomy. Clin Orthop Relat Res 1988;226:182–191.

procedures and mutually agreed on by patient/surgeon, an intraoperative algorithm can be applied on the hallux rigidus grade encountered, directly visualized during the surgical procedure (**TABLE 2**).

DIFFERENTIAL DIAGNOSIS

- Gout
- Other systemic arthritides (rheumatoid arthritis, psoriatic arthritis, seronegative arthropathy)
- Posttraumatic arthritis
- Arthritis associated with severe hallux valgus or sequelae status post hallux valgus surgery
- Central osteochondral defect, first metatarsal head
- Avascular necrosis of the metatarsal head
- Sesamoiditis or sesamoid-related pathology
- Septic arthritis
- Soft tissue or bone neoplasm

NONOPERATIVE MANAGEMENT

- Nonoperative management of hallux rigidus includes shoe wear modifications, use of anti-inflammatories, orthotics with a Morton extension or carbon fiber plate orthotic, and, rarely, intra-articular cortisone injections.

SURGICAL MANAGEMENT

- When nonoperative management fails to provide adequate symptom relief, the patient and surgeon are faced with choosing from an array of surgical procedures.

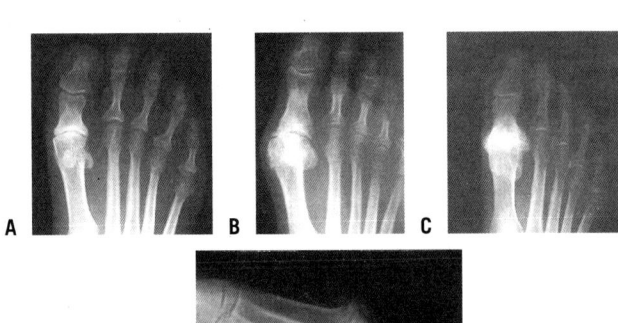

FIG 4 A. Grade 1 hallux rigidus. **B.** Grade 2 hallux rigidus. **C.** Grade 3 hallux rigidus. **D.** Lateral view of hallux rigidus.

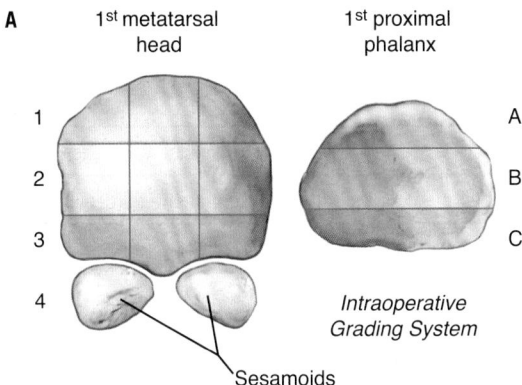

Metatarsal grade level assignment is determined by:
- Involvement of >50% of one segment within level
- Any involvement that crosses into two segments within level
- Grade 4 severe sesamoid involvement with full-thickness loss of articular surface

Proximal phalanx grade level assignment is determined by:
- Any involvement that crosses the border of each level

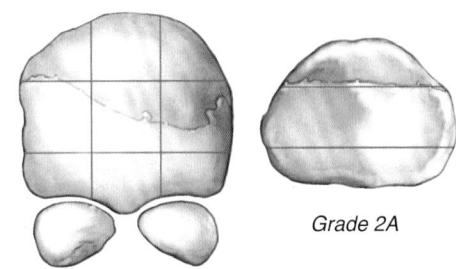

Grade 2A: Full-thickness articular cartilage loss extending to central aspect of metatarsal head and dorsal one-third of proximal phalanx articular surface.

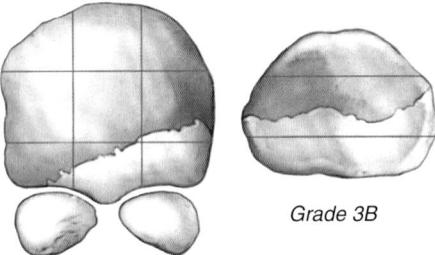

Grade 3B: Full-thickness articular cartilage loss extending to plantar aspect of metatarsal head and central one-third of proximal phalanx articular surface.

FIG 5 A. Intraoperative grading system for hallux rigidus. **B.** Examples of grading system. (From San Giovanni TP. Hallux Rigidus: Intraoperative grading system for accurate determination of articular cartilage loss and use for surgical outcome studies. Unpublished data.)

- The most common performed procedure for hallux rigidus is a cheilectomy.
- Simple cheilectomy has been proven successful for early stages of hallux rigidus,[3,4,7,12,14] although cheilectomy outcomes are less promising with advanced disease, particularly grade 3.[3,10,11] As articular cartilage loss extends to the central and plantar aspects of the joint, the joint deterioration progresses beyond that which a cheilectomy would be expected to adequately treat.
- Alternative or adjunctive procedures to cheilectomy include the following:
  - Moberg dorsal closing wedge phalangeal osteotomy[13,14,18]
  - Various first metatarsal decompression osteotomies[18]

Table 2 Intraoperative Grading System for Hallux Rigidus

Metatarsal Grade	Full-Thickness Articular Cartilage Loss
1	Dorsal one-third level
2	Central one-third level
3	Plantar one-third level
4	Sesamoid surface
Proximal Phalanx Grade	
A	Dorsal one-third level
B	Central one-third level
C	Plantar one-third level

- Soft tissue interposition arthroplasties and modified oblique Keller resection[1,4,9]
- Proximal phalangeal base hemiarthroplasty[12,21]
- Metatarsal head resurfacing hemiarthroplasty[2,6,8,16,17]
- Total great toe arthroplasty[9]
- First MTP arthrodesis[3,12,15]
- Historically, a first MTP arthrodesis has proven to be the most reliable procedure for providing pain relief in advanced stages (grade 3).[3,15] However, many patients find the thought of complete motion loss in exchange for pain relief unacceptable and prefer not to undergo a fusion procedure for this reason alone. This represents a rather large subset of the hallux rigidus patient population and has been the driving force behind the development of joint-sparing, motion-preserving procedures.
- Alternative surgical solutions that maintain some degree of motion and provide pain relief have been sought in an effort to address this patient subset with advanced disease who refuse to undergo fusion. This has led to the development of various arthroplasty techniques, including soft tissue interposition or implant arthroplasty.
- One such implant is the Arthrosurface HemiCAP DF which is a second generation metatarsal head resurfacing implant. The "DF" signifies dorsal flange which provides improved dorsal coverage and prevents reformation of dorsal osteophytes occasionally seen in the original HemiCAP design. In addition, the implant was designed with a unique geometric feature to the dorsal slope of the head where a double radii of curvature was built in. At a point which corresponds to 12 degrees dorsiflexion, the radii of curvature changes effectively, creating built-in dorsal decompression to the implant. The purpose of the double radii is to improve what the senior author calls "passive dorsal roll back" of the proximal phalanx, as it clears and glides over the metatarsal head upon ambulation, thereby reducing the cam effect may expect in a contracted first MTP joint on weight-bearing dorsiflexion (**FIG 6**). The HemiCAP DF more anatomically matches the first metatarsal head morphology and was based on a biomechanical study which demonstrates the center of rotation changes with varying degrees of dorsiflexion.[19] The technique for the HemiCAP DF first metatarsal head resurfacing procedure is described in the following text.

Preoperative Planning

- History and physical examination are performed with particular attention to the location of pain, midrange motion pain, or significant symptomatic sesamoid involvement.
- Range of motion and active and passive dorsiflexion and plantarflexion are recorded preoperatively.
- Routine weight-bearing radiographs are assessed for the presence of dorsal osteophytes, the degree of joint space narrowing, joint alignment and congruency, metatarsal length, and sesamoid pathology.
- Careful preoperative discussion regarding the patient's goals and expectations are paramount in determining whether individual goals will be met by the procedure. A discussion of the risks and alternative procedures, in particular discussion regarding arthrodesis, is important.

Positioning

- The patient is positioned supine with a bump under the ipsilateral hip to rotate the foot to neutral.
- A tourniquet is applied; however, we prefer not to use a tourniquet for this particular case if possible. Not using the tourniquet forces the surgeon to obtain excellent hemostasis during the first few minutes of the approach and leads to a drier wound on closure. We believe that postoperative swelling from hemarthrosis or hematoma formation contributes to some degree of the early motion loss seen during the early postoperative period.

Approach

- A dorsal longitudinal incision is made centered over the first MTP joint.
- The extensor hallucis longus tendon is identified and retracted laterally (**FIG 7**).
- Sharp dissection is carried down just medial to the extensor hallucis longus tendon, and a dorsal longitudinal capsulotomy is performed with soft tissue dissection performed subperiosteally along the medial and lateral aspects of the first metatarsal head.
- If a large proximal phalangeal base dorsal osteophyte is encountered upon approach, the phalangeal osteophyte is excised at this time. The metatarsal head osteophyte may be left at this time for it will be removed upon using the dorsal reaming jig, which gives accurate bone preparation for dorsal flange component of the HemiCAP DF. Alternatively, a small portion of the osteophyte can be excised at this time but not to the depth that it jeopardizes the bony contact of the implant.
- After adequate soft tissue releases are performed, the hallux is maximally plantarflexed to expose the joint. The extent of full-thickness cartilage loss is then assessed for the metatarsal side and phalangeal side. The intraoperative grade of hallux rigidus is then assigned and recorded based on a grading system devised by the senior author.
- To release the plantar capsular joint contracture, a curved elevator (McGlamry or flattened spoon-shaped spinal gouge) can be passed between the sesamoids and plantar aspect of the metatarsal head as long as this can be performed carefully without causing iatrogenic injury to the articular cartilage. An offset elevator is provided for this function on the Arthrosurface set. In particularly tight joints, the surgeon may find it easier to performed additional soft tissue release after joint decompression and the trial implant is in place.

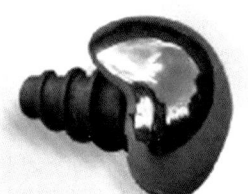

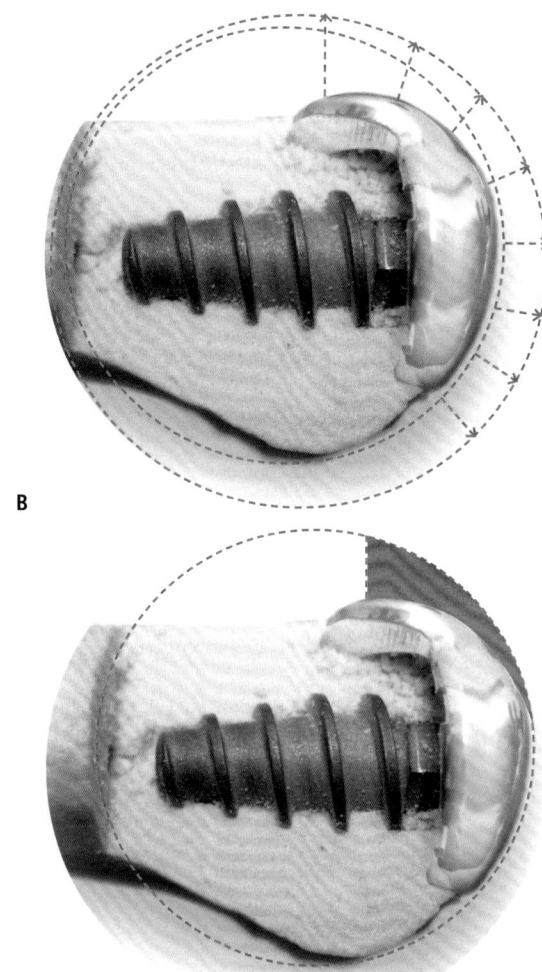

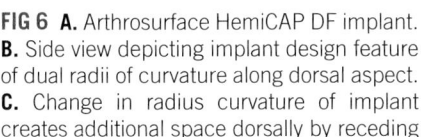

FIG 6 A. Arthrosurface HemiCAP DF implant. **B.** Side view depicting implant design feature of dual radii of curvature along dorsal aspect. **C.** Change in radius curvature of implant creates additional space dorsally by receding slope.

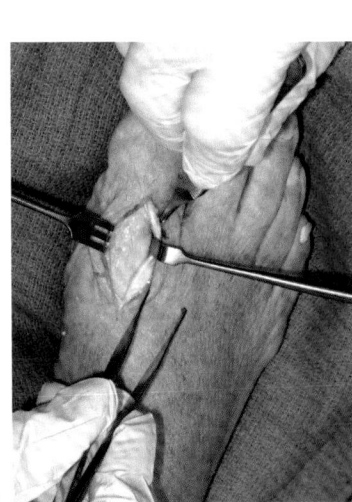

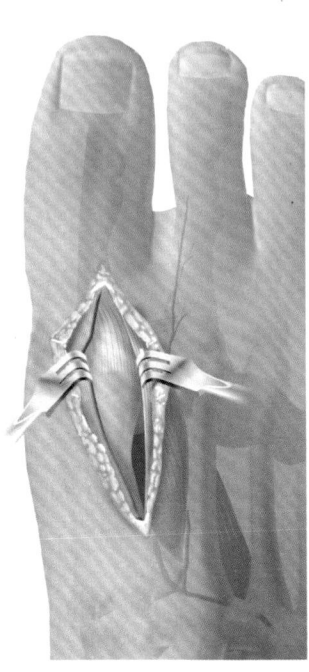

FIG 7 A,B. Dorsal longitudinal incision. The capsulotomy is done medial to the extensor hallucis longus tendon and the tendon is retracted laterally.

GUIDE PIN PLACEMENT FOR HEMICAP DF

- Obtain complete visualization of the metatarsal head with hallux plantarflexion.
- Place the centering spherical guide for the 15-mm HemiCAP on the metatarsal head with the feet of the guide in a supero-inferior position. A 15-mm guide is used typically; only on rare occasions is a 12-mm guide used as an alternative with an anatomically small head. Alternatively, the guide pin can be placed freehand on surgeon preference.
- During this step, particular importance should be paid to (1) location of the starting point and (2) pin trajectory on the AP and lateral views for ultimate alignment of the implant is based off of this first step. The importance of this step cannot be understated. We suggest entering the head only slightly and then checking AP and lateral fluoroscopic images, thereby making adjustments prior to committing. Note: Starting point is more plantar than what appears to be the center of the metatarsal head; also, the inclination angle of the metatarsal is greater than one would think so must drop hand while drilling.

- The perimeter of the guide should not violate the metatar-sosesamoid complex and its inferior border is generally seated just above the crista. Avoid malplacement of the guide pin by plantarflexing the guide as necessary to adjust for normal inclination of the metatarsal shaft. It is critical that this be in line with the long axis of the metatarsal shaft on the lateral fluoroscopic view.
- Place the centering guide pin on the metatarsal head in line with the long axis of the metatarsal shaft and verify its position on AP and lateral fluoroscopic views. Adjust the guide pin as necessary to obtain correct placement (**TECH FIG 1A–E**). Pay particular attention to the guide pin lateral view, for there is a tendency to underestimate the degree of inclination of the metatarsal shaft; parallel to the long axis of the shaft is the desired position. Adjust the pin before proceeding.
- Use a cannulated step drill over the guide pin and drill to depth so that the proximal shoulder of the drill bit is flush with the articular surface (**TECH FIG 1F–J**).

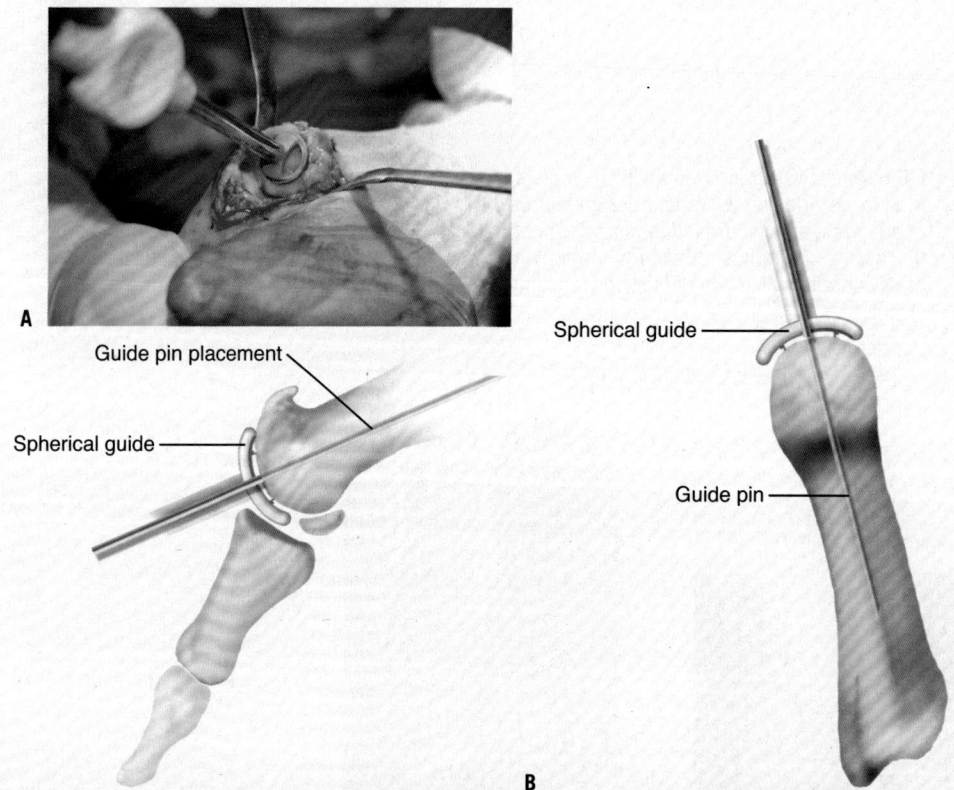

TECH FIG 1 Guide pin placement. **A.** Intraoperative picture of spherical guide placement just above the crista of the first metatarsal. **B.** AP view of pin placed in line with the long axis of the first MTP shaft. **C.** Lateral image of pin placed parallel to the long axis of the MTP shaft. The surgeon can drop his or her hand as necessary to match the inclination of metatarsal and midline within the shaft. *(continued)*

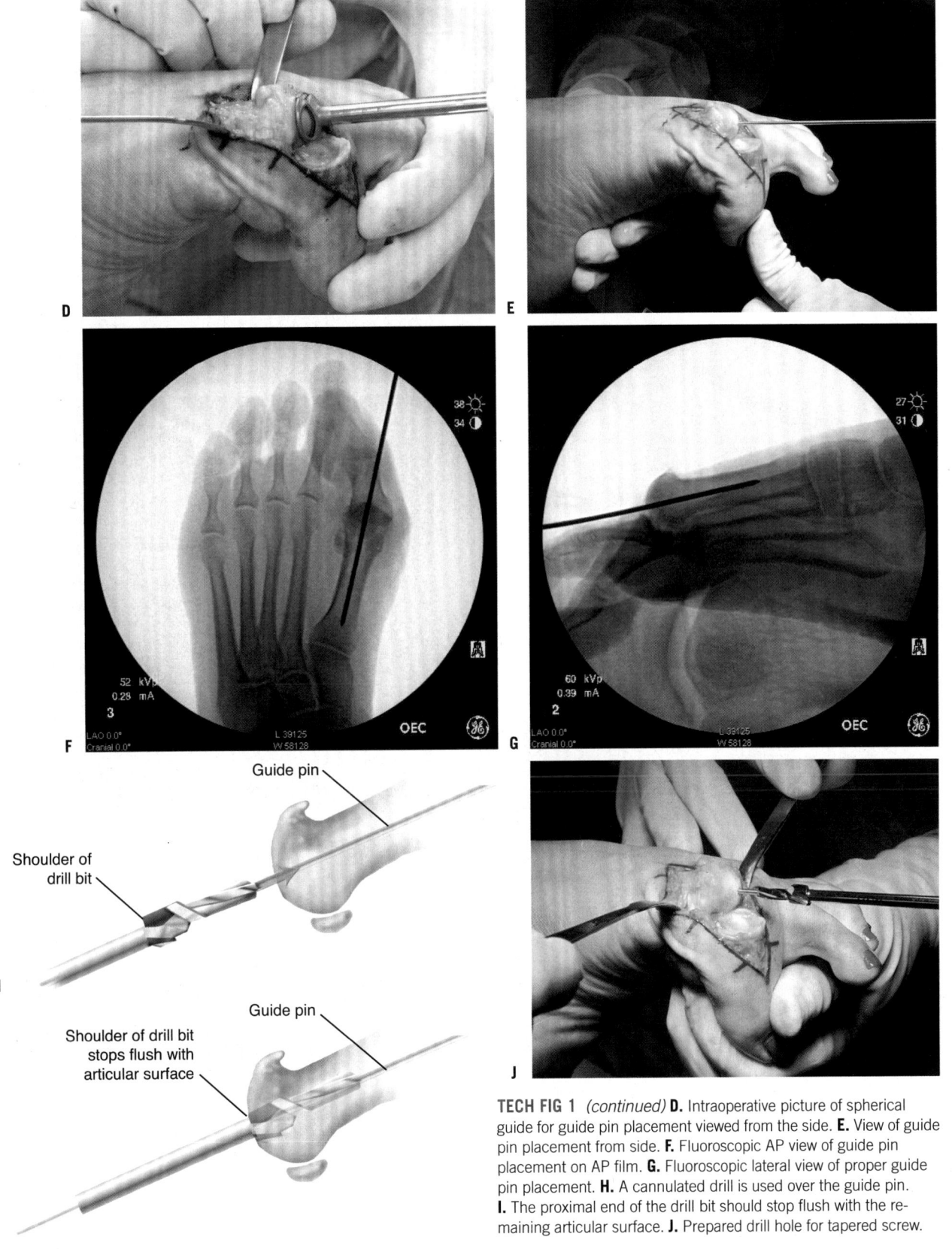

TECH FIG 1 *(continued)* **D.** Intraoperative picture of spherical guide for guide pin placement viewed from the side. **E.** View of guide pin placement from side. **F.** Fluoroscopic AP view of guide pin placement on AP film. **G.** Fluoroscopic lateral view of proper guide pin placement. **H.** A cannulated drill is used over the guide pin. **I.** The proximal end of the drill bit should stop flush with the remaining articular surface. **J.** Prepared drill hole for tapered screw.

DRILL HOLE AND PLACEMENT OF TAPER POST SCREW

- Tap the drill hole to the etched line (**TECH FIG 2A–C**).
- Place the tapered screw of the HemiCAP DF implant, gaining purchase within the distal metatarsal bone. Bring the line indicator on the screwdriver just flush with the depth of the remaining articular surface level (**TECH FIG 2D,E**).

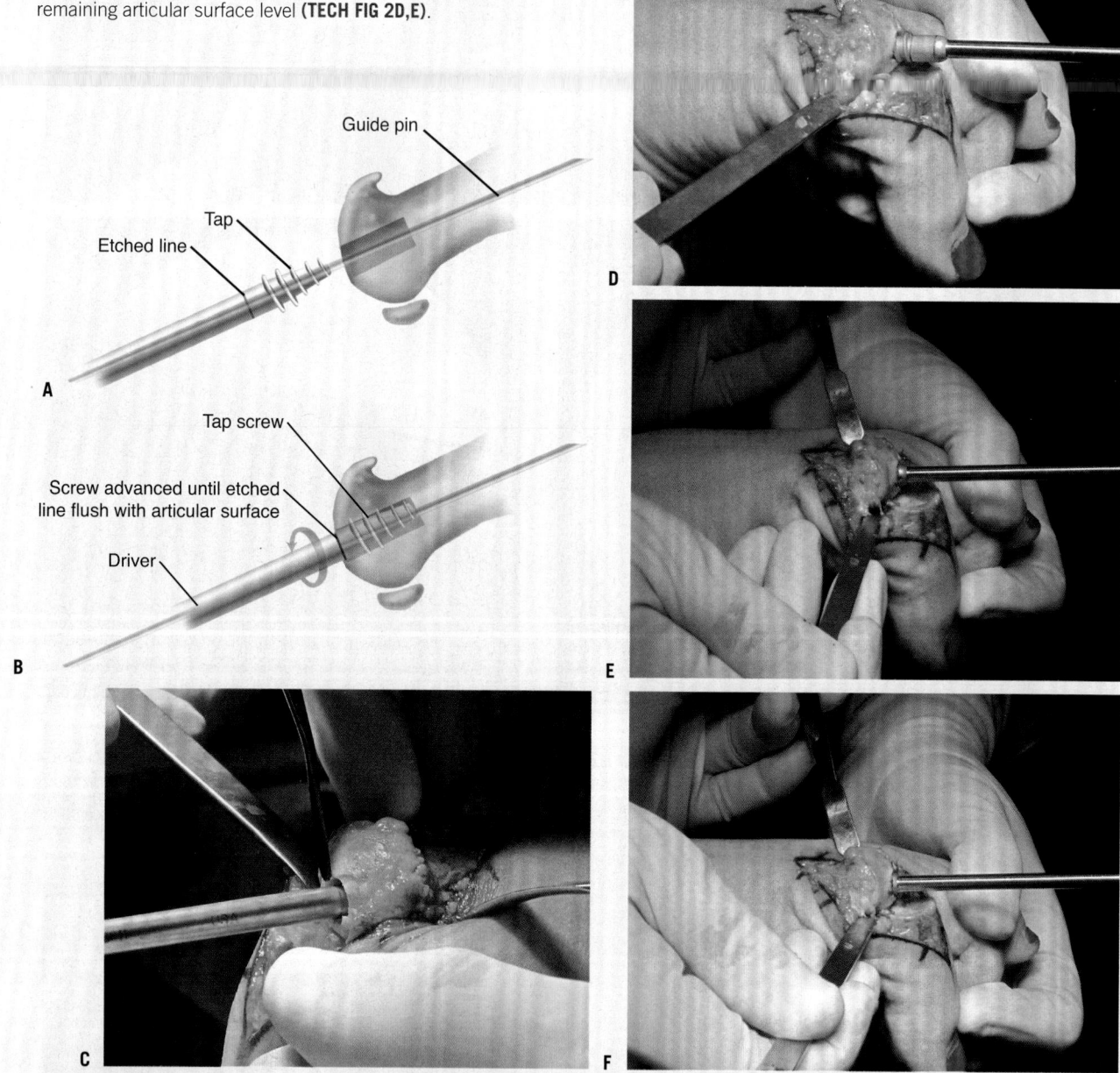

TECH FIG 2 A. A tap is used within the first metatarsal head, stopping at the etched line on the driver when flush with the plantar articular surface. **B.** A taper post screw is placed to the etched line when flush with the joint surface. **C.** Intraoperative use of tap to etched line using inferior aspect as reference point. **D.** Intraoperative screw placement. **E.** The screw is stopped when the etched line is flush with the remaining joint surface using the inferior aspect as the reference point. **F.** Screw can be advanced past etched line if bony decompression desired. Each one quarter-turn past the line equals 1 mm additional joint decompression. *(continued)*

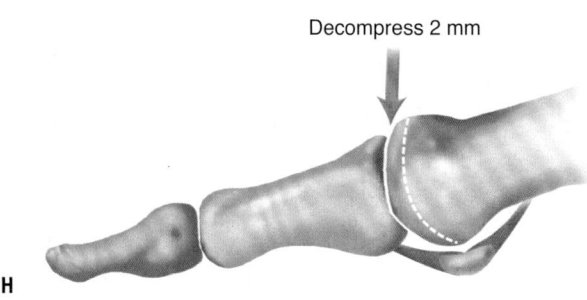

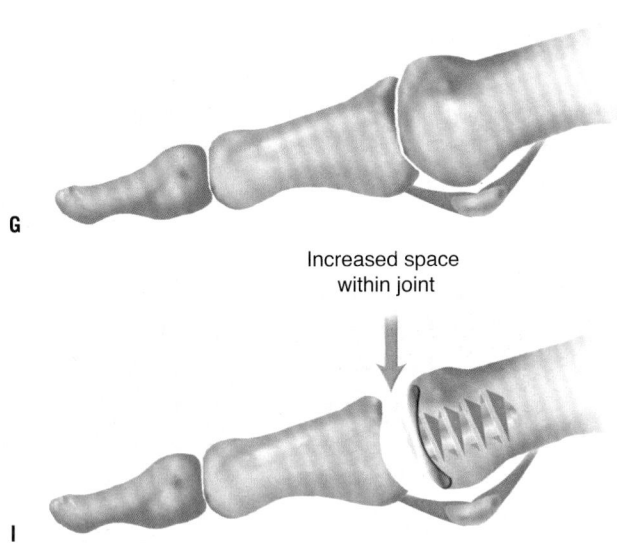

Increased space
within joint

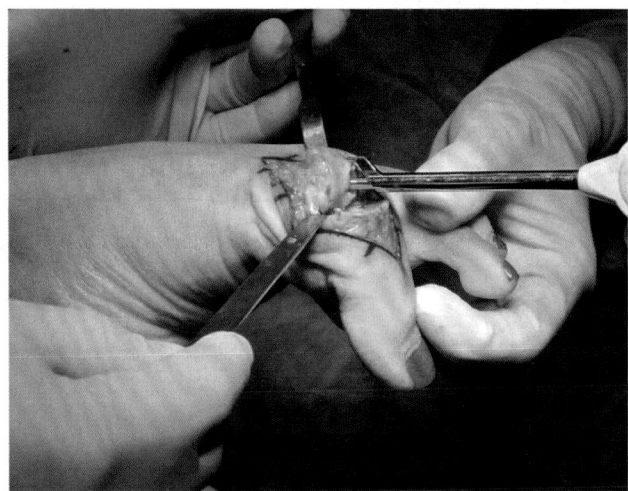

TECH FIG 2 *(continued)* **G–I.** Space can be created within joint by decompression of metatarsal side. Example depicts 2 mm additional decompression from previous joint line by advancement of screw by half turn past etched line, followed by surface reaming preparation and final impression following placement of implant.

DEPTH AND METATARSAL HEAD SURFACE MEASUREMENTS

- Remove the guide pin and place the trial button cap to confirm the correct depth of the screw. Place the peak height of the trial cap flush or slightly countersunk to the level of the existing articular cartilage surface. The depth can be adjusted simply by either advancing or backing out the screw, with each quarter-turn accounting for 1 mm.
- Note: With experience of the procedure, it has become more routine at this step to decompress at least 2 to 3 mm by advancing the screw one-half to three quarter-turns past the etched line **(TECH FIG 2F–I)**. This can be performed at this early step in the procedure particularly with very contracted joints and/or those with a long/equal length first metatarsal relative to the second metatarsal. This can also be performed later in the procedure with the trial in place upon assessing motion. If decompression is performed from the start, the implant will appear recessed upon placement of the trial component. Do not be concerned by this appearance; the excess bone medially, laterally, and plantarly is excised using a microsagittal saw blade (the crista may be excised if blocking fluid motion following decompression).
- Place the centering shaft pin through the cannulated portion of the screw to act as a centering point for measuring the radii of curvature of the metatarsal head at four index points. This measures the geometric shape of the metatarsal head, assessing superior, inferior, medial, and lateral dimensions.
- Slide the contact probe device through the centering pin; this measures the distance at these four points pivoting at 90-degree intervals **(TECH FIG 3)**. This should be measured at the 3 o'clock, 6 o'clock, 9 o'clock, and 12 o'clock positions. Of note, the probe is used to determine the articular joint line level. The superior 12 o'clock position may be inaccurate due to the degree cartilage loss. Upon measuring the inferior 6 o'clock position, the probe tip should be placed just to the side of the crista and not directly on top in order to give an

accurate reading. Record the numbers and choose the closest match to the provided implant size. Note: Choose the largest number measured in the superior and inferior and medial and lateral dimensions. In most cases, we tend to use the 4.5-mm surface reamer and place either a 1.5- × 4.5-mm or 2.5- × 4.5-mm implant. The 4.5 mm corresponds to the superoinferior geometry which slopes back further dorsally, creating an additional built-in dorsal decompression.
- Remove the centering shaft pin and place a standard guide pin back within the cannulated portion of the screw.

TECH FIG 3 The guide pin is replaced with a wider centering shaft pin. A contact probe is then used to measure the dimensions of the metatarsal head so the proper implant size can be chosen.

TECHNIQUES *(vertical text, left margin)*

SURFACE PREPARATION OF METATARSAL HEAD

- A circular surface reamer is then used **(TECH FIG 4)**. The proper size is the largest size measured in either the superoinferior or mediolateral dimensions. For example, if superoinferior measures 4.5 mm and mediolateral 2.5 mm, then use a 4.5-mm circular reamer. Note: It is important to start the reamer before contacting the bone to avoid the remote chance of uncontrolled metatarsal bone blowout if poor bone quality is noted. The depth of the reamer is controlled, for it will stop on its own when contacting the screw.

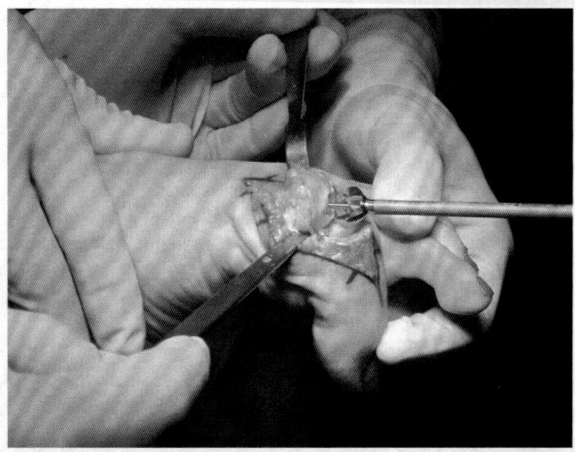
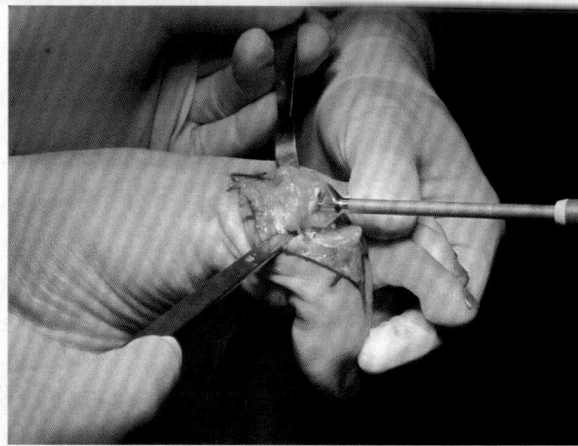
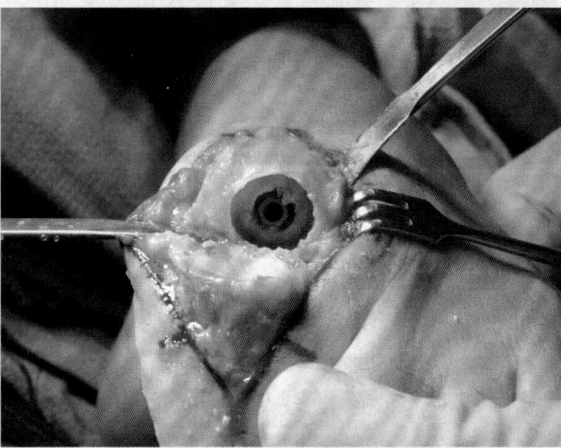

TECH FIG 4 A. A circular reamer is used over the guide pin. **B.** Start reamer prior to bone contact. There is a built-in stop when it reaches the edge of the screw. **C.** View after reaming for bone preparation for the HemiCAP. The screw is seen within the metatarsal head, for which the cap will mate with the Morse taper interlock.

SURFACE PREPARATION OF THE DORSAL FLANGE

- Place the appropriately size dorsal reamer guide into the cannulated portion of the taper post screw **(TECH FIG 5)**. This should match the same millimeter size used for the surface reaming of the metatarsal head in the prior step. Note: The 3.5-mm dorsal reamer will provide a lesser curvature and the 4.5-mm dorsal reamer will provide a more receding curvature over the dorsal flange.

- The guide should be oriented such that the dorsal reamer is at the 12 o'clock position. Be sure this is oriented correctly prior to reaming.
- Advance the dorsal reamer to the depth stop.
- Once the dorsal reamer has advanced to the handle, immediately stop the cannulated power drill and removed the dorsal reamer guide.

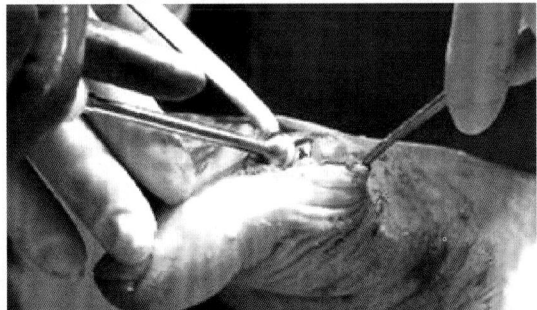

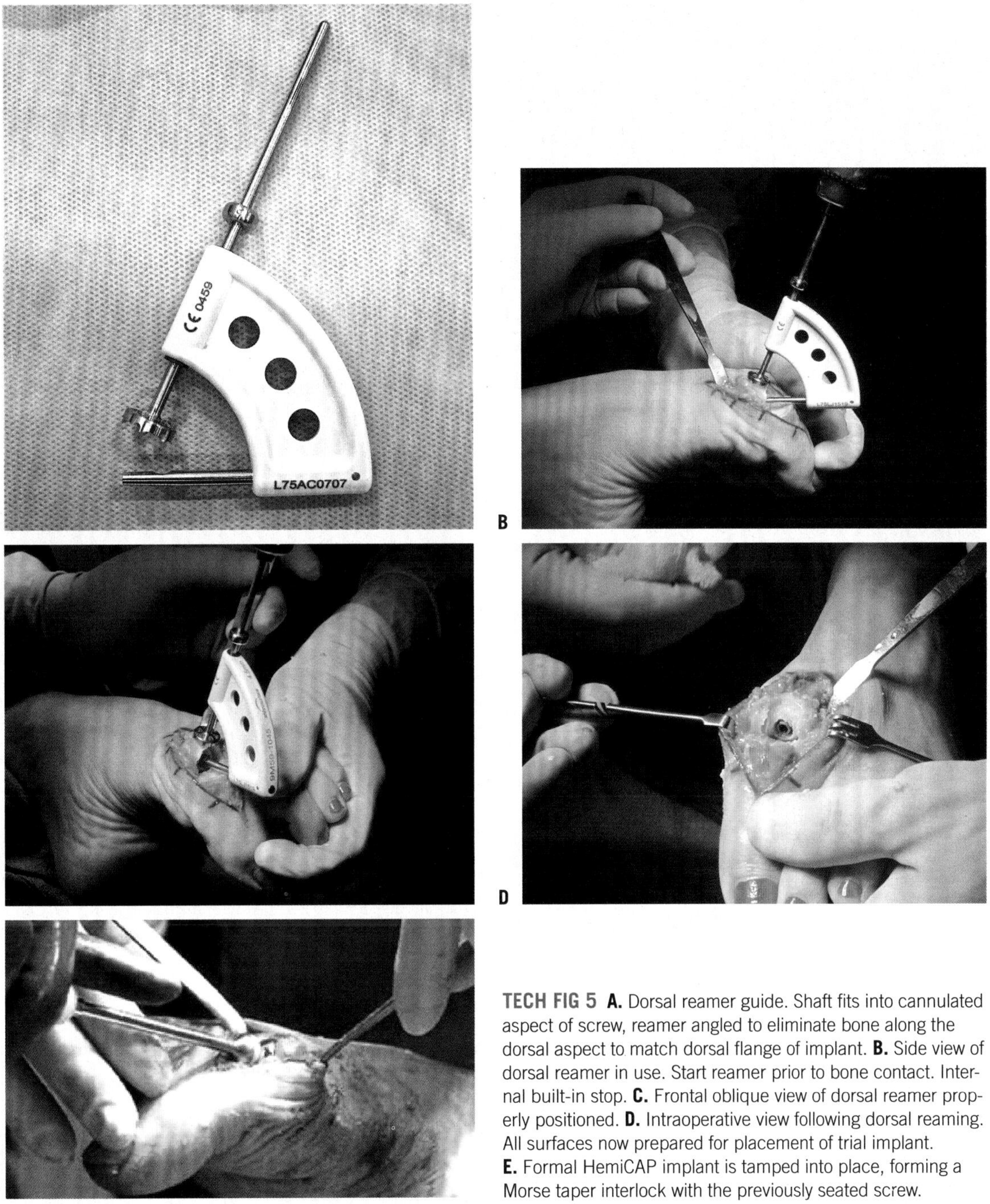

TECH FIG 5 A. Dorsal reamer guide. Shaft fits into cannulated aspect of screw, reamer angled to eliminate bone along the dorsal aspect to match dorsal flange of implant. **B.** Side view of dorsal reamer in use. Start reamer prior to bone contact. Internal built-in stop. **C.** Frontal oblique view of dorsal reamer properly positioned. **D.** Intraoperative view following dorsal reaming. All surfaces now prepared for placement of trial implant. **E.** Formal HemiCAP implant is tamped into place, forming a Morse taper interlock with the previously seated screw.

PLACEMENT OF TRIAL COMPONENT, BONE EXCISION, AND MOTION ASSESSMENT

- Confirm the trial size component so that it is congruent with the edge of the surrounding articular cartilage or slightly recessed (TECH FIG 6A).
- Remove excess bone around trial component using a micro-sagittal saw blade and/or rongeur. Any prominent bone along the dorsomedial/dorsolateral/medial/lateral and plantar aspects is removed in an effort to eliminate any source of bony impingement as the hallux is brought into dorsiflexion. Note: The author typically chamfers the medial eminence and lateral head using the trial component edge as its border. Often times, the crista

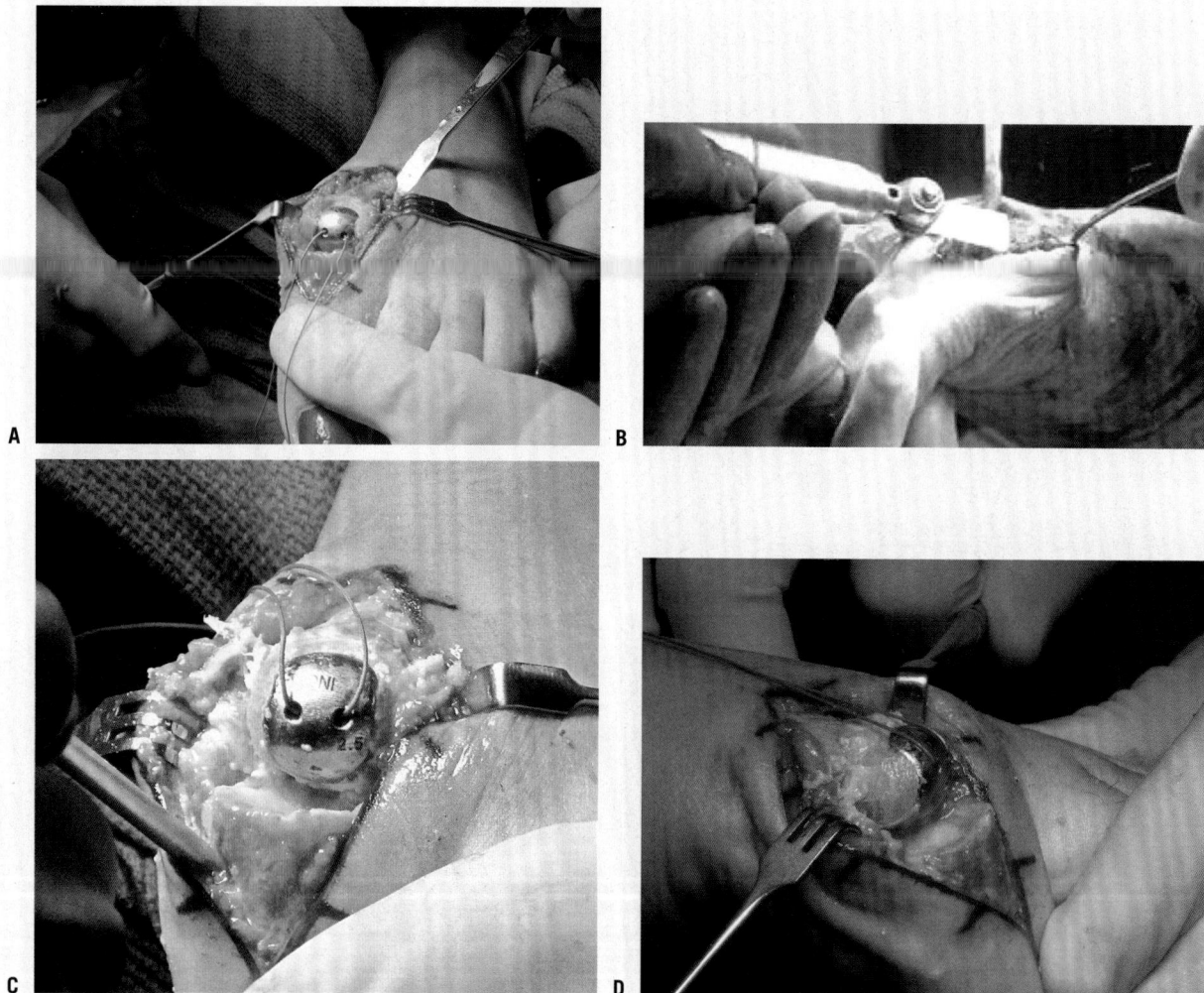

TECH FIG 6 A. Trial component placed. **B.** Excess bone along the dorsal, medial, lateral, and plantar aspects is removed with a microsagittal saw, osteotome, or rongeur, leaving an area of perimeter of bone to enclose the implant. **C,D.** Frontal and side view following excision of excess bone around perimeter of trial implant.

along the plantar aspect is excised as well for it may impede fluid motion (particularly if the joint has been decompressed) **(TECH FIG 6B–D)**.

- Assess dorsiflexion of the hallux with passive motion in the non–weight bearing and simulated weight-bearing mode by using a firm sterile surface. If motion still appears restricted, where the hallux cannot be dorsiflexed to 70 to 80 degrees relative to long axis of the first metatarsal, perform a gentle sustained dorsiflexion stretch to allow for soft tissue adaptation. This should be performed without considerable force. If still restricted, consider performing an additional soft tissue releases and/or bony decompression.
- With the trial implant in place to protect the bone preparation, soft tissue release of plantar joint contracture can be performed to gain additional motion in severely contracted joints. **(TECH FIG 7)**. In the space between the plantar aspect of the metatarsal head and the sesamoids, a McGlamry-type

elevator, flattened spoon-shaped spinal gouge, or Kapner gouge can be passed to free up the plantar contracture proximally. The motion is then reassessed. If required, the plantar joint contracture can be released distally along the base of the proximal phalanx in a similar manner by carefully elevating subperiosteally with care to stay directly against the bone. This may be used to "reset" the tension of the contracted plantar capsule and flexor hallucis brevis (FHB) tendon. If more dorsiflexion is required following plantar capsular release, consider additional joint decompression via bone decompression.

- Additional joint decompression can be performed by removal of the trial cap component, advancing the screw (each quarter-turn equals 1 mm additional decompression); repeat steps of using the appropriate-size surface reamer and dorsal reamer for bone preparation. Place the trial component again and reassess motion until desired motion is obtained.

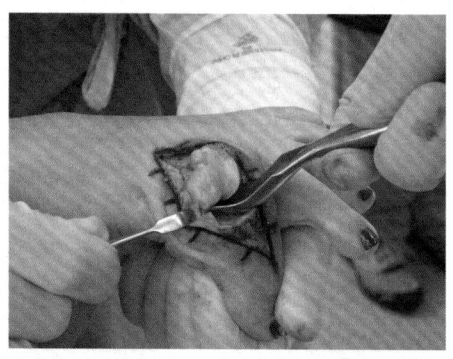
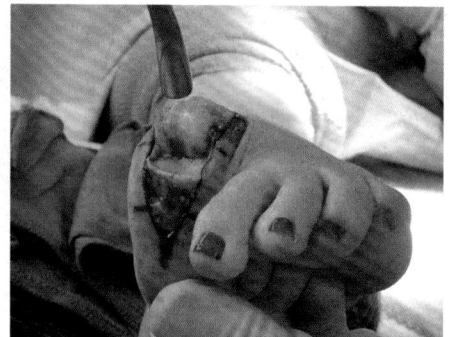
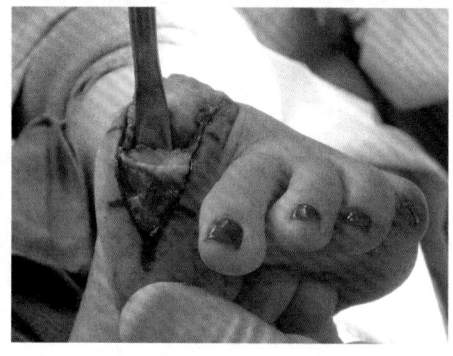

TECH FIG 7 A. Plantar soft tissue release is performed on metatarsal side using McGlamry elevator between metatarsal head and sesamoid. **B,C.** Hallux is maximally plantarflexed and soft tissue release performed along phalangeal side using blunt-tipped Kapner spinal gouge directly along bone of plantar aspect proximal phalangeal base.

PLACEMENT OF FORMAL METATARSAL HEAD HEMICAP COMPONENT

- The suction device hose is used to hold the implant to the delivery device with attached red suction cup. The suction tubing is detached once the formal component cap is properly positioned within the screw in the correct orientation **(TECH FIG 8A–D)**.
- Place the formal HemiCAP DF cap component by seating the cap using the impactor device as it forms a Morse taper interlock with the neck of the taper screw. A final check for any prominent bone edges may be excised. The final range of motion of the hallux

is assessed and recorded. An intraoperative lateral picture in maximal dorsiflexion may be taken and shown to patient in postoperative period. This demonstrates to them what was obtained in surgery and helps motivate them to perform aggressive motion exercises early in the postoperative period **(TECH FIG 8E–K)**.

- Obtain final AP and lateral fluoroscopic images to confirm alignment of the HemiCAP DF device. A maximally dorsiflexed lateral view may also be obtained **(TECH FIG 9)**.

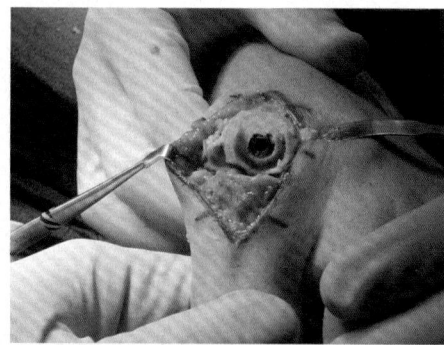
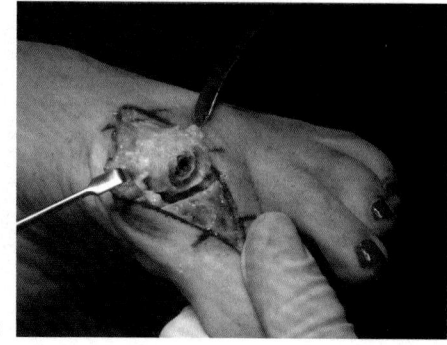
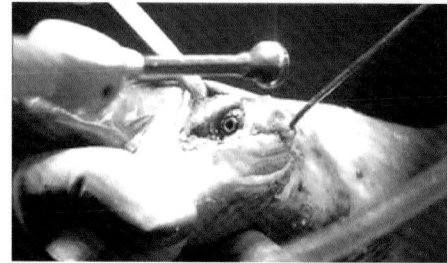

TECH FIG 8 A,B. Intraoperative views demonstrating complete bone preparation for implant following removal of trial component. **C.** The HemiCAP implant is placed in the suction delivery device.
(continued)

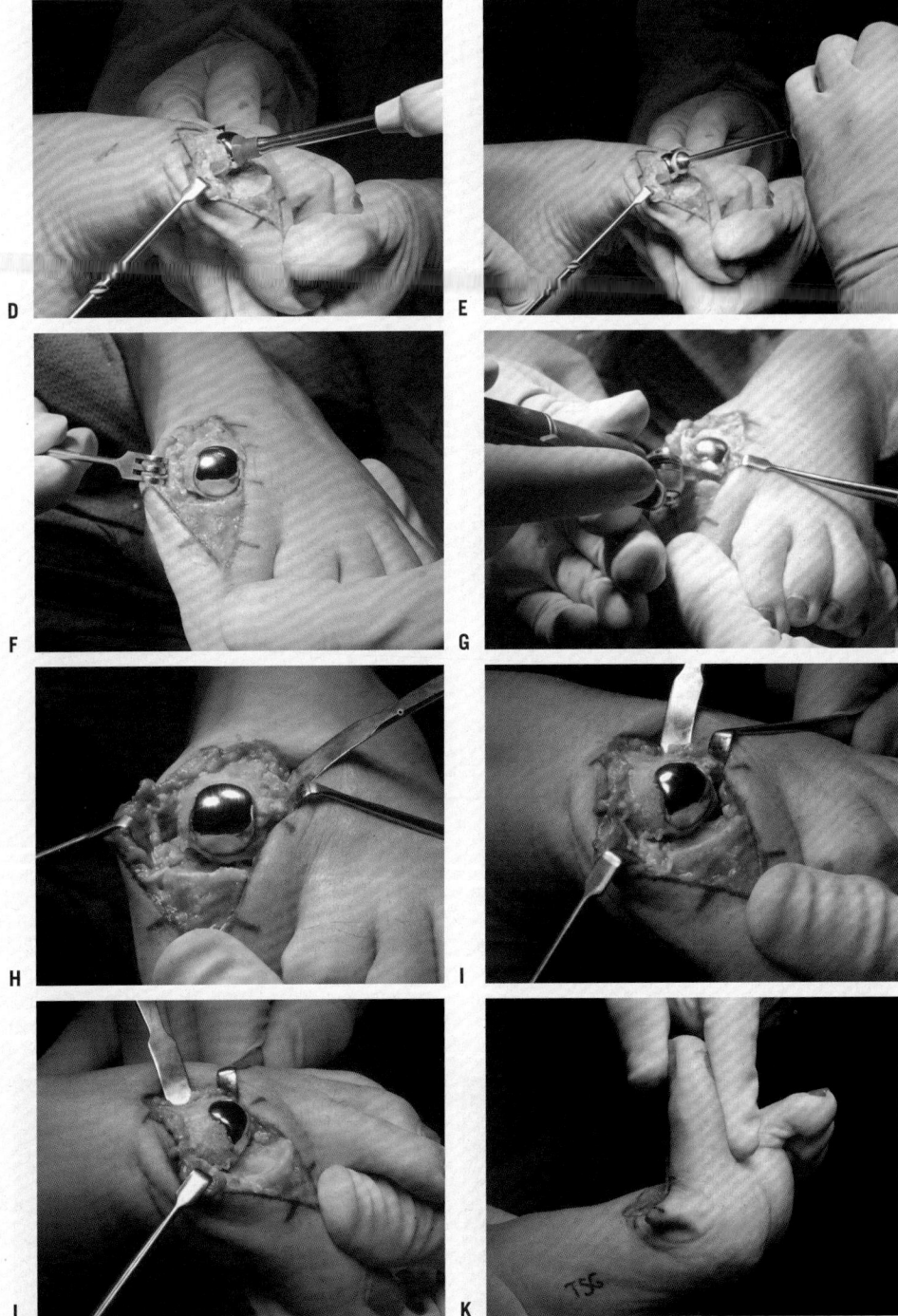

TECH FIG 8 *(continued)* **D.** Formal HemiCAP DF implant is placed within screw segment **E.** Impactor is used to seat and lock in Morse taper interlock between cap and screw. **F.** Formal HemiCAP DF implant. **G.** Excision of excess bone may need to be performed at times following seating of formal component. **H–J.** Frontal, medial, oblique, and side views of the DF implant. **K.** Dorsiflexion range of motion assess following placement of HemiCAP DF implant.

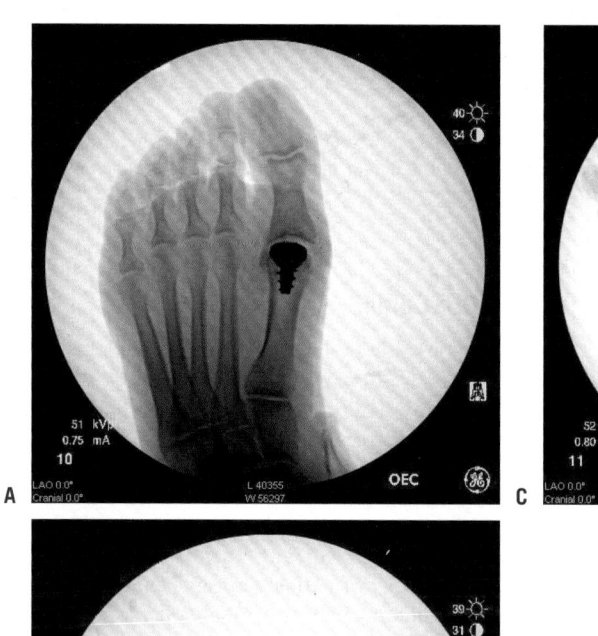

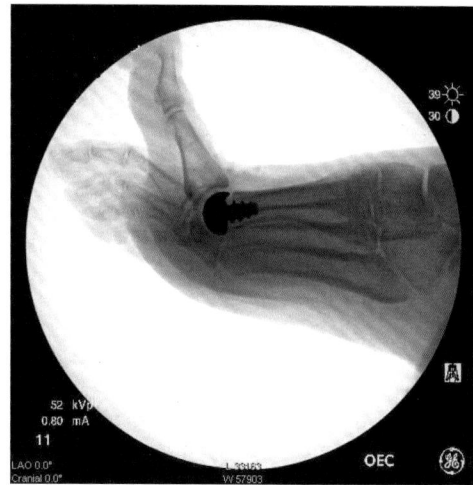

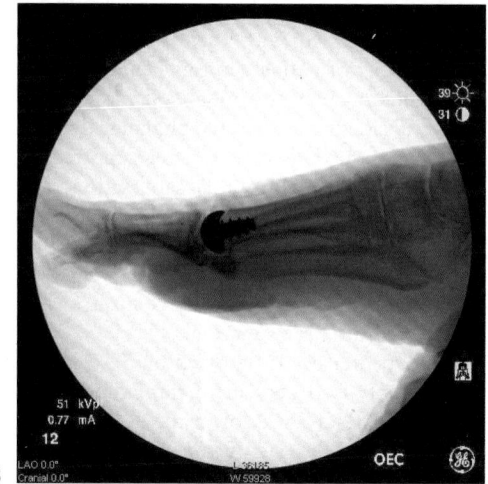

TECH FIG 9 Intraoperative fluoroscopic views following HemiCAP DF resurfacing. **A.** AP view. **B.** Lateral view neutral. **C.** Lateral view dorsiflexion.

TECHNIQUES

Pearls and Pitfalls

Indications	• Evaluate for advanced arthritis of the metatarsosesamoid articulation. Failure to recognize this may lead to a poor result with persistent plantar joint pain. This patient would be a better candidate for arthrodesis. • Carefully review the patient's expectations preoperatively. Although the patient's pain may be reduced from preoperative status, any joint-sparing procedure carries the risk of some degree of residual pain, whether occasional or daily. If the patient cannot accept the possibility of some degree of residual pain, he or she may be a better candidate for arthrodesis. It would be difficult for any joint-sparing procedure to reach the same predictability of pain relief that an arthrodesis delivers, yet an arthrodesis does not deliver any degree of motion preservation. Different patients have different goals and expectations; the varying importance that the patient place on pain relief and motion preservation can help determine whether they are a better arthroplasty or arthrodesis candidate.
Guide Pin Placement	• Avoid malposition of the implant by verifying that the guide pin placement is in line and parallel to the first metatarsal shaft axis on AP and lateral fluoroscopic views before drilling and placing the taper post screw. A common tendency is to underestimate the metatarsal inclination on the lateral view as well as making the starting point too dorsal.
Intraoperative Motion	• Soft tissue contracture: Release a plantar joint contracture with a curve elevator between the sesamoid and metatarsal region. Avoid iatrogenic injury to the sesamoid articular surface. Consider subperiosteal release along the plantar base of proximal phalanx, staying directly along bone with a small elevator. • Peri-implant bone excision: After placement of the HemiCAP DF, carefully excise all surrounding bone around the dorsal, medial, and lateral aspects of the implant for thorough bony decompression in an effort to lessen the chances of residual bony impingement against the proximal phalanx. Leave a small rim of bone along the implant perimeter for cap stability.

Postoperative Swelling and Hemarthrosis	• No tourniquet: Postoperative swelling and hemarthrosis tend to restrict early joint motion. Performing the case without a tourniquet forces the surgeon to obtain excellent hemostasis upon the approach and leads to a drier wound on closure. Less postoperative swelling may reduce the degree of motion lost commonly seen postoperatively by allowing for improved early range of motion.
Postoperative Motion	• Early range-of-motion exercises are initiated within days. • Exchange the initial postoperative dressing for a light waterproof OpSite dressing within 2 to 3 days postoperatively. Apply it along the dorsal incision site only, so as not to hinder early motion due to a bulky restrictive dressing.

POSTOPERATIVE CARE

- A compressive dressing is placed intraoperatively.
- The dressing is changed at 2 to 3 days postoperatively for a light dressing along the dorsal incision only with a waterproof OpSite **(FIG 8)**. This allows for less restriction due to the bandage and encourages early range of motion.
- Early range-of-motion exercises are emphasized in an effort to preserve the motion gained intraoperatively. Some degree of motion loss is anticipated postoperatively from its intraoperative measurements, although every effort is made to minimize this amount.
- We have found the first 2 to 3 weeks to be a critical period for maintaining motion. Swelling, hematoma, or hemarthrosis that occurs within the joint postoperatively contributes to the loss of motion seen after surgery. Recent attempts to minimize this with strict hemostasis and an early motion protocol are encouraged. Patients are instructed to begin toe motion exercises early at home several times per day, in addition to formal physical therapy. Physical therapy and rehabilitation continue until the patient reaches a normal gait pattern and range of motion is maximized.
- Patients are allowed to bear weight immediately on the heel of a rigid postoperative shoe or sandal. Between 3 and 4 weeks, the patient is transitioned to a running or jogging type of sneaker with a solid supportive sole.
- Radiographs are obtained at 1, 6, and 12 weeks postoperatively. Subsequent radiographs are obtained at 6 months, 1 year, and 2 years postoperatively.
- The patient should avoid placing high-impact stress on the joint, such as running, jogging, or sports involving pivoting and cutting, for at least the first 3 to 4 months postoperatively.

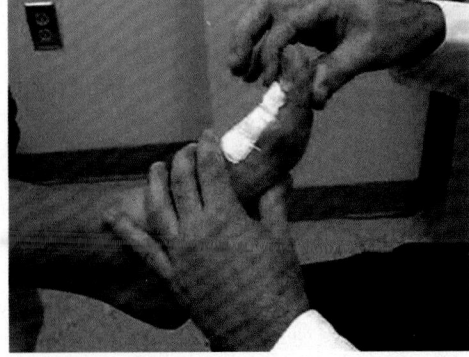

FIG 8 The initial dressing is changed to a light dorsal postoperative dressing so as not to restrict early motion. A waterproof sealed OpSite is used.

OUTCOMES

- A study by Hasselman and Shields[6] reported on 25 of their first 30 patients. At 20 months follow-up, the patients showed a postoperative motion increase of 42 degrees (from 23 degrees preoperatively to 65 degrees postoperatively). Significant improvement in visual analog scale, American Orthopaedic Foot and Ankle Society (AOFAS), and SF-36 scores were noted. All patients in this series claimed to be very satisfied with their results. Of note, an unspecified number of patients in this HemiCAP series underwent concomitant interpositional soft tissue grafting of the phalangeal side if considerable phalangeal involvement was noted. Kline and Hasselman[8] later reported on 26 implants (30 patients) with a 100% satisfaction rate at 60-month follow-up. No evidence of radiographic loosening or component subsidence was noted. Patients with greater than 50% phalangeal involvement underwent additional soft tissue interposition of the phalanx surface with a slip of extensor digitorum brevis tendon.
- Carpenter et al[2] reported on 32 implants and 30 patients. Seventy-two percent of implants were for grade 3 hallux rigidus and 28% for grade 2. At an average follow-up of 27.3 months, significant improvements in AOFAS scores were noted. No implants were had to be revised or removed, and all patients stated they were satisfied with the outcome. Carpenter et al[2] concluded that first metatarsal head resurfacing in combination with joint decompression, soft tissue mobilization, and débridement resulted in excellent satisfaction levels in patients with grades 2 and 3 hallux rigidus.
- The results of our follow-up study[17] on 36 patients using the first-generation HemiCAP at an average of 45 months were less favorable than those of the previously cited studies, although fair satisfaction rates were achieved in this patient population that had refused to consider fusion. Good to excellent results were noted in 76% of patients, 12% fair, and 12% poor. We found a modest increase in dorsiflexion motion averaging 26 degrees (from 20 degrees preoperatively to 46 degrees postoperatively), along with improvement in visual analog scale scores from an average before surgery of 6.3 to an average of 2.2 after surgery. Although complete pain relief was not noted in most patients, the reduction of pain in the majority of the patients led to an overall satisfaction rate of 80% for the procedure at a follow-up of nearly 4 years. Intermediate-term radiographic evaluation of the HemiCAP prosthesis in 56 patients demonstrated no significant evidence of loosening; it appeared to show superior radiographic results compared to those of other metallic implants using a stemmed design.[17]

- Occasional evidence of regrowth of bony osteophytes along the dorsal perimeter of the first-generation implant was noted. This issue was eliminated with the current second-generation HemiCAP DF due to the dorsal flange. Several patients displayed some degree of progressive chondral surface loss on the apposing proximal phalangeal base. Rather than loosening, progressive cartilage loss on the phalangeal surface remains the main issue associated with significant persistent pain and less-than-satisfactory results. Besides advanced metatarsal head involvement, if significant cartilage loss is noted on the phalanx at the time of the index procedure (intraoperative grades 2B, 2C or 3B, 3C), the use of a dermal allograft soft tissue interposition coverage of the phalangeal articular surface appears to add to the pain relief gained with the metatarsal head resurfacing. The authors have used this combination in recent years to improve patient satisfaction while awaiting for the release of the total toe arthroplasty design.
- When pain relief is the foremost goal of the patient, first MTP joint arthrodesis is the most predictable procedure for complete pain relief in advanced stages of hallux rigidus.
- When pain relief and preservation of motion are the desired goals, metatarsal head resurfacing can provide a reduction in pain and satisfactory outcome in a patient with modest expectations. We have found that the additional use of a dermal soft tissue allograft on the phalangeal side improves the pain reduction results when used with HemiCAP metatarsal resurfacing in those with phalangeal involvement of grades B or C. The U.S. Food and Drug Administration (FDA)-cleared Arthrosurface ToeMotion total toe arthroplasty implant may prove to provide predictable pain relief and low rates of loosening in the scenario of advanced involvement of both sides of the joint.
- It is critical to clearly explain to the patient preoperatively the differences between a fusion and an arthroplasty. As with all arthroplasty or joint-sparing procedures (whether soft tissue interposition or implant), if the patient is unwilling to accept less-than-complete pain relief as a risk, then continued nonoperative treatment should be considered until a more predictable option becomes available or the patient accepts a fusion. In their effort to avoid a fusion and maintain motion, if they do not appear to show a reasonable understanding of modest expectations preoperatively, then they will certainly not postoperatively.
- Unlike other metallic prosthetic implants or silastic implants, the HemiCAP did not display significant evidence of loosening. In fact, quite the opposite is evident on instances of removal, where the implant cap/screw will usually have excellent bio-ingrowth at times, making removal difficult. This should not be confused with failure secondary to loosening; rather, the mode of failure in cases in which patients were not satisfied proved to be secondary to persistence of pain or lack of adequate pain relief. The predominant mode of failure has been progressive chondral wear of the apposing phalangeal base which accounted for the residual pain seen in some patients. Given that this resurfaces only one side of the joint, certain obvious factors such as progressive changes to the surface not resurfaced (proximal phalanx) may lead to incomplete pain relief at the time of index procedure or gradual pain on disease progression. For instance, the implant may not fail, but the procedure

may fail to deliver the desired goal if significant phalangeal involvement is present or develops over time.

- Given the lack of significant rates of loosening seen with this implant, recent FDA approval has been obtained for a novel total toe arthroplasty design (Arthrosurface ToeMotion Total Toe Arthroplasty) using the same tapered screw fixation method within proximal phalanx **(FIG 9)**. A proximal phalangeal component with polyethylene insert was created as a complement to the metatarsal HemiCAP DF implant in an effort to address progressive arthritic changes of the proximal phalangeal articular surface. When significant involvement of both sides of the joint are seen at the time of the index procedure, use of the ToeMotion total toe arthroplasty design would be more appropriate than a hemiarthroplasty alone with the desired goal of providing a more predictable procedure for pain relief.
- Loosening and malalignment have been the main mechanisms of failure with other first MTP joint implants using stemmed or finned fixation methods. There are indeed perceivable differences of bone density and quality within the metatarsal head/neck compared with that of the proximal phalangeal base. Respecting these differences, secure rigid fixation within the first metatarsal and proximal phalanx that allows for early motion along with a more advanced understanding of first MTP joint kinematics should lead to lower rates of complications and higher rates of patient satisfaction than previously seen.
- Proper patient selection is paramount to the success of this procedure and adequate time should be given toward discussion of patient's goals and expectations. This joint can be very unforgiving, along with the patient attached to it, if their anticipated goals are set too high or expectations are unrealistic. Conversely, the senior author has found this to be a very rewarding procedure in properly selected patients when strict adherence to technique is followed and modest goals and expectations are set. The success of the procedure relies on placement of a "well-aligned implant in a well-aligned joint in a well-aligned patient."
- The lack of radiographic loosening is encouraging with this design. Having made significant strides in tackling the main issue of first MTP joint implant failure (implant loosening), the HemiCAP DF served as the model for design development of the FDA-cleared ToeMotion total toe arthroplasty. As long as loosening rates are kept at a minimum and proper alignment is maintained, resurfacing both sides of the arthritic first MTP joint should improve the predictability of pain relief and satisfaction rates in those patients with advanced hallux rigidus desiring preservation of motion as an alternative to joint fusion.

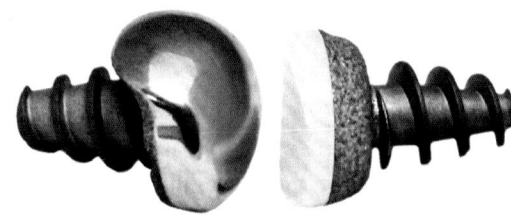

A

FIG 9 A. Arthrosurface ToeMotion total toe arthroplasty implant. Inlay arthroplasty using taper screw-based fixation and modular polyethylene insert. *(continued)*

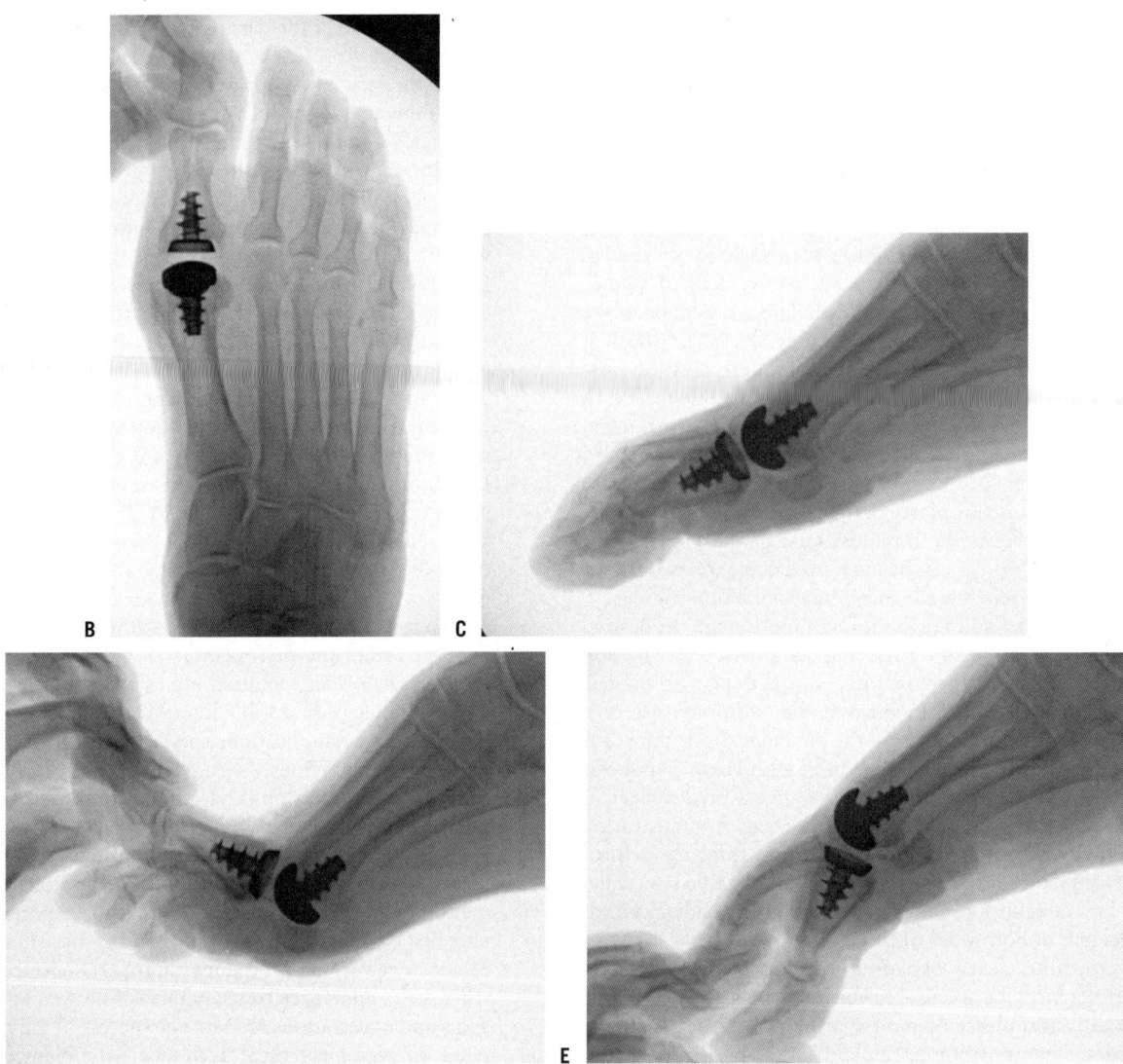

FIG 9 *(continued)* **B–E.** Radiographs of ToeMotion total toe arthroplasty.

COMPLICATIONS

Early Complications

- Delayed wound healing
- Deep infection
- Arthrofibrosis (not unique to procedure, seen as complication in many hallux rigidus procedures. Adequate soft tissue releases, bone–joint decompression, and early postoperative motion can lessen the incidence.)
- Residual joint pain (moderate to severe) which persists beyond the expected postoperative period. In our experience, the pain source in these patients has been due to the level and extent of the articular cartilage loss on the phalangeal side. Difficulty to manage a two-sided joint disease with a one-sided procedure. Significant residual joint pain may be present in some patients if extensive proximal phalangeal surface involvement extended to the central (grade level B) or plantar (level C). To minimize this occurrence and improve predictability of patient's pain relief, the author's suggestion is to discuss with patient preoperatively that if intraoperative grade 2C or 3C is encountered at the time of surgery, either perform a HemiCAP first metatarsal head resurfacing combined with soft tissue interposition resurfacing of the proximal phalangeal surface versus proceeding with a total toe arthroplasty in an effort to address both sides of the joint.
- Sesamoiditis (usually transient unless significant preexisting metatarsosesamoid arthritis; transient occurrence may be due to increased sesamoid motion stress as MTP joint dorsiflexion improved following years of long-standing restricted motion)
- Angular deformity (hallux valgus or hallux varus; can see extension deformity with dorsal capsular scarring or extensor tendon contracture)
- Lateral transfer metatarsalgia (avoid excessive shortening; can also be a late complication)

Late Complications

- Progressive arthritic changes proximal phalangeal articular surface
- Periprosthetic dorsal osteophyte formation (noted in first-generation HemiCAP implant, not noted in second-generation HemiCAP DF due to dorsal flange)

- Metallosis (can occur as a rare late complication if progressive phalangeal surface wears down and metatarsal resurfacing implant contacts a staple or screw used for an Akin or Moberg phalangeal osteotomy)
- Loosening (uncommon in early to intermediate follow-up studies)

SALVAGE OPTIONS FOR PAIN FOLLOWING METATARSAL RESURFACING

- First and foremost, determine the mode of failure and/or source of painful symptoms.
- Distinguish between implant failure versus failure of the procedure to result in the desired level of pain relief. In the latter, the implant may be stable and therefore can be retained while addressing the opposite side of the joint which is likely the painful source.
- The most common source of pain is progressive chondral loss on the phalangeal articular surface or pain from arthritic metatarsal sesamoid complex.
- Several intermediate-term follow-up studies have shown that loosening is an uncommon mode of failure with this implant design. In fact, in the majority of cases where the implant has been removed, the challenge has been significant bone ingrowth to the taper screw rather than loosening. Because of the ingrowth, attention must be given to careful removal of the screw, for significant torque can be generated on the first few back turns. If the implant is well

positioned and has no evidence of loosening, in certain salvage procedures, the implant may be retained.
- Dependent on the source of pain, stability of the implant, and the patient's desire to either retain or remove the implant; several surgical options exist presently.

SURGICAL OPTIONS

- Implant retained and soft tissue interposition coverage of arthritic phalangeal articular surface (**FIG 10**)
- Implant is retained and conversion to total toe arthroplasty by placing matching proximal phalangeal metal component with polyethylene insert. If first-generation design, will need to exchange to HemiCAP DF to match the phalangeal and polyethylene component (**FIG 11**).
- Implant removal and conversion to first MTP arthrodesis (**FIG 12**). Have freeze-dried allograft femoral head or iliac crest available. The author has had excellent results with intercalary allograft in the few instances where patients desired the implant to be removed due to pain. After implant removal and adequately preparing the joint, the approximate bone gap measured 2.0 to 2.5 cm. We have simply used a structural allograft (freeze-dried femoral head or iliac crest) cut to size and contoured using convex/concave reamer system to maintain hallux length on implant removal. In our experience, this has not been a complex procedure yet requires the appropriate graft and equipment for the case to flow smoothly.

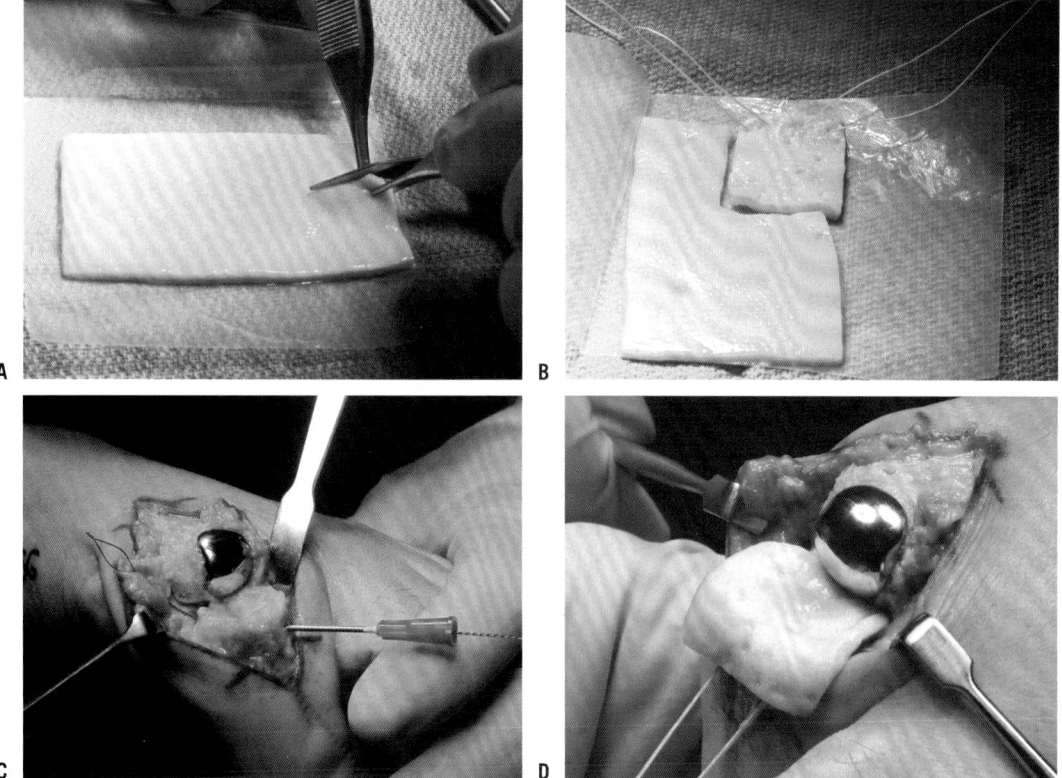

FIG 10 A,B. Dermal soft tissue allograft cut and mattress sutures placed. **C.** Criss-cross drill holes made with a K-wire at phalangeal base from dorsal to plantar. Suture passer passed through 18-gauge needle. **D.** Graft placed to cover articular surface of proximal phalanx, and sutures drawn up from plantar to dorsal through drill holes. *(continued)*

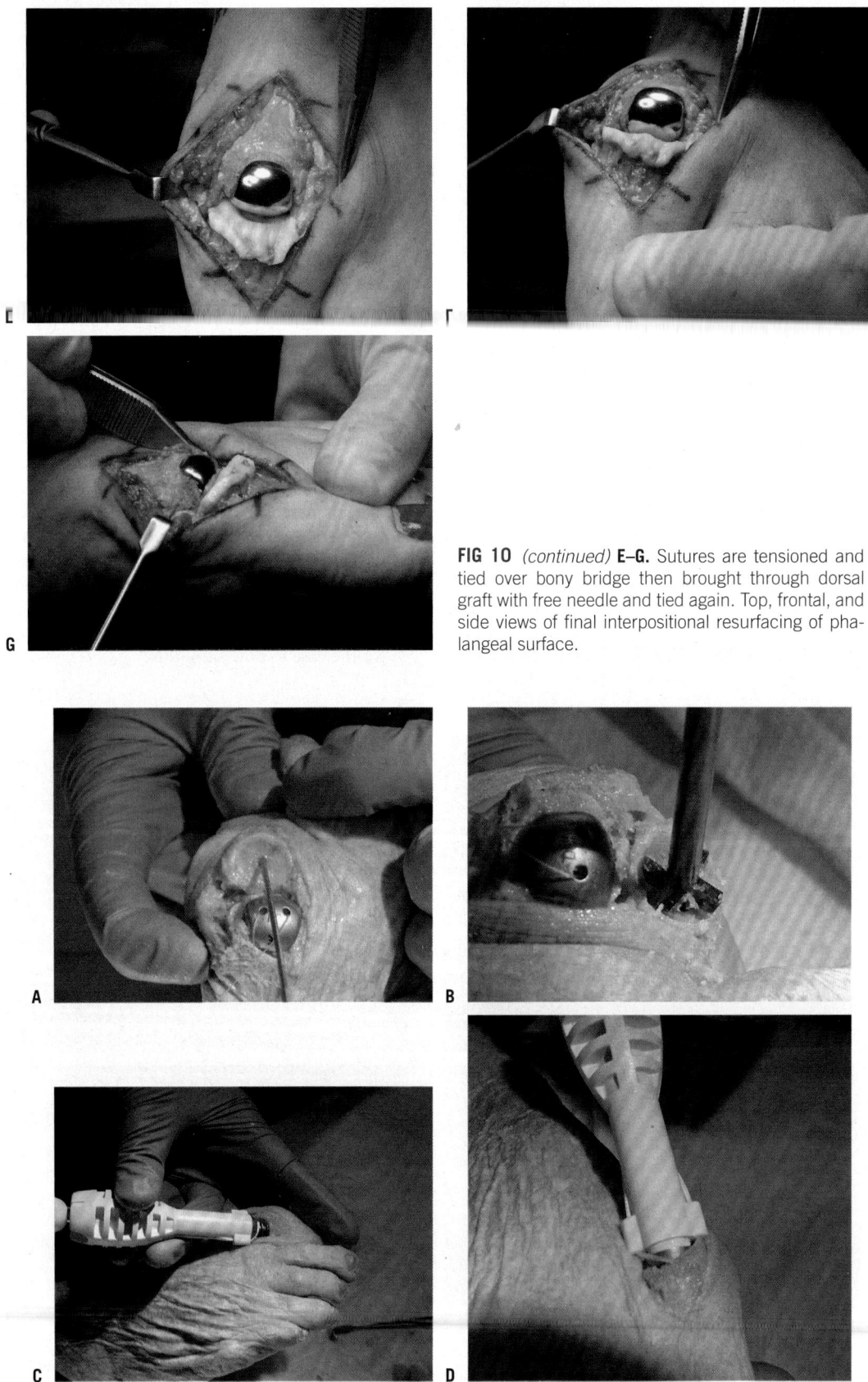

FIG 10 *(continued)* **E–G.** Sutures are tensioned and tied over bony bridge then brought through dorsal graft with free needle and tied again. Top, frontal, and side views of final interpositional resurfacing of phalangeal surface.

FIG 11 A. HemiCAP conversion to ToeMotion total toe arthroplasty. HemiCAP DF must be used on metatarsal side to match phalangeal component with polyethylene insert. Centralized pin is placed within proximal phalanx. **B.** Phalangeal reamer is used for inlay phalangeal component. **C,D.** Following tapping, taper screw-based phalangeal tray component is placed. *(continued)*

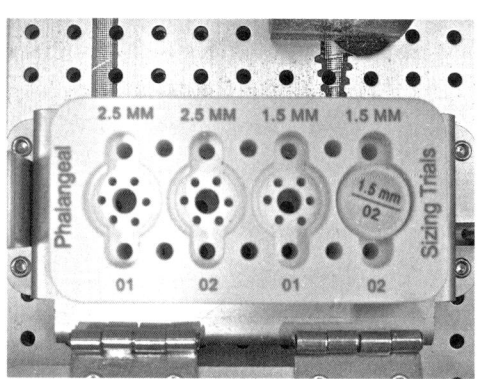
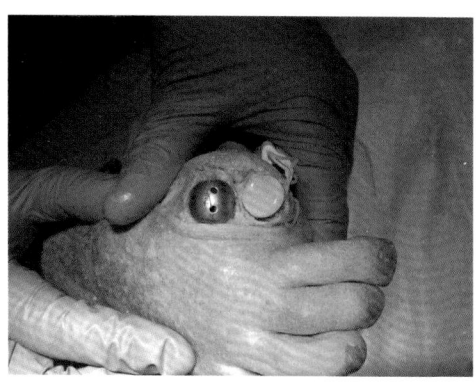
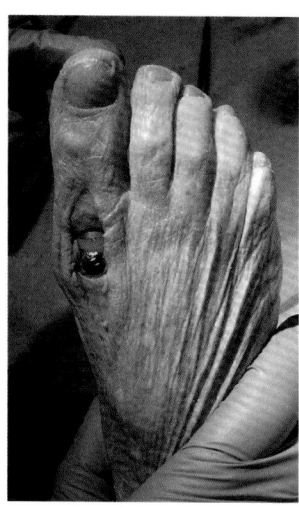

FIG 11 *(continued)* **E,F.** Following assessment with modular trials, polyethylene insert chosen and placed with delivery device which locks into phalangeal tray. **G.** Final components for ToeMotion implant.

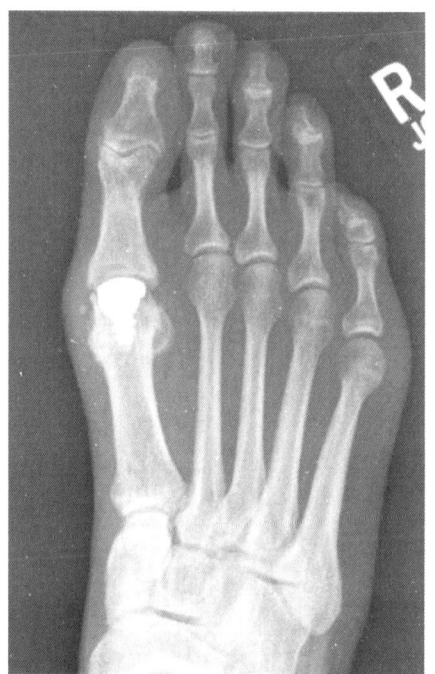
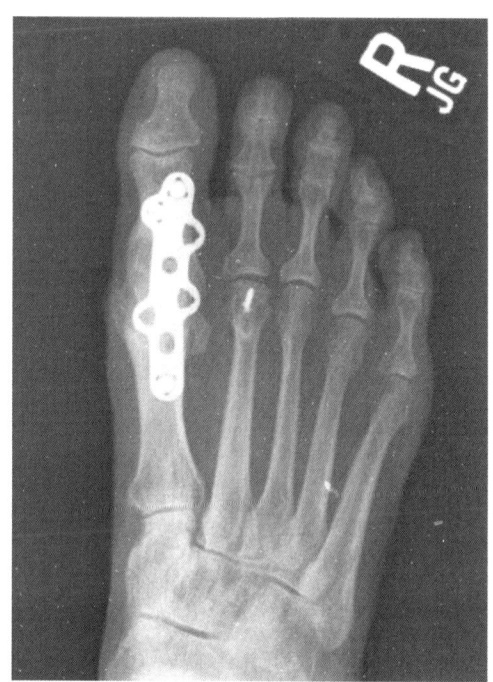
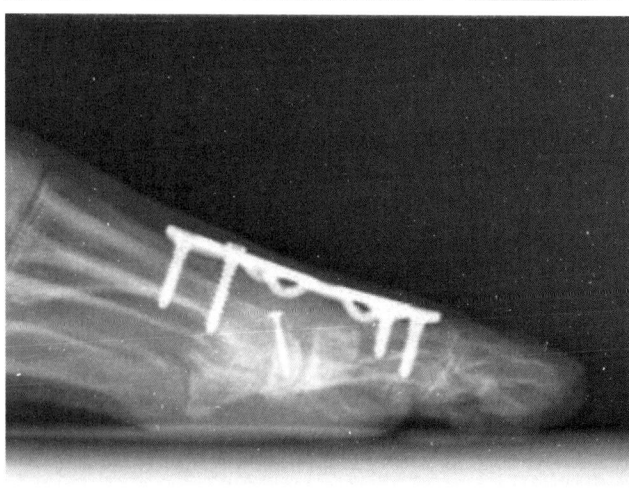

FIG 12 A. Patient developed arthrofibrosis and persistent pain despite proper implant alignment and no evidence of loosening. Elected for implant removal and conversion to fusion. **B,C.** Implant removed and intercalary allograft placed to maintain hallux length. Freeze-dried femoral head allograft used. Prepared with convex/concave reamers and stabilized with dorsal plate fixation. Solid bone fusion noted on AP and lateral radiographs. Weil osteotomy performed on second metatarsal and proximal interphalangeal (PIP) arthrodesis to address lateral transfer metatarsalgia and semirigid hammer toe deformity.

FINAL COMMENTS

- Given that this procedure only resurfaces one side of the joint, if significant cartilage loss is present opposite that of the implant, the predictability of pain relief would not be expected to reach that of an arthrodesis. However, pain relief alone is not the only thing that matters to this subset of hallux rigidus patients. Typically, these are the patients that outright refuse the option of an arthrodesis and would not be satisfied with the motion an arthrodesis provides. Pain relief and motion are the desired goals; a much different patient group than those willing to accept a fusion from the start. Extremely high percentages of pain relief satisfaction is more difficult to achieve in this group compared to arthrodesis patients, for these are truly two separate subgroups in terms of desired goals and expectations. Even if they have identical clinical or radiographic grades, the subject groups in comparative studies of arthrodesis versus joint-sparing procedures may never be truly comparable for this reason; this is rarely discussed when interpreting the results of these studies but is more obvious to those in clinical practice treating these two groups of patients. Similar to the resurgence of interest in total ankle arthroplasty, continued progress needs to be made for the development of predictable joint-sparing implant arthroplasty for hallux rigidus. As we gain better understanding of the nuances of the first MTP joint, this goal will be reached.

REFERENCES

1. Berlet GC, Hyer CF, Lee TH, et al. Interpositional arthroplasty of the first metatarsophalangeal joint using regenerative tissue matrix for the treatment of advanced hallux rigidus. Foot Ankle Int 2008;29:10–21.
2. Carpenter B, Smith J, Motley T, et al. Surgical treatment of hallux rigidus using a metatarsal head resurfacing implant: mid-term follow-up. J Foot Ankle Surg 2010;49:321–325.
3. Coughlin MJ, Shurnas PS. Hallux rigidus. Grading and long-term results of operative treatment. J Bone Joint Surg Am 2003;85-A(11):2072–2088.
4. Easley ME, Davis WH, Anderson RB. Intermediate to long-term follow-up of medial-approach dorsal cheilectomy for hallux rigidus. Foot Ankle Int 1999;20:147–152.
5. Hamilton WG, O'Malley MJ, Thompson FM, et al. Roger Mann Award 1995. Capsular interposition arthroplasty for severe hallux rigidus. Foot Ankle Int 1997;18:68–70.
6. Hasselman C, Shields N. Resurfacing of the first metatarsal head in the treatment of the hallux rigidus. Tech Foot Ankle Surg 2008;7:31–40.
7. Hattrup SJ, Johnson KA. Subjective results of hallux rigidus following treatment with cheilectomy. Clin Orthop Relat Res 1988;(226):182–191.
8. Kline AJ, Hasselman CT. Metatarsal head resurfacing for advanced hallux rigidus. Foot Ankle Int 2013;24(5):716–725.
9. Konkel KF, Menger AG, Retzlaff SA. Mid-term results of Futura hemi-great toe implants. Foot Ankle Int 2008;29:831–837.
10. Lau JT, Daniels TR. Outcomes following cheilectomy and interpositional arthroplasty and hallux rigidus. Foot Ankle Int 2001;22:462–470.
11. Mann RA, Clanton TO. Hallux rigidus: treatment by cheilectomy. J Bone Joint Surg Am 1988;70(3):400–406.
12. Mann RA, Coughlin MJ, DuVries HL. Hallux rigidus: a review of literature and a method of treatment. Clin Orthop Relat Res 1979;(142):57–63.
13. Moberg E. A simple operation for hallux rigidus. Clin Orthop Relat Res 1979;(142):55–56.
14. O'Malley MJ, Basran HS, Gu Y, et al. Treatment of advanced stages of hallux rigidus with cheilectomy and phalangeal osteotomy. J Bone Joint Surg Am 2013;95(7):606–610.
15. Raikin SM, Ahmad J, Pour AE, et al. Comparison of arthrodesis and metallic hemiarthroplasty of the hallux metatarsophalangeal joint. J Bone Joint Surg Am 2007;89(9):1979–1985.
16. San Giovanni TP, Botto-Van Bemden A. First metatarsal head resurfacing: a new technique for surgical management of advanced hallux rigidus. Presented at American Academy of Orthopedic Surgery Annual Meeting, 2006.
17. San Giovanni TP, Marx R, Botto-Van Bemden A, et al. Presented at American Orthopedic Foot and Ankle Society Specialty Day at American Academy of Orthopedic Surgeons Annual Meeting, May 2010, New Orleans, LA.
18. Seibert NR, Kadakia AR. Surgical management of hallux rigidus: cheilectomy and osteotomy phalanx and metatarsal. Foot Ankle Clin 2009;14:9–22.
19. Shereff MJ, Bejjani FJ, Kummer FJ. Kinematics of the first metatarsophalangeal joint. J Bone Joint Surg Am 1986;68:392–398.
20. Thomas PJ, Smith RW. Proximal phalanx osteotomy for surgical treatment of hallux rigidus. Foot Ankle Int 1999;20:3–12.
21. Townley CO, Taranow WS. A metallic hemiarthroplasty resurfacing prosthesis for the hallux metatarsophalangeal joint. Foot Ankle Int 1994;15:575–580.

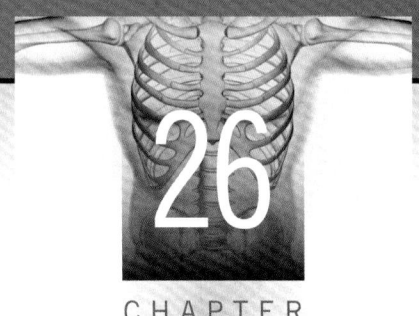

26
CHAPTER

First Metatarsophalangeal Joint Hemiarthroplasty

Michael S. Aronow

DEFINITION

- Hallux rigidus is arthritis of the first metatarsophalangeal (MTP) joint.
- The amount of arthritis can range from focal areas of cartilage injury or osteophyte formation without joint space narrowing to ankylosis with complete loss of the joint space. In one classification system proposed by Coughlin and Shurnas,[4] grade 1 has osteophyte formation with minimal first MTP joint space narrowing, grade 2 has mild to moderate joint space narrowing, grade 3 has significant narrowing of the joint space and pain at extremes of joint range of motion but not midrange, and grade 4 has severe arthritis with pain at midrange of passive motion.

ANATOMY

- The joint consists of the articulation of the first metatarsal head with the hallux proximal phalanx and the medial and lateral sesamoids (FIG 1).
- The flexor hallucis brevis contains the two sesamoids within its medial and lateral heads and inserts on the plantar base of the hallux proximal phalanx.
- The flexor hallucis longus runs between the medial and lateral sesamoids and inserts on the plantar base of the hallux distal phalanx.
- The extensor hallucis longus and the more lateral extensor hallucis brevis insert into the extensor mechanism of the great toe.
- The abductor hallucis and adductor hallucis insert on the medial and lateral sesamoids, respectively, along with the plantar base of the hallux proximal phalanx.

PATHOGENESIS

- Hallux rigidus may be secondary to primary osteoarthritis, systemic inflammatory arthritis, or less commonly septic arthritis.
- It may also be posttraumatic in nature, developing after a previous intra-articular fracture or significant turf toe injury to the ligamentous structures of the first MTP joint.
- Biomechanical factors such as a long, hypermobile, or dorsally elevated first metatarsal may lead to dorsal impingement of the proximal phalangeal base on the first metatarsal head with first MTP dorsiflexion.

NATURAL HISTORY

- The extent of arthritis often progresses with time, leading to increased osteophyte formation and joint space narrowing. This may occur with or without joint-sparing surgical intervention.

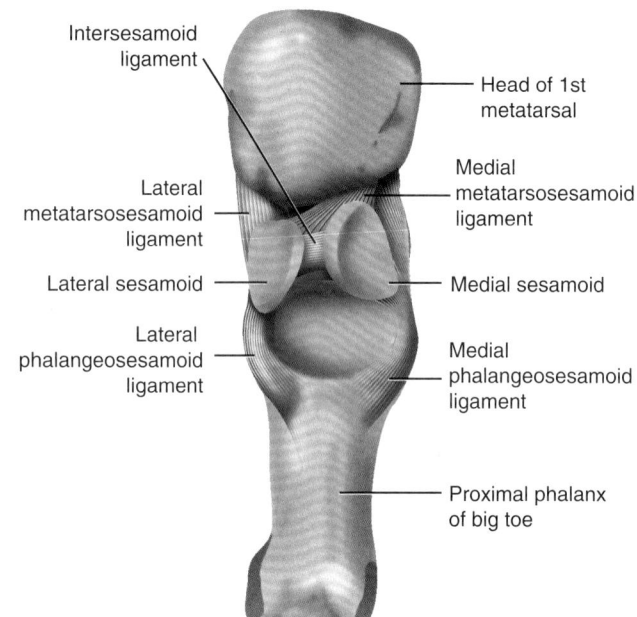

FIG 1 Anatomy of the first MTP joint.

Labels:
- Intersesamoid ligament
- Head of 1st metatarsal
- Lateral metatarsosesamoid ligament
- Medial metatarsosesamoid ligament
- Lateral sesamoid
- Medial sesamoid
- Lateral phalangeosesamoid ligament
- Medial phalangeosesamoid ligament
- Proximal phalanx of big toe

PATIENT HISTORY AND PHYSICAL FINDINGS

- Patients often complain of pain and stiffness in their first MTP joint. Symptoms may be exacerbated by shoes with a restrictive toe box and by walking barefoot or in shoes with a flexible forefoot.
- On examination, there may be a prominent first metatarsal head, a swollen first MTP joint, and tender osteophytes of the metatarsal head and phalangeal base.
  - First MTP joint motion may be limited and painful.
  - Dorsiflexion range of motion should also be assessed with the patient bearing weight or with dorsal translation applied to the first metatarsal head to simulate weight bearing to assess for "functional hallux rigidus."
    - In mild to moderate hallux rigidus, pain is principally with maximum joint dorsiflexion or plantarflexion secondary to dorsal osteophytes causing bone impingement or soft tissue tenting, respectively.
    - With severe arthritis, there may be pain throughout the entire arc of motion and a positive "grind test," in which midrange of motion with axial compression applied to the first MTP joint is painful.

IMAGING AND OTHER DIAGNOSTIC STUDIES

- Anteroposterior (AP), lateral, oblique, and sesamoid views of the foot should be obtained to assess the extent of arthritis in the first MTP, metarsosesamoid, and adjacent first tarsometatarsal and hallux interphalangeal joints.
- An assessment is also made for any concurrent hallux valgus or hallux varus deformity, osteopenia, avascular necrosis, or occult sesamoid fracture.
- If needed, magnetic resonance imaging and computed tomography scan can provide more detailed information, particularly with respect to sesamoid pathology, which is important, as this procedure leaves the metarsosesamoid joint intact.

DIFFERENTIAL DIAGNOSIS

- Osteochondral lesion
- Avascular necrosis
- Occult fracture

NONOPERATIVE MANAGEMENT

- Conservative treatment should always be offered before performing first MTP joint hemiarthroplasty.
- The principal goal is to limit painful motion of the first MTP joint and pressure on prominent osteophytes. An accommodative shoe with a soft upper and a stiff forefoot rocker may be worn. A rigid turf toe plate may be placed under a removable soft insole, or an orthotic with a Morton's extension may be worn. Doughnut pads may be placed over tender osteophytes.
- Medications such as nonsteroidal anti-inflammatories, glucosamine and chondroitin sulfate, and acetaminophen may be taken.
- Corticosteroid and possibly hyaluronic acid or biologic injections may be performed.

SURGICAL MANAGEMENT

- There are many surgical options for hallux rigidus including cheilectomy, metatarsal osteotomy, proximal phalangeal osteotomy, distraction arthroplasty, tissue interposition arthroplasty, implant arthroplasty, and arthrodesis.
- Of the many implants available, the author's preference is a cobalt-chrome proximal phalangeal hemiarthroplasty made by BioPro (**FIG 2**). The material does not break down with associated extensive bone destruction such as the silicone total and hemi implants; there are good long-term results published in the literature; and the amount of bone removed is small, making salvage of a failed prosthesis less challenging. The prosthesis is also available in titanium for patients with metal sensitivity.
- Unlike metal or hydrogel hemiarthroplasty implants that resurface only part of the metatarsal head, the BioPro implant replaces the entire articular surface of the proximal phalangeal base, which allows removal of sufficient bone to decompress the joint, and does not preclude an aggressive

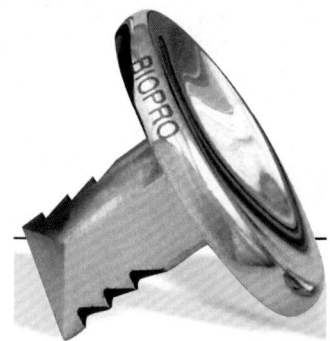

FIG 2 BioPro first MTP hemiarthroplasty implant.

dorsal metatarsal head cheilectomy without destabilizing the implant.

- The author's potential indications for performing a first MTP hemiarthroplasty are symptomatic grade 2 arthritis with loss of greater than 50% of the metatarsal head articular cartilage and grade 3 and 4 arthritis without severe involvement of the articulation between the metatarsal head and the sesamoids.
- The author is unaware of any literature comparing the results of any hemiarthroplasty implant on the market to cheilectomy for the above potential indications. In the author's experience, both procedures often provide good outcomes for grade 2 and 3 arthritis when performed appropriately. Cheilectomy is typically not recommended for stage 4 arthritis.[4]

Preoperative Planning

- History, physical examination, and radiographs are reviewed to confirm the appropriate indications for the procedure and determine if there are any concurrent deformities or biomechanical abnormalities that also need to be addressed.
- The patient needs to be told that based on the intraoperative findings, a decision may be made that hemiarthroplasty is not the best option and that a simple cheilectomy, arthrodesis, or tissue interposition arthroplasty may be preferable.
- The equipment to perform the hemiarthroplasty and the alternatives mentioned earlier should be readily available in the operating room.

Positioning

- The patient is placed in the supine position with a leg or thigh tourniquet.

Approach

- A dorsomedial approach is preferable, although a medial longitudinal approach can also be used in the presence of a previous incision there.
- Perioperative antibiotics and a regional anesthetic block are given.

EXPOSURE

- Make a longitudinal dorsomedial incision over the first MTP joint.
- Protecting the dorsomedial sensory nerve, expose the extensor digitorum longus tendon and dorsomedial joint capsule.
- Leaving a sufficient cuff of capsular tissue for subsequent repair, make a longitudinal capsulotomy medial to the extensor digitorum longus tendon.
- Using subperiosteal dissection and preserving the collateral ligaments, expose the dorsal aspect of the proximal phalanx and the dorsal, medial, and, if prominent, lateral aspect of the metatarsal head **(TECH FIG 1)**.
  - Release any adhesions between the sesamoids and the metatarsal head.
- Inspect the joint to determine the extent of articular cartilage damage.
  - If there is severe ankylosis and arthritis of the metatarsosesamoid joints, then a first MTP joint arthrodesis or tissue interposition arthroplasty is probably a better option.
  - If the cartilage of the proximal phalanx and the plantar half of the metatarsal head is in good condition, then a cheilectomy with or without a metatarsal or phalangeal osteotomy is usually sufficient.

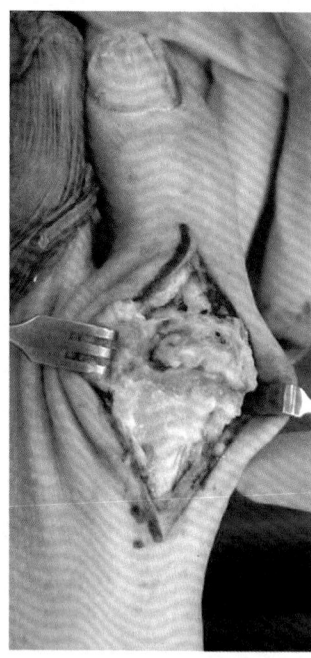

TECH FIG 1 Exposure of dorsal osteophytes after capsular incision.

SITE PREPARATION

- Using a rongeur or sagittal saw, remove osteophytes from the metatarsal head, proximal phalangeal base, and also circumferentially about the sesamoids.
  - Remove a prominent medial eminence of the metatarsal head if it is present.
- Make an adequate dorsal cheilectomy of the metatarsal head.
  - With dorsal stress applied to the metatarsal head, there should be at least 70 degrees and preferably 90 degrees of first MTP dorsiflexion relative to the axis of the first metatarsal shaft.
  - Make an initial cut parallel to the dorsal cortex of the first metatarsal head. However, after the trial and final prostheses have been inserted, range of motion is reassessed and, usually, additional dorsal bone resection (up to 25% to 40% of the normal metatarsal head) is required. The author's experience with this procedure and with isolated cheilectomy is that there is a higher rate of recurrent symptoms if less than 30% of the dorsal metatarsal head is removed.
- Débride loose chondral flaps and drill or microfracture areas of visible subchondral bone on the remaining metatarsal head to promote fibrocartilage ingrowth.

- Remove the base of the proximal phalanx using a sagittal saw, with the cut perpendicular to the axis of the proximal phalanx.
  - Take care to avoid injuring the flexor hallucis brevis insertion, which may occur with resection of too much bone (>6 mm or 20% of the total proximal phalangeal length) or overpenetration of the saw blade.
- The implant sizer is the same thickness as the prosthesis (2 mm) and can be used to guide the amount of bone resection.
  - If only 2 mm of bone is removed, then the joint is usually too tight and postoperative motion is restricted.
  - Usually, at least 3 to 4 mm of bone resection is required for adequate motion; this can be assessed by the amount of "shuck" with the trial implant inserted.
  - Ideally, the space between the trial or final implant and the metatarsal head should distract at least 3 mm with applied force.
  - Visualization of the plantar aspect of the joint may be easier after this cut has been made.

IMPLANT SIZING AND INSERTION

- Available BioPro implant diameters are 17 mm (small), 18.5 mm (medium/small), 20 mm (medium), 21.5 mm (medium/large), and 23 mm (large); these implants are either porous coated or nonporous coated.
  - With the toe plantarflexed 90 degrees to improve exposure, use the sizer guide to determine the largest size implant that does not extend beyond the margins of the proximal phalangeal cut.
  - With respect to orientation, the prosthesis is slightly wider in the mediolateral dimension than the dorsal–plantar dimension.
  - There is a hole in the center of the sizer that is used as a guide to drill or punch the proximal phalangeal base to accommodate the stem of the trial prosthesis. The hole needs to be in line with the long axis of the proximal phalanx.
- Insert the trial stem and evaluate the extent of phalangeal base coverage and joint range of motion and stability. If, as noted earlier, there is insufficient joint distraction or dorsiflexion, more bone can be removed from the phalangeal base or dorsal metatarsal head, respectively.
- Once satisfied with the implant size and bone cuts, center the chisel with its longer end in the mediolateral dimension on the trial hole and use it to create a channel for the stem of the final prosthesis.
- Impact the prosthesis into position.
  - It should be flush with the phalangeal base and should not extend beyond its margins **(TECH FIG 2A)**.
  - Joint motion should be smooth with dorsiflexion, and there should be at least 3 mm of shuck, as noted earlier.
- Use AP and lateral fluoroscopy or plain radiographs to confirm acceptable prosthesis position **(TECH FIG 2B)**.
  - If the patient is not allergic, place bone wax on the cut dorsal surface of the metatarsal head and irrigate the joint.

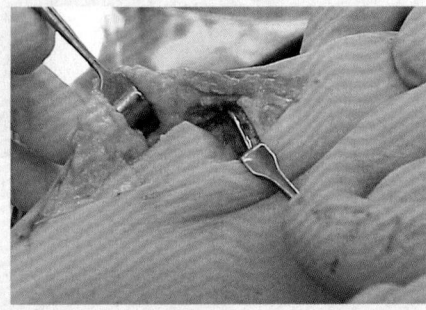 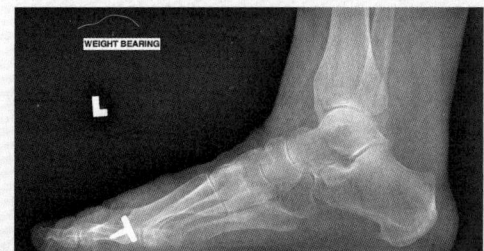

TECH FIG 2 A. Cheilectomy has been performed and implant inserted. **B.** Postoperative lateral radiograph showing component in place.

WOUND CLOSURE

- Close the joint capsule with absorbable suture.
  - If a large dorsal and medial eminence has been resected, then sometimes, the capsule needs to be imbricated or partially removed. However, take care not to make the closure too tight, which may restrict postoperative motion.
- Close the subcutaneous tissue and skin in layers and apply a sterile compressive dressing.

TECHNIQUES

Pearls and Pitfalls

- Failure to recognize and address concurrent deformity or potential causative biomechanical abnormalities may lead to progressive arthritis of the remaining metatarsal head and sesamoids, component loosening, and postoperative pain and stiffness.

- An adequate cheilectomy must be performed, particularly if there is residual elevation of the metatarsal head or hypermobility of the first tarsometatarsal joint. If not, there is more likely to be recurrent dorsal osteophyte formation and decreased postoperative range of motion.

- Sufficient bone must be removed from the proximal phalangeal base to decompress the joint without damaging the flexor hallucis brevis insertion.

- The stem of the prosthesis needs to press-fit tightly and be centered within the proximal phalangeal canal. An attempt to remove more dorsal than plantar phalangeal bone to "increase relative toe dorsiflexion" or protect the flexor hallucis brevis insertion risks having the tip of the stem abut or penetrate the plantar cortex and may lead to poorer results.

POSTOPERATIVE CARE

- Postoperatively, the patient may be progressive weight bearing as tolerated in an orthopaedic or regular shoe.
- Early first MTP joint range-of-motion and strengthening exercises should be initiated within the first few days after surgery.
- Sutures are removed at 10 to 21 days postoperatively.

OUTCOMES

- The developer of the BioPro prosthesis reported his results for 279 procedures with follow-up of 8 months to 33 years as 93.1% excellent, 2.2% good, and 4.7% unsatisfactory results.[13]
  - Twelve of the 13 unsatisfactory results underwent revision, including prosthesis removal.
  - A subsequent update on 468 procedures with follow-up of 2 months to 38 years noted no additional revisions and one case of radiographic loosening.[6]
- Seven patients (nine feet) underwent a BioPro resurfacing endoprosthesis, and at 1-year follow-up, there was an average increase on a modified American Orthopaedic Foot & Ankle Society (AOFAS) Hallux Metatarsophalangeal–Interphalangeal 100-point scale from 51.1 to 77.8, an average increase in first MTP joint dorsiflexion range of motion from 11.9 to 17.9 degrees, and no change in first MTP joint plantarflexion range of motion.[9]
- Another study evaluated 32 procedures in 28 patients with an average follow-up of 33 months.[12]
  - Foot Function Index pain, disability, and activity scores improved; 82% of patients were completely satisfied, and 11% were satisfied with reservations.
  - There were three cases of radiographic loosening or subsidence.
- The author performed 16 procedures in 15 patients with average follow-up of 49 months.[1] There was a 92% satisfaction rate and an 83% incidence of no or mild occasional pain for index procedures and a 50% satisfaction rate and 25% incidence of no or mild occasional pain for patients having had a previous failed first MTP joint cheilectomy or tissue interposition arthroplasty.
  - There were three revision procedures—one implant removal for postoperative infection and two revision cheilectomies for recurrent osteophytes, possibly secondary to inadequate initial cheilectomy.
- Twenty-three patients completed 1-year follow-up after BioPro hemiarthroplasty with an average American College of Foot and Ankle Surgeons (ACFAS) score increase from 41.2 to 80, an average first MTP joint dorsiflexion increase from 12.6 to 50 degrees, and an average first MTP joint plantarflexion increase from 8 to 17.5 degrees.[7]
- In a retrospective comparison study, 21 BioPro hemiarthroplasties and 27 first MTP arthrodeses were evaluated at mean final follow-up of 79.4 and 30 months, respectively.[8] Five (24%) of the hemiarthroplasties failed, 1 of them was revised, and 4 were converted to an arthrodesis. Eight of the feet in which the hemiprosthesis had survived had evidence of plantar cutout of the prosthetic stem on the final follow-up radiographs. The satisfaction ratings in the hemiarthroplasty group were good or excellent for 12 feet, fair for 2, and poor or failure for 7, with a mean pain score of 2.4 out of 10.

- Seventy-nine BioPro first MTP hemiarthroplasties were performed in 76 patients with mean of 2.91-year follow-up with 34 of the procedures also involving flexor hallucis longus transfer to the proximal phalanx.[10] Forty were done in first MTP joints with minimal adaptive arthritic changes and 10 in joints with ankylosis. The mean postoperative ACFAS score was 94, 42 (53%) had freedom from pain, and 45 (57%) had satisfaction or a high level of satisfaction with the outcome. There were eight complications: two patients with severe pain with one requiring implant removal, one sesamoiditis, one extensor hallucis longus contracture, one hallux subluxation, one hallux dislocation, and two misaligned implants.
- Twenty-two elective BioPro first MTP hemiarthroplasties were performed on 20 patients with grade III hallux rigidus with follow-up examination at 1 year and questionnaire at 2 years.[5] There was improvement in average range of motion of 15 degrees from 33 to 48 degrees, visual analogue scale pain score from 4.7 to approximately 1.0, and AOFAS forefoot score from 61 to 86. Painless ambulation occurred after 6 weeks. At 1 year, there was no radiographic loosening or subsidence of any implants. Three patients had postoperative stiffness requiring manipulation under anesthesia, and two patients underwent conversion to arthrodesis for pain attributed to sesamoid arthritis.
- Ninety-seven consecutive BioPro metallic hemiarthroplasties performed in 80 patients (mean age 55 years, range 22 to 74 years) for end-stage hallux rigidus were reviewed with a minimum follow-up of 5 years and no patients lost to follow-up.[3] Fifteen implants in 12 patients required a revision: 1 for infection, 2 for osteolysis, and 12 for pain. Younger age was a significant predictor of revision, and it was suggested that perhaps the use of this implant should be limited to older patients. Significant improvements were demonstrated at 5 years in the Manchester-Oxford Foot Questionnaire and in the physical component of the Short Form-12 score. The overall rate of satisfaction was 75%, and the procedure was found to be a cost-effective intervention.
- A retrospective comparison of 46 patients who had undergone BioPro first MTP hemiarthroplasties and 132 patients who had undergone arthrodesis was performed with median follow-up of 38.4 (range 12 to 96) months and 39.8 (range 12 to 96) months, respectively.[11] There were no statistically significant differences found in the satisfaction rate; the failure rate; or the Foot and Ankle Outcome Score, the Foot Function Index, and Numerical Rating Scale for pain and limitations questionnaires. Two (4.1%) hemiarthroplasties were converted to arthrodesis at 12 and 72 months for persistent pain, and 81.6% were satisfied with the procedure. Five (3.7%) arthrodeses required revision fusion for nonunion, 15 (11.1%) required hardware removal for pain or infection, and 64% were satisfied with the arthrodesis.
- A total of 47 primary arthrodeses and 31 BioPro hemiarthroplasties for Coughlin and Shurna's stage 3 and 4 hallux rigidus with less than 20 degrees of preoperative motion and at least 5-year follow-up were evaluated after a mean follow-up period of 8.6 and 7.7 years, respectively.[2] The mean AOFAS Hallux Metatarsophalangeal–Interphalangeal Scale scores after arthrodesis and hemiarthroplasty were 72.8 ± 14.5 and 89.7 ± 6.6, respectively ($p = .001$).

The patients were significantly more pleased after hemiarthroplasty ($p < .001$), and this procedure was recommended more often ($p < .001$). The number of unplanned repeat surgical procedures did not differ between the two groups. Two hemiarthroplasty patients underwent unplanned surgery for decreased range of motion (<30 degrees) and 1 for loosening while 4 arthrodesis patients underwent unplanned surgery for nonunion, although another 25 arthrodesis patients underwent what was considered planned surgery for hardware removal. Patients also resumed sports activities significantly sooner after hemiarthroplasty ($p = .002$).

COMPLICATIONS

- Infection
- Nerve injury
- Component loosening
- Recurrent pain and loss of motion

REFERENCES

1. Aronow MS, Leger R, Sullivan RJ. The results of first MTP joint hemiarthroplasty in grade 3 hallux rigidus. Presented at: American Orthopaedic Foot & Ankle Society 22nd Annual Summer Meeting; July 15, 2006; La Jolla, CA.
2. Beekhuizen SR, Voskuijl T, Onstenk R. Long-term results of hemiarthroplasty compared with arthrodesis for osteoarthritis of the first metatarsophalangeal joint. J Foot Ankle Surg 2018;57(3):445–450.
3. Clement ND, MacDonald D, Dall GF, et al. Metallic hemiarthroplasty for the treatment of end-stage hallux rigidus: mid-term implant survival, functional outcome and cost analysis. Bone Joint J 2016;98-B(7):945–951.
4. Coughlin MJ, Shurnas PS. Hallux rigidus. Grading and long-term results of operative treatment. J Bone Joint Surg Am 2003;85(11):2072–2088.
5. Giza E, Sullivan M, Ocel D, et al. First metatarsophalangeal hemiarthroplasty for hallux rigidus. Int Orthop 2010;34(8):1193–1198.
6. Goez JC, Townley CO, Taranow WS. An update on the metallic hemiarthroplasty resurfacing prosthesis for the hallux. Presented at: 56th Annual Meeting and Scientific Seminar of the American College of Foot and Ankle Surgeons; February 1998; Orlando, FL.
7. Kissel CG, Husain ZS, Wooley PH, et al. A prospective investigation of the BioPro hemi-arthroplasty for the first metatarsophalangeal joint. J Foot Ankle Surg 2008;47(6):505–509.
8. Raikin SM, Ahmad J, Pour AE, et al. Comparison of arthrodesis and metallic hemiarthroplasty of the hallux metatarsophalangeal joint. J Bone Joint Surg Am 2007;89(9):1979–1985.
9. Roukis TS, Townley CO. BIOPRO resurfacing endoprosthesis versus periarticular osteotomy for hallux rigidus: short-term follow-up and analysis. J Foot Ankle Surg 2003;42(6):350–358.
10. Salonga CC, Novicki DC, Pressman MM, et al. A retrospective cohort study of the BioPro hemiarthroplasty prosthesis. J Foot Ankle Surg 2010;49(4):331–339.
11. Simons KH, van der Woude P, Faber FW, et al. Short-term clinical outcome of hemiarthroplasty versus arthrodesis for end-stage hallux rigidus. J Foot Ankle Surg 2015;54(5):848–851.
12. Taranow WS, Moutsatson MJ, Cooper JM. Contemporary approaches to stage II and III hallux rigidus: the role of metallic hemiarthroplasty of the proximal phalanx. Foot Ankle Clin 2005;10:713–728.
13. Townley CO, Taranow WS. A metallic hemiarthroplasty resurfacing prosthesis for the hallux metatarsophalangeal joint. Foot Ankle Int 1994;15:575–580.

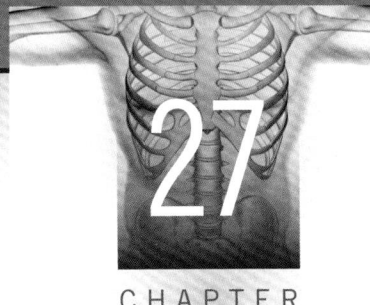

First Metatarsophalangeal Total Joint Arthroplasty with Roto-Glide

Martinus Richter

DEFINITION

- The Roto-Glide (Implants International, Thornaby-on-Tees, United Kingdom; distributed by Ten20 Medical, Dallas, TX) is a noncemented titanium-calcium-phosphate surfaced three-component device for total replacement of the first metatarsophalangeal (MTP-1) joint **(FIG 1)**. It allows for normal mobility in the joint.
- The metatarsal implant has a rather long intramedullary stem. The upper part of the metatarsal head has an anatomic flange. In the middle, it has a crest that corresponds to the natural crest in the lower part of the head. The phalangeal implant also has a stem. This stem is hollow and has a flat surface toward the metatarsal head. Between the metal pieces, a polymeniscus is inserted. This meniscus has a peg corresponding to the hollow phalangeal implant. The cranial surface of the meniscus is congruent with the metatarsal's surface. It should correspond to the crest for sideboard stability.
  - Thus, extension/flexion takes place between the meniscus and the metatarsal implant, whereas rotation takes place between the meniscus and the phalangeal implant.
- The prosthesis comes with different interchangeable sizes and a set of instruments for precise cutting and drilling.

ANATOMY

- The MTP-1 joint is a true synovial joint. It has a capsule and stabilizing elements such as collateral ligaments and tendon. Involved in the articulation are also the two sesamoids.
- Functions are dorsiflexion/plantar flexion, abduction/adduction, and rotation.
- Mobility is foremost dorsiflexion/plantar flexion (80/30) in combination with slight abduction/adduction and rotation

that secures an adaption of the great toe to the ground no matter the position of the foot.

PATHOGENESIS

- Forces during motion are increasing the more dorsiflexion the joint is loaded in and the forces are applied to the upper half of the metatarsal head and the phalangeal counterpart. These forces lead to degeneration of the cartilage over time that effect primarily the upper aspect of the metatarsal head.
- The lower part of the metatarsal head, the base of the phalanx, and the sesamoids are less likely affected.

NATURAL HISTORY

- Total replacement of the MTP-1 joint has been in use for about 35 years. It has never reached a standard where it could compete with other treatments such as osteotomy, cheilectomy, arthroplasty, or arthrodesis.[3]
- This chapter describes the evolution and suggests a new concept. Before going into the different prosthetic designs that have been tried, one should consider the facts about the anatomy, function, mobility, and forces applied to the MTP-1 joint during loading.

PATIENT HISTORY AND PHYSICAL FINDINGS

- Symptoms of arthrosis of the MTP-1 joint include pain in the joint, especially at the dorsal aspect. This gives pressure problems in shoe wear.
  - The other trouble is diminished mobility, especially in dorsiflexion.
- The contour of the metatarsal head is square. On physical examination, osteophytes can be palpated from lateral, over the dorsal aspect, and to the medial side of the metatarsal head.
  - There is a painful collision phenomenon in dorsiflexion.
  - The toe is in an anatomic position and the joint is stable.
  - There may also be distinct pain when moving the sesamoids, especially the tibial one.

IMAGING AND OTHER DIAGNOSTIC STUDIES

- Radiographically, arthrosis in MTP-1 joint is graded into four stages, as shown in **FIG 2**.
- Pedography
  - Unloading under the MTP-1 joint with decreased contact area and decreased force percentage
  - Lateral shift of the course of the center of gravity, especially during the second half of the gait stance phase

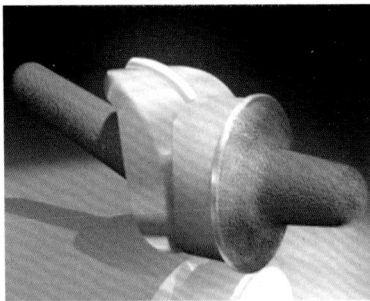

FIG 1 The Roto-Glide is a three-component noncemented device with a mobile bearing.

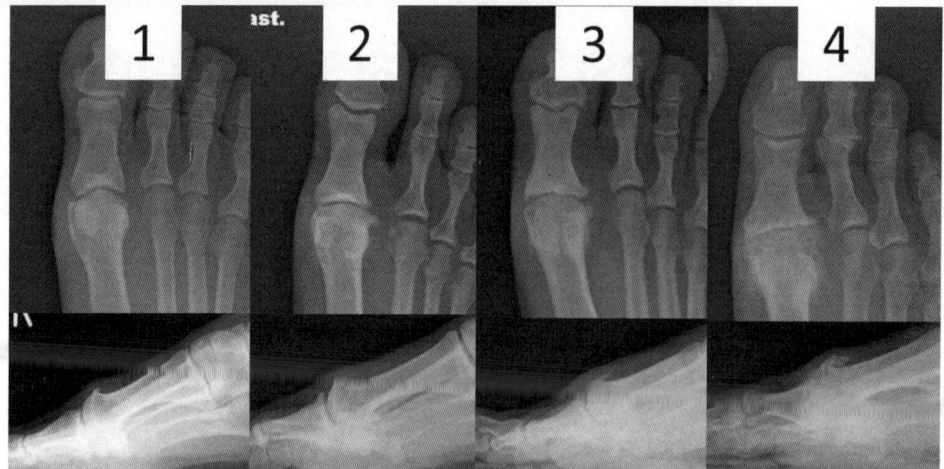

FIG 2 Grades of arthrosis in the MTP-1 joint. *1*, grade 1, dorsal osteophyte; *2*, grade 2, dorsal arthrosis; *3*, grade 3, obliterated joint; *4*, grade 4, ankylosis.

DIFFERENTIAL DIAGNOSIS

- Fracture or pseudarthrosis of the sesamoids
- Gout

NONOPERATIVE MANAGEMENT

- Nonoperative treatment includes stiffening of insole and/or shoe under the MTP-1 joint to decrease the motion of the joint.
- Pain medication, nonsteroidal anti-inflammatory drugs, rest, and complete unloading are other options for nonoperative treatment.

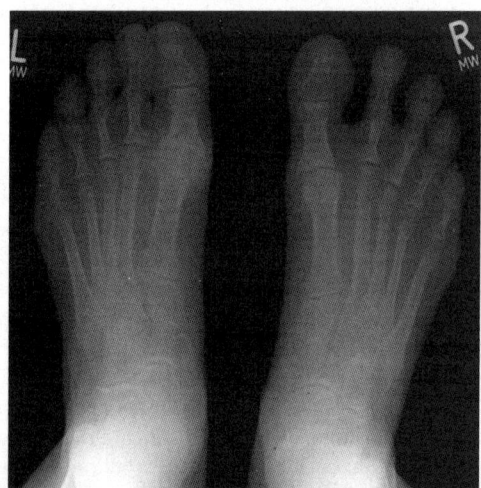

FIG 3 Preoperative radiographs. Dorsoplantar (**A**) and lateral (**B**) views with weight bearing showing a hallux rigidus grade 3.

- Physiotherapy has no proven effect.
- Injections (with corticosteroids) are not recommended due to limited effect and risk of infection.

SURGICAL MANAGEMENT

- Please note that insulin-dependent diabetes mellitus and missing flexor hallucis longus tendon/function are considered as absolute contraindications by the author. Deformities such as hallux valgus are considered as relative contraindications.

Preoperative Planning

- Dorsoplantar and lateral radiographs with weight bearing **(FIG 3)**
- Pedography
- Instruments **(FIG 4A)** with trial implants **(FIG 4B)**

Positioning

- Supine position with leg elevated **(FIG 5)**
- Tourniquet at the thigh

Approach

- Medial approach with straight incision

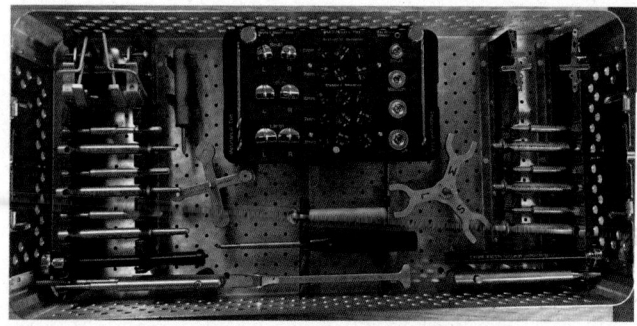

FIG 4 Instruments and trial implants used during the procedure.

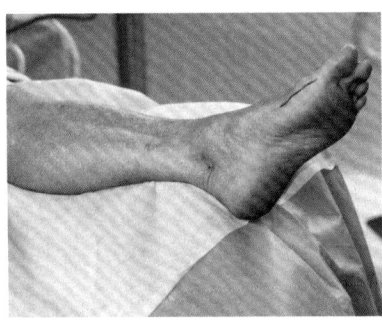

FIG 5 The patient is positioned supine with the leg elevated.

EXPOSURE AND JOINT PREPARATION

- The medial joint capsule is incised **(TECH FIG 1A)**.
- The entire joint, including the sesamoids, is exposed **(TECH FIG 1B)**.
- The flexor hallucis tendon is released but not cut. Synovectomy follows if needed.

- Osteophytes at the metatarsal head are removed dorsally, medially, and laterally.
- The osteophytes at the base phalanx do not need to be removed because they are cut away **(TECH FIG 1C)**.
- Osteophytes at the sesamoids should be removed if present.

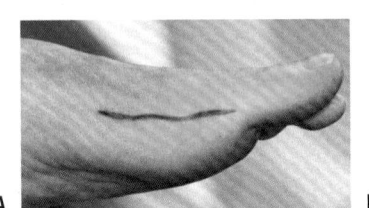
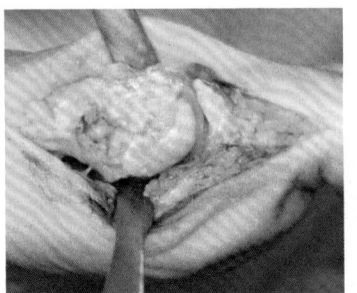
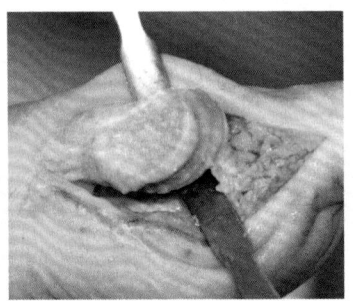

TECH FIG 1 A. A straight medial incision is used. **B.** MTP-1 exposed. **C.** The first metatarsal after resection of the medial pseudoexostosis.

METATARSAL AND PHALANGEAL CUTS

- The metatarsal jig is applied, taking care it is the normal rotation **(TECH FIG 2A)**.
- The angulated cut removes the dorsal osteophyte, and the upper half of the metatarsal head is sliced off at 60 degrees similar to a cheilectomy **(TECH FIG 2B)**.

- Another jig is applied for the cutting of the phalangeal joint surface **(TECH FIG 2C)**. Care must be taken to secure the plantar structures (capsule and the short flexor tendon).
- About 2 or 3 mm of the upper phalanx is resected perpendicular to the phalanx axis **(TECH FIG 2D)**.

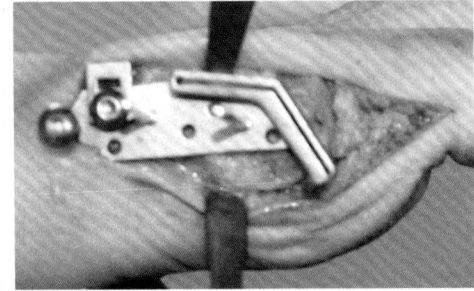
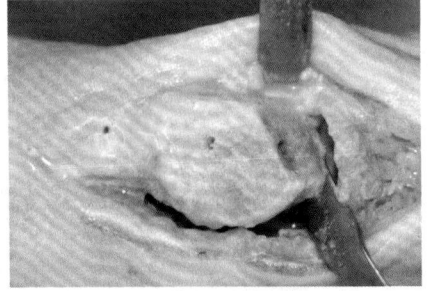

TECH FIG 2 A. Application of the metatarsal jig. **B.** The first metatarsal after dorsal and distal osteotomies. *(continued)*

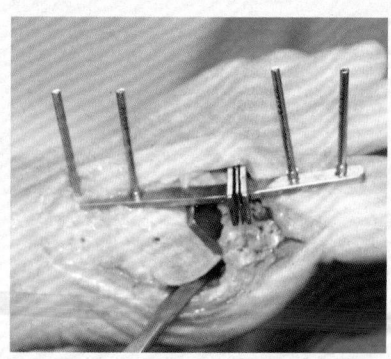
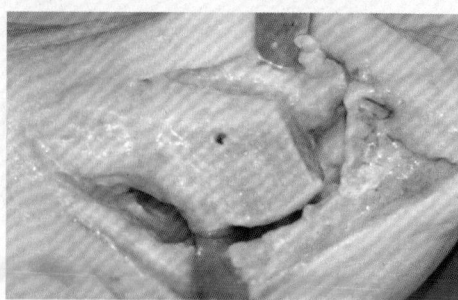

TECH FIG 2 *(continued)* **C.** Application of the jig for the cutting of the phalangeal joint surface. **D.** Phalanx and metatarsal after osteotomies.

PREPARATION OF INTRAMEDULLARY CANALS

- Instruments for drill guides to the medullary canals are used **(TECH FIG 3)**.
- Care must be taken to ensure the holes are centralized and that the hole in the metatarsal head corresponds to the crest.

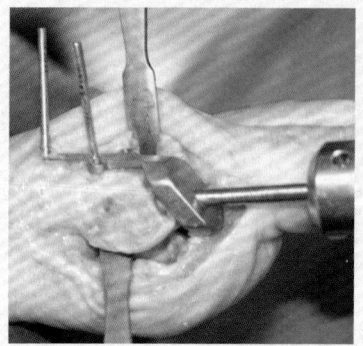
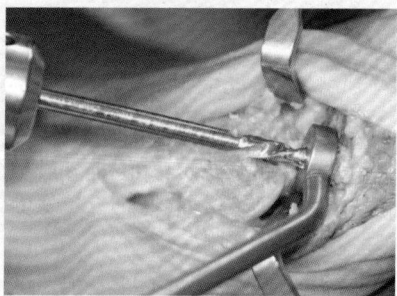

TECH FIG 3 A. Preparation of metatarsal canal. **B.** Preparation of phalangeal canal.

PROSTHESIS INSERTION

- Trial prostheses are inserted, and the best fitting meniscus is inserted and checked fluoroscopically **(TECH FIG 4A,B)**.
- The joint should be a little slack but not sideboard unstable **(TECH FIG 4C,D)**.

- The definite prosthesis is coated and the stems are minimally thicker than the trial prosthesis. This allows for press-fit fixation but might hinder the insertion.
- If the joint cannot move to 80-degree dorsiflexion, fasciotomy of the flexor muscles is performed.

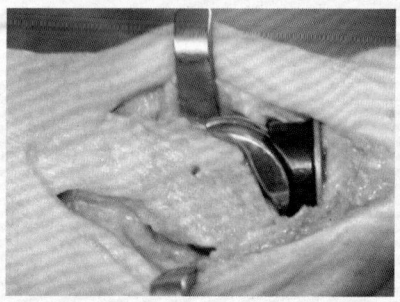
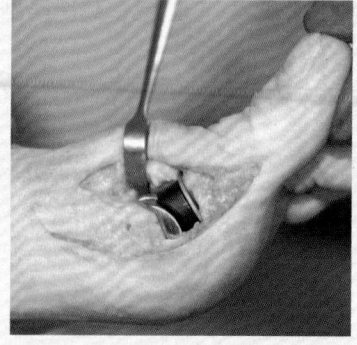

TECH FIG 4 A,B. The trial prosthesis is inserted and tested. *(continued)*

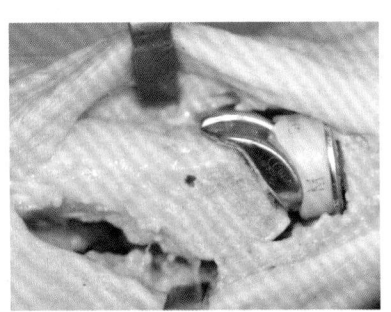

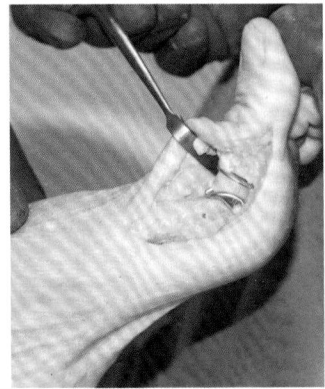

TECH FIG 4 *(continued)* **C,D.** The final prosthesis is inserted.

CLOSURE

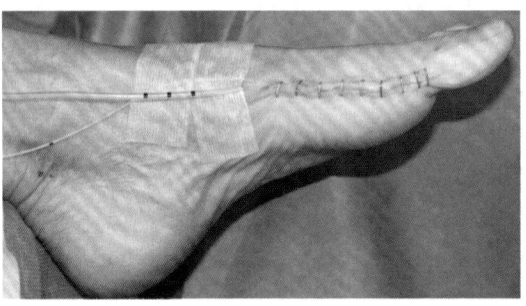

- The wound is closed in anatomic layers (joint capsule, subcutaneous, skin) following the local standard.
- A drainage and pain control catheter is inserted **(TECH FIG 5)**.
- A dressing is applied. No orthosis or cast is needed.

TECH FIG 5 Drain and pain control center inserted.

INTRAOPERATIVE FLUOROSCOPIC IMAGING

- Intraoperative imaging included dorsoplantar **(TECH FIG 6A)** and lateral **(TECH FIG 6B)** views and lateral view with dorsiflexion to confirm adequate range of motion and missing dorsal (sub) luxation during dorsiflexion **(TECH FIG 6C)**.

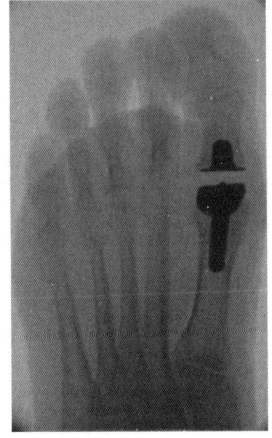

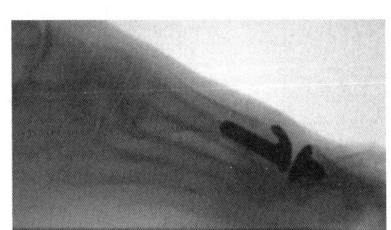

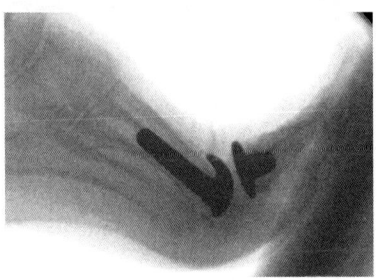

TECH FIG 6 Intraoperative imaging includes dorsoplantar (**A**) and lateral (**B**) views and lateral view with dorsiflexion to confirm adequate range of motion and missing dorsal (sub)luxation during dorsiflexion (**C**). (Same patient as in **FIGS 1–5**.)

Pearls and Pitfalls

Insufficient Flexor Hallucis Longus (Tendon) Function	• Leads to weak or missing push-off and might lead to dorsal (sub)luxation. Inspection and reconstruction if necessary could avoid malfunction/(sub)luxation.

POSTOPERATIVE CARE

- Full weight bearing is allowed in cases with normal bone situations, that is, normal or moderately decreased bone density. Partial weight bearing is safer in cases with significantly decreased bone density.
  - The same strategy is recommended for postoperative physiotherapy. In stable situations, the postoperative care includes direct toe standing exercises. In less stable situations, motion could be limited until osseous integration at 6 weeks.
- Radiographs are taken at 6 weeks to confirm osseous integration (FIG 6).
- The patient is also taught to load on the medial side of the foot over the hallux (the former habit of walking on the lateral side of the foot should be abandoned from day 1).
- Skin sutures or staples are removed 20 days postoperatively, and the instructions on how to walk correctly are reinstructed.
- Pedography at 3 months is recommended to confirm adequate loading of the first ray.

OUTCOMES

- Although stemmed silicone prostheses have been rather successful in hand surgery, it led to a significant number of failures in the great toe replacement. The reasons were the greater forces in the MTP-1 joint and the inability for the device to rotate the joint. This gave rise to breakage of the implant at the joint space level, followed by severe synovitis and eventually removal of the implant, leaving severe bone losses.
- Metal implants have been and are still used either as hemiprosthesis or total prosthesis. The total joints are all two-piece devices. Although uncemented hemiprosthesis may be useful in grades 1 and 2 arthrosis, they have no place in grades 3 and 4 arthrosis. Originally, the two-piece metal devices were cemented. Those with short pegs in the medullary canal loosened. The same has been reported about the uncemented device.[1,4,10] Modern two-piece devices have used metal on polyethylene.
- At 3 years of follow-up, Fuhrmann et al[5] found radiographic loosening in 33% of their cases. In a recent study, Bartak et al[1] found 16% failures after 24 months, which confirms the results of Kundert and Zollinger-Kies.[8]
  - Ceramics have no real long-term results, but the results that have been published are not encouraging with short-term loosening between 12.5% and 18% after 26 months and 3 years, respectively.[2,4]
- In the only attempt of a randomized prospective study, arthrodesis versus total replacement of the MTP-1 joint unfortunately had serious flaws.[6] There was change of the procedure in the replacement group from uncemented to cemented implantation because of loosening of the uncemented devices. The authors used the implant for arthrosis stages 1 to 3, and there were bilateral cases and cases that got both arthrodesis on one side and replacement on the other side. Furthermore, the authors claimed that the arthrodesis group got normal loading of the great toe.
  - This is contradictory to what all others have found, and at the same time, the replacement group did not get any loading on the great toe. Using the knowledge of the biomechanics of the different devices, there would be room for a new device which takes into consideration the failure modes of the current devices. The inventor of the Roto-Glide reported favorable results including improved pedobarographic patterns.[7,11]
- The author has used this prosthesis for 10 years. At present, 92 cases have been treated. A prospective study to compare with arthrodesis has been performed.[9] The aim of this study was to compare outcome (clinical and pedographic) of total joint arthroplasty (TJA) (Roto-Glide) and arthrodesis (A) of MTP-1. All patients that completed follow-up of at least 24 months after TJA and A of MTP-1 before November 5, 2018, were included in the study. Preoperatively and at follow-up, radiographs and/or weight-bearing computed tomographies were obtained. Degenerative changes were classified in four degrees. Standard dynamic pedography was performed (percentage force at first metatarsal head/first toe from force of entire foot). Visual-Analogue-Scale Foot and Ankle (VAS FA) and MTP-1 range of motion (ROM) for dorsiflexion/plantar flexion were registered and compared preoperatively and follow-up. From November 24, 2011, until October 31, 2016, 25 TJA and 49 A were performed that completed follow-up (TABLE 1). Six wound healing delays were registered (TJA, 2; A,4) as only complications. Parameters did not differ between TJA and A (each $p > .05$) except higher force percentage first toe and lower ROM for A at follow-up (each $p < .05$) (see TABLE 1). VAS FA and pedography parameters improved for TJA and A between

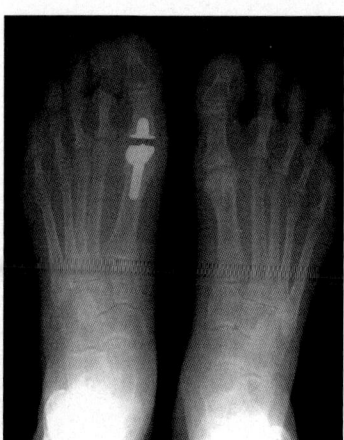

FIG 6 Postoperative radiograph.

TABLE 1 Study Results

	Roto-Glide	Arthrodesis	p
n	25	49	
Surgery			
Age at time of surgery (y)	59	60	.8
Male (%)	7 (28)	14 (29)	.9
Height (cm)	168.2	169.1	.9
Weight (kg)	71.4	72.1	.9
Hallux rigidus stadium (0–4)	3.3	3.1	.7
ROM dorsiflexion/ plantar flexion (degrees)	19.4/0/9.8	20.3/0/9.2	.9
Force percentage First metatarsal head/ sesamoids/great toe (%)	7.9/14.6	8.5/15.3	.8
VAS FA	45.9	46.2	.7
Wound healing delay	2 (8%)	4 (8%)	.9
Follow-up			
Revisions (*n*)	0	0	—
Follow-up time (mo)	45.7 (25.0-80.3)	46.3 (24.1-81.1)	.2
ROM dorsiflexion/ plantar flexion (degree)	35.6/0/10.5	10.5/0/0	.01
Force percentage First metatarsal head/ sesamoids/great toe (%)	15.8/5.8	12.3/10.8	.05
VAS FA	73.4	70.2	.8

ROM, range of motion; VAS FA, Visual-Analogue-Scale Foot and Ankle.

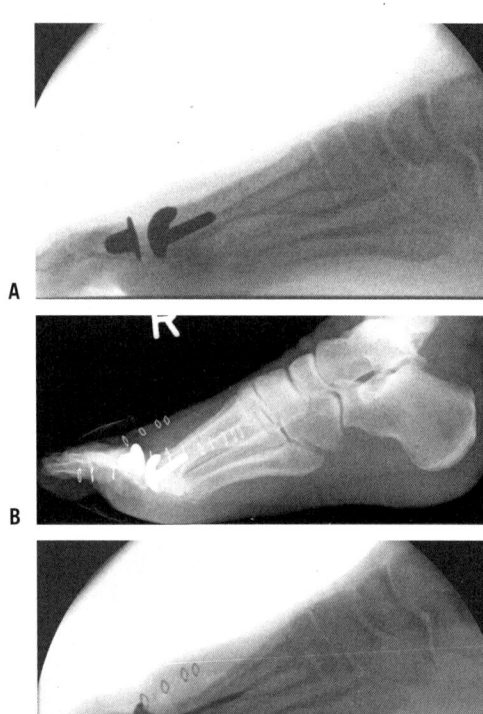

FIG 7 Insufficient flexor hallucis longus (tendon) function leads to weak or missing push-off and might lead to dorsal (sub)luxation. Revision, inspection, and reconstruction if necessary could avoid malfunction/(sub)luxation. If reconstruction is not possible, prosthesis removal and fusion are recommended. **A.** Intraoperative fluoroscopic image with correct position. **B.** Postoperative radiograph with dorsal subluxation. **C.** Intraoperative fluoroscopic image after prosthesis removal and fusion due to nonreconstructible flexor hallucis tendon rupture. The patient desired typical heel elevation of 2 cm, which is simulated intraoperatively to allow for correct positioning of the base phalanx (axis is desired to be parallel to simulated floor with simulated heel elevation).

preoperatively and follow-up, ROM increased for TJA and decreased for A (each *p* <.05) (see **TABLE 1**). In conclusion, TJA and A were performed in similar patient cohorts regarding demographic parameter, degree of degenerative changes, ROM, pathologic pedographic pattern, and VAS FA. TJA and A improved pathologic pedographic pattern and VAS FA at minimum follow-up of 24 months. TJA additionally improved ROM and showed better pedographic pattern (and not different to physiologic pattern) than A. Survival rate of TJA was 100% up to 6 years. In this study, TJA was a valuable alternative to A for treatment of severe MTP-1 osteoarthritis.

COMPLICATIONS

- Stiffness: Revision with arthrolysis and aggressive aftertreatment is recommended.
- Insufficient flexor hallucis longus (tendon) function: leads to weak or missing push-off and might lead to dorsal (sub)luxation. Revision, inspection, and reconstruction if necessary could avoid malfunction/(sub)luxation. If reconstruction is not possible, prosthesis removal and fusion are recommended **(FIG 7)**.
- Polyethylene component wear/disintegration: Revision with exchange of polyethylene component is recommended.
- Loosening: Prosthesis removal and fusion are recommended.
- Infection: Prosthesis removal, repetitive débridement, and staged fusion are recommended.

REFERENCES

1. Bartak V, Popelka S, Hromadka R, et al. Toe-Fit-Plus system for replacement of the first metatarsophalangeal joint. Acta Chir Orthop Traumatol Cech 2010;77(3):222–227.
2. Barwick TW, Talkhani IS. The MOJE total joint arthroplasty for 1st metatarso-phalangeal osteoarthritis: a short-term retrospective study. Foot (Edinb) 2008;18(3):150–155.
3. Brewster M. Does total joint replacement or arthrodesis of the first metatarsophalangeal joint yield better functional results? A systematic review of the literature. J Foot Ankle Surg 2010;49(6):546–552.
4. Brewster M, McArthur J, Mauffrey C, et al. Moje first metatarsophalangeal replacement—a case series with functional outcomes using the AOFAS-HMI score. J Foot Ankle Surg 2010;49(1):37–42.

5. Fuhrmann RA, Wagner A, Anders JO. First metatarsophalangeal joint replacement: the method of choice for end-stage hallux rigidus? Foot Ankle Clin 2003;8(4):711–721.

6. Gibson JN, Thomson CE. Arthrodesis or total replacement arthroplasty for hallux rigidus: a randomized controlled trial. Foot Ankle Int 2005;26(9):680–690.

7. Kofoed H. Is total replacement of the first MTP-joint for arthrosis an option? An overview. Fuss Sprungg 2011;9:39–45.

8. Kundert HP, Zollinger-Kies H. Endoprosthetic replacement of hallux rigidus. Orthopade 2005;34:748–757.

9. Richter M. Total joint replacement of the first metatarsophalangeal joint with Roto-Glide as alternative to arthrodesis. Fuss Sprungg 2019;17:42–50.

10. Sinka S, McNamara P, Bhatia M, et al. Survivorship of the bio-action metatarsophalangeal joint arthroplasty for hallux rigidus: 5-year follow-up. Foot Ankle Surg 2010;16(1):25–27.

11. Wetke E, Zerahn B, Kofoed H. Prospective analysis of a first MTP total joint replacement. Evaluation by bone mineral densitometry, pedobarography, and visual analogue score for pain. Foot Ankle Surg 2012;18(2):136–140.

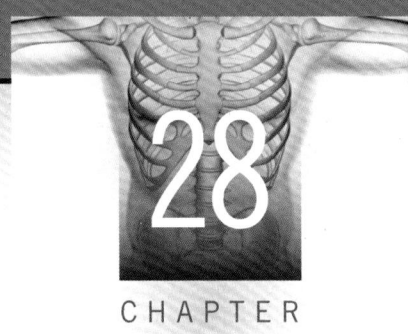

First Metatarsophalangeal Joint Arthrodesis:
Perspective 1

Michael M. Stephens and Ronan McKeown

DEFINITION

- Arthrosis of the first metatarsophalangeal (MTP) joint is commonly seen in osteoarthritis (hallux rigidus), rheumatoid disease, and gout.
- The indication for surgical treatment of the first MTP joint is pain where conservative treatment has failed.
- Arthrodesis of the first MTP joint is the surgical treatment of choice in rheumatoid disease and is indicated in hallux rigidus when the disease is advanced.
- Many techniques in preparation of the joint exist to provide good cancellous apposition:
  - Flat cuts: These make accurate positioning of the toe difficult.
  - Cone or peg socket: This leads to excessive shortening.
  - Ball and socket: This results in minimal shortening and has the additional benefit of ease of adjustment in positioning the toe.
- Various methods of fixation have been described. The most biomechanically advantageous method of fixation has been shown to be a dorsal plate and compression screw.[2,3]

ANATOMY

- The first MTP joint is a ball-and-socket joint.
- The normal hallux valgus angle is less than 15 degrees.
- The metatarsal inclination angle relative to weight bearing is usually 25 to 30 degrees but varies with foot type (greater for cavus, less for planus) (FIG 1).
- The final position of the arthrodesed first MTP joint must allow for heel rise during the late stance phase of gait (third rocker).
- The position can be checked by applying a flat surface to the sole of the foot. The tip of the toe should clear the surface with the interphalangeal joint in full extension and should touch the surface with the interphalangeal joint in 45 to 60 degrees of flexion.

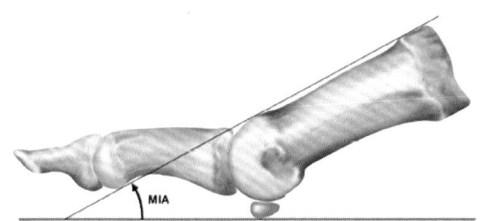

FIG 1 Metatarsal inclination angle (*MIA*).

PATHOGENESIS

- Primary osteoarthritis (hallux rigidus) and the inflammatory arthritides (rheumatoid, gout, psoriatic arthritis) account for the majority of causative factors.
- Secondary osteoarthritis arises from mechanical abnormalities (hallux valgus and varus) and trauma resulting in joint incongruity and excessive cartilage wear.

NATURAL HISTORY

- The natural history of first MTP joint arthrosis is related to its cause.
- Hallux rigidus is a progressive disease process and the joint will deteriorate with time, but the patient's symptoms may not show the same deterioration.
- Progression of arthrosis secondary to the inflammatory arthritides will be related to the activity of the disease.

PATIENT HISTORY AND PHYSICAL FINDINGS

- In true hallux rigidus, patients experience an insidious onset of pain, swelling, and stiffness in the first MTP joint that is aggravated by activity (eg, walking, running).
- Lateral forefoot pain due to overload may develop as the foot supinates to avoid dorsiflexion of the first ray just before and immediately after heel rise.
- A comprehensive physical examination is required to enable diagnosis and selection of correct surgical procedure.
- The physician should palpate the MTP joint for tenderness; dorsal or dorsolateral osteophytes (cheilus) may be palpable and tender.
- The physician should examine the range of motion of the MTP and interphalangeal joints. Restriction in dorsiflexion but full plantarflexion may indicate that a dorsiflexion osteotomy of proximal phalanx may improve the dorsiflexion arc.
- The grind test is not normally painful unless an osteochondral defect is present or degeneration is advanced. If painful, then an arthrodesis is indicated rather than a cheilectomy.
- The physician should observe the patient's walking gait. Avoidance of weight bearing on the hallux implies pain. Increased callus may be present under the lesser metatarsals.
- The physician should palpate for posterior tibial and dorsalis pedis pulses. Peripheral vascular disease is a contraindication to surgery. If suspected, vascular assessment and treatment is required first.

- The physician should palpate and move the tarsometatarsal joint. Arthrosis of the tarsometatarsal joint is a relative contraindication to arthrodesis of the first MTP joint. The examiner should also palpate and move the interphalangeal joint. Arthrosis of the interphalangeal joint is a contraindication to arthrodesis of the first MTP joint.

IMAGING AND OTHER DIAGNOSTIC STUDIES

- Weight-bearing anteroposterior and lateral radiographs should be obtained before surgery.
  - The severity of the arthrosis can be assessed and any co-existing forefoot pathology identified and addressed at the time of surgery.
  - The hallux valgus angle and the metatarsal inclination angle should be measured accurately.
  - The lateral radiograph shows the cheilus and any narrowing of the joint space (either dorsally or throughout).
- Hallux rigidus can be graded using the clinical and radiologic information obtained.
- We have created a seven-point clinicoradiologic grading system (adapted from Coughlin and Shurnas[1]) that correlates the severity of the disease (symptoms, clinical examination, and radiologic findings) with the appropriate surgical procedure (TABLE 1).

NONOPERATIVE MANAGEMENT

- Nonoperative management encompasses activity modification, weight loss, analgesic and anti-inflammatory medication (oral and intra-articular), physiotherapy (tendo Achilles and hamstring stretching), and shoe modification.

- Shoe modification can involve a carbon fiber extended insole with cutouts for the lesser toes, metal stiffeners in the last, and a forefoot rocker sole.

SURGICAL MANAGEMENT

- Arthrodesis of the first MTP joint does not restore normal anatomy or gait pattern. The patient should be counseled as to the surgical goals and optimal outcome in order to have realistic expectations of the surgery.
- Absolute contraindications to first MTP joint fusion include active infection, peripheral vascular disease, and arthrosis of the interphalangeal joint.
- Relative contraindications to first MTP joint fusion include degeneration of the first tarsometatarsal joint and peripheral neuropathy.

Preoperative Planning

- Initial assessment should include examination of circulation, sensation, the first tarsometatarsal joint, the interphalangeal joint, and any previous surgical incisions about the foot.
- It may be necessary to consult with the patient's rheumatologist to reduce or stop immunosuppressant drugs before surgery.
- Preoperative weight-bearing anteroposterior and lateral radiographs should be obtained.

Positioning

- We prefer to position the patient supine with the heels at the end of the operating table.

TABLE 1 Grading of Hallux Rigidus				
Grade	Dorsiflexion	Radiologic Findings	Clinical Findings	Treatment
0	>40 degrees, minimal loss compared to normal side	Normal	No pain, stiffness with decreased range of movement only	Conservative
1a	30–40 degrees, <50% loss compared to normal side but 40 degrees or more painless plantarflexion	Dorsal osteophyte, minimal joint space narrowing	Painful, limited dorsiflexion but large painless and normally unused plantarflexion arc	Moberg osteotomy and cheilectomy
1b	As earlier but minimal plantarflexion arc	As earlier	Occasional dorsal or dorsolateral pain; pain at extreme dorsiflexion (impingement) or plantarflexion (capsular tightening)	Cheilectomy
2a	10–30 degrees, <75% loss compared to normal side	Dorsal, lateral, and medial osteophytes; only the dorsal 25% joint space is narrowed on the lateral radiograph.	Moderate dorsal or dorsolateral pain, just before maximum dorsiflexion or plantarflexion	Cheilectomy
2b	As earlier	As earlier	Dorsal or dorsolateral pain throughout arc of motion (positive grind test)	Arthrodesis
3	<10 degrees, >75% compared to normal side	Cyst formation; on the lateral radiograph, >25% joint space is narrowed; sesamoid involvement	Stiffness and constant pain; extreme pain at end of plantarflexion and dorsiflexion but not at midrange	Arthrodesis
4	As grade 3	As grade 3	As grade 3 plus pain in midrange of motion	Arthrodesis

This grading system is an adaptation by the authors (Stephens and McKeown) from Coughlin M, Shurnas P. Hallux rigidus. Grading and long-term results of operative treatment. J Bone Joint Surg Am 2003;85-A(11):2072–2088. Copyright © 2003 by The Journal of Bone and Joint Surgery, Incorporated.

- A thigh tourniquet is inflated to 350 mm Hg after prophylactic intravenous antibiotics have been given and the limb has been exsanguinated.
- The foot and leg are then prepared and draped above the knee in a routine manner.
- The end of the table is dropped 20 to 30 degrees. The surgeon sits at the end of the table.

Approach

- A dorsal approach is recommended regardless of previous scars. Care should be taken to avoid the dorsal cutaneous nerve and extensor hallucis longus. The former is retracted medially and the latter laterally, so they are protected.

EXPOSURE

- Make a dorsal slightly curved incision just medial to the extensor hallucis longus tendon and lateral to the dorsal cutaneous nerve, extending from the middle of the shaft of the first metatarsal to the interphalangeal joint.
- Retract the extensor hallucis longus tendon laterally.
- Make a capsulotomy in the same plane and expose the joint.
- Perform a synovectomy.
- Release the medial and lateral soft tissues to allow maximum plantarflexion of the proximal phalanx, exposing both articular surfaces.

JOINT PREPARATION

- Excise any large medial eminence or osteophyte with an oscillating saw.
- Excise osteophytes on the proximal phalanx to find the true center and size of the articular surface.
- Size the articular surface of the proximal phalanx to determine the correct convex reamer required.
- Insert a 1.6-mm Kirschner wire through the center of the articular surface of the proximal phalanx and pass it in line with its long axis. In osteoporotic bone, the wire should cross the interphalangeal joint into the distal phalanx to prevent toggling of the wire, leading to eccentric reaming.
- Guide the sized convex reamer over the Kirschner wire and ream the surface sparingly to expose subchondral cancellous bone **(TECH FIG 1A)**.

- Remove the Kirschner wire. Remove any fine collar of cartilage remaining around the wire entry hole. Insert the wire into the center of the articular surface of the first metatarsal and advance it along its long axis. If the bone is osteoporotic, then the wire should cross the tarsometatarsal joint.
- Use the matched-sized concave reamer in a similar fashion to expose the subchondral cancellous bone of the metatarsal head **(TECH FIG 1B)**. Remove the wire and retain all fragments of bone in the reamer. Any areas of hard subchondral bone can be drilled with the Kirschner wire.

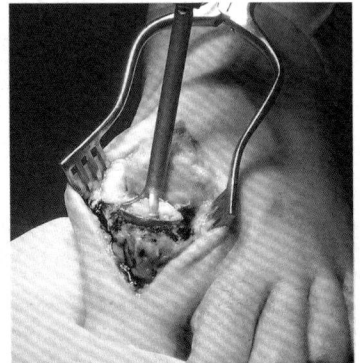
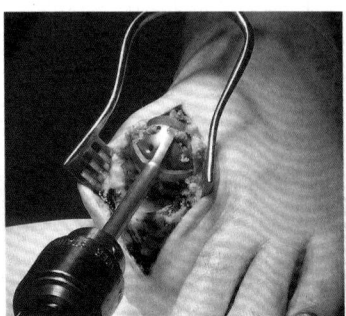

TECH FIG 1 A. Reaming the articular surface of the proximal phalanx. **B.** Reaming the articular surface of the metatarsal head.

TECHNIQUES

POSITIONING

- Approximate the position of the hallux in relation to the first metatarsal and fix the position temporarily with an obliquely directed 1.6-mm Kirschner wire.
  - The ideal position is 20 to 25 degrees of dorsiflexion of the proximal phalanx in relation to the first metatarsal axis.
  - The valgus angle should be 10 to 15 degrees.
  - However, a gap of 3 to 5 mm must be left between the hallux and the second toe.
  - The rotation of the hallux should be neutral so that the arc of rotation of the interphalangeal joint is at 90 degrees to the weight-bearing surface.
- Confirm the correct position of the hallux by placing a flat surface against the sole of the foot and bringing the ankle to 90 degrees. In this position, with the interphalangeal joint in full extension, the tip of the hallux lies about 1 cm from the flat surface. When the interphalangeal joint is flexed to 45 to 60 degrees, its tip comes in contact with the plantar surface. This enables the foot to have a third rocker on heel rise **(TECH FIG 2)**.

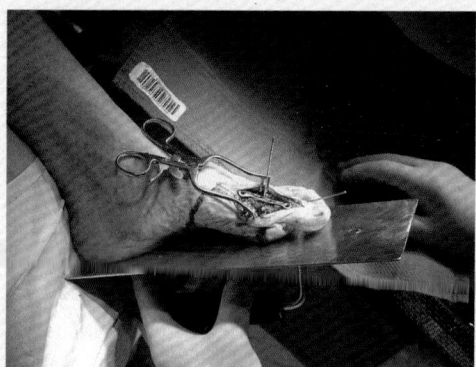

TECH FIG 2 Foot plate to check arthrodesis position.

FIXATION

- Insert an oblique 2.7-mm compression screw of appropriate length from distal medial to proximal lateral across the MTP joint.
- Size and secure the plate on the dorsal aspect of the joint with a Kirschner wire and fix it with six 2.7-mm self-tapping screws **(TECH FIG 3A,B)**. The Kirschner wires are then removed.
  - The plate is available in three side-specific (left and right) sizes (small for a small hallux, medium for a larger hallux, large for revision arthrodesis).
- Close the wound in layers over a drain.
- Apply a compression dressing.

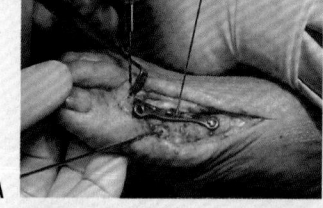
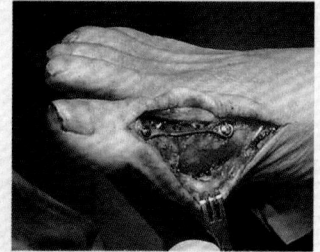

TECH FIG 3 A. Plate secured with temporary Kirschner wire. **B.** Screw fixation of plate.

TECHNIQUES

Pearls and Pitfalls

Clinical Examination	• Coexisting arthritis of the tarsometatarsal and interphalangeal joints should be excluded. • Plantarflexion of the first MTP joint is functionless in bipedal gait. When painless, a Moberg osteotomy is helpful in patients with a good plantarflexion arc, especially in athletes.
Final Arthrodesis Position	• Too dorsiflexed: A painful corn develops on the dorsum of the interphalangeal joint. • Too plantarflexed: Callosities may form under the condyles of the proximal phalanx. With time, a hyperextension deformity can arise in the interphalangeal joint (recurvatum). • Too varus: not a major concern but can cause problems with footwear • Too valgus: This can be a major problem and causes great irritation of the second toe due to impingement and the inability to cleanse the web space.

POSTOPERATIVE CARE

- If this technique is performed as an isolated procedure, we do not use a cast but a compressive dressing and a postoperative stiff-soled shoe to allow early mobilization. Active interphalangeal joint motion is encouraged immediately.
- Patients are kept non–weight bearing for 2 weeks and then encouraged to bear weight by heel walking for 2 weeks.
- Four weeks after surgery, a radiograph is taken (**FIG 2**). If there is evidence of consolidation, forefoot weight bearing is commenced in the postoperative shoe. Progression to full forefoot loading, assisted by crutches, follows over the next 4 weeks.
- Radiographs taken 8 weeks after surgery usually confirm consolidation. At this stage, flat shoes with cushioned, shock-absorbing soles are worn.

OUTCOMES

- Union rates for arthrodesis are quoted in the literature ranging from 80% upward. Using this technique, we have achieved 100% union. The average time for union to be visible radiologically is 6 weeks. All patients experienced significant improvement in their outcome scores.[2]

COMPLICATIONS

- Potential complications of first MTP joint arthrodesis include malunion, infection, delayed union, interphalangeal joint stiffness, extensor hallucis longus tenodesis (secondary to scarring), dorsal cutaneous nerve damage, and hardware problems.
- The incision described in this technique minimizes the risk to the extensor hallucis longus and dorsal cutaneous nerve while facilitating maximal plantarflexion to allow reaming.
- The ball-and-socket bone end preparation minimizes shortening and provides a large congruent cancellous area of contact, enabling easy positioning of the hallux and reducing consolidation time. Temporary Kirschner wire fixation facilitates correct alignment.
- Use of the compression screw followed by a dorsal neutralization plate ensures maximum stability.

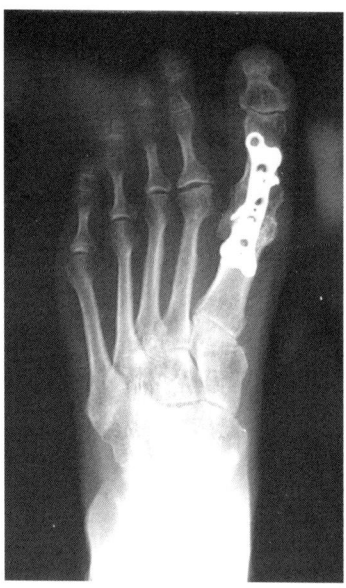

FIG 2 Radiograph taken 4 weeks after surgery.

- The low-profile precontoured titanium plate has inbuilt dorsiflexion and hallux valgus angles and is contoured to the specific shapes of the proximal phalanx and the first metatarsal. Depending on the metatarsal inclination angle, the degree of dorsiflexion on the plate can be adjusted. It acts as a neutralization plate and facilitates correct positioning. The differing screw axes increase pullout strength.
- These mechanical factors significantly reduce the risk of delayed union and nonunion.

REFERENCES

1. Coughlin M, Shurnas P. Hallux rigidus. Grading and long-term results of operative treatment. J Bone Joint Surg Am 2003;85(11):2072–2088.
2. Flavin R, Stephens MM. Arthrodesis of the first metatarsophalangeal joint using a dorsal titanium contoured plate. Foot Ankle Int 2004;25: 783–787.
3. Politi J, Hayes J, Njus G, et al. First metatarsal-phalangeal joint arthrodesis: a biomechanical assessment of stability. Foot Ankle Int 2003;24:332–337.

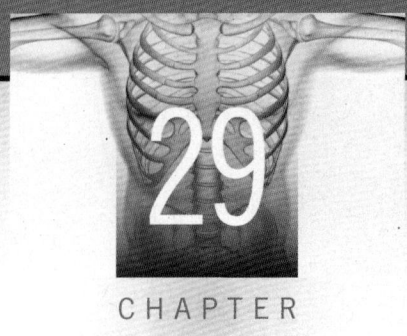
First Metatarsophalangeal Joint Arthrodesis: Perspective 2

James R. Jastifer, Bertil W. Smith, and Michael J. Coughlin

DEFINITION

- The term *hallux rigidus* refers to a painful condition of the first metatarsophalangeal (MTP) joint of the great toe that is characterized by restricted motion (mainly dorsiflexion) and periarticular bone formation.
- The basic pathologic entity is that of degenerative arthritis.
- Initially, hallux rigidus is characterized by pain, swelling, and MTP joint synovitis.
- As the degenerative process proceeds, proliferation of bony osteophytes on the dorsal and dorsolateral aspect of the first metatarsal head develop.
- With advanced disease, near-complete bony ankylosis may occur.

ANATOMY

- The round, cartilage-covered first metatarsal head articulates with the somewhat smaller, concave base of the proximal phalanx.
- Articulating on the plantar surface of the metatarsal head are the two sesamoids, which are contained in the tendon of the flexor hallucis brevis.
- Distally, the two sesamoids are attached by the plantar plate to the base of the proximal phalanx.
- The sesamoids are connected by the intersesamoidal ligament and protect, on their plantar surface, the tendon of the flexor hallucis longus within its tendon sheath.
- Dorsally, the extensor hallucis longus is anchored medially and laterally by the dorsal capsule and MTP joint hood ligaments.

- The tendons of the abductor and adductor hallucis pass medially and laterally but much closer to the plantar surface of the MTP joint (**FIGS 1** and **2**).

PATHOGENESIS

- The cause of hallux rigidus has not been determined, but joint trauma often is cited as a predisposing factor.
  - This may occur as a single episode, such as an intra-articular fracture, as a crush injury, or with repetitive microtrauma.
  - In a patient who sustains an acute injury to the MTP joint, forced hyperextension or plantarflexion may lead to an acute chondral or osteochondral injury.
- The only documented factors associated with the cause of hallux rigidus are a flat or chevron-shaped metatarsal articular surface, bilaterality in those with a positive family history, and female gender.
- Metatarsus primus elevatus typically is a secondary phenomenon related to the severity of the disease and restricted MTP joint motion and is not a primary cause of hallux rigidus (**FIG 3**).

NATURAL HISTORY

- A patient with hallux rigidus typically complains of stiffness with ambulation and pain localized to the dorsal aspect of the first MTP joint that is aggravated by walking, especially during toe-off.
- Patients tend to ambulate with an inverted foot posture to prevent stress on the first MTP joint.

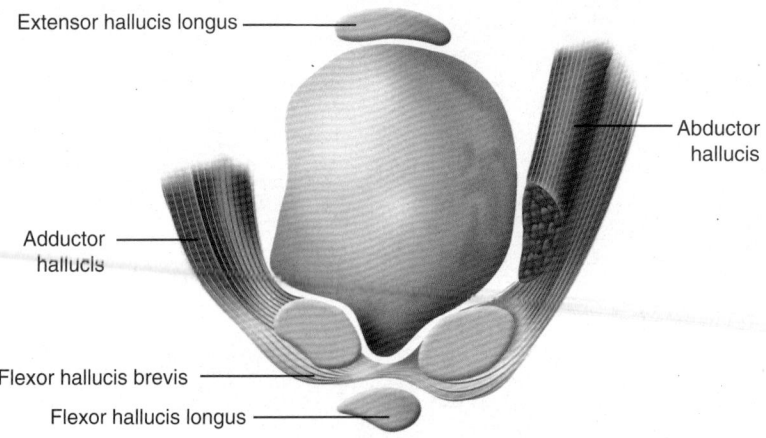

Extensor hallucis longus

Abductor hallucis

Adductor hallucis

Flexor hallucis brevis

Flexor hallucis longus

FIG 1 Axial drawing of the first MTP joint.

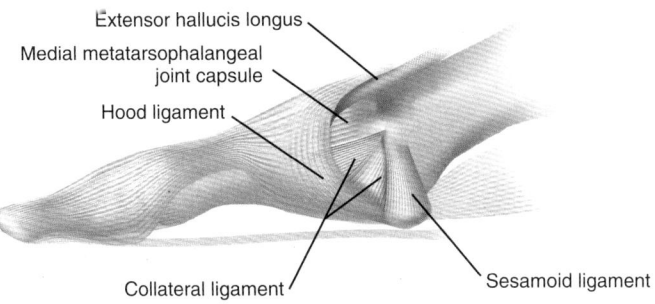

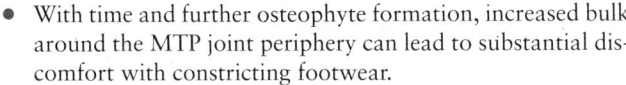

FIG 2 Lateral drawing of the first MTP joint.

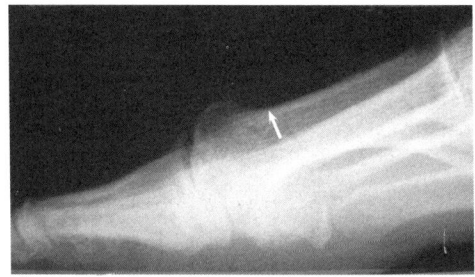

FIG 3 Lateral radiograph of a patient with hallux rigidus and notable metatarsus primus elevatus. The *arrow* shows the elevation of the first metatarsal relative to the second.

- With time and further osteophyte formation, increased bulk around the MTP joint periphery can lead to substantial discomfort with constricting footwear.
- More than 80% of patients, if followed long enough, will develop bilateral symptoms.
- Ninety-five percent of patients with bilateral symptoms have a positive family history.

PATIENT HISTORY AND PHYSICAL FINDINGS

- Patients will commonly report insidious onset pain with activity, which is relieved by rest.
- Pain is most commonly located dorsally as opposed to pain associated with hallux valgus, which is commonly over the medial eminence.
- Physical exam:
  - Patients often have pain and restricted first MTP joint motion with forced dorsiflexion.
  - There is commonly a dorsal ridge of bone on the distal first metatarsal and periarticular osteophytes.

- Other disease processes may be identified and must be considered including a gastrocnemius contracture, hammer toe deformity, and interdigital neuromas.

IMAGING AND OTHER DIAGNOSTIC STUDIES

- Weight-bearing radiographs (anteroposterior [AP], lateral, and sesamoid views) are obtained to evaluate the first MTP joint.
- The Coughlin/Shurnas classification of hallux rigidus **(TABLE 1)** is used to grade the severity of joint arthrosis.
- The AP radiograph often demonstrates nonuniform joint space narrowing with widening and flattening of the first metatarsal head.
- An oblique radiograph may demonstrate a well-preserved joint space, which is obscured on the AP radiograph by overlying osteophytes.
- On the lateral radiograph, with more severe disease, the dorsal metatarsal osteophyte resembles "dripping candle wax" as it courses proximally along the first metatarsal **(FIG 4)**.

TABLE 1 Coughlin/Shurnas Clinical and Radiographic Classification of Hallux Rigidus

Grade	Dorsiflexion	Radiograph[a]	Clinical
0	40–60 degrees and/or 10%–20% loss compared with normal side	Normal or minimal findings	No pain; only stiffness and loss of passive motion on examination
1	30–40 degrees and/or 20%–50% loss compared with normal side	Dorsal osteophyte is main finding; minimal joint space narrowing, minimal periarticular sclerosis, minimal flattening of metatarsal head	Mild or occasional pain and stiffness; pain at extremes of dorsiflexion and/or plantarflexion on examination
2	10–30 degrees and/or 50%–75% loss compared with normal side	Dorsal, lateral, and possible medial osteophytes giving flattened appearance to metatarsal head; no more than one-fourth of dorsal joint space involved on lateral radiograph; mild to moderate joint narrowing and sclerosis; sesamoids not usually involved but may be irregular in appearance	Moderate to severe pain and stiffness that may be constant; pain occurs just before maximum dorsiflexion and maximum plantarflexion on examination.
3	Less than or equal to 10 degrees and/or 75%–100% loss compared with normal side. There is notable loss of MTP plantarflexion as well (often 10 degrees or less plantarflexion).	As in grade 2 but with substantial narrowing, possible periarticular cystic changes, more than 25% dorsal joint may be involved on lateral side, sesamoids are enlarged and/or cystic and/or irregular.	Nearly constant pain and substantial stiffness at extremes of range of motion but not at midrange
4	Same as grade 3	Same as grade 3	Same as grade 3 but with definite pain at midrange of motion

[a]Weight-bearing anteroposterior and lateral radiographs are used.
MTP, metatarsophalangeal joint.
Reprinted with permission from Coughlin MJ, Shurnas PS. Hallux rigidus. Grading and long-term results of operative treatment. J Bone Joint Surg Am 2003;85-A(11): 2072–2088. Copyright © 2003 by The Journal of Bone and Joint Surgery, Incorporated.

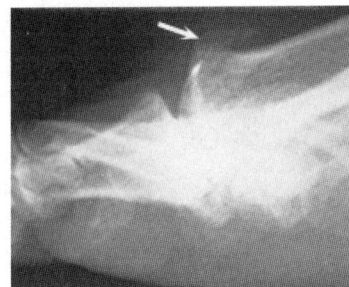

FIG 4 Lateral radiograph of a patient with hallux rigidus. The *arrow* points to a large dorsal metatarsal osteophyte.

- The lateral radiograph also may be used to evaluate for the presence of an elevated first metatarsal in relation to the lesser metatarsals. Up to 5 mm of elevation is considered normal (see **FIG 3**).
- Dorsal proximal phalangeal osteophytes and loose bodies also may be seen.
- Subchondral cysts and sclerosis in the first metatarsal head, widening of the base of the proximal phalanx, and hypertrophy of the sesamoids are characteristic findings in more advanced stages of hallux rigidus.
- Rarely, a magnetic resonance imaging scan may be necessary to identify an occult chondral or osteochondral injury in a younger patient with a history of an acute injury.

DIFFERENTIAL DIAGNOSIS

- MTP joint synovitis
- Osteochondral injury or loose body
- Gouty arthropathy
- Hallux rigidus
- Rheumatoid arthritis
- Turf toe or capsular ligamentous injury

NONOPERATIVE MANAGEMENT

- Conservative management of symptomatic hallux rigidus depends on a patient's symptoms and the magnitude of the articular degenerative process (see **TABLE 1**).
- Nonsteroidal anti-inflammatory drugs and a graphite insole or Morton extension to reduce MTP motion are the mainstays of conservative treatment (**FIG 5**).

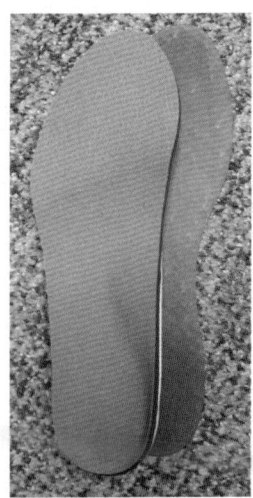

FIG 5 Graphite insole with liner used to restrict first MTP joint motion.

- Several commercially prefabricated orthoses provide rigidity to the forepart of the shoe and can be moved from shoe to shoe.
- The addition of an extended steel or fiberglass shank placed between the inner and outer sole may be effective in reducing MTP joint motion as well.
- Custom-made orthoses may be fabricated to reduce midfoot pronation, which also may help to reduce symptoms.
- Unfortunately, orthoses also diminish available room in the toe box of the shoe, which may, in turn, increase pressure on the dorsal exostosis.
- Occasionally, judicious use of an intra-articular corticosteroid injection may provide temporary relief of pain. Repeated injections, however, may accelerate the degenerative process and are discouraged.
- Synovitis and limited MTP joint motion without radiographic changes should be evaluated by ruling out an inflammatory or erosive joint process with the following laboratory tests: serum complete blood count, erythrocyte sedimentation rate, C-reactive protein, antinuclear antibody, rheumatoid factor, human leukocyte antigen B27, and uric acid tests.

SURGICAL MANAGEMENT

- Indications and contraindications for surgery are presented in **TABLE 2**.

TABLE 2 Indications and Contraindications for Surgery

Indications	Contraindications
Grade 4 hallux rigidus	Active infection
Grade 3 hallux rigidus with less than 50% metatarsal articular cartilage remaining at the time of surgery	Significant IP joint degenerative arthritis
Deformity associated with severe hallux valgus, recurrent hallux valgus, traumatic arthritis, and rheumatoid arthritis	Grades 1, 2, and 3 hallux rigidus (with >50% metatarsal articular cartilage remaining at the time of surgery) in younger athletic patients, in which case a cheilectomy is preferable.[10,15,17]
Neuromuscular disorder with instability	Severe osteoporosis, which can make it difficult to stabilize a fusion site with routine methods of internal fixation
Failed implant surgery of the first MTP joint	

IP, interphalangeal; MTP, metatarsophalangeal.

Preoperative Planning

- All imaging studies must be carefully evaluated.
- An arthrodesis provides stability to the first MTP joint, maintains length of the first ray, relieves pain, achieves permanent correction of any deformity of the hallux, and allows the use of ordinary shoes.
- For grade 4 hallux rigidus, salvage procedures in addition to MTP joint arthrodesis include excisional arthroplasty,[7,17] soft tissue interpositional arthroplasty,[8,17] and prosthetic replacement.[17]
- The Keller procedure may be considered in more sedentary patients or the household ambulator with a grade 3 or 4 hallux rigidus. However, Coughlin and Mann[7] reported significant postoperative metatarsalgia after excisional arthroplasty.

Positioning

- The patient is placed supine on the operating table with a bump beneath the ipsilateral buttock to align the foot in a neutral position (**FIG 6**).
- A popliteal, sciatic, or ankle block is used for anesthesia.
- An Esmarch bandage is used to exsanguinate the foot and ankle. It is applied as an ankle tourniquet and wrapped just above the malleoli with a thin layer of padding beneath the bandage (**FIG 7**).

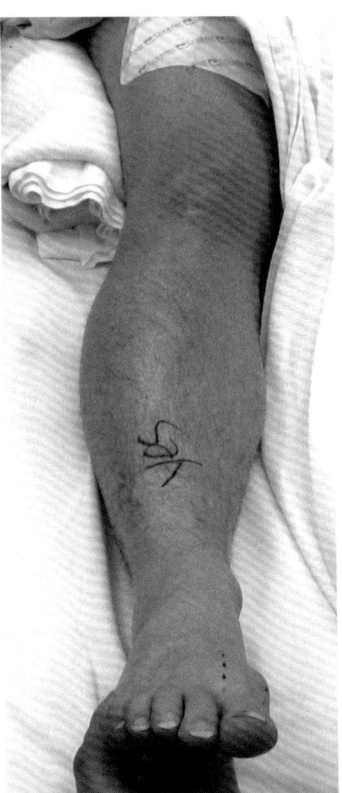

FIG 6 Patient is positioned supine with a bump under the ipsilateral hip allowing the foot to rest in a neutral position.

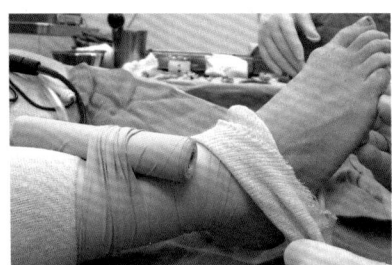

FIG 7 An Esmarch bandage is used as a tourniquet.

Approach

- Numerous surgical techniques have been proposed describing various approaches, techniques of joint preparation, and methods of internal fixation to improve both the alignment and the success rate of arthrodesis.
- Although the use of flat surfaces for MTP joint arthrodesis has been popular because of the simplicity of creating horizontal osteotomies of the proximal phalanx and metatarsal articular surfaces, this technique requires precision to obtain the desired alignment.
- The joint is prepared with a power reaming system coupled with internal fixation with a dorsal plate, providing a strong construct that "brings the bones to the plate," usually ensuring correct alignment.
- The convex male reamer excavates the proximal phalanx to a concave congruous surface, whereas the concave female portion of the reamer shapes the metatarsal surface to a matching uniform, curved hemisphere (**FIG 8**).
- The cup-shaped surfaces tend to resect less bone, reducing shortening of the first ray.
- The curved nature of the cup-shaped surfaces allows preparation without predetermination of the dorsiflexion or plantarflexion, rotation, and varus and valgus alignment.
- After the joint preparation is completed, the surgeon can then select the appropriate alignment for the MTP joint arthrodesis.

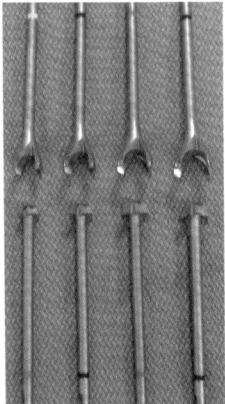

FIG 8 Four sizes of matched metatarsal and phalangeal reamers.

JOINT EXPOSURE

- A dorsal longitudinal incision is centered directly over the MTP joint in an interval between the medial and lateral common digital nerves.
- The incision is extended from a point just proximal to the interphalangeal joint of the hallux to a point 3 to 4 cm proximal to the MTP joint.
- The dissection is deepened along the medial aspect of the extensor hallucis longus tendon through the extensor hood and the joint capsule **(TECH FIG 1A)**.
- A thorough synovectomy is performed, and the MTP joint is inspected to locate osteophytes or loose bodies and to assess the extent of the articular cartilage damage **(TECH FIG 1B)**.

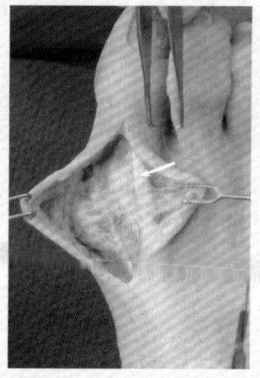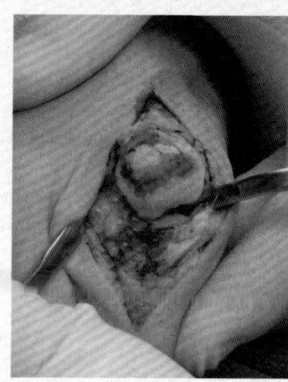

TECH FIG 1 A. Dissection is carried out medial to the extensor hallucis longus tendon (*arrow*). **B.** The extensor hallucis longus tendon has been retracted medially and a capsulotomy performed.

JOINT RESECTION AND DECOMPRESSION

- A thin section of the articular surfaces of the distal first metatarsal and proximal phalanx is removed using a sagittal saw **(TECH FIG 2A,B)**.
- If further shortening of the first ray is desired, more bone may be resected from the metatarsal head.

- By decompressing the MTP joint, increased exposure is achieved for the MTP joint surface preparation.
- A sagittal saw is also used to resect the medial eminence if the fusion is performed for a hallux valgus deformity **(TECH FIG 2C)**.

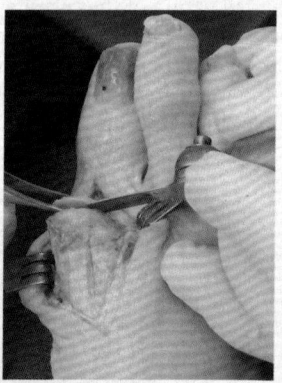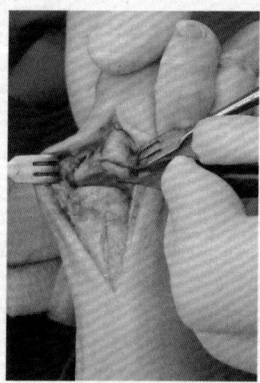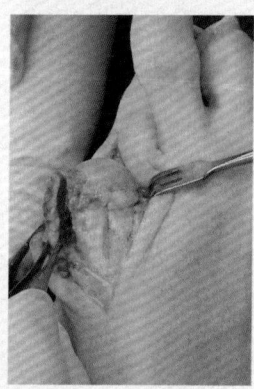

TECH FIG 2 A. A wafer of the distal first metatarsal is removed. **B.** A thin section of the base of the proximal phalanx is resected. **C.** The medial eminence is resected in a patient with a hallux valgus deformity.

METATARSAL HEAD PREPARATION

- A 0.062-inch Kirschner wire (K-wire) is driven in a proximal direction at the center of the metatarsal head **(TECH FIG 3A)**.
- The appropriate size of the reamer is chosen by comparing the diaphyseal width of the metatarsal to the inner size of the metatarsal reamer.
- The power reamer engages the K-wire and is then driven in a proximal direction, shaving the metatarsal subchondral

surface and metaphysis to a cup-shaped convex surface **(TECH FIG 3B)**.
- Any debris or excess bone along the periphery is removed with a rongeur.
- The K-wire is then removed and used to perforate the prepared metatarsal head in multiple places to increase the surface area for arthrodesis **(TECH FIG 3C)**.

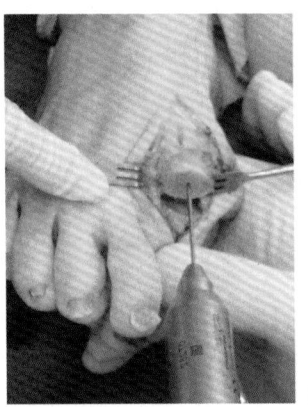 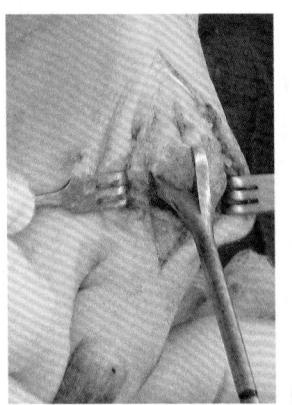 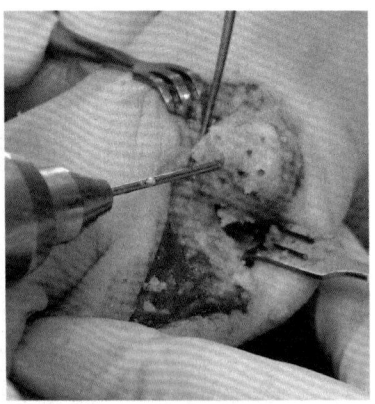

TECH FIG 3 A. A K-wire is placed in the center of the metatarsal head. **B.** Power reamers prepare the metatarsal joint surface. **C.** Multiple perforations in the prepared metatarsal head.

PROXIMAL PHALANGEAL PREPARATION

- A 0.062-inch K-wire is centered on the base of the proximal phalanx and driven distally **(TECH FIG 4A)**.
- The smallest of the convex cannulated phalangeal reamers is then chosen to prepare the phalangeal surface. Care must be taken to avoid "plunging" the reamer, as the proximal phalanx metaphyseal bone is often extremely osteoporotic beneath the subchondral bone.

- Each successively larger reamer is used to enlarge the phalangeal surface until it matches the size of the prepared metatarsal surface **(TECH FIG 4B)**.
- The K-wire is then removed and used to perforate the prepared phalangeal surface in multiple places to increase the surface area for arthrodesis **(TECH FIG 4C)**.
- Cancellous bone shavings are collected throughout the joint preparation process and saved in a small cup to form a slurry for use as an autograft as the surfaces are coapted.

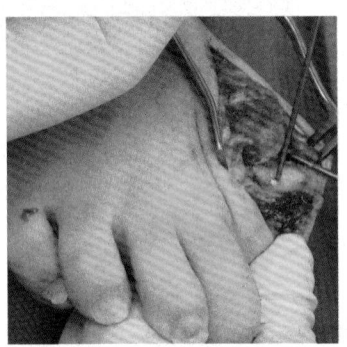 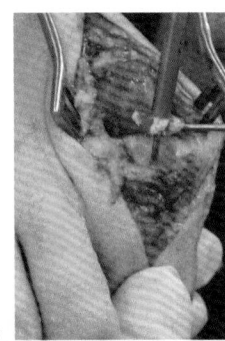 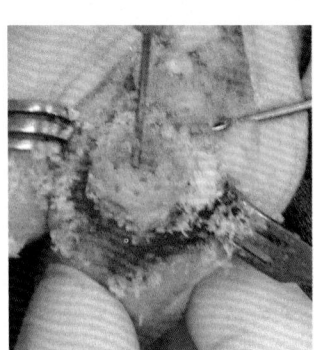

TECH FIG 4 A. A K-wire is placed in the center of the base of the proximal phalanx. **B.** Power reamers prepare the proximal phalangeal joint surface. **C.** Multiple perforations in the prepared base of the proximal phalanx.

JOINT ALIGNMENT

- The bone slurry saved from the reamings is placed between the joint surfaces **(TECH FIG 5)**.
- The congruous cancellous joint surfaces are coapted in the desired amount of varus and valgus, dorsiflexion and plantarflexion, and rotation.
- The desired position is 20 to 25 degrees of dorsiflexion, 10 to 15 degrees of valgus, and neutral rotation. For women who

prefer high-heeled shoes, increased dorsiflexion at the fusion site may be desirable.
- All angular measurements relate to the axis of the first metatarsal shaft.
- An advantage of using the ball-in-socket surface preparation technique is that any dimension may be adjusted without disturbing the other alignment variables.

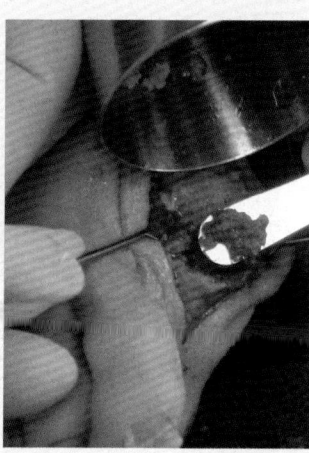

TECH FIG 5 Cancellous autograft bone reamings are placed between the prepared joint surfaces before fixation.

INTERNAL FIXATION

- After obtaining proper alignment, the arthrodesis site is temporarily stabilized with one or two crossed 0.062-inch K-wires (**TECH FIG 6**).
- A rongeur is used to smooth the dorsal aspect of the first metatarsal and proximal phalanx to allow the plate to sit flush against the bone.
- The primary arthrodesis plate comes prebent to the desired dorsiflexion and valgus angles and is placed over the dorsal aspect of the prepared metatarsal and proximal phalanx (**TECH FIG 7**).
- If more or less dorsiflexion is desired, the plate may be bent further to the desired dorsiflexion.
- If more or less valgus is desired, the plate may be offset slightly to accommodate MTP joint angulation.
- Bicortical self-tapping screws are used first to fix the plate to the proximal phalanx. Locking screws may be used in the presence of osteopenic bone, which is often the case.
- The plate is then affixed to the metatarsal, with the first screw placed in compression. There is usually no need for locking screws in the metatarsal because the bone quality is generally better (**TECH FIG 8A**).
- The K-wire is then removed, and a neutralization screw is placed to augment the fixation construct.
- The general philosophy is that in most cases, the plate can be trusted for appropriate alignment of the arthrodesis.

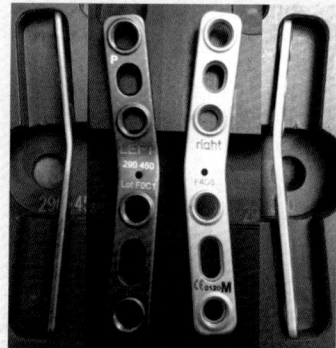

TECH FIG 7 Precontoured primary arthrodesis plates.

- Using the flat surface of an instrument cover is helpful to ensure the hallux is in appropriate and acceptable dorsiflexion alignment.
- The capsule and skin are then closed in a routine manner (**TECH FIG 8B**).

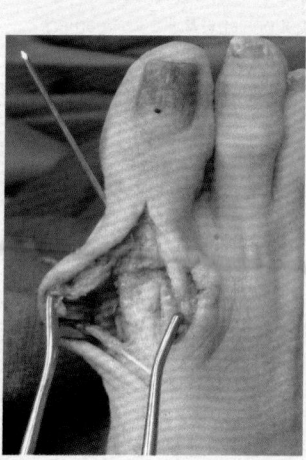

TECH FIG 6 Temporary fixation with a 0.062-inch K-wire.

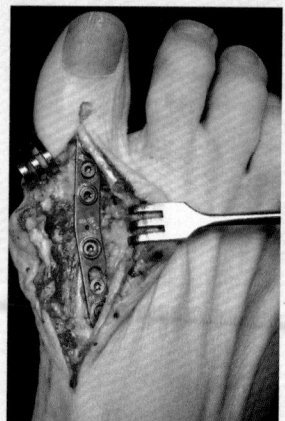 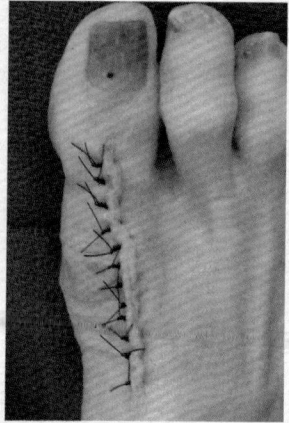

TECH FIG 8 A. Dorsal plate in place. The compression screw will augment the fixation construct. **B.** Final wound closure with interrupted mattress sutures.

Pearls and Pitfalls

Joint Preparation	• Results vary depending on the selected method of joint preparation. • An enlarged surface area is created by using the ball-and-socket–shaped reamers. • Coupled with this, multiple perforations of the prepared surfaces and the use of a bony slurry aid in increasing the rate of successful joint fusion.
Alignment	• If the MTP joint is fixed in a straight position (minimal valgus or slight varus), the medial border of the hallux may impact the toe box of the shoe. • Dorsiflexion of less than 10 degrees may cause a complaint of pressure at the tip of the toe. • Malrotation in either pronation or supination is poorly tolerated **(FIG 9)**. • The use of precontoured plates helps to minimize this type of complication.

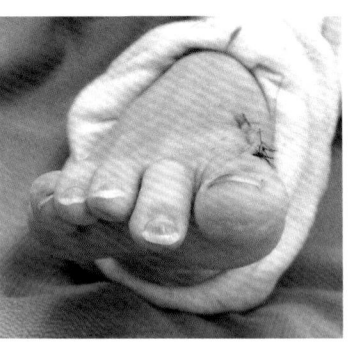

FIG 9 Neutral rotation of the final arthrodesis. Note that the toenail is parallel to the plantar surface of the foot.

Internal Fixation	• A variety of methods can be used to stabilize the arthrodesis, including K-wires, single or cross screws, staples, wire sutures, and plates. • We have demonstrated a high rate of successful fusion with dorsal plates and a cross-compression screw.
Radiographic Parameters	• Although preoperative radiographs may demonstrate an abnormally widened 1–2 intermetatarsal angle, a first metatarsal osteotomy is rarely, if ever, indicated in combination with a first MTP joint arthrodesis. • Typically, following decompression and arthrodesis of the first MTP joint, the 1–2 intermetatarsal angle will reduce substantially.

IMPLANT CONSIDERATIONS

- Ball-and-socket reaming followed by a dorsal plate and crossing screw has been shown to be biomechanically the strongest construct when compared to others; however, union rates are likely similar between different constructs.[16]
- The addition of the cross screw in this technique adds to the stability in the sagittal plane over a dorsal plate alone.[1]
- This biomechanical stability of this technique may be particularly useful in cases of severe hallux valgus when the deforming forces on the first ray may be increased.

POSTOPERATIVE CARE

- The foot is wrapped in a gauze-and-tape compression dressing following the surgery, and the dressing is changed weekly.
- The patient is allowed to ambulate in a postoperative shoe or short walking boot.
- Weight initially is borne on the heel and lateral aspect of the foot.
- Dressings are discontinued, and the patient is transitioned to normal shoe wear at 12 weeks after surgery with radiographic evidence of a successful MTP joint arthrodesis **(FIG 10)**.

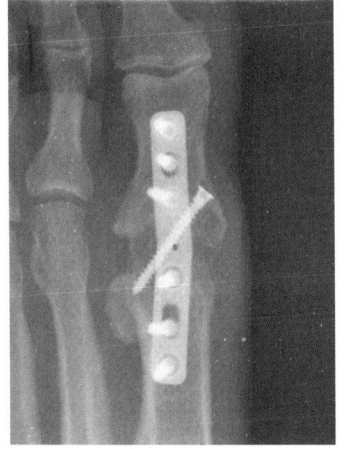

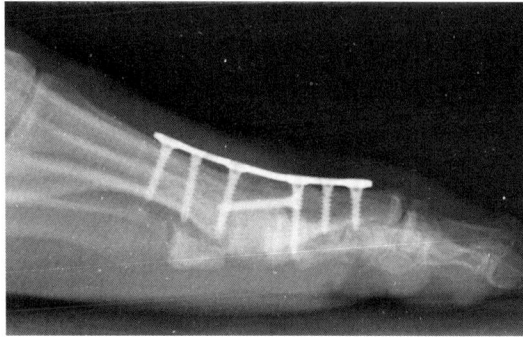

FIG 10 AP (**A**) and lateral (**B**) radiographs of a healed first MTP joint fusion.

OUTCOMES

- In seven published series on the use of conical joint preparation and dorsal plate fixation for MTP joint arthrodesis, we have achieved a 95% fusion rate (313/327 first MTP joint arthrodeses).[3–6,10,12–14]
- The preoperative diagnoses of this multiseries cohort included patients with hallux rigidus (28%); hallux valgus, as a primary, recurrent, or postoperative complication (41%); and rheumatoid arthritis (31%).
- Of the 14 nonunions in this multiseries analysis, only 5 were symptomatic.
- Although the concept of the ball-and-socket–shaped preparation of joint surfaces has changed little over the last two decades except for refinement of power reamer design,[2,3,5,9,13,17] the techniques and design of the dorsal plate fixation have changed dramatically.
- Our initial use of a stainless steel minifragment plate witnessed a 34% hardware removal rate (12/35) after fusion and occasional hardware failure.[3]
- More recently, the use of a precontoured low-profile titanium plate has demonstrated a significant reduction in the incidence of hardware removal to 2% (2/99 cases).[12,13]
- Subjective good and excellent results were noted in 92% of cases (301/327 feet).
- Overall, 48 patients were noted to have slight progression of interphalangeal joint arthritis, but only 6 were symptomatic.
- Return to sports is common. One study demonstrated 96% of patients were satisfied with the procedure regarding return to sports and activities and reached their maximal level of participation in 88.6% of physical activities.[11]

COMPLICATIONS

- Nonunion
- Malunion
- Hardware failure
- Interphalangeal joint arthritis

REFERENCES

1. Cone B, Staggers JR, Naranje S, et al. First metatarsophalangeal joint arthrodesis: does the addition of a lag screw to a dorsal locking plate influence union rate and/or final alignment after fusion. J Foot Ankle Surg 2018;57(2):259–263.
2. Coughlin MJ. Arthrodesis of the first metatarsophalangeal joint. Orthop Rev 1990;19:177–186.
3. Coughlin MJ. Arthrodesis of the first metatarsophalangeal joint with mini-fragment plate fixation. Orthopedics 1990;13:1037–1048.
4. Coughlin MJ. Rheumatoid forefoot reconstruction. A long-term follow-up study. J Bone Joint Surg Am 2000;82(3):322–341.
5. Coughlin MJ, Abdo RV. Arthrodesis of the first metatarsophalangeal joint with Vitallium plate fixation. Foot Ankle Int 1994;15:18–28.
6. Coughlin MJ, Grebing BR, Jones CP. Arthrodesis of the metatarsophalangeal joint for idiopathic hallux valgus: intermediate results. Foot Ankle Int 2005;26:783–792.
7. Coughlin MJ, Mann RA. Arthrodesis of the first metatarsophalangeal joint as salvage for the failed Keller procedure. J Bone Joint Surg Am 1987;69(1):68–75.
8. Coughlin MJ, Shurnas PJ. Soft-tissue arthroplasty for hallux rigidus. Foot Ankle Int 2003;24:661–672.
9. Coughlin MJ, Shurnas PS. Hallux rigidus. Bone Joint Surg Am 2004;86-A(suppl 2, pt 2):119–130.
10. Coughlin MJ, Shurnas PS. Hallux rigidus. Grading and long-term results of operative treatment. J Bone Joint Surg Am 2003;85(11):2072–2088.
11. Da Cunha RJ, MacMahon A, Jones MT, et al. Return to sports and physical activities after first metatarsophalangeal joint arthrodesis in young patients. Foot Ankle Int 2019;40(7):745–752.
12. Doty J, Coughlin MJ, Hirose CB, et al. Hallux metatarsophalangeal joint arthrodesis with a hybrid locking plate and a plantar neutralization screw: a prospective study. Foot Ankle Int 2013;34(11):1535–1540.
13. Goucher N, Coughlin M. Hallux metatarsophalangeal joint arthrodesis using dome-shaped reamers and dorsal plate fixation: a prospective study. Foot Ankle Int 2006;27:869–876.
14. Grimes JS, Coughlin MJ. First metatarsophalangeal joint arthrodesis as a treatment for failed hallux valgus surgery. Foot Ankle Int 2006;27:887–893.
15. Mann RA, Coughlin MJ, DuVries HL. Hallux rigidus: a review of the literature and a method of treatment. Clin Orthop Relat Res 1979;(142):57–63.
16. Politi J, John H, Njus G, et al. First metatarsal-phalangeal joint arthrodesis: a biomechanical assessment of stability. Foot Ankle Int 2003;24(4):332–337.
17. Shurnas P, Coughlin M. Arthritic conditions of the foot. In: Coughlin M, Mann R, Saltzman C, eds. Surgery of the Foot and Ankle, ed 8. Philadelphia: Elsevier, 2007:805–922.

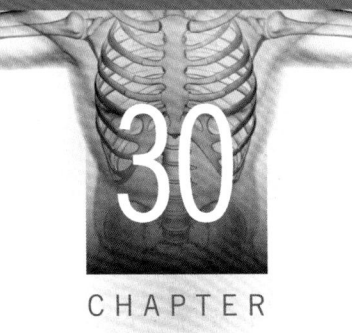

First Metatarsophalangeal Joint Arthrodesis:
Perspective 3

John T. Campbell and Kevin L. Kirk

DEFINITION

- Disorders of the first ray are a common cause of foot and ankle problems. Arthrodesis of the hallux metatarsophalangeal (MTP) joint is a utilitarian technique in contemporary foot and ankle surgery.
- Arthrodesis can effectively address a variety of conditions affecting the hallux, including deformity, inflammatory and degenerative arthritides, spasticity and neuromuscular disorders, and salvage of failed surgeries.
- The most important aspect of this procedure is optimal positioning of the toe during first MTP joint arthrodesis.

ANATOMY

- The bony anatomy of the first MTP joint includes the rounded first metatarsal head, which articulates with the concave, elliptically shaped base of the proximal phalanx.
- Two longitudinal grooves separated by the crista, a central prominence, are located on the plantar surface of the metatarsal head. The two sesamoid bones contained in the medial and lateral tendon slips of the flexor hallucis brevis articulate with their corresponding longitudinal grooves on the inferior surface of the first metatarsal head. The flexor

hallucis longus (FHL) tendon runs between the two sesamoids, bypassing the MTP joint to insert distally onto the distal phalangeal base.
- The extensor hallucis brevis tendon inserts into the dorsal MTP capsule and the extensor hallucis longus runs distally to insert onto the distal phalanx.
- The strong, fan-shaped collateral ligaments of the MTP joint originate medially and laterally from the metatarsal head and run distally and plantarward to the base of the proximal phalanx. The metatarsosesamoid ligaments fan out in a plantar direction to the margin of the sesamoid and the plantar capsule.
- Distally, the two sesamoids are attached by the fibrous plantar plate to the base of the proximal phalanx, stabilizing the joint plantarly (FIG 1).

PATHOGENESIS

- Common forms of degenerative arthritis that affect the hallux MTP joint include hallux rigidus and posttraumatic arthritis. Hallux rigidus may be the result of isolated trauma, with forced hyperextension and resultant chondral injury, or the result of repetitive microtrauma of the articular cartilage. Pathologic alteration in the kinematics of the first MTP joint also may lead to degenerative changes.

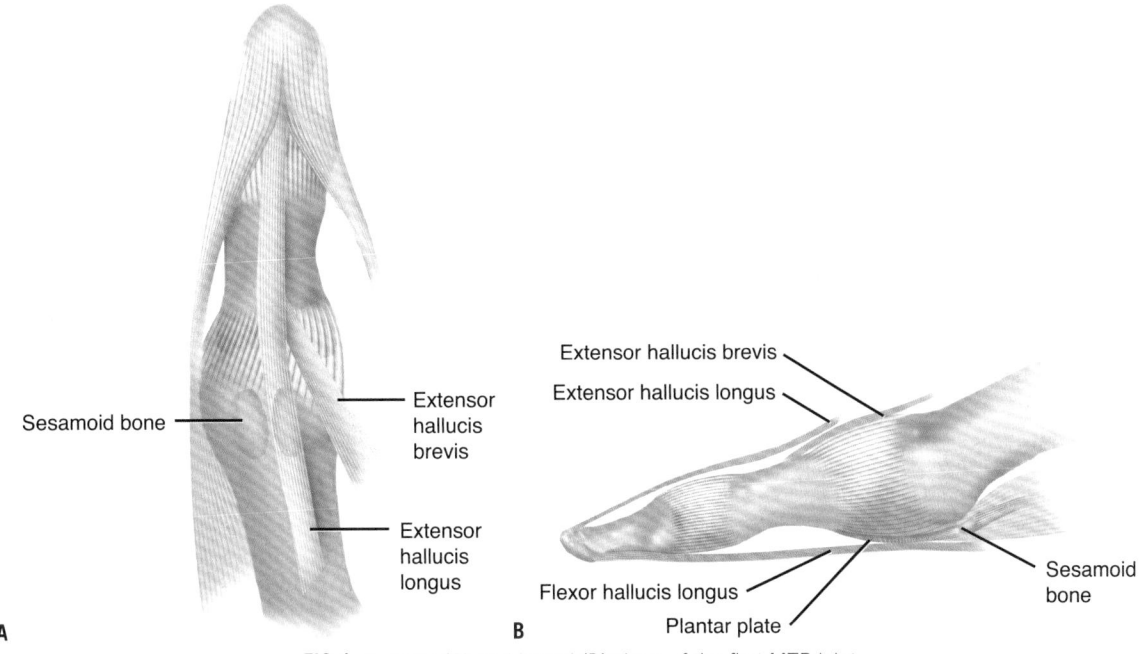

FIG 1 Anterior (**A**) and lateral (**B**) views of the first MTP joint.

- Chondral erosion or loss is seen dorsally on the metatarsal head and phalangeal base.
- Inflammatory arthropathies can affect the hallux MTP joint, necessitating fusion. Common causes include rheumatoid arthritis, gouty arthropathy, lupus, and seronegative spondyloarthropathies. Repetitive episodes of synovitis lead to chondral loss and joint narrowing.
- Progressive hallux valgus or hallux varus with severe deformity, spasticity (secondary to neurologic conditions), soft tissue contracture, or failed implant arthroplasty also may benefit from MTP arthrodesis.

NATURAL HISTORY

- Hallux rigidus and degenerative arthritis present with progressive pain, stiffness, and osteophyte formation of the MTP joint.
- Initial symptoms of inflammatory arthritides include pain and swelling from MTP synovitis; progressive disease is marked by worsening stiffness, pain, and deformity.
- Hallux valgus or hallux varus deformities typically are flexible in the early stage, but over time, these deformities tend to become progressively rigid secondary to joint contracture.
- All of these conditions can produce pain, difficulty with ambulation, and transfer metatarsalgia to the lesser toes.

PATIENT HISTORY AND PHYSICAL FINDINGS

- Patient history
  - Pain and mechanical symptoms on ambulation in hallux rigidus and degenerative arthritis
  - Pain at rest or in the morning with inflammatory arthritis
  - Pain with shoe wear over the hallux or medial eminence (bunion)
  - Some patients complain of the dorsal prominence over the first MTP joint.
- Physical findings
  - Careful interview of the patient to identify contributing medical conditions, shoe wear history, previous treatment methods, and previous surgical procedures

- Standing examination of the foot to assess for malalignment of the toe, including varus, valgus, or claw deformity
- Gait examination to identify dynamic deformity of the foot, including forefoot supination or generalized pes planovalgus
- Visible shortening of the hallux, failure of the toe to engage the ground, and lesser toe metatarsalgia or keratosis (callus) indicate mechanical unloading of the first ray.
- Examination of the seated patient allows observation for callus, skin irritation, or presence of dorsal or medial bunion.
- Palpation elicits tenderness about the joint. Hallux rigidus typically is tender dorsally, whereas the pain with hallux valgus is located medially over the bunion. Advanced degenerative or inflammatory arthritides exhibit diffuse tenderness about the MTP joint and axial grinding of the phalanx against the metatarsal elicits pain.
- Manipulation of the joint is performed to assess stability of the collateral ligaments and the relative flexibility or rigidity of varus or valgus toe deformity.
- Range-of-motion examination often shows limited passive MTP dorsiflexion, with normal or reduced plantar flexion.
- Skin irritation may be present over the dorsal exostosis or medial bunion.
- Tingling, hypesthesias, or a positive Tinel (percussion) sign over the dorsal hallucal nerve may indicate nerve compression from synovitis or dorsal osteophytes.

IMAGING AND OTHER DIAGNOSTIC STUDIES

- Standing anteroposterior (AP), lateral, and oblique radiographs are the standard views for evaluation. Additional views, such as a sesamoid view, sometimes are indicated.
  - The weight-bearing AP view is obtained to determine the overall alignment of the MTP joint. It also can be assessed for the extent of arthritic involvement, including joint narrowing; flattening of the metatarsal head; and the presence of subchondral sclerosis, erosions, or cystic changes within the metatarsal head, osteopenia, or bone loss (**FIG 2A**). This view can also facilitate evaluation of

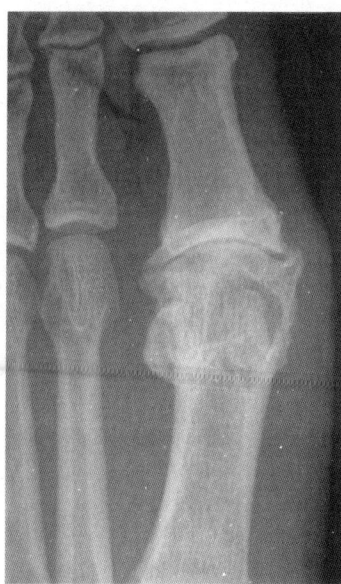

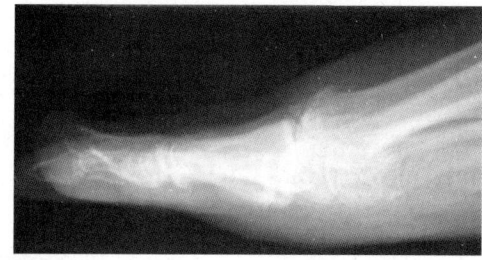

FIG 2 A. AP weight-bearing radiograph of the first MTP joint. Note the joint narrowing, extensive osteophytes, and the medial subchondral cyst. **B.** Lateral weight-bearing view of the first MTP joint. A large dorsal osteophyte and plantar joint space narrowing are noted.

shortening of the first ray relative to the lesser metatarsals. The oblique view also can illuminate these findings.

- The lateral weight-bearing view can show dorsal metatarsal or phalangeal osteophytes and can be used to evaluate the degree of joint narrowing (particularly plantarly) and the presence of an elevated first metatarsal **(FIG 2B)**. However, the plantar two-thirds of the joint can be obscured by overlapping shadows of the lesser metatarsals.
- An axial sesamoid view can be an adjunctive radiograph for evaluating the metatarsal–sesamoid articulation for narrowing or cystic changes, although involvement of the metatarsosesamoid joint occurs infrequently, except with severe arthrosis.
- Additional imaging studies, such as computed tomography (CT) or magnetic resonance imaging (MRI), are sometimes necessary. CT scan may be useful for defining the degree of bone loss, fracture, or cyst involvement in failed implant arthroplasty or inflammatory arthritis, whereas MRI can identify avascular necrosis of the metatarsal head; these can assist in preoperative planning such as the possible need for intraoperative bone grafting.

DIFFERENTIAL DIAGNOSIS

- Arthrodesis is appropriate for surgical correction of the following conditions[5,11,12,16]:
  - Osteoarthritis or posttraumatic arthritis
  - Hallux rigidus
  - Failed interpositional arthroplasty or implant arthroplasty (silastic, metallic, or polyvinyl alcohol)
  - Severe hallux valgus, particularly in elderly patients
  - Hallux varus caused by inflammatory disorders, iatrogenic deformity after previous surgery, or idiopathic involvement
  - Inflammatory arthropathies, including rheumatoid arthritis, lupus, gout, and seronegative spondyloarthropathies
  - Soft tissue contracture, as in scleroderma
  - Deformity secondary to neurologic conditions or spasticity, such as that occurring in patients with diabetes or those who have experienced a stroke

NONOPERATIVE MANAGEMENT

- Nonoperative measures to be attempted before MTP arthrodesis include the following:
  - Nonsteroidal anti-inflammatory drugs to decrease joint pain and inflammation
  - Judicious use of corticosteroid injections into the hallux MTP joint to relieve synovitis, although repeated injections are not advised
  - The use of silicone gel, cotton wool, or felt pads to relieve pressure from calluses or impingement against the shoe or adjacent toe

- Strapping or taping of the hallux may be useful for flexible deformities.
- Comfortable shoe wear with low heels and wide toe box; extra-depth shoes may allow use of an orthotic device. Shoe modifications, such as a stiff sole or metatarsal bar, may unload the forefoot during push-off.
- A full-length orthotic insole with a carbon fiber or stainless steel extension may limit the motion of a painful MTP joint in hallux rigidus.
- Custom accommodative orthotic insole with a buildup under the hallux may improve weight bearing of a shortened or dorsiflexed first ray to diminish transfer metatarsalgia.

SURGICAL MANAGEMENT

- In situ hallux MTP arthrodesis is a utilitarian technique with a wide range of indications.[2–5,10–13,16–18,20,21,27]
- Absolute contraindications include active infection of the MTP joint, severe peripheral vascular disease, and poor soft tissue envelope secondary to systemic disease or scar tissue.
- A relative contraindication to MTP arthrodesis is symptomatic interphalangeal joint arthritis; however, concurrent arthrodesis of both joints has been described.[24]

Preoperative Planning

- Radiographs are assessed for extensive bony lysis, erosions, or cysts that may require bone grafting.
- Severe bone loss, shortening, or failed implant arthroplasty may require distraction of MTP arthrodesis with bulk bone graft, discussed elsewhere.
- Standard arthrodesis can be performed under general, spinal, or regional anesthesia, such as a popliteal or ankle block.
  - We prefer to administer an ankle block in conjunction with intravenous sedation, using a 1:1 mixture of 2% lidocaine and 0.5% ropivacaine, via a 25-gauge needle.

Positioning

- The patient is positioned supine with a roll under the ipsilateral hip.
- Our preferred technique is use of an Esmarch tourniquet applied over cotton padding at the level of the supramalleolar ankle. Alternatively, the procedure can be performed without a tourniquet or with use of a pneumatic calf or thigh tourniquet.

Approach

- Our preferred approach is a dorsal incision centered over the MTP joint.
- An alternate approach is the medial midline incision, based on the surgeon's preference or if a previous medial surgical scar exists.

EXPOSURE

- Make a dorsal incision over the MTP joint just medial to the extensor hallucis longus tendon.[4,9–12,16,18,21]
- Carry the dissection down to the joint capsule, avoiding the dorsomedial cutaneous nerve, a terminal branch of the superficial peroneal nerve.[3]
- Retract the extensor hallucis longus tendon laterally and perform an arthrotomy directly over the MTP joint.[10–12,16,18]
- Perform subperiosteal dissection to raise medial and lateral flaps off the metatarsal head and base of the proximal phalanx, exposing the joint **(TECH FIG 1)**.[3,4,21]
- Release the collateral ligaments and the plantar portion of the joint by releasing the plantar plate with a Freer elevator.
- Remove large osteophytes and loose ossicles with a rongeur.
- Resect the medial eminence from a dorsal approach with a microsagittal saw or chisel.[11,16,21]

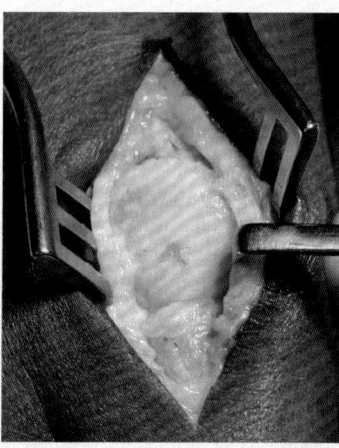

TECH FIG 1 Exposure of metatarsal head through dorsal approach. The extensor hallucis longus tendon is retracted laterally with the exposed metatarsal head, showing a large dorsal osteophyte and loss of articular cartilage.

JOINT PREPARATION

- Prepare the joint surfaces for arthrodesis with a power burr or specialized reamers.
  - Biomechanically, spherical surfaces provide for improved stability compared with flat cuts.[7] Hemispherical surfaces also provide more freedom for positioning the arthrodesis compared with flat saw cuts.
- We use specialized reamers that produce similar hemispheric surfaces **(TECH FIG 2A)**.[5,10–12,16,18]
- Insert a guidewire axially in the center of the metatarsal head. Use a cannulated, concave-shaped reamer to prepare the metatarsal head.
- Remove the wire and then insert it in the proximal phalanx and use a cannulated convex reamer while plantarflexing the proximal phalanx.[3,4]

- An alternative method of joint preparation is to use a power burr, preparing the joint surfaces in a ball-and-cup fashion by removing the chondral surfaces.
  - Shape the subchondral surface hemispherically, with the metatarsal head convex and the phalangeal base concave **(TECH FIG 2B)**.[27]
- Carefully avoid excessive bony resection, particularly in osteopenic or rheumatoid patients, to prevent additional shortening of the toe.
- Create multiple drill holes in the metatarsal head and phalangeal base with a Kirschner wire or small drill bit to augment bleeding and bony ingrowth.[11,16]

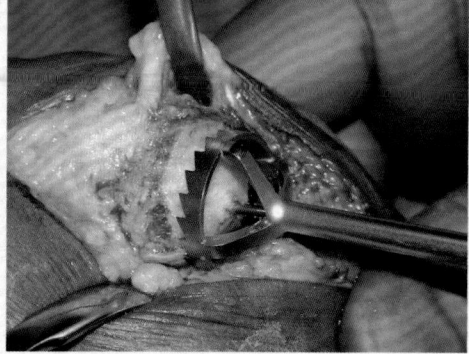

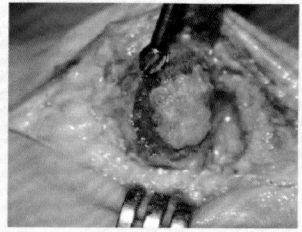

TECH FIG 2 A. Technique for joint preparation with specialized reamers. The Kirschner wire is placed in the center of the metatarsal head to ensure concentric joint preparation. **B.** Joint preparation with power burr. The metatarsal head is shaped hemispherically in a convex manner to fuse with the concave base of the proximal phalanx.

A   B

ARTHRODESIS POSITIONING AND FIXATION

- After preparing the joint surfaces, position the arthrodesis in 10 to 15 degrees of valgus, 10 degrees of dorsiflexion relative to the sole of the foot, and neutral pronation–supination.
- Because it can be difficult to determine the plane of the sole with the patient on the operative table, a more predictable method of positioning the toe is to determine dorsiflexion relative to the first metatarsal axis. In most cases, the appropriate angle is about 25 to 30 degrees of dorsiflexion.[3–5,14,19,21]
- The hallux is held provisionally with Kirschner wires or partially threaded guidewires from a cannulated screw set.
    - Confirm the positioning radiographically with a mini-fluoroscopy unit and clinically with use of a flat surface to simulate weight bearing (the cover of the screw set tray works nicely).[14,18,28]
    - The hallux should be slightly off the surface with the heel on the cover **(TECH FIG 3A)**.[11,28]
    - Placing a finger or screwdriver handle under the heel simulates a shoe with a small heel; in this case, the pulp of the distal hallux should just barely engage the surface.
- Cannulated or solid screws can be used per the surgeon's preference.[28] We use 4.0- or 4.5-mm cannulated screws in most patients. Solid 3.5-mm cortical screws are an alternative **(TECH FIG 3B)**.
- Insert one guidewire from the medial aspect of the phalangeal base just distal to the metaphyseal flare and advance it across the arthrodesis site through the dorsolateral cortex of the metatarsal neck.
    - If desired, a second screw can be considered if the first screw provides insufficient fixation in patients with osteopenia. Place the second wire from the medial aspect of the metatarsal neck, just proximal to the flare of the medial eminence; advance this wire distally and slightly plantarly across the arthrodesis site to engage the plantar–lateral cortex of the phalanx.

- Check wire position and length with fluoroscopy.
- Measure the wires percutaneously with the cannulated depth gauge and overdrill with the cannulated drill bit. Then, countersink the cortex carefully to prevent subsequent cracking with screw placement.[3]
- Place the partially threaded cannulated screw(s) over the guidewire(s) while compressing the hallux manually.
    - Alternatively, insert solid lag screws under fluoroscopic guidance.
- Our preferred technique also uses a supplementary dorsal plate, which has been shown to provide improved fixation.[11,16,25] This is particularly helpful if screws alone provide suboptimal fixation or in patients with osteopenic bone (eg, secondary to rheumatoid arthritis or chronic oral corticosteroid usage).[22]
- A precontoured locking hallux MTP fusion plate is selected and applied dorsally.[5,10–12,18] It may be necessary to débride any osteophytes that prevent adequate seating of the plate on the arthrodesis site.[18] Provisional fixation with pinning is performed and fluoroscopy confirms proper sizing and placement of the plate.
- The plate is then fixed with 2.7- or 3.5-mm nonlocking screws in the phalanx and metatarsal and augmented with 2.7- or 3.5-mm locking screws if bone quality is a concern.[10,16,22] Whether locking or nonlocking screws provide superior fixation remains controversial, with advocates for each **(TECH FIG 4A,B)**.[10,15,16,18,22]
    - Alternatively, a standard minifragment plate can be cut and contoured to fit and then affixed to the dorsal surface of the metatarsal and phalanx with small-diameter screws (eg, 2.7 or 3.5 mm).[22]
- Close the incision in layers with absorbable suture for the arthrotomy and subcutaneous layers and nonabsorbable monofilament for the skin.

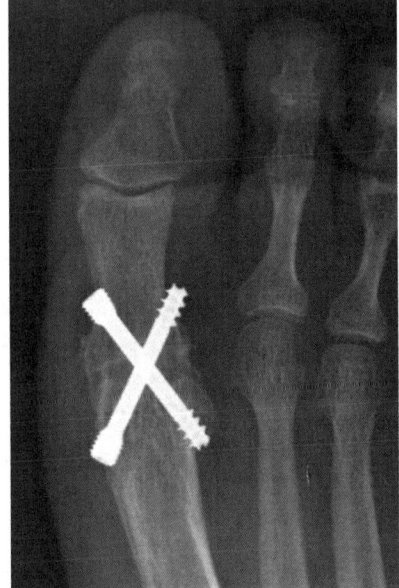
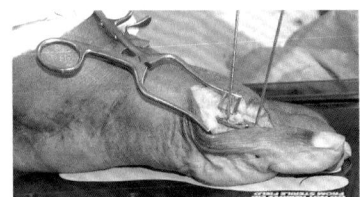

TECH FIG 3 **A.** Positioning of the first MTP joint. A flat surface is used to position the toe properly. Note the positioning of the toe to allow for adequate clearance during gait. **B.** Postoperative radiograph shows the crossed-screw technique.

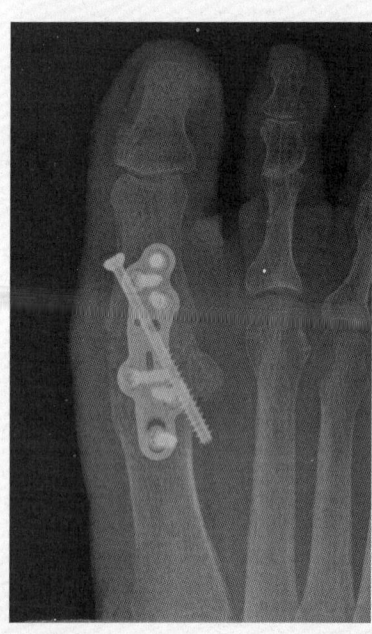

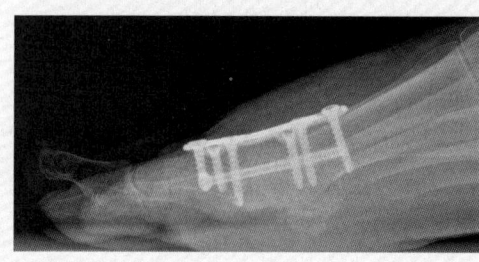

TECH FIG 4 Dorsal locking plate is used to augment the crossed-screw fixation. Anteroposterior **(A)** and lateral **(B)** views.

ALTERNATIVE TECHNIQUE: MEDIAL APPROACH

- A medial incision over the hallux MTP joint can be used in the presence of a previous surgical scar, severe soft tissue contracture about the joint, or at the surgeon's preference.[28]
- Carry out dissection at the level of the joint capsule, taking care to avoid the dorsomedial branch of the superficial peroneal nerve with elevation of the flap.
- Perform a midline arthrotomy to expose the metatarsal head and base of the proximal phalanx.
- Prepare the joint surfaces with a saw blade.[28]

- To allow for correct positioning, make the cut on the metatarsal head perpendicular to the sole of the foot and avoid resecting excessive bone when making the cut on the proximal phalanx. Then, position the hallux, with attention to all three planes as described earlier.
- Perform fixation with the crossed lag screw technique as described earlier, with supplemental dorsal plate fixation as needed.[28]

CASE EXAMPLE (COURTESY OF MARK E. EASLEY, MD)

Exposure

- Dorsomedial longitudinal incision over first MTP joint
  - Extensor hallucis longus tendon protected
  - Dorsomedial superficial nerve branch to hallux protected
- Longitudinal capsulotomy
- Capsule reflected
- Joint exposure optimized by release of flexor hallucis brevis from base of proximal phalanx while avoiding injury to the FHL tendon **(TECH FIG 5)**

Joint Preparation

- Cup-and-cone reamer system
- Optimally sized cone reamer for first metatarsal head may be centered over first metatarsal head and used to optimally center guide pin **(TECH FIG 6A,B)**.
- First metatarsal head reamed with soft tissues well protected **(TECH FIG 6C)**

- Guide pin centered in proximal phalanx **(TECH FIG 6D)**
- Proximal phalanx reamed with appropriately sized cup reamer **(TECH FIG 6E)**
- Subchondral bone drilled to optimize fusion, with cold saline irritation to limit heat necrosis **(TECH FIG 6F)**

Provisional Fixation

- MTP joint reduced
- Provisional fixation
- Toe rotated into neutral position
  - Pronation must be avoided **(TECH FIG 7A,B)**.
  - Err into slight supination to avoid pronation.
- Optimize sagittal plane toe position.
  - An instrument lid may be used to simulate weight bearing.
  - Ideally, with hallux in neutral position, hallux tuft should barely touch or be elevated 1 to 2 mm from the instrument lid that is simulating weight bearing **(TECH FIG 7C)**.

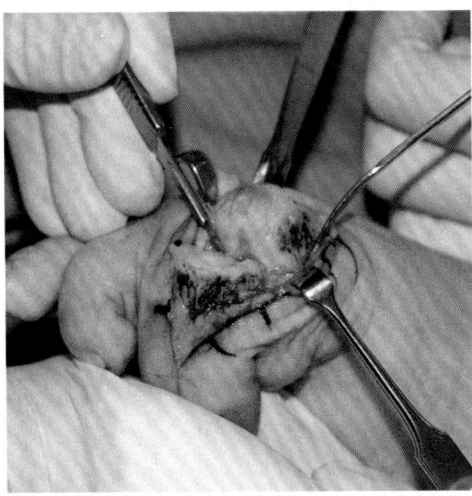

TECH FIG 5 A 40-year-old man with posttraumatic arthritis of the right first MTP joint. With soft tissues well protected, MTP joint is released, here showing release of flexor hallucis brevis tendon from base of proximal phalanx, to optimize exposure.

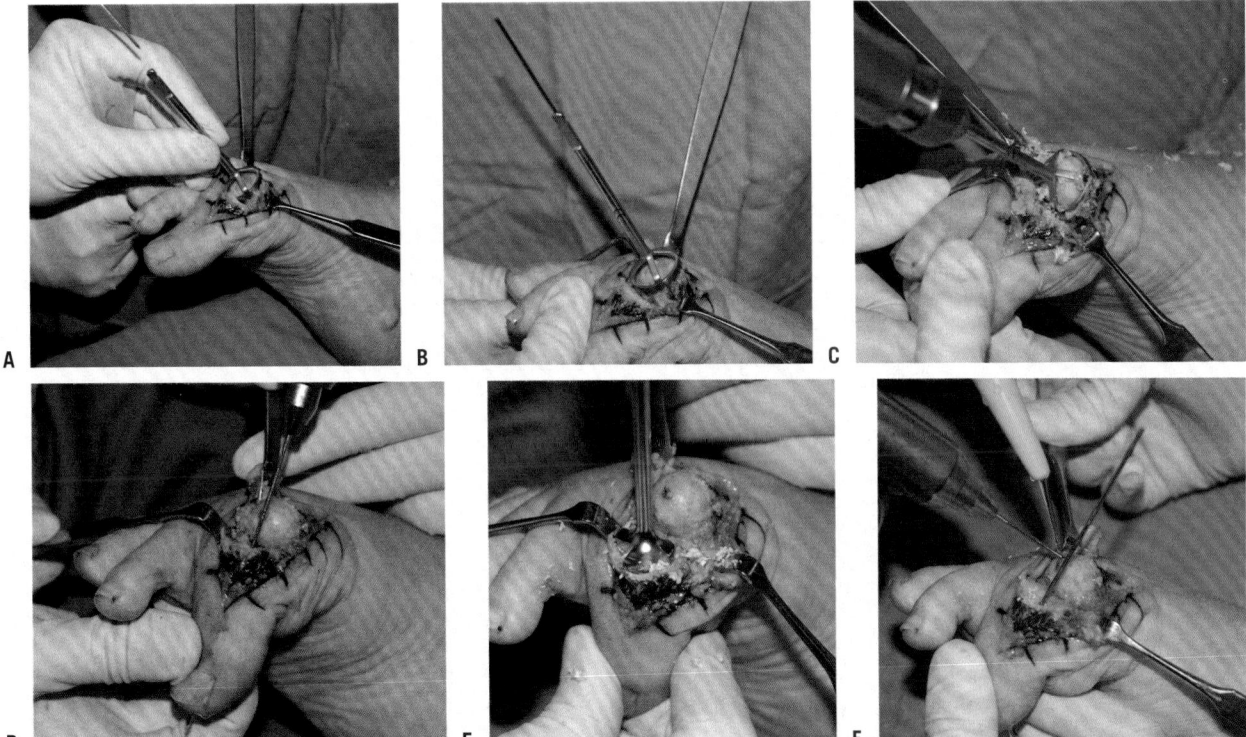

TECH FIG 6 A–C. Metatarsal head preparation. **A.** The dedicated cone reamer is optimally positioned on the metatarsal head. **B.** The guide pin is inserted after optimal reamer position is determined. **C.** With soft tissues well protected, metatarsal head is reamed over the guide pin. **D,E.** Proximal phalanx preparation. **D.** Insertion of the guide pin. **E.** With soft tissues well protected, the proximal phalanx is reamed with a dedicated metatarsal arthrodesis cup reamer. **F.** The subchondral surfaces are drilled to promote fusion. In this case, a Kirschner wire was used; however, a drill may be better, as it typically generates less heat. Cold saline irrigation may limit the risk of heat necrosis.

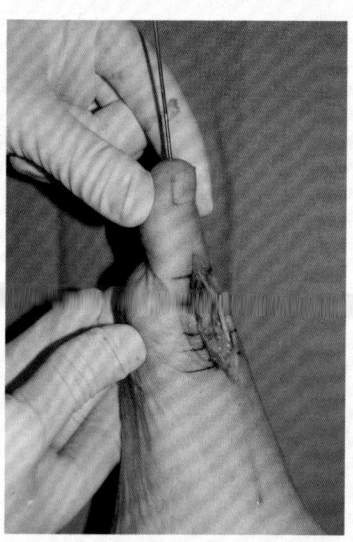 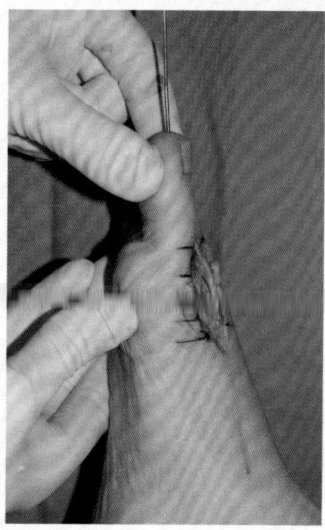 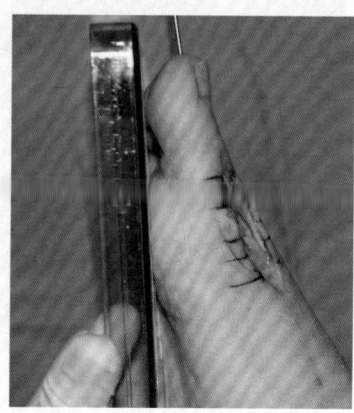

TECH FIG 7 A. Hallux pronation should be avoided. **B.** Hallux with optimal rotation. **C.** Ideally, with hallux in neutral position, the hallux tuft should barely touch or be elevated 1 to 2 mm from the instrument lid that is simulating weight bearing.

Definitive Fixation

- Lag screw
  - May be placed from distal–medial to proximal–lateral **(TECH FIG 8A)**
  - When protecting the dorsomedial sensory nerve, be sure that the hallux does not rotate into pronation.
  - If the screw has a head, be sure to countersink to distal aspect of the head to avoid proximal phalanx fracture when the screw head contacts the proximal phalanx.
- Hallux should be in neutral alignment **(TECH FIG 8B)**.
  - Although some authors recommend valgus position, neutral position will avoid impingement on the second toe.

- To optimize stability of the first MTP joint arthrodesis, a dorsal plate may be placed.
  - Numerous different plates are commercially available.
  - In this case, a simple small fragment plate was used **(TECH FIG 8C)**.

Postoperative Care

- Protective weight bearing avoiding forefoot loading for 6 weeks
- Short-leg cast versus cam boot for 4 weeks
- Postsurgical shoe for additional 2 to 4 weeks until patient can transition into stiffer-soled shoe

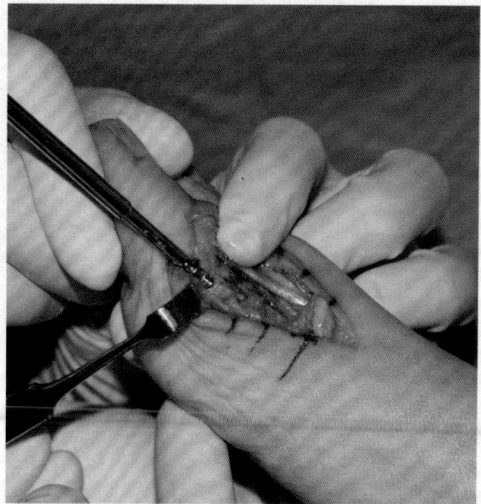 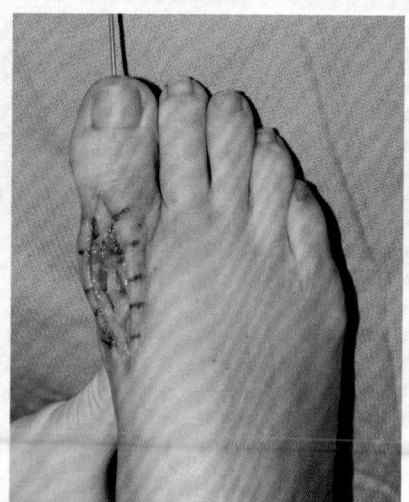 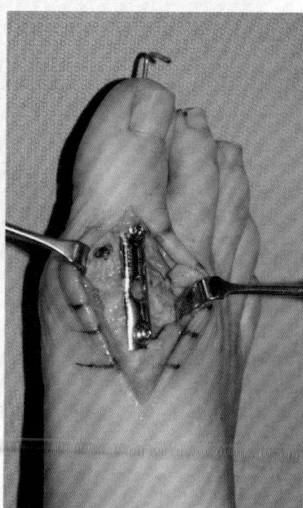

TECH FIG 8 A. Lag screw fixation. In this case, a fully threaded and headed screw was used. The proximal phalanx must be countersunk to avoid stress fracture when the head is fully seated. **B.** Assessing alignment after lag screw fixation. Although some authors recommend valgus position, neutral position will avoid impingement on the second toe. **C.** The MTP joint arthrodesis is stabilized with a dorsal plate. In this case, a simple small fragment plate was used. Note that the plate is straight, limiting the risk of dorsiflexion malunion. The provisional fixation Kirschner wire is removed after definitive fixation is complete.

Pearls and Pitfalls

Arthrodesis Preparation	• To prevent shortening, avoid excessive bone resection.
Hallux Positioning	• Intraoperatively, the position of the hallux is assessed fluoroscopically and clinically with a flat surface to simulate weight bearing. Proper positioning includes valgus of 10–15 degrees, dorsiflexion of 25–30 degrees relative to the metatarsal shaft (or 10 degrees relative to the sole of the foot), and neutral rotation. Clinically, the hallux should not impinge on the second toe and the nail plate should be aligned with the same plane as the lesser toes.
Guide Pin Breakage	• Maintain correct positioning of the hallux during insertion of the guide pin. Avoid bending and shearing of the wire during cannulated drilling.
Fixation Problems	• When arthrodesis is performed on osteopenic bone, requiring additional fixation with a dorsal locked plate,[5,15] additional Kirschner wires or threaded pins[3,12] may be necessary to supplement standard fixation.

POSTOPERATIVE CARE

- In patients with an isolated arthrodesis with good bone quality and solid fixation, weight bearing as tolerated on the heel and lateral border of the foot is allowed in a postoperative hard-soled shoe or fracture boot, restricting weight bearing on the forefoot.[11,16]
- If there are concerns about bone quality, suboptimal fixation, or potential noncompliance by the patient, strict non–weight bearing in a boot or below-the-knee cast is maintained for 6 weeks.
- After 6 weeks, partial weight bearing is advanced, based on evidence of clinical and radiographic healing.
- Full weight bearing usually is achieved by 8 to 10 weeks, at which time the patient transitions from the postoperative shoe or boot into sneakers, clogs, or comfortable, low-heeled walking shoes.
- At 12 to 16 weeks, with additional reduction in swelling, most patients can transition into unrestricted shoe wear; however, some individuals have permanent difficulty wearing fashion shoes or high heels.
- Prolonged walking and athletic activities usually resumes at 3 to 5 months.
- Custom-made orthotics with a buildup under the hallux to improve weight bearing of the first ray may dissipate forefoot stresses.

OUTCOMES

- The clinical results after hallux MTP arthrodesis usually are excellent, with high rates of bony union, patient satisfaction, and pain relief.
  - Union rates for in situ arthrodesis range from 77% to 100%.[4,5,10–13,16–18,21,28]
  - Patient satisfaction rates also are high, regardless of the indications.[4,5,8–12,16–18,21,28]
  - Patients also have excellent functional recovery including the ability to resume exercise or sports activities in most cases.[8]
- Hallux MTP arthrodesis not only improves hallux alignment but also leads to correction of the intermetatarsal[1,2] angle, obviating the need for proximal osteotomy despite severe preoperative deformity.[6,20,23,26]

- MTP arthrodesis causes a rigid lever arm, resulting in an earlier toe-off in the gait cycle and decreasing the stress on the lesser metatarsals.[4,9,21] This stiffness may result in increased stress across the hallux interphalangeal joint.[19]
- After arthrodesis, the first ray shows improved weight-bearing capacity, with the foot compensating for the relative stiffness during stance phase.[9] Formal gait analysis after fusion demonstrates improvements in propulsive power, weight-bearing function of the foot, and stability during gait.[1]

COMPLICATIONS

- Nonunion rates range from 5% to 22%.[5,9–13,16,17,21] Nonunion may not be symptomatic and may not require revision surgery.[17]
- Malunion after MTP arthrodesis can result in mild malalignment that is tolerated, but more severe malposition may be symptomatic.
  - Excessive dorsiflexion leads to unloading of the hallux and lesser toe transfer metatarsalgia.
  - Positioning the hallux in relative plantar flexion may lead to interphalangeal joint irritation, callus formation, and later interphalangeal arthritis.[27]
  - Valgus positioning can lead to painful impingement on the second toe, whereas varus positioning causes impingement of the hallux against the toe box of the shoe.
- Subsequent arthritis of the interphalangeal joint may occur in one-third of cases.[5,13]
  - Arthritis in the interphalangeal joint is more common than that of the first tarsometatarsal or other midfoot joints.[13]
  - However, symptoms may be mild despite radiographic involvement and may take 10 years to develop.
  - Severe symptoms may require secondary interphalangeal arthrodesis, which leads to extreme stiffness of the hallux.
- Iatrogenic nerve injuries of the dorsomedial cutaneous nerve are more common than injuries to the plantar nerves.
  - These may result in neuroma formation, mild numbness, or persistent dysesthesias that compromise an otherwise successful arthrodesis.
  - Prevention by proper incision placement and meticulous surgical dissection remains the best strategy.

REFERENCES

1. Brodsky JW, Baum BS, Polio FE, et al. Prospective gait analysis in patients with first metatarsophalangeal joint arthrodesis for hallux rigidus. Foot Ankle Int 2007;28:162–165.

2. Castro MD, Klaue K. Technique tip: revisiting an alternative method of fixation for first MTP joint arthrodesis. Foot Ankle Int 2001;22:687–688.

3. Conti SF, Dhawan S. Arthrodesis of the first metatarsophalangeal and interphalangeal joints of the foot. Foot Ankle Clin North Am 1996;1:33–53.

4. Coughlin MJ. Rheumatoid forefoot reconstruction. A long-term follow-up study. J Bone Joint Surg Am 2000;82:322–341.

5. Coughlin MJ, Grebing BR, Jones CP. Arthrodesis of the first metatarsophalangeal joint for idiopathic hallux valgus intermediate results. Foot Ankle Int 2005;26:783–792.

6. Cronin JJ, Limbers JP, Kutty S, et al. Intermetatarsal angle after first metatarsophalangeal joint arthrodesis for hallux valgus. Foot Ankle Int 2006;27:104–109.

7. Curtis MJ, Myerson M, Jinnah RH, et al. Arthrodesis of the first metatarsophalangeal joint: a biomechanical study of internal fixation techniques. Foot Ankle 1993;14:395–399.

8. Da Cunha RJ, MacMahon A, Jones MT, et al. Return to sports and physical activities after first metatarsophalangeal joint arthrodesis in young patients. Foot Ankle Int 2019;40:745–752.

9. DeFrino PF, Brodsky JW, Pollo FE, et al. First metatarsophalangeal arthrodesis: a clinical, pedobarographic and gait analysis study. Foot Ankle Int 2002;23:496–502.

10. Doty J, Coughlin M, Hirose C, et al. Hallux metatarsophalangeal joint arthrodesis with a hybrid locking plate and a plantar neutralization screw: a prospective study. Foot Ankle Int 2013;34:1535–1540.

11. Ellington JK, Jones CP, Cohen BE, et al. Review of 107 hallux MTP joint arthrodesis using dome-shaped reamers and a stainless-steel dorsal plate. Foot Ankle Int 2010;31:385–390.

12. Goucher NR, Coughlin MJ. Hallux metatarsophalangeal joint arthrodesis using dome-shaped reamers and dorsal plate fixation: a prospective study. Foot Ankle Int 2006;27:869–876.

13. Grimes JS, Coughlin MJ. First metatarsophalangeal joint arthrodesis as a treatment for failed hallux valgus surgery. Foot Ankle Int 2006;27:887–893.

14. Harper MC. Positioning of the hallux for first metatarsophalangeal joint arthrodesis. Foot Ankle Int 1997;18:827.

15. Hunt KJ, Barr CR, Lindsey DP, et al. Locked versus nonlocked plate fixation for first metatarsophalangeal arthrodesis: a biomechanical investigation. Foot Ankle Int 2012;33:984–990.

16. Hunt KJ, Ellington JK, Anderson RB, et al. Locked versus non-locked plate fixation for hallux MTP arthrodesis. Foot Ankle Int 2011;32:704–709.

17. Kitaoka HB, Patzer GL. Arthrodesis versus resection arthroplasty for failed hallux valgus operations. Clin Orthop Relat Res 1998;(347):208–214.

18. Kumar S, Pradhan R, Rosenfeld PF. First metatarsophalangeal arthrodesis using a dorsal plate and a compression screw. Foot Ankle Int 2010;31:797–801.

19. Mann RA. Surgical implications of biomechanics of the foot and ankle. Clin Orthop Relat Res 1980;(146):111–118.

20. Mann RA, Katcherian DA. Relationship of metatarsophalangeal joint fusion on the intermetatarsal angle. Foot Ankle 1989;10:8–11.

21. Mann RA, Schakel ME II. Surgical correction of rheumatoid forefoot deformities. Foot Ankle Int 1995;16:1–6.

22. Mayer SA, Zelenski NA, DeOrio JK, et al. A comparison of nonlocking semitubular plates and precontoured locking plates for first metatarsophalangeal joint arthrodesis. Foot Ankle Int 2014;35:438–444.

23. McKean RM, Bergin PF, Watson G, et al. Radiographic evaluation of intermetatarsal angle correction following first MTP joint arthrodesis for severe hallux valgus. Foot Ankle Int 2016;37:1183–1186.

24. Mizel MS, Alvarez RG, Fink BR, et al. Ipsilateral arthrodesis of the metatarsophalangeal and interphalangeal joints of the hallux. Foot Ankle Int 2006;27:804–807.

25. Politi J, Hayes J, Njus G, et al. First metatarsal-phalangeal joint arthrodesis: a biomechanical assessment of stability. Foot Ankle Int 2003;24:332–337.

26. Pydah SKV, Toh EM, Sirikonda SP, et al. Intermetatarsal angular change following fusion of the first metatarsophalangeal joint. Foot Ankle Int 2009;30:415–418.

27. Trnka HJ. Arthrodesis procedures for salvage of the hallux metatarsophalangeal joint. Foot Ankle Clin 2000;5:673–686.

28. van Doeselaar DJ, Heesterbeek PJ, Louwerens JW, et al. Foot function after fusion of the first metatarsophalangeal joint. Foot Ankle Int 2010;31:670–675.

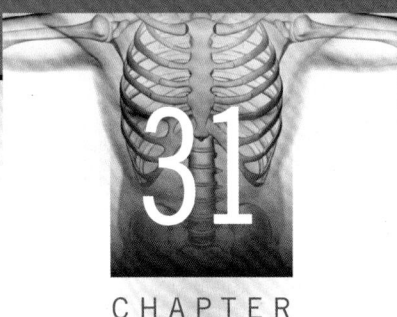

Hallux Interphalangeal Joint Arthrodesis

Glenn G. Shi and Mark E. Easley

DEFINITION

- Multiple potentially disabling disorders affect the hallux interphalangeal joint (IPJ).
- Symptomatic hallux IPJ arthritis and/or deformity may be effectively treated with hallux IPJ arthrodesis.
- The goal of hallux IPJ arthrodesis is to relieve intra-articular pain, dorsal IPJ and distal toe pressure due to flexion contracture, and/or resultant sesamoid pain due to chronic hallux metatarsophalangeal (MTP) joint extension and IPJ flexion contracture.

ANATOMY

- The hallux consists of two phalanges, proximal and distal.
- The hallux IPJ is the articulation of the proximal phalangeal head and the distal phalangeal base. This simple and stable hinge joint allows for motion up to 11.9 degrees of active extension and 46 degrees of flexion.
- The osteology of the proximal phalangeal head has been described as a large trochlear groove that is wider and more concave on the plantar side. The phalangeal head topography is congruently matched by the distal phalangeal base.
- Static stability is primarily created by the collateral ligaments originating from the superolateral aspect of the phalangeal head and inserting into the dorsal tubercle of the distal phalanx and augmented by the circumferential joint capsule that includes the plantarflexor plate. Dynamic support arises from the extensor and flexor hallucis tendons that cross the joint.

PATHOGENESIS

- Intra-articular fractures: Often, they are due to direct axial load/impact to the hallux. Treatment with rest and a period of immobilization may relieve symptoms in the acute setting for nondisplaced fractures. Patients with displaced intra-articular fractures may require open reduction and

internal fixation versus IPJ arthrodesis. Degenerative hallux IPJ arthritis is often attributed to trauma.
- Osteochondritis dissecans (OCD): OCD of the hallux IPJ is rare compared to that of the knee or talus. Case series of athletes with IPJ osteochondral fragments have been published.
  - Débridement and temporary Kirschner wire fixation have produced short-term symptomatic improvement of symptoms; to our knowledge, no long-term data are available (FIG 1A).
- Claw hallux deformity: Etiology comprises compartment syndrome of the foot, Charcot-Marie-Tooth disease, cerebral palsy, spina bifida, and other static or progressive neuromuscular diseases. The soft tissue imbalance produces hyperextension of the MTP joint and flexion of the hallux IPJ.
- Cock-up toe deformity: develops from chronic untreated turf toe (plantar plate) injuries. Likewise, when both the medial and lateral sesamoid are excised with inadequate repair of the residual flexor mechanism, a cock-up toe deformity may develop (FIG 1B).
- Inflammatory arthritis: In select cases, inflamed synovitis and progressive periarticular joint destruction of an inflammatory arthropathy may occur in the hallux IPJ.

PATIENT HISTORY AND PHYSICAL FINDINGS

- Occasionally, the patient recalls a traumatic inciting event such as stubbing of the great toe. However, the patient typically presents with an activity-related ache or pain in the hallux IPJ.
- Careful history should be directed to explore possible etiology of the pain or deformity.
- Physical examination
  - Patient may have an obvious deformity such as claw hallux, hyperextension, or hallux valgus interphalangeus. The clinician should examine the skin for associated soft tissue corns, plantar callosities, or even open ulcers in patients with severe deformities.

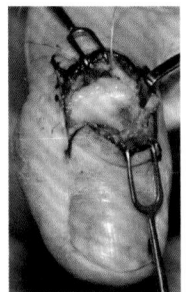
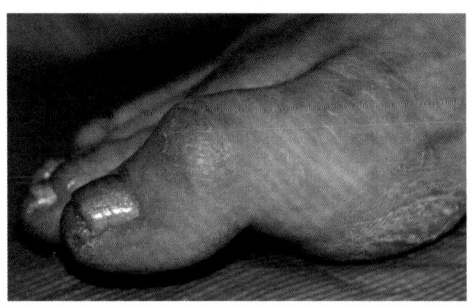

FIG 1 A. Osteochondral lesion on the proximal phalanx prior to hallux IPJ arthrodesis. B. Cock-up toe deformity in patient with chronically insufficient sesamoid complex.

- Tenderness is typically present directly over the IPJ.
- Patient usually experience discomfort with active and passive hallux IPJ range of motion.

IMAGING AND OTHER DIAGNOSTIC STUDIES

- Standard weight-bearing plain radiographs should include anteroposterior (AP), lateral, and oblique views.
- A radiographic grading system for hallux IPJ arthritis is available for reference:
  - Grade I: no degenerative change
  - Grade II: mild degenerative changes, less than 1 mm of chondrolysis
  - Grade III: moderate degenerative changes with 1 to 2 mm of chondrolysis
  - Grade IV: severe degenerative changes with joint space narrowing, periarticular cysts, and alignment deformity
- Computed tomography (CT) scan shows more detailed internal bony architecture. It may be used to evaluate the periarticular cystic lesions as well as estimate the bone stock available for IPJ arthrodesis.
- Thin cut magnetic resonance imaging (MRI) through the IPJ may be used as a screening test for osteochondral lesions.

DIFFERENTIAL DIAGNOSIS

- Intra-articular fracture
- Hallux IPJ dislocation
- Inflammatory arthritis
- Posttraumatic degenerative arthritis
- Hallux IPJ gout
- Osteochondral lesion
- Loose bodies
- Claw hallux
- Hallux valgus interphalangeus

NONOPERATIVE MANAGEMENT

- Activity modification
- Stiff-soled shoe modification
- Morton extension
- Wider toe box to the shoe
- Extra depth to the toe box
- Nonsteroidal anti-inflammatory medications
- Corticosteroid injection

SURGICAL MANAGEMENT

- Indications for hallux IPJ fusion include symptomatic individuals who have failed nonoperative management:
  - Posttraumatic degenerative IPJ arthritis
  - Inflammatory IPJ arthritides
  - IPJ varus or valgus deformity associated with hallux IPJ arthritis
  - Claw hallux
  - Cock-up toe deformity
  - Progressive neuromuscular diseases, typically leading to fixed hallux IPJ flexion contracture

Preoperative Planning

- Active and passive range of motion to determine if deformity is fixed or flexible (**FIG 2A,B**)
- Evaluation of rotational deformity, particularly with hallux pronation
- Three weight-bearing views of the foot; consideration may be given to cone-in detail views of the hallux (**FIG 2C,D**).
- Rarely is more detailed imaging necessary. High-resolution MRI may reveal cartilage damage not visible on plain radiographs, and CT may provide greater detail of subchondral bone irregularity.

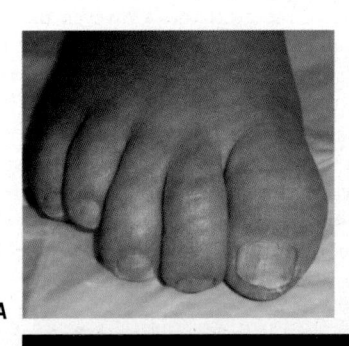
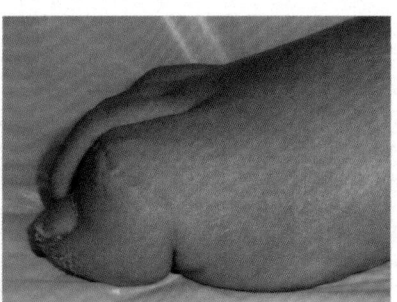
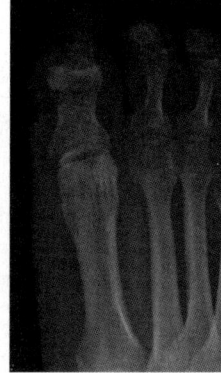
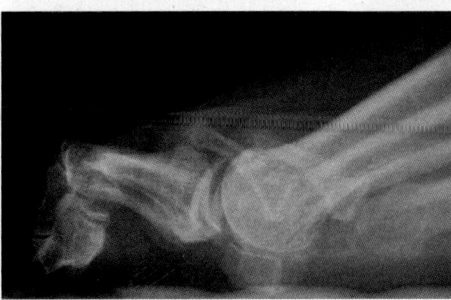

FIG 2 Fixed claw toe deformities, including a clawed hallux in a 50-year-old man. **A.** Dorsal view. **B.** Medial view. **C.** AP radiograph. **D.** Lateral radiograph.

Positioning

- This procedure is typically performed under a peripheral nerve block.
- The patient is placed in a supine position with a support under the ipsilateral hip so that the toes of the affected foot are pointed toward the ceiling.
- The tourniquet, if desired, may be used at the ankle or calf.

Approach

- We prefer to use a dorsal approach to the hallux IPJ.
- Although perhaps not universally used, we typically perform isolated hallux IPJ arthrodesis via an H-shaped incision. In our experience, this incision allows for optimal exposure and heals reliably.

INCISION

- The H-shaped incision is made with the transverse incision at the IPJ and the dorsomedial and dorsolateral longitudinal limbs extending approximately 1 cm distally and proximally to the transverse incision **(TECH FIG 1A)**.
- Full-thickness skin flaps including capsule and periosteum are raised; undermining of the skin layers should be limited **(TECH FIG 1B)**.
- Dissection is carried down to the terminal portion of the extensor hallucis longus (EHL) tendon. A transverse tenotomy is performed. The EHL tendon may be tagged to be reattached at the completion of the arthrodesis to reinforce toe extension that otherwise would be limited to the extensor hallucis brevis.
- With the full-thickness flaps elevated from the capsule distally and proximally, the IPJ is exposed along the path of the transverse joint line.

- Collateral ligaments are then freed from their periarticular attachments, thereby exposing the IPJ.

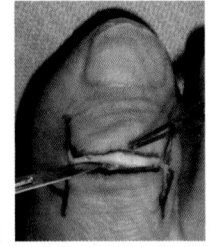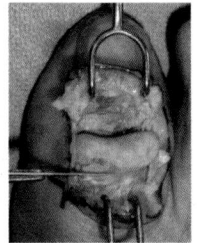

TECH FIG 1　A. Dorsal H-shaped incision. **B.** Capsular and subperiosteal elevation distal and proximal to the IPJ.

PREPARATION OF THE HALLUX INTERPHALANGEAL JOINT

- Using retraction on the deeper tissues to reflect the distal and proximal flaps, the distal articular surface of the proximal phalanx is exposed.
- With the soft tissues protected, we use a microsagittal to remove the residual articular surfaces. We minimize bone resection by initiating the saw cut immediately proximal to the articular surface.
- We prepare the arthrodesis of the hallux IPJ in slight plantarflexion by tilting the saw to remove slightly more bone from the plantar aspect than the dorsal aspect of the proximal phalanx at the IPJ **(TECH FIG 2A,B)**.
  - Avoid overpenetration of the saw blade as it may damage the flexor hallucis longus (FHL) tendon immediately plantar to the IPJ.

- The articular surface of the proximal aspect of the distal phalanx is prepared using a microsagittal saw and also with the cut made in slight plantarflexion (removing slightly more bone plantarly than dorsally) **(TECH FIG 2C,D)**.
  - Avoid overpenetration of the saw blade as it may damage the FHL tendon immediately plantar to the IPJ.
- Clinically and fluoroscopically, proper hallux alignment after bony preparation is confirmed **(TECH FIG 2E)**. If alignment is not optimal, the bone preparation should be repeated until alignment is ideal.
- Slight plantarflexion to both the proximal and distal preparations should place the hallux IPJ in approximately 5 degrees of flexion.

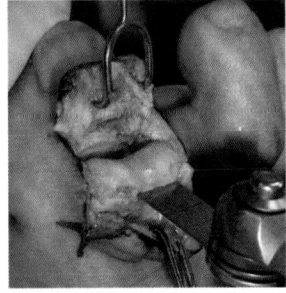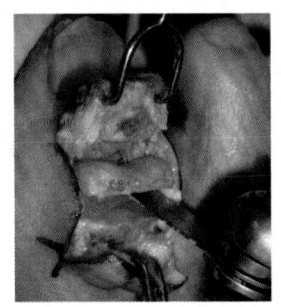

TECH FIG 2　A,B. Proximal phalanx preparation. **A.** The bone is cut immediately proximal to the articular surface. **B.** The cut is made in slight plantarflexion (more bone resected dorsally than plantarly). *(continued)*

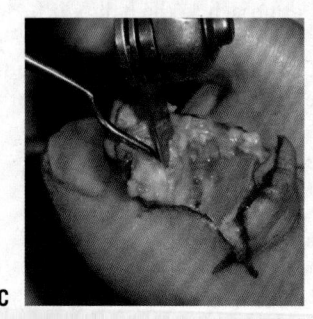
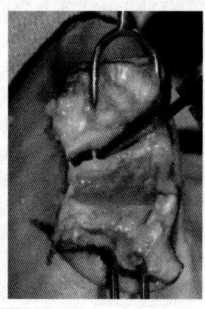
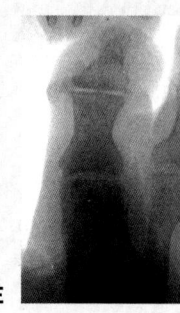

TECH FIG 2 *(continued)* **C,D.** Distal phalanx preparation. **C.** Relatively minimal bone resection. **D.** More bone is resected dorsally than plantarly to promote slight plantarflexion. **E.** Intraoperative fluoroscopy with prepared surfaces reduced to confirm satisfactory bony alignment prior to fixation.

GUIDEWIRE PLACEMENT

- A guidewire is placed in retrograde fashion from inside the joint through the center of the distal phalangeal base, aiming longitudinally with the exit point at the distal toe immediately inferior to the nail bed **(TECH FIG 3A)**.
- A small transverse incision is made at the exit point of the guidewire along the direction of Langer lines **(TECH FIG 3B)**.
- The guidewire is backed into the distal phalanx except for 1 or 2 mm **(TECH FIG 3C)**. This spike allows for anchoring into the center of proximal phalanx medullary canal.
  - The guidewire is advanced after the alignment, translation, and rotation of the hallux IPJ and is satisfactory clinically and fluoroscopically **(TECH FIG 3D)**.

- The depth to which the guidewire is advanced determines the screw length. The bony apposition, alignment, and translation are again confirmed under fluoroscopy. Care must be taken to leave adequate space for the screw to be inserted. Should the screw violate the nail matrix, it may create symptoms and potentially affect nail growth **(TECH FIG 3E)**.

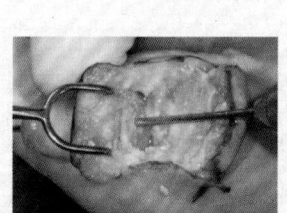
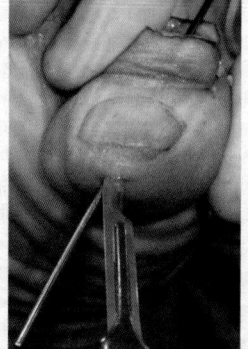
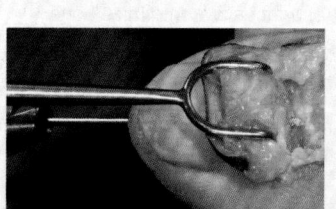
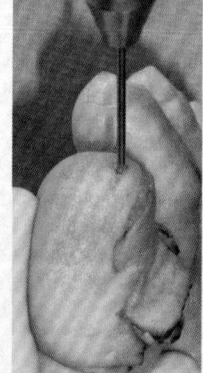
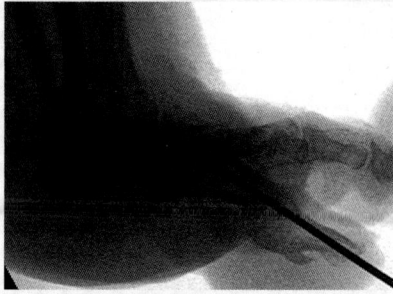

TECH FIG 3 A. The guide pin for the cannulated screw is first driven antegrade across the distal phalanx. **B.** Transverse stab incision at distal toe to allow depth gauge, drill, and screw to be placed. **C.** The guide pin is driven retrograde in preparation for reduction of the arthrodesis. **D.** With the arthrodesis reduced and the toe in satisfactory alignment and rotation, the guide pin is driven retrograde across the arthrodesis site into the proximal phalanx. **E.** Intraoperative fluoroscopy to confirm optimal guide pin position. On this lateral view, the pin is in satisfactory position within the distal phalanx so that the screw will not violate the nail matrix.

SCREW INSERTION

- After confirmation of satisfactory joint preparation and ideal guidewire position and determination of screw length using the dedicated depth gauge, the guidewire is overdrilled with a cannulated drill (**TECH FIG 4A**). We only drill to immediately across the arthrodesis site, not the full length of the proximal phalanx, in order to optimize screw purchase in the proximal phalanx.

- The screw of proper length is selected and inserted (**TECH FIG 4B,C**). The IPJ should be held securely in one hand as the screw is advanced with the other to be sure proper rotation and compression are maintained (**TECH FIG 4D,E**).

- Final AP, lateral, and oblique fluoroscopic images confirm sustained bony apposition, alignment, and screw position (**TECH FIG 4F**).

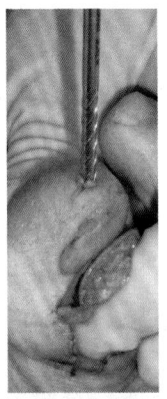 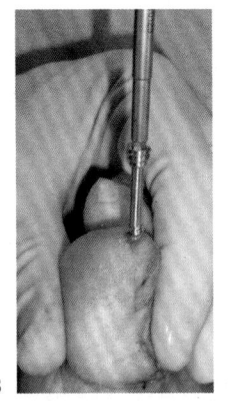 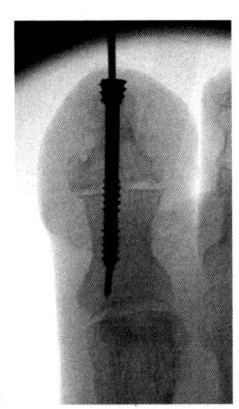 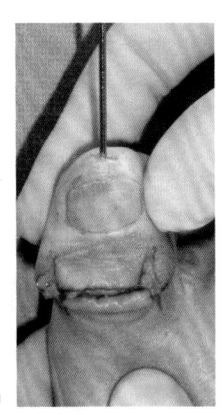 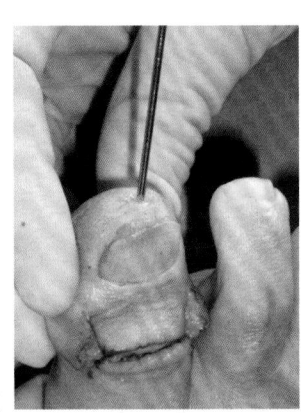

A   B   C   D   E

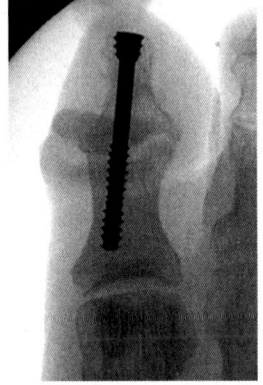

F

TECH FIG 4 **A.** The guide pin is overdrilled. **B.** With the arthrodesis being stabilized with one hand, the screw is advanced from the distal phalanx into the proximal phalanx. Note that rotation is controlled. **C.** Fluoroscopic visualization of the screw being advanced across the arthrodesis site. **D.** If the arthrodesis is not stabilized, the distal phalanx could rotate into pronation. **E.** Ideally, the hallux nail should be rotated to match the rotation of the second toe nail. **F.** Intraoperative fluoroscopy suggesting the screw should be advanced further to optimize compression. The screw head should be buried within the tip of the distal phalanx.

CLOSURE

- Wound closure starts with mattress closure of the residual capsule and transected EHL using 2-0 Vicryl (**TECH FIG 5A**).

- Subcutaneous tissue is closed with 3-0 Vicryl suture, and skin is reapproximated with 4-0 Nylon vertical mattress sutures to a tensionless closure (**TECH FIG 5B**).

- Sterile dressings are applied with abundant padding.

- If the patient can reliably protect the forefoot, a postoperative shoe that extends beyond the toes may be applied. If there is a concern that the patient may not be able to protect the forefoot, then we favor a short-leg splint with the ankle in neutral position, reinforced with a forefoot spica splint to protect the hallux.

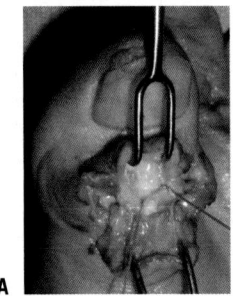 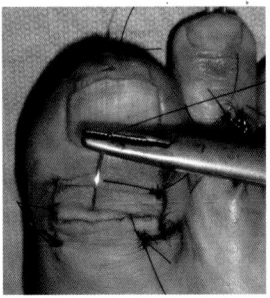

A   B

TECH FIG 5 **A.** The capsule and EHL tendon are reapproximated. **B.** The skin edges of the H-shaped incision are reapproximated to a tensionless closure.

TECHNIQUES

ADDITIONAL CASE

- A 55-year-old woman with cock-up toe deformity had status post forefoot reconstruction with excision of both sesamoids in two prior surgeries (**TECH FIG 6A**).
- Radiographs demonstrate residual hallux valgus, hallux IPJ arthritis, and cock-up toe deformity (**TECH FIG 6B,C**).
- We performed a dorsal approach to prepare the IPJ for arthrodesis.
- Through the joint, we identified the FHL tendon, released the tendon from the plantar distal phalanx, and placed a suture in the distal tendon (**TECH FIG 6D**).

- We performed the hallux IPJ arthrodesis but left the screw (and a pin to control rotation) slightly short within the proximal phalanx (**TECH FIG 6E**).
- By leaving the screw slightly short, enough space remained to create a drill hole in the base of the proximal phalanx to transfer the FHL tendon from plantar to dorsal. We secured the FHL tendon in the base of the proximal phalanx with an interference screw (**TECH FIG 6F,G**).

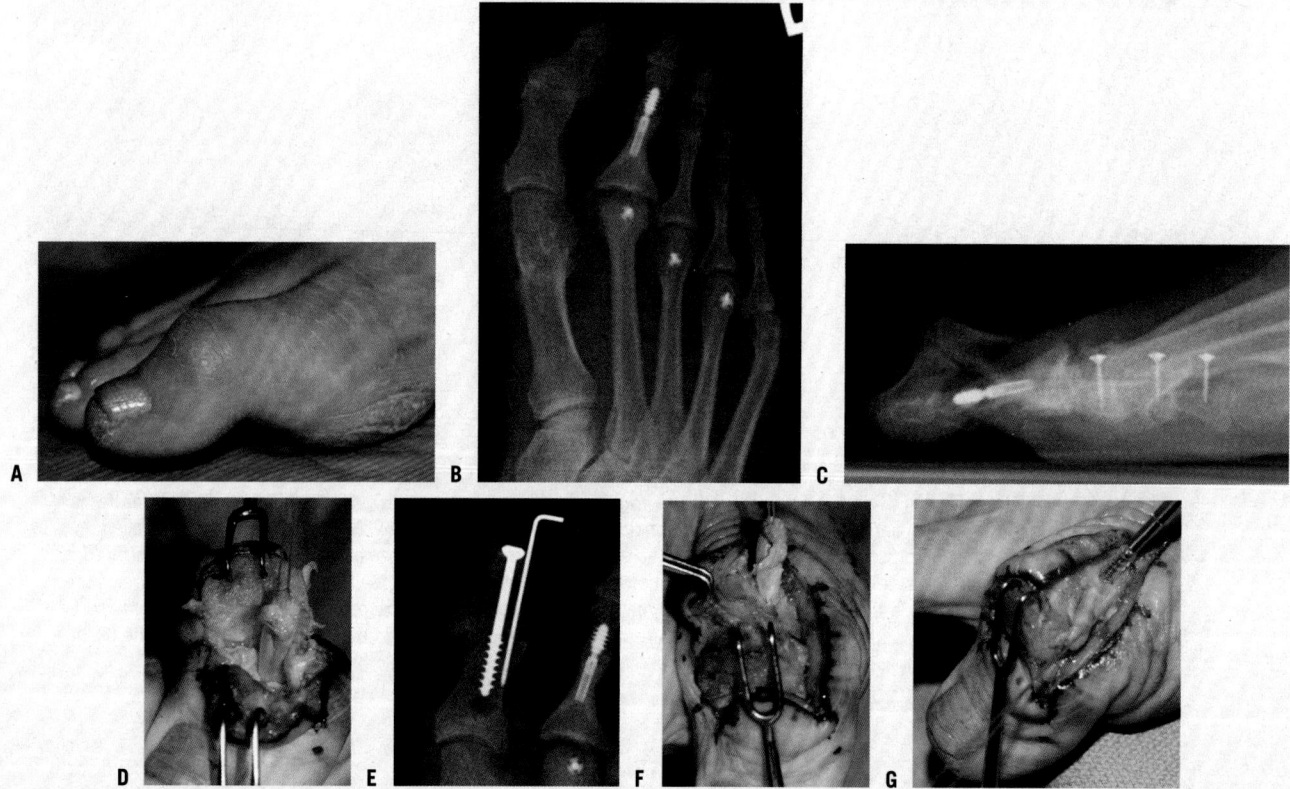

TECH FIG 6 A. Cock-up toe deformity in 55-year-old patient who had both sesamoids removed. AP (**B**) and lateral (**C**) radiographs. **D.** FHL tendon harvest through IPJ preparation. **E.** IPJ arthrodesis and drill hole proximal to fixation to allow for FHL tendon transfer to base of proximal phalanx. **F.** FHL tendon being transferred through base of proximal phalanx. **G.** FHL fixation with interference screw, prior to IPJ arthrodesis fixation.

Pearls and Pitfalls

Proper Guidewire Placement	• The starting point must be centered in the phalanges and directed along the center of the medullary canals. Deviating dorsally in the distal phalanx may cause the screw to violate the nail matrix, creating symptoms and potential aberrant nail growth. Wire and screw deviation in other directions may limit optimal compression and screw purchase.
Anatomic Hallux Rotation	• Proper distal phalanx rotation must be maintained until screw is fully seated and compression is applied. A reasonable reference point is the second toe nail: The hallux nail should have the same rotational alignment as the second toe. If any error is made, it should be into supination; pronation must be avoided.
Translation between the Two Phalanges	• Maximum fusion contact surface area is dependent on optimal alignment between the distal and proximal phalanges. At the arthrodesis site, the distal phalanx surface is usually greater than that of the proximal phalanx, so balance between the two is important to create ideal chance for fusion. Translation of the distal phalanx in relation to the proximal phalanx may also create symptomatic prominences.
Perform arthrodesis in slight flexion.	• Extension of the arthrodesis tends to create a callus under the hallux IPJ arthrodesis site.
Protect the flexor hallucis longus tendon.	• The FHL tendon lies immediately deep to the hallux IPJ, and overpenetration of the saw blade may damage the FHL.

POSTOPERATIVE CARE

• Until follow-up at 10 to 14 days, the patient maintains protected weight-bearing restrictions in either a postoperative shoe or a splint.

• Sutures are typically removed at first follow-up visit.

• We routinely continue protected weight bearing in a postoperative stiff-soled shoe for 6 weeks, with weight bearing allowed on the heel.

OUTCOMES

• Dhukaram et al reported a case series on 20 patients after hallux IPJ fusion using 3.5-mm screw fixation. All subjects were pain-free at the final mean follow-up of 19 months with fusion rate of 100%.

• Thitiboonsuwan et al reviewed a series of 42 patients, with or without previous first metatarsophalangeal joint arthrodesis, who underwent hallux IPJ fusion with a median follow-up of 9 months. Previous first metatarsophalangeal joint arthrodesis was a risk factor for IPJ nonunion and other complications.

• At 18-month follow-up of the patient in **TECH FIG 6**, after hardware removal, hallux alignment and function had improved (**FIG 3**).

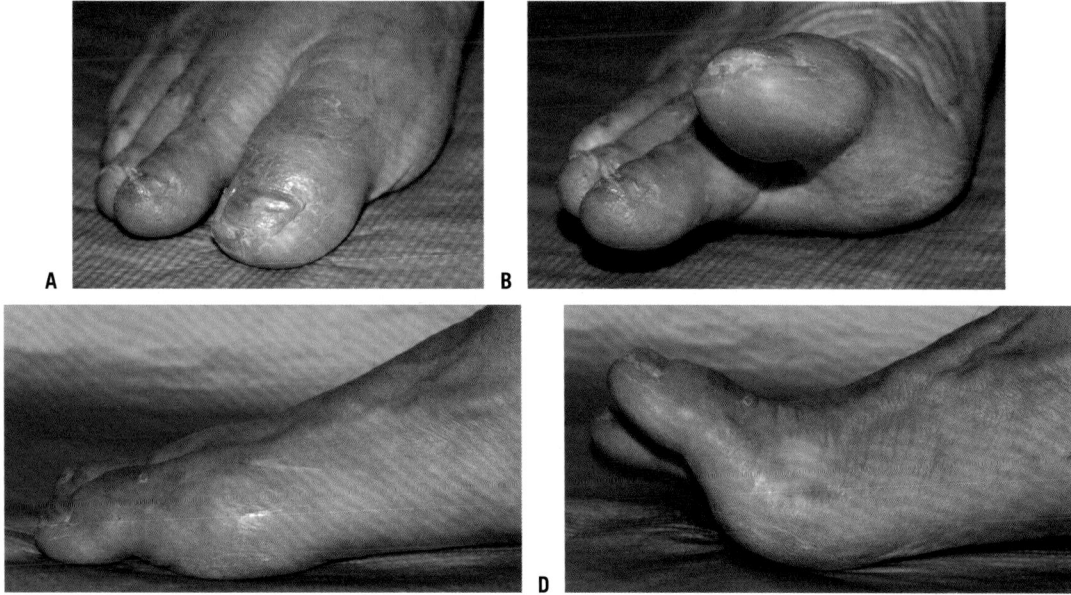

FIG 3 Follow-up of IPJ arthrodesis with FHL tendon transfer for cock-up toe deformity secondary to both sesamoids being excised (same patient as in **TECH FIG 6**). **A.** Toe neutral. **B.** MTP joint dorsiflexion. **C.** Lateral view of toe in neutral position (note intentional slight residual flexion of IPJ arthrodesis). **D.** Lateral view of MTP joint dorsiflexion. *(continued)*

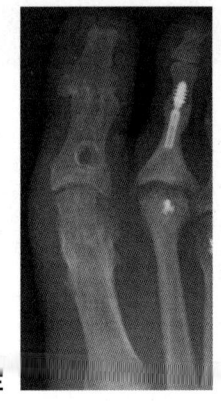
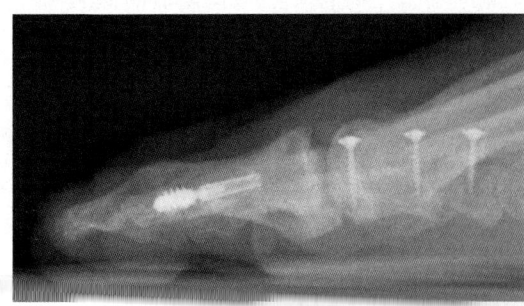

E   F

FIG 3 *(continued)* AP (**E**) and lateral (**F**) radiographs at 18-month follow-up and after removal of hardware.

COMPLICATIONS

- Wound complications
- Infection
- Malrotation
- Malunion
- Nonunion

SUGGESTED READINGS

Dhukaram V, Roche A, Walsh HPJ. Interphalangeal joint fusion of the great toe. Foot Ankle Surg 2003;9:161–163.

Salleh R, Beischer A, Edwards WH. Disorders of the hallucal interphalangeal joint. Foot Ankle Clin 2005;10(1):129–140.

Shives TC, Johnson KA. Arthrodesis of the interphalangeal joint of the great toe—an improved technique. Foot Ankle 1980;1(1):26–29.

Thitiboonsuwan S, Kavolus JJ II, Nunley JA II. Hallux interphalangeal arthrodesis following first metatarsophalangeal arthrodesis. Foot Ankle Int 2018;39(10):1178–1182.

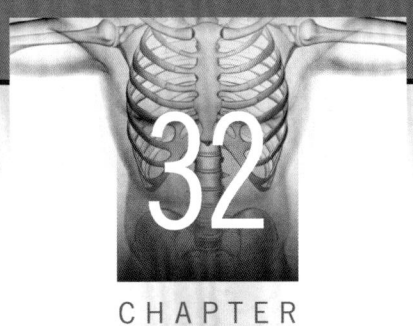

32

CHAPTER

Surgical Management of Turf Toe Injuries

Robert B. Anderson and Christopher Nicholson

DEFINITION

- Turf toe injuries involve the capsular–ligamentous–sesamoid complex of the hallux metatarsophalangeal (MP) joint.[1,2] They fall within a spectrum ranging from stable capsular sprains to unstable disruptions of the complex, often associated with a frank dislocation. The direction/force of the injury will dictate what structures are injured—most are hyperextension in nature.
- Turf toe injuries have become more prevalent with less forgiving playing surfaces (ie, artificial/infill turf) and less rigid shoe wear[7,10] and may be considered more disabling than ankle sprains.[5,9] The incidence is increasing as these injuries are better recognized and reported.[12]
- Turf toe can result in significant disability and loss of playing time in athletes, with long-term implications such as hallux rigidus. It must be diagnosed early and evaluated properly to restore function and improve outcome.[8]

ANATOMY

- The hallux MP joint is stabilized by adjacent capsular, ligamentous, tendinous, and osseous structures (FIG 1). Disruption of any part of this complex results in a turf toe injury.
- The plantar plate is composed of the joint capsule, with attachments to the transverse head of the abductor hallucis, to the flexor tendon sheaths, and to the deep transverse intermetatarsal ligament.
- The tibial and fibular sesamoids articulate with the metatarsal head. They are contained within the medial and lateral portions of the flexor hallucis brevis (FHB) tendons, respectively. Their relationship is maintained by the intersesamoid ligament. Ligamentous attachments also run between the sesamoids and the metatarsal head and proximal phalanx. The sesamoids may be bipartite, particularly the tibial.
- The FHB is located within the third plantar layer of the foot. It originates from the lateral cuneiform and the cuboid. It inserts into the proximal phalanx of the hallux and is innervated by the medial plantar nerve.
- Medially, in the first plantar layer of the foot, the abductor hallucis muscle originates from the medial process of the os calcis tuberosity. It inserts with the medial tendon of the FHB into the medial aspect of the base of the hallux proximal phalanx. It also is innervated by the medial plantar nerve.
- Laterally, also in the third plantar layer of the foot, the adductor hallucis has two heads. The oblique head originates from the base of metatarsals two through four, whereas the transverse head takes origin from the lateral fourth MP joint. The two heads unite and insert through the fibular

sesamoid into the lateral aspect of the base of the hallux proximal phalanx. Both heads are innervated by the lateral plantar nerve.

PATHOGENESIS

- The primary mechanism of injury involves a hyperextension force to the hallux MP joint. Most commonly, an axial load is applied to the heel of a foot fixed in equinus (FIG 2).

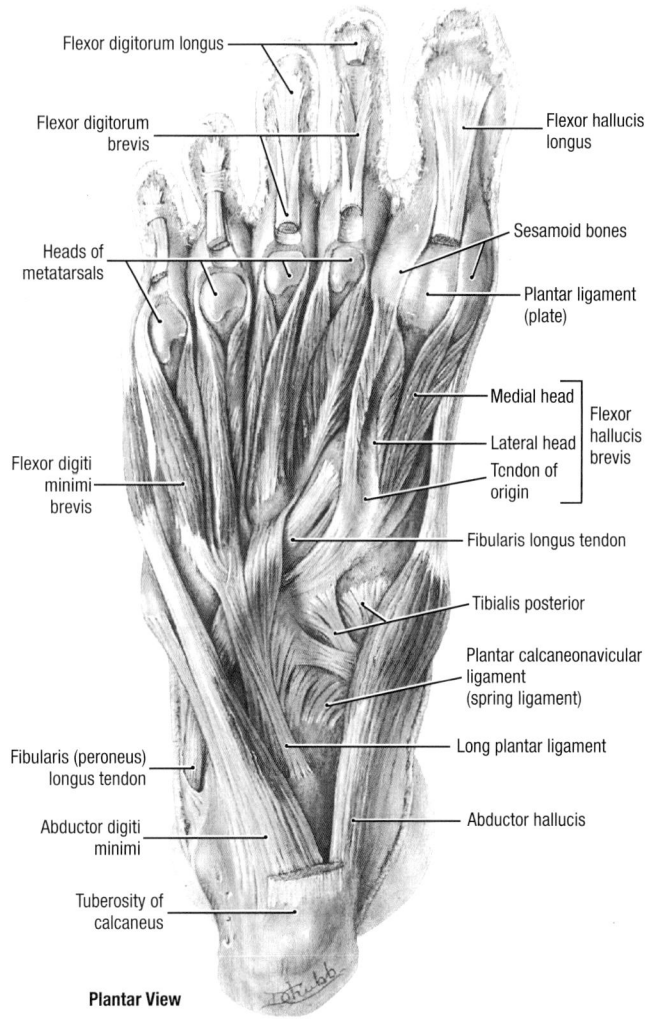

FIG 1 Normal plantar anatomy of the hallux MP joint. (Reprinted with permission from Agur AMR, Dalley AF. Grant's Atlas of Anatomy, ed 11. Philadelphia: Lippincott Williams & Wilkins, 2005.)

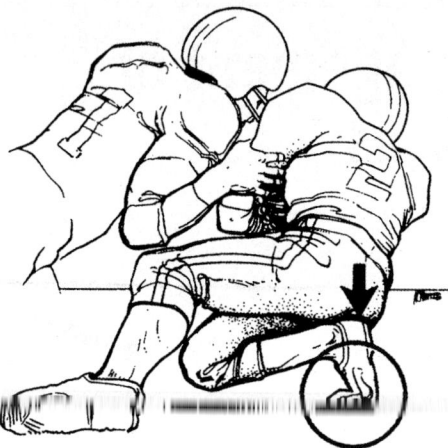

FIG 2 Typical mechanism of turf toe injury: A foot fixed to the ground is subjected to an axial load and creates a hyperextension force at the hallux MP joint.

- The most common variation is that created by a valgus-directed force, resulting in an injury to the medial collateral ligament, plantar medial complex, or tibial sesamoid that, if left untreated, may lead to a traumatic bunion and hallux valgus. A varus-directed force is much less common but can lead to a traumatic varus deformity.
- In our experience, limited ankle dorsiflexion (often from a tight Achilles tendon) places the hallux MP joint at greater risk for injury, although the literature is controversial on this mode of pathogenesis.

NATURAL HISTORY

- The natural history of turf toe depends on the degree of injury to the capsular–ligamentous–sesamoid complex. Simple, stable sprains usually heal uneventfully. Missed or untreated unstable injuries may lead to chronic pain and push-off weakness due to hallux limitus or rigidus and clawing (cock-up deformity).

PATIENT HISTORY AND PHYSICAL FINDINGS

- The history of this injury is particularly important. Useful information includes the type of shoe the patient was wearing and the circumstances of the injury (ie, the position of the foot at the time of injury, the direction of applied force, the type of athletic surface and shoe, any perceived "pop," and any initial obvious deformity, such as a dislocation that may have reduced spontaneously or required manual manipulation).
- In our experience, limited ankle dorsiflexion (often from a tight Achilles tendon) places the hallux MP joint at greater risk for injury, although the literature is controversial on this mode of pathogenesis.
- Relevant clinical findings include plantar swelling and ecchymosis about the hallux MP joint. Alignment of the hallux MP joint is noted and compared to the contralateral side. Asymmetric hallux valgus suggests a traumatic bunion, and asymmetric hallux varus implies traumatic injury to the lateral sesamoid complex. The hallux may be elevated off the ground, which may be indicative of a flexor hallucis longus (FHL) tendon disruption or significant loss of plantar restraints. Dorsal dislocation of the first MP joint is an obvious finding and may imply severe injury to the sesamoid complex.

TABLE 1 Classification of Turf Toe
Hyperextension (Turf Toe)
Grade 1: stretching of the plantar complex; localized tenderness, minimal swelling, no ecchymosis
Grade 2: partial tear; diffuse tenderness, moderate swelling, ecchymosis, restricted movement with pain
Grade 3: complete tear; severe tenderness to palpation, marked swelling and ecchymosis, limited movement with pain, positive vertical Lachman test; associated injuries possible (medial–lateral injury, sesamoid fracture/bipartite diastasis, articular cartilage–subchondral bone bruise)
Hyperflexion (Sand Toe)
Dislocation
Type I: dislocation of the hallux with the sesamoids, no disruption of the intersesamoid ligament, usually irreducible
Type II: IIA (associated disruption of intersesamoid ligament; usually reducible), IIB (associated transverse fracture of one of the sesamoids; usually reducible), IIC (complete disruption of intersesamoid ligament with fracture of one of the sesamoids; usually reducible)

- The examination will include the following:
  - Active and passive hallux MP range of motion. Hallux MP motion varies widely among individuals, with reported plantarflexion from 3 to 40 degrees and dorsiflexion from 40 to 100 degrees. Varus and valgus stressing is also performed. The best method to determine significance is to compare to the noninjured contralateral side.
  - The examiner should observe the patient's gait (specifically, the time between heel rise and toe-off). The patient will shorten time spent after heel rise because this concentrates pressure onto the injured hallux MP joint.
  - Vertical Lachman test. A positive test is any laxity greater than the contralateral side.
- Turf toe classification is shown in **TABLE 1**.

IMAGING AND OTHER DIAGNOSTIC STUDIES

- A thorough radiographic evaluation is mandatory (including weight-bearing views of the foot in the anteroposterior [AP], lateral, and oblique planes) **(FIG 3)**. Sesamoid axial views may also be helpful.
- Bilateral standing AP views are mandatory for comparison. Sesamoid station is assessed.
- Forced (stress) dorsiflexion lateral views are helpful to diagnose disruption/diastasis of a bipartite sesamoid or a sesamoid fracture **(FIG 4)**. It will also suggest a complete distal disruption of the FHB if the sesamoid(s) fails to migrate distally with dorsiflexion of the hallux. Studies suggest that more than 10.4 mm from the tip of the tibial sesamoid to the phalanx or more than 13.3 mm from the fibular sesamoid equates to a 99.7% chance for plantar complex rupture.[11] Compare the injured to uninjured side.
- Fluoroscopic evaluation has proven invaluable and is highly recommended when available. The hallux is dorsiflexed, and if the sesamoids do not migrate distally, a plantar plate disruption can be inferred.

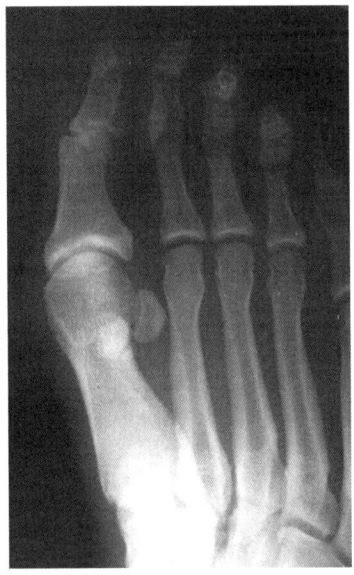

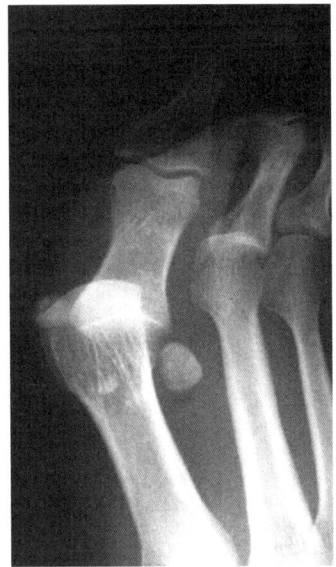

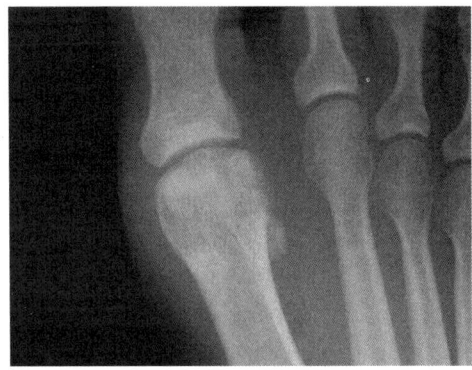

FIG 3 A. AP foot radiograph showing proximal migration of the tibial sesamoid suggestive of an unstable turf toe injury. **B.** AP foot radiograph showing a hallux MP dislocation with an associated sesamoid fracture. **C.** AP radiograph demonstrating diastased bipartite tibial and fibular sesamoids. The proximal poles of each sesamoid are retracted.

- Magnetic resonance imaging (MRI) is recommended for any patient with radiographic abnormalities and for those with significant swelling, any ecchymosis or limitation of motion, or a positive vertical Lachman test **(FIG 5)**. Osteochondral lesions and edema in the metatarsal head are often present and may be prognostic. Injury to the FHL tendon is also assessed.

DIFFERENTIAL DIAGNOSIS

- Chondral or osteochondral lesion of the hallux metatarsal head
- Hyperflexion injury (sand toe)[6]

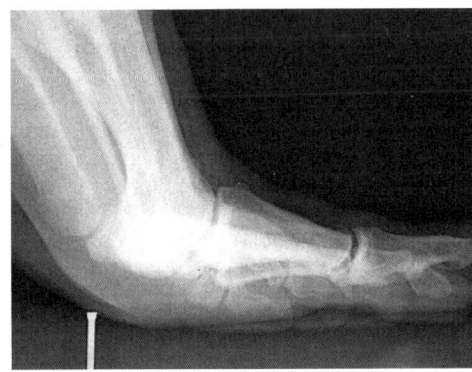

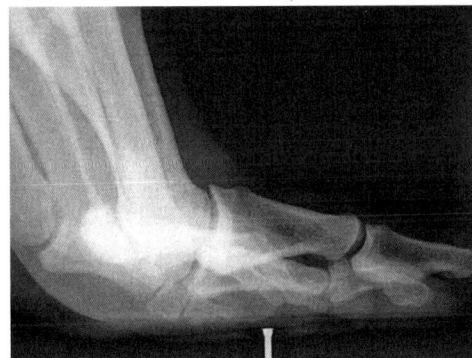

FIG 4 Dorsiflexion stress lateral radiographs. **A.** Normal. Note the position of the sesamoids. **B.** Abnormal. Note the proximal migration of the sesamoid complex.

- Fracture of the proximal or distal phalanx of the hallux
- Synovitis of the hallux MP joint

NONOPERATIVE MANAGEMENT

- Rest, ice, elevation, and nonsteroidal anti-inflammatories[4]
- Immobilization with a boot or cast. A toe spica cast with the hallux in plantarflexion relieves tension on the injured plantar complex **(FIG 6)**; found to be very helpful with a diastased bipartite or fractured sesamoid
- Corticosteroid and anesthetic injections are avoided, especially in the athlete, to avoid rupture or further weakening of the capsular–ligamentous complex. These injections can mask unstable injuries that, if not addressed, can lead to hallux deformity and permanent loss of push-off strength.
- Taping of the hallux to prevent excessive dorsiflexion
- Inserts: off-the-shelf orthoses with an aluminum or carbon "turf toe" plate or a custom device that includes the Morton extension to stiffen the first ray

SURGICAL MANAGEMENT

- Operative treatment should be considered for large capsular avulsions with an unstable joint; diastasis of a bipartite sesamoid or a sesamoid fracture; retraction of the sesamoids (single or both), traumatic bunion, or progressive hallux

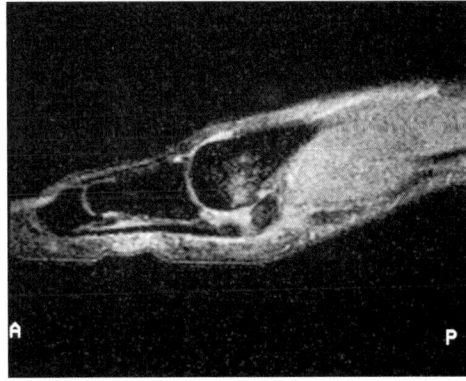

FIG 5 Sagittal T2-weighted MRI scan showing distal soft tissue defect and proximal position of the sesamoid.

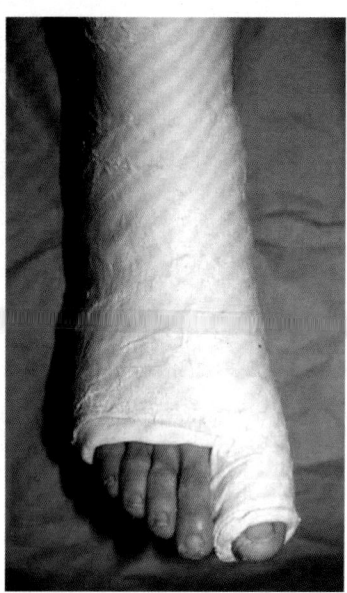

FIG 6 Plaster toe spica cast for conservative or postoperative care of a turf toe injury.

valgus; a positive vertical Lachman test; and the presence of a loose body or chondral injury. Progression of sesamoid diastasis or migration implies an unstable situation and one requiring surgery.

- Serial examinations may be needed to document progressive varus–valgus or cock-up deformities, but ideally, early diagnosis and appropriate surgical repair of the injury are performed before these late sequelae develop.

Preoperative Planning

- The degree and exact location of the injury are determined before surgery. MRI is a useful preoperative tool to ascertain the area of involvement but may exaggerate the true extent of the injury by revealing adjacent edema.

Positioning

- Although the patient may be placed prone for direct access to the sesamoid complex, we routinely perform surgical repair of turf toe injuries with the patient in the supine position. It is ideal to have the operative extremity in slight

external rotation because the approach is largely medial. If the patient's natural tendency is not external rotation, then a bump can be placed under the contralateral hip or the table can be tilted toward the operative side.

Approach

- Described approaches include a plantar medial, medial and plantar lateral, and the J configuration. Over the past 6 years, we have employed the combined medial and plantar lateral approach in patients suspected of having a complete plantar plate disruption. This approach allows for a more direct repair of the lateral structures without extensive skin and neurovascular dissection and retraction. Improved wound healing has been noted anecdotally (**FIG 7**).

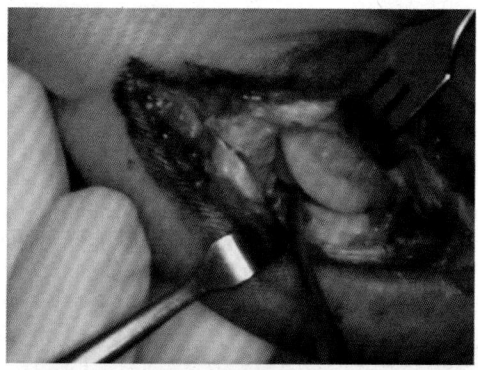

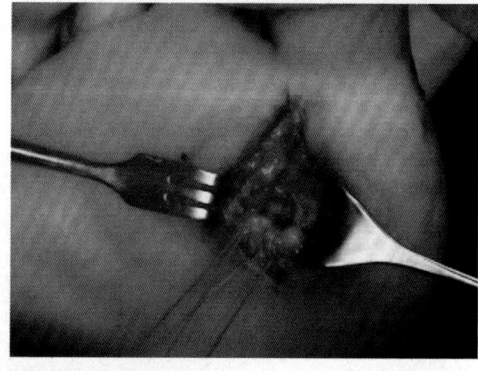

FIG 7 Intraoperative photograph of the medial (**A**) and plantar lateral (**B**) incisions about the hallux MP joint used for exposure and repair of the plantar plate rupture.

TECHNIQUES

INCISION

- In this example, the surgeon has elected to use the J incision, which extends plantar medial and then crosses plantarly along the flexor crease at the base of the phalanx (**TECH FIG 1A**).
- Take extreme care to identify and protect the plantar medial digital nerve (**TECH FIG 1B**).
- Make a longitudinal incision at the level of the abductor hallucis tendon (**TECH FIG 1C**). This allows both intra- and extra-articular examination of the plantar complex.
- Fully define the extent of the injury (**TECH FIG 1D**).
- Once the defect has been fully defined, distally mobilize the plantar plate and sesamoid complex.

- In complete plantar ruptures, both sesamoids will be proximally retracted but will slide distally around the FHL tendon.
- In chronic cases, this requires removal of fibrous scar tissue. Protect the FHL tendon while débriding the scar tissue.
- Thoroughly examine the FHL tendon for longitudinal tears (**TECH FIG 1E**). In our experience, longitudinal tears of the FHL tendon are most commonly associated with a late presentation of turf toe injury in which the FHL is subjected to frequent greater than physiologic stretching as a result of the lack of plantar restraint of the MP joint.

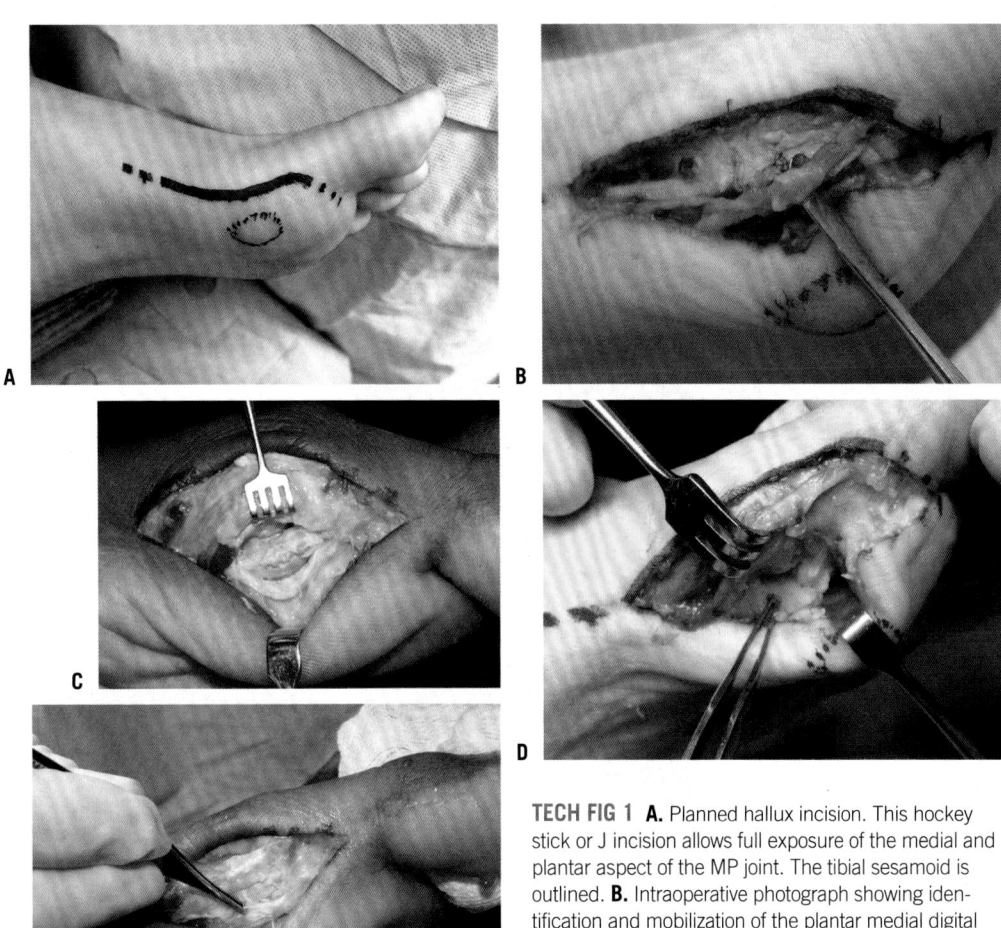

TECH FIG 1 A. Planned hallux incision. This hockey stick or J incision allows full exposure of the medial and plantar aspect of the MP joint. The tibial sesamoid is outlined. **B.** Intraoperative photograph showing identification and mobilization of the plantar medial digital nerve. **C.** Longitudinal incision at the abductor hallucis and capsule allows visualization of the joint. **D.** After exposure, the extent of the injury must be defined. This involves identifying each element of the plantar complex to determine its integrity. **E.** The FHL tendon is inspected for longitudinal tears and repaired primarily if necessary.

REPAIR OF DISTAL RUPTURES

- Make a J incision or dual incision and identify the plantar medial digital nerve where it crosses obliquely immediately deep to the planned incision. Once the nerve is identified, carefully retract it throughout the surgery but with intermittent relaxation to limit the risk of a traction neuralgia.
- Make an incision at the level of the abductor hallucis tendon to allow examination of the MP joint.
- Identify the components of the plantar complex, including FHB, FHL, sesamoids, intersesamoid ligament, transverse and oblique heads of adductor hallucis, and plantar capsule. This step may take some time, depending on the degree of disruption and the time from injury.
- In acute cases, a rim of stout capsule typically remains on the base of the proximal phalanx. In the chronic situation, the sesamoid complex may appear redundant, often due to intervening scar tissue or elongated, weakened soft tissues at the site of

injury (**TECH FIG 2A**). We recommend excising the redundant scar tissue sharply and advancing the proximal intact and healthy portion of the complex (**TECH FIG 2B**).
- Distal ruptures require primary repair of remnants from lateral to medial, working around the FHL tendon (**TECH FIG 2C**). The hallux is held in approximately 15 degrees of plantarflexion as sutures are secured.
- If the soft tissue is contracted and cannot be advanced to allow a primary repair, the FHB and abductor hallucis may be fractionally lengthened.
- If soft tissues are inadequate, suture anchors or drill holes to the plantar aspect of the base of the proximal phalanx may be used (**TECH FIG 2D,E**). A transverse drill hole can also be created in the distal pole of the tibial sesamoid if there is an absence of soft tissue for repair on the proximal aspect.
- Close the wound using standard techniques.

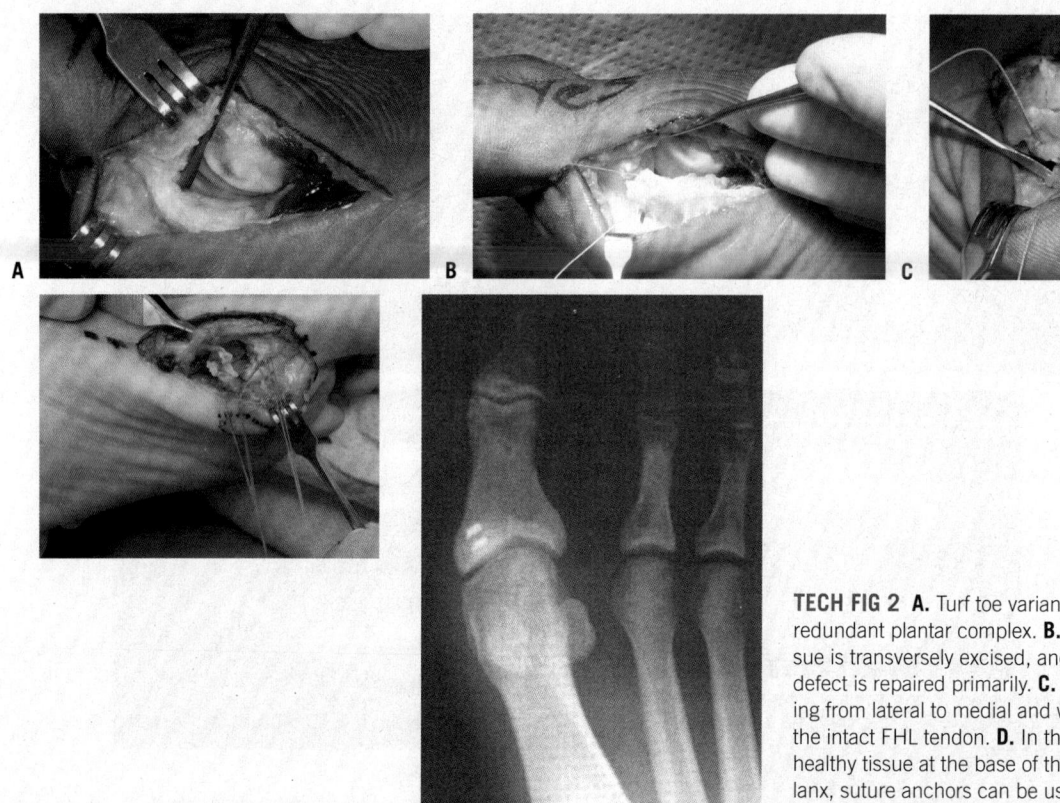

TECH FIG 2 A. Turf toe variant with intact but redundant plantar complex. **B.** Redundant tissue is transversely excised, and the remaining defect is repaired primarily. **C.** Repair proceeding from lateral to medial and working around the intact FHL tendon. **D.** In the absence of healthy tissue at the base of the proximal phalanx, suture anchors can be used to advance the plantar complex. **E.** Radiograph showing anchors in the proximal phalanx.

REPAIR OF DIASTASIS OR FRACTURE OF THE TIBIAL SESAMOID

- Make a J or dual incision and protect the plantar medial digital nerve. Retract the abductor superiorly.
- Identify the FHB with the associated tibial sesamoid.
- Diastasis or fracture of the tibial sesamoid may occasionally be repaired with a small-diameter cannulated screw. However, comminuted fractures, particularly those in chronic injuries, are, in our opinion, better treated with excision of both poles of the fractured sesamoid. Sharply excise each osseous fragment

from the FHB tendon. Repair the resulting soft tissue defect primarily (**TECH FIG 3A–C**). A grasping tendinous stitch or simply a figure-8 stitch will usually suffice. Take care to avoid incorporating the FHL tendon in the repair.

- We maintain a low threshold to transfer the abductor hallucis tendon to the resulting plantar defect (**TECH FIG 3D,E**). The distal aspect of the abductor hallucis tendon is easily elevated from its attachment on the proximal phalanx and rotated

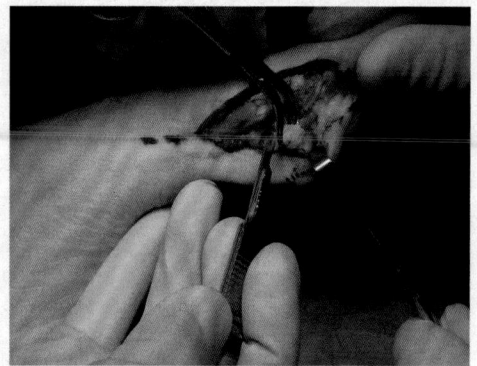

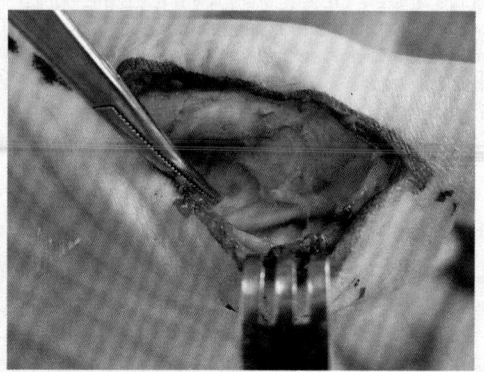

TECH FIG 3 Repair of injury involving a tibial sesamoid fracture. **A.** The fragments are excised. **B.** The remaining void is often significant. *(continued)*

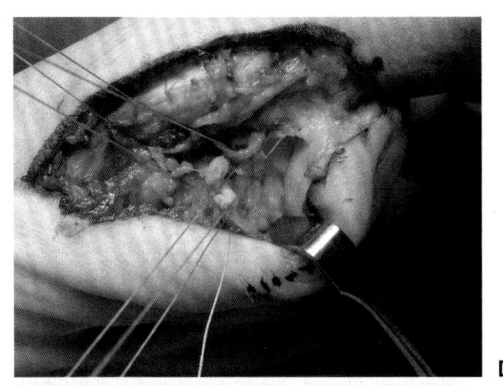

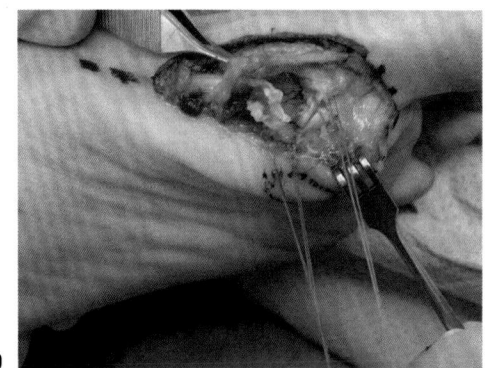

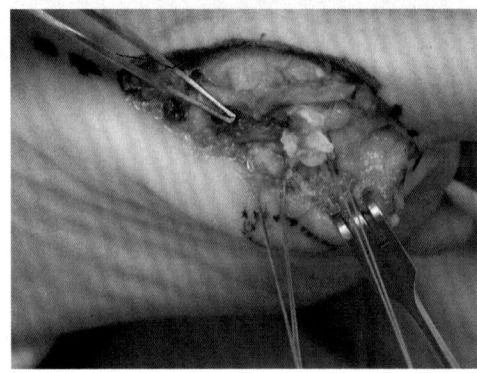

TECH FIG 3 *(continued)* **C.** An attempt is made to close the void primarily with approximation of adjacent tissue. **D.** Advancement of the abductor hallucis tendon into the defect after sesamoid excision. The rerouted abductor tendon now serves as a flexor tendon. **E.** The abductor tendon has been advanced and secured.

plantarly into the defect created by tibial sesamoid excision, where it is secured to the FHB tendon. This transfer affords not only an improved soft tissue closure of the defect but also, we believe, a dynamic component to strengthen the repair. When performed, we routinely release the adductor hallucis tendon

from its attachment to the proximal phalanx. This is accomplished via a dorsal first web space incision and will remove a potential deforming force from the unopposed abductor hallucis tendon.

- Perform routine closure.

REPAIR OF BOTH FIBULAR AND TIBIAL SESAMOIDS

- Use the standard J or dual incision and the aforementioned approach.
- Isolate each fragment of both the tibial and fibular sesamoids. Reduce the corresponding fragments with a pointed reduction forceps.
- Due to the small size of the sesamoids and because comminution is often present, internal fixation can be difficult, with resultant further fragmentation of the sesamoids.
- Therefore, cerclage the proximal and distal poles of the sesamoids using nonabsorbable suture **(TECH FIG 4)**. Then, repair the adjacent soft tissue.
- If the articular surface of the sesamoid is damaged or demonstrates significant cystic change or fragmentation within the sesamoid body, excise it. The defect is managed with an abductor tendon transfer as described earlier.
- If at all possible, avoid excising both sesamoids, as it may lead to a cock-up hallux toe deformity. If both sesamoids are painful and pathologic, it is best to stage the sesamoidectomies to lessen the risk for this complication.

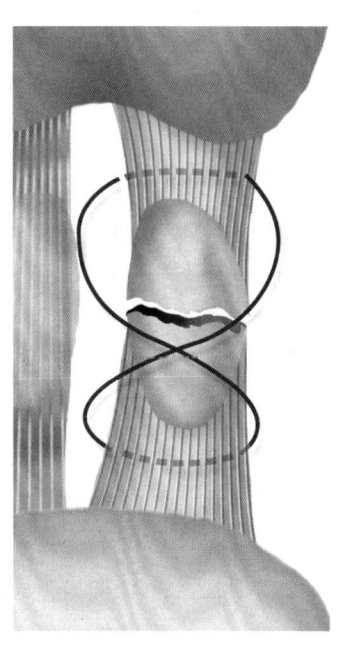

TECH FIG 4 Standard cerclage technique used to repair a fractured or diastased sesamoid.

TECHNIQUES

REPAIR OF TRAUMATIC BUNION

- In essence, this repair is a modified McBride bunionectomy with distal soft tissue realignment. Release the adductor hallucis tendon via a longitudinal incision in the dorsum of the first web space **(TECH FIG 5A)**. Transect it and elevate it off the lateral sesamoid.
- Make a medial incision and perform a longitudinal or V capsulotomy **(TECH FIG 5B)**. The incision may need to include a frank rupture of the capsule and medial collateral ligament.
- Perform a conservative excision of the medial eminence **(TECH FIG 5C)**. This assists with subsequent scarring of the medial soft tissue structures.
- Identify the medial defects and repair them primarily as described earlier, followed by routine closure **(TECH FIG 5D)**.

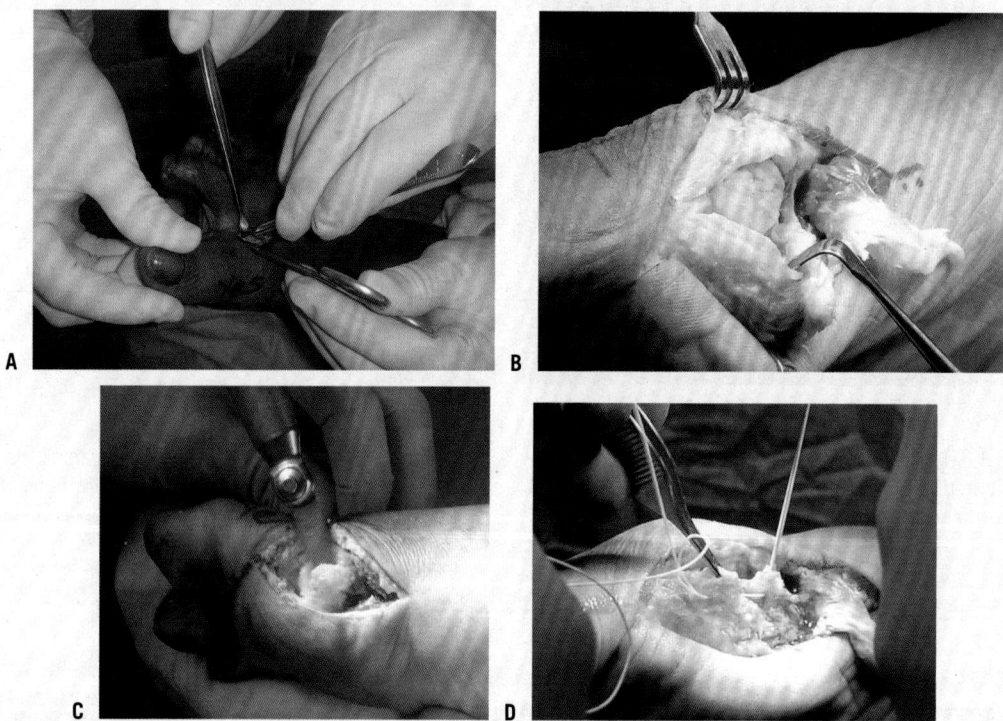

TECH FIG 5 A. Incision and release of adductor hallucis in a traumatic bunion. **B.** Standard J incision is performed followed by capsulotomy to expose the medial eminence. **C.** Intraoperative picture of a conservative medial eminence resection for a traumatic bunion. **D.** Primary capsular repair and advancement after medial eminence resection for a traumatic bunion.

CORRECTION OF LATE COCK-UP HALLUX DEFORMITY

- A sequela of untreated turf toe injury is the cock-up hallux deformity or hyperextension of the hallux MP joint and flexion at the hallux interphalangeal joint.
- Perform a medial incision.
- Often, the dorsal capsule and extensor hallucis longus and brevis are contracted and must be released. The extensors may need to be Z-lengthened.

- Release the FHL as far distal as possible at its insertion into the distal phalanx. Make a dorsal to plantar drill hole in the proximal phalanx toward its base. Route the FHL tendon from plantar to dorsal through the osseous tunnel and secure it dorsally. A small interference screw may be used, or the tendon can simply be secured with a nonabsorbable suture. Tensioning is done in 5 to 10 degrees of plantarflexion with full excursion on the tendon.

Pearls and Pitfalls

Proper Diagnosis	• Attention to history and physical examination is paramount. An MRI is ordered if any concern for an unstable situation exists.
Progressive Deformity	• With injuries managed nonsurgically, serial examinations allow the physician to appreciate a tendency for progressive deformity. Surgical repair is recommended before the deformity leads to late sequelae such as traumatic bunion or cock-up deformity.
Plantar Medial Soft Tissue Defects	• These defects, typically noted after medial sesamoid excision, may be augmented with transfer of the abductor hallucis tendon into the defect.

POSTOPERATIVE CARE

- Postoperative care is a delicate balance between soft tissue protection and early hallux MP range of motion, avoiding arthrofibrosis of the sesamoid–metatarsal articulation.
- Gentle passive range of motion (plantarflexion) is initiated under supervision in 5 to 7 days after surgery.
- The patient remains non–weight bearing in a removable splint or boot with the hallux protected for 4 weeks.
- At 4 weeks, the patient is allowed to initiate active motion of the joint and ambulate in a boot.
- Modified shoe wear consisting of a turf toe plate (aluminum or carbon fiber) is instituted at 2 months.
- Return to contact activity occurs at 3 to 4 months, with protection from excessive dorsiflexion. Return to play depends on the player's position, level of discomfort, and healing potential.
- Full recovery is expected to take 6 to 12 months. Shoe modifications are generally needed for at least 6 months after return to play. In general, this correlates to the presence of 50 to 60 degrees of painless passive range of motion of the hallux MP joint.

OUTCOMES

- Clanton et al[3] found that half of 20 athletes had persistent symptoms, including stiffness and pain, at 5-year follow-up.
- Warson et al[13] report that 17 of 19 college and professional athletes returned to full athletic activity with minimal residual discomfort after surgical repair of a turf toe injury.

COMPLICATIONS

- As with any surgery, infection and wound problems are potential complications. Athletes may be at increased risk if they attempt to initiate rehabilitation too early.
- Transient neuritis of the plantar medial digital nerve at the level of the hallux MP joint is common due to retraction of the nerve during surgery. However, a transection and secondary neuroma may result in significant discomfort and difficulty with shoe wear and push-off.
- Disruption of the repair may result with excessive dorsiflexion during the early rehabilitation process.
- Degeneration of the hallux MP joint (hallux rigidus) may occur despite appropriate treatment.
- A missed or delayed diagnosis can lead to progressive hallux varus or valgus or cock-up deformity **(FIG 8)**.

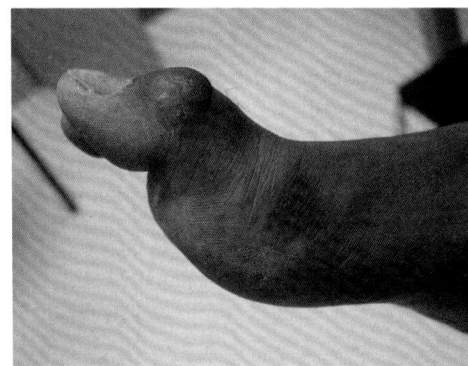

FIG 8 Hallux claw toe after a missed turf toe injury.

REFERENCES

1. Anderson RB. Turf toe injuries of the hallux metatarsophalangeal joint. Tech Foot Ankle Surg 2002;1:102–111.
2. Bowers KD Jr, Martin RB. Turf-toe: a shoe-surface related football injury. Med Sci Sports 1976;8:81–83.
3. Clanton TO, Butler JE, Eggert A. Injuries to the metatarsophalangeal joints in athletes. Foot Ankle 1986;7:162–176.
4. Clanton TO, Ford JJ. Turf toe injury. Clin Sports Med 1994;13:731–741.
5. Clough TM, Majeed H. Turf toe injury—current concepts and an updated review of literature. Foot Ankle Clin 2018;23(4):693–701.
6. Coker TP, Arnold JA, Weber DL. Traumatic lesions of the metatarsophalangeal joint of the great toe in athletes. Am J Sports Med 1978;6:326–334.
7. Frey C, Andersen GD, Feder KS. Plantarflexion injury to the metatarsophalangeal joint ("sand toe"). Foot Ankle 1996;17:576–581.
8. Jones DC, Reiner MR. Turf toe. Foot Ankle Clin 1999;4:911–917.
9. McCormick JJ, Anderson RB. The great toe: failed turf toe, chronic turf toe, and complicated sesamoid injuries. Foot Ankle Clin 2009;14:135–150.
10. Rodeo SA, O'Brien S, Warren RF, et al. Turf-toe: an analysis of metatarsophalangeal joint sprains in professional football players. Am J Sports Med 1990;18:280–285.
11. Rodeo SA, Warren RF, O'Brien SJ, et al. Diastasis of bipartite sesamoids of the first metatarsophalangeal joint. Foot Ankle 1993;14:425–434.
12. Smith K, Waldrop N. Operative outcomes of grade 3 turf toe injuries in competitive football players. Foot Ankle Int 2018;39(9):1076–1081.
13. Watson T, Anderson R, Davis W. Periarticular injuries to the hallux metatarsophalangeal joint in athletes. Foot Ankle Clin 2000;5:687–713.

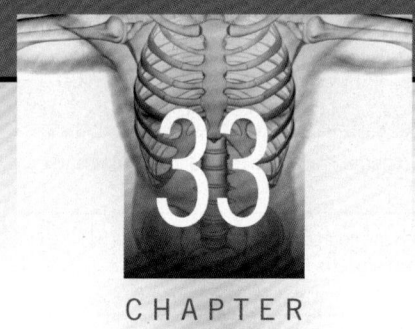

33

CHAPTER

Internal Fixation of Sesamoid Fractures

Geert I. Pagenstert, Victor Valderrabano, and Beat Hintermann

DEFINITION

- *Hallux sesamoid bone fracture* is a break through the sesamoid bone or cartilage. Medial sesamoid bone fractures are more common than lateral sesamoid bone fractures.[1,14]
- Fractures usually occur about perpendicular to the long axis of the elliptically shaped bone. Longitudinal and comminuted fractures are less common.[5,16]
- In partite or bipartite sesamoid bones, the fracture always occurs in the fibrocartilaginous junctional zone (most often perpendicular to the long axis), which can disguise the fracture.[14]

ANATOMY

- The hallux sesamoid bones usually are 13.5 ± 3 mm long. The sesamoid bones are larger in men than in women, and the medial sesamoid is more elliptically shaped and larger compared to the more circularly shaped lateral sesamoid.[13]
- The hallux sesamoid bones are invested in the tendon sheath of the flexor hallucis brevis. They connect with the intersesamoid ligament to form a solid pedestal to elevate the first ray and absorb stress during gait[2,3,13] (FIG 1A).
- The sesamoid complex acts as a fulcrum to the flexor hallucis brevis and longus tendons, increasing their lever arms and big toe push-off power, for example, the patella to the quadriceps tendon[2,3] (FIG 1B).

- Failure of the bone to ossify completely during childhood results in a multipart sesamoid bone. Bipartite sesamoids are much more common than those with three or more parts. Despite incomplete ossification, the sesamoid parts are firmly connected with fibrocartilaginous tissue to act as one bone. Spontaneous fusion can occur later in life.[9]
- Partite sesamoid bones are bilateral in only about 25% of cases; therefore, unilaterality cannot be relied on as a criterion of fracture.[9]
- The main blood supply is provided over the posterior tibial to the medial plantar artery to the sesamoids. Considerable variation exists, however, such as the main blood supply from the lateral plantar artery or even the dorsal arterial arch.[7,13]
- In general, only one major artery pierces the cortex of the sesamoid bone at the plantar aspect of the proximal pole. Small vessels also enter from the plantar nonarticular side and over the capsular attachments as a second source of vascularity.[7,13]

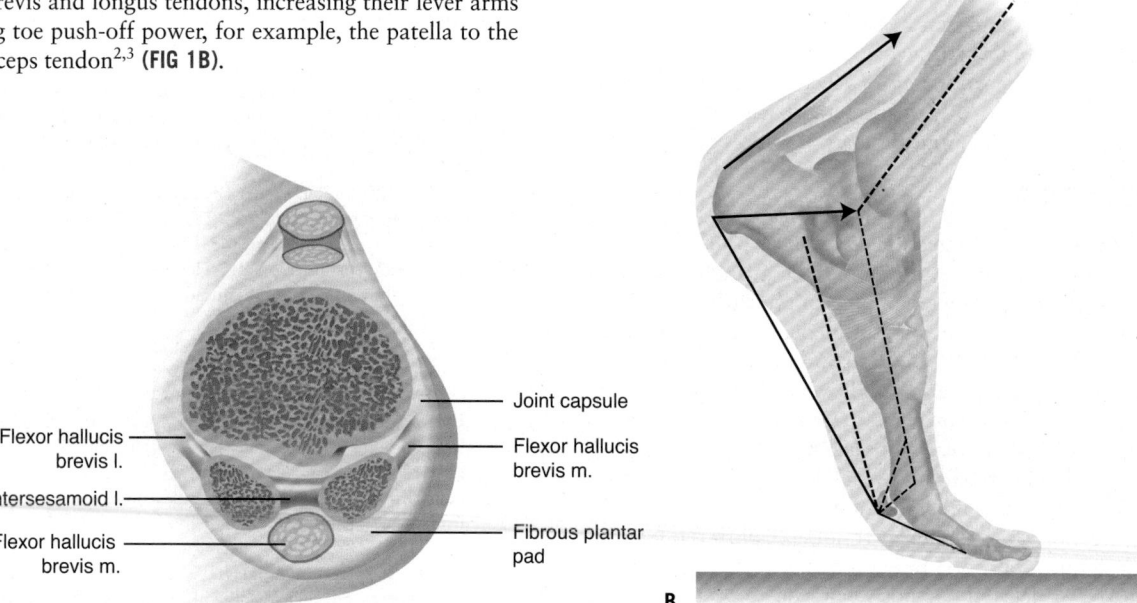

Flexor hallucis brevis l.

Intersesamoid l.

Flexor hallucis brevis m.

Joint capsule

Flexor hallucis brevis m.

Fibrous plantar pad

A

B

FIG 1 Anatomy and biomechanics of the hallux sesamoid complex. **A.** The sesamoids elevate the first metatarsal bone. Fifty percent or more of body weight is transferred over the first ray. With sesamoid excision, preloading of the metatarsal bone is decreased, transferring the load to the lesser toes. **B.** Sesamoid bones increase the lever arm of the hallucis brevis and hallucis longus flexor tendons. Sesamoid excision reduces this lever and subsequently reduces push-off power of the big toe.

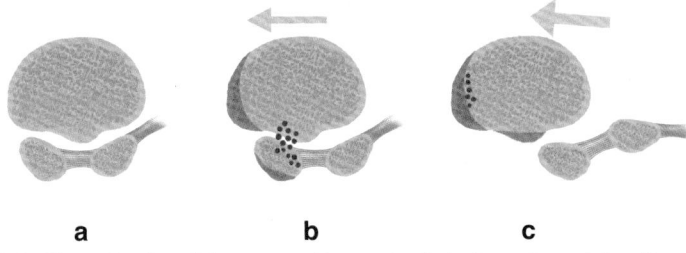

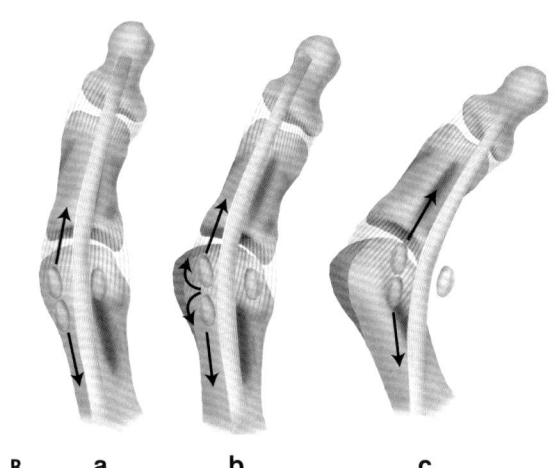

FIG 2 Biomechanics of the sesamoid complex in hallux valgus deformity. **A.** Varus subluxation of the first metatarsal bone causes pressure concentration to the medial sesamoid bone. The intersesamoid crista enhances friction to the sesamoid joint surface. **B.** After stress fracture occurs, hallux deviation will cause constant fragment displacement. Therefore, immobilization may not suffice. Sesamoid excision will enhance hallux deviation if the deformity is not addressed. (Reprinted with permission from Pagenstert GI, Valderrabano V, Hintermann B. Medial sesamoid nonunion combined with hallux valgus in athletes: a report of two cases. Foot Ankle Int 2006;27[2]:135–140. Copyright © 2006 SAGE Publications.)

PATHOGENESIS

- Acute trauma or chronic overuse leads to acute or stress fractures, respectively, of the sesamoid bones.[1,14]
- In the acute setting, the typical mechanism is excessive hyperextension of the big toe, also referred to as the *turf toe injury* seen in American football players. Disruption of the plantar joint capsule occurs as a transsesamoidal fracture-dislocation of the first metatarsophalangeal (MTP) joint.[14]
- Typically, in the chronic setting, no trauma is remembered. Pain and swelling increase insidiously over weeks, months, or years. Diagnosis is significantly delayed. Endurance sports such as running and dancing have shown to be associated with chronic stress fractures of the hallux sesamoid bones.[5,11]
- Foot deformities that concentrate pressure to the sesamoids increase the chance of suffering sesamoid stress fractures in both athletic and nonathletic persons. Cavus foot deformities with a steep plantarflexed first ray stress both sesamoid bones. Hallux valgus deformity with varus dislocation of the metatarsal head leads to pressure concentration at the medial sesamoid bone only[11,12] **(FIG 2)**.

NATURAL HISTORY

- Acute fractures without mild dislocation heal normally with little or even no treatment.[14]
- Chronic stress fractures usually do not heal without surgery, which is explained by the typical pathogenesis described earlier. During the prolonged time to diagnosis and the constant friction of fracture fragments, necrotic tissue accumulates at the fracture site and prevents healing. Brodsky et al,[6] Van Hal et al,[16] and Saxena and Krisdakumtorn[15] independently reported on consecutive series of athletes with chronic sesamoid fractures. None of the sesamoid fractures in their series healed, even with prolonged nonsurgical regimens. Histologic examination after sesamoid excision revealed accumulation of necrotic tissue at the fracture site.[6]
- Foot deformities can cause fragment separation and may prevent healing with immobilization.[11]

PATIENT HISTORY AND PHYSICAL FINDINGS

- The patient history and physical examination must rule out the differential diagnoses.
  - The typical patient history is discussed in the section Pathogenesis.
- The physical examination includes examination of areas of localized pain and swelling and hyperextension testing of the big toe.
- Patients have localized pain and swelling around the first MTP joint **(FIG 3)**.
- A complete examination of sesamoid status includes examination of the whole foot and ankle, with special attention to cavus deformity with a flexed first ray or hallux valgus deformity[11] (see **FIG 2B**).

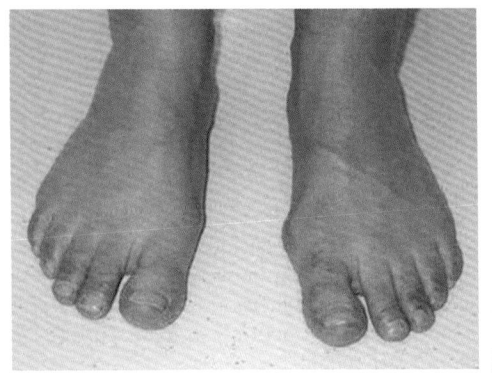

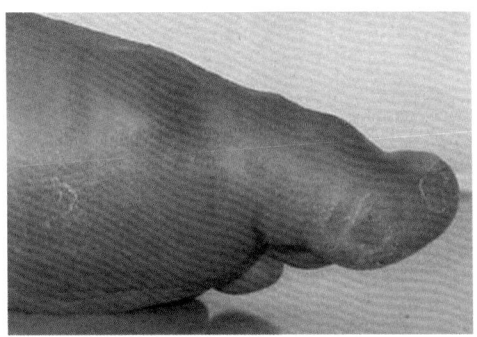

FIG 3 Clinical appearance of sesamoid stress fracture. **A.** Swelling of the MTP joint with localized tenderness at the medial sesamoid bone. **B.** Evaluate the hallux valgus deformity on the left. Progression of the deformity was noted by the patient within the preceding 3 months.

IMAGING AND OTHER DIAGNOSTIC STUDIES

- Sesamoid oblique and tangential ("skyline") views are useful to evaluate sesamoid fracture displacement (**FIG 4A**).
- Partite sesamoid bones are bilateral in only about 25% of cases.[9] Therefore, radiographs of the contralateral foot do not rule out fracture. In addition, fractures of bipartite sesamoid bones occur at the fibrocartilaginous junctional zone.[14]
- A longitudinal computed tomography (CT) scan of the foot has been shown to be very effective in demonstrating sesamoid stress fracture in difficult settings[4] (**FIG 4B**).
- Magnetic resonance imaging (MRI)[10] and bone scans[8] are nonspecific for diagnosing stress fracture or distinguishing between a traumatized bipartite sesamoid and a stress fracture. Bone edema is seen on MRI in bone contusion, inflammatory disease, avascular necrosis, and infection.[10] Localized sesamoid scintigraphic activity has been demonstrated in about 26% to 29% of cases in asymptomatic active and sedentary populations.[8]
- On full weight-bearing radiographs of the lateral whole foot, the angle between the talus and the first metatarsal is evaluated. In a normal foot, it is straight or in up to 10 degrees of flexion. A greater amount of flexion demonstrates a flexed first ray, whereas flexion of less than 0 degree demonstrates medial arch insufficiency, which is connected with hallux valgus formation.
- On full weight-bearing dorsoplantar radiographs of the foot, the hallux valgus, sesamoid position, metatarsus primus varus, and talo–first metatarsal angle are evaluated for stress concentration to the medial sesamoid bone. The talonavicular joint congruence is examined to identify excessive forefoot abduction with pes planovalgus or excessive adduction with neurogenic pes cavovarus.

DIFFERENTIAL DIAGNOSIS

- Hallux rigidus or sesamoid–first metatarsal bone osteoarthritis
- Hallux valgus
- First MTP joint capsuloligamentous disruptions (turf toe)

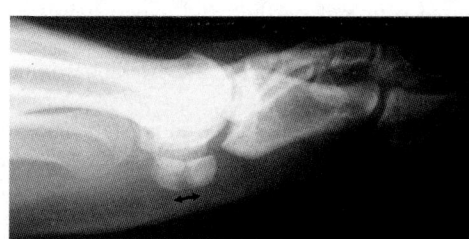

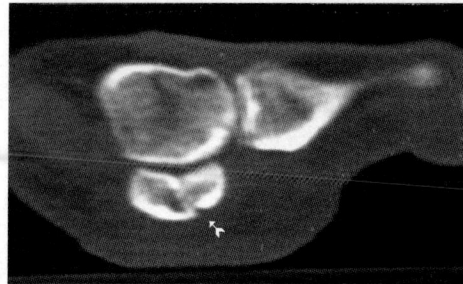

FIG 4 Radiologic examination of sesamoid fractures. **A.** Conventional radiographs demonstrating horizontal sesamoid fracture dislocation. **B.** CT scan shows fracture line of chronic painful sesamoid, which was not visible on conventional radiographs.

- Osteomyelitis and septic arthritis
- Podagra of gout and pseudogout
- Inflammatory arthritis
- Avascular necrosis of sesamoid or metatarsal head

NONOPERATIVE MANAGEMENT

- Acute fractures with up to 5-mm dislocation are treated with a forefoot immobilization shoe (stiff and convex sole) for 6 to 8 weeks.[14]
- Treatment of chronic fractures is controversial. Despite frequent failure after nonsurgical treatment attempts[5,6,11,12,15,16] and the already long time it takes to establish diagnosis, many physicians try immobilization with a shoe or cast, sometimes with the patient non–weight bearing on crutches. Recommendations for the duration of this approach before surgery is advocated range from 6 to 12 weeks.[15,16]
- If the diagnosis of stress fracture was established soon after the symptoms began, activity modification and use of a stiff-soled shoe for 6 weeks may be successful. Modification in athletic training and eating habits, with running on soft ground only, a change of sole stiffness in the athletic shoe, and increased intake of calcium and vitamin D$_3$ may be reasonable adjuncts in the future.

SURGICAL MANAGEMENT

- Severe (>5 mm) acute transsesamoidal fracture-dislocations of the first MTP joint require open repair of the capsule and flexor muscles.[14] The sesamoid bone fixation can be done with a compression screw or heavy no. 1 suture.
- Indications for percutaneous compression screw fixation include a transverse sesamoid stress fracture, transverse nonunion, or transverse symptomatic bipartite sesamoid. Fragments must be at least 3 mm to allow screw fixation.[12]
- Contraindications include infection, longitudinal sesamoid fractures, and comminuted fractures with multiple fragments that are too small for screw fixation. In these cases, partial or total sesamoid resection is indicated.
- Combined medial sesamoid fracture and hallux valgus deformity are best treated with conventional open correction of the hallux and open reduction and fixation of the sesamoid fracture by heavy no. 1 suture or compression screw.[11] Débridement of the necrotic fracture zone and grafting can be done to enhance healing.[1] In cases with less than 2-mm dislocation, the fracture zone can be stabilized by grafting only. The flexor brevis tendon sheath acts as tension band fixation.[1]
- In patients who are likely to be noncompliant, a temporary 2.5-mm Kirschner wire (K-wire) can be placed through the first MTP joint to prevent hallux dorsiflexion and stress to the fragments.
- Combined hindfoot and first ray deformities with chronic sesamoid fractures must be addressed in the same surgery.[11]

Preoperative Planning

- Acute transsesamoidal fracture-dislocations of the first MTP joint require open stabilization sometimes with an extended medioplantar L-shaped incision to reach the lateral aspect of the joint. Sesamoid fracture fixation is part of the plantar capsule or plate repair.[14]

- In chronic sesamoid fracture, preoperative planning should incorporate treatment of any underlying foot deformities.
  - A metatarsus primus flexus is treated with a dorsal extension osteotomy or arthrodesis.
  - A metatarsus primus varus and hallux valgus are addressed with appropriate osseous or soft tissue procedures.
  - Reduction of mechanical stress to the sesamoid bones is thought to be the main factor contributing to fracture healing. Surgical stress reduction alone may result in fracture healing even without sesamoid osteosynthesis in marked foot deformities.
- In the combined setting, medial sesamoid stress fractures are treated open because deformity correction is done at the same time as arthrotomy of the first MTP joint. Lateral sesamoid stress fractures are treated percutaneously because deformity correction does not include arthrotomy of the first MTP joint.
- The least invasive approach can be used in the absence of foot deformities.
  - Chronic sesamoid fractures can be addressed by percutaneous compression screw fixation alone.
  - Surgery can be performed under local anesthesia, and the stab incision of the skin can be closed with Steri-Strips.
  - Healing is thought to occur because of reaming (vitalizing) of the fracture zone and fracture stabilization. Ossification of the bipartite sesamoids occurs.[12]

- Grafting of sesamoid nonunions (bipartite sesamoids) is inherently stabilized by the flexor brevis tendon sheath.[1] In cases of persistent instability after grafting, additional suture or screw fixation is advisable.

Positioning

- The patient is placed in the supine position for isolated sesamoid bone fixation or combined deformity corrections. A tourniquet is needed, except in percutaneous fixation.

Approach

- A medial internervous or medioplantar L-shaped approach to the lateral aspect of the first MTP joint is used for acute turf toe repair, including sesamoid fracture fixation or partial removal.[14]
- A standard medial internervous approach is used for grafting of medial sesamoid nonunions and combined hallux correction.[11]
- In the case of percutaneous fixation, a stab incision is made distal to the pole of the fractured sesamoid bone and distal to the weight-bearing area of the first MTP joint. Lateral sesamoid fractures usually are treated with percutaneous screw fixation.[12]

ANDERSON-MCBRYDE TECHNIQUE OF GRAFTING SESAMOID NONUNIONS

- A medial internervous skin incision is made over the first MTP joint (**TECH FIG 1A**).
- Longitudinal capsulotomy and subperiosteal limited exposure of the medial sesamoid wall are done.
- Débridement of the necrotic tissue at the fracture site is performed with a small curette from an extra-articular medial approach (**TECH FIG 1B**).
- Fenestration of the metatarsal head is performed to enable autologous bone harvesting (**TECH FIG 1C**).
- The sesamoid fracture zone is grafted and stuffed, with care not to disrupt the fracture line in the joint surface.
- If stability is in doubt, fixation with no. 1 resorbable suture is performed to leave the least amount of foreign material in situ.

Cannulated compression screws are used as well and may provide higher compression. (Screw placement is described in the next section.)
- The suture needle is introduced from the proximal lateral pole along the internal lateral cortex to the distal lateral pole. Backstitching is done outside the bone under the medial sesamoid suspensory (capsule) ligament, back to the proximal medial pole, and knotted tight to stabilize the sesamoid joint line (**TECH FIG 1D**).
- The capsule and skin are closed as usual.
- A compressive dressing is applied with the foot in the neutral hallux position.

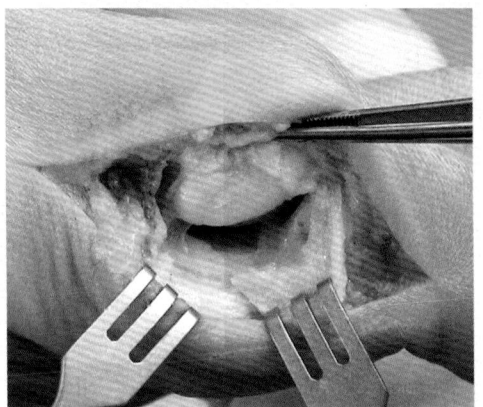
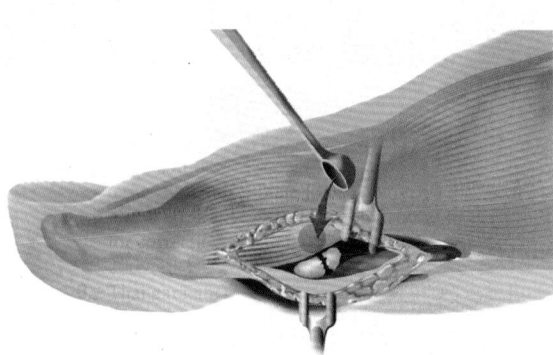

TECH FIG 1 **A.** Medial internervous approach. **B.** Débridement of the fracture with a small curette using an extra-articular approach to the necrotic tissue. *(continued)*

TECHNIQUES

TECHNIQUES

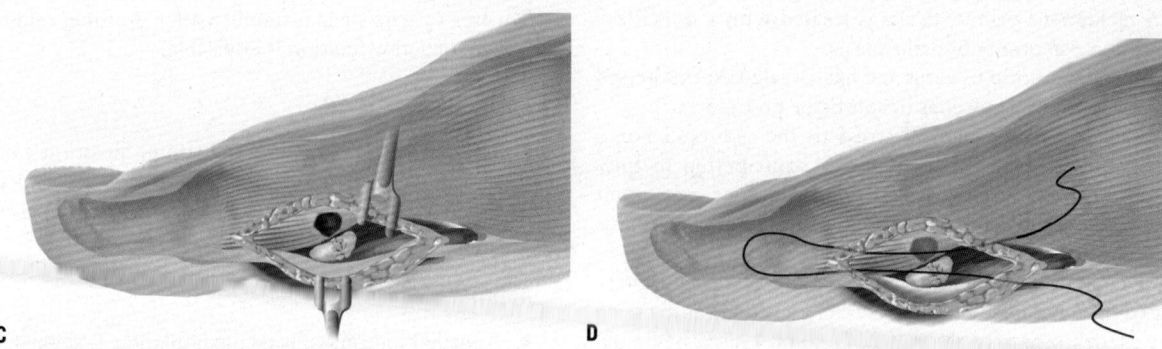

C   D

TECH FIG 1 *(continued)* **C.** Harvesting of autologous bone from the first metatarsal head. **D.** Suture cerclage of the fractured sesamoid.

PREFERRED TECHNIQUE OF PERCUTANEOUS SESAMOID SCREW FIXATION

- The hallux is held in dorsiflexion, and the sesamoid bone is pressed against the metatarsal head to level the fracture fragments against the joint line of the metatarsal head (**TECH FIG 2A**).
- One 3-mm stab incision is done distal to the fractured sesamoid bone and distal to the weight-bearing area of the first MTP joint (**TECH FIG 2B**).
- The guidewire (1.5-mm wire for 2.4-mm self-tapping Bold screws [Newdeal, Lyon, France]) is introduced under fluoroscopic control from the distal pole, perpendicular to the fracture line and subchondral to the sesamoid joint line (**TECH FIG 2C**).

- The length of the headless cannulated compression screw is measured as the difference to a second guidewire that is held next to the first and is advanced to the sesamoid cortex. The usual range is between 12 and 16 mm. The shortest screw available is 10 mm (Bold screws; **TECH FIG 2D,E**).
- The screw should pierce the proximal cortex to enhance stability (**TECH FIG 2F**).
- The stab incision is closed with sterile strips.
- Apply compression dressing in neutral hallux position.

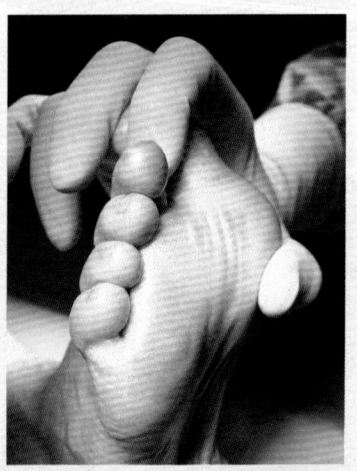 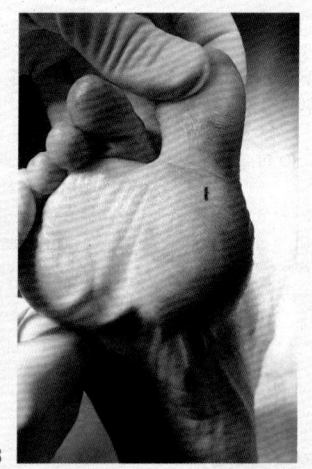 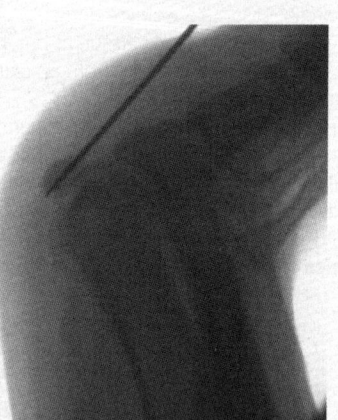

A   B   C

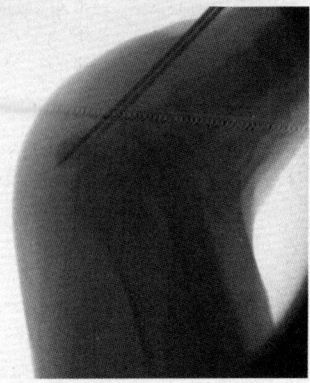

D

TECH FIG 2 A. Fixation of the hallux in hyperextension. Compress the sesamoid against the metatarsal head to level the fracture fragments against the joint line. **B.** Place the stab incision distal to the sesamoid outside the weight-bearing area of the MTP joint. **C.** Place the guidewire perpendicular to the fracture line, subchondral from proximal to distal. **D.** The guidewire should just pierce the proximal cortex. The second guidewire is advanced to the distal cortex for exact measurement. *(continued)*

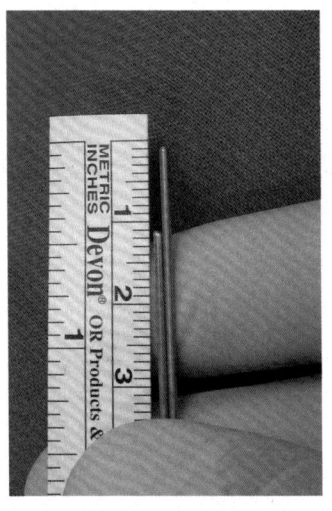
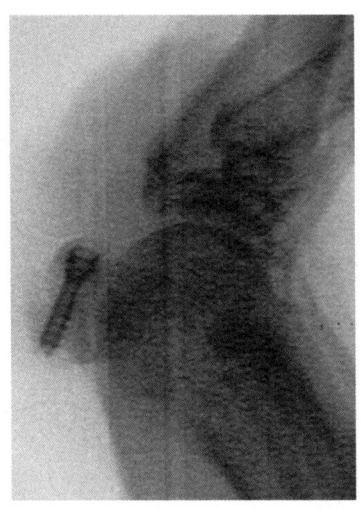

TECH FIG 2 *(continued)* **E.** Measurement using two K-wires. **F.** The definitive screw should incorporate both cortices for optimal compression. The usual length of the screw ranges between 12 and 16 mm.

CASE EXAMPLE (COURTESY OF MARK E. EASLEY, MD)

Background and Imaging

- A 22-year-old football player with a 6-month history of medial (tibial) sesamoid pain under first metatarsal head with weight bearing and push-off
- Physical examination
  - Tenderness under medial (tibial) sesamoid
  - Plantar pain with hallux MTP joint dorsiflexion
  - Negative first MTP joint Lachman test
- Radiographs suggest medial (tibial) sesamoid fracture **(TECH FIG 3A,B)**.
- CT scan demonstrates transverse fracture line with a subacute/chronic appearance **(TECH FIG 3C)**.

Exposure

- Prone position, which typically improves exposure, particularly if extensile excision becomes necessary

- Medial (and slightly plantar) longitudinal incision with extensile option by extending across plantar hallux proximal crease **(TECH FIG 4A)**
- Plantar medial sensory nerve to the hallux identified and protected **(TECH FIG 4B)**
- Longitudinal medial capsulotomy, slightly plantar to expose sesamoid with minimal periosteal stripping **(TECH FIG 4C)**
- Flexor hallucis longus (FHL) tendon identified and protected **(TECH FIG 4D)**

Fracture/Nonunion Site Preparation and Fixation

- Fracture/nonunion site identified intraoperatively and débrided of fibrous tissue and prepared for open reduction with internal fixation (ORIF) with careful medial sesamoid drilling (see **TECH FIG 4C**)
- Calcaneal bone graft harvested
- Bone graft morselized and placed within nonunion site **(TECH FIG 5)**

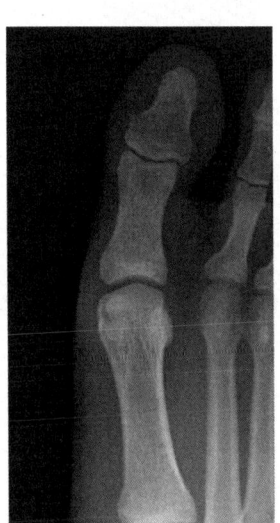
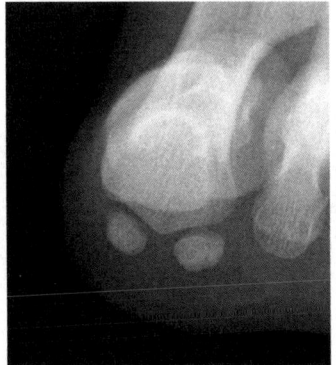
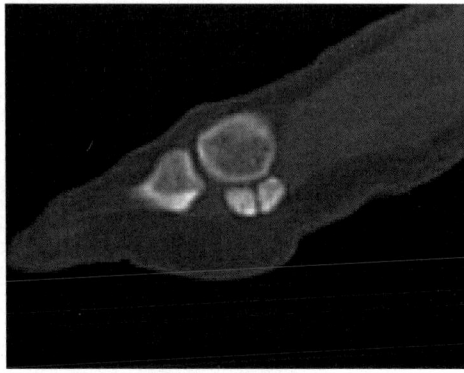

TECH FIG 3 A 22-year-old man with right medial (tibial) stress fracture failing to heal with nonoperative measures. **A.** AP view. Note medial (tibial) sesamoid with a gap and slight hallux valgus. **B.** Sesamoid view does not demonstrate this fracture. **C.** CT scan demonstrates transverse fracture line with a subacute/chronic appearance.

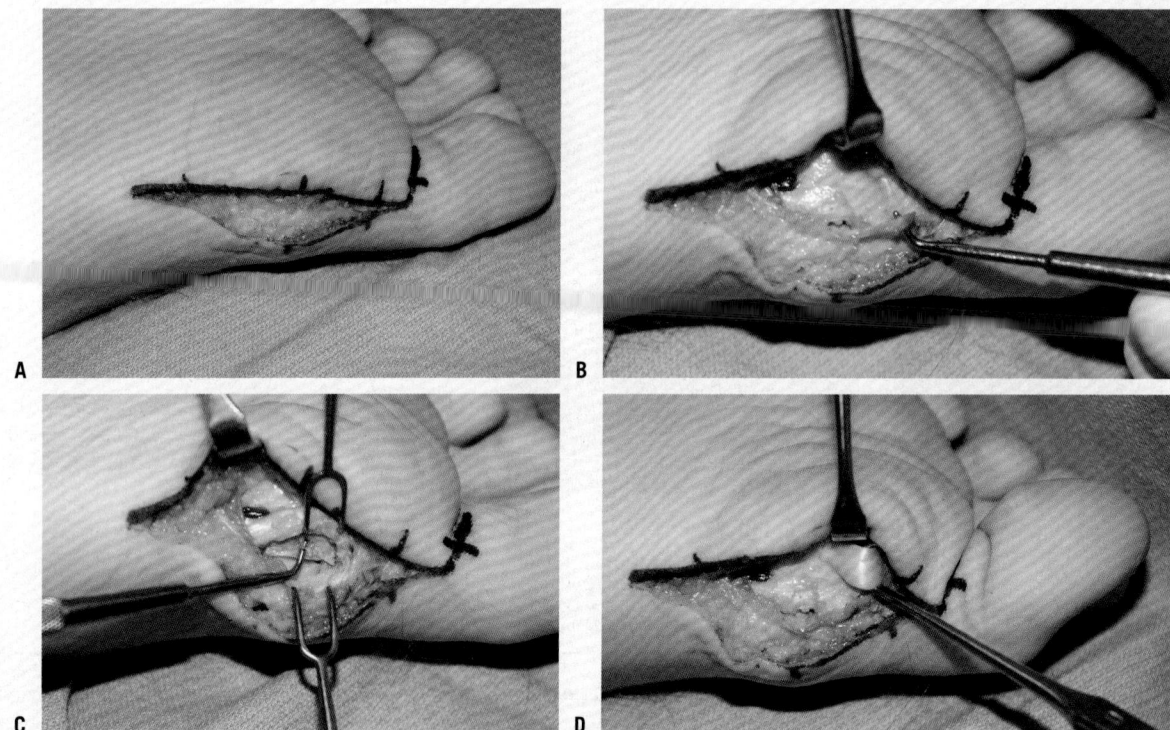

TECH FIG 4 **A.** Medial (and slightly plantar) longitudinal incision with extensile option by extending across plantar hallux proximal crease. **B.** Plantar medial sensory nerve to the hallux identified and protected. **C.** Through a medial longitudinal capsulotomy slightly plantar to the midaxial line, the medial sesamoid exposed. **D.** FHL tendon identified and protected.

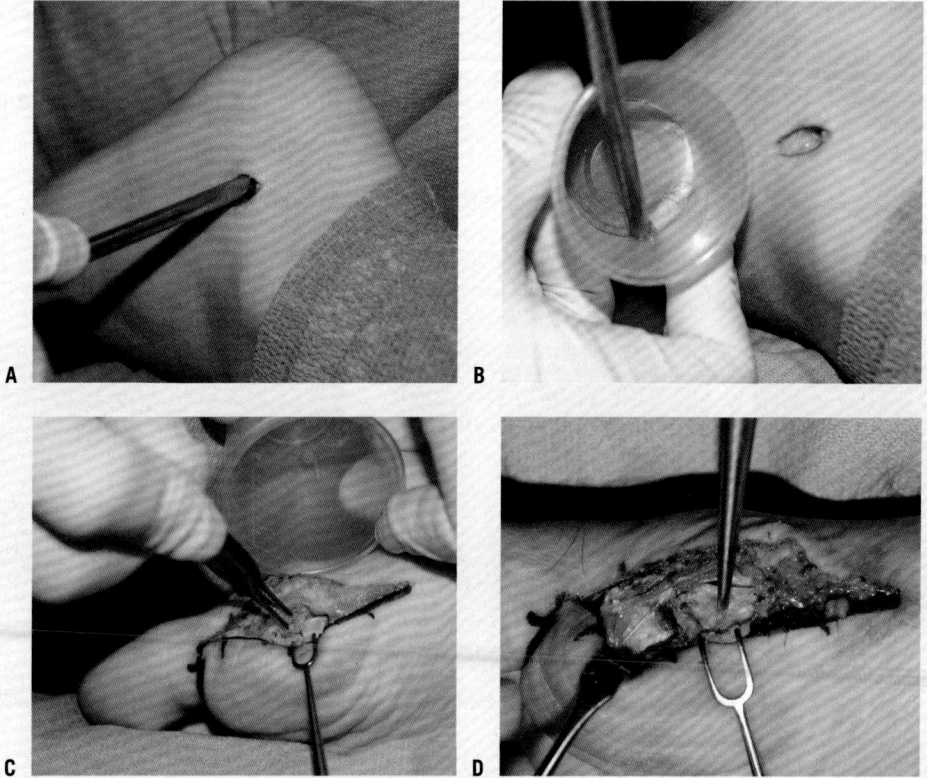

TECH FIG 5 Calcaneal autograft bone. **A.** Biopsy instrumentation used to harvest bone cylinders from the calcaneus. **B.** Bone graft cylinder within the collection cup. **C,D.** After fracture/nonunion débridement, the sesamoid fracture/nonunion is bone grafted.

Fracture Fixation

- Guide pin for cannulated screw inserted, from distal to proximal while protecting the soft tissues **(TECH FIG 6A)**
- Fluoroscopic confirmation of appropriate guide pin position
- Further calcaneal bone graft inserted into nonunion site
- Cannulated screw is placed over guide pin, with soft tissues well protected **(TECH FIG 6B,C)**.
- Clinical assessment of medial (tibial) sesamoid with hallux range of motion
- Fluoroscopic confirmation of proper screw position
- Routine closure including medial capsule
- Bunion strapping to limit risk of hallux valgus developing

Postoperative Care

- Bunion strapping to continue for minimum of 6 weeks
- Protected weight bearing on heel for 6 to 8 weeks
- Follow-up radiographs at 4- and 8-week follow-up, with the simulated weight bearing at 4 weeks and full weight bearing at 8 weeks
- If healing cannot be confirmed at 8 weeks, then CT scan of forefoot to confirm satisfactory healing and allow advancing weight bearing to the forefoot.
- Typically 3 months before return to full activities

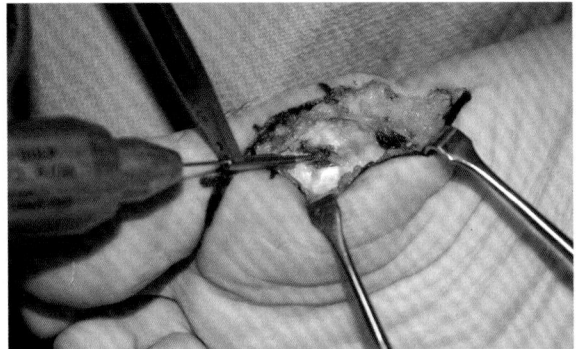
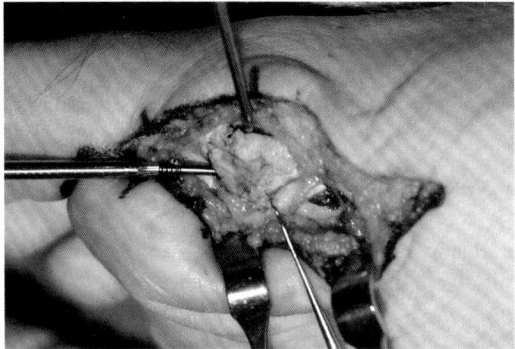

TECH FIG 6 A. Guide pin insertion while protecting the soft tissues. **B.** Cannulated medial (tibial) sesamoid screw being advanced from distal to proximal.

TECHNIQUES

Pearls and Pitfalls

Indications	• Look for foot deformities causing excessive stress to the sesamoid bones. Correction will promote sesamoid healing and prevent treatment failure.[11] • With late diagnosis of sesamoid stress fracture, early surgery will save time for the athlete.[11]
Postoperative Management	• In cases of uncertain patient compliance, temporary K-wire fixation of the first MTP joint will protect against early excessive MTP joint dorsiflexion.

POSTOPERATIVE CARE

- Full weight bearing over the heel is allowed immediately after surgery.
  - A shoe with a stiff and convex sole is used to prevent dorsiflexion of the first MTP joint for 6 weeks after surgery, after which time conventional shoes are allowed.
  - Return to full athletic activity is not recommended before 12 weeks after surgery.
- Anderson and McBryde[1] treated their patients with 4 weeks non–weight bearing and another 4 weeks with a weight-bearing cast. In our experience with the Anderson-McBryde procedure, hallux correction or turf toe repair requires no adaptations to the postoperative program outlined earlier.
- No suture removal or wound care is needed with percutaneous sesamoid fixation because the stab incision has been closed by a sterile strip.

- With combined deformity correction, the type of correction performed dictates postoperative management.

OUTCOMES

- Blundell and colleagues[5] repaired nine sesamoid fractures in athletes with percutaneous cannulated screws and achieved excellent results. All of the athletes returned to their previous level of activity, with no complications reported. Blundell et al[5] concluded that percutaneous screw fixation is a safe and fast procedure. They also questioned the importance of diagnosing the etiology of painful sesamoid fragments because treatment is the same regardless of the cause.
- Anderson and McBryde[1] performed autogenous bone grafting of medial sesamoid nonunions in 21 athletic and nonathletic patients. Of these, 19 grafts healed, whereas 2 grafts failed because the initial fracture dislocation was greater

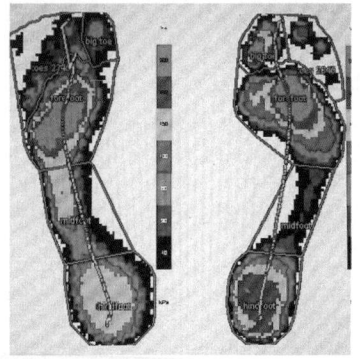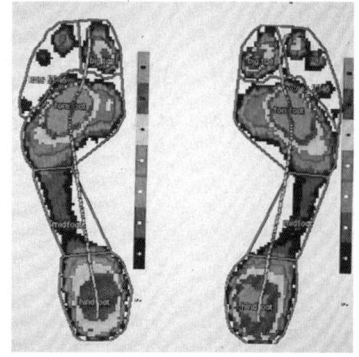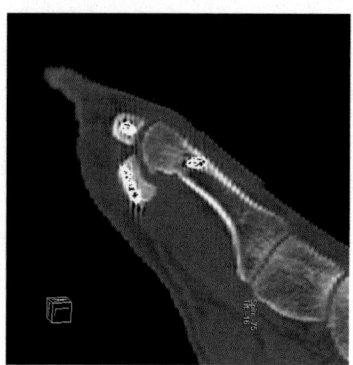

FIG 5 Postoperative clinical and radiographic results. **A.** Preoperative pedobarogram shows functional amputation of the first MTP joint as a result of painful sesamoid nonunion in the left foot. **B.** Pedobarogram 8 weeks postoperatively shows normalization of pressure distribution of the left foot after sesamoid screw fixation. **C.** CT scan 8 weeks postoperatively shows the healed sesamoid fracture with a screw in place.

than 2 mm. These two sesamoids were excised. All patients returned to their preinjury activity levels. No hallux deviations have been reported.

- At our institution, we performed screw fixation in eight athletes and suture fixation with grafting in two nonathletic women and had excellent results with full recovery.
  - The "athletic group" included six women and two men, all of whom were endurance athletes (eg, running, dancing).
  - We treated two lateral and eight medial sesamoid bone nonunions.
    - In one patient, an accompanying forefoot-driven pes cavovarus was corrected with extension osteotomy of the first metatarsus.
    - In four patients, concomitant hallux valgus deformity was corrected in combined open surgery. In two of these patients, screws were used, and in two other patients, sutures were used to stabilize the sesamoid bone during the open approach.
    - The rest of the patients were treated percutaneously. Local anesthesia was sufficient in one of these cases.

- All of the patients returned to their preinjury athletic or occupational activity level within 12 weeks after surgery.
- Clinical healing was documented with pedobarography (**FIG 5A,B**), and osseous healing of the fractures was proved by CT scan in three cases (**FIG 5C**). One screw had to be removed because of intermittent pain with exercise 1 year after surgery.
- Since then, we have used suture cerclage in open approaches, but we also continue to use percutaneous screw fixation.
  - No sesamoid has had to be excised, and no hallux deformity has occurred.
- **FIG 6** is 6-month follow-up radiographs of the patient in the case example.

COMPLICATIONS

- Persistent sesamoid pain may be caused by the following:
  - Unrecognized foot deformity and continuous stress to the hallux sesamoids
  - Development of arthritis or avascular necrosis

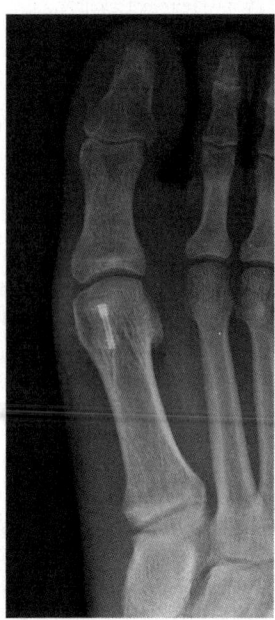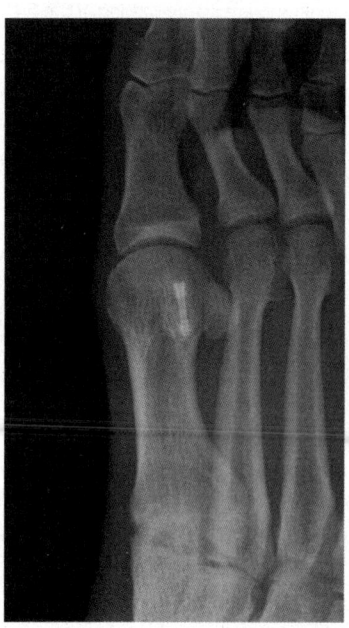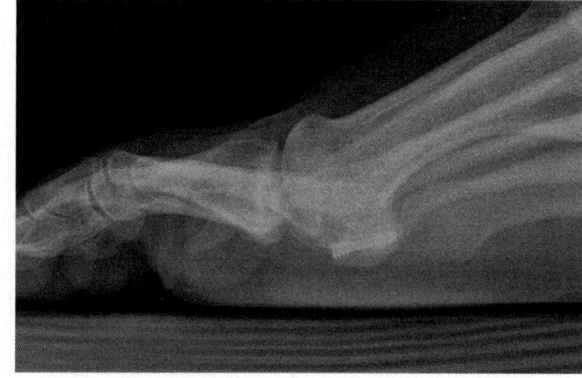

FIG 6 Six-month follow-up weight-bearing radiographs after ORIF of medial sesamoid fracture/nonunion (patient in **TECH FIGS 3** to **6**). **A.** AP view. **B.** Oblique view. **C.** Lateral view.

- Screw irritation
- Focused therapy (eg, deformity correction, screw removal) may prevent total excision as a definitive treatment of persistent sesamoid pain.
- Hallux varus after lateral sesamoid excision, hallux valgus after medial sesamoid excision, and cock-up deformity after both sesamoids were excised have been consistently described in 10% to 20% of cases in the current literature.[6,15,16] No hallux deviation has been described after fixation of sesamoid bone fractures.[1,5,11,12]
- A lever arm for flexor tendons and consecutive hallux push-off can be reconstructed with sesamoid fixation and may be important for the running athlete.[2,3]
- This biomechanical advantage has been proven in vitro[2,3] but has an uncertain use in praxis, given the excellent functional results if only one sesamoid bone is excised.[6,14–16]

REFERENCES

1. Anderson RB, McBryde AM Jr. Autogenous bone grafting of hallux sesamoid nonunions. Foot Ankle Int 1997;18:293–296.
2. Aper RL, Saltzman CL, Brown TD. The effect of hallux sesamoid excision on the flexor hallucis longus moment arm. Clin Orthop Relat Res 1996;325:209–217.
3. Aper RL, Saltzman CL, Brown TD. The effect of hallux sesamoid resection on the effective moment of the flexor hallucis brevis. Foot Ankle Int 1994;15:462–470.
4. Biedert R. Which investigations are required in stress fracture of the great toe sesamoids? Arch Orthop Trauma Surg 1993;112:94–95.
5. Blundell CM, Nicholson P, Blackney MW. Percutaneous screw fixation for fractures of the sesamoid bones of the hallux. J Bone Joint Surg Br 2002;84(8):1138–1141.
6. Brodsky JW, Robinson AHN, Krause JO, et al. Excision and flexor hallucis brevis reconstruction for the painful sesamoid fractures and non-unions: surgical technique, clinical results and histo-pathological findings. J Bone Joint Surg Br 2000;82B:217.
7. Chamberland PD, Smith JW, Fleming LL. The blood supply to the great toe sesamoids. Foot Ankle Int 1993;14:435–442.
8. Chisin R, Peyser A, Milgrom C. Bone scintigraphy in the assessment of the hallucal sesamoids. Foot Ankle Int 1995;16:291–294.
9. Inge GAL, Ferguson AB. Surgery of sesamoid bones of the great toe: an anatomic and clinical study, with a report of forty-one cases. Arch Surg 1933;27:466–489.
10. Karasick D, Schweitzer ME. Disorders of the hallux sesamoid complex: MR features. Skeletal Radiol 1998;27:411–418.
11. Pagenstert GI, Valderrabano V, Hintermann B. Medial sesamoid nonunion combined with hallux valgus in athletes: a report of two cases. Foot Ankle Int 2006;27:135–140.
12. Pagenstert GI, Valderrabano V, Hintermann B. Percutaneous screw fixation of hallux sesamoid fractures. In: Scuderi GR, Tria AJ, eds. Minimally Invasive Orthopaedic Surgery. New York: Springer Science+Business Media, 2009:501–504.
13. Pretterklieber ML. Dimensions and arterial vascular supply of the sesamoid bones of the human hallux. Acta Anat 1990;139:86–90.
14. Rodeo SA, Warren RF, O'Brien SJ, et al. Diastasis of bipartite sesamoids of the first metatarsophalangeal joint. Foot Ankle 1993;14:425–434.
15. Saxena A, Krisdakumtorn T. Return to activity after sesamoidectomy in athletically active individuals. Foot Ankle Int 2003;24:415–419.
16. Van Hal ME, Keene JS, Lange TA, et al. Stress fractures of the great toe sesamoids. Am J Sports Med 1982;10:122–128.

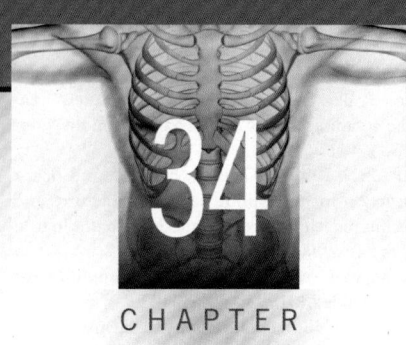

CHAPTER **34**

Sesamoidectomy

Christopher E. Gross, Simon Lee, Kamran Hamid, and George B. Holmes, Jr.

DEFINITION

- *Sesamoiditis* is a general term that indicates an injury to the sesamoid bone. There are multiple possible causes, such as trauma (fracture, contusion, repetitive stress), infection, arthrosis, osteonecrosis, and osteochondritis dissecans.[3,5,13,14,16]
- There are two sesamoid bones located plantar to the metatarsal head of the hallux: the lateral or fibular and the medial or tibial sesamoid.

ANATOMY

- The two sesamoid bones are located plantar to the metatarsal head within the tendon of the flexor hallucis brevis (FHB). They are held together by the intersesamoid ligament and plantar plate. Their dorsal surfaces articulate with the head of the first metatarsal articular facets and are separated by a crista. The sesamoids absorb the weight-bearing stress across the medial ray and protect the flexor hallucis longus (FHL) tendon that passes between them. The tibial

sesamoid is typically larger and located slightly more distal than the fibular sesamoid (**FIG 1**).
- During the stance phase of gait, the sesamoids are slightly proximal to the metatarsal head. With dorsiflexion of the hallux, the sesamoids are pulled distally, protecting the exposed surface of the metatarsal head (**FIG 2A**). During the act of heel raise, the sesamoids bear a significant amount of stress. This stress is typically concentrated more medially over the tibial sesamoid, thus accounting for the increased incidence of tibial sesamoid injuries.[14]
- Biomechanically, the sesamoids function as a fulcrum for the FHB tendon during metatarsal phalangeal joint plantarflexion as well as serving as the center of the insertional complex of the plantar fascia into the hallux.[8]
- Ossification of the sesamoids typically occurs from multiple centers and occurs during the 7th to 10th years of life. The multiple ossification centers may account for the incidence of bipartite and tripartite sesamoids.[5]
- The bipartite tibial sesamoid occurs in about 19% of the population and is bilateral in 25% (**FIG 2B**).[6]

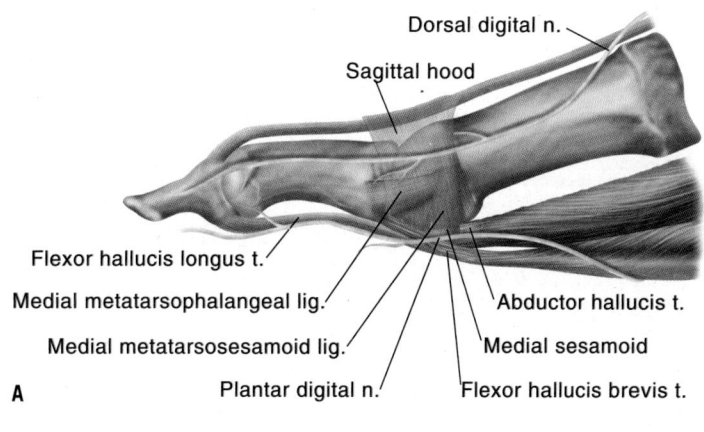

A

FIG 1 **A.** Medial view of relevant anatomy with special note of the adductor hallucis brevis and the relationship to the plantar cutaneous nerve. **B.** Plantar view of the sesamoid complex and the investing structures.

B

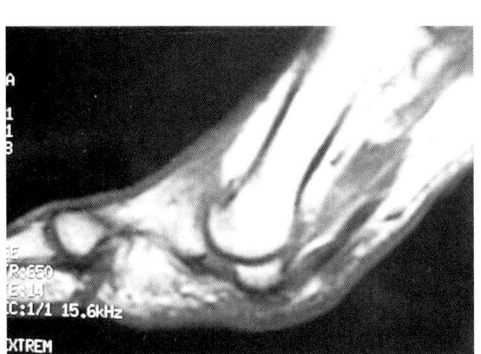 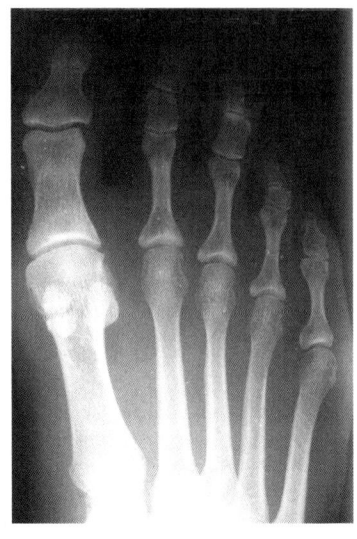

FIG 2 A. Sagittal MRI of the sesamoid–MTP complex showing the increased stress across the tibial sesamoid in MTP dorsiflexion. **B.** AP view of the foot showing a bipartite sesamoid. (**B:** Reprinted with permission from Lee S. Technique of isolated tibial sesamoidectomy. Tech Foot Ankle Surg 2004;3[2]:85–90.)

PATHOGENESIS

- Symptoms of sesamoiditis and sesamoid avascular necrosis mimic each other. These pathologies can arise from a single acute traumatic event, or, more commonly, there is a history of minor or repetitive trauma.
- Acute injuries typically occur with acute hyperextension to the hallux metatarsophalangeal (MTP) joint or a direct contusion to the sesamoid region of the forefoot. This can also result in a fracture or an injury to a bipartite sesamoid.
- In nonacute injuries, the patient often cannot remember a specific incident or injury and can only initially recall activity-related discomfort to the forefoot. This history is typically noted in cases of repetitive stress, osteochondritis dissecans, and arthrosis. A bipartite sesamoid can similarly be injured in this case.
- Neuritic pain has also been described with compression to the plantar medial cutaneous nerve underlying the tibial sesamoid.

NATURAL HISTORY

- Most sesamoid injuries resolve with appropriate nonoperative treatment.
- Sesamoiditis that does not resolve with conservative treatment is unlikely to improve significantly after 3 to 12 months.
- As a result, patients often have pain that prevents them from participating in everyday activities that involve a dorsiflexed MTP joint and in athletic activities.

PATIENT HISTORY AND PHYSICAL FINDINGS

- Most patients cannot remember a specific incident or injury, unless it was acute, and can only recall a gradual onset of discomfort to their forefoot. This pain is often generalized and localized to the great toe region. Some patients may complain of paresthesias as well.
- Pain is made worse with forced dorsiflexion of the hallux.
- Pain is localized more plantarward and is worse with weight-bearing activity. Patients will often prefer cushioned shoe wear versus barefooted activity.

- Performing activities that require a dorsiflexed MTP joint such as running, jumping, toe raising, or stair climbing can become very irritating to this region.
- Gait is often antalgic, specifically in the toe-off phase, and can also reveal evidence of medial offloading and lateral foot overload as the patient walks with the forefoot in pronation and the foot externally rotated.
- Clinical inspection will reveal swelling over the plantar aspect of the hallux MTP joint.
- In acute injuries or in patients with a bipartite sesamoid, a drawer test of the hallux MTP joint may also reveal laxity, indicating a fracture of the sesamoid or disruption of the synchondrosis of a bipartite sesamoid.
- Direct palpation over the tibial sesamoid may also reveal a positive Tinel sign or paresthesias distally, indicating a compression over the plantar medial cutaneous nerve.
- Assessment of hallux alignment is critical, as concomitant procedures may be necessary in those with hallux valgus or a cavus foot to prevent further migration after tibial sesamoidectomy.
  - Augmenting a tibial sesamoidectomy with a lateral capsular release, medial capsular reefing, or metatarsal or phalangeal osteotomy may be considered to prevent progressive deformity.[16]
- Methods for examining the tibial sesamoid include the following:
  - Direct palpation under the tibial sesamoid with the foot in neutral and with dorsiflexion of the MTP joint
  - Range of motion (ROM): One hand should be placed on the proximal phalanx with the other stabilizing the metatarsal. Dorsiflexion and plantarflexion ROM should be assessed. Symmetry between the right and left side should be noted.
  - Drawer test: The examiner grasps the proximal phalanx in one hand and the metatarsal head in the other and performs a dorsal to plantar stress of the MTP joint.
  - Toe raise: The patient is asked to do double-limb and single-limb toe raises.
  - Forced dorsiflexion of the great toe will result in the most pain.

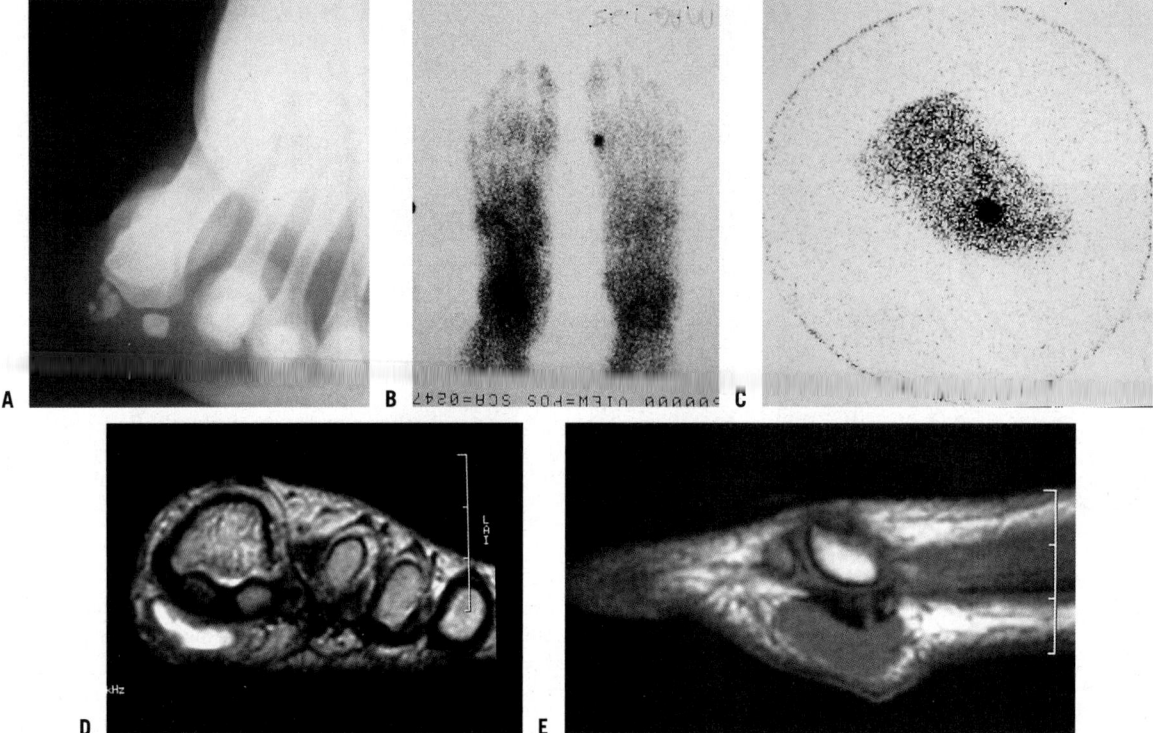

FIG 3 A. A sesamoid view of the foot. Note the significant fragmentation of the tibial sesamoid. **B.** Triple-phase bone scan showing increased uptake of the tibial sesamoid region in an AP view of bilateral feet. **C.** Collimated view showing the increased uptake of the tibial sesamoid. **D.** Coronal MRI view highlighting the signal change of the tibial sesamoid and reactive plantar bursitis, compared to the fibular sesamoid, indicating tibial sesamoid avascular necrosis. **E.** Sagittal MRI view of a tibial sesamoid fracture and subsequent reactive plantar bursitis. (Reprinted with permission from Lee S. Technique of isolated tibial sesamoidectomy. Tech Foot Ankle Surg 2004;3[2]:85–90.)

IMAGING AND OTHER DIAGNOSTIC STUDIES

- Routine radiographs should consist of standing anteroposterior (AP), lateral, oblique, and axial sesamoid views.
  - Plain radiographs will often be diagnostic in cases of arthrosis and osteochondritis dissecans if fragmentation is present (**FIG 3A**).
  - A bipartite tibial sesamoid may be distinguished from a fractured sesamoid in that an acutely injured sesamoid may have a sharp radiolucent line (irregular trabecular pattern) that may assist in differentiation.
  - AP radiographs in neutral and dorsiflexion may assist in evaluating separation of the sesamoid segments.
- A triple-phase bone scan or magnetic resonance imaging (MRI) is often required to confirm the diagnosis.
  - A triple-phase bone scan, with collimated views of the MTP joint, is very sensitive and may demonstrate increased uptake before radiographic changes become present (**FIG 3B,C**).
  - MRI allows the examiner to identify most causes of hallux MTP pathology in addition to sesamoiditis (**FIG 3D,E**).

DIFFERENTIAL DIAGNOSIS

- Infection, sesamoid–metatarsal or MTP arthrosis or chondromalacia, bursitis, flexor tendinosis, fracture, osteochondritis dissecans, intractable plantar keratosis, nerve compression, bi- or tripartite sesamoid, turf toe injury, sesamoid avascular necrosis

NONOPERATIVE MANAGEMENT

- Most patients respond to conservative therapy. This consists of nonsteroidal anti-inflammatory medication; rest or immobilization for 2 to 4 weeks; followed by protected weight bearing with an orthotic, walker boot, or cast for an additional 4 to 6 weeks.
- Typically, a hard-soled shoe decreases the dorsiflexion stresses across the MTP joint, and a negative heel shoe will decrease forefoot loading.
- An orthosis such as a turf toe plate or dancer's pad with a medial longitudinal arch support will decrease the stresses across the sesamoids (**FIG 4**).
- In athletes, taping the MTP joint to prevent dorsiflexion may allow continued participation.
- The judicious use of steroid injections for chronic sesamoiditis is also indicated.

SURGICAL MANAGEMENT

- Pain under the tibial sesamoid, unresponsive to conservative treatment, is the main indication for operative intervention. The presence of hallux MTP malalignment, a cavus foot, or stiffness requires careful evaluation and may require additional surgical procedures to improve clinical results.
- Previous excision of the fibular sesamoid or absence of the fibular sesamoid is the main contraindication to a tibial sesamoidectomy.[1,2] A tibial and fibular sesamoidectomy may result in a cock-up deformity of the great toe. A history

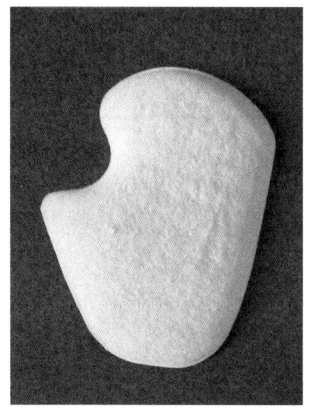 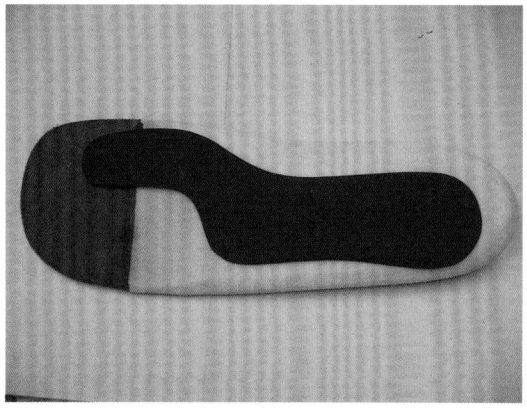

FIG 4 A. Dancer's pad with sesamoid cutout. **B.** Example of a Morton extension in an orthotic.

of peripheral vascular disease, soft tissue or wound healing problems, diabetes mellitus, and smoking are also relative contraindications that require proper evaluation and discussion with the patient before operative intervention.

Preoperative Planning

- The initial evaluation of hallux alignment is of utmost importance, as failure of reconstruction of the tibial FHB complex or failure to address preexisting hallux malalignment will compromise patient outcome.
- In general, any patient whose hallux alignment would be considered for surgical realignment without tibial sesamoiditis should have the malalignment corrected during the tibial sesamoidectomy.

Positioning

- Anesthesia should be similar to a bunion procedure.
- A single-shot popliteal or ankle block with some mild sedation is typically well tolerated.
- The patient should be placed on the operating table in a supine position.
- A well-padded Esmarch tourniquet is applied. However, an Esmarch tourniquet may limit excursion of the great toe due to tenodesis effect.
- The natural external rotation of the lower extremity allows excellent exposure to the medial aspect of the forefoot **(FIG 5)**.

Approach

- Dorsomedial, straight medial, and plantar medial incisions to approach the tibial sesamoid have been described. The most commonly used incision is a longitudinal medial skin incision that is slightly plantar to the standard incision for a bunion excision (see **FIG 5**).
- With the dorsomedial incision, it is difficult to obtain adequate exposure of the plantar aspect of the foot, whereas the plantar medial incision is typically directly over the plantar cutaneous nerve and near the weight-bearing surface of the foot, increasing wound complications.

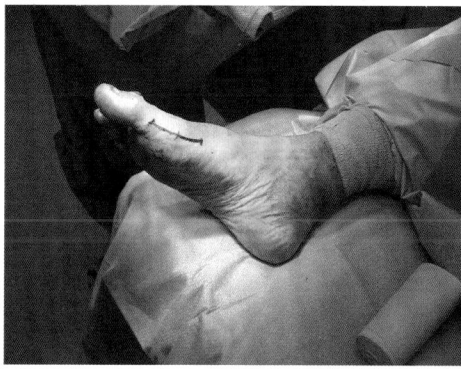

FIG 5 Patient positioning including the slightly plantar-planned incision and the natural externally rotated view of the foot.

TECHNIQUES

EXPOSURE

- The most commonly used incision is a 3-cm longitudinal medial skin incision that is slightly plantar to the standard incision for a bunion excision. The incision is started at the midshaft of the proximal phalanx and ends at the metatarsal metaphyseal flare.
- The plantar cutaneous nerve must be identified and mobilized inferiorly for protection during the procedure (**TECH FIG 1A**).
  - The nerve can usually be found along the inferior border of the abductor hallucis brevis tendon alongside the MTP joint.
  - A vessel loop can also be placed around the nerve to protect it.

- Make a longitudinal incision in the capsule in line with the skin incision in order to evaluate the MTP joint.
  - This incision is usually dorsal to the fibers of the insertion of the abductor hallucis tendon.
- Assess the sesamoid articular surface for significant displacement or step-off in acute fractures or bipartite sesamoids. In chronic cases, assess the sesamoid–metatarsal articular cartilage that may be damaged by osteonecrosis, osteochondritis dissecans, or arthrosis (**TECH FIG 1B**).

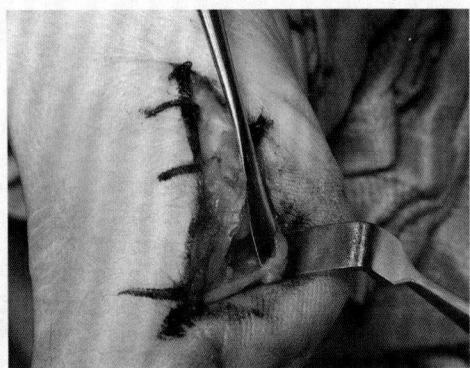 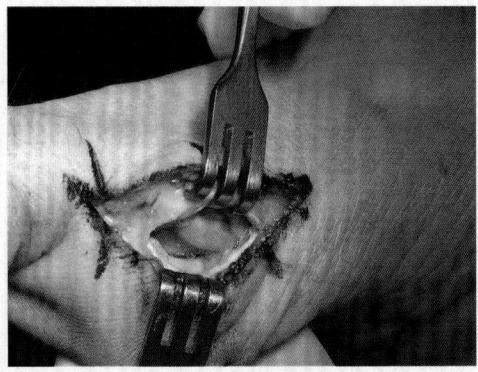

TECH FIG 1 A. The Freer elevator is underneath the plantar cutaneous nerve. **B.** Intracapsular view showing the articulation of the tibial sesamoid and the metatarsal head. (**B:** Reprinted with permission from Lee S. Technique of isolated tibial sesamoidectomy. Tech Foot Ankle Surg 2004;3[2]:85–90.)

TIBIAL SESAMOIDECTOMY

- Outline the tibial sesamoid with a Beaver blade from the intra-articular approach, as it will assist in its later removal.
- In an acute fracture or a bipartite sesamoid without articular damage, consider bone grafting of the defect and repair as opposed to performing a sesamoidectomy. This bone graft may come from the distal portion of the first metatarsal or calcaneus.
- At this time, a repair of the capsulotomy with a 2-0 nonabsorbable suture before proceeding with the sesamoidectomy exposure can be performed or deferred for visualization of the sesamoid from an intra-articular or plantar vantage point (**TECH FIG 2A**).
- Expose the tibial sesamoid through an extra-articular plantar medial incision in line with the FHB fibers.
  - The sesamoid is embedded within a dense fibrous sheath, and careful dissection out of the FHB and its soft tissue attachments is required (**TECH FIG 2B**).
  - This can be facilitated by the use of a Beaver mini-blade, using a pushing technique rather than a cutting motion, as

well as grasping the sesamoid with a small towel clamp or Kocher clamp for stability.
  - Take utmost care to protect the nerve medially as well as the FHL laterally to prevent injury.
- Once the sesamoid is removed, carefully assess the continuity of the FHB complex, as there are usually some remaining fibers of the FHB complex.
- Repair the plantar capsule defect with a 2-0 nonabsorbable suture in a triangular, figure-8, or purse-string fashion, with careful reapproximation of the FHB complex (**TECH FIG 2C**). The use of a UCL taper needle is recommended because it is noncutting and has a smaller radius of curvature, allowing easier manipulation.
- Assess the FHL tendon at this time.
- Once the FHB complex is reapproximated, take the hallux through an ROM to confirm that the FHB is intact and that the FHL tendon has not been inadvertently sutured. Stress fluoroscopy views may also be helpful.

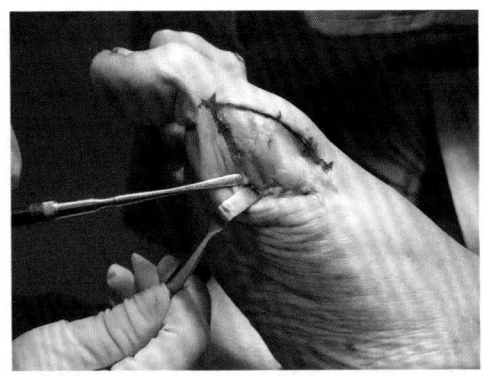
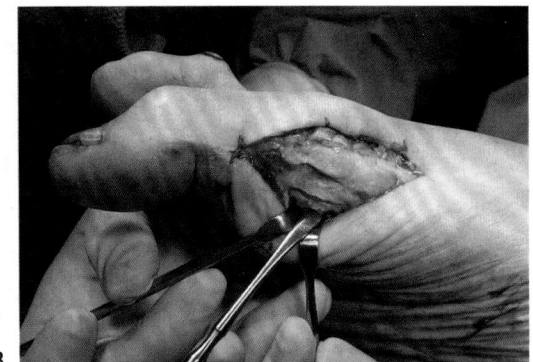
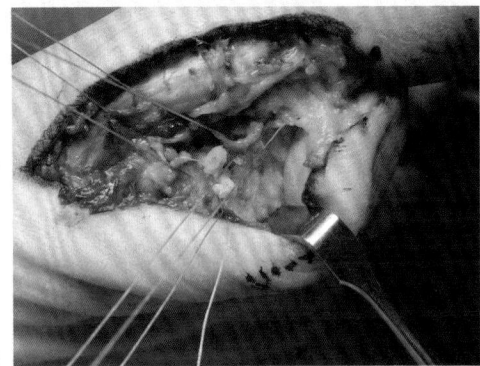

TECH FIG 2 A. The tip of the Freer elevator is underneath the tibial sesamoid before dissection of the FHB complex. Also, note the longitudinal capsulotomy and repair. **B.** After the initial incision to separate the FHB in line with its fibers. **C.** Note the FHL tendon deep to the operative incision as well as the subsequent purse-string repair of the FHB complex.

WOUND CLOSURE

- Complete the closure in standard fashion for a bunion procedure.
- Reapproximate the skin edges with a 3-0 nylon suture, and dress the wound with a bunion dressing, with the hallux protected in plantarflexion and in mild varus.

CASE EXAMPLE (COURTESY OF MARK E. EASLEY, MD)

Background and Imaging

- A 34-year-old man with 1-year history of right plantar first metatarsal pain
- Pain/ache with weight bearing and push-off during gait
- Physical examination
  - Tender under lateral (fibular) sesamoid
  - Plantar pain with hallux MTP joint dorsiflexion
  - Negative first MTP joint Lachman test
- Radiographs suggest lateral (fibular) sesamoid fracture **(TECH FIG 3A,B)**.
- Sesamoid view suggests some irregularity to lateral sesamoid **(TECH FIG 3C)**.
- Computed tomography scan demonstrates transverse fracture line with a subacute/chronic appearance **(TECH FIG 3D)**.
- T2-weighted MRI scan demonstrates signal change in lateral (fibular) sesamoid **(TECH FIG 3E)**.

Positioning and Exposure

- Prone position typically improves exposure and visualization **(TECH FIG 4A)**.
- Longitudinal plantar incision between lateral sesamoid and second metatarsal head **(TECH FIG 4B–E)**
- A hockey stick incision here may also be helpful.
- The plantar lateral sensory nerve to the hallux identified and protected **(TECH FIG 4F)**
- Longitudinal sharp division in periosteum over lateral sesamoid **(TECH FIG 4G,H)**
- FHL tendon identified and protected

Lateral Sesamoidectomy

- Fractured/nonunited area of lateral sesamoid identified **(TECH FIG 5A)**

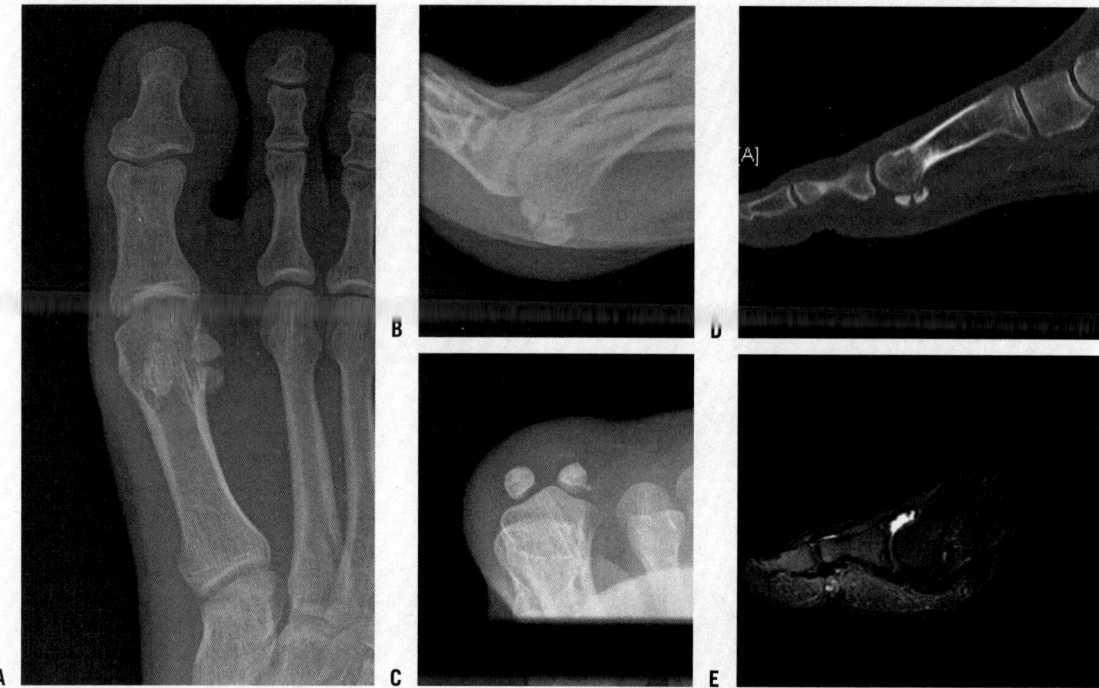

TECH FIG 3 A–C. Weight-bearing AP, lateral, and sesamoid radiographs, respectively, of a 34-year-old man with 1-year history of right lateral sesamoid fracture/nonunion. **D.** Computed tomography demonstrating fracture/nonunion and fragmentation of proximal pole of sesamoid. **E.** T2-weighted MRI demonstrates signal change in lateral sesamoid and dorsal first MTP joint effusion.

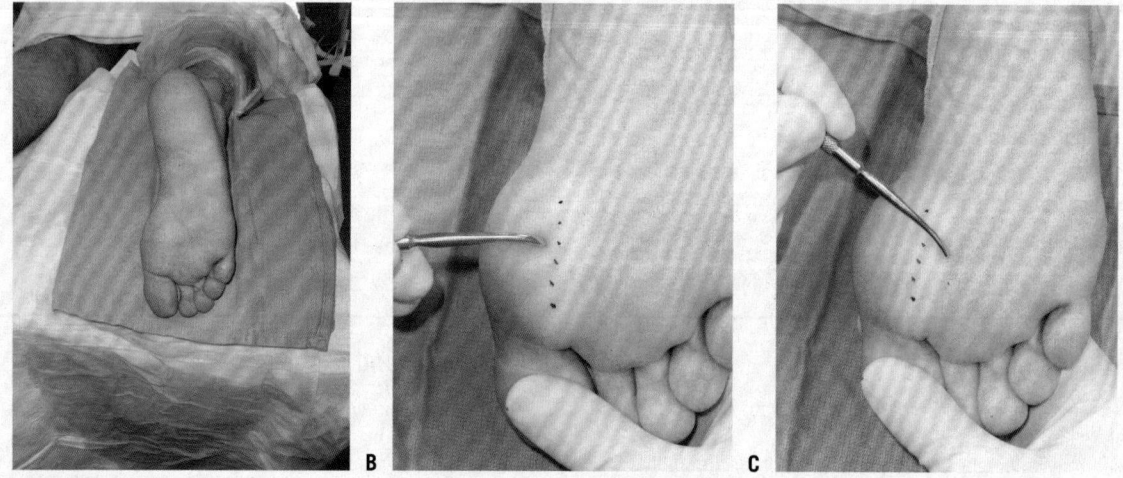

TECH FIG 4 A. Prone position is used to facilitate visualization and exposure. **B,C.** Planned longitudinal plantar incision between lateral sesamoid and second metatarsal head. **B.** Lateral sesamoid is medial. **C.** Second metatarsal head is lateral. *(continued)*

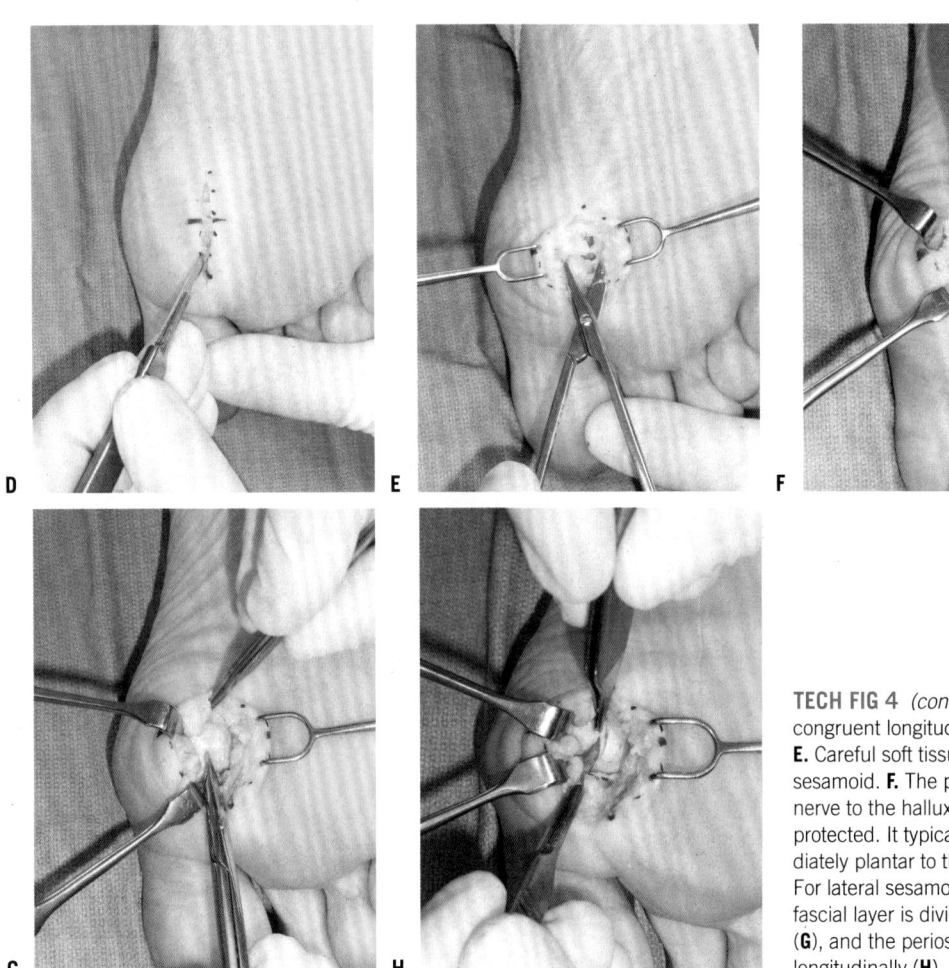

TECH FIG 4 *(continued)* **D.** Careful congruent longitudinal incision is made. **E.** Careful soft tissue dissection to lateral sesamoid. **F.** The plantar lateral sensory nerve to the hallux identified and protected. It typically courses immediately plantar to the lateral sesamoid. For lateral sesamoid exposure, the fascial layer is divided longitudinally (**G**), and the periosteum is divided longitudinally (**H**).

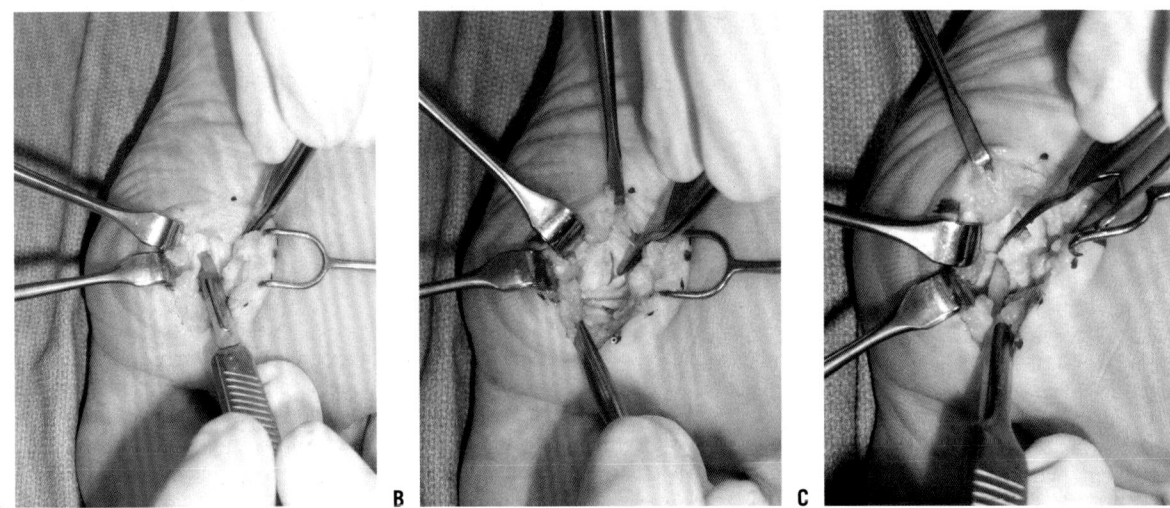

TECH FIG 5 A. Fracture/nonunion site identified. Note scalpel blade in the fracture/nonunion site. **B.** Careful elevation of periosteum from plantar lateral sesamoid. **C.** Distal pole gradually being separated from intersesamoidal ligament. *(continued)*

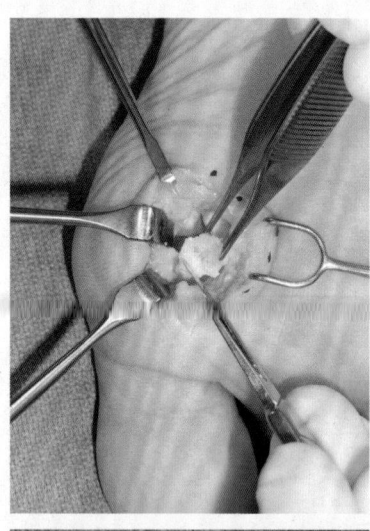

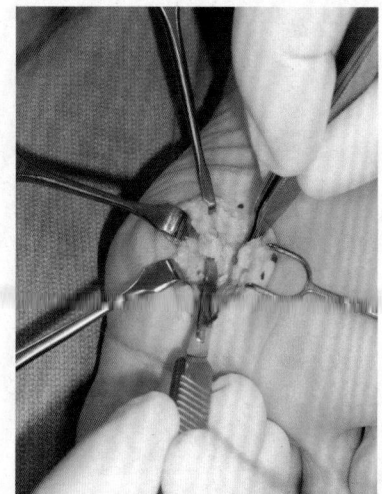

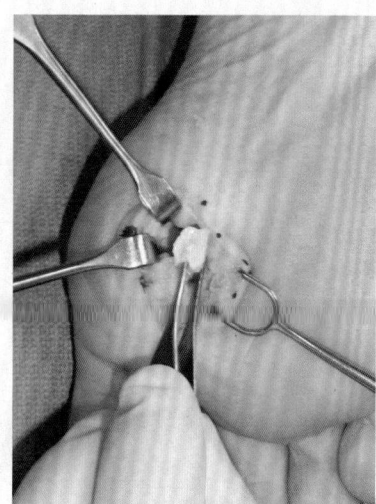

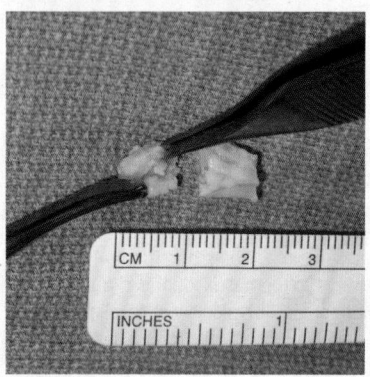

TECH FIG 5 *(continued)* **D.** Distal pole extracted. **E.** Proximal pole separated from sesamoid complex. **F.** Proximal pole extracted. **G.** Excised sesamoid inspected. Note fragmentation and degeneration of sesamoid, particularly the proximal pole, suggestive of avascular necrosis.

- Distal pole of lateral sesamoid enucleated from surrounding flexor mechanism/residual sesamoid complex (**TECH FIG 5B–D**)
- Proximal of lateral sesamoid enucleated from surrounding flexor mechanism/residual sesamoid complex (**TECH FIG 5E,F**)
- Excised sesamoid is inspected; in this case, cartilage degeneration, fragmentation, and suggestion of avascular necrosis are noted (**TECH FIG 5G**).

Flexor Mechanism/Residual Sesamoid Complex Repair

- Preserving the flexor mechanism/residual sesamoid complex allows for its optimal repair, improves hallux MTP joint plantarflexion, and limits risk of hallux varus developing.
- While protecting the FHL tendon, the residual intersesamoidal ligament (**TECH FIG 6A–C**) and periosteum (**TECH FIG 6D–F**) are reapproximated in layers to close the defect left by sesamoidectomy.
- Intraoperative fluoroscopy confirms complete lateral sesamoidectomy and satisfactory hallux MTP joint alignment (**TECH FIG 6G**).
  - In this case, because the patient was placed in prone position, the fluoroscopic image appears to be a left foot.

- Hallux MTP ROM is evaluated to make sure that the repair is not too tight (**TECH FIG 6H,I**).
- Hallux interphalangeal joint ROM is checked to ensure that the FHL tendon has not been trapped in the repair (**TECH FIG 6J,K**).
- The plantar wound is closed carefully to make sure the wound margins are congruent (**TECH FIG 6L,M**).

Postoperative Care

- A bunion dressing is placed to protect the lateral soft tissue repair and limit the risk of developing hallux varus; a lower profile bunion dressing should continue for 4 to 6 weeks (**TECH FIG 7**).
- Protected weight bearing on heel for 4 weeks
- Return to full activities limited for 8 to 10 weeks from surgery
- With careful lateral flexor mechanism, closure, and protected weight bearing postoperatively with bunion strapping, a patient's alignment, ROM, and push-off strength are typically well maintained (**TECH FIG 8A–C**).
- Plantar incision typically heals well, especially if it was performed between the weight-bearing surfaces (**TECH FIG 8D**).

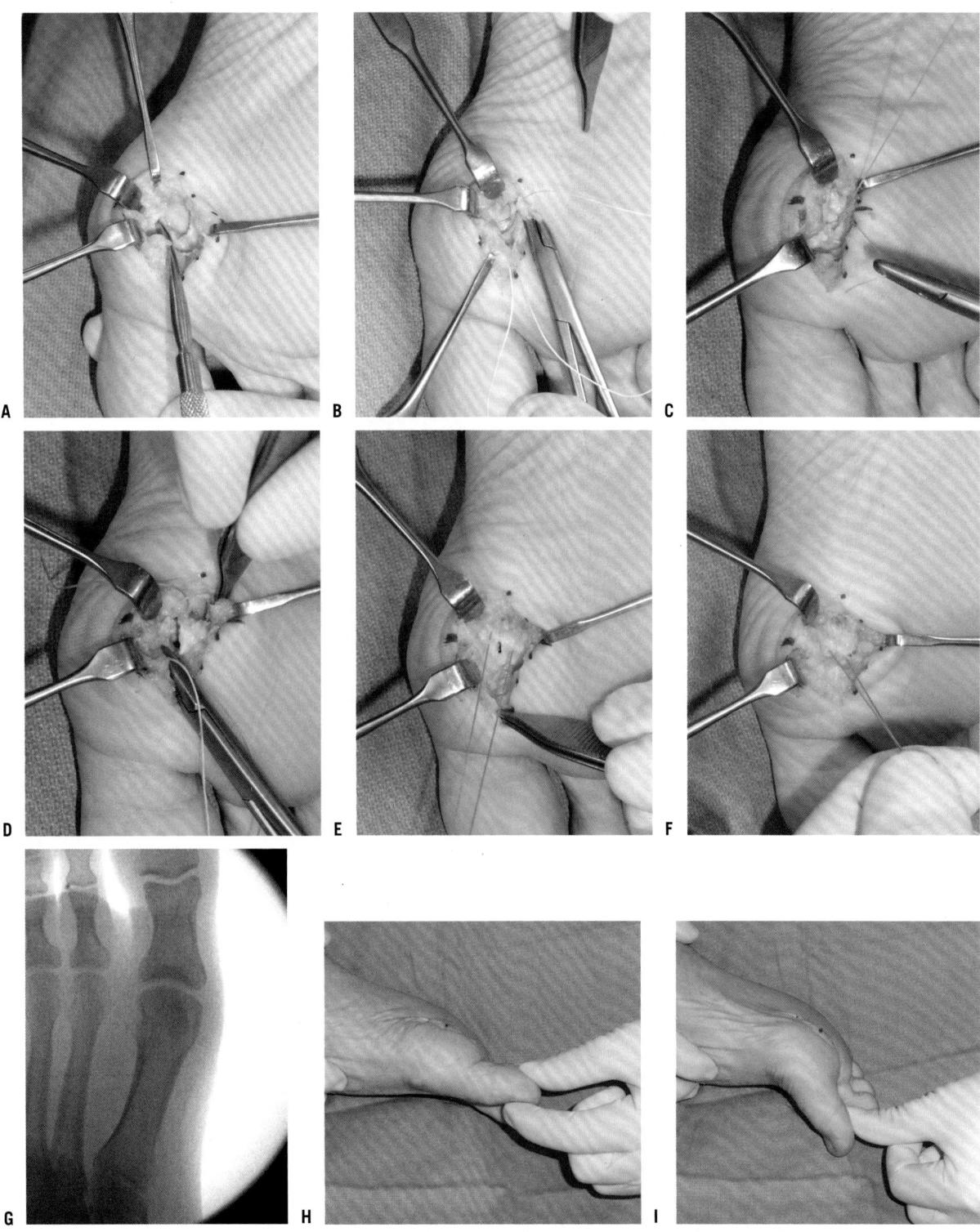

TECH FIG 6 A–C. Reapproximation of residual sesamoid complex. **A.** Defect left by excised lateral sesamoid assessed. **B.** With FHl tendon protected, intersesamoidal ligament reapproximated to lateral periosteum. **C.** Defect being closed. **D–F.** Plantar fascial layer reapproximation. **D.** Suture passed through lateral tissue. **E.** Suture passed through medial tissue while protecting the plantar lateral sensory nerve to the hallux. **F.** Layer closed. **G.** Intraoperative fluoroscopy confirms complete lateral sesamoidectomy and satisfactory hallux MTP joint alignment. In this case, because the patient was placed in prone position, the fluoroscopic image appears to be a left foot. Passive MTP joint motion confirms that the repair is not overtightened: neutral position (**H**) and dorsiflexion (**I**). *(continued)*

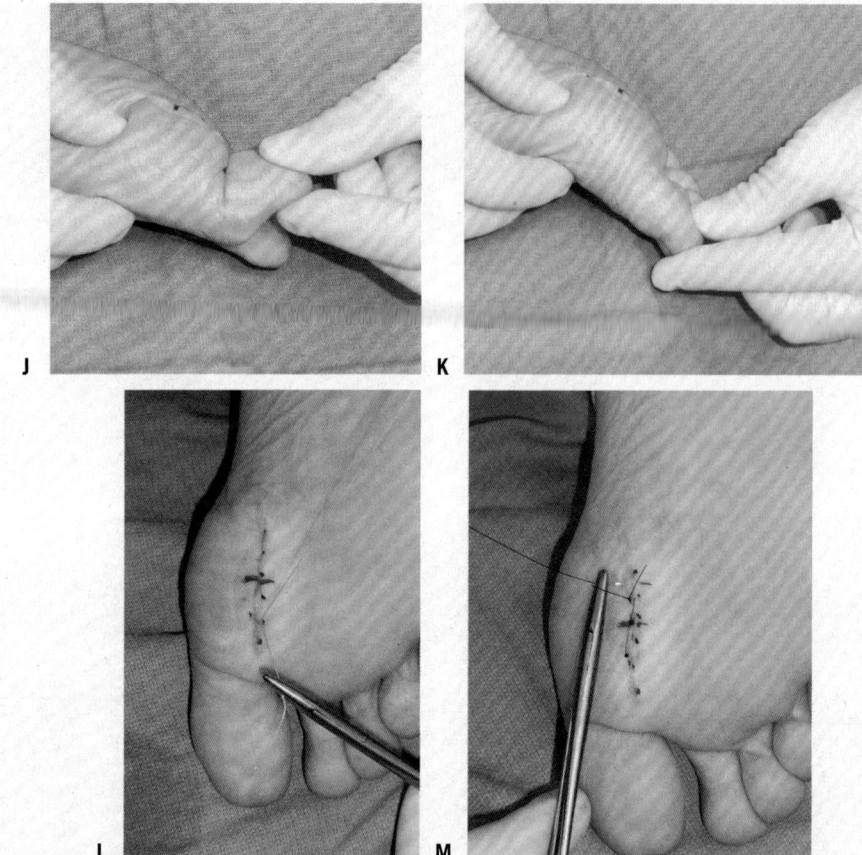

TECH FIG 6 *(continued)* Passive interphalangeal joint motion confirms that the FHL tendon is not trapped in the repair: neutral position (**J**) and dorsiflexion (**K**). **L.** Careful subcutaneous layer repair. **M.** Congruent plantar skin reapproximation.

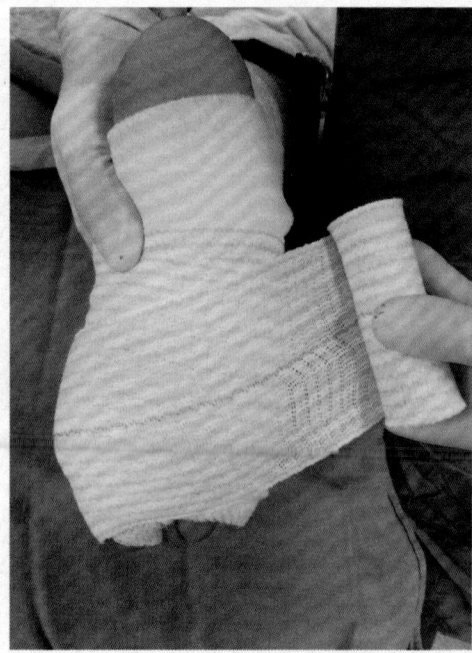

TECH FIG 7 Bunion dressing applied to limit risk of hallux varus developing.

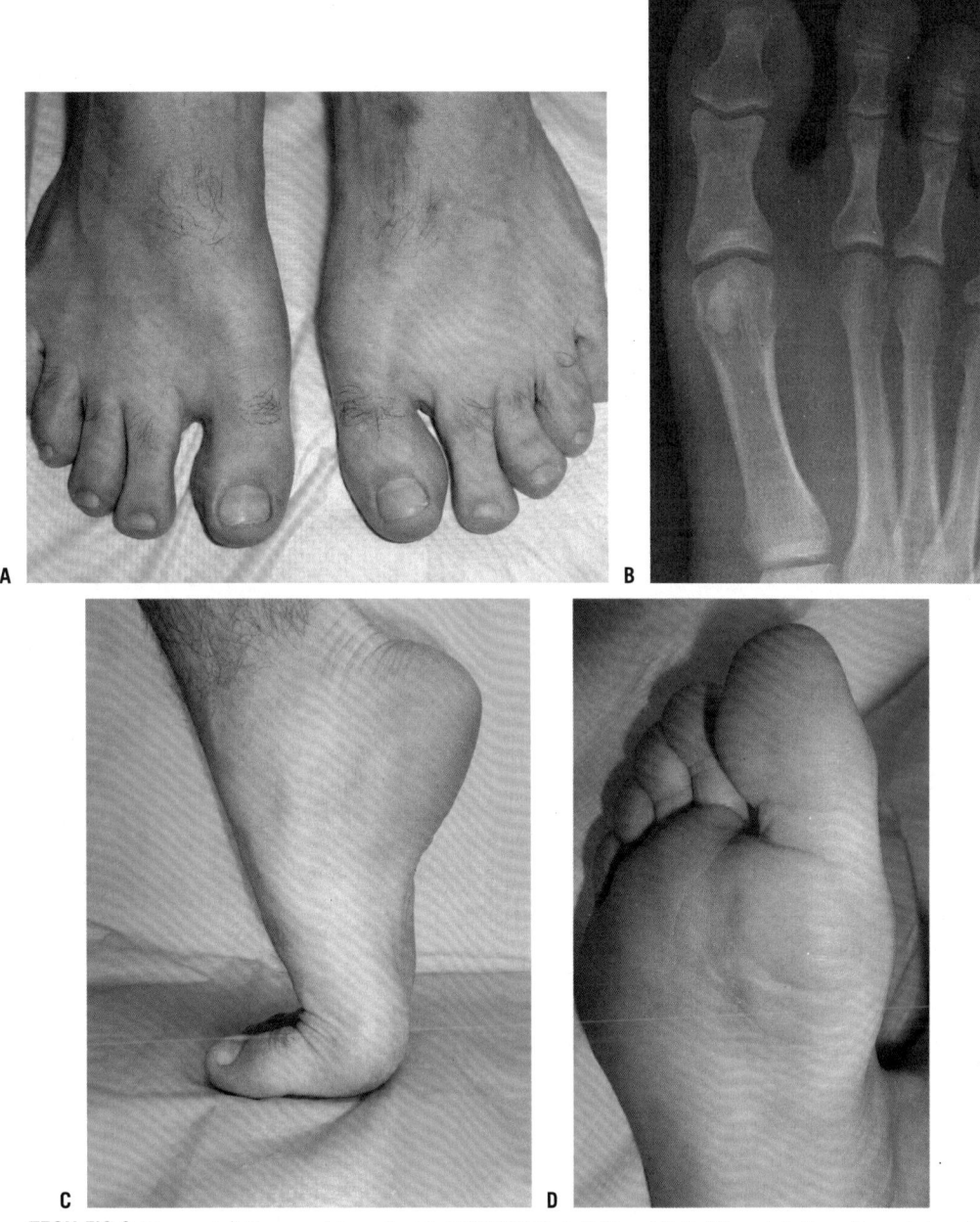

TECH FIG 8 Six-month follow-up of the patient in **TECH FIGS 3, 4, 5, 6,** and **7. A.** Although hallux with neutral position compared to contralateral hallux, alignment is satisfactory without suggestion of hallux varus. **B.** Weight-bearing AP radiograph demonstrating lateral sesamoid excision and satisfactory alignment. **C.** Dorsiflexion function well preserved. **D.** Plantar incision is well healed without thickened scar or symptoms.

Pearls and Pitfalls

Hallux Malalignment	• The presence of a cavus foot, hallux valgus, claw toe, cock-up deformity, or stiffness requires careful evaluation and may require additional surgical procedures to improve clinical results.
Plantar Cutaneous Nerve	• The nerve is most commonly located plantar to the inferior border of the abductor hallucis brevis tendon. This nerve should be visualized and protected throughout the case.
FHB Repair	• A UCL taper needle is easier to use in the limited surgical field. Careful and meticulous repair of the FHB complex is required to prevent the development of malalignment.

POSTOPERATIVE CARE

- The patient is provided with a firm-soled postoperative shoe or a short walker boot and allowed immediate heel weight bearing.
  - Patients are limited to heel weight bearing for 2 weeks.
- At the 2-week follow-up visit, stitches are removed, a toe spacer is placed, and patients are allowed to bear weight as tolerated in a postoperative shoe or a short walker boot.
  - Standing radiographs should be performed to confirm maintenance of hallux alignment.
  - The toe spacer should remain in place for 6 to 8 weeks postoperatively to prevent hallux valgus deformity.
- If a hallux realignment procedure was also performed, we use a taping technique for 6 weeks similar to a bunion procedure.
- Patients are encouraged to begin active and passive ROM exercises for the hallux MTP joint after stitches are removed.
- In active patients, formal physical therapy is warranted to monitor patient progress and to assist in ROM and soft tissue modalities.
- Patients return at 6 weeks postoperatively and are then allowed to progress to accommodative shoe wear and activity as tolerated.
- Patients may occasionally require continued short-term use of a sesamoid relief orthotic while returning to activity.

OUTCOMES

- **FIG 6** shows the case example at 6-month follow-up.
- Hallux malalignment with resultant claw toe and cock-up and hallux valgus deformity after tibial sesamoid excision have been described.[9,10,12]
  - Historical studies have found a 10% to 42% incidence of hallux valgus and a 33% to 60% incidence of loss of motion on follow-up.[9,12]
  - Kaiman and Piccora[10] also reviewed tibial sesamoidectomies and concluded that assessment of the osseous relationship was crucial to prevent hallux valgus deformity. Their average follow-up was only 13.2 months, and they found no evidence of valgus drift, but they recommended tendon balancing or capsulorrhaphy in conjunction with the tibial sesamoidectomy.
  - Lee et al[11] reported on 20 patients without preoperative malalignment and noted no significant difference in postoperative ROM or the development of subsequent hallux malalignment.

- Saxena and Krisdakumtorn[14] reported on active individuals who had isolated tibial sesamoidectomies.
  - One patient developed loss of hallux flexion after surgery.
  - Two patients with hallux valgus deformity were identified before surgery. One patient had a concomitant distal metatarsal osteotomy with no further drift, whereas the other patient did not have a concomitant procedure at the same time and went on to a bunion correction at a later date.
- Inge and Ferguson[9] found that 41% of their patients continued to have mild to severe pain after a tibial sesamoidectomy. More recently, however, Van Hal et al,[16] Saxena and Krisdakumtorn,[14] and Lee et al[11] have reported excellent pain relief in the majority of their patients with tibial sesamoidectomies in their athletic population.
- Ford et al[7] found that in 36 fibular sesamoidectomies, final postoperative hallux valgus and intermetatarsal angles did not change. The visual analog scale scores improved five points at final follow-up. Eighty-eight percent of patients would have surgery again. Hallux flexion strength did not differ relative to the contralateral foot.
- Aper et al[2] showed in two cadaveric studies that the FHB effective tendon moment arms are significantly decreased with the excision of both hallux sesamoids. However, FHL effective tendon moment arms are noted to be diminished with isolated sesamoid excisions as well.[1] However, Van Hal et al[16] and Saxena and Krisdakumtorn[14] did not find functional weakness of plantarflexion in any of their patients. Their patients were also able to return to their previous level of athletic participation with no functional deficit. Lee et al[11] also reported that 30% of their patients could not do a single-limb toe raise, indicating some plantarflexion weakness, but this did not affect any subsequent athletic activity.
- Tagoe et al[15] described 36 feet that underwent total sesamoidectomy for the management of hallux rigidus or limitus. No significant functional impairment or malalignment were found postoperatively. There were no patients with transfer metatarsalgia or pain with metatarsal compression. Postoperatively, the patients had a statistically significant improvement in their American Orthopaedic Foot and Ankle Society scores.
- Bichara et al[4] reported on 24 athletic patients (5 elite athletes) with sesamoid fractures that failed conservative management were treated surgically with an isolated sesamoidectomy. Twenty-two out of 24 patients (91.6%) returned to athletic activities at a mean of 11.6 weeks. Mean preoperative pain level decreased from 6.2 to a mean of 0.7 postoperatively. One patient developed a symptomatic hallux valgus deformity after tibial sesamoidectomy.

COMPLICATIONS

- Complications related to sesamoid excisions can be separated into intraoperative complications, insufficient pain relief, functional weakness, and hallux malalignment.
- The most common intraoperative complication reported is injury to the plantar digital nerve.
  - Patients typically complain of nerve irritation postoperatively. This generally responds well to observation or localized steroid injections. It occurs more commonly with fibular sesamoid excisions.
  - Complete laceration of the nerve has never been reported, and this nerve irritation appears to be the result of aggressive retraction during surgery. This can be avoided by using meticulous technique with identification and protection of the plantar digital nerve during surgery.
- Isolated complete sesamoidectomies are thought to alter the mechanical balance of the hallux MTP joint. Clinical studies have described stiffness, functional loss, cock-up deformity, claw toe deformity, and the development of a hallux valgus deformity after isolated tibial sesamoidectomies.[9-11]
  - As noted earlier, identifying and addressing any significant malalignment of the hallux MTP can decrease the rate of future deformities.
- The loss of single-limb toe raise has also been reported and may be related to the decreased moment arm and inadequate repair of the FHB complex.[11]

REFERENCES

1. Aper RL, Saltzman CL, Brown TD. The effect of hallux sesamoid excision on the flexor hallucis longus moment arm. Clin Orthop Relat Res 1996;(325):209–217.
2. Aper RL, Saltzman CL, Brown TD. The effect of hallux sesamoid resection on the effective moment of the flexor hallucis brevis. Foot Ankle Int 1994;15:462–470.
3. Beaman DN, Nigo LJ. Hallucal sesamoid injury. Oper Tech Sports Med 1999;7:7–13.
4. Bichara DA, Henn RF III, Theodore GH. Sesamoidectomy for hallux sesamoid fractures. Foot Ankle Int 2012;33:704–706.
5. Coughlin MJ. Sesamoid pain: causes and surgical treatment. Instr Course Lect 1990;39:23–35.
6. Dobas DC, Silvers MD. The frequency of partite sesamoids of the first metatarsophalangeal joint. J Am Podiatry Assoc 1977;67:880–882.
7. Ford SE, Adair CR, Cohen BE, et al. Efficacy, outcomes, and alignment following isolated fibular sesamoidectomy via a plantar approach. Foot Ankle Int 2019;40(12):1375–1381.
8. Helal B. The great toe sesamoid bones: the lus or lost souls of Ushaia. Clin Orthop Relat Res 1981;(157):82–87.
9. Inge GAL, Ferguson AB. Surgery of the sesamoid bones of the great toe: an anatomic and clinical study, with a report of forty-one cases. Arch Surg 1933;27:466–489.
10. Kaiman ME, Piccora R. Tibial sesamoidectomy: a review of the literature and retrospective study. J Foot Surg 1983;22:286–289.
11. Lee S, James WC, Cohen BE, et al. Evaluation of hallux alignment and functional outcome after isolated tibial sesamoidectomy. Foot Ankle Int 2005;26:803–809.
12. Nayfa TM, Sorto LA Jr. The incidence of hallux abductus following tibial sesamoidectomy. J Am Podiatry Assoc 1982;72:617–620.
13. Richardson EG. Hallucal sesamoid pain: causes and surgical treatment. J Am Acad Orthop Surg 1999;7:270–278.
14. Saxena A, Krisdakumtorn T. Return to activity after sesamoidectomy in athletically active individuals. Foot Ankle Int 2003;24:415–419.
15. Tagoe M, Brown HA, Rees SM. Total sesamoidectomy for painful hallux rigidus: a medium-term outcome study. Foot Ankle Int 2009;30:640–646.
16. Van Hal ME, Keene JS, Lange TA, et al. Stress fractures of the great toe sesamoids. Am J Sports Med 1982;10:122–128.

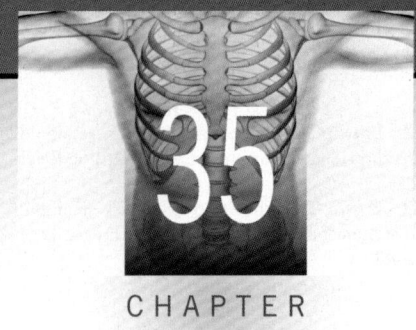

35

CHAPTER

Flexor to Extensor Tendon Transfer for Flexible Hammer Toe Deformity

Emilio Wagner

DEFINITION

- A hammer toe deformity is defined by a flexion deformity of the proximal interphalangeal (PIP) joint, typically with associated metatarsophalangeal (MTP) joint hyperextension. The distal interphalangeal (DIP) joint may be flexed, extended, or in a neutral position.[3]

ANATOMY

- The plantar plates of the MTP and PIP joints of the toes provide insertion points for ligaments, tendons, and soft tissue septa.
  - At the MTP joint, the plantar plate originates from the periosteum of the shaft of the metatarsal, and it inserts onto the base of the proximal phalanx. Plantar plate dysfunction has been associated with hammer toes and claw toes.[7,10]
  - At the PIP joint, the plantar plate also attaches in a similar way as in the MTP joint, lying immediately plantar to the joint.
  - The collateral ligaments insert to the plantar plate at both the PIP and MTP joints.
  - The final position of the toe depends on the delicate balance between the static stabilizers of the MTP and PIP joints (plantar plate, collateral ligaments) and the dynamic stabilizers (extrinsic and intrinsic tendons).
- The extensor digitorum longus (EDL) tendon is the primary extensor of the MTP joint; it attaches to the lateral four toes. The extensor digitorum brevis (EDB) tendon is the only dorsal intrinsic muscle of the foot, and it attaches to the medial four toes.
  - These two tendons maintain their orientation in part due to the fibroaponeurotic extensor hood. Its proximal segment, called the *extensor sling*, attaches to the plantar base of the proximal phalanx. It receives contributions from the interossei muscles. Its distal segment or extensor wing receives the insertion of the lumbrical muscles.
  - Extension of the PIP and DIP joints is achieved by the coordinated action of the extrinsic extensor tendons and the intrinsic flexor muscles; with paralysis of the intrinsic muscles, the extensor muscles would extend only the MTP joints.
- The extrinsic flexors are the flexor digitorum brevis (FDB) and flexor digitorum longus (FDL) muscles. The FDB and FDL tendons unite to the base of the middle and distal phalanx, respectively. They flex the PIP and DIP joints and are weak flexors of the MTP joint.
- The intrinsic flexors are the interossei and lumbrical muscles. The lumbricals flex the MTP joints and extend the interphalangeal (IP) joints; they have a stronger effect over the extension of the PIP and DIP joints due to their distal attachment compared to the interossei, which are weak extensors of the toes (FIG 1).[7]

PATHOGENESIS

- Any disruption of the foot's complex and delicate balance between the static stabilizers (ligaments, plantar plate) and dynamic stabilizers (intrinsic and extrinsic tendons) creates a lesser toe deformity.
  - With diminished intrinsic muscle flexion power, the extrinsic extensor tendons will extend the MTP joints. With MTP joint extension, the long flexor tendons flex the PIP and DIP joints, resulting in the intrinsic tendons being insufficient in flexing the MTP joint or extending the PIP or DIP joints. This imbalance creates deformity.
  - Plantar plate disruption may also compromise the balance of the toes and promote MTP joint hyperextension, thus leading to a similar chain of events to that described earlier (FIG 2).[10]

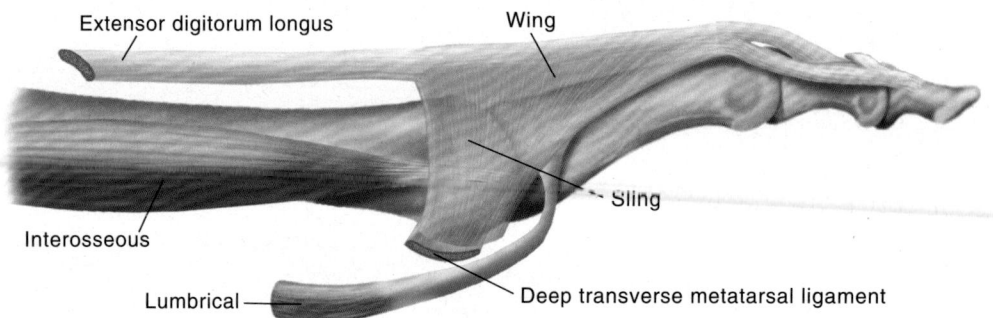

Extensor digitorum longus   Wing

Interosseous

Lumbrical

Sling

Deep transverse metatarsal ligament

FIG 1 Lateral view of the normal anatomy of the MTP and PIP joints of the lesser toes.

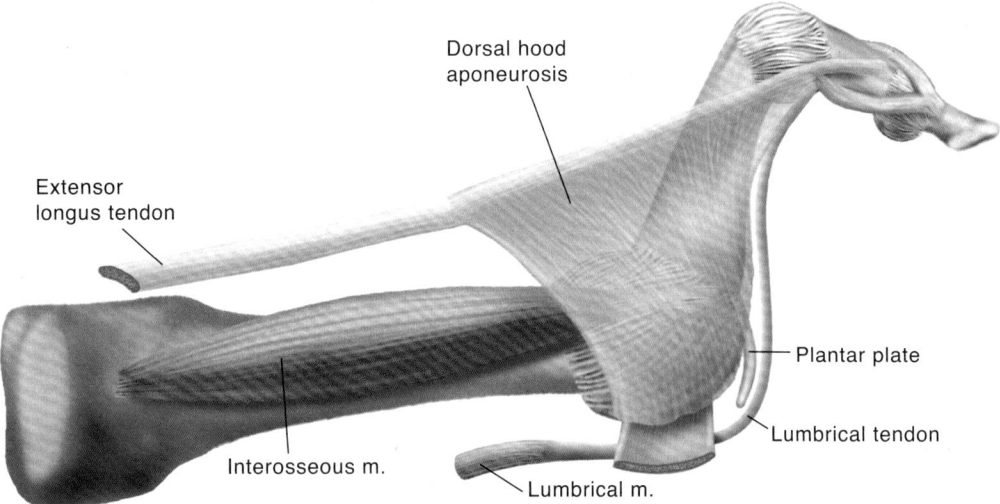

FIG 2 Lateral view of the pathologic anatomy of a hammer toe. Notice how the MTP extension renders insufficient the lumbricals and dorsally subluxates the interosseous tendon. The PIP flexion subluxates the extensor tendon, and continued pull of the extensor digitorum will increase the PIP flexion.

- The pathologic anatomy of claw toes and hammer toes has been investigated in cadaveric dissections.
  - In one of these studies,[8] contributions of various anatomic structures to the deformity were determined:
    - For MTP joint hyperextension deformity, the skin provided about 9% of total deformity, the extensor tendons (EDL + EDB) 25%, the dorsal capsule 19%, and the collateral ligaments 47%.
    - For PIP joint flexion deformity, the skin accounted for about 20% of deformity, the FDB tendon 40%, and the plantar capsule 40%; the FDL tendon had no contribution.
    - These numbers show the relative importance of the different anatomic structures in the deformity and suggest which structures to release in surgery.
  - With clawing (hyperextension of the MTP joint), the interossei become subluxated in relation to the MTP joint and their line of pull becomes dorsally situated in relation to the joint axis and center of MTP joint rotation.
    - This results in an increased deformity with interossei activity: Instead of plantarflexion, they provide dorsiflexion at the MTP joint.
    - The lumbricals normally have an angle of 35 degrees with respect to the metatarsal axis. With clawing, they can subtend an angle of 90 degrees with the metatarsal axis, rendering them insufficient to flex the MTP joint.[8]
- Causes for lesser toe deformity are posttraumatic, inflammatory, neurologic, congenital, postsurgical, and nonspecific in nature.
  - Posttraumatic deformities include sequelae of leg injuries, fractures, soft tissue injuries, and compartment syndromes.
    - In these cases, a scarring or contracture of the deep compartment of the leg can lead to flexion deformities of the toes.
    - A compartment syndrome after a calcaneal fracture, affecting the calcaneal compartment, will compromise the quadratus plantae muscle, thereby shortening the intrinsic musculature.
    - Damage to the tibial nerve due to these same reasons may also be responsible for loss of intrinsic

flexor action, resulting in an MTP joint extension deformity.
  - Inflammatory: in rheumatoid arthritis due to capsular inflammation and disruption
    - Plantar plate attenuation may lead to MTP joint hyperextension and nonphysiologic PIP joint flexion.
  - Neuromuscular and congenital causes may alter the foot's intrinsic and extrinsic muscle balance.
    - Neuromuscular causes of lesser toe deformities include cerebral palsy, Charcot-Marie-Tooth disease, Friedreich ataxia, spinal dysraphism, and polio, among others.
    - Congenital causes include idiopathic cavovarus foot, clubfoot sequelae, and arthrogryposis.[7]
- Postsurgical causes
  - Dorsiflexion of the metatarsal head after distal metatarsal osteotomies (to relieve metatarsalgia or synovitis)
  - Proximal metatarsal osteotomies with elevation of the distal fragment and secondary overpull of the flexor tendons[5]
  - Secondary to metatarsal lengthening due to undesired lengthening of the flexor and extensor tendons
- Nonspecific causes
  - Muscular imbalance, ineffectiveness of the intrinsic flexors, and age-related deficiencies of plantar structures[7]
  - Shoe wear has been implicated because of the buckling effect of the toes inside a short toe box, with resulting flexion of the PIP joint.

NATURAL HISTORY

- The natural history of this deformity is a slow progression to a claw toe, where extension of the MTP joint increases with an increase in PIP flexion.
- If the deformity is flexible, the prognosis is good, as a conservative option may be successful, or if surgery is deemed necessary, simple techniques typically meet with satisfactory outcomes.
- As the lesser toe deformity becomes fixed, the chance of a successful nonsurgical treatment decreases, and surgical treatment generally involves more complex reconstructive procedures with an increased risk for postoperative stiffness.

PATIENT HISTORY AND PHYSICAL FINDINGS

- The chief complaint is pain and tenderness on the dorsal PIP joint, typically due to pressure from the shoe.
- A progressive hammer toe deformity may lead to an extended MTP joint and eventually a plantar callus under the corresponding metatarsal head. Occasionally, with associated PIP and DIP flexion, a plantar callus at the tip of the toe will develop.
- Toe position must be evaluated with weight bearing to appreciate the full extent of the deformity. With the patient seated, the range of motion of the ankle and subtalar, transverse tarsal, and MTP joints is inspected.
- Flexibility of the MTP, PIP, and DIP joints must be determined as it influences surgical decision making.
- Inspection and palpation of the plantar foot may reveal calluses under the metatarsal heads and tips of the toes.
- A comprehensive neurovascular examination is performed. Correction of lesser toe deformities will place digital vessels and nerves on stretch; preoperative neurovascular compromise to the toes must be identified, particularly if surgical correction is considered.
- Examinations of the lesser toes' MTP and IP joints may include the following:
  - Push-up test (MTP): If the deformity is flexible, with the push-up test, the MTP joint will flex to its normal position. If not, it will remain extended, defining a fixed deformity. Semiflexible deformities are those that correct partially with the push-up test.
  - Evaluation of PIP joint stiffness: Fixed deformities are present if it is not possible to obtain full extension of the PIP joint. Flexible deformities allow the PIP joint to extend fully.
  - Evaluation of MTP joint stability: stage 0, no laxity to dorsal translation; stage 1, the base of the proximal phalanx can be subluxated with the dorsal stress; stage 2, the proximal phalangeal base can be dislocated and relocated; stage 3, the base of the proximal phalanx is fixed in a dislocated position.[15] A new classification for lesser toe MTP joint stability has been presented by Nery et al[10] where besides the drawer test clinical signs such as alignment, flexibility, pain, and loss of toe purchase have been included.

IMAGING AND OTHER DIAGNOSTIC STUDIES

- Plain radiographs
  - Inflammatory arthritis may be associated with periarticular erosions, and this may influence surgical management.
  - The extent of the deformity is characterized on plain radiographs: subluxation, dislocation, or medial or lateral deviation. Dislocation of the MTP joint is characterized by an overlap of the base of the proximal phalanx on the head of the metatarsal on the anteroposterior (AP) view and complete dorsal displacement of the proximal phalanx relative to the metatarsal head on the lateral view (**FIG 3**).
- Magnetic resonance imaging (MRI)
  - MRI evaluation of the extent of plantar plate damage has been reported to be reliable after adequate training.[11] Although not needed as a rule, MRI evaluation of plantar plate disruption can guide our efforts when deciding treatment alternatives of MTP instability.

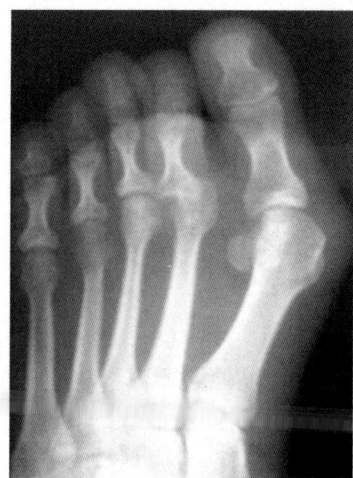

FIG 3 AP view of a foot with hammer toe deformity with MTP joint subluxation. Notice the overlap between the base of the proximal phalanx and the metatarsal head.

DIFFERENTIAL DIAGNOSIS

- Fixed hammer toe or claw toe deformities (not amenable to treatment with tendon transfer alone)
- MTP synovitis (absence of deformity warranting tendon transfer)
- Posttraumatic toe deformities
- Soft tissue tumors of the toes

NONOPERATIVE MANAGEMENT

- For flexible deformities, an initial conservative approach is recommended.
- Stretching exercises may help but have little proven benefit, as they do not alter the imbalance of extrinsic and intrinsic tendons.
- Shoe wear modifications: wider, deeper toe box to give more room to the toes
- Metatarsal pads to relieve metatarsal head pressure and toe sleeves to cushion pressure on the dorsum of the PIP joints. Orthotics with metatarsal padding must be used judiciously because they elevate the toes and may lead to greater dorsal PIP joint pressure.
- Hammer toe sling orthoses (or taping) are available that hold the proximal phalanx in a more physiologic position (**FIG 4**).
- The value of these measures depends to some degree on the degree of flexibility remaining in the deformity.

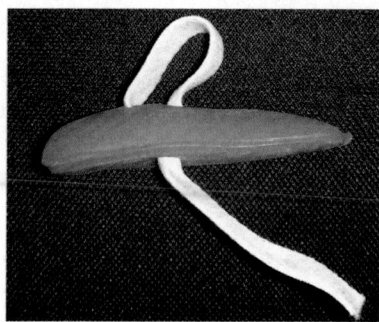

FIG 4 Hammer toe orthosis designed to hold the proximal phalanx in a plantarflexed position.

SURGICAL MANAGEMENT

- A toe flexor to extensor tendon transfer is rarely performed in isolation; typically, it is an adjunct to a more comprehensive correction of hammer toe and claw toe deformities.
- The goal of a flexor to extensor tendon transfer is to reposition the proximal phalanx into a more physiologic alignment, with realignment of the MTP and PIP joints. It is essentially "taping of the toe under the skin." Despite flexible deformity, tendon transfer may need to be performed with dorsal capsulotomy and collateral ligament release of the MTP joint. As the deformity becomes more fixed, a PIP arthroplasty or arthrodesis with or without metatarsal shortening osteotomy would typically be warranted, but a flexor to extensor tendon transfer may need to be added to avoid residual elevation of the toe ("floating toe"), one that does not touch the floor with weight bearing.

Preoperative Planning

- For MTP joint hyperextension deformity, a bone-shortening procedure can be performed. This procedure is commonly performed if associated metatarsalgia is present.[14]
  - Generally, a soft tissue procedure is chosen; the choice will vary depending on the amount of release needed.
  - Progressive releases have to be made, starting with the dorsal skin, followed by extensor tendons (tenotomy or lengthening), the dorsal capsule, and collateral ligaments, until an aligned MTP joint is obtained.
  - A plantar plate repair can be considered, depending on the MTP instability, the number of toes involved, and the extent of plantar plate damage. The authors would recommend adding a plantar plate repair when grade 1 and 2 MTP joint instability is present, one or two toes are involved, and preferably within an acute setting with recognizable plantar plate tissue left to repair, in contrast to a chronic instability where chronic damage to the plantar plate may render the tissue insufficient and unreliable to be fixed.
  - For further correction and stabilization, a flexor to extensor transfer should be added. In this case, the transfer should be done suturing the FDL to the EDL proximal to the middle of the proximal phalanx to obtain more flexion power over the MTP joint.
- For PIP joint flexion deformities, FDB releases are considered if the flexion contracture is not solved percutaneously.
  - If FDB tenotomy is not enough to treat the PIP deformity, a PIP joint arthroplasty or arthrodesis should be added.
  - A bone-shortening procedure can be also considered, typically a metatarsal-shortening osteotomy, if relevant clinical metatarsalgia is present. A resection of the proximal aspect of the proximal phalanx should be avoided due to a high prevalence of postoperative MTP joint instability.
  - The flexor to extensor transfer will correct the PIP joint flexion if flexible and will also stabilize the deformity if a FDB tenotomy or a PIP joint arthroplasty was performed.

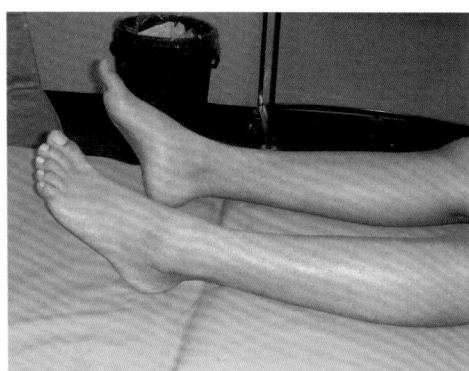

FIG 5 Positioning of the patient with adequate room for the surgeon to comfortably approach the toe distally.

In this case, the transfer should be done suturing the FDL to the EDL distal to the middle of the proximal phalanx to obtain more extension power over the PIP joint.

Positioning

- A supine position is preferred, with the involved foot on the same side as the surgeon.
- When performing the flexor to extensor transfer, as a plantar approach is needed, enough distance between the foot and the distal end of the table has to be available so that the surgeon can work comfortably (**FIG 5**).

Approach

- For the MTP approach, a longitudinal dorsal incision over the involved MTP joint is performed.
  - The incision can be performed in a curvilinear fashion to avoid skin contractures (a rare complication).
- For the PIP joint approach, a dorsal transverse approach over the PIP joint is performed, removing the hyperkeratotic skin with the incision.
  - It is also possible to perform a longitudinal incision after the tendon transfer incision, which may include the MTP incision when an additional procedure has been performed over the MTP joint.
- For the flexor to extensor transfer, a dorsal approach over the proximal phalanx must be made.
  - An extension deformity at the MTP joint is virtually always present, and therefore, a procedure over the MTP joint is commonly performed. This MTP approach can be used, extending it distally.
  - To gain access to the flexor tendons, two plantar incisions have to be made: one transverse along the proximal skin crease of the toe and the second oblique over the DIP joint.
  - This last incision can be made transverse, and a percutaneous FDL tenotomy can be performed.
  - There is a risk of damaging the plantar plate of the DIP joint, and hyperextension of the joint can be observed.

T E C H N I Q U E S

FLEXOR TO EXTENSOR TENDON TRANSFER

Exposure

- Make a plantar incision in a short transverse fashion along the proximal skin crease of the involved toe.
  - Carry the dissection through the subcutaneous layer. Identify the flexor tendon sheath and open it longitudinally with a blade (TECH FIG 1).
  - This incision can also be made longitudinally, as shown by Boyer and DeOrio,[1] which helps to avoid damage to the neurovascular structures.

Preparing the Flexor Digitorum Longus

- Identify the FDL tendon between the slips of the FDB (TECH FIG 2A) and retract it with a hemostat to the surface of the wound, placing it into traction (TECH FIG 2B). Keep the dissection central to avoid excursion to the adjacent medial and lateral digital neurovascular bundles.
- Place a second plantar incision oblique in orientation over the DIP, just proximal to the fat pad, and identify the plantar capsule of the joint to protect it.
- Detach the FDL from its insertion to the distal phalanx. As noted before, this incision can be made transversely and the FDL can be detached percutaneously (TECH FIG 2C).
- Keep the stab incision central to avoid damage to the digital neurovascular bundles. Although the incision is at the distal crease, direct the scalpel proximally at a 45-degree angle to ensure that the FDL tendon is transected and the DIP plantar plate is avoided.
- Pull the FDL tendon from the proximal incision and separate it into two slips along its midline raphe. Hold each half with a hemostat (TECH FIG 2D).

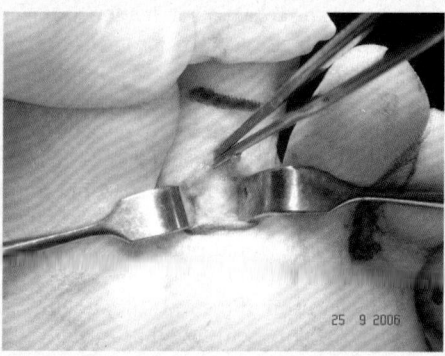

TECH FIG 1 Plantar view of the proximal plantar incision: flexor tendon sheath identification.

Preparing the Extensor Tendon

- Place a dorsal longitudinal incision over the dorsum of the proximal phalanx just distal to its midpoint to the proximal metaphyseal flare.
- Perform superficial dissection and identify the extensor tendon and split it in line with the long axis of the phalanx (TECH FIG 3). Carry the dissection in a subperiosteal manner deep to the neurovascular bundle.

Performing the Transfer

- Pass a small hemostat from the dorsal aspect of the toe through the extensor tendon, between the bone and the periosteum, to the plantar aspect of the toe. Identify the tip of the hemostat in the plantar incision. Take care to avoid pinching the bundle.

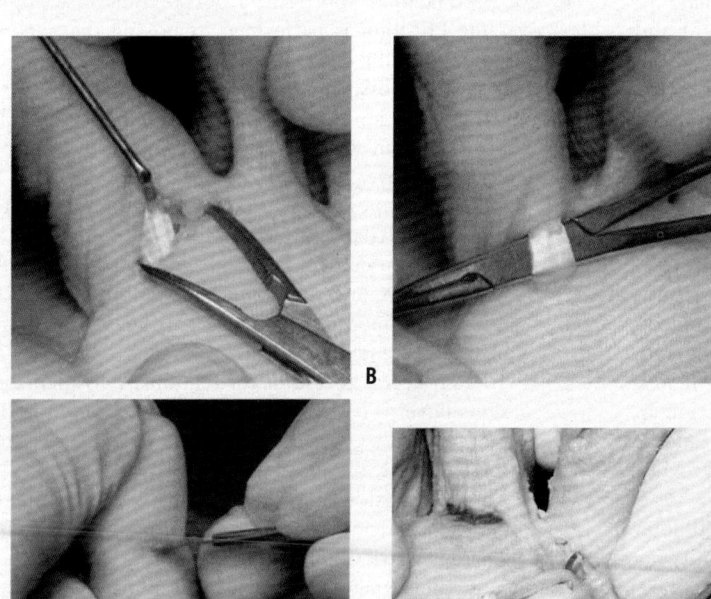

TECH FIG 2 **A.** The FDB appears dividing itself in two slips, and the FDL rests in between. The FDL possesses a midline raphe, which helps to identify it. **B.** The FDL is identified with a small hemostat, and traction is being placed on it. **C.** Detachment of the FDL through a transverse distal incision in a percutaneous way. **D.** Splitting of the FDL in two following the middle raphe.

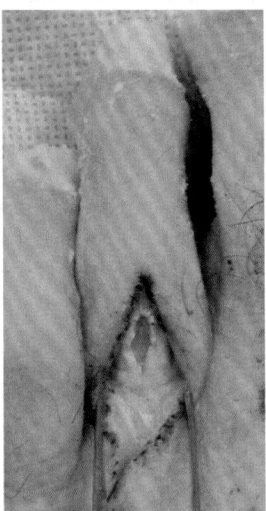

TECH FIG 3 Dorsal incision over the proximal phalanx, identifying the extensor tendon and splitting it following the longitudinal axis.

The tip of the hemostat must be passed through the slips of the FDB tendon **(TECH FIG 4)**.

- First, pull half of the FDL tendon from the plantar aspect of the toe to the dorsal aspect, keeping their relative position—in other words, the lateral one is pulled to the lateral dorsal aspect of the phalanx and vice versa.
- Then, with the ankle held in a neutral position, the MTP joint in 20 degrees of plantarflexion, and the PIP joint in neutral, secure both slips of the FDL over the extensor tendon with two or three separate stitches of 4-0 absorbable suture.
- Evaluate the MTP joint at this time to observe for continued extension at that joint. If any is present, alternative procedures will need to be performed.

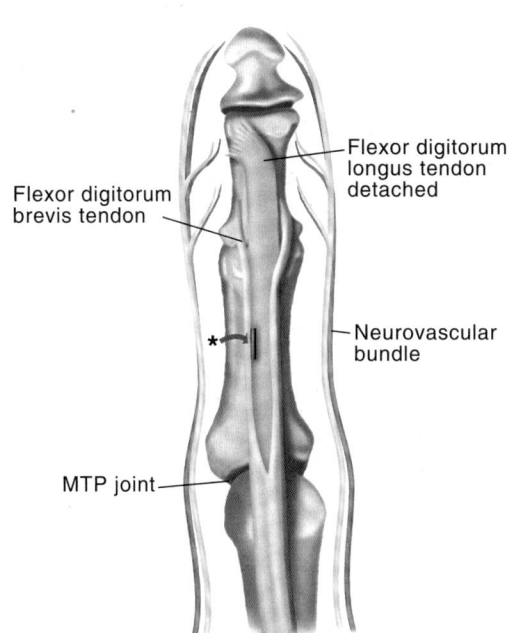

Flexor digitorum longus tendon detached

Flexor digitorum brevis tendon

Neurovascular bundle

*

MTP joint

TECH FIG 4 Plantar picture of the toe showing the place (marked with an *asterisk*) where a small hemostat should pass through from dorsal to plantar, deep to the neurovascular bundle, in between the slips of the FDB tendon to hold one of the divided halves of the detached FDL tendon.

- Close the wound with absorbable stitches on the plantar incisions and nylon dorsally.
- Before breaking sterility, deflate the tourniquet to ensure revascularization of the toe.

FLEXOR TO EXTENSOR TENDON TRANSFER THROUGH A DRILL HOLE

- The technique is as described earlier up to the step where the FDL is brought through the plantar aspect of the toe.
- Make a dorsal longitudinal incision over the proximal phalanx from just proximal to its midpoint to the distal metaphyseal flare.
- Take the dissection down to the extensor sheath and split the sheath and periosteum in line with the incision, exposing the dorsum of the phalanx.

- Place a drill hole dorsal to plantar large enough to allow passage of the tendon, in the junction of the middle and distal third of the proximal phalanx.
  - Generally, use a 2.0-mm drill and take care to avoid making a hole larger than one-third of the diameter of the bone.
- Pass the tendon between the short flexors and through the hole. Position the foot as described earlier and suture the tendon with 4-0 absorbable sutures to the extensor sheath.
- The rest of the procedure remains the same as described earlier.

Pearls and Pitfalls

Indications	• Evaluate the stiffness of the deformity preoperatively. It is important to inform the patient about the possible additional procedures needed and the corresponding outcome. The surgery for hammer toes is a step-by-step procedure: Additional surgery is commonly needed as the alignment is being corrected. Soft tissue procedures will be followed if needed by bone-shortening procedures and tendon transfers, depending on the alignment obtained.
Preoperative Planning	• Always correct the deformity going proximal to distal. Deciding to add a bone procedure is not always easy; it depends on how stiff the deformity is. If there is no metatarsalgia, prefer to do soft tissue procedures including a plantar plate repair when the deformity is isolated. If metatarsalgia is present, a Weil osteotomy will help in treating the metatarsal overload, but it may increase soft tissue imbalance at the MTP joint. This effect is due to the metatarsal shortening, which translates into a loss in plantar fascia tension,[13] which has to be considered if repairing the plantar plate. If after the bone-shortening and/or soft tissue repair the MTP is deemed unstable, a flexor to extensor transfer is indicated.[9]
PIP Resection Arthroplasty or Arthrodesis	• This is a common adjunct in hammer toe surgery. Failure to resect enough of the head of the proximal phalanx can lead to postoperative pain or recurrence of the deformity. Failure to perform the tenodesis and dermodesis adequately to stabilize the joint may also result in a recurrence.
Flexor to Extensor Transfer	• When performing the transfer, hold down the toe to 20 degrees of plantarflexion at the MTP joint and the ankle at 90 degrees. Adequate traction on the tips of the tendon will suffice to hold down the toe. Sometimes, half of the tendon can be stripped off before performing the transfer. In this case, it is possible to perform the transfer through a drill hole to achieve an adequate balance with just one slip of the tendon. If the tissues are of bad quality, then a Kirschner wire may be used to fix the joint and protect the repair.

POSTOPERATIVE CARE

- Individual soft compressive dressings are placed over each operated toe; sterile strips of adhesive bandage are commonly used to keep each toe aligned.
- Small "tie-down" straps are used to hold each toe in plantarflexion (the straps are placed around the proximal phalanx of each toe). These are kept in place for 6 weeks.
- A soft compressive dressing is placed over the foot, and the foot is placed in a postoperative shoe with a rigid rocker bottom sole.
- Immediate weight bearing as tolerated is allowed, with a plantigrade foot, keeping the MTP joints neutral inside the postoperative shoe.
- From weeks 2 to 4, once soft tissues allow mobilization and the stitches are removed, passive plantarflexion exercises at the level of the MTP joint are done to stretch the dorsal structures.
- From the sixth week on, depending on comfort and edema, a return to normal shoes is permitted.

OUTCOMES

- The first reports of this technique used both the FDL and FDB tendons in the transfer.
  - Parrish[12] in 1973 described the technique shown in this chapter, using only the FDL and splitting the tendon longitudinally and suturing each half to each other under the extensor tendon. Fifteen of 18 patients had good to excellent results (83%).
  - Barbari and Brevig[1] reported 89% patient satisfaction in 39 cases.
  - Cyphers and Feiwell[4] reported 95% good to excellent results in 20 patients with residual paralysis from myelomeningocele.

- Boyer and DeOrio[2] recently reported an 89% satisfaction rate, using the technique in fixed and flexible hammer toes. They reported better results for fixed deformities where a concomitant resection of the head of the proximal phalanx was performed.
- The author generally offers up to 85% of success rate to his patients when using this technique.
  - Most postoperative complaints are due to stiffness of the PIP joint and in relation to the MTP joint when a procedure was added at this level (osteotomy, tenotomy, or capsulotomy).
  - Recurrence of deformity has been noted in 9% of the cases.
  - Retrospective evaluation of our results has shown that incomplete evaluation of the preoperative stiffness at the MTP joint may explain most of the recurrences.

COMPLICATIONS

- Swelling and numbness
- These complications usually subside with time.[3]
- Loss of vascularity can occur due to traction on the neurovascular bundle or compression due to the transfer.
  - Waiting, using a warm gauze, modifying, or removing the Kirschner wire if used and redissecting to ensure that the neurovascular bundle is not compressed are useful measures to solve this problem.
  - A small amount of lidocaine around the bundle can assist in smooth muscle relaxation. Nitropaste can be applied to the toe, too.
- PIP stiffness
  - This has been reported in up to 60% of cases (excluding joint arthrodesis or arthroplasties).[6]
  - It is one of the main reasons for dissatisfaction, specifically in flexible hammer toe deformity correction.[4]

- In earlier studies, no mention was made of preoperative stiffness, so it is difficult to quantify the relative contribution of previous stiffness (in fixed hammer toes) versus stiffness due to the transfer itself.
- Hyperextension deformities
  - Hyperextension deformities at the DIP joint are the infrequent result of excessive dissection in the volar aspect of the DIP joint when harvesting the FDL tendon.
    - They can be avoided with careful dissection.
  - These deformities at the MTP joint are due to inadequate positioning of the transfer (too distal over the proximal phalanx) or preoperative stiffness not adequately evaluated, which may need, besides additional MTP joint releases, bone-shortening procedures.
- Recurrence of the deformity
  - This has been reported in up to 20% of cases.
  - Recurrence is due to inadequate tension of the transfer, preoperative stiffness not adequately evaluated requiring additional soft tissue releases or bone-shortening procedures, underlying neurologic causes, excessive dorsal soft tissue scarring, or failure of the transfer.

REFERENCES

1. Barbari SG, Brevig K. Correction of clawtoes by the Girdlestone-Taylor flexor-extensor transfer procedure. Foot Ankle 1984;5:67–73.
2. Boyer ML, DeOrio JK. Transfer of the flexor digitorum longus for the correction of lesser-toes deformities. Foot Ankle 2007;28:422–430.
3. Coughlin M. Lesser toes abnormalities. J Bone Joint Surg Am 2002; 84A:1446–1469.
4. Cyphers SM, Feiwell E. Review of the Girdlestone-Taylor procedure for clawtoes in myelodysplasia. Foot Ankle 1988;8:229–233.
5. Hurwitz S. Hammertoe deformity following forefoot surgery. Foot Ankle Clin 1998;3:269–277.
6. Kirchner J, Wagner E. Girdlestone-Taylor flexor-extensor tendon transfer. Tech Foot Ankle Surg 2004;3:91–99.
7. Marks R. Anatomy and pathophysiology of lesser toes deformities. Foot Ankle Clin 1998;3:199–213.
8. Myerson M, Shereff M. The pathological anatomy of claw and hammer toes. J Bone Joint Surg Am 1989;71(1):45–49.
9. Nery C, Baumfeld D. Lesser metatarsophalangeal joint instability: treatment with tendon transfers. Foot Ankle Clin N Am 2018;23: 103–126.
10. Nery C, Coughlin M, Baumfeld D, et al. Lesser metatarsophalangeal joint instability: prospective evaluation and repair of plantar plate and capsular insufficiency. Foot Ankle Int 2012;33(4): 301–311.
11. Nery C, Coughlin M, Baumfeld D, et al. MRI evaluation of the MTP plantar plates compared with arthroscopic findings: a prospective study. Foot Ankle Int 2013;34(3):315–322.
12. Parrish TF. Dynamic correction of clawtoes. Orthop Clin North Am 1973;4:97–102.
13. Perez H, Reber L, Christensen J. The role of passive plantar flexion in floating toes following Weil osteotomy. J Foot Ankle Surg 2008;47(6):520–526.
14. Schuh R, Trnka HJ. Metatarsalgia: distal metatarsal osteotomies. Foot Ankle Clin 2011;16:583–595.
15. Thompson FM, Hamilton WG. Problem of the second metatarsophalangeal joint. Orthopedics 1987;10:83–89.

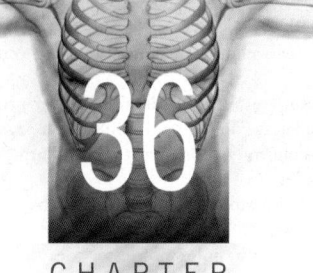

CHAPTER

Hammer Toe Correction

Lloyd C. Briggs, Jr.

DEFINITION

- Hammer toe deformity is one of the most common lesser toe disorders. Its severity can range the gamut from asymptomatic to disabling.
- Appropriate treatment of lesser toe disorders begins with determination of the exact joints involved and the plane of the primary and secondary deformities.
- Sagittal plane deformities of the lesser toes are generally classified as hammer toes (FIG 1A), claw toes (FIG 1B), and mallet toes (FIG 1C).
- Specifically, a hammer toe is a lesser toe deformity in which a sagittal plane, flexion contracture of the proximal interphalangeal (PIP) joint, is the primary deformity.
- A secondary, slight extension deformity of the metatarsophalangeal (MTP) joint may be present with a hammer toe, but this deformity is secondary and does not represent the primary deformity.

- The primary deformity being at the level of the PIP joint differentiates a hammer toe from a mallet toe or claw toe, in which case the primary deformity is located at the distal interphalangeal joint or the MTP joint, respectively.
- Hammer toe deformities are further classified as flexible or fixed depending on whether they completely correct with gentle, passive manipulation.

ANATOMY

- The lesser toes comprise three articulating phalanges (distal, middle, and proximal) that, at the proximal phalanx, articulate with the metatarsal head. The only exception to this pattern is the fifth toe, which in about 15% of individuals comprises just two phalanges (distal and proximal).
- The interphalangeal joints and their corresponding ligaments normally allow flexion but not extension past neutral, whereas the MTP joint complex allows both flexion and extension.

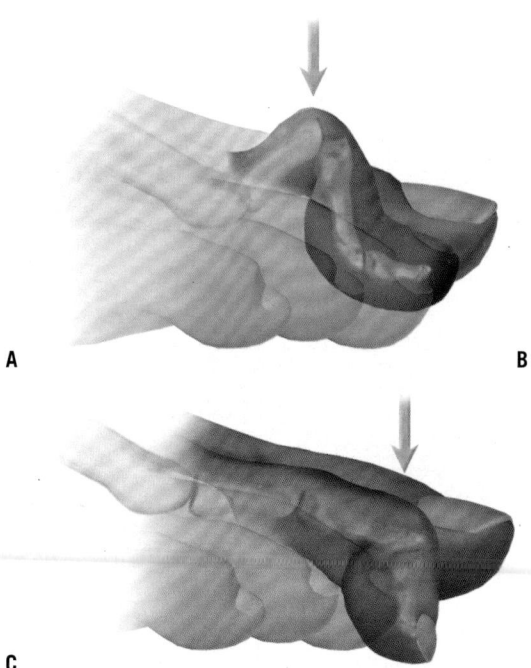

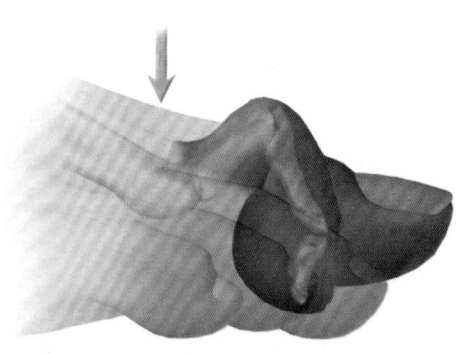

A

B

C

FIG 1 **A.** Hammer toe. The primary deformity is at the PIP joint. **B.** Claw toe. The primary deformity is at the MTP joint. **C.** Mallet toe. The primary deformity is at the distal interphalangeal joint.

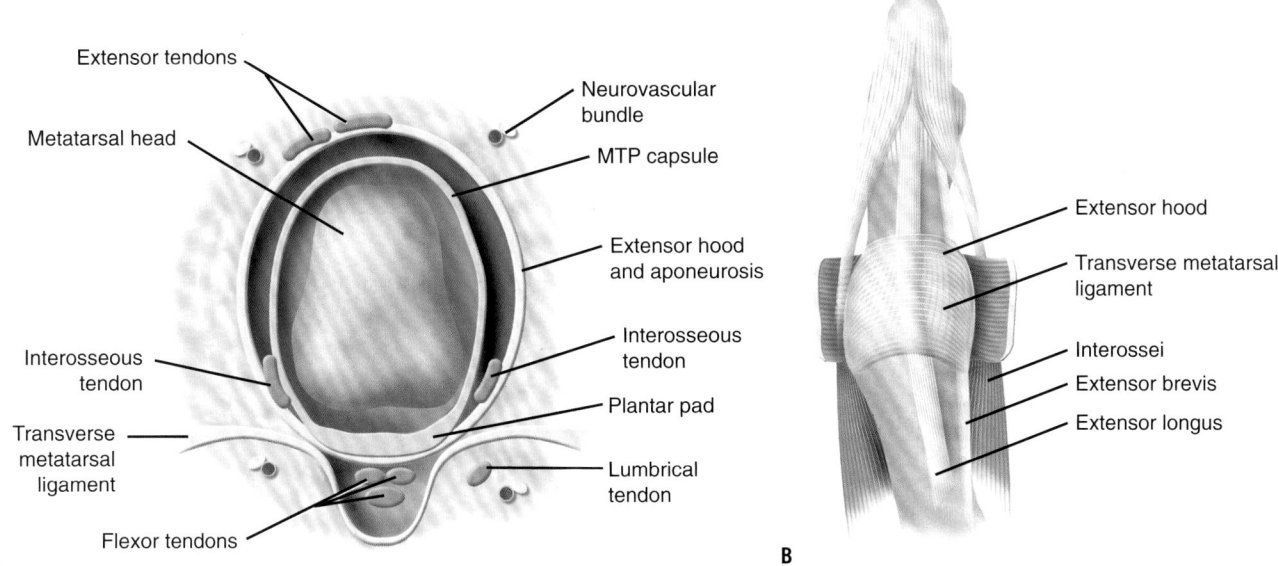

FIG 2 A. Cross-sectional anatomy of the lesser toe at the level of the metatarsal head. **B.** Dorsal view of a right lesser toe.

- Active motion and dynamic stability of the toe are achieved by both extrinsic muscles (originating in the leg) and intrinsic muscles (originating in the foot) **(FIG 2A)**.
- The extensor digitorum longus and flexor digitorum longus are the extrinsic muscles.
- The extensor digitorum longus invests the extensor hood over the proximal phalanx as well as inserting on the dorsal aspect of both the middle and distal phalanx **(FIG 2B)**, whereas the flexor digitorum longus inserts only on the distal phalanx.
- The intrinsic muscles of the toes include seven interosseous muscles, four lumbricals, the abductor digiti minimi, the flexor digitorum brevis, and the extensor digitorum brevis.

PATHOGENESIS

- Although the etiology of lesser toe deformities is multifactorial and includes neurologic, congenital, traumatic, and arthritic causes, the usual culprit for hammer toe deformity is restrictive shoe wear that does not provide sufficient room for the toes.
- Crowding of the toes in a shoe's toe box can be the result of poor shoe design, poor shoe fit, or a foot condition such as a hallux valgus deformity (and to a lesser degree, bunionette deformity) that crowds the toe box so that pressure is applied to the tips of the lesser toes and causes them to be passively flexed within the shoe for prolonged periods.
- As the extensor digitorum longus, the primary extensor of the PIP joint, simultaneously inserts on the middle and distal phalanx, the flexion of the PIP joint by the pressure of the toe box is reinforced by the inability of the extensor digitorum longus tendon to extend the PIP joint when the proximal phalanx is not neutrally aligned (ie, the MTP joint is dorsiflexed).
- This passive dorsiflexion at the MTP joint can occur from the pressure of the toe box on the toe as well as from elevation of the heel (eg, high-heeled shoe wear).

- As flexible hammer toe deformity is generally well tolerated, the patient does not usually seek treatment during the initial development of a hammer toe.
- With time, unless the factors that are stressing the toe are eliminated, the hammer toe will progress to a symptomatic fixed deformity.

NATURAL HISTORY

- Hammer toe deformity generally worsens with time if the causative factors are not mitigated. Over time, the PIP joint flexion deformity will tend to increase and the toe will eventually progress from a flexible to a fixed deformity.

PATIENT HISTORY AND PHYSICAL FINDINGS

- The most important information to elicit from the patient's history is whether the patient's complaints are solely resulting from the hammer toe deformity or whether other sources of pain are present.
- Occasionally, patients will present requesting surgery, having already made the diagnosis on their own. They experience pain in the foot and because the hammer toe deformity is the only abnormality they can see, they may conclude, sometimes mistakenly, that the hammer toe is the source of their pain.
- A good patient history includes the conservative treatment measures that have been tried, the types of shoes the patient wants to wear, the sorts of shoes the patient needs to wear for his or her occupation (ie, steel-toed shoes), and other patient factors that might be relative contraindications for surgery (eg, peripheral vascular disease) or would encourage you to pursue operative intervention (eg, history of ulceration).
- Typically, patients with a hammer toe deformity present with a complaint of pain centered over the PIP joint that is relieved with removal of their shoes.

- The degree of deformity generally corresponds to the degree of symptoms.
- Symptoms of numbness and tingling in the foot, diffuse pain, pain that occurs at night, or pain that does not improve with removal of shoes or shoe modifications raises concerns that the pain may be nonmechanical or emanating from a source other than the hammer toe.
- Attempts by the patient to try different toe pads or different shoes should be noted in the history, as improvements in the patient's pain with more reasonable shoe wear helps to clarify the diagnosis as well as direct efforts for nonoperative care.
- A history of neuropathy, peripheral vascular disease, systemic arthritides, and diabetes is important to elicit to assess for operative risk as well as to screen for other confounding sources of foot and toe pain.
- Finally, a history of ulceration or infection needs to be elicited, as this may indicate a need for more urgent operative correction of the deformity to prevent recurrence.
- The physical examination for hammer toe deformity, as with all foot and ankle examinations, begins with inspection of foot posture. Calluses, scars, and previous surgical incisions should be noted, as should the degree of the toe deformity.
- Hallux valgus deformity and bunionette deformity need to be assessed as to their contribution to the crowding of the toe box.
- With the patient standing, there must be enough room for the hammer toe to lie in the corrected position if surgically corrected. If a coexistent hallux valgus deformity prevents the hammer toe from being fully corrected, then the bunion must be surgically addressed at the same time as the hammer toe to avoid recurrence of the lesser toe deformity.
- Palpation of the foot and toes should reveal a point of maximal tenderness over the PIP joint, and the ability or inability to passively correct the hammer toe to neutral should be recorded.
- Finally, as with all foot examinations, pulses and foot sensation are assessed.
- Methods for examining a hammer toe deformity include the following:
  - Palpation of the distal interphalangeal, PIP, and MTP joints for points of maximal tenderness. The PIP joint should be the area of maximal tenderness, but the tip of the toe may be painful as well.
  - Gentle manual straightening of the toe to assess the ability of the toe to correct to neutral. If the toe completely corrects to neutral, it is considered a flexible deformity. If the toe does not completely correct, it is considered a fixed deformity. A flexible deformity can be addressed with a soft tissue procedure such as a flexor to extensor tendon transfer, but a fixed deformity will require bone resection for surgical correction.
  - Push-up test: With the patient seated and knee flexed, the examiner dorsiflexes the ankle to neutral by applying pressure under the metatarsal heads. The correction of the toe deformity with this maneuver is noted. This will determine whether the deformity is fixed versus flexible and is also useful in the operating room to assess residual MTP joint contracture after the hammer toe has been corrected at the PIP joint. Residual MTP joint contracture necessitates additional surgical correction at the MTP joint such as extensor tendon lengthening, capsular release, or collateral ligament release.

IMAGING AND OTHER DIAGNOSTIC STUDIES

- Standing radiographs of the foot (anteroposterior [AP] standing, lateral standing, and an oblique view) are helpful to assess alignment of the toes as well as to rule out arthritis of the various toe joints.
- Vascular studies of the lower extremity (transcutaneous P_{O_2} readings and arterial Doppler studies with waveforms and toe pressures) are essential if surgical intervention is contemplated and there is any question of vascular compromise.

DIFFERENTIAL DIAGNOSIS

- Claw toe
- Mallet toe
- Crossover toe deformity
- Degenerative joint disease
- Morton neuroma
- Neuropathy
- Radiculopathy
- Vascular insufficiency
- Metatarsal stress fracture
- MTP joint instability or synovitis

NONOPERATIVE MANAGEMENT

- Ultimately, the treatment of a hammer toe deformity involves "making the shoe fit the foot, or the foot fit the shoe."
- Conservative treatment for a symptomatic hammer toe involves accommodating the deformity with a shoe the patient finds acceptable. Generally, an athletic-type shoe with a soft toe box will accommodate many mild deformities, whereas a prescription extra-depth shoe with an extra wide toe box will be needed to accommodate others.
- Occasionally, softening of the leather upper of a shoe and stretching of the shoe over the area of the deformity will allow several millimeters of extra room for the toe, and in extreme cases, a "bubble patch" or cutout and elevation of a portion of the shoe toe box can give relief.
- Silicone toe sleeves or toe pads can help relieve symptoms in mild deformities, but they are not usually successful for the treatment of fixed deformities as they tend to "stuff" the already crowded toe box and make the deformity more symptomatic.

SURGICAL MANAGEMENT

- The primary indication for surgical correction of a hammer toe is a symptomatic (painful or preulcerative lesion) in a patient with adequate vascularity and realistic expectations who has failed to respond to conservative care.
- Generally, patients with these problems tend to present having already attempted some type of conservative treatment or change in shoe wear. If they have not, it is worthwhile to educate the patient concerning the nature of the problem and conservative treatment options.
- Generally, the most important determinant of postoperative patient satisfaction is a realistic preoperative expectation. When considering surgery, the patient should be told that by choosing surgery, he or she is electing to trade a painful, thin, deformed toe with some voluntary motion for a less painful (ideally pain-free), short, scarred, possibly numb, swollen toe with little volitional control. The patient should

not make the decision for surgery based on whether he or she wants a "normal" toe.

- If the patient's preoperative expectations are too high, he or she should be advised to maximize conservative care and avoid surgery, as most likely he or she would be disappointed with the surgical outcome.

- Preoperatively, the patient's shoe wear goals should be discussed, stressing that the goal of the operation is to allow the patient to wear "reasonable" shoes.

- A patient with a coexistent hallux valgus deformity that does not allow adequate space for the lesser toe to move down onto the floor with surgical correction will need to have the hallux valgus deformity corrected at the time of the lesser toe surgery to avoid recurrence of the hammer toe.

- In this situation, the hallux valgus deformity will have to be corrected even if it is asymptomatic. The patient needs to be counseled that correction of an asymptomatic hallux valgus deformity, to provide space for the hammer toe, may lead to a painful or numb great toe. ("It is difficult to make something that does not hurt better.") Patients need to be aware of this possibility before electing surgery and consider it in their decision to have surgery.

- With the decision made to proceed with fixed hammer toe deformity correction, there are primarily two surgical options: PIP joint resection arthroplasty and PIP joint arthrodesis.

- With either option, the fixed nature of the hammer toe deformity requires resection of bone to shorten the toe so that, as it is straightened, the contracted, plantar neurovascular structures are not injured, which would occur with simply forcibly straightening the toe and pinning it without bone resection.

- PIP joint resection arthroplasty involves resecting the distal condyles of the proximal phalanx, which relieves the deformity and often retains a small amount of motion at the PIP joint. This procedure has almost universally good results[5] and is generally regarded as the gold standard for the correction of the majority of hammer toe deformities.

- When it is desirable to have permanent, multiplanar stability at the PIP joint or to perform the procedure without the use of a postoperative stabilizing Kirschner wire, arthrodesis at the PIP joint may be a better option.

- PIP joint arthrodesis involves preparation of the adjacent middle and proximal phalanx articular surfaces and some type of fixation to create stability at the fusion site. Several methods of fixation have been advocated, including Kirschner wire fixation and preparing the bone so that it interdigitates, such as in a peg and dowel fusion,[1] intramedullary screw fixation,[3] or an interphalangeal implant[2,4,11] such as the Hat-Trick PIP joint implant (Smith & Nephew, Inc., Watford, United Kingdom) (**FIG 3**).

- The Hat-Trick PIP joint implant is designed for PIP joint arthrodesis. It is composed of two matching polyetheretherketone radiolucent, biocompatible, nonabsorbable polymer components that are individually inserted into the prepared middle and proximal phalanxes and then interlocked, creating stable PIP joint fixation.

- Arthrodesis is beneficial for patients for whom recurrence of deformity is likely, such as in severe deformity or revision hammer toe surgery. When a pin extending from the toe may pose an unacceptable infection risk—such as in a patient with diabetes mellitus, rheumatoid arthritis, or

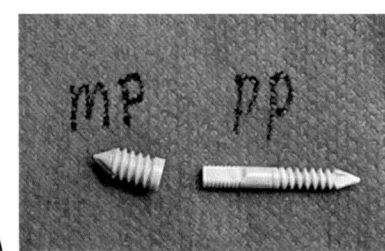

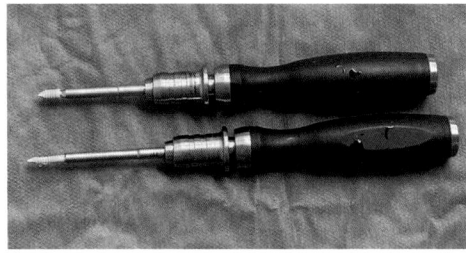

FIG 3 A. Hat-Trick implant. *MP*, middle phalanx. *PP*, proximal phalanx. **B.** Hat-Trick middle phalanx driver with implant inserted (*top*) and proximal phalanx driver with zero degree implant inserted (*bottom*). Proximal phalanx 10-degree driver not depicted.

compliance issues—an arthrodesis with an implant spanning the PIP joint can be beneficial.

- Fusion is also useful for crossover toe deformity correction, when destabilizing the PIP joint with a resection arthroplasty may result in a symptomatic angular deformity at the PIP joint, as crossover toe deformity invariably recurs with time.

- **TABLE 1** compares PIP joint resection arthroplasty and arthrodesis.

Preoperative Planning

- With any toe surgery, adequate vascularity must be ensured before proceeding with surgery.

- With lesser toe surgery, especially in the revision situation or if the patient has systemic conditions that might impair toe circulation, vascular injury to the toe and loss of the toe are possibilities and need to be discussed with the patient before the surgery.

- For PIP joint arthrodesis with use of the StayFuse implant, a preoperative AP radiograph of the foot is useful to determine whether the proximal phalanx and middle phalanx are of sufficient length and width to accommodate the implants.
  - The proximal phalanx implants are 15 mm in length with the narrowest implant being 2.7 mm in width.

TABLE 1 Proximal Interphalangeal Joint Resection Arthroplasty versus Arthrodesis

Arthroplasty indications

- Gold standard; the procedure of choice unless there is a special circumstance

Arthrodesis indications

- Situations with expected high recurrence rates (severe deformities and revision hammer toe surgery)
- Unacceptable elevated infection risk with external pin (diabetes, rheumatoid arthritis, or anticipated noncompliance)
- Need for multiplanar stability (crossover toe deformity)

TABLE 2 Hat-Trick Proximal Interphalangeal Implant Sizes	
Proximal Phalanx Size	**Middle Phalanx Size**
2.7 × 15 mm, 0 degree	4 × 9 mm
2.7 × 15 mm, 10 degree	4 × 9 mm
3.2 × 15 mm, 0 degree	4 × 9 mm
3.2 × 15 mm, 10 degree	4 × 9 mm
3.7 × 15 mm, 0 degree	4 or 5 × 9 mm
3.7 × 15 mm, 10 degree	4 or 5 × 9 mm
4.2 × 15 mm, 0 degree	4 or 5 × 9 mm
4.2 × 15 mm, 10 degree	4 or 5 × 9 mm

- The middle phalanx implants are shorter, 9 mm in length, but wider with the narrowest implant being 4 mm in width **(TABLE 2)**. Keep in mind that the middle phalanx will be a millimeter or two shorter after the bone resection. Ideally, the implants should just engage the cortex of the phalanx and not penetrate the MTP or distal interphalangeal joints.
- The goal is to select an implant that will fill the canal, but it is generally better to err on the side of a narrower implant to avoid breaking the phalanx cortex and decreasing fusion site stability.

Positioning

- Positioning of the patient is supine, with the patient's heel resting at the end of the operating table. A small, padded bump may be placed under the ipsilateral greater trochanter of the hip to internally rotate the foot to give better access to the dorsum of the foot.
- The procedure can be easily performed with an ankle block or forefoot block with or without a tourniquet.
- An ankle block is generally preferred in combination with an ankle Esmarch tourniquet if there are no vascular issues with regard to the toes; otherwise, the procedure is performed without a tourniquet.

Approach

- PIP joint resection arthroplasty and PIP joint arthrodesis are both performed through a dorsal approach to the PIP joint.
- A curvilinear incision is usually marked out over the MTP joint as well in case the extensor tendon or MTP joint capsule needs to be approached after the hammer toe correction to address any residual extension deformity at the MTP joint **(FIG 4)**.

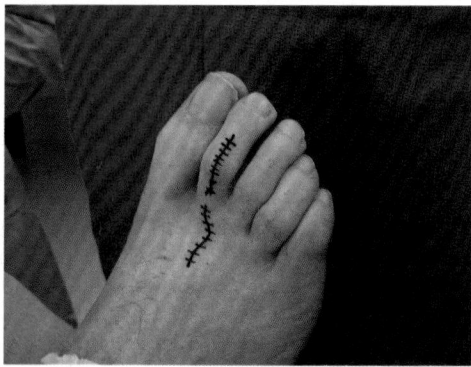

FIG 4 Skin markings for hammer toe surgery.

PROXIMAL INTERPHALANGEAL JOINT ARTHROPLASTY

Exposure

- Make a straight longitudinal dorsal approach through the skin overlying the PIP joint, exposing the extensor tendon overlying the joint. The incision is about 1.5 cm long.
- Generally, for hammer toe surgery, a longitudinal incision is utilized, but a transverse incision can be used **(TECH FIG 1A)**. With the toe flexed, remove a transverse-oriented ellipse of skin over the dorsum of the PIP joint. The size of the ellipse depends on the amount of redundant skin but is generally about 3 mm wide.
  - This incision has the benefit of removing some of the redundant tissue overlying the PIP joint and may be more cosmetic, but it can make the hammer toe correction more difficult if the incision is not placed directly over the proximal phalanx condyles.

- With either initial incision, the remainder of the procedure for PIP joint arthroplasty is the same.
- Retract the skin and expose the extensor tendon and cut it transversely over the joint as the toe is slightly flexed. Make a second parallel transverse cut in the extensor tendon to remove a 1-mm section of the tendon to account for the inevitable tendon redundancy one will encounter when closing the soft tissues after the bone resection.
  - Alternatively, the tendon can be addressed at the end of the case.
- Introduce a no. 15 blade into the joint between the collateral ligament and the underlying condyle of the proximal phalanx, releasing one side and then the other **(TECH FIG 1B)**.
- Direct the knife blade proximally, staying along the bone and not penetrating below the level of the plantar plate.

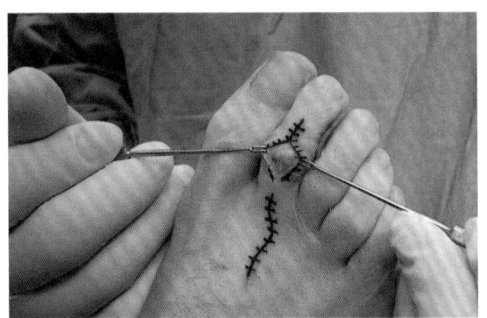

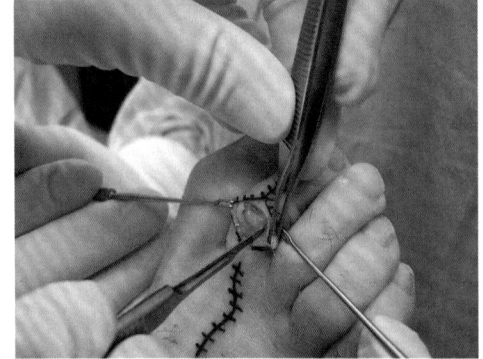

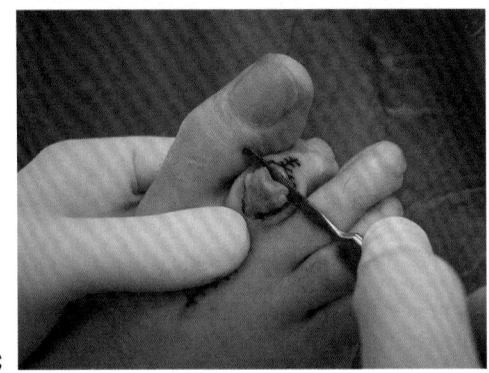

TECH FIG 1 **A.** Dorsal approach for PIP joint arthroplasty exposing the extensor digitorum longus tendon. **B.** Releasing the collateral ligaments from the proximal phalanx with retraction of the extensor digitorum longus tendon. **C.** Releasing the plantar plate and exposing the proximal condyles.

Progressively flexing the toe to keep the collateral ligaments under tension helps make them easier to cut.

- With the collateral ligaments released and the toe flexed, bluntly dissect the plantar plate off the neck of the proximal phalanx with a periosteal elevator to completely expose the proximal phalanx condyles (**TECH FIG 1C**).

Bone Resection

- Resect the condyles using a sagittal saw oriented at a 90-degree angle to the axis of the proximal phalanx in both the coronal and sagittal planes at the metaphyseal–epiphyseal junction. A Freer elevator is placed under the proximal phalanx condyles to aid exposure and protect the underlying soft tissues while the bone is being cut (**TECH FIG 2**).

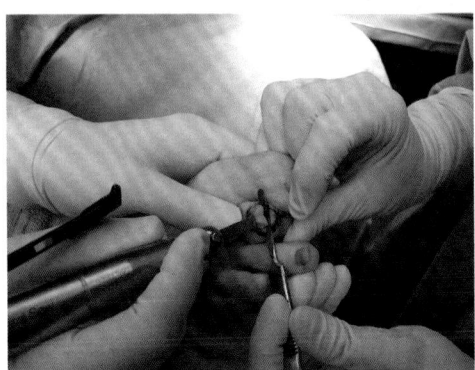

TECH FIG 2 The proximal phalanx is cut at right angles while protecting the plantar soft tissues.

- At this point, if one is attempting to achieve more of an arthrodesis as opposed to a "true" arthroplasty, a small osteotome can be used to remove the cartilage on the base of the middle phalanx so that the subchondral bone is exposed.

- Extend the toe to see if adequate bone has been resected. Ideally, gentle extension of the toe should bring the toe to neutral but not hyperextension. If the toe does not extend completely, if more than gentle extension is needed to do so, or if the toe seems to want to "spring back" to a more flexed position, additional bone can be resected, preferably a millimeter or two at a time until the toe is properly tensioned.

- The goal is to remove enough bone so that the toe straightens completely without residual tension on the plantar soft tissues so that the deformity is corrected and the soft tissues are balanced.
  - Excessive resection of the bone can lead to postcorrection hyperextension at the PIP joint, which can make the patient symptomatic at the poorly padded plantar aspect of the PIP joint.
  - In addition, excessive shortening of the bone will result in varus–valgus instability of the toe, especially as the proximal phalanx resection moves from the metaphysis into the shaft of the proximal phalanx.

- With adequate bone removed from the proximal phalanx, palpate the dorsal aspect of both the middle and proximal phalanges and smooth any bony prominences with a rongeur if necessary.

Kirschner Wire Insertion

- Place a 0.045-inch Kirschner wire (a 0.062-inch Kirschner wire is used if the MTP joint is to be pinned) in the center of the articular surface of the middle phalanx and pass it across the middle phalanx through the distal phalanx and out the tip of the toe.

- If one is trying to achieve an arthrodesis of the toe as opposed to a true arthroplasty and the cartilage has been removed from the base of the middle phalanx, a Kirschner wire is used to create 2-mm deep perforations in the subchondral bone of the middle phalanx in 3-mm increments to increase the likelihood of fusion, prior to placing the Kirschner wire centrally in the middle phalanx and advancing it out the tip of the toe.
- Advance the Kirschner wire through the toe until it extends only a millimeter or two from the surface of the middle phalanx. Reduce the PIP joint to its neutral position and then drive the Kirschner wire back through the proximal phalanx shy of the MTP joint.
- The pin position can be assessed with an AP fluoroscopic view (**TECH FIG 3**).
- Perform a push-up test and assess the corrected position of the toe at the MTP joint. If the MTP joint corrects to neutral, proceed to closure; but if there appears to be extension at the MTP joint, that is addressed with an MTP joint soft tissue release.

Metatarsophalangeal Joint Soft Tissue Release

- Make a curvilinear incision over the MTP joint about 2.5 cm long. Identify and lengthen the extensor digitorum longus tendon in a Z-fashion (**TECH FIG 4A**).
- Lengthen the extensor digitorum longus tendon by dissecting out the tendon and placing a sterile tongue depressor under the tendon to both protect the underlying soft tissues and assure that an adequate length of tendon has been exposed (about 2 cm).
- Divide the tendon first longitudinally in halves and then cut it proximally and distally to create a Z-pattern cut.
- Isolate the extensor digitorum brevis tendon, which travels lateral to the extensor digitorum longus tendon, and tenotomize it to further relieve any dorsiflexion contracture.
- Perform the push-up test again, and if additional extension of the proximal phalanx at the MTP joint remains, cut the

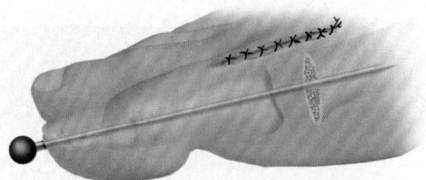

TECH FIG 3 Completed PIP joint resection arthroplasty hammer toe deformity correction. (Briggs LC Jr. Proximal interphalangeal joint arthrodesis using the StayFuse Implant. Tech Foot Ankle Surg 2004;3:77–84.)

capsule of the MTP joint transversely and release the dorsal third of the collateral ligaments on both sides of the metatarsal head in a similar fashion to how the PIP joint collateral ligaments were released in the initial part of the procedure (**TECH FIG 4B**).

- If the MTP joint has to be addressed, use a 0.062-inch Kirschner wire, instead of the 0.045-inch Kirschner wire, to pin the PIP joint and the MTP joint. The wire is usually placed 2 cm or more into the metatarsal, across the MTP joint to stabilize the joint. Pin the MTP joint while the ankle is held in neutral flexion and the toe is held in 5 degrees of flexion at the MTP joint.

Closure

- Close the PIP joint using a 4-0 plain suture to close the extensor tendon in one layer and then close the skin with simple 4-0 plain suture. If there is significant redundancy of the extensor tendon, a portion of it can be removed still allowing a loose closure over the PIP joint.
- Close the extensor tendon at the MTP joint with a 2-0 nonabsorbable suture, followed by a 4-0 absorbable subcuticular closure and 4-0 nylon skin closure.

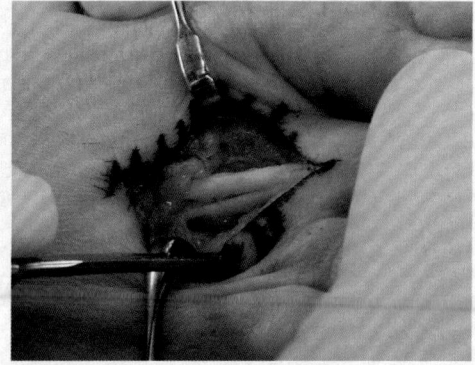
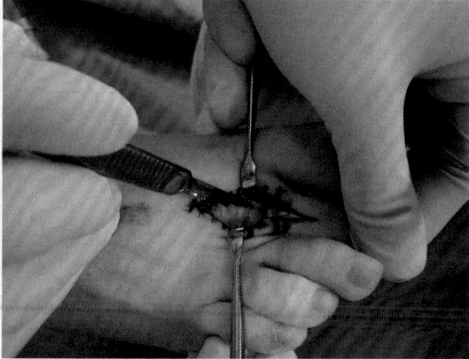

A **B**

TECH FIG 4 A. Exposure of the extensor digitorum longus and brevis over the MTP joint. **B.** Release of the dorsal portion of the collateral ligaments of the MTP joint after the extensor digitorum brevis has been tenotomized, the extensor digitorum longus Z-lengthened, and the MTP joint capsule released.

PROXIMAL INTERPHALANGEAL JOINT ARTHRODESIS

- The surgical technique for the arthrodesis is identical to that for the arthroplasty with regard to joint exposure.
- Having confirmed that the diameter and length of the proximal and middle phalanx will accommodate at least the smallest Hat-Trick implant, (2.7 × 15 mm and 4.0 × 9 mm, respectively), the surgeon must decide before making the bone cuts whether to use the standard 0-degree implant or a "flexed" 10-degree implant.
  - The 10-degree implant has the advantage of offering a more "natural" or cosmetic toe appearance.
  - If addressing the deformity of only one or two toes, the implant decision can be guided by observing the remaining unaffected toes.

Bone Resection

- After exposing the proximal phalanx condyles, use a sagittal saw to resect the proximal phalanx at the junction of the metaphyseal–epiphyseal junction as described previously for the standard 0-degree implant.
  - For the 10-degree implant, the saw blade will need to be angled off the perpendicular, to a small degree, to take off slightly more of the plantar proximal phalanx cortex to create the 10-degree cut at the arthrodesis site.
- In addition to exposing the proximal phalanx, arthrodesis requires exposure of the middle phalanx. This is exposed using sharp dissection to remove the soft tissue for a millimeter or two along the dorsal, medial, and lateral aspects of the middle phalanx (TECH FIG 5).
- With the middle phalanx exposed, use a narrow sagittal saw blade to resect the articular cartilage but no more than a millimeter or so of the subchondral bone. Be careful not to leave bony fragments or ledges in the depths of the wound, as these may later be prominent when the toe is fused.
- With both the proximal phalanx and the middle phalanx exposed, bring the toe into extension to see if the bony surfaces adequately align and if overall toe alignment is acceptable. If using

the 10-degree implant, there should be a slight, 10-degree flexion at the PIP joint with the cut, flush, bone surfaces opposed.
- Additional bony resection can be performed at this time.
  - Make sure enough bone has been removed to avoid excessive tension on the contracted plantar neurovascular bundles once the toe is realigned. Once the implant is engaged, it is difficult to remove it if the toe does not "pink up" after the removal of the tourniquet.
  - Although adequate bony resection is necessary, excessive bony resection should be avoided as it will lead to a cosmetically displeasing short toe.

Implant Site Preparation

- After the bone resection, place a 0.062-inch Kirschner wire or 1.6-mm drill tip wire down the center of the proximal phalanx to find the central axis of the bone. Use an AP fluoroscopic picture to confirm that the wire is centrally placed and perpendicular to the cut surface (TECH FIG 6A).
- Remove the wire, and starting with the smallest (2.7 mm) proximal phalanx tap, follow the path created by the wire, seating the tap to the top of the black laser line. When advancing the tap, watch closely for the development of stress riser on the dorsal cortex. When tapping, the goal is to engage the proximal phalanx cortex but not fracture the phalanx.
  - If, when seated, the 2.7-mm tap does not appear to demonstrate sufficient canal fill, progressively ream with the next size tap (3.2, 3.7, and 4.2 mm) stopping when the appropriate implant size has been determined by the "feel" of tap resistance aided by fluoroscopy if necessary (the implant size matches the tap diameter, 1:1) (TECH FIG 6B).
- After making the channel in the proximal phalanx, drill the same 0.062-inch or 1.6-mm wire down the axis of the middle phalanx starting at least 3 mm from the dorsal cortex and ideally 1 mm dorsal to the exact center of the of the middle phalanx cut bone surface.
  - This slight dorsal offset of the guidewire and subsequent slight dorsal starting point for the middle phalanx tap attempts to counteract the "natural" prominence of the dorsal middle phalanx after the implant is interdigitated and compressed.
- After the middle phalanx has been drilled, fluoroscopy can be used to check that the wire is centrally positioned. The middle phalanx is then tapped using the 4.0-mm tap.
  - Similarly, to the preparation of the proximal phalanx, if the cortex is not engaged by the implant, a 5.0-mm tap can be used if the proximal phalanx has been tapped to a 3.7- or 4.2-mm width.
  - If the proximal phalanx has only been tapped with one of the smaller two taps (2.7 or 3.2 mm), the 5.0-mm middle phalanx tap should *not* be used (TECH FIG 6C).

Implant Insertion

- With both sides prepared, insert the middle phalanx implant first to avoid interference with its placement by the protruding post of the proximal phalanx implant once it is inserted. Insert the middle phalanx implant flush with the cut surface (TECH FIG 7A).

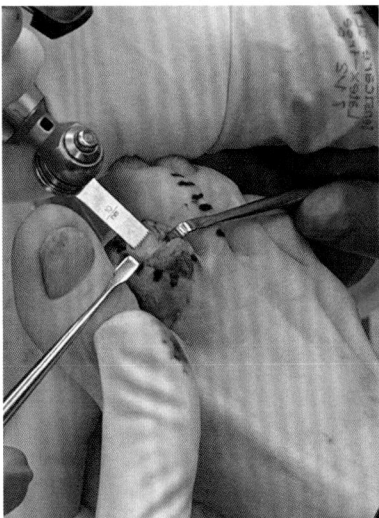

TECH FIG 5 Preparation of the middle phalanx with sagittal saw.

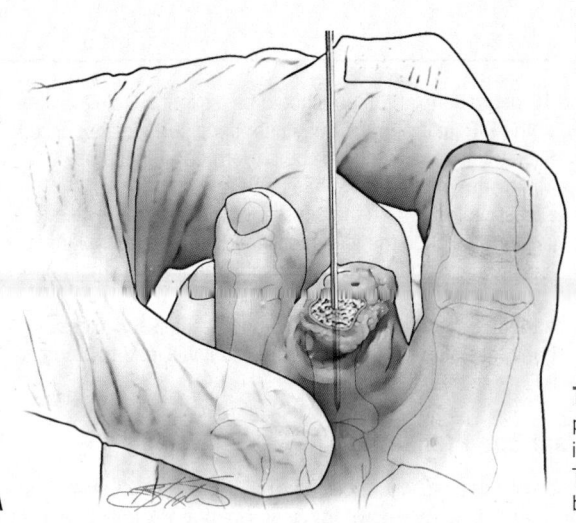

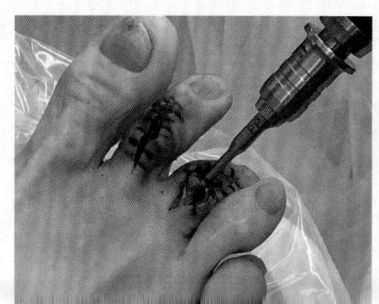

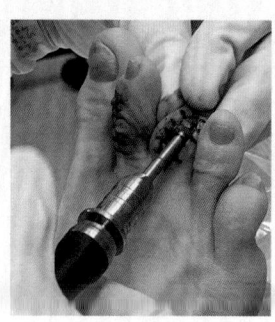

TECH FIG 6 A. Middle phalanx is prepared with the hand drill. **B.** Proximal phalanx tap is advanced down the canal until the black laser line (pictured) is below the surface of the cut bone. **C.** The middle phalanx is then tapped. The tap is advanced until the black laser line (still visible in the picture) travels below the cut surface of the bone.

- Place the proximal phalanx implant with the body of the implant flush with the cut surface of the bone and the post of the implant exposed.
  - If using the 10-degree implant (as opposed to the 0-degree implant), care must be taken to insert the implant so that the black laser line on the driver is oriented dorsally to properly orient the proximal phalanx component **(TECH FIG 7B).**
- The implants are then ready to be engaged. They are distracted and brought together, engaging the two components as horizontally as possible to avoid an iatrogenic fracture **(TECH FIG 7C).**
- It is important not to more than slightly lever the two components together, as this can fracture the bone or loosen the implant. It is recommended to grasp the toe with a 4 × 4 dressing sponge to give better hold of the toe as you manipulate it.[12]
- If the components are not aligning, or any more than gentle pressure has to be applied to position the post in the middle phalanx channel, the proximal phalanx driver can be reapplied and the implant advanced one additional turn to make it easier to engage the proximal phalanx post.

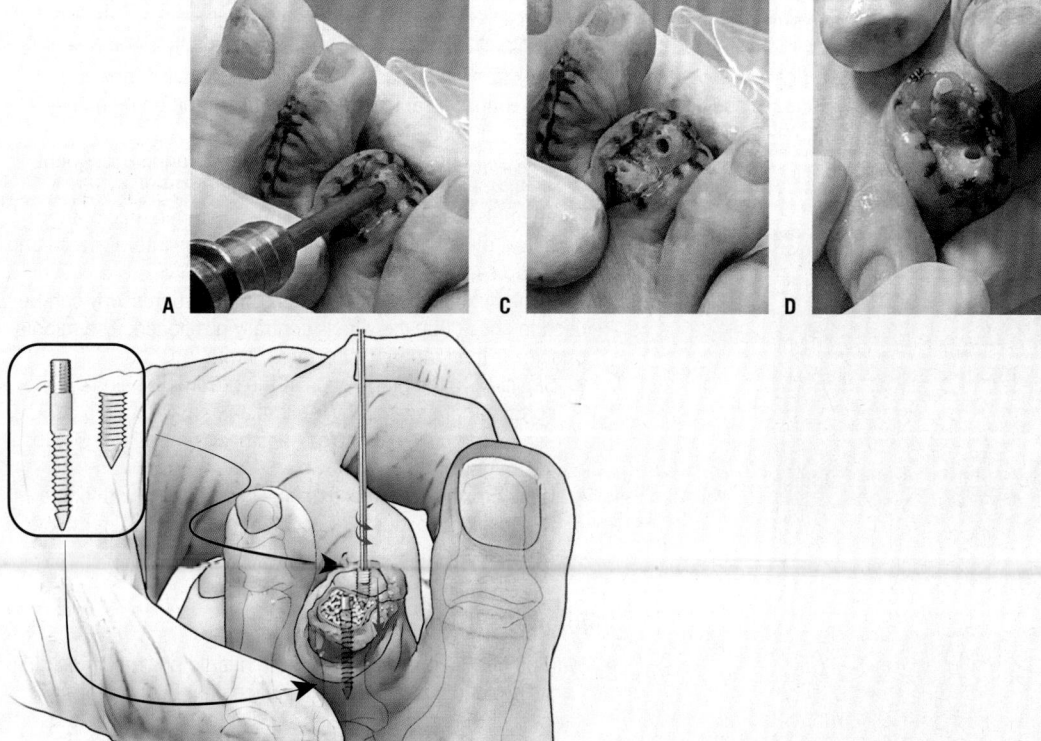

TECH FIG 7 A. Insertion of the middle phalanx implant. **B.** Fully inserted implant. **C.** Seating of the implant flush with the cut bony surface. **D.** Both the proximal and middle phalanx implants are seated. *(continued).*

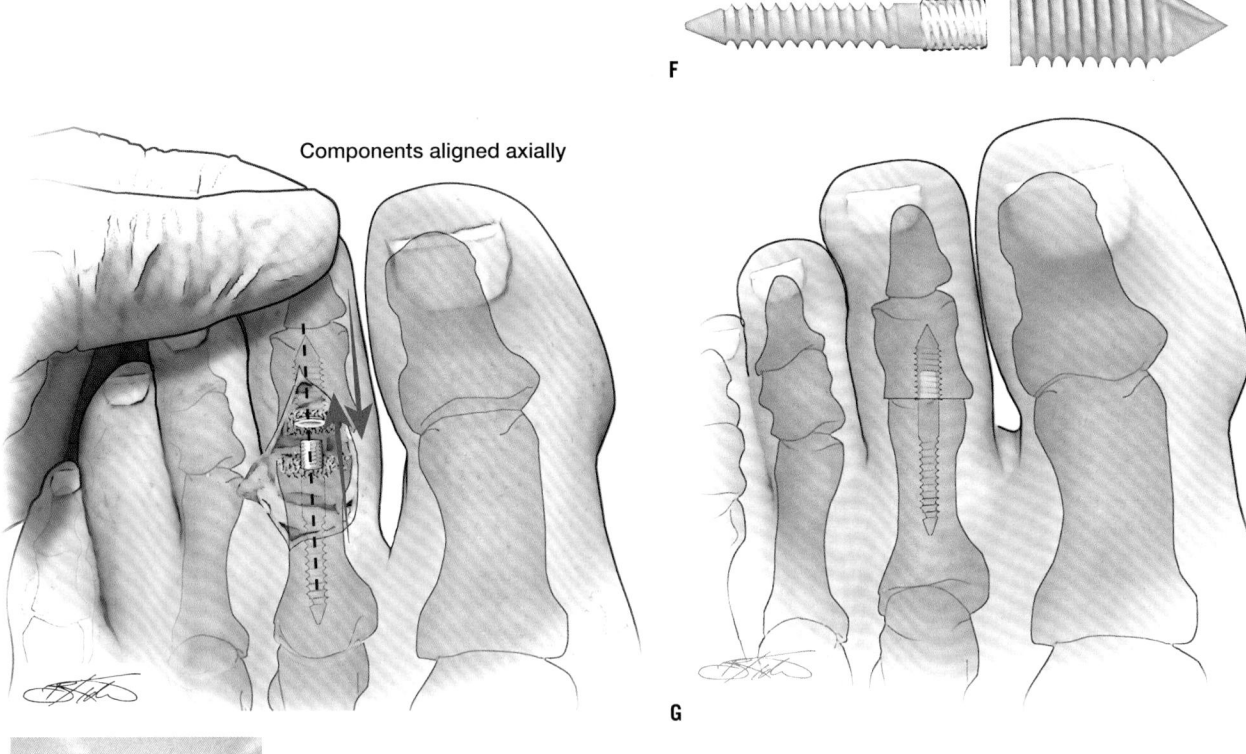

TECH FIG 7 *(continued)* **E.** The two implants are engaged with axial compression rather than levering the implants together. This avoids bending or breaking the implant. **F.** Proper alignment of implant. **G.** Implant securely engaged. **H.** AP fluoroscopic image of the second and third toes demonstrating proper implant engagement and good apposition of the bony surfaces.

- If the proximal phalanx implant appears to subside as the attempt is made to engage the post, stop the attempt at engaging the two components. At this point, there are two options depending on the implant "stability."
  - Remove the original implant and ream the phalanx to a larger size and place a larger implant.
  - Alternatively, pull the subsiding implant back to its original position and then drill a temporary Kirschner wire from dorsal to plantar across the phalanx just proximal to the implant to block the migration of the implant. This will prevent subsidence as the components of the implants are engaged. Following confirmation that the implants are engaged and fixation is adequate, the Kirschner wire is removed.
- As the post of the implant engages, a ratcheting sound will be audible. The components should be completely compressed and the bone surfaces come in contact with each other, which can be visually confirmed **(TECH FIG 7D)**.
- As the implant is fully interdigitated, the ends of the bones should visually come to rest together and the implant should fully engage **(TECH FIG 7E)**.
- A C-arm is usually used to confirm that the component is properly engaged and the toe is well aligned **(TECH FIG 7F,G)**.

- If there is a slight gap anywhere along the bone fusion site **(TECH FIG 7H)**, this is acceptable. The gap can be filled with some bone graft from the resected condyles.
- Finally, after engagement of the implant if visually there appears to be some malrotation of the toe, the toe can be gently twisted or "rotated" to achieve a neutral position and properly align the toe with the nail plate parallel to the plantar surface of the foot.
- With the toe implant inserted, palpate the bony dorsal surface of the toe at the PIP joint to make sure that there are no protrusions; remove any bony prominences with a rongeur to create a smooth surface.
- The remainder of the arthrodesis procedure is identical to the PIP joint arthroplasty, with the exception being that if the MTP joint must be addressed, it is done so without fixing it with a Kirschner wire, as the Hat-Trick PIP joint implant will not allow the Kirschner wire to pass down the toe.
  - In these cases, I extend the dressing sponges or ABD pads out over the toe with the dressing to block dorsiflexion of the toe. In this situation, in the immediate postoperative period, I initiate taping of the toe in neutral position at the first postoperative visit and continue it for up to 3 months.

Pearls and Pitfalls

Avoid vascular compromise	• Assess the circulation preoperatively. • Keep all dissection around the phalanxes subperiosteal. • Make sure there is adequate resection of bone at the PIP joint. The implant or Kirschner wire should only hold the correction that was obtained with the bone resection. • If the toe does not pink up at the end of the case after the tourniquet is let down, wait 10 minutes for reperfusion. If this does not resolve the problem, check to see if all constrictive dressings have been removed. • Next, apply warm saline-soaked sponges to the toe. • If this does not allow the toe to pink up, 1% lidocaine without epinephrine can be lavaged over the neurovascular structures. • Nitropaste applied to the toe has also been advocated in this situation. • Finally, in the case of PIP joint arthroplasty, removal of the Kirschner wire may be necessary. Slight bending (5–10 degrees) of the Kirschner wire to flex the PIP joint more or dorsiflex the MTP joint slightly is acceptable, although it makes taking the Kirschner wire out more difficult postoperatively. In the case of PIP joint arthrodesis, the implant might have to be removed, although we have not found this to be necessary.
Avoid pinning the toe too straight (PIP joint arthroplasty)	• When pinning the toe, try to start more plantarly on the middle phalanx and then exit the tip of the toe. When the pin is then driven back in a retrograde fashion, there is a slight flex at the PIP joint.
Properly remove the implant (If necessary)	• If after insertion a metallic implant has to be removed, the dorsal cortex of either middle or proximal phalanx must be partially removed. Whichever side of the implant is the narrower in relation to the canal diameter should be teased out by removing as little of the dorsal cortex as necessary. • After one end of the implant is removed, the implant can be grabbed and used to unscrew the implant from the opposite side. After this, one option is to insert another implant using one with a slightly larger diameter in the portion that has had the dorsal cortex partially removed. • The larger diameter of the implant will allow the implant to have some purchase in this situation. • If after insertion the Hat-Trick PIP joint implant has to be removed, it can be cut transversely at the arthrodesis site[8] and then removed in two pieces.
Avoid breaking or loosening the implant (PIP joint arthrodesis)	• Do not lever the implant together but distract, engage, and then bring the implant together with it axially aligned. • If necessary, the proximal phalanx implant can be screwed further into the canal to make it easier to engaging the implants.
Select the proper-sized implant (PIP joint arthrodesis)	• Progressively ream the proximal phalanx with the 2.7-, 3.2-, 3.7-, and 4.2-mm tap until resistance is encountered from the cortical bone. Seat the tap so that the top of the laser line is covered. Look for any sign of a stress riser forming on the dorsal cortex. Check the tap's fit in the canal with fluoroscopy if necessary. • The middle phalanx has two tap options, the standard 4.0 mm plus 5.0 mm, which can be used if the proximal phalanx is reamed to a 3.7- or 4.2-mm diameter. • The implant width will match the size of the tap. • The standard implant is not angled (0 degrees), but a 10-degree implant can be used and may give a more cosmetic appearing toe. • Most of the fifth toe phalanxes are too small for an implant.
Avoid incomplete engagement of the Hat-Trick PIP joint implant (PIP joint arthrodesis)	• Make sure the middle phalanx implant and the base of the proximal phalanx implant are flush with the bone cut. • If most of the post engages, but a portion does not, this is probably acceptable if the bone has been brought into proper apposition.

POSTOPERATIVE CARE

• Immediately postoperatively, the patient is advised to heel weight bear in a postoperative shoe.
• For the first 2 days, activity is limited as the patient is advised to spend the majority of time with the foot up and elevated above the heart, "toes above the nose" (23 out of 24 hours).
• After this, activity and elevation should be guided by swelling.
• Sutures are removed at 2 to 3 weeks, and any pins are removed at 3 weeks.
• At 3 weeks, the patient can attempt to get into a loose tennis shoe but should be encouraged to wear the postoperative shoe as needed for comfort.

• At 6 weeks, the patient can resume vigorous activity as tolerated.
• In the case of an arthrodesis with an implant, radiographs are obtained at the first postoperative visit and at 6 weeks. If the patient is asymptomatic at that time and radiographs do not show signs of arthrodesis, further radiographs are probably unnecessary.
• If the MTP joint has been addressed, we will strap the toe in a neutral position with cloth tape or a Budin splint for up to 12 weeks. We start this after the pin has been removed at week 3 or at the first postoperative visit if a pin has not been used.

OUTCOMES

- Large, long-term studies[4,10] on resection PIP joint arthroplasty and nonimplant arthrodesis have shown high satisfaction rates, in the range of 80% to 90%, with rare complications of infection, recurrent deformity, and problems inherent to Kirschner wire fixation.
- Studies involving the use of PIP joint arthrodesis implants have also shown equally high patient satisfaction rates. The largest study of 150 implants in 140 patients reported a 95% patient satisfaction rate, 73% fusion rate, with a 3.3% revision rate at 18-month follow-up.[7] Another PIP joint arthrodesis implant study of 38 implants reported similar findings.[6] A third study of only 28 implants reported significantly higher problems with implant failure both intraoperatively and postoperatively suggesting that use of PIP joint arthrodesis implant is technically more difficult to perform than traditional hammer toe resection arthroplasty.[9]
- Review of the current implant arthrodesis literature would suggest that strict adherence to proper technique is important and although the union rate is high, as with any fusion surgery, there is a risk of nonunion. A majority of the nonunions will be asymptomatic, but a few will go on to demonstrate implant failure, which may have symptoms sufficient to require further surgery.
- When selecting PIP joint arthroplasty or nonimplant arthrodesis versus an implant arthrodesis, the surgeon must weigh the risks and benefits of the two procedures both of which have overall good results. PIP joint arthroplasty and nonimplant arthrodesis are technically easier to perform but carry the potential for complications inherent with Kirschner wire fixation and loss of deformity correction. PIP joint implant arthrodesis such as with the Hat-Trick PIP joint implant while being more technically demanding has the advantage of more inherent stability at the fusion site but carries the disadvantage of the additional risk of implant failure as well as a significant expense for the implant itself.

COMPLICATIONS

- Neurovascular compromise
- Prolonged recovery
- Loss of volitional control
- Swelling
- Recurrence of deformity
- Toe "too straight"
- Infection
- Transfer lesion
- Nonunion
- Implant failure

REFERENCES

1. Alvine FG, Garvin KL. Peg and dowel fusion of the proximal interphalangeal joint. Foot Ankle Int 1980;1:90–94.
2. Briggs LC Jr. Proximal interphalangeal joint arthrodesis using the StayFuse implant. Tech Foot Ankle Surg 2004;3:77–84.
3. Caterini R, Farsetti P, Tarantino U, et al. Arthrodesis of the toe joints with an intramedullary cannulated screw for correction of hammertoe deformity. Foot Ankle Int 2004;25:256–261.
4. Coillard JY, Petri GJ, van Damme G, et al. Stabilization of proximal interphalangeal joint in lesser toe deformities with an angulated intramedullary implant. Foot Ankle Int 2014;35:401–407.
5. Coughlin MJ, Dorris J, Polk E. Operative repair of the fixed hammertoe deformity. Foot Ankle Int 2000;21:94–104.
6. Ellington MA, Anderson RB, Davis WH, et al. Radiographic analysis of proximal interphalangeal joint arthrodesis with an intramedullary fusion device for lesser toe deformities. Foot Ankle Int 2010;31:372–376.
7. Fazal MA, James L, Williams RL. StayFuse for proximal interphalangeal joint fusion. Foot Ankle Int 2013;34:1274–1278.
8. HAT-TRICK Lesser Toe Repair System [package insert]. Andover, MA: Smith & Nephew, Inc.; 2016.
9. Khan M, Walter RP, Loxdale P, et al. Early results of lesser toe proximal interphalangeal joint arthrodesis using an intramedullary device [abstract]. Bone Joint J 2013;95-B(suppl 9):10.
10. O'Kane C, Kilmartin T. Review of proximal interphalangeal joint excisional arthroplasty for the correction of second hammer toe deformity in 100 cases. Foot Ankle Int 2005;26:320–325.
11. Richman SH, Siqueria MB, McCullough KA, et al. Correction of hammertoe deformity with novel intramedullary PIP fusion device versus K-wire fixation. Foot Ankle Int 2017;38:174–180.
12. StayFuse Implant [package insert]. Montbonnot Saint Martin, France: Tornier, Inc.; 2011.

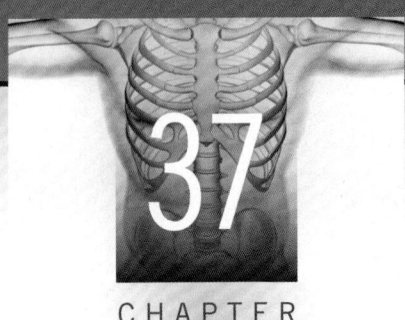

37
CHAPTER

Weil Lesser Metatarsal Shortening Osteotomy

Hans-Joerg Trnka

DEFINITION

- Subluxation or dislocation of the metatarsophalangeal (MTP) joints results in a disruption of the fibers of the plantar plate, which is the central structure of the MTP joint dislocation. The plate provides a cushion to the joint and weight-bearing forces.
- The key point in deciding how to treat this pathology is to determine whether the pathology leads to abnormal pressure distribution in the forefoot.

ANATOMY

- The proximal phalanx and the fibrocartilaginous plantar plate form an anatomic and functional unit at the MTP joint.
- The plate is the major factor of dorsoplantar stability.
- The plantar plate attaches to the proximal phalanx and the plantar fascia, but except for the two collateral ligaments, it is without substantial fibrous attachment to the metatarsal head.[18]
- The extensor digitorum longus tendon extends to the proximal phalanx and the proximal interphalangeal joint.
- Antagonists of the extensor mechanism are the flexor tendons and the plantar plate.
- The function of the interossei and lumbrical muscles is to hold the proximal phalanx in a neutral position.

PATHOGENESIS

- High functional stresses of weight bearing and repetitive hyperextension of the MTP joint can lead to attenuation or rupture of the plantar plate, followed by subluxation or dislocation of the toe.
- A hallux valgus deformity is often associated with a subluxated second MTP joint.[6,12]
- The hallux pushes the second toe laterally, which may lead to instability and maybe to subluxation.
- It may also result from an excessive length of the second or third metatarsal relative to the first metatarsal.
- The second MTP joint is then biomechanically more subject to the pressure of tight stockings or shoes.
- Once the plantar plate is elongated and ruptured, the dorsal capsule and the extensor tendon become contracted, leading to a chronically dislocated MTP joint.[18]
- The plantar plate significantly contributes to stabilize the sagittal plane of the lesser MTP joints.[3]

NATURAL HISTORY

- Weil presented in 1992 in Europe a joint-preserving, intra-articular shortening osteotomy, and Barouk[1] first published it in 1996.

- Researchers from Europe have shown in anatomic, clinical, and radiologic studies the advantages of the Weil osteotomy compared to alternative procedures.[11,18,19]
- A dorsal soft tissue release with pin fixation,[4] silicone implants,[5] metatarsal neck osteotomies without fixation (Helal osteotomy),[8,10,16,17,20] and MTP joint excisional arthroplasties[7] have been reported in the literature as surgical alternatives. However, a high rate of complications such as nonunions, malalignments, and transfer lesions are associated with these alternative surgical procedures.[17]

PATIENT HISTORY AND PHYSICAL FINDINGS

- Physical examination methods include the following:
  - Determining circulatory status is necessary to assess not only the feasibility of an individual procedure but also whether multiple procedures can be performed, if necessary.
  - Clinical examination of cutaneous sensory response may indicate a systemic disease such as diabetes.
  - The drawer test is used to evaluate the stability of all the MTP joints and the reducibility of lesser toe deformities in plantarflexion. How stable overall is the first ray?
  - Passive range of motion: Normal range of motion is 60 to 80 degrees full extension to 40 degrees full flexion; loss of flexion may be a result of the contracted extensor tendons or because the proximal phalanx lies dorsal to the second metatarsal head.
- Each patient must be analyzed individually, with attention to a detailed history and a careful clinical examination. Ruling out differential diagnosis is mandatory.
- History of painful forefeet over a long period of months or years
- The pain usually occurs dorsally over the toe and on the plantar side of the metatarsal head.
- Plantar keratosis: This callus is a circumscribed keratotic area under the metatarsal head that usually corresponds with the patient's complaints (FIG 1).
- Hammer toe: A hammer toe deformity may lead to MTP joint subluxation, dislocation, or both. However, MTP joint subluxation and dislocation can also lead to a hammer toe deformity.
- A simultaneous hallux valgus deformity may lead to dorsiflexion forces in the second MTP joint. The great toe may cross under the second toe ("crossover toe deformity").
- A prominent dorsal base of the proximal phalanx is easily palpated.

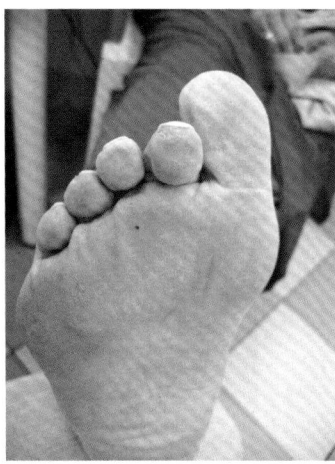

FIG 1 Plantar aspect of the foot with a hyperkeratotic area under the second metatarsal head.

- Tightness of extensor tendons: The toe cannot be plantar-flexed due to pain and to shortening of the extensor muscle and interosseous dorsalis muscle.
- Rarely, a third or fourth toe is subluxated.

IMAGING AND OTHER DIAGNOSTIC STUDIES

- Dorsoplantar and lateral weight-bearing radiographs should be obtained to rule out fractures or associated injuries and degenerative arthritic changes.
- All radiographs are examined for the length of the second and third toe relative to the first and the alignment (Maestro line).
- Radiographs must be obtained for subluxation or dislocation to assess joint congruency of the lesser MTP joints (**FIG 2**).
- A "gun barrel" sign may be seen on the anteroposterior radiograph. The diaphysis of the proximal phalanx projects as a round hole in the area of the distal condyle of the proximal phalanx.
- The articular cartilage of the adjoining surfaces leaves a "clear space" of 2 to 3 mm. This clear space diminishes with progression of the hyperextension of the MTP joint.
- Avascular necrosis of a lesser metatarsal head with infraction (Freiberg infraction) may be seen.
- The hallux valgus angle and the intermetatarsal angle are measured.

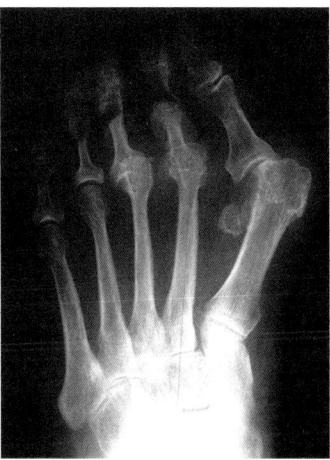

FIG 2 Severe subluxated second and third MTP joint with an associated hallux valgus deformity.

- Pedobarography is highly sensitive to peak pressures in the foot. It allows static and dynamic qualitative measurement of pedal pressures and load distribution for specific areas of the foot. Load imbalance may also be detected as well as insufficiency of the first ray.

DIFFERENTIAL DIAGNOSIS

- Morton neuroma
- Freiberg infraction (avascular necrosis of the metatarsal head)
- Rheumatoid arthritis
- Nonspecific synovitis
- Metatarsal head fracture

NONOPERATIVE MANAGEMENT

- Initial treatment options for metatarsalgia include shoe wear modifications, metatarsal pads, and custom-made orthoses.
- Trimming of the callus mechanically
- Orthotics for the foot
  - Reduce forefoot pressure.
  - Lower heel to reduce metatarsal head pressure (avoid high-heeled shoes).
  - Carefully placed metatarsal pad proximal to painful metatarsal head.
- If metatarsalgia is due to a ruptured volar plate (such as in rheumatoid arthritis), often a stiff, full-length insole that limits MTP hyperextension of the foot is useful.
- However, conservative treatment in an already existing dislocation is of no benefit, and surgical intervention is indicated.[14]

SURGICAL MANAGEMENT

- The Weil osteotomy is a joint-preserving, intra-articular shortening osteotomy and has been recommended for the treatment of metatarsalgia resulting from a dislocated or subluxated MTP joint.
- The goal of the Weil osteotomy is first to alter load transmission through the forefoot by shifting the plantar fragment proximal to the area of the lesion, where thicker and more compliant soft tissue is still present, and second to resolve the hammer toe deformity or MTP subluxations that are increasing or resulting in metatarsalgia.
- The flexor to extensor tendon transfer significantly stabilized the disrupted lesser MTP joints in both superior subluxation and in dorsiflexion. The flexor to extensor tendon transfer following a Weil osteotomy also significantly stabilized the disrupted lesser MTP joints in both superior subluxation and in dorsiflexion.[3] Surgeons using the Weil osteotomy for plantar plate deficient MTP joints may consider adding a flexor tendon transfer to the procedure despite that this technique is challenging. Nevertheless, more comparative clinical data is needed to support this additional technique.
- The direct plantar plate repair combined with a Weil osteotomy and lateral soft tissue reefing can restore the normal alignment of the MTP joint.[15] Fleischer et al[8] {Fleischer, 2020 392 /id} performed a comparative study of Weil osteotomies combined with direct plantar plate repair versus Weil osteotomies alone. There were no differences in alignment or complications rates, but the combined group demonstrated significant improvements preoperatively to postoperatively in four of the five Foot and Ankle Outcome Score (FAOS) subscales and had higher Quality of Life and Pain subscale scores at 1 year compared with those in the Weil osteotomy alone group.

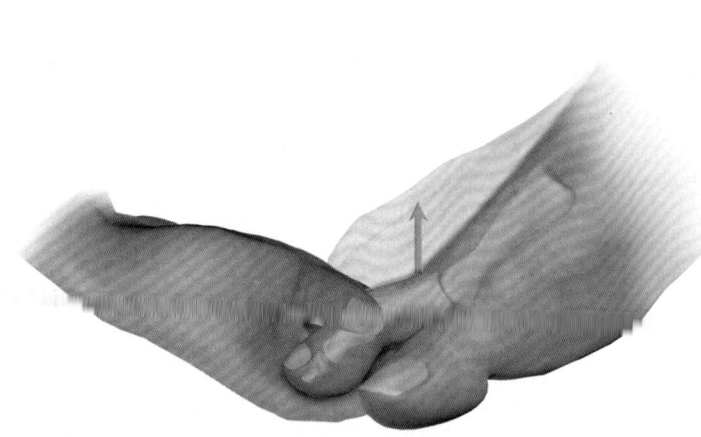
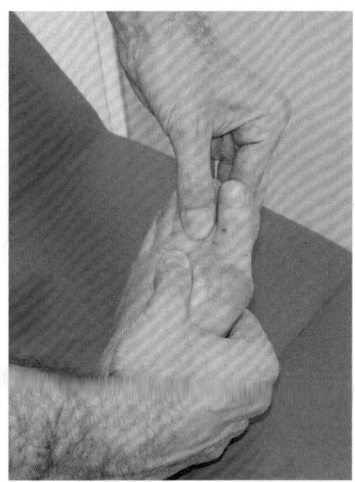

A   **B**

FIG 3 A,B. The surgeon grasps the base of the proximal phalanx and attempts to subluxate or dislocate the joint with a dorsally directed force.

Preoperative Planning

- All radiographic images are reviewed for subluxation or dislocation, alignment of the metatarsal heads, hallux valgus deformity, degenerative changes of the joints, and claw toes.
- If there is a hallux valgus deformity or a hypermobile first tarsometatarsal joint, this pathology should be corrected to achieve a satisfying result.
- The length of shortening is measured on the plain radiographs. The second metatarsal should be even with or shorter than the first, and the third should be shorter than the second metatarsal.
- During the preoperative physical examination, the surgeon must look for plantar keratotic disorders.
- The tightness of the extensor tendon is palpated.
- A drawer test of the dislocated MTP joint should be included in the examination under anesthesia (**FIG 3**).

Positioning

- The patient is positioned supine on the operating table.
- The surgery is performed either under general anesthesia or using a regional ankle block supplemented with intravenous or oral sedation.
- An Esmarch tourniquet may be used to obtain a bloodless field.

Approach

- A 3-cm longitudinal incision is made dorsal over the metatarsal for a single osteotomy, over the web space for a double osteotomy, and over two metatarsals for a triple osteotomy.
- A small amount of soft tissue dissection is done to identify the extensor tendons, which are lengthened in a Z fashion.
- A transverse or longitudinal capsulotomy of the MTP joint is used to identify the junction of the head and neck.

EXPOSURE OF METATARSAL

- Make a 3-cm longitudinal incision dorsal over the metatarsal for a single osteotomy (**TECH FIG 1A,B**) or over the web space for a double osteotomy.

- Perform a small amount of soft tissue dissection to identify the extensor tendons and lengthen them in a Z fashion (**TECH FIG 1C–E**).

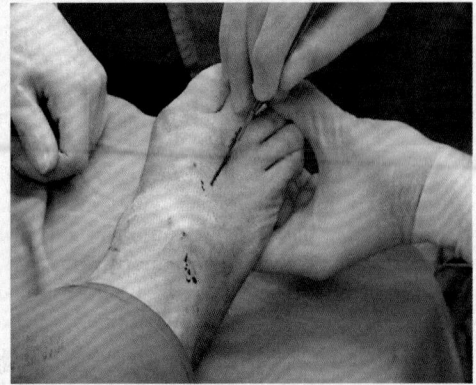
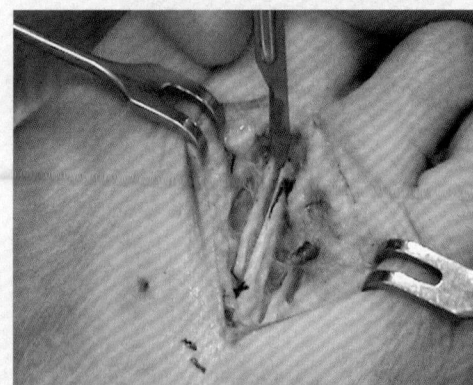

A   **B**

TECH FIG 1 A,B. Dorsal skin incision. *(continued)*

TECHNIQUES

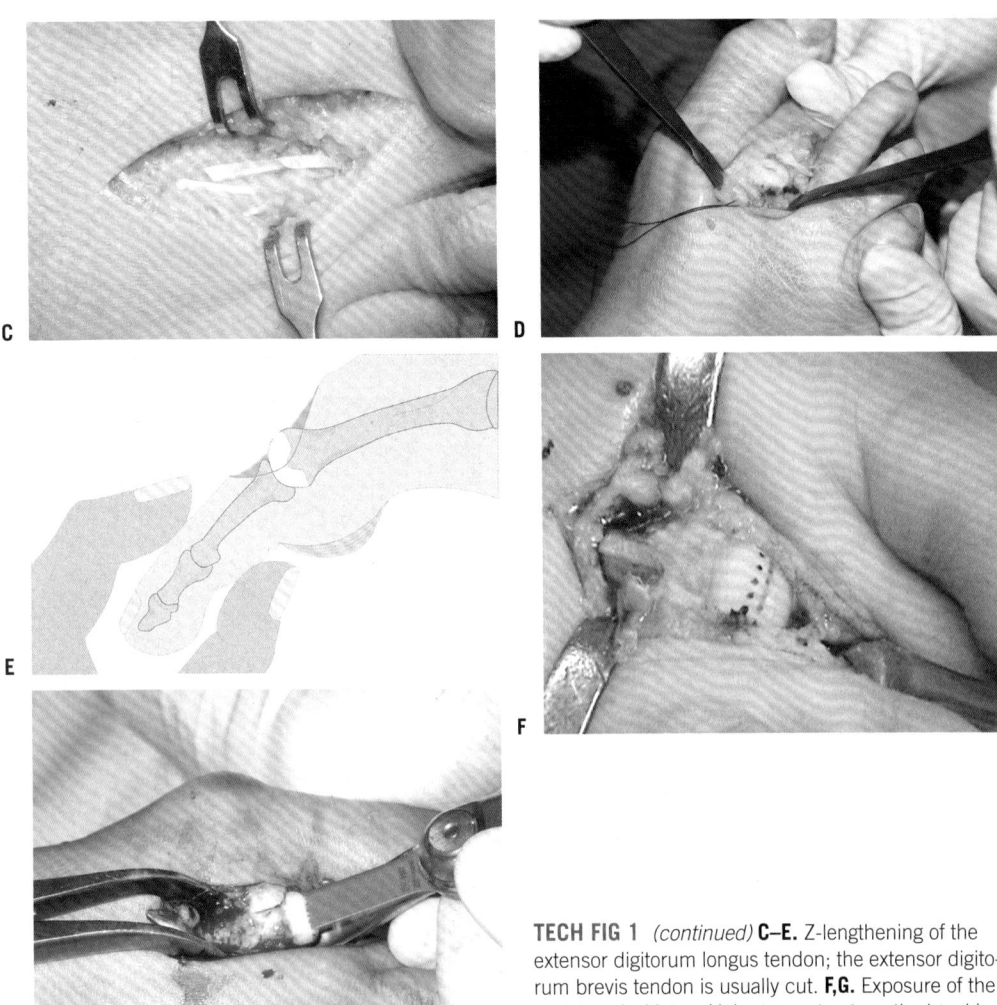

TECH FIG 1 *(continued)* **C–E.** Z-lengthening of the extensor digitorum longus tendon; the extensor digitorum brevis tendon is usually cut. **F,G.** Exposure of the metatarsal with two Hohmann retractors; the head is exposed using an elevator.

- Incise the joint capsule in a transverse fashion and release the collateral ligaments if necessary.
- Expose the metatarsal head with two small Hohmann retractors. Maximally plantarflex the toe and expose the metatarsal head with the help of an elevator (**TECH FIG 1F,G**).

- Take care not to strip the plantar soft tissue attachments to aid in stabilizing the osteotomy and maintain vascularity to the head.

OSTEOTOMY AND BONY SLICE EXTRACTION

- Use a 2-mm bony slice extractor to lift the plantar fragment because the axis of motion of the MTP joint has changed with plantarflexion of the metatarsal head.
- Expose the metatarsal head and mark the osteotomies (**TECH FIG 2A**).

- Use an oscillating saw to perform the osteotomy at the dorsal portion of the metatarsal head without finishing the second cortex totally to avoid a free-gliding plantar fragment (**TECH FIG 2B**).
- The second osteotomy through both cortices is 2 mm under the dorsal cut (**TECH FIG 2C,D**).
- The bony slice can now be easily removed (**TECH FIG 2E,F**).

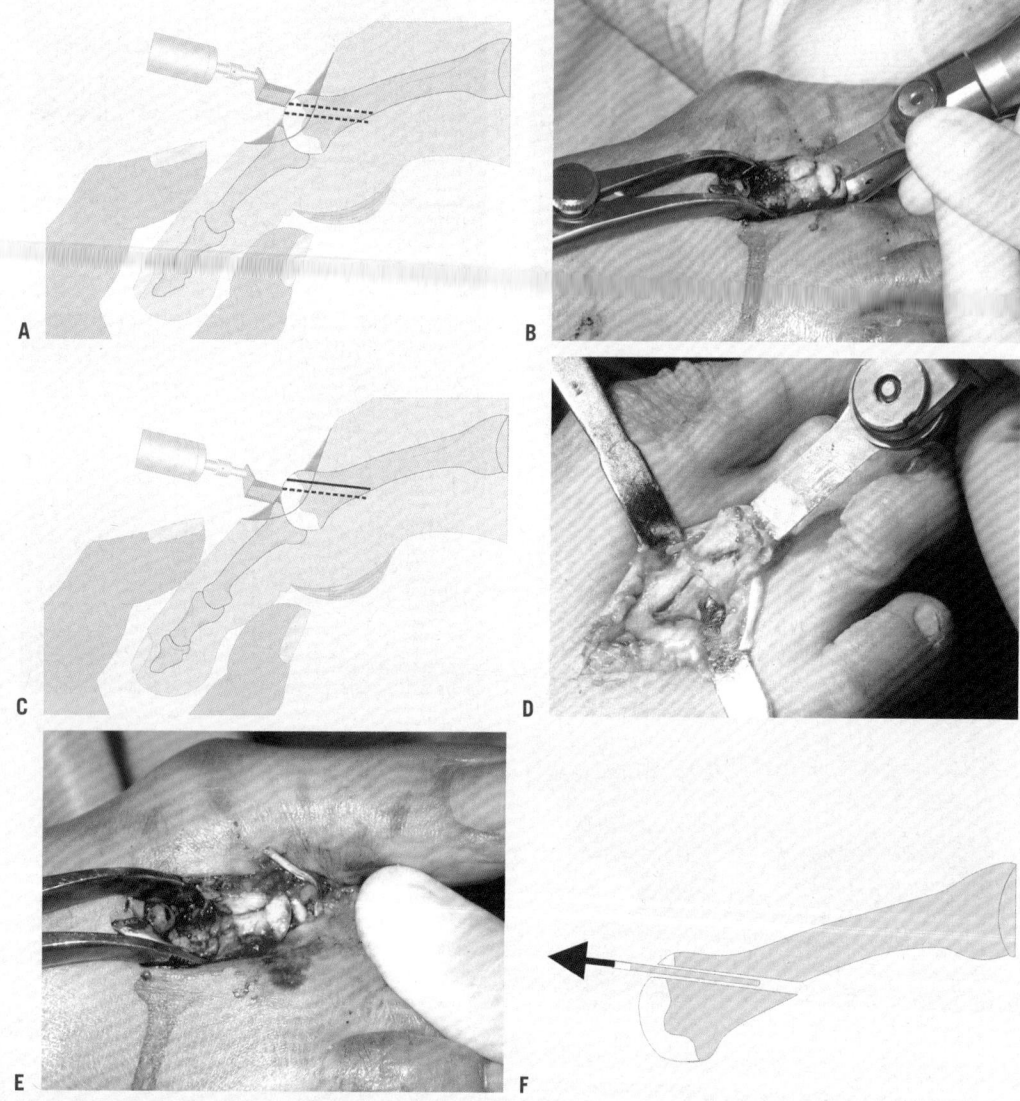

TECH FIG 2 A. Exposure of the metatarsal head and marking of the two osteotomy levels. **B.** Osteotomy at the dorsal aspect of the metatarsal head. **C,D.** Plantar osteotomy of the metatarsal head. **E,F.** Removal of the bony slice after the osteotomies.

FIXATION OF THE MOBILE FRAGMENT

- Grasp the plantar mobile fragment with a pointed reduction clamp and shift it proximally to achieve the requisite amount of shortening that was measured preoperatively on the dorsoplantar radiographs **(TECH FIG 3A)**.
- The second metatarsal should be even with or shorter than the first, and the third should be shorter than the second metatarsal.
- The plane of the osteotomy should be as parallel to the ground surface as possible. Secure the osteotomy with a special 2-mm

titanium "snap-off screw" (Wright Medical Technology, Inc., Arlington, TN) **(TECH FIG 3B)**. Use a 12-mm length for the second metatarsal and 11 mm for the other metatarsals.

- Remove the resulting dorsal protuberance over the metatarsal head remnant with a rongeur or the edge of the saw blade **(TECH FIG 3C,D)**.
- Repair the overlying Z-lengthened extensor tendon and suture the skin.

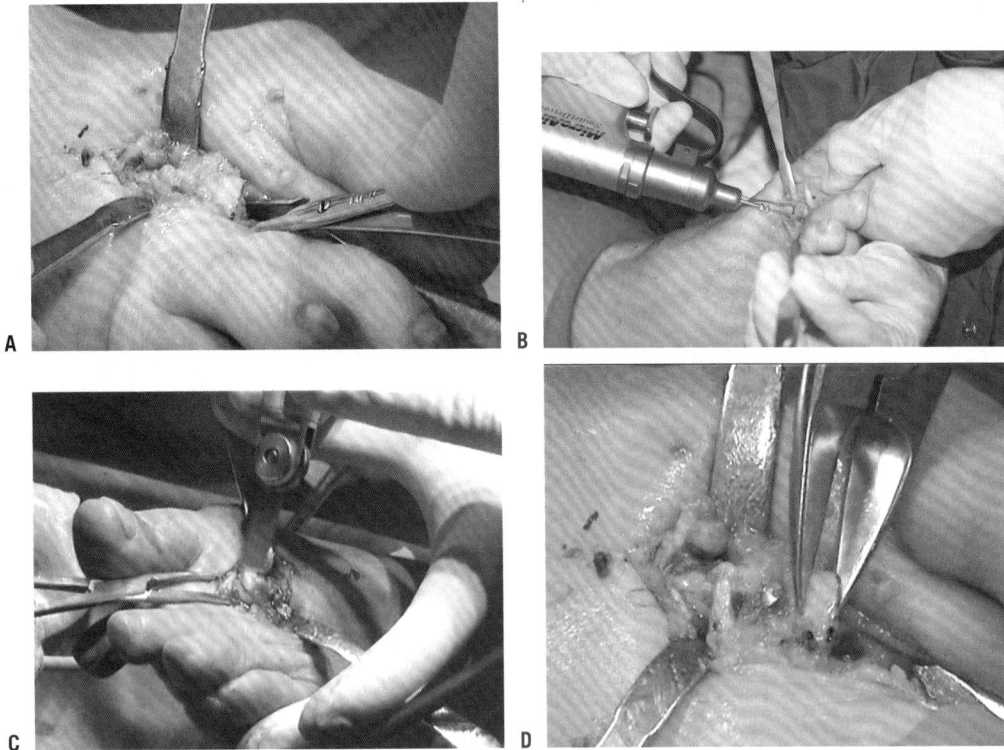

TECH FIG 3 A. Positioning of the plantar fragment. **B.** Fixation of the Weil osteotomy with a snap-off screw (Wright Medical Technology, Inc., Arlington, TN). **C,D.** Modeling of the dorsal protuberance with a rongeur or the edge of the saw blade.

MACEIRA MODIFICATION OF THE WEIL METATARSAL OSTEOTOMY (COURTESY OF MARK E. EASLEY, MD)

- The traditional Weil osteotomy often leaves a prominent rim of cortex immediately dorsal to the metatarsal head cartilage.
  - Even when the residual dorsal overhang of the traditional Weil metatarsal shortening osteotomy is resected, this rim of cartilage is present.
  - To eliminate this rim of cortex and create a more natural transition between the cartilage and dorsal metatarsal cortex, the Maceira modification may be considered.
- A dorsal skin incision is used and a capsulotomy performed, as for the Weil osteotomy.

Osteotomy

- Initial transverse osteotomy cut is made with the microsagittal saw blade similar to that for the Weil osteotomy **(TECH FIG 4A)**.
  - This initial cut is not completed so that control over the osteotomy is maintained.
- A vertical cut is made, removing the amount of dorsal cartilage and bone that would traditionally overhang in the Weil osteotomy once the metatarsal head is translated proximally **(TECH FIG 4B)**.
  - This leaves the rim of bone that would normally be seen in the traditional Weil osteotomy after the overhanging distal cortex is removed **(TECH FIG 4C)**.
- Immediately plantar to this rim of cortex, a second transverse osteotomy is created to converge with the initial transverse

osteotomy and completing the separation between the metatarsal head and shaft fragments **(TECH FIG 4D)**.
  - With this second cut, a wedge of bone is removed not only from the remaining distal cortex but also from the distal to proximal aspect of the osteotomy, thereby elevating the metatarsal head slightly **(TECH FIG 4E–G)**.
- The metatarsal head is then shifted proximally and aligned with the distal end of the metatarsal.

Fixation

- A screw dedicated for securing metatarsal shortening osteotomies may be used, as was used in this case.
  - Directing the screw slightly medially or laterally allows for a longitudinal Kirschner wire (K-wire) to be passed across the MTP joint, if necessary **(TECH FIG 5A,B)**.
  - If no K-wire is needed, the screw *can* be directed more vertically.
- If preoperatively medial or lateral deviation of the toe is being corrected, the metatarsal head may be shifted relative to the metatarsal shaft, as would be done for hallux valgus correction.
  - In this example case, the second toe deviated medially, so the metatarsal head was shifted slightly medially to promote more neutral second toe alignment **(TECH FIG 5B,C)**.

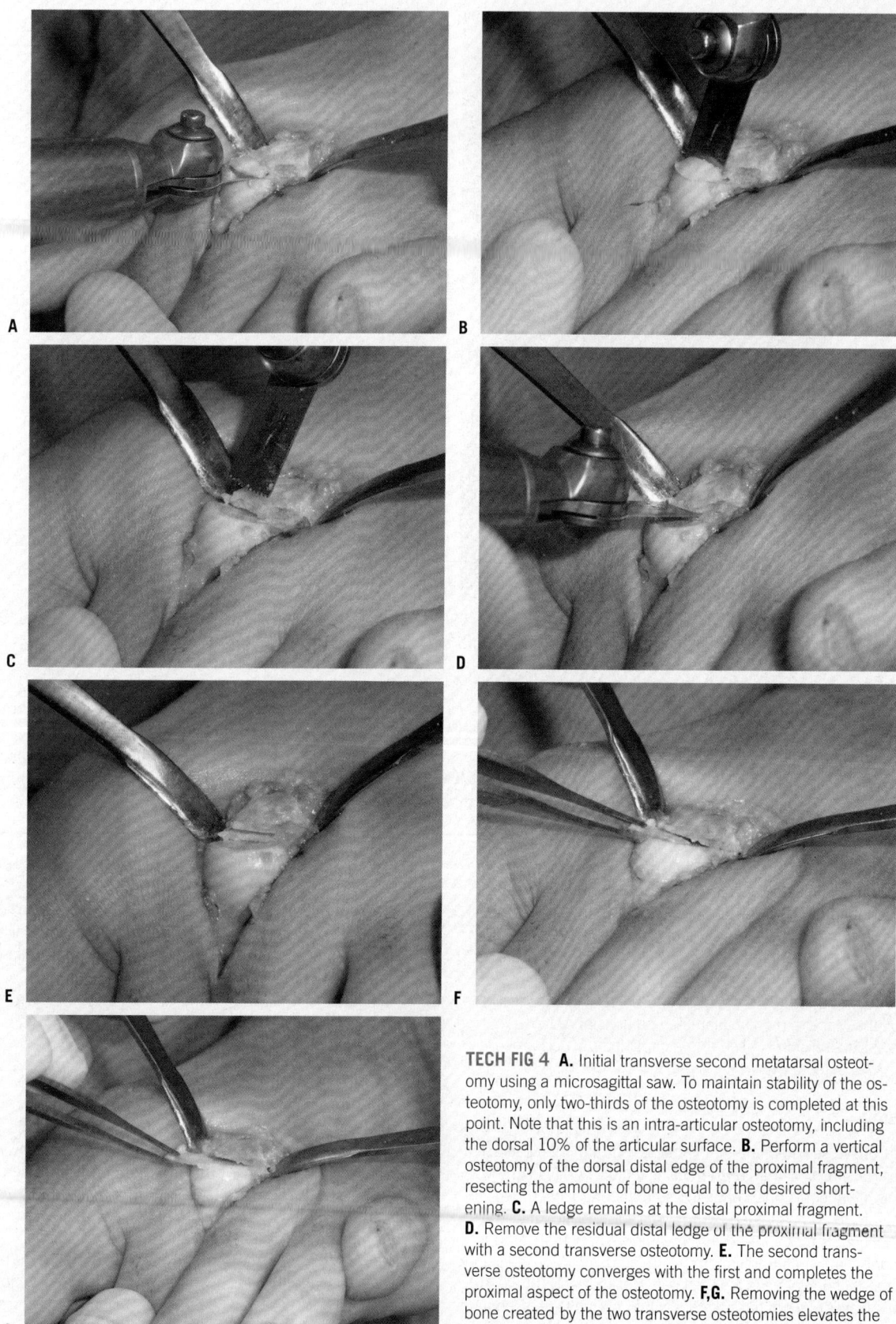

TECH FIG 4 A. Initial transverse second metatarsal osteotomy using a microsagittal saw. To maintain stability of the osteotomy, only two-thirds of the osteotomy is completed at this point. Note that this is an intra-articular osteotomy, including the dorsal 10% of the articular surface. **B.** Perform a vertical osteotomy of the dorsal distal edge of the proximal fragment, resecting the amount of bone equal to the desired shortening. **C.** A ledge remains at the distal proximal fragment. **D.** Remove the residual distal ledge of the proximal fragment with a second transverse osteotomy. **E.** The second transverse osteotomy converges with the first and completes the proximal aspect of the osteotomy. **F,G.** Removing the wedge of bone created by the two transverse osteotomies elevates the metatarsal head.

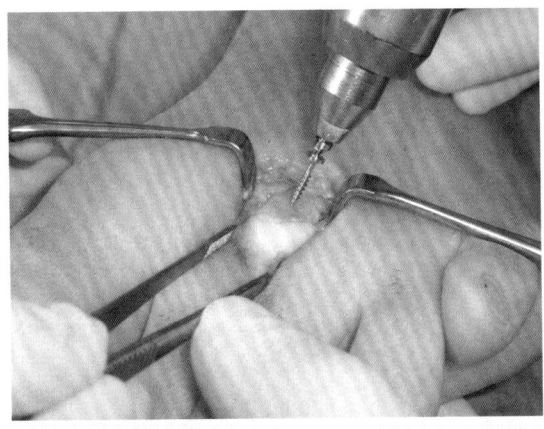

A

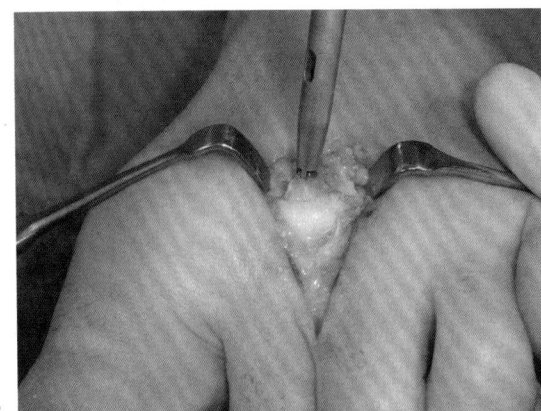

B

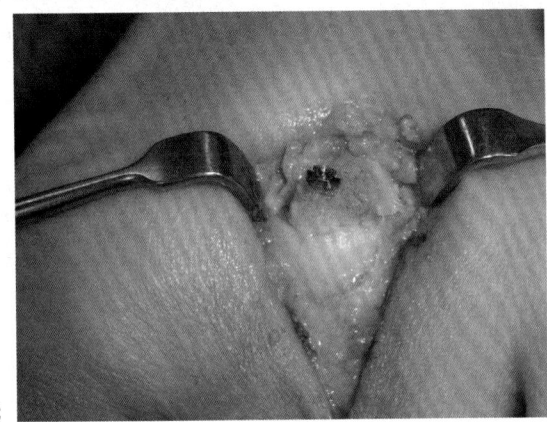

C

TECH FIG 5 A. With the metatarsal head translated prox-imally to shorten the metatarsal, a congruent transition is created between the dorsal aspects of the two fragments for fixation. **B.** The screw is directed slightly medially and secured. By directing the screw away from vertical leaves the option to safely pass a longitudinal pin across the MTP joint into the metatarsal without interference from the screw. **C.** Given preoperative medial deviation of the second toe, the metatarsal head was translated medially to promote a more neutral second toe alignment.

TECHNIQUES

Pearls and Pitfalls

Collateral Ligaments	• We do not routinely release the collateral ligaments when performing a Weil osteotomy. A substantial portion of the metatarsal head blood supply courses via delicate arteries in the collateral ligaments.
Orientation of the Saw Blade	• We dorsiflex the ankle and use the plantar heel as a guide to orient the saw blade in the sagittal plane and look at the whole forefoot to get the orientation in the transverse plane.
Wedge Resection	• We excise a wedge within the osteotomy in lieu of creating a single cut. Elevation is not important regarding loading of the head, but elevating the head will maintain a favorable center of rotation for the head. In theory, this will keep the intrinsic flexor tendons plantar to the center of rotation, thereby reducing the risk for postoperative toe elevation ("floating toe").

POSTOPERATIVE CARE

- Dressings and a tight bandage are used to protect the suture and to prevent swelling.
- The patient's toes are taped in slight plantarflexion.
- Weight bearing with a postoperative shoe is allowed after the first postoperative day (FIG 4A).
- Patients should wear the postoperative shoe for 6 weeks.
- Postoperative imaging includes dorsoplantar and lateral radiographs (FIG 4B–D).
- Passive motion (starting on the fifth postoperative day) of the MTP joint is indicated and necessary to prevent postoperative extension contracture.

- If swelling occurs, foot elevation, cryotherapy, and elastic stockings may keep the swelling down.

OUTCOMES

- Clinical results of the Weil osteotomy have been promising. Outcomes include a significant reduction of pain, a significant reduction in plantar callus formation, a low dislocation rate, and increased ambulatory capacity.
- No malunion or pseudarthrosis was documented in the literature.
- Bony and soft tissue modifications such as lengthening of the extensor tendon, 2-mm bony slice extraction, and

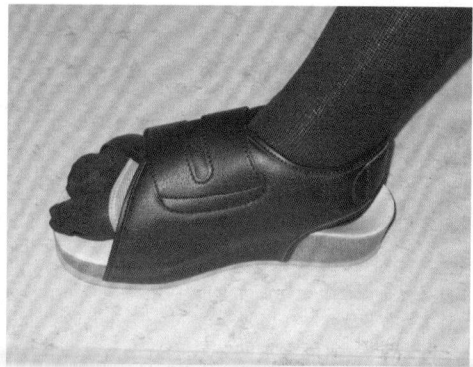

FIG 4 A. Postoperative shoe. **B.** Preoperative radiographs with hallux valgus deformity and subluxation of second and third MTP joint. **C.** Chevron osteotomy with pin fixation along with a Weil osteotomy on the second to fourth rays. **D.** Seven-year radiograph showing maintenance of corrected lesser MTP joints.

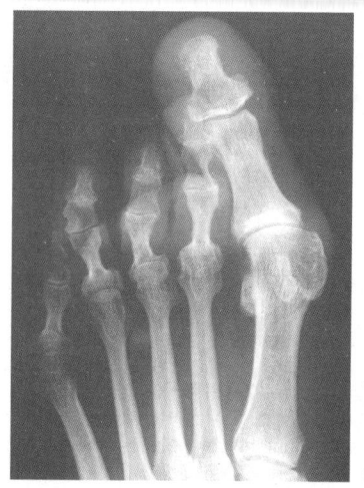
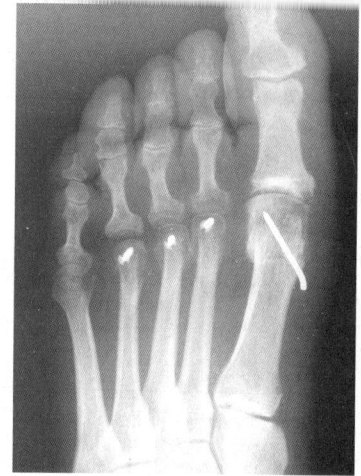
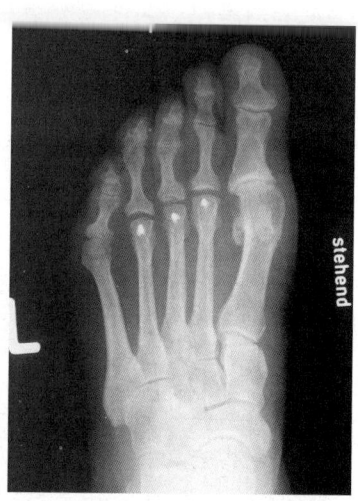

insertion of a K-wire from the tip of the toe across the MTP joint and the osteotomy into the metatarsal, in a position of 5 degrees plantarflexion (in severely subluxated contracted cases), may prevent postoperative dorsiflexion contracture.

- Boyer and DeOrio[2] described good results of a single-pin fixation for a combined metatarsal neck osteotomy with proximal interphalangeal joint resection arthroplasty and flexor digitorum longus transfer in severely dislocated MTP joints and severe hammer toe deformities.

- Fleischer et al[8] investigated whether a Weil osteotomy alone or a combination of Weil osteotomy with direct plantar plate repair was superior. The combined technique had superior Quality of Life and Pain subscale scores at 1-year follow-up.

COMPLICATIONS

- Reported complications in the literature are floating or stiff toes, a high rate of postoperative dorsiflexed contracture and transfer metatarsalgia in cases of excessive shortening with variable rates, and a limitation of the range of motion in the MTP joint.[9,11]

- The transfer of the flexor digitorum brevis tendon to the proximal interphalangeal joint might restore the windlass mechanism and decrease the incidence of floating toes. This was shown in a cadaveric study.[13] Clinical results in the future may support this interesting finding.

- The combined Weil osteotomy with direct plantar plate repair bears the risk of a stiff MTP joint.

REFERENCES

1. Barouk LS. Weil's metatarsal osteotomy in the treatment of metatarsalgia [in German]. Orthopade 1996;25:338–344.
2. Boyer ML, DeOrio JK. Metatarsal neck osteotomy with proximal interphalangeal joint resection fixed with a single temporary pin. Foot Ankle Int 2004;25:144–148.
3. Chalayon O, Chertman C, Guss AD, et al. Role of plantar plate and surgical reconstruction techniques on static stability of lesser metatarsophalangeal joints: a biomechanical study. Foot Ankle Int 2013;34(10):1436–1442.
4. Coughlin MJ. Subluxation and dislocation of the second metatarsophalangeal joint. Orthop Clin North Am 1989;20:535–551.
5. Cracchiolo A III, Kitaoka HB, Leventen EO. Silicone implant arthroplasty for second metatarsophalangeal joint disorders with and without hallux valgus deformities. Foot Ankle 1988;9:10–18.
6. Davies MS, Saxby TS. Metatarsal neck osteotomy with rigid internal fixation for the treatment of lesser toe metatarsophalangeal joint pathology. Foot Ankle Int 1999;20:630–635.
7. DuVries HL. Dislocation of the toe. JAMA 1956;160:728.
8. Fleischer AE, Klein EE, Bowen M, et al. Comparison of combination Weil metatarsal osteotomy and direct plantar plate repair versus Weil metatarsal osteotomy alone for forefoot metatarsalgia. J Foot Ankle Surg 2020;59(2):303–306.
9. Hart R, Janecek M, Bucek P. The Weil osteotomy in metatarsalgia [in German]. Z Orthop Ihre Grenzgeb 2003;141:590–594.
10. Helal B, Greiss M. Telescoping osteotomy for pressure metatarsalgia. J Bone Joint Surg Br 1984;66:213–217.
11. Hofstaetter SG, Hofstaetter JG, Petroutsas JA, et al. The Weil osteotomy: a seven-year follow-up. J Bone Joint Surg Br 2005;87(11):1507–1511.
12. Kitaoka HB, Patzer GL. Chevron osteotomy of lesser metatarsals for intractable plantar callosities. J Bone Joint Surg Br 1998;80:516–518.
13. Lee LC, Charlton TP, Thordarson DB. Flexor digitorum brevis transfer for floating toe prevention after Weil osteotomy: a cadaveric study. Foot Ankle Int 2013;34(12):1724–1728.

14. Mann RA. Metatarsalgia: common causes and conservative treatment. Postgrad Med 1984;75:150–163.

15. Nery C, Coughlin MJ, Baumfeld D, et al. Lesser metatarsophalangeal joint instability: prospective evaluation and repair of plantar plate and capsular insufficiency. Foot Ankle Int 2012;33(4):301–311.

16. Trnka HJ, Kabon B, Zettl R, et al. Helal metatarsal osteotomy for the treatment of metatarsalgia: a critical analysis of results. Orthopedics 1996;19:457–461.

17. Trnka HJ, Mühlbauer M, Zettl R, et al. Comparison of the results of the Weil and Helal osteotomies for the treatment of metatarsalgia secondary to dislocation of the lesser metatarsophalangeal joints. Foot Ankle Int 1999;20:72–79.

18. Trnka HJ, Nyska M, Parks BG, et al. Dorsiflexion contracture after the Weil osteotomy: results of cadaver study and three-dimensional analysis. Foot Ankle Int 2001;22:47–50.

19. Vandeputte G, Dereymaeker G, Steenwerckx A, et al. The Weil osteotomy of the lesser metatarsals: a clinical and pedobarographic follow-up study. Foot Ankle Int 2000;21:370–374.

20. Winson IG, Rawlinson J, Broughton NS. Treatment of metatarsalgia by sliding distal metatarsal osteotomy. Foot Ankle 1988;9:2–6.

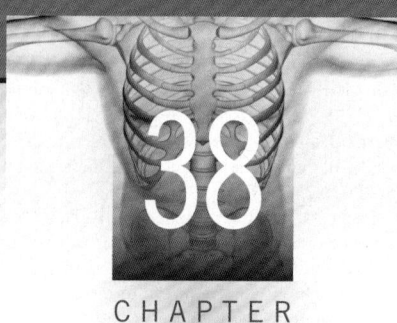

Second Metatarsal Shortening Osteotomy

John G. Anderson, Donald R. Bohay, and Omar Yaldo

CHAPTER 38

SURGICAL MANAGEMENT

- The main indication for a metatarsal shortening osteotomy is to relieve metatarsalgia (forefoot pain) caused by increased loading of the lesser metatarsal heads due to elongated metatarsals or altered biomechanics of the foot due to first ray insufficiency or shortened first ray.
- Surgical management should be withheld until trials of conservative treatments and nonoperative management have failed.
- Ankle equinus contracture should be considered as a contributing factor to the patient's metatarsalgia if gastrocnemius contracture or gastrocnemius-soleus complex contracture is present.
  - The authors believe that ankle equinus contracture, if present, must be addressed in conjunction with metatarsal shortening osteotomies to alleviate the patient's symptoms.
- This procedure is commonly paired with hallux valgus correction procedures as well as other pes planovalgus reconstructive procedures.
- There are multiple types of osteotomies with acceptable results; however, this chapter focuses on two types of osteotomies that are the authors' preferred techniques.[2]

Preoperative Planning

- Weight-bearing anteroposterior (AP) and lateral radiographs of the foot are evaluated to aid in the evaluation of metatarsalgia; metatarsal length comparison; plantar metatarsal head hypertrophy; and to evaluate for hallux valgus, pes planovalgus, and other contributing factors.
- Measurements can be made from the AP radiographs to determine the length of osteotomy needed; the second metatarsal length is typically 1 to 3 mm longer than the first metatarsal in patients with normal anatomy.
  - Alternatively, a line drawn from the first metatarsal head to the third metatarsal head can be drawn, and the second metatarsal head should be 1 to 3 mm distal to this line (FIG 1).

Positioning

- This procedure is typically accompanied by other procedures, and care should be taken to position the patient in a manner that allows for all concomitant procedures to be performed.

- The patient is positioned supine on a diving board table with a bump under the ipsilateral hip.
- A nonsterile tourniquet is applied to the ipsilateral thigh.
- Prophylactic antibiotics are given.
- Regional blocks can be administered for postoperative pain control if desired by the operating surgeon.

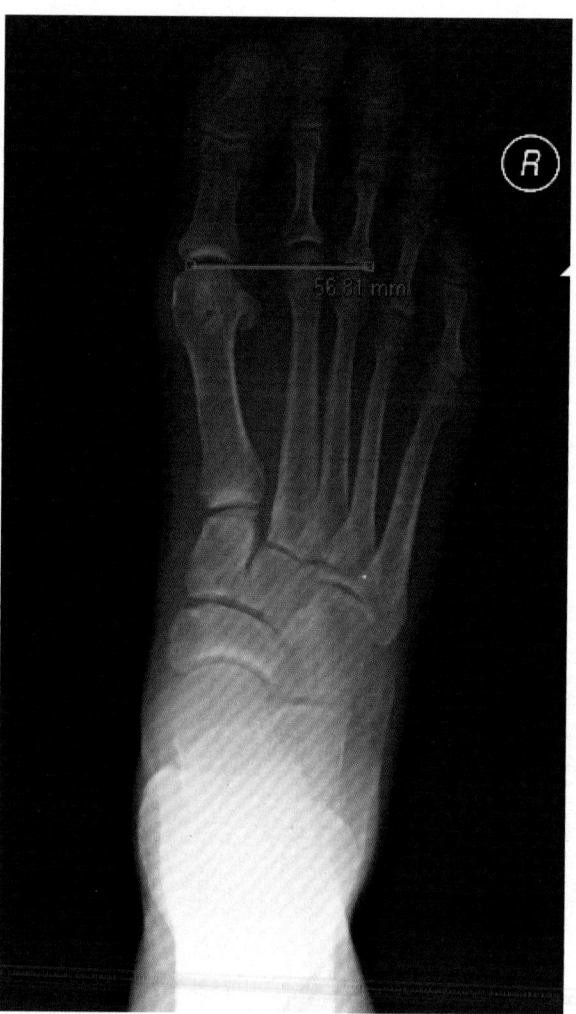

FIG 1 Weight-bearing AP radiograph of the right foot with line drawn from the first metatarsal head to the third metatarsal head demonstrates normal second metatarsal length.

TRANSVERSE DIAPHYSEAL METATARSAL SHORTENING OSTEOTOMY

Exposure

- The exposure in isolation is a 2- to 3-cm dorsal incision over the metatarsal shaft. However, this procedure is often undergone in conjunction with hallux valgus correction surgery, and the incision should be planned for in accordance with other concomitant procedures. For example, the incision for a Lapidus procedure can be made slightly lateral and extended distally to account for a second metatarsal shortening osteotomy.
- The dissection is carried bluntly down to the extensor tendons, which are then retracted away from the metatarsal. This is followed by sharp dissection down to periosteum. The dorsal neurovascular bundle lies just medial to the plane of dissection, and the neurovascular bundle should be protected during the dissection and osteotomy of the second metatarsal. Care should be taken to retract and protect the small sensory branches of the superficial peroneal nerve in the dorsal foot.
- A soft tissue elevator is used to dissect the periosteum from the dorsal metatarsal. This is done to create an area large enough to fit the one-quarter tubular plate.
- The desired resection segment may be marked on the diaphysis with either marking pen or by scoring with an oscillating saw.

Plate Preparation

- A one-quarter tubular plate with four holes is prebent with a slight convexity to help compress the plantar cortex of the osteotomy site. This plate is then placed centrally over the metatarsal and held in place with a mosquito hemostat.
- The most distal screw hole is drilled, and a 2.7-mm screw of appropriate length is placed.
- The second most distal screw hole is also drilled, and an appropriately length screw is placed and then immediately removed (**TECH FIG 1A**).

- The most distal screw at this point can be loosened and the plate rotated away from the metatarsal (**TECH FIG 1B**).

Osteotomy

- After preparation of the metatarsal with the two distal holes drilled, a microsagittal saw is used to remove the desired length of bone.
  - Care should be taken to account for the 1-mm width of the saw blade.
- The distal cut of the osteotomy is performed first as the distal metatarsal will become free floating after the first cut of the osteotomy.
- The first cut is placed just proximal to the most proximal screw hole.
  - Care is taken to make sure the osteotomy cuts are perpendicular to the long axis of the metatarsal shaft.
- The proximal osteotomy cut is then made 2 to 7 mm proximal to the initial cut depending on the desired length of shortening (**TECH FIG 2A**).
- The osteotomized segment of bone is removed (**TECH FIG 2B**).

Plate Placement

- The plate is then rotated back into place, and the distal screws are screwed back down into the plate and bone. The plate is used to help acquire reduction of the osteotomy fragments, often with the aid of a hemostat to hold the plate down to the proximal fragment (**TECH FIG 3A**).
  - Care is taken to ensure compression is applied across the osteotomy site.
- The next screw hole, which is immediately proximal to the osteotomy, is drilled eccentrically to add compression across the osteotomy site (**TECH FIG 3B**).
- The final most proximal screw hole is then drilled and placed with an appropriate length screw (**TECH FIG 3C**).

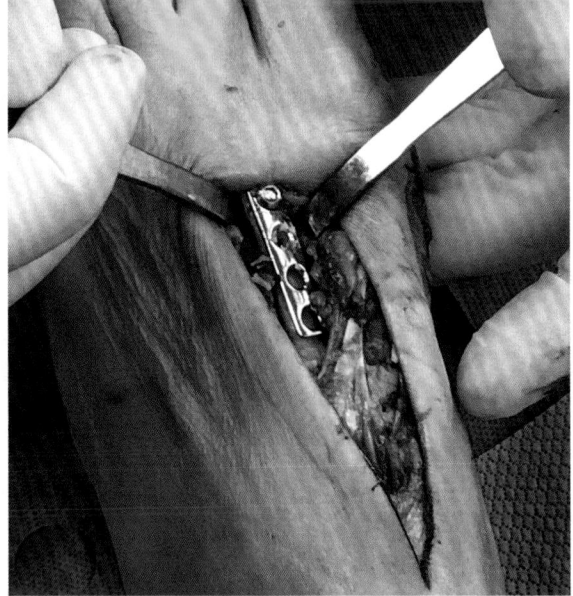
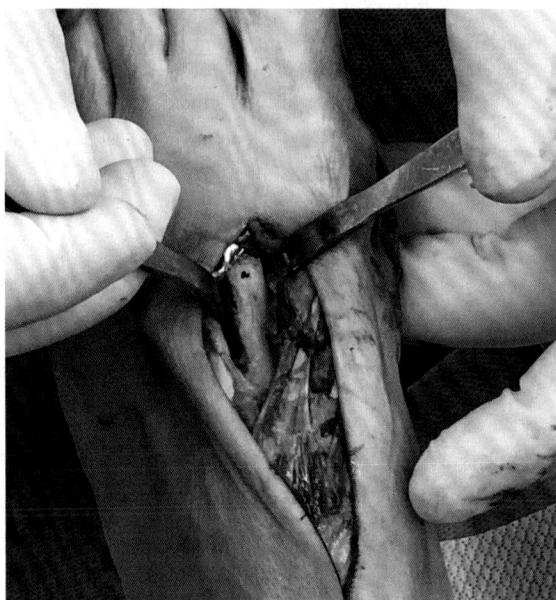

A　　　　　　　　　　　　　　　　　　　　　**B**

TECH FIG 1 A. The plate is placed onto the metatarsal, the most distal screw is placed, and the next screw is then placed and removed. **B.** The most distal screw is loosened to allow for plate rotation for visualization of the osteotomy site.

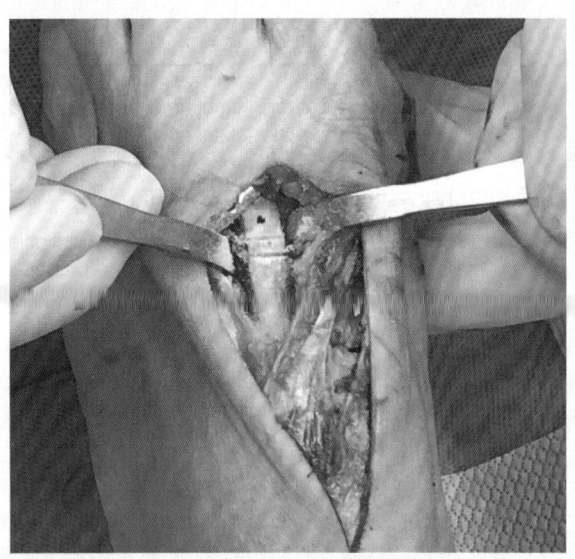
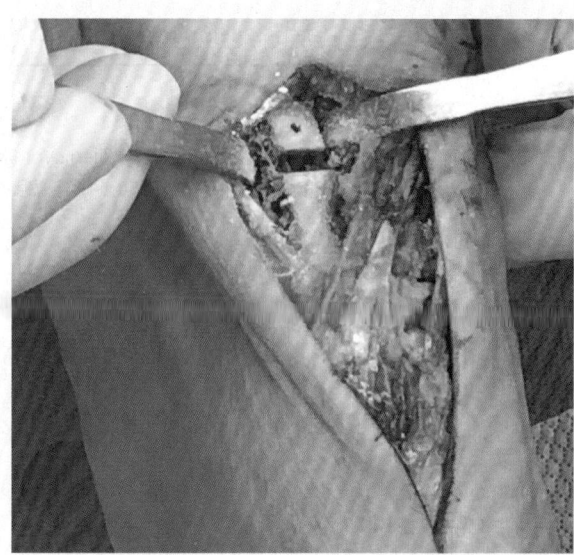

TECH FIG 2 **A.** First distal and then proximal osteotomy cuts are made. **B.** The osteotomized segment of bone is then removed.

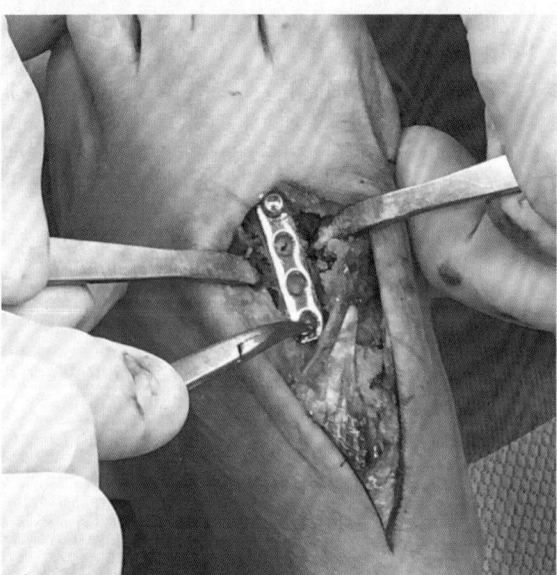
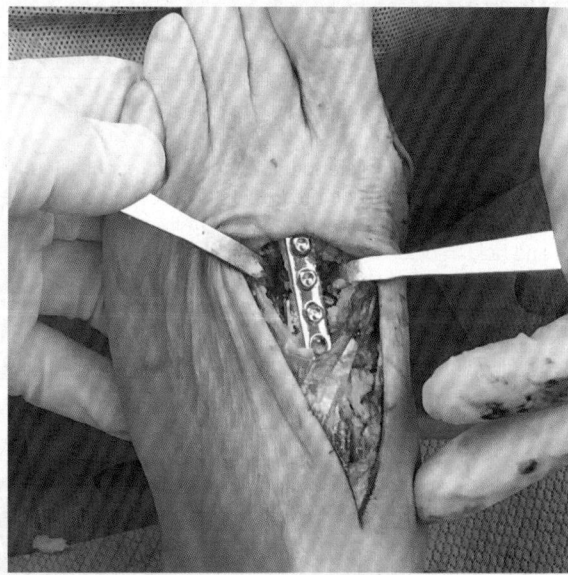

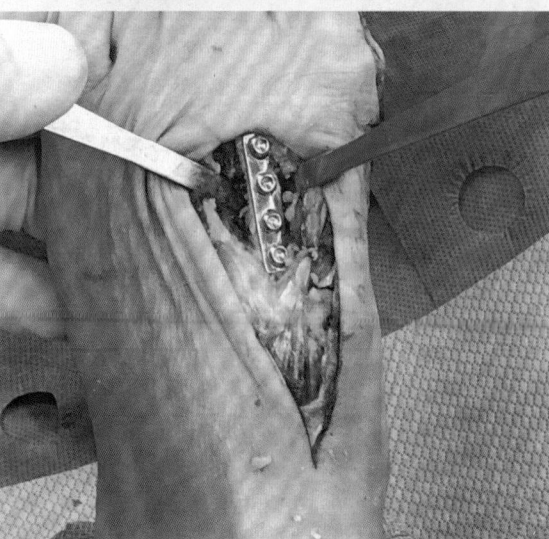

TECH FIG 3 **A.** The plate is rotated back onto the metatarsal, and compression is applied over the proximal portion of the plate with a hemostat. **B.** The next hole is drilled eccentrically to add compression across the osteotomy site. **C.** The final screw hole is drilled and screw placed. *(continued)*

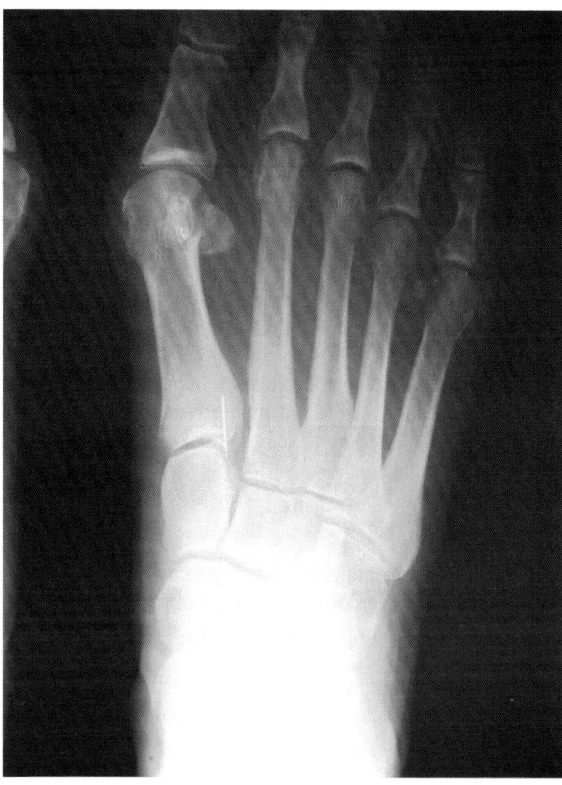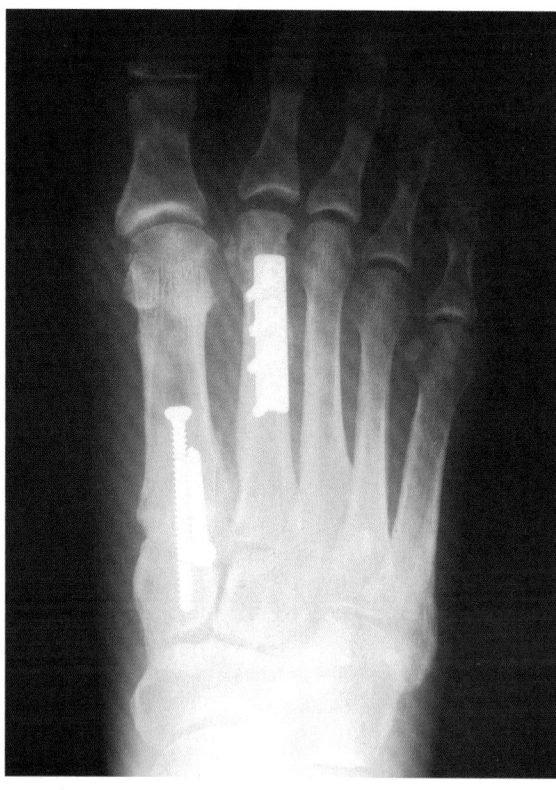

D   E

TECH FIG 3 *(continued)* **D.** Weight-bearing AP of the right foot with *line* drawn from the first metatarsal head to the third metatarsal head demonstrating elongated second metatarsal with associated hallux valgus deformity. **E.** Weight-bearing AP of the right foot after transverse second metatarsal osteotomy in conjunction with the Lapidus procedure for hallux valgus correction.

- A small area around the osteotomy site can be decorticated with a bur, and autogenous bone graft acquired from drill reamings can be packed around the osteotomy site.
- Intraoperative fluoroscopic images are taken to ensure appropriate metatarsal shortening, reduction of osteotomy, and placement of implants (**TECH FIG 3D,E**).

Wound Closure

- The wound is irrigated with sterile saline.
- The wounds are then closed in a layered fashion. The use of sutures, suture type, or staples is determined at the discretion of the surgeon.

OBLIQUE DIAPHYSEAL METATARSAL SHORTENING OSTEOTOMY USING THE MSP METATARSAL SHORTENING PLATE SYSTEM

Exposure

- The exposure in isolation is a 2- to 3-cm dorsal incision over the metatarsal shaft.
  - However, this procedure is often undergone in conjunction with hallux valgus correction surgery, and the incision should be planned for in accordance with other concomitant procedures. For example, the incision for a Lapidus procedure can be made slightly lateral to the first ray and extended distally to account for a second metatarsal shortening osteotomy.

- The dissection is carried bluntly down to the extensor tendons, which are then retracted away from the metatarsal. This is followed by sharp dissection down to bone.
  - The dorsal neurovascular bundle lies just medial to the plane of dissection, and the neurovascular bundle should be protected during the dissection and osteotomy of the second metatarsal.
- A soft tissue elevator is used to dissect the periosteum from the dorsal metatarsal (**TECH FIG 4**).

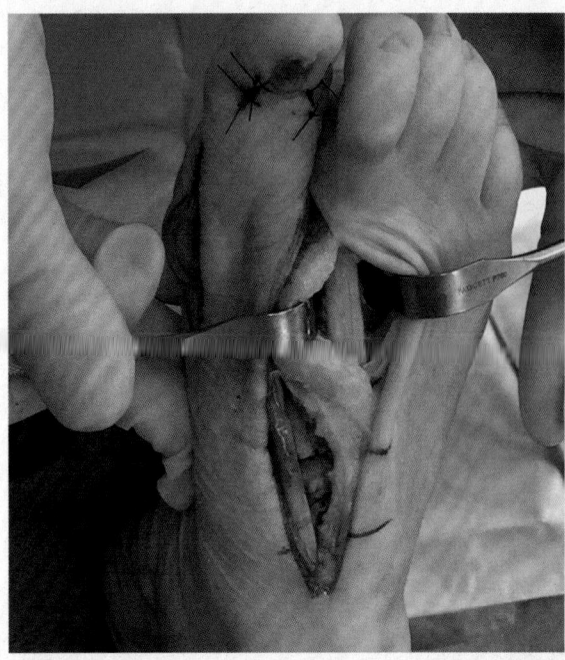

TECH FIG 4 The exposure of the metatarsal after periosteal dissection.

Plate Preparation

- This particular implant has separate right and left implant kits.
- The plate is placed directly onto the metatarsal shaft with the distal edge of the plate positioned approximately 5 mm proximal to the metatarsal head. It can be placed more proximal if desired.

- The bushing is screwed into the most distal hole and is pointed perpendicularly to the dorsal metatarsal cortex to ensure appropriate plate placement (**TECH FIG 5A**).
- The distal screw hole is then drilled through the bushing, and an appropriate length locking screw is placed in the distal hole. The bushing is then removed.
- The bushing is then placed onto the next hole, the proximal hole of the distal osteotomy fragment. This hole is drilled, an appropriate length locking screw is placed, and the bushing is removed (**TECH FIG 5B–E**).
- The plate must be positioned in a manner to ensure that the keel of the plate is in contact with the medial cortex of the metatarsal shaft.
- The proximal drill guide is used to aim for a hole in the most proximal aspect of the proximal screw slot. An appropriate length cortical screw is placed into the proximal slot but not fully tightened.

Osteotomy

- Using an oscillating saw, the osteotomy is made through the oblique cutting guide within the plate. Care must be taken to ensure the saw is held perpendicular to the dorsal cortex (**TECH FIG 6A,B**).
- The distal osteotomy fragment is then shifted proximally to acquire the desired length of shortening. This particular implant allows for up to 6 mm of shortening.
- When the desired shortening is confirmed, the most proximal screw is fully tightened (**TECH FIG 6C**).
- A clamp can be placed onto the medial keel of the plate and the lateral cortex of the metatarsal (perpendicular to the osteotomy) to allow for added compression if desired.

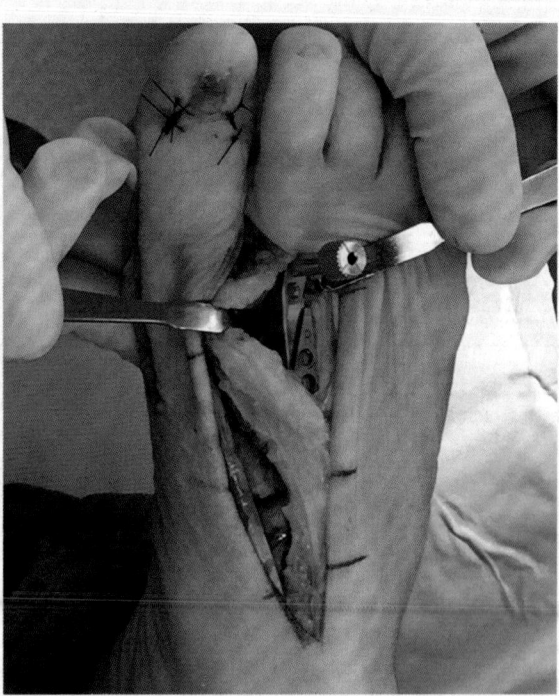

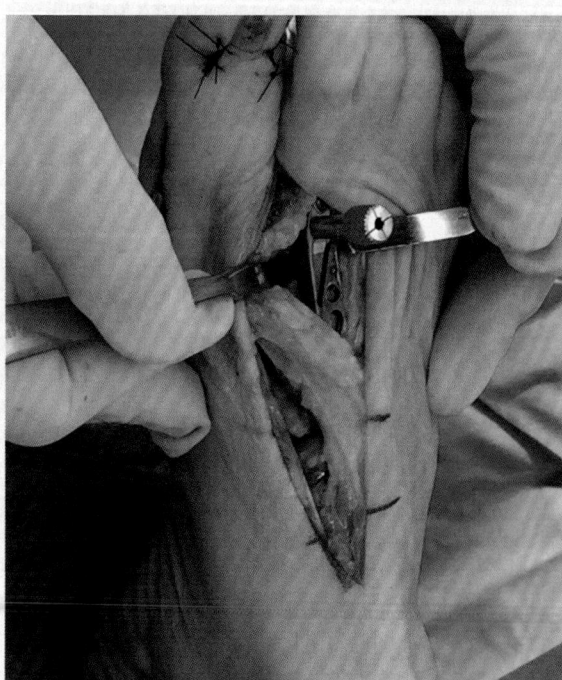

TECH FIG 5 A. The plate is placed, and the bushing is screwed into the most distal hole. **B.** The most distal screw is placed, and the bushing is moved to the next hole. *(continued)*

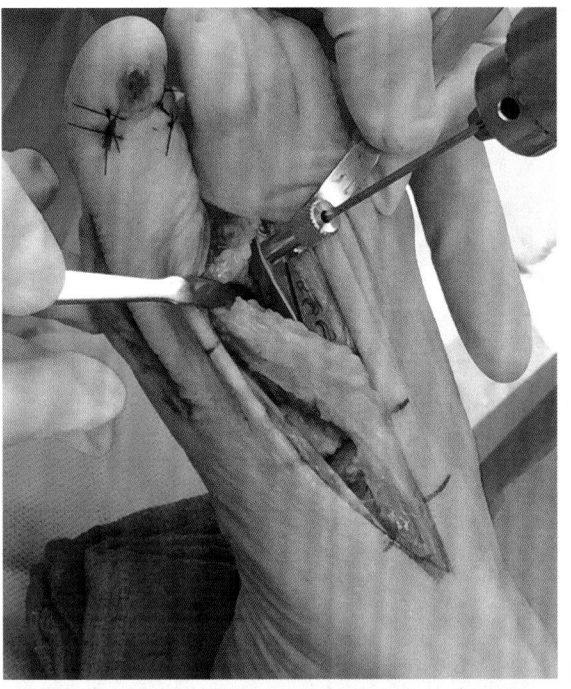

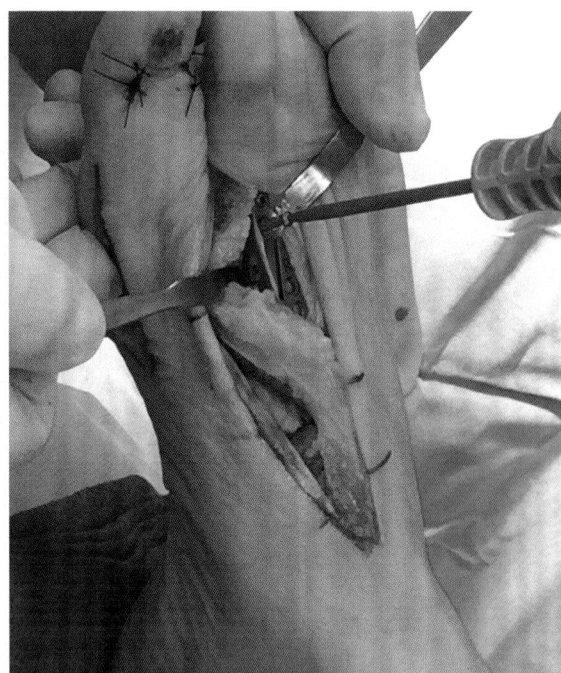

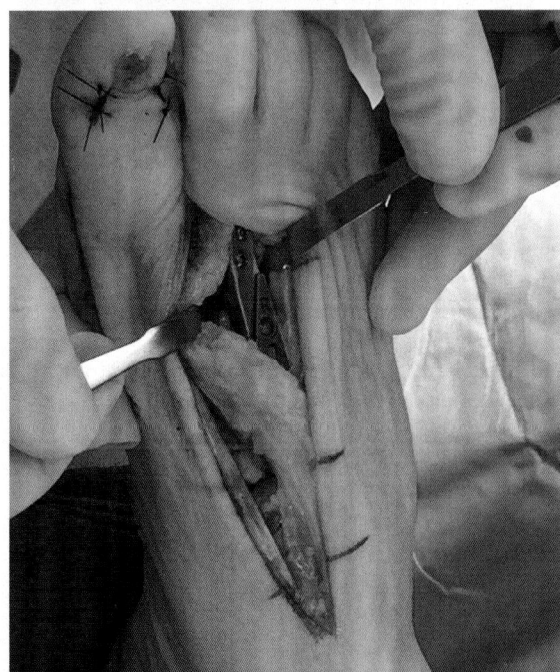

TECH FIG 5 *(continued)* **C.** The next screw hole is drilled through the bushing. **D.** The next screw is then placed. **E.** The plated metatarsal with distal screws in place.

- The remaining proximal screw hole is then drilled using the proximal drill guide, and an appropriate length cortical screw is placed (**TECH FIG 6D,E**).
- Intraoperative fluoroscopy images are taken to ensure adequate placement of implants (**TECH FIG 6F,G**).

Wound Closure

- The wound is irrigated with sterile saline.
- The wounds are then closed in a layered fashion. The use of sutures, suture type, or staples is determined at the discretion of the surgeon.

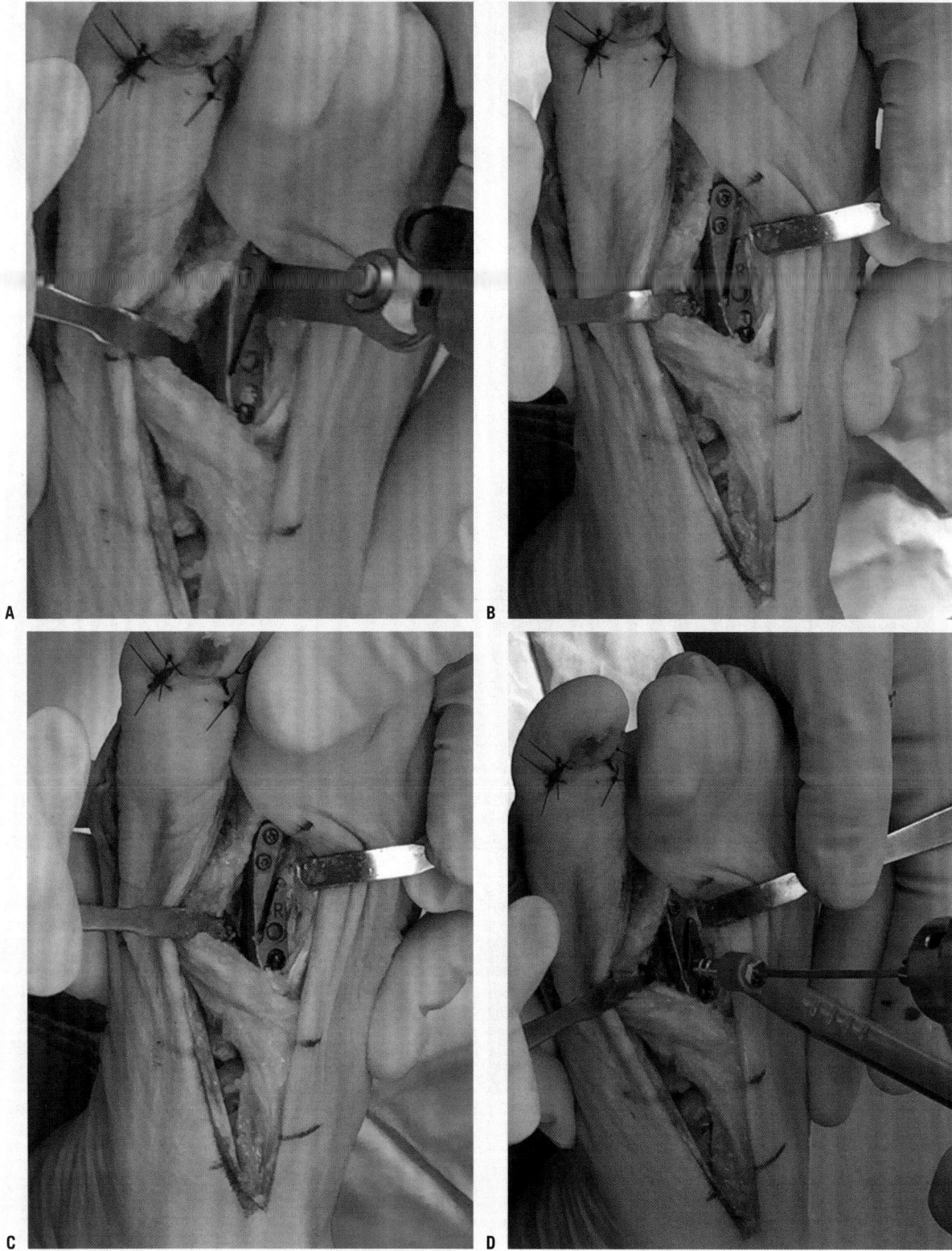

TECH FIG 6 **A.** The most proximal screw is placed but not fully tightened, and then an oscillating saw is used for the oblique osteotomy. **B.** The osteotomy has been made. **C.** The most proximal screw is then fully tightened. **D.** The final screw hole is then drilled through the proximal screw guide. *(continued)*

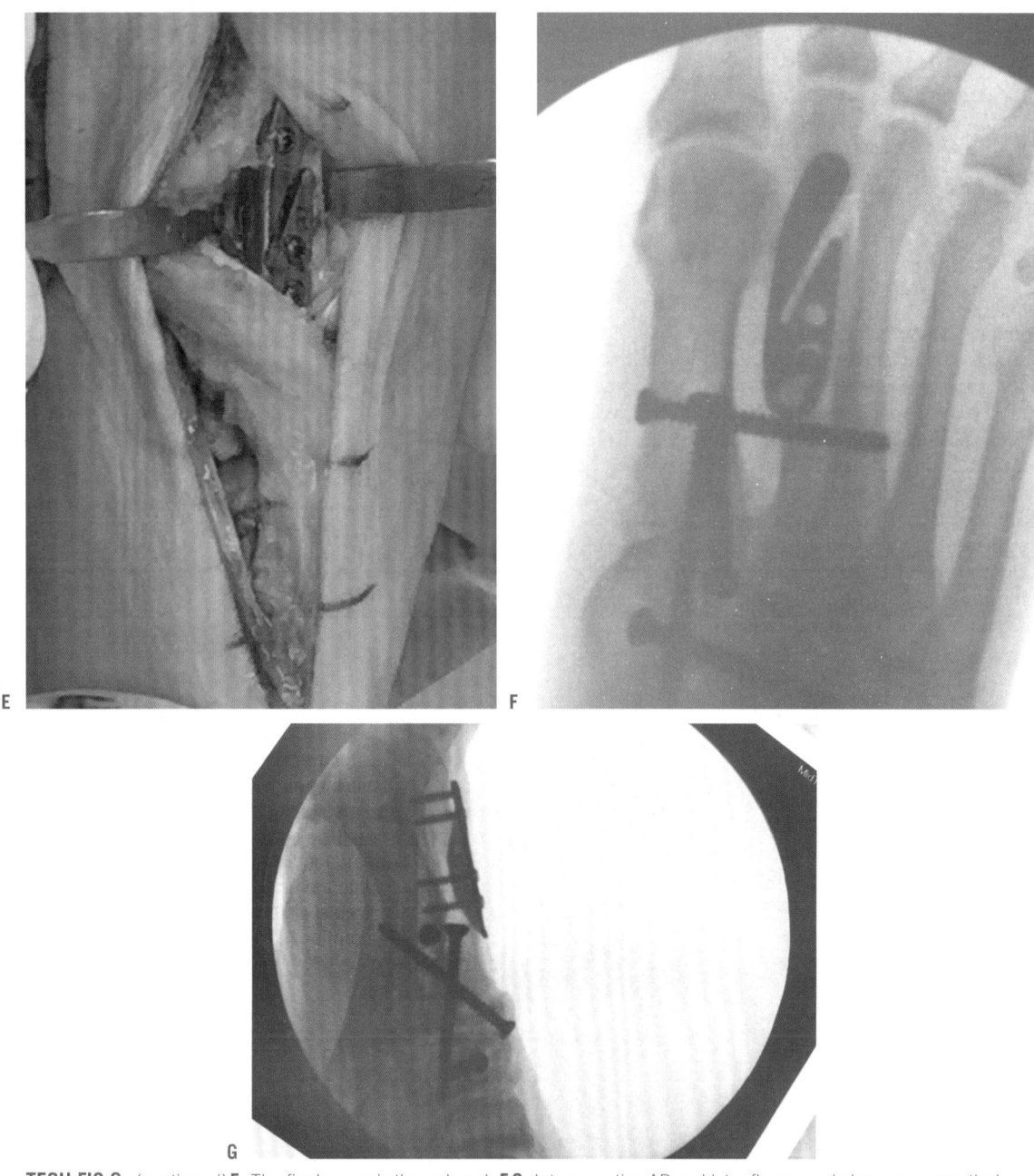

TECH FIG 6 *(continued)* **E.** The final screw is then placed. **F,G.** Intraoperative AP and later fluoroscopic images, respectively, of the right foot showing oblique second metatarsal shortening osteotomy undergone in conjunction with Lapidus procedure for hallux valgus correction.

Pearls and Pitfalls

Pearls	• Center the plate over the metatarsal to make sure reduction is appropriate. • Ensure bicortical purchase of all screws. • Osteotomy must be perpendicular to the long axis of metatarsal shaft to prevent angular deformity.
Pitfalls	• Plantar or dorsal translation of the metatarsal head • Overshortening of the lesser metatarsal • Not obtaining compression across osteotomy site

POSTOPERATIVE CARE

- The patient is placed in a short-leg splint postoperatively and is to remain non-weight bearing for 2 weeks.
- After 2 weeks, the splint is removed and the patient is placed in a short-leg cast or boot, depending on surgeon preference, and is allowed to bear weight through the heel of the cast.
- If the metatarsal shortening osteotomy is done in isolation, the patient is allowed bear weight through a forefoot offloading orthosis at 2 weeks.
- At 8 weeks postoperatively, the cast or boot is removed and the patient can begin a graduated weight-bearing progression protocol and transition to shoe wear when swelling allows.
- Any alteration of the weight-bearing protocol is dependent on the concomitant procedures at the time of surgery.

OUTCOMES

- These osteotomies provide a simple and reproducible technique aimed at treating the symptoms of metatarsalgia.
- The transverse diaphyseal metatarsal shortening osteotomy has had a 99.2% union rate reported by the senior authors (JA and DB),[1] and similar techniques have had reproducible results with 92% union rate reported elsewhere.[3]
  - The authors hold strong beliefs that addressing equinus contracture, when present, has aided in the achievement of high union rates.

- In a small series of 60 patients by the senior authors (JA and DB), the MSP plate system was used for second metatarsal shortening osteotomy in conjunction with tarsometatarsal arthrodesis for hallux valgus and had a 100% union rate with 5% delayed unions.[3]

COMPLICATIONS

- Reported complications include painful nonunion, nerve damage, infection, failure to relieve initial symptoms, transfer lesions, and painful hardware necessitating hardware removal.
- Transfer lesions may be caused by failure to address all the involved lesser metatarsals that are prominent or by overshortening the lesser metatarsal that has undergone the osteotomy.

REFERENCES

1. Galluch D, Bohay D, Anderson J. Midshaft metatarsal segmental osteotomy with open reduction and internal fixation. Foot Ankle Int 2007;28(2):169–174.
2. Hamilton K, Anderson J, Bohay D. Current concepts in metatarsal osteotomies. Techn Foot Ankle Surg 2009;8(2):77–84.
3. Nemec SA, Habbu RA, Anderson JG, et al. Outcomes following midfoot arthrodesis for primary arthritis. Foot Ankle Int 2011;32(4):355–361.

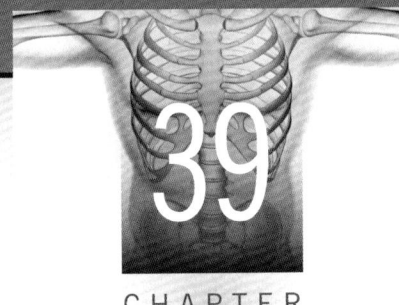

CHAPTER 39

Lesser Toe Plantar Plate Repair

Caio Nery and Daniel Baumfeld

DEFINITION

- The plantar plate is a fibrocartilaginous structure that provides metatarsophalangeal (MTP) joint stability.[15]
- The progressive instability of the MTP joint can result from different patterns of plantar plate tears.[12]
- Each type of plantar plate tear has a particular treatment and different postoperative results.[12]

ANATOMY

- The lesser MTP joint is statically stabilized by the plantar plate, the main collateral ligaments, and the accessory collateral ligaments (**FIG 1**). The plantar plate provides the major stabilizing force in dorsal/plantar direction.[11,15]
- This fibrocartilaginous structure originates on the metaphysis of the metatarsal head via a thin synovial attachment. The strongest insertion is at the base of the proximal phalanx through its two bundles that derives directly from the two major bands of the plantar fascia. Between these two bundles, a small V-shaped synovial recess can be found.[1,15]
- The length of the plantar plate ranges from 16 to 23 mm, and the width ranges from 8 to 13 mm.[9] The borders are thicker than the central region, and it is mainly composed by type 1 collagen (75%) and type 2 collagen (21%) fibers. The collagen fibers of the plantar plate runs in a longitudinal direction, with oblique bundles interspersed at regular intervals.[4,5]
- The plantar plate serves as an attachment for important structures, including the distal fibers of the plantar fascia,

collateral ligaments, transverse metatarsal ligaments, interosseous tendons, and the fibrous sheath of the flexor tendons.[14]

- The tendon of the lumbrical muscle runs plantar and medial to the plantar plate just beneath the deep transverse intermetatarsal ligament (DTIL). The interossei tendons are dorsal to the DTIL and run adjacent to the plantar plate; the plantar interossei are medially located, whereas the dorsal interossei are laterally situated.[1]

PATHOGENESIS

- Lesser MTP instability can occur after acute trauma or secondarily to a chronic inflammation of the joint.
- Synovitis, lesser metatarsal overload, or inflammatory arthropathy can lead to this chronic inflammation.
- Overloading of the lesser MTP joint can result from a long metatarsal, disruption of the metatarsal parabola, hypermobility of the first ray, hallux valgus, flatfeet, or genetic predisposition.
- The use of high-heeled shoes is believed to cause repetitive hyperextension forces on the lesser MTP joints, which in time may lead to attenuation or rupture of the plantar plate, followed by subluxation or dislocation of the toe.

NATURAL HISTORY

- Lesser MTP joint instability with plantar plate tear occur more frequently in women aged older than 40 years and often in association with hallux valgus.

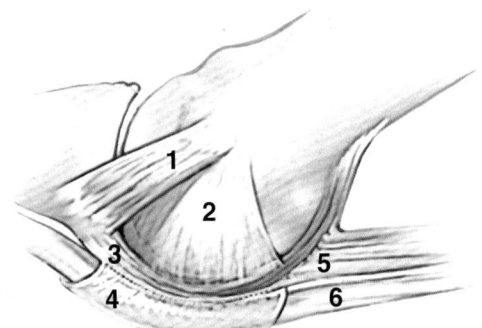
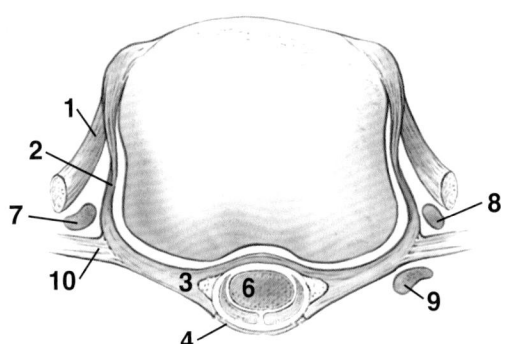

FIG 1 Stabilizers of the lesser MTP joints: proper collateral ligament (*1*), accessory collateral ligament (*2*), plantar plate (*3*), fibrous flexor tendons sheath (*4*), plantar fascia insertion to the plantar plate (*5*), flexor tendons (*6*), dorsal interosseus tendon (*7*), plantar interosseus tendon (*8*), lumbrical tendon (*9*), and deep transversal intermetatarsal ligament (*10*).

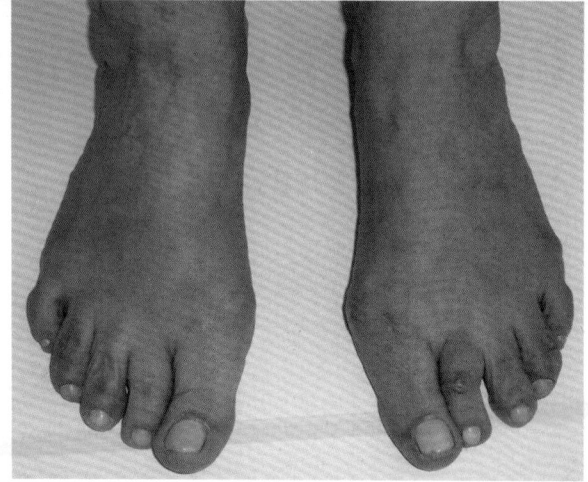
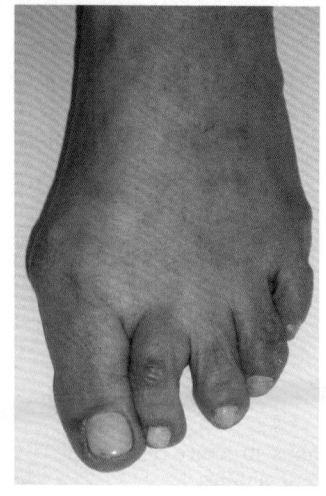

FIG 2 Widening of the left second web space after the "inflammatory" phase of the MTP plantar plate lesion. **A.** Comparison of both feet. **B.** Detail of the left forefoot.

- The clinical symptoms of the patients can be minimal in the early stages and incapacitating with chronic disease.
- Observation of clinical signs and physical examination findings provide a specific diagnosis.
- The use of local anesthetic injections can help to differentiate from other pathologies.

PATIENT HISTORY AND PHYSICAL FINDINGS

- Pain under the affected metatarsal head is the most prevalent and significant complaint.
- Initial observation reveals swelling or thickening of the MTP joint with no other deformities.
- When the first inflammation subsides, the affected toe lightly deviates from its natural axis, creating a wider interdigital space in comparison with the other foot **(FIG 2)**.
- As the disease progresses, dorsal, dorsomedial, or dorsolateral deviation of the toe occurs, followed by the loose of contact of the toe with the ground and a loss of power of the toe (digital purchase); a flexible or fixed hammertoe

may develop with time and, at the end, the classic "crossover toe" can be found.
- Objective physical findings include swelling, malalignment of the toe, positive drawer test, loss of digital purchase, and dysfunction in the normal biomechanics of toe motion.[6]
- The MTP joint drawer test (also known as *Hamilton-Thompson test*) is the first objective sign of MTP joint instability **(FIG 3)**. The involved toe should be plantarflexed 20 degrees during the MTP joint drawer test. Comparison with the normal foot is mandatory to value the physical findings. The stability of the joint is rated as follows:
  - G0 = stable joint
  - G1 = light instability (<50% subluxable)
  - G2 = moderate instability (>50% subluxable)
  - G3 = gross instability (displaceable joint)
  - G4 = dislocated joint
- Ground touch signal is the ability of the toe to keep its pulp pressed in a normal fashion to the ground while standing. It is better evaluated in the podoscope or in a podography.

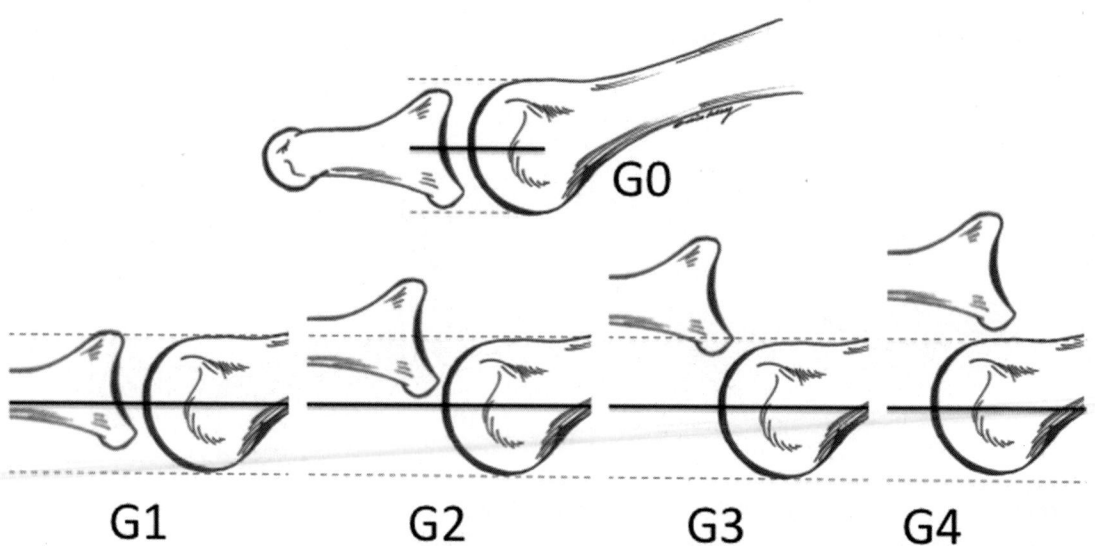

FIG 3 Hamilton-Thompson MTP "drawer" test: *G0* = stable joint, *G1* = light instability (<50% subluxable), *G2* = moderate instability (>50% subluxable), *G3* = gross instability (dislocatable joint), and *G4* = dislocated joint.

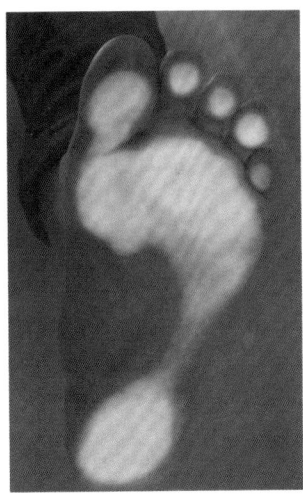 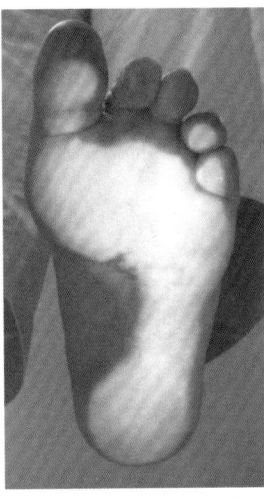

A   B

FIG 4 Podoscopic images showing the ground touch signal. **A.** Normal appearance. **B.** Patient with complains on the second and third toes, loosening of the ground touch ability of both toes.

With the progressive deviation of the toe, this ground touch ability disappears (**FIG 4**).

- Digital purchase is the ability of the toe to pressure the ground. The toe purchase depends on the stability of the MTP joint. It can be evaluated with the Bouché and Heit[2] "paper pullout test."
  - A thin strip of paper is placed under the affected toe pulp. The examiner attempts to pull the paper strip out while the patient resists with toe pressure against the ground.
  - Results are positive when there is no toe purchase present, reduced when the purchase is present but not powerful enough to resist the paper strip to being pulled out, and negative when the toe is able to prevent the paper strip to being pulled out.
- Intractable plantar keratosis beneath the metatarsal head is another common finding.

- A comprehensive review of MTP joint instability reported that a high percentage of patients presents a hammertoe deformity, hallux valgus, hallux rigidus, and hallux varus.[17]
- The clinical staging system for lesser metatarsal instability grades the evolution of the deformity in five stages—0 to 4 (**TABLE 1**).

IMAGING AND OTHER DIAGNOSTIC STUDIES

- The diagnosis of lesser MTP joint instability is most often based on the history and physical examination.[18]
- Standing anteroposterior (AP), lateral, and oblique radiographs are necessary to evaluate the MTP joint and exclude osseous pathology (**FIG 5A,B**). AP and lateral radiographs can demonstrate the magnitude of the MTP joint angular deformity, joint incongruity, the presence of MTP joint arthritis, and determining the metatarsal parabola.[10]
- In a normal AP radiograph, the normal articular cartilage has clear space of 2 to 3 mm. As hyperextension of the MTP joint progresses, the clear space disappears and the base of the proximal phalanx subluxates dorsally over the metatarsal head. With frank dislocation, the base of the proximal phalanx can lie dorsally over the metatarsal head.
- Ultrasonography is a very good method to identify the MTP plantar plate tears. As always, the accuracy and specificity of this diagnostic tool depends on the experience of the examiner, and this could be an obstacle to its use.
- Magnetic resonance imaging (MRI) is essential to some differential diagnosis and to confirm the initial stages of the pathology (**FIG 5C,D**). The sensitivity of MRI is up to 87%, and this finding can be upgraded with the use of intra-articular contrast or an MRI combined with sonographic evaluation.[8]
- Although MRI may aid in the diagnosing and grading of MTP plantar plate pathology, it is paramount the previous knowledge of each type of plantar plate tear to improve description and correlation between the images and the anatomy.[13]

TABLE 1 Clinical Staging System for the Metatarsophalangeal Joint Instability

Grade	Alignment	Physical Examination
0	MTP joint aligned Pain but no deformity	MTP plantar pain, thickening and swelling, reduced toe purchase, negative MTP drawer test
1	Widening of the web space Mild medial deviation of the toe	MTP plantar pain, swelling of MTP joint, loss of toe purchase, mild positive MTP drawer test (<50% subluxable)
2	Moderate MTP malalignment Medial, lateral, dorsal, or dorsomedial deformity Hyperextension of the toe	MTP plantar pain, reduced swelling, no toe purchase, moderate positive MTP drawer test (>50% subluxable)
3	Severe MTP malalignment Dorsal or dorsomedial deformity Overlap of the toes Flexible hammer toe	Joint and toe pain, little swelling, no toe purchase, very positive MTP drawer test (dislocatable joint), flexible hammer toe
4	Dorsomedial or dorsal dislocation Severe deformity with joint dislocation Fixed hammer toe	Joint and toe pain, little or no swelling, no toe purchase, dislocated MTP joint, fixed hammer toe (crossover toe)

MTP, metatarsophalangeal.
From Coughlin MJ, Baumfeld DS, Nery C. Second MTP joint instability: grading of the deformity and description of surgical repair of capsular insufficiency. Phys Sportsmed 2011;39[3]:132–141. Reprinted by permission of Taylor & Francis Ltd, http://www.tandfonline.com.

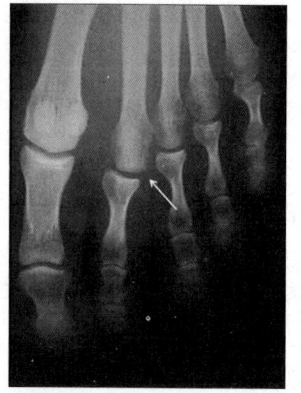 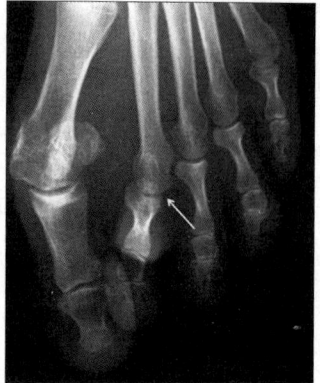 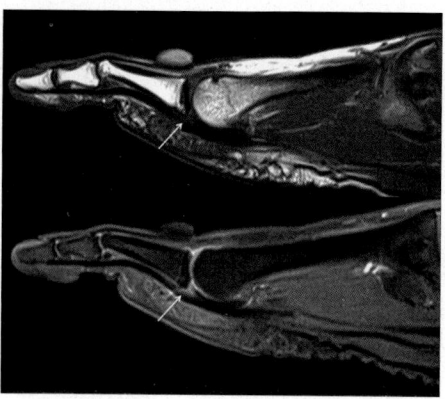

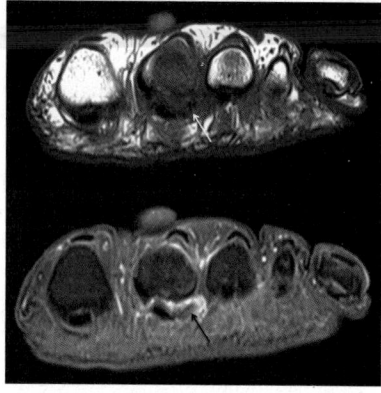

FIG 5 **A,B.** AP plain radiographs of the left forefoot of two patients with different stages of plantar plate lesions. **A.** An initial lesion with a light medial deviation of the second toe. The asymmetric articular space is noted by the *arrow*. **B.** A late lesion with severe dislocation of the second MTP joint and a crossover toe deformity. Note the overlap of the images of the base of the proximal phalanx and the second metatarsal head (*arrow*). **C,D.** Coronal and sagittal MRI scans, respectively, of a patient with second MTP plantar plate lesion (*arrows*).

- MRI can present an eccentric pericapsular soft tissue thickening, increase of lesser metatarsal supination, and rupture of the plantar plate in sagittal and coronal images.
- There are reproducible differences in the measurement of metatarsal axis rotation and second metatarsal protrusion and their relationship with plantar plate tears. Lesser metatarsal supination greater than 36 degrees or second metatarsal protrusion greater than 4-mm trend toward a correlation with plantar plate tear. Lesser metatarsal supination less than 24 degrees is a strong negative predictor, and second metatarsal protrusion greater than 4.5 mm is a strong positive predictor of plantar plate tear.

DIFFERENTIAL DIAGNOSIS

- MTP joint synovitis
- Morton interdigital neuroma
- Mechanical metatarsalgia
- Freiberg infraction
- Degenerative arthritis
- Systemic arthritis localized at the lesser MTP joint
- Stress fracture of the metatarsal neck
- Intermetatarsal bursitis
- Synovial cyst formation

NONOPERATIVE MANAGEMENT

- Nonsurgical treatment of lesser MTP joint instability is generally unsuccessful. It may eliminate the symptoms but do not achieve correction or realignment of the toe.[3,6]
- Conservative management can include nonsteroidal antiinflammatory drugs (NSAIDs), orthotics, tapping, and physical therapy.[3,16]

- The objective of taping is to hold the toe into a neutral position, provide external stability, and help to decrease the inflammation. Prolonged taping does not correct the digital deformity and may lead to chronic edema.
- The use of NSAIDs can decrease discomfort from inflammation at a symptomatic lesser MTP joint.
- Orthotics can relieve metatarsal head pressure and alleviate plantar discomfort by redistributing the body weight on the plantar surface of the foot. A rigid rocker bottom sole may help to improve the gait and relieve dorsiflexion stress to the forefoot.
- Physical therapy can decrease inflammation, improve forefoot load with stretching of the posterior muscular chain, and reduce local edema.

SURGICAL MANAGEMENT

- After the history, clinical, and radiologic evaluation, each involved digit is classified according to the clinical staging system (see **TABLE 1**).
- Each type of plantar plate tear has a particular treatment. The anatomic grading system is a classification that addresses plantar plate dysfunction and matches the clinical staging system. This anatomic grading helps the surgical planning and management of plantar plate ruptures (**FIG 6**).
- The surgery indication is failure of conservative treatment in a patient who has appropriate vascular status and no comorbidities that contraindicate surgery.

Preoperative Planning

- The surgery can be done under regional block anesthesia and lower thigh tourniquet.

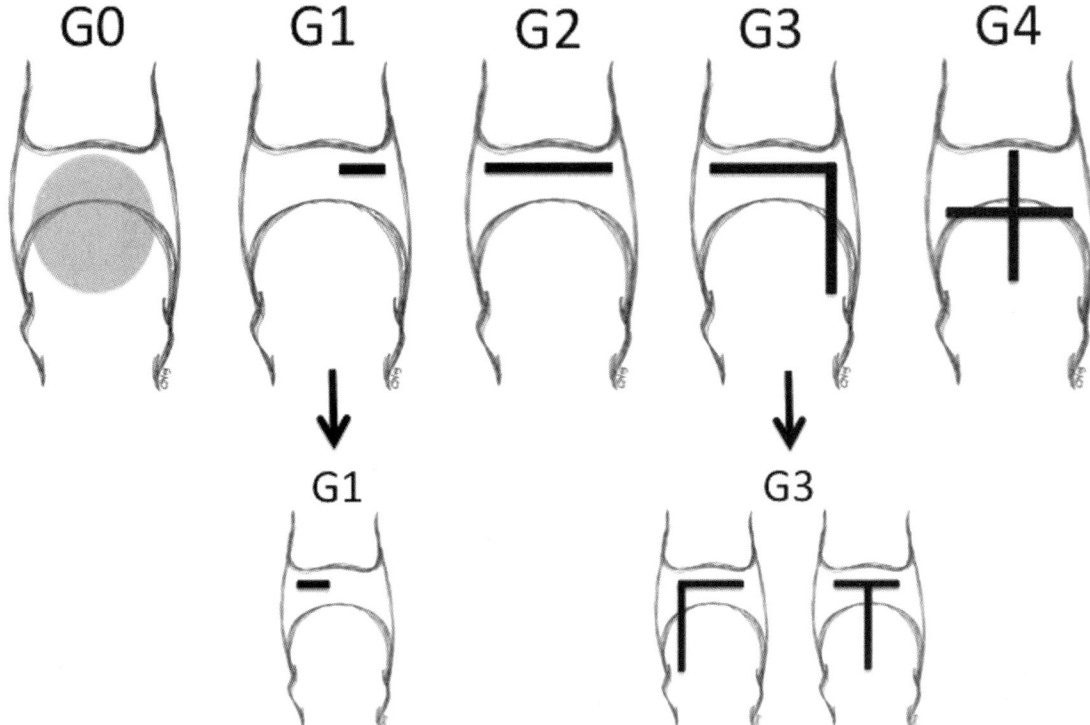

FIG 6 Schematic representation of a right second MTP joint with the anatomic grading system of plantar plate lesions.

- The examination under anesthesia allows for better evaluation of the MTP joint drawer test.
- In our routine, we start the surgical procedure with an MTP arthroscopy that has two distinct objectives:
  - The first is to confirm our clinical assessment of the plantar plate tears.
  - The second is to remove the intra-articular hypertrophic and inflamed synovial tissue and the fringes of fibrous tissue from the torn plantar plate tears. With the help of microshaving instruments (2 mm), one can regularize both the free border of the plantar plate created by the lesion and the plantar rim of the proximal phalanx where the plantar plate will be reattached.
- In our treatment algorithm, the grades 0 and 1 plantar plate lesions were treated through the radiofrequency shrinkage of the attenuated or partially torn tissue followed by a Weil metatarsal osteotomy, whereas the grade 4 lesions was treated through the combination of a Weil metatarsal osteotomy and the flexor digitorum longus (FDL) tendon transfer technique. Tendon transfer is not discussed in this chapter.

Positioning

- The patient is placed supine on the operating table. The surgeon starts the procedure facing the dorsal aspect of the forefoot, whereas its first assistant faces the sole of the foot. In some steps of the procedure, they will change their positions to make feasible the surgical maneuvers.

Approach

- Two dorsal arthroscopic portals are used to perform the lesser MTP joints: the dorsomedial and dorsolateral portals.
  - Both are placed at or slightly distal to the MTP articular joint line, medially, and laterally 4 to 5 mm equidistant from the extensor digitorum longus (EDL) tendon **(FIG 7)**.
- To perform the open repair of the lesser MTP plantar plate through the dorsal approach, we can use
  - A dorsal longitudinal incision centered over the MTP joint (especially when the arthroscopic step of the procedure is not performed)
  - An S-shaped dorsal incision that encompasses the arthroscopic portals **(FIG 8)**

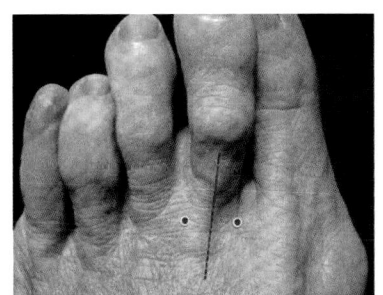 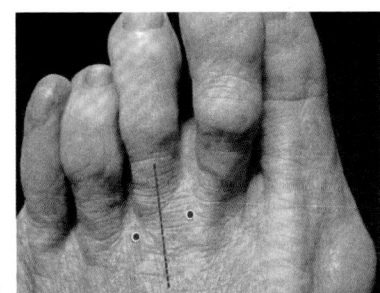 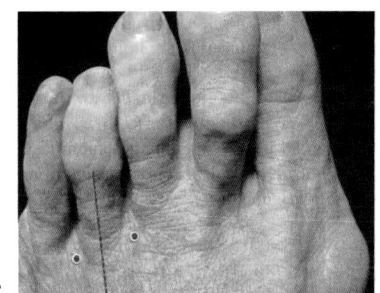

FIG 7 Arthroscopic dorsal (medial and lateral) portals (*red dots*) for the second (**A**), third (**B**), and fourth (**C**) MTP joints. The *red lines* are indicating the EDL tendons of each lesser toes.

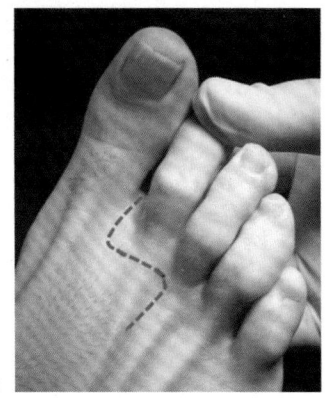
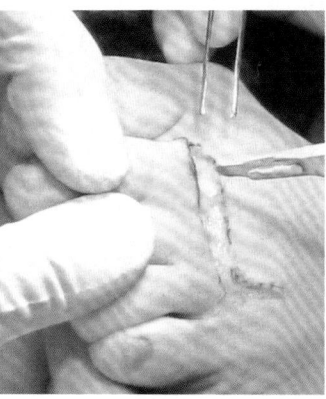

FIG 8 A. S-shaped dorsal incision encompassing the arthroscopic portals made over the involved digit. **B.** Long S-shaped dorsal incision encompassing all the arthroscopic portals when more than one MTP joint are involved.

METATARSOPHALANGEAL JOINT ARTHROSCOPY AND PLANTAR PLATE RADIOFREQUENCY

- Arthroscopic evaluation of the involved lesser MTP joint is performed through two dorsal portals (medial and lateral portals placed over the MTP articular space), and a 2.7- or 1.9-mm, 30-degree arthroscope is used.
- With an 18-gauge needle, the adequate penetration point was marked, and 2 to 3 mL of saline solution was injected into the joint to confirm the proper placement. A no. 11 scalpel blade was used to incise the skin only, and a mosquito clamp is used to enter the joint, preventing injury to the neurovascular structures.
- A pump system is used to provide adequate intra-articular saline flow and joint distention. We assumed the small joint arthroscopy levels of 35 mm Hg and 100% flow rate.

- Pressure and flow levels may be adjusted during the procedure to ensure good visibility of the anatomic structures.
- Light manual traction was applied to the toe so that the central and distal portions of the plantar plate could be visualized, inspected, and then palpated with a probe.
- Synovectomy of the affected joint is performed, and the plantar plate lesions grades 0 and 1 were treated with radiofrequency (ArthroCare Short Bevel 25 degrees 2.3 mm, Andover, MA) shrinkage. The unit was automatically set to deliver a temperature of 60° C.
- After the arthroscopic radiofrequency shrinkage and sealing of the plantar plate lesions, a Weil osteotomy through a dorsal approach using a sagittal saw is performed.

WEIL METATARSAL OSTEOTOMY

- A Weil distal metatarsal osteotomy is performed using a sagittal saw.
  - The saw cut is made parallel to the plantar aspect of the foot, starting at a point 2 to 3 mm below the top of the metatarsal articular surface.
  - In the presence of a plantar keratosis beneath the metatarsal head, a small slice of bone is removed to achieve a subtle elevation of the metatarsal head **(TECH FIG 1A)**.

- The capital fragment is pushed proximally as far as possible (8 to 10 mm) and held in this position temporarily with a small vertical Kirschner wire (K-wire) **(TECH FIG 1B)**.
  - It is recommended to resect 2 or 3 mm of the distal metaphyseal flare to improve the plantar plate visualization **(TECH FIG 1C)**.
- Longitudinal traction to the toe helps to distract the joint, creating space to the next steps of the procedure.

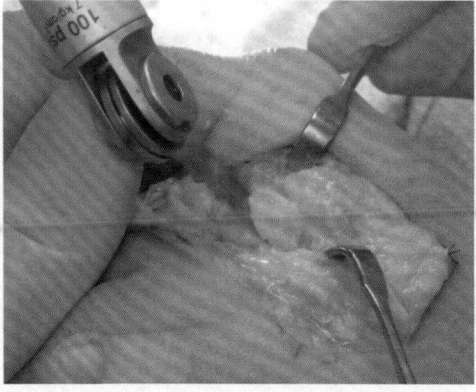
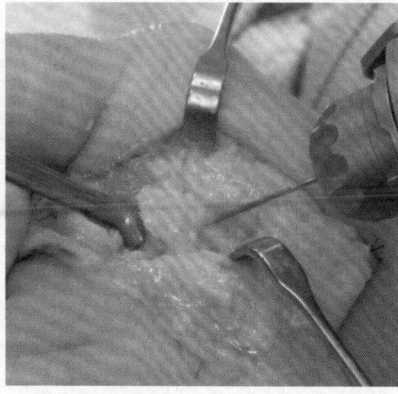

TECH FIG 1 A. Performing the distal Weil osteotomy. **B.** The capital fragment is pushed proximally as far as possible. *(continued)*

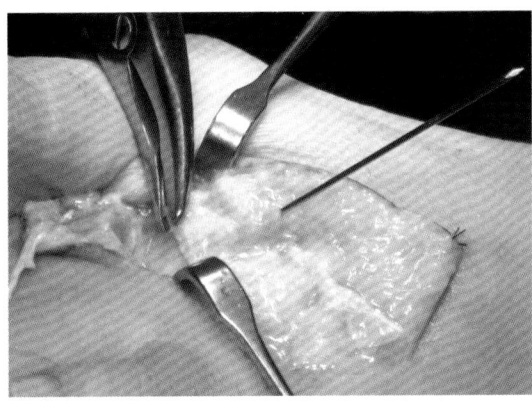

C

TECH FIG 1 *(continued)* **C.** Resection of the distal margin of the proximal fragment, 2 to 3 mm.

PREPARING THE PLANTAR PLATE AND THE PHALANX

- The plantar plate is then inspected, and the type of lesion is confirmed.
  - If some portion of the plantar plate remains connected to the inferior border of the proximal phalanx, it is cut carefully with a small scalpel avoiding lesions to the FDL tendon.
  - It is important to release the distal margin of the plantar plate from any soft tissue adhesions especially at the plantar surface, creating space for the instruments and the sutures.
  - The MTP plantar plate is 2.0 to 2.5 mm thick in its anterior border, and care must be taken not to delaminate the plantar plate during the intent to free the margins of the lesion.
- Any residual tissue is excised from the plantar margin of the proximal phalanx with a small rongeur or curette, creating a roughened surface for optimal attachment of the plantar plate.
- If a longitudinal tear of the plantar plate is detected (grade 3 T- or 7-shaped lesion), it can be repaired through interrupted nonabsorbable 3-0 sutures placed with the help of a small needle holder (**TECH FIG 2**).

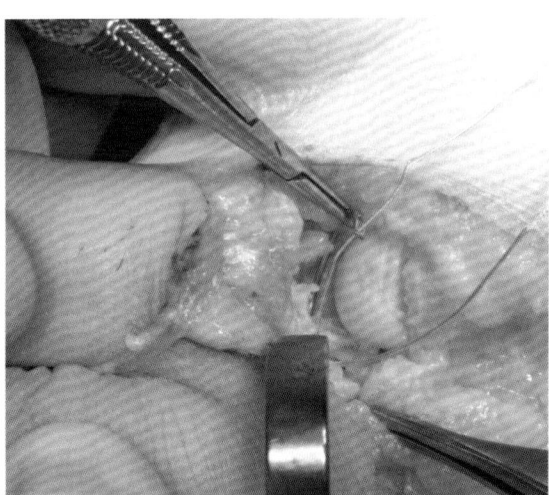

TECH FIG 2 Suturing a longitudinal tear of the plantar plate.

SUTURE PASSING THROUGH THE PLANTAR PLATE

- There are different and efficient ways to suture the distal border of plantar plate, in all of them, the main objective is to attach the sutures in a viable tissue as proximal as possible at the free border of the PP.
- A joint distractor can be used to help the visualization of the plate. It is placed over the proximal phalanx and the retracted metatarsal head with K-wires to support the distraction.
- To perform the suture, one can use a mechanical suture passer or a micro "pig-tail" suture passer (Mini SutureLasso [Arthrex, Inc., Naples, FL]), and with those, we can easily and safely place horizontal or longitudinal mattress sutures in the plantar plate.
- The horizontal mattress stitch may be the biomechanically superior configuration in plantar plate repairs. The mattress and luggage-tag configuration demonstrated better peak load-to-failure force compared with the Mason-Allen suture.
- The mechanical suture passer that can be used are the Mini Scorpion or the Viper suture passer from Arthrex, Inc., Naples, FL.

- When the mechanical or manual suture passer is not available, there is an alternative surgical technique that has been called the *ugly technique*.
- With this technique, before starting to pass the main sutures to the anterior border of the plantar plate, we have to construct a "snakehead" NINJA instrument with a 1.0-mm K-wire (**TECH FIG 3A**).
- The head of the NINJA instrument is positioned under the anterior border of the plantar plate, in its lateral or medial half, taking care to avoid injuries to the flexor tendons. To pass the suture into a healthy tissue, it is important to reach the plantar plate as proximal as possible (**TECH FIG 3B,C**).
- A straight handheld suture passer (SutureLasso [Arthrex, Inc., Naples, FL]) or an 18-gauge needle is passed from dorsal to plantar through the plantar plate, into the snakehead of the NINJA instrument, and through the soft tissue of the sole until it exteriorizes at the plantar face of the foot (**TECH FIG 3D–F**).

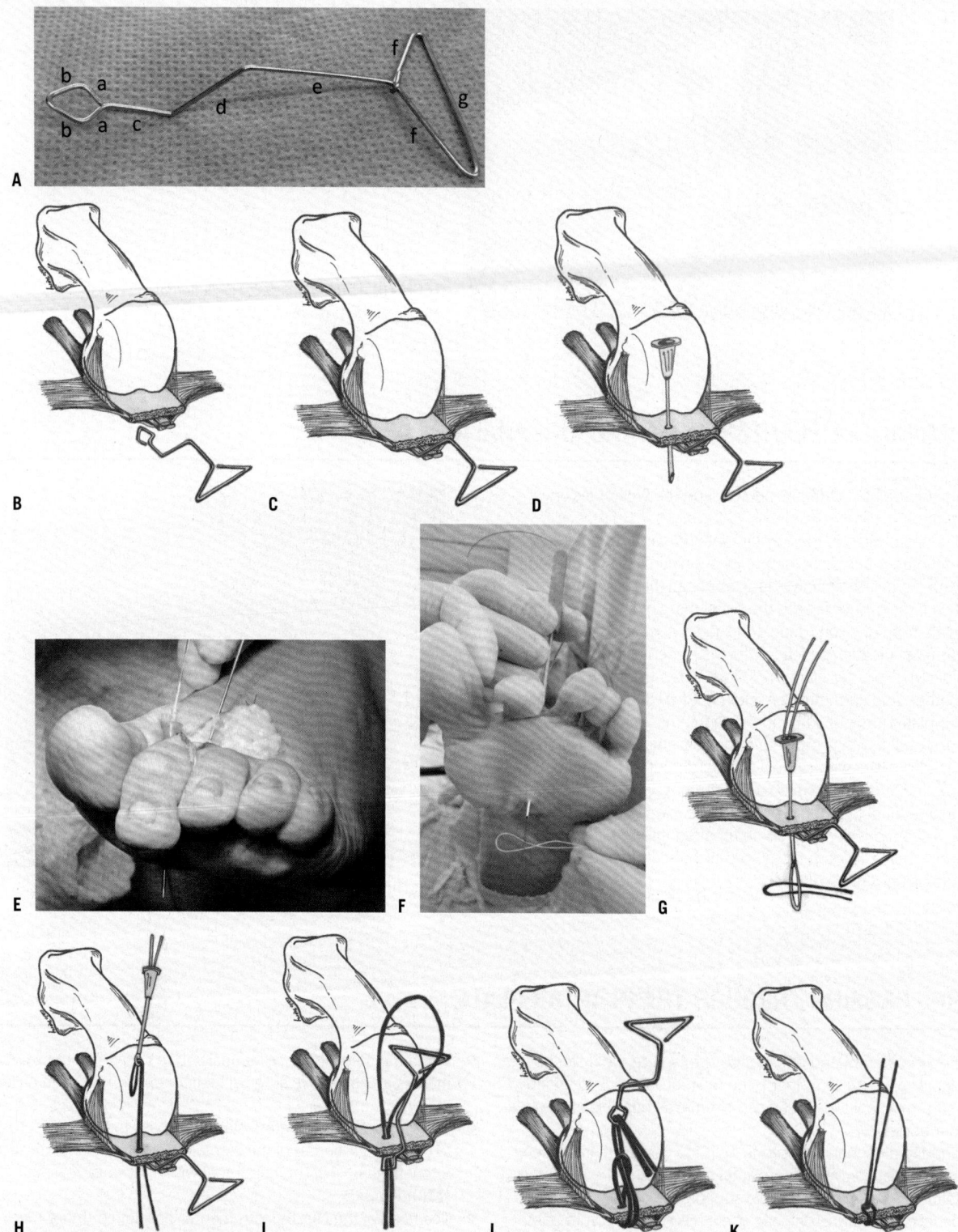

TECH FIG 3 A. The snakehead NINJA instrument is made by bending a 1.0-mm K-wire with a delicate pair of pliers or a strong surgical needle holder: head (*a* = 3 mm; *b* = 5 mm), neck (*c* = 10 mm), step 1 (first step angle = 45 degrees), bridge (*d* = 15 mm); step 2 (second step angle = 45 degrees), stem (*e* = 20 mm), handle (*f* = 15 mm; *g* = 20 mm). **B.** Positioning of the NINJA head under the plantar plate. **C.** The NINJA head must be positioned as proximal as possible. **D.** An 18-gauge needle is passed through the plantar plate and the snakehead of the NINJA instrument. **E,F.** Two different instruments are used to pass the sutures through the plantar plate—an 18-gauge needle (**E**) and a straight SutureLasso (Arthrex, Inc., Naples, FL) (**F**). **G.** A flexible wire loop is introduced into the needle, and a folded suture is passed through the wire loop. **H.** The needle is pulled up through the plantar plate. **I.** The loop of the suture involves the handle of the NINJA instrument. **J.** A lace is created, and the NINJA instrument is pulled out. **K.** The suture firmly locks into the distal margin of the plantar plate.

- A flexible wire loop is introduced into the needle or suture passer from dorsal to plantar. A folded 2-0 nonabsorbable suture (Fiber-Wire [Arthrex, Inc., Naples, FL]) is passed through the wire loop and pulled up through the plantar plate (**TECH FIG 3G,H**).
- The loop of the suture involves the handle of the NINJA instrument while the free suture tails are firmly kept in the plantar face of the foot by the assistant.
  - With this maneuver, a lace will be created while the NINJA instrument is pulled out of the surgical field at the same

time that the suture tails are released by the assistant (**TECH FIG 3I,J**).
- Pulled tight, the suture firmly locks in to the distal margin of the plantar plate (**TECH FIG 3K**).
- The same sequence is repeated for the other half of the plantar plate.
- At the end, we have two sutures firmly passed through the remaining healthy tissue from the MTP plantar plate.

PASSING SUTURES THROUGH THE BASE OF THE PROXIMAL PHALANX

- With use of a 1.5-mm K-wire or a drill bit, two vertical drill holes are made medially and laterally in the base of the proximal phalanx from the dorsal cortex to the plantar rim of the proximal phalanx, matching the sutures placed over the plantar plate (**TECH FIG 4A,B**).

- The same flexible wire loop used in the previous steps is passed from dorsal to plantar through the holes of the phalanx base and then used to catch and pull the sutures through the dorsal side (**TECH FIG 4C–E**).

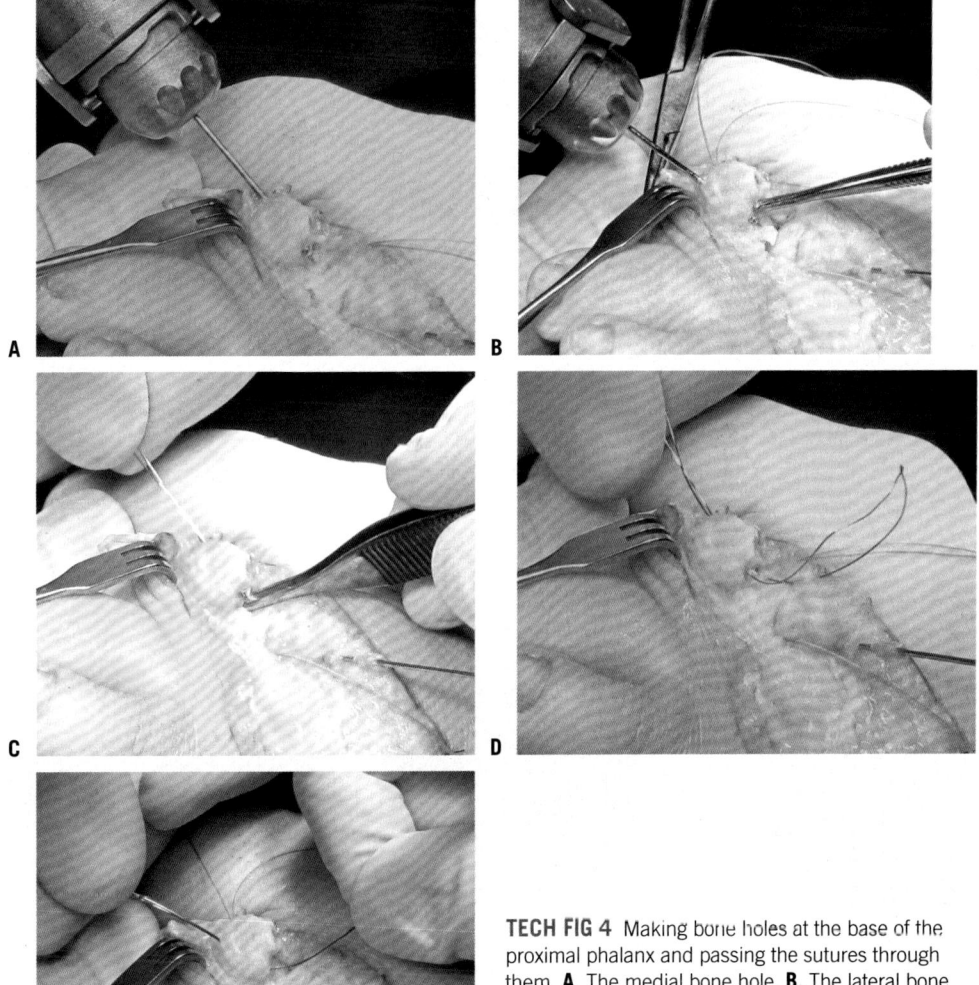

TECH FIG 4 Making bone holes at the base of the proximal phalanx and passing the sutures through them. **A.** The medial bone hole. **B.** The lateral bone hole. **C.** A wire loop is passed through the bone hole. **D.** The suture is introduced into the wire loop. **E.** Pulling the wire loop out, the suture passes through the bone hole. The procedure is repeated for the other suture and bone hole.

FIXING THE WEIL OSTEOTOMY AND FINISHING

- The Weil osteotomy is fixed in the desired position with one small snap-off self-tapping vertical screw.
- The metatarsal shortening is determined in the preoperative planning to achieve a regular metatarsal parabola. Normally, only 2 or 3 mm of metatarsal shortening is required.
- Once the Weil osteotomy is fixed, the sutures are tied over the bone bridge at the proximal phalanx, attaching the plantar plate at the base of the phalanx while the toe is held in 20 degrees of plantarflexion (**TECH FIG 5A**).
- Lateral soft tissue reefing is performed to repair any lateral collateral ligamentous insufficiency and transverse plane deformities.

- The articular capsule is closed, and the EDL tendon is sutured in the appropriate length if elongation was performed.
- At this moment, it is important to release the tourniquet and to proceed to a careful hemostasis of the dorsal region of the MTP joints.
  - Substantial bleeding can result from the small dorsal vessels, and the hematoma formed can compromise the skin coverage of the region with potential skin and soft tissue necrosis with dehiscence of the surgical incision.
- After routine wound closure, a postoperative compression dressing is applied with the affected toes held in 20 degrees of plantarflexion (**TECH FIG 5B,C**).

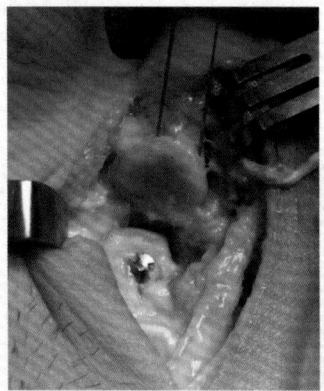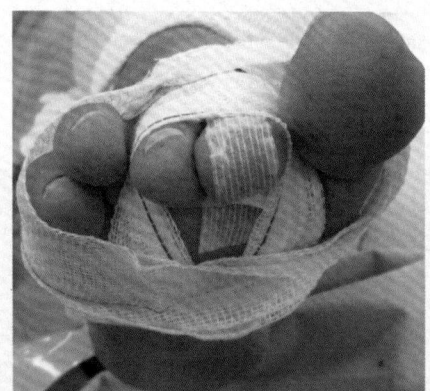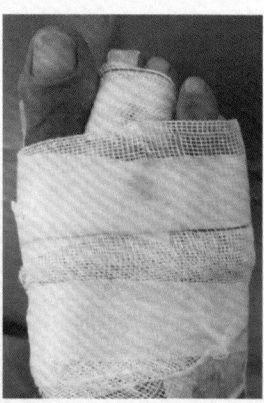

TECH FIG 5 A. Gross aspect of the MTP joint just before the finalization of the dorsal knots. **B,C.** Dressing with the operated toes held in 20 degrees of plantarflexion.

PLANTAR PLATE REPAIR ADDITIONAL CASE

- **TECH FIGS 6** and **7** show plantar plate repairs undertaken according to the description used in this chapter.

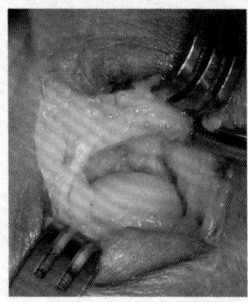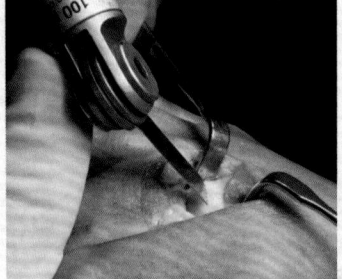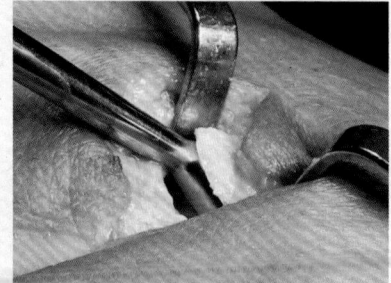

TECH FIG 6 A. The exposition of a grade 3 seven-type second MTP joint plantar plate lesion. **B.** The Weil osteotomy starts at a point 2 mm below the dorsal border of the articular surface. **C.** The metatarsal head is retracted proximally. *(continued)*

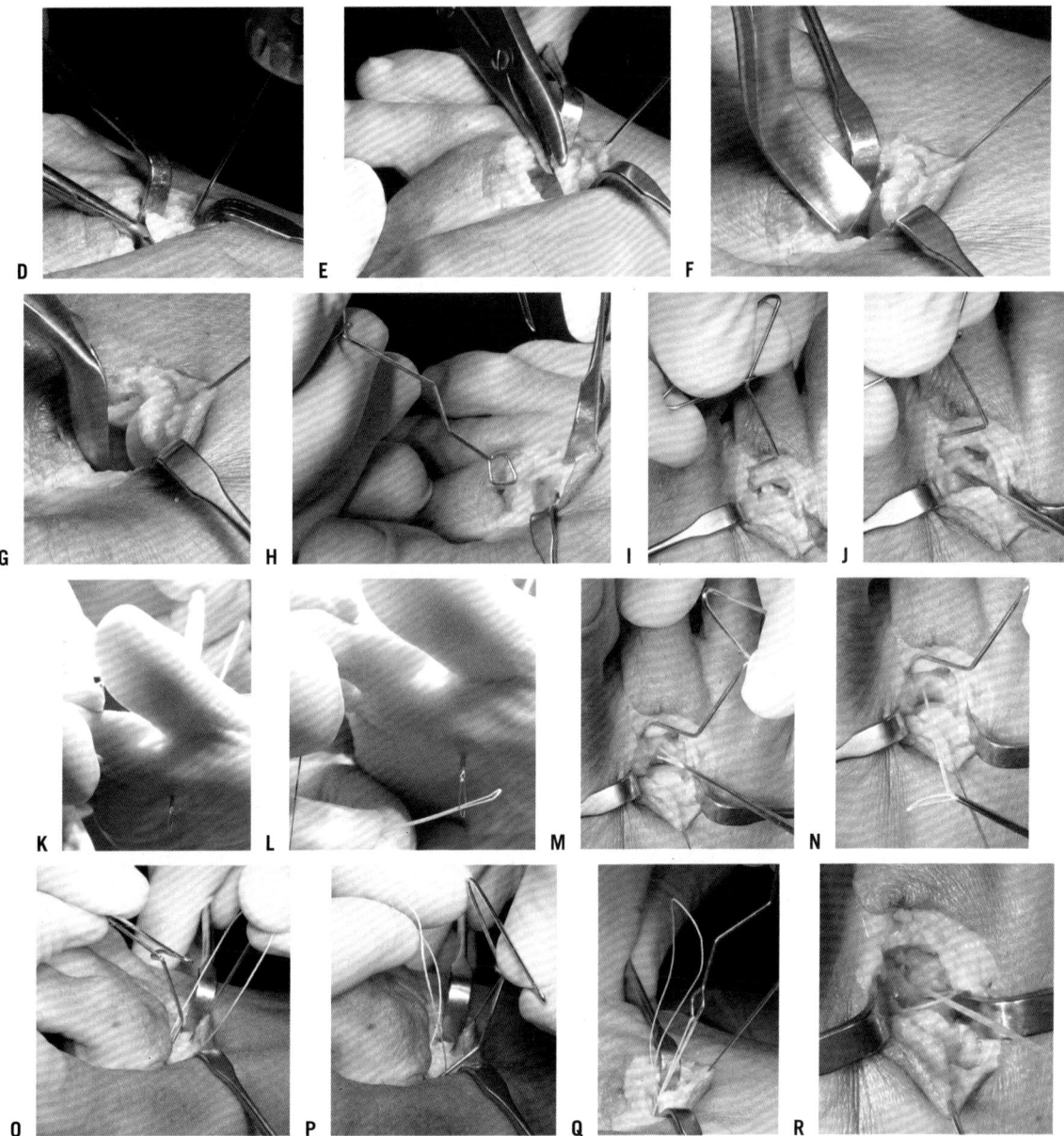

TECH FIG 6 *(continued)* **D.** The metatarsal head is temporarily fixed with a K-wire. **E.** Resection of the distal border of the proximal fragment—2 to 3 mm. **F,G.** A McGlamry elevator is introduced under the metatarsal head to free all adhesions to the plantar plate. **H,I.** The snakehead NINJA instrument is introduced under the plantar plate. **J.** The suture passer is introduced through the plantar plate and the snakehead of the NINJA instrument. **K.** A flexible wire loop appears at the plantar aspect of the foot. **L.** A folded 2-0 suture is passed through the wire loop. **M,N.** The suture passer is pulled up. **O–Q.** The loop involves the handle of the NINJA instrument. **R.** At the end, a firm suture locks in the margin of the plantar plate.

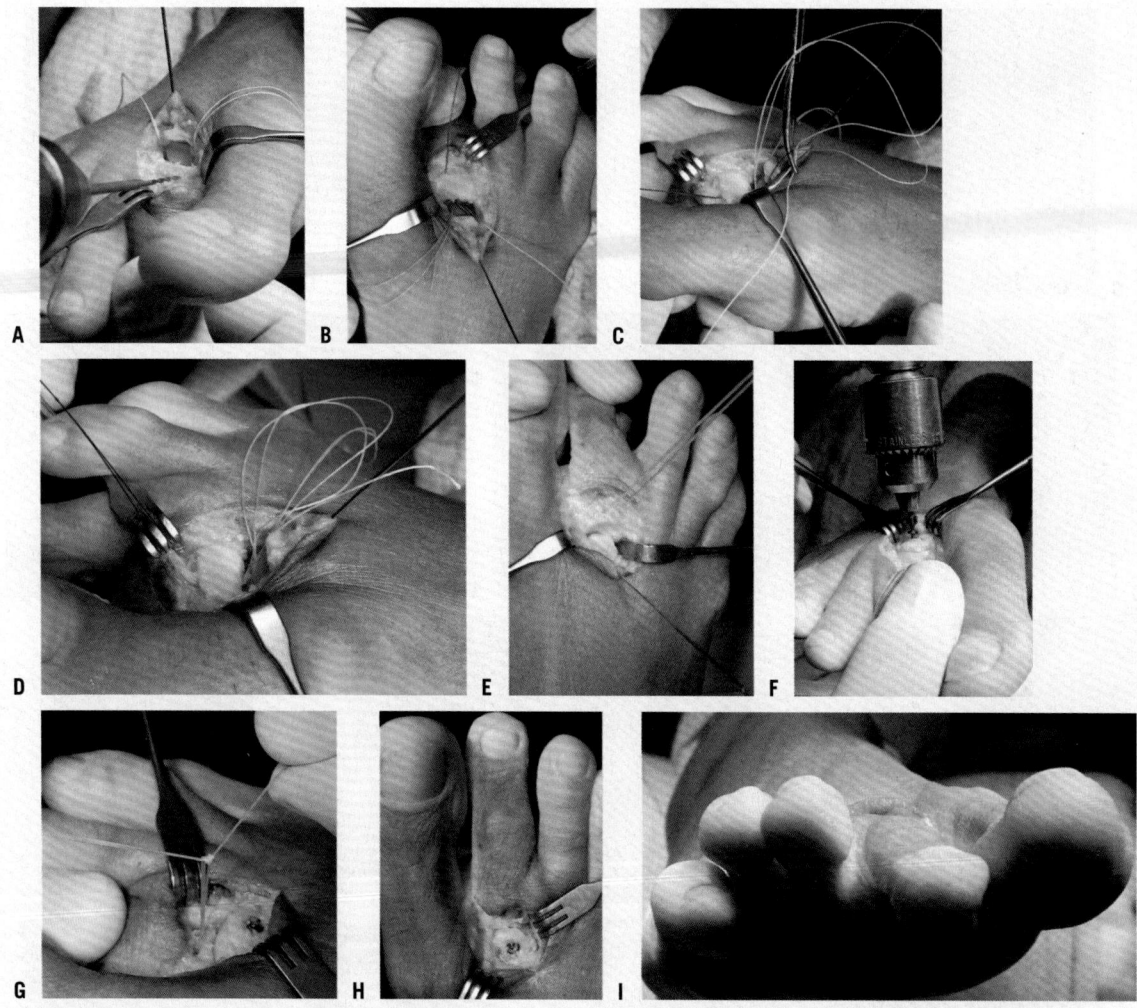

TECH FIG 7 **A.** With a drill bit, two bone holes are made at the base of the proximal phalanx. **B–E.** The sutures are passed through the bone holes with the help of the flexible wire loop. **F.** The Weil osteotomy is fixed in the desired position. **G.** The sutures are tied, bringing the plantar plate to the base of the proximal phalanx. **H,I.** Final aspect of the corrected toe. Note the plantarflexion of the MTP joint resulting from the reinsertion of the plantar plate at the base of the proximal phalanx.

TECHNIQUES

Pearls and Pitfalls

Diagnosis	• "Think plantar plate lesion" is the first step to diagnose correctly.
	• Intimacy with the regional anatomy is paramount to understand and propose the right treatment regimen.
	• Acute pain under the affected metatarsal head, widening of the web space, and the positive MTP drawer test are the most important and reliable findings in MTP joint instability.
	• The clinical staging system and its correlation with the anatomic grading system for the MTP plantar plate lesions proved to be very important in the treatment decision-making process.
Skin Incision	• The S-shaped dorsal incision can be elongated to expose two or three MTP joints at the same time.
Extensor Digitorum Longus Tendon	• Depending on the amount of the toe deformity, consider elongating the EDL tendon.
Weil Osteotomy	• Try to keep the osteotomy as parallel as possible with the sole, avoiding the descending of the metatarsal head.
	• Take off a thin slice of bone if you pretend to elevate the metatarsal head and reduce its overloading.
	• Beware of metatarsal shortenings greater than 3 mm.

Plantar Plate Repair	• Remove all fibrous tissue from the free border of the plantar plate lesion. • Be sure to free the plantar plate from its adhesions to the plantar fat pad before passing the sutures. • Be sure to pass the sutures in a healthy tissue. • Be sure to identify and suture any longitudinal tear of the plantar plate.
Preparing the Phalanx	• Be extremely careful when orienting the K-wire or the drill bit to make the bone holes at the base of the proximal phalanx. • Leave, at least, 1 mm of bone between the articular cartilage and the bone hole. • Take care not to jeopardize the metatarsal head while doing the phalangeal bone holes.
Fixing the Weil Osteotomy	• Beware of rotational deviation of the metatarsal head while fixing the osteotomy. Use two screws if you feel it is necessary. • Be gentle while bending the screwdriver of the powered machine at the end of the screw insertion. You can cause a bone fracture at this moment.
Tie the Sutures	• Keep the toe in a 20-degree plantarflexion at the MTP joint while fixing the sutures over the proximal phalanx. • Be sure that the MTP joint is stable and aligned at the end of this step. • If not, complete the procedure by reefing the collateral ligaments and the articular capsule. • Suture the tendons at the appropriate length.
Before Closing	• Caution with the hemostasis before closing the wound
Dressing	• Keep the affected toes in 20 degrees of plantarflexion for 6 weeks after the surgery.

POSTOPERATIVE CARE

- The operated toe is held in 20 degrees of plantarflexion to provide adequate healing of the repaired plantar plate during the first 6 weeks.
- The patient is allowed to ambulate in a postoperative shoe for 6 weeks with no weight bearing on the forefoot (**FIG 9**).
- After 6 weeks, dressings are discontinued, and comfortable shoes are permitted.
- An exercise program to condition the extrinsic and intrinsic muscles of the lesser toes is then initiated.

OUTCOMES

- The objective of plantar plate repair is to restore the stability of the MTP joint and preserve the joint function and motion.
- Surgical repair of the plantar plate thought dorsal approach has a reported success rates of 68% to 93%.[7,12,17]
- With the combination of plantar plate repair and a Weil metatarsal osteotomy, over 63% of the patients have the ability to perform digital purchase.[12]
- Regarding the stability, some authors found that 68% of the patients were completely stable after this treatment (grade 0 of the stability classification), and 32% had an unstable MTP joint grade 1 or mild instability with no clinical implications.[12]

COMPLICATIONS

- Recurrence of symptoms: This may be due to incorrect diagnosis, incomplete repair of the plantar plate, or true incorrect alignment of the metatarsal parabola.
- Painful prominent hardware can occur after fixation of the Weil osteotomy.[17]
- Dorsal hematoma formation and healing skin problem
- Scaring and retraction of the surgical incisions
- Persisting edema (long lasting)
- Elevated and insufficient toes

REFERENCES

1. Armen K. Sarrafian's Anatomy of the Foot and Ankle: Descriptive, Topographic, Functional, ed 3. Philadelphia: Lippincott Williams & Wilkins, 2011.
2. Bouché RT, Heit EJ. Combined plantar plate and hammertoe repair with flexor digitorum longus tendon transfer for chronic, severe sagittal plane instability of the lesser metatarsophalangeal joints: preliminary observations. J Foot Ankle Surg 2008;47:125–137.
3. Coughlin MJ, Baumfeld DS, Nery C. Second MTP joint instability: grading of the deformity and description of surgical repair of capsular insufficiency. Phys Sportsmed 2011;39:132–141.
4. Deland JT, Lee KT, Sobel M, et al. Anatomy of the plantar plate and its attachments in the lesser metatarsal phalangeal joint. Foot Ankle Int 1995;16:480–486.

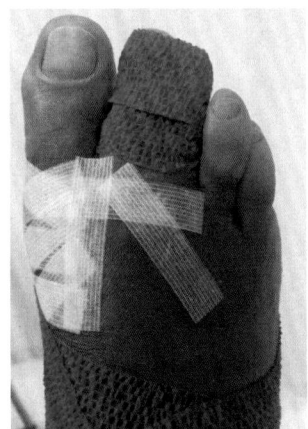
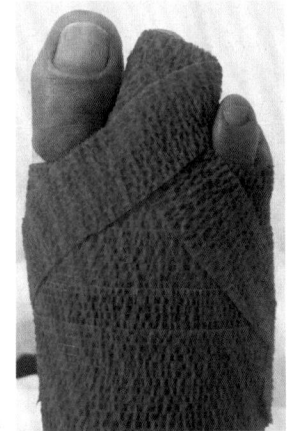
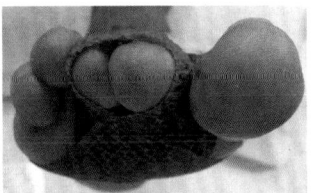
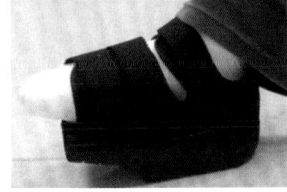

FIG 9 Postoperative dressing and postoperative shoe. **A.** Tapping the operated toes in 20 degrees of plantarflexion. **B.** Frontal view of the same patient at the same moment. **C.** At the end of the tapping procedure. **D.** The Barouk postoperative shoe with a reduced forefoot platform to permit the toes to be held in plantarflexion.

5. Deland JT, Sung IH. The medial crosssover toe: a cadaveric dissection. Foot Ankle Int 2000;21:375–378.

6. Doty JF, Coughlin MJ. Metatarsophalangeal joint instability of the lesser toes. J Foot Ankle Surg 2014;53(4):440–445. doi:10.1053/j.jfas.2013.03.005.

7. Ford LA, Collins KB, Christensen JC. Stabilization of the subluxed second metatarsophalangeal joint: flexor tendon transfer versus primary repair of the plantar plate. J Foot Ankle Surg 1998;37:217–222.

8. Gregg J, Silberstein M, Schneider T, et al. Sonographic and MRI evaluation of the plantar plate: a prospective study. Eur Radiol 2006;16:2661–2669.

9. Johnston RB III, Smith J, Daniels T. The plantar plate of the lesser toes: an anatomical study in human cadavers. Foot Ankle Int 1994;15:276–282.

10. Kaz AJ, Coughlin MJ. Crossover second toe: demographics, etiology, and radiographic assessment. Foot Ankle Int 2007;28:1223–1237.

11. Mendicino RW, Statler TK, Saltrick KR, et al. Predislocation syndrome: a review and retrospective analysis of eight patients. J Foot Ankle Surg 2001;40:214–224.

12. Nery C, Coughlin MJ, Baumfeld D, et al. Lesser metatarsophalangeal joint instability: prospective evaluation and repair of plantar plate and capsular insufficiency. Foot Ankle Int 2012;33:301–311.

13. Nery C, Coughlin MJ, Baumfeld D, et al. MRI evaluation of the MTP plantar plates compared with arthroscopic findings: a prospective study. Foot Ankle Int 2013;34:315–322.

14. Sarrafian SK, Topouzian LK. Anatomy and physiology of the extensor apparatus of the toes. J Bone Joint Surg Am 1969;51:669–679.

15. Suero EM, Meyers KN, Bohne WH. Stability of the metatarsophalangeal joint of the lesser toes: a cadaveric study. J Orthop Res 2012;30:1995–1998.

16. Trepman E, Yeo SJ. Nonoperative treatment of metatarsophalangeal joint synovitis. Foot Ankle Int 1995;16:771–777.

17. Weil L Jr, Sung W, Weil LS Sr, et al. Anatomic plantar plate repair using the Weil metatarsal osteotomy approach. Foot Ankle Spec 2011;4:145–150.

18. Yu GV, Judge MS, Hudson JR, et al. Predislocation syndrome. Progressive subluxation/dislocation of the lesser metatarsophalangeal joint. J Am Podiatr Med Assoc 2002;92:182–199.

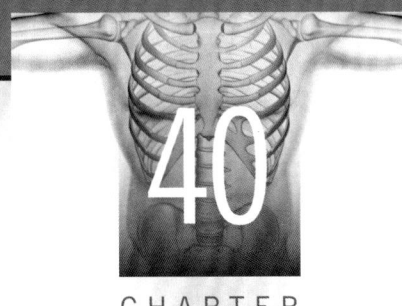

Chapter 40

Angular Deformity of the Lesser Toes

Amanda M. Holleran, Joshua G. Hunter, Brian D. Giordano, and
Adolph S. Flemister, Jr.

BACKGROUND

- Varus or valgus angulation of the lesser toes can result in significant pain and disability and can be grouped broadly into the following subcategories:
  - Crossover or crossunder second toe
  - Isolated metatarsophalangeal (MTP) joint angular deformity
  - Clinodactyly
  - Congenital crossover fifth toe
  - Curly toe deformity
- Understanding the cause behind each type of angular toe deformity is crucial for determining whether surgical or nonsurgical management is appropriate.
- Angular toe deformities can occur as the result of a variety of intrinsic or extrinsic factors, including inflammatory arthritis, trauma, congenital abnormalities, neuromuscular disorders, and poorly fitting shoe wear.
- Surgical management options are based on the severity of the deformity, degree of response to nonsurgical management, and underlying cause of the deformity. A variety of surgical procedures have been proposed to address angular deformity of the lesser toes:
  - Tenodesis
  - Tenotomy
- Tendon transfer
- Soft tissue release
- Soft tissue lengthening
- Proximal basilar osteotomy
- Resection arthroplasty
- Interphalangeal fusion
- Outcomes are predicated on the degree of return to full activity, pain relief, and recurrence of deformity.

DEFINITIONS

- *Crossover second toe deformity* (**FIG 1A**) is characterized by a second toe that lies dorsomedially relative to the hallux.
- *Isolated MTP angular deformity* (**FIG 1B**) is varus or valgus angulation of the lesser toes occurring solely through the MTP joint. This often occurs in conjunction with great toe varus or valgus deformity.
- *Clinodactyly* (**FIG 1C**) is varus or valgus deviation of a toe caused by angulation within the phalanx itself. This condition is more commonly seen in the fingers and is often associated with a syndrome (eg, symphalangism) or chromosomal disorder.
- *Congenital crossover fifth toe* (**FIG 1D**) represents a variable congenital anomaly involving the fifth MTP joint in which the small toe deviates medially and superiorly relative to the

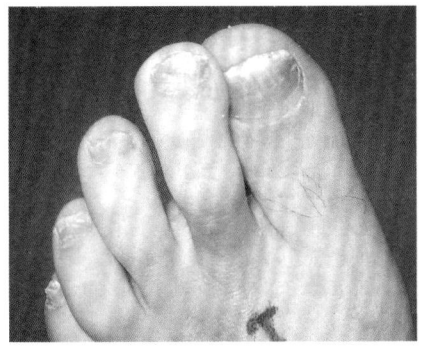
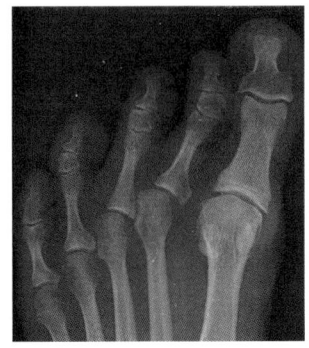
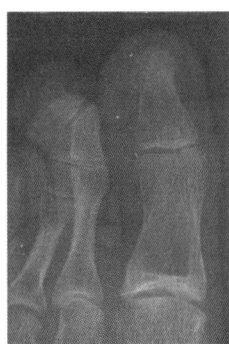
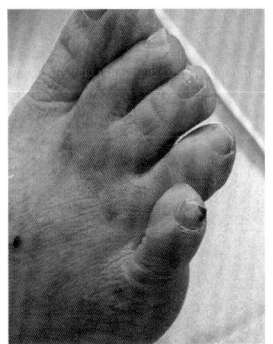
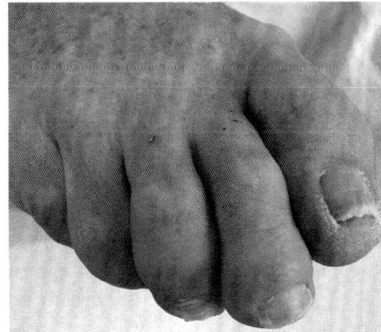

FIG 1 Deformities of the lesser toes. **A.** Crossover second toe deformity. **B.** Isolated MTP angular deformity. **C.** Clinodactyly. **D.** Congenital crossover of the fifth toe. **E.** Curly toe deformity.

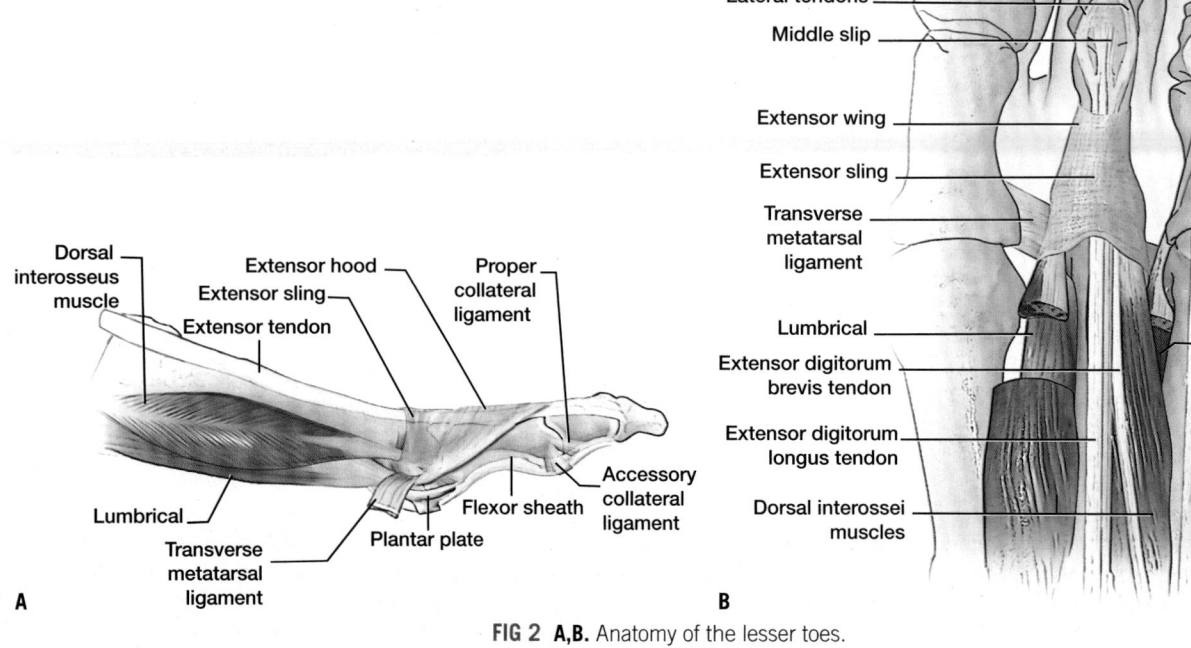

FIG 2 A,B. Anatomy of the lesser toes.

fourth toe. Patients typically complain of discomfort and irritation over the dorsum of the fifth toe, especially when wearing constrictive footwear.

- *Curly toe deformity* (**FIG 1E**) is a relatively common congenital anomaly, usually found in children, that may be related to intrinsic muscle paresis, although this relationship has not been clearly established. The deformity usually involves the fourth or fifth toe, or both, and is characterized by a flexible flexion deformity of the proximal interphalangeal (PIP) and distal interphalangeal (DIP) joints with underlapping of the fourth toe on the third and of the fifth toe on the fourth.

ANATOMY

- The extensor digitorum longus (EDL) forms three tendinous slips on the dorsum of each toe—the first inserts into the middle phalanx, and the other two merge and insert on the distal phalanx (**FIG 2**).
- In concert, the EDL and extensor digitorum brevis (EDB) extend the MTP, PIP, and DIP joints through their pull on the extensor hood.
- The flexor digitorum longus (FDL) courses deep to the flexor digitorum brevis (FDB) on the plantar surface of the toe and acts as a powerful flexor at the DIP joint.
- The PIP and MTP joints are flexed through the combined action of the FDL and FDB tendons.
- The intrinsics first pass plantar to the axis of MTP joint rotation and then dorsal to the axis of motion of the PIP and DIP joints. This anatomic relationship allows the intrinsics to act as flexors at the MTP joint and extensors at the PIP and DIP joints.
  - Disruption of this delicate balance can lead to problematic disequilibrium between the intrinsics and extrinsics,

which in turn can result in characteristic lesser toe deformities and associated pressure phenomena.

- The plantar plate originates on the metatarsal head and inserts on the proximal phalanx on the plantar surface. It is arguably the most important stabilizer, as it is centrally located and has multiple attachments. The plantar plate resists tensile loads in the sagittal plane as the joint goes into dorsiflexion.[4]
- The medial collateral ligament (MCL) and lateral collateral ligament (LCL) play a vital role in stabilizing the MTP joint by acting as static constraints to joint subluxation or dislocation. The collaterals originate from the dorsal aspect of the metatarsal head and insert distally both at the base of the proximal phalanx and at the plantar plate.
- In addition to providing stability in the transverse plane, the collaterals resist dorsal subluxation of the proximal phalanx on the metatarsal head. Laxity of the collaterals is commonly noted intraoperatively with angular lesser toe deformities and, in some cases, is thought to play a causative role in the development of these deformities.

CROSSOVER DEFORMITY OF THE SECOND TOE

PATHOGENESIS

- Crossover second toe deformity most commonly occurs as the result of attritional rupture of plantar plate, the LCL, and lateral capsule of the second toe.
  - Pathology in the plantar plate tends to occur at its distal attachment on the base of the proximal phalanx due to its attachment with loose synovial tissue.[4]
- Frequently, this specific type of lesser toe deformity occurs in association with long-standing hallux valgus.

- Association with a long second metatarsal and attenuation of the first dorsal interosseous tendon and plantar plate is also common.
- Destabilization of the second MTP joint can also occur as the result of trauma, synovitis related to underlying inflammatory arthritides such as rheumatoid arthritis, nonspecific or chronic synovitis, overloading of the second ray, constriction from narrow toe box shoes, or connective tissue diseases such as systemic lupus erythematosus.
- Neuromuscular disorders such as diabetic neuropathy, Charcot-Marie-Tooth disorder, poliomyelitis, or Friedreich ataxia can also disrupt the dynamic stability of the foot and, subsequently, that of the lesser toes.
- Often, medial soft tissue such as the MCL, medial capsule, and interosseous and lumbrical tendons are contracted at the MTP joint.

NATURAL HISTORY

- Early synovitis, then subluxation, and finally dorsomedial or inferomedial dislocation are the characteristic stages in the natural progression of this coronal plane deformity.

PATIENT HISTORY AND PHYSICAL FINDINGS

- Crossover second toe deformity presents either as a dorsomedially subluxated second toe that crosses up and over the hallux or as an inferomedially subluxated second toe that crosses under the great toe.
- There is often associated hyperextension or hyperflexion at the proximal phalanx at the MTP joint and adduction of the second ray from the midline.
- A painful intractable plantar keratotic lesion beneath the second metatarsal head or dorsal corn over any portion of the second phalanges (particularly over the PIP joint) may be due to impingement of the toe box of the shoe.
- Instability of the plantar plate can be evaluated by the drawer test applied in the sagittal plane, and a positive test is pathognomonic for an unstable MTP joint.

IMAGING AND DIAGNOSTIC STUDIES

- All angular deformities involving the lesser toes can be appropriately studied by examining standard anteroposterior (AP), lateral, and oblique radiographs of the affected foot.
- Magnetic resonance imaging (MRI) can be helpful in diagnosing a plantar plate rupture. They have been useful in identifying the location and severity of the tearing in the plantar plate as well as damage to adjacent soft tissues.

NONOPERATIVE MANAGEMENT

- In general, conservative measures are more effective for treatment of subluxation of the second MTP joint versus dislocation.
- Activity modification is usually necessary to resolve underlying second MTP synovitis.
- Some degree of relief is usually afforded by avoidance of shoes with a tight, narrow toe box and by modification of shoe wear to include a broad toe box with extra depth.
- Splinting or taping the second toe in plantarflexion may relieve symptoms but does not correct deformity. This is most helpful early on in the disease process when the deformity is mild to moderate.[5]

- Placing a metatarsal pad in the shoe may help relieve pressure on the plantar plate.
- Wearing a shoe with a firm sole may prevent propagation of synovitis and further attenuation of the plantar plate.
- Metatarsal bars or a full-length rocker bottom sole with metal inlay may provide additional means of relieving pressure at the second MTP joint.

SURGICAL MANAGEMENT

Preoperative Planning

- All radiographs should be carefully examined to evaluate the degree of deformity of the hallux and surrounding lesser toes.
- Clinical examination should determine whether the deformities at the interphalangeal and MTP joints are flexible or rigid.
- Hallux valgus deformity, which does not allow for correction of the second toe, must be corrected.
- PIP deformity should be corrected with an interphalangeal joint fusion or arthroplasty.

Surgical Options and Indications

- Dorsal capsular release and repair of the LCL is a soft tissue realignment procedure that is indicated for mild crossover toe deformities without MTP joint subluxation or dislocation.
- The Girdlestone-Taylor procedure, or transfer of the split FDL tendon to the dorsum of the proximal phalanx, is a well-established procedure.[6,17] All grades of second toe deformity may benefit from it.
  - Initially described for the correction of flexible lesser toe deformities in patients with underlying neuromuscular disorders, this procedure has undergone various modifications throughout the years.
  - A PIP resection can be performed simultaneously for correction of rigid deformity.
- The EDB tendon transfer was originally described by Haddad et al[7] and is most appropriate in patients with mild to moderate deformity. Benefits include better control of sagittal plane motion and less stiffness than is associated with an FDL transfer.
- A modification of the EDB transfer, as popularized by Lui and Chan,[11] attempts to reduce the supination force of the transferred EDB as well as to provide a more robust side-to-side suture repair.
- Recently, several authors have described direct repair of the plantar plate for surgical correction of instability.[13] This correction addresses subluxation and dislocation of the MTP joint.
- Proximal phalanx basilar osteotomy is indicated for resistant angular deformities of the lesser toes and for failure to achieve multiplanar correction after complete soft tissue release at the MTP joint.
- The Weil osteotomy can be used to shorten the second metatarsal as well as to decrease the overall prominence of the second metatarsal head **(FIG 3)**.
  - This procedure is used for persistent subluxation of the second MTP joint after adequate soft tissue procedures have been performed.
  - It may be used as an alternative to a flexor to extensor transfer.
  - A flexor to extensor transfer can be performed simultaneously for additional correction in refractory cases.

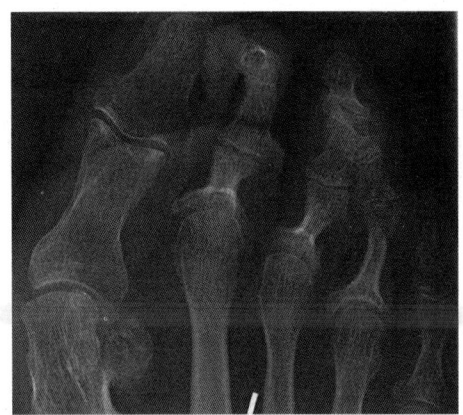 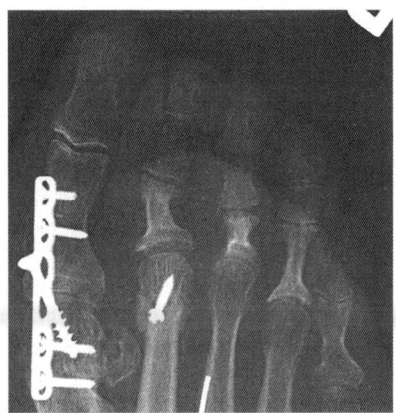

FIG 3 A,B. The Weil osteotomy can be used to shorten the second metatarsal as well as to decrease the overall prominence of the second metatarsal head.

DORSAL CAPSULAR RELEASE AND REPAIR OF THE LATERAL COLLATERAL LIGAMENT

- The second MTP joint is approached via a 3-cm longitudinal, curved, or Z-shaped incision.
- A dorsal incision in the adjacent web space is also appropriate.
- The EDL and EDB are sectioned, and the dorsal capsule is opened **(TECH FIG 1A)**.
- Release of the EDL, EDB, and dorsal capsule allows the sagittal plane deformity to be addressed **(TECH FIG 1B)**.

- Balancing the MCL and the LCL is required to address coronal plane deformity.
  - The contracted MCL is released off the metatarsal and the phalanx from dorsal to plantar.
  - The attenuated LCL is then repaired in a shortened fashion **(TECH FIG 1C)**.
- For added stabilization, the MTP joint is pinned from distal to proximal using a 0.054- or 0.062-inch Kirschner wire (K-wire).

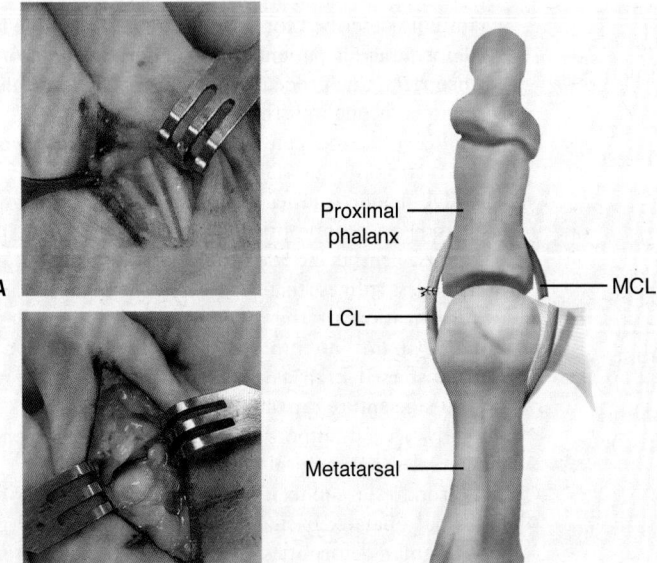

Proximal phalanx

MCL

LCL

Metatarsal

TECH FIG 1 A. The EDL and the EDB are sectioned, and the dorsal capsule is opened. **B.** The EDL, EDB, and dorsal capsule are released. **C.** Repair of the LCL in a shortened fashion and release of the MCL off the metatarsal and phalanx.

FLEXOR TO EXTENSOR TENDON TRANSFER (GIRDLESTONE-TAYLOR PROCEDURE)

- The second MTP joint is approached through a longitudinal dorsal incision extending from the MTP joint to the PIP joint.
- The extensor tendons are retracted laterally, and the MTP joint is entered through a dorsal capsulotomy.

- The MCL is then sectioned.
- In patients with more advanced deformity, further correction may be obtained with EDL lengthening and EDB tenotomy as well as a release of the interosseous and lumbrical tendons.

TECHNIQUES

- A small transverse plantar incision is then made at the level of the proximal flexion crease, and the FDL tendon is identified using blunt dissection (TECH FIG 2A).
- The FDL tendon is released from its insertion onto the distal phalanx via a percutaneous tenotomy at the level of the DIP joint.
- The released FDL tendon is brought into the proximal wound and split centrally along the median raphe (TECH FIG 2B).
- Each limb is then passed from plantar to dorsal on either side of the proximal phalanx, avoiding injury to adjacent neurovascular structures.
- When a fixed contracture of the PIP is present, resection of the distal one-fourth of the proximal phalanx can be performed after the extensor hood and collateral ligaments are incised.

- The limbs of the split FDL are then passed over the extensor hood, tensioned (with the ankle held in a neutral or slightly dorsiflexed position), and sutured to each other with 4-0 nonabsorbable sutures (TECH FIG 2C).
- Manual manipulation of the proximal phalanx can be performed to assess the tensioning of the transferred tendons. The MTP joint should remain slightly mobile, not overly tight, when correct tensioning is achieved.
- A 0.062-inch K-wire is driven, in retrograde fashion, from the base of the proximal phalanx distally through the tip of the toe and then antegrade across the MTP joint with the toe held parallel to the floor or weight-bearing surface of the foot.
- The incisions are then closed in a layered fashion (TECH FIG 2D).

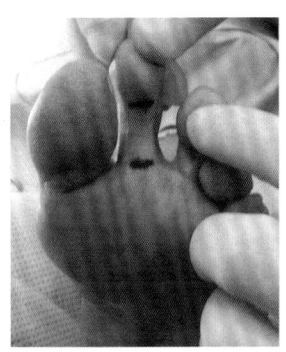 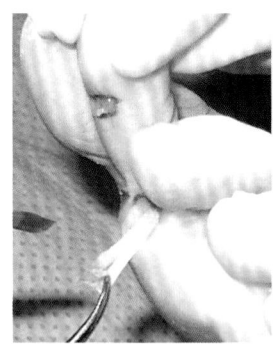 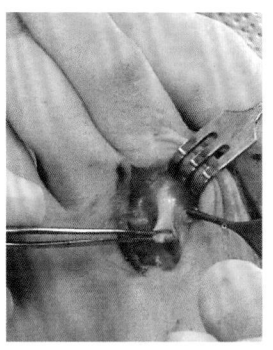 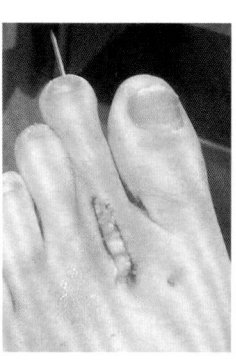

TECH FIG 2 A. A small transverse plantar incision is then made at the level of the proximal flexion crease. **B.** The released FDL tendon is brought into the proximal wound and split centrally along the median raphe. **C.** The limbs of the split FDL are passed over the extensor hood, tensioned, and sutured. **D.** The incisions are then closed in a layered fashion.

EXTENSOR DIGITORUM BREVIS TENDON TRANSFER

- A dorsal approach similar to that used for a flexor to extensor transfer is used to perform an EDB tendon transfer.
- The EDB tendon is identified and freed proximally after dissection and release of the MTP joint capsule and Z lengthening of the EDL tendon.

- After two 4-0 stay sutures have been placed longitudinally into the tendon 4 cm proximal to the MTP joint, the tendon is transected between these two sutures (TECH FIG 3A).
- Care is taken to maintain the integrity of the distal EDB tendon insertion, and the distal EDB tendon stump is then passed

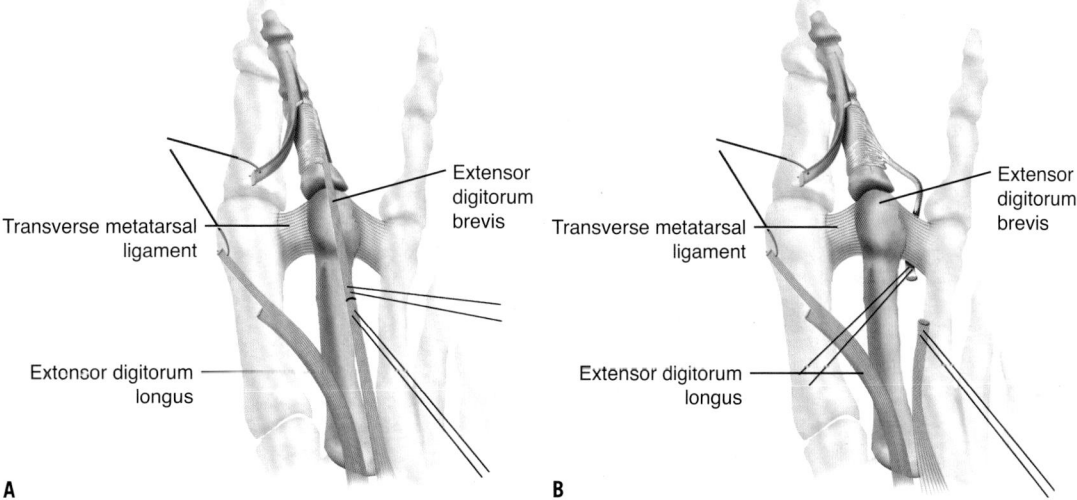

TECH FIG 3 A. Stay suture placement along the EDB tendon and transaction point identified by *dashed line* between the two sutures. The EDL tendon is also shown after Z-lengthening. **B.** Transfer of distal EDB stump plantar to transverse metatarsal ligament and lateral to second metatarsal. *(continued)*

TECHNIQUES

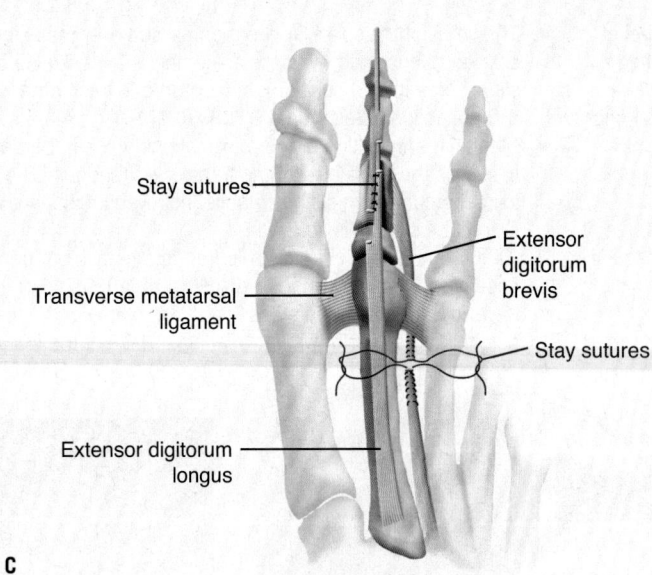

Stay sutures

Extensor digitorum brevis

Transverse metatarsal ligament

Stay sutures

Extensor digitorum longus

C

TECH FIG 3 *(continued)* **C.** End-to-end repair of the EDB tendon with the toe pinned in a corrected position. The Z-lengthened EDL tendon is also shown following repair.

from distal to proximal underneath the transverse metatarsal ligament and lateral to the MTP joint **(TECH FIG 3B)**.
- A 0.062-inch K-wire is placed across the MTP joint with the toe held in a corrected position.

- The passed distal limb of the EDB is then tensioned and secured by a direct end-to-end tendon repair to the proximal stump, with the joint held in congruity **(TECH FIG 3C)**.

MODIFIED EXTENSOR DIGITORUM TENDON TRANSFER

- Under tourniquet control, a lazy S incision is used to expose the EDL and EDB of the second toe.
- A long Z incision of the EDL is made, and the EDB is released at the distal metatarsal level **(TECH FIG 4A)**.
- The MTP joint is entered transversely, and the MCL is sectioned.
- A transverse bone tunnel is placed through the proximal aspect of the proximal phalanx using a 2.5-mm drill.
- The distal stump of the EDL is passed through the bone tunnel from medial to lateral. The passed tendon is then shuttled from

distal to proximal, plantar to the transverse metatarsal ligament between the second and third metatarsals.
- The transferred tendon is tensioned, and a 0.062-inch K-wire is inserted across the MTP joint to hold the toe in a corrected position **(TECH FIG 4B)**.
- The distal stump of the EDL is then repaired side to side with the proximal stump of the EDB.
- The proximal stump of the EDL is then sutured to the distal stump of the EDB in side-to-side fashion.

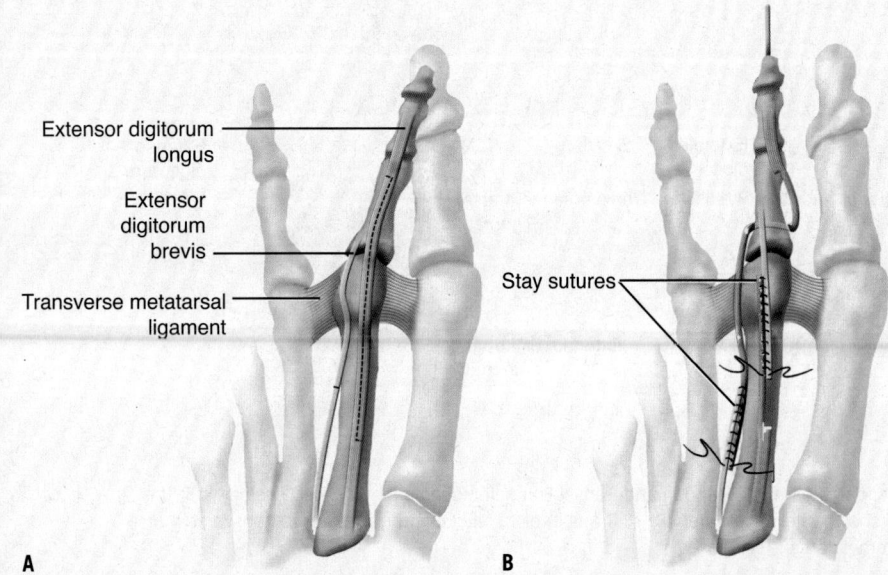

Extensor digitorum longus

Extensor digitorum brevis

Transverse metatarsal ligament

Stay sutures

A   B

TECH FIG 4 A. Long Z incision through the EDL tendon. EDB transected at the level of the distal metatarsal shaft. **B.** Correction of deformity and pinning. The distal EDL stump has been shuttled through the transverse drill tunnel and anastomosed to the proximal stump of the EDB tendon. The proximal stump of EDL has been repaired side to side with the distal stump of the EDB.

PROXIMAL PHALANX BASILAR OSTEOTOMY

- An oblique incision is made over the MTP joint extending longitudinally onto the dorsum of the base of the proximal phalanx.
- Extensor tenotomy or lengthening and dorsal capsular incision with collateral release can all be added for further soft tissue correction.
- If complete correction is not attainable following these soft tissue releases, the approach can be extended to the base of the proximal phalanx, where a proximal phalanx basilar osteotomy can subsequently be performed.

- Davis et al[3] described using a small awl to make multiple perforations at the base of the proximal phalanx opposite the direction of toe deviation (**TECH FIG 5A**).
- After penetrating the appropriate cortex multiple times, taking care not to perforate the opposite cortex, finger pressure alone is used to complete the osteotomy and correct the underlying deformity (**TECH FIG 5B**).
- A 0.062-inch K-wire is placed percutaneously if added stability is needed.

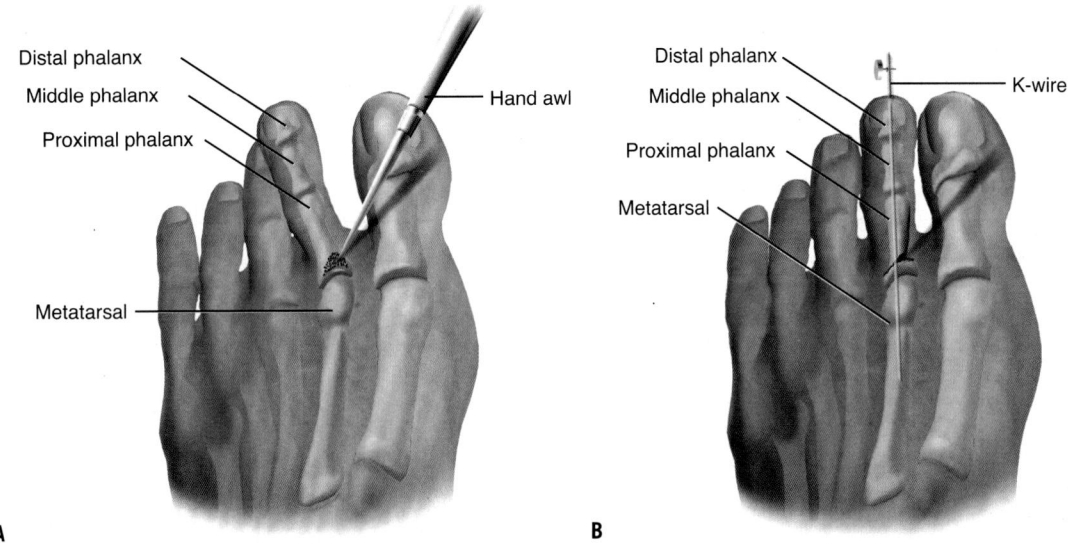

TECH FIG 5 A. A hand awl is used to make multiple perforations in the medial cortex of the proximal phalanx. **B.** K-wire stabilization after osteotomy completion and positional correction.

DISTAL HORIZONTAL METATARSAL OSTEOTOMY (WEIL OSTEOTOMY)

- A dorsal 3-cm longitudinal incision is made over the second MTP joint, the extensor tendons are retracted, and the capsule is incised to expose the MTP joint.
- Collaterals are then released to facilitate delivery of the second metatarsal head dorsally out of the wound.
- Plantarflexion at the MTP allows for optimal exposure of the articular surface of the second metatarsal.
- With use of an oscillating saw, a cut is initiated at the articular surface of the most dorsal aspect of the second metatarsal head.

- The cut is carried proximally and parallel to the plantar plane of the foot (**TECH FIG 6A**).
- The plantar osteotomy fragment is then grasped with a pointed reduction clamp and slid proximally to achieve the desired amount of shortening (**TECH FIG 6B**).
- The osteotomy is finally secured with a compression screw placed in lag fashion from dorsal to plantar (**TECH FIG 6C**).
- The excess dorsal bony prominence is shaved to a smooth surface.

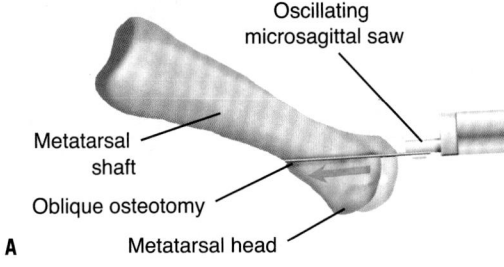

TECH FIG 6 A. Diagram of osteotomy plane, made using an oscillating saw. Care must be taken to initiate the saw cut at the dorsal most aspect of the second metatarsal head. *(continued)*

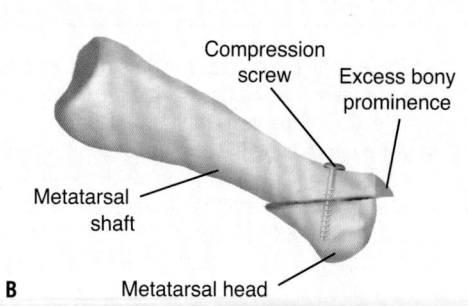

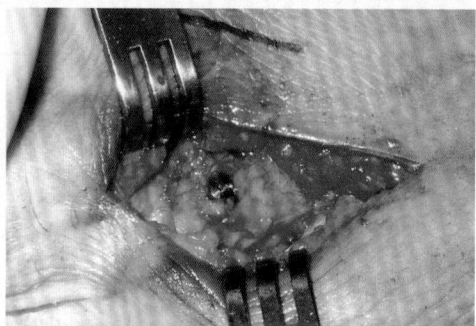

TECH FIG 6 *(continued)* **B.** The osteotomy is slid proximally and fixed with a compression screw from dorsal to plantar. **C.** The osteotomy is finally secured with a compression screw placed in lag fashion from dorsal to plantar.

DIRECT REPAIR OF THE PLANTAR PLATE WITH WEIL OSTEOTOMY

- Diagnostic arthroscopy prior to repair of the plantar plate has been described. This allows for confirmation of the plantar plate tear with clinical exam and MRI findings.[13]
- Two small dorsal incisions on either side of the MTP joint may be used if a diagnostic arthroscopy is performed prior to repair and can then be incorporated into an "S-shaped" incision when performing the open repair.
- If no diagnostic arthroscopy is performed, a dorsal 3-cm longitudinal incision is made over the second MTP joint, the extensor tendons are retracted or elongated (Z-plasty), and the capsule is incised to expose the MTP joint. A Weil osteotomy is then performed as described earlier to allow full visualization of the plantar plate.
- Visualization of the plantar plate can be further enhanced with longitudinal traction or various other distraction techniques **(TECH FIG 7A)**.
- Completion of the plantar plate tear may be necessary if a direct repair of the partial tear is possible. This should

be performed as close to the phalanx as possible when needed.
- The plantar surface of the proximal phalanx is roughened with a rongeur or curette to facilitate healing of the repair to the bone.
- The plantar plate tear is then identified **(TECH FIG 7B)**, and the plate needs to be mobilized to allow for repair with longitudinal or transverse sutures in mattress fashion based on the orientation of the tear.
- Two vertical holes are then drilled using a K-wire in the proximal phalanx from dorsal to plantar **(TECH FIG 7C)**. These should exit the plantar phalanx just below the plantar surface.
- The sutures from the plantar plate repair are then shuttled through these holes from plantar to dorsum and tied over the top for fixation with the toe held in 20 degrees of plantarflexion.
- The Weil osteotomy is then stabilized as described earlier **(TECH FIG 7D)**, and any soft tissue corrections may also be performed at this time.

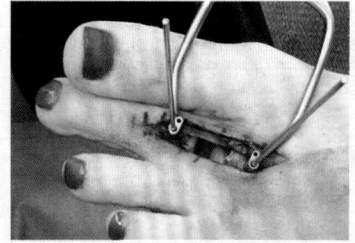

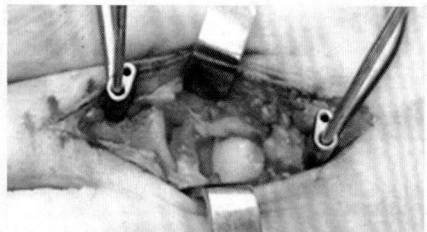

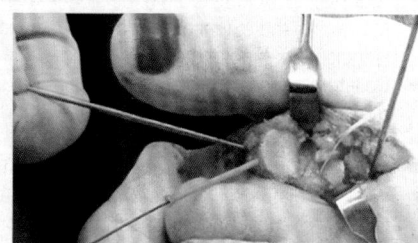

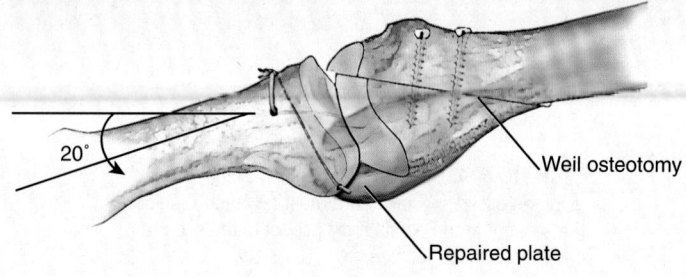

TECH FIG 7 A. Distraction across the MTP joint after performing a Weil osteotomy. **B.** Identification of the plantar plate rupture at the base of the proximal phalanx. **C.** Suture is passed through the plantar plate, and the bone tunnels are prepared in the proximal phalanx. **D.** The completed plantar plate repair with fixation of the Weil osteotomy.

Pearls and Pitfalls

Dorsal Capsular Release and Repair of the LCL	• Procedure is best used to correct mild or early deformities. • Before pinning the second toe, the surgeon should ensure that the toe is able to passively lie in a corrected position after adequate dorsal capsular release and LCL repair. There is a high probability that if the surgeon has to rely on pin fixation to maintain the second toe in a corrected position, this correction will be lost over time.
Flexor to Extensor Tendon Transfer	• Procedure should be used for correction of moderate crossover toe deformity or for toes that display a tendency to resublux after initial correction. • When passing the FDL through the proximal plantar incision, flexing the toe will further relax the flexor and facilitate delivery of the tendon to the proximal plantar incision. • Overtensioning either limb of the FDL prior to repair can result in further malalignment of the toe and shift the toe into even greater varus or valgus deformity. • Rapid postoperative mobilization and early K-wire removal (2 weeks postoperatively) are crucial to preventing uncomfortable postoperative stiffness.
EDB Tendon Transfer	• Rapid postoperative mobilization and K-wire removal (2 weeks postoperatively) are crucial to preventing uncomfortable postoperative stiffness. • For advanced deformity (rigid stage 3 or 4), FDL transfer may be more appropriate. • Anchoring the brevis tendon into a metatarsal head drill hole may lead to a higher recurrence rate than an end-to-end transfer. • Supination of the second toe may result from overpull of the EDB.
Modified EDB Tendon Transfer	• The Z-lengthening of the EDL should be long enough to permit passage through the bone tunnel and eventual anastomosis of the transfer. • The EDB is cut at the distal metatarsal level to preserve adequate length to facilitate the transfer. • Drill tunnel placement is critical. The tunnel should be placed close to the longitudinal axis of the proximal axis and not too dorsal or plantar. • Correction of the hyperextension deformity relies mainly on adequate soft tissue release. Reflection of the plantar capsule and plate off the metatarsal head using an elevator may be necessary to accomplish adequate soft tissue release. • Placing the drill tunnel too dorsal will lead to residual supination; locating it too plantar will lead to hyperextension of the MTP joint.
Proximal Phalanx Basilar Osteotomy	• If complete correction of the crossover toe deformity is not attainable following initial soft tissue releases, the approach can be extended to the base of the proximal phalanx, where a proximal phalanx basilar osteotomy can be performed. • Care should be taken to prevent perforation of the far cortex when performing the osteotomy, or instability and delayed bony union may result.
Weil Osteotomy	• The distal fragment of the osteotomy can be preliminarily secured with a K-wire prior to completion of the dorsal to plantar compression screw fixation. • Pinning across the MTP joint will decrease the risk of floating toe deformity. • Avoid securing the distal osteotomy fragment in plantarflexion; if anything, err on the side of dorsiflexion if accepting mild angular deformity in the sagittal plane.
Plantar Plate Repair	• A flexor to extensor transfer in addition to the Weil osteotomy has been shown to increase the stability of the toe in the sagittal plane.[2] • It is important to hold the foot in 20 degrees of flexion as the sutures are being tied to appropriately tension the plantar plate.

POSTOPERATIVE CARE

• Dorsal capsular release and repair of the LCL
   • The pin is left in for approximately 3 to 4 weeks.
   • Immediate ambulation is allowed in a stiff postoperative shoe.
   • Once the pin is removed, the toe is taped in plantarflexion for another 3 to 4 weeks.
   • The patient is progressed into normal shoe wear once the pin is removed.
• Girdlestone-Taylor procedure
   • Ambulation in a hard-soled shoe using only the heel is permitted immediately following surgery.

   • The K-wire is removed between 2 and 3 weeks postoperatively.
   • The patient is instructed to adhere to 6 additional weeks of taping the toe in slight plantarflexion and lateral deviation.
• EDB tendon transfer
   • Postoperative care is essentially identical to that used for a flexor to extensor transfer.
   • The percutaneously placed K-wire is maintained for 2 to 3 weeks, followed by an additional 6 weeks of taping the corrected toe to maintain alignment.
• Modified EDB tendon transfer: The pin is kept in place for 3 to 6 weeks followed by 6 additional weeks of toe taping.

- Proximal phalanx basilar osteotomy
  - After surgery, dressings are placed with the toe maintained in an overcorrected position.
  - The patient is placed in a hard-soled shoe, and dressing changes are performed weekly.
  - At 6 weeks postoperatively, the patient is advanced to a soft-soled shoe as tolerated.
  - K-wire is removed at 4 weeks postoperatively.
  - Postoperative radiographs are assessed at 4 to 6 weeks to evaluate for bony healing at the osteotomy site.
- Weil osteotomy
  - Sterile dressings are placed intraoperatively, and the toe is taped down in an overcorrected position.
  - Dressings are changed weekly until drainage ceases.
  - Weight bearing in a postoperative shoe is resumed immediately after surgery.
- Plantar plate repair
  - A period of protected weight bearing through the heel is recommended immediately after surgery for a period of 6 weeks. This can be progressed as tolerated into athletic shoes at this time point.
  - Dressings changed as needed until no drainage is present.
  - Physical therapy may be needed to facilitate conditioning of the extrinsic flexors of the lesser digits.

OUTCOMES

- Girdlestone-Taylor procedure
  - Thompson and Deland[18] performed FDL flexor to extensor tendon transfers on 13 feet in 11 patients and reported that at an average follow-up of 33.4 months, all patients had substantial pain relief, with 8 of 13 becoming completely pain free.
  - They concluded that although flexor to extensor tendon transfer is successful in reestablishing MTP joint congruity and relieving pain due to instability, rapid postoperative mobilization and early K-wire removal (2 weeks postoperatively) are crucial to preventing uncomfortable postoperative stiffness.
- EDB tendon transfer
  - Haddad and colleagues[7] performed either flexor to extensor or EDB tendon transfer on 38 patients (42 feet) with an average follow-up of 51.6 months.
  - Of the 31 patients (35 feet) followed until their final examination, 24 were satisfied with their surgical correction, 6 were satisfied with reservations, and 1 was dissatisfied.
  - No statistical significance in clinical outcome was demonstrated between patients who underwent FDL tendon transfer and those who underwent EDB tendon transfer, but Haddad et al[7] recommended the technique because they believed that it demonstrated better patient satisfaction and improved flexibility compared with the FDL transfer.
  - Other advantages favoring EDB transfer over FDL transfer that were cited were better postoperative range of motion (78 degrees for EDB vs. 62 degrees for FDL) and hence better patient satisfaction, decrease in recurrence of deformity (14%), and better pain control (71% asymptomatic; 26% mild pain).
- Weil osteotomy
  - Hofstaetter and colleagues[9] analyzed their results at 1 and 7 years in 25 feet using the Weil osteotomy for treatment of instability at the MTP joint.

- Good to excellent results were obtained in 21 feet (84%) after 1 year and in 22 (88%) after 7 years.
  - The authors demonstrated marked improvement in pain, diminished plantar callus formation, and an increase in walking capacity.
  - Adverse results included recurrent instability, floating toes, and restricted motion at the MTP joint, but these complications were often not clinically significant.
- Plantar plate repair
  - Nery and colleagues[13] reported that 77% of their prospective cohort of 55 plantar plate repairs had improvement of their American Orthopaedic Foot and Ankle Society (AOFAS) scores and reduction of visual analog scale (VAS) from 8 to 1 at 17 months postoperatively.
  - The authors also reported that all surgically repaired toes were congruent at 17 months with weight-bearing films.
  - Weil et al[20] similarly reported a significant improvement in VAS from 7.3 to 1.7 postoperatively at 22.5 months in a retrospective group of 15 feet.
  - The authors reported that 77% (10 of 13) of their patients were either satisfied or very satisfied with their outcome.
  - Flint et al[5] reported a prospective case series evaluating the results of plantar plate repair from a dorsal approach with a Weil osteotomy in 97 feet with 138 plantar plate tears. They were followed for 12 months and had "good" to "excellent" satisfaction scores. They demonstrated an improvement in the VAS pain scale, AOFAS score, and decreased MTP joint motion.

COMPLICATIONS

- Dorsal capsular release and repair of the LCL
  - Recurrence
  - MTP stiffness
  - Persistent swelling
  - Failure to achieve correction
- Girdlestone-Taylor procedure
  - Swelling
  - Recurrent deformity
  - Stiffness
  - Hyperextension
- EDB tendon transfer
  - Recurrent crossover toe deformity or failure to achieve complete correction of deformity
  - Infection
  - Symptomatic incisional scar formation
  - Stiffness of the MTP joint, especially with flexor to extensor tendon transfer
- Proximal phalanx basilar osteotomy
  - Infection
  - Loss of correction with persistent angular deformity
  - Failure of union at the osteotomy site
- Weil osteotomy
  - Persistent dorsiflexion at the MTP joint (floating toe deformity)
  - Claw toe
  - Nonunion or malunion at the osteotomy site
  - Stiffness at the MTP joint due to incorporation of articular surface into osteotomy cut
  - Overcorrection with excessive shortening of the second metatarsal
  - Hardware failure or prominence

- Infection
- Neurovascular insult
- Plantar plate repair
  - Recurrence of the crossover deformity
  - MTP hyperextension
  - Metatarsalgia
  - Infection

ISOLATED METATARSOPHALANGEAL ANGULAR DEFORMITY

PATHOGENESIS

- Isolated MTP angular deformity of the lesser toes is defined as varus or valgus deformity exclusively at the MTP joint relative to the normal anatomic axis of the toe due to attritional rupture of the plantar plate, collaterals, and capsule.
- Second to fifth toes are usually involved.
- This type of deformity characteristically follows abnormal deviation of the hallux, which is frequently in a position of varus or valgus.

SURGICAL MANAGEMENT

- To achieve successful correction of the lesser toes, it is usually necessary to address any varus or valgus deformity of the hallux concomitantly.
- Procedures that are used to correct isolated MTP angular deformity are similar to those used for surgically treating mild or moderate crossover second toe deformities and are described earlier in this chapter.
- MTP joint subluxation has been treated in various ways, including synovectomy, soft tissue release, tendon transfers, and bony decompression; however, plantar plate repair has become more frequent in the literature.[13]

Pearls and Pitfalls

Isolated MTP Angular Deformity	• Deviations in the lesser toes tend to follow angular deformities of the hallux. To create lasting correction of the lesser toes, the surgeon must address deformity of the hallux concomitantly.
	• Failure to address associated deformity of the hallux can result in early loss of successful lesser toe correction.

CLINODACTYLY

PATHOGENESIS

- Clinodactyly refers to the medial or lateral deviation of a toe caused by true angulation within a phalanx.
- This type of lesser toe deformity is thought to result from a failure of segmentation between the normally transverse epiphysis and metaphysis.
- Often bilateral and familial, clinodactyly most frequently involves the DIP joint of the fourth and fifth digits, although any digit may be involved.

- There is also a strong predilection for involvement of the fingers with this lesser toe deformity.
- A variety of syndromes and chromosomal disorders have been linked to clinodactyly of the lesser toes (symphalangism, brachydactyly, trisomy 21, Turner syndrome, Holt-Oram syndrome, Marfan syndrome).
- An associated "delta phalanx," or a triangular middle phalanx, is sometimes associated with clinodactyly.

NATURAL HISTORY

- Clinodactyly is usually nonprogressive and no more than a cosmetic concern, although overlapping or underlapping of adjacent toes may occur.
- If significant overlap or underlap is present, impingement on adjacent digits may cause the patient to be symptomatic.

PATIENT HISTORY AND PHYSICAL FINDINGS

- The affected toe is deviated medially or laterally relative to the normal longitudinal axis of the toe.
- The DIP of the involved toe is the most common site of angulation.
- A complete physical examination should be performed because of the prevalence of clinodactyly with associated syndromes and chromosomal disorders.
- Impingement on adjacent toes due to overlapping or underlapping may cause indentation on the toes, local irritation, corns, or callosities at variable locations from associated pressure phenomenon.

IMAGING AND DIAGNOSTIC STUDIES

- All angular deformities involving the lesser toes can be appropriately studied by examining standard AP, lateral, and oblique radiographs of the affected foot.

NONOPERATIVE MANAGEMENT

- For symptomatic toes, strategic padding, stretching, taping, and accommodative shoe wear may temporarily alleviate certain components of a patient's discomfort. These conservative approaches are often ineffective, however.

SURGICAL MANAGEMENT

- Surgical options include wedge osteotomies, arthrodesis, and soft tissue lengthening procedures.[12]
- Both opening and closing wedge osteotomies can effectively address angulation at the affected joint.
- Closing wedge osteotomy or arthrodesis is indicated for the treatment of symptomatic clinodactyly of any severity grade.
- A closing wedge osteotomy can be performed at the middle or distal phalanx through a small transverse dorsal incision.
- Intercalary allograft can be used to perform an opening wedge osteotomy and thereby preserve much of the length of the digit, but Z-plasty of the skin must also be performed for added soft tissue correction.
- A closing wedge arthrodesis of the affected joint is an acceptable treatment method provided that excessive shortening of the digit is not present.
- Skin dermodesis may be added for further acceptability of correction.

CLOSING WEDGE OSTEOTOMY OR ARTHRODESIS

- The skin over the affected middle or distal phalanx is incised through a dorsal incision. Redundant skin, equal to the planned osteotomy, is carefully removed (**TECH FIG 8A**).
- Subperiosteal exposure is obtained at the apex of the deformity (**TECH FIG 8B**).
- A microsagittal saw is used to create the desired cut at an appropriate angle to facilitate a satisfactory correction.
- Care should be taken to preserve a small bridge of bone at the for portor

- The osteotomy fragment is removed, and the wedge is closed with manual manipulation (**TECH FIG 8C**).
- If an arthrodesis is desired, the closing wedge may be removed through the interphalangeal joint.
- Dermodesis is then performed, incorporating skin into the closure.
- Alternatively, a K-wire can be placed percutaneously in retrograde fashion for added stability.
- Sterile dressings are placed, emphasizing overcorrection of the affected toe

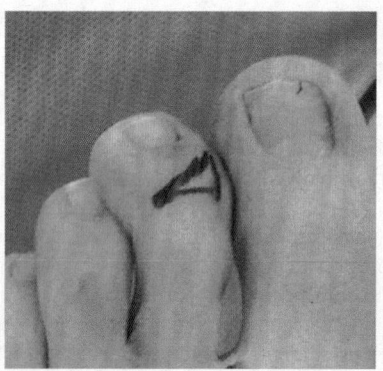 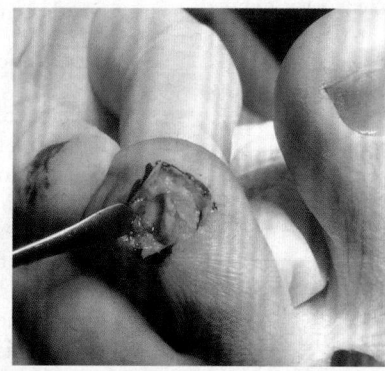 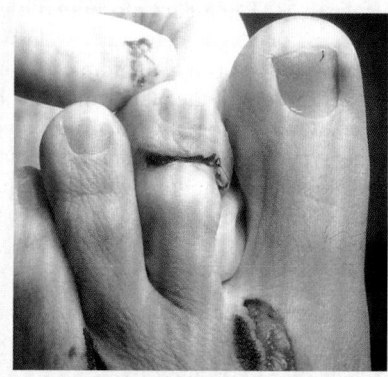

TECH FIG 8 A. The affected middle or distal phalanx is approached through a dorsal incision. **B.** Subperiosteal exposure is obtained at the apex of the deformity. **C.** The osteotomy fragment is removed, and the wedge is closed with manual manipulation.

TECHNIQUES

POSTOPERATIVE CARE

- If a K-wire is placed, it should be removed by 4 weeks postoperatively.
- Weight bearing in a postoperative shoe is permitted to tolerance immediately after surgery.
- Dressings should be changed until drainage subsides, with continued emphasis on maintaining an overcorrected position of the toe.

OUTCOMES

- Reports are largely anecdotal but overall have been favorable and support the continued use of the procedure.

COMPLICATIONS

- Neurovascular insult due to an overaggressive exposure
- Loss of reduction due to inadequate stabilization
- Wound healing problems
- Violation of the dorsal extensor structures
- Failure of bony healing at the osteotomy site

CONGENITAL CROSSOVER OF THE FIFTH TOE

PATHOGENESIS

- Although the underlying cause is unknown, congenital crossover fifth toe is widely recognized as a familial problem with an equal gender predilection.

- Often bilateral (20% to 30% of cases), congenital crossover fifth toe (or congenital overriding fifth toe) deformity causes pain with restrictive shoe wear and other symptoms in about half of all patients.[12]
- Pathoanatomy includes dorsomedial subluxation and adduction at the fifth MTP joint, with external rotation of the toe.
- There is associated contracture of the fifth toe EDL tendon, skin of the dorsal fourth web space, MCL, and dorsomedial MTP joint capsule.
- Often, impingement lesions at the base of the adjacent fourth toe identify the compressive influence of the overriding fifth toe due to its subluxated position.
- Furthermore, dorsal subluxation of the fifth toe at the MTP joint causes excessive pressure on the metatarsal head. This abnormal pressure distribution can lead to painful plantar callosity under the metatarsal head.
- When the fifth toe crosses *under* the fourth toe, painful callosity may develop under any portion of the toe that comes in abnormal contact with the ground surface during weight bearing.

NATURAL HISTORY

- Crossover fifth toe deformity is almost always present from birth and therefore is usually nonprogressive with respect to its degree of deformity.
- As stated, a painful callosity of either the fourth or fifth toes may develop over time because of pressure phenomenon in cases of long-standing deformity.
- Also, abnormal pressure distribution due to subluxation at the fifth MTP joint can eventually lead to pain

at the plantar surface of the fifth metatarsal head and metatarsalgia.
- Approximately half of all patients experience symptoms due to an overriding fifth toe.

PATIENT HISTORY AND PHYSICAL FINDINGS

- On examination, the fifth toe is noted to override the fourth toe to a variable degree.
- The interphalangeal joints are usually in normal full extension.
- There is often mild dorsiflexion at the MTP joint as well as malalignment and contracture of the skin at the fourth web space.
- In patients with long-standing deformity, the toe may assume a flattened, paddle-shaped appearance in the AP plane that is usually the result of years of compression by constrictive shoe wear.
- The toenail usually appears normal, and the toe is able to participate in active flexion and extension.
- A hard corn of the fifth toe or a soft corn between the fourth and fifth toes may also develop because of pressure phenomenon.

IMAGING AND DIAGNOSTIC STUDIES

- All angular deformities involving the lesser toes can be appropriately studied by examining standard AP, lateral, and oblique radiographs of the affected foot.
- Radiographs show dorsolateral subluxation at the MTP joint.

NONOPERATIVE MANAGEMENT

- Reliably ineffective, conservative treatment modalities include splinting, taping, accommodative shoe wear, and protective padding.

SURGICAL MANAGEMENT

- Many surgical approaches have been advocated for correction of crossover fifth toe deformity, and many modifications of these have been subsequently developed.
- The type of procedure selected is based on the severity of deformity encountered.
- Soft tissue procedures such as dorsal skin lengthening with Z-plasty of contracted skin, dermodesis of redundant skin, EDL tendon transfer, EDL lengthening or release, syndactylization of the fourth and fifth toes, and dorsal and medial capsular release have all been described and proved effective.[1,8,10–16,19,21]
- Bony resection, performed in isolation or in conjunction with any of the aforementioned soft tissue procedures, has also been successful in correcting crossover fifth toe deformity.
- The DuVries technique can be used to correct mild to moderate deformities.
- The Lapidus procedure can be used to address moderate to severe deformities.
  - In this technique, the EDL is isolated and rerouted under the MTP joint and attached to the abductor digiti quinti muscle or lateral joint capsule.
  - Unlike other procedures, the Lapidus technique allows for rotational correction, expanding the indications for its use.
- Proposed salvage operations include the so-called Ruiz-Mora procedure (proximal phalangectomy via a plantar elliptical incision with soft tissue realignment and plantar dermodesis) with or without syndactylization of the fifth toe to the fourth and even amputation.

DUVRIES TECHNIQUE

- A longitudinal incision is made over the fourth web space.
- An extensor tenotomy is performed, followed by dorsal capsulotomy and MCL release (**TECH FIG 9A**).
- The toe is plantarflexed, bringing the skin along the lateral margin of the incision distally (**TECH FIG 9B**).
- Layered suture closure is performed with the toe held in an overcorrected position of plantarflexion and lateral deviation to maximize the degree of soft tissue correction afforded by this technique (**TECH FIG 9C**).
- Soft tissue release and skin advancement alone are usually sufficient to hold the toe in an adequately corrected position. Otherwise, a K-wire can be placed percutaneously for added stabilization and correction.

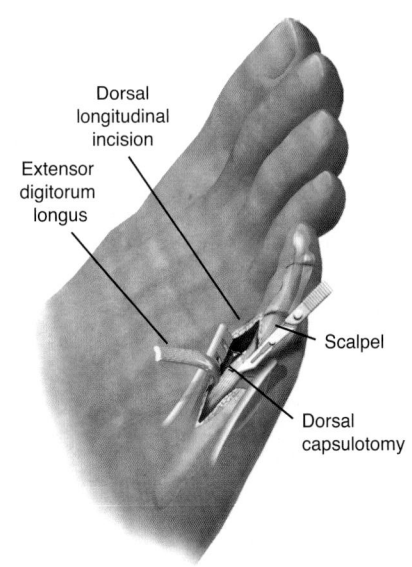

Dorsal longitudinal incision

Extensor digitorum longus

Scalpel

Dorsal capsulotomy

TECH FIG 9 A. A longitudinal incision is made over the fourth metatarsal interspace and extensor tenotomy is performed. *(continued)*

A

TECHNIQUES

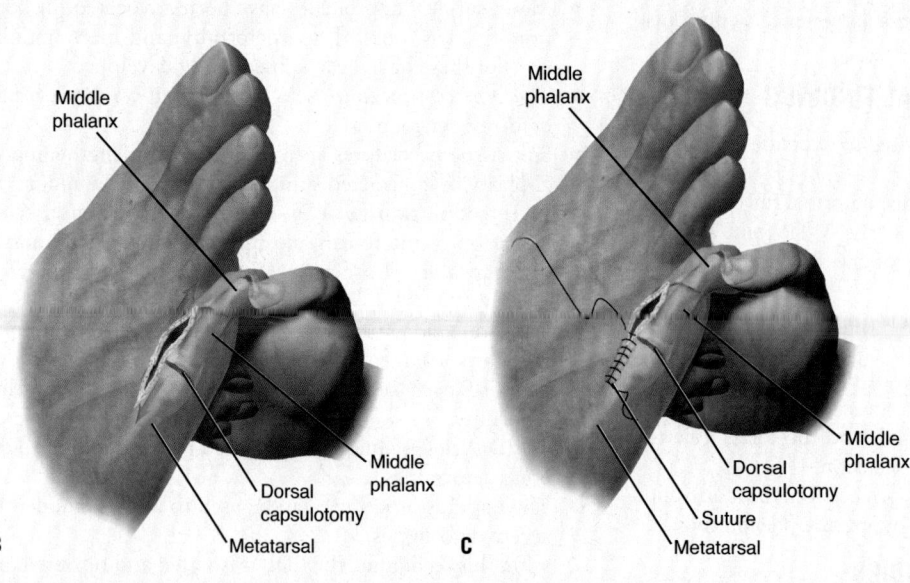

TECH FIG 9 *(continued)* **B.** Plantarflexion of the fifth toe brings the lateral margin of the incision distally and the medial margin proximally. **C.** Layered closure is undertaken with the toe held in an overcorrected position.

LAPIDUS PROCEDURE

- A longitudinal hockey stick–shaped or curvilinear incision is carried along the dorsomedial border of the fifth toe, from the level of the medial DIP joint distally to the fourth web space proximally.
- Through this incision, a thorough dorsomedial capsulotomy of the fifth MTP joint is made.
- Any adhesions encountered between the plantar capsule and metatarsal head should be released with a curved elevator to prevent hyperextension deformity of the MTP joint after capsular release.

- The hook of the hockey stick incision is then created by extending the incision over the dorsum of the fifth MTP joint laterally and proximally to the lateral aspect of the fifth MTP head.
- The extensor tendon is carefully exposed, maintaining the extensor hood expansion, and the fifth toe is forcibly plantarflexed, causing the extensor tendon to become taut.
- A second 1-cm incision is made transversely over the taut EDL tendon at the mid-diaphyseal level of the fifth metatarsal **(TECH FIG 10A)**.

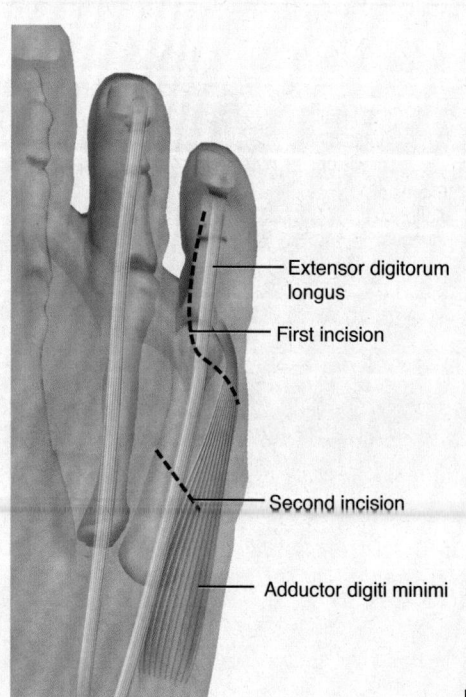

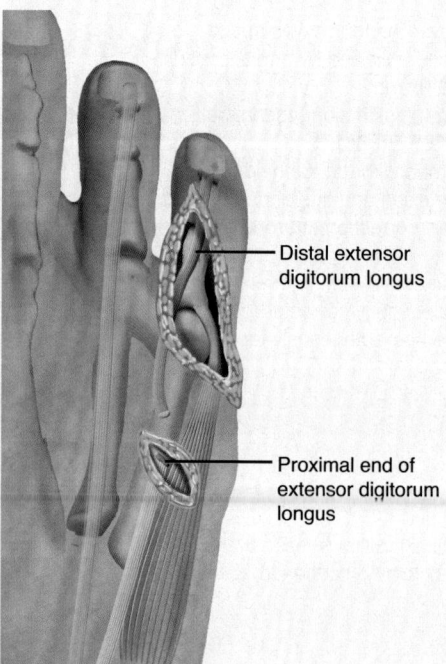

TECH FIG 10 A. Incisions for the Lapidus technique. **B.** EDL tenotomy using the more proximal of the two incisions. *(continued)*

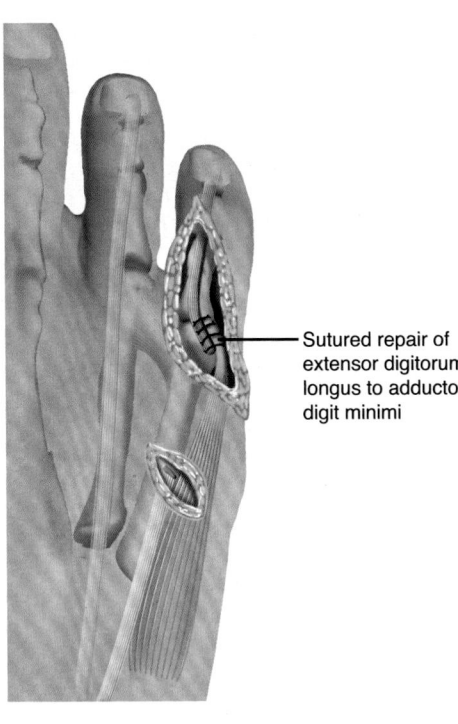

- Using this incision, an EDL tenotomy is performed (TECH FIG 10B).
- The distal limb of the EDL tendon is retrieved and then passed beneath the plantar aspect of the fifth toe from the dorsomedial DIP joint to the lateral aspect of the fifth MTP joint.
- The passed extensor tendon is then sutured to the conjoined tendon of the abductor and short flexor of the fifth toe (TECH FIG 10C).
- The fifth toe is held in an overcorrected position, and the transplanted extensor tendon is placed under slight tension prior to suture fixation.
- Skin is closed with interrupted sutures or with advancement techniques if significant skin contractures are present.

Sutured repair of extensor digitorum longus to adductor digit minimi

C

TECH FIG 10 *(continued)* **C.** Transfer of the distal EDL limb beneath the fifth toe and repair to the conjoined tendon.

TECHNIQUES

Pearls and Pitfalls

DuVries Technique	• Procedure is best used for mild deformities without associated rotational deformity of the toe. If any substantial rotational deformity is present, the Lapidus procedure is a more appropriate surgical solution. • Failure to hold the toe in an overcorrected position while performing soft tissue advancement and layered closure will result in a higher recurrence rate.
Lapidus Procedure	• Following dorsomedial capsulotomy, any adhesions encountered between the plantar capsule and metatarsal head should be released with a curved elevator to prevent hyperextension deformity of the MTP joint after capsular release. • If the toe is not held in an overcorrected position during repair, or if transplanted extensor tendon is incorrectly tensioned, early recurrence is common.

POSTOPERATIVE CARE

- DuVries technique
  - The toe is taped in a slightly overcorrected (plantarflexed and lateral) position for 6 weeks in a hard-soled postoperative shoe, after which unrestricted weight bearing is permitted.
  - If a pin is placed, it should be removed at 4 weeks postoperatively and the toe taped for a total of 6 weeks.
- Lapidus procedure
  - Postoperatively, the toe is dressed in a corrected position and weight bearing in a postoperative shoe is allowed. Sutures are removed at 2 weeks, and the toe is then taped in a corrected position for another 4 to 6 weeks. Regular shoe wear is allowed at 4 to 6 weeks.
  - Alternatively, if there is concern about the strength of the repair, the operative foot is maintained in a splint

for a total of 3 to 4 weeks and progression to full weight bearing and activity in a wide toe box shoe is gradually allowed.

OUTCOMES

- In his original description, Lapidus[10] notes that his experience with the procedure that bears his name resulted in satisfactory outcomes in all cases.

COMPLICATIONS

- A 5% to 10% recurrence rate has been reported using the DuVries technique. Mild swelling and clinically insignificant postoperative edema have also been reported.
- Circulatory insult and wound healing problems are potential risks of the Lapidus procedure but were not reported by Lapidus[10] in his original description. Recurrence of deformity has also been reported.

CROSSUNDER OF THE FIFTH TOE DEFORMITY (CONGENITAL CURLY TOE OR UNDERLAPPING FIFTH TOE)

PATHOGENESIS

- Although the cause of curly toe deformity is unknown, it is thought to be familial in nature, with a high instance of bilaterality.
- Frequently, this type of lesser toe deformity involves both fourth *and* fifth toes and is usually symmetric.
- Hypoplasia of the intrinsic musculature has been proposed as a causative influence on the development of curly toe deformity, but this notion has not been substantiated in the literature.
- The fifth toe is flexed, deviated plantarward in varus, and is laterally rotated at the DIP joint.
- The EDL and dorsal capsule are often attenuated, in contrast to overlapping fifth toe deformity.
- The plantar MTP joint capsule and FDL tendon are often contracted and shortened also.

NATURAL HISTORY

- As curly toe deformity is frequently congenital, progression is limited, and cosmesis is the major concern of parents and caretakers.
- The deformity is often asymptomatic in children and may improve without intervention.
- With initiation of weight bearing and different stages of shoe wear, chronic skin irritation can develop, the toenail may become short and flattened, and other pressure phenomena such as corns and callosities may develop.

PATIENT HISTORY AND PHYSICAL EXAMINATION

- As previously stated, the fifth toe is flexed, deviated plantarward in varus, and is laterally rotated at the DIP joint.
- The distal phalanx or the distal and middle phalanges underride the more medial toe as a result of these anatomic abnormalities.
- The deformity is usually flexible in childhood but may become rigid as an adult.

- In contrast to crossover fifth toe deformity, the skin in the web spaces is normally aligned, but it can become hyperemic from chronic irritation.
- Patients usually present with varying degrees of symptoms caused by pressure on the weight-bearing surface of the curly toe.
- Callosities, corns, or nail deformities can all develop and cause discomfort with curly toe deformities.

IMAGING AND DIAGNOSTIC STUDIES

- All angular deformities involving the lesser toes can be appropriately studied by examining standard AP, lateral, and oblique radiographs of the affected foot.
- Imaging of the curly toe is usually unnecessary and does not contribute significantly to management strategies.

NONOPERATIVE MANAGEMENT

- Conservative treatment modalities, including splinting, taping, accommodative shoe wear, and protective padding, may relieve symptoms but are usually ineffective for correcting the deformity.

SURGICAL MANAGEMENT

- For flexible deformities, FDL and FDB tenotomy have been recommended in the pediatric population.
- Flexor to extensor transfer, syndactylization with or without partial proximal phalangectomy, middle phalangectomy, and derotational procedures have all been proposed as surgical options to address the underlying pathoanatomy.
- A simple flexor tenotomy can be used to correct mild underlapping fifth toe deformity.
- Originally described by Taylor[17] and credited to Girdlestone[6] in 1951, the flexor to extensor tendon transfer is based on the premise that curly toe deformity results from weakness of the intrinsic musculature. This technique is described earlier in this chapter.
- The Thompson technique uses resection arthroplasty of the proximal phalanx in combination with Z-plasty of the skin to achieve derotation of the toe and correction of the deformity.[19] This technique is useful for addressing more rigid, severe crossunder fifth toe deformities.

TECHNIQUES

FLEXOR TENOTOMY

- Various surgical incisions have been successfully used to perform open flexor tenotomy, including a longitudinal incision proximal to the proximal flexor crease, a longitudinal incision distal to the proximal flexor crease, and a transverse incision 1 mm from the proximal flexor crease.
- It is important not to violate the proximal flexor crease with the incision, or scar formation may occur and recurrent deformity can develop.
- The flexor sheath is incised longitudinally, long and short flexor tendons are carefully exposed, and tendons are then transected at the same level (**TECH FIG 11**).
- Manual manipulation may be used to improve the adequacy of correction.
- The wound is closed with interrupted 3-0 absorbable sutures.

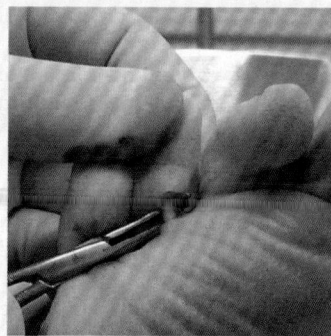

TECH FIG 11 The flexor sheath is incised longitudinally, the long and short flexor tendons are carefully exposed, and the tendons are then transected at the same level.

THOMPSON PROCEDURE

- A laterally based Z-type or elliptical incision is made over the proximal phalanx.
- Subperiosteal dissection is used to expose the distal half of the proximal phalanx.
- Partial phalangectomy of the distal 25% to 50% of the proximal phalanx or complete phalangectomy is then performed using a microsagittal saw.
- If persistent flexion contracture exists at the level of the PIP, a flexor tenotomy can be added for further correction.

- The digit is manually derotated, and a 0.045-inch K-wire is placed in a retrograde fashion across the PIP joint for stabilization.
- Additional soft tissue correction is obtained by using a reverse Z closure with 4-0 nylon vertical mattress sutures.
- If an elliptical incision was used initially, full-thickness closure is performed with the toe derotated using a dermodesis.

TECHNIQUES

Pearls and Pitfalls

Flexor Tenotomy	• Failure to transect all three plantar tendons can lead to an incomplete correction of the deformity. • It is important not to violate the proximal flexor crease with the incision, or scar formation may occur and recurrent deformity can develop.
Girdlestone-Taylor Procedure	• Isolated flexor tenotomy and flexor to extensor transfer appear to be equally efficacious. However, it is thought that the long flexor tenotomy represents the essential portion of either procedure and that flexor to extensor transfer is unnecessary.
Thompson Procedure	• If persistent flexion contracture exists at the level of the PIP, a flexor tenotomy can be added for further correction. • Overresection of the proximal phalanx can lead to a "floppy," unstable toe as well as a transfer lesion beneath the fourth metatarsal.

POSTOPERATIVE CARE

- Flexor tenotomy: Sterile dressings and elastic straps are applied to maintain correction, and the wound is inspected 10 days postoperatively.
- Girdlestone-Taylor procedure: Sterile dressings are applied, and full weight bearing is permitted in a short-leg plaster splint with an extended toe box. Splinting is maintained for 4 to 6 weeks.
- Thompson procedure: The foot is placed in a hard-soled shoe postoperatively, and pins are removed at 4 weeks. Using taping techniques, the toe is maintained in a derotated position for 6 additional weeks.

OUTCOMES

- Flexor tenotomy
  - Ross and Menelaus[15] reviewed their long-term outcome data on open flexor tenotomy performed in 62 children (188 toes) and found that at an average follow-up of 9.8 years, 95% of the toes examined had maintained satisfactory correction, and no patients were aware of any loss of toe function.
  - The fourth and fifth toes had significantly more fair and poor results, hypothesized to be due to greater rotational deformity of these toes, especially the fifth.
  - Overall, the authors concluded that open flexor tenotomy is a safe, reliable, and effective method for correcting curly toes in children and is preferable to flexor to extensor transfer.

- Girdlestone-Taylor procedure
  - In a double-blind randomized prospective trial, Hamer and colleagues[8] studied long-term data from 46 toes (19 patients) randomly assigned to either flexor tenotomy or flexor to extensor tendon transfer for operative correction of curly toe deformity.
    - In general, results were good, with all patients remaining symptom-free at final follow-up.
    - The authors concluded that neither procedure was clearly superior to the other, that long flexor tenotomy was the essential portion of either procedure, and that flexor to extensor transfer was unnecessary.
  - Biyani and colleagues[1] reviewed 130 curly toes in 43 children that were treated with flexor to extensor tendon transfer over a period of 24 years.
    - At an average follow-up of 8 years (range 1 to 25 years), good to excellent results were obtained in 95 toes (73%), fair results in 25 toes (19%), and poor results in 10 toes (8%).
  - In general, results of the Thompson procedure have been acceptable.

COMPLICATIONS

- Flexor tenotomy
  - When performing longitudinal skin incision, care should be taken to avoid crossing the flexion creases because scar formation and skin contracture have been reported.

- Ten of 188 patients in Ross and Menelaus's[15] study were found to have tethering of the plantar skin as a result of violating some aspect of the flexor crease.
- Stiffness has also been reported as a complication of flexor tenotomy.
- Neurovascular compromise has not been reported but, in theory, represents a significant potential complication with this procedure.
- Recurrent deformity, failure to achieve full correction, and infection are all potential complications of the Girdlestone-Taylor procedure.
- Thompson procedure
  - Digital edema from resection arthroplasty can result as well as neurovascular insult to the digital bundle.
  - Recurrence in single or multiple planes can also result from attempts at derotation.
  - Overresection can lead to a floppy, unstable toe as well as a transfer lesion beneath the fourth metatarsal.

REFERENCES

1. Biyani A, Jones DA, Murray JM. Flexor to extensor tendon transfer for curly toes. 43 children reviewed after 8 (1–25) years. Acta Orthop Scand 1992;63:451–454.
2. Chalayon O, Chertman C, Guss AD, et al. Role of plantar plate and surgical reconstruction techniques on static stability of lesser metatarsophalangeal joints: a biomechanical study. Foot Ankle Int 2013;34:1436–1442.
3. Davis WH, Anderson RB, Thompson FM, et al. Proximal phalanx basilar osteotomy for resistant angulation of the lesser toes. Foot Ankle Int 1997;18:103–104.
4. Deland JT, Lee KT, Sobel M, et al. Anatomy of the plantar plate and its attachments in the lesser metatarsal phalangeal joint. Foot Ankle Int 1995;16(8):480–486.
5. Flint WW, Macias DM, Couhglin MJ, et al. Plantar plate repair for lesser metatarsophalangeal joint instability. Foot Ankle Int 2017;38(3):234–242.
6. Girdlestone GR. Physiology for hand and foot. Physiotherapy 1947;32:167–169.
7. Haddad SL, Sabbagh RC, Resch S, et al. Results of flexor-to-extensor and extensor brevis tendon transfer for correction of the crossover second toe deformity. Foot Ankle Int 1999;20:781–788.
8. Hamer AJ, Stanley D, Smith TW. Surgery for curly toe deformity: a double-blind, randomised, prospective trial. J Bone Joint Surg Br 1993;75(4):662–663.
9. Hofstaetter SG, Hofstaetter JG, Petroutsas JA, et al. The Weil osteotomy: a seven-year follow-up. J Bone Joint Surg Br 2005;87(11):1507–1511.
10. Lapidus PW. Transplantation of the extensor tendon for correction of the overlapping fifth toe. J Bone Joint Surg Am 1942;24:555–559.
11. Lui TH, Chan KB. Technique tip: modified extensor digitorum brevis tendon transfer for crossover second toe correction. Foot Ankle Int 2007;28:521–523.
12. Myerson MS. Foot and Ankle Disorders. Philadelphia: WB Saunders 2000.
13. Nery C, Coughlin MJ, Baumfeld D, et al. Lesser metatarsophalangeal joint instability: prospective evaluation and repair of plantar plate and capsular insufficiency. Foot Ankle Int 2012;33:301–311.
14. Paton RW. V-Y plasty for correction of varus fifth toe. J Pediatr Orthop 1990;10:248–249.
15. Ross ER, Menelaus MB. Open flexor tenotomy for hammer toes and curly toes in childhood. J Bone Joint Surg Br 1984;66(5):770–771.
16. Stamm TT. Minor surgery of the foot: elevated fifth toe. In: Carling ER, Ross JP, eds. British Surgical Practice, vol 4. London: Butterworth, 1948:161–162.
17. Taylor RG. The treatment of claw toes by multiple transfers of flexor into extensor tendons. J Bone Joint Surg Br 1951;33-B(4):539–542.
18. Thompson FM, Deland JT. Flexor tendon transfer for metatarsophalangeal instability of the second toe. Foot Ankle 1993;14:385–388.
19. Thompson TC. Surgical treatment of disorders of the fore part of the foot. J Bone Joint Surg Br 1964;46(5):1117–1128.
20. Weil L Jr, Sung W, Weil LS Sr, et al. Anatomic plantar plate repair using the metatarsal osteotomy approach. Foot Ankle Spec 2011;4(3):145–150.
21. Wilson JN. V-Y correction for varus deformity of the fifth toe. Br J Surg 1953;41:133–135.

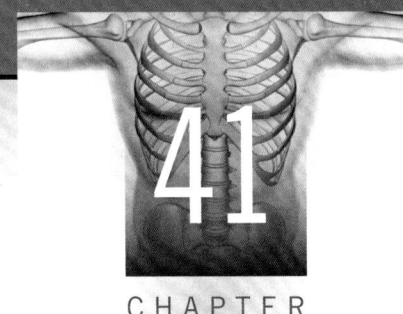

41

CHAPTER

Surgical Management of Freiberg Infraction

Richard W. Rutherford and Mark E. Easley

DEFINITION

- Freiberg infraction is an osteochondrosis of a lesser metatarsal head, most commonly involving the second metatarsal.
- In 1913, Freiberg originally documented six cases and used the term *infraction* to indicate incomplete fracture.

ANATOMY

- An osteochondrosis is an insult to the blood supply to the epiphysis. In Freiberg infraction, it leads to avascular necrosis.
- Freiberg disease is characterized by collapse of the dorsal articular surface, with relative preservation of the plantar surface of the involved metatarsal head.

PATHOGENESIS

- Not fully understood but most likely multifactorial
- Proposed etiologies include vascular insufficiency and potential genetic predisposition.
- Thought to involve repetitive microtrauma and altered biomechanics
- In our opinion, may be loosely compared to femoral head osteonecrosis

NATURAL HISTORY

- Peak onset is between ages 11 and 17 years.
- Incidence is uncertain but occurs in a 5:1 female-to-male ratio.
- Typically unilateral but occurs bilaterally in 7% of cases

PATIENT HISTORY AND PHYSICAL FINDINGS

- The classic presentation is activity-related pain and an antalgic gait, often worse when barefoot.
- Tenderness to palpation, classically at the dorsal metatarsal head and metatarsophalangeal (MTP) joint
- Decreased MTP joint range of motion, particularly with dorsiflexion
- Pain and impingement with forced MTP joint dorsiflexion
- Pain may also be present with forced MTP joint plantarflexion.
- Periarticular hypertrophy with palpable dorsal metatarsal head bony prominence
- MTP joint effusion, indicative of synovitis

IMAGING AND OTHER DIAGNOSTIC STUDIES

- Although the aforementioned clinical findings are highly suggestive of Freiberg infraction, routine weight-bearing foot radiographs are recommended to confirm the diagnosis.

- The radiographic Smillie classification remains a widely used staging system representing the spectrum of metatarsal head degeneration/collapse, from minimal involvement (simple dorsal metatarsal head flattening) to advanced disease (complete metatarsal head collapse and MTP joint destruction), which may be loosely compared to femoral head osteonecrosis.
- Mild to moderate disease may be manifest only radiographically as flattening of the metatarsal head's subchondral architecture.
- In our experience, symptomatic patients most commonly present with intermediate stages, with the observed radiographic appearance being collapsed with or without fragmentation of the dorsal one-third to half of the metatarsal head; the plantar articular surface is typically preserved (**FIG 1A,B**).
- Should plain radiographs fail to confirm a history and clinical examination suggestive of Freiberg infraction or if the diagnosis remains in question, magnetic resonance imaging (MRI) may prove useful.
- MRI for Freiberg infraction generally demonstrates a dorsal metatarsal head with a hypointense signal on T1-weighted images and mixed signals on T2-weighted images.
- MRI may also suggest metatarsal head flattening and dorsal osteophyte formation (**FIG 1C**).
- Similar to MRI, technetium bone scans may detect early disease not evident on plain radiographs. With technetium bone scanning, Freiberg infraction typically appears as a photopenic center ringed by an area of hyperactivity on the involved metatarsal head. In our opinion, isolated technetium bone scanning is not indicated for Freiberg infraction.
- Computed tomography may provide greater detail of subchondral collapse and dorsal metatarsal head prominence but is generally not indicated in the evaluation of Freiberg infraction (**FIG 1D**).

DIFFERENTIAL DIAGNOSIS

- Metatarsal neck stress fracture
- MTP joint synovitis (without suggestion of metatarsal head avascular necrosis and subchondral collapse)
- MTP joint arthritis (without suggestion of metatarsal head avascular necrosis and subchondral collapse)
- Neuroma, lipoma, ganglion cyst, or other soft tissue tumor

NONOPERATIVE MANAGEMENT

- Limited weight bearing, with forefoot unloading and immobilization for 4 to 6 weeks
- Gradually advance to a semirigid longitudinal arch support, with metatarsal support fitted in a stiffer-soled shoe to continue unloading of the involved MTP joint.

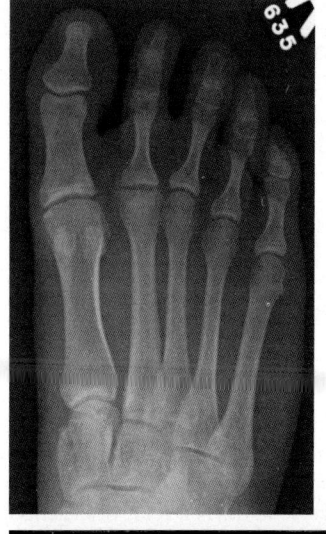
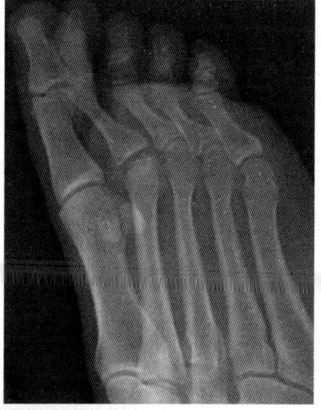
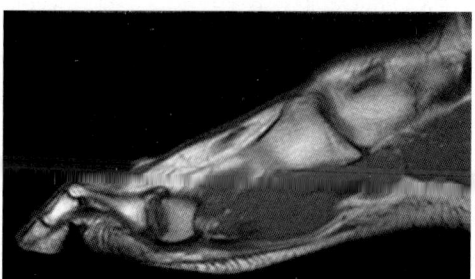
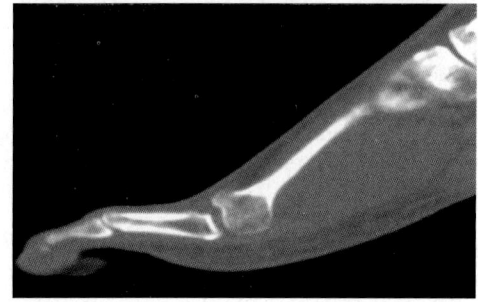

FIG 1 A. Right foot AP radiograph showing central subchondral collapse of the second metatarsal head. **B.** Oblique radiograph of same right foot demonstrating flattening of the dorsal second metatarsal head; note preservation of the plantar subchondral architecture. **C.** Sagittal T1-weighted MRI scan demonstrating articular and subchondral flattening of the second metatarsal head. **D.** Sagittal computed tomography detailing dorsal metatarsal head osteophyte formation.

- Progressive return to activities, with aforementioned orthotic and shoe modifications, as symptoms allow
- Nonsteroidal anti-inflammatory drugs may diminish associated symptoms related to MTP joint synovitis.
- Intra-articular corticosteroid injection should be used cautiously, as it may harm the residual articular cartilage or compromise the MTP joint's ligamentous integrity.
- Gait training may permit safe ambulation/running while compensating for the involved MTP joint's stiffness; however, aggressive range-of-motion exercises for the affected MTP joint may aggravate impingement. We typically reserve physical therapy for patients who have had surgical management to improve the joint's mechanics and to relieve mechanical impingement.

SURGICAL MANAGEMENT

- Nonoperative treatment is first line. For patients who fail conservative treatment, the stage of disease generally dictates the planned surgical procedure.
- For metatarsal heads with Freiberg infraction that have not progressed to dorsal subchondral bone collapse, with or without dorsal osteophyte formation, a joint synovectomy, dorsal cheilectomy, and/or decompression with bone grafting of the affected metatarsal head should be undertaken.
- For patients who have gone on to subchondral bone collapse of the dorsal metatarsal head, with or without fragmentation, we typically perform a (subcapital) dorsiflexion osteotomy, bringing the healthier plantar articular surface dorsally to improve joint function.

- For patients who have severe subchondral bone collapse and advanced MTP joint degeneration, consideration may be given to salvage procedures such as partial versus complete metatarsal head resection arthroplasty, or a soft tissue interpositional arthroplasty may be considered.

Preoperative Planning

- Standard weight-bearing anteroposterior (AP), lateral, and oblique radiographs and potentially MRI are useful in assessing the severity of disease and determining the planned procedure.

Positioning

- The patient is positioned supine on the operating room table with a support under the ipsilateral hip to limit external rotation of the leg.
- We typically use a calf tourniquet.

Approach

- The approach for all techniques involves a dorsal longitudinal incision overlying the affected (usually second) metatarsal. A curvilinear incision may also be used.
- Careful soft tissue handling is maintained. The extensor tendon is retracted, and the capsule overlying the MTP joint is split longitudinally.
- The capsule is elevated from the proximal phalanx and metatarsal to expose the joint.
- The proximal phalanx is then maximally plantarflexed to expose the metatarsal head.
- For all cases of Freiberg infraction that we have treated operatively, we have performed a comprehensive synovectomy.

DORSAL CHEILECTOMY

- With the metatarsal head fully exposed, the articular surface is examined. If the cartilage is preserved in the presence of a dorsal osteophyte, as in this case, dorsal cheilectomy alone is performed.
- The microsagittal saw is used to remove the osteophyte from distal to proximal, along with any diseased dorsal metatarsal head articular cartilage, similar to the surgical management of the first metatarsal head in hallux rigidus (**TECH FIG 1**).
- Range of motion is checked, particularly forced dorsiflexion after removing the osteophyte, to ensure impingement has been eliminated and satisfactory range of motion has been reestablished. As with hallux rigidus, a blunt elevator may be used to mobilize plantar capsular contractures to further improve dorsiflexion.

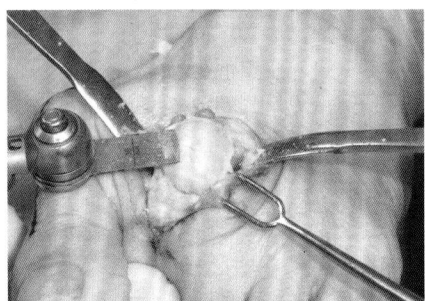

TECH FIG 1 Resection of the dorsal osteophyte with microsagittal saw.

BONE GRAFTING OF METATARSAL HEAD

- Albeit relatively rare, MRI scanning may demonstrate precollapse Freiberg disease involving a symptomatic subchondral cyst and relative preservation of metatarsal head.
- In select cases, we have been successful in relieving symptoms by decompressing and bone grafting the cyst without disrupting the intact subchondral bone.

- If the cartilage is found to be intact after exposure, a dorsal drill hole is created, and the metatarsal cyst is evacuated with a curette (**TECH FIG 2A,B**).
- Calcaneal bone graft is harvested from the ipsilateral foot and packed densely into the cyst (**TECH FIG 2C,D**).

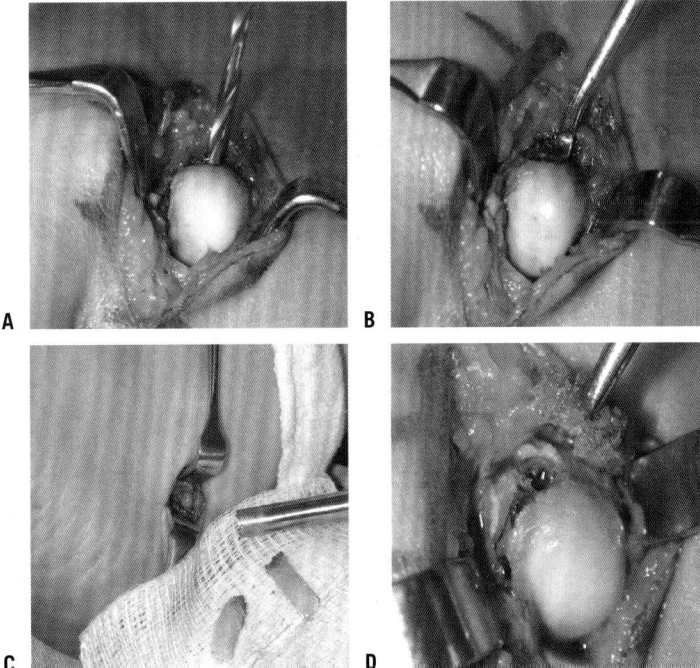

TECH FIG 2 A. Drilling of the involved metatarsal head from a dorsal approach. **B.** Decompression of the cyst with a small curette. **C.** Harvest of calcaneal bone graft from the ipsilateral calcaneus. **D.** Autograft is packed into the defect in the metatarsal head.

DORSAL (SUBCAPITAL) DORSIFLEXION OSTEOTOMY

Osteotomy

- For patients with collapse of the articular surface, we favor a subcapital dorsiflexion metatarsal head/neck osteotomy (**TECH FIG 3A,B**).
- This technique uses a dorsal closing wedge osteotomy to excise the unhealthy cartilage and rotate the intact healthy plantar articular cartilage to replace it.
- After dorsal longitudinal approach to the MTP joint, the metatarsal head is inspected (**TECH FIG 3C**).
- The dorsal osteophyte is removed, either with a microsagittal saw or with a rongeur (**TECH FIG 3D**).
- If upon inspection the dorsal articular surface is collapsed and the plantar cartilage is preserved, we perform a dorsally based wedge osteotomy, removing the diseased cartilage with extraction of the wedge (**TECH FIG 3E,F**).
- Ideally, the dorsally based wedge osteotomy should not penetrate the plantar cortex. Instead, both limbs of the osteotomy should meet at or immediately short of the plantar cortex.
  - This way, the osteotomy may be collapsed dorsally, maintaining plantar periosteum and stability.

- Prior to closing osteotomy, the bony surfaces may be carefully drilled to facilitate healing.
- With closure of the osteotomy, the intact plantar cartilage is rotated into position to articulate with the proximal phalanx.

Kirschner Wire Stabilization

- The osteotomy may be stabilized with a Kirschner wire (K-wire) placed across the osteotomy from proximal to distal. Because the plantar cortex remains intact and stable, we typically suture the wedge into place with one or two sutures (**TECH FIG 4A**).
- In this case, in which considerable correction was required, we opted to add a temporary longitudinal K-wire first placed antegrade from the MTP joint across the toe and then retrograde across the MTP joint into the metatarsal (**TECH FIG 4B**).
  - The K-wire's position is confirmed fluoroscopically.
  - When using a K-wire, we generally leave it in place for 4 weeks.
- Aggressive rotation of the metatarsal head (ie, a large wedge resection) increases the risk for transfer metatarsalgia.

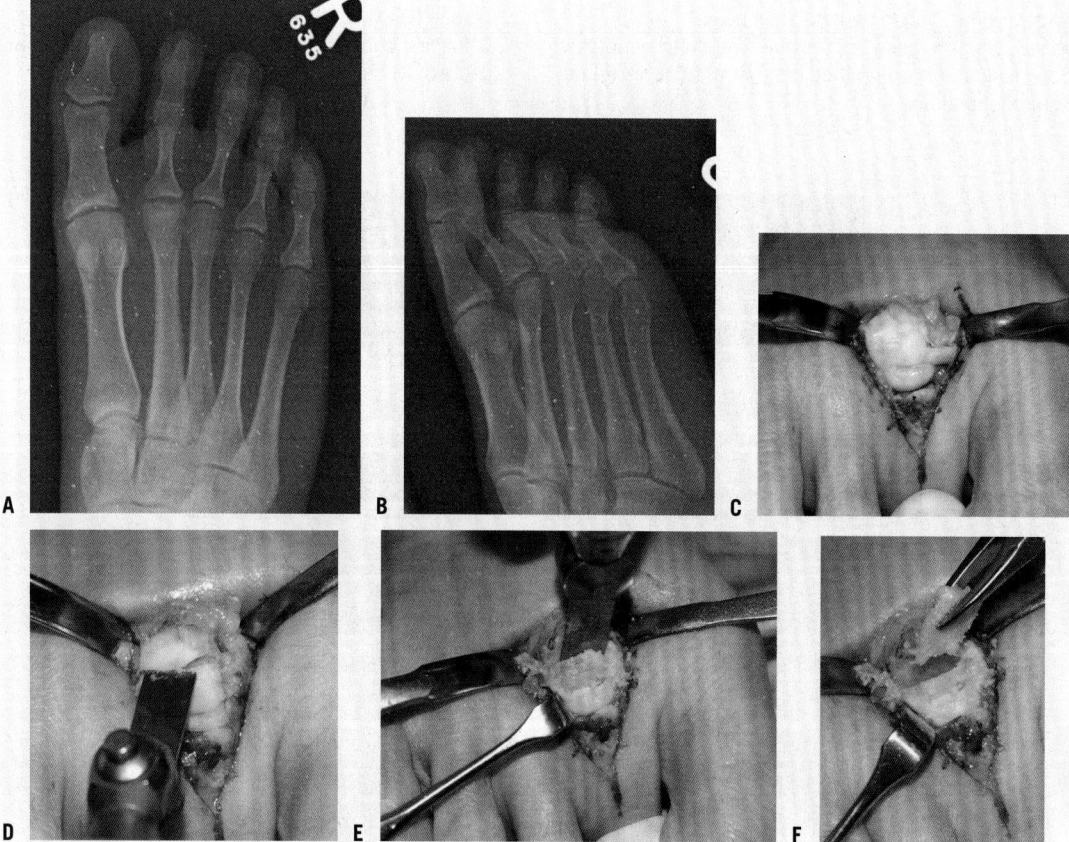

TECH FIG 3 **A.** Preoperative AP right foot radiograph in a 19-year-old female college basketball player, with a symptomatic second MTP joint. **B.** Oblique radiograph. Note dorsal osteophyte versus dorsal osteophyte and preserved plantar subchondral bone architecture. **C.** Full exposure of the involved metatarsal head. **D.** Dorsal prominence removal with a microsagittal saw. **E.** Dual converging osteotomies, creating the dorsal closing wedge osteotomy using the microsagittal saw to excise the diseased dorsal distal aspect of the metatarsal head. **F.** Extraction of the diseased portion of metatarsal head.

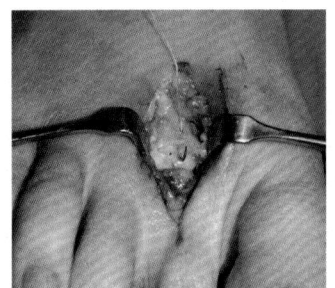 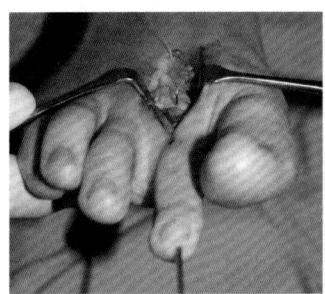

TECH FIG 4 A. Elevation of the plantar articular surface and fixation with nonabsorbable sutures. **B.** Given considerable correction and potential for instability, K-wire is placed across MTP joint to further stabilize the osteotomy.

METATARSAL HEAD ARTHROPLASTY VERSUS CAPSULAR INTERPOSITIONAL ARTHROPLASTY

Metatarsal Head Reshaping

- Even with severe metatarsal head degeneration **(TECH FIG 5A–D)**, we recommend against complete metatarsal head excision, as it may lead to transfer metatarsalgia.
- We favor reshaping and partial excision of the involved lesser metatarsal head without capsular interposition **(TECH FIG 5E)**. Although this procedure does not fully relieve symptoms, in our experience, it often leads to less pain, less impingement, and improved function with little risk of creating transfer metatarsalgia **(TECH FIG 5F,G)**.

Capsular Interpositional Arthroplasty

- Interpositional arthroplasty for Freiberg infraction has not, in our hands, been as successful as when it is performed for first MTP joint arthritis **(TECH FIG 6)**.
- Adequate decompression is necessary because the joint will remain symptomatic if too little bone is resected. However,

overzealous metatarsal head bone resection to accommodate the capsular interposition may lead to transfer metatarsalgia.
- Capsular interpositional arthroplasty for hallux rigidus also includes excision of the proximal phalanx base; given poor results with lesser toe proximal phalanx base excision for claw toe correction, we advise against excision of the lesser toe proximal phalanges to accommodate a lesser MTP joint capsular interpositional arthroplasty.

Closure and Aftercare

- Both the capsule and subcutaneous layers are closed with 3-0 absorbable suture.
- The tourniquet is released, and meticulous hemostasis is obtained.
- Care is taken to ensure that the toes are well perfused.
- The skin is reapproximated with 4-0 monofilament suture to a tensionless closure.
- A sterile dressing is used to protect the wound, and a mildly compressive dressing is placed.

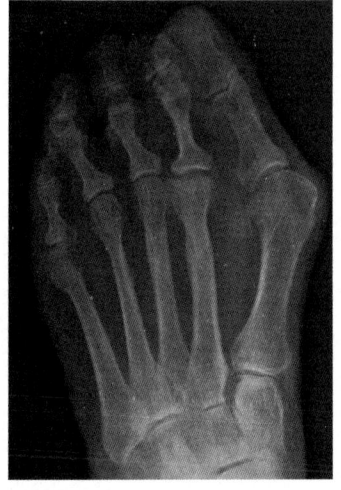 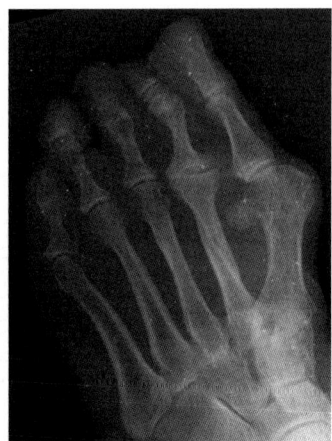 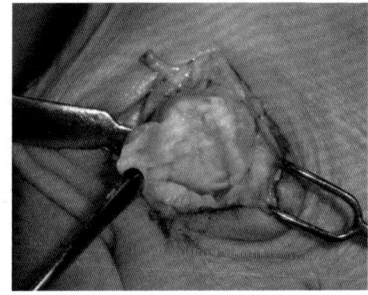

TECH FIG 5 A 67-year-old woman with left hallux valgus, long-standing second metatarsal head Freiberg infraction, and more advanced second MTP joint arthritis. **A.** AP left foot radiograph; note advanced metatarsal head collapse and joint arthrosis. **B.** Same patient's oblique left foot radiograph. **C.** Intraoperative image demonstrating same patient's severe, advanced metatarsal head collapse and joint degeneration. *(continued)*

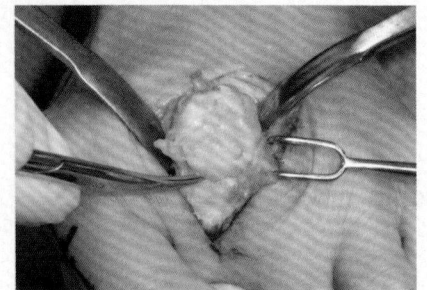 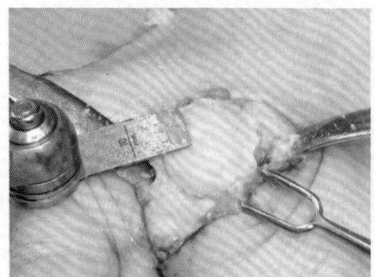 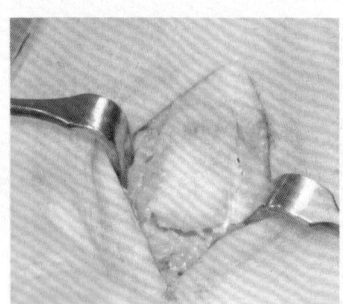

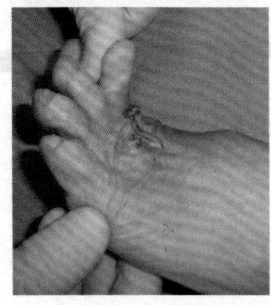

TECH FIG 5 *(continued)* **D.** There is some intact residual plantar articular cartilage but not enough to consider subcapital osteotomy. **E.** Metatarsal head is reshaped, accepting minimal residual metatarsal head cartilage but eliminating impingement and decompressing the joint. **F.** Note limited intact residual plantar cartilage. **G.** Satisfactory passive MTP joint dorsiflexion without impingement demonstrated.

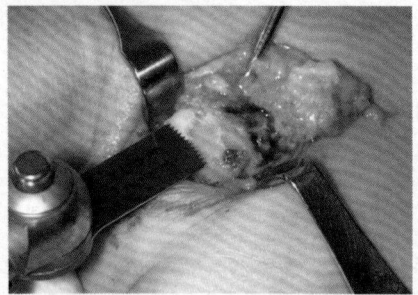 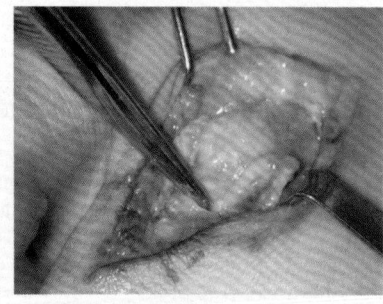 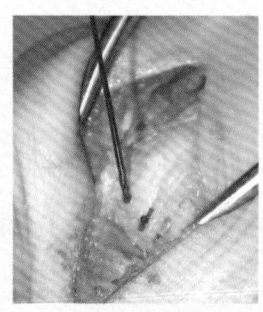

TECH FIG 6 Capsular interpositional arthroplasty. **A.** Essentially, no residual metatarsal head articular cartilage noted on direct inspection. Dorsal cheilectomy performed. **B.** Dorsal capsule preserved to allow for an interpositional arthroplasty. Important to ensure that this MTP joint is relatively loose and is not overstuffed with capsule, which will create impingement symptoms. **C.** Dorsal capsule is sutured to plantar plate.

TECHNIQUES

Pearls and Pitfalls

Instability of the Dorsiflexion Osteotomy	• Remember to avoid violating the plantar cortex during the wedge resection. • Use a dorsal suture to approximate the osteotomy. If necessary, place a longitudinal K-wire.
Transfer Metatarsalgia	• Avoid being overly aggressive in the dorsal wedge resection; otherwise, transfer metatarsalgia may result. • In advanced disease, avoid complete resection of the metatarsal head; instead, perform a partial metatarsal head resection arthroplasty only.

POSTOPERATIVE CARE

- If we did not perform an osteotomy, weight transfer to the forefoot progresses relatively rapidly over the first 2 weeks in a stiffer-soled postsurgical shoe, and transition to regular shoe and physical therapy is permitted when the wound is stable.
- Suture removal is typically at 10 to 14 days.
- If an osteotomy was performed, we typically splint the patients with the ankle in neutral position, particularly if

the toe has been stabilized with a K-wire. The splint protects against inadvertent displacement of the osteotomy and/or K-wire.
- The patient returns to the office at 10 to 14 days for possible suture removal and another splint. If the patient is capable of remaining off of the forefoot, a boot may be placed in which the patient may weight bear through the heel.
- The pin is removed in the office at 4 to 5 weeks (**FIG 2**).

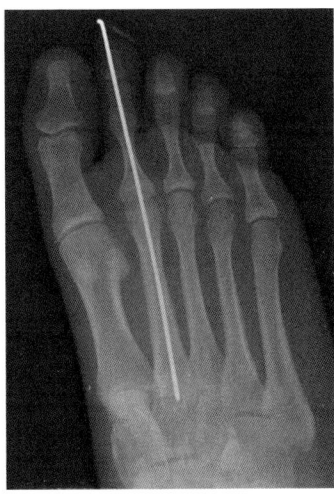

FIG 2 Early radiographic follow-up suggests improved metatarsal head architecture.

- We routinely obtain simulated weight-bearing foot radiographs at 4 weeks.
  - Even if the radiographs suggest satisfactory bony apposition at the osteotomy site, we recommend restricting weight transfer to the forefoot for a full 6 weeks.
- At 6 weeks, the patient may transfer to a boot or postoperative shoe and gradually progress to full weight bearing over the subsequent 2 weeks.
- We recommend that the patient be fitted for an offloading orthotic with metatarsal support as he or she transitions to a regular shoe between 6 and 8 weeks.

- Our standard postoperative protocol for forefoot surgery is Xeroform over the incision, soft dressing, and immediate weight bearing in a hard-soled postoperative shoe.
- If an osteotomy is performed, the patient is placed into a well-padded posterior/sugar-tong splint with no pressure on the involved toe, and weight bearing is protected. The pin remains for 6 weeks.
- We recommend return to full activities only with resolved MTP joint symptoms and radiographic improvement in involved metatarsal head's radiographic appearance.

OUTCOMES

- There is a lack of meaningful data that goes beyond simple case series regarding outcomes after treatment of Freiberg disease, with much of the recommendations based on anecdotal experience.
- **FIGS 3** and **4** show follow-up after dorsiflexion osteotomy for second metatarsal head Freiberg infraction in two patients.

COMPLICATIONS

- Infection, wound complications, and nerve deficit are no more prevalent than in other forefoot procedures.
- Vascular compromise is possible yet rare. In our hands, delayed capillary refill may occur if the toe is pinned in too much plantarflexion.
- Joint stiffness typically persists after surgery, albeit without dorsal impingement pain provided the dorsal metatarsal head prominence is removed.
  - Physical therapy may help to improve motion but rarely can regain physiologic motion.

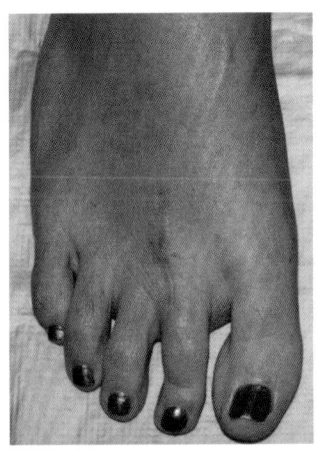
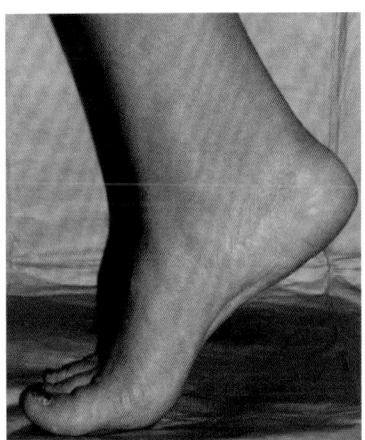
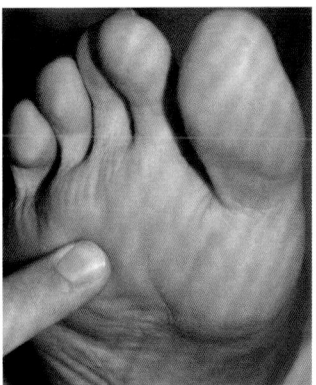
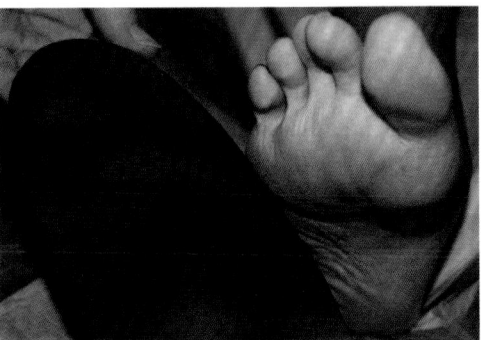

FIG 3 Same patient as **TECH FIG 3**. A 19-year-old female basketball player at 2-year follow-up after dorsiflexion osteotomy for second metatarsal head Freiberg infraction. **A.** Healed dorsal incision. **B.** Satisfactory forefoot range of motion. **C.** She developed transfer metatarsalgia of the third metatarsal head. **D.** This was effectively treated conservatively with semirigid longitudinal arch support and metatarsal support to unload the third metatarsal head.

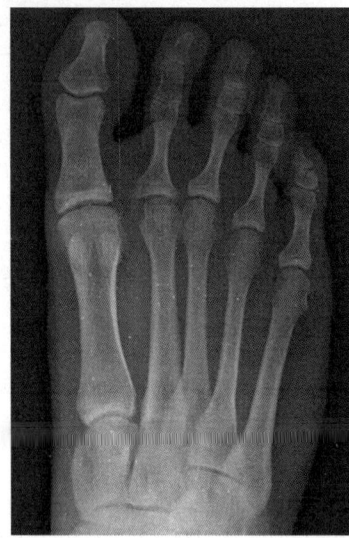
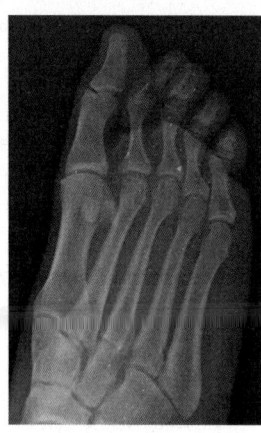

A   **B**

FIG 4 Two-year follow-up after dorsiflexion osteotomy for second metatarsal head Freiberg infraction. **A.** AP view. Note marked improvement and restoration of near-anatomic joint congruency. **B.** Oblique view of left foot.

- In our experience, the most common complication after dorsiflexion osteotomy is transfer metatarsalgia. Fortunately, the overload of the adjacent metatarsal head is rarely as bothersome as was the untreated Freiberg infraction.
  - Transfer metatarsalgia is generally well managed with a semirigid longitudinal arch support with metatarsal support and that unloading of the affected adjacent metatarsal heads.

SUGGESTED READINGS

Freiberg AH. Infraction of the second metatarsal bone: a typical injury. Surg Gynecol Obstet 1914;19:191–193.

Gauthier G, Elbaz R. Freiberg's infraction: a subchondral bone fatigue fracture. A new surgical treatment. Clin Orthop Relat Res 1979;(142):93–95.

Katcherian D. Treatment of Freiberg's disease. Orthop Clin North Am 1994;25:69–81.

Mandell GA, Harke HT. Scintigraphic manifestations of infraction of the second metatarsal (Freiberg's disease). J Nucl Med 1987;28(2):249–251.

Seybold JD, Zide JR. Treatment of Freiberg disease. Foot Ankle Clin 2018;23(1):157–169.

Smillie IS. Treatment of Freiberg's infraction. Proc R Soc Med 1967;60(1):29–31.

Smith TW, Stanley D, Rowley DI. Treatment of Freiberg's disease. A new operative technique. J Bone Joint Surg Br 1991;73:129–130.

Talusan PG, Diaz-Collado PJ, Reach JS Jr. Freiberg's infraction: diagnosis and treatment. Foot Ankle Spec 2014;7(1):52–56.

Trnka HJ, Lara JS. Freiberg's infraction: surgical options. Foot Ankle Clin 2019;24(4):669–676.

Viladot A, Sodano L, Marcellini L. Joint debridement and microfracture for treatment late-stage Freiberg-Kohler's disease: long-term follow-up study. Foot Ankle Surg 2019;25(4):457–461.

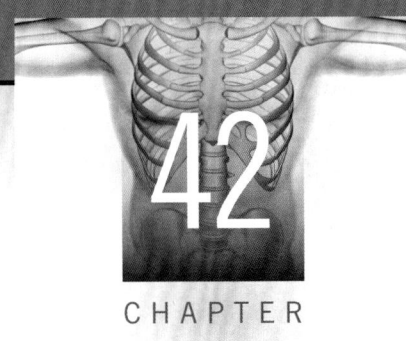

42

CHAPTER

Percutaneous Management of Bunionette Deformity and Fifth Metatarsalgia

Amanda N. Fletcher, Jonathan Day, A. Holly Johnson, and Oliver N. Schipper

DEFINITION

- Bunionette deformity, historically known as *tailor's bunion*, is a painful prominence of the lateral fifth metatarsal head.
- Fifth metatarsalgia refers to pain due to overload of the fifth metatarsal head and soft tissue structures.
- Minimally invasive surgeries (MIS) for the management of bunionette deformities and fifth metatarsalgia were recently introduced and are becoming increasingly popular.
- Early to midterm outcomes for MIS bunionette correction are promising. Although the literature is limited to small retrospective case series,[7,9,11–13,15,19] there is evidence of significant improvements in patient-reported functional outcomes, pain scores, radiographic alignment, and an overall low complication rate.

ANATOMY

- The bunionette deformity often consists of both abnormal fifth metatarsal morphology and abnormal overlying soft tissue structures.
- Most commonly, bunionettes are the result of a widened intermetatarsal angle (IMA) between the fourth and fifth rays with associated varus of the fifth metatarsophalangeal joint. However, a congenital deformity of the fifth metatarsal or wide fifth metatarsal head may also be present.
- Severity of bunionette deformity can be classified as type I to III based on anteroposterior (AP) radiographs as described by Coughlin[4]:
  - Type I: enlarged fifth metatarsal head or a prominent lateral condyle/lateral exostosis
  - Type II: congenital lateral bow of distal aspect of the fifth metatarsal; normal 4-5 IMA
  - Type III: increased 4-5 IMA
- Fifth metatarsal MIS osteotomies can place the dorsolateral sensory nerve branch of the fifth toe at risk, and safe zones lie between 10 and 2 o'clock position.[14]

PATHOGENESIS

- Bunionette deformity can be caused by multiple anatomic and biomechanical factors[1]:
  - Anatomic: constrictive shoe wear, abnormal loading of the lateral aspect of the foot (ie, when tailors historically sat with their legs crossed), prominent fifth metatarsal head, soft tissue hypertrophy of overlying soft tissue, congenital fifth ray deformities including a dumbbell-shaped fifth metatarsal or lateral bowing, supernumerary ossicles at the lateral fourth metatarsal, increased 4-5 IMA (splaying), and an abnormal transverse metatarsal ligament

  - Biomechanical: hypermobility of the fifth metatarsal causing excessive pronation, pes planus
- Fifth metatarsalgia may be caused by tight or ill-fitting shoe wear, use of heels, gastrocnemius contracture, and/or altered gait. The prevalence of metatarsalgia is about 10% in the general population and more common in females.[6]

NATURAL HISTORY

- Generally, bunionette deformities are progressive deformities of multifactorial etiology. The deformity of the fifth ray may progress to subluxation of the metatarsophalangeal joint when severe. Most commonly, a painful callus or bursa forms at the dorsolateral aspect of the fifth metatarsal head and becomes increasingly symptomatic with the risk of ulceration if not addressed.
- Bunionette deformity has an estimated prevalence of 13.8% with a female predominance and positive family history in 61.2% of patients.[17] Bilateral deformities are common.
  - It is commonly seen in adolescents and adults with a peak incidence during the fourth and fifth decades, frequently becoming more symptomatic with age.
- When symptomatic, bunionette deformities often respond successfully to nonsurgical methods including wider shoes and padding. Sometimes, physical therapy for gastrocnemius and soleus stretching, gait evaluation, and foot intrinsic strengthening may be helpful adjuncts. Metatarsal pads or orthotics may be used to offload the fifth metatarsal head. Surgical management is an option when patients fail nonoperative management.

PATIENT HISTORY AND PHYSICAL FINDINGS

- The most common chief complaint related to bunionette deformity is increased pressure and pain over the lateral condyle of the fifth metatarsal head with constrictive shoe wear.
- Cosmetic concerns include medial deviation of the fifth toe and prominence of the fifth metatarsal head.
- Patients complain of swelling, pain with ambulation that is aggravated by shoe wear and activity, and callus formation over the dorsolateral fifth metatarsal head.
- Patients with fifth metatarsalgia complain of pain and swelling over the fifth metatarsal head that is worse with weight bearing and improved with rest.
- Physical exam should begin with inspection of both feet. Note obvious deformities, including lateral prominence of the metatarsal head (**FIG 1**), curvature of the metatarsal, wide 4-5 IMA, and varus deformity at the metatarsophalangeal joint. Lateral, dorsolateral, or plantar hyperkeratosis about the fifth metatarsal head is commonly found.

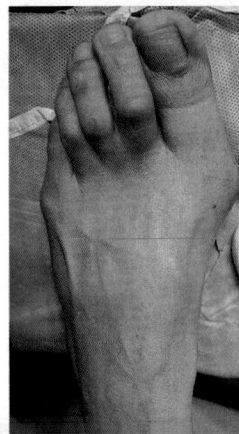

FIG 1 Clinical photograph of a bunionette deformity demonstrating prominence of the lateral fifth metatarsal head.

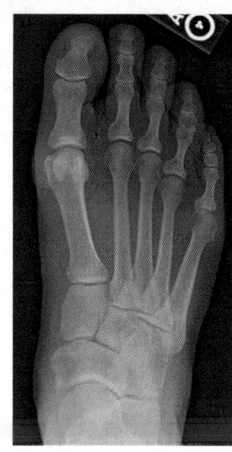

FIG 2 AP radiograph of Type II bunionette deformity.

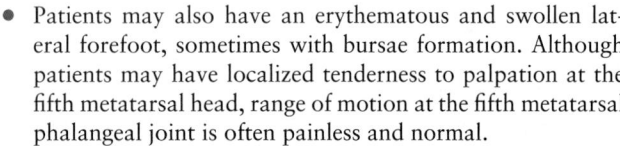

- Patients may also have an erythematous and swollen lateral forefoot, sometimes with bursae formation. Although patients may have localized tenderness to palpation at the fifth metatarsal head, range of motion at the fifth metatarsal phalangeal joint is often painless and normal.

IMAGING AND OTHER DIAGNOSTIC STUDIES

- Standard weight-bearing radiographs are recommended including AP, lateral, and oblique films. Advanced imaging is rarely required.
- Characteristic imaging findings of bunionette deformity are as follows (FIG 2):
  - Bony prominence at the lateral aspect of the fifth metatarsal head
  - Lateral bowing of the fifth metatarsal bone
  - Increased width of the metatarsal head (normal <13 mm)[16]
  - Increased 4-5 IMA (normal 6.5 to 8 degrees)[2]
  - Increased lateral deviation angle (normal 0 to 7 degrees)[3]
  - Increased fifth metatarsophalangeal angle (normal <10 degrees)[18]

DIFFERENTIAL DIAGNOSIS

- Inflammatory arthritis
- Fifth metatarsal fracture
- Hammer toe, curly toe, claw toe

NONOPERATIVE MANAGEMENT

- Nonoperative management is always the first line of management for bunionettes with only 10% to 23% of cases requiring surgery.[5,16] Conservative management includes:
  - Anti-inflammatories
  - Activity modification (Avoid activities and positions that place pressure on the lateral forefoot.)
  - Shoe wear modification: larger shoes, wider toe box, cutouts
  - Orthotics: semirigid shoe inserts, metatarsal bars, metatarsal pads, other off-loading devices
  - Shaving keratotic lesions
  - Physical therapy for gastrocnemius and soleus stretching and foot intrinsic strengthening

SURGICAL MANAGEMENT

- Operative correction of a symptomatic bunionette or fifth metatarsalgia is indicated if conservative treatment has failed to relieve patient symptoms.
- Indications
  - Type I bunionette deformity
  - Type II bunionette deformity with IMA less than 12 degrees
  - Type III bunionette deformity with IMA less than 12 degrees
- Fifth metatarsalgia
- Contraindications
  - Type II bunionette deformity with IMA greater than 12 degrees
  - Type III bunionette deformity with IMA greater than 12 degrees
  - Cases of severe deformity warrant open techniques previously described.[10]

Preoperative Planning

- Begin with a thorough history and physical exam; ensure conservative measures have been exhausted prior to surgical planning.
- Standard weight-bearing radiographs including AP, lateral, and oblique views should be obtained and reviewed to assess deformity severity and ensure indications are met.
- Concomitant deformities and abnormalities should be assessed including hallux valgus and pes planus, which are commonly associated with bunionette deformity, to determine whether these pathologies warrant concomitant correction.
- Consider any prior surgeries including location of incisions or presence of hardware.

Positioning

- The patient is positioned supine in 10 to 20 degrees of Trendelenburg with the operative foot off of the bed.
- A bump is placed under the hip on the operative side to prevent external rotation of the lower extremity.
- The operative leg is elevated on a bump or blankets secured to the bed.

- The nonoperative leg may be frog-legged away from the operative field and secured to the bed.
- It is recommended to position the mini C-arm to the right of the patient for right-handed surgeons and to the left of the patient for left-handed surgeons; however, this is based on surgeon preference.

Approach

- In general, MIS bunionette correction procedures include an osteotomy of the fifth metatarsal without internal fixation (**FIG 3**).
- Most of the procedure is performed through percutaneous dorsolateral and/or dorsomedial incisions.

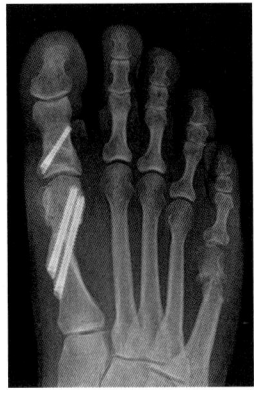 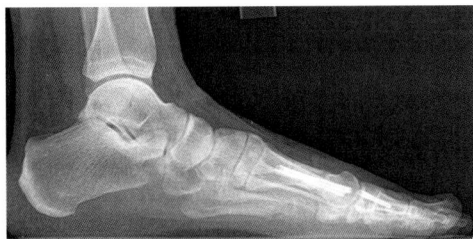

FIG 3 Postoperative AP (**A**) and lateral (**B**) radiographs demonstrating a healing 5th metatatarsal osteotomy with correction of bunionette deformity. Also shown is a percutaneous chevron-akin bunionectomy.

TYPE I BUNIONETTE DEFORMITY: LATERAL FIFTH METATARSAL HEAD OSTECTOMY

- The standard working approach is through a dorsolateral incision.
- A 2- to 3-mm incision is made over the dorsolateral fifth metatarsal at the distal metaphyseal region, approximately 1 cm proximal to the fifth metatarsal head.
- Blunt dissection is carried down to the lateral fifth metatarsal head, and an elevator is then used to create a working space over the lateral fifth metatarsal head. Care should be taken to avoid injuring the dorsolateral sensory nerve branch to the fifth toe.

- Under AP fluoroscopic guidance, the 3-mm wedge burr or 2- × 12-mm Shannon burr is introduced into the lateral fifth metatarsal head.
- The lateral fifth metatarsal head is then shaved down using a sweeping motion in both the plantar-dorsal and proximal-distal directions. This is carried out until the lateral fifth metatarsal head prominence is flush with the metadiaphysis both clinically and on AP fluoroscopic views.
- An angiocatheter is then used to irrigate the incision with normal saline to remove any bone debris.
- The incision is closed with Steri-Strips. A small soft dressing and firm postoperative shoe are applied.

TYPE II/III BUNIONETTE DEFORMITY: LATERAL FIFTH METATARSAL HEAD OSTECTOMY AND DISTAL METATARSAL OSTEOTOMY

- For type II and III bunion deformities, begin by following the earlier technique for type I bunionette deformities. The procedure begins by creating the dorsolateral working space and performing the lateral fifth metatarsal head ostectomy.
- The surgeon then stands distal to the foot.
  - Right-handed surgeon: For a left foot, the same dorsolateral incision created for the lateral fifth metatarsal head ostectomy may be used. For a right foot, a separate dorsomedial incision is made at the distal metaphyseal region of the fifth metatarsal, mirroring the dorsolateral incision.
  - Left-handed surgeon: For a right foot, the same dorsolateral incision created for the lateral fifth metatarsal head ostectomy may be used. For a left foot, a separate dorsomedial incision is made at the distal metaphyseal region of the fifth metatarsal, mirroring the dorsolateral incision.

- The 2- × 12-mm Shannon burr is then introduced through the incision. With the use of lateral and oblique fluoroscopic views, the distal fifth metatarsal metaphysis is localized, just outside of the fifth metatarsophalangeal joint capsule.
- The burr is positioned at a 45-degree angle from dorsal-distal to plantar-proximal (**TECH FIG 1A**).
- Maintaining this angle, a sweeping motion of the hand is used from dorsal-distal to plantar-proximal in retrograde fashion. The distal fifth metaphyseal osteotomy is completed and confirmed under lateral and slight oblique fluoroscopy (**TECH FIG 1B**).
- In the case of bunionette deformity correction, the metatarsal head is then shifted medially relative to the diaphysis, although this often occurs spontaneously due to soft tissue tension (**TECH FIG 1C**).

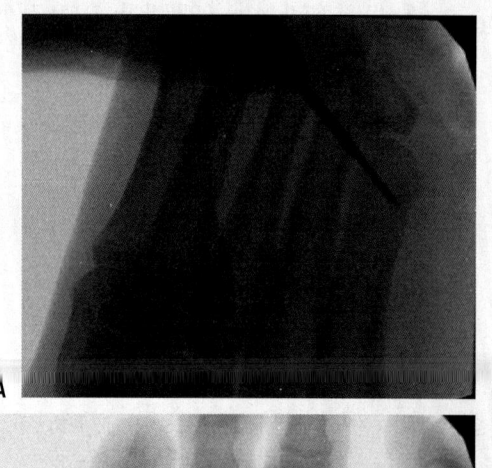
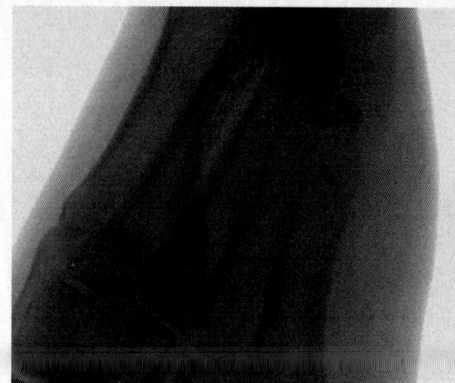
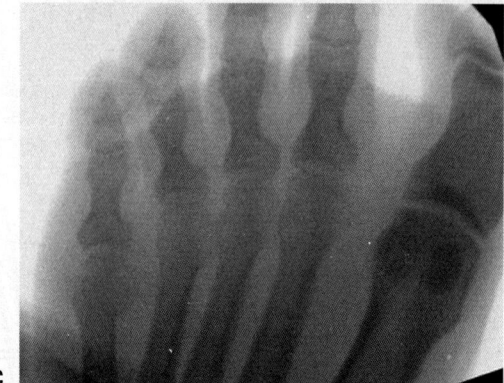

TECH FIG 1 **A.** Lateral fluoroscopic view demonstrating proper position and trajectory of the Shannon burr at a 45-degree angle from dorsal-distal to plantar-proximal. **B.** Lateral fluoroscopy demonstrating a complete fifth metatarsal head osteotomy. **C.** Intraoperative AP fluoroscopic view demonstrating a medial shift of the fifth metatarsal head.

- After the medial shift of the metatarsal head, a prominent lateral fifth metatarsal metadiaphyseal cortical spike may be present. This may then be shaved down through the preestablished portal(s) with a 3-mm wedge burr or 2- × 8-mm Shannon burr under AP fluoroscopy.

- This technique requires no fixation.
- An angiocatheter is then used to irrigate the incision with normal saline to remove any bone debris.
- The incision is closed with Steri-Strips. A small soft dressing and firm postoperative shoe are applied.

FIFTH METATARSALGIA: DISTAL METATARSAL SHORTENING OSTEOTOMY

- The standard working approach is through a dorsolateral or dorsomedial incision depending on laterality and surgeon handedness.
- The surgeon stands at the foot of the bed.
  - Right-handed surgeon: For a right foot, a dorsomedial incision is made at the distal metaphyseal region of the fifth metatarsal. For a left foot, a dorsolateral incision is made.
  - Left-handed surgeon: For a left foot, a dorsomedial incision is made at the distal metaphyseal region of the fifth metatarsal. For a right foot, a dorsolateral incision is made.
- Blunt dissection is carried down to the bone, and an elevator is then used to create a working space over the lateral fifth metatarsal head.
- The 2- × 12-mm Shannon burr is then introduced through the incision. With the use of lateral and oblique fluoroscopic views,

the distal fifth metatarsal metaphysis is localized, just outside of the fifth metatarsophalangeal joint capsule.
- The burr is positioned at a 45-degree angle from dorsal-distal to plantar-proximal.
- Maintaining this angle, a sweeping motion of the hand is used from dorsal-distal to plantar-proximal in retrograde fashion. The distal fifth metaphyseal osteotomy is completed and confirmed under lateral and slight oblique fluoroscopy.
- The fifth metatarsal head is then shifted proximally to shorten and elevate by 2 mm, equivalent to the width of the burr. No fixation is necessary for this technique.
- An angiocatheter is then used to irrigate the incision with normal saline to remove any bone debris.
- The incision is closed with Steri-Strips. A small soft dressing and firm postoperative shoe are applied.

Pearls and Pitfalls

Preoperative Counseling for Postoperative Swelling	• Although these are minimally invasive techniques, it is important to counsel patients preoperatively and set appropriate expectations that the forefoot swelling may take 3–6 months to resolve completely.
Tourniquet Use	• A tourniquet is not recommended in order to reduce the risk of thermal injury and bone necrosis. Placing the patient in a slight Trendelenburg may help reduce bleeding during the procedure.
Avoiding Vascular Damage	• When using blunt dissection and the elevator, care should be made to elevate tissue dorsally rather than plantarly to avoid damaging the blood supply to the metatarsal head.
Avoiding Nerve Damage	• Fifth metatarsal MIS osteotomies can place the dorsolateral sensory nerve branch of the fifth toe at risk. The safe zone lies between 10 and 2 o'clock position.[14]
Preventing Thermal Skin Injury	• Copious irrigation should be used whenever the burr is active to minimize risk of thermal injury to the skin or bone necrosis.

POSTOPERATIVE CARE

• The operative dressing is left in place for the first 2 weeks, and then removed at the two week postoperative visit.
• In type II and III bunionette cases requiring a distal metatarsal osteotomy, the fifth toe may be taped to the fourth toe for an additional 3 weeks to maintain correction.
• The patient is allowed to weight bear as tolerated in a firm postoperative shoe for the first 4 weeks postoperatively, followed by transition into normal shoe wear and increased activity as tolerated at 4 weeks postoperatively.

OUTCOMES

• MIS techniques to correct bunionette deformities have limited but positive outcomes thus far, with correction, complication rates, and patient-reported outcomes comparable to traditional open techniques. At this time, the literature is limited to small case series[7,9,11–13,15,19] with no direct comparison of open and MIS techniques.
• Patients have shown an average improvement of 31.2 to 46.5 points in American Orthopaedic Foot and Ankle Society (AOFAS) score with the average postoperative AOFAS scores ranging from 94 to 100.[7,9,11–13,15] Additional patient-reported outcomes include improvements in the Manchester–Oxford Foot Questionnaire (MOXFQ)[19] and visual analog scale (VAS) for pain.[9,19] Overall, 94% to 100% of patients reported good to excellent results.
• All series also report improvements in both the 4-5 IMA angle (average of 3.4- to 15-degree reduction) and fifth metatarsophalangeal angle (average 7.9- to 17.1-degree reduction).[7,9,11–13,15,19]
• Of important note, earlier case series included Kirschner wire fixation,[7,11,13] whereas more recent literature has favored the no fixation technique as described earlier.[12,15,19]
• The minimally invasive distal metatarsal metaphyseal osteotomy for lesser toe metatarsalgia has also demonstrated improvements in MOXFQ and VAS scores with good patient satisfaction, functional improvement, and low complication rates in most cases.[8]

COMPLICATIONS

• In general, complications with MIS surgery are similar to traditional open surgery, including the risk of infection and nonunion.
  • Operative irrigation and débridement are recommended for deep infections.
  • Full radiographic bony union may take up to 3 to 6 months. In patients with persistent pain and equivocal radiographs, a computed tomography scan should be considered for the evaluation of a nonunion. Revision surgery with a compression plate and/or screws is recommended for cases of nonunion.
• Thermal burns to the skin are unique to MIS techniques.
  • To prevent thermal injury, it is recommended to avoid use of a tourniquet and thoroughly irrigate the active burr.
• The two most prevalent complications reported specific for MIS bunionette correction in the literature include hypertrophic dorsal callus formation in 10% to 12% of cases[9,15,19] and superficial infection in 2% to 5% of cases.[7,11,13]
  • Other less common complications include fourth transfer metatarsalgia,[11] plantar callus,[7] dorsolateral sensory neurapraxia, wound dehiscence,[12] complex regional pain syndrome,[9] and delayed union.[9]

REFERENCES

1. Bertrand T, Parekh SG. Bunionette deformity: etiology, nonsurgical management, and lateral exostectomy. Foot Ankle Clin 2011;16(4):679–688.
2. Bishop J, Kahn A III, Turba JE. Surgical correction of the splayfoot: the Giannestras procedure. Clin Orthop Relat Res 1980;146:234–238.
3. Cohen BE, Nicholson CW. Bunionette deformity. J Am Acad Orthop Surg 2007;15(5):300–307.
4. Coughlin MJ. Treatment of bunionette deformity with longitudinal diaphyseal osteotomy with distal soft tissue repair. Foot Ankle 1991;11(4):195–203.
5. Diebold PF. Basal osteotomy of the fifth metatarsal for the bunionette. Foot Ankle 1991;12(2):74–79.
6. Fadel GE, Rowley DI. Metatarsalgia. Curr Orthop 2002;16:193–204.
7. Giannini S, Faldini C, Vannini F, et al. The minimally invasive osteotomy "S.E.R.I." (simple, effective, rapid, inexpensive) for correction of bunionette deformity. Foot Ankle Int 2008;29(3):282–286.

8. Haque S, Kakwani R, Chadwick C, et al. Outcome of minimally invasive distal metatarsal metaphyseal osteotomy (DMMO) for lesser toe metatarsalgia. Foot Ankle Int 2016;37(1):58–63.

9. Laffenêtre O, Millet-Barbé B, Darcel V, et al. Percutaneous bunionette correction: results of a 49-case retrospective study at a mean 34 months' follow-up. Orthop Traumatol Surg Res 2015;101(2):179–184.

10. Lau J, Henderson B, Yee G. Surgical correction of bunionette deformity. In: Easley ME, Wiesel SW, eds. Operative Techniques in Foot and Ankle Surgery. Philadelphia: Lippincott Williams & Wilkins, 2010:250–255.

11. Legenstein R, Bonomo J, Huber W, et al. Correction of tailor's bunion with the Boesch technique: a retrospective study. Foot Ankle Int 2007;28(7):799–803.

12. Lui TH. Percutaneous osteotomy of the fifth metatarsal for symptomatic bunionette. J Foot Ankle Surg 2014;53(6):747–752.

13. Magnan B, Samaila E, Merlini M, et al. Percutaneous distal osteotomy of the fifth metatarsal for correction of bunionette. J Bone Joint Surg Am 2011;93(22):2116–2122.

14. Malagelada F, Dalmau-Pastor M, Sahirad C, et al. Anatomical considerations for minimally invasive osteotomy of the fifth metatarsal for bunionette correction: a pilot study. Foot (Edinb) 2018;36:39–42.

15. Michels F, Van Der Bauwhede J, Guillo S, et al. Percutaneous bunionette correction. Foot Ankle Surg 2013;19(1):9–14.

16. Nestor BJ, Kitaoka HB, Ilstrup DM, et al. Radiologic anatomy of the painful bunionette. Foot Ankle 1990;11(1):6–11.

17. Şayli U, Altunok EC, Güven M, et al. Prevalence estimation and familial tendency of common forefoot deformities in Turkey: a survey of 2662 adults. Acta Orthop Traumatol Turc 2018;52(3):167–173.

18. Steel MW III, Johnson KA, DeWitz MA, et al. Radiographic measurements of the normal adult foot. Foot Ankle 1980;1(3):151–158.

19. Teoh KH, Hariharan K. Minimally invasive distal metatarsal metaphyseal osteotomy (DMMO) of the fifth metatarsal for bunionette correction. Foot Ankle Int 2018;39(4):450–457.

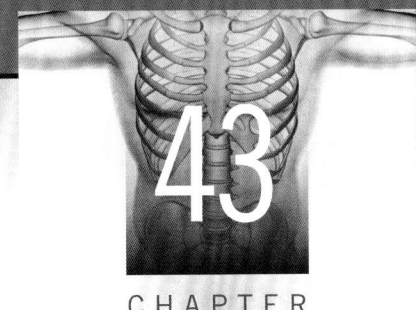

43

CHAPTER

Surgical Correction of Bunionette Deformity

Sahil Kooner, Andrew Marsh, and Johnny T.C. Lau

DEFINITION

- A bunionette deformity is a painful prominence on the lateral aspect of the fifth metatarsal head. This is usually caused by a prominent lateral metatarsal condyle, lateral bowing of the fifth metatarsal, or increased intermetatarsal angle (IMA). This is often associated with varus deformity of the fifth toe as well.

ANATOMY

- The Coughlin[4] classification illustrates the pertinent anatomic differences between the different types of bunionette deformities:
  - In type I, a prominent lateral condyle may be noticeable under the callus.
  - In type II, a curvature in the metatarsal shaft may be evident.
  - In type III, there is a wider than expected angle between the fourth and fifth metatarsal.
- All may be associated with an inflamed bursa or callus, depending on the chronicity of the problem.

PATHOGENESIS

- This was historically named a *tailor's bunionette* because tailors spent long hours with crossed legs, causing pressure over the fifth metatarsal head and resulting in local pressure and formation of a callus and occasionally a painful bursa.
- Local pressure can also be increased by a larger-than-normal lateral metatarsal condyle, angulation in the shaft of the metatarsal, or a wide intermetatarsal space, resulting in local tissue inflammation, pain, and swelling.

NATURAL HISTORY

- It has a female-to-male ratio of between 1:1 and 10:1.[7]
- The natural history is increasing formation of painful callus and bursae over the area.
- It can result in ulceration if proper foot care is not instituted or if underlying neuropathy is present.
- Surgery is reserved for recalcitrant cases, as it is usually responsive to conservative therapies including regular paring of callosities, wide toe box shoes, orthotics, and toe spacers.

PATIENT HISTORY AND PHYSICAL FINDINGS

- Patients complain of pain and tenderness over the lateral aspect of the foot over the fifth metatarsal head.

- Symptoms are usually worse with activity, especially any position causing increased pressure over the metatarsal head.
- Enclosed shoes will exacerbate symptoms when causing local pressure. Hence, it is often described as improved in the summer, with less restrictive footwear and perhaps reduced work hours.
- The examiner should view both feet simultaneously while standing.
- The examiner should look for a prominent lateral metatarsal condyle, an obvious curvature in the metatarsal shaft, or a wide IMA.
- The examiner should note any hard or soft callus over the lateral or plantar aspect of the fifth metatarsal.
- The examiner should look for any ulceration over the callus or between the fourth and fifth toes.

IMAGING AND OTHER DIAGNOSTIC STUDIES

- Standing plain radiographs (anteroposterior [AP], lateral, and oblique views) are necessary.
- For all views, the radiographs are evaluated for osteoarthritis, narrow joint space, subchondral sclerosis, osteophyte formation, enlarged metatarsal condyle, curvature of metatarsal shaft, or a wide IMA between the fourth and fifth metatarsal shafts.
- Oblique radiographs may give a better view of the metatarsal head profile.
- On the lateral radiograph, the surgeon should look for any flexion or extension of the interphalangeal joints suggestive of claw or hammer toes.

DIFFERENTIAL DIAGNOSIS

- Curly toe
- Claw toe
- Hammer toe
- Stress fracture of the fifth metatarsal
- Fifth metatarsal fracture with prominent fracture callus

NONOPERATIVE MANAGEMENT

- Nonoperative management focuses on decreasing pressure.
- It is very important for the patient to avoid sitting positions that place lateral-sided pressure on the fifth metatarsal.
- Placing lamb's wool or cotton between the fourth and fifth toes to act as a toe spacer and reduce varus deviation of the fifth toe can reduce lateral-sided pressure.
- Proper-fitting wide toe box or orthopaedic shoes can alleviate pressure caused by footwear.

SURGICAL MANAGEMENT

Preoperative Planning

- The surgeon should take into consideration any previous scars, edema, or skin abnormalities that would affect incision placement.
- Plain weight-bearing films are reviewed to determine which type of bunionette is present. Soft tissue balancing or osteotomy is based on the type of deformity.
- The more proximal the osteotomy, the higher the degree of correction that can be attained. This must be weighed with the potential risk associated with proximal osteotomies, including delayed union and nonunion.[9]
- Type I deformity is treated with excision of the lateral metatarsal condyle in conjunction with soft tissue balancing and lateral capsular reefing.
- Type II deformity can be treated with a proximal, diaphyseal, or distal metatarsal osteotomy depending on the center of rotation of angulation and the magnitude of deformity. We describe the chevron type of osteotomy to correct the lateral deviation in the distal metatarsal shaft. The lateral deviation angle measures the degree of lateral bowing and is measured off the medial aspect of the fifth metatarsal shaft base to the center of the metatarsal head. The normal value is 2.6 degrees (range 0 to 7 degrees).[4]
- In type III deformity, a wide IMA between the fourth and fifth metatarsal is noted, with the mean angle being 6.5 degrees (range 3 to 11 degrees), whereas an angle of 9.6 degrees or higher is correlated with a symptomatic bunionette.[5,11] Similarly, this is best treated with a proximal, diaphyseal, or distal metatarsal osteotomy depending on the severity of deformity and amount of correction desired. We describe a Ludloff diaphyseal osteotomy to correct a bunionette secondary to a widened IMA.
- Minimally invasive and percutaneous procedures are gaining in popularity due to decreased risk of infection and wound healing problems.[10] These procedures can be used for the same indications as open osteotomies, depending on surgeon's preference and availability of specialized equipment and imaging. We describe both a percutaneous osteotomy and a mini-open technique for bunionette correction that can be modified depending on bunionette morphology.
- Fixation of osteotomies can vary from Kirschner wires, minifragment screws, or minifragment plates to no fixation and stabilization with an external splint.
- Metatarsal head resection and ray amputation should only be used as a last resort in a salvage situation.

Positioning

- The patient is positioned supine on a radiolucent operating table. A small lift is placed under the buttock on the operative side. A tourniquet is placed on the upper thigh or a sterile Esmarch tourniquet is placed above the ankle.

Approach

- All skin incisions should be lateral, with caution to avoid any digital nerves on the lateral aspect of the fifth toe (FIG 1).
- This approach allows for bunionectomy and osteotomy of the shaft with screw, pin, or plate fixation, and the approach can be extended proximally or distally if needed.

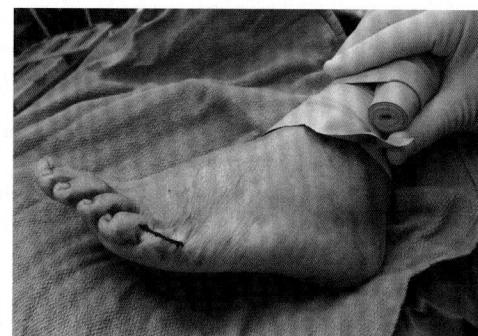

FIG 1 Lateral incision over bunionette.

LATERAL METATARSAL CONDYLECTOMY WITH CAPSULAR PLICATION

Exposure

- Use a lateral approach, making an incision down to the capsule.
- Free the soft tissue between the capsule and the overlying skin to expose the lateral aspect of the metatarsal head (TECH FIG 1A,B).
- Make a V-shaped capsulotomy with the proximal apex to allow for plication on closure (TECH FIG 1C,D).

Bunionectomy

- Expose the enlarged lateral condyle of the fifth metatarsal. Place small Hohmann retractors below and above the metatarsal head to protect both flexor and extensor tendons (TECH FIG 2A).
- With a small saw, excise the prominent lateral condyle head parallel to the shaft of the metatarsal (TECH FIG 2B,C).
- Pull the distal part of the V-shaped capsulotomy proximally to the desired amount of tension and sew with a heavy nonabsorbable suture (TECH FIG 2D).
- Close the subcutaneous tissue with small absorbable suture and the skin with small nonabsorbable suture.
- Place a small amount of gauze between the fourth and fifth toes to keep the fifth toe from deviating medially while it heals.

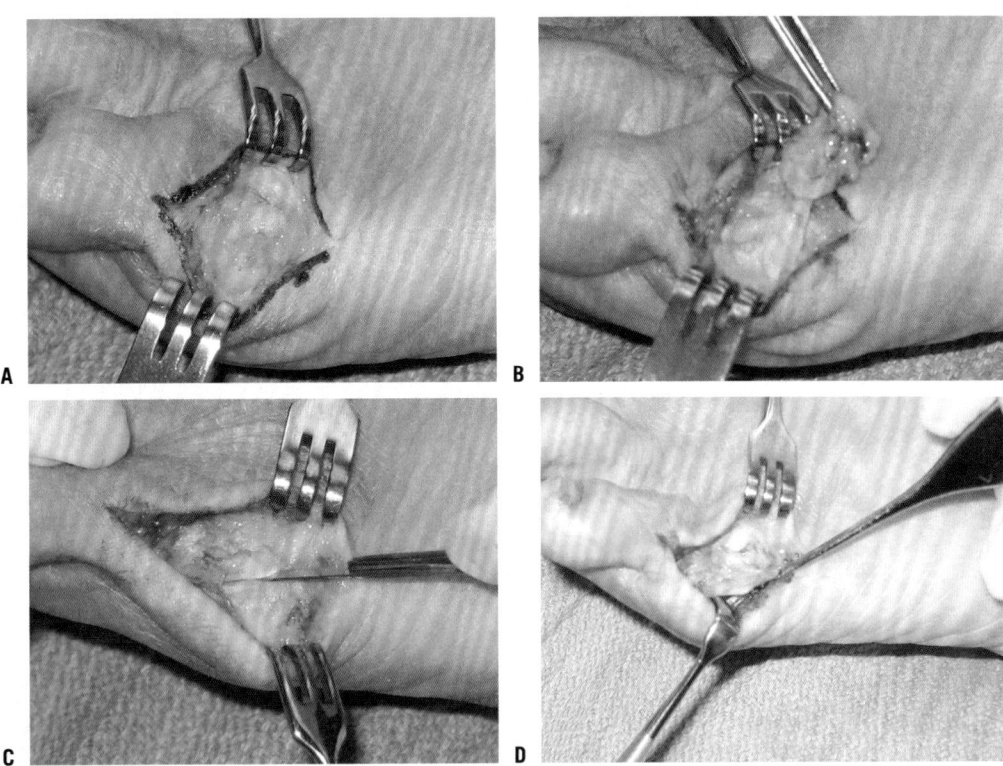

TECH FIG 1 A. Dissection through subcutaneous tissue to bursa. **B.** Excision of bursa over bunionette. **C,D.** V-shaped capsulotomy performed to expose bunionette.

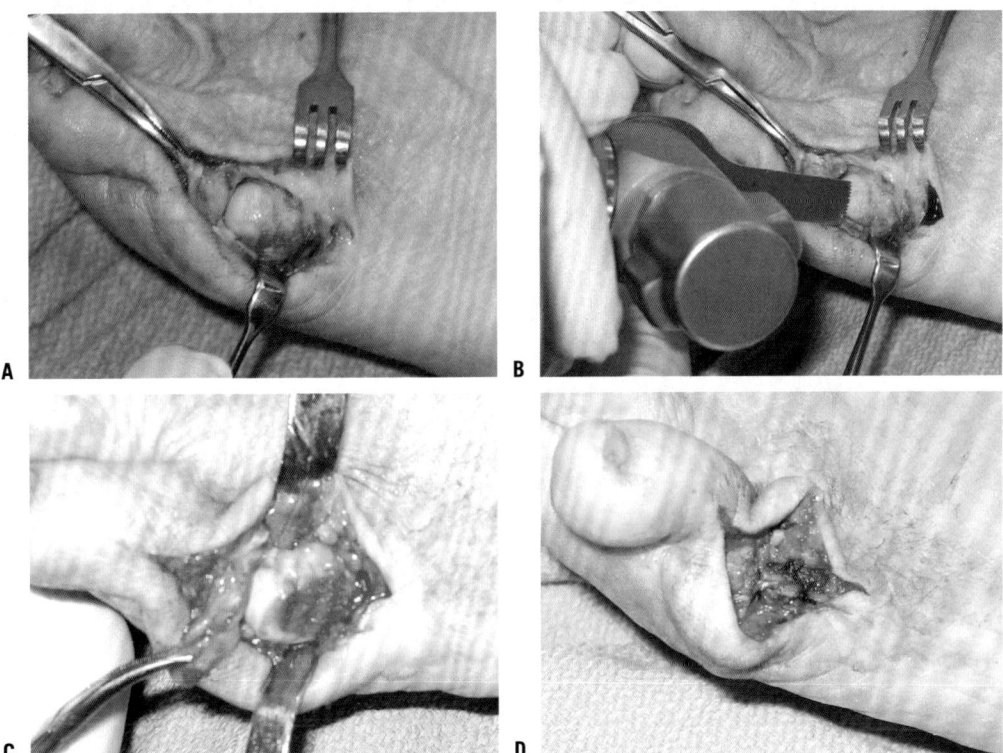

TECH FIG 2 A. Bunionette exposed through capsulotomy. **B,C.** Bunionette excised with saw. **D.** V-shaped capsulotomy repaired with proximal advancement to correct deformity.

CHEVRON OSTEOTOMY OF THE FIFTH METATARSAL

Exposure and Bunionectomy

- Make a lateral incision down to the capsule.
- Free the soft tissue between the capsule and the overlying skin to expose the lateral aspect of the metatarsal head.
- Make a V-shaped capsulotomy with the proximal apex to allow for plication on closure.
- Expose the enlarged lateral condyle of the fifth metatarsal and perform excision of the lateral metatarsal condyle as described previously (**TECH FIG 3**).

Osteotomy

- Mark the center of the freshly cut lateral aspect of the metatarsal head with a sterile marker (**TECH FIG 4A**).
- The limbs of the chevron osteotomy are 60 degrees.

- Use your free hand to palpate the plane of the metatarsal heads and make the chevron osteotomy parallel to the plantar surface of the foot (**TECH FIG 4B,C**).
- Shift the metatarsal head medially, leaving 3 to 4 mm of exposed metatarsal shaft (**TECH FIG 4D–G**).
- Cut the residual lateral bone with the saw again parallel to the metatarsal shaft.

Fixation

- Secure the osteotomy with a minifragment screw inserted from proximal to distal fixing the osteotomy site (**TECH FIG 5**). Alternatively, a Kirschner wire can be used to secure the osteotomy site.
- Close the capsule with a heavy nonabsorbable suture.
- Close the subcutaneous tissue with small absorbable suture and the skin with small nonabsorbable suture.

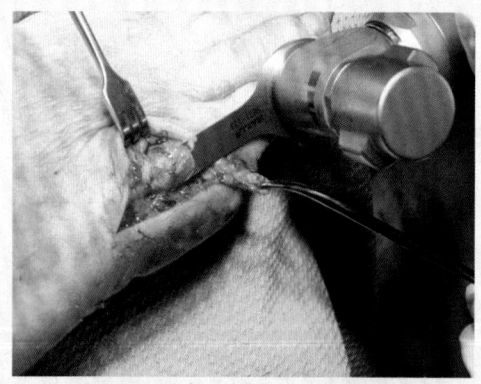

A

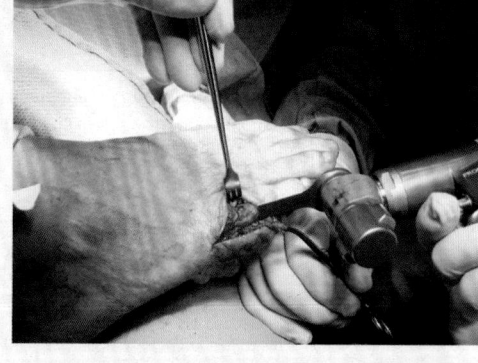

B

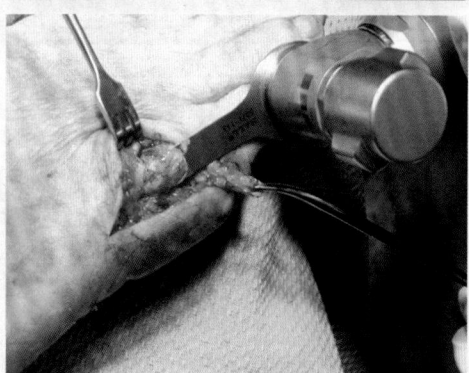

C

TECH FIG 3 A. Bunionette exposed through lateral approach and V-shaped capsulotomy. **B,C.** Bunionette excision performed with saw.

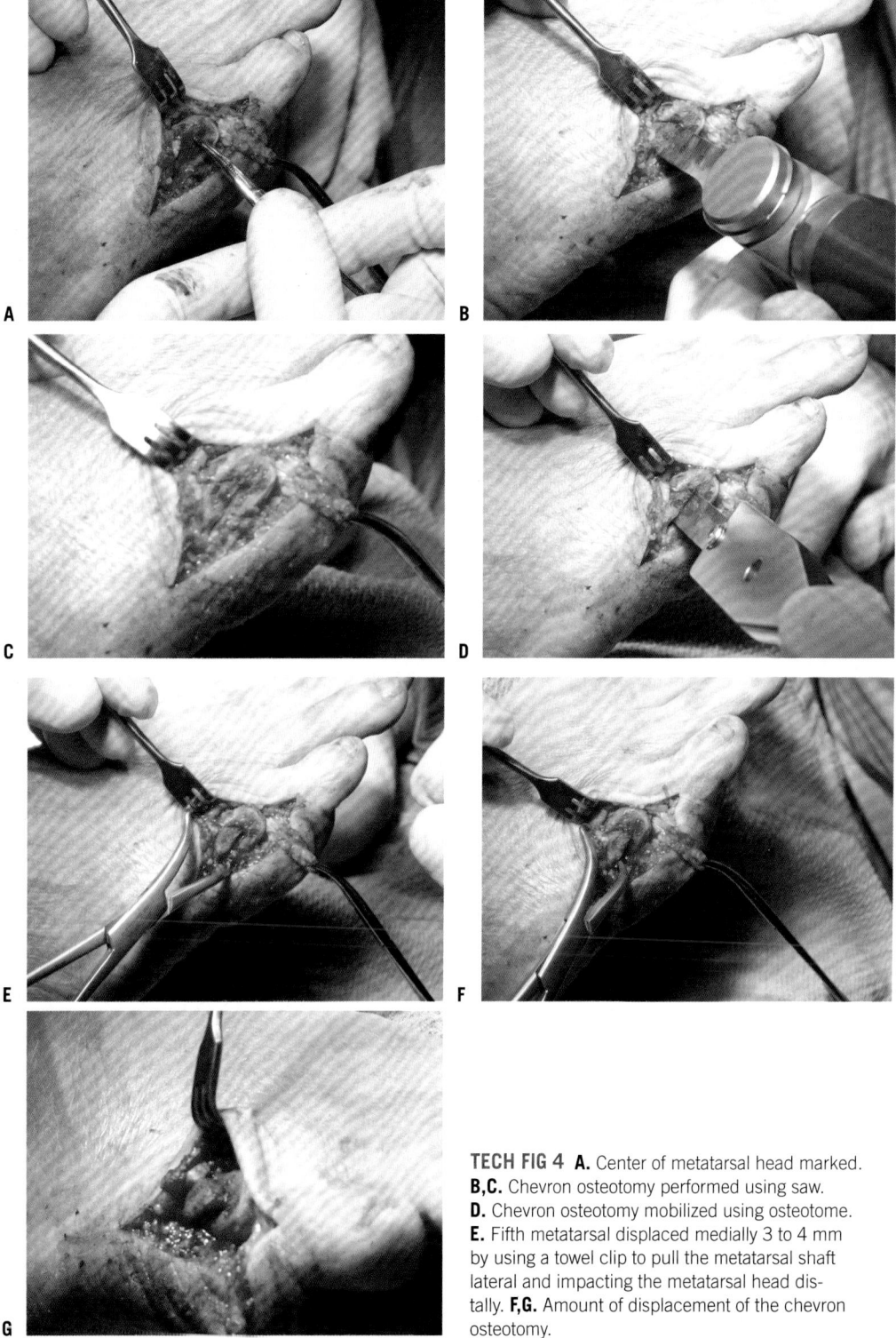

TECH FIG 4 A. Center of metatarsal head marked.
B,C. Chevron osteotomy performed using saw.
D. Chevron osteotomy mobilized using osteotome.
E. Fifth metatarsal displaced medially 3 to 4 mm
by using a towel clip to pull the metatarsal shaft
lateral and impacting the metatarsal head distally. **F,G.** Amount of displacement of the chevron
osteotomy.

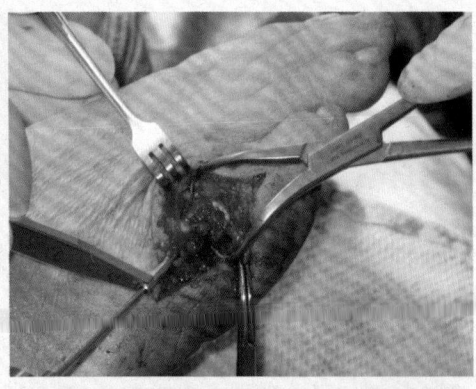

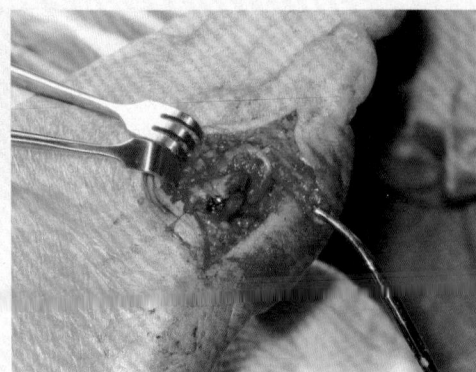

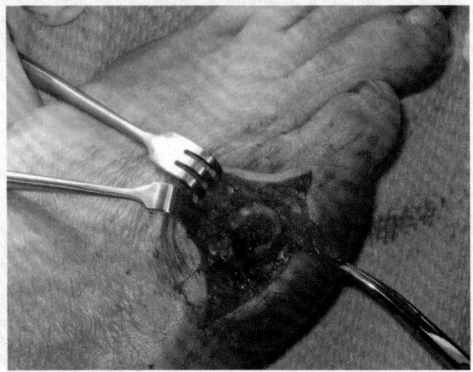

TECH FIG 5 A,B. Metatarsal head is stabilized with a towel clip and fixed using a minifragment screw. **C.** Overhanging bone on the proximal and lateral aspect of the metatarsal shaft is excised.

OBLIQUE METATARSAL SHAFT OSTEOTOMY (COUGHLIN)

Exposure

- Make a lateral skin incision and carry it down to the capsule.
- Free the soft tissue between the capsule and the overlying skin to expose the lateral aspect of the metatarsal head.
- With a sterile marker, mark the plantar aspect of the metatarsal where the capsule meets the metatarsal neck. Then mark the osteotomy on the dorsal proximal aspect.
- Place Hohmann retractors above and below to protect the extensor and flexor tendons.

Osteotomy

- Cut the osteotomy two-thirds of the way, leaving the plantar third intact.
- Insert a minifragment screw (2.0 or 2.7 mm) in the proximal portion of the osteotomy. Tighten the screw completely and then loosen it before completing the osteotomy.
- Complete the osteotomy.
- Swing the distal portion medially to the desired amount of correction and tighten the proximal screw. Insert another 2.0- or 2.7-mm screw more distally to supplement fixation.
- Cut the excess bone from the proximal osteotomy site with the saw.
- Close the subcutaneous tissue with small nonabsorbable suture and the skin with nonabsorbable suture.

CASE EXAMPLE (COURTESY OF MARK E. EASLEY, MD)

Background and Imaging

- A 37-year-old man with symptomatic right bunionette deformity who had failed nonoperative measures including shoe wear modifications
  - Wide forefoot
  - Tenderness over fifth metatarsal head
  - Medial deviation of fifth toe

- Weight-bearing AP radiograph of the right foot demonstrated a wide fourth to fifth IMA and medial deviation of the fifth toe (TECH FIG 6).

Exposure

- Longitudinal approach over the dorsolateral fifth metatarsal is used.
- Sural nerve and extensor digitorum longus tendon are identified and protected.

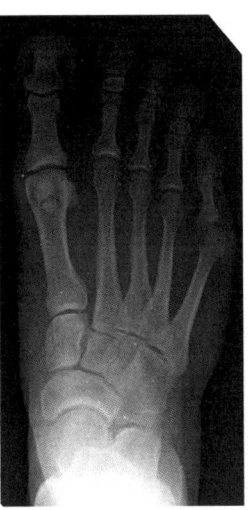

TECH FIG 6 Weight-bearing AP radiograph of the right foot demonstrated a wide fourth to fifth IMA and medial deviation of the fifth toe.

Distal Soft Tissue Procedure

- Lateral fifth metatarsophalangeal (MTP) joint capsule is exposed.
- Lateral capsulotomy and capsule is reflected.
  - A simple longitudinal lateral midaxial capsulotomy is usually all that is required, provided the bony correction is adequate.
  - Through the joint, the medial capsule can be released.

Fifth Metatarsal Osteotomy and Fixation

- Lateral fifth metatarsal is exposed with minimal periosteal stripping.
- The long oblique osteotomy is similar to the long oblique Ludloff first metatarsal osteotomy described for hallux valgus correction.
- Using a microsagittal saw, the dorsal/proximal two-thirds of the osteotomy is completed, leaving the plantar/distal one-third intact.
- A lag screw is placed across the proximal completed aspect of the osteotomy, tightened to confirm compression, and then the screw is loosened slightly, maintaining osteotomy stability and allowing for completion of the distal aspect of the osteotomy.
- The distal osteotomy is completed using the microsagittal saw **(TECH FIG 7A)**.
- With one hand applying tension on a towel clip attached to the proximal fragment and the other hand applying pressure to the lateral metatarsal head, the distal fragment is rotated to correct the IMA **(TECH FIG 7B)**.
- The screw in the proximal osteotomy is tightened to secure the osteotomy and maintain correction **(TECH FIG 7C)**.
- Fluoroscopic confirmation that the IMA is appropriately corrected
- A second lag screw is placed from plantar to dorsal to fully stabilize the osteotomy **(TECH FIG 7D)**.

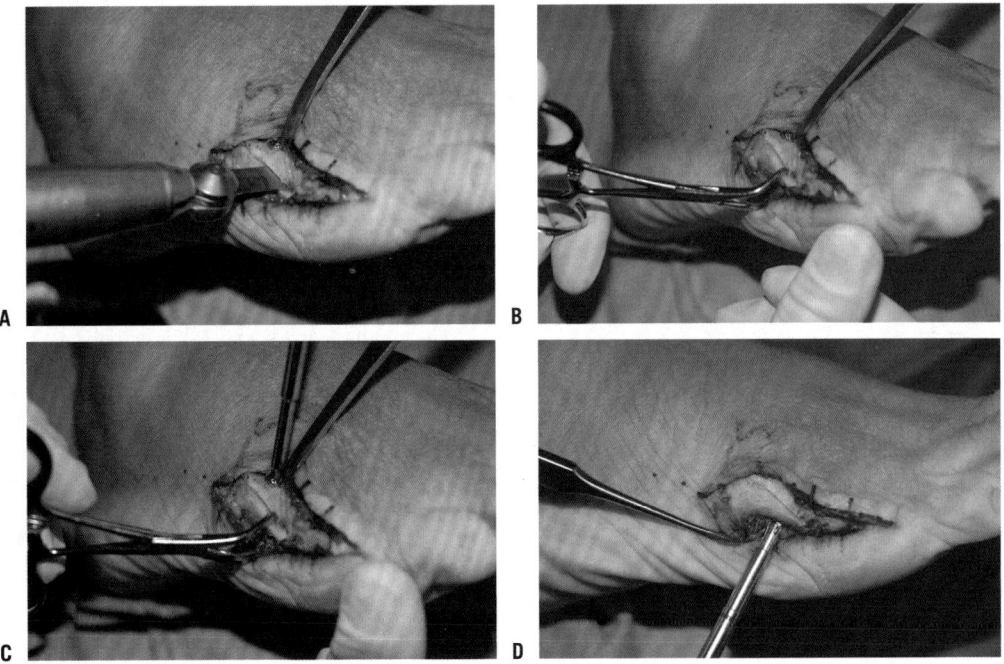

TECH FIG 7 Long oblique metatarsal osteotomy. **A.** After performing the dorsal/proximal two-thirds of the osteotomy and stabilizing it with a proximal lag screw, the long oblique osteotomy is completed using the microsagittal saw. **B.** With one hand applying tension on a towel clip attached to the proximal fragment and the other hand applying pressure to the lateral metatarsal head, the distal fragment is rotated to correct the IMA. **C.** The screw in the proximal osteotomy is tightened to secure the osteotomy and maintain correction. **D.** A second lag screw is placed from plantar to dorsal to fully stabilize the osteotomy.

TECHNIQUES

Closure

- The medial eminence is excised with the microsagittal saw (TECH FIG 8).
- The medial capsule is imbricated.
- Final intraoperative fluoroscopy to confirm appropriate correction of the IMA and hallux valgus angle (HVA)
- The tourniquet is released, and meticulous hemostasis is achieved.
- Subcutaneous layer and skin are reapproximated.
- Bunion-type dressing is applied to the fifth toe.

Postoperative Care

- Protected weight bearing on the heel for 4 to 6 weeks
- Bunion-type dressings are maintained for 4 to 6 weeks (TECH FIG 9).
- Provided follow-up weight-bearing radiographs suggest satisfactory healing, the patient can return to full activities at 3 months.

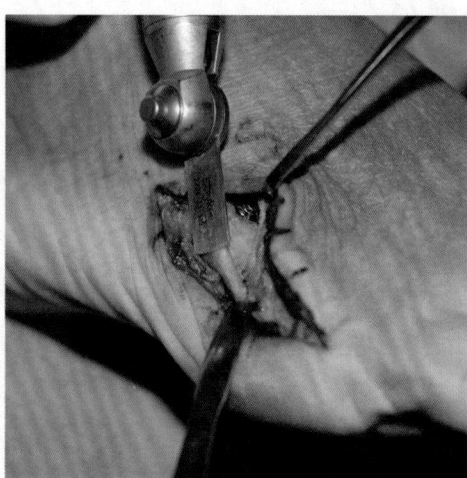

TECH FIG 8 The medial eminence is excised with the microsagittal saw.

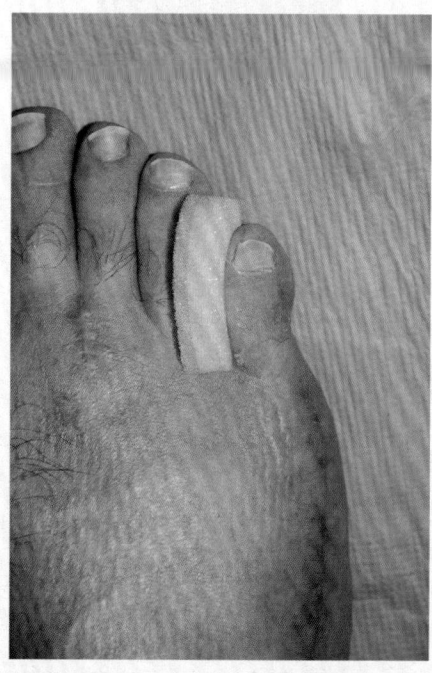

TECH FIG 9 Bunion-type dressing to be maintained for 4 to 6 weeks. The larger bunion-type dressing may be eventually replaced with a toe spacer.

MINIMALLY INVASIVE OSTEOTOMY (SERI OSTEOTOMY)[6]

Exposure

- 1- to 2-cm longitudinal incision centered over the lateral aspect of the fifth metatarsal neck
- Blunt dissection down to bone with a small Hohmann retractor placed inferior and superior to metacarpal shaft

Osteotomy

- Use a microsagittal saw to make a complete transverse or oblique osteotomy just proximal to metacarpal neck depending on the magnitude of metatarsal shortening desired.
- A transverse osteotomy perpendicular to metatarsal shaft will maintain length, whereas a 25-degree oblique osteotomy from distal lateral to proximal medial will facilitate shortening to decompress the joint.
- Mobilize the osteotomy using an osteotome to lever the head and stretch the adjacent soft tissues.
- Translate the metatarsal head 2 to 4 mm medially and confirm appropriateness of correction with fluoroscopy.

Fixation

- Insert and advance a small 1.6 Kirschner wire in an antegrade direction through the small incision adjacent to the metatarsal, exiting just lateral to the lateral border of fifth-digit nail.
- After ensuring bunionette correction is satisfactory, advance the wire retrograde to achieve fixation into the shaft, advancing the wire to the level of the fifth TMT joint.

Postoperative Care

- Protected weight bearing on the heel for 4 to 6 weeks
- Bunion-type dressings are maintained for 4 to 6 weeks.
- Remove Kirschner wire at 4 to 6 weeks.
- Provided follow-up weight-bearing radiographs suggest satisfactory healing; the patient can return to full activities at 3 months.

PERCUTANEOUS OSTEOTOMY

Exposure and Bunionectomy

- Make a small stab incision 1 cm proximal to the lateral aspect of the fifth metatarsal head using a no. 11 blade. Advance the blade in line with the metatarsal shaft until bone is felt.
- Use a periosteal elevator or small rasp to bluntly dissect to the level of the lateral metatarsal head and create space for your burr.
- Insert your burr and ensure it is lateral to the metatarsal head under fluoroscopic guidance. Ensure you can see the fluoroscopic monitor easily at the base of the bed while burring.
- Using a glancing continuous movement, gently burr away the lateral one-third of the metatarsal head under generous fluoroscopic guidance to avoid overresection.
- Remove the resulting bone paste by compressing it out of the incision and irrigating.
- A single simple interrupted suture is used to approximate the wound.

Medial Closing Wedge Osteotomy

- Confirm the level of your proximal, diaphyseal, or distal osteotomy under fluoroscopic guidance, depending on the apex of the deformity and the amount of correction desired.
- Make a small stab incision dorsal and lateral to the fifth extensor tendon.
- Use a periosteal elevator or small rasp to dissect bluntly in an oblique direction to the medial metatarsal cortex and create space for your burr.

- Insert your burr to the level of the medial metatarsal cortex at the level of the osteotomy site and confirm with fluoroscopy.
- Under fluoroscopic guidance, start your burr and continue burring alongside the medial cortex in a distal dorsal to proximal plantar direction. Ensure you burr in a gentle back-and-forth sweeping motion at approximately 45 degrees, ensuring you maintain the integrity of lateral cortical hinge. While burring, use the skin incision site as a guide to prevent burring the lateral cortical hinge.
- Stop burring once a small medial wedge has been removed.
- Gently reposition the metatarsal to "close" your osteotomy using a push–pull maneuver where you push the metatarsal head medially into varus using your thumb while pulling the fifth toe into valgus.
- Confirm adequate correction using fluoroscopy.
- A single simple interrupted suture is used to approximate the wound.

Stabilization and Postoperative Care

- No fixation is required as this is a stable osteotomy.
- A tensor or wrap dressing may be placed snugly around the distal forefoot to hold the varus metatarsal correction, and a toe spacer or cotton padding may be used between the fourth and fifth toe to hold the fifth toe straight.
- Protected weight bearing on the heel for 4 to 6 weeks

TECHNIQUES

Pearls and Pitfalls

Lateral Metatarsal Head Excision	• Avoid excising too much metatarsal because it can result in joint instability. • The osteotomy should be directed away from the metatarsal shaft to avoid splitting the metatarsal with the osteotomy.
Chevron Osteotomy	• The apex of the osteotomy should be located at the center of the metatarsal head. If it is too distal, it can fracture the head. If it is too proximal, the location of the osteotomy is diaphyseal bone, which may take longer to heal. • If the plane of the osteotomy is not parallel to the plantar aspect of the foot, it will prevent shifting of the metatarsal head.
Oblique Osteotomy	• A long oblique osteotomy is needed to achieve better correction and more stable fixation. • Screw placement for the osteotomy is important. If it is too close to the end of the osteotomy, it will fracture the osteotomy. If it is too distal to the end of the osteotomy, it limits the correction because the point of rotation is more distal than the apex of the osteotomy. • Stable fixation is key to union and maintaining the correction.

POSTOPERATIVE CARE

- The wound is checked at 1 week postoperatively to examine for any evidence of infection.
- Sutures are removed at 2 weeks.
- If a pin was used, it is removed at 6 weeks.

- Heel walking only is permitted for 6 weeks.
- In the oblique metatarsal osteotomy, a postoperative fiberglass splint is applied in the operating room and is changed to an air cast at 2 weeks. This is continued for 6 weeks.
- **FIG 2** is the case example at 6-week follow-up.

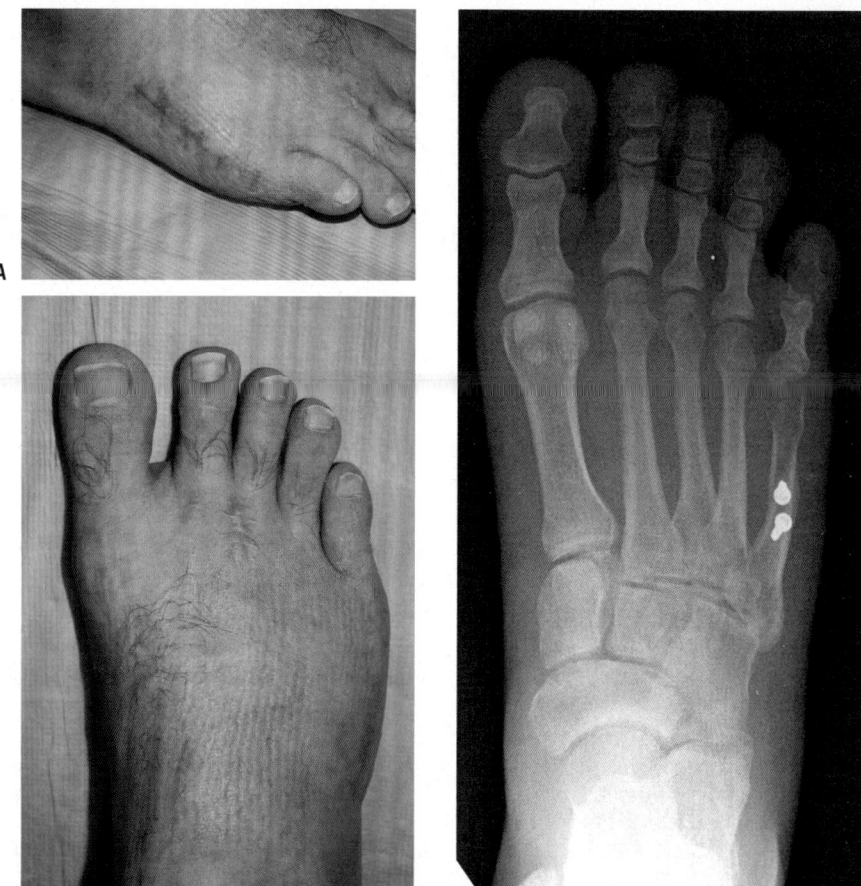

FIG 2 Patient in **TECH FIGS 6**, **7**, and **8** at 6-week follow-up. **A.** Lateral view. **B.** Dorsal view. **C.** Weight-bearing radiograph suggest satisfactory correction: narrowed forefoot with corrected IMA and HVA.

OUTCOMES

- Although the bunionette deformity is common, it is rarely symptomatic enough to warrant surgical intervention. This is reflected by the small numbers found in case studies reported in the literature.
- A recent systematic review of 28 studies demonstrated that proximal and diaphyseal osteotomies provided a significantly greater IMA correction than distal osteotomies. Nonetheless, distal osteotomies had the lowest complication rate (11%), which was nearly half the complication rate associated with diaphyseal and proximal osteotomies (21% and 22%, respectively). All osteotomies had a satisfaction rate of 92% to 100%.[5]
- Kitaoka and Holiday[7] reported results on 21 feet (16 patients) who underwent lateral condylar resection for bunionette. The overall results were considered good in 15 feet, fair in 3, and poor in 3. However, 23% of the patients had recurrent or persistent lateral forefoot pain. They attributed the failures to an inadequate amount of resection, MTP joint subluxation, and severe forefoot splaying. Limitations of the procedure included lack of deformity correction, a significant incidence of residual lateral forefoot pain, and difficulty treating bunionettes with intractable plantar keratosis.

- Several studies have reported good results in the surgical treatment of bunionette with chevron osteotomies.[2,8,11]
- Moran and Claridge[11] felt that stabilization of the osteotomy site with fixation was necessary to minimize the risk of displacement.
- One study reported that Kirschner wire fixation led to less dorsal displacement of the distal fragment.[13]
- Kitaoka et al's[8] series of 19 chevron osteotomies for bunionettes reported a satisfaction rate of 89.5%. They used Kirschner wire fixation in only 1 of 19 patients due to intraoperative instability at the osteotomy site; however, they did note postoperative displacement in another patient.
- No incidence of displacement was found in series that routinely used fixation.[2,11]
- Limited correction of the fourth to fifth IMA was seen, where 1 mm of translation results in a decrease of that angle of only 1 degree.[3,8]
- The fifth metatarsal head can be shifted only by 33% to 40% of its width, generally in the range of 3 to 4 mm.[2,3,8,11]
- Kitaoka et al[8] noted that neither the preoperative nor the postoperative intermetatarsal fourth to fifth angle correlated with the postoperative foot score.

- Oblique metatarsal diaphyseal osteotomies have been shown to provide a large correction for a type II or III deformity with a high IMA.[4,14,17] Coughlin[4] found that the IMA decreased from an average of 16 degrees preoperatively to 0.5 degrees postoperatively. Results have shown a reliable improvement in postoperative subjective scores.[4,14,17] With the use of internal fixation, there was only one report of delayed union.[4,14,17] This is compared to other series reporting rates of delayed union of up to 11% without fixation.[16] However, prominent hardware can be an issue, and in one study, 87% of patients required later removal.[4] Proximal osteotomies are not recommended due to the poor blood supply in the region and the higher risk of delayed or nonunion.[1,15]
- Proximal or base or fifth metatarsal osteotomies have been used to address primarily large type III deformities with an increased IMA. Okuda et al[12] reported a case series on 10 patients treated with proximal osteotomies and found an IMA correction from 12.2 degrees to 4.8 degrees postoperatively. These osteotomies are losing favor as they are associated with the highest rate of nonunion secondary to disruption of the nutrient artery, which enters the medial aspect of the metatarsal 2 cm from its base.[12]
- Metatarsal head resection is used as a salvage option due to unacceptably high rates of complications. Kitaoka and Holiday[7] reported a series of 11 patients treated with head resection and reported a 64% complication rate, including metatarsalgia and progressive toe deformity.

COMPLICATIONS

- Infection
- Recurrent deformity
- Digital nerve injury
- Nonunion of the osteotomy
- Delayed union
- Displacement of the osteotomy
- Avascular necrosis of the fifth metatarsal head
- Transfer metatarsalgia

REFERENCES

1. Baumhauer JF, DiGiovanni BF. Osteotomies of the fifth metatarsal. Foot Ankle Clin 2001;6:491–498.
2. Boyer ML, Deorio JK. Bunionette deformity correction with distal chevron osteotomy and single absorbable pin fixation. Foot Ankle Int 2003;24:845–857.
3. Cooper PS. Disorders and deformities of the lesser toes. In: Myerson MS, ed. Foot and Ankle Disorders. Philadelphia: WB Saunders, 2000:335–358.
4. Coughlin MJ. Treatment of bunionette deformity with longitudinal diaphyseal osteotomy with distal soft tissue repair. Foot Ankle 1991;11:195–203.
5. Fallat LM, Buckholz J. An analysis of the tailor's bunion by radiographic and anatomical display. J Am Podiatry Assoc 1980;70:597–603.
6. Giannini S, Faldini C, Vannini F, et al. The minimally invasive osteotomy "S.E.R.I." (simple, effective, rapid, inexpensive) for correction of bunionette deformity. Foot Ankle Int 2008;29(3):282–286.
7. Kitaoka HB, Holiday AD Jr. Lateral condylar resection for bunionette. Clin Orthop Relat Res 1992;(278):183–192.
8. Kitaoka HB, Holiday AD Jr, Campbell DC II. Distal chevron metatarsal osteotomy for bunionette. Foot Ankle Int 1991;12:80–85.
9. Martijn HA, Sierevelt IN, Wassink S, et al. Fifth metatarsal osteotomies for treatment of bunionette deformity: a meta-analysis of angle correction and clinical condition. J Foot Ankle Surg 2017;57(1):140–148.
10. Michels F, Van Der Bauwhede J, Guillo S, et al. Percutaneous bunionette correction. Foot Ankle Sur 2013;19(1):9–14.
11. Moran MM, Claridge RJ. Chevron osteotomy for bunionette. Foot Ankle Int 1994;15:684–688.
12. Okuda R, Kinoshita M, Morikawa J, et al. Proximal dome-shaped osteotomy for symptomatic bunionette. Clin Orthop Relat Res 2002:(396):173–178.
13. Pontious J, Brook JW, Hillstrom HJ. Tailor's bunion. Is fixation necessary? J Am Podiatr Med Assoc 1996;86:63–73.
14. Radl R, Leithner A, Koehler W, et al. The modified distal horizontal metatarsal osteotomy for correction of bunionette deformity. Foot Ankle Int 2005;26:454–457.
15. Shereff MJ, Yang QM, Krummer FJ. Vascular anatomy of the fifth metatarsal. Foot Ankle Int 1991;11:350–353.
16. Sponsel KH. Bunionette correction by metatarsal osteotomy: preliminary report. Orthop Clin North Am 1976;7:808–819.
17. Vienne P, Oesselmann M, Espinosa N, et al. Modified Coughlin procedure for surgical treatment of symptomatic tailor's bunion: a prospective follow-up study of 33 consecutive operations. Foot Ankle Int 2006;27:573–580.

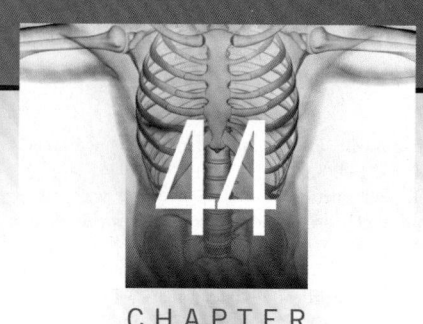

CHAPTER 44

Rheumatoid Forefoot Reconstruction

Thomas G. Padanilam

DEFINITION

- Rheumatoid arthritis is an inflammatory condition of synovial joints that usually presents as a symmetric polyarthropathy.
- Ninety percent of patients with chronic rheumatoid arthritis have involvement of the foot; the forefoot is the most commonly involved area of the foot.

ANATOMY

- The metatarsophalangeal (MTP) joint of the foot is stabilized by the plantar plate, the collateral ligaments, the capsule, and a dynamic balance between the intrinsic and extrinsic muscles of the foot.
- The intrinsic muscles are plantar to the MTP joint axis and help to plantarflex the joint.
- The proximal phalanx of the hallux has a valgus orientation of 0 to 15 degrees at the MTP joint.
- A plantar fat pad normally provides cushioning and protection for the metatarsal heads.

PATHOGENESIS

- Unrelenting synovitis leads to a painful and swollen joint. This causes a stretching of the ligamentous structures surrounding the MTP joint.
- Ligament stretching combined with forces of walking leads to soft tissue instability, articular cartilage destruction, and subchondral bone resorption.
- Residual laxity leads to subluxation and dislocation of the lesser MTP joints. This allows the metatarsal head to protrude through the plantar plate and capsule.
- The hallux most commonly develops a hallux valgus deformity, with an occasional hallux varus developing.
- MTP instability leads to intrinsic muscles becoming dorsal to the MTP axis, which leads to loss of active MTP flexion and interphalangeal extension. This leads to a claw toe deformity.
- Dislocation of the metatarsal lesser MTP joints leads to a distal migration of the fat pad, which exposes the metatarsal heads, increasing pressure in this area.

NATURAL HISTORY

- Rheumatoid arthritis initially presents in the foot in about 17% of patients.
- It is a progressive disorder that may start as synovitis and progress to dislocations and degeneration of the joint.
- The longer active rheumatoid disease is present, the greater the likelihood the patient will develop deformities as a result of the associated synovitis.

PATIENT HISTORY AND PHYSICAL FINDINGS

- Initially, patients often complain of an insidious onset of poorly defined forefoot pain and difficulty with ambulation. As synovitis leads to deformity within the forefoot, the symptoms then become more localized.
- Patients will often have shoe wear–related irritation along the medial eminence of the hallux and along the dorsal aspects of the proximal interphalangeal (PIP) joints of the lesser toes.
- With the development of the lesser toe MTP dislocation, pain on the plantar aspect of the metatarsal heads is present.
- Hallux valgus: The examiner should look for the degrees of valgus orientation and its impingement on lesser toes. Patients often have pain along the medial eminence and from pressure on the toes (FIG 1).
- Lesser MTP dislocation and plantar callus: The examiner should inspect and palpate the dorsal and plantar aspects of the forefoot. MTP instability can vary from subluxation to dislocation. Increased pressure under the metatarsal heads is a common source of pain (FIG 2).
  - Examination should include range of motion for the ankle, subtalar, and MTP joints.
- The examiner should perform a complete vascular and neurologic examination of the foot.

IMAGING AND OTHER DIAGNOSTIC STUDIES

- Plain radiographs will often show periarticular osteopenia, symmetric joint space narrowing, marginal cortical erosions, and subchondral cysts (FIG 3).
- The severity of hallux valgus and the presence of MTP dislocation can be evaluated.

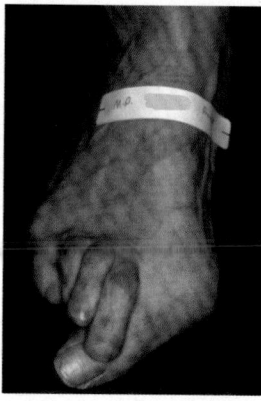

FIG 1 Hallux valgus: The examiner should inspect the foot with the patient standing.

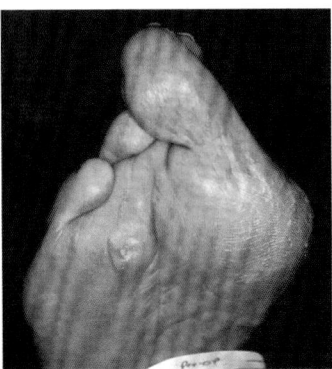

FIG 2 Lesser MTP dislocation and plantar callus: The examiner should inspect and palpate the dorsal and plantar aspects of the forefoot.

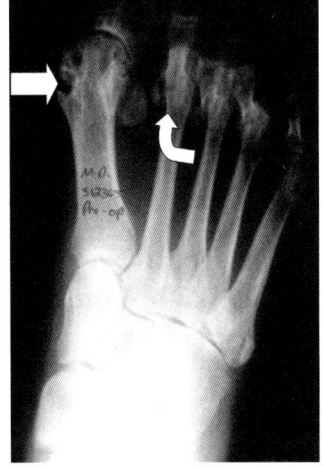

FIG 3 Loss of joint space, severe hallux valgus, and associated osteopenia. The *straight arrow* shows marginal cortical erosion. The *curved arrow* shows the overlap between the proximal phalanx and the metatarsal head seen with dislocation of the joint.

DIFFERENTIAL DIAGNOSIS

- Inflammatory arthritides such as psoriatic arthritis, Reiter syndrome (reactive arthritis), and ankylosing spondylitis
- Gout and pseudogout
- Connective tissue disorders (ie, lupus)
- Inflammatory bowel disease (Crohn disease or ulcerative colitis)
- Neurologic disorders
- Osteoarthritis

NONOPERATIVE MANAGEMENT

- New pharmacologic agents that can control synovitis have the potential for minimizing the severity and frequency of deformities seen.
- Shoe wear modifications such as extradepth shoes decrease shoe wear irritation.
- Custom inserts can help relieve pressure from painful areas.
- Plantar calluses may benefit from periodic shaving.

SURGICAL MANAGEMENT

- Surgical treatment is indicated for patients whose pain is unrelieved by nonoperative treatment or those with ulcerative lesions due to their deformity.
- The goals of surgical treatment include the following:
  - Restoration of the weight-bearing function of the first ray
  - Relocation of the plantar fat pad
  - Reduction of pressure under the lesser metatarsal heads
  - Correction of claw toe or hammer toe deformities
- Mild deformities may be amenable to joint-preserving surgery in patients with excellent medical control of their disease, but probably the most reliable method for accomplishing these goals is with fusion of the first MTP joint, resection of the lesser metatarsal heads, and either osteoclasis or open hammer toe repair.

Preoperative Planning

- These patients have a relatively poor soft tissue envelope, and this may compromise wound healing.
- There is no perioperative standard as to whether to continue the use of disease-modifying antirheumatic drugs.
- Consideration should be given regarding the need for cervical spine evaluation before general anesthesia.

Positioning

- The patient is placed supine on the operating table, with the foot positioned near the distal end of the table (**FIG 4**).

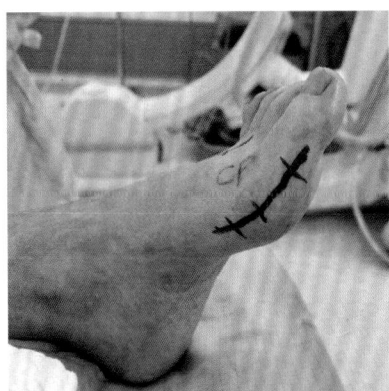
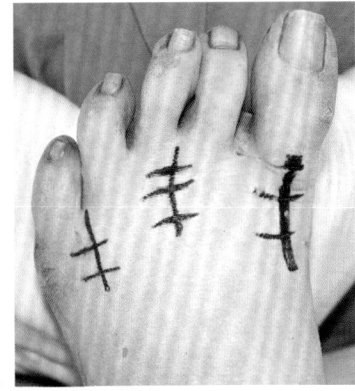

FIG 4 A. The patient is placed supine with the foot near the distal end of the table. **B.** The foot is positioned so that the dorsal aspect can be visualized. This may require the use of a blanket roll or sandbag under the ipsilateral hip.

A   B

Approach

- The first MTP joint can be exposed through a dorsal or medial approach. Both provide adequate exposure, but the medial approach may provide a greater skin bridge between incisions. Incisions from previous procedures may dictate the approach used.

- Lesser metatarsal head resection can be performed through dorsal longitudinal incisions or a plantar incision. Although the plantar approach may provide more direct access to the metatarsal head when the MTP joint has been dislocated for a while, there is more of a risk of problems with wound healing.

HAMMER TOE CORRECTION

Closed Correction

- If the deformity at the PIP joint of the lesser toes is not severe, the contractures at the joint can be corrected by closed manipulation **(TECH FIG 1)**.
  - Grasp the toe distal and proximal to the PIP joint and hyperextend it until the joint is resting in a neutral position.

Open Correction

- If the deformity is severe, an open hammer toe correction is performed **(TECH FIG 2)**.
  - Make an elliptical incision along the PIP joint.
  - Remove an elliptical portion of skin over the PIP joint and open the capsule over the joint.
  - Release the collateral ligaments and expose the head of the proximal phalanx.
  - Resect the proximal phalanx at the metaphyseal–diaphyseal junction.
  - Stabilize the area with a Kirschner wire after performing metatarsal head resections.

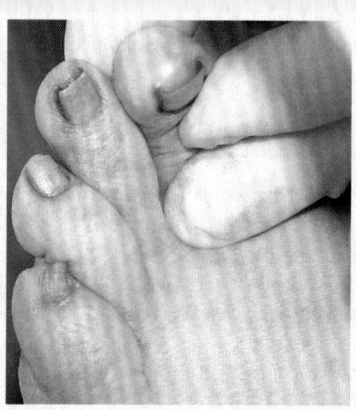

TECH FIG 1 Performance of osteoclasis, in which the PIP joint is passively manipulated to break up contracture.

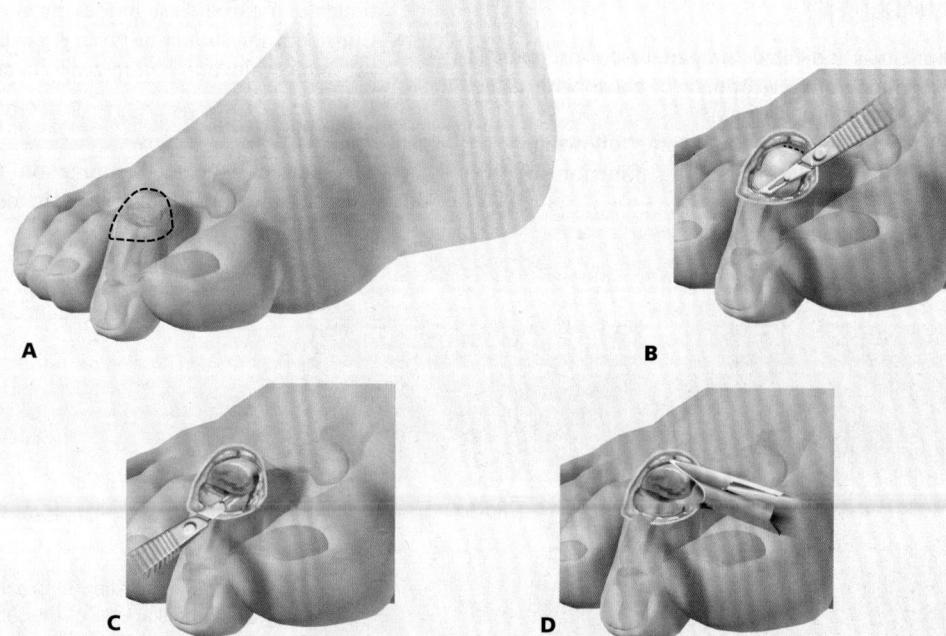

TECH FIG 2 An open hammer toe repair is performed with an elliptical incision over the PIP joint (**A**), followed by capsular release (**B**), exposure (**C**), and resection (**D**) of the head of the proximal phalanx.

LESSER METATARSAL HEAD RESECTION

- Make longitudinal incisions over the second and fourth intermetatarsal spaces **(TECH FIG 3A)**.
  - Blunt dissection is recommended to minimize trauma.
- Identify the extensor digitorum longus and retract it to one side **(TECH FIG 3B)**.
- Release the dorsal capsule and collateral ligaments off the metatarsal head **(TECH FIG 3C)**.
- Bring the metatarsal head into the dorsal aspect of the incision.
- A curved retractor can be useful in obtaining exposure of the metatarsal head **(TECH FIG 3D)**.
- Use a sagittal saw to resect the metatarsal head. The blade is oriented in an oblique fashion from dorsal-distal to plantar-proximal **(TECH FIG 3E,F)**.

- Remove the metatarsal head as one fragment if possible. Take care to avoid leaving any bone fragments **(TECH FIG 3G)**.
  - Make sure the plantar aspect of the metatarsal is smooth and does not have a sharp edge.
- The metatarsal head resection usually starts on the second metatarsal and moves laterally **(TECH FIG 3H)**.
  - Leave the third metatarsal slightly shorter than the second and the fourth shorter than the third metatarsal. This creates a smooth cascade from medial to lateral.
- Pass 0.625-mm Kirschner wires from the base of the proximal phalanx to the tip of the toes **(TECH FIG 3I)**.
- Pass the wires retrograde down the metatarsal shaft **(TECH FIG 3J)**.

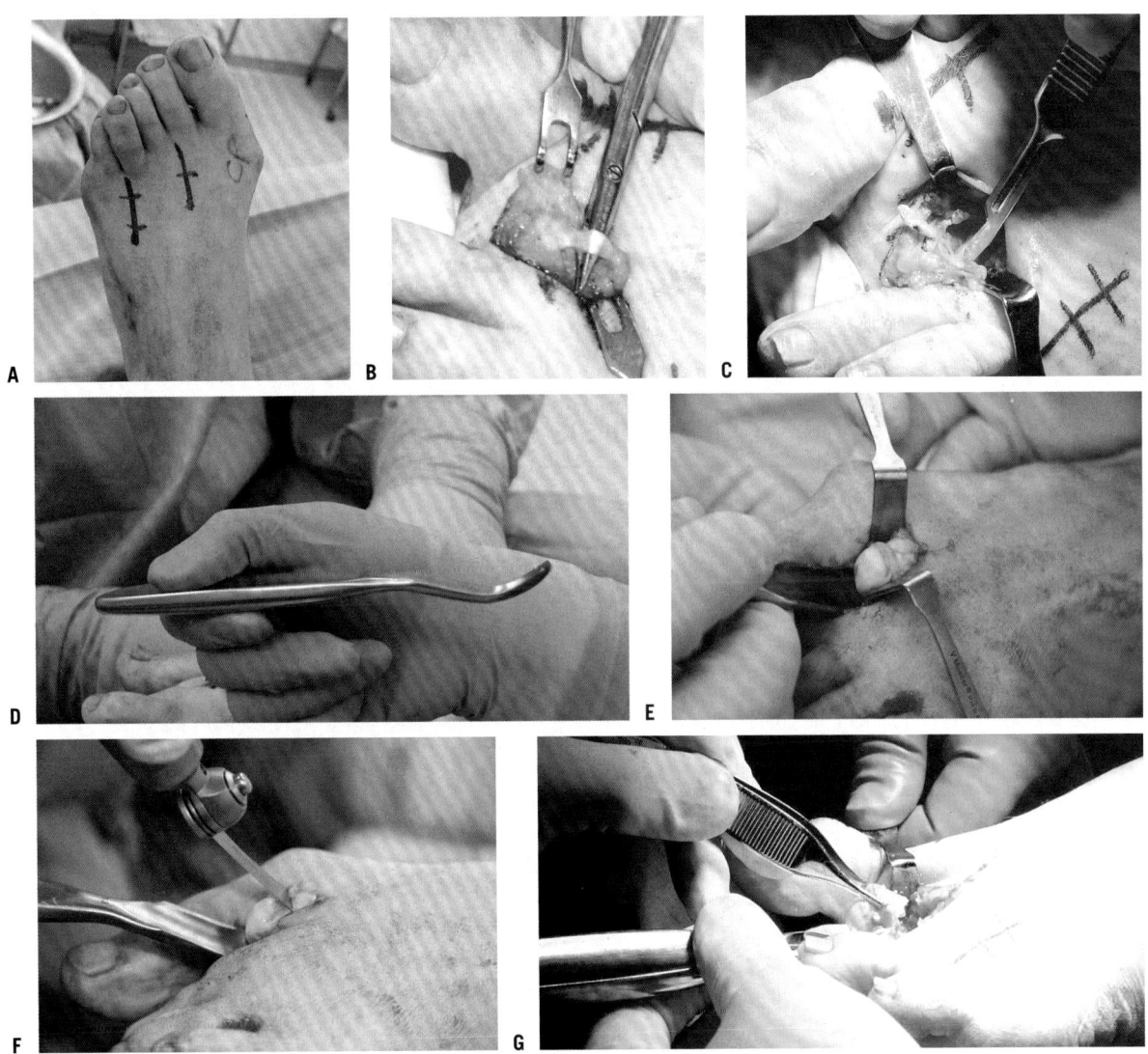

TECH FIG 3 A. Dorsal, longitudinal incisions are made in the second and fourth intermetatarsal spaces. **B.** The extensor tendon is identified and retracted to one side. **C.** The dorsal capsule and collateral ligaments are released off the metatarsal head. **D.** A curved retractor can be helpful in exposure of the metatarsal head. **E.** The metatarsal head is brought into the dorsal aspect of the incision. **F.** Metatarsal head resection is oriented in an oblique fashion from dorsal-distal to plantar-proximal. **G.** The metatarsal head is removed as one fragment if possible. *(continued)*

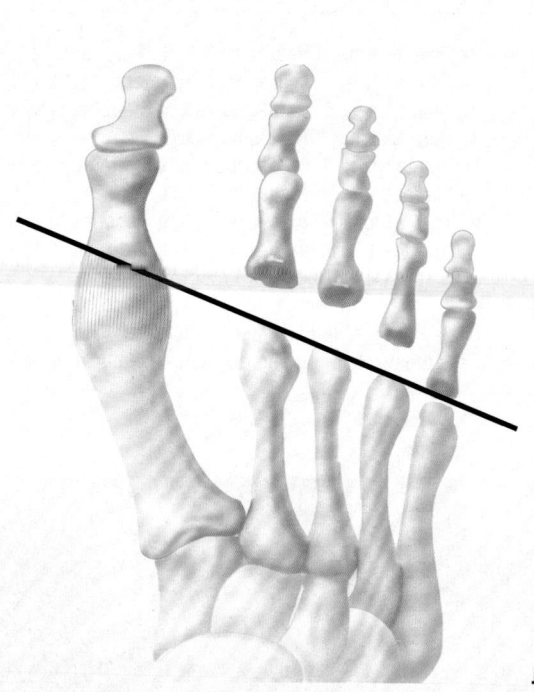

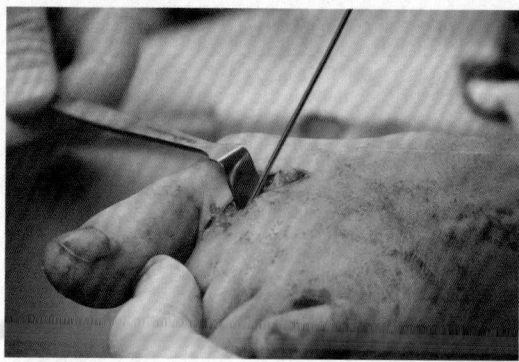

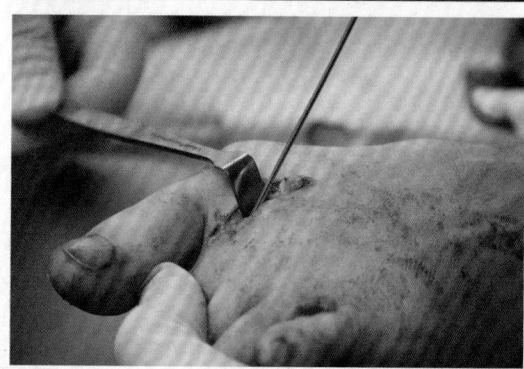

TECH FIG 3 *(continued)* **H.** Progressive resection from the second to fifth metatarsal is performed, creating a smooth cascade. **I.** Kirschner wires are passed from the base of the proximal phalanx to the tip of the toes. **J.** The wires are then passed retrograde down the metatarsal shaft.

HALLUX METATARSOPHALANGEAL ARTHRODESIS

- Make a medial incision along the MTP joint (**TECH FIG 4A**).
- Incise the capsule and expose the metatarsal head and proximal phalanx (**TECH FIG 4B**).
- Prepare the joint surfaces by removing the remaining articular cartilage and exposing the underlying bone.
  - This can be done with the use of a cup and cone reamer system (**TECH FIG 4C**) or with rongeurs and curettes.
  - Flat cuts using a saw can also be used (**TECH FIG 4D**), but it is slightly more difficult to orient the cuts such that the correct alignment of the joint is obtained.
  - Multiple drill holes are placed in both articular surfaces to penetrate subchondral bone to encourage fusion of the joint.

- Place the MTP joint in 10 to 15 degrees of valgus and 20 to 25 degrees of dorsiflexion relative to the metatarsal shaft.
  - The correct dorsiflexion can be approximated by using a flat tray as a guide and keeping the pulp of the hallux 5 to 10 mm off the surface of the tray (**TECH FIG 4E**).
- The position is held temporarily with a Kirschner wire (**TECH FIG 4F**).
- Perform definitive fixation with cross screws or a dorsal plate or, in salvage cases, threaded pins (**TECH FIG 4G–I**).
- Close the wounds and apply a forefoot dressing (**TECH FIG 4J**).

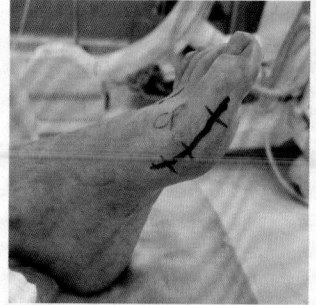

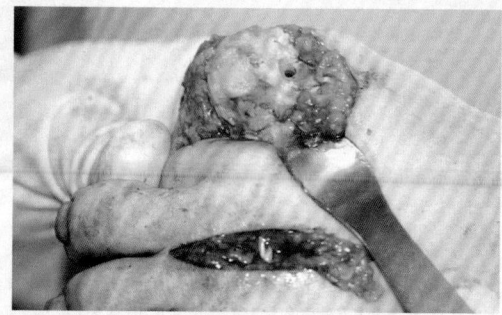

TECH FIG 4 A. Medial incision for exposure of hallux MTP. **B.** The proximal phalanx and metatarsal head articular cartilage are exposed. *(continued)*

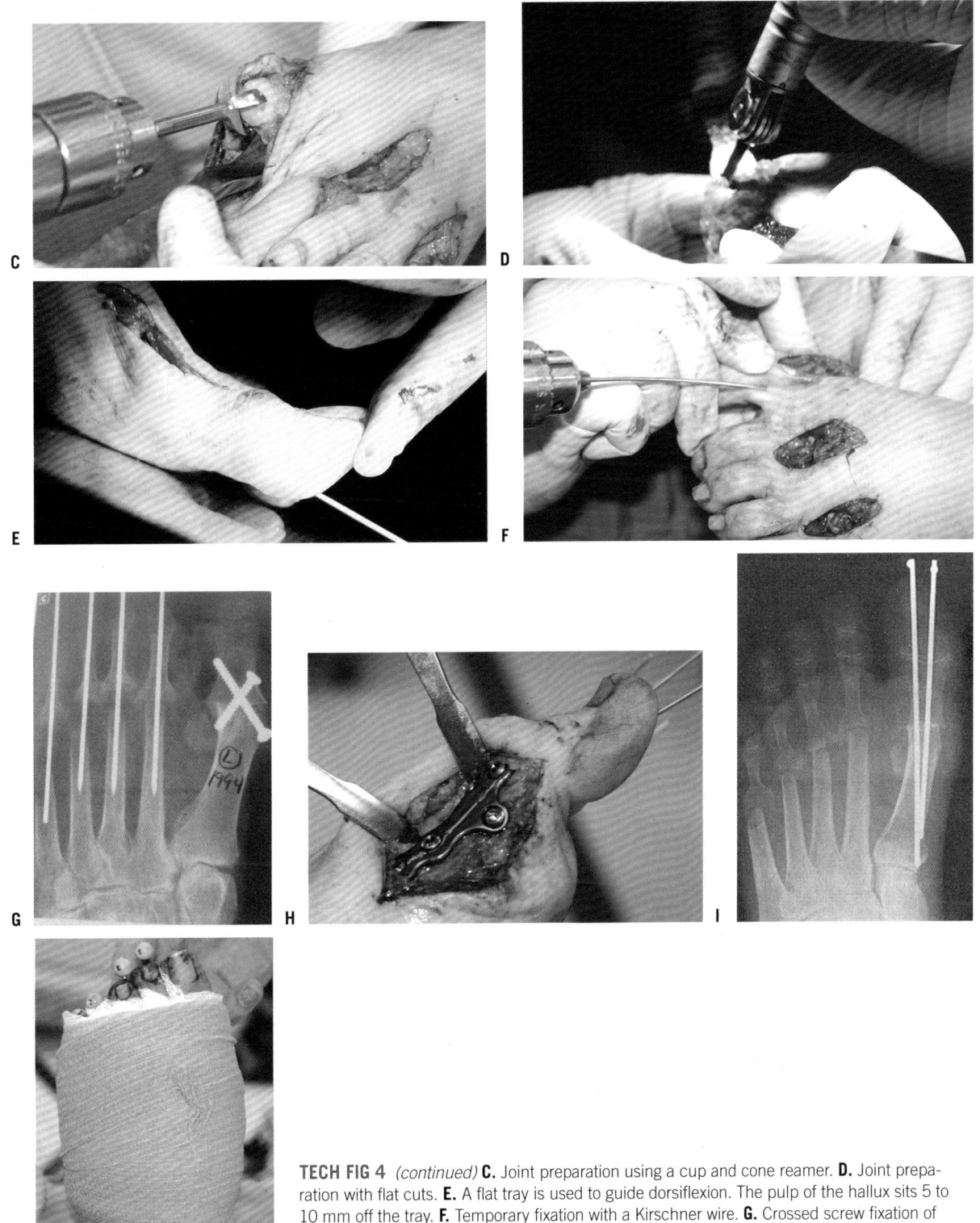

TECH FIG 4 *(continued)* **C.** Joint preparation using a cup and cone reamer. **D.** Joint preparation with flat cuts. **E.** A flat tray is used to guide dorsiflexion. The pulp of the hallux sits 5 to 10 mm off the tray. **F.** Temporary fixation with a Kirschner wire. **G.** Crossed screw fixation of fusion. **H.** Dorsal plate fixation. **I.** Fixation with threaded pins. **J.** Postoperative forefoot dressing.

Pearls and Pitfalls

Hammer Toe Correction	• Fixed deformities often require an open correction.
	• Failure to correct the deformity can lead to recurrent deformity.
Metatarsal Head Resection	• Oblique orientation of the resection helps decrease plantar pressure and sharp plantar edges.
	• Loose fragments can lead to recurrent callus formation and should be avoided.
	• Adequate decompression of the lesser MTP joint is seen with about 1 cm of space between the base of the phalanx and remaining metatarsal.
	• Progressive shortening of the metatarsals from medial to lateral allows better stress transfer.
	• After pin fixation, check the vascularity of the toe, as compromise occasionally requires pin removal.
Hallux MTP Fusion	• This is performed after the lesser metatarsal head resection to prevent an excessively long first ray.
	• Excessive dorsiflexion can cause pain over the interphalangeal joint and under the metatarsal head.
	• Fusion in greater than 20 degrees of valgus can increase the incidence of interphalangeal joint arthritis.
	• Care must be taken to prevent excessive pronation or supination of the toe.

POSTOPERATIVE CARE

- After placement of the forefoot dressing, a walking boot is applied **(FIG 5)**.
- Patients are instructed to bear weight on the heel of the foot.
- Sutures are removed 10 to 14 days after surgery.
- A forefoot dressing is used for the first 6 weeks.
- Kirschner wires are removed at 6 weeks.
- A walking boot is used for 8 to 10 weeks, based on healing of the first MTP fusion.

OUTCOMES

- Most studies have noted a significant improvement in ability to ambulate and in shoe wear options.
- Patient satisfaction rates are high and seem to hold up over time.
- Patients should be aware that the lesser toes are unlikely to touch the floor and can be floppy, there may be a change in shoe size, and toes may develop a rotational deformity.

COMPLICATIONS

- Recurrent intractable plantar keratosis
- Recurrent toe deformities
- Wound healing problems
- Nonunion of MTP fusion
- Infection

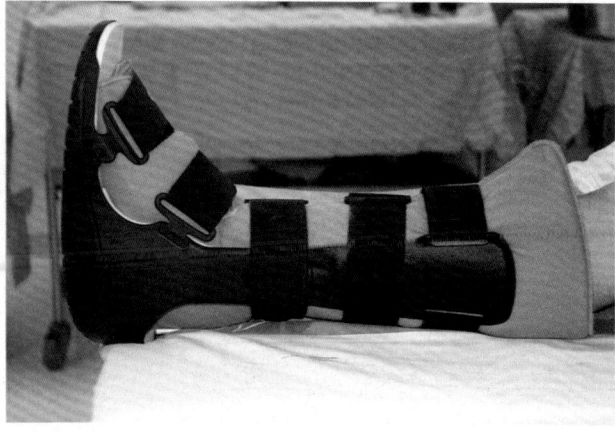

FIG 5 Postoperative walking boot.

SUGGESTED READINGS

Abdo RV, Iorio LJ. Rheumatoid arthritis of the foot and ankle. J Am Acad Orthop Surg 1994;2:326–332.

Beauchamp CG, Kirby T, Rudge SR, et al. Fusion of the first metatarsophalangeal joint in forefoot arthroplasty. Clin Orthop Relat Res 1984;(190):249–253.

Clayton ML, Leidholt JD, Clark W. Arthroplasty of rheumatoid metatarsophalangeal joints. An outcome study. Clin Orthop Relat Res 1997;(340):48–57.

Coughlin MJ. Rheumatoid forefoot reconstruction. A long-term follow-up study. J Bone Joint Surg Am 2000;82(3):322–341.

Fukushi J, Nakashima Y, Okazaki K, et al. Outcome of joint-preserving arthroplasty for rheumatoid forefoot deformities. Foot Ankle Int 2016; 37(3):262–268.

Garner RW, Mowat AG, Hazleman BL. Wound healing after operations of patients with rheumatoid arthritis. J Bone Joint Surg Br 1973; 55(1):134–144.

Hamalainen M, Raunio P. Long-term followup of rheumatoid forefoot surgery. Clin Orthop Relat Res 1997;(340):34–38.

Jaakkola JI, Mann RA. A review of rheumatoid arthritis affecting the foot and ankle. Foot Ankle Int 2004;25:866–874.

Lipscomb PR, Benson GM, Sones DA. Resection of proximal phalanges and metatarsal condyles for deformities of the forefoot due to rheumatoid arthritis. Clin Orthop Relat Res 1972;82:24–31.

Mann RA, Schakel ME II. Surgical correction of rheumatoid forefoot deformities. Foot Ankle Int 1995;16:1–6.

Mann RA, Thompson FM. Arthrodesis of the first metatarsophalangeal joint for hallux valgus in rheumatoid arthritis. J Bone Joint Surg Am 1984;66(5):687–692.

McGarvey SR, Johnson KA. Keller arthroplasty in combination with resection arthroplasty of the lesser metatarsophalangeal joints in rheumatoid arthritis. Foot Ankle 1988;9:75–80.

Nassar J, Cracchiolo A III. Complications in surgery of the foot and ankle in patients with rheumatoid arthritis. Clin Orthop Relat Res 2001;(391):140–152.

Schrier J, Keijsers N, Matricali G, et al. Resection or preservation of the metatarsal heads in rheumatoid forefoot surgery? A randomised clinical trial. Foot Ankle Surg 2019;25:37–46.

Spiegel TM, Spiegel JS. Rheumatoid arthritis in the foot and ankle—diagnosis, pathology, and treatment. The relationship between foot and ankle deformity and disease duration in 50 patients. Foot Ankle 1982;2:318–324.

Thomas S, Kinninmonth AW, Kumar S. Long-term results of the modified Hoffman procedure in the rheumatoid forefoot. J Bone Joint Surg Am 2005;87(4):748–775.

Thordarson DB, Aval S, Krieger L. Failure of hallux MP preservation surgery for rheumatoid arthritis. Foot Ankle Int 2002;23:486–490.

Trieb K. Management of the foot in rheumatoid arthritis. J Bone Joint Surg Br 2005;87(9):1171–1177.

Vandeputte G, Steenwerckx A, Mulier T, et al. Forefoot reconstruction in rheumatoid patients: Keller-Lelievre-Hoffman versus arthrodesis MTP1-Hoffman. Foot Ankle Int 1999;20:438–443.

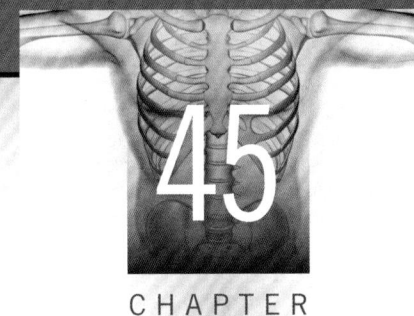

45
CHAPTER

Morton Neuroma and Revision Morton Neuroma Excision or Endoscopic Decompression

David R. Richardson and Steven L. Shapiro

DEFINITION

- Morton neuroma was first described in 1845 by Lewis Durlacher, a chiropodist to the Queen of England.
- A primary interdigital (Morton) neuroma is in fact not a neuroma, as it does not involve the haphazard proliferation of axons seen in a traumatic nerve injury.
  - Instead, this condition is best described as an interdigital perineural fibrosis.
- Recurrent neuromas are true histopathologic (haphazard proliferation of axons) amputation stump neuromas.
- Eighty-five percent to 90% of nontraumatic neuromas are found in the third web space. The rest are found in the second web space.

ANATOMY

- The medial plantar nerve supplies sensation to the first to third digits and the medial aspect of the fourth digit. It emerges plantar and medial to the flexor digitorum brevis, coursing obliquely across the plantar surface of the muscle.
- The lateral plantar nerve supplies sensation to the lateral half of the fourth and the fifth digits.
- Both are branches of the tibial nerve and terminate with digital branches that course plantarly deep to the transverse metatarsal ligament (FIG 1).
- The lumbrical tendon appears lateral and superficial to the digital nerve, as it attaches to the medial aspect of the extensor expansion of the digit and may be mistaken for nerve.
- In a cadaveric study, Levitsky et al[6] found that 27% of specimens had a communicating branch connecting the medial and lateral plantar nerves. They also noted that the second and third interspaces were significantly narrower than the first and fourth.
- Changes in the nerve itself involve perineural fibrosis, demyelinization and degeneration of nerve fibers, endoneural edema, and the absence of inflammatory changes.
- Plantar-directed nerve branches may tether the common digital nerve to the plantar skin.
- These nerve branches are present up to 4 cm proximal to the transverse metatarsal ligament.

PATHOGENESIS

- All histologic changes in a primary interdigital neuroma occur distal to the transverse metatarsal ligament, as shown in studies by Lassmann[5] and Graham et al.[3]
- The cause is unclear but is thought to evolve as an entrapment neuropathy.

- The second and third intermetatarsal spaces are narrower than the first and fourth.
- Mobility between the medial three rays and the lateral two rays may contribute to the high number of primary neuromas in the third interspace.
- In a limited number of patients (about 27%), the common digital nerve to the third interspace consists of branches from the medial and lateral plantar nerves, which perhaps increases the size of the nerve and predisposes it to entrapment (see FIG 1).
- A "recurrent interdigital neuroma" may be due to several factors, including failure to make the correct diagnosis originally.[11]
- Neurogenic pain may be due to causes other than perineural fibrosis, such as neuropathy and radiculopathy. Also, neuroma-like symptoms may be due to nerve irritation from local synovitis or bursitis.

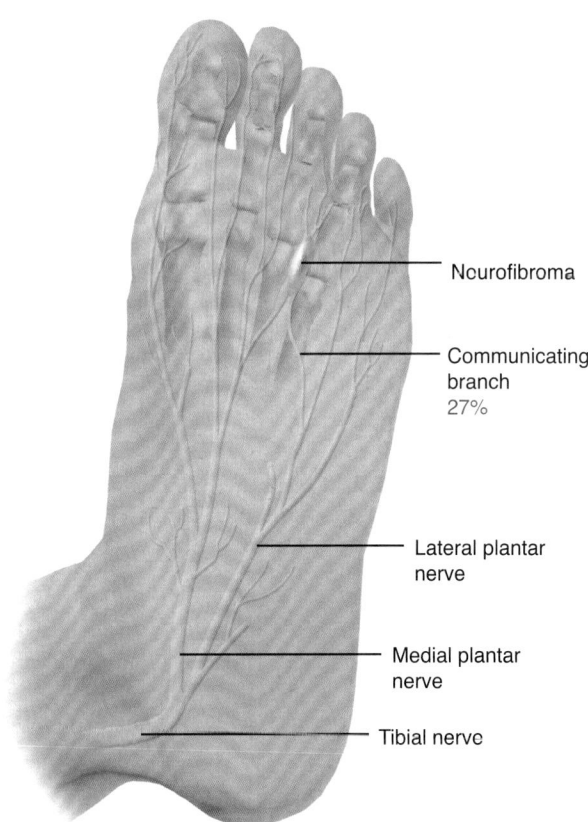

Neurofibroma

Communicating branch 27%

Lateral plantar nerve

Medial plantar nerve

Tibial nerve

FIG 1 Course of medial and lateral plantar nerves. A communicating branch of the lateral plantar nerve occurs in about 27% of patients.

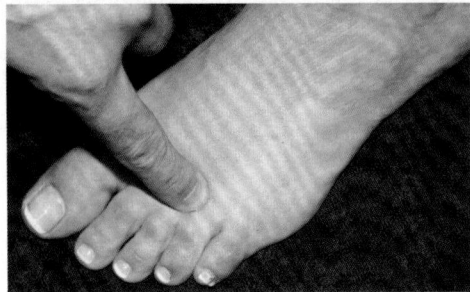

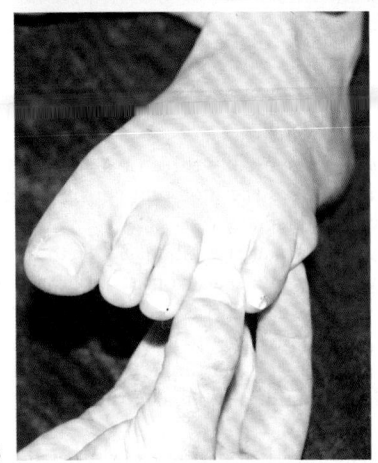

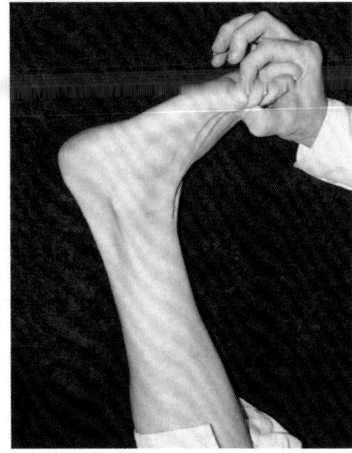

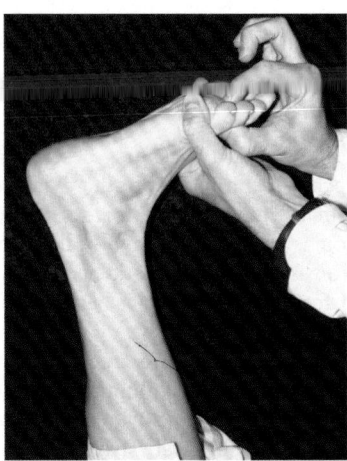

FIG 2 A. Standing palpation of the web space. **B.** MTP joint plantar-flexion stress test. **C.** Mulder test: The examiner places the thumb on the dorsal surface and the index finger on the plantar surface in the affected web space and applies gentle pressure. **D.** With the opposite hand, the examiner applies a gentle squeeze to the forefoot in a mediolateral direction. A clicking sensation that reproduces the patient's pain will often be appreciated.

- Beskin and Baxter[2] found that in patients with recurrent symptoms of interdigital neuroma, about two-thirds presented within 12 months and one-third had recurrence 1 to 4 years after primary surgery.
- Those with "recurrence" within the first 12 months probably represent patients who were originally misdiagnosed.
- Those presenting after 12 months probably represent patients with a true bulb neuroma at the cut end of the common digital nerve. It probably requires at least this length of time for a neuroma to grow big enough to cause symptoms.
- Formation of a recurrent neuroma after primary surgery is usually due to inadequate resection.
- Plantar-directed nerve branches may tether the common digital nerve to the plantar skin and not allow for retraction of the nerve after it is cut. These nerve branches may occur up to 4 cm proximal to the transverse metatarsal ligament.

NATURAL HISTORY

- Interdigital neuromas occur more commonly in females.
- The primary symptom of an interdigital neuroma is pain, most often described as burning, aching, or cramping.
- The pain often radiates to the toes or proximally along the plantar aspect of the foot.
- Relief usually occurs with removing narrow toe box shoes.
- Walking barefoot on soft surfaces often produces no symptoms.
- Recurrent neuromas usually occur within 12 months of index resection.[11]

PATIENT HISTORY AND PHYSICAL FINDINGS

- In patients with an interdigital neuroma, the most common complaint is plantar pain, which is often increased by walking.
- Pain is often relieved by resting and removing shoes.

- Often, there are no symptoms with barefoot walking on a soft surface.
- About half of patients describe pain radiating to the toes.
- The duration of pain varies from a few weeks to many years.
- Plantar tenderness in the web space is the most common physical examination finding.
- The examiner should inspect for deviation or subluxation of the toes or fullness of the web space. This is best done with the patient standing (**FIG 2A**).
- Palpating the web space proximal to the metatarsal heads and proceeding distally will usually reproduce the patient's symptoms.
- It is often difficult to differentiate adjacent metatarsophalangeal (MTP) joint synovitis from a neuroma.
  - Plantarflexion of the corresponding MTP joint may help with the diagnosis (**FIG 2B**). This maneuver often causes little increased pain in those with an interdigital neuroma but is quite painful in those with MTP joint synovitis.
  - Difficulty in making a diagnosis may arise when primary synovitis causes secondary neuritic symptoms.
- The Mulder test is also useful.
  - Pain may be present on the asymptomatic contralateral side but is usually not as painful and the "click" not as striking.
  - This test is best performed with the patient lying prone and the knee flexed 90 degrees. The examiner places the thumb on the dorsal surface and the index finger on the plantar surface in the affected web space and applies gentle pressure (**FIG 2C**). With the opposite hand, the examiner applies a gentle squeeze to the forefoot in a mediolateral direction (**FIG 2D**). A clicking sensation that reproduces the patient's pain will often be appreciated.
- Recurrent neuromas produce localized pain that is more proximal and plantar than a primary neuroma (**FIG 3**).

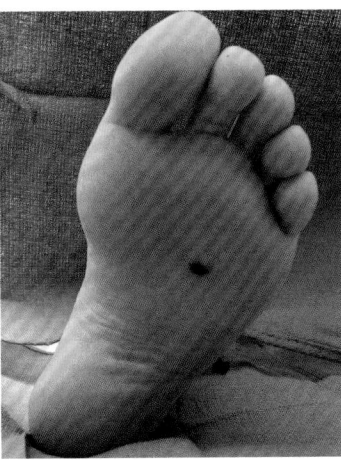

FIG 3 As noted by the mark above, localized pain from recurrent neuroma is more proximal and plantar than that caused by a primary neuroma.

IMAGING AND OTHER DIAGNOSTIC STUDIES

- The diagnosis of an interdigital neuroma is most often made solely on the basis of the history and physical examination.
- Standing anteroposterior, lateral, and oblique radiographs are necessary to exclude osseous pathology and to assess the MTP joint.
- The use of nerve conduction testing has not been shown to be beneficial, as findings often are abnormal in patients without symptoms of an interdigital neuroma.
- Studies differ as to the benefit of ultrasonography or magnetic resonance imaging (MRI). If necessary, ultrasonography appears to be more useful than MRI in cases with a questionable diagnosis.[12]
- A diagnostic injection may be helpful, although other pathology in the area may improve with this local anesthetic. There is questionable benefit to adding ultrasound guidance.[8,10]
  - Two milliliters of lidocaine are placed in the symptomatic web space through a dorsal approach.
  - The needle must be plantar to the transverse metatarsal ligament.

DIFFERENTIAL DIAGNOSIS

- Adjacent web space neuroma
- MTP joint synovitis

- Freiberg osteochondrosis
- Stress fracture of the metatarsal neck
- Tarsal tunnel syndrome
- Peripheral neuropathy
- Lumbar radiculopathy
- Unrelated soft tissue tumor (eg, ganglion, synovial cyst, lipoma)

NONOPERATIVE MANAGEMENT

- Although reported results of conservative treatment vary, it is still worthwhile to try, as 30% to 40% of patients may avoid surgery.
- The patient should be fitted with a wide, soft, laced shoe with a low heel.
- A soft metatarsal support should be added just proximal to the metatarsal heads (**FIG 4A**).
- An injection of steroids with anesthetic may be both diagnostic and possibly therapeutic, although recent literature calls into question the therapeutic value of corticosteroids over local anesthetic alone.[7] For there to be diagnostic value, however, the anesthetic must be directed to the common digital nerve in the affected web space and not into the MTP joint. A combination of 40-mg methylprednisolone acetate (Depo-Medrol) and 1-mL 0.25% bupivacaine (Marcaine) is used for the injection (**FIG 4B**).
  - Thirty percent of patients may have relief for 2 years or longer. Steroids should be used with caution as fat pad atrophy, skin discoloration, or MTP joint capsule laxity may result and create a new problem for the patient.

SURGICAL MANAGEMENT

- The indication for excision surgery is failure of conservative treatment in a patient who is healthy enough to undergo forefoot surgery and who has appropriate vascular status.
- For endoscopic decompression, the advantage of dividing the transverse intermetatarsal ligament (TIML) without excising the interdigital neuroma is that there is no loss of sensation or possible formation of a stump neuroma, which may produce symptoms worse than those with which the patient originally presented. Barrett and Pignetti[1] introduced endoscopic decompression of the intermetatarsal nerve, a procedure that offers several advantages over

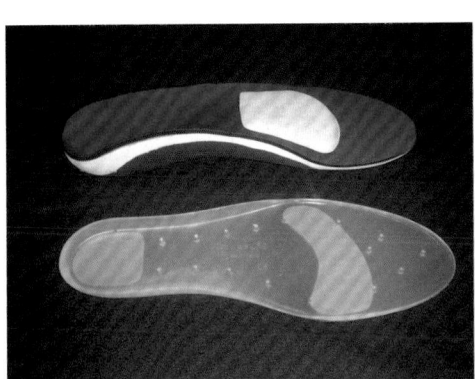

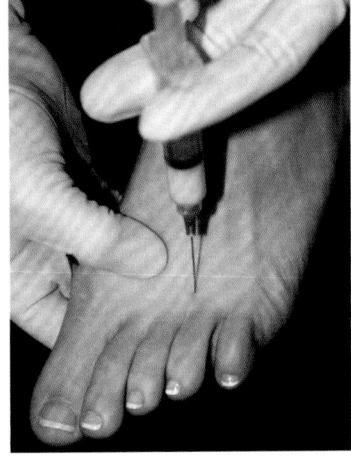

FIG 4 A. Soft inserts and metatarsal support should be the first line of treatment. **B.** Steroid injection may improve symptoms and help with diagnosis.

an open procedure, including a smaller incision, faster postoperative recovery, and a reduced incidence of hematoma and infection.

- Although these authors reported good and excellent results in 88% of patients, the original technique was difficult, with a steep learning curve.
- They have since modified their technique, changing from two portals to a single portal.

Preoperative Planning

Excision

- A forefoot or ankle block may be used. Twenty to 30 mL of a 50% mixture of a short- and long-acting anesthetic (eg, lidocaine and bupivacaine [Marcaine]) without epinephrine is recommended.
- An examination under anesthesia allows for better appreciation of an interspace mass and often will produce a more striking Mulder click.
- Instruments needed include a Weitlaner or neuroma retractor (FIG 5), small tenotomy scissors, a Senn retractor, and a Freer elevator.
- An ankle tourniquet is used with cast padding and an Esmarch bandage.
- If a plantar approach is being used (recurrent neuroma), the surgeon should palpate and outline with a sterile marker the metatarsal heads corresponding to the web space being explored.

Endoscopic Decompression

- All patients should have plain films preoperatively to rule out other diagnoses, in particular stress fracture or Freiberg infraction.
- In our experience, preoperative ultrasound is valuable in confirming the diagnosis.
- Without ultrasound, simple palpation of the web space is typically accurate in determining which web space is most tender.
- Diagnostic lidocaine injection may also pinpoint the appropriate web space. However, if both the second and third web spaces are symptomatic, the surgeon should consider endoscopy on both spaces.

Positioning

Excision

- The patient is placed supine with a 3-inch bump under the distal leg just proximal to the heel. The heel should be floating just off the bed.

Endoscopic Decompression

- The patient is positioned supine on the operating table with a bump under the ipsilateral buttock and thigh if the leg tends to externally rotate.
  - The toes should extend just beyond the end of the table, with the heel firmly resting on the table.
- Anesthesia may be general or regional (popliteal or ankle block).
- Local anesthesia should be avoided, as it may distort the endoscopic anatomy.
- Prophylactic intravenous antibiotics are given when the patient comes to the operating room.
- We routinely use an ankle tourniquet inflated to 250 mm Hg.
- Equipment required includes the AM Surgical set and a 30-degree 4-mm scope. The AM Surgical system includes an elevator, slotted cannula and obturator, locking device, and disposable knife blade.
- Presented here is a technique originally designed by Dr. Ather Mirza for endoscopic carpal tunnel release. The instrumentation has been adapted for uniportal endoscopic decompression of the intermetatarsal nerve (FIG 6).[14]

Approach

Excision

- A dorsal approach is used for primary neuromas. The surgeon should sit proximal to the foot with the assistant positioned at the end of the table to assist with retraction (FIG 7A).
- For recurrent neuroma excision, either a plantar longitudinal incision or a plantar transverse incision is used.[4] The surgeon sits at the end of the table facing the plantar aspect of the foot (FIG 7B).

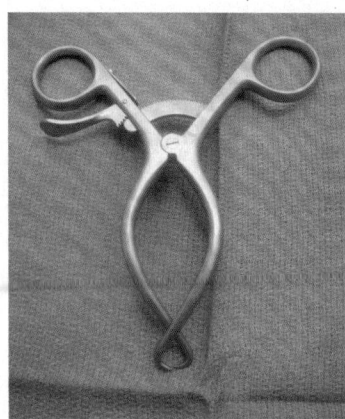

FIG 5 A neuroma retractor may help with exposure during surgery.

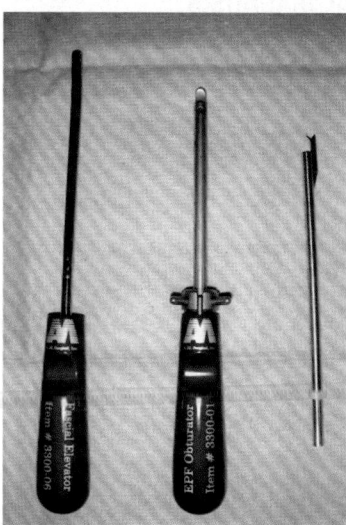

FIG 6 *Left* to *right*: elevator, cannula and obturator, and disposable knife.

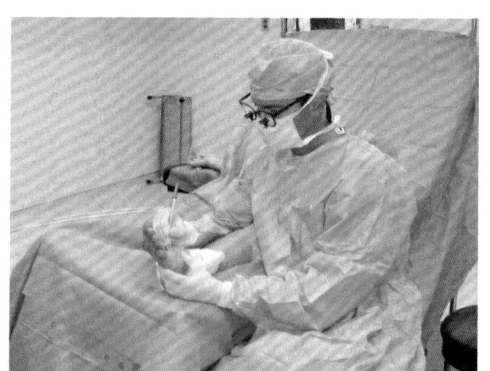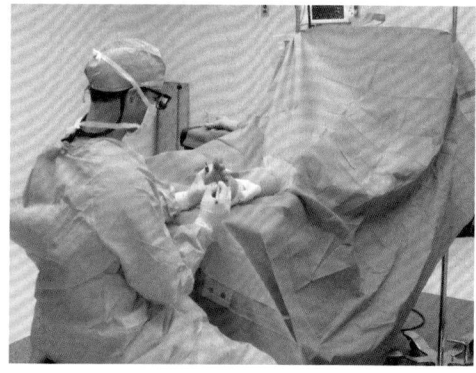

FIG 7 A. Surgeon position for primary neuroma excision. Magnifying loupes are beneficial. **B.** Surgeon position for revision neuroma excision.

PRIMARY INTERDIGITAL NEUROMA EXCISION

Incision and Exposure

- A dorsal incision is made 3 cm proximal to the web, extending distally to the edge of the web space (**TECH FIG 1**).
- The incision is slightly oblique and medial to the extensor tendons. It is important not to follow the tendons themselves, as they will take a more lateral direction.
- The dissection is deepened, and the dorsal sensory nerves are retracted to the side of least resistance.
- The lumbrical tendon is lateral to the dissection.
- The surgeon should proximally identify the dorsal interosseous fascia and muscle belly and follow it distally to the bursa overlying the transverse metatarsal ligament.
- The surgeon should place a Weitlaner retractor, lamina spreader, or neuroma retractor between the metatarsals and spread them apart.
- The bursa is opened to identify the transverse metatarsal ligament.
- Web space fat is retracted using a Senn retractor, and the distal aspect of the intermetatarsal ligament is identified.

- A Freer elevator is placed beneath the transverse metatarsal ligament from distal to proximal, protecting the underlying structures.
- The transverse metatarsal ligament is incised with a no. 15 blade knife, staying on top of the Freer elevator.
- The lumbrical tendon is in the lateral aspect of the dissection just plantar to the intermetatarsal ligament.
- The neurovascular bundle is identified medial and plantar to the lumbrical.

Excision

- Once the approach has been completed, the nerve should be identified in the wound. It is usually easier to identify the nerve proximally and dissect distally (**TECH FIG 2A**).
- Manually palpate the wound to be sure the transverse metatarsal ligament has been completely transected, as this is essential to a successful outcome.
- Despite the size of the nerve or the obvious presence of a neuroma, the nerve should be resected as planned.

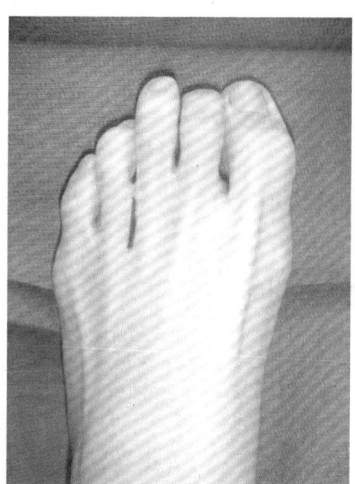

TECH FIG 1 For a primary interdigital neuroma, a 3-cm incision is made in the affected web space just medial to the extensor tendons.

TECHNIQUES

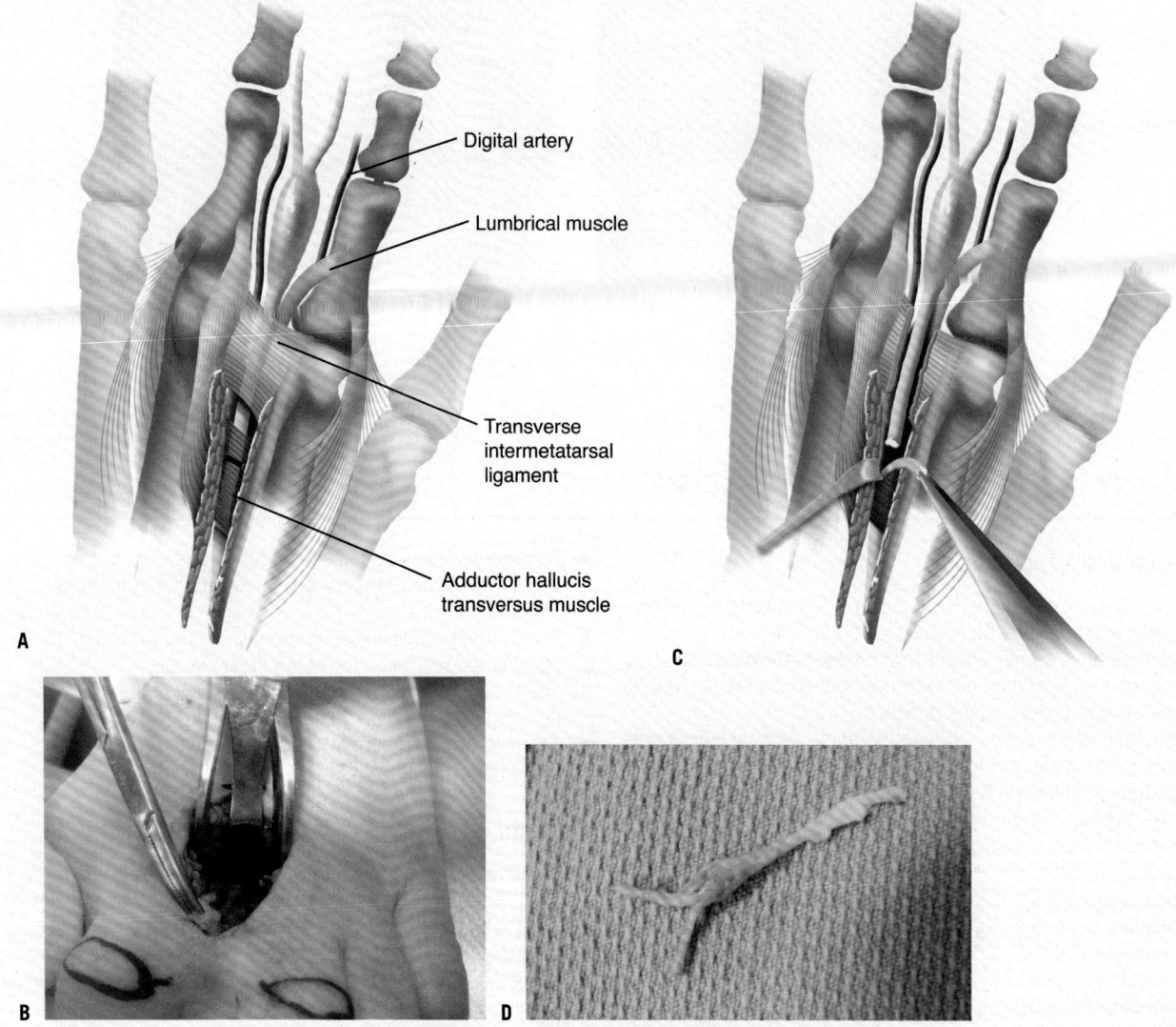

Digital artery

Lumbrical muscle

Transverse intermetatarsal ligament

Adductor hallucis transversus muscle

A

C

B

D

TECH FIG 2 A. The TIML must be divided. **B.** The neuroma is visualized and the common digital nerve transected 4 cm proximal to the TIML and allowed to retract proximal to the weight-bearing pad of the forefoot. **C.** After transection of the intermetatarsal ligament, the nerve is transected proximally (the transverse head of the adductor hallucis muscle often must be retracted) and dissected distally past the bifurcation. **D.** The specimen is sent for pathologic examination.

- Structures that may be mistaken for the nerve include the lumbrical tendon, which passes to the medial portion of the adjacent proximal phalanx (extensor expansion) and therefore is lateral to the nerve. The common digital artery usually crosses proximal-medial to distal-lateral lying dorsally over the nerve. The artery often emerges from under the metatarsal neck and if identified needs to be dissected away from the nerve and preserved.
- Using gentle traction **(TECH FIG 2B)**, transect the nerve about 4 cm proximal to the transverse intermetatarsal ligament (TIML).
- The transverse head of the adductor hallucis may need to be retracted dorsally to identify the plantar-directed branches of the common digital nerve. Divide these branches to allow the proximal aspect of the nerve to retract at least 1 to 2 cm proximal to the weight-bearing pad of the forefoot **(TECH FIG 2C)**.
- Use a hemostat to place the remaining nerve stump well proximal and dorsal into the interosseous muscles.

- Circumferentially dissect the nerve distally to the bifurcation of the proper digital branches.
- Divide the proper digital nerve just distal to the bifurcation.
- The necessity of sending the specimen **(TECH FIG 2D)** for pathologic examination has been called into question in the recent literature.[9,10]

Completion and Closure

- With the Weitlaner or neuroma retractor still in place, release the ankle tourniquet. Use cautery to obtain hemostasis.
- Irrigate the wound with sterile saline.
- Close the wound with 4-0 nylon suture in a running locking fashion.
- If subcutaneous suture is desired, use a 3-0 Monocryl, taking care not to include the dorsal sensory nerves.
- Place a mildly compressive dressing over a Xeroform gauze covering the wound **(TECH FIG 3)**.

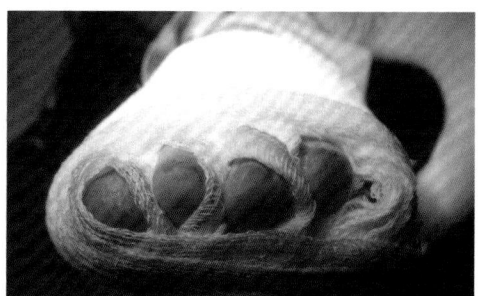

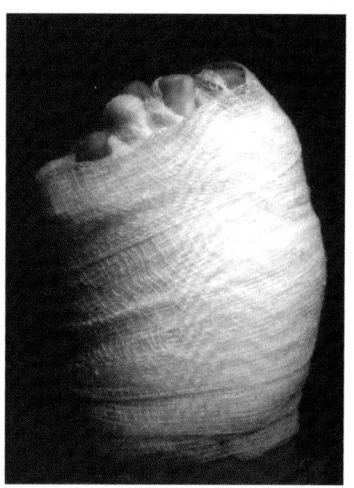

TECH FIG 3 A,B. For a primary neuroma excision, a mildly compressive dressing is placed and the patient is allowed to bear weight as tolerated in a postoperative shoe.

REVISION INTERDIGITAL NEUROMA EXCISION

Plantar Longitudinal Incision Approach

- A longitudinal plantar incision is made 4 cm proximal to the web, extending distally to within 1 cm of the web space.
- The incision is made between the metatarsal heads (which have been identified and marked before making an incision) and proceeds just distal to this area **(TECH FIG 4)**.
- A small Weitlaner retractor is placed to retract the fat overlying the plantar aponeurosis.
- Using a no. 15 blade knife, the aponeurosis is incised in line with the skin incision.
- A tenotomy scissors is used to bluntly spread until the common digital nerve is identified proximally.
- The surgeon dissects distally to identify the stump neuroma.

Plantar Transverse Incision Approach

- Alternatively, 3- to 4-cm transverse plantar incision is made over the affected interspace just proximal to the weight-bearing pad and parallel to the natural crease **(TECH FIG 5)**.
- The metatarsal heads are continually palpated to provide a reference point to the appropriate interspace to be explored.
- The dissection is carefully deepened with scissors to expose the septa of the plantar fascia.
- The interval between the longitudinal limbs of the plantar fascia septa is opened with scissors.
- The bands of the plantar fascia are retracted medially and laterally with a Senn retractor, and the interspace is carefully

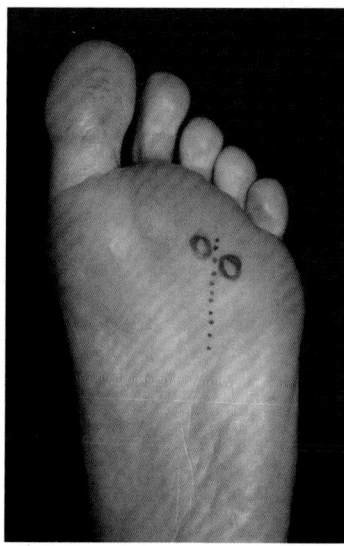

TECH FIG 4 For recurrent interdigital neuromas, a 4-cm longitudinal plantar incision is made proximal to the web extending distally to within 1 cm of the web space.

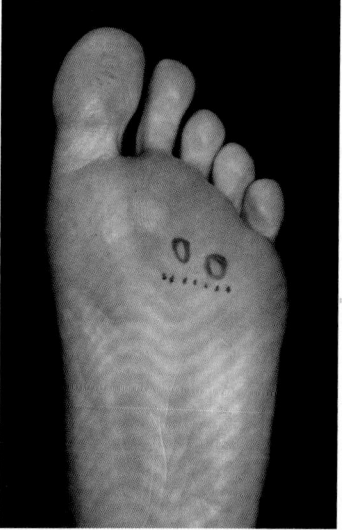

TECH FIG 5 Alternatively, one may use a 3- to 4-cm transverse plantar incision. The incision is placed over the affected interspace just proximal to the weight-bearing pad and parallel to the natural crease.

TECHNIQUES

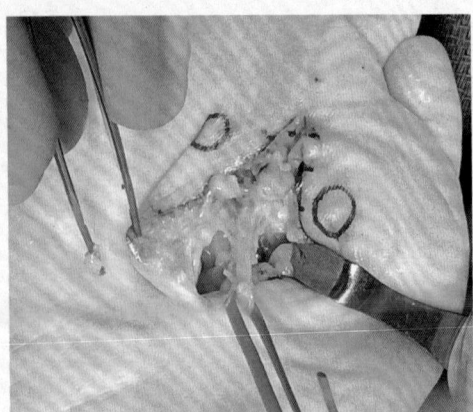

TECH FIG 6 Stump neuroma usually is located on the tibial (medial) side of the interspace.

explored with blunt dissection to identify the common digital nerve and vessel.
- The nerve (neuroma) will lie superficial (plantar) to the flexor digitorum brevis muscle or tendon and immediately deep (dorsal) to the plantar fascia.
- The surgeon dissects distally to identify the stump neuroma.

Excision

- The neuroma is identified just deep to the distal extensions of the plantar fascia that fan out to attach to the plantar aspects of the MTP joints and just superficial (plantar) to the flexor digitorum brevis.
- The intermetatarsal ligament is often scarred in but does not need to be transected, as it is distal and dorsal to the neuroma
- The stump neuroma usually is found on the tibial (medial) side of the interspace and often is adherent to the lumbrical muscle, flexor tendon, or lateral aspect of third metatarsal **(TECH FIG 6)**.
- Place gentle traction on the common digital nerve **(TECH FIG 7A)**. Identify and excise the neuroma **(TECH FIG 7B)**.
- Allow the common digital nerve to retract proximally as far as possible.
- Release the ankle tourniquet and obtain hemostasis.
- Irrigate the wound with sterile saline.
- Close the wound with interrupted 3-0 nylon suture in a vertical mattress fashion.
- Place a mildly compressive dressing over a Xeroform gauze on the wound.
- Place the patient in a short-leg posterior splint.

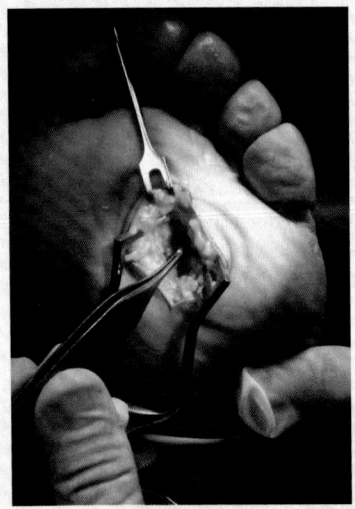

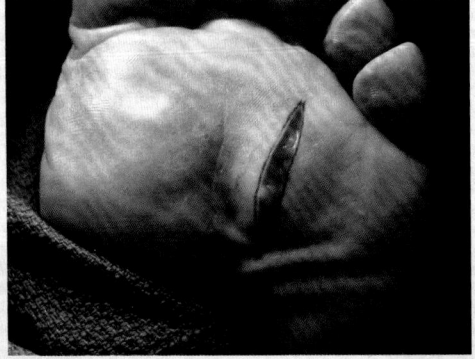

TECH FIG 7 A. The plantar longitudinal incision is shown with gentle traction placed on the common digital nerve. **B.** Excision of the recurrent neuroma through a plantar longitudinal incision.

UNIPORTAL ENDOSCOPIC DECOMPRESSION OF THE INTERDIGITAL NERVE

Port Creation

- Make a 1-cm vertical incision in the appropriate web space and spread the subcutaneous tissue gently with blunt tenotomy scissors.
- Use the AM Surgical elevator to palpate and separate the TIML from the surrounding soft tissues. Scrape the elevator both dorsal and plantar to the TIML.
- Place the slotted cannula and obturator through the same path, just plantar to and scraping against the TIML. The slot should face dorsally at the 12 o'clock position **(TECH FIG 8A,B)**.

- Remove the obturator from the cannula and remove any fat or fluid from the cannula with absorbent cotton-tipped applicators.
- Insert a short, 4-mm 30-degree scope into the cannula.
- Visualize the entire TIML by advancing the scope. The ligament is dense and white. The lumbrical tendon can often be seen just lateral to the TIML.
- The intermetatarsal nerve can be visualized by rotating the cannula 180 degrees so that the slot is facing plantar at 6 o'clock position. The nerve can often be seen unless obscured by fat.

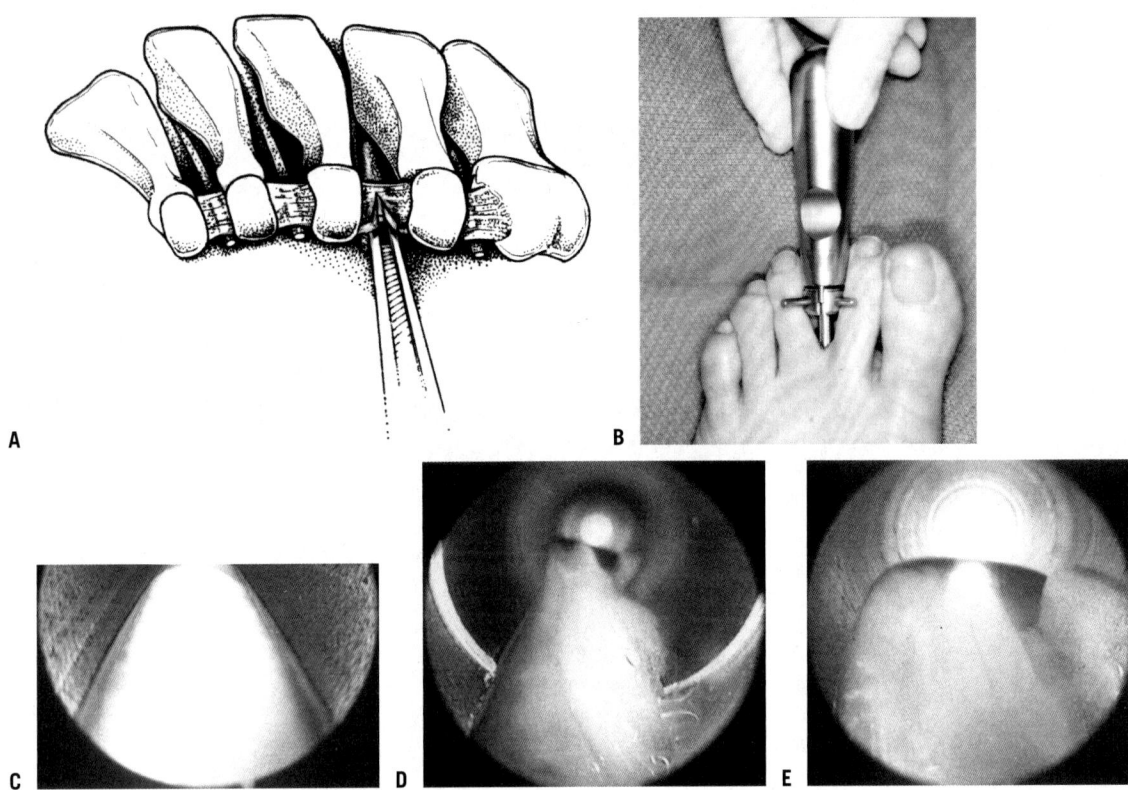

TECH FIG 8 A. Surgical technique for uniportal endoscopic decompression of the intermetatarsal nerve. Cannula is in the interspace just plantar to the TIML and dorsal to the intermetatarsal (interdigital) nerve. The TIML is being transected from distal to proximal. **B.** Intraoperative view of insertion of cannula and obturator into second web space, notch at 12 o'clock, positioned to view the TIML. **C.** Endoscopic view of TIML. **D.** Normal interdigital nerve. **E.** Thickened interdigital nerve (neuroma). (**A:** Courtesy of AM Surgical, Inc.)

It is often thickened distally, tapers, and becomes normal proximally **(TECH FIG 8C–E)**.

- Return the cannula to the 12 o'clock position and remove the scope from the cannula.

Transverse Intermetatarsal Ligament Transection

- Slide the disposable endoscopic knife onto the locking device with the lever in the open position.
- Insert the knife and locking device assembly into the scope and advance the knife blade until it nearly touches the lens. The blade should also be parallel to the lens. Push the lever of the locking device forward until finger tight **(TECH FIG 9A)**.
- Advance the scope and knife assembly through the cannula. Visualize the knife blade transecting the TIML from distal to proximal **(TECH FIG 9B–E)**.
- While cutting the TIML, maintain the cannula tight against the ligament. Place more tension on the TIML by placing a finger of the nondominant hand between the adjacent metatarsal necks.

- Withdraw the scope and knife assembly and remove the knife from the scope. Reinsert the scope to confirm complete transection of the TIML. The divided edge of the ligament can be observed to further separate by applying manual digital pressure between the adjacent metatarsal heads.
- Irrigate the wound through the cannula.
- Remove the cannula, insert the elevator into the wound, and palpate the interspace. The taut TIML should no longer be palpable.

Completion and Closure

- Deflate the tourniquet; irrigate and close the wound with one or two interrupted mattress sutures.
- Apply a soft compression dressing and postoperative shoe.
- If the surgeon chooses to perform a neurectomy in cases in which the nerve is very large and bulbous, the incision can be extended proximally 1 to 2 cm and neurectomy can be performed in routine fashion.

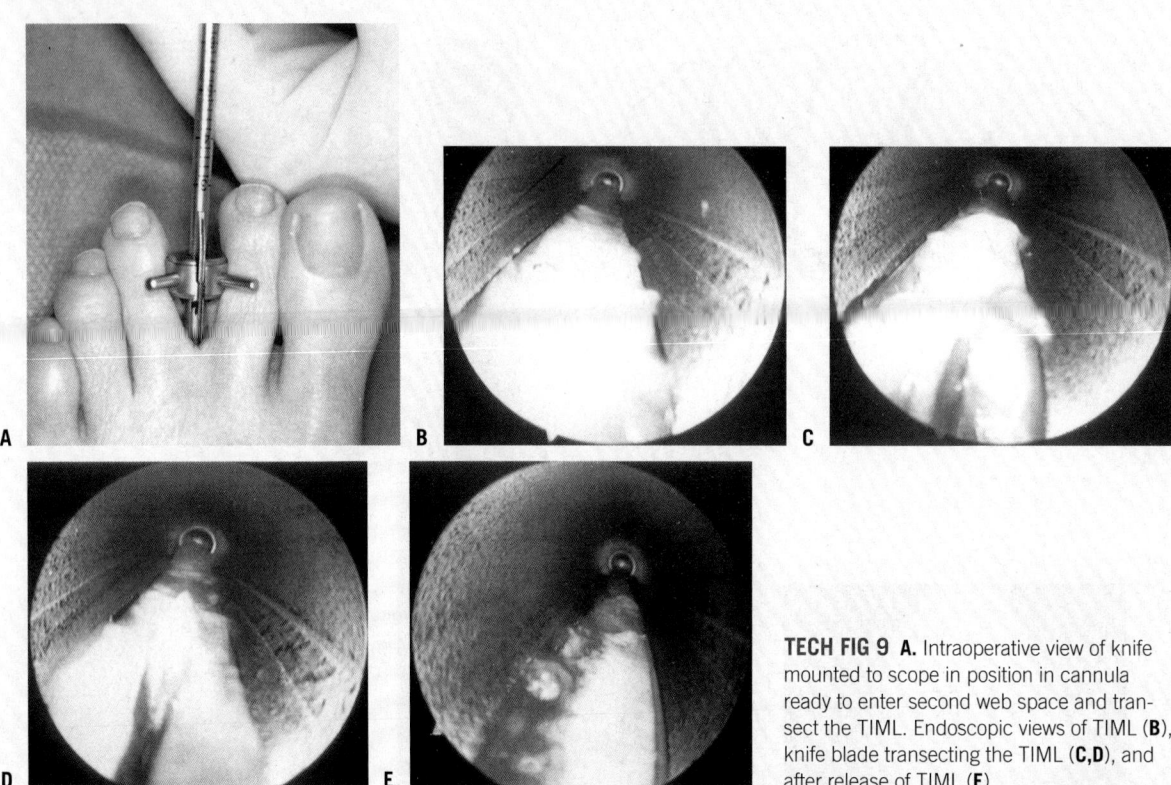

TECH FIG 9 A. Intraoperative view of knife mounted to scope in position in cannula ready to enter second web space and transect the TIML. Endoscopic views of TIML (**B**), knife blade transecting the TIML (**C,D**), and after release of TIML (**E**).

TECHNIQUES

Pearls and Pitfalls

Always perform a thorough history and physical examination. This is the primary basis of diagnosis and treatment.	• Perform standing, sitting, and prone examination of the foot and ankle.
Attempt conservative treatment before surgery.	• Discuss with the patient possible complications of surgery, especially incomplete relief and recurrence.
Transect the common digital nerve at least 3–4 cm proximal to the transverse metatarsal ligament.	• Grasp the nerve and with gentle traction, pull it distally. Transect and allow the nerve to retract.
Release the tourniquet and obtain hemostasis before closure.	• Hematoma formation increases the risk of slow wound healing and infection.
The key to the endoscopic procedure is isolating and separating the TIML from the soft tissues.	• Developing these tissue planes with the elevator is the critical step; everything else follows. • Hugging the TIML with the cannula while cutting is very important. • If unable to visualize the TIML, abort the procedure and perform the procedure open.

POSTOPERATIVE CARE

Excision

- For 24 hours, the operative extremity is maximally elevated and the patient ambulates only for bathroom privileges.
- For a primary excision (dorsal approach), the patient is then allowed to ambulate with weight bearing as tolerated in a hard-soled postoperative shoe for 4 weeks.

- For a revision excision (plantar approach), the patient is kept non–weight bearing on crutches for 2 weeks and then transitioned into a stiff-soled postoperative shoe for another 2 weeks with weight bearing as tolerated.
- Sutures are removed at 2 weeks, and Steri-Strips are placed on the wound.
- At 4 weeks after surgery, the patient is allowed into a wide toe box, soft-vamp comfortable shoe and progressed as tolerated.

Endoscopic Decompression

- Ice and elevation are recommended for the first 48 to 72 hours.
- Weight bearing as tolerated is permitted in a surgical shoe. Crutches or a walker should be provided as needed.
- Sutures are removed in 12 to 14 days. A comfortable shoe or sandal may then be worn.
- Vigorous activities such as running or racquet sports should be avoided for 4 to 6 weeks.
- Patients should be advised that complete resolution of symptoms may take up to 4 months.

OUTCOMES

- Surgical excision of a primary neuroma has a reported success rate of 51% to 90%, although results tend to diminish with time. A study by Womack et al[15] suggests long-term pain relief is not as significant as once thought.
  - These results seem to be similar for both second and third web space neuroma excisions.
  - Rungprai et al[13] compared simple neurectomy to neurectomy with intramuscular implantation of the proximal nerve stump and concluded that the intramuscular implantation technique might offer superior pain relief.
- After reexploration for a recurrent neuroma, less than complete satisfaction can be expected in 20% to 40% of individuals.

COMPLICATIONS

- Recurrence of symptoms may be due to incorrect diagnosis, incomplete resection, or true recurrence.
  - Recurrence of symptoms due to incorrect diagnosis and incomplete resection usually occurs within the first 12 months.
  - Recurrence after 1 year is more likely related to the formation of a stump neuroma.
- Significant wound complications are rare, but slow wound healing and superficial cellulitis are more common.
- Incisional tenderness after a plantar approach is less common than one may suppose but may occur if placed under a weight-bearing portion of the forefoot.

REFERENCES

1. Barrett SL, Pignetti TT. Endoscopic decompression for intermetatarsal nerve entrapment—the EDIN technique: preliminary study with cadaveric specimens; early clinical results. J Foot Ankle Surg 1994;33(5):503–508.
2. Beskin JL, Baxter DE. Recurrent pain following interdigital neurectomy—a plantar approach. Foot Ankle 1988;9(1):34–39.
3. Graham CE, Johnson KA, Ilstrup DM. The intermetatarsal nerve: a microscopic evaluation. Foot Ankle 1981;2(3):150–152.
4. Kundert HP, Plaass C, Stukenborg-Colsman C, et al. Excision of Morton's neuroma using a longitudinal plantar approach: a midterm follow-up study. Foot Ankle Spec 2016;9(1):37–42.
5. Lassmann G. Morton's toe: clinical, light and electron microscopic investigations in 133 cases. Clin Orthop Relat Res 1979;(142):73–84.
6. Levitsky KA, Alman BA, Jevsevar DS, et al. Digital nerves of the foot: anatomic variations and implications regarding the pathogenesis of interdigital neuroma. Foot Ankle 1993;14(4):208–214.
7. Lizano-Díez X, Ginés-Cespedosa A, Alenton-Geli E, et al. Corticosteroid injection for the treatment of Morton's neuroma: a prospective, double-blinded, randomized, placebo-controlled trial. Foot Ankle Int 2017;38(9):944–951.
8. Mahadevan D, Attwal M, Bhaatt R, et al. Corticosteroid injection for Morton's neuroma with or without ultrasound guidance: a randomised controlled trial. Bone Joint J 2016;98-B(4):498–503.
9. O'Connor KM, Johnson JE, McCormick JJ, et al. Correlation of clinical, operative, and histopathologic diagnosis of interdigital neuroma and the cost of routine diagnosis. Foot Ankle Int 2016;37(1):70–74.
10. Raouf T, Rogero R, McDonald E, et al. Value of preoperative imaging and intraoperative histopathology in Morton's neuroma. Foot Ankle Int 2019;40(9):1032–1036.
11. Richardson DR, Dean EM. The recurrent Morton neuroma: what now? Foot Ankle Clin 2014;19(3):437–449.
12. Ruiz Santiago F, Prados Olleta N, Tomás Munoz P, et al. Short term comparison between blind and ultrasound injection in Morton neuroma. Eur Radiol 2019;29(2):620–627.
13. Rungprai C, Cychosz CC, Phruetthiphat O, et al. Simple neurectomy versus neurectomy with intramuscular implantation for interdigital neuroma: a comparative study. Foot Ankle Int 2015;36(12):1412–1424.
14. Shapiro SL. Endoscopic decompression of the intermetatarsal nerve for Morton's neuroma. Foot Ankle Clin 2004;9(2):297–304.
15. Womack JW, Richardson DR, Murphy GA, et al. Long-term evaluation of interdigital neuroma treated by surgical excision. Foot Ankle Int 2008;29(6):574–577.

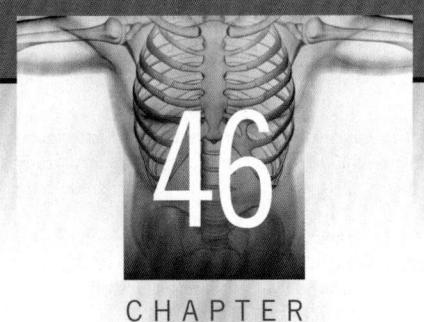

46

CHAPTER

Midfoot
Medial Cuneiform Osteotomy

Jeffrey E. Johnson, Jonathon D. Backus, and J. Jordan Stivers

DEFINITION

- Forefoot varus is a component of the multiplanar pes planovalgus deformity that occurs as a result of posterior tibial tendon insufficiency.
- In addition to being a component of adult acquired flatfoot deformity, forefoot varus is also present in some cases of congenital pes planus and posttraumatic deformities of the first tarsometatarsal joint.
- In 1936, Cotton[4] described an adjunctive procedure for the operative treatment of flatfoot deformity using an opening wedge plantarflexion medial cuneiform osteotomy to restore what he termed the *triangle of support* of the static foot.

ANATOMY

- The medial cuneiform is well vascularized from multiple sources. The deep/superficial medial plantar arteries, dorsalis pedis, and plantar medial artery contribute to the blood supply of the medial cuneiform. This extensive network of anastomoses allows for sufficient bony healing in the setting of midsection osteotomy of the medial cuneiform.[6]
- Forefoot varus deformity may occur through a dorsiflexion angulation or rotation at the talonavicular, naviculocuneiform, or tarsometatarsal joints.
- These joints are supported by the spring ligament and the plantar intertarsal ligaments, including the long plantar ligament.
- In addition, the naviculocuneiform and tarsometatarsal joints are supported by their relatively constrained joint architecture, which in the normal state allows only a few degrees of motion in the sagittal plane.
- Medial displacement calcaneal osteotomy, lateral column lengthening, and subtalar fusion all provide correction of heel valgus; lateral column lengthening will correct forefoot abduction, but none of these procedures adequately addresses the fixed forefoot varus component of the pes planovalgus deformity.

PATHOGENESIS

- The pathogenesis of forefoot varus in association with an adult acquired flatfoot deformity secondary to posterior tibial tendon insufficiency is not well understood.
- Forefoot varus is presumed to develop when the posterior tibialis tendon can no longer provide dynamic support to the medial column of the midfoot. In the absence of the posterior tibialis tendon acting as a dynamic stabilizer, the static ligamentous stabilizers (spring ligament complex and the plantar supporting intertarsal ligaments) stretch out due to the repetitive dorsally directed weight-bearing forces on the medial column of the foot and the dorsally directed force of the anterior tibialis muscle.

- Lateral column-lengthening procedures, in conjunction with a flexor digitorum longus (FDL) transfer, are commonly used to address flatfoot deformity but can result in lateral column overload. Medial cuneiform osteotomy helps to correct lateral column overload by shifting forefoot pressures from lateral to medial.[3,8]
- Several patterns of medial column "sag" have been described, although the understanding of why some patients have dorsal instability at the first tarsometatarsal joint, the naviculocuneiform joint, or the talonavicular joint is not well understood. The differences in the magnitude and location of the dorsal sag may be related to bony anatomy, generalized ligamentous laxity, the presence or absence of gastrocnemius–soleus contracture, and the existence of an underlying congenital pes planovalgus deformity.

NATURAL HISTORY

- The natural history of forefoot varus associated with an acquired adult flatfoot deformity has not been studied. It is presumed that the severity of the forefoot varus deformity progresses as the underlying pes planovalgus deformity progresses. Long-standing instability and subluxation at the first tarsometatarsal joint or naviculocuneiform joint may result in localized osteoarthritis of these joints.
- Some acquired adult flatfeet develop a fixed forefoot varus without osteoarthritis when the deformity has been long-standing and capsular stiffness holds the joint in the deformed position.

PATIENT HISTORY AND PHYSICAL FINDINGS

- Forefoot varus is one of the components of a pes planovalgus deformity that is determined primarily by radiographic and physical examination findings.
- In the patient history, there may be complaints of localized pain to the dorsal medial column of the midfoot, either the tarsometatarsal joint or the naviculocuneiform joint.
- Patients may complain of pressure-related discomfort beneath the base of the first metatarsal or cuneiform due to excessive weight bearing at the apex of the plantar medial column sag.
- The presence and the magnitude of forefoot varus are determined on physical examination by placing the hindfoot

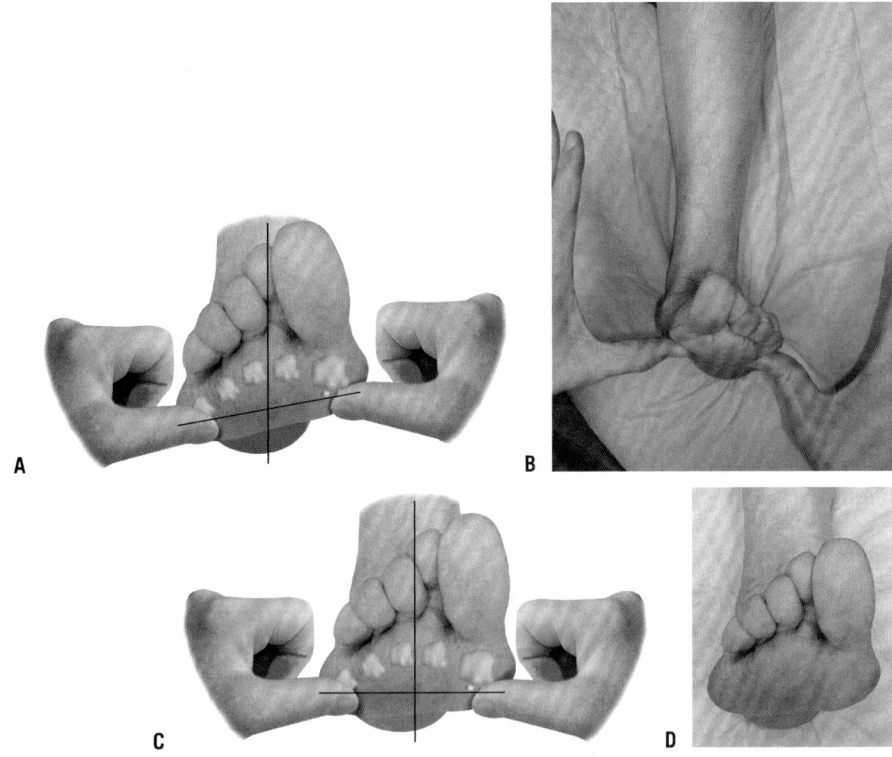

FIG 1 Placing the hindfoot into the subtalar neutral position allows the examiner to determine the presence and the magnitude of a forefoot varus deformity that may accompany pes planovalgus. **A,B.** The forefoot is in varus alignment relative to the neutral heel as evidenced by the examiner visualizing and palpating the first metatarsal head dorsally translated relative to the fifth metatarsal head. **C,D.** The forefoot and hindfoot alignment are both in neutral position with the first and fifth metatarsal heads in the same plane. This is the position desired after the appropriate-sized bone wedge has been placed into the first cuneiform osteotomy.

into the "subtalar neutral" position with the patient seated (**FIG 1**).

- With the hindfoot held in neutral position and with the talonavicular joint congruent, a dorsally directed force is applied to the fourth and fifth metatarsal heads until the ankle is dorsiflexed to the neutral position. If the first metatarsal head rests above the transverse plane of the fifth metatarsal, then forefoot varus is present.
  - Forefoot varus is quantified clinically by the degree to which the first metatarsal rests above the transverse plane of the forefoot as a mild, moderate, or severe deformity.
- The deformity is further characterized by whether the forefoot varus deformity is passively correctable by manual pressure to bring the first ray back down to the level of the other metatarsals or whether it is fixed in this position.

IMAGING AND OTHER DIAGNOSTIC STUDIES

- Standing anteroposterior (AP) and lateral radiographs with a medial oblique view of the involved foot will determine the presence of subluxation or osteoarthritis at the first tarsometatarsal or naviculocuneiform joint.
- The lateral standing radiograph will quantify the amount of dorsiflexion based on the measurement of the lateral talo–first metatarsal angle (Meary's angle).
- The apex of the deformity may be at the talonavicular joint, the naviculocuneiform joint, or the first tarsometatarsal joint.
- Preoperative measurement of the cuneiform articular angle (CAA) can help guide graft size selection intraoperatively. Each millimeter of graft size corresponds to a 2.1-degree decrease of the CAA.[7]

- In the case of an acquired flatfoot deformity superimposed on a congenital pes planovalgus deformity, comparison measurements of the opposite foot standing radiograph may help determine what amount of deformity is a result of posterior tibial tendon insufficiency.
- A weight-bearing AP radiograph of the involved ankle will determine the presence of a valgus tilt of the talus within the ankle joint mortise secondary to deltoid insufficiency.
- Additional procedures to address medial ankle instability due to deltoid ligament insufficiency may be needed to fully correct the valgus hindfoot deformity.

DIFFERENTIAL DIAGNOSIS

- Forefoot varus secondary to instability or osteoarthritis at the first tarsometatarsal joint
- Global forefoot varus associated with supination of the first, second, and third metatarsals

NONOPERATIVE MANAGEMENT

- If the deformity is passively correctable, a custom-molded total contact foot orthosis is fabricated with posting under the medial aspect of the hindfoot and midfoot to correct heel valgus and additional posting placed under the lateral aspect of the forefoot to promote plantarflexion of the first ray with weight bearing.
- If the forefoot varus is fixed, an accommodative total contact foot orthosis would be fabricated with medial posting under the entire hindfoot and midfoot or a medial wedge could be added to the sole of the shoe.
- If pain symptoms are not controlled with foot orthoses alone, a custom-made leather and polypropylene-molded

gauntlet-style brace or a polypropylene custom-molded short articulated ankle–foot orthosis would be indicated.[1,2]

- Because forefoot varus is only one component of a complex multiplanar pes planovalgus deformity, decision making about conservative versus operative treatment will most likely depend on the characteristics of the hindfoot valgus deformity rather than solely on the forefoot varus component alone.

SURGICAL MANAGEMENT

- Both opening and closing wedge osteotomies of the medial cuneiform have been described in the literature.[4,9-11]
- More commonly, a plantarflexion opening wedge medial cuneiform osteotomy is performed. This helps to correct the fixed forefoot varus associated with a flatfoot deformity. This osteotomy is rarely performed in isolation and typically is performed as a component of multiple procedures to correct a given flatfoot deformity.
- Typically, the surgeon begins with bony correction of the foot, followed by soft tissue reconstruction and tendon transfers.
- The reconstructive procedure begins in the proximal aspect of the foot and ankle and proceeds distally because each level of correction is determined by aligning it to the next most proximal segment. Therefore, the forefoot varus is often the last portion of the bony deformity to be corrected during the realignment portion of the procedure.
- Occasionally, once the hindfoot deformity correction has been performed, the apparent forefoot varus that was present preoperatively has been improved sufficiently that osteotomy of the first cuneiform is not required.

Preoperative Planning

- Traditionally, the opening wedge osteotomy requires interposition of some type of bone graft material. Therefore, the surgeon should be prepared to harvest a bone graft or have an allograft or synthetic bone graft material available.
  - We have used exclusively frozen tricortical iliac crest allograft bone fixed with a single Kirschner wire for this interposition osteotomy without complication.

- Trabecular metal wedges or an opening wedge "Puddu" style plate offer an alternative to traditional bone grafting techniques.[8,12,13] Potential advantages include no donor site morbidity seen with autograft and no potential risk of disease transmission with allograft.[12,13] However, plates and screws may create a painful prominence on the dorsum of the foot, and metal wedges may confound any future revision surgery. Long-term studies evaluating the durability of these nonbiologic implants are lacking.
- Alternatively, a closing wedge osteotomy does not involve interposition of bone graft or synthetic material but requires careful preoperative planning and measurement of bony resection to ensure accurate angular correction.
  - Although it is not the authors' preferred technique, potential advantages of a closing wedge osteotomy include direct bone healing without a need for graft, no implant interposition, ability to perform the procedure through a single incision,[9] and the ability to slightly adduct the foot through the osteotomy.

Positioning

- The patient is positioned supine with a small pad placed under the ipsilateral buttock to internally rotate the foot to the neutral position.

Approach

- The opening wedge osteotomy opens dorsally; therefore, the approach is over the dorsal aspect of the first cuneiform.
- If procedures are performed on the medial side of the midfoot, the incisions should be kept at least 3 cm apart to minimize undermining.
- Performing this open wedge osteotomy through a medial approach would significantly increase the difficulty, would require significant additional soft tissue dissection, and would require retraction of the anterior tibialis tendon near its insertion.
- The closing wedge osteotomy technique is performed through a medial incision, which is the distal extension of an incision used for a medial soft tissue procedure for posterior tibial tendon reconstruction.

TECHNIQUES

OPENING WEDGE MEDIAL CUNEIFORM OSTEOTOMY

Exposure

- Under tourniquet control, make a dorsal longitudinal skin incision over the medial cuneiform and the base of the first metatarsal.
- Carry dissection through the skin and subcutaneous tissue to develop the interval between the extensor hallucis longus tendon (retracted medially) and the extensor hallucis brevis tendon (retracted laterally).
- Free up and retract any crossing cutaneous branches of the superficial peroneal nerve.
- Expose the dorsal portion of the medial cuneiform with identification of the first tarsometatarsal joint and the joint between the medial and middle cuneiform. It is not necessary to open the joint capsule of the first tarsometatarsal joint.

Osteotomy

- With fluoroscopic guidance, identify the midportion of the cuneiform and place a Kirschner wire from dorsal to plantar to identify the saw cut line on the bone. Usually, this line is at or just proximal to the plane of the second tarsometatarsal joint (TECH FIG 1A).
- With a small microsagittal saw, make a transverse osteotomy in the dorsal to plantar direction following the guide wire through the midportion of the medial cuneiform by cutting down to, but not through, the plantar cortex (TECH FIG 1B).
- Use a thin osteotome to complete the osteotomy, leaving the plantar cortex and periosteum intact.

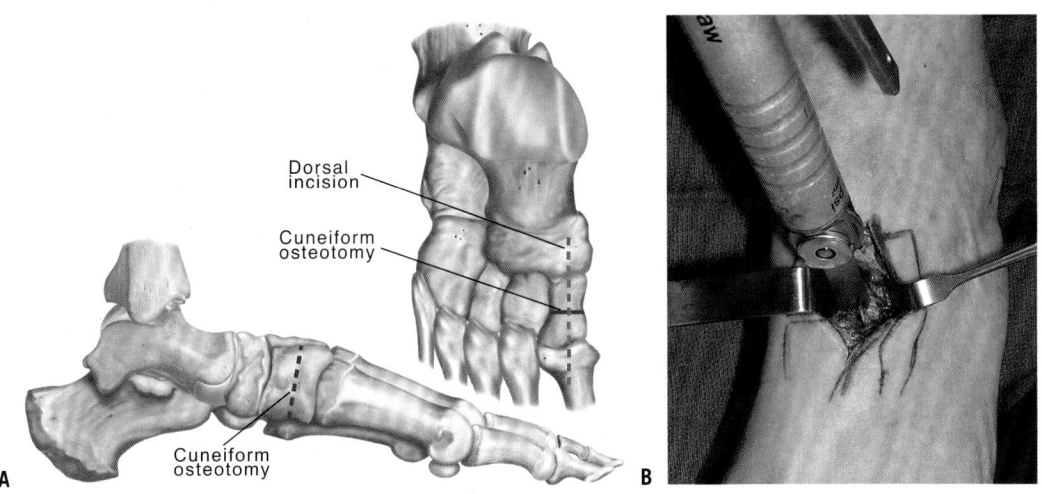

TECH FIG 1 A. Location of first cuneiform osteotomy. **B.** The osteotomy is made dorsal to plantar across the mid-portion of the first cuneiform. A narrow elevator or retractor is placed into the first and second intercuneiform joint to prevent inadvertent osteotomy of the second cuneiform.

Bone Wedge

- Pull the osteotome distally to lever open the medial cuneiform osteotomy and plantarflex the first ray **(TECH FIG 2A)**.
  - Using a ruler, measure the amount of opening of the cuneiform osteotomy needed to achieve the desired plantarflexion of the first ray.
  - On average, a 5- to 8-mm wedge of bone graft is needed to plantar-angulate the first metatarsal to the desired level of the other metatarsal heads (especially the fifth metatarsal) in order to restore Cotton's normal "tripod" configuration.
- A wedge of iliac crest bone graft is harvested either from the patient or obtained from the bone bank.

- Use a microsagittal saw to shape this bone into a wedge, with the dorsal cortex of the iliac crest wedge cut to the width of the dorsal opening gap that was measured previously and oriented so that the exposed cancellous bone surfaces of the iliac wedge will be adjacent to the exposed cancellous surfaces of the osteotomized cuneiform.
- Use a distractor with a pin on either side of the osteotomy or a narrow osteotome to lever open the cuneiform osteotomy while an assistant places plantar-directed pressure on the first metatarsal to help open the osteotomy maximally while the bone graft wedge is impacted from dorsal to plantar into the medial cuneiform osteotomy using a bone tamp **(TECH FIG 2B,C)**.

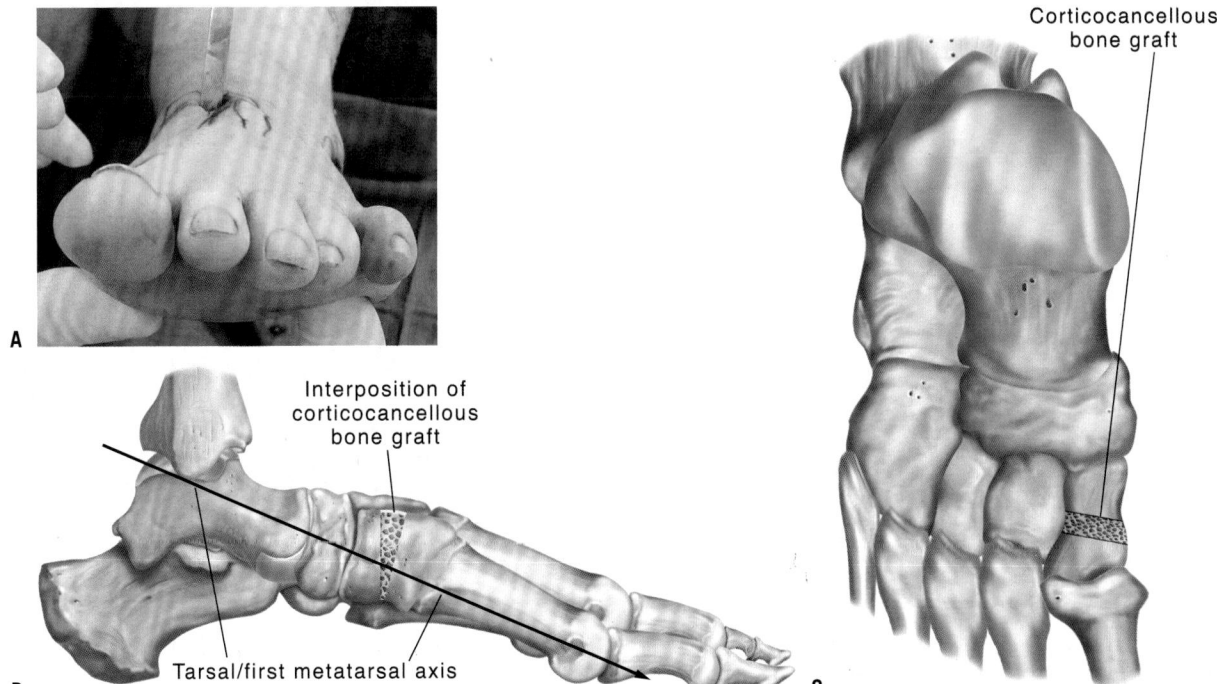

TECH FIG 2 A. An assistant levers the osteotomy open to depress the first metatarsal head while the surgeon determines when the forefoot varus deformity has been adequately corrected. **B,C.** The interposition bone graft wedge is placed into the dorsal opening in the first cuneiform to depress the first metatarsal and correct the forefoot varus deformity.

- Place small amounts of morselized cancellous bone graft, as autograft either from adjacent osteotomies of the hindfoot or from the piece of allograft, medially and laterally around the bone wedge to fill whatever gap remains in the cuneiform.

Kirschner Wire Fixation

- The osteotomy is stable due to the surrounding ligamentous support and the compression across the bone wedge created by tamping the bone wedge into the osteotomy and some authors have advocated that internal fixation is not necessary.[14] We use percutaneous fixation across the osteotomy to prevent dorsal displacement of the bone block until early healing has occurred **(TECH FIG 3)**.
- Bend to 90 degrees the percutaneous pin protruding from the dorsal medial aspect of the first cuneiform and apply a pin cap.
- Irrigate the wound and close it in layers.

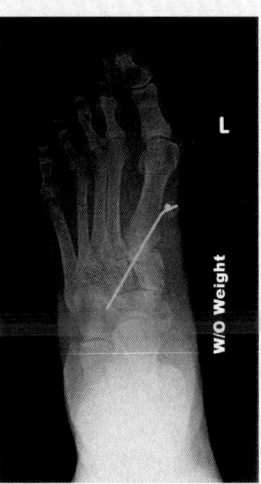

TECH FIG 3 Fixation of the osteotomy with a 0.62-inch Kirschner wire placed from the distal portion of the first cuneiform obliquely into the second cuneiform.

CLOSING WEDGE MEDIAL CUNEIFORM OSTEOTOMY[9]

Exposure

- If a hip bump is in place from prior portions of the procedure, this should be removed to allow the leg to externally rotate.
- Under tourniquet control, make a medial, curvilinear incision centered over the naviculocuneiform joint. *It is possible to perform an FDL transfer through this same incision if indicated.*
- Carry dissection through the skin and subcutaneous tissue to expose the medial cuneiform.
- On the plantar aspect, approximately 20% of the insertion of the tibialis anterior should be reflected to perform the osteotomy.

Osteotomy

- With fluoroscopic guidance, identify the midportion of the cuneiform on the medial side and draw a saw cut line on the bone **(TECH FIG 4)**.
- Using a microsagittal saw from medial to lateral, take a wedge of 2 mm in width, which will result in approximately a 4-mm wedge of removed bone.

- Both the medial and lateral cortices should be cut, but the dorsal cortex should be left intact.

Kirschner Wire Fixation

- The void left behind should be closed by manual compression and a temporary Kirschner wire driven across the osteotomy site.
- The position of the first ray should then be checked clinically and fluoroscopically. The first metatarsal head should be level with the fifth metatarsal head in the coronal plane in order to restore Cotton's "triangle."
- If insufficient correction has been obtained, then the temporary Kirschner wire should be removed and additional plantar-based wedges should be removed in increments of 1 mm.
- Once adequate correction has been achieved, the osteotomy may be fixed with two staples—one plantar and one plantar-medial **(TECH FIG 5)**.
- The temporary Kirschner wire should be removed at this time.

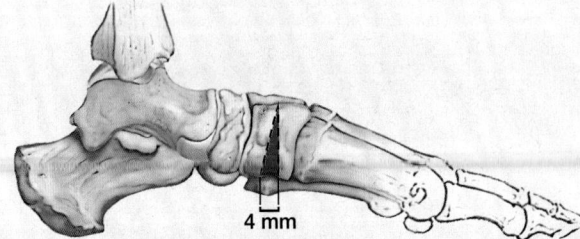

TECH FIG 4 Location of closing wedge first cuneiform osteotomy as viewed from medial approach. Removal of a 2-mm wedge of bone will result in approximately a 4-mm plantar gap to be closed. More bone is removed as needed to achieve desired correction.

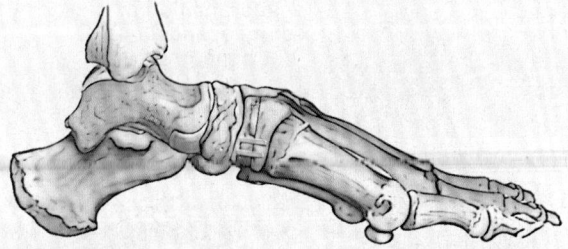

TECH FIG 5 Closing wedge osteotomy is fixed with two staples inserted into the plantar surface of the first cuneiform.

Pearls and Pitfalls

Graft Placement	• Avoid placing the graft too far laterally, which would cause impingement of the graft against the second cuneiform.
Fixation Problems	• Dorsal screw or plate fixation is not usually necessary, and the prominence of the dorsal hardware often requires hardware removal. • A second Kirschner wire, staple, or dorsal plate could be employed if the surgeon desires additional fixation. • Plantar closing wedge osteotomies require more fixation due to the inherent instability of this osteotomy. The authors of the clinical study cited here recommend two 10-mm staples.
Contouring Bone	• After opening wedge graft fixation, the microsagittal saw or a power rasp is used to smooth down any portions of the graft that extend beyond the surface of the cuneiform either medially or dorsally and to reduce any prominence of the cuneiform that may have been created by the osteotomy.

POSTOPERATIVE CARE

- The pin site is dressed along with the other wounds, and a compressive, bulky Robert Jones type of dressing is applied with medial lateral and posterior plaster slab splints covered with an elastic wrap.
- If a tendon transfer has been performed as part of the reconstructive procedure, the foot is positioned as needed for proper soft tissue healing.
- At 10 to 14 days after surgery, the splint, dressings, and sutures are removed.
- A dressing is placed around the pin site, which is then padded with a small felt doughnut, and a short-leg fiberglass cast is applied in neutral or whatever position is needed for proper soft tissue healing if a tendon transfer has been performed.
- The cast is removed at 6 weeks after surgery.
- Radiographs are obtained to ensure early incorporation of the graft without displacement.
- The percutaneous pin is removed, and full weight bearing as tolerated is allowed in a removable walker boot (FIG 2). Joint and muscle rehabilitation, as indicated by the other operative procedures performed in addition to cuneiform osteotomy, is begun.

OUTCOMES

- Outcomes of this procedure have shown predictable healing. In a review of 16 feet (15 patients) by Hirose and Johnson,[5] there were no malunions or nonunions. All patients at follow-up described mild to no pain with ambulation.

In a small series of medial closing wedge osteotomies, all patients went on to union as well. They also noted statistically significant improvements in Foot and Ankle Outcome Score and 12-Item Short Form Survey scores.[9]
- Average improvement in the first metatarsal–medial cuneiform angle as measured on the lateral radiograph was 9 degrees.[5]
- Because of the variety of hindfoot procedures performed in patients undergoing the cuneiform osteotomy, the degree of hindfoot correction contributed by the cuneiform osteotomy alone is difficult to determine.[5]
- This procedure combined with hindfoot reconstruction for flatfoot provides superior correction of the flatfoot deformity (as evidenced by the lateral talo–first metatarsal angle and the medial cuneiform to floor distance) compared to FDL tendon transfer with subtalar joint arthrodesis or medial displacement calcaneal osteotomy.[5,9,12,13]

COMPLICATIONS

- Few complications have been described in the literature on this procedure. They include the need for hardware removal due to a prominent screw head or staple.[5,9]
- Structures at risk during the exposure include the extensor hallucis longus or the extensor digitorum brevis tendon and the superficial and deep peroneal nerves. In the closing wedge medial cuneiform osteotomy, the tibialis anterior is at risk and is partially excised.
- Although predictable healing has been noted, nonunion, overcorrection, and undercorrection could occur. In a series of patients where trabecular metal wedges were used,

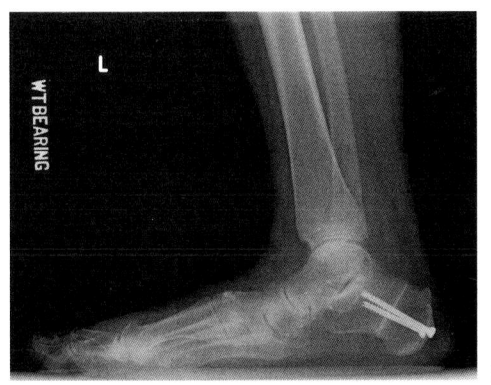 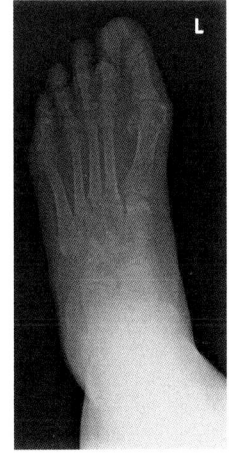

FIG 2 Lateral (**A**) and AP (**B**) radiographs at 10 weeks after acquired flatfoot deformity correction with first cuneiform osteotomy. The allograft bone wedge has healed.

two nonunions were identified, but only one was found to be symptomatic at 35.4 months follow-up.[13]

• When a dorsal screw is used for fixation, removal of the hardware is often required due to dorsal shoe pressure or irritation of the overlying nerve or tendon.

REFERENCES

1. Alvarez RG, Marini A, Schmitt C, et al. Stage 1 and II posterior tibial tendon dysfunction treated by a structured nonoperative management protocol: an orthosis and exercise program. Foot Ankle Int 2006;27:2–8.
2. Augustin JF, Lin SS, Berberian WS, et al. Nonoperative treatment of adult acquired flat foot with the Arizona brace. Foot Ankle Clin 2003;8.431–501.
3. Benthien RA, Parks BG, Guyton GP, et al. Lateral column calcaneal lengthening, flexor digitorum longus transfer, and opening wedge medial cuneiform osteotomy for flexible flatfoot: a biomechanical study. Foot Ankle Int 2007;28(1):70–77.
4. Cotton FJ. Foot statics and surgery. N Engl J Med 1936;214:353–362.
5. Hirose CB, Johnson JE. Plantarflexion opening wedge medial cuneiform osteotomy for correction of fixed forefoot varus associated with flatfoot deformity. Foot Ankle Int 2004;25:568–574.
6. Kraus JC, Mckeon KE, Johnson JE, et al. Intraosseous and extraosseous blood supply to the medial cuneiform. Foot Ankle Int 2013;35(4):394–400.
7. Kunas GC, Do HT, Aiyer A, et al. Contribution of medial cuneiform osteotomy to correction of longitudinal arch collapse in stage IIb adult-acquired flatfoot deformity. Foot Ankle Int 2018;39(8):885–893.
8. League AC, Parks BG, Schon LC. Radiographic and pedobarographic comparison of femoral head allograft versus block plate with dorsal opening wedge medial cuneiform osteotomy: a biomechanical study. Foot Ankle Int 2008;29(9):922–926.
9. Ling JS, Ross KA, Hannon CP, et al. A plantar closing wedge osteotomy of the medial cuneiform for residual forefoot supination in flatfoot reconstruction. Foot Ankle Int 2013;34(9):1221–1226.
10. Mosca VS. Flexible flatfoot in children and adolescents. J Child Orthop 2010;4(2):107–121.
11. Rathjen KE, Mubarak SJ. Calcaneal-cuboid-cuneiform osteotomy for the correction of valgus foot deformities in children. J Pediatr Orthop 1998;18(6):773–782.
12. Romeo G, Bianchi A, Cerbone V, et al. Medial cuneiform opening wedge osteotomy for correction of flexible flatfoot deformity: trabecular titanium vs. bone allograft wedges. Biomed Res Int 2019;2019:1–7.
13. Tsai J, McDonald E, Sutton R, et al. Severe flexible pes planovalgus deformity correction using trabecular metallic wedges. Foot Ankle Int 2018;40(4):402–407.
14. Wang C-S, Tzeng Y-H, Lin C-C, et al. Comparison of screw fixation versus non-fixation in dorsal opening wedge medial cuneiform osteotomy of adult acquired flatfoot. Foot Ankle Surg 2019;26(2):193–197.

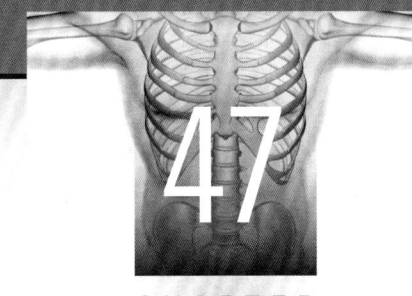

47

CHAPTER

Midfoot Arthrodesis

Ian L. D. Le, Jonathan Bourget-Murray, Jeannie Huh, and Mark E. Easley

DEFINITION

- A midfoot arthrodesis is a procedure where the separate bones that make up the midfoot are fused together—eliminating all motion. The operation is most commonly used to treat midfoot arthritis with or without deformity.

ANATOMY

- Midfoot joints include the following:
  - Tarsometatarsal (TMT) joints
  - Intercuneiform joints
  - Naviculocuneiform joint
- Together, these articulations form the transverse (roman) arch of the foot in the axial plane and the medial longitudinal arch in the sagittal plane.
- The base of the second cuneiform acts as a keystone to the transverse arch.
  - The plantar surface of the arch is narrower than the dorsal surface.
- The three columns of the midfoot
  - Medial column
    - First metatarsal
    - Medial cuneiform
    - Navicular
  - Middle column
    - Second and third metatarsals
    - Middle cuneiform
    - Lateral cuneiform
  - Lateral column
    - Fourth and fifth metatarsals
    - Cuboid
- The medial and middle columns are the least mobile.
  - The rigidity serves as a lever during push-off and throughout the gait cycle.
  - In contrast, the lateral column is supple, allowing to accommodate to uneven surfaces.
- Given the lack of motion across the medial and middle midfoot, fusing these joints does not generally cause noticeable loss of motion, thus creating few functional deficits.
- In contrast, fusing the lateral column is generally contraindicated, as doing so eliminates the midfoot's ability to accommodate to uneven surfaces.

PATHOGENESIS

- Etiology
  - Idiopathic
    - Osteoarthritis is most common.

- Posttraumatic arthritis
    - For example, a chronic Lisfranc fracture-dislocation
  - Inflammatory arthropathy
  - Charcot neuroarthropathy
- Pathoanatomy
  - When the normal anatomy of the midfoot is compromised, the relationship of the talo–first metatarsal is disrupted. The foot loses its mechanical advantage during standing and push-off.
    - In the sagittal (lateral) plane, this can be appreciated with a loss of the medial longitudinal arch height, and a midfoot sag.
    - In the coronal (anteroposterior [AP]) plane, the midfoot becomes abducted at the transverse tarsal joint, with uncovering of the talar head.
  - In a normal plantigrade foot, weight is normally evenly distributed across the "tripod of the foot," which includes the first metatarsal head, the fifth metatarsal head, and the calcaneus.
  - With progressive midfoot collapse, the tripod of the foot is disrupted, and the medial longitudinal arch can eventually reverse, causing a "rocker bottom deformity."
  - Consequently, the hindfoot may eventually develop excessive valgus deviation.
  - Progressive stretching of the medial soft tissue structures further accentuates this deformity. Ultimately, this can lead to shortening of the Achilles tendon and equinus contracture.
  - In extreme cases, the ankle may become incongruent.

NATURAL HISTORY

- An injury to the midfoot joints or ligaments, particularly the "Lisfranc ligament" between the first cuneiform and the base of the second metatarsal, leads to destabilization of the midfoot's biomechanics and a tendency toward gradual collapse of the medial longitudinal arch and abduction of the transverse tarsal joint with progressive hindfoot valgus deformity.

PATIENT HISTORY AND PHYSICAL FINDINGS

- History
  - Often (but not always), a history of midfoot trauma is reported.
    - Caution is warranted in patients with peripheral neuropathy, as trauma may have occurred but due to their lack of sensation, may not have been appreciated.
  - Primary and inflammatory arthritis may be responsible without trauma.

- Patients experience pain in their midfoot with weight bearing, especially with push-off.
- Patients may also note a loss of medial longitudinal arch height and/or new difficulty with shoe wear.
- Physical examination
  - The patient must be examined while weight bearing.
  - Comparison to the contralateral foot is often useful and should be assessed for the following:
    - Pain with palpation or stress of the midfoot
    - Pain with weight bearing
    - Medial longitudinal arch height loss
    - Forefoot abduction
    - Hindfoot valgus deformity
    - Equinus contracture
  - Special tests
    - The "piano key test" isolates the focus of the pathology to the specific TMT joint.
- Neurologic examination
  - If there is a concern for underlying neuropathy, cutaneous sensation should be assessed.
    - Semmes-Weinstein monofilament test
    - If the patient can sense the 5.07 monofilament, protective sensation is deemed intact.

IMAGING AND OTHER DIAGNOSTIC STUDIES

- Plain weight-bearing three view series of the foot should be obtained: AP, lateral, and oblique views.
- Angular deformity of the midfoot is simplest to assess on weight-bearing films:
  - AP radiographs
    - The talo–first metatarsal axis (Meary line) should be collinear.
    - Abduction of the midfoot
    - Uncovering of the talar head
  - Lateral radiographs
    - The talo–first metatarsal axis should be congruent.
      - Is the apex of deformity at the level of the midfoot?
  - Collapse of the medial longitudinal arch
- Rarely is a computed tomography (CT) scan required for assessment or preoperative planning.
- To identify which specific midfoot joint is symptomatic, ultrasound-guided corticosteroid injections may be used—these can serve as a diagnostic and possibly therapeutic modality.
- A single-photon emission CT/CT may be used for enhancing diagnostic specificity.

NONOPERATIVE MANAGEMENT

- Activity modification
- Nonsteroidal anti-inflammatory drugs
- Intra-articular corticosteroid injections
- Mechanical support
  - Longitudinal arch support
  - Stiffer-soled shoe with or without a low-profile rocker bottom
    - With midfoot arthritis with little deformity, a rocker may be placed on a sensible regular shoe; it need not be a big cumbersome shoe.
    - However, with progressive deformity, the shoe may need to be accommodative.
  - Bracing
    - A double upright brace or ankle–foot orthosis
      - This can be worn in addition to wearing a stiffer-soled shoe.

- Diabetics with peripheral neuropathy or neuroarthropathy require a stiffer-soled shoe with a rocker modification in combination with a total contact insert.

SURGICAL MANAGEMENT

- Surgical management is warranted with failure of nonoperative measures.
- In addition to a midfoot arthrodesis, a realignment midfoot osteotomy, Achilles tendon lengthening, and/or hindfoot realignment may need to be done concomitantly.
- Contraindications
  - Active infection
  - Patient's health is too poor to undergo surgery
- Relative contraindications
  - Advanced osteoporosis
  - Poor skin quality
  - Smoking
    - Increases the risk of nonunion

Preoperative Planning

- Preoperative weight-bearing radiographs of the foot are essential for preoperative planning.
  - The goal of surgery is to restore congruency of the talo–first metatarsal alignment.
  - The apex of deformity must be determined in order for proper realignment.
  - The degree of destruction or distortion of the midfoot anatomy (more commonly seen with inflammatory arthropathies) is important and factors in how to best to proceed with reconstruction.
  - Range of motion should be thoroughly assessed to identify an underlying equinus contracture.
    - Often, an Achilles tendon lengthening, either with a triple cut or gastrocnemius–soleus recession, is necessary to realign the foot. Doing so will serve to unload undue stress on the midfoot.
  - Hindfoot deformity and alignment must be appreciated and to determine the need for a hindfoot realignment.
- Equipment
  - Various screw and plating systems exist, some are even dedicated to the midfoot.
  - Depending on the planned reconstruction, the following options exist:
    - Standard screws and plates
    - Locking midfoot screws and plates
    - Intramedullary screws
    - Compression staples
    - Compression plates

Positioning

- The patient is positioned supine on the operating table.
- We routinely use a tourniquet.

Approach

- Dual longitudinal approach over the midfoot
  - One dorsal and one medial incision
- Transverse approach
  - Has been used by many surgeons but is not universally accepted

TECHNIQUES

SCREW AND COMPRESSION PLATE FIXATION

Background

- The patient was a 38-year-old woman with posttraumatic midfoot arthritis following a chronic Lisfranc fracture-dislocation.
- She also had a "nutcracker" injury to her cuboid with some degenerative changes to her lateral column (**TECH FIG 1**).

Exposure and Joint Preparation

- Dual dorsal longitudinal incisions with an adequate skin bridge
- Medial incision
  - Extensor hallucis brevis is exposed (**TECH FIG 2A**).

- Deep neurovascular bundle is found deep to the extensor hallucis longus muscle–tendon (**TECH FIG 2B**).
- First and second TMT joint preparation
  - Particularly deep joint (2.5 to 3.0 mm)
  - Use an oblong curette to ensure there is no residual plantar lip and cartilage in order to avoid dorsiflexion malunion (**TECH FIG 2C**).
  - It is important to remove scar tissue between the base of the second metatarsal and first cuneiform to allow anatomic reduction of the second metatarsal base (**TECH FIG 2D**).

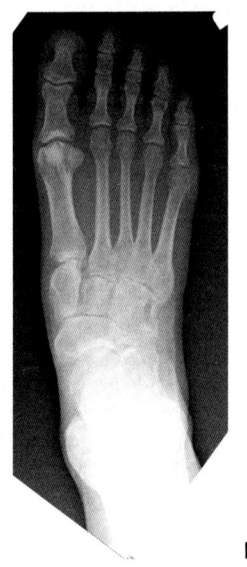 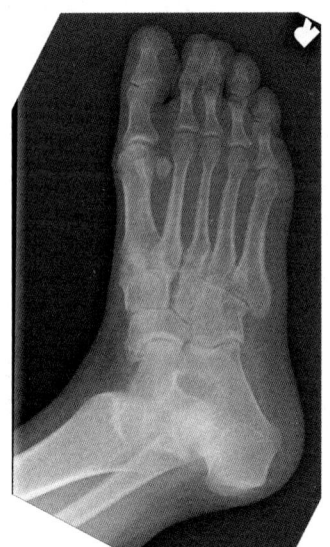 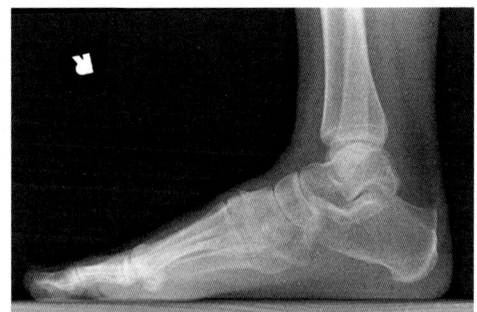

TECH FIG 1 Preoperative radiographs of 38-year-old woman with postoperative midfoot arthritis secondary to chronic Lisfranc injury. **A.** AP view. **B.** Oblique view (note distortion to cuboid: chronic nutcracker injury). **C.** Lateral view.

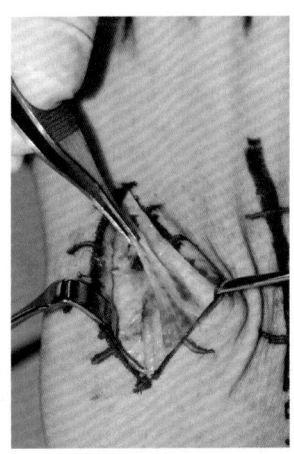 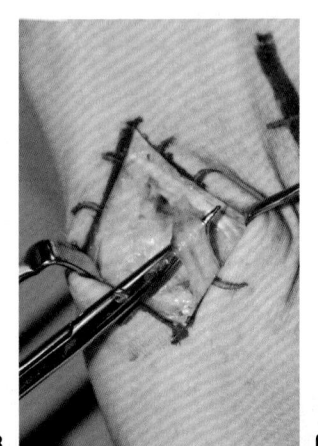 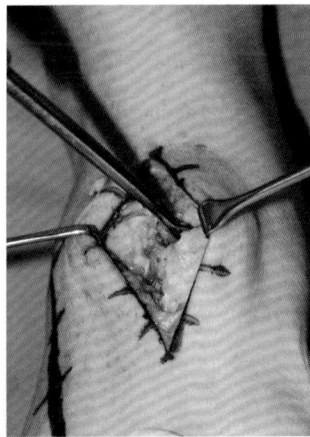

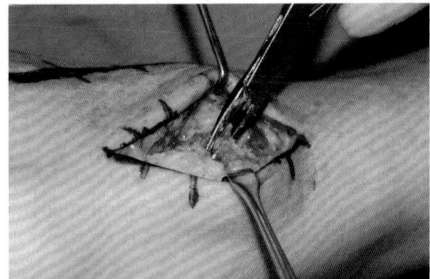 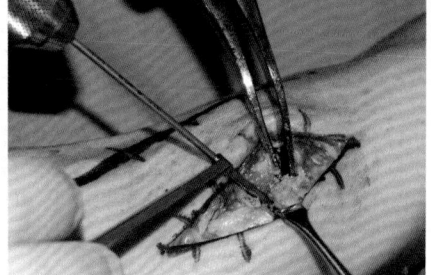

TECH FIG 2 Dorsal medial approach. **A.** Extensor hallucis brevis (EHB) muscle elevated. **B.** Immediately deep to EHB is the deep neurovascular bundle. **C–E.** Preparing medial aspect of TMT joints. **C.** Sharp elevator for first TMT joint. (Note the toes at top of **A** to **C**.) **D.** Rongeur in junction between base of second metatarsal and first cuneiform (it is important to be sure the second metatarsal fully reduces). **E.** Drill to penetrate subchondral bone. The second TMT joint is prepared in a similar manner. Dorsolateral approach. *(continued)*

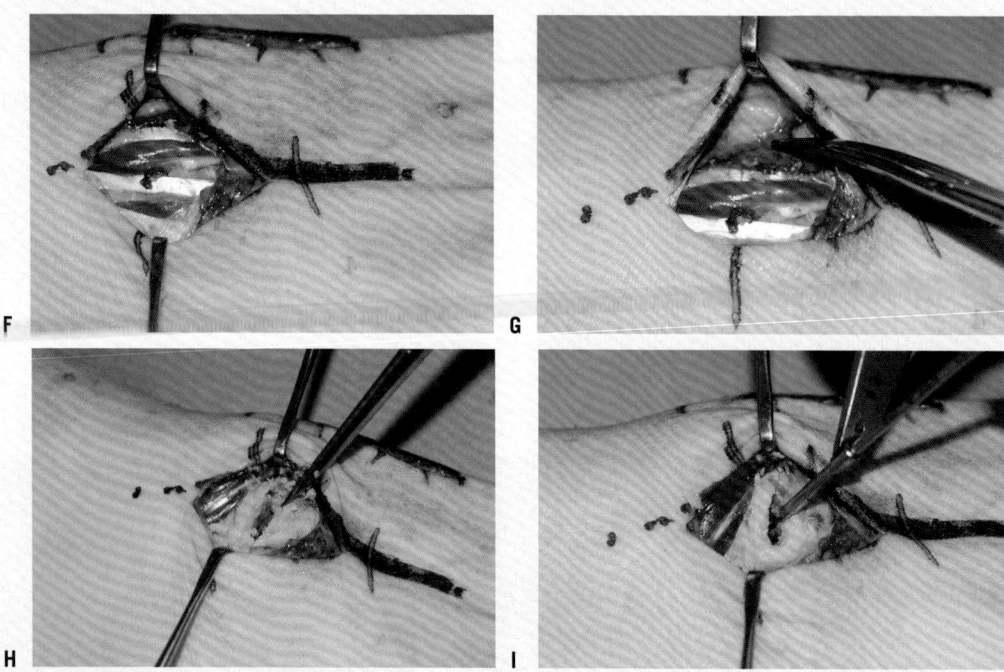

TECH FIG 2 *(continued)* **F.** Interval identified. **G.** Superficial peroneal nerve branches are identified and protected. **H,I.** Preparation of third TMT joint. **H.** Sharp elevator to remove residual cartilage. **I.** Drilling subchondral bone. (Note the toes at right side of **F** to **I**.)

- Fenestrate the subchondral bone multiple times with a 2.0-mm drill to improve angiogenic and osseous growth to the arthrodesis site **(TECH FIG 2E)**.
- Lateral incision (with adequate skin bridge) **(TECH FIG 2F)**
  - Protect the superficial peroneal nerve branch or branches **(TECH FIG 2G)**.
  - Third TMT joint preparation: Remove residual cartilage and fenestrate the subchondral bone **(TECH FIG 2H,I)**.
- Add bone graft as necessary.

Reducing the Deformity

- The "windlass" mechanism may be useful in reducing the TMT joints and particularly in avoiding dorsiflexion malunion. Moreover, it compresses the joints **(TECH FIG 3A)**.

- We maintain dorsiflexion of the toes (activates windlass mechanism) while we place the provisional fixation **(TECH FIG 3B,C)**.
- Using a bone reduction clamp the second metatarsal base is reduced. We then place a guide pin to drill with a cannulated drill the path for a classic "Lisfranc screw" **(TECH FIG 3D)**.

Provisional Fixation

- Guide pins are placed for provisional fixation of the middle column **(TECH FIG 4A)**.
- Thin guide pins for cannulated drills are fragile. We measure the desired screw length and then pass the wires all the way through the foot. That way, if the guide pin should break, we can retrieve both ends and not leave a pin in the foot **(TECH FIG 4B,C)**.

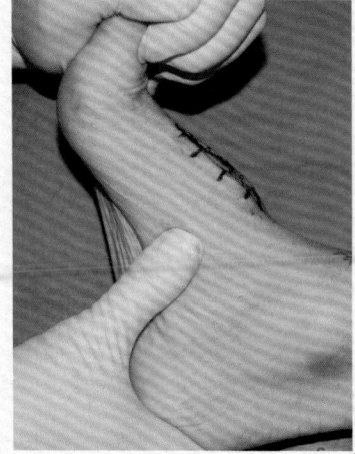

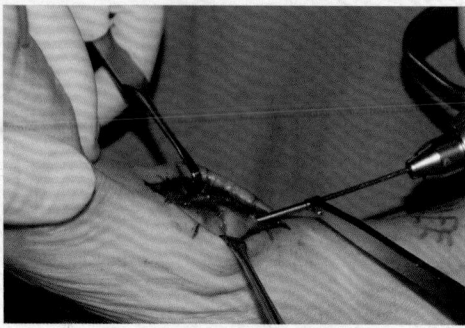

TECH FIG 3 A. Use the windlass mechanism to assist in reduction and promote proper alignment of the TMT joints. Note dorsiflexion of the toes and ankle to tighten plantar soft tissues; this compresses the TMT joints and keeps them from dorsiflexing. **B,C.** Provisional fixation of first TMT joint. **B.** Proximal to distal pin. *(continued)*

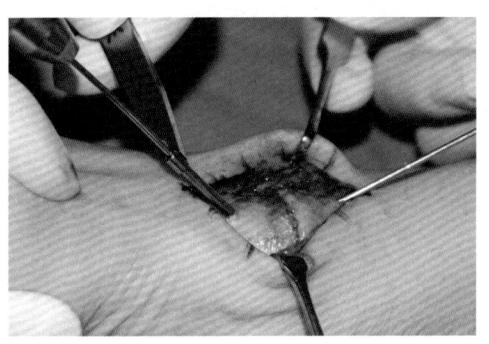

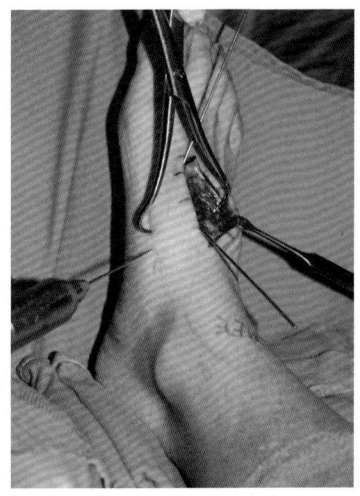

C   D

TECH FIG 3 *(continued)* **C.** Distal to proximal pin. Note that the windlass mechanism is still being maintained with dorsiflexion of the toes. **D.** Large bone reduction clamp to ensure that the second metatarsal base is reduced, much like open reduction and internal fixation of an acute Lisfranc fracture-dislocation. Provisional pin to fix second metatarsal base.

- Balancing the forefoot is essential. While performing provisional fixation, keep in mind that the metatarsal heads need to be balanced.
  - Typically, that means that the sesamoids are slightly more plantar than the second and third metatarsal heads **(TECH FIG 4D)**.

Lisfranc Screw Placement

- The Lisfranc screw stabilizes the base of the second metatarsal, and it will limit dorsiflexion of the second TMT joint if a compression plate is used dorsally.
- We routinely use solid screws but may initiate the drill hole with a cannulated system.
- For the placement of a Lisfranc screw from the first cuneiform to the base of the second metatarsal, we overdrill the guide pin but only to the medial cortex of the second metatarsal base.

- We remove the guide pin and complete the drill hole through the second metatarsal base.
- We then overdrill the first cuneiform.
- We place a fully threaded cortical screw in lag fashion. We typically use a washer for this screw **(TECH FIG 5)**.

Final Fixation

- We routinely use two lag screws to stabilize the first TMT joint **(TECH FIG 6A–F)**.
- It is important to use a countersink on the distal to proximal screws so that the dorsal cortex of the first metatarsal base does not fracture when the screw is fully seated (see **TECH FIG 6E**).
- The middle column may be further stabilized with a lag screw **(TECH FIG 6G–J)**.

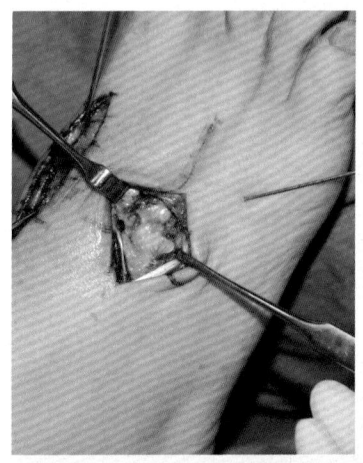

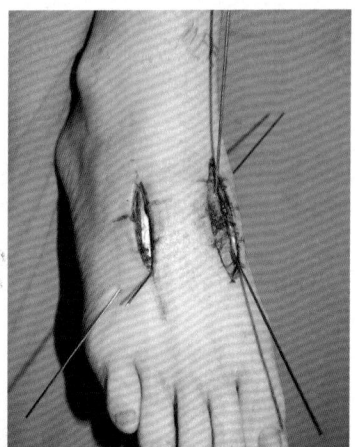

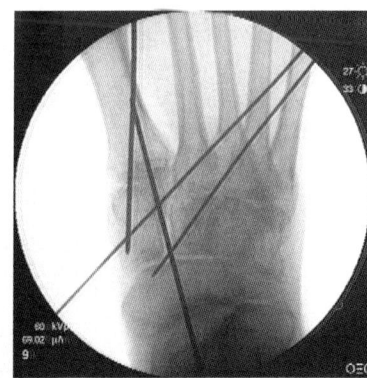

A   B   C

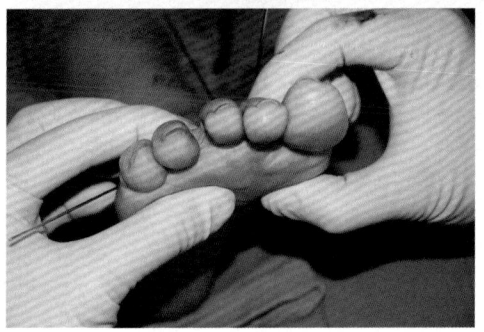

D

TECH FIG 4 A. Provisional lateral fixation. **B,C.** Provisional fixation for second metatarsal is the guide pin for the drill for the screw to be placed from the first cuneiform to the second metatarsal base, a traditional Lisfranc screw. **B.** Clinical view. **C.** Fluoroscopic view. Note that the guide pin position was checked on fluoroscopy and measured to determine optimal screw length and then the guide pin was driven fully through the second metatarsal to exit the lateral wound. This way, when the guide pin is drilled and potentially sheared by the drill, both ends of the guide pin may still be retrieved. **D.** Before placing definitive fixation, the surgeon should check the balance of the forefoot (metatarsal heads). Metatarsal heads should be well balanced, with the sesamoids slightly more plantar than the second and third metatarsal heads.

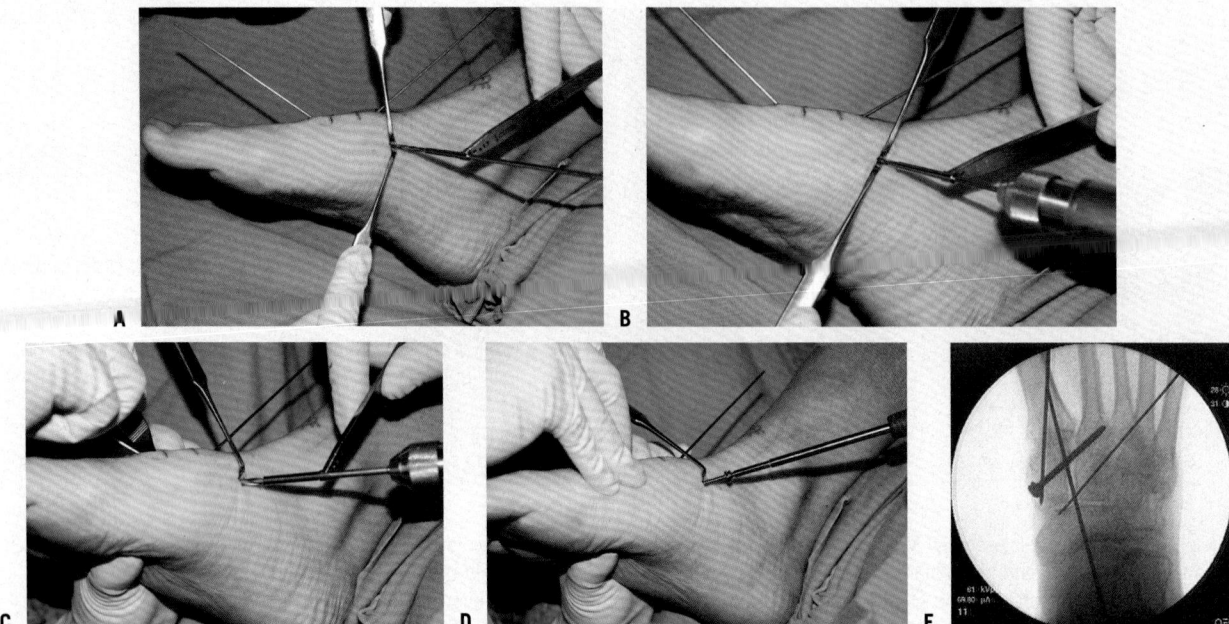

TECH FIG 5 Placing the Lisfranc screw. **A.** Initiating the drill hole with a cannulated drill over the guide pin. **B.** Guide pin is removed and drill hole completed with a solid drill. **C.** Proximal cortex (first cuneiform) is overdrilled to create lag effect. **D.** Solid screw is placed. **E.** Fluoroscopic view.

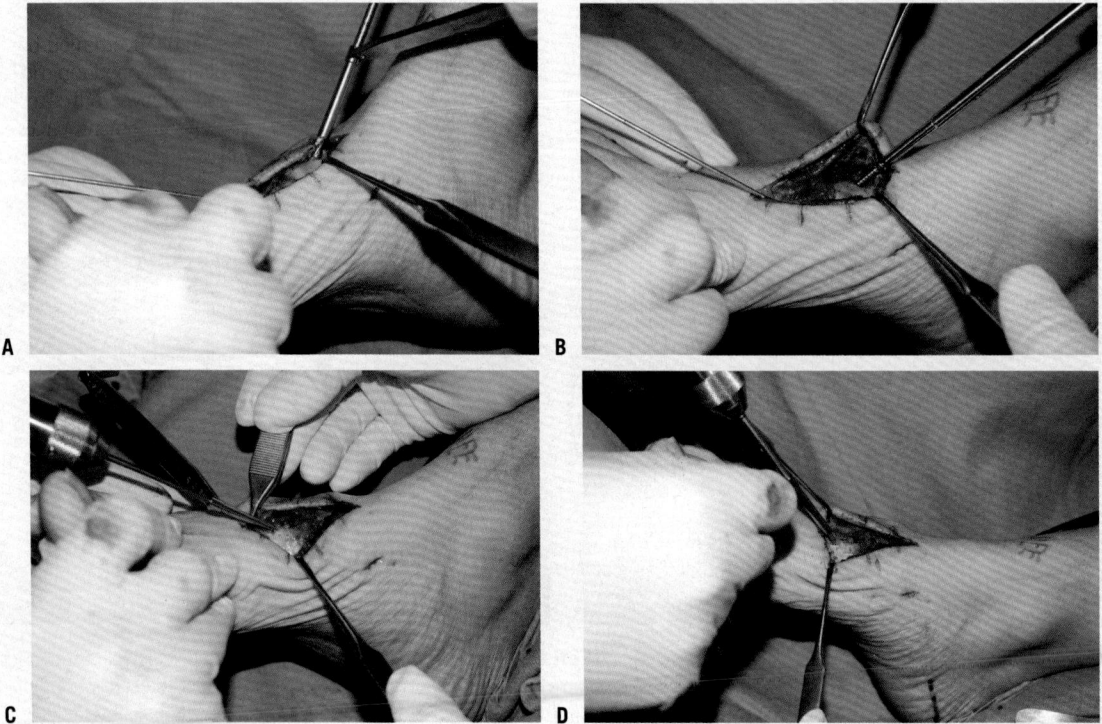

TECH FIG 6 A,B. Proximal to distal lag screw across first TMT joint. **A.** After removal of provisional fixation, overdrilling proximal cortex. **B.** Solid screw placement. **C–F.** Distal to proximal screw across the first TMT joint. **C.** After removal of provisional fixation, solid drill. **D.** Overdrill near cortex (first metatarsal). *(continued)*

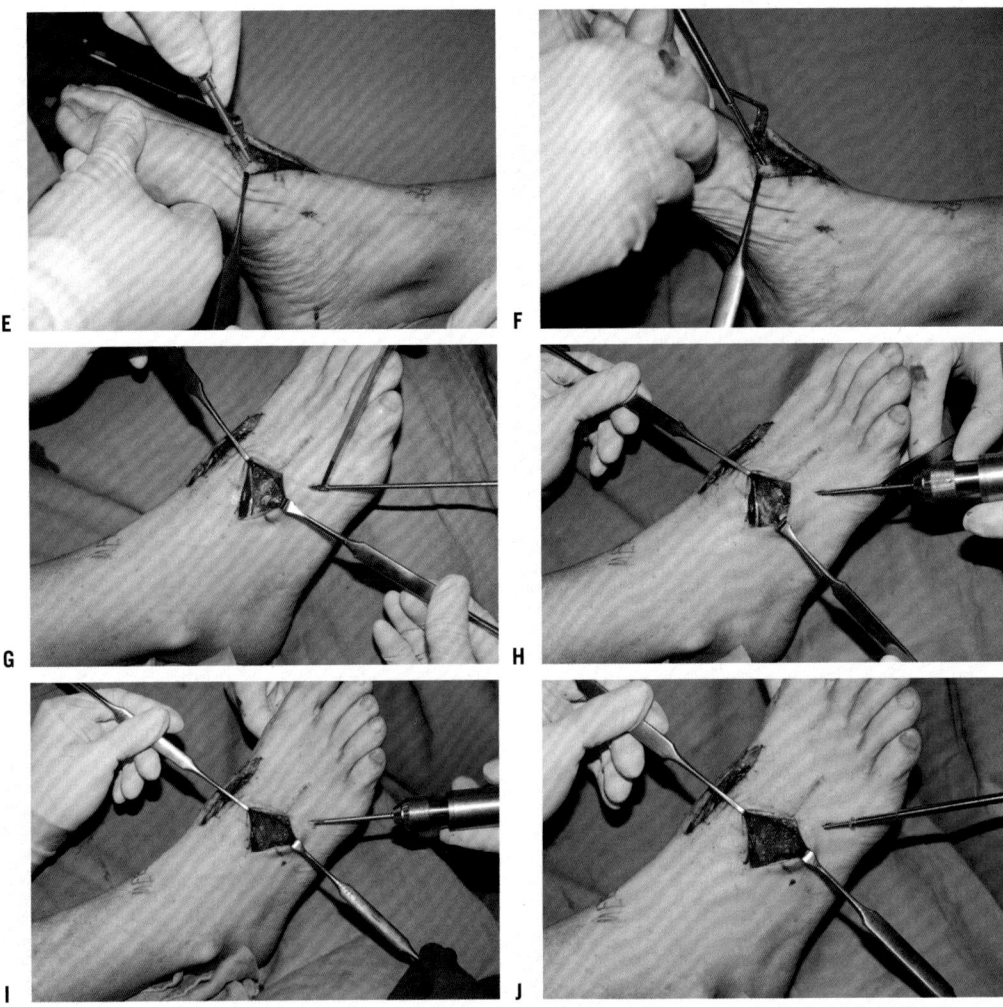

TECH FIG 6 *(continued)* **E.** Countersink (essential so that dorsal first metatarsal cortex does not fracture). **F.** Solid screw placement. **G–J.** Lateral screw placement. **G.** Overdrill guide pin with cannulated drill (pin is measured and then driven through medial foot so that both ends of the wire may be retrieved should the pin break). **H.** Drill with solid drill bit. **I.** Overdrill. **J.** Solid screw placed.

Dorsal Compression Plate Application

- We secure the third TMT joint with a dorsal compression plate; with the lag screw already placed, excessive dorsiflexion of the third TMT joint is avoided **(TECH FIG 7A–F)**.
- We also use a dorsal compression plate on the second TMT joint **(TECH FIG 7G–M)**. Because the Lisfranc screw has already been placed, dorsiflexion can be avoided.
- Precontouring the plate also prevents dorsiflexion.

Completion

- Intraoperative fluoroscopy of the construct confirms reduction and that dorsiflexion has been avoided **(TECH FIG 8A,B)**.
- The hardware is often close to the deep neurovascular bundle **(TECH FIG 8C)**.
- A drain may be used for this procedure **(TECH FIG 8D)**.

Postoperative Care

- Follow-up radiographs suggest satisfactory reduction.
- The patient had some residual lateral column symptoms, so we opted to add a subtalar arthroereisis implant to correct hindfoot alignment and perhaps unload some lateral column stress. Fortunately, that was a satisfactory solution in this case **(TECH FIG 9)**.
- The first through third TMT articulations have little physiologic motion, so arthrodesing them leaves little functional deficit.
- To avoid loss of the midfoot's accommodative capacity, we rarely, if ever, fuse the lateral side.

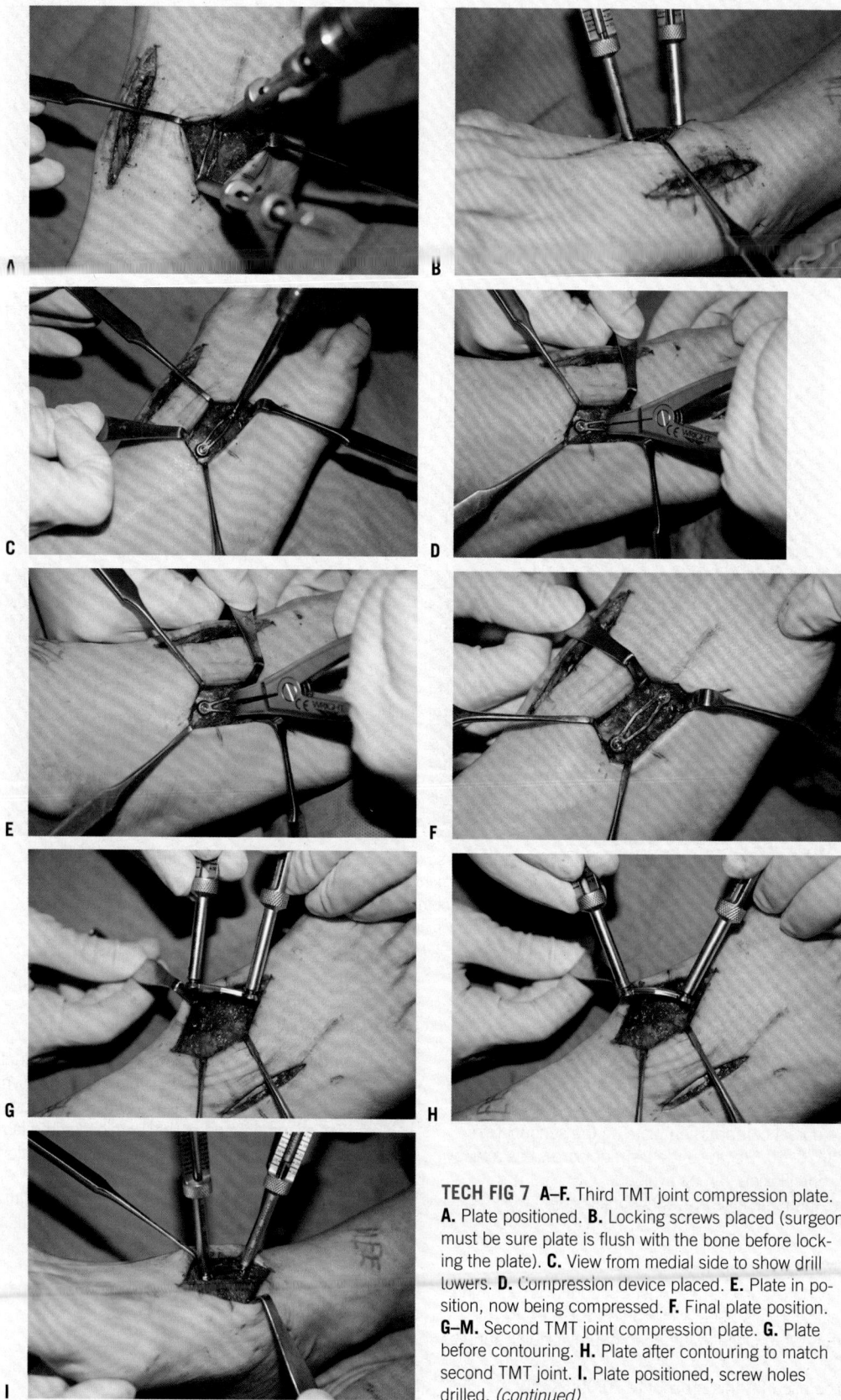

TECH FIG 7 A–F. Third TMT joint compression plate.
A. Plate positioned. **B.** Locking screws placed (surgeon must be sure plate is flush with the bone before locking the plate). **C.** View from medial side to show drill lowers. **D.** Compression device placed. **E.** Plate in position, now being compressed. **F.** Final plate position. **G–M.** Second TMT joint compression plate. **G.** Plate before contouring. **H.** Plate after contouring to match second TMT joint. **I.** Plate positioned, screw holes drilled. *(continued)*

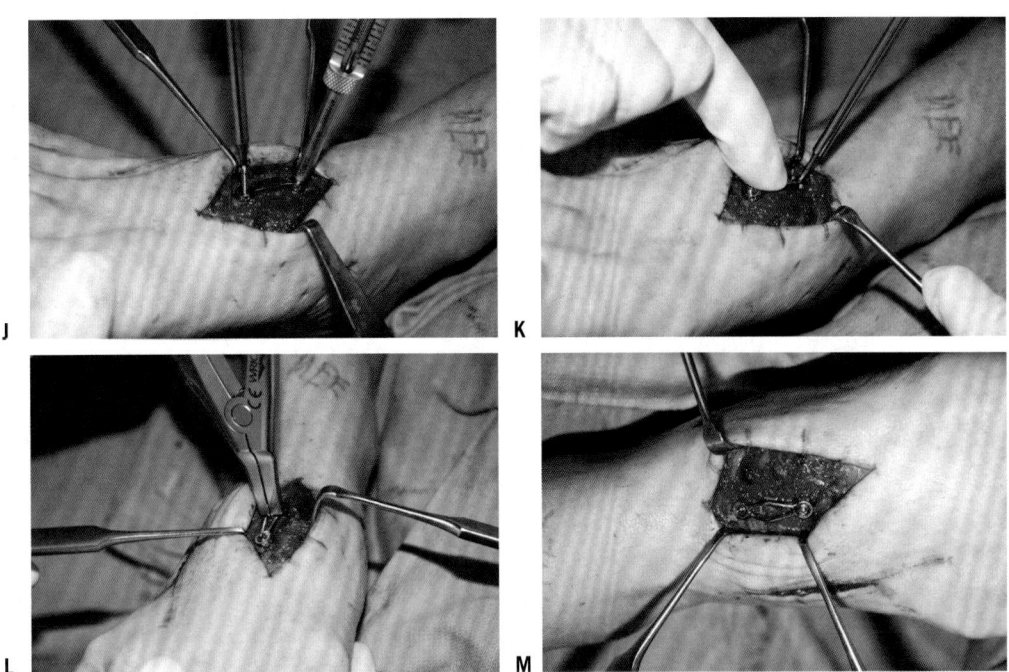

TECH FIG 7 *(continued)* **J.** Locking screw being inserted. **K.** Surgeon must be sure that plate is flush with bone before fully seating the locking screws. **L.** Compression device. **M.** Final plate position.

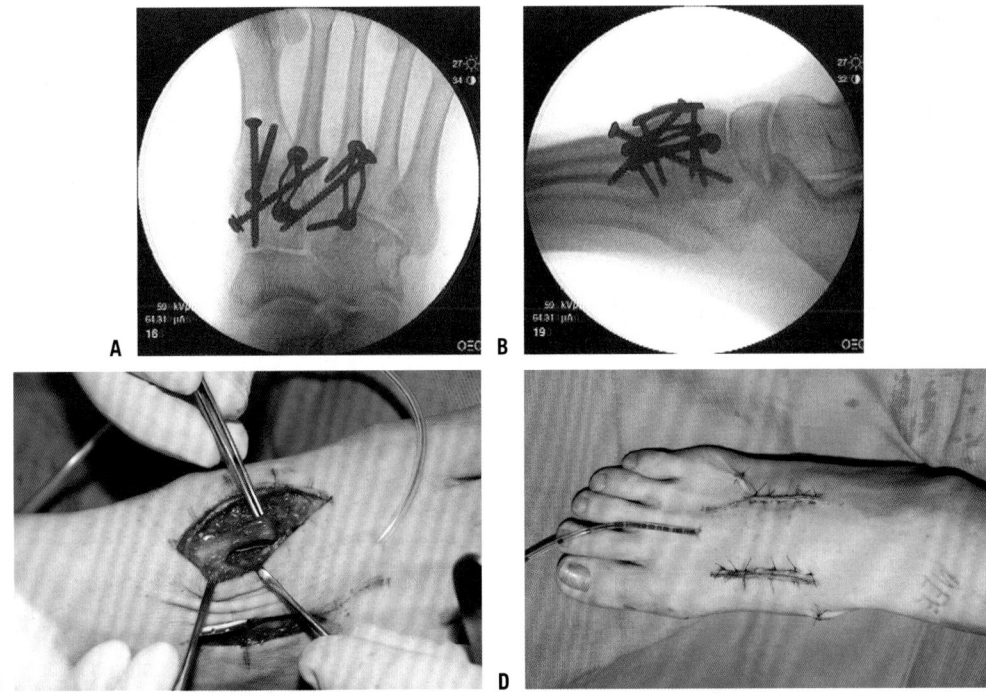

TECH FIG 8 AP (**A**) and lateral (**B**) fluoroscopic views of final construct. Note that first metatarsal is not elevated. **C.** Deep neurovascular bundle intact but will lie directly on second TMT joint compression plate. Note use of a drain (author's preference). **D.** Wounds closed without tension on skin bridge.

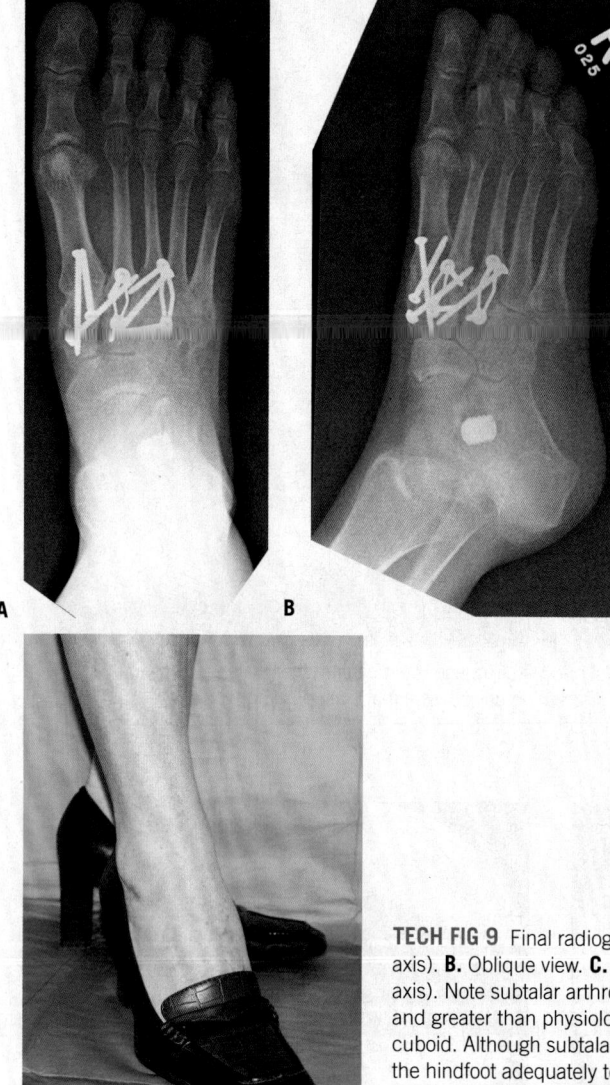

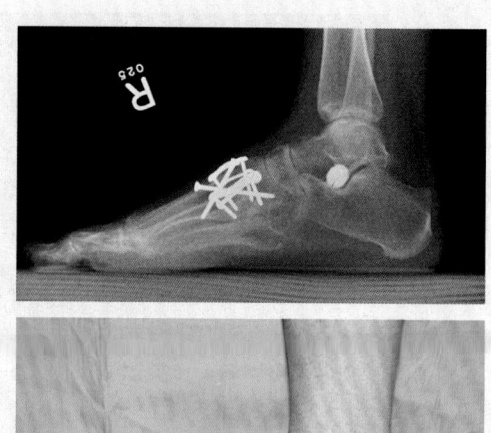

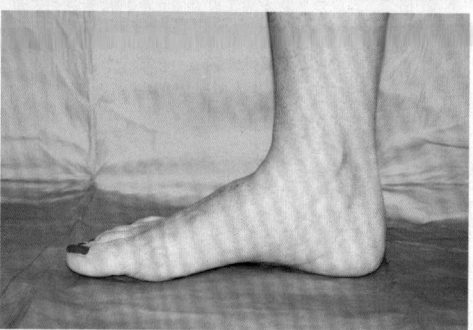

TECH FIG 9 Final radiographs. **A.** AP view (note restoration of talo–first metatarsal axis). **B.** Oblique view. **C.** Lateral view (also with restoration of talo–first metatarsal axis). Note subtalar arthroereisis. This patient had some residual lateral foot pain and greater than physiologic hindfoot valgus, probably secondary to the injury to the cuboid. Although subtalar arthroereisis does not address this directly, it reoriented the hindfoot adequately to relieve the lateral column stress. **D.** Clinical view of arch. **E.** The midfoot articulations normally have limited motion, so fusion of these joints does not restrict the foot substantially.

PLATE FIXATION WITH DEDICATED MIDFOOT PLATING SYSTEM

Background

- The patient was a 48-year-old woman with midfoot Charcot neuroarthropathy who has failed bracing (TECH FIG 10).
- She had severe distortion of the midfoot anatomy and loss of her medial longitudinal arch.

Medial Midaxial Approach to Allow for Medial Plating

- A medial midaxial incision is made, and the tibialis anterior tendon is retracted to expose the TMT joint (TECH FIG 11A–C).

- Should the tendon become detached, it can be sutured securely to the appropriate soft tissues during closure, and with prolonged immobilization to allow the midfoot to heal, the patient typically will retain full active dorsiflexion.
- Residual articular cartilage is removed and subchondral bone drilled to prepare the joint and promote fusion (TECH FIG 11D).

Dorsal Longitudinal Approach

- A dorsal longitudinal midfoot incision is made (TECH FIG 12A).
- The deep neurovascular bundle is immediately deep to the extensor hallucis brevis tendon. It must be identified and protected throughout the procedure (TECH FIG 12B–D).

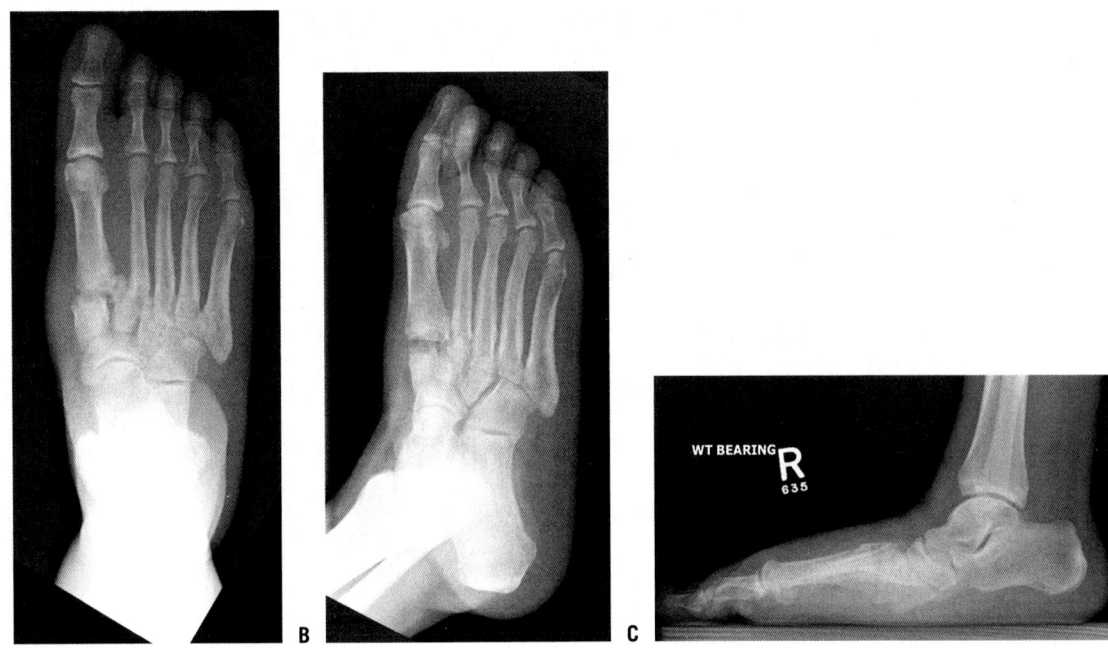

TECH FIG 10 Preoperative weight-bearing radiographs of 48-year-old patient with midfoot Charcot neuroarthropathy. **A.** AP view. **B.** Oblique view. **C.** Lateral view.

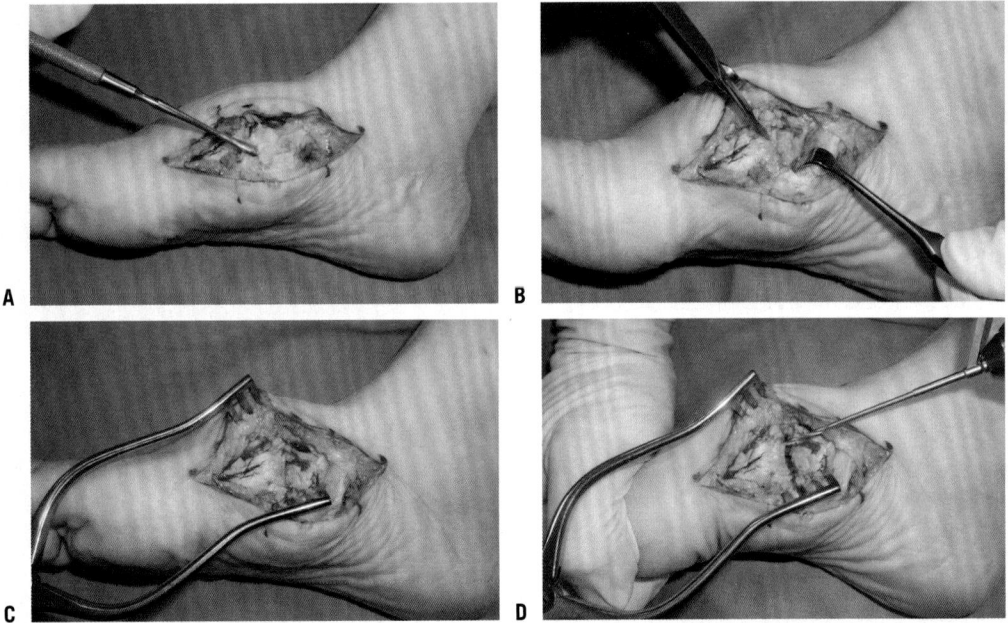

TECH FIG 11 Direct medial midaxial approach. **A.** Exposure. **B.** Reflecting tibialis anterior tendon to expose first TMT joint. **C.** Full exposure. **D.** After removing residual cartilage, subchondral bone is drilled to promote fusion.

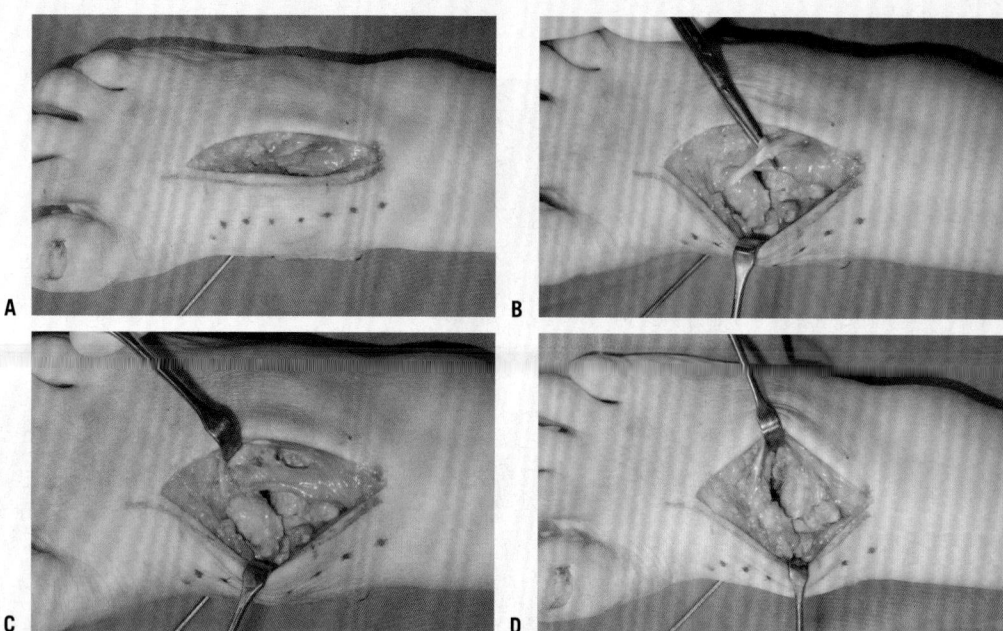

TECH FIG 12 Dorsal approach. **A.** Approach. **B.** Extensor hallucis brevis (EHB) tendon directly over deep neurovascular bundle. **C.** EHB tendon retracted to expose deep neurovascular bundle. **D.** Neurovascular bundle protected and second and third TMT joints exposed to prepare for arthrodesis (note eccentric joint deformity secondary to Charcot neuroarthropathy).

Joint Preparation

- Joint preparation can be interesting, given the distortion of the anatomy as a result of the Charcot process.
- For an acute Lisfranc fracture-dislocation, a bone reduction clamp from the first cuneiform to the base of the second or third metatarsal is helpful (**TECH FIG 13**).
- Once the reduction is confirmed fluoroscopically, provisional fixation can be placed.

Medial Plating

- Modern dedicated midfoot fusion plates have a contour that matches, for the most part, physiologic anatomy. If the plate fits well, the reduction is typically acceptable (**TECH FIG 14**).
- Also, if the plate is positioned properly on the first cuneiform, the first metatarsal can be reduced to the plate, and the reduction is typically satisfactory.
- A lag screw can be added to the medial column construct, but often, there is little room for such a screw and the plate, unless a headless screw is placed deep to the plate.

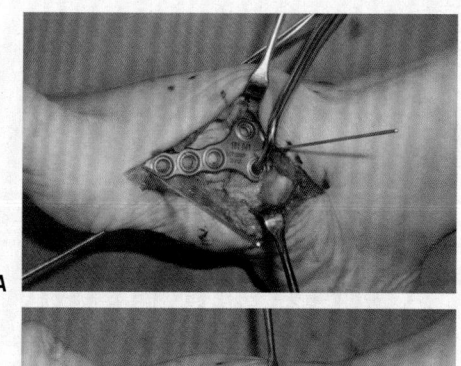
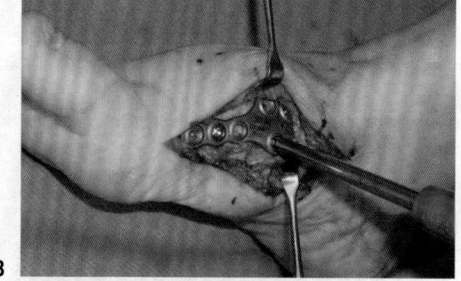
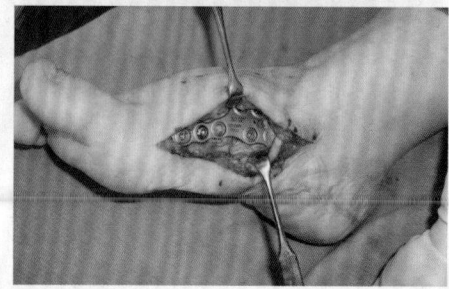

TECH FIG 14 A–C. Medial plate. The plate is designed to restore physiologic alignment; therefore, it may be used as a reduction tool. Occasionally, we fix the plate to the first cuneiform and then "bring" the first metatarsal to the plate.

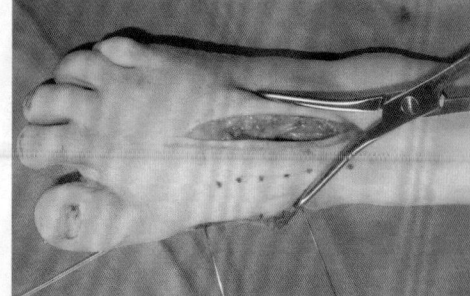

TECH FIG 13 Bone reduction clamp used to reduce medial and middle columns of the foot after joint preparation (and bone grafting) performed.

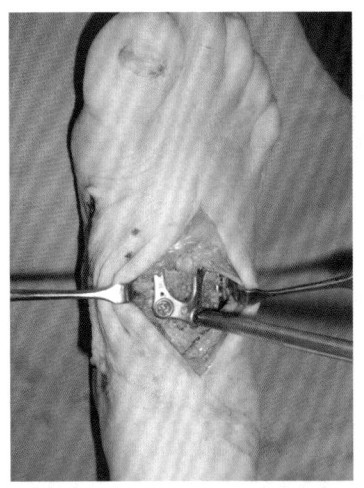
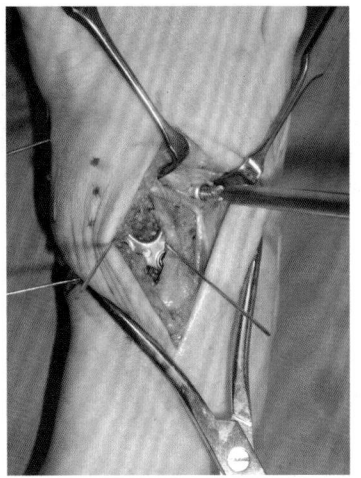
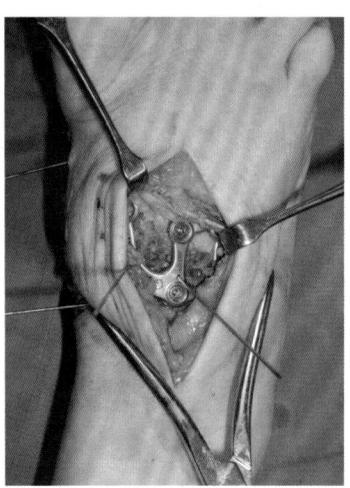
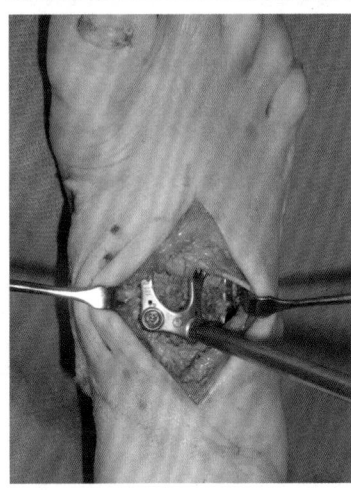

TECH FIG 15 A–D. Dorsal plate. The plate extends from the first TMT joint to the third TMT joint, so it must be carefully positioned under the deep neurovascular bundle and the extensor tendons.

Dorsal Plating

- Dedicated dorsal plating systems are now also available. These locking plates secure the first through third TMT joints **(TECH FIG 15)**.
- Alternatively, individual plates may be used on each TMT joint; however, if a single plate can be used to stabilize all three TMT joints, the construct tends to be stronger.
  - With the distortion of anatomy from Charcot neuroarthropathy, plates designed for physiologic anatomy sometimes are difficult to place perfectly on all three TMT joints.
  - Take care to protect the deep neurovascular bundle (in neuropathy, obviously the artery only matters) and the extensor tendons.

Postoperative Care

- Follow-up radiographs for the patient are shown in **TECH FIG 16**.
- In this case of Charcot neuroarthropathy and dislocation of the fourth and fifth TMT joints, we opted to also arthrodese the lateral column.
- Only in this situation of neuroarthropathy do we attempt to fuse the lateral column. Typically, we do not wish to sacrifice the midfoot's ability to accommodate.

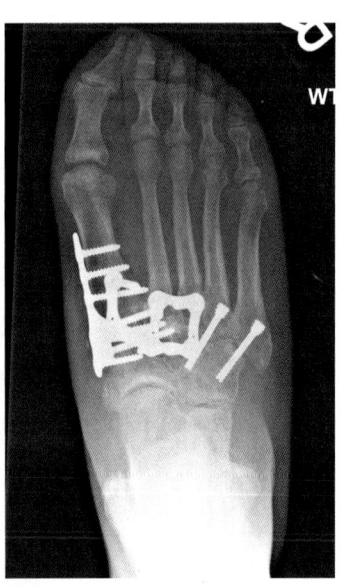

TECH FIG 16 Follow-up radiographs. **A.** AP view. *(continued)*

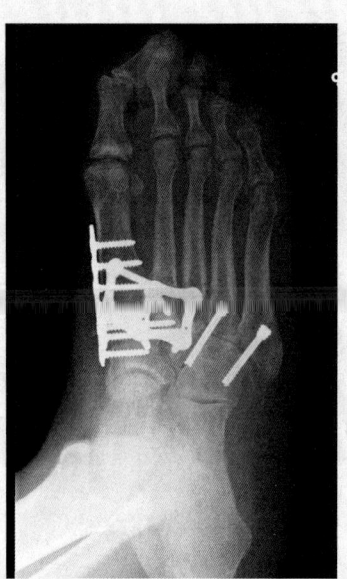

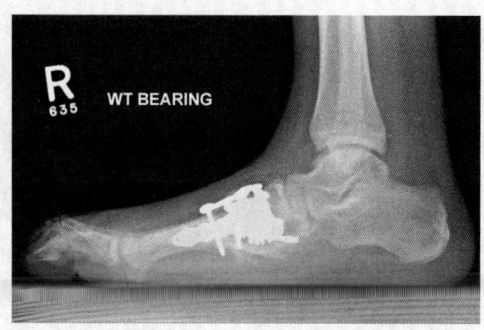

TECH FIG 16 *(continued)* **B.** Oblique view. **C.** Lateral view. In this patient with Charcot neuroarthropathy, the lateral column of the foot was also arthrodesed. We do not routinely arthrodese the lateral column but make an exception in select cases of Charcot neuroarthropathy where added stability may be needed for preoperative first and fifth TMT joint dislocation.

EXTERNAL FIXATION

Background

- The patient was a 44-year-old woman with midfoot sag and a forefoot abduction deformity and has failing nonoperative treatment **(TECH FIG 17)**.

Medial Midaxial Approach

- Medial approach for midfoot biplanar osteotomy is undertaken.
- Two reference pins serve to mark the desired osteotomy (confirmed fluoroscopically) **(TECH FIG 18)**.

Applying the External Fixator

- The saw is shown positioned for the osteotomy in **TECH FIG 19A**; but to maintain stability of the foot, we routinely apply the external fixator first and then complete the osteotomy.
- In this case, a "butt frame" construct was used.
- The hindfoot component of the frame stabilizes the hindfoot with two U rings.
  - The frame is first secured with thin wires **(TECH FIG 19B,C)**.
  - Next, half-pins are added for further stability **(TECH FIG 19D)**.
  - We usually tension the thin wires after the half-pins have been inserted **(TECH FIG 19E,F)**.

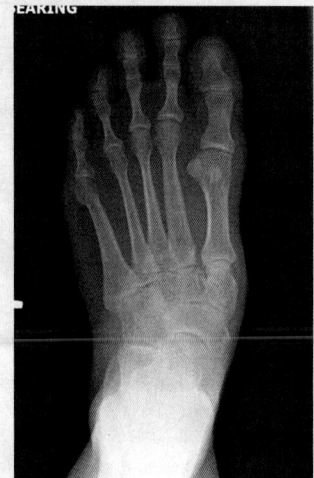

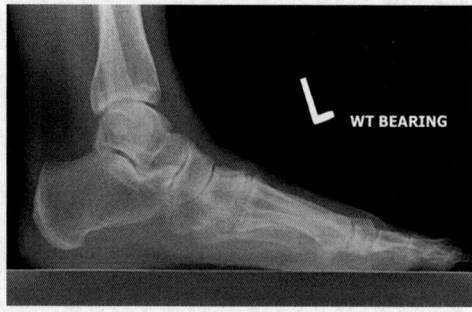

TECH FIG 17 Preoperative weight-bearing radiographs of 44-year-old woman with midfoot deformity leading to forefoot abduction and midfoot sag, failing nonoperative measures. **A.** AP view. **B.** Lateral view.

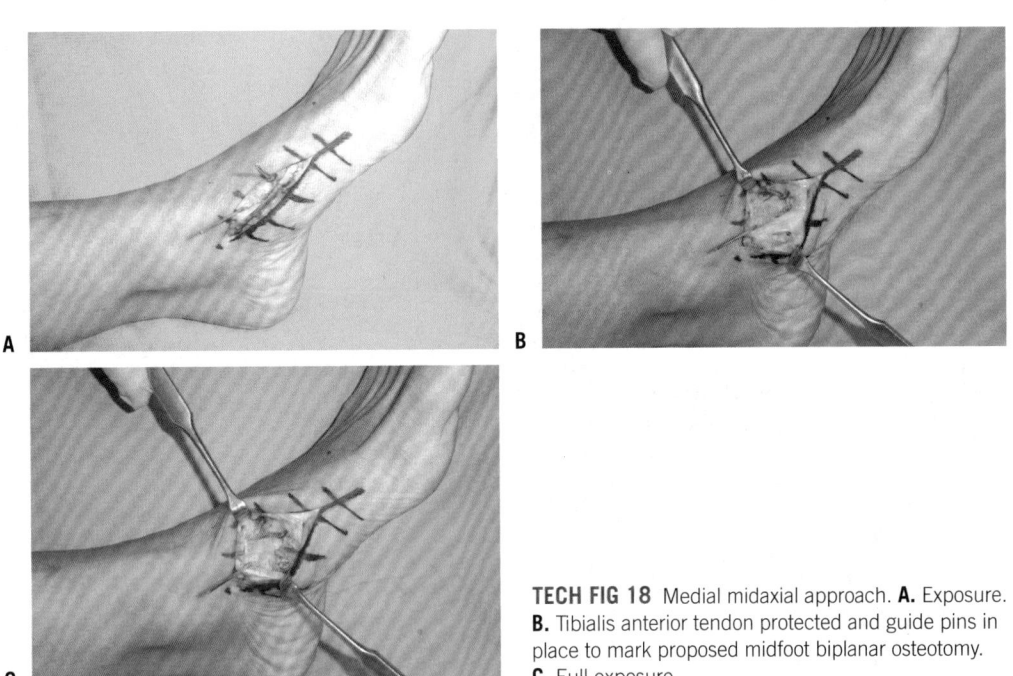

TECH FIG 18 Medial midaxial approach. **A.** Exposure. **B.** Tibialis anterior tendon protected and guide pins in place to mark proposed midfoot biplanar osteotomy. **C.** Full exposure.

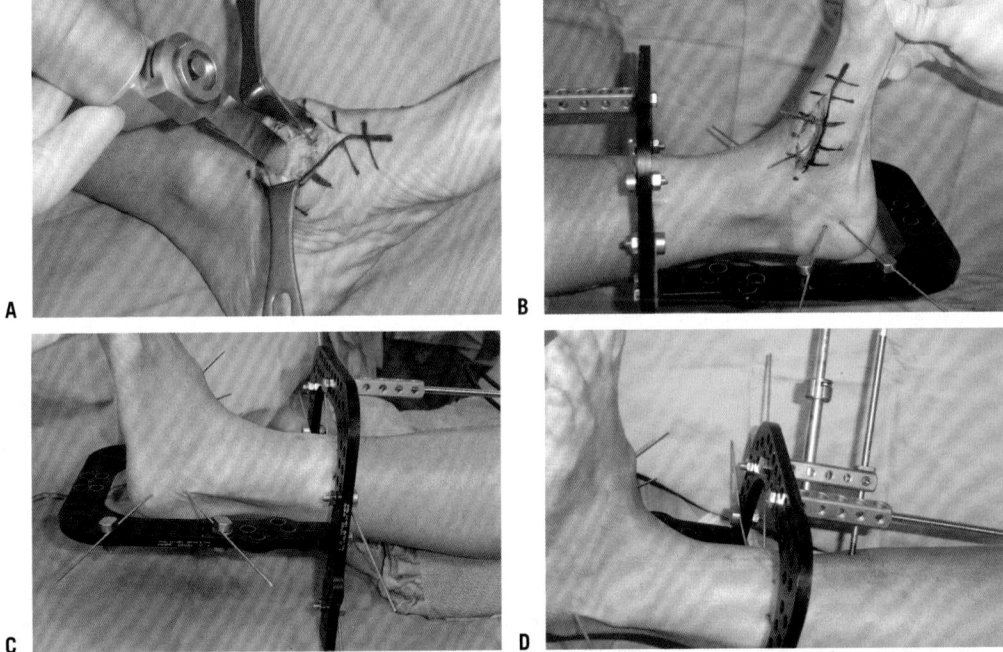

TECH FIG 19 A. Saw blade in position for proposed osteotomy. **B,C.** Butt frame applied before osteotomy, initially with thin wires. **B.** Medial view. **C.** Lateral view. Note U ring like a stirrup in coronal plane to stabilize hindfoot. Attached to this is second U ring to provide further support in tibia. **D.** Frame stabilized further with half-pins from proximal U ring into tibia. *(continued)*

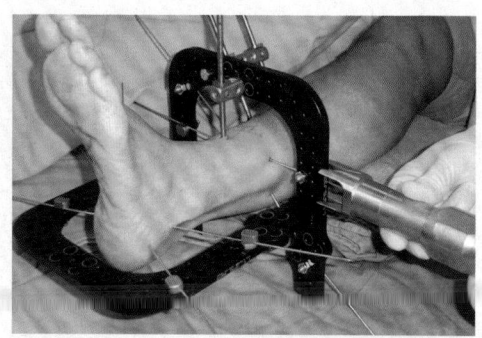

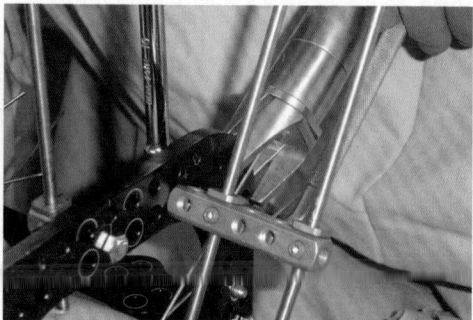

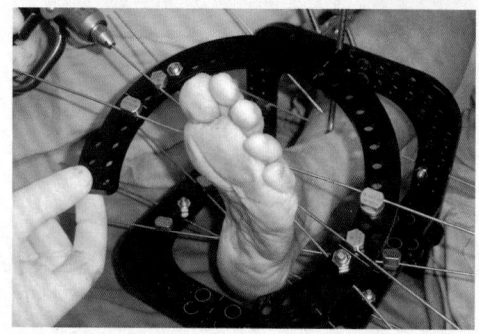

TECH FIG 19 *(continued)* **E,F.** Tensioning thin wires. **G.** Applying the forefoot ring, primarily with tensioned thin wires, but we routinely add one small-diameter half-pin to augment the ring's stability.

- For the forefoot component, a partial ring is added to the forefoot, which is first stabilized with three tensioned thin wires **(TECH FIG 19G)**.
  - We typically add a half-pin to the forefoot–midfoot after we have performed the osteotomy and then know exactly where the struts connecting the forefoot to the hindfoot rings will be positioned.

Midfoot Osteotomy

- We use an oscillating saw, but a Gigli saw may be used as well **(TECH FIG 20A)**.
- We create a biplanar wedge with a medial and plantar base to correct abduction and promote plantar flexion in order to recreate the arch.
- We complete the osteotomy with an osteotome **(TECH FIG 20B)**.
- Remove the wedge of bone **(TECH FIG 20C)**.
- The osteotomy can then be closed **(TECH FIG 20D,E)**.
  - If it should not close congruently, protect the soft tissues, place the saw in the osteotomy, close the osteotomy as much as possible, and run the saw gently to remove any irregularities. This trick tends to make the osteotomy appose well.

- Through this osteotomy, the forefoot may also be derotated.
  - We often "spin" the forefoot out of varus, a common forefoot deformity associated with a flatfoot.
- Place the struts to connect the hindfoot frame to the forefoot ring **(TECH FIG 20F–I)**.
- Add compression. With the system's computer program, further correction can be added now or even postoperatively.
- We routinely reduce the deformity as much as possible intraoperatively, always ensuring appropriate bony apposition at the arthrodesis site, and then compress further to promote stability and healing.

Postoperative Care

- Follow-up radiographs with frame in place are shown in **TECH FIG 21A–C**.
- Final follow-up after frame removal is shown in **TECH FIG 21D–H**.
- Often, after flatfoot correction for midfoot collapse, the first ray may appear short.
- As long as the first ray is adequately plantarflexed and dorsiflexion of the medial column is avoided, transfer metatarsalgia is rarely a problem.

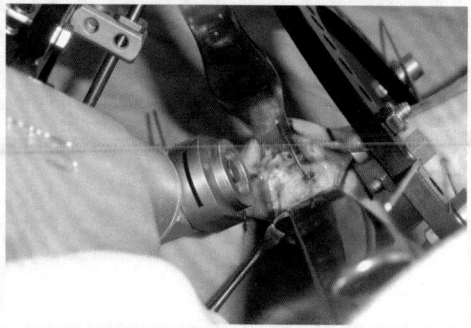

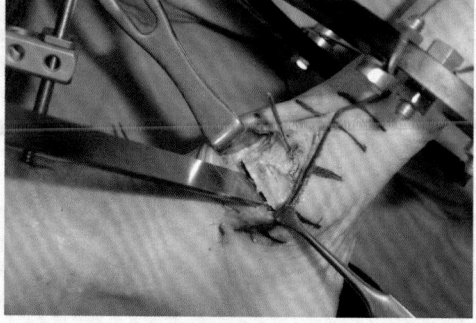

TECH FIG 20 A–C. Midfoot biplanar osteotomy at planned osteotomy site after application of external fixator (butt frame). **A.** Saw cut. **B.** Completion of osteotomy with an osteotome. *(continued)*

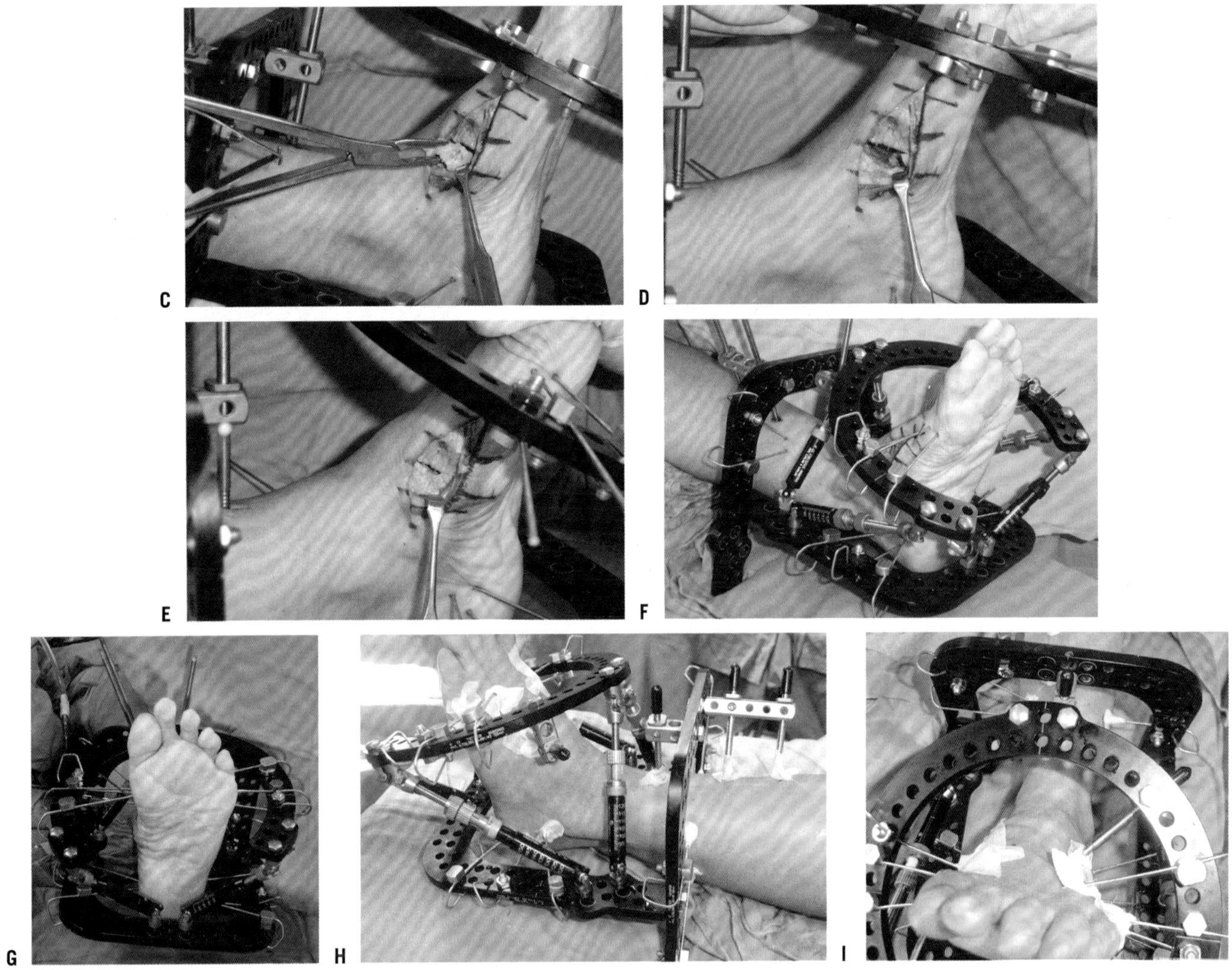

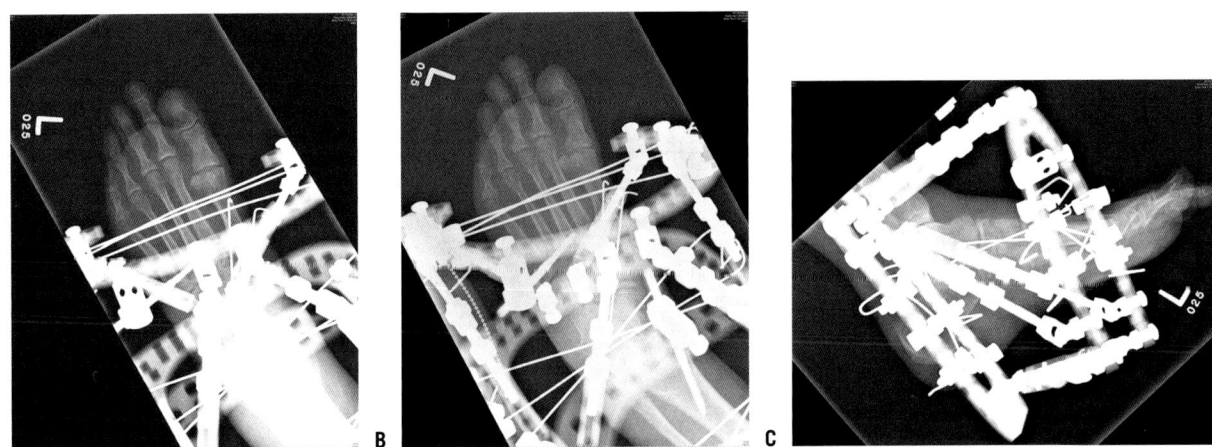

TECH FIG 20 *(continued)* **C.** Removal of bone wedge with a rongeur. **D,E.** Reducing the deformity. **D.** Osteotomy open. **E.** Osteotomy closed medially and plantarly. **F,G.** Frame in place, with struts attached and osteotomy compressed. **F.** Medial view. **G.** Plantar foot view, demonstrating recreation of the arch and correction of abduction deformity. **H,I.** Dressings placed on wires and pins. Note the half-pin added to dorsolateral forefoot. **H.** Lateral view. **I.** AP view.

TECH FIG 21 A–C. Postoperative radiographs. **A.** AP view. **B.** Oblique view. **C.** Lateral view. Note supplemental wires placed across osteotomy site for initial stabilization. With external fixation, further correction and compression may be performed after the index procedure. *(continued)*

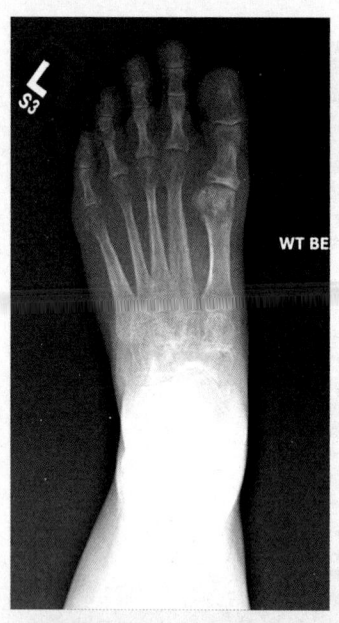
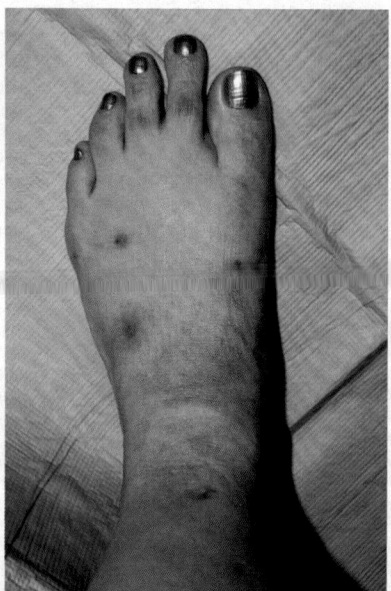
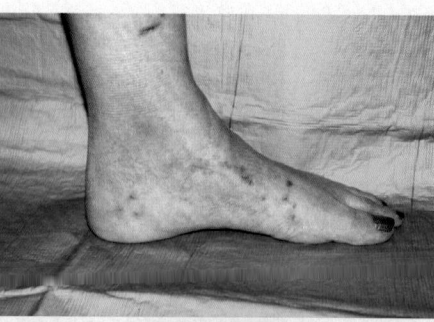
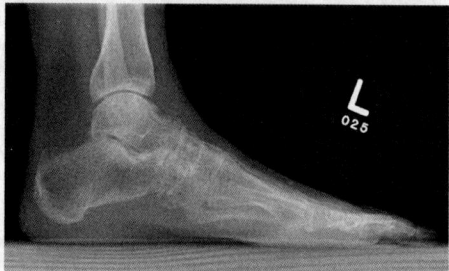
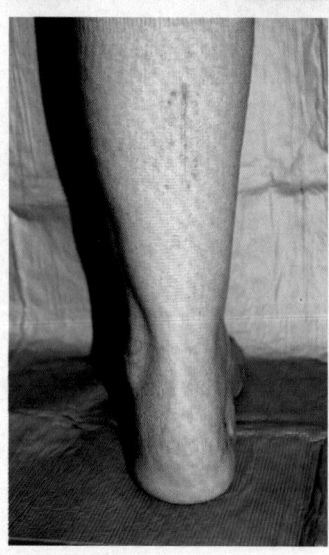

TECH FIG 21 *(continued)* **D,E.** Clinical and radiographic follow-up after external fixator removal. **D.** Weight-bearing AP radiograph. **E.** Clinical view. The first ray appears short, which is common after correction of abduction deformity with internal or external fixation. However, provided the first ray is adequately plantarflexed and bears weight, the foot functions well with little risk of transfer metatarsalgia despite a relatively long second metatarsal. **F–H.** Clinical and radiographic follow-up after external fixator removal. **F.** Lateral clinical view. **G.** Lateral weight-bearing radiograph (note restoration of arch). **H.** Hindfoot clinical view (note healed incision for gastrocnemius–soleus recession).

ADDITIONAL CASE

Background

- This 32-year-old man had undergone open reduction and internal fixation of a Lisfranc fracture-dislocation and subsequent hardware removal at an outside institution (**TECH FIG 22A–C**). He had failed further nonoperative measures.

- We performed a midfoot medial column plantar plating in combination with middle column dorsal plating after attempted deformity correction (**TECH FIG 22D–G**).
- Follow-up radiographs (**TECH FIG 22H–J**) show that although his longitudinal arch appears corrected, his forefoot still remains in abduction and he remains symptomatic.
- Further nonoperative care failed.

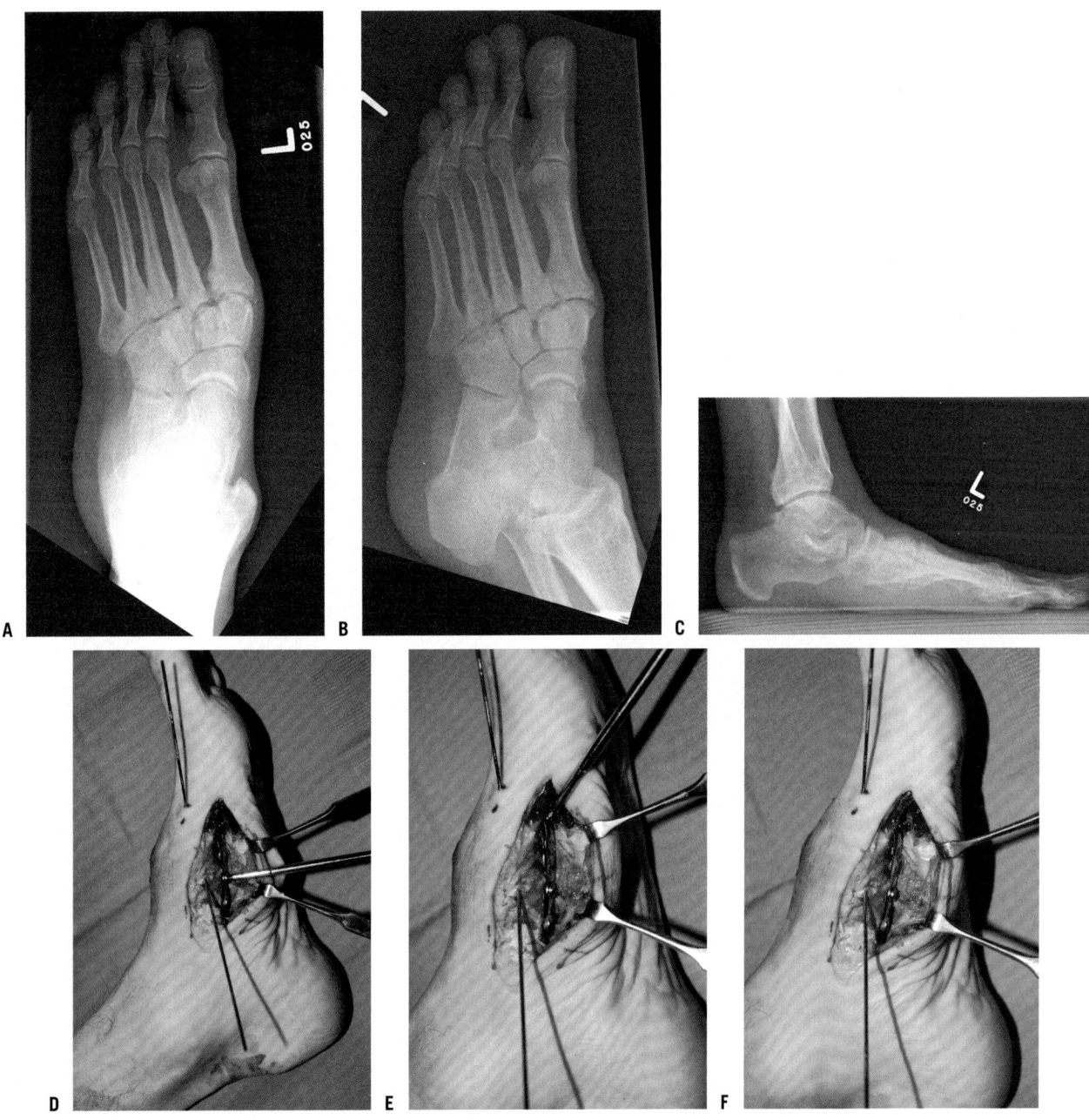

TECH FIG 22 Preoperative weight-bearing radiographs of a 32-year-old man with chronic Lisfranc fracture-dislocation that had undergone prior open reduction and internal fixation of the injury and subsequent hardware removal. **A.** AP view. **B.** Oblique view. **C.** Lateral view. Revision surgery with medial plantar plating and middle column plating was undertaken through dual longitudinal approaches after attempted reduction of severe abduction deformity and midfoot collapse. **D–F.** Screw fixation of medial column plantar plate. Note provisional wire fixation. *(continued)*

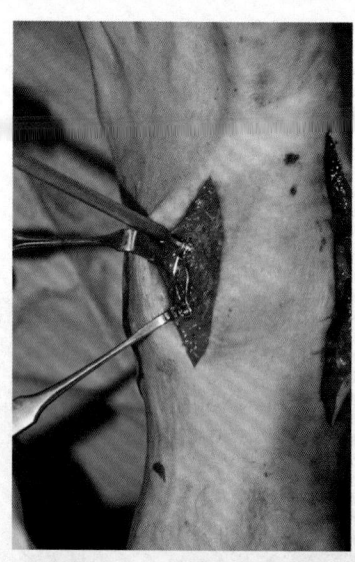

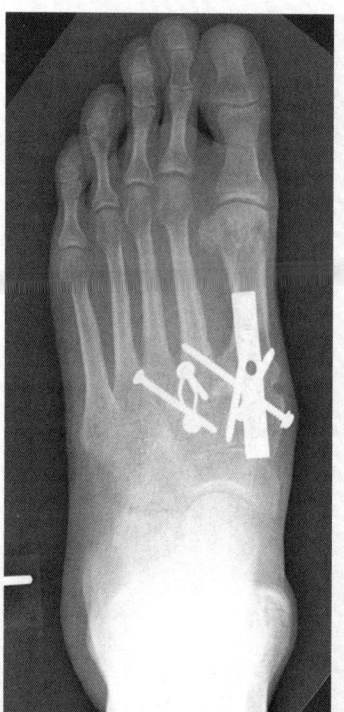

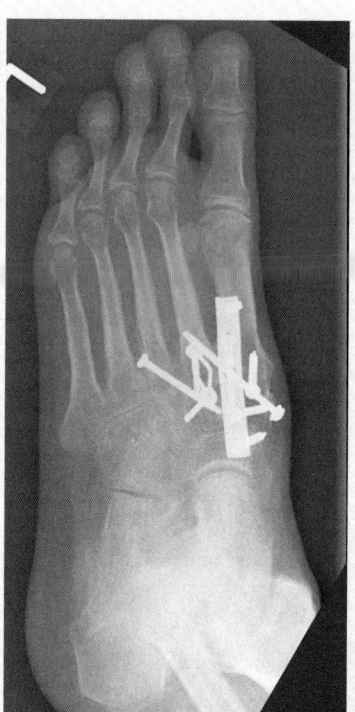

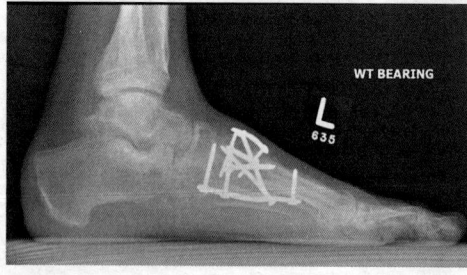

TECH FIG 22 *(continued)* **G.** Dorsal approach to middle column for compression plating. **H–J.** Follow-up weight-bearing radiographs. Although arch is restored, forefoot abduction is incompletely corrected. **H.** AP view. **I.** Oblique view. **J.** Lateral view. Patient was improved but remained symptomatic and failed orthotic management.

Revision Surgery

- Medial biplanar wedge osteotomy after hardware removal (**TECH FIG 23A–C**)
- Further correction of abduction deformity and more plantar flexion to the medial column
- We was able to reuse the plantar plate (**TECH FIG 23D,E**).
- We performed two adjunctive hindfoot procedures:
  - Medial displacement calcaneal osteotomy (**TECH FIG 23F**)
  - Subtalar arthroereisis (**TECH FIG 23G**)

Postoperative Care

- Follow-up weight-bearing radiographs suggest improved alignment, particularly with respect to the talo–first metatarsal axis in the AP plane (**TECH FIG 24A,B**).
- Clinically, alignment and function were improved. In fact, he had perhaps better alignment in his operated foot than his contralateral foot (remains to be seen if this is advantageous but anecdotally appears to be the case) (**TECH FIG 24C–E**).

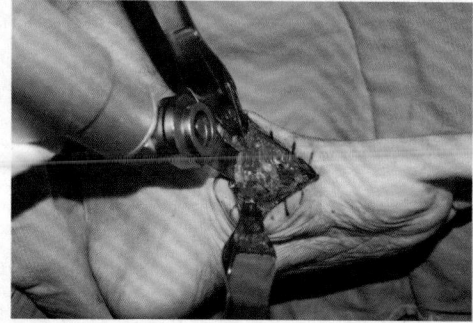

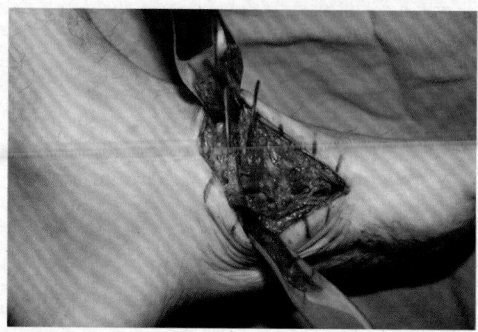

TECH FIG 23 A–C. Re-revision surgery with removal of plantar plate and medial approach biplanar midfoot osteotomy to correct residual abduction deformity and promote even further plantar flexion of the medial column. **A.** Saw to create biplanar osteotomy along reference pins marking proposed osteotomy. **B.** Wedge resected. *(continued)*

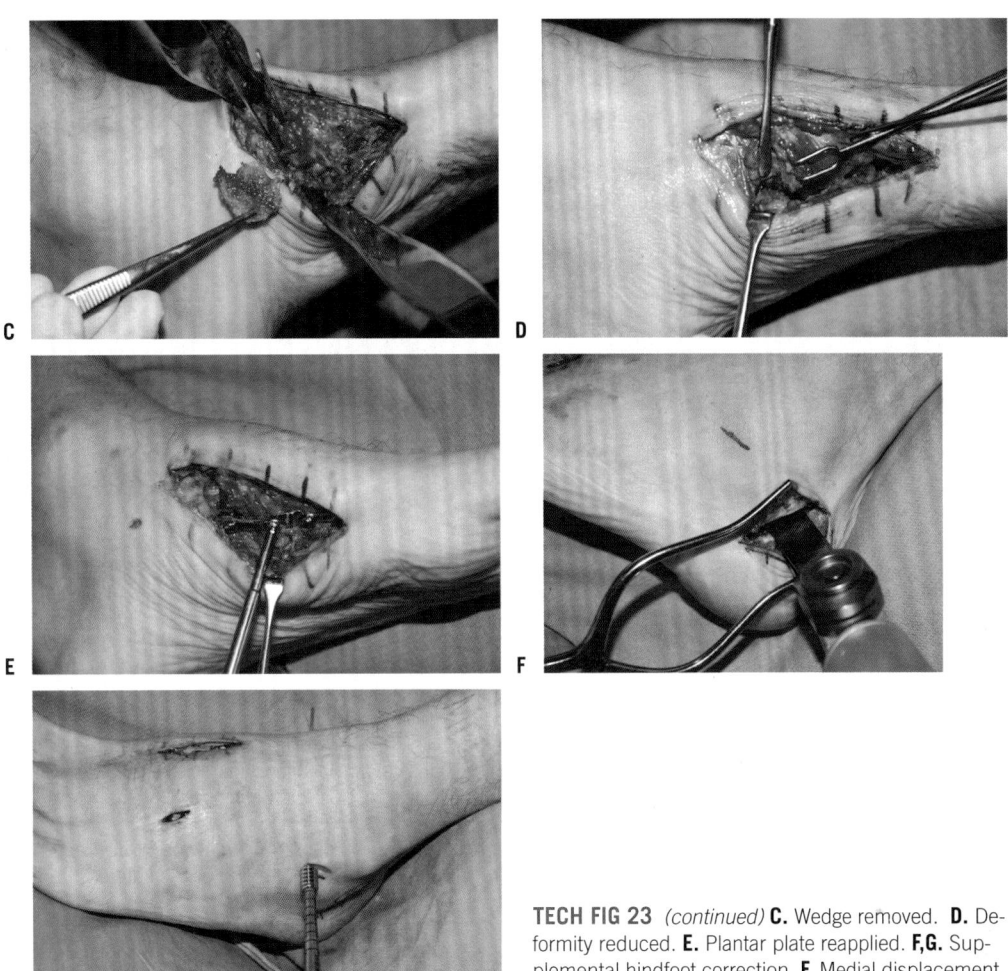

TECH FIG 23 *(continued)* **C.** Wedge removed. **D.** Deformity reduced. **E.** Plantar plate reapplied. **F,G.** Supplemental hindfoot correction. **F.** Medial displacement calcaneal osteotomy. **G.** Subtalar arthroereisis.

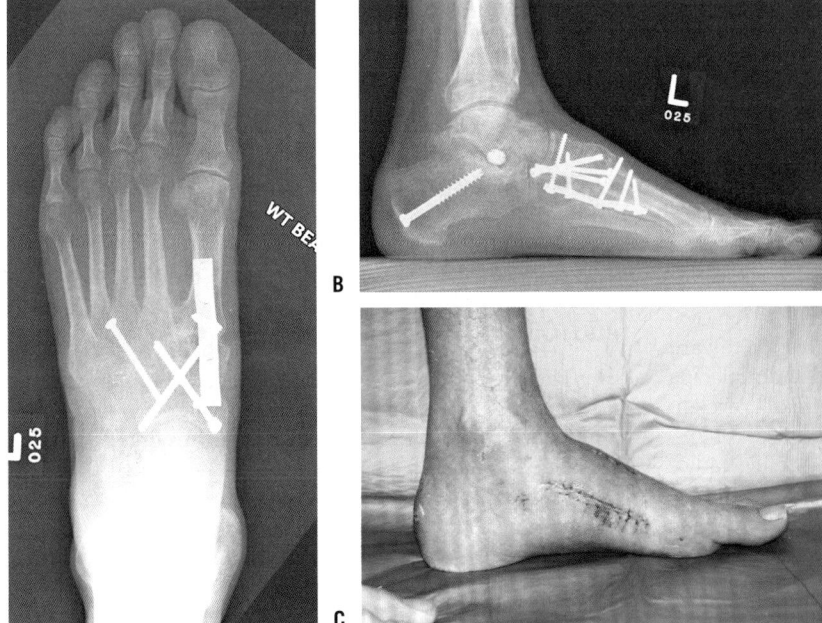

TECH FIG 24 A,B. Follow-up weight-bearing radiographs. **A.** AP view (note correction of abduction) and near-anatomic restoration of congruent talo–first metatarsal axis. **B.** Lateral view, also with restoration of talo–first metatarsal axis. **C–E.** Clinical follow-up. **C.** Lateral view. *(continued)*

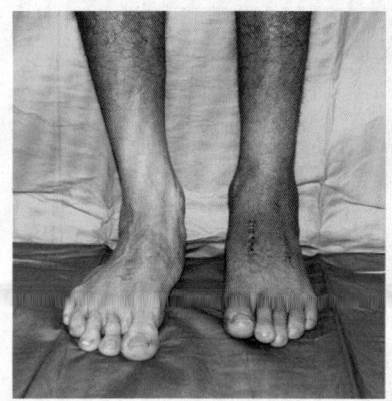
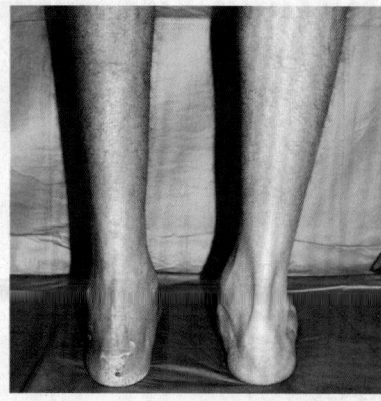

TECH FIG 24 *(continued)* **D.** AP view. **E.** Hindfoot view. Operated foot is in a more physiologically normal position than contralateral foot.

TECHNIQUES

Pearls and Pitfalls

Deformity Correction	• Realign talo–first metatarsal axis in both the AP and lateral planes; undercorrection rarely leads to satisfactory outcome.
TMT Joint Anatomy	• The TMT joints are quite deep (2.5–3.0 cm).
Avoid dorsiflexion or elevated malpositioning.	• Be sure to prepare the TMT joints to their bases; leaving plantar bone and cartilage will lead to a dorsiflexion malunion. Also, do not take any dorsal bone from the TMT joints.
Correct Abduction	• The physiologically normal medial aspect of the medial column of the foot is relatively straight; with severe midfoot deformity, the first metatarsal must really be swung around to align anatomically; then, the lesser metatarsals should follow.
Forefoot Balance	• When arthrodesing the TMT joints, be sure to check the relative position of the metatarsal heads. The first metatarsal head and sesamoids should be slightly plantar to the lesser metatarsal heads. Palpate this balance as the midfoot is provisionally stabilized.
Tricks to Correcting Abduction	• In severe deformity, avoid first metatarsal elevation and attempt to reduce the abduction deformity. Fix the plate to the medial aspect of the first cuneiform and then reduce the first metatarsal to the plate. • As for a reduction of a Lisfranc fracture-dislocation, use a large bone reduction clamp to reduce the base of the second metatarsal by spanning the course of the first cuneiform–second metatarsal base.

POSTOPERATIVE CARE

- A splint is used that extends beyond the toes with the ankle in neutral position for 2 weeks.
- The patient returns to clinic at 2 weeks for suture removal and application of a short-leg cast. Feather weight bearing is permitted.
- The patient returns to clinic at 6 weeks for cast removal and imaging (three views of the foot). If progression toward healing is suggested, the surgeon should consider placing the patient in a CAM boot. Once again, only feather weight bearing is permitted.
- At 10 weeks, the patient returns for weight-bearing radiographs (three views of the foot).
  - If there is radiographic evidence of progressive healing, the patient is encouraged to gradually progress from feather to full weight bearing in the CAM boot over the ensuing 3 weeks. Once this is achieved, the patient can transition

into wearing regular shoes. We often recommend a longitudinal arch support and a relatively stiff-soled shoe.
- If no progression toward healing is seen, the patient is returned to the CAM boot, with limited weight bearing, and the boot is used for an additional 3 to 4 weeks, at which time new imaging is done and patient is reassessed.

OUTCOMES

- There are limited level IV studies for midfoot arthrodesis, but there are reasonable functional outcomes and improvement in pain scores for midfoot arthrodesis based on the weak literature.
- Results are generally better when restoration of physiologically normal alignment is achieved.
- There are virtually no reported outcomes for modern dedicated midfoot plating systems.
- More information and higher level evidence are needed.

COMPLICATIONS

- Undercorrection
- Overcorrection
- Surgical site infection
- Wound dehiscence
- Nonunion
- Malunion
  - Greater than physiologic elevation of one or more metatarsals
  - Imbalance of the metatarsal heads

SUGGESTED READINGS

Coetzee JC, Ly TV. Treatment of primarily ligamentous Lisfranc joint injuries: primary arthrodesis compared with open reduction and internal fixation. Surgical technique. J Bone Joint Surg Am 2007;89(suppl 2, pt 1): 122–127.

Ferris LR, Vargo R, Alexander IJ. Late reconstruction of the midfoot and tarsometatarsal region after trauma. Orthop Clin North Am 1995;26: 393–406.

Greisberg J, Assal M, Hansen ST Jr, et al. Isolated medial column stabilization improves alignment in adult-acquired flatfoot. Clin Orthop Relat Res 2005;(435):197–202.

Horton GA, Olney BW. Deformity correction and arthrodesis of the midfoot with a medial plate. Foot Ankle 1993;14:493–499.

Jung HG, Myerson MS, Schon LC. Spectrum of operative treatments and clinical outcomes for atraumatic osteoarthritis of the tarsometatarsal joints. Foot Ankle Int 2007;28:482–489.

Komenda GA, Myerson MS, Biddinger KR. Results of arthrodesis of the tarsometatarsal joints after traumatic injury. J Bone Joint Surg Am 1996; 78(11):1665–1676.

Raikin SM, Schon LC. Arthrodesis of the fourth and fifth tarsometatarsal joints of the midfoot. Foot Ankle Int 2003;24:584–590.

Rammelt S, Schneiders W, Schikore H, et al. Primary open reduction and fixation compared with delayed corrective arthrodesis in the treatment of tarsometatarsal (Lisfranc) fracture dislocation. J Bone Joint Surg Br 2008;90(11):1499–1506.

Sammarco VJ, Sammarco GJ, Walker EW Jr, et al. Midtarsal arthrodesis in the treatment of Charcot midfoot arthropathy. J Bone Joint Surg Am 2009;91(1):80–91.

Sammarco VJ, Sammarco GJ, Walker EW Jr, et al. Midtarsal arthrodesis in the treatment of Charcot midfoot arthropathy. Surgical technique. J Bone Joint Surg Am 2010;92(suppl 1, pt 1):1–19.

Suh JS, Amendola A, Lee KB, et al. Dorsal modified calcaneal plate for extensive midfoot arthrodesis. Foot Ankle Int 2005;26:503–509.

Toolan BC. Midfoot arthrodesis: challenges and treatment alternatives. Foot Ankle Clin 2002;7:75–93.

Vertullo CJ, Easley ME, Nunley JA. The transverse dorsal approach to the Lisfranc joint. Foot Ankle Int 2002;23:420–426.

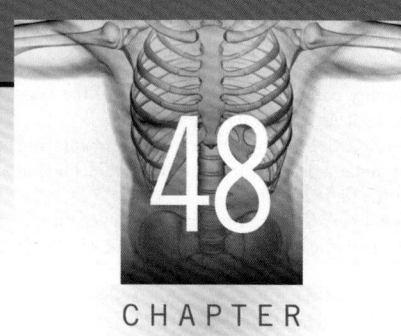

48
CHAPTER

Percutaneous Lesser Toe Correction

Jonathan Day, Amanda N. Fletcher, A. Holly Johnson, and Oliver N. Schipper

DEFINITION

- Percutaneous correction of lesser toe deformities includes a variety of soft tissue procedures and osteotomies that offer an attractive alternative to traditional open approach procedures with quicker recovery while reducing the risk for scar tissue and wound complications.
- Extensor digitorum longus (EDL) tendon Z-lengthening and extensor digitorum brevis (EDB) tenotomy are used to address dorsiflexion deformities of the metatarsophalangeal (MTP) joint.
- Flexor digitorum longus (FDL) and flexor digitorum brevis (FDB) tenotomies are used to correct plantarflexion deformities of the distal and proximal interphalangeal (IP) joints, respectively.
- Extra-articular proximal phalanx osteotomies are used to correct varus, valgus, or dorsiflexion deformities of the MTP joint.

ANATOMY

- The lesser toes consist of a distal, middle, and proximal phalanx.
- Each toe has two flexor tendons and two extensor tendons:
  - The FDL inserts onto the plantar aspect of the base of the distal phalanx, whereas the FDB travels plantar to the FDL and splits to insert onto the middle phalanx. The FDL and FDB flex the distal and proximal IP joints, respectively.
  - The EDL travels dorsally and is joined by the EDB at the level of the MTP joint before trifurcating into a central

tendon that inserts onto the middle phalanx and medial/lateral tendons that insert onto the base of the distal phalanx.

PATHOGENESIS

- Lesser toe deformities are categorized based off the relative alignment of the MTP and IP joints. Deformities tend to be flexible in early stages and may progress to rigidity over time.
- A hammertoe describes a deformity in which the proximal IP joint is plantarflexed and the distal IP joint is extended (FIG 1A). Concurrent hallux valgus and trauma are commonly cited causes of this deformity.[5]
- A mallet toe describes a deformity in which there is isolated plantarflexion deformity of the distal IP joint. It is caused by tightening of the FDL or injury to the EDL insertion.
- A claw toe describes a deformity in which the MTP joint is hyperextended and both the proximal and distal IP joints are plantarflexed. It is caused by unopposed extension at the MTP with tightening of the FDL and FDB at the distal and proximal IP joints.[2]
- A crossover toe describes deviation of the toe in the axial plane with hyperextension of the MTP joint (FIG 1B). It commonly occurs in the second toe with medial deviation and is caused by a progressive tearing and attenuation of the plantar plate with weakening of the collaterals.[4]
- Concurrent hallux valgus is often associated with lesser toe deformities and may be due to altered dynamics of the plantar fascia causing failure of the collaterals and supporting structures of the lesser toes.[9]

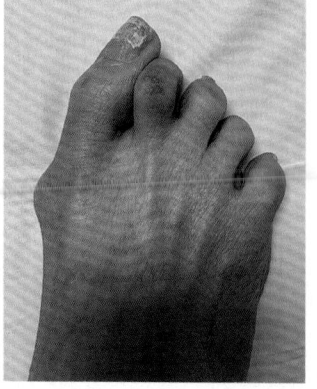

A   **B**

FIG 1 A. Hammertoe deformity. **B.** Crossover toe deformity.

NATURAL HISTORY

- Lesser toe deformity is common and affects up to 60% of the older adult population.[6]
- Generally, lesser toe pathology is considered progressive with multifactorial etiology. Commonly cited risk factors include genetics, ill-fitting (ie, high-heeled, tight) footwear, pes planus and cavus deformity, and concurrent hallux valgus deformity.[2,3,10]

PATIENT HISTORY AND PHYSICAL FINDINGS

- Pertinent details to elicit when gathering patient history include history of trauma, diabetes, inflammatory arthritis, neuromuscular disorders, previous surgeries, family history, and footwear.
- Physical examination should include evaluation of the resting position and standing posture of the toes. An assessment should be performed to rule out hallux valgus deformity and plantar plate pain and swelling. The IP joints should be examined with the MTP joint in neutral. A Lachman test (dorsal plantar drawer) should be performed to rule out MTP joint instability.[9]
- In addition to the characteristic findings in alignment of the IP and MTP joints, additional physical exam findings may further define the type of lesser toe deformity. For example, due to the flexion deformity of the distal IP joint, patients with mallet toe may have calluses at the distal aspect of the toe.[12]

IMAGING AND OTHER DIAGNOSTIC STUDIES

- Radiographic assessments with weight-bearing plain anteroposterior (AP), oblique, and lateral views are the gold standard.
- Magnetic resonance imaging can be used to rule out a suspected plantar plate tear.

DIFFERENTIAL DIAGNOSIS

- Autoimmune disorders
- Metatarsalgia
- Gout

NONOPERATIVE MANAGEMENT

- In general, conservative management includes a trial of footwear modification (ie, switching to shoes with a wider/taller toe box), gel toe sleeves, and Budin splint.

SURGICAL MANAGEMENT

Preoperative Planning

- Standard weight-bearing radiographs of the AP, lateral, and oblique views should be reviewed prior to surgery to assess severity of the lesser toe deformity. Oftentimes, multiple concurrent deformities and/or multiple toes are involved, and therefore, careful assessment should be made.
- Bone quality should be considered prior to surgery as well as the presence of any prior hardware in or around the joint.
- If an osteotomy is planned, the power box for the burr should be capable of delivering high torque at a low speed (four-in-one reducer) in order to efficiently cut through bone while minimizing heat production and soft tissue injury.

Positioning

- Place the patient supine on the operating table with the operative foot extending off the bed distally to allow accessibility for AP and lateral fluoroscopy of the forefoot.
- Elevate the operative leg using blankets or a bump. Secure the nonoperative leg away from the operative field in the frog-leg position to allow easier access to the operative foot.
- Position the mini C-arm adjacent to the patient, ipsilateral to the surgeon's dominant hand.
- A tourniquet is not recommended as this can increase risk for thermal injury to the soft tissue and bone necrosis.

Approach

- The approach varies by tenotomy and osteotomy procedure.
- For a tenotomy or Z-lengthening of the extensor tendons, approach should be made dorsally where the tendons are anatomically separated at the level of the MTP joint.
- For a tenotomy of the flexor tendons, approach should be made medially or laterally at the level of the proximal IP joint (FDB) or plantarly at the level of the distal IP joint (FDL).
- For extra-articular proximal phalanx osteotomies, approach should be made at the proximal metadiaphyseal region of the proximal phalanx.
- A 2- × 8-mm Shannon burr is used to perform all lesser toe osteotomies. The senior author (O.S.) recommends 4000 rpm for lesser toe osteotomies.

EXTENSOR DIGITORUM LONGUS Z-LENGTHENING AND EXTENSOR DIGITORUM BREVIS TENOTOMY

- Used for hyperdorsiflexion deformities of the MTP joint
- Perform the EDL Z-lengthening and EDB tenotomy through a dorsal incision at the MTP joint, where the two tendons are separated.
- Assess for correction of hyperdorsiflexion of the MTP joint.

- If extensor lengthening/tenotomy are insufficient or if there is residual dorsal subluxation/dislocation of the MTP joint, a dorsal MTP joint capsule release may be performed. Use traction to distract the joint and release the dorsal capsule using a no. 15 blade or beaver blade.

FLEXOR DIGITORUM LONGUS AND FLEXOR DIGITORUM BREVIS TENOTOMIES

- Used to correct hyperplantarflexion deformities of the proximal and distal IP joints
- Perform the FDL tenotomy using the beaver blade through a plantar approach with simultaneous dorsiflexion of the distal IP joint.

- Perform the FDB tenotomy using the beaver blade through either a medial or lateral approach just proximal to the proximal IP joint with simultaneous plantarflexion to avoid injuring the plantar nerve. Release the proximal IP joint capsule and then release the two FDB insertions at the base of the middle phalanx.

EXTRA-ARTICULAR PROXIMAL PHALANX OSTEOTOMY

- Both methods described here are performed at the level of the metadiaphysis of the proximal phalanx.

Plantar Closing Wedge Osteotomy

- Used to correct hyperdorsiflexion deformity of the MTP joint
- A 3-mm longitudinal incision is made midaxially over the medial or lateral proximal metadiaphyseal region of the proximal phalanx using a no. 15 blade.
  - Preference for a medial or lateral approach depends on surgeon's hand dominance.
  - A plantar approach may also be employed, but disadvantages include having to avoid the flexor tendons and inability to use AP fluoroscopic guidance.
- Under AP fluoroscopic guidance, the 2- × 8-mm Shannon burr (4000 rpm) is inserted slightly more dorsal than plantar bicortically at the proximal metadiaphysis of the proximal phalanx.
- Complete the osteotomy plantarly by rotating the hand plantarly, leaving the dorsal cortex intact **(TECH FIG 1)**.
- Plantarflex the osteotomy. If unsuccessful, continue to carefully feather the remaining dorsal cortex using the 2- × 8-mm

Shannon burr until plantarflexion of the osteotomy can be achieved.
- No fixation is used for the osteotomy. A soft dressing followed by a toe splint and/or taping are used to maintain lesser toe deformity correction.

Akinette Osteotomy

- Used to correct varus or valgus deformities of the MTP joint
- Under AP fluoroscopic guidance, insert a 2- × 8-mm Shannon burr dorsally at the level of the proximal metadiaphysis of the proximal phalanx.
- To correct a valgus deformity, complete the osteotomy medially while leaving the lateral cortex intact **(TECH FIG 2)**. To correct a varus deformity, complete the osteotomy laterally while leaving the medial cortex intact.
- If closure of the osteotomy is initially unsuccessful, continue to feather the remaining cortex using the 2- × 8-mm Shannon burr until closure is successful.
- No fixation is used for the osteotomy. A soft dressing followed by a toe splint and/or taping are used to maintain lesser toe deformity correction.

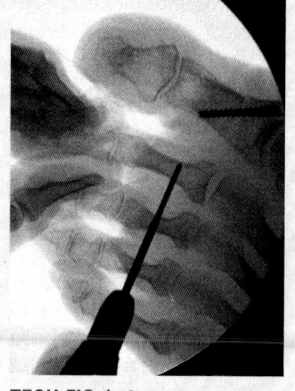 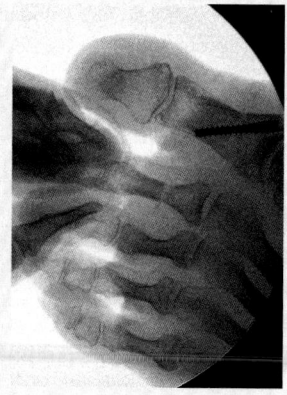

A **B**

TECH FIG 1 A. Intraoperative fluoroscopy demonstrating lateral approach of the burr at the metadiaphysis of the proximal phalanx. **B.** Completion of the osteotomy plantarly, leaving the dorsal cortex intact.

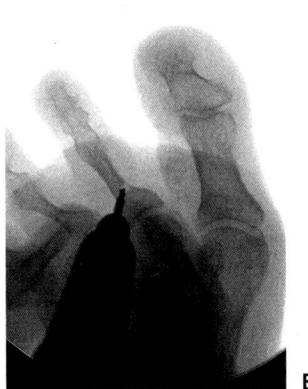 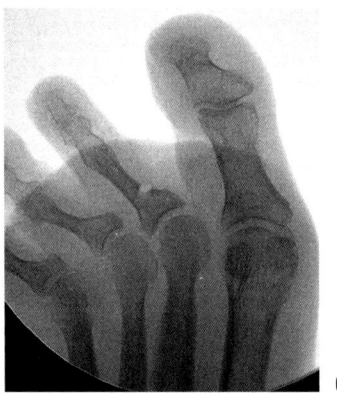 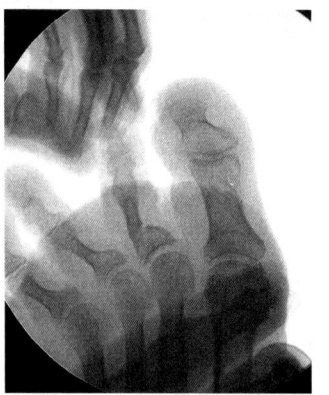

TECH FIG 2 **A.** Intraoperative fluoroscopy demonstrating medial starting location of the burr for an Akinette osteotomy in the correction of second toe valgus deformity. **B.** Completion of the medial-based osteotomy with the lateral cortex intact. **C.** Closure of the medial osteotomy to correct a valgus deformity of the second toe.

PROXIMAL PHALANX OSTEOTOMY FOR MEDIAL CROSSOVER TOE DEFORMITY

- A stab incision with blunt dissection down to bone is made just proximal to the proximal IP joint, at the medial edge of the distal aspect of the proximal phalanx.
- The 2- × 8-mm Shannon burr is then used to make an oblique osteotomy across the phalanx, aiming to exit proximal laterally toward the base of the phalanx. Complete the osteotomy plantarly and dorsally using a sweeping motion with the distal medial fulcrum maintained **(TECH FIG 3)**.

- When the osteotomy is complete, the phalanx will close down, shortening the toe and moving the toe to a neutral position.
- Any overhanging or sharp edges from the osteotomy should be smoothed down using the burr.
- The wound and osteotomy site are copiously irrigated using an angiocatheter, and the incision should be closed with a small suture or Steri-Strip.

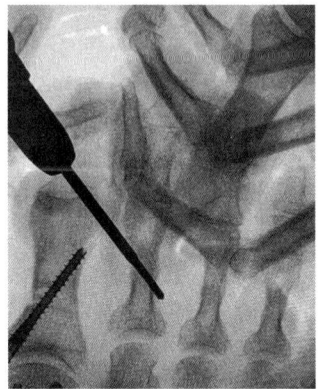 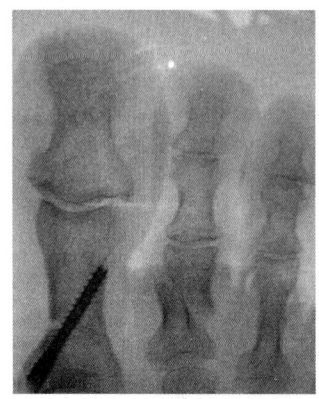

TECH FIG 3 Intraoperative photographs of the proximal phalanx osteotomy for medial crossover toe deformity correction. **A.** The Shannon burr is used to create the oblique osteotomy across the phalanx, aiming toward the base of the phalanx. **B.** Closing of the phalanx shortens the toe by moving it to a neutral position.

Pearls and Pitfalls

Indications	• Percutaneous correction is indicated in a wide spectrum of lesser toe pathologies, including flexible or rigid deformity, IP joint instability, and arthritis.
Contraindications	• Infection, avascular necrosis, poor bone stock
Tourniquet Use	• A tourniquet is not required and may even increase the chance of thermal injury and bone necrosis. Placing the patient in the Trendelenburg position may reduce bleeding.
Preventing Thermal Skin Injury	• We recommend copious irrigation whenever using the burr, inserting wires, or overdrilling guidewires to minimize risk of thermal injury to the skin or bone necrosis.
Pinning	• If close patient follow-up is not possible, temporary pinning across the osteotomy sites to hold the toe in position may be desirable **(FIG 2)**.

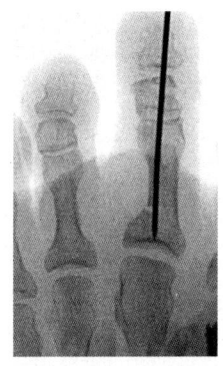 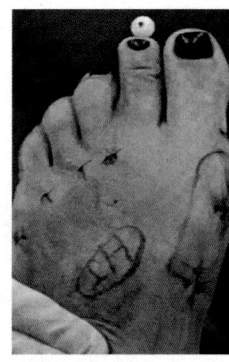

A   B

FIG 2 A. Intraoperative photograph showing pin fixation across the osteotomy site. **B.** Postoperative clinical photograph showing temporary pin fixation to hold the desired toe position.

POSTOPERATIVE CARE

- It is important to strap the toes in the desired position postoperatively to prevent recurrence of deformity for 5 weeks **(FIG 3)**. The surgical dressing is generally left in place for the first 2 weeks, at which time the patient is transitioned to a removable toe splint or instructed on taping of the toe for another 3 weeks.
- Immediate weight bearing in a rigid postoperative shoe is allowed as tolerated for the first 5 weeks, followed by transition into a supportive shoe.

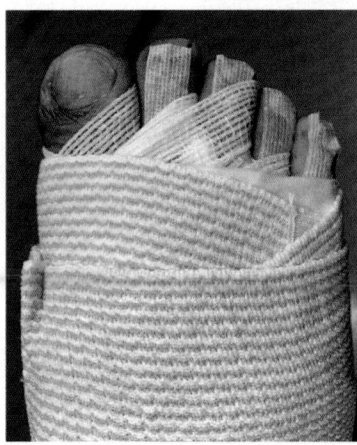

FIG 3 Postoperative strapping and dressing to keep the toes in the desired position for proper healing.

- Physical therapy can be initiated at 4 to 5 weeks postoperatively, or the patient may be instructed on MTP capsular stretching exercises to prevent recurrence of deformity.

OUTCOMES

- **FIG 4** shows outcomes in two patients.
- In a retrospective study of 675 hammertoes that underwent either open correction with resection arthroplasty and Kirschner wire fixation (n = 454) or percutaneous correction with 3M Coban dressings (3M, St. Paul, MN) (n = 221), the authors noted that at an average of 6 months postoperatively, patients who underwent percutaneous correction had a significantly lower incidence of infection (2.2% vs. 5.3%) and significantly greater improvement in postoperative pain. However, there was no significant difference in rates of malalignment or patient satisfaction observed.[13]
- In a study of 54 patients (57 feet) who underwent percutaneous proximal phalanx osteotomy with or without associated extensor tendon tenotomy (n = 24) for correction of flexible or rigid proximal phalanx deformity of the second toe, results demonstrated an overall patient satisfaction rate of 89.5%, which included cosmetic (98%) and pain relief satisfaction (81%). The mean follow-up was 30.7 months. Complication rate was 5.2%, with two cases of revision arthrodesis (3.5%) due to anatomic failure.[8] The results of this study are similar to those in the literature for traditional open approaches, which cite a satisfaction rate ranging from 80% to 90%.[1,7,11]

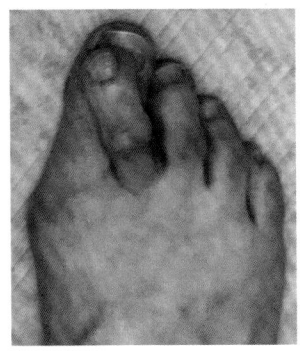 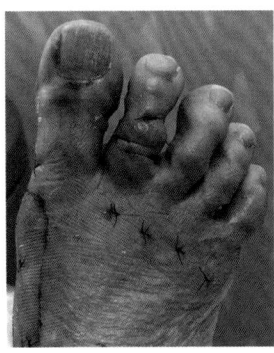 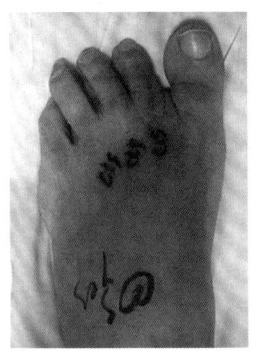 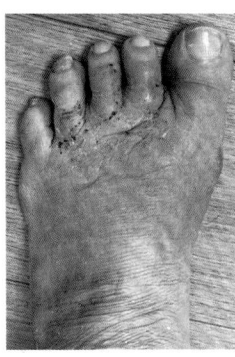

FIG 4 A. Preoperative clinical photograph of a crossover toe deformity. **B.** Postoperative photograph showing restoration of neutral alignment following proximal phalanx osteotomy. **C.** Preoperative clinical photograph of a different patient demonstrating valgus deformity of the second through fourth toes. **D.** Two weeks postoperative photograph demonstrating good correction of valgus deformity. The percutaneous incisions are healing well.

COMPLICATIONS

- Infection
- Nonunion
- Malunion
- Skin thermal burn

REFERENCES

1. Boyer ML, DeOrio JK. Transfer of the flexor digitorum longus for the correction of lesser-toe deformities. Foot Ankle Int 2007;28(4):422–430.
2. Coughlin MJ. Lesser-toe abnormalities. J Bone Joint Surg Am 2002;84(8):1446–1469.
3. Coughlin MJ. Mallet toes, hammer toes, claw toes, and corns. Causes and treatment of lesser-toe deformities. Postgrad Med 1984;75(5):191–198.
4. Coughlin MJ. Subluxation and dislocation of the second metatarsophalangeal joint. Orthop Clin North Am 1989;20(4):535–551.
5. Coughlin MJ. Lesser toe deformities. In: Coughlin MJSC, Anderson RB, eds. Mann's surgery of the foot and ankle. Ninth ed Elsevier; 2014:322–424.
6. Dunn JE, Link CL, Felson DT, et al. Prevalence of foot and ankle conditions in a multiethnic community sample of older adults. Am J Epidemiol 2004;159(5):491–498.
7. Errichiello C, Marcarelli M, Pisani PC, et al. Treatment of dynamic claw toe deformity flexor digitorum brevis tendon transfer to interosseous and lumbrical muscles: a literature survey. Foot Ankle Surg 2012;18(4):229–232.
8. Frey S, Hélix-Giordanino M, Piclet-Legré B. Percutaneous correction of second toe proximal deformity: proximal interphalangeal release, flexor digitorum brevis tenotomy and proximal phalanx osteotomy. Orthop Traumatol Surg Res 2015;101(6):753–758.
9. Malhotra K, Davda K, Singh D. The pathology and management of lesser toe deformities. EFORT Open Rev 2017;1(11):409–419.
10. Menz HB, Morris ME. Footwear characteristics and foot problems in older people. Gerontology 2005;51(5):346–351.
11. O'Kane C, Kilmartin T. Review of proximal interphalangeal joint excisional arthroplasty for the correction of second hammer toe deformity in 100 cases. Foot Ankle Int 2005;26(4):320–325.
12. Shirzad K, Kiesau CD, DeOrio JK, et al. Lesser toe deformities. J Am Acad Orthop Surg 2011;19(8):505–514.
13. Yassin M, Garti A, Heller E, et al. Hammertoe correction with K-wire fixation compared with percutaneous correction. Foot Ankle Spec 2017;10(5):421–427.

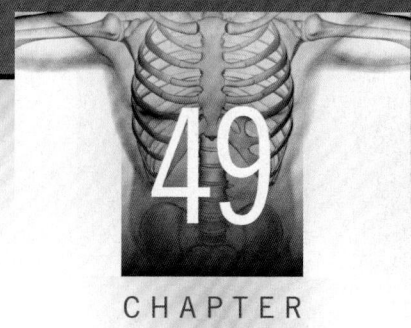

49

Surgical Stabilization of Nonplantigrade Charcot Arthropathy of the Midfoot

Michael S. Pinzur

DEFINITION

- Charcot foot arthropathy is an inflammatory disease process that primarily affects the foot and ankle of patients with long-standing diabetes (10-plus years) and diabetic peripheral neuropathy (PN).[3,4,7,24]
- The destructive inflammatory process often leads to bone destruction and joint subluxation or dislocation. The hallmark clinical deformity is known as a *rocker bottom deformity*.
- The resulting disabling deformity impairs walking, can be painful, and makes patients prone to develop overlying pressure-induced wounds, which lead to deep infection and the eventual need for lower extremity amputation.[26]
- Treatment has historically involved immobilization in a total contact non–weight-bearing cast during the acute destructive phase, followed by longitudinal management with accommodative shoes, foot orthoses, and ankle–foot orthoses.[13]
- Even when this treatment is successful, the negative impact on health-related quality of life has been demonstrated to be similar to lower extremity amputation.[6,17]
- This observation has led most experts to currently recommend surgical correction of the acquired deformity to avoid skin breakdown and deep infection, allow use of commercially available therapeutic footwear, avoid amputation, and maintain walking independence.[15,24,25]
- This chapter presents an evidence-based algorithm for use in the management of Charcot foot arthropathy at the level of the midfoot.

ANATOMY

- The foot is a unique terminal end organ adapted for weight bearing.
- The multiple-linked small bones of the normal foot allow prepositioning of the durable plantar soft tissue envelope to accept the loading forces associated with weight acceptance and then become a stable launching platform for push off.
- The bone and joint destructive associated with Charcot foot arthropathy impairs the capacity to orient the foot in the optimal position to perform these tasks.
- The ensuing deformity induces weight bearing through less durable tissues, leading to soft tissue failure, ulceration overlying bony prominences, destructive osteomyelitis, and ending with systemic sepsis or need for lower extremity amputation.

PATHOGENESIS

- The key clinical risk factor associated with the development of Charcot foot arthropathy is long-standing diabetic PN as

measured by insensitivity to 10 g of applied pressure with the Semmes-Weinstein 5.07 monofilament (**FIG 1**).
- Peripheral neuropathy associated with alcohol abuse has been suggested as an initiator of the destructive disease process; however, many of these patients are eventually confirmed to be diabetic. Patients with PN secondary to chemotherapy or other drugs are unlikely to develop Charcot foot arthropathy.
- The true pathophysiology of Charcot foot arthropathy is likely a combination of both neurotraumatic and neurovascular theories. The inciting trauma can be a single event, that is, fracture or dislocation or repetitive microtrauma combined with the neuropathy-induced motor imbalance that creates an

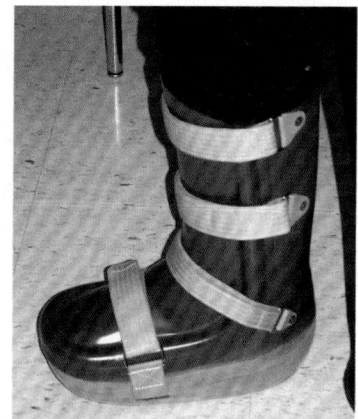
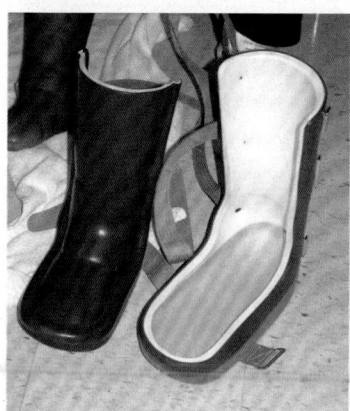

FIG 1 A,B. The Semmes-Weinstein 5.07 monofilament applies 10 g of pressure. The inability to "feel" this amount of pressure appears to be the threshold of peripheral neuropathy associated with the development of the two major foot morbidities associated with diabetes: diabetic foot ulcers and Charcot foot arthropathy.

equinus moment at the midfoot level. Arteriovenous shunting in the bone of patients that have been demonstrated to be vitamin D deficient and osteoporotic leads to mechanical failure. Loss of protective sensation allows morbidly obese patients to continually load the mechanically weak bone, which fails, depending on the direction of the applied force vectors, leading to a clinical scenario that mimics hypertrophic nonunion or malunion.

- Trauma appears to be the trigger that initiates the destructive inflammatory process.[24] The high association of morbid obesity in symptomatic patients would suggest a mechanical component.[18]
- Although the presence of sensory PN is well recognized, the accompanying motor and vasomotor neuropathies are often overlooked. The motor neuropathy affects the smaller nerves and muscles of the anterior leg (foot and ankle dorsiflexors) earlier in the disease process than the posterior leg compartments, leading to a motor imbalance and an equinus-induced bending moment at the level of the midfoot. The autonomic neuropathy leads to increased swelling, making the tissues less resistant to the applied shearing forces during walking.
- Baumhauer et al[1] has demonstrated, via histochemical studies, the cytokines involved with the initiation of the destructive inflammatory process.[24]

NATURAL HISTORY

- It is currently estimated that Charcot foot arthropathy occurs at a rate of approximately 0.3% per year in the overall diabetic population.[8] Many patients are misdiagnosed with gout, tenosynovitis, cellulitis, or deep infection.[20] The symptoms will spontaneously resolve in many of these patients, making determination of the true incidence difficult.[8] It is likely that those patients who are morbidly obese are more likely to become symptomatic.
- Eichenholtz[7] in 1966 published a detailed monograph based on his observations in 66 patients over a 30-plus year career. This clinical, radiographic, and histologic observational monograph provides valuable benchmark information on the development and progression of this destructive disease process.[7]
- Longitudinal data would suggest that the health-related quality-of-life impact of Charcot foot arthropathy is similar to that of a transtibial amputation.[6,17,23]

PATIENT HISTORY AND PHYSICAL FINDINGS

- The classic presentation is a grossly swollen, painless foot, without a history of trauma, in a mid-50s to mid-60s morbidly obese long-standing diabetic. Many patients remember a specific traumatic event, although it might be trivial **(FIG 2)**.[14,18,21] It is common for Charcot foot arthropathy to develop following fracture or dislocation.
- The key element appears to be the presence of PN as measured by insensitivity to the Semmes-Weinstein 5.07 (10 g) monofilament (see **FIG 1**).
- Classically described as painless, many patient have pain associated with the onset.
- Many describe a feeling of clicking or "crunching" at the involved site, associated with the development of instability. Palpable, painless joint instability is present at this time.
- The foot is typically swollen, erythematous, and warm.

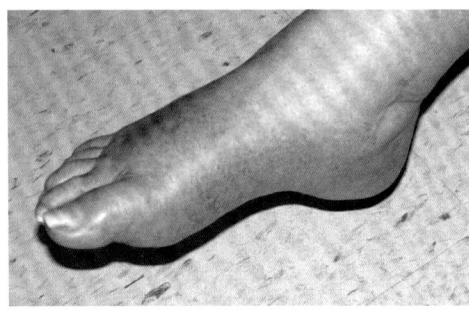

FIG 2 Patients classically present with a grossly swollen, nonpainful foot without a history of trauma. In fact, most remember an episode of trauma, often trivial, and many are painful. Patients generally do not have a draining wound, supporting the presence of a diabetic foot abscess. The erythema is generally greatly lessened with elevation, which clinically differentiates it from infection.

IMAGING AND OTHER DIAGNOSTIC STUDIES

- Treatment can be determined based on clinical examination and plain weight-bearing radiographs.
- Eichenholtz[7] arbitrarily categorized the timeline of the disease process into three stages.
  - Stage I is the early active stage of the disease process. The foot is swollen, warm, and erythematous. Radiographs are normal.
  - Stage II is entered when there is sufficient destruction of the ligamentous structures of the involved joints or bony weakness to allow joint dislocation and/or periarticular fracture. A healing response will often develop during this destructive phase of the disease process, prompting other authors to divide the disease process into more stages. This is when the radiographs take on the characteristic appearance of hypertrophic destruction with or without bony repair. One can conceptualize this stage somewhat similar to that of a hypertrophic nonunion.
  - Stage III is the consolidation of the destructive process. The resultant deformity will develop based on the mechanical loading during the active phase. Radiographs will assume a classic posture of deformity and/or hypertrophic nonunion.[7]
- Nuclear scanning is rarely helpful in distinguishing acute Charcot foot arthropathy from diabetic foot infection or abscess.
- Magnetic resonance imaging is occasionally beneficial when it demonstrates bony destruction contiguous to a wound.

DIFFERENTIAL DIAGNOSIS

- In the least destructive presentations of the disease process, patients are frequently misdiagnosed with a deep venous thrombosis, cellulitis, acute gout, or tenosynovitis.[20]
- Although patients have evidence of peripheral arterial disease, as evidenced by calcified pedal or leg arteries, pedal pulses are generally bounding and ultrasound Doppler studies are normal.
- The critical differential is foot abscess.
  - Patients with Charcot foot arthropathy do not respond to antibiotic therapy. Patients with a diabetic foot abscess, or infective cellulitis, will admit to malaise as opposed to

those with Charcot foot arthropathy who do not demonstrate constitutional symptoms.

- The first sign of occult infection in the diabetic is increasing blood sugar or increasing insulin demand. White blood cell count may not increase, as these patients are often poor hosts and are not capable of mounting a normal immune response.
- Patients with deep infection will generally have an entry portal for infection, which might be as simple as an infected ingrown toe nail or a crack or pinhole between the toes.
- Patients with acute Charcot foot arthropathy will have normal blood sugar levels (for the individual patient) and will not have open wounds or purulent drainage.
- The erythema that is present in the diabetic patient with acute Charcot arthropathy will disappear with elevation, in contrast to the patient with an abscess or deep infection.

NONOPERATIVE MANAGEMENT

- Classically, treatment has been accommodative with a non–weight-bearing total contact cast during the acute phase. Long-term management has been accomplished with accommodative bracing. Surgery was only advised for bony infection or when orthotic management could not accommodate the acquired deformity.
- Patients who are clinically and radiographically plantigrade can be treated with a weight-bearing total contact cast during the active phase of the disease process.[5,21] The cast should be changed every 2 weeks until the volume of the limb stabilizes and the foot is sufficiently stable to transition to therapeutic footwear **(FIG 3)**.[5,21]
- When followed longitudinally, patients who are clinically nonplantigrade, that is, have a noncolinear lateral talar–first metatarsal axis, as determined from weight-bearing dorsal–plantar

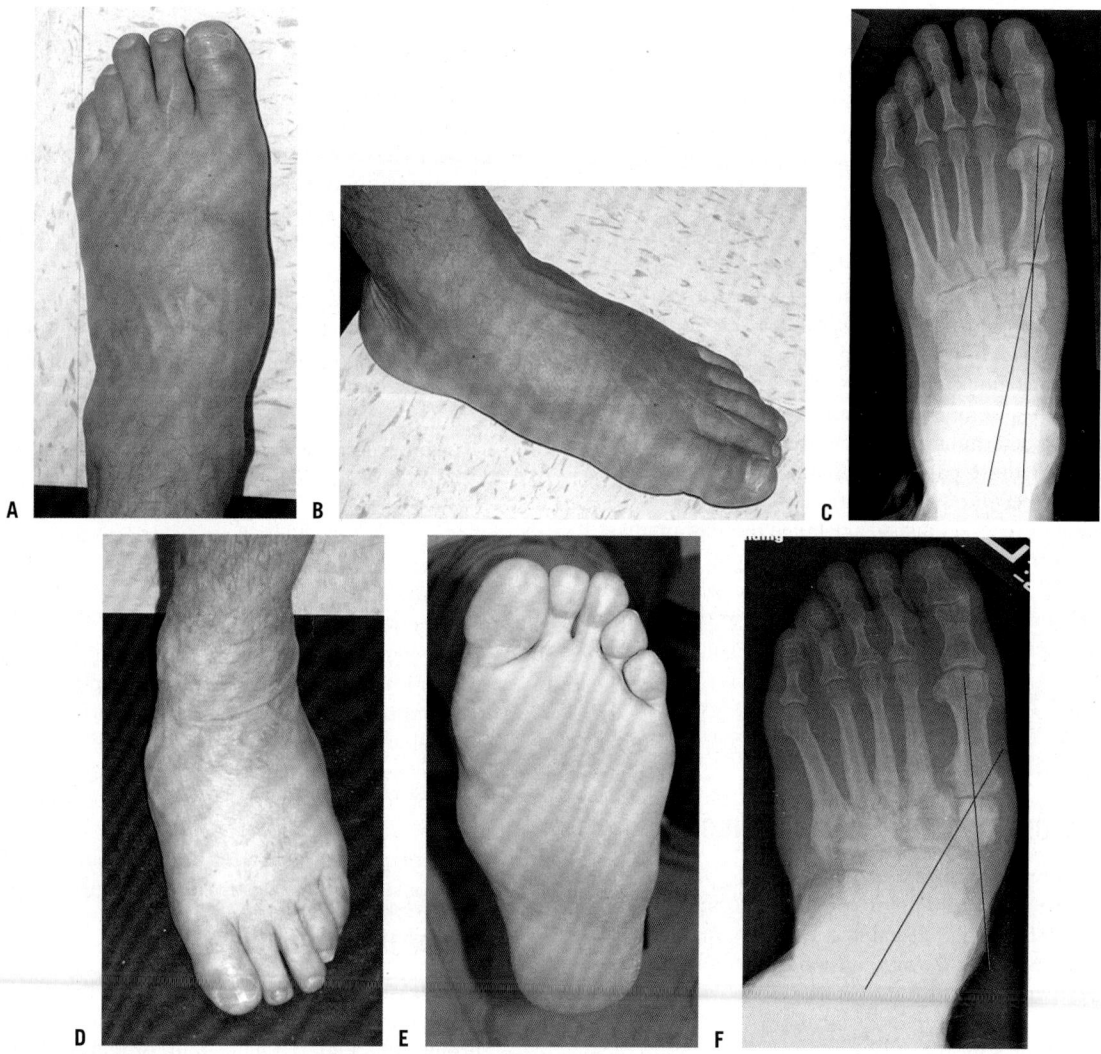

FIG 3 A,B. Weight-bearing photographs of a 55-year-old diabetic male of normal body size. **FIG 3B** demonstrates that he is clinically plantigrade, that is, he is bearing weight on plantar skin designed for weight bearing. **C.** Weight-bearing anteroposterior radiograph demonstrating a relatively colinear talar–first metatarsal axis. Patients who are clinically and radiographically plantigrade are unlikely to develop tissue breakdown and can be managed longitudinally with therapeutic footwear. **D,E.** Clinical photographs 2 years following clinical presentation with active Charcot arthropathy. The foot is clinically plantigrade and capable of being managed longitudinally with commercially available therapeutic footwear (depth-inlay shoes) with custom accommodative foot orthoses. **F.** Weight-bearing radiograph at follow-up. Although the radiograph demonstrates progression of the deformity between hindfoot and forefoot, the foot remained clinically plantigrade and has been successfully managed with commercially available therapeutic footwear.

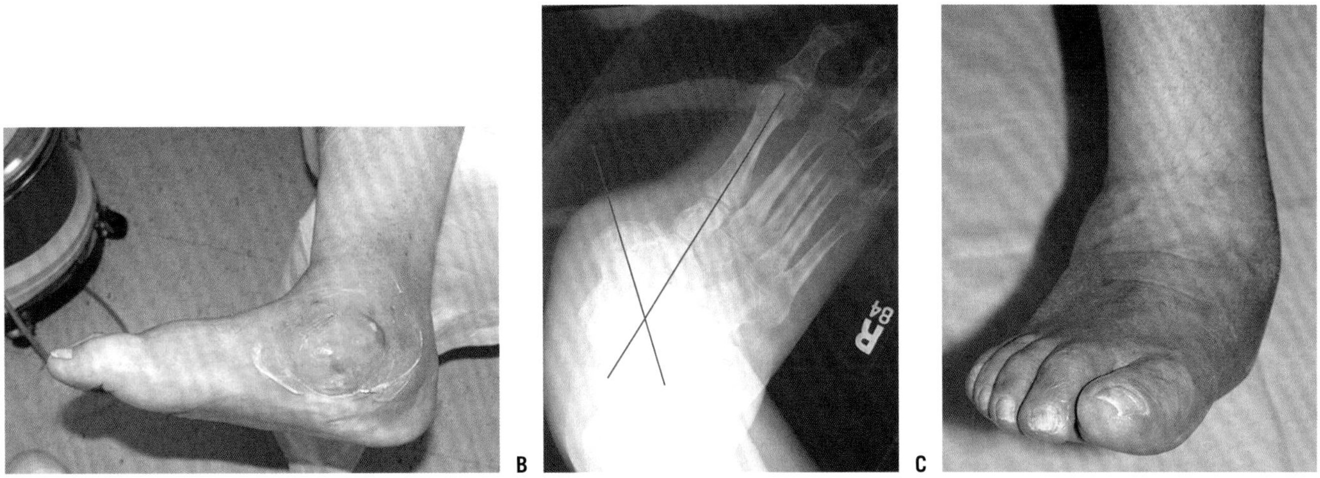

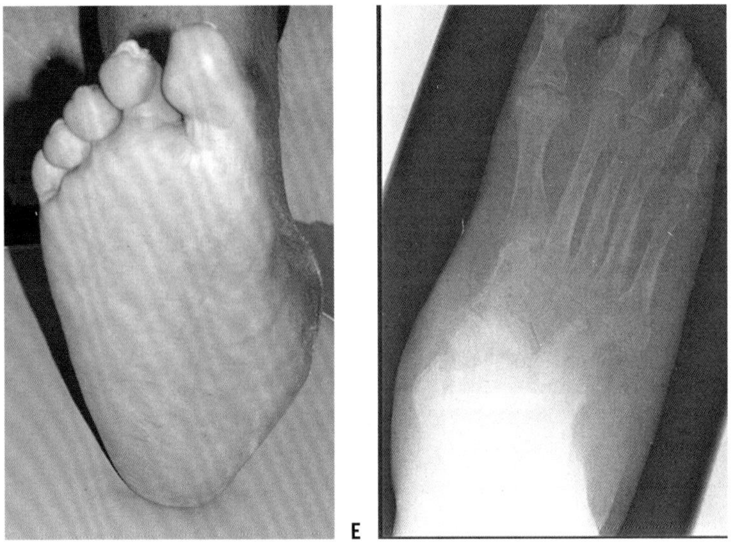

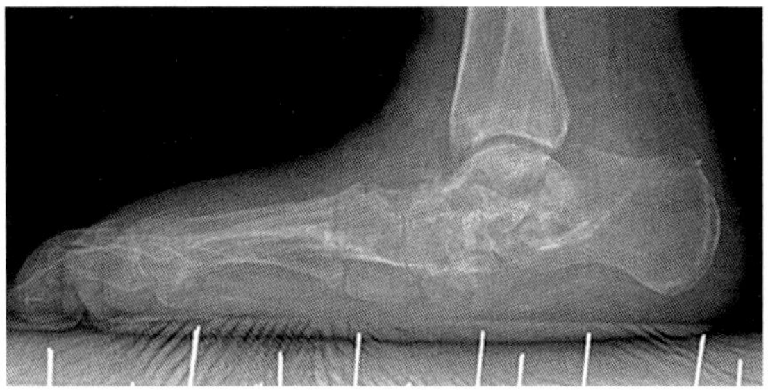

FIG 4 A. This 58-year-old, morbidly obese diabetic accountant is clinically bearing weight on the medial skin overlying the uncovered talar head. **B.** The talar–first metatarsal axis is noncolinear. Patients who are both radiographically and clinically nonplantigrade are likely to develop skin breakdown through nonplantar skin overlying bony deformity. **C,D.** The patient was successfully treated with surgical correction of the deformity and longitudinal management with therapeutic footwear. **E,F.** Clinical photographs and weight-bearing radiographs 2 years following surgery.

radiographs, are likely to develop foot ulcers overlying the deformity over time.[2,16] These patients are best treated with surgical correction of their acquired deformity (**FIG 4**).

- This extremely cooperative patient demonstrates the difficulties in longitudinal management of the nonplantigrade patient without correction of the deformity. The acute destructive process was successfully treated with a total contact cast. The patient carefully followed instructions, wearing the therapeutic footwear full time and returning for scheduled visits to both the physician and pedorthist. Despite close monitoring, the patient developed an ulcer in the skin overlying the head of the talus. When multiple surgical attempts failed, a transtibial amputation was necessary because of infection (**FIG 5**).

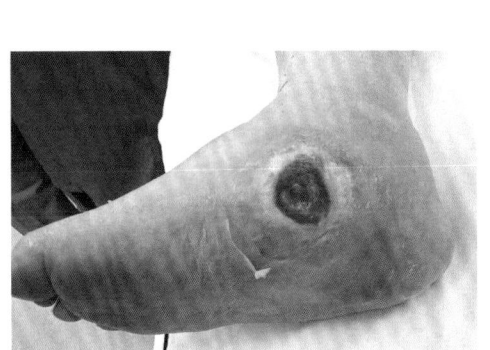
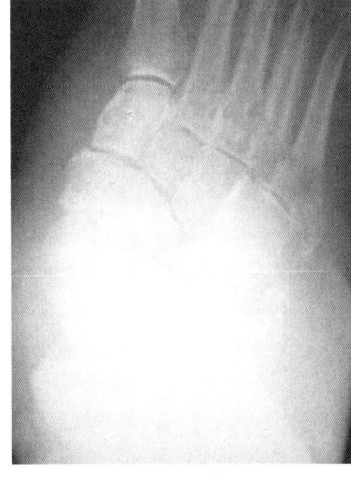

FIG 5 A,B. This 55-year-old, extremely cooperative patient was successfully treated with a total contact cast, progressing to therapeutic footwear. Despite very careful attention by the patient and close monitoring by the patient's physicians, patient developed this ulcer using therapeutic footwear 2.5 years after the development of a Charcot foot deformity.

SURGICAL MANAGEMENT

- The midfoot is the most common location for the development of Charcot foot arthropathy. This is likely due to the applied mechanical bending forces produced by either intrinsic contracture of the gastrocnemius–soleus muscle–tendon complex limiting passive ankle dorsiflexion or the motor imbalance between the neuropathy-weakened ankle dorsiflexors and the strong ankle plantarflexors.[11,12]
- The first step in surgical treatment is a lengthening of the gastrocnemius–soleus motor group to create balance between ankle flexors and extensors. This is accomplished either by gastrocnemius recession (musculotendinous lengthening of the gastrocnemius) or percutaneous Achilles tendon lengthening
- In most patients, the progressive deformity is biplanar. Correction of the bony deformity can generally be achieved by

- removing a sufficient wedge of bone at the apex of the deformity to create a plantigrade foot **(FIG 6)**.
- Patients who are clinically good biologic hosts have no evidence of open wounds overlying bony deformity and no deep infection and appear to have a reasonable quality of bone density and can have surgical stabilization achieved with augmented methods of internal fixation.
- The two most common methods of internal fixation currently employed are large beaming intramedullary screws or rigid medial plate and screw constructs **(FIG 7)**.[22,25]
- In patients who clinically appear to be poor surgical hosts or have wounds or skin ulceration overlying bony deformity, deep infection, or poor-quality osteopenic bone, surgical stabilization is accomplished with a three-level ring external fixator.[9,15]

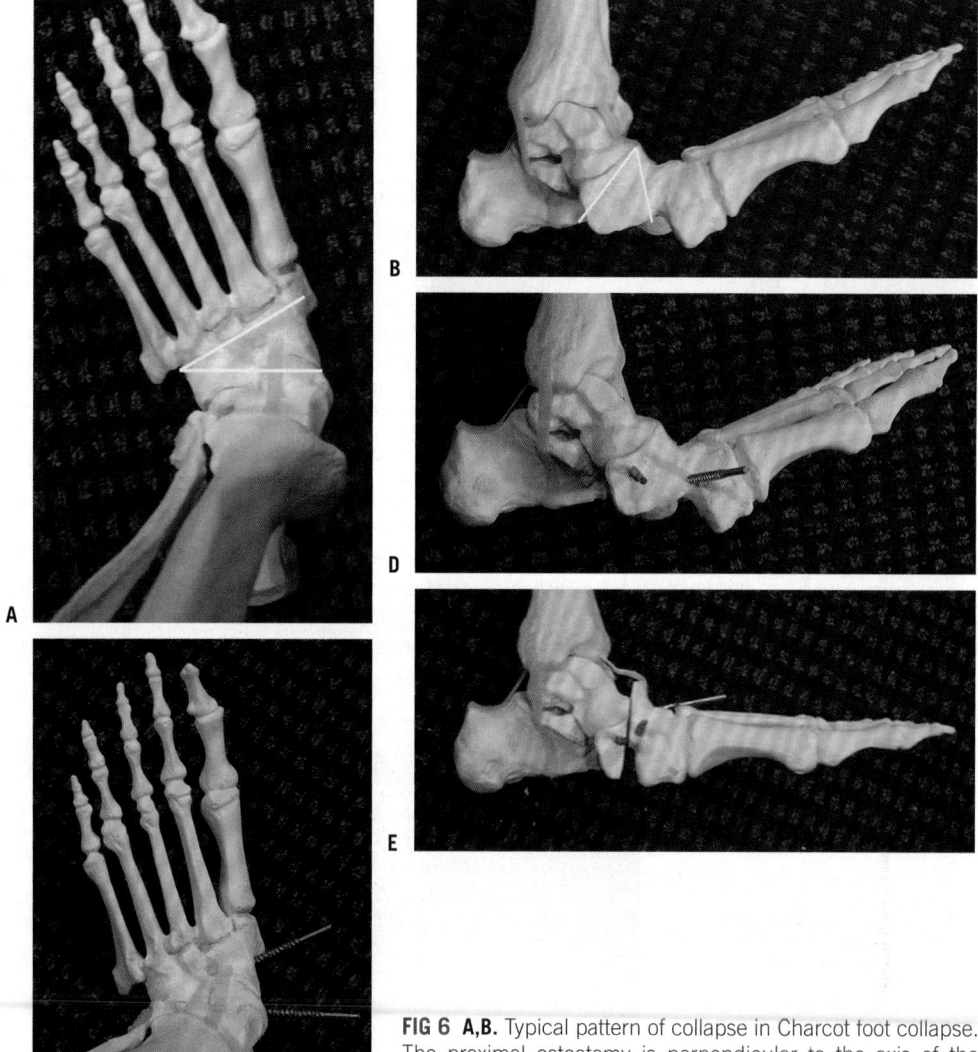

FIG 6 A,B. Typical pattern of collapse in Charcot foot collapse. The proximal osteotomy is perpendicular to the axis of the hindfoot in both planes and perpendicular to the axis of the forefoot distally in both planes. **C–E.** A wedge of bone that is larger at the apex of the deformity, that is, dorsal and medial, is resected to achieve surgical correction of the deformity. *(continued)*

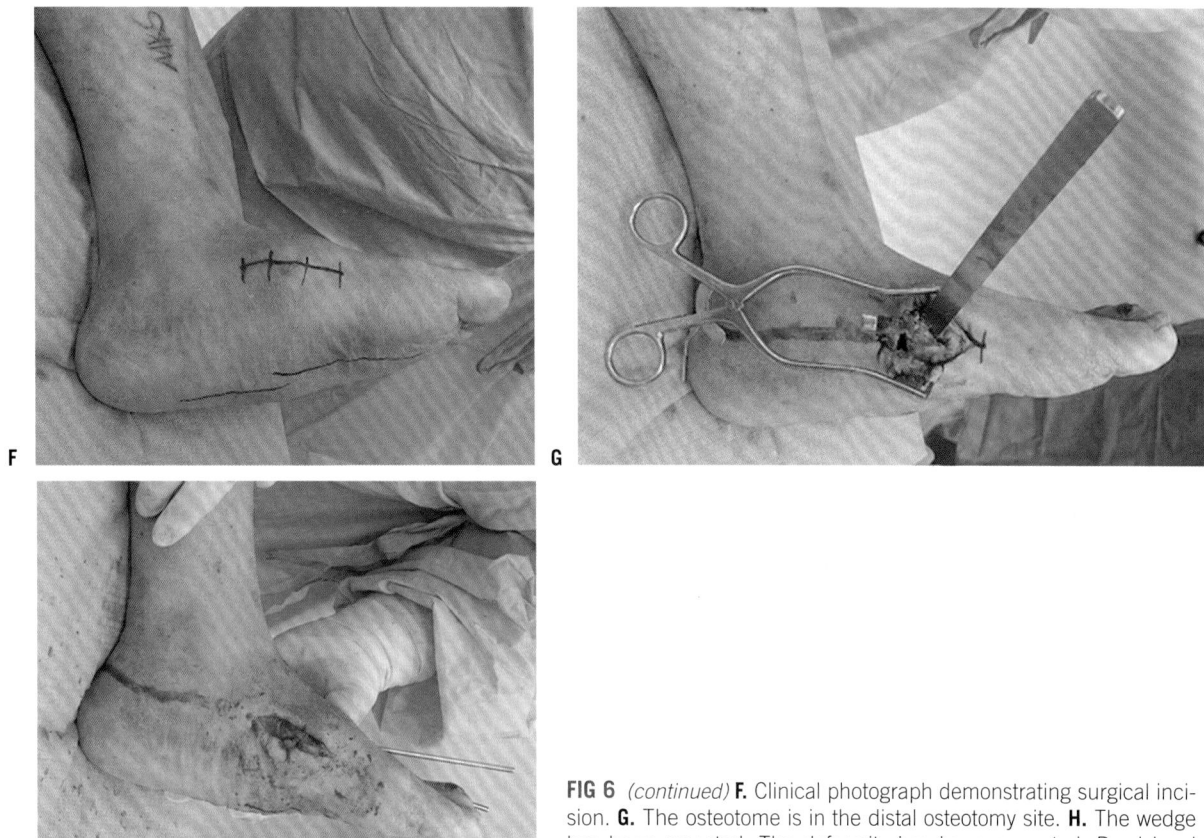

FIG 6 *(continued)* **F.** Clinical photograph demonstrating surgical incision. **G.** The osteotome is in the distal osteotomy site. **H.** The wedge has been resected. The deformity has been corrected. Provisional fixation is accomplished with large smooth K-wires.

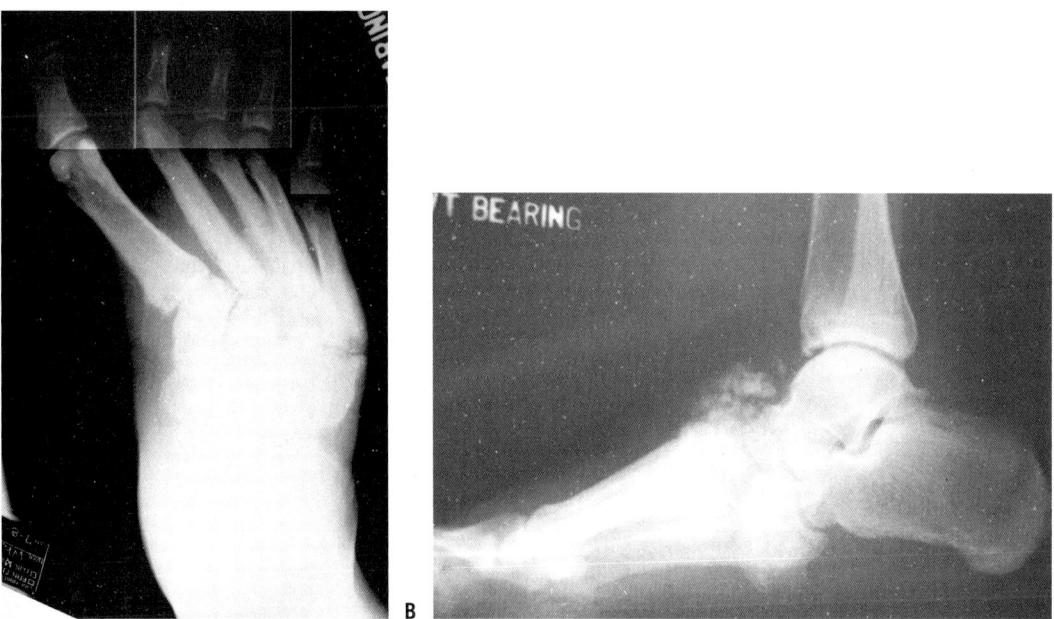

FIG 7 A,B. Preoperative weight-bearing radiographs on a 57-year-old diabetic female with no open wounds. She underwent correction of the deformity followed by internal fixation with super construct *beaming* screws. *(continued)*

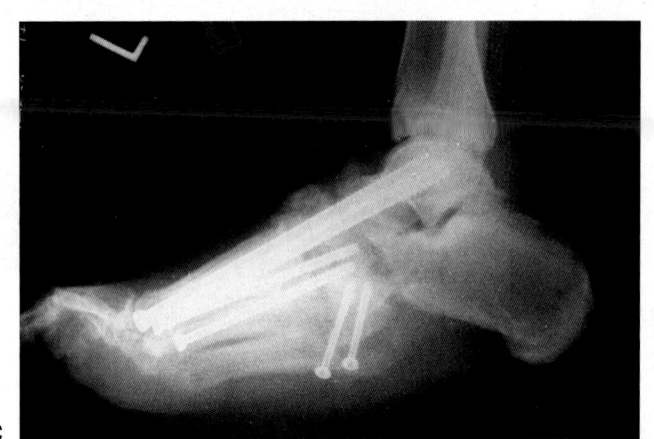
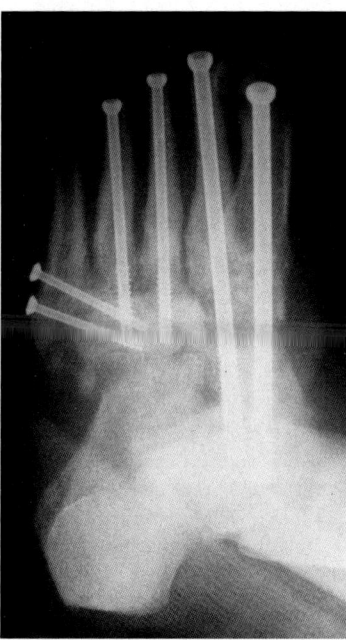

FIG 7 *(continued)* **C,D.** Radiographs at 1 year, demonstrating successful union.

LENGTHENING AND CORRECTION OF BONE DEFORMITY

- The first step is a lengthening of the gastrocnemius musculotendinous unit by either percutaneous triple hemisection of the Achilles tendon or fractional muscle lengthening of the gastrocnemius (Strayer procedure).

- Correction of the bony deformity is accomplished through an incision placed directly over or just inferior to the apex of the deformity.
- A biplanar wedge of bone is resected at the apex of the deformity, allowing correction of the deformity and creation of a plantigrade foot.

INTERNAL FIXATION

- Internal fixation can be achieved with either intramedullary screws or a large medial screw–plate construct.
- Beaming is accomplished by passing large intramedullary screws from the metatarsophalangeal joints of the first and fourth metatarsals across the osteotomy and into the talus.

This superstructure concept theoretically behaves much like an intramedullary nail.
- Several device manufacturers have developed large medial plates that can be used with "osteoporosis" large threaded screws to optimize stabilization in this patient population with poor bone quality.[22,25]

EXTERNAL FIXATION

- The application of external fixation to the Charcot foot is accomplished with a static ring technique. When this technique is employed, correction is obtained at the time of surgery and the external fixator is employed to maintain the correction.
- Provisional fixation is accomplished with large percutaneous smooth wires.
- A three-level static neutral ring external fixation frame is assembled before surgery. The frame has limited adjustability to increase frame stability and minimize the risk for bolt or screw loosening.

Note that the proximal ring can be "upsized" by one ring diameter size to accommodate the calf muscles **(TECH FIG 1A)**.
- The foot is centered within the closed foot ring with a two-fingerbreadth clearance between the foot and the foot ring. Two olive wires are drilled through the calcaneus at a 30-degree angle to each other and parallel with the weight-bearing surface of the heel. The wires are tensioned from 90 to 120 mm of tension and attached to the closed foot ring **(TECH FIG 1B)**.

- Two (three in large patients) olive wires are then drilled through the metatarsals at a 30-degree angle to each other and parallel with the weight-bearing surface of the foot. To avoid flattening the arch, each of these wires generally passes through only three metatarsals. The forefoot is compressed to the hindfoot by arch wire technique, where the wires are tensioned and then attached to the foot ring one ring hole posterior to where they naturally lie **(TECH FIG 1C)**.

- Two olive wires are then drilled through the tibia at a 60-degree angle to each other, perpendicular to the weight-bearing axis of the tibia, at the level of the proximal ring. To avoid neurovascular injury, the wires are drilled through the bone and then carefully tapped through the soft tissues. With the tibia centered in the proximal ring, the wires are tensioned to 120 mm and attached to the proximal and middle rings. Smooth wires are used in the center ring **(TECH FIG 1D,E)**.

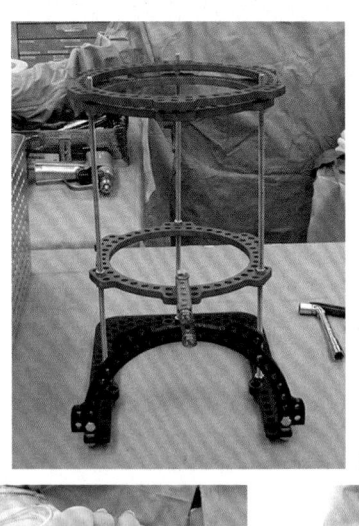
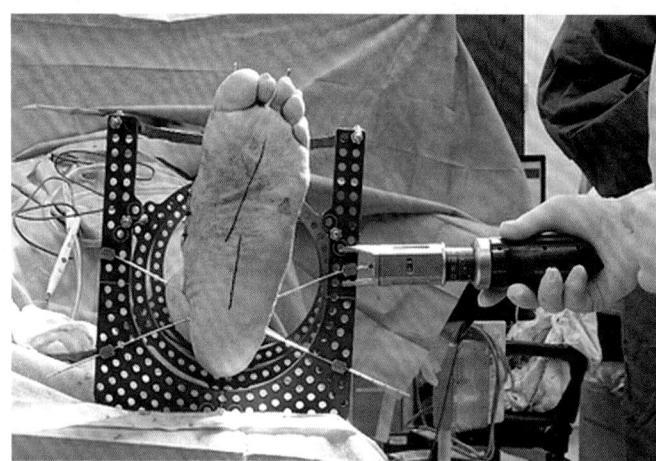
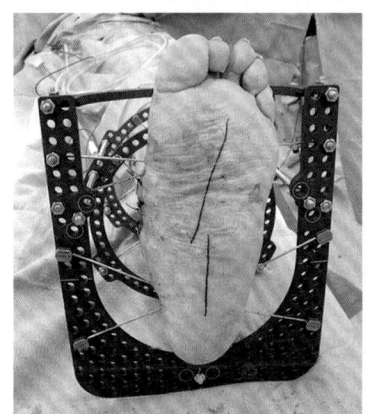
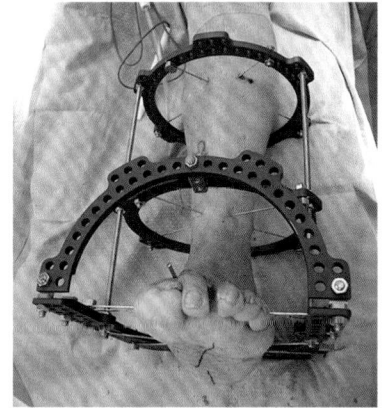
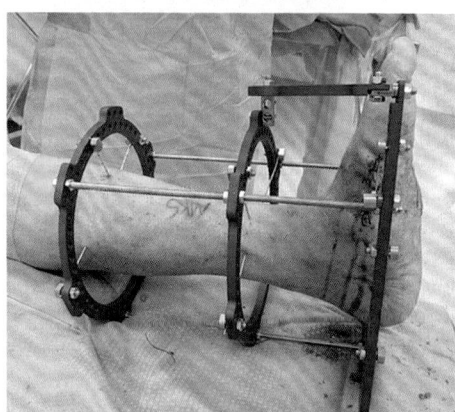

TECH FIG 1 A. A three-level static neutral ring external fixation frame is assembled before surgery. The frame has limited adjustability to increase frame stability and minimize the risk for bolt or screw loosening. Note that the proximal ring can be upsized by one ring diameter size to accommodate the calf muscles. **B.** The foot is centered within the closed foot ring with a two-fingerbreadth clearance between the foot and the foot ring. Two olive wires are drilled through the calcaneus at a 30-degree angle to each other and parallel with the weight-bearing surface of the heel. The wires are tensioned from 90 to 120 mm of tension and attached to the closed foot ring. **C.** Two (three in large patients) olive wires are then drilled through the metatarsals at a 30-degree angle to each other and parallel with the weight-bearing surface of the foot. To avoid flattening the arch, each of these wires generally passes through only three metatarsals. The forefoot is compressed to the hindfoot by arch wire technique, where the wires are tensioned and then attached to the foot ring one ring hole posterior to where they naturally lie. **D,E.** Two olive wires are then drilled through the tibia at a 60-degree angle to each other, perpendicular to the weight-bearing axis of the tibia, at the level of the proximal ring. To avoid neurovascular injury, the wires are drilled through the bone and then carefully tapped through the soft tissues. With the tibia centered in the proximal ring, the wires are tensioned to 120 mm and attached to the proximal and middle rings. Smooth wires are used in the center ring.

TECHNIQUES

Pearls and Pitfalls

- Most of these patients are morbidly obese and have poor balance due to their PN.[10,15,19] We therefore allow them partial weight bearing with a modified "frame shoe."

- Whether using internal or external fixation, large soft tissue stripping wounds should be avoided to decrease the risk for deep infection and wound failure.

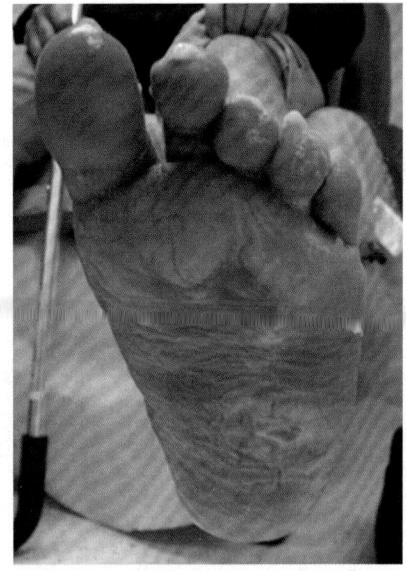

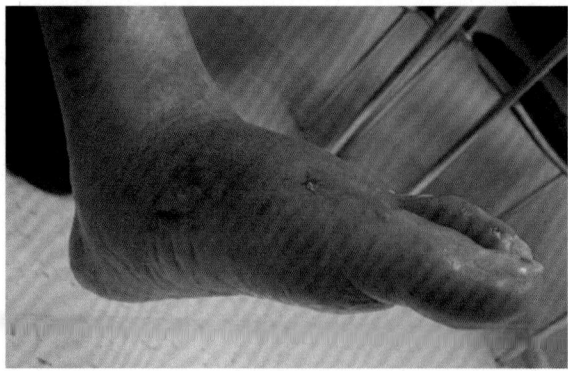

FIG 8 A,B. Clinical photographs at 8 weeks postoperative on the day of external fixator removal.

POSTOPERATIVE CARE

- Patients undergoing surgical correction and maintenance with internal fixation are initially immobilized with a posterior plaster splint.
- Weight bearing is initiated when the surgeon feels that the fixation construct is secure.
- The cast is maintained for 6 to 8 weeks, when patients are transitioned to a commercially available pneumatic diabetic walking boot until limb volume is sufficiently stable to allow fitting with commercially available depth-inlay shoes and custom accommodative foot orthoses in a similar fashion to the nonoperative group.
- Patients treated surgically with a neutral external fixator are allowed partial weight bearing with an adapted frame shoe.
- The external fixator is removed at 8 to 12 weeks (**FIG 8A,B**), at which point a weight-bearing total contact cast is applied for 4 to 6 weeks.
- Progression to therapeutic footwear is accomplished in a similar fashion to the other groups.

OUTCOMES

- Very few clinically and radiographically plantigrade patients will require surgery if successfully treated initially.[18]
- Walking independence and quality of life can be accomplished in over 90% of patients with a low risk for complications with well-planned surgery.[10,15,19,22,25]
- The initial complication rate in the surgical patients was high compared with current standards. Infection rates have been greatly reduced with the use of minimal soft tissue dissection and the use of circular external fixation.
- Similar successful outcomes can be achieved with single-stage resection of the infection, correction of the deformity, and maintenance of the correction with static circular external fixation.[9,19]
- Surgical correction of the deformity is accomplished before application of the external fixator, so the frame construct need not be adjustable. This absence of multiple connections appears to be responsible for the limited frame-associated morbidity.

COMPLICATIONS

- Early attempts at surgical treatment in the complex patient population were fraught with wound infection, wound failure, and loss of mechanical fixation.
- Newer methods of internal fixation designed specifically for this complex patient population and the use of static circular external fixation have greatly decreased morbidity and improved outcomes.

REFERENCES

1. Baumhauer JF, O'Keefe R, Schon L, et al. Cytokine-induced osteoclastic bone resorption in Charcot arthropathy: an immunohistochemical study. Foot Ankle Int 2006;27:797–800.
2. Bevan WP, Tomlinson MP. Radiographic measure as a predictor of ulcer formation in midfoot Charcot. Paper presented at: The Annual Meeting of the American Orthopaedic Foot and Ankle Society; July 2004; Seattle, WA.
3. Charcot JM. Lecons sur les maladies nerveux. New Sydenham Series, 4th Lesson. Paris, France: Aux Bureaux du Progrès Medical, 1868.
4. Charcot JM. Sur quelques arthropathies qui paraissant dependre d'une lesion du cerveau ou de la maelle epiniere. Arch Physiol Norm Path 1868;1:161–178.
5. de Souza L. Charcot arthropathy and immobilization in a weight-bearing total contact cast. J Bone Joint Surg Am 2008;90(4):754–759.
6. Dwahan V, Spratt K, Pinzur MD, et al. Reliability of AOFAS diabetic foot questionnaire in Charcot arthropathy: stability, internal consistency, and measurable difference. Foot Ankle Int 2005;26:717–731.
7. Eichenholtz SN. Charcot Joints. Springfield, IL: Charles C. Thomas, 1966.
8. Fabrin J, Larsen K, Holstein PE. Long-term follow-up in diabetic Charcot feet with spontaneous onset. Diabetes Care 2000;23(6):796–800.
9. Farber DC, Juliano PJ, Cavanagh PR, et al. Single stage correction with external fixation of the ulcerated foot in individuals with Charcot neuroarthropathy. Foot Ankle Int 2002;23:130–134.
10. Gil J, Schiff AP, Pinzur MS. Cost comparison: limb salvage versus amputation in diabetic patients with Charcot foot. Foot Ankle Int 2013;34(8):1097–1099.
11. Ledoux WR, Shofer JB, Ahroni JH, et al. Biomechanical differences among pes cavus, neutrally aligned, and pes planus feet in subjects with diabetes. Foot Ankle Int 2003;24:845–850.
12. Mueller MJ, Sinacore DR, Hastings MK, et al. Effect of Achilles tendon lengthening on neuropathic plantar ulcers. A randomized clinical trial. J Bone Joint Surg Am 2003;85(8):1436–1445.

13. Myerson M, Papa J, Eaton K, et al. The total-contact cast for management of neuropathic plantar ulceration of the foot. J Bone Joint Surg Am 1992;74(2):261–269.

14. Pinzur MS. Benchmark analysis of diabetic patients with neuropathic (Charcot) foot deformity. Foot Ankle Int 1999;20:564–567.

15. Pinzur MS. Neutral ring fixation for high-risk nonplantigrade Charcot midfoot deformity. Foot Ankle Int 2007;28:961–966.

16. Pinzur MS. Surgical versus accommodative treatment for Charcot arthropathy of the midfoot. Foot Ankle Int 2004;25:545–549.

17. Pinzur MS, Evans A. Health-related quality of life in patients with Charcot foot. Am J Orthop (Belle Mead NJ) 2003;32:492–496.

18. Pinzur MS, Freeland R, Juknelis D. The association between body mass index and foot disorders in diabetic patients. Foot Ankle Int 2005;26:375–377.

19. Pinzur MS, Gil J, Belmares J. Treatment of osteomyelitis in Charcot foot with single-stage resection of infection, correction of deformity, and maintenance with ring fixation. Foot Ankle Int 2012;33:1069–1074.

20. Pinzur MS, Kernan-Schroeder D, Emanuele NV, et al. Development of a nurse-provided health system strategy for diabetic foot care. Foot Ankle Int 2001;22:744–746.

21. Pinzur MS, Lio T, Posner M. Treatment of Eichenholtz stage I Charcot foot arthropathy with a weightbearing total contact cast. Foot Ankle Int 2006;27:324–329.

22. Pinzur MS, Sammarco VJ, Wukich DK. Charcot foot: a surgical algorithm. Instr Course Lect 2012;61:423–438.

23. Raspovic KM, Wukich DK. Self-reported quality of life in patients with diabetes: a comparison of patients with and without Charcot neuroarthropathy. Foot Ankle Int 2014;35(3):195–200.

24. Rogers LC, Frykberg RG, Armstrong DG, et al. The Charcot foot in diabetes. Diabetes Care 2011;34:2123–2129.

25. Sammarco VJ, Sammarco GJ, Walker EW Jr, et al. Midtarsal arthrodesis in the treatment of Charcot midfoot arthropathy. J Bone Joint Surg Am 2009;91(1):80–91.

26. Sohn MW, Stuck RM, Pinzur M, et al. Lower-extremity amputation risk after Charcot arthropathy and diabetic foot ulcer. Diabetes Care 2010;33(1):98–100.

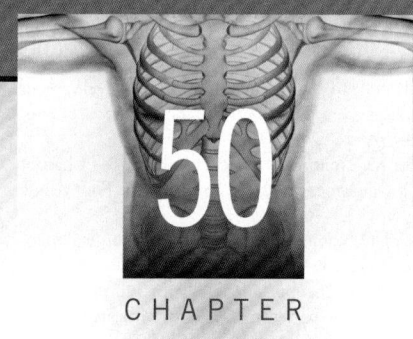

50

CHAPTER

Hindfoot

Flexor Digitorum Longus Transfer and Medial Displacement Calcaneal Osteotomy

Gregory P. Guyton

DEFINITION

- The posterior tibial tendon undergoes tearing and degeneration, and as it fails, the foot falls into a planovalgus configuration. Posterior tibial tendon dysfunction (PTTD) is the most common cause of an adult acquired flatfoot deformity.
- Most cases occur spontaneously without known antecedent trauma. Women are much more commonly affected than men, with a typical age range older than 50 years.
- With time, a rigid deformity develops. The degree and flexibility of the deformity play a key role in determining treatment.

ANATOMY

- The posterior tibialis typically degenerates in an area underneath the medial malleolus and distally to its insertion. The process is not inflammatory but is rather characterized by replacement of the normal collagen fibers with amorphous scar and mucinous degeneration.[6]
- As the arch falls, the hindfoot will fall into valgus relative to the leg, whereas the forefoot will abduct through the talonavicular joint. Uncovering of the talar head results as the forefoot pivots laterally.
- The sag of the arch and the abduction of the forefoot can be described in terms of the loss of alignment of the first metatarsal and the talus. The long axes of these bones should normally be colinear. A sag of the arch is seen by an angulation in this line on the standing lateral radiograph, whereas abduction of the forefoot is seen by lateral angulation of this line on the anteroposterior (AP) view.

PATHOGENESIS

- In most cases, the cause of PTTD is unknown and is not associated with a clear antecedent trauma.
- The collapse of the arch is the result of a tendon imbalance. The antagonists to the posterior tibialis are the peroneals, and they must be functional for the deformity to develop.
- A single study has suggested a correlation of PTTD with the human leukocyte antigen B27 genotype, typically associated with seronegative arthropathies.[9]
- Cumulative mechanical factors likely play a role in the development of the disorder; a preexisting planovalgus deformity presumably places extra stress on the tendon and is thought to be a risk factor for degeneration.

- The presence of an accessory navicular ossicle within the tendon substance at its insertion into the medial pole of the navicular is also a risk factor for tendon degeneration, likely from local mechanical stress (**FIG 1**).

NATURAL HISTORY

- Dysfunction of the posterior tibialis is thought to be the initiating event in the collapse of the arch.[2]
- Early in the course of the disease, pain along the course of the posterior tibialis or weakness of its function will be present without any arch collapse. This is called *stage I disease*.
- With time, a planovalgus foot deformity develops. Initially, this deformity is flexible and is called *stage II disease*.
- A fixed deformity eventually results; this is called *stage III disease*. The first component of the deformity to become fixed is usually an elevation of the first ray relative to the fifth ray. This is the result of a compensation of the forefoot for the hindfoot valgus and is called a *fixed forefoot varus*. Later, the valgus alignment of the calcaneus through the subtalar joint becomes contracted and irreducible.
- Rarely, a secondary failure of the deltoid ligament along the medial aspect of the hindfoot develops as the mechanical stresses placed on it by the flattened arch increase. This is called a *stage IV deformity*.

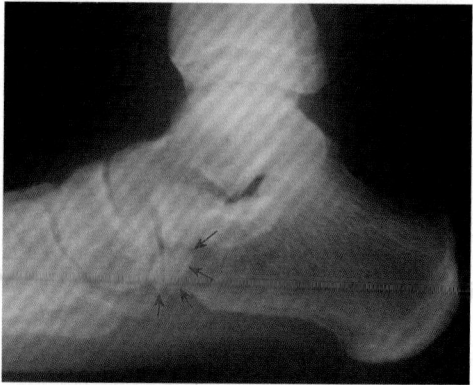

FIG 1 The accessory navicular (*arrows*) may be subtle and can usually be seen on the lateral or AP radiographs. To better visualize the accessory navicular and external oblique, radiograph should be obtained.

TABLE 1	Stages of Posterior Tibial Tendon Dysfunction
Stage	**Description**
I	Tenosynovitis and tear without arch collapse
II	Tenosynovitis and tear with flexible deformity
III	Fixed deformity present
IV	Additional deltoid ligament insufficiency with tibiotalar tilt

- Achilles tendon contracture is commonly seen in association with PTTD. As the planovalgus deformity develops, the foot collapses through the arch and the Achilles is no longer stretched to its normal length in a standing or walking posture.
- **TABLE 1** details the PTTD stages.

PATIENT HISTORY AND PHYSICAL FINDINGS

- Most, but not all, patients present with pain along the medial arch.
- In some cases, lateral impingement develops as the valgus posture of the hindfoot becomes extreme. The calcaneus impinges against the inferior border of the fibula. This is usually a late finding and is often intractable to conservative management.
- The most painful phase of PTTD is usually as the tendon is actively degenerating. Some patients will note a history of intense pain that diminishes once the tendon finally ruptures completely. They may present with deformity or lateral pain as their primary complaint.
- Other deformities may coexist, most significantly hallux valgus or midfoot arthritis.
- Methods for examining the foot for PTTD include the following:
  - The single-leg toe rise. The examiner should note the ability to perform the maneuver, the presence of inversion, and the presence or absence of pain. This is a critical and sensitive screening test. Action of the posterior tibialis is required to invert and lock the hindfoot, allowing the foot to act as a rigid lever through which the Achilles powers the ankle into plantar flexion.
  - The "too many toes" sign. The examiner observes the standing patient from behind. The more abducted forefoot will show more toes visible on the lateral side of the leg. The examiner also notes the presence of forefoot abduction. Abduction of the forefoot occurs as the posterior tibialis fails and must be corrected in treatment.
  - Power of the posterior tibialis. The examiner isolates the tendon by resisted inversion past the midline with the foot held in plantar flexion. Typical muscle strength grading is used. The result can be normal early in the disease. The patient may attempt to substitute the anterior tibialis; it is also an invertor but will dorsiflex the ankle as well.
  - Fixed forefoot varus. The examiner holds the calcaneus in a neutral position (out of valgus) and notes any fixed elevation of the first ray relative to the fifth. The severity

of deformity is noted in degrees. Fixed forefoot varus must be accounted for in any treatment algorithm and is usually the first component of the deformity to become rigid.
  - Achilles contracture. The examiner holds the calcaneus in a neutral position and notes dorsiflexion of the ankle, with the knee both flexed and extended (the Silfverskiöld test). The result is measured in degrees of ankle dorsiflexion. A significant Achilles contracture limits the degree of correction possible with bracing and may require surgical correction.

IMAGING AND OTHER DIAGNOSTIC STUDIES

- Plain radiographs should be obtained with weight bearing to adequately describe the alignment of the foot. The talo–first metatarsal angle describes the sag of the arch when drawn on the lateral view and the abduction of the forefoot when drawn on the AP view.
- Plain foot radiographs should also be examined for the presence of hindfoot arthritis, midfoot arthritis or instability, and an accessory navicular.
- A standing ankle mortise view should be obtained to rule out deltoid laxity (stage IV disease).
- Magnetic resonance imaging (MRI) is not routinely necessary and may underestimate the severity of disease, but it may be useful in ruling out other pathologies. Findings of PTTD typically include fluid in the sheath, dramatic thickening of the tendon, and a heterogeneous signal within the tendon substance indicating the presence of interstitial tears **(FIG 2)**.

DIFFERENTIAL DIAGNOSIS

- Midfoot arthritis resulting in pes planus through tarsometatarsal joint collapse
- Medial ankle arthritis
- Medial osteochondral lesion of the talus
- Neurogenic failure of the posterior tibialis through spinal or central pathology

NONOPERATIVE MANAGEMENT

- The flatfoot that results from posterior tibial tendon failure is irreversible, but symptoms may be controllable in many patients by nonoperative means.
- A simple in-shoe semirigid or rigid foot orthotic may provide sufficient arch support to reduce symptoms in some patients.
- The gold standard for nonoperative management is the use of a cross ankle brace. This allows direct control of the tendency of the calcaneus to fall into valgus. The most commonly used and best tolerated is a leather ankle lacer with an incorporated custom-molded plastic stirrup, often referred to as an *Arizona brace* after a common brand name.[1]
  - Other options that may be suitable for higher demand situations or patients with edema control problems include a hinged molded ankle–foot orthosis or a conventional double metal upright ankle–foot orthosis with a leg strap.

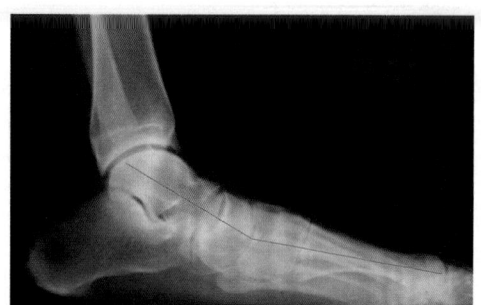
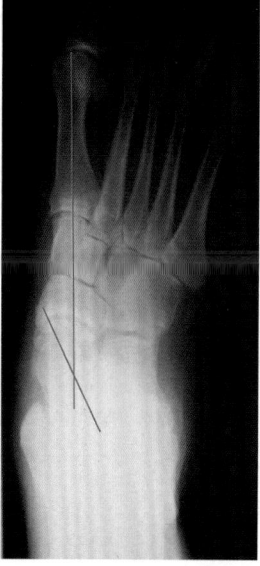
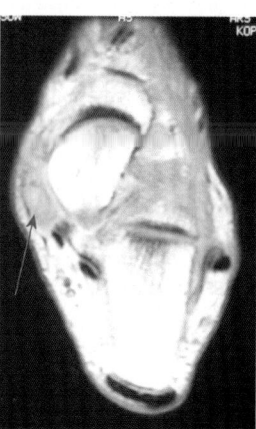

FIG 2 The talo–first metatarsal angle is drawn down the long axis of the talus and the first metatarsal on both lateral (**A**) and AP (**B**) radiographs. Any break from a *straight line* demonstrates both sag and abduction of the arch. **C.** MRI finding may demonstrate posterior tibial tendon edema and enlargement (*arrow*). Physiologic, nonedematous tendon appearance is demonstrated by the homogenous black signal of the FDL and FHL tendons immediately posterior to the diseased posterior tibial tendon.

- Steroid injections into the posterior tibial tendon sheath are contraindicated, as they may directly or indirectly precipitate frank rupture and further collapse.
- No brace, physical therapy regimen, or medication has been shown to modify the course of the disease or the ultimate outcome for the tendon. These are all best thought of as modalities to control the symptoms.

SURGICAL MANAGEMENT

- Surgery is indicated when the symptoms cannot be controlled by a nonoperative means acceptable to the patient. An active patient in his or her 50s, for instance, may find the use of an Arizona brace for the remainder of his or her life to be intolerable and may choose to pursue a surgical remedy.

Preoperative Planning

- The patient's size must be considered before any motion-sparing tendon reconstruction in the hindfoot is considered. Although not rigorously proven in the literature, the morbidly obese patient with an acquired pes planus deformity is at greater risk to break down the repair and may be better served by a triple arthrodesis.
- The presence of hindfoot arthritis similarly requires a fusion rather than an osteotomy and tendon reconstruction.
- A fixed forefoot varus should be addressed, either as part of the procedure through a medial column osteotomy or by a triple arthrodesis if severe.
- Tightness of the gastrocnemius should also be assessed to determine if a fractional lengthening of the gastrocnemius (Strayer procedure) will be required.

Positioning

- The patient is positioned supine with a bolster under the ipsilateral hip. This internally rotates the leg to allow access to the lateral aspect of the calcaneus, which is addressed first. The bolster may then be removed to allow the leg to externally rotate and allow access to the medial aspect of the foot.
- A tourniquet is applied to the thigh.

Approach

- The posterior tibial tendon is débrided directly and augmented or replaced by transferring the flexor digitorum longus (FDL) to the navicular. This procedure alone was first described in the 1980s and proved quite effective at pain control in most cases, although static correction of the arch was minimal.[2,5]
- A medial displacement calcaneal osteotomy is then used to provide a measure of arch correction, directly addressing the hindfoot valgus. Indirectly, this raises the sag along the medial column of the foot as well and helps correct the talo–first metatarsal angle. Correcting the mechanics of the arch is thought to confer an element of protection to the FDL transfer.[3,7,8,11]
- If necessary, up to about 20 degrees of forefoot varus may be corrected by a plantar flexion osteotomy of the medial column through the medial cuneiform (the Cotton procedure). This allows the indications for a motion-sparing procedure to be expanded to a wider patient population, and the need for this step is assessed after the other components of the correction are complete.[4]
- Once the arch is corrected, a final check of the tightness of the gastrocsoleus complex is made to ensure that a lengthening is not required.

MEDIAL DISPLACEMENT CALCANEAL OSTEOTOMY

- Make a 4-cm oblique incision over the lateral aspect of the calcaneal tuberosity behind the peroneal sheath **(TECH FIG 1A)**.
- Carefully avoid the sural nerve during dissection down to the periosteum **(TECH FIG 1B)**.
- Pass a small elevator above and below the calcaneal tuberosity. Ensure that inferiorly the cut will be anterior to the origin of the plantar fascia.
- Place small retractors superiorly and inferiorly and place a low-profile self-retainer in the center of the wound.
- Use a narrow microsagittal saw to cut the tuberosity from lateral to medial. Using a narrow handheld blade provides greater tactile feedback to avoid overpenetration on the medial side **(TECH FIG 1C)**.

- Lever the osteotomy free with a large osteotome or elevator.
- Place a lamina spreader in the osteotomy and leave it for about 1 minute to allow for stress relaxation of the tissues on the medial side. If necessary, a Cobb elevator can be used to gently strip the area **(TECH FIG 1D,E)**.
- Displace the tuberosity fragment medially, usually by about 1 cm. Fix it with one or two 5.0- to 6.5-mm screws placed percutaneously from the posterior tuberosity **(TECH FIG 1F)**.
- Obtain lateral and axial calcaneal fluoroscopy shots to confirm displacement of the tuberosity and confinement of the screws within bone.
- With a rongeur, smooth any sharp step-off on the lateral side of the osteotomy **(TECH FIG 1G,H)**.

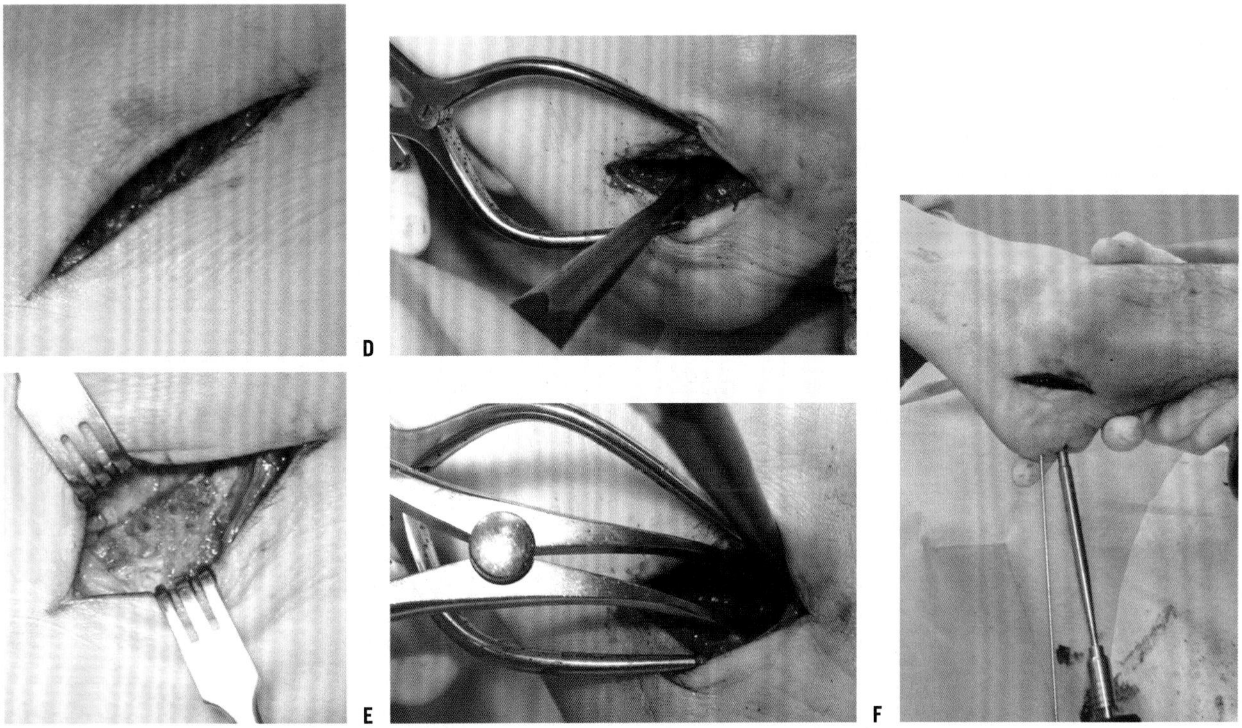

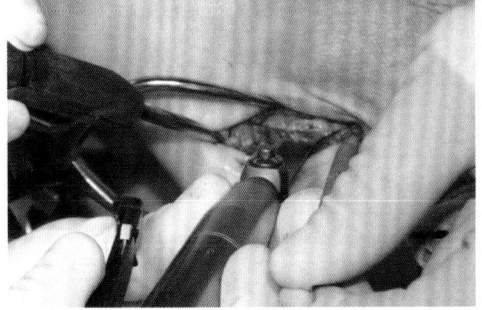

TECH FIG 1 A. Oblique incision for the calcaneal osteotomy. **B.** Careful dissection to the periosteum is made, avoiding the sural nerve. **C.** Dorsal and plantar retractors are placed, and a microsagittal saw is used to make the cut. **D.** A Cobb elevator is used to free up the osteotomy. **E.** A lamina spreader is placed to provide further stress relaxation of the tissues. **F.** After displacement, retrograde screws are used to provide fixation. *(continued)*

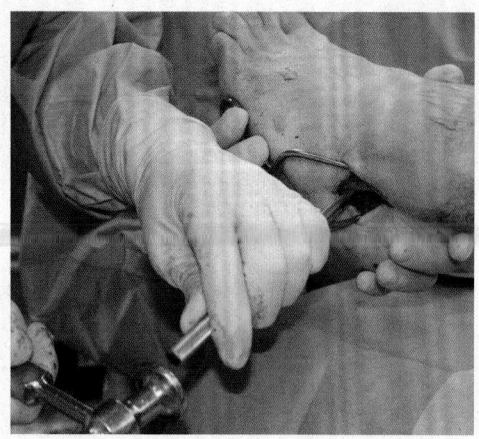
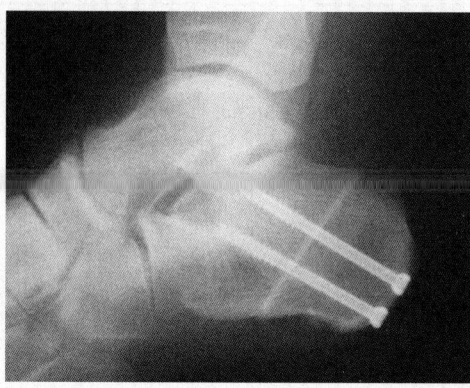

TECH FIG 1 *(continued)* **G.** The sharp margin of the osteotomy is impacted to form a smooth contour. **H.** Radiographic appearance after fixation with two 5.0 screws.

ALTERNATIVE MINIMALLY INVASIVE TECHNIQUE

- A safe zone can be defined for the osteotomy projected anteriorly 11 mm from a line connecting the plantar fascia origin to the posterosuperior apex of the calcaneus on a perfect lateral image of the foot. This reliably avoids the primary branches of the sural nerve and the tibial neurovascular bundle **(TECH FIG 2A)**.
  - Make a 7-mm oblique incision at the anterior margin of this zone in the middle of tuberosity on the lateral side. Spread bluntly down to bone **(TECH FIG 2B)**.
  - Pass a narrow periosteal elevator along the anticipated path of the osteotomy dorsally and plantarly **(TECH FIG 2C)**.
  - Place a 0.062-inch Kirschner wire in the center of the osteotomy normal to the surface of the calcaneus. Confirm the appropriate placement on lateral and axial calcaneal fluoroscopy images **(TECH FIG 2D–F)**.

- Use a narrow microsagittal saw to make an initial entry 2 to 3 mm deep into the bone along the expected obliquity of the osteotomy. Remove the handpiece, leave the blade in place, and confirm the appropriate obliquity on a lateral x-ray along its axis **(TECH FIG 2G–J)**.
- Replace the handpiece onto the microsagittal blade and complete the passage across the calcaneus to complete an appropriately oriented channel in the center of the planned osteotomy **(TECH FIG 2K)**.
- Remove the microsagittal blade and insert a microreciprocating saw into the channel. Complete the osteotomy plantarly and dorsally. The flat blade will template itself along the already created channel to create a clean, regular cut with minimal kerf **(TECH FIG 2L)**.
- Displace the osteotomy medially and complete the fixation per surgeon preference **(TECH FIG 2M)**.

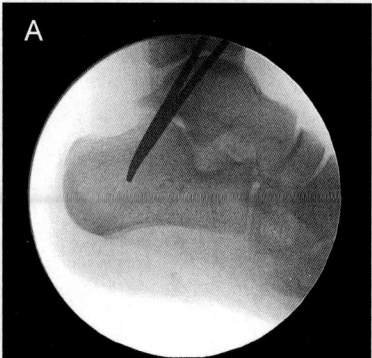
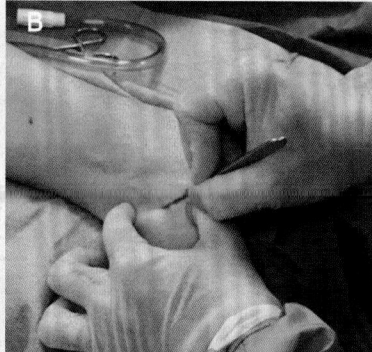
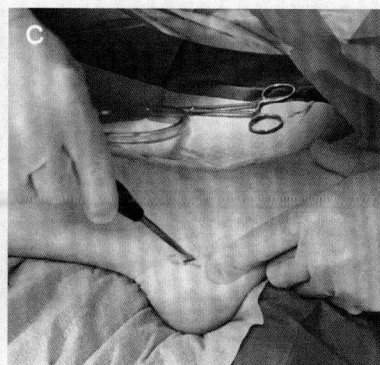

TECH FIG 2 A. The safe zone on lateral x-ray used to avoid the sural nerve. **B.** Use a 7-mm oblique incision. **C.** Elevate the periosteum with a narrow elevator. *(continued)*

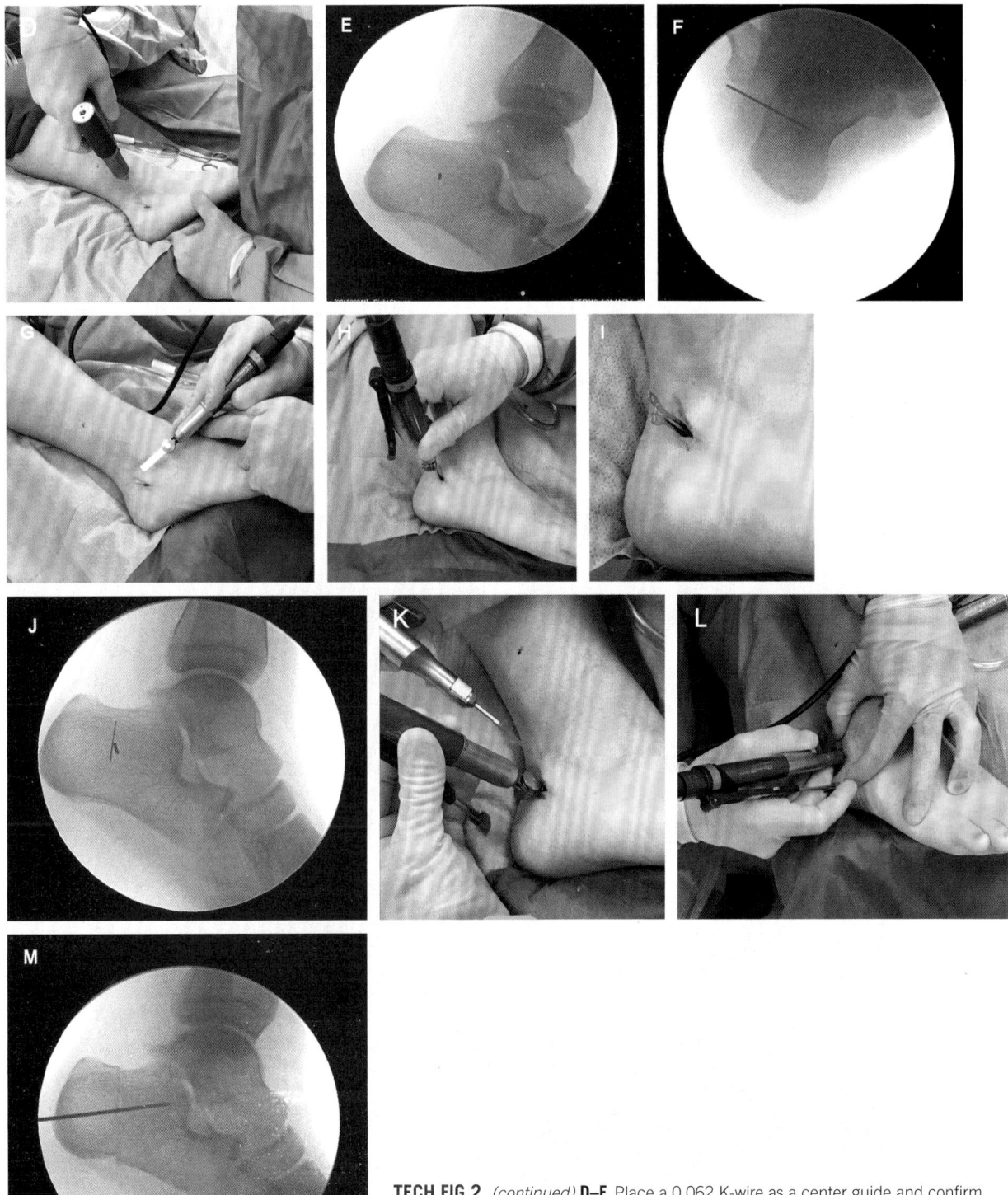

TECH FIG 2 *(continued)* **D–F.** Place a 0.062 K-wire as a center guide and confirm position. **G–J.** Make a shallow entry with a narrow microsagittal saw and confirm the obliquity. **K.** Complete a center channel with the microsagittal saw. **L.** Place a microreciprocating saw in the channel and complete dorsal and plantar cuts. **M.** Displace and fix the osteotomy as desired.

POSTERIOR TIBIAL TENDON DÉBRIDEMENT AND FLEXOR DIGITORUM LONGUS TRANSFER

- Make a longitudinal incision down the medial column of the foot, beginning behind the medial malleolus, passing over the navicular tuberosity, and following the inferior border of the first metatarsal **(TECH FIG 3A)**.
- Open the posterior tibialis sheath and débride the tendon. Complete tendon resection is appropriate in the vast majority of cases, as any remaining diseased tendon is a potential source of pain. Leave roughly a 1-cm stump of tendon attached to the navicular tuberosity to facilitate reconstruction **(TECH FIG 3B)**.
- Identify the FDL sheath and open it just below the medial malleolus. It is located inferior to the posterior tibialis sheath and lies superficial to the sustentaculum tali **(TECH FIG 3C)**.
- Trace the FDL sheath distally to about 2 to 3 cm distal to the navicular tuberosity. To achieve this, develop the plane between the abductor hallucis and the first metatarsal periosteum and take down a portion of the tendinous origin of the

flexor hallucis brevis. This reveals the decussation of the flexor hallucis longus (FHL) and FDL, also called the *knot of Henry* **(TECH FIG 3D)**.
- The FDL is optionally tenodesed to the FHL at the distal aspect of the incision and any evident juncturae between the two tendons are resected. Although small toe function is theoretically aided by this tenodesis, there appears to be little clinically recognizable effect from its omission **(TECH FIG 3E)**.
- Drill a 4- to 5-mm hole through the navicular tuberosity and apply a lead stitch to the FDL tendon. Pass it through the hole from plantar to dorsal and suture it into the deep periosteum at both entrance and exit. If possible, pass it back upon itself. Hold the foot in about 20 degrees of equinus and 20 degrees of inversion during this maneuver **(TECH FIG 3F–I)**.
- Any evident defects or redundancy in the plantar talonavicular ligament (spring ligament) can be imbricated at this time.

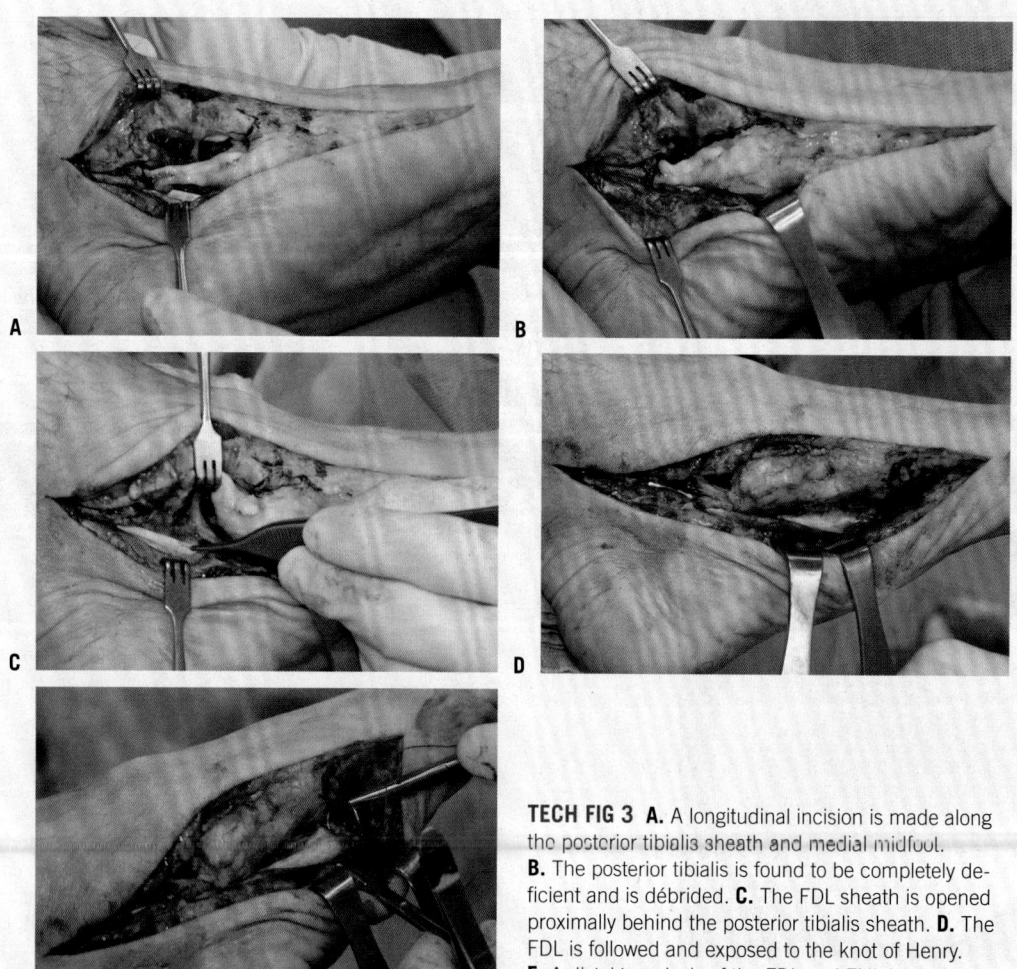

TECH FIG 3 A. A longitudinal incision is made along the posterior tibialis sheath and medial midfoot. **B.** The posterior tibialis is found to be completely deficient and is débrided. **C.** The FDL sheath is opened proximally behind the posterior tibialis sheath. **D.** The FDL is followed and exposed to the knot of Henry. **E.** A distal tenodesis of the FDL and FHL is made; the FDL is then cut. *(continued)*

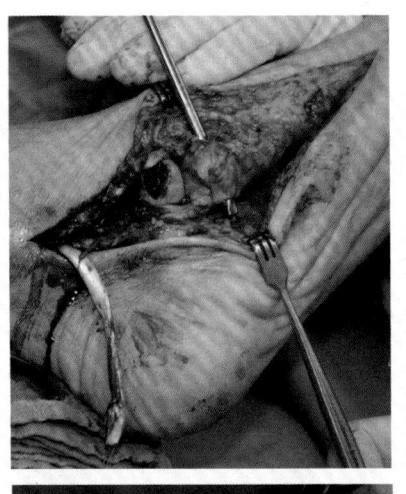
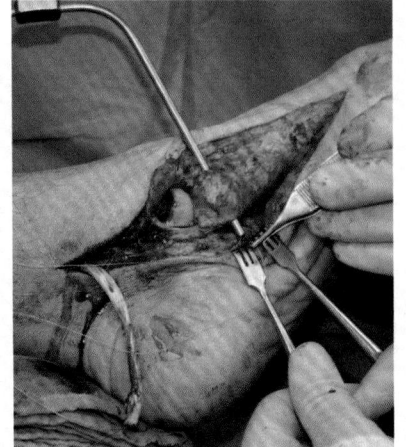
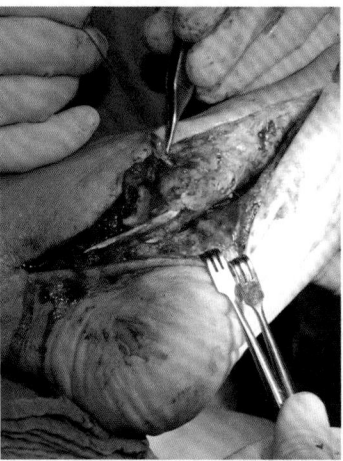
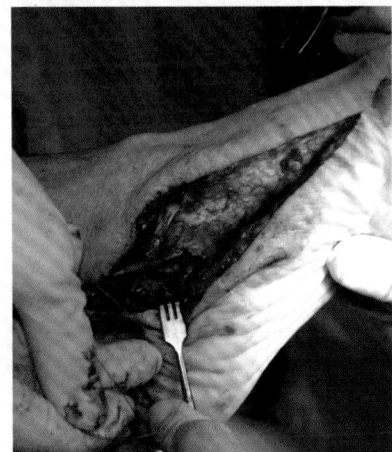

TECH FIG 3 *(continued)* **F.** A dorsal to plantar drill hole is made in the navicular tuberosity. **G.** Placing a sucker tip to suck the sutures through the drill hole allows for easy passage. **H.** The FDL is passed through the navicular from plantar to dorsal. **I.** The FDL is turned back on itself and sutured in place, and the spring ligament is repaired.

PLANTAR FLEXION OSTEOTOMY OF THE MEDIAL CUNEIFORM (COTTON PROCEDURE)

- Make a 4-cm incision centered over the medial cuneiform. This should be a separate incision from that used for the posterior tibialis reconstruction, and usually, a 3- to 4-cm skin bridge can be achieved **(TECH FIG 4A)**.
- Identify the central portion of the medial cuneiform, essentially even with the base of the second metatarsal. Drive a Kirschner wire in to template the desired location of the osteotomy **(TECH FIG 4B,C)**.
- Use a microsagittal saw to create a transverse osteotomy through the medial cuneiform only, taking care to avoid penetrating the plantar cortex **(TECH FIG 4D)**.

- Hinge open the osteotomy with a small osteotome. Kirschner wires drilled on either side of the osteotomy spread with a lamina spreader can facilitate access **(TECH FIG 4E,F)**.
- Insert a tapered piece of graft into the osteotomy to complete the correction. A piece from the calcar of a femoral head allograft or iliac crest allograft may be used. Proximal tibial autograft is also suitable. The piece is sized depending on the degree of correction required; typically, a wedge measuring 5 to 7 mm at its base is used **(TECH FIG 4G,H)**.
- Fixation is not usually necessary. If the graft is not felt to be stable, a dorsal three-hole 2.0- or 2.4-mm plate can be contoured to fit **(TECH FIG 4I,J)**.

TECHNIQUES

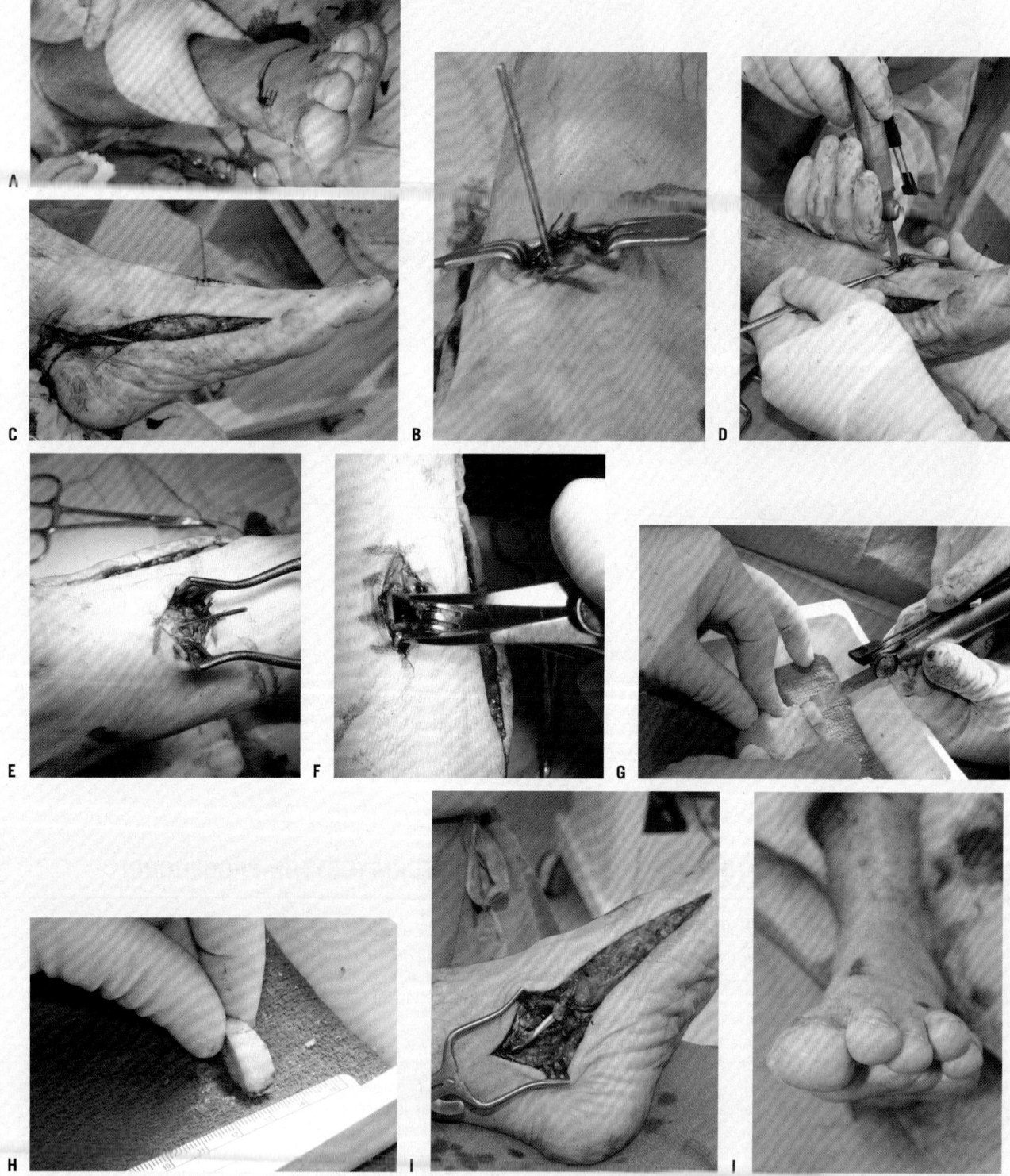

TECH FIG 4 **A.** Residual forefoot varus is noted after the other components of the reconstruction are done. **B,C.** A longitudinal incision is made over the medial cuneiform, and a Kirschner wire is placed to mark the center of the bone. The position is then checked fluoroscopically. **D.** A microsagittal saw is used to create the osteotomy, leaving the plantar cortex intact as a hinge. **E.** Temporary Kirschner wires are placed on either side of the osteotomy. **F.** A lamina spreader is used against them to lever the osteotomy open, dropping the medial column. **G.** A femoral head allograft is used to provide a wedge of bone (**H**), which typically measures 5 to 7 mm at its base. **I,J.** After impaction of the allograft, the medial column has been plantarflexed, and the forefoot varus has been corrected.

Pearls and Pitfalls

Indications	• Excessive forefoot varus (>30 degrees) cannot be accommodated. • Hindfoot arthritis must be carefully ruled out using weight-bearing films.
Medial Displacement Calcaneal Osteotomy	• The sural nerve must be carefully protected; sural neuritis is a common issue postoperatively. • Avoid placing the osteotomy cut too far posteriorly into the origin of the plantar fascia. • Adequate displacement is achievable, only if the tuberosity can be adequately distracted before attempting the medial shift. • Confirm screw placement with an axial fluoroscopic image.
Posterior Tibial Tendon Reconstruction	• Have a low threshold for complete resection of the posterior tibial tendon. • Be prepared for vascular perforators overlying the approach to the knot of Henry. • Suture anchors may provide a salvage if the FDL is harvested too short or if tunnel problems occur.
Cotton Osteotomy	• Be sure the osteotomy will be parallel to the first tarsometatarsal joint by checking the templating Kirschner wire position on the lateral fluoroscopic image. • Slight overcorrection is usually well tolerated.

POSTOPERATIVE CARE

- A bulky postoperative splint is initially applied.
- The patient is transferred to a removable boot at 10 to 14 days and allowed gentle active foot motion only.
- Weight bearing may commence at 1 month for the calcaneal osteotomy alone, 6 weeks if a cuneiform osteotomy has been performed.
- Physical therapy for hindfoot motion and posterior tibialis strengthening commences with weight bearing and is continued for at least 6 weeks. Thera-Band exercises are particularly useful.
- Regular shoe wear is initiated at 2.5 to 3 months depending on swelling. Postoperative compression stockings may be useful in some patients.
- Patients should be warned that the full effect of surgery may take up to 1 year to occur. This time is required for the small cross-sectional area of the transferred FDL tendon to hypertrophy into its new expanded role.

OUTCOMES

- Initial reports of FDL transfer with posterior tibialis débridement alone demonstrated excellent pain relief but little lasting correction of the arch.[2,5]
- The FDL transfer in combination with a calcaneal osteotomy has demonstrated lasting radiographic arch correction and the functional ability to perform a single-leg toe rise. Three-year to 5-year follow-up studies have shown success rates of 90% or greater.[3,7,8,11]
- Long-term follow-up of the medial cuneiform osteotomy in this setting is not yet available. One short-term study detailing its use in a variety of foot deformity corrections in adults demonstrated no nonunions in 16 feet.[4]
- Dramatic hypertrophy of the FDL muscle occurs over the first year after transfer.[10] No clinical difference in ultimate strength has been noted between patients in whom the diseased posterior tibialis was excised versus débrided and retained.

COMPLICATIONS

- Sural nerve injury
- Navicular tunnel failure or early FDL pullout
- Hardware tenderness from the posterior calcaneal screws
- Nonunion
- Deep venous thrombosis

REFERENCES

1. Augustin JF, Lin SS, Berberian WS, et al. Nonoperative treatment of adult acquired flat foot with the Arizona brace. Foot Ankle Clin 2003;8:491–502.
2. Funk DA, Cass JR, Johnson KA. Acquired adult flat foot secondary to posterior tibial-tendon pathology. J Bone Joint Surg Am 1986;68(1):95–102.
3. Guyton GP, Jeng C, Krieger LE, et al. Flexor digitorum longus transfer and medial displacement calcaneal osteotomy for posterior tibial tendon dysfunction: a middle-term clinical follow-up. Foot Ankle Int 2001;22:627–632.
4. Hirose CE, Johnson JE. Plantarflexion opening wedge medial cuneiform osteotomy for correction of fixed forefoot varus associated with flatfoot deformity. Foot Ankle Int 2004;25:568–574.
5. Mann RA, Thompson FM. Rupture of the posterior tibial tendon causing flatfoot. Surgical treatment. J Bone Joint Surg Am 1985;67(4):556–561.
6. Mosier SM, Pomeroy G, Manoli A II. Pathoanatomy and etiology of posterior tibial tendon dysfunction. Clin Orthop Relat Res 1999;(365):12–22.
7. Myerson MS, Badekas A, Schon LC. Treatment of stage II posterior tibial tendon deficiency with flexor digitorum longus tendon transfer and calcaneal osteotomy. Foot Ankle Int 2004;25:445–450.
8. Myerson MS, Corrigan J. Treatment of posterior tibial tendon dysfunction with flexor digitorum longus tendon transfer and calcaneal osteotomy. Orthopedics 1996;19:383–388.
9. Myerson MS, Solomon G, Shereff M. Posterior tibial tendon dysfunction: its association with seronegative inflammatory disease. Foot Ankle 1989;9:219–225.
10. Rosenfeld PF, Dick J, Saxby TS. The response of the flexor digitorum longus and posterior tibial muscles to tendon transfer and calcaneal osteotomy for stage II posterior tibial tendon dysfunction. Foot Ankle Int 2005;26:671–674.
11. Wacker JT, Hennessy MS, Saxby TS. Calcaneal osteotomy and transfer of the tendon of flexor digitorum longus for stage-II dysfunction of tibialis posterior. Three- to five-year results. J Bone Joint Surg Br 2002;84(1):54–58.

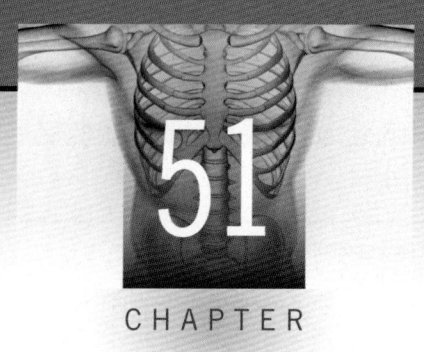

51

CHAPTER

Lateral Column Lengthening

Thomas B. Bemenderfer, Bryan L. Witt, Donald R. Bohay, and John G. Anderson

DEFINITION

- Posterior tibial tendon (PTT) deficiency is a common pathologic foot and ankle deformity encountered by orthopaedic foot and ankle surgeons.
- This insufficiency is described as a painful flatfoot deformity secondary to an incompetent PTT leading to hindfoot valgus and forefoot abduction.
- An equinus contracture, forefoot supination, and medial column instability can also be associated with PTT insufficiency.
- PTT deficiency has several classification systems. The most common classification system is the Johnson and Strom classification with Myerson modification (TABLE 1).[26,35]
- Bluman et al[6] further subclassified stage II PTT deficiency based on clinical examination (TABLE 2).
- Deland et al[12] used radiographic criteria to subclassify stage II PTT deficiency. Stage IIA is characterized by less than 30% of talar head uncoverage, whereas stage IIB is classified as having greater than 30% of talar head uncoverage.[12]
- Lateral column lengthening was incidentally discovered by Dillwyn Evans in 1961 while treating relapsed clubfeet. Evans[18] noted that overcorrected clubfeet had a short lateral column and placing a wedge bone graft into the anterior process of the calcaneus equalized the length of the medial and lateral columns that corrected the forefoot abduction deformity.
- Lateral column lengthening procedures include lengthening through the anterior process of the calcaneus (Evans procedure), calcaneocuboid distraction arthrodesis, or Z calcaneal osteotomy are commonly used to correct forefoot abduction and hindfoot valgus in patients with PTT deficiency.[32,33]
- Interposition grafts used to maintain lateral column lengthening include tricortical iliac autograft, allograft, porous coated titanium wedge, and plate interposition fixation.[14,19,20,30,31,34]

ANATOMY

- The PTT originates from the posterior aspect of the proximal tibia and fibula and interosseous membrane and courses distally through the tarsal tunnel with the flexor digitorum tendon as well as the posterior tibial artery, nerve, vein, and flexor hallucis longus tendon.[40]
- The PTT inserts onto the navicular tuberosity, cuneiform bones, and second to fourth metatarsals.[40]
- This tendon is responsible for ankle plantarflexion and midfoot supination and adduction.
- The lateral column is composed of the calcaneus, cuboid, and fourth and fifth metatarsals. It also encompasses the calcaneocuboid joint as well as the fourth and fifth tarsometatarsal joints.
- The peroneal brevis tendon attaches to the base of the fifth metatarsal and acts as an antagonist to the PTT.
- The PTT functions during the stance phase of gait from heel strike to toe-off.
- During heel strike, this tendon eccentrically contracts to decelerate subtalar joint pronation.
- At heel lift-off, the PTT locks the transverse tarsal joint, allowing the gastrocnemius and soleus muscles to maximize plantarflexion power.
- By locking the talonavicular joint in adduction and plantarflexion, the mechanical axis of the Achilles tendon is shifted medially, causing the subtalar joint to invert and thereby creating a rigid lever for propulsion.
- The PTT also acts as a dynamic support structure for the medial longitudinal arch by acting to adduct and plantarflex the navicular bone around the talar head.

TABLE 1 Johnson and Strom Classification of Posterior Tibial Tendon Deficiency with Myerson Modification

Stage	Description
I	Posterior tibial tendon tenosynovitis and/or tear without arch collapse
II	Posterior tibial tendon tenosynovitis and/or tear with flexible flatfoot deformity
III	Fixed flatfoot deformity
IV	Stage I–III with deltoid ligament insufficiency and/or lateral talar tilt

Based on data from Johnson KA, Strom DE. Tibialis posterior tendon dysfunction. Clin Orthop Relat Res 1989;(239):196–206; Myerson MS. Adult acquired flatfoot deformity: treatment of dysfunction of the posterior tibial tendon. Instr Course Lect 1997;46:393–405.

TABLE 2 Bluman et al. Subclassification of Stage II Posterior Tibial Tendon Deficiency

Stage	Description
IIA	Hindfoot valgus
IIB	Forefoot abduction
IIC	Medial column instability

Based on data from Bluman EM, Title CL, Myerson MS. Posterior tibial tendon rupture: a refined classification system. Foot Ankle Clin 2007;12(2):233–249, v.

- The medial longitudinal arch is also statically supported by the plantar calcaneonavicular (spring) ligament and the plantar fascia through a windlass mechanism.

PATHOGENESIS

- The exact cause of PTT failure is unknown but most likely is multifactorial.
- Most common plausible explanation is repetitive microtrauma causing tenosynovitis, longitudinal splint tears, and eventual rupture.
- An accessory navicular is commonly associated with PTT pathology.
- Spontaneous and traumatic ruptures are infrequently associated with PTT insufficiency.

NATURAL HISTORY

- As the PTT decompensates and fails, the dynamic support of the medial longitudinal is lost.
- The unopposed peroneal brevis tendon, which is the antagonist to the PTT, pulls the hindfoot into valgus and abducts the midfoot.
- Failure of the powerful ankle invertor causes the mechanical axis of the Achilles tendon to move laterally, accentuating the hindfoot valgus deformity keeping the transverse tarsal joint unlocked during toe-off.
- In addition, the Achilles tendon acts to plantarflex the talus through the talonavicular joint.
- These events place increased stress across the static restraints of the medial longitudinal arch, causing attenuation and tearing of the spring ligament.
- This results in a loss of the medial longitudinal arch, dorsolateral peritalar subluxation, and hindfoot valgus.
- The functionally shortened lateral column secondary to the dorsolateral peritalar subluxation creates sinus tarsi impingement and increases pressure through the calcaneocuboid joint.[21]
- Further stress on the medial soft tissues leads to attenuation of the deltoid ligaments and ankle valgus deformity and resultant ankle arthritis.
- Subfibular impingement occurs as the calcaneus falls further into valgus, abutting against the tip of the fibula.
- Finally, chronic shortening of the gastrocnemius or Achilles tendon leads to an equinus contracture.

PATIENT HISTORY AND PHYSICAL FINDINGS

- Examination of PTT insufficiency includes a standing, seated, and ambulatory evaluation.
- On standing examination, note any deformity about the knee including genu varum, valgum, or recurvatum.
- Inspect for medial longitudinal arch collapse and forefoot abduction.
- Evaluate for fullness or swelling along the course of the PTT.
- Standing from behind assess for hindfoot valgus deformity. This is commonly represented as "too many toes" sign (**FIG 1**).
- A double and single heel rise is done to evaluate the competency of the PTT. A normal tendon will invert the heel with a double- or single-leg heel raise. Inability to perform

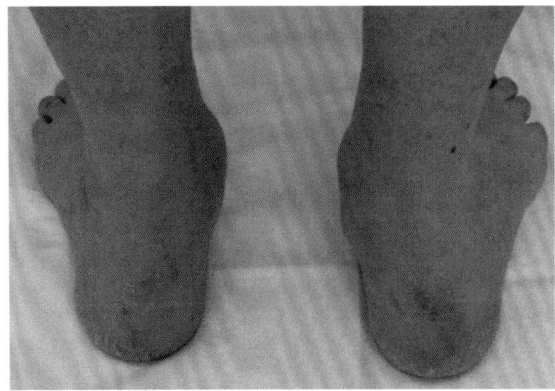

FIG 1 Hindfoot valgus and too many toes sign in a patient with PTT deficiency.

a single or double heel rise is commonly seen with posterior tibial insufficiency.

- Frequently, there is tenderness to palpation, swelling, and warmth over the medial aspect of the ankle over the course of the PTT.
- If the hindfoot valgus deformity is severe, the patient may have tenderness to palpation over the lateral aspect of the ankle. This discomfort is caused by impingement between the calcaneus and distal tip of the fibula termed *subfibular impingement*. A stress fracture of the distal fibula can occur with chronic subfibular impingement.
- It is important to determine if the deformity is passively correctable. In a flexible PTT deficiency, the reestablishment of a plantigrade foot is achieved by manually reducing the hindfoot valgus, forefoot abduction, and forefoot supination. When the foot is rigid, not passively correctible, a triple arthrodesis instead of joint-preserving procedures is warranted.
- Excessive mobility at the first tarsometatarsal joint is assessed by stabilizing the hindfoot in the neutral position and testing the mobility both in the sagittal and coronal plane. When excessive motion is noted on examination, a first tarsometatarsal joint arthrodesis is necessary in order to obtain a stable medial column for weight transfer from heel strike to toe-off.
- A Silfverskiöld test is performed to evaluate an Achilles tendon or gastrocnemius contracture. A Achilles tendon lengthening or gastrocnemius recession is merited if there is a contracture especially if a lateral column lengthening procedure is performed.
- Finally, evaluate for forefoot supination on seated examination; this is a result of compensated hindfoot valgus and will determine if a plantarflexion osteotomy of the first ray is necessary.

IMAGING AND OTHER DIAGNOSTIC STUDIES

- PTT insufficiency is mostly a clinical diagnosis; however, foot and ankle radiographs can guide surgical decision making. Advanced diagnostic imaging such as ultrasonography and magnetic resonance imaging (MRI) can more specifically evaluate the disease severity of the PTT, spring ligament, or calcaneocuboid degenerative joint changes, yet its usefulness in diagnosing and surgical decision making is limited.

- Obtain bilateral weight-bearing anteroposterior (AP), lateral, and oblique foot radiographs. These images, in general, should be evaluated for subtalar, talonavicular, or calcaneocuboid arthritis as well as first tarsometatarsal joint instability, naviculocuneiform collapse, tarsal coalition, or an accessory navicular.
- Also, obtain bilateral weight-bearing AP, lateral, and mortise ankle radiographs to evaluate for ankle instability (dorsal talar beaking and distal tibial exostoses), valgus tilt of the talus (deltoid laxity), tibiotalar joint arthritis, and subfibular impingement **(FIG 2A)**.
  - Four radiographic parameters of forefoot abduction may be measured: talonavicular coverage angle,[25,39] talonavicular uncoverage percentage,[13,17] talus–first metatarsal angle,[25] and lateral incongruency angle.[17]
  - The talonavicular coverage angle can be measured on the AP foot radiographs. This angle is measured between a line drawn parallel to the articular of the talus and a second line drawn parallel the articular surface of the navicular on the AP radiograph **(FIG 2B)**. This represents the amount of forefoot abduction through the talonavicular joint.
  - The talonavicular uncoverage percentage can be measured on the AP foot radiographs. This percentage is measured as the percentage of talar head articular surface uncovered by navicular **(FIG 2C)**.[13,17]
  - The lateral incongruency angle can be measured on the AP foot radiographs. This angle is determined by the intersection of two lines: (1) a line drawn between the most lateral extent of the articular surfaces of both

the navicular and talus and (2) a line connecting the lateral aspect of the talar neck at its most visibly narrow segment and the lateral extent of the talar articular surface **(FIG 2D)**. The normal lateral incongruency angle ranges from −5 to 20 degrees.[17]
  - The lateral talus–first metatarsal angle can be measured on lateral foot radiographs and determines the amount of collapse about the medial column through the talonavicular joint.[25] This is measured as the angle between a line drawn down the longitudinal axis of the talus and a line drawn down the longitudinal axis of the first metatarsal **(FIG 2E)**. The normal lateral talus–first metatarsal angle ranges from 4 to 24 degrees.
- The calcaneal pitch angle can be measured on lateral foot radiographs. This measurement evaluates the amount of pes cavus or planus. The calcaneal pitch is measured as the angle between a line tangent the inferior aspect of the calcaneus to the inferior aspect of the medial sesamoid and a second line drawn tangent to the inferior aspect of the calcaneus and the most inferior aspect of the anterior calcaneus **(FIG 2F)**. Normal values range from 10 to 30 degrees, with a calcaneal pitch ankle less than 10 degrees representing a flatfoot deformity and more than 30 degrees representing a cavus foot deformity.
- MRI is often used to rule out other causes of medial foot and ankle pathology.
  - MRI findings include increased fluid on T2-weighted and short T1 inversion recovery (STIR) imaging within the PTT sheath and/or thickening of the PTT on T1- or T2-weighted images represented posterior tibial tenosynovitis.

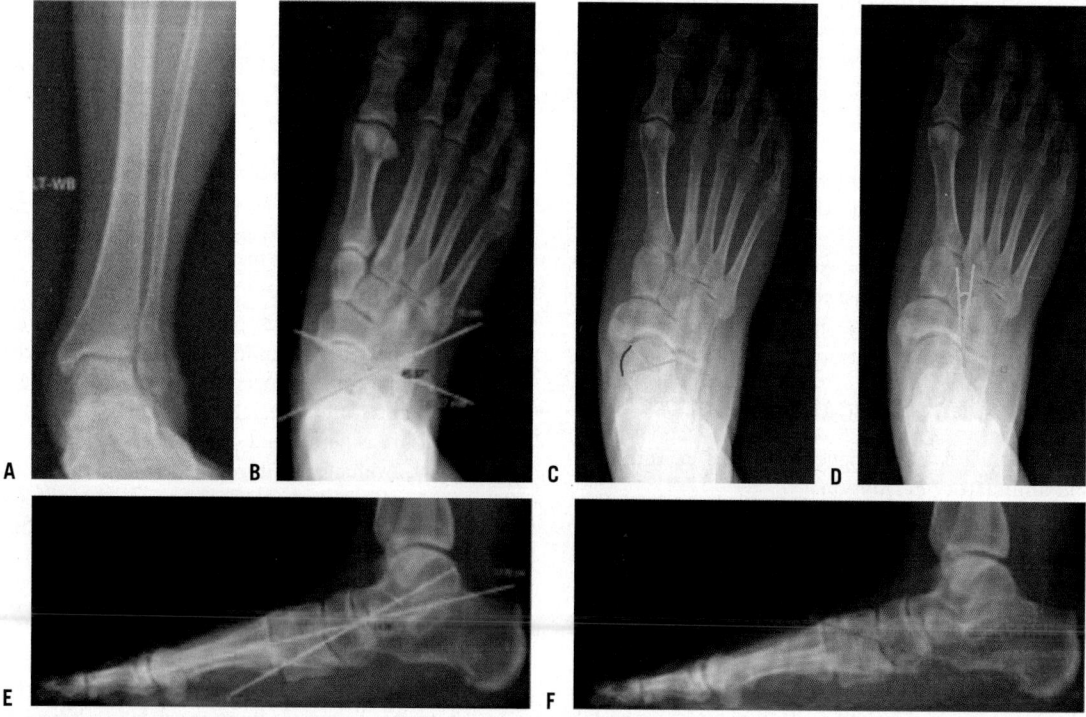

FIG 2 A. AP radiograph of the ankle demonstrating subfibular impingement with an associated lateral malleolus fracture in a patient with PTT deficiency. **B.** AP radiograph of the foot measuring the talonavicular coverage angle. **C.** AP radiograph of the foot measuring the talonavicular uncoverage percentage. **D.** AP radiograph of the foot measuring the lateral incongruency angle. **E.** Lateral radiograph of the foot measuring the talus–first metatarsal angle. **F.** Lateral radiograph of the foot measuring the calcaneal pitch angle.

- Furthermore, a heterogenous signal within the PTT on T2 or STIR imaging signifies longitudinal split tearing of the tendon.
- A spring (plantar calcaneonavicular) ligament tear or rupture, however difficult, can be identified using T2 or STIR imaging.

DIFFERENTIAL DIAGNOSIS

- Tarsal coalition
- Accessory navicular
- Naviculocuneiform degenerative joint disease with joint collapse
- Midfoot degenerative joint disease with collapse through tarsometatarsal joint
- Medial ankle degenerative joint disease
- Osteochondral lesion talus
- Charcot neuroarthropathy
- Neurogenic arthropathy (spinal cord lesion or central nervous system pathology)

NONOPERATIVE MANAGEMENT

- Conservative therapy regarding PTT insufficiency aims at decreasing pathologic symptoms such as pain and inflammation as well as correcting the associated foot deformities, including hindfoot valgus, forefoot abduction, and equinus contracture.
  - Unfortunately, nonoperative management will not permanently correct the foot deformities, restore the pathologic PTT, or change the natural history of the disease.
- Braces, walking boots, and short-leg casts theoretically limit the amount of PTT excursion allowing the tendon to rest, thus decreasing inflammation and pain.
  - A controlled ankle motion or fixed ankle support device is used for acute episode of posterior tibial tendinopathy and Johnson and Strom stage I PTT deficiency **(FIG 3A)**. The walking boot is worn for a short period of time or until the symptoms of pain and swelling have dissipated. Thereafter, an orthotic or brace is used to offload the PTT.
  - A short-leg walking cast is used if there are compliance problems wearing the walking boot.

- If the symptoms are mild, a lace-up ankle brace (Swede-O or ankle stabilizing orthosis) will decrease that amount of inversion about the midfoot and ankle while being less cumbersome than a walking boot or cast. However, the lace-up ankle brace is less effective at limiting the excursion of the PTT compared to the walking boot or cast.
- Nonsteroidal anti-inflammatory medications are used alone or in conjunction with other treatment modalities to manage inflammation and pain.
- Corticosteroid injections within the PTT sheath are contraindicated and can weaken or rupture the tendon, leading to further deformity and pain.[28]
- Physical therapy includes stretching, strengthening, and therapeutic modalities.
- Stretching a tight heel cord or gastrocnemius contracture will improve the hindfoot valgus deformity, alleviating the stress placed on the PTT.
- Strengthening the PTT aids in inversion power of the midfoot during gait and also helps support the static restraints of the medial longitudinal arch (spring ligament). However, vigorous strengthening exercises should be avoided until pain and swelling associated with PTT deficiency is controlled or alleviated.
- Therapeutic modalities such as ultrasound, phonophoresis, transcutaneous neuromuscular stimulation, iontophoresis, and cryotherapy aid to control inflammation and pain.
- There are several orthotic devices made to correct foot deformities associated with PTT dysfunction or to stabilize the affected joint alleviating symptoms.
  - For mild deformities, such as stage I disease, a semirigid orthotic with a ¼-inch medial heel wedge and medial posting can help alleviate the tension on the PTT and spring ligament.
  - The University of California Biomechanical Laboratory (UCBL) brace is commonly employed in patients with flexible but more advanced deformities, such as stage II disease. The UCBL brace aims to reestablish the medial longitudinal arch by holding the hindfoot in neutral and preventing forefoot abduction.[24]
  - Another orthotic option includes the cross ankle brace or more formally known as the *Arizona brace* **(FIG 3B)**.

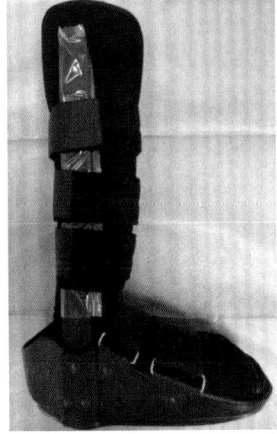 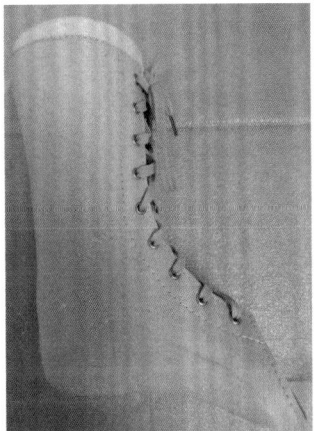 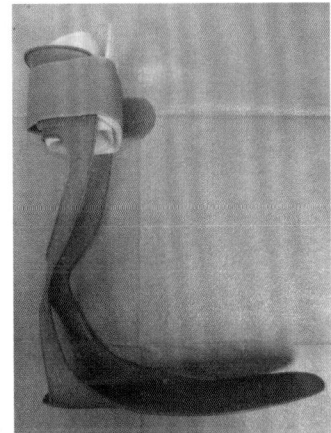

FIG 3 A. Fixed ankle support device. **B.** Arizona brace. **C.** AFO.

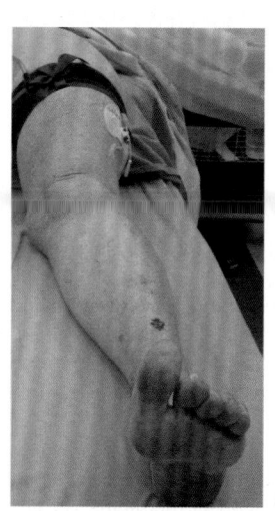

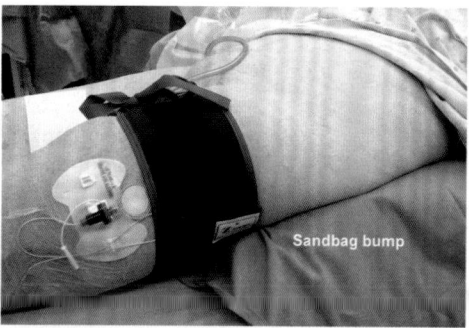

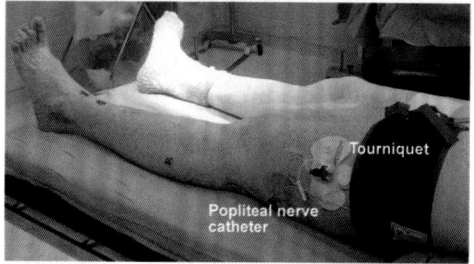

FIG 4 A,B. The patient is positioned supine on the operating table with a tourniquet secured to ipsilateral thigh and a bump beneath it. **C.** Placement of popliteal nerve catheter.

This brace does not correct hindfoot valgus deformity; however, it does reestablish the medial longitudinal arch. This brace has been used for stage I to III PTT deficiency; however, because of its cumbersome nature, its compliance in stage I and II disease is poor.[3]

- For fixed deformities, stage III PTT deficiency, an articulating ankle–foot orthosis (AFO) may be used for pain relief. However, because this deformity is fixed, the AFO will not correct any hindfoot or forefoot deformities.
- In stage IV deformity, which includes ankle valgus deformity and arthritis, a nonarticulating AFO is used for comfort and pain relief **(FIG 3C)**.

SURGICAL MANAGEMENT

Preoperative Planning

- The surgeon should obtain and review appropriate bilateral weight-bearing foot and ankle radiographs, assess comorbidities, and whether adjunctive procedures are needed.
- The surgeon should decide whether to use tricortical iliac crest allograft, tricortical iliac crest autograft, or tantalum wedges for the lateral column lengthening.

- The surgeon should note the presence or absence of calcaneocuboid joint arthritis. Symptomatic calcaneocuboid joint arthritis is an indication to perform the lateral column lengthening through a calcaneocuboid joint distraction arthrodesis.

Positioning

- The patient is positioned in the supine position with a bump underneath the ipsilateral hip, so the toes are perpendicular to the ceiling and with a tourniquet around the ipsilateral thigh **(FIG 4A,B)**.
- Fluoroscope is positioned on the side opposite of the surgical site.
- A popliteal nerve block with or without catheter placement is frequently used to control postoperative pain and decrease narcotic use **(FIG 4C)**.

Approach

- A longitudinal lateral incision is made either centering over the calcaneocuboid joint (calcaneocuboid arthrodesis) or starting at the calcaneocuboid joint and proceed proximally to the sinus tarsi (Evans procedure).
- The lateral malleolus, calcaneocuboid joint, and peroneal tendons are palpated and outlined **(FIG 5)**.

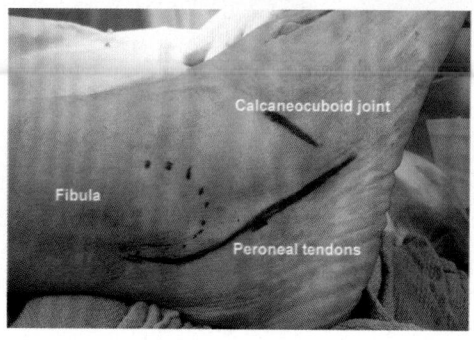

FIG 5 Landmarks for the lateral approach for lateral column lengthening including the distal tip of the fibula, peroneal tendons, and calcaneocuboid joint.

LATERAL COLUMN LENGTHENING VIA ANTERIOR CALCANEUS (EVANS)

Exposure

- Make a standard lateral incision measuring 6 to 8 cm centered over the calcaneocuboid joint and extended proximally to the sinus tarsi **(TECH FIG 1A)**.
- The incision is parallel to the plantar aspect of the foot and perpendicular to the calcaneocuboid joint.
- Identify the sural nerve and peroneal tendons and carefully retract them plantarly **(TECH FIG 1B)**.
- Elevate the extensor digitorum brevis muscle from the anterior process of the calcaneus to expose the superior corner of the calcaneocuboid joint and the sinus tarsi at the angle of Gissane **(TECH FIG 1C)**.
- Place two small Hohmann retractors, one in the sinus tarsi and the other plantar to the anterior calcaneus, after subperiosteal dissection to enhance exposure to the lateral column.

Osteotomy

- Use electrocautery or a marking pen to mark a point on the lateral calcaneus, approximately 13 mm proximal to the superior corner of the calcaneocuboid joint **(TECH FIG 2A)**.
- The osteotomy is performed with a small oscillating saw beginning posterolaterally and aiming slightly anteromedially to avoid the subtalar joint. Irrigation is used to avoid thermal damage to bone.
- Ensure peroneal tendons are retracted plantarly to avoid inadvertent damage with the oscillating saw **(TECH FIG 2B)**.
- Complete the osteotomy with an osteotome, leaving the medial hinge intact **(TECH FIG 2C)**. AP and oblique intraoperative fluoroscopy can be used to make sure the osteotome does not completely break through the medial cortex.

- Place a small lamina spreader in the osteotomy **(TECH FIG 2D)** and gently open until the desired correction of forefoot adduction is achieved.
- Intraoperative fluoroscopic imaging of the foot with the use of a lamina spreader is useful in determining the amount of correction by facilitating visualization of the restoration of the talar head coverage by the navicular on AP view.
- Remove the lamina spreader without changing the amount of "spread" on the lamina; the lamina spreader can be used as a caliper to measure the size of the graft **(TECH FIG 2E)**.
- The distance between the teeth of the lamina determines the graft size **(TECH FIG 2F)**.
- When using allograft, use at least a 15-mm wide iliac crest wedge. Mark the wedge size with a marking pen from the measurements obtained earlier and then carefully cut the block in a "pie" or wedge shape, with the widest side being the cortical side **(TECH FIG 3A,B)**.
- When using autograft bone, use a standard approach to the iliac crest. Avoid the superficial branch of the femoral nerve and make an incision approximately 6 cm long. Expose the anterior iliac crest using subperiosteal dissection and Taylor retractors. Mark the size of the graft from the measurements previously obtained and score the margins with a curved osteotome.
- Cut the block as a pie or wedge in situ or remove a standard block and trim to a pie or wedge on the back table.
- Place block into the lateral column osteotomy and tamp it in securely with a bone tamp and mallet. The graft should be flush with the margins of the osteotomy **(TECH FIG 3C–E)**.
- Use caution to avoid fracturing the graft. The senior authors use a small lamina spreader and place it in the far dorsal edge of the osteotomy to provide distraction. Avoid striking the allograft centrally and rather strike graft on the cortical edges.

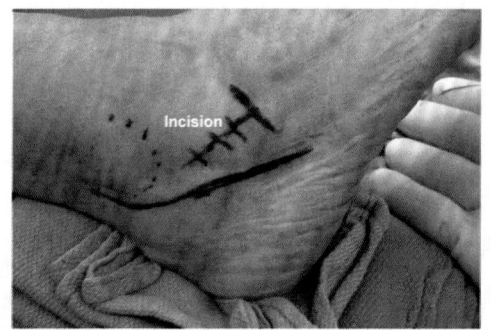
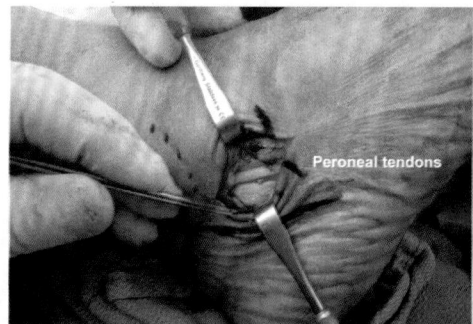
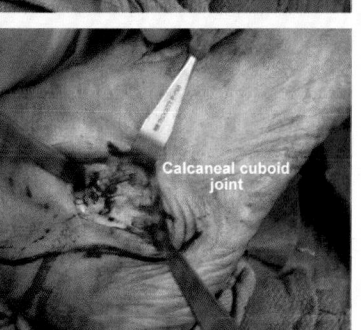

TECH FIG 1 A. Incision site for the lateral approach. **B.** Lateral incision showing exposure of the peroneal tendons. **C.** Elevation of the extensor digitorum brevis and retraction of the peroneal tendons with small Hohmann retractors.

TECHNIQUES

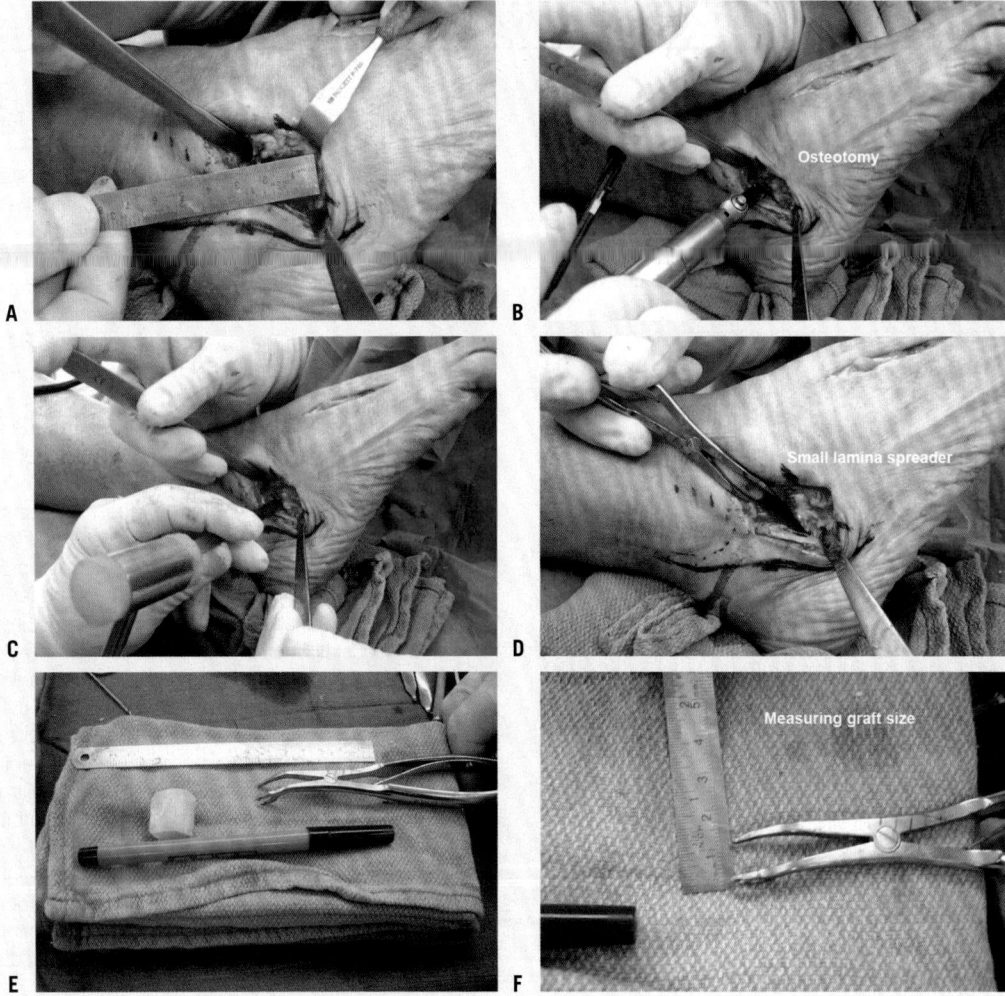

TECH FIG 2 A. Measuring 1.5 to 2.0 cm proximal from the calcaneocuboid joint. **B.** Osteotomy of the anterior os calcis using a small oscillating saw. **C.** Completion of the osteotomy using an osteotome. **D.** Small lamina spreader is used to distract the osteotomy appropriately. **E.** Note the open lamina spreader on the back table to be used as a caliper to measure the bone graft size. **F.** Measuring the distance between the teeth of the lamina spreader for bone graft size.

- Avoid subluxation of the calcaneocuboid joint. Occasionally, the senior authors (DRB, JGA) temporarily fix the calcaneocuboid joint in its anatomic position with a 0.062-inch Kirschner wire before implanting graft.
- Next, secure the graft with a single 3.5-mm fully threaded cortical screw from the anterosuperior corner of the calcaneocuboid joint across the graft into the proximal calcaneus **(TECH FIG 3F–I)**.
- Avoid using a partially threaded screw or placing a screw by lag technique. The additional compression of the lag screw, in combination with the compression provided by the distracted osteotomy, may cause crushing of the graft and a loss of lateral column length.

- Use the additional cancellous allograft or autograft bone to supplement the lateral column osteotomy.
- Check the alignment clinically.
- Use AP and lateral fluoroscopic images to confirm position and restoration of the lateral column height, the talus–first metatarsal angle, and the talonavicular coverage angle **(TECH FIG 3J,K)**.
- Undercorrection to residual deformity or overcorrection to an adductus deformity can be avoided by checking for desired alignment with the lamina spreader in place, before sizing and inserting graft.
- The subcuticular layer of skin is closed using a 3-0 Monocryl suture, and the skin is approximated using a 3-0 nylon suture.

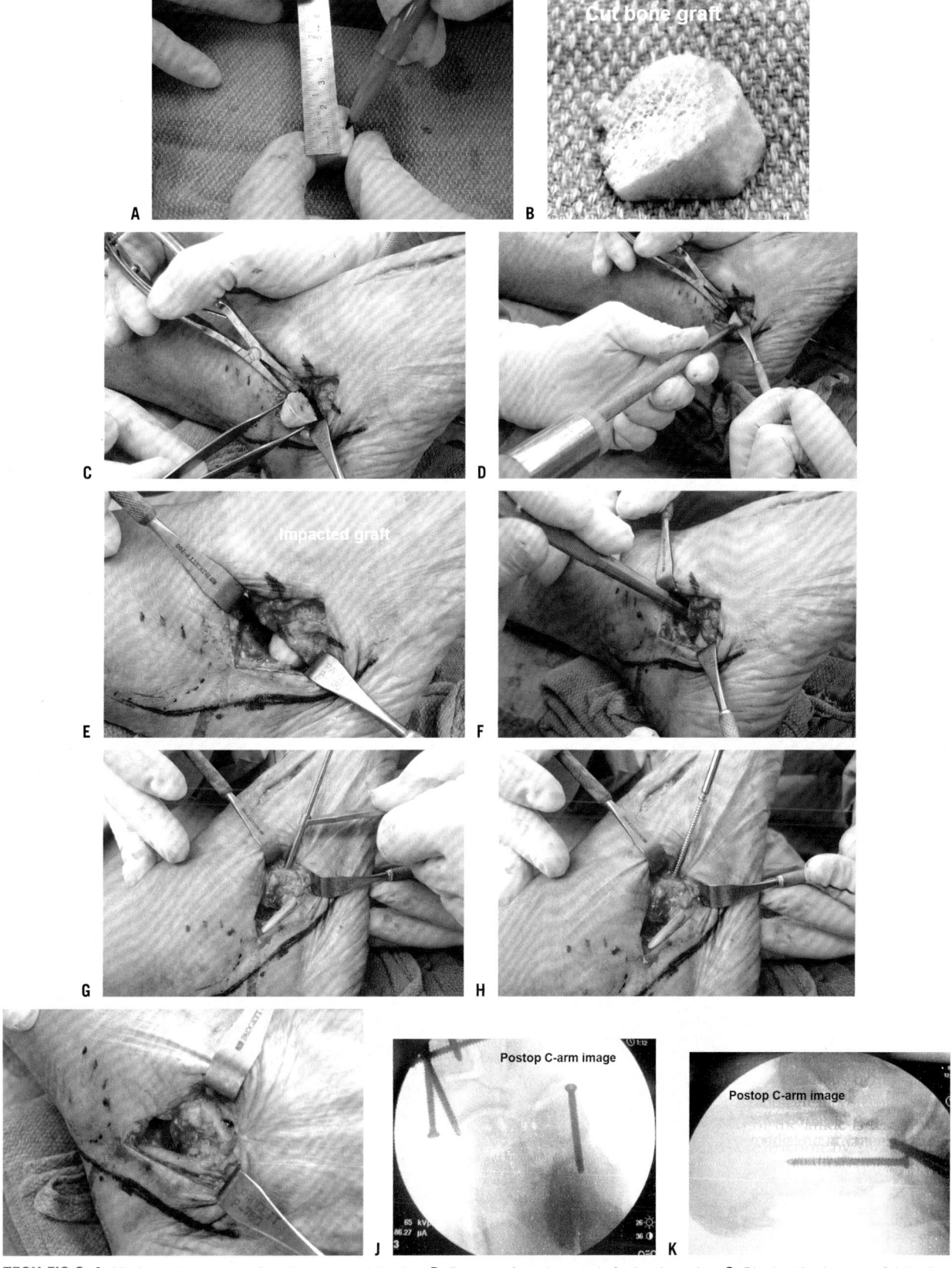

TECH FIG 3 A. Marking the bone graft to the appropriate size. **B.** Bone graft wedge ready for implantation. **C.** Placing the bone graft into the osteotomy site. **D.** Tamping the bone graft into place. **E.** Impacted iliac crest wedge. **F–I.** Securing the graft with a single 3.5-mm screw from the anterosuperior corner of the calcaneocuboid joint through the graft and into the os calcis. **J.** AP C-arm image after procedure to confirm graft and screw position. **K.** Lateral C-arm image.

TECHNIQUES

LATERAL COLUMN LENGTHENING VIA CALCANEOCUBOID JOINT DISTRACTION ARTHRODESIS

Approach

- Approach the calcaneocuboid joint through a standard lateral approach centered over the calcaneocuboid joint and extending a total length of 6 to 8 cm, slightly more distal than the approach for lateral column lengthening via the anterior process of the calcaneus.
- Identify the peroneal tendons and sural nerve and retract them plantarward and elevate the extensor digitorum brevis muscle dorsally.
- Distract the calcaneocuboid joint with a small lamina spreader and remove the articular cartilage from both sides of the joint.
- Drill the subchondral bone with a 2.0-mm drill or a 0.062-inch Kirschner wire to provide vascular channels.
- Distract the calcaneocuboid joint using the small lamina spreader until the desired correction is obtained.
- Check AP and lateral fluoroscopy images with the lamina spreader in place. The AP image confirms that the navicular is reduced on the talar head, and the lateral view confirms that subluxation of the calcaneocuboid joint is avoided.
- Remove the lamina spreader without changing the amount of spread on the lamina, so it can be used as a caliper to measure the size of the graft.
- The distance between the teeth of the lamina determines the graft size.
- When using allograft, use at least a 15-mm wide iliac crest wedge or patellar wedge. Mark the wedge size from the measurement obtained earlier and then carefully cut the block in a pie or wedge shape, with the cortical side widest.
- When using autograft, use a standard approach to the iliac crest, avoiding the superficial branch of the femoral nerve, and make an incision about 6 cm long. Expose the anterior iliac crest using subperiosteal dissection and Taylor retractors. Mark the size of the graft from the measurement previously obtained and score the margins with a curved osteotome. Cut the block as a pie or wedge in situ or remove a standard block and trim it to a pie or wedge on the back table.
- Insert the graft in the calcaneocuboid joint, as flush as possible with the lateral column of the foot, and confirm correction clinically and fluoroscopically.
- Maintain congruent alignment of the cuboid and calcaneus during graft insertion.
- Secure the arthrodesis with a small H plate, cervical plate, or semitubular plate **(TECH FIG 4)**.
- Avoid overcompression and shortening of the lateral column.
- Augment the fusion with further bone graft.
- Check overall clinical correction.
- AP and lateral fluoroscopy images serve to confirm restoration of lateral column height, talus–first metatarsal angle, and dorsolateral peritalar subluxation.
- By checking realignment with the lamina spreader before contouring or inserting the graft, overcorrection to adductus deformity and undercorrection with residual abduction is avoided.
- We routinely close the wound with 3-0 Monocryl and 3-0 nylon.

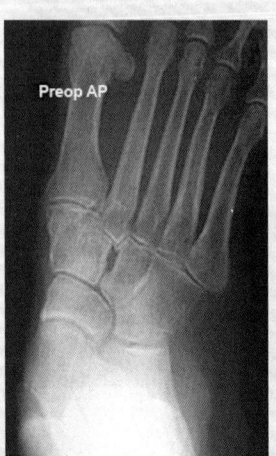

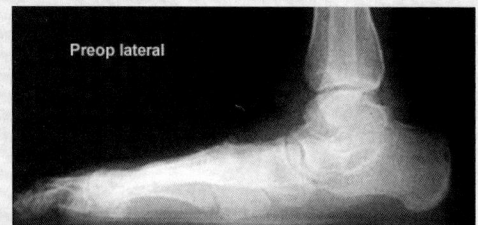

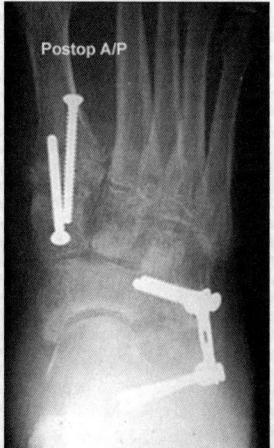

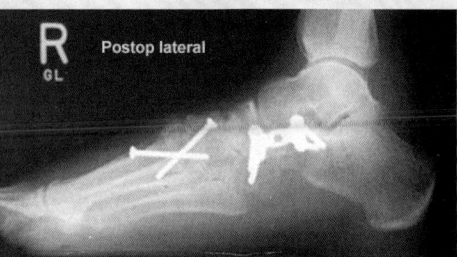

TECH FIG 4 Preoperative AP (**A**) and lateral (**B**) radiographs. Postoperative AP (**C**) and lateral (**D**) radiographs after lateral column lengthening through the calcaneocuboid joint. (Courtesy of Bruce Sangeorzan, MD.)

LATERAL COLUMN LENGTHENING VIA Z CALCANEAL OSTEOTOMY

Exposure

- Make a 5-cm longitudinal incision through the skin centered over the peroneal tubercle with a no. 15 blade scalpel.
- Use tenotomy scissors to dissect through the subcutaneous tissue, taking care to identify the sural nerve.
- Identify the peroneal tendon sheath and carefully open with tenotomy scissors, taking care not to injury the peroneal tendons.
- Retract the peroneal tendons plantarly out of the surgical field using retractors.
- Bluntly dissect the soft tissue more distally so the calcaneocuboid joint can be identified.

Osteotomy

- Start the dorsal limb of the Z osteotomy 1.5 cm from the calcaneocuboid joint and mark with a surgical marking pen **(TECH FIG 5A)**.
- Mark the transverse limb of the Z osteotomy using a pen and starting at the end of the most plantar aspect of the dorsal limb and continue proximally approximately 2.0 cm.
- Finally, mark the plantar limb with a surgical pen and start from the proximal aspect of the transverse limb and proceed to the plantar surface of the calcaneus.
- Retract the peroneal brevis tendon dorsally while the peroneal longus tendon is retracted plantarly, gaining visualization to the transverse limb.
- Using an oscillating saw, initially cut the transverse limb while taking care not to injure any medial structures.
- Retract the peroneal brevis tendon plantarly with the peroneal longus tendon and place a small Hohmann retractor within the sinus tarsi.

- Using the oscillating saw, cut the dorsal limb of the Z osteotomy.
- Retract the peroneal longus and brevis tendons dorsally and place a small Hohmann retractor on the plantar surface of the calcaneus.
- With an oscillating saw, cut the plantar limb of the Z osteotomy.
- A straight osteotome is commonly needed to complete the osteotomy.
- Place a small, smooth lamina spreader in the plantar limb of the Z osteotomy and gently open until the desired correction of forefoot adduction is achieved.
- Intraoperative fluoroscopic imaging of the foot with the lamina spreader in place is useful in determining the amount of correction by appreciating the restoration of the talar head coverage by the navicular on AP view.
- Place trial metal wedges in the dorsal limb of the Z osteotomy for best fit.
- Once the correct wedge size is determined, the appropriately sized graft can be placed into the dorsal limb of the osteotomy **(TECH FIG 5B)**.
- Remove the lamina spreader from the plantar limb. A similar size graft as the dorsal limb can then be placed into the plantar limb **(TECH FIG 5C)**.
- Tantalum, allograft, or autograft wedges can be used for graft placement within the Z osteotomy.
- Often, the compression through the distraction Z osteotomy provides enough stability without further stabilization. However, a plate and screws can be used to secure the graft within the osteotomy.
- The subcuticular layer of skin is closed with a 3-0 Monocryl suture, and the skin edges are approximated with a 3-0 nylon suture.

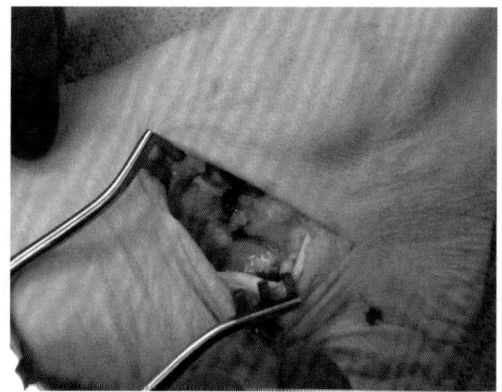
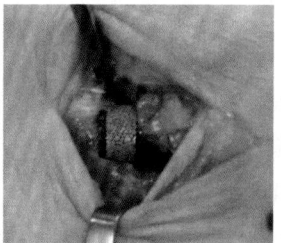
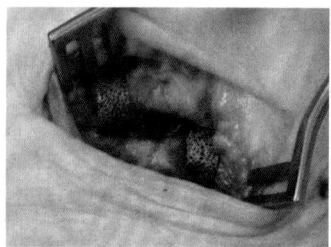

TECH FIG 5 A. Incision showing where dorsal limb of the Z calcaneal osteotomy will be made. **B.** Placement of tantalum wedge in the dorsal limb of Z calcaneal osteotomy. **C.** Placement of tantalum wedge in plantar limb of the osteotomy.

Pearls and Pitfalls

Physical Examination	• Examine the patient in the sitting position with the knee bent and the hindfoot reduced to evaluate Achilles tendon contracture and with the knee straight and the hindfoot reduced to evaluate gastrocnemius contracture. • Watch for the peroneal spastic flatfoot and evaluate appropriately for tarsal coalition. • Evaluate for ipsilateral ankle instability. • Assess the foot for fixed forefoot supination. Even when the hindfoot is supple and can be passively corrected, the forefoot may have compensatory supination that does not correct spontaneously. Lateral column lengthening may correct the hindfoot but could worsen the relative forefoot supination. An adjunctive medial column stabilization procedure to plantarflex the first ray may be necessary (Lapidus procedure or plantarflexion osteotomy of the medial cuneiform).
Approach	• Evaluate and be prepared to treat any concomitant peroneal tendon pathology, such as splits or contracture.
Osteotomy	• Take care not to place the osteotomy too far distal and destabilize the calcaneocuboid joint. • Take care not to place the osteotomy too far proximal and violate the middle or posterior facet of the subtalar joint. • If the calcaneocuboid joint is unstable, secure the joint with a 0.062-inch Kirschner wire before distracting the osteotomy. • Retract the peroneal tendons with a small Lambotte osteotome under the inferior edge of the calcaneus and watch carefully to avoid accidental laceration of the tendons by the oscillating saw. • Angle the fixation screw slightly plantar to avoid placing the screw in the subtalar joint **(FIG 6)**. • Calcaneal osteotomy should be parallel to calcaneocuboid joint and directed from posterolateral to anteromedial to minimize risk of violating middle or posterior subtalar joint facets.[8] • Lateral column lengthening should attempt to redirect proximal aspect of calcaneus medially and plantar. Do not remove the marginal spurs. Rather, the osteophytes are maintained to provide an area to insert a retrograde fixation screw.[29] 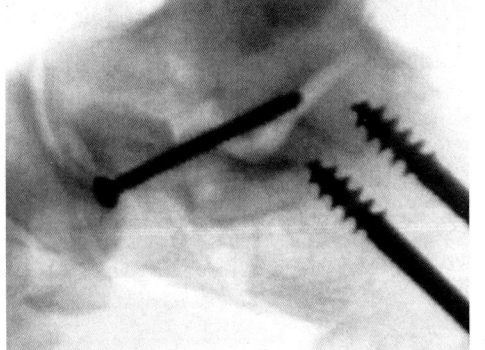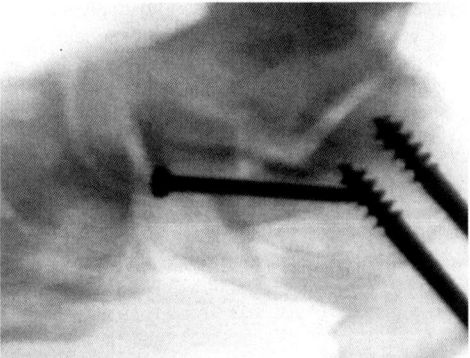 **FIG 6 A.** Misplaced lateral column screw. **B.** Corrected position.
Graft Size	• Graft is usually close to 10 mm. • Ensure that the allograft has been soaked in normal saline for approximately 20 minutes prior to cutting the block to prevent iatrogenic graft fracture. • Dial your correction by placing small lamina spreader (or alternatively trial metal wedges)[15] in the osteotomy and open and close the device to find the appropriate amount of correction.

POSTOPERATIVE CARE

- Patient is placed into a bulky short-leg posterior splint after surgery for 2 weeks.
- At 2 weeks after the date of surgery, the sutures are removed and simulated weight-bearing radiographs (AP, lateral, oblique, and Harris axial heel views) are obtained **(FIG 7)**.
- Patient is placed into a toe-touch weight-bearing short-leg cast.
- At 6 weeks after surgery, the patient is transitioned from a short-leg cast into a fixed ankle support device and allowed to start partial weight bearing. Over the next 4 weeks, the patient is allowed to progress to full weight bearing in the walking boot.
- Physical therapy is initiated working on gait training, strengthening, stretching, and therapeutic modalities.
- Typically, patients are allowed to return to a well-supportive lace-up tennis shoe at 10 weeks postoperatively.

OUTCOMES

- Nonoperative management for mild stage I to II deformity should be attempted first as success has been described in less severe stages of deformity. Nonoperative management consisting of a structured nonoperative protocol (ie, an orthosis, aggressive exercise/stretching with high-repetition exercises, and home regimen) resulted in improved function and satisfaction in nearly 90% of patients with only 11% to 12.5% requiring surgery at approximately 2 years.[1,27]

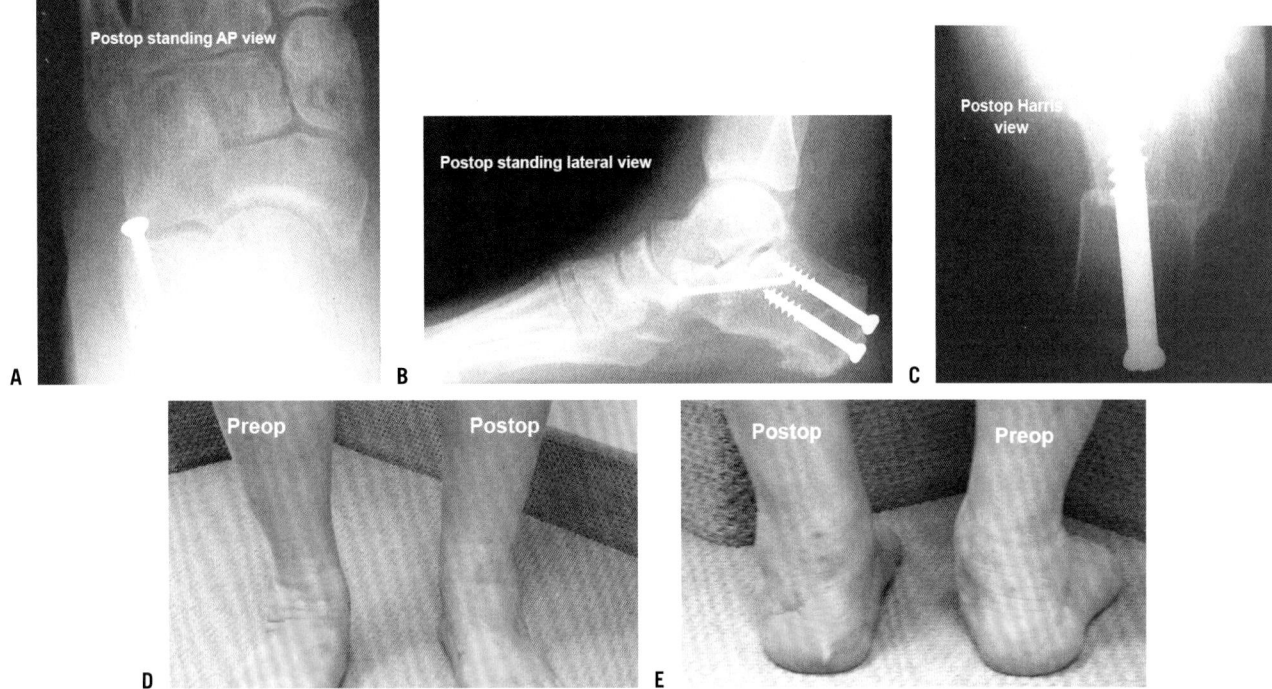

FIG 7 A–C. Postoperative standing AP foot, lateral foot, and Harris view of the os calcis. **D.** Clinical photograph of the patient viewed from the front, comparing the unoperated side with PTT insufficiency and the corrected side. Note the corrected longitudinal height and forefoot abduction. **E.** Clinical photograph of the patient viewed from behind, comparing the unoperated side with PTT insufficiency and the corrected side. Note the corrected hindfoot valgus and the absence of a too many toes sign.

- Although there are four primary radiographic parameters of forefoot abduction may be measured: talonavicular coverage angle,[25,39] talonavicular uncoverage percentage,[13,17] talus–first metatarsal angle,[25] and lateral incongruency angle,[17] the literature is controversial with respect to most accurate and predictive measure for preoperative and postoperative forefoot measurement for identifying necessary graft size for lateral column lengthening.[9,16,43,46]
- Studies have demonstrated less postoperative morbidity, higher or equal union rates, and lower complication rates using tricortical iliac crest allograft bone for lateral column lengthening in adult acquired flatfoot deformity when compared to autograft bone.[14,20,34]
- A cadaveric study demonstrated that using a starting point of 1.3 cm proximal to the calcaneocuboid joint and directed slightly posterolateral to anteromedial avoided violating the sustentaculum tali and anterior and middle facet more often than performing an Evans osteotomy perpendicular to the plantar surface of the foot.[8,23]
- Lateral column lengthening provides greater correction of the medial longitudinal arch, including talonavicular coverage angle and lateral talus–first metatarsal angle, than a medial displacement calcaneal osteotomy alone. However, after lateral column lengthening, the nonunion rate and radiographic progression of degenerative joint disease of the calcaneocuboid joint was more common.[7,45]
- In a recent retrospective case series, it was determined that a combination of medial displacement calcaneal osteotomy and lateral column lengthening procedures resulted in greater improvement in lateral talus–first metatarsal angle and talonavicular coverage angle compared to performing a medial displacement calcaneal osteotomy alone.[25,38]

- A single retrospective case series suggested faster healing times and fewer nonunions, similar outcomes scores, and equivalent correction of deformity with step cut lengthening calcaneal osteotomy compared to traditional Evans osteotomy for lateral column lengthening.[41]
- The Evans lateral column lengthening and calcaneal distraction arthrodesis can lead to pain and increased lateral column pressure secondary to forefoot supination. A Cotton (plantarflexion) first metatarsal osteotomy or first tarsometatarsal joint arthrodesis may need to be added to correct forefoot supination.[16,43,46]
- Lengthening of the lateral column through the calcaneus may increase calcaneocuboid contact pressure[10] and potentiate or accelerate arthrosis developing in the adjacent calcaneocuboid joint.[37]
- Although lateral column pain is a known complication following correction of the painful flexible flatfoot deformity correction, there is little clinical evidence to demonstrate a difference in lateral column pain following deformity correction with or without lateral column lengthening.[44]
- Increased lateral column lengthening greater than 6 to 8 mm can lead to lateral column pressures greater than those of a plantigrade foot, causing lateral column overload and lateral foot pain.[36,47]
- There is no difference in ankle and subtalar motion following Evans lateral column lengthening compared to calcaneal distraction arthrodesis.[5]
- Arthrodesis of the calcaneocuboid joint has no impact on subtalar joint motion and decreases talonavicular joint motion by one-third.[2]
- Although review of the literature fails to provide any consistent preoperative predictors of length of lateral column

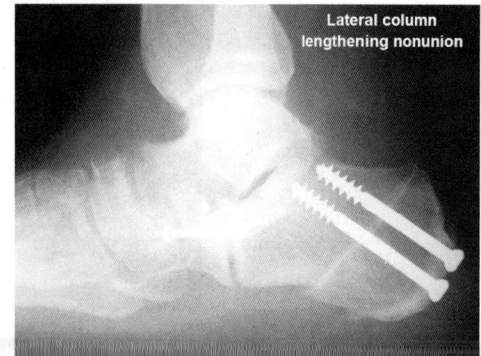
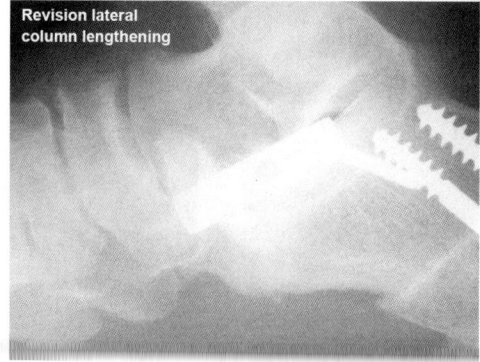

FIG 8 A. Radiograph of late graft nonunion and hardware failure. **B.** Radiograph showing healed revision with plate fixation.

lengthening necessary, two small case series reported that (1) a 1 mm lateral column lengthening corrects the forefoot abduction deformity by 1 degree[42] and (2) corresponds to a 6.8-degree change in lateral congruency angle.[9]

- There is cadaveric evidence that graft shape had no effect on the correction of talonavicular abduction or dorsiflexion but does influence coronal plane motion and forefoot loading mechanics suggesting that a graft with a larger taper may lower the incidence of lateralized forefoot pressure following correction.[4]
- In the pediatric population, a retrospective comparative study suggests that lateral column lengthening through the neck of the calcaneus may provide a more durable correction than lengthening with calcaneocuboid joint fusion (29.3% vs. 0% collapse).[11]
- In cadaveric models, tightening of the plantar fascia did not occur with lateral column lengthening (or medial calcaneal displacement osteotomy).[22]
- Porous titanium wedges in lateral column lengthening can achieve good radiographic and clinical correction of adult-acquired flatfoot deformity with a low rate of nonunion and other complications.[30,31]
- We recommend against lateral column lengthening through the cuboid until higher level of evidence is available.[48]

COMPLICATIONS

- Nonunion **(FIG 8)** or malunion
- Graft fracture or displacement
- Painful retained deep hardware
- Undercorrection or overcorrection
- Peroneal tendon irritation or injury
- Sural nerve irritation or injury
- Lateral column overload and pain
- Calcaneocuboid degenerative joint disease

REFERENCES

1. Alvarez RG, Marini A, Schmitt C, et al. Stage I and II posterior tibial tendon dysfunction treated by a structured nonoperative management protocol: an orthosis and exercise program. Foot Ankle Int 2006;27(1):2–8.
2. Astion DJ, Deland JT, Otis JC, et al. Motion of the hindfoot after simulated arthrodesis. J Bone Joint Surg Am 1997;79(2):241–246.
3. Augustin JF, Lin SS, Berberian WS, et al. Nonoperative treatment of adult acquired flat foot with the Arizona brace. Foot Ankle Clin 2003;8(3):491–502.
4. Baxter JR, Demetracopoulos CA, Prado MP, et al. Graft shape affects midfoot correction and forefoot loading mechanics in lateral column lengthening osteotomies. Foot Ankle Int 2014;35(11):1192–1199.
5. Beimers L, Louwerens JW, Tuijthof GJ, et al. CT measurement of range of motion of ankle and subtalar joints following two lateral column lengthening procedures. Foot Ankle Int 2012;33(5):386–393.
6. Bluman EM, Title CI, Myerson MS. Posterior tibial tendon rupture: a refined classification system. Foot Ankle Clin 2007;12(2):233–249, v.
7. Bolt PM, Coy S, Toolan BC. A comparison of lateral column lengthening and medial translational osteotomy of the calcaneus for the reconstruction of adult acquired flatfoot. Foot Ankle Int 2007;28(11):1115–1123.
8. Bussewitz BW, DeVries JG, Hyer CF. Evans osteotomy and risk to subtalar joint articular facets and sustentaculum tali: a cadaver study. J Foot Ankle Surg 2013;52(5):594–597.
9. Chan JY, Greenfield ST, Soukup DS, et al. Contribution of lateral column lengthening to correction of forefoot abduction in stage IIb adult acquired flatfoot deformity reconstruction. Foot Ankle Int 2015;36(12):1400–1411.
10. Cooper PS, Nowak MD, Shaer J. Calcaneocuboid joint pressures with lateral column lengthening (Evans) procedure. Foot Ankle Int 1997;18(4):199–205.
11. Danko AM, Allen B, Pugh L, et al. Early graft failure in lateral column lengthening. J Pediatr Orthop 2004;24(6):716–720.
12. Deland JT, de Asla RJ, Sung IH, et al. Posterior tibial tendon insufficiency: which ligaments are involved? Foot Ankle Int 2005;26(6):427–435.
13. Deland JT, Page A, Sung I-H, et al. Posterior tibial tendon insufficiency results at different stages. HSS J 2006;2(2):157–160.
14. Dolan CM, Henning JA, Anderson JG, et al. Randomized prospective study comparing tri-cortical iliac crest autograft to allograft in the lateral column lengthening component for operative correction of adult acquired flatfoot deformity. Foot Ankle Int 2007;28(1):8–12.
15. Ellis SJ, Williams BR, Garg R, et al. Incidence of plantar lateral foot pain before and after the use of trial metal wedges in lateral column lengthening. Foot Ankle Int 2011;32(7):665–673.
16. Ellis SJ, Yu JC, Johnson AH, et al. Plantar pressures in patients with and without lateral foot pain after lateral column lengthening. J Bone Joint Surg Am 2010;92(1):81–91.
17. Ellis SJ, Yu JC, Williams BR, et al. New radiographic parameters assessing forefoot abduction in the adult acquired flatfoot deformity. Foot Ankle Int 2009;30(12):1168–1176.
18. Evans D. Relapsed club foot. J Bone Joint Surg Br 1961;43(4):722–733.
19. Foster JR, McAlister JE, Peterson KS, et al. Union rates and complications of lateral column lengthening using the interposition plating technique: a radiographic and medical record review. J Foot Ankle Surg 2017;56(2):247–251.
20. Grier KM, Walling AK. The use of tricortical autograft versus allograft in lateral column lengthening for adult acquired flatfoot deformity: an analysis of union rates and complications. Foot Ankle Int 2010;31(9):760–769.

21. Hansen SJ. Functional Reconstruction of the Foot and Ankle. Philadelphia: Lippincott Williams & Wilkins, 2000.
22. Horton GA, Myerson MS, Parks BG, et al. Effect of calcaneal osteotomy and lateral column lengthening on the plantar fascia: a biomechanical investigation. Foot Ankle Int 1998;19(6):370–373.
23. Hyer CF, Lee T, Block AJ, et al. Evaluation of the anterior and middle talocalcaneal articular facets and the Evans osteotomy. J Foot Ankle Surg 2002;41(6):389–393.
24. Imhauser CW, Abidi NA, Frankel DZ, et al. Biomechanical evaluation of the efficacy of external stabilizers in the conservative treatment of acquired flatfoot deformity. Foot Ankle Int 2002;23(8):727–737.
25. Iossi M, Johnson JE, McCormick JJ, et al. Short-term radiographic analysis of operative correction of adult acquired flatfoot deformity. Foot Ankle Int 2013;34(6):781–791.
26. Johnson KA, Strom DE. Tibialis posterior tendon dysfunction. Clin Orthop Relat Res 1989(239):196–206.
27. Kulig K, Reischl SF, Pomrantz AB, et al. Nonsurgical management of posterior tibial tendon dysfunction with orthoses and resistive exercise: a randomized controlled trial. Phys Ther 2009;89(1):26–37.
28. Mann RA. Adult acquired flatfoot deformity. Treatment of dysfunction of the posterior tibial tendon. J Bone Joint Surg Am 1997;79(9):1434.
29. Manoli A. Remodeling of the calcaneocuboid joint in the acquired flatfoot. J Surg Orthop Adv 2018;27(3):237–245.
30. Matthews M, Cook EA, Cook J, et al. Long-term outcomes of corrective osteotomies using porous titanium wedges for flexible flatfoot deformity correction. J Foot Ankle Surg 2018;57(5):924–930.
31. Moore SH, Carstensen SE, Burrus MT, et al. Porous titanium wedges in lateral column lengthening for adult-acquired flatfoot deformity. Foot Ankle Spec 2018;11(4):347–356.
32. Moseir-LaClair S, Pomeroy G, Manoli A II. Intermediate follow-up on the double osteotomy and tendon transfer procedure for stage II posterior tibial tendon insufficiency. Foot Ankle Int 2001;22(4):283–291.
33. Mosier-LaClair S, Pomeroy G, Manoli A II. Operative treatment of the difficult stage 2 adult acquired flatfoot deformity. Foot Ankle Clin 2001;6(1):95–119.
34. Müller SA, Barg A, Vavken P, et al. Autograft versus sterilized allograft for lateral calcaneal lengthening osteotomies: comparison of 50 patients. Medicine (Baltimore) 2016;95(30):e4343.
35. Myerson MS. Adult acquired flatfoot deformity: treatment of dysfunction of the posterior tibial tendon. Instr Course Lect 1997;46:393–405.
36. Oh I, Imhauser C, Choi D, et al. Sensitivity of plantar pressure and talonavicular alignment to lateral column lengthening in flatfoot reconstruction. J Bone Joint Surg Am 2013;95(12):1094–1100.
37. Phillips GE. A review of elongation of os calcis for flat feet. J Bone Joint Surg Br 1983;65(1):15–18.
38. Ruffilli A, Traina F, Giannini S, et al. Surgical treatment of stage II posterior tibialis tendon dysfunction: ten-year clinical and radiographic results. Eur J Orthop Surg Traumatol 2018;28(1):139–145.
39. Sangeorzan BJ, Mosca V, Hansen ST. Effect of calcaneal lengthening on relationships among the hindfoot, midfoot, and forefoot. Foot Ankle 1993;14(3):136–141.
40. Sarrafian S. Anatomy of the Foot and Ankle. Philadelphia: JB Lippincott, 1983:217–219.
41. Saunders SM, Ellis SJ, Demetracopoulos CA, et al. Comparative outcomes between step-cut lengthening calcaneal osteotomy vs traditional Evans osteotomy for stage IIB adult-acquired flatfoot deformity. Foot Ankle Int 2018;39(1):18–27.
42. Saxena A. Evans calcaneal osteotomy. J Foot Ankle Surg 2000;39(2):136–137.
43. Scott AT, Hendry TM, Iaquinto JM, et al. Plantar pressure analysis in cadaver feet after bony procedures commonly used in the treatment of stage II posterior tibial tendon insufficiency. Foot Ankle Int 2007;28(11):1143–1153.
44. Tellisi N, Lobo M, O'Malley M, et al. Functional outcome after surgical reconstruction of posterior tibial tendon insufficiency in patients under 50 years. Foot Ankle Int 2008;29(12):1179–1183.
45. Thomas RL, Wells BC, Garrison RL, et al. Preliminary results comparing two methods of lateral column lengthening. Foot Ankle Int 2001;22(2):107–119.
46. Tien TR, Parks BG, Guyton GP. Plantar pressures in the forefoot after lateral column lengthening: a cadaver study comparing the Evans osteotomy and calcaneocuboid fusion. Foot Ankle Int 2005;26(7):520–525.
47. Xia J, Zhang P, Yang Y-F, et al. Biomechanical analysis of the calcaneocuboid joint pressure after sequential lengthening of the lateral column. Foot Ankle Int 2013;34(2):261–266.
48. Zhou H, Ren H, Li C, et al. Biomechanical analysis of cuboid osteotomy lateral column lengthening for stage II B adult-acquired flatfoot deformity: a cadaveric study. Biomed Res Int 2017;2017:4383981.

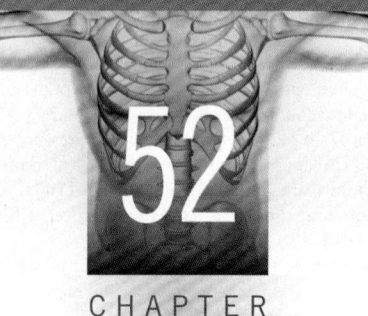
Spring Ligament Reconstruction

Jonathan T. Deland

DEFINITION

- Spring ligament failure consists of lengthening or disruption of the spring ligament complex resulting in subluxation at the talonavicular joint.
- Spring ligament failure is commonly associated with considerable degeneration of the ligament. The ligament complex may have tears or large defects, or it may just be attenuated.
- Tears most commonly occur in the superomedial portion of the spring ligament complex, adjacent to the posterior tibial tendon, but can occur in the inferior portion as well.
- It is necessary to look at the alignment of the foot to determine how to treat failure in the spring ligament. If a flatfoot is present with increased heel valgus or abduction (or both) through the midfoot and there is a full tear of more than 30% of the ligament or severe attenuation, the risk of progression of deformity is high.

ANATOMY

- The spring ligament is actually a complex of ligaments composed primarily of a superomedial portion and an inferior portion. The deltoid ligament blends in with the superomedial portion.[1]
- The superomedial portion is medial to the posterior tibial tendon. It originates from the superomedial aspect of the sustentaculum tali and the anterior facet of the calcaneus to insert on the medial navicular adjacent to its articular surface (**FIG 1A**).
- The inferior portion originates from the notch between the anterior and medial calcaneal facets. It inserts on the inferior surface of the midnavicular, just lateral to the insertion of the superomedial portion of the spring ligament (**FIG 1B**).
- Because of location, failure of the superomedial portion results in primarily medial migration of the talar head, whereas that of the inferior portion results in primarily plantar migration. Most commonly, the migration is both medial and plantar (**FIG 2**).

PATHOGENESIS

- Spring ligament failure is usually due to the repetitive stresses of a flatfoot causing increased strain on the medial ligaments of the foot.

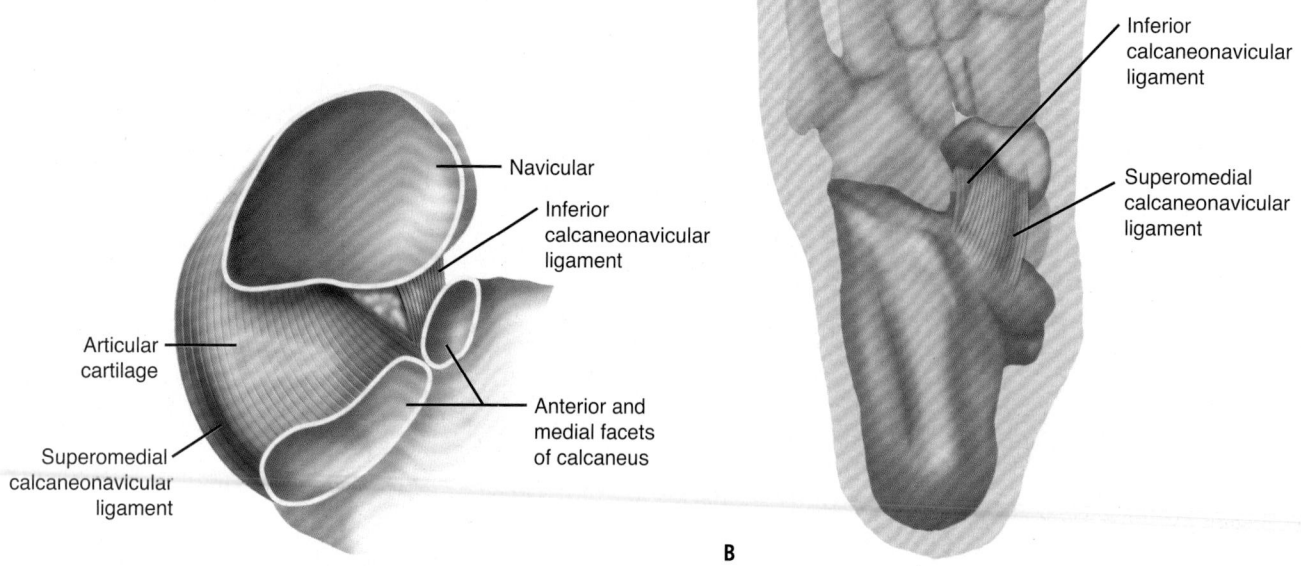

FIG 1 A. Anatomy of the spring ligament complex (dorsal view with talar head removed). Note the location of the superomedial and inferomedial positions. The superomedial portion is medial to the posterior tibial tendon. It originates from the superomedial aspect of the sustentaculum tali and anterior facet of the calcaneus to insert on the medial navicular adjacent to its articular surface. **B.** Anatomy of the spring ligament complex seen from the plantar view. The inferior portion originates from the notch between the anterior and medial calcaneal facets. It inserts on the inferior surface of the midnavicular, just lateral to the insertion of the superomedial portion of the spring ligament.

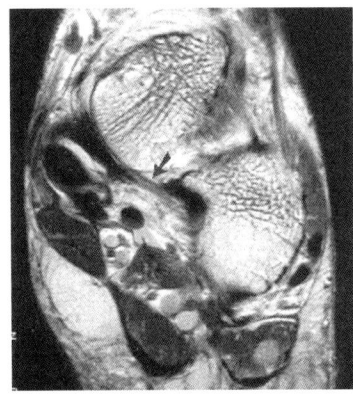

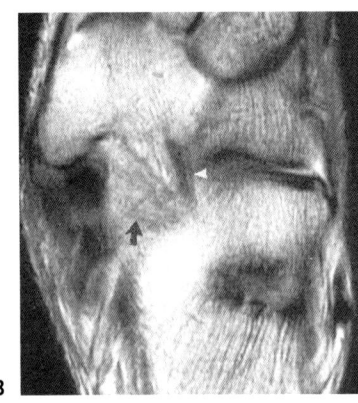

FIG 2 Because of its location, failure of the superomedial portion should result in primarily medial migration of the talar head, whereas failure of the inferior portion results in primarily plantar migration. Most commonly, the migration is both medial and plantar. **A.** MRI scan with severe degeneration and attenuation (grade III/IV) of the superomedial portion of the spring ligament complex. **B.** MRI with a severely frayed and degenerated (grade IV/IV) plantar portion of the spring ligament complex.

- Failure most often occurs in the setting of a degenerated ligament, but it can be associated with an acute episode.
- Although spring ligament failure is associated with a preexisting flatfoot, once spring ligament failure occurs, it frequently results in progressive deformity of the foot at the talonavicular joint and hindfoot. Because the foot progresses out from under the talar head dorsally and laterally, the talar head migrates medially and plantarly in relation to the rest of the foot.

NATURAL HISTORY

- Failure of the spring ligament complex most commonly occurs along with posterior tibial tendon insufficiency.[3]
- With or without tendon insufficiency, spring ligament failure places the patient at risk for progressive subluxation at the talonavicular joint. If subluxation is already present, progression of the subluxation is highly likely.[4]
- Progressive subluxation at the talonavicular joint eventually can cause enough deformity in the triple joint complex (ie, the talonavicular, calcaneocuboid, and subtalar joints) to result in lateral impingement and pain in the hindfoot, a collapsed foot.

PATIENT HISTORY AND PHYSICAL EXAMINATION

- Patients present with medial pain, which usually is associated with the failure of the posterior tibial tendon rather than the spring ligament. Isolated traumatic injuries to the

spring ligament do occur but are uncommon. Later in the course of the condition, if enough deformity has occurred, pain occurs in the lateral hindfoot from impingement secondary to subluxation in the triple joint complex.
- Depending on the presence and amount of deformity, the patient may or may not notice the weakness or collapse in the arch. Most patients notice some weakness.
- Physical examination should evaluate the posterior tibial tendon and alignment of the foot with the patient letting the arch sag fully when standing.
- The posterior tibial tendon should be palpated for tenderness. Inversion strength should be tested from an everted position to a plantarflexed and inverted position.
- Clinical alignment should be checked for midfoot abduction and height of the arch as noted on the frontal standing view. The degree of heel valgus is assessed from the posterior standing view.
- Physical examination should also include the following steps:
  - Palpate the medial talonavicular joint and posterior tibial tendon to check any tenderness.
  - Tenderness on the tendon indicates tendon involvement and often masks tenderness from a ligament tear.
  - Evaluate range of motion. Compare the arc of motion (maximum eversion to maximum inversion) to the other foot. The arc of motion may be categorized as follows: full, some inversion present, motion only to neutral, or joint contracted in eversion. The joint must be mobile into inversion for tendon repair or reconstruction.
  - Evaluate inversion strength. Start with the foot in eversion and have the patient push against the examiner's hand to inversion and plantarflexion. Do not be misled by combined dorsiflexion and inversion strength, which is from the anterior tibial tendon and muscle.

IMAGING

- The anteroposterior (AP) and lateral foot radiographs should be obtained standing with the patient told to let the arch sag. An AP standing radiograph of the ankle also should be performed to rule out valgus deformity at the ankle joint.
  - On the AP view of the foot, abduction at the talonavicular joint can be measured with the talonavicular uncoverage angle (ie, the amount of talar head not covered by the navicular; **FIG 3A**).
  - On the lateral view, plantar migration of the talar head in relation to the navicular can be checked (**FIG 3B**). The lateral talometatarsal angle, although a useful measurement, includes deformity at the naviculocuneiform and metatarsal–tarsal joints.
  - Radiographs are not diagnostic tools but are helpful in assessing deformity—as long as the patient is standing, letting the arch sag with weight bearing.
- A magnetic resonance imaging (MRI) scan visualizing the spring ligament complex of the ligament tear and amount of degeneration can indicate the amount of degeneration or tear in the complex and is useful for diagnosis if it is of good quality and if it is read by an experienced examiner (see **FIG 2**).

DIFFERENTIAL DIAGNOSIS

- Degeneration or tear of the posterior tibial tendon without spring ligament failure
- Congenital flatfoot

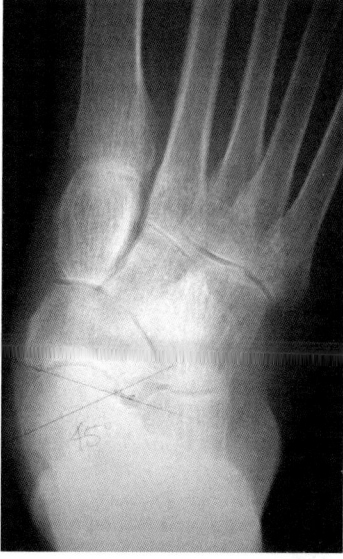

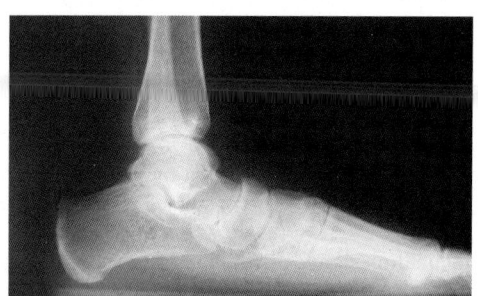

A   B

FIG 3 The lateral and AP radiographic views of the foot should be obtained with the patient standing and told to let the arch sag. **A.** Standing lateral view of the foot showing a flat medial longitudinal arch with an increased talometatarsal angle on the lateral view. **B.** The AP view shows increased uncoverage of the medial talar head. These findings are characteristic—but not diagnostic—of a flatfoot associated with spring ligament pathology. Standing AP radiograph of the ankle also should be performed to rule out valgus deformity at the ankle joint.

NONOPERATIVE MANAGEMENT

- Nonoperative management is particularly appropriate for those patients for whom the tear and alignment are thought to have a low probability of progression. These are patients with no or minimal flatfoot deformity and not a large tear. Conservative treatment may also be used for those patients who wish to delay surgery, but they must be informed of the risk of progression of deformity.
- Nonoperative management consists of support for the medial longitudinal arch with one of the following devices. (They do not at all guarantee stopping the progression of deformity.)
  - A removable boot is helpful for initial management. A medial longitudinal arch support inside the boot is advised.
  - A short, articulated ankle–foot orthosis is less cumbersome and allows ankle motion with a customized arch support.
  - A custom orthotic with a medial longitudinal arch support and medial heel wedge is the least cumbersome but also provides the least support.
  - A solid leather gauntlet or Arizona brace allows minimal motion. It is best for those patients with considerable deformity and limited function.
  - Patients receiving conservative care should be monitored for progression of flatfoot deformity.

SURGICAL MANAGEMENT

- Surgery is the best choice for patients with progression of flatfoot deformity associated with failure of the spring ligament complex or patients whose alignment places them at high risk for progressive deformity.[4]
- Relative contraindications include medical conditions that adversely affect healing such as diabetes, corticosteroid use, and neuropathy.
- Reconstruction of the spring ligament is not useful in those patients with rigid hindfoot deformity and is not necessary in those patients with small tears or good correction of alignment with bony procedures.

Preoperative Planning

- Standing clinical alignment and standing AP and lateral radiographs of the foot and ankle should be carefully reviewed to plan for correction of alignment as well as repair or reconstruction of the spring ligament. A heel alignment (Saltzman view) is also helpful to assess amount of calcaneal valgus.
- Surgeons should be prepared to deal with large tears or significant tissue loss in the spring ligament complex.
  - This will often necessitate the use of tendon graft, most commonly allograft tendon.
  - Possible Achilles contracture should be assessed.
  - Correction of the foot alignment should be considered a critical part of the procedure.
  - Remember that repair or reconstruction of the spring ligament on its own has yet to be shown to correct bony malalignment and that a flatfoot deformity places strain on the spring complex.
  - Alignment correction is achieved by spring ligament reconstruction if osteotomies are performed at the same time and the foot is placed near the corrected position (>50% corrected) by the osteotomies. Although spring ligament reconstruction cannot give correction on its own, it can add correction to what is achieved by the bony procedures.
  - Spring ligament reconstruction is the most logical choice for large tears and is performed along with bony realignment of deformity.[2,5,6]

Positioning

- The patient is placed in the supine position with a bolster under the greater trochanter so that the lower leg is neither internally or externally rotated. This allows good access to both sides of the foot.
- In this position, exposure of the spring ligament, posterior tibial tendon, and lateral hindfoot is possible.

Approach

- A medial incision is made from the tip of the medial malleolus to 2 cm distal to the navicular to inspect the posterior tibial tendon and expose the spring ligament complex by retracting the tendon.
- Lateral hindfoot incisions are used as necessary for calcaneal osteotomies.

PRIMARY SUPEROMEDIAL SPRING LIGAMENT REPAIR

- Primary repair rather than reconstruction is done when good tissue for repair is present and ends can be well apposed. Foot deformity is corrected at the same time by the bony procedures.
- Figure-8 or horizontal mattress sutures are placed to appose both ends of the ligament with the foot in neutral position. Knots are placed to avoid impingement against the posterior tibial tendon **(TECH FIG 1)**.
- If the ligament cannot be apposed with the foot in neutral or the tissue is attenuated, then reconstruction of the ligament is necessary for large tears. The reconstruction is performed together with osteotomies to correct bony alignment.

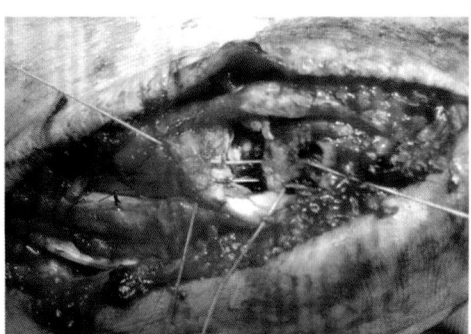

TECH FIG 1 Operative photograph of repair of spring ligament. This repair was accompanied by a medial slide calcaneal osteotomy to address the deformity. Figure-8 or horizontal mattress sutures are placed to appose both ends with the foot in neutral position. Knots are placed to avoid impingement against the posterior tibial tendon.

SUPEROMEDIAL SPRING LIGAMENT RECONSTRUCTION

- Tendon graft is used to replace insufficient ligament tissue and block medial migration of the talar head.
- Achilles or peroneus longus allograft is used most commonly, although peroneus longus autograft can be used if both the longus and brevis are in good condition and overcorrection of bony realignment is avoided.
- Because the superomedial spring ligament blends in with the anterior deltoid ligament, which also can be attenuated, reconstruction of the anterior deltoid and superomedial spring ligaments is commonly performed together **(TECH FIG 2A)**.
- Bone tunnels in the navicular and tibia are used to create a ligament path to support the medial talar head **(TECH FIG 2B)**.

- The navicular tunnel is placed from dorsal to plantar/medial over a cannulated drill. The graft is to exit plantar medially and cross the medial talar head.
- A tibial tunnel beginning at the most inferior midportion of the medial malleolus tip is used.
  - The tibial tunnel exits medially 5 to 9 cm above the ankle joint line.
  - A medial longitudinal incision over the tibia is used to access the medial tibia for drilling of the tunnel.
- Given the size of the foot, the largest drill hole in the navicular is used, so a large tendon graft (6 to 8 mm) is possible.

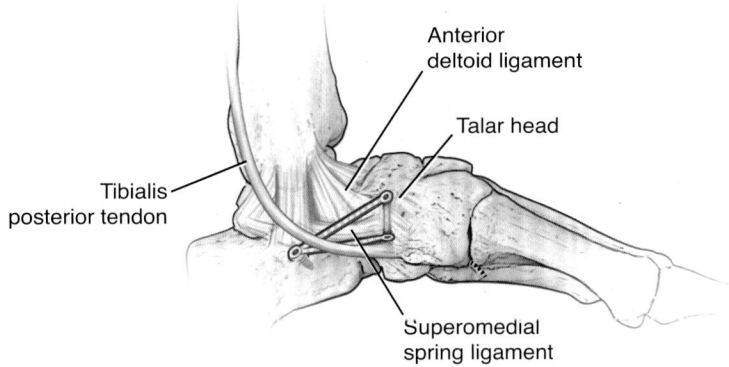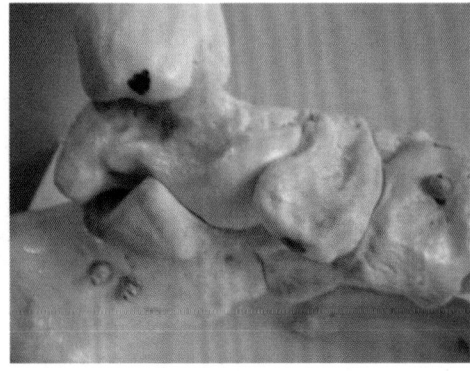

TECH FIG 2 A. Diagram of superomedial spring ligament reconstruction. The repaired ligament crosses the medial aspect of the talar head to block medial migration of the head. **B.** Exit hole of the graft at the inferior navicular and corresponding entrance hole into the tibia at the midportion of the tip of the medial malleolus. The navicular hole is drilled from dorsal to plantar and the tibial hole from the medial malleolus up through the medial tibial metaphysis above the ankle. Bone tunnels in the navicular and tibia are used to create a ligament path to support the medial talar head. Screw placement is not chosen until the graft is tensioned. An alternative to the tibial drill hole is a drill hole to the medial calcaneus at the sustentaculum to fixate the graft at that location after it has passed through the navicular drill hole and then along both the medial and more plantar aspect of the talar head.

- The graft is fixed at the navicular first and tensioned at the proximal exit of the tibial drill hole. The graft is tightened with the talonavicular joint in neutral to slight adduction.
- Fixation of the graft is with whipstitch using no. 2 nonabsorbable suture tied at each end and tied to a dorsal screw in the navicular and a medial screw on the tibial shaft.
  - With the navicular end tied down first, the foot is placed in neutral to slight adduction and the ligament graft tensioned. The screw's position is then chosen such that the graft can be properly tensioned. Tension the graft, place the screw, and then tie down the graft and place the bone graft in the tunnels.

- Alternative fixation is interference screws at the distal tibia, but the fixation may not be as strong with this technique. Placing an interference screw on the navicular risks fracture.
- Spring ligament reconstruction alone cannot be expected to hold correction and should, based on my experience, be used as a supplement to a lateral column lengthening procedure.
- Lateral column lengthening is done to place the talonavicular joint in neutral alignment.
- The lateral column lengthening procedure should allow a minimum of 5 degrees of passive eversion to avoid excessive lateral tightness and adequate eversion motion remaining should be in the operating room by everting the foot.

INFERIOR SPRING LIGAMENT RECONSTRUCTION

- Tendon grafting also is used but for deformity that is primarily plantar migration of the talar head.
- Graft is used to replace attenuated or degenerated tissue in combination with bony procedures to correct flatfoot deformity **(TECH FIG 3A)**.
- Bone tunnels are used in the navicular and calcaneus **(TECH FIG 3B)**.
  - The navicular tunnel is made from dorsal to plantar medial.
  - The calcaneal tunnel is drilled from just underneath the sustentaculum tali and exits out the lateral calcaneus. The lateral exit point is exposed using the standard oblique incision for a posterior calcaneal osteotomy.
  - The graft is fixed first at the navicular, with the foot placed in 5 degrees of inversion with the calcaneus out of

valgus (neutral). A medializing calcaneal osteotomy is commonly performed to address valgus deformity and is fixed before the calcaneal drill hole is made.
- The graft is pulled through the calcaneal tunnel and tensioned with the talus out its plantarflexed position ("slight dorsiflexion"). Temporary pinning of the talonavicular joint can be done in the position described, and the graft is then tensioned and fixed. Fixation of the graft is with nonabsorbable suture sewn into the ends of the graft and tied down to screws in the dorsal navicular and lateral calcaneus. Alternative or supplemental fixation is done with interference screws.
- The calcaneus cannot be left in valgus or excessive strain on the graft will result.

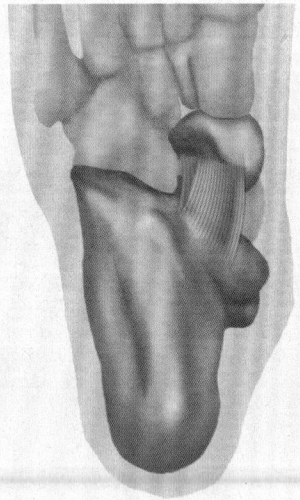

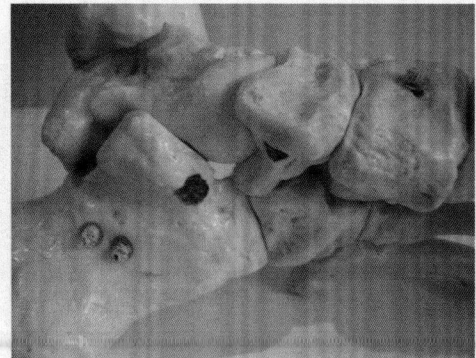

TECH FIG 3 A. Diagram of plantar spring ligament reconstruction with the graft extending from the drill hole in the navicular to the calcaneus. **B.** Navicular exit hole and calcaneal entrance for the graft. A drill hole is made dorsal (dorsal portion not shown) to plantar in the navicular and medial to lateral (not shown) in the calcaneus.

COMBINED SUPEROMEDIAL AND PLANTAR SPRING LIGAMENT RECONSTRUCTION

- Combined superomedial and plantar spring ligament reconstruction is done for patients with considerable abduction of the talonavicular joint and plantar migration of the head.
- Two tendon grafts or a large tendon graft that is split at the plantar medial navicular tunnel is used **(TECH FIG 4B,C)**.
- The navicular tunnel is made as large as possible without fracturing the navicular to enable placement of large grafts. If allograft tendon is used, Achilles allograft with a bone block in the navicular tunnel is suggested **(TECH FIG 4D)**.
- The talonavicular joint is pinned in the corrected position (ie, 5 degrees of inversion and the calcaneus in neutral) after any bony procedures are fixed.

- Depending on the technique, the graft is fixed first at the navicular (split technique) or passed from the first metatarsal to the calcaneus. Once the free ends are passed into the tibia or calcaneus, the final fixation to screw posts is done after tensioning the graft to the screw in the tibia or at the navicular. At the calcaneus, interference screws can be used.
- Reconstruction with combined techniques is intended not to replace bony procedures but to supplement them when considerable tissue loss in the spring ligament complex is noted and correction of bony alignment has been gained at or near neutral position.
  - Commonly, a posterior osteotomy and lateral column lengthening are performed.

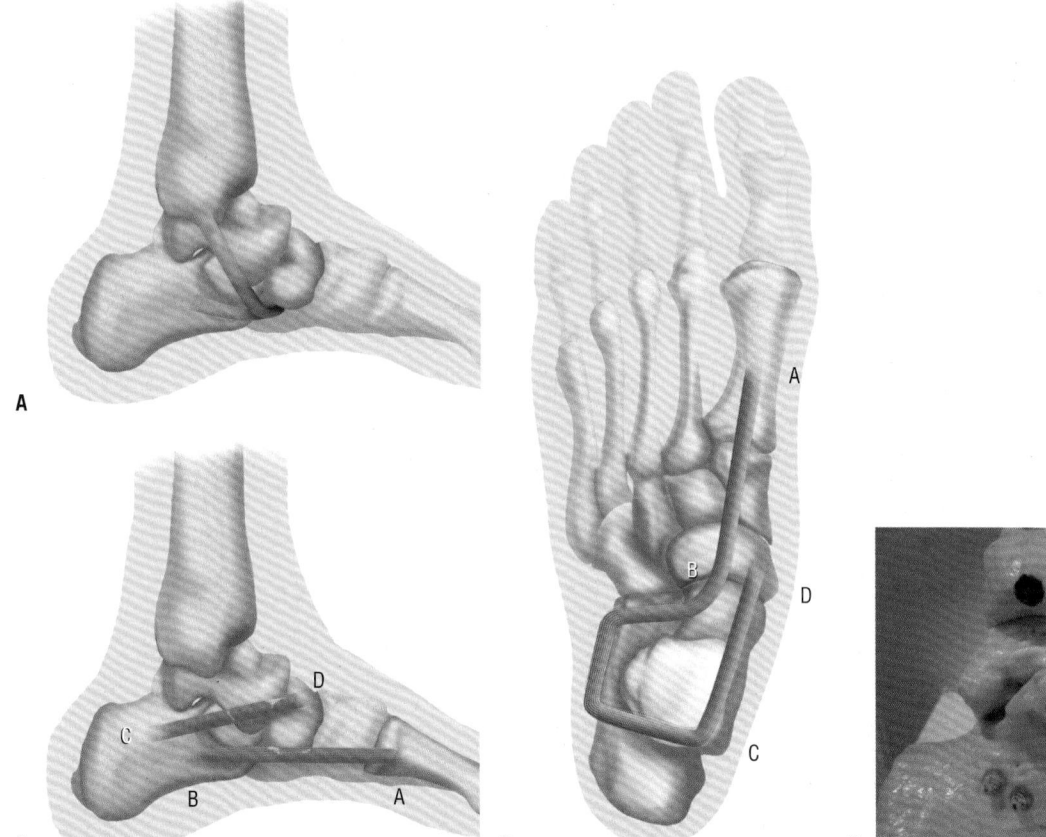

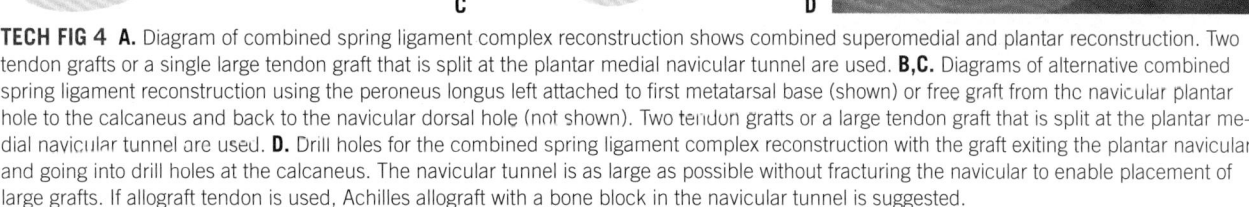

TECH FIG 4 A. Diagram of combined spring ligament complex reconstruction shows combined superomedial and plantar reconstruction. Two tendon grafts or a single large tendon graft that is split at the plantar medial navicular tunnel are used. **B,C.** Diagrams of alternative combined spring ligament reconstruction using the peroneus longus left attached to first metatarsal base (shown) or free graft from the navicular plantar hole to the calcaneus and back to the navicular dorsal hole (not shown). Two tendon grafts or a large tendon graft that is split at the plantar medial navicular tunnel are used. **D.** Drill holes for the combined spring ligament complex reconstruction with the graft exiting the plantar navicular and going into drill holes at the calcaneus. The navicular tunnel is as large as possible without fracturing the navicular to enable placement of large grafts. If allograft tendon is used, Achilles allograft with a bone block in the navicular tunnel is suggested.

Pearls and Pitfalls

Do not expect soft tissue reconstruction to correct bony malalignment.	• The foot must be well aligned without excessive calcaneal valgus (≤5 degrees) and without excessive abduction through the talonavicular joint (<40% uncoverage).
Avoid over- and undercorrection of deformity.	• Correct bony malalignment first. Then, pin or hold the talonavicular joint in neutral position before tensioning the reconstruction.
Do not use lateral column lengthening unless necessary.	• Bony procedures, although necessary to correct malalignment, have morbidity. For lateral column lengthening, good eversion motion should remain after the bony procedures and fixing the tendon grafts.
Avoid weakening of tendon grafts	• Fix bony procedures first to avoid crossing bony tunnels with screws, and use sizers to avoid multiple passage of the tendon grafts in tunnels.
Avoid unnecessary spring ligament reconstruction.	• Small tears and mild to moderate deformity do not necessitate spring ligament reconstruction.

POSTOPERATIVE CARE

- Touchdown weight bearing is allowed at 2 weeks and progressive weight bearing from 8 to 10 weeks.
- In reliable patients, a cast boot can be used instead of a cast beginning at 4 weeks.
- Full weight bearing without a boot is allowed at 12 to 16 weeks.
- Active inversion and eversion can be started at 6 weeks.

OUTCOMES

- Because spring ligament reconstructions are commonly combined with other procedures, it is difficult to define the contribution of these procedures to patient outcomes, and no reports have done so until recently.
- In our experience, spring ligament reconstruction does contribute to correction of deformity but only when most of the correction has been achieved through the bony procedures. I would use the superomedial spring ligament reconstruction for those feet with more of an abduction deformity and the plantar for those with more of a plantar sag deformity at the talonavicular joint. The superomedial may adequately correct combined deformity; if not, use the combined superomedial and spring ligament reconstruction.

COMPLICATIONS

- Failure of the graft can occur, particularly when a soft tissue procedure is used to try to correct large amounts of deformity without adequate bony correction of deformity.

- Failure of fixation of the graft. Interference screws are helpful, but the fit must be tight and tunnels must be made at somewhat of an angle to avoid straight pullout of the graft. Large grafts combined with interference screws are not recommended because of the risk of fracture.
- Overcorrection with lateral weight bearing can occur, either with a medial slide osteotomy or, more commonly, if lateral column lengthening is used. Normal eversion motion should be maintained.
  - The heel should be in alignment with the lower leg (clinically straight), and passive eversion into at least 5 degrees should be present after all the procedures are fixed.
  - The lateral column should not feel tight on range-of-motion testing in the operating room after the bony correction; eversion should be present.

REFERENCES

1. Davis WH, Sobel M, Deland JT, et al. Gross, histological and microvascular anatomy and biomechanical testing of the spring ligament complex. Foot Ankle Int 1996;17:95–102.
2. Deland JT. The adult acquired flatfoot and spring ligament complex. Pathology and implications for treatment. Foot Ankle Clin 2001;6:129–135.
3. Deland JT, de Asla RJ, Sung IH, et al. Posterior tibial tendon insufficiency: which ligaments are involved? Foot Ankle Int 2005;26:427–435.
4. Deland JT, Page A, O'Malley MJ, et al. Posterior tibial tendon insufficiency results at different stages. HSS J 2006;2:157–160.
5. Hiller L, Pinney S. Surgical treatment of acquired adult flatfoot deformity: what is the state of practice among academic foot and ankle surgeons in 2002? Foot Ankle Int 2003;24:701–705.
6. Pinney SJ, Lin SS. Current concept review: acquired adult flatfoot deformity. Foot Ankle Int 2006;27:66–75.

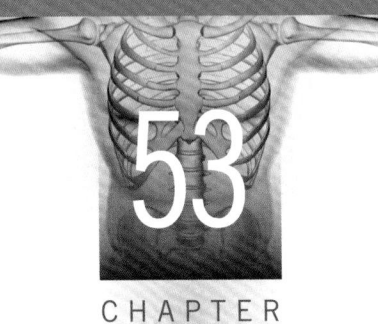

53

CHAPTER

Tarsal Coalition Resection in the Adult Patient

Aaron T. Scott and H. Robert Tuten

DEFINITION

- A tarsal coalition is an abnormal fusion between two adjacent tarsal bones.
- Less than 2% of the general population is affected, and there appears to be no gender or racial predisposition.[2,6,10]
- Nearly 90% of all tarsal coalitions involve either the subtalar joint or the intervening space between the calcaneus and the navicular, with nearly an equal distribution between these two areas.[1]
- Although most calcaneonavicular coalitions are identified in children or adolescents, there does exist a subset of patients who become symptomatic in adulthood.

ANATOMY

- Unlike other tarsal coalitions, the calcaneonavicular coalition forms between two bones that normally do not articulate with each other.
- A calcaneonavicular coalition generally occurs between the anterior process of the calcaneus and the inferolateral aspect of the navicular.
- Histologically, these coalitions may be fibrous, cartilaginous, or osseous in nature and may progress through these stages as the patient matures.

PATHOGENESIS

- Tarsal coalitions are most likely secondary to a failure of segmentation of the primitive mesenchyme.[2,3]
- In adolescents and young adults, the time at which the coalition becomes symptomatic appears to coincide with its ossification.[5]
- Although most coalitions are idiopathic, a dominant trait has been suggested.[10]

NATURAL HISTORY

- The natural history of a calcaneonavicular coalition is one of progressive disability.
- As the coalition ossifies in adolescence, the lack of subtalar range of motion may lead to hindfoot or midfoot pain, recurrent ankle sprains, and difficulty ambulating on uneven surfaces.
- In long-standing coalitions, the increased stresses imposed on the remaining mobile tarsal joints secondary to absent subtalar inversion and eversion may contribute to degenerative arthritic changes elsewhere in the foot.

PATIENT HISTORY AND PHYSICAL FINDINGS

- Symptomatic adults with calcaneonavicular coalitions generally present with hindfoot or midfoot pain, recurrent ankle sprains, or difficulty ambulating on uneven surfaces.
- In contrast to the often insidious onset of symptoms in adolescents with a calcaneonavicular coalition, onset in adults with this condition is abrupt and often coincides with a specific traumatic event, such as a severe ankle sprain.
- Other adults may simply present with a planovalgus foot deformity.
- Physical examination findings consistent with a calcaneonavicular coalition may include the following:
  - Planovalgus foot deformity (rarely, a cavovarus deformity)
  - Decreased or absent subtalar and transverse tarsal joint range of motion
  - Tenderness in the region of the coalition
  - Pain with inversion or eversion of the hindfoot
  - Antalgic gait
  - Instability secondary to multiple ankle sprains (as determined by anterior drawer testing)

IMAGING AND OTHER DIAGNOSTIC STUDIES

- Plain radiographs should be obtained in every patient suspected of having a tarsal coalition and should include anteroposterior, lateral, 45-degree oblique, and axial views of the foot.
- The 45-degree oblique view of the foot is the most useful plain radiograph for identifying a calcaneonavicular coalition. On this oblique view, the coalition may be seen as a discrete bony bridge between the calcaneus and the navicular, or this may simply be suggested by the presence of an extended, narrow beak of bone projecting from the anterior process of the calcaneus in the direction of the navicular (the "anteater sign"; **FIG 1A**).
- An axial view is important because it may aid in the identification of a talocalcaneal coalition.
- Computed tomography (CT) scans should be obtained in all patients preoperatively to rule out a concomitant talocalcaneal coalition and to further evaluate for degenerative changes that may alter the surgical plan **(FIG 1B)**.
- Magnetic resonance imaging may help identify a fibrous or cartilaginous coalition but is not necessary in the workup and treatment of most calcaneonavicular coalitions in adults.

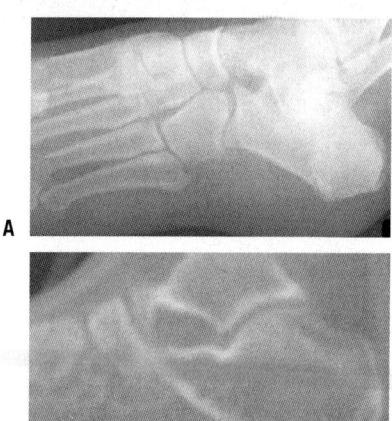

FIG 1 A. A 45-degree oblique radiograph depicting a calcaneonavicular coalition (the anteater sign). **B.** CT showing an isolated calcaneonavicular coalition.

DIFFERENTIAL DIAGNOSIS

- Talocalcaneal (subtalar) coalition
- Trauma or fracture of the hindfoot
- Arthritis (primary osteoarthrosis, posttraumatic arthritis, or inflammatory arthritis)
- Flatfoot secondary to posterior tibial tendon (PTT) insufficiency
- Chronic ankle instability

NONOPERATIVE MANAGEMENT

- Initially, all patients with symptomatic calcaneonavicular coalition should be managed nonoperatively.

- Patients are first treated with nonsteroidal anti-inflammatory medications and custom orthotics that support the medial longitudinal arch.
- The UCBL brace is another orthotic option that acts to limit hindfoot motion.
- If patients fail this early conservative treatment, they are immobilized in a fiberglass short-leg walking cast for 4 to 6 weeks.
- Symptomatic coalitions that are recalcitrant to casting in feet that display no degenerative changes may require surgical resection for relief of symptoms.

SURGICAL MANAGEMENT

- For patients who do not achieve relief with an adequate trial of nonoperative management, surgical intervention is warranted.

Preoperative Planning

- Plain radiographs, as well as CT or magnetic resonance imaging scans, are reviewed.
- All images are evaluated for additional pathology, including concomitant coalitions or degenerative arthritic changes that may alter the surgical treatment plan.

Positioning

- Thirty to 90 minutes before the incision is made, the patient is given an appropriate intravenous antibiotic.
- The patient is placed supine on the operating table, and a bump is placed under the ipsilateral sacrum to internally rotate the foot.
- A pneumatic tourniquet is placed around the upper thigh, and the extremity is prepped and draped in a standard, sterile fashion.

TECHNIQUES

INCISION AND EXPOSURE

- After exsanguination with an Esmarch bandage and inflation of the tourniquet, a standard Ollier incision is created.
- This incision is centered directly over the dorsal aspect of the coalition and extends along a transverse Langer line plantarly to the peroneal tendon sheath and dorsally to the most lateral of the extensor digitorum longus tendons **(TECH FIG 1A)**.
- Preemptive cauterization of any crossing vessels is performed.
- The sural cutaneous nerve and dorsal intermediate branch of the superficial peroneal nerve are identified and protected, as are the peroneal tendons.

- The extensor digitorum brevis muscle is visualized in the depths of the wound and subsequently elevated as a distally based flap using a scalpel and a Cobb elevator, with great care taken to preserve the overlying fascia, which will increase the suture-holding capacity of the flap **(TECH FIG 1B)**.
- The elevated origin of the brevis is then grasped with a modified Mason-Allen stitch using 0 Vicryl **(TECH FIG 1C)**.
- As the flap is retracted distally, the calcaneonavicular coalition is easily identified **(TECH FIG 1D)**.

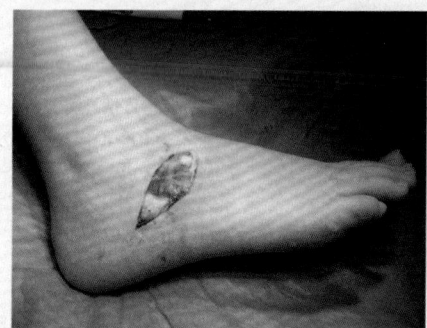
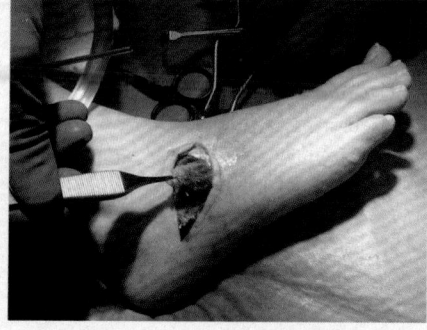

TECH FIG 1 A. Incision. **B.** Elevation of the extensor digitorum brevis flap. *(continued)*

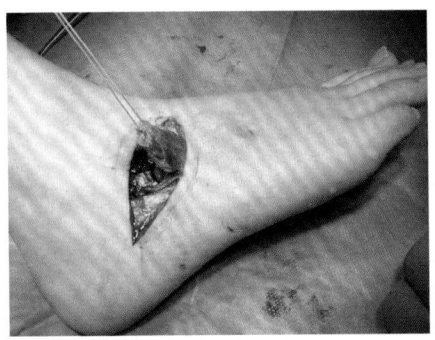
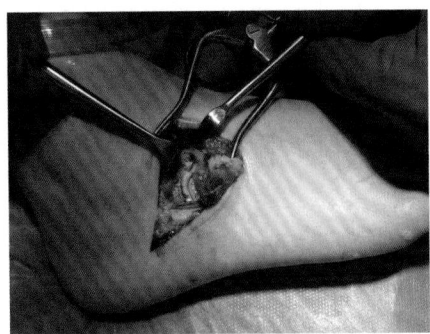

TECH FIG 1 *(continued)* **C.** Grasping of the extensor digitorum brevis with Vicryl suture. **D.** Flap retraction and visualization of calcaneonavicular coalition.

RESECTION OF CALCANEONAVICULAR COALITION WITH INTERPOSITION OF THE EXTENSOR DIGITORUM BREVIS

- After adequate visualization of the coalition, a straight osteotome is used to remove a 1-cm block to include the entire coalition.
- The osteotome cuts are made parallel to prevent the removal of a convergent, trapezoidal block of bone **(TECH FIG 2A)**.
- Any remaining soft tissue within the resection site is cleared with a rongeur.
- The two limbs of the previously placed Vicryl suture attached to the extensor digitorum brevis flap are passed through the void created by coalition resection with the use of a free Keith needle **(TECH FIG 2B)**.
- The tips of the Keith needles should pass just dorsal to the glabrous skin of the medial arch **(TECH FIG 2C)**.
- The two limbs of the Vicryl suture are then tied over a soft dental bolster (no button; **TECH FIG 2D**).

- Alternatively, the raw bony surfaces of the resection site may be covered with bone wax, the void filled with Gelfoam or autologous fat graft, and the brevis reattached to its origin.
- Radiographs are taken to confirm the adequacy of the resection **(TECH FIG 2E)**.
- The wound is thoroughly irrigated, the tourniquet is released, and hemostasis is secured.
- Closure of the wound is performed using 2-0 Vicryl for the deep subcutaneous layer and 4-0 nylon horizontal mattress sutures for the skin **(TECH FIG 2F)**.
- Finally, the wound is covered with a nonadherent dressing, sterile gauze, sterile cast padding, and a short-leg fiberglass walking cast.

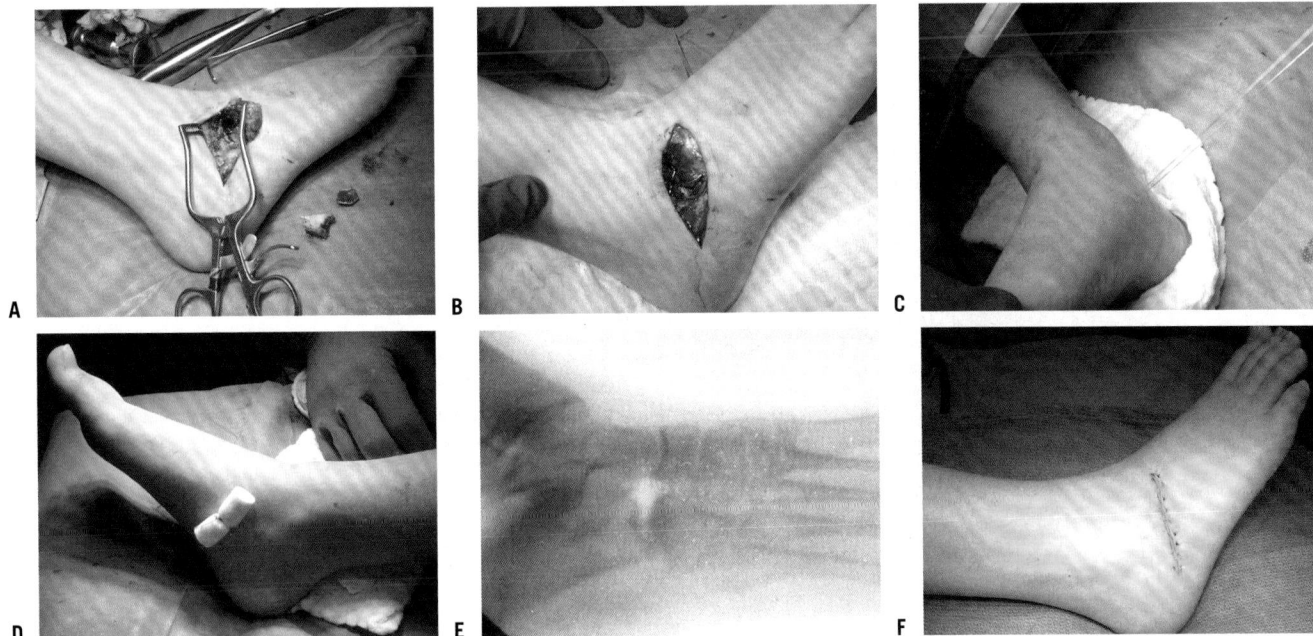

TECH FIG 2 Resection and interposition. **A.** Removal of a rectangular block of bone using parallel osteotome cuts. **B.** Interposition of the extensor digitorum brevis flap into the void created by the resection. **C.** Passage of Keith needles through the skin of the medial arch. **D.** Flap sutures tied over soft dental bolster. **E.** Intraoperative radiographs to confirm the adequacy of the resection. **F.** Wound closure.

CALCANEONAVICULAR COALITION RESECTION (COURTESY OF MARK E. EASLEY, MD)

Exposure

- Make a longitudinal incision from the tip of the fibula toward the base of the fifth metatarsal.
- Identify and protect the sural nerve and peroneal tendons.
- Retract the extensor hallucis brevis (EHB) muscle after carefully releasing its overlying fascia.
  - The fascia may be released where it attaches immediately deep to the peroneal tendons.
- Expose the dorsal aspect of anterior process of calcaneus and lateral navicular (**TECH FIG 3**).
  - Coalition may be bony, cartilaginous, or fibrous.
  - Confirm coalition on intraoperative fluoroscopy; oblique view is most helpful.

Coalition Resection

- Protect the soft tissues.
- Use a chisel to resect medial aspect of coalition, which is the lateral aspect of the navicular (**TECH FIG 4A**).
  - Avoid injury to the lateral talar head.
- Reposition chisel to resect lateral aspect of coalition, which is the anterior process of the calcaneus (**TECH FIG 4B**).
  - Avoid injury to the calcaneocuboid joint.
- Create a wide and congruent resection.
  - Although some convergence of the two resection planes is unavoidable, the two resection planes should be nearly parallel.
  - Converging the resections creates a wedge resection with a wide dorsal base and a narrow plantar aspect that may not allow for full separation of the coalition planes.
  - The resection should be generous but without violating the lateral talar head or the medial calcaneocuboid joint.
  - At the most plantar aspect of the coalition, the planar talar head's articulation with the anterior calcaneal facet should also be protected.

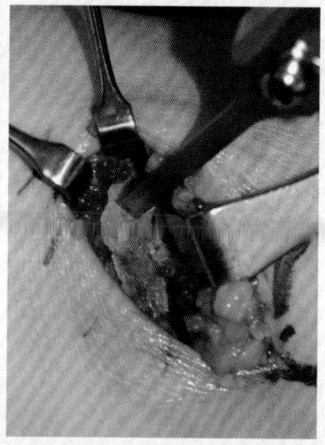

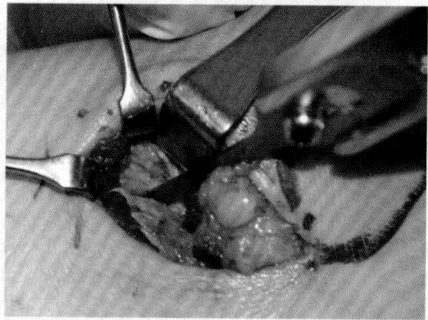

TECH FIG 4 Calcaneonavicular coalition. **A.** Use a chisel to create a resection plane on the lateral aspect on the navicular. **B.** Create the second resection plane on the medial anterior process of the calcaneus. Note that the resection demonstrated here is inadequate and needs to widen with nearly parallel resection planes, creating a trapezoidal or even rectangular resection not a wedge.

Confirm Adequate Resection

- Clinically, hindfoot motion should be reestablished.
- Fluoroscopically, in the oblique plane, there should be a generous gap with complete separation of the navicular from the anterior process of the calcaneus.
  - Also, confirm that no bone fragments remain.

Closure

- Irrigate the wound thoroughly with sterile saline to remove any smaller residual bone fragments (**TECH FIG 5A**).
- Limit bone regrowth into the coalition resection by placing bone wax on both the navicular and calcaneal cancellous (**TECH FIG 5B**).
- The EHB muscle is released from retraction and repositioned in its anatomic position and its overlying fascia is reapproximated if possible.
  - The fascia and muscle may have some damage from retraction, but typically, the fascia may still be reapproximated in a satisfactory manner.
- The subcutaneous layer and skin are carefully closed.

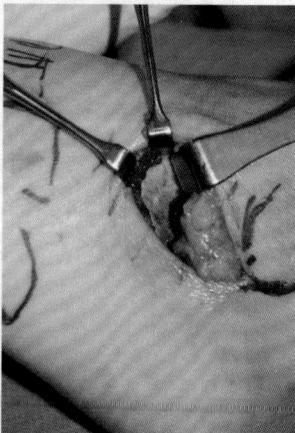

TECH FIG 3 Expose dorsal aspect of anterior process of calcaneus and lateral navicular through a longitudinal incision from the anterior distal fibula toward the base of the fourth metatarsal. Protect the sural nerve and peroneal tendons and retract the EHB muscle.

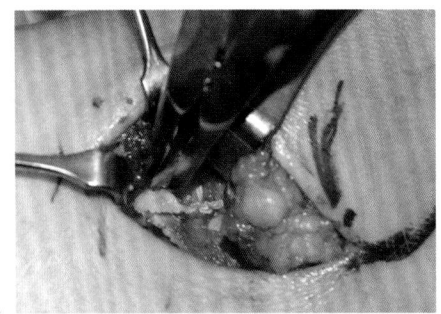 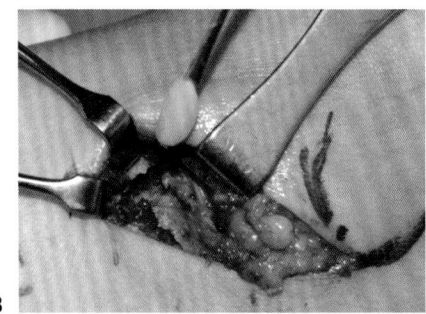

TECH FIG 5 A. Be sure to remove all bone fragments from deep within the resection. **B.** Bone wax can be used within the coalition, on the exposed cancellous surfaces, to limit bone reformation of the coalition.

MIDDLE FACET (SUBTALAR) COALITION RESECTION (COURTESY OF MARK E. EASLEY, MD)

Exposure

- Obtain a preoperative CT to assist in guiding the middle facet coalition resection.
- Medial approach directly over the middle facet coalition **(TECH FIG 6)**
    - In most patients, the prominent coalition can be palpated. It is confluent with the sustentaculum tali.
    - Palpate the medial malleolus and the medial navicular and then identify the sustentaculum tali inferior to the medial malleolus and proximal to the navicular.
    - The dorsomedial aspect of the calcaneus is also palpable.
- Course of the incision
    - Start at the dorsomedial aspect of the calcaneus, anterior to the Achilles tendon, immediately posterior to the medial malleolus.
    - Continue the incision immediately dorsal to the sustentaculum tali, over the prominent coalition and inferior to the medial malleolus.
    - Complete the incision immediately proximal to the navicular.

Exposing the Coalition

- After the skin incision, carefully divide the flexor retinaculum.
    - Lift the retinaculum as it is divided so that the underlying tendons and neurovascular structures are not injured.
- Interval to access the coalition
    - In most cases, the flexor digitorum longus (FDL) tendon courses directly over the coalition.

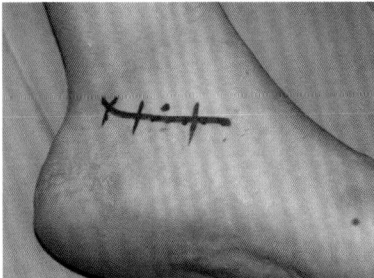

TECH FIG 6 From the dorsomedial aspect of the calcaneus, make the incision immediately dorsal to the palpable sustentaculum tali, directly over the prominent coalition and inferior to the medial malleolus, ending immediately proximal to the navicular.

- The posterior aspect of the coalition is accessed between the FDL and flexor hallucis longus (FHL) tendon.
- The anterior aspect of the coalition is accessed between the FDL and the PTT.

Identifying the Coalition

- The coalition is often difficult to identify, particularly when a complete bone bridge is present.
- Incomplete coalitions (cartilaginous or fibrous) are sometimes easier to identify.
    - Preoperative imaging, especially CT, is useful in determining the coalition orientation.
    - The coalition may not be transverse, instead having a more vertical orientation, and the preoperative CT should be used to locate the incomplete coalition.
- The medial aspect of the posterior subtalar joint, immediately posterior to the middle facet coalition, is typically easy to identify **(TECH FIG 7)**.
    - In the posterior aspect of the incision, identify and carefully retract the neurovascular bundle (tibial nerve, posterior tibial artery and veins) posteriorly and inferiorly.
    - The interval will be between the FDL tendon dorsally and the FHL tendon inferiorly.
    - The medial aspect of the posterior subtalar joint may be visualized (cartilage surfaces of the inferior talus and calcaneal posterior facet).
    - Carefully place a hypodermic needle in the joint.
        - If desired, fluoroscopically confirm that the needle is in the subtalar joint.
    - To outline the planned course of coalition resection, a hypodermic needle may also be placed between the talar head and the anterior calcaneal facet.
        - This is sometimes more difficult to identify but is useful in complete bony coalitions were identifying the optimal course of resection from proximal to distal cannot be readily determined.

Resection

- Begin the coalition resection proximally, starting at the posterior calcaneal facet and advancing distally.
    - Use the preoperative CT to help guide the resection in the plane of an incomplete coalition.

TECHNIQUES

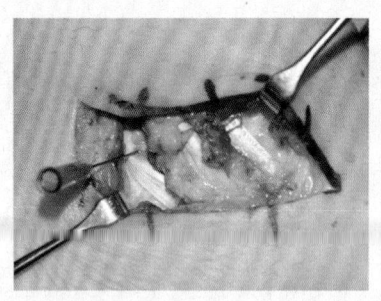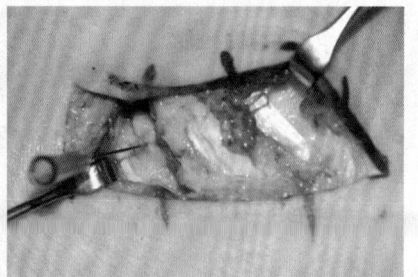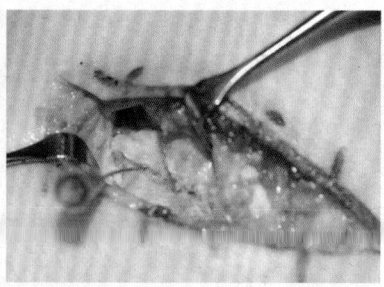

TECH FIG 7 Identify the posteromedial subtalar joint. **A.** The posterior subtalar joint may be identified between the FDL and FHL tendons. **B.** Note that the posteromedial neurovascular bundle is retracted posteriorly and inferiorly. **C.** The hypodermic needle is used as a guide in the posterior subtalar joint.

- For complete bony coalitions, intraoperative fluoroscopy may be useful to guide the resection.
- Incomplete coalitions may be identified using a curette on the coalition's medially aspect until the coalition's plane is determined.
- On the proximal aspect, the FDL is retracted dorsally **(TECH FIG 8A)**.
- To advance distally, the FDL should be retracted plantarly **(TECH FIG 8B)**.
- Once the coalition plane is determined, a chisel is used **(TECH FIG 8C–E)**.
  - From medial to lateral, the coalition is typically quite deep, often 2 or 3 cm.
  - Confirm the coalition resection has been completed anteriorly by stressing the subtalar joint and demonstrating motion.
- The resection should be generous to optimize motion and avoid recurrence **(TECH FIG 9)**.
  - If possible, preserve the inferior aspect of the sustentaculum tali so that the FHL maintains its anatomic course.

- Confirm that there is no impingement medially and that inversion is reestablished.
- Once a generous amount of bone has been resected from the coalition, thoroughly irrigate the wound and place bone wax to limit bone regrowth.

Closure and Postoperative Care

- After thorough irrigation with sterile saline, release the tourniquet and perform hemostasis.
- The extensor retinaculum does not need to be closed.
- Use a drain to limit formation of a hematoma over the neurovascular bundle.
- Close the subcutaneous layer and skin.
- The ankle and foot should be immobilized in a CAM boot or splint to allow the wound to heal.
- As soon as the soft tissues are stable, range of motion should be initiated to optimize hindfoot motion.
- Weight bearing may be initiated when the wound is stable, but full weight bearing may not be tolerated for 4 to 6 weeks.
- Consider physical therapy to optimize outcome.

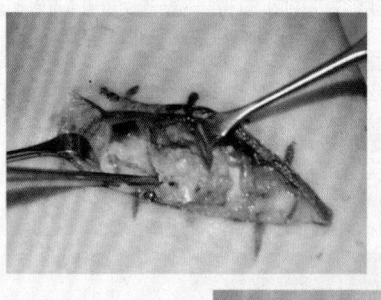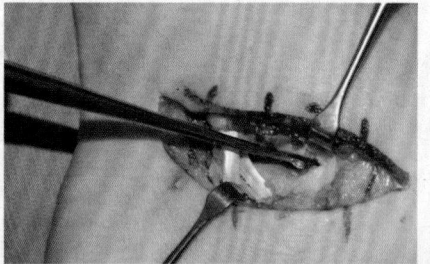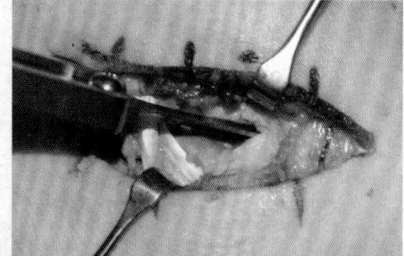

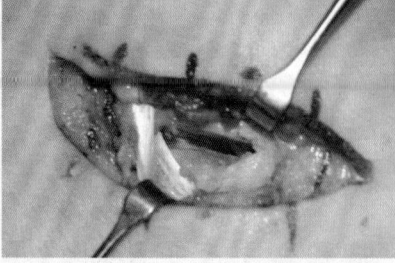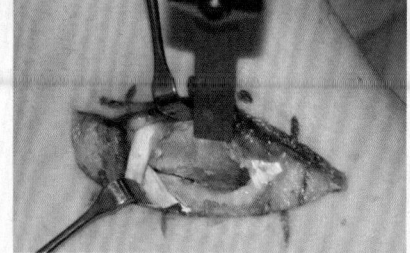

TECH FIG 8 A,B. Initiating the middle facet coalition resection using a curette. **A.** The posterior aspect of the coalition is accessed with the FDL tendon retracted dorsally. **B.** The anterior aspect of the coalition is accessed with the FDL tendon retracted inferiorly. **C–E.** Deepening the middle facet coalition resection. **C.** A chisel is used to perform the deeper (more lateral) coalition resection. **D.** With most of the middle facet coalition resected, the posterior calcaneal facet is exposed. **E.** The resection should be generous to limit risk of coalition reformation.

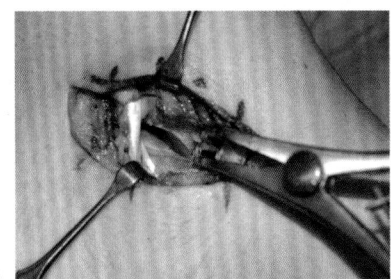
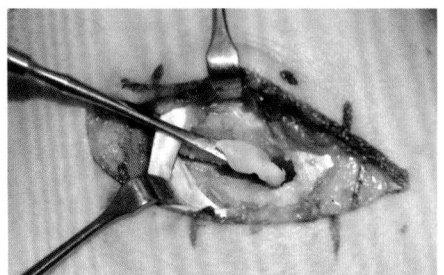

TECH FIG 9 Completing the middle facet coalition resection. **A.** A lamina spreader is used to demonstrate complete separation of the talus from the calcaneus. **B.** Bone wax may be used on the exposed cancellous surfaces to limit the risk of coalition reformation.

TECHNIQUES

Pearls and Pitfalls

Preoperative Workup	• Evaluate plain radiographs for the presence of significant degenerative changes, which would necessitate an appropriate arthrodesis. • Review available CT or magnetic resonance imaging scans for the presence of any concomitant coalitions.
Coalition Resection	• Osteotome cuts made in a parallel fashion will remove a rectangular block of bone rather than a convergent, trapezoidal segment, which may lead to recurrent pain secondary to an inadequate medial excision of the coalition.
Interpositional Graft	• Preserve the fascia overlying the extensor digitorum brevis to increase the holding power of the Vicryl stitch.
Deformity Correction	• Consider adding a lateral column lengthening procedure in the face of a significant pes planus.

POSTOPERATIVE CARE

• The patient is allowed to bear weight as tolerated in the cast on postoperative day 1.
• At 3 weeks, the patient returns to clinic for removal of the cast, wound sutures, and bolster stitch. At this point, the patient is placed in a walking boot.
• Following removal of the cast, physical therapy is initiated for ankle and hindfoot range-of-motion exercises.

OUTCOMES

• In the absence of significant degenerative changes that may necessitate an appropriate arthrodesis, resection of a cal-caneonavicular coalition can be a successful procedure in symptomatic adults or adolescents.
• Cohen et al[1] reviewed results of calcaneonavicular coalition resection in 12 adult patients. Subjective relief was attained in 10 patients, and the average increase in total subtalar range of motion was 10 degrees.[1]
• In a group of 48 child and adolescent patients, Gonzalez and Kumar[4] achieved 77% good to excellent results following cal-caneonavicular coalition resection with interposition of the extensor digitorum brevis. The results did not deteriorate with time in those patients followed up for more than 10 years.[4]

• The importance of using an interpositional material has been reinforced in several publications.
• No recurrences of a calcaneonavicular coalition were noted by Moyes et al[8] on oblique radiographs when an extensor digitorum brevis interposition was performed. However, in this same study, three of seven patients who underwent resection without interposition displayed radiographic evidence of a recurrence.[8]
• Swiontkowski et al[9] used an interpositional material (fat or muscle) in 38 of 39 feet undergoing calcaneona-vicular coalition resection and found no radiographic recurrences.
• Mitchell and Gibson,[7] on the other hand, found a recurrence of the coalition in nearly two-thirds of their 41 patients who had undergone a simple coalition resection without interposition of the extensor digitorum brevis.

COMPLICATIONS

• Superficial or deep infection
• Wound dehiscence[1]
• Recurrence of the coalition[7]
• Nerve damage
• Inadequate resection[3]
• Reflex sympathetic dystrophy[1]

REFERENCES

1. Cohen BE, Davis WH, Anderson RB. Success of calcaneonavicular coalition resection in the adult population. Foot Ankle Int 1996; 17:569–572.
2. Cooperman DR, Janke BE, Gilmore A, et al. A three-dimensional study of calcaneonavicular tarsal coalitions. J Pediatr Orthop 2001; 21:648–651.
3. Ehrlich MG, Elmer EB. Tarsal coalition. In: Jahss M, ed. Disorders of the Foot and Ankle, ed 2. Philadelphia: Saunders, 1991:921–938.
4. Gonzalez P, Kumar SJ. Calcaneonavicular coalition treated by resection and interposition of the extensor digitorum brevis muscle. J Bone Joint Surg Am 1990;72(1):71–77.
5. Jayakumar S, Cowell HR. Rigid flatfoot. Clin Orthop Relat Res 1977;(122):77–84.
6. Kulik SA Jr, Clanton TO. Tarsal coalition. Foot Ankle Int 1996; 17:286–296.
7. Mitchell GP, Gibson JM. Excision of calcaneo-navicular bar for painful spasmodic flat foot. J Bone Joint Surg Br 1967;49(2):281–287.
8. Moyes ST, Crawfurd EJ, Aichroth PM. The interposition of extensor digitorum brevis in the resection of calcaneonavicular bars. J Pediatr Orthop 1994;14:387–388.
9. Swiontkowski MF, Scranton PE, Hansen S. Tarsal coalitions: long-term results of surgical treatment. J Pediatr Orthop 1983;3:287–292.
10. Vincent KA. Tarsal coalition and painful flatfoot. J Am Acad Orthop Surg 1998;6:274–281.

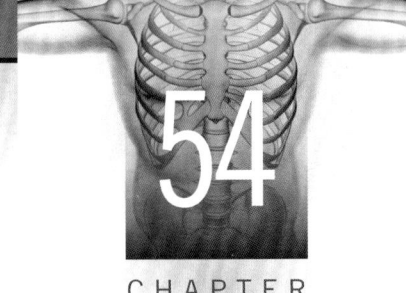

54

CHAPTER

Treatment of the Accessory Navicular

Christopher E. Gross and Mark E. Easley

DEFINITION

- An accessory navicular is an osseous abnormality that is caused by a secondary ossification center that fails to unite during maturation.
- Roughly 5% to 14% of all feet have this accessory bone, which is likely an autosomal dominant trait.[2,4]
- Up to 38.6% of feet with an accessory navicular have a pes planovalgus deformity.[5]

ANATOMY

- The tuberosity of the navicular forms from a secondary ossification center.
  - This ossification center normally does not ossify until 9 years old.
- There are three types of accessory naviculars[4]:
  - Type I: small round or ovoid sesamoid within the posterior tibialis tendon (PTT) that is typically located at the plantar aspect of the tendon adjacent to the spring ligament
    - Two to 3 mm in diameter
    - No bony attachment
    - Rarely symptomatic
  - Type II: connected by a synchondrosis of less than 2 mm between the ossicle and the navicular (FIG 1)
    - Usually 9 to 12 mm in diameter
    - Typically becomes symptomatic with relatively minor trauma to the foot that stresses the previously stable synchondrosis

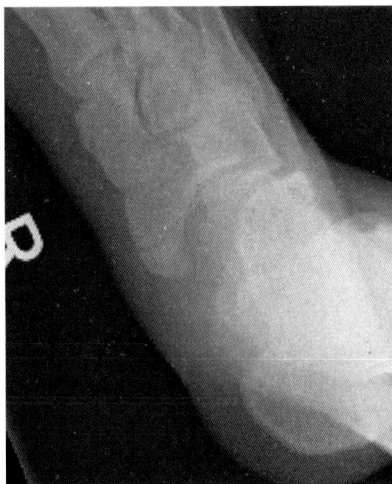

FIG 1 External oblique view of a right foot demonstrating a type II accessory navicular, with the navicular attached by a synchondrosis.

- IIA: less acute angle (tension force)
  - More at risk for an avulsion injury
- IIB: more inferior (shear force)
- Type III: united by a bony bridge
  - Produces a cornuate navicular
  - Occasionally symptomatic

PATHOGENESIS

- Kidner[7] described the relationship of the accessory navicular with pes planus:
  - The accessory navicular alters the pull and leverage of the PTT, forcing it to become more of an adductor than a supinator.
  - As the foot adducts, the talus impinges on the medial malleolus.
  - The abnormal pull of the PTT interferes with normal foot mechanics and can cause a weakness of the medial arch and may lead to pes planus.

NATURAL HISTORY

- Pain is likely due to pressure from shoes in children.
- At times, it is associated with flattening of the longitudinal arch due to an abnormal insertion of the PTT.
- Symptoms can develop after relatively minor ankle sprains, other trauma, or chronic overuse/repetitive stress.
- Tension, shearing, and compressive forces are transmitted via the PTT to the synchondrosis.

PATIENT HISTORY AND PHYSICAL FINDINGS

- The patient may complain of an insidious onset of medial foot pain often experienced only during activities or with certain types of shoe wear.
- On examination, the patient will have a normal neuromuscular examination with minimal to no limitations in ankle or foot range of motion. Subtalar motion is typically well preserved.
- There may be a prominence over the medial forefoot (FIG 2).
  - Tenderness to palpation and edema over the prominence
- Unilateral pes planus may be present in patients with a symptomatic accessory navicular.
  - PTT strength should be tested (plantarflexion and inversion against resistance to isolate the PTT): symptoms usually directly at accessory navicular.
  - Single-limb heel rise to isolate PTT function: symptoms usually experienced directly over the accessory navicular

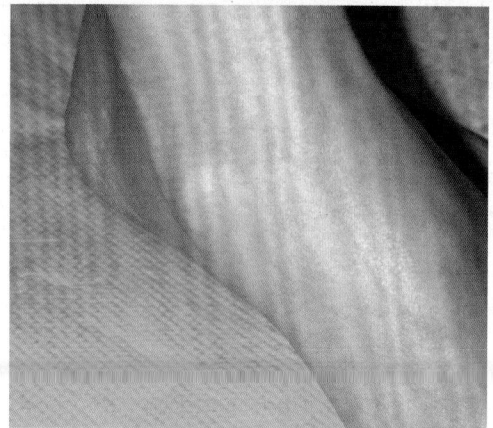 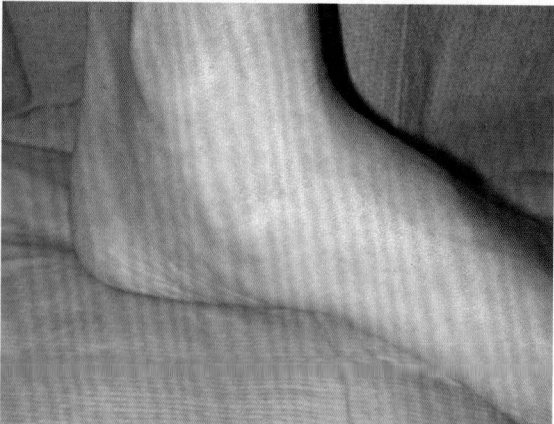

FIG 2 A. Medial prominence. **B.** Note PTT attaching to prominent accessory navicular.

- The examiner should assess the patient's gait and overall alignment to look for hindfoot valgus and a pes planus deformity.

IMAGING AND OTHER DIAGNOSTIC STUDIES

- Standard anteroposterior (AP), lateral, and external oblique x-rays can help determine the type and potential size of the accessory bone **(FIG 3A–C).**
  - A routine internal oblique does not allow visualization of the medial navicular.
  - The external oblique radiograph (opposite of the internal oblique view) is usually not included in a routine radiographic series of the foot (see **FIG 3C**).
- Magnetic resonance imaging (MRI) may suggest a symptomatic synchondrosis with bony edema surrounding the synchondrosis **(FIG 3D,E).**
  - Can be useful in ruling out other potential pathology with similar symptoms, including spring ligament pathology, posterior tibial tendinopathy, and navicular stress fracture
- Bone scan is highly sensitive for symptomatic accessory navicular but not specific.[3]
- Single-photon emission computed tomography/computed tomography scans may also be useful in the aid of diagnosis.[1]

DIFFERENTIAL DIAGNOSIS

- PTT tear or tendinopathy
- Spring ligament tear
- Navicular stress fracture

NONOPERATIVE MANAGEMENT

- Acute phase (after recent injury)
  - CAM boot to limit PTT tension on synchondrosis between accessory navicular and main body of navicular
    - If severe, temporary short-leg cast
  - Avoid boot or cast pressure over tender medial accessory navicular.
- Chronic phase (removed from acute onset of symptoms)
  - Shoe wear modification with improved longitudinal arch support and relatively stiff sole
  - Felt or gel doughnut over the medial prominence to potentially reduce pressure on the prominent accessory navicular
  - Semirigid longitudinal arch support
    - Will need a relief area directly at accessory navicular
    - Although arch support is recommended to relieve stress from the PTT on the synchondrosis, direct pressure on the accessory navicular may cause pain from a high medial arch support, may create more symptoms from

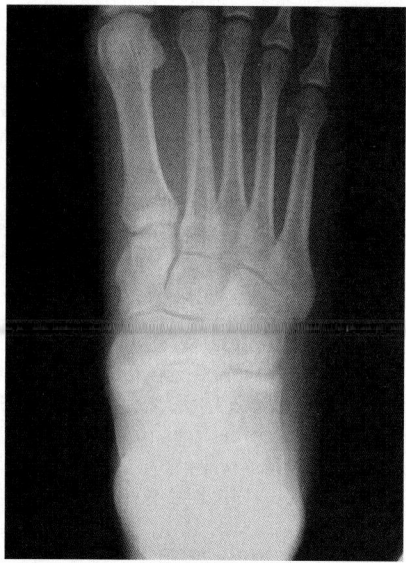 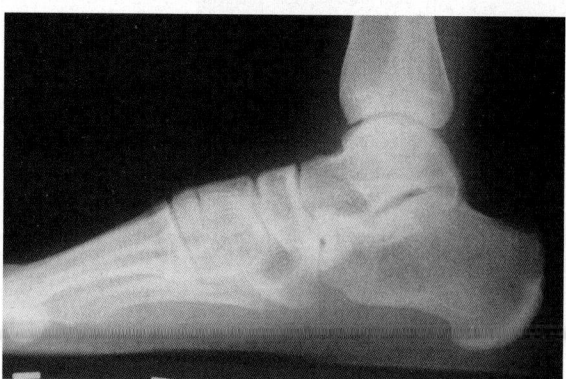

FIG 3 A. Weight-bearing AP foot radiograph suggests accessory navicular but provides little detail. **B.** Weight-bearing lateral radiograph also suggests accessory navicular but with little detail. Note that arch is relatively well preserved in this patient. *(continued)*

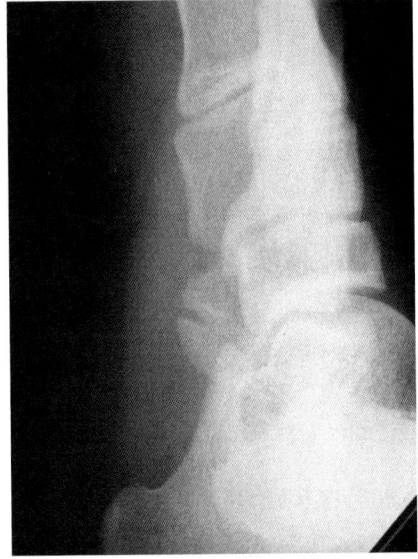

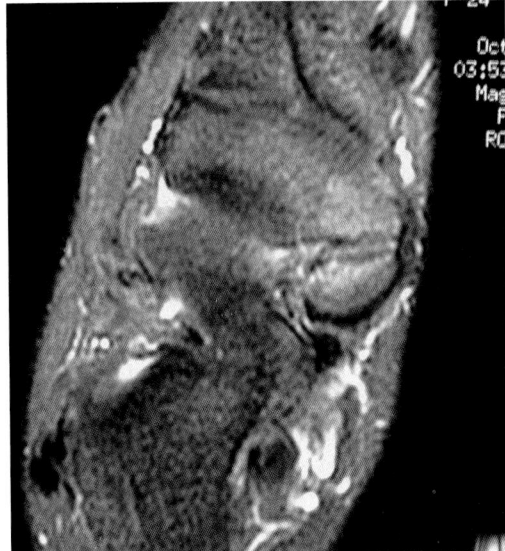

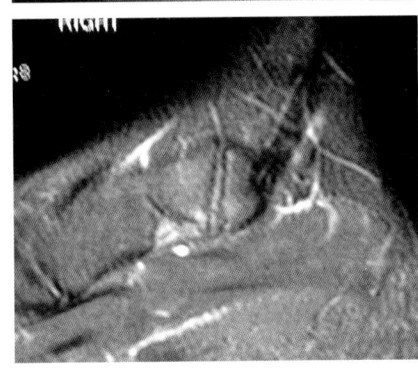

FIG 3 *(continued)* **C.** External oblique view offers best view of the accessory navicular. Note that this is a type II accessory navicular, separated from the main body of the navicular by a synchondrosis. **D.** Axial MRI suggests edema at the synchondrosis. **E.** Sagittal MRI demonstrates synchondrosis and the attachment of the PTT on the accessory navicular.

direct pressure; therefore, a modified orthotic with relief directly over the prominent accessory navicular is recommended.

- Physical therapy
  - Exercises that place high demand on the PTT should be avoided.
    - Will place more stress on the symptomatic synchondrosis
  - Modalities to calm irritation at the synchondrosis may be of benefit.
    - Ultrasound and/or iontophoresis
- External bone stimulation
  - Because a symptomatic type II accessory navicular is due to injury/stress on a cartilaginous/fibrous synchondrosis and is not a fracture, external bone stimulation has no role in management.

SURGICAL MANAGEMENT

Preoperative Planning

- Foot alignment, based on weight-bearing clinical and radiographic evaluation, must be understood.
  - With a well-preserved arch, surgery may be limited to the accessory navicular.
  - With pes planus, consideration may need to be given to correct hindfoot alignment in addition to surgical management of the accessory navicular.
- Characteristics of the type II accessory navicular
  - If the accessory navicular is large, consideration may be given to excision of the synchondrosis, preparation of the opposing navicular surfaces, and arthrodesis of the accessory navicular to the main body of the navicular.
  - If the accessory navicular is small, then excise and reattach the PTT to the medial aspect of the navicular.
- Detailed review of the imaging studies, including MRI and/ or computed tomography scan
  - Identify associated pathology such as PTT pathology or spring ligament pathology that may need to be addressed surgically.
  - Further define the accessory navicular.
- Anesthesia per the anesthesia team. Although an ankle block is probably sufficient, consideration may be given to a popliteal block. If a tourniquet is used, it may have less propensity to trap the PTT if it can be used higher in the calf (popliteal block) than if used at the ankle (ankle block).

Positioning

- The patient is placed supine on a radiolucent operating room table.
- The leg should be allowed to externally rotate to facilitate access to the medial navicular.
  - Often, a support (bump) under the contralateral hip promotes ideal leg rotation for the operating on the medial foot.
- Neutral leg alignment is recommended if concomitant foot realignment for pes planus is planned.
  - Thereby, access for medial (accessory navicular) and lateral (calcaneal osteotomy) procedures is facilitated.

TECHNIQUES

EXPOSURE AND APPROACH

- A 4-cm longitudinal medial incision is made dorsomedially over the accessory navicular and distal PTT at its insertion on the accessory navicular (**TECH FIG 1A**).
- The distal PTT tendon sheath is opened to directly expose the PTT's insertion on the accessory navicular. The PTT is inspected with a tenosynovectomy performed when necessary (**TECH FIG 1B**).
- The synchondrosis is identified.
  - Preoperative imaging is useful in determining the orientation of the synchondrosis.
  - If arthrodesis of the accessory navicular to the main body of the navicular is being considered, minimize periosteal stripping and maintain the PTT insertion on the accessory navicular.
  - A 25-gauge needle and fluoroscopy may be used as a probe to find the synchondrosis between the accessory navicular and the navicular body (**TECH FIG 1C**).

Excision of the Synchondrosis

- With the interval between the two bones identified from the dorsal aspect the synchondrosis, the cartilaginous and fibrous tissue is sharply excised without compromising the PTT or adjacent spring ligament.
- The two opposing surfaces of the main body of the navicular and accessory navicular should be fully exposed.

Consideration for Arthrodesis of the Accessory Navicular to the Main Body of the Navicular

- If the accessory bone is large enough to support one and preferably two 3-mm cannulated screws, an arthrodesis may be performed.
  - Two screws afford more stable fixation and control rotation of the accessory navicular, thereby potentially increasing the chance for healing.

- In larger patients, larger cannulated screws may be feasible; however, care must be taken to avoid fracturing the accessory navicular.
- If the accessory bone is too small to support screw fixation, then a modified Kidner procedure (excision of the accessory navicular) is performed.
- If the main navicular bone is prominent even without the accessory navicular, a microsagittal saw can be used to remove some the main navicular.
  - This may provide a better ingrowth surface for the PTT or for arthrodesis of the accessory navicular.

Advancing the Posterior Tibialis Tendon

- Kidner procedure: Kidner originally described accessory navicular excision and advancing the PTT to the residual medial navicular.
- Modified Kidner procedure: Other authors have described accessory navicular excision and attaching the PTT to the medial navicular at its resting tension without advancing the PTT.
- Although it may appear that advancing the PTT to the medial navicular, that is, adding more tension, may provide a mechanical advantage, there is no evidence to suggest improved clinical outcome over simply attaching the PTT to the medial navicular at its resting tension.
- In our experience, after excising the accessory navicular, the PTT must be advanced to some degree to allow satisfactory attachment to the navicular.

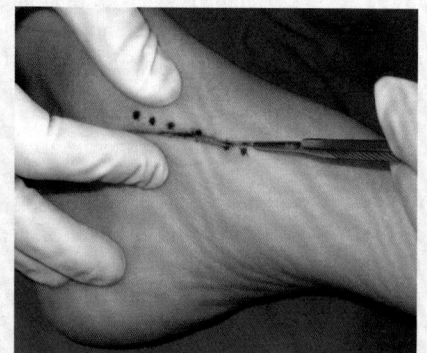
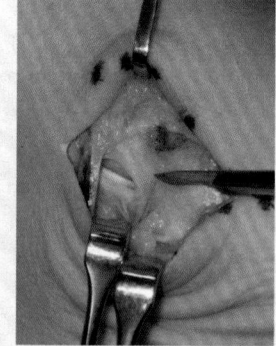
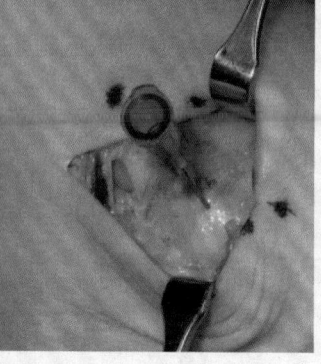

TECH FIG 1 A. Medial longitudinal incision over dorsal aspect of navicular and PTT at insertion on navicular. **B.** Dorsal aspect of PTT sheath opened. **C.** Hypodermic needle used to identify synchondrosis.

MODIFIED KIDNER PROCEDURE

- The accessory navicular and the synchondrosis are identified within the distal medial PTT **(TECH FIG 2A)**.
- While protecting all of the PTT fibers, including the ones coursing toward the plantar foot, the accessory navicular is excised by elevating the PTT attachment directly from the accessory navicular **(TECH FIG 2B–D)**.
- The PTT tendon fibers should be maintained in continuity, essentially elevated as a sleeve, so that they may be effectively attached to the medial navicular.
- The synchondrosis needs to be identified and mobilized to separate the accessory navicular.
- The medial talonavicular capsule and spring ligament must be protected from inadvertent injury during accessory navicular removal.

- The residual synchondrosis should be removed from the medial navicular and the medial navicular should be prepared to expose a bony surface conducive to tendon attachment.
  - If the residual medial navicular is prominent, it may be shaved with a microsagittal saw **(TECH FIG 2E–G)**.
- The PTT is attached to the plantar medial aspect of the navicular using a one or two bone suture anchors (3.0 or 3.5 mm) **(TECH FIG 2H,I)**.
- The PTT attachment to the medial navicular periosteum is reinforced with a combination of absorbable and nonabsorbable 0-0 or 2-0 sutures to the periosteum **(TECH FIG 2J–L)**.
- The PTT tendon sheath is closed and the subcutaneous layer and skin are reapproximated.

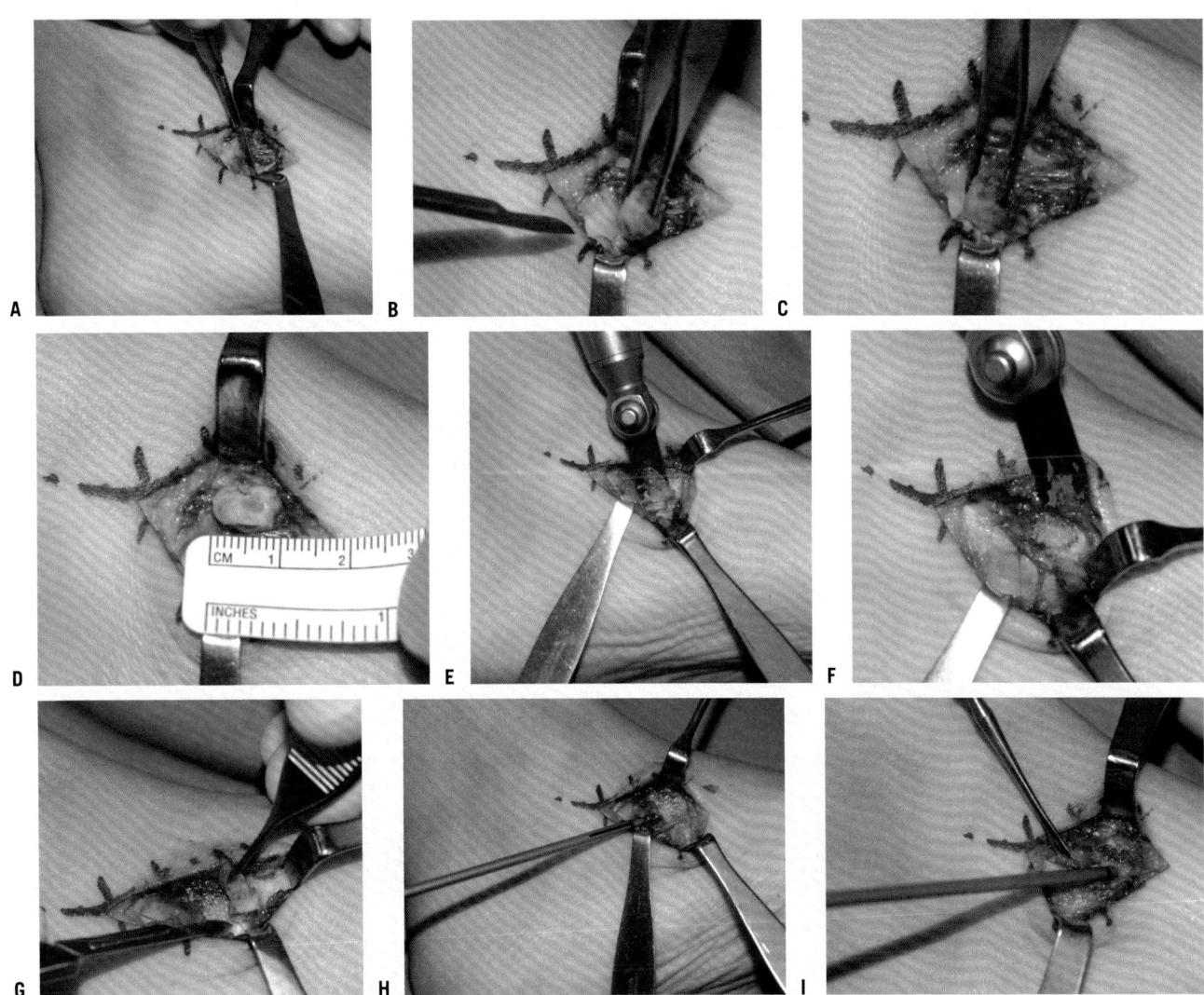

TECH FIG 2 A. The accessory navicular and the synchondrosis are identified within the distal medial PTT. **B.** The accessory navicular is excised by elevating the PTT attachment directly from the accessory navicular. **C.** Accessory navicular extracted from PTT and separated from synchondrosis. **D.** In this case, relatively small accessory navicular. **E.** Microsagittal saw to shave medial navicular. **F.** Exposes more cancellous surface for PTT reattachment healing. **G.** Sharp resection of residual resected bone. **H.** Suture anchor being inserted. Recommend fluoroscopic guidance to ensure talonavicular joint not violated. **I.** Anchor seated fully in medial navicular. *(continued)*

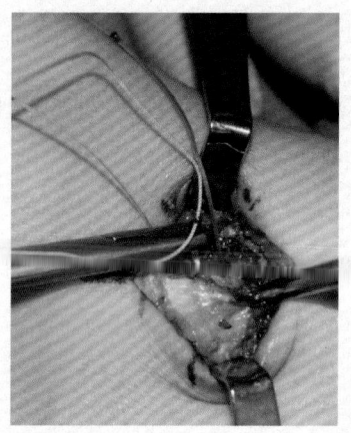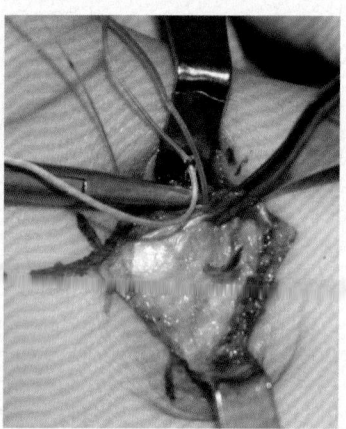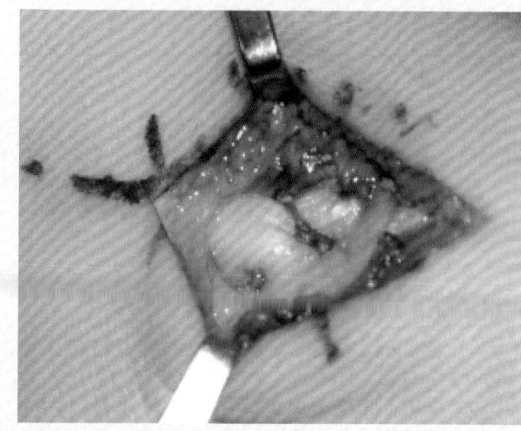

TECH FIG 2 *(continued)* **J.** Anchor sutures being passed through PTT. **K.** PTT may be advanced to enhance tension, but this is not necessary. **L.** PTT secured to navicular.

ACCESSORY NAVICULAR AND NAVICULAR ARTHRODESIS/ OPEN REDUCTION AND INTERNAL FIXATION

- The accessory navicular and synchondrosis are exposed **(TECH FIG 3A–C)**.
- It typically is obvious where the PTT attaches to the unstable accessory navicular **(TECH FIG 3D)**.
- With the opposing surface of the accessory navicular fully exposed, a microsagittal saw is used to create a flat surface at the medial aspect of the main body of the navicular, where once

the synchondrosis was attached, to create a satisfactory healing surface **(TECH FIG 3E)**.
- The distal aspect of the accessory bone is prepared in a similar manner to optimize the healing surface **(TECH FIG 3F)**.
- If desired, more medial navicular may be removed to create a lower profile with reattachment of the accessory navicular.

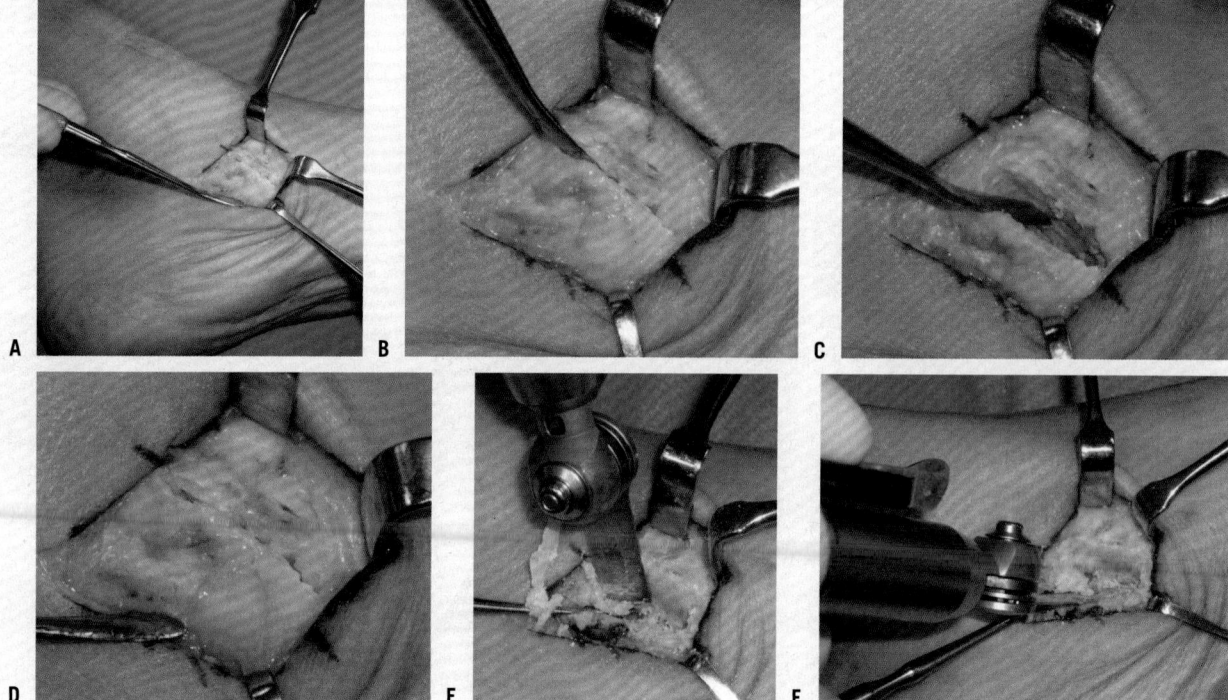

TECH FIG 3 A. Medial navicular exposed. **B.** Synchondrosis identified. **C.** Synchondrosis opened. **D.** PTT fibers attaching to accessory navicular. With unstable synchondrosis, symptoms are produced with PTT tension on accessory navicular. Preparation for arthrodesis with microsagittal saw to remove residual synchondrosis on the medial **(E)** and accessory **(F)** naviculars. *(continued)*

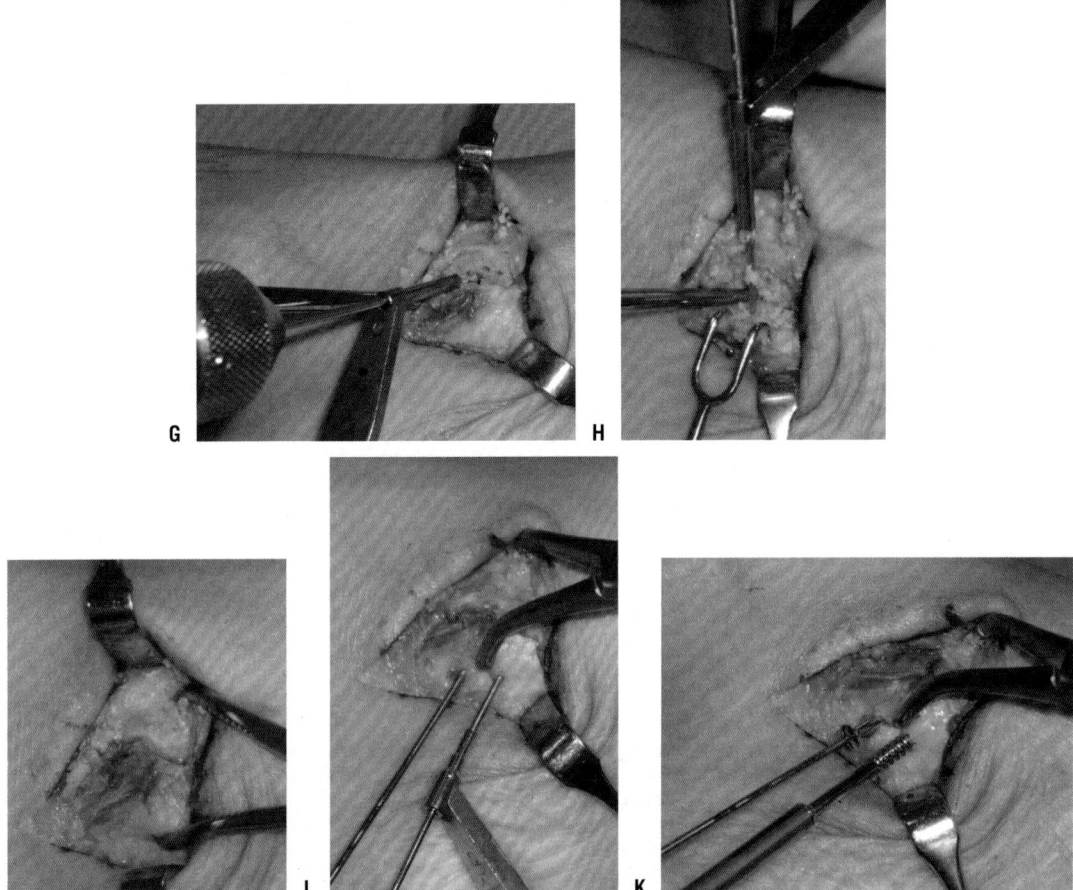

TECH FIG 3 *(continued)* The medial (**G**) and accessory (**H**) navicular surfaces are prepared with small-diameter drill to increase surface area for healing. The drill holes in the accessory navicular are superficial to limit risk for stress fracture when screws inserted. **I–K.** Accessory navicular fixation. **I.** Reduction with bone clamp, optimizing bony apposition. **J.** Guidewire insertion for cannulated screw placement. Note that the clamp is placed centrally on the accessory navicular to facilitate placing two screws for definitive fixation. **K.** Screw placement.

- Similar to any other arthrodesis, the surfaces are drilled to increase surface area to optimize chance for fusion **(TECH FIG 3G,H)**.
  - The accessory navicular's healing surface should be drilled carefully and only superficially to limit risk of stress fracture when screws are inserted.
- The accessory navicular is advanced to the prepared surface of the navicular.
  - To facilitate approximation of the accessory navicular on the medial navicular, ankle plantarflexion and hindfoot inversion is recommended (relieves tension from the PTT).
  - A bone reduction clamp may be used, best centered on the accessory navicular so that two screws may be inserted, on either side of the clamp **(TECH FIG 3I)**.
- The guide pins for the cannulated screws are placed through the PTT attachment on the accessory navicular **(TECH FIG 3J)**.
  - Using a scalpel blade, creating careful longitudinal slits within the tendon limits damage to the PTT insertion during pin insertion, drilling, and screw placement.

- Fluoroscopic evaluation in more than one plane is important to confirm satisfactory bony opposition in multiple planes and optimal position of the guide pins.
- After overdrilling the guidewires, the cannulated screws are carefully advanced through the PTT attachment on the accessory navicular **(TECH FIG 3K)**.
  - Typically, the screw heads will need to advance under the tendon to effectively engage the cortex of the accessory navicular.
  - The slits made sharply in the PTT tendon insertion may need to be carefully enlarged to accommodate the screw heads.
  - Compression of the accessory navicular to the navicular is desired, but overcompression that may lead to accessory navicular stress fracture must be avoided.
- Closure is similar to that described for the modified Kidner procedure earlier.

ADDITION OF SUBTALAR ARTHROEREISIS (EXTRA-ARTICULAR SUBTALAR/SINUS TARSI IMPLANT)

Background

- Patients with a symptomatic accessory navicular may have an associated flexible pes planovalgus deformity. Although this deformity may not need to be corrected, consideration may be given to foot realignment in combination with surgical management of the accessory navicular.
- Some surgeons recommend an extra-articular subtalar arthroereisis (subtalar/sinus tarsi implant) to realign the foot; subtalar arthroereisis has been used in combination with surgical management of the symptomatic accessory navicular.[5,8]
- In the pediatric patient population, subtalar arthroereisis has been used in isolation.
  - In skeletally immature patients with flexible pes planovalgus, the implant may realign the foot in anticipation that bone growth in the foot will adjust to a more neutral position.
  - Once the patient reaches skeletal maturity, the subtalar arthroereisis implant may be removed, and because bone growth has been modified with the implant, foot alignment will remain improved.

- In skeletally mature patients with symptomatic flexible pes planovalgus, subtalar arthroereisis is rarely effective as a stand-alone procedure to correct deformity.
- Most surgeons that use subtalar arthroereisis to treat their patients recommend that the implant is used as an adjunct to correct flexible pes planovalgus.
- Procedures that may be used in combination with subtalar arthroereisis are as follows:
  - Tendo Achilles lengthening versus gastrocnemius recession (TECH FIG 4)
  - Medial displacement calcaneal osteotomy
  - Plantarflexion medial cuneiform osteotomy (Cotton osteotomy)
- Although perhaps feasible, lateral column lengthening through the anterior calcaneus (Evans procedure) probably should not be used in combination with subtalar arthroereisis because the implant would rest directly on the calcaneal osteotomy, potentially negatively influencing its healing and effectiveness.

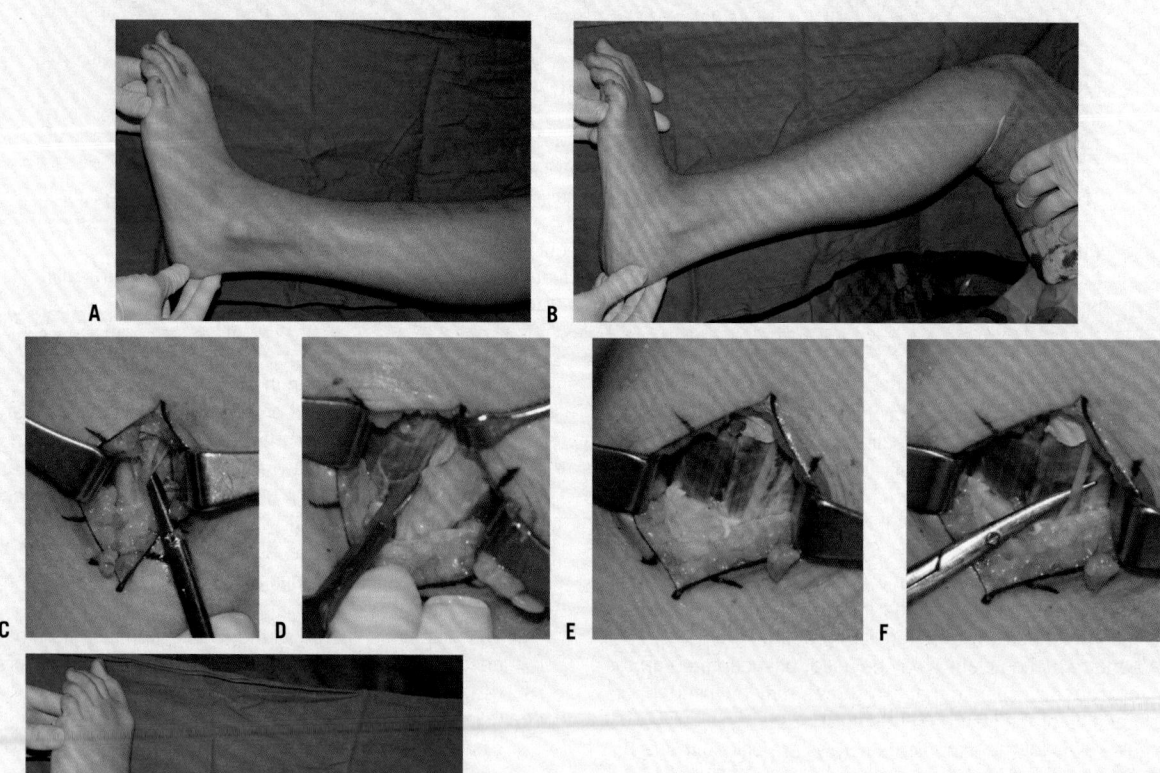

TECH FIG 4 A,B. Silfverskiöld test demonstrating isolated gastrocnemius contracture. **A.** Equinus with knee in extension. **B.** No equinus with knee in flexion. **C–F.** Gastrocnemius–soleus recession. **C.** Posterior approach at musculotendinous junction. Note sural nerve. **D.** Gastrocnemius tendon release. **E.** Gastrocnemius released with soleus fibers remaining intact. **F.** Sural nerve intact. **G.** Equinus contracture corrected.

Exposure

- Because the subtalar/sinus tarsi implant is inserted from the lateral foot, the foot should be positioned in neutral position on the operating room table to allow access to both the medial and lateral aspects.
- The sinus tarsi is palpated distal and inferior to the tip of the lateral malleolus.
- A 1- to 2-cm oblique incision, parallel to the typical course of the sural nerve, is created over the sinus tarsi, dorsal to the peroneal tendons.
- A hemostat is used to bluntly dissect to the tarsal canal, avoiding the sural nerve and the lateral dorsal cutaneous nerve.

Guidewire Placement

- A blunt guidewire is passed through the sinus tarsi and tarsal canal from lateral to medial **(TECH FIG 5A)**.

- Provided it is oriented properly, the smooth and blunt guidewire should pass relatively readily through the tarsal canal to the medial foot, anterior to the calcaneal posterior facet, and dorsal to the middle calcaneal facet.
- The desired medial exit point is immediately distal and inferior to the medial malleolus and dorsal to the PTT **(TECH FIG 5B)**.
- The path of least resistance is usually the correct one and has an oblique axis: anterolateral to posteromedial.
- Once the wire passes to the medial skin, immediately dorsal to the PTT, a superficial incision is made at the tip of the wire to allow the wire to be passed through the skin **(TECH FIG 5C,D)**.
- Optimal wire position should be confirmed fluoroscopically **(TECH FIG 5E)**.
  - In the AP plane, the wire should pass from anterolateral to more posteromedial, directly under the neck of the talus **(TECH FIG 5F)**.
  - In the lateral plane, the wire should be inferior to the talar neck and anterior to the calcaneal posterior facet **(TECH FIG 5G)**.

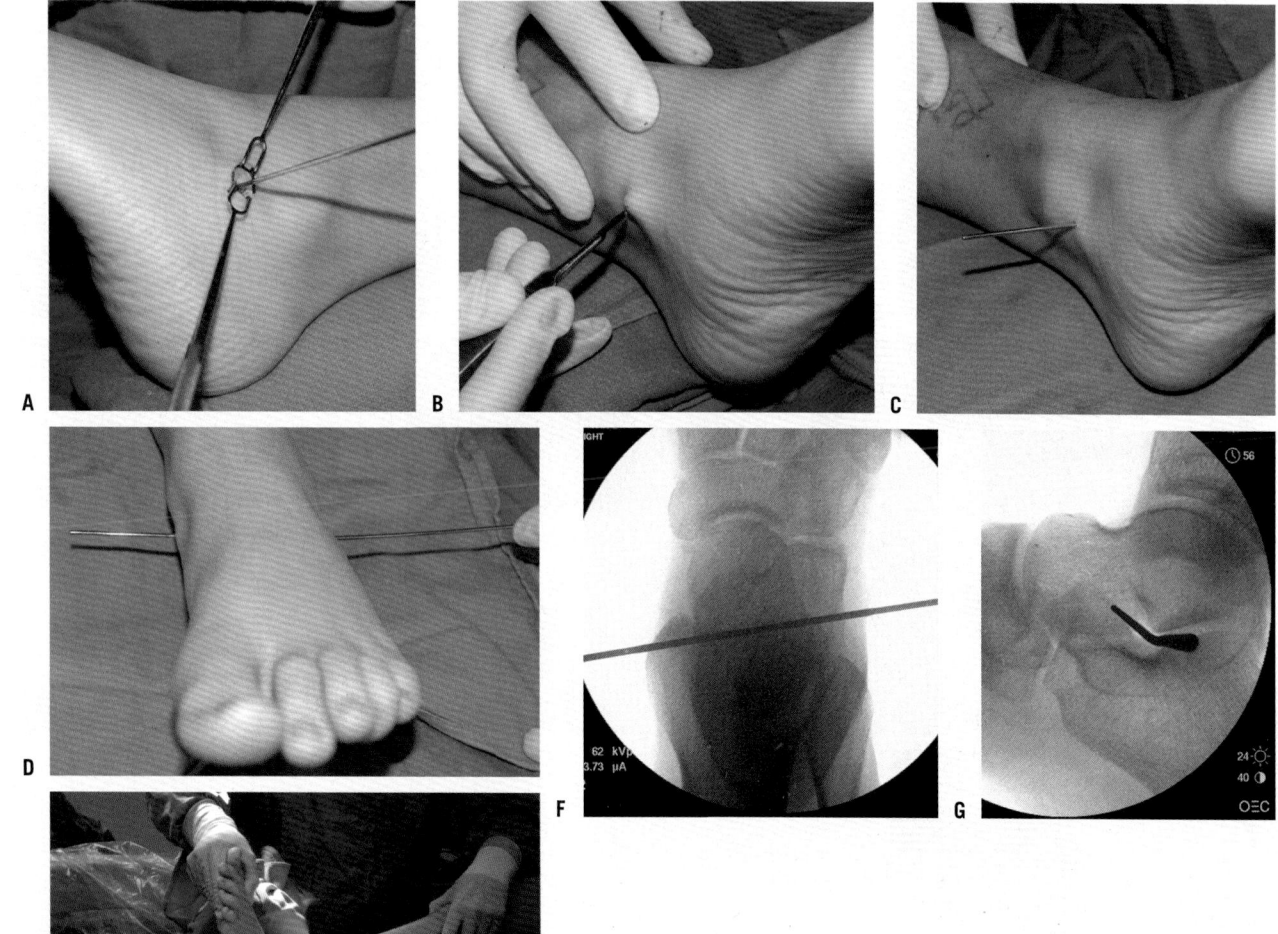

TECH FIG 5 A. A 1-cm incision is made over sinus tarsi to insert guidewire. **B.** Guidewire passed through sinus tarsi and exiting medial subtalar joint anterior and distal to medial malleolus and dorsal to PTT; stab incision to pass wire through skin. **C,D.** Guidewire passed through medial skin. **E.** Foot positioned for fluoroscopic confirmation of proper guidewire position fluoroscopy. **F.** AP view. **G.** Lateral view.

Sizing

- Most commercially available subtalar arthroereisis systems have sizing guides in 1- or 2-mm diameter increments.
- With fluoroscopic confirmation of proper wire position successively, larger subtalar/sinus tarsi sizing guides are inserted until the optimal guide is determined **(TECH FIG 6A)**.
- The goal of the sizing guide, trial, and implant is to correct deformity by blocking hindfoot eversion but without overcorrection into valgus.
- With the proper size determined with the guide, the optimal trial is placed over the guidewire **(TECH FIG 6B–D)**.
- The optimally sized trial is identified.
  - Valgus hindfoot stress should block valgus to a physiologic hindfoot position, preventing excessive valgus hindfoot position **(TECH FIG 6E)**.

- Varus hindfoot position suggests that the trial implant diameter is too great.
- Proper trial position should be confirmed fluoroscopically.
- Ideally, the implant's leading edge will approach the midaxis of the talar neck (AP fluoroscopic view), and its opposite end will not be completely recessed under the lateral talar neck cortex **(TECH FIG 6F)**.
- The implant should have a slight anterolateral to posteromedial orientation.
- In our experience, 9- and 10-mm implants are most commonly used.
- Lateral fluoroscopy should also be obtained to confirm that the implant is in optimal position, immediately inferior to the talar neck and anterior to the calcaneal posterior facet **(TECH FIG 6G)**.

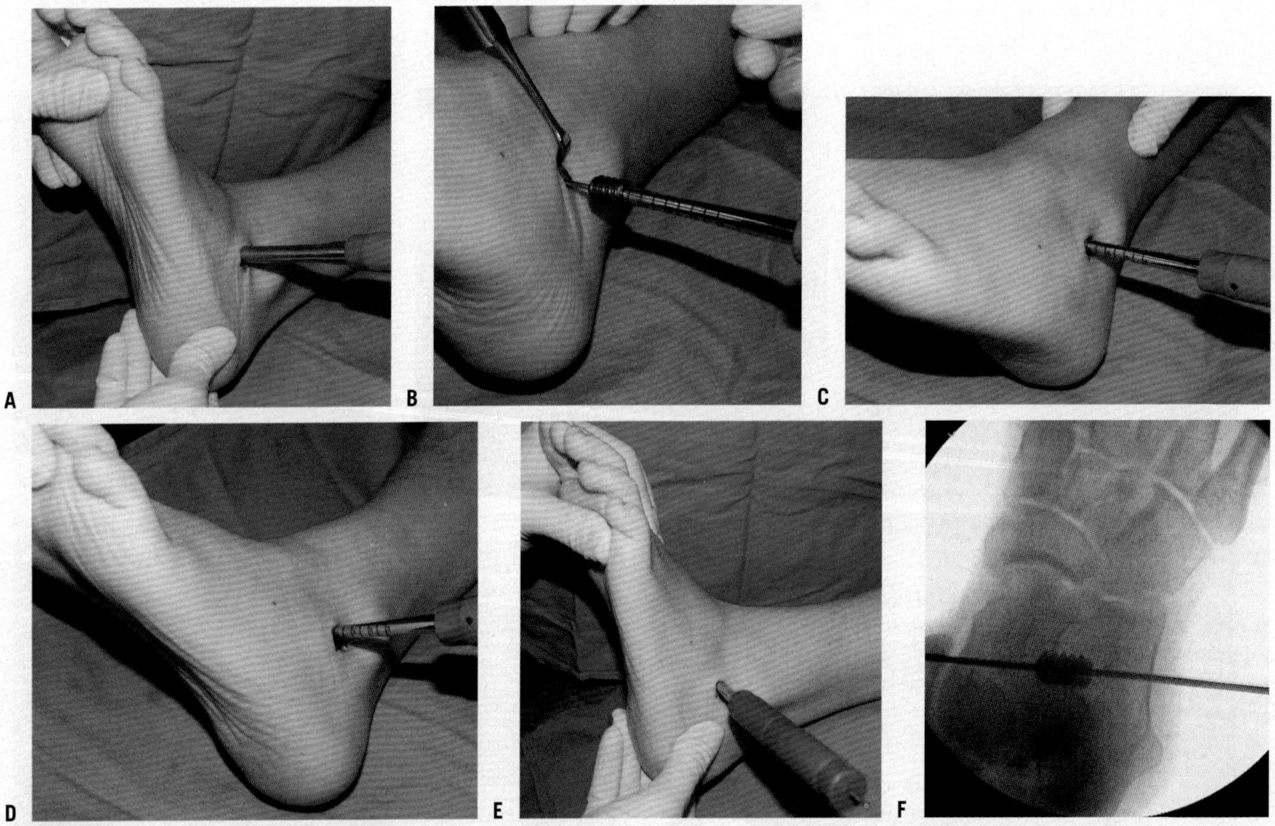

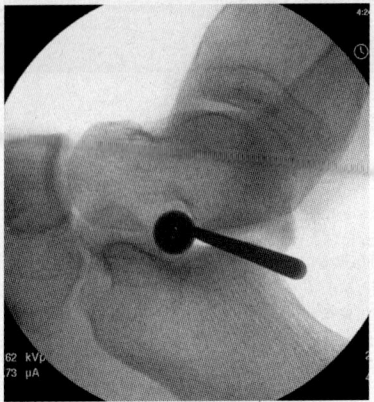

TECH FIG 6 A. Sizing guide to determine optimal implant diameter. With cannulated sizing guide placed over guidewire into sinus tarsi to lateral talar neck and dorsal anterior calcaneus, optimal elimination of excessive hindfoot valgus is determined without overcorrection into varus. **B.** Trial implant being placed over guide pin. **C.** Trial implant insertion. The incision must be large enough to avoid soft tissue and nerve injury with trial (and eventual final implant) insertion. **D.** Full insertion. **E.** Confirming optimal hindfoot valgus with trial in place. **F.** Ideally, an AP fluoroscopic view is obtained to determine ideal implant position; this oblique view does not afford ideal view. **G.** Lateral view.

Implant Placement

- With the optimal size determined clinically and proper trial position confirmed fluoroscopically, the trial is removed and the final implant is placed over the guidewire **(TECH FIG 7A–C)**.
  - The implant should be advanced to the point that it appropriately blocks eversion without overcorrecting the hindfoot into varus **(TECH FIG 7D,E)**.
  - Fluoroscopic confirmation of proper implant position should be performed, as described for the trial earlier.

- Ideally, the implant's leading edge approaches the midaxis of the talar neck (AP fluoroscopic view) without its opposite end completely recessed under the lateral talar neck cortex **(TECH FIG 7F–H)**.
- The guidewire is removed from the medial side to limit the risk of implant displacement **(TECH FIG 7I–L)**.

Completion

- Final fluoroscopic confirmation in the AP and lateral planes to confirm the implant is in the optimal position **(TECH FIG 8)**
- Routine wound closure

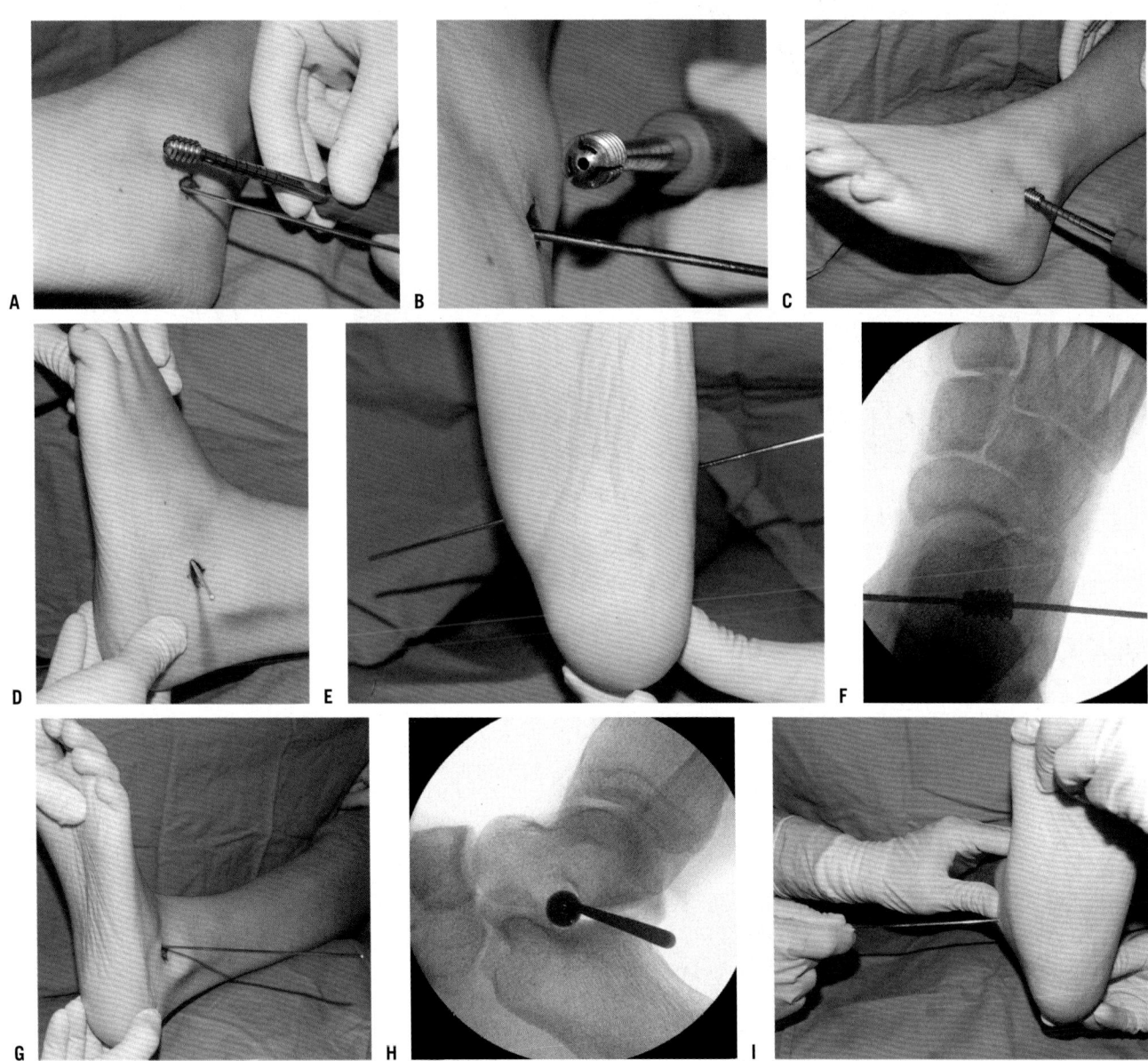

TECH FIG 7 A. The final implant is threaded to provide stability. It is also fluted to absorb shock. **B.** End-on view to show fluted design. **C.** Final implant insertion. **D,E.** Confirming proper heel position with final implant in place. **D.** Valgus heel stress. **E.** Heel position evaluated. **F.** AP fluoroscopic view to confirm proper final implant position. Ideally, the implant's leading edge approaches the midaxis of the talar neck without its opposite end completely recessed under the lateral talar neck cortex. **G,H.** Optimal position based on lateral view with guide pin still in place. **I.** Guidewire extracted medially. By removing it medially, the implant has less chance of dislodging from its ideal position. *(continued)*

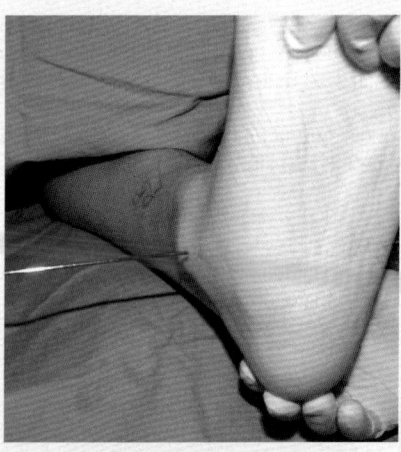
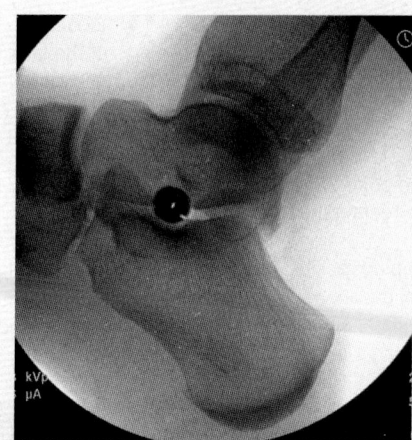
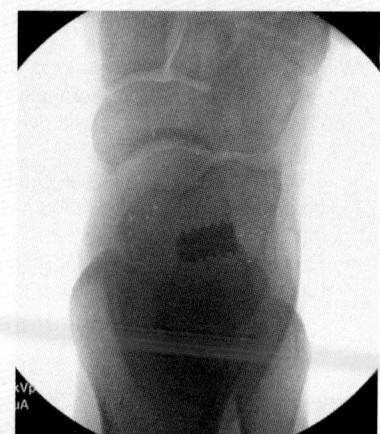

TECH FIG 7 *(continued)* **J.** Guidewire fully extracted. **K.** Final lateral fluoroscopic view. **L.** Final AP fluoroscopic view. Note that the implant's leading edge approaches the midaxis of the talar neck without crossing it, and the trailing edge is not fully buried under the lateral talar neck.

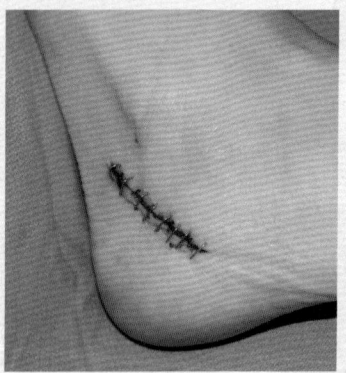
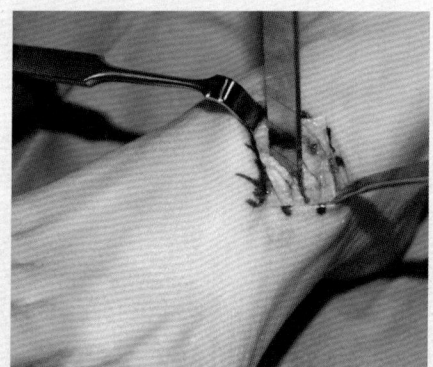
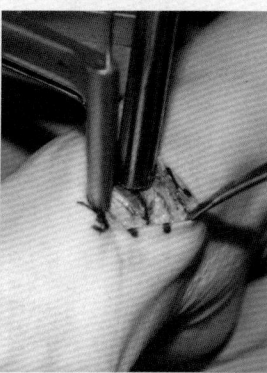

TECH FIG 8 Associated foot realignment. **A.** Medial displacement calcaneal osteotomy completed prior to subtalar arthroereisis in this case. **B.** Plantarflexion osteotomy of first cuneiform. **C.** Graft insertion into medial cuneiform.

CASE EXAMPLE

- In our experience, isolated subtalar arthroereisis does not afford adequate correction in skeletally mature patients with flexible pes planovalgus deformity.
  - In this particular case, the 26-year-old woman had better correction on the right foot, where foot realignment procedures were added to subtalar arthroereisis, than in the left

foot, where subtalar arthroereisis was performed with only gastrocnemius–soleus recession **(TECH FIG 9A–F)**.
- Weight-bearing radiographs of the same patient's right foot with subtalar arthroereisis performed with gastrocnemius–soleus recession, medial displacement calcaneal osteotomy, and plantarflexion osteotomy of the first cuneiform **(TECH FIG 9G,H)**

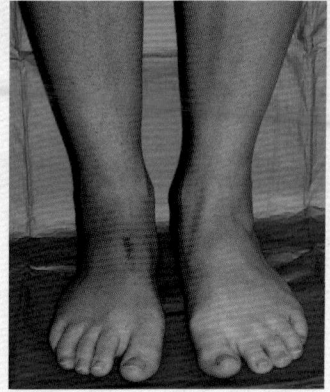
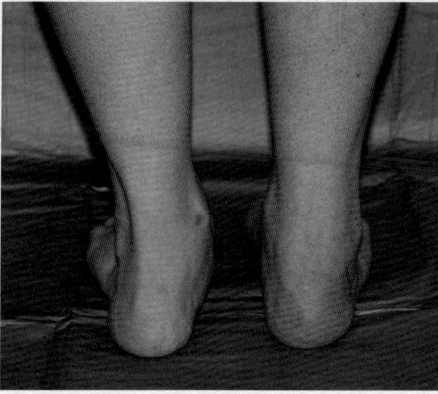

TECH FIG 9 Example case of a 26-year-old woman with better correction on right foot where foot realignment procedures were added to subtalar arthroereisis when compared to left foot where subtalar arthroereisis was performed with only gastrocnemius–soleus recession. **A.** AP view. **B.** Posterior view. *(continued)*

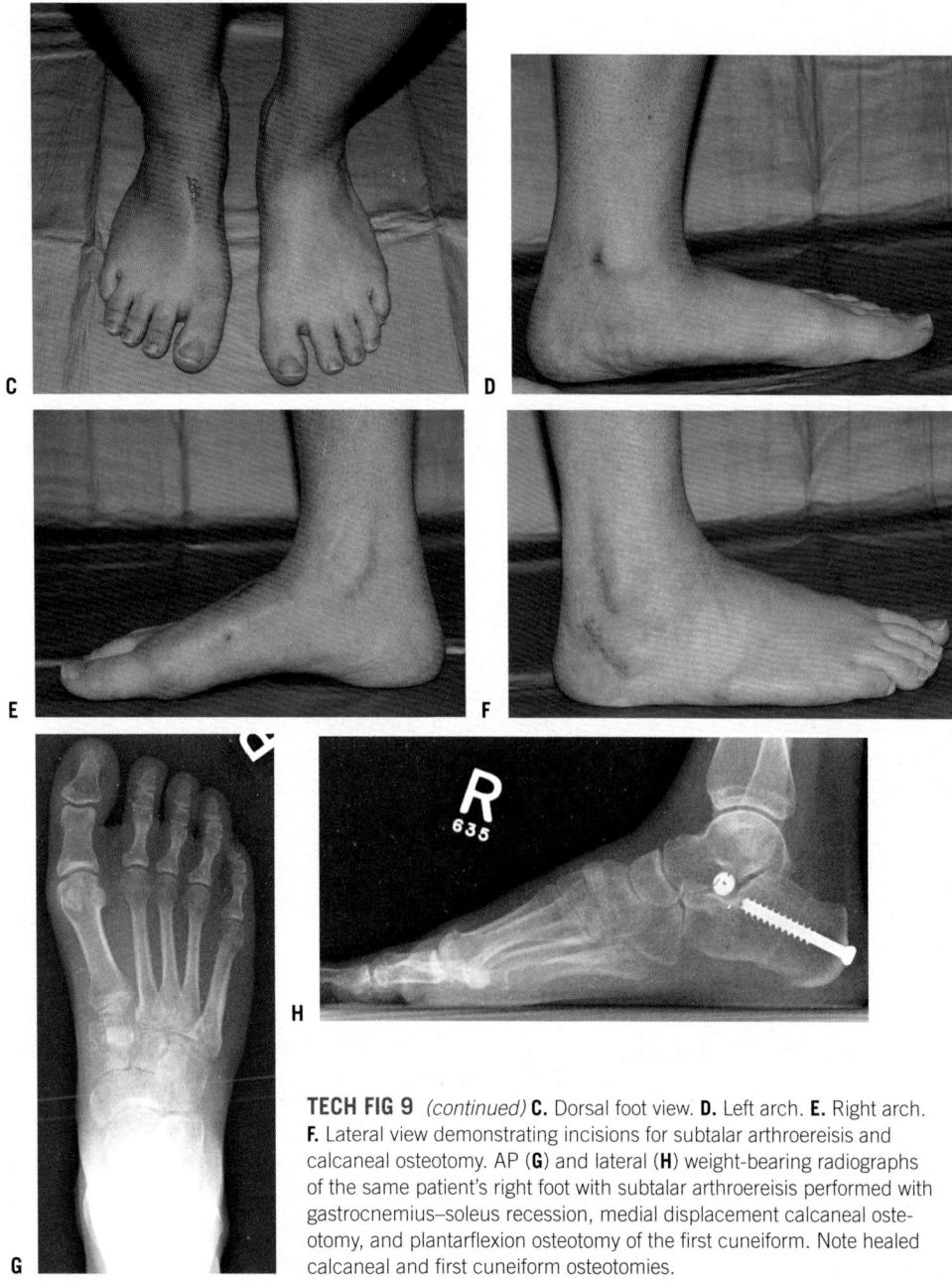

TECH FIG 9 *(continued)* **C.** Dorsal foot view. **D.** Left arch. **E.** Right arch. **F.** Lateral view demonstrating incisions for subtalar arthroereisis and calcaneal osteotomy. AP (**G**) and lateral (**H**) weight-bearing radiographs of the same patient's right foot with subtalar arthroereisis performed with gastrocnemius–soleus recession, medial displacement calcaneal osteotomy, and plantarflexion osteotomy of the first cuneiform. Note healed calcaneal and first cuneiform osteotomies.

SUBTALAR ARTHROEREISIS WITH FOOT REALIGNMENT AND ACCESSORY NAVICULAR EXCISION

- Flexible pes planus with forefoot supination (**TECH FIG 10A**)
- Equinus contracture (**TECH FIG 10B,C**)
- Gastrocnemius–soleus recession (**TECH FIG 10D**)
- Plantarflexion osteotomy of the first cuneiform to correct forefoot supination (**TECH FIG 10E–I**)
- Subtalar arthroereisis performed
  - Guidewire placed (**TECH FIG 10J–L**)
  - Trial and final implant insertion over guidewire (**TECH FIG 10M,N**)

- Fluoroscopic confirmation of proper implant position (**TECH FIG 10O**)
- Guide pin removed medially (**TECH FIG 10P**)
  - Guide pin typically exits in planned medial approach for modified Kidner procedure.
- Modified Kidner procedure performed (**TECH FIG 10Q**)

TECHNIQUES

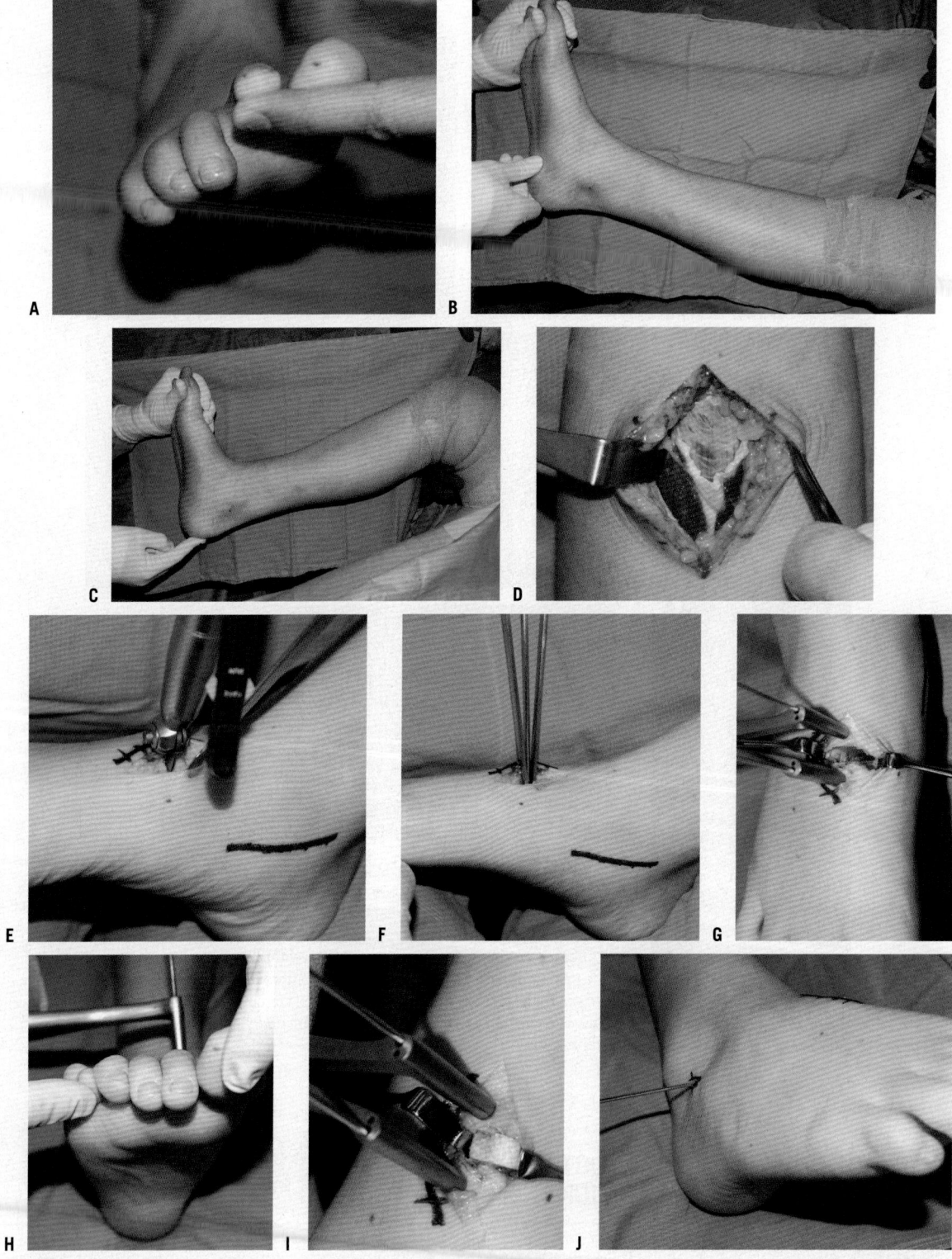

TECH FIG 10 A. Patient with symptomatic flexible pes planus and forefoot supination. Gastrocnemius contracture demonstrated with Silfverskiöld test: equinus with knee in extension (**B**) and no equinus with knee in flexion (**C**). **D.** Gastrocnemius–soleus recession. **E.** Osteotomy with microsagittal saw. **F.** Triple osteotome technique to gradually open osteotomy, leaving plantar cortex intact. **G.** Dorsal distraction. **H.** Forefoot supination corrected. **I.** Graft inserted. **J.** Guidewire insertion into sinus tarsi. *(continued)*

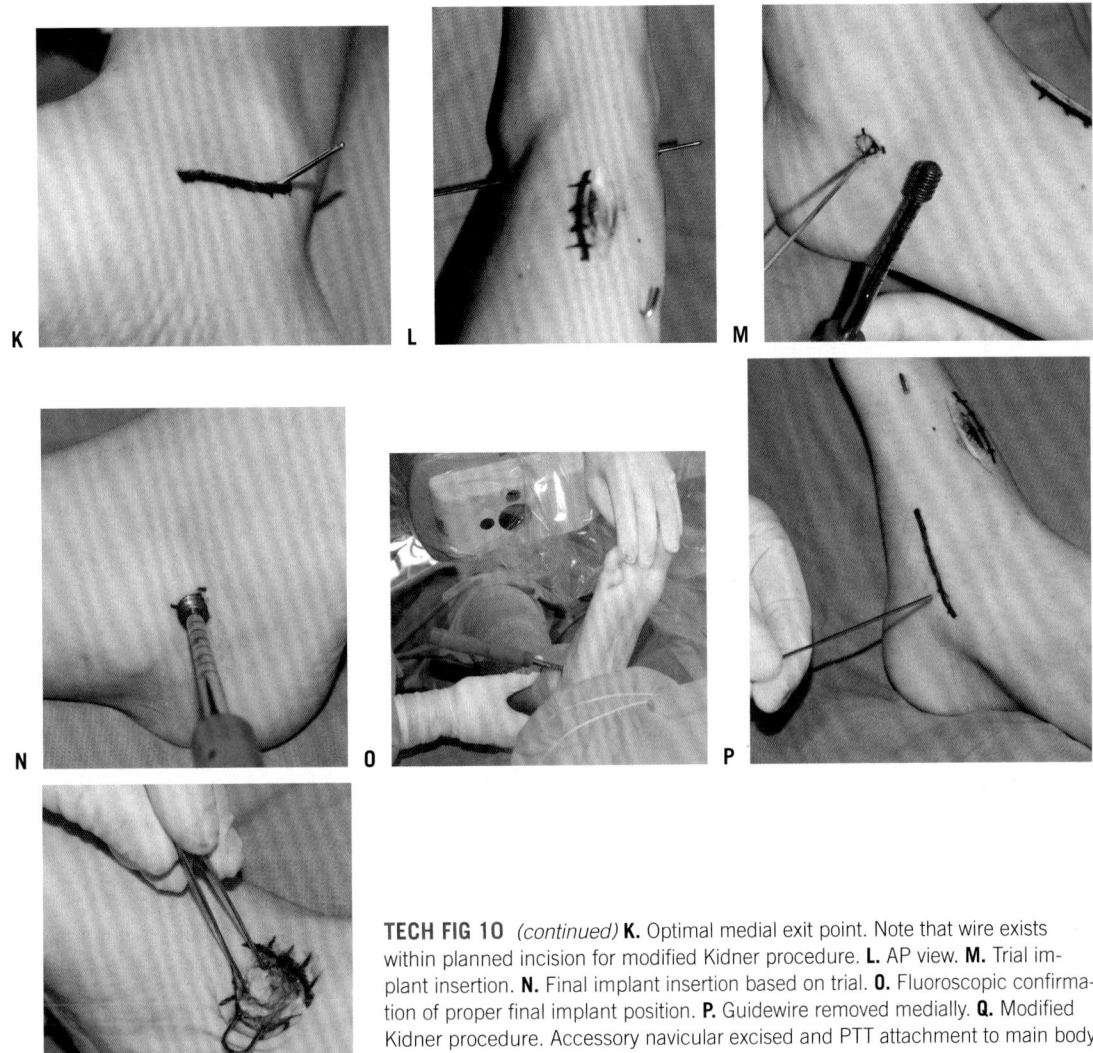

TECH FIG 10 *(continued)* **K.** Optimal medial exit point. Note that wire exists within planned incision for modified Kidner procedure. **L.** AP view. **M.** Trial implant insertion. **N.** Final implant insertion based on trial. **O.** Fluoroscopic confirmation of proper final implant position. **P.** Guidewire removed medially. **Q.** Modified Kidner procedure. Accessory navicular excised and PTT attachment to main body of navicular.

TECHNIQUES

Pearls and Pitfalls

Imaging the Accessory Navicular	• The external oblique radiograph, different from the internal oblique obtained in routine three views of the foot, provides the best perspective on the accessory navicular.
Excising the Accessory Navicular	• Preserve as much as the medial PTT tendon fibers as possible. • Preserve the plantar PTT fibers that course to the plantar midfoot. • Avoid injury to the spring ligament
Arthrodesis of the Accessory Navicular to the Main Body of the Navicular	• Prepare the synchondrosis like any other arthrodesis. • Remove all fibrous and cartilaginous tissue and prepare the bony surfaces of the navicular and the accessory navicular. • Oppose the prepared bony surfaces and secure with one or two screws.
Subtalar Arthroereisis	• The implant should not be used as a stand-alone device. • The guidewire should be removed from the medial side to avoid displacing the implant.

POSTOPERATIVE CARE

- Sterile dressings are applied to the wounds.
- With satisfactory stability of the PTT or accessory navicular to the medial navicular, the ankle and hindfoot may be splinted in neutral position.
  - Slight ankle plantarflexion and hindfoot inversion relieves tension at the repair site but should not be excessive, as it could lead to contracture and be counterproductive if concomitant tendo Achilles lengthening was performed.
- A subtalar arthroereisis implant is typically stable and does not warrant special consideration in the postoperative management.
- Follow-up in 2 to 3 weeks for suture removal and short-leg cast versus cam boot. We favor casting for an additional 3 to 4 weeks to protect the medial repair.
  - The ankle and hindfoot are generally placed in neutral at this time, but if there is any concern about the stability, then slight hindfoot inversion may be maintained.
- Touchdown weight bearing is maintained for 6 weeks.
- At the 6-week follow-up, the patient may typically begin gentle range-of-motion exercises and gradually advance weight bearing in a cam boot to advance to full weight bearing by 10 weeks.
  - If an accessory navicular arthrodesis was performed, then an external oblique radiograph should be obtained to confirm satisfactory healing of the accessory navicular to the navicular.
    - If healing is delayed, then casting and limited weight bearing must be continued.
  - If a subtalar arthroereisis was performed, then routine weight-bearing radiographs of the foot should be obtained to confirm appropriate implant position and foot realignment.
- To optimize return to full function, consideration may be given to physical therapy at 10 to 12 weeks.
- In general, return to full activities including athletic activities takes 4 to 6 months.
- The subtalar implant may be eventually removed (>6 months), but in our experience, if left in place to afford more favorable foot alignment and support for the medial repair, it typically does not cause symptoms.

OUTCOMES

- Prospective evaluation of 20 patients with a symptomatic type II accessory navicular[9]
  - Ten patients had a modified Kidner, and 10 patients had an open reduction and internal fixation (ORIF) of the accessory navicular.
  - After an average follow-up of 35 months, the 10 patients who underwent ORIF had a significant improvement in their American Orthopaedic Foot and Ankle Society (AOFAS) scores (greater improvement than the Kidner group, but the postoperative scores were not significantly different).
    - One patient had to return to the operating room for painful hardware.
    - Two others had nonunion, and one had symptoms. There were no signs of medial arch collapse.

- The 10 patients who underwent the modified Kidner had a significant improvement in their AOFAS scores.
  - Three of 10 showed progressive loss of medial arch.
- Retrospective study of 23 feet with painful type II accessory naviculars who underwent a combined modified Kidner and subtalar arthroereisis with planovalgus deformity at 53.9 months and average age of 18 years
  - Significantly improved AOFAS scores
  - Significantly decreased visual analog scale pain scores
  - Improvement in Meary angle and talar head uncoverage
  - Three patients had the implant removed for pain. Deformity correction was maintained after removal.
  - Nineteen had good or excellent results.
- Seventy-nine patients with accessory navicular syndrome were analyzed.[6] Significantly, less athletes (6.9%) improved after conservative treatment versus nonathletes (34%). Athletes were significantly younger with a higher likelihood of a history of trauma. Radiographically, more athletes had movement of the accessory navicular and the navicular during a forefoot eversion stress test.

COMPLICATIONS

- Modified Kidner procedure
  - Incomplete to the medial navicular
    - May warrant PTT healing revision surgery
  - Development/progression of symptomatic pes planovalgus
    - May warrant bracing versus flatfoot corrective surgery
  - Prominent symptomatic medial suture anchor knots
    - Once tendon has healed to medial navicular, these knots may be excised.
    - Ideally, the suture knots are buried as deep as possible.
- ORIF of the accessory navicular
  - Loss of fixation/delayed union/nonunion
    - May warrant revision surgery or conversion to modified Kidner procedure
  - Development/progression of symptomatic pes planovalgus
    - May warrant bracing versus flatfoot corrective surgery
  - Prominent hardware
    - May warrant removal of hardware once arthrodesis has progressed to fusion
- Subtalar arthroereisis
  - Impingement pain
    - Sinus tarsi pain with eversion
    - May warrant implant removal
  - Subtalar stiffness
    - May warrant implant removal
  - Forefoot supination
    - In patients with long-standing pes planovalgus, the forefoot may have subtle fixed deformity.
    - Subtalar arthroereisis may exacerbate forefoot supination, creating symptomatic lack of loading on the medial column of the foot and potential lateral column overload.
  - Implant migration
    - If inserted properly and used with proper indications, typically, the implant does not migrate.
  - Subtalar arthritis
    - Rare
    - Typically, only occurs if implant placed incorrectly

REFERENCES

1. Bae S, Kang Y, Song YS, et al. Maximum standardized uptake value of foot SPECT/CT using Tc-99m HDP in patients with accessory navicular bone as a predictor of surgical treatment. Medicine (Baltimore) 2019;98(2):e14022.
2. Bennett GL, Weiner DS, Leighley B. Surgical treatment of symptomatic accessory tarsal navicular. J Pediatr Orthop 1990;10(4):445–449.
3. Chiu NT, Jou IM, Lee BF, et al. Symptomatic and asymptomatic accessory navicular bones: findings of Tc-99m MDP bone scintigraphy. Clin Radiol 2000;55(5):353–355.
4. Coughlin M. Sesamoids and accessory bones of the foot. In: Coughlin M, Mann R, Saltzman C, eds. Surgery of the Foot and Ankle, ed 8. Philadelphia: Mosby, 2007:531–610.
5. Garras DN, Hansen PL, Miller AG, et al. Outcome of modified Kidner procedure with subtalar arthroereisis for painful accessory navicular associated with planovalgus deformity. Foot Ankle Int 2012;33(11):934–939.
6. Jegal H, Park YU, Kim JS, et al. Accessory navicular syndrome in athlete vs general population. Foot Ankle Int 2016;37(8):862–867.
7. Kidner FC. The prehallux (accessory scaphoid) in its relation to flatfoot. J Bone Joint Surg Am 1929;11:831–837.
8. Schon LC. Subtalar arthroereisis: a new exploration of an old concept. Foot Ankle Clin 2007;12(2):329–339.
9. Scott AT, Sabesan VJ, Saluta JR, et al. Fusion versus excision of the symptomatic type II accessory navicular: a prospective study. Foot Ankle Int 2009;30:10–15.

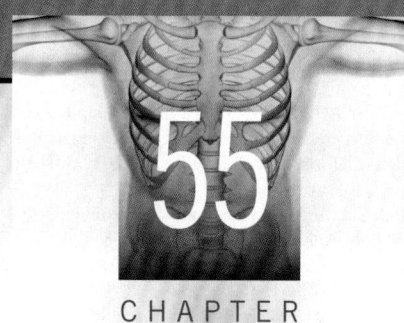

55

CHAPTER

Isolated Subtalar Arthrodesis

Aaron T. Scott and Robert S. Adelaar

DEFINITION

- An isolated subtalar arthrodesis can be used in the treatment of a myriad of different hindfoot conditions, including primary arthrosis of the subtalar joint, posttraumatic arthritis secondary to a talar or complex calcaneal fracture, rheumatoid arthritis, and talocalcaneal coalition.
- Other indications include posterior tibial tendon insufficiency and any neuromuscular disorder presenting with instability of the subtalar joint.
- When the pathologic process resides solely in the talocalcaneal articulation, isolated subtalar arthrodesis is preferred over a triple arthrodesis for its preservation of hindfoot motion, its decreased potential for development of degenerative changes in neighboring joints, its relative simplicity, and its lower potential for pseudarthrosis of the talonavicular and calcaneocuboid joints.

ANATOMY

- The term *subtalar* refers to the articulation between the anterior, middle, and posterior facets of the inferior talus and the corresponding anterior, middle, and posterior facets located on the superior aspect of the calcaneus.
- The subtalar joint is a "plane type" synovial joint with a weak fibrous capsule supported by medial, lateral, and posterior talocalcaneal ligaments as well as an interosseous talocalcaneal ligament.
- This important articulation provides for inversion and eversion of the hindfoot, which is critical for proper adaptation of the foot during ambulation on uneven terrain and for dissipation of heel-strike forces.
- Isolated fusions of the subtalar joint have been shown to reduce talonavicular joint motion by 74% and calcaneocuboid joint motion by 44%.[1]

PATHOGENESIS

- Numerous causes of subtalar joint arthritis exist, including the following:
  - Primary osteoarthrosis: articular cartilage degeneration of unknown etiology
  - Secondary arthritis: caused by either traumatic articular cartilage damage or increased joint stresses following an arthrodesis of an adjacent joint
  - Inflammatory arthritis: autoimmune joint destruction (eg, rheumatoid arthritis, psoriatic arthritis)

- Other etiologies that may necessitate an isolated subtalar arthrodesis include the following:
  - Talocalcaneal coalition: abnormal fusion between the talus and calcaneus, most likely secondary to a failure of segmentation of the primitive mesenchyme
  - Instability or deformity secondary to muscular imbalance (eg, posterior tibial tendon insufficiency, Charcot-Marie-Tooth disease, poliomyelitis)

NATURAL HISTORY

- Depends on specific etiology
- In general, the various forms of subtalar arthritis are progressive in nature.
- Despite waxing and waning of symptoms, no spontaneous resolution of the pathologic process is noted.

PATIENT HISTORY AND PHYSICAL FINDINGS

- A problem-focused history should include direct questioning regarding the exact nature of the symptoms, specific location, duration and progression of symptoms, aggravating or alleviating factors, prior therapeutic interventions, and functional disability.
- Patients often complain of lateral ankle pain and difficulty ambulating on uneven terrain.
- The pain often gets better with rest and may be mitigated by wearing high-top shoes.
- Physical examination findings consistent with subtalar joint arthritis may include the following:
  - Hindfoot swelling
  - Tenderness within the sinus tarsi
  - Pain with inversion and eversion of the hindfoot
  - Limited range of motion of the subtalar joint
  - Antalgic gait
- To help localize the pathology to the subtalar joint complex, palpate and observe the sinus tarsi (the soft tissue depression just anterior and slightly distal to lateral malleolus) for swelling.
- Passively dorsiflex the ankle to neutral to lock the talus within the mortise. Descriptions of normal subtalar range of motion vary widely. Therefore, it is useful to describe the range as a fraction of the asymptomatic, contralateral side. Pain and decreased range of motion may be indicative of subtalar joint arthritis. Complete loss of range of motion is consistent with a tarsal coalition.

IMAGING AND OTHER DIAGNOSTIC STUDIES

- Plain radiographs should include standing anteroposterior (AP), lateral, and oblique views of the foot and standing AP, lateral, and mortise views of the ankle.
- Additional plain radiographs may include a Broden view (lower extremity internally rotated 45 degrees; x-ray tube angled 10 to 40 degrees cephalad) to evaluate the posterior subtalar facet and a Canale view (AP view of the foot in 15 degrees of pronation with tube angled 75 degrees from the horizontal) to evaluate the sinus tarsi.
- Radiographic findings consistent with a degenerative process include joint space narrowing, osteophytes, and subchondral cysts or sclerosis (**FIG 1**).
- Computed tomography (CT) and magnetic resonance imaging offer little additional information about the arthritic process involving the subtalar joint, but they may identify a previously undiagnosed tarsal coalition or concomitant soft tissue pathology.
- A diagnostic injection of a local anesthetic into the subtalar joint may help localize the patient's complaints, and if a corticosteroid is added to the injection, this procedure may provide significant short-term relief.

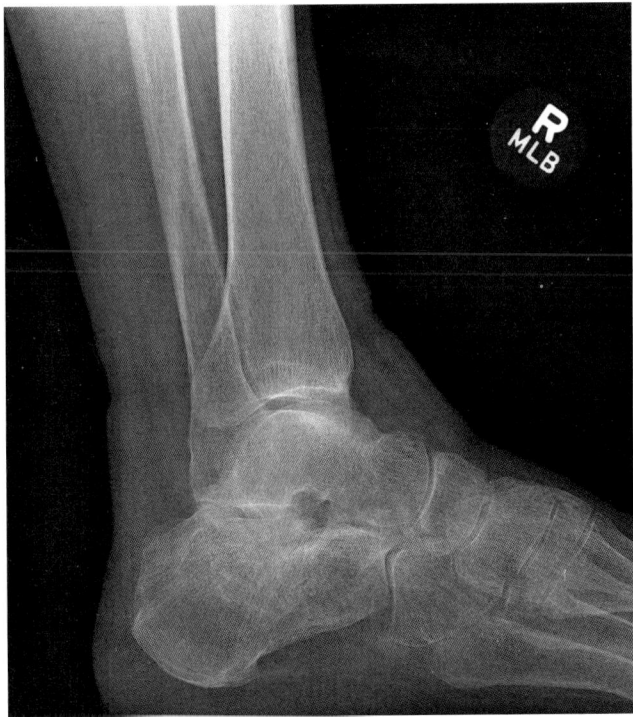

FIG 1 Preoperative plain radiograph demonstrating flattening of Bohler angle and posttraumatic arthrosis of the subtalar joint.

DIFFERENTIAL DIAGNOSIS

- Primary osteoarthrosis
- Posttraumatic arthritis
- Inflammatory arthritis
- Acute fracture
- Sinus tarsi syndrome
- Instability of the subtalar joint or subtalar sprain
- Fibrous or cartilaginous talocalcaneal coalition
- Subtalar loose body

NONOPERATIVE MANAGEMENT

- Subtalar joint arthritis is initially managed nonoperatively in all patients.
- Nonoperative management strategies may include the following:
  - Activity modification
  - Nonsteroidal anti-inflammatory medications
  - Intra-articular corticosteroid injection
  - Use of an ankle–foot orthosis or University of California Biomechanics Laboratory (UCBL) orthosis to limit hind-foot motion. Other options include an air stirrup or high-top boot.
  - Patellar tendon–bearing brace to unload the subtalar joint
- Conservative treatment may also be indicated in patients with significant peripheral vascular disease, active infection, inability to comply with the postoperative regimen, or a severe sensory neuropathy.

SURGICAL MANAGEMENT

- For patients who do not achieve relief with an adequate trial of nonoperative management, surgical intervention is warranted.

Preoperative Planning

- Plain radiographs are reviewed for deformity or malalignment, loose bodies, or retained hardware from a prior surgery.
- CT or magnetic resonance imaging scans are reviewed, if available.

Positioning

- The patient is placed supine on the operative table, and the sole of the foot is aligned with the end of the bed to facilitate later screw insertion into the heel.
- A pneumatic tourniquet is placed around the upper thigh, and a soft bump is placed beneath the ipsilateral sacrum to internally rotate the operative extremity. Placement of the bump beneath the sacrum, rather than beneath the buttock, will prevent any undue pressure on the sciatic nerve. Alternatively, the patient may be placed semilateral on a bean bag.
- The fluoroscopy unit is brought in from the contralateral side of the bed.
- The tourniquet is elevated to a pressure 100 mm Hg greater than the patient's systolic pressure.

EXPOSURE

- The incision begins approximately 1 cm below the tip of the lateral malleolus and progresses distally to a point just shy of the base of the fourth metatarsal **(TECH FIG 1A)**. Alternatively, a modified Ollier incision may be used.
- The subcutaneous tissue is incised in line with the skin incision, and preemptive hemostasis of any crossing vessels is performed using electrocautery. The sural nerve is identified and protected.
- The origin of the extensor digitorum brevis muscle is identified and elevated along with the sinus tarsi fat pad as a distally

based flap. A small cuff of tissue is preserved proximally for later reattachment of this flap.
- Deep dissection is carried in the interval between the peroneal tendons and the sinus tarsi fat pad **(TECH FIG 1B)**. A small Hohmann retractor is placed posterior to the posterior facet of the calcaneus and a lamina spreader is placed into the sinus tarsi **(TECH FIG 1C)**.
- At this point, the subtalar joint is well visualized.

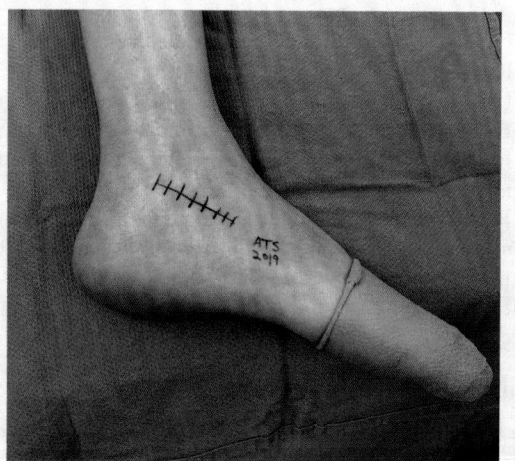

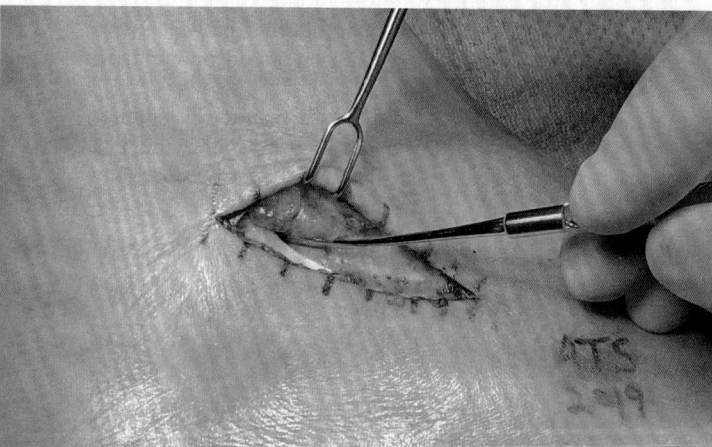

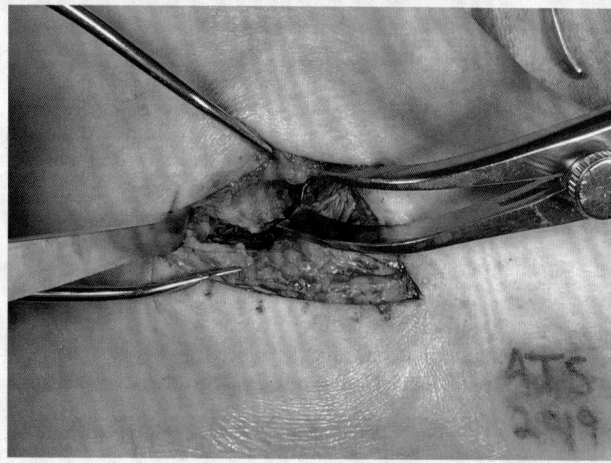

TECH FIG 1 A. Surgical incision. **B.** Deep dissection is carried in the interval between the peroneal tendons and the sinus tarsi fat pad. **C.** Small Hohmann retractor placed posterior to the posterior facet of the calcaneus and lamina spreader placed into the sinus tarsi.

PREPARATION OF THE ARTHRODESIS SITE

- After adequate visualization of the lateral aspect of the posterior facet of the subtalar joint has been attained, any remaining fatty or ligamentous tissue is removed from the joint with a rongeur. Care is taken to protect the interosseous talocalcaneal ligament and, thus, avoid damaging the plantar blood supply to the talar body.
- Using a sharp osteotome, the articular cartilage is removed from the inferior talus and superior aspect of the calcaneal facets **(TECH FIG 2A,B)**. Note that the goal is to maintain the normal, curved contours of the articular facets.
- Residual cartilage remnants are removed with a sharp periosteal elevator **(TECH FIG 2C)**. Curved curettes and a rongeur are also utilized as necessary.

Implant Placement

- With the optimal size determined clinically and proper trial position confirmed fluoroscopically, the trial is removed and the final implant is placed over the guidewire (**TECH FIG 7A–C**).
  - The implant should be advanced to the point that it appropriately blocks eversion without overcorrecting the hindfoot into varus (**TECH FIG 7D,E**).
  - Fluoroscopic confirmation of proper implant position should be performed, as described for the trial earlier.

- Ideally, the implant's leading edge approaches the midaxis of the talar neck (AP fluoroscopic view) without its opposite end completely recessed under the lateral talar neck cortex (**TECH FIG 7F–H**).
- The guidewire is removed from the medial side to limit the risk of implant displacement (**TECH FIG 7I–L**).

Completion

- Final fluoroscopic confirmation in the AP and lateral planes to confirm the implant is in the optimal position (**TECH FIG 8**)
- Routine wound closure

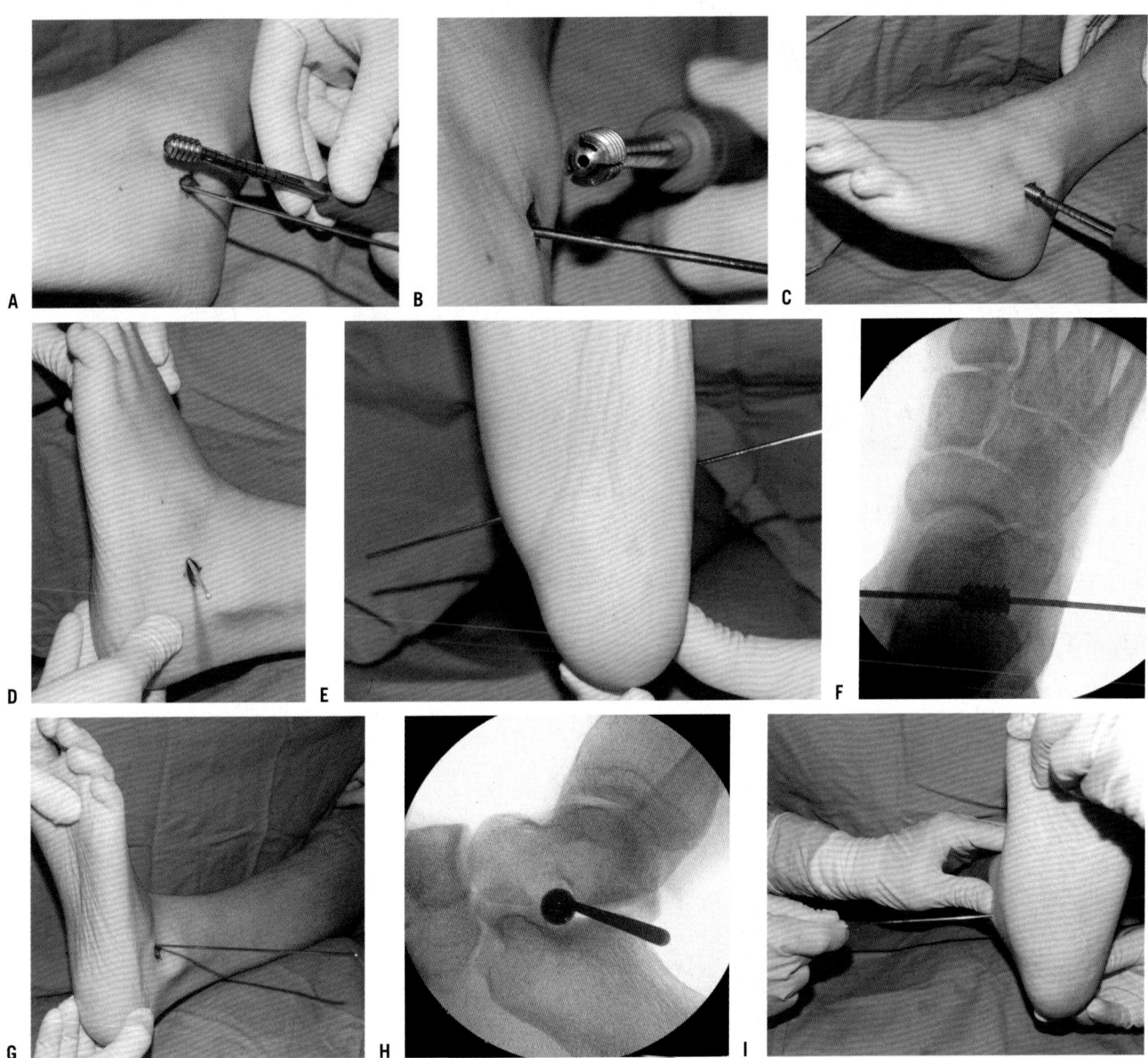

TECH FIG 7 A. The final implant is threaded to provide stability. It is also fluted to absorb shock. **B.** End-on view to show fluted design. **C.** Final implant insertion. **D,E.** Confirming proper heel position with final implant in place. **D.** Valgus heel stress. **E.** Heel position evaluated. **F.** AP fluoroscopic view to confirm proper final implant position. Ideally, the implant's leading edge approaches the midaxis of the talar neck without its opposite end completely recessed under the lateral talar neck cortex. **G,H.** Optimal position based on lateral view with guide pin still in place. **I.** Guidewire extracted medially. By removing it medially, the implant has less chance of dislodging from its ideal position. *(continued)*

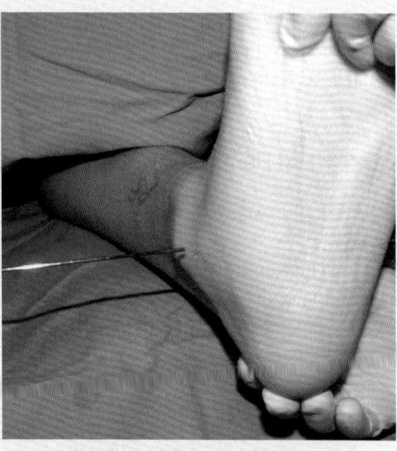
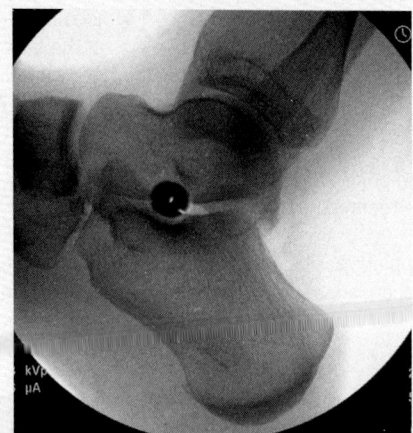
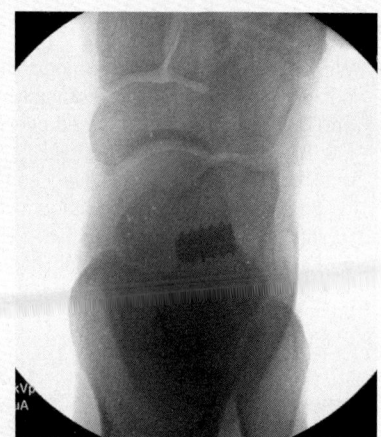

TECH FIG 7 *(continued)* **J.** Guidewire fully extracted. **K.** Final lateral fluoroscopic view. **L.** Final AP fluoroscopic view. Note that the implant's leading edge approaches the midaxis of the talar neck without crossing it, and the trailing edge is not fully buried under the lateral talar neck.

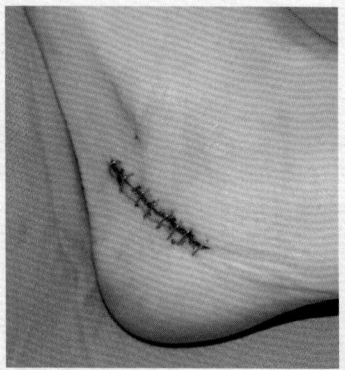
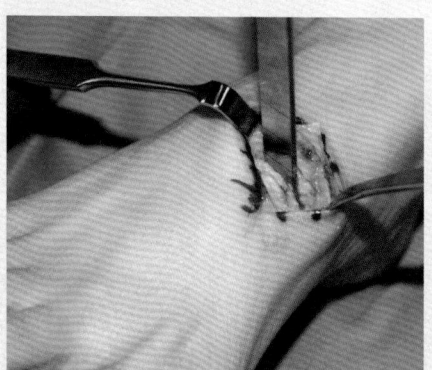
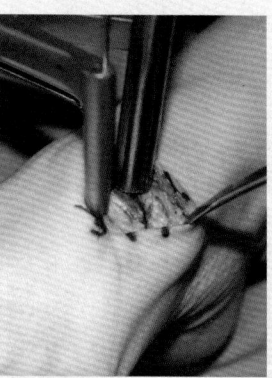

TECH FIG 8 Associated foot realignment. **A.** Medial displacement calcaneal osteotomy completed prior to subtalar arthroereisis in this case. **B.** Plantarflexion osteotomy of first cuneiform. **C.** Graft insertion into medial cuneiform.

CASE EXAMPLE

- In our experience, isolated subtalar arthroereisis does not afford adequate correction in skeletally mature patients with flexible pes planovalgus deformity.
  - In this particular case, the 26-year-old woman had better correction on the right foot, where foot realignment procedures were added to subtalar arthroereisis, than in the left foot, where subtalar arthroereisis was performed with only gastrocnemius–soleus recession **(TECH FIG 9A–F)**.
- Weight-bearing radiographs of the same patient's right foot with subtalar arthroereisis performed with gastrocnemius–soleus recession, medial displacement calcaneal osteotomy, and plantarflexion osteotomy of the first cuneiform **(TECH FIG 9G,H)**

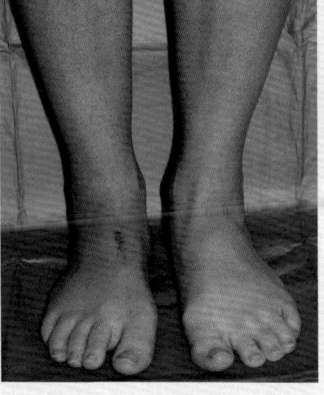
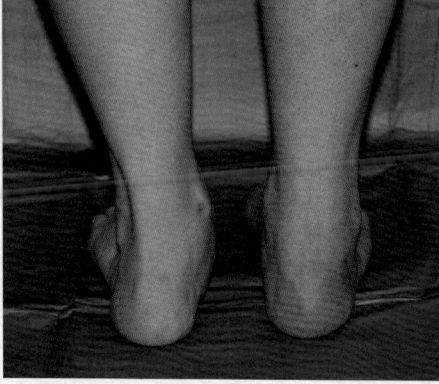

TECH FIG 9 Example case of a 26-year-old woman with better correction on right foot where foot realignment procedures were added to subtalar arthroereisis when compared to left foot where subtalar arthroereisis was performed with only gastrocnemius–soleus recession. **A.** AP view. **B.** Posterior view. *(continued)*

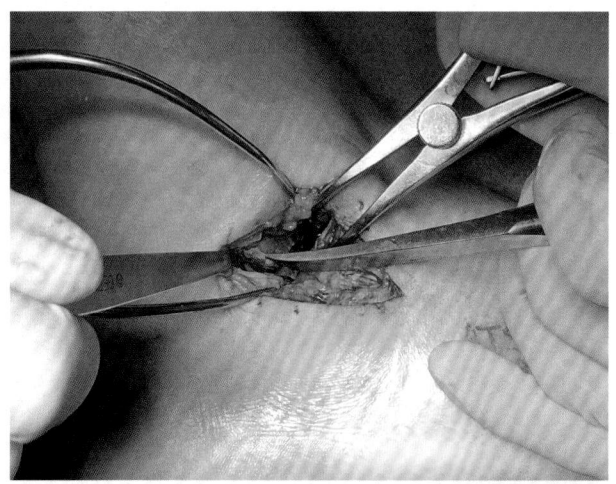

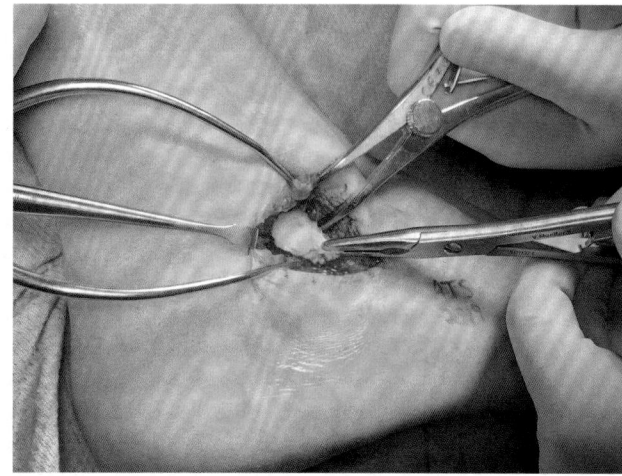

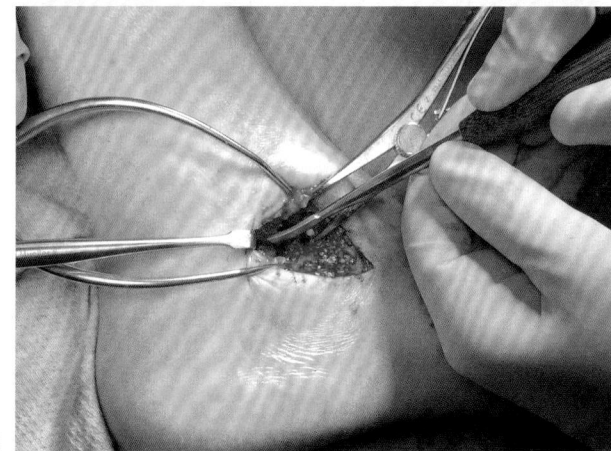

TECH FIG 2 A. Articular cartilage removed with a sharp curved osteotome. **B.** Large sheet of cartilage retrieved from the joint with a rongeur. **C.** Any residual cartilage remnants are removed using a sharp periosteal elevator.

- After complete removal of all articular cartilage, a sharp 0.25-inch osteotome is utilized to "feather" the subchondral bone of the inferior surface of the talus and superior surface of the calcaneus. It is imperative that the sharp edge of the osteotome penetrates the subchondral plate to allow for adequate communication of the talar and calcaneal marrow contents **(TECH FIG 3)**.
- Cancellous autograft obtained from the proximal tibia (see Harvesting of Tibial Bone Graft in the Techniques section) is mixed with demineralized bone matrix and is inserted into the subtalar joint **(TECH FIG 4)**, and the extensor digitorum brevis muscle is reattached to its site of origin to seal the arthrodesis site.

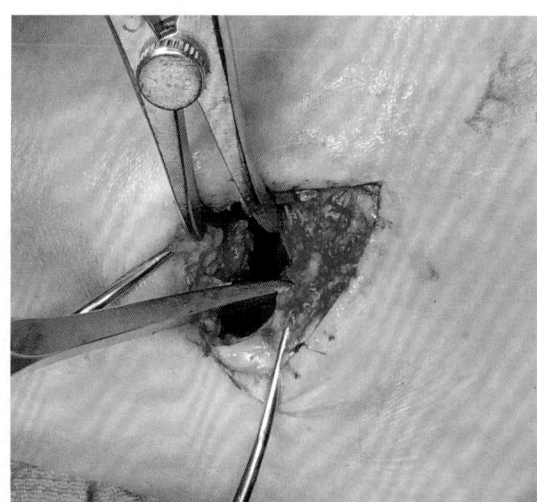

TECH FIG 3 Subchondral bone is feathered with a sharp 0.25-inch osteotome.

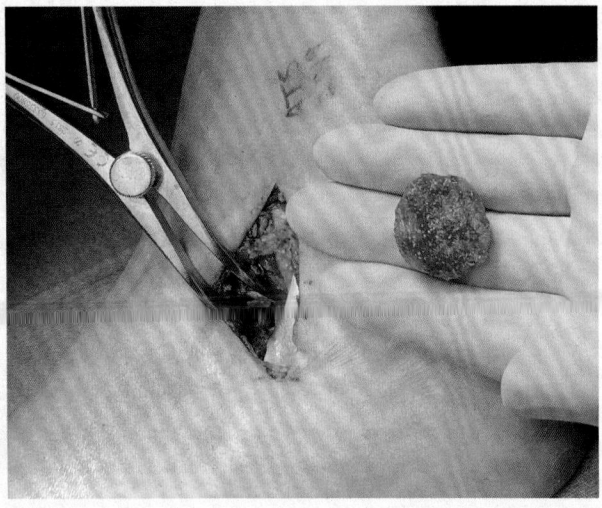
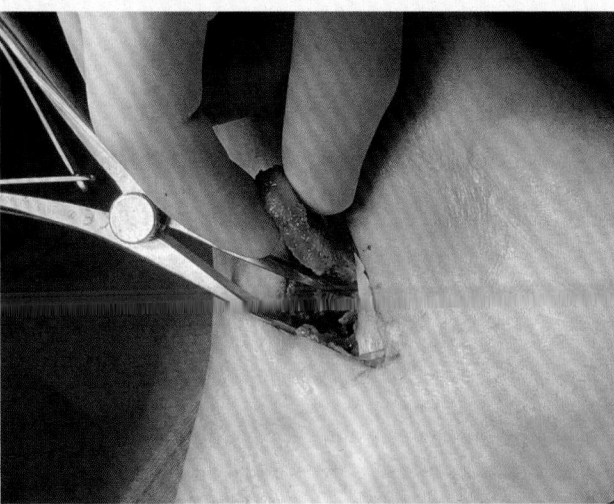

TECH FIG 4 **A.** Harvested cancellous bone graft is mixed with demineralized bone matrix and formed into a patty. **B.** Bone graft mixture is then inserted into the posterior facet of the subtalar joint.

INSERTION OF HARDWARE

- At this point, the subtalar joint is positioned into 5 degrees of valgus.
- A 1-cm incision is created at the apex of the heel for insertion of a guide pin, which is subsequently driven through the posterior tuberosity, across the subtalar joint, and into the talar body–neck junction **(TECH FIG 5)**. This guide pin is placed under fluoroscopic guidance using lateral, Broden, axial (Harris) heel views **(TECH FIG 6)**. After lodging the tip of the pin into the dorsal talar cortex, a measurement is obtained using the cannulated depth gauge **(TECH FIG 7)**. At least 5 mm should be subtracted from the measured length to account for compression at the level of the joint.

- The guide pin is then overreamed with the cannulated drill bit. The tip of the drill is advanced across the subtalar joint until it just penetrates the subchondral bone of the talus **(TECH FIG 8)**.
- The cannulated compression screw of an appropriate length is then inserted **(TECH FIG 9)** over the guide pin, and the depth of the insertion is confirmed with fluoroscopy. In this case, the selected screw was a 7.5-mm headless, variable pitch screw.
- Final fluoroscopic images are obtained to verify proper screw position **(TECH FIG 10)**.
- The tourniquet is released, and hemostasis is secured.
- The wound is, subsequently, closed using 2-0 Vicryl for the deep fascial layer and 3-0 nylon horizontal mattress sutures for the skin.

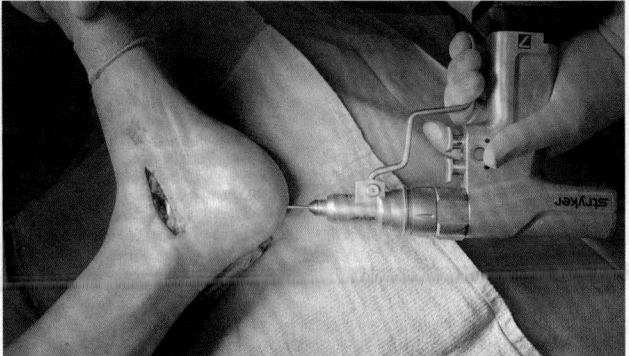

TECH FIG 5 After positioning the hindfoot into 5 degrees of valgus, the guide pin for the cannulated compression screw is inserted into the posteroinferior apex of the calcaneal tuberosity.

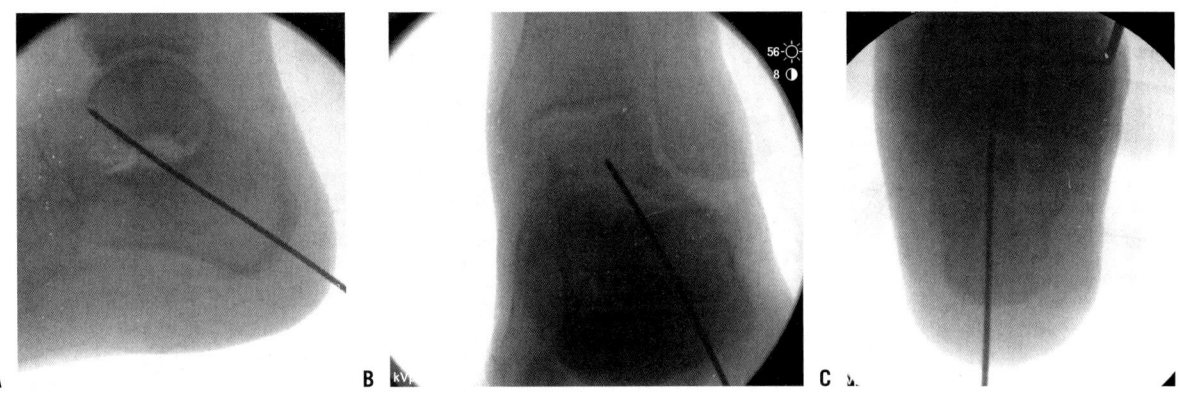

TECH FIG 6 Proper position of the guide pin as seen on lateral (**A**), Broden (**B**), and axial calcaneal (**C**) views.

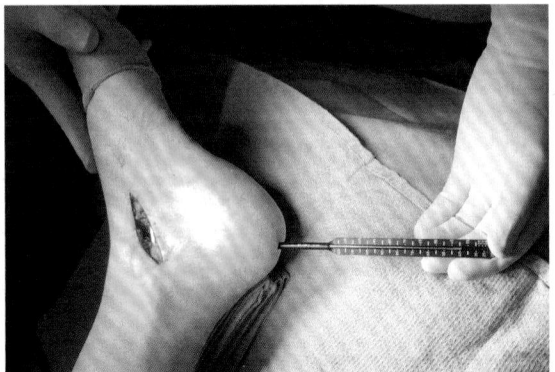

TECH FIG 7 Use of cannulated depth gauge.

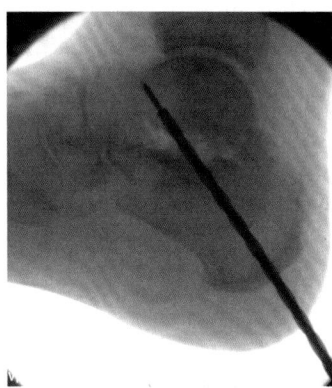

TECH FIG 8 Cannulated drilling. Drill tip must penetrate plantar cortex of the talus.

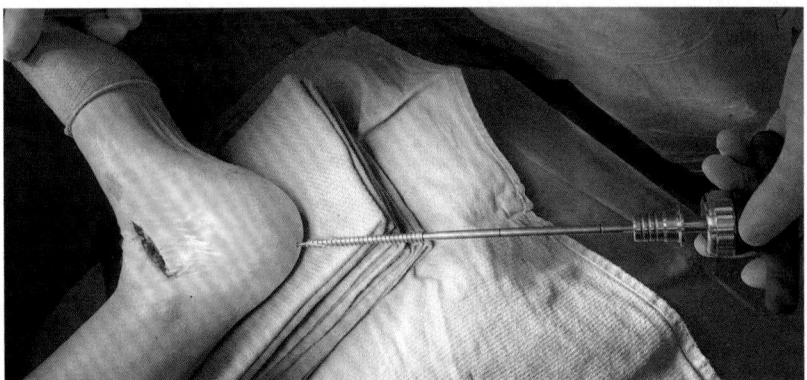

TECH FIG 9 Screw insertion.

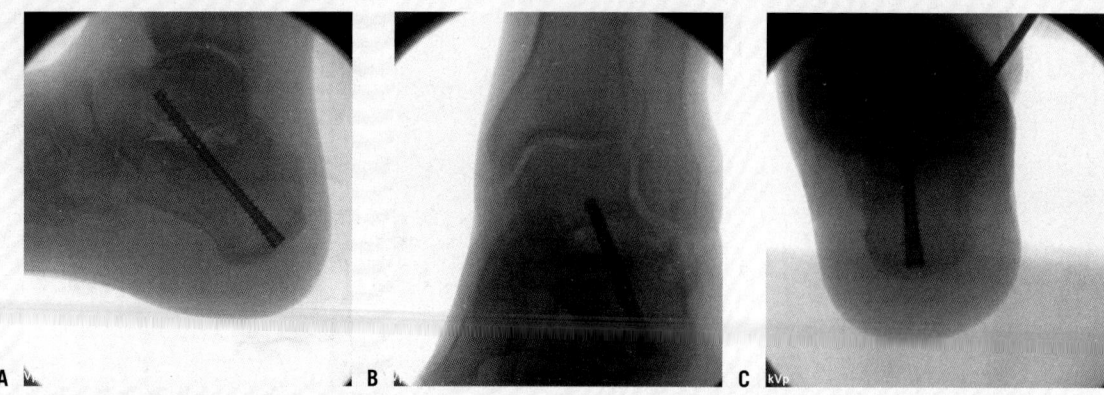

TECH FIG 10 Final position of the compression screw on lateral (**A**), Broden (**B**), and axial calcaneal (**C**) views.

HARVESTING OF TIBIAL BONE GRAFT

- An incision beginning 1 cm distal to the distal aspect of the tibial tubercle and 1 cm lateral to the anterior tibial crest is carried distally for a length of 4 cm (**TECH FIG 11A**).
- The fascia overlying the anterior compartment musculature is divided in line with the skin incision.
- Muscle and periosteum overlying the anterolateral face of the tibia is elevated using a periosteal elevator, thus exposing the anterolateral cortex (**TECH FIG 11B**).

- A 1- × 1-cm cortical window is created in the center of the anterolateral face, and a curette is inserted into the window for removal of cancellous graft (**TECH FIG 11C,D**).
- After an adequate amount of cancellous graft is harvested, the window is sealed with the previously removed square plug of bone and a layered closure of the fascia, subcutaneous tissue, and skin is performed.
- Time from graft harvest to insertion into the fusion site should be less than 30 minutes.

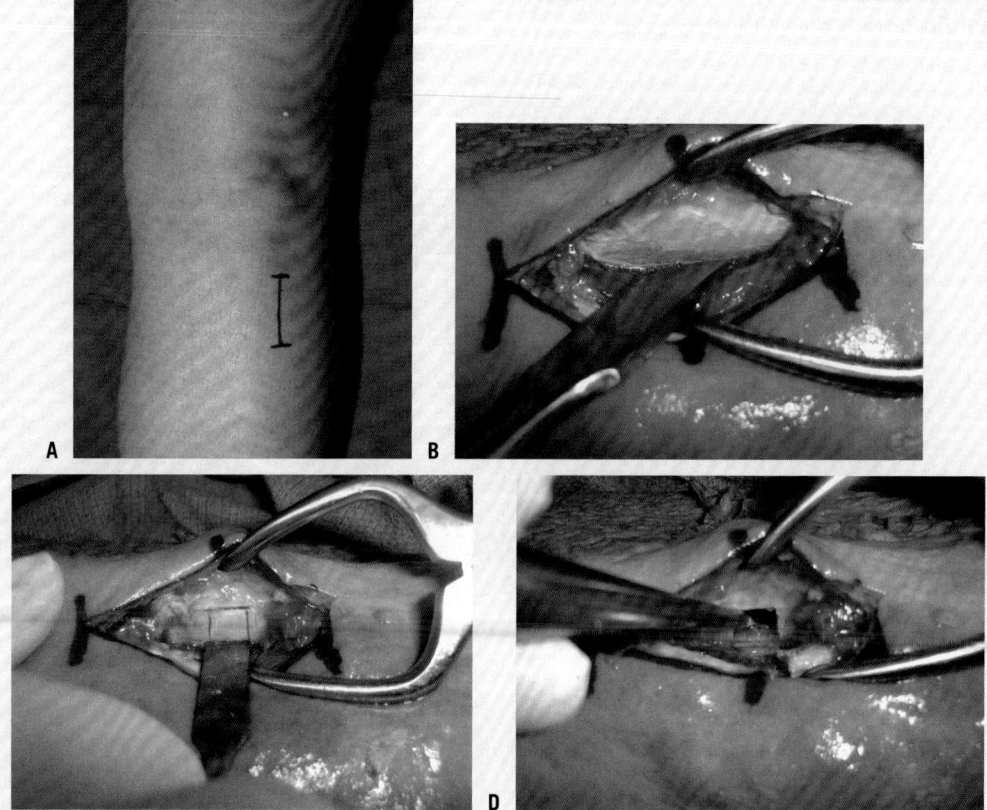

TECH FIG 11 Harvesting of tibial bone graft. **A.** Incision. **B.** Periosteal elevation along the anterolateral cortex. **C.** Creation of 1- × 1-cm cortical window. **D.** Removal of cancellous autograft with a curette.

Pearls and Pitfalls

Preparation of Joint Surfaces	• Remove articular cartilage only. • Preservation of subchondral bone will provide structural support and will allow for better coaptation.[9] • Use of a sharp 0.25-inch osteotome to perforate the residual subchondral bone of the talus and calcaneus will allow communication between the marrow cavities and the arthrodesis site and will aid in the fusion.
Positioning of Arthrodesis	• The arthrodesis is ideally placed in 5 degrees of valgus.[6] • Fusing the subtalar joint in varus will lock the transverse tarsal joint, leading to increased lateral forefoot pressures with weight bearing.[10] • Fusing the subtalar joint in excessive valgus can potentially lead to subfibular impingement and medial knee pain.[10]
Internal Fixation	• Use of a headless compression screw will reduce the likelihood of hardware irritation at the posterior heel. • Penetration of the plantar cortex of the talus with the cannulated drill bit will reduce the tendency of the screw to distract the arthrodesis site.

POSTOPERATIVE CARE

- The extremity is placed in a well-padded, non–weight-bearing short-leg fiberglass cast prior to leaving the operating room.
- The patient is seen in clinic at 2 to 3 weeks postoperatively, at which point the initial cast and sutures are removed.
- A new short-leg fiberglass cast is applied, and the patient is kept nonweight bearing.
- At the 6-week mark, radiographs are obtained, and the patient is converted to a walking boot. Full weight-bearing and gentle ankle range-of-motion exercises are allowed at this juncture.
- If radiographic union is appreciated at the 12-week appointment, the patient may transition out of the boot and into regular shoes.

OUTCOMES

- At an average of nearly 5 years of follow-up, Mann et al[12] reported a 93% satisfaction rate with isolated subtalar arthrodesis.
- In another study by Mann and Baumgarten,[11] subtalar joint fusion in 6 degrees of valgus resulted in the maintenance of approximately 50% of the transverse tarsal joint motion as compared with the unaffected, contralateral extremity. In this same study, minimal degenerative changes were noted at the talonavicular and calcaneocuboid joints, a finding that was not clinically significant.[11]
- In a retrospective study, Dahm and Kitaoka[3] demonstrated a 96% union rate in 25 adult feet.
- Similarly, Easley et al[4] demonstrated a 96% subtalar fusion rate after excluding smokers, revision arthrodeses, fusions using a structural graft, and subtalar fusions performed in an extremity with a previously fused tibiotalar joint.

COMPLICATIONS

- Infection[8]
- Nonunion[4,7,10]
- Malalignment
  - Varus leading to increased lateral column forefoot pressures[6,10]
  - Valgus leading to subfibular impingement[6,10]
- Symptomatic hardware[4]
- Superficial wound breakdown[2]
- Reflex sympathetic dystrophy[5]

REFERENCES

1. Astion DJ, Deland JT, Otis JC, et al. Motion of the hindfoot after simulated arthrodesis. J Bone Joint Surg Am 1997;79(2):241–246.
2. Chandler JT, Bonar SK, Anderson RB, et al. Results of in situ subtalar arthrodesis for late sequelae of calcaneus fractures. Foot Ankle Int 1999;20:18–24.
3. Dahm DL, Kitaoka HB. Subtalar arthrodesis with internal compression for posttraumatic arthritis. J Bone Joint Surg Br 1998;80(1):134–138.
4. Easley ME, Trnka HJ, Schon LC, et al. Isolated subtalar arthrodesis. J Bone Joint Surg Am 2000;82(5):613–624.
5. Flemister AS Jr, Infante AF, Sanders RW, et al. Subtalar arthrodesis for complications of intra-articular calcaneal fractures. Foot Ankle Int 2000;21:392–399.
6. Kile TA, Bouchard M. Degenerative joint disease of the ankle and hindfoot. In: Thordarson DB, ed. Orthopaedic Surgery Essentials: Foot and Ankle. Philadelphia: Lippincott Williams & Wilkins, 2004:195–220.
7. Kitaoka HB. Talocalcaneal (subtalar) arthrodesis. In: Kitaoka HB, ed. Master Techniques in Orthopaedic Surgery: The Foot and Ankle, ed 2. Philadelphia: Lippincott Williams & Wilkins, 2002:387–399.
8. Lin SS, Shereff MJ. Talocalcaneal arthrodesis: a moldable bone grafting technique. Foot Ankle Clin 1996;1:109–131.
9. Lippert FG, Hansen ST. Subtalar arthrodesis. In: Lippert FG, Hansen ST, eds. Foot and Ankle Disorders: Tricks of the Trade. New York: Thieme, 2003:133–139.
10. Mann RA. Arthrodesis of the foot and ankle. In: Coughlin MJ, Mann RA, eds. Surgery of the Foot and Ankle, ed 7. St Louis: Mosby, 1999:651–699.
11. Mann RA, Baumgarten M. Subtalar fusion for isolated subtalar disorders. Preliminary report. Clin Orthop Relat Res 1988;(226):260–265.
12. Mann RA, Beaman DN, Horton GA. Isolated subtalar arthrodesis. Foot Ankle Int 1998;19:511–519.

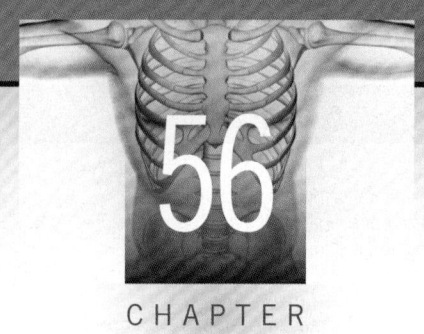

Surgical Management of Calcaneal Malunions

Michael P. Clare and Roy W. Sanders

DEFINITION

- A calcaneal malunion refers to residual bony malalignment and associated clinical sequelae resulting from inadequate treatment of a displaced intra-articular calcaneal fracture.

ANATOMY

- The calcaneus is an odd-shaped bone which supports full body weight and provides a lever arm through which the powerful gastrocsoleus complex assists with forward propulsion during gait (FIG 1).
- The calcaneus also provides articulations for the subtalar and calcaneocuboid joints and thus is integral to function of the triple joint complex of the hindfoot for normal ambulation and accommodation to uneven ground (FIG 2).
- The normal orientation of the calcaneus is reflected radiographically as calcaneal pitch, calcaneal height, and calcaneal length, which directly affect the three-dimensional alignment of the hindfoot and midfoot and indirectly affect ankle dorsiflexion (FIG 3).

PATHOGENESIS

- In the event of a displaced intra-articular calcaneal fracture, there is typically not only intra-articular displacement of the posterior facet but also loss of calcaneal height, shortening and varus angulation of the calcaneal tuberosity, extension into the anterior process or calcaneocuboid joint, and expansion of the lateral calcaneal wall.
- Nonoperative treatment, or inadequate operative treatment, of a displaced intra-articular calcaneal fracture results in a calcaneal malunion, which affects function of the ankle,

subtalar, and calcaneocuboid joints and leads to pain and disability.[4,15,16] Associated sequelae include the following:
- Posttraumatic subtalar and calcaneocuboid arthritis due to residual articular incongruity[8,17]
- Lateral subfibular impingement from residual lateral wall expansion and heel widening[3,10]
- Peroneal tendon stenosis, tenosynovitis, or subluxation/dislocation as a result of adjacent bony prominence[2,5,13]
- Anterior ankle impingement and loss of ankle dorsiflexion due to loss of calcaneal height, resulting in relative dorsiflexion of talus[3]
- Hindfoot malalignment (typically varus) affecting gait pattern and shoe wear and potentially producing a leg length discrepancy[14]

NATURAL HISTORY

- Patients with displaced intra-articular calcaneal fractures that go on to malunion typically have a poor result, including pain with weight bearing, limitations in shoe wear, secondary gait alterations, and progressive posttraumatic subtalar arthritis.[6,12]

PATIENT HISTORY AND PHYSICAL FINDINGS

- History of prior calcaneal fracture (displaced intra-articular fracture)—note prior method of treatment (operative or nonoperative)
- Pain with weight bearing (standing or walking, particularly on uneven terrain)
- Thorough examination of the ankle and hindfoot should also include assessment of the following:
  - Skin and soft tissue envelope, including location of previous surgical incisions, overall mobility of lateral hindfoot skin, swelling, or any dystrophic changes where present
  - Neurovascular status (particularly the presence or absence of palpable pulses)

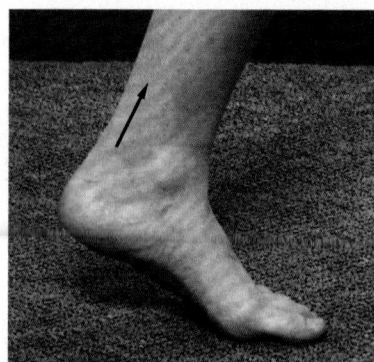

FIG 1 The calcaneus serves as a lever arm for the powerful gastrocsoleus complex.

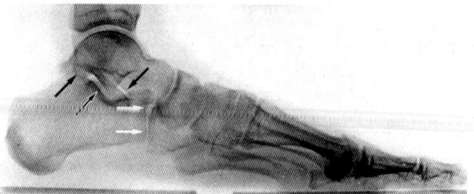

FIG 2 Normal weight-bearing lateral radiograph demonstrating posterior and middle facets of subtalar joint (black arrows) and calcaneocuboid joint (white arrows).

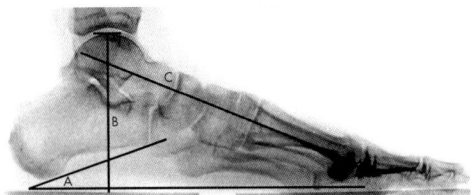

FIG 3 Normal weight-bearing lateral radiograph. Note downward orientation of talus. (*A*) Calcaneal pitch angle. (*B*) Calcaneal height. (*C*) Talo–first metatarsal angle.

- Hindfoot malalignment: Excessive hindfoot varus or valgus relative to uninvolved limb represents malalignment.
- Subtalar range of motion: Decreased subtalar range of motion may result from posttraumatic arthritis.
- Subtalar arthritis: Tenderness to palpation suggests articular degeneration.
- Subfibular impingement, bony prominence, and tenderness suggest peroneal stenosis or tenosynovitis from residual lateral wall expansion. Peroneal tendons may actually be subluxed or dislocated in severe cases.
- Ankle range of motion: Decreased dorsiflexion compared to uninvolved limb may indicate anterior impingement from relative dorsiflexion of talus and loss of calcaneal height.

IMAGING AND OTHER DIAGNOSTIC STUDIES

- Standard weight-bearing radiographs of the ankle and foot, in addition to a Harris axial view of the calcaneus, reveal the calcaneal malunion.
- The lateral view of the hindfoot demonstrates loss of calcaneal height and relative dorsiflexion of the talus (**FIG 4**).
- The mortise view of the ankle demonstrates residual lateral wall expansion and degenerative changes in the subtalar joint as well as a fracture-dislocation variant fragment where present (**FIGS 5** and **6**).
- The axial view shows residual shortening of the calcaneus and any hindfoot malalignment were present (**FIG 7**).
- Once the diagnosis is established, a computed tomography (CT) scan of the calcaneus, including axial, sagittal, and 30-degree semicoronal images, further delineates the extent of subtalar and calcaneocuboid arthritic change, hindfoot

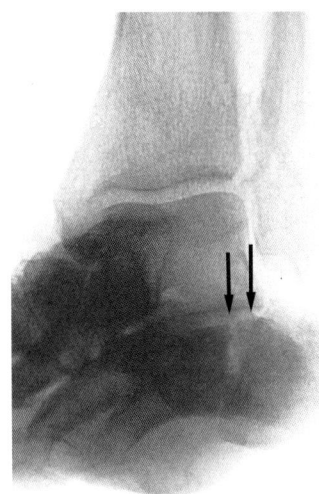

FIG 5 Weight-bearing mortise radiograph of calcaneal malunion. Note residual intra-articular step-off and associated degenerative changes (*black arrows*).

malalignment, lateral wall exostosis, subfibular impingement, as well as any associated talar or other ankle joint pathology (**FIGS 8–10**).

DIFFERENTIAL DIAGNOSIS

- Posttraumatic subtalar arthritis (without malunion)
- Subtalar osteoarthritis
- Calcaneal fracture nonunion
- Lateral ankle instability or peroneal tendon pathology

NONOPERATIVE MANAGEMENT

- Nonoperative treatment options are limited but consists primarily of supportive modalities to lessen inflammation and painful motion through the hindfoot.
- A lace-up ankle brace, University of California at Berkeley Laboratory, ankle–foot orthosis, or Arizona-type brace may

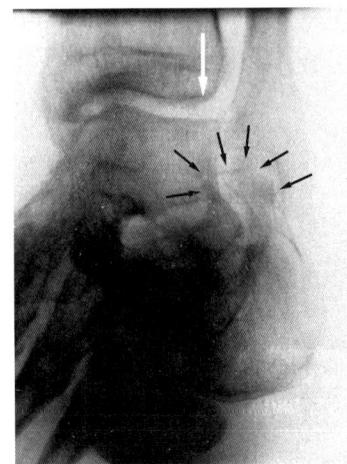

FIG 6 Weight-bearing mortise radiograph of calcaneal malunion from fracture-dislocation variant pattern. Note residually dislocated posterolateral fragment wedged within talofibular joint (*black arrows*) and subtle varus tilt within ankle mortise (*white arrow*), suggesting incompetence of lateral ligamentous complex.

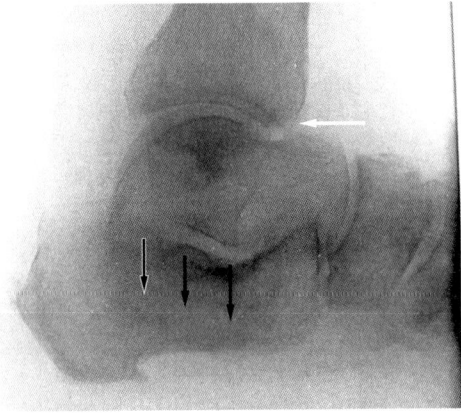

FIG 4 Weight-bearing lateral radiograph of calcaneal malunion. Note loss of calcaneal height (*black arrows*), producing relative dorsiflexion of talus and anterior impingement at ankle joint (*white arrow*).

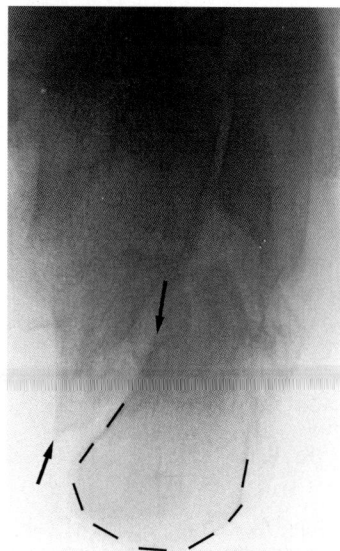

FIG 7 Axial radiograph of calcaneal malunion. Note marked residual shortening (*black arrows*) and varus angulation of calcaneal tuberosity (*dashed lines*).

be beneficial in limiting painful subtalar motion and providing symptomatic relief. A prefabricated fracture boot may be used intermittently for episodes of arthritic flare-up.

- Intermittent use of nonsteroidal anti-inflammatory medication can also be beneficial in disrupting the inflammatory cycle.
- Activity modification, such as limited standing and walking, particularly on uneven terrain, may also lessen symptoms.

SURGICAL MANAGEMENT

- We use the Stephens-Sanders classification system and treatment protocol for calcaneal malunions, which is based on CT evaluation.[17] Type I malunions include a large lateral wall exostosis, with or without far lateral subtalar arthrosis. Type II malunions include a lateral wall exostosis and subtalar arthrosis involving the entire width of the joint. Type III

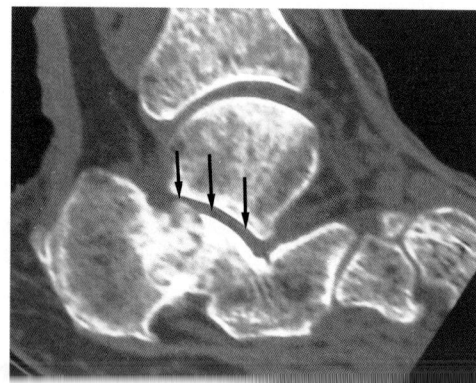

FIG 9 Sagittal CT image demonstrating loss of calcaneal height (*black arrows*).

malunions include a lateral wall exostosis, subtalar arthrosis, and malalignment of the calcaneal body resulting in significant hindfoot varus or valgus angulation (**FIG 11A–C**).

Preoperative Planning

- The calcaneal malunion is evaluated with plain radiographs and CT scan and classified according to the Stephens-Sanders classification.[17] Treatment is based strictly on malunion type:
  - Type I malunions are managed with a lateral wall exostectomy and a peroneal tenolysis.[2,5,13]
  - Type II malunions are managed with a lateral wall exostectomy, peroneal tenolysis, and a subtalar bone block arthrodesis, using the excised lateral wall as autograft.[11]
  - Type III malunions are managed with a lateral wall exostectomy, peroneal tenolysis, subtalar bone block arthrodesis, and a calcaneal osteotomy to correct hindfoot malalignment.[7]
- The procedure requires use of a radiolucent table and a standard C-arm.
- A pneumatic thigh tourniquet is used. The procedure should be completed within 120 to 130 minutes of tourniquet time to minimize potential wound complications.

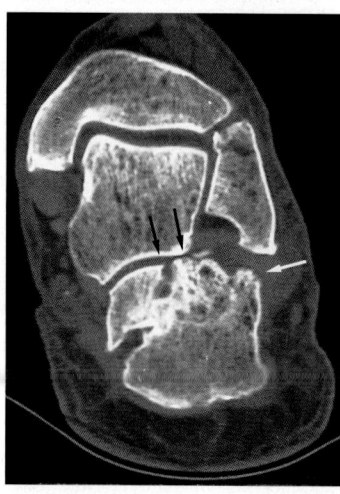

FIG 8 Semicoronal CT image demonstrating subfibular impingement (*white arrow*) and posttraumatic arthritic changes in posterior facet (*black arrows*).

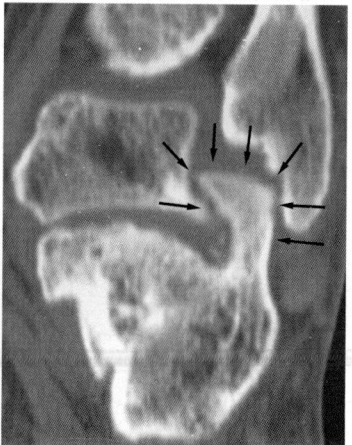

FIG 10 Semicoronal CT image of calcaneal malunion from fracture-dislocation variant pattern (*black arrows*). This 25-year-old laborer had unfortunately been treated nonoperatively and rapidly developed posttraumatic arthritis.

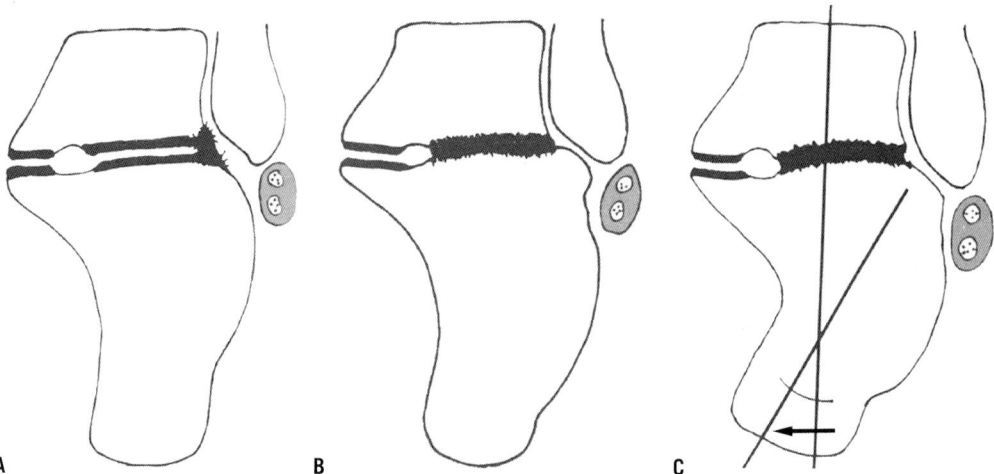

FIG 11 Stephens-Sanders classification of calcaneal malunions. **A.** Type I malunion. **B.** Type II malunion. **C.** Type III malunion.

Positioning

- The patient is placed in the lateral decubitus position on a bean-bag. The lower extremities are positioned in a scissor configuration, such that the operative ("up") limb is flexed at the knee and angles toward the distal posterior corner of the operating table, whereas the nonoperative ("down") limb is extended at the knee and lies away from the eventual surgical field, which facilitates intraoperative fluoroscopy without interference from the nonoperative limb. Protective padding is placed beneath the contralateral limb for protection of the peroneal nerve, and an operating "platform" is created with blankets and foam padding to elevate the operative limb (**FIG 12**).
- Alternatively, the prone position may be used in the event of bilateral procedures.

Approach

- We use the extensile lateral approach for surgical management of the calcaneal malunion, regardless of malunion type. The lateral calcaneal artery, typically a branch of the peroneal artery, supplies the majority of the full-thickness flap.[1] Thus, strict attention to detail with respect to placement of the incision and gentle handling of the soft tissues is of paramount importance.
- The planned extensile lateral approach is then outlined on the skin:
  - The incision begins approximately 2 cm proximal to the tip of the lateral malleolus, just lateral to the Achilles tendon and thus posterior to the sural nerve and the lateral calcaneal artery, and the vertical limb extends toward the plantar foot
  - The horizontal limb is drawn along the junction of the skin of the lateral foot and heel pad; this skin demarcation can be identified by compressing the heel. We substitute a gentle curve where these two lines combine to form a right angle, primarily to avoid apical necrosis. The horizontal limb also includes a gentle anterior curve along the skin creases distally, ideally ending over the calcaneocuboid articulation (**FIG 13**).

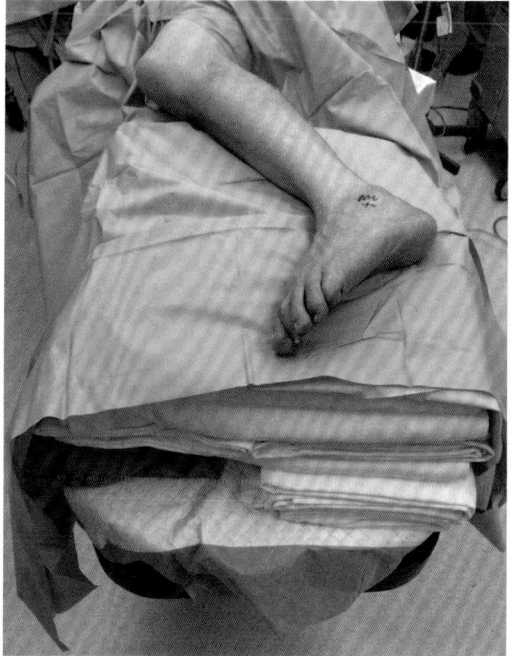

FIG 12 Lateral decubitus position. Note scissor configuration of limbs to facilitate intraoperative fluoroscopy.

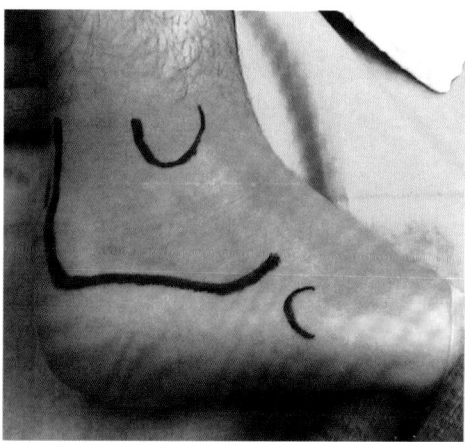

FIG 13 Planned incision for extensile lateral approach.

TECHNIQUES

EXTENSILE LATERAL APPROACH

- The limb placed on a sterile bolster and the incision begins at the proximal portion of the vertical limb, becoming full thickness at the level of the calcaneal tuberosity—literally "straight to bone" while avoiding any beveling of the skin.[9] Scalpel pressure is again lessened beyond the apical curve of the incision, and a layered incision is developed along the horizontal limb of the incision.
- A full-thickness, subperiosteal flap is then raised starting at the apex, specifically avoiding use of retractors until a considerable subperiosteal flap is developed, in order to prevent separation of the skin from the underlying subcutaneous tissue **(TECH FIG 1A)**.
- The calcaneofibular ligament is sharply released from the lateral wall of the calcaneus, and the adjacent peroneal tendons are released from the peroneal tubercle through the cartilaginous "pulley" to avoid iatrogenic injury **(TECH FIG 1B)**.

- A periosteal elevator is then used to gently mobilize the tendons along the distal portion of the incision, which then exposes the anterolateral calcaneus. Thus, the peroneal tendons and sural nerve are contained entirely within the flap, and devascularization of the lateral skin is minimized **(TECH FIG 1C)**.
- Deep dissection continues to the sinus tarsi and anterior process region anteriorly, calcaneocuboid joint distally, and to the superior most portion of the calcaneal tuberosity posteriorly.
- Three 1.6-mm Kirschner wires (K-wires) are placed for retraction of the subperiosteal flap: one into the fibula as the peroneal tendons are slightly subluxed anterior to the lateral malleolus, a second wire is placed in the talar neck, and a third wire is placed in the cuboid as the peroneal tendons are levered away from the anterolateral calcaneus with a periosteal elevator. Thus, each K-wire retracts its respective portions of the peroneal tendons and full-thickness skin flap **(TECH FIG 1D)**.

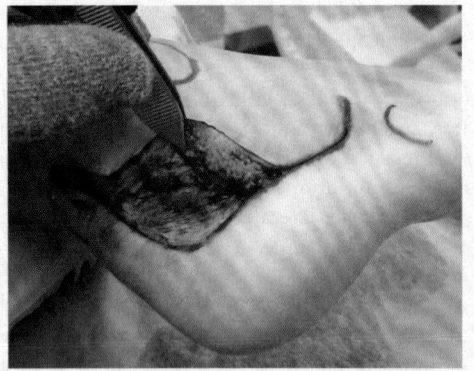
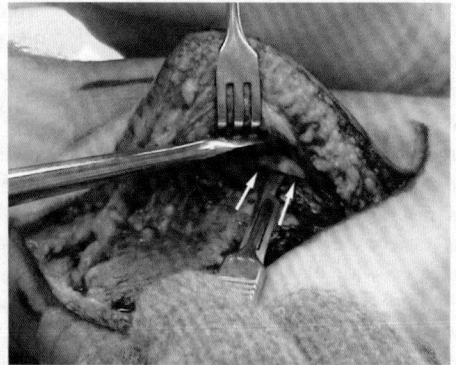
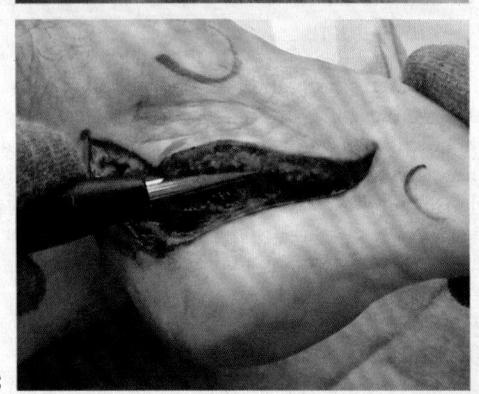
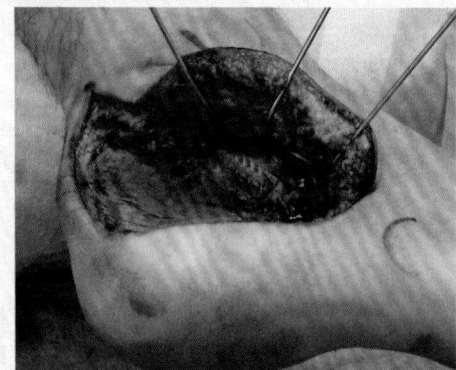

TECH FIG 1 Extensile lateral approach. **A.** Note absence of retractors until a sizeable subperiosteal flap has been raised. **B.** Mobilization of peroneal tendons (*white arrows*). **C.** Gentle mobilization of flap along anterolateral wall of calcaneus. **D.** 1.6-mm K-wire retractors.

LATERAL WALL EXOSTECTOMY

- A lateral wall exostectomy is completed for all three malunion types.
- Starting posteriorly, the A/O osteotomy saw blade is angled slightly medially relative to the longitudinal axis of the calcaneus, preserving more bone plantarly and thereby providing decompression of the subfibular impingement **(TECH FIG 2A,B)**.
- Care is taken throughout the exostectomy to avoid violation of the talofibular joint: A small Bennett-type retractor is placed at the level of the posterior facet **(TECH FIG 2B)**.

- The exostectomy is continued to the level of the calcaneocuboid joint and is completed with an osteotome. The fragment is removed en bloc as a single fragment and is preserved in saline on the back table for later use as autograft **(TECH FIG 2C)**.
- The width of the exostectomy fragment is variable (~10 to 15 mm) but is generally proportional to the extent of loss of calcaneal height and lateral wall expansion from the original injury, which reflects the amount of initial energy involved.

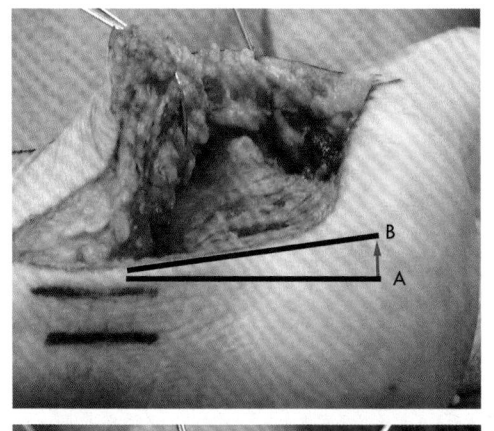

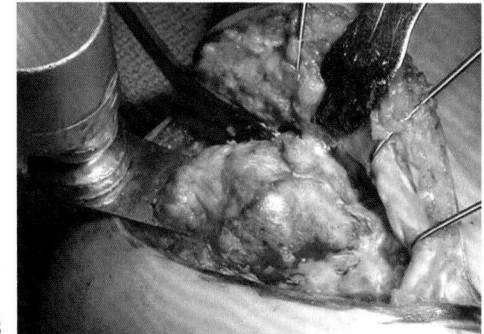

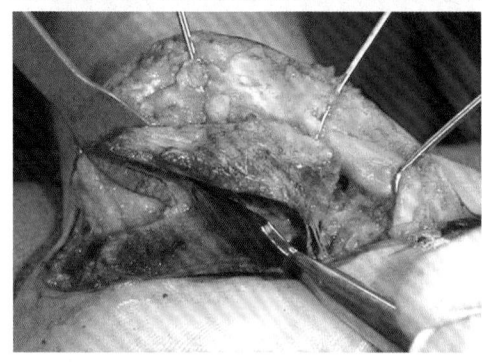

TECH FIG 2 Lateral wall exostectomy. **A.** Intraoperative photo demonstrating vertical axis of limb (*line A*) and plane of lateral wall exostectomy (*line B*). **B.** Use of A/O osteotomy saw; note presence of small Bennett retractor protecting talofibular joint. **C.** Exostectomy fragment is removed en bloc for later use as autograft.

SUBTALAR BONE BLOCK ARTHRODESIS

- In patients with a type II or III malunion, the subtalar joint is gently mobilized with a small osteotome, carefully identifying the plane of the posterior facet.
- A laminar spreader is then placed and joint is meticulously débrided of any residual articular surface while preserving the underlying subchondral bone; we prefer to use a sharp periosteal elevator and pituitary rongeur.
- The joint is irrigated and multiple perforations are made in the subchondral surface with a 2.5-mm drill bit to stimulate vascular ingrowth. Highly concentrated platelet aspirate is then placed both within the joint and on the previously resected lateral wall fragment.
- The lateral wall fragment is placed within the subtalar joint as an autograft bone block; we prefer to place the laminar spreader posteriorly to better facilitate bone block placement **(TECH FIG 3A)**.

- The fragment is positioned such that the widest portion of the autograft is oriented posteromedially to avoid varus malalignment **(TECH FIG 3B)**.
- Any remaining voids within the subtalar joint are filled with supplemental allograft.
- With the subtalar joint held in neutral to slight valgus alignment, definitive stabilization is obtained with two large (6.5 to 8.0 mm) partially threaded cannulated screws placed from posterior to anterior in diverging fashion: The more lateral screw is placed in the talar dome, whereas the more medial screw is placed in the talar neck.
- A third screw may be placed extending from the anterior process region into the talar neck and head, avoiding violation of the talonavicular articulation **(TECH FIG 4A–D)**.

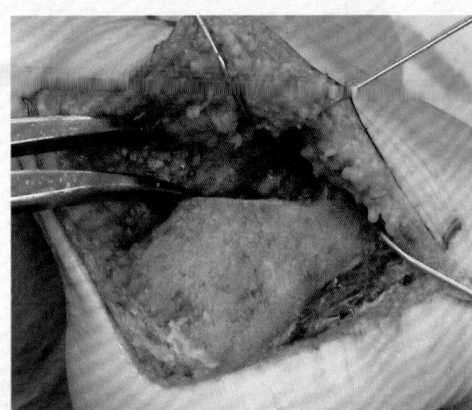

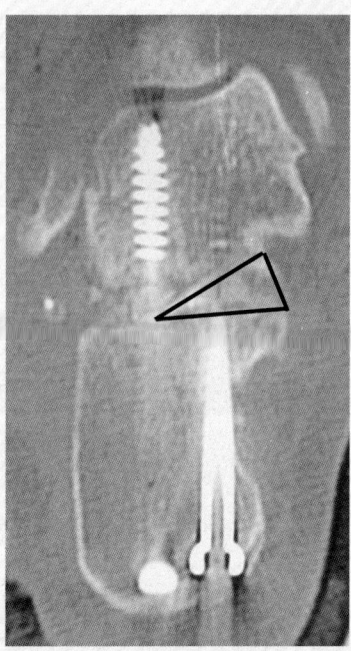

TECH FIG 3 Placement of autograft bone block. **A.** Note position of laminar spreader within subtalar joint posteriorly. **B.** Postoperative semicoronal CT image demonstrating proper orientation of autograft bone block (*black triangle*), with widest portion placed posteromedially.

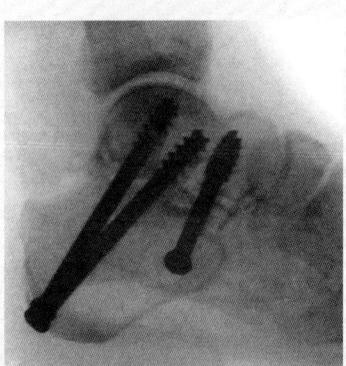

TECH FIG 4 Definitive stabilization. **A.** Intraoperative fluoroscopic lateral view demonstrating diverging orientation of large cannulated screws posteriorly and supplemental screw traversing middle facet. **B.** Intraoperative fluoroscopic mortise view; note slight medial angulation to avoid violation of talofibular joint. **C.** Intraoperative fluoroscopic anteroposterior view; note transverse orientation of anterior screw avoiding violation of talonavicular joint (*black arrows*). **D.** Intraoperative fluoroscopic axial view; note neutral hindfoot alignment.

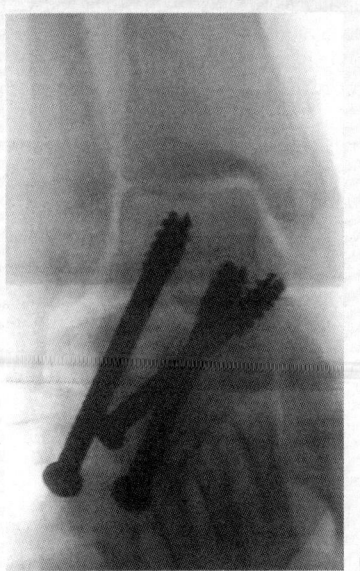

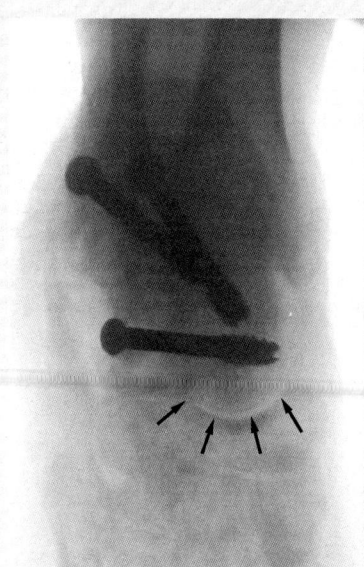

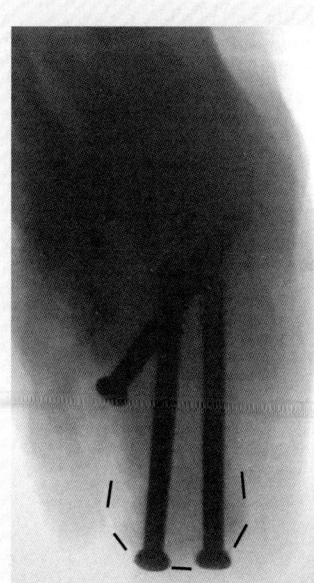

CALCANEAL OSTEOTOMY

- For those patients with a type III malunion, correction of angular malalignment in the calcaneal tuberosity is performed prior to implant placement.
- A Dwyer-type closing wedge osteotomy is performed for those with varus malalignment **(TECH FIG 5)**.
- A medial displacement calcaneal osteotomy is used for those with valgus malalignment (rare).
- Because the plane of the osteotomy is nearly parallel to the plane of the posterior facet, the osteotomy and subtalar joint are stabilized simultaneously as described earlier.

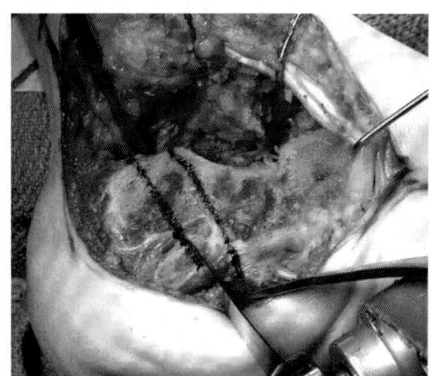

TECH FIG 5 Calcaneal osteotomy. Dwyer closing wedge osteotomy for correction of varus malalignment in calcaneal tuberosity.

PERONEAL TENOLYSIS

- The K-wire retractors are removed, and the peroneal tendon sheath is incised along the undersurface of the subperiosteal flap over a length of 2 to 3 cm. A peroneal tenolysis is then completed.
- A Freer elevator is advanced within the tendon sheath to the level of the lateral malleolus proximally, thereby mobilizing the peroneal tendons.

- The competence of the superior peroneal retinaculum (SPR) is assessed by gently levering the Freer elevator forward while observing the overlying skin. The presence of an end point is indicative of an intact retinaculum; in the event of an incompetent SPR, the elevator will easily slide anterior to the lateral malleolus, with no demonstrable end point.
- The Freer elevator is then advanced within the tendon sheath distally to the cuboid tunnel.

SUPERIOR PERONEAL RETINACULUM REPAIR

- In the event of an incompetent SPR, a separate 3 cm incision is made along the posterior border of the lateral malleolus, exposing the tendon sheath.
- With the peroneal tendons held reduced in the peroneal groove, one to two suture anchors are used to secure the detached SPR to bone **(TECH FIG 6)**.
- Tendon stability is then reassessed using a Freer elevator in the same manner.

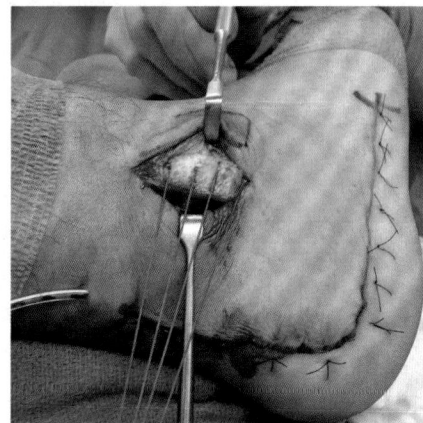

TECH FIG 6 SPR repair. Suture imbrication of incompetent SPR.

CLOSURE

- A deep drain is placed exiting proximally in line with the vertical limb of the incision.
- Deep no. 0 absorbable sutures are placed in interrupted, figure-of-eight fashion, beginning with the apex of the incision and progressing to the proximal and distal ends. The sutures are temporarily clamped until all sutures have been passed, then hand tied sequentially, starting at the proximal and distal ends, and working toward the apex of the incision, so as to eliminate tension at the apex of the wound **(TECH FIG 7)**.

- Because of the lateral decompression from the exostectomy, the flap should close fairly easily with minimal tension (despite restoration of calcaneal height).
- The skin layer is closed with 3-0 monofilament suture using the modified Allgöwer-Donati technique, again starting at the ends and working toward the apex **(TECH FIG 7B)**.
- The tourniquet is deflated, and sterile dressings are placed, followed by a bulky Jones dressing and Weber splint.

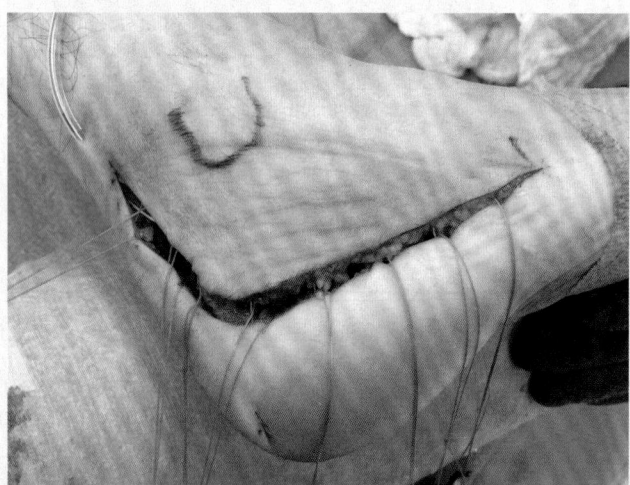 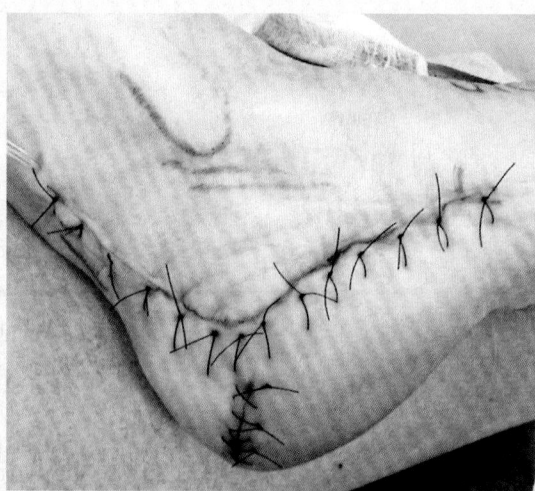

A **B**

TECH FIG 7 Flap closure. **A.** Deep absorbable sutures placed and temporarily clamped. **B.** Skin closure using modified Allgöwer-Donati technique.

TECHNIQUES

Pearls and Pitfalls

Lateral Wall Exostectomy	• Avoid violation of talofibular joint during lateral wall exostectomy. • Gently place small Bennett-type retractor within subtalar joint at level of posterior facet to protect talofibular joint.
Placing Autograft Bone Block	• Use of an additional lamina spreader at crucial angle of Gissane may be helpful in facilitating graft placement. • Release of deltoid ligament should be strictly avoided, as this destabilizes the ankle joint. • The peripheral margin of the fragment may need to be shaped slightly to prevent overhang and prominence laterally.

Definitive
Stabilization

- Avoid violation of talofibular joint by angling slightly medially during placement of guide pins **(FIG 14A)**.
- Fluoroscopic visualization of ankle joint prior to screw placement is of paramount importance **(FIG 14B)**.

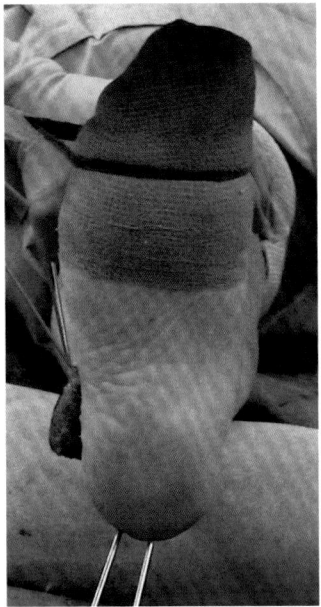 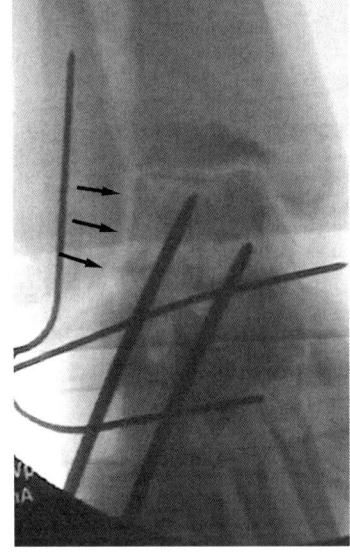

A   **B**

FIG 14 Axial orientation of guide pins traversing posterior facet of subtalar joint. **A.** Intraoperative photo. **B.** Intraoperative fluoroscopic view. Note slight medial angulation to avoid violation of talofibular joint.

Fracture-
dislocation Variant
Patterns

- With fracture-dislocation variant patterns, posterolateral fragment is typically wedged within talofibular joint and is often associated with secondary lateral ankle instability.
- Mobilize subtalar joint prior to lateral wall exostectomy and excise prominent portion of posterolateral fragment flush with remaining posterior facet articular surface.
- At conclusion of procedure, ankle joint should be stressed (varus force) under live fluoroscopy and lateral ligament reconstruction completed where necessary.

POSTOPERATIVE CARE

- For type I malunions, the patient is converted to a prefabricated fracture boot at 2 weeks postoperatively. Weight bearing and range-of-motion exercises are initiated once the incision has fully sealed.
- For type II or type III malunions, the patient is converted to a short-leg non–weight-bearing cast at 2 to 3 weeks and again at 6 to 7 weeks postoperatively. Weight bearing is not permitted until 10 to 12 weeks postoperatively, at which point radiographic union is confirmed.
- The patient is then converted to a prefabricated fracture boot, and weight bearing is initiated. The patient is gradually transitioned to regular shoe wear and activity is advanced as tolerated thereafter.

OUTCOMES

- Outcomes following open reduction and internal fixation (ORIF) of displaced intra-articular calcaneal fractures (when properly performed) are superior to those following initial nonoperative management of the fracture, even in the event of late posttraumatic subtalar arthritis.[15]
- Surgery for a calcaneal malunion is therefore intended as a salvage procedure for pain relief and restoration of alignment.

- We previously reported our intermediate- to long-term results of this protocol[4]:
  - Ninety-three percent initial arthrodesis union rate
  - Ninety-three percent had neutral or slight valgus hindfoot alignment; 100% had plantigrade foot
  - No statistical difference in outcome scores among the three malunion types
  - Significantly greater restoration of talocalcaneal height among type III malunions

COMPLICATIONS

- Delayed wound healing, wound dehiscence, deep infection
- Arthrodesis delayed union or nonunion
- Postoperative ankle stiffness
- (Late) Lateral ankle ("sprain") pain from coronal plane stresses applied to ankle joint
- (Late) Compensatory ankle joint arthritis (theoretical)

REFERENCES

1. Borrelli J Jr, Lashgari C. Vascularity of the lateral calcaneal flap: a cadaveric injection study. J Orthop Trauma 1999;13:73–77.
2. Braly WG, Bishop JO, Tullos HS. Lateral decompression for malunited os calcis fractures. Foot Ankle 1985;6:90–96.
3. Carr JB, Hansen ST, Benirschke SK. Subtalar distraction bone block fusion for late complications of os calcis fractures. Foot Ankle 1988;9:81–86.

4. Clare MP, Lee WE III, Sanders RW. Intermediate to long-term results of a treatment protocol for calcaneal fracture malunions. J Bone Joint Surg Am 2005;87:963–973.

5. Cotton FJ. Old os calcis fractures. Ann Surg 1921;74:294–303.

6. Crosby LA, Fitzgibbons T. Computerized tomography scanning of acute intra-articular fractures of the calcaneus. A new classification. 1990;72:852–859.

7. Dwyer FC. Osteotomy of the calcaneum for pes cavus. J Bone Joint Surg Br 1959;41:80–86.

8. Gallie WE. Subastragalar arthrodeses in fractures of the os calcis. J Bone Joint Surg 1943;25:731–736.

9. Gould N. Lateral approach to the os calcis. Foot Ankle 1984;4: 218–220.

10. Isbister JF. Calcaneo-fibular abutment following crush fracture of the calcaneus. J Bone Joint Surg Br 1974;56:274–278.

11. Kalamchi A, Evans J. Posterior subtalar fusion. A preliminary report on a modified Gallie's procedure. J Bone Joint Surg Br 1977;59: 287–289.

12. Kitaoka HB, Schaap EJ, Chao EY, et al. Displaced intra-articular fractures of the calcaneus treated non-operatively. Clinical results and analysis of motion and ground-reaction and temporal forces. J Bone Joint Surg Am 1994;76:1531–1540.

13. Magnuson PB. An operation for relief of disability in old fractures of the os calcis. JAMA 1923;80:1511–1513.

14. Myerson M, Quill GE Jr. Late complications of fractures of the calcaneus. J Bone Joint Surg Am 1993;75:331–341.

15. Radnay CS, Clare MP, Sanders RW. Subtalar fusion after displaced intra-articular calcaneal fractures: does initial operative treatment matter? J Bone Joint Surg Am 2009;91:541–546.

16. Sanders R, Fortin P, DiPasquale T, et al. Operative treatment in 120 displaced intraarticular calcaneal fractures. Results using a prognostic computed tomography scan classification. Clin Orthop Relat Res 1993;(290):87–95.

17. Stephens HM, Sanders R. Calcaneal malunions: results of a prognostic computed tomography classification system. Foot Ankle Int 1996;17:395–401.

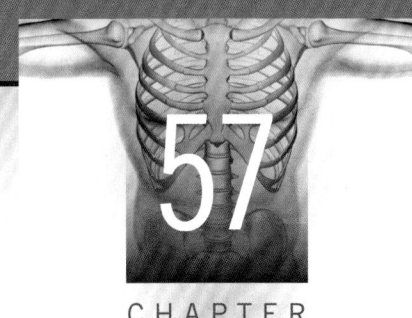

57

CHAPTER

Traditional Triple Arthrodesis

Mark E. Easley

DEFINITION

- Triple arthrodesis is a procedure performed to restore and maintain physiologic hindfoot alignment.
- It is typically reserved for the following:
  - Severe fixed deformity not amenable to joint-sparing procedures
  - Inflammatory arthropathy of the hindfoot

ANATOMY

- The hindfoot comprises the talus, calcaneus, navicular, and cuboid.
- Physiologic alignment is generally defined as a congruent talar–first metatarsal alignment in both the anteroposterior (AP) and lateral planes with weight bearing.
- The talar–calcaneal articulation is referred to as the *subtalar joint*.
- The combination of the talonavicular and calcaneocuboid articulations is known as the *transverse tarsal joint*.
- Multiple ligamentous static restraints support the hindfoot. In fact, in stance phase, the physiologically normal foot is balanced and plantigrade without any dynamic muscle forces acting on it.
- Physiologic hindfoot alignment is influenced by the ankle, midfoot, and forefoot.
- The hindfoot is a component of the ankle–hindfoot complex. To an extent, ankle malalignment can be compensated by the hindfoot.
- The foot is balanced when there is relatively even pressure distribution on the heel, first metatarsal–sesamoid complex, and the fifth metatarsal (ie, a plantigrade foot).
- Physiologically normal hindfoot alignment can be distorted by ankle, midfoot, and forefoot deformity.
- Although the ankle is primarily responsible for dorsiflexion and plantarflexion, the hindfoot has some capacity to compensate in the sagittal plane with ankle stiffness, as evidenced by residual dorsiflexion and plantarflexion following ankle arthrodesis.
- Ambulation
  - With transition from heel strike to stance phase, the hindfoot becomes accommodative to the surface it contacts by "unlocking" the hindfoot joints.
  - With push off, the posterior tibial tendon (PTT) inverts the hindfoot, thereby locking the transverse tarsal joints and hindfoot.
    - This converts the foot's accommodative function to one of biomechanical advantage with creation of a rigid lever arm for the Achilles tendon.

PATHOGENESIS AND NATURAL HISTORY

- Hindfoot alignment is easily distorted by imbalance of its dynamic stabilizers, in particular, the posterior tibial and peroneal tendons.
  - If the imbalance persists and becomes chronic, the hindfoot's static ligamentous restraints may weaken, creating a hindfoot deformity that ultimately may become fixed.
  - PTT dysfunction leads to a flatfoot deformity with attenuation of the medial static restraints (spring ligament complex, medial talonavicular capsule) and pes planovalgus (flatfoot) deformity.
  - Peroneal tendon dysfunction may lead to lateral ankle–hindfoot attenuation and a pes cavovarus (hindfoot varus) deformity.
- Posttraumatic or inflammatory arthritis may also create a stiff and painful hindfoot, with or without deformity.

PATIENT HISTORY AND PHYSICAL FINDINGS

- The patient typically describes aching in the hindfoot, particularly in the sinus tarsi area, with weight bearing.
- There may be a report of a progressive deformity.
- Stiffness and swelling are common complaints.
- It is important to elicit a history of an inflammatory arthropathy.
- A neurologic and vascular examination is required.
- The patient should be examined while standing and ambulating.
  - The deformity may not be obvious with the patient non–weight bearing.
  - Typically, the patient will walk with a limp.
  - A single limb heel rise for a patient with pes planovalgus deformity, if possible, will determine if the deformity is flexible and if the PTT is functional.
- With the patient seated, range of motion (ROM) is assessed.
  - Inversion and eversion are almost always restricted in patients being considered for triple arthrodesis.
  - The talus can be stabilized with a thumb on the talar neck to determine dorsiflexion and plantarflexion in the hindfoot.
  - Ankle ROM and stability also should be evaluated.
  - An equinus contracture may be present and is important when considering surgery. Achilles tendon lengthening may be required to reposition the hindfoot anatomically. Many hindfoot deformities result in Achilles tendon contractures.

IMAGING AND OTHER DIAGNOSTIC STUDIES

- Plain radiographs of the weight-bearing foot in the AP, lateral, and oblique views **(FIG 1)**
- Occasionally, contralateral foot radiographs are useful in understanding what is physiologically normal for an individual.
- I routinely obtain ipsilateral ankle radiographs as well.
- In severe deformity, there may be a preexisting talar tilt.
  - If this is the case, proper operative realignment of the hindfoot may be compromised by the more proximal deformity.
  - One needs to be aware of preexisting talar tilt or ankle malalignment to ensure that the hindfoot deformity is corrected appropriately.
  - I will check the ankle alignment fluoroscopically while realigning the hindfoot in surgery.
- Rarely is computed tomography or magnetic resonance imaging necessary.

NONOPERATIVE MANAGEMENT

- Activity modification
- Nonsteroidal anti-inflammatory agents

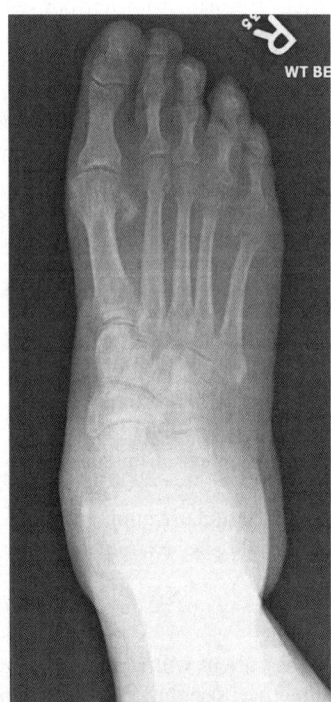

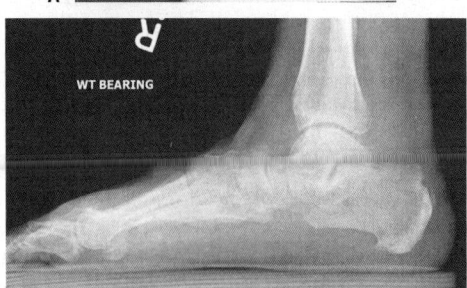

FIG 1 Weight-bearing radiographs of patient with PTT dysfunction and fixed hindfoot deformity. **A.** AP view demonstrates forefoot abduction and talonavicular joint uncovering (note divergence of talar and first metatarsal longitudinal axes, rather than the congruence/parallelism seen in patients without PTT dysfunction). **B.** Lateral view. Note the severe talonavicular sag (suggestive of spring ligament attenuation/incompetence).

- Corticosteroid injection
- Bracing
  - Lace-up brace
  - Hinged or fixed ankle–foot orthosis

SURGICAL MANAGEMENT

- A spectrum of pathologies may warrant triple arthrodesis:
  - Stage III posterior tibial tendinopathy
  - Chronic peroneal tendinopathy
  - Posttraumatic hindfoot arthritis
  - Inflammatory arthritis
  - Charcot neuroarthropathy
  - Chronic spring ligament rupture
- If a joint-sparing procedure can be performed, it should be favored over triple arthrodesis.
- Selective hindfoot arthrodesis may also be considered.
- There has been a trend toward double arthrodesis in lieu of triple arthrodesis.
  - The concept is to preserve the accommodative effect of the calcaneocuboid joint when possible and only perform talonavicular and subtalar joint arthrodeses.
  - Isolated talonavicular joint arthrodesis restricts hindfoot motion by 90%.

Preoperative Planning

- The preoperative deformity needs to be assessed to determine what correction is warranted.
  - If there is a severe pes planovalgus deformity, consider a single-incision medial approach double arthrodesis to eliminate the risk of lateral wound problems that may occur with a lateral approach in such deformity.
- Equinus contracture: It may be necessary to lengthen the Achilles tendon to correct the deformity.
- Equipment
  - Fluoroscopy unit to confirm reduction and hardware placement
  - Preferred screw (and plating or staple) system
  - Bone graft is not required but may be useful to fill any voids or gaps with deformity correction.

Positioning

- With a traditional triple arthrodesis, the patient is placed on the operating table in a modified lateral decubitus position ("sloppy lateral position"; **FIG 2**). This allows access to the lateral and medial hindfoot.

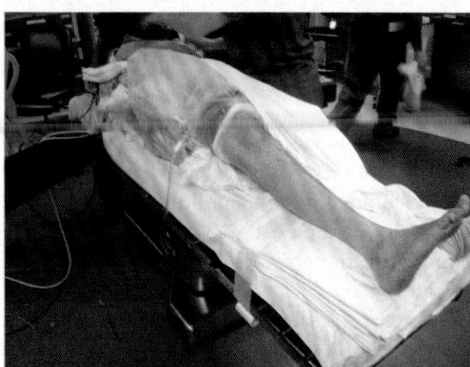

FIG 2 The patient is placed on a beanbag in a modified lateral position that allows access to the medial and lateral foot. A stack of folded sheets is placed under foot to be operated.

- The patient's torso is supported with a beanbag.
- An axillary roll is usually indicated.
- The contralateral hip is flexed slightly to make room for a stack of folded sheets on which the operative leg is placed.
  - The opposite leg must be padded if it contacts the beanbag.
- I routinely use a thigh tourniquet if I am considering an Achilles tendon lengthening.
  - If an Achilles tendon lengthening is unnecessary, a calf tourniquet is adequate.

Approach

- The traditional utilitarian lateral approach uses a 7- to 8-cm incision from the tip of the fibula toward the base of the fourth metatarsal.
- The traditional utilitarian dorsomedial approach uses a 7- to 8-cm incision from the anterior aspect of the anterior medial malleolus toward the dorsomedial base of the first metatarsal.
- If equinus contracture is present, I first perform an Achilles tendon lengthening.

LATERAL EXPOSURE

- Create a lateral longitudinal incision **(TECH FIG 1A)**.
- Protect the sural nerve **(TECH FIG 1B)**.
- Create the interval between the peroneal tendons and the extensor digitorum brevis (EDB) muscle.
- Elevate the EDB muscle with its fascia dorsally **(TECH FIG 1C)**.
  - Avoid "shredding" the muscle and fascia, as it will be used as the deep layer closure at the completion of the surgery.
- Release the bifurcate (calcaneonavicular and calcaneocuboid) ligament that lies deep to the EDB muscle.

- Release the calcaneocuboid capsule also **(TECH FIG 1D)**.
- Place a blunt retractor between the lateral subtalar joint and the calcaneofibular ligament **(TECH FIG 1E)**.
- Use a distractor to expose the subtalar joint first **(TECH FIG 1F,G)** and then the calcaneocuboid joint.
- The lateral talonavicular joint may also be accessed through this approach.

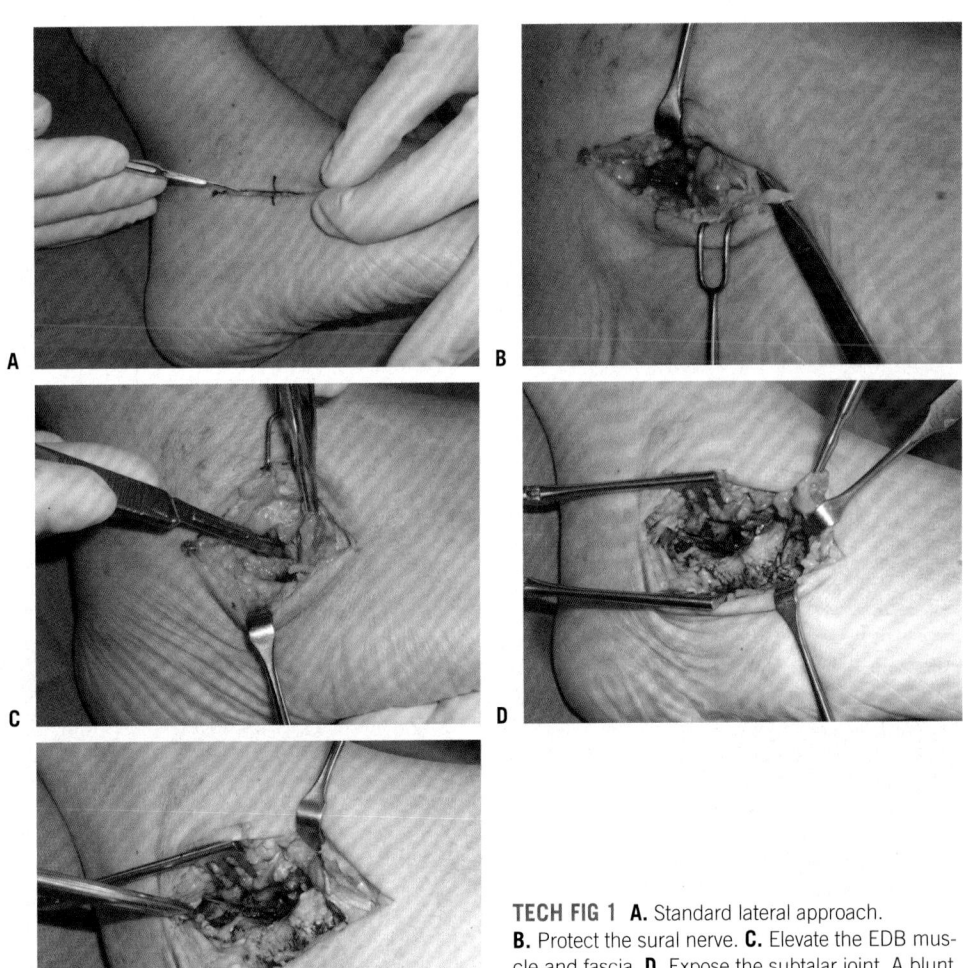

TECH FIG 1 A. Standard lateral approach. **B.** Protect the sural nerve. **C.** Elevate the EDB muscle and fascia. **D.** Expose the subtalar joint. A blunt retractor may be placed deep to the calcaneofibular ligament. **E.** Identify the calcaneocuboid joint. In this patient with an inflammatory arthropathy, the joint is distorted. *(continued)*

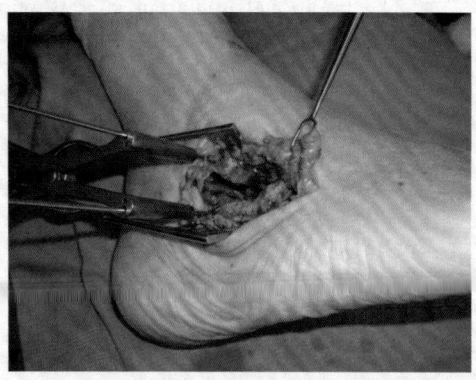 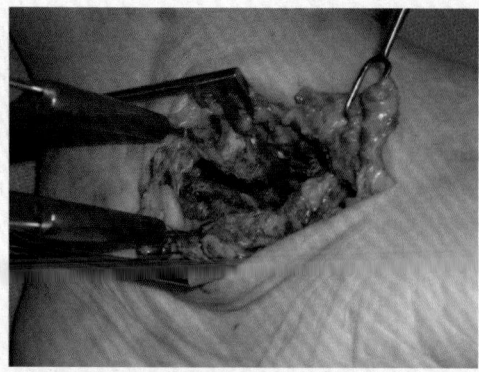

TECH FIG 1 *(continued)* **F,G.** Subtalar joint exposed with a distraction device.

SUBTALAR, CALCANEOCUBOID, AND LATERAL TALONAVICULAR JOINT PREPARATION

- The preparation is the same for all three joints.
- Remove residual articular cartilage with a sharp elevator or chisel **(TECH FIG 2A)**.
- Preserve the native subchondral bone architecture.
- Drill or chisel ("feather") the subchondral bone to allow for vascular channels to form at the arthrodesis surfaces while maintaining subchondral bone architecture **(TECH FIG 2B,C)**.
- For the subtalar joint, include not only the posterior facet but also the middle and anterior facets.
  - However, be careful to not disrupt the delicate vasculature on the undersurface of the talar neck, if possible.

- The calcaneocuboid joint is a "saddle" joint, so avoid simply driving a chisel directly across the joint surfaces as it may result in more than desired bone removal, particularly when correcting pes planovalgus **(TECH FIG 2D,E)**.
- The lateral talonavicular joint is often difficult to reach from the medial approach, but the lateral exposure affords satisfactory access to prepare this aspect of the talonavicular joint **(TECH FIG 2F,G)**.
- I irrigate the joint before drilling the subchondral bone. Drilling creates reamings that serve as bone graft, and I do not want to wash the reamings away.

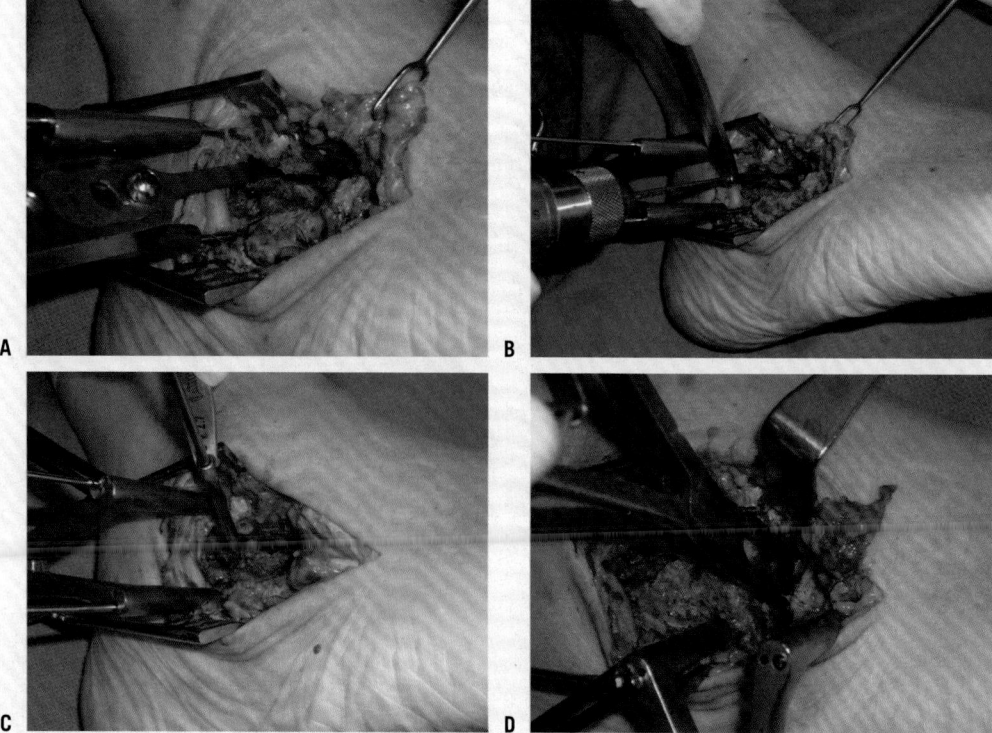

TECH FIG 2 **A.** Chisel being used to remove residual cartilage. **B,C.** Preparing the subtalar joint. **B.** Drill being introduced. **C.** The reamings created will serve as bone graft. **D,E.** Preparing the calcaneocuboid joint. **D.** Chisel being used to remove residual cartilage. *(continued)*

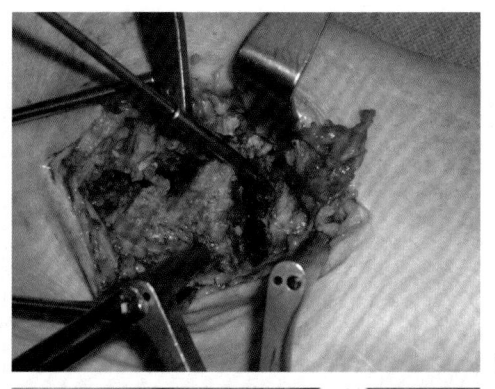

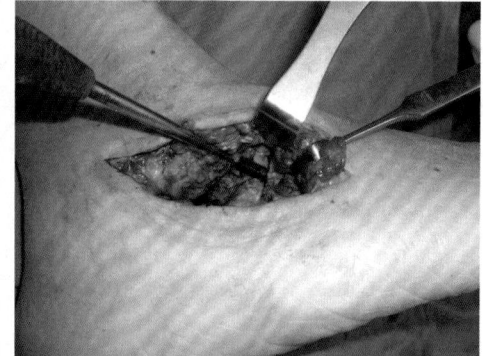

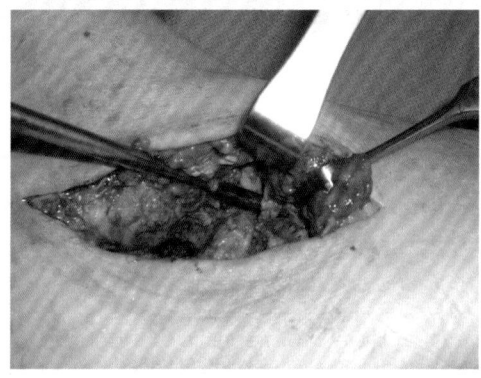

TECH FIG 2 *(continued)* **E.** Drilling the subchondral bone to promote fusion and adding reamings that serve as bone graft. **F,G.** Exposure of the lateral talonavicular joint.

MEDIAL EXPOSURE

- Create a longitudinal incision **(TECH FIG 3A)**.
- Cauterize connecting branches of the saphenous vein, so the vein can be mobilized.
- Identify the tibialis anterior tendon and protect it throughout the procedure **(TECH FIG 3B)**.
  - Typically, fibers of the extensor retinaculum must be released to access the tibialis anterior tendon.

- Perform a longitudinal capsulotomy **(TECH FIG 3C,D)**.
  - The spring ligament may need to be divided, and the PTT tendon may need to be released from the navicular to improve access to the talonavicular joint.

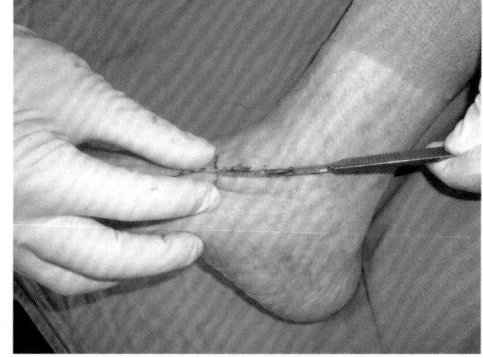

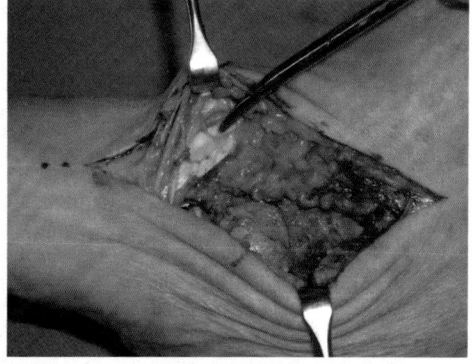

TECH FIG 3 A,B. Medial approach to the talonavicular joint. *(continued)*

TECHNIQUES

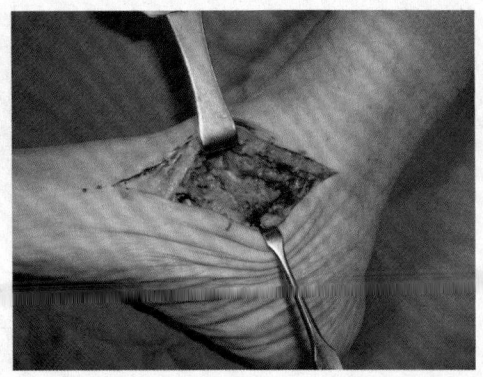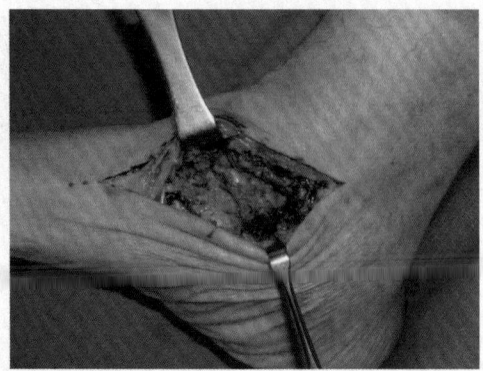

TECH FIG 3 *(continued)* **C.** Medial exposure after capsulotomy. **D.** Close-up demonstrating erosive changes in the talonavicular joint in a patient with an inflammatory arthropathy.

TALONAVICULAR JOINT PREPARATION

- Use a distractor to gain full exposure to the talonavicular joint **(TECH FIG 4A,B)**.
  - In brittle bone, be careful when applying pressure to the navicular as it may fracture.
- Remove the residual articular cartilage from the talonavicular joint **(TECH FIG 4C)**.
  - In pes planovalgus deformity, the talar head may be weak, so be careful not to gouge the talar head when attempting to delaminate the residual articular cartilage.

- The lateral talar head should have already been prepared from the lateral approach.
- Remove cartilage from the navicular.
- Penetrate the subchondral bone to promote fusion.
  - The talus is relatively easy to access with a small-diameter drill bit **(TECH FIG 4D)**. Be careful using a chisel on the talar head as it may fracture.
  - The navicular can also be readily drilled.

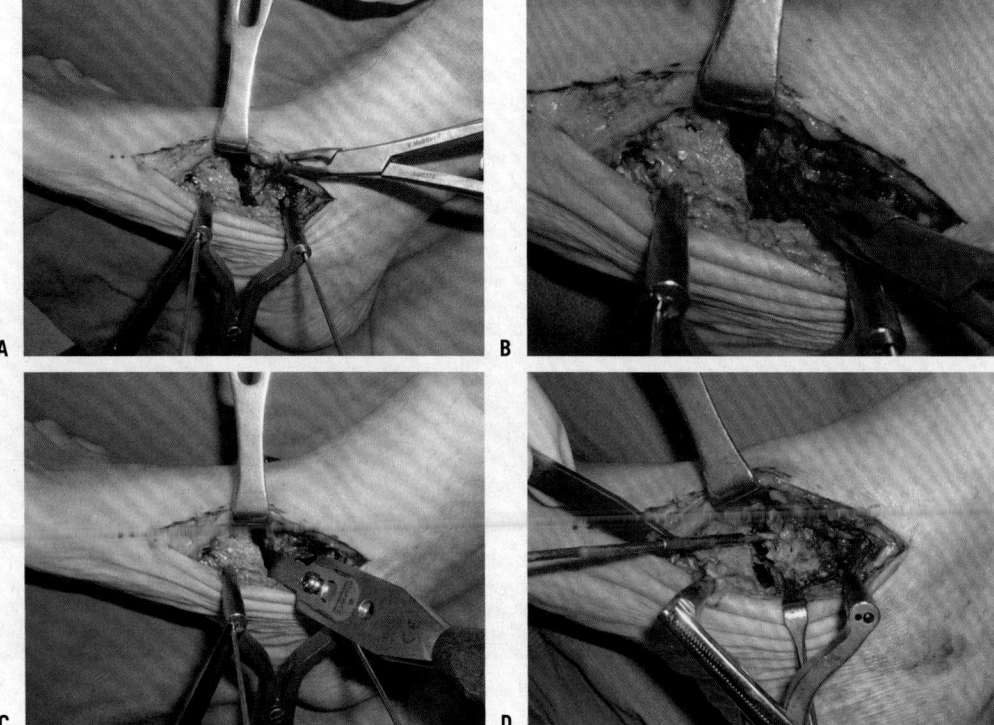

TECH FIG 4 A. Talonavicular joint distracted. **B.** Débriding the joint with a rongeur. **C.** A chisel is used to remove residual articular cartilage. **D.** Drilling the subchondral bone to promote fusion.

- I do not often use a burr to prepare subchondral bone for fusion, but on the navicular, it is sometimes very effective, provided cold water or saline irrigation is used simultaneously to limit bone necrosis. However, this may wash away desirable reamings that could serve as bone graft.

- As for the preparation of the other joint surfaces, I irrigate the talonavicular joint before drilling and then try to maintain the reamings, so they can be used as bone graft.

HINDFOOT REDUCTION

- Place bone graft in the arthrodesis sites at this time, before the reduction is performed.
  - I routinely use bone graft to fill voids at the surfaces to be fused. Although this is not mandatory, I believe that filling the voids enhances the body's ability to form bridging trabeculations.
- The calcaneus must be centered properly under the talus.
  - Through the lateral wound, the optimal relationship of the posterior facet can be assessed and controlled (**TECH FIG 5A,B**).

- Physiologically, there is a gap between the anterolateral talus and the anterior calcaneal process, and this should be recreated.
- In correcting severe pes planovalgus, I aim to overcorrect the calcaneus beneath the talus (**TECH FIG 5C**).
- Once the optimal subtalar relationship established, I provisionally pin the subtalar joint.
  - I use a guide pin for the intended cannulated screw and try to place the pin in the intended trajectory for the screw (**TECH FIG 5D,E**).

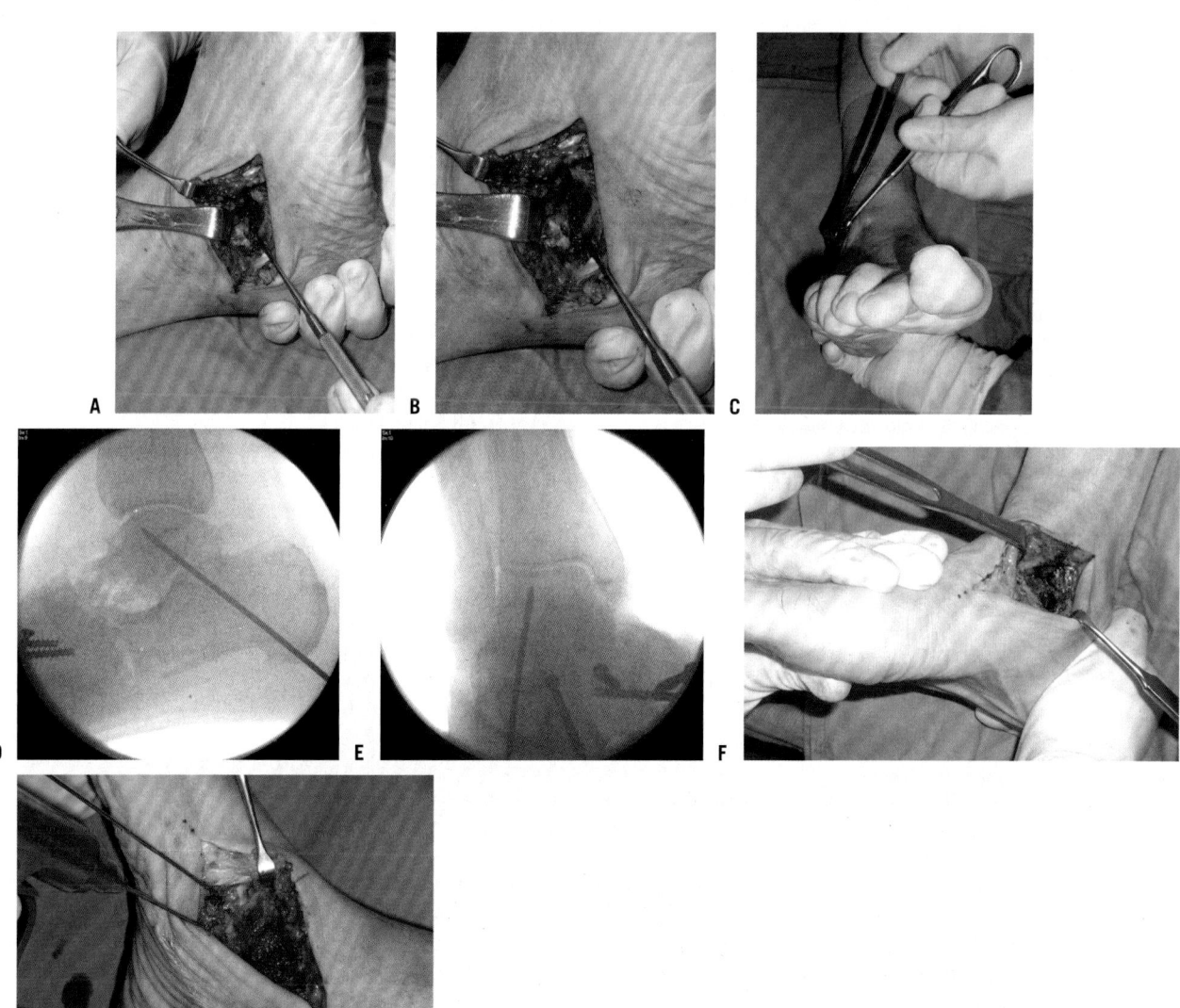

TECH FIG 5 Reducing the hindfoot. **A,B.** Checking the subtalar joint reduction. **C.** The hindfoot is maintained in the corrected position. Lateral (**D**) and mortise (**E**) fluoroscopic views after a guide pin was placed across the reduced subtalar joint. **F.** Reduction of talonavicular joint. **G.** Guide pins placed across talonavicular joint.

- Typically, I have an assistant working with me, so I hold the reduction while the assistant places the guide pin from the calcaneal tuberosity into the talar body.
- The dual-incision approach affords the surgeon the ability to palpate the talonavicular and calcaneocuboid joint reductions simultaneously.
  - With the subtalar joint reduced, I then attempt to reduce the talonavicular joint to an anatomic position. I can palpate both sides of the talonavicular joint by having two incisions **(TECH FIG 5F)**.
  - When correcting pes planovalgus deformity, I err on the side of overcorrection of the navicular on the talar head.
- Once I have the talonavicular joint reduced, I protect the tibialis anterior tendon and have my assistant drive two guide pins, appropriately spaced from one another, from the navicular into the talar head **(TECH FIG 5G)**.
  - I attempt to place the screw from the most distal aspect of the navicular, even reaming the medial wall of the first

cuneiform slightly, so the pin needs to be flush against the medial aspect of the first cuneiform.
- Finally, I provisionally pin the calcaneocuboid joint.
- To create a relief area on the anterior process of the calcaneus for the screw insertion, I remove a small wedge of bone from the anterior process using a rongeur.
- I routinely push up on the cuboid and down on the anterior process of the calcaneus to reduce the joint.
- Despite the lateral approach, optimal longitudinal orientation of the guide pin across the calcaneocuboid joint is not possible.
  - I sometimes create a stab incision behind the peroneal tendons; dissect carefully deep to the sural nerve and tendons, creating a soft tissue tunnel; insert a drill sleeve; and then deliver the guide pin safely to the anterior process of the talus.
- The guide pin is driven across the joint.

HINDFOOT STABILIZATION

- The reduction and the position of the guide pins are checked fluoroscopically **(TECH FIG 6A)**.
  - Adjustments are made as necessary.
  - At this stage, I also routinely check the ankle fluoroscopically to be sure there is no ankle deformity that may distort the true hindfoot alignment.
- I determine proper screws lengths and overdrill the guide pins but only to the initial aspect of the second bone.
  - Most modern screws are self-drilling and self-tapping; however, particularly in the navicular, I prefer to predrill to diminish the risk of navicular fracture.
  - By not drilling the full length of the planned screw, purchase of the screw is typically improved.
- I first place the subtalar screw as a compression screw **(TECH FIG 6B,C)**.
- Next, I place the two talonavicular screws **(TECH FIG 6D–F)**.
  - The first screw is a compression screw.
  - I use a positional screw for the second screw.

- If greater talonavicular stability is needed, I create a small dorsal incision over the midfoot; protect the superficial peroneal nerve, extensor tendons, and the deep neurovascular bundle; and using a drill sleeve, place a guide pin from the centrolateral navicular into the talar body or sometimes through the inferior talar body and into the calcaneus. Over this, I place a third talonavicular screw, either positional or compression; although with two screws medially, further compression is generally not possible.
- For the calcaneocuboid joint, I protect the soft tissues and overdrill only the anterior calcaneal process. Then I insert a compression or positional screw across the calcaneocuboid joint **(TECH FIG 6G,H)**.
  - If the joint is well reduced, I tend to use a positional screw; if the joint could stand to be compressed for better bony apposition, however, I place a compression screw.

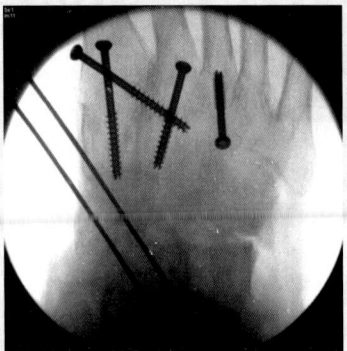
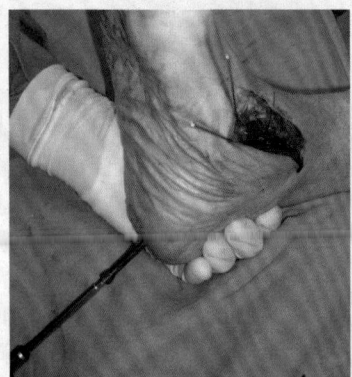
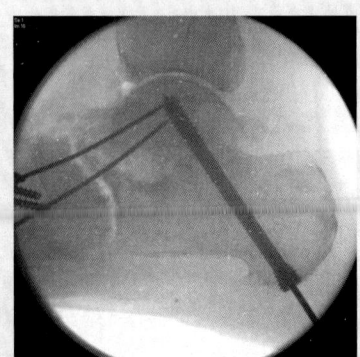

TECH FIG 6 **A.** Fluoroscopic confirmation of the guide pins placed across the talonavicular joint (this patient had undergone prior midfoot arthrodesis). **B,C.** Clinical and fluoroscopic views of the subtalar screw in place. *(continued)*

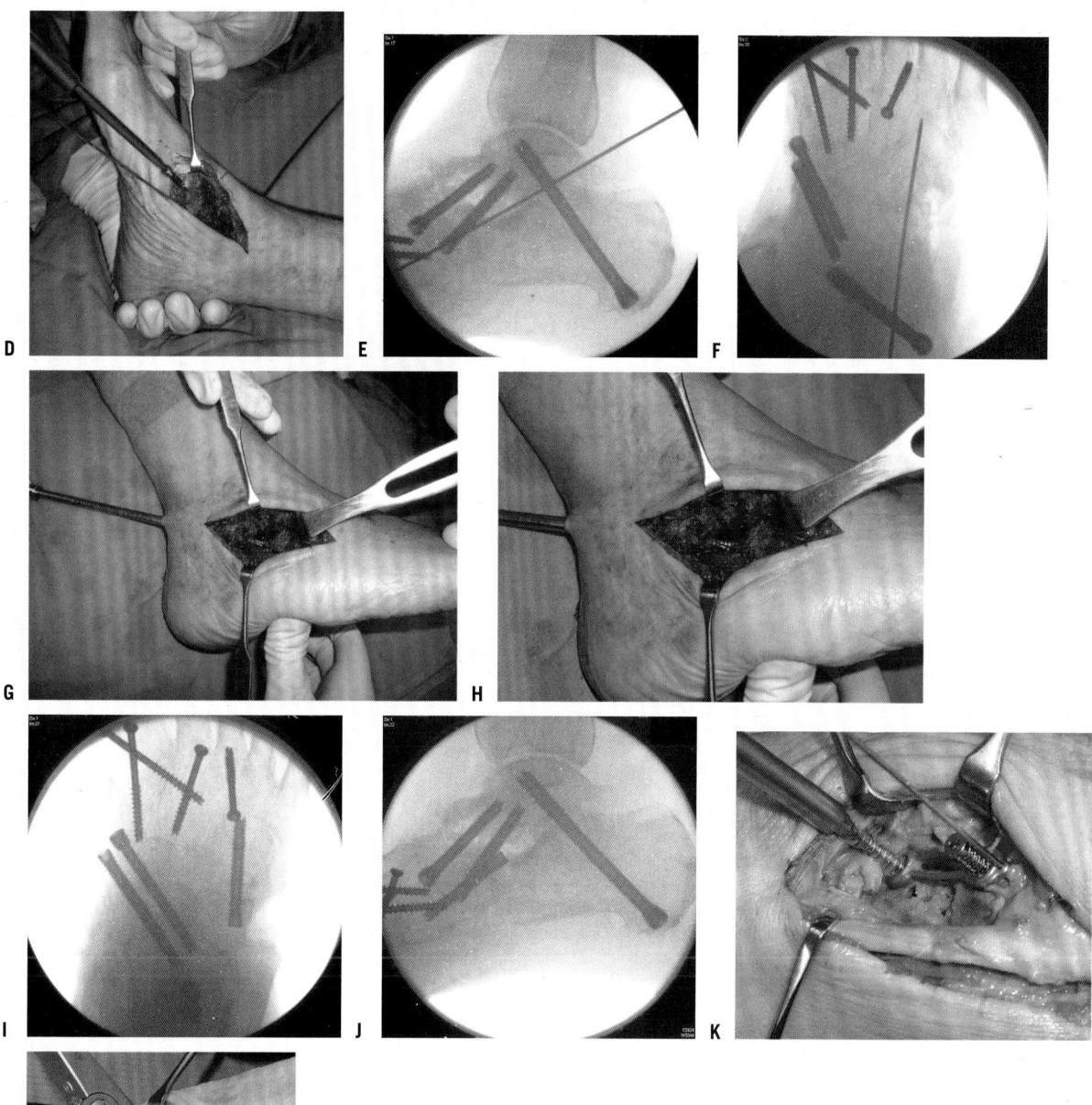

TECH FIG 6 *(continued)* **D–F.** Clinical and fluoroscopic views of the talonavicular screws in place. One partially threaded compression screw is placed first, and one fully threaded positional screw is placed second. **G,H.** Calcaneocuboid screw. A separate stab incision is made with a carefully prepared soft tissue tunnel under the sural nerve and peroneal tendons. Note thumb pressure pushing up on the cuboid to maintain joint reduction and a more favorable position of the cuboid. **I,J.** Final AP and lateral fluoroscopic views confirming appropriate reduction, bony apposition at the arthrodesis sites, and proper hardware position. **K.** Different patient in whom a compression plate was used at the dorsolateral talonavicular joint. **L.** Note compression being applied uniformly across the talonavicular joint by simultaneous compression with medial compression screw and dorsolateral compression plate.

- As mentioned earlier, I push up on the cuboid and down on the anterior calcaneal process to maintain the reduction and to make sure the cuboid does not sag, occasionally leaving it prominent postoperatively. However, with an anatomic reduction, this is rarely an issue.

- I get final fluoroscopic confirmation of alignment, bony apposition at the arthrodesis sites, and hardware position **(TECH FIG 6I,J)**.
- Alternatively, I may use compression plates or staples across the talonavicular and/or calcaneocuboid joints to augment the fixation **(TECH FIG 6K,L)**.

CLOSURE

- I routinely pack bone graft at the "quadruple arthrodesis" site, where talus, calcaneus, navicular, and cuboid meet at the lateral aspect of the talonavicular joint **(TECH FIG 7)**.
- Medially, the capsule is reapproximated.
- Laterally, the fascia overlying the EDB muscle can usually be re-approximated to soft tissues adjacent to the peroneal tendons.
- Any bone graft in the soft tissues is irrigated away, as it may interfere with wound healing.
- Next, the subcutaneous tissues are closed.
- The skin incisions are then reapproximated to tensionless closures.
- I routinely release the tourniquet prior to subcutaneous layer closure.
- I also routinely use a lateral drain.
- The stab incisions for screw placement are closed.
- Sterile dressings and a posterior or sugar-tong splint are placed over adequate padding, with the ankle in neutral position.

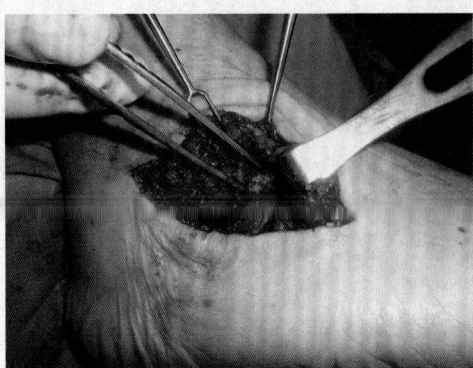

TECH FIG 7 Bone grafting the confluence of all four hindfoot bones at the "quadruple arthrodesis" site.

TECHNIQUES

Pearls and Pitfalls

Achilles Tendon	• If an equinus contracture is not corrected, anatomic reduction will be difficult or impossible.
Severe Pes Planovalgus Deformity	• This is perhaps more safely corrected with a single-incision medial approach double arthrodesis. A traditional dual-incision triple arthrodesis may lead to a lateral wound complication when correcting severe flatfoot deformity.
Ankle	• In severe deformity, be sure to check the ankle preoperatively. With preexisting ankle deformity, a triple arthrodesis is sure to fail.
Sequence of Reduction	• Although the talonavicular joint may be reduced first, the most important correction of deformity, in my opinion, is the centering of the calcaneus anatomically under the talus.
Talonavicular Joint Preparation	• If a traditional dual-incision triple arthrodesis is performed, use the lateral access to prepare the lateral talonavicular joint because it is difficult to reach the lateral talar head from the medial approach.

POSTOPERATIVE CARE

- I routinely keep patients overnight for pain control, nasal oxygen (which may improve wound healing), and limb elevation.
  - Although I recognize that some of my colleagues perform this surgery as a pure outpatient procedure, I believe that one night (which still qualifies as an outpatient procedure) is in the patient's best interest after major hindfoot surgery.
- The patient wears a splint for 2 weeks.
- The patient returns to the clinic at 2 weeks for suture removal and short-leg cast.
- The patient returns to the clinic at 6 weeks after surgery for radiographs out of cast and repeat casting.
- Touchdown weight bearing is the rule for a full 10 weeks.
- The patient returns to the clinic at 10 weeks, and if repeat simulated weight-bearing radiographs suggest healing and no complications, he or she can be placed in a cam boot with gradual progression to full weight bearing by 12 to 14 weeks.

- The patient returns to the clinic at 14 to 16 weeks for full weight-bearing radiographs **(FIG 3)** and then gradual progression to full activities.

OUTCOMES

- Patients are generally improved with an appropriately performed triple arthrodesis.
- At intermediate to long-term follow-up, patients are functional in their activities of daily living, but few are able to perform demanding recreational activities.
- With time, patients tend to develop adjacent joint arthritis, but it is unclear if this causes functional deficits.
- "Triple arthrodesis" performed through a single medial incision and including only the subtalar and talonavicular joints is gradually displacing the traditional triple arthrodesis. Results of this procedure are promising, but it is not clear if they are more favorable than those of the traditional triple arthrodesis.

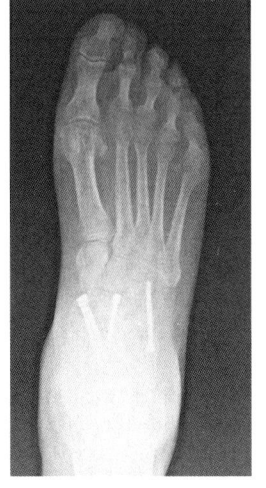
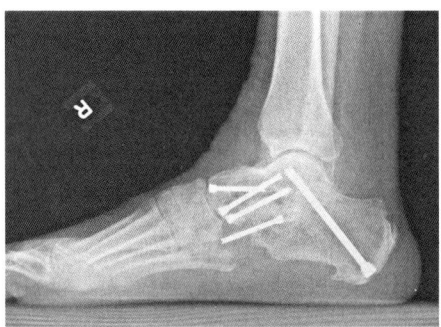
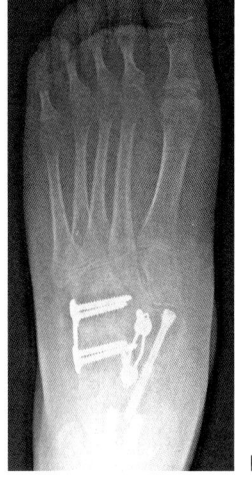
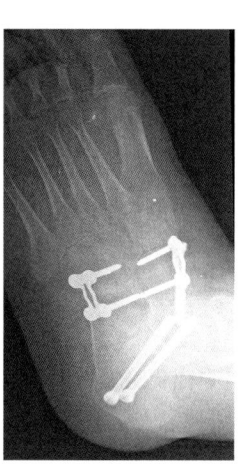

A B C D

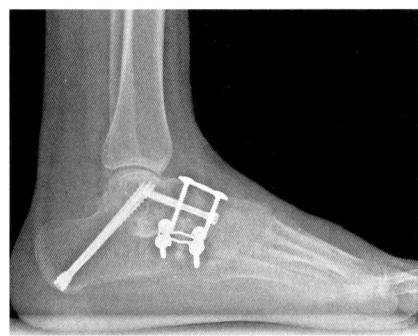

E

FIG 3 A,B. Follow-up weight-bearing radiographs of the patient with fixed hindfoot deformity secondary to PTT dysfunction and spring ligament tear. Note the congruent alignment of the talar–first metatarsal axis in both the AP (**A**) and lateral (**B**) views. **C–E.** Follow-up weight-bearing radiographs of a different patient who underwent triple arthrodesis with combination of screw and compression plate fixation. Note compression plates across dorsal talonavicular and lateral calcaneocuboid joints. Alternatively, compression staples may be used in lieu of compression plates. **A.** AP view with compression plates. **B.** Oblique view. **C.** Lateral view.

COMPLICATIONS

- Nonunion
- Malunion
- Wound dehiscence
- Infection
- Sural neuralgia
- Prominent hardware
- Persistent pain despite appropriate management and satisfactory clinical and radiographic findings

SUGGESTED READINGS

Bednarz PA, Monroe MT, Manoli A II. Triple arthrodesis in adults using rigid internal fixation: an assessment of outcome. Foot Ankle Int 1999;20:356–363.

Haritidis JH, Kirkos JM, Provellegios SM, et al. Long-term results of triple arthrodesis: 42 cases followed for 25 years. Foot Ankle Int 1994;15:548–551.

Klerken T, Kosse NM, Aarts CAM, et al. Long-term results after triple arthrodesis: influence of alignment on ankle osteoarthritis and clinical outcome. Foot Ankle Surg 2019;25(2):247–250.

Knupp M, Skoog A, Törnkvist H, et al. Triple arthrodesis in rheumatoid arthritis. Foot Ankle Int 2008;29:293–297.

Pell RF IV, Myerson MS, Schon LC. Clinical outcome after primary triple arthrodesis. J Bone Joint Surg Am 2000;82:47–57.

Rosenfeld PF, Budgen SA, Saxby TS. Triple arthrodesis: is bone grafting necessary? The results in 100 consecutive cases. J Bone Joint Surg Br 2005;87:175–178.

Saltzman CL, Fehrle MJ, Cooper RR, et al. Triple arthrodesis: twenty-five and forty-four-year average follow-up of the same patients. J Bone Joint Surg Am 1999;81:1391–1402.

Sangeorzan BJ, Smith D, Veith R, et al. Triple arthrodesis using internal fixation in treatment of adult foot disorders. Clin Orthop Relat Res 1993;(294):299–307.

Schipper ON, Ford SE, Moody PW, et al. Radiographic results of nitinol compression staples for hindfoot and midfoot arthrodesis. Foot Ankle Int 2018;39(2):172–179.

Seybold JD, Coetzee JC. Primary triple arthrodesis for management of rigid flatfoot deformity. JBJS Essent Surg Tech 2016;6(3):e29.

Smith RW, Shen W, Dewitt S, et al. Triple arthrodesis in adults with non-paralytic disease. A minimum ten-year follow-up study. J Bone Joint Surg Am 2004;86:2707–2713.

Song SJ, Lee S, O'Malley MJ, et al. Deltoid ligament strain after correction of acquired flatfoot deformity by triple arthrodesis. Foot Ankle Int 2000;21:573–577.

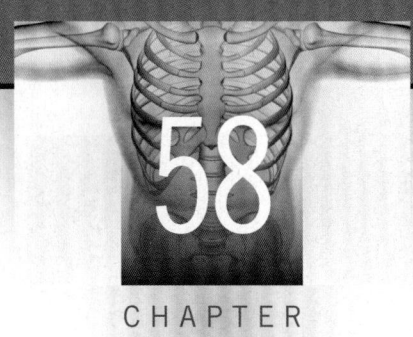

58

CHAPTER

Comprehensive Correction of Cavovarus Foot Deformity

Robert B. Lewis and Gregory C. Pomeroy

DEFINITION AND PATHOGENESIS

- Cavovarus foot deformity is defined as a high arch foot with a hindfoot that is in a varus position.
  - This may be neuromuscular in etiology or nonneuromuscular.
    - Typically, nonneuromuscular is more subtle and does not require a neurologic workup. Subtle cavovarus feet are very common in the general population and are often missed.[4]
    - Neuromuscular cavovarus foot deformity requires a complete neurologic workup. Unilateral cavovarus foot deformity also requires a neurologic workup.

NONOPERATIVE MANAGEMENT

- Subtle cavovarus foot deformity may be corrected in a full length over-the-counter orthotic such as an Arch Rival that has only a recessed first ray.
- More severe deformities often require a custom orthotic.
  - The orthotic should be full length and have a recessed first ray with a lower medial arch, which does not support the existing cavus deformity and a lateral heel post. Often, in a severe cavovarus foot, there needs to be a recessed area under the fifth metatarsal base.
- Peroneal tendon pathology is often present and may require physical therapy (PT) after an orthotic has corrected the underlying foot deformity.

SURGICAL MANAGEMENT

Preoperative Planning

- Physical examination should be done to test for motion at the subtalar joint and hypermobility at the first tarsal metatarsal joint. Presence of the "peek-a-boo" heel sign is noted. A Silfverskiöld test is performed as well as a complete neurologic exam. Coleman block testing confirms forefoot-driven hindfoot varus or primary hindfoot varus.
- Plain radiographs should be examined for arthritic changes, with triple arthrodesis reserved for severe, rigid deformity.[7]
- Computed tomography scanning can aid in determining arthritis when plain radiographs are unclear, but suspicion is high.
- A tight Achilles tendon should be addressed during the same procedure (gastrocnemius recession, percutaneous, or open Achilles lengthening). Concurrent problems, such as lateral ankle instability and peroneal tendon pathology, should be addressed during the same procedure.

- Regional anesthesia for postoperative pain control, including single-shot or continuous nerve block, should be considered.

Positioning

- The patient is positioned supine on the table with the heel resting at the end of the bed (**FIG 1**).
- Thigh tourniquets are used and well padded.
- A bump is placed beneath the ipsilateral hip until the foot is perpendicular to the table to facilitate medial and lateral exposures if needed.
- The leg is prepared to the knee.

Approach

- Achilles tendon pathology is addressed first, so this will minimize the deforming force on the heel when shifted.
  - Lengthening of the Achilles in a neuromuscular patient can cause significant weakness with ankle plantarflexion postoperatively and should be performed with caution.
- A dorsiflexion osteotomy of the first ray is performed until the first ray is out of plantarflexion.
  - This is the most common location needing an osteotomy in our practice.
- Either a lateral displacement or Dwyer-type osteotomy is performed, depending on the surgeon's preference, if rigid heel varus is still present.
  - In order to assess the hindfoot position, the surgeon places himself at the foot of the bed and holds the foot up to eye level while loading the forefoot evenly with one hand.

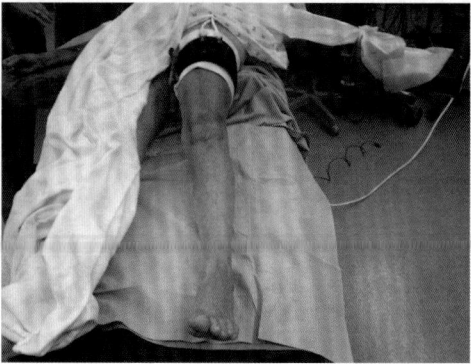

FIG 1 Positioning for cavovarus reconstruction. The patient is supine with a bump under the ipsilateral hip. The foot is placed perpendicular to the floor to facilitate medial and lateral foot access.

- In the setting of a subtle hindfoot varus, after a gastrocnemius recession and first ray osteotomy, there may not be a need for a calcaneal osteotomy.
- The lateral displacement osteotomy is used for most adult cases, as the Dwyer weakens the moment arm of the Achilles and often cannot achieve the desired correction.[8]
- Through the same incision, a peroneus longus to brevis transfer is done if appropriate.
- For more severe cases, multiple metatarsal dorsiflexion osteotomies may be required in a similar fashion.[6]
- More advanced cases with extensive cavus through the midfoot and forefoot may require dorsal wedge osteotomies at more proximal levels, as described by multiple authors.[2,3]

- Adequate preoperative planning should alert the surgeon to the need for these more advanced procedures.
- A plantar fascia release is useful as an adjunct when midfoot flexion is severe and prevents adequate reduction of the forefoot after osteotomy.
  - This can also be done first in deformities associated with increased calcaneal pitch, where a proximal slide of the calcaneus is being done to lower the arch.
- A Jones procedure can be used to correct residual claw hallux with Girdlestone and Taylor hammer toe procedures for the lesser toes if required.
- Transfer of the tibialis posterior to the lateral cuneiform is a useful adjunct in cases of Charcot-Marie-Tooth associated with dorsiflexion weakness of the ankle.[5]

GASTROCNEMIUS RECESSION

- Isolate the gastrocnemius fascia through a longitudinal incision just distal to the musculotendinous junction of the gastrocnemius on the medial side of the leg **(TECH FIG 1)**.
- Identify the deep fascia of the leg and incise it in line with the incision, revealing the muscle and tendon structures beneath.
- The plantaris tendon will be visible along the medial border of the tendons and may be cut.
- Using blunt dissection, the separation of the deep soleus and the more superficial gastrocnemius can be recognized.

- The gastrocnemius fascia is easily isolated using a pediatric vaginal speculum, but various retraction techniques may be employed.
  - Retraction helps protect the sural nerve, which lies adjacent to the gastrocnemius at this level near the midline.
- Once isolated, cut the entire fascia transversely using tenotomy scissors.
- Fifteen to 20 degrees of increased ankle dorsiflexion with the knee extended can usually be obtained.
- Reapproximate the deep fascia using 3-0 absorbable sutures.

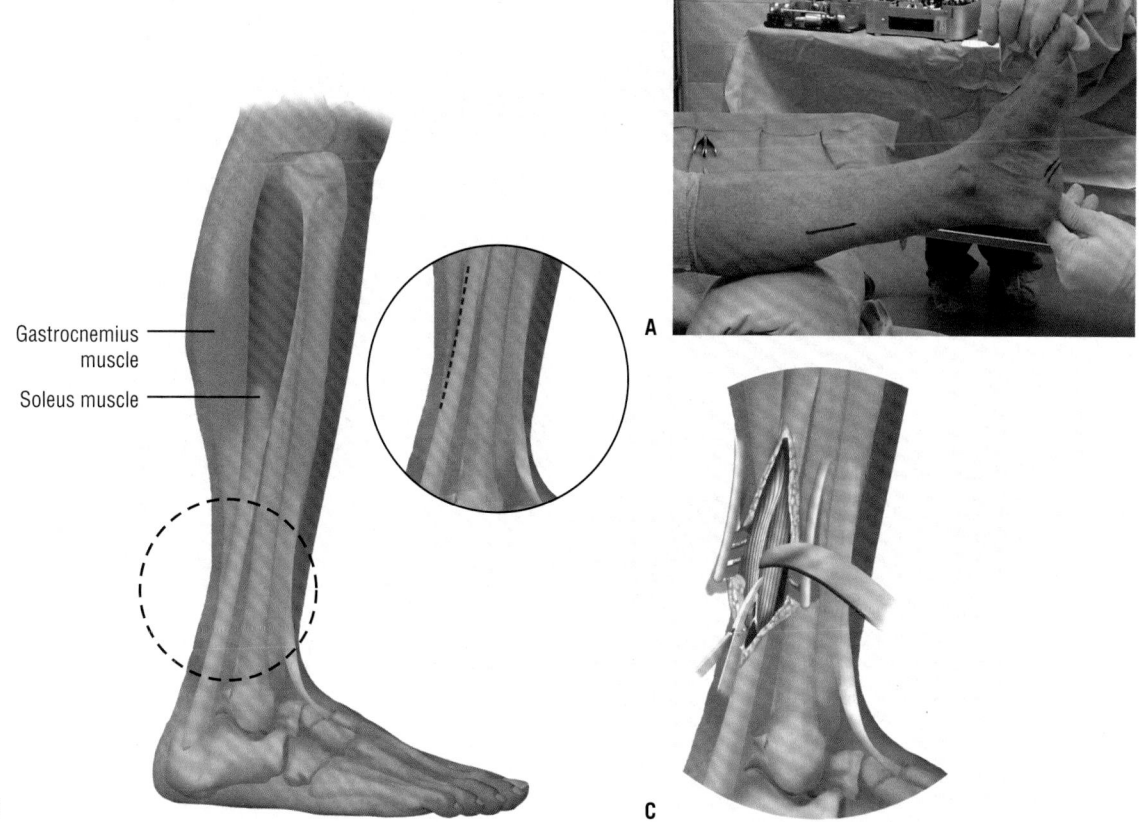

Gastrocnemius muscle

Soleus muscle

TECH FIG 1 A. Location of incision along medial leg. **B.** Deep fascia has been incised, revealing division of gastrocnemius and soleus fascias. **C.** Gastrocnemius fascia is isolated and cut from medial to lateral using tenotomy scissors. This protects the overlying sural nerve and saphenous vein.

TECHNIQUES

LATERAL DISPLACEMENT CALCANEAL OSTEOTOMY AND PERONEUS LONGUS TO BREVIS TRANSFER

- The incision to accomplish both of these procedures is made inferior to but parallel to the peroneus longus tendon **(TECH FIG 2)**.
- Deepen the dissection from the original incision until the peroneal tendons are identified.
- Enter the sheaths for the length of the incision, making sure to preserve the superior peroneal retinaculum (SPR).
  - The SPR may be taken down directly off the posterior fibula and reattached with a suture anchor if tendon pathology exists such as tears or instability, such as in our example.
  - Otherwise, the tendons can be sutured together, preserving this structure.
- Remove a section of the peroneus longus with a knife.
- Reapproximate the longus and brevis tendons proximally and hold them together with figure-8 no. 0 nonabsorbable suture, making sure the knot does not impinge below the SPR.
- Carry dissection inferior to the sural nerve, taking care to identify and protect it.

- Once the calcaneus is reached, carry the subperiosteal dissection inferior.
- Place small Hohmann retractors superior and anterior to the calcaneal tuberosity, protecting the insertion of the Achilles tendon and the origin of the plantar fascia, respectively.
- With soft tissues protected, use a sagittal saw to make the osteotomy perpendicular to the axis of the calcaneus.
- Shift the free tuberosity piece lateral until a physiologic valgus position of 5 degrees is obtained (usually 8 to 10 mm).
- Make a midline longitudinal incision just off the posterior plantar heel pad.
- Carry dissection straight through subcutaneous fat to bone.
- An assistant or Kirschner wire holds the heel shift in the corrected position while two 6.5-mm partially threaded cancellous screws are placed in lag fashion.
- The screws should be off the posterior weight-bearing surface of the heel and should not penetrate the subtalar joint.
- Use a rasp to smooth down the prominent lateral bone after the heel shift.

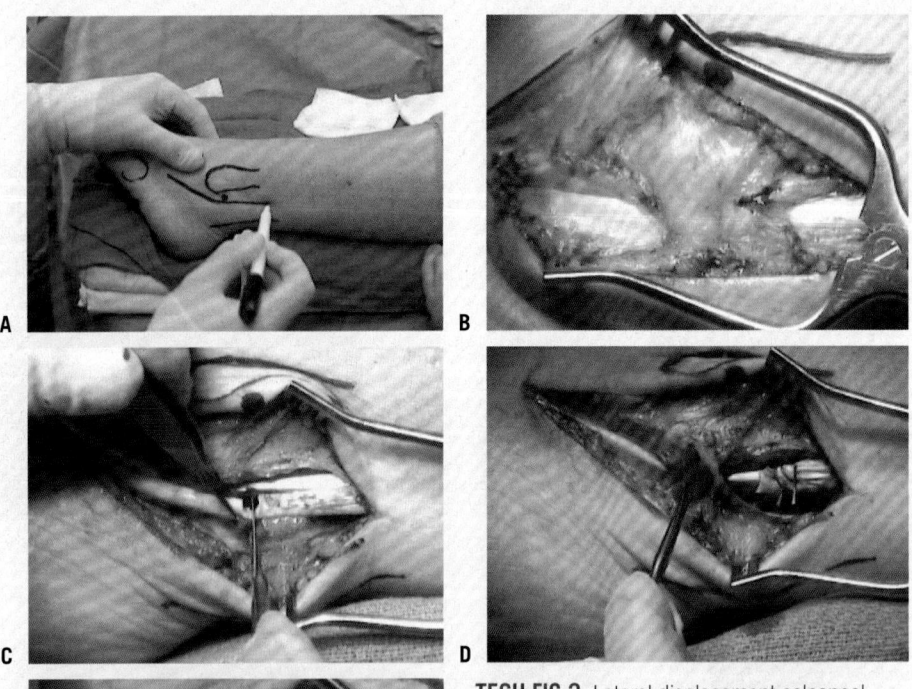

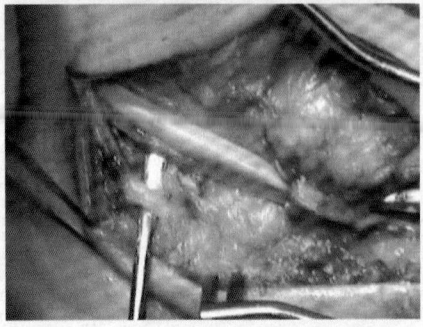

TECH FIG 2 Lateral displacement calcaneal osteotomy and peroneus longus to brevis transfer. **A.** Lateral incision over hindfoot just posterior to peroneal tendons. **B.** Dissection carried down to the peroneal tendons, with the SPR still intact. **C.** With the SPR flap taken posterior, a section of the peroneus longus is removed. **D.** The peroneus longus has been sutured to the brevis, making sure the knot does not impinge under the SPR through range of motion of the tendon. **E.** Sural nerve is identified as dissection is carried inferior. *(continued)*

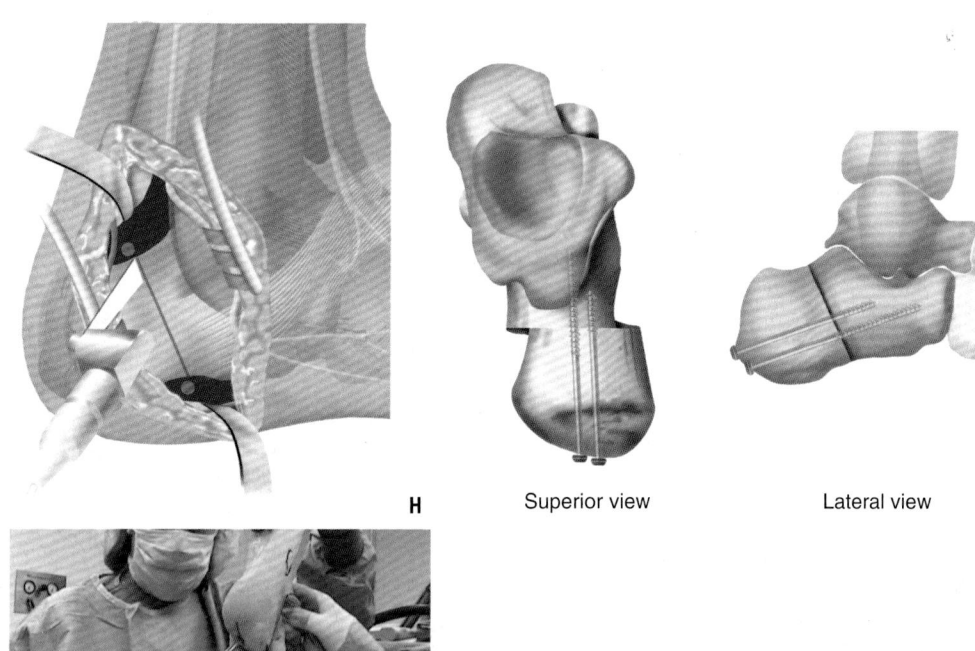

Superior view　　　Lateral view

F　　　　　　　H

G

TECH FIG 2 *(continued)* **F.** A saw is used to cut across the calcaneus, perpendicular to its long axis, protecting the Achilles and plantar fascia. **G.** An assistant holds the lateral shift while two 6.5-mm partially threaded cancellous screws are placed across the osteotomy. **H.** Final screw positioning as seen from lateral and superior views.

DWYER LATERAL CLOSING WEDGE CALCANEAL OSTEOTOMY

- Use the approach outlined earlier for the lateral sliding calcaneal osteotomy.
- Instead of a transverse cut with a shift, remove a wedge of bone, based laterally, using a sagittal saw **(TECH FIG 3)**.
- The size of the wedge depends on the desired correction but should bring the heel to a physiologic valgus position.
- Once the bone is removed, dorsiflex the foot to close the wedge and proceed with fixation as described previously.[1]

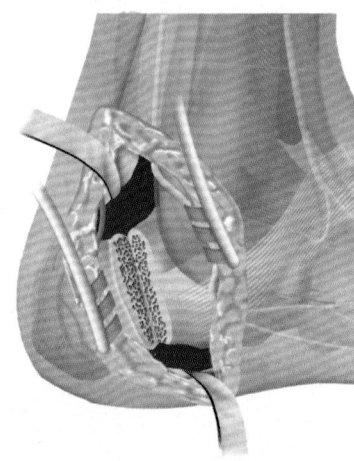

TECH FIG 3 Dwyer calcaneal osteotomy. Instead of a straight cut through bone, a lateral-based wedge is removed.

TECHNIQUES

FIRST METATARSAL DORSIFLEXION OSTEOTOMY

- Make a dorsal incision over the proximal first metatarsal and carry dissection down to the extensor tendons **(TECH FIG 4)**.
  - Retract them lateral, so dissection can be carried down to bone.
- Subperiosteal dissection allows exposure of the proximal metatarsal to the first tarsometatarsal joint.
- Mark a line transversely on the bone 1 cm from the joint for the bone cut.
- Place small Hohmann retractors around the bone to protect the soft tissues and perform a dorsal closing wedge osteotomy using a sagittal saw.
- The first cut is through 90% of the bone and perpendicular to the diaphysis.
- The second cut is 2 to 3 mm distal and angled back toward the plantar end point of the first cut.

- Complete the first cut and remove the bone wedge. Take enough bone to restore anatomic alignment of the talus and first metatarsal on the lateral radiograph (about 0 degree).
- Use a small burr to make a shallow hole in the dorsal bone to recess the screw head.
- Reduce the first metatarsal and place a 3.5-mm lag screw from the burr hole across the osteotomy, taking care not to enter the first tarsometatarsal joint.
- If the surgeon is having difficulty closing the osteotomy, check that the osteotomy is completely through the plantar cortex. Avoid disrupting the plantar periosteum as this will destabilize the osteotomy and make fixation more difficult. If there is still difficulty, consider peroneal longus spasticity and subsequently perform a peroneal longus tenotomy.

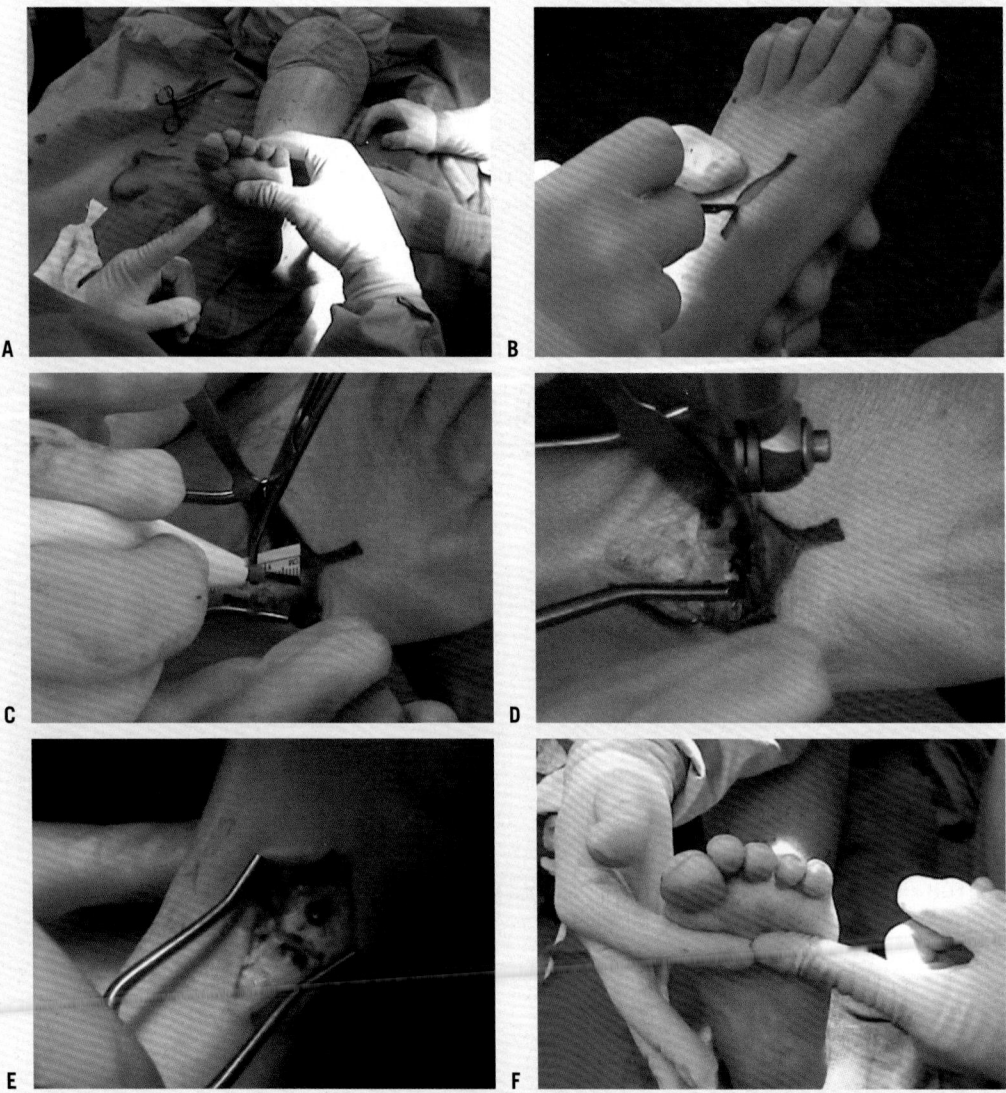

TECH FIG 4 First metatarsal dorsiflexion osteotomy. **A.** Plantarflexed first ray. **B.** Incision over first metatarsal. **C.** Measuring 1 cm from first tarsometatarsal joint. **D.** A small dorsally based wedge is removed. **E.** The wedge is closed and held with a screw recessed in the first metatarsal. **F.** Final first ray position.

PARTIAL PLANTAR FASCIOTOMY

- Make an incision just distal and parallel to the plantar heel pad **(TECH FIG 5)**.
- Dissection through subcutaneous fat exposes the plantar fascia.
- When the medial and lateral borders of the fascia are identified, partial or complete release may be undertaken.
- Begin transection 1 cm from the origin on the calcaneus and proceed medial to lateral.
- More severe deformities may require more of a release.

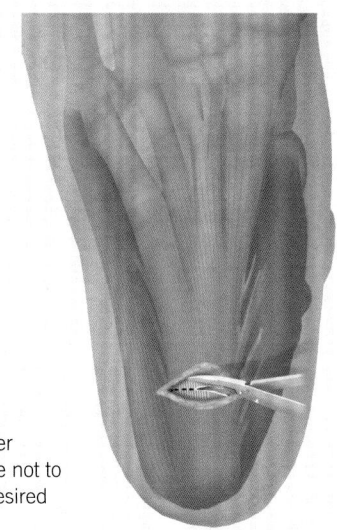

TECH FIG 5 Partial plantar fasciotomy. Incision is made over medial hindfoot, off the weight-bearing surface, making sure not to disturb nerves. The plantar fascia is cut transversely until desired correction is achieved.

JONES PROCEDURE

- The interphalangeal (IP) fusion of the great toe begins with a transverse incision over the IP joint dorsally **(TECH FIG 6)**.
- Cut the extensor hallucis and make an arthrotomy in the joint, freeing up the collateral ligaments.
- Use curettes to remove the articular cartilage and use a 2-mm drill bit to fenestrate both sides of the joint.
- Place a Kirschner wire from proximal to distal through the distal phalanx and out the tip of the toe just under the nail, leaving minimal wire within the joint.
- Place the wire retrograde across the IP joint while holding it reduced.
- Make a transverse incision at the toe tip to allow drilling over the wire.

- Measure the length of screw, so it does not penetrate the metatarsophalangeal joint.
- Place a 4.0-mm partially threaded cannulated screw over the wire for compression.
- Confirm the position on fluoroscopy and remove the wire.
- Center a dorsal midline incision over the first metatarsal neck.
- Identify the extensor hallucis longus (EHL) and bring its distal end into the wound.
- Make 4.0-mm drill holes on the medial and lateral aspects of the metatarsal neck and connect them using a curette.
- Pass the tendon from lateral to medial through the hole and suture it back on to itself using nonabsorbable suture while holding the ankle in a neutral to slightly dorsiflexed position.

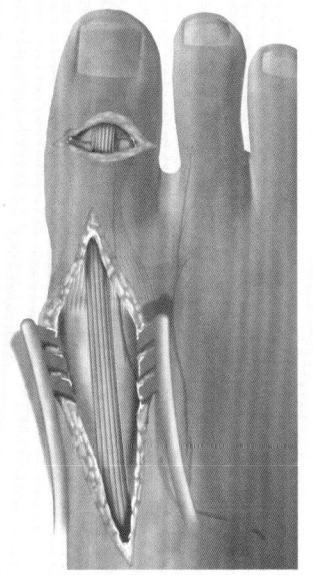
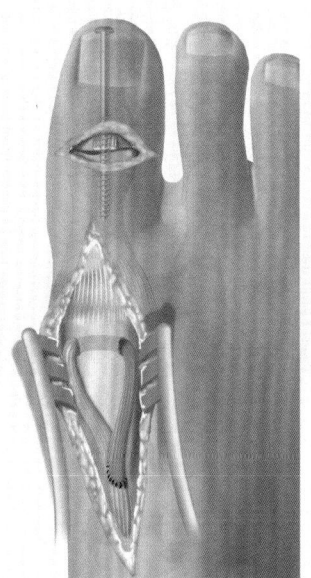

A   B

TECH FIG 6 Jones procedure of first toe. **A.** Incision is made transversely over the IP joint to remove cartilage and harvest EHL tendon. **B.** Incision is made longitudinally over the first metatarsal, transferring the tendon to the neck, and a screw is placed across the IP joint in lag mode.

TECHNIQUES

EXAMPLE CASE (COURTESY OF MARK E. EASLEY, MD)

Background, Physical Examination, and Imaging

- A 36-year-old man with progressive hereditary sensory motor neuropathy
  - Left cavovarus foot symptomatic despite bracing
  - Flexible hindfoot deformity: nearly fully passively correctable
  - Some fixed plantarflexion of the first ray
  - Some clawing of the toes, including the hallux
- Cavovarus foot alignment with weight bearing
  - Overload of lateral border of the foot **(TECH FIG 7A)**
  - High arch **(TECH FIG 7B)**
  - Heel varus: Be sure to observe patient weight bearing **(TECH FIG 7C)**.
- Fixed or flexible
  - If deformity is flexible, joint-sparing realignment is feasible.
  - If deformity is fixed, hindfoot arthrodesis should be considered.
- Motor function deficits
  - Sagittal plane motion
    - Limited ankle dorsiflexion
      - ❑ Lack of tibialis anterior muscle function
      - ❑ Compensation with toe extensors and peroneus tertius
    - Typically associated with an equinus contracture: intact gastrocnemius–soleus function
  - Coronal plane motion (hindfoot motion)
    - Limited eversion/forefoot abduction: lack of peroneus brevis tendon function
    - Hindfoot varus /forefoot adduction due to unopposed intact posterior tibialis function
  - Often associated with clawing of the toes
- Evaluate the ankle radiographically because there may be associated talar tilt.
  - In this case, the ankle is congruent, but hindfoot is obviously in varus through the subtalar and transverse tarsal joints **(TECH FIG 7D)**.

- Evaluate the foot.
  - Anteroposterior (AP) foot radiograph: forefoot abduction with stacking of the lesser metatarsals
  - Lateral foot radiograph: cavus alignment with stacking of the lesser metatarsals and plantarflexed first ray **(TECH FIG 7E)**; clawing of toes often observed

Tendo Achilles Lengthening

- Favor gastrocnemius recession over lengthening the Achilles tendon
- Triple cut hemisection **(TECH FIG 8)**
  - Goal is to lengthen and not completely release
  - Three percutaneous hemisections
    - Two toward the medial side
    - One toward the lateral side between the two toward the medial side
    - Hemisections spaced approximately 2.5 to 3 cm apart
- Gentle dorsiflexion force to lengthen the tendon but maintain its continuity

Plantar Fascia Release

- Unlike the partial release (rarely) performed for recalcitrant plantar fasciitis, the release performed for symptomatic cavus foot malalignment is complete.
- Make a longitudinal 3- to 4-cm incision immediately medial to the tight plantar fascia.
- Dorsiflex the toes to activate the windlass mechanism, putting the plantar fascia on stretch, making it easier to palpate.
- Careful dissection to expose and isolate the plantar fascia completely on its dorsal and plantar aspects.
- Perform a complete plantar fascia release with a scalpel blade **(TECH FIG 9)**.

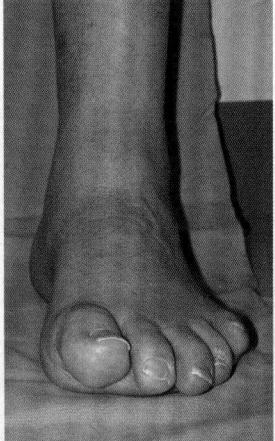
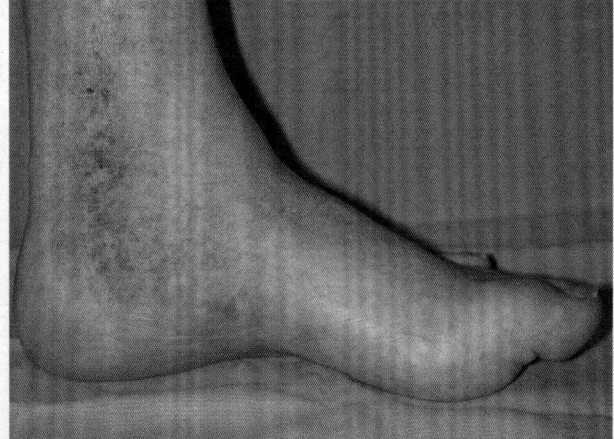
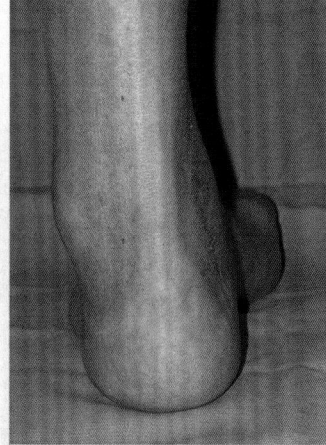

TECH FIG 7 A 36-year-old man with a progressive hereditary sensory motor neuropathy and right cavovarus foot deformity. **A.** Note peek-a-boo heel on visualization from anterior perspective and clawing of the hallux. **B.** High arch and clawed hallux on lateral perspective. **C.** Heel varus on posterior perspective. *(continued)*

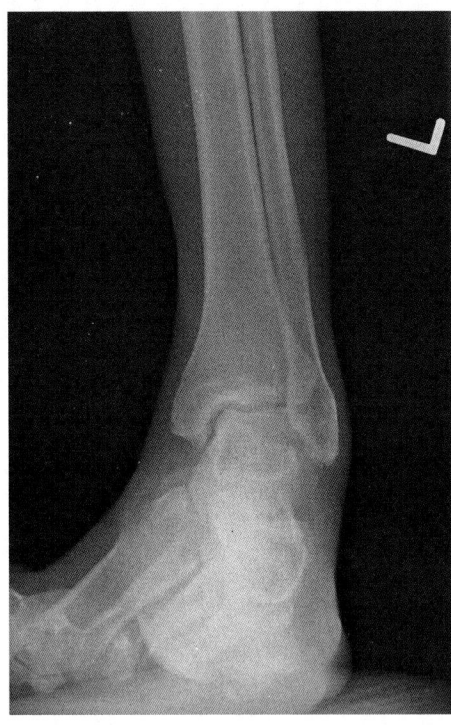

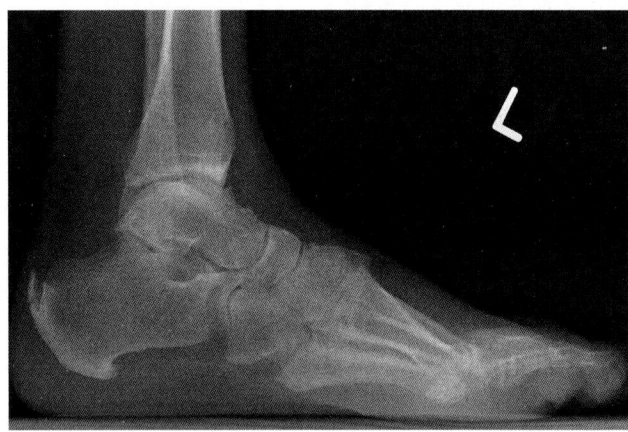

TECH FIG 7 *(continued)* **D.** Weight-bearing AP ankle view suggests that mortise is congruent, and varus deformity is in the hindfoot. **E.** Weight-bearing lateral view does not give full appreciation of cavovarus noted clinically; however, plantarflexed first ray is evident.

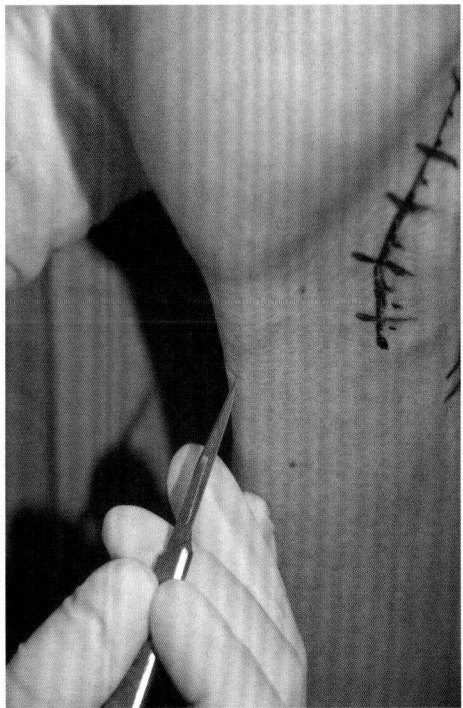

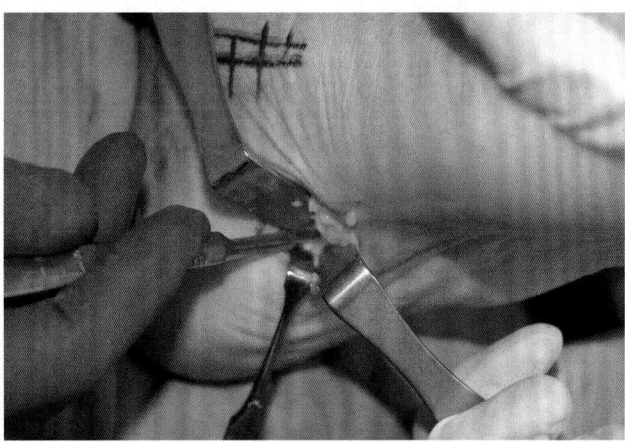

TECH FIG 8 Tendo-Achilles lengthening via percutaneous hemisection technique.

TECH FIG 9 Plantar fascia release. As opposed to the partial release recommended for plantar fasciitis, in cavovarus foot deformity, the plantar fascia is completely released through an incision more distal than the one used for traditional plantar fascia release.

Posterior Tibial Tendon Transfer

- Make a longitudinal 5-cm incision directly over the posterior tibial tendon (PTT) insertion at the navicular.
- Incise the PTT sheath to expose the tendon.
- Release the tendon from the insertion on the navicular, including as much distal tendon as possible to optimize the tendon length for the planned transfer **(TECH FIG 10A).**
- Place a suture in the distal (released) tendon to facilitate in tendon transfer.
- While protecting the plantar medial venous plexus and the spring ligament, release as distal as possible the portion of the PTT that courses plantar to the foot.
- Mobilize the released tendon for transfer.
- Make an incision over the posteromedial tibial cortex 10 to 12 cm proximal to the medial malleolus.
- Release the retinaculum from the posteromedial tibia.
- Expose the PTT.
  - Typically, the first tendon encountered is the flexor digitorum longus tendon; this tendon needs to be retracted to access the PTT.
- With the distal PTT released, pull the PTT through the more proximal medial wound **(TECH FIG 10B).**
  - It may bind where the tendon passes posterior to the medial malleolus.

- This is typically mitigated by spreading within the PTT sheath at the distal medial malleolus with a blunt scissor from the distal incision.
- Pass the PTT posterior to the tibia, from the medial wound, immediately adjacent to the posterior tibia, through the interosseous membrane, and through a lateral wound created anterior to fibula **(TECH FIG 10C,D).**
- The interosseous membrane should be carefully spread to create enough space to avoid tendon binding.
- Alternatively, the tendon may be passed anterior to the tibia.

Peroneal Tendon Transfer

- Transfer the peroneus longus to the peroneus brevis tendon.
- Make a standard utilitarian lateral curvilinear incision over the peroneal tendons.
  - Protect the sural nerve.
  - Open the peroneal tendon sheaths for both peroneal tendons.
  - Release the more inferior peroneus longus tendon **(TECH FIG 11A).**
  - Transfer the peroneus longus tendon to the peroneus brevis tendon.
    - Side-to-side repair
    - Tendon weave **(TECH FIG 11B)**

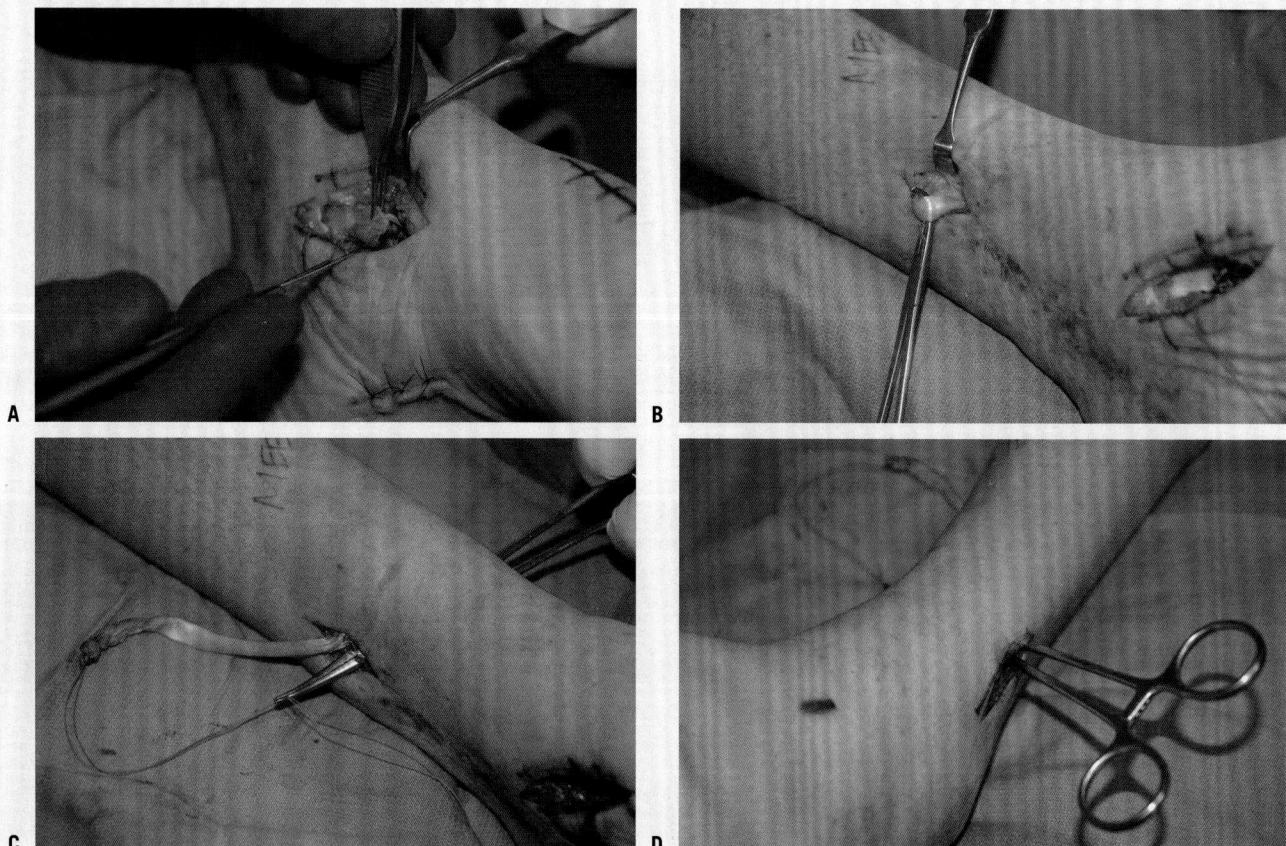

TECH FIG 10 PTT release. **A.** Release of the PTT from the medial navicular and plantar arch. **B.** Identifying the PTT through a medial incision 10 to 12 cm proximal to the medial malleolus. **C.** Delivering the PTT to the proximal medial wound and preparing for anterior transfer through interosseous membrane. **D.** The clamp is passed from the anterolateral wound, immediately posterior to the tibia.

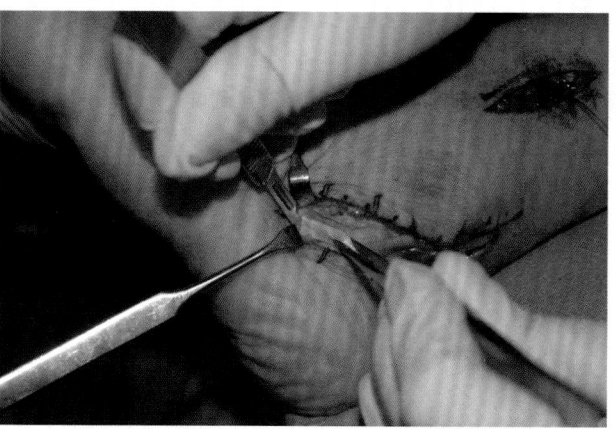 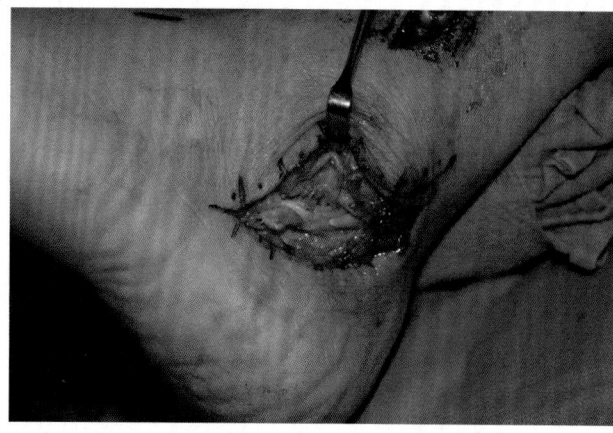

TECH FIG 11 Peroneus longus to brevis tendon transfer. **A.** Through approach on lateral aspect of foot, peroneus longus is transected. **B.** Weave the peroneus longus into the peroneus brevis.

Calcaneal Osteotomy

- Use the same utilitarian lateral incision.
- Retract the peroneal tendons anteriorly and protect soft tissues.
- Calcaneal osteotomy pattern (surgeon's preference)
  - Lateral closing wedge (Dwyer)
  - Lateral calcaneal tuberosity translation
  - Combination **(TECH FIG 12A)**
  - Z-osteotomy
- Fixation is with one or two axial screws from the posterior calcaneus perpendicular to the osteotomy without violating the subtalar joint.
  - Obtain fluoroscopic confirmation **(TECH FIG 12B)**.

Transfer of Posterior Tibial Tendon to the Dorsum of the Midfoot

- Make a 2- to 3-cm dorsolateral midfoot incision over the lateral cuneiform.
- Protect the superficial peroneal nerve.
- Create a subcutaneous tunnel with a long clamp, carefully spreading to limit binding of tendon **(TECH FIG 13A)**.

- Pull the distal end of tendon to be transferred through subcutaneous tunnel and have it ready to be secured to the lateral cuneiform.
- Drill a hole in the lateral cuneiform.
  - Use careful soft tissue dissection to protect superficial peroneal nerve, extensor tendons, and neurovascular structures.
  - Place a guide pin in the lateral cuneiform and confirm its appropriate orientation and position fluoroscopically.
  - Overdrill the guide pin to gradually enlarge to tunnel so that it may accommodate the tendon **(TECH FIG 13B)**.
  - Use fluoroscopy to confirm appropriate tunnel **(TECH FIG 13C)**.
- Pass the tendon into the tunnel.
  - Attach the suture to a long needle.
  - Pass the needle through the bone tunnel in the lateral cuneiform and carefully pass it through the arch **(TECH FIG 13D)**.
  - Pull the suture on the plantar foot and advance the tendon into the tunnel to confirm that it will easily fit into the tunnel without binding **(TECH FIG 13E)**.
  - Delay PTT fixation to cuneiform until end of procedure.
    - Securing it at this point risks weakening the fixation prior to closure and casting.

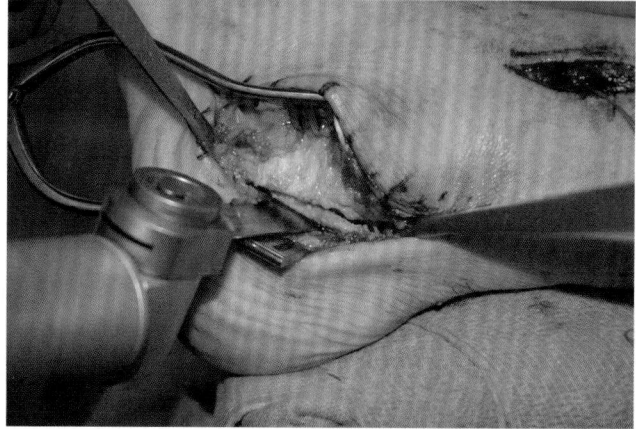 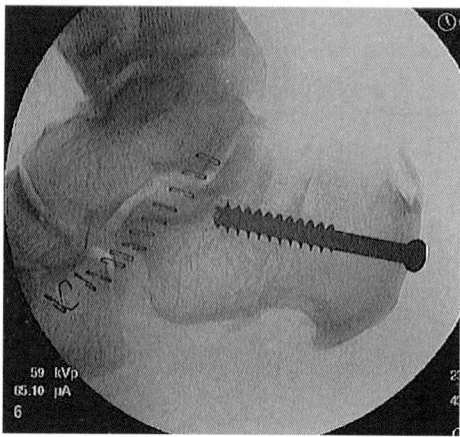

TECH FIG 12 Lateralizing/lateral closing calcaneal osteotomy. **A.** Through the same utilitarian lateral approach, with the peroneal tendons elevated, carefully expose the lateral calcaneus to perform the osteotomy. **B.** Intraoperative fluoroscopy confirming satisfactory bony apposition of the osteotomy and proper position of hardware.

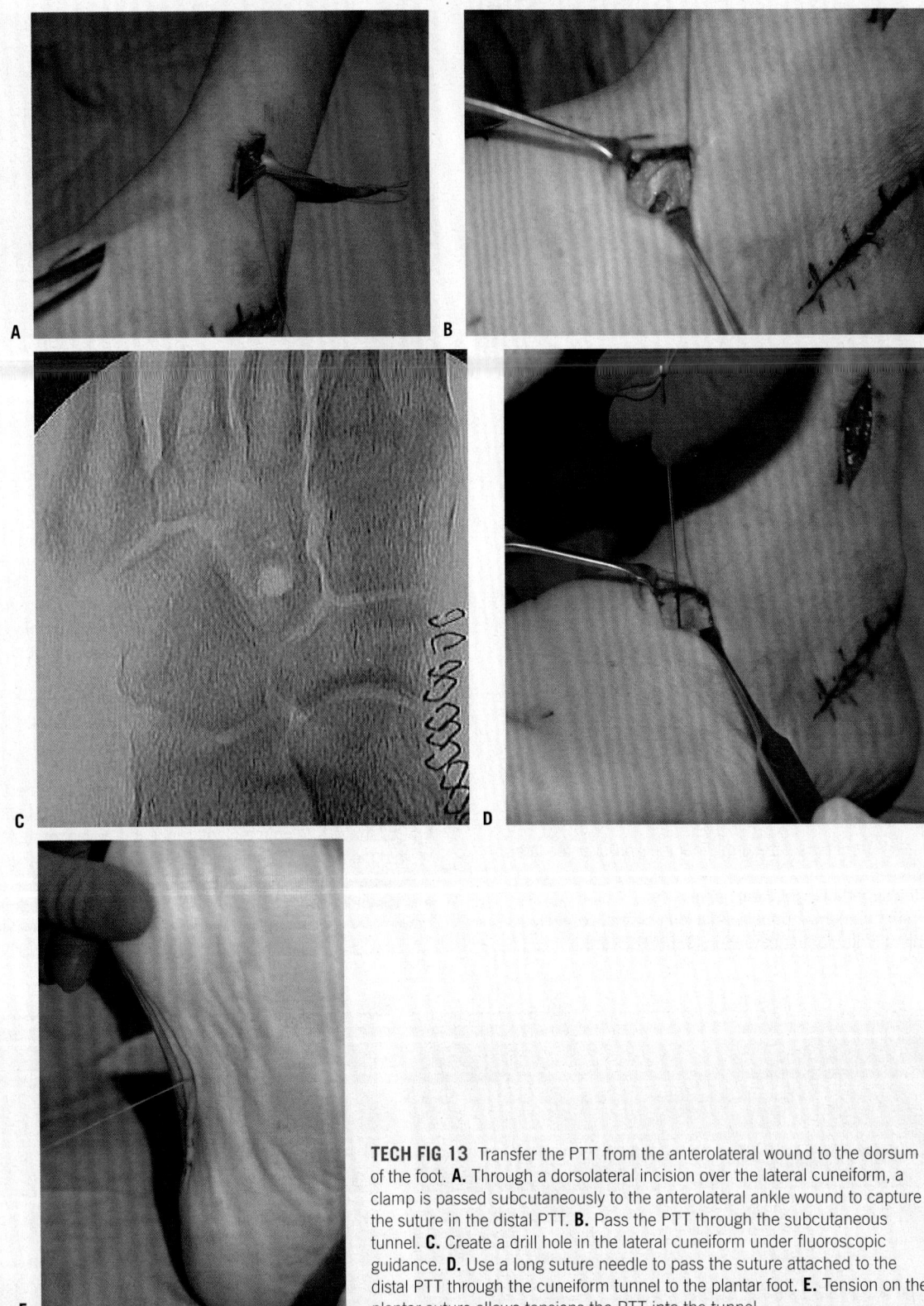

TECH FIG 13 Transfer the PTT from the anterolateral wound to the dorsum of the foot. **A.** Through a dorsolateral incision over the lateral cuneiform, a clamp is passed subcutaneously to the anterolateral ankle wound to capture the suture in the distal PTT. **B.** Pass the PTT through the subcutaneous tunnel. **C.** Create a drill hole in the lateral cuneiform under fluoroscopic guidance. **D.** Use a long suture needle to pass the suture attached to the distal PTT through the cuneiform tunnel to the plantar foot. **E.** Tension on the plantar suture allows tensions the PTT into the tunnel.

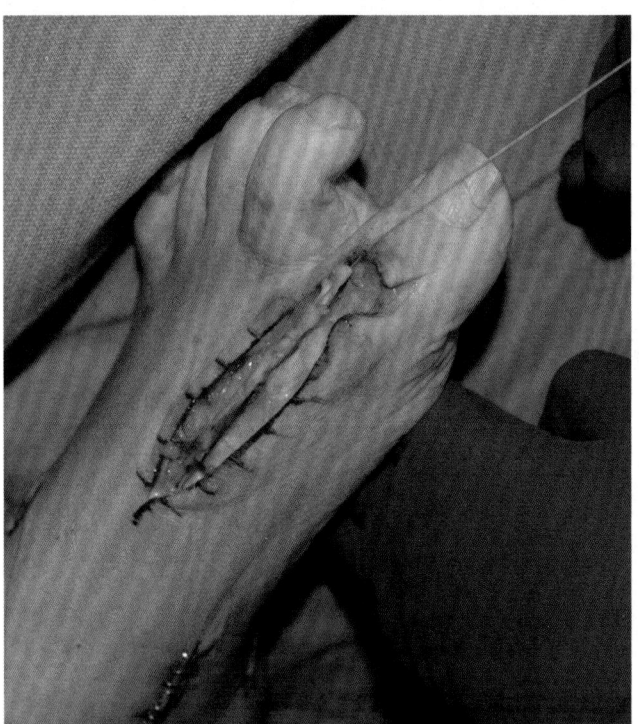

TECH FIG 14 Through a longitudinal incision over the first ray, release the EHL tendon from its insertion on the distal phalanx.

First Metatarsal Elevation and Correction of Clawed Hallux (Jones Procedure)

- Make a dorsal longitudinal incision over the first ray.
- Over the hallux IP joint, the incision may be continued as a Z in order to improve access to the joint.
- Release the EHL tendon from the hallux distal phalanx.
- Place a tagging suture in the EHL tendon **(TECH FIG 14)**.

Dorsiflexion Osteotomy of the First Metatarsal

- Limit periosteal stripping of the first metatarsal.
- Identify optimal position for dorsiflexion osteotomy of first metatarsal **(TECH FIG 15A)**.
- Dorsal wedge resection in the proximal metatarsal can be either vertical or oblique, depending on surgeon preference.
  - Maintain plantar cortex to create a stable closing wedge osteotomy **(TECH FIG 15B)**.
  - Stabilize the osteotomy with a low-profile dorsal compression plate **(TECH FIG 15C)**.

Correction of Clawed Hallux (Jones Procedure)

- Create tunnel in first metatarsal head–shaft junction from medial to lateral **(TECH FIG 16A,B)**.
- Delay EHL tendon transfer (and the PTT transfer) to the first metatarsal until the completion of the surgery.
  - Complete all bony correction.
  - Perform tendon transfers as last step to obtain proper tension and balance and to protect tendon fixation to bone.
- Prepare the hallux IP joint for arthrodesis.
  - Remove cartilage surfaces and prepare subchondral bone.
  - Maintain slight plantarflexion of the IP joint and avoid removing too much dorsal bone that may create hyperextension.
  - Secure the hallux IP joint arthrodesis with a longitudinal compression screw placed from the tip of the toe through a transverse stab incision 2 mm plantar to the hallux nail **(TECH FIG 16C,D)**.

Complete the Tendon Transfers

- Delay EHL tendon transfer (and the PTT transfer) to the first metatarsal until the completion of the surgery.
  - Complete all bony correction.
  - Perform tendon transfers as last step to obtain proper tension and balance and to protect tendon fixation to bone.

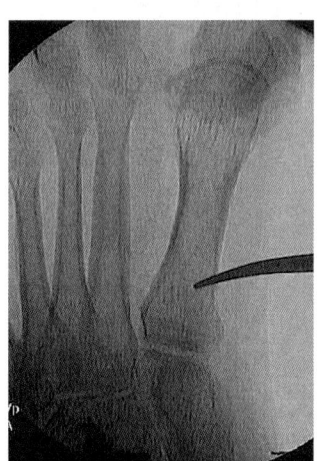
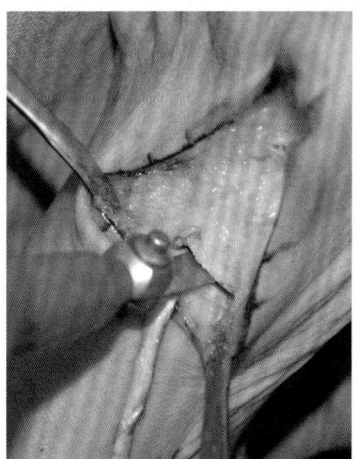
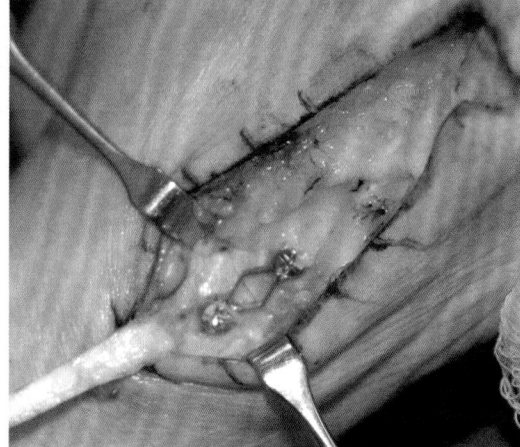

A   B   C

TECH FIG 15 First metatarsal dorsiflexion osteotomy. **A.** Fluoroscopic confirmation of proper position for osteotomy, leaving adequate space for proximal fixation in the metatarsal without violating the tarsometatarsal joint. **B.** Dorsal wedge resection osteotomy, with minimal periosteal stripping and leaving the plantar cortex intact. **C.** Osteotomy fixation with a dorsal compression plate.

TECHNIQUES

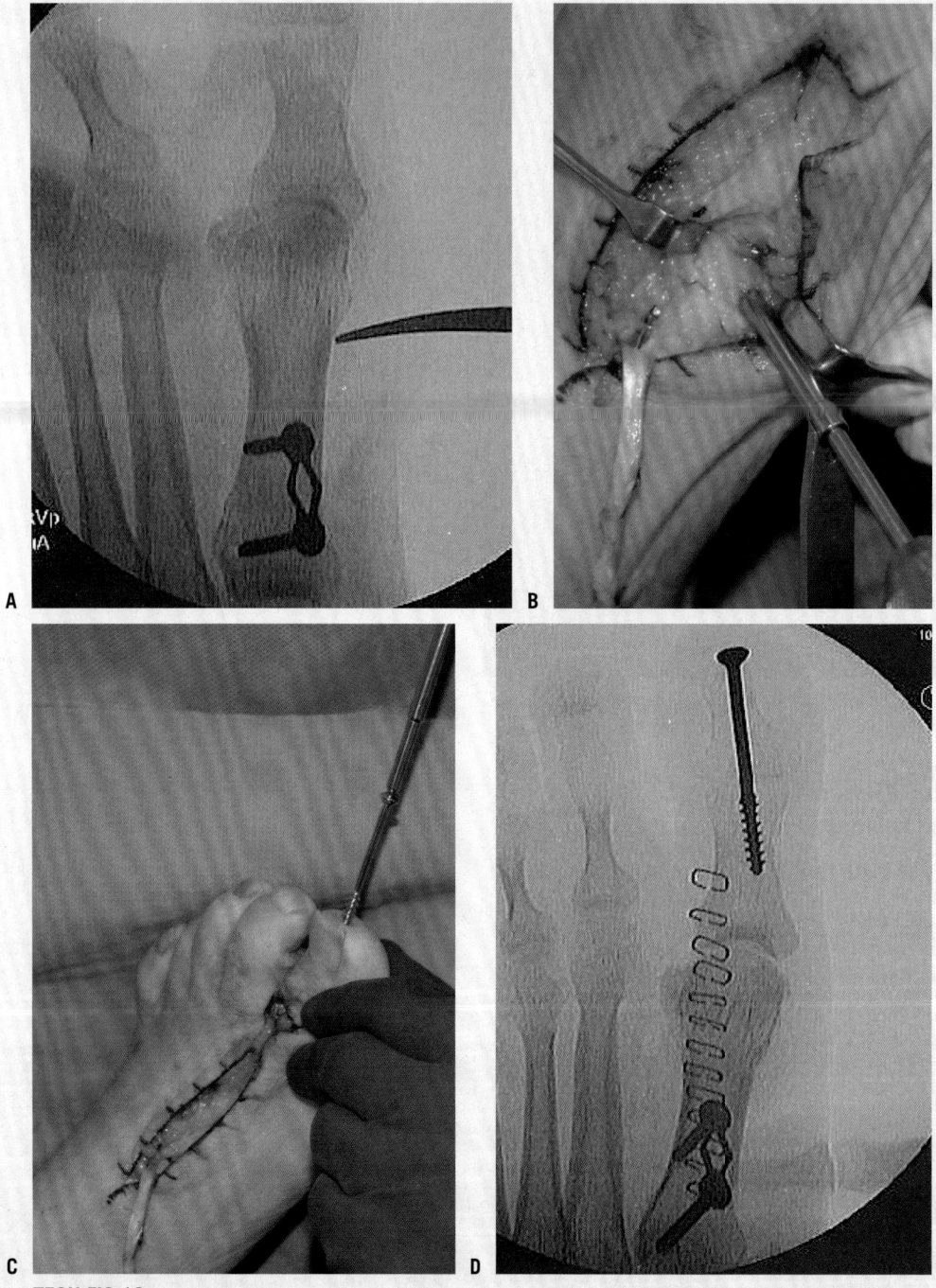

TECH FIG 16 Drill hole in metatarsal neck for Jones procedure. **A.** Identifying optimal position for drill hole in metatarsal neck to transfer the EHL tendon. **B.** Drill hole in first metatarsal created. **C.** After preparation of hallux IP joint for arthrodesis, axial screw is placed, with toe in proper rotation. **D.** Intraoperative fluoroscopic image demonstrating metatarsal and hallux IP joint fixation and satisfactory bony apposition.

- With the ankle in slight dorsiflexion, secure the PTT tendon to the lateral cuneiform.
  - Suture anchors can be used, even within the tunnel created in the cuneiform.
  - Currently, available interference screws offer satisfactory stability.
  - If concern for fixation, consideration may be given to using a combination of the interference screw and suture anchors.

- Pass the EHL tendon through the metatarsal neck tunnel and secure it to itself after passing through the tunnel.
- The EHL transfer, if functional, will add dynamic elevation to the first ray rather than promote clawing of the hallux.

Closure and Casting

- Routine closure (sutures or staples)
- With the ankle in slight dorsiflexion, place a well-padded short-leg cast that extends beyond the toes.

Postoperative Care

- 3 weeks of non–weight-bearing short-leg cast and then suture/stable removal
- 4 more weeks of new short-leg cast partial weight bearing permitted
- At 7 weeks, surgeon decision is based on stability of tendon fixation and osteotomies and evaluation of follow-up radiographs.
  - If stable fixation and satisfactory healing on radiographs, consider cam boot and gradually advance weight bearing.
  - Patient should maintain dorsiflexion when boot is removed to clean leg/foot and should sleep in boot.

- If more healing deemed necessary, then new short-leg cast and gradually advance weight bearing
- At 10 to 11 weeks
  - Fit for hinged ankle–foot orthosis (AFO) that has a plantar-flexion stop at neutral
  - Initiate PT program for training for PTT to dorsiflex the ankle, generalized conditioning and gait training.
  - Gradually transfer from cam boot to hinged AFO.
- Continue PT and hinged AFO for 8 weeks.
- At 18 to 20 weeks, after satisfactory progression with PT program, transition to regular shoe (see **FIG 2**)

TECHNIQUES

Pearls and Pitfalls

Preoperative Assessment	• A neurologic workup is indicated if no identifiable neurologic cause for deformity is known, as a progressive muscle imbalance may cause recurrence.
Heel Screw Placement	• With a lateral heel shift, the tendency is to place screws too far lateral. • The drill should be angled slightly medial to ensure entering the remaining calcaneus. • Aiming toward the lateral malleolus distal tip will ensure appropriate slope.
First Metatarsal Osteotomy	• The tendency is to take too much of a dorsal wedge, making the first metatarsal too dorsiflexed. • Always perform this first and then the calcaneal osteotomy.
Plantar Fascia Release	• The medial calcaneal branch of the tibial nerve and the intrinsic musculature of the foot are at risk, so careful dissection is warranted.

POSTOPERATIVE CARE

- Posterior sugar-tong splinting is used immediately postoperatively with the ankle in neutral dorsiflexion.
- Skin staples are removed at 2 weeks.
- Patients are kept immobilized and non–weight bearing for a total of 8 weeks, and weight bearing is begun when bony healing has occurred.
- PT is prescribed as needed for gait training and scar mobilization and to increase foot and subtalar motion.

- **FIG 2** shows 6-month follow-up of the patient in the Example Case.

OUTCOMES

- Long-term studies of cavovarus correction in adults are lacking, likely given the varied presentation and multiple modes of treatment for the disorder.
- Early treatment while feet are flexible is advised to prevent more extensive procedures required for rigid deformities and complications from progressive arthrosis.

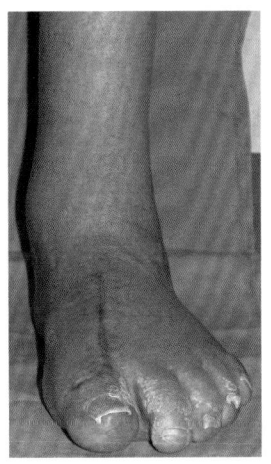
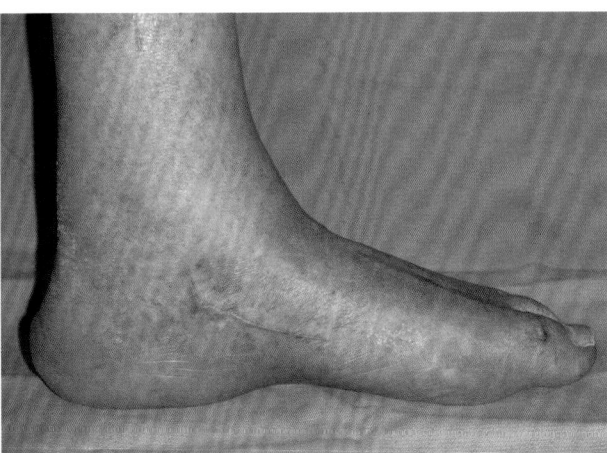
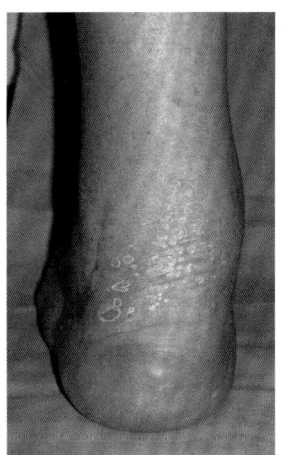

FIG 2 Six-month follow-up of the patient in **TECH FIGS 7** to **16**. **A.** Anterior perspective. The "peek-a-boo" heel is no longer present. **B.** Lateral perspective demonstrates more physiologic arch and correction of the hallux claw toe deformity. **C.** Posterior perspective demonstrates correction of heel varus. (continued)

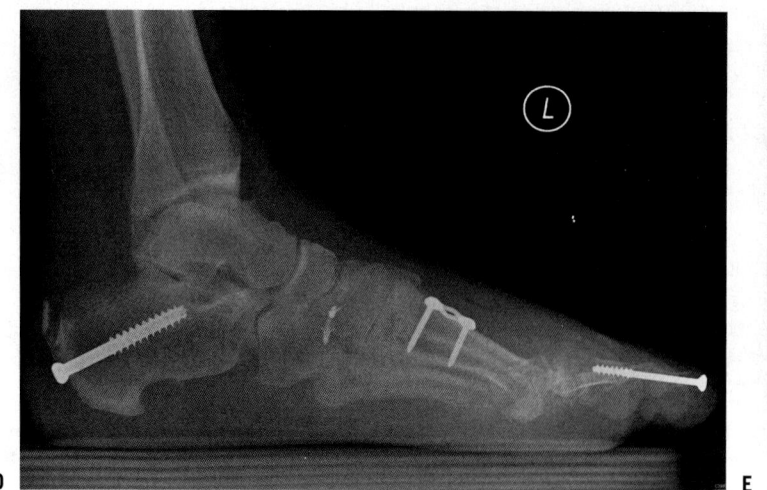 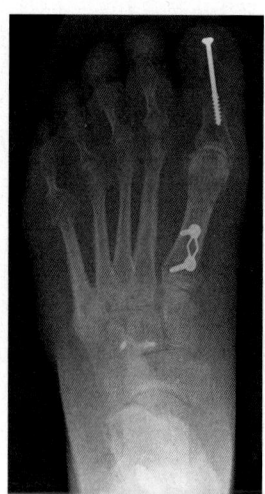

FIG 3 *(continued)* Lateral (**D**) and AP (**E**) weight-bearing follow-up radiographs.

COMPLICATIONS

- Painful hardware especially over the heel
- Infection
- Recurrence of deformity particularly with neuromuscular etiology
- Wound dehiscence
- Nonunion
- Undercorrection of deformity
- Ankle plantarflexion weakness after Achilles lengthening in a neuromuscular patient

ACKNOWLEDGMENT

- The authors would like to thank Michael Barnett, Arthur Manoli, Bruce J. Sangeorzan, and Brian C. Toolan for their outstanding work on the previous edition chapter.

REFERENCES

1. Dwyer FC. The present status of the problem of pes cavus. Clin Orthop Relat Res 1975;(106):254–275.
2. Jahss MH. Tarsometatarsal truncated-wedge arthrodesis for pes cavus and equinovarus deformity of the fore part of the foot. J Bone Joint Surg Am 1980;62(5):713–722.
3. Japas LM. Surgical treatment of pes cavus by tarsal V-osteotomy. Preliminary report. J Bone Joint Surg Am 1968;50(5):927–944.
4. Manoli A II, Graham B. The subtle cavus foot, "the underpronator." Foot Ankle Int 2005;26(3):256–263.
5. McCluskey WP, Lovell WW, Cummings RJ. The cavovarus foot deformity. Etiology and management. Clin Orthop Relat Res 1989;(247):27–37.
6. Sammarco GJ, Taylor R. Cavovarus foot treated with combined calcaneus and metatarsal osteotomies. Foot Ankle Int 2001;22:19–30.
7. Wetmore RS, Drennan JC. Long-term results of triple arthrodesis in Charcot-Marie-Tooth disease. J Bone Joint Surg Am 1989;71(3):417–422.
8. Younger AE, Hansen ST Jr. Adult cavovarus foot. J Am Acad Orthop Surg 2005;13:302–315.

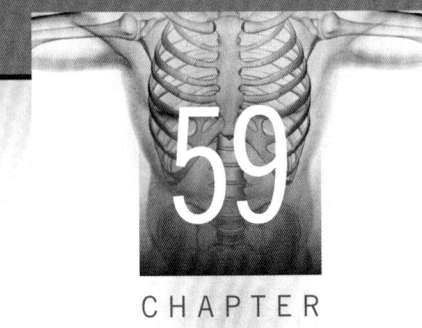

59 CHAPTER

Management of Equinocavovarus Foot Deformity

Wolfram Wenz and Thomas Dreher

DEFINITION

- Pes cavus is characterized by increased plantarflexion of the forefoot and midfoot in relation to the hindfoot. An isolated pes cavus is rare; it is commonly accompanied by other deformities of the foot. Therefore, pes cavus should be classified in different groups: pes cavovarus, pes equinocavus, pes calcaneocavus, and pes valgocavus (**FIG 1**). In many cases, a combination of the first two types occurs, called the *pes equinocavovarus*.

- The equinocavovarus foot describes a mostly acquired foot deformity consisting of an increased arch of the foot (forefoot and midfoot equinus), a limited dorsiflexion of

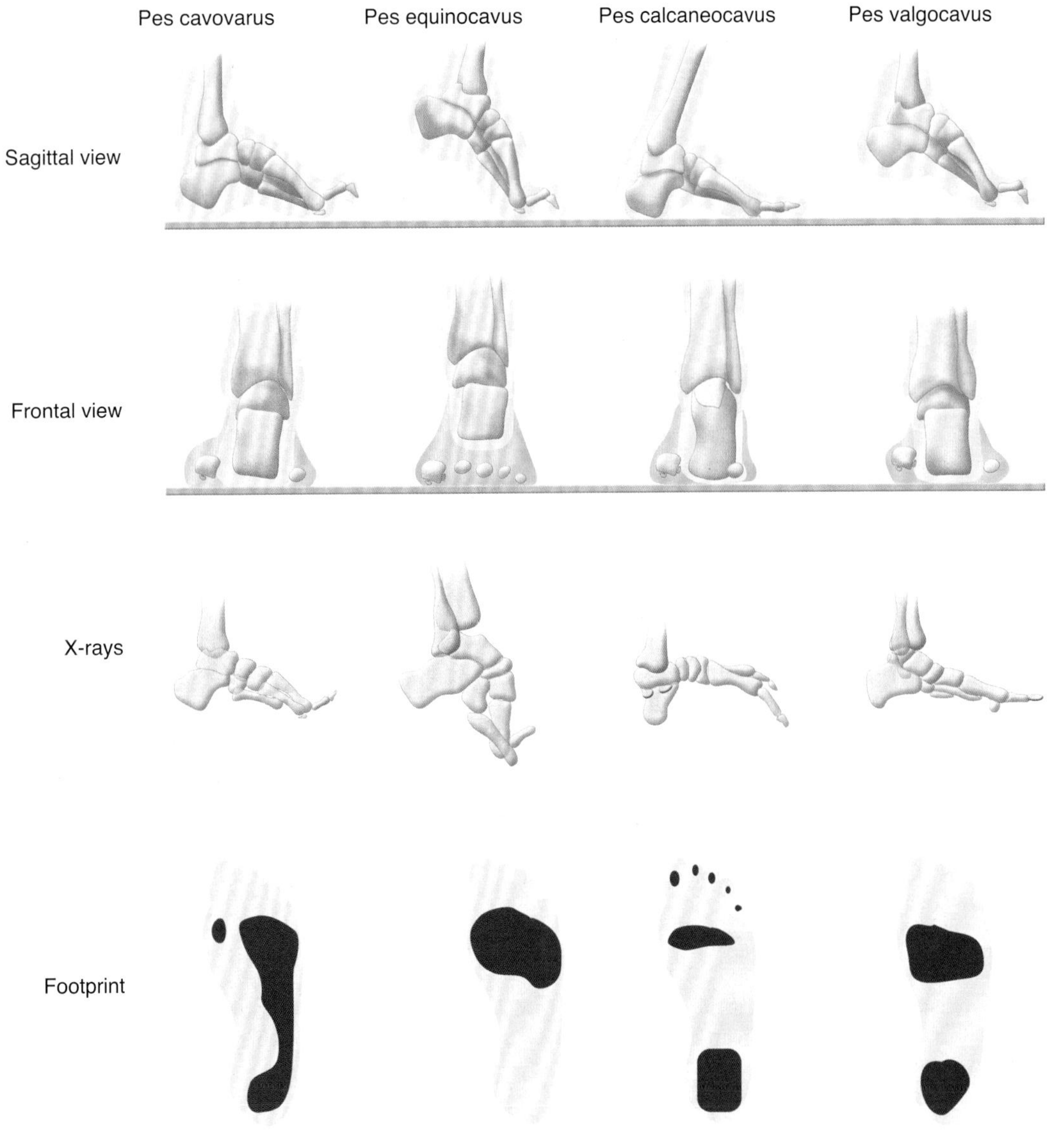

| Pes cavovarus | Pes equinocavus | Pes calcaneocavus | Pes valgocavus |

Sagittal view

Frontal view

X-rays

Footprint

FIG 1 Cavus foot deformities.

the ankle joint (hindfoot equinus), and a hindfoot varus. A concomitant forefoot and midfoot adductus, supinatus, or pronatus can occur, depending on the underlying pathology.

- "The cavovarus foot is one of the most perplexing and challenging of all foot deformities."[2]
- "The literature on pes cavus is extremely confusing."[15]

ANATOMY

- Equinus deformity of the ankle (limited dorsiflexion)
- Hindfoot in varus position (inversion of the calcaneus, flexible or rigid)
- External rotation of the talus and retraction of the lateral malleolus
- Medial dislocation of the navicular and the cuboid bone in the Chopart joint
- Cavus deformity medially (flexible or rigid)
- Plantarflexed position of the first metatarsal bone (flexible or rigid)
- Pronation and adduction of the forefoot (flexible or rigid)
- Claw toes, isolated to the hallux or involving all five toes (flexible or fixed)

PATHOGENESIS

- "[A] story of repeated failure to comprehend the basic pathogenesis and mechanics of a deformity which remains a mystery to this day, comparable only to problems such as scoliosis."[6]
- There are various theories concerning the pathogenesis of pes equinocavovarus:
  - "There is little doubt that the condition is caused by a muscle imbalance, involving both the intrinsic and the extrinsic muscles of the foot."[15]
  - Weakness of the anterior tibial muscle (progressive plantarflexion of the first metatarsal bone) because of relative overactivity of the long peroneal muscle; the long toe extensors try to compensate the reduced dorsiflexion force of the anterior tibial muscle. This results in an overbalance of the extrinsic extensor muscles in comparison to the intrinsic extensor muscles. The toes are hyperextended in the metatarsophalangeal joints. At the same time, the long toe flexors pull the end phalangeal bone into plantarflexion. Both mechanisms result in increased cavus (forefoot and midfoot equinus).
  - Weakness of the short peroneal muscle (peroneus brevis). Relative overactivity of the posterior tibial muscle forces the hindfoot into varus position. The force of the long toe flexors (increased flexion of the metatarsophalangeal joints) is antagonized by increased activity of the long peroneal muscle (peroneus longus) that also pulls the first metatarsal bone into plantarflexion. Because of its limited effects on the hindfoot, the peroneus longus cannot antagonize the overactivity of the posterior tibial muscle.

NATURAL HISTORY

- One functionally relevant consequence of the deformity is the limited ankle dorsiflexion. Its causes can be an isolated shortened Achilles tendon, which is rare. An acquired horizontal position of the talus resulting from hindfoot supination can cause a limited dorsiflexion. The cavus deformity itself may be responsible for limited ankle dorsiflexion.

- The limited ankle dorsiflexion in pes equinocavovarus may cause a genu recurvatum. Another consequence is toe walking with excessive load transfer to the metatarsophalangeal joints and a reduced stance phase of gait.
- Pronation in the subtalar joint is inhibited, potentially causing impingement between the medial malleolus and the talus, similar to the impingement in severe clubfoot deformity.
- Another consequence is the medialization of the navicular, which migrates toward the medial malleolus to cause additional bony impingement. Osteophytes often develop at the talar neck.
- In the case of a concomitant hindfoot equinus and subtalar joint compensation, the acquired varus stress in the subtalar joint frequently cannot be compensated by the ankle joint, leading to eventual varus talar tilt in the ankle mortise.

PATIENT HISTORY AND PHYSICAL FINDINGS

- A characteristic description of a patient with pes equinocavovarus can be found in the book by Tubby and Jones[24] for Charcot-Marie-Tooth (hereditary motor sensory neuropathy):
  - "The patient was a healthy-looking country-woman, aged fifty-six years, practically free from any disability from this condition. The patient stated that when about seven years old she found that her ankles, especially the right, easily 'turned in', and that consequently she often suffered from sprains. She was unaware that there was anything unusual about her hands. The muscles of the rest of the upper extremity and of the shoulder girdle did not appear to be in any way affected. In the lower extremity deformity was more advanced and unequally developed on either side. On the right the foot was hollowed and inverted, and also somewhat dropped. The tendon of the tibialis anticus stood out as a taut cord. The toes and ankle joint could be freely moved in all directions except that of eversion, owing to complete paralysis of the peronei muscles. In addition to pes cavus there was some equinovarus. The other muscles of the lower extremity were capable of causing powerful movements. The knee jerks could not be obtained."
  - "A man, aged thirty-one years, the third child of the above patient showed a marked club-foot on both sides, and the feet were inverted and dropped, but without any contracture of tendons. The power of dorsiflexion and of eversion was completely lost. The toes were in the characteristic position."

Dynamic Examination

- Problems during stance phase of the gait cycle
  - Initial contact with the toes (toe walking, hindfoot equinus, limited dorsiflexion)
  - Hyperextension of the knee (genu recurvatum due to equinus) and proximal compensatory mechanisms
  - Overload of the lateral border of the foot (varus deformity)
  - Instability in loading response of the gait cycle
  - Main load on the first and fifth metatarsal head, in some cases with ulceration
  - Limited roll-off movement due to reduced dorsiflexion in midstance
  - Internal rotation moment due to rolling off over the lateral border of the foot and the forefoot
  - Missing load bearing of the toe tips due to claw toe deformity

- Problems during swing phase of the gait cycle
  - Drop foot (weak extensor muscles, primarily the anterior tibial muscle) with foot clearance problems; this is aggravated by hindfoot equinus
  - Compensatory mechanisms for drop foot (eg, increased knee or hip flexion, circumduction of the leg)
  - Equinus foot at the end of the swing phase, which leads to forefoot initial contact
  - Overactivity of the long toe extensors to compensate for decreased dorsiflexion force with consecutive claw toe deformity

Methods for Examining the Equinocavovarus Foot Deformity

- In stance: medial view. The examiner inspects the medial aspect of the foot, evaluating for elevated heel, increased medial arch, plantarflexion of the first metatarsal bone, and claw toe deformity of the first column of the foot.
- In stance: lateral view. The examiner inspects the lateral aspect of the foot, evaluating for posterior shift of the lateral malleolus, convexity of the lateral border of the foot, prominent basis of the fifth metatarsal bone, and prominent head of the talus on the lateral dorsum of the foot.
- In stance: dorsal view. The examiner inspects the posterior aspect of the foot, evaluating for varus deformity of the heel, elevation of the heel, prominent lateral malleolus, pronation of the forefoot, and "hello big toe" sign (normally, the hallux cannot be seen from posterior view, but in case of forefoot adduction, it may be visible).
- In stance: plantar view. The examiner inspects the plantar aspect of the foot, evaluating for convex lateral border of the foot and prominent basis of the fifth metatarsal bone, increased weight bearing of the heads of the first and fifth metatarsal bones, increased skin wheal (in severe cases, the heads of all metatarsal bones are involved), and hindfoot equinus (lack of weight bearing on the heel).
- In stance: anterior view. The examiner inspects the ventral aspect of the foot, evaluating for lateral prominence of the talar head, convex lateral border of the foot, forefoot adduction, and clawing of the first through fifth toes.
- Coleman block.[3] With a block placed under the hindfoot and the second through fifth toes, the examiner tests the compensability of the hindfoot in fixed forefoot pronation and compensation of the plantarflexion of the first metatarsal bone.
- Silfverskiöld test.[20] Dorsiflexion is examined in knee flexion and knee extension. This test is important for detecting equinus deformity and differentiating between the involvement of gastrocnemius and soleus muscles.

- "Trying to assess actions of individual muscles is a trap for the unwary because muscle action is so much one of synergism and unassessable motive power that it becomes impossible to apportion with any accuracy the actions of single muscles."[6]

Problems Due to Footwear

- Ulcerations over the interphalangeal (IP) joints of the toes
- The foot is broad and short (problems wearing regular shoes).
- Wearing out of the lateral border of the shoes or the forefoot, respectively

Further Problems

- Cosmetically disturbing
- Rapid fatigue
- Progressive deformities

IMAGING AND OTHER DIAGNOSTIC STUDIES

Conventional Radiographs

- Lateral view (standing) **(FIG 2A)**
  - Posterior shift of the lateral malleolus
  - The longitudinal axis of the talus is parallel to the axis of the calcaneus.
  - The calcaneus seems to be shortened due to varus position.
  - There is decreased distance between the navicular and the medial malleolus.
  - The calcaneocuboid joint is visible; it is normally obscured by the talonavicular joint.
  - The first metatarsal is plantarflexed and its head has a plantar prominence.
  - Claw toes
  - The posterior subtalar joint is projected horizontally.
  - Opened sinus tarsi ("sinus tarsi window")
- Anteroposterior (AP) view (standing) **(FIG 2B)**
  - Longitudinal axes of the talus and calcaneus are parallel.
  - There is a medial shift of the talonavicular joint and, in some cases, the calcaneocuboid joint.
  - The first metatarsal seems to be shortened due to its plantarflexed position.
  - There is overlapping of the metatarsal bones, especially the fourth and fifth.
- AP view of the ankle joint (standing) **(FIG 2C)**
  - Varus deformity of the ankle joint
  - Hindfoot varus

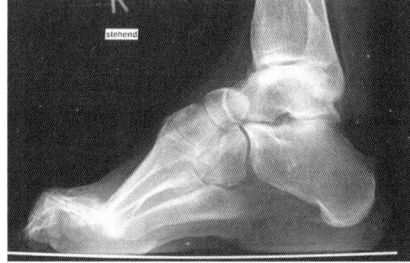
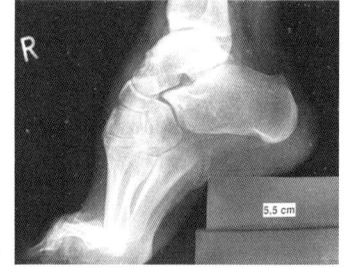

FIG 2 Conventional radiograph. **A,B.** Lateral view with and without correction of the forefoot equinus. *(continued)*

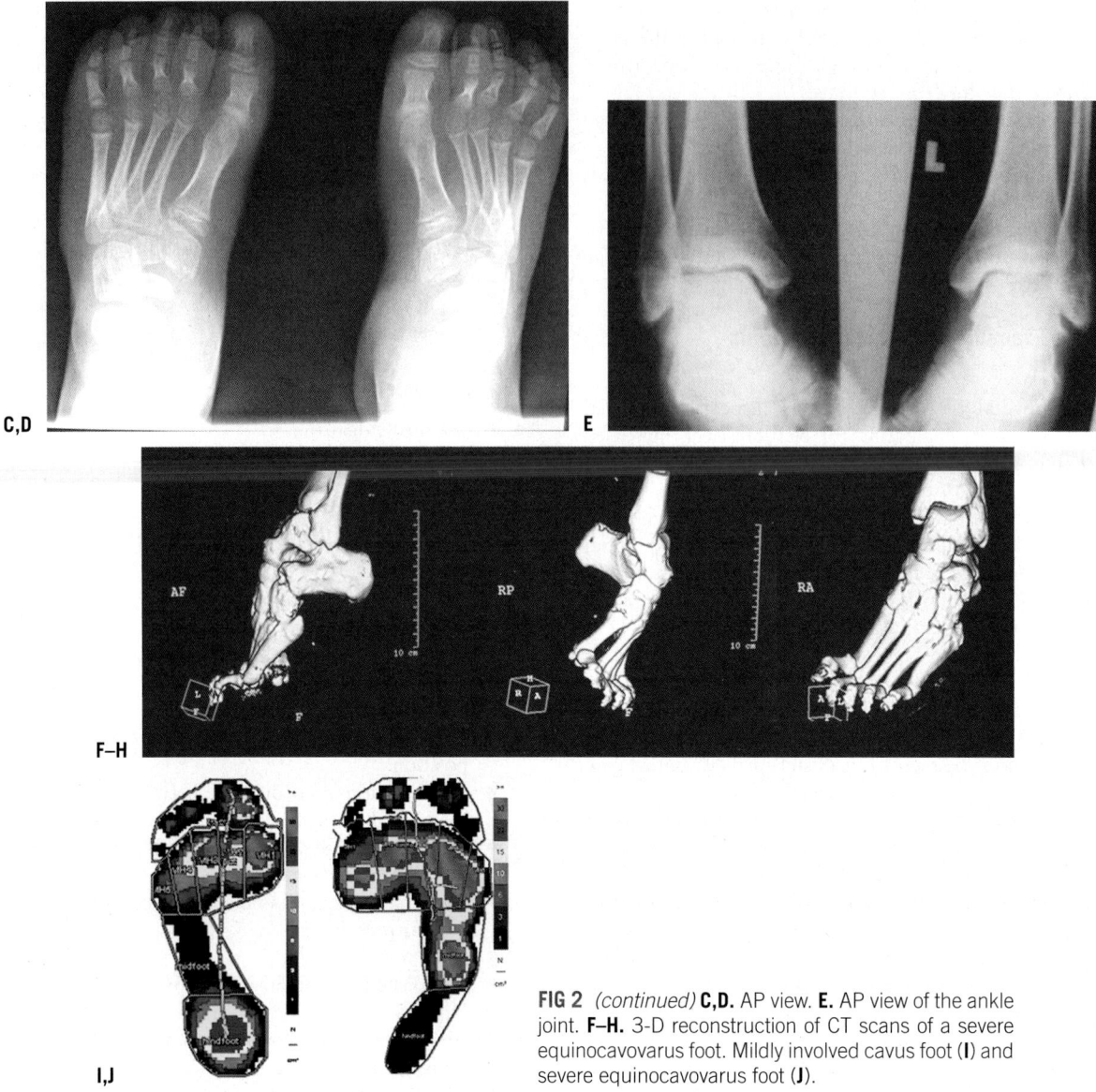

FIG 2 *(continued)* **C,D.** AP view. **E.** AP view of the ankle joint. **F–H.** 3-D reconstruction of CT scans of a severe equinocavovarus foot. Mildly involved cavus foot (**I**) and severe equinocavovarus foot (**J**).

Computed Tomography with Three-dimensional Reconstruction

- In severe cases, computed tomography (CT) imaging with three-dimensional (3-D) reconstruction may be needed (**FIG 2D**).

Dynamic Pedobarography

- An objective method to measure the pressure distribution pattern is the dynamic pedobarography EMED examination.
- It is used to identify the imbalance of the major pressure points of the foot due to the deformity.
- A mildly involved footprint is shown in comparison with the typical pattern for a severe equinocavovarus foot (**FIG 2E**).

Three-dimensional Foot and Gait Analysis (Heidelberg Foot Model)

- This objective and computer-assisted method records movements between single segments of the foot in all three planes (sagittal, frontal, transverse) during walking.

- The foot and shank are equipped at typical anatomic landmarks with 17 reflective markers (**FIG 3**).[16] Special cameras send and record reflected ultrared light while the patient walks over a defined distance.
- After processing by dedicated software, characteristic segment movements in all three planes can be visualized.

DIFFERENTIAL DIAGNOSIS

- Pes equinocavovarus can occur in different primary diseases:
  - Central nervous system
    - Progressive diseases
      - Increased muscle tone (eg, multiple sclerosis)
      - Reduced muscle tone (eg, tethered cord syndrome)
      - Diastematomyelia, syringomyelia, intraspinal tumor
    - Limited diseases
      - Increased muscle tone (cerebral palsy, traumatic brain injuries, stroke)
      - Reduced muscle tone (eg, spina bifida)
      - Lipoma, angioma
      - Encephalitis

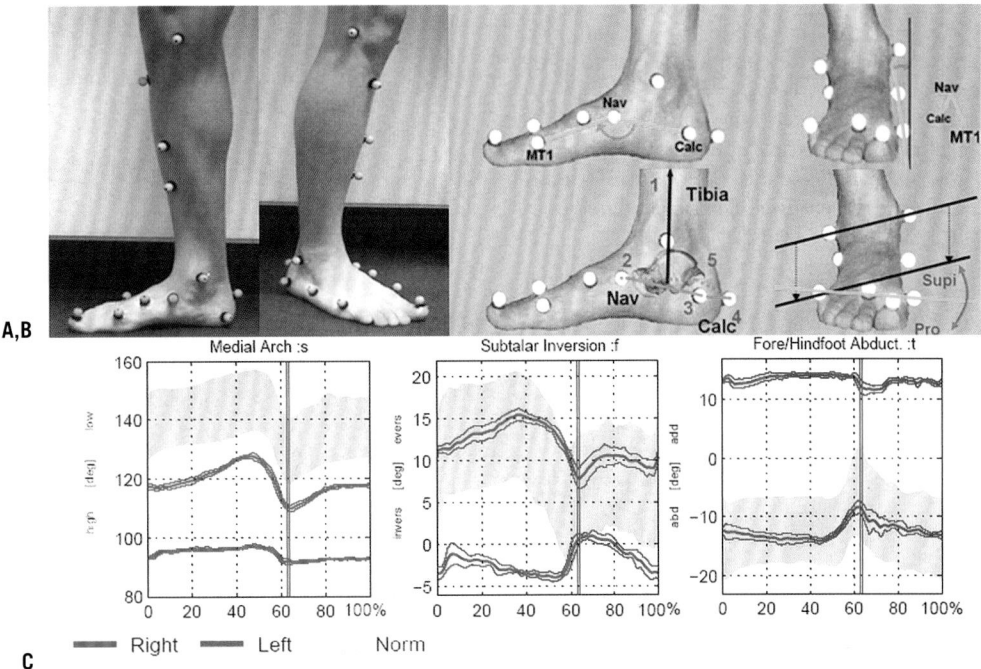

FIG 3 Heidelberg foot motion measurement. **A.** Marker placement and angle calculation. **B.** Examples of motions in different planes for an equinocavovarus foot. **C.** *Left*, increased medial arch; *middle*, increased subtalar inversion; *right*, increased forefoot adduction.

- Peripheral nervous system
  - Progressive diseases
    - Hereditary sensory motor neuropathy (Charcot-Marie-Tooth disease)
    - Spinal muscular atrophy
    - Polyneuropathy
  - Limited diseases
    - Poliomyelitis
    - Arthrogryposis multiplex congenita
- Other causes
  - Compartment syndrome
  - Burn injuries
  - Inflammatory arthritides
  - Diabetic neuropathy

NONOPERATIVE MANAGEMENT

- "Nonsurgical management of cavus, cavovarus, and calcaneocavus is uniformly unsuccessful in the long run."[22]
- "Nonoperative measures generally do not stop progression or prevent deformity, therefore their role is extremely limited."[17–19]
- Nonoperative treatment can only compensate for the functional problems in pes equinocavovarus; it cannot stop its progression.

- Possible nonoperative treatment methods are as follows:
  - Orthopaedic arch support (reduced head of the first metatarsal bone and smooth bedding)
  - Orthopaedic shoes

SURGICAL MANAGEMENT

Preoperative Planning

- "Muscle balance is the key to understanding the production of pes cavus."[12]
- "A foot will deform in the presence of a solid, well-performed triple arthrodesis when the foot is not in gross muscular balance . . . When definite muscular imbalance is evident, tendon transfer is mandatory."[10]
- Preoperative clinical examination, radiographs, EMED, dynamic foot analysis (instrumented foot gait analysis), and clinical examination (Silfverskiöld test[20]) under anesthesia represent optimal preoperative planning.

Positioning

- The patient is placed supine on the operating table. We routinely drape the iliac crest into the operative field when there may be a need for iliac crest bone harvest **(FIG 4)**.

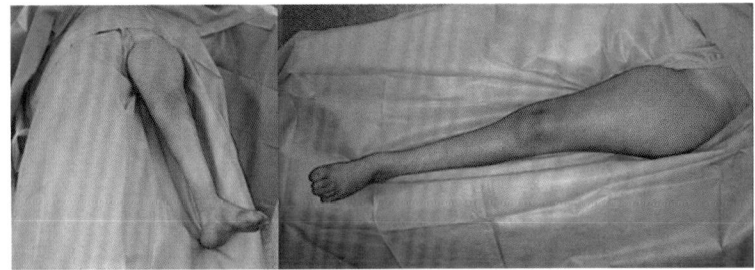

FIG 4 Positioning in the operating room.

Approach

- The different approaches that we consider in equinocavovarus deformity correction are shown in **FIG 5**.
  - Dorsal incision for the modified Jones procedure[4]
  - Lateral–dorsal incision for the triple or Lambrinudi arthrodesis[14] or the Cole procedure[1] and the posterior tibial tendon (PTT) transfer as well as the Russel-Hibbs procedure[8]
  - Ventral incision for the PTT transfer[21]
- Distal medial shank incision for the open Achilles tendon lengthening, the PTT transfer, and, if needed, the intramuscular lengthening of the long toe flexors
- Skin incision for the triple or Lambrinudi arthrodesis,[14] the Cole procedure,[1] and the PTT transfer; this incision can be connected with the previous one (distal medial shank) if needed
- Skin incision for the Steindler procedure[21]

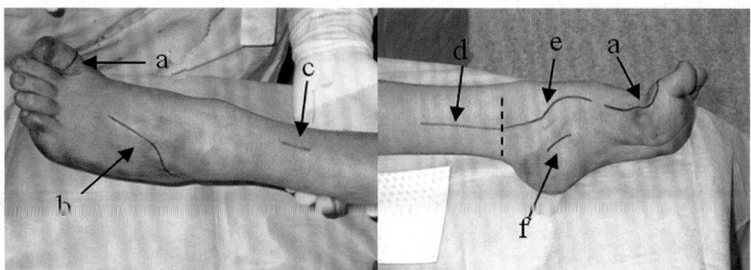

FIG 5 Approaches for foot deformity correction. (*a*) Dorsal incision for the modified Jones[13] procedure. (*b*) Lateral/dorsal incision for the triple/Lambrinudi arthrodesis[14] or the Cole procedure[1] and the PTT transfer as well as the Russel-Hibbs procedure.[8] (*c*) Ventral incision for the PTT transfer.[17–19] (*d*) Distal medial shank incision for the open Achilles tendon lengthening, the PTT transfer, and, if needed, the intramuscular lengthening of the long toe flexors. (*e*) Skin incision for the triple/Lambrinudi arthrodesis,[14] the Cole procedure,[1] and the PTT transfer; incision (*d,e*) can be connected if needed. (*f*) Skin incision for the Steindler[21] procedure.

OVERVIEW

- The first step is the Steindler procedure.[21] In mildly involved cases, it is possible to correct the cavus deformity with this procedure. In most cases, however, a total correction is not possible and this procedure is followed by bony correction of the cavus component.
- After the Steindler procedure, the tendon transfers are prepared (split posterior tibialis transfer,[21] modified Jones procedure[4]).
  - Important: Tendon transfers and Achilles tendon lengthening are only *prepared* at this point; they are eventually secured with suture during the final stages of the reconstruction.
- Next, we correct the clawed hallux (modified Jones procedure[4]).
  - Important: The tendon transfer of the extensor hallucis longus (EHL tendon) is sutured at the end of all procedures.
- Bony correction of the midfoot and hindfoot is performed next. Depending on the severity of deformity, an arthrodesis of the Chopart joint or triple arthrodesis may be required. In cases of dorsal impingement of the talus on the tibia with limited dorsiflexion or extreme hindfoot equinus, we recommend adding a modified Lambrinudi procedure.[14]
- In select cases, an extra-articular correction of the cavus (Cole procedure[1]) and the hindfoot varus (Dwyer osteotomy[5]) are indicated.
- To correct hindfoot equinus, an intramuscular lengthening of the calf muscles or an open or percutaneous Achilles tendon lengthening is carried out. In cases of severe equinus tested in knee flexion and extension, proximal or distal Achilles tendon lengthening (open or percutaneous) is considered. The choice of open or percutaneous lengthening depends on the surgeon's preference. A percutaneous Achilles tendon lengthening is more prone to overcorrection, whereas with an open technique, tension can be more easily controlled. In mildly involved cases, intramuscular calf muscle lengthening is done (eg, Baumann procedure).
- After correction of the hindfoot and midfoot, we typically reassess the forefoot. In the case of shortened long toe flexors (masked on initial examination by the equinus deformity), an intramuscular lengthening of the long digitorum and hallucis flexor (extensor digitorum longus [EDL] and EHL) tendons can be done through the same approach used for the open Achilles tendon lengthening.
- When satisfactory correction of first metatarsal plantarflexion is not possible with the modified Jones procedure alone, we routinely add a first metatarsal dorsiflexion osteotomy.[11]
- The final step before wound closure is securing all tendon transfers. We do not routinely use bone anchors, but instead, suture tendons directly to target other tendons or soft tissues at the site of desired transfer (EHL, tibialis posterior) and the lengthened Achilles tendon slips.

STEINDLER PROCEDURE (TRANSECTION OF THE PLANTAR APONEUROSIS)

- Although an important step is the correction of the equinocavovarus foot deformity, our experience is that it does not afford much correction if used in isolation. In our hands, this technique represents the first step in the treatment of pes equinocavovarus. It is a simple method for correcting flexible forefoot and midfoot cavus deformity.
- Make a slightly dorsal convex, 3- to 4-cm long incision at the medial border of the foot directly above the origin of the plantar aponeurosis at the calcaneus (TECH FIG 1).

- Carefully divide the subcutaneous tissue and retract it with Langenbeck retractors. Expose the origin of the plantar aponeurosis at the calcaneus as far proximally as possible. Sharply transect the aponeurosis as well as the origin of the short flexor digitorum muscle with the strong preparation scissors.
- It is important to stay directly at the bone and to feel for the peak of the scissors at the lateral border of the foot. After the transection, use a clamp to create the lengthening effect.

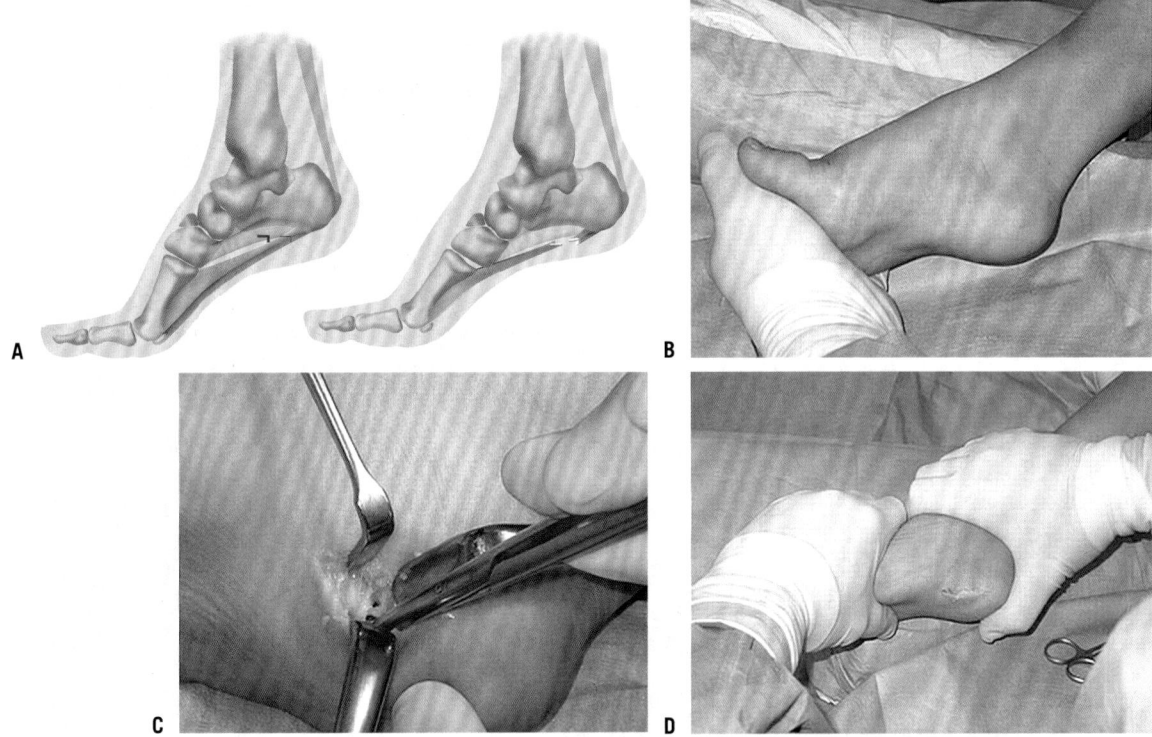

TECH FIG 1 A–D. Steindler procedure.

TOTAL SPLIT POSTERIOR TIBIAL TENDON TRANSFER (MODIFIED SPOTT)

- The purpose of the modified SPOTT[21] is the augmentation of the attenuated ankle dorsiflexor muscles that are often compromised by long-standing hindfoot equinus deformity. Furthermore, it eliminates the function of the posterior tibial muscle on the hindfoot position.
- Make a 3- to 4-cm incision over the insertion of the PTT at the navicular. After dividing the subcutaneous tissue, incise the flexor retinaculum and PTT sheath. Tension the tendon using an Overholt clamp and release it at its insertion point with the scalpel as distally as possible.
- Make another skin incision (3 cm) at the distal medial calf, three to four fingerbreadths proximally to the ankle, directly behind the posterior edge of the tibia.

- After dividing the subcutaneous tissue, incise the fascia and retract it with Langenbeck retractors. Identify and retract the tendon of the long toe flexor muscle (flexor hallucis longus [FHL] tendon). Immediately deep to the FHL tendon, identify the PTT. Expose it with an Overholt clamp and pull it out (TECH FIG 2).
- Bisect the tendon and tag both halves with atraumatic 1-0 Vicryl sutures.
- Make a third skin incision 3 cm in length on the lateral side of the shank on the same height directly ventrally to the fibular bone. Beneath the subcutaneous tissue, incise and retract the fascia.

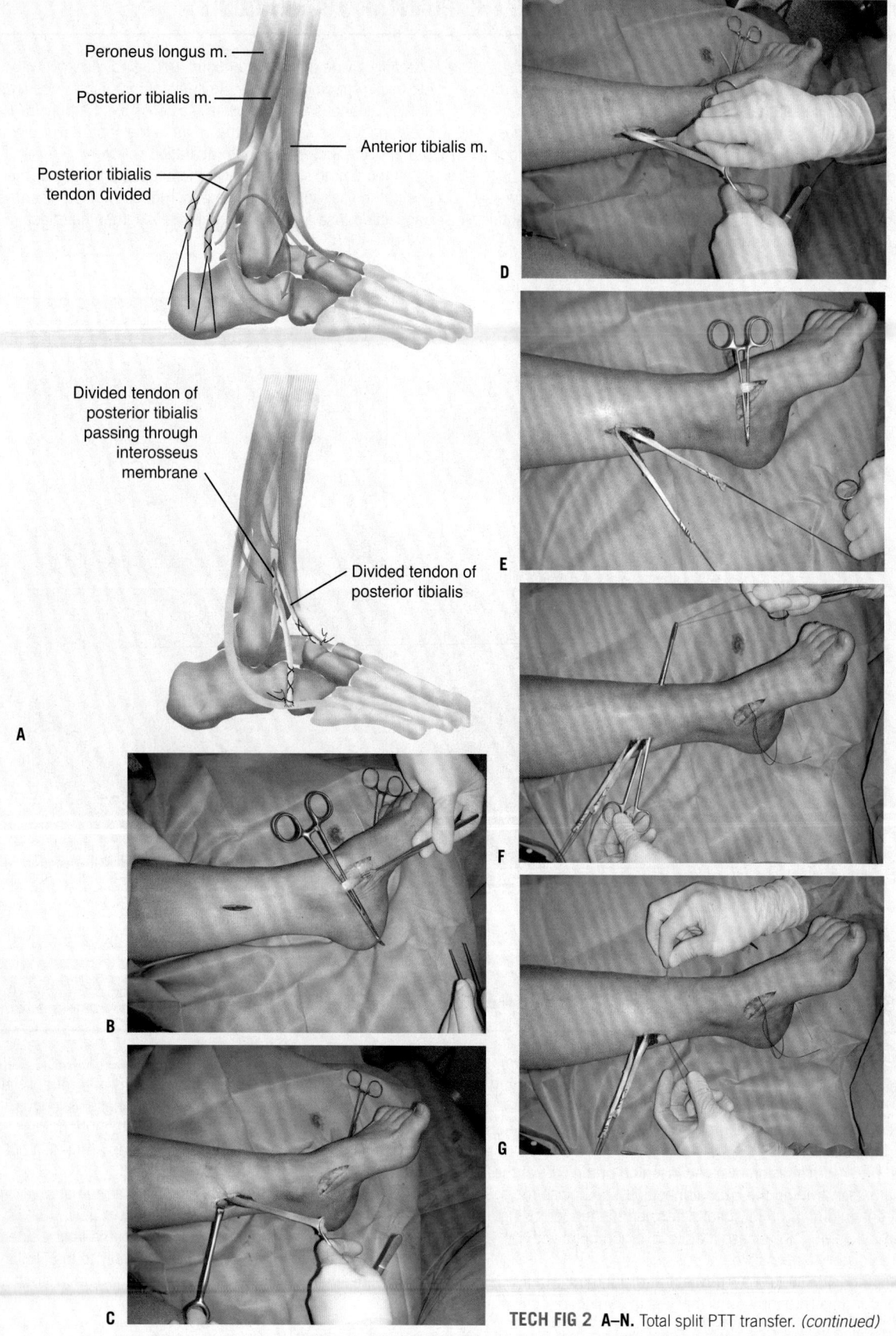

Peroneus longus m.

Posterior tibialis m.

Anterior tibialis m.

Posterior tibialis tendon divided

Divided tendon of posterior tibialis passing through interosseus membrane

Divided tendon of posterior tibialis

A

B

C

D

E

F

G

TECH FIG 2 **A–N.** Total split PTT transfer. *(continued)*

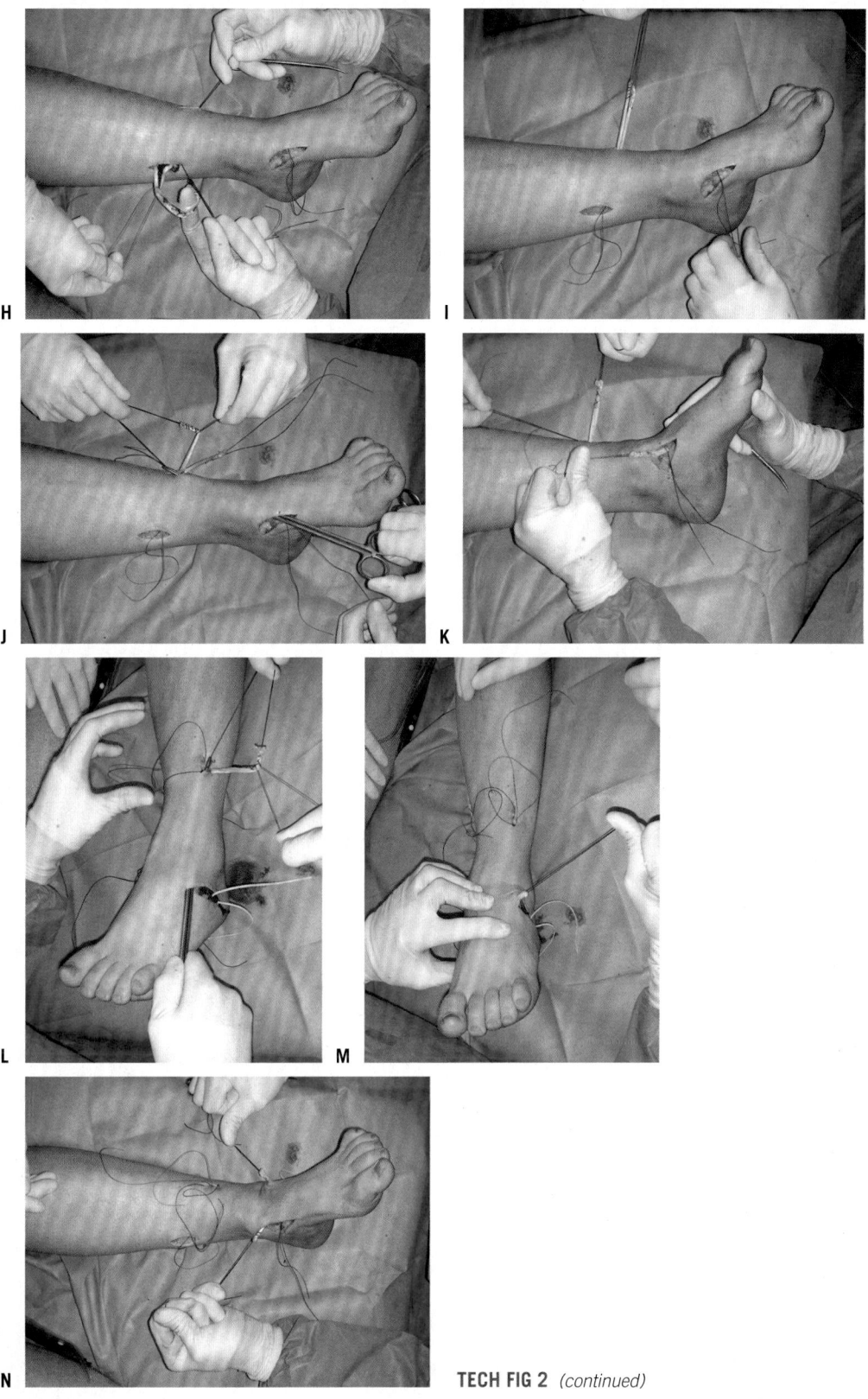

TECH FIG 2 *(continued)*

- Perform the following preparation of the interosseous membrane with caution because of the superficial peroneal nerve. Carefully direct a narrow forceps through the interosseous membrane from the medial wound to lateral wounds.
- Grab a single thread with the forceps and pull it through the medial wound. Capture the tag sutures of the two halves of the PTT in the loop. Transfer the split PTT to the lateral wound by pulling the end of the single thread.
- To maintain the ability to pull back the transferred tendons, loop another single thread around the tendons.
- Expose the anterior tibial tendon by making a 2- to 3-cm skin incision. When planning this incision, take into consideration the possible need for an arthrodesis of the talonavicular joint. If it is needed, the incision should be in line with the previous incision made to expose the PTT.
- After dissecting the subcutaneous tissue, incise the sheath of the anterior tibial tendon and pass the forceps through its

sheath to the extensor compartment, where the two halves of the PTT were transferred before.
- There, grab the tagged suture of one-half and transfer it distally. For the transfer of the second half of the tendon, make an additional skin incision on the dorsal foot.
- Expose the tendons of the long toe extensors (EDL) and incise their sheath. The same technique is used for the distal transfer of the other half of the PTT. Perform any other concomitant procedures now, before securing the tendon transfers.
- At the end of the operation, suture the medial half of the PTT to the anterior tibial tendon and suture the lateral half to the peroneus brevis tendon, which is previously exposed.
- When tensioning the tendon transfers, we routinely position the ankle in neutral and avoid not only undercorrection but also overcorrection of the foot.
- After suturing the transfers, the foot should rest in the corrected position. Therefore, hindfoot equinus must be corrected before suturing the tendon transfers.

MODIFIED JONES PROCEDURE (ROBERT JONES, 1916)

- The purpose of the modified Jones procedure[4] is to eliminate the overactive EHL muscle and to correct the clawed hallux.

Exposure

- Make an S-shaped skin incision from the proximal first metatarsal to the first IP joint.
- After careful soft tissue dissection and protection of the dorsomedial sensory nerve to the hallux, tag the EHL tendon distally with a 0 Vicryl suture.

- Release the tendon as far distally as possible and perform an arthrotomy of the first IP joint **(TECH FIG 3)**.

Hallux Interphalangeal Joint Arthrodesis

- We use a rongeur to remove cartilage at the hallux IP joint **(TECH FIG 4A–C)**.
- We then place two crossing Kirschner wires (1.4 mm for children, 1.8 mm for adults) through the distal fragment, antegrade from proximal to distal.

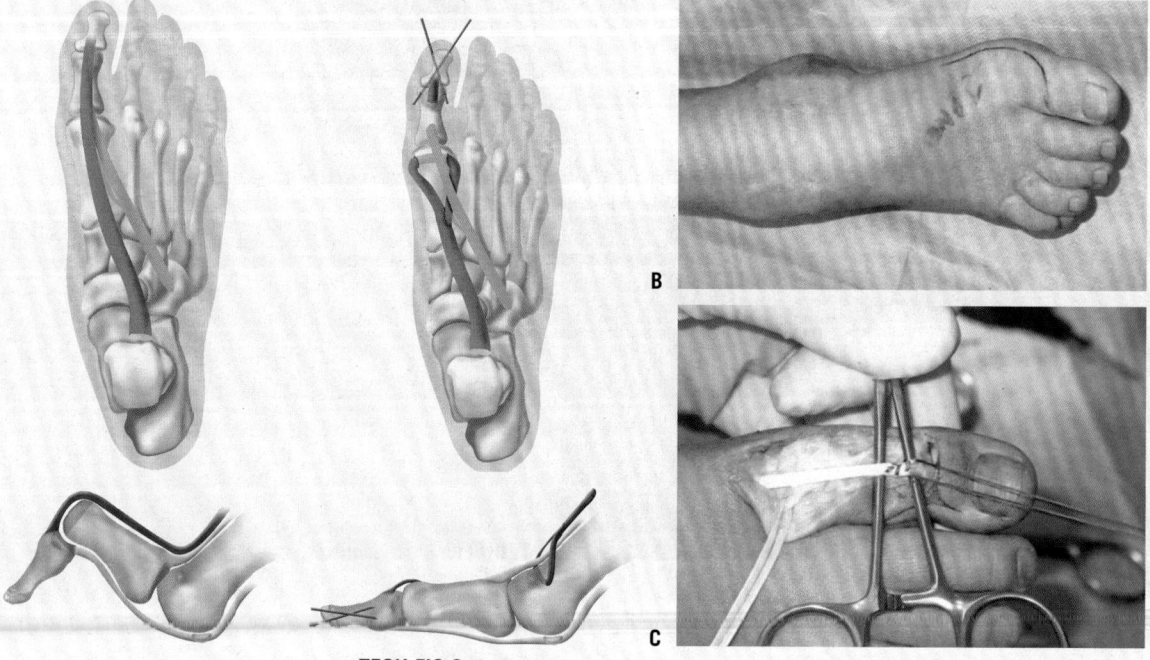

TECH FIG 3 A–C. Modified Jones procedure.

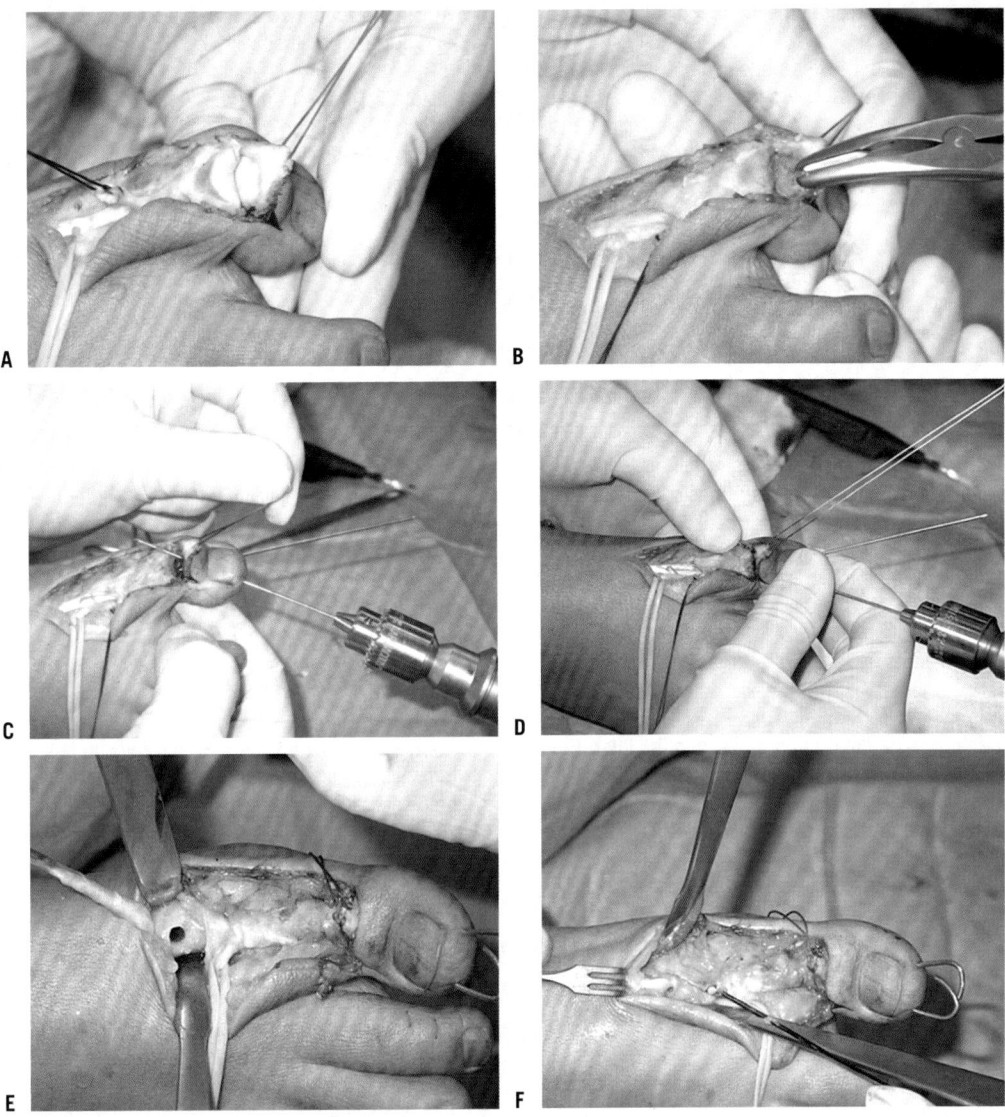

TECH FIG 4 A–F. Modified Jones procedure.

- Using the wire driver on the distal aspect of the wires, retract the Kirschner wires from the IP joint arthrodesis site, reduce the IP joint, and advance the Kirschner wires retrograde across the IP arthrodesis site **(TECH FIG 4D–F)**.
- Avoid excessive IP joint extension because it may lead to problems with shoe wear.
- Confirm proper toe rotation after placing the first wire and then advance the second wire.
- We routinely use two Kirschner wires for fixation; however, the combination of one longitudinal screw and a derotational Kirschner wire is a reasonable alternative. We caution against using only a single screw because this fixation may prove rotationally unstable.

Extensor Hallucis Longus Tendon Transfer (with or without Dorsiflexion Osteotomy of the First Metatarsal)

- Expose the first metatarsal to the proximal third of its shaft. If the plantarflexion of the first metatarsal bone cannot be corrected by soft tissue correction alone, a dorsiflexion osteotomy of the first metatarsal must be performed. (The technique will be described in greater detail later.)
- Extend the approach a few more centimeters proximally.
- Perform the dorsiflexion osteotomy with an oscillating saw, removing a dorsal wedge of bone in the proximal third of the metatarsal and leaving the plantar cortex intact.

- Secure it with Kirschner wires, a small dorsal plate, or a screw and tension band technique.
- For the EHL tendon transfer, use a periosteal elevator to expose the bone at the first metatarsal head–neck junction.
- Place two Hohmann retractors to protect the soft tissues and drill a hole centrally in the first metatarsal bone with sequentially larger diameter drill bits: first, 2.0 mm; then, 2.7 mm; followed by 3.2 mm.

- Advance the tagged EHL tendon through the hole with a needle and suture it to itself with 1-0 Vicryl.
- If the hallux tends to plantarflex after the tendon transfer, the distal end of the transferred EHL tendon or its suture tags may be reattached to the periosteum of the distal phalanx as a tenodesis to avoid undesirable postoperative flexion of the first toe.

FUSION OF THE CHOPART JOINT, TRIPLE FUSION (HOKE, 1921), AND LAMBRINUDI FUSION (LAMBRINUDI, 1927)

- Fixed hindfoot cavus deformity may warrant talonavicular and calcaneocuboid joint (Chopart joint) arthrodesis. However, when the deformity is isolated to a fixed, plantarflexed first ray, a dorsiflexion first metatarsal osteotomy may be adequate. Likewise, global cavus of the entire forefoot may be effectively treated with a dorsiflexion midfoot osteotomy (Cole procedure).
- In select cases of flexible hindfoot varus, a Dwyer lateral closing wedge calcaneal osteotomy (see in the following text) may be performed in lieu of hindfoot arthrodesis.
- The lateral approach is performed with an S-shaped skin incision, beginning 2 cm distally and dorsally to the lateral malleolus, proceeding in an arch shape to the navicular, distally to the palpable talar head.
- Expose the sural nerve in the proximal wound edge with its accompanying vessels and retract it.
- The preparation leads to the peroneal tendon sheath and the origin of the extensor digitorum brevis (EDB) muscle at the anterior processes of the calcaneus.
- With an L-shaped incision, release the EDB. Using a concave chisel, detach its origin from the anterior processes of the calcaneus bone. Expose the calcaneocuboid joint by inserting a Vierstein retractor.
- Use an additional Vierstein retractor to expose the talonavicular joint.
- The hindfoot arthrodesis may be performed with preservation of the subchondral bone architecture or as a corrective wedge resection. If cavus was not corrected by the Steindler procedure, a dorsally based wedge must be taken from the Chopart joint.
- With extreme forefoot and midfoot adduction, the dorsal wedge resection may need to include an additional lateral-based wedge resection.
- The more conservative arthrodesis that maintains subchondral bone architecture of the joints is reserved for mild to moderate deformity. Remove the cartilage and penetrate the subchondral bone with a chisel or drill to promote fusion.
- If a wedge resection is required to correct the deformity, we prefer to use an oscillating saw.
- After the complete release of the Chopart joint, the cavus foot can be manually corrected and the navicular centered on the talar head.
- We routinely stabilize the reduced joints with Kirschner wires (two through the talonavicular joint, two through the calcaneocuboid joint). Alternatively, the fixation can be done with screws.

- If a satisfactory deformity correction is not possible by Chopart arthrodesis, especially with severe hindfoot varus, the hindfoot arthrodesis must be extended to the subtalar joint to complete the triple arthrodesis (Hoke[9]).
- In severe deformity, a laterally based wedge can be removed from the subtalar joint. Dorsal impingement of the talus on the tibia, in cases with limited ankle dorsiflexion or extreme hindfoot equinus, may warrant a modified Lambrinudi procedure.[7,14]
- For both the triple arthrodesis and modified Lambrinudi procedure, the sinus tarsi is freed from all soft tissue structures (interosseous ligaments and fat). The most important structure to be dissected is the interosseous ligament between the talus and calcaneus. To expose the subtalar joint, use a lamina spreader in the subtalar joint and place a Vierstein retractor below the apex of the lateral malleolus.
- Prepare the surfaces at the arthrodesis site with a concave chisel or with the oscillating saw, depending on the amount of correction needed.
- A severe hindfoot varus is corrected by removing a lateral-based wedge from the subtalar joint (**TECH FIG 5**). If a Lambrinudi fusion is needed, a dorsally based wedge is taken out of the subtalar joint.
- The determination of the osteotomy lines is important for the size of the remaining bone. The first osteotomy runs parallel to the ankle joint line and through the talar head. It should not take more than 50% of the talus head.
- The osteotomy ends dorsally in the posterior edge of the subtalar joint. The second osteotomy runs parallel to the subtalar joint line and through the calcaneal bone. Both osteotomies unite in the posterior edge of the subtalar joint, forming a dorsally based wedge with its apex in the posterior aspect of the subtalar joint.
- After resecting the cartilage or the bony wedge, assess the effect of correction by the reposition of the talocalcaneal and the Chopart joint. In addition to the correction of the cavus hindfoot varus components, it is very important that the foot can be repositioned in a plantigrade position.
- The osteosynthesis can be done with six Kirschner wires (2.2 to 2.5 mm, two for the talonavicular joint, two for the calcaneocuboid joint, and two for the subtalar joint). Alternatively, the fixation may be performed with screws or a locking plate.

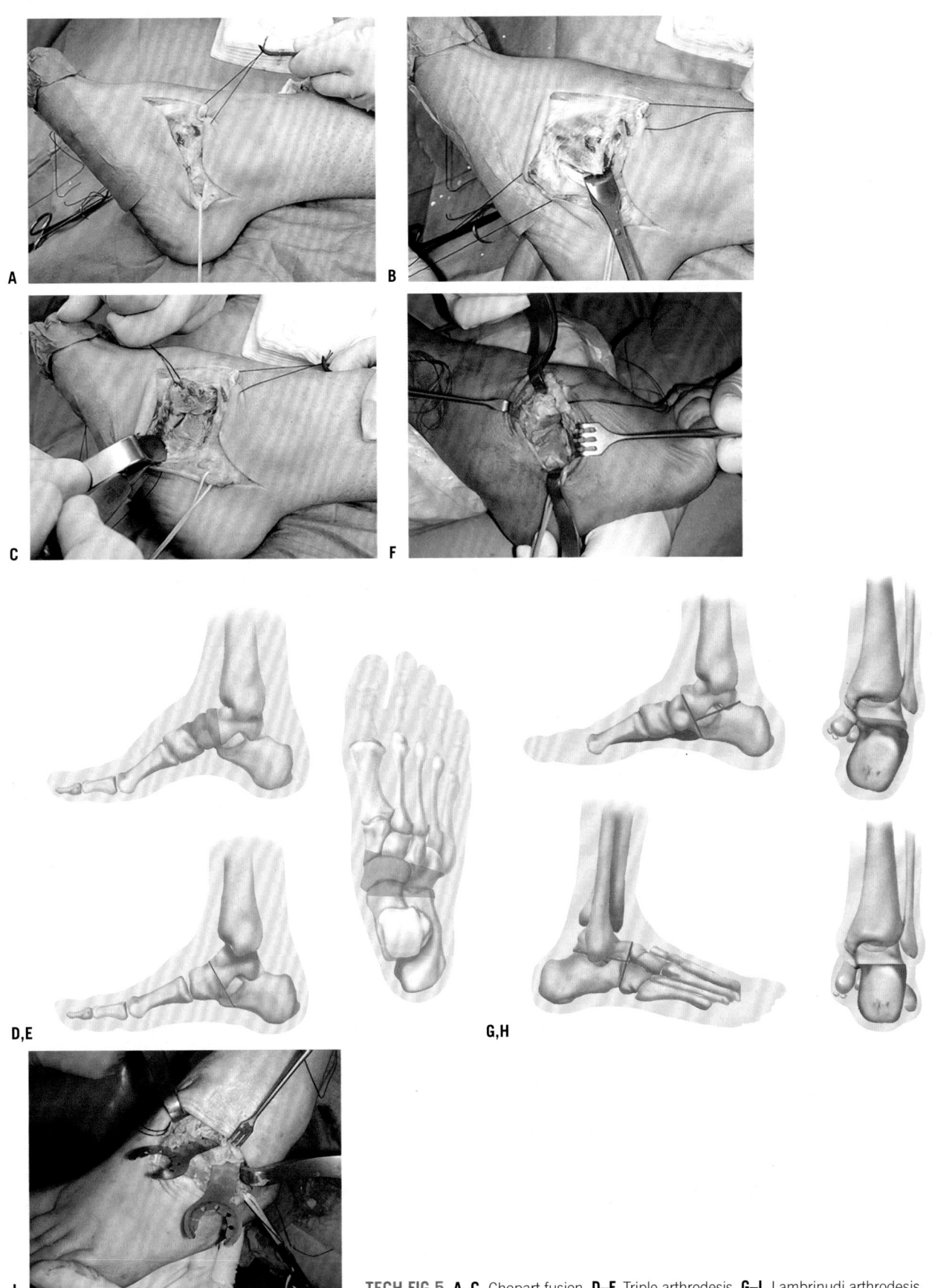

TECH FIG 5 **A–C.** Chopart fusion. **D–F.** Triple arthrodesis. **G–I.** Lambrinudi arthrodesis.

COLE OSTEOTOMY

- The Cole osteotomy[1] is used for bony correction of cavus deformity when the talonavicular and calcaneocuboid joints can be reduced. A dorsally based wedge is removed from the navicular–cuneiform joints and the cuboid.
- We perform this procedure through a lazy S incision at the lateral midfoot. Expose the sural nerve in the subcutaneous tissue and retract it.
- Make an incision between the sheath of the peroneal tendons and the EDB to expose the cuboid. Perform the osteotomies with an oscillating saw or osteotome.

- The distal osteotomy should be driven exactly through the cuneiforms and the cuboid; the proximal osteotomy runs through the cuboid and navicular. At least 0.5 cm of bone must be preserved between the proximal osteotomy and the talonavicular joint.
- These osteotomies converge on the plantar aspect of the midfoot. Remove a dorsal-based bony wedge **(TECH FIG 6)**.
- After the resection, the osteotomy can be closed and fixed with two to four Kirschner wires (talonavicular and calcaneocuboid joint, Chopart fusion). Alternatively, screws or locking plates can be used.

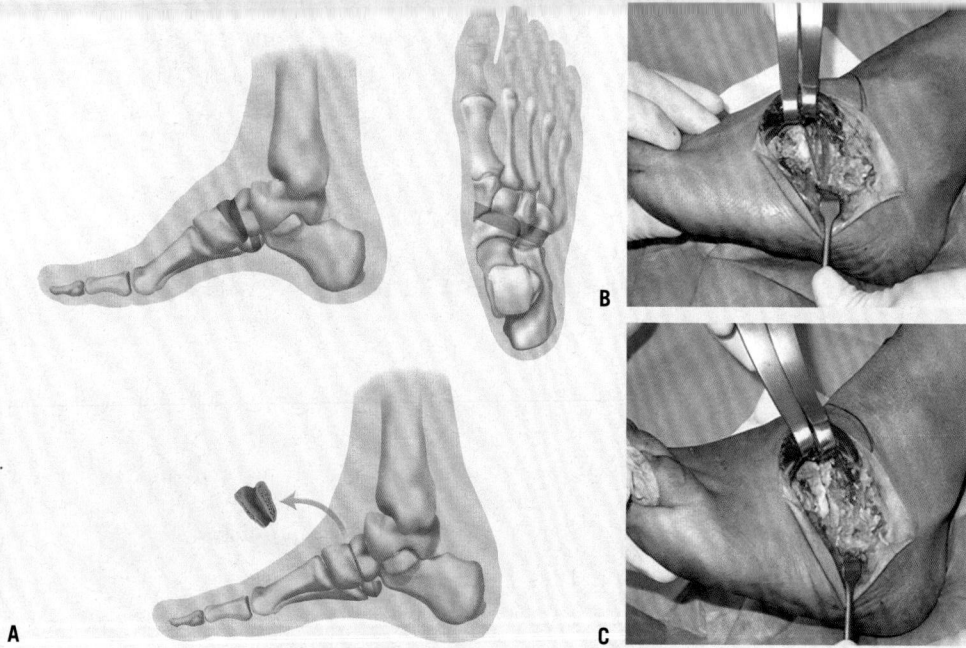

TECH FIG 6 A–C. Cole procedure.

DWYER OSTEOTOMY

- The Dwyer osteotomy[5] is used for bony correction of hindfoot varus deformity, when subtalar joint fusion is not indicated, the hindfoot cannot be completely reduced, and a correction of the hindfoot varus cannot be achieved by tendon transfer alone.
- Make a skin incision (about 5 cm) at the lateral border of the hindfoot above the peroneal tendons, vertical to the longitudinal axis of the calcaneus. Expose the sural nerve in the subcutaneous tissue and retract it.
- Expose the neck of the calcaneus subperiosteally by two Hohmann retractors.

- A laterally based bony wedge may be resected from the calcaneal neck with the oscillating bone saw if greater correction is required **(TECH FIG 7)**.
- Avoid overpenetration of the medial calcaneal cortex with the saw blade, which may injure the medial neurovascular bundle.
- The osteotomy can be opened with a straight chisel. The osteotomy is then closed holding the hindfoot into slight valgus position.
- Use two crossing Kirschner wires inserted from posterior for transfixion.

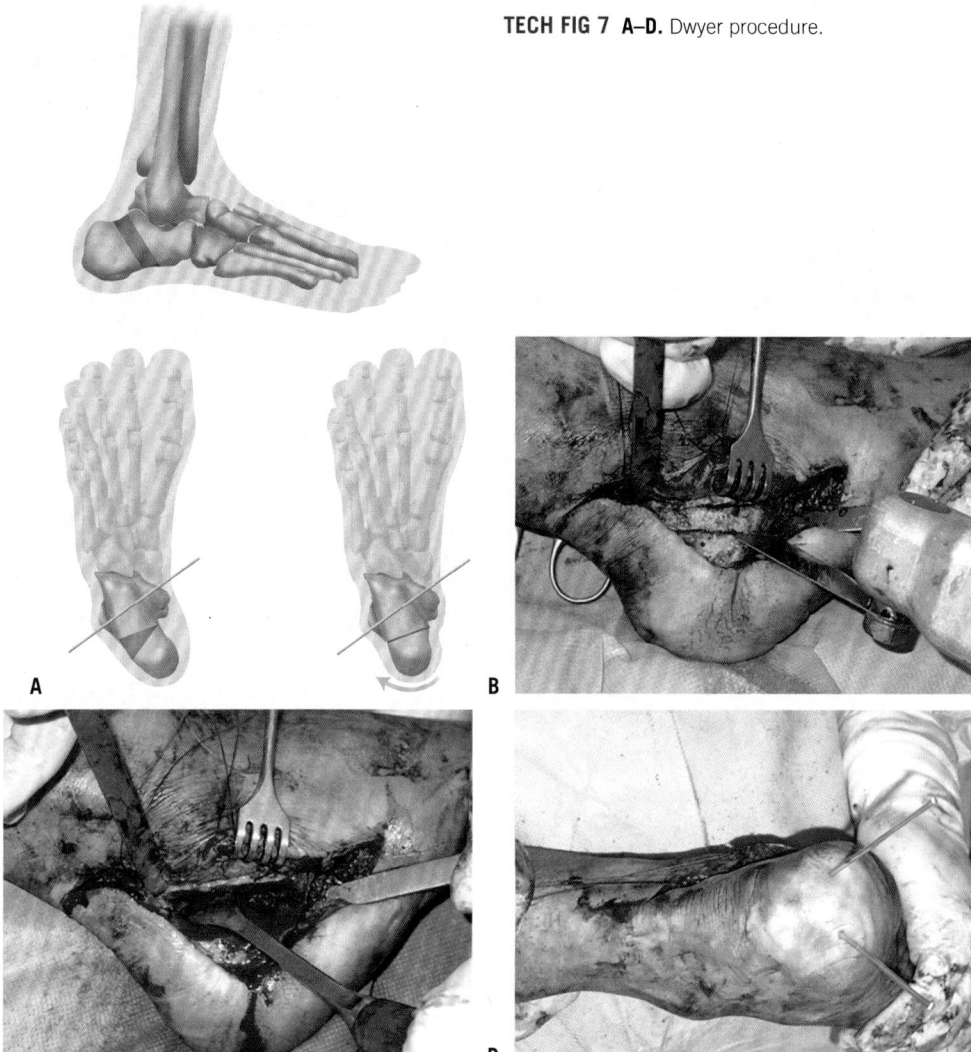

TECH FIG 7 A–D. Dwyer procedure.

SOFT TISSUE CORRECTION OF HINDFOOT EQUINUS
(BAUMANN PROCEDURE, ACHILLES TENDON LENGTHENING)

- Achilles tendon lengthening is done when both calf muscles are shortened and the equinus is severe and fixed. In case of a flexible and mild equinus, intramuscular recession (Baumann technique) is done.
- The approach for an open Achilles tendon lengthening is done through a 6- to 10-cm skin incision made at the medial distal calf, about 3 to 4 cm above the ankle joint, running proximally. The length of the skin incision varies with the amount of Achilles tendon lengthening needed for equinus correction.
- After identifying and retracting the saphenous nerve and vein, expose the fascia and incise and divide it proximally and distally. Beneath the fascia, identify the Achilles tendon and elevate it with two Langenbeck hooks, inserted under the tendon proximally and distally.
- Perform the Z-lengthening with a small scalpel over the entire tendon **(TECH FIG 8A–C)**.

- In hindfoot varus deformity, we prefer to preserve the lateral half of the tendon distally. Do not dissect the underlying muscle tissue.
- Tag both tendon slips with 1-0 Vicryl sutures.
- The ankle joint can now be reduced to 10 to 20 degrees of dorsiflexion, so that both tendon slips slide apart. With the ankle joint in neutral position, suture together both tendon slips with atraumatic 1-0 Vicryl suture.
- For the Baumann procedure, make a 4- to 5-cm skin incision in the medial aspect of the proximal third of the calf. Expose and incise the fascia after tagging it with two sutures.
- Open the interval between the gastrocnemius and the soleus muscle and insert two broad Langenbeck retractors.
- Perform an intramuscular recession of the aponeurosis of the gastrocnemius, soleus, or both **(TECH FIG 8D–H)** based on an intraoperative Silfverskiöld test.
- After recession, the ankle can be redressed. The aponeurosis will slide apart.

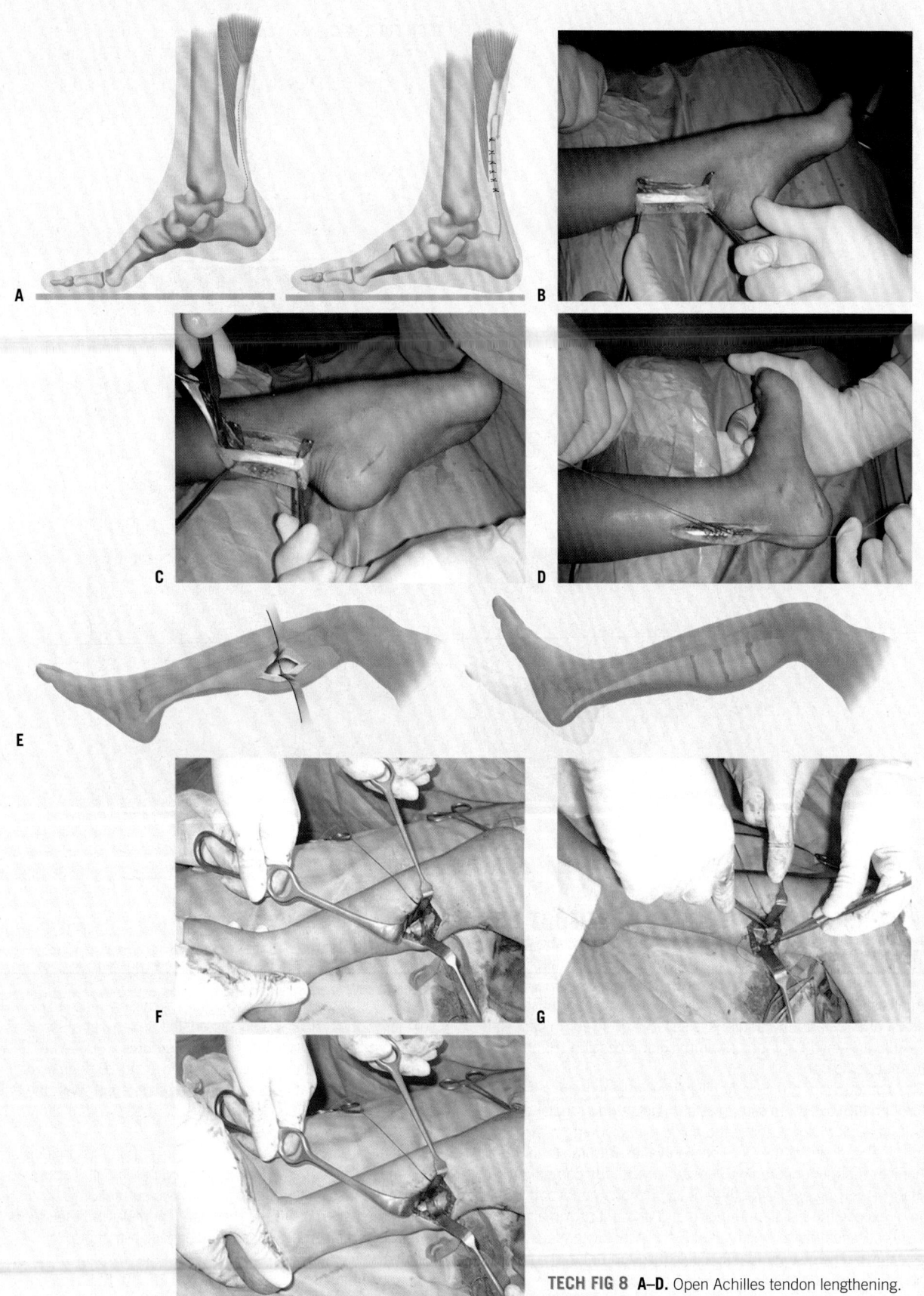

TECH FIG 8 A–D. Open Achilles tendon lengthening.
E–H. Baumann procedure.

DORSIFLEXION FIRST METATARSAL OSTEOTOMY (A. H. TUBBY, 1912)

- The dorsiflexsion first metatarsal osteotomy (Tubby[23]) is one of the final steps in the surgical correction of pes equinocavovarus. It is warranted when fixed plantarflexion of the first metatarsal fails to correct with the modified Jones procedure alone.
- The approach is easily done by lengthening the incision for the Jones procedure proximally to the first metatarsal base.
- Sharply incise the periosteum over the dorsal first metatarsal lengthwise approaching the first tarsometatarsal joint, protecting the soft tissues with two Hohmann retractors.
- Perform the proximal limb of the osteotomy with an oscillating saw, vertical to the first metatarsal, about 0.5 cm distal to the first tarsometatarsal joint in adults and the growth plate

in children. It is important to keep the plantar cortex intact to control rotation error.

- The distal osteotomy converges with the first osteotomy at the plantar cortex, creating a dorsal wedge **(TECH FIG 9A)**.
- The width of the dorsal wedge is determined by the planned correction; in our experience, bone resection of 2 to 3 mm is appropriate.
- Close the osteotomy with plantar pressure on the head of the first metatarsal **(TECH FIG 9B)**.
- We routinely secure the osteotomy with two crossing Kirschner wires **(TECH FIG 9C)**. Alternatively, a dorsal locking plate or screw and tension band technique may be used to stabilize the osteotomy.

TECH FIG 9 A–D. Extension osteotomy of the first metatarsal bone.

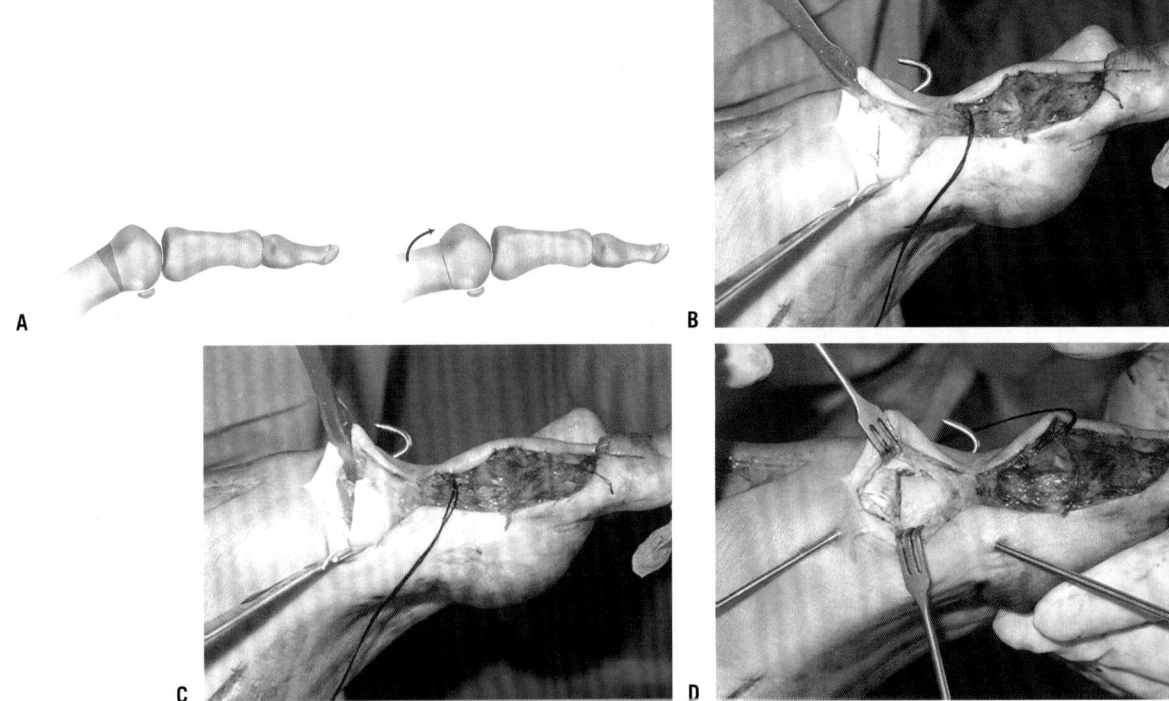

A   B   C   D

RUSSEL-HIBBS PROCEDURE (1919)

- The Russell-Hibbs procedure[8] corrects claw toes secondary to overactivity of the extrinsic (long extensor and flexor digitorum muscles) relative to the intrinsic muscle groups.
- We use a convex lateral 4-cm incision over the fourth metatarsal. Identify and retract the superficial peroneal nerve.
- Expose the EDL tendons of the second through fourth toes and tag them together proximally and distally **(TECH FIG 10)** with atraumatic 1-0 Vicryl sutures.
- Cut the tendons between the two sutures.

- Dissect the EDB muscle carefully and expose the underlying bone.
- In children, the proximal endings of the tendons can be sutured to the periosteum. The foot should come into neutral position spontaneously after the suture.
- In adults, a tendon anchor is secured to the underlying bone (intermediate cuneiform body) and the tendons are secured to the anchor. The distal part of the tagged tendons should also be sutured to periosteum or the anchor to create a distal tenodesis.

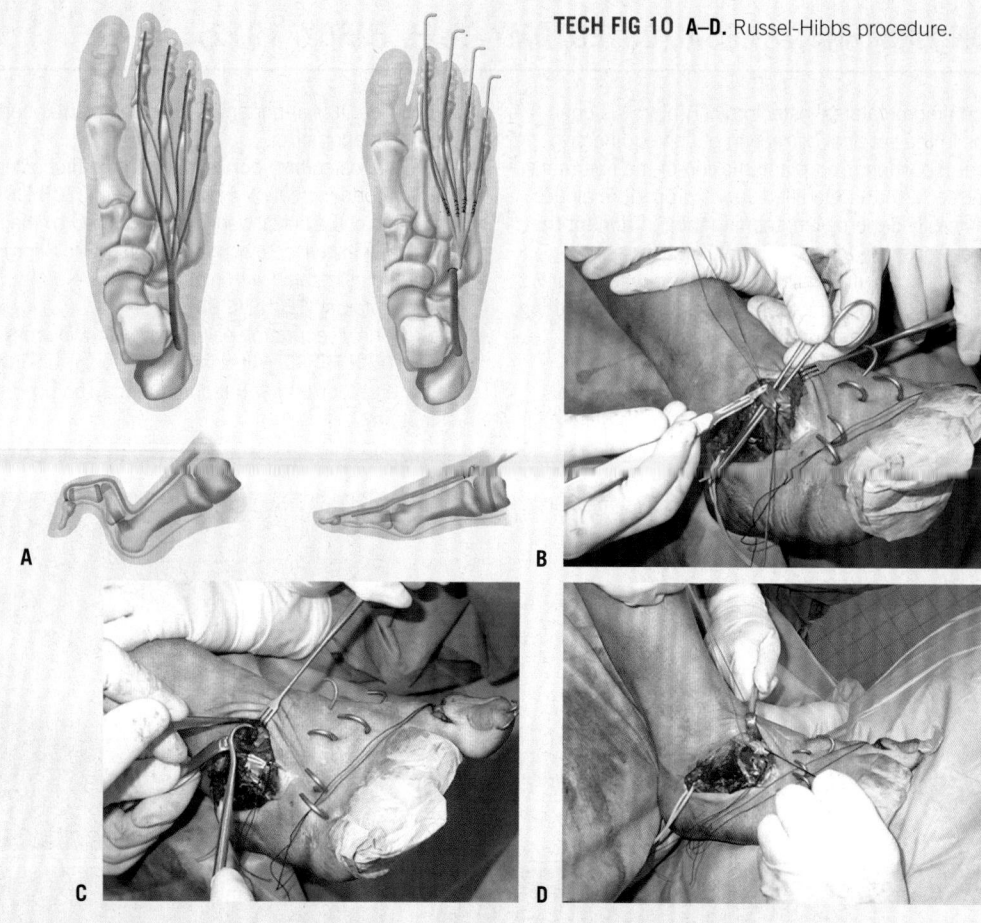

TECH FIG 10 A–D. Russel-Hibbs procedure.

WOUND CLOSURE

- Tendon transfers and lengthened Achilles tendon are sutured with atraumatic 1-0 Vicryl. All wounds are closed in layers.
- At the calf, the fascial incisions are sutured with 0 Vicryl.
- If removed, the anterior processes of the calcaneus are reattached with 1-0 Vicryl.

- Afterward, the subcutaneous tissue is closed (2-0 Vicryl).
- We routinely use a simple suture technique (and occasionally, the Allgöwer-Donati technique) for skin closure on the foot (3-0 Ethilon) and we use an intracutaneous technique for skin closure on the calf.

TECHNIQUES

Pearls and Pitfalls

Indications	• A detailed clinical examination is the basis for the correct indication and a good outcome. Concomitant deformities should be considered when planning the treatment.
Order of Procedures	• Begin with soft tissue procedures before performing bony procedures. This may decrease the extent of bony wedge resection. Sutures of soft tissue procedures are done after the bony correction.
Joint Fusion	• Ensure that all cartilage is removed from the resection areas to avoid nonfusion.
Overcorrection	• Avoid overcorrection; start with small wedges and extend the resection if needed.
Wound Closure Problems	• In severe cases that demand significant correction, skin closure can be difficult. This should be considered before performing skin incisions. The problem often can be solved with S-shaped incisions.

POSTOPERATIVE CARE

- In the operating room, we apply a short-leg cast with the ankle in neutral ankle position and the hindfoot in slight eversion.
- On postoperative day 1, we routinely obtain a radiograph and change the plaster cast.
- With bony procedures, weight bearing is restricted for 6 and 4 weeks for adults and children, respectively. At the subsequent follow-up, new radiographs are obtained; the Kirschner wires are removed; and a short-leg, weight-bearing plaster cast is applied for an additional 6 weeks and 4 weeks for adults and children, respectively.
- In contrast, without bony procedures, the weight-bearing plaster cast is applied immediately after the operation for 6 (adults) or 4 (children) weeks.
- The stitches are removed 14 days postoperatively, when we perform a routine cast change. After the removal of the final plaster cast, we advise our patients to use a brace for 6 months to a year, depending on the severity of deformity and correction required.

OUTCOMES

- References concerning long-term outcomes after complex foot reconstruction surgery in pes equinocavovarus are rare. Controlled outcome studies, based on clinical, radiographic, and functional data (3-D foot analysis, EMED), are needed.

Case 1

- This 16-year-old patient with tethered cord syndrome and myelolysis suffered from a painful equinocavovarus foot on the right side with hindfoot varus and equinus, cavus deformity, plantarflexion of the first metatarsal, and claw toes **(FIG 6A–I)**.

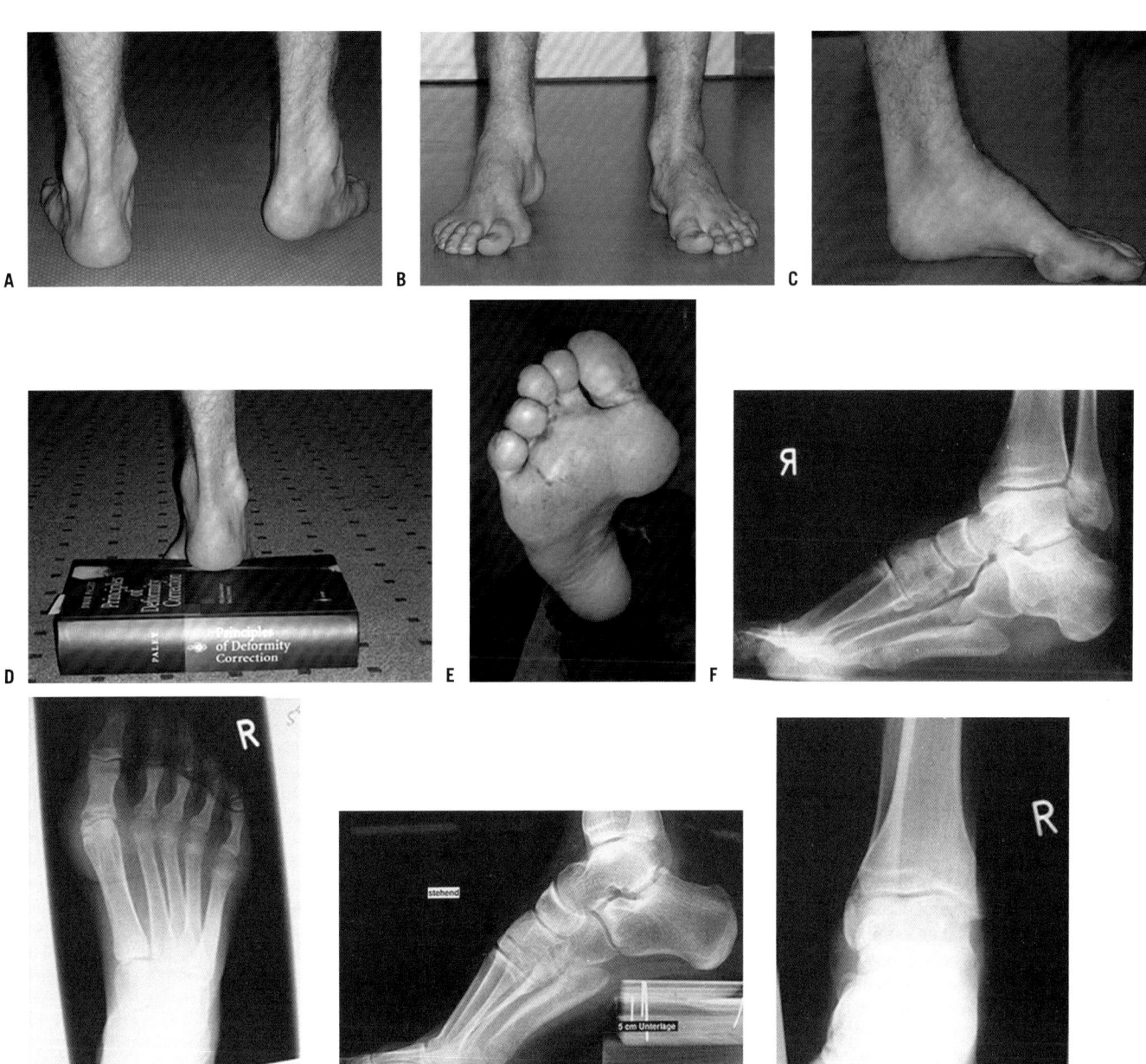

FIG 6 A–I. Preoperative clinical and radiographic findings of a 16-year-old patient with tethered cord syndrome, myelolysis, and an equinocavovarus foot deformity on the right side. *(continued)*

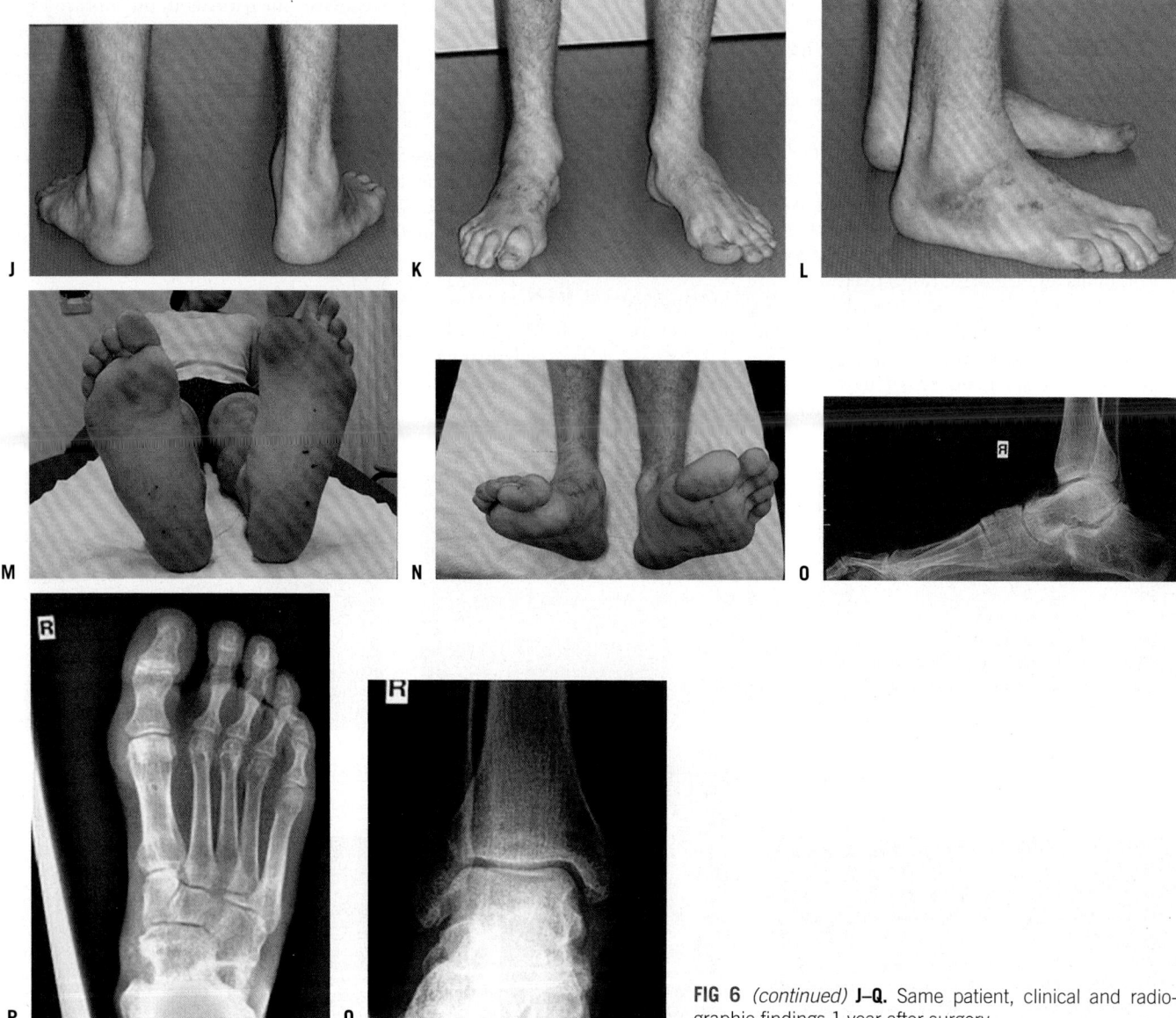

FIG 6 *(continued)* **J–Q.** Same patient, clinical and radiographic findings 1 year after surgery.

- He was treated with a Steindler procedure, a Jones procedure, a PTT transfer, a Chopart fusion, an Achilles tendon lengthening, and a dorsiflexion first metatarsal osteotomy. The postoperative results are shown in **FIG 6J–Q.**
- After his foot deformity correction, he is now able to work as a roof tiler without functional limitations or pain.

Case 2

- A 32-year-old man with severe equinocavovarus had his major problems combined forefoot and hindfoot equinus, hindfoot varus, a cavus component, and clawing of the toes.
- After Achilles tendon lengthening, a split PTT transfer, a Steindler procedure, a Chopart fusion, a dorsiflexion first metatarsal osteotomy, and a modified Jones procedure, a plantigrade functional foot was restored.
- **FIG 7A,B** shows preoperative findings and **FIG 7C,D** shows findings 1 year postoperatively.

COMPLICATIONS

- Infection
- Vessel or nerve bundle injury
- Nonunion
- Overcorrection (flatfoot, valgus foot, calcaneus foot)
- Undercorrection
- Recurrence
- Ulceration due to plaster casting
- Pin tract infection from the Kirschner wires

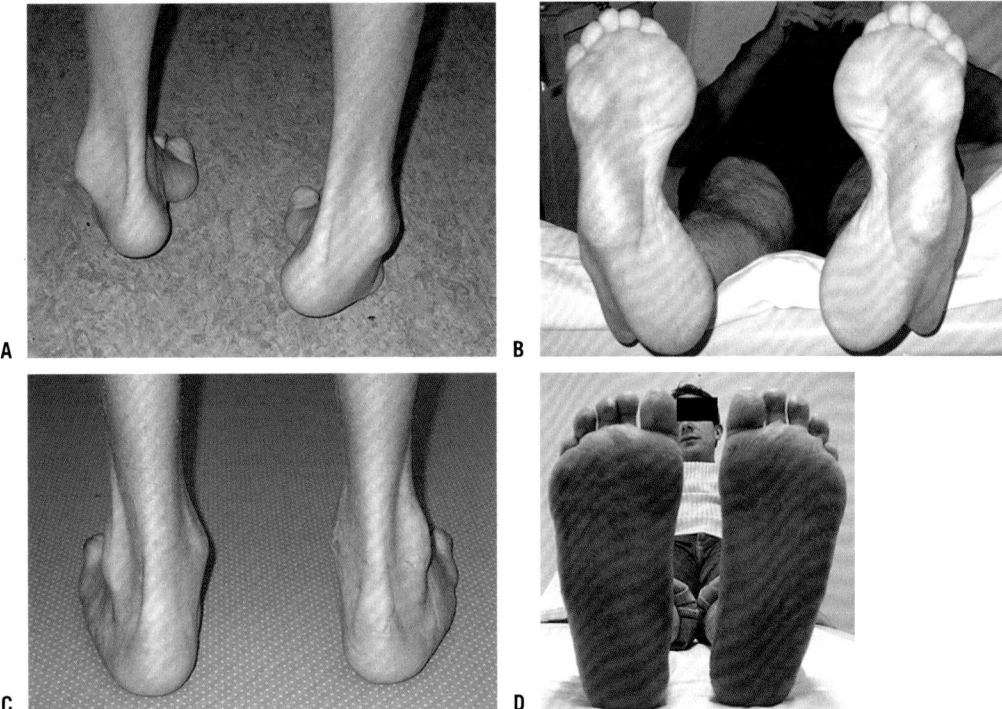

FIG 7 Preoperative (**A,B**) and postoperative (**C,D**) clinical and radiographic findings of a 32-year-old patient with severe equinocavovarus foot deformity bilaterally.

REFERENCES

1. Cole WH. The treatment of claw-foot. J Bone Joint Surg Am 1940;22:895–908.
2. Coleman SS. Complex Foot Deformities in Children. Philadelphia: Lea & Febiger, 1983.
3. Coleman SS, Chesnut WJ. A simple test for hind-foot flexibility in the cavo-varus foot. Clin Orthop Relat Res 1977;(123):60–62.
4. de Palma L, Colonna E, Travasi M. The modified Jones procedure for pes cavovarus with claw hallux. J Foot Ankle Surg 1997;36:279–283.
5. Dwyer FC. Osteotomy of the calcaneum for pes cavus. J Bone Joint Surg Br 1959;41(1):80–86.
6. Dwyer FC. The present status of the problem of pes cavus. Clin Orthop Relat Res 1975;(106):254–275.
7. Hall JE, Calvert PT. Lambrinudi triple arthrodesis: a review with particular reference to the technique of operation. J Pediatr Orthop 1987;7:19–24.
8. Hibbs RA. An operation for "claw foot." JAMA 1919;73:1583–1585.
9. Hoke M. An operation for stabilizing paralytic feet. Am J Orthop Surg 1921;3:494–507.
10. Hsu JD, Hoffer MM. Posterior tibial tendon transfer anteriorly through the interosseous membrane. Clin Orthop Relat Res 1978;(131):202–204.
11. Imhäuser G. Treatment of severe concave clubfoot in neural muscular atrophy [in German]. Z Orthop Ihre Grenzgeb 1984;122:827–834.
12. Jahss MH. Evaluation of the cavus foot for orthopedic treatment. Clin Orthop Relat Res 1983;(181):52–63.
13. Jones R. An operation for paralytic calcaneo-cavus. Am J Orthop Surg 1908;4:371–376.
14. Lambrinudi C. New operation for drop foot. Br J Surg 1927;15:193.
15. Mann RA. Pes cavus. In: Mann RA, Coughlin MJ, eds. Surgery of the Foot and Ankle, vol 1, ed 6. St. Louis: Mosby, 1993:785–801.
16. Samilson RL, Dillin W. Cavus, cavovarus and calcaneocavus: an update. Clin Orthop Relat Res 1983;(177):125–132.
17. Shapiro F, Bresnan MJ. Orthopaedic management of childhood neuromuscular disease. Part I: spinal muscular atrophy. J Bone Joint Surg Am 1982;64(5):785–789.
18. Shapiro F, Bresnan MJ. Orthopaedic management of childhood neuromuscular disease: Part II: peripheral neuropathies, Friedrich's ataxia, and arthrogryposis multiplex congenita. J Bone Joint Surg Am 1982;64(6):949–953.
19. Shapiro F, Bresnan MJ. Orthopaedic management of childhood neuromuscular disease. Part III: diseases of muscle. J Bone Joint Surg Am 1982;64(7):1102–1107.
20. Simon J, Doederlein L, McIntosh AS, et al. The Heidelberg foot measurement method: development, description and assessment. Gait Posture 2006;23:411–424.
21. Steindler A. The treatment of pes cavus (hollow claw foot). Arch Surg 1921;2:325–337.
22. Thometz JG, Gould JS. Cavus deformity. In: Drennan JC, ed. The Child's Foot and Ankle. New York: Raven Press, 1992:343–353.
23. Tubby AH. Deformities Including Diseases of Bones and Joints, ed 2. London: Macmillan, 1912.
24. Tubby AH, Jones R. Modern Methods in the Surgery of the Paralysis. London: Macmillan, 1902.

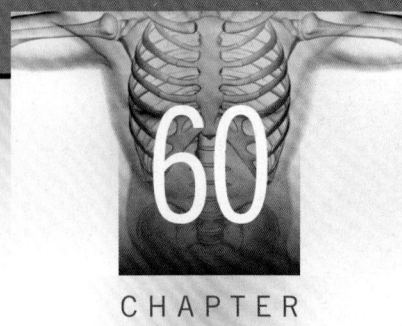

60
CHAPTER

Plantar Fascia Release in Combination with Proximal and Distal Tarsal Tunnel Release

Benedict F. DiGiovanni, Irvin C. Oh, and John S. Gould

DEFINITION

- Chronic plantar fasciitis with distal tarsal tunnel syndrome is an underrecognized disorder in which the patients with the typical enthesopathy of plantar fasciitis develop neurogenic symptoms and signs, becoming recalcitrant to the usual management of the initial condition.[6]
- This chapter concentrates on the most common type of distal tarsal tunnel syndrome: chronic plantar fasciitis associated with the involvement of the lateral plantar nerve and the first branch of the lateral plantar nerve.

ANATOMY

- Proximal or classic tarsal tunnel syndrome was first described by Kopell and Thompson[17] in 1960. It was subsequently named by Keck[16] and Lam[19] in two independent reports in 1962. Entrapment of the entire tibial nerve as it courses beneath the flexor retinaculum behind the medial malleolus defines proximal tarsal tunnel syndrome (FIG 1A). The flexor retinaculum or laciniate ligament is formed by

joining the deep and superficial aponeurosis of the leg, and it is closely attached to the sheaths of the posterior tibial, flexor digitorum longus, and flexor hallucis tendons.

- Distal tarsal tunnel syndrome, proposed by Heinkes et al[11] in 1987, results from irritation of one or more of the terminal branches of the tibial nerve. The three terminal branches are the medial plantar nerve, lateral plantar nerve, and medical calcaneal nerve.
- The first branch of the lateral plantar nerve occurs just after the lateral plantar nerve branches from the posterior tibial nerve (FIG 1B). The first branch travels between the abductor hallucis muscle deep fascia and the medial fascia of the quadratus plantae muscle. It then changes direction and travels laterally in a horizontal plane between the quadratus plantae and the flexor digitorum brevis muscles, sending a sensory branch to the central heel pad, and terminates as motor branch to the abductor digiti quinti muscle. (The "first branch" may, in some patients, emerge from the tibial nerve itself but then passes under the abductor hallucis and follows the usual course of the nerve.)[7,22]

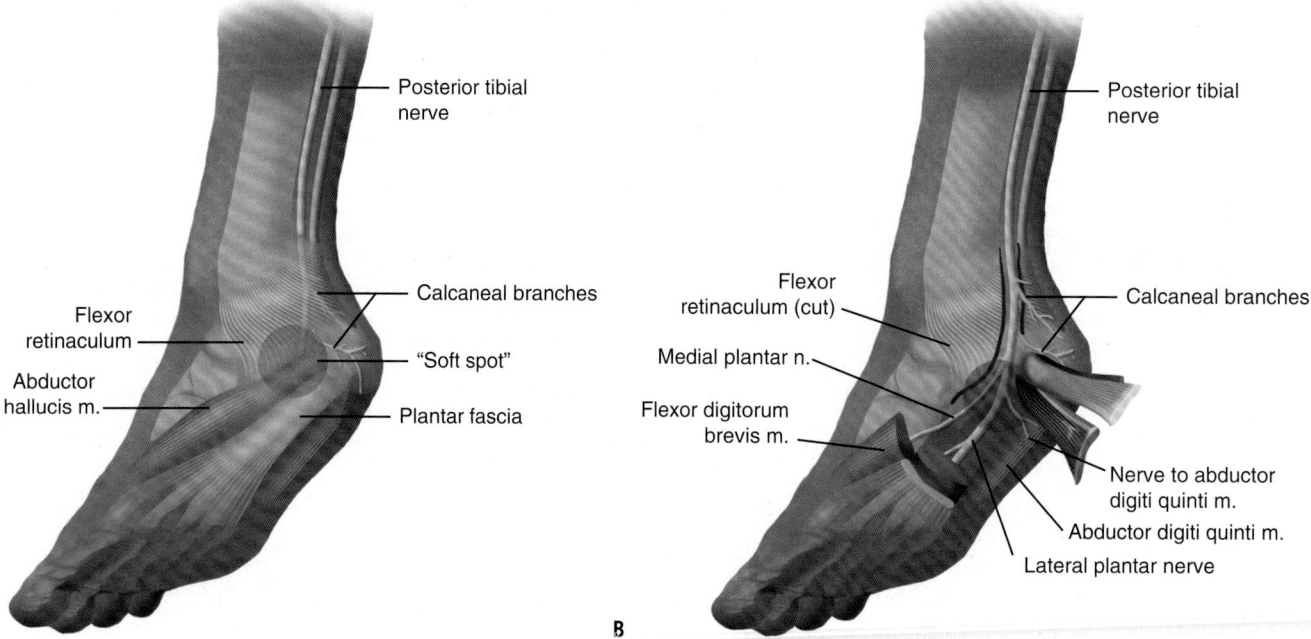

FIG 1 A. The laciniate ligament, three branches of the tibial nerve, and the classic tarsal tunnel. B. Detailed anatomy of the tibial nerve and branches.

- The lateral plantar nerve follows the same course initially, passing under the deep fascia of the abductor hallucis muscle and the medial edge of the plantar fascia and over the quadratus plantae fascia, and then turns distally under the flexor digitorum brevis, emerging distally just under the plantar fascia to form the intermetatarsal nerves to the 4–5 interspace and contributing to the 3–4 intermetatarsal nerve as well.
- The medial plantar nerve leaves the tibial nerve just proximal to or just under the abductor hallucis muscle and travels under the abductor hallucis muscle, innervating it and forming the intermetatarsal nerves to the 1–2, 2–3, and 3–4 interspaces. Both the medial and lateral plantar nerves provide innervation to the interossei and lumbrical muscles.
- The medial calcaneal nerves may be multiple and emerge from the tibial nerve proximal to the upper edge of the abductor hallucinating muscle. (On occasion, the calcaneal branch[s] may emerge from the tibial nerve under the abductor hallucis muscle, split the fibers of the abductor hallucis muscle and its fascia, and then continue subcutaneously to innervate the medial skin of the heel.)
- The plantar fascia or aponeurosis arises from the os calcis and is composed of three segments—the central, medial, and lateral portions.
  - Clinically, the central portion is considered to be the plantar fascia and originates from the medial tuberosity of the os calcis and inserts into all five toes.
  - Extension of the toes and the metatarsophalangeal (MTP) joints tightens the plantar aponeurosis, elevates the longitudinal arch, and inverts the hindfoot. This mechanism, which is entirely passive and depends on bony and ligamentous stability, is referred to as the *windlass mechanism.*

PATHOGENESIS

- Plantar fasciitis is thought to be a result of repetitive microtearing of the origin of the central band of the plantar aponeurosis.
  - This repetitive trauma results in inflammation and persistent pain, especially pain with the first steps in the morning or with the first steps after periods of inactivity.
- Chronic symptoms of plantar fasciitis develop in about 10% of patients with plantar heel pain.
  - We believe that these patients experience partial ruptures or attenuation of the plantar fascia as suggested by clinical findings in which the medial border of the fascia becomes less distinct than the normal side when the ankle and toes are dorsiflexed.[7,9]
  - A subset of these patients has chronic, disabling plantar heel pain with associated neurogenic symptoms of distal tarsal tunnel syndrome.

NATURAL HISTORY

- In 1986, Rondhuis and Huson[22] described compression of the first branch of the lateral plantar nerve and its association with heel pain.
- Baxter et al[1] further studied and reported on the principle of isolated compression of the first branch and its association with chronic plantar fasciitis.
- Further studies by Lau and Daniels[20] demonstrated that increased traction in the lateral plantar nerve and in its first branch is noted as the supporting structures of the longitudinal arch are selectively divided, including the plantar fascia, which could result in a "traction neuritis" of the nerves.
- Inflammatory conditions and local edema affect the nerve as it travels in the hindfoot. Entrapment, or *traction irritation*, of the lateral plantar nerve and its first branch is thought to occur between the abductor hallucis muscle deep fascia, the medial border of the plantar fascia, and the medial caudal margin of the quadratus plantae muscle.
  - Electrodiagnostic evidence of compression of the lateral plantar nerve first branch and its association with chronic plantar fasciitis have been reported by Schon et al.[24]

PATIENT HISTORY AND PHYSICAL FINDINGS

- Patients with chronic proximal plantar fasciitis with distal tarsal tunnel syndrome have signs and symptoms typical of both plantar fasciitis and neuritis.
- We believe that chronic plantar heel pain that does not respond to a standard nonoperative protocol is the result of attenuated or significant partial plantar fascia rupture, in addition to some degree of neuritis or nerve entrapment.
- The patient population is diverse, with a wide age range and varied activity levels, and includes both nonathletes and elite competitive athletes. Occupations are also diverse, although many patients are employed in vocations that require prolonged standing or walking.

Plantar Fasciitis

- Plantar fasciitis symptoms are considered chronic when they persist for at least 3 months and more typically 9 months or longer.[7,9]
  - Typically, symptoms include plantar heel pain that is most severe with the first steps in the morning or with the first steps after prolonged sitting. This pain disappears relatively quickly after walking for a few moments and is relieved immediately upon non–weight bearing. It does not become increasingly painful with increased walking or at rest.
- Tenderness is noted at the medial tubercle of the calcaneus, which correlates with the origin of the plantar fascia. This area of tenderness is focal and reproducible and is located at the plantar medial heel.
  - Most patients in the chronic state have evidence of attenuation of the plantar fascia and probable biomechanical incompetence.
  - This asymmetry between the two feet in terms of firmness of the plantar fascia is noted when recreating the windlass mechanism (ankle dorsiflexion and first to fifth metatarsophalangeal joint dorsiflexion) and palpating the plantar fascia medial border. This difference is thought to represent a significant chronic partial plantar fascia tear.
  - Significant attenuation of the plantar fascia was noted at preoperative evaluation in 15 of 22 patients in the series reported by DiGiovanni et al.[4]

Neuritis/Distal Tarsal Tunnel Syndrome

- Neuritic symptoms and signs may be subtle and not appreciated unless the examiner is aware of their potential presence and checks for their possible existence.

- Neuritic symptoms typically include reports of an "after-burn" rather than instant relief of heel pain with non–weight bearing after prolonged activity.
  - Patients may also describe radiation of pain in the posteromedial ankle, medial hindfoot, and distal plantar foot, often, but not always, with numbness or burning and often worse with prolonged standing or when resting after prolonged activity.
  - Neuritis pain may radiate up the medial aspect of the leg, a condition known as the *Valleix phenomenon.*
  - Radiation of the neuritic pain may occur along the lateral aspect of the plantar heel, following the course of the lateral plantar nerve first branch. This pain may be experienced in the center of the heel ("central heel pad syndrome") or along the lateral heel border and also attributable to the first branch or "nerve to the abductor digiti quinti."
  - In many cases, the patient will have difficulty describing the exact nature of the pain but may report diffuse tingling, burning, or numbness.
- The medial hindfoot tenderness is located over the abductor hallucis muscle at a position approximately 5 cm anterior to the posterior border of the heel at the intersection of the plantar and medial skin.
  - If one palpates the medial border of the heel, the examiner's digit will suddenly feel a "soft spot," which corresponds with the course of the lateral plantar nerve and its first branch as they pass from the ankle into the foot at the lower edge of the fascia of the abductor hallucis, an area that is associated with nerve entrapment or neuritis.
  - This is a separate area from the medial tubercle of the calcaneus tenderness associated with plantar fasciitis.
- In athletes (especially basketball players) or individuals whose occupations involve prolonged standing, enlargement or hypertrophy of the abductor hallucis muscle may be appreciated.
- Patients with such irritation of the tibial nerve and its branches may also be tender over the nerves in the arch, noted with the plantar fascia relaxed by passively plantar-flexing the ankle and toes.
  - These patients have been diagnosed with so-called distal plantar fasciitis, an entity which is much less common than classic or proximal plantar fasciitis, except with acute midsubstance ruptures of the plantar fascia.
  - These patients with tarsal tunnel syndrome may also have tenderness in the intermetatarsal spaces, suggesting intermetatarsal neuritis, Morton neuroma, or a "double crush" syndrome. This is usually not the case, however, as patients with primary pathology proximally in the distal tarsal tunnel and plantar fascia complain of heel, arch, and posteromedial ankle pain, whereas those with primary disease distally complain of metatarsal pain (metatarsalgia) and may incidentally also have tenderness over the nerves proximally.

IMAGING AND OTHER DIAGNOSTIC STUDIES

- Electrodiagnostic studies are considered before surgical intervention, but decision to obtain or not is patient-case specific. Most are aimed at ruling out associated pathology, such as radiculopathy and generalized peripheral neuropathy.
  - If diffuse peripheral neuropathy rather than localized nerve entrapment is suspected, screening for diabetes, thyroid dysfunction, or alcoholism may be indicated.

- Lower extremity electrodiagnostic studies are known to be less reproducible than upper extremity studies and are also dependent on the expertise and skill of the electrodiagnostician in performing detailed foot and ankle studies. The studies should evaluate potential entrapment of both the lateral and medial plantar nerves.
  - Electromyelographic results for the abductor hallucis muscle or abductor digiti quinti muscle are more likely to be abnormal than are nerve conduction studies.[23]
  - A positive result adds confirmation to the clinical diagnosis. However, since the neuritic component is thought to be a traction neuropathy,[20] and is believed to be most evident in the dynamic situation, a negative result does not rule out the diagnosis. Accordingly, it is not uncommon to have negative electrodiagnostic studies despite signs and symptoms of neuritis.
- Serologic studies may be indicated to evaluate for possible inflammatory arthritis in patients with bilateral heel pain of simultaneous onset and similar severity.
- Weight-bearing foot radiographs are obtained to rule out such associated pathology as calcaneal stress fracture and hindfoot degenerative joint disease.
  - Patients with subtalar and sometimes ankle arthrosis or with tenosynovitis of the posterior tibial, flexor digitorum longus, and flexor hallucis tendons may have sufficient swelling to irritate the tibial nerve.
  - A subset of patients with posterior tibial tendon dysfunction may also have symptoms of tarsal tunnel syndrome.[18]
  - If there is a history of previous fracture or significant trauma, radiographs of both the ankle and foot should be obtained to rule out external sources of nerve compression such as exostosis.
- Computed tomography has a limited role but may be helpful if there is a prior history of trauma with posttraumatic changes to assess for bony exostosis and deformity.
- Technetium 99 bone scans have a poor specificity and are rarely indicated.
- Magnetic resonance imaging is sensitive for detecting frank fascial rupture and confirming proximal plantar fasciitis, but it is not indicated in most cases.
  - Magnetic resonance imaging can demonstrate occult pathology, such as a space-occupying lesion in the proximal or distal tarsal tunnel or a subtle calcaneal stress fracture.
- Ultrasonography can be helpful to determine pathology in the tarsal tunnel, a site of external compression or changes in the size and character of the nerve in the area of compression or traction.[21]

DIFFERENTIAL DIAGNOSIS

- Diffuse peripheral neuropathy (diabetes mellitus, thyroid dysfunction, alcoholism)
- Lumbar radiculopathy
- Inflammatory arthritis
- Calcaneal stress fracture, hindfoot degenerative joint disease

NONOPERATIVE MANAGEMENT

- Initial nonoperative treatment includes relative rest, plantar fascia and Achilles tendon stretching exercises, ice, and nonsteroidal anti-inflammatory drugs.

- Physical therapy modalities that involve or promote heating of the tissues, such as whirlpool baths, hydrocollator packs, diathermy, ultrasound, or phonophoresis, seem to irritate the neuritic symptoms and increase rather than decrease symptoms.
  - Iontophoresis, which diffuses steroid with electrolysis, is typically well tolerated and may be beneficial.
- Steroid injections into the plantar fascia or along the nerve itself are discouraged.
  - Many patients present with a history of earlier episodes of plantar fasciitis that responded to steroid injections. These patients are now unresponsive to injection and have an obviously attenuated plantar fascia. This suggests an association of steroid injection with plantar fascia rupture and the ensuing chronicity.
- Inexpensive, over-the-counter orthotics are prescribed to support the arch and cushion the heel. With chronicity, a semirigid, accommodative, custom orthotic is prescribed. These are cork based and triple layered and include a "nerve relief channel" made of viscoelastic polymer, which is placed along the path of the lateral plantar nerve beginning at the proximal abductor hallucis muscle belly and extending to the soft spot.[12]
  - If the patient has more symptoms in the central heal pad, which involves the first branch of the lateral plantar, the channel is carried more posteriorly and onto the plantar heel to include the painful central area.
  - The same orthotic devices are used postoperatively if the patient requires surgery.
- Studies with extracorporeal shock wave lithotripsy, of both low and high intensity, for chronic plantar fasciitis report a positive response and the modality appears to be safe and effective.[5,15]
  - In the authors' experience, individuals with chronic plantar fasciitis and associated signs and symptoms of neuritis has the potential to further aggravate the neurogenic symptoms and therefore should be used with caution.

SURGICAL MANAGEMENT

- In the late 1980s and early 1990s, Baxter and colleagues[1] reported on and popularized their surgical approach to painful heel syndrome in athletes with entrapment of the first branch of the lateral plantar nerve. This approach includes partial release of the plantar fascia combined with release of the first branch of the lateral plantar nerve and removal of a heel spur if present. The investigators have reported a high success rate, particularly in the athletic population.
  - More recent reports using this approach in a more general patient population have noted mixed results, however, with Davies et al[2] in 1999 reporting less than 50% of patients with complete satisfaction as a result of persistent symptoms.
- DiGiovanni and colleagues[3,4] have devised and reported on a modified surgical approach based partially on the work of Baxter and colleagues.[1] The approach is also based on the observation that patients with plantar fascia rupture and chronic pain who do not have neurogenic symptoms respond to a complete surgical release of the plantar fascia.
  - Patients who had the release described by Baxter et al[1] and continued to be symptomatic responded to the complete release and neurolysis as described in the following text.

- The more extensile approach is used to allow the release of all potential sources of entrapment of the tibial nerve and its branches and thus allow for improved rates of complete resolution of pain and elimination of activity limitations.
- This technique combines a complete plantar fascia release with a proximal and distal tarsal tunnel release, without bone spur removal.
- The philosophy behind a complete release of the plantar fascia rather than a partial release is as follows:
  - The literature does not provide information about the optimal amount of partial release to perform to allow for reproducible resolution of plantar heel pain. The amount is probably highly variable from patient to patient and depends on a number of factors, including the type of foot arch.
  - Patients with chronic heel pain commonly have evidence of attenuation of their plantar fascia and probably have preexisting biomechanical incompetence. A further partial release in feet with preexisting plantar fascia attenuation has not consistently led to resolution of plantar heel symptoms.
  - Complete release of the plantar fascia from the abductor hallucis to the abductor digiti quinti has resulted in high rates of elimination of the pain experienced after the first step in the morning or after in recumbence in primary and revision surgery after previous partial plantar fascia release.
- The nerve component of the pathology is also specifically addressed. In our experience, release of the plantar fascia alone in patients with chronic plantar fasciitis often leads to increased neuritic symptoms. Consequently, the nerve procedure is typically performed in addition to the plantar fascia release.
  - Rather than an isolated release of the first branch of the lateral plantar nerve, a proximal (or classic) as well as a distal tarsal tunnel release is performed to address all potential sites of nerve entrapment.
  - Proximal tarsal tunnel syndrome may coexist with distal and can be difficult to differentiate and isolate.
  - In addition, more than one branch of the terminal tibial nerve branches may be entrapped.

Preoperative Planning

- Good history taking, specifically to determine when and in which anatomic location symptoms occur, is essential. We cannot emphasize enough that the history will differentiate metatarsalgia, pure plantar fasciitis, radiculopathy, and neuropathy.
- A careful physical examination must be done as indicated previously.
- Electrodiagnostic testing is useful when the history and physical have not clearly ruled out generalized peripheral neuropathy in particular or radiculopathy.
  - Tibial nerve entrapment may coexist with neuropathy, but the prognosis for a good result with this surgery is guarded, and we believe such a combination accounts for less than optimal results.

Positioning

- The patient is positioned supine without a bump under the hip, allowing the leg to externally rotate.
  - When we move around to the plantar side, we ask the anesthetist to place the foot of the bed in Trendelenburg to improve access.

Approach

- We use a posteromedial and plantar approach to fully visualize the anatomy.
- The procedure is done with high thigh tourniquet control after exsanguination of the leg.
- Bipolar cautery is used for minimal tissue necrosis.
- There are circumstances when division of the abductor hallucis is required—abnormal or confusing anatomy and

bleeding from small vessels. Consequently, a unipolar cautery with grounding is always in place to use in the cutting mode, and vessel ligation clips of small and medium size are available in the operating room.

- Loupe magnification is recommended, with a preference of 3.5 to 4.5 magnification.

T E C H N I Q U E S (V i d e o)

COMPLETE RELEASE OF THE PLANTAR FASCIA AND TARSAL TUNNEL[6]

- The midpoint between the posterior border of the medial malleolus and the medial border of the Achilles tendon is marked. The medial edge of the heel is palpated beginning posteriorly and moving distally until the palpating finger feels the soft spot where the neurovascular bundle enters the foot, and this point is marked as well.

- The midpoint of the malleolar–tendon interval is marked proximally, and the incision extends plantarward and curves distally to cross the soft spot, continuing onto the plantar skin at the distal portion of the heel pad, and extending transversely about three quarters of the width of the heel skin **(TECH FIG 1A)**.

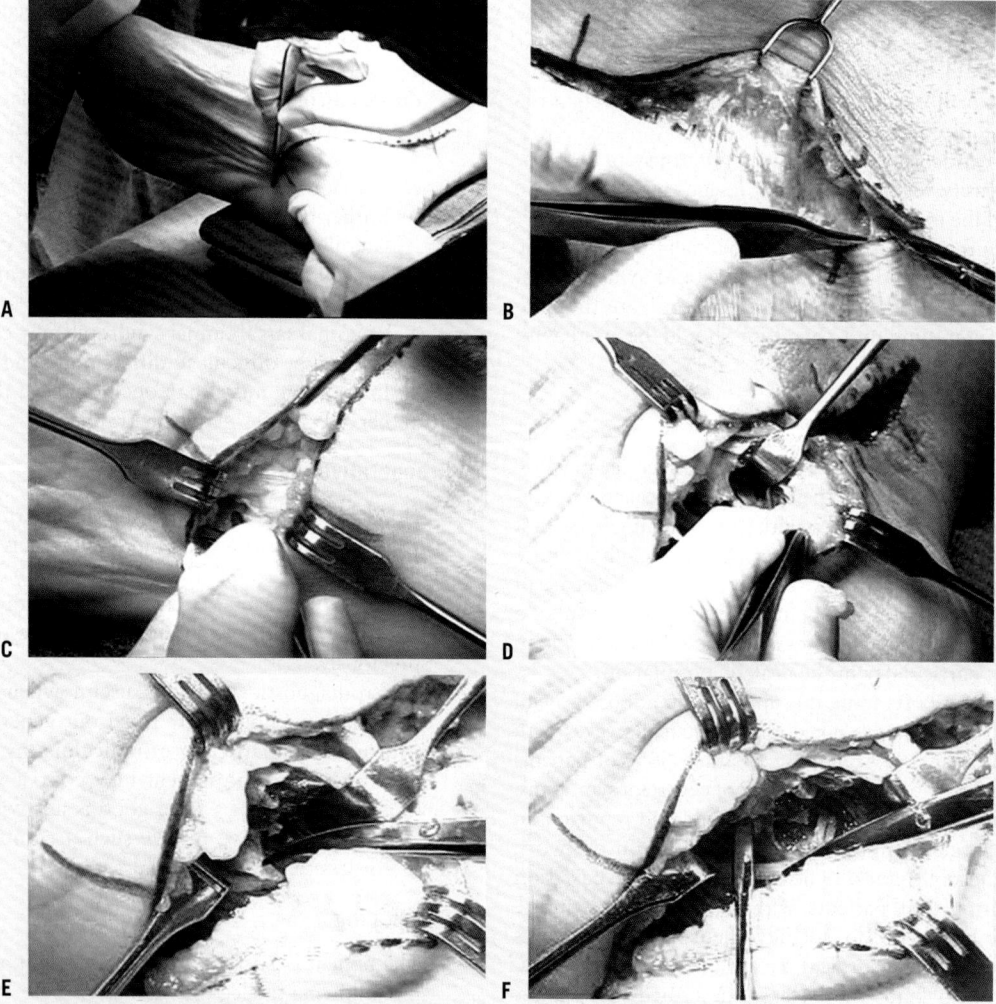

TECH FIG 1 A. The skin incision for the complete release. **B.** Dividing the laciniate ligament. **C.** Dividing the entire plantar fascia. **D.** Dividing the deep fascia of the abductor hallucis. **E.** The abductor hallucis and flexor digitorum brevis interval. **F.** Lateral plantar nerve overlying the quadratus plantae fascia.

- The entire skin incision is made following the skin marking.
- The proximal subcutaneous tissue is separated bluntly to identify the superficial vessels, and a double skin hook is placed on the far side of the surgeon and lifted away from the ankle.
- The surgeon easily spreads, cuts, and cauterizes superficial vessels and identifies the flexor retinaculum (laciniate ligament). This layer is divided directly over visible posterior tibial veins distally to the level of the abductor hallucis muscle. No attempt is made to isolate the tibial nerve **(TECH FIG 1B)**.
- The superficial fascia of the abductor hallucis is divided sharply with a no. 15 surgical scalpel or no. 64 Beaver blade.
- The hooks are now moved distally to the plantar surface, and spreading and cutting is done with a long-handled tenotomy scissors down to the plantar fascia. Two sharp Senn retractors are now used, which gather the fat away from the abductor hallucis fascia and improve visualization.
- A Meyerding retractor is placed at the distal extent of the incision to expose the fascia overlying the abductor digiti quinti.
- The plantar fascia is divided 2 to 4 cm distal to its origin. The knife blade is used to sharply cut the plantar fascia from its lateral extent, at the edge of the abductor digiti quinti fascia, progressing medially to the abductor hallucis fascia, fully exposing the underlying flexor digitorum brevis muscle **(TECH FIG 1C)**.
  - The plantar fascia surface is actually convex and meets each of the abductor fascias more deeply or dorsally than at its midpoint.
- As right-handed surgeons, we release this deep fascia on the right foot from the laciniate ligament distally. On the left foot, we begin from the plantar fascia side. In either case, we now place a self-retaining retractor in the wound to allow the assistant to help with the next step **(TECH FIG 1D)**.
- The blades of the tenotomy scissors are spread between the muscle of the abductor hallucis and its deep fascia to initiate its exposure. The Meyerding retractor is used to further tease the muscle off the fascia and enhance and complete its visualization.
- The fascia is divided under the muscle, exposing the neurovascular structures and the tarsal tunnel. We divide the deep fascia as far as we can see it and then expose the structure from the opposite side (either proximally or distally) and complete the release.

- The muscle of the flexor digitorum brevis is then retracted laterally, and the fine fascia overlying the neurovascular structures is divided.
- The interval between the abductor hallucis and the flexor brevis is then exposed. The self-retaining retractor is placed on the skin and subcutaneous fat at this interval. One Meyerding (or similar right angle) retractor is placed under the abductor hallucis muscle, retracting it proximally. Another right angle retracts the flexor digitorum brevis muscle laterally **(TECH FIG 1E)**.
- The posterior tibial artery and veins are easily seen. Parallel to them but slightly more anterior is the lateral plantar nerve, often with a little fat around it. The first branch is not specifically exposed but lies more posteriorly.
- The nerve is carefully teased from its surrounding tissues and gently retracted, and the underlying quadratus plantae fascia is observed.
  - If no further tenting or compression is noted along the lateral plantar nerve, then the procedure is complete.
  - If compression is noted, one should proceed with further release. A small vessel may obscure visualization of the nerve in some patients. In such cases, with the power of the bipolar cautery turned down, we carefully cauterize and cut it to provide the needed exposure. The quadratus fascia is often a dense band over which the nerve is obviously tented. In other cases, the white bands of fascia are visible but less dense. They are cut sharply with the scissors to expose the muscle. The nerve now lies under no tension **(TECH FIG 1F)**.
- With the confluence of the superficial and deep abductor fascias distally and the medial border of the plantar fascia, a dense band of fascia overlies the lateral plantar nerve, and with the dense band of the quadratus fascia below, it is easy to visualize a pincer effect on the nerve at this point with weight bearing and particularly when the plantar fascia is less taut.
- Closure is carried out after irrigation of the wound. The ankle subcutaneous tissue is closed with 4-0 absorbable suture and the skin with 4-0 nonabsorbable suture. The glabrous plantar skin is closed with only 3-0 or 4-0 skin permanent suture using locking horizontal mattress sutures, with no subcutaneous suture.
- A soft bulky dressing is applied and the tourniquet released. Sterility is not broken until the toes show good perfusion.

COMPLETE PLANTAR FASCIA AND TARSAL TUNNEL RELEASE FOR PRIOR INCOMPLETE AND FAILED RELEASES[10]

- The same basic approach is used as just described but with several additions to the technique.
- The new incision begins proximal to the original one to start in normal tissue.
- The old incision is incorporated into the new, ensuring access to the soft spot.
- When the laciniate ligament is divided, the tibial nerve is exposed and a vessel loop is placed around the nerve and a tie is placed on the loop as opposed to a hemostat to avoid any traction on the nerve.

- As the release proceeds, external neurolysis of the tibial nerve and of the medial and lateral plantar branches is carried out. The calcaneal nerves are identified and protected. The first branch of the lateral plantar nerve is identified.
- The muscle belly of the abductor hallucis is often divided with a cutting cautery with careful blunt dissection to protect the underlying critical structures. The muscle of the flexor digitorum brevis may also be partially or fully divided to achieve adequate exposure.
- If there is no evidence of damage to the nerves or marked wound scar or scar around the nerves, the wounds are closed as in the primary procedure.

COMPLETE PLANTAR FASCIA AND TARSAL TUNNEL RELEASE WHEN EXTENSIVE SCARRING OF THE NERVE IS PRESENT, WITH THE USE OF BARRIER WRAPPING OF THE NERVE

- The senior author, JSG, a microvascular-trained surgeon, used greater saphenous vein wrapping or commercially available collagen tubes and reported his experience with addressing scarred mixed nerves that must be preserved. The following are the description of his techniques.[10,13]
- The complete release as described earlier is performed.

Use of the Greater Saphenous Vein

- The greater saphenous vein is harvested with a longitudinal incision beginning in the midpoint between the crest of the tibia and its posteromedial margin. One usually has to harvest a length of vein three times the length of nerve to be wrapped.
    - At harvest, metal Ligaclips are used for the branches, which are few in number in the distal vein. Double medium clips are used at either end of the vein, and one is left on the proximal end of the harvested proximal vein to indicate the orientation of the vein.
- The vein is placed in lidocaine to relax the smooth muscle component. It is then dilated from distal to proximal either with mechanical dilators or hydrostatically with lidocaine inserted under pressure with a syringe, using a vein plastic adaptor fitted to the syringe.
- All metal clips are then removed and the vein divided longitudinally.
- The vein is then curled around the involved nerve in barber pole fashion with the venous intima adjacent to the nerve. The vein is wrapped without tension, and each end is attached to surrounding tissues so as not to have a closed loop at either end. The coils are attached to each other with two 7-0 Prolene sutures placed about 180 degrees apart **(TECH FIG 2)**.
- The medial and lateral plantar nerves are wrapped separately.
    - The tibial nerve may be wrapped, and then the surgeon may continue down one or the other of the branches.
    - The wrap of the other plantar nerve joins the initially wrapped portion.

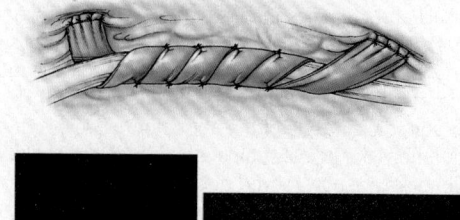
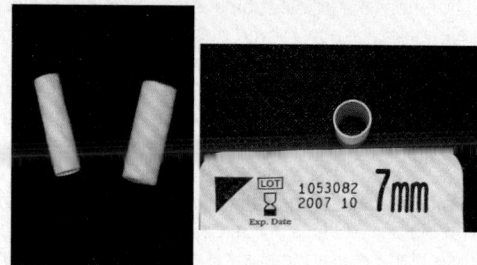

TECH FIG 2 A. Vein wrapping. **B.** Bovine collagen longitudinally split tubes for wrapping.

- The first branch of the lateral plantar may be initially wrapped with the lateral plantar and then allowed to travel independently distally.
- The calcaneal branches are allowed to escape between the coils and must not be entrapped in the procedure.

Use of Commercial Collagen Tubes[10,13]

- Use of the commercially available collagen tubes simplifies the process. The tubes come in diameters ranging from 2 to 10 mm and lengths of 2.5 to 5 cm. The tubes are provided longitudinally divided.
- The size to be used is determined by the surgeon's estimation of the needed diameter and lengths. Several lengths may be joined or a slightly long segment may be trimmed.
- The slit in the tube is closed, not too tightly, with a few interrupted 6-0 nylon sutures. Some of the commercially available wraps have enough material overlap to obviate the need for any suturing.

USE OF CONDUITS FOR NEUROMAS OF THE CALCANEAL BRANCHES[8,11,13,25]

- A neuroma of a calcaneal branch is treated with either a vein or a collagen conduit.
- The neuroma is exposed and excised.
- A conduit of at least 2 cm should be used. (Bovine collagen conduits are 2.5 cm in length and start at the 2.0 mm diameter with availabilities of increasing diameters at 0.5 mm increments.)
    - Collagen tubes of a proper diameter to loosely enclose the nerve are available, and the 5 cm lengths may be trimmed as needed.
    - When using a vein, the diameter must also be large enough to loosely accommodate the nerve, and the lumen diameter may need to be narrowed a bit so that it fits a little more closely around the nerve end.

- A nylon suture is placed through the end of the nerve, the needle is removed, and the two ends of the suture are grasped with a hemostat.
- A suture passer (Hewson) is placed through the conduit, and the nylon suture attached to the nerve is placed through the suture passer loop.
- The conduit is slid over the nerve, overlapping by 5 mm to 1 cm, and 8-0 sutures are used to attach the conduit lumen to the epineurium of the nerve. Typically, two sutures at 180 degrees are placed. The nylon suture used to draw the nerve into the conduit is removed **(TECH FIG 3)**.
- The nerve and its "conduit to nowhere" is buried posteromedially, often into the retrocalcaneal space.

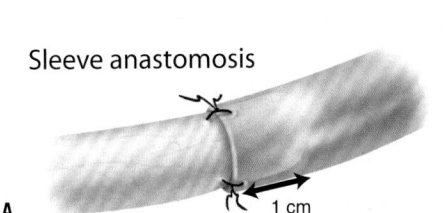

Sleeve anastomosis

A   1 cm

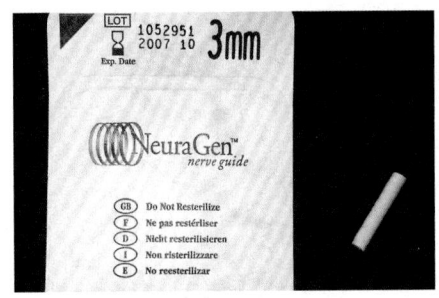

B

TECH FIG 3 A. Vein conduits. **B.** Bovine collagen conduits for neuromas (or nerve guide for repairs).

T E C H N I Q U E S

CASE EXAMPLE (COURTESY OF MARK E. EASLEY, MD)

Combined Proximal and Distal Tarsal Tunnel Release

- Approach for both proximal and distal tarsal tunnel release
- Oblique vertical incision over posteromedial foot and ankle **(TECH FIG 4A)**
- Avoid transverse incision (for plantar fascia release), which may injure superficial medial calcaneal branches.
- Exposure for tarsal tunnel release:
  - Release the flexor retinaculum.
  - Tibial nerve branches exposed **(TECH FIG 4B–F)**

Distal Tarsal Tunnel and Partial Plantar Fascia Release

- In the absence of proximal tibial nerve compression and plantar fascia attenuation, some surgeon may elect to perform distal tarsal tunnel and partial plantar fascia release.
- Oblique incision over posteromedial foot **(TECH FIG 5A)**
- Release the superficial fascia over abductor hallucis muscle.
- Expose the abductor hallucis muscle **(TECH FIG 5B,C)**.

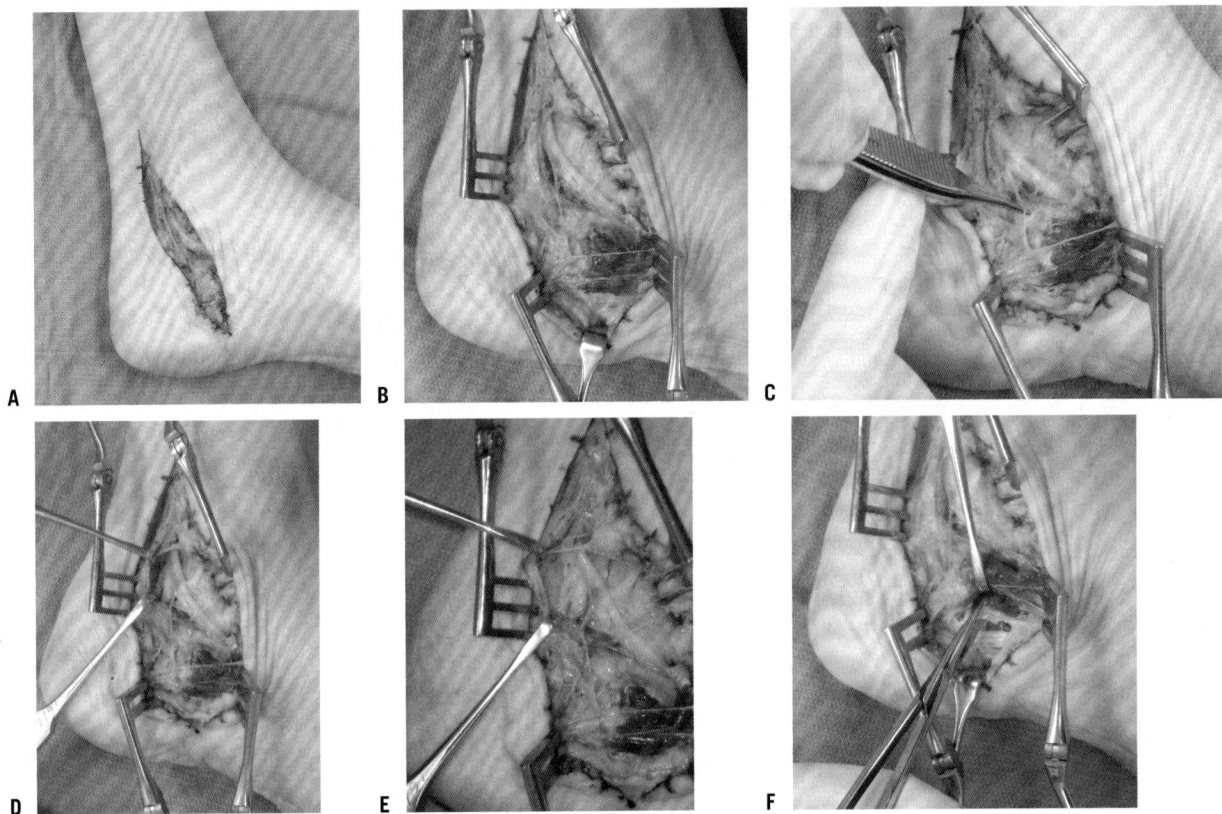

TECH FIG 4 A. Oblique vertical incision for proximal and distal tarsal tunnel release. **B.** With the flexor retinaculum released, tibial nerve branches exposed. **C.** Superficial medial calcaneal branch identified. Medial calcaneal branches may be injured if transverse incision has been traditionally used for plantar fascia release. **D,E.** Medial and lateral tibial nerve branching. **F.** Distal tarsal tunnel exposed to release deep fascia of the abductor hallucis muscle. Note the plantar fascia immediately plantar to the inferior margin of the deep abductor hallucis fascia.

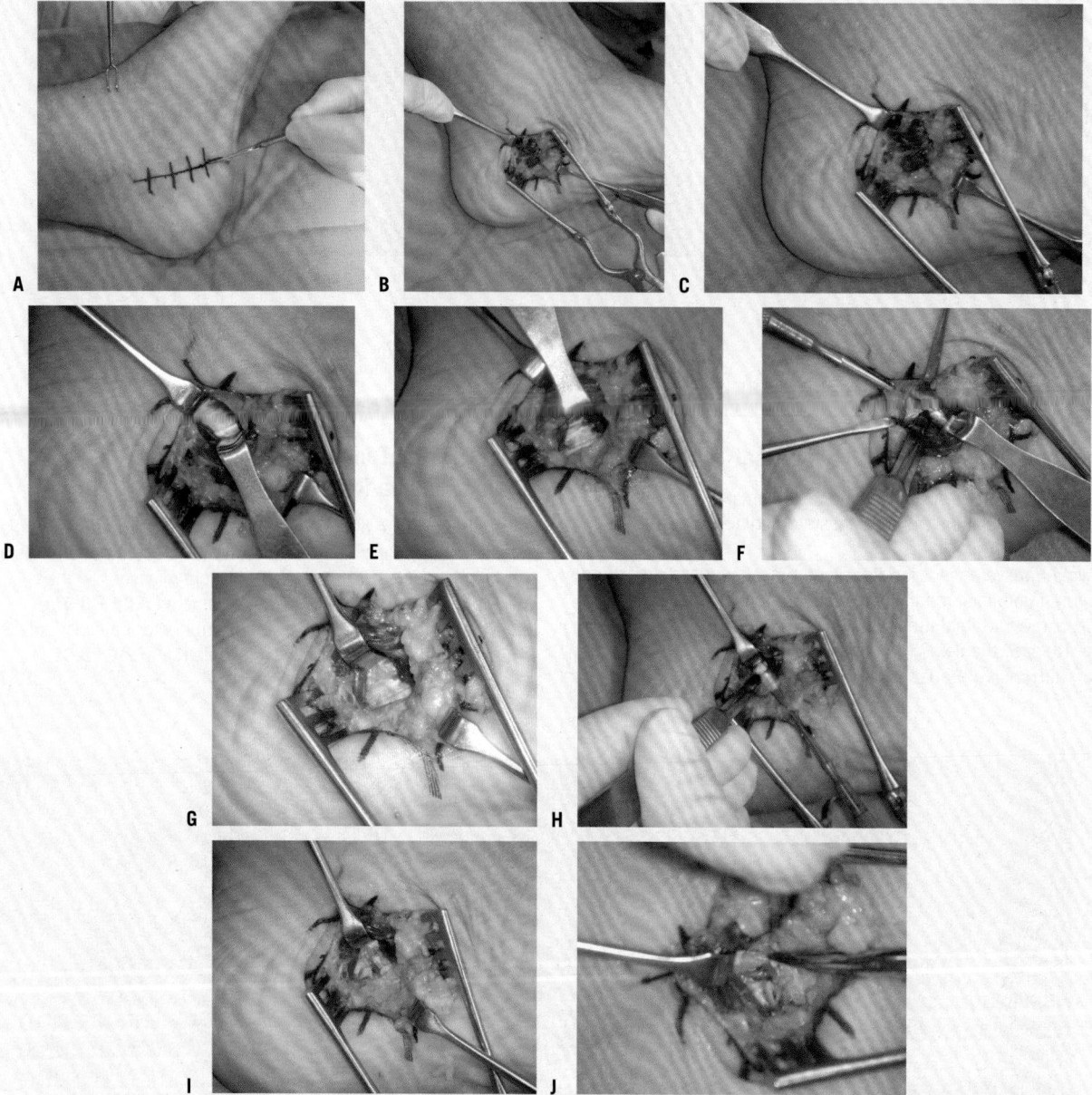

TECH FIG 5 A. Approach for distal tarsal tunnel and plantar fascia. With superficial abductor hallucis fascia release, the abductor muscle is exposed. **B,C.** A 4- to 5-cm oblique incision is made over the posteromedial heel. **D.** With plantar retraction of the abductor muscle, the superior aspect of the deep fascia is exposed. **E.** With dorsal retraction, the inferior aspect of the deep fascia is exposed. It is important to release the entire deep abductor fascia so that no residual bands compress the nerves. **F.** Release of the superior aspect of the deep fascia. **G.** With elevation of the abductor muscle, the inferior aspect of the completed superior release of deep abductor hallucis fascia is identified. **H.** The inferior deep fascia is released, directly extending from the identified completed portion of the deep fascia release. **I.** Completed deep abductor hallucis fascia release. Note that immediately plantar to the inferior border of the deep fascia lies the medial border of the plantar fascia. **J.** Note neurovascular structures exposed with release of the deep abductor hallucis fascia.

- Release the deep fascia of abductor hallucis muscle.
  - The tibial nerve branches course directly under this fascia.
  - A tight deep fascia creates compression on the nerve branches.
  - A complete release of the deep fascia is important.
    - Any residual intact fibers of the deep fascia may continue to create nerve compression.
    - A potential error is to incompletely release the most distal fascia fibers.

- Retract the abductor muscle inferiorly to expose the superior aspect of the deep fascia **(TECH FIG 5D)**.
- Retract the abductor muscle superiorly to expose the inferior aspect of the deep fascia **(TECH FIG 5E)**.
- First, release the superior aspect of the deep fascia **(TECH FIG 5F)**.

- Retract the abductor muscle superiorly to identify the inferior aspect of the completed superior release of deep fascia **(TECH FIG 5G)**.
- Complete the inferior release of the deep fascia **(TECH FIG 5H)**.
- With complete release, the tibial nerve branches are typically decompressed **(TECH FIG 5I,J)**.

Partial Plantar Fascia Release

- Immediately inferior to the inferior border of the deep abductor hallucis fascia is the medial border of the plantar fascia **(TECH FIG 6A)**.
- Relax the medial plantar fascia.
  - A section of medial plantar fascia is resected to take tension off of the tight and most symptomatic aspect of the plantar fascia **(TECH FIG 6B,C)**.

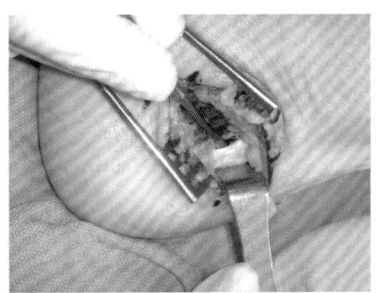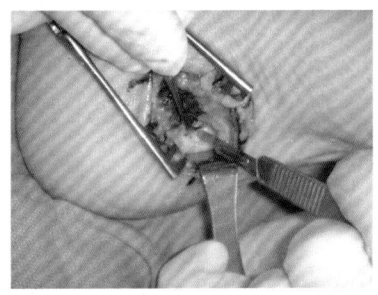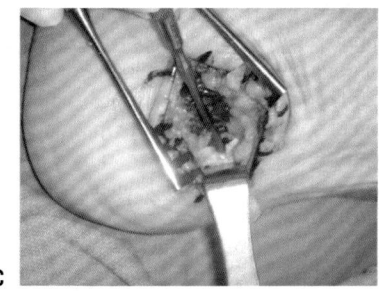

A   B   C

TECH FIG 6 A. Medial border of plantar fascia is identified. **B.** Medial plantar fascia partial resection. **C.** A section of plantar fascia is released to ensure that the medial plantar fascia cannot reconstitute.

TECHNIQUES

Pearls and Pitfalls

Indications	• It is essential that the patient's history is compatible with the diagnosis and that he or she is tender or has a Tinel sign at the soft spot.
	• If the history and physical examination do not correlate, look elsewhere for the diagnosis.
Accuracy of the Skin Incision	• The skin incision must be accurate and the anatomy clearly seen.
	• If the entrance of the neurovascular bundle to the foot is not accurately located, the release will be unsuccessful.
	• If there is difficulty finding the nerve in the interval between the abductor and the flexor brevis, divide the muscle of the abductor hallucis and find the nerve more proximally and follow it through the interval.
	• If you are lost, find the nerve under the laciniate ligament (it is posterior to the vessels and more lateral) and follow it and the lateral plantar branch more distally to carry out a proper release.
Bleeding	• Use of loupes and careful hemostasis will prevent bleeding, which prevents accurate visualization of the structures.
	• Postoperative bleeding will irritate the nerve and create more scarring and can compromise the result.
	• Make sure the tourniquet is of proper size for the size of the thigh, and exsanguination must be right up to the tourniquet. This may necessitate the use of a sterile tourniquet applied after draping. At times, with a very obese thigh, a double width or two tourniquets in succession may be helpful or a calf tourniquet may be used.
	• We cannot emphasize enough the importance of excellent visualization of the anatomy.
Completeness of the Release	• All structures noted in the description must be fully released.

POSTOPERATIVE CARE

- The patient is placed in a soft bulky dressing at surgery, and crutches are used for non–weight bearing. From immediately after the operation, motion of the foot and ankle is encouraged.
- Sutures are removed at 2 weeks, and a light dressing is applied. Gentle range-of-motion exercise of the ankle is reemphasized to promote gliding of the nerve but non–weight bearing continues for 2 more weeks.

- At 4 weeks, the patient is allowed to bear weight using the custom orthotic described earlier.
  - The orthotic is used for at least 9 months and then may be phased out.
  - If the patient fails to comply, pain will be experienced, usually on the dorsum and lateral border of the foot, presumably from "arch strain."

OUTCOMES

Primary Surgery

- DiGiovanni et al[3,4] reported an 82% rate of total satisfaction in primary surgery patients, with a marked decrease in pain to a level of no pain or mild, intermittent pain. This is a significant improvement over the less than 50% total satisfaction reported in most recent studies of limited plantar fascia release with a limited nerve release or nerve release without plantar fascia release.
- The improved rate of total satisfaction is reflective of the lower rates of residual pain and activity limitations. Improved surgical results in primary surgery patients are thought to be due to the comprehensive surgical approach with the goal of addressing all potential sites of pathology—nerve and plantar fascia.
- Our unreported data from more than 100 cases followed for over 2 years indicate that patients take varying periods of time to reach a steady state of complete relief of all symptoms. This averaged about 18 months and varied from 6 months to 2.5 years
- The surgical technique described here is highly recommended in patients with chronic plantar fasciitis and neuritic signs and symptoms, without prior surgery.

Revision Surgery

- Less predictable results have been reported for revision surgery. Although 73% of patients indicated they were better off than before surgery, total satisfaction was reported by only 27%, and 36% were dissatisfied with the procedure. There was a much higher incidence of residual pain and activity limitation.
- In revision situations, patients with evidence of inadequate prior distal tarsal tunnel release and those with persistent mechanical plantar fasciitis are most likely to have good resolution of their symptoms.
- Although the results for barrier wrapping and of the use of conduits for neuromas are less certain than those for the primary releases, successful results have been reported by Gould and colleagues.[13]

COMPLICATIONS

- A low rate of complications, both intra- and postoperatively, can be expected with this technique.
- Meticulous technique is needed to avoid potential complications, which include wound dehiscence, perineural scarring, and direct nerve injury. We recommend using bipolar electrocautery and surgical loupe magnification.
- Development of complex regional pain syndrome is possible postoperatively. Early diagnosis and aggressive treatment improve the prognosis.

REFERENCES

1. Baxter DE, Pfeffer GB, Thigpen M. Chronic heel pain. Treatment rationale. Orthop Clin North Am 1989;20:563–569.
2. Davies MS, Weiss GA, Saxby TS. Plantar fasciitis: how successful is surgical intervention? Foot Ankle Int 1999;20:803–807.
3. DiGiovanni BF, Abuzzahab FS Jr, Gould JS. Plantar fascia release with proximal and distal tarsal tunnel release: a surgical approach to chronic, disabling plantar fasciitis with associated nerve pain. Tech Foot Ankle Surg 2003;2:254–261.
4. DiGiovanni BF, Rodriguez del Rio FA, Gould JS. Chronic, disabling heel pain with associated nerve pain: primary and revision surgery results. Paper presented at: 17th Annual Summer Meeting of the American Orthopaedic Foot & Ankle Society; July 19–21, 2001; San Diego, CA.
5. Gollwitzer H, Saxena A, DiDomenico LA, et al. Clinically relevant effectiveness of focused extracorporeal shock wave therapy in the treatment of chronic plantar fasciitis: a randomized, controlled multicenter study. J Bone Joint Surg Am 2015;97(9):701–708.
6. Gould JS. Chronic plantar fasciitis. Am J Orthop (Belle Mead J) 2003;32:11–13.
7. Gould JS. Entrapment syndromes. In: Gould JS, ed. The Handbook of Foot and Ankle Surgery: An Intellectual Approach to Complex Problems. New Delhi, India: Jaypee Brothers, 2013:247–272.
8. Gould JS. Neuromas—acute and chronic or recurrent. In: Gould JS, ed. The Handbook of Foot and Ankle Surgery: An Intellectual Approach to Complex Problems. New Delhi, India: Jaypee Brothers, 2013:242–246.
9. Gould JS. Plantar heel pain. In: Chou LB, ed. Orthopaedic Knowledge Update: Foot and Ankle, ed 5. Rosemont, IL: American Academy of Orthopaedic Surgeons, 2014:237–247.
10. Gould JS. Recurrent tarsal tunnel syndrome. Foot Ankle Clin 2014;19(3):451–467.
11. Gould JS, Florence MN. Neuromas of the foot and ankle. Foot Ankle 2014;12.
12. Gould JS, Ford D. Orthoses and insert management of common foot and ankle problems. In: Porter DA, Schon LC, eds. Baxter's The Foot and Ankle in Sport, ed 2. Philadelphia: Mosby Elsevier, 2008: 585–593.
13. Gould JS, Naranje SM, McGwin G Jr, et al. Use of collagen conduits in management of painful neuromas of the foot and ankle. Foot Ankle Int 2013;34(7):932–940.
14. Heimkes B, Posel P, Stotz S, et al. The proximal and distal tarsal tunnel syndromes. An anatomical study. Int Orthop 1987;11:193–196.
15. Ibrahim MI, Donatelli RA, Hellman M, et al. Long-term results of radial extracorporeal shock wave treatment for chronic plantar fasciopathy: a prospective, randomized, placebo-controlled trial with two years follow-up. J Orthop Res 2017;35(7):1532–1538.
16. Keck C. The tarsal-tunnel syndrome. J Bone Joint Surg Am 1962;44:180–182.
17. Kopell HP, Thompson WA. Peripheral entrapment neuropathies of the lower extremity. N Engl J Med 1960;262:56–60.
18. Labib SA, Gould JS, Rodriguez-del-Rio FA, et al. Heel pain triad (HPT): the combination of plantar fasciitis, posterior tibial tendon dysfunction and tarsal tunnel syndrome. Foot Ankle Int 2002;23: 212–220.
19. Lam SJ. A tarsal-tunnel syndrome. Lancet 1962;2:1354–1355.
20. Lau JT, Daniels TR. Effects of tarsal tunnel release and stabilization procedures on tibial nerve tension in a surgically created pes planus foot. Foot Ankle Int 1998;19:770–777.
21. Lopez-Ben R. Imaging of nerve entrapment in the foot and ankle. Foot Ankle Clin 2011;16(2):213–224.
22. Rondhuis JJ, Huson A. The first branch of the lateral plantar nerve and heel pain. Acta Morphol Neerl Scand 1986;24:269–279.
23. Roy PC. Electrodiagnostic evaluation of lower extremity neurogenic problems. Foot Ankle Clin 2011;16(2):225–242.
24. Schon LC, Glennon TP, Baxter DE. Heel pain syndrome: electrodiagnostic support for nerve entrapment. Foot Ankle 1993;14: 129–135.
25. Wagner E, Ortiz C. The painful neuroma and the use of conduits. Foot Ankle Clin 2011;16(2):295–304.

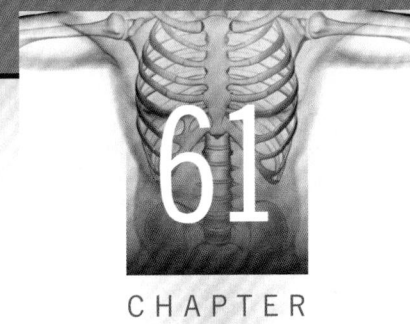

61
CHAPTER

Ankle
Supramalleolar Osteotomy with Internal Fixation:
Perspective 1

Emmanouil D. Stamatis

DEFINITION

- Ankle arthritis is characterized by loss of joint cartilage and joint narrowing.
- Primary ankle arthritis is relatively rare; most commonly, ankle arthritis is posttraumatic in origin. Inflammatory arthritides may also involve the ankle. Although ankle arthrodesis and total ankle arthroplasty are accepted surgical treatments for advanced ankle arthritis, joint-preserving supramalleolar osteotomy is an attractive alternative in select patients with advanced ankle arthritis, particularly in ankle arthritis associated with malalignment.[21]
- Supramalleolar osteotomy, whether opening or closing wedge, redistributes stresses on the ankle, transferring weight from an overloaded arthritic portion of the joint to a healthier aspect of the joint.[4,18,22,24] In theory, realignment also improves the biomechanics of the lower extremity[23] and may improve function and delay the progression of the degenerative process. Despite the fact that the later theoretical hypothesis sounds reasonable, Knupp et al[8] demonstrated, using an experimental cadaveric model, that the isolated supramalleolar varus or valgus deformities did not inevitably lead to a medial or lateral overload, respectively. They concluded that the alterations of force transmission and intra-articular pressure in the ankle joint occur with the combined alteration in both the bony alignment and the congruency of the ankle joint.[8]

ANATOMY

- The ankle joint is the articulation formed by the mortise (tibial plafond–medial malleolus and the distal part of the fibula) and the talus.
- The ankle is a modified hinge joint with a slight oblique orientation in two planes: (1) posterior and lateral in the transverse plane and (2) lateral and downward in the coronal plane.
- This sagittal plane orientation affords about 6 degrees of rotation and 45 to 70 degrees in the flexion–extension motion arc.
- The tibiotalar joint functions as part of the ankle–subtalar joint complex during gait; portions of the medial and lateral collateral ligaments cross both the ankle and subtalar joints. The blood supply is provided by the anterior and posterior tibial arteries and the peroneal artery as well as their branches and anastomoses, forming a rich vascular ring.
- The distal tibial plafond is slightly valgus oriented, in the coronal plane, with respect to the tibial diaphysis, forming an angle called the *tibial ankle surface* (TAS) with a value of 93 degrees.[13]

- The same angle in the sagittal plane, with its apex posteriorly, is called the *tibial lateral surface* (TLS), with a value of 80 degrees.[13]

PATHOGENESIS

- Idiopathic (primary) arthritis, or osteoarthrosis, is relatively rare in the ankle. The exact mechanism of cartilage degeneration and loss has not been clearly defined, although several theories have been proposed.
- Secondary arthritic involvement is mainly posttraumatic, occurring after intra-articular fractures, chondral or osteochondral injuries, and chronic instability.
- Other causes of ankle arthritis include peripheral neuropathy (neuroarthropathy) and various inflammatory disorders (such as rheumatoid arthritis, mixed connective tissue disorders, gout, and pseudogout), primary synovial disorders (pigmented villonodular synovitis), and septic arthritis as well as seronegative arthritides associated with psoriasis, Reiter syndrome, and spondyloarthropathy.
- Distal tibial deformity may be a result of malunion of a distal tibial or pilon fracture, physeal disturbance from adjacent osteochondromata, physeal dysplasia, and so forth.

NATURAL HISTORY

- Untreated ankle arthritis typically progresses, with worsening pain that eventually interferes with daily activities. Gradually, ankle stiffness in addition to pain leads to a disturbance of physiologic heel-to-toe gait.
- Low-demand patients with isolated ankle arthritis may function surprisingly well because of the adaptive effect of the healthy subtalar and transverse talar joints. However, obesity, high-demand activity levels, and concomitant subtalar or transverse tarsal joint pathology typically contribute to the morbidity of ankle arthritis.
- To our knowledge, there are no absolute numbers for tibiotalar angular alignment that predispose an ankle to the development of arthritis. Several authors have reported that angulation exceeding 10 degrees was compatible with long-term normal function and absence of pain in the ankle joint,[9,14] whereas biomechanical studies on cadavers have shown that there is a decrease of the contact surface area in the ankle joint of up to 40% in the presence of malalignment,[25,26] with the distal tibial deformities significantly altering total tibiotalar contact area, contact shape, and contact location.[25]

PATIENT HISTORY AND PHYSICAL FINDINGS

- A complete examination of the ankle and hindfoot joints should include the following:
  - Soft tissue condition: previous scars, callosities, ulcers, fistulas, and so forth
  - Vascular status: peripheral pulses, microcirculation (capillary refill), ankle–brachial index
  - Sensation: light touch and, if indicated, Semmes-Weinstein monofilament testing to rule out a peripheral neuropathy. A joint-preserving realignment supramalleolar osteotomy is feasible in select patients with peripheral neuropathy, but the potential for Charcot neuroarthropathy and failure of the procedure must be considered.
  - Stability: Anterior drawer test and inversion and eversion stress evaluations are performed to evaluate the integrity of the ankle and hindfoot ligaments. Realignment osteotomy with unstable or incompetent ankle or hindfoot ligaments may fail to improve function.
  - Motor strength: Manual motor testing of the major muscle groups is performed. Realignment in patients lacking essential motor function at the ankle will improve function in stance phase but will typically necessitate bracing for effective gait.
  - Alignment: The angle made by the Achilles and the vertical axis of the calcaneus is normally 5 to 7 degrees of valgus. Altered alignment to varus or increased valgus position indicates either abnormal tilt of the talus within the ankle mortise (eg, unicompartmental cartilage wear) or abnormality of the subtalar joint.
  - Effusion testing: Elimination or fullness of the gutters indicates intra-articular fluid accumulation or hypertrophied capsular tissue.
  - Normal ankle and hindfoot range of motion (ROM) in the sagittal plane is 20 degrees of dorsiflexion to 50 degrees of plantarflexion. Normal values of hindfoot motion are difficult to measure because the motion is triplanar. A reasonable reference is 5 degrees of eversion and 20 degrees of inversion.
    - Isolated supramalleolar osteotomy for a stiff ankle rarely improves ROM; a stiff, diffusely arthritic and malaligned ankle may be best treated with realignment.
- Hindfoot stiffness must also be documented. In patients with malaligned ankles, the hindfoot compensates. For example, a varus ankle will generally be associated with a compensating hindfoot in excessive valgus. If the hindfoot has lost its flexibility due to long-standing compensation for ankle malalignment, then supramalleolar osteotomy may realign the tibiotalar joint but create hindfoot malalignment. With a flexible hindfoot, this is generally not a problem.
- Colin et al[3] reported that the clinical "sidewalk sign" could be of significant preoperative predictive value. It is considered positive if pain improves when patient walks on a surface slope that is tilted in opposite direction of deformity.

IMAGING AND OTHER DIAGNOSTIC STUDIES

- Weight-bearing anteroposterior (AP), lateral, and mortise ankle and foot radiographs determine the extent of arthritic involvement, deformity, bone defects in the distal tibial plafond or talus, and the presence of arthritis in the adjacent hindfoot articulations. Radiographs may also suggest avascular necrosis (AVN) of the talus or distal tibia.
- With deformity, a minimum of full-length, weight-bearing AP and lateral tibial radiographs must be obtained. If more proximal deformity is suspected, then mechanical axis, full-length hip-to-ankle radiographs should be considered to accurately plan realignment. More comprehensive full-length, weight-bearing radiographs are required to measure the TAS and TLS angles, the level of center of rotation of angulation (CORA) in case of existing deformity, and the preoperative leg length discrepancy because any substantial discrepancy may have an impact to the choice of osteotomy.
- Combined single-photon emission computed tomography (SPECT) and conventional computed tomography (CT) is a rather recent imaging modality that shows a combination of metabolic and structural information about the ankle, including arthritis. Gross et al[5] reported that uptake in specific locations within the ankle joint could be associated with both clinical outcomes and might help predict which patients would have a successful supramalleolar osteotomy. Based on their findings, they cautioned against performing a supramalleolar osteotomy in patients with bipolar activation kissing lesion on both tibia and talus on a preoperative SPECT-CT scan.
- Diagnostic injection. If there is uncertainty over whether the pain is originating from the ankle or hindfoot, selective injections may be of use in distinguishing the source of pain.

DIFFERENTIAL DIAGNOSIS

- Bone marrow edema
- Soft tissue pathology
- Distal tibial plafond or talar AVN
- Osteochondritis

NONOPERATIVE MANAGEMENT

- Nonoperative treatment of ankle arthritis includes pharmacologic agents, intra-articular corticosteroid injections, shoe wear modifications, and orthoses.
- Nonsteroidal anti-inflammatory drugs (NSAIDs) are widely used and have proven efficacy in the management of arthritis, including ankle arthritis. In select patients with gastrointestinal irrigation, cyclooxygenase-2 inhibitors may offer a reasonable alternative to NSAIDs. Inflammatory arthritides are managed with immunosuppressive agents.
- Judicious use of intra-articular corticosteroid injections may temporize inflammation associated with intra-articular ankle pathology. Moreover, initial injections of the ankle or hindfoot may serve a diagnostic purpose to distinguish ankle from hindfoot pain. Indiscreet use of corticosteroid injections may have a deleterious effect on the residual joint cartilage as a result of the steroid, the anesthetic, or perhaps the accompanying preservative.
- Bracing to immobilize and support the arthritic ankle may provide some pain relief with weight bearing and ambulation. Specifically, polypropylene ankle–foot orthoses, double metal upright braces, and lace-up braces, combined with the use of a stiff-soled rocker bottom shoe, may be of benefit. Bracing tibial and tibiotalar malalignment is challenging. With a flexible hindfoot, some axial realignment may be feasible, but correction is generally not possible at the focus of deformity.

SURGICAL MANAGEMENT

- We use the supramalleolar osteotomy for the following indications[20]:
  - Realignment of distal tibia fracture malunion without or with mild osteoarthritic changes of the ankle joint
  - Realignment of distal tibia malunion with mild to moderate osteoarthritic changes of the ankle joint
  - Ankle fusion malunion
  - Ankle arthritis with deformity secondary to intra-articular trauma or AVN of the distal tibia
  - Correction of valgus deformity associated with a ball-and-socket ankle joint configuration secondary to tarsal coalition
  - Tibiotalar osteoarthritis resulting from chronic lateral ankle instability or a cavovarus foot deformity
  - Restoration of a plantigrade foot position in ankle deformity resulting from Charcot neuroarthropathy to create ankle and hindfoot alignment that may be safely braced
  - Correction of limb alignment in adolescents and young adults due to growth plate injury
  - Correction of lower limb alignment as staged planning for a total ankle replacement
- As a rule, we reserve supramalleolar osteotomy using internal fixation for mild to moderate angular deformities in the coronal or the sagittal plane. Severe angular deformities with concomitant translation of the distal segment or shortening are, in our opinion, better managed using external fixation and the principles of Ilizarov.[6]
- Moreover, gradual correction of severe deformity with formation of a regenerate avoids large plates under a wound and typically thin soft tissues that would be under tension with acute correction using internal fixation.
- Lee et al[12] warned out that a supramalleolar osteotomy is indicated for the treatment of ankle osteoarthritis in patients with minimal talar tilt and neutral or varus heel alignment.
- Comparing closing and opening wedge supramalleolar osteotomies: A closing wedge osteotomy may result in limb shortening when compared to opening wedge osteotomies. Conflicting reports exist regarding healing rates between the two methods. Studies suggest that closing wedge osteotomies exhibit delayed healing when compared to opening wedge osteotomies,[23] but other reports demonstrate more rapid healing using a closing wedge osteotomy.[18-20] One advantage of a closing wedge osteotomy is that it does not necessitate incorporation of cancellous or structural interpositional graft. Although an opening wedge osteotomy may preserve limb length, resultant skin tension from acute correction may create problems with wound healing and potential vascular compromise if the vessels are put on sudden stretch. Gradual correction with external fixation may be a safer option in cases with severe deformity.
- In the absence of appreciable preoperative leg length discrepancy, we recommend correcting distal tibial varus deformities with a medial opening wedge osteotomy and valgus deformities with a medial closing wedge osteotomy.
- Knupp et al[7] reported that the decision for the type of osteotomy was based on the amount of correction needed. Thus, in the presence of severe varus deformities, the authors preferred a lateral closing osteotomy instead of a medial opening wedge because the fibula, in the late scenario, would restrict the potential for adequate correction.[7]

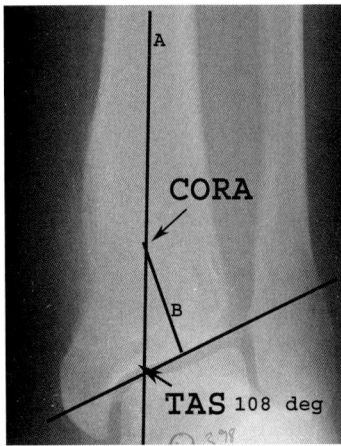

FIG 1 Preoperative AP radiograph of a patient with severe valgus malalignment of the distal tibia due to physeal disturbance from adjacent osteochondroma that was excised in a previous procedure. Note the location of center of rotation of angulation (*CORA*) at the intersection of two lines that represent the mechanical axes of the proximal (*line A*) and distal segments (*line B*). Line A, also representing the tibial mechanical axis (which in the case of the tibia coincides with the anatomic axis), and another line that is drawn to represent the distal tibial articular surface form the tibial ankle surface (*TAS*) angle on the AP view with a magnitude of 108 degrees.

Preoperative Planning

- We routinely obtain bilateral, full-length, weight-bearing radiographs of the tibia including the knee and ankle joints.
- We draw two lines on the preoperative radiographs: (1) the tibial mechanical axis (which for the tibia coincides with the anatomic axis) and (2) the distal tibial articular surface. On the AP view, the angle formed by these lines is the TAS angle (**FIG 1**). On the lateral view, these lines form the TLS angle.
- Ideally, we define the physiologic TAS and TLS angles for each patient using radiographs of the healthy contralateral limb. The goal of surgery is to realign the TAS and TLS to physiologic values and perhaps add a few degrees of (slight) overcorrection to compensate for anticipated minor subsidence during healing of the osteotomy.
- The full-length, weight-bearing radiographs serve to determine preoperative leg length discrepancy, which may influence the choice between opening and closing wedge osteotomies.
- Determining the CORA of the deformity (see **FIG 1**): The CORA is the intersection of the two lines that define the deformity, lines that are drawn to represent the mechanical axes of the proximal (line A) and distal segments (line B).
- With isolated angular deformity, the CORA is at the apex of the deformity. When translation is also present, the CORA is located proximal to the deformity.
- In very distal tibial deformities or ankle deformities with minor to moderate alterations of the TAS angle, the CORA is at the level of the ankle joint line.
- With distal tibial procurvatum deformity (malunion) or ankle fusion malunion in equinus, the CORA is the intersection of the tibial mechanical axis and a line representing the ankle's center of rotation. Typically, in such cases, the CORA is the level of the lateral process of the talus.

- Significance of the CORA: An osteotomy made at the level of the CORA, whether closing or opening, will predictably realign the ankle without translation of the distal segment and center of the ankle. If the osteotomy is not performed at the CORA, the center of the ankle will translate relative to the mechanical axis of the tibia, creating undesirable malalignment of the two segments and an unnecessary shift of loads to the ankle joint. To avoid secondary translational deformity when the osteotomy is intentionally made at a different level than the CORA, the distal segment must be translated relative to the proximal segment. These osteotomy rules apply irrespective of the method of fixation chosen.[17]

- The size of the opening wedge or closing wedge resection can be determined by drawing the desired correction angle on the preoperative radiographs and measuring the wedge size on a template, taking magnification into account.[1]

- The final step in preoperative planning is to determine the extent of compensation that is achieved by the subtalar joint before correction of the deformity. Deformities in the coronal plane are well compensated for by the subtalar joint, unless there is preoperative stiffness in the hindfoot.

- For example, a varus deformity of the tibia is compensated for by eversion of the subtalar joint. In cases of chronic deformity, this attempt to compensate and maintain the foot plantigrade may become fixed at the subtalar joint. Moreover, other adaptive changes may occur including the transverse tarsal joint or midfoot, creating a fixed forefoot deformity. These secondary fixed deformities may also require surgical correction after the ankle is realigned in order to create a functional, plantigrade foot.

- Knupp et al[7] grouped several types of asymmetric ankle arthritis into classes, depending on the degree of talar tilt in the ankle mortise, the degree of narrowing of the joint space, and the presence or not of anterior extrusion of the talus.

- Their classification along with the proposed treatment algorithm are useful in the clinical practice by means of dictating the choice of type of supramalleolar osteotomy and any concomitant procedures as well as predicting the risk factors for treatment failure. Thus, according to their algorithm, a supramalleolar osteotomy should be biplane (including an anterior opening or posterior closing wedge) in cases with anterior talar extrusion, whereas in cases with talar tilt greater than 4 degrees, additional procedures, such as soft tissue reconstruction, calcaneal osteotomy, and fibula osteotomy, are mandatory.[7]

Positioning

- The supramalleolar osteotomy is performed with the patient supine.
- A bump under the ipsilateral hip prevents the natural tendency of the lower extremity to fall into external rotation.

Approach

- The fibular osteotomy is performed first, using a small lateral incision, protecting the lateral branch of the superficial peroneal nerve.
- For the supramalleolar osteotomy, a medial skin incision is made, and periosteal elevation is performed only to the extent needed to perform the osteotomy.

MEDIAL CLOSING WEDGE SUPRAMALLEOLAR OSTEOTOMY

- Perform the fibular osteotomy first, using a small lateral incision. The osteotomy is oblique, located at the same level with the planned tibial cut. Some surgeons prefer to make the fibular osteotomy at a different level from the supramalleolar osteotomy.
- We do not routinely apply fixation to the fibular osteotomy, except in cases where it is felt that additional stability is required.
- When correcting tibial deformity, perform the osteotomy at the CORA (**TECH FIG 1**).

- In select cases, the supramalleolar osteotomy is not performed at the CORA. In some distal tibial deformities, the CORA may be located at the ankle joint, where the osteotomy is not feasible, and the translational component must be compensated. Also, in ankle deformity with only minor alterations of the TAS angle and when detrimental translation of the distal fragment is not a major concern, we generally perform the osteotomy 4 to 5 cm proximal to the medial malleolar tip.

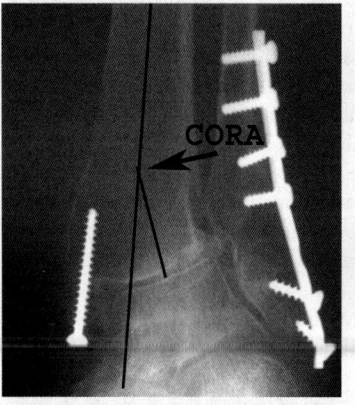
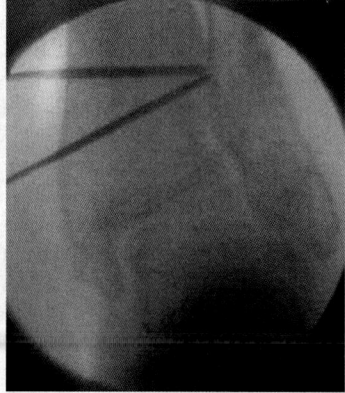

TECH FIG 1 Medial closing wedge supramalleolar osteotomy. **A.** Using a preoperative radiograph, the center of rotation of angulation (*CORA*) is located at the intersection of two lines that represent the mechanical axes of the proximal and distal segments. **B.** Under fluoroscopy, a Kirschner wire is inserted to the tibia perpendicular to the mechanical axis, and a second Kirschner wire is inserted parallel to the ankle joint line intersecting the first wire, ideally at the apex of the deformity. *(continued)*

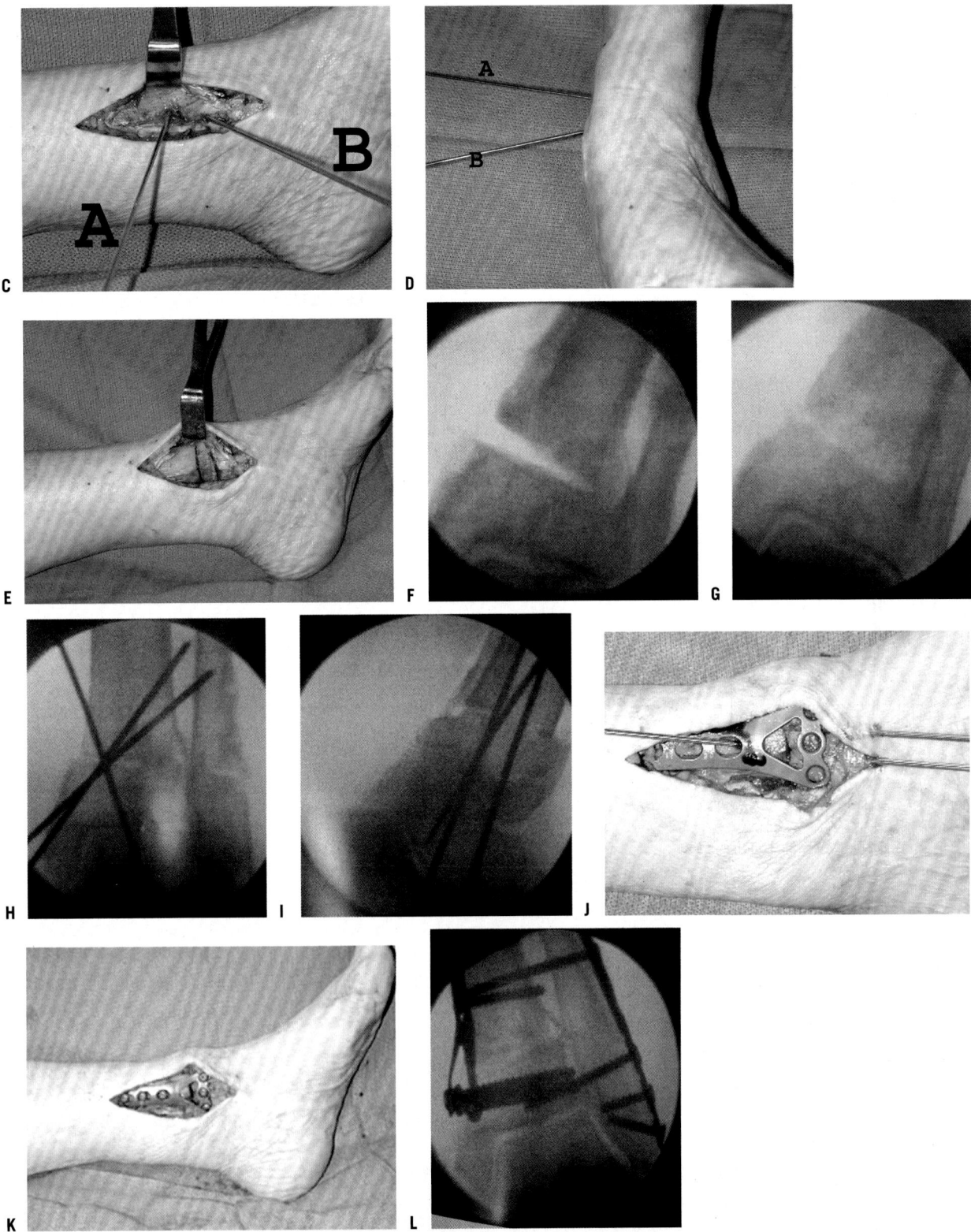

TECH FIG 1 *(continued)* **C,D.** Guide pin wires used to perform a closing medial wedge osteotomy. *Pin A* has been inserted to the tibia perpendicular to the mechanical axis, and *pin B* has been inserted parallel to the ankle joint line, intersecting *pin A* at the apex of the deformity. **E.** The cut wedge. The pins have been used as a guide for the tibial cuts, whereas the size of the wedge has been determined during the preoperative planning. **F.** Fluoroscopic view of the resected wedge. **G.** Fluoroscopic view of the closed osteotomy. **H,I.** Fluoroscopic AP and lateral views of the provisionally fixed osteotomy with Kirschner wires. **J.** Photo of the applied periarticular plate. Note the excellent fit on the distal tibia. **K.** The applied periarticular plate after completion of fixation with three screws in the distal segment. **L.** Fluoroscopic view of the osteotomy after completion of fixation.

- We routinely use Kirschner wires to define our proposed osteotomy; for an opening wedge osteotomy, we use a single Kirschner wire, but for the medial closing wedge osteotomy, two Kirschner wires are required to define the tibial wedge resection. Under fluoroscopic guidance, insert the first Kirschner wire perpendicular to the mechanical axis and the second parallel to the ankle joint, intersecting the first Kirschner wire at the apex of the deformity. The size of the wedge has been determined during the preoperative planning, and the Kirschner wires are positioned 1 to 2 mm wider than the proposed osteotomy, so they can be left in place as a guide for the saw cuts. Although the Kirschner wires define the osteotomy in one plane, the surgeon must also orient the saw blade perpendicular to the tibial shaft axis when performing the osteotomy. With the anterior and posterior soft tissue and neurovascular structures protected, we routinely use a broad oscillating saw, constantly irrigating the blade with cooled sterile saline or water to limit osteonecrosis. Ideally, a thin cortical bridge and periosteal sleeve on the opposite cortex will be preserved to allow for a greenstick-like closure of the osteotomy that facilitates maintenance of alignment and enhances stability. However, when the osteotomy is intentionally performed at a level different than that of CORA, then the opposite cortex must be violated to allow the distal segment to be translated.
- After removing the resected wedge and performing appropriate translation of the distal segment, close the osteotomy and

provisionally fix it with Kirschner wires. The provisional fixation may be guidewires for intended cannulated screws or it must be positioned so as not to interfere with the definitive fixation. Assess alignment of the tibia and ankle fluoroscopically, in both the AP and lateral planes.

- Several dedicated low-profile periarticular plating systems for the distal tibia are marketed, both locking and nonlocking. The majority of these plates were designed for the contours of the physiologic tibia. With a wedge resection, the fit is typically acceptable but may not be perfect. Locking plates may provide optimal stability, but if the osteotomy is not fully closed, these may in fact delay or even hinder healing. Nonlocking plates, in our opinion, allow for a small amount of settling at the osteotomy with weight bearing, potentially facilitating healing. (If additional stability is required, then cannulated or solid screws may be used from the tip of the medial malleolus across the osteotomy. Alternatively, a second plate may be added anteriorly on the tibia to provide rotational control to the tibia; however, this requires greater soft tissue dissection.)
- We do not routinely apply fixation to the fibula, but if additional stability is required, then we apply a low-profile fibular plate.
- Final fluoroscopic images in the AP and lateral planes confirm proper alignment, apposition of the osteotomy, and position of hardware.

MEDIAL OPENING WEDGE SUPRAMALLEOLAR OSTEOTOMY

- Again, the osteotomy is ideally located at the level of the CORA **(TECH FIG 2)**. If the CORA is located at the ankle joint level or if only minor correction is required and translation of the distal segment is of little concern, then we perform the osteotomy 4 to 5 cm proximal to the medial malleolar tip.
- We perform either a horizontal or slightly oblique (proximal medial to distal lateral) tibial osteotomy with a broad oscillating saw, preserving the opposite cortex and periosteal sleeve

to serve as a fulcrum for the opening wedge and to enhance stability. If translation is necessary (the osteotomy is intentionally performed at a level different than that of CORA), then the opposite cortex is cut completely to allow the distal segment to move.

- Under fluoroscopy, gently distract the tibial osteotomy using a lamina spreader or alternative distraction system until desired correction is achieved.

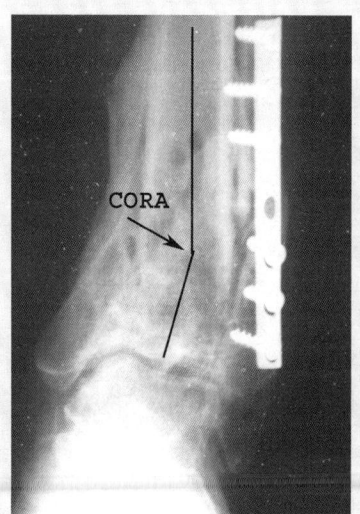
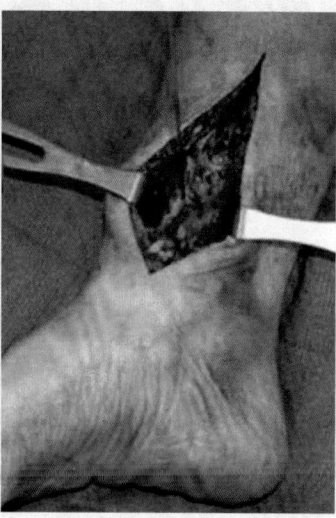

CORA

A   B

TECH FIG 2 Medial opening wedge supramalleolar osteotomy. **A.** Using a preoperative radiograph, the center of rotation of angulation (*CORA*) is located at the intersection of two lines that represent the mechanical axes of the proximal and distal segments. **B.** Under fluoroscopy, a Kirschner wire is used to mark the osteotomy site at the CORA level. *(continued)*

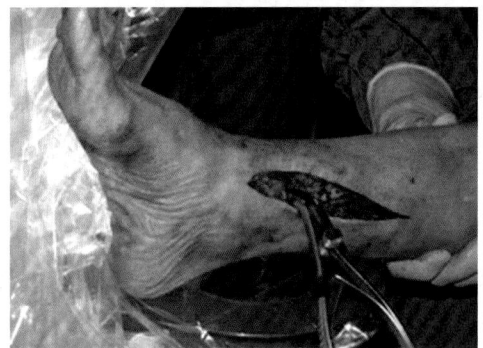

C

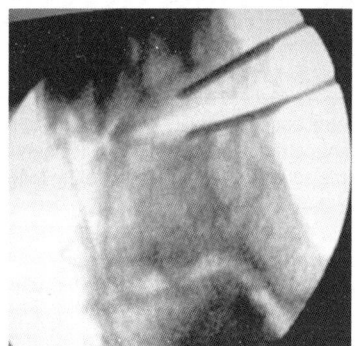

D

TECH FIG 2 *(continued)* **C,D.** Under fluoroscopy, the tibial osteotomy is gently distracted using a lamina spreader until desired correction is achieved. (**A,C,D:** Reprinted from Myerson MS. Osteotomy of the tibia and fibula. In: Myerson MS, ed.Reconstructive Foot and Ankle Surgery. Philadelphia: Elsevier, 2005:254. Copyright © 2005 Elsevier. With permission.)

- We routinely use contoured structural graft (generally, the neck portion of a femoral head allograft) to fill the osteotomy.
- After correcting the deformity, provisionally fix the osteotomy with Kirschner wires in a manner that does not interfere with the definitive fixation. Assess the alignment using fluoroscopy, both in the AP and lateral planes.
- Several dedicated low-profile periarticular plating systems for the distal tibia are marketed, both locking and nonlocking. The majority of these plates were designed for the contours of the physiologic tibia. With an opening wedge osteotomy, the fit is typically acceptable but may not be perfect. Locking plates may provide optimal stability, but if the osteotomy is not fully closed, these may in fact delay or even hinder healing. Nonlocking plates, in our opinion, allow for a small amount of settling at the osteotomy with weight bearing, potentially facilitating incorporation of the interpositional graft. (If additional stability is required, then cannulated or solid screws may be used from the tip of the medial malleolus across the osteotomy. Alternatively, a second plate may be added anteriorly on the tibia to provide rotational control to the tibia; however, this requires greater soft tissue dissection.)

WOUND CLOSURE

- After completing the fixation, close the wound routinely in layers. With opening wedge osteotomies, the skin tension is typically greater than before surgery, but with longitudinal incisions, this is rarely problematic. Use of a drain is at the discretion of the surgeon; we do not routinely use a drain.

TECHNIQUES

Pearls and Pitfalls

Fixation	• We recommend internal fixation for supramalleolar osteotomies in mild to moderate corrections. Complex and severe deformity may be best managed with external fixation and Ilizarov principles. Multiplanar correction with external fixation effectively manages angular and translational deformity and simultaneously compensates for potential loss of limb length. If there is no significant preoperative leg length discrepancy, then all varus deformities are corrected using a medial opening wedge osteotomy, whereas the valgus deformities are corrected with a medial closing wedge osteotomy.
Exposure	• Minimal periosteal elevation preserves vascularity at the osteotomy site.
Osteotomy Level	• A closing or opening wedge osteotomy at the level of the CORA will lead to complete realignment of the foot and ankle. If the osteotomy is made proximal or distal to the CORA, the distal segment and center of the ankle will translate relative to the mechanical axis of the tibia. When the osteotomy must be performed at a level different than the CORA, then the osteotomy must be completed on the lateral cortex and translated along with the angular correction. These osteotomy rules apply irrespective of the method of fixation chosen.
Fixation of the Osteotomy	• In our experience, medial plating is typically adequate for fixation of opening or closing wedge supramalleolar osteotomies. However, additional stability may be gained with (1) screws from the tip of the medial malleolus that cross the osteotomy or (2) supplemental anterior plating. No fixation is applied to the fibular osteotomy, except in cases where it is felt that additional stability is required.

Graft Choice	• The graft alternatives are to harvest it from the ipsilateral iliac crest or the proximal tibia or to use tricortical allograft.[2] The two basic types of bone grafts are structural and cancellous. A structural bone graft is one that alters the shape during a reconstruction procedure by virtue of its size and dimension. The structural bone graft provides immediate mechanical support, with little likelihood of collapse even after the resorption that occurs during revascularization. Some structural integrity remains during the process of bone graft incorporation to allow the graft to withstand loads.
Locked versus Nonlocked Plates	• Locked plating affords optimal stability; however, if the plate is locked with suboptimal bony contact at the osteotomy site, then there may be a delay in osteotomy healing or incorporation of a structural graft. Nonlocked plating permits some settling during weight bearing that may promote healing of the osteotomy, provided stability is satisfactory.

POSTOPERATIVE CARE

- The procedure may be performed on an outpatient basis, but we routinely keep the patient overnight for monitoring and pain control (23-hour observation status).
- Although rare, a tibial osteotomy, albeit distal to the lower leg muscles, could potentially create a compartment syndrome, and therefore, overnight monitoring is prudent. All patients are discharged with a non–weight-bearing postoperative splint, are instructed to maintain elevation of the extremity, and are to return to the clinic 2 weeks after surgery for suture removal.
- At 2 weeks, we routinely place the patient in a removable, prefabricated cam walker boot. If we have concern for the osteotomy stability or patient compliance, we obtain radiographs at this time to ensure satisfactory alignment and fixation, and place the patient into a short-leg non–weight-bearing cast.
- The patient returns at 6 weeks from surgery, at which time we routinely obtain simulated weight-bearing radiographs of the ankle. Depending on the stability of fixation and evidence for progression toward healing, we allow the patient to progressively advance weight bearing in the cam walker boot.
- Typically, with follow-up at 10 weeks from surgery, full weight bearing is permitted in the cam walker boot, with a rapid transition to a regular shoe, provided that weight-bearing radiographs of the ankle suggest satisfactory healing. Early ROM exercises without resistance are initiated early (at 2 weeks), when osteotomy fixation is deemed stable and if there is no concomitant procedure[10] (eg, ligament reconstruction or tendon transfer) dictating adjustment of the rehabilitation protocol.

OUTCOMES

- Several studies have shown that the overall outcome of supramalleolar osteotomy is very good in terms of pain relief, correction of any existing mechanical malalignment, and the arresting of arthritic changes in the ankle joint.[4,11,15,16,18,22,23]
- The type of osteotomy (opening vs. closing wedge) does not influence the final outcome, even though a closing wedge osteotomy may lead to leg length discrepancy or decreased strength.[18]
- The type of osteotomy (opening vs. closing wedge) has no influence on the time of osseous healing.[18]

COMPLICATIONS

- Nonunion
- Delayed union

- Over- or undercorrection of the deformity
- Decreased postoperative ROM
- Failure to perform the osteotomy at the level of CORA, thus translating the distal fragment and center of the ankle away from the mechanical axis
- Failure to perform the appropriate translation of the distal segment, in cases where the osteotomy is intentionally performed at a different level than that of CORA (such as when the CORA is at the level or distal to the ankle joint), leading to mechanical axis shifting

ACKNOWLEDGMENT

- I would like to thank my mentor Mark S. Myerson for his enlightening training, friendship, and help for the preparation of this chapter.

REFERENCES

1. Acevedo JI, Myerson MS. Reconstructive alternatives for ankle arthritis. Foot Ankle Clin 1999;4:409–430.
2. Borrelli J Jr, Leduc S, Gregush R, et al. Tricortical bone grafts for treatment of malaligned tibias and fibulas. Clin Orthop Relat Res 2009;476:1056–1063.
3. Colin F, Bolliger L, Horn Lang T, et al. Effect of supramalleolar osteotomy and total ankle replacement on talar position in the varus osteoarthritic ankle: a comparative study. Foot Ankle Int 2014;35(5):445–452.
4. Graehl PM, Hersh MR, Heckman JD. Supramalleolar osteotomy for the treatment of symptomatic tibial malunion. J Orthop Trauma 1987;1:281–292.
5. Gross CE, Barfield W, Schweizer C, et al. The utility of the ankle SPECT/CT scan to predict functional and clinical outcomes in supramalleolar osteotomy patients. J Orthop Res 2018;36(7):2015–2021.
6. Horn DM, Fragomen AT, Rozbruch SR. Supramalleolar osteotomy using external fixation with six-axis deformity correction of the tibia. Foot Ankle Int 2011;32:986–993.
7. Knupp M, Stufkens SA, Bolliger L, et al. Classification and treatment of supramalleolar deformities. Foot Ankle Int 2011;32:1023–1031.
8. Knupp M, Stufkens SA, van Bergen C, et al. Effect of supramalleolar varus and valgus deformities on the tibiotalar joint: a cadaveric study. Foot Ankle Int 2011;32:609–615.
9. Kristensen KD, Kiaer T, Blicher J. No arthrosis of the ankle 20 years after malaligned tibial-shaft fracture. Acta Orthop Scand 1989;60:208–209.
10. Lee HS, Wapner KL, Park SS, et al. Ligament reconstruction and calcaneal osteotomy for osteoarthritis of the ankle. Foot Ankle Int 2009;30:475–480.
11. Lee KB, Cho YJ. Oblique supramalleolar opening wedge osteotomy without fibular osteotomy for varus deformity of the ankle. Foot Ankle Int 2009;30:565–567.
12. Lee WC, Moon JS, Lee K, et al. Indications for supramalleolar osteotomy in patients with ankle osteoarthritis and varus deformity. J Bone Joint Surg Am 2011;93:1243–1248.
13. Mangone PG. Distal tibial osteotomies for the treatment of foot and ankle disorders. Foot Ankle Clin 2001;6:583–597.

14. Merchant TC, Dietz FR. Long-term follow-up after fractures of the tibial and fibular shafts. J Bone Joint Surg Am 1989;71(4): 599–606.
15. Neumann HW, Lieske S, Schenk K. Supramalleolar, subtractive valgus osteotomy of the tibia in the management of ankle joint degeneration with varus deformity [in German]. Oper Orthop Traumatol 2007;19:511–526.
16. Pagenstert GI, Hintermann B, Barg A, et al. Realignment surgery as alternative treatment of varus and valgus ankle osteoarthritis. Clin Orthop Relat Res 2007;462:156–168.
17. Paley D, Herzenberg JE, Tetsworth K, et al. Deformity planning for frontal and sagittal plane corrective osteotomies. Orthop Clin North Am 1994;25:425–465.
18. Stamatis ED, Cooper PS, Myerson MS. Supramalleolar osteotomy for the treatment of distal tibial angular deformities and arthritis of the ankle joint. Foot Ankle Int 2003;24:754–764.
19. Stamatis ED, Myerson M. Supramalleolar osteotomy for the treatment of distal tibial angular deformities and arthritis of the ankle joint. Tech Foot Ankle Surg 2004;3:138–142.
20. Stamatis ED, Myerson MS. Supramalleolar osteotomy: indications and technique. Foot Ankle Clin 2003;8:317–333.
21. Swords MP, Nemec S. Osteotomy for salvage of the arthritic ankle. Foot Ankle Clin 2007;12:1–13.
22. Takakura Y, Takaoka T, Tanaka Y, et al. Results of opening-wedge osteotomy for the treatment of a post-traumatic varus deformity of the ankle. J Bone Joint Surg Am 1998;80(2):213–218.
23. Takakura Y, Tanaka Y, Kumai T, et al. Low tibial osteotomy for osteoarthritis of the ankle. Results of a new operation in 18 patients. J Bone Joint Surg Br 1995;77(1):50–54.
24. Tanaka Y, Takakura Y, Hayashi K, et al. Low tibial osteotomy for varus-type osteoarthritis of the ankle. J Bone Joint Surg Br 2006;88(7): 909–913.
25. Tarr RR, Resnick CT, Wagner KS, et al. Changes in tibiotalar joint contact areas following experimentally induced tibial angular deformities. Clin Orthop Relat Res 1985;(199):72–80.
26. Ting AJ, Tarr RR, Sarmiento A, et al. The role of subtalar motion and ankle contact pressure changes from angular deformities of the tibia. Foot Ankle 1987;7:290–299.

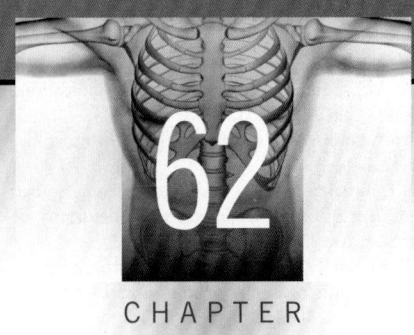

62
CHAPTER

Supramalleolar Osteotomy with Internal Fixation:
Perspective 2

Markus Knupp and Beat Hintermann

DEFINITION

- A supramalleolar osteotomy is an osteotomy at the level of the distal tibia with or without osteotomy of the fibula.
- The correction is intended to normalize altered load distribution across the joint and may be indicated in cases of asymmetric osteoarthritis, malunited fractures of the distal tibia, osteochondral lesions, and recurrent instability with deformity.

ANATOMY

- Trauma and neurologic disorders leading to varus or valgus alignment around the ankle joint predispose to asymmetric joint load.
- This causes cartilage wear, in particular in the presence of associated ligamentous instability and muscular imbalance.

PATHOGENESIS

- Various conditions such as neurologic disorders, congenital and acquired foot deformities, posttraumatic malunions, and instability may be associated with malalignment of the ankle joint complex.

NATURAL HISTORY

- Malalignment of the hindfoot may result from bony deformities above or below the level of the ankle joint.
- Ligamentous instability or muscular imbalance of the ankle or the adjacent joints may be a contributing or even an initiating factor in the natural history of malalignment around the ankle joint.

PATIENT HISTORY AND PHYSICAL FINDINGS

- A thorough medical history should be taken.
  - Systemic diseases such as diabetes mellitus (Charcot arthropathy), rheumatoid arthritis, and neurovascular disorders need to be assessed carefully.
  - Tobacco use should be considered a relative contraindication to supramalleolar osteotomy.
  - Disorders that alter the bone quality and healing capacity (medication, osteoporosis, age) should be assessed carefully.
- Physical examination should include the following:
  - Drawer test and talar tilt test to assess ankle joint stability
  - Assessment of the inversion and eversion force to exclude peroneal tendon insufficiency
  - Subtalar range of motion
  - Coleman block test to exclude a forefoot-driven hindfoot varus

IMAGING AND OTHER DIAGNOSTIC STUDIES

- Weight-bearing radiographs of the entire foot, the ankle, the tibial shaft (full-length radiographs), and a hindfoot alignment view are necessary to assess the nature and location of the deformity. Unless deformity at the level of the knee joint or the femur can be excluded clinically, whole lower limb radiographs are obtained.
- Next to conventional radiography, computed tomography and magnetic resonance imaging are not routinely required. However, they could be of value when assessing rotational malalignment, osteochondral lesions, and peroneal tendon disorders or evaluating the aspect of the ligament insufficiency.
- Combined single-photon emission and conventional computed tomography has been found to be a valuable tool for the assessment and staging of osteoarthritis in asymmetric osteoarthritis of the ankle joint.

DIFFERENTIAL DIAGNOSIS

- Symmetric or end-stage osteoarthritis
- Muscular imbalance (eg, in neurologic disease)
- Forefoot-driven hindfoot deformities

NONOPERATIVE MANAGEMENT

- Asymptomatic, moderate malalignment usually is treated conservatively.
- Malalignment that is due to forces from the neighboring structures, such as plantarflexed first metatarsal or unbalanced muscle forces, can be treated with physiotherapy or shoe wear modifications. Deforming forces, such as forefoot abnormalities or muscular imbalance, may require surgical procedures other than supramalleolar osteotomies.
- Recommendations whether surgical or conservative therapy should be aimed for in asymptomatic but severe malaligned hindfeet are controversial. Because the deformity is likely to lead to excessive wear, surgery should be considered.
- An alternative surgical treatment is the calcaneal displacement osteotomy (medial or lateral). Commonly, however, correction of malalignment is best performed at the level of the deformity.

SURGICAL MANAGEMENT

- Supramalleolar osteotomies are divided into opening/closing wedge osteotomies and dome-shaped osteotomies.
- Ideally, the correction is carried out at the center of rotation of angulation (CORA), preferably in the metaphyseal bone.
- For deformities that cannot be corrected at the CORA as well as for large corrections, a dome-shaped osteotomy should be considered in order to avoid excessive translation of the distal fragment.
- Congruent joints should be considered for dome-shaped osteotomies; incongruent joints usually qualify for wedge osteotomies.
- In case of a wedge osteotomy
  - Valgus deformities are usually addressed with a medial closing wedge osteotomy.
  - Varus malalignment is corrected with a medial opening wedge osteotomy or a lateral closing wedge osteotomy.
- For all corrections of the distal tibia, a correction of the length and position of the fibula must be considered in order to preserve ankle joint congruency.

Preoperative Planning

- The most important aspect of the preoperative planning is the assessment of the origin of the deformity. Different entities need to be distinguished, and it is mandatory to separate single-plane deformities from combined deformities in the sagittal, frontal, and transverse plane with or without muscular dysfunction and imbalanced ligamentous structures.
- In frontal plane deformities distinction of congruent and incongruent joints **(FIG 1)** is helpful in determining the type of osteotomy performed (tibia only vs. tibia and fibula; wedge osteotomy vs. dome-shaped osteotomy).
- To determine the size of the wedge that should be added or removed to restore anatomic alignment in the ankle, the tibiotalar angle should be measured.
  - On a standard anteroposterior image of the ankle joint, the tibiotalar angle is the angle between the tibial axis and the tibial joint surface. The wedge to be corrected can be measured out of the radiographs or calculated with the mathematical formula tan α = H / W, where α is the angle to be corrected, H is the wedge height in millimeters, and W is the tibial width **(FIG 2)**.
  - An overcorrection of 3 to 5 degrees is recommended by most authors for asymmetric osteoarthritis.
- Additional deviation (eg, rotational or translational deformities) must be taken into consideration during the planning of the osteotomy.

Positioning

- Positioning of the patient depends on the surgical approach:
  - Anterior approach: supine position
  - Lateral approach: lateral decubitus position or supine with a sandbag under the buttock of the affected limb
  - Medial approach: supine, ipsilateral knee in slight flexion with a sandbag under the calf

Approach

- An anterior, lateral, or medial approach can be chosen to correct the deformity. The choice depends on the nature of the deformity, the local soft tissue conditions, and previous approaches.

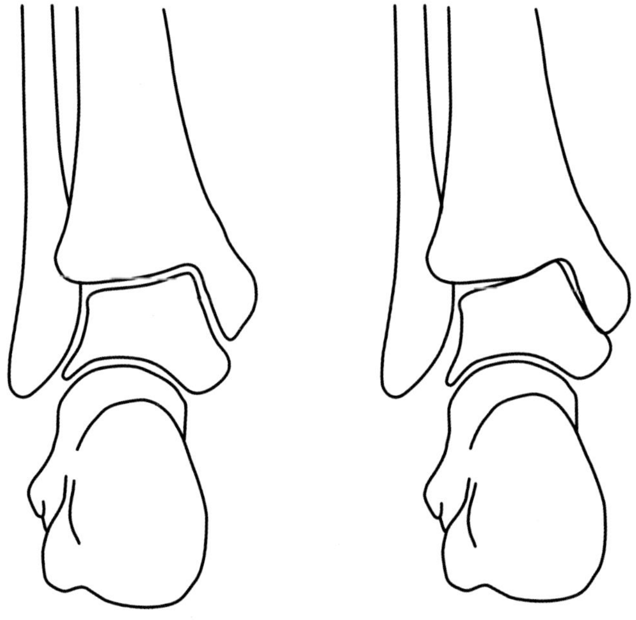

FIG 1 An illustration of a congruent (*left*) and an incongruent (*right*) joint. In congruent joints, the joint space between tibia and talus is parallel despite the distal tibial joint surface angle being in a varus or valgus deviation. In incongruent joints, the talus is tilted within the ankle mortise.

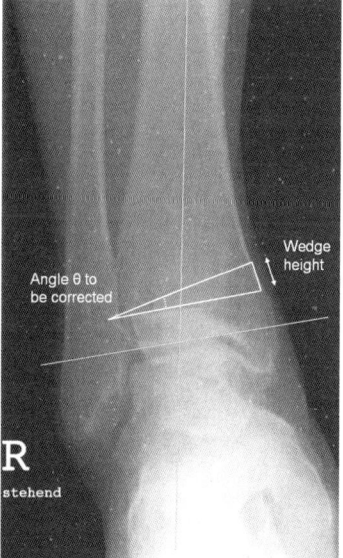

FIG 2 Planning of the correction: measuring the deformity and planning the wedge size that should be inserted (*lower line of the white triangle* indicating the level of the osteotomy).

LATERAL CLOSING WEDGE OSTEOTOMY TO CORRECT VARUS

Exposure

- After exsanguination of the leg, a pneumatic tourniquet is inflated on the thigh.
- A 10-cm longitudinal, slightly curved incision is made along the anterior margin of the distal fibula. If the incision needs to be extended distally, it is curved ventrally to end just distal to and anterior of the lateral malleolus **(TECH FIG 1)**.
- The fibula and the tibia are then exposed laterally. To avoid devascularization of the bone, stripping of the periosteum is not performed.
- At the distal end of the incision, the anterior syndesmosis is exposed.
- The lateral branch of the sural nerve and the short saphenous vein run dorsal to the line of incision and are usually not seen during this procedure. However, extended proximal dissection may require identification, exposure, and protection of the branches of the superficial peroneal nerve. Cauterization of some of the branches of the peroneal artery, which lie deep to the medial surface of the distal fibula, may be necessary.

Fibular Osteotomy

- In most cases in which a varus deformity is addressed with a lateral closing wedge osteotomy, the fibula needs to be shortened to preserve the congruency in the ankle joint. The shortening can be done by simple bone block removal or a Z-shaped osteotomy. Alternatively, an oblique osteotomy (distal anterior to proximal posterior) can be used, although the Z-shaped fibular osteotomy confers greater control of rotation and primary stability compared to a block resection for fibular shortening.
- The length of the Z-shaped fibular osteotomy is approximately 2 to 3 cm, starting distally at the level of the anterior syndesmosis.
- Kirschner wires (K-wires) can be placed as a reference at the level of the transverse cuts to confirm the location of the osteotomy fluoroscopically.
- The osteotomy is then carried out with an oscillating saw.
- After the fibula has been mobilized, bone blocks are resected on both ends of the Z based on the amount of the planned shortening **(TECH FIG 2)**.

- To avoid interference from the dense syndesmotic ligaments when performing the Z-osteotomy, we routinely direct the proximal transverse cut anteriorly and the distal cut (which typically sits at the syndesmosis) posteriorly.

Lateral Closing Wedge Tibial Osteotomy

- To define the desired osteotomy, two K-wires are drilled through the tibia, with the tips converging at the medial cortex, making sure that the angle between the K-wires corresponds with the preoperative planning (see **TECH FIG 2**).
  - Unless the deformity is located proximal to the supramalleolar area, the wires are directed from proximal to the anterior syndesmosis to the medial physeal scar **(TECH FIG 3A)**.
- After fluoroscopic verification of the location of the wires **(TECH FIG 3B)**, the periosteum is incised only at the level of the planned osteotomy and carefully mobilized with a scalpel or periosteal elevator.
- The osteotomy is then performed using an oscillating saw cooled with saline or water irrigation to limit thermal injury to bone.
- Placing the K-wires accurately avoids cutting through the medial cortex; ideally, the medial cortex should serve as a hinge.
- Correction of the deformity must be performed at the CORA of the deformity to avoid relative translational malpositioning of the distal (ankle) and proximal (tibial shaft) fragments.
- The gap is then closed and the osteotomy is secured with a plate. We prefer locking plates that afford optimal primary stability; however, it is imperative that the osteotomy is completely closed when employing locking plate technology **(TECH FIG 3C,D)**.

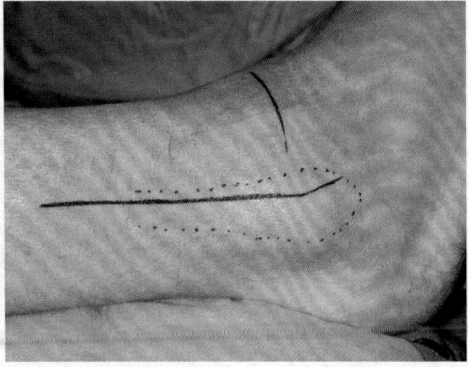

TECH FIG 1 Lateral approach to the distal fibula and tibia.

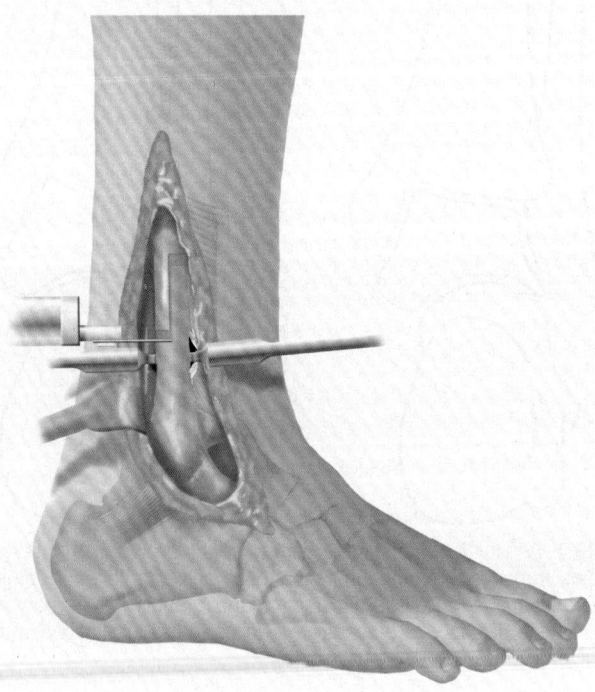

TECH FIG 2 Drawing illustrating the Z-shaped osteotomy to shorten the fibula.

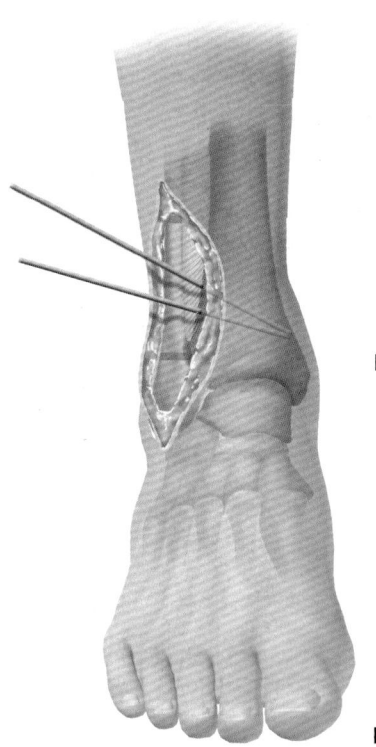

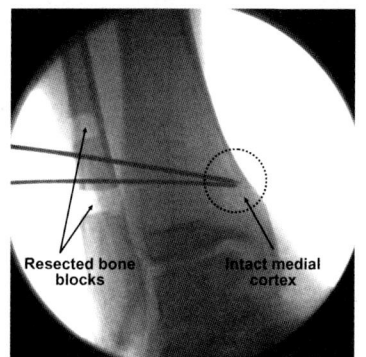

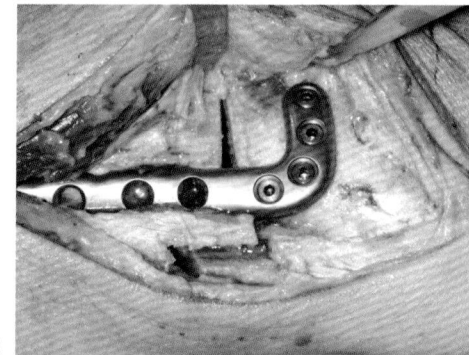

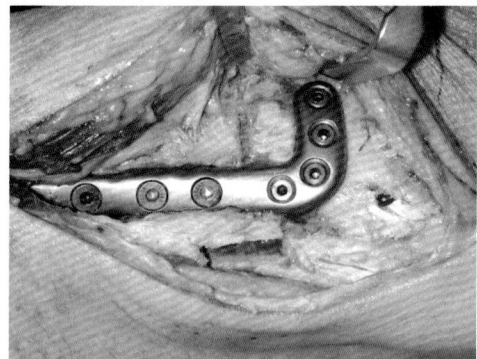

TECH FIG 3 A. Placement of the K-wires for guidance of the osteotomy. **B.** Intraoperative radiograph showing the guidewires for the tibial osteotomy after the Z-shaped fibula osteotomy. Distal tibia/fibula before (**C**) and after (**D**) closure of the osteotomy. Note the shortening of the fibula.

- Prior to locking the plate both proximal and distal to the osteotomy, we use a tensioning device to optimally compress the osteotomy.
- We routinely close the periosteum over the osteotomy with 2-0 absorbable sutures.

Optimizing Joint Congruity and Securing the Fibula

- Fluoroscopically, optimal tibiotalar joint congruity and fibular osteotomy reduction are determined.
- Once the joint is congruent, the fibula is secured with screws (in the longitudinal limb of the Z-osteotomy) or a one-third tubular plate (**TECH FIG 4**).
- The subcutaneous tissues and the skin are closed with interrupted sutures.

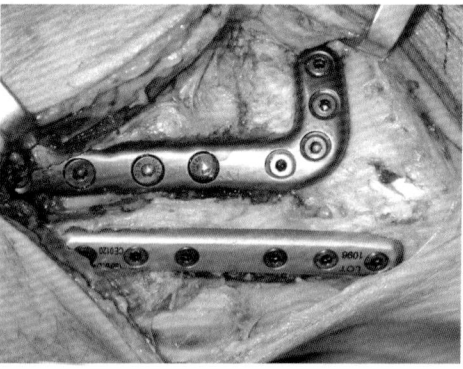

TECH FIG 4 Fixation of the fibula with a plate.

MEDIAL OPEN WEDGE OSTEOTOMY FOR CORRECTION OF VARUS DEFORMITY

Exposure

- The limb is exsanguinated and the thigh tourniquet is inflated.
- The anterior incision is made anteriorly over the distal tibia and ankle, immediately lateral to the tibial crest. The superficial peroneal nerve crosses the distal aspect of the incision and must be protected.
- The extensor retinaculum is then divided longitudinally to expose the extensor tendons. The approach uses the interval between the tibialis anterior and extensor hallucis longus tendons.

- A longitudinal incision in the extensor retinaculum is made between the anterior tibial tendon and the extensor hallucis longus tendon, starting 10 cm proximal to the joint, about midway between the malleoli (**TECH FIG 5**).
- The anterior tibial tendon is retracted medially and the tendon of the extensor hallucis longus is retracted laterally, if possible, without opening the tendon sheaths.
- The deep neurovascular bundle (anterior tibial artery and deep peroneal nerve), located in the lateral aspect of the approach, must be identified and protected.

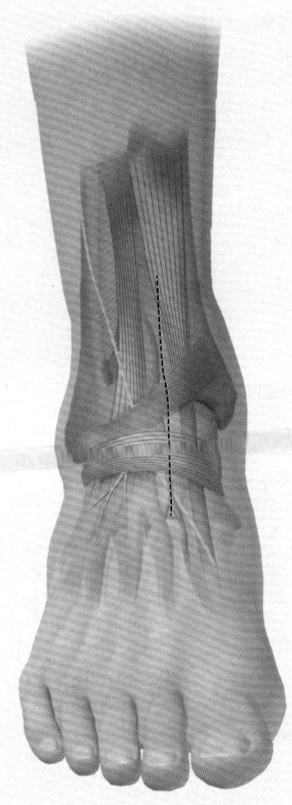

TECH FIG 5 Anterior approach to the distal tibia with the interval between the extensor hallucis longus and the anterior tibial tendon and the neurovascular bundle lying lateral to it.

- The ankle joint is covered by an extensive fat pad that contains a venous plexus and requires partial cauterization.
- If tibiotalar joint débridement or exostectomy is required, we make an anterior capsulotomy at this time. If only a supramalleolar osteotomy is planned, however, there is no need to expose the joint.
- With all soft tissues and neurovascular structures protected, the anterior surface of the tibia can be exposed. To promote healing of the osteotomy, periosteal stripping should be limited to the osteotomy site.
- The osteotomy is carried out as described in the Tibial Osteotomy section

Medial Approach

- The patient is positioned supine on the operating table; a bump placed under the contralateral hip may improve exposure.
- The limb is exsanguinated, and the tourniquet is inflated.
- The great saphenous vein and the saphenous nerve usually lie anterior to the incision. A 10-cm longitudinal incision is made, beginning over the medial malleolus and extending proximally over the distal tibia **(TECH FIG 6A)**.
- The skin flaps are mobilized, with care taken not to damage the neurovascular bundle, which runs along the anterior border of the medial malleolus **(TECH FIG 6B)**.
- The posterior tibial tendon, which lies immediately on the posterior aspect of the medial malleolus, must be identified and retracted posteriorly. It needs to be exposed, its sheath incised, and the tendon retracted posteriorly to visualize the dorsal surface of the distal tibia.

Tibial Osteotomy

- The tibia is exposed with minimal periosteal stripping **(TECH FIG 7A)**.
- The plane of the osteotomy is determined under image intensification, and a K-wire is placed from the medial cortex into the physeal scar or, in case of a malunion, at the apex of the deformation **(TECH FIG 7B)**.
- The periosteum is then incised at the level of the osteotomy and elevated off the bone using a scalpel or a periosteal elevator. The osteotomy must be planned carefully because placing it inaccurately may lead to relative translation of the distal and proximal fragments, resulting in malalignment of the ankle joint under the tibial shaft axis.

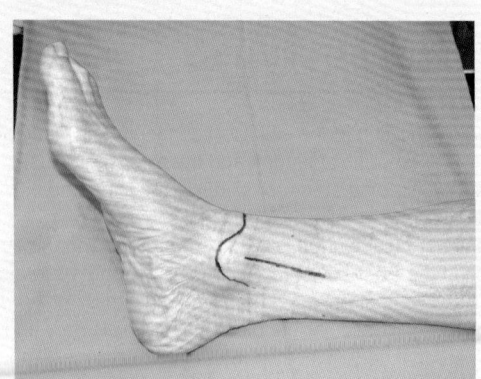

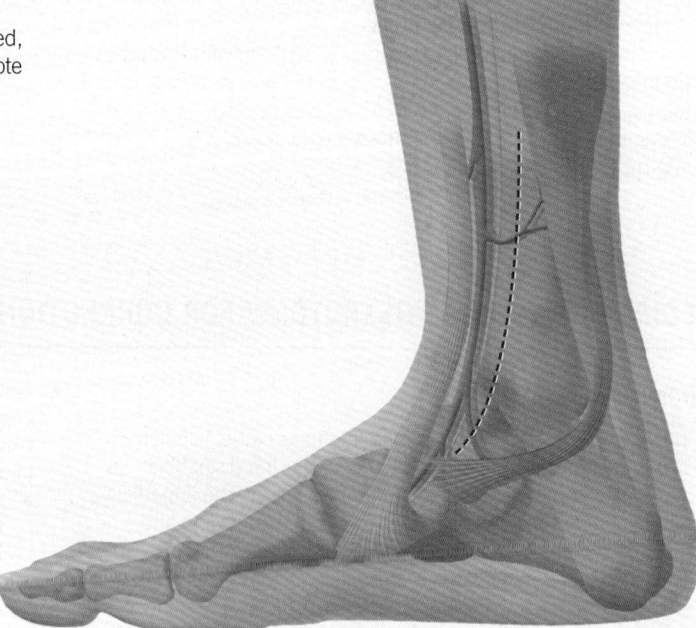

A   B

TECH FIG 6 A,B. Medial approach to the distal tibia.

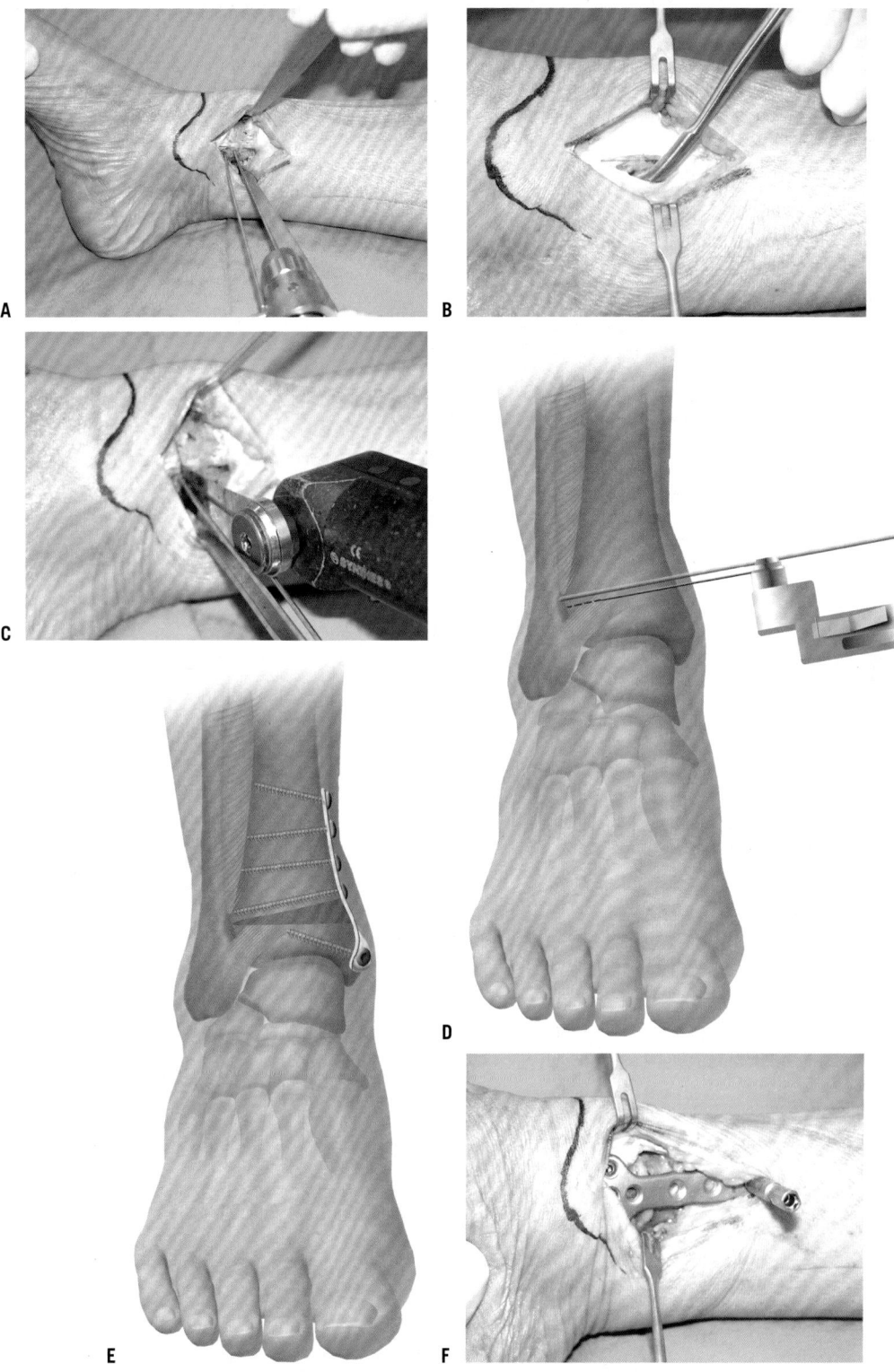

TECH FIG 7 A. Intraoperative picture of the K-wire placement. **B.** Incision and careful stripping of the periosteum. **C.** Osteotomy of the tibia with an oscillating saw. **D.** Drawing of the saw cut for a medial opening wedge osteotomy. **E.** Fill the gap. **F.** Plate fixation of the osteotomy.

TECHNIQUES

- We recommend using a wide saw blade to create a congruent osteotomy **(TECH FIG 7C,D)**.
  - Alternatively, a chisel or osteotome may be used instead of the oscillating saw to limit thermal injury to bone.
- The correction is based on preoperative planning.
- The gap can be filled with allograft (we use Tutoplast Spongiosa [Tutogen Medical GmbH, Neunkirchen, Germany]) or autograft iliac crest bone **(TECH FIG 7E)**.
- We typically secure the osteotomy with a medial locking plate, but plates with an integrated spacer (eg, Puddu plate [Arthrex, Inc., Naples, FL]) can be used instead **(TECH FIG 7F)**.
- Fixation of the osteotomy is as described earlier in the Lateral Closing Wedge Osteotomy to Correct Varus section.
- The tendon sheath of the posterior tibial tendon is reapproximated with 2-0 absorbable sutures, and the subcutaneous tissues and the skin are closed with interrupted sutures. Do not overtighten the posterior tibial tendon sheath because it may create stenosing flexor tenosynovitis.
- Case results are shown in **TECH FIG 8**.

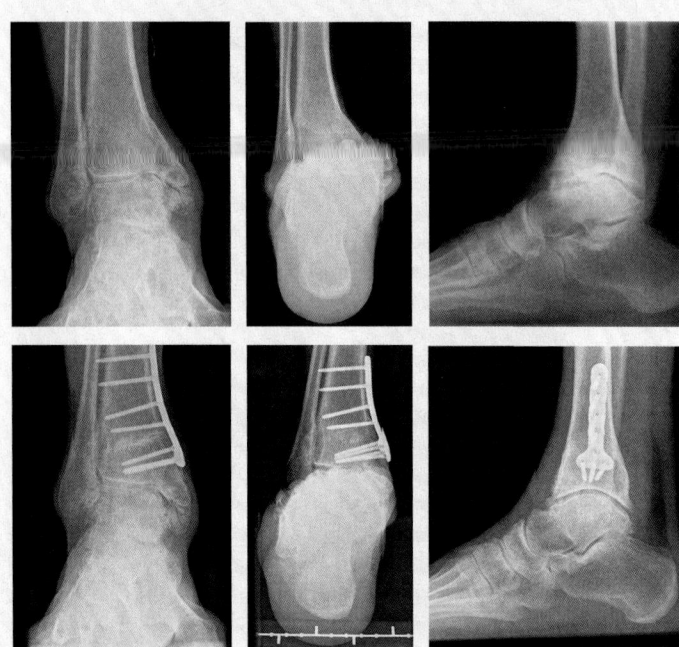

TECH FIG 8 Pre- and postoperative radiographs (weight-bearing anteroposterior, lateral, and Saltzman views, respectively) of a 62-year-old male patient with varus osteoarthritis of his ankle joint. The postoperative images are made 1 year after a medial opening wedge osteotomy.

MEDIAL CLOSING WEDGE OSTEOTOMY FOR CORRECTING VALGUS MALALIGNMENT

- The technique essentially is the same as for the opening wedge osteotomy described in the previous section with removal of a bone wedge.
- K-wire placement is done according to the planned correction **(TECH FIG 9A)**.
- The bone wedge is then removed **(TECH FIG 9B)** and the correction secured with a medial plate.
- A clinical example is shown in **TECH FIG 10**.

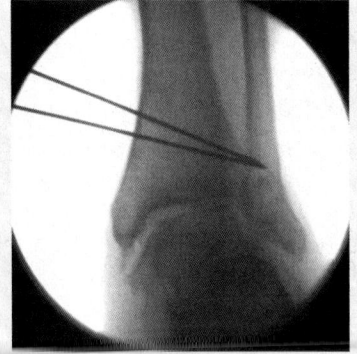
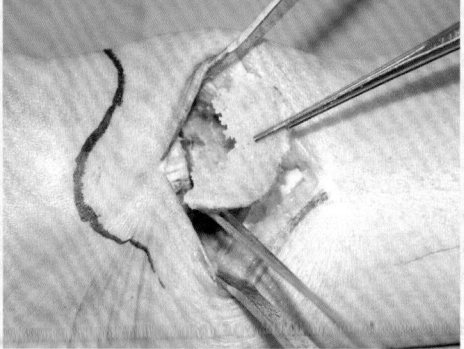

TECH FIG 9 A. K-wire placement for a medial closing wedge osteotomy. **B.** Wedge removal in a medial closing osteotomy.

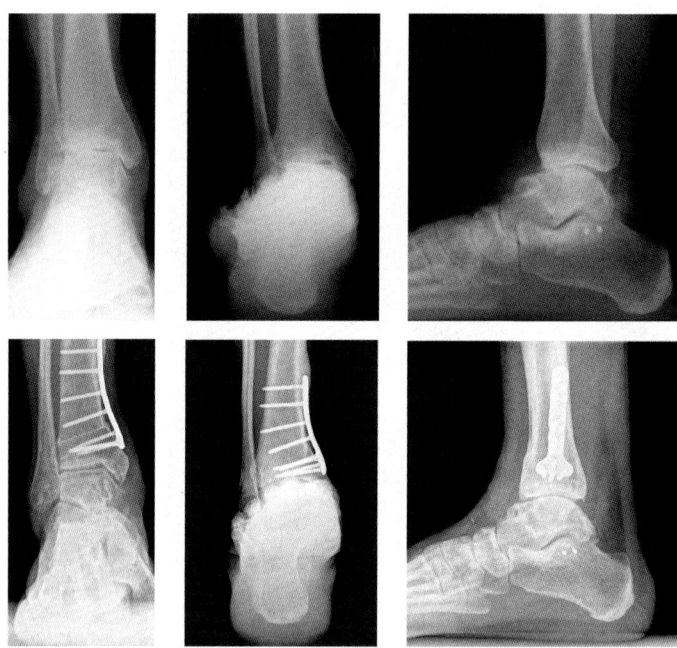

TECH FIG 10 Pre- and postoperative radiographs (weight-bearing anteroposterior, lateral, and Saltzman views, respectively) of a 58-year-old male patient with valgus osteoarthritis of his ankle joint. The postoperative images are made 1 year after a medial closing wedge osteotomy.

DOME-SHAPED OSTEOTOMY

- An anterior approach is used.
- The level of the osteotomy usually lies at the metaphyseal level, above the tibiofibular syndesmosis.
- A marking pen can be used to mark the osteotomy of the tibia and the planned angular correction.
- Multiple 2-mm drill holes along the osteotomy line are made **(TECH FIG 11A)**. The osteotomy is then completed with a 5-mm chisel **(TECH FIG 11B)**.
- Prior to mobilization of the osteotomy, the original position of the distal fragment in relation to the proximal fragment is marked on the anterior surface of the tibia (use a marking pen or the electrocautery to mark the bone) **(TECH FIG 11C)**.

- The fibula is exposed through a separate lateral incision and then osteotomized as described in the Fibular Osteotomy section.
- The osteotomy is mobilized, the deformity corrected as preoperatively planned, and a 2.5-mm K-wire introduced from the medial malleolus to preliminarily secure the correction.
- The correction of the tibia is secured with one T-shaped plate or two straight (one medial and one lateral plate) plates with interlocking screws.
- The length and position of the fibula is then adjusted under fluoroscopic control and the fibula secured with an additional plate or with two screws **(TECH FIG 11D)**.

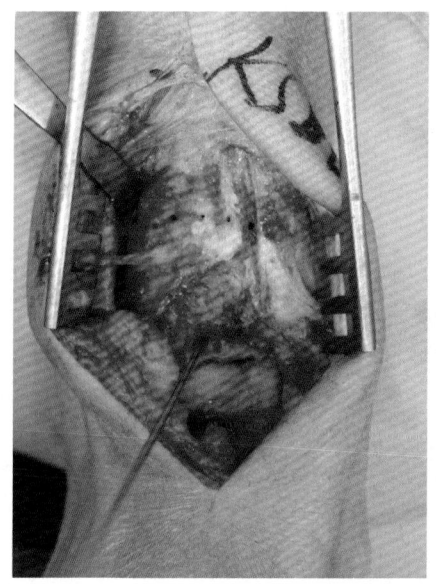

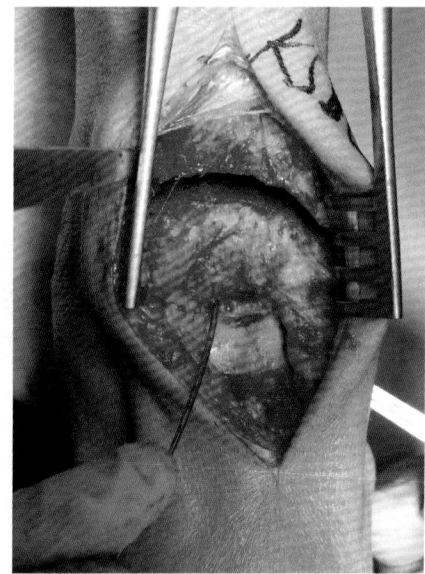

TECH FIG 11 A. Intraoperative image showing the marking of the center of rotation (K-wire) and the drill holes along the osteotomy line. **B.** Image after completion of the osteotomy with a chisel. *(continued)*

A   B

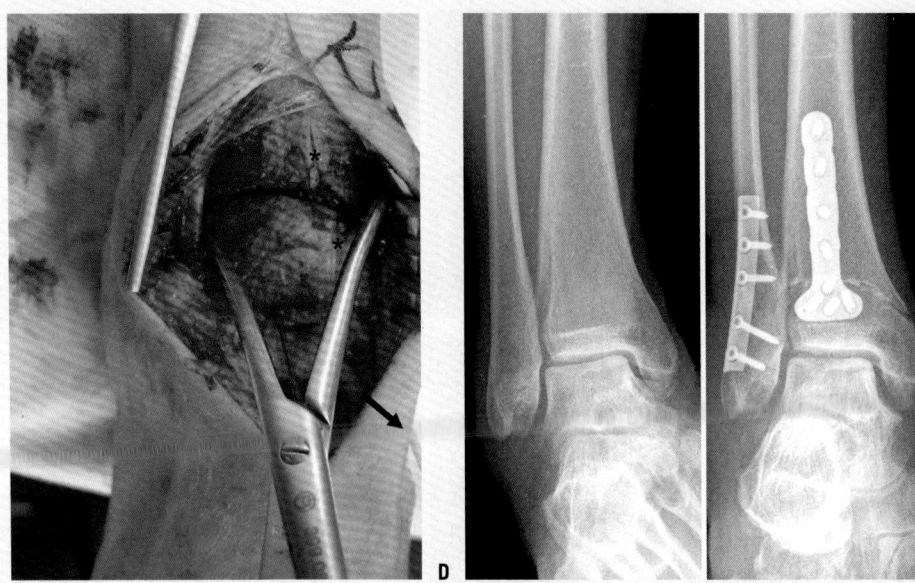

TECH FIG 11 *(continued)* **C.** Image after correction of the deformity. Note the electrocautery markings on the tibial cortex *(asterisks)* and the 2.5-mm K-wire in the medial malleolus *(arrow)*, which was used as a joystick to correct the deformity and then for preliminary fixation of the correction. **D.** Preoperative *(left)* and postoperative *(right)* radiographs of a 46-year-old patient with congruent varus arthritis of his ankle joint. The correction was fixed with a T-shaped plate for the tibia and a third tubular plate for the fibula.

SUPRAMALLEOLAR OSTEOTOMY FOR SAGITTAL PLANE CORRECTION

- Correction can be done by a wedge osteotomy through an anterior approach or a lateral approach. Alternatively, a dome-shaped osteotomy is done through a combined medial (tibia) and a lateral (fibula) approach.
- The level of the osteotomy is at the CORA or in the metaphyseal area in wedge osteotomies.
- In a sagittal dome-shaped osteotomy, the center of correction is chosen according to the desired correction (isolated

sagittal plane correction vs. sagittal plane correction with anterior/posterior translation). Most commonly, it lies close to the rotational center of the talus.
- Anterior opening wedge osteotomy
  - The level is marked with a K-wire **(TECH FIG 12A)**.
  - The osteotomy is carried out with an oscillating saw. Care is taken not to violate the posterior cortex.

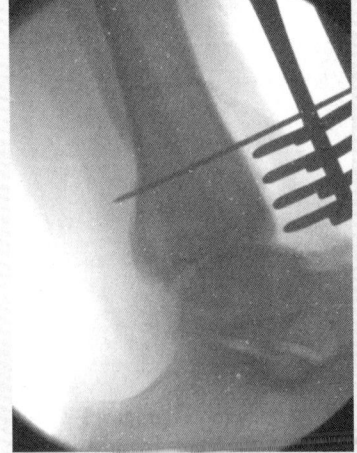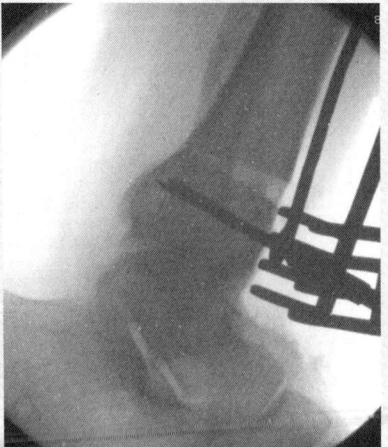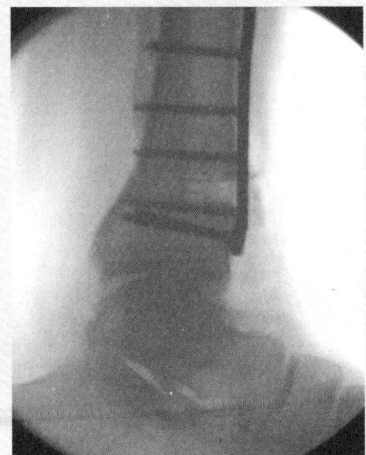

TECH FIG 12 A. Intraoperative image showing the marking of the center of rotation (K-wire). **B.** Image after the osteotomy and anterior wedge impaction. **C.** Anterior plate fixation of the correction. *(continued)*

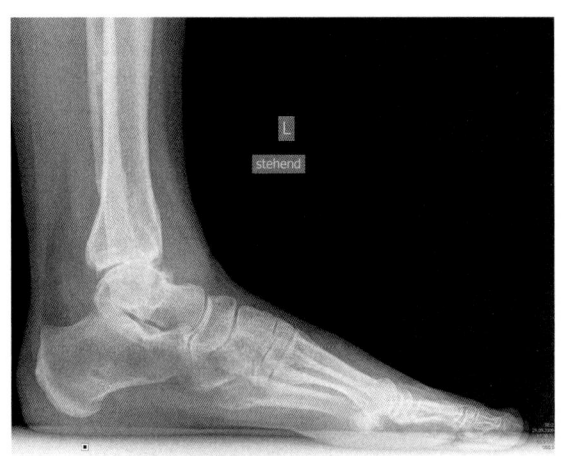

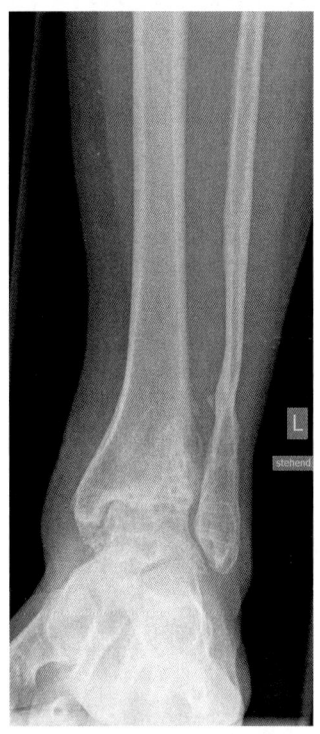

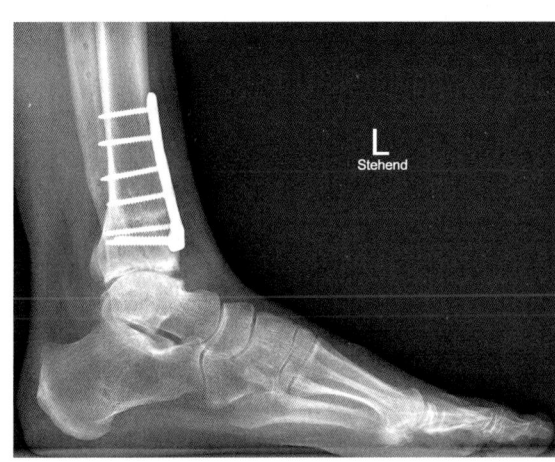

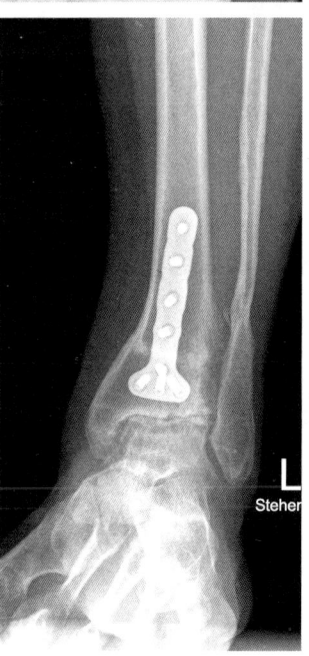

TECH FIG 12 *(continued)* Preoperative (**D,E**) and 1-year postoperative images (**F,G**) of a 48-year-old lady with posttraumatic anterior ankle arthritis and a recurvatum of the distal tibia.

- The osteotomy is carefully opened with a chisel or with a Hintermann spreader (**TECH FIG 12B**).
- The void can be filled with cancellous bone graft or allograft (**TECH FIG 12C**).
- The correction is secured with an anterior plate (**TECH FIG 12D–G**).

- Correction of the fibula usually is necessary in all dome-shaped osteotomies and may be necessary in wedge osteotomies.
- The fibula is exposed through a separate lateral incision and is osteotomized as described in the Fibular Osteotomy section.
- Appropriate length and positioning are verified under fluoroscopy and the fibula subsequently secured with screws or a plate.

Pearls and Pitfalls

Laceration of the Posterior Tibial Tendon	• For lateral osteotomies and dome-shaped osteotomies in posttraumatic cases with extensive scarring on the posteromedial aspect of the ankle, it may be necessary to expose the tendon through a minimal incision to protect it.
Accidental Cutting through the Entire Tibia in Wedge Osteotomies	• This loss of the hinge mechanism of the far cortex introduces the risk for rotational or translational malpositioning and postoperative displacement of the osteotomy. • Consider additional fixation with a second plate in a second plane.
Mobilization of the Syndesmosis	• In select cases, the syndesmosis needs to be mobilized to maintain congruent tibiotalar joint alignment. We do this by releasing the anterior syndesmotic ligaments from the anterolateral distal tibia, immediately proximal to the ankle joint. The ligaments are released by removing Chaput tubercle from the anterolateral distal tibia using an osteotome or chisel. Once the osteotomy is secured and the fibula is reduced to the desired position to create a congruent ankle joint, the syndesmosis is stabilized at its new resting tension by reattaching Chaput tubercle with a screw and a washer or with transosseous sutures.
Loss of Reduction of the Osteotomy	• The risk can be lowered by using implants that provide angular stability and by leaving a hinge of bone and periosteum at the far cortex when performing the tibial osteotomy to achieve a controlled correction in the desired plane.

POSTOPERATIVE CARE

- The leg is elevated in the immediate postoperative period.
- A compressive dressing and splint are maintained for 2 days to diminish swelling.
- A short-leg non–weight-bearing cast is used for 6 to 8 weeks.
- If radiologic evidence of consolidation is present after 6 weeks, partial weight bearing is allowed for 2 weeks, after which the patient advances gradually to full weight bearing.
- A rehabilitation program for strengthening, gait training, and range of motion is prescribed 8 weeks after surgery, with gradual return to full activities as tolerated.

OUTCOMES

- We have been observing our first series of 94 patients with a varus or valgus deformity of the ankle joint for 43 months (range of 12 to 126 months).
- At the radiographic assessment after 12 months, all osteotomies showed complete consolidation. Pain reduction was found in all patients, which is similar to earlier reports. Improved radiographic osteoarthritis scores were noted in 75% of the patients. Additionally, patients exhibited a trend toward normalization of gait and function.

COMPLICATIONS

- Apart from perioperative complications such as delayed wound healing problems or infection, postoperative concerns include delayed union or nonunion of the osteotomy.
- Another potential complication is malunion, resulting from inaccurate alignment of the osteotomy at the time of surgery or postoperative loss of position.
- Intraoperative complications include nerve or tendon injury. We ensure that all adjacent neurovascular structures and tendons are identified and protected.

SUGGESTED READINGS

Knupp M. The use of osteotomies in the treatment of asymmetric ankle joint arthritis. Foot Ankle Int 2017;38(2):220–229.

Knupp M, Stufkens SA, Bolliger L, et al. Classification and treatment of supramalleolar deformities. Foot Ankle Int 2011;32(11):1023–1031.

Knupp M, Stufkens SA, van Bergen CJ, et al. Effect of supramalleolar varus and valgus deformities on the tibiotalar joint: a cadaveric study. Foot Ankle Int 2011;32(6):609–615.

Krähenbühl N, Zwicky L, Bolliger L, et al. Mid- to long-term results of supramalleolar osteotomy. Foot Ankle Int 2017;38(2):124–132.

Myerson MS, Zide JR. Management of varus ankle osteoarthritis with joint-preserving osteotomy. Foot Ankle Clin 2013;18(3):471–480.

Pagenstert GI, Hintermann B, Barg A, et al. Realignment surgery as alternative treatment of varus and valgus ankle osteoarthritis. Clin Orthop Relat Res 2007;462:156–168.

Pagenstert GI, Knupp M, Valderrabano V, et al. Realignment surgery for valgus ankle osteoarthritis. Oper Orthop Traumatol 2009;21(1):77–87.

Scheidegger P, Horn Lang T, Schweizer C, et al. A flexion osteotomy for correction of a distal tibial recurvatum deformity: a retrospective case series. Bone Joint J 2019;101-B(6):682–690.

Stamatis ED, Cooper PS, Myerson MS. Supramalleolar osteotomy for the treatment of distal tibial angular deformities and arthritis of the ankle joint. Foot Ankle Int 2003;24(10):754–764.

Stufkens SA, van Bergen CJ, Blankevoort L, et al. The role of the fibula in varus and valgus deformity of the tibia: a biomechanical study. J Bone Joint Surg Br 2011;93(9):1232–1239.

Takakura Y, Takaoka T, Tanaka Y, et al. Results of opening-wedge osteotomy for the treatment of a post-traumatic varus deformity of the ankle. J Bone Joint Surg Am 1998;80(2):213–218.

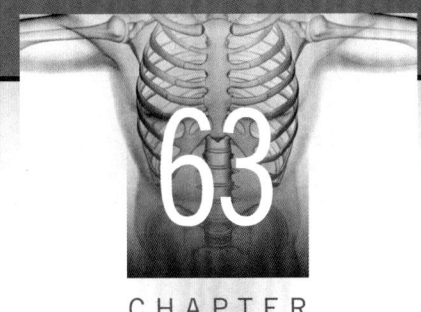

63 CHAPTER

Total Ankle Shell Allograft Reconstruction

Michael E. Brage and Joan R. Williams

DEFINITION

- Articular defects of the tibiotalar joint, posttraumatic arthritis, and osteoarthritis can limit activity, make walking difficult, and lead to severe pain.
- Unlike the knee and hip, primary arthritis rarely affects the ankle. The most common causes of degenerative changes in the ankle are secondary to trauma and abnormal ankle mechanics. Posttraumatic arthritis is correlated to the severity of the fracture pattern and nonanatomic reduction of articular surfaces.[20]
- Rheumatoid or other inflammatory arthropathies and infection can also cause significant ankle pain, deformities, and arthritis.
- Osteoarthritis is described by degradation of the articular cartilage, subchondral sclerosis, and subchondral cyst and osteophyte formation. Changes seen on radiographs include joint space narrowing, osteophytes, and subchondral bone sclerosis.
- Treatment options for patients who fail to respond to conservative treatment for ankle arthrosis are tibiotalar arthrodesis, total ankle arthroplasty, and fresh ankle osteochondral shell allografts.[1,2,10,12,13,18] Tibiotalar osteochondral shell allografts are a reasonable alternative to tibiotalar arthrodesis and total ankle arthroplasty in young patients with posttraumatic ankle arthropathy.[10,13,18]

ANATOMY

- The ankle joint is complex, but its complexity may be simplified if the ankle is thought of as a single-axis joint in an oblique path from medial to lateral and oriented downward and backward. The main motion is dorsiflexion and plantarflexion, with some inversion and eversion of the tibiotalar joint.[3]
- The bones that make up the ankle joint are the tibia, fibula, and talus. The tibia plafond is concave anteroposteriorly and mediolaterally.
- The talus has no muscular or tendinous attachments, and 60% of its surface is covered by articular cartilage.
- In addition to the bony support of the ankle, the medial and lateral ligamentous complexes provide stability to the ankle and hindfoot.

PATHOGENESIS

- The predominant collagen in articular cartilage is type II collagen. Articular cartilage has limited blood supply, cannot proliferate, and has little reparative potential.

- Type 1 injury to articular cartilage involves microscopic disruption of chondrocytes and the extracellular matrix, whereas type 2 injuries involve macroscopic damage to the surface. Because the subchondral bone is not involved in these injuries, there is little inflammatory response and therefore poor healing of these injuries. Type 3 injuries involve the subchondral bone as well as the surface and thus heal with a fibrocartilage, consisting mainly of type I collagen.[16]
- Ankle arthritis may cause loss of motion, pain, deformity, and instability.

NATURAL HISTORY

- Tibiotalar arthritis may result from trauma, inflammatory diseases, and osteoarthritis. Posttraumatic arthritis is the most common cause of ankle arthritis despite advances in open reduction and internal fixation of ankle and pilon fractures. Most likely, the tibiotalar chondral surfaces are injured at the time of injury and do not have the capacity to heal.
- Posttraumatic tibiotalar arthrosis often fails to respond to nonoperative management, and definitive surgical treatment has been ankle arthrodesis in a majority of patients and total ankle arthroplasty in select patients.[1,2,6,8,12,18]
- Ankle arthrodesis has been shown to alleviate pain in the arthritic ankle. However, loss of range of motion, functional limitation, and secondary progressive arthritis in the hindfoot and midfoot have been found in long-term follow-up studies on patients with isolated ankle arthrodesis.[2,7]
- Current total ankle prosthetic designs are a promising alternative to arthrodesis, but the patient's age has an adverse effect on the risk of failure and reoperation rate.[11,17,18]
- Osteochondral shell allografting, in which the tibial plafond and talar dome are replaced with a donor ankle matched for size, affords relief of pain, congruent articular surfaces, maintenance of bone stock, and preservation of surrounding joints. Recent improvements in surgical techniques and experience with allografts have improved short-term outcomes with this technique. Recent studies advocate the use of fresh osteochondral allografting as an alternative treatment for selected individuals with end-stage tibiotalar arthrosis.[10,13,21]

PATIENT HISTORY AND PHYSICAL FINDINGS

- A thorough history and physical examination of both lower extremities must be performed for any deformities or malalignment to identify multiple joint involvement, symmetric involvement, family history, and a history of trauma. The function and stability of the ligaments and tendons surrounding the ankle should be tested. This includes assessment for an equinus contracture or pes planus or pes cavus deformities. A neurovascular examination must also be performed before surgery.

- Physical examination methods include the following[15]:
  - Anterior drawer test to evaluate the anterior talofibular ligament and ankle stability. The surgeon should look for a difference of 3 to 5 mm in the relationship between the lateral talus and the anterior aspect of the fibula.
  - Inversion stress test to evaluate talar instability (somewhat difficult due to subtalar motion). Compared to the contralateral ankle, a difference of more than 15 degrees is significant.
  - Equinus contracture assessment. A gastrocnemius recession or Achilles lengthening procedure may be required concomitantly if there is 5 degrees of equinus in the ankle.
  - Range of motion. Normal total range of motion of the tibiotalar joint is from 20 degrees of dorsiflexion to 50 degrees of plantarflexion. Normal subtalar joint motion is about 20 degrees from maximal inversion to eversion.
- Contraindications for shell allograft ankle reconstruction are as follows:
  - Diminished peripheral pulses
  - Varus or valgus malalignment of the tibiotalar joint of more than 10 degrees
  - Instability of the ankle joint

IMAGING AND OTHER DIAGNOSTIC STUDIES

- Weight-bearing radiographs of the ankle, including anteroposterior (AP), lateral, and mortise views, are obtained (**FIG 1**).
- When indicated, AP stress radiographs may be obtained to confirm instability. Anterior translation between the talus and tibia of 3 to 5 mm greater than the contralateral ankle indicates instability.[3]
- Talar tilt on stress radiographs with the ankle internally rotated 30 degrees: A difference greater than 15 degrees compared to the contralateral ankle indicates instability.[3]

DIFFERENTIAL DIAGNOSIS

- Ankle instability or deformities
- Anterior or posterior impingement syndrome
- Osteochondritis dissecans (OCD) lesions of talus or tibia
- Subtalar joint osteoarthritis
- Sinus tarsi syndrome

NONOPERATIVE MANAGEMENT

- Conservative treatment includes mechanical aids (such as ankle–foot orthoses and shoe modifications), anti-inflammatories, and intra-articular steroid injections.

SURGICAL MANAGEMENT

- For young healthy individuals who need alleviation of pain and retention of motion and function, osteochondral shell allografts represent an alternative to ankle arthrodesis and total ankle replacement.

Preoperative Planning

- Standard radiographs on the ankle are needed for preoperative planning. In our opinion, an external fixator or distraction device is useful during the operation. We routinely use the DePuy Agility (DePuy, Warsaw, IN) ankle arthroplasty cutting block to increase the precision of cuts.
- Size-matched osteochondral allografts, based on radiographs, are procured from one of several regional tissue banks.

Positioning

- The patient is supine on a radiolucent operating table.

Approach

- A standard anterior approach to the ankle is used between the tibialis anterior and extensor hallucis longus tendons while protecting the superficial peroneal nerve. The deep neurovascular bundle (deep peroneal nerve and anterior tibial and dorsalis pedis artery) is retracted laterally and dissection is carried through the joint capsule to expose the ankle.

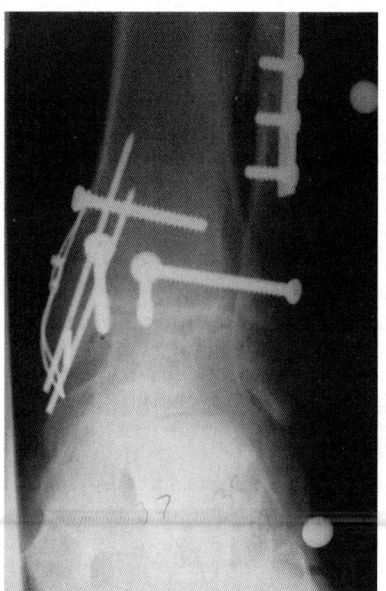 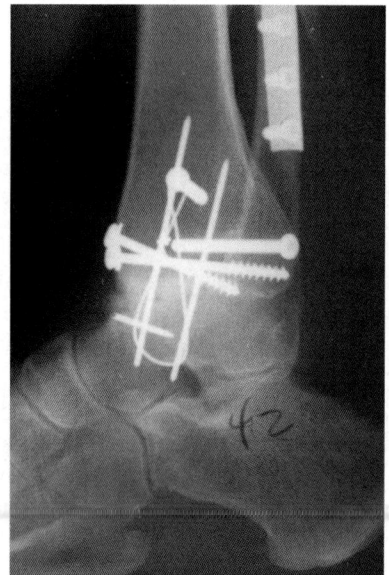 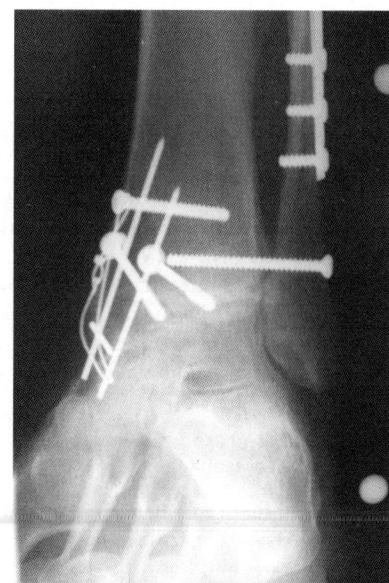

A   **B**   **C**

FIG 1 **A.** Preoperative AP radiograph. **B.** Lateral view. **C.** Mortise view. (Courtesy of Dr. Michael Brage.)

DÉBRIDEMENT AND DISTRACTION OF THE ANKLE JOINT

- Through the anterior approach, excise synovitis and remove osteophytes using rongeurs and osteotomes. Next, apply an external fixator to distract the joint symmetrically about 1 cm (**TECH FIG 1**).

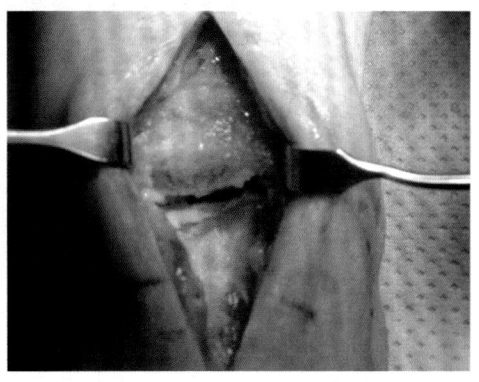

TECH FIG 1 Débridement and distraction of the ankle joint. (Courtesy of Dr. Michael Brage.)

TIBIAL AND TALAR CUTS

- Although we always procure a complete ankle joint, careful inspection of the arthritic ankle may indicate that complete joint replacement may not be warranted. Occasionally, we perform only hemi-joint resurfacing but with the disadvantage of loss of optimal articular congruency afforded by a complete or bipolar joint replacement. We determine the ideal Agility cutting block by templating the ankle radiographs. Pin the corresponding Agility ankle arthroplasty cutting block into place over the anterior ankle (**TECH FIG 2A**). Confirm placement and size with intraoperative fluoroscopy (**TECH FIG 2B**).

- Using a blunt reciprocating saw, resect the tibial plafond and talar dome to a thickness of about 7 to 10 mm.
- Remove an articular portion of the medial malleolus (about 3 to 4 mm) as well.
- Take extreme care as the posterior tibial neurovascular bundle is close to the posteromedial corner of the ankle joint.
- On the lateral aspect of the tibial cut, take care to avoid contact with the fibula to keep it fully preserved.

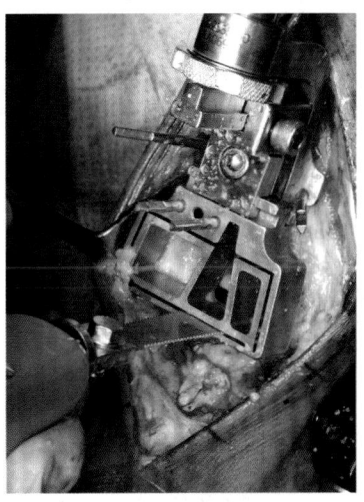
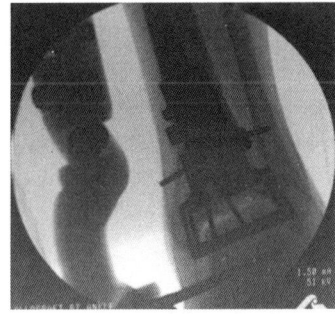

A   B

TECH FIG 2 Tibial and talar cuts. **A.** Ankle arthroplasty jig is placed over tibia and pinned into place. **B.** Cutting jig size and placement are confirmed with fluoroscopy before cuts are made. (Courtesy of Dr. Michael Brage.)

ALLOGRAFT PREPARATION AND CUTS

- The Agility ankle cutting block for the tibial cut of the donor graft is one size larger than the block used on the recipient tibia. Pin the cutting block onto the graft using fluoroscopy and make the cut with an oscillating saw (**TECH FIG 3A,B**).

- Cut the talus graft freehand using an oscillating saw. The cut is made at the interface between the anterior neck and cartilage. We routinely lavage both the tibial and talar grafts to remove immunogenic marrow elements (**TECH FIG 3C,D**).

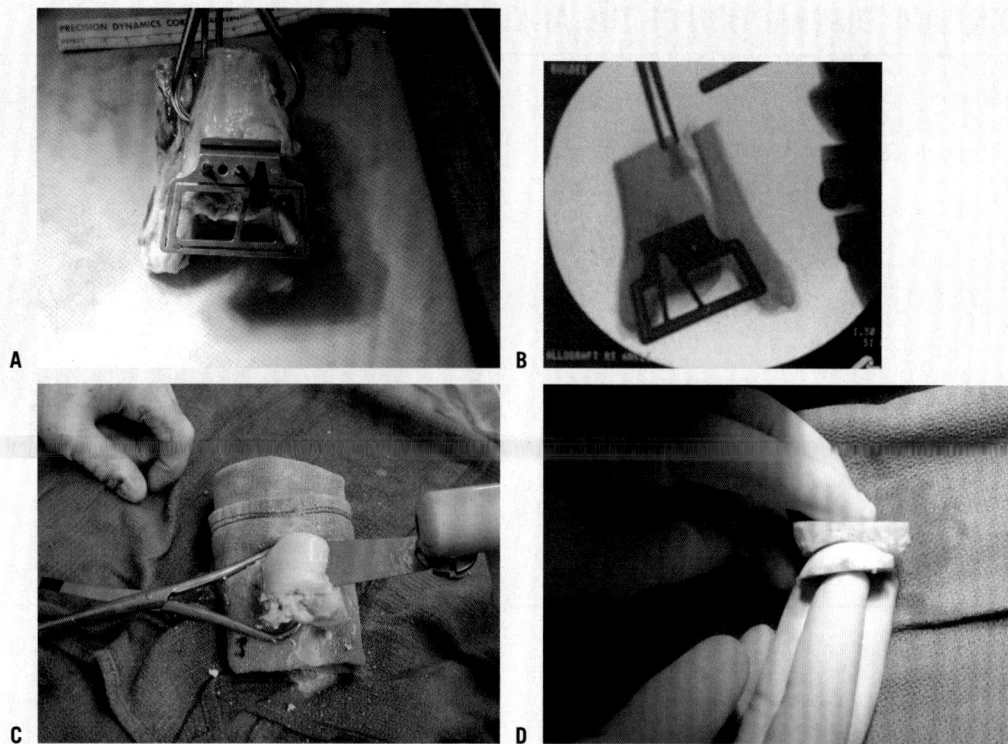

TECH FIG 3 Allograft preparation and cuts. **A.** Cutting jig is pinned onto tibia. **B.** Size and position are confirmed with fluoroscopy. **C.** Talus allograft is cut freehand. **D.** Articulating tibial and talar allografts. (Courtesy of Dr. Michael Brage.)

PLACEMENT AND FIXATION OF THE GRAFTS

- With the ankle in plantarflexion, seat the grafts into the recipient mortise. We remove the external fixator and take the ankle through a range of motion to confirm graft and ankle stability.
- Imaging in the AP, mortise, and lateral planes confirms that the grafts have satisfactory apposition to the host bone and that the anatomy of the tibiotalar joint has been restored.

- Place two parallel 3.0-mm cannulated screws into each graft for fixation. Place them from the anterior portion of the tibial graft while aiming superiorly and posteriorly.
- Place two fixation screws on the anterior portion of the talar graft through the most anterior portion of the articular cartilage. Countersink these screws into subchondral bone (**TECH FIG 4**).

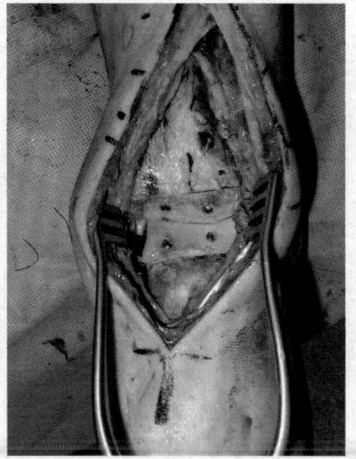
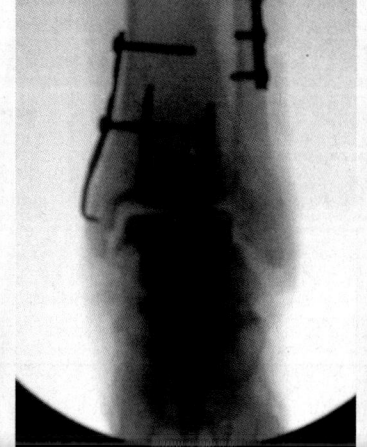
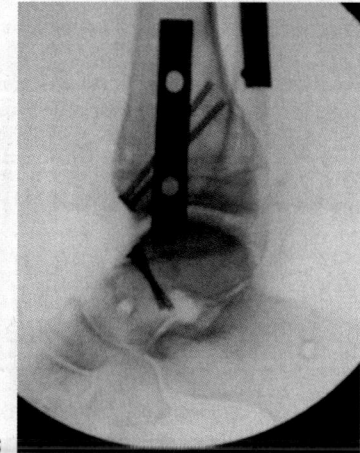

TECH FIG 4 Placement and fixation of graft. **A.** Grafts are placed and fixed with two countersunk cannulated screws. **B.** AP fluoroscopic view of grafts with fixation. **C.** Lateral fluoroscopic view. (Courtesy of Dr. Michael Brage.)

CLOSURE

- Perform copious irrigation and routine wound closure and place the patient in a bulky cotton splint **(TECH FIG 5)**.

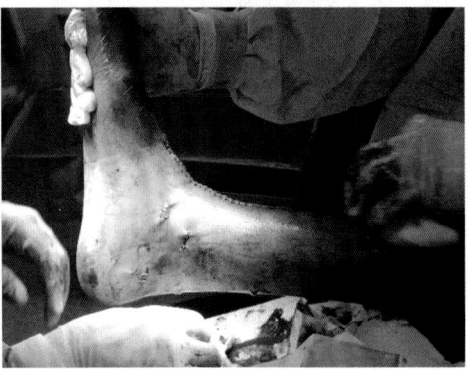

TECH FIG 5 Wound is closed, and range of motion is checked. (Courtesy of Dr. Michael Brage.)

TECHNIQUES

Pearls and Pitfalls

Indications	• Perform a complete history and physical examination.
	• Address associated pathology such as an equinus contracture, pes planus, or pes cavus deformity.
Intraoperative Fracture	• Take care when making cuts to avoid fracture of the lateral or medial malleolus.
Graft Preparation	• Take care when preparing the allografts.
	• Use cutting guides to improve precision of cuts. Improper graft cuts may result in graft failure.
Neurovascular Bundle	• Avoid injury to the posterior tibial neurovascular bundle at the posteromedial corner of the ankle joint.

POSTOPERATIVE CARE

- Perioperative antibiotics and pain control are at the surgeon's discretion. The patient is placed in a bulky cotton splint with the ankle in neutral to slight dorsiflexion postoperatively.
- Range-of-motion exercises are started when the wound has sealed, typically at postoperative day 10.
- We routinely keep the operated extremity at touchdown weight bearing for 3 months and then progress to weight bearing as tolerated as long as there are satisfactory radiographs that suggest progression toward graft incorporation.

OUTCOMES

- Promising case series have reported on total ankle osteochondral shell allograft replacement of the tibiotalar joint as a viable alternative for posttraumatic ankle arthritis in young patients **(FIGS 2 and 3)**.[10,13,21]

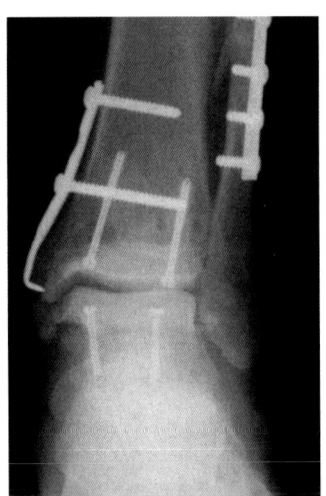
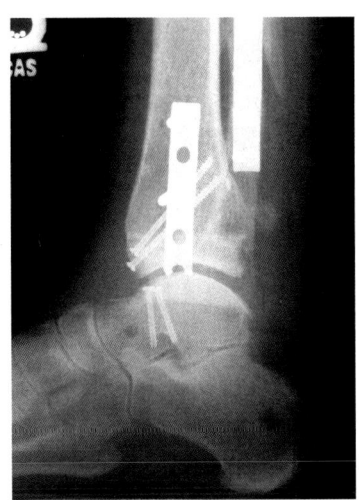

FIG 2 A. Four-month follow-up radiograph. **B.** Lateral view. (Courtesy of Dr. Michael Brage.)

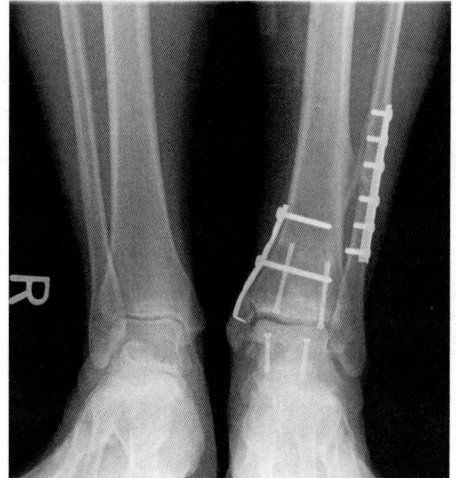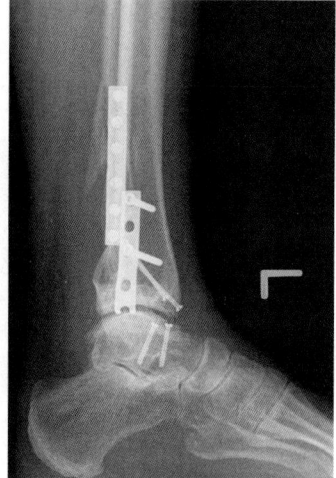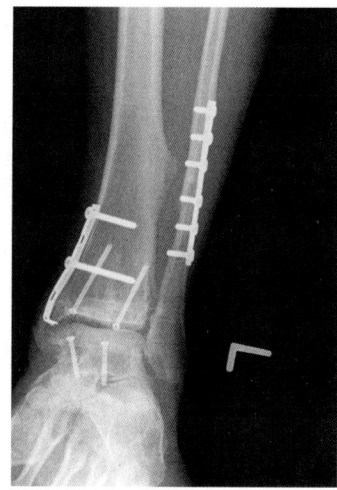

FIG 3 Three year follow up radiograph. **A.** AP view. **B.** Lateral view. **C.** Mortise view. (Courtesy of Dr. Michael Brage.)

- A large case series reports 6 out of 11 successful grafting procedures at a minimum follow-up of 24 months. Of the other five patients, three had revision allografting and one was revised to total ankle arthroplasty. The last patient did not have any further surgery.[13]
- Jeng et al[9] reported that 14 of 29 fresh osteochondral shell allograft transplants had been revised to a repeat ankle transplant/arthrodesis. Six of the remaining 15 allografts were radiographic failures with progressive loss of joint space but did not require revision surgery. The remaining 9 allografts (31%) were deemed a success. The authors concluded that patients with a lower body mass index (BMI) and less angular deformity and who refused arthrodesis did better. These authors did not use an external fixator during the procedure and did not use a cutting block one size bigger for the allograft as suggested in this chapter. Therefore, their grafts may have been small/thin. Grafts should be at least 7 mm thick to prevent collapse.[9]
- Gross et al[6] reported on nine patients treated with large fresh allografts of the talus to treat OCD lesions. Of the nine patients, six had successful procedures and remained in situ with a mean survival of 11 years. Three patients had fragmentation and collapse of the grafts and were converted to arthrodeses.[6]
- Giannini et al[5] reported on 32 patients treated with bipolar allografts via a lateral transmalleolar approach. Of the 32 patients, 9 required revision at the time of the latest follow-up of 31 months. They also examined cartilage samples from 7 of the patients at 1 year of follow-up finding hyaline-like histology with normal collagen; however, it was more disorganized than native cartilage and had less proteoglycan content. They also delayed weight bearing for 6 months, which they believe may have increased their success rate.[5]
- Neri et al[14] examined the genotypic and phenotypic characterizations of transplanted osteochondral allograft in 17 patients and found prevalence of host DNA in retrieved allografts suggesting incorporation.[13]
- Multiple studies have listed graft–host size mismatch, excessively thin cuts, elevated BMI, and degree of preoperative deformity as risk factors for graft failure. They have also

discussed that decreased time between harvesting of the allograft and implantation may increase success.[9,19,21,22]
- Gaul et al[4] recently examined outcomes for salvage arthrodesis or arthroplasty after failed osteochondral allograft transplantation and found that these procedures had higher revision and reoperation rates than primary ankle arthrodesis or ankle arthroplasty.

COMPLICATIONS

- Intraoperative fracture
- Graft collapse
- Poor graft fixation
- Nonunion
- Need for additional débridement postoperatively

REFERENCES

1. Abidi NA, Gruen GS, Conti SF. Ankle arthrodesis: indications and techniques. J Am Acad Orthop Surg 2000;8:200–209.
2. Coester LM, Saltzman CL, Leupold J, et al. Long-term results following ankle arthrodesis for post-traumatic arthritis. J Bone Joint Surg 2001;83-A(2):219–228.
3. Coughlin MJ, Mann RA. Surgery of the Foot and Ankle. St. Louis: Mosby, 1999.
4. Gaul F, Barr CR, McCauley JC, et al. Outcomes of salvage arthrodesis and arthroplasty for failed osteochondral allograft transplantation of the ankle. Foot Ankle Int 2019;40(5):537–544.
5. Giannini S, Buda R, Grigolo B, et al. Bipolar fresh osteochondral allograft of the ankle. Foot Ankle Int 2010;31(1):38–46.
6. Gross AE, Agnidis Z, Hutchison CR. Osteochondral defects of the talus treated with fresh osteochondral allograft transplantation. Foot Ankle Int 2001;22(5):385–391.
7. Haddad SL, Coetzee JC, Estok R, et al. Intermediate and long-term outcomes of total ankle arthroplasty and ankle arthrodesis a systematic review of the literature. J Bone Joint Surg 2007;89:1899–1905.
8. Hansen ST. Functional Reconstruction of the Foot and Ankle. Philadelphia: Lippincott Williams & Wilkins, 2000.
9. Jeng CL, Kadakia A, White KL, et al. Fresh osteochondral total ankle allograft transplantation for the treatment of ankle arthritis. Foot Ankle Clin North Am 2008;29:554–560.
10. Kim CW, Jamali A, Tontz W Jr, et al. Treatment of post traumatic ankle arthrosis with bipolar tibiotalar osteochondral shell allografts. Foot Ankle Int 2002;23:1091–1102.

11. Kitaoka HB, Patzer GL, Ilstrup DM, et al. Survivorship analysis of the Mayo total ankle arthroplasty. J Bone Joint Surg 1994;76-A(7):974–979.
12. Mann RA, Rongstad KM. Arthrodesis of the ankle: a critical analysis. Foot Ankle Int 1998;19:3–9.
13. Meehan R, McFarlin S, Bugbee W, et al. Fresh ankle osteochondral allograft transplantation for tibiotalar joint arthritis. Foot Ankle Int 2005;26:793–802.
14. Neri S, Vannini F, Desando G, et al. Ankle bipolar fresh osteochondral allograft survivorship and integration: transplanted tissue genetic typing and phenotypic characteristics. J Bone Joint Surg 2013;95:1852–1860.
15. Reider B. The Orthopaedic Physical Examination. Philadelphia: Elsevier, 2005.
16. Richardson EG. Orthopaedic Knowledge Update: Foot and Ankle 3. Rosemont, IL: American Academy of Orthopaedic Surgeons, 2003.
17. SooHoo NF, Zingmond DS, Ko CY. Comparison of reoperation rates following ankle arthrodesis and total ankle arthroplasty. J Bone Joint Surg 2007;89:2143–2149.
18. Spirt AA, Assal M, Hansen ST Jr. Complications and failure after total ankle arthroplasty. J Bone Joint Surg 2004;86-A(6):1172–1178.
19. Strauss EJ, Sershon R, Barker JU, et al. The basic science and clinical applications of osteochondral allografts. Bull NYU Hosp Jt Dis 2012;70(4):217–223.
20. Thomas RH, Daniels TR. Ankle arthritis. J Bone Joint Surg 2003;85-A(5):923–936.
21. Tontz WL Jr, Bugbee WD, Brage ME. Use of allografts in the management of ankle arthritis. Foot Ankle Clin North Am 2003;8:361–373.
22. Winters BS, Raikin SM. The use of allograft in joint-preserving surgery for ankle osteochondral lesions and osteoarthritis. Foot Ankle Clin Am 2013;18:529–542.

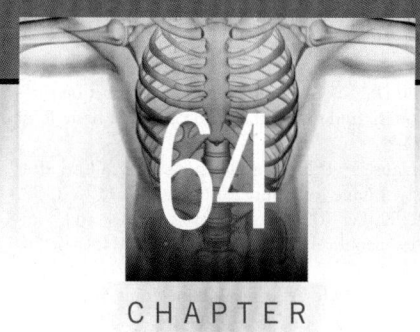

64

CHAPTER

The STAR (Scandinavian Total Ankle Replacement)

Mark E. Easley, James A. Nunley II, and James K. DeOrio

DEFINITION

- End-stage ankle arthritis failing to respond to nonoperative treatment

ANATOMY

- Ankle
  - Tibial plafond with medial malleolus
    - Articulations with dorsal and medial talus
    - In sagittal plane, slight posterior slope
    - In coronal plane, articular surface is 88 to 92 degrees relative to lateral tibial shaft axis.
  - Fibula
    - Articulation with lateral talus
    - Responsible for one-sixth of axial load distribution of the ankle
  - Talus
    - Sixty percent of surface area covered by articular cartilage
    - Dual radius of curvature
  - Distal tibiofibular syndesmosis
    - Anteroinferior tibiofibular ligament
    - Interosseous membrane
    - Posterior tibiofibular ligament
- Ankle functions as part of the ankle–hindfoot complex much like a mitered hinge.

PATHOGENESIS

- Posttraumatic arthrosis
  - Most common etiology
  - Intra-articular fracture
  - Ankle fracture-dislocation with malunion
  - Chronic ankle instability
- Primary osteoarthrosis
  - Relatively rare compared to hip and knee arthrosis
- Inflammatory arthropathy
  - Most commonly rheumatoid arthritis
- Other
  - Hemochromatosis
  - Pigmented villonodular synovitis
  - Charcot neuroarthropathy
  - Septic arthritis

NATURAL HISTORY

- Posttraumatic arthrosis
  - Malunion, chronic instability, intra-articular cartilage damage, or malalignment may lead to progressive articular cartilage wear.

- Chronic lateral ankle instability may eventually be associated with the following:
  - Relative anterior subluxation of the talus
  - Varus tilt of the talus within the ankle mortise
  - Hindfoot varus position
- Primary osteoarthrosis of the ankle is rare and poorly understood.
- Inflammatory arthropathy
  - Progressive and proliferative synovial erosive changes failing to respond to medical management
  - May be associated with chronic posterior tibial tendinopathy and progressive valgus hindfoot deformity, eventual valgus tilt to the talus within the ankle mortise, potential lateral malleolar stress fracture, and compensatory forefoot varus

PATIENT HISTORY AND PHYSICAL FINDINGS

- Patient history
  - Often a history of ankle trauma
    - Ankle fracture, particularly intra-articular
    - Ankle fracture with malunion
    - Chronic ankle instability (recurrent ankle sprains)
  - Chronic anterior ankle pain, primarily with activity and weight bearing
  - Ankle stiffness, particularly with dorsiflexion
  - Ankle swelling
  - Progressively worsening activity level
- Physical findings
  - Limp
  - Patient externally rotates hip to externally rotate ankle to avoid painful push-off.
  - Painful and limited ankle range of motion (ROM), particularly limited dorsiflexion
  - Mild ankle edema
  - Potential associated foot deformity
    - Posttraumatic arthrosis secondary to chronic instability may be associated with varus ankle and hindfoot and compensatory forefoot varus.
    - Inflammatory arthritis may be associated with progressively worsening flatfoot deformity, valgus tilt to the ankle and hindfoot, and equinus.

IMAGING AND OTHER DIAGNOSTIC STUDIES

- Weight-bearing anteroposterior (AP), lateral, and mortise views of the ankle (FIG 1)
- Weight-bearing AP, lateral, and oblique views of the foot, particularly with associated foot deformity

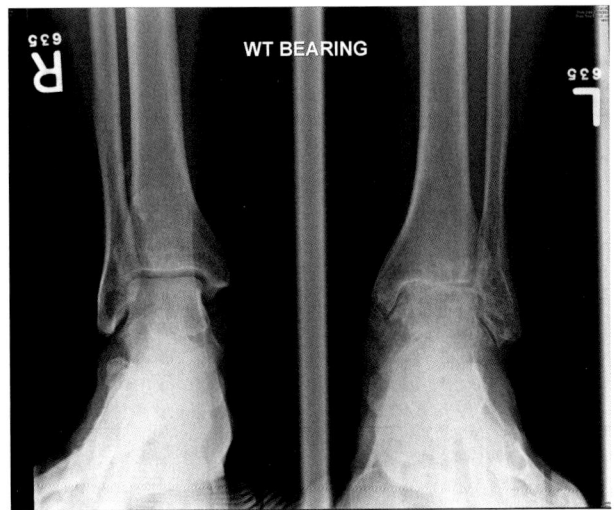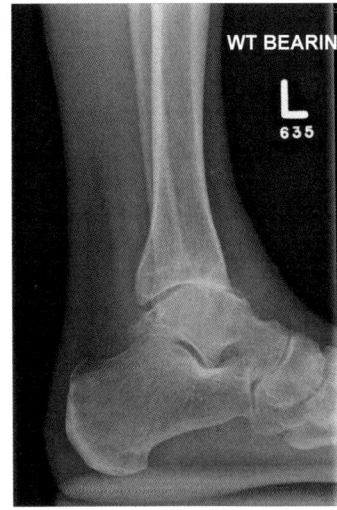

FIG 1 Weight-bearing ankle radiographs of a 60-year-old woman with end-stage posttraumatic left ankle arthritis. **A.** AP view (note slight varus talar tilt). **B.** Lateral view.

- With associated or suspected lower leg deformity, we routinely obtain weight-bearing AP and lateral tibia–fibula views.
- With deformity in the lower extremity, we routinely obtain weight-bearing mechanical axis (hip-to-ankle) views of both extremities.
- We typically evaluate complex or ill-defined ankle–hindfoot patterns of arthritis with or without deformity using computed tomography (CT) of the ankle and hindfoot.
- If we suspect avascular necrosis of the talus or distal tibia, we obtain a magnetic resonance imaging (MRI) of the ankle.

DIFFERENTIAL DIAGNOSIS

- See the section on Pathogenesis.

NONOPERATIVE MANAGEMENT

- Activity modification
- Bracing
  - Ankle–foot orthosis (AFO)
  - Double upright brace attached to shoe
- Stiffer-soled shoe with a rocker bottom modification
- Nonsteroidal anti-inflammatories or COX-2 inhibitors
- Medications for systemic inflammatory arthropathy
- Corticosteroid injection
- Viscosupplementation

SURGICAL MANAGEMENT

Preoperative Planning

- The surgeon must be sure the patient has satisfactory perfusion to support healing and is not neuropathic.
  - Noninvasive vascular studies and potential vascular surgery consultation should be obtained if necessary.
- The surgeon should inspect the ankle for prior scars or surgical approaches that need to be considered in planning the surgical approach for total ankle arthroplasty (TAA).
- The surgeon must understand the clinical and radiographic alignment of lower extremity, ankle, and foot.
  - The surgeon must be prepared to balance and realign the ankle. Occasionally, this necessitates corrective osteotomies of the distal tibia or foot, hindfoot arthrodesis, ligament releases or stabilization, or tendon transfers.

- The surgeon should determine whether coronal plane alignment is passively correctable; this provides some understanding of whether ligament releases will be required.
- Ankle ROM should be determined.
  - Ankle stiffness, particularly lack of dorsiflexion, needs to be corrected:
    - Anterior tibiotalar exostectomy
    - Posterior capsular release
    - Occasionally, tendo Achilles lengthening
- Instrumentation
  - These instruments facilitate TAA:
    - Small oscillating saw to fine-tune cuts, resect prominences with precision, and easily morselize large bone fragments to be evacuated from the joint
    - A rasp for final preparation of cut bony surfaces
    - An angled curette, particularly to separate bone from the posterior capsule
    - A toothless lamina spreader to judiciously distract the ankle to improve exposure even after preparing the surfaces of the tibia and talus

Positioning

- The patient is positioned supine with the plantar aspect of the operated foot at the end of the operating table.
- The foot and ankle are well balanced, with toes directed to the ceiling.
- A bolster placed under the ipsilateral hip prevents undesired external rotation of the hip.
- We routinely use a thigh tourniquet and regional anesthesia.
  - A popliteal block provides adequate pain relief postoperatively, particularly if a regional catheter is used. Moreover, hip and knee flexion–extension is not forfeited, facilitating safe immediate postoperative mobilization.
  - However, using a thigh tourniquet with a popliteal block typically requires a supplemental femoral nerve block (patient forfeits knee extension) or general anesthesia.

Approach

- An anterior approach to the ankle is made, using the interval between the tibialis anterior (TA) tendon and the extensor hallucis longus (EHL) tendon.

EXPOSURE

- Make a longitudinal midline incision over the anterior ankle, starting about 10 cm proximal to the tibiotalar joint and 1 cm lateral to the tibial crest (**TECH FIG 1**).
- Continue the incision midline over the anterior ankle just distal to the talonavicular joint.
- At no point should direct tension be placed on the skin margins; we perform deep, full-thickness retraction as soon as possible to limit the risk of skin complications.
- Identify and protect the superficial peroneal nerve by retracting it laterally.
  - In our experience, there is a consistent branch of the superficial peroneal nerve that crosses directly over or immediately proximal to the tibiotalar joint.
- We then expose the extensor retinaculum, identify the course of the EHL tendon, and sharply but carefully divide the retinaculum directly over the EHL tendon.
  - We always attempt to maintain the TA tendon in its dedicated sheath.
  - Preserving the retinaculum over the TA tendon:
    - This prevents bowstringing of the tendon and thereby reduces the stress on the anterior wound.

- Should there be a wound dehiscence, then the TA is not directly exposed.
- Preserving the retinaculum over the TA tendon is not always possible; some patients do not have a dedicated sheath for the TA.
- The interval between the TA and EHL tendon is used, with the TA and EHL tendons retracted medially and laterally, respectively.
- Identify and carefully retract the deep neurovascular bundle (anterior tibial–dorsalis pedis artery and deep peroneal nerve) laterally throughout the remainder of the procedure.
- Perform an anterior capsulotomy along with elevation of the tibial and dorsal talar periosteum to about 6 to 8 cm proximal to the tibial plafond and talonavicular joint, respectively.
- Elevate this separated capsule and periosteum medially and laterally to expose the ankle, to access the medial and lateral gutters, and to visualize the medial and lateral malleoli.
- Remove anterior tibial and talar osteophytes to facilitate exposure and avoid interference with the instrumentation.

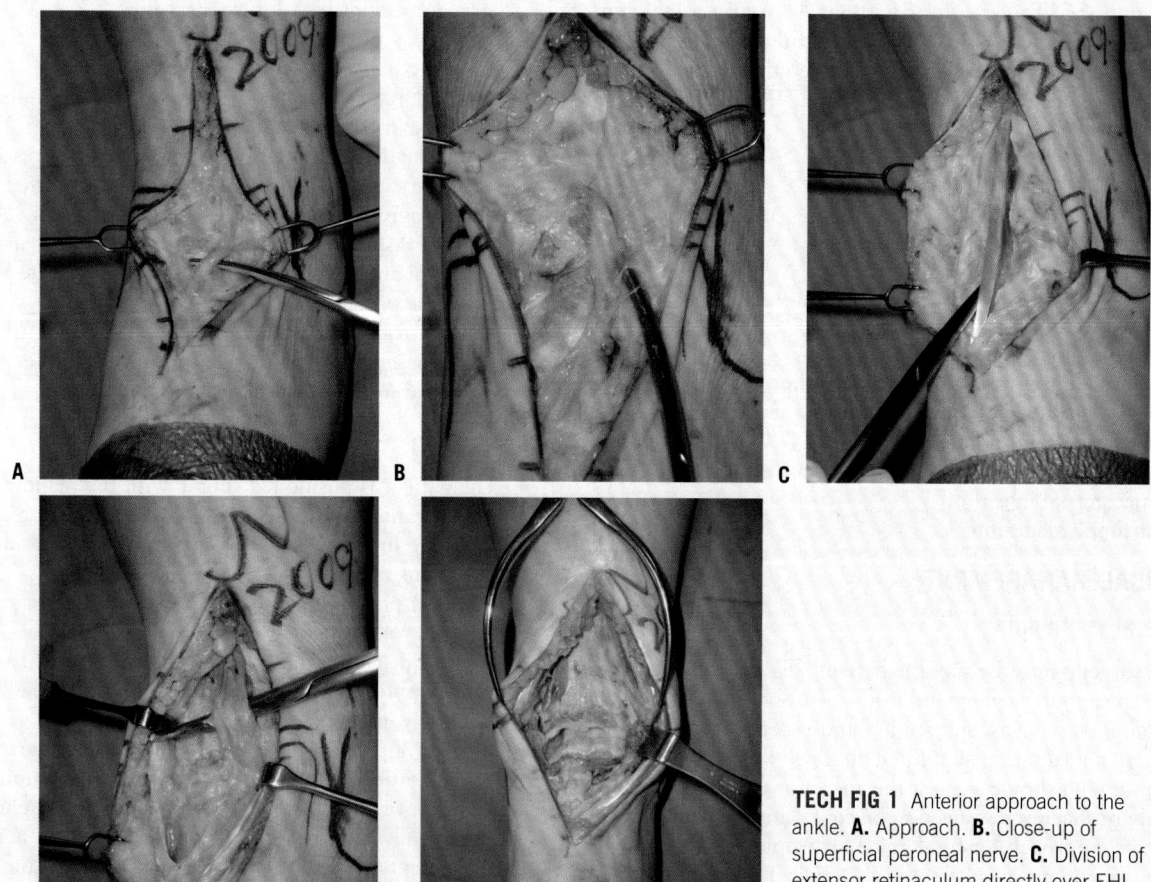

TECH FIG 1 Anterior approach to the ankle. **A.** Approach. **B.** Close-up of superficial peroneal nerve. **C.** Division of extensor retinaculum directly over EHL tendon. **D.** Deep neurovascular bundle is identified and protected. **E.** After anterior capsulotomy, with ankle exposed.

TIBIAL PREPARATION

Positioning the External Tibial Alignment Guide

- An osteotome placed in the medial gutter serves as a reference for optimal rotation for the tibial preparation (TECH FIG 2).
- Place a pin in the proximal tibia via a 1-cm incision over the tibial tubercle.
  - When viewed in the AP plane, this pin is oriented parallel to the reference osteotome in the medial gutter.
  - When viewed in the lateral plane, the pin should be perpendicular to the tibial shaft axis if the physiologic 3 to 5 degrees of posterior slope to the tibial component is desired. We prefer to implant the tibial component perpendicular to the longitudinal tibial shaft axis (no posterior slope), aiming the pin slightly proximally. The external tibial alignment guide directs the initial tibial cut into 3 degrees of posterior slope; we aim to eliminate this slope.
- Suspend the external tibial alignment guide from the proximal pin. To further promote a perpendicular tibial preparation

relative to the tibial shaft axis, we raise the proximal aspect of the external tibial alignment guide two to three fingerbreadths above the tibial spine before securing it to the proximal pin.
- Set the rotation of the cutting block for tibial preparation based on the reference osteotome set in the medial gutter. A dedicated T guide temporarily attached to the distal aspect of the guide facilitates setting proper rotation. Lock the rotation of the distal block with the knob connecting the telescoping rods of the guide.
- While controlling rotation, set the proper length of the guide via the telescoping rods.
- Fine-tuning of the distal block's lateral plane position is possible. We routinely separate the distal block of the guide from the portion of the guide used to pin it to the tibia by at least 10 mm.
- If the initial position of the distal block is set at the apex of the plafond, the desired 5 mm of resection may be easily set and even greater resection is possible in a tighter ankle.

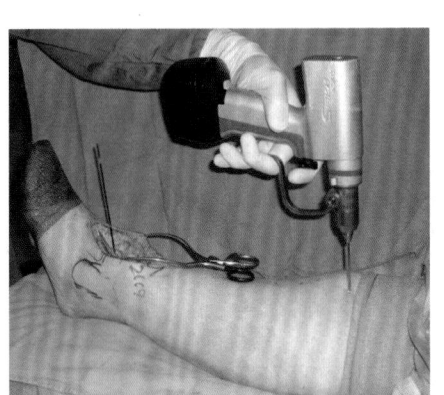
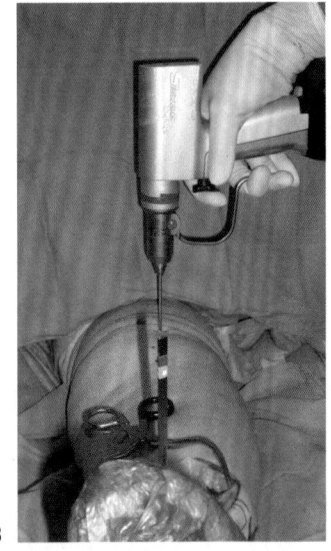
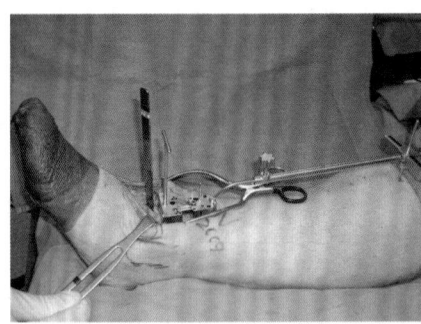
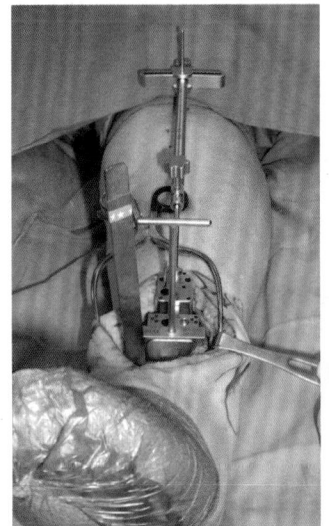
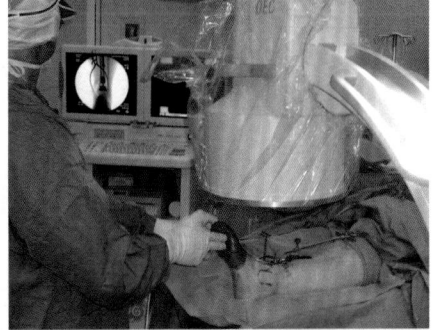
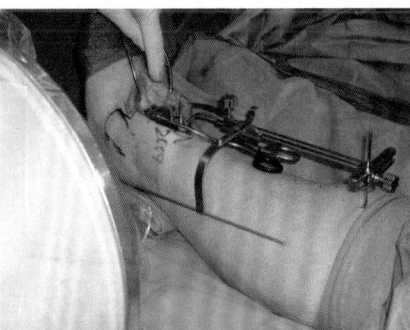

TECH FIG 2 Positioning the external tibial alignment guide. **A,B.** Positioning the proximal pin relative to a reference osteotome placed in the medial gutter. **C,D.** Setting rotation of the distal cutting block of the guide relative to the medial gutter reference osteotome. **E,F.** Fluoroscopic confirmation of proper guide position in the AP and lateral planes.

TECHNIQUES

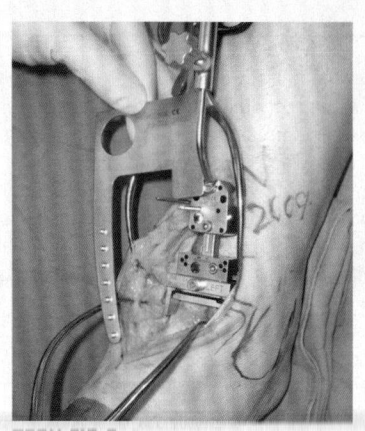
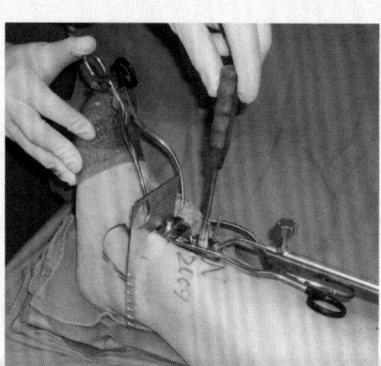
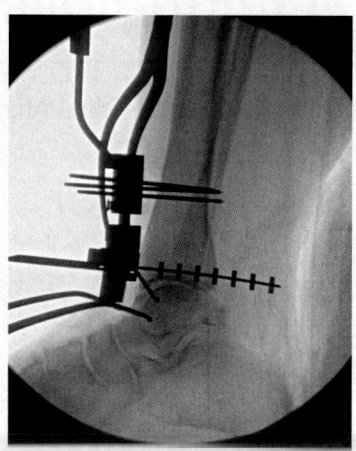

TECH FIG 3 Determining tibial plafond resection level. **A.** Angel wing about to be inserted into capture guide attached to distal tibial cutting block. **B.** Angel wing in capture guide with height adjustment being made under fluoroscopy. **C.** Fluoroscopic image of angel wing confirming tibial resection level.

- We make sure that the block is positioned at the tibial plafond's apex, that it is properly rotated, and that we are able to fine-tune the block's proximal–distal position before pinning the guide to the tibia.
  - Multiple options exist to pin the guide to the tibia. We recommend using pins at different levels rather than pins in a single plane (risks creating a stress riser).

Determining Tibial Plafond Resection Level

- Attach the cutting capture guide to the distal block and insert an angel wing resection guide in the capture guide. Use fluoroscopy in the lateral plane to determine the proper resection level for the tibial cut **(TECH FIG 3)**.
- Adjust the cutting guide in the coronal plane to ensure that the malleoli are protected with tibial resection.
  - There is only a single capture guide size.
  - We routinely set the guide based on a pin placed loosely in the medial aspect of the capture guide.
  - We aim to position the guide so that the medial extent of tibial preparation is directly proximal from the transition of tibial plafond to medial malleolus.

- Drive the pin used as a reference into the tibia through the medial aspect of the capture guide to protect the medial malleolus.
- Similarly, place a lateral pin in the lateral aspect of the capture guide and advance it into the lateral gutter.
- The capture guide has several options to place the lateral pin to accommodate any coronal plane dimension of the tibial plafond.

Initial Tibial Resection

- With the soft tissues protected, particularly the deep neurovascular bundle, make the distal tibial cut with an oscillating saw through the horizontal portion of the capture guide. To complete the cut, use a reciprocating saw along the medial border of the capture guide, extending proximally from the medial gutter **(TECH FIG 4)**.
- Remove the capture guide and evacuate the resected bone.
  - A toothless lamina spreader may be placed judiciously on the prepared tibial surface and dorsal talus to facilitate evacuation of bone from the posterior ankle.
  - We routinely use a small reciprocating saw to morselize the posterior fragments and a combination of curved curette

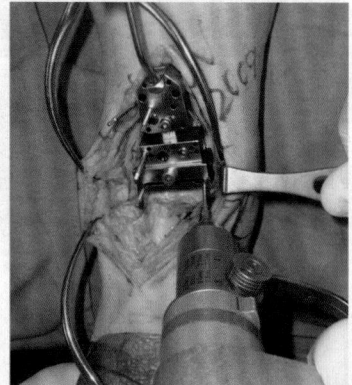
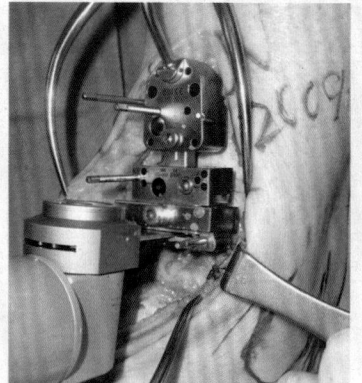
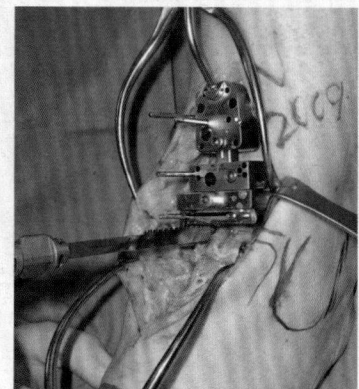

TECH FIG 4 A. After determining proper coronal placement of the tibial cutting block, the capture guide is pinned, with the pins used to protect the malleoli. **B.** Saw in the capture guide. **C.** Medial resection with a reciprocating saw to complete the initial tibial preparation. *(continued)*

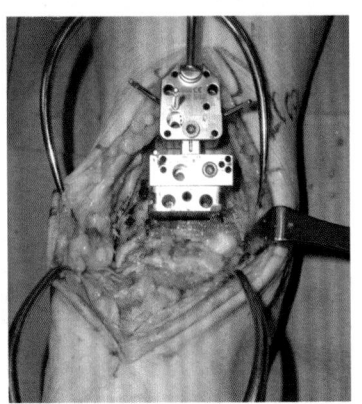 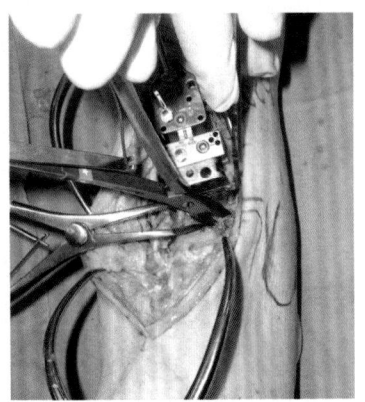 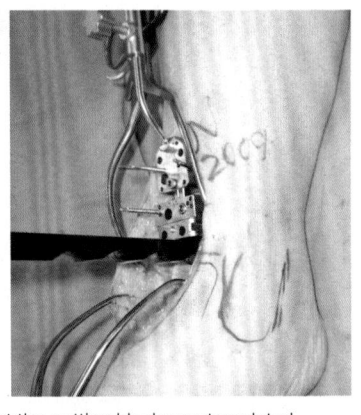

D **E** **F**

TECH FIG 4 *(continued)* **D.** Tibial resection after removal of the capture guide (note that the cutting block was translated slightly medial for optimal positioning). **E.** Removal of the resected tibial bone (note the judicious use of a toothless lamina spreader to facilitate access to the posterior ankle). **F.** Confirming adequate tibial resection with plastic spacer (9 mm).

and rongeur to retrieve the fragments that need to be separated from the posterior capsule.
- ■ The curette is used directly vertically in the ankle and never levered against a malleolus.
- We routinely perform a posterior capsular resection to optimize dorsiflexion.

- To ensure that the tibial resection is adequate, use the system's plastic spacer as a sizing guide. The 9-mm end of this sizing guide equals the combined height of the tibial component (3 mm) and the thinnest polyethylene component (6 mm).

TALAR PREPARATION

Initial Talar Preparation

- Residual articular cartilage must be removed from the dorsal talar dome so that the talar cutting guide may be properly balanced on the dorsal talus. We routinely use a thin oscillating saw to remove residual cartilage.
- Position the talar guide within the ankle joint and secure it to the distal block of the external alignment guide.
- We then hold the ankle in neutral dorsiflexion–plantarflexion.
  - Excessive dorsiflexion risks talar preparation, leading to anterior translation and tilt of the talar implant. Moreover, an exaggerated notch will be created in the dorsal talar neck.
  - Excessive plantarflexion risks talar preparation, leading to posterior translation and tilt of the talar implant. In addition, too much posterior talus will be removed.
  - Excessive plantarflexion may be a result of fixed equinus. If the talus cannot be brought to a neutral position (confirm with an intraoperative radiograph), then consider a tendo Achilles lengthening rather than risk resecting too much of the posterior talus.
- With perfect contact of both the medial and lateral talar dome on the intra-articularly placed paddle of the talar cutting guide and a neutral sagittal plane alignment maintained, pin the talar guide.
- Place the angel wing resection guide in the talar cutting guide and use lateral plane fluoroscopy to confirm proper resection level and desired orientation for the guide.
- Place two more pins in the talar guide to protect the malleoli and further stabilize the guide.

- Make the initial talar cut using an oscillating saw, remove the guide, and evacuate the resected bone from the joint (**TECH FIG 5A–E**).
- To ensure that a balanced resection was performed on the tibia and talus and that the resection levels are appropriate, use the plastic spacer–sizing guide impactor and confirm proper alignment and resection levels on intraoperative fluoroscopy (**TECH FIG 5F,G**).

Sizing the Talus and Positioning the 4-in-1 Talar Reference Guide ("Datum")

- Position a sizing guide on the dorsal prepared talar surface and properly rotate it with the second metatarsal. The proper sizing guide matches the dimensions of the true talar implant and therefore should be placed in the desired position for the talar component (**TECH FIG 6A**).
- With the sizing guide in the appropriate position, drive the central pin through the guide into the talus (**TECH FIG 6B**).
- Confirm proper sagittal plane guide position on the lateral fluoroscopic view: The nob on the guide should center over the lateral process of the talus (**TECH FIG 6C**).
- With the sizing guide removed, position the 4-in-1 talar reference guide (datum) over the central pin and flush onto the prepared talar surface (**TECH FIG 6D**).
  - Be sure the guide is rotated in line with the second metatarsal. Coronal plane position of the datum is dictated by the central pin position; often, the datum position may appear slightly lateral.
  - Secure the 4-in-1 guide to the talus with dedicated pins (**TECH FIG 6E,F**).

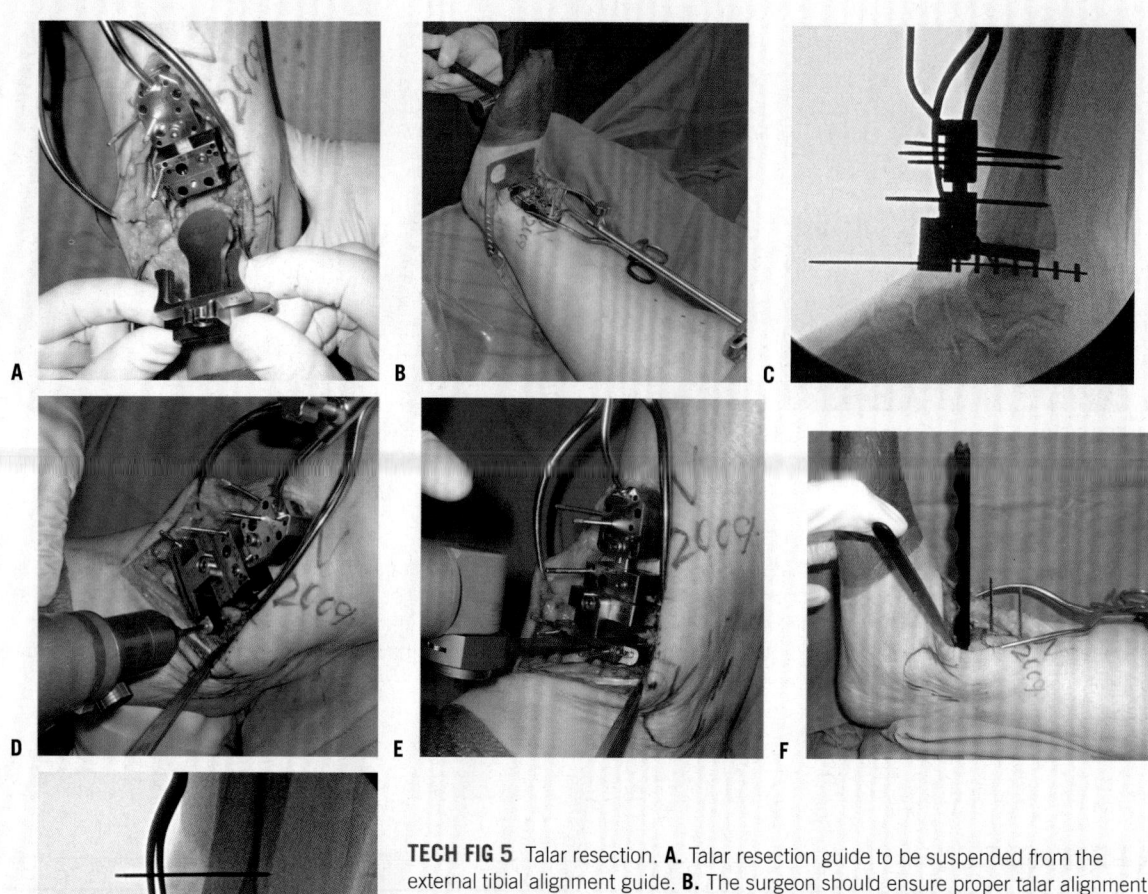

TECH FIG 5 Talar resection. **A.** Talar resection guide to be suspended from the external tibial alignment guide. **B.** The surgeon should ensure proper talar alignment (patient had an equinus contracture, and gastrocnemius–soleus recession was required to obtain optimal talar position). **C.** Intraoperative fluoroscopic view confirming resection level. Note the gap between intra-articular paddle of talar resection guide, suggesting some residual articular cartilage on talar dome and leaving talar resection too shallow. This prompted removal of residual talar cartilage to obtain optimal talar resection. **D.** Pinning the talar cutting guide. **E.** Talar resection with soft tissues protected. **F.** Plastic spacer confirms adequate resection (12-mm gap). **G.** Fluoroscopy confirms that the resections are balanced.

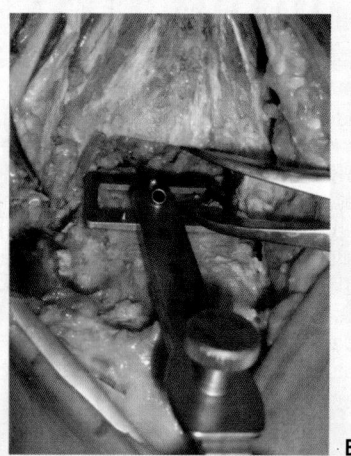
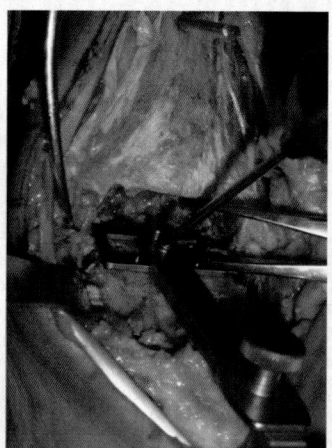
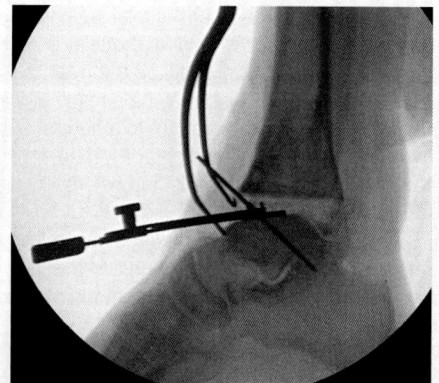

TECH FIG 6 Talar sizing (different patient). **A.** Talar sizing guide being used to determine ideal talar size. **B.** Talar sizing guide properly positioned on the prepared talar surface with proper rotation, aligned with the second metatarsal axis, and with the central pin positioned. **C.** Fluoroscopic confirmation of proper sagittal plane position. Note that the nob on the guide is directly over the lateral process of the talus. *(continued)*

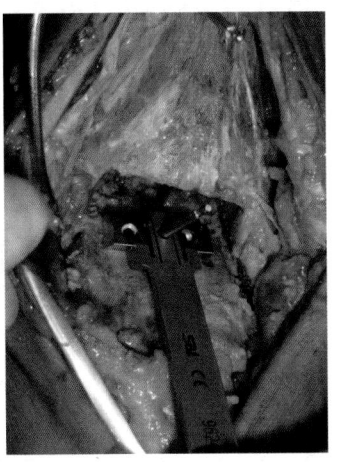
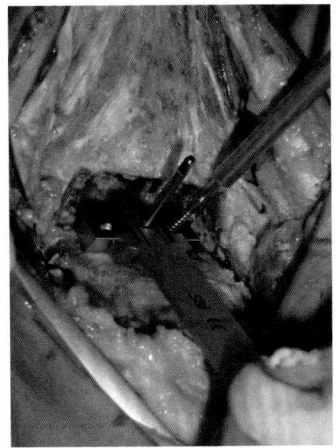
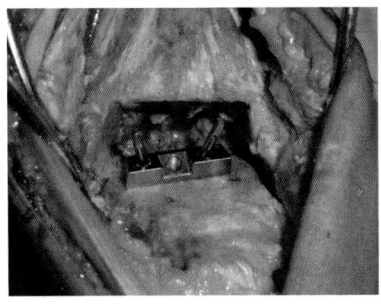

TECH FIG 6 *(continued)* **D.** The 4-in-1 reference guide is positioned on the prepared talar surface over the central pin. Guide positioned on the prepared talar surface with the handle that may be used to avoid posterior lift-off. **E.** Threaded pin fixation of the 4-in-1 guide to the talus. **F.** The 4-in-1 guide properly positioned and secured, with handle removed.

- Confirm proper position of the 4-in-1 guide with lateral fluoroscopy. Ideally, the center point of the undersurface of the guide rests directly over the lateral talar process. Another rough estimate of proper position is that the guide is centered under the tibia.
  - Full dorsiflexion of the talus is not possible due to impingement of the pins securing the guide to the talus.

- If this position cannot be confirmed, then the 4-in-1 talar guide must be repositioned and repinned.
  - This may be difficult because, typically, only a subtle move of the guide is necessary and securing a pin immediately adjacent to a previous pin position is possible but challenging.

COMPLETING THE TALAR PREPARATION AND IMPLANTING THE TALAR COMPONENT

Anteroposterior Talar Chamfer Cutting Guide

- Secure the anteroposterior talar chamfer cutting guide to the 4-in-1 talar reference guide and place an additional pin in the guide to stabilize it to the talus **(TECH FIG 7A)**.
- Cut the posterior talar chamfer using an oscillating saw in the posterior capture guide.
- Mill the anterior chamfer with the soft tissues and deep neurovascular bundle protected **(TECH FIG 7B)**.

- Remove the AP chamfer guide, leaving the 4-in-1 guide in place **(TECH FIG 7C)**.

Mediolateral Chamfer Cutting Guide

- Secure the mediolateral chamfer cutting guide to the 4-in-1 talar reference guide **(TECH FIG 8)**.
  - Two additional smooth pins may be placed through this guide to further stabilize the guide to the talus.

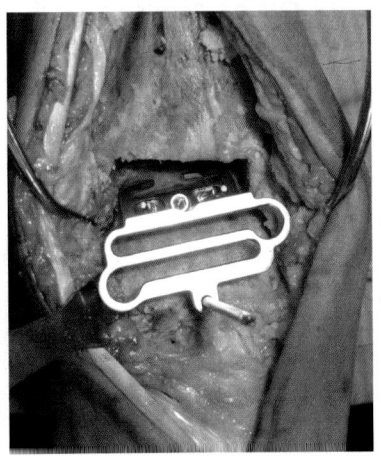
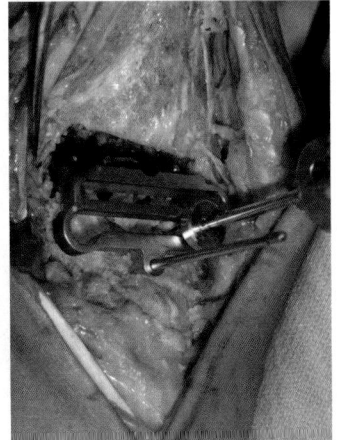
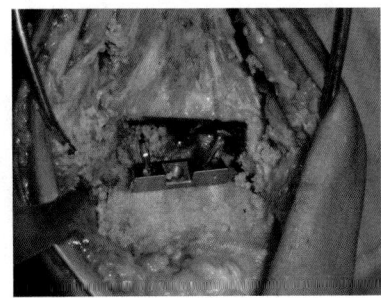

TECH FIG 7 Anterior and posterior talar chamfer preparation. **A.** Posterior chamfer bone resection; note the AP chamfer guide has a posterior capture guide. **B.** Anterior chamfer milling. **C.** Talus with 4-in-1 reference guide in place and with prepared anterior and posterior chamfers.

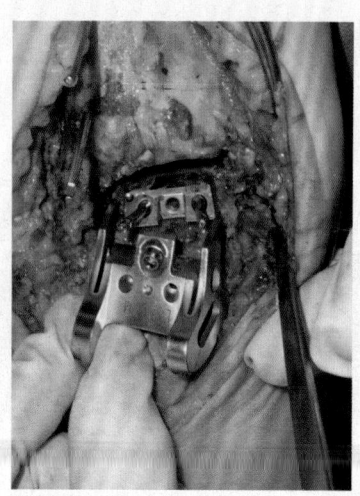 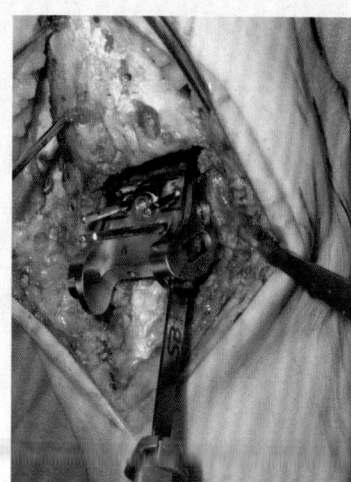 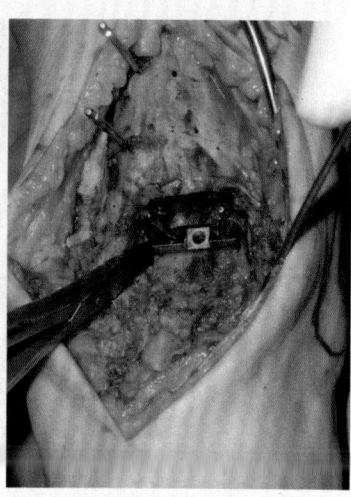

TECH FIG 8 Mediolateral talar chamfer preparation. **A.** The mediolateral chamfer guide. **B.** Guide attached to the 4-in-1 reference guide and lateral chamfer being prepared with reciprocating saw (note protection of soft tissues with retractor). **C.** Talus after mediolateral chamfer resection and rongeur used to evacuate resected bone from medial gutter.

- With the soft tissues and neurovascular structures protected, make the medial and lateral chamfer cuts with a reciprocal saw.
  - To accommodate the talar implant:
    - Medial cut is made to a depth of 10 mm.
    - Lateral cut is made to a depth of 15 mm.
- Remove the mediolateral chamfer and 4-in-1 reference guides.
- Evacuate the resected bone with the following:
  - A thin osteotome
  - A curved curette
  - A rongeur
- Inspect the prepared talus for any uneven surfaces or residual bony prominences, which may be removed judiciously with a small reciprocal saw and a rasp.

The "Window" Talar Trial

- Position the window talar trial on the prepared talus **(TECH FIG 9A–C)**.

- Often, any incongruencies or prominences still need to be addressed to ensure that the guide rests completely flush on all prepared surfaces of the talus.
  - Because the guide is a window, proper fit can be confirmed for the true implant that is resurfacing without any means of determining the actual bony contact between bone and implant.
- Pin the talar trial.
- Use a router to create the slot in the talus to accommodate the talar implant's fin **(TECH FIG 9D–F)**.
- Use a stem punch to finish preparing the talar fin slot.

Implanting the Talar Component

- Orient the properly sized talar component with the longer side placed laterally (to articulate with the fibula) **(TECH FIG 10)**.
- Gently tap the prosthesis posteriorly with the set's plastic spacer–sizer impactor to rest in the optimal position over the fin slot.

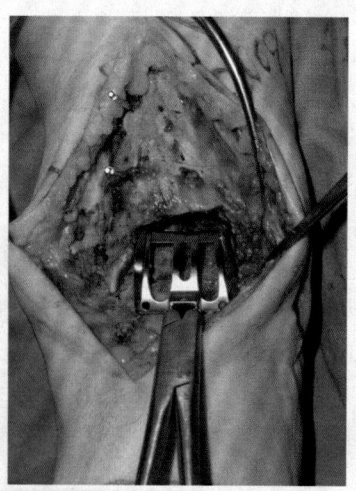 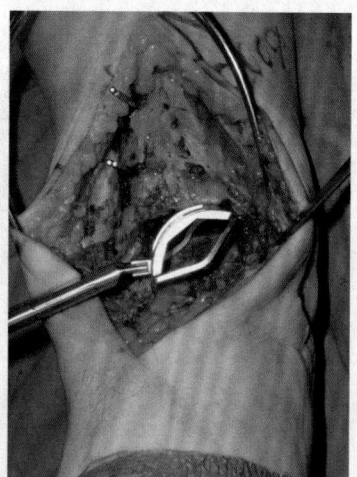 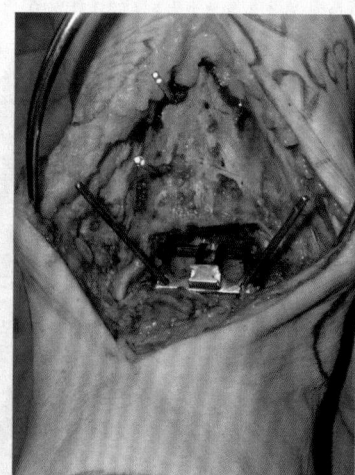

TECH FIG 9 Trial talus (window trial). **A.** Lateral view of trial. **B.** AP view of trial. **C.** Trial pinned to talus; note congruent fit on all prepared surfaces. *(continued)*

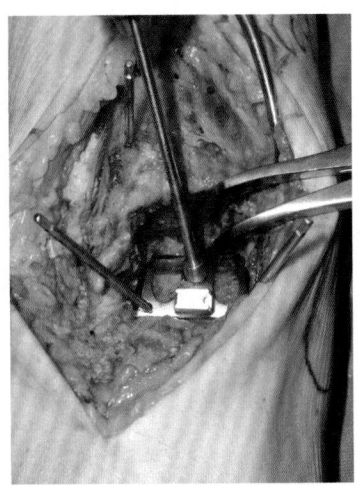
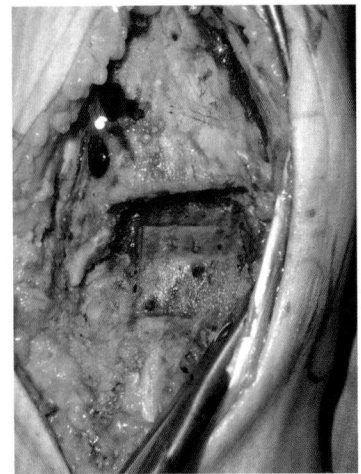
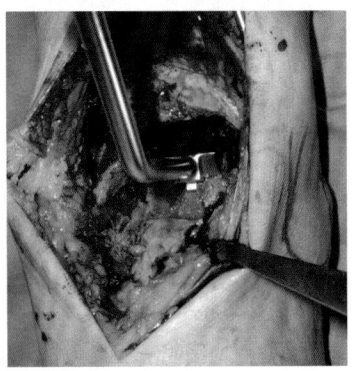

TECH FIG 9 *(continued)* **D–F.** Preparing the fin slot for the talar stem. **D.** Using the router in the trial talus (note the judicious use of a toothless lamina spreader to afford greater support to the trial during talar stem preparation). **E.** Talus after removal of talar trial and fin slot preparation. **F.** Stem punch is used to complete preparation of fin slot.

- Use the talar dome impaction device to impact the talar component.
  - The anterior tibial cortex must be protected.
- We make sure that despite proper initial positioning the talar component does not tilt anteriorly, which it will tend to do given the limited access to the natural talus.
- Fully seat the talar component.

Final Preparation of the Tibial Plafond and Tibial Component Implantation

- Measure the AP dimensions of the tibia.
- Select the corresponding tibial component.
- If the mediolateral dimensions of the tibial plafond do not accommodate this component, then judiciously remove one or two more millimeters of medial bone to safely position the tibial trial.
- Also, all syndesmotic soft tissue impinging in the joint must be removed.
- The tibial trial should align with the center of the tibial shaft axis **(TECH FIG 11A–D)**.
  - It should not be tilted in varus or valgus.

- It should not be lateral to the longitudinal center of the tibial shaft.
- After positioning the proper size of tibial component and confirming its position on intraoperative fluoroscopy, pin the tibial trial.
- Temporarily insert a trial polyethylene insert to maintain pressure on the tibial trial and therefore optimal bony apposition of the tibial trial base plate and prepared tibial surface.
- On intraoperative fluoroscopy, there should not be any posterior tibial tray lift-off from the prepared tibial surface and the tibial trial should be well aligned with the tibial shaft axis on the AP view.
- Prepare the barrel holes with the corresponding drill and chisel and remove the tibial trial and trial polyethylene. Leave the pin placed to secure the tibial trial as a reference.
- Irrigate the joint.
- Using the dedicated tibial impaction device, impact the tibial component almost fully **(TECH FIG 11E–G)**.
- Use the plastic spacer–sizer impactor to advance the tibial component to its final position.
  - Again, use a trial polyethylene to afford further stability to the tibial trial as the final impaction is performed **(TECH FIG 11H,I)**.

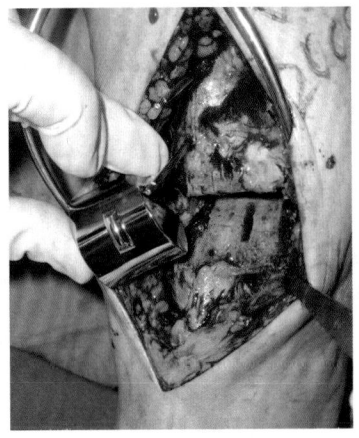
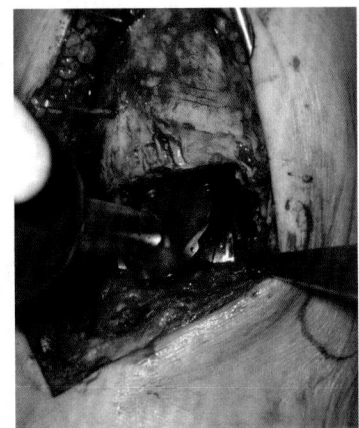

TECH FIG 10 Inserting talar component. **A.** Talar component properly oriented. **B.** Impacting the talar component (note that the ankle is plantarflexed and the impactor is not contacting the anterior tibia).

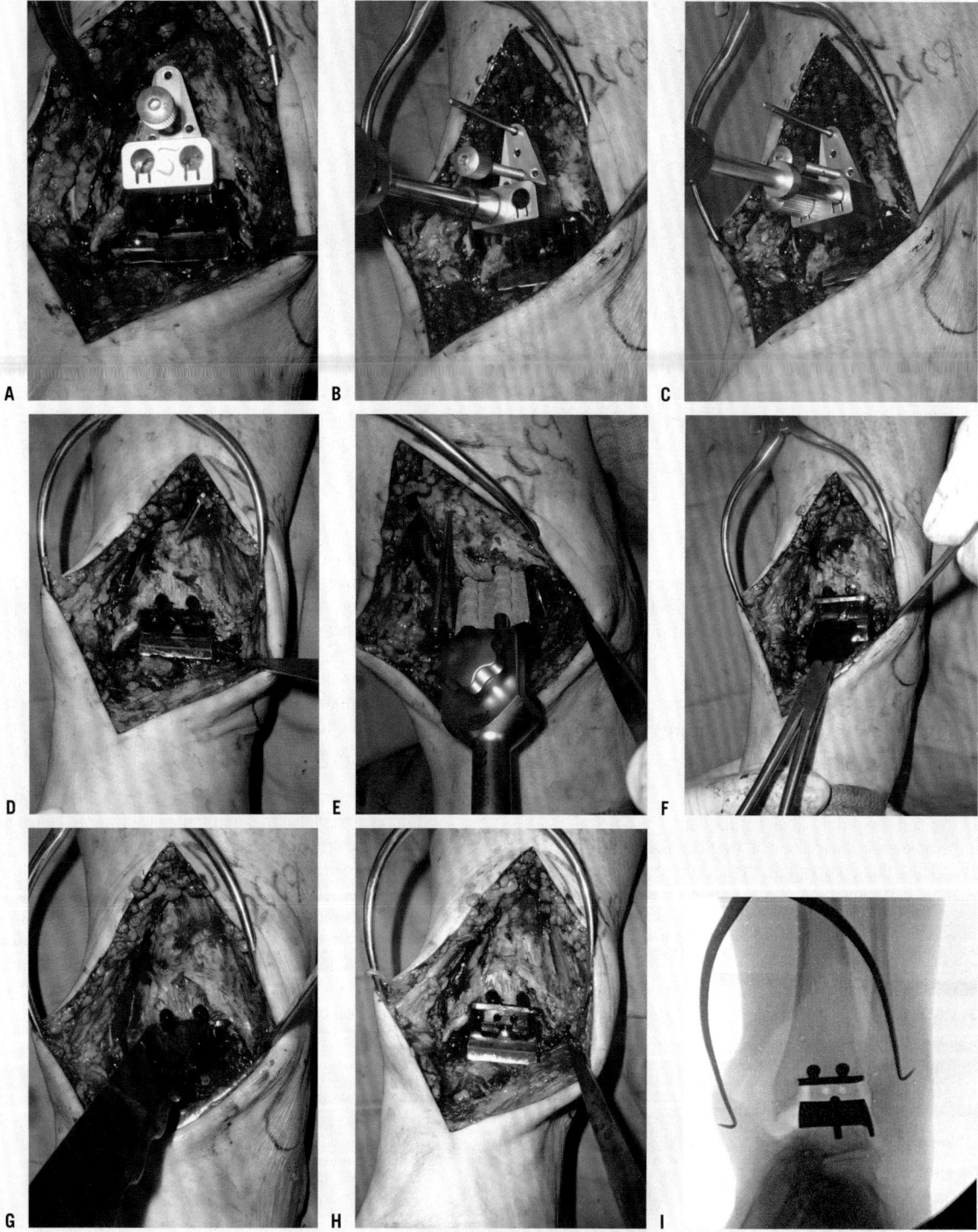

TECH FIG 11 Final tibial preparation and insertion. **A.** Properly sized tibial trial in place, with trial polyethylene for support (we routinely obtain fluoroscopic confirmation in the lateral plane that the tibial trial is flush on the prepared tibial surface). **B.** Reaming the barrel holes. **C.** Using the dedicated chisel to complete the barrel hole preparation. **D.** Prepared tibia. **E.** Tibial component being advanced with insertion device. **F.** With tibial component nearly fully seated, trial polyethylene is inserted to support posterior tibial component. **G.** Final impaction of tibial component. Trial polyethylene clinical (**H**) and fluoroscopic (**I**) views.

Final Polyethylene Implantation

- With the true tibial and talar components implanted, determine the optimal polyethylene size based on the trial polyethylenes **(TECH FIG 12A–D)**.
- With the ankle in neutral position, there should be virtually no lift-off at the two polyethylene–prosthesis interfaces when a varus or valgus stress is applied.

- ROM must allow dorsiflexion to at least 5 to 8 degrees, preferably more.
  - Occasionally, tendo Achilles lengthening is required. In these select situations, we routinely perform a gastrocnemius–soleus recession.
- Contain the polyethylene meniscus under the tibial component during ROM **(TECH FIG 12E,F)**.

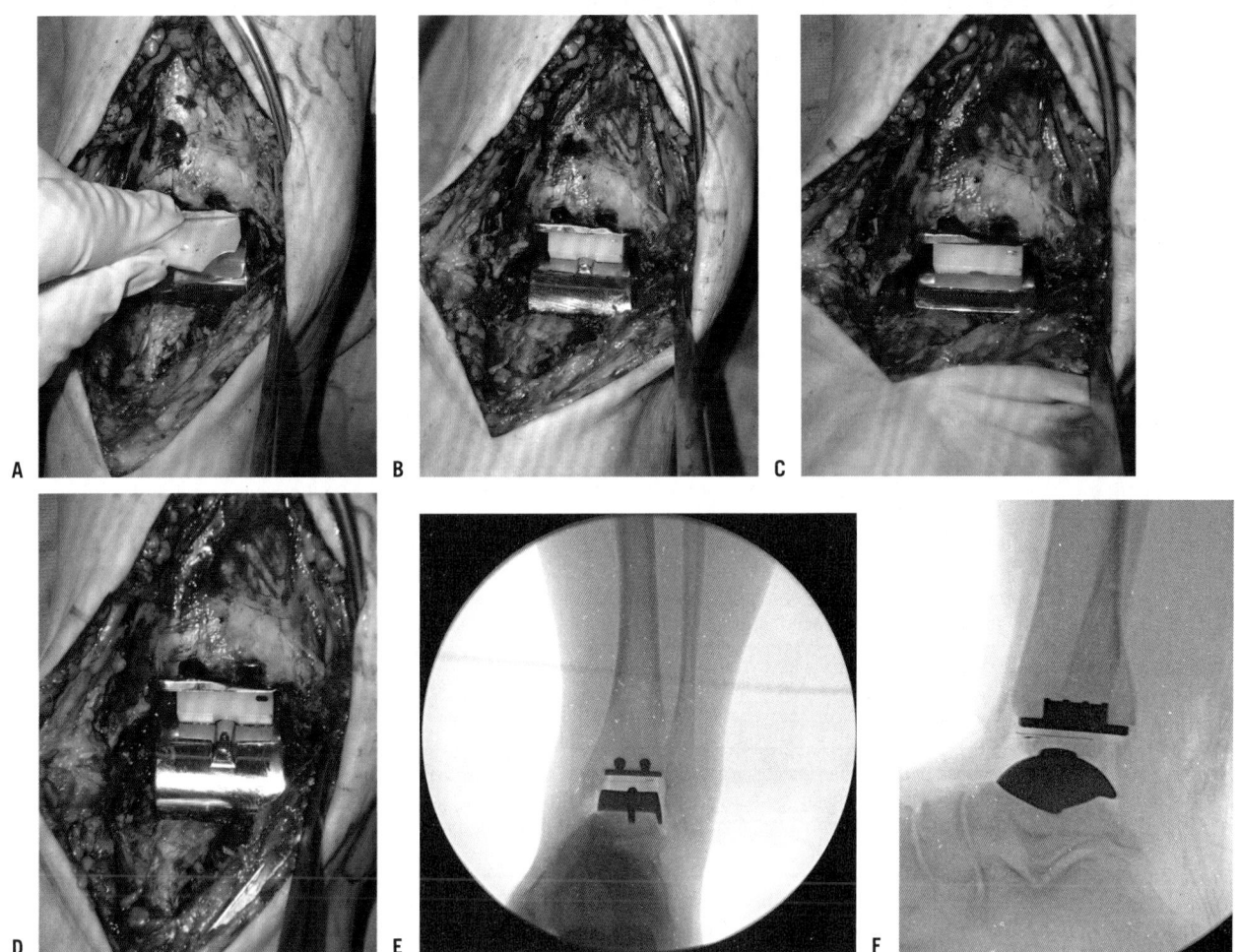

TECH FIG 12 Insertion of final polyethylene. **A.** Manual insertion. **B.** Polyethylene in place. **C.** Dorsiflexion. **D.** Plantarflexion. Final fluoroscopic AP (**E**) and lateral (**F**) views. The talus is proud posterior because of a relatively conservative initial talar cut. In our experience, the component will settle (not subside) into a stable position.

CLOSURE AND CASTING

- Thoroughly irrigate the joint and implant with sterile saline.
- While protecting the prosthesis, fill the anterior barrel holes with bone graft from the resected bone **(TECH FIG 13)**.
- Remove the pin from the proximal tibia.
- Reapproximate the capsule.
- We routinely use a drain.
- The tourniquet is released and meticulous hemostasis is obtained.

- Reapproximate the extensor retinaculum while protecting the deep and superficial peroneal nerves.
- Irrigate the subcutaneous layer with sterile saline and then reapproximate it.
- Reapproximate the skin to a tensionless closure.
- Place sterile dressings on the wounds, and apply adequate padding and a short-leg cast with the ankle in neutral position.

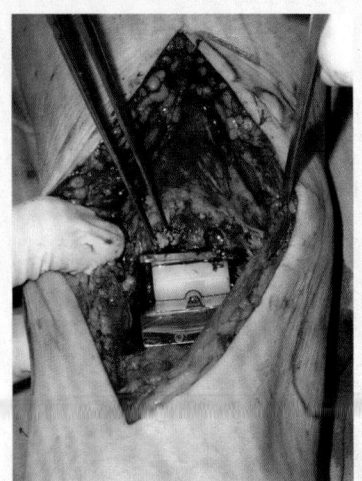 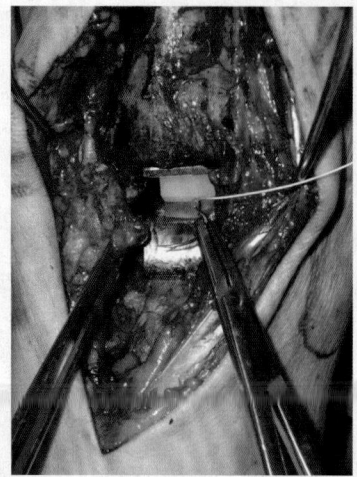

TECH FIG 13 Bone grafting and closure. **A.** Bone grafting the anterior cortex at the barrel holes. **B.** Capsular closure.

TECHNIQUES

Pearls and Pitfalls

Tibial Preparation	• Although traditionally up to 7 degrees of posterior slope was recommended, we favor 0 degree of posterior slope. In our opinion, the mobile bearing will be more stable with a more uniform load distribution across the ankle.
Talar Preparation	• Confirm fluoroscopically that the talus is in neutral dorsiflexion–plantarflexion in the sagittal plane so that the talar component will be in optimal position. If there is residual equinus despite anterior osteophyte removal, perform a tendo Achilles lengthening or gastrocnemius–soleus recession to position the talus correctly. • Remove residual cartilage from the dome of the talus to ensure an adequate talar resection level. The distance between the cutting slot and paddle that rests on the talar dome is fixed. Therefore, if there is residual talar dome cartilage or a prominence that tilts the cutting guide, the initial talar cut will be less than desired or asymmetric.
Use of the 4-in-1 Talar Reference Guide (Datum)	• Confirm its proper AP position with a lateral fluoroscopic view.
Impacting the Talar Component	• Because of the limited access to the ankle, the talar component tends to tilt anteriorly when impacted, even with optimal talar preparation. Be sure it is positioned properly in the sagittal plane over the talus (inserted posteriorly enough) before it is impacted. During impaction, carefully place a small osteotome under the anterior edge of the prosthesis to limit the anterior tilt.
Coronal Plane Position of the Tibial Component	• The tibial component must be centered under the tibial shaft axis. If performed judiciously, one or two more millimeters of medial tibial bone may be resected with a small reciprocating saw to translate the tibial component more medially, without compromising the medial malleolus.
Impacting the Tibial Component	• The tibial component is wider anteriorly than posteriorly. The medial malleolus must be carefully monitored during tibial component impaction. If the component begins to impinge on the medial malleolus, the reciprocating saw may be used to perform an anterior "relief" cut to relieve stress on the malleolus. With proper reaming of the barrels in the trial component, this is rarely an issue, but it may be encountered.

POSTOPERATIVE CARE

- Overnight stay
- Nasal oxygen while in the hospital
- Touchdown weight bearing on the cast is permitted, but elevation is encouraged as much as possible.
- The patient returns in 2 to 3 weeks for cast change and suture removal.
- The patient then returns at 6 weeks postoperatively for removal of cast and weight-bearing radiographs of the ankle.

- If there is no evidence of a stress fracture or failure of the procedure, then the patient can progress to a regular shoe and full weight bearing **(FIG 2)**.

OUTCOMES

- Although some recently reported outcomes are based on high-level evidence, results of TAA are almost uniformly derived from level IV evidence. Two recent investigations of the Scandinavian total ankle replacement are level I[5] and level II[3] but with short- to intermediate-term follow-up only.[2,4]

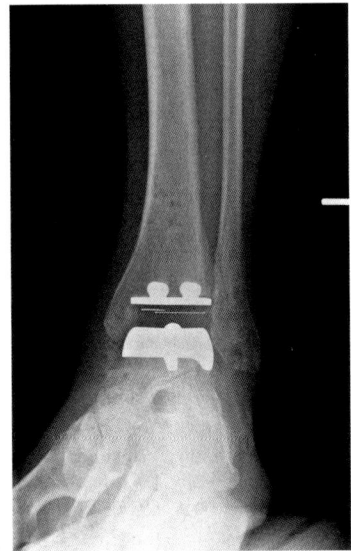
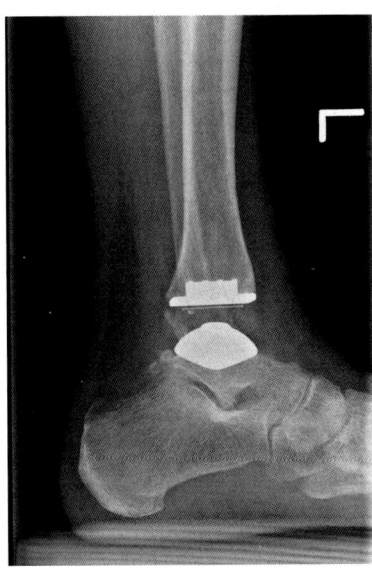

FIG 2 Weight-bearing radiographs of same patient in **FIG 1. A.** AP view. **B.** Lateral view (note that talus has assumed anatomic position under tibial shaft axis).

- Functional outcome using commonly used scoring systems for TAA (American Orthopaedic Foot and Ankle Society [AOFAS],[1] Mazur, and New Jersey Orthopaedic Hospital [NJOH] [Buechel-Pappas]) suggest uniform improvement in all studies, with follow-up scores ranging from 70 to 90 points (maximum 100 points).
- Patient satisfaction rates for TAA exceed 90%, although follow-up for the patient satisfaction rating often does not exceed 5 years.
- Overall survivorship analysis for currently available implants, designating removal of a metal component or conversion to arthrodesis as the end point, ranges from about 90% to 95% at 5 to 6 years, 80% to 92% at 10 to 12 years, and 73% to 75% at 15 to 19 years.

COMPLICATIONS

- Infection (superficial or deep)
- Neuralgia (superficial or deep peroneal nerve; rarely tibial nerve)
- Delayed wound healing
- Wound dehiscence
- Persistent pain despite optimal orthopaedic examination and radiographic appearance of implants
- Osteolysis
- Subsidence
- Malleolar or distal tibial stress fracture
- Implant fracture (including polyethylene)

REFERENCES

1. Kofoed H. Scandinavian total ankle replacement (STAR). Clin Orthop Relat Res 2004;(424):73–79.
2. Nunley JA, Caputo AM, Easley ME, et al. Intermediate to long-term outcomes of the STAR Total Ankle Replacement: the patient perspective. J Bone Joint Surg Am 2012;94(1):43–48.
3. Saltzman CL, Mann RA, Ahrens JE, et al. Prospective controlled trial of STAR total ankle replacement versus ankle fusion: initial results. Foot Ankle Int 2009;30:579–596.
4. Wood PL, Prem H, Sutton C. Total ankle replacement: medium-term results in 200 Scandinavian total ankle replacements. J Bone Joint Surg Br 2008;90(5):605–609.
5. Wood PL, Sutton C, Mishra V, et al. A randomised, controlled trial of two mobile-bearing total ankle replacements. J Bone Joint Surg Br 2009;91(1):69–74.

SUGGESTED READINGS

Daniels TR, Mayich DJ, Penner MJ. Intermediate to long-term outcomes of total ankle replacement with the Scandinavian Total Ankle Replacement (STAR). J Bone Joint Surg AM 2015;97(11):895–903.

Frigg A, Germann U, Huber M, et al. Survival of the Scandinavian Total Ankle Replacement (STAR): results of ten to nineteen years follow-up. Int Orthop 2017;41(10):2075–2082.

Loewy EM, Sanders TH, Walling AK. Intermediate-term experience with the STAR Total Ankle in the United States. Foot Ankle Int 2019;40(3):268–275.

Palanca A, Mann RA, Mann JA, et al. Scandinavian Total Ankle Replacement: 15-year follow-up. Foot Ankle Int 2018;39(2):135–142.

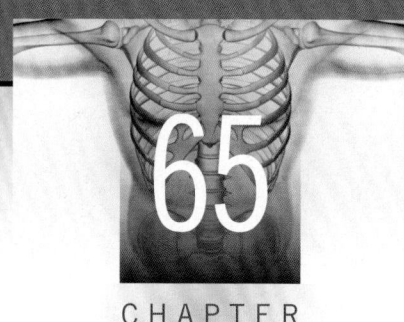

The Hintermann Series H2 and H3 Total Ankle Arthroplasty

Beat Hintermann and Roxa Ruiz

DEFINITION

- The Hintermann Series (former HINTEGRA) Total Ankle Prosthesis (DT MedTech, LLC [Towson, MD]) is available in two versions:
  - H3: an unconstrained, three-component system that provides inversion–eversion stability (introduced to market 2000, U.S. Food and Drug Administration [FDA] approved 06/2019) **(FIG 1A)**. Axial rotation and normal flexion–extension mobility are provided by a mobile-bearing element.[9,12,17–19]
  - H2: a semiconstrained, two-component system that provides inversion–eversion stability and allows for free adaption to individual axis of rotation (introduced to market 2018, FDA approved 11/2017) **(FIG 1B)**. It is basically a three-component system that is converted into a two-component system after insertion of components, allowing them to adapt to the given anatomy of the osteoarthritic ankle and its individual axis of rotation.
- The H3 ankle includes a metal tibial component, an ultra-high-density polyethylene bearing, and a metal talar component, all of which are available in six sizes, whereas the H2 ankle includes a capture mechanism with a locking piece and screw to fix the polyethylene bearing in the given position. The metal components are made up of a cobalt-chromium

alloy and coated with a 200-μm porous titanium and hydroxyapatite coating where osteointegration is necessary. The remaining metallic surfaces are highly polished.

- The Hintermann Series ankle uses all available bone surfaces for support. The anatomically shaped, flat tibial and talar components essentially resurface the tibia and the talar dome, respectively, and the wings hemiprosthetically replace degenerate medial and lateral facets (a potential source of pain and impingement).
- The Hintermann Series ankle uses a sophisticated press-fit concept for optimal primary stability: on tibial side, by six pyramidal peaks and the anterior shield and on talar side, by curved wings and two pegs. With this, it allows for immediate full weight bearing of the ankle after surgery without fear of hindering osteointegration process. In addition, it minimizes stress shielding to occur over time.
- The Hintermann Series ankle provides 50 degrees of congruent contact flexion–extension and 50 degrees of congruent contact axial rotation. This provides congruent contact surfaces for normal load-bearing activities, even in the case of a distinct implantation error or preexisting deformity. Limits of motion depend on natural soft tissue constraints: With the Hintermann Series ankle, no mechanical prosthetic motion constraints are imposed for any natural ankle movement.

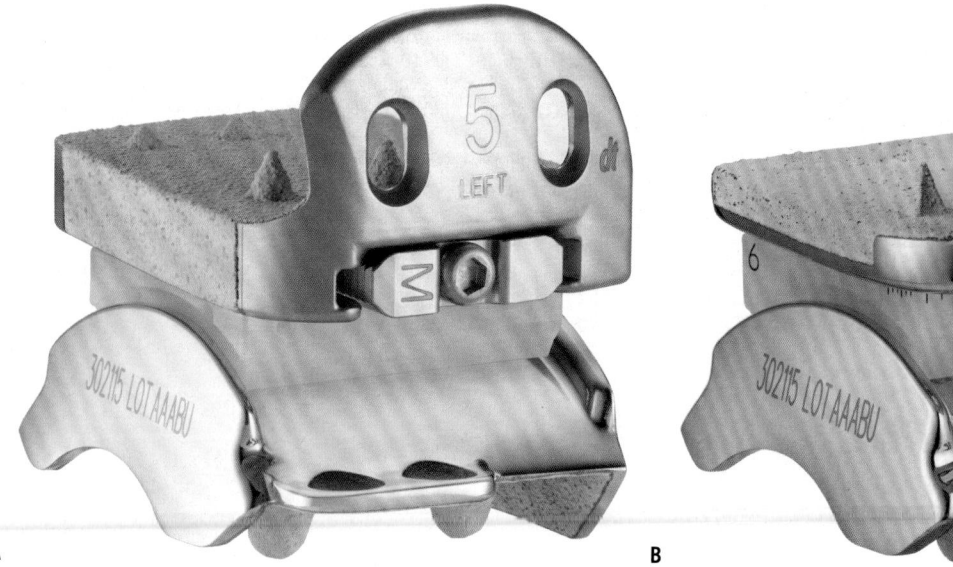

A   **B**

FIG 1 A. The H3 ankle consists of three components. **B.** The H2 ankle consists of two components; after insertion of components, the polyethylene insert is locked to the tibial component in its given position by the individual anatomy.

The H3 Ankle

- The tibial component consists of a flat 4-mm-thick loading plate with six pyramidal peaks facing the resection surface of tibia and an anterior shield facing the anterior surface of tibia to provide maximal stability against rotational and translational forces. In critical bone conditions as it may be the case in revision arthroplasty, the two holes in the anterior shield serve for additional screw fixation. The anatomically shaped flat surface ensures optimal contact with the subchondral bone, as well as optimal support of the cortical bone ring, providing a maximal load-transfer area. It further allows minimal resection (2 to 3 mm) of the subcortical bone to insert the implant. This fixation concept prevents stress shielding from occurring and ensure long-term stability by osteointegration in three planes (eg, flat resection surface, medial malleolus, and anterior cortex).
- The talar component is conically shaped, with a smaller radius on the medial side. The articular surface is highly polished and has a 2.5-mm-high rim on the medial and lateral side, which ensures a stable position and guided rotation of the polyethylene bearing (flexion–extension). The medial and lateral talar surfaces are covered by two wings, which through their anatomic shape cover the original cartilage-covered surface and allow press-fit of the component to the bone. Furthermore, the anterior shield increases the bone support on the weaker bone at the talar neck to increase stability in the sagittal plane and to prevent the adherence of scar tissue that might restrict motion. The current design, introduced in 2004, includes two pegs, which facilitate the insertion of the talar component and provide additional stability. With its coat, the whole undersurface provides osteointegration.
- The high-density polyethylene mobile bearing (ultra-high-molecular-weight polyethylene) consists of a flat surface on the tibial side and a concave surface that perfectly matches the talar surface. It has a minimum thickness of 5 mm but is also available in thicker sizes (6, 7, and 9 mm). The size of the polyethylene bearing corresponds to the talar size. It fully covers the talar component and therefore ensures optimal stability against valgus–varus forces and minimal contact stress on both the primary and secondary articulating surfaces. The bearing is restrained by the compressive action of the collateral ligaments and adjacent tissues. Furthermore, compressive muscle forces and gravitational loads across the joint hold the bearing against the metallic articulating surfaces. Thus, when properly positioned, dislocation of the bearing is unlikely.

The H2 Ankle

- The tibial component has the same configuration as the H3 tibial component but has a thickness of 6.5 mm and includes a capture mechanism for the polyethylene insert on its undersurface. This is a slot to receive the upper ring of the polyethylene insert and locking piece for fixation of it.
- The talar component is the same as that of the H3 ankle.
- The polyethylene insert has the same configuration as that of the H3 ankle but includes a mushroom-like ring on its upper surface that fits exactly into the slot on undersurface of tibial component. The metallic ring contains teeth on its anterior surface to receive the teeth of the locking piece to provide rotational stability once the locking pressure is applied by the screw.

The Revision Ankle

- The tibial component is available with an additional thickness of 4 and 8 mm to compensate for bone loss of distal tibia.
- The talar component provides a flat undersurface to compensate bone loss of talar body and longer pegs to enhance primary stability.

SELECTION OF IMPLANTS

- The selection of implants can be done preoperatively (based on clinical and imaging evaluation) or intraoperatively (based on bone stock and condition, ligament competence) as
  - The H3 (mobile-bearing) and H2 (fixed-bearing) ankle use the same resection cut on both the tibial and talar side
- The revision talus needs just adding a flat cut of talus along the anteroinferior border (eg, anterior shield).
- The H3 ankle may be selected for
  - An osteoarthritic joint with preserved congruency
  - A well-aligned and stable ankle
  - Well-preserved bone stock of tibia allowing for minimal bone resection
- The H2 ankle may be selected for
  - An osteoarthritic joint with loss of congruency
  - A maligned and unstable ankle
  - Bad bone stock of tibia needing higher amount of bone resection
- The revision talar component may be selected for
  - Loss of bone stock (eg, apex of talar body)
  - Avascular necrosis of talus
  - Flat talar configuration

ANATOMY

- The superior extensor retinaculum is a thickening of the deep fascia above the ankle, running from tibia to fibula.
- It includes, when looking from medial to lateral, the tendons of the tibialis anterior, the extensor hallucis longus, and the extensor digitorum longus.
- The anterior neurovascular bundle lies roughly halfway between the malleoli; it can be found consistently between the extensor hallucis longus and the extensor digitorum longus tendons.
- The neurovascular bundle contains the anterior tibial artery and the deep peroneal nerve. The nerve innervates the extensor digitorum brevis, the extensor hallucis brevis, and the sensory space interdigital I–II.
- On the height of the talonavicular joint, the medial branches of the superficial peroneal nerve cross from lateral to medial. It supplies the skin of the dorsum of the foot.
- On the posterior aspect of the ankle, the medial neurovascular bundle is located behind its posteromedial corner and the flexor hallucis longus tendon on its posterior aspect.
- On medial side, the deltoid ligament is a multibanded complex with superficial and deep components that provides stability to the talus against eversion and external rotation forces.
- The lateral ankle ligaments provide stability to the talus against inversion and internal rotation forces.

PATHOGENESIS

- Primary osteoarthritis of the ankle joint is rare; degenerative disease of the ankle is more often seen after trauma and systemic diseases (eg, rheumatoid arthritis).[1,2,4,5]
- Osteoarthritis of the ankle joint is often associated with malalignment, deformities, instabilities, and stiffness of the foot, particularly in posttraumatic ankles.[11,16]

NATURAL HISTORY

- Development of osteoarthritis of the ankle joint can take years, particularly in posttraumatic ankles (eg, after fractures and sprains).
- Once symptomatic, osteoarthritic changes usually progress, resulting in pain under loading conditions and finally at rest as well.
- If associated with instability or muscular dysfunction, misalignment and deformity may occur.

PATIENT HISTORY AND PHYSICAL FINDINGS

- A careful history is taken to assess the following:
  - Previous trauma
  - Previous infections
  - Underlying diseases
  - Actual pain
  - Limitations in daily and sports activities
- While the patient is standing, a thorough clinical investigation of both lower extremities is done to assess the following:
  - Alignment
  - Deformities
  - Foot position
  - Muscular atrophy
- While the patient is sitting with free-hanging feet, the examiner assesses the following:
  - The extent to which a deformity is correctable
  - Preserved joint motion at the ankle and subtalar joints
  - Ligament stability of the ankle and subtalar joints with anterior drawer and tilt tests
  - Supination and eversion power (eg, function of posterior tibial and peroneus brevis muscles)

IMAGING AND OTHER DIAGNOSTIC STUDIES

- Plain weight-bearing radiographs, including anteroposterior (AP) views of the foot and ankle, a lateral view of the foot, and an alignment view of the hindfoot (**FIG 2**),[14] are obtained to assess the following:
  - Extent of destruction of the tibiotalar joint (eg, tibia, talus, and fibula)
  - Status of neighboring joints (eg, associated degenerative disease)
  - Deformities of the foot and ankle complex (eg, heel alignment, foot arch, talonavicular alignment)
  - Tibiotalar malalignment (eg, varus, valgus, recurvatum, and antecurvatum)
  - Bony condition (eg, avascular necrosis, bony defects)
- A weight-bearing computed tomography (CT) scan (**FIG 3**) may be used for assessment of the following:
  - Destruction of joint surfaces and incongruency
  - Bony defects
  - Segmental instability (eg, tibiotalar and peritalar joints)
  - Avascular necrosis
- Single-photon emission computed tomography combined with CT (SPECT-CT) with a superimposed bone scan (**FIG 4**) may be used to visualize the following:
  - Morphologic pathologies and associated activity process
  - Biologic bone pathologies and associated activity process
- Magnetic resonance imaging may be used to show the following:
  - Injuries to ligament structures
  - Morphologic changes of tendons
  - Avascular necrosis of bones (eg, talar body and tibial plafond)
- Gait analysis[20]

NONOPERATIVE MANAGEMENT

- Although nonoperative management is controversial, patients with less debilitating pain and dysfunction may be treated nonoperatively.
- Nonoperative treatment may consist of the following:
  - Shoe modifications to facilitate gait
  - Physiotherapy to decrease inflammatory response
  - Anti-inflammatory medicine for acute pain

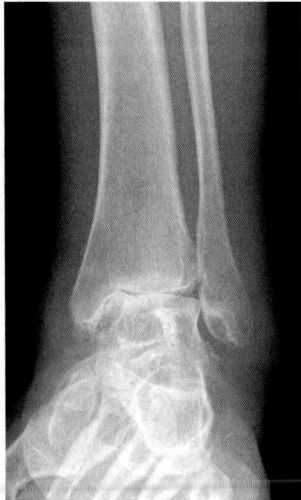 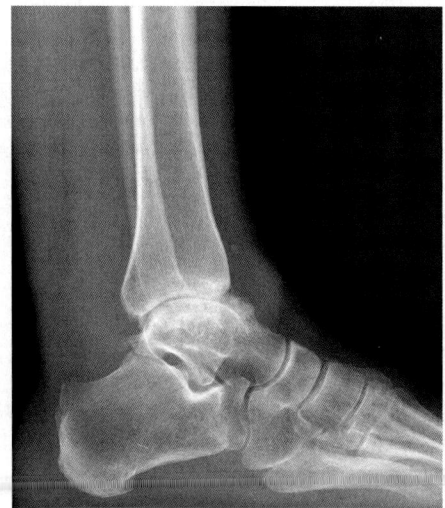 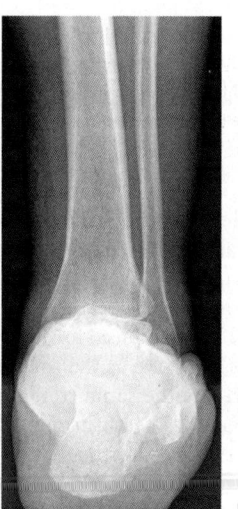 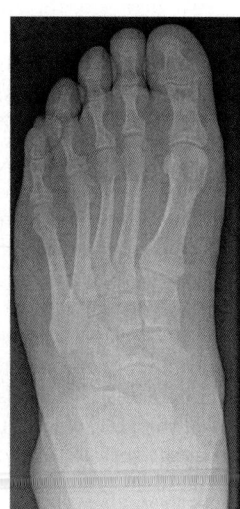

A   B   C   D

FIG 2 Preoperative assessment includes weight-bearing standard radiographs as follows: AP view of the ankle (**A**), lateral view of the foot (**B**), Saltzman alignment view (**C**), and AP view of the foot (**D**).

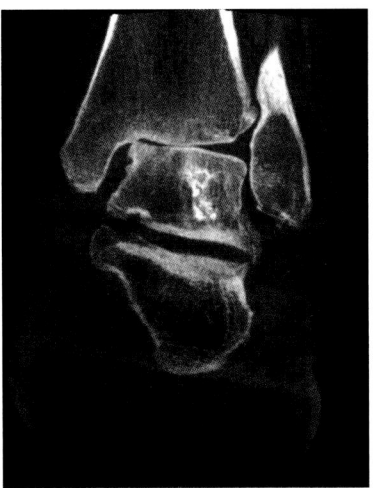 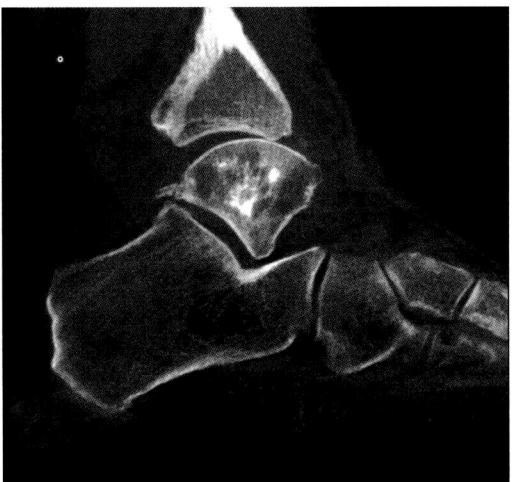 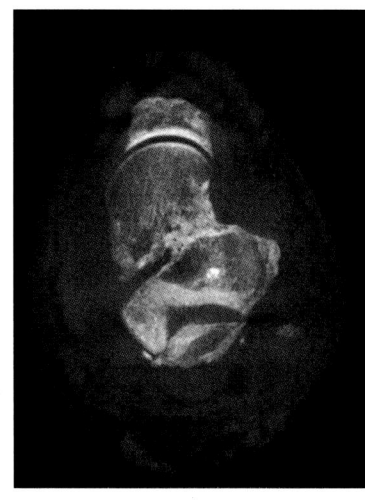

FIG 3 Weight-bearing CT in a patient with varus deformity showing the wear process in the medial tibiotalar joint, the varus tilt of talus, and the valgus tilt of calcaneus subsequently to the peritalar instability: AP coronal plane (**A**), sagittal plane (**B**), and AP horizontal plane (**C**).

SURGICAL MANAGEMENT

- Successful total ankle arthroplasty demands thorough preoperative planning to address all associated pathologies.
- During surgery, the surgeon must continuously check whether these associated pathologies are sufficiently addressed. For instance:
  - Whether preexisting deformities are sufficiently corrected
  - Whether the foot is properly aligned
  - Whether soft tissues are sufficiently balanced
- Indications
  - Primary osteoarthritis (eg, degenerative disease)
  - Systemic arthritis (eg, rheumatoid arthritis, hemochromatosis,[2] hemophilia,[1] gout[4])
  - Posttraumatic osteoarthritis (if instability and malalignment are manageable)
  - Secondary osteoarthritis (eg, infection, avascular necrosis) (if at least two-thirds of the talar surface is preserved)
  - Salvage for failed total ankle replacement (if bone stock is sufficient)[13]
  - Salvage for nonunion and malunion of ankle fusion (if bone stock is sufficient)[7]
  - Low demands for physical activities (hiking, swimming, biking, golfing)
- Relative indications
  - Severe osteoporosis
  - Immunosuppressive therapy
  - Increased demands for physical activities (eg, jogging, tennis, downhill skiing)
  - Bony avulsion fracture of medial malleolus (with or without fracture of the fibula–syndesmotic disruption)
- Contraindications
  - Infection
  - Avascular necrosis of more than one-third of the talus
  - Unmanageable instability
  - Unmanageable malalignment
  - Neuromuscular disorder
  - Neuroarthropathy (Charcot)
  - Diabetic syndrome

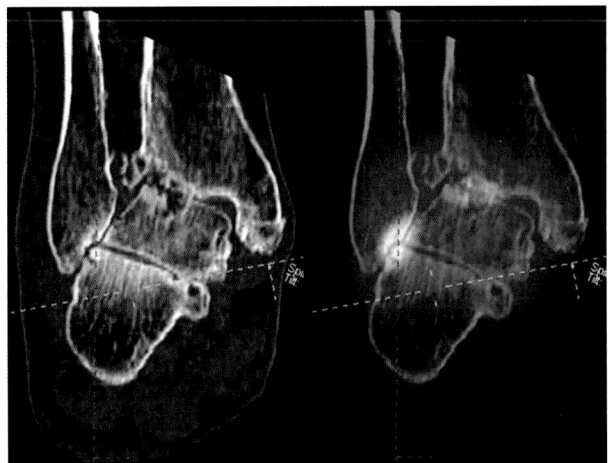 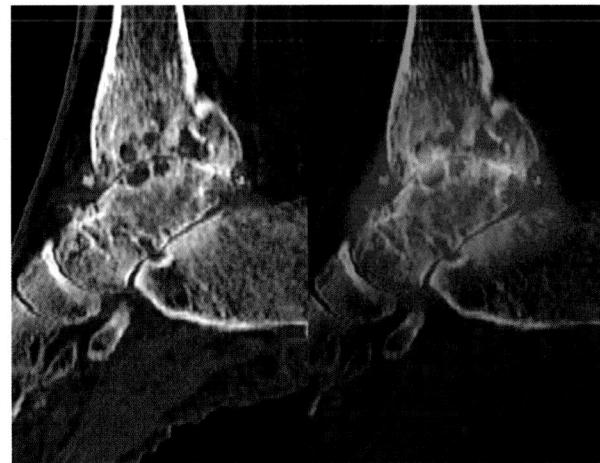

FIG 4 SPECT-CT in a patient with valgus deformity showing the pathologic process in the lateral tibiotalar and fibulotalar joints. **A.** AP view. **B.** Lateral view.

- Suspected or documented metal allergy or intolerance
- Highest demands for physical activities (eg, contact sports, jumping)
- Controversial indications
  - Diabetic syndrome without polyneuropathy
  - Avascular necrosis of talus
  - Obesity[3]

Preoperative Planning

- All imaging studies are reviewed.
- Plain films should be reviewed to identify possible coexisting arthritis of adjacent joints as well as varus and valgus of the hindfoot and the longitudinal arch.
- Associated foot deformity, malalignment, and instability should be addressed concurrently.
- Examination under anesthesia should be accomplished to compare with the contralateral ankle.

Positioning

- The patient is positioned with the feet on the edge of the table.
- The ipsilateral back is lifted until a strictly upward position of the foot is obtained.
- A block is placed under the affected foot to facilitate fluoroscopy during surgery.
- The contralateral (nonaffected) leg is also draped if significant deformity is to be corrected.
- A tourniquet is applied on the ipsilateral thigh.

Approach

- An anterior longitudinal incision 10 to 12 cm long is made to expose the retinaculum.

- The retinaculum is dissected along the lateral border of the anterior tibial tendon, and the anterior aspect of the distal tibia is exposed.
- While the soft tissue mantle is dissected with the periosteum from the bone, attention is paid to the neurovascular bundle that lies behind the long extensor hallucis tendon.
- Capsulotomy and capsulectomy are done, and a self-retaining retractor is inserted to carefully keep the soft tissue mantle away (FIG 5).
- Osteophytes on the tibia are removed, particularly on the anterolateral aspect.
- Osteophytes on the talar neck and the anterior aspect of medial malleolus are also removed.
- The fibula usually cannot be fully visualized at this stage.

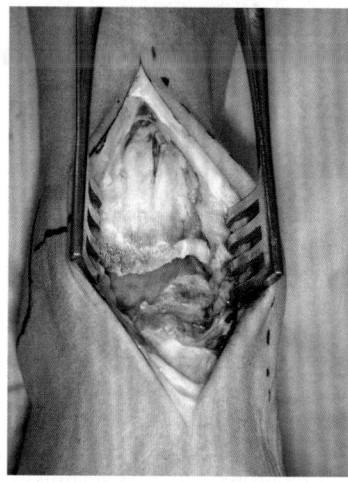

FIG 5 The ankle joint is exposed through an anterior approach.

TIBIAL RESECTION

- Position the tibial cutting block with its alignment rod using the tibial tuberosity (eg, the anterior cresta iliaca of pelvis in the case of leg deformity) (TECH FIG 1A) as the proximal reference and the anterior border of the ankle (eg, the center of the resection block is supposed to be at intermediate line of the tibiotalar joint) as the distal reference.
- Make the final adjustment as follows:
  - Sagittal plane: Move the rod until a parallel position to the anterior border of the tibia has been achieved (TECH FIG 1B).
  - Frontal (coronal) plane: Frontal plane position is given by the position of the rod (eg, there is a fixed 90-degree angle between the resection surface and the rod). Once the rod is proximally centered to tibial tuberosity (TECH FIG 1C), two pins are used for fixation.
  - Vertical adjustment: Move the tibial resection block proximally until the desired resection height is achieved. Usually, resection of about 2 to 3 mm (for H2 ankle, 2 mm more) on the apex of the tibial plafond is desired. In varus ankles, more tibial resection is usually needed, whereas in valgus ankles or in presence of high joint laxity, less bone resection is advised.

- Rotational adjustment: Rotate the tibial resection block to get a parallel position of its medial surface to the medial surface of the talus (eg, to avoid damaging the malleoli with the saw blade during resection).
- Slide the tibial cutting guide into the cutting block, creating a slot in which the saw blade will be guided. The width of the slot limits the excursion of the saw blade, thereby protecting the malleoli from being hit and fractured.
- Once the tibial cut is made, a reciprocating saw might be used to finalize the cuts, particularly for the vertical cut on the medial side (TECH FIG 1D).
- Remove the remaining bone with a rongeur (TECH FIG 1E), including the posterior capsule.
- Use the measuring gauge to determine the size of the implant. In doubt (eg, if the anterior border of the tibia is projected onto the gauge between two markers), select the bigger size (TECH FIG 1F).
- Remove the depth gauge and, if necessary, smooth the anterior border of the tibial resection with an oscillating saw or rongeur according to the shape of the indicated resection.
- Insert the tibial trial. Try to get the tibial component in close contact with the medial malleolus and the anterior surface of tibia (TECH FIG 1G).

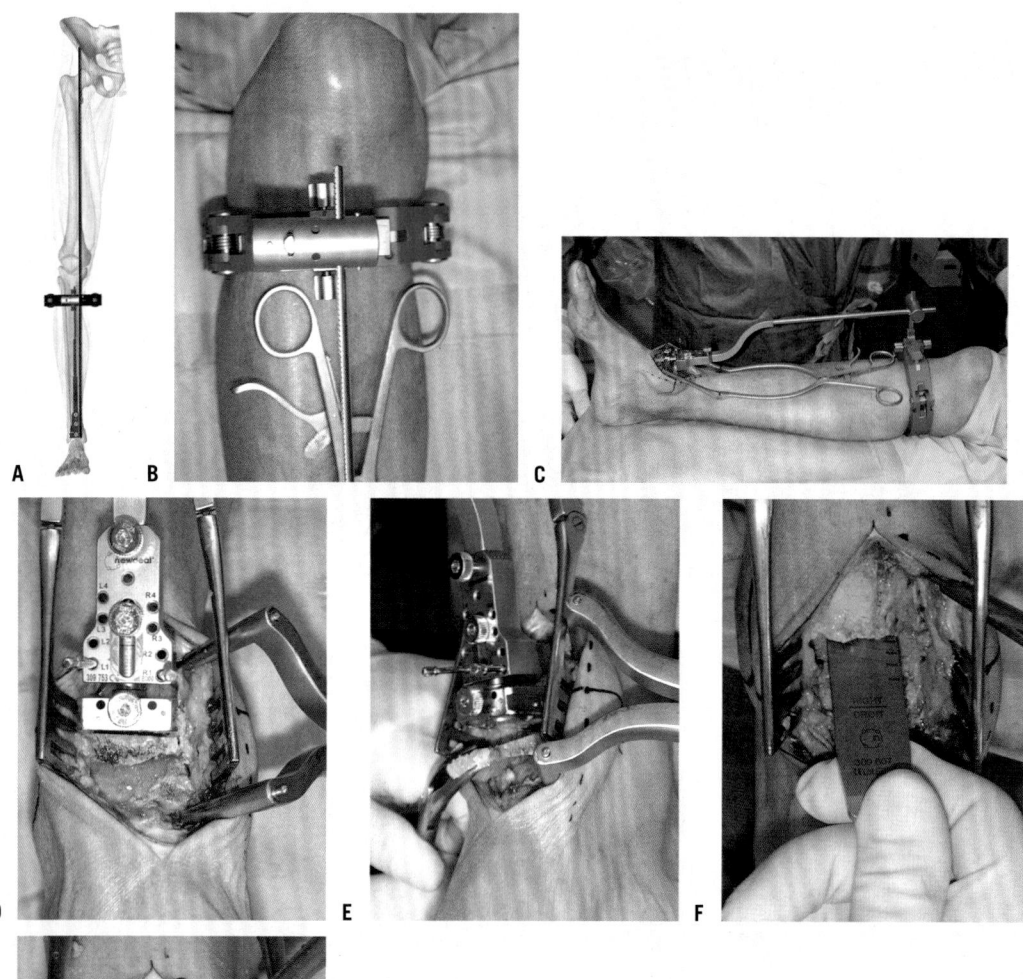

TECH FIG 1 Tibial resection. Tibial resection block is adjusted taking the tibial tuberosity or the anterior spina of iliac crest as the reference in the frontal plane (**A,B**) and the anterior tibia in the sagittal plane (**C**). **D.** Two to 3 mm of bone is removed, as measured at the apex of the tibial plafond. **E.** Bone is removed, and resection is finalized at the lateral side, paying attention not to damage the integrity of the fibula and at the medial side to get a sharp perpendicular cut along the medial malleolus. **F.** The tibial depth gauge is inserted, and the size of tibial implant is determined. **G.** The tibial trial implant is inserted making sure that the tibial component is in close contact with the medial malleolus and the anterior surface of tibia. If necessary, the anterolateral tibia has to be smoothed.

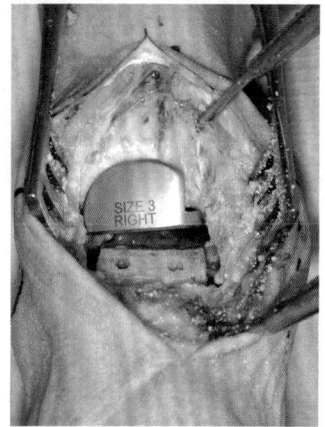

TALAR RESECTION (FOR STANDARD TALAR COMPONENT)

Positioning the Resection Block

- Insert the talar resection block into the tibial cutting block.
- Move the resection block as far distal as possible to properly tension the collateral ligaments **(TECH FIG 2A)**.
- Remove all distractors and spreaders before the foot is moved to a neutral position (eg, with respect to dorsiflexion–plantarflexion and pronation–supination).

- Once the foot is in a neutral position, fix the resection block with two pins (medially and laterally) **(TECH FIG 2B)**.
- The hindfoot alignment should now be neutral, indicating that no inframalleolar correction will be necessary **(TECH FIG 2C)**.

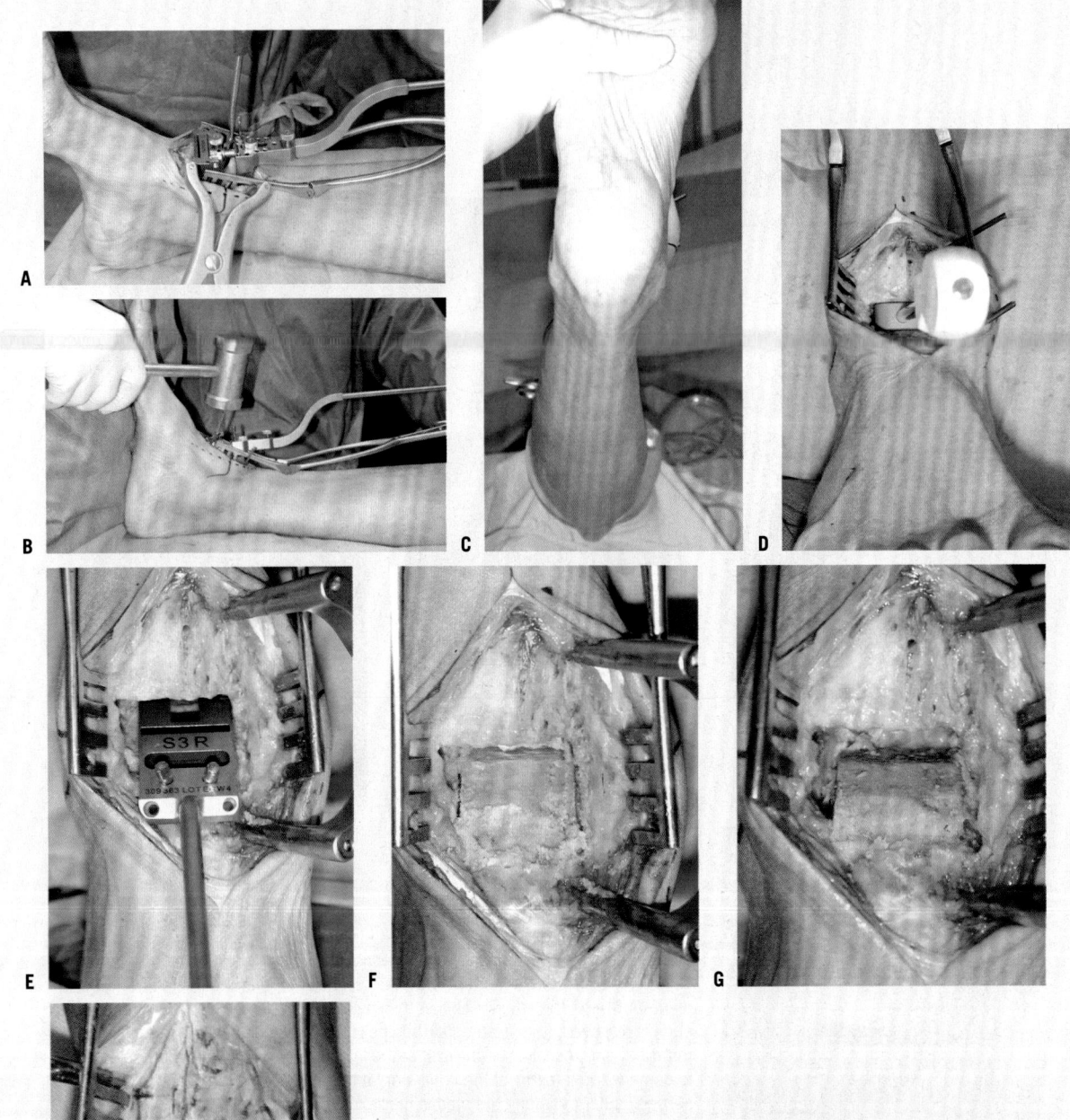

TECH FIG 2 Talar resection. **A.** After insertion of talar resection block, the whole block is moved distally until collateral ligaments of the ankle are fully tensioned. **B.** The talar resection block is fixed by pins to the talus while the foot is held in a neutral position. **C.** Alignment of the hindfoot is carefully checked. **D.** After the horizontal cut is made by the saw through the slot and the resection block is removed, the spacer is inserted to check alignment and stability of the ankle. **E.** The appropriate size of the talar resection block is fitted to the bone using the medial border of the talus as a reference. **F.** After posterior, medial, lateral, and anterior cuts are made, the block is removed. **G.** Bone stock of the talus after careful débridement of the medial, lateral, and posterior compartment as well as complete resection of the posterior capsule of the ankle joint. **H.** While the foot is held strictly in the neutral position, a strictly parallel cut to the tibial resection is done on remaining talar bone stock, paying attention to preserve as much bone as possible.

Making the Horizontal Cuts

- Resect the talar dome with the oscillating saw through the slot of the talar cutting block.
- Remove the tibial and talar resection block and again, mount the distractor (Hintermann Series spreader) to distract the joint.
- Remove the posterior capsule completely until fat tissue and tendon structures are visible to achieve full dorsiflexion.
- Insert the 12- (H3) or 15.5-mm (H2) thick spacer representing the thickness of the tibial and talar components and the thinnest 5-mm inlay into the created joint space (**TECH FIG 2D**). While the foot is held in neutral flexion position, the surgeon should check the following:
  - Whether an appropriate amount of bone has been resected
  - Whether the achieved alignment is appropriate
  - Whether the medial and lateral stability are ensured
- If the spacer cannot be properly inserted into the joint space and if there is no obvious contracture of the remaining posterior capsule present, additional bony resection might be considered. In most instances, such additional resection should be done on the tibial side. Reposition the tibial cutting block using the same fixation holes for the pins. Move the distal resection block proximally as desired and make a new cut with the saw blade.
- If the alignment is not appropriate and if an associated deformity of the foot itself (eg, varus, valgus heel) can be excluded, consider a corrective cut.
- If the ankle is not stable on both sides, consider using a thicker inlay. If the ankle is not stable on one side, consider a release of the contralateral ligaments or ligament reconstruction on the affected side. Ligament reconstruction should be done once the definitive implants have been inserted and an obvious instability still exists.
- Remove the spacer and mount the distractor (Hintermann Series spreader) using the same pins.

Making the Final Cuts of Talus (TECH FIG 2E)

- Select the size of talar resection according to the selected size of tibial component.
- Use the medial side of the talus as the reference; position the resection block along the medial border of the talus so that 1 to 2 mm of bone will be removed from the medial side of the talus.
- On the lateral side, the resection block is supposed to remove as little bone as possible on its posterior aspect; usually, more bone will need to be removed on the lateral aspect of the talus, as osteophytes are more common there.
- If the selected resection block overpasses the lateral border of resection surface, a smaller size is selected. Downsizing of talar component may be done as much as needed.

- If, with the selected resection block, greater than 3 mm of bone will remain to be removed along the whole lateral aspect of talus, a one size larger resection block is selected. Upsizing of talar component greater than 1 size is critical as the polyethylene insert would risk overpassing the tibial component, thus causing edge load.
- On the posterior side, the resection block is supposed to remove 2 to 3 mm of bone in addition to the remaining cartilage; this is given by the distance of the posterior hooks of the resection block that aim to be in strong contact with the posterior surface of the talus.
- After having positioned the talar cutting block properly, fix it with two or three pins. While the foot is brought to a neutral position, its handle should meet the second ray (eg, the longitudinal axis of the foot).
- Perform the posterior resection of the talus with an oscillating saw that is guided through the posterior slot of the talar cutting block.
- Perform the medial and lateral resections of the talus with a reciprocating saw that is guided along the talar cutting block. Make the cut as following:
  - Medial side: 6 mm deep; the reference is the upper surface of the talus.
  - Lateral side: 8 mm deep; the reference is the upper surface of the talus.
- Perform the anterior resection of the talus with a drill that is guided through the anterior slot of the talar cutting block.

Finishing the Resection

- Remove the talar cutting block (**TECH FIG 2F**).
- On the medial and lateral sides, the cuts are finalized by using a chisel to make an almost horizontal cut along the base of the cuts previously made, thereby avoiding extended loss of bone stock and potential damage to the vascular supply of the talus.
- Clean the medial and lateral gutters using a rongeur.
- Remove the remaining bone and capsule of the posterior compartment (**TECH FIG 2G**).

Talar Resection (for Revision Talar Component)

- If the upper contour of remaining talus is somehow preserved, allowing the talar resection block with its tongue to keep the talus in an appropriate position, the cut is done accordingly with the oscillating saw through the provided slot.
- If there is substantial bone loss, the talus should be held in its desired position to the tibia while holding the Hintermann Series distractor that tensions the ligaments. Then, a freehand flat cut is made parallel to the tibial resection surface for minimal resection of additional bone on talar side, aiming to start at anteroinferior border of former joint surface (**TECH FIG 2H**).

INSERTING TRIAL IMPLANTS AND FINALIZING CUTS

- Talar trial (for standard talar component)
  - Insert the talar trial using the given impactor. The window on the posterior aspect of the trial allows the surgeon to check its proper fit to the posterior resection surface of the talus (**TECH FIG 3A**).
  - If proper position of the talus has been achieved, resect the anterior surface of the talus using a rongeur or the oscillating saw.
  - Fix the drill guide onto the talar trial (**TECH FIG 3B**).

- Make two drill holes with the provided 4.5-mm drill and remove the trial (**TECH FIG 3C**).
- Talar trial (for revision talar component)
  - Mount the resection block (**TECH FIG 3D**) and make the cut with the small saw is done along the lateral and medial border.
  - Remove the resected bone in the medial and lateral gutter and resect dorsal scarred capsular.

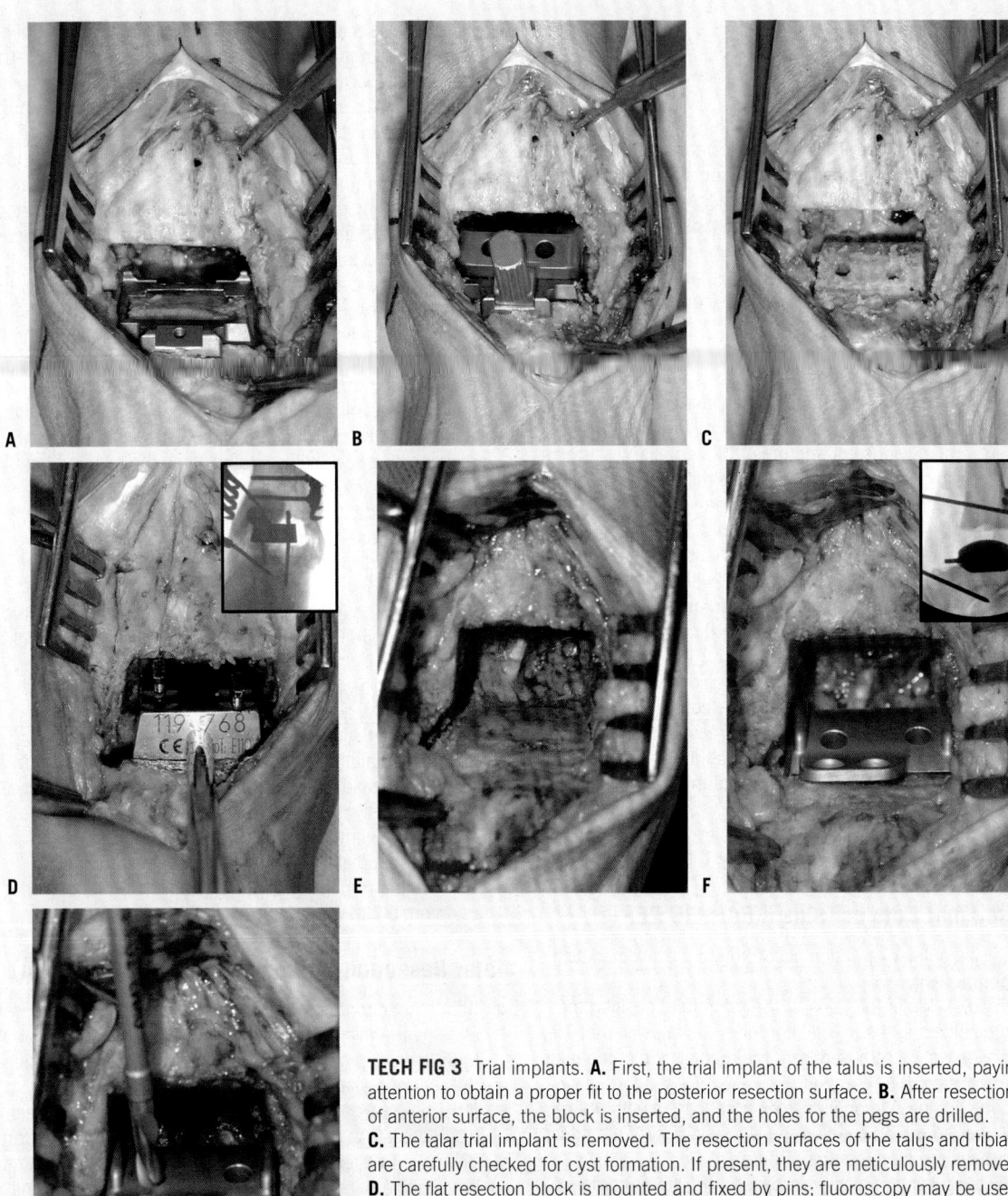

TECH FIG 3 Trial implants. **A.** First, the trial implant of the talus is inserted, paying attention to obtain a proper fit to the posterior resection surface. **B.** After resection of anterior surface, the block is inserted, and the holes for the pegs are drilled. **C.** The talar trial implant is removed. The resection surfaces of the talus and tibia are carefully checked for cyst formation. If present, they are meticulously removed. **D.** The flat resection block is mounted and fixed by pins; fluoroscopy may be used to check the position before the medial and lateral cuts are made with the use of a reciprocal saw. **E.** Allograft is used to fill the defects, and a flat spreader is used to impact the allograft; some bone matrix maybe added to fill the remaining defects. **F.** The tibial trial component is inserted and moved posteriorward until it has reached the appropriate position, as checked by fluoroscopy. **G.** The drill holes for the pegs are made.

- Fill the defects with allograft and add, if necessary, some bone matrix to get a solid resection surface **(TECH FIG 3E)**.
- Insert the trial talar component and make sure, that its AP position is appropriate **(TECH FIG 3F)**. Check by fluoroscopy.
- Drill the holes for the pegs **(TECH FIG 3G)**.
- Tibial trial
  - Insert the tibial trial.
- Trial inlay
  - Insert the 5-mm inlay trial and remove the distractor (Hintermann Series spreader).

- If not enough soft tissue tension can be achieved, insert the 6-, 7-, or 9-mm trial.
- The use of fluoroscopy is highly recommended to check the position of implants while the foot is held in neutral position, particularly the following (lateral view):
  - Appropriate length of the tibial component: Its posterior border should be in line with the posterior aspect of the tibia so that the tibial surface is fully covered.
  - Proper fit of the tibial component to the tibial surface

- Proper fit of the posterior edge of the talar component to the posterior surface of the talus
- Point of contact of the talar component to the tibial component. This contact point should be between 40% and 45% of the tibial component when the anterior border is taken as 0% and the posterior border as 100%, respectively. If the point of contact is too posterior, ligament balance will not be achieved.

- AP view:
  - Appropriate position of tibial and talar component on resection surfaces
  - Alignment of tibial and talar component
  - Remaining bone in the medial and lateral gutter

FINAL PREPARATION

- Carefully check the bony surfaces.
  - Any cysts need to be cleaned with a curette; furthermore, filling with cancellous bone taken from the removed bony material or with bone matrix is recommended.

- If there is sclerotic bone left on the surface, drilling with a 2.0-mm drill is recommended.

INSERTION OF IMPLANTS (H3 ANKLE)

- Insert the final implants previously selected as follows:
  - Insert the talar component so that the pegs can glide into the two drilled holes; use a hammer and impactor to obtain a proper fit of the component to the bone **(TECH FIG 4A)**.
  - Insert the tibial component along the medial malleolus until proper fit to the anterior border of the tibia is achieved **(TECH FIG 4B)**.

- Insert the inlay (same size as the talar component) of selected thickness. Remove the distractor (Hintermann Series spreader).
- Hammer and impactor might be used for appropriate fit to the bone **(TECH FIG 4C)**.
- Check stability and motion clinically.

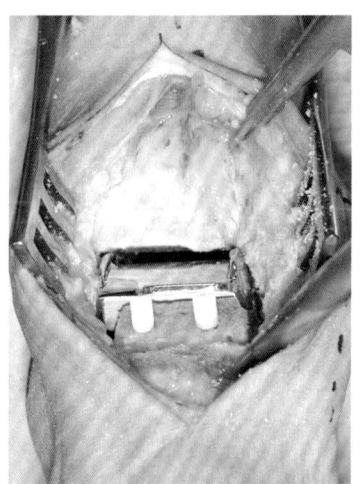 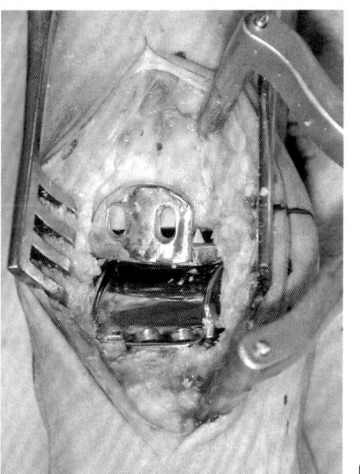 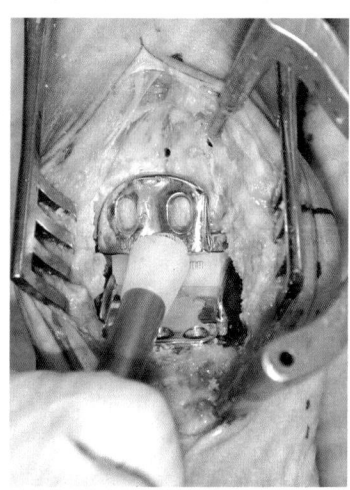

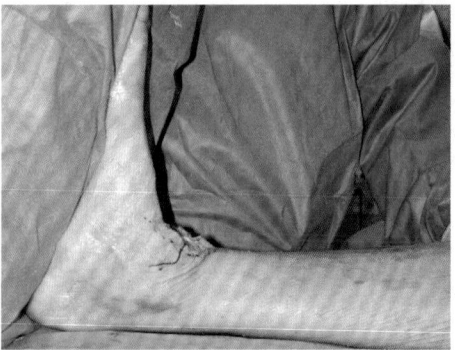

TECH FIG 4 Insertion of definitive implants for the H3 ankle. **A.** The talar component is impacted first. **B.** After insertion of the tibial component and the polyethylene insert (**C**), the tibial component is impacted to obtain a proper fit to the tibial resection surface. **D.** The foot is moved in dorsiflexion with the surgeon's maximal power, hereby settling of the implant might be improved and remaining soft tissue contracture on the posterior aspect of the ankle might be released. *(continued)*

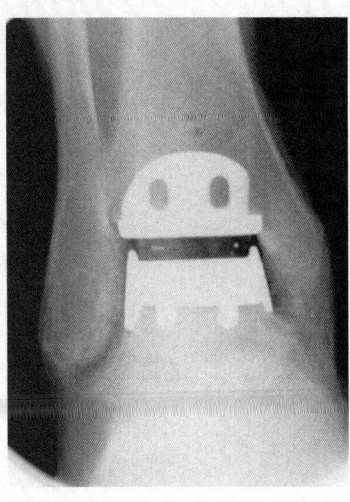

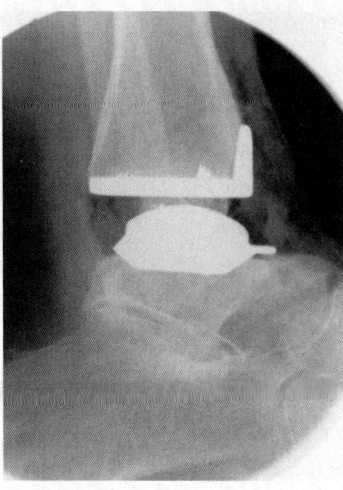

E

F

TECH FIG 4 *(continued)* **E.** Final check of the position of the implants using fluoroscopy. On the AP view, the surgeon checks the position of the implants for any misalignment that may cause edge load of the polyethylene insert, overall alignment in the frontal (coronal) plane, distraction of the ankle (gap between the fibula and talus), and medial and lateral gutters for any bone left that may cause bony impingement. **F.** On the lateral view, the surgeon checks the position of the implants with regard to the bone surfaces (proper fit) and alignment of the implants with regard to contact area (usually, the apex of the talar component should meet the tibial component 3 to 5 mm anterior to its midpoint).

- While the foot is moved in dorsiflexion with the surgeon's maximal power, settling of the implant might be improved and remaining soft tissue contracture on the posterior aspect of the ankle might be released **(TECH FIG 4D)**.
- If the tibial component is seen not to be stable during this maneuver, screw fixation of the tibial component may be considered; however, this is very seldom necessary, as proper

fit and the pyramidal peaks and anterior shield usually provide sufficient primary stability.
- It is furthermore highly recommended to check the position of the implants by fluoroscopy, as described earlier for the trial implants **(TECH FIG 4E,F)**. This allows the surgeon to verify appropriate position of components and to detect any remaining bony fragments or osteophytes that could be a potential source of pain or motion restriction.

INSERTION OF IMPLANTS (H2 ANKLE)

- Insert the final implants previously selected as follows:
  - Insert the talar component so that the pegs can glide into the two drilled holes; use a hammer and impactor to obtain a proper fit of the component to the bone (see **TECH FIG 4A**).
  - Insert the tibial component along the medial malleolus until proper fit to the anterior border of the tibia is achieved **(TECH FIG 5A)**.
  - Insert the trial inlay offset measurement tool to verify the relative AP position of the talar and tibial components **(TECH FIG 5B)**.

- While the foot is held in neutral position, letters are used on the tool to indicate offset:
  - A: anterior position
  - N: neutral position
  - P: posterior position
- Insert the inlay (same size as the talar component) of selected thickness. Positioning a support beneath distal tibia will avoid that the foot/talus is not moved toward anterior, thus hindering insertion of polyethylene insert **(TECH FIG 5C)**.

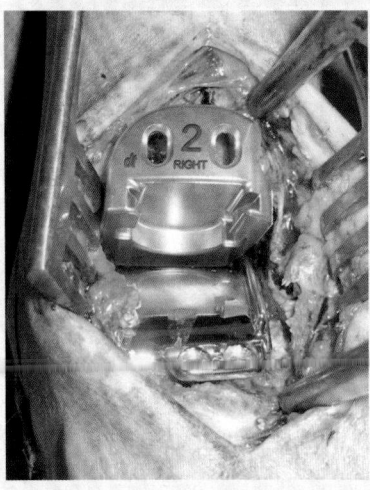

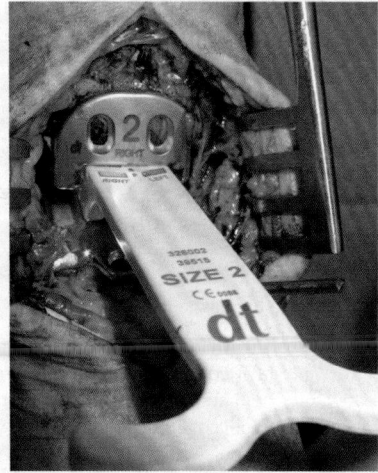

A

B

TECH FIG 5 A. After insertion of the tibial component, the trial inlay offset measurement tool is inserted to verify the relative AP position of the talar and tibial components and to determine the thickness needed to get a well-balanced and stable ankle (**B**). *(continued)*

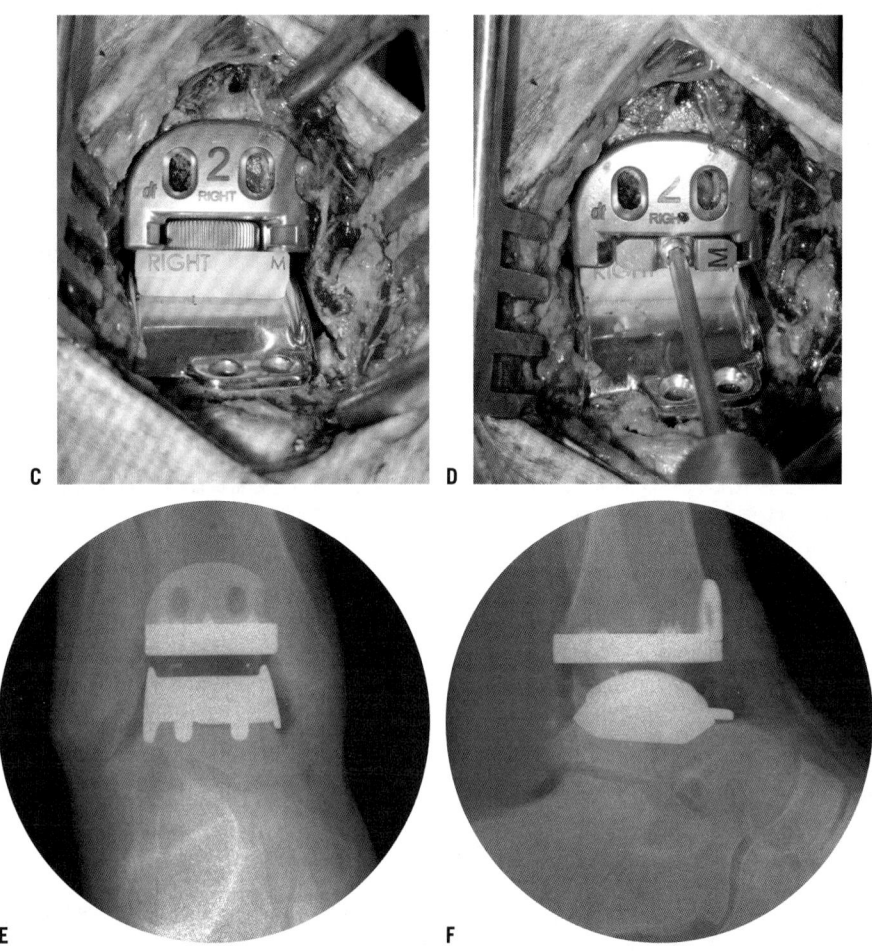

TECH FIG 5 *(continued)* **C.** Thereafter, the polyethylene insert (same size as the talar component) of selected thickness is inserted. The locking piece is inserted with its marker M on medial side and thereafter tightens with the use of a torque screwdriver (**D**). **E,F.** The position of the components is checked by fluoroscopy.

- Remove the distractor (Hintermann Series spreader).
- While the foot is moved into maximal dorsiflexion, thereby improving settling of the implant might be improved and remaining soft tissue contracture on the posterior aspect of the ankle might be released.
- As the polyethylene insert is now seen not to move anymore while moving the foot into dorsiflexion and plantarflexion, the locking piece is inserted with its marker M on medial side.

- The insert is locked into place with the aid of the torque limiting screwdriver that is turned clockwise until the clutch mechanism disengages at its predetermined level (**TECH FIG 5D**).
- After locking the inlay, the ankle should be flexed to its maximum allowable range of motion while observing congruency of the implants and proper tensioning of the joint.
- The position of the components is checked by fluoroscopy (**TECH FIG 5E,F**).

WOUND CLOSURE

- The wound is closed by suturing the tendon sheath, the retinaculum (**TECH FIG 6A**), and the skin (**TECH FIG 6B**).
- Dress the wound, taking care to avoid any pressure to the skin (**TECH FIG 6C**).

- A splint is used to keep the foot in neutral position (**TECH FIG 6D**)

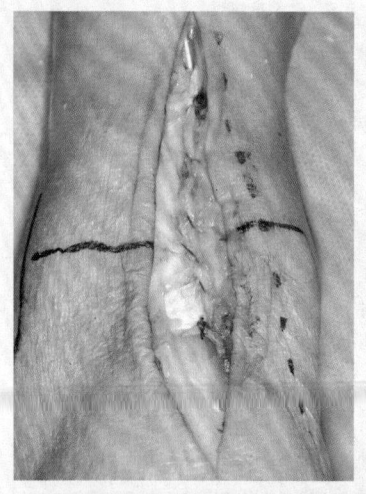
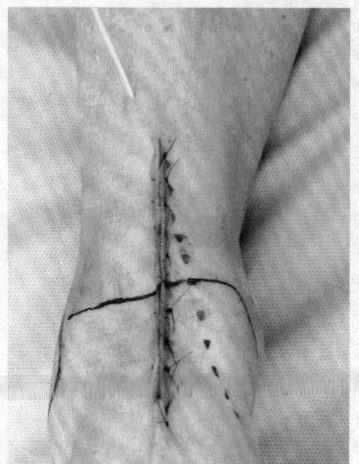
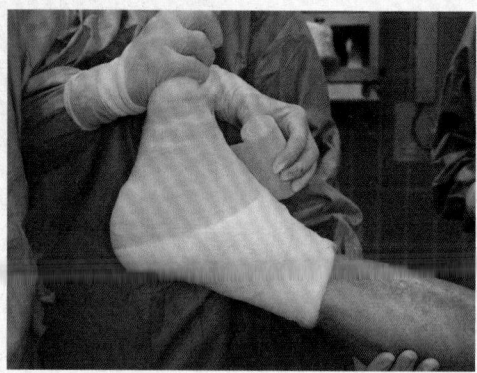

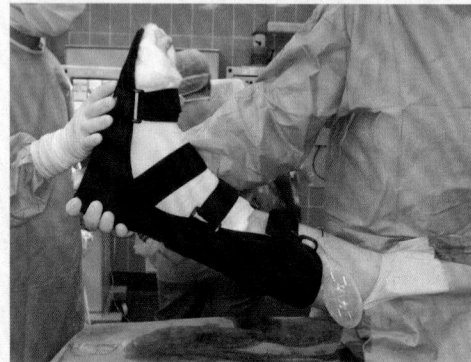

TECH FIG 6 Wound closure and dressing. **A.** The extensor retinaculum is closed first. **B.** Then, the skin is closed by interrupted sutures. **C.** A compressive dressing is used to avoid swelling and hematoma formation. **D.** A splint is used to keep the foot in neutral position.

TECHNIQUES

Pearls and Pitfalls

Malalignment or Malunion above the Ankle Joint	• Above the ankle joint
	  • Supramalleolar osteotomy[6,8]
	• At the ankle joint
	  • Corrective tibial cut
	  • Osteotomy of fibula or medial malleolus
	• Beneath the ankle joint
	  • Calcaneal osteotomy

Adjacent Osteoarthrosis	• Subtalar joint
	  • Subtalar arthrodesis[15]
	• Talonavicular joint
	  • Talonavicular arthrodesis

Fixed Deformity	• Valgus deformity
	  • Triple arthrodesis
	  • Medial sliding osteotomy of calcaneus
	• Varus deformity[10]
	  • Release of medial ankle ligaments or a tilting osteotomy of medial malleolus
	  • Reconstruction of lateral ankle ligaments
	  • Peroneus longus to brevis tendon transfer
	  • Lateral sliding osteotomy of calcaneus
	  • Dorsiflexion osteotomy of first ray

Ligamentous Instability	• Lateral ankle ligaments
	• Lateral ligament reconstruction
	• Medial ankle ligaments
	• Tibiotalar tilt of less than 10 degrees: medial ligament reconstruction
	• Tibiotalar tilt of more than 10 degrees: ankle arthrodesis
Muscular Dysfunction	• Peroneus brevis
	• Peroneus longus to brevis tendon transfer
	• Tibialis posterior
	• Diple or triple arthrodesis

POSTOPERATIVE CARE

- The wound dressing and splint are removed and changed after 2 days.
- When the wound is dry and proper, typically 2 to 4 days after surgery, the foot is placed in a stabilizing cast or walker that protects the ankle against eversion, inversion, and plantarflexion movements for 6 weeks.
- Active motion and lymphatic drainage may support recovery of the soft tissues during the first 6 weeks. However, overly aggressive motion during the first postoperative days may lead to breakdown of soft tissues.
- Weight bearing is allowed as tolerated. Usually, full weight bearing is achieved after 1 week.
- In case of an additional fusion of adjacent joints, immobilization for 8 weeks is advised.
- In case of an additional supramalleolar osteotomy, the patient should remain non–weight bearing for 8 to 10 weeks.
- A rehabilitation program should be started for the foot and ankle after cast or walker removal, including stretching and strengthening of the triceps surae.[21]
- First clinical and radiologic follow-up is done at 6 weeks to check the wound site, osteointegration, and position of the implants.
- The patient is advised to wear a compression stocking for a further 4 to 6 months to avoid swelling.

OUTCOMES

- Between May 2000 and July 2019, 1768 total ankle arthroplasties were performed in 1725 patients: primary arthroplasties with the H3, 1285 (72.7%), and with the H2, 75 (4.2%), takedown of fusion with ankle arthroplasties, 88 (5.0%), and revision arthroplasties, 320 (18.1% [H3, 278; H2, 42]) **(TABLE 1)**.
- Out of the 1609 ankles with a minimal follow-up of 1 year (91%), the mean American Orthopaedic Foot & Ankle

Society hindfoot score improved from 43.4 ± 17.8 preoperatively to 72.4 ± 18.6 at latest follow-up and the mean pain (visual analog scale for pain) improved from 6.7 ± 1.8 to 2.4 ± 2.3.
- At latest follow-up, the mean plantarflexion was 26.8 ± 9.8 degrees, and the mean dorsiflexion was 7.8 ± 6.5 degrees. Overall, motion was slightly higher after primary arthroplasties (35.5 degrees) than after revision arthroplasties (33.9 degrees), and it was significant less after takedown a fusion with arthroplasties (23.4 degrees).
- A 1271 patients (75.2%) were satisfied/very satisfied with their ankle, whereas 146 patients (9.0%) were not satisfied. To note that patient's satisfaction was highest after takedown a fusion and ankle arthroplasty despite of significant lowest gain of motion.

COMPLICATIONS

- Early complications included malleolar fractures intraoperatively, 62 ankles (3.5%); wound healing problems, 48 ankles (4.4%); infection, 67 ankles (3.7%); and polyethylene dislocation, 23 ankles (1.3%).
- Late complications needing a revision of arthroplasty included loosening of components, 87 ankles (4.9%); polyethylene dislocation/fracture, 17 ankles (1.0%); polyethylene wear, 9 ankles (0.5%); progressive cyst formation, 21 ankles (1.2%); progressive loss of motion, 19 ankles (1.1%); progressive instability/misalignment, 32 (1.8%); chronic pain syndrome, 34 ankles (1.9%); infection, 9 (0.5%); and others, 27 (1.5%).
- Taking revision of a metallic implant or conversion into ankle arthrodesis as the end point, overall survivorship of both components at 10 years was 86.1% (89.9% for the talar component and 91.8% for the tibial component).
- While 212 ankles were revised to total ankle arthroplasty (161 [74.5%]) or to ankle arthrodesis (51 [32.6%]), 4 patients (1.9%) underwent below-knee amputation (see **TABLE 1**).

TABLE 1 Casuistic, Etiology, Results and Failures with the H2 and H3 Ankle from 2000 to 2019[a]

Casuistic		Primary TAR				Takedown Fusion and TAR		Revision TAR		Total TAR	
		H3		H2							
		n	%	n	%	n	%	n	%	n	%
Numbers	N	1285		75		88		320		1768	
Gender	M	715	55.6	44	58.7	45	51.1	175	54.7	979	55.4
	F	570	43.4	31	41.3	43	48.9	145	45.3	789	44.6
Age	At time of TAR	62.0		62.6		57.0		61.9		61.9	
	Range	17.0–90.0		31.0–86.7		21–83.7		26.9–93.8		17.0–93.8	
Etiology	Primary	129	10.0	4	5.3			31	9.7		
	Systemic	123	9.6	10	13.3			12	3.8		
	Posttraumatic	987	76.8	53	70.7			268	83.8		
	Others	46	3.6	8	10.7			9	42.8		
Results	>1 year FU	1213	94.4	34	45.3	76	86.4	268	83.8	1609	91.0
Satisfaction	Very satisfied	524	43.2	18	53.0	25	32.9	95	35.4	662	41.1
	Satisfied	413	34.1	6	17.6	27	35.5	102	38.1	548	34.1
	Somehow Satisfied	179	14.8	10	29.4	12	15.8	34	12.7	238	14.8
	Not satisfied	97	7.9	0	0.0	12	15.8	37	13.8	146	9.0
Function	AOFAS score	74.9		78.8		63.5		66.3		72.4	
Pain	VAS	2.3		2.1		2.9		3.2		2.4	
Failures		163	12.6	1	1.3	15	17.0	37	11.6	216	12.2
Component	Tibia	48	3.7	1	1.3	3	3.5	17	5.3	69	3.9
	Talus	27	2.1	0	0.0	2	3.1	4	1.3	33	1.9
	Tibia and talus	88	6.8	0	0.0	10	11.4	16	5.0	114	6.4
Revised to	Tar	130	79.8	1	100.0	10	58.8	20	54.1	161	74.5
	Arthrodesis	31	19.0	0	0.0	4	23.5	16	43.2	51	32.6
	Amputation	2	1.2	0	0.0	1	5.7	1	1.7	4	1.9

AOFAS, American Orthopaedic Foot & Ankle Society; FU, follow-up; TAR, total ankle replacement; VAS, visual analog scale.
[a]At author's institution.

REFERENCES

1. Barg A, Elsner A, Hefti D, et al. Haemophilic arthropathy of the ankle treated by total ankle replacement: a case series. Haemophilia 2010;16(4):647–655.
2. Barg A, Elsner A, Hefti D, et al. Total ankle arthroplasty in patients with hereditary hemochromatosis. Clin Orthop Relat Res 2011;469(5):1427–1435.
3. Barg A, Knupp M, Anderson AE, et al. Total ankle replacement in obese patients: component stability, weight change, and functional outcome in 118 consecutive patients. Foot Ankle Int 2011;32(10):925–932.
4. Barg A, Knupp M, Kapron AL, et al. Total ankle replacement in patients with gouty arthritis. J Bone Joint Surg Am 2011;93(4): 357–366.
5. Barg A, Zwicky L, Knupp M, et al. HINTEGRA total ankle replacement: survivorship analysis in 684 patients. J Bone Joint Surg Am 2013;95(13):1175–1183.
6. Deforth M, Krähenbühl N, Zwicky L, et al. Supramalleolar osteotomy for tibial component malposition in total ankle replacement. Foot Ankle Int 2017;38(9):952–956.
7. Hintermann B, Barg A, Knupp M, et al. Conversion of painful ankle arthrodesis to total ankle arthroplasty. J Bone Joint Surg Am 2009;91(4):850–858.
8. Hintermann B, Knupp M, Barg A. Supramalleolar osteotomies for the treatment of ankle arthritis. J Am Acad Orthop Surg 2016;24(7): 424–432.
9. Hintermann B, Ruiz R. HINTEGRA total ankle system. In: Raikin S, ed. Foot and Ankle Surgery: Tricks of the Trade. New York: Thieme, 2018:351–357.
10. Hintermann B, Ruiz R. Total replacement of varus ankle: three-component prosthesis design. Foot Ankle Clin 2019;24(2):305–324.
11. Hintermann B, Ruiz R, Barg A. Dealing with the stiff ankle: preoperative and late occurrence. Foot Ankle Clin 2017;22:425–453.
12. Hintermann B, Valderrabano V, Dereymaeker G, et al. The HINTEGRA ankle: rationale and short-term results of 122 consecutive ankles. Clin Orthop Relat Res 2004;(424):57–68.
13. Hintermann B, Zwicky L, Knupp M, et al. HINTEGRA revision arthroplasty for failed total ankle prostheses. J Bone Joint Surg Am. 2013;95(13):1166–1174.
14. Saltzman CL, el-Khoury GY. The hindfoot alignment view. Foot Ankle Int 1995;16:572–576.
15. Sokolowski M, Krähenbühl N, Wang C, et al. Secondary subtalar joint osteoarthritis following total ankle replacement. Foot Ankle Int 2019;40(10):1122–1128.
16. Valderrabano V, Hintermann B, Horisberger M, et al. Ligamentous posttraumatic ankle osteoarthritis. Am J Sports Med 2006;34: 612–620.
17. Valderrabano V, Hintermann B, Nigg BM, et al. Kinematic changes after fusion and total replacement of the ankle: part 1: range of motion. Foot Ankle Int 2003;24:881–887.
18. Valderrabano V, Hintermann B, Nigg BM, et al. Kinematic changes after fusion and total replacement of the ankle: part 2: movement transfer. Foot Ankle Int 2003;24:888–896.
19. Valderrabano V, Hintermann B, Nigg BM, et al. Kinematic changes after fusion and total replacement of the ankle: part 3: talar movement. Foot Ankle Int 2003;24:897–900.
20. Valderrabano V, Nigg BM, von Tscharner V, et al. Gait analysis in ankle osteoarthritis and total ankle replacement. Clin Biomech (Bristol, Avon) 2007;22:894–904.
21. Valderrabano V, Pagenstert G, Horisberger M, et al. Sports and recreation activity of ankle arthritis patients before and after total ankle replacement. Am J Sports Med 2006;34:993–999.

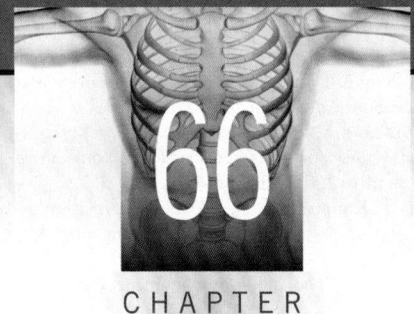

66

CHAPTER

The Salto and Salto Talaris Total Ankle Arthroplasty

Jean Langlois, Michel Bonnin, Brian Donley, Thierry Judet, and
Jean-Alain Colombier

DEFINITION

- The Salto Talaris Total Ankle Prosthesis (Tornier SA, Saint-Ismier, France) are cementless resurfacing-type implants that are intended to restore near-normal joint kinematics. Fixation is achieved through bone ingrowth.
- The surgical technique is critical to a successful outcome, and some criteria are essential:
  - Tight fit of the components and extended contact area with bone to achieve good primary stability, which is a prerequisite for secondary biologic fixation
  - Restoration of the mechanical axis of the ankle
  - Accurate restoration of the joint line (proper level and strict horizontal plane)
  - Preservation or restoration of the soft tissue balance
  - Adequate soft tissue release and appropriately sized implants to achieve good range of motion (ROM) intraoperatively

ANATOMY

The Mobile-Bearing Salto Prosthesis

- The Salto Total Ankle Prosthesis was developed between 1994 and 1996 and has been used clinically since January 1997.
- Based on experience with the third-generation cementless meniscal-bearing designs, this system was designed to restore nearly normal kinematics of the ankle (**FIG 1**).
- A dedicated instrument system was developed to achieve optimal positioning of the components, and the design of the implant was optimized to better restore the natural anatomy and obtain an optimal primary fixation of the components while retaining a minimally invasive resurfacing concept.
- The tibial component accommodates the superior flat surface of the mobile bearing. Its smooth surface allows free translation and rotation of the mobile bearing. The 3-mm medial rim protects the polyethylene from impingement with the medial malleolus.
- The specific shape (segment of a cone of revolution) of the talar component replicates the anatomy of the talar dome without overstressing the deltoid ligament. It is broader anteriorly than posteriorly, and the lateral condyle has a larger radius of curvature than the medial condyle (**FIG 2**).
  - As a result, the axis of flexion and extension of the talar component, under the polyethylene, is aligned with the physiologic axis.

- The lateral aspect of the talus is resurfaced, allowing articulation with the lateral malleolus.
- Primary fixation to the tibia is ensured by close match of the tibial component to the epiphysis and enhanced by an anteroposterior (AP) keel and a tapered cylindrical plug.
- Stability of the talar component is provided by three bone cuts and insertion of an 11-mm diameter hollow fixation peg into the body of the talus.
- Secondary fixation is provided by bone ingrowth into a dual coating of hydroxyapatite applied to a 200-γm thick layer of plasma-sprayed titanium.

The Fixed-Bearing Salto Talaris Prosthesis

- Experience with the Salto prosthesis has led the conceptors to revise the concept of mobile bearing. Because of the anatomic design of the implant, the precision of the bone cuts, the accuracy in component positioning, and the need for and the potential problems associated with postoperative motion of the polyethylene bearing during flexion–extension movements have been almost completely eliminated. This

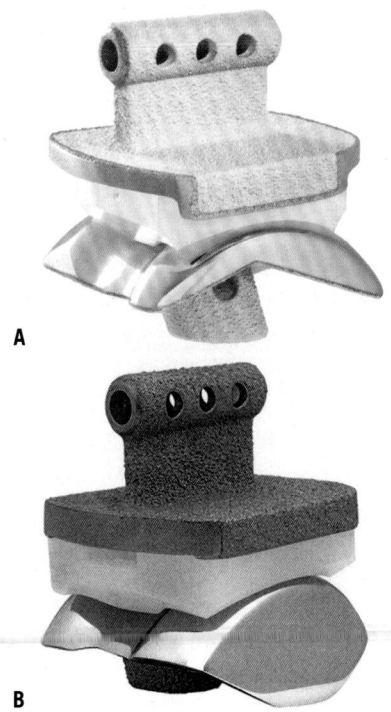

A

B

FIG 1 A. Oblique view of the Salto Total Ankle Prosthesis. **B.** Oblique view of the Salto Talaris Total Ankle Prothesis (fixed-bearing).

Dr. Donley is a paid consultant for Tornier, Inc., the company that makes the Salto Talaris Anatomic Ankle.

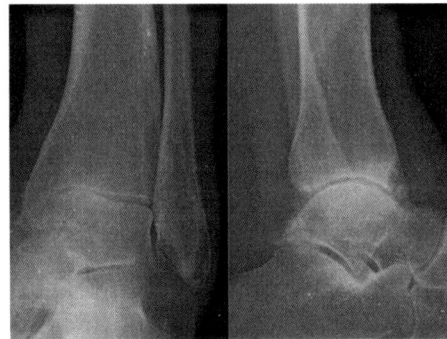

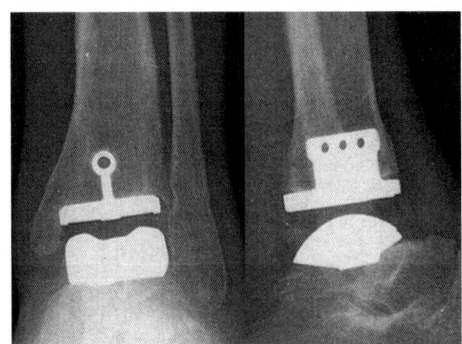

FIG 2 Preoperative (**A**) and postoperative (**B**) AP and lateral radiographs of the Salto Talaris prosthesis.

has been confirmed in clinical studies based on standing dynamic views.
- On the other hand, intraoperative motion of the tibial component assembly is most helpful in allowing self-positioning of the bearing with respect to the talar component before the tibial keel preparation is completed.
- Launched in 2006, the Salto Talaris components and instrument system are the same as those of the Salto prosthesis, except that the tibial component is a fixed-bearing design (**FIG 3**).
  - Polyethylene is attached to tibial component prior to insertion.
  - The final position of the tibial component is fine-tuned at the end of the procedure to achieve perfect alignment with the talar component. In this manner, the self-positioning feature of the mobile-bearing insert has been retained.
  - The tibial base can be the same or one size larger than the talar component allowing for mismatching based on patient anatomy.

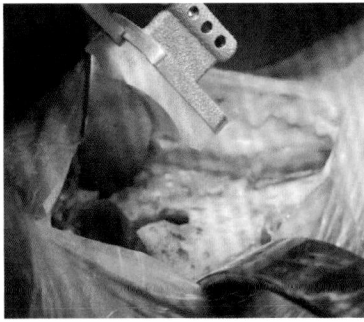

FIG 3 The Salto Talaris components and instrument system are the same as those of the Salto prosthesis, except that the tibial component is a fixed-bearing design.

PATHOGENESIS

- In general, our indications for total ankle arthroplasty (TAA) are end-stage ankle osteoarthritis (OA) and rheumatoid arthritis (RA).
  - In OA, degeneration may be due to sequelae of trauma, chronic ankle instability, and rarely primary OA.
  - In our experience, RA occurs relatively infrequently in the ankle when compared to the hip or knee. However, there is no consensus on the actual rate of ankle joint involvement in RA patients, with figures ranging from 9% to 40%, depending on the selection criteria and the studies.
- Occasionally, end-stage erosive or degenerative changes of the ankle may develop secondary to osteochondromatosis, pigmented villonodular synovitis, hemochromatosis, or osteochondritis dissecans.
- Ankle joint involvement in RA tends to occur late in the disease process, with symptoms not occurring until a mean disease duration of 17 to 19 years.
- Because the tibiotalar joint is rarely affected in isolation, treatment will need to be systemic and not only for the ankle.

NATURAL HISTORY

- Progressive tibiotalar arthritis typically is accompanied by progressive ankle stiffness. Loss of ankle ROM, particularly dorsiflexion, results from tibiotalar osteophytes and less resilience in the distal tibiofibular syndesmosis.
- Over time, the patient may develop an equinus gait with resultant Achilles tendon contracture, posterior capsular adhesions, and, occasionally, tibialis posterior adhesions.

PATIENT HISTORY AND PHYSICAL FINDINGS

- Silfverskiöld test
  - Passive ankle ROM with the patient supine and the knee flexed and extended
  - Physiologic ROM with this examination is 15 degrees dorsiflexion or 0 to 40 degrees plantarflexion.
  - An isolated gastrocnemius contracture is present when lack of dorsiflexion with the knee in extension is eliminated with knee flexion.
- Evaluation of ankle ROM with the patient standing and walking
- Visualizing the gait pattern. The patient may externally rotate the extremity, or female patients may be able to walk in high heels to mask the lack of ankle dorsiflexion.
- Hindfoot ROM
  - We use three grades of hindfoot motion: physiologic, diminished, or stiff. We favor TAA over ankle arthrodesis in patients with a stiff hindfoot.
- Hindfoot alignment with the patient standing or ambulating
  - Hindfoot malalignment (varus or greater than physiologic valgus) may be most pronounced with the patient walking.
- Hindfoot alignment with the patient supine
- We typically assess passive hindfoot motion to determine if the deformity can be reduced to a physiologic position. In our hands, this examination determines the type of

hindfoot realignment that will be performed concomitant to TAA.

- Tibiotalar instability
  - The examiner successively assesses coronal plane and sagittal plane stability with varus–valgus stress and anterior drawer testing, respectively. In our hands, varus instability or fixed varus ankle requires careful ligament balancing.

IMAGING AND OTHER DIAGNOSTIC STUDIES

- In our preoperative assessment, we not only determine the extent of deformity and instability at the ankle but also assess any concomitant ipsilateral lower extremity malalignment that may have a bearing on the outcome of TAA.
- We routinely obtain weight-bearing AP, mortise (ie, an AP view with 30 degrees of internal rotation, exposing the tibiofibular joint space), and straight lateral (evaluating the anterior osteophytic margin, the talar dome morphology, and the talar positioning beneath the pilon) radiographs of both ankles (with maximum dorsiflexion and plantarflexion); radiographs of the uninvolved ankle typically provide some understanding of what is physiologic for the patient.
  - Weight-bearing mechanical axis hip-to-ankle radiographs are required if there is associated deformity, such as malunion responsible for malalignment, of the ipsilateral lower extremity.
  - Weight-bearing hindfoot alignment views (Cobey-Saltzman or Meary) of both ankles are also critical in the evaluation of varus–valgus deformities.
- We recommend obtaining computed tomography (CT) scans of the ankle and hindfoot, particularly to review coronal sections, to further evaluate tibial or talar bone loss or cysts not fully defined on plain radiographs, and to anticipate the need for an associated procedure, such as a subtalar fusion.

NONOPERATIVE MANAGEMENT

- We have had limited success with nonoperative management in active patients with end-stage ankle arthritis.
- Activity modification, rocker bottom shoe modification, and bracing offer some relief.
- We reserve nonoperative management for low-demand patients who are poor surgical candidates.

SURGICAL MANAGEMENT

- Prudent patient selection is key to a successful outcome and avoidance of complication.

Contraindications

- Septic arthritis
- Charcot neuroarthropathy—insufficient bone stock or poor skin coverage

Total Ankle Arthroplasty versus Ankle Arthrodesis

- In general, arthrodesis is favored over TAA because of the following:
  - Lower risk of mechanical implant failure; no risk of implant wear
  - Lower risk of infection

- Less chance of skin necrosis when the ankle has been previously operated on
- In our hands, lower incidence of residual pain
- In general, TAA is favored over ankle arthrodesis because of the following:
  - Less risk of developing adjacent (hindfoot) joint arthritis
  - In our hands, more favorable functional outcome
  - In our opinion, malunion or development of adjacent joint arthritis makes revision surgery more difficult after arthrodesis.

Preoperative Planning

- Preoperative evaluation of weight-bearing radiographs and CT scan to:
  - Anticipate the optimal implant size, with the use of available templates. This is important because an oversized prosthesis will alter the center of rotation, giving rise to pain and stiffness.
    - If the talus is particularly deformed, the template should be applied to the contralateral, unaffected ankle.
  - Determine the reference for establishing the ideal tibial resection level, taking into account the extent of wear in the tibial plafond.
  - Analyze tibiotalar joint alignment relative to the tibial shaft axis. This allows differentiation between axial deviations:
    - Resulting from asymmetric wear of the tibial plafond that may be corrected with tibial preparation
    - Because of malunion that may require corrective osteotomy, simultaneous to or staged with TAA
  - Analyze the residual talar body.
    - Asymmetry needs to be balanced in the talar preparation.
  - Evaluate the hindfoot.
    - A joint-sparing calcaneal osteotomy may be necessary to realign the hindfoot.
    - In the face of hindfoot arthritis or hindfoot instability, a subtalar or even triple arthrodesis may be warranted.

Positioning

- The patient is positioned supine on the operating table, with a pad under the ipsilateral hip to promote a neutral tibial and foot alignment with the foot pointing to the ceiling.
- The plantar aspect of the foot should be flush with the end of the table.
- Placing a rolled towel under the ankle facilitates subtle adjustments in ankle positioning.
- We routinely use a thigh tourniquet.
- Include the knee in the sterile field so that the limb can be positioned more freely and so that the patella and tibial tubercle can be used to confirm optimal alignment. The surgeon stands at the foot of the table, with the assistant at the lateral side of the operative leg.
- We recommend using a fluoroscope in the early experience or for difficult cases, ensuring proper positioning and sizing of the cutting guides and implants before each critical step.

EXPOSURE

- The tibiotalar joint is approached through an anterior midline incision (facing the lateral border of the tibialis anterior tendon) starting 8 to 10 cm proximal to the joint line and extending to the midfoot.
- The soft tissues must be handled carefully, especially in patients being managed with systemic steroid treatment.
  - The surgeon should avoid undermining the skin.
  - The surgeon should maintain deep retraction only and avoid tension directly on the skin edges.
  - Extending the skin incision will further diminish skin tension.
- Although we maintain meticulous hemostasis, we ligate vessels whenever possible and use electrocautery sparingly to diminish the risk of skin burns. We typically incise the crural fascia and extensor retinaculum along the lateral border of the tibialis anterior tendon, using the interval between the tibialis anterior and extensor hallucis longus (EHL) tendons.
  - Whenever possible, the tibialis anterior tendon should remain protected in its individual sheath throughout the procedure (this also separates the tendon from the anterior incision during closure).
- Alternatively, the extensor retinaculum may be incised at the lateral border of the EHL tendon, using the interval between the EHL and extensor digitorum longus tendons. The tendons are retracted with angled retractors, and the deep neurovascular bundle (anterior tibial artery and deep peroneal nerve) is identified in the proximal wound and carefully reflected laterally.
- The periosteum and joint capsule are incised longitudinally. The medial and lateral flaps are elevated using a scalpel and an elevator to expose the tibiotalar joint to the anterior margins of the malleoli.
- To avoid direct tension on the skin margins, we use deep retractors, one at the proximal aspects of each malleolus.
- Anterior osteophytes are removed with an osteotome, and the talar facets are cleared with a rongeur.

- We then define the physiologic aspects of both malleoli, removing any osteophytes, ossifications, and loose bodies that obscure visualization of the medial and lateral ankle gutters, distort the natural anatomy, or impinge on the talus (**TECH FIG 1**).
- Upon completion of these steps, the talus should be mobile, and the medial and lateral gutters should be fully exposed.

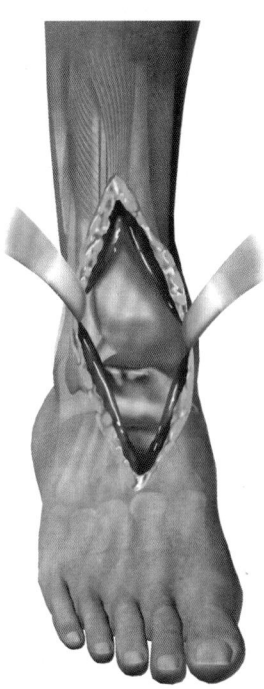

TECH FIG 1 A lateral retractor is placed against the lateral malleolus and a medial retractor against the upper part of the medial malleolus. Anterior osteophytes are removed with an osteotome, and the talar facets are cleared with a rongeur.

TIBIAL RESECTION

- The goal is to restore a physiologic tibiocalcaneal axis. Ideally, implant position should produce a joint line at right angles to the mechanical tibial axis in the coronal plane and set a 3- to 7-degree posterior slope in the sagittal plane.
- Align the extramedullary guide with the anterior tibial crest or a line joining the center of the knee and the midpoint of the distal tibial surface.
  - Proximally, secure the alignment guide to the anterior tibial tuberosity with a self-drilling pin, roughly perpendicular (in the sagittal plane) to the malleolar tips and distal medial tibial metaphysis in the sagittal plane (**TECH FIG 2**).
- We then perform five sequential adjustments.

Orientation in the Coronal Plane

- Provided there is anatomic or near-anatomic overall alignment of the lower extremity, the tibial cut should be horizontal and perpendicular to the tibial axis (**TECH FIG 3**).

- Perform resection using the extramedullary guide referencing off the anterior tibial border.
- A few degrees of coronal plane deviation proximal to the ankle or at the knee is readily compensated by realigning the proximal aspect of the external tibial alignment guide on the pin placed in the tibial tubercle. However, in our experience, moderate to severe deformity proximal to the ankle should be corrected before TAA, typically in a staged fashion.

Orientation in the Sagittal Plane

- The external tibial alignment guide, when positioned parallel to the anterior tibial cortex, establishes a physiologic posterior slope of 3 degrees (or 7 degrees, depending on the cutting guide selected and how the extramedullary guide rest parallel to the tibia) for the tibial cut.
- In our experience, to achieve final ROM, a 3-degree posterior slope is adequate in most cases.

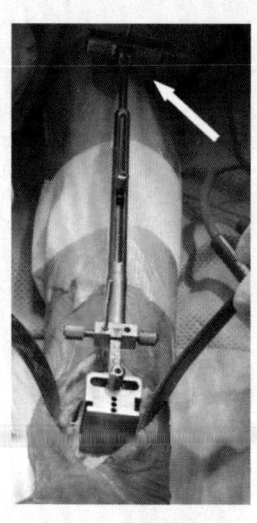

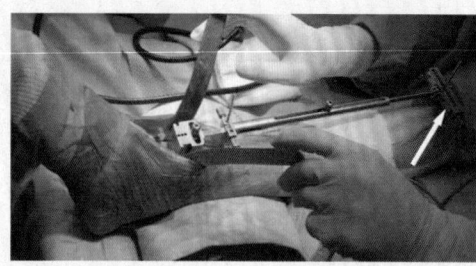

TECH FIG 2 A,B. Left ankle. The extramedullary guide is aligned with the anterior tibial crest. It is attached with self-drilling pins at the anterior tibial tuberosity, roughly perpendicular (in the sagittal plane) to the malleolar tips, and then at the distal medial metaphysis of the tibia. Resection is performed using the extramedullary guide, referencing off the anterior tibial border. A few degrees of axial deviation of the knee joint in the coronal plane can be compensated for by using the proximal holes (*arrows*) to obtain a perfect adjustment and to perform a bone cut that will be almost horizontal.

Resection Level

- The goal is to restore an anatomic joint line level. When the subchondral architecture of the tibial plafond is intact, the amount of distal tibial resection should match the metal tibial baseplate plus the polyethylene insert.
- We use the apex of the tibial plafond as the reference point for tibial resection. To expose this apex, we resect the anterior margin of the tibial plafond using an osteotome. With clinical inspection or fluoroscopic confirmation in the sagittal plane, the resection level is determined from this reference point (**TECH FIG 4**).
- For the Salto Talaris (two-part fixed-bearing) prosthesis, the minimum resection is 8 mm (4 mm for the thickness of the metal baseplate plus 4 mm for the minimum thickness of the polyethylene).

- We modify the tibial cut based on the ligamentous tension in the ankle. In stiff ankles, we typically resect 1 to 2 mm more than the minimal resection; in ankles with instability, we generally resect 2 mm less than the minimal resection.
- Bone loss in the tibia may warrant adjusting the tibial cut to reestablish the proper joint line.

Orientation in Rotation

- Because both the tibial and initial talar cutting guides are suspended from the tibial alignment guide, thus linking the tibial and initial talar resection, proper rotational alignment is critical. Malrotation of the components may interfere with the implant's kinematics, create malleolar impingement, risk edge loading, and lead to increased constraint (**TECH FIG 5**).
- Every effort should be made to orient the implant on the center bisecting line of the talus in the coronal plane, the line that is parallel with the talus when it is taken through its motion arc. We rotate the cutting guide until it is centered on the line bisecting the space between the medial and lateral talar facets.
  - Rotational alignment of the cutting guide may be adjusted using pins inserted in each malleolar groove. The guide is therefore set along the bisector axis of the two groove pins.

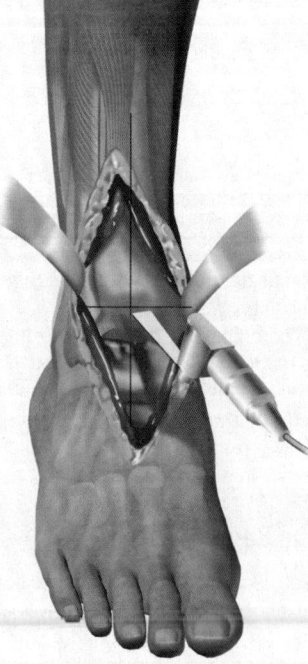

TECH FIG 3 In the coronal plane, provided there is a good overall alignment of the lower extremity, the tibial cut should be horizontal and perpendicular to the tibial axis.

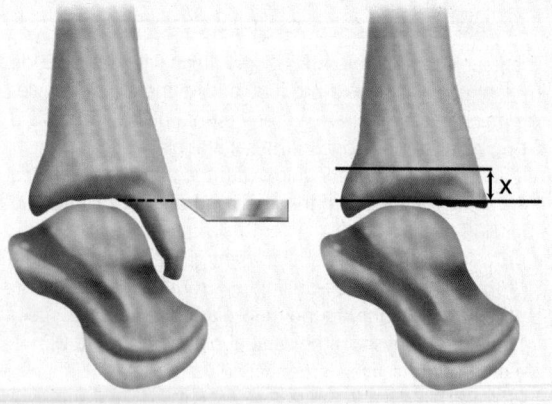

TECH FIG 4 A. The goal with the Salto Talaris prosthesis is to restore an anatomic joint line level. Then, in the absence of significant bone wear, the amount of bone resection on the tibia must fit exactly with the thickness of the tibial components. *x*, metal baseplate plus polyethylene. *(continued)*

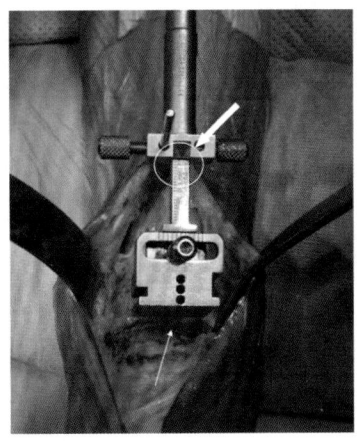

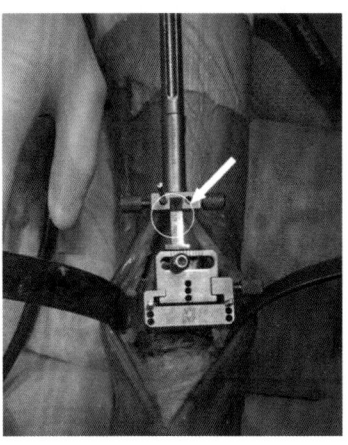

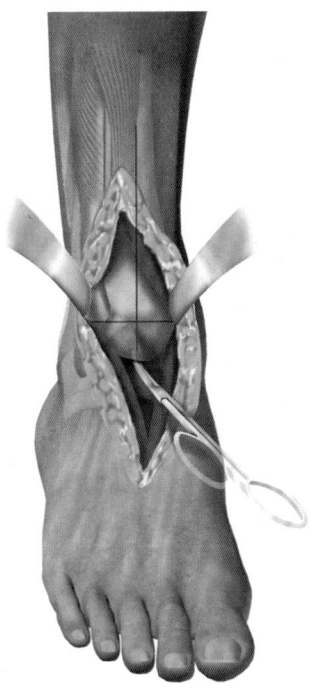

B

TECH FIG 4 *(continued)* **B.** The only reliable landmark is the plafond of the tibial pilon. The anterior margin of the tibial pilon is resected using an osteotome. This will provide direct exposure of the joint surface. From this reference level, the required cut is determined, aiming to remove as little bone as possible. **C.** Left ankle. The guide is adjusted at the level of the tibial pilon (*small arrow*) and this level is observed on the scale on the tibial alignment jig (*large arrow* and *circle*). **D.** Then, from the initial reference position, the guide is adjusted proximally from 7 to 9 mm according to the desired amount of resection (*arrow* and *circle*).

- Orienting the implant in line with the second metatarsal may be useful but introduces errors with associated midfoot or forefoot deformity.

Coronal Plane Positioning

- The final adjustment is to center the cutting block on the tibial plafond, often necessitating medial or lateral translation of the cutting block relative to the tibial alignment guide. The proper-size cutting block must be selected; the reference landmarks for sizing are the medial axilla and the lateral edge of the tibia.
  - Set the guide to avoid compromise of the malleoli. Using dedicated talar gauges, preselection of the talar implant size can also be performed at this stage. Secure pins within the cutting block at the level of resection to protect the malleoli from inadvertent saw blade excursion (**TECH FIG 6A**).
- Bone resection
  - Before making the sagittal bone cuts (medial and lateral), drill holes through the appropriate-size cutting block and fully insert two short pins through the superior holes to

protect the malleoli during resection. Before placing the protective pins, an AP fluoroscopic image may be obtained to confirm proper position and sizing of the cutting block in the coronal plane.
- When implanting a Salto Talaris prosthesis, the rotational alignment is established using the trials and ranging the ankle to allow the tibial base and insert assembly to self-center with respect to the trial talar component.
- The capture guide on the cutting block guides the saw blade.
- The tibial resection must be completed through the posterior cortex of the distal tibia, without plunging the saw blade into the posterior soft tissues.
- We typically use a saw blade of adequate length and limited excursion.
- Removing the resected bone
  - Remove the tibial cutting block but leave the external tibial alignment guide in position.
  - With a thin osteotome or small reciprocating saw, complete the two sagittal cuts through the predrilled holes created using the cutting block.

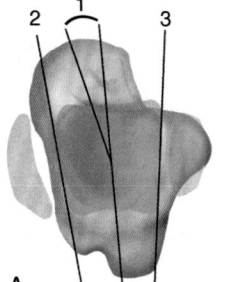

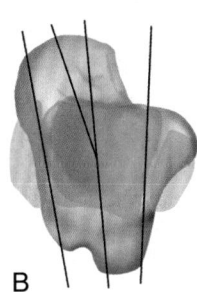

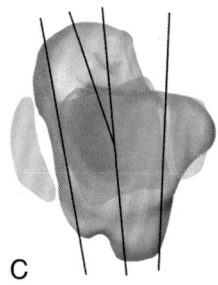

A   **B**   **C**

TECH FIG 5 The rotational alignment is of critical importance even more so as the tibial and talar resections are linked. **A.** The talar component must be aligned with the axis of the talar dome (*1*) and is centered on the line bisecting the space between the medial and lateral talar facets (*2* and *3*). External (**B**) or internal (**C**) rotational malpositioning of the components will result in increased stress being placed on the fixation system, impingement with the malleoli, and may interfere with the kinematics of the joint replacement.

TECHNIQUES

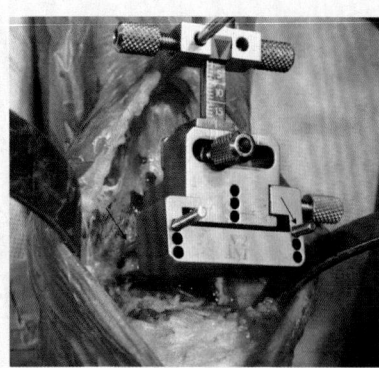

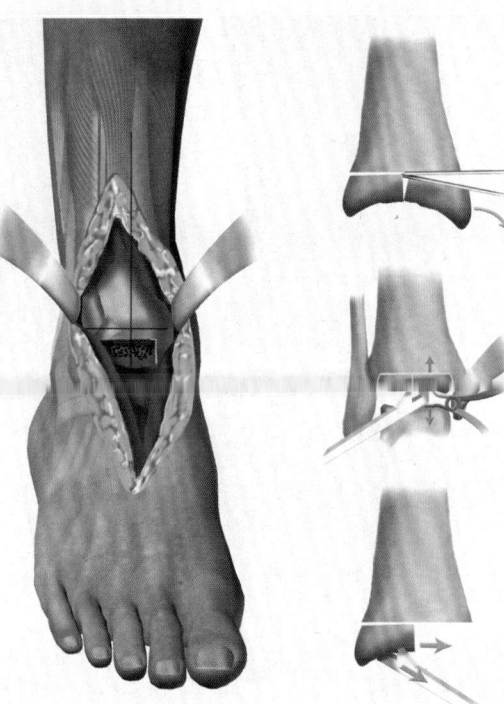

TECH FIG 6 **A.** The instrument system provides accurate component positioning through adjustment of the resection level, translation, and rotation. Pins can be inserted in the medial and lateral holes of the guide to visualize the limits of the tibial cut with respect to the malleoli. Before the tibial cut is performed, holes are drilled through the appropriate-size cutting block and two short pins are fully inserted through the superior holes to protect the malleoli during resection. **B.** The removal of the distal tibial resection is rarely done in one piece; usually, piecemeal removal is required. The anterior half is removed and then removal of the posterior portion can be delayed until after the posterior talar cut is completed.

- Remove the resected bone wafer.
- The resected bone must be fully mobilized before attempting to extract it from the joint; abrupt mobilization of this bone may result in a fracture of the medial malleolus if the cut is not complete, especially in an ankle with an equinus contracture. The removal of the distal tibial resection

is rarely done in one piece; usually piecemeal removal is required.
- Remove the anterior half. With the Salto Talaris prosthesis, removal of the posterior portion may be delayed until after the posterior talar cut is completed **(TECH FIG 6B)**.

TALAR PREPARATION

- Talar preparation requires that the ankle can be dorsiflexed to at least 90 degrees.
  - This angle is almost always obtained at this stage because the removal of bone from the tibia (anterior part of tibial resection) will have created more space, even in a stiff ankle.
  - In the rare case that it is not achieved, then an Achilles tendon lengthening or gastrocnemius–soleus recession may need to be considered.
- Talar preparation comprises three cuts: posterior, anterior, and lateral. The native medial talar dome is left intact with this technique.

Posterior Talar Chamfer Cut

- To position the talar component properly on the prepared talar dome, the posterior talar cut must be inclined 20 degrees posteriorly.
- With the ankle maintained at 90 degrees of dorsiflexion and the hindfoot in physiologic valgus position, suspend the talar guide

from the external tibial alignment guide and insert a pin into the talus **(TECH FIG 7A)**.
- This pin dictates the sagittal orientation of the talar component.
- This reference pin must be placed with the ankle in a strictly neutral position between flexion and extension **(TECH FIG 7B)**.
- Excessive plantarflexion tilts the implant backward **(TECH FIG 7C)**.
- Excessive dorsiflexion will lead to anterior and flexed positioning of the talar component **(TECH FIG 7D)**.
- Secure the posterior chamfer talar cutting block on this reference pin.
- Talar styli are available to determine the level for an anatomic resection that corresponds to the thickness of the talar component.
- In case of severe flattening of the talar dome, this resection level may need to be adjusted. The talar resection level depends on having satisfactory fixation of the implant in healthy

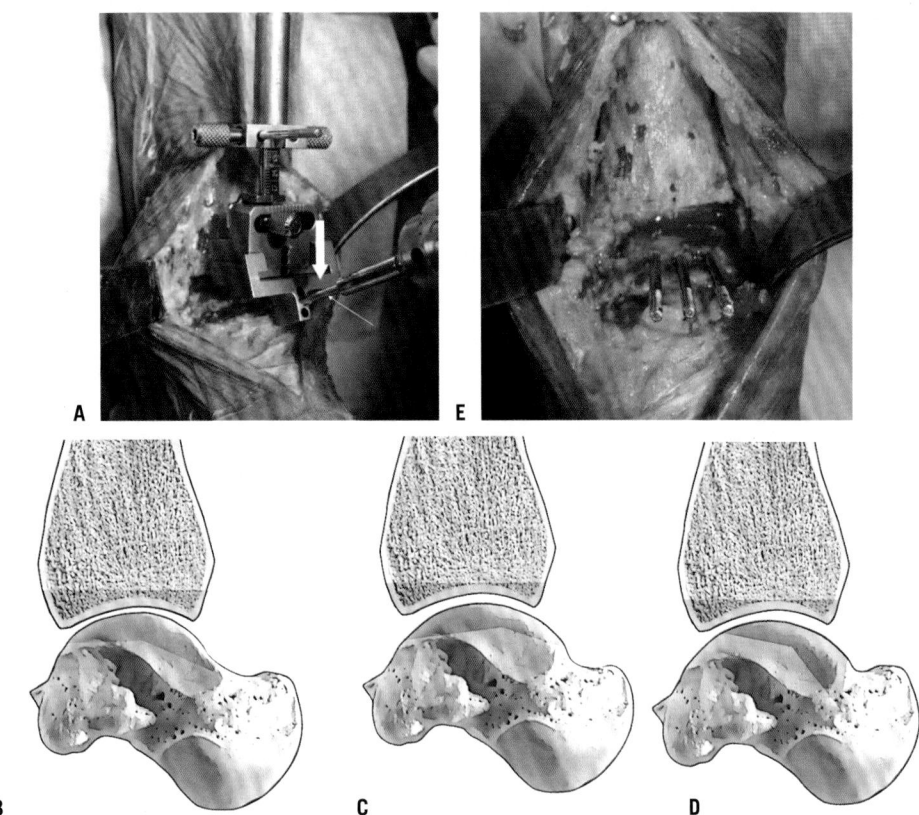

TECH FIG 7 A. The talar pin setting guide is positioned on the distal end of the tibial guide. With the ankle positioned in neutral flexion, a pin is inserted through the hole into the talus (left ankle). **B.** This reference pin must be placed with the ankle in a strictly neutral position between flexion and extension. **C.** Excessive plantarflexion of the ankle tilts the implant backward. **D.** Excessive dorsiflexion of the ankle will lead to anterior and plantarflexed positioning of the talar component. **E.** The pin-guided resection is performed with an oscillating saw, taking care to keep the saw blade flat against the pin surface during resection.

bone while simultaneously trying to preserve as much talar bone stock as possible.

- The posterior chamfer cut of the talus should be anatomic, parallel to the superior margin of the talar dome.
- Asymmetric wear must be recognized and the posterior talar chamfer cut adjusted appropriately; shims are available to make such adjustments.
- We do not recommend compensating extra-articular or hindfoot deformity by means of an asymmetric posterior talar chamfer cut; instead, simultaneous or staged hindfoot correction should be performed.
- The talar guide orients the placement of four pins in the talus that are then used to guide the talar resection. Maintain the oscillating saw flush with the dorsal aspects of the pins while protecting the malleoli from injury **(TECH FIG 7E)**.

- The residual tibial bone is relatively easy to extract at this point, along with the resected portion of talus. A lamina spreader without teeth, used judiciously, usually improves exposure, using ribbon retractors if available.
- Posterior arthrolysis can be completed at this stage if needed.

Anterior Talar Chamfer Preparation

- Anterior talar preparation contributes to the correct AP and rotational positioning of the talar component.
- Perform the anterior chamfer cut with a milling device controlled by the anterior talar cutting guide, secured on the posterior resected surface **(TECH FIG 8)**.
- The AP position of the guide should be carefully adjusted, with the anterior cortex of the tibia being tangent to the calibration line tagged on the guide.

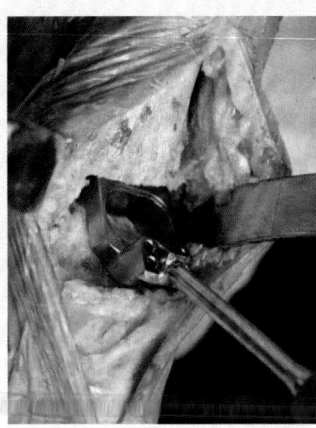

TECH FIG 8 The anterior chamfer cut is performed with an end mill cutter controlled by the anterior talar cutting guide, which is positioned on the posterior resected surface.

- Adequate anterior resection is essential to avoid an anterior talar position relative to the tibia, a situation that may lead to increased anterior contact stresses and potential edge loading.
  - In our experience, the threshold to deepen the anterior chamfer preparation should be low.
  - Removing anterior talar neck osteophytes allows the guide to be properly seated on the talus.

- Appropriate anterior chamfer preparation is determined using the talar gauge.
- With respect to rotation, the guide must be perfectly aligned with the axis of the talar body. The second metatarsal may be used as a reference provided there is no associated foot malalignment.

Lateral Chamfer and Talar Stem Preparation

- Proper positioning is essential.
  - In the sagittal plane, the guide should be positioned flush with the two previously resected surfaces, with no anterior overhang.
  - In the horizontal plane, rotation is determined with reference to the axis of the talar body.
  - In the coronal plane, correct mediolateral position is referenced from the lateral margin of the prepared talar dome.
  - Once correctly positioned, pin the cutting guide to the bone.
- First, prepare the talar stem recession using the bell saw. Then, insert a dedicated metal peg into this prepared portion of talus to afford greater stability to the lateral talar chamfer cutting guide. Prepare the lateral chamfer using an oscillating or reciprocating saw.
- The most recent instrumentation also integrates a preliminary talar trial to set the correct position of the implant before performing the plug and the lateral chamfer.

INSERTION OF TRIAL COMPONENTS

- The appropriate-size talar trial is one that provides good coverage of the talus in the mediolateral plane, without medial overhang.
- The talar trial lacks the plasma spray coating and thus lacks the interference fit of the actual talar implant; therefore, the talar trial may appear loose. To determine optimal polyethylene thickness and ligament balance, the talar trial remains in situ during insertion of the tibial trials.
- Insertion of tibial trials
  - First, thoroughly irrigate the ankle joint and remove any debris.
  - Push the trial tibial base and insert assembly into position; it is free to rotate relative to the tibia.
  - As the ankle is ranged from flexion to extension, the tibial trial locates and translates its ideal position and rotation with respect to the talus, unless the tibial trial has essentially the same dimensions as the prepared tibial surface.

- When this automatic adjustment is obtained, the definitive position is determined.
- Perform preparation for the press-fit hole for the tapered cylindrical plug.
- Note the line on the superior surface of the base trials should align with the anterior tibial cortex.
  - A lateral fluoroscopic view can confirm at this stage the congruity between the tibial trial and the distal part of the tibia.
- Range the joint and check stability. The implant should be stable in the coronal plane, without any residual laxity; dorsiflexion greater than 10 degrees should be readily obtained.
  - If not, consider a thinner polyethylene insert or an additional soft tissue procedure (eg, deep deltoid ligament release, lateral ligament reconstruction, Achilles tendon lengthening, or gastrocnemius recession).

INSERTION OF THE DEFINITIVE COMPONENTS

- Insert the definitive components.
  - Be sure you maintain a good contact between the upper side of the tibial implant and the tibial resection to prevent any risk of posterior gap.
- The prosthesis must have sound initial stability, indicating appropriate ligament balance.
- Check the final fluoroscopic views while reassessing ankle motion and stability.

- Before impacting the components, any tibial or talar subchondral cysts or other bone defects may be filled with bone graft.
- Insert the talar component first.
- After inserting the tibial component, fill the anterior opening of the cortex with bone graft obtained from the bone cuts to prevent any ingress of joint fluid (**TECH FIG 9**), which may lead to osteolysis.

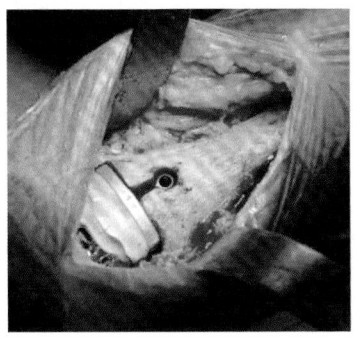
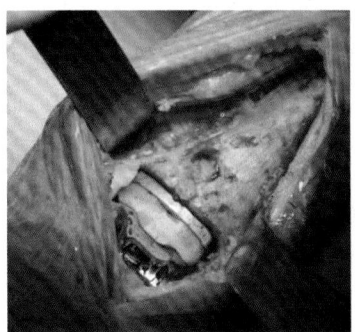

TECH FIG 9 After insertion of the tibial component, the anterior opening of the cortex (**A**) is filled with bone graft obtained from the bone cuts to prevent any ingress of joint fluid (**B**).

CLOSURE

- Because the skin over the ankle is very delicate, closure must be meticulous.
- Close the wound over an intra-articular drain. Whenever possible, close the capsule with absorbable sutures.
- Suture the fascia and retinaculum. Isolate the toe extensor tendons and particularly the tibialis anterior tendon from the fascial suture line.

- Close the loose subcutaneous tissue and the skin with interrupted sutures.
- Apply a below-knee, well-padded cast with the ankle in neutral position.

SALTO TALARIS CASE EXAMPLE (COURTESY OF MARK E. EASLEY, MD)

Background

- A 62-year-old woman with right ankle arthritis failed appropriate nonoperative treatment.
    - Ankle/hindfoot alignment in neutral; lacking physiologic valgus
    - Some associated hindfoot stiffness
- Weight-bearing radiographs
    - Suggested slight varus at the ankle (**TECH FIG 10A**)
    - End-stage ankle arthritis with loss of the joint space (**TECH FIG 10A–C**)

- Large anterior osteophytes and suggestion of talar cysts (see **TECH FIG 10C**)
- Hindfoot alignment in neutral (**TECH FIG 10D**)
- CT suggested end-stage ankle arthritis with medial joint wear pattern (**TECH FIG 10E**).
    - Despite radiographic appearance, no large talar cysts suggested (**TECH FIG 10E,F**)

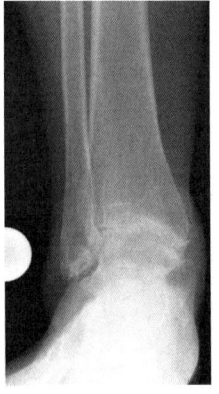
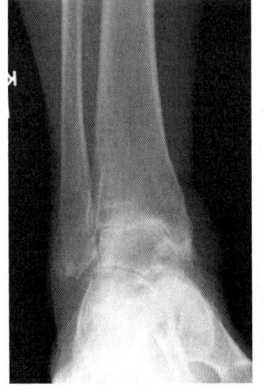
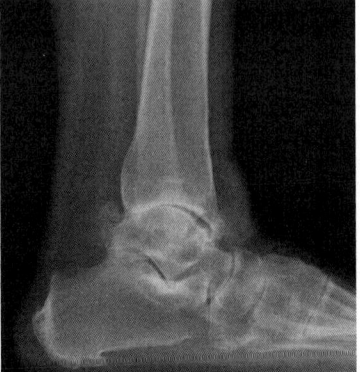
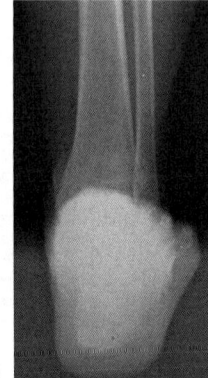

TECH FIG 10 A 62-year-old woman with end-stage right ankle arthritis. **A–D.** Weight-bearing radiographs. **A.** AP view. **B.** Mortise view. Note medial ankle joint wear pattern with some varus malalignment. **C.** Lateral view. Note large anterior osteophytes and question of talar cyst formation. **D.** Hindfoot alignment view suggesting neutral heel position. *(continued)*

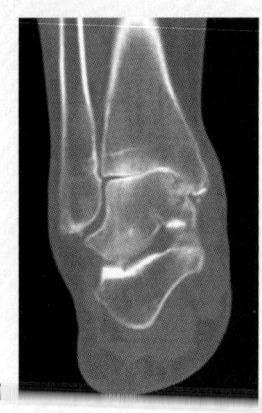
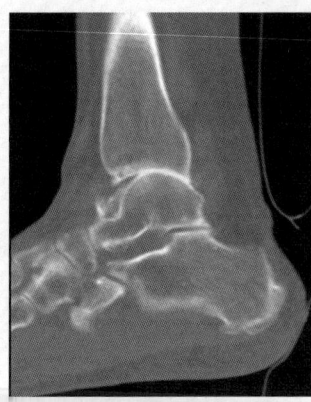

TECH FIG 10 *(continued)* **E.** Coronal CT demonstrates end-stage ankle arthritis and medial wear pattern. **F.** Sagittal view shows no obvious talar cysts, and no advanced subtalar arthritis is suggested.

Exposure

- Longitudinal anterior incision over ankle **(TECH FIG 11A)**
  - Starting 1 cm lateral to tibial crest, approximately 8 cm proximal to ankle
  - Extending to central midfoot approximately 4 cm distal to joint
- Superficial peroneal nerve identified and protected throughout procedure **(TECH FIG 11B)**
  - Occasionally, there is one medial crossing branch immediately anterior to the ankle that needs to be sacrificed because it would be under tension and at risk for injury.

- Extensor retinaculum exposed
- Extensor retinaculum opened longitudinally over EHL tendon **(TECH FIG 11C)**
- Deep neurovascular bundle identified, mobilized laterally, and protected throughout procedure **(TECH FIG 11D,E)**

Joint Preparation

- Osteophytes removed **(TECH FIG 12A,B)**
- Distal anterior tibial resection
  - Osteophytes removed **(TECH FIG 12C)**
  - Congruent resection recommended
    - Perpendicular to tibial shaft axis to facilitate orthogonal positioning of external tibial alignment guide **(TECH FIG 12D,E)**
    - Cutting the anterior distal tibial preparation to expose the tibial plafond in varus may promote varus positioning of the external tibial alignment guide.
  - Tibial plafond exposed **(TECH FIG 12F)**

Placing the External Tibial Alignment Guide

- An osteotome may be placed in the medial gutter to use as a reference to align the proximal tibial (tubercle) pin from which the external tibial alignment guide will be suspended **(TECH FIG 13A)**.
- External tibial alignment guide positioned, centered over the tibial crest **(TECH FIG 13B)**
- External tibial alignment guide secured in distal medial tibia **(TECH FIG 13C)**

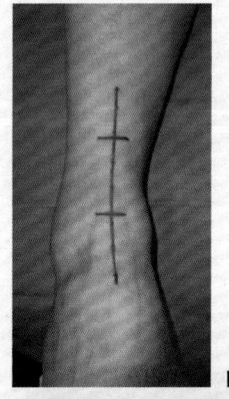
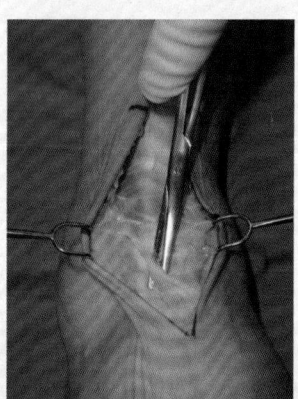
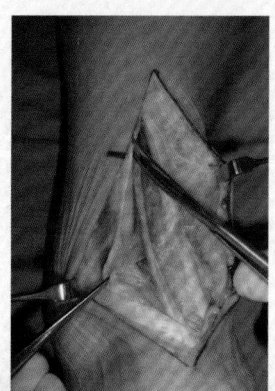
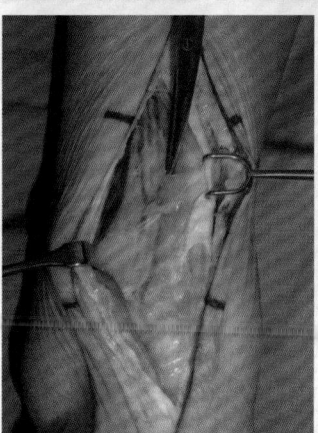
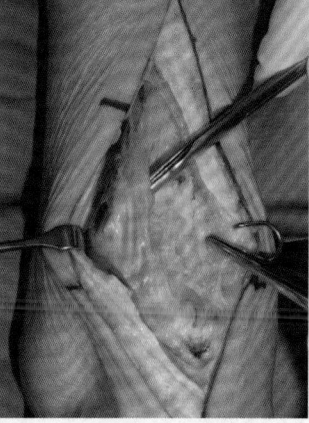

TECH FIG 11 A. Longitudinal anterior incision over ankle. **B.** Superficial peroneal nerve identified and protected throughout procedure. **C.** Extensor retinaculum opened longitudinally over EHL tendon. **D.** Deep neurovascular bundle identified. **E.** Deep neurovascular bundle mobilized laterally and protected.

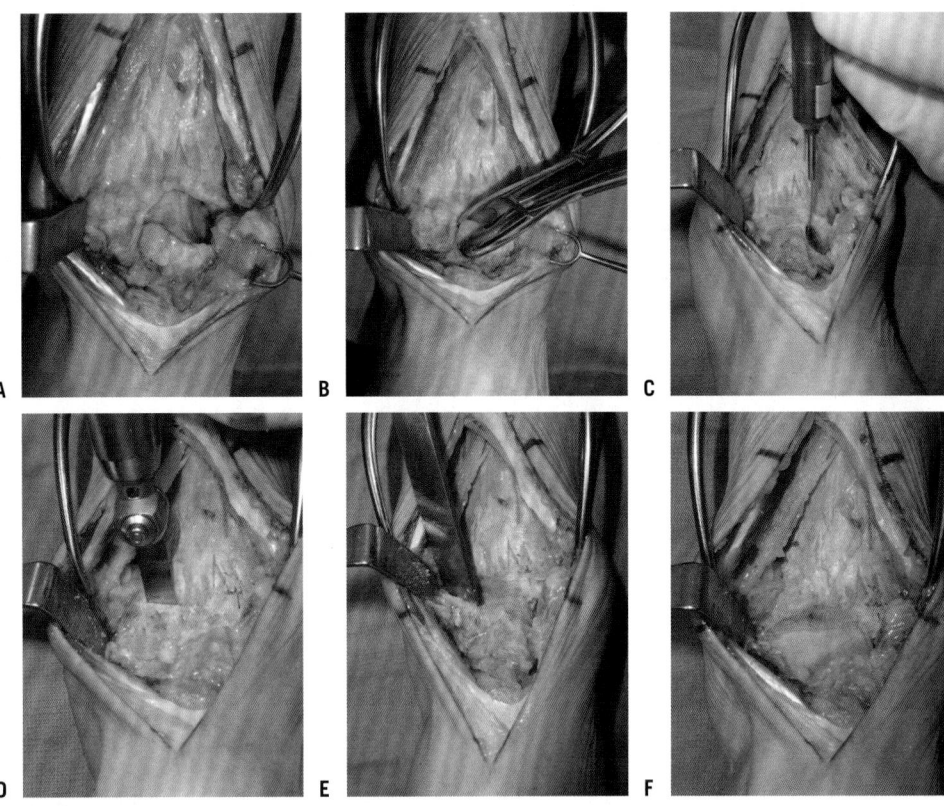

TECH FIG 12 A. Anterior osteophytes. **B.** Osteophytes removed with a rongeur. **C–F.** Anterior distal tibial preparation. **C.** Osteophytes removed. **D.** Reciprocating saw used to create a vertical relief cut. **E.** Anterior bone/osteophyte resection to expose ankle. **F.** Tibial plafond exposed.

- Slope properly adjusted
  - Traditional guide has 7 degrees of anterior opening if alignment guide placed parallel to tibial shaft axis.
    - Elevating the alignment guide proximally removes some of this slope to neutralize the tibial plafond cut (**TECH FIG 13D**).
  - Newer instrumentation will have less than 7 degrees of slope built into the system.

- Rotation properly adjusted
  - With the talus moved in the sagittal plane, a reference pin suspended from the tibial alignment guide is used to orient the cutting block to match the talar axis (**TECH FIG 13E**).
  - Ideally, this will determine optimal rotation for the tibial cutting block.

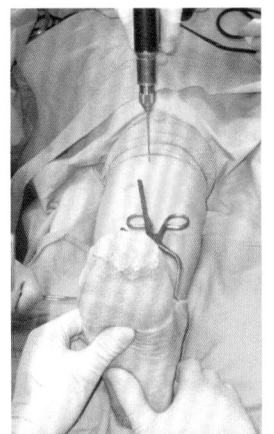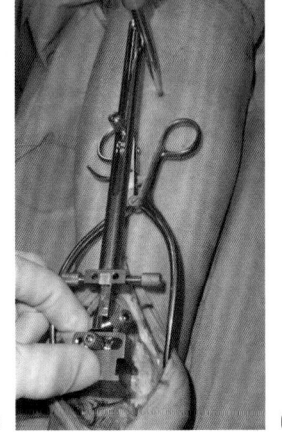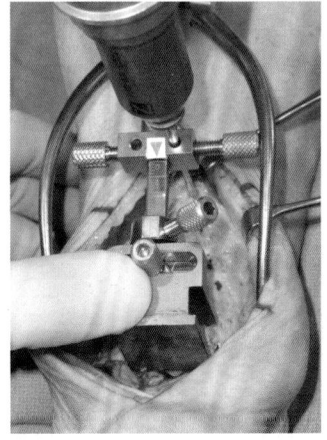

TECH FIG 13 External tibial alignment guide. **A.** Osteotome may be placed in medial gutter, serves as a reference to align proximal tibial (tubercle) pin from which external tibial alignment guide is suspended. **B.** External tibial alignment guide centered over tibial crest. **C.** External tibial alignment guide secured in distal medial tibia. *(continued)*

TECHNIQUES

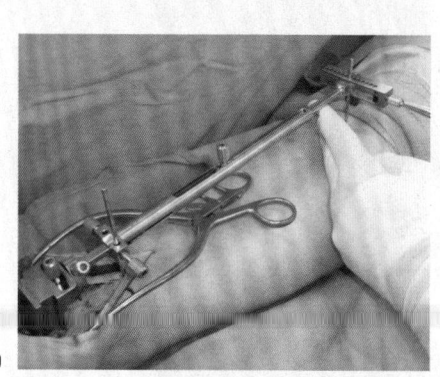

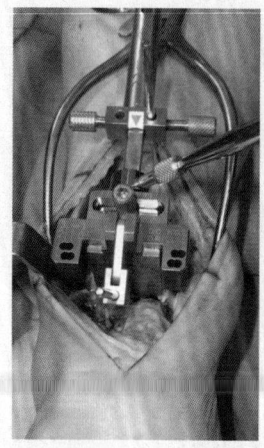

TECH FIG 13 *(continued)* **D.** Elevating the alignment guide proximally removes some of this slope to neutralize the 7 degrees of anterior opening (slope) built into the traditional alignment guide (a new guide with less slope is to be released). **E.** Setting tibial cutting block rotation. With the talus moved in the sagittal plane, a reference pin suspended from the tibial alignment guide used to orient the cutting block's rotation to match the talar axis.

Setting the Tibial Cutting Block

- The tibial cut is set for 8 to 9 mm from the apex of the tibial plafond (**TECH FIG 14A,B**).
- Proper tibial cutting block positioning confirmed fluoroscopically (**TECH FIG 14C–E**)
- Provisionally, a pin is manually placed in the proximal medial aspect of the cutting guide to ensure that the cutting block is not placed too medially, risking weakening medial malleolar support (**TECH FIG 14F**).
  - Even if fluoroscopy suggests optimal position, clinical confirmation is recommended.
  - A simple lateral shift of the cutting block or downsizing the block protects the malleolus.

- With the tibial cutting block in place, the two proximal pins are placed to protect the malleoli (**TECH FIG 14G**).
- The additional holes are drilled to weaken the bone planned for resection, thereby facilitating the bone's removal (**TECH FIG 14H**).
- Careful tibial preparation with the oscillating saw (**TECH FIG 14I**).
  - Avoid overpenetration with the saw blade posteriorly, as it will potentially risk injury to the flexor hallucis longus tendon and the posteromedial neurovascular bundle.
- With the cutting block removed, the medial and lateral drill holes are connected with a small reciprocating saw (**TECH FIG 14J**).
- The tibial plafond resection is mobilized and removed.
  - Rarely can the resected distal tibial bone be removed as one piece (**TECH FIG 14K**).

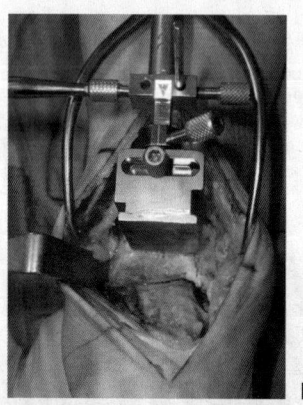

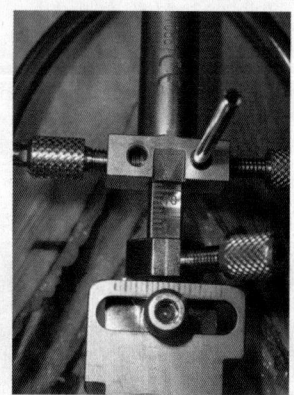

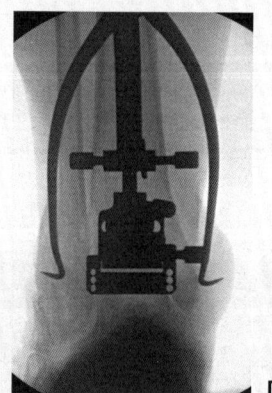

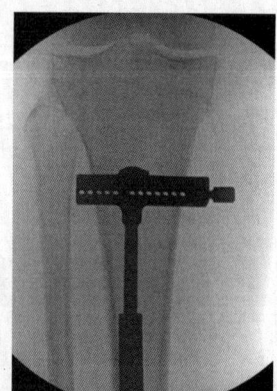

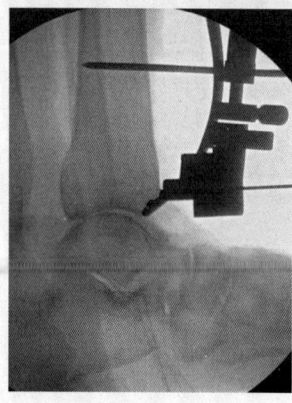

TECH FIG 14 Setting the tibial cutting block. **A.** The tibial cut is set for 8 to 9 mm. **B.** Note that the resection level is set for 8 mm (moved from zero position that was positioned at the apex of the tibial plafond). **C–E.** Fluoroscopic confirmation of optimal tibial cutting block position. **C,D.** In the AP plane, the external tibial alignment guide should be parallel to the tibial shaft axis, and the cutting block should be oriented with the joint without violating the malleoli. **E.** In the lateral plane, the resection will ideally be nearly perpendicular to the tibial shaft axis and resecting approximately 8 to 9 mm of bone from the apex of the tibial plafond. *(continued)*

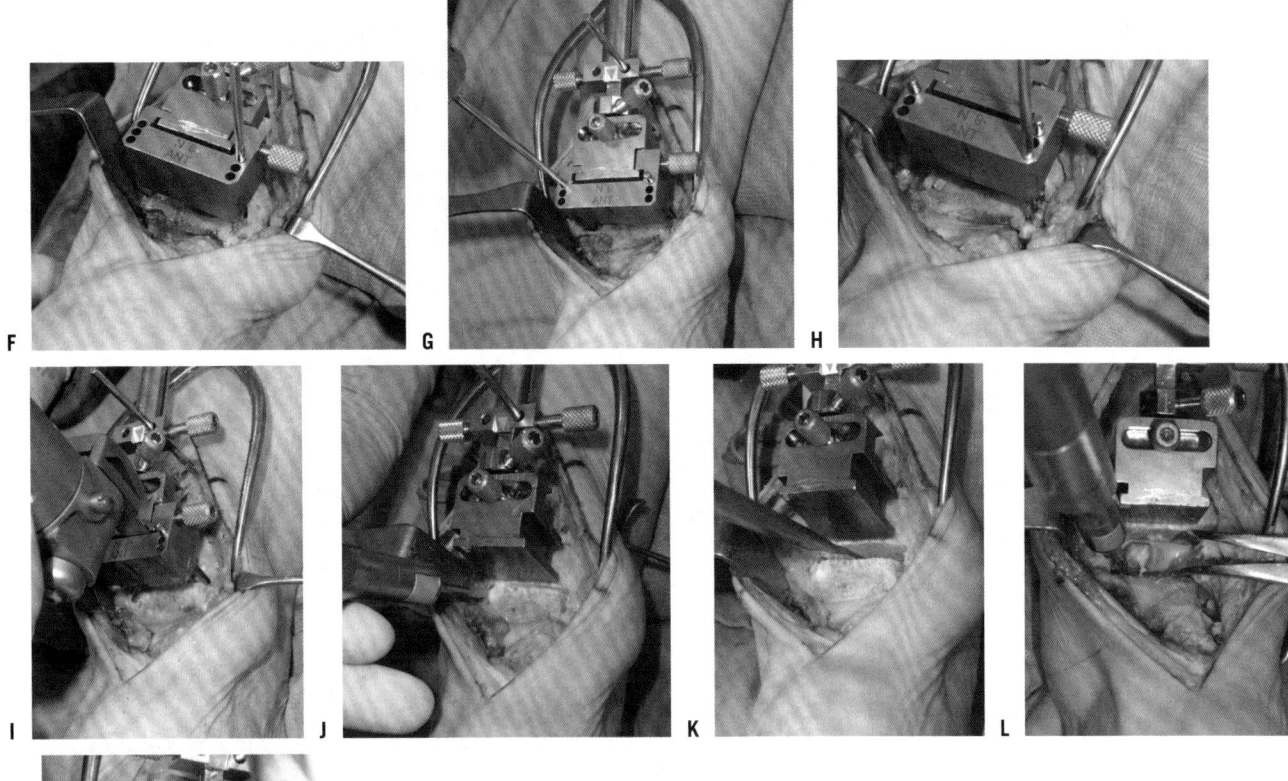

TECH FIG 14 *(continued)* **F.** A pin is manually placed in the proximal medial aspect of the cutting guide to ensure that the cutting block is not placed too medially, risking weakening medial malleolar support. **G.** Pins serve to protect malleoli. **H.** The additional holes are drilled to weaken the bone planned for resection, thereby facilitating the bone's removal. **I.** Careful tibial preparation with the oscillating saw, avoiding overpenetration of the posterior cortex that may risk flexor hallucis longus or posteromedial neurovascular bundle injury. **J.** With cutting block removed, the medial and lateral drill holes are connected with small reciprocating saw. **K.** Rarely can the resected distal tibial bone be removed as one piece. **L.** Using lamina spreader (without teeth so the prepared tibial surface is protected), residual posterior bone may be carefully morselized with the small reciprocating saw. **M.** Fragments removed using a 90-degree curette and rongeur.

- Using a lamina spreader (without teeth so the prepared tibial surface is protected), the residual posterior bone may be carefully morselized with the small reciprocating saw and the fragments removed using a 90-degree curette and rongeur (**TECH FIG 14L,M**).

Initial Talar Preparation

- Through a dedicated drill guide suspended from the external tibial alignment guide, a reference hole is drilled in the anterior talus with (**TECH FIG 15A,B**) the following:
  - Ankle held in neutral sagittal plane position
  - Hindfoot held in physiologic valgus
- Drill guide removed (**TECH FIG 15C**)
- Pin placed in reference drill hole (**TECH FIG 15D**)
- External tibial alignment guide removed (**TECH FIG 15E**)
- Posterior talar chamfer cutting guide placed (**TECH FIG 15F**)

- Four drill holes through posterior chamfer guide and four pins placed through the guide, serving as reference for the posterior chamfer cut (**TECH FIG 15G,H**)
  - In narrow ankles, sometimes, only three pins gain purchase in the talar dome.
- With malleoli protected, posterior chamfer cut made directly on the four pins and resected bone removed (**TECH FIG 15I–L**)

Anterior Talar Chamfer Preparation

- Residual anterior osteophytes removed, so there is no impingement on the guide (**TECH FIG 16A**)
- Anterior chamfer milling guide properly positioned and secured with dedicated lamina spreader(s) (**TECH FIG 16B–D**)
- Guide should align with second metatarsal when foot is positioned for simulated weight bearing.
  - The anterior chamfer will dictate talar component rotation.

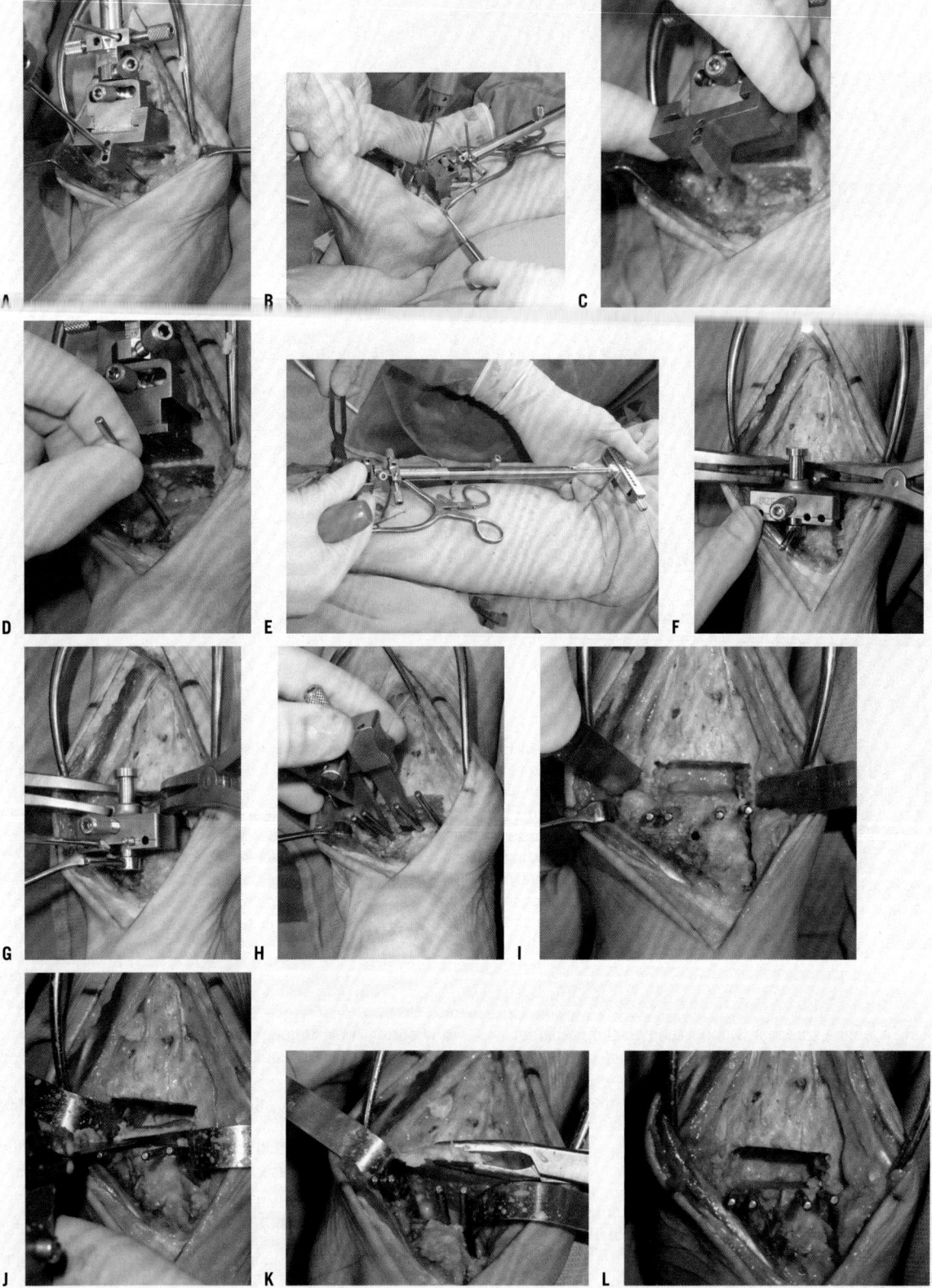

TECH FIG 15 A. Through a dedicated drill guide suspended from the external tibial alignment guide, a reference hole is drilled in the anterior talus. **B.** Ankle held in neutral position and hindfoot supported in slight valgus. **C.** Drill guide removed. **D.** Pin placed in reference drill hole. **E.** External tibial alignment guide removed. **F.** Posterior talar chamfer cutting guide placed on reference pin, with paddles flush on posterior talar dome. Note use of dedicated lamina spreaders to keep paddles flush. **G.** Four drill holes through posterior chamfer guide and four pins placed through the guide. **H.** Posterior chamfer guide removed. **I.** Four pins serve as reference for posterior chamfer cut. **J.** Posterior chamfer cut with oscillating saw. Note ribbon retractors to protect malleoli. **K.** Resected bone removed. **L.** Posterior chamfer cut complete.

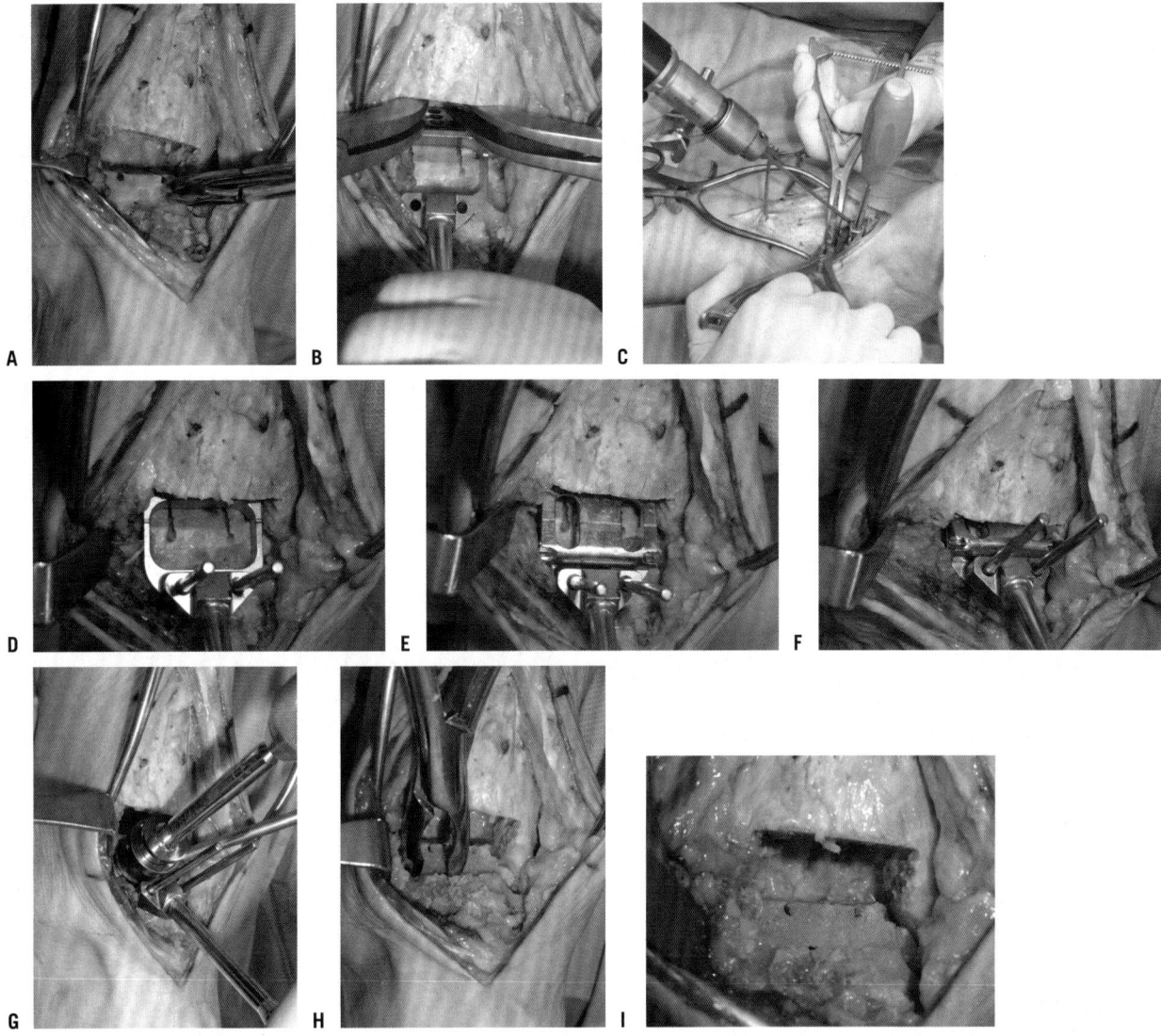

TECH FIG 16 A. Residual anterior osteophytes removed. **B.** Anterior talar chamfer guide properly positioned, aligned with second metatarsal. **C.** Guide secured with anterior pins and lamina spreader(s). **D.** Guide in proper position. **E.** AP reference guide placed. **F.** With ankle dorsiflexion, AP reference guide confirms satisfactory anterior chamfer guide position. **G.** Anterior chamfer milled. **H.** Anterior chamfer completed with rongeur. **I.** Completed anterior chamfer.

- Proper position confirmed with dedicated AP reference guide **(TECH FIG 16E,F)**
- Anterior chamfer milled **(TECH FIG 16G)**
- Anterior chamfer preparation completed with a rongeur **(TECH FIG 16H,I)**

Lateral Chamfer and Stem Relief Preparation

- Lateral chamfer guide properly positioned on prepared anterior and posterior chamfer cuts
- Guide pinned in place **(TECH FIG 17A)**
- Confirm proper position clinically.
  - Stem preparation should be situated directly over crest, where two chamfers meet **(TECH FIG 17B)**.
  - Avoid posterior lift-off of the lateral chamfer guide.

- Stem relief drilled with dedicated bell saw that leaves central core of bone for larger sizes **(TECH FIG 17C,D)**
  - For smallest size, the central core is forfeited.
- Stabilizing plug placed through lateral chamfer cutting guide into prepared stem relief area to further stabilize guide for lateral chamfer preparation **(TECH FIG 17E)**
- Lateral chamfer preparation **(TECH FIG 17F)**
  - Protect anterior neurovascular bundle and EHL tendon.
  - Avoid violating anterior tibial cortex with edge of saw.
- Central stabilizing plug removed and lateral chamfer cutting guide removed **(TECH FIG 17G)**
- Resected lateral chamfer bone removed **(TECH FIG 17H)**
- Gutters inspected to ensure no impinging bone present **(TECH FIG 17I)**

TECHNIQUES

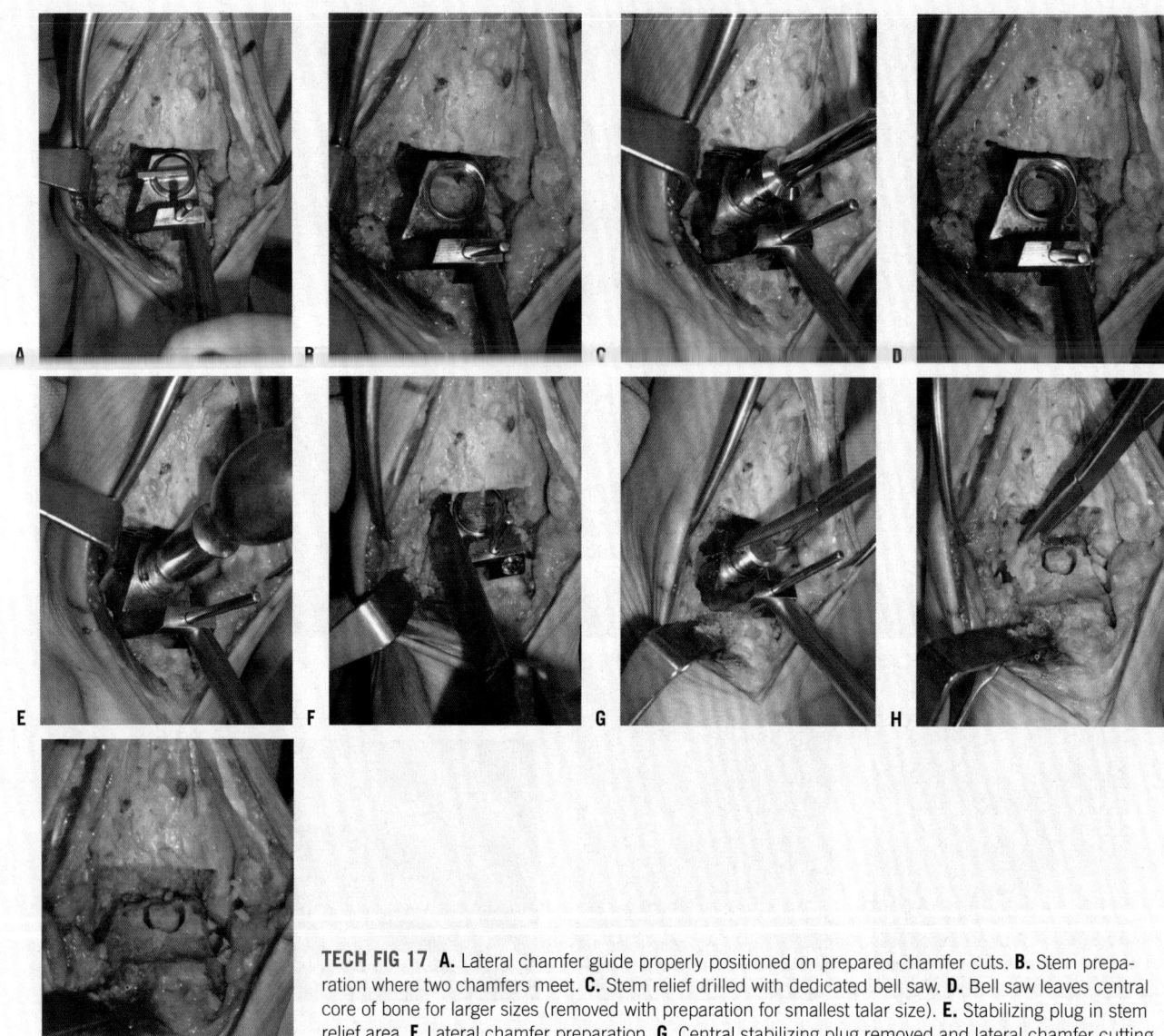

TECH FIG 17 A. Lateral chamfer guide properly positioned on prepared chamfer cuts. **B.** Stem preparation where two chamfers meet. **C.** Stem relief drilled with dedicated bell saw. **D.** Bell saw leaves central core of bone for larger sizes (removed with preparation for smallest talar size). **E.** Stabilizing plug in stem relief area. **F.** Lateral chamfer preparation. **G.** Central stabilizing plug removed and lateral chamfer cutting guide removed. **H.** Resected lateral chamfer bone removed. **I.** Gutters inspected to ensure no impinging bone present.

Trial Components

- Talar trial placed and fully seated **(TECH FIG 18A,B)**
- Tibial trial with attached polyethylene trial placed with careful axial distraction placed on the joint **(TECH FIG 18C,D)**
- Clinical assessment
  - Satisfactory ROM, especially dorsiflexion
  - Satisfactory stability in the coronal plane; assess with the ankle in neutral position.
- Fluoroscopic assessment
  - Confirm proper alignment **(TECH FIG 18E)**.
  - Confirm proper bony apposition of tibial component, particularly posteriorly; no posterior "lift-off"

- Assess posterior tibial component coverage **(TECH FIG 18F)**.
- Tibial component may be upsized **(TECH FIG 18G–J)**.
  - If posterior coverage based on intraoperative fluoroscopy is not ideal, then the tibial component may be upsized one size from that of the talar component.
    - The polyethylene size will remain the same, so it continues to match the talus.
- Once optimal combination of trial components determined, open true components.
  - In this case, a size 2 tibial component is used with a size 1 talar component, and a 10-mm polyethylene was used to optimize coronal plane stability.

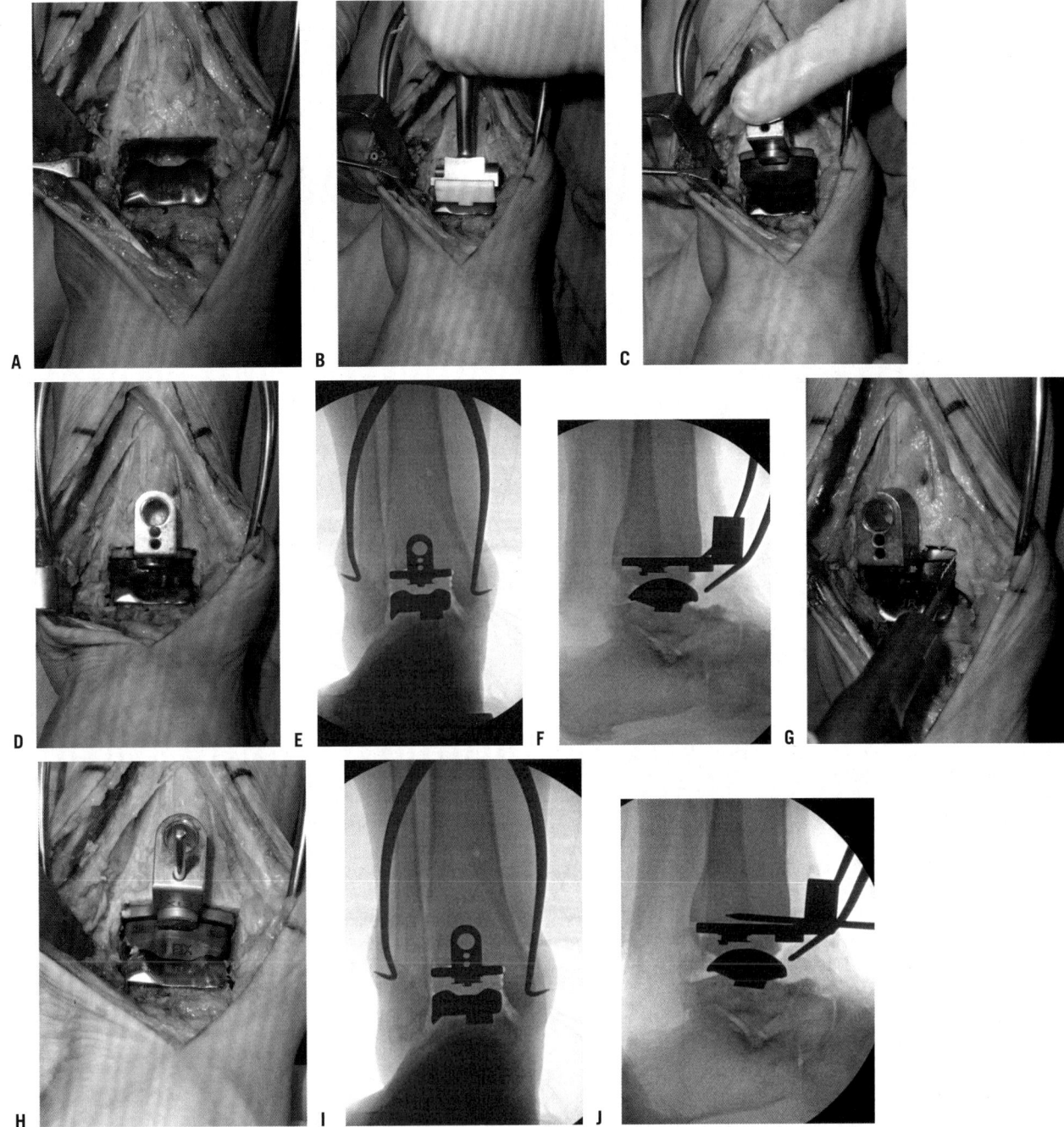

TECH FIG 18 **A.** Talar trial placed. **B.** Talar trial impacted. **C.** Tibial trial with attached polyethylene trial placed with careful axial ankle distraction. **D.** Tibial trial fully seated. **E,F.** Fluoroscopic assessment of trial components. **E.** AP view suggesting satisfactory alignment. **F.** Lateral view. Note that posterior tibial coverage could be improved. **G–J.** Upsizing tibial component. **G.** Judiciously, the tibial preparation is widened to accommodate a size 2 tibial component. **H.** Size 2 tibial component with size 1 polyethylene (to match unchanged talar component) placed. **I.** AP view suggests widening tibial preparation and upsizing tibial trial without compromising malleoli. **J.** Posterior tibial coverage improved; no posterior tibial lift-off and tibial trial pinned.

Final Tibial Preparation

- Preparing the tibial stem relief area does not require violating the posterior tibial cortex.
- With proper trial components in place, tibial trial is pinned.
- Fluoroscopic confirmation that there is indeed no posterior tibial component lift-off (see **TECH FIG 18J**)
- Second, more proximal, tibial drill hole made to create relief area for tibial component stem

- Proximal tibial reaming performed **(TECH FIG 19A)**
- Tibial stem relief area preparation completed
  - Drill holes connected with a small reciprocating saw **(TECH FIG 19B)**
  - Dedicated chisel used to the proper depth without violating the posterior tibial cortex **(TECH FIG 19C)**
  - Dedicated tibial rasp used to ensure transition from prepared tibial surface to prepared relief area for the stem

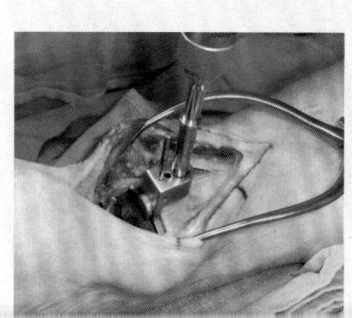 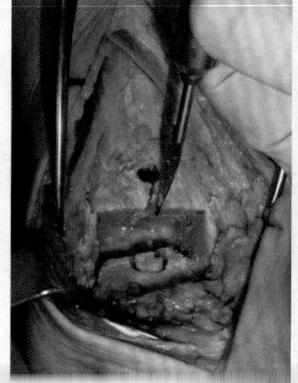 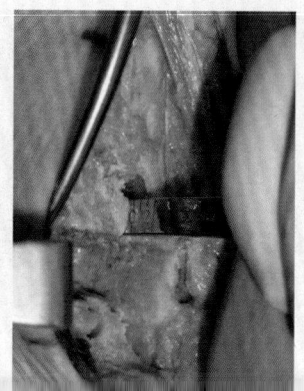

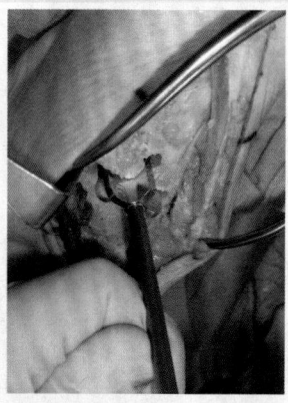

TECH FIG 19 A. With tibial trial pinned and second drill hole prepared, tibia reamer used. Note that posterior cortex is not violated with this preparation. **B.** Drill holes connected with a small reciprocating saw. **C.** Dedicated chisel used to the proper depth without violating the posterior tibial cortex. **D.** Dedicated tibial rasp used to ensure transition from prepared tibial surface to prepared relief area for the stem is appropriate.

is appropriate and limits risk of component lift-off during insertion **(TECH FIG 19D)**.

Final Implants

- Locking polyethylene to tibial component
  - On the back table, the polyethylene is attached to the true tibial component **(TECH FIG 20A,B)**.
  - A dedicated device may be used to facilitate locking the polyethylene to the tibial component **(TECH FIG 20C)**.
- Talar component insertion
  - Talus carefully positioned to preserve central core of bone for the stem **(TECH FIG 21A,B)**

- Impactor used
  - Avoid impinging the impactor handle on the anterior tibia **(TECH FIG 21C)**.
- Tibial component insertion
  - Assistant applies axial traction.
  - Surgeon "drives" tibia up into prepared tibia in proper rotation with the goal to avoid posterior lift-off **(TECH FIG 21D)**.
    - Requires and upwardly directed force with the dedicated insertion device **(TECH FIG 21E)**
    - If any concern that lift-off occurs, then a lateral fluoroscopy image should be obtained before fully inserting tibial component **(TECH FIG 21F)**.

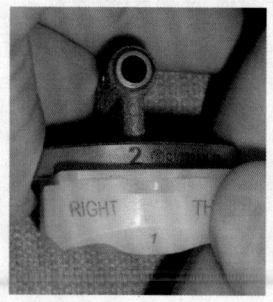 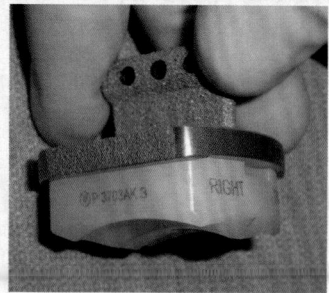 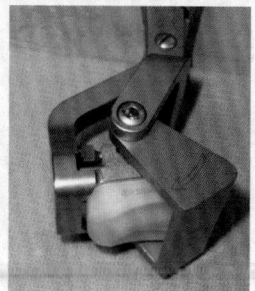

TECH FIG 20 A. Manually, polyethylene inserted into locking mechanism on tibial component. A size 2 tibial component was used with size 1 polyethylene. **B.** Polyethylene locked to tibial component. **C.** A dedicated device may be used to facilitate locking the polyethylene to the tibial component.

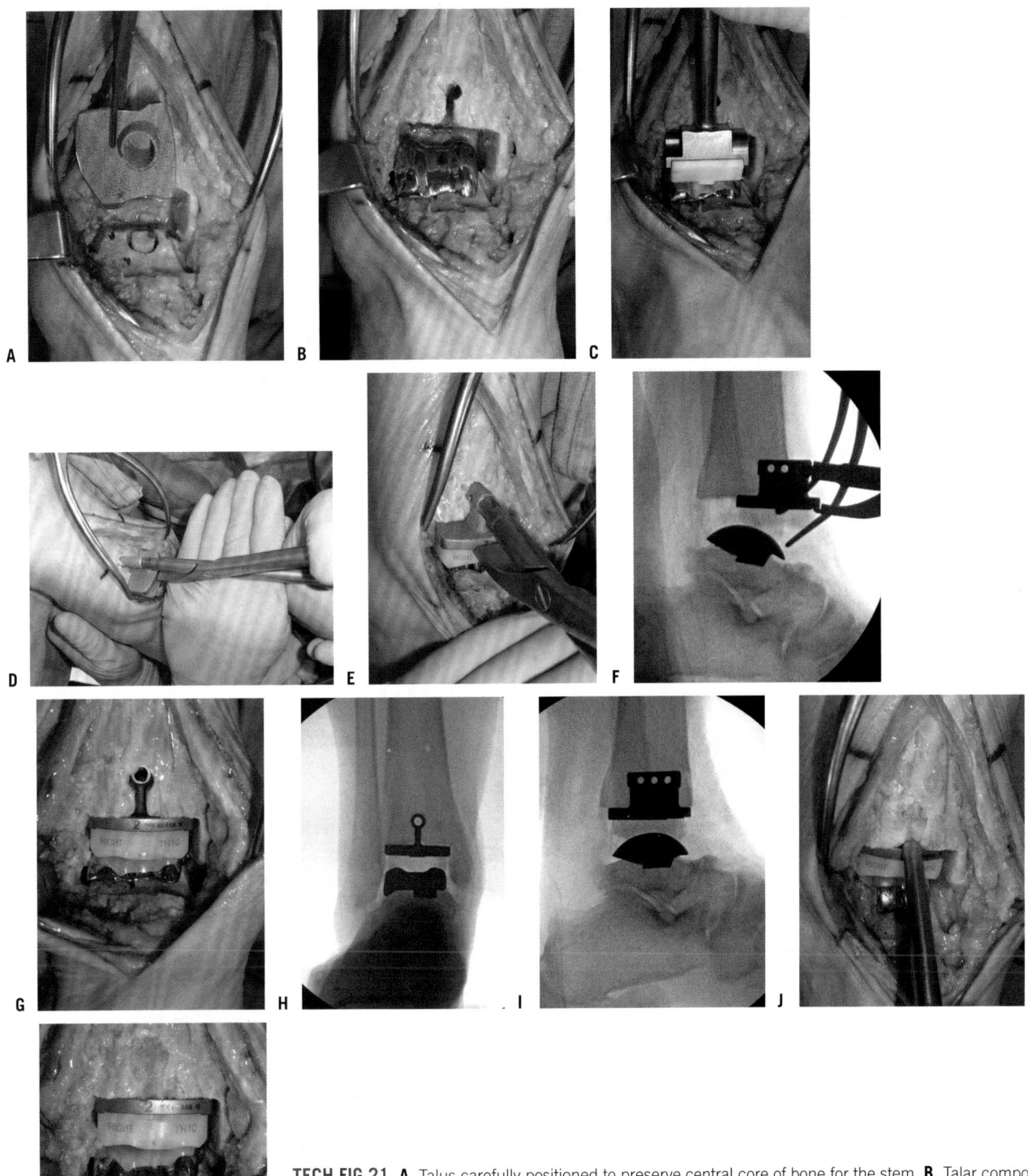

TECH FIG 21 A. Talus carefully positioned to preserve central core of bone for the stem. **B.** Talar component properly positioned. **C.** Talar component impacted with dedicated impactor. **D.** Tibial component is driven up into prepared tibia in proper rotation, with the goal to avoid posterior lift-off. **E.** This requires an upwardly directed force with the dedicated insertion device. **F.** If any concern that lift-off occurs, a lateral fluoroscopy image should be obtained before fully inserting tibial component. **G.** Final tibial component is fully seated to same depth as tibial trial. **H,I.** Fluoroscopic confirmation of proper component position and alignment. **H.** AP view. **I.** Lateral view confirming no posterior lift-off of final components. **J.** Morselized bone graft form distal tibial resection. **K.** Anterior defect filled.

TECHNIQUES

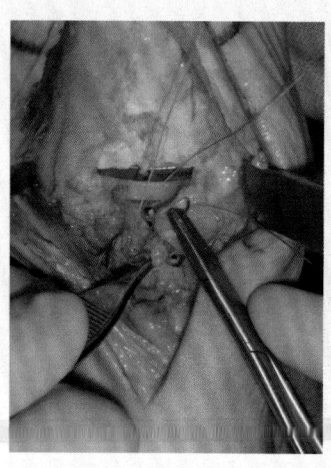
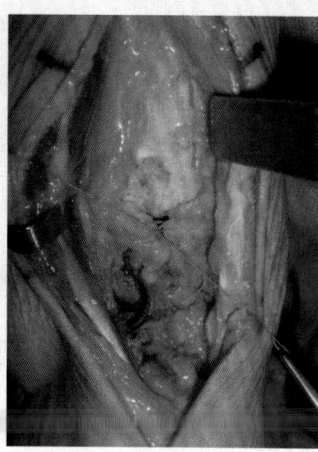

TECH FIG 22 Capsular closure. **A.** Capsule reapproximated over components. **B.** Deep neurovascular bundle protected during capsular closure.

- • Fully seat final tibial component to same depth as tibial trial (**TECH FIG 21G**)
- • Fluoroscopic confirmation
  - • Proper component position (**TECH FIG 21H**)
  - • No posterior tibial lift-off (**TECH FIG 21I**)
  - • No stress fracture
- • Clinical evaluation
  - • Satisfactory ROM
  - • Satisfactory balance/stability
- • Irrigation
- • Bone graft anterior tibial defect (**TECH FIG 21J,K**)
  - • Use morselized bone from tibial resection.

Closure and Postoperative Care

- • Capsule (**TECH FIG 22**): Protect deep neurovascular bundle.
- • Extensor retinaculum: Protect superficial peroneal nerve.
- • Routine subcutaneous layer and skin closure
  - • Over a drain
  - • Avoid pinching skin edges with forceps.
- • Recommend well-padded cast with ankle in neutral position.
- • Protected weight bearing for approximately 6 weeks
- • Regular follow-up recommended at 6 weeks, 3 months, 6 months, 1 year, and every year thereafter (**TECH FIG 23**)

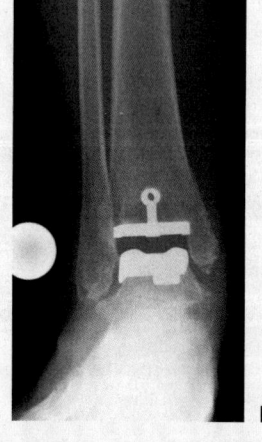
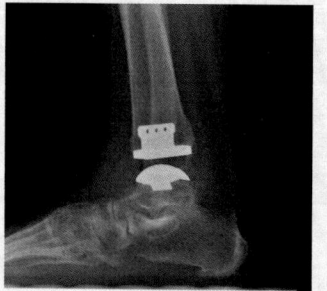
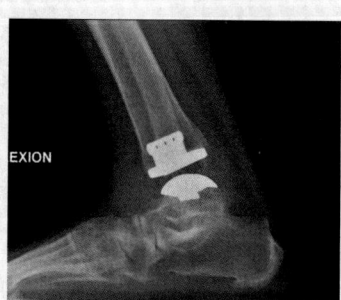
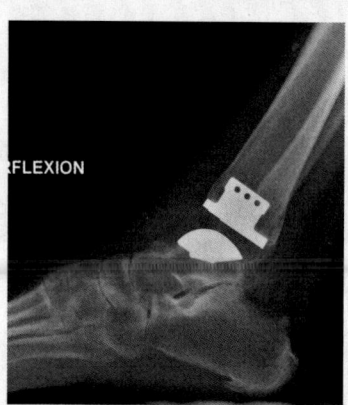
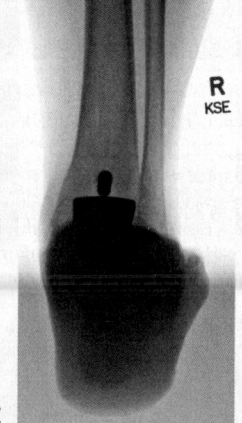

TECH FIG 23 One-year follow-up. **A.** AP view. **B.** Lateral view. **C.** Dorsiflexion view. **D.** Plantarflexion view. **E.** Hindfoot alignment view suggesting improved hindfoot position from preoperative alignment.

Pearls and Pitfalls

Impossible to Insert Even the Thinnest Bearing	• Tibial side will need to be reresected.
Dorsiflexion Unobtainable	• Check the size and the positioning of the talar component. • Check that the posterior capsular structures and the medial and lateral talar margins have been adequately cleared. • Reresect the tibia. • Perform percutaneous lengthening of the Achilles tendon or gastrocnemius release.
Lateral Residual Laxity	• Perform medial collateral ligament release and use a thicker polyethylene component. • Consider lateral ligament reconstruction.
Absolute Contraindications for TAA	• Active infection • Poor anterior skin (multiple scars, previous graft) • Risk factors for skin necrosis • Major bone loss • Diffuse (as opposed to focal) osteonecrosis of the talus • Nonreconstructable ankle ligamentous instability
Relative Contraindications for TAA	• Eradicated tibiotalar infection • Previous medial or lateral surgical approaches to the ankle (TAA incision will be anterior and central.) • Multiple prior surgeries to the ankle • High body mass index • High-demand patient (eg, construction work) • Unrealistic patient expectations

POSTOPERATIVE CARE

• The drain is removed the day after the operation.
• Once the swelling has subsided, a below-knee removable semirigid boot is applied.
• Partial to total weight bearing may be resumed immediately if no additional procedure performed.
• Patients who have undergone Achilles tendon lengthening will be non–weight bearing for 3 weeks.
• Where there has been a malleolar fracture, the period of non–weight bearing will be 45 days.
• Boot cast is removed after 45 days and physiotherapy is commenced, based mainly on self-rehabilitation exercises.

OUTCOMES

• Bonnin et al reported the results of a consecutive series of the first 98 mobile-bearing initial Salto prostheses implanted between 1997 and 2000.
  • Of those, 87 prostheses had a mean follow-up of 8.9 years (range, 6.8 to 11.1 years).
  • The survival rate was 65% (95% confidence interval [CI], 50 to 80) with any reoperation of the ankle and 85% (95% CI, 75 to 95) with revision of a component as the end points. Six prostheses were removed for arthrodesis, and 18 ankles underwent reoperation without arthrodesis. Symptomatic cysts grafting was the main cause for reoperation.
  • The mean American Orthopaedic Foot & Ankle Society ankle–hindfoot score preoperatively was 32 (standard deviation [SD] 10) and 79 (SD 12) at last follow-up.

• Hofmann et al reported the clinical results of the "modern" fixed-bearing Salto Talaris with a mean of 5.2 years.
  • Reviewing 81 consecutive ankles, they reported a 97.5% implant survivorship at 5.2 years.
  • There was one revision of a tibial component and one revision of a talar component.
  • Concurrent procedure at the time of the index surgery (mostly removal of previous hardware) were performed in 46% of the cases and additional procedures following the index surgery in 22% of the cases (mostly for gutter debridement).

COMPLICATIONS

• Technical difficulties in TAA may arise from a number of factors.

Failure to Reestablish the Physiologic Joint Line

• The final level of the implant joint line will depend on the level of the tibial cut.
• The level is determined with reference to the preoperative radiographs. Depending on the status of the tibial plafond, the anatomy of the malleoli, and lateral talomalleolar congruency, four different patterns may be encountered (FIG 4):
  • The ankle mortise is intact, with symmetric wear of the tibial plafond. The procedure should be a simple resurfacing, with the metal tibial component and polyethylene thickness replacing exactly what is resected.
  • The ankle mortise is intact, but the tibial plafond is asymmetrically worn. This pattern is seen in advanced RA, especially in the wake of long-term steroid therapy.

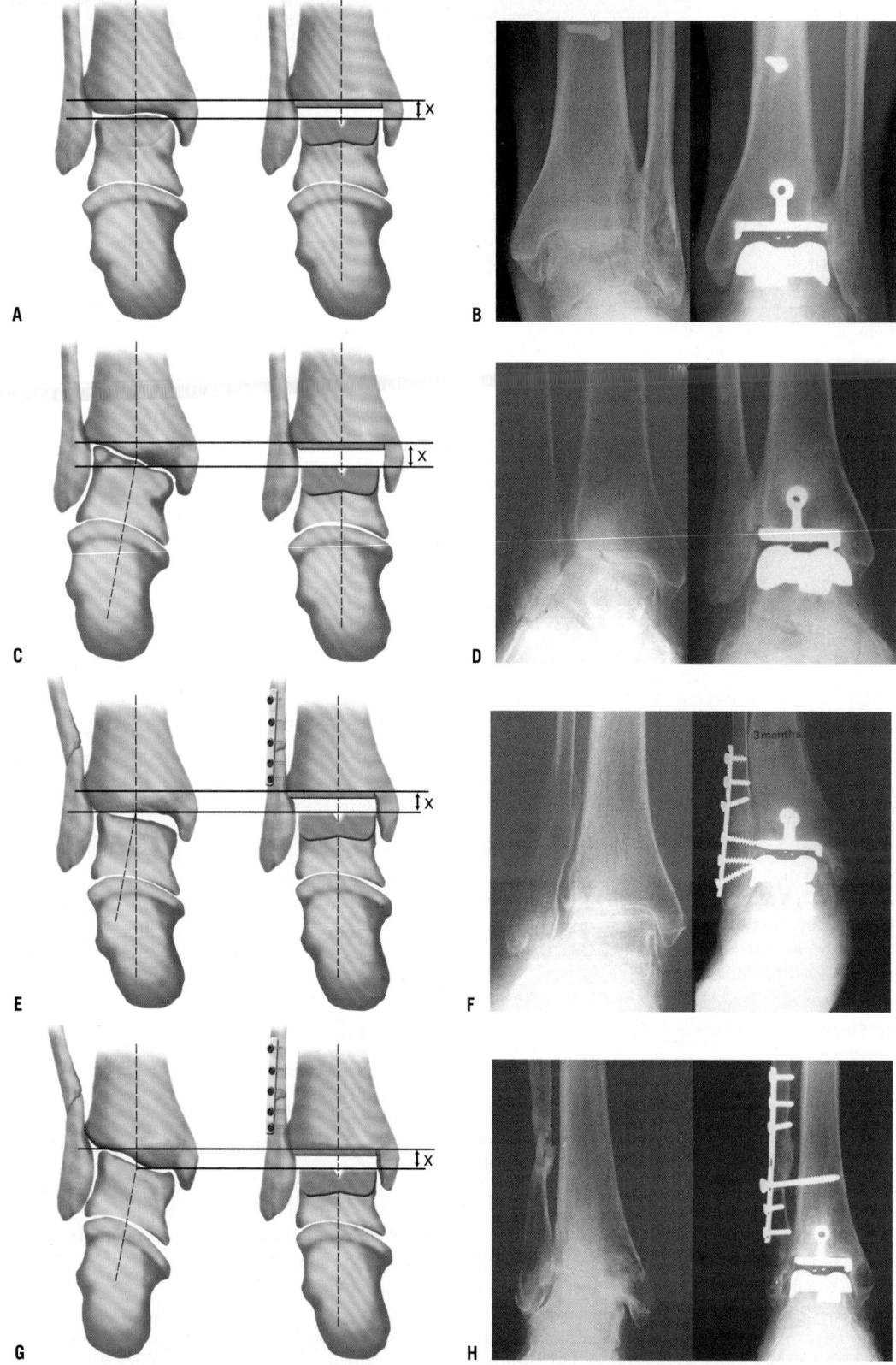

FIG 4 A,B. Ankle mortise intact, no asymmetric wear of the tibial pilon. **C,D.** Ankle mortise intact, tibial pilon asymmetrically worn. **E,F.** Malleoli deformed, tibial pilon intact. **G,H.** Malleoli deformed, tibial pilon worn. *x*, metal baseplate plus polyethylene.

In this case, a reasonable and balanced distal tibial resection level will need to be determined during preoperative planning.

- The malleoli are deformed, but the tibial plafond is intact. In our experience, this deformity involves the lateral malleolus. This pattern is seen in RA with severe hindfoot valgus that has resulted in a fatigue fracture of the fibula. In this case, the lateral malleolus will need to be managed with malleolar osteotomy and plating before TAA.
- The malleoli are deformed, and the tibial plafond is worn or depressed. These cases will need to be managed with a combination of the principles discussed earlier: First, a normal ankle mortise pattern will have to be created and then, a resection level will need to be determined, taking into account the extent of loss of tibial bone stock.

Extra-articular Deformity

- The physiologic ankle joint line is perpendicular to the axis of the tibia, and the hindfoot axis is in slight (5 to 10 degrees) valgus in relation to the tibial axis. To promote long-term implant survival, physiologic alignment will need to be restored.
- Inserting a TAA prosthesis into a malaligned tibia or hindfoot is a recipe for early loosening and failure.
- Correction of deformities may be difficult in sequelae of trauma or RA. Preoperative evaluation should allow the determination of whether these deformities have an intra-articular or extra-articular origin.
- In our experience, most intra-articular deformities resulting from wear or laxity (including varus position caused by OA in chronic instability) can be corrected from within the joint with the prosthesis.
- In contrast, most extra-articular deformities cannot be corrected from within the joint with the prosthesis and must be treated independently with supramalleolar osteotomy, performed either staged or simultaneous to TAA (**FIG 5A**).

- In our opinion, hindfoot malalignment associated with arthritis must be corrected by performing a calcaneus osteotomy, a subtalar fusion, or a triple arthrodesis before or after TAA (**FIG 5B**).
  - We recommend performing staged triple arthrodesis and TAA to reduce the potential for skin problems and edema. In our hands, triple arthrodesis is usually done as a first-stage procedure 45 days before TAA, which avoids prolonged cast immobilization.
  - We perform the triple arthrodesis by what would be an extension of the anterior approach to the ankle to prepare the talonavicular joint and a limited lateral–subfibular approach to the subtalar joint. We avoid dissection under the talar head to minimize the risk of necrosis of the talar body.
  - Fixation is achieved using a talocalcaneal screw and two talonavicular and calcaneocuboid staples.
  - The TAA prosthesis must be positioned on a properly aligned hindfoot.
    - In RA patients with a valgus deformity and severe lateral bone loss, bone grafting is the rule. Graft material is harvested from a local donor site (bone slices taken from the midtarsal joint, sometimes bone material taken from the proximal tibial metaphysis) and, in some cases, from the ipsilateral iliac crest in case of severe deformity.
- We stage the TAA 45 days after triple arthrodesis using the proximal extension of the same anterior approach. The talocalcaneal screw is removed.

Bone Loss

- Implant fixation requires sufficient tibial and talar bone stock and an intact ankle mortise.
- In RA patients or in posttraumatic OA, there may be major bone loss, and defects may have to be grafted. In particularly severe cases, TAA may be contraindicated.

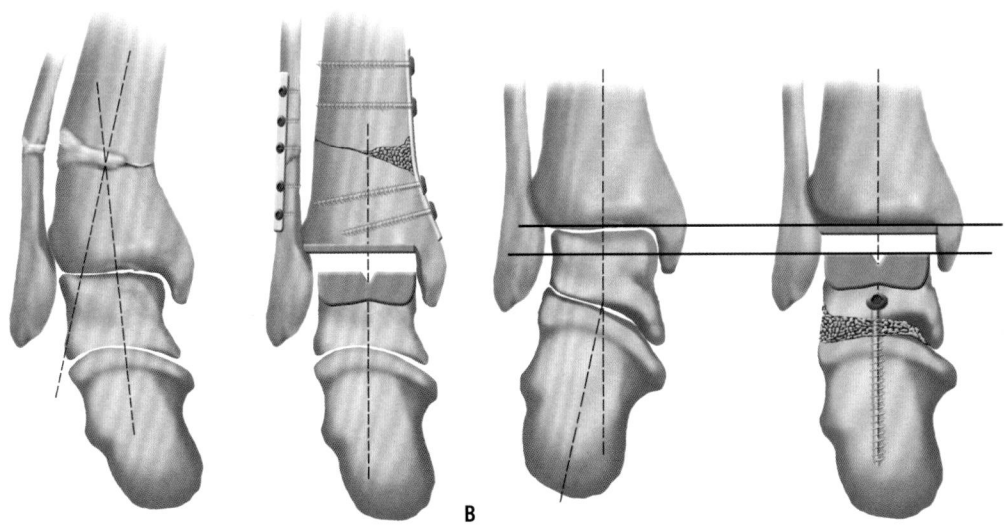

A   **B**

FIG 5 A. In case of tibial malunion, a correction via a supramalleolar osteotomy must be associated with the ankle prosthesis. **B.** In case of hindfoot deformity, a correction via a subtalar or triple arthrodesis or calcaneal osteotomy must be done in association with the ankle prosthesis.

Ankle Instability

- OA secondary to chronic lateral laxity is technically challenging because the persistence of lateral laxity may cause rapid deterioration of the prosthesis.
- In our experience, most cases can be balanced with TAA. We routinely restore the ankle's soft tissue balance with TAA and comprehensive soft tissue release on the concave side of the deformity.
  - Medial release in a varus deformity is challenging and involves the entire deltoid ligament, which is first released subperiosteally from its malleolar attachment and then detached from the talus. We have been satisfied with this balancing technique, which, in our hands, eliminates the need for the medial malleolar osteotomy technique to rebalance the deltoid ligament.
  - With comprehensive and satisfactory medial release, we rarely need to perform a ligament reconstruction on the convex side of the deformity (**FIG 6**). Occasionally, however, for severe varus malalignment, we perform a lateralizing and valgus-producing calcaneal osteotomy to further realign the hindfoot.

Ankle Stiffness

- End-stage tibiotalar joint arthritis almost always leads to stiffness of the tibiotalar joint.
- Stiffness with equinus deformity requires sequential steps to regain dorsiflexion, beginning with excision of anterior ossifications, then freeing of talomalleolar adhesions, and finally posterior capsulectomy from within the joint.
  - The use of a lamina spreader greatly facilitates capsulectomy. However, great caution should be used to avoid avulsion of the medial malleolus and accidental penetration of the prepared tibial surface.

- In particular, the surgeon must make sure that complete capsulectomy is performed at the posteromedial corner, flush with the tibialis posterior tendon.
- Freeing up adhesions to this tendon is important, as they may cause postoperative pain, particularly in patients who have previously undergone a procedure through a posteromedial approach.
- In this case, tenolysis of the tibialis posterior tendon with opening of its retinaculum through a limited posteromedial approach may be useful. This approach makes posterior capsular release and even repair of associated fissures much easier.
- Last, contracture of the triceps surae and Achilles tendon is often responsible for a deficit of dorsiflexion. Therefore, lengthening should be considered whenever dorsiflexion is less than 10 degrees after insertion of the trials. Release of flexors may be achieved through either tendon lengthening or fasciotomy of the triceps surae.
- Achilles tendon lengthening
  - This simple procedure has little influence on the postoperative course, but it is associated with long-term persistence of posterior discomfort and sometimes with permanent loss of plantarflexion strength and ROM.
  - Lengthening technique consists of making two or three percutaneous staged incisions with a fine scalpel; each incision should involve slightly more than half of the tendon.
  - The most distal incision may be performed on either side, depending on the fibers to be lengthened—laterally for a valgus deformity in order to preserve varus-oriented fibers and medially for a varus hindfoot.
  - While making incisions, the ankle should be held in forced dorsiflexion with the trial components in place.

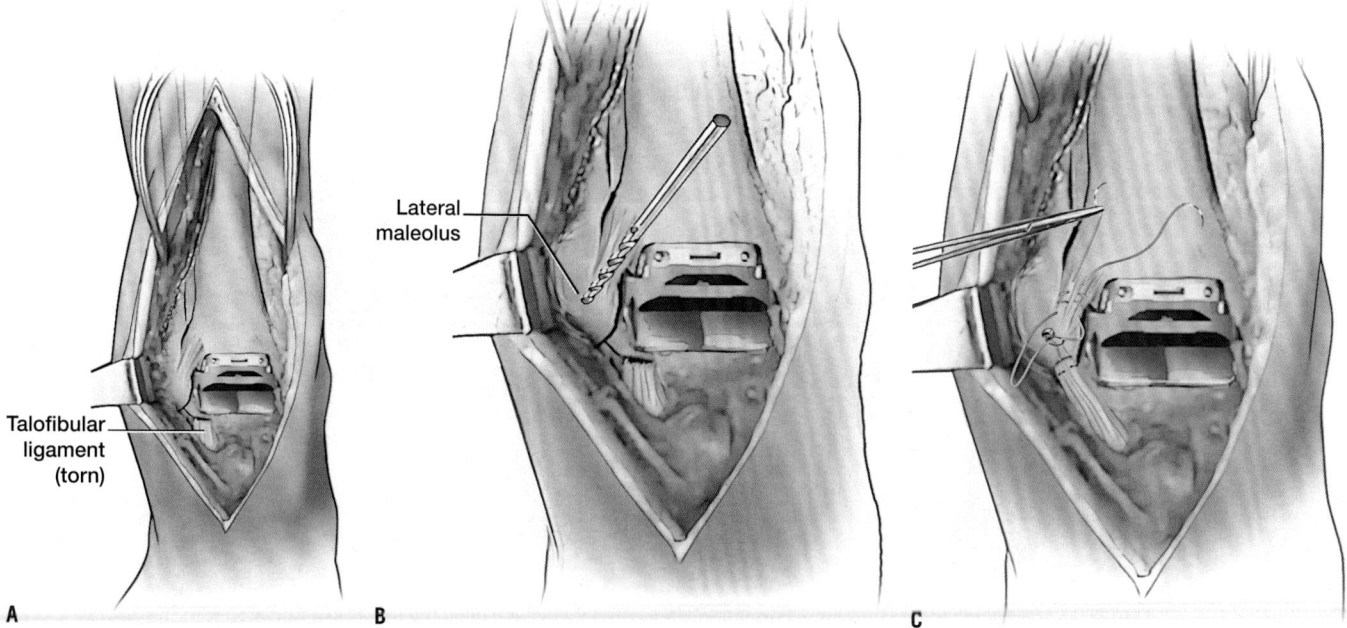

Talofibular ligament (torn)

Lateral maleolus

A   B   C

FIG 6 A. Ankle instability repaired by lateral ligament reconstruction (plication) using a suture anchor technique. A hole is drilled into the fibula (**B**), a suture anchor is inserted, and sutures are passed through the anterior talofibular ligament distally and through the anterior inferior tibiofibular ligament proximally (**C**) and then tightened before the repair is tested.

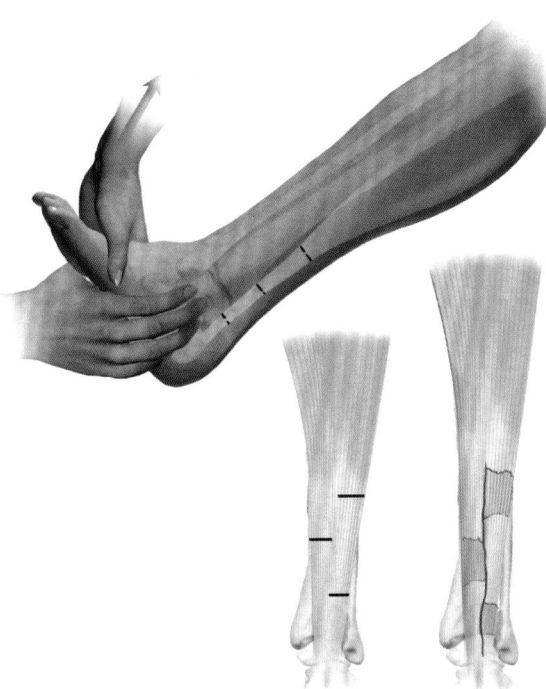

FIG 7 Percutaneous lengthening of the Achilles tendon. Lengthening technique consists of making two or three percutaneous staged incisions with a fine scalpel; each incision should involve slightly more than half of the tendon.

Dorsiflexion suddenly increases as fibers slide over one another (**FIG 7**).

- Fasciotomy of the triceps surae usually does not cause postoperative pain; it is performed through a limited midline posterior approach at the middle third of the leg. The sural vein is preserved.
- The insertional fascia of the gastrocnemius is sectioned in a V-shaped fashion, and the underlying soleus fascia is sectioned in line with the muscle fibers. The postoperative course is the same as for Achilles tendon lengthening.

Anterior Translation of Talus

- Anterior translation of the talus must always be corrected to restore normal kinematics and avoid early wear due to overloading in a fixed-bearing prosthesis.
- Repositioning of the talar component requires complete soft tissue release (ie, talomalleolar compartment, posterior capsule) as well as correction of equinus deformity (if any) through Achilles tendon lengthening.
- Should these procedures prove ineffective, the talar component will have to be moved posteriorly, which means recutting the anterior chamfer.
- In our experience, the tibial component will have to be positioned as far anteriorly as possible beneath the distal tibia.

SUGGESTED READINGS

Bonnin M. La prothèse totale de cheville. Techn Chir Orthopéd Traumatol 2002;10:44–903.

Bonnin M, Bouysset M, Tebib J, et al. Total ankle replacement in rheumatoid arthritis: treatment strategy. In: Bouysset M, Tourné Y, Tillmann K, eds. Foot and Ankle in Rheumatoid Arthritis. Paris, France: Springer-Verlag, 2006:207–219.

Bonnin M, Gaudot F, Laurent JR, et al. The Salto total ankle arthroplasty: survivorship and analysis of failures at 7 to 11 years. Clin Orthop Relat Res 2011;469:225–236.

Bonnin M, Judet T, Siguier T, et al. Total ankle replacement. History, evolution of concepts, design and surgical technique. In: Bouysset M, Tourné Y, Tillmann K, eds. Foot and Ankle in Rheumatoid Arthritis. Paris, France: Springer-Verlag, 2006:179–200.

Hofmann KJ, Shabin ZM, Ferkel E, et al. Salto Talaris total ankle arthroplasty: clinical results at a mean of 5.2 years in 78 patients treated by a single surgeon. J Bone Joint Surg Am 2016;98(24):2036–2046.

Jakubowski S, Mohing W, Richter R. Operationen am rheumatischen Fuss. Therapiewoche 1970;220:762–768.

Judet T, Piriou P, Elis JB, et al. Total endoprothese des oberen Sprunggelenks. Konzepte und Indikationen der Saltoprothese. In: Imhoff AB, Zollinger-Jies H, eds. Fubchirurgie. Stuttgart, Germany: Georg Thieme Verlag, 2003:241–245.

Schweitzer KM, Adams SB, Viens NA, et al. Early prospective clinical results of a modern fixed-bearing total ankle arthroplasty. J Bone Joint Surg Am 2013;95:1002–1011.

Stewart MG, Green CL, Adams SB, et al. Midterm results of the Salto Talaris total ankle arthroplasty. Foot Ankle Int 2017;38(11):1215–1221.

Weber M, Bonnin M, Colombier JA, et al. Erste Ergebnisse der Salto-Sprunggelenkendopprothese Eine französische Multizenterstudie mit 115 Implantaten. Fub Sprunggelenk 2004;2:29–37.

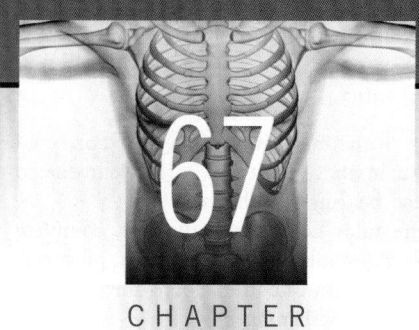

67
CHAPTER

The INBONE Total Ankle Arthroplasty

James K. DeOrio, Mark E. Easley, James A. Nunley II, and Mark A. Reiley

DEFINITION

- The INBONE II (Wright Medical Technology, Arlington, TN) total ankle system, like other total ankle systems, is indicated for end-stage ankle arthritis failing to respond to nonoperative intervention.
- In contrast to essentially all other total ankle systems, however, the INBONE II total ankle system uses intramedullary rather than extramedullary referencing.
- Although the intramedullary alignment guide passes through the plantar foot, calcaneus, talus, and tibia, it does so anterior to the posterior facet of the calcaneus and does not violate any articulations of the subtalar joint. It may, however, interfere with the vascularity of the talus.[1]
- To achieve reliable intramedullary alignment, the INBONE II total ankle system uses a leg frame that is initially cumbersome, demands more preincision preparation, and requires greater fluoroscopy time than other total ankle systems. However, with experience, this technique becomes manageable and allows the user to correct deformities prior to making bone cut.
- The design of the INBONE I has been changed and is now called *INBONE II*.
  - The talus now has a sulcus designed superior surface with a V groove in the center and a corresponding matching polyethylene.
  - The talar component has two more anterior pegs on its inferior surface in addition to the central stem.
  - The tibial baseplate is now available as a long and a standard length.
- The INBONE II has virtually completed replaced INBONE I because of the increased options for fixing the talar component to the talus, the increased stability with the V sulcus in the coronal plane, and the increased coverage of the tibia when necessary.
  - Additionally, to obviate need of the leg holder, a new INBONE II is available, called the *Prophecy*. With this ankle, a computed tomography (CT) scan is sent to the manufacturer preoperatively and molds are created which allow placement of pins. Over these pins are placed the cutting blocks for the talus and tibia. This also allows separation of the cutting blocks to be placed individually on the tibia and talus. Otherwise, the actual ankle replacement, INBONE II, is the same.

ANATOMY

- Ankle
  - Tibial plafond with medial malleolus
    - Articulations with dorsal and medial talus
      - In sagittal plane, slight posterior slope
      - In coronal plane, articular surface is 88 to 92 degrees relative to lateral tibial shaft axis.
  - Fibula
    - Articulation with lateral talus
    - Responsible for one-sixth of axial load distribution of the ankle
  - Talus
    - Sixty percent of surface area covered by articular cartilage
    - Dual radius of curvature
  - Distal tibiofibular syndesmosis
    - Anterior inferior tibiofibular ligament
    - Interosseous membrane
    - Posterior tibiofibular ligament
- Ankle functions as part of the ankle–hindfoot complex much like a mitered hinge.

PATHOGENESIS

- Posttraumatic arthrosis
  - Most common cause
  - Intra-articular fracture
  - Ankle fracture-dislocation with malunion
  - Chronic ankle instability
- Primary osteoarthrosis
  - Relatively rare compared to hip and knee arthrosis
- Inflammatory arthropathy
  - Most commonly rheumatoid arthritis
- Other
  - Hemochromatosis
  - Pigmented villonodular synovitis
  - Charcot neuroarthropathy
  - Septic arthritis
  - Hemophilia

NATURAL HISTORY

- Posttraumatic arthrosis
  - Malunion, chronic instability, intra-articular cartilage damage, or malalignment may lead to progressive articular cartilage wear.
  - Chronic lateral ankle instability may eventually be associated with the following:
    - Relative anterior subluxation of the talus
    - Varus tilt of the talus within the ankle mortise
    - Hindfoot varus position
- Primary osteoarthrosis of the ankle is rare and poorly understood.

- Inflammatory arthropathy
  - Progressive and proliferative synovial erosive changes failing to respond to medical management
  - May be associated with chronic posterior tibial tendinopathy and progressive valgus hindfoot deformity, eventual valgus tilt to the talus within the ankle mortise, potential lateral malleolar stress fracture, and compensatory forefoot varus

PATIENT HISTORY AND PHYSICAL FINDINGS

- Patient history
  - Often a history of ankle trauma
    - Ankle fracture, particularly intra-articular
    - Ankle fracture with malunion
    - Chronic ankle instability (recurrent ankle sprains)
  - Chronic anterior ankle pain, primarily with activity and weight bearing
  - Ankle stiffness, particularly with dorsiflexion
  - Ankle swelling
  - Progressively increased pain with activity
- Physical findings
  - Limp
  - Patient externally rotates hip to externally rotate ankle to avoid painful push-off.
  - Painful and limited ankle range of motion (ROM), particularly limited dorsiflexion
  - Mild ankle edema
  - Potential associated foot deformity
    - Posttraumatic arthrosis secondary to chronic instability may be associated with varus ankle and hindfoot and compensatory forefoot varus.
    - Inflammatory arthritis may be associated with progressively worsening flatfoot deformity, valgus tilt to the ankle and hindfoot, and equinus.

IMAGING AND OTHER DIAGNOSTIC STUDIES

- Weight-bearing anteroposterior (AP) with contralateral ankle included lateral and mortise views of the ankle.
- Weight-bearing AP with contralateral foot included lateral and oblique views of the foot, particularly with associated foot deformity.
- With associated or suspected lower leg deformity, we routinely obtain weight-bearing AP and lateral tibia–fibula views.
- With deformity in the lower extremity, we occasionally obtain weight-bearing mechanical axis (hip-to-ankle) views of both extremities.
- We occasionally evaluate complex or ill-defined ankle–hindfoot patterns of arthritis with or without deformity using CT of the ankle and hindfoot.
- If we suspect avascular necrosis of the talus or distal tibia, we obtain a magnetic resonance imaging of the ankle.

DIFFERENTIAL DIAGNOSIS

- See the Pathogenesis section.

NONOPERATIVE MANAGEMENT

- Activity modification
- Bracing
  - Ankle–foot orthosis
  - Double upright brace attached to shoe
- Stiffer soled shoe with a rocker bottom modification
- Nonsteroidal anti-inflammatories drugs (NSAIDs)
- Medications for systemic inflammatory arthropathy
- Corticosteroid injection
- Viscosupplementation

SURGICAL MANAGEMENT

- In contrast to essentially all other total ankle systems, the INBONE II total ankle system uses intramedullary rather than extramedullary referencing.
- Although the intramedullary alignment guide passes through the plantar foot, calcaneus, talus, and tibia, it does so anterior to the posterior facet of the calcaneus and does not violate any articulations of the subtalar joint, albeit the vascularity of the talus has been shown to be at risk from the 6-mm drill hole from the calcaneus through the talus and into the tibia.[3]
- To achieve reliable intramedullary alignment, the INBONE II total ankle system uses a leg frame that is initially cumbersome, demands more preincision preparation, and requires greater fluoroscopy time than other total ankle systems. However, with experience, this technique becomes manageable and allows the user to correct deformities prior to making bone cut. As mentioned, there is now the option of obtaining a preoperative CT of the ankle, which can obviate use of the leg holder.
- In our opinion, the INBONE II total ankle system is perhaps more stout than some other systems.
  - We have been able to correct coronal and sagittal plane deformities through the tibiotalar joint with appropriate soft tissue balancing and corrective osteotomies relying also on the durability of the implants, particularly the broad talar component and the tibial stem extensions to maintain correction.

Preoperative Planning

- The surgeon must be sure the patient has satisfactory perfusion to support healing and is not neuropathic.
  - Noninvasive vascular studies and potential vascular surgery consultation if necessary
- The surgeon must inspect the ankle for prior scars or surgical approaches that need to be considered in planning the surgical approach for total ankle arthroplasty.
- The surgeon must understand the clinical and radiographic alignment of the lower extremity, ankle, and foot.
  - The surgeon must be prepared to balance and realign the ankle. Occasionally, this necessitates corrective osteotomies of the distal tibia or foot, hindfoot arthrodesis, ligament releases or stabilization, and tendon transfers.
  - The surgeon should determine whether coronal plane alignment is passively correctable; this provides some understanding as to whether ligament releases will be required.
- Ankle ROM is determined.
  - Ankle stiffness, particularly lack of dorsiflexion, needs to be corrected.
    - Anterior tibiotalar exostectomy
    - Posterior capsular release
    - Frequently, tendo Achilles lengthening or gastrocnemius tendon lengthening
- Instrumentation
  - These instruments facilitate total ankle arthroplasty:
    - Small oscillating and reciprocating saws for fine cuts as well as larger oscillating saw for broad bone cuts. The smaller saws make it easier to resect prominences

with precision and easily morselize large bone fragments to be evacuated from the joint.

- A rasp for final preparation of cut bony surfaces
- A 90-degree angled curette, particularly to separate tibial bone from the posterior capsule
- A lamina spreader to distract the joint and aid in realignment of preoperative ankle deformity. Because the INBONE II prosthesis uses a monoblock cutting guide for tibial and talar resection, an intra-articular lamina spreader assists in limiting bone resection. A lamina spreader placed on the concave side of the joint also assists in realignment.
- A toothless lamina spreader to judiciously distract the ankle to improve exposure even after preparing the surfaces of the tibia and talus
- Large fluoroscopic scanner
  - Fluoroscopy confirms proper alignment of the cutting guide to the ankle.
    - The leg holder maintains the leg in position relative to the alignment guides and reference drill.
  - With the leg holder, the large scanner is necessary to straddle the leg and leg holder.
  - Fluoroscopy through the operating table is necessary, so a mini fluoroscopy unit is inadequate.
- Foot pedals to make adjustments to the table position
  - With the foot secured in the leg holder, subtle adjustments to the table's rotation confirm ideal alignment relative to the alignment guides.

- Subtle adjustments to the alignment guides relative to the ankle allow fine-tuning for the reference drill trajectory.

Positioning

- The patient is placed supine with the plantar aspect of operated foot at end of operating table.
- Foot and ankle well balanced with toes directed to the ceiling
- A bolster under the ipsilateral hip prevents undesired external rotation of the hip.
- We routinely use a thigh tourniquet and regional anesthesia.
  - A popliteal block provides adequate pain relief postoperatively, particularly if a regional catheter or lipsomal bupivacaine is used. Moreover, hip and knee flexion–extension is not forfeited, facilitating safe immediate postoperative mobilization.
  - However, using a thigh tourniquet with a popliteal block typically requires a supplemental femoral nerve block (patient temporarily forfeits knee extension in the immediate postoperative period) or general anesthesia.
- The operative extremity needs adequate space for the INBONE II leg holder. The surgeon should be sure the opposite extremity is not secured too close to the operative extremity.

Approach

- Anterior approach to the ankle, using the interval between the tibialis anterior (TA) tendon and the extensor hallucis longus (EHL) tendon

EXPOSURE

- Make a longitudinal midline incision over the anterior ankle, starting about 10 cm proximal to the tibiotalar joint and 1 cm lateral to the tibial crest.
- Continue the incision midline over the anterior ankle just distal to the talonavicular joint.
- At no point should direct tension be placed on the skin margins; we perform deep, full-thickness retraction as soon as possible to limit the risk of skin complications. Placing a Gelpi retractor deep within the wound can be helpful.
  - Identify and protect the superficial peroneal nerve by retracting it laterally.
  - In our experience, there is a consistent branch of the superficial peroneal nerve that crosses directly over or immediately proximal to the tibiotalar joint. This is cut.
- We then expose the extensor retinaculum, identify the course of the EHL tendon, and sharply but carefully divide the retinaculum directly immediately lateral to the anterior tibialis tendon.
  - Some surgeons incise the retinaculum directly over the EHL tendon. However, that does not protect the neurovascular bundle from the deep retractor, and we believe it is better to leave a little retinaculum protecting the neurovascular bundle.
  - We always attempt to maintain the TA tendon in its dedicated sheath if present.
  - Preserving the retinaculum over the TA tendon prevents bowstringing of the tendon and thereby reduces the

stress on the anterior wound. Should there be a wound dehiscence, then the TA is not directly exposed.
  - However, preserving the retinaculum over the TA tendon is not always possible. Frequently, only the retinaculum is present over the TA tendon and it will be free with the EHL tendon (TECH FIG 1).
- Use the interval between the TA and EHL tendons, with the TA and EHL tendons retracted medially and laterally, respectively.
- Identify the deep neurovascular bundle (anterior tibial–dorsalis pedis artery and deep peroneal nerve) and carefully retract it laterally throughout the remainder of the procedure.
- Perform an anterior capsulotomy and elevate the tibial and dorsal talar periosteum to about 6 to 8 cm proximal to the tibial plafond and to the talonavicular joint, respectively.
- Elevate this separated capsule and periosteum medially and laterally to expose the ankle, access the medial and lateral gutters, and visualize the medial and lateral malleoli.
- Remove anterior tibial and talar osteophytes to facilitate exposure and avoid interference with the instrumentation.
- At this point, it is advisable to take a long 4-mm wide rongeur down the gutters. This will take away a little bone from the talus and malleoli and help prevent impingement and oversizing of the talar component.

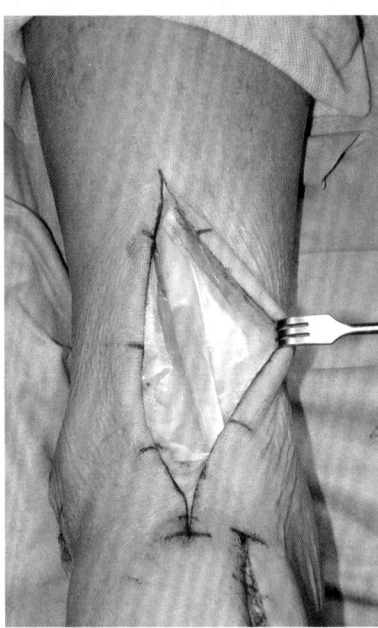

TECH FIG 1 In this case, there is no separate sheath for the TA tendon. Nonetheless, the retinaculum was opened lateral to the tendon, and upon closure, the TA will not be immediately up against the suture line.

TIBIOTALAR ALIGNMENT

- Before placing the lower leg in the INBONE foot and ankle holder, we optimize ankle soft tissue balance and alignment.

Varus Malalignment

- We routinely perform a comprehensive medial release for moderate to severe varus malalignment. This means peeling off all tissue from the medial malleolus circumferentially and not making a transverse cut in the deltoid ligament.
- The concept is similar to balancing the varus knee for total knee arthroplasty and was well described by Bonnin et al[2] in their 2004 report of the Salto prosthesis.
- We routinely subperiosteally raise a continuous soft tissue sleeve from the distal medial tibia to the medial talus.
- There is no need to be aggressive on the medial talus as this could compromise the deltoid branch of the posterior tibial artery that perfuses the medial talar dome.
- The superficial deltoid (medial collateral) ligament is elevated but left intact proximally and attached distally. The release of these fibers is complete when the posterior tibial tendon can be visualized.
- The deep deltoid (medial collateral) ligament may be peeled off the medial malleolus to balance the ankle appropriately. In severe varus deformity, the entire deep deltoid ligament must be released to achieve tibiotalar balance (**TECH FIG 2A**). Overrelease is theoretically possible, but in our experience, with severe varus deformity, the ankle will not collapse into valgus even with a complete release.
- In our experience, with an appropriate medial release, optimal bony resection and metal component alignment, and proper sizing of the polyethylene, a lateral ligament reconstruction is only occasionally necessary. One exception is when there

has been an avulsion fracture of the tip of the fibula: In that instance, it is difficult to obtain any ability to rotate the ankle against the lateral tissue, and a Brostrom ligament reconstruction can be done at the beginning of the case (**TECH FIG 2B–D**). This marks a significant change from our initial practices in rebalancing the varus ankle. Doing the ligament reconstruction early allows the lamina spreader placed medially to rotate the talus.
- A lamina spreader placed in the medial tibiotalar joint maintains the correction.

Valgus Malalignment

- Likewise, a valgus malalignment must be rebalanced.
- We seldom need to perform a ligament release. If, however, the patient has anterior subluxation of the talus on the preoperative lateral standing x-ray, the lateral ligament may indeed be incompetent. Doing a modified Brostrom procedure is usually all that is required to balance the ankle.
- Often, valgus malalignment is secondary to lateral ankle joint collapse and some medial (deltoid) ligament attenuation. This may involve a component of lateral ankle ligament instability as well.
  - Although the latter portion of this statement seems counterintuitive, this has been our experience in treating many patients with end-stage ankle arthritis and valgus malalignment.
  - Moreover, lateral release in such situations may lead to paradoxical lateral instability.
- We use a lateral lamina spreader to realign the ankle and regain functional tension in the medial ligaments (**TECH FIG 2E,F**).

TECHNIQUES

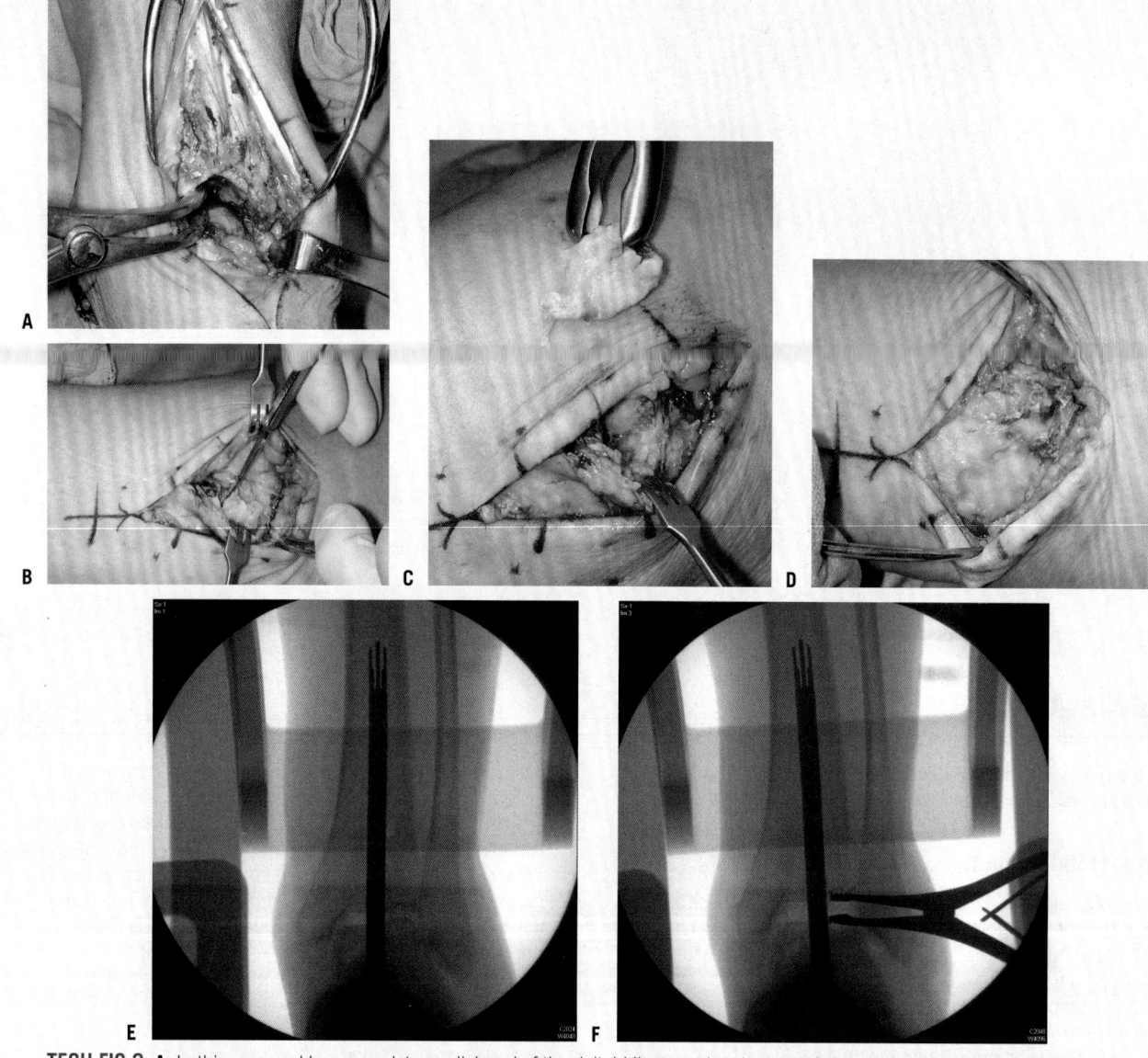

TECH FIG 2 **A.** In this varus ankle, a complete medial peel of the deltoid ligament has been performed, and the ankle can be opened up with the lamina spreader. **B.** There was a large ossicle at the tip of the fibula representing an old avulsion fracture containing the anterior talofibular ligament. Hence, the bone was removed (**C**) and a Brostrom ligament reconstruction was performed (**D**). **E.** Valgus ankle with AP alignment guide properly rotated. However, the talus is not orthogonal to the guide or the tibia. **F.** In this view, the lamina spreader has been placed laterally on the concave side, and now, the talus is orthogonal to the tibia and the alignment guide.

INTRAMEDULLARY ALIGNMENT

- Be sure the foot and ankle frame is properly assembled and the alignment drill guide trajectory is calibrated. If unsure, you can assemble the cannula into the holder, put the drill in, and take a fluoroscopic view to make sure they coincide (**TECH FIG 3A**).
- The foot and lower leg are secured in the leg holder.
  - With correction of the preoperative deformity, we transfer the leg into the foot and ankle holder with the lamina spreader in place (**TECH FIG 3B**).
    - If the foot and ankle are secured first, it may be difficult to position the lamina spreader effectively.

- Proper rotation
  - We use a small, straight osteotome in the medial gutter as a reference. The foot is rotated until the osteotome is parallel with the leg holder foot plate.
- Plantigrade foot
  - The heel must be flush with the foot plate of the guide and at a 90-degree angle to the leg.
  - If it is dorsiflexed, then the talar cut will have a posterior slope, removing an excessive amount of the talar body and increasing the risk of posterior talar component

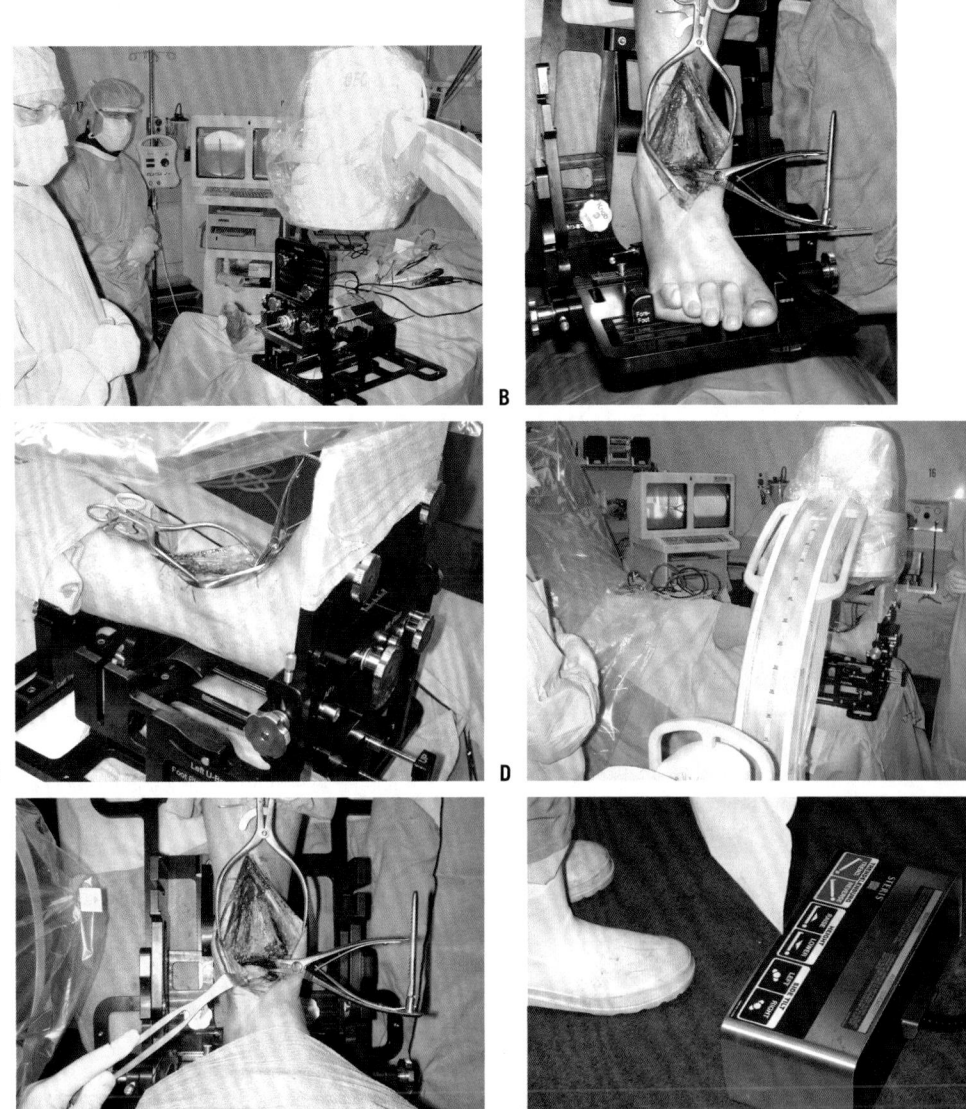

TECH FIG 3 **A.** Fluoroscopic view being obtained of leg holder with cannula and drill in place to ensure correct assembly of leg holder. **B.** Gelpi retractor holding deep tissue aside with lamina spreader on concave medial side of varus ankle. **C.** Leg positioned in leg holder with Achilles and calf rests supporting leg. **D.** C-arm coming in to obtain AP view of ankle on ipsilateral side. **E.** Overhead view of lamina spreader in place and deep Gelpi retractor holding deep tissue apart. C-arm to the left is coming in for lateral view. **F.** Foot pedals are used to control tilting of the table to get the alignment sites exactly parallel to one another.

subsidence. If it is plantar flexed, too high a cut will be made on the posterior talus, and the cut of the tibia will have a posterior opening cut. Be sure all anterior tibiotalar osteophytes are removed. Perform a gastrocnemius release or tendo Achilles lengthening if necessary.

- Coronal plane alignment
  - In the mediolateral plane, center the heel over the starting point for the reference drill.
  - We use the AP alignment guides to grossly set this alignment.

- This position should also be in line with the tibial shaft axis so that minimal adjustments will be necessary.
- Preoperative deformity complicates such preliminary alignment.
- Sagittal plane alignment
  - We use the lateral alignment guides to grossly set this alignment.
  - The calf and Achilles rests need to be adjusted to optimize the lower leg's position relative to the foot (talus) **(TECH FIG 3C)**.

- In our experience, proper heel position, optimal tibial alignment, and ideal rotation may make the foot appear internally rotated relative to the lower leg.
- Fluoroscopic confirmation of proper alignment
  - ▪ A large fluoroscopic scanner is needed **(TECH FIG 3D,E)**.
- Foot pedals to make adjustments to the table position **(TECH FIG 3F)**
  - ▪ With the foot secured in the leg holder, subtle adjustments to the table's rotation confirm ideal alignment relative to the alignment guides.
- Subtle adjustments to the alignment guides relative to the ankle to allow fine-tuning for the reference drill trajectory may be made with the foot pedal.
- Reference drill
  - ▪ Make a horizontally oriented 1-cm incision in the plantar foot, directly in the opening in the foot frame for passing the reference drill. Placing marker ink on the trocar and inserting it and pushing on the skin to leave a mark gives you the exact entry point of the drill.
    - ▪ One centimeter allows for subtle adjustments to the medial and lateral position of the reference drill, even when its drill sleeve has been positioned on the plantar calcaneus.

- ▪ The incision should not be more than a 5 mm deep because, otherwise, it could injure the lateral plantar nerve.
- Insert the drill guide to contact the plantar calcaneus.
  - ▪ Avoid holding the frame while inserting this guide, as this could allow the drill to bend, achieving a different trajectory than the guide.
- Secure the drill guide.
- Advance the reference drill from calcaneus to tibia.
  - ▪ Because the trajectory may change when the drill hits the plantar medial calcaneus, we typically start the drill in reverse and "peck drill" (tap drill) to gradually penetrate the plantar calcaneal cortex without veering from the planned trajectory.
  - ▪ Once the plantar cortex is penetrated, the drill is run in forward.
- Because drilling may shift the frame slightly, fluoroscopic confirmation of proper alignment must be reestablished, after which proper alignment of the reference drill may be confirmed.
- Advance the drill into the distal tibia, about 8 to 10 cm.
- Confirm appropriate reference drill position fluoroscopically in both the coronal and sagittal planes.

TIBIOTALAR JOINT PREPARATION

Sizing

- Approximate sizing for the component may be performed on preoperative radiographs of either the involved side or the uninvolved opposite ankle.
- Position the cutting block in roughly the correct position by using the reference drill guide to estimate its position.
- Fine-tune the cutting block using the reference drill guide under fluoroscopy.
  - In the AP plane, we align the cutting guide with the reference drill guide **(TECH FIG 4A)**.

- In the lateral plane, we use saw blades through the cutting guide to determine the resection level **(TECH FIG 4B)**. Cutting too low on the talar head may also damage the vascularity to the head of the talus.
- The position of the cutting block should be finalized only if proper alignment has been confirmed fluoroscopically with the alignment guides.
- It is important that the guide is centered medially and laterally and no more than 1 mm of bone is removed from the medial malleolus.

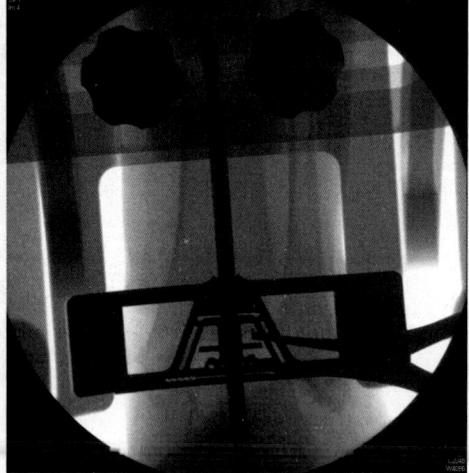 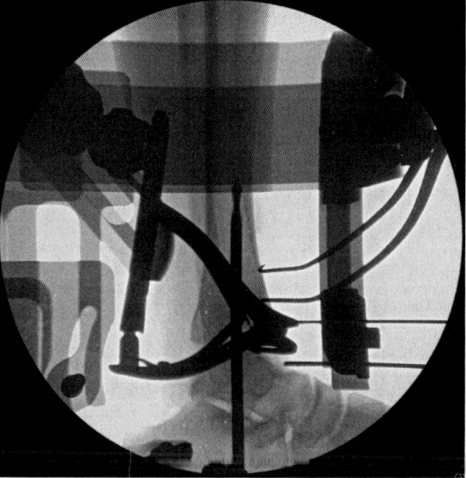

A   B

TECH FIG 4 **A.** The cutting guide has been placed over the ankle and centered on the drill. **B.** A lateral view of the cutting guides with the saw and "dummy" blade in place gives the surgeon the amount of bone resected on the top of the talus and the bottom of the tibia.

Pinning the Cutting Block

- Once proper position of the cutting block is established, the block is pinned, tibial pins first and talar pins next.
- Occasionally, the talar pins will skive and not engage the talus, particularly if a lamina spreader is being used to distract the joint or if the talar dome is sclerotic.
- A toothless lamina spreader may be used to gently keep the talar pins in position as they are driven into the bone, but do this carefully because too much pressure may cause the pins to permanently bind in the cutting guide.
- Two more pins are placed in the medial and lateral gutter.
  - Their mediolateral position is determined on the fluoroscopic image of the final cutting block position.
  - These pins protect the malleoli.
- If a lamina spreader was used to distract the joint, it will interfere with the pin placement.
  - Try to keep it in place long enough to get enough pins in so that when the lamina spreader is removed, the correction is maintained.
- Withdraw the axial reference drill.
- The antirotation drill corresponding to the cutting block is used to drill the antirotation slot in the tibia (the sagittal prominence on the tibial baseplate). Make sure you drill the posterior cortex. Otherwise, when you are inserting the baseplate, the ridge going from anterior to posterior can split the posterior cortex.

Bone Resection

- With the soft tissues protected, make the tibial and talar cuts.
- The bone resection should go all the way through the posterior cortex for each cut.
  - It may not be possible on the initial pass, depending on the height of the cutting block and the particular saw used. After the initial cut, the cutting block can typically be lowered to complete the cuts or the cuts can be freehand after the initial cuts. Obviously, avoid plunging the saw blade.
  - Release the Achilles support to help prevent the flexor hallucis longus from being forced anteriorly and cut with the saw. Gently tapping the saw on the posterior cortex is usually possible to confirm that there is still cortex in place.
  - Beware of the length of the saw, as it may cut posterior structures especially when the cutting block is removed. It is now considered safe practice to make an vertical incision on the posterior medial malleolus at the beginning of the case allowing the surgeon to insert a 1-inch malleable retractor to protect the posterior structures.
- Once the posterior cortex has been penetrated for all cuts, the cutting guide and its pins can be removed.
- The resected bone is evacuated from the joint.
  - A toothless lamina spreader may be used to facilitate accessing the most posterior bone.
  - Avoid levering on the malleoli with the instruments, as they may break.
  - A rongeur and an angled curette are ideal to remove the bone.
  - A fine reciprocating saw may be necessary to morselize the resected bone to facilitate removing all of the bone. Avoid cutting into the prepared tibial and talar surfaces with this saw and protect the malleoli.

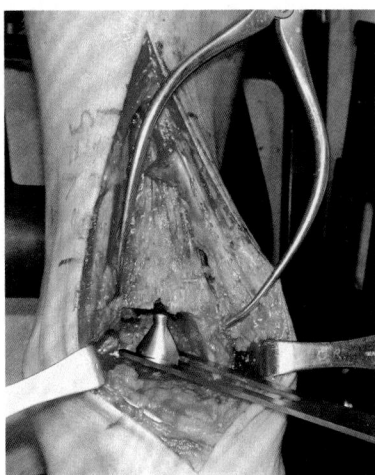

TECH FIG 5 Reamer tip being assembled onto reamer to ream out distal tibia.

Tibial Reaming

- Secure the reamer tip to the drilling shaft within the joint (**TECH FIG 5**). A toothless lamina spreader may be required to open the joint to facilitate securing the reamer tip within the ankle opening.
- Advance the reamer. We typically use four segments for the stem extension; this requires reaming 55 mm into the tibia. However, the INBONE prosthesis is now cleared by the U.S. Food and Drug Administration for the use of two to eight segments of the tibial stem.
- Extract the reamer tip from the joint. When the wrench is placed on the reamer tip, avoid activating the driver, as it will spin the reamer and the wrench, which then may fracture a malleolus. Keep your fingers off the trigger during this portion. With the wrench secured to the reamer tip and firmly held with one hand, set the driver for reverse and disengage the shaft from the tip, thereby protecting the malleolus. Extract the reamer tip from the joint, and withdraw the reamer shaft from the plantar foot.

Talar Preparation

- Secure the talar alignment guide sleeve to the plantar aspect of the foot plate.
- Advance the talar positioning guide through this sleeve to the prepared talar surface.
- Secure the talar pin guide to the positioning guide and place the talar pin. Check to see if the pin will be appropriately placed in the prepared talar surface; if not, then the talar pin guide affords multiple options for pin positioning. Alternatively, the pin may be placed in the "O" position and then the talar pin guide may be used over that initial pin to position a second, more appropriately positioned pin.
- We have also used the talar trial to determine optimal pin position. The talar trial may be positioned in the ideal mediolateral position and on the posterior cortex (**TECH FIG 6A**).
  - Two Kirschner wires (K-wires) are placed to secure the talar trial.
  - Once ideal talar trial position is confirmed clinically and fluoroscopically, the central pin for the stem may also be placed through the talar trial (**TECH FIG 6B**).

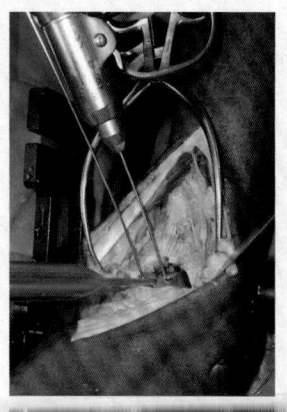
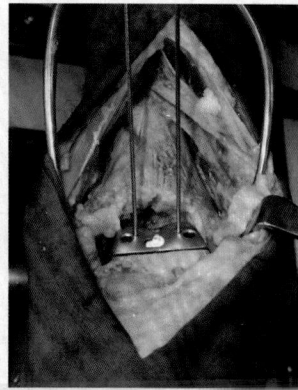
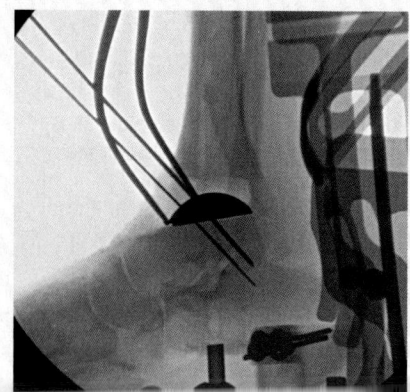

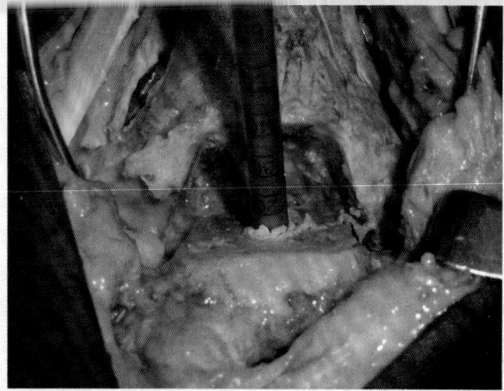
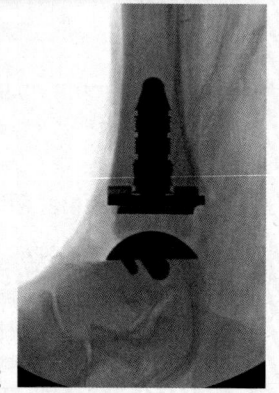

TECH FIG 6 A. Talar trial component positioned and pinned with two K-wires. Central pin for talar stem may also be placed through the guide, but because the INBONE II talar component has two anterior pegs, some surgeons implant the talar component without the stem. **B.** Talar trial component pinned in proper position in AP plane. **C.** Lateral fluoroscopic image demonstrating satisfactory sagittal plane talar position. In addition to the anterior K-wires, the central pin was inserted in preparation for using the stem. **D.** With trial talus removed, central pin overdrilled for placing the talar stem. **E.** Final fluoroscopic image demonstrating satisfactory component positioning in the sagittal plane.

- The fluoroscopic view confirms that the talar component will be in the desired position (**TECH FIG 6C**).
- The anterior peg holes are reamed.
- Optimally, the talar pin (which is the drill guide for the talar stem) is just posterior midpoint to the center of the calcaneal posterior facet.
- The 10-mm stem can typically be attached to the talar component on the back table, and the talar dome–stem combination may be inserted simultaneously. The 14-mm stem, which we rarely use, requires placing the stem first and attaching the talar component on the stem in situ. Increasingly, we have been

using only the anterior pegs on the talar component to avoid taking away too much bone from the talus. Additionally, we have begun bone grafting the calcaneal talar hole to prevent ingress of synovial fluid from the subtalar joint.
- With the talar trial component removed and the talar stem to be used, the central pin is overdrilled with the acorn reamer to create a relief area for the talar stem (**TECH FIG 6D**).
- Final fluoroscopic view demonstrating proper component position. Note that the central stem was used in this case. As mentioned, some surgeons advocate only using the anterior pegs for talar implant stability (**TECH FIG 6E**).

COMPONENT IMPLANTATION

Tibial Stem Assembly within the Joint

- We routinely leave the ankle plantar flexed, assemble the first two segments of the tibial stem on the back table, and insert them into the reamed tibia with the corresponding wrench (**TECH FIG 7A**).
- Return the ankle to the neutral position in which the tibia was reamed and introduce the "X screwdriver" from the plantar foot while the next tibial stem segment is positioned within the joint using the corresponding clip (**TECH FIG 7B**). A toothless lamina spreader is used to gently distract the joint to introduce the next segment, especially if you have used the lamina spreader to balance the joint.

- Using the X screwdriver and while securing the wrench holding the other two segments in the tibia, secure the third segment to the stem (**TECH FIG 7C**). Be sure to hold the wrench that is stabilizing the two segments already in the tibia; if the third segment is advanced and secured and then turned, the wrench could impact the malleolus and break it.
- Remove the X screwdriver and place the rod impactor from the plantar foot to advance the three-segment stem into the tibia (**TECH FIG 7D**). Obtaining a radiograph at this point can help ensure the correct angle of placement in this varus ankle (**TECH FIG 7E**). Be sure to attach the appropriate wrench to the third segment while impacting the stem to avoid having the stem advance too far into the tibia.

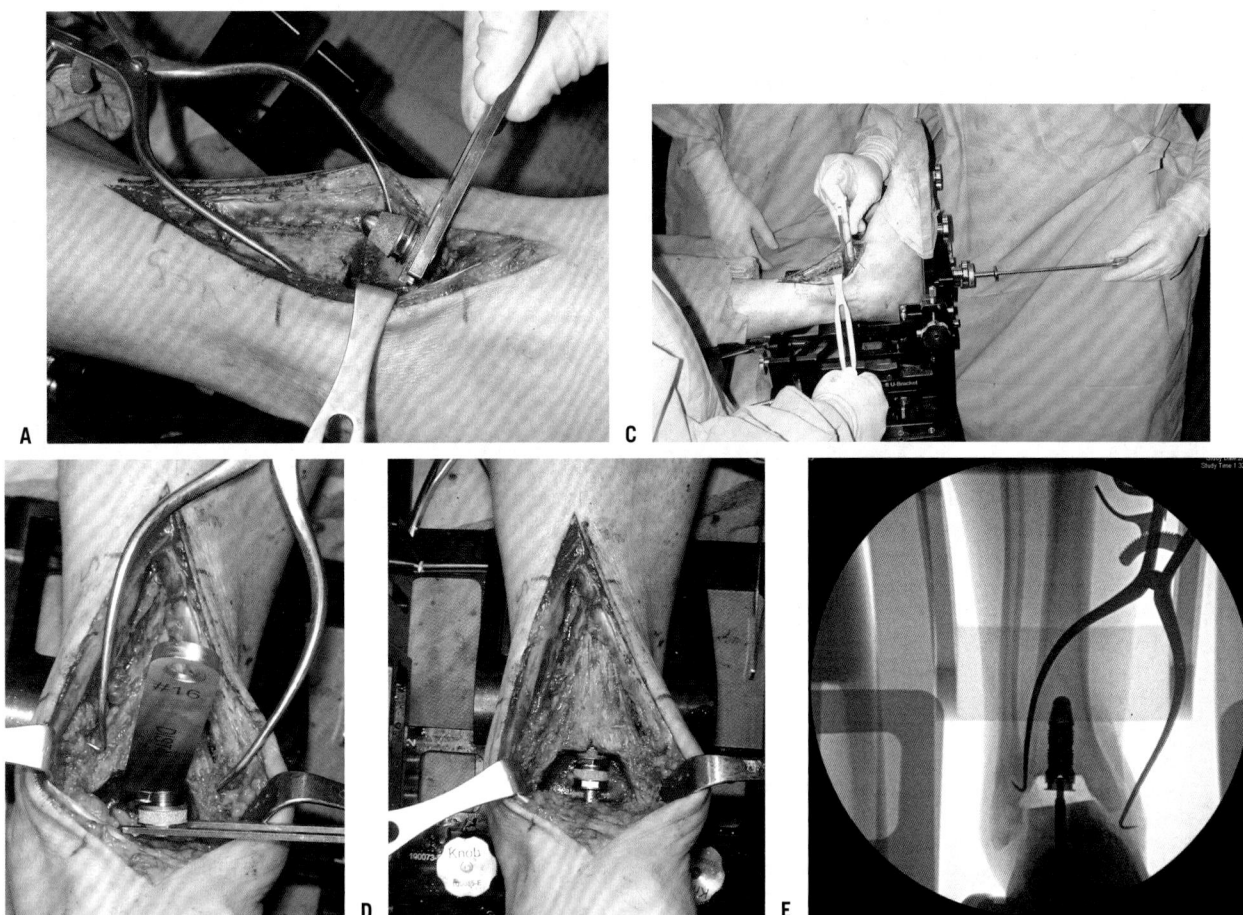

TECH FIG 7 A. The foot is plantar flexed to allow insertion of the cone piece with one midstem cylinder attached. **B.** Wrench holding already inserted pieces in place while another midstem component is being inserted. **C.** An X screwdriver being inserted into stem component to screw it in place. **D.** Stem components inserted, waiting for wrench to be attached before tapping stem up into tibia. **E.** AP view of stem just before wrench is attached and stem is pushed up into tibia.

- Repeat the steps to attach the fourth segment to the third segment. Add additional segments as needed. We typically use four segments.
- The final segment is different from the others in that it houses the female portion of the Morse taper. It also has a small hole that indicates proper rotation. Be sure this segment is aligned and rotated properly and faces anteriorly. Then, the entire stem is fully seated with its corresponding wrench using the rod impactor.

Tibial Baseplate

- Introduce the tibial baseplate into the joint (**TECH FIG 8A**).
- Withdraw the rod impactor from the stem slightly, allowing the tibial baseplate to be positioned, and then use the rod impactor to secure the baseplate to the stem. The tibial baseplate is secured to the stem by means of a Morse taper (see **TECH FIG 8A**).
- Once the Morse taper is secured, remove the wrench on the stem and the composite baseplate and stem combination is ready to be fully seated. Make sure there is enough room for the baseplate, and trim out any bone on the sides, which could lead to a malleolus fracture (**TECH FIG 8B**).

- During this step, rotation of the tibial component must be controlled. A narrow handle attaches to the anterior aspect of the baseplate to control rotation as the tibial component is impacted. When the component is fully seated, it should rest snugly in the mortise (**TECH FIG 8C**).
  - If the stem is not in the proper varus–valgus orientation, the small reciprocating saw may be taken and a small sliver of bone removed from the concave side (the side to which the stem is leaning). Then, the impactor can be used to impact that side superiorly, correcting any malalignment. Hint: Removal of the trocar will allow you to insert the impactor at a slightly increased angle to facilitate this impaction.

Talar Component

- This may be the most challenging step of the procedure, particularly if the joint was distracted to minimize bone resection or to correct deformity. In this situation, the joint space is quite tight by design to achieve optimal soft tissue balance and ligament tension.
- We routinely assemble a 10-mm stem to the talar dome component on the back table for the size 2 and 3 prosthesis, using the dedicated assembly device to secure the Morse taper.

TECHNIQUES

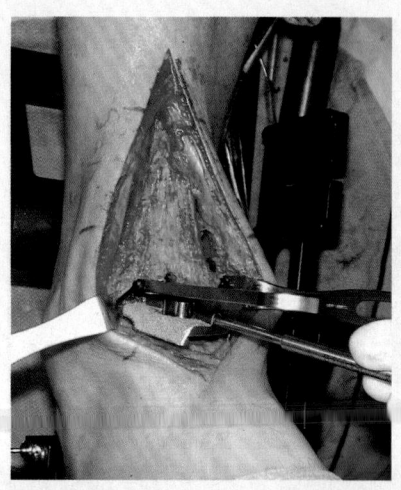
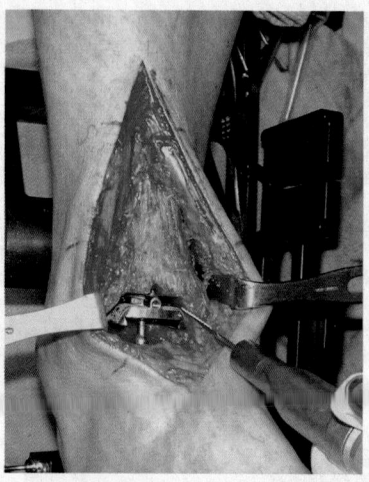
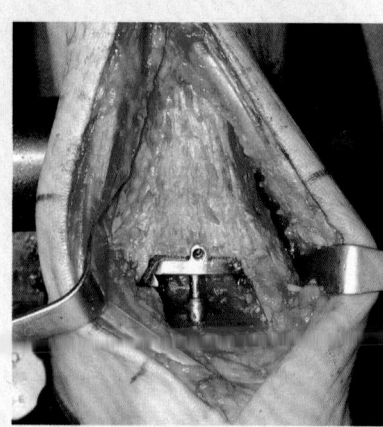

TECH FIG 8 **A.** Baseplate of tibial component being inserted onto base of stem. Note male Morse taper. **B.** Trimming away of bone using small reciprocating saw to ensure final fit. **C.** Baseplate with stem being tapped up into tibia.

- Typically, a 14-mm stem is too long to be connected to the talar dome component before implantation. Therefore, we place the 14-mm talar stem first for size 4 and up if there is enough depth to the talus and seat it to the thin rib wrench that is flush with the prepared talar surface. Because the Morse taper has not been secured, the rib wrench must remain under the 14-mm talar stem.
- The joint must then be gently distracted with a lamina spreader, followed by insertion of the talar dome component. A protective plastic sleeve inserted onto the tibial baseplate protects the talar dome from being scratched (**TECH FIG 9A**). The toothless lamina spreader may need to go under the talar dome component to obtain the distraction while the talar component is carefully

forced posteriorly into position. A handle attached to the talar dome component facilitates driving the talar dome posteriorly (**TECH FIG 9B**).
- Once the talar dome component seats on the pegs and with or without the stem, the talar dome impactor is used to fully seat the talar component (**TECH FIG 9C,D**).
- Remove the rib wrench and inspect the interface between talar dome and stem to ensure that the two talar components are securely attached. Use the impactor to fully seat the talar component.
- While impacting the talar component, use the handle that inserts into the talar dome to control subtle changes in rotation of the talar component.

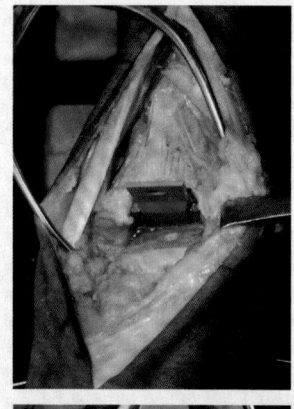
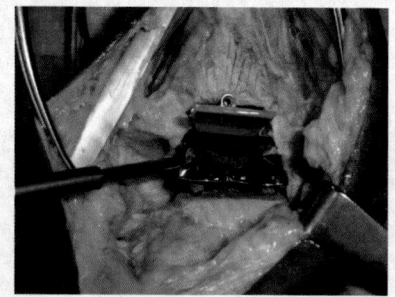
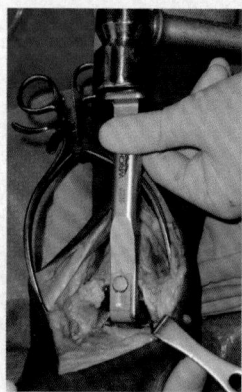
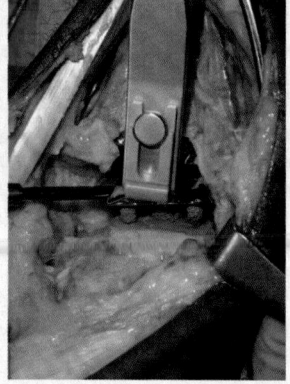

TECH FIG 9 Talar component insertion. **A.** Protective sleeve placed to protect tibial component. **B.** Talar component insertion with dedicated handle. **C.** Talar impactor. **D.** Note that in this case, the 10-mm stem (attached to the talar component on the back table) is used to optimize talar component stability. Some surgeons do not use the central stem, relying solely on the two anterior pegs for talar component stability.

Polyethylene Insertion

- The polyethylene trials determine optimal polyethylene thickness (**TECH FIG 10**).
- We routinely remove the leg from the leg holder and obtain AP and lateral fluoroscopic images at this stage to confirm proper position and balance of the components.
- With the ankle in neutral position, there should be a balance with varus and valgus stress. If not, the polyethylene thickness may be inappropriate or, more likely, balance needs to be established. Typically, the medial joint (deltoid ligament) is too tight. Traditionally, we have performed a lateral ligament reconstruction (modified Brostrom or Brostrom-Evans technique); however, in our more recent experience, we have been successful in rebalancing the ankle with a deltoid ligament release (described earlier) and increasing the polyethylene thickness.
- The ankle should dorsiflex to at least 5 degrees, preferably 10 degrees beyond neutral. If not, the polyethylene thickness may be too thick. If the polyethylene thickness is appropriate and the foot cannot be dorsiflexed to 90 degrees, consider a gastrocnemius recession or percutaneous tendo Achilles lengthening.
- Using the dedicated polyethylene insertion device (**TECH FIG 11A**), insert the polyethylene. In our experience, the polyethylene will engage the tibial baseplate's locking mechanism most effectively with the following maneuvers:
  - Have an assistant or co-surgeon distract the joint. During the initial portion of the insertion, gently pull the insertion device into slight plantarflexion, thus driving the polyethylene into the tibial baseplate's locking mechanism (**TECH FIG 11B**).

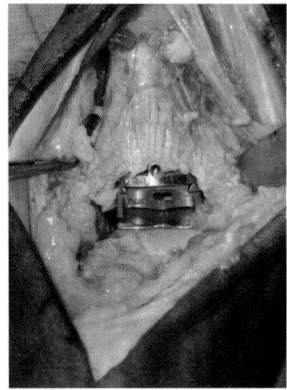

TECH FIG 10 Polyethylene trial placed to determine optimal final thickness of final polyethylene component to provide satisfactory coronal plane stability and sagittal plane motion.

- Once the polyethylene has cleared the superior dome of the talar component, ease off on the plantarflexion of the insertion device and have the assistant or co-surgeon compress the joint, thereby forcing the polyethylene into the locking mechanism (**TECH FIG 11C**).
- Remove the insertion device and fully seat the polyethylene with the dedicated impactor. With that accomplished, the prosthesis should be fully seated (**TECH FIG 11D**).
- Obtain final AP and lateral fluoroscopic views of the valgus ankle (**TECH FIG 11E,F**).

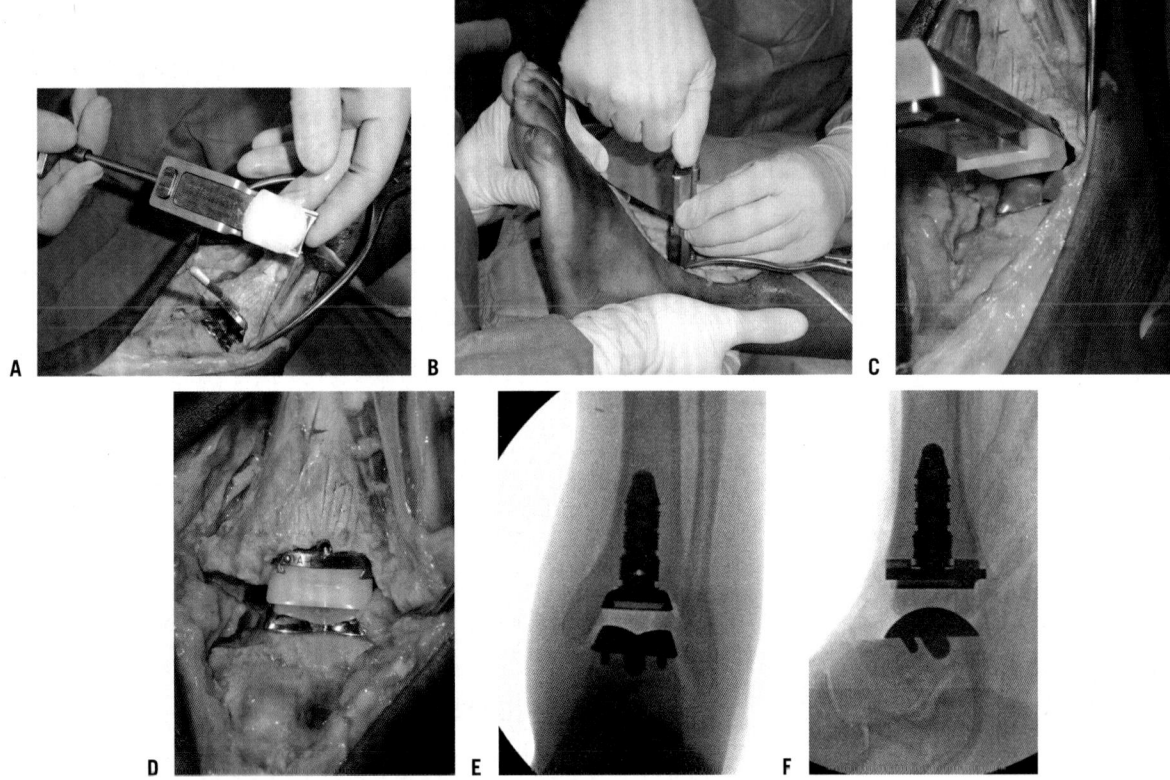

TECH FIG 11 Final polyethylene insertion. **A.** Temporary stem attached to tibial component and polyethylene positioned on dedicated insertion device. **B.** With assistant applying joint distraction, surgeon inserts polyethylene with dedicated insertion device. **C.** Close-up view of polyethylene insertion. **D.** Final components in place. Final fluoroscopic AP (**E**) and lateral (**F**) views.

CLOSURE

- Thoroughly irrigate the joint and implant with sterile saline.
- Reapproximate the capsule. We routinely use a drain.
- Release the tourniquet and obtain meticulous hemostasis.
- Reapproximate the extensor retinaculum while protecting the deep and superficial peroneal nerves.

- Irrigate the subcutaneous layer with sterile saline and then reapproximate it.
- Reapproximate the skin to a tensionless closure.
- Apply sterile dressings on the wounds, adequate padding, and a short-leg cast with the ankle in neutral position.

TECHNIQUES

Pearls and Pitfalls

Equinus Contracture	• Because the initial tibial and talar preparation is performed using a single monoblock cutting guide, an equinus contracture will lead to excessive and undesired resection from the posterior talus. Therefore, perform a gastrocnemius recession or tendo Achilles lengthening to get the talus in a neutral position before securing the leg in the leg holder. If the heel does not rest fully on the leg holder's foot plate with the toes touching the foot plate, there is equinus.
Rotation	• The foot and leg may be well positioned in the leg holder and fluoroscopy may suggest proper alignment, but the ankle may still be malrotated, leading to symmetric but malrotated tibial and talar preparation. Place a thin osteotome in the medial gutter of the tibiotalar joint to determine optimal rotation; the osteotome should be parallel to the side of the leg holder.
Varus Ankle and Valgus Malalignment	• Balance the ankle before placing it into the leg holder. For varus, perform the medial release; for valgus, the ankle is usually loose and simply needs the lamina spreader to realign the talus within the ankle mortise.
Place the ankle at the center of the fluoroscopic monitor.	• The ankle must be in the center of the monitor or alignment cannot be accurately determined. Therefore, first place the ankle in the center of the fluoroscopic beam and then make adjustments. Note also that as adjustments are made to the operating table to optimize alignment, the ankle may "drift" from the center of the monitor and will need to be recentered in the fluoroscopic beam while alignment is being set.
Be sure alignment is proper before any reading is made off the fluoroscopy.	• Assessing the position of any instrument fluoroscopically demands that proper alignment has been confirmed first. For example, when positioning the cutting block relative to the reference drill, first check that alignment is perfect, and then assess the cutting block position.
Returning the Ankle to Neutral Position while It Is in the Leg Holder	• The stop on the side of the leg holder must be set before the ankle is plantar flexed with the frame or else it is difficult to return to the same neutral position.
Morse Taper	• The tibial baseplate and the talar dome components attach to their respective stems with Morse tapers; be sure these are fully secured before seating either composite (combination main component and stem) fully.
Insertion of Talar Component	• May be difficult when joint distraction with lamina spreaders was used to minimize bone resection. However, judicious use of lamina spreaders is again possible to facilitate insertion of the talar component. When using a 10-mm talar stem, we typically have ample room to insert the combination of talar dome and stem composite that was attached on the back table; however, we usually have to independently insert the 14-mm stem followed by the talar dome component, securing the Morse taper within the joint. With the decreased working space necessitated by the anterior prongs on INBONE II, we rarely, if ever, use the 14-mm stem and, as already mentioned, have eliminated the talar stem completely in some situations.

POSTOPERATIVE CARE

- Overnight stay
- Nasal oxygen while in hospital
- Touchdown weight bearing on the cast is permitted, but elevation is encouraged as much as possible. We tell patients to keep their "toes above their nose" to encourage proper elevation.
- Follow-up in 2 to 3 weeks for cast change and suture removal. If the wound looks good, we advance patients to a removable boot with partial weight bearing.

- The patient returns 6 weeks after surgery for cast removal if it was reapplied and weight-bearing radiographs of the ankle as well as 1-year follow-up (**FIG 1**).

OUTCOMES

- Although some recently reported outcomes based on high-level evidence, results of total ankle arthroplasty are almost uniformly derived from level IV evidence.
- Functional outcome using commonly used scoring systems for total ankle arthroplasty (American Orthopaedic Foot

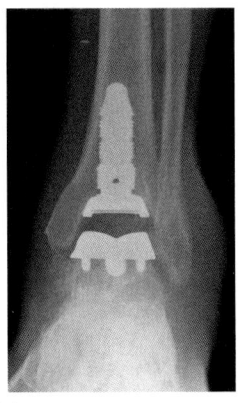
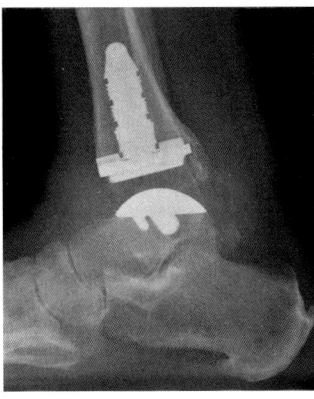

FIG 1 One-year follow-up weight-bearing radiographs. **A.** Mortise view. **B.** Lateral view demonstrating ankle dorsiflexion.

and Ankle Society [Kofoed, Mazur] and New Jersey Orthopaedic Hospital [Buechel-Pappas]) suggests uniform improvement in all studies, with follow-up scores ranging from 70 to 90 points (maximum 100 points).

- Patient satisfaction rates for total ankle arthroplasty exceed 90%, although follow-up data for patient satisfaction often do not exceed 5 years.
- Our study on the INBONE ankle replacement showed a 93.8% survival, mean 3.7-year follow-up, designating removal of a metal component or conversion to arthrodesis as the end point.[1]
  - There was a direct correlation of avascular collapse of the talus in association with previous subtalar arthrodesis and concomitant subtalar and talonavicular arthrodesis. Many of these cases were done with the screws brought from anterior to posterior. Now, when a concomitant

subtalar arthrodesis is warranted, we recommend preparation of the posterior facet of the subtalar joint only and using screws from posterior to anterior avoiding the talar vascularity in the sinus tarsi.
  - We also noticed cases of avascular collapse of the talus in which the only factor for injuring the blood supply to the talus was the 6-mm drill hole.

COMPLICATIONS

- Infection (superficial or deep)
- Neuralgia (superficial or deep peroneal nerve; rarely tibial nerve)
- Delayed wound healing
- Wound dehiscence
- Persistent pain despite optimal orthopaedic examination and radiographic appearance of implants
- Osteolysis
- Subsidence
- Malleolar or distal tibial stress fracture
- Implant fracture (including polyethylene)

REFERENCES

1. Adams SB Jr, Demetracopoulos CA, Queen RM, et al. Early to mid-term results of fixed-bearing total ankle arthroplasty with a modular intramedullary tibial component. J Bone Joint Surg Am 2014;96(23): 1983–1989.
2. Bonnin M, Judet T, Colombier JA, et al. Midterm results of the Salto total ankle prosthesis. Clin Orthop Relat Res 2004;(424):6–18.
3. Tennant J, Rungprai C, Pizzimenti M, et al. The effect of current total ankle arthroplasty methods on blood supply of the talus: a latex injection cadaver study with computed tomography and dissection analysis poster presentation. Paper presented at: American Orthopaedic Foot and Ankle Society Summer Meeting; July 17–20, 2013; Hollywood, FL.

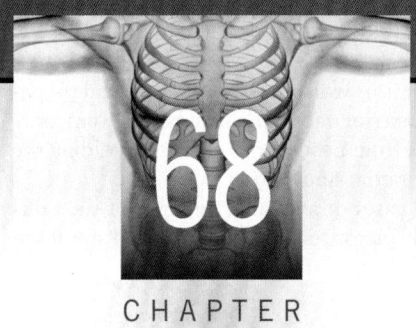

68

CHAPTER

PROPHECY Infinity Total Ankle Replacement

Craig C. Akoh, Karl M. Schweitzer, Jr., Andrew Hsu, Hodges Davis, and Robert B. Anderson

DEFINITION

- The PROPHECY™ Infinity total ankle replacement (TAR) system is a computed tomography (CT) based, computer constructed system that was developed and made commercially available in the United States through Wright Medical Technology (Memphis, TN).
- It uses the patient's exact osseous anatomy and surgeon-set preferences, combined with computer virtual analysis of the patient's anatomic and mechanical alignment axes in the coronal and sagittal planes, along with rotational considerations, to create a patient-specific preoperative plan that optimizes bone coverage and minimizes bone resection.
- The basis for PROPHECY technology use in TAR is the knowledge that appropriate implant sizing, positioning, and alignment is essential in TAR success and patient outcomes.

ANATOMY

- The tibiotalar joint is a highly constrained, hinged articulation composed of osseous and ligamentous stabilizers.
- Osseous stabilizers
  - Tibial plafond
  - Medial malleolus
  - Lateral malleolus
  - Talus: Sixty percent of talar surface area is covered by articular cartilage. The talar dome has a double radius of curvature.
- Ligamentous stabilizers
  - Lateral ligamentous structures
  - Distal tibiofibular syndesmosis
    - Anterior inferior tibiofibular ligament
    - Posterior tibiofibular ligament
    - Interosseous membrane
  - Deltoid ligament
    - Superficial deltoid ligament
    - Deep deltoid ligament

PATHOGENESIS

- Posttraumatic arthritis: This is the most common cause (70%).[9] This type is often associated with rotational ankle injuries.
- Inflammatory arthropathy (12%): This includes arthritis resulting from rheumatoid, psoriatic, and other inflammatory conditions.
- Primary osteoarthritis: This is less common in the foot ankle (7%) compared to the hip and knee.
- Septic/postinfectious arthritis
- Charcot neuroarthropathy
- Others
  - Osteonecrosis
  - Hemophilia
  - Crystalline arthropathy
  - Joint dysplasias

NATURAL HISTORY

- Posttraumatic arthritis
  - An ankle fracture can be a source of initial chondral damage and potentially initiate a pathway of inflammatory mediator production in the joint that can lead to progressive stiffness and further chondral damage.[1]
  - Ankle fracture malunion can lead to altered and increased contact stresses across the ankle joint. This can lead to progressive cartilage damage and the development of end-stage arthritis of the ankle.
  - Ligamentous instability of the ankle can lead to abnormal talar subluxation, increased contact stresses across the ankle, and subsequent development of ankle arthritis.
  - Patient's suffering from posttraumatic ankle arthritis are often significantly younger than those patients dealing with primary osteoarthritis.
- Inflammatory osteoarthritis: An inflammatory, autoimmune-mediated pannus can lead to diffuse articular joint destruction and periarticular osteopenia.
- Primary osteoarthritis: This is certainly less understood in the ankle joint. The native anatomy and structure of the ankle joint is protective of primary osteoarthritis, due to greater osseous congruency and articular cartilage tensile stiffness.
- Septic arthritis: This is attributed to a downstream cascade of proteolytic enzyme release from proinflammatory cells and subsequent cartilage destruction. Although active septic arthritis is an obvious contraindication to TAR, prior history of septic ankle arthritis that is cured should not preclude consideration for a TAR.[10]
- Charcot neuroarthropathy: This is thought to be due to neurotraumatic destruction and cumulative trauma related to the lack of protective sensation. This leads to an increase in proinflammatory cytokines, dysregulated blood flow, and subsequent destructive bony changes. This process in the ankle represents a contraindication to TAR.
- Sequelae: reduced ankle motion, reduced plantarflexion moment, and reduced power generated during gait

PATIENT HISTORY AND PHYSICAL FINDINGS

- Most patients present with a history of chronic ankle instability or previous ankle fracture.
- Patients usually describe progressive activity-related anterior ankle pain and swelling that progresses to diffuse ankle discomfort and stiffness.
- A thorough medical history should be obtained from the patient, specifically inquiring about current or past nicotine usage, presence of diabetes mellitus and associated glycemic control, neuropathy, history of thromboembolic event, and any history of immunosuppressive agent usage.
- A social history should be obtained to determine the patient's current work requirements, recreational activity, and activities of daily living.
- Alignment
  - Genu varum and valgum
  - Cavovarus: peek-a-boo heel sign
  - Pes planovalgus: too many toes sign
  - Assess patient shoe wear for established wear patterns (ie, lateral wear in subtle cavus alignment).
- Gait
  - Antalgic gait
  - Patient may externally rotate the ankle to avoid painful push-off and in presence of limited ankle dorsiflexion.
- Skin
  - Evaluate for previous surgical incisions, wounds, and generalized skin condition.
- Tenderness
  - Assess areas over the tibiotalar and hindfoot joints.
- Neuromuscular exam
  - Motor strength
  - Sensation
    - Perform Semmes-Weinstein 5.07 filament (10 g) test in diabetics to assess for protective sensation.
  - Vascular
    - Evaluate posterior tibialis and dorsalis pedis pulses. Poor vascularity warrants further workup, starting with noninvasive arterial studies. Furthermore, assess for presence of chronic venous insufficiency or lymphedema that may negatively affect healing potential around the ankle and require preoperative optimization/treatment.
- Range of motion (ROM)
  - In addition to assessing ankle (dorsi-/plantarflexion) and hindfoot (inversion/eversion) mobility, the hip and knee should also be checked to assure no proximal contractures/stiffness that might impact the ankle/foot and gait.
  - Silfverskiöld test to evaluate for isolated gastrocnemius versus combined (gastrosoleus complex/Achilles) contracture

IMAGING AND OTHER DIAGNOSTIC STUDIES

- Weight-bearing ankle plan radiographic series (standing anteroposterior [AP], lateral, and mortise) should be performed on all patients, along with a Saltzman hindfoot alignment view.
  - Osteophyte formation and joint-space narrowing are often present.
  - Evidence of talar tilt and subluxation indicate sequelae of ligamentous instability.
- Previous hardware and overall talar morphology should also be noted.
- Assess for presence of cystic changes at distal tibia and dorsal talus.
- A foot series (standing AP, lateral, and oblique) should be considered in patients with associated foot deformities, such as cavovarus or hindfoot pronation from posterior tibialis tendon dysfunction.
- The hip-to-ankle alignment views should be obtained if proximal malalignment is seen on clinical exam or in a patient with a history of lower extremity fracture.
- In general, a preoperative ankle CT scan is important to evaluate for evidence of adjacent hindfoot arthritis, the presence of periarticular cystic changes that may impact total ankle implant selection, placement, and further planning.
- More specifically, when planning to perform a PROPHECY Infinity TAR, a PROPHECY protocol CT of the extremity (knee/distal femur through ankle/foot) is completed. To ensure the PROPHECY specifications are complete and appropriate, and to allow for adequate time for production of the alignment guides, it is typically expected that the company receive the PROPHECY CT at least 4 weeks prior to planned surgery date. For accuracy of patient-specific anterior distal tibial and dorsal landmarks that the guides are built to precisely fit onto, it is recommended that the PROPHECY CT is performed within 4 to 6 months of planned surgery. The PROPHECY CT protocol, which is available on the company website, is worth reviewing and providing to the radiology department performing the protocoled CT scan to assure completeness and adequacy of the study.
- A magnetic resonance imaging (MRI) may be obtained in patients with suspected osteonecrosis of the talus or distal tibial plafond.
  - Using MRI in combination with CT, the amount and pattern/distribution of avascular bone and subchondral collapse should be assessed to determine the feasibility of performing a TAR, and furthermore, which particular TAR implant system may be most appropriate, depending on particular bone resection/cuts (ie, use of INFINITY™, INBONE II™, or even INVISION™ [Wright Medical Technology, Memphis, TN] talar component, which are all compatible with the Infinity tibial component and polyethylene liner). PROPHECY preoperative planning can be immensely helpful here to determine and plan for appropriate resection of avascular bone segments in conjunction with the particular implants selected for use.

DIFFERENTIAL DIAGNOSIS

- Posttraumatic arthritis
- Inflammatory osteoarthritis
- Primary osteoarthritis
- Septic arthritis
- Charcot neuroarthropathy

NONOPERATIVE MANAGEMENT

- Activity modification
- Nonsteroidal anti-inflammatory drugs
- Intra-articular injections
  - Corticosteroid
  - Viscosupplementation

- Orthotics/bracing
  - Ankle brace
  - Solid ankle cushion heel
  - Single rocker sole shoes
  - Unloading ankle–foot orthotic brace

SURGICAL MANAGEMENT

- The goals for a TAR are to provide a well-aligned, stable joint that allows for pain-free motion, gait, and function for the patient.
- A general indication for surgery includes patients with symptomatic, end-stage ankle arthritis that is recalcitrant to conservative treatment.
- Absolute contraindications to TAR include patients with an acute or unresolved chronic ankle joint infection, Charcot neuroarthropathy, peripheral neuropathy with lack of protective sensation in feet, arterial insufficiency not correctable by vascular intervention, and inadequate ankle soft tissue envelope to support TAR that is not addressable via soft tissue coverage procedure.

Preoperative Planning

- Patient preoperative medical optimization prior to TAR is essential for achieving successful perioperative and postoperative outcomes. As an example, glycemic control should be optimized (hemoglobin A1c <7.5) prior to surgery.
- Vascular studies, as applicable, including potentially arterial noninvasive studies to start, should be obtained in patients with poor pulses or other signs of arterial insufficiency. Furthermore, patients with signs of venous insufficiency should undergo further assessment via venous ultrasound evaluation.
  - In either circumstance of vascular insufficiency, vascular surgery consultation is warranted prior to surgery.
- Patients with poor skin/soft tissue envelope around the ankle, multiple prior incisions, soft tissue contracture, or any concerning soft tissue lesion should undergo further evaluation typically with a plastic surgeon. In some cases, collaboration with a plastic surgeon adept in free tissue transfer is critical, in cases of severely compromised or contracted ankle soft tissue envelope, in order to perform preoperative free flap placement or other soft tissue coverage procedure, or potentially guide the surgical approach/incision.
- The treating surgeon should take into careful consideration the overall limb alignment. Patients with symptomatic knee osteoarthritis with genu varum or valgus should likely undergo their proximal surgery (ie, knee) prior to undergoing TAR in order to account for compensatory hindfoot valgus or varus alignment and potentially prevent TAR failure resulting from significant proximal deformity.[5]
- The PROPHECY CT scan should be scrutinized, in particular for tibial or talar bone cysts that may impact implant selection, osseous resections, and implant placement **(FIG 1)**. In select cases with large distal–tibial cysts or avascular segments that will not be removed with typical Infinity bone resection levels, an intramedullary stemmed component should be considered for improved implant stability.
- Preoperative passive ankle dorsiflexion and plantarflexion can help to determine the need for an isolated gastrocnemius recession or percutaneous triple Achilles tendon

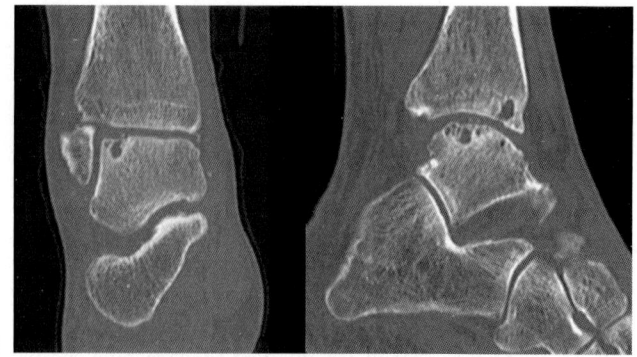

FIG 1 Coronal (**A**) and sagittal (**B**) preoperative ankle CT scans. Note the moderate-sized distal tibial and dorsal talar dome cysts present. Cystic lesions of this size and in this location would typically be resected with the Infinity TAR system, and PROPHECY guidance can help the surgeon intraoperatively.

hemisection (Hoke) lengthening to achieve adequate ROM, particularly dorsiflexion.
  - Although this step can be performed at the beginning of the TAR procedure if needed, this step is typically performed at the time of implant trialing, to assure that a patient's equinus contracture is properly addressed with the appropriate amount of equinus release.
  - Of note, the latter step is possible with the Infinity TAR because the distal tibial and talar cuts are decoupled and do not require the ankle to be in a neutral or 90-degree position prior to completion of these bone resections.
- Patients should be counseled that undergoing a TAR does not drastically improve ankle ROM or make it "normal motion" by any means. Rather, TAR maintains or slightly improves ankle ROM following TAR compared to the patient's preoperative ROM.

PROPHECY Preoperative Navigation and Patient-Specific Alignment Guides

- The basis for PROPHECY technology use in TAR is the knowledge that appropriate implant sizing, positioning, and alignment is essential in TAR success and patient outcomes.
- Most TAR systems use an external alignment guide in order to establish appropriate resection levels, along with implant placement, alignment, and rotation. As such, a similar type of external alignment guide is available for use with the Infinity TAR system. Please refer to the company's published surgical technique on proper usage of this guide. If the surgeon prefers at any time during the procedure to abandon the use of the PROPHECY alignment guides, it is certainly possible to do so, with utilization of the standard external alignment guide.
- The PROPHECY Infinity TAR system uses the patient's exact osseous anatomy, surgeon-set preferences, combined with computer virtual analysis of the patient's anatomic and mechanical alignment axes in the coronal and sagittal planes, along with rotational considerations, to create a patient-specific preoperative plan **(FIG 2)** that optimizes bone coverage and minimizes bone resection.
  - The surgeon reviews online the preoperative plan, including deformity analysis, planned resections, and implant specifics (sizing, positioning, and alignment).

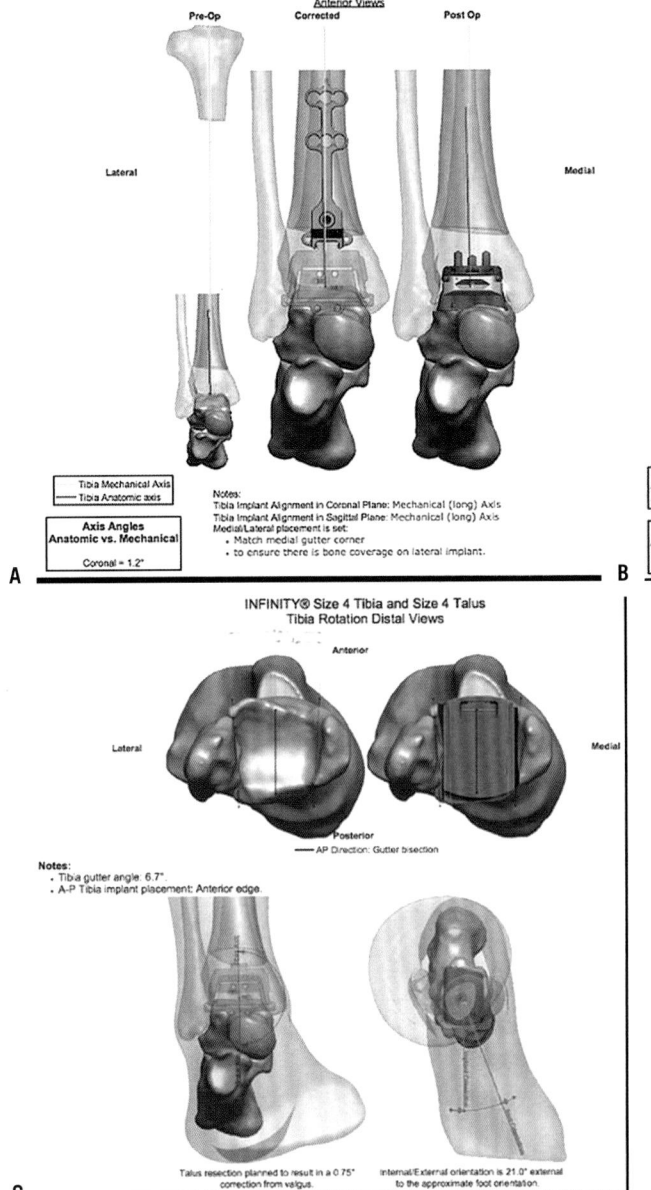

FIG 2 Preoperative PROPHECY template. Example of the preoperative planning for the PROPHECY Infinity TAR system with coronal (**A**), sagittal (**B**), and axial (**C**) alignment details of the components. *Sz*, size; *AP*, anteroposterior. (Courtesy of Wright Medical Group N.V.)

- This plan is then accepted or altered as needed by the surgeon (eg, a surgeon may choose to set the distal tibial/dorsal talar cuts to be a few millimeters underresected, in cases of global ligamentous laxity or anterior talar subluxation to potentially minimize eventual polyethylene thickness), and once finalized, is then used to produce patient-specific alignment guides for the distal tibia and dorsal talus, that will be used intraoperatively to guide the appropriate placement of cut guides to perform the Infinity TAR, in decoupled fashion.
- The thorough preoperative plan established with the PROPHECY Infinity TAR system and patient-specific alignment guides used in surgery are intended to make the process of establishing the appropriate implant positioning and alignment more reliable and reproducible for the surgeon. This in effect is then intended to reduce surgical time, reduce the use of intraoperative fluoroscopic exposure, and reduce procedural costs.[3,4] Early studies have shown some of these goals have been realized.

Positioning

- Regional anesthesia is performed utilizing a popliteal-saphenous nerve block.
- The patient is placed onto the operative table in the supine position with the heels flush at the distal end of the bed.
- A bump is placed under the ipsilateral buttock in order to prevent external rotation of the hip, keeping the anterior ankle positioned perpendicular to the bed for ease of operating.
- A nonsterile, well-padded thigh tourniquet is placed onto the operative extremity.
- Appropriate preoperative intravenous (IV) antibiotics are administered no longer than 60 minutes prior to making surgical incision.
- The operative extremity is prepped and draped in standard, sterile fashion.
- The extremity is elevated and Esmarch exsanguinated prior to incision.

TECHNIQUES

EXPOSURE

- A 10-cm anterior ankle incision is made about 1 cm lateral to the anterior tibial crest. The incision extends from the distal tibia to the talonavicular joint.
- A standard anterior ankle approach is made, protecting the superficial peroneal nerve, entering the interval between the anterior tibialis and extensor hallucis longus tendons, and protecting the deep anterior neurovascular bundle. An anterior ankle arthrotomy is made and the ankle joint is exposed.
- Because the PROPHECY CT effectively "sees" only bone, it is critical to remove all overlying soft tissue and periosteum where the PROPHECY alignment guides will fit, to improve accuracy of guide placement. In the case of the talar alignment guide, it is also critical to carefully remove any residual cartilage on the anterior talar dome where the guide will sit.
- The soft tissues are sharply released from the anterior distal tibia and retracted to expose from the medial malleolus over to the anterior inferior tibiofibular ligament laterally.
- Distally, the dissection is carried down to the dorsal talonavicular joint to allow for proper talar alignment guide fitting and placement.
  - One should be able to visualize the lateral talar neck and talonavicular joint.
- Place a deep self-retaining retractor avoiding any retraction on the skin.
- Any residual periosteum and soft tissue in the areas where the PROPHECY guides are placed is removed using Bovie electrocautery and a wet sponge to remove any soft tissue debris **(TECH FIG 1)**. The PROPHECY report details, which loose osteophytes (loose bodies) should be removed and which osteophytes to leave intact in order to assure proper alignment guide fit. It is critical not to remove stable osteophytes, as these are the exact landmarks the PROPHECY guides are built to fit directly onto. Again, the surgeon should refer to the PROPHECY report for full specifics and details.

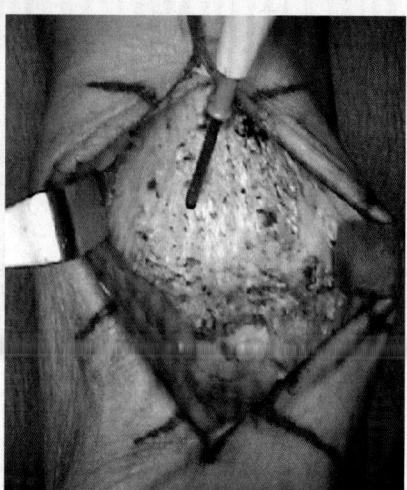

TECH FIG 1 Standard anterior ankle approach. It is important to completely remove overlying soft tissue, periosteum, and loose bodies from the portion of the anterior distal tibia that the PROPHECY alignment guide will fit over to ensure proper seating and fit of the guide onto the native bone.

- Ligament balancing is not performed at this time, which is different than most other TAR systems in which the ankle needs to be corrected to neutral prior to performing any bone resections. The PROPHECY system corrects identified malalignment through osseous resection, more specifically, via the talar resection.
  - Typically, once these planned resections are made, it is uncommon to need to perform additional ligament balancing about the ankle because it was addressed via the planned talar resection.

ALIGNMENT AND DISTAL TIBIAL RESECTION

- Place the patient-specific tibial alignment guide onto the distal tibia model to confirm the location of the landmark osteophytes, alignment, and general "fit and feel" (using tactile and visual confirmation) of the guide, prior to placement on the patient's anterior distal tibia **(TECH FIG 2A–C)**. At this time, the PROPHECY report can be referenced to confirm any details of this patient-specific "fit."
- Once accurate placement of the patient-specific tibial alignment guide is confirmed on the distal tibial model, the alignment guide is then properly placed onto the patient's anterior distal tibia in similar fashion. Make sure there is nothing impeding proper guide placement, such as osteophytes on the dorsal talus. If this is the case, place a towel bump under the distal tibia and allow the talus to fall posteriorly and the ankle to plantarflux to prevent this interference with the guide.
- While carefully maintaining this proper tibial alignment guide position, place a single guide pin bicortically into one of the proximal holes in the guide.

- Place two small cut guide pins and a long guide pin into the coronal alignment slots within the tibial alignment guide.
- With the ankle centered on the fluoroscopic image, obtain an AP ankle view. To ensure proper AP ankle image, the long pin should be positioned directly between/bisecting the two short pins **(TECH FIG 2D–F)**.
  - Check the PROPHECY report to ensure that the tibial alignment matches the preoperative templating prior to definitive guide pinning with remaining pins. It is important to recognize that there may be some parallax seen at the proximal aspect of the guidewire on the fluoroscopic image. Assuring the precise tibial alignment guide placement and resulting alignment is arguably the most critical portion of the entire procedure, and time should be taken here to assure accuracy of this step.
- Once the proper position of the patient-specific tibial alignment guide is confirmed, place the remaining 2.4-mm Steinmann pins in bicortical fashion through the guide and distal tibia to secure its final position.

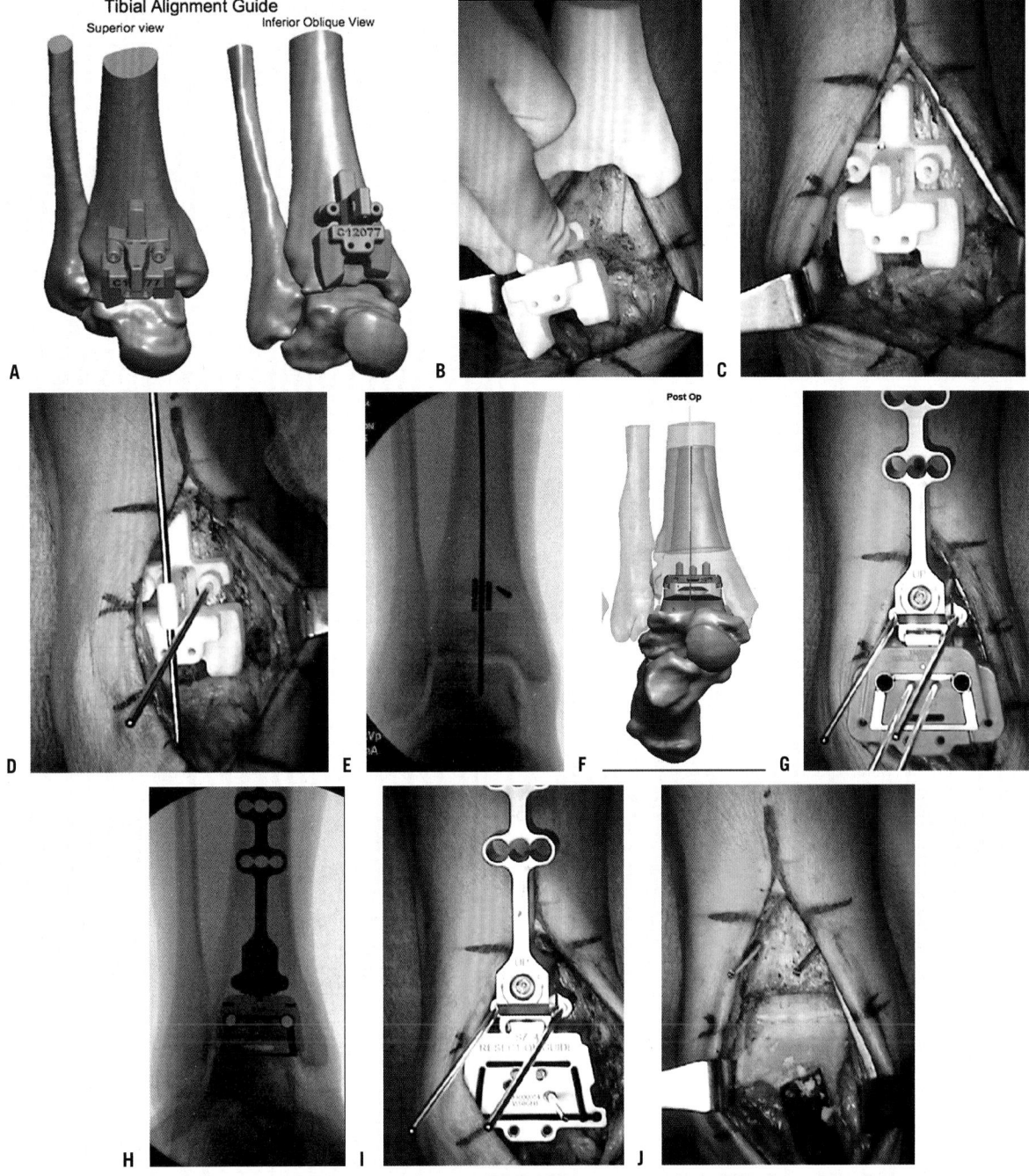

TECH FIG 2 Comparing the preoperative planning (**A**) with the distal tibial model (**B**) allows for the proper placement of the tibial alignment guide onto the patient's anterior distal tibia (**C**). Intraoperative placement of the tibial alignment guide (**D**) should be confirmed with an AP view of the ankle (**E**) and compared directly to the preoperative PROPHECY plan (**F**) prior to placement of all guide pins. Placement of the coronal sizing guide (**G**) is confirmed with a perfect pin in circle view on the AP ankle fluoroscopic image (**H**). The tibial cutting guide is then placed (**I**), and the tibial resection is performed (**J**).

- Remove the patient-specific tibial alignment guide over the distal tibial pins and place the appropriate coronal sizing guide (refer to PROPHECY report) over the anterior tibial pins, which dovetails into the proximal conversion instrument and tightens with a hex driver.
- Confirm that the selected tibial coronal guide is the appropriate size by first obtaining a perfect "pin-in-circle" view on fluoroscopy. Also, confirm that the alignment of the coronal sizing guide matches the preoperative template (**TECH FIG 2G,H**).

- Obtain a lateral view of the ankle with the medial and lateral distal pins superimposed (ie, coplanar) to ensure the correct tibial resection slope, which should be perpendicular to the mechanical axis of the tibia to produce a neutral slope.
- Place a sterile bump under the heel to allow for the posterior soft tissues and neurovascular structures to fall away from the posterior tibia during the bone resection.
- Drill the proximal tibial corner holes bicortically with the tibial corner drill from anterior to posterior.

- Exchange the coronal guide for the proper tibial resection guide over the tibial pins, which can be cut at staggered levels to ease guide placement. Double-check that the resection guide is the appropriate, intended size.
  - Further secure the resection guide with the medial oblique, divergent pin.
  - Cut the Steinmann pins flush with the resection guide, except for the oblique pin, which should be cut long enough for removal, but short enough for saw passage around it medially (usually 1.5 to 2 cm in length).
- Complete the three distal tibial resections using a thin sagittal saw blade through the proximal tibial transverse, medial, and lateral cut slots in the resection guide. Typically, a narrow saw blade is used for the Infinity size 1 through 3 resection guides and a wide saw blade used for Infinity size 4 and 5 resection guides. Do not complete the distal talar cut at this time as the decoupled resection will be made later **(TECH FIG 2I,J)**.

- Remove the distal three pins from the cutting block. The oblique pin needs to be removed prior to attempting removal of the resection guide. Leave the two proximal tibial pins in place in case there is a need to revisit the tibial cut.
- Use a small reciprocating saw and corner chisel to complete the medial and lateral gutter cuts while protecting the malleoli.
- Use a threaded Schanz pin and osteotome to carefully remove the tibial resection from the ankle joint. You may have to carefully release the adherent posterior capsule with the capsular release tool. It is important to not lever off of the malleoli to prevent iatrogenic fracture, particularly of the medial malleolus. If the tibial resection is unable to be removed in this fashion, then use an osteotome to carefully remove the anterior portion for now to allow enough space for the talar preparation and resection. The rest can be removed more easily after completing the talar resection.

DORSAL TALAR RESECTION

- Similar to the distal tibial preparation, confirm that all of the soft tissue and periosteum is removed from the talar neck with Bovie electrocautery. Be sure to keep the talar neck osteophytes intact for proper seating of the patient-specific talar alignment guide. A portion of the guide sits on the anterior talar dome, therefore it is important to remove any residual cartilage present in these areas for proper guide fit.
- Assess the surface match and fit of the talar alignment guide on the talar three-dimensional (3-D) model prior to placement on the patient's native dorsal talus **(TECH FIG 3A)**. There tend to be less available landmarks for surface matching of the talar alignment guide compared to the distal tibial guide, therefore it is critical to take time to assure precise and proper fit.
- Once accurate placement of the patient-specific talar alignment guide is confirmed on the talar model, then place the talar alignment guide onto the patient dorsal talus.
- Once satisfied with the talar alignment guide placement, secure the guide with three 2.4-mm Steinmann pins **(TECH FIG 3B)**, the first of which is placed from dorsal to plantar in oblique fashion followed by anterior to posterior pin placement.
  - The talar bone may be sclerotic and may cause the anterior to posterior talar guide pins to skive proximally during

placement. It may be helpful to use a smooth lamina spreader applied between the top of the guide and distal tibial resection surface to prevent this from occurring.
- Confirm proper placement of the patient-specific talar alignment guide with a lateral ankle fluoroscopic image. The proximal Infinity talar resection will be 2 mm proximal to and parallel to the top of the anterior to posterior pins.
- Remove talar alignment guide and place the appropriate talar resection guide over the talar pins.
  - Gutter pins can be placed if needed for additional resection guide stability, but care must be used during their placement, as they can introduce rotation or shifting of the talar resection guide.
  - At this point, the surgeon still has the option to switch to an Inbone II talar cut (flattop cut) if necessary. If this is the case, an appropriate Inbone resection guide can be used and pins switched accordingly. For the purposes of this technique chapter, we proceed with the description for performing a chamfered talar cut for the Infinity talus.
- Use a thin sagittal saw to make the proximal talar resection. Be sure to keep the saw oriented straight anterior to posterior to prevent iatrogenic injury to the malleoli.

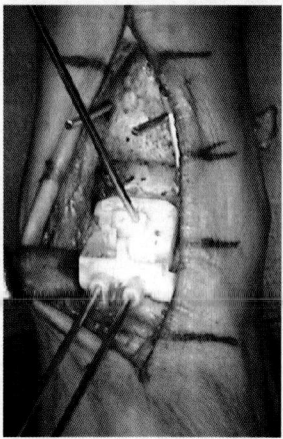
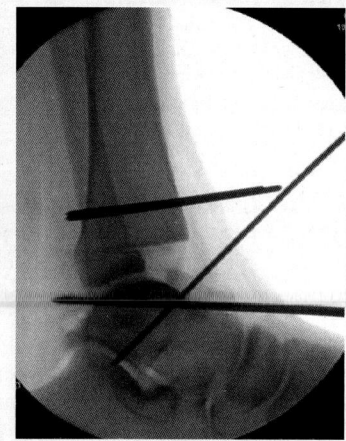

A   B

TECH FIG 3 Talus alignment guide. Intraoperative placement **(A)** of the talus alignment guide is confirmed on a lateral ankle fluoroscopic image **(B)** to confirm the resection level of the talus.

- Complete the talar resection with a small reciprocating saw if needed. Remove the talar bone resection with a rongeur.
- If not done so already, complete the removal of all resected bone from the joint space, including the posterior portion of the distal tibial resection.

- Irrigate the wound and directly inspect the joint space and resections to assure they are complete and appropriate. Remove any residual bone fragments that remain. Confirm appropriate initial joint resections and bone removal via AP and lateral ankle fluoroscopy as well.

TIBIAL IMPLANT ANTEROPOSTERIOR SIZING

- Place the appropriate tibial tray trial onto the distal tibial resection surface over the two remaining proximal tibial pins.
  - Ensure that the tibial tray trial is sitting flush with the distal tibial cut (TECH FIG 4A). A smooth lamina spreader should be used here to assure no posterior lift-off of this trial on the distal tibia.
- Check anterior and posterior tibial tray coverage with a lateral ankle fluoroscopic image.
  - For tibial tray sizes 3 through 5, there is a standard and long AP-sized option. For those respective trials, the posterior notch denotes the standard tray AP size, and the most posterior portion of trial represents the long tray AP sizing option. Tibial tray sizes 1 and 2 have the same medial to lateral width, and each has only one AP sizing option, therefore they share the same trial, and the posterior notch represents

a size 1 AP length, and the most posterior aspect of the trial demonstrates the size 2 AP length.
  - It is most ideal to have full anterior and posterior coverage and to avoid excessive posterior overhang. Slight adjustments in the AP component placement can be made using the anterior set screw to offset the tibial guide by up to 3 mm to avoid excessive tibial component posterior overhang.
- Once the tibial tray trial position is finalized on the distal tibia and lamina spreader is placed, set the posterior T-handle tibial peg broach in the posterior peg hole site and mallet to the laser line. Leave the posterior broach in place until the anterior pegs are broached.
- Place and mallet the anterior peg broach into the anterior two peg hole sites (TECH FIG 4B). Remove all broaches and leave the tibial tray trial in place.

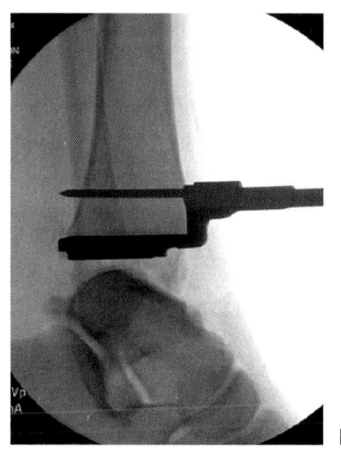
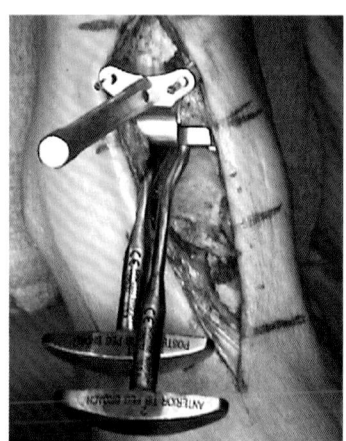

TECH FIG 4 Component sizing and trial component insertion. **A.** Tibial tray sizing should be confirmed on a lateral ankle fluoroscopic image to confirm appropriate AP coverage and minimizing posterior overhang. The tibial tray should be flush with the distal tibial resection prior to peg preparation, which can be assisted with use of a smooth lamina spreader. **B.** The tibial pegs are then prepared.

TALAR COMPONENT SIZING AND POSITIONING

- Place a polyethylene trial into the tibial tray (6 mm thickness for tibial sizes 1 to 3, size 8 mm for the larger sizes).
- Place the appropriate talar dome trial onto the resected proximal talar surface.
  - The talar component can match the tibial component size or be one size smaller. Both of these sizes should be assessed in the AP and lateral fluoroscopic views to determine the most optimal talar sizing to maximize coverage but minimize potential overhang and resulting medial/lateral gutter impingement.

- Ensure that the proper rotation is set to the talar trial using the second ray as a guide with the ankle held in a neutral position.
- If an equinus ankle position is still present, then perform either a gastrocnemius recession or percutaneous triple Achilles lengthening to improve ankle dorsiflexion. If the ankle remains tight in dorsiflexion with the smallest polyethylene liner, then consider recutting the talus by 2 mm at this time.
- Obtain AP and mortise ankle fluoroscopic images to confirm appropriate medial and lateral talar coverage as well as ensuring

- no implant overhang that may cause impingement in the medial and lateral gutters.
  - The surgeon may opt to downsize the talar component by one size if a substantial gutter débridement needs to be performed.
- Obtain a lateral fluoroscopic view to ensure proper talar trial positioning and fit (**TECH FIG 5**).
  - Specifically, ensure that the posterior portion of the talar trial is resting flush along the posterior cortex of the proximal resected talar surface for proper congruence.
  - Check that the location of the posterior chamfer cut is appropriate using the posterior slot on the guide as a reference.
- Once the appropriately sized talar trial and component position are confirmed, place two 2.4-mm Steinmann pins through the talar dome trial handle to secure it into place.
- Use the polyethylene insert trial holder to remove the polyethylene insert.
- Remove the talar dome and tibial tray trials over the 2.4-mm Steinmann pins and prepare for the talar chamfer resection.

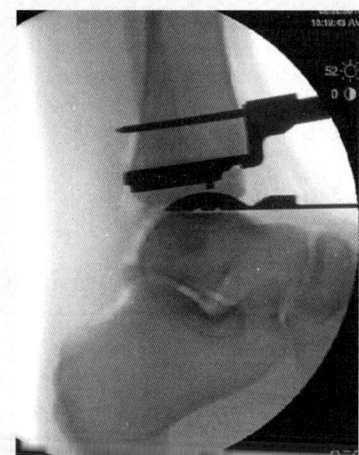

TECH FIG 5 The trial polyethylene and talus are inserted, and a lateral image is obtained to confirm the overall talar trial AP position and posterior talar chamfer cut prior to resection.

TALAR CHAMFER RESECTION AND FINAL TALAR PREPARATION

- Slide the talar chamfer resection guide base over the two 2.4-mm talar Steinmann pins.
- Place two temporary fixation screws (medial and lateral) into the talar chamfer resection guide base. Avoid excessive torqueing and improper shifting of the guide base position.
- Use a thin sagittal saw to perform the posterior talar chamfer cut.
- Remove the two 2.4-mm talar Steinmann pins and place one pin through the anterior central pin hole in the resection base and cut the pin flush.
- Place the anterior talar pilot guide with the pegs facing down onto the anterior face of the talar resection guide base.
- Ream the four pilot holes flush within the anterior pilot guide.
- Remove the pilot guide and place the anterior talar finish guide.
- With the talar reamer flush in the finishing slot, ream the talus from side to side.
  - Be careful not to dislodge the finishing guide during reaming.

- Remove the finishing guide and rotate the pilot guide 180 degrees so that the pegs are placed into the posterior face of the talar resection guide.
- Repeat the pilot hole and finishing guide steps to complete the anterior talar chamfer preparation. Remove all fixation pins and the resection base.
- Remove the posterior chamfer cut and other bone fragments with a small osteotome and rongeur. Inspect the chamfer cuts to make sure all excess bone is carefully removed that would prevent proper talar implant placement.
- Thoroughly irrigate the wound and joint space of any bone debris.
- Place the appropriately sized tibial tray trial and polyethylene insert, followed by the talar peg drill guide (**TECH FIG 6**). Recheck AP and lateral fluoroscopy to make sure all trials are seated and positioned appropriately. Check the talar peg drill guide position in terms of medial to lateral coverage.

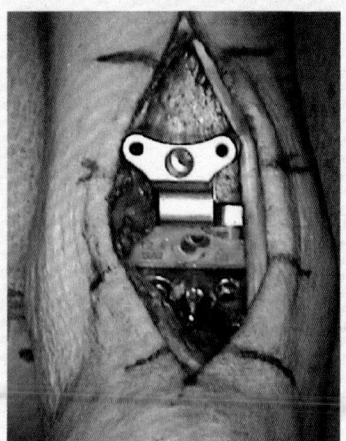 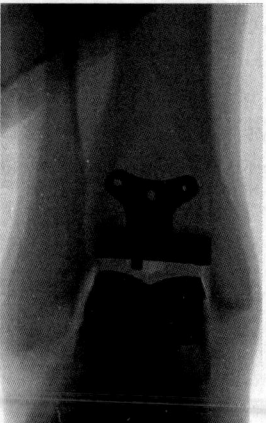 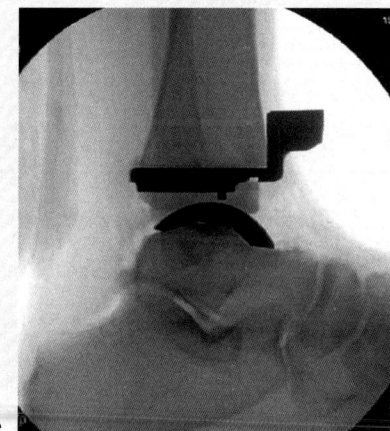

A   B   C

TECH FIG 6 A. The tibial tray, polyethylene, and talar trials are inserted after the posterior and anterior talar chamfer cuts are performed. AP (**B**) and lateral (**C**) fluoroscopic images are obtained of the trial components to confirm adequate alignment and component positioning.

Although its overall medial–lateral position is basically set at this point by the articulating tibial tray trial and polyethylene liner, subtle adjustments can be made.

- Secure the talar guide with a single 2.4-mm Steinmann pin anteriorly and drill the anterior peg holes with the 4-mm peg drill.
- Remove all trials and thoroughly irrigate out the joint space and wound of any residual debris.

INSERTION OF DEFINITIVE COMPONENTS

- Dry all resected joint surfaces well. As specified in the surgical technique, place a thin layer of cement onto the top (back side) and side walls of the final tibial tray component being held on the impaction insert.
- Using the tibial tray impaction insert, place the posterior peg into the prepared posterior hole site on the distal tibia.
  - Rotate the component so that the anterior two pegs are in line with the prepared anterior peg holes.
  - Manually seat the tibial pegs into the peg holes before impaction
- Using the offset tibial tray impactor and mallet, and while an assistant firmly holds the insertion handle to the impaction insert with an upward/proximal directed force, uniformly impact the tibial tray into its final position. Obtain a lateral fluoroscopic image to confirm the complete seating of the tibial tray **(TECH FIG 7A)**.
  - Avoid using the impactor back and forth between the posterior and anterior recesses on the tibial impaction insert,

as this may create a "rocking horse" phenomenon with the tibial tray, widening the peg holes, and ultimately compromising tibial component stability.
- Remove the impaction insert from the tibial tray and place the tibial tray protector while working on the talar side.
- Place a thin layer of cement on the underside of the final talar component and impact the talar component into the peg holes with the talar dome impactor.
  - Be careful to not lever the talar impactor into the tibial tray component. With the ankle plantarflexed, use the impactor posteriorly first and then orient impaction more vertically to final impact the talar component into place.
  - Obtain a lateral fluoroscopic image to confirm appropriate talar component seating.
- Remove the tibial tray protector and insert the appropriate trial polyethylene liner. Assess ankle ROM and varus–valgus stability with the ankle held in a neutral (90-degree) position. The PROPHECY system builds some joint alignment correction

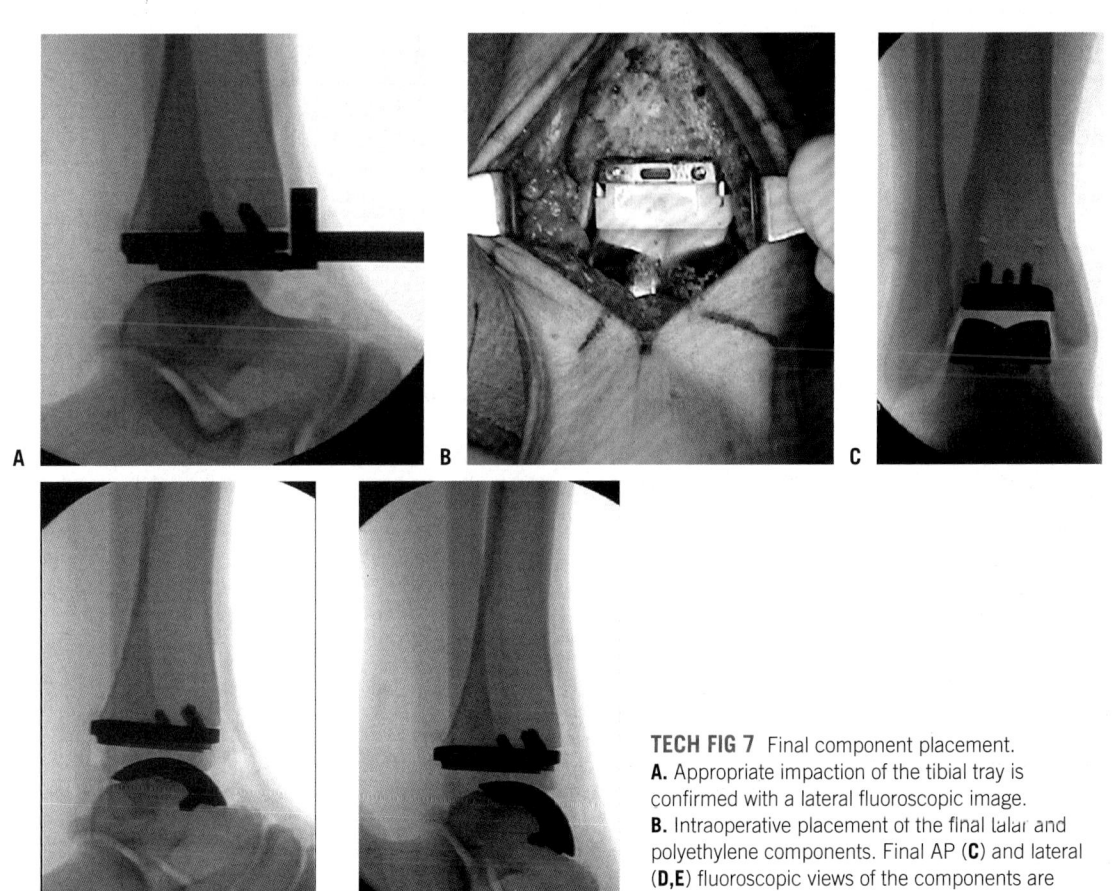

TECH FIG 7 Final component placement. **A.** Appropriate impaction of the tibial tray is confirmed with a lateral fluoroscopic image. **B.** Intraoperative placement of the final talar and polyethylene components. Final AP (**C**) and lateral (**D,E**) fluoroscopic views of the components are obtained prior to wound closure.

TECHNIQUES

into the plan with the talar resection; however, it is critical to assess the need for further ligamentous balancing.

- To improve ankle ROM, minimize gutter impingement, and potentially help with ligament balancing/tensioning, a small reciprocating saw is used to remove any excess bone medially and laterally. This is typically performed on the talar side; however, small resections can be carefully performed on the distal tibial/medial malleolar and lateral malleolar sides if necessary.
- If needed, further ligament balancing is performed in standard fashion, using selective ligamentous releases medially or laterally, and/or reconstructive procedure to imbricate tissue, such as performing a modified Brostrom ligament reconstruction for residual lateral ankle instability, followed by polyethylene retrialing to confirm a stable and well-balanced TAR. A modified Brostrom procedure would be performed in standard fashion via separate short, lateral incision with the trial polyethylene liner removed to assure appropriate imbrication of lateral tissues.
- Once satisfied with the ankle joint stability and polyethylene liner sizing, remove the poly trial liner and irrigate the ankle space to remove any final pieces of debris that may be present throughout the joint.
- To insert the final polyethylene liner, screw in the two attachment posts into the anterior face of the tibial component.

- Once the final polyethylene liner is loaded correctly onto the poly inserter and rail guide, then carefully slide the whole assembly over the two attachment posts. Confirm that the inserter is sitting flush against the anterior portion of the tibial component, use an attachment nut over each attachment post to secure the entire assembly into place.
- Final tighten the two small nuts over the posts using a needle driver. Performing this step can help avoid the need for final polyethylene impaction after insertion, as it usually will fully seat through the insertion process.
- Unlock the plunger and push it forward until it engages the inserter housing. Then, turn the plunger clockwise all the way down until it reaches the final depth, in order to advance the final polyethylene liner into the tibial tray.
- Disassemble the entire poly inserter assembly by first loosening the attachment nuts, then removing the inserter, followed by attachment rail removal. Inspect the final polyethylene seating into the tibial component. If not fully seated, then use the impactor and mallet to gently final seat the polyethylene liner into place (**TECH FIG 7B**).
- Check final AP, mortise, and lateral ankle fluoroscopic images to ensure that all components are properly aligned, positioned, and seated. Perform a final check of the medial and lateral gutters. Confirm TAR stability and adequate ROM (**TECH FIG 7C–E**).

CLOSURE

- Thoroughly irrigate the wound.
- Close the anterior ankle joint capsule and extensor retinaculum with 2-0 Vicryl suture.
- Release the tourniquet and assure hemostasis is achieved. Place a deep drain if deemed necessary.

- Close the subcutaneous tissue with 3-0 Vicryl suture.
- Close the skin in interrupted fashion with 3-0 nylon suture.
- Place the patient into a well-padded short-leg splint with the ankle in neutral position.

TECHNIQUES

Pearls and Pitfalls

Residual Deltoid Ligament Contracture and Lateral Ankle Ligament Laxity	• Perform a medial deltoid release/peel and trial a slightly thicker polyethylene liner. If this does not adequately balance the ankle joint, then remove the trial polyethylene line and perform a modified Brostrom lateral ankle ligament reconstruction, which should then restore joint stability and usually allow for a thinner polyethylene line.
Patient-specific alignment guides are not properly aligning and fitting with the preoperative template.	• Make sure that all of the periosteum and soft tissue are removed in the affected areas to ensure complete surface matching and congruency. • Remove any loose bodies as indicated in the PROPHECY report. • Ensure that the custom guide is resting on the correct osseous landmarks. Use the 3-D distal tibial and talar models to check this as well. • Slightly plantarflex the foot and place a towel bump under the distal tibia to allow the talus to fall out of the way for tibial alignment guide placement.
Difficulty Removing the Resected Tibial Bone	• Use a threaded Schanz pin to remove the resected bone in one piece if possible. • If the bone cannot be removed, then first remove the anterior portion with an osteotome. This should allow enough space to perform the talar work. Once the talar resection is performed, it will be easier to remove the remaining posterior tibial bone, often using a reciprocating saw and rongeur/curette to remove it in smaller pieces.

Tibial tray is not fully seated posteriorly.	• Check to ensure that the tibial resection is completely flat and perpendicular to the shaft of the tibia. The presence of an anterior or posterior tibial resection slope can prevent the tibia peg from fully seating. Any irregularities in the tibial cut can prevent proper seating as well. When preparing to broach the three peg holes, make sure to use a lamina spreader to keep the tibial tray trial flush with the distal tibial surface. • When placing the final tibial component, impact the posterior aspect of the tibial tray to ensure that it engages into the posterior peg before impacting anteriorly.
The talar component is not fully seated.	• Remove any bony debris from the talar surface and palpate the chamfer cuts to make sure there are no improper ridges or uneven cuts. • Remove any anterior talar neck osteophytes or overhanging anterior talar bone that may be blocking the talar component from fully seating.
Lack of Ankle Dorsiflexion	• Check the medial and lateral gutters for osseous impingement. • Downsize the polyethylene liner as long as varus–valgus stability is maintained. • Consider the need to perform a gastrocnemius recession of Hoke Achilles lengthening. Carefully perform a posterior ankle capsular release if contracted. • If a lack of dorsiflexion persists, it is possible that the initial resections were undercut. Consider recutting the talus by 2 mm and retrialing.

POSTOPERATIVE CARE

- Overnight hospitalization for pain control and non–weight-bearing mobilization training by physical therapy; completion of perioperative IV antibiotics
- Unless specific patient risk factors dictate more aggressive treatment, we advise use of a full-strength, enteric-coated aspirin taken once daily, along with regular mobilization and extremity elevation as appropriate for deep venous thrombosis prophylaxis.
- Maintain non–weight-bearing precautions on the operative extremity in a short-leg splint for 2 weeks.
  - Concomitant reconstructive/realignment procedures, such as osteotomies and/or arthrodesis will necessitate a longer period of offloading.
- Suture removal at 2 to 3 weeks if appropriate and placement into short-leg cast for an additional 2 weeks if needed for soft tissue healing
- Transition into a pneumatic walking boot and weight bearing as tolerated around 4 weeks
- Transition into normal shoe wear and ankle stabilizing orthosis (ASO) brace (as needed) around 8 to 10 weeks
- Return to activities as tolerated by 12 weeks

OUTCOMES

- Although there has been recent literature on the benefits of total ankle arthroplasty, most of the current literature is based on level IV evidence.
- Although there have been some favorable short-term benefits in regards to costs,[3] improved alignment,[4,8] and patient outcomes[2,6,7] following patient-specific total ankle arthroplasty, long-term follow-up is needed for patient-specific Infinity total ankle arthroplasty.

COMPLICATIONS

- Wound dehiscence
- Infection (superficial or deep)
- Periprosthetic fracture
- Osteolysis
- Component subsidence
- Avascular necrosis of the talus
- Complex regional pain syndrome

REFERENCES

1. Adams SB Jr, Nettles DL, Jones LC, et al. Inflammatory cytokines and cellular metabolites as synovial fluid biomarkers of posttraumatic ankle arthritis. Foot Ankle Int 2014;35(12):1241–1249.
2. Cody EA, Taylor MA, Nunley JA II, et al. Increased early revision rate with the INFINITY total ankle prosthesis. Foot Ankle Int 2019;40(1):9–17.
3. Hamid KS, Matson AP, Nwachukwu BU, et al. Determining the cost-savings threshold and alignment accuracy of patient-specific instrumentation in total ankle replacements. Foot Ankle Int 2017;38(1):49–57.
4. Hsu AR, Davis WH, Cohen BE, et al. Radiographic outcomes of preoperative CT scan-derived patient-specific total ankle arthroplasty. Foot Ankle Int 2015;36(10):1163–1169.
5. Norton AA, Callaghan JJ, Amendola A, et al. Correlation of knee and hindfoot deformities in advanced knee OA: compensatory hindfoot alignment and where it occurs. Clin Orthop Relat Res 2015;473(1):166–174.
6. Penner M, Davis WH, Wing K, et al. The Infinity total ankle system: early clinical results with 2- to 4-year follow-up. Foot Ankle Spec 2019;12(2):159–166.
7. Saito GH, Sanders AE, de Cesar Netto C, et al. Short-term complications, reoperations, and radiographic outcomes of a new fixed-bearing total ankle arthroplasty. Foot Ankle Int 2018;39(7):787–794.
8. Saito GH, Sanders AE, O'Malley MJ, et al. Accuracy of patient-specific instrumentation in total ankle arthroplasty: a comparative study. Foot Ankle Surg 2019;25(3):383–389.
9. Saltzman CL, Salamon ML, Blanchard GM, et al. Epidemiology of ankle arthritis: report of a consecutive series of 639 patients from a tertiary orthopaedic center. Iowa Orthop J 2005;25:44–46.
10. Shi GG, Huh J, Gross CE, et al. Total ankle arthroplasty following prior infection about the ankle. Foot Ankle Int 2015;36(12):1425–1429.

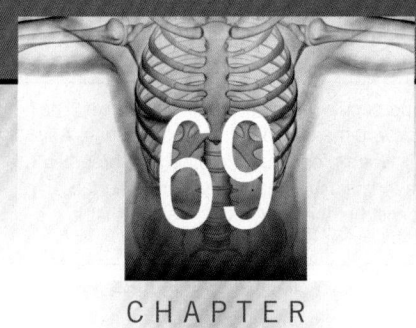

69

CHAPTER

The Cadence Total Ankle Arthroplasty

Akhil Sharma and Selene G. Parekh

DEFINITION

- The ankle is the most commonly injured joint in the body subjected to more weight-bearing force per square centimeter than any other joint.[18]
- There is an inverse relationship between articular cartilage thickness and its compressive modulus—thus, the thin ankle cartilage (1 to 1.7 mm) has a high compressive modulus relative to the thick knee (1 to 6 mm).[3,18]
- Treatment modalities for ankle arthritis must take into account personal choice, age, occupation, desired activities, comorbidities, and prior history of infection.[5]

ANATOMY

- The medial anatomy of the ankle joint is composed of the distal tibia, the talar dome, the medial malleolus, and the deltoid ligament.[1,7]
- The lateral anatomy of the ankle joint includes the distal anterior border of the tibia, the talus, the lateral ligament complex, and the lateral malleolus.[1,7]
- The central anatomy of the ankle joint is made up of the tibial plafond, the talar dome, and the incisura where the fibula nestles against the tibia.[1,7]
- In both males and females, the left tibia is slightly longer on average.[9]
  - The average anteroposterior (AP) diameter at the mid-tibia is 3.13 cm in males and 2.64 cm in females.[9]
  - In males, the tibia has an average lateral diameter of 2.22 cm. In females, the lateral diameter is approximately 1.95 cm.[9]
- Both the length and width of the talus is larger in males than females.[19]
  - Average talar width in males is 54.4 mm, whereas it is 48.3 mm in females.
  - Average talar length in males is 44.4 mm, and in females it is 38.8 mm.
- Blood supply to the posterior and proximal ankle joint occurs via the tibial nutrient artery, a branch of either the posterior tibial artery or the popliteal artery.[6]
- The medial third of the ankle joint is supplied by the fibular nutrient artery, coming from the peroneal artery.[6]
- The distal tibia and fibula receive vascular supply from the perimalleolar arterial ring, connected by the anterior tibial, posterior tibial, and peroneal arteries.[6]
- Nervous supply to the ankle joint comes from the deep peroneal, saphenous, sural, and tibial nerves.[4]

PATHOGENESIS

- The most common causes of degenerative changes to the ankle joint result from trauma, abnormal ankle mechanics, or both.[10]
- Examples of traumatic injuries that contribute to ankle arthritis include fractures of the malleoli, tibial plafond, and talus.[18]
- Tibial plafond fractures are caused by high-energy forces. The arthritis that results from these forces is often complicated by articular damage, avascular necrosis, postoperative infection, and inadequate reduction.[18]
- Instability of the ankle joint can be caused by chronic laxity of the lateral ligament, which then predisposes degenerative changes on the medial side.[18]

NATURAL HISTORY

- Ankle arthritis that is not managed will progress with pain that gets exacerbated by daily activities.[17]
- Heel-to-toe gait is affected as the ankle joint becomes stiff in addition to pain.[17]
- Morbidity is amplified by factors such as obesity, high activity level, and pathology in the subtalar or transverse talar joint.[17]
- According to research by Agel and colleagues, patients with end-stage ankle arthritis scored three times worse than normal patients on the Musculoskeletal Functional Assessment.[5]
- Long-term durability of the ankle joint depends heavily on proper alignment and function of the subtalar joint.[16]

PATIENT HISTORY AND PHYSICAL FINDINGS

- Patient history may include the following:
  - Prior ankle fracture that was followed by a nonanatomic reduction (as opposed to a rigid anatomic fixation)[3]
  - Ankle joint angle greater than 10 degrees of equinus, leading to a vaulting gait and slower walking speed, predisposing to laxity of the medial collateral ligament and posterior capsule of the knee[3]
  - Family history of autoimmune disease, such as rheumatoid arthritis
- Physical examination methods include the following:
  - Joint effusion: Patients who have acute inflammatory ankle arthritis often have involvement of soft tissue swelling in adjacent structures, such as the flexor hallucis longus, flexor digitorum longus, tibialis posterior, and subtalar joint.[12]
  - Physical appearance: Changes may occur in the shape of the patient's foot, such as the presence of bunions or hammertoe.[15]

- Range of motion: Patients experience an overall reduced range of motion, and their ankle joints undergo less gliding and rotational motion compared to normal subjects.[8]
- Limited and painful ankle dorsiflexion and plantarflexion are appreciated, although isolated movements of the hindfoot and forefoot are not limited and are pain-free.[13]
- A complete examination of the ankle should also include evaluation of associated injuries:
  - Chondrocyte cell death may occur following direct injuries to cartilage after trauma.[13]
  - Even with appropriate open reduction and internal fixation, one must still look for structural changes to the ankle joint.[13]
  - Arthritis in the setting of trauma can lead to an asymmetrical pattern of wearing in the ankle joint, and associated changes include malalignment, altered weight-bearing forces, and incongruent joint loading.[13]
  - It is important to check for ligamentous injuries at the ankle joint as they can predispose to abnormal joint loading.[13]

IMAGING AND OTHER DIAGNOSTIC STUDIES

- Plain radiographs, including AP, lateral, and mortise views (three view series of the distal tibia, distal fibula, talus, and proximal metatarsals) in weight bearing[13]
- X-ray findings may include subchondral sclerosis, osteophytes, and asymmetrical joint space narrowing.[13]
- Having multiple weight-bearing views on plain radiograph may allow one to see varus or valgus tilt in the subtalar or ankle joint.[13]
- Other imaging modalities that may be helpful in diagnosing ankle arthritis include computed tomography (CT) scan and magnetic resonance imaging (MRI).
- CT scans have been shown to help in diagnosing occult arthritis in joints below the ankle; these findings have then led to bias in management by replacement or joint fusion.[13] Additionally, a weight-bearing CT can provide information on alignment.
- MRI is less useful in diagnosis but can help affect management because it can help to rule out stress fractures, soft tissue infections, and tumors.[13]

DIFFERENTIAL DIAGNOSIS

- Mechanical versus inflammatory pathology
- Malignancy
- Inflammatory arthropathy
- Stress fracture

NONOPERATIVE MANAGEMENT

- Combination therapy is indicated initially, which includes medications, orthotic devices, and footwear modifications.[18]
- Corticosteroid injections are sometimes used intra-articularly to help alleviate symptoms of pain and inflammation, although this effect has only proven to be effective up to 8 weeks. It is recommended to limit injections to two times per year.[15,18]
- Lifestyle modification in the form of weight loss is counseled among obese patients.[15,18]

- Orthotic shoe inserts help with pain relief in ankle arthritis by redistribution of stress of the foot to areas that are less arthritic.[15]
- Gait pattern can be improved with addition of a rocker bottom sole and solid ankle cushion heel to the shoe, as it improves forward progression of the tibia during gait.[18]
- Braces may also be used as an attempt to immobilize the ankle joint in cases where orthotics have either failed or were deemed inappropriate. These may be used in patients who are not surgical candidates.[5,15]
- Platelet-rich plasma and stem cells have been used and are seeing increasing interest. Success is mostly anecdotal at this time.

SURGICAL MANAGEMENT

Design of Cadence

- The Cadence Total Ankle System (Integra LifeSciences Corp., Princeton, NJ) was designed to treat ankle arthritis by reducing pain, restoring alignment of the ankle joint, and allowing for improved movement.[11]
- This system is predicated around a prosthetic model for total ankle replacement composed of a tibial tray, a talar dome, and an insert.[11]
- There are many advantages of the Cadence method:
  - The tibial component is sided, as it recreates the incisura, allowing for a resting place for the fibula.
  - Patient anatomy is preserved with specific implant designs to recreate optimal conical flexion and extension of the ankle and minimize resection of the talus and risk of injury to malleoli.[11]
  - Prosthetic alignment and symmetry are enhanced through a poly that comes in a neutral, anterior, or posterior bias. This allows for the treatment of patients with subluxation of the talus as well as ensure the final talar implant is appropriately aligned on the sagittal view.[11]
  - Polyethylene survivorship is optimized with an ultra-high-molecular-weight-bearing material, thereby reducing wear.[11]
  - The technique is easy to reproduce and allows for anatomic diversity among patients, with many multipurpose instruments and a single alignment guide (**FIG 1**).[11]

Preoperative Planning

- Weight-bearing radiographic imaging is evaluated for the foot and ankle.
- Images are investigated for presence of fractures, articular malalignment, loose bodies, and non-native material (hardware, foreign bodies).
- Any incidental lesions or injuries found on imaging or physical exam should also be addressed during the procedure, if possible.

Positioning

- The patient should be placed in the supine position, with the foot at the edge of the operating table.[11]
- Neutral rotation of the operative extremity is obtained by the placement of a bump under the ipsilateral hip of the affected extremity.[11]
- The ipsilateral tibia is also elevated by a bump in order to ensure that the affected heel is off the table.[11]

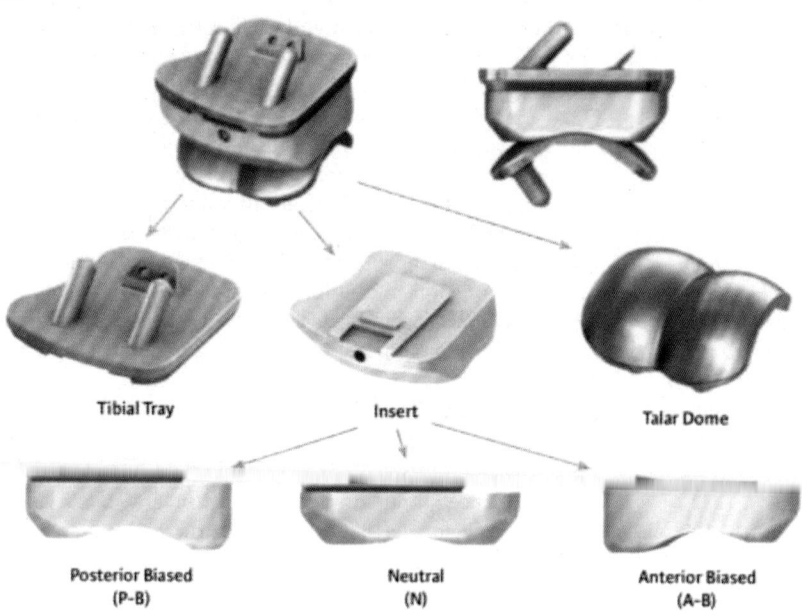

FIG 1 The Integra Cadence Total Ankle System caters to a diverse array of anatomic variability to best suit a patient's individual needs.

(labels within figure: Tibial Tray, Insert, Talar Dome, Posterior Biased (P-B), Neutral (N), Anterior Biased (A-B))

Approach

- An anterior longitudinal incision is created lateral to the subcutaneous border of the tibia proximally.
- The incision should extend across the midline of the ankle joint all the way to the dorsal medial border of the midfoot.
- As the dissection is carried down beneath the anterior tibia tendon bed, it is crucial to protect the anterior neurovascular bundle by mobilizing it laterally, along with the tendon of the extensor hallucis longus.

- Dissection parameters are as such:
  - Medially as far as the medial gutter in order to best visualize the medial malleolus
  - Laterally as far until the anterior inferior tibiofibular syndesmotic ligament and tubercle of Chaput become visible
- Contraindications for the Cadence system include active infection; skeletal immaturity; pregnancy; severe avascular necrosis of the talus/tibia; neurologic/musculoskeletal diseases, which can affect gait; and poor bone stock.

TECHNIQUES

INITIAL POSITIONING OF TIBIAL ALIGNMENT GUIDE

- Prior to positioning on the patient, assemble the tibial alignment guide—this consists of the proximal tibial clamp, the rod connector, and the proximal translation block (**TECH FIG 1**).
- The proximal translation block needs to be fixed to the center of the proximal tibial clamp with the aid of a hex screwdriver, and the anterior end of the proximal translation block must slide through the mating hole in the rod connector at the proximal end of the tibial rod.
- At the distal end, lock the tibial rod into the distal tibial alignment block and ensure neutrality of starting positions.
- For positioning purposes, the proximal tibial clamp must be adjusted to the patient's tibial tuberosity, whereas the distal tibial alignment block is placed on the center of the tibial metaphysis. The tibial rod should be parallel to the tibia in the sagittal plane, about 6 to 7 cm apart.
- Initial resection height is set by aligning the gap sizer with the joint line and then bringing the distal tibial alignment block into contact with the proximal part of the gap sizer.
- The tibial alignment guide is then held in place with a shoulder pin.
- Fluoroscopy is performed to ensure the distal block is in neutral to slight valgus orientation (**TECH FIG 2**). This can be adjusted with the proximal set screw in the rod connector.
- A lateral view is obtained, and the height of the tibial resection is set to the most distal aspect of the distal pegs on the angel wing.
- At this time, the slope of the cut is evaluated with the same angel wing. The external cutting jig is adjusted proximally to provide more plantarflexion or dorsiflexion as required.

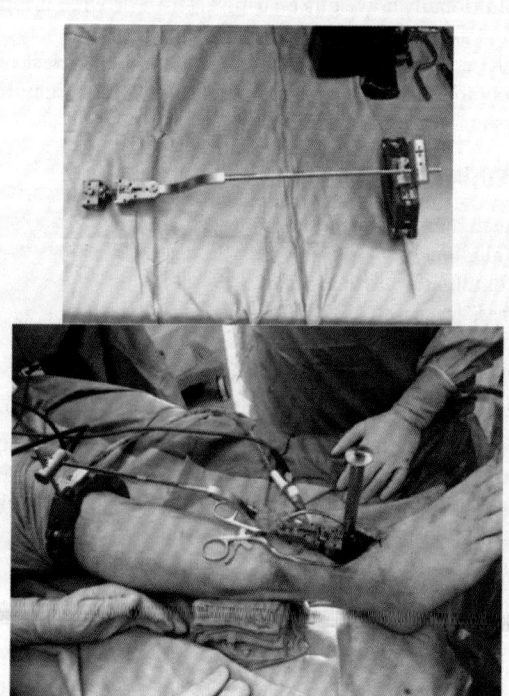

TECH FIG 1 Complete assembly of the tibial alignment guide.

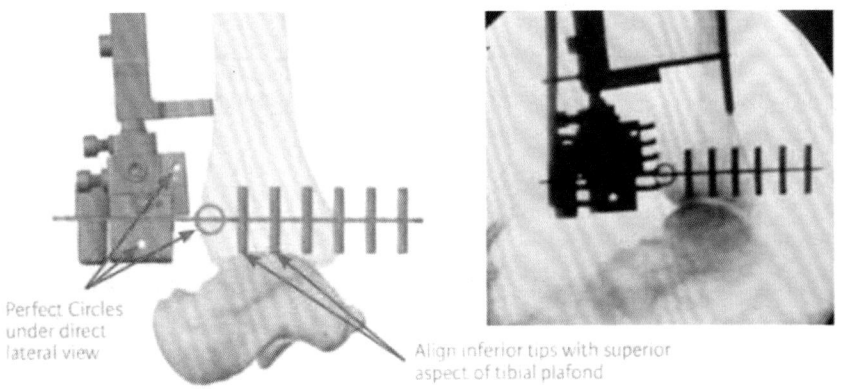

Perfect Circles
under direct
lateral view

Align inferior tips with superior
aspect of tibial plafond

TECH FIG 2 Ensuring proper amount of tibial resection.

TIBIAL ALIGNMENT GUIDE ADJUSTMENT

- An angle bisector is then placed into the center of the distal tibial alignment block and adjusted so that it points between the second and third metatarsal.
- At this point, the main priority for resection is to create adequate medial/lateral positioning, which is achieved by utilizing the adjustment screw on the distal tibial alignment block.
- Under fluoroscopy, the medial three holes in the cutting guide and aligned with the medial gutter or medial talar dome, as required by the patient's medial tibial and malleolar bone stock
- Once placed, under fluoroscopy, an initial size of the tibia can be determined by the lateral holes in the cutting jig. The correct tibial size is the one that is just medial to the medial fibular cortex.
- Without hitting the fibula, a straight bone pin with trocar tip is placed in the most lateral bone pin position that the tibial cut guide will allow.

- Next, it is important to protect the malleoli by marking the medial resection line of the distal tibia.
  - This is achieved by placing a straight bone pin adjacent to the saw slot and then drilling bicortically through each of the three medial distal holes on the tibial cut guide.
- A 1.27-mm thick saw blade is used for resection and extends to the posterior cortex of the tibia (**TECH FIG 3**).
- Medial resection is achieved by first removing the tibial cut guide and straight bone pins to access the resected tibial bone and then using either a corner osteotome or a reciprocating saw to cut the bone remaining between holes drilled previously.
- Finally, the resected bone is removed with the use of osteotomes or rongeurs.
  - At this time, only the anterior 60% of the tibial plafond needs to be removed.
  - Because internal and external rotation levering puts the malleoli at risk for fracture, one must apply only anteriorly directed force to remove bone.

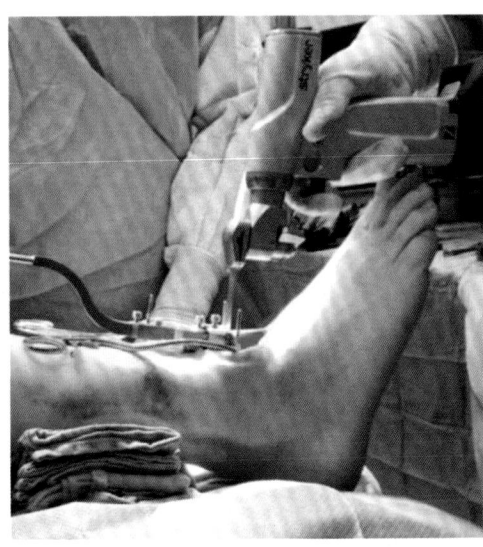

TECH FIG 3 Cutting bone during tibial resection.

TENSIONING OF THE TALUS

- Depending on the patient's anatomy and talar size, select the appropriate talar cut guide—defined by the lateral most hole overlapping the lateral gutter.
- The talar cut guide is then guided into position on the distal tibial alignment block until it comes into contact with the talus. The locking screw must then be secured on the cut guide.
- To increase tension on the talus, the locking screw on the distal tibial alignment block should be loosened, and lamina spreaders can be used to extend the talar cut guide as far distally as possible (**TECH FIG 4**).
  - The goal of this step is to tighten the collateral ligaments and compress the talar cut guide against the talus underneath it.
- Lastly, the distal/proximal locking screw on the distal tibial alignment block is locked, and lamina spreaders are removed in preparation for resection of the talus.

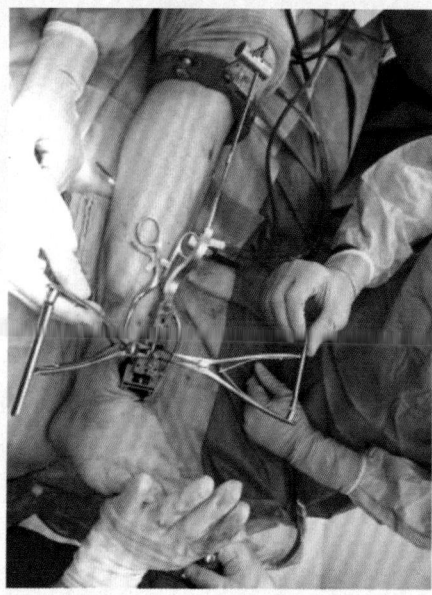

TECH FIG 4 Extension of talar cut guide via lamina spreaders to tighten collateral ligaments.

INITIAL TALAR BONE RESECTION

- The talus should be held in neutral plantigrade position. Next, a long shouldered bone pin should be inserted through the talar cut guide and into the talus after proper positioning is obtained.
- To protect the malleoli during talar resection, straight bone pins with trocar tips are inserted on both the medial and lateral sides of the saw slot for the talar cut guide (**TECH FIG 5**).

- A narrow width 1.27-mm thick saw blade is recommended for resection while ensuring that this procedure extends to the posterior cortex of the talus (**TECH FIG 6**).
- The tibial alignment guide assembly is detached, along with the talar cut guide and all bone pins.
- The resected bone is removed with the use of osteotomes or rongeurs.

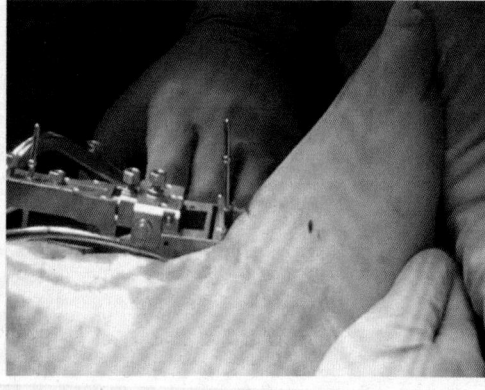

TECH FIG 5 Protecting the malleoli during initial talar resection by use of straight bone pins.

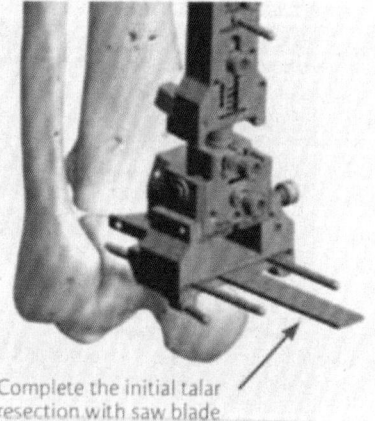

Complete the initial talar resection with saw blade

TECH FIG 6 Resecting the talus.

VERIFICATION OF THE REQUIRED IMPLANT GAP

- The gap sizer is used to ensure sufficient resection of tibial and talar bone—15 mm is the minimum amount of space required for positioning of the tibial and talar implant components (TECH FIG 7).

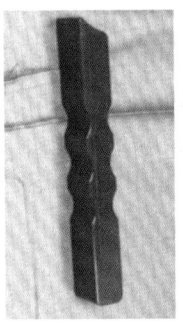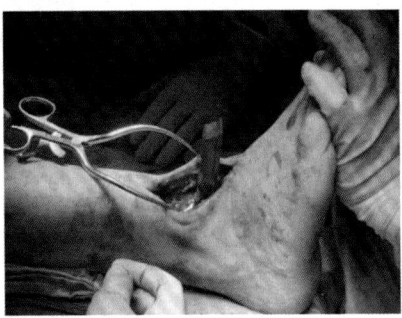

TECH FIG 7 Checking the resulting size with gap sizer.

- If the gap sizer is tight or does not fit, this indicates that not enough bone has resected.
  - Use the 2-mm tibial cut guide to resect additional tibial bone, as needed.
  - This is done in the same way as described previously.

Selection of Talar Dome Size

- A talar sizer is selected based on the individual patient's anatomy.
  - If a patient is in between two sizes, select the smaller size.
- The talar sizer is then inserted into the talar sizer holder—sliding until it "clicks."
- The selected talar sizer and holder are then placed onto the cut surface of the talus, taking care to match the outline of the sizer with the posterior edge of the talar bone, and centered medially and laterally.
  - The outline of the talar sizer corresponds to the outline of the talar implant component.

FINAL PREPARATION OF THE TALAR BONE

- Proper rotational alignment of the selected talar sizer must be attained; this is done by aligning the handle of the talar sizer holder with the patient's second to third metatarsal.
- The talar sizer holder is then expanded against the distal tibia to maintain proper medial/lateral, AP, and rotational alignment of the talar sizer.
- AP alignment of the talar sizer must be visualized with fluoroscopy (TECH FIG 8). The radius of curvature of the simulated articular surface should be contiguous with the posterior radius of curvature of the natural talus.
  - The AP center point of the talar sizer is represented by the point at the top of the triangle containing the saw slot.
  - The trajectory of the saw slot is represented by the small slot toward the posterior aspect of the talar sizer (this is seen well in the lateral view).

- A short shouldered bone pin and a straight bone pin with drill tip should be inserted into the bone pin holes to hold the location in place.
- The talar sizer holder is then removed from the talar sizer so that a narrow width saw blade (1.27 mm thick) can be placed in the saw slot and resect the posterior chamfer (TECH FIG 9).
- Following resection, the location of the talar sizer is maintained by reengagement of the talar sizer holder with the talar sizer and expansion against the distal tibia.
- The short shouldered bone pin from the previous step is then removed and replaced with another straight bone pin with drill tip.
- As the bone pins are left in position in the talus, the talar sizer is slid off over the pins in order to be removed.

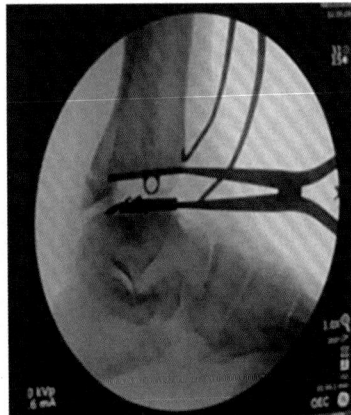

TECH FIG 8 Alignment of talar sizer with AP center of the distal tibia.

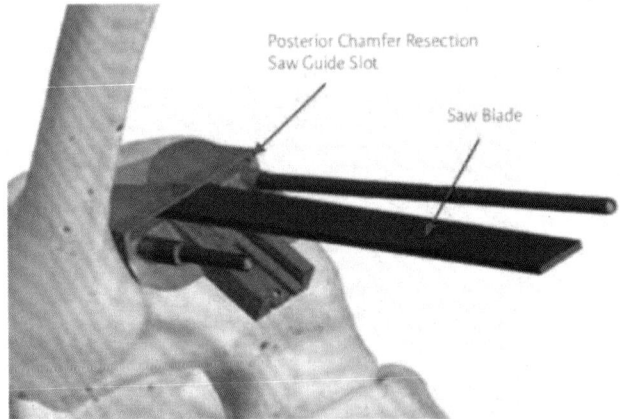

Posterior Chamfer Resection
Saw Guide Slot

Saw Blade

TECH FIG 9 Posterior chamfer resection.

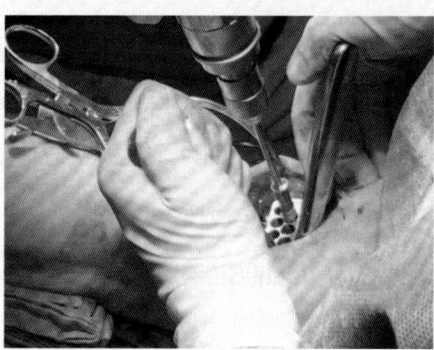

TECH FIG 10 Reaming the anterior chamfer.

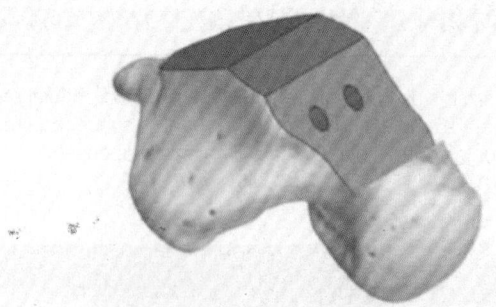

TECH FIG 12 Chamfer preparation for talar trial.

- The talar sizer is replaced with the anterior talar chamfer cut guide, which must first have its holes aligned with the two straight bone pins and is then slid into position until the cut guide rests on the initial flat surface of the proximal talus.
- Depending on the size of the talar sizer, the talar chamfer cut guide is then aligned with either the inside or outside holes.
  - If a size 1 or 2 talar sizer was selected, the inside holes will be used.
  - If a size 3, 4, or 5 talar sizer was selected, the outside holes will be used.
- Medium shoulder bone pins are then placed through each of the top holes of the chamfer cut guide prior to reaming the chamfer.
- The talar chamfer cut guide must be secured to the bone, resting on the flat surface created on the proximal talus; this can be ensured with the use of long shoulder bone pins for additional fixation.
- The two straight bone pins with drill tip are then removed from the talar chamfer cut guide.
- The talar chamfer reamer guide is then placed into the chamfer cut guide in the proper orientation, such that the "no. 1" markings are in the top left and top right hand corners of the reamer guide.
- Reaming occurs by initially securing the talar chamfer reamer guide against the cut guide and then placing the talar reamer down through the holes of the reamer guide into the anterior surface of the talus **(TECH FIG 10)**.
  - The shoulder of the reamer should come into contact with the face of the reamer guide.
  - The trajectory of the talar reamer should be perpendicular to the talar chamfer reamer guide, as reaming off-axis can damage instrumentation.

- Next, the reamer guide is removed and rotated 180 degrees before it is replaced into the cut guide, such that the "no. 2" markings should be in the top left and top right hand corners of the reamer guide.
  - Reaming then occurs in all nine holes of the reamer guide, using the same steps as described previously.
- The talar chamfer reamer guide is then removed from the cut guide.
- In preparation for drilling the talar post holes, the talar chamfer drill guide must be placed into the talar chamfer cut guide while ensuring that the "TOP/PROXIMAL" and "BOTTOM/DISTAL" markings are oriented properly **(TECH FIG 11)**.
- The post drill is then placed down through the holes in the drill guide, where it is used to drill implant post holes into the talus. Sufficient depth of drill is gauged by advancement of post drill until the shoulder of the drill contacts the bottom of the hole in the drill guide.
- After the chamfer cut guide, chamfer drill guide and both bone pins are removed from the talus, resected bone is removed from the chamfers and the remaining tibial plafond **(TECH FIG 12)**.

Placement of the Talar Trial

- The talar trial is first selected on the basis of the way in which it corresponds to the talar sizer chosen in prior steps.
- The posts of the talar trial are then placed into the post holes already prepared in the talus.
- The talar impactor is used to fully seat the trial **(TECH FIG 13)**.

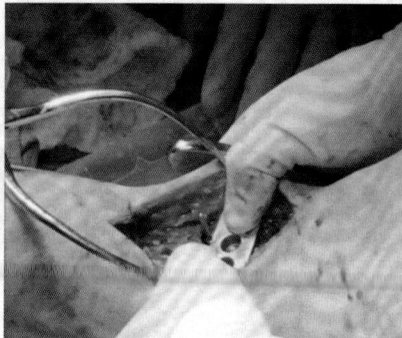

TECH FIG 11 Preparation for drilling of talar post holes.

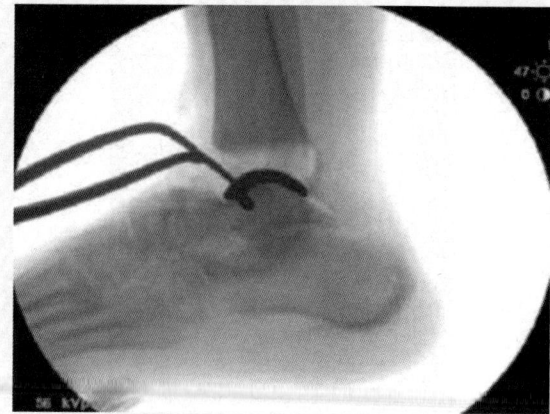

TECH FIG 13 Confirming the proper placement of chamfer and full seating of talar trial.

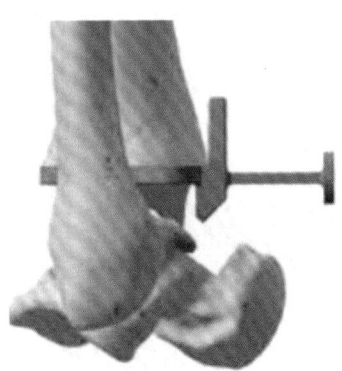

TECH FIG 14 Tibial tray sizing.

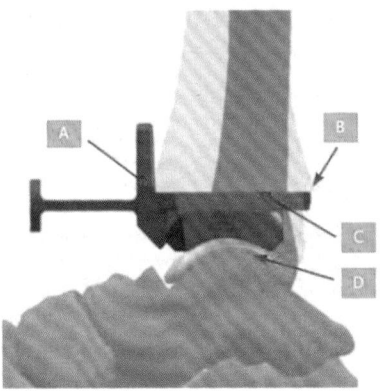

TECH FIG 16 Verifying proper placement of tibial and talar trials via visualization of four checkpoints.

Selection of Tibial Tray Size

- The depth of the tibia is measured. The tibial implant sizer is hooked onto the posterior cortex of the distal tibia, and the line on the tibial implant sizer that most closely approximates the anterior cortex of the distal tibia is determined **(TECH FIG 14)**.
- The selected tibial trial is then placed into the joint space, with precaution taken to avoid oversizing **(TECH FIG 15)**.

Placement of Tibial Tray with Insert Trials

- The size of the talar trial that was placed on the talus in a previous step dictates the corresponding size of the polyethylene insert trial.
  - The insert trials are reversible and can therefore be used as either right-handed ("RIGHT" and "R" markings face anteriorly) or left-handed ("LEFT" and "L" markings face anteriorly).
  - Insert trials are offered in 6 to 12 mm thicknesses in 1-mm increments—start with 6 mm.
  - Insert trials can also have an anterior or posterior attachment to help reduce the talus under the tibia on a sagittal view.
- The insert trial is then attached to the dovetail of the tibial trial.

- The tibial trial and insert trial assembly is placed into position on the distal tibia, with a goal of mating the articular surfaces of the two trials with each other.
- Joint kinematics and tension are evaluated via dynamic flexion/extension tests on the foot.
  - Tibial trial should find its optimal position on the frontal, sagittal, and rotational planes.
  - During evaluation, it may be determined that the joint is too loose—in this case, the assembly is removed, and the insert trial is replaced with incrementally thicker trials until proper joint kinematics and tension are attained.
- Visual and/or fluoroscopic verification is required to determine proper placement of the tibial trial on the resected tibia and talar trial on the resected talus **(TECH FIG 16)**.
  - The anterior aspect of the tibial trial should be flush against the anterior cortex of the distal tibia.
  - The posterior aspect of the tibial trial should extend to, but not past, the posterior cortex of the distal tibia.
  - The proximal surface of the tibial trial should sit flush across the entire distal surface of the tibia.
  - The chamfered surfaces of the talar trial should sit flush with the resected chamfered surfaces of the proximal talus.

Selected Talar implant size			M/L Width Determined by Tibial Tray Trial	A/P Length Determined from Tibial Implant Sizer	Recommended Tibial Tray Implant size
			1	1	1
1			1	1x or 2	1x
			2	1x or 2	2
	2		2	2x or 3	2x
			3	2x or 3	3
	3		3	3x or 4	3x
			4	3x or 4	4
	4		4	4x or 5	4x
		5	5	4x or 5	5

TECH FIG 15 Choosing the proper tibial implant size. *M/L*, Medial/Lateral; *A/P*, Anterior/Posterior.

FINAL PREPARATION OF THE TIBIAL BONE

- After proper placement of the tibial trial is determined, positioning is maintained by placement of two short shouldered bone pins through the two bone pin holes in the anterior face of the tibial trial.
- The post drill or flex shaft drill is used next in order to drill tibial implant post holes into the tibia through the tibial trial.
  - Correct depth is measured by ensuring that the shoulder of the drill comes into contact with the face of the tibial trial.
- Finally, the two short shouldered bone pins, tibial trial, and insert trial are removed.

Securing the Tibial Tray

- The talar trial is initially removed from the talus.
- Based on the size of the tibial trial, a corresponding tibial tray implant is selected, and bone cement is applied to the flat, titanium plasma–sprayed surface of the tray.
  - Bone cement must not be applied to the posts or to the posterior wedge.
- The tibial impactor handle is then screwed into the tibial impactor tip, and the dovetail of the impactor tip is slid into the dovetail of the tibial implant until it "clicks"—this signifies full engagement of the tibial tray.
  - To prevent overinsertion, the tibial impactor stop can be attached to the impactor tip.
- The anterior peg tips of the tray are engaged gently into the prepared peg holes.
- Prior to impaction, the foot is plantarflexed as is necessary to achieve proper positioning of the tibial tray.
- Fluoroscopic confirmation is used to ensure that the implant is parallel to the tibial cut while being impacted in place.
  - If the tray is not parallel to the resected tibia, impaction can result in posterior tibial fractures.
- Impaction (guided by fluoroscopy) continues until the implant is fully seated (**TECH FIG 17**).
  - The gap sizer can be inserted at an angle to help gently impact the posterior end of the tibial tray until it is fully seated.
- Once the tibial tray is fully seated, it is disengaged as the thumb lever on the tibial impactor tip is depressed.

Securing the Talar Dome

- Prior to placement of the talar dome, it is imperative to protect both the tibial tray and the talar dome implants from damage.
  - Therefore, the implant protector is slid into the dovetail of the tibial tray such that the implant protector covers the entire distal face of the tibial tray implant (**TECH FIG 18**).
- The talar dome implant that corresponds to the talar trial chosen previously is then selected, and bone cement is applied to the flat, titanium plasma–sprayed surfaces.
- Next, the posts of the talar dome implant are placed into the post holes prepared into the anterior chamfer of the talus.
- In order to fully seat the talar dome implant, the talar impactor is used to selectively apply posterior and interior impaction as it rotates.

Securing the Insert

- The implant protector is first removed from the tibial tray implant.
- The polyethylene inserter is then prepared as the top portion of the instrument is slid forward until it is flush with the etched line, which corresponds to the selected insert trial size.

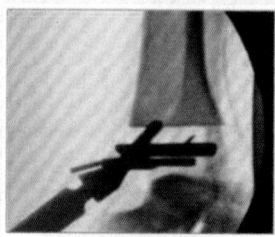
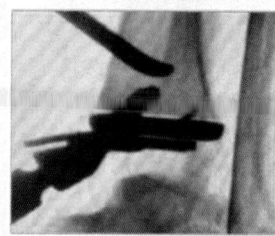
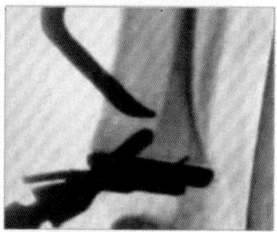

TECH FIG 17 Visualizing that the tibial implant is fully seated.

- Based on the size and thickness of the insert trial that was chosen previously, the corresponding insert implant is selected and loaded into the dovetail of the insert inserter.
- The exposed posterior portion of the dovetail of the insert implant is placed into the dovetail of the tibial tray implant.
  - The tip of the insert inserter should contact the anterior face of the implant.
  - If the posterior portion of the dovetail feature is not engaged, later impaction by the mallet may prevent proper securing of the insert.
- Insert implant must then be pushed as far possible manually into the tibial tray implant.
- For full seating of the insert implant into the tibial tray implant, a mallet can be used to gently impact the handle of the insert inserter until an audible click occurs.

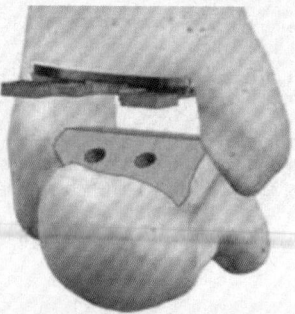

TECH FIG 18 Sliding the implant protector into tibial implant dovetail.

VERIFICATION OF THE FINAL IMPLANT

- Lateral fluoroscopic guidance is required to ensure the following criteria are met:
  - The proximal surface of the tibial implant sits flush across the entire distal surface of the tibia.
  - The posterior aspect of the tibial implant extends to, but not past, the posterior cortex of the tibia.
  - The chamfered surfaces of the talar implant sit flush with the resected chamfered surfaces of the talus.
- The next step requires visual verification of proper seating for all the implants (**TECH FIG 19**).
  - The anterior aspect of the tibial implant is flush against the anterior cortex of the tibia.
  - The insert implant is seated fully in the tibial implant, with no gap between the anterior surfaces of the two implants.
- Finally, functionality of the procedure is again tested with a dynamic flexion/extension test on the foot to evaluate the joint's kinematics and tension.

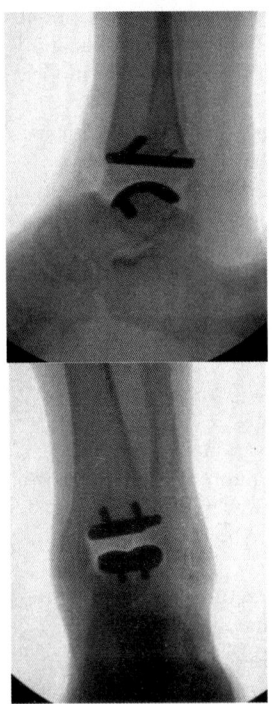

TECH FIG 19 Fluoroscopic confirmation of the proper placement of the final implant.

TECHNIQUES

SPECIAL CONSIDERATIONS

- Biased inserts
  - For patients with either an anterior or posterior sub-luxed talus, the Integra Cadence Total Ankle System also features anterior biased insert and posterior biased insert implants for additional joint constraint/support.
  - Lateral fluoroscopic evaluation of implant trials relative to patient anatomy can determine that the patient would benefit from the use of a biased insert.
  - Biased insert trial extensions can be used to evaluate their benefit and make a final determination as to their utility in each individual patient scenario.
  - The post of the biased insert trial extension is pushed into the threaded hole in the center of the insert trial until the mating surfaces of the two components are flush.
  - For simulation of anterior biased insert implant, the extension should be placed on the anterior surface of the insert trial and conversely to simulate posterior bias.
- Relative outcomes
  - Based on recent studies looking at Cadence versus other systems of total ankle arthroplasty, there appears to be no difference among implants in complication rates or other outcome measures.[14]

POSTOPERATIVE CARE

- Plain radiographs are used to ensure full seating of implants and proper alignment of unit.
- A hospital stay of 0 to 3 days may be needed.
- Ambulation directly following surgery will be restricted, with specific limitations left up to the protocol of the surgeon based on each individual patient scenario.
  - Restrictions on ambulation generally last 3 to 6 weeks following operation.
- Achieving early range of motion is encouraged.
- Rehabilitation therapy is typically started 6 to 8 weeks after surgery, but normal activities of daily living can usually be resumed within the first 2 weeks.[10]
- The main factors in determining a patient's ability to return to work are accommodations for transportation, parking, office access, and ability to rest and keep elevation on the foot.
  - If these resources are provided, the patient typically returns to work in 2 to 3 weeks postoperatively.
  - Patients who have more physical demands in their work will typically return 3 to 4 months postoperatively, once they have recovered endurance for standing and walking.

OUTCOMES

- Recovery of full ankle function may take as long as 12 months and is contingent on patient adherence to postoperative rehabilitation and physical therapy.
- Residual swelling persists for 6 to 12 months.
- The postoperative rates of complications are the same for Cadence as it is with other models of total ankle arthroplasty.
- Success of the surgery depends on patient's age, baseline activity level, and other factors.
- Outcomes are improved if patients do not bear weight on the affected ankle joint immediately after surgery and follow-up regularly with the surgeon after operation.

COMPLICATIONS

- Complications for the Cadence system are the same as they are for other modalities of total ankle arthroplasty, which include the following[2]:
  - Injury to neurovascular structures
  - Malpositioning/improper sizing of prosthetic components
  - Malleolar fractures
  - Infection/impaired wound healing
  - Stress fractures
  - Periprosthetic fractures
  - Aseptic loosening
  - Heterotopic bone formation

REFERENCES

1. Andrews JR, Previte WJ, Carson WG. Arthroscopy of the ankle: technique and normal anatomy. Foot Ankle 1985;6(1):29–33.
2. Bestic JM, Peterson JJ, DeOrio JK, et al. Postoperative evaluation of the total ankle arthroplasty. AJR Am J Roentgenol 2008;190(4):1112–1123.
3. Daniels T, Thomas R. Etiology and biomechanics of ankle arthritis. Foot Ankle Clin 2008;13:341–352.
4. De Maeseneer M, Madani H, Lenchik L, et al. Normal anatomy and compression areas of nerves of the foot and ankle: US and MR imaging with anatomic correlation. Radiographics 2015;35(5):1469–1482.
5. Gentile MA. Nonsurgical treatment of ankle arthritis. Clin Podiatr Med Surg 2017;34:415–423.
6. Giebel GD, Meyer C, Koebke J, et al. The arterial supply of the ankle joint and its importance for the operative fracture treatment. Surg Radiol Anat 1997;19:231–235.
7. Golanó P, Vega J, de Leeuw PA, et al. Anatomy of the ankle ligaments: a pictorial essay. Knee Surg Sports Traumatol Arthrosc 2010;18:557–569.
8. Greaser M, Ellington JK. Ankle arthritis. J Arthritis 2014;3(2):1–5.
9. Hrdlicka A. Study of the normal tibia. Am Anthropol 1898;11(10):307–312.
10. Integra®. Cadence® Total Ankle System: Patient Information. Austin, TX: Ascension Orthopedics, 2017.
11. Integra®. Cadence® Total Ankle System: Surgical Technique. Austin, TX: Ascension Orthopedics, 2017.
12. Lee IM, Chung CT, Wolf JH, et al. Adjacent tissue involvement of acute inflammatory ankle arthritis on magnetic resonance imaging findings. Int Orthop 2013;37:1943–1947.
13. Martin RL, Stewart GW, Conti SF. Posttraumatic ankle arthritis: an update on conservative and surgical management. J Orthop Sports Phys Ther 2007;37(5):253–259.
14. Mulligan RP, Parekh SG. Safety of outpatient total ankle arthroplasty vs traditional inpatient admission or overnight observation. Foot Ankle Int 2017;38(8):825–831.
15. NYU Langone Health. Diagnosing foot & ankle arthritis. NYU Langone Health Website. Available at: https://nyulangone.org/conditions/foot-ankle-arthritis-in-adults/diagnosis. Accessed May 24th, 2019.
16. Saltzman CL, Salamon ML, Blanchard GM, et al. Epidemiology of ankle arthritis: report of a consecutive series of 639 patients from a tertiary orthopaedic center. Iowa Orthop J 2005;25:44–46.
17. Stamatis ED. Supramalleolar osteotomy with internal fixation. In: Easley ME, Wiesel SW, eds. Operative Techniques in Foot and Ankle Surgery. Philadelphia: Wolters Kluwer, 2016:473.
18. Thomas RH, Daniels TR. Ankle arthritis. J Bone Joint Surg Am 2003;85(5):923–936.
19. Zhao DH, Huang DC, Zhang GH, et al. Gender variation in the shape of superior talar dome: a cadaver measurement based on Chinese population. Biomed Res Int 2018;2018:6087871.

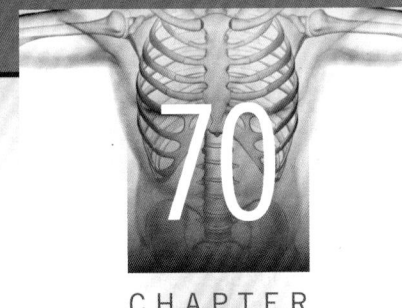

70 CHAPTER

Vantage Total Ankle Replacement

Jie Chen, James K. DeOrio, Victor Valderrabano, and Mark E. Easley

DEFINITION

- The Vantage (Exactech, Gainesville, FL) total ankle prosthesis is one of the newest total ankle systems on the market.
- Design features include the following:
  - Tibial fixation with three vertical pegs to allow axial loading and immediate weight bearing
  - Central fenestrated tibial cage to allow for bony ingrowth
  - Posterolateral cutout of the tibial component to allow space for the fibula and prevent impingement
  - Anatomically curved talus to allow for minimal bone resection and increase anteroposterior (AP) stability
  - Anterior flange of the talar component to prevent subsidence
  - Unique locking clip mechanism to facilitate easy polyethylene insertion and removal
  - The ability to match any size talus with any size tibia
- The Vantage total ankle system is available as a two-component semiconstrained fixed-bearing system or a three-component unconstrained mobile-bearing system.

ANATOMY

- The ankle is a unique joint made up of articulations between the distal tibia, the fibula, and the talus with multiple ligaments providing static constraint.
  - The cartilage found in the ankle has greater stiffness and decreased permeability compared to cartilage found elsewhere.[1] Chondrocytes synthesize proteoglycans at an increased rate, leading to increased repair capacity.
  - Normal range of motion is 20 degrees of dorsiflexion and 50 degrees of plantarflexion with minimal degrees of inversion and eversion.
- The tibial plafond and medial malleolus
  - Dorsal and medial articulations with the talus
  - Slight posterior slope of the plafond in the sagittal plane
  - Tibial plafond articular surface is 88 to 92 degrees relative to the lateral tibial shaft axis in the coronal plane
- The talus
  - A 60% of the articular surface is covered by articular cartilage.
  - Central trochlea for tibial articulation allows for increased stability.
- The fibula
  - Articulates with the lateral talus and provides lateral buttress
  - Responsible for one-sixth of axial load distribution of the ankle
  - Attachment point of several important ligaments

- The distal tibiofibular syndesmosis
  - Anterior inferior tibiofibular ligament
  - Interosseous membrane
  - Transverse tibiofibular ligament
  - Posterior tibiofibular ligament
- Lateral ankle ligaments
  - Anterior talofibular ligament
  - Calcaneofibular ligament
  - Posterior talofibular ligament

PATHOGENESIS

- Posttraumatic arthritis: most common cause by far
  - Intra-articular fracture
  - Ankle fracture-dislocation with malunion
  - Chronic ankle instability
  - Stage IV posterior tibial tendon dysfunction
- Primary osteoarthritis: relatively uncommon compared to primary osteoarthritis of the hip and knee
- Inflammatory arthropathy: most commonly rheumatoid arthritis
- Other
  - Hemochromatosis
  - Pigmented villonodular synovitis
  - Charcot neuroarthropathy
  - Septic arthritis
  - Tibial shaft fracture leading to altered ankle biomechanics

NATURAL HISTORY

- Ankle fractures and fractures to the articular surface of the tibial plafond lead to malunion, cartilage damage, or malalignment, which lead to progressive cartilage wear. Altered joint loading forces are found with even minor articular incongruity.
- Chronic lateral ankle instability or disruption to the syndesmosis or medial deltoid ligament leads to altered gait mechanics of the ankle which are associated with
  - Widened tibiofibular distance
  - Varus tilt of the talus within the ankle mortise
  - Relative anterior subluxation of the talus relative to the tibia
- Stage IV posterior tibial tendon dysfunction can lead to valgus tilt of the talus within the ankle mortise and arthritis of the ankle, the potential for a lateral malleolar stress fracture, and compensatory forefoot varus.
- Primary osteoarthrosis of the ankle is rare and poorly understood.

- Inflammatory arthropathy
  - Progressive and proliferative synovial erosive changes failing to respond to medical management

PATIENT HISTORY AND PHYSICAL FINDINGS

- Patients often present with a history of trauma to the ankle
  - Ankle fractures, particularly intra-articular
  - Unstable ankle fractures with malunion
  - Ankle fractures anatomically fixed may still develop posttraumatic arthritis.
  - Chronic ankle instability and a history of recurrent ankle sprains
  - History of long-standing painful flatfoot deformity, tibial shaft fracture, rheumatoid arthritis, or ankle infection
  - Ankle pain worse with weight bearing may be particularly painful going up hills or stairs due to anterior impingement with dorsiflexion.
  - Swelling and stiffness
  - Progressively worsening activity level
- Physical examination
  - Antalgic gait
  - Obligatory hip external rotation to externally rotate the ankle and avoid painful push-off
  - Tenderness to palpation at the anterior ankle joint, medial, or lateral gutters
  - Edema about the ankle
  - Decreased range of motion with crepitation and painful range of motion, particularly dorsiflexion
  - Can have visible varus or valgus deformity secondary to chronic instability
    - Ankles with arthritis due to long-standing chronic instability are usually stable to anterior drawer examination.

IMAGING AND OTHER DIAGNOSTIC STUDIES

- Weight-bearing radiographs including AP, lateral, and mortise views of the ankle (**FIG 1**).
- If there is associated hindfoot or leg deformity, obtain weight-bearing AP and lateral views of the tibia-fibula and also hindfoot alignment views. Weight-bearing full leg-length views bilaterally are useful for significant lower extremity deformity.
- Obtain weight-bearing foot AP, lateral, and oblique views if there is associated foot deformity, which may need to be addressed.
- Weight-bearing computed tomography scans of the ankle are used to evaluate bone stock, hindfoot alignment, and the presence of cysts.
- Magnetic resonance imaging is used to evaluate the viability of the talus or distal tibia if there is concern for avascular necrosis.

DIFFERENTIAL DIAGNOSIS

- Subtalar arthritis
- Ankle instability
- Osteochondral defect
- Peroneal tendonitis
- Posterior tibialis tendon dysfunction
- Painful os trigonum

NONOPERATIVE MANAGEMENT

- Activity modification
- Shoe wear modification including stiffer-soled shoe and rocker-bottom modification
- Bracing
  - Ankle–foot orthosis
  - Double-upright brace attached to shoe

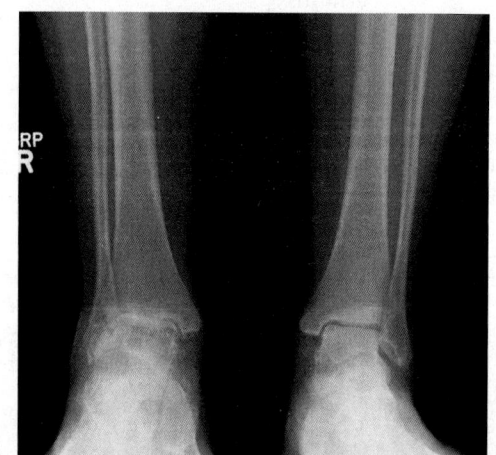
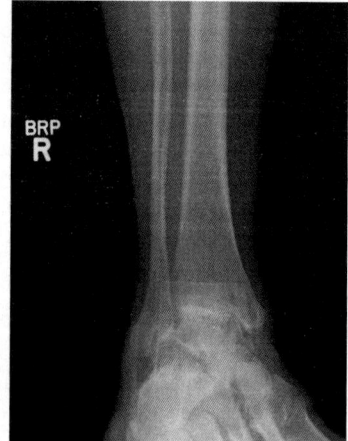
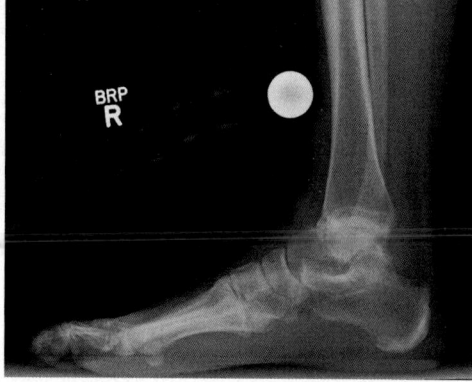

FIG 1 Preoperative weight-bearing x-rays of a 60-year-old male patient with end-stage right-ankle arthritis. **A.** AP view. **B.** Mortise view. **C.** Lateral view.

- Nonsteroidal anti-inflammatories
- Topical analgesics
- Systemic inflammatory or immune modulators for inflammatory arthropathy
- Intra-articular corticosteroid injections
- Viscosupplementation

SURGICAL MANAGEMENT

- Surgery is indicated when a prolonged period of nonoperative management fails.
- Consideration should be paid to the following risk factors:
  - Young age
  - Obesity
  - Diabetes mellitus
  - Neuropathy
  - History of smoking
  - History of depression
  - Preexisting deformity
  - Current range of motion
  - Poor bone stock

Preoperative Planning

- The surgeon should perform a diligent physical examination with significant attention to the following:
  - Location of surgical scars indicating previous incisions in order to plan the approach
  - Deformity of the ankle, which may require additional procedures to balance the ankle
  - Compensatory hindfoot or foot deformities, which may need to be addressed
  - Neurovascular examination to assess for adequacy of perfusion and for neuropathy
  - Range of motion
  - History of previous ipsilateral knee, leg, and foot procedures. In particular, a total knee arthroplasty in place may interfere with the tibial tubercle pin, and any hardware about the leg or ankle should be identified in the preoperative planning stage.
- Additional procedures may include the following:
  - Medial release
  - Lateral ligament reconstruction
  - Cotton osteotomy

- First metatarsal dorsiflexion osteotomy
- Gastrocnemius release or tendo-Achilles lengthening
- Tendon transfers or lengthening
- Subtalar arthrodesis
- Calcaneus slide osteotomy
- Posterior capsule release
- Anterior tibiotalar exostectomy
- Instrumentation
  - Small oscillating and small reciprocating saw
  - V. Mueller bone impactor set
  - Angled curette to separate tibial bone from posterior capsule
  - Toothless lamina spreader to distract the ankle when additional exposure is needed
  - Set of osteotomes

Positioning

- Patient is positioned supine with the foot at the edge of the operating room table.
- A bump is placed under the ipsilateral hip so that the patella is facing directly up, and the toes are directed to the ceiling.
- Side railings are placed on the bed in case the table needs to be tilted for additional procedures such as a lateral ligament reconstruction.
- A well-padded unsterile thigh tourniquet is placed.
- We routinely use regional anesthesia with a popliteal block. We have found that long-acting bupivacaine works well and can routinely provide 3 days of relief.
  - A regional catheter, which is pulled by the patient in the postoperative period, is another option.
  - A femoral block can be given as a supplement, but the patient will forfeit active knee extension, which may hinder immediate postoperative mobilization. General anesthesia can be used as well.
- A large C-arm is used for fluoroscopy.

Approach

- An anterior approach to the ankle is made, using the interval between the tibialis anterior (TA) tendon and the extensor hallucis longus (EHL) tendon.
- Incision can be cheated slightly medial or lateral to incorporate previous incisions.

EXPOSURE

- Midline incision is made centered approximately 1 cm lateral to the anterior border of the tibial crest (**TECH FIG 1A**).
- Incision is approximately 15 cm long centered on the ankle joint.
- Once through skin, scissors are used to mobilize the superficial peroneal nerve laterally, which may cross from lateral to medial in the distal part of the incision (**TECH FIG 1B**).
- Full-thickness dissection is taken down to the extensor retinaculum. The EHL and the TA tendons are visualized through the sheath.
- The EHL sheath and retinaculum is incised along the extent of the incision, with care to preserve the TA tendon sheath.

Alternatively, some surgeons prefer to incise the retinaculum just lateral to the TA tendon, which is directly in line with the deeper dissection plane.
- The EHL and TA tendons are retracted laterally and medially, and scissors are used to spread longitudinally down to bone medial to the deep anterior neurovascular bundle.
- Once on bone, capsule and periosteum is sharply incised and elevated with full-thickness flaps medially and lateral to expose the medial and lateral gutters and malleoli.
- Self-retaining Gelpi retractor is inserted deep with handle facing proximal at this stage to retract the neurovascular bundle laterally and maintain exposure (**TECH FIG 1C**).

TECHNIQUES

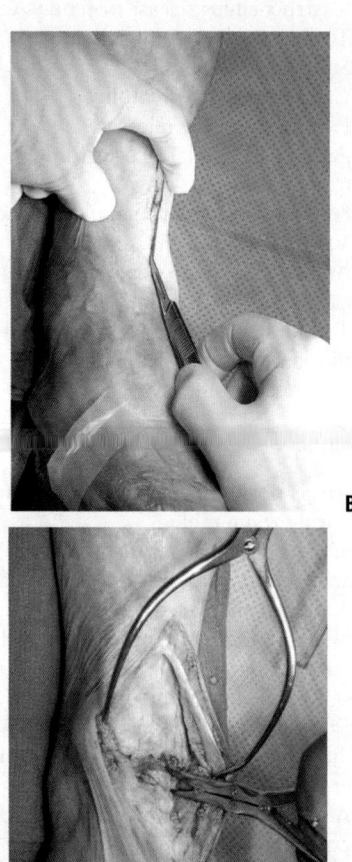
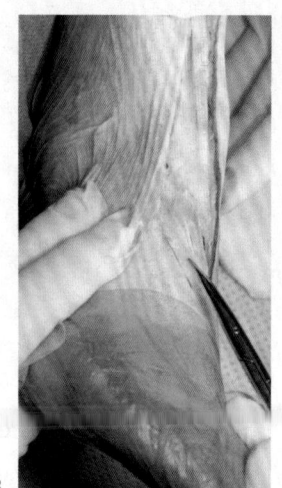
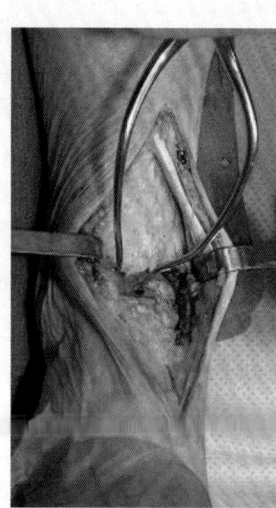

TECH FIG 1 **A.** Anterior incision centered 1 cm lateral to the tibial crest. **B.** Scissors used to dissect out the superficial peroneal nerve. **C.** Gelpi retractor placed between EHL and TA tendons at the level of the ankle. **D.** Rongeur used for osteophyte removal to expose the tibiotalar joint.

- Remove anterior tibial and talar osteophytes with a small oscillating saw or osteotome and rongeur to identify joint level and allow instrumentation guide to sit flush on bone (TECH FIG 1D).
- Use a curved osteotome to remove any remaining cartilage on the talar dome so that the talar guide will sit flush on the prepared bony surface.

- Use a 4-mm wide skinny rongeur to débride the medial and lateral gutters of any loose bodies, scar tissue, and other potentially impinging debris.

ANKLE ALIGNMENT AND TIBIAL PREPARATION

- Place medial shim (sword) into medial gutter in order to guide rotational placement of the proximal tibial tubercle pin (TECH FIG 2A).
- Place the 5-mm threaded tubercle pin into the tibial tubercle with care to match the rotation of the medial shim and perpendicular to the tibial bone in the sagittal plane.
- Place the anterior alignment guide with the tibial cutting block attached over the pin so that the rod is about two fingerbreadths off of the anterior skin.

- Gross adjustments are made by placing the anterior alignment guide into valgus, centering the distance of the tibial cut guide over the ankle joint. Proximally, move the guide into valgus halfway. Place the flag in the anterior guide slot and adjust rotation using the screwdriver in the rotation slot so that the flag is parallel to the sword. You should also match the rotation of the flag with the second ray of the foot.
- Once rotation is adjusted, drive a flexible thin pin into the large pinhole at the top of the anterior guide through just the anterior tibial cortex (TECH FIG 2B).

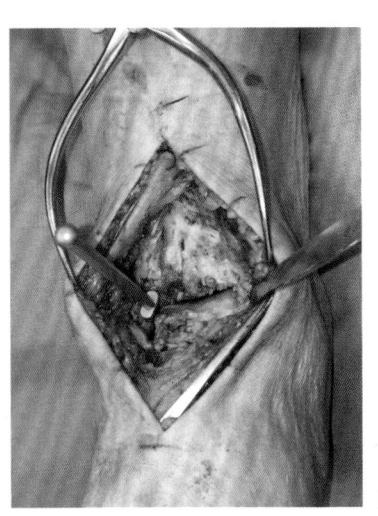
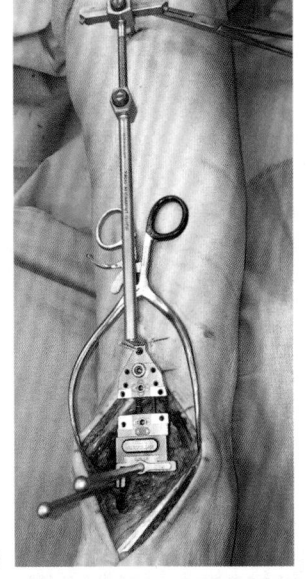
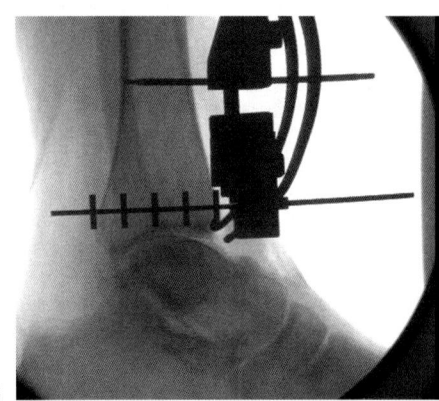

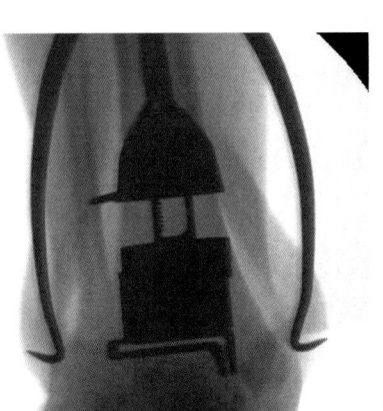
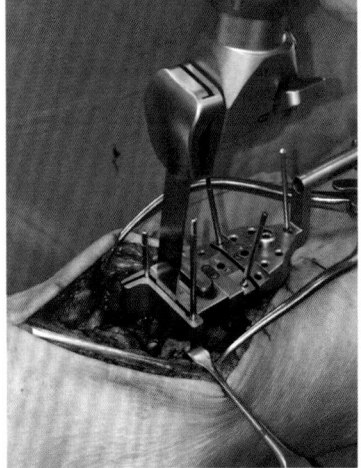

TECH FIG 2 A. Medial shim placed into the medial gutter following exposure. **B.** Anterior alignment guide with flexible pin in place following gross adjustment of proximal to distal length and placement of the flagpole to match the medial shim alignment. **C.** Lateral x-ray taken demonstrating thinning out of the angel wing and appropriate resection level and slope. **D.** AP x-ray of the ankle showing appropriate tibial cutting block size and appropriate medial to lateral placement. **E.** Oscillating saw to make tibial cut with protection pins in place.

- Under AP fluoroscopy, adjust the varus–valgus position of the anterior alignment rod so that it is parallel to the slope of the lateral cortex of the tibial shaft.
- Place the angel wing into the tibial cutting block laterally and on lateral fluoroscopy, abduct or adduct the leg so that the angel wing is parallel to the x-ray beam as indicated by thinning out of the wing.
- Finely move the guide proximally or distally using the hex screwdriver so that the 7-mm tabs hit the bottom of the tibial plafond with the angel wing parallel to the x-ray beam.
- Adjust the slope by moving the proximal alignment rod up or down the tibial tubercle pin so that the tibial cut is perpendicular to the distal tibia on lateral fluoroscopy **(TECH FIG 2C).**
- Place one pin into the proximal block and one into the distal block of the cutting guide unicortically.
- Use the smaller tibial cutting block with size 1 or 2 for smaller individuals and the larger cutting guide with size 3 or 4 for medium or larger individuals. Place into the distal portion of the anterior guide and adjust the medial to lateral position using the screwdriver under fluoroscopy so that the distal fibula and medial malleolus are not compromised **(TECH FIG 2D).**
- Place protection pins bicortically into the medial and lateral corners of the tibial cutting block.
- Use the larger oscillating saw to cut the distal tibia between the protection pins, with care not to plunge into the posterior neurovascular bundle **(TECH FIG 2E).**
  - Some surgeons open the posteromedial ankle and place a malleable retractor behind the tibia and in front of the posterior tibial tendon to protect the posterior structures.
- Use the large reciprocating saw to cut the distal tibia in the vertical slot of the tibial cutting block.
- Attempt to remove the cut bone in one piece. If the piece breaks, use a reciprocating saw to cut the remaining bone into smaller fragments, which can be removed using a rongeur and right angle curette.

TALAR PREPARATION

- Remove the distal tibial cutting block and insert the talar cutting guide. Choose a 2-mm cut guide if there is loss of talar height or the joint appears to be loose and a 4-mm cut guide for a talus with normal height.
- Remove the pin from the distal portion of the anterior alignment guide to allow for proximal movement of the talar guide.
- Dorsiflex the ankle to 90 degrees and slight valgus, use the screwdriver to drive the talar guide into the talar dome surface in order to tension the ligaments, and pin the distal block in place (TECH FIG 3A).
- Check a lateral x-ray with the angel wing inserted into the talar cutting guide to ensure an appropriate resection level perpendicular to the tibia with the ankle at 90 degrees of dorsiflexion (TECH FIG 3B).
- Use the oscillating saw in the middle of the guide slot to resect the top of the talar dome. Do not veer too far medially or laterally as the malleoli are not protected with capture guide pins.
- Remove the talar cutting block and complete the resection using the oscillating or small reciprocating saw to finish the cut if not complete.
- With all bone removed, insert the size specific gap spacer to ensure adequate resection (TECH FIG 3C).
- Remove all guides and pins at this point. The proximal tibial tubercle pin must be removed in reverse.
- Use the tibial measuring guide to measure the AP tibial size at this step by hooking the posterior cortex of the tibia.
- Choose a talar sizing guide ("lollipop") that sufficiently covers the talar surface without overhang. Place the talar lollipop onto the cut talar surface with attention to AP position and rotation down the second metatarsal.
- Place the distraction tool to hold the lollipop in place and check a perfect lateral x-ray of the lollipop by abducting and adducting the leg and rotating the foot and ankle until the center hole in the lollipop is a perfect circle (TECH FIG 3D).

- On this perfect lateral, ensure that the hole in the lollipop is directly above the lateral process of the talus (TECH FIG 3E).
- Place two pins into the talar lollipop. Remove the lollipop and the distraction tool by sliding over the pins.
- Place the corresponding talar chamfer block over the alignment pins until down on bone. Pin into place with two oblique pins (TECH FIG 3F).
- Use the oscillating saw to cut the posterior chamfer through the posterior slot, making sure to stay centered as the malleoli are not protected. Cut no more than ½ inch deep to avoid posterior structures. Do not cut deeper than ¼ inch. You can remove additional bone under direct vision using the small reciprocating saw.
- Use the anterior mill tool to remove talar bone through the two anterior slots. Do this by making two middle holes and then a medial and lateral hole on the sides of the slot. Then, run the router diagonally to connect the holes and then medial to lateral while aiming vertically at the bone (TECH FIG 3G).
- Remove the two anterior pins to make room for the second posterior chamfer cut. Use the oscillating saw to make this cut, making sure to stay centered as the malleoli are not protected.
- Remove the chamfer guide and remove any cut bone. Any incomplete cuts can be completed with a small reciprocating saw.
- Use a Cushing rongeur to remove the anterior talar bone directly distal to the cut surface of the top of the talus in order to make room for the dome rasp. Use a small rasp to flatten out the bone.
- Use the large rasp that corresponds to the size of the talus to rasp the talus forward and backward with care to rasp all the way anterior and posterior until high spots are removed (TECH FIG 3H).

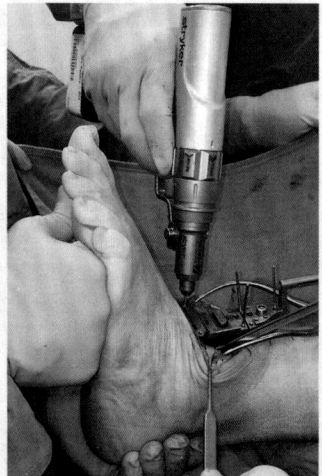 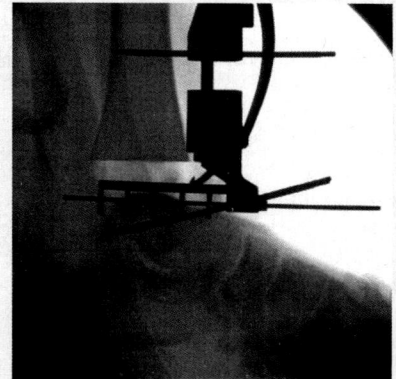 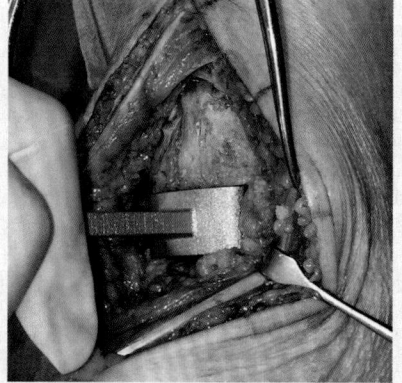

TECH FIG 3 A. Foot in optimal position for pinning of the talar cutting guide. **B.** Lateral x-ray showing appropriate talar resection level with the foot at 90 degrees of dorsiflexion. **C.** Gap sizing block to check adequateness of tibial and talar resection. *(continued)*

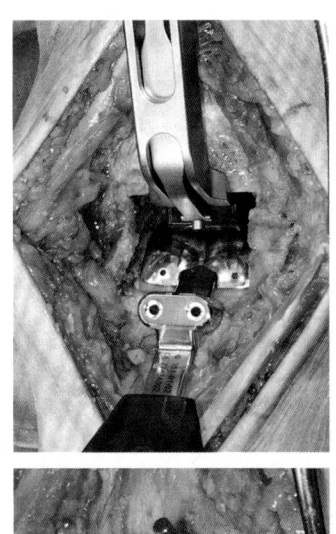

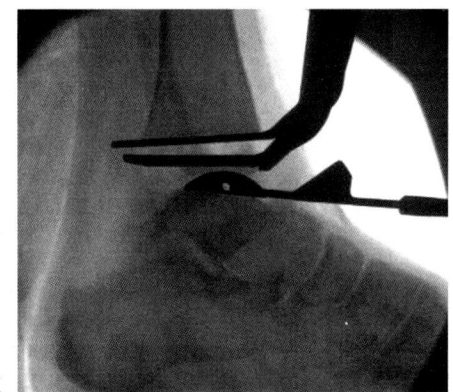

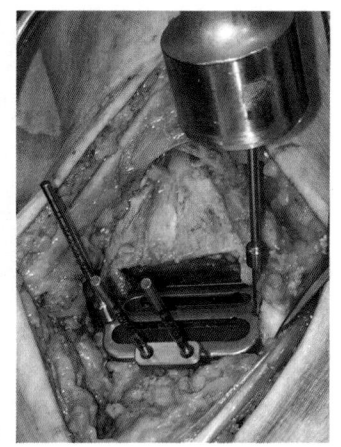

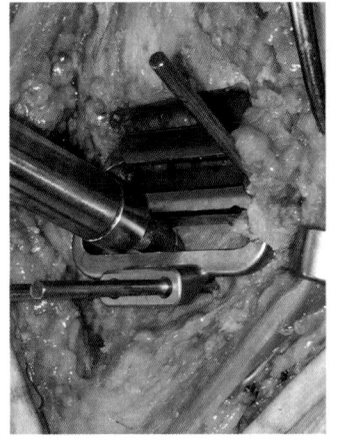

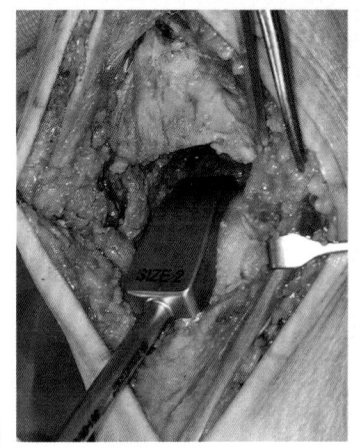

TECH FIG 3 *(continued)* **D.** Talar lollipop in place with distraction tool. **E.** Lateral x-ray showing talar lollipop with perfect circle directly over lateral process of talus. **F.** Talar chamfer cut guide placed onto bone and pinned into place. **G.** Milling of the slots on the talar chamfer guide with router. **H.** Large rasp to even the bone surface.

TRIAL PLACEMENT

- Place the talar trial on the cut talus with care taken to ensure correct medial–lateral and AP position and rotation. Insert the screw to hold it in place (TECH FIG 4A).
- Place the appropriately sized tibial trial and the appropriate punch liner and take an AP and lateral x-ray to ensure appropriate position of the trials (TECH FIG 4B).
  - The central cutouts of the talar trial should align on a perfect lateral x-ray and be centered over the lateral process of the talus (TECH FIG 4C).
- Once satisfied with the position, drill the two anterior holes through the talar trial.
- The tibial trial should sit flush on the bone surface without significant overhang. The thumb screw can be used to bring the anterior edge of the tibial trial flush with the bone. At this point, the punch liner and talar trial can be removed and a laminar spreader used to push the tibial trial flush against the bone. Check the range of motion.

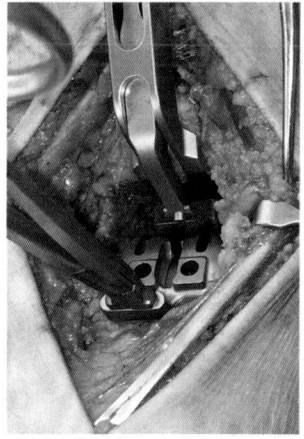

A

TECH FIG 4 A. Talar trial in place with center slot for a screw. *(continued)*

TECHNIQUES

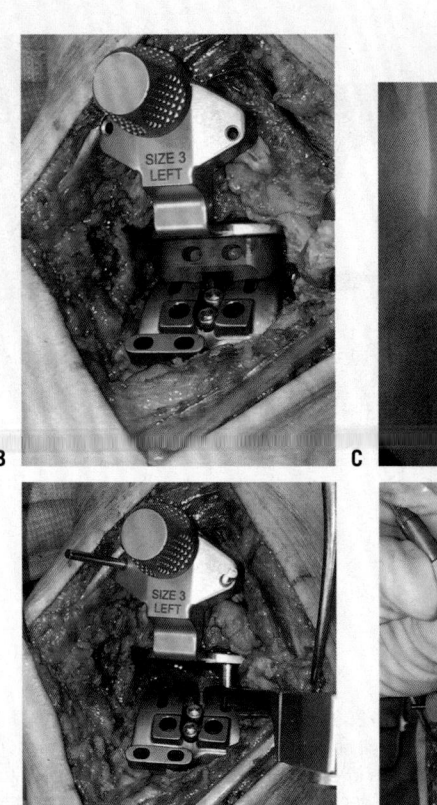

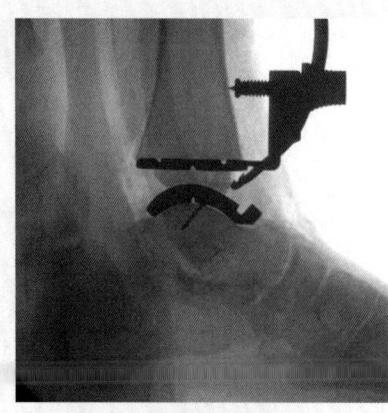

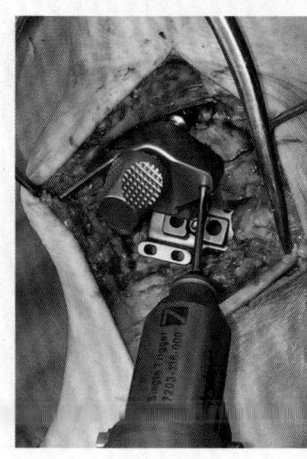

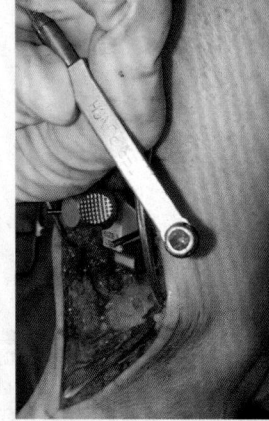

TECH FIG 4 *(continued)* **B.** Talar trial in place with tibial trial and punch liner. **C.** Perfect lateral x-ray of the trials with visible slots demarking the tibial pegs and the talar trial sitting centered over the lateral process. **D.** Pinning of the tibial trial in place. **E.** Small punch lined up with a small peg hole in the tibial trial. **F.** Bone removed with the central cage punch.

- It is critical to check the position of the tibial trial on x-ray. The anterior and posterior slots demark where the pegs will be positioned.
  - Once satisfactory, the tibial trial is pinned in place. If not done already, the punch liner and talar trial are removed **(TECH FIG 4D)**.
- Guide the peripheral punch into the ankle and use the mallet to impact the punch into the three small peg holes until flush **(TECH FIG 4E)**. Be sure that the punch is directed exactly perpendicular to the tibial trial.
- Impact the central cage punch into the central hole of the tibial trial until fully seated. As for the pegs, it is imperative to direct the central cage punch perpendicular to the tibial trial.

Do not angle this punch during insertion. With harder bone, stronger impaction will be necessary, but be sure not to angle the punch; keep it perpendicular to the prepared tibial surface and the tibial trail. Once fully impacted, do not angle or rock the punch; gently twist it as it is extracted perpendicular to the bone and trial. The central core of bone within the cage punch will most likely extract with the punch as it is withdrawn. This bone may be removed from the punch and impacted into the central cage of the final tibial implant **(TECH FIG 4F)**.

- Remove the tibial trial.
- Some surgeons elect to punch the holes again without the tibial trial in place to facilitate the implant sitting flush with the tibial bone.

FINAL PREPARATION AND IMPLANTATION

- Copiously irrigate the wound and suction clean of all bony and cartilaginous debris.
- Use a marking pen to ink the outline of the talar and tibial holes to facilitate identification of them when inserting the final components.
- Insert the tibial component by hand, focusing on the central cage being directed exactly perpendicular to the prepared tibial bone surface. Align the pegs with the respective prepared peg holes using the spatula ("paddle") impactor to rotate the tibial component into optimal position. Then, use the spatula impactor to drive the tibial component flush with the bone. It is imperative that the tibial component be impacted exactly perpendicular

to the bone until it is fully seated. We recommend obtaining a perfect lateral fluoroscopy spot image as the component is being impacted; the tendency is for the tibial component to seat anteriorly first, thereby creating posterior component lift-off and weakening the ideal tibial preparation for the pegs and particularly the cage. If the fluoroscopic spot image suggests a tendency toward posterior lift-off, then place the impactor on the posterior edge of the implant and favor posterior impaction to align the tibial component congruently with the prepared tibial surface to ensure uniform bone–prosthesis interface contact. Ensure the tibial component is flush on lateral fluoroscopy **(TECH FIG 5A)**.

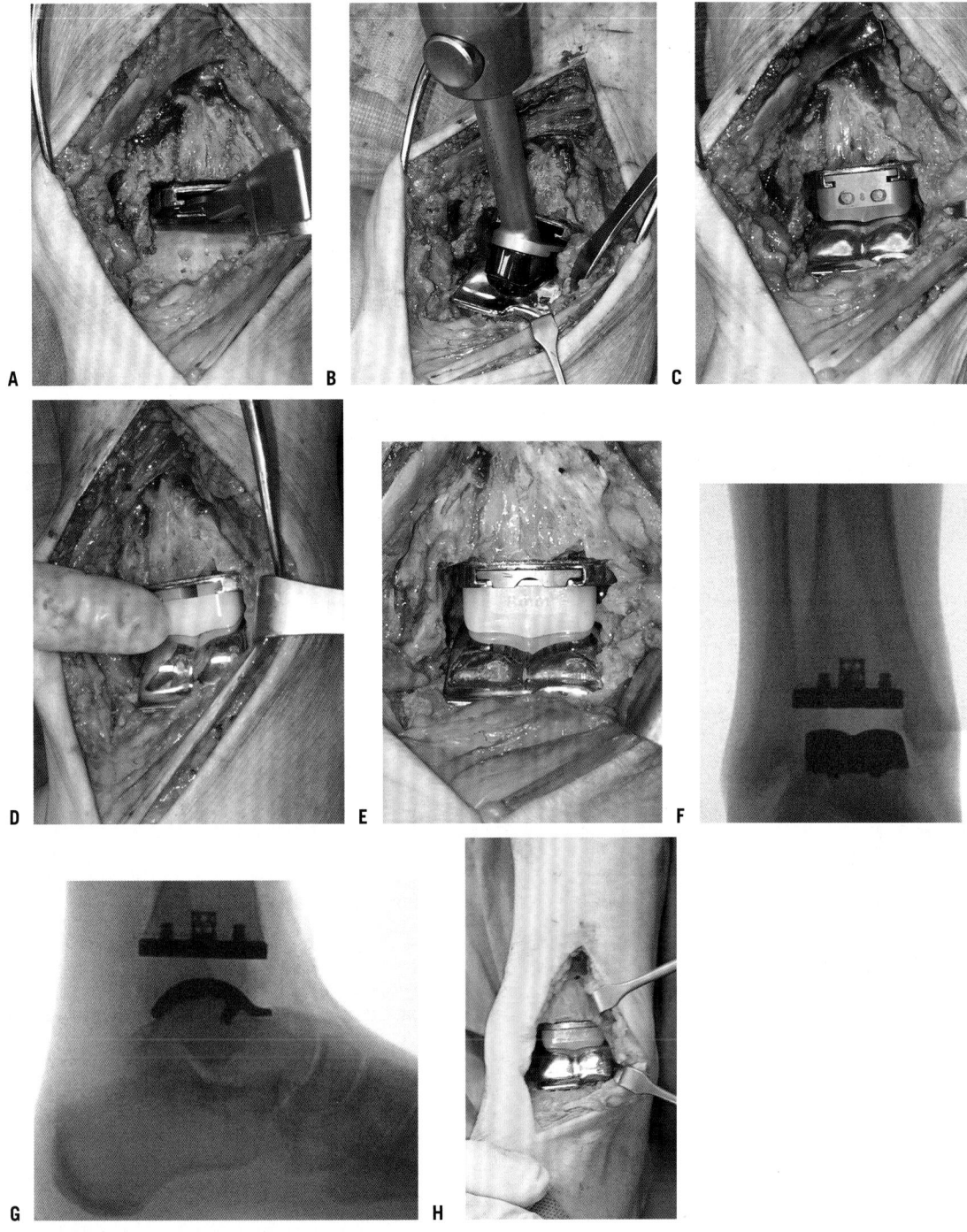

TECH FIG 5 **A.** Spatula impactor placed on the tibial component. **B.** Talar impactor for the talar component. **C.** Polyethylene trial in place. **D.** Finger pressure on the polyethylene to push into place. **E.** Locking clip engaged to lock the polytheylene in place. **F,G.** Final fluoroscopic AP and lateral images. **H.** Final implantation of the mobile-bearing system.

- Place the talar component with the pegs lined up with the holes by hand. Use the talar impactor to drive the component flush with bone **(TECH FIG 5B)**.
- Trial an appropriately sized polyethylene **(TECH FIG 5C)**.
  - Distract ankle with straight pull traction on the heel to ensure no gapping exists.
  - Test varus and valgus stability with the ankle in neutral position, that is, simulated weight-bearing position.

- Test range of motion to ensure the ankle dorsiflexes beyond neutral.
- Consider a gastrocnemius recession or tendo-Achilles lengthening if dorsiflexion is limited to less than 5 to 10 degrees.
- If varus instability exists, consider performing a medial capsular (deltoid ligament) release and use of a larger polyethylene with or without lateral ankle ligament tightening (modified Brostrom ligament reconstruction).

- Once the appropriate polyethylene thickness is chosen, place the true polyethylene with the etched in number facing anteriorly by hand. Apply thumb pressure to fully seat the polyethylene within the tibial tray so that it is posterior to the notches in the tibial tray rails. Your assistant may need to distract the ankle to facilitate inserting the polyethylene (**TECH FIG 5D**).
- Insert the tibial locking clip all the way until the bar drops down, often with an audible click (**TECH FIG 5E**). The clip will only lock if the polyethylene is fully seated posterior to the notches in the rails of the tibial tray.
- If the clip is not able to be seated, take an impactor and drive the polyethylene posteriorly to make sure it is fully seated. Place the clip to lock.

- To remove the locking clip, insert a #15 blade or threaded K-wire underneath the clip to lift it up. Then use a small right-angled curette to scrape the clip anteriorly or a pointed reduction clamp to pull it anteriorly.
- Obtain final AP and lateral x-rays (**TECH FIG 5F,G**).
- In the mobile-bearing system, there is no locking clip mechanism, and the implantation is finished with insertion of the polyethylene (**TECH FIG 5H**).
- Irrigate the wound, close the deep capsule, the extensor retinaculum, the subcutaneous tissue, and finally the skin. A drain can be placed below the extensor retinaculum and pulled the next day. A well-padded short-leg cast can be placed and immediate partial weight bearing can be started.

T E C H N I Q U E S

Pearls and Pitfalls

Removal of Tibial Resection in One Piece	• After making the tibial cut and removing the tibial cutting block, a ½-inch curved osteotome can be inserted into the tibial cut site one-third of the way down the bone and used to push the bone distally. Lever the handle of the osteotome against the distal block of the alignment guide and with sustained force, gently pry the bone away from the posterior capsule.
Prophylactic Medial Malleolus Fixation	• In patients with soft bone, or if after tibial resection there appears to be compromised bone stock of the medial malleolus, a fully threaded cannulated 4.0-mm screw is placed under fluoroscopy for prophylactic fixation.
When the Talar Trial Does Not Sit Flush on the Lateral X-ray	• Remove the talar trial and make sure that adequate bone was removed from the anterior talar neck with the cushing rongeur to facilitate the use of the large rasp. Rerasp the talar surface until smooth, with care to rasp all the way anterior and posterior without lifting the rasp off the bone.
When the Tibial Trial Does Not Slide All the Way Posterior	• The trial may be impinging on the medial malleolus, which may lead to a stress reaction. A small reciprocating saw can be used to make a "relief cut" to remove a small amount of the impinging bone.
When the Tibial Component Does Not Sit Flush with Bone	• A square-nosed impactor can be used against the central portion of the piece to impact the component into the bone. Because the polyethylene is fixed onto the tibial piece, this does not accelerate wear.
When the Talar Component Does Not Align beneath the Tibial Component	• It is possible that impinging bone or debris in the gutter is preventing the talar component from sitting directly beneath the tibial component. Use a small reciprocating saw to resect a minimal vertical sliver of overhanging bone from the impinging gutter to allow the talus freedom of movement necessary to sit under the tibia.

POSTOPERATIVE CARE

- Patients are observed overnight in the hospital.
- Immediate partial weight bearing is allowed in the cast.
- Aspirin 325 mg twice a day is prescribed to prevent deep vein thrombosis and pulmonary embolism.
- The drain is pulled on postoperative day 1, and the patient is discharged if he has cleared physical therapy.
- Follow-up is at 2 to 3 weeks, and the cast and sutures are removed. The patient is placed in a boot.
- Next, follow-up is at 6 weeks postoperative, at which a full series of ankle x-rays is obtained, and the patient is placed into a regular shoe and allowed to partake in all low-impact activities as tolerated.
- Patients are then followed at 3 months, 6 months, 1 year, and every year after (**FIG 2**).
- Patients are given a prescription for one dose of oral amoxicillin for use 1 hour prior to invasive dental procedures.

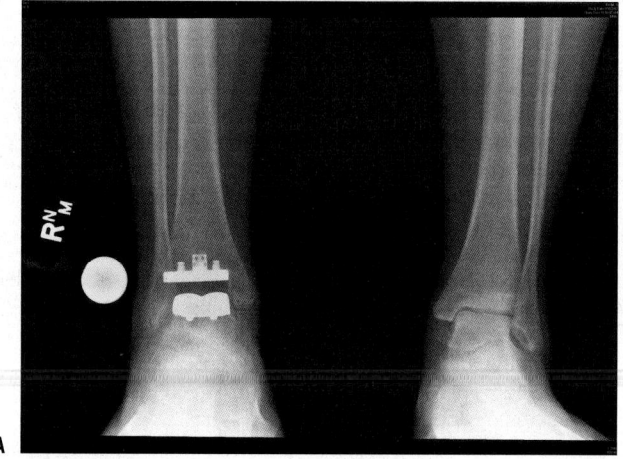

FIG 2 A–C. One-year follow-up weight-bearing radiographs. **A.** AP view. *(continued)*

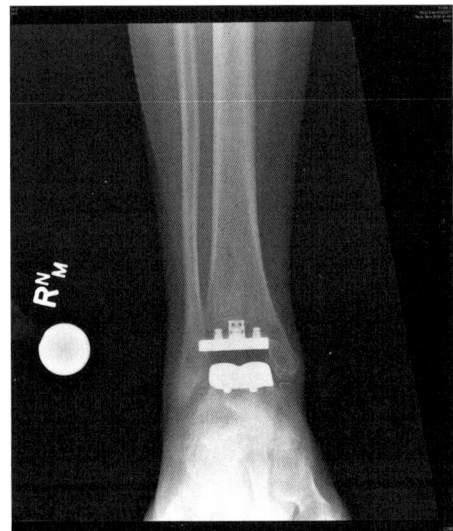

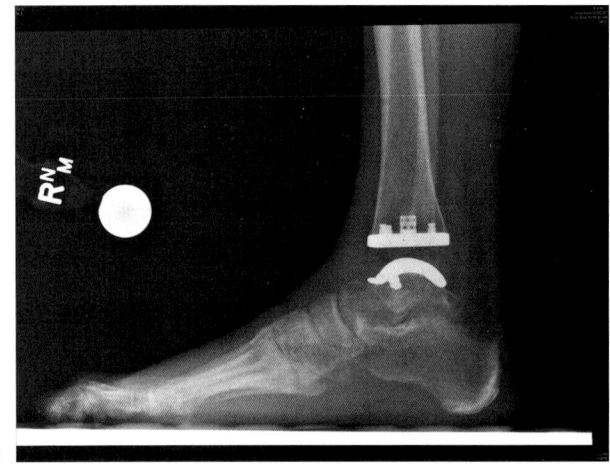

FIG 2 *(continued)* **B.** Mortise view. **C.** Lateral view.

OUTCOMES

- As of now, there are no published data on the outcome of the Vantage total ankle system.
- However, current generation total ankle systems have greater than 85% mid to long-term survival on multiple clinical series.[2–4]

COMPLICATIONS

- Infection (superficial or deep)
- Neuralgia (superficial or deep peroneal nerve, rarely tibial nerve)
- Wound complications
- Iatrogenic malleolar fracture or late-presenting malleolar stress fractures
- Flexor hallucis longus laceration

- Osteolysis
- Subsidence
- Cyst formation
- Gutter impingement
- Persistent pain without positive radiographic findings

REFERENCES

1. Kraeutler MJ, Kaenkumchorn T, Pascual-Garrido C, et al. Peculiarities in ankle cartilage. Cartilage 2017;8(1):12–18.
2. Lee GW, Lee KB. Outcomes of total ankle arthroplasty in ankles with >20° of coronal plane deformity. J Bone Joint Surg Am 2019;101(24):2203–2211.
3. Palanca A, Mann RA, Mann JA, et al. Scandinavian total ankle replacement: 15-year follow-up. Foot Ankle Int 2018;39(2):135–142.
4. Stewart MG, Green CL, Adams SB Jr, et al. Midterm results of the Salto Talaris total ankle arthroplasty. Foot Ankle Int 2017;38(11):1215–1221.

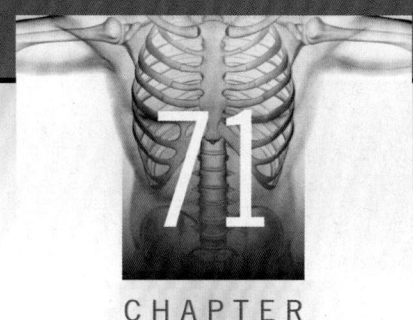

71

CHAPTER

Trabecular Metal Total Ankle Arthroplasty

Anna-Kathrin Leucht, Alastair Younger, Lew Schon, and Charlie Saltzman

DEFINITION

- Ankle arthritis is less common than hip and knee arthritis.[14]
- In 70% to 80%, the etiology is posttraumatic, evolving from a previous ankle fracture or a chronic ligament instability. Secondary osteoarthritis is found in 12% to 13% predominantly due to rheumatoid arthritis, primary osteoarthritis in 7% to 9%, respectively.[7,23,28]
- Ankle osteoarthritis results in the similar reduction of health-related quality of life and function as hip arthritis.[12]
- Due to the high percentage of posttraumatic osteoarthritis, younger patient are affected than in hip or knee osteoarthritis, resulting in a higher impact on inability to work and unemployment and subsequent economic burden.[11]
- Radiographic classification of ankle osteoarthritis is not standardized in the literature. The Kellgren-Lawrence classification primary known from knee osteoarthritis is widely used. We prefer the Canadian Orthopaedic Foot and Ankle Society (COFAS) system, which differentiates between an isolated arthritis and arthritis with intra- or extra-articular deformity, instability, or adjacent joint arthritis **(TABLE 1)**.[16,17]

ANATOMY

- The ankle joint forms a hinge, in which the trochlea tali correspond with the mortise formed by the distal tibia and fibula, but the biomechanics of the ankle are more complex than a simple hinge. The oblique sagittal rotation axis through the malleoli and the complex talar anatomy with different radial curvature medial and lateral imply a changing axis of rotation throughout ankle dorsiflexion/plantarflexion.[6]
- Due to congruent bony structure and the correspondent ligaments, the ankle is a highly stable joint, in which the load is mainly transmitted through the tibiotalar joint.
- The ankle has to withstand forces up to five times bodyweight during stance and 13 times bodyweight while running, respectively.
- The ankle joint has a higher joint congruency but a lower contact area than the knee joint, which results in a higher contact force per area in the ankle.[9] This contact force increases furthermore with ankle motion from dorsiflexion into plantarflexion, as the total contact area decreases.[8]

TABLE 1 Canadian Orthopaedic Foot and Ankle Society System

	Type 1	Type 2	Type 3	Type 4
Preoperative Classification	Isolated ankle arthritis	Ankle arthritis with intra-articular varus or valgus deformity, ankle instability, and/or a tight heel cord	Ankle arthritis with hindfoot deformity, tibial malunion, midfoot ab- or adductus, supinated midfoot, plantarflexed first ray, etc.	Types 1–3 plus subtalar, calcaneocuboid, or talonavicular arthritis
Postoperative Classification	AA or TAR with no procedure requiring a second incision except syndesmosis fusion	AA or TAR with a soft tissue procedure requiring a separate incision	AA or TAR with an additional osteotomy including midfoot arthrodesis	AA or TAR with an additional hindfoot arthrodesis
Concurrent Procedures	None, hardware removal	Deltoid ligament release, ligament reconstruction, tendo-Achilles lengthening, gastrocnemius recession, tendon transfer, capsule release, forefoot reconstruction, metatarsal osteotomy, dissection of neurovascular structures, plantar fascia release, syndesmosis reconstruction	Fibular osteotomy, calcaneal osteotomy, tibial osteotomy, midtarsal arthrodesis	Arthrodesis: triple, subtalar, talonavicular, calcaneocuboid

AA, total ankle; TAR, ankle arthrodesis.

- To resist this forces, the talar cartilage shows a higher dynamic stiffness, due to denser extracellular matrix, lower water content, and higher sulfated glycosaminoglycan content in contrast to the knee.[25] Furthermore, the cartilage of the ankle joint is thinner (0.7 to 1.62 mm) compared to the knee.[1,9,24]

PATHOGENESIS

- A 70% to 80% of all ankle arthritis are posttraumatic,[7,23,28] either triggered by an irreversible injury to the cartilage during the trauma or caused by incongruency or instability of the joint leading to chronic cartilage overload.[2,19–21]
- Significant risk factors for the development of posttraumatic ankle osteoarthritis are fibular fractures type Weber C or associated medial malleolar fractures. Fracture-dislocation, obesity, age older than 30 years as well as length of time till surgery increase the risk of development of arthritis.[18]
- Secondary arthritis is related to different comorbidities such as rheumatoid arthritis, hemochromatosis, hemophilia, gout, etc.[23,28]
- Obese patients have an increased likelihood to develop ankle osteoarthritis.[10]

NATURAL HISTORY

- Posttraumatic osteoarthritis develops with an average latency of 20.9 years in ankle fractures. This time differs largely depending on the fracture type, with talus fracture having the shortest time interval (9.3 years) to develop posttraumatic osteoarthritis.[13]
- The mean latency to develop a posttraumatic ankle arthritis after an ankle ligament injury is 34.3 years, with a shorter latency time of 25.7 years following a single severe ankle sprain compared to 38.0 years in recurrent ankle sprains.[27]

PATIENT HISTORY AND PHYSICAL FINDINGS

- The assessment of the patient starts with a thorough assessment. This includes the symptoms of the patients, for example, swelling, stiffness, blocking, or catching and detailed evaluation of the pain, for example, area of maximal discomfort, pain with activity, pain with starting while resting or night time.
- Additional relevant facts are previous trauma to the ankle like ligament sprains, ankle/pilon fractures, or lower leg fractures.
- The medical history, former surgeries, allergies, medications, as well as job and hobbies are questioned.
- The examination starts with observation of the patients' gait and the alignment of the leg, the hindfoot, and the foot while standing barefoot.
- The range of motion of the ankle as well as the subtalar and the transverse tarsal joints are determined (**FIG 1**). Any rigid deformity is recognized.
- Points of tenderness around the ankle joint as well as the subtalar, calcaneocuboidal, talonavicular, naviculocuneiform, and tarsometatarsal joints are localized. Pain on palpation and during resisted testing of the peroneal tendon and the tibialis posterior tendon are noted.
- The ligamentous integrity of the ankle joint and the subtalar joint is determined.

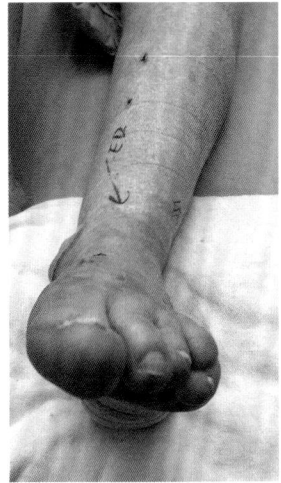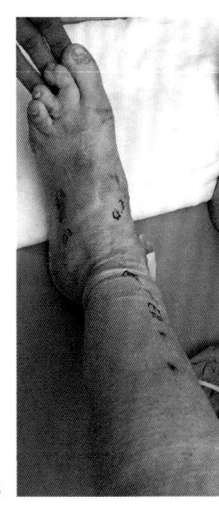

FIG 1 Assessment of alignment preoperatively. In this case, the forefoot was externally rotated, in varus and the hindfoot in valgus. The patient had undergone an arch reconstruction, and a poorly reduced bimalleolar fracture 3 years later caused the ankle to collapse into valgus.

- Finally, the skin status and previous surgical approaches are noted and the neurovascular status examined.

IMAGING AND OTHER DIAGNOSTIC STUDIES

- A standard x-rays series includes weight-bearing ankle anteroposterior (AP) and mortise views, foot and ankle lateral, foot AP, and a hindfoot alignment view (**FIG 2A–C**).
- To rule out any bony deformity above the ankle joint, a full leg alignment view can be helpful.
- Imaging modalities like computed tomography (CT) and single-photon emission computed tomography are helpful in evaluating the degree of adjacent joint arthritis especially subtalar arthritis and detecting possible bone loss due to cyst or deformity. If there is considerable deformity a three-dimensional reconstruction can be performed to assess the position of the forefoot and hindfoot (**FIG 2D–G**).
  - A weight-bearing CT is valuable to understand complex deformities.
- The magnetic resonance imaging assesses soft tissue pathologies and cartilage defects and degeneration.

DIFFERENTIAL DIAGNOSIS

- Inflammatory arthritis
- Reactive arthritis
- Pigmented villonodular synovitis
- Gout
- Pseudogout

NONOPERATIVE MANAGEMENT

- The primary goal of nonoperative treatment is pain relief, which can be partially achieved by offloading of the ankle joint. A single cane used on the contralateral side can reduce the peak vertical force around 11%.[3]
- Patients with ankle osteoarthritis should try to modify their activity. In general, high-impact sports such as running should be avoided and changed to low-impact activities like swimming and biking.

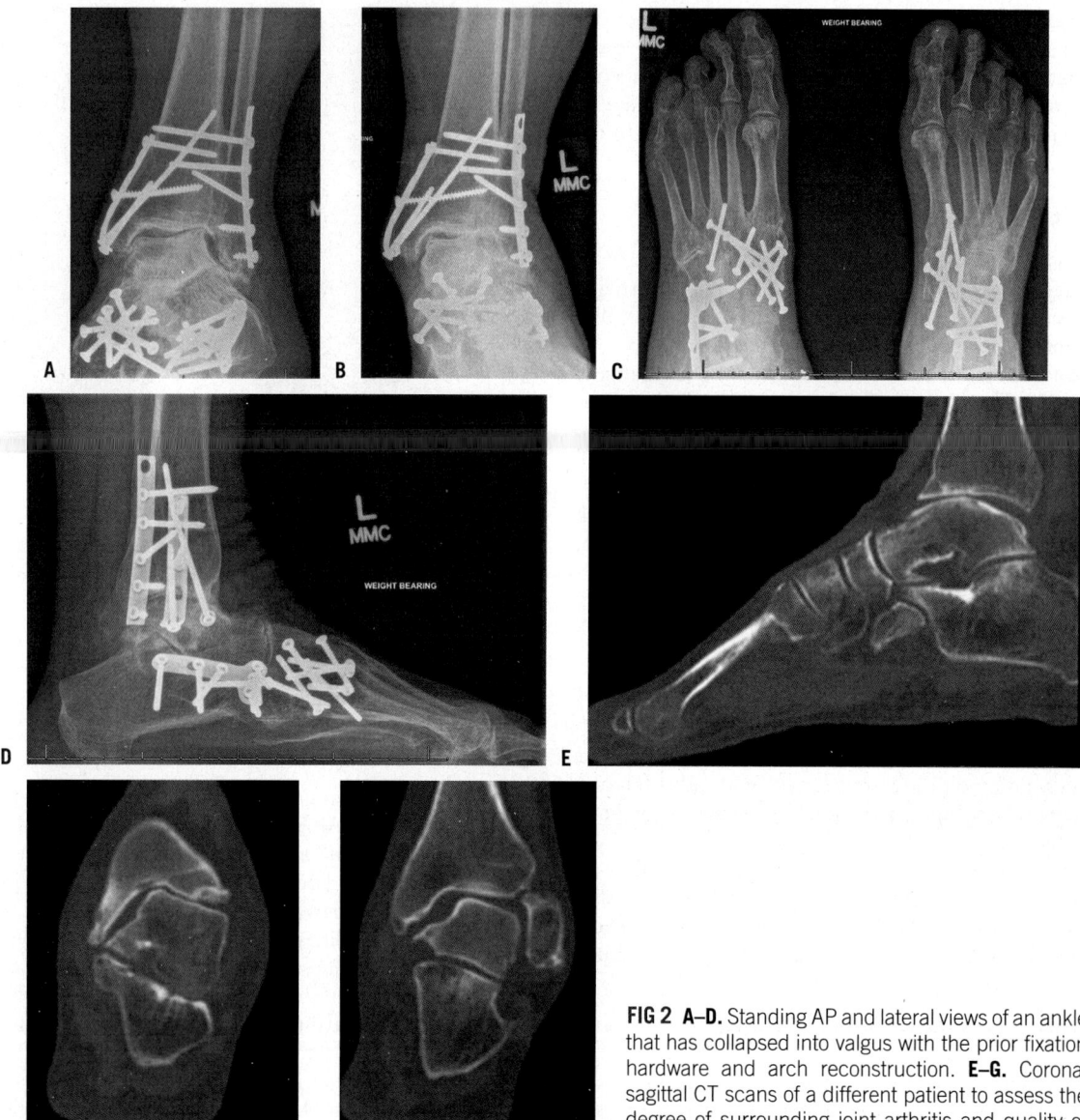

FIG 2 A–D. Standing AP and lateral views of an ankle that has collapsed into valgus with the prior fixation hardware and arch reconstruction. **E–G.** Coronal sagittal CT scans of a different patient to assess the degree of surrounding joint arthritis and quality of remaining bone.

- Physiotherapy can be beneficial in earlier stages of ankle osteoarthritis to maintain range of motion and flexibility as well as strengthening the ankle stabilizing muscles.
- Shoe wear modifications like a rocker bottom sole shoe with heel cushion reduces ankle motion during the gait cycle as well as the ground reaction force at heel strike. In addition, flexible deformities of the ankle can be aligned with orthotics with heel wedges.
- To limit the range of motion through the ankle joint and therefore limit the pain while ambulating, braces like a lazed up Arizona brace or orthoses ankle foot orthosis (AFO) can be used.
- Intra-articular corticosteroid injection can reduce symptoms of ankle osteoarthritis temporarily due to the anti-inflammatory effect. There is a lack of evidence in the current literature to show a beneficial effect of intra-articular platelet-rich plasma injection in ankle osteoarthritis. Five weekly intra-articular injections of sodium hyaluronate provide pain reduction and improve function as has been shown

in a randomized, controlled double-blind study.[22] Nevertheless, a Cochrane review concluded that there is insufficient data to support the effectiveness of hyaluronic acid.

- Nonsteroidal anti-inflammatory drugs (NSAIDs) can provide pain relief and reduce swelling, but comorbidities must be considered in prescribing NSAID, especially in older patient.

SURGICAL MANAGEMENT

- A lateral based ankle replacement is used as a primary ankle based on surgeon preference and training.
- Benefits resulting from the lateral approach include avoidance of anterior wound healing problems and lower risk for neurovascular damage with the approach.
- Furthermore, using the lateral approach results in lesser bone resection and more surface area contact because the design of the implant copies the bended shape of tibia and talus.

Preoperative Planning

- Supramalleolar alignment is evaluated with the medial distal tibia angle,[15] intra-articular deformity with the talar tilt, and hindfoot alignment in the hindfoot alignment view.
- If there is significant deformity of the tibia that cannot be corrected through the ankle joint, then consideration should be given to a tibial osteotomy prior to the ankle replacement being performed.
- Hindfoot alignment and foot alignment can be assessed using standing AP and lateral views of both the ankle and foot. The hindfoot position can be seen on the AP view of the ankle and the foot position assessed on AP and lateral views with respect to cavus and planus. If required, imaging of the opposite leg can be performed at the same time.
- A talar tilt of up to 10 degrees can be corrected with the surgery, in larger talar tilts, a prior correction is needed.
- Preoperative sizing of the implant can be determined using templates. A maximum coverage with minimal overhang and minimal talar notching needs to be achieved.

Positioning

- The patient is placed in supine position on a radiolucent table (FIG 3).
- A beanbag or a large bump is used under the ipsilateral hip to internally rotate the leg, resulting in a vertical foot position.
- A wide thigh tourniquet is applied, and the leg is prepped and draped up to above the knee joint. A contoured cuff is preferable.
- Ensure enough space is available to position the alignment stand.

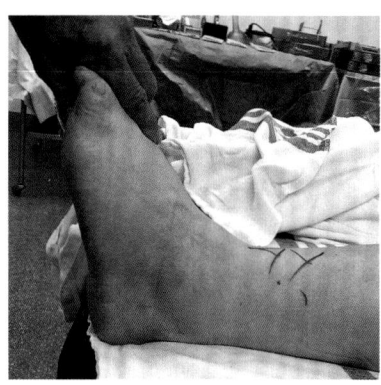

FIG 3 Positioning of the patient on the operating room (OR) table. The patient is brought distal to the edge of the OR table, and the operative hip bumped up to ensure that the ankle is correctly aligned. The large C-arm will need to be brought in from the opposite side of the bed. A small C-arm can be used from the foot of the bed.

- A regional nerve block is beneficial for postoperative pain relief.
- A large C-arm is used for imaging and brought in from the opposite side of the operative leg. If required, the room is reversed to allow ease of imaging.
  - Alternatively, the frame will fit within a well-padded small C-arm, but the dimensions should be checked prior to beginning surgery.

Approach

- A lateral and medial approach is required. The medial side is needed for a complete medial gutter débridement.

INCISION AND JOINT PREPARATION

- The lateral approach is centered over the fibula proximally. The distal end curves forward to allow access to the anterior side of the tibia and talus for reaming. The lateral collateral ligaments will require repair at the end of the procedure.
- A medial malleolar osteotomy may be required to allow correction of varus deformity.
- The proximal end of the lateral incision needs to be approximately 15 cm above the ankle. Care is taken not to damage the superficial branch of the peroneal nerve (TECH FIG 1A).
- The fibula is transected approximately 5 cm above the joint line. We prefer to use a fibular nail to transfix the osteotomy and to rotate the fibula posteriorly rather than distally. This allows exposure so long as the peroneal tendons are detensioned with the foot in plantarflexion (TECH FIG 1B).
- After the osteotomy, the lateral collateral ligaments are transected (anterior talofibular and calcaneal fibular) and the fibula

rotated posteriorly. The posterior talofibular and tibiofibular ligaments may need to be mobilized to allow appropriate external rotation of the fibula. This is then held in place with Kirschner wires (K-wires). If hindfoot correction is required in the frame, the fixation is to the tibia only.

- Anterior osteophytes of the tibia are removed, and the medial débridement is also performed at this time. If required, the medial malleolar osteotomy is performed prior to frame application as this will need to be released to allow a neutral position of the talus on the tibia.
- The ankle can be sized at this point. The sizer is placed from the lateral side and imaging used to confirm it is seated on the medial side appropriately (TECH FIG 1C). If between sizes, it is preferable to upsize the component. A lateral view and sizer can also be used to assess the position of the components and confirm the size.

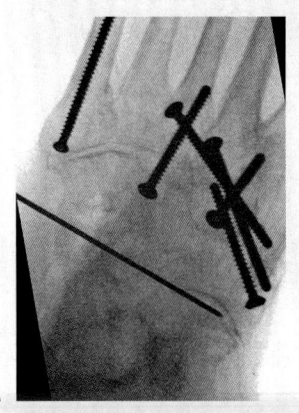
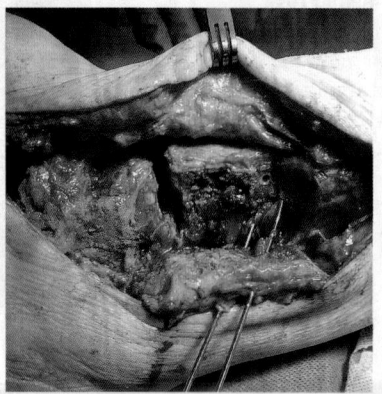
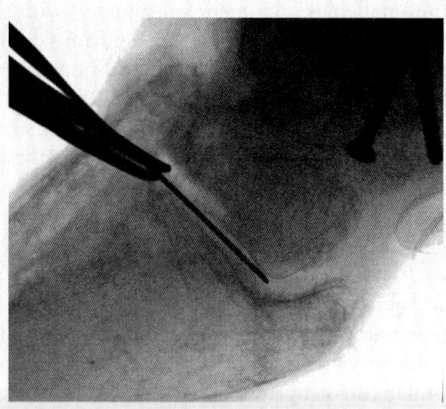

TECH FIG 1 **A.** K-wire positioning to determine the position of the calcaneal osteotomy and talonavicular fusion. This is to correct the forefoot position on the hindfoot and is performed prior to the placement in the jig, but fixation performed at the end of the procedure once the correction of the hindfoot has been achieved through the ankle. **B.** The lateral collaterals have been sectioned and the fibula osteotomized. Because the ankle will be pulled into varus to correct the hindfoot valgus, the K-wire fixation is into the tibia only to ensure that the relationship between the talus, calcaneus, and tibia is not held fixed through the K-wires in the fibula. The calcaneocuboid fusion site can be seen. In this case, the talonavicular fusion was achieved through the same lateral incision. **C.** A sizing jig is placed into the ankle. In this case, the ankle was sized for a no. 3 component. Final size choice can be made by comparing arcs of the talus and tibia. It is better in general to oversize rather than undersize. A plastic template is also within the set and can be used to determine coverage.

FRAME APPLICATION

- The frame is assembled on the back table. All components are checked before the frame is applied.
- The frame is applied with the ankle in 10 degrees of plantarflexion if the fibula is rotated posteriorly. The added benefit is the rotation of the fibula prevents posterior sag of the tibia.
- The heel is placed in the heel cup. Rotation of the foot on the footplate is checked. The transverse access of the ankle should match the axis of the frame.
- Fixation is first achieved with the calcaneus. A partial thread cancellous pin is placed through the calcaneus and fixed to the frame medially and laterally. A second pin is placed on the talus with it being transfixed to the frame using the medial post. These two pins will transfix the foot to the frame.

- The knee is then elevated or lowered by inserting or removing blocks for the knee rest. The frame is pointed toward the knee and the tibial pins placed **(TECH FIG 2A,B)**.
- The position of the ankle and its axis is then checked on the AP view of the ankle, with the alignment rod in place. A lateral view is also obtained to ensure that the tibia is concentric with the talus. The tibia should not be anteriorly or posteriorly displaced on the tibia. Equally, the tibia should not be medially or laterally displaced on the talus. This should be corrected prior to milling **(TECH FIG 2C–E)**.
- Further immobilization is then achieved by placing a rod between the bottom tibial pin and the talar pin. All pins and rods are then confirmed to be firmly fixed and solid.

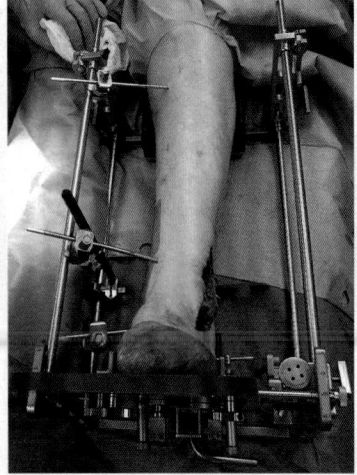
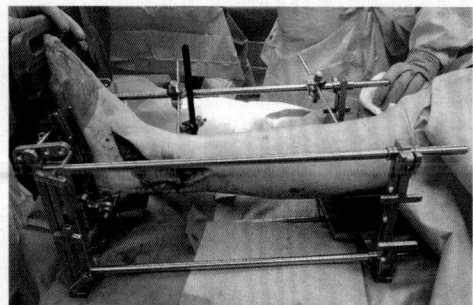

TECH FIG 2 A,B. Placement in the frame. The foot is held in plantarflexion. The foot is neutrally aligned. The foot is transfixed using a talar pin and a calcaneal pin. Two pins are used in the tibia. The foot is aligned on the long axis of the leg. Distraction and correction of varus is achieved through the ankle. Additional rods are applied between the talar pin and distal tibia to improve rigidity of the frame. *(continued)*

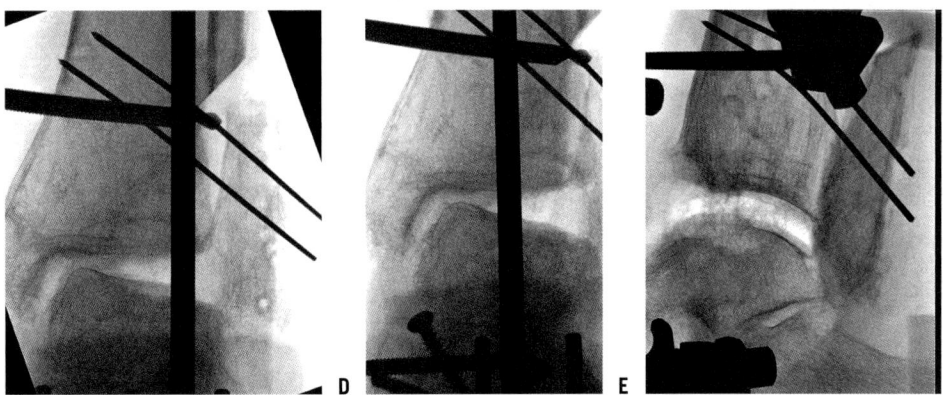

TECH FIG 2 *(continued)* **C.** Initial alignment of the ankle. The correction of hindfoot varus is good, but the talus is laterally translated compared to the tibia. This therefore is corrected. **D,E.** AP and lateral views showing alignment of the tibia and talus after correction of the translation by lateral translation of the tibia. The lateral view shows congruency of the tibial and talar surfaces. There is a tendency for the tibia to fall posterior on the talus on the lateral view.

IDENTIFYING THE CENTRAL AXIS OF THE ANKLE

- Identifying the correct AP position of the central axis of milling as well as the proximal to distal positioning of the cut is a critical next step. Once milling has been started, the position of the ankle cannot be changed.
- Using the correct size of jig (ie, if a size 4 was measured, use the size 4 jig). On the jig is a positioning hole and three reaming holes. Place the narrow end of the sizer into the positioning hole and bring the milling apparatus proximal or distal until the sizer is approximately on the joint line. The anterior and posterior position is then adjusted until the arc of the sizer follows the tibia and talus approximately **(TECH FIG 3A)**.
- Imaging is used extensively at this point **(TECH FIG 3B)**. If an error is made, the center of rotation should be slightly anterior to the midpoint of the tibia as this will preserve posterior tibial bone. However, the position should also allow a full cut of bone off the talus such that there is a solid bed and not deficiencies

on the talar side. If need be, (depending on the arc of the cut) the size can be upsized or downsized one size at this point. The pointer is reversed and placed into the talar cutting hole and the tibial no. 1 cutting hole. This will outline the extent of the cut using the reamer. In the illustrated case, the talus and tibia were in valgus from a prior ankle fracture. Care was therefore taken to ensure that the talus was completely covered with the cut.
- Prior to reaming, the same-sized drill guide is placed. A final check on position is achieved by determining the position of the drill on the anterior and posterior holes of the drill guide. These should not be excessively anterior or posteriorly placed on the tibia or talus. The drill holes are then made on the tibia and talus to the depth of the component using the trial. The drill should be cleaned of bone debris to prevent heating. The drill holes are pilot holes for the reamer.

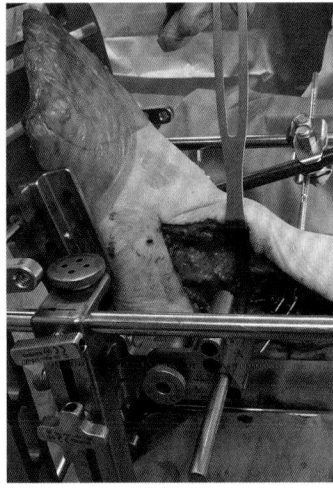 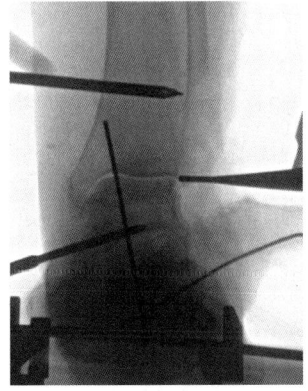

TECH FIG 3 Finding the joint center. **A.** This is a critical step to ensure that the center of rotation is correctly placed proximal to distal and anterior to posterior. Once the center of rotation is identified, it cannot be changed once milling has begun. **B.** In this case, a proximal joint line will result in too little talus being cut and an incomplete bed for the talus. A distal joint line will result in removal of too much talus. A posterior position will result in removal of too much talar neck and posterior tibia and an anterior position removal of too much posterior talus and anterior tibia. The joint replacement is a surface replacement, so incorrect position of the center of rotation will also compromise range of motion (in this case a separate patient).

MILLING THE TIBIA AND TALUS

- Once the surgeon is certain the position of the cuts are correctly positioned anterior to posterior and proximal to distal, the reaming is performed. The reamer will cut differently going clockwise and counterclockwise. For this reason, all cuts are made clockwise on the talus and anticlockwise on the tibia.
  - A final check is made with the first cuts on the tibia and talus to ensure that the arcs are appropriate.
- The depth of the reamer is restricted by a clamp on the shaft of the reamer. This is matched to the depth of the trial components and the final medial extent of the prosthesis is achieved using C-arm control.
- The talus is reamed first **(TECH FIG 4A)**. The reamer should not be allowed to overheat on the bone. An appropriate anterior to posterior extent of the cut is required to allow seating of the

components. Care needs to be taken with the medial posterior cut on the talus and tibia as this comes close to the neurovascular bundle.
- Anteriorly, the talar cut may need to be advanced down into the talar neck area. This may be into osteophyte. It should not extend too deep into the talar neck area.
- The first tibial cut is made counterclockwise. Anteriorly, care is taken not to damage the soft tissues. Posteriorly, the cut should be completed to ensure that the tibial component is not proud **(TECH FIG 4B)**.
- Debris can be removed using a pituitary rongeur. The final medial cut is made using the tibia no. 2 cutter to ensure that there is no medial ridge. The milling is confirmed by palpation **(TECH FIG 4C)**.

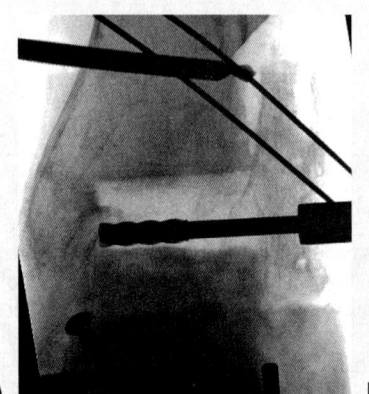 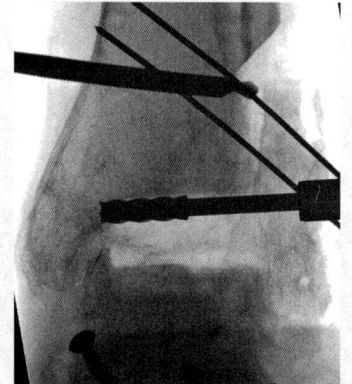 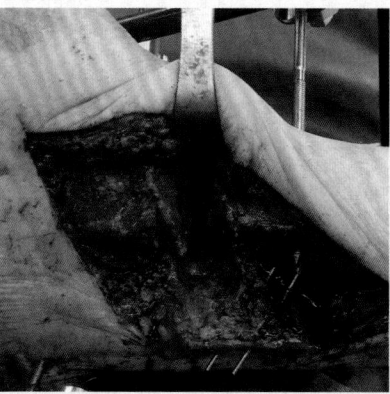

TECH FIG 4 A,B. Final milling of the tibia and talus. The medial extent should be appropriate to ensure capping of the tibia and talus without removing so much bone as to weaken the medial malleolus. **C.** Clinical appearance of final milling. The tibia and talus should feel smooth with no rough areas and no raised area. The cut should extend anteriorly and posteriorly enough to seat the entire component. Sometimes, repeat milling has to be performed after placement of the rail guides.

PREPARATION OF THE TIBIAL AND TALAR RAILS

- The talar and tibial cutting jigs are first placed individually to ensure that the cuts are complete anteriorly and posteriorly and that they will sit appropriately. If they do, they can be placed and a distracting clip placed.
  - A lateral view and an AP view are obtained to ensure that the jigs are medially placed and are correctly seated as seen on the lateral view. The rail holes need to be appropriately placed on the tibia so that they do not cause a fracture of the tibia anteriorly or posteriorly. Therefore, central placement on the tibia is important. Anterior or posterior placement of the talus will result in liftoff of the components.

- The jigs can be changed before the distraction clip is placed. The talus can be placed anterior or posterior on the tibia. If the jigs will not seat, further milling is likely required. Occasionally, a small resection of the tibia or talus laterally is required.
- K-wire fixation is used once the jigs are correctly seated.
- A 5-mm drill is then used to drill the rail holes, and a plug is placed in each hole to prevent migration as the other holes are drilled.
- The jigs are then removed and the implants are placed **(TECH FIG 5)**. The implants can be placed with the frame on or after removal from the frame.

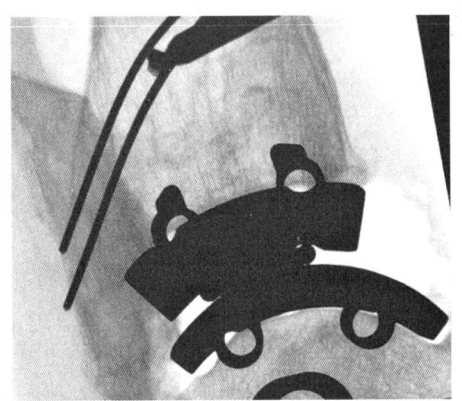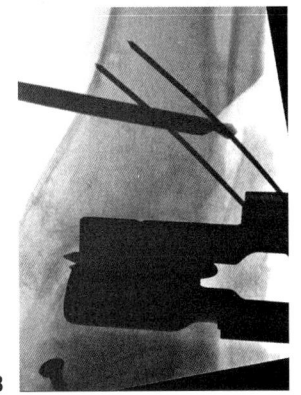

TECH FIG 5 A,B. Placement and confirmation of seating of the tibial and talar rail guides. These are used to drill the holes for the rails of the components. A true lateral radiograph of each component is required to ensure seating as well as medial placement. A distraction clip is placed to force the guides onto bone. Confirmation of the drill hole position is required on the tibial side to ensure that neither the anterior tibia nor the posterior tibia fractures because the drill hole is too close to bone.

PLACEMENT OF THE IMPLANTS

- The trial components can be placed and the footplate released if the surgeon chooses **(TECH FIG 6A)**. Alternatively, the final components can be placed. Consideration is given to the thickness of the polyethylene to be used.
- The talar component is first placed **(TECH FIG 6B)**. The holding jig can be used. The tibial trial of the correct size is placed first. The rails of the component will be undersized on the rail drill holes and so will need to cut a track into the drill holes. The rails will therefore need to be carefully started. Gradual impaction is then performed to seat the component completely. This is then

checked on the AP and lateral view. Care should be taken to ensure that the components follow the rails as they are seated.
- The tibial trial is then removed and the process repeated on the tibial side. The tibial component will overall be easier to insert because the bone is softer. The tibial polyethylene is inserted prior to insertion of the component.
- Cement is then added if licensing or surgeon choice dictates it **(TECH FIG 6C,D)**.
- Once seated, the frame is removed carefully (if not already removed) and range of motion checked.

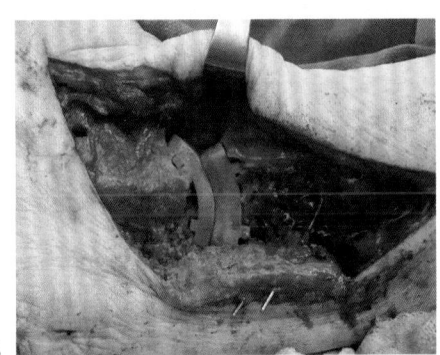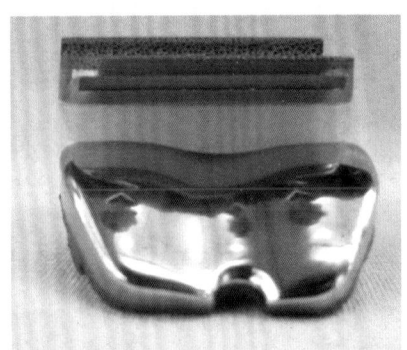

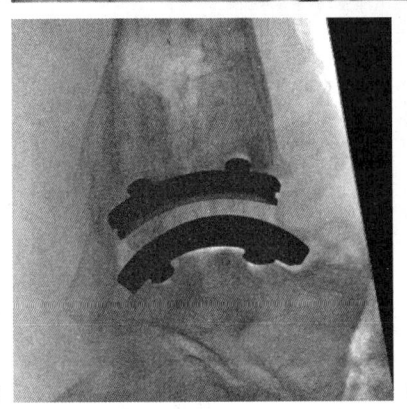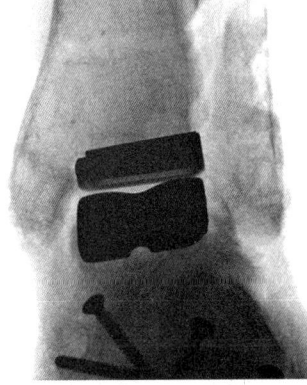

TECH FIG 6 A. After removal of the frame and assessment of thickness of components. Because of a lateral defect in the talus, we elected to cement the components on the rails and over the lateral side of the talus using low-viscosity cement. **B.** The trabecular metal (TM) implant ankle prior to insertion. **C,D.** The osteopenic bone on both the talus and the tibia failed to hold the components so cement was added.

REPAIR OF THE FIBULA

Repair Using a Plate

- The fibular K-wires are removed and the fibula rotated back.
- The fibula can then be held in place using a five-hole locking plate.
- The fibula should be appropriately reduced.
- On occasion, the lateral side of the talus may require trimming, or parts of the fibula.
- Once the plate is in the correct position, screws are placed (TECH FIG 7).

Repair Using a Fibular Rod

- The authors prefer to use a fibular nail, which gives more flexibility in the position of the fibula on the talus, reduces the bulk of fixation, and takes less proximal dissection and time (TECH FIG 8).
- Because changing to the fibular nail, the number of wound complications has reduced dramatically.

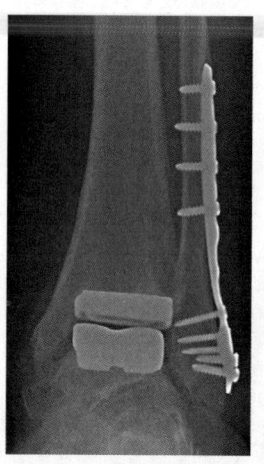
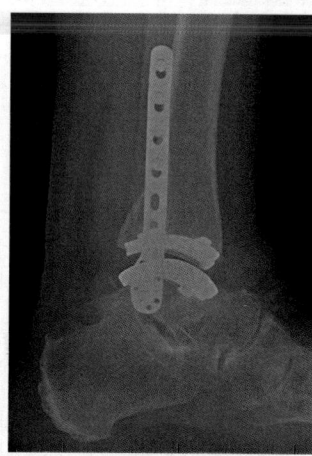

A   B

TECH FIG 7 Plate fixation of the fibula.

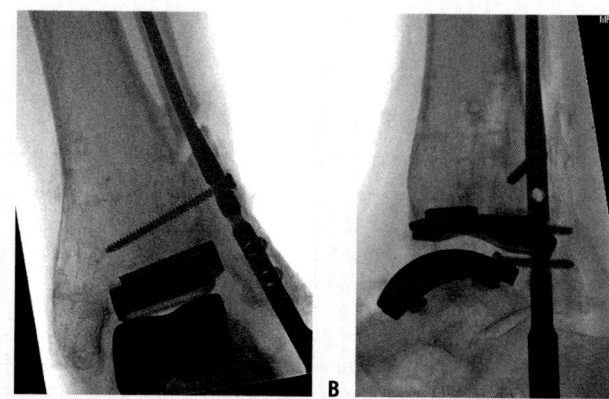

A   B

TECH FIG 8 Placement of the fibular rod.

REPAIR OF THE LATERAL COLLATERALS AND CLOSURE

- After plate or nail fixation, the lateral collateral ligaments are repaired. Drill holes into the fibula can be used. A Brostrom-style technique can be used.
- If necessary, further surgical correction can be undertaken to correct lingering varus (TECH FIG 9A–D).

- Closure of all approaches and stab incisions is performed, a sterile dressing is applied, and the ankle is placed in a well-padded plaster cast (TECH FIG 9E–I).

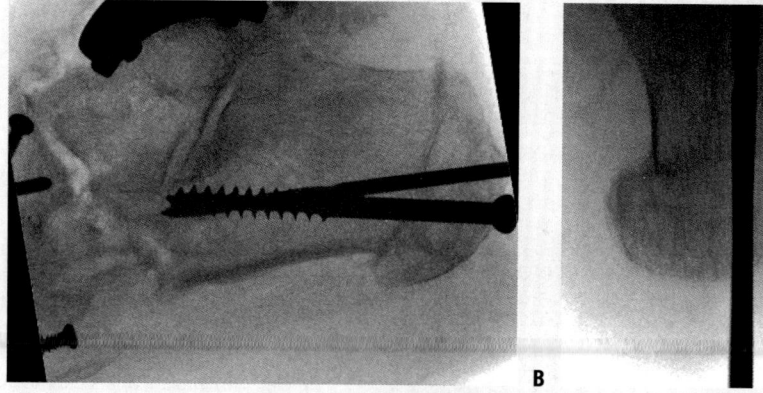

A   B

TECH FIG 9 A,B. After the placement of the components and lateral ligament repair, the heel was still felt to be in too much varus so a medializing calcaneal osteotomy was added. *(continued)*

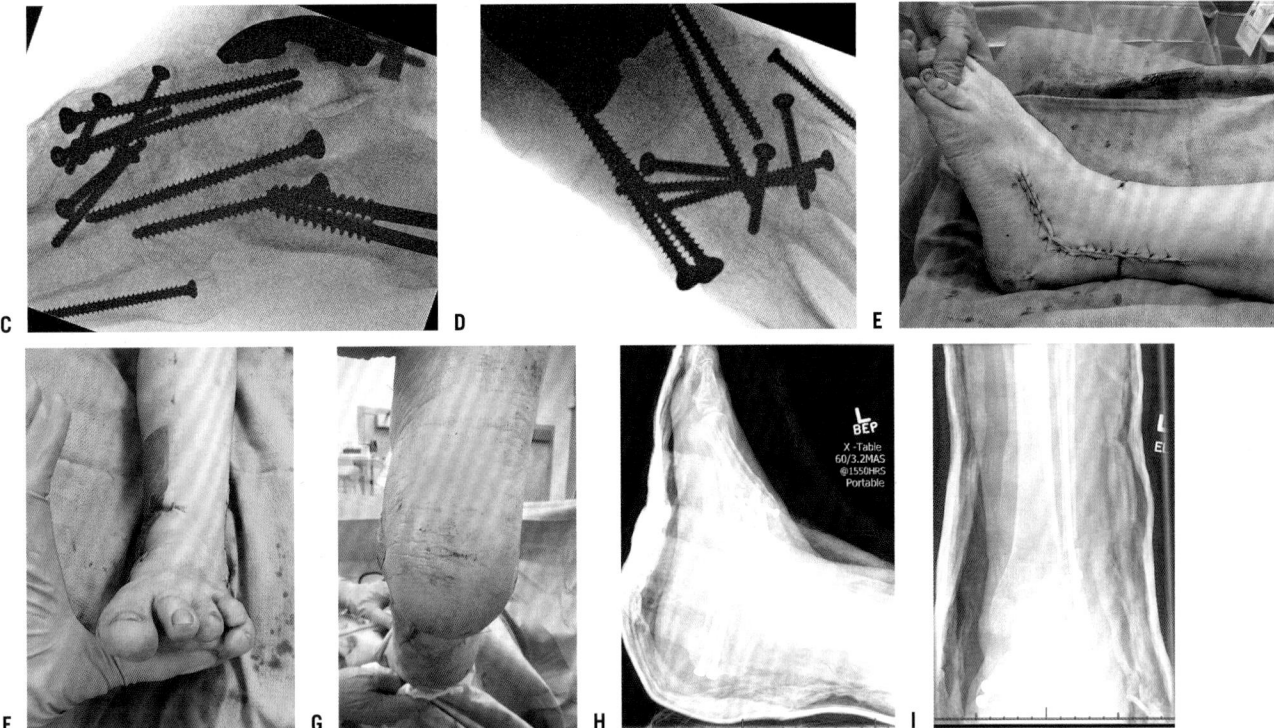

TECH FIG 9 *(continued)* **C,D.** Fixation of the forefoot was also performed to correct the forefoot varus and external rotation. This will reduce the valgus moment arm on the ankle and reduce the tension load on the deltoid ligament. **E.** Interrupted nylon sutures are used for closure and Steri-Strips are placed. **F.** Alignment of the forefoot after correction. **G.** Alignment of the heel after correction through the ankle and medializing calcaneal osteotomy. **H,I.** Postoperative AP and lateral views.

TECHNIQUES

Pearls and Pitfalls

Positioning	• Supine position on a radiolucent table. The ankle has to be positioned on the table with sufficient space both to the lateral side and distally that the frame can be placed in a stable position.
Approach	• A lateral approach of approximately 15 cm is performed. A medial approach is required for the débridement of the medial gutter.
Frame Application	• After the application of the frame, anterio-posterior and lateral fluoroscopy should confirm a concentric position of the ankle.
Identifying the Central Axis of Ankle	• Identifying the AP position of the central axis of milling and the proximal to distal positioning of the cuts is a critical step. Time should be spent to determine this correct position.
Milling the Tibia and Talus	• Cuts on the talus are performed clockwise and cuts on the tibia anticlockwise. The talus is reamed first. Avoid heat generation.
Preparation of Rails	• Correct placement of the drill guides is important to ensure the proper implant position. • Implant AP position is defined by the rail holes.
Inserting the Prosthesis	• A reduction with trial components assesses appropriate joint tension. • The talar component is inserted first with the tibial trial component in place. • The tibial component is assembled and then inserted.
Repairing the Fibula	• Repairing the fibula with a fibular nail seems to reduce the postoperative wound infections and complications.
Repairing the Lateral Collaterals	• A Brostrom-style technique is an appropriate way to repair the lateral ligaments.
Closure	• After closure of the skin, a well-padded plaster cast is applied.

POSTOPERATIVE CARE

- The ankle is placed in a plaster cast at the end of surgery.
- The splint and the sutures are removed at 2 weeks. The foot is then positioned in a walker boot. Ankle range-of-motion exercises supervised by physiotherapy are initiated at this time.
- At 4 weeks, the patients are allowed to bear weight as tolerated.
- At 6 weeks, a follow-up appointment with x-rays is planned.
- Walker boot for a total of 10 weeks, afterward transition to normal shoe

OUTCOMES

- In our opinion, the reoperating rate in total ankle replacement should be consequently documented in the COFAS reoperating coding system **(TABLE 2)**.[29]
- There are only a few studies so far reporting of the results of the Zimmer Biomet Trabecular Metal Total Ankle with a mean follow-up of at least 12 months.
- In 2018, Barg et al[4] published a short-term outcome of 55 primary total ankle arthroplasties with a mean follow-up of 26.6 months and an implant survivorship of 93%. Three revisions were required for aseptic loosening of the tibial component and 10 of 55 patients needed a secondary procedure in the follow-up period. The postoperative outcome was good with a significant increase of range of motion and significant decrease of the pain score. Nonunions of the fibula were not observed.
- As well in 2018, Usuelli et al[26] reported of their case series with 89 patients and a minimum follow-up of 24 month. They noticed a statistically significant improvement in the American Orthopaedic Foot & Ankle Society (AOFAS) score, Ankle–Hindfoot Score, visual analog scale (VAS), and Short Form 12 Physical and Mental Composite Scores. Once more, a significant increase of range of motion was documented. Seven of 89 patients needed repeated surgery for hardware removal, 2 patients had a delayed wound healing, and 1 patient developed a deep infection with subsequent removal of the implants.
- Bianchi et al[5] published their early results of a case series of 30 patients with a follow-up of 12 months in 2019. They showed a significant improvement in the AOFAS score as well as in the Foot Function Index and a significant decrease in the VAS score.

COMPLICATIONS

- Wound healing problem, superficial infection
- Deep infection
- Aseptic loosening
- Heterotopic ossifications
- Intraoperative/postoperative fracture
- Malunion or nonunion of fibula
- Malpositioning/technical error

TABLE 2 Canadian Orthopaedic Foot and Ankle Society Reoperating Coding System			
Type	**Code**	**Description of Reoperation**	**Applicable Procedure**
Nil	1	No reoperation within or surrounding the ankle	Ankle replacement or arthrodesis
Reoperation surrounding primary operative site	2	Isolated hardware removal around the ankle	Ankle replacement or arthrodesis
	3	Repeat operation outside the ankle replacement or arthrodesis (eg, osteotomy, fusion, or ligament repair) but related to the replacement or arthrodesis	Ankle replacement or arthrodesis
Reoperation within primary operative site	4	Ankle gutter or heterotopic ossification débridement without exchange of metal components, with or without intact polyethylene exchange	Ankle replacement only
	5	Exchange of polyethylene liner as a result of polyethylene liner failure	Ankle replacement only
	6	Débridement of an osteolytic cyst without exchange of metal components, with or without intact polyethylene exchange	Ankle replacement only
	7	Deep infection or wound complication requiring operative débridement (without exchange of metal components in ankle replacement), with or without intact polyethylene exchange	Ankle replacement or arthrodesis
	8	Revision of arthrodesis due to malposition or nonunion (no infection)	Ankle arthrodesis only
	9	Implant failure leading to revision of metal components due to aseptic loosening, component fracture, or malposition (no infection)	Ankle replacement only
	10	Revision of metal component(s) secondary to infection	Ankle replacement only
Amputation	11	Amputation above the level of the ankle	Ankle replacement or arthrodesis

REFERENCES

1. Adam C, Eckstein F, Milz S, et al. The distribution of cartilage thickness in the knee-joints of old-aged individuals—measurement by A-mode ultrasound. Clin Biomech (Bristol, Avon) 1998;13(1):1–10.
2. Anderson DD, Chubinskaya S, Guilak F, et al. Post-traumatic osteoarthritis: improved understanding and opportunities for early intervention. J Orthop Res 2011;29(6):802–809.
3. Aragaki DR, Nasmyth MC, Schultz SC, et al. Immediate effects of contralateral and ipsilateral cane use on normal adult gait. PM R 2009;1(3):208–213.
4. Barg A, Bettin CC, Burstein AH, et al. Early clinical and radiographic outcomes of trabecular metal total ankle replacement using a transfibular approach. J Bone Joint Surg Am 2018;100(6):505–515.
5. Bianchi A, Martinelli N, Hosseinzadeh M, et al. Early clinical and radiological evaluation in patients with total ankle replacement performed by lateral approach and peroneal osteotomy. BMC Musculoskelet Disord 2019;20(1):132.
6. Brockett CL, Chapman GJ. Biomechanics of the ankle. Orthop Trauma 2016;30(3):232–238.
7. Brown TD, Johnston RC, Saltzman CL, et al. Posttraumatic osteoarthritis: a first estimate of incidence, prevalence, and burden of disease. J Orthop Trauma 2006;20(10):739–744.
8. Calhoun JH, Li F, Ledbetter BR, et al. A comprehensive study of pressure distribution in the ankle joint with inversion and eversion. Foot Ankle Int 1994;15(3):125–133.
9. Delco ML, Kennedy JG, Bonassar LJ, et al. Post-traumatic osteoarthritis of the ankle: a distinct clinical entity requiring new research approaches. J Orthop Res 2017;35(3):440–453.
10. Frey C, Zamora J. The effects of obesity on orthopaedic foot and ankle pathology. Foot Ankle Int 2007;28(9):996–999.
11. Gagné OJ, Veljkovic A, Glazebrook M, et al. Prospective cohort study on the employment status of working age patients after recovery from ankle arthritis surgery. Foot Ankle Int 2018;39(6):657–663.
12. Glazebrook M, Daniels T, Younger A, et al. Comparison of health-related quality of life between patients with end-stage ankle and hip arthrosis. J Bone Joint Surg Am 2008;90(3):499–505.
13. Horisberger M, Valderrabano V, Hintermann B. Posttraumatic ankle osteoarthritis after ankle-related fractures. J Orthop Trauma 2009;23(1):60–67.
14. Huch K. Knee and ankle: human joints with different susceptibility to osteoarthritis reveal different cartilage cellularity and matrix synthesis in vitro. Arch Orthop Trauma Surg 2001;121(6):301–306.
15. Knupp M, Ledermann H, Magerkurth O, et al. The surgical tibiotalar angle: a radiologic study. Foot Ankle Int 2005;26(9):713–716.
16. Krause FG, Di Silvestro M, Penner MJ, et al. Inter- and intraobserver reliability of the COFAS end-stage ankle arthritis classification system. Foot Ankle Int 2010;31(2):103–108.
17. Krause FG, Di Silvestro M, Penner MJ, et al. The postoperative COFAS end-stage ankle arthritis classification system: interobserver and intraobserver reliability. Foot Ankle Spec 2012;5(1):31–36.
18. Lübbeke A, Salvo D, Stern R, et al. Risk factors for post-traumatic osteoarthritis of the ankle: an eighteen year follow-up study. Int Orthop 2012;36(7):1403–1410.
19. McKinley TO, Borrelli J Jr, D'Lima DD, et al. Basic science of intra-articular fractures and posttraumatic osteoarthritis. J Orthop Trauma 2010;24(9):567–570.
20. McKinley TO, Rudert MJ, Koos DC, et al. Pathomechanic determinants of posttraumatic arthritis. Clin Orthop Relat Res 2004; (427 suppl):S78–S88.
21. McKinley TO, Rudert MJ, Tochigi Y, et al. Incongruity-dependent changes of contact stress rates in human cadaveric ankles. J Orthop Trauma 2006;20(10):732–738.
22. Salk RS, Chang TJ, D'Costa WF, et al. Sodium hyaluronate in the treatment of osteoarthritis of the ankle: a controlled, randomized, double-blind pilot study. J Bone Joint Surg Am 2006;88(2):295–302.
23. Saltzman CL, Salamon ML, Blanchard GM, et al. Epidemiology of ankle arthritis: report of a consecutive series of 639 patients from a tertiary orthopaedic center. Iowa Orthop J 2005;25:44–46.
24. Shepherd DE, Seedhom BB. Thickness of human articular cartilage in joints of the lower limb. Ann Rheum Dis 1999;58(1):27–34.
25. Treppo S, Koepp H, Quan EC, et al. Comparison of biomechanical and biochemical properties of cartilage from human knee and ankle pairs. J Orthop Res 2000;18(5):739–748.
26. Usuelli FG, Maccario C, Granata F, et al. Clinical and radiological outcomes of transfibular total ankle arthroplasty. Foot Ankle Int 2019;40(1):24–33.
27. Valderrabano V, Hintermann B, Horisberger M, et al. Ligamentous posttraumatic ankle osteoarthritis. Am J Sports Med 2006;34(4):612–620.
28. Valderrabano V, Horisberger M, Russell I, et al. Etiology of ankle osteoarthritis. Clin Orthop Relat Res 2009;467(7):1800–1806.
29. Younger AS, Glazebrook M, Veljkovic A, et al. A coding system for reoperations following total ankle replacement and ankle arthrodesis. Foot Ankle Int 2016;37(11):1157–1164.

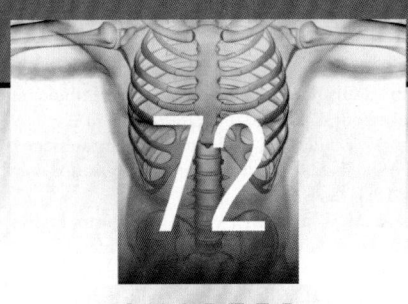

72

CHAPTER

Ankle Arthrodesis

Mark E. Easley

DEFINITION

- The procedure to fuse the tibiotalar joint for isolated end-stage tibiotalar arthrosis

ANATOMY

- Ankle
  - Tibial plafond with medial malleolus
    - Articulations with dorsal and medial talus
    - In sagittal plane, slight posterior slope
    - In coronal plane, articular surface is 88 to 92 degrees relative to lateral tibial shaft axis.
  - Fibula
    - Articulation with lateral talus
    - Responsible for one-sixth of axial load distribution of the ankle
  - Talus
    - 60% of surface area covered by articular cartilage
    - Dual radius of curvature
  - Distal tibiofibular syndesmosis
    - Anterior inferior tibiofibular ligament
    - Interosseous membrane
    - Posterior tibiofibular ligament
- Ankle functions as part of the ankle–hindfoot complex much like a mitered hinge.

PATHOGENESIS

- Posttraumatic arthrosis
  - Most common cause
  - Intra-articular fracture
  - Ankle fracture-dislocation with malunion
  - Chronic ankle instability
- Primary osteoarthrosis
  - Relatively rare compared to hip and knee arthrosis
- Inflammatory arthropathy
  - Most commonly rheumatoid arthritis
- Other
  - Hemochromatosis
  - Pigmented villonodular synovitis
  - Charcot neuroarthropathy
  - Septic arthritis

NATURAL HISTORY

- Posttraumatic arthrosis
  - Malunion, chronic instability, intra-articular cartilage damage, or malalignment may lead to progressive articular cartilage wear.

- Chronic lateral ankle instability may eventually be associated with
  - Relative anterior subluxation of the talus
  - Varus tilt of the talus within the ankle mortise
  - Hindfoot varus position
- Primary osteoarthrosis of the ankle is rare and poorly understood.
- Inflammatory arthropathy
  - Progressive and proliferative synovial erosive changes failing to respond to medical management
  - May be associated with chronic posterior tibial tendinopathy and progressive valgus hindfoot deformity, eventual valgus tilt to the talus within the ankle mortise, potential lateral malleolar stress fracture, and compensatory forefoot varus

PATIENT HISTORY AND PHYSICAL FINDINGS

- History
  - Typically, history of trauma to the ankle
    - Intra-articular ankle fracture (bi- or trimalleolar ankle fracture; tibial plafond [pilon] fracture)
    - Chronic ankle instability
  - Inflammatory arthropathy
  - Primary ankle arthritis
- Symptoms and complaints
  - Pain in anterior ankle with weight bearing and particularly with forced dorsiflexion
  - Often relieved by rest, but patient may have pain even at rest after vigorous activity or prolonged standing
  - Ankle swelling
  - Ankle stiffness
- Medications
  - If patient is taking anti-inflammatory agents, these will need to be stopped preoperatively to limit the risk of perioperative bleeding.
  - Rheumatoid medications may need to be stopped perioperatively to optimize wound and bone healing.
- Physical examination
  - Alignment
    - Ipsilateral limb alignment (not simply ankle alignment). The surgeon should examine the lower extremity from the hip to the foot. Optimal limb alignment is essential for the ankle arthrodesis to function well. Any ability for the lower limb to compensate for malalignment through the ankle is forfeited with ankle arthrodesis.
  - Ankle–foot alignment
    - The ankle functions as part of an ankle–subtalar joint complex.

- Ankle fusion must be positioned on a sufficiently supportive and plantigrade foot.
- Hindfoot, midfoot, and even forefoot malalignment may need to be addressed simultaneous to or staged with ankle arthrodesis.
- Range of motion (ROM)
  - Ankle ROM is not critical because the ankle will be stiff following arthrodesis.
  - Hindfoot ROM is essential for successful ankle arthrodesis. A stiff hindfoot and fused ankle allows very little accommodation and functions as a tibiotalocalcaneal or even pantalar arthrodesis. Ankle arthritis associated with hindfoot stiffness, particularly if due to hindfoot arthritis, may be better treated with total ankle arthroplasty (TAA).
- Soft tissues
  - An intact, relatively healthy soft tissue envelope surrounding the ankle is less likely to have soft tissue complications postoperatively, provided careful soft tissue handling is maintained.
  - Previous surgical scars must be considered. Either they can be incorporated into the surgical approach or the surgical approach may be modified to limit postoperative wound complications.
  - Vascular status: Intact pulses and satisfactory refill must be confirmed; if not, a Doppler ultrasound or noninvasive vascular studies must be performed before considering surgery.
  - Neurologic status: A peripheral neuropathy is a relative contraindication for TAA; in my opinion, well-controlled diabetes without neuropathy is not. However, if there is any question about risks, then arthrodesis should be considered in lieu of arthroplasty for end-stage ankle arthritis. Established neuropathy and either existing or high risk of Charcot neuroarthropathy is a contraindication for TAA. Ankle arthrodesis or even tibiotalocalcaneal arthrodesis is favored over TAA for end-stage ankle arthritis associated with a dense peripheral neuropathy and risk of or existing Charcot neuroarthropathy.
  - Motor function: Intact motor function of the ankle and foot is essential to successful ankle arthrodesis. Lack of active dorsiflexion, plantarflexion, inversion, or eversion is a relative contraindication to ankle arthrodesis. Tibialis anterior (TA) function is still required to dorsiflex the foot at the transverse tarsal (talonavicular and calcaneocuboid) joints. Gastrocnemius–soleus function is needed to plantarflex the hindfoot. Posterior tibial and peroneal tendon function is necessary to maintain a dynamic balance of the foot under the ankle arthrodesis. Without these functioning muscle groups, a tibiotalocalcaneal or pantalar arthrodesis or possibly a bridle tendon transfer may be warranted.

IMAGING AND OTHER DIAGNOSTIC STUDIES

- Weight-bearing anteroposterior (AP), lateral, and mortise views of the ankle
- Weight-bearing AP, lateral, and oblique views of the foot, particularly with associated foot deformity

- With associated or suspected lower leg deformity, I routinely obtain weight-bearing AP and lateral tibia–fibula views.
- With deformity in the lower extremity, we routinely obtain weight-bearing mechanical axis (hip-to-ankle) views of both extremities.
- We typically evaluate complex or ill-defined ankle–hindfoot patterns of arthritis with or without deformity using computed tomography of the ankle and hindfoot.
- If we suspect avascular necrosis of the talus or distal tibia, we obtain a magnetic resonance imaging of the ankle.

DIFFERENTIAL DIAGNOSIS

- See Pathogenesis.

NONOPERATIVE MANAGEMENT

- Activity modification
- Bracing
  - Ankle–foot orthosis
  - Double upright brace attached to shoe
- Stiffer-soled shoe with a rocker bottom modification
- Nonsteroidal anti-inflammatories or cyclooxygenase-2 inhibitors
- Medications for systemic inflammatory arthropathy
- Corticosteroid injection
- Viscosupplementation

SURGICAL MANAGEMENT

- The trend is to perform ankle arthrodesis through an anterior approach with preservation of the malleoli.
  - Recently, there have been favorable outcomes in conversion of ankle fusion to TAA.
    - Although ankle arthrodesis is typically successful in relieving symptoms related to end-stage ankle arthritis, over time, the hindfoot may develop compensatory degenerative changes (ie, adjacent joint arthritis).
  - If one or both of the malleoli are sacrificed, then this potential conversion is compromised.
  - The anterior approach is also used for the majority of TAA cases.

Preoperative Planning

- Vascular and neurologic examination
  - It is easy to focus on the patient's symptoms and radiographs demonstrating end-stage ankle arthritis.
  - Satisfactory circulation is essential to allow wound healing and fusion.
  - A neuropathy may warrant a more extensive ankle–hindfoot stabilization.
- Deformity correction
  - A sound preoperative plan facilitates effective intraoperative deformity correction.
- The surgeon should evaluate the contralateral extremity and ankle to have an understanding of what is physiologic for that patient.

Positioning

- Supine
- Plantar aspect of operated foot at end of operating table

- Foot and ankle well balanced, with toes directed to the ceiling
- A bolster under the ipsilateral hip prevents undesired external rotation of the hip.
- We routinely use a thigh tourniquet and regional anesthesia.
  - A popliteal block provides adequate pain relief postoperatively, particularly if a regional catheter is used. Moreover, hip and knee flexion–extension is not forfeited, facilitating safe immediate postoperative mobilization.

- However, to use a thigh tourniquet with a popliteal block typically requires a supplemental femoral nerve block (patients temporarily forfeit knee extension postoperatively) or general anesthesia.

Approach

- Anterior approach to the ankle, using the interval between the TA tendon and the extensor hallucis longus (EHL) tendon

EXPOSURE

- Make a longitudinal midline incision over the anterior ankle, starting about 10 cm proximal to the tibiotalar joint and 1 cm lateral to the tibial crest (**TECH FIG 1A**).
- Continue the incision midline over the anterior ankle just distal to the talonavicular joint.
- At no point should direct tension be placed on the skin margins; we perform deep, full-thickness retraction as soon as possible to limit the risk of skin complications.
- Identify and protect the superficial peroneal nerve by retracting it laterally.
  - In our experience, there is a consistent branch of the superficial peroneal nerve that crosses directly over or immediately proximal to the tibiotalar joint.
- We then expose the extensor retinaculum, identify the course of the EHL tendon, and sharply but carefully divide the retinaculum directly over the EHL tendon (**TECH FIG 1B,C**).
  - We always attempt to maintain the TA tendon in its dedicated sheath.
  - Preserving the retinaculum over the TA tendon
    - Prevents bowstringing of the tendon and thereby reduces the stress on the anterior wound

- Should there be a wound dehiscence, then the TA is not directly exposed.
    - Preserving the retinaculum over the TA tendon is not always possible; some patients do not have a dedicated sheath for the TA.
- Use the interval between the TA and EHL tendon, with the TA and EHL tendons retracted medially and laterally, respectively.
- Identify the deep neurovascular bundle (anterior tibial–dorsalis pedis artery and deep peroneal nerve) and carefully retract it laterally throughout the remainder of the procedure (**TECH FIG 1D**).
- Perform an anterior capsulotomy along with elevation of the tibial and dorsal talar periosteum to about 6 to 8 cm proximal to the tibial plafond and talonavicular joint, respectively (**TECH FIG 1E**).
- Elevate this separated capsule and periosteum medially and laterally to expose the ankle, access the medial and lateral gutters, and visualize the medial and lateral malleoli (**TECH FIG 1F,G**).
- Remove anterior tibial and talar osteophytes to facilitate exposure and avoid interference with the instrumentation (**TECH FIG 1H,I**).

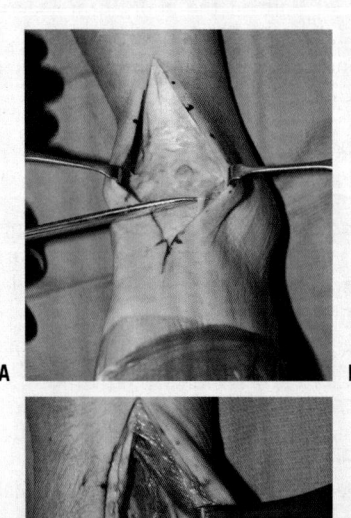
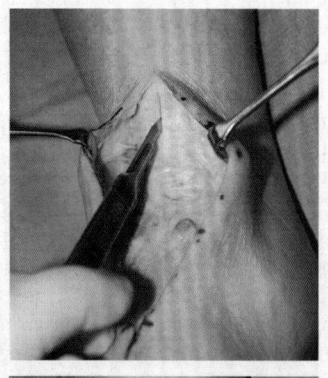
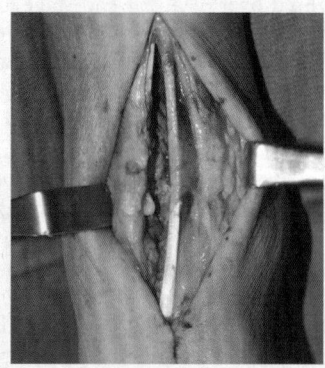
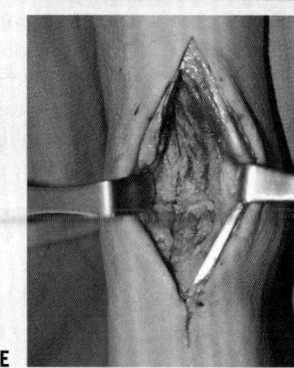

TECH FIG 1 A. Anterior approach to ankle (note sural nerve). **B,C.** The extensor retinaculum is divided. **B.** Initiating the longitudinal incision in the retinaculum immediately superficial to the EHL tendon. **C.** EHL tendon exposed. **D.** The deep neurovascular bundle must be identified and protected. **E.** Tibiotalar joint exposed after arthrotomy. *(continued)*

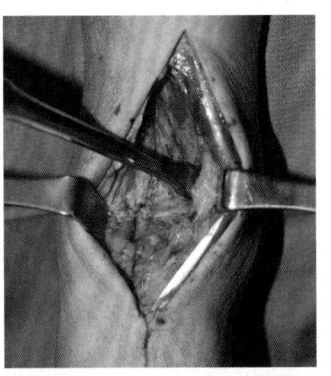
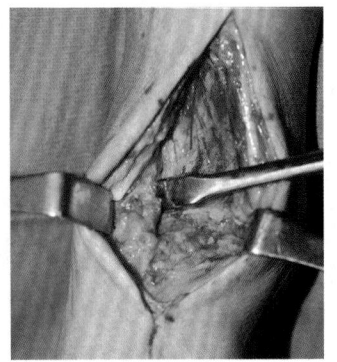
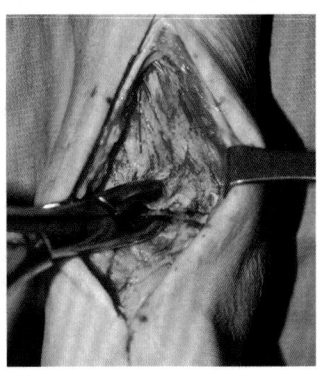
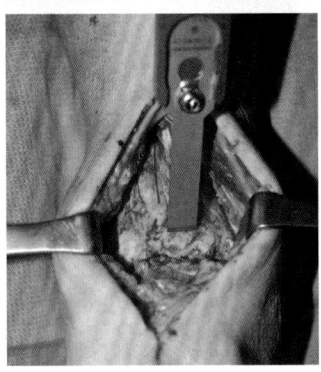

TECH FIG 1 *(continued)* **F,G.** Exposure improved with capsular and periosteal elevation at the joint line. **F.** Laterally. **G.** Medially. **H,I.** Distal anterior tibial exostectomy. **H.** Rongeur. **I.** Chisel.

TIBIOTALAR JOINT PREPARATION

- I routinely use joint distraction **(TECH FIG 2A,B)**.
- I prefer to maintain the subchondral bone architecture.
  - In preserving the essential anatomy of the talar dome and tibial plafond, I have the ability to adjust dorsiflexion–plantarflexion without compromising limb length or bony apposition at the arthrodesis site.
    - Flat cuts tend to forfeit limb length and the ability to adjust alignment without forfeiting optimal bony apposition.
  - Obviously, with deformity correction through the joint, some of the subchondral architecture may need to be sacrificed.
- I remove the residual cartilage with a sharp elevator or chisel (see **TECH FIG 2A**).

- While preserving the subchondral architecture as best as possible, I penetrate the subchondral bone with a drill bit, a narrow chisel, or both **(TECH FIG 2C–E)**.
  - This increases surface area and promotes fusion.
- Although careful to preserve the malleoli, I still prepare the tibiotalar joint gutters to further increase the surface area for fusion **(TECH FIG 2F,G)**.
- Use of bone graft is at the surgeon's discretion.
  - I routinely use bone graft to fill any voids at the arthrodesis site.
  - Avoid excessive use of bone graft; the best chance for fusion is if the physiologic surfaces are appropriately prepared and well apposed.

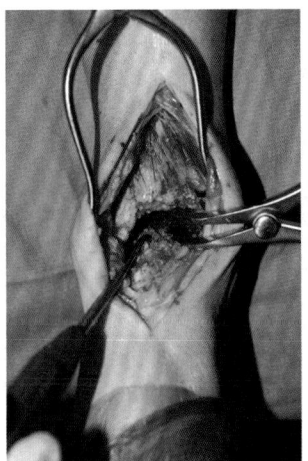
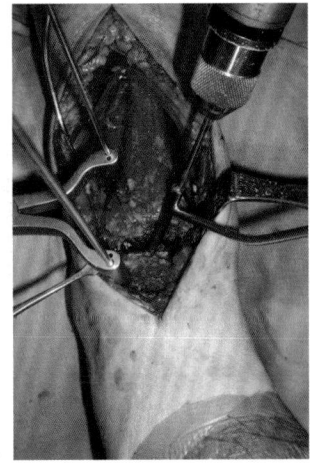

TECH FIG 2 A,B. Tibiotalar joint preparation. **A.** Using a lamina spreader for distraction and a sharp elevator to delaminate residual cartilage. **B.** Alternatively, an invasive joint distractor may be used, here with drilling of the subchondral bone to promote healing. Tibiotalar joint preparation. *(continued)*

TECHNIQUES

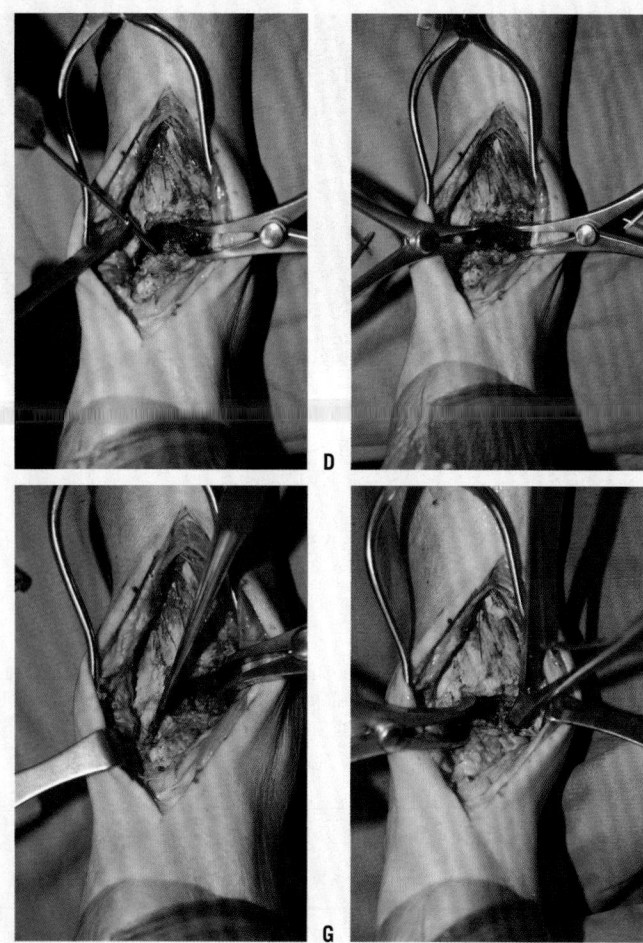

TECH FIG 2 *(continued)* **C.** Lateral lamina spreader with medial talar dome subchondral bone drilling. **D.** Dual lamina spreaders to switch to using only the medial lamina spreader. **E.** Medial lamina spreader with sharp elevator to remove residual lateral talar dome cartilage. **F,G.** Preparation of the tibiotalar gutters. **F.** Medial gutter with sharp elevator. **G.** Lateral gutter using a rongeur.

TIBIOTALAR JOINT REDUCTION

- For me, optimal tibiotalar joint alignment for arthrodesis is as follows:
  - Neutral dorsiflexion–plantarflexion **(TECH FIG 3A)**
    - Many years ago, there was a tendency to fuse women's ankles in plantarflexion to facilitate wearing a heel. This is an idea that should be abandoned.
    - The tendency is to underestimate how much dorsiflexion is needed to get the ankle to neutral. Therefore, I typically dorsiflex the talus within the mortise just slightly more than what I think it may need. This usually results in neutral dorsiflexion–plantarflexion.
  - Slight hindfoot valgus
    - Balance the talus within the ankle mortise, but be sure that the hindfoot is in slight valgus.
    - If not, then contour the tibiotalar preparation to get the hindfoot in slight valgus.
    - A reasonable landmark is to have the lateral bony aspect of the calcaneus be in line with the fibula; if it is medial to the fibula, then a neutral to varus position is inappropriately set.
  - Rotation
    - Align the second metatarsal with the anterior tibial crest.
    - When the malleoli are preserved, rotation is often auto-adjusted.

- External rotation is recommended by some authors, but I consider this only if the contralateral extremity dictates this position.
  - The goal is to avoid internal rotation.
- Sagittal plane relationship of the talus to the tibia
  - Avoid anterior translation of the talus relative to the tibia. This places the ankle and foot at a biomechanical disadvantage.
  - With some deformity, it may be difficult to translate the talus posteriorly to a more physiologic position. In some cases, I have had to resect some of the posterior malleolus (through the joint from the anterior approach with joint distraction) to allow such posterior translation **(TECH FIG 3B)**. Also, judiciously, the deltoid ligament may need to be partially released to allow posterior translation. Perform this cautiously, though, as some of the talar dome blood supply travels through the deltoid branch off the posterior tibial artery.
- I routinely obtain intraoperative fluoroscopic views in the AP and lateral planes to confirm appropriate alignment and bony apposition.

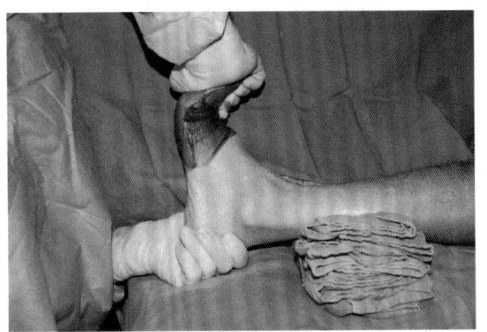
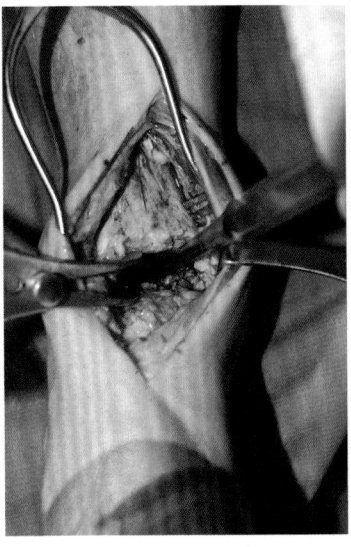

TECH FIG 3 A. Tibiotalar joint reduction, with neutral dorsiflexion–plantarflexion, slight hindfoot valgus, and second metatarsal rotated to anterior tibial crest. **B.** If the talus fails to translate posteriorly in the ankle mortise, then the posterior malleolus may need to be weakened to allow the talus to reduce under the tibial axis.

INTERNAL FIXATION WITH ANTERIOR PLATING–SCREW FIXATION

- Internal fixation is contraindicated or less than optimal in the face of the following:
  - Infection
  - Osteopenic bone
- Traditionally, I performed screw fixation and added an anterior plate for further stability; more recently, I have switched to a technique where anterior plating is the primary technique, and I supplement with screws (other than those in the plate) only if I feel further stability is needed.
- Provisional fixation once optimal reduction is achieved

Traditional Screw Fixation and Supplemental Anterior Plate

- Case: 55-year-old man high-demand patient with anterior translation of the talus within the ankle mortise **(TECH FIG 4A–C)**
- Patient is positioned supine on the operating table with a bump under the ipsilateral hip to resist external rotation of the extremity.
- I typically use a medial screw first **(TECH FIG 4D).**

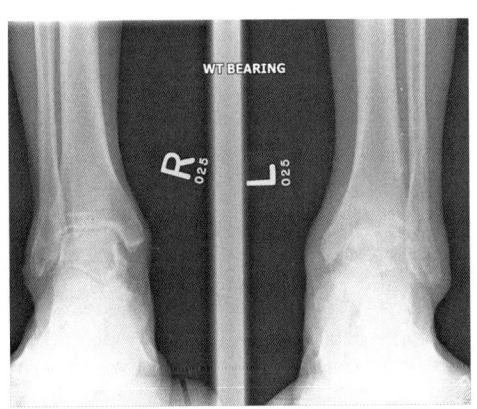
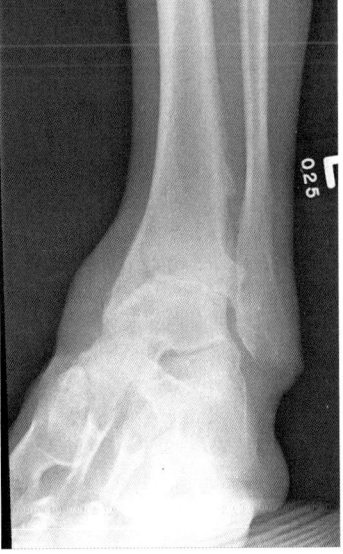
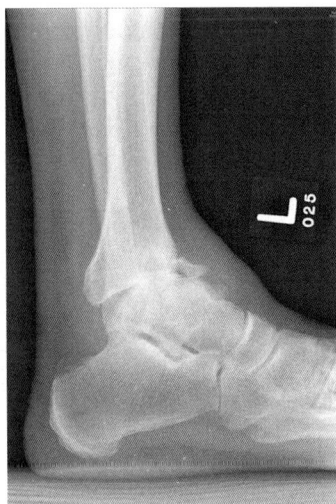

TECH FIG 4 A–C. A 55-year-old man with chronic instability and posttraumatic arthritis. **A.** AP view with comparison to contralateral ankle. **B.** Mortise view. **C.** Lateral view. There is considerable anterior translation of the talus from the ankle mortise. *(continued)*

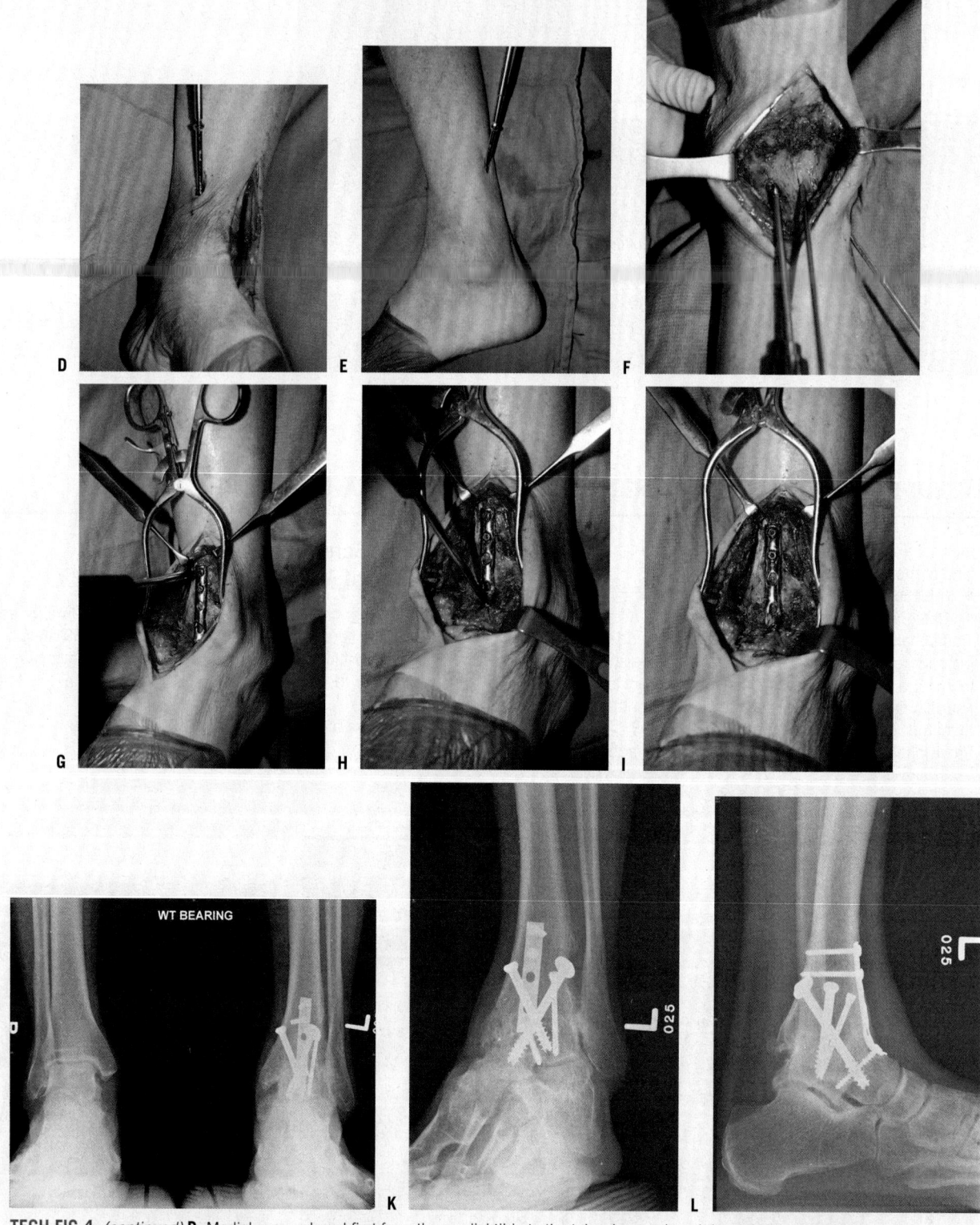

TECH FIG 4 *(continued)* **D.** Medial screw placed first from the medial tibia to the talar dome, placed through a medial stab incision.
E. Traditional posterior to anterior screw, placed via a posterolateral stab incision (care must be maintained to avoid injury to the sural nerve).
F. Anterolateral screw placed through the anterior approach. Provisional fixation was placed adjacent to this screw. **G–I.** Anterior plating.
G. Proximal screw fixation. **H.** Talar screw fixation. **I.** Final view of plate before closure. **J–N.** Postoperative weight-bearing radiographs of
example patient with traditional screw fixation and supplemental anterior plate. **J.** AP radiograph. **K.** Mortise view. **L.** Lateral view (talus is
reduced under tibial axis). *(continued)*

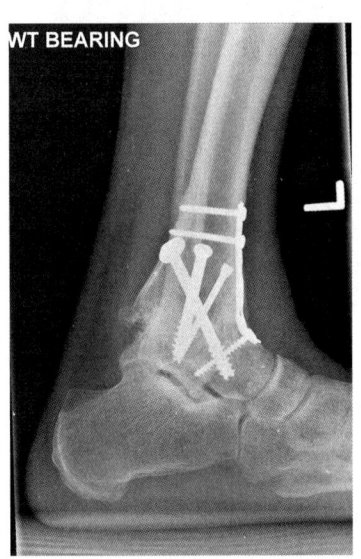

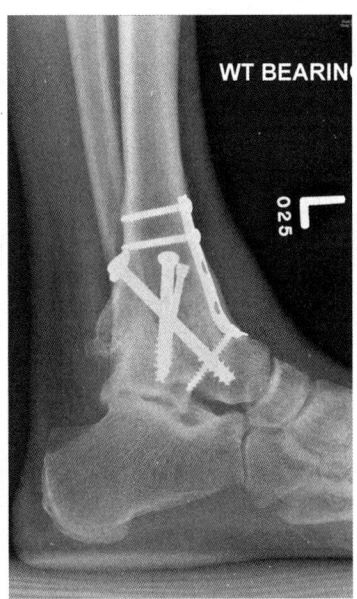

TECH FIG 4 *(continued)* **M.** Dorsiflexion view. **N.** Plantarflexion view. The patient lacks some hindfoot compensation for dorsiflexion and plantarflexion.

- Next, I place the posterior to anterior screw, the "home-run" screw.
  - With the newer anterior plating techniques that provide satisfactory stability, this screw has been largely abandoned; it is awkward to place and equally difficult to remove **(TECH FIG 4E)**.
- I add an anterolateral screw, one that is relatively vertical **(TECH FIG 4F)**.
- Finally, I augment the fixation with an anterior plate. In this case, a small fragment, nonlocking plate was used **(TECH FIG 4G–I)**.
  - In my experience, adding a supplemental anterior plate to an ankle arthrodesis construct adds considerable stability.
- Follow-up radiographs **(TECH FIG 4J–N)**
  - Patient returned to full activities, even playing doubles tennis.
  - He lacks some plantarflexion; time will tell what effect this will have on the hindfoot articulations that are attempting to compensate.
  - The talus is again in a physiologic relationship with the tibia, improving his biomechanics despite ankle arthrodesis.

Plate Fixation as the Primary Fixation

- Case: 33-year-old man with posttraumatic ankle arthritis and syndesmotic disruption **(TECH FIG 5A–C)**
- Same joint preparation as described earlier
- Provisional fixation with desired joint reduction
- Plate locked to the dorsolateral talar neck with locking screws
- Plate is precontoured based on average anterior ankle morphology.

- Compression device is secured, and compression is applied, thereby approximating the arthrodesis surfaces **(TECH FIG 5D–F)**.
  - Although the locking plate creates axial compression, a mild but desirable valgus moment may be introduced because the lateral plate is being used for compression.
  - To obtain optimal compression, provisional fixation is removed before compression is applied but after the screws are locked into the talar neck and the compression device is secured proximally.
- After performing compression and securing the lateral plate in the tibia, the medial plate is applied **(TECH FIG 5G,H)**.
  - Because compression has already been performed, this medial plate, which is also precontoured, serves to statically lock the arthrodesis.
- Each plate has a screw hole to allow nonlocking screw fixation from the plate to the posterior talar body **(TECH FIG 6A,B)**.
- Follow-up of case example **(TECH FIG 6C–G)**
- A supplemental screw may be added from the medial tibia to the talar body, but often, this is unnecessary **(TECH FIG 6H,I)**.

Closure

- I use a drain for 24 hours.
- Standard wound closure
  - I routinely close the capsule, extensor retinaculum, subcutaneous layer, and skin (to a tensionless closure).
  - The deep neurovascular bundle, extensor tendons, and superficial peroneal nerve need to be protected during closure.
- Sterile dressings on wound
- Padding
- Posterior sugar-tong splint

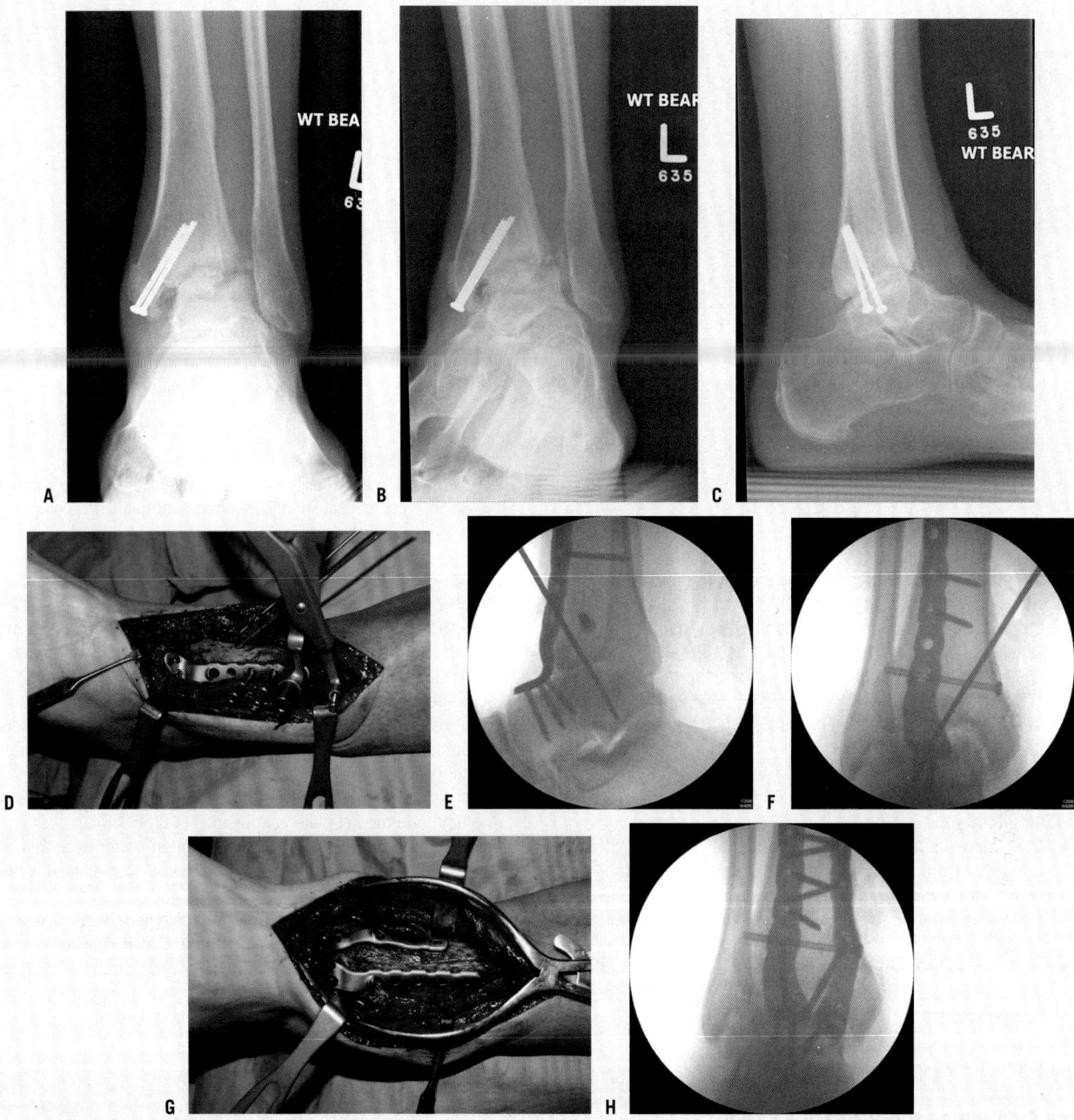

TECH FIG 5   A–C. Preoperative radiographs of patient undergoing double anterior plating arthrodesis technique. **A,B.** AP and mortise views with end-stage ankle arthritis and chronic syndesmosis disruption. **C.** Lateral view. **D.** Lateral anterior plate applied and secured to talus and proximal compression device in place. **E,F.** Intraoperative fluoroscopic views of ankle of a different patient undergoing dual anterior plating, with provisional fixation and lateral plate in place. **E.** Lateral view. **F.** AP view. **G.** Example patient with both plates in place. **H.** Intraoperative fluoroscopic view of different patient with both plates in place.

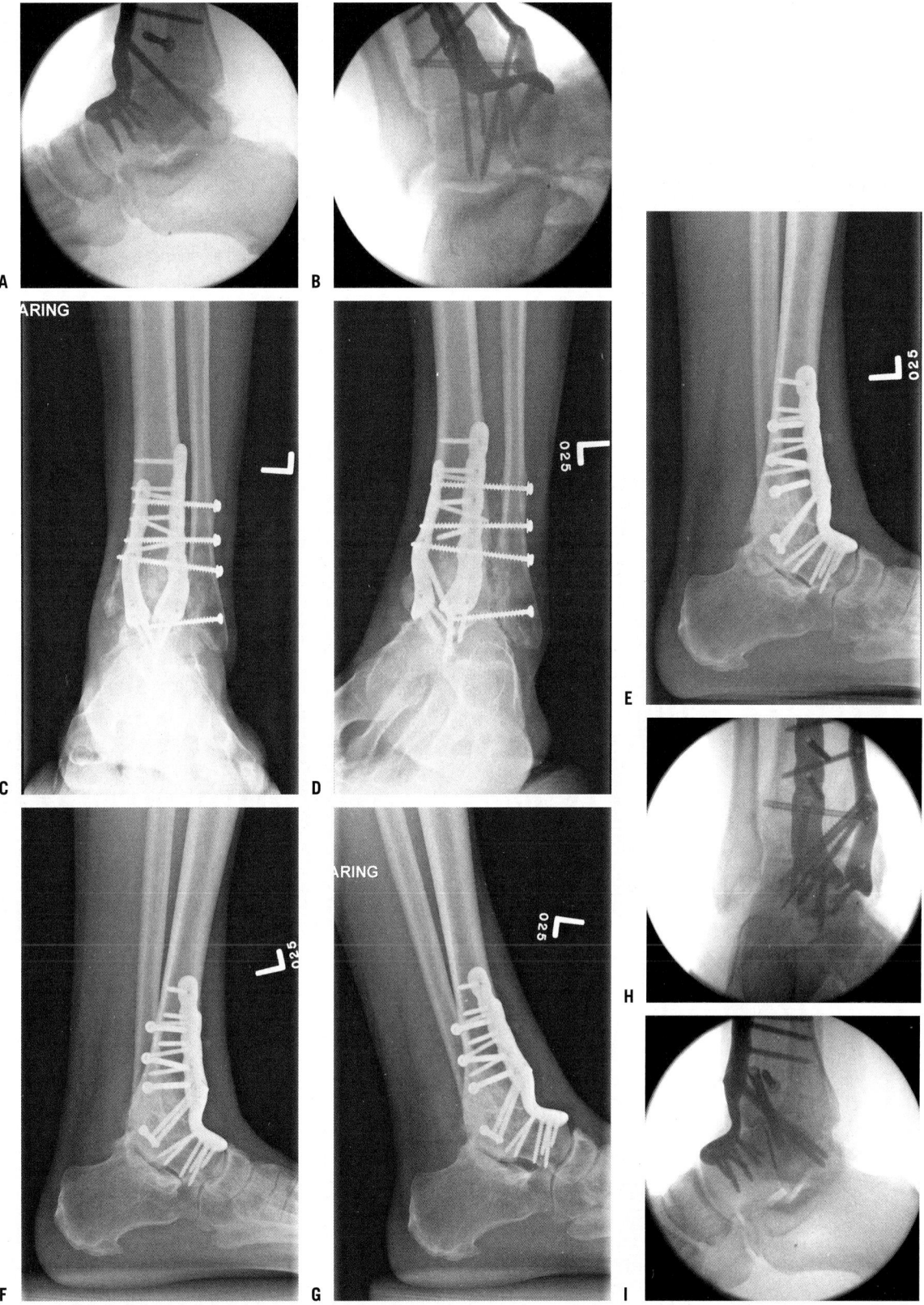

TECH FIG 6 **A,B.** Intraoperative fluoroscopic views of two screws placed through the plate into the posterior talus for additional stability. **A.** Lateral view. **B.** Broden view to confirm that screws do not violate the subtalar joint. **C–G.** Postoperative radiographs of example patient for dual anterior plating. **C.** AP view. **D.** Mortise view. **E.** Lateral view. **F.** Dorsiflexion view. **G.** Plantarflexion view. **H,I.** Intraoperative fluoroscopic views of different patient with supplemental screw to anterior plating. **H.** AP view. **I.** Lateral view (note broken guide pin; it is important to follow the exact trajectory of the guide pin with cannulated screw systems).

EXTERNAL FIXATION

- Infection is not a contraindication for external fixation.
  - There will be no implant directly at the tibiotalar joint.
  - In some cases, I have performed a staged arthrodesis, with initial débridement and antibiotic bead placement. The external fixator may be placed at that initial procedure or at the definitive procedure when the antibiotic beads are removed and the joint is reduced and compressed with the external fixator.
- Case: 45-year-old patient with posttraumatic arthritis and deformity of the ankle, failing to respond to a prior attempt at ankle arthrodesis.

- Radiographs demonstrate nonunion and residual deformity **(TECH FIG 7A–C)**.
  - Clinically, there are poor soft tissues anteriorly and a prior medial incision that will need to be incorporated into the surgical approach **(TECH FIG 7D,E)**.
    - A standard anterior approach is too risky and, in my opinion, would leave an insufficient skin bridge to the prior incision.
- Patient is positioned supine on the operating table, again with a bolster under the ipsilateral hip to direct the ankle anteriorly.
  - This patient also had a distal tibial external rotation malunion and an ankle nonunion with residual ankle external rotation **(TECH FIG 7F)**.
- Hardware is removed.

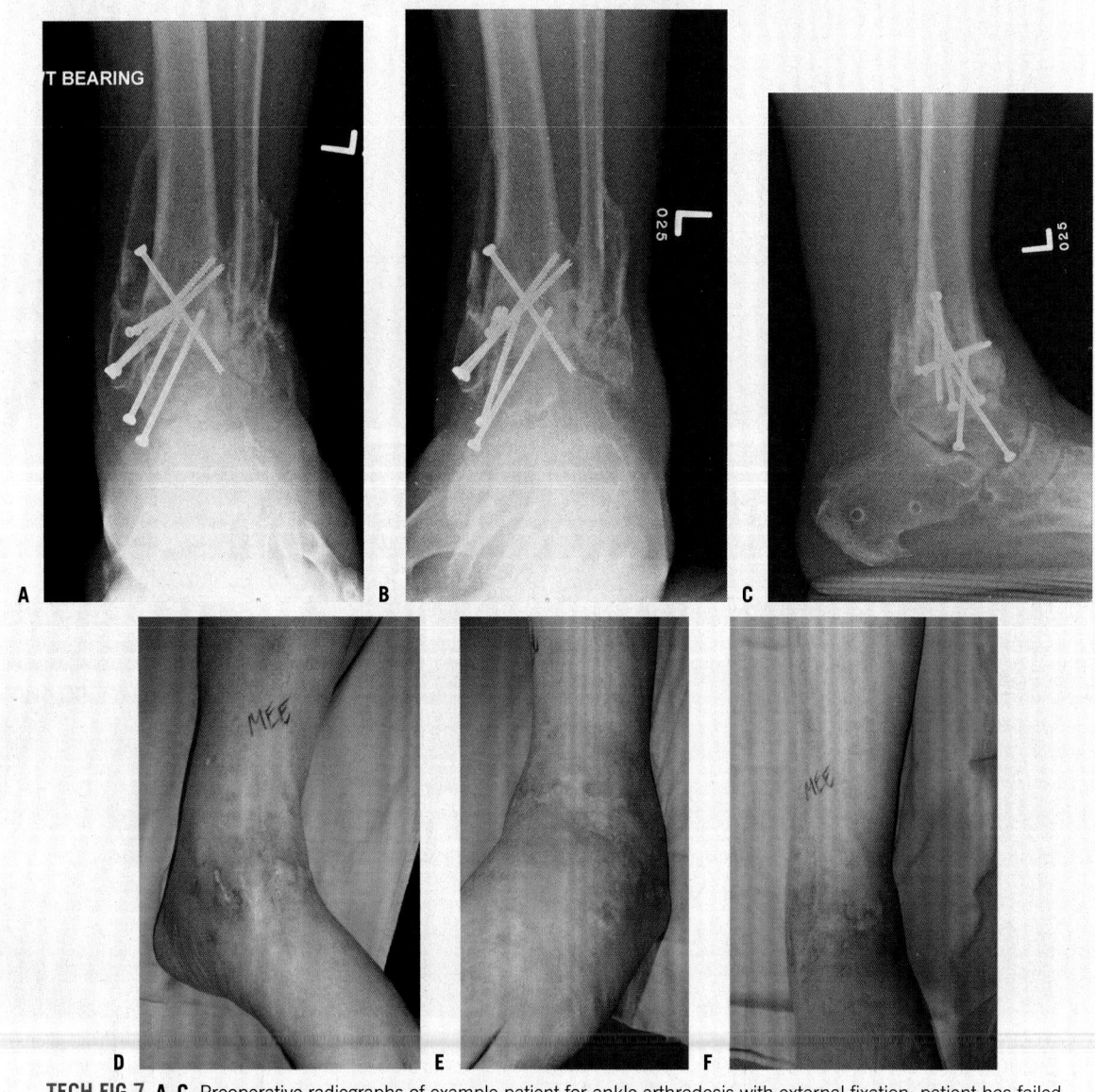

TECH FIG 7 A–C. Preoperative radiographs of example patient for ankle arthrodesis with external fixation; patient has failed ankle arthrodesis with internal fixation. **A.** AP view. **B.** Mortise view. **C.** Lateral view. **D,E.** Poor skin condition. **D.** Medial ankle with prior anteromedial approach. **E.** Dorsolateral aspect with residual scarring. **F.** Patient positioned supine on the operating table. The external rotation malunion of the distal tibia creates excessive external rotation of the foot relative to the tibial axis.

Approach

- I used the prior incision and added another "miniarthrotomy" incision laterally, thereby avoiding the unhealthy skin directly anteriorly over the ankle **(TECH FIG 8A)**.
- I prepared the joint through the medial incision and used the lateral incision to provide joint distraction **(TECH FIG 8B)**. I also switched the lamina spreader to the medial wound so that I could prepare the remainder of the joint via the lateral incision.
- From the preoperative radiographs, it is obvious that there is distal tibial deformity and nonanatomic malleolar anatomy **(TECH FIG 8C,D)**.
  - For this reason, the talus is not locked within the ankle mortise, and rotation will need to be carefully controlled. However, this is more important with internal fixation; with external fixation, such malrotation could still be corrected postoperatively with external fixator frame adjustment.

Joint Reduction and Provisional Fixation

- Neutral dorsiflexion–plantarflexion
- Slight hindfoot valgus
- Correct malrotation
  - Align second metatarsal with the anterior tibial crest.
- Provisionally pin the joint.
  - I usually place two Steinmann pins axially. Although this violates the subtalar joint, I do not believe that this has significant consequences in these patients with deformity, severe ankle arthritis, and compensatory hindfoot alignment.

- I routinely close the wounds at this point because once the external fixator is in place, suturing is particularly tedious.
  - However, if you prefer to delay the wound closure until the external fixator is in place, one or two struts can easily be reflected to allow adequate access to the wound or wounds.

Proximal Ring Block

- I place the proximal ring block (I usually use two rings to create the "block") orthogonally to the tibia **(TECH FIG 9A)**.
- Initially, I stabilize the rings with two thin wires but do not tension them at this point.
- I supplement the proximal ring block fixation with three half-pins **(TECH FIG 9B)**.
- Once the half-pins are secured, I tension the thin wires **(TECH FIG 9C)**.

Foot Plate

- I suspend the foot plate ("horseshoe") from a transverse forefoot wire. This way, I can control the foot's position within the foot plate **(TECH FIG 10A)**.
- Once I am satisfied with the foot's position relative to the foot plate, I secure the hindfoot with two crossed thin wires, making sure the plantar surface of the foot is distal to the foot ring **(TECH FIG 10B)**.
- I typically place a midfoot wire as well.

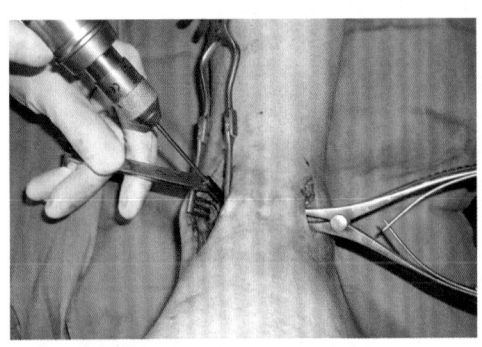
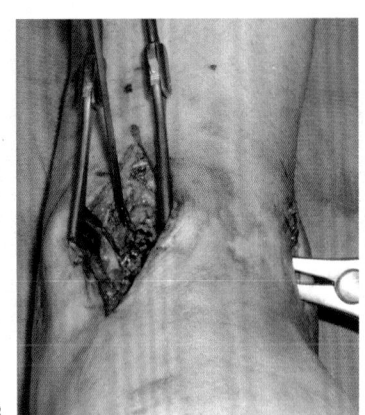
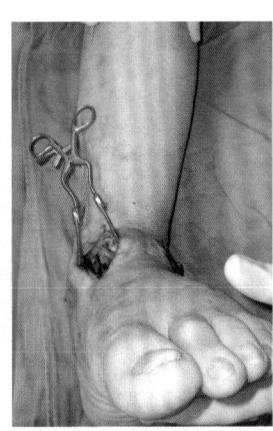
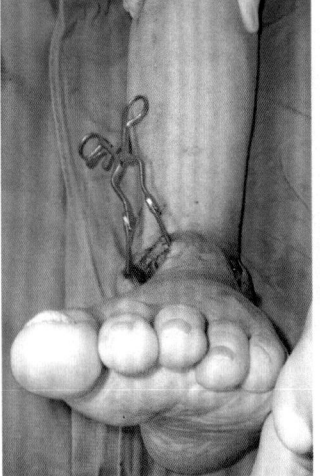

TECH FIG 8 **A.** Modified "mini-open" arthrotomy approach to ankle arthrodesis. Previous medial incision used and a separate mini-lateral incision. Medial incision is being used for joint preparation while joint is being distracted by lamina spreader placed via lateral incision. Skin bridge between two wounds is adequate, and previously compromised skin is not violated. **B.** Medial joint preparation. **C,D.** With distortion of the malleolar anatomy, the talus is not "locked" within the ankle mortise. **C.** Ankle tends to externally rotate. **D.** Ankle can be manually reduced to a physiologic position with the second metatarsal aligned to the anterior tibial shaft axis.

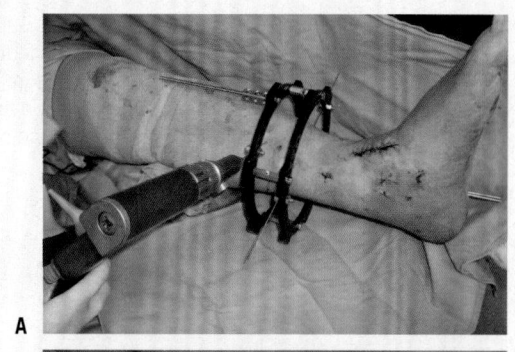

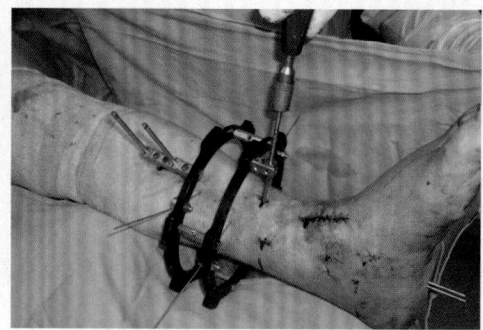

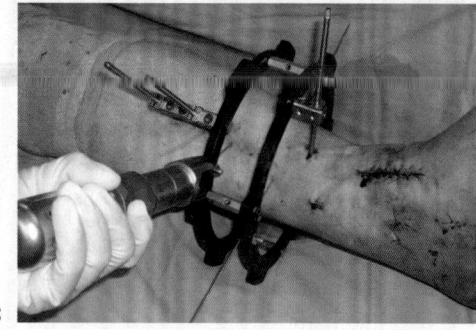

TECH FIG 9 A. Building the proximal ring block, first with thin wires. Wounds were closed before applying external fixator. **B.** Half-pins added to stabilize the proximal ring block. **C.** Thin wires are tensioned within the proximal ring block.

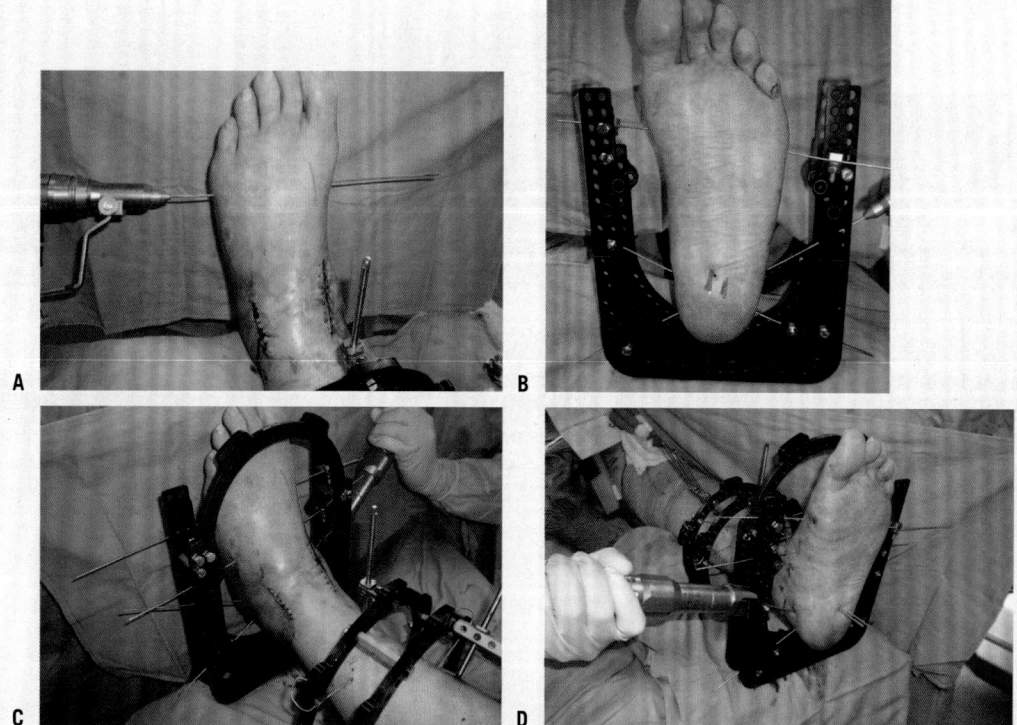

TECH FIG 10 A. Forefoot wire placed to suspend the foot plate. **B.** Foot balanced within the foot plate. Foot plate suspended from forefoot wire and calcaneal wires being passed to stabilize the hindfoot. **C.** Tensioning the thin wires in the foot. The ring has been closed on the foot frame so that tension in all wires can be effectively maintained. **D.** In this case, two rings were used for the foot plate portion of the frame. Closing the top ring allows the foot frame to be closed even without placing a half-ring on the anterior portion of the "horseshoe." *(continued)*

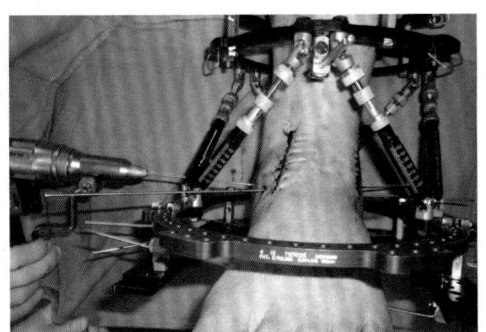
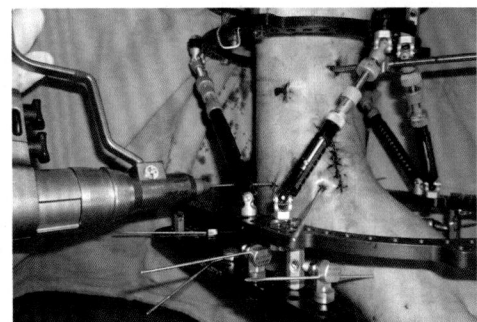

E   F

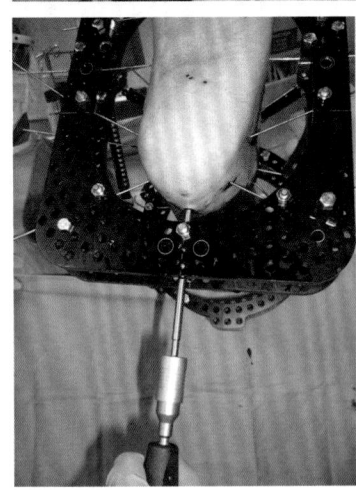

G

TECH FIG 10 *(continued)* **E,F.** Two talar wires are passed. Without talar wires, compression would be placed not only on the tibiotalar joint but also on the subtalar joint. **G.** Calcaneal half-pin for added foot frame stability.

- Before tensioning the thin wires, I close the horseshoe-shaped foot plate anteriorly.
  - This can be done by adding a half-ring to the anterior foot plate, or I can have a double-decker foot plate and close the more proximal of the two foot plates **(TECH FIG 10C)**.
  - Having two foot plate components affords less interference between the struts (that will connect the proximal ring block to the foot plate) and the thin wires to be passed through the foot from the foot plate.
- I then tension the thin wires in the foot **(TECH FIG 10D)**.
- I also place one or two talar wires to provide greater support and to protect the subtalar joint **(TECH FIG 10E,F)**.
  - These two wires either need to be built up from a single foot plate or connected to the proximal component of a two-ring foot plate setup.
  - This is also essential to protect the subtalar joint from compression. If fixation from the foot plate to the foot is limited to the forefoot, midfoot, and calcaneus and no fixation is added to the talus, then axial compression will not be isolated to the tibiotalar joint but will also include the subtalar joint (with potential detrimental effects to the subtalar joint cartilage and motion). A perhaps more sophisticated (but not more complicated) construction of the foot plate is to distract between the two components of the foot plate so that the subtalar joint is distracted while the tibiotalar joint is compressed. Although unproven, this may have a protective effect on the subtalar joint.
- I routinely add a calcaneal half-pin for added foot plate stability **(TECH FIG 10G)**.

Adding the Struts

- Connect the proximal ring block and foot plate by struts and apply tibiotalar compression **(TECH FIG 11A)**.
- I make subtle adjustments at this point, which sometimes warrants removing one or both of the provisional fixation pins **(TECH FIG 11B)**.
- If the alignment is optimal, then I can leave one provisional pin in place (provided it is truly axial) to act as a rail as I compress the tibial talar joint with the external fixator.
  - If no translation, angulation, or rotation is required, which is often the case if the initial reduction was appropriate, then simply tightening the struts uniformly leads to satisfactory axial compression **(TECH FIG 11C,D)**.
- If adjustments need to be made, the computer program may be used to run an effective correction at this time. However, on the operating table, the struts may simply be loosened, a gross manual adjustment can be made (with the provisional fixation removed), and the struts again are secured. Then, uniform tightening of all struts can be performed.
- Final fluoroscopic views in the AP and lateral planes are sometimes difficult to interpret with an external fixator in place, but with subtle rotation of the limb, appropriate alignment and bony apposition can be confirmed.
- Final check is made to be sure that all bolts and connections are stable.

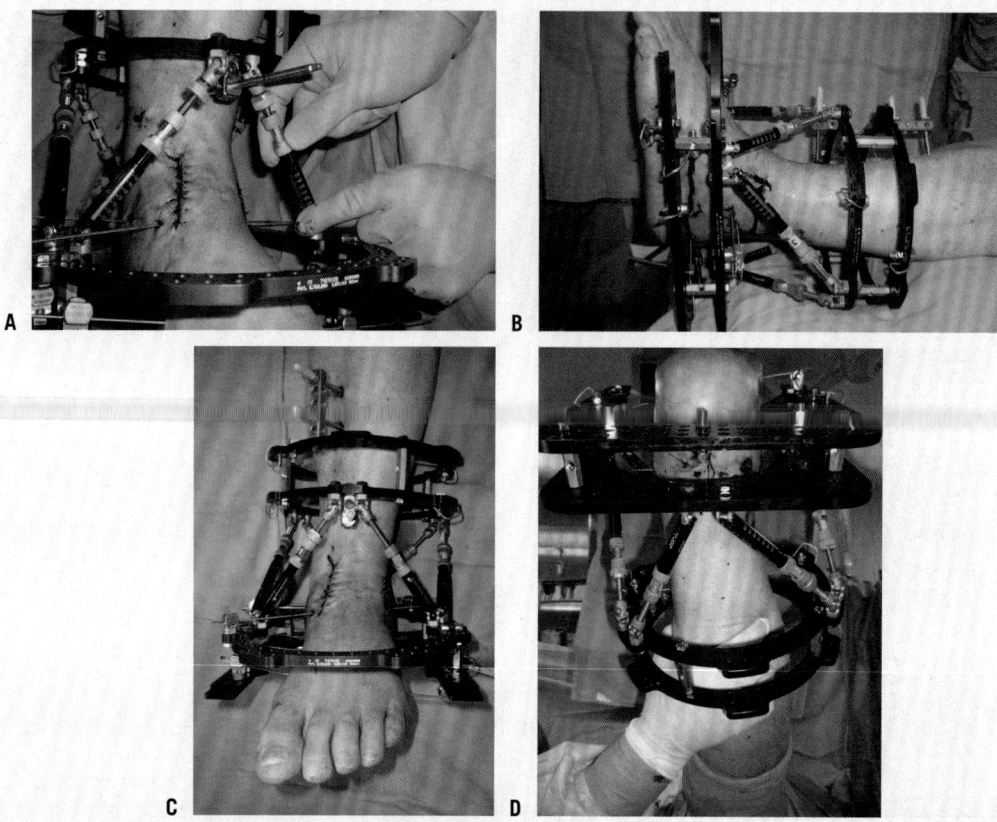

TECH FIG 11 A. Adding struts to be used for compression between the proximal ring block and the foot frame.
B. Proper position of the foot and leg within the external fixator. Ankle with neutral dorsiflexion–plantarflexion and plantar foot is distal to most distal ring plate. The provisional fixation was removed for compression.
C,D. Physiologic hindfoot valgus, with varus avoided. **C.** AP view. **D.** Posteroanterior view.

Wound Dressing and Follow-up

- Sterile dressings are placed on the wound.
- Sterile dressings are placed on the wires and half-pins.
  - Pin irritation typically occurs because of skin motion or tension about the half-pins or thin wires.
  - I routinely place thick dressings around the thin wires and half-pins, creating moderate pressure from the dressing on the skin immediately adjacent to the half-pin or wire and thereby stabilizing the skin.
- Prefabricated bolsters are also available to stabilize the skin around the pins.
- Final follow-up for this case shows that alignment has been restored. Fusion is apparent despite distorted distal tibial alignment (TECH FIG 12).

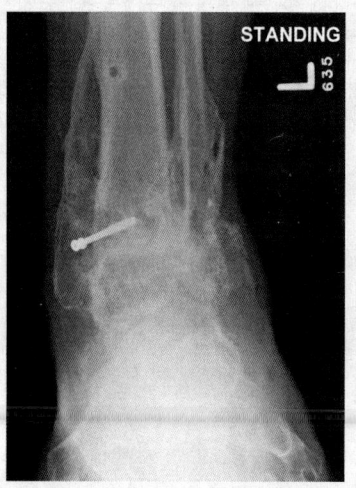
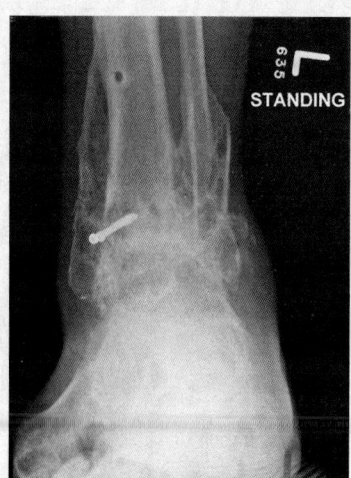
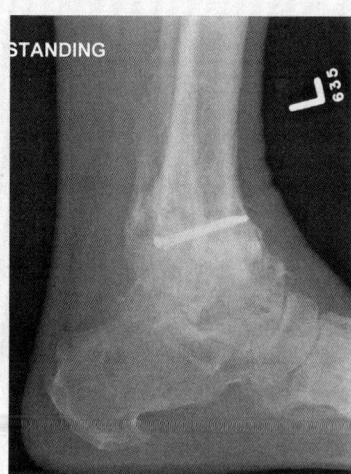

TECH FIG 12 Follow-up radiographs suggesting successful revision ankle arthrodesis using external fixation. **A.** AP view. **B.** Mortise view. **C.** Lateral view.

Pearls and Pitfalls

Position of Arthrodesis	• Avoid varus and internal rotation. Optimal position is neutral dorsiflexion–plantarflexion, slight hindfoot valgus, and the second metatarsal aligned with the anterior tibial crest.
Prior or Active Infection	• Internal fixation for ankle arthrodesis is probably contraindicated; however, arthrodesis is still possible with external fixation.
Joint Preparation	• Internal and external fixation may stabilize the joint, but satisfactory joint preparation for arthrodesis is essential for fusion to occur.
Preservation of Subchondral Bone Architecture	• If possible, maintain the subchondral bone architecture. This allows adjustments in dorsiflexion–plantarflexion position without forfeiting bony apposition at the arthrodesis site before fixation.
Potential Advantages of Internal Fixation over External Fixation	• No need for pin care; perhaps less intimidating to the patient
Potential Advantages of External Fixation over Internal Fixation	• Further compression and adjustments at the arthrodesis site are possible postoperatively; perhaps earlier weight bearing

POSTOPERATIVE CARE

- With advances in anesthesia, ankle arthrodesis may be performed on an outpatient basis.
- However, we typically keep these patients at least overnight for pain control, nasal oxygen (which may have some positive effect on anterior wound healing), and prophylactic intravenous antibiotics.
- Follow-up in 10 to 14 days
  - Internal fixation
    - Suture removal
    - Short-leg, touchdown weight-bearing cast
  - External fixation
    - Suture removal
    - Radiographs to assess bony apposition at the arthrodesis site and alignment. If a subtle adjustment needs to be made, it is done at this time, typically with the computer program.
    - We routinely add more compression to the arthrodesis site at this and subsequent visits. Simple axial compression does not require use of the computer program; instead, uniform tightening of all struts creates axial compression at the arthrodesis site. This is a major advantage of external fixation over internal fixation. With internal fixation, bony apposition at the arthrodesis site cannot be altered after the index procedure.
    - The patient is instructed how to perform pin care. We do not usually have the patient perform pin care in the first 10 to 14 days in order to protect the wound. My routine pin care includes once-a-day pin cleaning with a sponge moistened with a 50-50 mixture of sterile saline and hydrogen peroxide. I instruct the patients to "shoeshine" the pins with the sponge so that the debris is removed at the pin–skin interface. If a pin is irritated, then we recommend placing an antibiotic ointment at that pin's interface with the skin and to continue to stabilize that particular pin with dressings that stabilize the skin adjacent to the pin. Oral antibiotics may be required in some situations.
    - We have the orthotist create a tread for the foot plate. Once the wounds have healed adequately and edema

is controlled, the tread can be added and weight bearing through the external fixator is possible—another potential advantage of external over internal fixation.
- Follow-up at about 6 weeks
  - Internal fixation
    - Ankle radiographs
    - If healing is progressing well, the patient is progressed to a cam boot.
    - If more healing is necessary, a short-leg cast is continued.
    - Weight bearing may be progressively increased if healing is progressing, but we typically restrict the patient from full weight bearing until 10 weeks (longer if healing is delayed).
  - External fixation
    - Radiographs
    - We routinely add more axial compression.
    - Pin care is reinforced.
    - Weight bearing is encouraged with the tread on the foot plate.
- Follow-up at 10 to 12 weeks and beyond
  - Internal fixation
    - Radiographs
    - If healing is suggested, then the patient can progress to full weight bearing, first in the cam boot and then transitioning to a regular shoe by 12 to 14 weeks. If healing is delayed, then this protocol is delayed.
  - External fixation
    - Radiographs
    - More axial compression is added.
    - If healing is suggested radiographically, then the surgeon should plan for external fixator removal between 12 and 16 weeks.
    - If healing is delayed, more axial compression is added, and follow-up is set for 3 to 4 more weeks. External fixator removal is delayed until healing is suggested.
    - Frame removal may be performed in the office, but removal of half-pins may be particularly uncomfortable for the patient (especially if hydroxyapatite-coated pins are used).

■ A short operating room procedure should be considered for frame removal with the patient under anesthesia.

■ We routinely add a short-leg walking cast for an additional 2 to 4 weeks, then transition to a cam boot and regular shoe.

OUTCOMES

- The literature suggests favorable outcomes of ankle arthrodesis, with good relief of ankle pain and high rates of patient satisfaction (mostly level IV retrospective studies without standardized foot and ankle outcome measures).
- At intermediate follow-up, good to excellent results have been reported in 66% to 90% of patients (mostly level IV retrospective studies without standardized foot and ankle outcome measures).
- In long-term follow-up, a considerable number of patients with ankle arthrodesis develop adjacent joint (subtalar and, to a lesser degree, transverse tarsal joint) arthrosis.
- Although most patients with arthrodesis report satisfactory pain relief, functional outcome, particularly gait analysis, is not physiologic.

COMPLICATIONS

- Both internal and external fixation
  - Infection
  - Wound dehiscence or delayed wound healing
  - Nonunion
  - Malunion
  - Late development of subtalar (and, to a lesser degree, transverse tarsal joint) arthritis (adjacent joint arthritis)
- Internal fixation
  - Prominent hardware
  - Residual gapping at tibiotalar arthrodesis site that cannot be compressed postoperatively
- External fixation
  - Pin tract infection

SUGGESTED READINGS

Agel J, Coetzee JC, Sangeorzan BJ, et al. Functional limitations of patients with end-stage ankle arthrosis. Foot Ankle Int 2005;26:537–539.

Anderson T, Montgomery F, Besjakov J, et al. Arthrodesis of the ankle for non-inflammatory conditions—healing and reliability of outcome measurements. Foot Ankle Int 2002;23:390–393.

Coester LM, Saltzman CL, Leupold J, et al. Long-term results following ankle arthrodesis for post-traumatic arthritis. J Bone Joint Surg Am 2001;83:219–228.

Colman AB, Pomeroy GC. Transfibular ankle arthrodesis with rigid internal fixation: an assessment of outcome. Foot Ankle Int 2007;28:303–307.

Easley ME, Montijo HE, Wilson JB, et al. Revision tibiotalar arthrodesis. J Bone Joint Surg Am 2008;90:1212–1223.

Eylon S, Porat S, Bor N, et al. Outcome of Ilizarov ankle arthrodesis. Foot Ankle Int 2007;28:873–879.

Fuchs S, Sandmann C, Skwara A, et al. Quality of life 20 years after arthrodesis of the ankle. A study of adjacent joints. J Bone Joint Surg Br 2003;85:994–998.

Glazebrook M, Daniels T, Younger A, et al. Comparison of health-related quality of life between patients with end-stage ankle and hip arthrosis. J Bone Joint Surg Am 2008;90:499–505.

Greisberg J, Assal M, Flueckiger G, et al. Takedown of ankle fusion and conversion to total ankle replacement. Clin Orthop Relat Res 2004;(424):80–88.

Haddad SL, Coetzee JC, Estok R, et al. Intermediate and long-term outcomes of total ankle arthroplasty and ankle arthrodesis. A systematic review of the literature. J Bone Joint Surg Am 2007;89:1899–1905.

Hintermann B, Barg A, Knupp M, et al. Conversion of painful ankle arthrodesis to total ankle arthroplasty. J Bone Joint Surg Am 2009;91:850–858.

Holt ES, Hansen ST, Mayo KA, et al. Ankle arthrodesis using internal screw fixation. Clin Orthop Relat Res 1991;(268):21–28.

Johnson EE, Weltmer J, Lian GJ, et al. Ilizarov ankle arthrodesis. Clin Orthop Relat Res 1992;(280):160–169.

King HA, Watkins TB Jr, Samuelson KM. Analysis of foot position in ankle arthrodesis and its influence on gait. Foot Ankle 1980;1:44–49.

Kovoor CC, Padmanabhan V, Bhaskar D, et al. Ankle fusion for bone loss around the ankle joint using the Ilizarov technique. J Bone Joint Surg Br 2009;91:361–366.

Kusnezov N, Dunn JC, Koehler LR, et al. Anatomically contoured anterior plating for isolated tibiotalar arthrodesis: a systematic review. Foot Ankle Spec 2017;10(4):352–358.

Mann RA, Rongstad KM. Arthrodesis of the ankle: a critical analysis. Foot Ankle Int 1998;19:3–9.

Monroe MT, Beals TC, Manoli A II. Clinical outcome of arthrodesis of the ankle using rigid internal fixation with cancellous screws. Foot Ankle Int 1999;20:227–231.

Muir DC, Amendola A, Saltzman CL. Long-term outcome of ankle arthrodesis. Foot Ankle Clin 2002;7:703–708.

Myerson MS, Quill G. Ankle arthrodesis. A comparison of an arthroscopic and an open method of treatment. Clin Orthop Relat Res 1991;(268):84–95.

Nielsen KK, Linde F, Jensen NC. The outcome of arthroscopic and open surgery ankle arthrodesis: a comparative retrospective study on 107 patients. Foot Ankle Surg 2008;14:153–157.

Ogut T, Glisson RR, Chuckpaiwong B, et al. External ring fixation versus screw fixation for ankle arthrodesis: a biomechanical comparison. Foot Ankle Int 2009;30:353–360.

Plaass C, Knupp M, Barg A, et al. Anterior double plating for rigid fixation of isolated tibiotalar arthrodesis. Foot Ankle Int 2009;30:631–639.

Salem KH, Kinzl L, Schmelz A. Ankle arthrodesis using Ilizarov ring fixators: a review of 22 cases. Foot Ankle Int 2006;27:764–770.

Saltzman CL, Mann RA, Ahrens JE, et al. Prospective controlled trial of STAR total ankle replacement versus ankle fusion: initial results. Foot Ankle Int 2009;30:579–596.

Sealey RJ, Myerson MS, Molloy A, et al. Sagittal plane motion of the hindfoot following ankle arthrodesis: a prospective analysis. Foot Ankle Int 2009;30:187–196.

SooHoo NF, Zingmond DS, Ko CY. Comparison of reoperation rates following ankle arthrodesis and total ankle arthroplasty. J Bone Joint Surg Am 2007;89:2143–2149.

Takakura Y, Tanaka Y, Sugimoto K, et al. Long-term results of arthrodesis for osteoarthritis of the ankle. Clin Orthop Relat Res 1999;(361):178–185.

Tarkin IS, Mormino MA, Clare MP, et al. Anterior plate supplementation increases ankle arthrodesis construct rigidity. Foot Ankle Int 2007;28(2):219–223.

Thomas RH, Daniels TR. Ankle arthritis. J Bone Joint Surg Am 2003;85:923–936.

Thomas RH, Daniels TR, Parker K. Gait analysis and functional outcomes following ankle arthrodesis for isolated ankle arthritis. J Bone Joint Surg Am 2006;88:526–535.

Trouillier H, Hänsel L, Schaff P, et al. Long-term results after ankle arthrodesis: clinical, radiological, gait analytical aspects. Foot Ankle Int 2002;23:1081–1090.

Wesley WF, Hirose CB, Coughlin MJ. Ankle arthrodesis using an anterior titanium dual locked plating construct. J Foot Ankle Surg 2017;56(2):304–308.

White AA III. A precision posterior ankle fusion. Clin Orthop Relat Res 1974;(98):239–250.

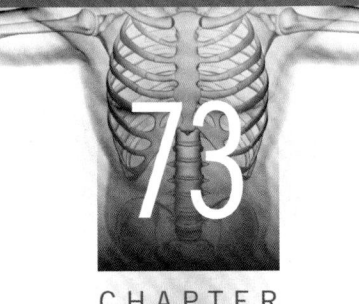

CHAPTER

Arthroscopic Ankle Arthrodesis

James P. Tasto

DEFINITION

- Arthritis of the ankle can evolve from multiple causes, including, but not limited to, osteoarthritis, rheumatoid arthritis, and posttraumatic conditions. As the condition progresses, it generally leads to increased pain, gait abnormalities, and diminished function.
- Surgical remedies are employed when conservative measures fail; they consist of the time-honored tibiotalar arthrodesis as well as total ankle replacement.
- We are discussing and illustrating the technique of arthroscopic ankle arthrodesis (AAA).

ANATOMY

- The ankle joint is composed of the tibiotalar and fibulotalar articulations, with the fibula bearing about one-fifth of the weight-bearing stress across the ankle joint (**FIG 1**).

PATHOGENESIS

- As with any condition, when articular cartilage is destroyed, either by systemic or local disease, the progression of arthritis may be unpredictably slow or rapid. If malalignment is an accompanying factor, the progression and pain are usually more pronounced.

NATURAL HISTORY

- Once the breakdown of the articular surface has begun, it will progress at a rate that is not always predictable. Radiographic changes will not always reflect the degree of pain that the patient presents with. Some patients will come to surgery early, whereas others may languish for decades without needing surgical intervention.

PATIENT HISTORY AND PHYSICAL FINDINGS

- Generally, the patient will complain of pain with weight bearing, usually lateral more than medial. Generally, it localizes anteriorly in a band from the lateral to the medial side of the ankle. There may be associated swelling and occasional night pain. The symptoms may in part be relieved by nonsteroidal anti-inflammatory drugs (NSAIDs), acetaminophen, crutches, bracing, and activity modification. When other joints are involved, such as the knee and the hip, the discomfort in these areas may overshadow the ankle symptomatology.
- The patient will generally walk with an antalgic gait, and if there is any leg length discrepancy, there may be a short-leg component to it. Gait will generally improve with the assistance of crutches or a cane.
- Stability is assessed with talar tilt and anterior drawer tests.
- Standing evaluation is critical in determining the feasibility of arthroscopic technique versus open as well as necessary osteotomies.
- Range of motion will be restricted in all planes, and pain will be elicited at the extremes of range of motion.
- Loss of dorsiflexion with plantarflexion contracture needs to be addressed at surgery.
- Careful isolation of ankle joint motion during the examination is critical so as not to confuse it with pathologic changes in the subtalar or midtarsal joints.
- There will usually be associated swelling about the ankle joint. Synovial hypertrophy, osteophytes, and generalized enlargement of the ankle will present rather than a frank effusion, which could indicate a systemic component.

IMAGING AND OTHER DIAGNOSTIC STUDIES

- Standing anteroposterior (AP), lateral, and mortise radiographs are necessary to determine the extent of arthritis, alignment, presence of osteophytes, and the presence or absence of avascular necrosis of the talus (**FIG 2**). Minor degrees of malalignment may be corrected up to 7 degrees, varus being the most important element to reverse to neutral.
- Magnetic resonance imaging scans may be helpful if avascular necrosis is suspected.
- Computed tomography may be indicated if bone loss needs to be addressed.
- Should there be questions on the circulatory status, a vascular workup may be necessary.

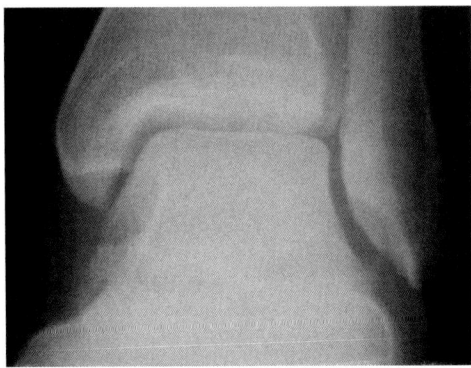

FIG 1 Mortise view of right ankle.

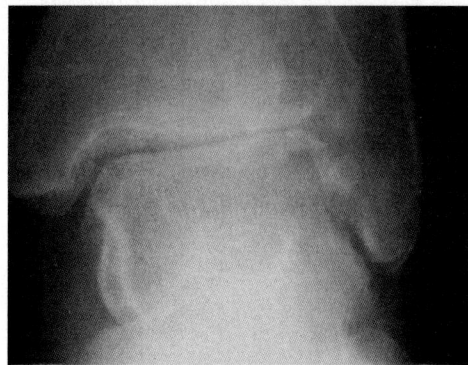

FIG 2 Standing AP radiograph showing degenerative arthritis of the ankle.

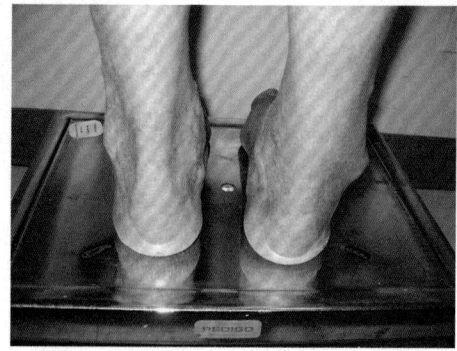

FIG 3 Posterior view of varus malalignment, right ankle.

DIFFERENTIAL DIAGNOSIS

- Infection
- Charcot joint
- Pseudogout and gout
- Osteochondral lesions of the talus
- Impingement
- Inflammatory synovitis

NONOPERATIVE MANAGEMENT

- As with most arthritic conditions, a wide variety of nonoperative measures can be employed. Medication in the form of NSAIDs, acetaminophen, and glucosamine sulfate can be used with careful monitoring for side effects. Bracing with simple soft tissue supports or a custom-made ankle–foot orthosis (AFO) can be effective. Cortisone injections, if used sparingly, can offer short-term pain relief. Off-label hyaluronic acid injections have been used with some reported success.

SURGICAL MANAGEMENT

- When patients fail to respond to conservative care, a number of procedures can be undertaken for isolated end-stage ankle arthritis. The time-honored procedure is an open ankle arthrodesis, but over the past 15 years, some surgeons have come to prefer AAA.
- Total ankle arthroplasty has been popularized recently and has the obvious advantage of motion preservation at the cost of a more challenging technical procedure and a higher complication rate.
- AAA is discussed in detail in the following section.

Preoperative Planning

- We cannot overstress the need for a thorough evaluation of alignment before AAA is undertaken (FIG 3). The films must be done in a standing position and compared to the opposite side. Often, patients will present with outside films showing a pseudovarus deformity, but when a weight-bearing film is taken, the alignment is satisfactory.

- All medical conditions must be addressed. Vascular status needs to be examined as well as the skin condition. Patients need to stop smoking 3 months before the operative procedure and must stay off NSAIDs 5 days before and 3 months after the surgery.
- Perioperative antibiotics are used as well as postoperative deep venous thrombosis prophylaxis in high-risk patients.

Positioning

- The patient is placed in a supine position.
- The use of a leg holder and tourniquet allows the extremity to be placed in a neutral position so that both the anteromedial and anterolateral aspects of the ankle can be easily accessed.
- The foot of the table is dropped about 30 degrees.
- The ankle is placed in a sterile traction device using a tensiometer, controlling traction to about 25 lb (FIG 4).

Approach

- The approach that is described is that of an AAA.
- Generally, a two-portal technique can be used with anteromedial and anterolateral portals, and on occasion, accessory portals located anterolateral, anteromedial, or posterolateral for additional flow or drainage (FIG 5).

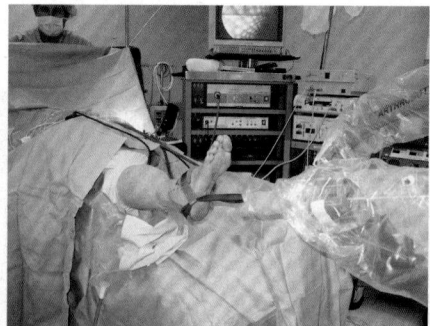

FIG 4 Sterile traction device with tensiometer applied to right ankle.

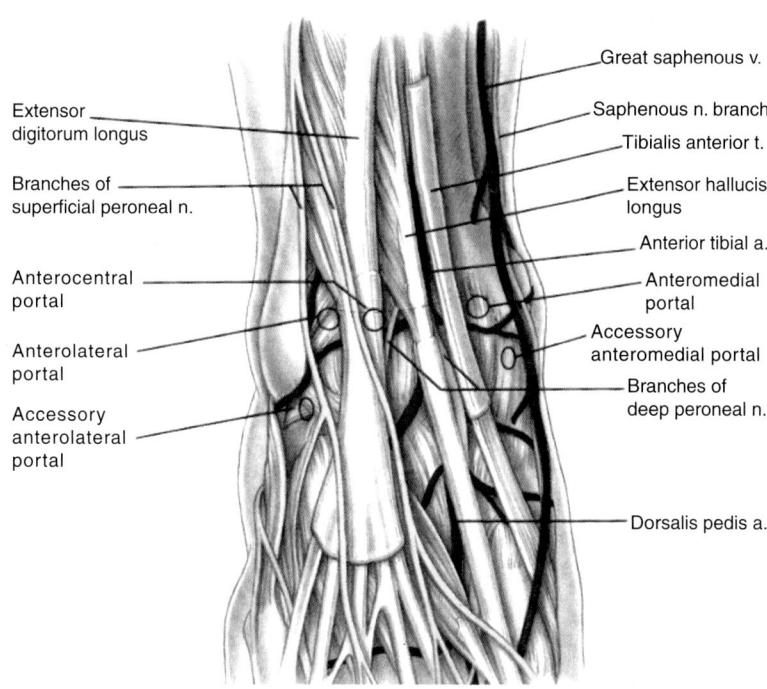

Great saphenous v.

Extensor digitorum longus

Branches of superficial peroneal n.

Anterocentral portal

Anterolateral portal

Accessory anterolateral portal

Saphenous n. branch

Tibialis anterior t.

Extensor hallucis longus

Anterior tibial a.

Anteromedial portal

Accessory anteromedial portal

Branches of deep peroneal n.

Dorsalis pedis a.

A

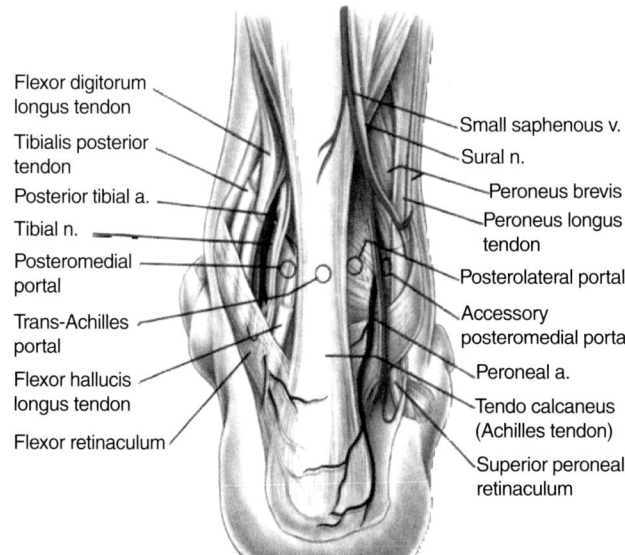

Flexor digitorum longus tendon

Tibialis posterior tendon

Posterior tibial a.

Tibial n.

Posteromedial portal

Trans-Achilles portal

Flexor hallucis longus tendon

Flexor retinaculum

Small saphenous v.

Sural n.

Peroneus brevis

Peroneus longus tendon

Posterolateral portal

Accessory posteromedial portal

Peroneal a.

Tendo calcaneus (Achilles tendon)

Superior peroneal retinaculum

B

FIG 5 A,B. Standard and accessory anterior portals for ankle arthroscopy.

TRACTION AND EXPOSURE

- Delineate anatomic landmarks with a marking pencil **(TECH FIG 1A)**.
- Apply a traction device after thoroughly preparing and draping the ankle.
- Apply traction to about 25 lb **(TECH FIG 1B)**.
- Countertraction is effective with the use of a tourniquet and leg holder.
- Dorsiflexion and plantarflexion are facilitated by the design of the traction strap.
- Instill 8 mL of normal saline into the ankle joint.
- Using a "nick and spread" technique, create the anteromedial portal with a no. 11 blade.

- Use a hemostat to bluntly dissect down to the capsule.
- Introduce a 2.7-mm wide-angled and small joint arthroscope through the anteromedial portal **(TECH FIG 1C)**.
- Establish drainage through the anterolateral portal.
- Use a pump to control pressure at about 30 mm Hg.
- Take care, as with any infusion technique, to avoid excessive pressure and fluid extravasation.
- Anterior osteophytes may impede entry and visualization in the joint **(TECH FIG 1D)**.
  - Osteophytes can be removed anteriorly to create a space for visualization and performance of the arthrodesis.

TECHNIQUES

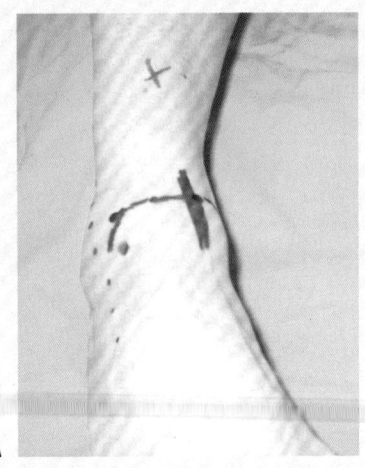

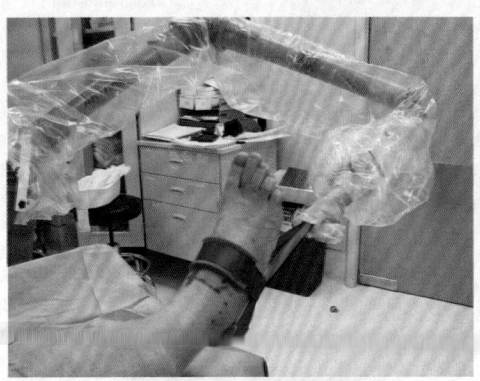

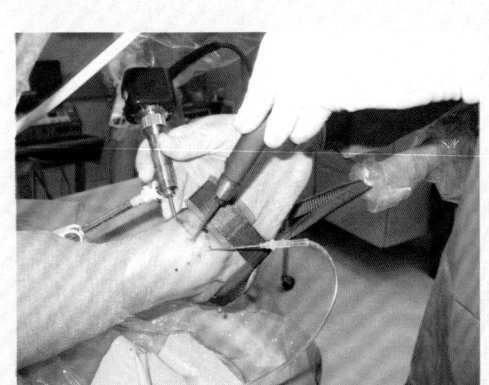

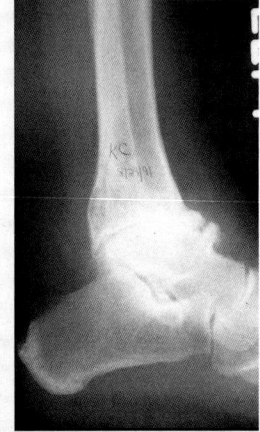

TECH FIG 1 A. Anatomic landmarks consisting of the superficial peroneal nerve and anterior tibial tendon, right ankle. **B.** Soft tissue traction device for the ankle with 25 lb of traction applied. **C.** A camera and small arthroscope are introduced through the anteromedial portal, the shaver is introduced through the anterolateral portal, and drainage is introduced through an accessory inferior anterolateral portal, right ankle. **D.** Lateral radiograph of an ankle with prominent tibial and talar osteophytes that need to be resected for access to the ankle joint during arthroscopy.

ARTHRODESIS

- Perform a synovectomy with a 3.5-mm resection blade **(TECH FIG 2A)**.
- Use a soft tissue motorized blade and a burr to remove the articular cartilage.
- One to 2 mm of subchondral bone is generally removed with the burr **(TECH FIG 2B)**.
- Spinal curettes can be used to débride the medial and lateral gutters as well as the posterior tibial plafond and posterior talus **(TECH FIG 2C)**.
- A radiofrequency device can be used for débridement in some areas where access is limited.

- During débridement, maintaining the normal architecture of the tibiotalar joint is imperative.
- Medial and lateral gutters need to be débrided thoroughly, removing 1 to 2 mm of subchondral bone as well **(TECH FIG 2D)**.
- Débriding the gutters allows for coaptation of the tibiotalar surfaces **(TECH FIG 2E)**.
- Multiple spot welds placed on the tibiotalar surfaces will allow increased vascularity **(TECH FIG 2F)**.
- Release the tourniquet and visualize the vascularity of both surfaces **(TECH FIG 2G)**.
- Further débridement may be necessary if diminished vascularity is encountered in any one particular area.

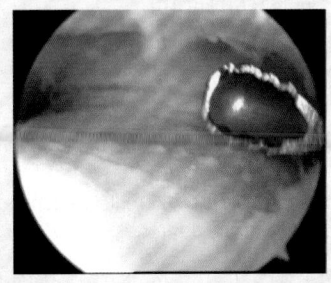

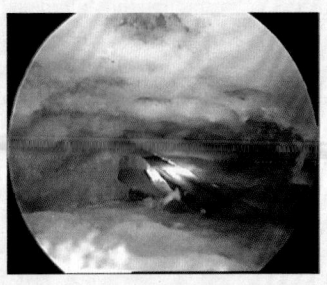

TECH FIG 2 A. A soft tissue resection blade is being used to perform a synovectomy in the ankle joint. **B.** One to 2 mm of subchondral bone is removed with a burr, and spot welds are created. *(continued)*

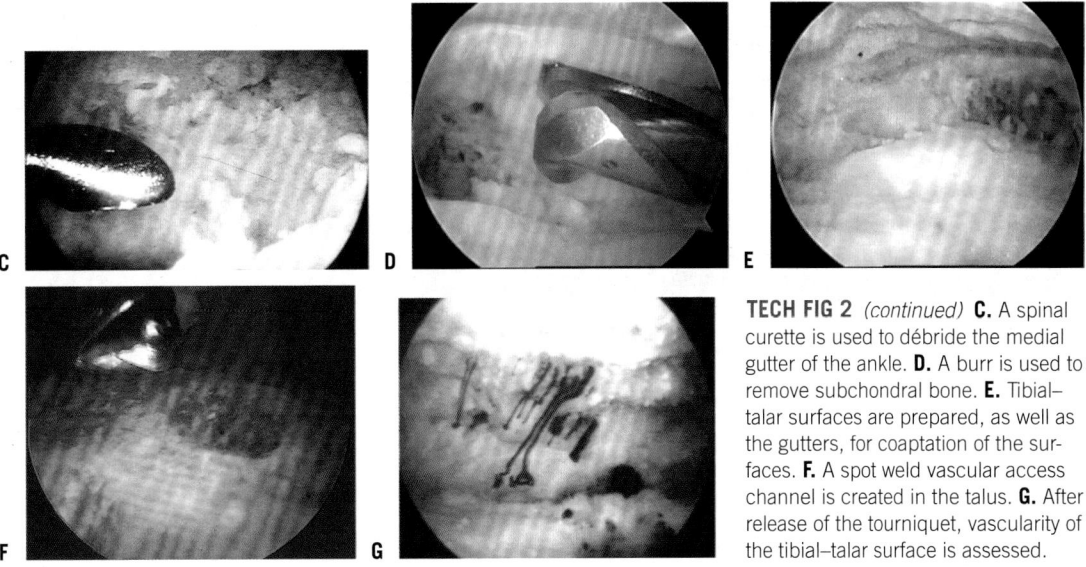

TECH FIG 2 *(continued)* **C.** A spinal curette is used to débride the medial gutter of the ankle. **D.** A burr is used to remove subchondral bone. **E.** Tibial–talar surfaces are prepared, as well as the gutters, for coaptation of the surfaces. **F.** A spot weld vascular access channel is created in the talus. **G.** After release of the tourniquet, vascularity of the tibial–talar surface is assessed.

STABILIZATION, FIXATION, AND CLOSURE

- Hold the ankle in the acceptable corrected neutral position and insert guidewires.
- Use two 7.3-mm Arbeitsgemeinscha fuer Osteosynthesefragen (AO) cannulated cancellous screws to stabilize the tibiotalar joint.
- Place screws parallel and obliquely from the medial tibia into the lateral talus **(TECH FIG 3)**.
- Perform fixation under fluoroscopic control to avoid any potential encroachment on the subtalar joint.

- Apply compression alternately to each screw.
- Check the final position both clinically and under fluoroscopy.
- Close the arthroscopic portals with Steri-Strips and close the operative site for screw insertion with 3-0 nylon sutures.
- Apply a local anesthetic and incorporate the leg into a bulky dressing and a bivalve cast.

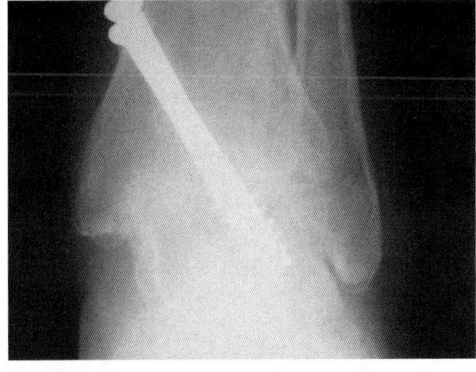
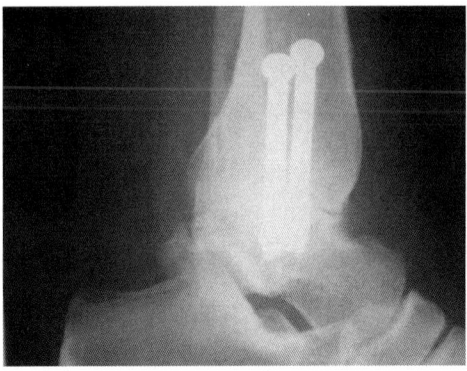

TECH FIG 3 A. AP radiographs showing two parallel oblique screws used for fixation of the arthroscopic fusion. **B.** Lateral radiographs showing two parallel oblique screws fixing the ankle fusion.

Pearls and Pitfalls

Indications	• If possible, avoid operating on smokers and patients with Charcot joints and avascular necrosis of the talus. • Carefully explain to the patient what the associated stiffness and lack of motion of the ankle will involve. • Avoid noncompliant patients.
Arthroscopic Procedure	• Use careful fluid management to avoid extravasation and compartment syndrome. • Do not exceed 25–30 lb of traction. • Have the appropriate small joint arthroscopy system available.
Surgical Technique	• Early removal of the anterior osteophytes will aid in visualization. • Do not remove excessive amounts of subchondral bone. • Spot weld technique will increase the vascular access. • Medial and lateral gutters need to be débrided for better coaptation. • Guide pins need to be checked carefully under fluoroscopy. • Avoid violating the subtalar joint with screws.

POSTOPERATIVE CARE

- Patients are placed in a bulky dressing with a bivalve cast in the operating room. Circulatory checks are done in the recovery room and 24 hours postoperatively.
- The cast is removed and the wounds are inspected at 7 days postoperatively. The patient is then fitted for an AFO brace **(FIG 6)**.
- The patient is allowed touch weight bearing the first few days after surgery, with progressive weight bearing, and may attain a full weight-bearing status as soon as tolerated.
- Generally, the patient will use crutches for 2 to 3 weeks. Full weight bearing is encouraged.
- The patient is allowed to remove the AFO for bathing and range-of-motion exercises. Range of motion and weight bearing reduce stress deprivation. The patient is allowed to remove the AFO and walk with normal shoe wear when radiographic union has taken place, there is no motion at the screw sites, and the patient is essentially pain-free.

OUTCOMES

- Fusion rates for AAA are generally in the range of 90% to 95%.

- There is definitely less pain after the arthroscopic procedure than with the open procedure.
- The operation is generally done as an outpatient procedure.
- Alignment is thought to be easier to obtain because of the maintenance of the normal architecture and geometry of the tibiotalar joint.

COMPLICATIONS

- The complication rate from ankle arthroscopy has been reported to be about 9%.
- Infection
- Synovial fistula **(FIG 7A)**
- Delayed union **(FIG 7B)**
- Nonunion
- Charcot joint
- Secondary degenerative changes, subtalar and midfoot
- Equinus or dorsiflexion malposition
- Residual varus malalignment
- Fibular–talar and fibular–calcaneal impingement **(FIG 7C)**
- Neurapraxia and nerve injuries
- Vascular injuries
- Skeletal traction complications **(FIG 7D)**
- Screw encroachment in subtalar joint **(FIG 7E)**

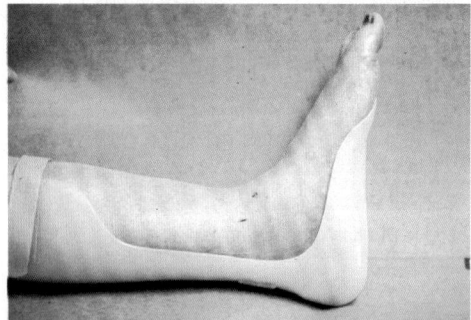

FIG 6 An AFO brace is used for immobilization, postoperative week 1.

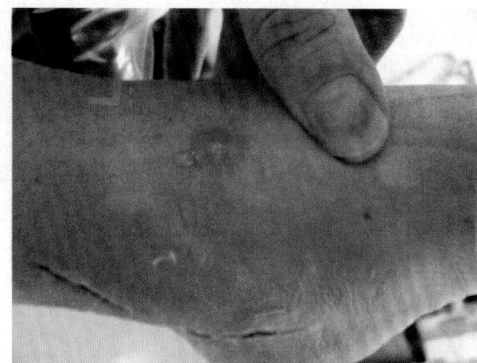

A
FIG 7 A. Synovial fistula after ankle arthroscopy. *(continued)*

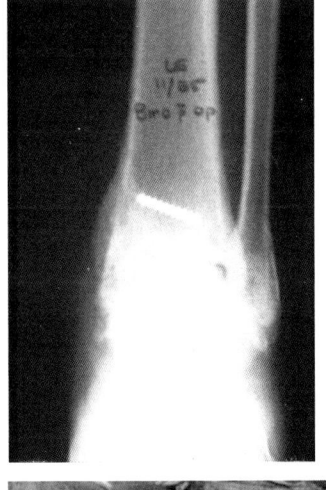

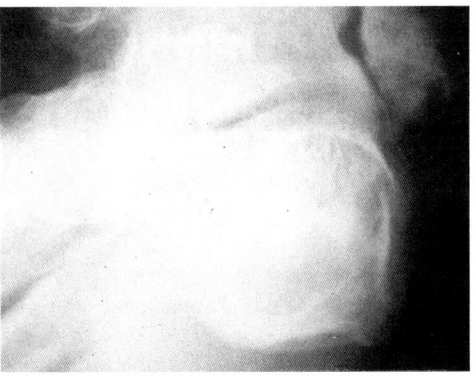

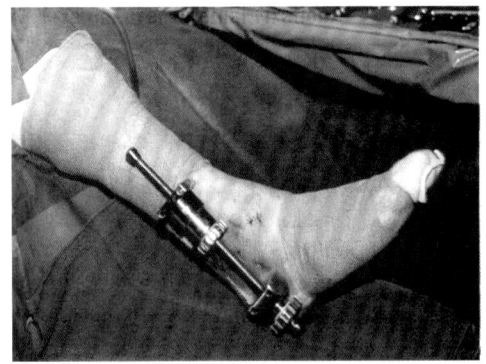

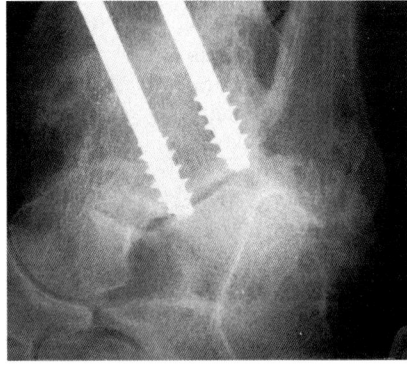

FIG 7 *(continued)* **B.** AP radiographs showing delayed union–nonunion of open ankle arthrodesis. **C.** AP radiograph in 40 degrees of internal rotation, showing fibular–talar and fibular–calcaneal impingement. **D.** Skeletal traction device previously used for ankle arthroscopy. **E.** Screw encroachment on the subtalar joint as seen with a 40-degree internal rotation and plantarflexion view.

SUGGESTED READINGS

Chen YJ, Huang TJ, Shih HN, et al. Ankle arthrodesis with cross screw fixation. Good results in 36/40 cases followed 3-7 years. Acta Orthop Scand 1996;67:473–478.

Cobb TK, Gabrielsen TA, Campbell DC II, et al. Cigarette smoking and nonunion after ankle arthrodesis. Foot Ankle Int 1994;15:64–67.

Collman DR, Kaas MH, Schuberth JM. Arthroscopic ankle arthrodesis: factors influencing union in 39 consecutive patients. Foot Ankle Int 2006;27:1079–1085.

Corso SJ, Zimmer TJ. Technique and clinical evaluation of arthroscopic ankle arthrodesis. Arthroscopy 1995;11:585–590.

Crosby LA, Yee TC, Formanek TS, et al. Complications following arthroscopic ankle arthrodesis. Foot Ankle Int 1996;17:340–342.

Dohm M, Purdy BA, Benjamin J. Primary union of ankle arthrodesis: review of a single institution/multiple surgeon experience. Foot Ankle Int 1994;15:293–296.

Elmlund AO, Winson IG. Arthroscopic ankle arthrodesis. Foot Ankle Clin 2015;20(1):71–80.

Ferkel RD, Hewitt M. Long-term results of arthroscopic ankle arthrodesis. Foot Ankle Int 2005;26:275–280.

Frey C, Halikus NM, Vu-Rose T, et al. A review of ankle arthrodesis: predisposing factors to nonunion. Foot Ankle Int 1994;15:581–584.

Glick JM, Morgan CD, Myerson MS, et al. Ankle arthrodesis using an arthroscopic method: long-term follow-up of 34 cases. Arthroscopy 1996;12:428–434.

Huang YZ, Zeng XT, Wang J, et al. Arthroscopic versus open ankle arthrodesis. Arthroscopy 2018;34(7):2010.

Jerosch J. Arthroscopic in situ arthrodesis of the upper ankle [in German]. Orthopade 2005;34:1198–1208.

Jerosch J, Steinbeck J, Schroder M, et al. Arthroscopically assisted arthrodesis of the ankle joint. Arch Orthop Trauma Surg 1996;115:182–189.

Jones CR, Wong E, Applegate GR, et al. Arthroscopic ankle arthrodesis: a 2-15 year follow-up study. Arthroscopy 2018;34(5):1641–1649.

Mann RA, Van Manen JW, Wapner K, et al. Ankle fusion. Clin Orthop Relat Res 1991;(268):49–55.

Morgan CD, Henke JA, Bailey RW, et al. Long-term results of tibiotalar arthrodesis. J Bone Joint Surg Am 1985;67:546–550.

Muir DC, Amendola A, Saltzman CL. Long-term outcome of ankle arthrodesis. Foot Ankle Clin 2002;7:703–708.

Papa J, Myerson M, Girard P. Salvage, with arthrodesis, in intractable diabetic neuropathic arthropathy of the foot and ankle. J Bone Joint Surg Am 1993;75:1056–1066.

Park JH, Kim HJ, Suh DH, et al. Arthroscopic versus open ankle arthrodesis: a systematic review. Arthroscopy 2018;34(3):988–997.

Quayle J, Shafafy R, Khan MA, et al. Arthroscopic versus open ankle arthrodesis 2018;24(2):137–142.

Stone JW. Arthroscopic ankle arthrodesis. Foot Ankle Clin 2006;11:361–368.

Winson IG, Robinson DE, Allen PE. Arthroscopic ankle arthrodesis. J Bone Joint Surg Br 2005;87:343–347.

Yasui Y, Vig KS, Murawski CD, et al. Open versus arthroscopic ankle arthrodesis: a comparison of subsequent procedures in a large database. J Foot Ankle Surg 2016;55(4):777–781.

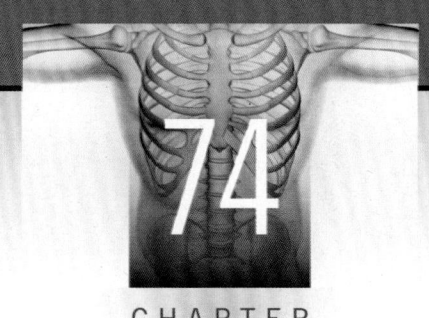

74

CHAPTER

Tibiotalocalcaneal Arthrodesis Using a Medullary Nail

George E. Quill, Jr. and Stuart D. Miller

DEFINITION

- Tibiotalocalcaneal arthrodesis is the surgical procedure to simultaneously fuse the ankle and the subtalar joints.
- In cases of posttraumatic, neuropathic, or avascular talar body bone loss, tibiocalcaneal arthrodesis may be indicated. The term *pantalar arthrodesis* refers to the surgical procedure to fuse all bones that articulate with the talus: the distal tibia, calcaneus, navicular, and cuboid. In essence, this is a combined ankle and triple arthrodesis.
- In our opinion, the term *medullary* refers to the inner marrow cavity of a long bone and the word *intramedullary* is a redundant, less useful term.
- The goal of tibiotalocalcaneal arthrodesis is to create a pain-free ankle and hindfoot that are biomechanically stable and fused in functional position.
- In our hands, tibiotalocalcaneal arthrodesis is a salvage operation performed for severe ankle and hindfoot deformity, bone loss, and pain.

ANATOMY

- Tibiotalocalcaneal arthrodesis aims to recreate physiologic ankle and hindfoot alignment with a plantigrade foot position (the foot is at a 90-degree angle to the long axis of the tibia) and about 5 to 7 degrees of hindfoot valgus.[6,14]
- In general, rotation of the foot relative to the longitudinal axis of the tibia in the coronal plane is congruent with the anterior tibia—that is, the second ray of the foot is usually in line with the anteromedial crest of the tibia.
- Hindfoot position influences forefoot position. With long-standing ankle and hindfoot deformity, forefoot pronation, supination, adduction, and abduction may be affected. Proper positioning of a tibiotalocalcaneal arthrodesis must take forefoot position into account. Ideally, in stance phase, the foot has near-equal pressure distribution under the heel and first and fifth metatarsal heads.[15]

NATURAL HISTORY

- Severe ankle and hindfoot deformities and pathologic processes result in disabling pathomechanics and, when left untreated, often confine patients to cumbersome brace use, limited ambulation with assistive devices, or a wheelchair.[10]
- Tibiotalocalcaneal arthrodesis is a major reconstructive process usually applied to otherwise disabling conditions.[9,11]
  - Gellman et al[4] noted that the dorsiflexion and plantarflexion deficits after ankle fusion compared to the nonfused contralateral ankle were 51% and 70%, respectively. Surprisingly, for tibiotalocalcaneal arthrodesis,

dorsiflexion and plantarflexion deficits were 53% and 71%, respectively.
- This same study concluded, however, that inversion and eversion were 40% less after tibiotalocalcaneal fusion than after tibiotalar fusion alone.

PATIENT HISTORY AND PHYSICAL FINDINGS

- The patient being considered for tibiotalocalcaneal arthrodesis with a medullary nail presents with a myriad of orthopaedic pathology affecting gait, weight bearing, and ability to earn a living.
- This patient may present with limited mobility, an equinus posture associated with genu recurvatum, and transverse plane deformity ranging from severe varus and instability of the hindfoot through profound valgus and ulceration over the medial structures (FIG 1).[11,13]

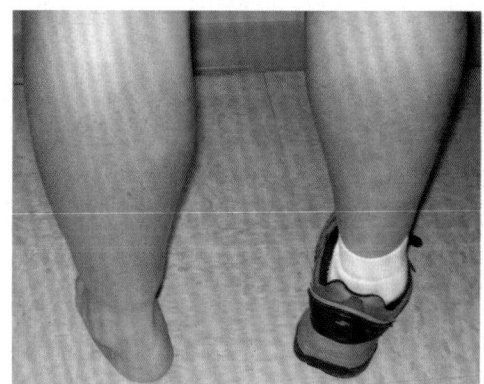

A

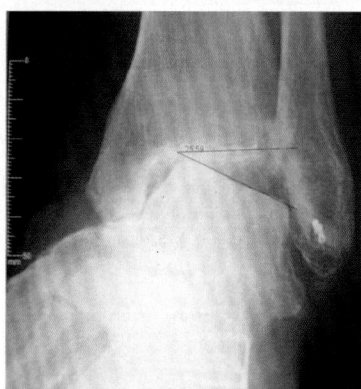

B

FIG 1 Weight-bearing clinical photograph (A) and weight-bearing AP radiograph (B) of a 53-year-old laborer with persistent ankle and hindfoot varus instability after prior attempt at calcaneal osteotomy and lateral ligament reconstruction.

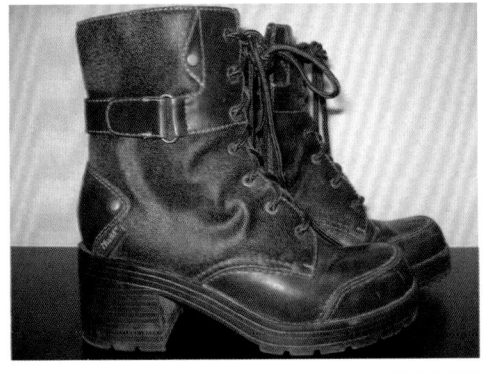
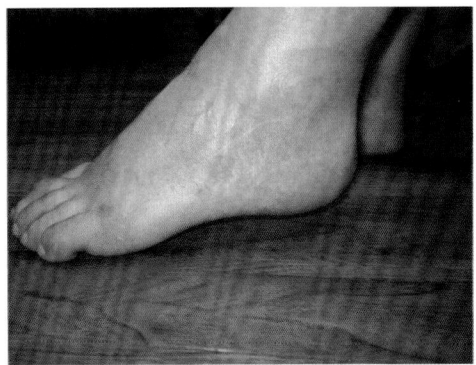

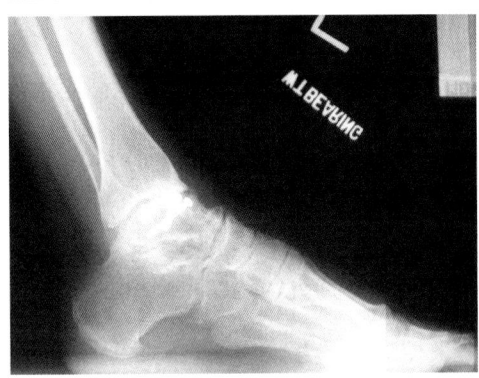

FIG 2 A. Reportedly, the only pair of high-heeled, high-topped boots that this 42-year-old woman was comfortable wearing 2 years after sustaining bilateral talus fractures malunited in equinus. **B.** Clinical appearance of this woman's foot in maximal passive left ankle dorsiflexion. **C.** Weight-bearing lateral radiograph of same woman. Note plantarflexion talus fracture malunion and posttraumatic osteoarthritis after open reduction and internal fixation.

- The neuromuscular or neuropathic patient may present with ulceration, intrinsic muscle loss, and multiple fractures in various stages of healing.[11]
- The posttraumatic patient often has a compromised soft tissue envelope, previously placed hardware, and already medullary canal sclerosis that must be considered in preoperative planning **(FIG 2)**.[10] Evaluation must include gait and weight-bearing posture, assessment of the soft tissue envelope, and a thorough neuromuscular examination.

IMAGING AND OTHER DIAGNOSTIC STUDIES

- We routinely obtain three weight-bearing radiographs of the ankle and foot. As many of these patients have deformity, we often obtain additional long-cassette radiographs of the ankle or even mechanical axis views of the lower leg from the hip to the foot.

- Posttraumatic and osteoarthritis
- Radiographs may reveal joint space narrowing, osteophyte formation, and subchondral sclerosis and cysts, all characteristic of osteoarthritis. Posttraumatic deformity and retained hardware may be identified and must be considered in preoperative planning **(FIG 3)**.[10,12,13]
- Rheumatoid arthritis and other inflammatory arthritides
  - Radiographs typically identify periarticular erosions and osteopenia.[7]
- Neuropathic arthrosis or Charcot neuroarthropathy
  - In our experience, this presentation is radiographically characterized by numerous fractures or microfractures in various stages of healing, hypertrophic new bone formation, and loss of normal weight-bearing architecture.
  - Bone resorption may be seen, along with vascular calcification and joint subluxation or dislocation.[11,17]

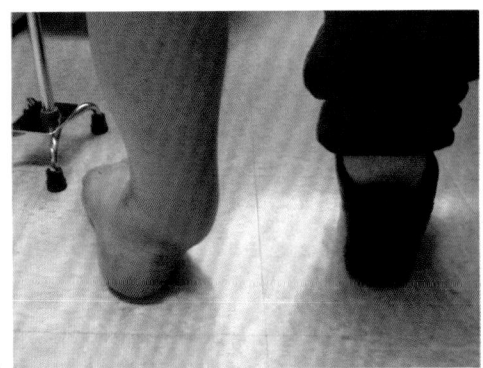
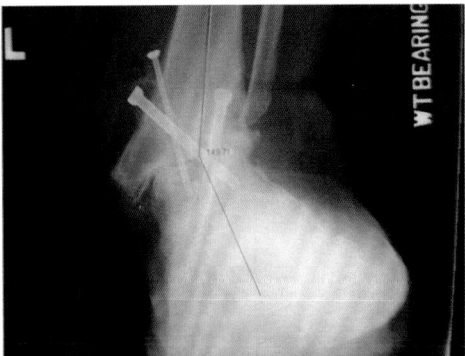

FIG 3 Preoperative weight-bearing clinical appearance **(A)**, AP radiograph **(B)**, and *(continued)*

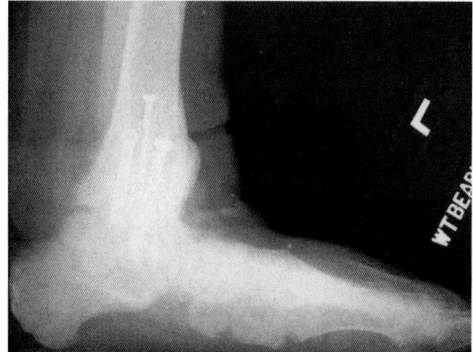

FIG 3 *(continued)* lateral radiograph (**C**) of an 69-year-old obese man after valgus nonunion of attempted tibiotalar arthrodesis.

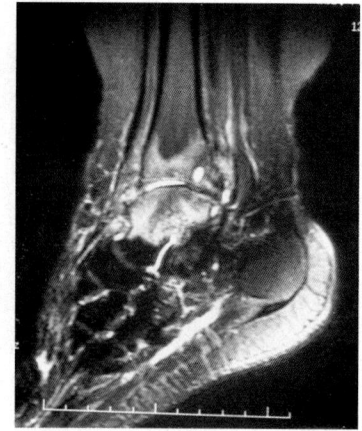

FIG 5 MRI demonstrating extensive bone involvement of the talus.

- Plain tomography or computed tomography (CT) may further define deformity, arthritis, bone loss, and prior malunion or nonunion (**FIG 4**).
  - We have not found three-dimensional CT reconstructions helpful in the routine setting.
  - CT is also useful in assessing progression toward union following tibiotalocalcaneal arthrodesis.
- Magnetic resonance imaging (MRI) may complement CT by evaluating for fluid in and around the joints, bone marrow edema, talar vascularity, infection, and periarticular tendon and ligament pathology (**FIG 5**).
- Technetium 99 bone scans may be useful in the evaluation of osteonecrosis after talus fracture, arthritic involvement of one or several joints, stress fracture, or neoplasm.
- Indium-labeled white blood cell scans can be helpful in the diagnosis of osteomyelitis or septic arthritis.

DIFFERENTIAL DIAGNOSIS

- Primary and secondary osteoarthrosis, including posttraumatic osteoarthritis
- Rheumatoid arthritis and other inflammatory arthritides (gout, pseudogout, pigmented villonodular synovitis, septic arthritis, psoriatic arthritis, spondyloarthropathy, Reiter syndrome)
- Neuropathic arthropathy (diabetes mellitus, spinal cord injury, hereditary sensory and motor neuropathy, syringomyelia, congenital indifference to pain, alcoholism, peripheral nerve disease, tabes dorsalis, and leprosy)
- Infectious arthritis (sepsis, open trauma, or previous surgical procedure for fixation of fractures)
- Arthritis and joint subluxation resulting from generalized ligamentous laxity, mixed connective disease, posterior tibial tendinopathy, spring ligament insufficiency

NONOPERATIVE MANAGEMENT

- Selective (diagnostic) injection of local anesthetic may help locate the exact anatomic source of the patient's pain.
- Tibiotalar arthritis may be associated with a stiff, painful subtalar joint that has a relatively normal radiographic appearance.
- The injection of 5 to 10 mL of 1% lidocaine into the subtalar joint can clarify whether the pain may not be isolated to the ankle but in fact be generated in both the ankle and subtalar joints.
- This has important implications when considering isolated tibiotalar versus tibiotalocalcaneal arthrodesis. We do not routinely incorporate the subtalar joint into the arthrodesis when performing an ankle arthrodesis. In select cases of end-stage ankle arthritis associated with severe deformity and talar bone loss, we consider including an otherwise

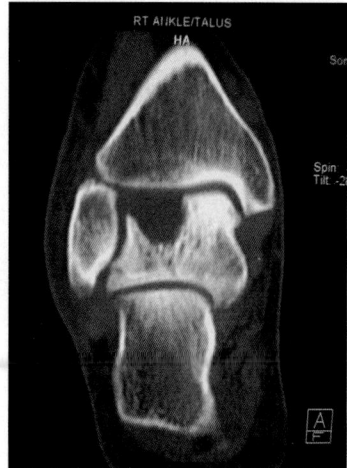

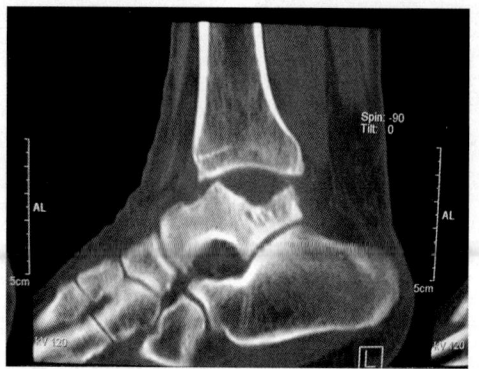

FIG 4 Coronal (**A**) and lateral (**B**) CT images of a 48-year-old man with massive osteochondral talar insufficiency.

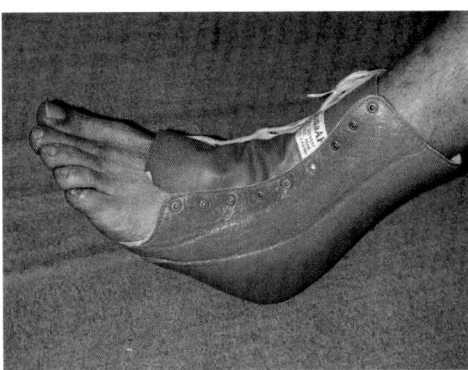

FIG 6 Molded AFO can provide stability and serve as an alternative to operative intervention.

normal asymptomatic subtalar joint in the fusion mass achieved for tibiotalocalcaneal fusion. Alternatively, an injection carefully placed in the peroneal tenosynovial sheath may prove that pain may be related to the tendons rather than the joint.

- Although often challenging for the patient with deformity, we recommend bracing for the patient with prohibitive medical illness or a dysvascular extremity, particularly for the patient with a nonfixed, passively correctible deformity. A custom-molded polypropylene ankle–foot orthosis (AFO) or a supramalleolar AFO with Velcro closures may be considered as an alternative to tibiotalocalcaneal arthrodesis in poor surgical candidates **(FIG 6)**.[11]
- For the neuropathic patient in whom bracing can achieve a relatively plantigrade posture for the hindfoot and ankle, we prescribe a double metal upright AFO attached to an Oxford shoe that includes Plastazote liners (total contact inserts).
- In our experience, polypropylene in-shoe braces lead to ulceration in these patients with complex deformity.
- In severe deformity, a Charcot retention orthotic walker may prove effective.
- Although we favor tibiotalocalcaneal arthrodesis for patients with posttraumatic arthritis and deformity, we have had some success in relieving pain and improving function with a patellar tendon–bearing brace for poor surgical candidates.

SURGICAL MANAGEMENT

Indications and Contraindications

- Indications for tibiotalocalcaneal arthrodesis
  - Sequelae of degenerative, posttraumatic, or inflammatory arthritis
  - Avascular necrosis of the talus
  - Severe instability or paralytic ankle and hindfoot weakness
  - Neuropathic arthropathy
  - Failed ankle arthroplasty with subtalar intrusion
  - Failed ankle arthrodesis with insufficient talar body
  - Severe deformity of talipes equinovarus
  - Neuromuscular disease

- Skeletal defects after tumor resection
- Pseudarthrosis
- Flail ankle
- Absolute contraindications for tibiotalocalcaneal arthrodesis with internal fixation
  - Dysvascular extremity
  - Active infection
- Relative contraindication to tibiotalocalcaneal arthrodesis with closed nailing techniques
  - Severe, fixed deformity that precludes a colinear reduction of the tibia, talus, and calcaneus for rod placement

Preoperative Planning

- We glean essential information for preoperative planning from a thorough history and physical examination of the soft tissue envelope, vascular status, degree of deformity, and assessment of the entire limb and contralateral limb.
- We review all imaging studies, including long-standing radiographs of the lower extremity. Many of these patients have comorbidities, so we ensure that medical clearance is obtained.
- The availability of implant and instruments is ascertained, and arrangements for perioperative care are confirmed.
  - Over the past 25 years, the simplicity and mechanical strength of tibiotalocalcaneal arthrodesis with a nail has proven successful.[8]
  - With the anterior ankle approach popular with several total ankle replacement procedures, this fusion can also be accomplished from the front. A separate incision will be needed to prepare the subtalar joint. Although an anterior plate is a popular option for the fusion hardware, many prefer the nail, especially in cases of neuropathy.[5,16]
  - A recent development of an ankle arthrodesis nail with an elastic (nitinol) internal compression device has enjoyed popularity and may offer further treatment options to the solid nail.[3]
  - The nail has also proven useful for fusion after failed total ankle arthroplasty (TAA), especially when a cage has been needed to fill a large gap.[2]

Positioning

- The patient with severe preoperative valgus deformity is positioned supine on a radiolucent operating table with a well-padded bump under the ipsilateral buttock to rotate the involved extremity internally **(FIG 7A)**. Another pad can be placed under the heel to facilitate cross-table fluoroscopic imaging.
- Alternatively and preferably, the patient with neutral to varus deformity is positioned in the lateral position with the affected extremity up **(FIG 7B)**.[1,10,11]
- We pad bony prominences and use an axillary roll in the recumbent axilla.
- The patient is usually fastened to the table with a beanbag and chest brace devices, and pneumatic tourniquet control at the level of the thigh is used.
- Parenteral, prophylactic antibiotics are administered before the tourniquet is inflated.

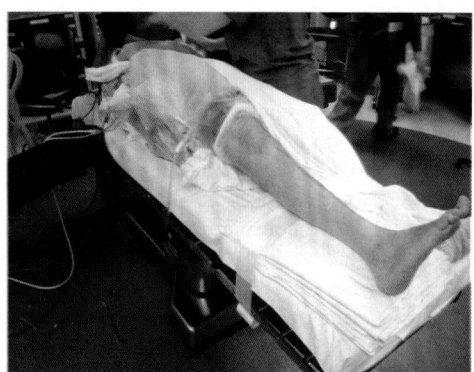 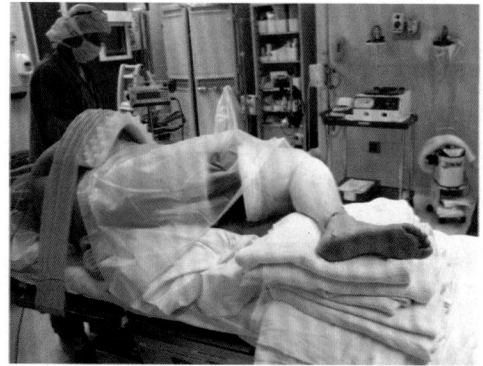

FIG 7 **A.** Patient is positioned on a beanbag in a modified lateral position that allows access to the medial and lateral foot. Note stack of folded sheets under foot to be operated. **B.** Lateral position on blankets to level the leg with the pelvis; this position still allows for external hip rotation to see the medial ankle joint.

EXPOSURE

- For the patient with severe preoperative valgus, we make a longitudinally oriented incision over the medial malleolus starting just at the supramalleolar level and carried 2 to 3 cm distal to the tip of the medial malleolus.
  - This allows a subperiosteal approach to the ankle and the removal of medially based closing wedge osteotomies of diseased tibiotalar bone and cartilage to correct the preoperative valgus deformity.
- We identify and protect the medial neurovascular structures during this approach.
- For all patients other than those who present with severe preoperative valgus, we routinely use a lateral transfibular approach through a longitudinal incision over the distal fibula carried onto the sinus tarsi, curving slightly anteriorly as one extends beyond the distal end of the fibula.
  - This approach affords wide access to both the ankle and subtalar joints and eliminates the possibility of the lateral malleolus rubbing in normal shoe wear postoperatively, and the fibula serves as a source of abundant cancellous and corticocancellous bone graft material during the case **(TECH FIG 1)**.
  - Fibular osteotomy should be especially considered at the time of hindfoot fusion if there is significant varus deformity or loss of tibial length relative to the fibula.
  - Resect the distal fibula in a beveled fashion with a micro-sagittal saw no more than 3 cm proximal to the level of the tibiotalar joint to preserve the distal tibiofibular syndesmosis

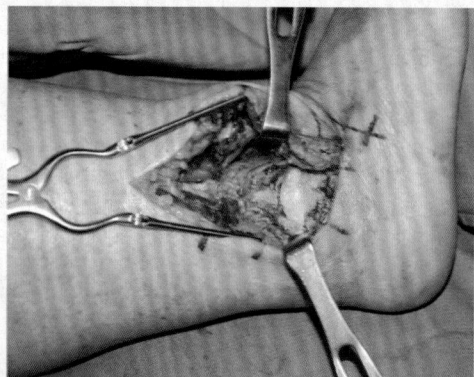

TECH FIG 1 Lateral approach to the tibiotalar and subtalar joint after distal fibulectomy.

and thereby minimize postoperative discomfort caused by distal tibiofibular movement and crepitus.
- We would like to clarify that the transfibular approach with or without fibulectomy is reserved for patients with severe deformity who are not candidates, nor will ever be candidates, for future ankle fusion takedown and conversion to TAA. For patients who may be considered for future TAA, every attempt should be made to preserve anatomy, especially the fibula—that is, the arthrodesis should be performed via an anterior or posterior approach.

ANKLE ARTHROTOMY

- We use a lateral ankle arthrotomy with the incision carried over the sinus tarsi and subtalar joint to correct any deformity that may be present across the tibiotalar and subtalar joints and to prepare the joint surfaces by removing what is left of the diseased articular cartilage **(TECH FIG 2)**.
- Small wedges of bone may be removed to obtain the appropriate plantigrade postoperative posture for the foot and ankle.
- These arthrotomies also leave space for insertion of bone graft as needed.

- Often, combined medial and lateral arthrotomies are needed to achieve the appropriate plantigrade posture of the foot and to remove medial malleolar prominence.
- In the case of the ankle with preoperative valgus deformity, we use a medial approach to the tibiotalar joint in combination with a limited lateral exposure to decorticate and decancellate the subtalar joint via a separate lateral incision over the sinus tarsi.

TECHNIQUES

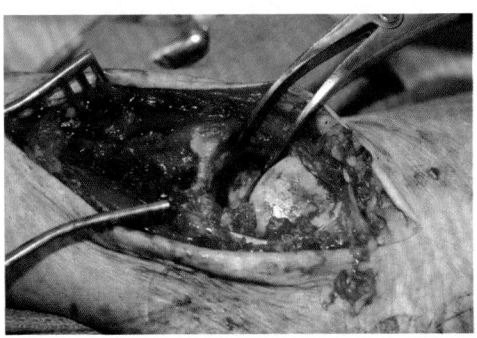

TECH FIG 2 The lateral arthrotomy, with removal of fibula, allows easy access to the ankle joint as well as extending to the subtalar joint.

PLANTAR INCISION FOR GUIDEWIRE INSERTION AND REAMING

- As is true with all other medullary fixation procedures, the starting point for insertion of the guidewire and subsequent medullary rod is critical to the success of the case.
- The correct starting point is midway between the tips of the medial and lateral malleoli, anterior to the subcalcaneal heel pad, and about 2.5 cm posterior to the transverse tarsal joints, in line with the longitudinal axis of the tibia **(TECH FIG 3A)**.
  - Make a 2-cm, longitudinally oriented plantar incision just anterior to the weight-bearing subcalcaneal heel pad.
  - After the incision is carried through dermis sharply, blunt dissection only is taken down to the plantar fascia, which is split longitudinally.
  - The intrinsic muscles can be swept aside and the neurovascular bundle protected and retracted with the intrinsic flexors.
  - Place a smooth Steinmann pin or a guidewire, over which is passed a cannulated drill to provide access to the talus

and tibial medullary canal after calcaneal corticotomy **(TECH FIG 3B)**.
- Confirm optimal insertion of the cannulated drill, which passes sequentially through the inferior cortex of the calcaneus, the calcaneal body, the subtalar joint, the talar body, across the ankle, and finally into the distal tibial canal, using intraoperative fluoroscopic views in both the anteroposterior (AP) and lateral planes.
- After removing the cannulated drill, pass a bulb-tipped guidewire through the calcaneus and talus into the distal tibial medullary canal.
- Pass a series of progressively larger, flexible reamers over the guidewire and use them to enlarge the tibiotalocalcaneal canal.
- We recommend that the final reamer diameter is a full 0.5 to 1 mm larger than the anticipated implant's diameter.
  - In our experience, overreaming avoids the risk of intraoperative and postoperative fracture at the proximal tip of the rod without compromising the construct's stability.

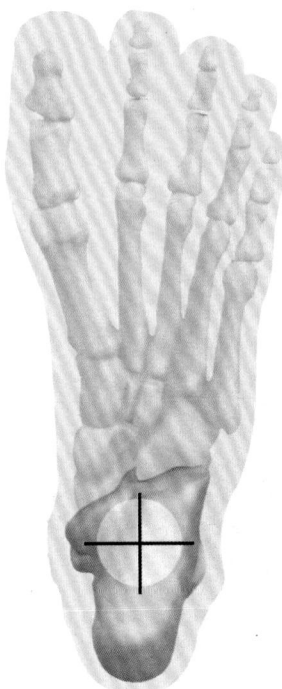

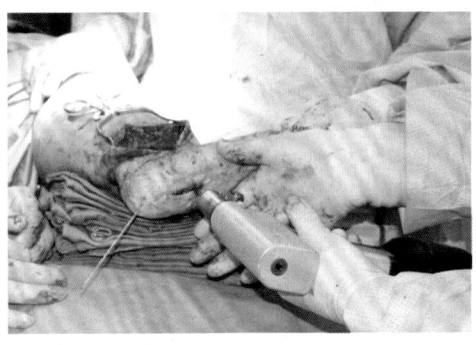

TECH FIG 3 A. Desired starting point for the guide pin and medullary nail. With deformity, establishing this starting point's relationship to the talus and tibia may require some manipulation of the subtalar and ankle joints, but it is generally attainable. **B.** The guidewire should align with the tibial shaft.

- Overzealous reaming in osteopenic bone may result in an intraoperative tibial fracture that then warrants using a longer medullary nail for spanning the fracture. When in doubt, check the reamer position with the fluoroscope.
- We are aware of several articles reporting fractures of the tibia at the proximal portion of the medullary nail when the nail

is left at the relatively sclerotic distal tibial diametaphyseal isthmus.
- When closing the plantar wound, use simple interrupted or horizontal mattress sutures for a flat rather than inverted skin edge closure.

NAIL SELECTION

- In most cases, a nail length of 15 to 18 cm suffices for tibio-talocalcaneal arthrodesis with the proximal extent of the nail in metaphyseal bone, distal to the diametaphyseal isthmus, where the risk of tibia fracture is greatest.
- Nail diameter (Phoenix Ankle Arthrodesis Nail, ZimmerBiomet, Warsaw, Indiana) is dictated by the size of the native tibia.
  - In most cases, a 10-mm-diameter nail affords satisfactory stability to allow progression toward fusion.
  - Although we acknowledge that an increase in nail diameter affords greater strength to the construct, we caution that

aggressive overreaming of the cortex to place a larger diameter nail may compromise the cortex, leading to a stress fracture.
- In profoundly neuropathic patients, we have used a long tibiotalocalcaneal nail that bypasses the distal tibial isthmus by a length equal to at least three times the diameter of the tibial canal measured at the level of the isthmus. A longer nail generally reduces the possibility of a distal tibial stress fracture, albeit by requiring more reaming of the tibia.

NAIL PLACEMENT ACROSS THE ARTHRODESIS SITE

- We find that locking the nail to its targeting arm, with each of two drill bits inserted through the drill guides and the two proximal most screw holes in the nail before the nail and its targeting arm are tightened, ensures optimal alignment before placement.
- The medullary nail is attached to its alignment and targeting guide. As it is inserted in retrograde fashion at plantar foot, it is slightly internally rotated so that when the locking screws

are passed from lateral to medial, they will pass into the tibia without impingement on the distal fibula **(TECH FIG 4A)**.
- During insertion, the distal aspect of the nail should be countersunk at least 5 mm cephalad to the plantar surface of the os calcis or at least countersunk the same distance that the surgeon anticipates achieving axial compression across the ankle and subtalar fusion sites. Be sure not to leave the nail prominent on the plantar aspect of the foot **(TECH FIG 4B)**.

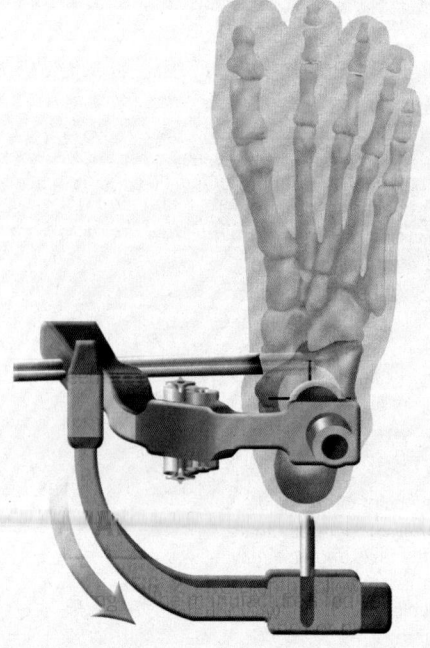

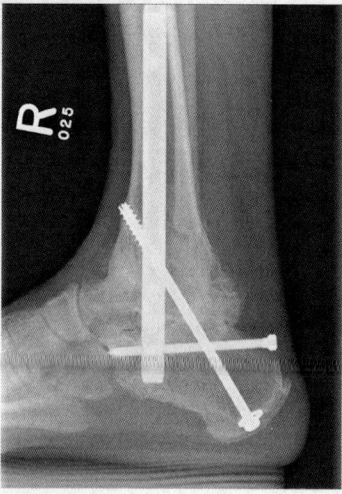

TECH FIG 4 A. In our experience, internally rotating the nail and the guide slightly, posterior to anterior screws placed through the guide and the nail, tends to align optimally with the calcaneus. **B.** Follow-up radiograph demonstrating that the nail is slightly countersunk to avoid being prominent on the plantar surface of the foot. A nail that is slightly proud rarely creates a problem because that portion of the calcaneus is not weight bearing; in fact, it may afford some further support with the end of the nail engaged in the calcaneal cortex.

A   B

SCREW PLACEMENT IN THE INTRAMEDULLARY NAIL

- When determining the final position for the nail, we simultaneously estimate the position of locking holes in the nail relative to the distal tibia, the talar body, and the calcaneal body.
- It is preferable but not necessary to fill all the locking holes.
- Nail failure is likely to occur in the heavyset or neuropathic patient if locking holes are left open at the level of either the ankle or subtalar fusion site. Early reports of nail failure at the subtalar joint often noted failure to fuse the subtalar joint.
- An advantage of modern nail design includes placement of locking screws at various angles to one another.
- The position of the nail for the proximal screws into the tibia will dictate the final rotation; thus, the guide for the posteroanterior screw may be applied and used to check (including fluoroscopy) the later position for the posteroanterior screw in the calcaneus as well as the talar screws **(TECH FIG 5A)**.
- A posterior to anterior calcaneal locking screw increases the torsional rigidity of the nail construct by at least 40% and improves purchase of the calcaneal bone exponentially when compared to simply locking in one plane relative to the long axis of the nail **(TECH FIG 5B)**.
- Further manual compression and impaction can be done across the arthrodesis sites before the proximal interlocking screws are inserted. Some nails use an extramedullary compression device, whereas others use compression of the heel against the tibial screws.
- Some medullary rods include an in-line compression device that can provide up to 15 mm of compression across the ankle and subtalar fusion sites **(TECH FIG 5C)**.
- Some nails also provide for compression of the talar screw proximally toward the tibial screws, further compressing the ankle joint 7 mm **(TECH FIG 5D)**.
- Do not remove this compression until the rod is locked both in the talus and the calcaneus so that the benefits of compression across both fusion sites (ankle and subtalar) can be achieved.

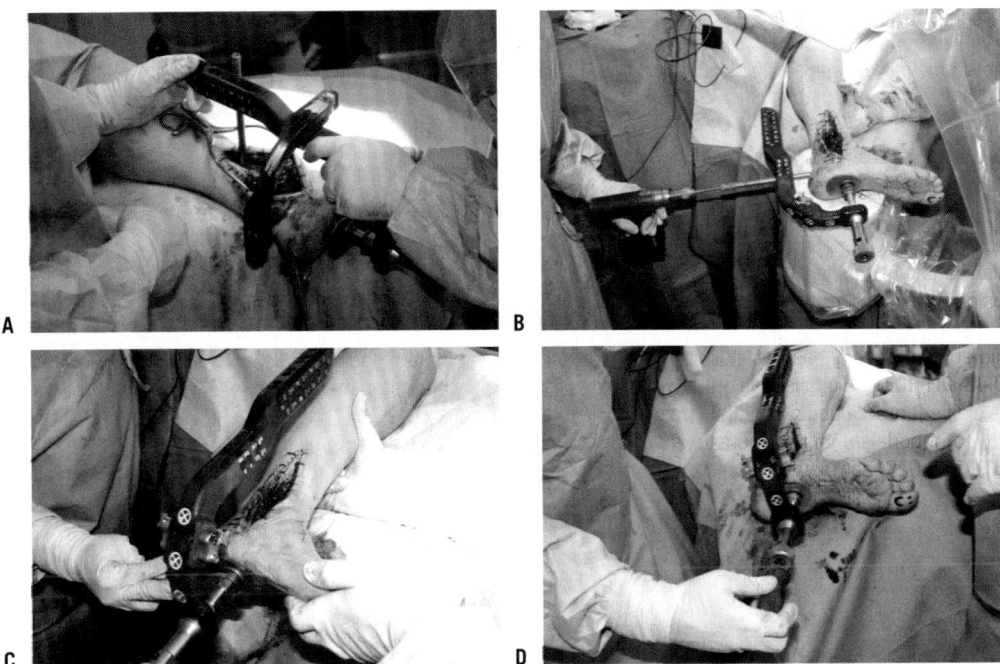

TECH FIG 5 A. The alignment guide provides a quick check of overall positioning before drilling the proximal tibial screws. The surgeon should make sure the posteroanterior screw will be hitting the posterior calcaneus at an appropriate height. **B.** The posteroanterior screw is predrilled and measured via the C-arm to discern the length, usually just posterior to the calcaneal cuboid joint. **C.** A wrench is used to tighten the bolt compressing the heel plate toward the tibial screws; this intramedullary compression force is then held with distal screws through talus and calcaneus. **D.** Intraoperative view of gold screwdriver advancing the talar screw 7 mm proximally to augment ankle compression.

END CAP INSERTION

- Although some surgeons consider the end cap optional, we routinely secure it to the distal end of the nail after removal of the targeting arm. It restricts medullary bleeding, limits heterotopic calcification, and protects the threads of the nail should extraction be needed later.
- Permanent radiographs may be obtained in the operating room, both with AP and lateral projection, to ascertain appropriate alignment, position, and fixation.

BONE GRAFTING

- Autogenous or allograft bone grafting is done to improve healing rates.
- Medullary reamings can be mixed with a fibular autograft and inserted at the tibiotalar and subtalar fusion sites even before placement of the nail.
- After insertion of the nail, place bone graft anterior, lateral, and posterior to the fusion sites.
- For large defects, such as removal of ankle prostheses, a femoral head allograft may be cut to fit the large defect, and then the nail can be placed directly through the allograft (**TECH FIG 6**).

- Because of the bleeding, cancellous surfaces of bone achieved at surgery, and the large amounts of bone graft employed, closed suction drainage is recommended.
- Some surgeons and investigators advocate internal or external electrical bone stimulators for improving healing rates in neuropathic, multiply operated patients or smokers.
- We have also used bone stimulation for patients with preexisting avascular necrosis at the arthrodesis site.

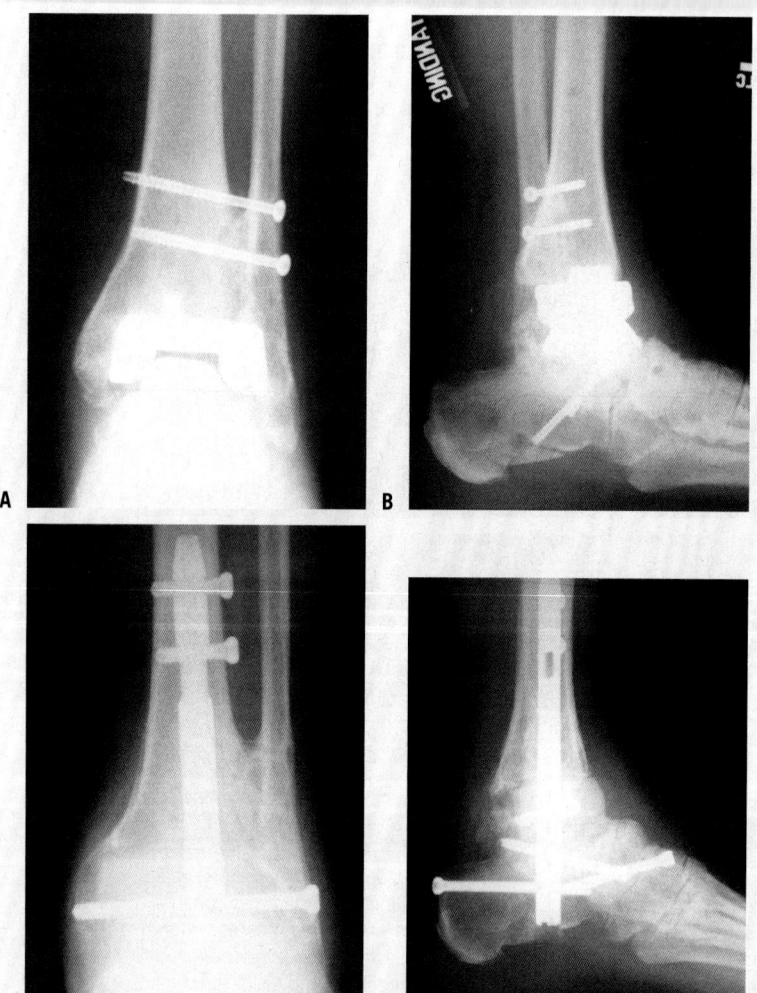

TECH FIG 6 A,B. Preoperative AP and lateral views of failing Agility total ankle prosthesis. **C,D.** Postoperative AP and lateral views after placement of femoral head allograft (soaked in concentrated bone marrow aspirate) demonstrate the excellent stability of an intramedullary device in a complicated revision situation.

WOUND CLOSURE

- Take care to approximate the tissues in the ankle region. A layered closure is preferable.
- Apply a sterile, nonadherent dressing with adequate padding from the tips of the toes to just below the knee.

- This dressing includes a posterior plaster splint with the ankle and foot at neutral position and a gentle compressive wrap over padding.

CASE EXAMPLE

- The patient was a 58-year-old man with posttraumatic talar avascular necrosis who failed brace wear.
- Preoperative radiographs are shown in **TECH FIG 7A** to **C**. The patient had pain from tibiotalar arthritis due to talar dome collapse. With increasing talar collapse, the foot gradually migrated anterior to the tibia, a biomechanically unfavorable position.
- Postoperative radiographs are shown in **TECH FIG 7D** and **E**. Tibiotalocalcaneal arthrodesis with a medullary nail was performed.

The anatomic relationship of the foot to the tibia has been reestablished. The nail is not proud on the plantar foot. Despite the relatively large diameter of the nail, a supplemental cannulated screw can be placed adjacent to the nail from the calcaneus to the anterior tibia to provide further support to the construct. Also, a large buttress (much like the flying buttress on a French cathedral) was placed on the posterior tibia and dorsal calcaneus to increase the surface area for fusion.

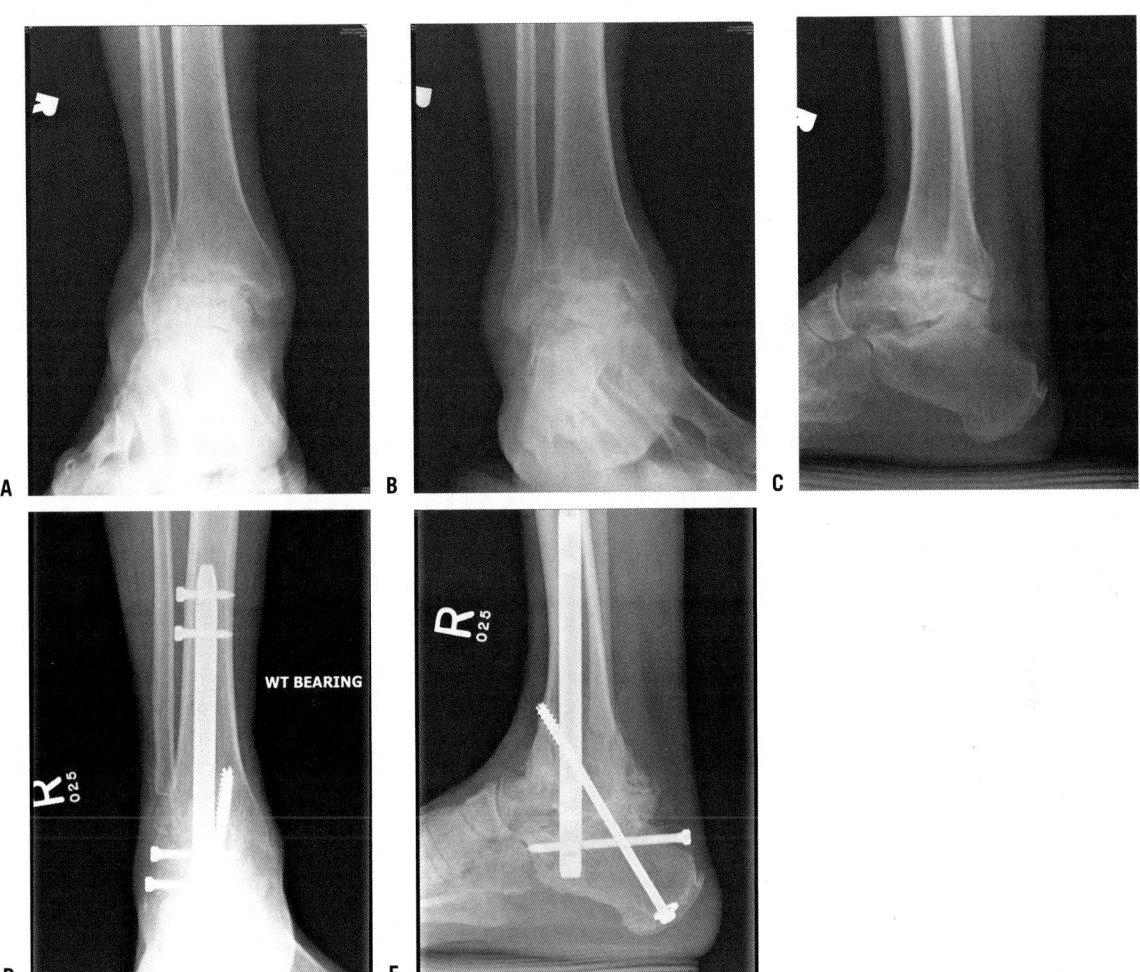

TECH FIG 7 A–C. Preoperative weight-bearing ankle radiographs with avascular necrosis of the talar dome and some degree of anterior translation of the talus relative to the tibial axis. **A.** AP view. **B.** Mortise view. **C.** Lateral view. **D,E.** Postoperative weight-bearing ankle radiographs of the same patient after tibiotalocalcaneal arthrodesis. Fusion appears to have been successful based on the bridging trabeculation at the arthrodesis sites. In our experience, the increased surface area afforded by the bone graft to the prepared posterior tibia and dorsal calcaneus increases the chance of fusion. Note that the physiologic relationship of talus to tibial shaft axis has been reestablished. Despite the nail's relatively large diameter, a supplemental cannulated screw could be passed adjacent to the nail to provide greater stability to the construct. **D.** AP view. **E.** Lateral view.

Pearls and Pitfalls

- The most important goal of tibiotalocalcaneal arthrodesis with medullary nail fixation is achieving satisfactory pain-free union of the ankle and hindfoot with the foot in optimal plantigrade posture.
- In our experience, radiographic and clinical assessment on the operating table before completion of the case is most important in achieving plantigrade posture.
- Intraoperative pearls include the need for appropriate positioning so that full access to the entire lower extremity is obtained.
  - We recommend that the patient with limited internal and external hip rotation should be positioned in slightly less-than-extreme lateral position to facilitate access to the medial malleolar side of the ankle and optimize AP imaging with a C-arm fluoroscope.
- The optimal insertion point for the nail is immediately lateral to the plantar calcaneus' midpoint and in line with the longitudinal tibial axis.
- Nail and targeting arm
  - Be sure that the targeting arm is rigidly coupled to the nail. Rigid coupling of the nail to its targeting arm in the appropriate position and alignment will save the surgeon a lot of effort and frustration in locking the nail proximally.
- Medullary nailing for tibiotalocalcaneal arthrodesis in the face of open ulcers or wounds is not absolutely contraindicated, but ulcers or wounds should be clean, noncellulitic, and granulating before medullary nail fixation is considered.
- Rotational alignment of the tibiotalocalcaneal arthrodesis: Satisfactory rotational alignment is most readily achieved by comparison to the contralateral uninvolved limb and by preserving the natural concave–convex relationship of the tibiotalar and subtalar fusion sites at the time of removal of diseased cartilage and subchondral bone.
- Performing tibiotalocalcaneal arthrodesis with limited assistance: A holding pin from the calcaneus to the posterior tibia can help hold alignment during the reaming process **(FIG 8)**.

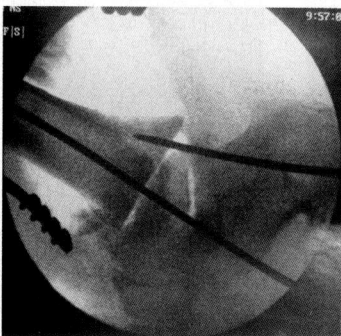

FIG 8 A holding pin from the calcaneus to the posterior tibia can help hold position when reaming and placing the nail as long as the pin remains out of the reamer's path.

POSTOPERATIVE CARE

- Most patients undergoing tibiotalocalcaneal arthrodesis with medullary nail fixation can be discharged the day after surgery with oral analgesics and after having received 24 hours of parenteral antibiotics.
- The typical case will require non–weight-bearing protection in a short-leg splint or cast for 6 weeks, followed by 4 to 6 weeks of weight bearing to tolerance in a short-leg walking cast.
- At 10 to 12 weeks postoperatively, the patient is fitted with a removable fracture orthosis equipped with a rocker bottom sole to ease the transition to weight bearing in more normal shoe wear by 12 to 16 weeks postoperatively.
- Less than half of the patients fused in the appropriate plantigrade posture with otherwise normal neuromuscular function will have a noticeable limp by 6 to 12 months postoperatively.
- Those requiring shoe wear modification are often best treated with a rocker bottom sole or a cushioned heel to make up for the rigidity of the fused joints.
- Heel lifts can be employed to equalize limb lengths to within 10 to 15 mm; the side undergoing tibiotalocalcaneal fusion desirably being the short one to allow for toe clearance during the swing phase of gait.
- The vast majority of our patients are ambulatory postoperatively in a noncustom, off-the-shelf shoe.
- Rod removal has been required in less than 1% of Dr. Quill's operative series.

OUTCOMES

- Medullary nail advantages over traditional fixation for arthrodesis of the ankle and hindfoot include the fact that a medullary nail is a load-sharing device that is especially indicated for the osteopenic or neuroarthropathic patient.
- Dr. Quill's personal clinical series includes a 93% union rate in an average of 12.2 weeks postoperatively (range 10 to 20 weeks).[14]
  - Delayed nonunions have occurred in neuropathic patients, but most are asymptomatic.
  - Mean improvement in the American Orthopaedic Foot & Ankle Society clinical scores for this series of patients has been 52 points.
  - Nail-related problems include the removal of 17 of 932 locking screws for fracture or local irritation.
  - There have been two fractured nails, both of which were in the face of severe persistent valgus and subtalar nonunion in neuropathic, obese patients.
  - One tibial fracture was sustained intraoperatively in an osteopenic rheumatoid patient. It was incomplete and healed during routine casting.
- Excellent early stability and rigid early fixation are achieved and maintained, providing for less perioperative morbidity and discomfort and shorter casting.
- The medullary nail ensures position and alignment from the immediate postoperative time frame, and the patients often require less activity restriction postoperatively.

- Medullary nail fixation for tibiotalocalcaneal arthrodesis has filled a particular niche in treating patients with severe deformities, disabilities, and bone loss who otherwise would have been severely disabled or would have needed to undergo limb amputation.

COMPLICATIONS

- We have not encountered plantar wound healing problems in any patient when the procedure is done as described earlier.
- Damage to the medial and lateral plantar nerves can be avoided by following the technique mentioned earlier and by dissecting with nothing sharper than a large key elevator deep to the dermis on the plantar aspect of the foot.
  - A three-quarter-inch key elevator can be used to bluntly spread the fibers of the plantar fascia and the intrinsic flexor muscles in line with the incision and to sweep soft tissues medially and laterally before inserting the guidewire through the sole of the foot.
- Complications of medullary nail fixation for ankle and hindfoot fusion include those germane to any orthopaedic procedure, such as infection, medical illness, and anesthetic perioperative complication as well as hardware prominence.
- The complications unique to medullary nail fixation for tibiotalocalcaneal arthrodesis include delayed union, nonunion, and malunion and can be minimized by adhering to the technique described.
- The proximal dissection for screw fixation may encounter the superficial peroneal nerve and the distal dissection may expose the sural nerve; care must be taken to avoid damage. In cases in which the medial malleolus is removed, the tibial nerve can be exposed to injury very easily.

REFERENCES

1. Adams JC. Arthrodesis of the ankle joint: experiences with the transfibular approach. J Bone Joint Surg Br 1948;30-B(3):506–511.
2. Bullens P, de Waal Malefijt M, Louwerens JW. Conversion of failed ankle arthroplasty to an arthrodesis. Technique using an arthrodesis nail and a cage filled with morsellized bone graft. Foot Ankle Surg 2010;16(2):101–104.
3. Ford SE, Kwon JY, Ellington JK. Tibiotalocalcaneal arthrodesis utilizing a titanium intramedullary nail with an internal pseudoelastic nitinol compression element: a retrospective case series of 33 patients. J Foot Ankle Surg 2019;58(2):266–272.
4. Gellman H, Lenihan M, Halikis N, et al. Selective tarsal arthrodesis: an in vitro analysis of the effect on foot motion. Foot Ankle 1987;8:127–133.
5. Gharehdaghi M, Rahimi H, Mousavian A. Anterior ankle arthrodesis with molded plate: technique and outcomes. Arch Bone Jt Surg 2014;2(3):203–209.
6. Hefti FL, Baumann JU, Morscher EW. Ankle joint fusion—determination of optimal position by gait analysis. Arch Orthop Trauma Surg 1980;96:187–195.
7. Iwata H, Yasuhara N, Kawashima K, et al. Arthrodesis of the ankle joint with rheumatoid arthritis: experience with the transfibular approach. Clin Orthop Relat Res 1980;(153):189–193.
8. Jehan S, Shakeel M, Bing AJF, Hill SO. The success of tibiotalocalcaneal arthrodesis with intramedullary nailing—a systematic review of the literature. Acta Orthop Belg 2011;77:644–651.
9. Kile TA, Donnelly RE, Gehrke JC, et al. Tibiocalcaneal arthrodesis with an intramedullary device. Foot Ankle Int 1994;15:669–673.
10. Papa JA, Myerson MS. Pantalar and tibiotalocalcaneal arthrodesis for post-traumatic osteoarthrosis of the ankle and hindfoot. J Bone Joint Surg Am 1992;74(7):1042–1049.
11. Papa JA, Myerson MS, Girard P. Salvage, with arthrodesis, in intractable diabetic neuropathic arthropathy of the foot and ankle. J Bone Joint Surg Am 1993;75(7):1056–1066.
12. Quill GE. An approach to the management of ankle arthritis. In: Myerson M, ed. Foot and Ankle Disorders. Philadelphia: WB Saunders, 2000:1059–1084.
13. Quill GE. Pantalar arthritis. In: Nunley JA, Pfeffer GB, Sanders RW, et al, eds. Advanced Reconstruction Foot and Ankle. Rosemont, IL: American Academy of Orthopaedic Surgeons, 2004:209–213.
14. Quill GE. Tibiotalocalcaneal and pantalar arthrodesis. Foot Ankle Clin 1996;1:199–210.
15. Quill GE. Tibiotalocalcaneal arthrodesis. Tech Orthop 1996;11:269–273.
16. Siebachmeyer M, Boddu K, Bilal A, et al. Outcome of one-stage correction of deformities of the ankle and hindfoot and fusion in Charcot neuroarthropathy using a retrograde intramedullary hindfoot arthrodesis nail. Bone Joint J 2015;97-B(1):76–82.
17. Stuart MJ, Morrey BF. Arthrodesis of the diabetic neuropathic ankle. Clin Orthop Relat Res 1990;(253):209–211.

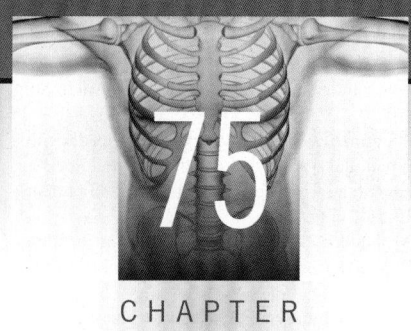

75

CHAPTER

Tibiotalocalcaneal Fusion Using an Intramedullary Nail

James K. DeOrio

DEFINITION

- A surgical procedure in which the ankle and the subtalar joint are arthrodesed simultaneously

ANATOMY

- The tibiotalar joint is bound by the medial malleolus, the fibula (lateral malleolus), anterior retinaculum and tendinous structures with the neurovascular bundle, and posteriorly by the flexor hallucis longus (FHL) and Achilles tendon.
- The posterior tibial nerve lies immediately adjacent to the FHL tendon on the medial side.

PATHOGENESIS

- Any trauma or inflammatory process that affect the ankle and subtalar joint simultaneously can cause pain in both of these joints. So too can the ankle be irreparably damaged with a failed total ankle with so much fibrosis and so little motion in the subtalar joint that it is not appropriate to preserve it.
- Because the rod stabilizes both the ankle and subtalar joint, it may be used in paralytic conditions and when the talus is avascular and both the ankle and subtalar joints have been affected. The avascular bone is often resected and replaced with a femoral head, talar allograft, or three-dimensional (3-D) printed metallic filler.

NATURAL HISTORY

- The natural history is for the pain to increase because of increasing damage and loss of motion in these two joints. The prognosis is poor without surgery.

PATIENT HISTORY AND PHYSICAL FINDINGS

- The patient complains of generalized pain across the anterior aspect of the ankle (ankle joint) and in the sinus tarsi (subtalar joint).
- They have a limited range of motion in these joints and they are often painful on attempted manipulation and deep palpation.

IMAGING AND OTHER DIAGNOSTIC STUDIES

- Diagnostic imaging consists of standard standing anteroposterior (AP), lateral, and mortise views of the ankle.
- Additional standing full foot films are necessary, including a calcaneal view to ensure that the patient does indeed have a problem in the ankle and subtalar joints.
- Frequently, a computed tomography (CT) scan of the ankle is necessary to confirm this fact.

DIFFERENTIAL DIAGNOSIS

- Inflammatory arthropathy (rheumatoid arthritis, gout, hemosiderosis, etc), trauma, failed ankle replacement, avascular necrosis of the talus and/or tibia, spastic paralysis, Charcot arthropathy, failed ankle fusion with subtalar arthritis, and resectable tumor with bone loss

NONOPERATIVE MANAGEMENT

- Nonoperative treatment included bracing, orthotics, nonsteroidal anti-inflammatory drugs, and injections of steroid and narcotic medication.

SURGICAL MANAGEMENT

- The indications for surgery are coexisting painful inflammation in the ankle and subtalar joints simultaneously. This procedure is indicated when it is believed that neither ankle fusion nor subtalar fusion alone would suffice in producing a relatively painless functional limb.
- It must be discussed with the patients that for whatever reason, they are not a good candidate for ankle replacement and subtalar fusion to deal with this problem (FIG 1).
- Preoperative physical examination is mandatory to ensure that the approach is appropriate when considering previous incisions, trauma, free flaps, wound healing problems, and deformity.

Positioning

- Although a tibiotalocalcaneal (TTC) arthrodesis may be accomplished in a supine and even lateral position, because insertion of the calcaneal screws is best done posterior to anterior, the prone position of the patient is desired. This position allows the leg to be shifted off the table for easy AP and, by rotating the leg, a lateral x-ray with fluoroscopy. The tibial screws are inserted with the knee flexed 90 degrees.
- Be careful to avoid the side paddle on the table near the thigh because this will prevent the leg from being shifted off the table.

Approach

- Approach can be anterior, lateral, and posterior.
  - The disadvantage of the anterior approach is the need to make a separate incision for preparation of the subtalar joint. It does, however, make removal of the avascular talus more manageable.

5500

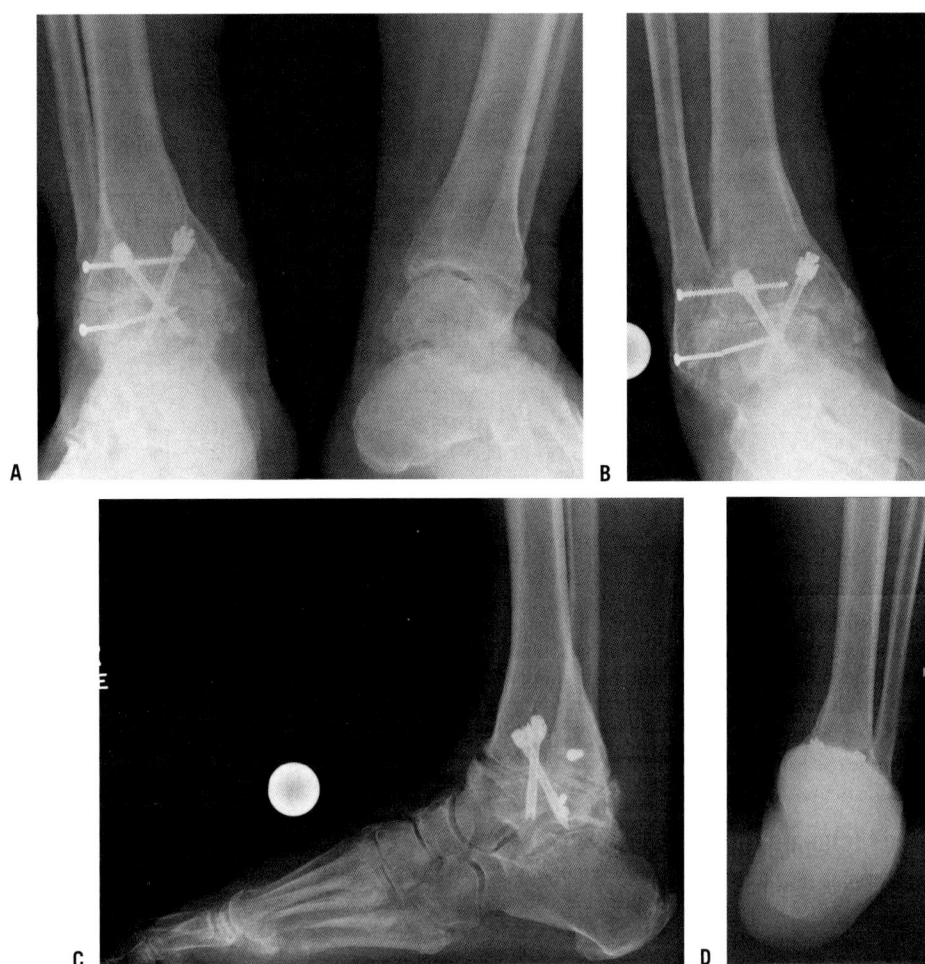

FIG 1 AP (**A**), lateral (**B**), mortise (**C**), and Saltzman (**D**) radiographs of 65-year-old man weighing 270 lb, who had undergone attempted fusion of right ankle after trauma 10 years earlier. He presented with a nonunion of his ankle joint and severe subtalar arthrosis.

- The lateral approach is discouraged because of the need to resect the fibula, a technique that is believed to be outmoded and contributes to subsequent valgus deformities of the ankle or subtalar joint that do not heal.[1] Nowhere else in orthopaedics do we remove a vascularized bone that can contribute to the construct.
- The posterior approach allows preparation of the ankle and subtalar joint simultaneously and has an angiosomic pattern that is ideal for healing.

EXPOSURE

Superficial Incision

- The incision can be made just lateral to the Achilles but I prefer a midline, longitudinal Achilles tendon approach (**TECH FIG 1**).[4,8]
- It begins 8 cm above the posterosuperior aspect of the calcaneus and extends to the inferior surface of the calcaneus.
- The tendon is split down the middle, and the attachment on the calcaneus is relieved both medially and laterally. Remember, this is where the posterior to anterior screws are inserted anyway, and this increased release facilitates exposure of the ankle and subtalar joint simultaneously.
- In extreme cases of equinus, one can do a Z-lengthening of the Achilles or completely remove the attachment onto the calcaneus.

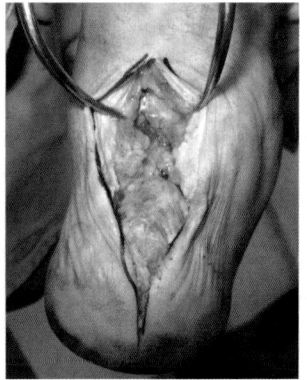

TECH FIG 1 After an anterior exposure to remove his previous hardware, the patient is opened straight posteriorly through the Achilles tendon to expose his ankle and subtalar joint.

Deep Incision

- Once through the Achilles tendon, the deep retinaculum is cut and the flexor hallucis muscle belly is visualized.
- The muscle belly is followed distally, and the FHL tendon is freed from the lateral calcaneus for mobility. The muscle belly is free and retracted medially. Use of the Henley retractor can assist with the visualization.

Ankle Exposure and Subtalar Exposure

- Now, the posteroinferior tibial lip is exposed and removed to facilitate entry into the ankle joint. Using a blunt periosteal elevator, the ankle joint and subtalar joint are freed from any adhesions. Exposed cartilage is removed from both joints. It helps to use a lamina spreader or pin distractor both medium and extra large to be able to open these joints.

- If there is a total ankle in place, the polyethylene is removed first. Then remove the talar component first and then the tibial component. A small reciprocating and oscillating saw is used to cut free any bony attachment to the prosthesis to preserve maximum bone stock.
- If there is an intramedullary (IM) tibial component, it may be necessary to window the posterior tibia for exposure. This way, the reciprocating saw can maneuver around the stem and free up most of the ingrowth bone.
- For the INBONE prosthesis, the baseplate can be removed with an impactor and the wrench can be inserted around the last stem piece and then impaction begins on the wrench. A large bone hook placed within the INBONE stem can help to counteract the posterior impaction force to keep the tibia from breaking anteriorly at the level of the ankle

DÉBRIDING THE ANKLE AND SUBTALAR JOINT

- Removal of the cartilage and/or soft tissue debris can be accomplished with curettes, rongeurs, sharp dissection with a knife, a burr, a saw to cut the talar surface slightly, or even a small acetabular reamer (38 mm) to speed up the process.[2]
- Remember to protect the posterior tibial nerve and leave a concavity in the tibia into which a femoral head can be inserted if necessary.
- If there is complete avascular necrosis of the talus, I like to remove the posterior half of the talus and replace that with a femoral head or allograft talus trimmed to fit. One can now also have 3-D printed cages to fill the defect.[6] These can be similarly bone grafted before insertion.
- If there is eburnated bone present, drilling the bone extensively with a 4.5-mm drill will break down the bone to allow vascular ingress more easily (**TECH FIG 2**).

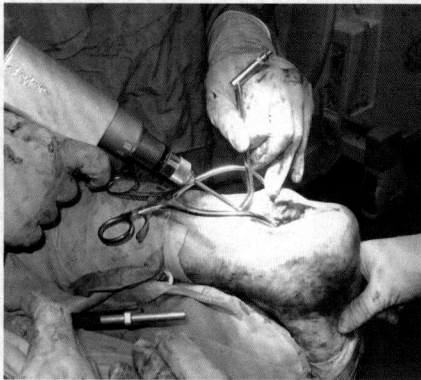

TECH FIG 2 Once any remaining cartilage and/or fibrous tissue is removed, the surfaces of the ankle and subtalar joints should be drilled with a 4.5-mm drill bit to break up the subchondral bone.

BONE GRAFTING

- Once the joint is cleaned and the surface prepared, bone graft is added. One can use bone morphogenetic protein (BMP) sheets laid anteriorly, medially, and laterally.[3] Other BMPs can be used instead. Onto this is laid up to 40 mL of thawed frozen cancellous bone. This is followed by a trimmed femoral head or allograft talus to fit the space or, as mentioned, a premade 3-D cage. Previously, vancomycin was added to the bone graft. However, this has been shown to inhibit osteoblasts and is no longer used.[11]

- I usually trim the sides and the base of the head to make it fit and then impact it into position.
  - This may also be done after preparing the leg for the rod because the head will want to spit out posteriorly as you prepare leg for the rod. The 3-D printed cages are made with a hole for the rod.
  - You can also put some posterior Steinmann pins into the head and surrounding bone to get it to stay in place while you ream.

PREPARATION OF THE LEG FOR THE NAIL

- Depending on the manufacture's rod you are using, preparation of the leg for the nail may vary. For purposes of detailing the surgical procedure here, I will use the A3 nail.[10]

- Place a guide pin into the calcaneal fat pad using the pin placement guide (**TECH FIG 3A–D**) or place it freehand parallel to the

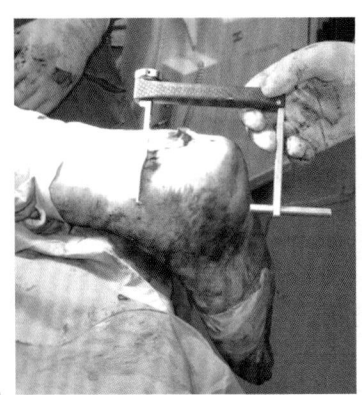
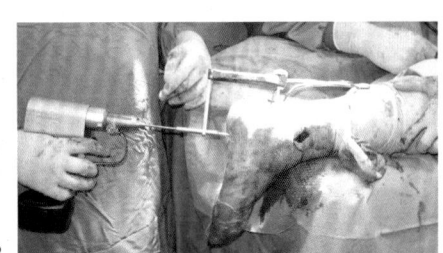
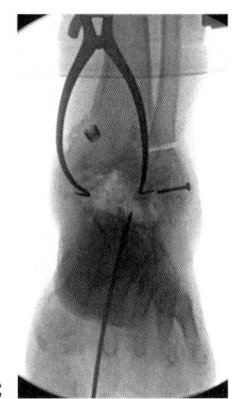
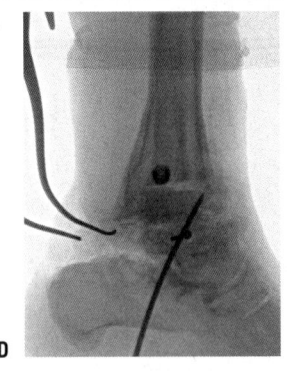

TECH FIG 3 A. A pin placement guide is now inserted into the ankle joint with its distal tip just anterior and lateral to talar dome center. **B.** The guide pin is now placed through the guide until it reaches the tibial plafond. It is then sitting in the calcaneus and talus. **C,D.** Checking the guide pin placement on AP and lateral x-rays, respectively. Note how the guide pin is situated anterolateral to the talar dome. Then, when the foot is brought into dorsiflexion and valgus, the rod will go up the tibia and place the foot in the proper position.

calcaneal cuboid (CC) joint, about 20 mm posterior to the joint and in the middle of the calcaneal fat pad.

- If you aim just slightly laterally and anteriorly, when the rod is placed, you will force the foot into dorsiflexion and valgus and help void plantarflexion and varus. The more varus the hindfoot is in, the more laterally you should place the guide pin. The more plantarflexed the foot, the more anteriorly you should place the guide pin.
- Note that in **TECH FIG 3C**, you see an osteotomy in the fibula. This was done to reduce the patient into a hindfoot valgus position.

Failure to do so would have caused the patient to walk on the side of his foot. However, it has never been necessary to remove the fibula which adds to the support of the final construct.

- The angulated drill sleeve is used to find the place laterally and posteriorly to place the incision for the reamers.
- Once the guide pin is in place, ream the guide pin starting with fixed reamers to the tibiotalar joint **(TECH FIG 4A–G)** and then insert a longer ball-tipped guide rod up the tibia and ream ½ mm larger than the intended rod for the shorter rod (150 to 180 mm) and 1 mm larger for the larger rods (210 mm) **(TECH FIG 4H–K)**.

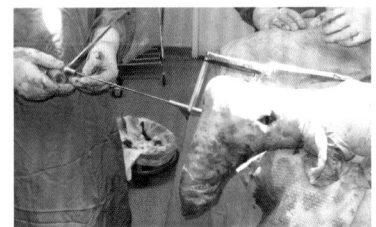
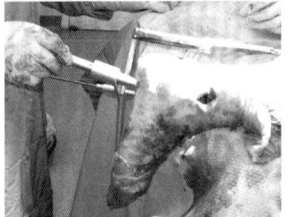
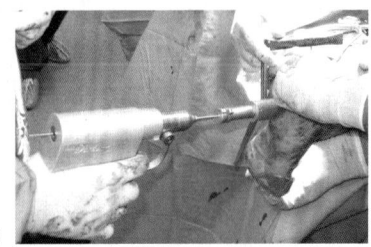
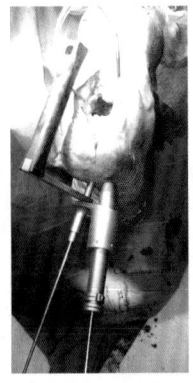
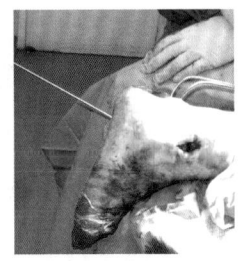

TECH FIG 4 A. Using the central pin already in place, an additional guide is placed over that pin to provide direction for the posterolateral bend in the A3 nail. **B.** The guide for the posterolateral pin is set in place. **C.** The posterolateral guide pin is being placed. **D.** Axial photo showing how both pins are now sitting in the ankle. The C-arm is brought over the top of the leg to ensure the two pins are in the correct position. **E.** The guide pin is directed anteriorly so that when the foot is dorsiflexed, the rod will go into the tibia. The first guide pin is then removed, and the posterolateral guide pin is reamed to accommodate the rod. *(continued)*

TECHNIQUES

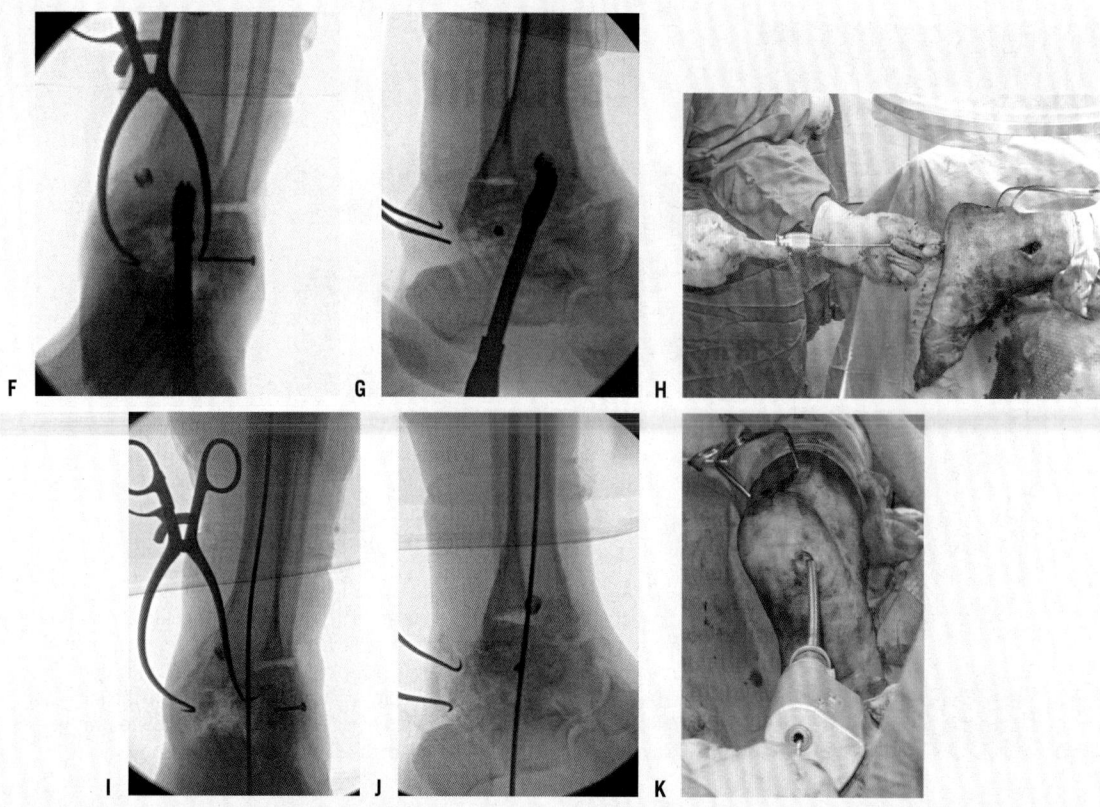

TECH FIG 4 *(continued)* **F,G.** AP and lateral x-rays, respectively, showing the extent of the first reaming over the guide rod. **H.** The reamer has now been removed and a ball-tipped guide is being inserted into the tibia to lie in the calcaneus, talus, and tibia. **I,J.** AP and lateral x-rays, respectively, showing the placement of the ball-tipped guide in the ankle and leg. **K.** Over this rod, sequentially ream up to ½ to 1 mm greater than the diameter of the rod intended for shorter or longer rods, respectively.

In patients with Charcot foot, it is best to use the longest rod possible up to 300 mm.

- Add the femoral head allograft and additional cancellous bone, insert the guide pin again, check its position with the fluoroscope **(TECH FIG 5)**, and then ream a hole into the bone graft to accommodate the rod. If using a 3-D printed cage, just make sure the rotation of the cage is correct, so the rod will go through the cage.

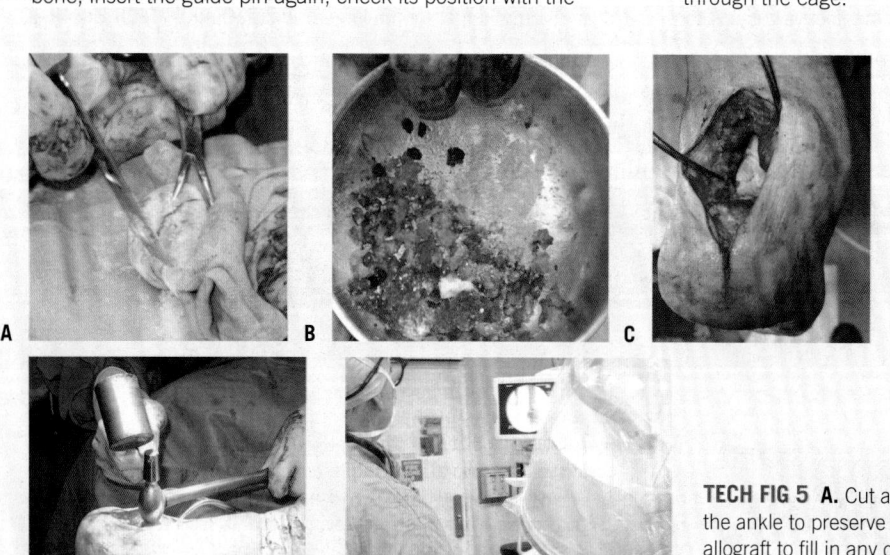

TECH FIG 5 A. Cut a femoral head to fill any major defect in the ankle to preserve leg length. **B.** Add plenty of thawed frozen allograft to fill in any defect. I usually add some form of BMP. **C.** Add enough bone graft to fill the defect while leaving room for the femoral head or 3-D printed cage. **D.** Impact the femoral head so it stays in place and add more bone graft to fill in any remaining defects and impact it into position. **E.** Replace the guide pin through the femoral head and check its position using the C-arm. Then, while holding the femoral head in position, ream over the guide rod to create a hole in the femoral head for the nail.

ROD INSERTION

- Assemble the rod according to the manufacture's specifications with the inserter.
- Remove the ball-tipped guide and push the rod into position.
- Check the lateral x-ray to ensure that the rod is deep enough but not too deep, usually just past the cortex of the calcaneus.

- Mark the rod holder so that you can see if this position is changed during insertion of the screws (**TECH FIG 6**).
- If the foot is not in proper position, remove the rod and ream the calcaneus and talus to 13.5 mm to give yourself some leeway to push the rod eccentrically into the hole and get more dorsiflexion or valgus.

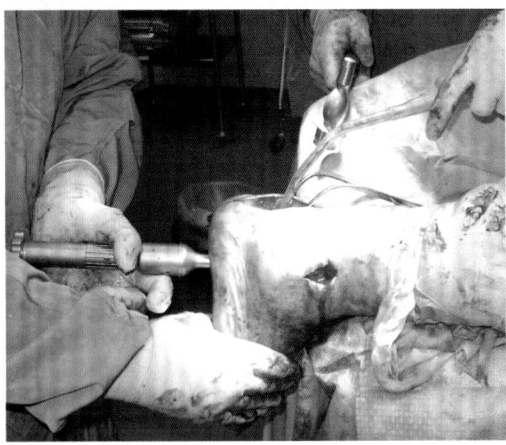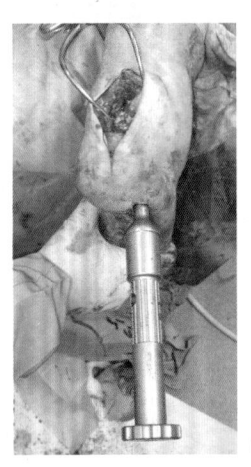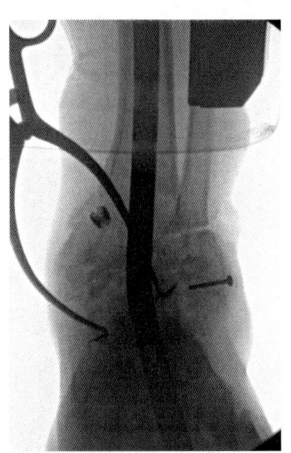

TECH FIG 6 A. Now, pull out the reamer and the guide pin out and insert the TTC A3 nail. **B.** The nail is in the hindfoot and leg, coming in from the posterior lateral side of the calcaneus in order to capture as much of the calcaneus as possible. **C.** The position of the nail is now checked on fluoroscopy to ensure the nail is inserted to its proper depth.

INTERLOCKING SCREWS

- Using the holder, rotate the guide into the C position.
- With the rod inserted to the correct depth, drill the calcaneal screw holes, usually in the compression position. Leave a drill in place and check the length of the intended screw on fluoroscopy.
- Insert the second drill; again, verify its position to ensure it has not gone through the CC joint.
- Insert the two calcaneal screws (**TECH FIG 7A–C**).
- Rotate the holder to the T position and insert the talar screw in the same manner (**TECH FIG 7D,E**).

- Rotate the rod to the M position. Make sure the holder is tight and drill one hole through the tibia from medial to lateral, measure its length and insert the screw, and again in the compression mode if you plan on trying to close down the space at the tibiotalar and subtalar joints. Add the second screw (**TECH FIG 7F**).
- Check to ensure correct positioning of the rod and add some compression to the construct (**TECH FIG 7G,H**).
- Let the tourniquet down to ensure return of vascularity to the leg (**TECH FIG 7I,J**).

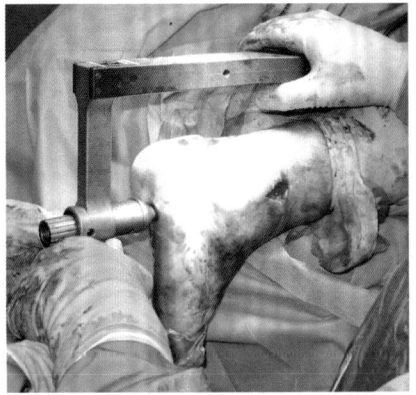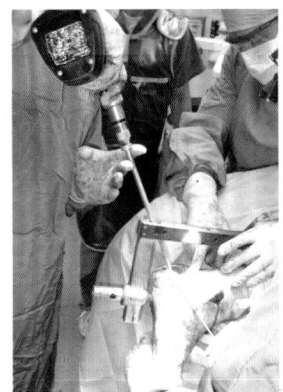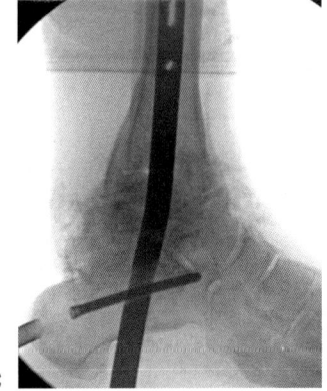

TECH FIG 7 A. The calcaneus, talar, and tibial screw guide is now locked in place. **B.** Drill a hole for the calcaneal screw first and insert that screw. **C.** Check its position as it goes into the calcaneus. Now, switch the guide to T for the talar screw. *(continued)*

TECHNIQUES

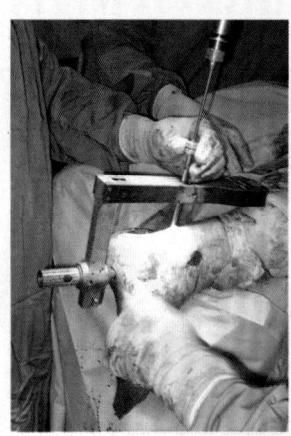
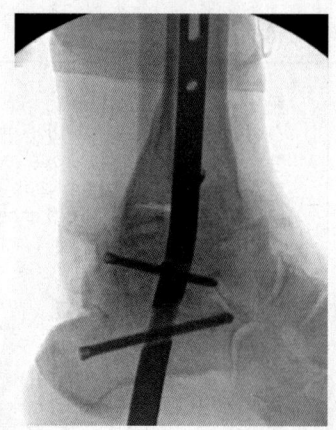
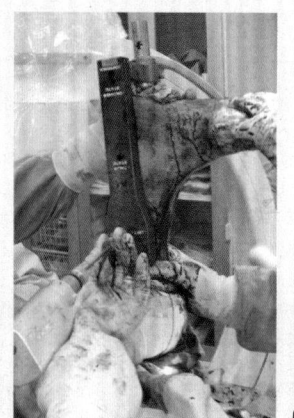
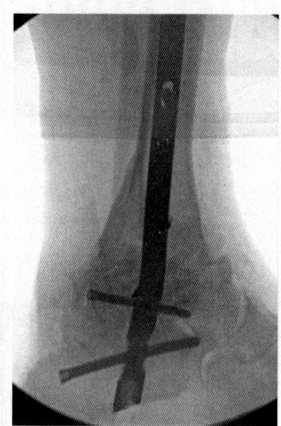

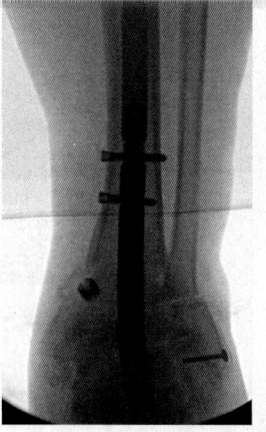
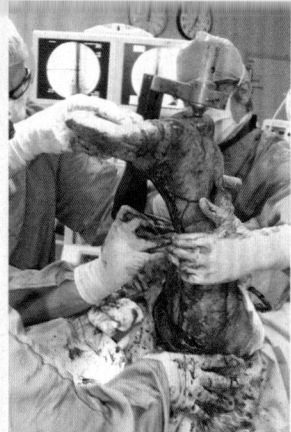
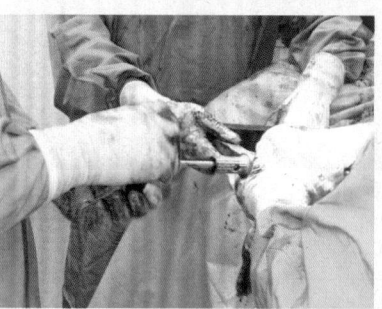

TECH FIG 7 *(continued)* **D.** Drill the talar screw hole and insert the talar screw. **E.** Check its position on fluoroscopy. **F.** Move the guide to the M position, drill one tibial hole, and insert the tibial screw, checking it fluoroscopically. **G,H.** Final lateral and AP x-rays, respectively, showing placement of the A3 nail. **I.** The tourniquet has been let down while the other tibial screw hole is prepared. **J.** Use screwdriver to exert final compression within the rod.

ADDITIONAL BONE GRAFTING

- Add more thawed cancellous chips over the femoral head or cage and pack it into position, being careful not to compress the posterior tibial nerve.

- Prepare the top of the calcaneus to allow bone ingrowth if not already done.
- Place BMP sheets posteriorly or add BMPs to the bone graft before insertion.

CLOSURE

- Use a running 2-0 absorbable stitch in the Achilles tendon over a drain. Using a drain obviates having the patients and/or the nurses to tell you the patient is bleeding out of the cast.

- Add some 3-0 absorbable stitches to the subcutaneous tissue.
- Close the skin with 3-0 nylon in a vertical mattress fashion.

TECHNIQUES

CASTING

- Apply two stacks of 4- × 8-inch gauze to the anterior ankle transversely, with the crack between them at the level of the ankle. Add two more 4- × 8-inch gauze packs each on the lateral and posterior sides (three 4- × 8-inch gauze packs altogether split in half).

- Apply soft roll so that there are five sheets countable proximally and distally.
- Apply three 4-inch rolls of fiberglass, being careful not to exceed the top of the cast padding.

CASE EXAMPLE (COURTESY OF MARK E. EASLEY, MD)

Background and Imaging

- A 65-year-old man with chronic right ankle/hindfoot pain
  - Remote history of severe ankle sprain
  - Failed course of bracing
- Physical examination
  - Hindfoot with neutral position
  - Ankle and hindfoot stiffness
  - Pain with ankle and hindfoot stress/motion
- Radiographs
  - Ankle with early arthritis and irregular lateral talar dome (**TECH FIG 8A**)
  - Hindfoot arthritis and loss of heel height and anterior ankle impingement (**TECH FIG 8B**)
  - Hindfoot alignment view suggests neutral heel alignment (**TECH FIG 8C**).

- CT
  - Coronal plane (**TECH FIG 8D**)
    - Advanced subtalar joint arthritis
    - Chronic anterolateral talar body nonunion
    - Subfibular impingement
  - Sagittal plane (**TECH FIG 8E**)
    - Advanced subtalar joint arthritis
    - Undersurface of talar body erosion/fragmentation
    - Anterior ankle impingement suggested

Intramedullary Tibiotalocalcaneal Arthrodesis

- Prone position
- Posterior approach (**TECH FIG 9A**)
- Achilles tendon Z-lengthening
- Protect posteromedial neurovascular bundle.

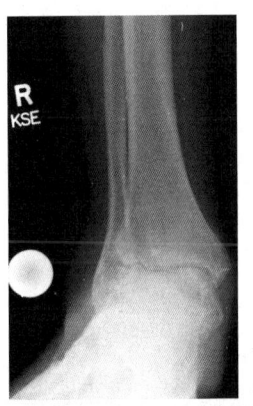
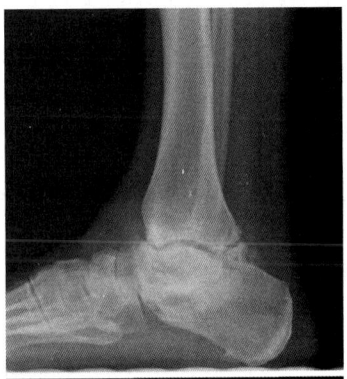
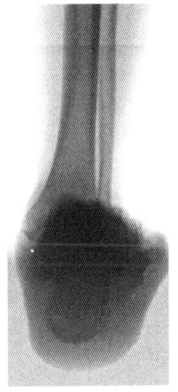
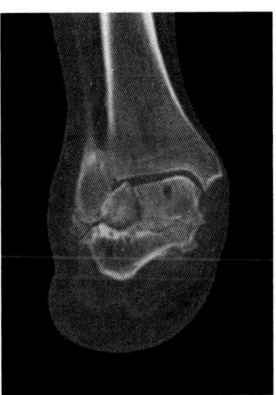
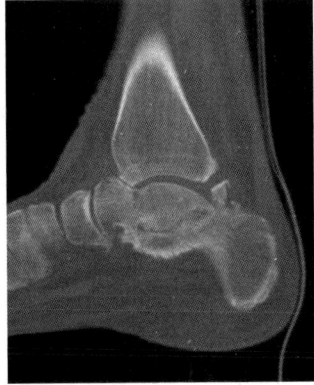

TECH FIG 8 A 65-year-old man with right ankle and hindfoot pain. **A.** Weight-bearing AP ankle view suggests irregular lateral talar dome. **B.** Severe loss of heel height and subtalar arthritis. **C.** Neutral heel alignment based on hindfoot alignment view. **D.** Coronal CT suggests severe subtalar arthritis and nonunion of anterolateral talar dome. **E.** Sagittal CT with severe subtalar arthritis, anterior ankle impingement, and loss of heel height.

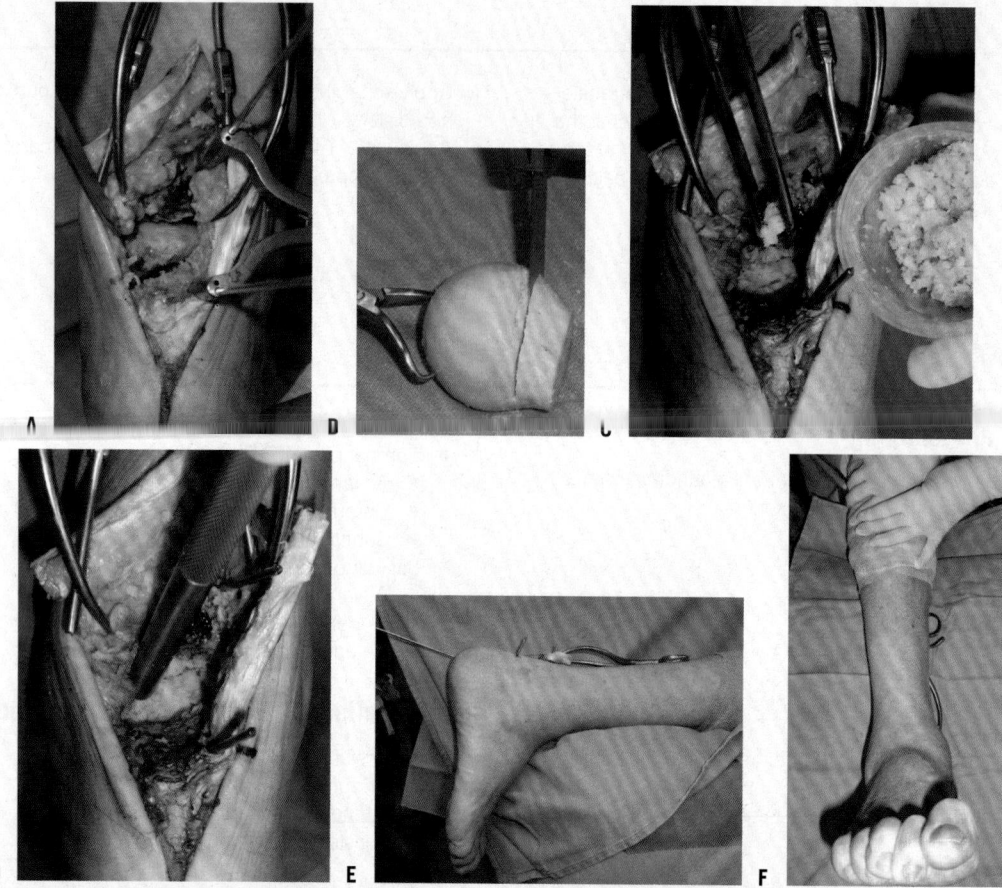

TECH FIG 9 A. Posterior approach with Z-lengthening of the Achilles tendon. **B.** Femoral head allograft. Using the neck portion of the structural graft to reestablish heel height and rebuild débrided avascular portion of talar dome. **C.** Augmenting structural graft with cancellous graft. **D.** Impacting the graft fully. **E,F.** Optimal alignment with provisional fixation. **E.** Neutral sagittal plane position. **F.** Neutral rotation. Note second metatarsal aligned with tibial crest. Also assess heel valgus.

- Joint distraction
  - Joint preparation
  - Joint reduction
  - Improve joint access for joint preparation for arthrodesis.
- Joint preparation
  - Débridement of unhealthy/avascular bone
  - Preparation of residual ankle and subtalar joints
- Bone grafting
  - Structural allograft: calcar of a femoral head allograft to compensate for loss of talar height **(TECH FIG 9B)**
  - Cancellous bone **(TECH FIG 9C,D):** fills voids and augments arthrodesis
- Provisional fixation and confirm satisfactory alignment and bony apposition
  - Clinical evaluation
    - Neutral dorsiflexion/plantarflexion **(TECH FIG 9E)**
    - Second metatarsal aligned with the tibial crest **(TECH FIG 9F)**
    - Heel valgus: Avoid heel varus.
  - Confirm optimal position fluoroscopically.

Definitive Fixation: Intramedullary Nail

- Properly place and align guide pin.
  - From plantar foot
  - Confirm proper position of pin on AP and lateral intraoperative fluoroscopy.
- Ream over guide pin **(TECH FIG 10A).**
  - Retrograde from calcaneus through talus and structural allograft into center of distal tibia
  - Determine optimal IM nail diameter and length.
- Place IM nail with guide/insertion device **(TECH FIG 10B).**
  - Maintain proper ankle and foot alignment.
  - Fluoroscopically confirm proper IM nail position, including appropriate depth to which the nail is inserted.
- Insert distal calcaneal interlocking screws, placed from posterior to anterior.
- Place provisional dynamic proximal fixation.
- Through the system, apply compression at the arthrodesis sites **(TECH FIG 10C).**
- Insert the proximal interlocking screws **(TECH FIG 10D).**
- Remove the insertion device.

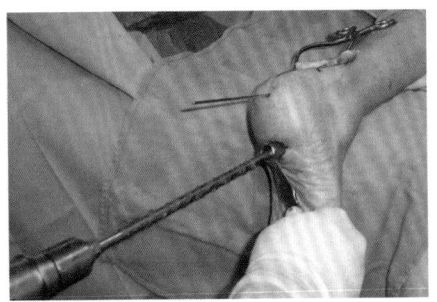 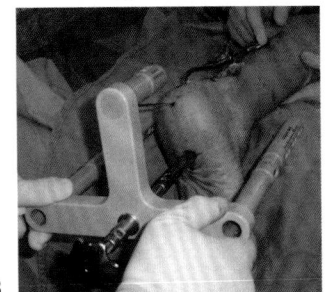 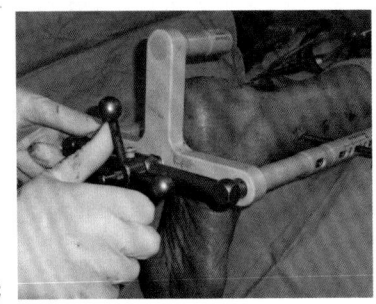

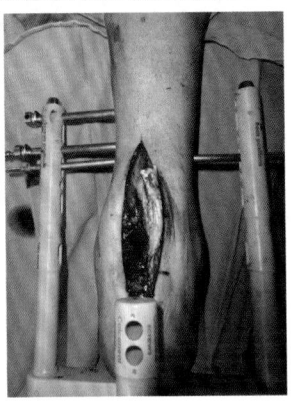

TECH FIG 10 A. Reaming from the calcaneus through talar body and structural graft into the tibia over guidewire. Note supplemental provisional fixation from calcaneus into posterior tibia to maintain reduction during reaming. Fluoroscopic evaluation to ensure optimal reaming. **B.** IM nail inserted with insertion device. Optimal rotation for the insertion device and IM nail is maintained. **C.** Once IM nail properly seated and provisional support pin placed proximally, compression is applied. **D.** Proximal interlocking screws inserted. Note compression through provisional proximal fixation.

Supplemental Fixation (at Surgeon's Discretion)

- Screw fixation from medial distal tibia into medial talar body (**TECH FIG 11A,B**)
- Posterior plate (**TECH FIG 11C**)
- Final intraoperative fluoroscopic views
- In this case, note 4 to 6 cm of Achilles lengthening suggesting that the heel height improved (**TECH FIG 11D**).

Postoperative Care

- Protected weight bearing for 8 weeks in short-leg cast (SLC)
- After 8 weeks, gradually advance weight bearing in SLC or cam boot.
- At 12 weeks, gradually transition to stiffer soled shoe with slight rocker bottom and ankle–foot orthosis with a fixed ankle.
- Gradual transition to full weight bearing in stiffer soled shoe with rocker bottom modification
- Consider CT scan at 12 to 16 weeks to assess incorporation of structural graft (**TECH FIG 12**).

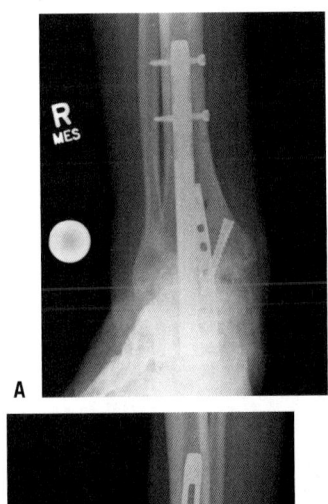 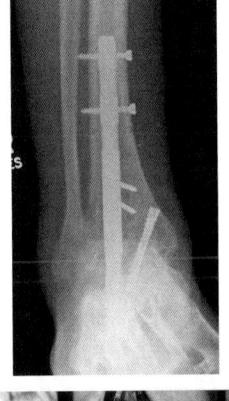

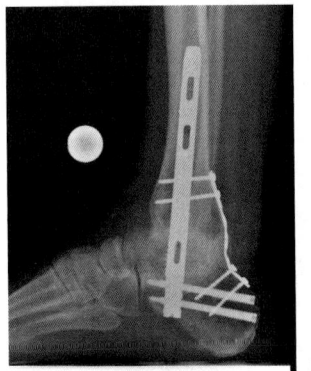 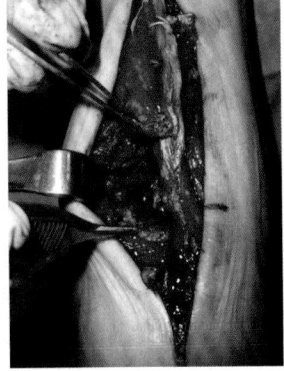

TECH FIG 11 A. Weight-bearing AP ankle view. **B.** Mortise view. Note supplemental medial screw. **C.** Lateral view. Note supplemental posterior plate. **D.** Considerable heel height restoration suggested with Achilles being lengthened approximately 4 to 5 cm.

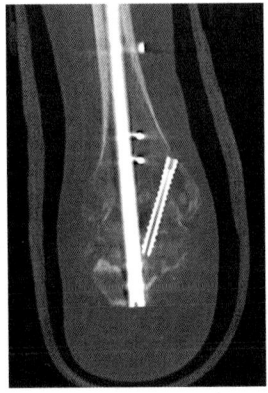

TECH FIG 12 CT scan coronal view at 12 weeks suggests satisfactory early bridging trabeculation at arthrodesis sites.

TECHNIQUES

Pearls and Pitfalls

Position the rod centrally in the calcaneus 20 mm from the joint and aim the guide pin slightly 3–4 mm laterally and anteriorly to get the nail in the correct position.	• If the rod leaves the leg in too much plantarflexion or varus, the patient will not be happy. Remove the rod and overream the calcaneus and talus to shift the foot into more dorsiflexion and valgus.
Avoid compression of the posterior tibial nerve.	• If the patient has dysesthesias in the foot postoperatively, obtain an electromyography and consider a tarsal tunnel release.
Do not leave the rod sticking out the plantar calcaneal cortex.	• Use fluoroscopy and constantly check to make sure the rod end is at the level of the plantar calcaneus.
Ensure the holder is fixed tightly to the rod.	• Leaving the holder even a little loose can result in the screw holes missing the rod.
Insert the calcaneal screws deep enough (5 mm past the cortex) as they do not bother the patient postoperatively.	• Visualize the end of the screw to make sure it is deep enough.
If the patient has a severe deformity and is being blocked from correction by the fibula, simply cut the fibula posteriorly so that it can angulate it the way you want it to. Do not remove it.	• Removing of the fibula was a technique done in the past to avoid the fibula hitting the counter of the shoes. Now that we add femoral head or 3-D printed cages to the construct, this is no longer a problem.

POSTOPERATIVE CARE

- The patients are usually done with an overnight stay only. They are discharged the next morning with instructions to keep their "toes above their nose" 23 hours per day, get up once an hour during the day, and do not put body weight on their leg. For prophylactic deep vein thrombosis (DVT) protection, they are placed on a full 325-mg acetylsalicylic acid twice per day beginning the day after surgery. If they have increased risk factors like prior DVT or pulmonary embolism, are using birth control pills, or have a history of cancer, they are placed on fractionated heparin 40 mg subcutaneously once a day.
- They are seen for the first time at 3 weeks postoperatively, the cast removed, stitches removed, and recasted for another 3 weeks with the same instructions.
- At 6 weeks, a standing x-ray is obtained and patients are allowed to begin weight bearing in a removable boot.

- They wear the boot for 4 weeks when up walking and then remove it and advance to shoes and compression hose if needed.
- Full healing takes about 6 months with continued remodeling of the bone graft for 2 years (**FIG 2**).

OUTCOMES

- In a retrospective case series of 32 patients, all of whom required a femoral head bulk allograft, there were only 50% successful fusions, albeit a 71% functional salvage rate and a 19% amputation rate.[7] All 9 diabetics in this case series developed a nonunion.
- In another series of 30 cases with less severe diagnoses, the patients experienced an 86% and 74% fusion rate of the tibiotalar and subtalar joints, respectively.[5]
- Finally, in multicenter European study, the union rate of TTC arthrodesis was 84%, with all 13 of the patients who were working prior to surgery returning to work after surgery.[9]

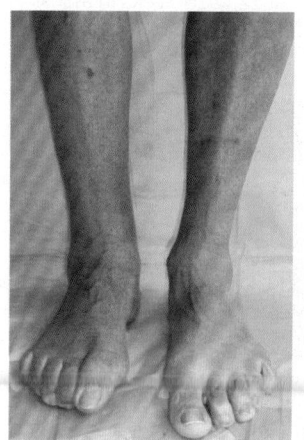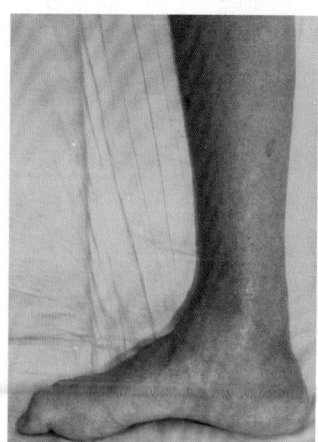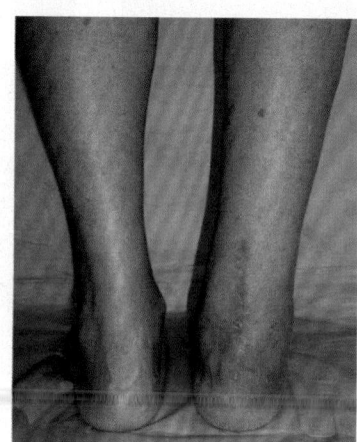

FIG 2 Five-month follow-up of the patient in **TECH FIGS 8** to **11**. **A.** Anterior view. **B.** Lateral perspective. **C.** Posterior view.

COMPLICATIONS

- Nonunion from inadequate preparation of the bone, not enough bone graft, poor stability
- Infection. I use double antibiotics on these big cases, that is, cefazolin × 24 hours and one dose gentamicin (80 mg) pre-operatively. I use antibiotic irrigation 1-g Ancef in 1-L normal saline. Vancomycin in the bone graft is no longer used because it has been shown to impede the osteoblasts.
- Improper positioning. See aforementioned information for pin insertion in slight (3 to 4 mm) anterior and lateral position to get the foot dorsiflexed and in valgus.
- Posterior tibial nerve irritation. Always keep in mind the closeness of the posterior tibial nerve by knowing it is just medial to the FHL.

REFERENCES

1. Berkowitz MJ, Clare MP, Walling AK, et al. Salvage of failed total ankle arthroplasty with fusion using structural allograft and internal fixation. Foot Ankle Int 2011;32(5):S493–S502.
2. Cuttica DJ, Hyer CF. Femoral head allograft for tibiotalocalcaneal fusion using a cup and cone reamer technique. J Foot Ankle Surg 2011;50(1):126–129.
3. DeVries JG, Nguyen M, Berlet GC, et al. The effect of recombinant bone morphogenetic protein-2 in revision tibiotalocalcaneal arthrodesis: utilization of the Retrograde Arthrodesis Intramedullary Nail database. J Foot Ankle Surg 2012;51(4):426–432.
4. Fetter NL, DeOrio JK. Posterior approach with fibular preservation for tibiotalocalcaneal arthrodesis with an intramedullary nail. Foot Ankle Int 2012;33(9):746–749.
5. Gross JB, Belleville R, Nespola A, et al. Influencing factors of functional result and bone union in tibiotalocalcaneal arthrodesis with intramedullary locking nail: a retrospective series of 30 cases. Eur J Orthop Surg Traumatol 2014;24(4):627–633.
6. Hsu AR, Ellington JK. Patient-specific 3-dimensional printed titanium truss cage with tibiotalocalcaneal arthrodesis for salvage of persistent distal tibia nonunion. Foot Ankle Spec 2015;8(6):483–489.
7. Jeng CL, Campbell JT, Tang EY, et al. Tibiotalocalcaneal arthrodesis with bulk femoral head allograft for salvage of large defects in the ankle. Foot Ankle Int 2013;34:1256–1266.
8. Pellegrini MJ, Schiff AP, Adams SB Jr, et al. Outcomes of tibiotalocalcaneal arthrodesis through a posterior Achilles tendon-splitting approach. Foot Ankle Int 2016;37(3):312–319.
9. Rammelt S, Pyrc J, Agren PH, et al. Tibiotalocalcaneal fusion using the hindfoot arthrodesis nail: a multicenter study. Foot Ankle Int 2013;34(9):1245–1255.
10. Richter M, Evers J, Waehnert D, et al. Biomechanical comparison of stability of tibiotalocalcaneal arthrodesis with two different intramedullary retrograde nails. Foot Ankle Surg 2014;20(1):14–19.
11. Zhang Y, Shen L, Mao Z, et al. Icariin enhances bone repair in rabbits with bone infection during post-infection treatment and prevents inhibition of osteoblasts by vancomycin. Front Pharmacol 2017;8:784.

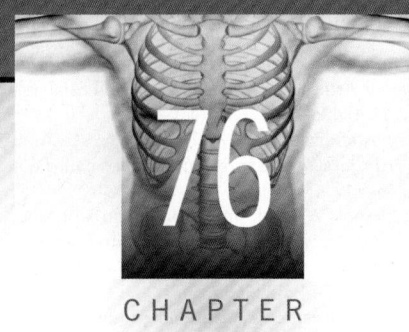

76
CHAPTER

Tibiotalocalcaneal Arthrodesis Using Lateral Fixed Angle Plate Fixation

Christopher P. Chiodo, Catherine E. Johnson, and Kimberly K. Broughton

DEFINITION

- Tibiotalocalcaneal arthritis is formally defined as the loss of cartilage from both the tibiotalar (ankle) and the talocalcaneal (subtalar) joints. This may be associated with secondary deformity.
- Tibiotalocalcaneal arthritis can cause substantial disability in terms of pain and limitation of function. Nonoperative treatment options are often limited, as in most instances, they only partially relieve pain and usually cannot correct deformity.
- The goal of tibiotalocalcaneal arthrodesis is to produce a stable, plantigrade, and pain-free foot and ankle.[1,13]
- Achieving stable fixation can be challenging in osteopenic bone and may preclude the use of intramedullary devices. Blade plate fixation of the tibiotalocalcaneal joint has been shown in biomechanical studies to have substantial initial and final stiffness.[2] Lateral locking plate plus screw augmentation is another biomechanically proven construct in tibiotalocalcaneal arthrodesis.[3,12]

ANATOMY

- The ankle joint is composed of the articulation between the talus and tibial plafond. The body of the talus is saddle-shaped dorsally and fits congruently within the mortise created by the distal tibia and fibula. In addition, the talus and the tibial plafond are narrower posteriorly to accommodate rotation with ankle dorsiflexion and plantarflexion.
- The subtalar joint is composed of the inferior talus and the calcaneus as they articulate through anterior, middle, and posterior facets.
- The talus is divided into head, body, and neck. Roughly 70% of the bone is covered with cartilage, and there are no muscular or tendinous attachments. The main blood supply of the talar body enters retrograde through the neck of the talus via the deltoid and tarsal canal branches of the posterior tibial artery. Subsequently, the talus body is prone to avascular necrosis in the case of displaced talar neck fractures.
- The lateral aspect of the foot is innervated by the superficial peroneal and sural nerves. The superficial peroneal nerve typically exits the crural fascia 10 to 12 cm proximal to the tip of the lateral malleolus. The nerve then courses anteriorly to give sensation to the dorsal aspect of the foot.
- The sural nerve has contributions from branches of both the tibial and common peroneal nerves. It courses lateral to the Achilles tendon and is found about 1 cm distal to the tip of the fibula at the level of the ankle.

PATHOGENESIS

- Arthritis of the tibiotalar and subtalar joints has multiple causes, including primary osteoarthritis, trauma, chronic instability, inflammatory disease, neuroarthropathy, infection, and avascular necrosis.
- Patients typically complain of diffuse ankle pain and usually cannot differentiate tibiotalar from subtalar symptoms. Although it is preferable to fuse only one joint to retain an adjacent motion segment, such isolated fusion in the setting of residual arthrosis can result in persistent pain.
- In posttraumatic cases, articular incongruency can result in increased contact stresses, with resultant cartilage wear and the development of arthritis.

NATURAL HISTORY

- Hindfoot arthritis is usually a progressive disorder, although the rate of progression can vary. Arthritis due to malalignment, trauma, and avascular necrosis of the talus can progress relatively rapidly.
- Nonoperative treatment of hindfoot arthritis in an ankle–foot orthosis (AFO) likely does not prevent or slow progression of the disease but merely decreases symptoms.[4]

PATIENT HISTORY AND PHYSICAL FINDINGS

- Physical examination should include the following:
  - Gait. The surgeon should watch the patient walking both toward and away from him or her and should clinically determine whether gait is normal or antalgic on both sides. The examiner should look for any assistive devices. Patients with painful arthritis will have an antalgic gait on the affected side. The patient may require the use of a cane or a walker.
  - Hindfoot alignment. The hindfoot is examined from behind. The surgeon should determine whether the hindfoot is in varus or valgus.
  - Tibiotalar range of motion. Active and passive sagittal plane motion is assessed. Normal ankle motion is approximately 50 degrees of plantarflexion and 10 to 20 degrees of dorsiflexion. Tibiotalar motion is usually decreased compared to the unaffected side.
  - Subtalar range of motion. Active and passive coronal plane motion through the subtalar joint is assessed. Normal motion is about 10 to 20 degrees of inversion and 5 to 10 degrees of eversion. Subtalar motion is usually decreased compared to the unaffected side.

- Past medical history may be significant for antecedent ankle or hindfoot trauma, talar osteonecrosis, diabetes, neuroarthropathy, osteochondral defect, or recurrent ankle instability.
- Past surgical history may include previous ankle or hindfoot surgery, including open reduction and internal fixation (ORIF), total ankle arthroplasty, and previous arthrodesis.
- Patients usually complain of pain and possibly instability with weight bearing. Selective anesthetic injections into the ankle or subtalar joints can be extremely helpful when determining which joints are symptomatic.
- Upon examination, hindfoot swelling and tenderness are usually evident. Most patients have decreased passive range of motion in both joints. Malalignment is also often present.

IMAGING AND OTHER DIAGNOSTIC STUDIES

- Weight-bearing plain radiographs including anteroposterior (AP), lateral, and mortise views of the ankle and AP, lateral, and oblique views of the foot are standard.
- A weight-bearing lateral radiograph should be performed to assess talocalcaneal and talo–first metatarsal angles (**FIG 1**).
- Computed tomography (CT) is often helpful preoperatively to assess bony anatomy, alignment, and articular integrity in greater detail. Weight-bearing CT is an evolving technology that may offer even greater bony detail in the loaded condition.

DIFFERENTIAL DIAGNOSIS

- Talar avascular necrosis
- Talar osteochondral injury
- Isolated ankle arthritis
- Isolated subtalar arthritis
- Ankle instability
- Foreign body

NONOPERATIVE MANAGEMENT

- Nonoperative treatment is aimed primarily at alleviating symptoms rather than correcting deformity. The patient is placed in a robust brace such as an AFO or Arizona brace in an attempt to provide support and limit motion.

- Bracing may not always be possible depending on the severity of the deformity. In addition, bracing typically does not prevent progression of disease.
- Corticosteroid injections may also be considered. Image guidance should be considered to improve accuracy and reliability.

SURGICAL MANAGEMENT

- Surgical management is generally indicated when nonoperative modalities have failed to provide adequate relief or are impractical (eg, a nonbraceable deformity).
- Tibiotalocalcaneal fusion is indicated in patients with arthritis in both the tibiotalar and subtalar joints. The goal of surgical intervention is to obtain a stable, plantigrade, and pain-free foot and ankle.
- Blade plate or locking plate fixation can be used primarily or in instances when the surgeon feels that intramedullary rod fixation is contraindicated. The latter may include poor bone stock or advanced osteopenia, a distal tibia deformity greater than 10 degrees, or significant loss of calcaneal height.[11]
- The main two contraindications to this procedure are (1) the presence of active infection and (2) destruction of calcaneal bone stock to the extent that purchase with the implant is compromised. In these instances, the use of a small wire ring fixator should be considered.

Preoperative Planning

- A full patient assessment is made before the operation. Smokers should be counseled regarding smoking cessation because in this population, as a 14-fold increase in the nonunion rate has been documented.[5]
- If active infection is suspected, an appropriate workup should be performed. This may include laboratory studies, magnetic resonance imaging with contrast, and nuclear imaging. If there is still uncertainty despite these tests, a bone biopsy or joint aspirate may be necessary.
- Disease-modifying antirheumatic drugs should be held preoperatively, typically for 2 weeks or a period determined in conjunction with a rheumatologist.
- Patients with significant comorbidities such as diabetes, cardiovascular disease, and nephropathy should be medically optimized by their primary care doctor before surgical intervention.

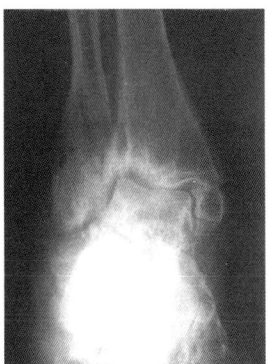
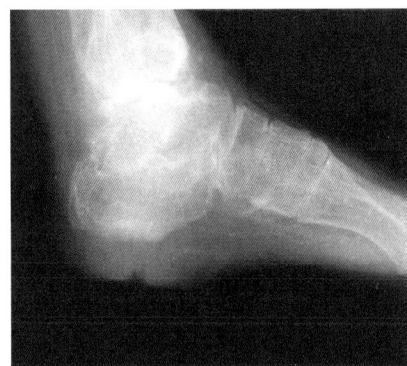

A   **B**

FIG 1 Preoperative AP (**A**) and lateral (**B**) radiographs of the ankle.

Positioning

- The patient is placed supine on the operating table with a bump under the ipsilateral buttock to maintain the foot in neutral or such that it is slightly rotated internally.
- The extremity is prepared and draped, including the iliac crest if structural autograft is desired. An alternative bone graft harvest site is the proximal tibia. A thigh tourniquet is used **(FIG 2)**.

Approach

- Traditionally, an extensile lateral approach to the ankle and subtalar joints is used, although a posterior approach has also been described.[9]

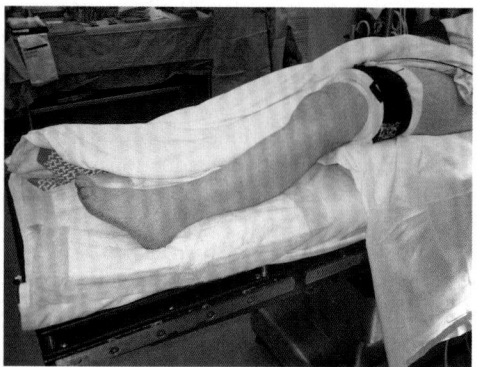

FIG 2 Preoperative positioning of the patient.

EXPOSURE

- A 15- to 20-cm curvilinear incision is made through the skin centered over the fibula shaft proximally and then curving toward the base of the fourth metatarsal distally.
- With deep dissection, care is taken to avoid injury to the superficial peroneal nerve, which exits the fascia about 10 to 12 cm proximal to the fibular tip. Distally, the surgeon must take care to avoid injury to the sural nerve along its course lateral to the fifth metatarsal **(TECH FIG 1)**.
- Distally, the extensor digitorum brevis is elevated to expose the subtalar joint.
- In some instances, a medial (longitudinal) incision may be necessary. These include the following: (1) to remove medial bony prominences and debris and (2) to assist in resection of medial bone when advanced varus deformity precludes reduction of the foot to neutral.

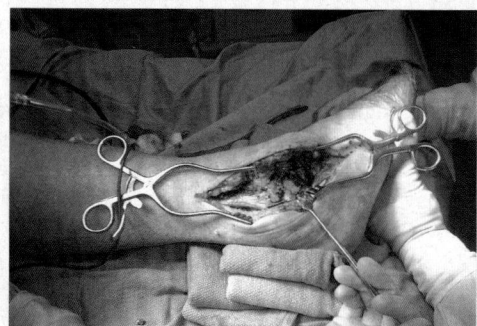

TECH FIG 1 The ankle and subtalar joints are approached through an extensile curvilinear incision.

OSTEOTOMY OF THE FIBULA AND PREPARATION OF THE TIBIOTALAR JOINT

- Make an osteotomy of the fibula approximately 8 to 10 mm proximal to the tip of the lateral malleolus **(TECH FIG 2A)**.
- Resect the distal section of the fibula.
  - The distal fibula can be readily morselized into autogenous bone graft using a small acetabular reamer before resection **(TECH FIG 2B)**.[14]
- Retract the peroneal tendons posteriorly and protect them.
- Enter the ankle joint sharply and fully expose it by releasing the lateral ligaments and anterior and posterior capsule.

- Distract the joint using a lamina spreader.
- Remove any remaining cartilage with a curette.
- After removing the cartilage, prepare the joint surface with flexible chisels or a small, low-speed burr. If using a burr, use copious irrigation and a speed of 20,000 revolutions/minute to avoid thermal necrosis. Burr holes should be just through the subchondral bone and immediately adjacent to each other creating dimpling reminiscent of a golf ball surface.

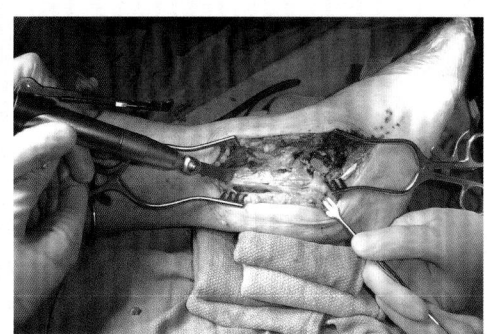 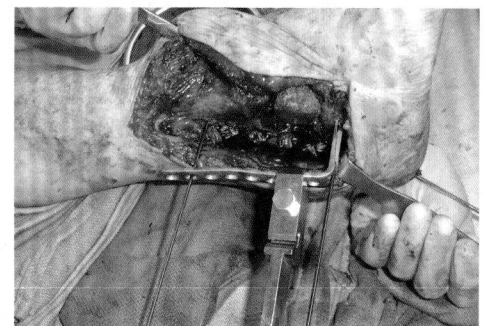

TECH FIG 2 A. An osteotomy of the fibula is performed about 8 to 10 mm proximal to the tip of the bone. **B.** The fibula can be morselized for bone graft using an acetabular reamer.

PREPARATION OF THE SUBTALAR JOINT

- Enter the subtalar joint sharply with release of the lateral ligaments, capsule, and the talocalcaneal intraosseous ligament.
- Maintain distraction of the joint using a lamina spreader.
- Curette the remaining cartilage off the joint surface and prepare the subchondral bone with flexible chisels or a burr as described earlier.
- If there is substantial bone loss or fragmentation of the talus, the tibia may have to be fused directly to the calcaneus. In this case, the calcaneal articular processes will need to be removed with an osteotome to create a flat surface that will lie flush with the tibial plafond.
- Bone graft can be packed into the subtalar and ankle joints. If there is a large bony deficit with substantial loss of limb length, structural graft in the form of iliac crest autograft or femoral head allograft can be used to restore height.

INSERTION OF THE BLADE PLATE

- After preparing the joint surfaces, insert a 90- or 95-degree fixed-angle blade plate for fixation. The use of both an adolescent blade plate and a humeral blade plate have been described. The length of the blade is typically 40 mm. The side plate can range from five to eight holes based on the size of the patient and the surgeon's preference.
- Ensure that the hindfoot is positioned in neutral to 5 degrees of valgus and the ankle is in neutral dorsiflexion and plantarflexion. External rotation should approximate that of the contralateral extremity, usually 5 to 10 degrees.
- The ankle and subtalar joints must be held rigidly during insertion of the blade plate. Provisional fixation can be obtained with guidewires or a Schanz pin.
- Use a 2.0-mm guidewire to facilitate insertion of the blade plate. The guidewire should be inserted such that 5 to 10 mm of calcaneal bone will remain plantar to the blade. Place the guidewire through the middle hole of the blade plate drill guide **(TECH FIG 3A)**. The lateral calcaneal cortex may then be further prepared for blade insertion by predrilling with a 4.5-mm drill bit (through appropriate holes in the drill guide).

- Remove the drill guide and insert the blade plate over the guidewire using the inserter–extractor handle **(see TECH FIG 3B)**. Impact the blade until it is flush with the lateral cortex of the tibia. Rotational control is best achieved by using a slotted hammer.
- Once the blade engages the calcaneus, the position of the plate proximally cannot be changed. To avoid sagittal plane malalignment (ie, the plate coming off the tibia anteriorly or posteriorly), consider using another guidewire through the most proximal hole of the plate as the blade plate construct is inserted **(see TECH FIG 3C)**.
- Contour the plate to the lateral aspect of the tibia and fill the screw holes sequentially. Use 4.5-mm cortical screws proximally and 6.5-mm cancellous screws distally.
- A single 6.5- or 7.3-mm cortical screw can be used to augment the blade plate fixation. Place the screw under fluoroscopic guidance from the calcaneal tuberosity into the anterior tibial cortex at roughly a 60-degree angle.

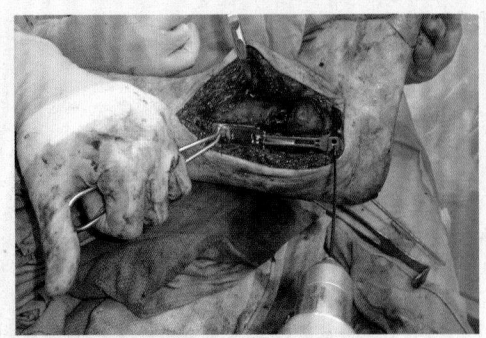
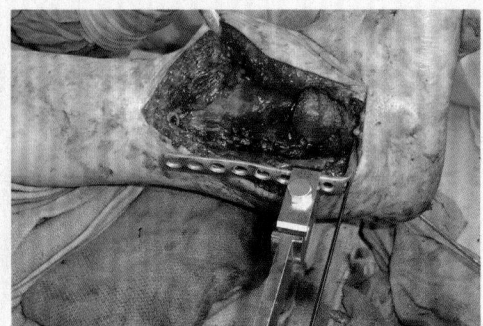
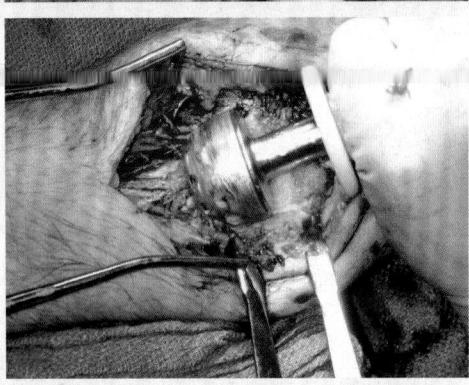

TECH FIG 3 A. A 2.0-mm guidewire is inserted through the drill guide into the calcaneus. **B.** The blade plate is inserted over the guidewire using the insertion handle. **C.** Sagittal plane malalignment can be avoided using a proximal guidewire.

CLOSURE

- Given the large amount of bleeding cancellous bone exposed during the procedure, a meticulous layered closure should be performed. Further steps that will aid in the prevention of a postoperative hematoma include releasing the tourniquet and assessing hemostasis before closure, the use of drains, and the use of a compression dressing.

CASE EXAMPLE (COURTESY OF MARK E. EASLEY, MD)

Background, Imaging, and Preoperative Planning

- A 47-year-old, 6 years after ORIF of right talar neck fracture
  - Severe pain in right ankle and hindfoot with weight bearing
  - Failed nonoperative management, including use of a patellar tendon–bearing brace
- Hindfoot alignment in slight varus
- Stiff ankle and hindfoot
- Pain with stress of ankle and hindfoot
- Ambulates with severe limp
- Radiographs (TECH FIG 4)
  - Retained hardware
  - Ankle and subtalar arthritis
  - Suggestion of (at least) partial talar body avascular necrosis
- Given talar body avascular necrosis, patient not a candidate for total ankle replacement
  - Fibular preservation therefore is less important.

- Favor tibiotalocalcaneal arthrodesis because both ankle and subtalar joint arthritis and stiffness are present.
  - Intramedullary nail
  - Lateral plating
  - In this case, lateral plating is performed.

Exposure

- Lateral longitudinal incision (TECH FIG 5A)
- Because the implant chosen has a posterior limb to fit on the calcaneus, the approach was not curved anteriorly but instead made straight vertically to allow access to the lateral calcaneal wall.
- Sural nerve protected
- Distal fibula excised (TECH FIG 5B); bone morselized and used as bone graft

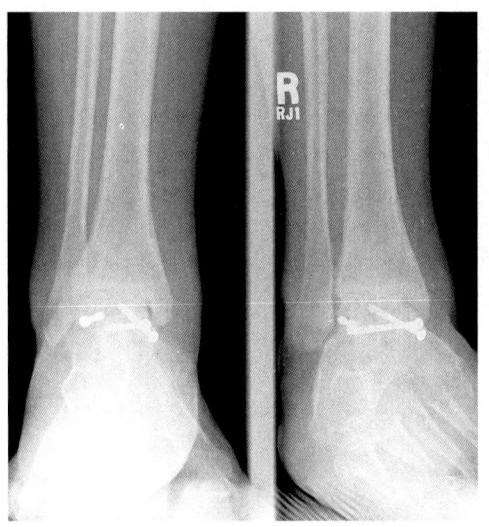
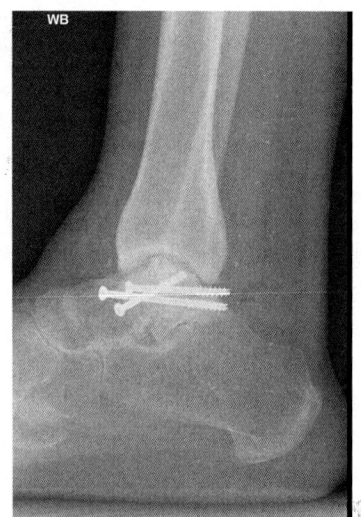

TECH FIG 4 Weight-bearing ankle radiographs in a 47-year-old woman with right ankle and hindfoot pain and stiffness 6 years after ORIF of talar neck fracture, with some concern for talar body avascular necrosis. **A.** AP and mortise views. **B.** Lateral view.

Preparation for Arthrodesis

- Hardware removed
- Ankle and subtalar joint
  - With preoperative varus, more bone is removed laterally to promote hindfoot valgus position **(TECH FIG 6A)**.
  - Drilling and chiseling to increase surface area and promote healing
- Bone graft is placed within the ankle and subtalar joints **(TECH FIG 6B)** as well as posteriorly along the tibia, talus, and dorsal calcaneus.
  - Acts as a posterior buttress
  - Augments arthrodesis
  - Promotes fusion

Provisional Fixation

- Proper alignment confirmed both clinically and fluoroscopically
- Sagittal plane: neutral ankle position; plantarflexion/equinus avoided

- Rotation: second metatarsal aligned with tibial crest
  - Coronal plane: heel valgus maintained; varus corrected/avoided
  - Guidewire placed retrograde as shown in **TECH FIG 6B**

Definitive Fixation

- Template is used to determine optimal plate position **(TECH FIG 7A,B)**.
- Lateral plate is positioned and provisionally secured, and position is confirmed fluoroscopically.
- Locking plate technology: This particular plate is initially secured as a nonlocking plate so that plate has satisfactory contact with bone **(TECH FIG 7C,D)** and then converted to locking plate with locking washers placed over screw heads, converting the plate to a fixed-angle device **(TECH FIG 7E,F)**.
- Distal fixation in calcaneus performed first
- Compression device used proximally **(TECH FIG 7G)**
  - After distal fixation
  - Prior to proximal fixation
  - Promotes compression at the arthrodesis sites

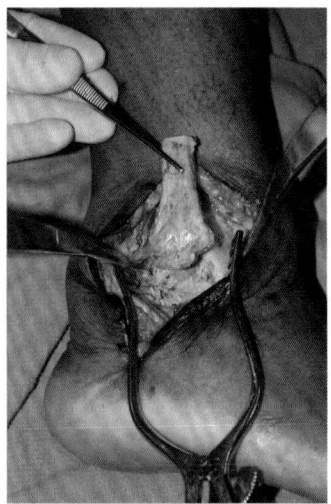
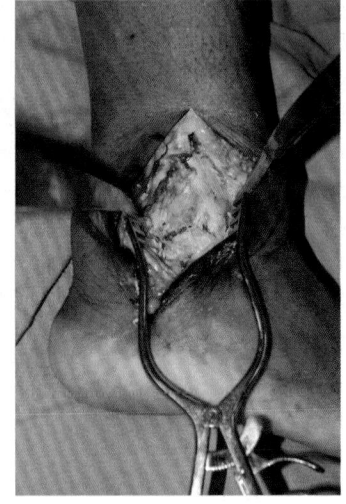

TECH FIG 5 Lateral approach. **A.** Fibula excised (and used as bone graft). **B.** Lateral ankle and subtalar joints exposed.

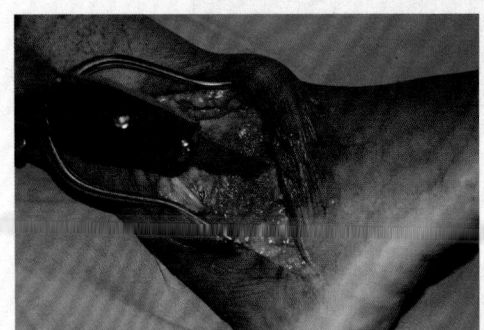

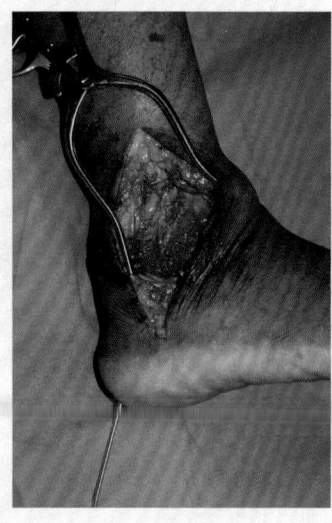

TECH FIG 6 Joint preparation and bone grafting. **A.** Chisel used to increase surface area and to remove more lateral bone to promote hindfoot valgus. **B.** Bone graft packed at arthrodesis sites and posterior to tibia, talus, and dorsal calcaneus.

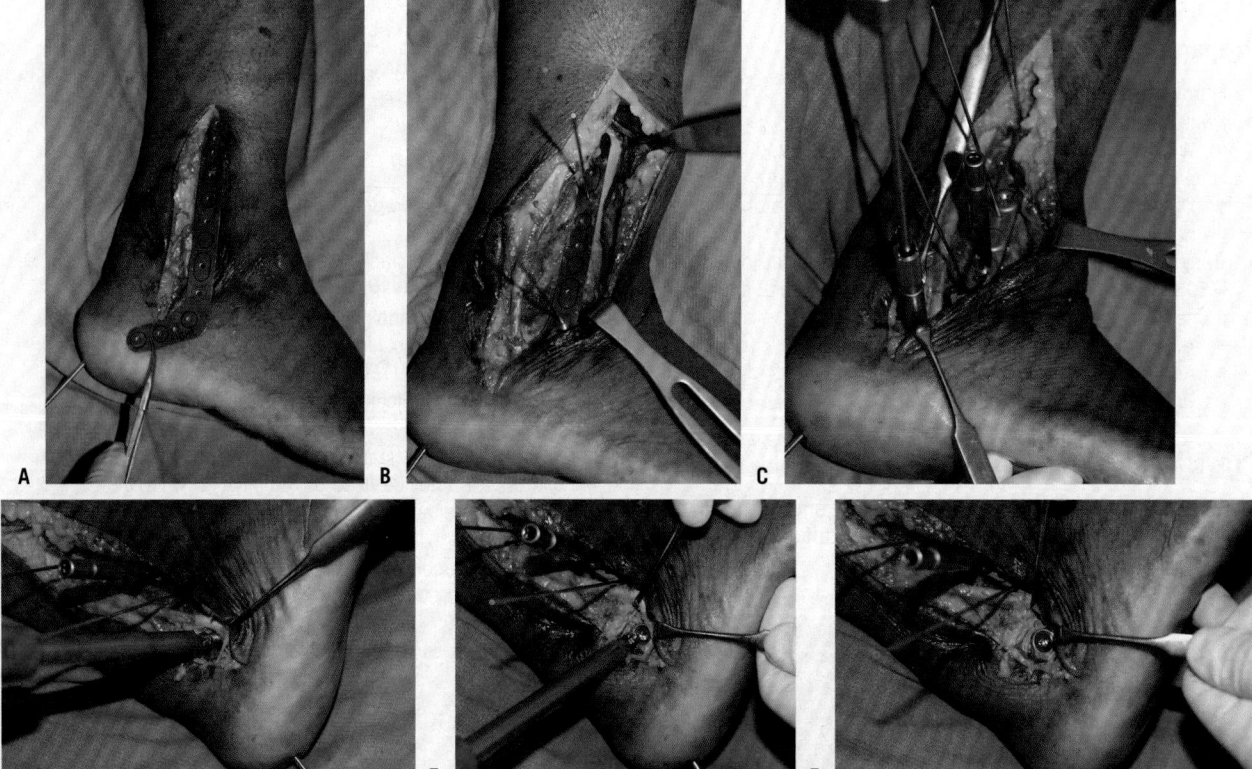

TECH FIG 7 **A.** Template for lateral plating being inserted. Note that this particular plate extends over lateral calcaneus posteriorly, and therefore, a vertical longitudinal incision was made rather than curving the distal incision anteriorly. **B.** Template in place with provisional fixation. **C.** Lateral plate in proper position based on template, clinical assessment, and intraoperative fluoroscopy. Distal screw hole being drilled with soft tissues and sural nerve protected. **D.** Screw inserted. Note that this nonlocking screw allows the plate to be fully secured to bone. **E.** After the locking screw is fully seated and plate is secured to the calcaneus, a locking washer is placed. **F.** Locking washer fully seated over nonlocking screw, creating the fixed-angle construct. *(continued)*

TECHNIQUES

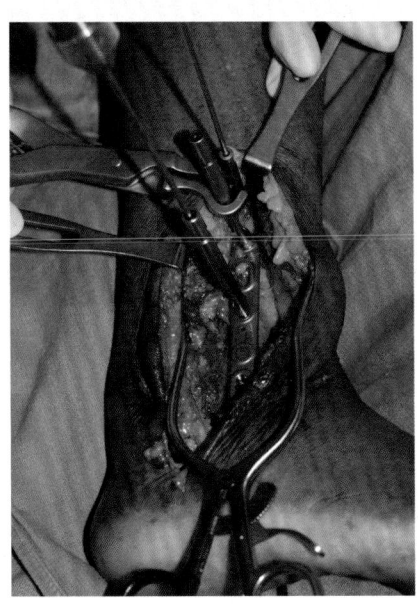

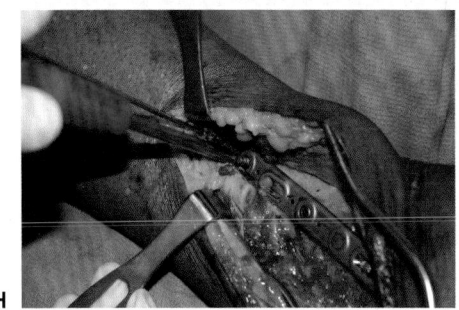

TECH FIG 7 *(continued)* **G.** After distal fixation, proximal compression applied to the plate and proximal fixation drill hole created. **H.** Proximal fixation completed after compression applied. Locking washers may also be placed on proximal screws to create the fixed-angle construct.

- Promotes heel valgus
  - Ideally, the provisional fixation is in neutral to slight valgus, and the compression then sets optimal heel valgus.
  - If necessary, the plate may be carefully bent prior to being inserted in order to create more valgus.
- Proximal screws placed after compression applied **(TECH FIG 7H)**
- Proximal locking washers convert entire construct to a fixed-angle device.

Supplemental Fixation

- Two additional cannulated screws to augment the construct
- First screw from the posterolateral tibia into the talar neck
- Second screw from posterolateral and inferior calcaneal tuberosity into anteromedial tibia

Postoperative Care

- Protected weight bearing for 6 weeks in a splint and then short-leg cast
- If wound stable, allow partial weight bearing for next 6 weeks; short-leg cast versus CAM boot
- At 12 weeks, recommend CT scan to confirm adequate healing at both arthrodesis sites.
  - If healed, advance to full weight bearing.
  - If delay in healing, then continue protected weight bearing in CAM boot.
- During transition from CAM boot to shoe wear, recommend stiffer-soled shoe, rocker bottom modification, and fixed ankle brace to extend to above the ankle.
- Long-term management **(TECH FIG 8)**
  - Although many patients eventually function without the ankle brace, a stiffer-soled shoe and rocker bottom modification are usually recommended.
  - There is a risk of potential stress fracture at the proximal end of the plate unless some of the stresses are dissipated.

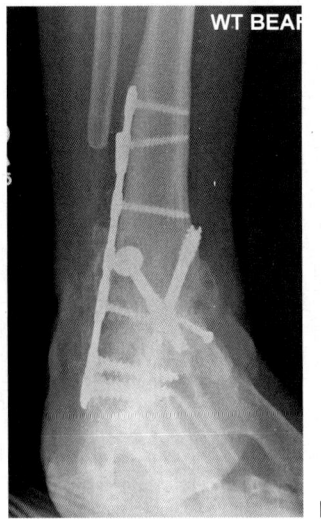

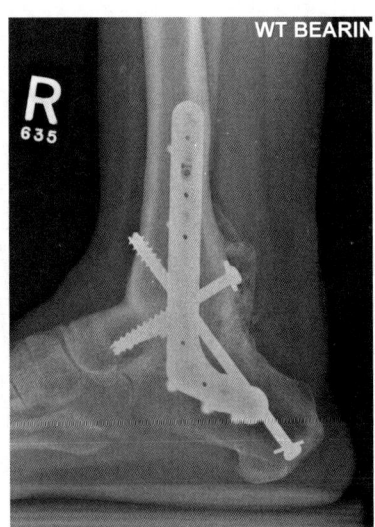

TECH FIG 8 Six-month follow-up. **A.** Weight-bearing mortise view radiograph. Note that lateral plate dictates proper hindfoot alignment. **B.** Weight-bearing lateral radiograph. Note supplemental cannulated screw fixation and bridging trabeculation suggested. Also note posterior buttress of bone augmenting fusion.

Pearls and Pitfalls

Maintain sagittal plane alignment.	• Use a proximal guidewire.
Bone Graft	• Use the resected fibula for autogenous bone graft.
Avoid the tendency of hindfoot to fall into valgus.	• As the plate is screwed down to the tibia, there is a tendency for the hindfoot to be pulled into valgus, given the normal contour of the lateral tibia. To avoid this, the blade plate should be carefully contoured before insertion. Resecting a groove for the plate in the most distal portion of the tibia using a chisel or burr may also be helpful.
Avoid the tendency of hindfoot to fall into varus.	• Failure to contour the blade plate when necessary can sometimes push the hindfoot into varus. Incorporating a small lateral "bow" distally will avert this.
Avoid prominence of the blade plate if not fully seated.	• If the blade plate does not lie flush with the lateral calcaneus, the blade plate may be prominent, causing potential difficulties with wound closure and healing.
Avoid dorsiflexion malunion with talectomy.	• In cases of talectomy, the foot must be aligned with the leg, as alignment of the distal tibia to the posterior calcaneal facet can result in a dorsiflexion malunion. The fused surfaces should be contoured accordingly.

POSTOPERATIVE CARE

- Postoperatively, patients are placed in a splint and admitted for 24 hours of intravenous antibiotics.
- After 10 to 14 days, patients return to the office for evaluation of the wound and suture removal. At this visit, patients are placed in a non–weight-bearing short-leg cast.
- Patients remain non–weight bearing in a short-leg cast for 6 to 12 weeks based on radiographic healing.
- Thereafter, patients are transitioned to a short-leg walking cast or boot and progressive weight bearing is begun.
- The fusion is protected until sufficient clinical and radiographic healing is obtained **(FIG 3)**. A CT scan may be needed to assess the adequacy of the fusion.

OUTCOMES

- A successful outcome is usually the norm for tibiotalocalcaneal fusion.
- Most studies report combined results of different approaches to fusion. In studies examining the use of blade plate fixation exclusively, the reported fusion rates have ranged from 90% to 100%.[2,9,11]

COMPLICATIONS

- Overall complication rates for tibiotalocalcaneal fusion have been as high as 50% in some series.[4,6] The most common complications include nonunion, malunion, infection, and neuroma. This correlates with the reported complication profile for tibiotalar arthrodesis.[7,8,10]

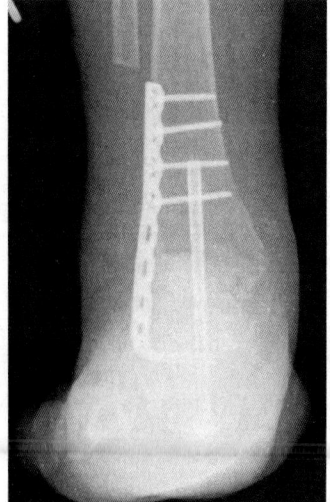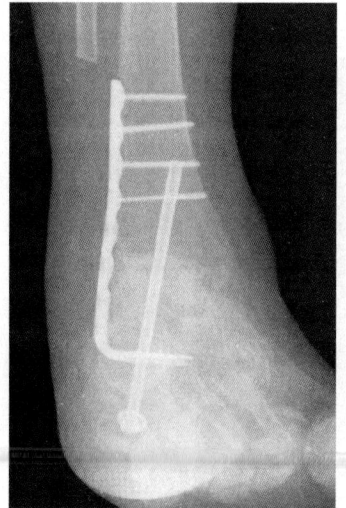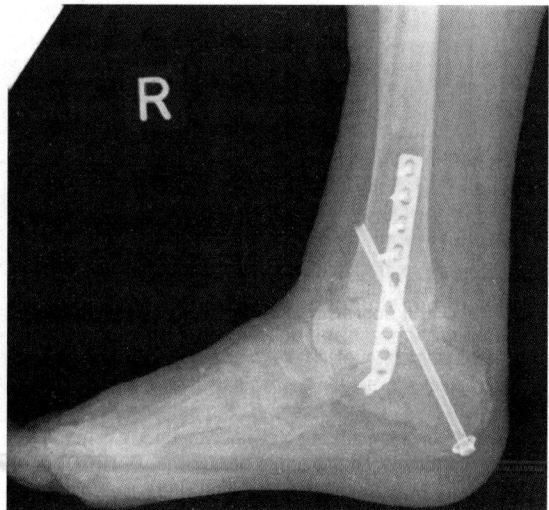

FIG 3 A–C. Postoperative radiographs showing healing. In this case, the talus was "replaced" with a carefully contoured femoral head allograft.

- In patients undergoing tibiotalocalcaneal fusion (regardless of fixation technique), the nonunion rate ranges from 0% to 40%. This is most common when there is avascular necrosis of the talus. In this patient population, the nonunion rate has been as high as 89%.[6] Nonunion rates are also significantly higher in smokers and patients with neuroarthropathy (33% to 75%).[5,6]
- Superficial and deep wound infections can be minimized through the use of appropriate perioperative antibiotics, meticulous soft tissue handling, a layered wound closure, avoidance of hematoma formation, and postoperative elevation. Placing vancomycin powder in the wound increases local antibiotic levels.
- Peripheral neuroma of either the sural or superficial peroneal nerves can be minimized by careful incision placement and gentle retraction and soft tissue handling. In patients with neuroarthropathy, there is usually decreased if not absent distal sensation. In these patients, peripheral nerve injury is usually clinically insignificant.

REFERENCES

1. Alvarez RG, Barbour TM, Perkins TD. Tibiocalcaneal arthrodesis for nonbraceable neuropathic ankle deformity. Foot Ankle Int 1994;15: 354–359.
2. Chiodo CP, Acevedo JI, Sammarco VJ, et al. Intramedullary rod fixation compared with blade-plate-and-screw fixation for tibiotalocalcaneal arthrodesis: a biomechanical investigation. J Bone Joint Surg Am 2003;85-A(12):2425–2428.
3. Chodos MD, Parks BG, Schon LC, et al. Blade plate compared with locking plate for tibiotalocalcaneal arthrodesis: a cadaver study. Foot Ankle Int 2008;29(2):219–224.
4. Chou LB, Mann RA, Yaszay B, et al. Tibiotalocalcaneal arthrodesis. Foot Ankle Int 2000;21:804–808.
5. Cobb TK, Gabrielsen TA, Campbell DC II, et al. Cigarette smoking and nonunion after ankle arthrodesis. Foot Ankle Int 1994;15: 64–67.
6. Cooper PS. Complications of ankle and tibiotalocalcaneal arthrodesis. Clin Orthop Relat Res 2001;(391):33–44.
7. Crosby LA, Yee TC, Formanek TS, et al. Complications following arthroscopic ankle arthrodesis. Foot Ankle Int 1996;17:340–342.
8. Frey C, Halikus NM, Vu-Rose T, et al. A review of ankle arthrodesis: predisposing factors to nonunion. Foot Ankle Int 1994;15: 581–584.
9. Hanson TW, Cracchiolo A III. The use of a 95 degree blade plate and a posterior approach to achieve tibiotalocalcaneal arthrodesis. Foot Ankle Int 2002;23:704–710.
10. Morrey BF, Wiedeman GP Jr. Complications and long-term results of ankle arthrodesis following trauma. J Bone Joint Surg Am 1980;62(5):777–784.
11. Myerson MS, Alvarez RG, Lam PW. Tibiocalcaneal arthrodesis for the management of severe ankle and hindfoot deformities. Foot Ankle Int 2000;21:643–650.
12. O'Neill PJ, Logel KJ, Parks BG, et al. Rigidity comparison of locking plate and intramedullary fixation for tibiotalocalcaneal arthrodesis. Foot Ankle Int 2008;29(6):581–586.
13. Papa JA, Myerson MS. Pantalar and tibiotalocalcaneal arthrodesis for post-traumatic osteoarthritis of the ankle and hindfoot. J Bone Joint Surg Am 1992;74(7):1042–1049.
14. Raikin SM, Myerson MS. A technique for harvesting bone graft for arthrodeses around the ankle. Foot Ankle Int 2000;21:778–779.

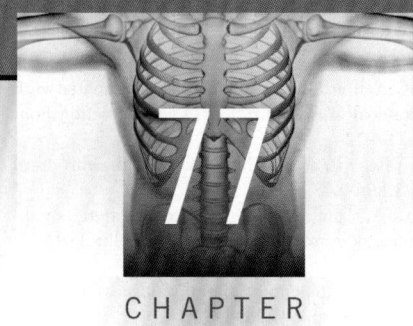

CHAPTER 77

Treatment of Bone Loss, Avascular Necrosis, and Infection of the Talus with Circular Tensioned Wire Fixators

Stephen M. Quinnan, James J. Hutson, Jr., and Chloe Shields

DEFINITION

- Talus fractures are high-energy fractures that can have traumatic bone loss, avascular necrosis (AVN), and infected nonunion as the outcome of the injury.[8]
  - Acute talar bone loss and subsequent AVN and infection will present a cascade of hindfoot reconstruction problems **(FIG 1)**.
  - Excision of the talus causes 3 to 4 cm of leg length discrepancy **(FIG 2)**.
  - Loss of the talus and subsequent bone defect can be reconstructed with internal fixation and bone grafting to maintain leg length.[9]
  - Traumatic loss of the talus or AVN is also treated with tibiocalcaneal arthrodesis using internal fixation without reconstruction of leg length.[4,7,11]
  - Replacement of the traumatic extrusion of the talus has had a high level of infection in case studies.[8]
  - There has been success in reimplanting extruded talar body fractures without a high incidence of infection.[12]
  - If there is severe comminution of the talus, contamination from extrusion, infection, or a compromised soft tissue envelope, massive bone grafting, and internal fixation has a high risk of failure and infection.
  - Half-pin fixators with a calcaneal tibial Steinmann pin also have had a poor rate of arthrodesis.

- Circular fixation provides an alternative to amputation in these complex cases.[1,6,10,13,14]
  - Because the pins and wires used in circular fixation are not in the zone of injury, a carefully débrided arthrodesis site can be compressed to achieve arthrodesis without foreign body internal fixation.
  - Wounds can heal by secondary intention over many weeks, and the foot can be salvaged.
  - For patients with appropriate physiology, a proximal leg lengthening can be added to the reconstruction to equalize leg length.
  - The reconstructed extremity requires shoe modifications to improve gait.
  - With a well-aligned tibiocalcaneal arthrodesis, the patient may participate in an active life without the problems and expense of a below-knee prosthesis.

ANATOMY

- The talus has a precarious blood supply because approximately two-thirds of the surface area is covered by articular cartilage.
- The ankle articulation, talar navicular joint, and the three facets of the subtalar joint leave limited areas on the neck of the talus and inferior surface for penetration of blood vessels into the dense bone of the talus.

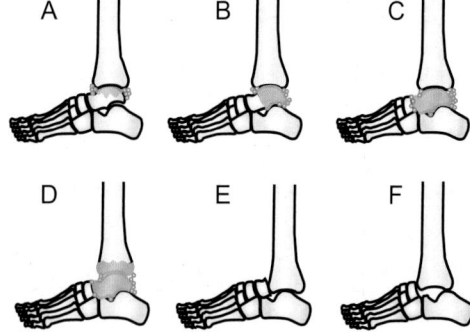

FIG 1 The extent of bone loss and infection will determine the reconstruction. **A.** Extensive infection of the talar dome compromising tibial talar arthrodesis. **B.** Complete necrosis of the talar body. **C.** Necrosis of the entire talus. **D.** Necrosis of the plafond and talus. **E.** Traumatic ejection or crushing of the talar body. **F.** Traumatic ejection or crushing of the talus.

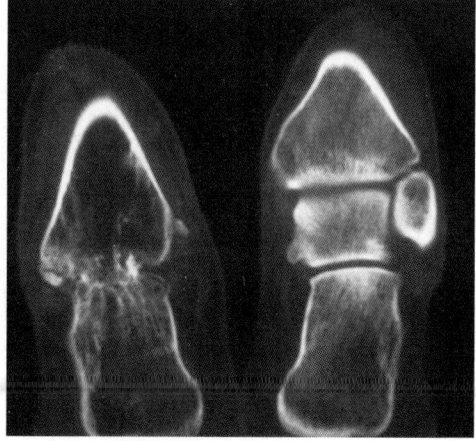

FIG 2 CT scan of tibiocalcaneal arthrodesis. The excision of the talus creates a 3- to 4-cm bone defect.

- The talus has no muscular attachments and is surrounded by the joint capsules of the multiple joints and a thin layer of soft tissue with bypassing tendons, vessels, and nerves.
- Open fracture-dislocations of the talus are high-energy injuries that cause disruption of the blood supply by dislocation, ejection of fragments, and fracture through the neck of the talus. This causes AVN of the body or entire talus, which is susceptible to infection (see **FIG 1**).

PATHOGENESIS

- High-energy ankle trauma
- Postoperative infection of open reduction and internal fixation of talus fractures
- Postoperative infection of ankle arthrodesis and ankle replacement
- Avascular necrosis of the talus with or without subsequent infection

PATIENT HISTORY AND PHYSICAL FINDINGS

- Painful ankle with swelling and local inflammation
- Ankylosis of the hindfoot and ankle
- Shortening of the extremity
- A draining sinus indicates a deep infection.

IMAGING AND OTHER DIAGNOSTIC STUDIES

- An ankle series of radiographs will reveal the extent of the bone loss, the extent of AVN, and the location of internal fixation hardware in the talus and plafond (**FIG 3**).
- There may be local bone erosion of the talus, plafond, and malleoli from the chronic infection in the joint.
- A white blood cell count, erythrocyte sedimentation rate, and C-reactive protein study are screening tests that will indicate the possibility of a deep infection.
- Aspiration of the ankle joint under fluoroscopic guidance is indicated if there is suspicion of an infection.
- Computed tomography (CT) scanning will define the fragmentation of the talus and may reveal erosions of the plafond and malleoli compatible with infection.
- Magnetic resonance imaging will have diffuse signals caused by the fracture and inflammation that will provide little additional useful data in making the diagnosis.

DIFFERENTIAL DIAGNOSIS

- Charcot joint

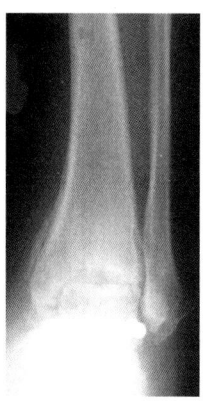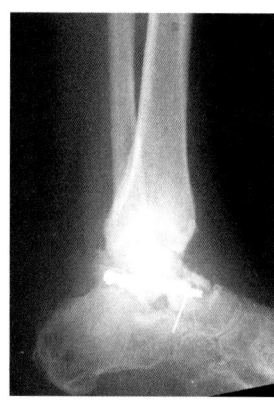

FIG 3 A,B. Anterior and lateral x-ray of ankle with infected nonunion of talus. The ankle had a draining sinus. The talar body is avascular, and the talar head has bone lysis around the two fixation screws. The plafond has erosion and destruction of the cartilage. There is reactive bone on the medial malleolus compatible with infection.

NONOPERATIVE MANAGEMENT

- The patient may use a cane and ankle brace to improve gait.
- There will be chronic pain with AVN of the talus, infection, or traumatic ejection of the talus.
- There is no conservative treatment for an infected nonunion of the talus.
- Treatment with oral or intravenous antibiotics will only suppress the infection.

SURGICAL MANAGEMENT

Preoperative Planning

- Infection of the talus is treated with aggressive débridement.
- Oral antibiotics should be discontinued 2 weeks before the débridement to obtain accurate cultures.
- If there is infection and drainage that requires emergent débridement, the patient is taken to surgery and deep cultures are obtained before starting intravenous antibiotics.
- It is essential to identify the infecting organism.
  - *Mycobacterium*, yeast, and aerobic organisms may be the source of an infection, and cultures should be obtained.
  - The organisms cultured in our series include methicillin-resistant *Staphylococcus aureus*, *Enterobacter cloacae*, *Escherichia coli*, *S. aureus*, *Streptococcus* (nonhemolytic), *Alcaligenes xylosoxidans*, and *Pseudomonas aeruginosa*.

TALAR PREPARATION

Débridement of Infection

- Use an anteromedial approach located medial to the anterior tibial tendon to explore the talus (**TECH FIG 1A**).
- Before making the incision, elevate the leg for 3 minutes to drain blood from the extremity.
- Do not use an elastic compression bandage when there is a deep infection.
- Use a tourniquet during the initial excision of bone. Without a tourniquet, the field would be flooded with blood, obscuring the appearance of the infected bone.
- Carefully explore the infected talus.

- The necrotic bone will have a discolored avascular consistency.
  - Necrotic bone tends to have a brittle consistency compared to viable bone.
- Excise the bone in small fragments, carefully observing for vascularity and the transition from necrotic infected bone to viable bone.
- The preoperative radiographic evaluation may not clearly identify the extent of infection.
  - The talar head may be necrotic without the appearance of AVN on the radiograph.
- Remove all hardware as the talus is débrided.

TECHNIQUES

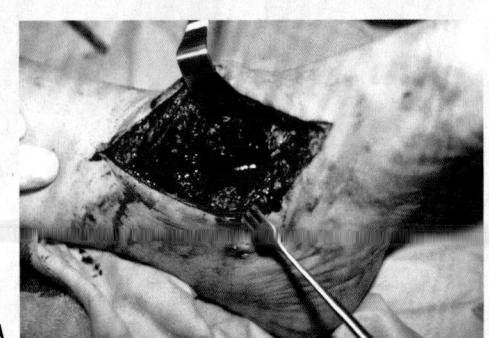 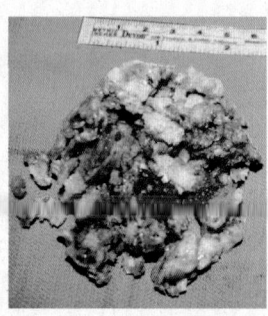 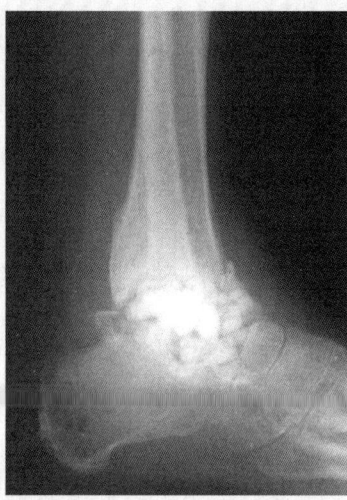

TECH FIG 1 **A.** Anteromedial approach with excision of the entire talus. **B.** The talus is excised in small fragments using a ¼-inch osteotome and pituitary rongeurs. This allows the entire talus to be removed without an extensive exposure. The bone is removed by working through the infected talus until the joint margins are cleared of all bone and cartilage. **C.** Débridement of the talus and distal plafond created a 5-cm bone gap. Antibiotic beads are placed in the ankle débridement.

- Take cultures from an area clearly involved with purulence and make certain to send tissue cultures for *Mycobacterium* and fungus.
- The infection and necrotic bone may be limited to the body of the talus, or the infection may have spread to the head of the talus, requiring excision of the entire talus **(TECH FIG 1B)**.
- There may be a posteromedial section of the talus that is viable bone, but it is not large enough to be used for a pantalar arthrodesis.
- Once all necrotic bone is removed, lavage the joint with low-pressure saline and deflate the tourniquet.[2]
- Viable bone will have punctate bleeding.
  - If the margin of the bone resection does not bleed, excise the bone until bleeding is encountered.
  - This may lead to excision of the talar head.
- The tibial plafond can have invasion of infection and require removal of the joint surface and metaphysis for several centimeters **(TECH FIG 1C)**.

Antibiotic Beads

- Antibiotic beads are manufactured on the back table.
  - The beads should have a small diameter (7 mm) to maximize antibiotic elusion and there should be an adequate amount to allow complete filling of the irregular volume created by the excision of the necrotic bone.
  - A 2.4 g of tobramycin powder is dry mixed with 1.0 g of vancomycin and crushed with the rounded end of a Cobb elevator until there is a fine powder.
  - The antibiotics are dry mixed with 20 g of methylmethacrylate cement before adding the liquid monomer.
- Using this large amount of antibiotics causes the cement to mix poorly, and it must be mashed into a paste before making the beads.
  - The cement is rolled into long 1-cm cylinders and cut into small pieces, which will form small-diameter beads.
  - The beads are formed and placed on a no. 2 nylon suture that has had the heavy needle straightened.
  - Fifteen to 20 minutes of drying time is needed for the beads.

- Once the beads have cooled, they are carefully packed into the wound to fill all of the space created by the talus excision (see **TECH FIG 1C**).
- The beads can be divided into two strings.
- A half string usually fills the defect.
- The remaining beads are placed in a sterile container for repeat débridement if needed.

Wound Closure

- Close the wound with 2-0 nylon suture.
- Because of the thorough débridement, the wound can be closed primarily.
- Copious postoperative hemorrhage will drain through the single-layer closure.
- If the wound is left open, the edges will retract, and a large open wound will develop that will take weeks to months to heal by secondary intention.
- If the infection was virulent, the patient is returned to surgery 24 to 48 hours later for a repeat débridement and bead exchange.
- The fibula is not excised at this time.
- With beads filling the defect and the fibula intact, the extremity is placed in a splint or fracture boot.

Postoperative Care

- Broad-spectrum antibiotics that cover methicillin-resistant *S. aureus* and gram-negative rods are administered until the cultures have identified the infecting organism.
- The extremity and surgical wound are examined daily.
- If the wound does not rapidly improve, a second débridement is indicated.
- After a week of intravenous antibiotics, the ankle is ready for tibiocalcaneal arthrodesis.
- Extending the intravenous antibiotic course for 2 to 3 weeks and further observation may be indicated if the condition of the extremity requires further time to be ready for surgery or there is a high suspicion of fastidious organisms (*Mycobacterium*).

TIBIOCALCANEAL ARTHRODESIS

- Technically, the most difficult aspect of the surgery is fitting the concave surface of the plafond to the asymmetric surface to the posterior facet of the calcaneus, anterior calcaneus, and neck of the talus or the navicular **(TECH FIG 2A)**.
- Cut the bone away in small shavings, with multiple trial fittings until the plafond fits securely into the calcaneus and talus or navicular.
- Approach the plafond and calcaneus from the lateral and medial sides of the ankle.
- Retention of the lateral malleolus is of no benefit.
- Excise the lateral malleolus through a lateral excision and perform an osteotomy 5 to 6 cm proximal with an oblique cut superolateral to inferomedial.
- Carefully elevate the fascia overlying the lateral malleolus from the surface.
  - This fascia provides a deep closure of the lateral tissues after completion of the osteotomy.
- The lateral approach exposes the posterior facet of the calcaneus, lateral calcaneus, and anterior process.
  - Do not extend the vertical excision past the level of the peroneal tendons to prevent injury to the sural nerve.
- The anteromedial approach exposes the navicular, talar neck, and medial facets of the calcaneus.
- Evaluate the plafond and posterior facets of the calcaneus.
  - If the posterior facet is intact, excise the cartilage and expose the subchondral bone to bleeding bone.

- Débride the medial facet of cartilage and level the facet with the middle and anterior calcaneus.
- Cut the posterior plafond at an angle to match the posterior facet and remove the cartilage from the central plafond.
- If the talar neck is viable, cut the anterior plafond away to match the plane of the talar neck and flatten the underside of the anterior plafond to match the contour of the middle and anterior calcaneus **(TECH FIG 2B)**.
- Cut away small amounts of bone from the tibia and calcaneus until there is a good fit between the tibia and calcaneus.
- Assess the alignment of the calcaneus with the tibia.
  - With the tibia compressed onto the calcaneus, the sole of the foot and heel should be in a foot-flat position.
  - The foot should be rotated straightforward or in slight external rotation.
  - Equinus must be avoided.
  - Neutral plantarflexion and slight dorsiflexion are functional positions.
  - If the arthrodesis is in equinus, the patient must wear shoes with a heel wedge to accommodate this malposition.
- The osteotomies of the tibia plafond and calcaneus must be fitted so that when the tibia is compressed onto the calcaneus, the fit of the osteotomy forces corrects alignment of the foot.
  - If the osteotomies are not correct, the compression applied by the circular fixation will malalign the arthrodesis.

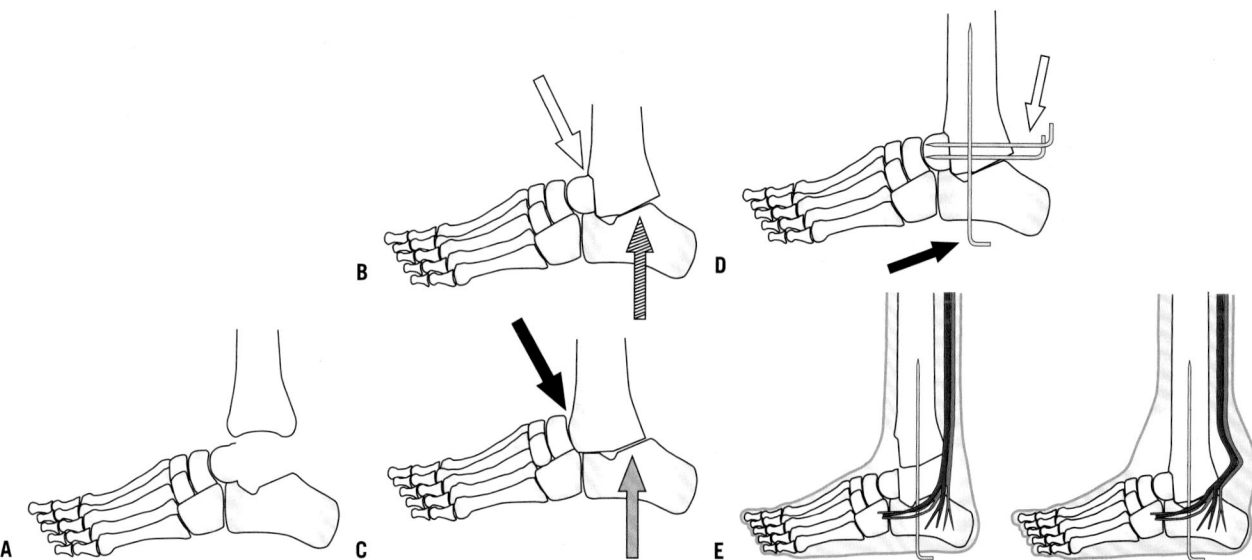

TECH FIG 2 A. Fitting the incongruent surfaces of the tibial plafond to the calcaneus and talar neck or navicular requires craftsmanship. The osteotomy cuts are made with small cuttings until a stable compression surface is created. **B.** The anterior plafond is cut to align with the talar neck when the talar head is viable (*white arrow*). The posterior plafond osteotomy requires an oblique osteotomy to fit the posterior facet of the calcaneus (*striated arrow*). **C.** The anterior prominence of the tibial plafond is not removed when the talar head has been excised (*black arrow*). The anterior cortex is prepared to bleeding bone. The bone resection of the posterior plafond is shaped to fit the posterior facet (*gray arrow*). The resection of the posterior plafond is less because the tibia is located anteriorly with the talar head excised. The anterior process of the calcaneus is leveled to allow the tibia to compress onto the calcaneus. **D.** An inferior to superior Steinmann pin is placed to align the calcaneus with the tibial shaft after the arthrodesis osteotomies have been completed (*black arrow*). One or two Steinmann pins are placed from posterolateral through the plafond into the head of the talus to improve stability of the fixation if talar head is preserved in the reconstruction (*white arrow*). **E.** Acute shortening causes the soft tissues to bulge in the horizontal plane. After the calcaneal tibial pin is in place, the wounds can be closed with the extremity distracted. The tibia is compressed to the calcaneus after closure. Shortening causes distortion of the blood vessels crossing the ankle. Vascular flow must be carefully monitored after shortening. *(continued)*

TECHNIQUES

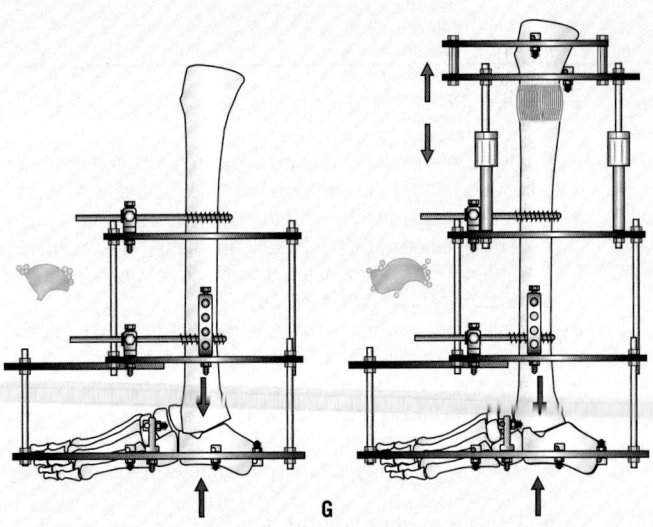
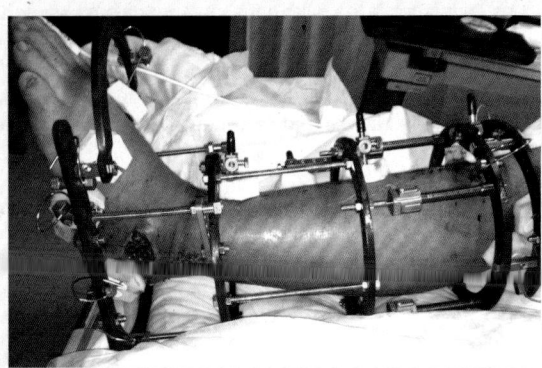

F   G   H

TECH FIG 2 *(continued)* **F.** Monofocal tibiocalcaneal talar head arthrodesis circular fixator. The frame consists of a double-ring fixation block and a foot fixation ring. The fixator is used to compress the arthrodesis. This illustration represents reconstruction of a talus with a viable talar head. *Red arrows* indicate direction of compression. **G.** Bifocal tibiocalcaneal navicular arthrodesis circular fixator. The frame incorporates a proximal ⅝-full ring block and corticotomy to combine proximal lengthening with distal compression. The illustration depicts reconstruction after complete excision of the talus. *Red arrows* indicate direction of compression, and proximal *red shaded area* represents new regenerate bone. **H.** Clinical photograph of bifocal fixator. Observe proximal ⅝-full ring block connected to double-ring midtibia fixation block with distraction clickers. The foot frame is compressed with square nuts. Observe open lateral traumatic wound, which will heal by secondary intention.

- The bone cuts of the anterior plafond are modified if the talar head has been excised because of infection **(TECH FIG 2C)**.
- Denude the navicular of cartilage to bleeding bone.
- Shape the bone contour of the anterior plafond to match the navicular concave surface.
- Flatten the anteroinferior plafond to fit the anterior calcaneus.
- The tibia is located in an anterior position toward the midfoot compared to the arthrodesis position if the talar head is present.
- Because of this anterior position, the osteotomy of the posterior plafond may require less bone resection.
  - Always align the plafond over the calcaneus and slowly cut away bone until there is a good fit of the bone surfaces.
- After completing the osteotomies, copiously lavage the operative field with low-pressure bulb irrigation to remove debris before closure.
  - The use of high-pressure pulsed irrigation destroys the exposed trabecular bone.[2]
- Deflate the tourniquet and examine the bone surfaces for punctate bleeding.
- If there is no bleeding, further bone resection is needed until viable bone is observed.
- Compress the calcaneus and align it manually and drill a smooth Steinmann pin through the plantar surface into the tibial shaft **(TECH FIG 2D)**.
  - This pin will help assure proper alignment during fixator application in order to guide the calcaneus to the correct position during compression with the circular fixator later on during the technique.
- Close the medial and lateral incisions with a deep layer of absorbable antibacterial plus suture and the skin with vertical nylon mattress sutures.
- The sutures may need to be in place for 3 to 4 weeks before there is adequate wound healing.
  - Never use staples for the skin closure.

- The shortening of the calcaneus onto the tibia will cause the soft tissues to expand in the horizontal plane (compression of a cylinder causes expansion of the diameter of the cylinder) **(TECH FIG 2E)**.
- To facilitate closure, distract the calcaneus on the Steinmann pin and close the wounds with the foot out to length.
  - The amount of edema and fibrosis of the soft tissue will affect the ability to acutely shorten the arthrodesis.[3]
  - If there is severe edema and fibrosis, an acute shortening may not be possible, and a delayed shortening may be required to compress the arthrodesis.
  - The surgeon will gauge the effect of the shortening.
- If the calcaneus is compressed against the plafond and the foot becomes cyanotic or there is a loss of pulses, a delayed shortening will be needed for the reconstruction.
- The circular fixator is constructed as a monofocal frame or as a bifocal frame **(TECH FIG 2F,G)**.
  - The circular rings are sized to provide 2 cm of soft tissue clearance.
  - Most frames are constructed with 160- or 180-mm rings.
- If the patient is a candidate for proximal distraction osteogenesis, the frame is assembled with a proximal ⅝-full ring block, a midtibial double-ring fixation block, and a foot fixation block.
- If the patient has poor physiology for lengthening (end-stage diabetes, tobacco abuse, ischemic vascular disease, steroid dependency, or psychosis), the frame is assembled as a monofocal frame with a two-ring tibial fixation block and a foot fixation block.
- Carefully assess the ability of the patient to undergo distraction histogenesis.
- If there is failure of the arthrodesis, the salvage is a below-knee amputation.
- If a proximal corticotomy has been done on a patient with poor physiology, the below-knee level of salvage could be lost.

PROXIMAL LENGTHENING

- The proximal and midtibial ring blocks are assembled as a unit.
  - The proximal ring block is constructed with a ⅝ or ⅔ ring connected to a full ring with three 3.0-cm hexagonal sockets (**TECH FIG 3A**).
  - The midtibial ring block is constructed with two rings connected with four 120- or 150-mm threaded rods (**TECH FIG 3B,C**).
  - The proximal and midtibial ring blocks are connected with four 40-mm distraction telescopic rods (clickers).
  - A horizontal reference olive wire is placed 15 mm below the tibial plateau with a 3-degree varus alignment orthogonal to the tibial shaft.
- The varus of the reference wire aligns the frame with the axis of the tibia shaft when the wire is tensioned to the ring (**TECH FIG 3D**).
  - The frame is aligned and centered on the tibia with adequate soft tissue clearance (**TECH FIG 3E**).
  - Observe the posterior gastrocsoleus muscle to ensure proper clearance.
- Tension the horizontal reference wire to 110 kg.
- The center frame should be parallel to the longitudinal axis of the tibial shaft.
  - If the alignment is not axial, washers can be placed under the lateral or medial reference wire to correct the alignment.
- During this phase of the procedure, an assistant must support the distal leg and foot to prevent distorted positions, which could injure the soft tissues.
  - A towel block under the heel also prevents displacement.
- Align the distal tibial ring block with the tibia and place a 5-mm half-pin in the anteroposterior (AP) plane. Secure it with a universal Rancho cube on the distal ring (**TECH FIG 3F**).
  - The universal cube allows the ring to be aligned on the lateral view in an orthogonal position to the long axis of the tibia.

- Alternatively, a transverse olive wire may be used to align the distal fixation block (see **TECH FIG 3C**).
- Once the frame is aligned, place a second AP 5-mm half-pin on the midtibial fixation block.
- Place a medial half-pin between the rings aligned 90 degrees to the two AP pins.
  - Place a second medial pin for large patients.
- Further stabilize the proximal ⅝-full ring block with a medial face olive wire on the inferior face of the full ring and place a smooth wire through the fibula head, exiting the anteromedial tibial plateau.
- Connect the footplate to the midtibial fixation block with two threaded rods placed in the posteromedial and posterolateral ring (**TECH FIG 3G**).
  - The rods should have about 50 mm of excess length.
- Place a horizontal reference wire in the tuberosity of the calcaneus from lateral to medial.
- Compress the foot on the Steinmann pin until the calcaneus is in alignment with the tibia.
- Manipulate the foot on the footplate to control rotational alignment and align the arthrodesis.
  - Close the footplate anteriorly with a half-ring before tensioning.

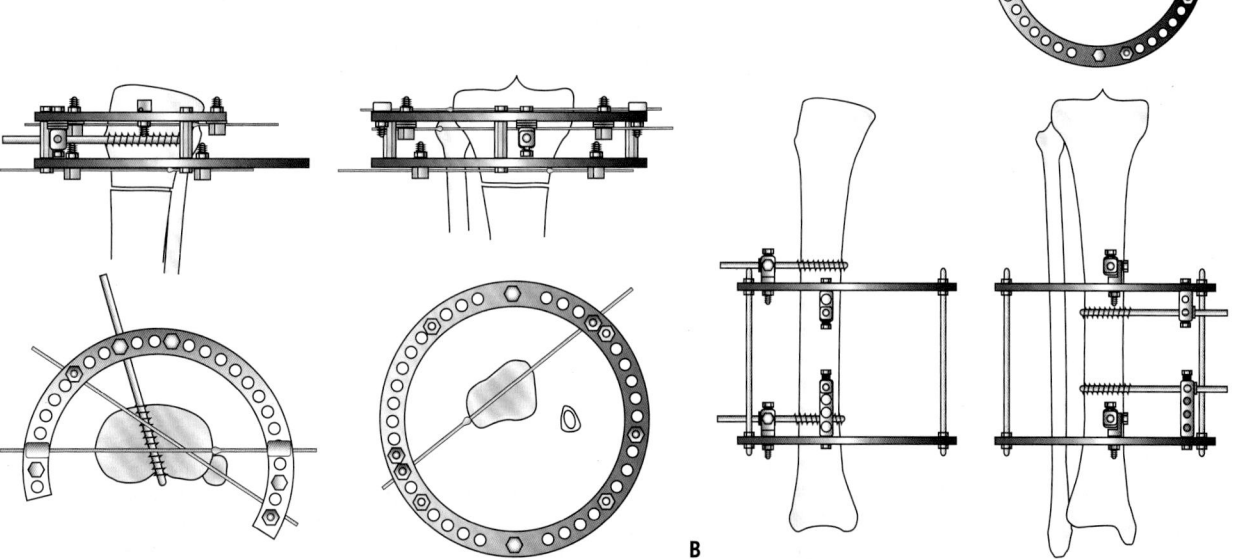

A   B

TECH FIG 3 A. The ⅝-full ring proximal fixation block. The ⅝ ring is connected to the full ring by three 3-cm hexagonal sockets. The horizontal reference wire is 15 mm below the joint in 3 degrees of varus. A smooth wire is placed into the fibula head. If the fibula head is not fixated, the fibula will be dragged down the leg with lengthening. A medial face wire is placed on the inferior surface of the full ring. A 5-mm half-pin is placed anteromedial after completion of the corticotomy. The ⅝ ring is rotated to the lateral side to allow placement of the fibula head wire. **B.** The tibial shaft double-ring fixation block is aligned orthogonally on the tibia with two AP 6-mm half-pins mounted on universal Rancho cubes. The Rancho cube mountings allow the fixation block to be aligned orthogonally. One or two medial pins are added once the fixation block is aligned. The distal ring is located about 6 cm superior to the arthrodesis. *(continued)*

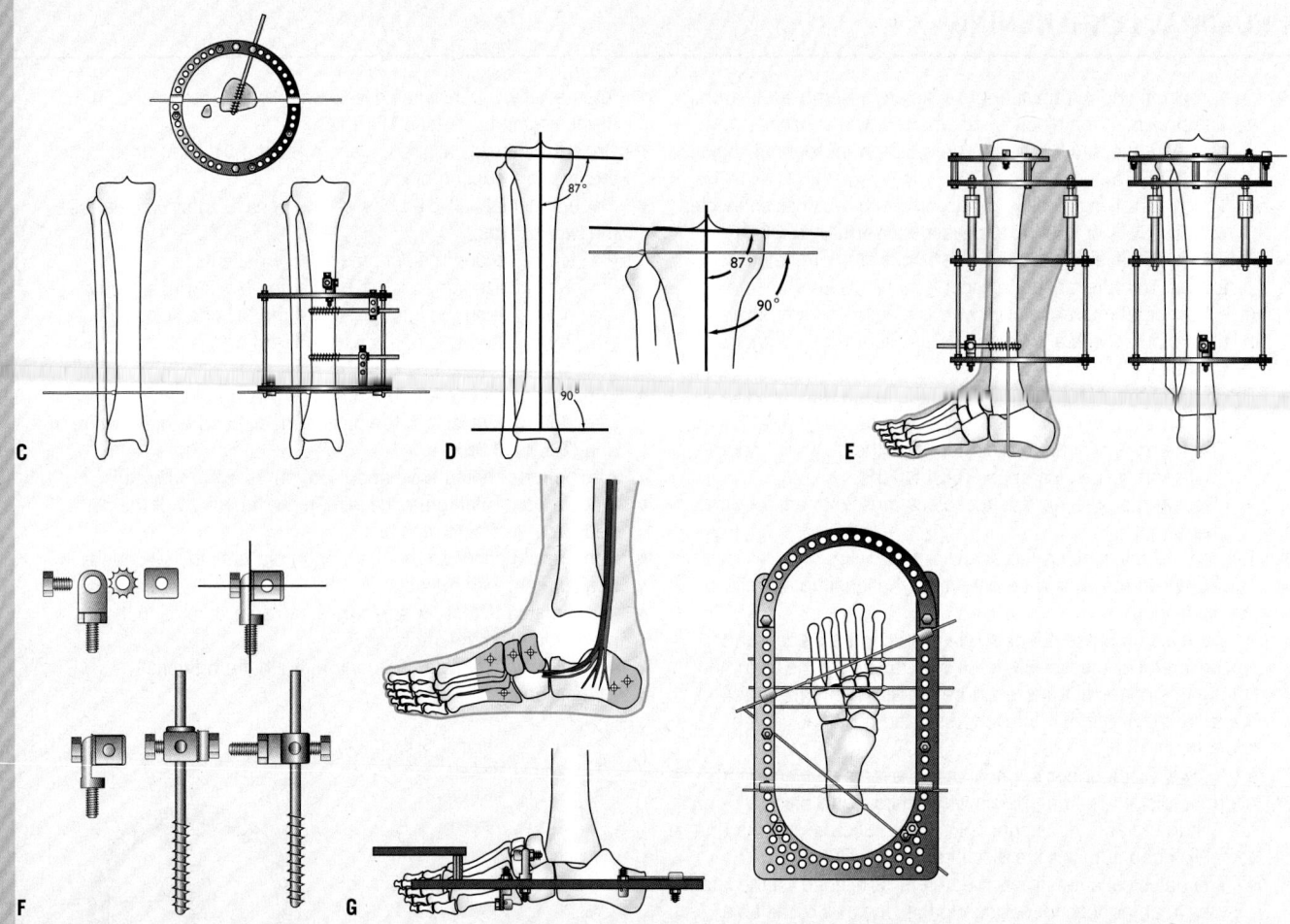

TECH FIG 3 *(continued)* **C.** An alternative method to align the stable base is to place a horizontal reference above the plafond. The wire should be placed posterior on the shaft to avoid the anterior tibial artery. The distal wire is located about 6 cm proximal to the arthrodesis. **D.** The joint surface of the plateau forms a varus 87-degree angle with the shaft. A horizontal reference wire placed 90 degrees to the shaft will be slightly closer to the medial plateau compared to the lateral. **E.** The proximal ⅝ ring block and the tibial shaft double-ring block are connected by 40-mm distraction rods. The frame is aligned on the proximal reference wire followed by a 5-mm half-pin placed on the distal ring. Manipulating these two fixation points aligns the frame orthogonally on the tibia. The rings must have soft tissue clearance at the posterior gastrocnemius muscle and anterior ankle soft tissue prominence. **F.** Universal Rancho cube pin fixation. Three-axis adjustment of the pin alignment allows the frame to be aligned orthogonally with the tibia. Rancho cubes bolted directly to the ring; fix the ring in the alignment of the half-pin. If the half-pin is not perfect, the ring block will be malaligned. **G.** The foot fixation block is constructed with a long footplate closed on the anterior open end with a half-ring. The ring extends above the toes to keep bed linen from irritating the toes. The surgeon should avoid wires that could penetrate the posterior tibial or plantar nerve. Two opposed olive wires are placed in the calcaneus, and two opposed olive wires are placed in the forefoot.

- Tension the wire to 100 kg and tighten the slotted fixation bolts.
- If the alignment is not satisfactory, repeat the process.
- Connect two threaded rods to the anterior footplate using extension plates from the stable base on the tibia.
- Stabilize the forefoot with opposed olive wires through the cuneiform row and metatarsals.
- Place a second wire from the posteromedial calcaneal tuberosity to the anterolateral calcaneal wall on the superior side of the footplate.
- Assess the vascularity of the foot with the foot in the acutely shortened position.
  - There should be brisk capillary refill.
- Use a Doppler device to verify pulsatile flow in the dorsalis pedis and posterior tibial artery.
  - If the vascular flow is good, maintain the foot in the acutely shortened position.

- If the foot is cyanotic and no pulses are detected with the Doppler, slowly distract the foot by lengthening the threaded rods between the tibial fixation block and the foot ring.
- Once pulsatile flow is detected, lock the threaded rod position in place.
- This position will create a gap between the tibia and calcaneus.
  - A delayed shortening is used to close this gap slowly over days or weeks **(TECH FIG 4)**.
  - The gap is closed at a rate of 1 mm four times per day until the arthrodesis is compressed.
- If the distal tibia plafond has extensive bone loss creating a bone deficit greater than 5 cm, the tibiocalcaneal arthrodesis can be accomplished with an intercalary transport **(TECH FIG 5)**.
- Complete a corticotomy using an osteotome or a Gigli saw.
- After the corticotomy, place a 6-mm half-pin on the medial side of the tibial tubercle from anterior to posterior.

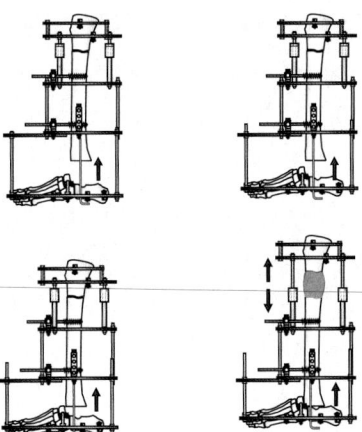

TECH FIG 4 The technique of delayed shortening. The foot fixation block is compressed at a rate of 1 mm four times a day until the tibiocalcaneal arthrodesis is compressed. The calcaneal tibial Steinmann pin aligns the foot during the compression. The proximal tibia is lengthened to equalize leg lengths. *Red arrows* indicate direction of ring movement. *Shaded red area* represents new regenerate bone.

- The Steinmann pin is maintained for 6 weeks after surgery, which stabilizes the arthrodesis site.
- Place two more Steinmann pins from the posteromedial plafond into the talar head or navicular after compressing the arthrodesis (see **TECH FIG 2D**).
  - These pins stabilize motion between the talar head and tibia, increasing arthrodesis between these structures.

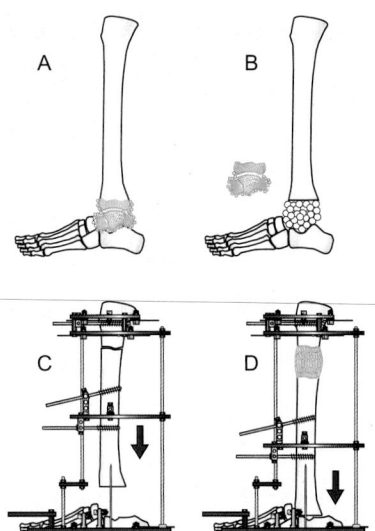

TECH FIG 5 The technique of intercalary transport to arthrodesis. **A.** Infection of plafond and talus. **B.** Excision with bone gap greater than 5 cm. **C.** Ilizarov frame maintaining leg length before transport. *Red arrows* indicate direction of ring movement. **D.** Intercalary transport to docking. A revision of the docking site will improve alignment. A spatial frame could also be used in this configuration. Large defects can also be closed with an acute shortening of 3 cm combined with an intercalary transport to close the gap. The circular fixator is converted to a lengthening frame to equalize the leg length. *Red arrows* indicate direction of ring movement. *Shaded red area* represents new regenerate bone.

TECHNIQUES WITHOUT LENGTHENING

- Apply a stable base to the distal tibia (see **TECH FIG 3B**).
- Place two AP half-pins on universal Rancho cubes and align the ring block orthogonally.
- The distal ring is located about 6 cm above the arthrodesis site.
  - The ring is further stabilized with one or two 5-mm half-pins placed into the medial tibia.
  - An alternative method is to place a horizontal reference wire 6 cm above the ankle and align the double-ring fixation on

the wire and place two AP pins and a medial face half-pin on the ring block (see **TECH FIG 3C**).
- In patients with osteopenia, the entire fixation block can be fixated to the tibia with four olive wires placed in safe corridors.
- Complete the arthrodesis of the tibia to the calcaneus as described in the prior section.

TECHNIQUES COMBINED WITH INTRAMEDULLARY FIXATION

- Intramedullary fixation from the hindfoot to the tibia with or without antibiotic polymethylmethacrylate coating in combination with circular external fixation is an alternative to external fixation alone (**TECH FIG 6A,B**).
- This integrated approach decreases time in the external fixator and may improve union rates.
- The arthrodesis is prepared, and then a hindfoot fusion nail is passed from the calcaneus to the tibia (**TECH FIG 6C,D**).
  - The arthrodesis is compressed initially in surgery and then 1 to 2 mm per week for the next 4 weeks (**TECH FIG 6E,F**).

- The fixator is removed at 4 to 6 weeks in the operating room after a proximal locking screw is placed in the nail (**TECH FIG 6G,H**).
- The patient remains non–weight bearing for a total of 3 months after the initial surgery.

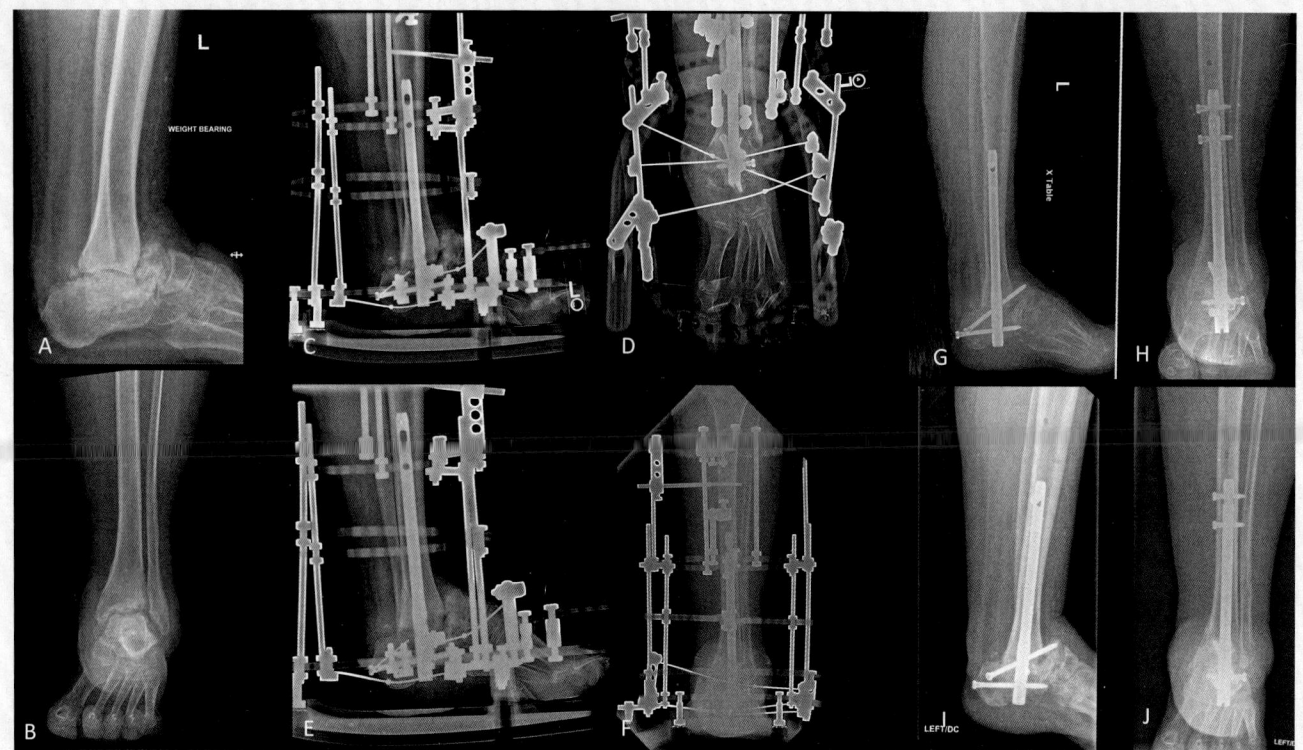

TECH FIG 6 A,B. AP and lateral x-rays of a Charcot ankle with complete destruction of the talar body. **C,D.** AP and lateral x-rays of Ilizarov compression frame with hindfoot fusion nail. **E,F.** AP and lateral radiographs at week 4 postoperatively after 6 mm of compression at 2 mm per week and then 1 mm per week. **G,H.** One month after initial procedure, the proximal locking screws are placed as well as the distal screw spanning from the calcaneus to the talus and the fixator removed. **I,J.** AP and lateral x-rays 3 months after initial operation showing solid healing at both the tibiocalcaneal and tibiotalar sites.

TECHNIQUES

Pearls and Pitfalls

Foot Position

- The arthrodesis must be in a plantar neutral position. A fusion with the foot in equinus will severely compromise the functional outcome **(FIG 4)**.

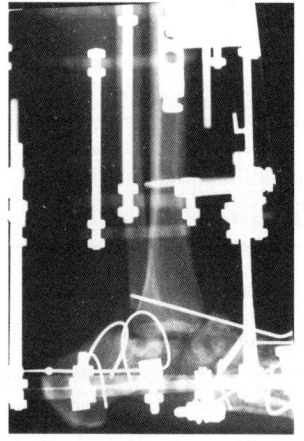

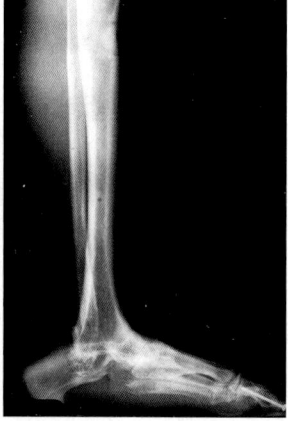

FIG 4 A. Tibiocalcaneal arthrodesis with loss of talar head and navicular in crush injury of foot. **B.** Full lateral x-ray of tibia and foot is accurate method to evaluate foot position. With no ankle motion and compromised forefoot motion, aligning the foot in plantar neutral position and correct forefoot rotation is essential for a functional result. Observe mature proximal bone transport to equalize leg length.

POSTOPERATIVE CARE

- The foot is observed for blood flow every 4 hours for the first 2 postoperative days.
  - If the foot becomes ischemic, the threaded rods connecting the foot frame to the tibia fixation block are lengthened until the blood flow improves.
  - A delayed shortening is then carried out until the arthrodesis is compressed **(FIG 5)**.
  - The patient is encouraged to mobilize the forefoot and toes and knee.
  - Toe loops on rubber bands are placed on a wire scaffold to prevent toe flexion contractures by the physical therapy service.
  - There will be significant bloody drainage, and the bulky dressing placed in surgery may need to be changed on the first postoperative day.
  - Open wounds are treated with normal saline wet-to-dry dressings until closure by secondary intention.
  - Vacuum dressings are an alternative to wet-to-dry dressings.
  - The sutures are left in place for at least 2 weeks.
  - Many patients will require 3 to 4 weeks of suture closure before it is possible to remove the sutures.
- Intravenous antibiotics are administered for 2 days in patients without infections.
  - If the wounds are complex, the intravenous antibiotics will be continued for 7 days.
  - Patients with infected talus nonunions will be treated for additional weeks using intravenous antibiotics appropriate for the infecting organism.
  - There is debate on whether the antibiotics need to be given for an additional week or continued for a total of 6 weeks during the treatment course.
- The dressing sponges are removed 2 weeks after surgery, and the pin sites are cleaned daily.
- Once the surgical wounds are healed, the leg is washed in the shower with soap and water, removing all dried secretions from the pins and wires.
  - Hydrogen peroxide 3% solution is used only occasionally to clean crust that cannot be removed with soap and water.
  - Cephalexin, trimethoprim–sulfamethoxazole (Septra DS), and ciprofloxacin are used if needed to control local pin or wire skin infections.

- Some patients will need only occasional use of antibiotics, whereas others will require constant oral antibiotic coverage while the circular fixator is on the leg.
- Rarely, a more aggressive pin or wire infection will develop.
  - The infecting organism is most commonly methicillin-resistant *S. aureus*.
  - A 1-week course of intravenous vancomycin will be needed to control the wire infection.
  - If this is not successful, the wire is removed.
- The plantar calcaneotibial, talar neck–tibia, and naviculotibial Steinmann pins are removed in the clinic 6 weeks after surgery.
  - The patient is started on partial weight bearing, increasing to 50% weight over the following month.
  - A shower sandal is placed over the toes when walking.
  - The sandal is elevated with a full sole elevation to equalize the leg lengths, and the sole is cut down as the lengthening progresses.
  - Most patients cannot tolerate full weight with wires in their foot.
- Lengthening proximally is at a rate of 0.25 mm (one quarter turn) twice a day in most patients.
  - The lengthening is started after a latency period of 7 to 10 days postoperatively.
  - The starting rate is always 0.25 mm twice a day.
    - If the patient forms robust new bone, this can be increased to 0.25 mm every 8 hours or even every 6 hours.
    - Most of these patients are of older age with multiple medical comorbidities that affect bone healing, thus requiring the slower speed of distraction that is recommended.
    - Younger patients with no comorbidities can distract at a rate of 0.25 mm every 6 hours.
  - The leg is lengthened until the leg length is equal (see **FIG 4**).
  - Given the choice, most patients request equal leg length rather than on to 2 cm of shortening.
  - The distraction index is between 1.5 and 2.0 months per centimeter.
  - For a patient with tibial bone loss, the lengthening required can exceed 5 cm, resulting in 10 or more months in the circular fixator.
  - Some patients will heal the arthrodesis before the lengthening is mature.

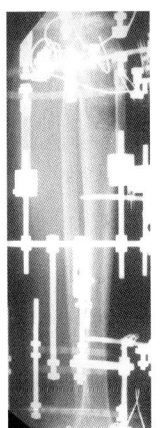 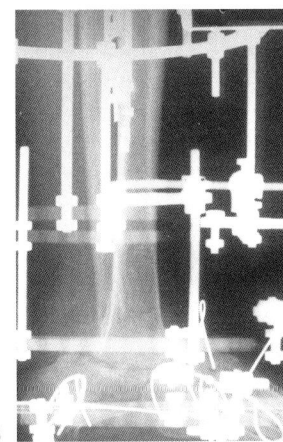 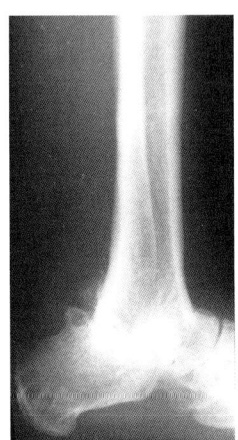 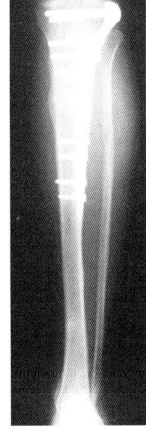

A   B   C   D

FIG 5 A. Lateral x-ray of bifocal external fixator. The proximal tibia has been lengthened between the ⅝-full ring block and the double-ring block on the midtibia. **B.** Lateral x-ray of the tibiocalcaneal arthrodesis with compression between the midtibia and the footplate. The foot is in plantar neutral alignment. **C.** Mature tibiocalcaneal arthrodesis with the plafond fused to the calcaneus and navicular. **D.** AP x-ray with axial alignment of arthrodesis. The patient had a valgus deformity after frame removal of the transport. The tibia was realigned with a lateral locked plate.

- The foot frame can be removed before the proximal transport is mature if the arthrodesis is complete.
- The tibiocalcaneal arthrodesis requires 6 months for union.
  - The footplate is compressed 1 or 2 mm at each clinic visit to maintain compression and retension of the wires over the course of treatment.
  - The fixator is removed under anesthesia, especially if hydroxyapatite pins are used.
  - A short-leg walking cast is applied, and the patient walks with partial weight bearing.
  - The patient continues partial weight gait until there is defined bone healing at the tibiocalcaneal arthrodesis and the proximal bone transport has a well-developed medial, lateral, and posterior cortex.
  - Often, patients will return to the clinic stating that they have advanced to full weight bearing around the house walking in the frame.
  - To increase the force transmitted across the transport, the frame is neutralized before frame removal.
  - This is accomplished by loosening the distraction clickers and allowing the distraction force to become neutral.
  - The rods are bolted in this neutral position, and the patient is observed for several weeks to see if the cortex of the regenerate is strong enough to prevent collapse.
  - The fixator is removed under general anesthesia.
  - The leg is casted for 2 weeks after frame removal.
  - The radiograph out of plaster in the office with the Ilizarov fixator removed is analyzed for healing of the transport bone and arthrodesis.
  - A fracture walking boot with a rocker bottom sole is applied.
  - The patient walks 50% weight bearing for 4 weeks.
  - The patient advances to full weight bearing with a cane and gradually increases his or her activity over the following year.
  - Activity is limited to walking on flat surfaces and light stress on the extremity.
  - The force applied to the leg is gradually increased with mature healing of the bone transport and arthrodesis observed at 1 year after fixator removal (see **FIG 5C,D**).
  - The patient self-selects walking and training shoes that have cushioned heels with a rounded radius heel.
  - Patients who do not have proximal bone transport to equalize leg length have full sole elevations of 3 to 5 cm added to their walking shoes (shoe prosthesis) with a rocker sole.
  - If the patient has mild valgus or varus foot alignment, an orthotic is prescribed that improves their foot loading when standing and walking.
  - Long-term follow-up reveals osteophyte development at the talar navicular joint, which is associated with arthritic pain.

OUTCOMES

- The average American Orthopaedic Foot and Ankle Society Ankle-Hindfoot Score was 65 for the 11 patients in our case series.[5]
  - We have reconstructed five further patients with good result for total of 16 cases.
  - Patients lose the ability to participate in sports and work as laborers.

- The work status is reduced to light or sedentary work.
- They can still ride motorcycles and drive cars.
- Patients are aware of the asymmetry of their legs from atrophy of the muscles motorizing the foot and ankle.
- When queried, no patient to date has considered having an amputation.
- The long-term follow-up will probably reveal progression of midfoot arthritis.

COMPLICATIONS

- Failure of the bone transport to mature is a major complication.
  - The distraction index is between 1.5 and 2.0 months per centimeter of lengthening.
  - Bone growth is stimulated by weight bearing, so during the treatment course, the patient is encouraged to place 50% partial weight on the extremity.
  - An EXOGEN bone stimulator (Smith & Nephew, Memphis, TN) can be used once the distraction is completed.
  - Bone grafting of the distraction can also stimulate maturation if poor bone formation is observed.
- If deformation of the transport occurs after frame removal, this problem can be treated by several methods.
  - If there is less than 5 degrees of angulation, the patient is treated with a knee brace and non–weight bearing for 6 weeks.
  - If greater deformity is observed, a second circular fixator is applied with angular correction and further time in the frame is indicated.
  - An alternative is to place a locked plate spanning the transport on the medial or lateral tibial shaft (see **FIG 5D**).
  - An intramedullary nail can also be used to allow fixator removal and stimulate healing for bone transport with poor bone formation.
  - The pin and wire tracks must be free of infection to use internal fixation after external fixation.
  - The patients walk 50% partial weight with crutches until healing of the transport if a plate is applied.
  - The patient can walk with partial weight for 1 month and then can weight bear as tolerated with an intramedullary nail in place.
- Failure to achieve arthrodesis is directly related to the physiologic status of the patient.
  - If union has not occurred by 6 months of frame time, further time in the frame will not alter the outcome.
  - If the patient is not on steroids and is in reasonable health, a revision arthrodesis is attempted. The docking site is explored, and fibrous tissue is removed. The bone surfaces are revised to bleeding bone (**FIG 6**).
  - Patients with rheumatoid arthritis who are using steroids chronically are prone to nonunion of their tibiocalcaneal arthrodesis.
  - Patients with rheumatoid arthritis are placed in a cast and encouraged to walk.
  - The mobile nonunion forms a pseudojoint similar to fascial arthroplasty that allows them to walk independently (**FIG 7**).
  - We have observed four patients who have maintained this pseudojoint for years and are able to participate in activities of daily living.

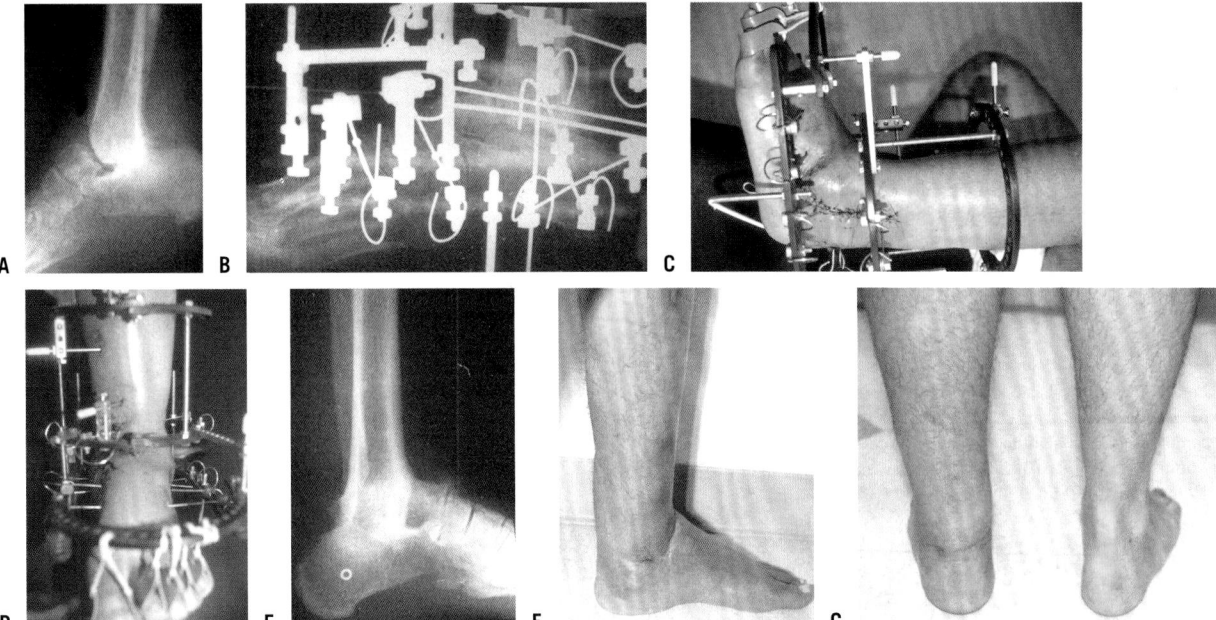

FIG 6 A. Nonunion of tibia metaphysis to calcaneus and talar head remnant following Ilizarov compression. **B.** Revision of docking site with Steinmann pin fixation through calcaneus into tibia and Steinmann pin fixation of talar head to anterior metaphysis of tibia. **C.** Revision frame with two-ring fixation block on distal tibia and foot fixation ring. Distal closing ring on footplate is offset with hexagonal socket to clear toes. Rubber band stirrups prevent flexion contracture of toes. **D.** Foot is aligned in frame plantar neutral. Wire pathways through foot illustrated. **E.** Seven-year follow-up of tibiocalcaneal arthrodesis. Observe reactive bone at talar navicular joint. **F.** Ninety-degree foot alignment and healed complex wound. It is essential to avoid any equinus position of the foot. **G.** Alignment of foot with the floor. Slight varus of heel. Ideal position equally loads first and fifth metatarsal heads.

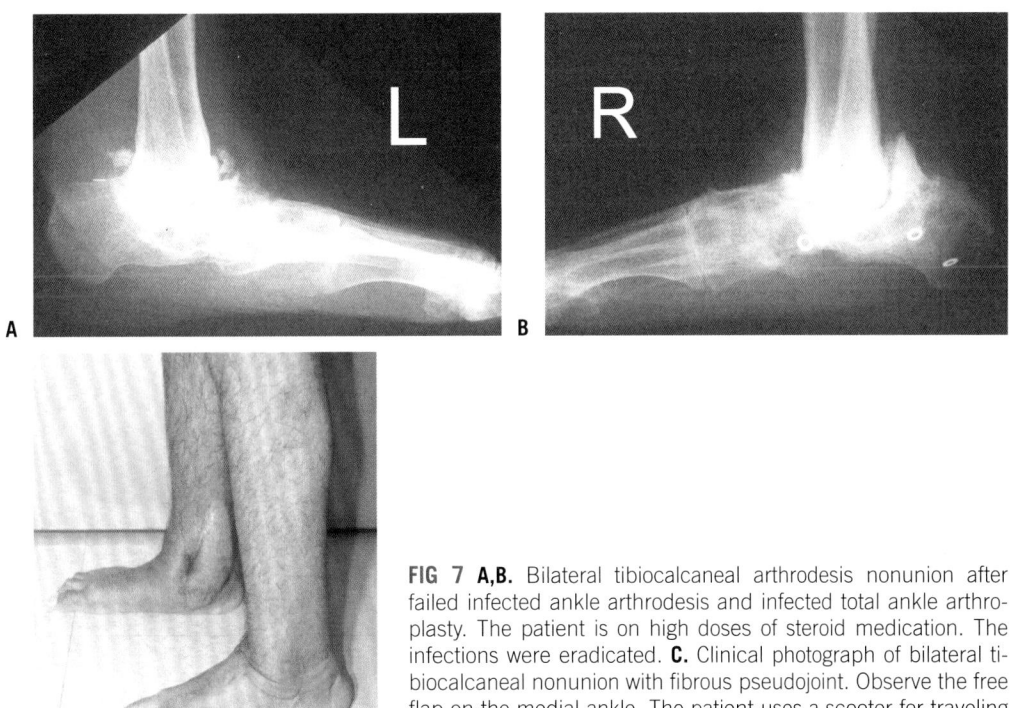

FIG 7 A,B. Bilateral tibiocalcaneal arthrodesis nonunion after failed infected ankle arthrodesis and infected total ankle arthroplasty. The patient is on high doses of steroid medication. The infections were eradicated. **C.** Clinical photograph of bilateral tibiocalcaneal nonunion with fibrous pseudojoint. Observe the free flap on the medial ankle. The patient uses a scooter for traveling distances but can walk independently and is independent in activities of daily living.

REFERENCES

1. Dennison MG, Pool RD, Simonis RB, et al. Tibiocalcaneal fusion for avascular necrosis of the talus. J Bone Joint Surg Br 2001;83(2):199–203.
2. Dirschl DR, Duff GP, Dahners LE, et al. High pressure pulsatile lavage irrigation of intraarticular fractures: effects on fracture healing. J Orthop Trauma 1998;12:460–463.
3. Hutson JJ. Appendix 2: acute shortening to reconstruct fractures and post traumatic deformities with Ilizarov fixators. Tech Orthop 2002;17:110–111.
4. Kile TA, Donnelly RE, Gehrke JC, et al. Tibiotalocalcaneal arthrodesis with an intramedullary device. Foot Ankle Int 1994;15:669–673.
5. Kitaoka HB, Alexander IJ, Adelaar RS, et al. Clinical rating systems for the ankle-hindfoot, midfoot, hallux, and lesser toes. Foot Ankle Int 1994;15:349–353.
6. Lou TF, Hamushan M, Li H, et al. Staged distraction osteogenesis followed by arthrodesis using internal fixation as a form of surgical treatment for complex conditions of the ankle. Bone Joint J 2018;100-B(6):755–760.
7. Mann RA, Chou LB. Tibiocalcaneal arthrodesis. Foot Ankle Int 1995;16:401–405.
8. Marsh JL, Saltzman CL, Iverson M, et al. Major open injuries of the talus. J Orthop Trauma 1995;9:371–376.
9. Ptaszek AJ. Immediate tibiocalcaneal arthrodesis with interposition fibular autograft for salvage after talus fracture: a case report. J Orthop Trauma 1999;13:589–592.
10. Rochman R, Jackson Hutson J, Alade O. Tibiocalcaneal arthrodesis using the Ilizarov technique in the presence of bone loss and infection of the talus. Foot Ankle Int 2008;29(10):1001–1008.
11. Sanders DW, Busam M, Hattwick E, et al. Functional outcomes following displaced talar neck fractures. J Orthop Trauma 2004;18:265–270.
12. Smith CS, Nork SE, Sangeorzan BJ. The extruded talus: results of reimplantation. J Bone Joint Surg Am 2006;88(11):2418–2424.
13. Tomczak C, Beaman D, Perkins S. Combined intramedullary nail coated with antibiotic-containing cement and ring fixation for limb salvage in the severely deformed, infected, neuroarthropathic ankle. Foot Ankle Int 2019;40(1):48–55.
14. Weber M, Schwer H, Zilkens KW, et al. Tibio-calcaneo-naviculo-cuboidale arthrodesis: 6 patients followed for 1–8 years. Acta Orthop Scand 2002;73:98–103.

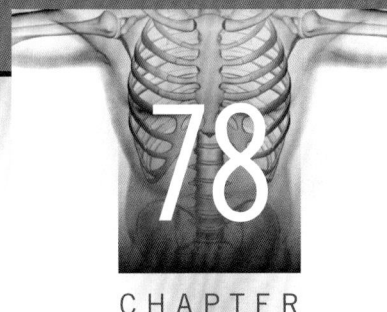
Femoral Head Allograft for Large Talar Defects

Bryan D. Den Hartog

INDICATIONS

- Talar body avascular necrosis with collapse or infection **(FIG 1A)** is one indication for femoral head allograft.
- Failed total ankle arthroplasty with insufficient bone remaining for revision **(FIG 1B)** also warrants a femoral head allograft.
- Use of a femoral head graft for those patients with severe (>25 degrees) hindfoot valgus may not be appropriate because correction of the deformity can cause significant lateral soft tissue tension and lead to tissue necrosis and poor

wound healing. In those cases, a tibiocalcaneal fusion with shortening of the medial ankle may be more appropriate.

POSITIONING

- Under a general or spinal anesthetic block, the patient is placed in a supine position on the operating table with the ipsilateral hip bumped to facilitate internal rotation of the leg.
- The lower extremity is prepped and draped in the usual fashion, and a thigh tourniquet inflated to 250 mm Hg is applied after exsanguination of the leg with an Esmarch bandage.

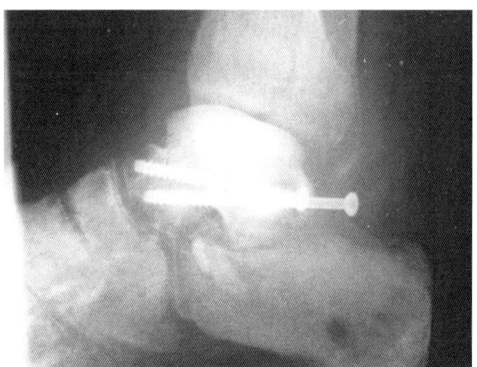

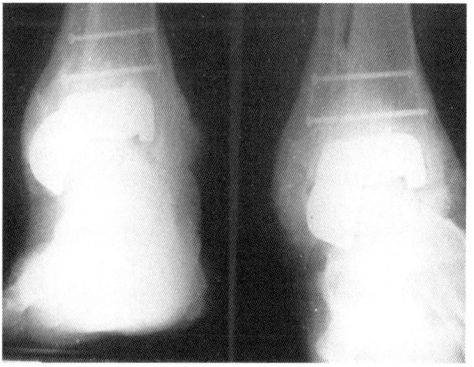

A   B

FIG 1 **A.** Lateral radiograph demonstrating avascular necrosis and infection of the talar body after open fracture-dislocation. **B.** Radiographs of a failed total ankle arthroplasty with severe loss of talar bone stock.

PREPARATION FOR ALLOGRAFT[4]

- A 12- to 14-cm lateral incision is made along the distal fibula, starting 6 cm above the ankle joint and extending distally along the anterior border of the peroneal tendons to the peroneal tubercle **(TECH FIG 1A)**.
- The tendons are carefully retracted posteriorly to expose the distal fibula, lateral ankle, and subtalar joints.
- The fibula is osteotomized 6 cm above the joint (or as high as necessary to allow placement of the blade or locking plate on the tibia) and then excised and morcellized for later grafting **(TECH FIG 1B)**.
- Débridement of avascular bone and removal of osteophytes or implant are performed until only viable bone surfaces remain (ie, distal tibial plafond, talar head and neck, and posterior facet of the subtalar joint).
- Determine the size of acetabular reamer from the total hip arthroplasty set that best fits the defect **(TECH FIG 1C)**.

- Only enough subchondral bone is removed from the tibia, talar neck, and calcaneus to expose viable, softer cancellous bone for fusion to the femoral head graft.
  - If an assistant holds the foot and ankle in the desired position, the surgeon can ream the defect safely, without the ankle bouncing around.
  - No provisional fixation is necessary: The ankle is still relatively stable even after the ankle implant or necrotic bone is removed.
- With the ankle and hindfoot held in neutral, the defect is reamed **(TECH FIG 1D)**. The desired position of fusion is with the ankle in neutral plantar-/dorsiflexion and the hindfoot in approximately 5 degrees of valgus in relation to the distal tibia.
- It is critical to protect the soft tissue about the ankle with either Army-Navy or Hohmann retractors while the acetabular reamers are used.
  - Bone shavings are saved and mixed with the morcellized fibular graft.

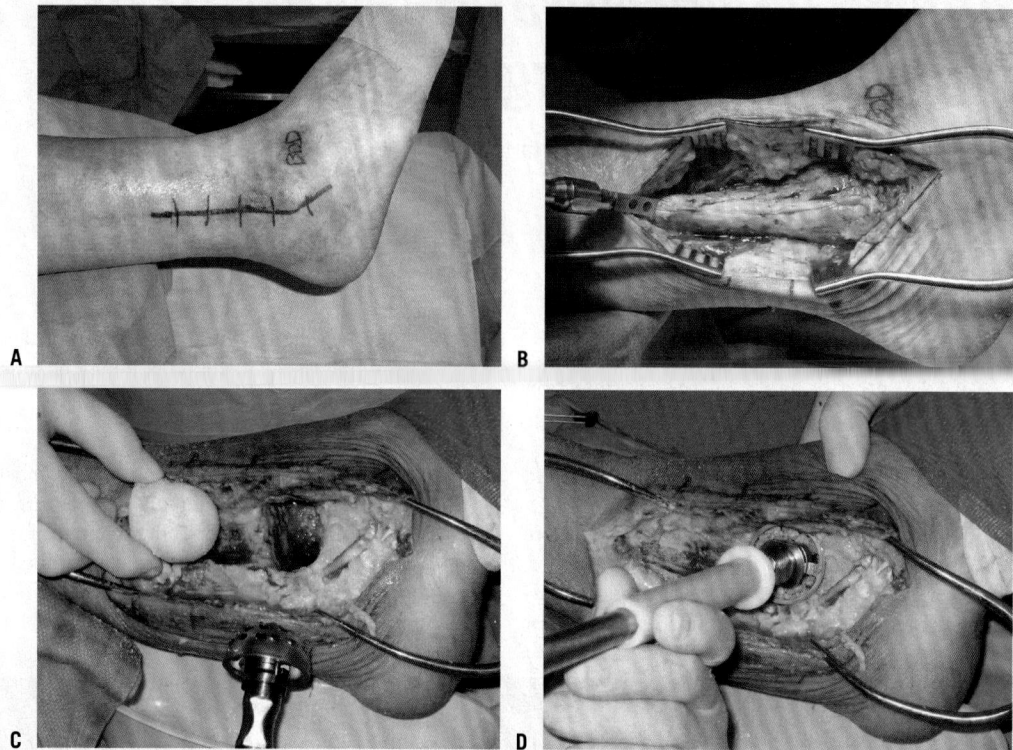

TECH FIG 1 A. Patient positioned supine on the operating table. A lateral incision is made over the distal fibula and lateral hindfoot. **B.** A fibulectomy is performed to expose the ankle and subtalar joints and lateral calcaneus. **C.** The defect remaining after talectomy is sized with the male reamers from the hip arthroplasty set. **D.** The bone surrounding the defect is reamed until cancellous bone is exposed on the distal tibia, talar neck, and calcaneus.

PREPARATION AND PLACEMENT OF ALLOGRAFT[4]

- An allograft femoral head is thawed in a warm saline bath at the beginning of the procedure and placed in the bone vice (Allogrip Bone Vise, [Synthes DePuy, Warsaw, IN]), with the three limbs of the vice gripping the femoral neck.
- The female reamer corresponding to the same size male reamer used for reaming the defect is used to decorticate the allograft.
  - It is optimal to ream only 2 or 3 mm of bone from the head to avoid significantly weakening the compressive strength of the graft **(TECH FIG 2A–C)**.
- The head can be drilled multiple times in areas that still contain hard sclerotic bone to facilitate fusion.
- The appropriately sized and decorticated femoral head allograft is then placed in the defect **(TECH FIG 2D)**.
  - Ankle and foot position is then checked for neutral position (ie, neutral ankle dorsiflexion–plantarflexion, 5 degrees of hindfoot valgus, and neutral rotation of the foot on the tibia). Because the femoral head graft is spherical, it

is relatively easy to dial in the correct position of the ankle and hindfoot.
- The femoral neck is marked flush with the lateral tibia, the graft is removed, and the femoral neck is cut with a large oscillating saw.
- A bone slurry graft, made up of the autograft from the fibula and male reamers, is then placed in the defect to fill any voids around the fusion site **(TECH FIG 2E)**.
- The male reamers can again be placed and used in reverse to evenly spread the graft.
- The femoral head graft is placed back in the defect, and alignment is checked to ensure that it sits flush with the lateral fusion surface.
  - Again, no provisional fixation is needed, as the interference fit between the femoral head and the recipient site is very stable.
  - This will allow unimpeded placement of the lateral plate or intramedullary fusion rod.

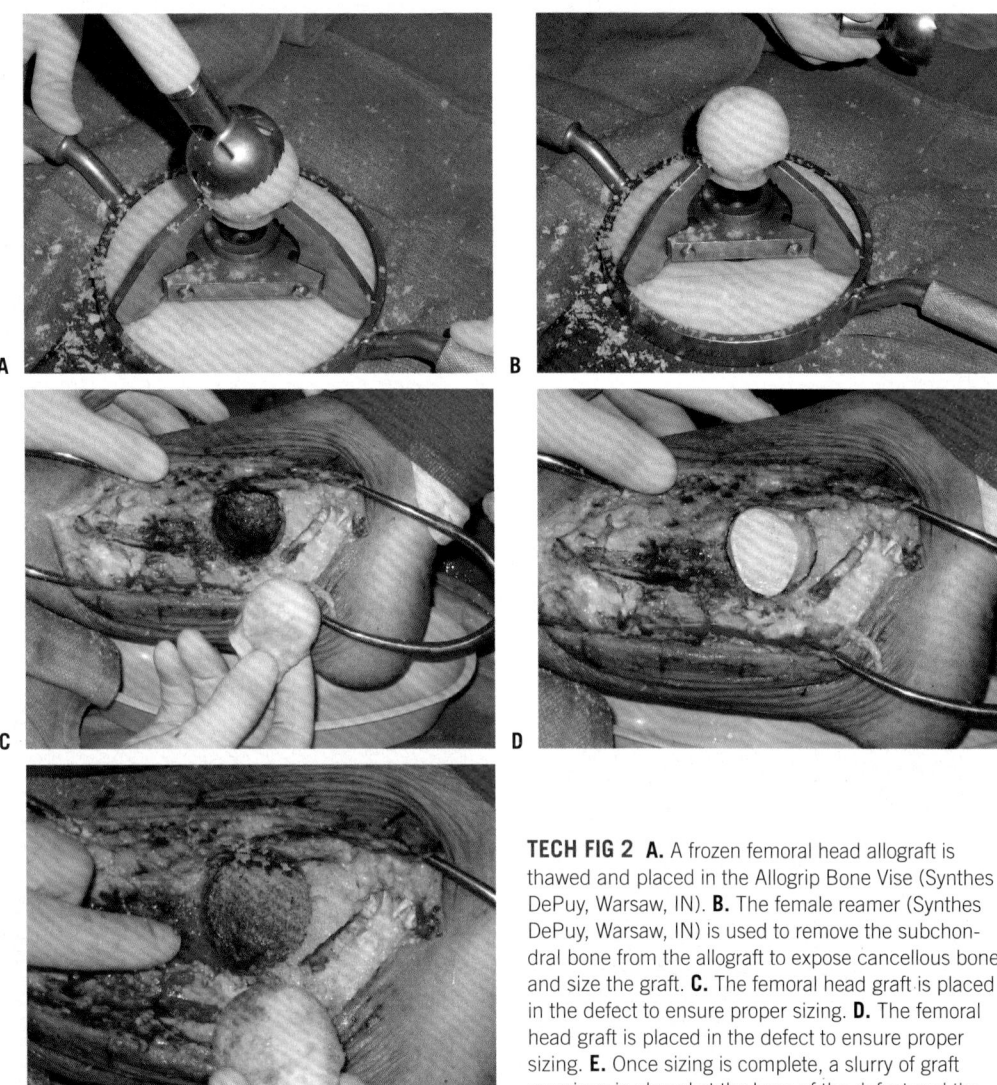

TECH FIG 2 A. A frozen femoral head allograft is thawed and placed in the Allogrip Bone Vise (Synthes DePuy, Warsaw, IN). **B.** The female reamer (Synthes DePuy, Warsaw, IN) is used to remove the subchondral bone from the allograft to expose cancellous bone and size the graft. **C.** The femoral head graft is placed in the defect to ensure proper sizing. **D.** The femoral head graft is placed in the defect to ensure proper sizing. **E.** Once sizing is complete, a slurry of graft reamings is placed at the base of the defect and the reamers placed in reverse to spread the graft.

PLACEMENT OF PLATE AND SCREWS[4]

- The 90-degree blade plate is then sized by placing it along the lateral fusion surface equidistant between the anterior and posterior surfaces of the tibia and femoral head graft.
- In my experience, fixation with six to eight cortical screws in the tibia proximal to the femoral head allograft is desirable; therefore, a blade plate of appropriate length is required. The decision depends on the quality of bone.
  - Typically, for six cortical screws to be positioned in the tibia above the graft, a nine-hole blade plate will be needed.
- The distal end of the plate (the blade end) should line up with the center of the calcaneal body to ensure maximum hold and minimize the chance of fracturing the calcaneus with insertion.
  - Usually, a six- to eight-hole plate with the short blade fits well.

- Once the plate size has been selected, place the plate "backward" along the lateral fusion area, so the blade is pointing lateral **(TECH FIG 3A)**. This technique allows for proper angle of insertion of the guidewire and, therefore, the blade of the plate.
- Check the hole alignment to ensure that at least one screw hole is over the calcaneus, one in the femoral head allograft, and two or three in the distal tibia.
- Drive the guidewire through the cannulated hole in the blade to the distal cortex of the calcaneus.
  - Pull the plate off the wire.
  - Because the plate could theoretically still rotate on the distal guide pin in the calcaneus, I often place a second wire through the plate. I use one of the screw holes proximally to

ensure that when I flip the plate and impact it, there is no chance that it will lose its desired proximal position on the tibia and potentially throw off the sagittal alignment or not be seated ideally on the tibia.

- Attach the driving device onto the plate and insert the blade plate over the guidewire **(TECH FIG 3B,C)**. The 30-mm blade is most commonly used because the 40-mm blade can easily penetrate the medial cortex and injure the neurovascular bundle.
  - Be sure to have an assistant apply counterpressure with a padded bolster while driving the plate into the calcaneus.
  - A separate guidewire driven through a proximal hole in the plate may help avoid unwanted twisting or rotation of the plate during insertion.
- Once the plate is seated, the position of the blade is checked to make sure it has not penetrated the medial cortex of the calcaneus. Again, if the 30-mm blade is used, penetration of the medial cortex should not occur.
- The screws (cancellous or cortical, depending on the type and quality of bone) are then inserted **(TECH FIG 3D)**. In addition to the blade in the calcaneus, I like to have one additional screw

through a distal hole in the plate, immediately above the blade, to enhance fixation in the calcaneus.

- A 7-mm cannulated screw is then placed from the posterolateral side of the distal tibia through the femoral head graft into the talar head and neck.
  - Fluoroscopy is used to check guidewire placement.
  - Avoid penetration into the talonavicular joint.
- A second cannulated screw can be placed from the calcaneal tuberosity into the femoral head graft if the blade plate fixation to the calcaneus is not stable, as indicated by visible micromotion at the fusion interface or if the patient's bone is osteoporotic. In about half of my patients, this second screw is needed to gain adequate stability of fixation.
- Use the remaining autograft to fill any remaining gaps at the fusion sites anteriorly, posteriorly, and laterally. It is helpful to use a high-speed burr to partially decorticate the anterior and posterior tibia, superior neck of the talus, and calcaneus before applying the bridge graft to better prepare the graft bed.
- A layered closure over a drain is done, and a bulky Jones dressing is applied.

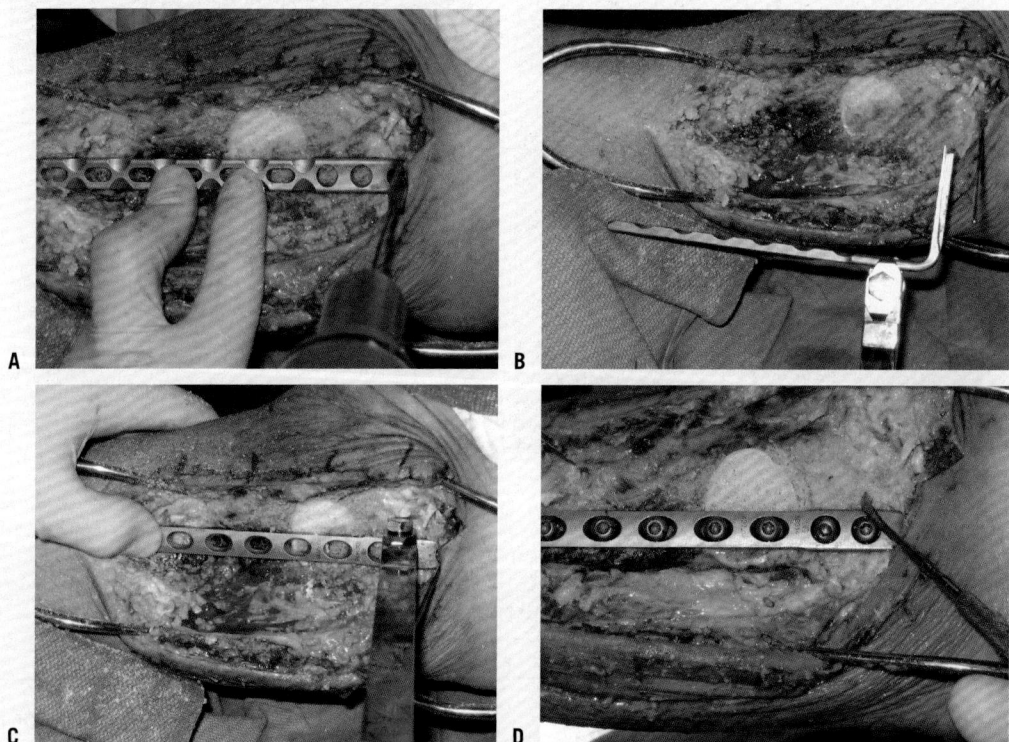

TECH FIG 3 A. The blade plate is placed in a backward position along the fusion site for sizing. A guidewire is passed through the hole in the blade into the calcaneus. **B.** The blade is pulled off the wire and the driving device attached. **C.** The blade is driven into the calcaneus over the guidewire. **D.** Appropriate length screws are applied.

LOCKING AND COMPRESSION PLATE TECHNIQUE[4]

- The contoured locking plate was applied to lateral tibial, femoral head, and calcaneal surfaces. Care is taken to excise the peroneal tubercle to allow better apposition of the plate to the lateral calcaneal bone surface. The alignment jig for the guidewire attached to the plate before the plate is positioned (**TECH FIG 4A**).
- The first compression screw (7 mm cannulated) is inserted over the guidewire placed by using the alignment jig and through the distal hole of the contoured plate (**TECH FIG 4B**).
- The screw threads should engage the metaphyseal flare of the medial tibia.

- Using a second guidewire jig, a second 7-mm cannulated lag screw is placed from the posterior inferior calcaneus through the graft into the metaphysis of the anterior distal tibia (**TECH FIG 4C,D**).
- The remaining screw holes are filled with either locking or nonlocking screws, depending on the need for rigidity of fixation (see **TECH FIG 4D**).
- The same bridge grafting technique is used as described earlier.
- Finalize the construct with completed screw placement (**TECH FIG 4E**).

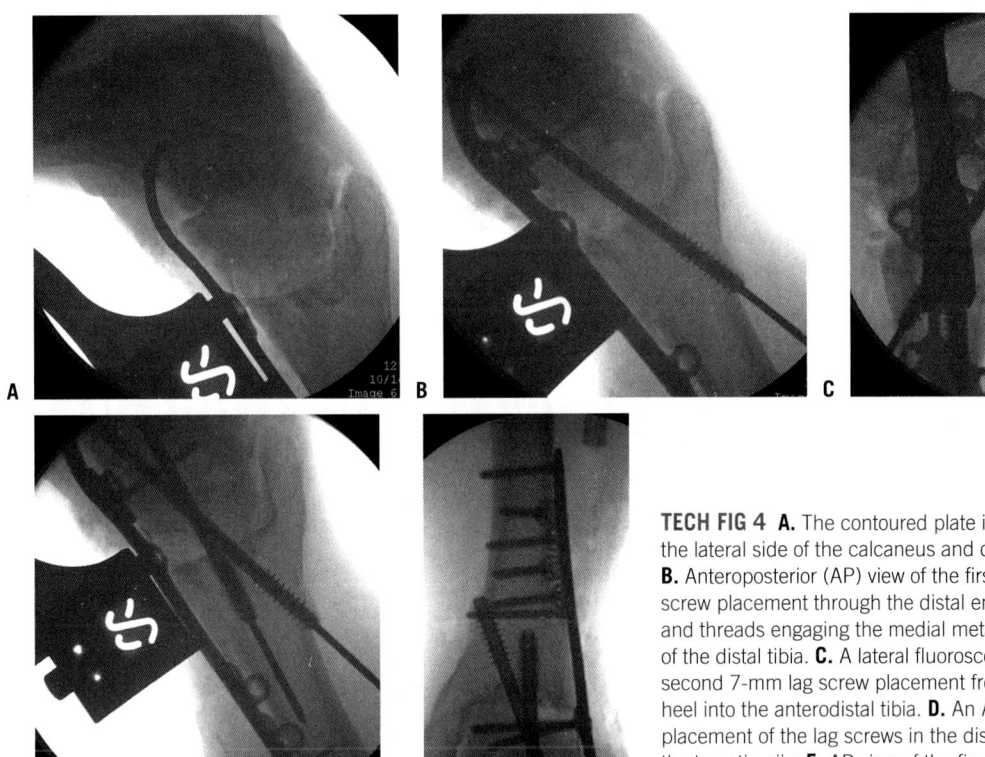

TECH FIG 4 A. The contoured plate is placed along the lateral side of the calcaneus and distal tibia. **B.** Anteroposterior (AP) view of the first 7-mm lag screw placement through the distal end on the plate and threads engaging the medial metaphyseal flare of the distal tibia. **C.** A lateral fluoroscopy view of the second 7-mm lag screw placement from the posterior heel into the anterodistal tibia. **D.** An AP view of the placement of the lag screws in the distal tibia using the targeting jig. **E.** AP view of the final construct with completed screw placement.

TECHNIQUES

POSTOPERATIVE CARE

- The bulky dressing is removed 10 to 14 days after surgery.
- The patient is in a short-leg cast for 6 to 8 weeks, with touchdown weight bearing permitted.
- The patient can begin weight bearing in a cam-soled walker at 2.5 to 3 months postoperatively if radiographs show signs of incorporation of the bone graft placed about the femoral head and fusion between the graft and the surrounding cancellous bone (**FIG 2A,B**).
- A computed tomography (CT) scan is recommended at 3 months postoperatively to assess the degree of spot welding of the fusion surfaces (**FIG 2C,D**).

- We recommend that all of our patients use a nonhinged, lightweight, plastic ankle–foot orthosis in a shoe with a soft anatomic cushioned heel indefinitely to protect the remaining joints of the foot.

OUTCOMES

- The lateral or anterior plate–screw construct for stabilizing tibiotalocalcaneal (TTC) fusions has been previously described as a method to gain exceptional stability in patients with Charcot ankle fracture who had unbraceable deformity and severe instability of the ankle.[1] This fixation construct has been found to be

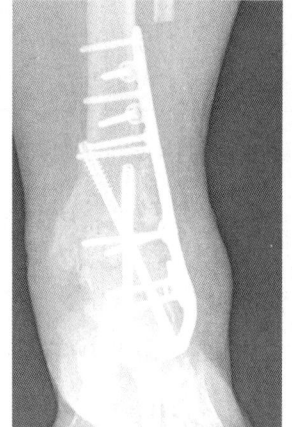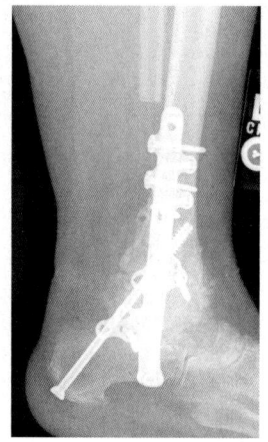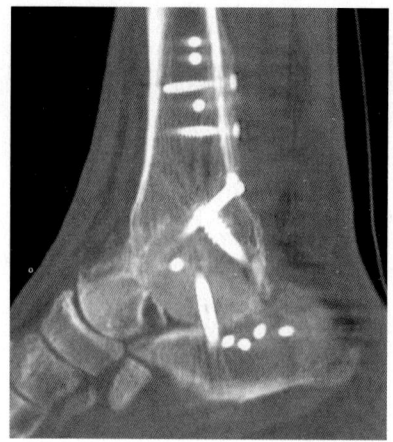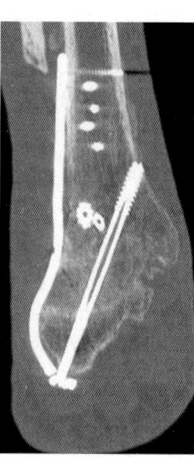

FIG 2 Patient in **TECH FIG 4** 3 months postoperatively. **A,B,** Radiographs showing progressive healing at the fusion sites. **C,D,** Sagittal and coronal CT scans, respectively, of the spot welding between the femoral head graft and the tibia, talus, and calcaneus at 3 months postoperatively.

biomechanically superior to an intramedullary rod for this type of fusion.[3]

- Myerson et al[6] have previously described the use of femoral head grafts through an anterior approach to fill large defects of the talar body. They have found them useful for filling large defects and avoiding severe limb shortening.
  - Jeng et al[5] reported a 50% nonunion rate with femoral head allograft, but this technique did not incorporate the use of a more stable locking plate.
  - Despite the high nonunion rate, most patients (70%) reported a significant improvement in pain and function.
  - High nonunion/collapse rates reported for bulk allografts (15% to 52%)[2]
- Our clinical results at Twin Cities Orthopedics as of year-end 2019 experience with 44 (43 patients) bulk allograft reconstructions of large talar defects for ankle or TTC fusion

with an anterior or lateral plate or TTC fusion intramedullary rod.

- All patients were followed for a minimum of 12 months postoperatively.
- Mean visual analog scale improved 66.4 to 28.7 ($P < .001$)
- Patients overly satisfied at latest follow-up at 80%
- Ninety percent of the bulk allografts healed.
- Of the five patients that didn't fuse, they underwent revision surgery at an average of twenty-four months (7.2 to 58.8 months) **(FIG 3)**.
- No significant difference in outcomes/fusions rates whether plates or rods were used.
- In all patients with rigid fixation and good apposition of fusion, surfaces with a successful bridge graft to reduce rotational, bending, and axial load on the bulk graft healed their fusions.

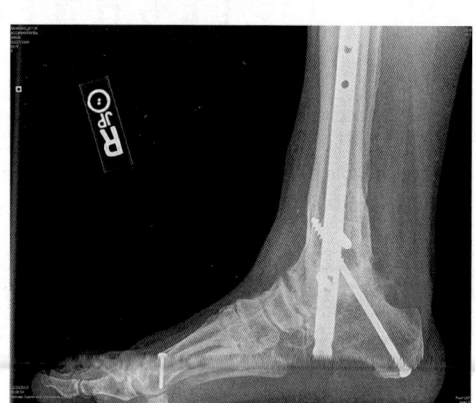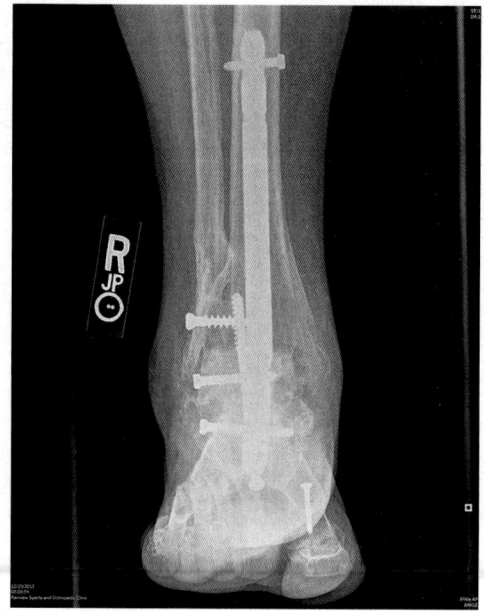

FIG 3 Revision of a failed total ankle arthroplasty with a femoral head bulk allograft and intramedullary rod. Lateral (**A**) and AP (**B**) views.

REFERENCES

1. Alvarez RG, Barbour TM, Perkins TD. Tibiocalcaneal arthrodesis for nonbraceable ankle deformity. Foot Ankle Int 1994;15:354–359.
2. Bussewitz B, DeVries JG, Dujela M, et al. Retrograde intramedullary nail with femoral head allograft for large deficit tibiotalocalcaneal arthrodesis. Foot Ankle Int 2014;35(7):706–711.
3. Chiodo CP, Acevedo JI, Sammarco VJ, et al. Intramedullary rod fixation compared with blade-plate-and-screw fixation for tibiocalcaneal arthrodesis: a biomechanical investigation. J Bone Joint Surg Am 2003;85(12):2425–2428.
4. Den Hartog BD, Palmer DS. Femoral head allografts for large talar defects. Tech Foot Ankle Surg 2008;7:264–270.
5. Jeng CL, Campbell JT, Tang EY, et al. Tibiotalocalcaneal arthrodesis with bulk femoral head allograft for salvage of large defects in the ankle. Foot Ankle Int 2013;34(9):1256–1266.
6. Myerson MS, Alvarez RG, Lam PW. Tibiocalcaneal arthrodesis for the management of severe ankle and hindfoot deformities. Foot Ankle Int 2000;21:643–650.

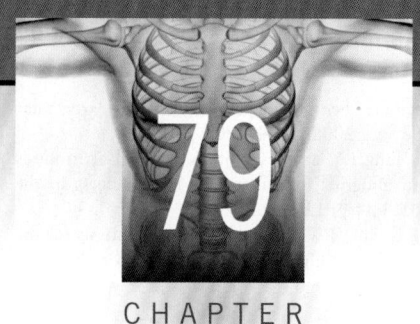

CHAPTER

79

Sports-Related Procedures for Ankle and Hindfoot
Arthroscopy of the Ankle

Jorge I. Acevedo and Peter Mangone

DEFINITION

- Arthroscopy of the ankle has become an invaluable tool for evaluating and treating pathology in the ankle joint.
- Arthroscopy allows a minimally invasive approach to the structures of the ankle with a magnified view.
- Detailed knowledge of the anatomy surrounding the ankle joint as well as the different structural variations is key to avoiding complications.

ANATOMY

- The anteromedial portal is located medial to the tibialis anterior tendon at the level of the ankle joint **(FIG 1)**. Care should be taken to avoid injury to the long saphenous vein and nerve usually located medial to the portal.
- The anterolateral portal lies on the anterior joint line just lateral to the peroneus tertius tendon or alternatively lateral to the extensor digitorum longus tendons. The intermediate cutaneous branch of the superficial peroneal nerve lies in close proximity to this portal.

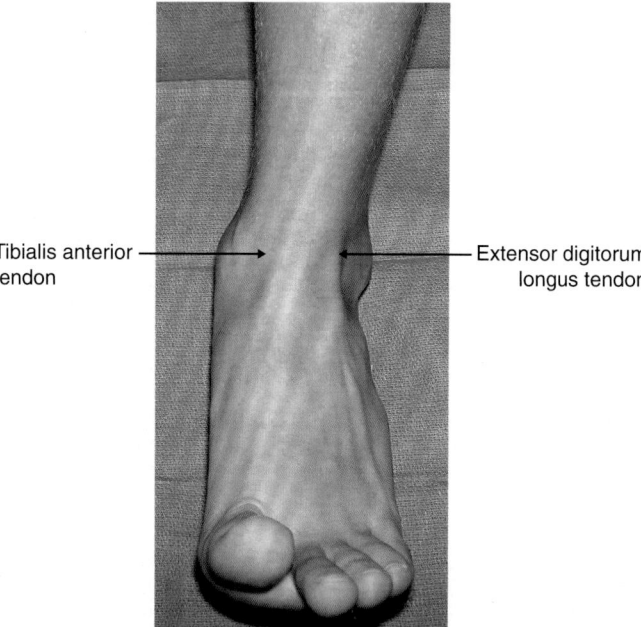

Tibialis anterior
tendon

Extensor digitorum
longus tendon

FIG 1 Anatomic landmarks for anterior ankle arthroscopy. At the joint line, the anteromedial portal is made immediately medial to the tibialis anterior tendon and the anterolateral portal is created lateral to the extensor digitorum longus tendon.

- Posteromedial and posterolateral coaxial portals lie parallel to the bimalleolar axis **(FIG 2A)**.
- The posterolateral coaxial portal **(FIG 2B)** is located immediately posterior to the peroneus longus tendon, and the posteromedial coaxial portal **(FIG 2C)** ideally lies between the posterior colliculus (of the medial malleolus) and the posterior tibial tendon. (Placement between the flexor digitorum longus and the posterior tibial tendon is also acceptable.)
- The sural nerve is located an average of 6.6 mm from this posterolateral portal, whereas the posterior tibial nerve is found an average of 5.7 mm from the posteromedial portal.
- For advanced arthroscopic ligament reconstruction, an anatomic safe zone exists between the intermediate branch of the superficial peroneal nerve and the sural nerve.

DIFFERENTIAL DIAGNOSIS

- Anterior ankle impingement
- Ankle arthritis or arthrofibrosis
- Osteochondral tibial or talar defects
- Lateral ankle instability
- Ankle fractures
- Recalcitrant ankle synovitis (often seen in patients with systemic inflammatory disease)

NONOPERATIVE MANAGEMENT

- In general, conservative treatment will include a trial with activity modification, immobilization with a brace, and nonsteroidal anti-inflammatory drugs.
- Physical therapy using modality treatment, range-of-motion exercises, neuromuscular coordination training (eg, balance board), and strengthening of the secondary or dynamic stabilizing muscles surrounding the ankle is a useful adjunct to most conditions.

SURGICAL MANAGEMENT

Preoperative Planning

- Imaging studies are reviewed to determine ideal portals to be used.
- Standard anteromedial and anterolateral portals are sufficient to access the anterior and central tibiotalar pathology.
- Posterior portals are considered when drilling posterior talar lesions or when it is necessary to address pathology (eg, synovitis, loose bodies) within the posterior capsule.
- A preoperative popliteal block may be placed by anesthesia. Over the past 10 years, we have been able to perform 75%

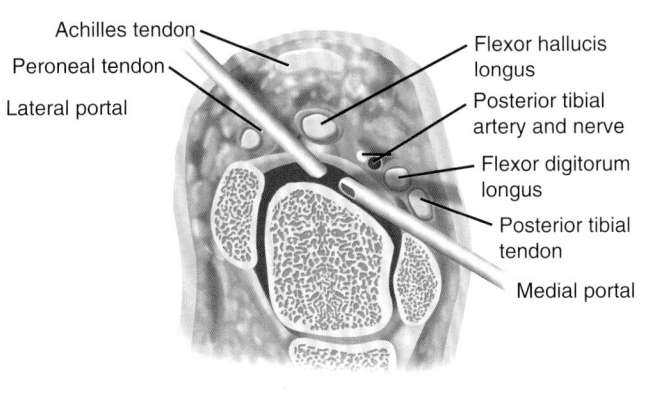

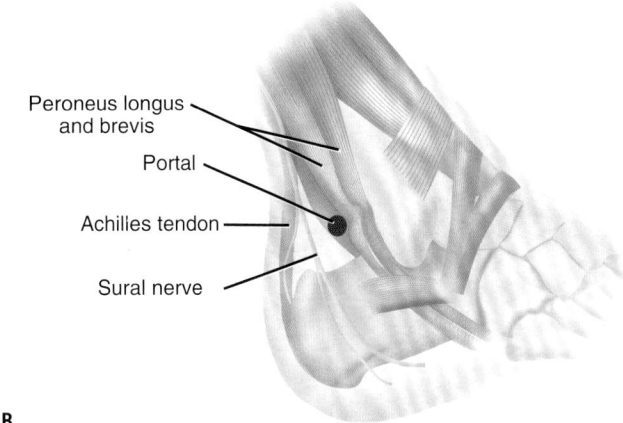

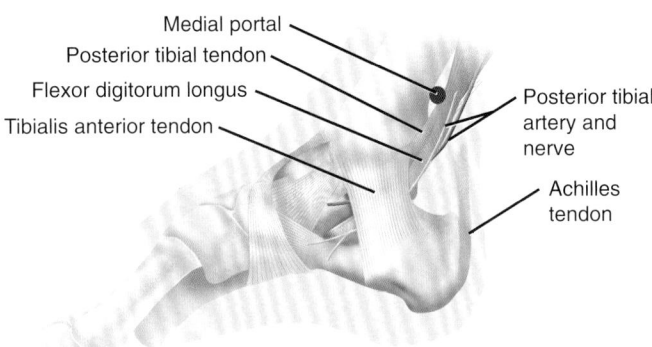

FIG 2 Coaxial portal anatomy: cross-sectional (**A**), posterolateral (**B**), and posteromedial (**C**).

of ankle arthroscopies with regional anesthesia and light sedation.

- An examination under anesthesia including anterior drawer as well as a talar tilt test should be performed before positioning.
- Examination under anesthesia is extremely helpful in determining the degree of medial and lateral instability, and thus, stabilization procedure will suffice.

Positioning

- The patient is placed on a regular operating table with a well-padded tourniquet on the proximal thigh.

- The supine position with a towel roll placed underneath the ankle is used when only anterior portals are necessary. In this situation, the tourniquet may be placed on the proximal calf.
- If access to posterior portals is likely, then we lower the leg extension of the bed and use a standard arthroscopy knee holder (**FIG 3A**). This restricts thigh motion but allows free leg motion and access to the posterior hindfoot (**FIG 3B**). The contralateral leg is placed in a well-padded holder or pillow (**FIG 3C**).
- Alternatively, a noninvasive ankle distractor is used with a triangle bump or thigh holder to maintain knee flexed (see Ankle Distractor Placement section or **TECH FIG 3**).

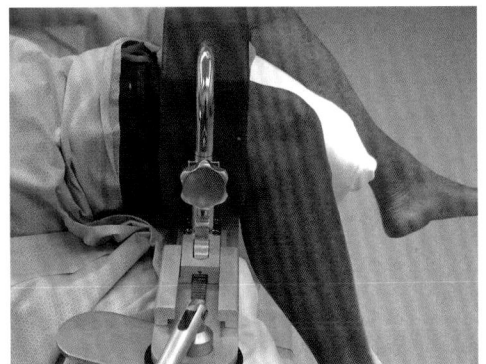

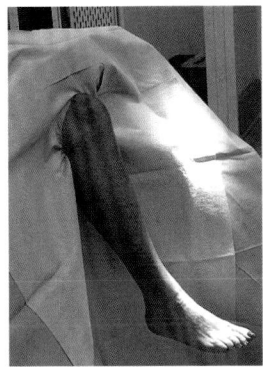

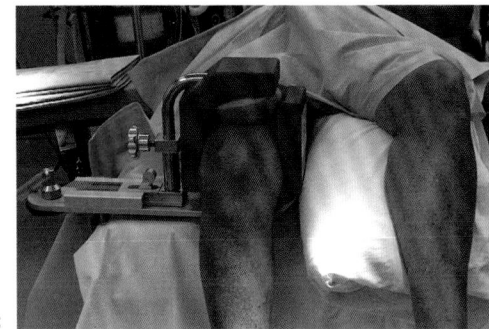

FIG 3 **A,B.** Leg holder and bed positions, respectively, for posterior portal access. **C.** Position of operative leg and padded contralateral limb.

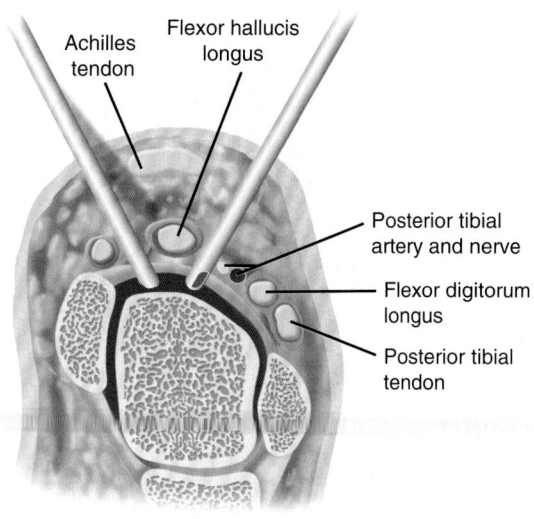

Achilles tendon

Flexor hallucis longus

Posterior tibial artery and nerve

Flexor digitorum longus

Posterior tibial tendon

FIG 4 Conventional posterior portal cross-sectional anatomy.

Approach

- The standard working approaches are the anteromedial and anterolateral portals.
- Auxiliary anterior portals (such as the anterocentral) should be used with caution because of the high incidence of neurovascular injury.
- The standard posteromedial and posterolateral portals should also be used with extreme caution due to the close proximity of neurovascular structures **(FIG 4)**.
- We prefer to use posterior coaxial portals parallel to the bimalleolar axis when addressing the posterior ankle joint.
- Although the standard 4-mm arthroscope may be used, we prefer to use 2.7-mm arthroscopic instruments, which facilitate access and simplify the approach to the anterior ankle.
- Instruments usually include 2.5 mm shaver, 2.5 mm shaver, thermal ablation device (this is especially helpful for synovectomy and débridement of the joint; however, care must be taken to avoid articular cartilage damage), and small arthroscopic biter and grabber devices.
- When addressing posterior tibiotalar pathology, endoscopic portals are used with the patient in the prone position (see Chap. FA-82).
- The 4-mm arthroscope offers a larger field of view and is preferred for posterior endoscopy.

ANTERIOR PORTAL PLACEMENT

- Preoperatively, the operative leg is identified and marked as well as washed with antiseptic scrub brush.
- The patient is placed supine on the operating table.
- Surgical timeout is performed.
- Inject the ankle with 10 mL of sterile saline via the anteromedial ankle. This step also allows identification of the correct orientation and location for the anteromedial arthroscopy portal.
- Make a 5-mm vertical skin incision and spread the subcutaneous tissue down to and then through the capsule with a small hemostat. A small gush of fluid confirms the intra-articular location.
- Use the blunt-tip trocar with the arthroscopic cannula to enter the joint. Insert the arthroscope, and start the water flow. Place the water pressure at about 35 mm Hg. This significantly reduces bleeding, which often obscures the view.

- Unless there is severe arthrofibrotic tissue in the anterior ankle, the anterolateral ankle is easily visualized upon introducing the arthroscope **(TECH FIG 1)**.
- Introduce an 18-gauge needle from the anterolateral portal location. This serves two purposes: (1) It allows for water flow through the needle, allowing for better visualization, and (2) it identifies the correct location of the portal incision in order to access the joint properly.
- Inspect the joint. Distraction allows for much greater joint inspection than otherwise would be possible.
- Make the anterolateral portal in a similar fashion to the anteromedial portal just lateral to the peroneus tertius (safest location).
- Using both portals, various arthroscopic instruments are used to address the individual patient's pathology.

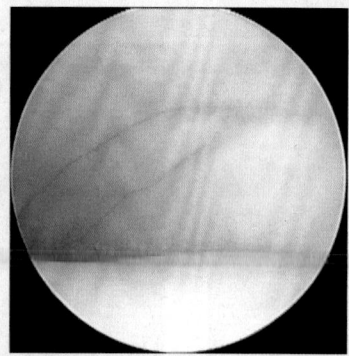
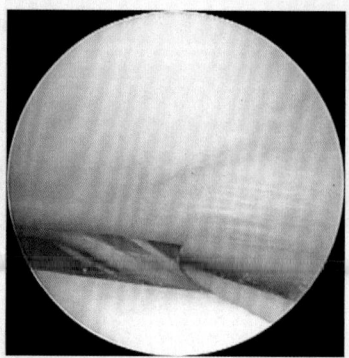

A   B

TECH FIG 1 View of anterolateral (**A**) and posterolateral (**B**) gutter using simple distraction with towel roll underneath ankle.

TECHNIQUES

- The addition of an anteromedial inferior portal is helpful when dealing with synovitis near the deltoid insertion.
  - This is performed by visualizing the medial gutter with the arthroscope through the anteromedial portal.
  - An 18-gauge needle is introduced under arthroscopic visualization into the inferior medial gutter (usually about 10 mm inferior to the normal anteromedial portal location).

- Once the needle is confirmed to be in the proper position, a new portal is then made as described earlier.
- This portal, in combination with the conventional anteromedial portal, can be used to first inspect and then débride the far inferomedial ankle joint and deltoid insertion.

POSTERIOR COAXIAL PORTALS

- With the arthroscope and inflow in the anterolateral portal, make the posterolateral portal with a small, vertical skin incision immediately posterior to the peroneal tendon sheath and 1.5 cm proximal to the tip of the fibula **(TECH FIG 2A)**.
- While holding the ankle in neutral dorsiflexion, insert the arthroscopic sheath and blunt trocar anterior and slightly inferior on a plane parallel to the bimalleolar axis.
  - Confirm intracapsular placement by briefly inserting the arthroscope.
- Insert a long switching rod through the cannula and direct it toward the medial malleolus.
  - Use the rod to palpate the posterior colliculus and penetrate just anterior to the posterior tibial tendon **(TECH FIG 2B)**.

- Tent and incise the skin over the posteromedial ankle. Subsequently, pass a second cannula over the switching stick into the posterior ankle recess.
- Alternatively, the medial portal can be made directly using a small, vertical skin incision posterior to the medial malleolus (posterior colliculus).
  - The arthroscopic sheath and blunt trocar are inserted anterior and slightly inferior on a plane parallel to the bimalleolar axis. Intracapsular placement is confirmed by briefly inserting the arthroscope **(TECH FIG 2C–F)**.
- For synovectomies or posteromedial osteochondral lesions, the arthroscope is placed in the posterolateral cannula while the posteromedial cannula is used as the working portal.

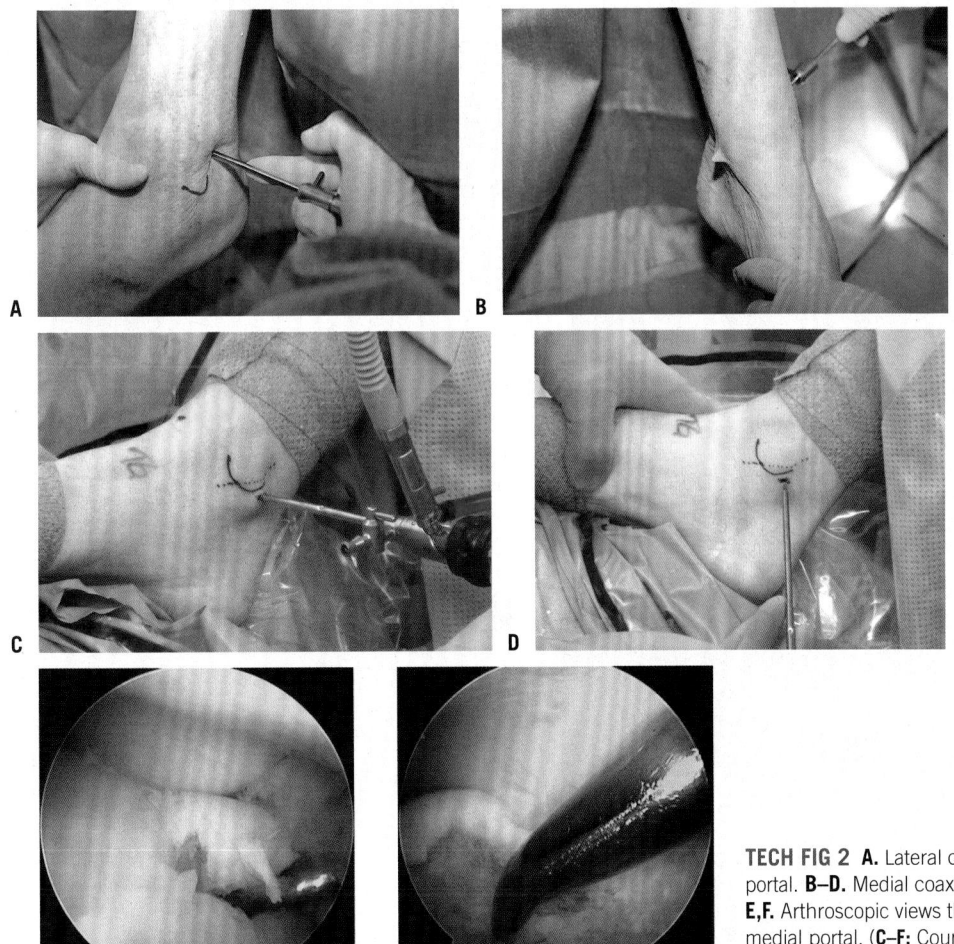

TECH FIG 2 A. Lateral coaxial portal. **B–D.** Medial coaxial portal. **E,F.** Arthroscopic views through medial portal. (**C–F:** Courtesy of M. T. Busch, MD.)

TECHNIQUES

ANKLE DISTRACTOR PLACEMENT

- Inspect all instruments and confirm that all parts of the noninvasive external distractor are sterile and on the operative field **(TECH FIG 3A)**.
- The patient is placed supine on the operating table so the foot rests within 10 cm of the end of the bed.
- A bump (made from a rolled blanket) is placed under the hip to rotate the leg so the toes point straight up.
- A tourniquet is placed on the calf below the level of the fibular head to prevent peroneal nerve impingement **(TECH FIG 3B)**.
- The hip is flexed 60 degrees, and the posterior thigh is placed in a padded thigh holder and secured with straps.
  - It is important that the thigh holder be placed so that the leg rests in the holder and does not rest in the popliteal fossa. If the thigh holder rests in the popliteal fossa, the pressure on the popliteal vein will increase bleeding throughout the case and make arthroscopic visualization much more difficult.
  - With limited pressure on the popliteal space, the tourniquet is rarely needed during the arthroscopic portion of the case **(TECH FIG 3C)**.
- The operative leg and ankle region are prepared and then draped using a standard arthroscopy drape.
- The distal portion of the arthroscopy drape is pulled off the end of the foot to allow for the distractor placement.

- The bed clamp is placed as far distal on the bed as possible. For the clamp to fit properly, the circulating nurse should make sure all of the underlying drapes except the top layer are moved away from the clamp attachment site **(TECH FIG 3D)**.
- The external distractor strap is placed with the foam portions over the posterior inferior heel and on the dorsal foot. After creating equal lengths on the medial and lateral sides of the foot, the hook–loop is pulled distally with manual distraction.
- The L-shaped metal post is placed and secured.
- The foot is then pulled manually via the strap and connected to the threaded attachment rod.
  - We recommend the initial placement requires moderate effort to get the hook–loop secured so that initial manual distraction provides most of the distraction.
  - Once this is connected, use the threaded rod to provide further distraction to the ankle **(TECH FIG 3E)**.
- The joint can be flexed or extended while in the distraction device to allow for complete evaluation of the joint.
- Some cases of pure anterior pathology can be performed with either minimal or no ankle distraction using a towel roll underneath the ankle. However, one must be careful when introducing the trocar and dorsiflex the ankle to avoid damaging the articular cartilage of the talus.

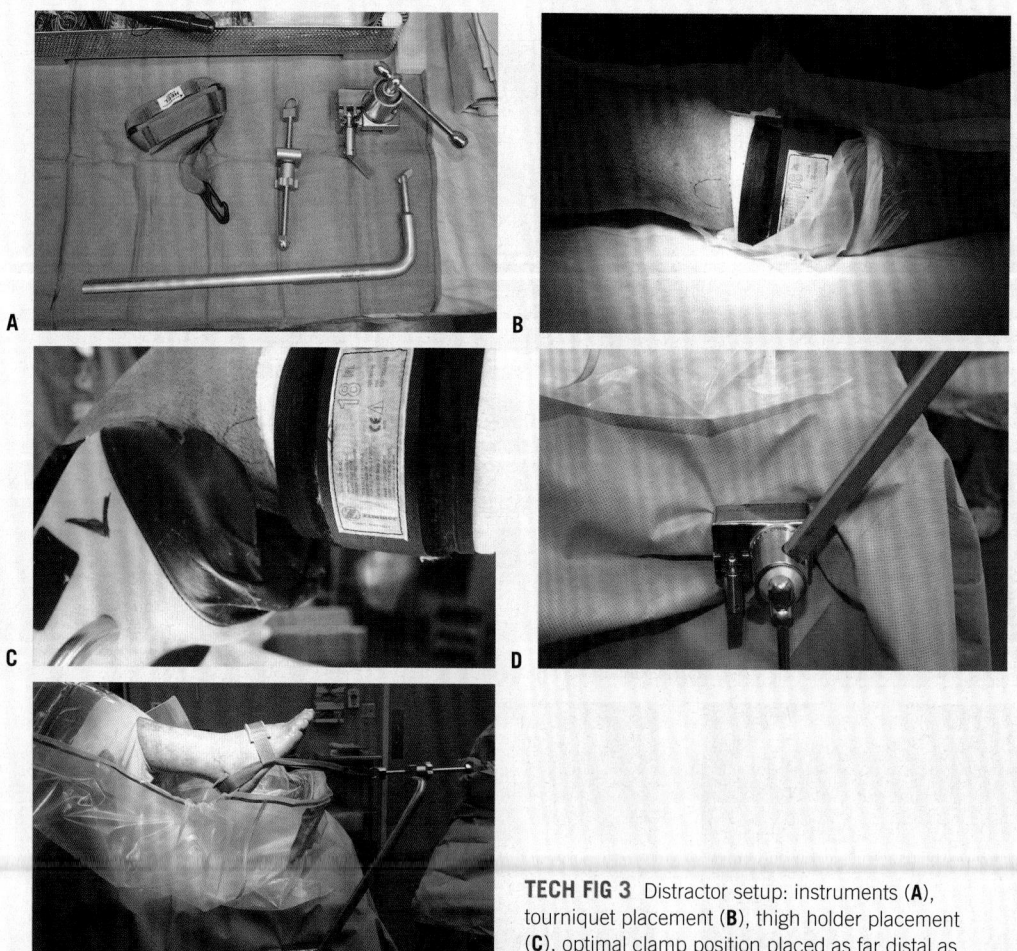

TECH FIG 3 Distractor setup: instruments (**A**), tourniquet placement (**B**), thigh holder placement (**C**), optimal clamp position placed as far distal as possible (**D**), and final ankle setup with manual tensioning (**E**).

Pearls and Pitfalls

Indications	• Careful analysis of preoperative films will allow proper planning of necessary portals (anterior only vs. both anterior and posterior).
Coaxial Portal Placement	• Spread soft tissues laterally directly behind the peroneals to avoid sural nerve injury. • Palpate the posterior colliculus medially with a switching stick before penetrating between the posterior tibial tendon and medial malleolus. • Occasionally, the medial coaxial portal will occur between the posterior tibial tendon and the flexor digitorum longus. • Avoid forceful medial penetration, which can result in tendon splitting. • When exposing the medial portal directly, posteromedial skin incision lies along the course of the posterior tibial tendon behind the posterior colliculus. The posterior tibial tendon can be retracted anteriorly or posteriorly to visualize bulging capsule.
Additional Equipment Needed for Posterior Portals	• One additional scope cannula with inflow port (total of two scope cannulas) • Small (about 2.5 mm) blunt-tip switching stick
Intra-articular Confirmation	• After joint injection, several factors indicate intra-articular placement: (1) inflow of saline without resistance, (2) ballooning of the anterolateral joint capsule, and (3) passive dorsiflexion of the ankle with insufflation of the joint.
Limiting Time Needed for Tourniquet Using Ankle Distraction	• Care should be taken to avoid thigh holder placement such that direct pressure occurs into the popliteal space when distraction is applied. Direct pressure in the popliteal space decreases outflow through the popliteal vein and will increase venous pressure and intra-articular bleeding. • Limit distraction time (<2 hours with <23-kg force) to avoid complications.
Arthroscopic Ankle Fracture Management	• Use conventional anteromedial and anterolateral portals. • Assess for osteochondral lesions. • Direct evaluation of syndesmotic instability • Allows direct assessment of deltoid ligament injury and medial gutter • Allows direct visualization of fracture reduction

Arthroscopic Lateral Ligament Reconstruction	• ArthroBrostrom technique: Use standard anterior portals.
	   • Other techniques require accessory anterolateral portal.
	   • May decrease operative time
	   • Biomechanically equivalent to open techniques
	   • Follow anatomic safe zones **(FIG 5)**.

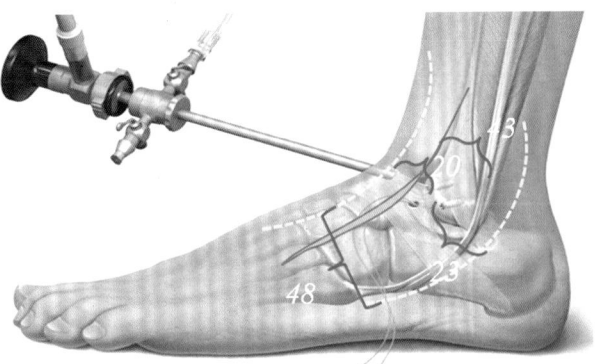

FIG 5 ArthroBrostrom safe zones (mean distances): internervous safe zone = 51 mm, intertendinous safe zone = 43 mm; medial suture to superficial peroneal nerve = 20 mm; inferior suture to sural nerve = 23 mm; and inferior suture to peroneal tendons = 19 mm. *Yellow dashed lines* indicate SPN and sural nerves.

"Don'ts"	• Avoid the following:
	   • Prolonged distraction or tourniquet use
	   • Sharp trocars
	   • Intra-articular bupivacaine (chondrotoxic)
	   • Immediate mobilization (immobilize 1–2 weeks)
	   • Surgical tape strips for wound closure

POSTOPERATIVE CARE

- For most conditions addressed with ankle arthroscopy, patients are placed in a well-padded short-leg splint.
  - Five to 7 days postoperatively, the splint is removed and patients are allowed weight bearing as tolerated in a brace.
- In cases in which drilling, microfracture, or retrograde bone grafting of an osteochondral lesion is performed, a period of non–weight bearing is emphasized.
- Early range of motion after 1 to 2 weeks of immobilization is always encouraged unless a fusion is performed.

OUTCOMES

- Ankle arthroscopy allows the surgeon to address a myriad pathology with a minimally invasive technique.
  - Success of outcomes varies according to underlying pathology but is generally in the range of 85% good to excellent.
- The complication rate ranges from 0.7% to 17%, with neurologic injuries accounting for most of these problems.
  - The superficial peroneal nerve is the most commonly injured nerve, followed by the sural nerve and then the saphenous nerve.
- In one study using the posterior coaxial portals in 29 ankles, no complications were observed at an average 45 months of follow-up.

COMPLICATIONS

- Neurovascular injury
- Cartilage damage
- Reflex sympathetic dystrophy
- Sinus tract formation
- Infection
- Skin necrosis

SUGGESTED READINGS

Acevedo JI, Busch MT, Ganey TM, et al. Coaxial portals for posterior ankle arthroscopy: an anatomic study with clinical correlation on 29 patients. Arthroscopy 2000;16(8):836–842.

Acevedo JI, Mangone PG. Arthroscopic lateral ankle ligament reconstruction. Tech Foot Ankle Surg 2011;10(3):111–116.

Acevedo JI, Ortiz C, Golano P, et al. ArthroBrostrom lateral ankle stabilization technique: an anatomical study. Am J Sports Med 2015;43(10):2564–2571.

Corte-Real NM, Moreira RM. Arthroscopic repair of chronic lateral ankle instability. Foot Ankle Int 2009;30(3):213–217.

Drakos M, Behrens SB, Mulcahey MK, et al. Proximity of arthroscopic ankle stabilization procedures to surrounding structures: an anatomic study. Arthroscopy 2013;29(6):1089–1094.

Ferkel RD, Heath DD, Guhl JF. Neurological complications of ankle arthroscopy. Arthroscopy 1996;12(2):200–208.

Ferkel RD, Hewitt M. Long-term results of arthroscopic ankle arthrodesis. Foot Ankle Int 2005;26(1):275–280.

Giza E, Shin EC, Wong S, et al. Arthroscopic suture anchor repair of the lateral ligament ankle complex: a cadaveric study. Am J Sports Med 2013;41(11):2567–2572.

Golanó P, Vega J, Pérez-Carro L, et al. Ankle anatomy for the arthroscopist. Part I: the portals. Foot Ankle Clin 2006;11(2):253–273.

Lui TH, Chan WK, Chan KB. The arthroscopic management of frozen ankle. Arthroscopy 2006;22(3):283–286.

Maiotti M, Massoni C, Tarantino U. The use of arthroscopic thermal shrinkage to treat chronic lateral ankle instability in young athletes. Arthroscopy 2005;21:751–757.

Nihal A, Rose DJ, Trepman E. Arthroscopic treatment of anterior ankle impingement syndrome in dancers. Foot Ankle Int 2005;26:908–912.

Sim J, Lee B, Kwak J. New posteromedial portal for ankle arthroscopy. Arthroscopy 2006;22:799.e1–799.e2.

Vega J, Dalmau-Pastor M, Malagelada F, et al. Ankle arthroscopy: an update. J Bone Joint Surg Am 2017;99(16):1395–1407.

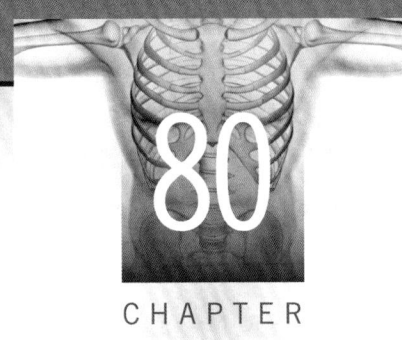

80
CHAPTER

Microfracture for Osteochondral Lesions of the Talus:
Perspective 1

Hajo Thermann and Christoph Becher

DEFINITION

- The terminology of osteochondral lesions is not uniform. Transchondral fractures, osteochondral fractures, flake fractures, or osteochondritis dissecans are used to describe the same entity.
- Osteochondral lesions are characterized by aseptic separation of a fragment of articular cartilage, with or without attached subchondral bone.
- The causes for osteochondral lesions of the talus remain controversial. The most important distinction to make is if the lesion is acute or chronic.

ANATOMY

- The talar body is trapezoidal in shape. The anterior surface is on average 2.5 mm wider than the posterior surface. The dome is covered by the articular surface, which articulates with the tibial plafond. The medial and lateral facet articulate with the medial and lateral malleoli.
  - Approximately 60% of the talar surface is covered by articular cartilage.
  - Most of the blood supply enters through the neck of the talus via the sinus tarsi.
- Biomechanical studies have shown that the talar cartilage is softest at the posteromedial part, whereas the maximum thickness is found at the posterolateral corner. The tibial cartilage is 18% to 37% stiffer than the corresponding sites on the talus.[2]

PATHOGENESIS

- Lateral lesions are most frequently caused by acute trauma. Common mechanism is a dorsiflexed ankle forced to inversion. This results in impaction of the talus on the fibula.
  - Lateral lesions are located more commonly in the anterior part of the talar dome.
  - They tend to be shallower than medial lesions.
- Medial lesions are often associated with repetitive traumatic events and chronic instability. Impaction of the medial talus on the tibia with a plantarflexed ankle forced to inversion and external rotation is regarded the etiologic mechanism.
  - Medial lesions are more common than lateral lesions and occur mostly in the middle or posterior third of the talus.
  - These lesions appear cup shaped and deeper than lateral lesions.
- Traumatic events appear to compromise perfusion in respected parts of the talus with subsequent separation of an osteochondral fragment. Other proposed mechanisms are genetic predisposition and endogenous factors. Medial

lesions are often detected bilaterally, often by coincidence after an ankle sprain.

NATURAL HISTORY

- Many chronic lesions are detected by coincidence after acute ankle distortion traumas that have been asymptomatic for many years.
- Other than in osteochondral lesions in the knee, the natural history of degenerative joint disease after osteochondral lesions of the talus has not been defined. No evidence exists that untreated lesions will subsequently result in osteoarthritis of the ankle.
- McCullough and Venugopal[12] found that in five of six patients treated conservatively for osteochondritis dissecans tali, radiologic assessment showed that the lesion had failed to heal, but nevertheless in each instance, the ankle joint was relatively asymptomatic after a mean period of follow-up of 15 years and 11 months (range, 7 to 28 years).

PATIENT HISTORY AND PHYSICAL EXAMINATION FINDINGS

- Acute lesions have to be ruled out after traumatic events when an osteochondral lesion is suspected.
- In most cases, patients complain about chronic ankle pain on or after activity. Swelling and stiffness are frequently accompanied with the pain. Other symptoms include catching, locking, and giving way.
- The severity of symptoms may not be related to the severity of the lesion.
- Physical examination is relatively unspecific in osteochondral lesions of the talus.
  - By having the patient plantarflex the foot and ankle, the anterior parts of the talar dome can be palpated at the anteromedial and anterolateral joint space. Tenderness in the specific area may indicate an osteochondral lesion.
  - Tenderness behind the medial malleolus by having the patient dorsiflex the ankle may indicate a posteromedial lesion.
  - Range of motion (ROM) of the ankle is tested with the knee flexed to eliminate restriction by shortened flexor muscles. ROM is often limited in because of synovitis and effusion.
- The examination should also include evaluation of associated pathology and ruling out differential diagnosis.
  - Osseous structures, tendons, ligaments and soft tissue structures should be palpated to discern tenderness of the specific anatomic part.

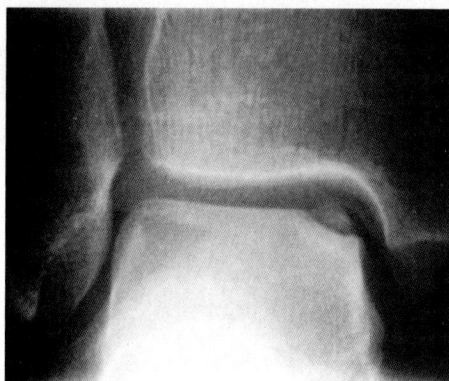

FIG 1 Osteochondral lesion stage III following Berndt and Harty classification.

- Ligamentous instability or laxity is assessed with the anterior drawer test and passive inversion or eversion stress.
- Pushing the ankle against resistance helps identifying inflammation or partial tears of tendons of the contracted muscles.
- Palpation of pulses and neurologic assessment should be part of every examination.

IMAGING AND OTHER DIAGNOSTIC STUDIES

- Standard ankle plain film radiographs should include anteroposterior, lateral, and mortise views. However, only 50% to 66% of osteochondral defects can be visualized by plain film radiographs alone.[10] The radiologic signs vary from a small area of compression of subchondral bone to a detached osteochondral fragment.
- The four-stage classification system by Berndt and Harty[6] is still the gold standard based on radiologic appearance.
  - Stage I: compression lesion; no visible fragment
  - Stage II: fragment attached
  - Stage III: nondisplaced fragment without attachment **(FIG 1)**
  - Stage IV: displaced fragment

- Stress view radiographs are frequently recommended if instability is suspected. However, a thorough clinical examination is more essential and in most cases sufficient for assessment.
- Computed tomography scan offers more accurate staging and characterization of the lesion. However, exposure to radiation is high. Therefore, the application should be limited to special indications.
- Magnetic resonance imaging (MRI) is regarded as the method of choice for all patients with suspected osteochondral lesions. MRI can identify occult injuries of the subchondral bone and cartilage that may not be detected with routine radiographs.
- Dipaola et al[7] developed a classification system on the basis of Berndt and Harty[6] radiographic system.
  - Stage I: thickening of articular cartilage and low-signal changes
  - Stage II: articular cartilage breached; low-signal rim behind fragment indicating fibrous attachment
  - Stage III: articular cartilage breached, high-signal changes behind fragment indicating synovial fluid between fragment and underlying subchondral bone **(FIG 2)**
  - Stage IV: loose body

DIFFERENTIAL DIAGNOSIS

- Degenerative joint disease
- Soft tissue impingement
- Ankle instability
- Subtalar joint dysfunction
- Tendinitis or partial rupture of the tibialis posterior, tibialis anterior, or the peroneal tendons
- Tarsal coalition

NONOPERATIVE MANAGEMENT

- Nonoperative treatment for osteochondral lesions is considered in stage I and II lesions with an intact chondral surface. Two months of conservative treatment is generally recommended before approaching the defect surgically. It usually consists of immobilization and physical therapy.[6,8]
  - Cast immobilization appears to result in inferior results than only restricting the activity of the patient by partial

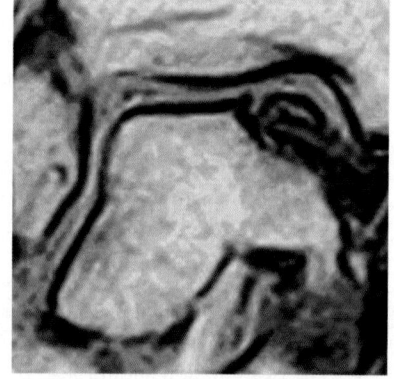
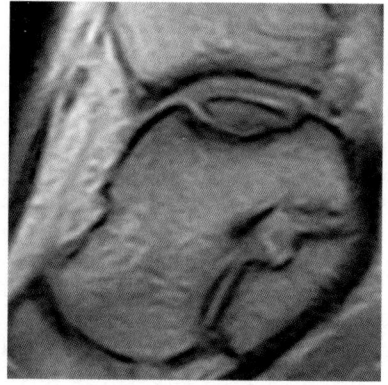

FIG 2 A. Coronal MRI (T1-SE-540 × 20) showing an osteochondral lesion stage III. **B.** Sagittal MRI (T2-SE-2000 × 90) showing an osteochondral lesion stage III with synovial fluid between the fragment and the underlying subchondral bone.

weight bearing.[17] Flick and Gould[8] concluded that therapy of 4 to 6 weeks with cast immobilization is inadequate immobilization resulting in poor results for most transchondral fractures. Berndt and Harty[6] reported in their early work in 1959 of 75% poor results after nonoperative treatment.

- In summary, it appears to be difficult to recommend conservative treatment. My algorithm is the following:
  - Primary conservative approach if the cartilage surface appears to be intact on MRI and the patient appears not to be willing to have surgery.
  - Activity allowed as tolerated by the patient. Immobilization with partial weight bearing has only healing potential for fresh traumatic osteochondral lesions. In an area with little perfusion, some contact pressure is necessary to create a healing response.
  - If no improvement is evident after a 2-month period or symptoms have worsened, diagnostic arthroscopy with probing of the cartilage surface should be considered to better define the lesion and perform an adequate surgical procedure.

SURGICAL MANAGEMENT

- The most important message in the treatment of osteochondral lesions of the talus is the following: Never treat asymptomatic lesions! Many chronic lesions are detected by coincidence after acute ankle distortion traumas that have been asymptomatic for many years. I have to be very cautious in being too aggressive in such findings.
- However, if the lesion appears to be the origin of discomfort and conservative treatment has failed, arthroscopic surgery is indicated for further management.
- Retrograde drilling might be considered if the chondral surface is found intact and detachable with a probe.
  - However, computer navigation should be used for the exact location of the lesion.
- If the chondral surface is found to be softened and is easily detachable, instable cartilage and fibrous tissue have to be débrided.
- Method of first choice in lesions stage II to IV is microfracture technique to stimulate fibrocartilage formation. Awls of different angles are penetrated into the subchondral bone to open the zone of vascularization. Blood enters the joint and leads to clot formation in the lesion. This clot contains pluripotent, marrow-derived mesenchymal stem cells, which produce a fibrocartilage repair with varying amounts of type II collagen content.[9,16]
  - Advantages over other marrow stimulation techniques such as abrasion or drilling include the avoidance of thermal damage, and all lesions can be accessed without more invasive steps such as transtibial drilling and osteotomy of the medial malleolus.
- In revision cases after failed treatment by microfracture, matrix-based autologous chondrocyte transplantation should be considered.
  - First-generation results after injecting the cultured cells under a periosteal flap appeared to be a viable alternative when treating osteochondral or chondral lesions of the talus.[3,11]

- Matrix-based autologous chondrocyte transplantation with cultured cells in scaffolds seems to be more promising and technically less demanding with good and excellent short-term results.[5]
- However, costs for the procedure are high, the approach is more invasive, and longer term results remain to be evaluated to prove superiority over microfracture technique.
- Osteochondral grafting or mosaicplasty is an option in the repair of severe osteochondral lesions with a significant lack of subchondral bone or in cystic lesions.[1]
  - The osteochondral plugs can either be harvested by open arthrotomy or arthroscopy of the knee. Local osteochondral grafting is also an option.
- Microfracture alone has shown limited success in lesions bigger than 2 × 2 cm.
  - The indication for bigger lesions is microfracturing with additional implantation of an acellular matrix scaffold derived from hyaluronic acid or collagen.
  - Autologous Matrix-Induced Chondrogenesis (AMIC) is a technique developed within the past 20 years to help heal cartilage damage. After microfracture, porcine collagen membrane is placed on the bleeding bone surface to encourage development of mesenchymal stem cells to stimulate chondrocyte growth and cartilage regeneration.

Preoperative Planning

- Review of all imaging studies, especially MRI evaluation, is most important for preoperative planning. Determinations of the size of the defect, location, topical geography, and depth of the defect have to be considered for choosing the correct approach and technique.
- Ankles have to be inspected for severe swelling, warmth, or erythema. Elevated parameters indicating acute inflammation processes have to be considered as a contraindication.
- In most cases, all locations of the ankle can be treated arthroscopically with standard portals.
  - However, in some posterior defects, a posterolateral approach is necessary, which demands different positioning of the patient.
- Examination under anaesthesia allows for better assessment of coexisting ankle instability.
  - In case of lateral ligamentous instability, lateral stabilization techniques have to be considered.

Positioning

- The procedure is performed under general anaesthesia with a tourniquet placed at the thigh.
- The patient is preferably positioned with a hanging leg in a manner that the flexor muscles are fully relaxed (**FIG 3A**).
- If a posterolateral approach is considered, the patient should be positioned in lateral position (**FIG 3B**).
- Atraumatic distraction can be performed using bandages (**FIG 3C**).
  - However, in most cases, no distraction is necessary to treat the lesion.

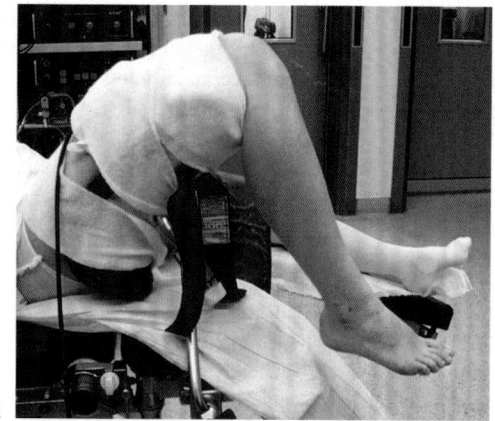
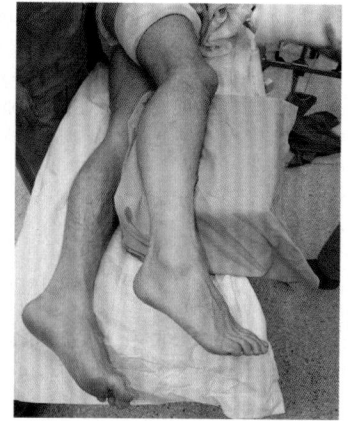
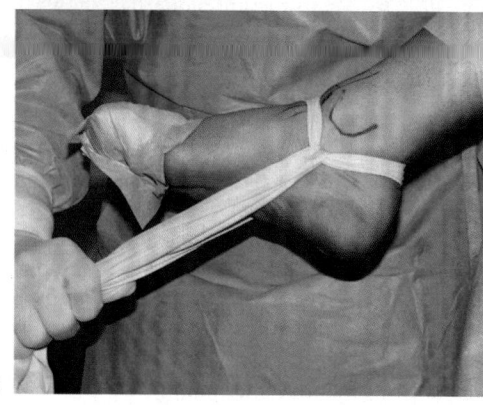

FIG 3 **A.** Positioning of the patient for ankle arthroscopy. **B.** Positioning of the patient if a posterolateral approach is necessary. **C.** Atraumatic distraction of the ankle with bandages.

PORTALS

- Standard anteromedial and anterolateral arthroscopic portals are employed. The anteromedial portal enters the ankle between the medial malleolus and the talar dome 0.5 to 1 cm distal to the joint line and just medial to the anterior tibial tendon. The anterolateral portal enters the joint between the fibula and talus at the same height lateral to the common extensor tendon.
- If necessary, the posterolateral portal is placed adjacent to the Achilles tendon and behind the peroneal tendon, slightly below the level of the joint line. A Kirschner wire can be directed under vision of the scope from the anteromedial portal posteriorly to find the same location (Wissinger rod technique). The patient must be fully relaxed and the joint adequately distracted and distended.
- In addition, a superomedial portal located 1 cm above the joint line, medial to tibialis anterior tendon might be helpful to achieve more perpendicular angles for the microfracturing (**TECH FIG 1**).

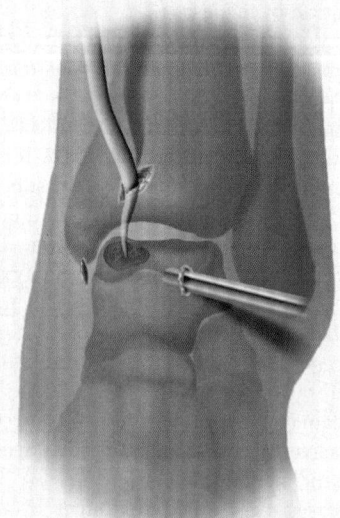

TECH FIG 1 Superomedial portal for better angles for microfracturing.

ARTHROSCOPY

- The joint is filled up with 20-mL saline solution through the anteromedial portal **(TECH FIG 2A)**.
- A 2.5- or 2.7-mm arthroscope is necessary to have the possibility to assess and treat defects in all areas of the joint **(TECH FIG 2B)**.
- A limited synovectomy should be performed in all cases. This allows better visibility during the procedure and inflamed synovia as a cause of pain and swelling can be removed.

- The ankle is systematically inspected and all pathology being documented.
- Loose bodies are removed if they are identified.
- Careful assessment and probing of the articular surface is performed. The medial and lateral malleolus and the tibial plafond have also to be considered.

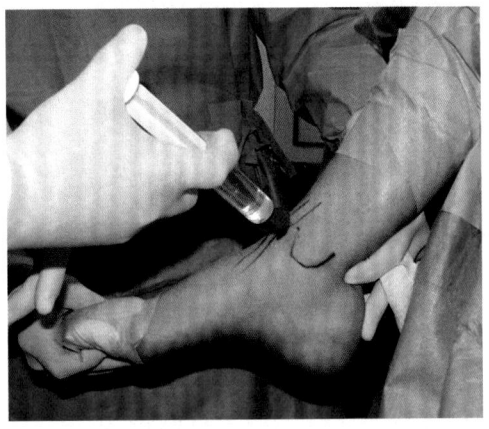
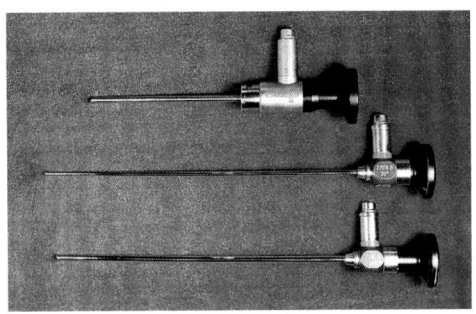

TECH FIG 2 A. Filling the joint with 20 mL of saline solution. **B.** A 2.7-mm arthroscope inserted in the medial portal.

PREPARATION OF THE LESION

- The lesion is identified with a probe **(TECH FIG 3A)**.
- All instable cartilage and fibrous tissue of the lesion and the surrounding area are addressed with débridement and curettage **(TECH FIG 3B)**.

- Sharp, perpendicular margins are created to optimize conditions for the attachment of the marrow clot **(TECH FIG 3C)**.
- The calcified cartilage layer is completely removed with a burr **(TECH FIG 3D)**.

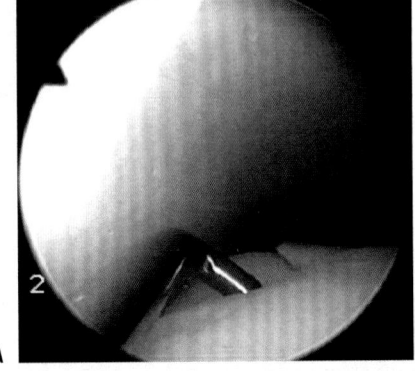
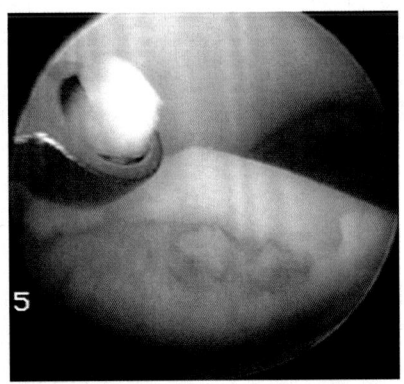

TECH FIG 3 A. Probing of the lesion. **B.** Débridement and curettage. *(continued)*

TECHNIQUES

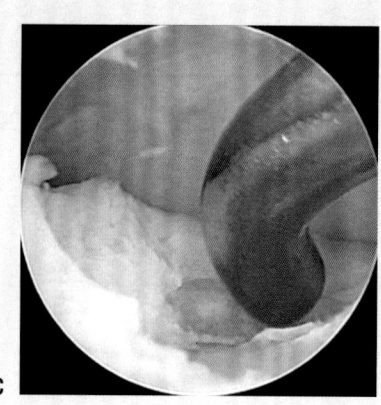
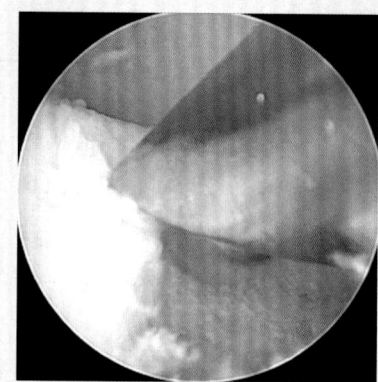

TECH FIG 3 *(continued)* **C.** Preparation of perpendicular margins. **D.** Removal of calcified layer.

MICROFRACTURE

- Microfracture technique is performed if the subchondral bone layer is healthy and intact. Cystic defects are excluded.
- With the arthroscopic awls of different angles, the microfractures are placed approximately 3 to 4 mm apart and 2 to 4 mm deep until fat droplets are present.

- Care is to be taken that the awl is placed perpendicular to the surface and that the subchondral bone–plate integrity is maintained **(TECH FIG 4A)**.
- When the tourniquet is released, blood enters the joint through the microfractures **(TECH FIG 4B)**.
- No drain is inserted; closure of the portals in standard techniques

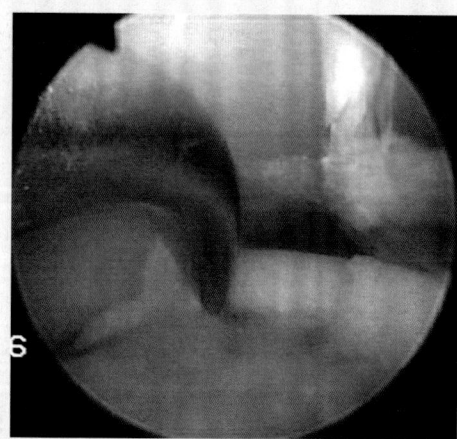
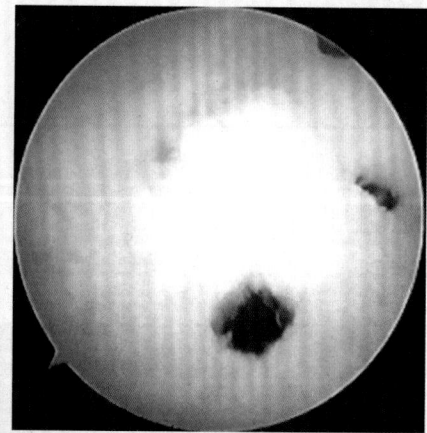

TECH FIG 4 **A.** Microfracture. **B.** Release of the tourniquet.

AUTOLOGOUS MATRIX-INDUCED CHONDROGENESIS PROCEDURE

- The preparation of the "scaffold bed" is more aggressive.
  - In chondral lesions, the subchondral surface is prepare by a 3.5-mm burr in an irregular fashion to increase surface area. Bone marrow aspirate is taken by a Jamshidi needle from the iliac crest.
  - The prepared lesion is covered with bone marrow, and the matrix scaffold is placed at the subchondral surface **(TECH FIG 5)**.
  - For a better fixation and an improvement of the biologic activity, fibrin glue, and Platelet-Rich Plasma (PRP) is applied.

- Osteochondral lesions are débrided until normal subchondral bone is visible. Additional microfracturing is not necessary as the lesion is mostly deep in the subchondral bone.
- The defect is filled with bone marrow and the matrix up to the chondral layer. A fibrin glue fixation stabilizes the implant.

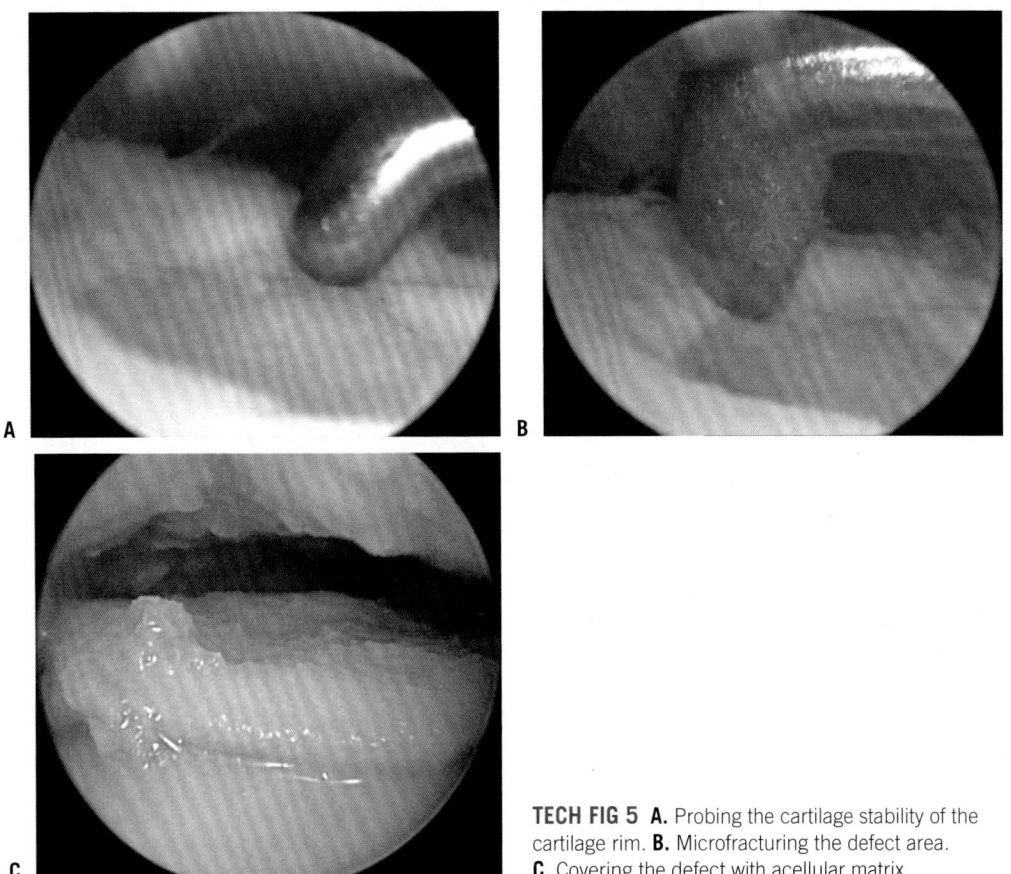

TECH FIG 5 A. Probing the cartilage stability of the cartilage rim. **B.** Microfracturing the defect area. **C.** Covering the defect with acellular matrix.

TECHNIQUES

Pearls and Pitfalls

Indications	• Care must be taken to address associated pathology.
	• In case of lateral ligament instability, a stabilizing procedure has to be added for success of the microfracture.
Technique	• Posterolateral approach with the Wissinger rod technique: A rod is inserted through the anteromedial portal in posterolateral direction to designate the optimal entry for the posterolateral portal.
	• The calcified cartilage layer has to be thoroughly removed to provide optimal amount and attachment of repair tissue.

POSTOPERATIVE CARE

- Compressive bandaging is performed up to the thigh. Elevation of the ankle and immediate cryotherapy is applied.
- Continuous passive motion from the first day as tolerated by pain and swelling for 6 to 8 hours per day for 4 to 6 weeks.
- Partial weight bearing to no more than 15 kg for the first 4 weeks. Partial weight bearing to no more than 30 kg for the next 2 weeks. If the ankle is pain-free, then weight bearing can be advanced as tolerated.
- No impact sports earlier than 6 months after surgery
- Dietary supplements (glucosamine and chondroitin sulphate) may have beneficial effects for cartilage regeneration.

OUTCOMES

- Results revealed significant improvement 2 years after microfracture of the talus.[4,5]
  - Ninety-five percent ankles with osteochondral defect had excellent or good results.
  - Patients older than 50 years had no significant difference outcome results compared with younger patients.
  - Location and grading of the defect showed no statistical importance on the obtained results.
  - MRI studies showed regeneration of tissue in the microfractured area. Subchondral signal changes were observed in almost all postoperative images.
  - A distinct correlation between clinical and imaging results could not be detected.

- The AMIC procedure has its indication of the consensus meeting[14,15] in bigger lesion and revision cases. Midterm results showed in these more challenging case comparable results to "simple" microfracture cases.[13,15,18]

COMPLICATIONS

- Development of ossifications with following restriction in dorsiflexion
- Damage to the deep peroneal nerve with following hyposensitivity in the distribution area
- Infection
- Deep vein thrombosis
- Arthrofibrosis

REFERENCES

1. Assenmacher JA, Kelikian AS, Gottlob C, et al. Arthroscopically assisted autologous osteochondral transplantation for osteochondral lesions of the talar dome: an MRI and clinical follow-up study. Foot Ankle Int 2001;22(7):544–551.
2. Athanasiou KA, Niederauer GG, Schenck RC Jr. Biomechanical topography of human ankle cartilage. Ann Biomed Eng 1995;23(5):697–704.
3. Baums MH, Heidrich G, Schultz W, et al. Autologous chondrocyte transplantation for treating cartilage defects of the talus. J Bone Joint Surg Am 2006;88(2):303–308.
4. Becher C, Driessen A, Hess T, et al. Microfracture for chondral defects of the talus: maintenance of early results at midterm follow-up. Knee Surg Sports Traumatol Arthrosc 2010;18(5):656–663.
5. Becher C, Thermann H. Results of microfracture in the treatment of articular cartilage defects of the talus. Foot Ankle Int 2005;26(8):583–589.
6. Berndt AL, Harty M. Transchondral fractures (osteochondritis dissecans) of the talus. J Bone Joint Surg Am 1959;41(6):988–1020.
7. Dipaola JD, Nelson DW, Colville MR. Characterizing osteochondral lesions by magnetic resonance imaging. Arthroscopy 1991;7(1):101–104.
8. Flick AB, Gould N. Osteochondritis dissecans of the talus (transchondral fractures of the talus): review of the literature and new surgical approach for medial dome lesions. Foot Ankle 1985;5(4):165–185.
9. Knutsen G, Engebretsen L, Ludvigsen TC, et al. Autologous chondrocyte implantation compared with microfracture in the knee. A randomized trial. J Bone Joint Surg Am 2004;86(3):455–464.
10. Loomer R, Fisher C, Lloyd-Smith R, et al. Osteochondral lesions of the talus. Am J Sports Med 1993;21(1):13–19.
11. Mandelbaum BR, Gerhardt MB, Peterson L. Autologous chondrocyte implantation of the talus. Arthroscopy 2003;19(suppl 1):129–137.
12. McCullough CJ, Venugopal V. Osteochondritis dissecans of the talus: the natural history. Clin Orthop Relat Res 1979;(144):264–268.
13. Richter M, Zech S. Matrix-associated stem cell transplantation (MAST) in chondral defects of foot and ankle is effective. Foot Ankle Surg 2013;19:84–90.
14. Rothrauff BB, Murawski CD, Angthong C, et al. Scaffold-based therapies: proceedings of the International Consensus Meeting on Cartilage Repair of the Ankle. Foot Ankle Int 2018;39:41S–47S
15. Shimozono Y, Yasui Y, Ross AW, et al. Scaffolds based therapy for osteochondral lesions of the talus: a systematic review. World J Orthop 2017;8:798–808.
16. Steadman JR, Rodkey WG, Singleton SB, et al. Microfracture technique for full-thickness chondral defects: technique and clinical results. Oper Tech Orthop 1997;7(4):300–304.
17. Tol JL, Struijs PA, Bossuyt PM, et al. Treatment strategies in osteochondral defects of the talar dome: a systematic review. Foot Ankle Int 2000;21(2):119–126.
18. Usuelli FG, D'ambrosi R, Maccario C, et al. All-arthroscopic AMIC® (AT-AMIC®) technique with autologous bone graft for talar osteochondral defects: clinical and radiological results. Knee Surg Sports Traumatol Arthrosc 2018;26:875–881.

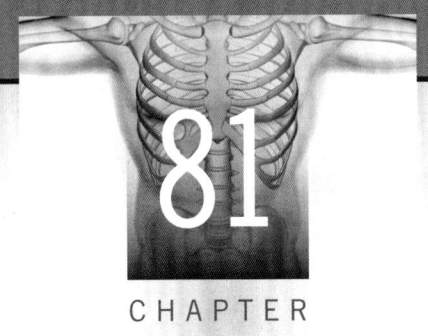

81 CHAPTER

Microfracture for Osteochondral Lesions of the Talus:
Perspective 2

Raymond J. Walls, Keir A. Ross, Yoshiharu Shimozono, and John G. Kennedy

DEFINITION

- Osteochondral lesions of the talus (OLT) are common conditions that can involve both the cartilage and underlying bone of the talar dome and have the propensity to degrade and lead to osteoarthritis if left untreated.[2,12] Cartilage injuries have a poor inherent healing response.
- Bone marrow stimulation (BMS), initiating fibrocartilage through microfracture or microdrilling, is a commonly used technique for small, noncystic lesions.
- The objective is to create multiple breaches in the subchondral plate to facilitate the flow of marrow with mesenchymal stem cells (MSCs) from the underlying bone.

ANATOMY

- The talus articulates with the tibial plafond superiorly as well as the medial and lateral malleoli to form the ankle mortise.
- Approximately 60% of talar surface is covered by cartilage.
- It has no muscular attachments, and thus, its blood supply is derived from branches of the posterior tibial artery (artery of the tarsal canal and deltoid branches), the peroneal artery (artery of the tarsal sinus), and the dorsalis pedis.

PATHOGENESIS

- The etiology is primarily traumatic with an incidence of between 50% and 70% following ankle sprains and fractures.[8,13,17]
- Repetitive microtrauma leading to OLTs is often associated with ankle instability.[13]
- Impaction, crush, and shearing injuries occur with the location of the OLT dependent on the position of the ankle at time of injury.

NATURAL HISTORY

- Smaller lesions can occasionally heal with nonoperative management, although this is more commonly seen in a pediatric population.[24]
- Theoretically, OLTs tend to progress, as highly pressurized fluid invades the subchondral plate through cartilaginous defects and eventually infiltrates subchondral bone.
- Spontaneous healing is uncommon, and there is a propensity for further degeneration.
- Prevention of disease progression is aimed at repair of the subchondral plate and alignment of the joint.
- Surgical intervention can be considered as reparative (BMS) or replacement (autologous chondrocyte implantation, autologous osteochondral transplantation, juvenile particulate cartilage).

PATIENT HISTORY AND PHYSICAL FINDINGS

- OLTs may be asymptomatic.
- Patients often, but not always, will recall an acute injury.
- Activity-related deep anterior ankle pain is the typical complaint.
- Mechanical symptoms such as clicking or locking of the ankle joint are less common and may indicate a loose fragment.
- Clinical examination may reveal swelling and localized tenderness along the joint line.
- Chronic cases with associated synovitis and joint effusions can have limited ankle motion.
- As many cases occur with concomitant pathology, such as ankle instability, detailed clinical examination of the ankle osseous, ligamentous, and tendinous structures is advocated.

IMAGING AND OTHER DIAGNOSTIC STUDIES

- Imaging studies are useful to assess lesion location, size, and depth as well as the presence of subchondral cysts preoperatively. This will determine the most appropriate treatment strategy.
- Standard weight-bearing plain radiographs (anteroposterior [AP], lateral, and mortise views) **(FIG 1A)**
  - May miss up to 50% of OLTs, especially if very small or isolated cartilage lesions[11]
  - Useful to assess lower limb, ankle, and hindfoot alignment
- Computed tomography (CT) **(FIG 1B,C)**
  - Permits further evaluation of osseous morphology and dimensions, especially depth
  - Only gives information about the osseous structure; no information regarding overlying chondral loss or damage
- Magnetic resonance imaging (MRI) **(FIG 1D,E)**
  - Recommended for a definitive diagnosis and evaluation
  - Evaluation of articular cartilage and the degree of subchondral involvement/bone edema
  - T2 mapping sequences provide increased sensitivity for cartilage architecture and quality.
  - Can also assess for concomitant pathology (ligamentous injury, tendinous injury, loose bodies, etc.)

DIFFERENTIAL DIAGNOSIS

- Anteromedial or anterolateral ankle impingement
- Chronic ankle instability
- Tendinopathy (peroneals, tibialis posterior, tibialis anterior)
- Early posttraumatic osteoarthritis
- Inflammatory arthropathy
- Stress response or fracture

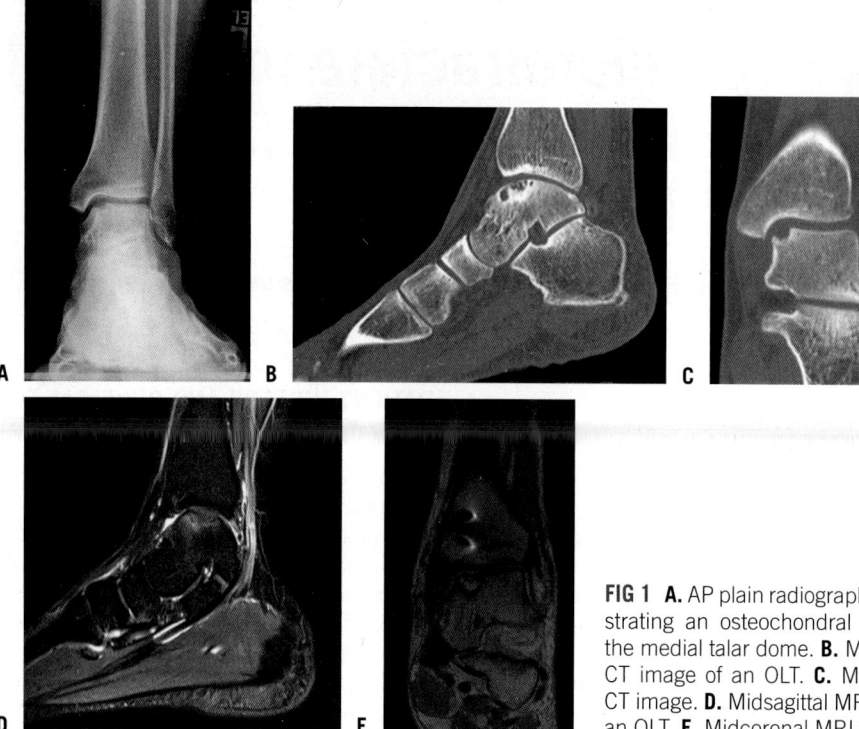

FIG 1 A. AP plain radiograph demonstrating an osteochondral lesion of the medial talar dome. **B.** Midsagittal CT image of an OLT. **C.** Midcoronal CT image. **D.** Midsagittal MRI scan of an OLT. **E.** Midcoronal MRI scan.

NONOPERATIVE MANAGEMENT

- Indicated for minimally symptomatic, smaller, stable lesions that involve cartilage alone
- A period of immobilization and restricted weight bearing followed by progressive weight bearing and physical therapy. Range-of-motion exercises are encouraged to preserve cartilage nutrition.
- Pharmacotherapy (oral nonsteroidal anti-inflammatory drugs and intra-articular steroid injection)
- Nonoperative management has traditionally shown high failure rates.[5,19,26]
- The role of biologic adjuncts such as platelet-rich plasma, concentrated bone marrow aspirate, and hyaluronic acid are under investigation.

SURGICAL MANAGEMENT

- Microfracture was first described by Steadman et al[22] and has gained widespread popularity, as it is marginally technically demanding, minimally invasive with minimal postoperative pain, is low cost, and is associated with low complication rates.
- Indications
  - Primary noncystic lesions[3,4] that are less than 10 mm in diameter or have a less than 100 mm² in area[16]
  - Failed conservative management
  - Consider retrograde drilling or lift-and-fill technique[9] for subchondral bone lesions where the overlying cartilage is intact.
- Absolute contraindications include severe degenerative joint disease and infection. Caution is recommended in the setting of active inflammatory arthropathy, especially if the patient is on long-term oral steroids.

Preoperative Planning

- Based on clinical examination and preoperative imaging outlined earlier
- The lesion location will determine surgical approach, whereas lesion size determines the technique.
- Anterior arthroscopy is used for most lesions through standard anteromedial and anterolateral portals. Accessory posteromedial portals are also employed on occasion.
- In our experience, approximately 75% of the ankle joint is accessible with the anterior approach.
- Posterior arthroscopy is used for the most posterior of lesions. The original two-portal technique is safe and provides access not only to an OLT but also to other hindfoot, posterior ankle, subtalar joint, and extra-articular pathologies.[21]
- Retrograde drilling is used for lesions in which the overlying cartilage is preserved and is performed under fluoroscopic navigation.[14]
- If concomitant ankle stabilization is to be performed, we evaluate the ankle while the patient is anesthetized to help determine the corrective procedure of choice.
- If necessary, additional corrective osteotomies to address mechanical deformity should be performed concurrently.

Positioning

- Preoperatively, we identify and initial the correct limb.
- The procedure is typically performed under regional anesthesia (combined spinal anesthesia and popliteal block), although a general anesthesia can be performed if preferred.
- For anterior arthroscopy, the patient is positioned supine on a standard operating table with a well-padded thigh tourniquet. A towel roll ("bump") is placed under the ipsilateral

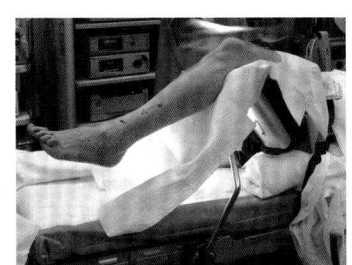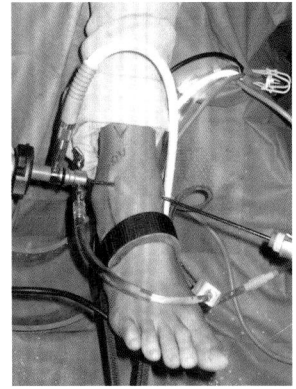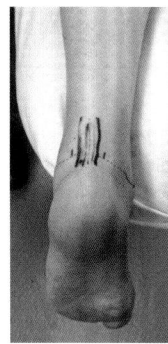

FIG 2 A. The patient is positioned supine on a standard operating table with a well-padded thigh tourniquet. A towel roll (bump) is placed under the ipsilateral buttock to improve lower limb orientation with the foot perpendicular to the floor. **B.** A noninvasive ankle distractor is fastened to the operating table and secured to the ankle with the ankle joint in plantarflexion. **C.** Posterior ankle arthroscopy positioning with the patient's foot overhanging the edge of operating table.

buttock to improve lower limb orientation with the foot perpendicular to the floor (**FIG 2A**).

- A padded thigh holder is placed proximal to the popliteal fossa so that the hip is flexed at 60 degrees and the knee can be easily positioned at 90 degrees with gentle traction.
- Standard prepping and draping of the limb is performed.
- A noninvasive ankle distractor is fastened to the operating table and secured to the ankle with the ankle joint in plantarflexion (**FIG 2B**). Approximately 15 lb of distraction force is appropriate for most cases to expand the joint and improve access.
- If a posterior approach is selected, the patient is placed prone with the ankle overhanging the end of the operating table (**FIG 2C**).
  - Alternatively, a triangular cushion can be placed under the distal tibia.

Approach

- Anterior arthroscopic procedures typically use anterolateral and anteromedial portals.
  - Inject 10 mL of saline into the ankle from an anteromedial direction. There should be easy insufflation of fluid with correct intra-articular placement with bulging of the anterolateral joint capsule noted.
  - The anteromedial portal is placed 5 mm distal to the joint line and just medial to the tibialis anterior tendon. We recommend incising only the skin and carefully form a path through the subcutaneous tissue by gently spreading a mosquito forceps. Outflow of saline confirms the capsule has been breached and a blunt trocar inserted (2.7-mm arthroscopic instrumentation).
  - The anterolateral portal is created in a similar fashion, also at a level of 5 mm below the joint line. The approach

is just lateral to peroneus tertius tendon with care taken to avoid the superficial peroneal nerve that we identify and mark preoperatively where possible.

- For posterior ankle arthroscopy, standard posteromedial and posterolateral portals are used (**FIG 3**).
  - A line is drawn from the tip of the medial malleolus to the tip of the lateral malleolus parallel to the sole of the foot.
  - The posterolateral portal is created 5 mm anterior to the lateral border of the Achilles tendon immediately proximal to the aforementioned line. Care is required to avoid the sural nerve when creating the subcutaneous tunnel.
  - The posteromedial portal is also created 5 mm anterior to the medial border of the Achilles tendon and just proximal to the drawn line. The medial neurovascular bundle is at risk, so great care must also be employed when creating a path through the soft tissues.

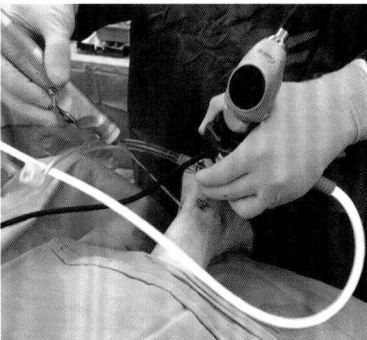

FIG 3 Posterior ankle arthroscopy with standard posteromedial and posterolateral portals.

ANTERIOR ANKLE ARTHROSCOPY

- Once the anteromedial portal has been created, standard 2.7-mm arthroscopic instrumentation is used with a 30-degree arthroscope. A water pump with inflow and outflow is attached to the arthroscopic port with a pressure of 40 mm Hg adequate for most cases.
- Full evaluation of the ankle joint is necessary; in pathologic joints, débridement of scar tissue and diseased hypertrophic synovium is frequently required for adequate visualization **(TECH FIG 1A)**.

- A limited resection of the anterior tibial margin may also be required with the use of an arthroscopic burr **(TECH FIG 1B)**.
- All concomitant intra-articular pathology such as synovectomy and loose body retrieval should be addressed prior to microfracture so that the induced marrow clot will not be disrupted.
- A systematic approach should be employed in all cases to ensure all aspects of the joint are formally evaluated (medial and lateral gutters; talar dome and tibial plafond). We advocate the 21-point systematic Ferkel evaluation.[6]

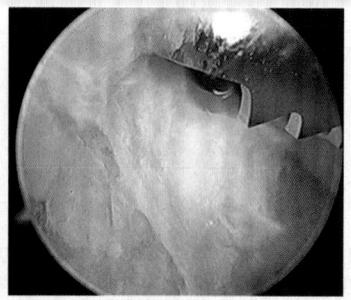 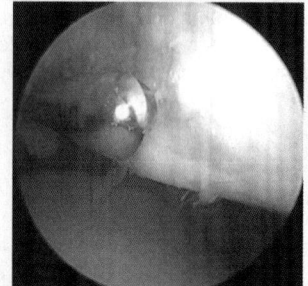

TECH FIG 1 A. Débridement of scar tissue and diseased hypertrophic synovium is often required for complete visualization of the ankle joint. **B.** A limited resection of the anterior tibial margin may be necessary for which we use an arthroscopic burr.

IDENTIFICATION, EVALUATION, AND PREPARATION OF THE OSTEOCHONDRAL LESION OF THE TALUS

- The location of the lesion should be localized and identified based on preoperative imaging studies.
- Careful probing of the cartilage is performed, and softened pathologic areas of cartilage should be identified in ankles where no loose cartilaginous flaps exist **(TECH FIG 2A)**.
- A curette is used to remove pathologic cartilage until a smooth rim of stable healthy cartilage is created **(TECH FIG 2B)**.
- A shaver is used to help remove loose fragments **(TECH FIG 2C)**.
- All delaminated cartilage should also be removed, as the cartilage lesion can extend beyond the margins indicated by preoperative imaging.

- Where a subchondral cyst is present, the associated pathologic bone and cystic lining must be removed.
- The calcified cartilage layer is removed with careful curettage to facilitate clot adhesion and repair.
- Additional manual plantarflexion from an assistant may be required to obtain adequate exposure of the OLT.
- The exact dimensions can be determined using a graduated probe to establish both transverse dimensions and lesion depth.

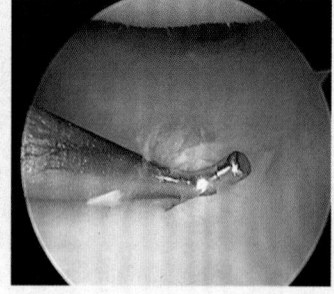 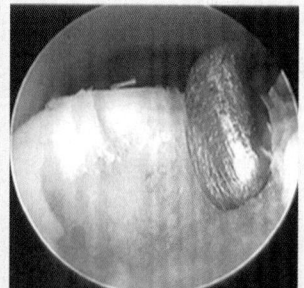 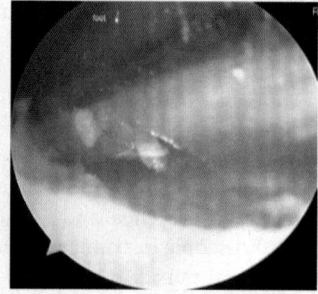

TECH FIG 2 A. Careful probing of the articular cartilage is performed to identify softened pathologic lesions or unstable cartilaginous flaps. **B.** A curette is used to remove pathologic cartilage until a smooth rim of stable healthy cartilage is created. **C.** A shaver is used to remove additional small loose fragments of cartilage and bone.

BONE MARROW STIMULATION/MICROFRACTURE TECHNIQUE

- Microfracture is performed only when complete removal of the OLT has been achieved, leaving a smooth, perpendicular rim of stable, healthy, and native cartilage.
- Commonly used techniques include drilling with a Kirschner wire or breaching the subchondral bone with a microfracture awl.
- Awls with various angulations are available and should be used judiciously depending on the location of the lesion to ensure the subchondral bone is penetrated perpendicular to the OLT base.
- The subchondral bone is breached to a depth of 2 to 4 mm, with the depth usually indicated on the awl (TECH FIG 3A,B).
- The emergence of fat droplets indicates adequate penetration has been achieved for subsequent subchondral bleeding and recruitment of MSCs from the marrow (TECH FIG 3C).
- Each microfracture should be separated by 3 to 4 mm.

- Ensure that BMS is also performed at the periphery of the OLT to improve fibrocartilage integration.
- The subchondral bone plate is damaged by the procedure and is not likely to adequately remodel. Therefore, microfracture should be performed with a small-diameter awl or microdrilling to reduce the damage of the subchondral bone, resulting in the improvement of the quality and longevity of the cartilage repair tissue.
- Final evaluation and lavage of the joint are performed and all loose bodies are removed.
- The water pump is turned off, and if a tourniquet is used, it can be deflated to confirm the presence of fat droplets and blood emerging from each BMS breach (TECH FIG 3D).
- The wounds are closed with 3-0 nylon and a sterile dressing applied.

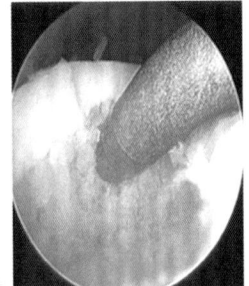 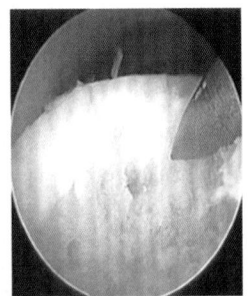 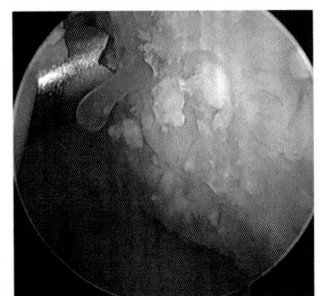 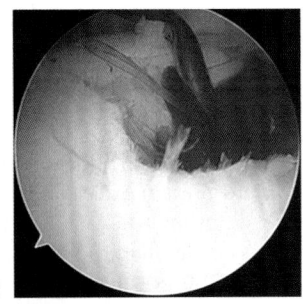

A   B   C   D

TECH FIG 3 A,B. The subchondral bone is breached to a depth of 2 to 4 mm with the depth usually indicated on the awl. **C.** Fat droplets emerging from the cancellous bone indicate adequate penetration through the subchondral plate. **D.** Turning off the water pump allows marrow blood to emerge from each BMS breach.

POSTERIOR ANKLE ARTHROSCOPIC MICROFRACTURE

- A systematic four-quadrant approach is used to address associated hindfoot pathologies (TECH FIG 4).[21]
- Adequate visualization of the posterior OLT can be achieved with manual ankle dorsiflexion.
- BMS is subsequently performed as outlined earlier.

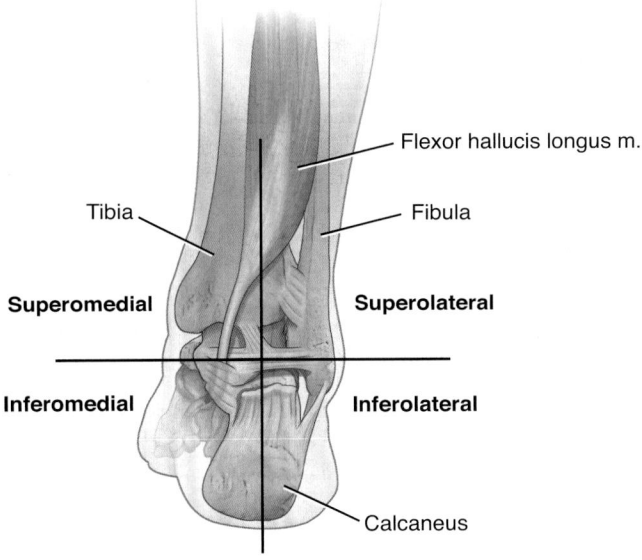

Flexor hallucis longus m.

Tibia

Fibula

Superomedial

Superolateral

Inferomedial

Inferolateral

Calcaneus

TECH FIG 4 A systematic four-quadrant approach to posterior ankle arthroscopy is used to address associated hindfoot pathologies.

TECHNIQUES

Pearls and Pitfalls

Neurovascular Injury	• Avoid overzealous distraction and take great care when creating arthroscopic portals. Always use a blunt trocar when switching between portal sites. Ensure the thigh holder is proximal to the popliteal fossa.
Incomplete Débridement	• Fully evaluate the rim for loose flaps or delaminated cartilage. This is particularly important for anterior margins, which may not be easily visualized.
Loose Body Fragments	• Always perform a thorough evaluation and lavage of the entire ankle joint at the end of débridement.
"Kissing" Tibial Lesions	• Coexisting lesions of the tibia should be evaluated, and we recommend concomitant management where appropriate.
Perpendicular Orientation of BMS Technique	• Be prepared to use awls with different angles and have a full selection ready preoperatively. It is advisable to have an assistant stabilize the ankle if controlled application of force is required to breach the subchondral bone and prevent iatrogenic injury to native, intact cartilage. Maximal plantarflexion of the ankle, again with the use of an assistant can increase the exposure.
Proper Awl Size	• It is important that the correct awl size is used. Compression of subchondral bone caused by a large awl can lead to closing of trabecular channels and creates a pore size too small to allow neovascularization.

POSTOPERATIVE CARE

• A well-padded soft dressing is applied for 14 days.

• Ankle pump exercises commence at 72 hours postoperatively and are continued for 4 weeks. Controlled ankle plantarflexion and dorsiflexion is performed for 20 minutes each day to prevent adhesion formation and stiffness and through diffusion will facilitate nutrition of the cartilage from the synovial fluid.

• At 2 weeks postoperatively, the sutures are removed and the patient progressed to a controlled ankle movement boot.

• At 4 weeks postoperatively, weight bearing commences starting at 10% of the patient's body weight and commencing by 10% each day so that full weight bearing is achieved by 6 weeks postoperatively.

• At 6 weeks postoperatively, we commence formal physical therapy rehabilitation focusing on reestablishing balance, proprioception, and stabilization.

• At 10 weeks postoperatively, rehabilitation focuses on strengthening and sport-specific training. Return to full contact sport must be evaluated continuously as the patient's symptoms improve.

OUTCOMES

• The aim of BMS is for pluripotent MSCs within the marrow to coagulate and form a fibrin clot in the defect. An inflammatory cascade should ensue with the ultimate outcome being stimulation of tissue healing.

• Although it is hoped that differentiation from MSCs into a chondrocyte-like cells occurs with the ability to synthesize a cartilaginous matrix including type II collagen, there is evidence that formation of fibrocartilage occurs.[18] This is of concern as fibrocartilage has inferior mechanical and biologic properties compared to hyaline cartilage.

• Nonetheless, the clinical results of BMS are generally good in the short to medium term with a recent systematic review citing an overall success rate of 85%.[25]

• The longest follow-up study reported 12-year clinical outcomes in 50 patients and demonstrated a median American Orthopaedic Foot & Ankle Society ankle–hindfoot score of 88 and overall 78% good to excellent Ogilvie-Harris scores. One-third of patients progressed ankle arthritis by one grade on plain radiograph.[23] Another study of 82 patients at 10 years follow-up reported that 57.4% of patients were symptomatic.[15]

• Concern exists regarding the long-term quality of fibrocartilage to sustain mechanical load. Deterioration of clinical outcome scores was found in 35% of patients within 5 years.[7]

• Fibrocartilage deterioration at 5 years using MRI evaluation and a lack of integration with native cartilage seen arthroscopically has been reported.[1,10]

• Subchondral bone was not restored at midterm after microfracture. In addition, subchondral bone damage at midterm follow-up was associated with poorer clinical outcomes.[20]

• In recent years, there has been growing interest in the use of biologic adjuncts such as hyaluronic acid, concentrated bone marrow aspirate, and platelet-rich plasma as well as the use of scaffolds/BioCartilage to augment repair.

COMPLICATIONS

• The overall complication rate after anterior ankle arthroscopic microfracture is as low as 3.5% with noninvasive distraction when great care is taken.[27] The rate after posterior arthroscopy is also low at 2.3%.[27]

• Nerve injury is the most commonly reported complication, although most resolve within 6 months.

• Vascular injury

• Infection

• Synovial fistula

• Loose bodies

• Arthrofibrosis, stiffness

• Iatrogenic cartilage injury

• Chronic regional pain syndrome

REFERENCES

1. Becher C, Driessen A, Hess T, et al. Microfracture for chondral defects of the talus: maintenance of early results at midterm follow-up. Knee Surg Sports Traumatol Arthrosc 2010;18:656–663.
2. Buckwalter JA, Mankin HJ. Articular cartilage: degeneration and osteoarthritis, repair, regeneration, and transplantation. Instr Course Lect 1998;47:487–504.
3. Choi WJ, Park KK, Kim BS, et al. Osteochondral lesion of the talus: is there a critical defect size for poor outcome? Am J Sports Med 2009;37:1974–1980.
4. Chuckpaiwong B, Berkson EM, Theodore GH. Microfracture for osteochondral lesions of the ankle: outcome analysis and outcome predictors of 105 cases. Arthroscopy 2008;24:106–112.
5. Easley ME, Scranton PE Jr. Osteochondral autologous transfer system. Foot Ankle Clin 2003;8:275–290.
6. Ferkel RD, Fischer SP. Progress in ankle arthroscopy. Clin Orthop Relat Res 1989;(240):210–220.
7. Ferkel RD, Zanotti RM, Komenda GA, et al. Arthroscopic treatment of chronic osteochondral lesions of the talus: long-term results. Am J Sports Med 2008;36(9):1750–1762.
8. Hintermann B, Regazzoni P, Lampert C, et al. Arthroscopic findings in acute fractures of the ankle. J Bone Joint Surg Br 2000;82(3):345–351.
9. Kerkhoffs GM, Reilingh ML, Gerards RM, et al. Lift, drill, fill and fix (LDFF): a new arthroscopic treatment for talar osteochondral defects. Knee Surg Sports Traumatol Arthrosc 2016;24(4):1265–1271.
10. Lee KB, Bai LB, Yoon TR, et al. Second-look arthroscopic findings and clinical outcomes after microfracture for osteochondral lesions of the talus. Am J Sports Med 2009;37(suppl 1):63S–70S.
11. Loomer R, Fisher C, Lloyd-Smith R, et al. Osteochondral lesions of the talus. Am J Sports Med 1993;21:13–19.
12. McCullough CJ, Venugopal V. Osteochondritis dissecans of the talus: the natural history. Clin Orthop Relat Res 1979;(144):264–268.
13. O'Loughlin PF, Heyworth BE, Kennedy JG. Current concepts in the diagnosis and treatment of osteochondral lesions of the ankle. Am J Sports Med 2010;38(2):392–404.
14. O'Loughlin PF, Kendoff D, Pearle AD, et al. Arthroscopic-assisted fluoroscopic navigation for retrograde drilling of a talar osteochondral lesion. Foot Ankle Int 2009;30:70–73.
15. Polat G, Erşen A, Erdil ME, et al. Long-term results of microfracture in the treatment of talus osteochondral lesions. Knee Surg Sports Traumatol Arthrosc 2016;24(4):1299–1303.
16. Ramponi L, Yasui Y, Murawski CD, et al. Lesion size is a predictor of clinical outcomes after bone marrow stimulation for osteochondral lesions of the talus: a systematic review. Am J Sports Med 2017;45(7):1698–1705.
17. Saxena A, Eakin C. Articular talar injuries in athletes: results of microfracture and autogenous bone graft. Am J Sports Med 2007;35(10):1680–1687.
18. Shapiro F, Koide S, Glimcher MJ. Cell origin and differentiation in the repair of full-thickness defects of articular cartilage. J Bone Joint Surg Am 1993;75:532–553.
19. Shearer C, Loomer R, Clement D. Nonoperatively managed stage 5 osteochondral talar lesions. Foot Ankle Int 2002;23:651–654.
20. Shimozono Y, Coale M, Yasui Y, et al. Subchondral bone degradation after microfracture for osteochondral lesions of the talus: an MRI analysis. Am J Sports Med 2018;46(3):642–648.
21. Smyth NA, Murawski CD, Levine DS, et al. Hindfoot arthroscopic surgery for posterior ankle impingement: a systematic surgical approach and case series. Am J Sports Med 2013;41:1869–1876.
22. Steadman JR, Rodkey WG, Singleton SB, et al. Microfracture technique for full-thickness chondral defects: technique and clinical results. Oper Tech Orthop 1997;7:300–304.
23. van Bergen CJ, Kox LS, Maas M, et al. Arthroscopic treatment of osteochondral defects of the talus: outcomes at eight to twenty years of follow-up. J Bone Joint Surg Am 2013;95:519–525.
24. van Dijk CN, Reilingh ML, Zengerink M, et al. The natural history of osteochondral lesions in the ankle. Instr Course Lect 2010;59:375–386.
25. Zengerink M, Struijs PA, Tol JL, et al. Treatment of osteochondral lesions of the talus: a systematic review. Knee Surg Sports Traumatol Arthrosc 2010;18:238–246.
26. Zengerink M, Szerb I, Hangody L, et al. Current concepts: treatment of osteochondral ankle defects. Foot Ankle Clin 2006;11:331–359.
27. Zengerink M, van Dijk CN. Complications in ankle arthroscopy. Knee Surg Sports Traumatol Arthrosc 2012;20:1420–1431.

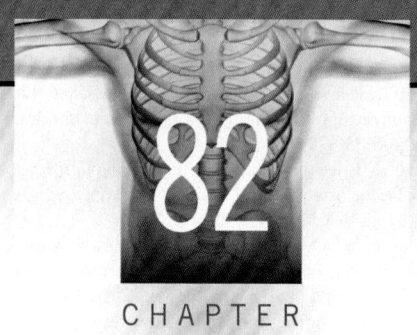

Posterior Ankle Arthroscopy and Hindfoot Endoscopy

C. Niek van Dijk and Tahir Ögüt

DEFINITION

- Because of their nature and deep location, posterior ankle problems pose a diagnostic and therapeutic challenge.
- Arthroscopic evaluation of posterior ankle problems by means of routine ankle arthroscopy using an anteromedial, anterolateral, and posterolateral portal is difficult because of the shape of the ankle joint. In cases in which the ankle ligaments are lax, it is possible to visualize and treat the pathology of the ankle joint itself, but pericapsular or extracapsular posterior pathologic conditions are not accessible through conventional arthroscopic portals.
- A two-portal posterior endoscopic approach with the patient in the prone position affords excellent access to the posterior ankle, the subtalar joint, and the pericapsular and extra-articular structures.[22]

ANATOMY

- Posterior ankle arthroscopy and hindfoot endoscopy enable visualization and accessibility to the posterior half of the tibiotalar joint, the subtalar joint, and extra-articular structures such as the os trigonum, the flexor hallucis longus (FHL) tendon, and the posterior syndesmotic ligaments.
- The posterior intermalleolar ligament, also called the *tibial slip* or *marsupial meniscus*, is a structure with consistent location but varying size and width. It is distinct from the posteroinferior tibiofibular ligament and separated from it by a small gap filled with synovial tissue.[2]
- The os trigonum is a secondary center of ossification of the talus. It is present in 1.7% to 7% of normal feet.[4] When this ossification center remains separate from the posterolateral process of the talus (the trigonal process or the Stieda process), it is referred to as the *os trigonum*. The prevalence of unilateral and bilateral (ununited) os trigona is 10% and 1.4%, respectively.[4,17]
- The FHL tendon originates in the posterior leg then runs within a tendon sheath that begins 1 cm proximal to the subtalar joint and binds the tendon to the posterior talus and calcaneus, forming the fibro-osseous tunnel, which may restrict FHL motion.[6,10]
- The posteromedial neurovascular bundle (tibial nerve and posterior tibial artery) are consistently medial to the FHL tendon throughout its course. Instruments introduced from the posteromedial portal do not risk injuring the neurovascular bundle provided they remain lateral to the FHL.[7] Sitler et al[15] dissected 13 cadavers and found that the tibial nerve was located posterior to the FHL tendon in two specimens.
- A posteromedial portal located 1 cm proximal to the level of the tip of the lateral malleolus is on average 2.9 mm

further removed from the medial neurovascular bundle than a portal placed 1 cm more proximally.[7]

PATHOGENESIS

- Posterior ankle pain may be a result of the following:
  - Posterior ankle impingement or os trigonum syndrome
  - FHL, posterior tibial, or peroneal tendinopathy
  - Posttraumatic calcifications or exostoses
  - Bony avulsions
  - Tibiotalar or subtalar loose bodies
  - Tibiotalar or subtalar osteochondral lesions or arthrosis
  - Any combination of these entities
- Overuse injuries play an important role in the pathogenesis of posterior ankle pain.
- Repetitive minor trauma in the ankle, as seen in athletes, can induce posterior ankle and/or hindfoot osteophyte formation.[18]
- Typically, to produce symptoms, an os trigonum must be disturbed by some traumatic event, such as a supination or forced plantarflexion injuries, dancing on hard surfaces, or pushing beyond physiologic limits.[18]
- The pain is thought to be a result of the following:
  - Symptomatic motion between the relatively unstable os trigonum and talus
  - Compression of thickened joint capsules (intermalleolar ligament)[1]
  - Impinging scar tissue between the os trigonum and tibia
  - Compression between os trigonum and calcaneus (referred to as *dancer's heel*)
  - Irritation of the FHL tendon that courses between the os trigonum and the medial tubercle of the talus[6,18]
- FHL tendinopathy is usually attributable to stenosing tenosynovitis rather than tendinosis or rupture[3]; it has only rarely been reported at sites other than the posteromedial ankle.[3,10] However, immunohistochemical studies have suggested an avascular zone of the tendon in the segment of tendon that passes behind the talus.[14]

NATURAL HISTORY

- Patients present with posterior ankle pain.
- Posterior ankle impingement can be caused by overuse (chronic pain) or trauma (acute pain). It is important to differentiate between these two because posterior impingement from overuse has a better prognosis.[18]
- Overuse injuries typically occur in ballet dancers, soccer players, and downhill runners.[3,21]
- In chronic conditions, stenosing tenosynovitis of the FHL tendon may coexist with os trigonum syndrome; this leads to poorer outcome if surgical treatment is delayed.[4]

- Nonsurgical treatment for os trigonum syndrome is successful in approximately 60% of patients.[8]

PATIENT HISTORY AND PHYSICAL FINDINGS

- Patients experience deep pain in the posterior aspect of the ankle joint, mainly with forced plantarflexion.
- On examination, there is pain on palpation of the posterior aspect of the talus.
- During the passive forced plantarflexion test, the investigator can apply a rotational movement on the point of maximal plantarflexion, thereby "grinding" the posterior talar process or os trigonum between the tibia and the calcaneus.
- A positive test result, in combination with pain on posterolateral palpation, should be followed by a diagnostic infiltration of an anesthetic (with or without corticosteroid).
- Posteromedial pain on palpation does not necessarily indicate impingement.[18]
- Tenderness on palpation over the musculotendinous junction of the FHL is diagnostic for FHL tendinitis; pain can be elicited by forced simultaneous ankle and first metatarsophalangeal joint dorsiflexion.[3,10]
- "Pseudo hallux rigidus" may coexist with posteromedial ankle pain. Hallux dorsiflexion may be limited with ankle dorsiflexion but restored with ankle plantarflexion. This examination finding/phenomenon has been reported to be secondary to nodular thickening of the proximal FHL that impinges within the fibro-osseous tunnel on the posteromedial ankle.[10]
- Palpation of posterior talar process is a sensitive test for posterior ankle impingement. A positive test should be followed by a hyperplantarflexion test.
- The hyperplantarflexion test is positive when the patient experiences recognizable pain at the moment of impact. It is a highly sensitive test for posterior ankle impingement. A negative test rules out a posterior ankle impingement syndrome.
- If the pain on forced plantarflexion disappears, the diagnosis is confirmed.
- Posteromedial ankle palpation is sensitive for FHL tendinitis.

IMAGING AND OTHER DIAGNOSTIC STUDIES

- In patients with posterior ankle impingement, the anteroposterior (AP) ankle view typically fails to demonstrate abnormalities **(FIG 1A)**.
  - On the lateral view, a prominent posterior talar process or os trigonum can sometimes be recognized.
  - As the posterolaterally located posterior talar process or os trigonum is often superimposed on the medial talar

tubercle, detection of an os trigonum on a standard lateral view is often not possible **(FIG 1B)**.
  - For the same reason, calcifications can sometimes not be detected by this standard lateral view.
  - We recommend lateral radiographs with the foot in 25 degrees of external rotation in relation to the standard lateral radiographs **(FIG 1C)**.
- Bone scintigraphy effectively localizes talar and peritalar injuries.[5]
- Computed tomography defines the exact size and location of calcifications, bony fragments, osteochondral lesions, or intraosseous talar cysts **(FIG 1D)**.
- Magnetic resonance imaging (MRI) is useful for detection of bone contusions, edema, posterior capsular or ligament thickening,[1] talar osteochondral lesions, and FHL tenosynovitis.
  - MRI has been reported to accurately identify FHL tendinitis in 82% of patients,[10] represented by intermediate or low-signal intensity on T2-weighted images.[4]
  - Fluid in the FHL tendon sheath is frequently seen in MRI without clinical signs of FHL tendinitis. Fluid in the tendon sheath of the FHL must be combined with changes in the tendon itself to be a sign of a tendinitis.
- Bone edema in the os trigonum is an important diagnostic finding.
  - It is a sign of chronic compression of the os trigonum between distal tibia and calcaneus.
  - It can be a sign of degeneration of the cartilage of the undersurface of the os trigonum. In these cases, the bone edema is combined with bone edema of the calcaneus.
  - It can also be a sign of movement between the os trigonum and the talus. In these cases, there is bone edema in the posterior talus as well. These cases represent a pseudoarthrosis type of lesion.

DIFFERENTIAL DIAGNOSIS

- Tarsal tunnel syndrome
- Plantar fasciitis
- Peroneal tenosynovitis
- Posterior tibial tenosynovitis
- Pseudo hallux rigidus (in FHL tenosynovitis)
- Bony avulsions
- Ankle and subtalar arthrosis

NONOPERATIVE MANAGEMENT

- Initial treatment of os trigonum syndrome consists of rest, ice, anti-inflammatory medication, avoidance of forced

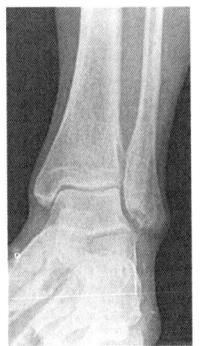 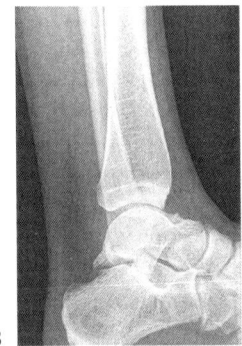 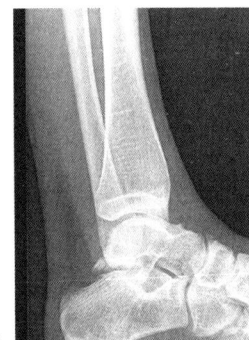 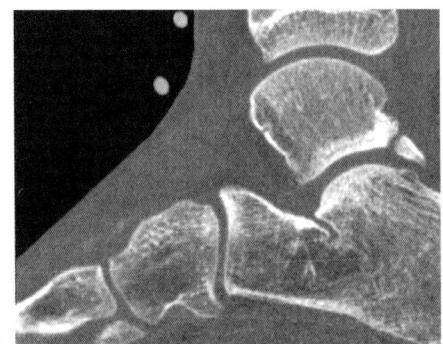

FIG 1 Imaging of posterior ankle impingement. **A.** AP ankle view showing no abnormalities. **B.** Standard lateral view. **C.** Lateral radiograph with the foot in 25 degrees of external rotation. **D.** Sagittal computed tomography scan showing os trigonum.

TABLE 1 Indications for Posterior Ankle Arthroscopy and Hindfoot Endoscopy

Articular Pathology

Posterior compartment ankle joint
Débridement and drilling of osteochondral defects
Removal of loose bodies, ossicles, calcifications, avulsion fragments
Resection of posterior tibial rim osteophytes
Treatment of chondromatosis and chronic synovitis
Posterior compartment subtalar joint
Removal of osteophytes and loose bodies
Subtalar arthrodesis
Treatment of intraosseous talar ganglions by retrograde curetting and drilling

Periarticular Pathology

Posterior ankle impingement
Deep portion of deltoid ligament: removal of posttraumatic calcifications or ossicles
Flexor hallucis longus stenosing tenosynovitis: débridement of flexor retinaculum, posterior talofibular ligament, prominent talar process, and opening the sheath of the tendon
Posterior syndesmotic ligaments: Hypertrophic ligaments can be excised.

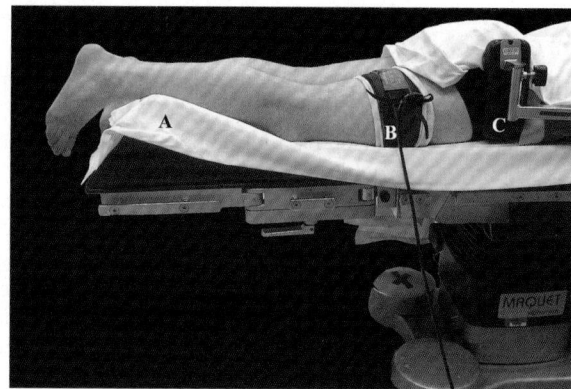

FIG 3 Positioning for hindfoot endoscopy. Small leg support (**A**), tourniquet (**B**), and leg holder (**C**).

plantarflexion, and, occasionally, ankle immobilization for 4 to 6 weeks. If there is an established nonunion, immobilization with casting is not recommended.[8]

- Physical therapy, such as progressive resistive exercises and strengthening, may be helpful.[8]
- Corticosteroid injection for os trigonum syndrome can effectively provide temporary pain relief.[4,8]
- Nonsurgical treatment for FHL tenosynovitis includes rest, ice, anti-inflammatories, longitudinal arch supports, standard physical therapy, and stretching exercises.[8,10]

SURGICAL MANAGEMENT

- Indications for posterior ankle arthroscopy and hindfoot endoscopy are listed in **TABLE 1**.
- The procedure is performed as outpatient surgery with the patient under general or epidural anesthesia.[20]

Preoperative Planning

- All imaging studies are reviewed to address not only the individual pathology but also the associated bone, cartilage, or ligament injuries as well as osteophytes, loose bodies, accessory muscles, and calcifications (**FIG 2**).
- Ankle and subtalar joint stability, stability of the peroneal tendons, and Achilles tendon tightness should be determined by examination under anesthesia.
  - Instability is a clinical diagnosis, and these patients are identified by their symptoms. They complain of recurrent

giving way. Laxity can be present without clinical symptoms of giving. If laxity is detected without clinical symptoms of giving way, it is not an indication for lateral ligament reconstruction.

- For irrigation, a single bag of normal saline with gravity flow can be used.
- A 4.0-mm arthroscope with a 30-degree angle is routinely used for posterior ankle arthroscopy.
- For posterior ankle arthroscopy, a noninvasive distraction device can be used when the ankle joint has to be entered for the diagnosis and treatment of an intra-articular pathology.
- A 4-mm chisel and a periosteal elevator may be needed during posterior arthroscopy for excision of osteophytes and ossicles.

Positioning

- The patient is placed in a prone position. The patient should be placed properly to avoid tension on the brachial plexus, avoid pressure on the ulnar nerve at the elbow, and protect the genitalia.
- A tourniquet is applied around the upper leg, and a small support is placed under the lower leg, making it possible to move the ankle freely (**FIG 3**).
- The foot is placed at the very end of the operating table so that the surgeon can fully dorsiflex the ankle.

Approach

- The landmarks on the ankle are the lateral malleolus, medial and lateral border of the Achilles tendon, and the sole of the foot. With a marking pen, a line is drawn as a reference from the tip of the lateral malleolus to the Achilles tendon, parallel to the sole of the foot.
- Posterolateral and posteromedial portals are made just above this line, at the same level in the horizontal plane, and just lateral and medial to the Achilles tendon (**FIG 4**).

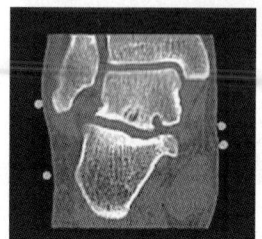
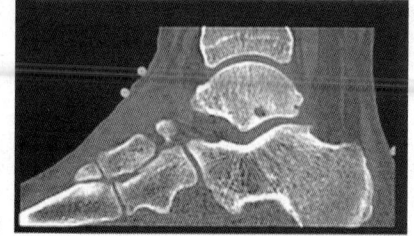
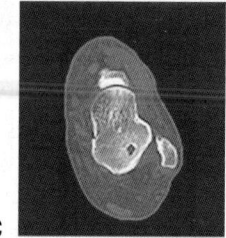

FIG 2 Preoperative planning for débridement and drilling of a subtalar osteochondral cyst lesion in a right ankle. Coronal (**A**), sagittal (**B**), and axial (**C**) computed tomography images showing the subtalar osteochondral defect and secondary cyst lesion.

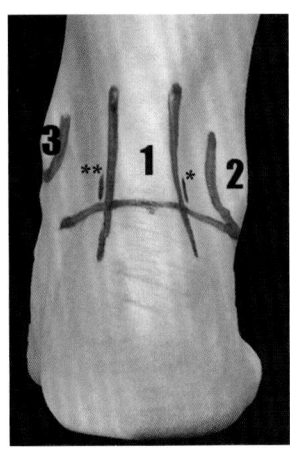
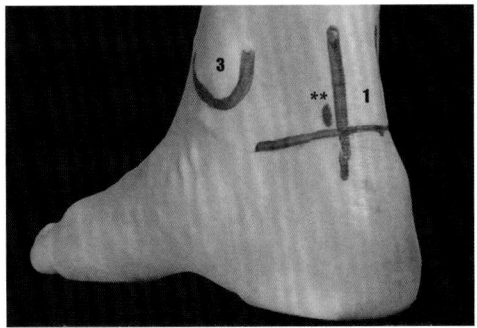
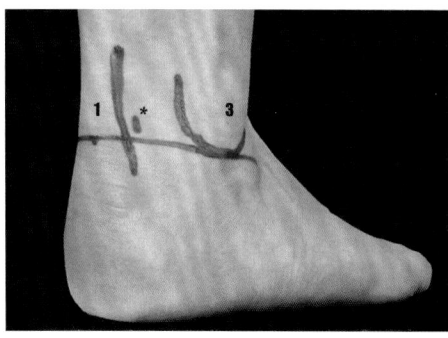

FIG 4 Posterior (**A**), posteromedial (**B**), and posterolateral (**C**) views of foot and ankle with the cutaneous landmarks for posterior ankle arthroscopy and hindfoot endoscopy. *1*, Achilles tendon; *2*, lateral malleolus; *3*, medial malleolus; *asterisk*, posterolateral portal; *double asterisks*, posteromedial portal.

CREATION OF THE POSTEROLATERAL PORTAL

- A vertical stab incision is made for posterolateral portal.
- The subcutaneous layer is split by a mosquito clamp that is directed anteriorly in the direction of the interdigital web space between the first and second toes (**TECH FIG 1A**).
- When the tip of the clamp touches the bone, it is exchanged for a 4.5-mm arthroscope shaft with the blunt trocar pointing in the same direction (**TECH FIG 1B**).
- The level of the ankle joint and subtalar joint can be distinguished by palpating the bone in the sagittal plane because the prominent posterior talar process or os trigonum can be felt as a posterior prominence between the two joints.
- The trocar is positioned extra-articularly at the level of the ankle joint.
- The trocar is exchanged for the 4-mm arthroscope; the direction of view is 30 degrees to the lateral side.

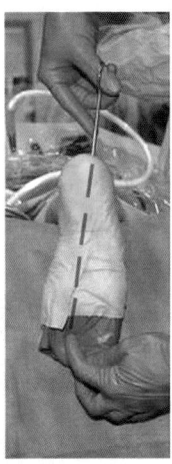
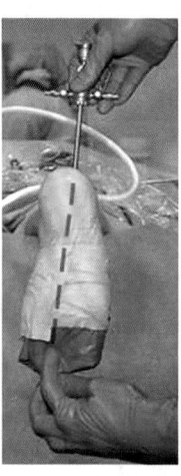

TECH FIG 1 Creation of the posterolateral portal. **A.** Subcutaneous tissue is dissected by a mosquito clamp in the direction of the first interdigital web space (*dashed line*). **B.** When the tip of the clamp touches the posterior talar process, it is exchanged for a 4.5-mm arthroscope shaft with the blunt trocar pointing in the same direction.

CREATION OF THE POSTEROMEDIAL PORTAL

- A vertical stab incision is made for the posteromedial portal.
- A mosquito clamp is introduced and directed toward the arthroscope shaft at a 90-degree angle (**TECH FIG 2A**).
- When the mosquito clamp touches the shaft of the arthroscope, the shaft is used as a guide for the clamp to move anteriorly in the direction of the ankle joint, touching the arthroscope shaft until it reaches the bone (**TECH FIG 2B**).
- Next, the arthroscope is withdrawn slightly, directly over the mosquito clamp until the tip of the mosquito clamp is visualized (**TECH FIG 2C**).

- The clamp is used to spread the extra-articular soft tissue in front of the tip of the lens.
- In situations in which scar tissue or adhesions are present, the mosquito clamp is exchanged for a 5-mm full-radius shaver.
- The tip of the shaver is directed in a lateral and slightly plantar direction toward the posterolateral aspect of the subtalar joint.
- When the tip of the shaver has reached this position, shaving can begin.

T E C H N I Q U E S

TECHNIQUES

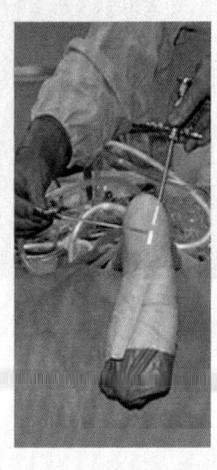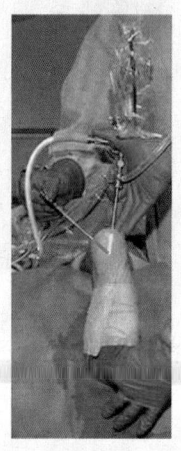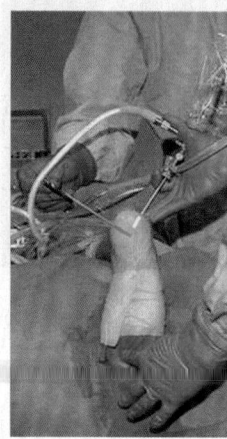

TECH FIG 2 Creation of the posteromedial portal. **A.** A mosquito clamp is introduced and directed toward the arthroscope shaft at a 90-degree angle. **B.** Touching the arthroscope shaft, the mosquito clamp is slid anteriorly until it reaches the bone. **C.** The arthroscope is now withdrawn slightly and slides over the mosquito clamp until the tip of the mosquito clamp comes into view. *White lines* indicate direction of the arthroscope shaft. *Red lines* indicate direction of the mosquito clamp.

WORKING POSTERIOR TO THE ANKLE

- The joint capsule and adipose tissue can be removed. The adipose tissue is removed first and with it the very thin joint capsule.
- The subtalar joint can now be recognized. The posterior talar fibular ligament that attaches to the talus at this level can be recognized as well.

- After removal of the thin joint capsule, the posterior subtalar joint can be inspected **(TECH FIG 3A)**.
- At the level of the ankle joint, the posterior tibiofibular and talofibular ligaments are identified and the posterior ankle joint can be visualized **(TECH FIG 3B)**.

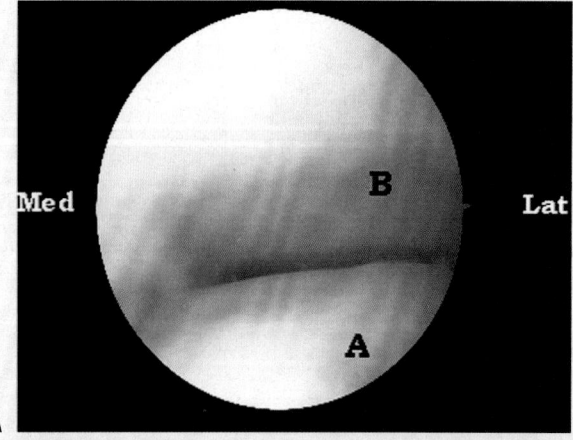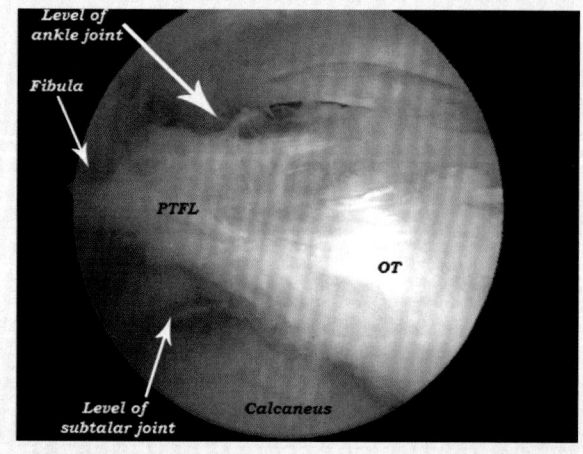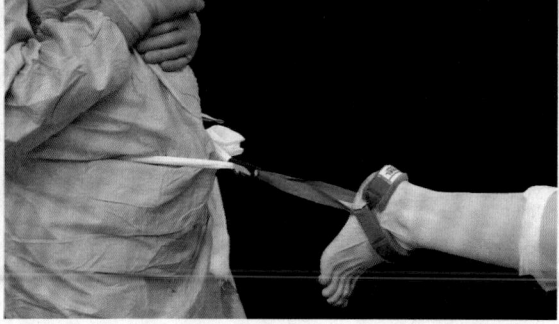

TECH FIG 3 A. Arthroscopic views of the posterior compartment of the subtalar joint showing the calcaneus (*A*) and the talus (*B*). **B.** Endoscopic overview of the posterolateral aspect of the ankle joint. Os trigonum (*OT*) and its connection to the posterior talofibular ligament (*PTFL*). **C.** Application of the soft tissue distractor.

- The posterior talar process can be freed of scar tissue, and the FHL tendon, an important landmark, is identified. Motion of the hallux helps isolate the fibers of the FHL tendon in the posterior ankle.
- The shaver should never be used medial to the FHL tendon because of the proximity of the posteromedial neurovascular bundle.
- After removal of the thin posterior ankle joint capsule, the ankle joint is entered with the arthroscope and inspected.
- On the medial side, both the tip of the medial malleolus and the deep portion of the deltoid ligament are visualized.

- By opening the joint capsule from inside out at the level of the medial malleolus, the tendon sheath of the posterior tibial tendon can be opened.
- With manual distraction on the os calcis, the posterior aspect of the ankle joint is opened, and the shaver can be introduced into the tibiotalar joint.
- For greater distraction, a noninvasive ankle distractor can be applied **(TECH FIG 3C)**.
- A total synovectomy or capsulectomy can be performed. In our experience, nearly the entire talar dome tibial plafond can be visualized via this posterior approach.
- An osteochondral defect or subchondral cystic lesion can be identified, débrided, and drilled **(TECH FIG 4)**.

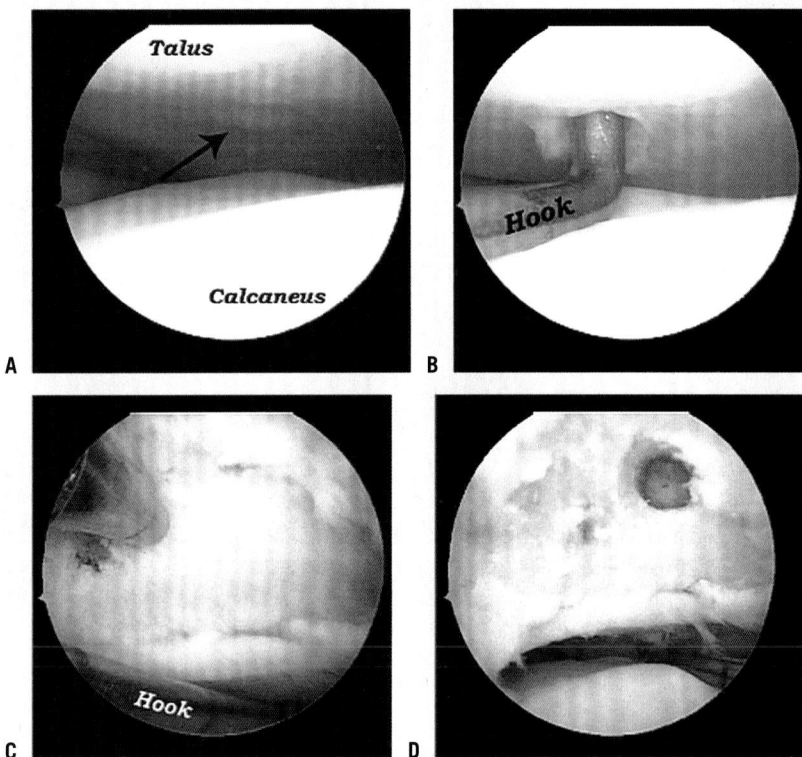

TECH FIG 4 Endoscopic procedure for débridement and drilling of a subtalar osteochondral cyst lesion in a right ankle (same patient as in **FIG 2**). **A.** Endoscopic image with an *arrow* indicating the defect. **B.** A hook is introduced via the posteromedial portal and penetrates the osteochondral defect up to the cyst. **C.** By retrograde drilling, the cyst is reached. The hook is used for guiding the exact direction of the drill. **D.** Postoperative overview.

REMOVAL OF AN OS TRIGONUM

- The posterior syndesmotic ligaments are inspected and, if hypertrophic, are partially resected.
- Removal of a symptomatic os trigonum (**TECH FIG 5**), a non-united fracture of the posterior talar process, or a symptomatic

large posterior talar prominence requires partial detachment of the posterior talofibular ligament and release of the flexor retinaculum, both of which attach to the posterior talar prominence.

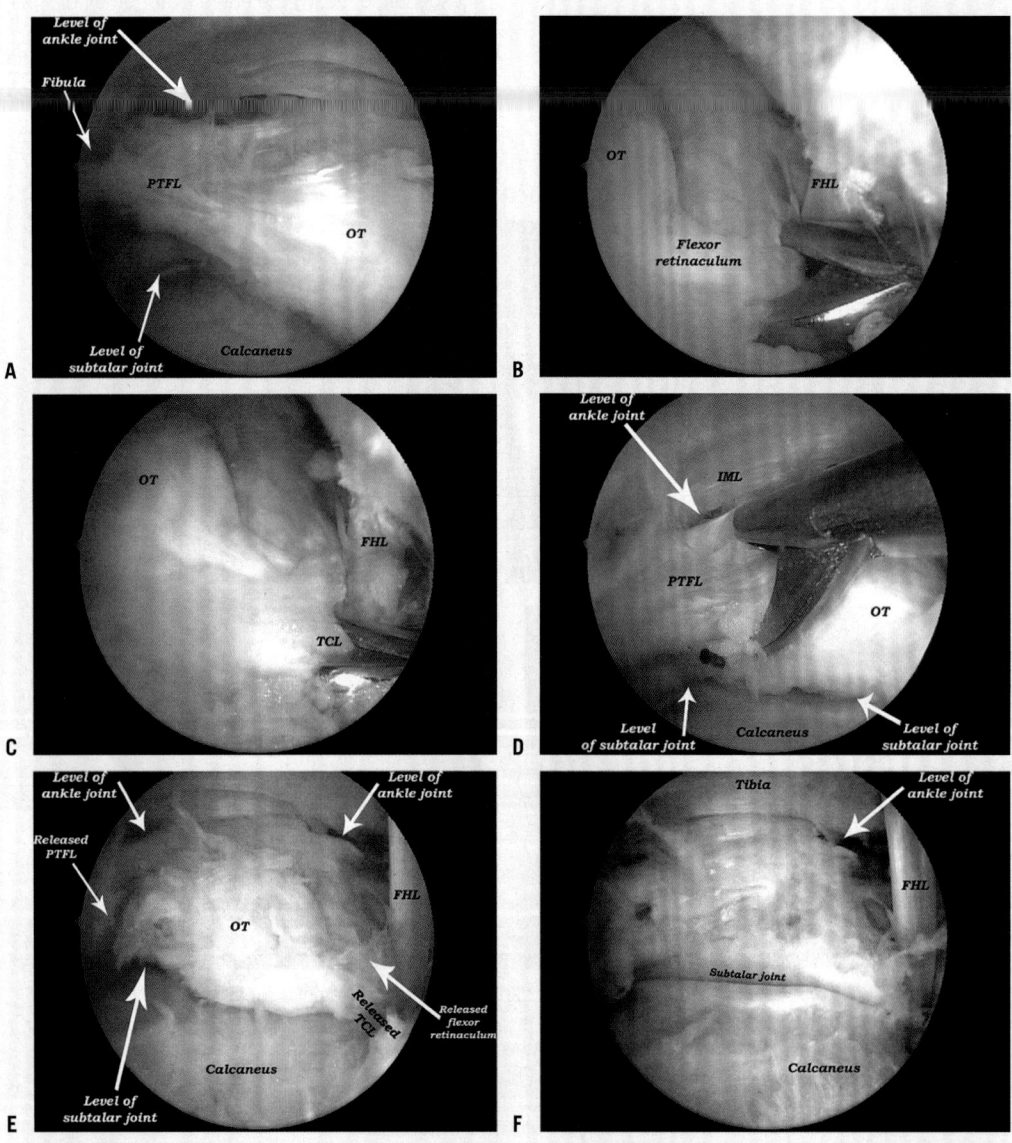

TECH FIG 5 Endoscopic procedure for removing an os trigonum and releasing the flexor hallucis longus (*FHL*) in a left ankle. **A.** Os trigonum (*OT*) with its connection to the posterior talofibular ligament (*PTFL*), flexor retinaculum, and talocalcaneal ligament (*TCL*). **B.** Cutting through the flexor retinaculum. **C.** Cutting through the TCL. **D.** Releasing the PTFL. **E.** Overview of the os trigonum released from its related anatomic structures. **F.** Postoperative overview. *IML*, intermalleolar ligament.

RELEASE OF THE FLEXOR HALLUCIS LONGUS TENDON

- Release of the FHL tendon involves detachment of the flexor retinaculum from the posterior talar process by means of a punch **(TECH FIG 6)**.
- A tight, thick crural fascia, if present, can hinder the free movement of instruments. It is helpful to enlarge the hole in the fascia using a punch or shaver.

- Bleeding is controlled by electrocautery at the end of the procedure.

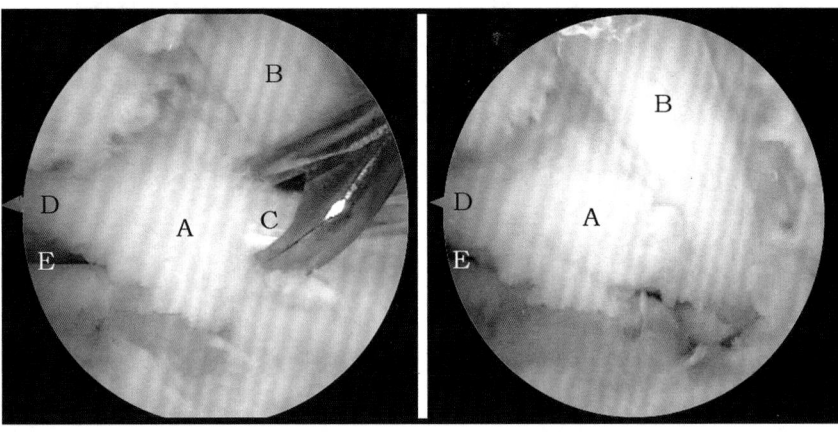

TECH FIG 6 Endoscopic procedure for releasing of the FHL tendon (*B*) involves detachment of the flexor retinaculum (*C*) from the posterior talar process (*A*) by means of a punch. *D*, talus; *E*, subtalar joint.

WOUND CLOSURE AND DRESSING

- After removal of the instruments, the stab incisions are closed with 3-0 nylon to prevent sinus formation.
- A sterile compression dressing is applied.
- In patients with combined anterior and posterior symptoms, the posterior pathology is addressed by means of the two-portal hindfoot approach, and the anterior pathology is approached by a two-portal anterior approach.

- This can be done in two ways. The anterior arthroscopy can be performed with the knee flexed and the foot upside down, but we typically prefer a two-stage procedure. First, the two-portal hindfoot approach is finished. The patient is then turned and a routine anterior ankle arthroscopy is performed.

TECHNIQUES

Pearls and Pitfalls

Position of the Arthroscope	• The direction of view should always be lateral.
Rouvière Ligament	• This ligament runs to the FHL retinaculum. • It can be attached to the posterior talar process. • An arthroscopic punch or scissors can be used to enlarge the entry through this ligament. • Usually, it has to be detached from the posterior talar process to get to the ankle joint.
Safe Areas	• The arthroscope should point into the direction of the web space between the first and second toes. • It should be positioned lateral to the FHL tendon. It can be positioned medial to the FHL tendon only when a release of the neurovascular bundle is required (posttraumatic tarsal tunnel syndrome).

| Removing the Hypertrophic Posterior Talar Process Using the Chisel | • Care should be taken not to place the chisel too far anterior to avoid entering the subtalar joint **(FIG 5)**. |

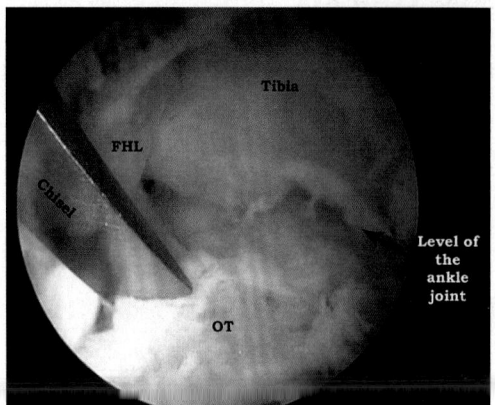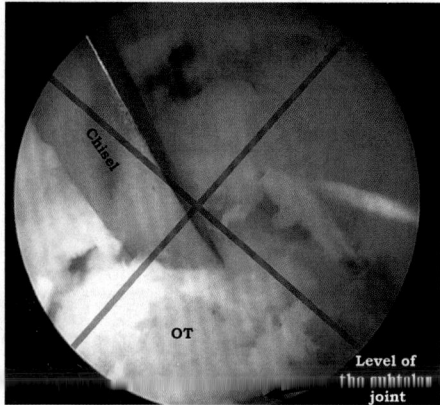

FIG 5 A,B. Removal of the hypertrophic posterior talar process using the chisel. Care should be taken not to place the chisel too far anterior to avoid entering the subtalar joint. *FHL*, flexor hallucis longus; *OT*, os trigonum.

| How to Initially Visualize or Gain Proper Orientation in the Posterior Ankle | • The most important trick is to start shaving at the level of the subtalar joint on the lateral side. This is an area in which it is relatively safe to start shaving. The opening of the shaver is directed toward the joint.
• Once the subtalar joint has been identified, the posterior talofibular ligament is identified. This ligament attaches to the lateral surface of the talus in this area.
• If we move the scope and shaver proximal from the posterior fibular ligament, we are at the level of the os trigonum. The soft tissue in this posterolateral area can now be removed.
• The ankle joint usually can now be identified by applying some traction to the calcaneus. Dorsiflexing the foot can also help.
• Part of the posterior ligaments can be removed to enter the ankle joint when desired.
• From the posterolateral corner, the instruments now can be moved over the posterior talar process or os trigonum to the medial side while staying in contact with the posterior ankle ligaments and the proximal surface of the os trigonum all the way. The FHL then comes into view. |

POSTOPERATIVE CARE

- As soon as possible after surgery, the patient is advised to start range-of-motion exercises as tolerated. It is not necessary to immobilize the ankle postoperatively to prevent sinus formation. The posterior ankle joint has a good soft tissue covering. The advantage of the procedure is that patients can start to move the ankle directly postoperatively.
- Postoperatively for 2 or 3 days, the patient is allowed weight bearing on crutches as tolerated.
- The dressing can be removed after 3 days. We remove the sutures 2 weeks postoperatively.
- The patient is reevaluated 1 week postoperatively. If necessary, physical therapy can be prescribed for range of motion, strengthening, and stability.

OUTCOMES

- In a consecutive series of 146 posterior ankle arthroscopies (136 patients) performed at the Academic Medical Center University of Amsterdam between 1994 and 2002, all patients were satisfied postoperatively. There were no complications other than 2 patients who experienced a small area of diminished sensation over the heel pad of the hindfoot.

- The main indication was a posterior ankle impingement syndrome. Procedures, all carried out by the same surgeon, were as follows:
  - Removal of a bony impediment (os trigonum or hypertrophic posterior talar process; n = 52)
  - Additional release of the FHL tendon (n = 37)
  - Removal of a soft tissue impediment by a shaver (n = 8)
  - Isolated release of the FHL tendon (n = 7)
  - Débridement and drilling of an osteochondral defect at the posteromedial talar dome (n = 7), in the tibial plafond (n = 4), or in the posterolateral talar dome (n = 2)
  - Removal of calcifications (n = 5)
  - Total synovectomy (the knee was flexed and an anterior synovectomy was performed by means of the standard anterolateral and anteromedial approach; n = 9)
  - Arthroscopic débridement of degenerated subtalar joint (n = 10)
  - Removal of a loose body from the subtalar joint (n = 1)
  - Curettage, drilling, and grafting of a large intraosseous talar ganglion (n = 3)
- Combined procedures did not cause any technical problems and were successful in most patients. Patients who were treated for a bony impingement did better than patients who were treated for a soft tissue impingement.

- None of these patients had deterioration of the result over time.[19]
- Marumoto and Ferkel[9] treated 11 patients with painful os trigonum by arthroscopic removal of the os trigonum. The average postoperative American Orthopaedic Foot & Ankle Society (AOFAS) scale was 86.4 points 3 years postoperatively.
  - Jerosch and Fadel[4] applied the same treatment method to 10 patients with symptomatic os trigonum; 9 of them were symptom-free 4 weeks postoperatively, and the average AOFAS scale increased from 43 preoperatively to 87 at a mean follow-up time of 25 months. They observed no complications in these 10 patients.
  - Tey et al[16] endoscopically treated 15 patients with posterior ankle impingement and reported that all but 1 patient (7%) improved at an average 3 years of follow-up.
  - Willits et al[23] performed 24 posterior ankle arthroscopies with an indication of posterior ankle impingement. The average time to return to work was 1 month and to sports was 5.8 months. Mean score on the AOFAS scale was improved to 91 at a mean follow-up time of 32 months postoperatively.
  - Ögüt et al[12,13] used the two-portal hindfoot endoscopy technique successfully in a variety of indications, including intraosseous cysts of talus, talar fracture, pigmented villonodular synovitis, synovial osteochondromatosis, talar osteochondral lesions, and peroneal tenosynovitis. FHL tenosynovitis and posterior ankle impingement syndrome were the most common indications. In their series of 60 feet, they noted only two complications (3.3%) of sural nerve damage.
  - Zwiers et al[24] reviewed 16 papers that report the results of surgical treatment for posterior ankle impingement syndrome. Of these 16 papers; 6 reported on open surgical techniques and 10 evaluated endoscopic techniques. The compared results for patient satisfaction did not differ in between the groups, but major complication rates and return to sports were significantly better for the endoscopically treated group (13.8% vs. 5.4%, and mean 7.8 weeks vs. 16.0 weeks, respectively).

COMPLICATIONS

- Potential complications of this technique include tibial nerve and vascular injury, FHL tendon injury, and sural nerve injury.
- To prevent sural nerve injury, it is important to create the posterolateral portal as described previously, close to the Achilles tendon, first making a stab incision and then continuing with blunt dissection by a mosquito clamp.
- Avoiding the potential complications of working through a posteromedial portal, the trick is to angle the instrument (shaver, burr, punch) in the posteromedial portal at 90 degrees to the arthroscope shaft.
- The arthroscope shaft subsequently is used as a guide for the instrument to travel into the direction of the joint. All the way, the mosquito clamp should be felt to touch the arthroscope shaft. In this manner, the neurovascular bundle is passed without problem.
- Precise control of the aspirator and shaver is mandatory to prevent tibialis posterior nerve and vessel injury and to

prevent damage to the FHL tendon. In areas close to the neurovascular bundle, the aspirator should be set to a minimum amount of suction.
  - In their case series of 189 ankles, Nickisch et al[11] found the complication rate as 8.5% (16 ankles); four patients had plantar numbness, three had sural nerve dysesthesia, four had Achilles tendon tightness, two had complex regional pain syndrome, two had infection, and one had a cyst at the posteromedial portal.
- We have applied this technique since 1994 without any complications other than two patients who experienced a small area of diminished sensation over the heel pad of the hindfoot.
- When performed in the manner described earlier, hindfoot endoscopy is a safe and reliable method of diagnosing and treating a variety of posterior ankle problems.
- The decision to treat posterior as well as anterior pathology is made preoperatively. If preoperatively it is decided to treat both anterior and posterior pathology, we start with addressing the posterior pathology by means of the two-portal hindfoot approach. After finishing the posterior procedure, the portals are sutured, and the patient is turned, and the anterior procedure is performed.

ACKNOWLEDGMENT

- The authors would greatly like to thank P. A. J. de Leeuw from the Department of Orthopaedic Surgery in the Academic Medical Center in Amsterdam, The Netherlands, for providing all the images for this chapter.

REFERENCES

1. Fiorella D, Helms CA, Nunley JA II. The MR imaging features of the posterior intermalleolar ligament in patients with posterior impingement syndrome of the ankle. Skeletal Radiol 1999;28:573–576.
2. Golanò P, Mariani PP, Rodríguez-Niedenfuhr M, et al. Arthroscopic anatomy of the posterior ankle ligaments. Arthroscopy 2002;18: 353–358.
3. Hamilton WG, Geppert M, Thompson FM. Pain in the posterior aspect of the ankle in dancers. J Bone Joint Surg Am 1996;78: 1491–1500.
4. Jerosch J, Fadel M. Endoscopic resection of a symptomatic os trigonum. Knee Surg Sports Traumatol Arthrosc 2006;14:1188–1193.
5. Johnson RP, Collier D, Carrera GF. The os trigonum syndrome: use of bone scan in the diagnosis. J Trauma 1984;24:761–764.
6. Kolettis G, Michell L, Klein JD. Release of the flexor hallucis longus tendon in ballet dancers. J Bone Joint Surg Am 1996;78:1386–1390.
7. Lijoi F, Marcello L, Baccarani G. Posterior arthroscopic approach to the ankle: an anatomic study. Arthroscopy 2003;19:62–67.
8. Maquirriain J. Posterior ankle impingement syndrome. J Am Acad Orthop Surg 2005;13:365–371.
9. Marumoto JM, Ferkel RD. Arthroscopic excision of the os trigonum: a new technique with preliminary clinical results. Foot Ankle Int 1997;18:777–784.
10. Michelson J, Dunn L. Tenosynovitis of the flexor hallucis longus: a clinical study of the spectrum of presentation and treatment. Foot Ankle Int 2005;26:291–303.
11. Nickisch F, Barg A, Saltzman CL, et al. Postoperative complications of posterior ankle and hindfoot arthroscopy. J Bone Joint Surg Am 2012;94:439–446.
12. Ögüt T, Ayhan E, Irgit K, et al. Endoscopic treatment of posterior ankle pain. Knee Surg Sports Traumatol Arthrosc 2011;19: 1355–1361.
13. Ögüt T, Seker A, Ustunkan F. Endoscopic treatment of posteriorly localized talar cysts. Knee Surg Sports Traumatol Arthrosc 2011;19:1394–1398.

14. Petersen W, Pufe T, Zantop T, et al. Blood supply of the flexor hallucis longus tendon with regard to dancer's tendinitis: injection and immunohistochemical studies of cadaver tendons. Foot Ankle Int 2003;24:591–596.

15. Sitler DF, Amendola A, Bailey CS, et al. Posterior ankle arthroscopy: an anatomic study. J Bone Joint Surg Am 2002;84:763–769.

16. Tey M, Monllau JC, Centenera JM, et al. Benefits of arthroscopic tuberculoplasty in posterior ankle impingement syndrome. Knee Surg Sports Traumatol Arthrosc 2007;15:1235–1239.

17. Uzel M, Cetinus E, Bilgic E, et al. Bilateral os trigonum syndrome associated with bilateral tenosynovitis of the flexor hallucis longus muscle. Foot Ankle Int 2005;26:894–898.

18. van Dijk CN. Anterior and posterior ankle impingement. Foot Ankle Clin 2006;11:663–683.

19. van Dijk CN. Hindfoot endoscopy. Foot Ankle Clin 2006;11:391–414.

20. van Dijk CN. Hindfoot endoscopy for posterior ankle pain. Instr Course Lect 2006;55:545–554.

21. van Dijk CN, Lim LS, Poortman A, et al. Degenerative joint disease in female ballet dancers. Am J Sports Med 1995;23:295–300.

22. van Dijk CN, Scholten PE, Krips R. A 2-portal endoscopic approach for diagnosis and treatment of posterior ankle pathology. Arthroscopy 2000;16:871–876.

23. Willits K, Sonneveld H, Amendola A, et al. Outcome of posterior ankle arthroscopy for hindfoot impingement. Arthroscopy 2008;24:196–202.

24. Zwiers R, Wiegerinck JI, Murawski CD, et al. Surgical treatment for posterior ankle impingement. Arthroscopy 2013;29(7):1263–1270.

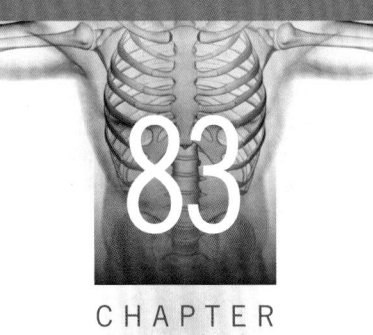

Endoscopic Treatment of Posterior Ankle Impingement through a Posterior Approach

Phinit Phisitkul and Annunziato Amendola

DEFINITION

- *Posterior ankle impingement syndrome* is a clinical disorder characterized by posterior ankle pain that occurs in forced plantarflexion. It can be caused by an acute or chronic injury, with the os trigonum or trigonal process of the talus as the most offending structure.[10,19]
- Synonyms used for posterior ankle impingement syndrome include *posterior block of the ankle, posterior triangle pain, talar compression syndrome, os trigonum syndrome, os trigonum impingement, posterior tibiotalar impingement syndrome,* and *nutcracker-type syndrome.*[4,11,20,38]
- The os trigonum is a secondary ossification center of the talus. It mineralizes between the ages of 11 and 13 years in boys and 8 and 11 years in girls. It fuses with the posterior talus within 1 year, forming the posterolateral process, often called the *Stieda* or *trigonal process*. The os trigonum remains as a separate ossicle in 1.7% to 7% of normal feet, twice as often unilaterally as bilaterally.[3,8,16,24]

ANATOMY

- The posterior process of the talus is composed of a smaller posteromedial process and a larger posterolateral or trigonal process flanking the sulcus for the flexor hallucis longus (FHL) tendon.
- The os trigonum may be found in connection with the posterolateral tubercle **(FIG 1)**. It is completely corticalized and has three surfaces: anterior, inferior, and posterior.

- The anterior surface connects to the posterolateral tubercle via fibrous, fibrocartilaginous, or cartilaginous tissue. The inferior surface forms the posterior part of the talocalcaneal joint.
- The posterior surface is nonarticular and has the attachments of posterior talofibular ligament, posterior talocalcaneal ligament, deep layer of the flexor retinaculum, and the talar component of the fibuloastragalocalcaneal ligament of Rouviere and Canela Lazaro.[30]
- The tibialis posterior tendon, the flexor digitorum longus tendon, and the FHL tendon situate in their own fibrous tunnels in continuity with the fascia of the deep posterior compartment.
- The neurovascular bundles are just medial and posterior to the FHL tendon at the level of the ankle joint, with the tibial nerve as the most lateral structure **(FIG 2)**. Peroneocalcaneal internus muscle, known as a *false FHL*, can mimic the FHL leading to a potential neurovascular injury.[28]
- In some variants, the posterior tibial artery can be thin or absent (0% to 2%), with the dominant peroneal artery traversing across the posterior ankle toward the tarsal tunnel.[2,6]

PATHOGENESIS

- Most cases of posterior ankle impingement syndrome occur in athletes such as ballet dancers or soccer players who have sustained acute or repetitive injuries with the ankle in forced plantarflexion, causing the "nutcracker effect" **(FIG 3)**.[12,20] Ankle sprain may cause avulsion fracture of the posterior talofibular ligament and secondary impingement.[15,21,25,36]

FIG 1 Os trigonum.

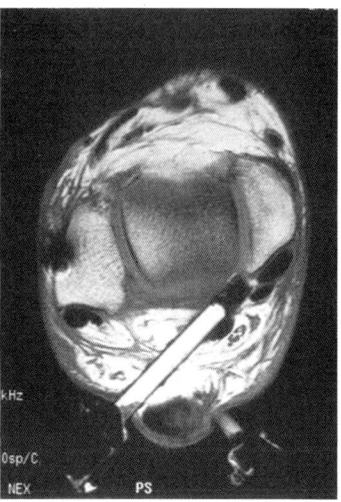

FIG 2 Neurovascular bundle posteromedial to the FHL tendon.

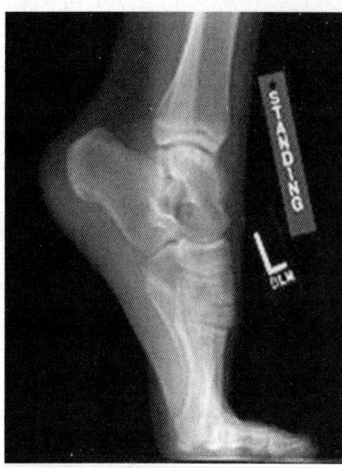

FIG 3 Forced plantarflexion as a cause of the nutcracker effect in the os trigonum.

- Symptoms can be aggravated by any structures localized between the posterior tibial plafond and the calcaneal facet of the posterior subtalar joint, such as the os trigonum; long trigonal process; FHL tendon; posterior inferior tibiofibular ligament; intermalleolar ligament; and any osseous, articular cartilage, capsule, or synovial lesions of the posterior ankle or subtalar joint.
- FHL tenosynovitis is commonly associated with posterior ankle impingement due to the intimate relationship between the tendon and the os trigonum or the trigonal process at the posterior aspect of the talus. This lesion can be an associated injury or secondary to the inflamed surrounding structures.[17,27,32]

NATURAL HISTORY

- The natural history of posterior ankle impingement is currently unknown. Os trigonum is a benign condition and usually is asymptomatic.
- When symptomatic, nonoperative treatment has been found to be successful in 60% of cases. However, Hedrick and McBryde[10] reported that only 40% of those successfully treated patients could achieve full preinjury activity levels. The prognosis with nonoperative treatment is generally poor in high-activity patients such as ballet dancers.[20]

PATIENT HISTORY AND PHYSICAL FINDINGS

- The routine history should include sex, age, occupation, sports activities, and mechanism of the injury.
- Patients should be asked for the description of pain, its location, and any aggravating positions or activities. Pain from the impingement usually is directly posterior or posterolateral to the ankle joint. Pain in the posteromedial aspect may be associated with tenosynovitis of the FHL tendon, which is usually described as pain along the tendon longitudinally. Aggravation of the symptoms with the ankle in full plantarflexion is essential to the diagnosis.
- Examination must be performed to rule out other pathologies causing posterior ankle and hindfoot pain, such as Achilles tendinopathy, Haglund syndrome, "pump bump" syndrome, tibialis posterior tendinitis, and peroneal tendon injuries. Diligent palpation of the described structures for pain is recommended.

- The physical examination should include the following:
  - Examination for retromalleolar swelling. Mild swelling occurs in posterior ankle impingement syndrome. Significant swelling should raise the suspicion of peroneal or tibialis posterior tenosynovitis.
  - Passive ankle plantarflexion. In a positive test, sharp pain or crepitus is produced at full plantarflexion.
  - In FHL tenosynovitis, pain is produced with active/passive motion of the hallux while a thumb palpates the tendon for tenderness and crepitus. The presence of FHL tenosynovitis should be documented, and it should be treated accordingly.
  - Tenderness from FHL tenosynovitis is produced with active/passive motion of the hallux while a thumb palpates the tendon for tenderness and crepitus. The presence of FHL tenosynovitis should be documented, and it should be treated accordingly.
  - Tenderness of other posterior ankle structures. Individual palpation of the peroneal tendons, tibialis posterior tendon, Achilles tendon, and posterior aspect of the calcaneal tuberosity is essential to exclude other pathologies. Palpation of the os trigonum itself is difficult due to its depth. Other diagnoses should be considered if there is no pain with passive ankle plantarflexion and the positive test for other possible lesions in spite of the presence of the os trigonum on radiographs.

IMAGING AND OTHER DIAGNOSTIC STUDIES

- A lateral radiograph of the ankle usually demonstrates the osseous lesions sufficiently (**FIG 4A**). Lateral radiographs can be taken in full ankle plantarflexion and slight external rotation of the limb to visualize impingement from the os trigonum.[9]
- Bone scanning has been reported to identify the symptomatic os trigonum. It is not routinely obtained, however, and does not replace accurate history taking and physical examination (**FIG 4B**). False-positive results in patients with high activity levels make this study less useful.[31]
- Computed tomography (CT) scan can help clarify osseous or osteochondral lesions, especially when the posteromedial facet fracture is suspected.[7]
- Magnetic resonance imaging (MRI) is the most useful imaging examination for posterior ankle impingement syndrome (**FIG 4C**). Anatomic variants and a range of osseous and soft tissue abnormalities have been found to be associated with this condition. Posterior tibiotalar synovitis and marrow edema within one or more of the tarsal bones were found in all cases. In contrast, os trigonum was found in only 30% of cases.[5,23,27]
- Diagnostic injection can be helpful when the signs and symptoms are inconclusive.[14,25] The postinjection symptoms have been shown to be parallel to results after surgical excision of the os trigonum. However, injection directly into the junction between the os trigonum and the talus is difficult and must be done under fluoroscopic guidance in experienced hands.

DIFFERENTIAL DIAGNOSIS

- Haglund syndrome
- Tendinitis (Achilles tendon, peroneal tendons, posterior z tendons)
- Loose bodies
- Ankle or subtalar arthritis

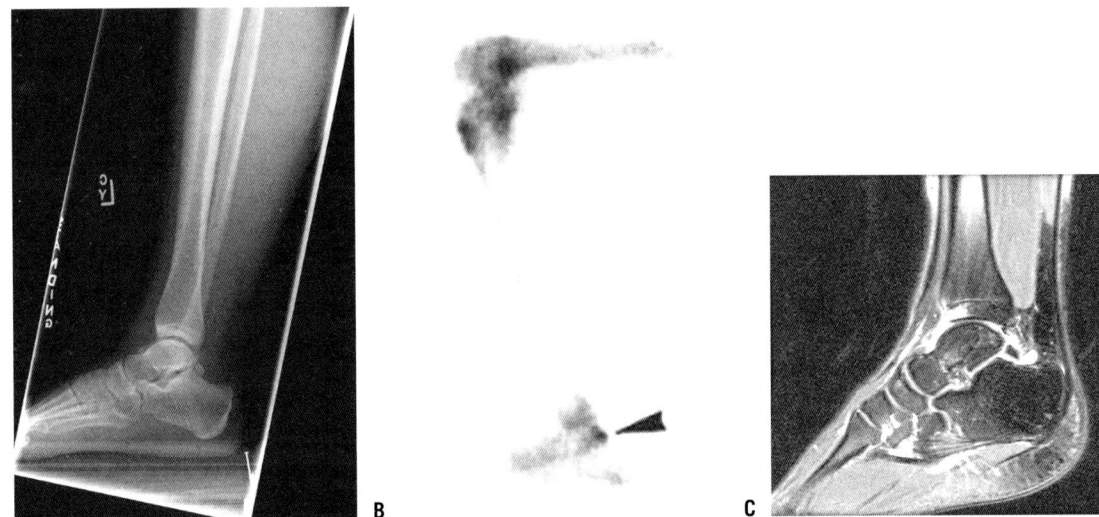

FIG 4 A. Lateral radiograph of the ankle. **B.** Positive bone scan. **C.** MRI examination for posterior ankle impingement syndrome.

NONOPERATIVE MANAGEMENT

- Nonoperative treatment is always the first approach. However, it has shown less than optimal results in the published literature, with, at best, a 60% rate of improvement plus long-term modification of activities.[10]
- Avoidance of aggravating activities such as forced plantar-flexion is the most important factor because it will avoid impingement and aggravation of the inflammatory response. This measure may not be tolerable in athletes who routinely require this position, such as ballet dancers and soccer players.
- Supportive treatments include rest, ice, anti-inflammatory medications, and immobilization in a short-leg walking cast.
- One or two cortisone injections under fluoroscopic guidance have shown more than 80% response rate at 2 years.[25] Its use was not routinely recommended due to the risk of FHL tendon rupture and potential disabilities especially in ballet dancers.
- Physical therapy can be instituted as symptoms improve. It consists of phonophoresis, isometric exercises, heel cord stretching, and selected isometric strengthening.

SURGICAL MANAGEMENT

- Indications
  - Failure of nonoperative treatment after at least 3 months
  - Inability to return to required activities after nonoperative treatment

Preoperative Planning

- All imaging studies are reviewed. MRI is helpful in the evaluation of associated lesions.
- All the pathologies should be carefully detected. Surgical steps with informed consent can be added accordingly, such as loose body removal, treatment for osteochondritis dissecans lesions, or an open FHL repair.
- When surgery is indicated, the treatment for an os trigonum, an acute or chronic fracture of the trigonal process, or an intact large trigonal process is virtually the same. Further studies, for example, CT scan, to distinguish them may not be necessary.
- If arthroscopic or open surgery is planned, the posterior tibial pulse must be palpable in the soft spot posterior to

the medial malleolus because an absence or a minor artery may be associated with a dominant peroneal artery. This artery traverses across the posterior ankle and is at high risk during arthroscopy.

Positioning

- The patient is placed in the prone position with standard padding (**FIG 5A,B**).
- The patient's ankles are at the level just distal to the end of the bed to leave enough room for possible anterior or lateral arthroscopic portals.

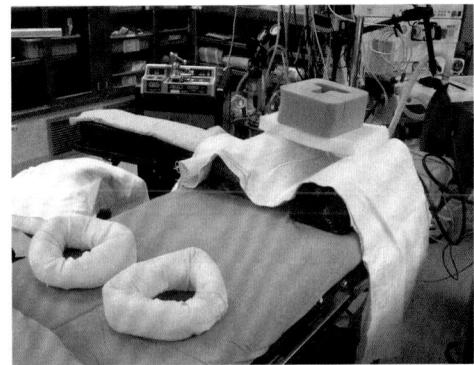

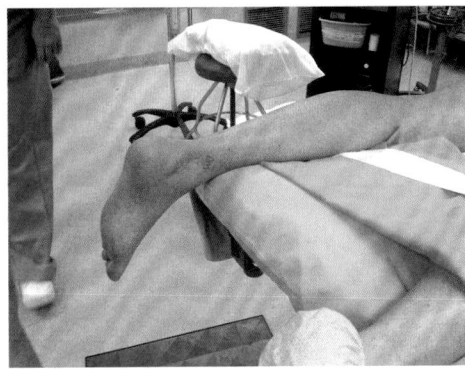

FIG 5 A. Prone positioning. **B.** Ensure adequate padding of all surfaces.

- The surgeon's body can be used to dorsiflex the ankle by leaning forward.

Approach

- The posterior aspect of the ankle and subtalar joints can be accessed open or arthroscopically.
- Open approaches can be posteromedial or posterolateral, on either side of the Achilles tendon.
  - The posteromedial approach is recommended by the authors. When the bony impingement is accompanied by pathologies in the neurovascular bundles or lesions in the FHL tendon that may require a repair, a posteromedial approach is advantageous.

- The posterolateral approach also may be used for cases that require only excision of the os trigonum and trigonal process or release of the FHL tendon.
- The arthroscopic approach has advantages over open surgeries in terms of minimizing surgical injury, postoperative pain, and early return to activities.
- We prefer the prone over the supine or lateral decubitus position because it provides a more direct approach, minimizing the risk of instrument skiving off toward the neurovascular bundles.
- Apart from the magnification advantage, we have found that this method also aids in visualization of intra-articular pathologies.[29]
- This technique requires familiarity with the hindfoot anatomy and arthroscopic skills.

ESTABLISHMENT OF PORTALS

- The anatomic landmarks of the posterior ankle are drawn, including the Achilles tendon, the medial and lateral malleoli, and the superior aspect of the calcaneal tuberosity.
- The posterolateral and the posteromedial portals are located 1.5 cm proximal to the superior aspect of the calcaneal tuberosity on either side of the Achilles tendon **(TECH FIG 1A,B)**.
- Ankle joint injection can be performed through the posterolateral portal, but it is not necessary because the joint will be

inspected easily after the os trigonum or the trigonal process has been removed.
- The posterolateral portal is established first with a vertical skin incision, followed by blunt dissection with a straight hemostat. The tip of the hemostat should be kept just next to the Achilles tendon laterally to minimize injury to the sural nerve.
- The dissection proceeds through a fat layer directly anteriorly.
- The os trigonum usually is palpable, and a blunt trocar is inserted toward its superior aspect.

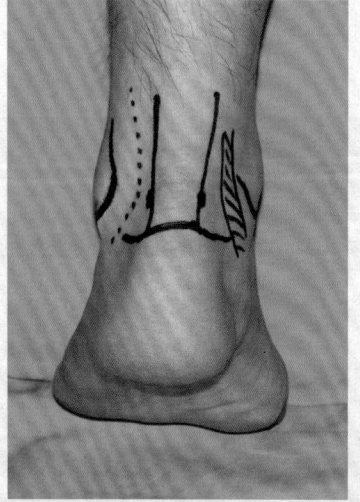
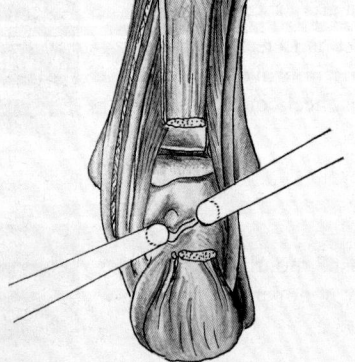
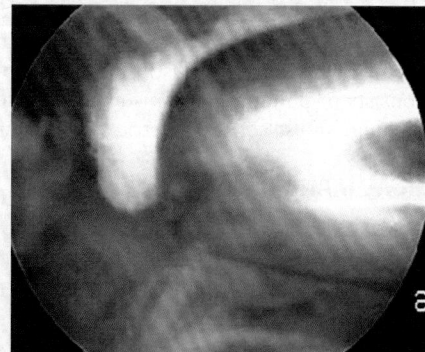
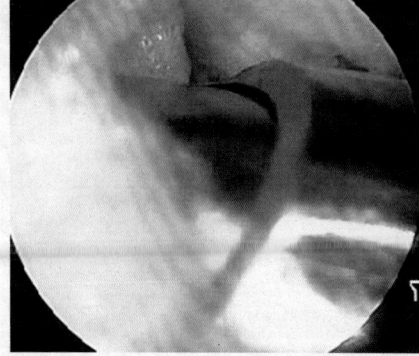

TECH FIG 1 **A.** Placement of posteromedial and posterolateral portals with the patient in the prone position. **B.** Topographical landmarks of the pertinent structures. **C.** The hemostat is visualized when creating the second portal. **D.** The 3.5-mm shaver is visualized through the second portal.

- A 4-mm arthroscope is inserted through the cannula.
- Next, the posteromedial portal is established at the same level just medial to the Achilles tendon.
- A straight hemostat is used to dissect into the same soft tissue tunnel as the arthroscope. The hemostat is advanced while it

is kept in contact with the arthroscopic cannula until the tip is seen by the arthroscope.
- The soft tissue is gently dilated. A full-radius 3.5-mm shaver is inserted into the posteromedial portal until the tip is seen **(TECH FIG 1C,D)**.

DÉBRIDEMENT OF THE SOFT TISSUE

- The initial débridement of the fatty tissue is performed first to make room for the arthroscopic maneuvers. This step will improve visualization tremendously.
- The shaver is kept deep just above or below the os trigonum, with its cutting surface turned laterally.
- The shaver is gradually moved medially until the FHL tendon is seen. The FHL tendon indicates the location of the neurovascular bundles, which lie medial and superficial to it.
- The os trigonum is débrided off all the attached soft tissue circumferentially **(TECH FIG 2A)**.

- Medially, the retinaculum of the FHL is released off the os trigonum with a shaver or arthroscopic scissors **(TECH FIG 2B)**.
- Tenosynovitic lesions of the FHL, if seen, may require a release and débridement further distally. Great care is taken to release the fibrous sheath from only the posterior attachment on the calcaneal wall. A partial tear of the FHL can be débrided, but a tear greater than 50% may require an open repair.
- The posterior talofibular ligament attached on the lateral aspect of the os trigonum is released.

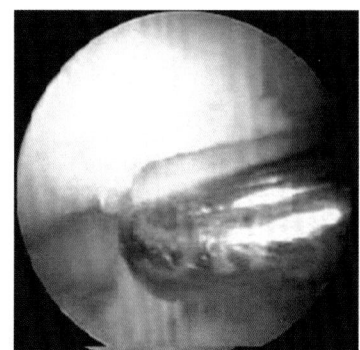

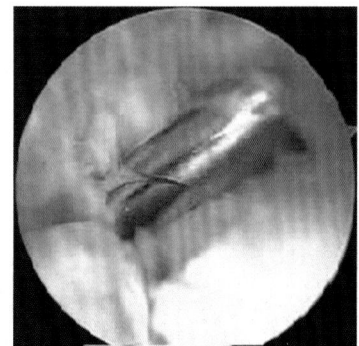

A   B

TECH FIG 2 A. The os trigonum is débrided of soft tissue attachments with a shaver circumferentially. **B.** The FHL is visualized and released from its soft tissue attachments to the os trigonum.

RESECTION OF THE OS TRIGONUM AND TRIGONAL PROCESS

- The synchondrosis is palpated by a Freer elevator coming from the superior aspect.
- Next, the tip of the instrument is pushed into the synchondrosis.
- Cracking of the synchondrosis is performed by levering maneuvers from either the superior or inferior surface **(TECH FIG 3A)**.

- The os trigonum is removed as a whole using a grasper **(TECH FIG 3B)**. In the presence of an intact enlarged trigonal process, it is removed entirely with a burr.
- The posterior aspect of the talus is evaluated, and any sharp bony edges are rounded off **(TECH FIG 3C)**.
- The most posterior aspect of the articular cartilage of the posterior talar facet of the subtalar joint is always removed together with the os trigonum.

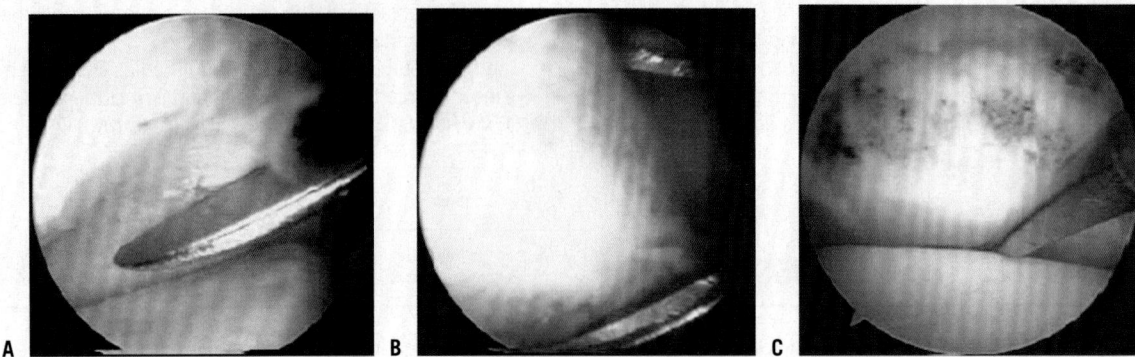

TECH FIG 3 A. Lever the os trigonum loose from its talar attachments with a Freer elevator. **B.** The os trigonum is removed as a whole using a grasper. **C.** The posterior aspect of the talus is evaluated and rounded off, particularly around the FHL tendon.

EVALUATION OF ASSOCIATED LESIONS

- The posterior aspect of the ankle joint is evaluated. Synovitis or a thickened intermalleolar ligament is débrided. Stay lateral to the FHL tendon. Loose bodies are removed if present. Intra-articular views of the ankle joint are best achieved with a 2.7-mm arthroscope.
- The subtalar joint is evaluated in the same manner **(TECH FIG 4)**. The dynamic view of the hindfoot is inspected when the ankle is manipulated into full plantarflexion.

- There should be no impingement at the completion of the procedure.
- If arthroscopic evaluation or treatment of the anterior ankle joint is required, it can be performed in two ways.
  - The first way is to reposition the patient into the supine position and redrape the limb.
  - The second way is to bend the knee to 90 degrees and perform the anterior ankle arthroscopy in the upside-down manner. This requires experience and familiarity of the ankle anatomy.

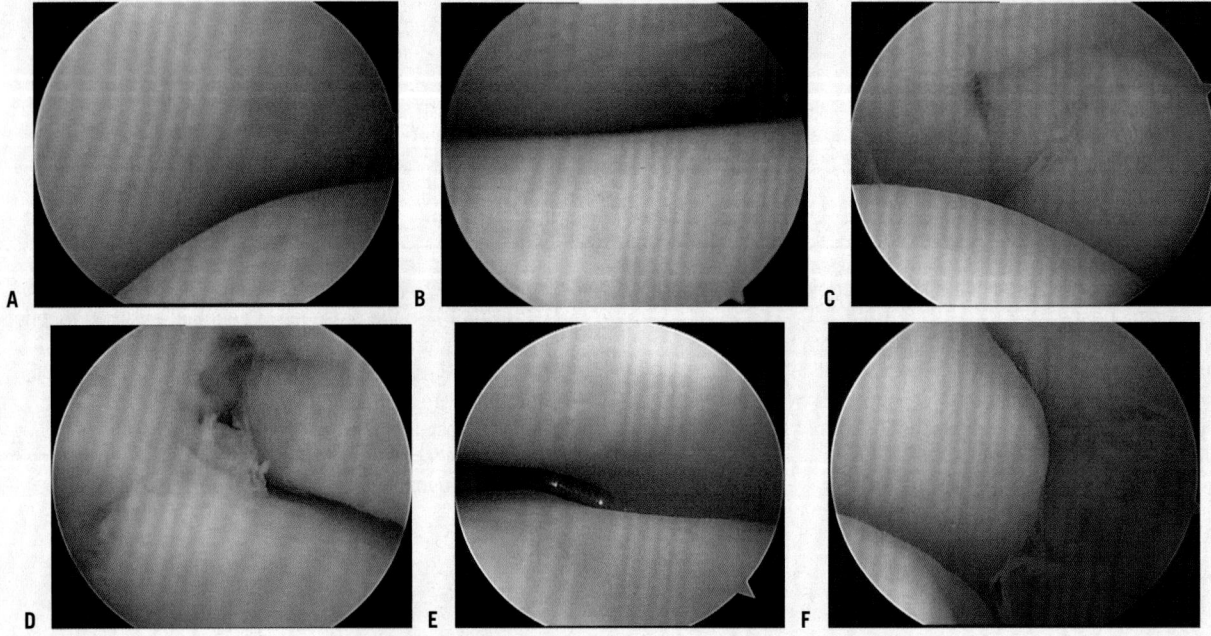

TECH FIG 4 A–F. Multiple views of the ankle and subtalar joint.

Pearls and Pitfalls

Diagnosis	• Good history taking and physical examination are paramount. • MRI and diagnostic injection can help in questionable cases.
Preoperative Planning	• Open surgery is preferred when the posterior tibial pulse is not palpable behind the ankle joint. This approach is limited in its access to anterior ankle lesions and may require redraping. However, simple ankle procedures can be performed when the knee is flexed to 90 degrees and the foot held by an assistant. • Patients should be informed of the possibility of conversion to open surgery, especially when a complete rupture of the FHL tendon is anticipated.
Portal Placement	• The ankle is placed firmly on the bed in true anteroposterior or slight external rotated alignment. The incision is made through the skin only. Blunt dissection is used to dissect through the soft tissue planes.
Débridement of Soft Tissue	• The shaver is kept deep on the joint capsule and lateral to the FHL. Beware of anatomic variations such as a peroneocalcaneus internus muscle, which can mimic the FHL.
Resection of the Os Trigonum and Trigonal Process	• Palpation with a Freer elevator to identify the synchondrosis. • "Death roll maneuver" is performed before removal of the bony fragment. Adequate portal size is needed.

POSTOPERATIVE CARE

• Portal incisions routinely are left unsutured.
• A compressive soft dressing is applied. The patient is informed about the possibility of some drainage in the first couple of postoperative days. The dressing can be changed if necessary.
• Leg elevation is encouraged.
• No immobilization is required.
• Patients can bear weight as tolerated in a postoperative shoe.
• When acute pain subsides, usually 2 to 3 days postoperatively, patients can begin early range-of-motion and strengthening exercise.
• Full activities are allowed gradually as tolerated.

OUTCOMES

• Nonoperative treatment has not shown promising results, especially in high-demand athletes, but a success rate of more than 80% could be achieved when cortisone injections are routinely given under fluoroscopic guidance.[10,25]
• When nonoperative treatment has failed, excellent outcomes have been reported with either open or arthroscopic resection of the os trigonum.[1,13,18,20,22,34,35]
• Arthroscopic techniques can help minimize morbidities associated with open dissection, such as a painful scar, severe postoperative pain, and wound complications. It requires arthroscopic skills and familiarity with hindfoot anatomy.[33,37]

COMPLICATIONS

• Neurovascular injuries are possible with either arthroscopic or open approaches. Neurapraxia of the tibial, peroneal, and sural nerves has been reported; most patients recovered spontaneously. Permanent sensory deficit and neuroma formation have occurred when the nerves were transected, especially the sural nerve when the open posterolateral approach is used.[1]

• Other possible complications include Achilles tendon tightness, complex regional pain syndrome, infection, and cyst at the posteromedial portal.[26]
• Symptoms can persist after operative treatment. Correct diagnosis and adequate treatment of all associated pathologies are the keys.

REFERENCES

1. Abramowitz Y, Wollstein R, Barzilay Y, et al. Outcome of resection of a symptomatic os trigonum. J Bone Joint Surg Am 2003;85-A(6): 1051–1057.
2. Adachi B. Das Arteriensystem der Japaner. Kyoto, Japan: Maruzen, 1928:215–291.
3. Bizarro A. On sesamoid and supernumerary bones of the limbs. J Anat 1921;55:256–268.
4. Brodsky AE, Khalil MA. Talar compression syndrome. Am J Sports Med 1986;14:472–476.
5. Bureau NJ, Cardinal E, Hobden R, et al. Posterior ankle impingement syndrome: MR imaging findings in seven patients. Radiology 2000;215:497–503.
6. Dubreuil-Chambardel L. Variations des arteres du pelvis et du membre inferieur. Paris, France: Masson et Cie, 1925:191–271.
7. Giuffrida AY, Lin SS, Abidi N, et al. Pseudo os trigonum sign: missed posteromedial talar facet fracture. Foot Ankle Int 2003;24: 642–649.
8. Grogan DP, Walling AK, Ogden JA. Anatomy of the os trigonum. J Pediatr Orthop 1990;10:618–622.
9. Hamilton WG. Stenosing tenosynovitis of the flexor hallucis longus tendon and posterior impingement upon the os trigonum in ballet dancers. Foot Ankle 1982;3:74–80.
10. Hedrick MR, McBryde AM. Posterior ankle impingement. Foot Ankle Int 1994;15:2–8.
11. Howse AJ. Posterior block of the ankle joint in dancers. Foot Ankle 1982;3:81–84.
12. Iovane A, Midiri M, Finazzo M, et al. Os trigonum tarsi syndrome. Role of magnetic resonance [in Italian]. Radiol Med 2000;99:36–40.
13. Jerosch J, Fadel M. Endoscopic resection of a symptomatic os trigonum. Knee Surg Sports Traumatol Arthrosc 2006;14:1188–1193.
14. Jones DM, Saltzman CL, El-Khoury G. The diagnosis of the os trigonum syndrome with a fluoroscopically controlled injection of local anesthetic. Iowa Orthop J 1999;19:122–126.
15. Karasick D, Schweitzer ME. The os trigonum syndrome: imaging features. AJR Am J Roentgenol 1996;166:125–129.

16. Lawson JP. International Skeletal Society Lecture in honor of Howard D. Dorfman. Clinically significant radiologic anatomic variants of the skeleton. AJR Am J Roentgenol 1994;163:249–255.

17. Lohrer H. Flexor hallucis longus tendon rupture as an impingement lesion induced by os trigonum instability [in German]. Sportverletz Sportschaden 2006;20:31–35.

18. Lombardi CM, Silhanek AD, Connolly FG. Modified arthroscopic excision of the symptomatic os trigonum and release of the flexor hallucis longus tendon: operative technique and case study. J Foot Ankle Surg 1999;38:347–351.

19. Maquirriain J. Posterior ankle impingement syndrome. J Am Acad Orthop Surg 2005;13:365–371.

20. Marotta JJ, Micheli LJ. Os trigonum impingement in dancers. Am J Sports Med 1992;20:533–536.

21. Martin BF. Posterior triangle pain: the os trigonum. J Foot Surg 1989;28:312–318.

22. Marumoto JM, Ferkel RD. Arthroscopic excision of the os trigonum: a new technique with preliminary clinical results. Foot Ankle Int 1997;18:777–784.

23. Masciocchi C, Catalucci A, Barile A. Ankle impingement syndromes. Eur J Radiol 1998;27(suppl 1):S70–S73.

24. McDougall A. The os trigonum. J Bone Joint Surg Br 1955;37-B(2):257–265.

25. Mouhsine E, Crevoisier X, Leyvraz PF, et al. Post-traumatic overload or acute syndrome of the os trigonum: a possible cause of posterior ankle impingement. Knee Surg Sports Traumatol Arthrosc 2004;12:250–253.

26. Nickish F, Barg A, Saltzman CL, et al. Postoperative complications of posterior ankle and hindfoot arthroscopy. J Bone Joint Surg Am 2012;94(5):439–446.

27. Peace KA, Hillier JC, Hulme JC, et al. MRI features of posterior ankle impingement syndrome in ballet dancers: a review of 25 cases. Clin Radiol 2004;59:1025–1033.

28. Phisitkul P, Amendola A. False FHL: a normal variant posing risks in posterior hindfoot endoscopy. Arthroscopy 2010;26(5):714–718.

29. Phisitkul P, Tochigi Y, Saltzman CL, et al. Arthroscopic visualization of the posterior subtalar joint in the prone position: a cadaver study. Arthroscopy 2006;22:511–515.

30. Sarrafian S. Anatomy of the Foot and Ankle: Descriptive Topographic Functional, ed 2. Philadelphia: JB Lippincott, 1993.

31. Sopov V, Liberson A, Groshar D. Bone scintigraphic findings of os trigonum: a prospective study of 100 soldiers on active duty. Foot Ankle Int 2000;21:822–824.

32. Uzel M, Cetinus E, Bilgic E, et al. Bilateral os trigonum syndrome associated with bilateral tenosynovitis of the flexor hallucis longus muscle. Foot Ankle Int 2005;26:894–898.

33. van Dijk CN, de Leeuw PA, Scholten PE. Hindfoot endoscopy for posterior ankle impingement. Surgical technique. J Bone Joint Surg Am 2009;91(suppl 2):287–298.

34. van Dijk CN, Scholten PE, Krips R. A 2-portal endoscopic approach for diagnosis and treatment of posterior ankle pathology. Arthroscopy 2000;16:871–876.

35. Veazey BL, Heckman JD, Galindo MJ, et al. Excision of ununited fractures of the posterior process of the talus: a treatment for chronic posterior ankle pain. Foot Ankle 1992;13:453–457.

36. Wenig JA. Os trigonum syndrome. J Am Podiatr Med Assoc 1990;80:278–282.

37. Willits K, Sonneveld H, Amendola A, et al. Outcome of posterior ankle arthroscopy for hindfoot impingement. Arthroscopy 2008;24:196–202.

38. Zeichen J, Schratt E, Bosch U, et al. Os trigonum syndrome. Unfallchirurg 1999;102:320–323.

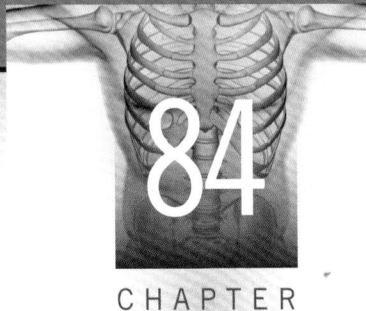

84
CHAPTER

Subtalar Arthroscopy:
Perspective 1

Carol Frey

DEFINITION

- The subtalar joint is a complex and functionally important joint of the lower extremity. It plays a major role in inversion and eversion of the foot.
- Subtalar arthroscopy can be applied as a diagnostic and therapeutic instrument.
- Subtalar arthroscopy includes arthroscopy of the sinus tarsi and posterior and anterior subtalar joints.
- Arthroscopic techniques have advanced and indications for subtalar arthroscopy have evolved to include loose body removal, synovectomy, resection fibrosis, resection os trigonum, treatment of osteochondral lesions, and resection of tarsal coalition.

ANATOMY

- For arthroscopic purposes, the subtalar joint is divided into anterior (talocalcaneonavicular) and posterior (talocalcaneal) articulations (FIG 1).
- The anterior and posterior articulations are separated by the tarsal canal, which has a large lateral opening called the *sinus tarsi*. The tarsal canal is filled with a thick interosseous

ligament. Because of this ligament, there is usually no connection between the anterior and posterior joint complex.
- Within the tarsal canal and sinus tarsi are found the interosseous talocalcaneal ligament, the medial and intermediate roots of the inferior extensor retinaculum, the cervical ligament, fatty tissue, and blood vessels.[5,6,8,12]
- The lateral ligamentous support of the subtalar joint consists of the lateral talocalcaneal ligament, the posterior talocalcaneal ligament, the lateral root of the inferior extensor retinaculum, and the calcaneofibular ligament (FIG 2).
- The anterior subtalar joint is generally thought to be inaccessible to arthroscopic visualization because of the thick interosseous ligament that fills the tarsal canal and the ligaments that insert on the floor of the sinus tarsi.[2-4,18] However, when there is a tear of the ligaments or they are débrided, the anterior joint can be visualized.
- The posterior subtalar joint has a synovial lining. This joint has a posterior capsular pouch with small lateral, medial, and anterior recesses.
- The posterior talar and subtalar anatomy has confusing nomenclature. The flexor hallucis longus runs in a fibro-osseous tunnel between the posterior medial tubercle

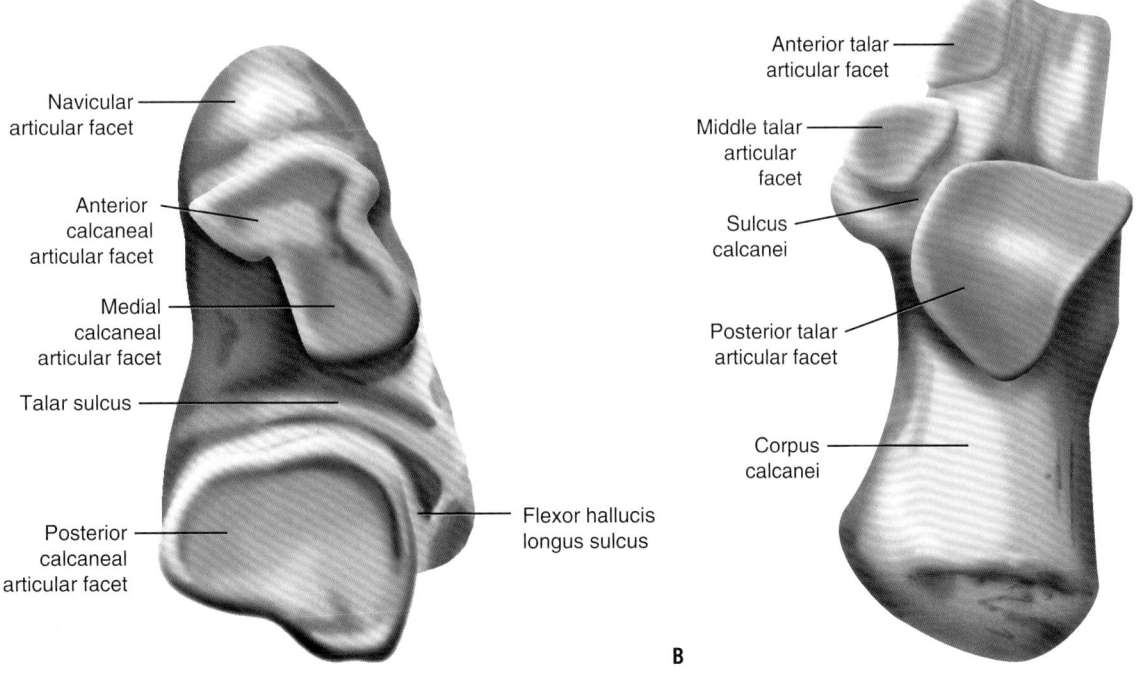

A   B

FIG 1 **A,B.** The subtalar joint is divided into the anterior (talocalcaneonavicular) and posterior joints (talocalcaneal).

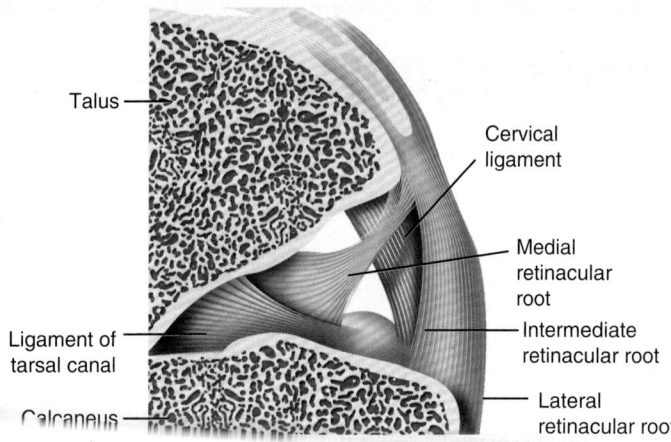

Talus

Cervical
ligament

Medial
retinacular
root

Intermediate
retinacular root

Ligament of
tarsal canal

Lateral
retinacular root

Calcaneus

FIG 2 The ligaments of the subtalar joint.

(process) and the posterior lateral tubercle (process) of the talus. The posterior lateral process is often called *Stieda process*, which can have an accessory ossicle known as the *os trigonum*. In some cases, the os trigonum unites with the Stieda process and is called the *trigonal process*.

PATHOGENESIS

- One of the most common indications for subtalar arthroscopy is chronic pain in the sinus tarsi, historically referred to as *sinus tarsi syndrome*.[2]
- Sinus tarsi syndrome has been described as persistent pain in the tarsal sinus secondary to trauma (80% of the cases reported).[2]
- There are no specific objective findings in this condition.
- The exact etiology is not clearly defined, but scarring and degenerative changes to the soft tissue structure of the sinus tarsi are thought to be the most common cause of pain in this region.
- Therefore, *sinus tarsi syndrome* is an inaccurate term that should be replaced with a specific diagnosis, as it can include many other pathologies, such as interosseous ligament tears, arthrofibrosis, and joint degeneration.

PATIENT HISTORY AND PHYSICAL FINDINGS

- Patients with subtalar joint pathology often present with lateral ankle pain that is aggravated by standing and walking activities, particularly on uneven terrain.
  - Walking on uneven terrain can result in a feeling of instability.
- Motion of the subtalar joint is not simple inversion and eversion.[8,12] However, motion is best tested by holding the left heel in the right hand and vice versa and then using the opposite hand to hold the forefoot and move the foot from inversion to eversion. This motion should be smooth and painless.
- Inversion and eversion are coming primarily from the talocalcaneal (subtalar) joint. Exact measurements are difficult using standard techniques. Restricted motion may be seen with acute ankle sprain, arthritis, posterior tibial tendon dysfunction, tarsal coalition, fracture, chondral injury, adhesions, synovitis, and inflammatory conditions.
- There may be swelling or stiffness in the joint.
- Subtalar stiffness and pain indicate pathology in and around the subtalar joint but are not specific to one diagnosis.

- Clinical examination reveals pain on the lateral aspect of the hindfoot aggravated by firm pressure over the lateral opening of the sinus tarsi.
- Relief of symptoms with injection of local anesthetic directly into the sinus tarsi confirms the diagnosis of pain or dysfunction in the sinus tarsi.
- Pathology of the interosseous ligaments of the subtalar joint usually is associated with focal pain over the lateral entrance to the sinus tarsi. Patients often have slight restriction and discomfort with passive subtalar motion.

IMAGING AND OTHER DIAGNOSTIC STUDIES

- Differential injections may be required to confirm pathology in the subtalar joint.
- Anteroposterior, lateral, and modified anteroposterior views of the foot are necessary to identify the subtalar joint.
- The lateral and posterior processes are better seen on hindfoot oblique views.
- The oblique 45-degree foot films show the anterior portion of the subtalar joint.
- Broden view shows the posterior facet of the subtalar joint. This view is obtained by rotating the foot medially 45 degrees with dorsiflexion. The x-ray beam is pointed at the lateral malleolus and angled 10 degrees cephalad. Different views are obtained by changing the angle of the x-ray beam from 10 to 40 degrees.
- Computed tomography (CT) scans in the coronal plane are best for visualizing the talar body or posterior and lateral processes of the talus. CT can be used to show intra-articular pathology.
- CT scans in the transverse or sagittal planes are best to visualize the talar neck and dome.
- Magnetic resonance imaging may detect chronic inflammation or fibrosis within the subtalar joint. Ligament injury, bone contusions, osteochondral lesions, chondral injury, impingement, synovitis, and fibrous or cartilaginous coalitions can be well demonstrated on magnetic resonance imaging.
- The preoperative imaging studies predict subtalar cartilage damage less accurately than does arthroscopy.

DIFFERENTIAL DIAGNOSIS

- Chronic lateral ankle pain
- Chronic ankle instability
- Peroneal tendon pathology
- Posterior tibial tendon dysfunction
- Superficial peroneal nerve pathology
- Fracture of the anterior process of the calcaneus
- Fracture of the lateral process of the talus
- Fracture of the posterior process of the talus
- Navicular fracture
- Calcaneal cuboid arthrosis/subluxation
- Calcaneus fracture
- Tarsal coalition
- Posterior ankle impingement including flexor hallucis longus tenosynovitis
- Os trigonum
- Osteochondral lesion
- Degenerative joint disease

NONOPERATIVE MANAGEMENT

- Injection of anesthetic agent or corticosteroid
- Foot orthosis, including a UCBL
- Anti-inflammatory medication
- Ankle brace with a hindfoot lock
- Peroneal tendon strengthening

SURGICAL MANAGEMENT

- Indications for subtalar arthroscopy include chondromalacia, subtalar impingement lesions, osteophytes, lysis of adhesions with posttraumatic arthrofibrosis, synovectomy, and the removal of loose bodies.[1,2,4,7,11]
- Other therapeutic indications include instability, débridement and treatment of osteochondral lesions, retrograde drilling of cystic lesions, resection of coalition (especially fibrous type), removal of a symptomatic os trigonum, evaluation and excision of fractures of the anterior process of the calcaneus and lateral process of the talus, and subtalar fusion.[9,10,15,16]

Preoperative Planning

- Confirm the diagnosis with testing, including differential injections to exclude ankle pathology.
- The absolute contraindications to subtalar arthroscopy must be ruled out. These include localized infection leading to a potential septic joint and advanced degenerative joint disease, particularly with deformity.
- Relative contraindications include severe edema, poor skin quality, and poor vascular status.

Positioning

- The patient is placed in the lateral decubitus position with the operative extremity draped free (**FIG 3**). Padding is placed between the lower extremities as well as under the contralateral extremity to protect the peroneal nerve.
- A thigh tourniquet is recommended.

Approach

Lateral Approach

- Three standard portals are recommended for visualization and instrumentation of the subtalar joint (**FIG 4**).

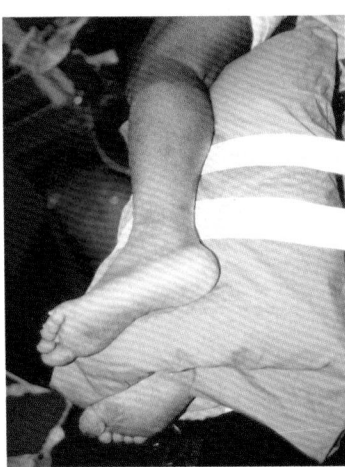

FIG 3 The patient is placed into the lateral decubitus position with the operative limb draped free.

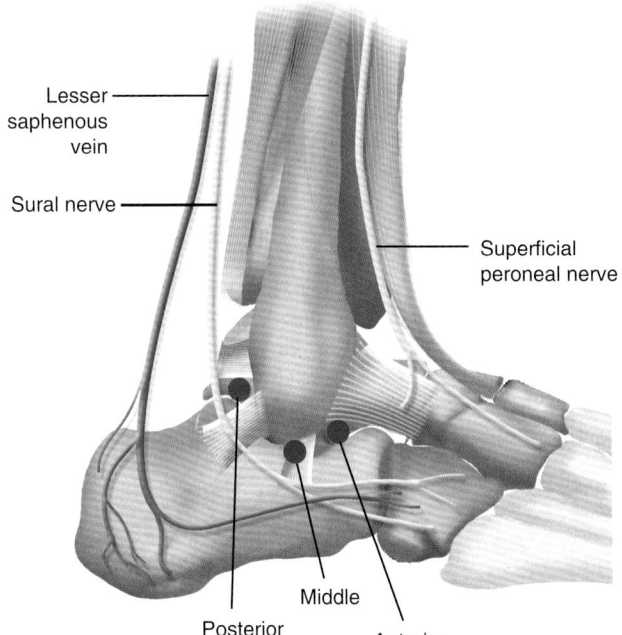

FIG 4 Standard portals and their positions.

The anatomic landmarks for lateral portal placement are the lateral malleolus, the sinus tarsi, and the Achilles tendon.

- Careful dissection and portal placement help avoid the superficial peroneal nerve branches (anterior portal) and the sural nerve and peroneal tendons (posterior portal).
- The anterior portal is established approximately 1 cm distal to the fibular tip and 2 cm anterior to it (**FIG 5**).
- The middle portal is just anterior to the tip of the fibula, directly over the sinus tarsi.

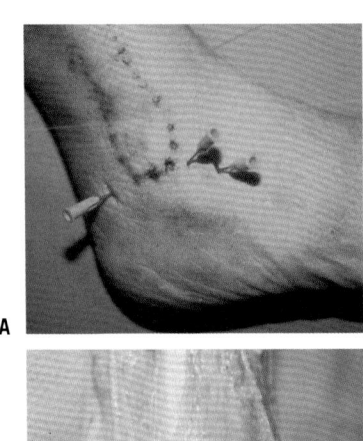

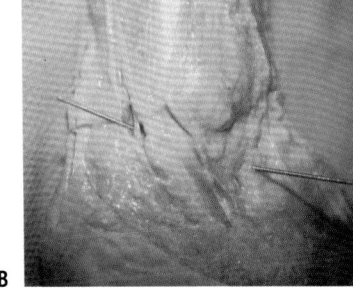

FIG 5 A. Standard subtalar arthroscopic portals demonstrated on a cadaver. **B.** Anterior and posterior portals with the skin stripped away. Note the proximity of the sural nerve to the posterior portal.

- The posterior portal is at or approximately one finger width proximal to the fibular tip and 2 cm posterior to the lateral malleolus.
- The posterior portal is usually safe when placed behind the saphenous vein and sural nerve and anterior to the Achilles tendon. With placement of the posterior portal, care must be taken to avoid the sural nerve.

Posterior Approach

- Posterior subtalar arthroscopy can be performed using a posterolateral and a posteromedial portal. This two-portal endoscopic approach to the hindfoot with the patient in the prone position has been credited with offering better access to the medial and anterolateral aspects of the posterior subtalar joint **(FIG 6)**.[13,14,17]

- The main difference between the two techniques is that the lateral approach for posterior subtalar arthroscopy is a true arthroscopy technique in which the arthroscope and the instruments are placed within the joint, whereas the two-portal posterior technique (using posterolateral and posteromedial portals) starts as an extra-articular approach.
- With the two-portal posterior technique, a working space is first created adjacent to the posterior subtalar joint by removing the fatty tissue overlying the joint capsule and the posterior part of the ankle joint.
- The joint capsule is then partially removed to enable inspection of the joint from the outside-in, with the arthroscope positioned at the edge of the joint without actually entering the joint space.
- The maximum size of the intra-articular instruments depends on the available joint space.

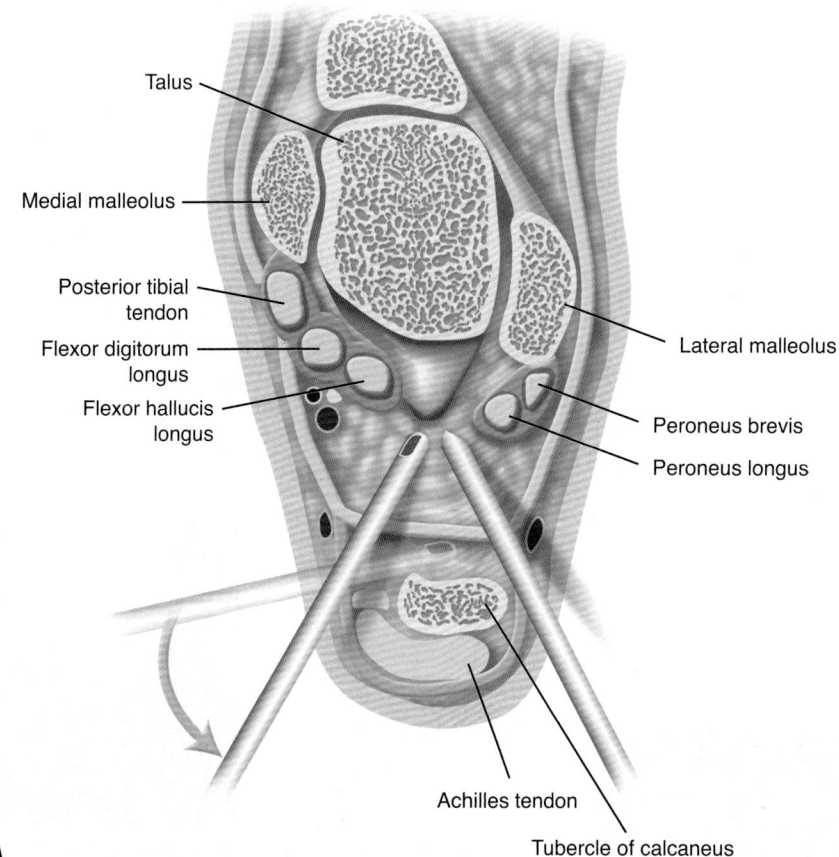

A

FIG 6 A–C. Posterior endoscopic technique with the use of two portals. *(continued)*

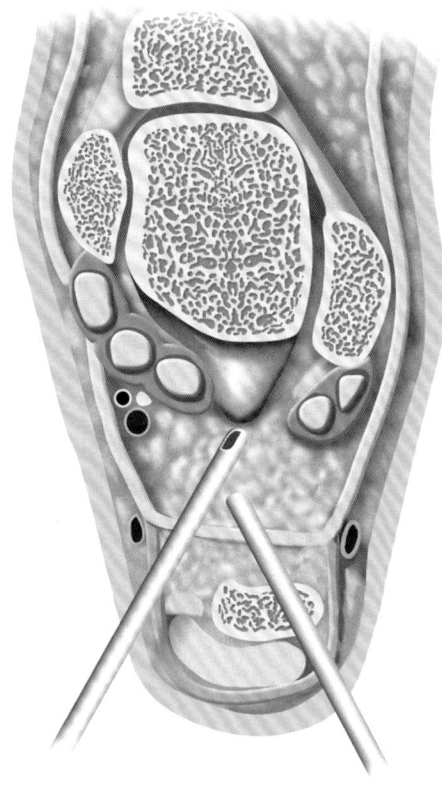

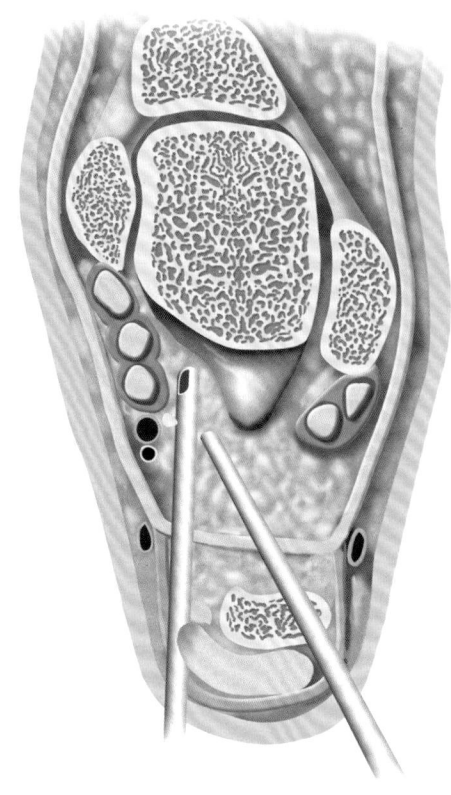

B   **C**   **FIG 6** *(continued)*

PORTAL PLACEMENT

- Local, general, spinal, or epidural anesthesia can be used for this procedure.
- The anterior portal is identified first with an 18-gauge spinal needle, and the joint is inflated with a 20-mL syringe (**TECH FIG 1**).
- A small skin incision is made, and the subcutaneous tissue is gently spread using a straight mosquito clamp.

- A cannula with a semiblunt trocar is then placed, followed by a 2.7-mm 30-degree oblique arthroscope.
- The middle portal is placed under direct visualization using an 18-gauge spinal needle and outside-in technique.
- The posterior portal can be placed at this time using the same direct visualization technique. The trocar is placed in an upward and slightly anterior manner.

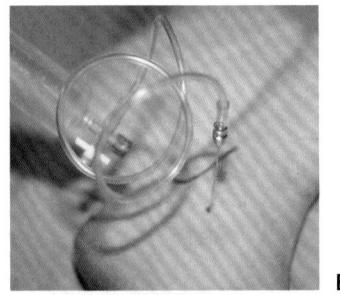

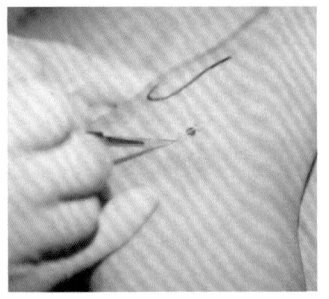

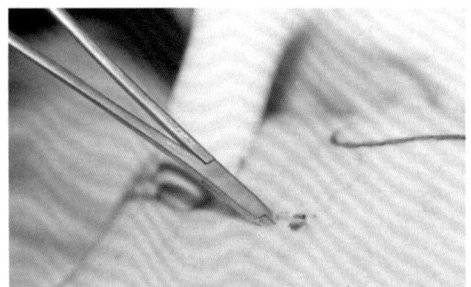

A   **B**   **C**

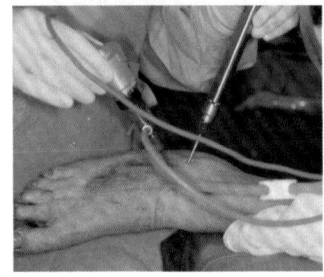

D

TECH FIG 1 The subtalar joint is entered using an 18-gauge spinal needle. The joint is inflated (**A**) and an incision is made (**B**), followed by blunt dissection (**C**) and entry into the subtalar joint (**D**). The middle portal is made using direct visualization techniques.

TECHNIQUES

INSPECTION FROM THE ANTERIOR PORTAL

- Diagnostic subtalar arthroscopy examination begins with the arthroscope viewing from the anterior portal (**TECH FIG 2A,B**). The ligaments that insert on the floor of the sinus tarsi are visualized. It is easy to get disoriented, as the ligaments are closely packed and cross over one another in the sinus tarsi.
- More medially, the deep interosseous ligament (**TECH FIG 2C**) is observed to fill the tarsal canal.
- The arthroscope should now be slowly withdrawn and the arthroscopic lens rotated to view the anterior process of the calcaneus (**TECH FIG 3A,B**).
- The arthroscopic lens is then rotated in the opposite direction to view the anterior aspect of the posterior talocalcaneal articulation (**TECH FIG 3C**).

- Next, the anterolateral corner of the posterior joint is examined, and reflections of the lateral talocalcaneal ligament and the calcaneofibular ligament are observed (**TECH FIG 3D**). The lateral talocalcaneal ligament is noted anterior to the calcaneofibular ligament.
- The arthroscopic lens may then be rotated medially and the central articulation observed between the talus and the calcaneus (**TECH FIG 3E**). The posterolateral gutter may be seen from the anterior portal.
- It is often possible to advance the scope along the lateral and posterolateral gutter and visualize the posterior pouch and Stieda process (or os trigonum; **TECH FIG 3F**).

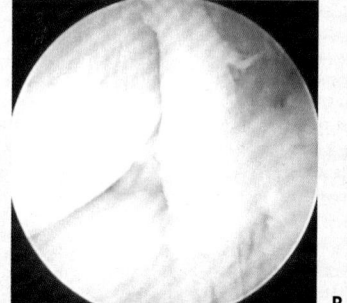
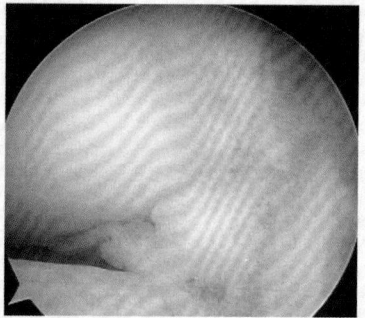
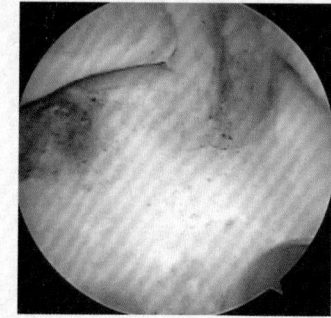

TECH FIG 2 With the arthroscope in the anterior portal, the ligaments that insert on the floor of the sinus tarsi can be visualized. It is often difficult to tell one from the other, especially if they are injured. **A,B.** Examples of a torn interosseous ligament that is impinging into the anterior aspect of the posterior facet of the subtalar joint. This impingement lesion is referred to as the *subtalar impingement lesion*. **C.** The interosseous ligament of the tarsal canal fills the canal and can be seen with the scope in the anterior portal. The anterior (*left*) and the posterior (*right*) facets are well seen.

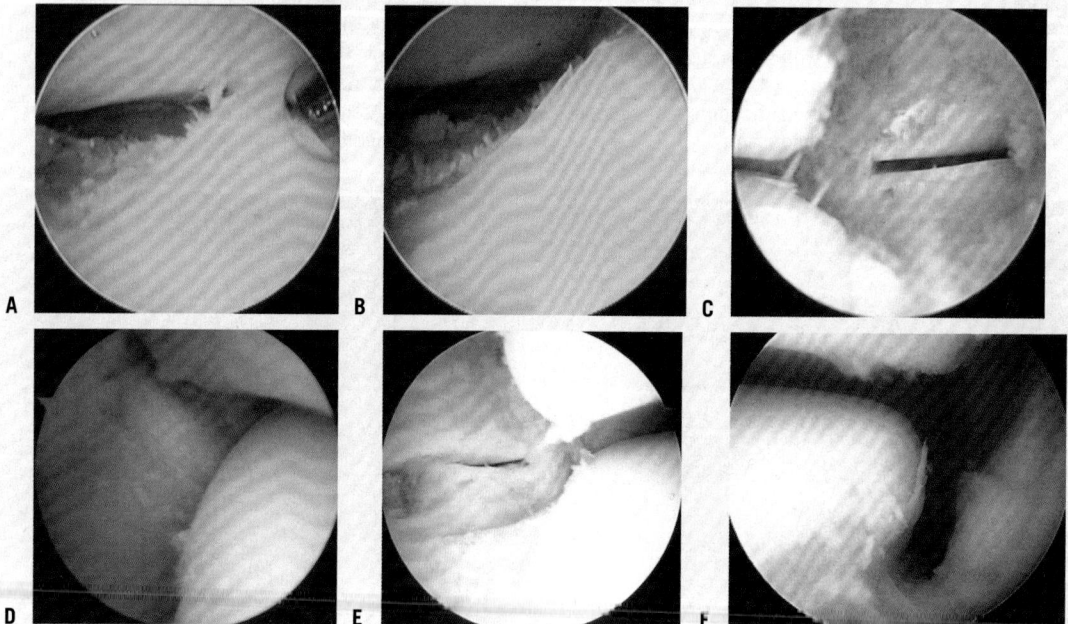

TECH FIG 3 Views with the arthroscope in the anterior portal. **A.** Anterosuperior process of the calcaneus. This view is useful for inspection and débridement or resection of a fracture in this location. **B.** Closer view of the anterior process. **C.** Anterior aspect of the posterior facet (*to the right*). **D.** Lateral gutter and lateral talocalcaneal and calcaneofibular ligaments. **E.** Anterior and central aspects of the posterior talocalcaneal articulation (*to the right*). **F.** It is possible to advance the scope from the anterior portal and visualize the lateral aspect of the posterior capsule and Stieda process or os trigonum.

INSPECTION FROM THE POSTERIOR PORTAL

- The arthroscope is then switched to the posterior portal. From this view, the interosseous ligament may be seen anteriorly in the joint. As the arthroscopic lens is rotated laterally, the lateral talocalcaneal ligament and calcaneofibular ligament reflections again may be seen.
- The central talocalcaneal joint may then be seen from this posterior view and the posterolateral gutter examined **(TECH FIG 4A)**.

- The posterolateral recess, posterior gutter, and posterolateral corner of the talus are visualized **(TECH FIG 4B)**. The posteromedial recess and posteromedial corner of the talocalcaneal joint can also be seen from the posterior portal.

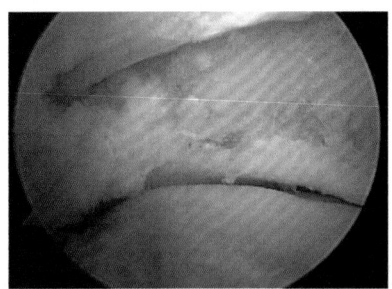 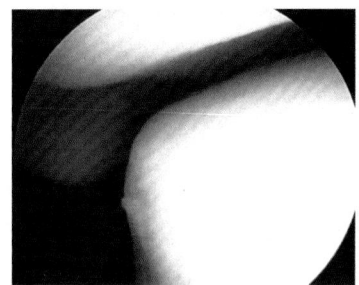

A   B

TECH FIG 4 Views with the arthroscope in the posterior portal. **A.** Posterior and central aspects of the posterior talocalcaneal joint can be seen to the *right*. The posterior capsule is to the *left*. **B.** Lateral aspect of the posterior capsule and Stieda process or the os trigonum.

SINUS TARSI PATHOLOGY

- The best portal combination for the evaluation and débridement of pathology in the sinus tarsi is the arthroscope in the anterior portal and the instruments in the middle portal.

- One can débride torn interosseous ligaments, remove loose bodies, and perform lysis of adhesions. A radiofrequency wand is a useful tool to access the hard-to-get-to spots in the sinus tarsi and subtalar joint.

OS TRIGONUM PATHOLOGY

- The best portal combination for evaluation and removal of the os trigonum is the arthroscope in the anterior portal and the instrumentation in the posterior portal.
- The os trigonum or a symptomatic Stieda process can be débrided with a burr or shaver and removed through an

arthroscopic portal using a standard arthroscopic grabber **(TECH FIG 5)**.
- Rarely, it is necessary to enlarge the portal for delivery of the os trigonum.

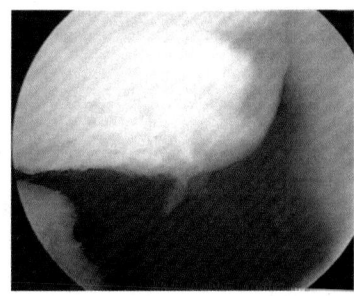

TECH FIG 5 A fracture of Stieda process or an injured os trigonum can be removed using standard arthroscopic grabbers. Rarely, the incision must be expanded to deliver the fragment.

ARTHROSCOPIC SUBTALAR ARTHRODESIS

- Both the anterior and posterior portals are used in an alternating fashion during the procedure for viewing and for instrumentation.
- It is important to obtain a fusion of the posterior facet. The anterior facet is generally not fused. A primary synovectomy and débridement are necessary for visualization.
- Débridement and complete removal of the articular surface of the posterior facet of the subtalar joint down to subchondral bone is the next phase of the procedure.
- Once the articular cartilage has been resected, approximately 1 to 2 mm of subchondral bone is removed to expose bleeding cancellous bone.

- Spot weld holes measuring approximately 2 mm in depth are created on the surfaces of the calcaneus and talus to create vascular channels.
- The posteromedial corner is inspected to ensure adequate débridement.
- The guidewire for a large cannulated screw (6.5 to 7 mm) can be visualized as it enters the posterior facet.
- The foot is then put in about 0 to 5 degrees of valgus, the guidewire is advanced, and the screw is placed.
- Screw position and length are confirmed with fluoroscopy.
- Postoperative care is similar to open techniques.
- In general, no autogenous bone graft or bone substitute is needed.

TECHNIQUES

Pearls and Pitfalls

The subtalar joint can be difficult to distract, especially the posterior joint.	• Use of a distraction device is not necessary or very useful for improving visualization of the subtalar joint. A high-flow system and an arthroscopic pump will improve visualization. • Rarely, invasive joint distraction, using talocalcaneal distraction with pins inserted from laterally, or tibiocalcaneal distraction can be used in a patient with a tight posterior subtalar joint. The disadvantage of using an invasive distractor is the potential damage to soft tissues (especially the lateral calcaneal branch of the sural nerve) and ligamentous structures and the risk of infection and fracturing the talar neck or body.
Visualization of the anterior joint and sinus tarsi can be difficult. It is easy to get disoriented, as the ligaments are closely packed and cross over one another in the sinus tarsi.	• The structures in the sinus tarsi, the anterior process of the calcaneus, and, occasionally, the anterior joint can be visualized best by placing the arthroscope through the anterior portal and instrumentation through the middle portal. This portal combination is recommended for visualization and instrumentation of the sinus tarsi and anterior aspects of the posterior subtalar joint. If the ligaments that insert on the floor of the sinus tarsi are torn or damaged or need débridement, the anterior joint can be visualized and accessed with this portal combination. Furthermore, this portal combination allows excellent visualization and access to the anterior process of the calcaneus.
Visualization of the posterior joint and lateral capsule and access to Stieda process (os trigonum) may be difficult.	• The best portal combination for access to the posterior joint is placement of the arthroscope through the anterior portal and instrumentation through the posterior portal. This allows direct visualization and access of nearly the entire surface of the posterior facet, the posterior aspect of the ligaments in the sinus tarsi, the lateral capsule and its small recess, Stieda process (os trigonum), and the posterior pouch of the posterior joint with its synovial lining.
Posterior ankle impingement syndrome may be difficult to treat and access.	• Posterior ankle impingement syndrome may be treated with a posterior two-portal endoscopic/arthroscopic technique that allows safe and better access to the posterior structures. The posterior anatomy of both the ankle and subtalar can be visualized with this technique. Small portals for the 2.7-mm 30-degree arthroscope are made on either side of the Achilles tendon.

POSTOPERATIVE CARE

- After completing the procedure, the portals are closed with sutures.
- A compression dressing is applied from the toes to the mid-calf. Ice and elevation are recommended until the inflammatory phase has passed.
- The patient is allowed to ambulate with the use of crutches, and weight bearing is permitted as tolerated.

- The sutures are removed approximately 10 days after the procedure.
- The patient should begin gentle active range-of-motion exercises of the foot and ankle immediately after surgery. Once the sutures are removed, if indicated, the patient is referred to a physical therapist for supervised rehabilitation.
- The patient should be able to return to full activities at 6 to 12 weeks postoperatively.

OUTCOMES

- Compared with open techniques, arthroscopy of the subtalar joint has advantages for the patient, including a faster postoperative recovery period, decreased postoperative pain, and fewer complications.
- Frey et al[2] demonstrated a success rate of 94% good and excellent results in the treatment of various types of subtalar pathology using arthroscopic techniques.
  - All of 14 preoperative diagnoses of sinus tarsi syndrome were changed at the time of arthroscopy.
  - The most common finding in these cases was a tear of the interosseous ligaments.
- In a more recent study of 126 cases followed for more than 2 years, a significant improvement (61 to 84) was noted using both the American Orthopaedic Foot & Ankle Society and Karlsson scores. Williams and Ferkel[19] reported on the 32-month (average) follow-up of 50 patients with hindfoot pain who underwent simultaneous ankle and subtalar arthroscopy.
  - Preoperative diagnoses included degenerative joint disease, sinus tarsi dysfunction, and os trigonum.
  - Good to excellent results were noted in 86% of the patients.
  - Overall, less favorable results were noted with associated ankle pathology, degenerative joint disease, increased age, and activity level of the patient.
  - No operative complications were reported.
- Goldberger and Conti[4] retrospectively reviewed 12 patients who underwent subtalar arthroscopy for symptomatic subtalar pathology with nonspecific radiographic findings.
  - The preoperative diagnoses were subtalar chondrosis in 9 patients and subtalar synovitis in 3 patients.
  - At 17.5 months (average) of follow-up, the postoperative American Orthopaedic Foot & Ankle Society hindfoot score was 71 (range 51 to 85) compared with a preoperative score of 66 (range 54 to 79). All patients stated that they would have the surgery again.
- Surgical removal of the contents of the lateral half of the sinus tarsi improves or eradicates symptoms in roughly 90% of cases of patients with sinus tarsi pain or dysfunction.[2]

COMPLICATIONS

- Although rare, the most likely complication to occur after subtalar arthroscopy is injury to any of the neurovascular structures in the proximity of the portals, including the sural nerve and superficial peroneal nerve.
- Other possible complications following subtalar joint arthroscopy include infection, instrument breakage, and damage to the articular cartilage.

REFERENCES

1. Beimers L, Frey C, van Dijk CN. Arthroscopy of the posterior subtalar joint. Foot Ankle Clin 2006;11:369–390.
2. Frey C, Feder KS, DiGiovanni C. Arthroscopic evaluation of the subtalar joint: does sinus tarsi syndrome exist? Foot Ankle Int 1999;20:185–191.
3. Frey C, Gasser S, Feder K. Arthroscopy of the subtalar joint. Foot Ankle Int 1994;15:424–428.
4. Goldberger MI, Conti SF. Clinical outcome after subtalar arthroscopy. Foot Ankle Int 1998;19:462–465.
5. Harper MC. The lateral ligamentous support of the subtalar joint. Foot Ankle 1991;11:354–358.
6. Inman VT. The subtalar joint. In: Inman VT, ed. The Joints of the Ankle. Baltimore: Williams & Wilkins, 1976:35–44.
7. Jaivin JS, Ferkel RD. Arthroscopy of the foot and ankle. Clin Sports Med 1994;13:761–783.
8. Lapidus PW. Subtalar joint, its anatomy and mechanics. Bull Hosp Joint Dis 1955;16:179–195.
9. Lundeen RO. Arthroscopic fusion of the ankle and subtalar joint. Clin Podiatr Med Surg 1994;11:395–406.
10. Mekhail AO, Heck BE, Ebraheim NA, et al. Arthroscopy of the subtalar joint: establishing a medial portal. Foot Ankle Int 1995;16:427–432.
11. Parisien JS. Posterior subtalar joint arthroscopy. In: Guhl JF, Parisien JS, Boynton MD, eds. Foot and Ankle Arthroscopy, ed 3. New York: Springer-Verlag, 2004:175–182.
12. Perry J. Anatomy and biomechanics of the hindfoot. Clin Orthop Relat Res 1983;(177):9–15.
13. Scholten PE, Altena MC, Krips R, et al. Treatment of a large intraosseous talar ganglion by means of hindfoot endoscopy. Arthroscopy 2003;19:96–100.
14. Sitler DF, Amendola A, Bailey CS, et al. Posterior ankle arthroscopy: an anatomic study. J Bone Joint Surg Am 2002;84(5):763–769.
15. Tasto JP. Arthroscopic subtalar arthrodesis. Tech Foot Ankle Surg 2003;2:122–128.
16. Tasto JP, Frey C, Laimans P, et al. Arthroscopic ankle arthrodesis. Instr Course Lect 2000;49:259–280.
17. van Dijk CN, Scholten PE, Krips R. A 2-portal endoscopic approach for diagnosis and treatment of posterior ankle pathology. Arthroscopy 2000;16:871–876.
18. Viladot A, Lorenzo JC, Salazar J, et al. The subtalar joint: embryology and morphology. Foot Ankle 1984;5:54–66.
19. Williams MM, Ferkel RD. Subtalar arthroscopy: indications, technique, and results. Arthroscopy 1998;14:373–381.

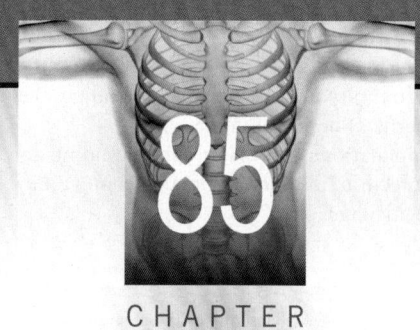

85 CHAPTER

Subtalar Arthroscopy:
Perspective 2

Christopher E. Gross and Mark E. Easley

DEFINITION

- Lateral or posterior subtalar arthroscopy confers diagnostic and potentially therapeutic value in treating subtalar trauma, arthrofibrosis, impingement, arthritis, and osteochondral lesions.
- One must establish a definitive diagnosis of subtalar pathology based on physical examination and detailed imaging studies to improve the likelihood of successful outcome with subtalar arthroscopy.
- Exploratory, or diagnostic, subtalar arthroscopy is rarely indicated.
- Based on preoperative physical examination and detailed imaging, determination may be made if lateral or posterior subtalar arthroscopy is favored to access subtalar pathology.

ANATOMY

- The subtalar joint comprises the talus and three facets of the superior articular surface of the calcaneus: anterior, middle, and posterior facet.
  - Functionally, the subtalar joint is separated into an anterior (anterior and middle articular surfaces, often confluent) and posterior portion. The posterior facet is the largest and bears the majority of the body weight.
- The tarsal canal (contents: talar body blood supply, talocalcaneal interosseous, inferior extensor retinaculum, and cervical ligaments) separates the anterior and posterior portions of the subtalar joint. Its lateral opening is the sinus tarsi.
- The anterior and middle facets are usually inaccessible unless the interosseous ligament is torn.
- Subtalar motion is not pure inversion and eversion the subtalar joint's coupling with the ankle.

PATHOGENESIS

- Not much literature is dedicated to osteochondral lesions of the subtalar joint.
- Snowboarders, with their hindfoot held in place with stiff boots during a fall, in addition to lateral talar process fractures, may experience injury to the middle facet of the subtalar joint.
  - The sustentaculum tali and middle facet are impacted.[1]
- Sinus tarsi syndrome is clinically described as lateral pain over the sinus tarsi.
- Although the etiology of sinus tarsi syndrome is unknown, several theories exist[3]:
  - Scarring and fibrosis of interosseous or cervical ligament
  - Subtalar synovitis
  - Sinus fat pad alterations and scarring

- Subtalar arthritis is most commonly posttraumatic, although it may be inflammatory or idiopathic.

PATIENT HISTORY AND PHYSICAL FINDINGS

- Commensurate with the patient's complaint of hindfoot soreness, stiffness, and, occasionally, physical examination of the hindfoot demonstrates pain and limited motion.
- The patient may have a sense of instability, particularly while walking on uneven surfaces.
- By stabilizing the ankle, typically with thumb support on the medial talar neck, some sense of subtalar inversion/eversion compared to the contralateral hindfoot should identify pain and restriction of motion.
- The patient often describes diffuse hindfoot pain, medially, laterally, and posteriorly.
- Sinus tarsi tenderness is a consistent finding suggestive of anterior subtalar pathology, often due to interosseous ligament sprain or lateral process avulsion injury.
- Pain with forced eversion may suggest lateral subtalar gutter impingement and is generally the most sensitive area on examination of a patient with subtalar pathology.
- Pain with forced plantarflexion is not definitive for the ankle or subtalar joint but may be due to posterior subtalar impingement.
- Due to the coupled ankle and subtalar mechanism, subtalar and ankle instability are often difficult to distinguish from ankle instability. Reliable and reproducible stress maneuvers that isolate subtalar motion have not been developed.
- Although invasive, perhaps the best test to isolate subtalar pathology is local anesthetic subtalar injection via the sinus tarsi.

IMAGING AND OTHER DIAGNOSTIC STUDIES

- Radiographs
  - May not reveal diagnosis
  - Anteroposterior, lateral, and oblique weight-bearing views of the foot
    - 45-degree oblique view: anterior portion of the subtalar joint (FIGS 1A and 2A)
  - Broden view: posterior facet (FIG 1B)
    - The foot is placed in neutral flexion, and the leg is internally rotated 30 to 40 degrees. The x-ray beam is centered over the lateral malleolus, and four x-rays are made with the tube angled 40-, 30-, 20-, and 10-degree cephalic tilt. The 10-degree view shows the posterior portion of the posterior facet and the 40-degree view shows the anterior portion.

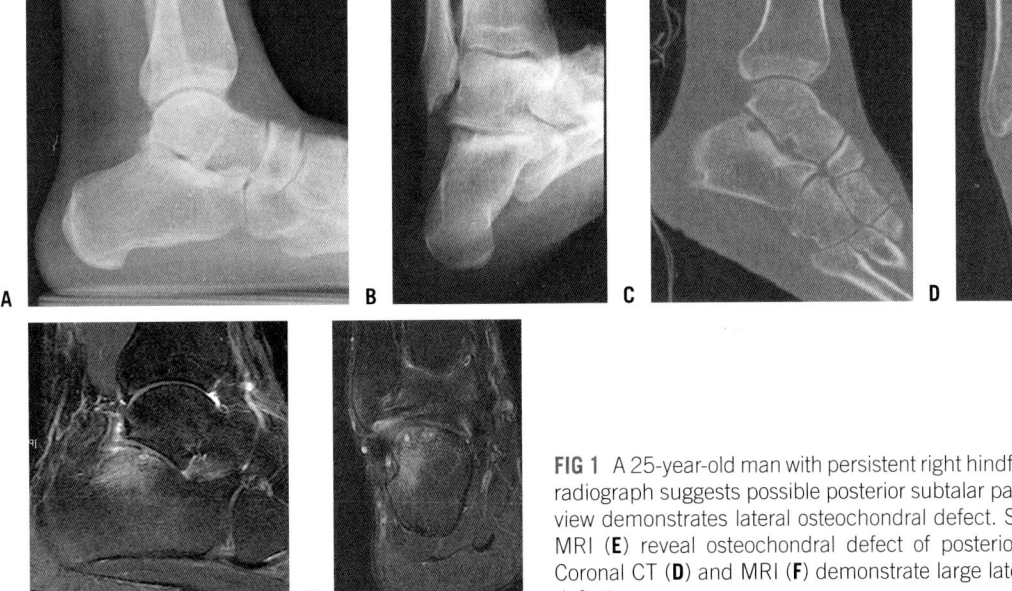

FIG 1 A 25-year-old man with persistent right hindfoot pain. **A.** Lateral radiograph suggests possible posterior subtalar pathology. **B.** Broden view demonstrates lateral osteochondral defect. Sagittal CT (**C**) and MRI (**E**) reveal osteochondral defect of posterior calcaneal facet. Coronal CT (**D**) and MRI (**F**) demonstrate large lateral osteochondral defect.

- Lateral oblique: posterior facet
  - Foot is dorsiflexed, everted, and externally rotated to 60 degrees.
  - Beam is centered 2 cm below medial malleolus with 10-degree cephalic tilt.
- Computed tomography (CT)
  - Cystic component of osteochondral lesions of the subtalar joint (**FIGS 1C,D** and **2B,C**)
  - Subchondral sclerosis, cystic changes consistent with arthritis
- Magnetic resonance imaging (MRI)
  - Cartilage or osteochondral defects (**FIGS 1E,F** and **2D,E**)
  - Edema associated with osteochondral lesions
  - Sinus tarsi pad fat changes
    - Interosseous or cervical ligament tears
  - Stress reactions

- Fibrosis within subtalar joint
- Cartilaginous coalitions

DIFFERENTIAL DIAGNOSIS

- Lateral ankle instability
- Peroneal tendon pathology
- Fractures of
  - Lateral talar process
  - Anterior beak of the calcaneus
  - Stieda process
  - Navicular
  - Calcaneus
- Osteochondral lesions of the inferior surface of talus or posterior facet of calcaneus
- Edema associated with osteochondral lesions

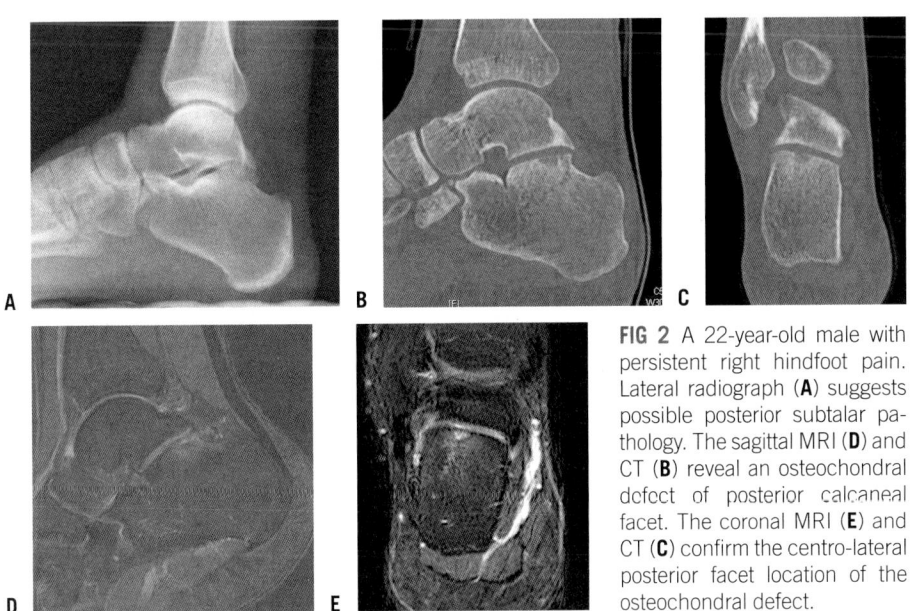

FIG 2 A 22-year-old male with persistent right hindfoot pain. Lateral radiograph (**A**) suggests possible posterior subtalar pathology. The sagittal MRI (**D**) and CT (**B**) reveal an osteochondral defect of posterior calcaneal facet. The coronal MRI (**E**) and CT (**C**) confirm the centro-lateral posterior facet location of the osteochondral defect.

- Subtalar arthritis
- Stress reactions
- Fibrosis within subtalar joint
- Cartilage coalitions

NONOPERATIVE MANAGEMENT

- Functional rehabilitation includes range of motion for the ankle and hindfoot, concentric and eccentric muscle strengthening, endurance training with particular attention to the peroneal musculature, and proprioceptive exercises.
- Anesthetic (with or without corticosteroid) injection into the sinus tarsi
- UCBL orthosis to limit inversion/eversion
- Nonsteroidal anti-inflammatory agents

SURGICAL MANAGEMENT

Indications

- Sinus tarsi syndrome with identifiable pathology
- Chondral and osteochondral lesions
- Chronic synovitis
- Adhesions, arthrofibrosis
- Loose bodies
- Mild arthritis
- Impingement (os trigonum)
- Preparation of the subtalar joint for fusion

- Assist in reduction of the posterior facet during a calcaneus open reduction internal fixation

Contraindications

- Local soft tissue/bone infection
- Severe deformity
- Poor vascular status
- Edema
- Chronic regional pain syndrome

Preoperative Planning

- Imaging studies must be reviewed so that the location of the lesion is identified.
- Plain films must be reviewed for degenerative changes, malalignment, and fractures.
- Physical examination, combined with preoperative imaging, typically directs if lateral or posterior subtalar arthroscopy is favored to access the specific subtalar pathology.
  - In general, lateral subtalar arthroscopy is favored for sinus tarsi and anterior pathology, including the anterior one-half of the subtalar joint.
  - Posterior arthroscopy is favored for posterior hindfoot impingement and pathology isolated to the posterior half of the subtalar joint.
  - Lateral subtalar and lateral gutter pathology may be better accessed with the lateral subtalar arthroscopy.
  - Medial subtalar pathology is difficult to access from either lateral or posterior portals.

LATERAL ARTHROSCOPY FOR ANTERIOR AND LATERAL SUBTALAR PATHOLOGY

Background

- A 25-year-old man with a 6-month history of hindfoot pain after inversion ankle/hindfoot injury, failing nonoperative measures
- Physical examination and imaging studies (see **FIG 1**) suggested lateral gutter impingement, sinus tarsi pathology, and lateral osteochondral lesion of the posterior calcaneal facet.

Positioning

- A well-padded thigh tourniquet is placed.
- Lateral subtalar arthroscopy setup for anterior and/or lateral subtalar gutter pathology **(TECH FIG 1)**
  - The patient is maintained in a lateral decubitus position.
  - In general, a beanbag or dedicated lateral positioning device is preferred to maintain the patient in proper position for lateral subtalar arthroscopy.
    - Positioning the patient in less than the full lateral decubitus position will limit satisfactory access to the posterior portal for the lateral approach.
  - A support placed under the medial malleolus allows the subtalar joint to fall open and improve access.

Establishing Portals

- Mark the three portals **(TECH FIG 2)**.
  - Anterior portal
    - 2 cm anterior and 1 cm distal lateral malleolus tip (distal portion of the sinus tarsi)
    - Mostly a viewing portal

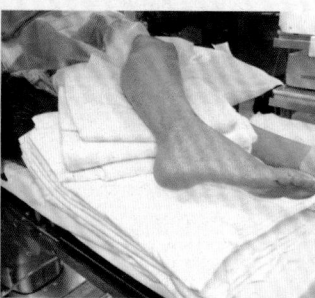

TECH FIG 1 Lateral subtalar arthroscopy is facilitated with the patient in the lateral decubitus position and the operated ankle suspended from a support under the lower leg to open the subtalar joint.

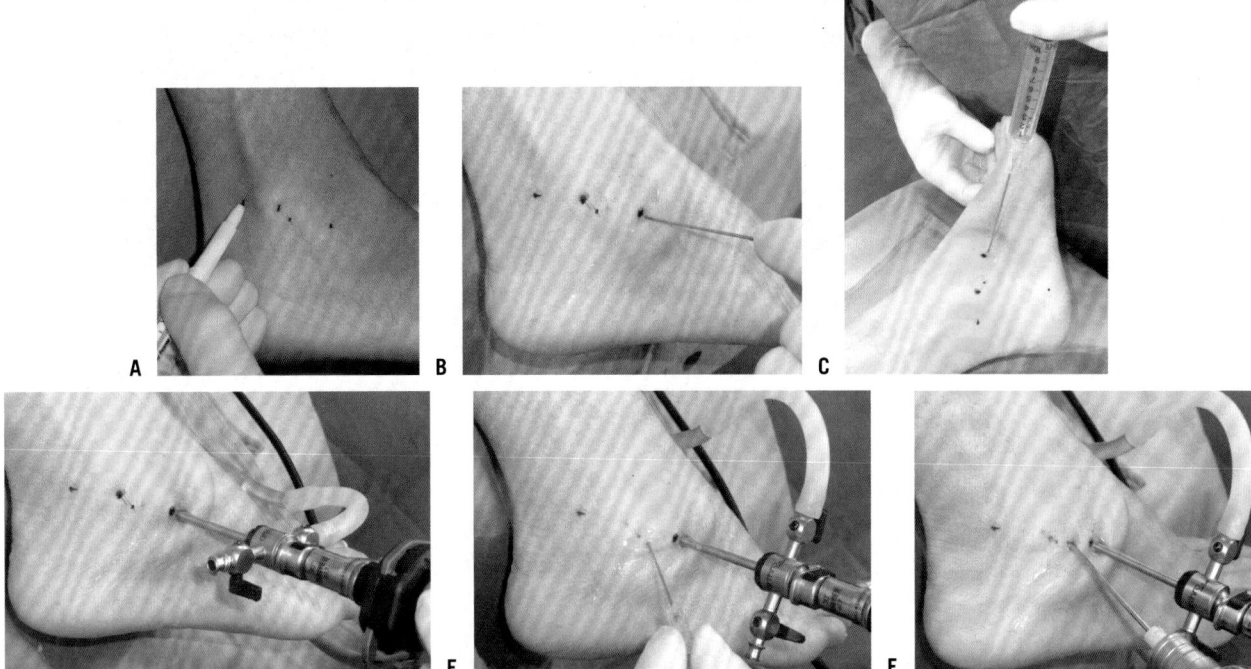

TECH FIG 2 A. Lateral subtalar joint arthroscopy portals. Tip of fibula marked. Middle portal, immediately distal and inferior to the tip of the fibula. Anterior portal, 1 cm inferior and 2 cm anterior to the tip of the fibula. The posterior portal is just proximal to the tip of the fibula and immediately posterior to the peroneal tendons. **B.** To determine the anterior portal, a spinal needle is placed into sinus tarsi immediately superior to anterior calcaneus at the angle of Gissane. **C.** Sterile saline is introduced to expand the anterior subtalar joint. **D.** Introduction of the arthroscope into the anterior portal. Note skin tension due to anterior portal made too proximally; ideally, portal should be created at the proper location without tensioning the skin. **E.** To create the middle portal, a spinal needle is introduced to determine the ideal trajectory for instrumentation. Direct visualization is possible with the anterior arthroscope. **F.** Shaver introduced in trajectory determined with spinal needle.

- Middle portal
  - Just distal and inferior lateral malleolus tip
  - Mostly an instrument portal; best for sinus tarsi pathology
- Posterior portal
  - 1 cm proximal lateral malleolus tip and anterior to Achilles
  - Just distal and inferior lateral malleolus tip
  - Mostly an instrument portal
  - From this portal, one can débride hypertrophic or inflamed synovium, remove impinging structures, and remove an os trigonum.
- The location for the anterior portal is first identified with palpation, dorsal to the calcaneal angle of Gissane in the sinus tarsi. Prior to creating the portal, the proper trajectory for passing anterior portal instrumentation is confirmed with a spinal needle **(TECH FIG 2B)**.
- The subtalar joint is insufflated with 10 mL of saline **(TECH FIG 2C)**.
- A stab incision is made with a no. 10 blade.
  - Protect the sural nerve by making only a superficial skin incision and perform blunt dissection to the subtalar joint.
- The subcutaneous tissue is spread with a hemostat clamp.
  - This nick-and-spread technique helps to avoid sural nerve injury.
- The trocar, followed by the arthroscope and camera with a fluid inflow source, is inserted **(TECH FIG 2D)**.

- The middle portal is created.
  - A spinal needle may be inserted to determine the optimal trajectory based on direct visualization within the joint **(TECH FIG 2E)**.
  - The shaver is introduced into the anterior subtalar joint under direct visualization from within the joint **(TECH FIG 2F)**.

Viewing from the Anterior Portal and Working from the Middle Portal

- Viewing from the anterior portal, inspect the floor of the sinus tarsi.
  - Approximately 75% of the posterior facet may be visualized from this position.
    - The initial view may be obscured by sinus tarsi scar or inflammatory tissue **(TECH FIG 3A)**.
    - With an arthroscopic shaver introduced through the middle portal, the reactive synovium and scar may be débrided to expose the anterior aspect of the posterior subtalar joint **(TECH FIG 3B)**.
- Medially, the talocalcaneal interosseous ligament fills the tarsal canal.
  - Medial scar tissue may be visualized medial to the ligament **(TECH FIG 3C)** and débrided under direct visualization **(TECH FIG 3D)**.
  - The lens is rotated to visualize the middle facet medially and anterior calcaneal process laterally.

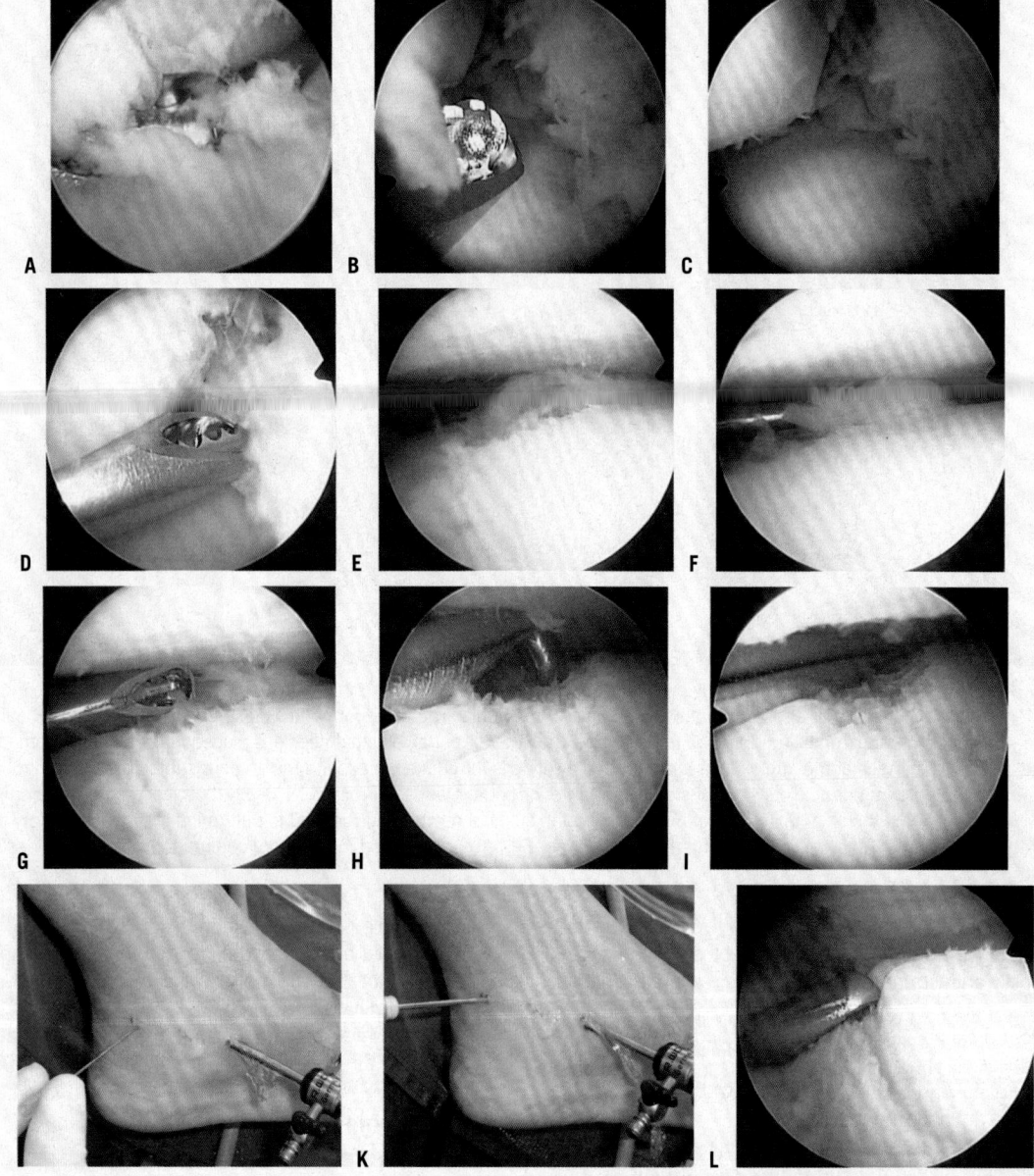

TECH FIG 3 **A.** Shaver initially obscured by sinus tarsi scar tissue. **B.** Débridement to expose anterior subtalar joint. **C.** Scarring noted medial and deep to the anterior aspect of the posterior facet and interosseous ligament. **D.** Débridement of the medial scar tissue. **E.** Visualizing of the osteochondral defect from the anterior portal. **F.** Probing the defect to identify unstable cartilage in the defect with probe through the middle portal. **G.** Débridement of the defect with the shaver introduced through the middle portal. **H.** The small joint awl introduced through the middle portal to perform microfracture of the defect. **I.** Further débridement after microfracture. **J.** With the arthroscope in the anterior portal, the spinal needle is directly visualized entering the posterolateral joint. **K.** Shaver introduced posteriorly. **L.** Visualization from anterior arthroscope of lateral gutter débridement with shaver introduced into the posterolateral portal.

- Occasionally, more anterior débridement may be facilitated by placing the arthroscope in the middle portal and the shaver in the anterior portal.
- After anterior débridement, the camera is rotated to inspect the posterior subtalar joint and the posterior calcaneal facet.
  - In this case, the lateral posterior facet osteochondral defect is noted and the unstable cartilage is mobilized with a probe **(TECH FIG 3F)**.

- With the camera in the anterior portal and the shaver in the middle portal, the osteochondral defect can be effectively débrided **(TECH FIG 3E–G)**.
- After débridement is complete, a dedicated small joint awl may be substituted for the shaver to perform microfracture of the osteochondral defect **(TECH FIG 3H)** followed by further débridement **(TECH FIG 3I)**.

- With the camera still in the anterior portal, a posterior portal may be created by directing the arthroscope into the lateral subtalar gutter and directly visualizing the spinal needle inserted from the intended posterior portal **(TECH FIG 3J)**.
- To protect the sural nerve, the posterior portal should be created with a superficial stab incision in the skin and blunt dissection through the posterolateral subtalar capsule.
- The shaver is then introduced through the posterior portal **(TECH FIG 3K)**.
- Scar tissue in the lateral gutter may be readily débrided **(TECH FIG 3L)**.

Viewing from the Posterior Portal

- The arthroscope is removed from the anterior portal, and the trocar and camera are introduced into the posterior portal **(TECH FIG 4A)**.
- The subtalar joint may be visualized, and in this case, the débrided lateral osteochondral defect may be inspected **(TECH FIG 4B)**.
- The lateral gutter may also be viewed from the posterior portal and further débridement is possible by introducing the shaver from the middle or anterior portal **(TECH FIG 4C)**.

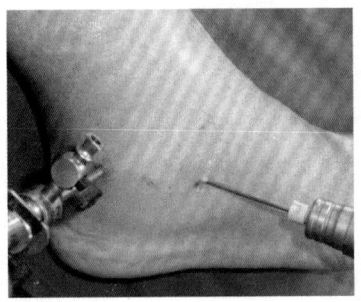 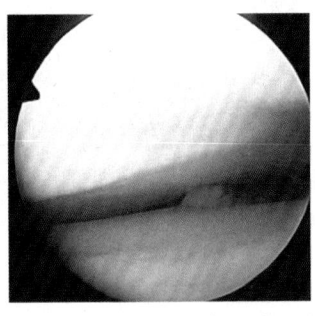 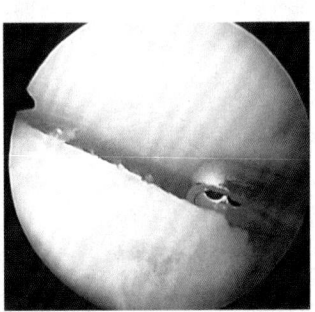

TECH FIG 4 A. Arthroscope introduced from posterior portal with shaver in anterior portal. **B.** Visualization of subtalar joint and débrided osteochondral defect from posterior portal. **C.** Further lateral gutter débridement with visualization from posterior portal and shaver introduced from middle portal.

POSTERIOR ARTHROSCOPY FOR ISOLATED POSTERIOR SUBTALAR PATHOLOGY

Background

- A 22-year-old man presented with a 6-month history of persistent hindfoot symptoms after inversion ankle/hindfoot injury
- Physical examination and imaging suggested posterior hindfoot pathology.
  - Although forced plantarflexion reproduced the symptoms, imaging suggested that the symptoms were due to a central and posterior osteochondral lesion of the posterior calcaneal facet (see **FIG 2**).

Positioning

- The patient is positioned prone with the chest and iliac crest well padded.
- A support is placed immediately proximal to the ankle so the tibiotalar joint can plantarflex and dorsiflex.
- Airway is well maintained.
- No tension on the brachial plexi; ulnar nerves at the elbows free of pressure
- All bony prominences well padded

Approach

- Two small skin incisions are made at the level of the fibula 1 cm from the medial and lateral border of the Achilles tendon.
  - These incisions should not be made too close to the Achilles tendon, as this can cause overcrowding and difficulties maneuvering the instrumentation.

- The skin incisions should be superficial only, and blunt dissection is carried through the posterior soft tissues to the posterior subtalar joint.
  - Laterally, the sural nerve is at risk.
  - Medially, the posteromedial neurovascular bundle is at risk.

Viewing from the Posterolateral Portal and Working from the Posteromedial Portal

- The arthroscope is routinely placed in the posterolateral portal **(TECH FIG 5A,B)**.
  - The camera should be directed medially to visualize the instrumentation.
- The shaver is introduced into the medial portal.
- Routinely, considerable adipose and fibrous tissue must be removed from the space immediately posterior to the subtalar joint **(TECH FIG 5C)**.
- Before any pathology is addressed, the flexor hallucis longus (FHL) tendon must be identified, as it serves as the medial reference point to protect the posteromedial neurovascular bundle **(TECH FIG 5D)**.
- One of the most common indications for posterior hindfoot arthroscopy is to remove a symptomatic os trigonum.
- In this case, inspection of the posterior facet demonstrates a central posterior osteochondral lesion with unstable cartilage **(TECH FIG 5E–G)**.
- Débridement of unstable cartilage from the posterior facet osteochondral defect **(TECH FIG 5H,I)**

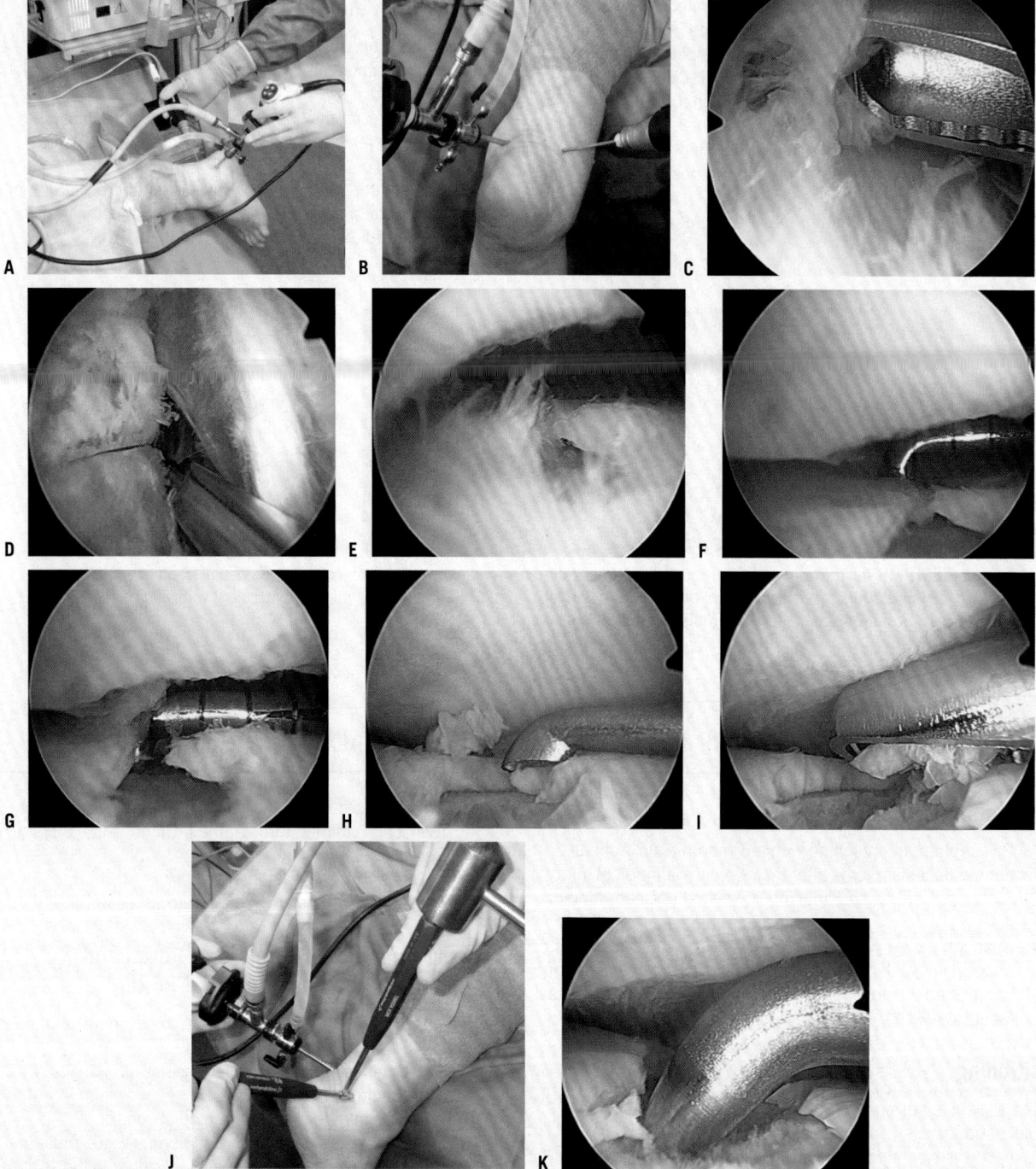

TECH FIG 5 A. Patient prone and posterior hindfoot portals created. **B.** Arthroscope posterolateral and instrumentation posteromedial so that the instrumentation and FHL tendon (reference structure to posteromedial neurovascular bundle) may be simultaneously
and safely visualized. **C.** Arthroscope viewing from posterolateral portal and shaver introduced from posteromedial portal. **D.** Posterior
subtalar joint visualized with shaver immediately anterior and medial to the FHL tendon. **E.** Identifying unstable posterior facet cartilage. **F.** Probe introduced through posteromedial portal. **G.** Unstable cartilage assessed. **H.** Débridement of unstable cartilage using
curette introduced through posteromedial portal. **I.** Shaver from posteromedial portal to remove débrided unstable cartilage fragments.
J,K. This small joint microfracture awl system uses a tamp that directly impacts on the dorsal aspect of the awl. *(continued)*

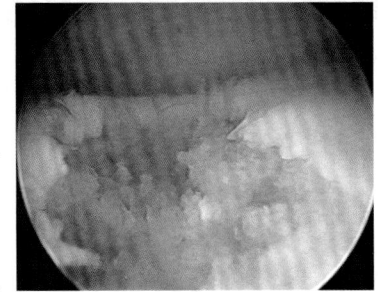
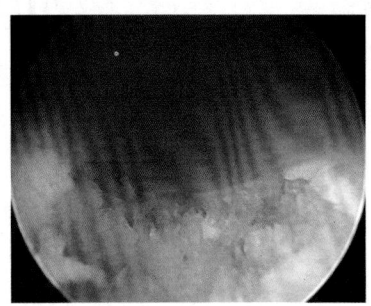

TECH FIG 5 *(continued)* **L.** At the conclusion of microfracture, the tourniquet is released and inflow discontinued to determine bleeding from the microfractured osteochondral defect. **M.** In this case, bleeding from the microfractured area serves as an indicator for a favorable healing potential.

- Microfracture using dedicated small joint microfracture instrumentation
  - In this case, two different systems are demonstrated. The external images demonstrate a system that includes a tamp to impact more vertically on the awl. The internal images demonstrate a more traditional awl where the impact

occurs directly on the proximal aspect of the awl handle **(TECH FIG 5J,K)**.

- At the conclusion of microfracture, the tourniquet is released and inflow discontinued to demonstrate bleeding from the microfractured osteochondral defect, in anticipation that bleeding is an indicator for a favorable healing potential **(TECH FIG 5L,M)**.

TECHNIQUES

Pearls and Pitfalls

Anterior or Lateral Subtalar Pathology	• Consider using lateral subtalar arthroscopy technique.
Posterior Subtalar Pathology	• Favor using posterior subtalar arthroscopy technique.
Medial Subtalar Pathology	• Accessing medial subtalar pathology is difficult from either the lateral or posterior subtalar arthroscopic technique.
Nerve Injury	• Superficial skin incisions only and blunt dissection to enter the subtalar joint

POSTOPERATIVE CARE

- Early range of motion is possible, but if an osteochondral defect was managed surgically, consideration may want to be given to protected weight bearing for 4 weeks.
- An initial CAM boot is recommended to protect the foot while the portal sites are healing.
- Partial weight bearing is allowed immediately and continued for to 4 weeks if microfracture performed.
- Consideration may be given to physical therapy to be started after portal sites are healed.
- Initial follow-up at approximately 7 to 10 days for wound inspection and possible suture removal
- Return to full activity may take 3 months or more.
- With an osteochondral defect, recommend low-impact exercise.

OUTCOMES

- Data on the 45-month follow-up of 49 patients was published by Frey et al.[2]
  - These patients had subtalar arthroscopic débridement for various pathologies including arthrofibrosis, sinus tarsi syndrome, interosseous ligament tears, coalition, and osteochondral lesion of the subtalar joint.

- Of the patients who had a preoperative diagnosis of sinus tarsi syndrome, all of their postoperative diagnoses changed to either interosseous ligament injury, arthrofibrosis, or arthritis.
- Ninety-four percent of patients had excellent/good results, which meant that they had, at the very most, some pain or lifestyle restrictions.

COMPLICATIONS

- Wound complications
- Sural or tibial nerve injury
- Persistent pain
- Iatrogenic cartilage damage

REFERENCES

1. Clanton TO, Chacko AK, Matheny LM, et al. Magnetic resonance imaging findings of snowboarding osteochondral injuries to the middle talocalcaneal articulation. Sports Health 2013;5(5):470–475.
2. Frey C, Feder KS, DiGiovanni C. Arthroscopic evaluation of the subtalar joint: does sinus tarsi syndrome exist? Foot Ankle Int 1999;20(3):185–191.
3. Lee KB, Bai LB, Song EK, et al. Subtalar arthroscopy for sinus tarsi syndrome: arthroscopic findings and clinical outcomes of 33 consecutive cases. Arthroscopy 2008;24(10):1130–1134.

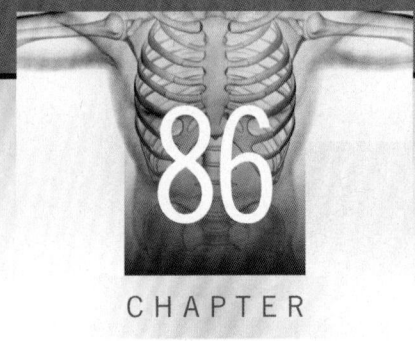

CHAPTER 86

Particulated Juvenile Cartilage Allograft Transplantation for Osteochondral Lesions of the Talus

Samuel B. Adams and Mark E. Easley

DEFINITION

- The term *osteochondral lesion of the talus* (OLT) refers to any pathology of the talar articular cartilage and corresponding subchondral bone. A variety of names have been given to these lesions, including osteochondritis dissecans, osteochondral fracture, transchondral fracture, and osteochondral defect, but currently, OLT is the preferred nomenclature.
- Particulated juvenile cartilage allograft transplantation (PJCAT) is a new technique of transplantation of multiple fresh juvenile cartilage allograft tissue pieces, containing live cells within their native extracellular matrix, with fibrin adhesive securing the tissue pieces firmly inside the OLT.
- This technique is in many ways similar to the osteochondral autograft transfer with the following differences: transplantation of particulated cartilage pieces instead of osteochondral plugs, the use of juvenile cartilage instead of adult cartilage, and graft fixation with fibrin adhesive instead of bony press-fit.
- The advantages of this technique are that it is a surgically simple procedure without the need for graft press-fitting/contouring (as needed for osteochondral autograft or allograft transplantation), it does not require osteotomy in most cases (as often needed for osteochondral autograft transfer or allograft transplantation), it is a single-stage procedure, there is no donor site morbidity, and there is a minimal chance for immunologic reaction (cartilage is considered immune privileged).
- The disadvantages of this technique are the fact that it is a relatively new procedure with limited patient data, there is a limited supply of juvenile donor cartilage, it is a relatively expensive treatment option compared to other techniques, and as with any allograft tissue, disease transmission concerns exist.
- Currently, the only graft material available for this procedure is DeNovo NT Natural Tissue Graft (Zimmer, Inc., Warsaw, IN). The cartilage pieces of this product are obtained, in compliance with good tissue practice, from donors ranging in age from newborn to age 13 years; however, it is typically obtained from neomorts younger than the age of 2 years.[1] No stillborn or fetal tissue is used. Standard disease screening is performed on each lot (one lot of tissue comes from a single donor).

ANATOMY

- Tol et al[16] reported that 56% of OLTs were located medially and 44% were located laterally. Of the medial lesions, trauma was implicated in only 62%, whereas trauma was implicated in 94% of the laterally located lesions.
- Elias et al[8] reported similar results regarding location in a magnetic resonance imaging (MRI) examination of 424 OLTs. The talar dome was divided into nine equal sizes zones. Sixty-two percent of lesions were located medially, whereas 34% were located laterally. In the sagittal plane, 80% of lesions were located centrally. The medial–central zone was the most common location for lesions (53%). The authors also reported that medial lesions were significantly larger and deeper.

PATHOGENESIS

- Kappis[9] initially described this pathology as osteochondritis dissecans, suggesting spontaneous necrosis of bone as the primary etiology.
- However, contemporary data support trauma as the cause of most OLTs, with repetitive microtrauma, avascular necrosis, and congenital factors as the remaining etiologies.[5]

NATURAL HISTORY

- There is debate as to whether a symptomatic OLT will increase in size or progress to ankle arthritis.

PATIENT HISTORY AND PHYSICAL FINDINGS

- An OLT should be suspected in anyone presenting after acute traumatic injury to the ankle, chronic ankle sprains, or chronic instability. Patients may complain of pain, stiffness, catching, and swelling of the ankle.[12] However, none of these complaints are specific to OLTs.
- Often, in the acute setting, a detailed examination is limited secondary to pain and swelling.
- In chronic cases, the ankle should be palpated for areas of tenderness. Specifically, the ankle should be plantarflexed, partially uncovering the talar dome, and deep palpation of the anteromedial and anterolateral corners can elicit pain in the presence of an OLT.
- Ankle range of motion (ROM) should be recorded and compared to the contralateral extremity. Ankle stability, including the anterior drawer and talar tilt tests should be performed and compared to the contralateral extremity.

IMAGING AND OTHER DIAGNOSTIC STUDIES

- Every patient should have weight-bearing anteroposterior (AP), lateral, and mortise radiographic views of the ankle joint.
- A debate exists as to the choice of MRI or computed tomography (CT) following negative plain radiographs in a patient with a suspected OLT. We routinely perform an MRI first, as this modality has been shown to be more accurate[3] in diagnosing OLTs in the setting of negative plain radiograph, and an MRI may identify other bony or soft tissue pathology involved in a painful ankle.
- Stroud and Marks[15] proposed an algorithm regarding OLTs diagnosed on plain radiographs. If the OLT is nondisplaced, an MRI is recommended to evaluate the integrity of the articular cartilage and assess the true stability of the lesion. If the lesion appears displaced on plain radiographs, a CT scan is preferred to accurately assess the lesion size and location.
- In some cases in which an OLT is diagnosed on MRI, a CT scan can be beneficial for determining the treatment modality, as estimation of the size and stage of the lesion can be obscured by bone marrow edema on MRI.[10] We routinely obtain both an MRI and a CT scan in large or cystic lesions to aid in treatment decision making.

DIFFERENTIAL DIAGNOSIS

- Occult fracture of the talus
- Syndesmosis injury
- Synovitis
- Degenerative arthrosis
- Peroneal tendonitis
- Soft tissue or bony impingement
- Ankle instability
- Subtalar arthritis

NONOPERATIVE MANAGEMENT

- The initial treatment for a newly diagnosed OLT should be based on the patient's age, symptoms, chronicity, and stage of the lesion.
- Incidentally found asymptomatic lesions do not need treatment but should be followed with serial radiographs.
- For symptomatic, nondisplaced lesions, some authors recommend a trial of conservative management for a period of 3 to 6 months.[4,11,14]
- Nonoperative modalities include protected weight bearing, physical therapy, and nonsteroidal anti-inflammatory drugs. Protected weight bearing can range from cast immobilization and non–weight-bearing status to weight bearing as tolerated in a walking boot.

SURGICAL MANAGEMENT

Arthrotomy

- Indications for PJCAT include a primary OLT that is larger than 15 mm in one dimension and/or that has previous failed a marrow stimulation technique with continued symptoms and an OLT as evidenced on MRI. Shoulder and cystic lesions are not excluded.
- Contraindications to surgical management of OLTs include infection, medical comorbidities that preclude a surgical procedure, diffuse ankle arthritis, or uncorrected ankle malalignment.
  - Specific recommended contraindications to PJCAT include large cystic or necrotic bony defects. Small cystic lesions with bony defects can be managed with concomitant bone grafting with PJCAT. In these instances, the authors have performed local bone grafting from the calcaneus, tibia, or iliac crest with application of the PJCAT graft in the same surgical setting.
- PJCAT delivers 1 mm^3 of fresh juvenile cartilage, containing live cells in their native extracellular matrix, that are secured into the osteochondral defect with the use of a fibrin adhesive. Because of the particulated nature, perpendicular access to the OLT is not needed. Therefore, an osteotomy is often not necessary. Here, we discuss the use of an anterior arthrotomy.

Arthroscopic

- Performing all-arthroscopic PJCAT can be challenging.
- The diagnostic arthroscopy serves to ensure that complete access to the OLT can be obtained.
- We have a low threshold to move to an extended portal approach or arthrotomy if OLT access or instrument working room is limited.

Preoperative Planning

- Preoperative planning is the same for open or arthroscopic surgery.
- Confirmation of the location and size of the OLT is absolutely necessary.
- Determination of the appropriate amount of graft to be preordered is necessary. Per the manufacturer, one pack of De-Novo NT Natural Tissue Graft (Zimmer) is recommended to treat each 2.5 cm^2 of lesion surface area, with a recommended fill ratio of at least 50% of the lesion size (eg, each pack of tissue graft will cover 1.25 cm^2 of surface area). In practice, attempts are made to completely fill the lesion's surface area to the depth of the surrounding healthy cartilage while allowing fibrin adhesive to interpose between cartilage pieces for good tissue fixation.
- Fibrin glue (5 to 10 mL) will be needed. Typically, this is stored frozen. It has been our experience that rapid thawing alters the workability of the fibrin glue. Therefore, the fibrin glue should be opened at the start of the case and placed in a warm saline bath according to the manufacturer's recommendations.
- Inspect the PJCAT product for the expiration date prior to starting the procedure.

Positioning

Arthrotomy

- The patient is positioned supine. An ipsilateral proximal thigh bump is used to point the toes to the ceiling.
- Often, even for the open approach, we perform a diagnostic arthroscopy to confirm the size and location of the lesion. The location of the lesion is assessed while the ankle joint is ranged. This allows a better assessment as to whether the lesion can be approached through an arthrotomy with or without plafondplasty versus a medial or lateral malleolar osteotomy. The technique for standard arthroscopy is beyond the scope of this chapter but is detailed elsewhere.

Arthroscopy

- The patient is placed supine on the operating room table with the foot at the end of the bed. The operative leg is placed in a leg holder to keep the hip and knee flexed.
- We recommend using noninvasive distraction to allow working room for graft application.

Approach

Arthrotomy

- The approach is based on the location of the lesion. An anteromedial arthrotomy is used for medial dome lesions, an anterolateral arthrotomy used for lateral dome lesions, and a direct anterior arthrotomy is used for central lesions.
- An anterior plafondplasty may be used for more posterior lesions when using an anterior approach. Peters et al,[13] using a limited anterior plafondplasty, were able to visualize all but the central 10% of the posterior talar dome.

Arthroscopy

- Standard anteromedial and anterolateral portals are used and routine arthroscopic examination of the ankle joint is performed.

ANTEROMEDIAL, ANTEROLATERAL, OR DIRECT ANTERIOR ARTHROTOMY

Exposure

- Make a longitudinal incision centered over the ankle joint and just medial to the tibialis anterior tendon for an anteromedial arthrotomy and just lateral to the peroneus tertius tendon for an anterolateral arthrotomy.
- Carefully dissect, identify, and protect any branches of the superficial peroneal nerve that may cross the incision for an anterolateral arthrotomy.
- Incise the extensor retinaculum in line with the skin incision.
- Retract the tibialis anterior tendon laterally or the peroneus tertius tendon medially to expose the joint capsule.
- Incise the joint capsule in line with the skin incision and place a deep retractor.

Plafondplasty (Optional)

- Plantarflex the foot to assess the visibility of the OLT. If the entire lesion is not visible, an anterior tibial plafondplasty is performed, but it is important to remember that perpendicular access is not needed for PJCAT **(TECH FIG 1A)**.
- Using a curved one quarter-inch osteotome, the superior and medial or lateral aspect of the anterior tibial plafond is removed **(TECH FIG 1B)**.
  - Place a Joker or Freer retractor into the joint space to protect against further damage to the talar cartilage **(TECH FIG 1C)**.

- Careful attention should be made not to remove more than 1 cm of the nonarticular tibia in any dimension. Only the minimal amount of tibia necessary to débride and fill the lesion should be removed. Smaller plafondplasties are generally not repaired.
  - If the plafondplasty approaches 1 cm in any dimension or loss of structural integrity is a concern, consideration should be given to small fragmentary screw or bioabsorbable pin fixation.

Osteochondral Lesion of the Talus Débridement

- Visualization may be further enhanced with use of a Hintermann-style distractor or a lamina spreader secured to the tibia and talus with pins.
- Débride the lesion until stable margins are achieved on all sides using a combination of a no. 15 blade and small curette **(TECH FIG 2A)**.
- Careful attention should be paid to the shoulder of the talus. If it is felt that the shoulder is not involved in the OLT, every attempt should be made to leave the medial or lateral cartilage border at the shoulder **(TECH FIG 2B)**. This will help to contain the cartilage/fibrin mixture in the lesion and not have it spill into the medial or lateral gutter.
- There is debate as to the preparation of the base of the lesion with regard to the addition of marrow stimulation (microfracture) by violating the subchondral plate. In all reality, with adequate débridement, the subchondral plate is often penetrated in at

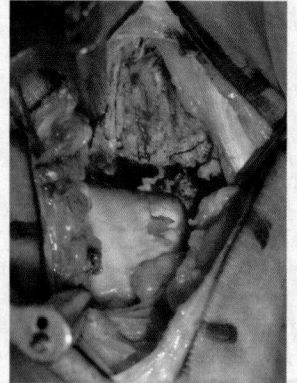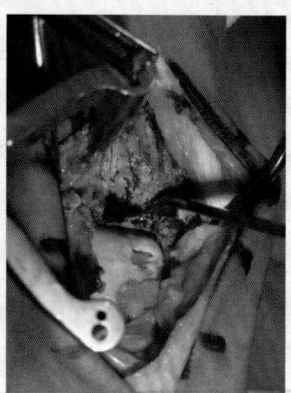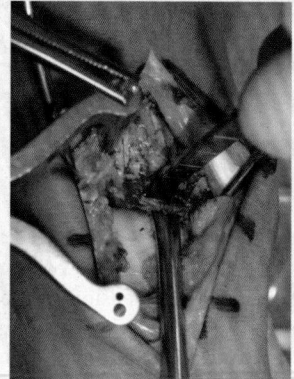

TECH FIG 1 **A.** Plantarflexed foot demonstrating anteromedial osteochondral lesion. The back of the lesion cannot be visualized. **B.** A curved osteotome is used to create the plafondplasty. **C.** A smooth elevator is placed in the joint space to protect the surrounding talar cartilage from injury during the plafondplasty.

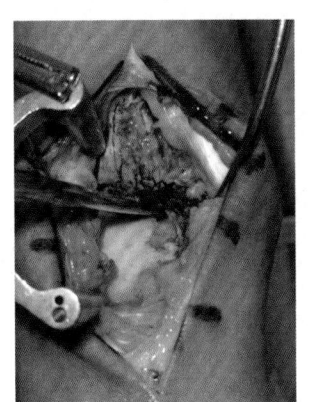 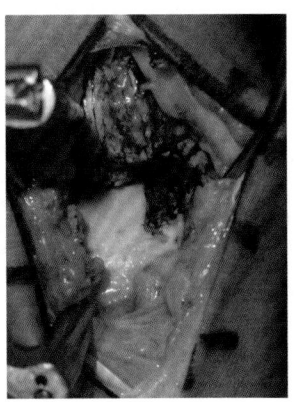

TECH FIG 2 A. A curette is used to débride the lesion to stable margins. **B.** The lesion has been débrided. Notice bleeding bone base.

least one location. We routinely perform microfracture at the base of the lesion.
- Irrigate the joint.
- If, after débridement, the base of the OLT requires bone grafting, the bone from the plafondplasty can be used. Alternatively, trephine obtained bone from the calcaneus, tibia, or iliac crest can be used.

Graft Preparation and Insertion

- Leave a sponge in the joint while preparing the graft to ensure a dry lesion base.
- Take the DeNovo NT Graft packet and turn it so that the pointed end of the plastic well faces the ground to allow the cartilage pieces to settle to the bottom.

- Insert a 21-gauge, 1.5-inch needle connected to a 10-mL syringe through the top of the plastic and carefully aspirate the medium without removing any of the cartilage pieces (the cartilage pieces are larger than the needle diameter) **(TECH FIG 3A,B)**.
- Peel back the foil (do not discard).
- Cut the foil lid a strip and bend in the center to create a trough. Alternatively, the plastic packaging can be cut to a point **(TECH FIG 3C,D)**.
- Use a Freer elevator to scoop the cartilage pieces into the trough and deliver to the joint space **(TECH FIG 3E)**.
- Next, use an elevator or equivalent instrument to push the cartilage pieces into the bed of the lesion until particulated cartilage completely covers the base.

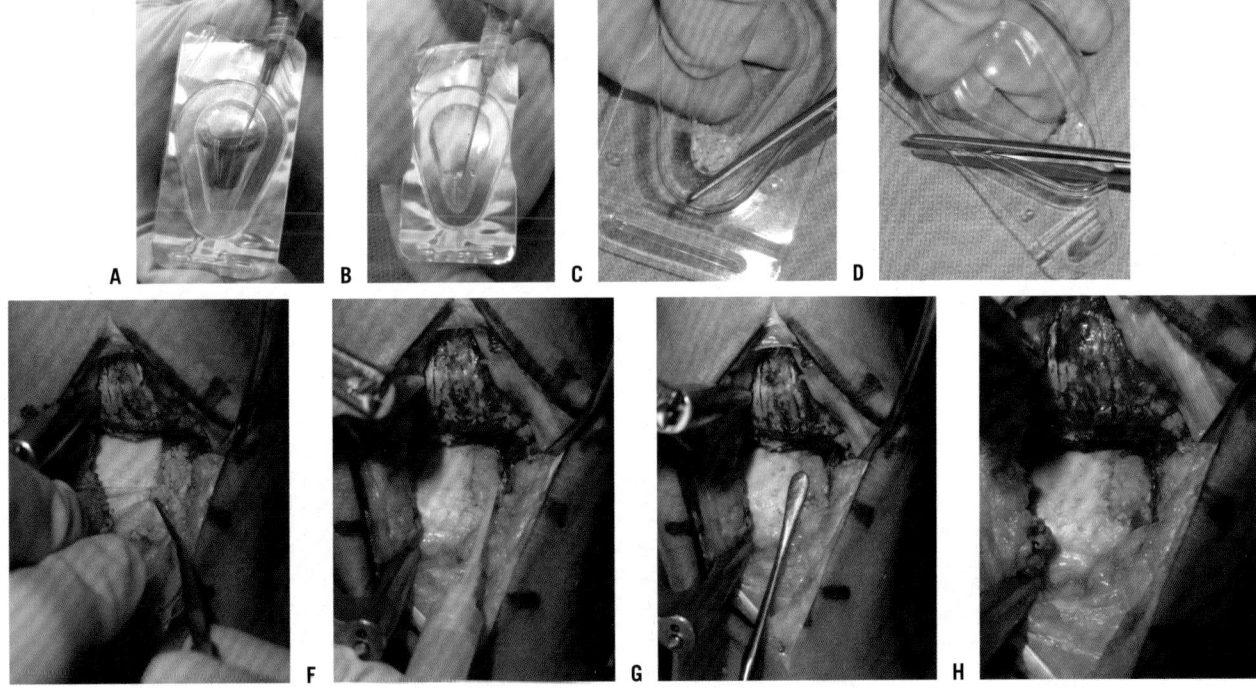

TECH FIG 3 A. A needle is introduced through the plastic to remove the support media. **B.** All of the media has been removed. The cartilage pieces are larger than the needle diameter and will not be aspirated. **C.** The plastic reservoir is being cut. **D.** The point of the plastic reservoir will be used to deliver the chips to the lesion. **E.** The chips are evenly delivered to the lesion using an elevator. **F.** Fibrin glue is applied to the lesion, and the cartilage chips are completely covered. **G.** An elevator is used to contour the lesion and remove and loose chips. **H.** The final covered lesion after being contoured to the tibial plafond.

- Apply a small amount of fibrin glue over the cartilage pieces (**TECH FIG 3F**).
- Additional particulated cartilage pieces are added in layered fashion until the depth of the lesion is completed filled without the construct being proud. An additional amount of fibrin glue is applied to the lesion to complete the particulated cartilage/fibrin glue construct.
- It is important to have extra fibrin delivery tips available, as they can become clogged in between applications of fibrin glue to the defect.
- Use a Freer elevator to remove any excess pieces and contour the surface of the lesion (**TECH FIG 3G**).
- Before the fibrin glue has completely set up, dorsiflex the ankle until the lesion is completely covered. Apply axial compression to use the contour of the tibial articular surface to mold the superior surface of the talar lesion. Maintain compression for 5 minutes.
- Plantarflex the ankle and assess the lesion for areas that require additional graft material (**TECH FIG 3H**).

Closure and Application of the Dressing

- Have an assistant keep the foot dorsiflexed during the closure and application of the splint. This will keep the lesions covered under the tibia.
- Close the capsule, retinaculum, and skin in layered fashion.
- Apply splint.

ARTHROSCOPIC TECHNIQUE

Osteochondral Lesion of the Talus Débridement

- Débride the synovium to prevent obstruction of the camera or passage of instruments and graft.
- Define the lesion with an arthroscopic probe. Measure the lesion to ensure there is adequate graft available (**TECH FIG 4A**).
- Use various arthroscopic cup and ring curettes to débride the cartilage back to a circumferential stable margin with vertical walls to contain the graft (**TECH FIG 4B**). Every attempt is made to leave a peripheral vertical wall for shoulder lesions (**TECH FIG 4C**).
- Temporarily shut off the inflow, as graft delivery occurs in this setting. This allows the surgeon to assess for soft tissue invagination at the working portal site that might interfere with graft insertion. Inflow is restored for further soft tissue débridement.
- If cancellous bone graft is needed at the base of the lesion, it can be applied in the same manner as described for cartilage graft insertion (see the following text). Bone graft can be obtained from the calcaneus using a trephine.

Joint Preparation

- Again, shut off the inflow and evacuate the joint of fluid with the use of a small suction catheter and the arthroscopic shaver (**TECH FIG 5A**).

- The lesion bed can be further dried with an epinephrine-soaked Weck-Cel sponge or cotton-tipped applicator to achieve hemostasis followed by a dry cotton-tipped applicator to soak up the excess fluid (**TECH FIG 5B–D**). Profuse bleeding at the base of the lesion can be addressed using a small amount of fibrin glue.

Graft Preparation and Insertion

- Take the DeNovo NT Graft packet and turn it so that the pointed end of the plastic well faces the ground to allow the cartilage pieces to settle to the bottom.
- Insert a 21-gauge, 1.5-inch needle connected to a 10-mL syringe through the top of the plastic and carefully aspirate the medium without removing any of the cartilage pieces (the cartilage pieces are larger than the needle diameter).
- Peel back the foil (do not discard).
- Load one-half to one-third of the graft material in a retrograde fashion into the tip of a 2.7-mm arthroscopic cannula using a Freer elevator (**TECH FIG 6A**).
- Do not load all of the pieces at once. We routinely make two or three passes per package of DeNovo NT.
- Recess the graft pieces into the cannula, using the corresponding trocar, so they are not exposed, as they can become entrapped in soft tissue when introduced into the joint (**TECH FIG 6B,C**).

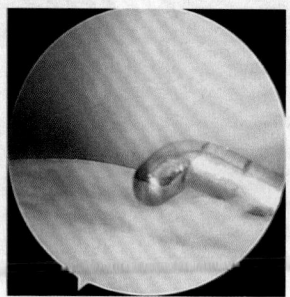 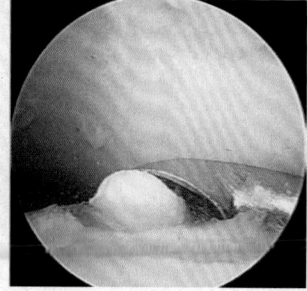 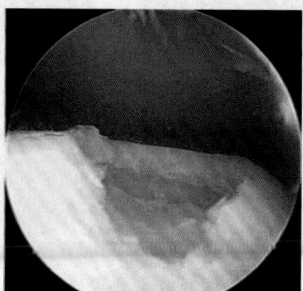

A   B   C

TECH FIG 4 A. A probe is used to assess the size of the lesion. **B.** A curette is used to débride the lesion. **C.** The lesion is débrided to stable cartilage margins.

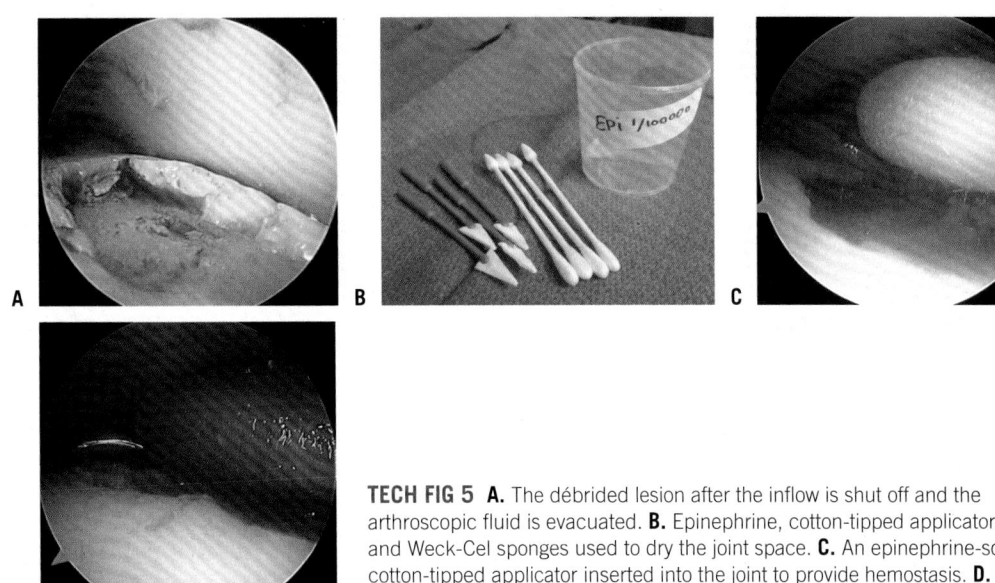

TECH FIG 5 A. The débrided lesion after the inflow is shut off and the arthroscopic fluid is evacuated. **B.** Epinephrine, cotton-tipped applicators, and Weck-Cel sponges used to dry the joint space. **C.** An epinephrine-soaked cotton-tipped applicator inserted into the joint to provide hemostasis. **D.** A dry applicator was inserted into the joint to absorb the remaining blood and fluid.

- Place the cannula, with the bevel down, at the near edge of the lesion and slowly push the pieces into the lesion using the trocar **(TECH FIG 6D,E)**.
- Remove the cannula and insert a Freer or probe to distribute the graft uniformly throughout the base of the lesion **(TECH FIG 6F,G)**.
- Insert the fibrin glue tip through the arthroscopic portal and apply a small amount of fibrin. Occasionally, the tip provided with the fibrin glue is too short, and an angiocatheter or a needle can be used **(TECH FIG 6H)**.
- Insert a Freer elevator or probe to mold the pieces uniformly in the lesion while the fibrin becomes more viscous **(TECH FIG 6I)**.

- Repeat these steps until the lesion is completely filled.
- Allow the fibrin glue to set for 5 to 10 minutes until opaque **(TECH FIG 6J)**.

Closure and Application of the Dressing

- Have an assistant keep the foot dorsiflexed during the closure and application of the splint. This will keep the lesions covered under the tibia.
- The arthroscopic portals are closed with nylon, and a well-padded splint is placed with the ankle in a position to fully contain the lesion under the tibia plafond.

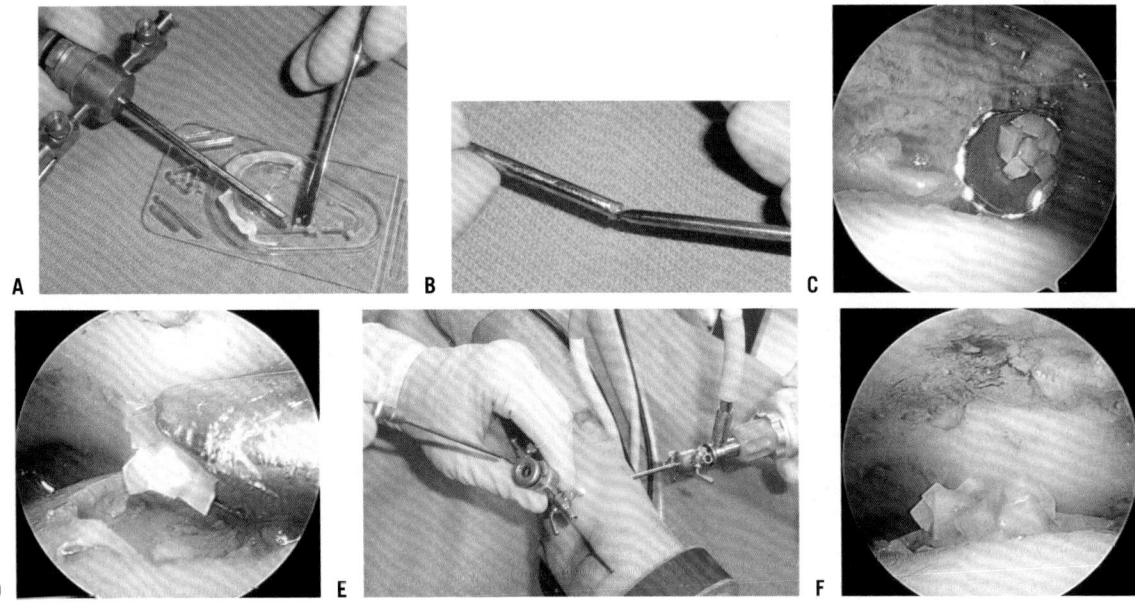

TECH FIG 6 A. A Freer is used to retrograde load the cartilage pieces into a 2.7-mm cannula. **B.** The trocar is used to recess the cartilage pieces. **C.** The cannula is inserted into the joint. Notice the cartilage pieces are recessed. **D.** The cannula is advanced to the lesion with the bevel side down, and the pieces are deployed to the lesion using the trocar. **E.** The trocar is inserted into the cannula to deploy the cartilage pieces to the lesion. **F.** The cartilage pieces have been placed into the lesion. *(continued)*

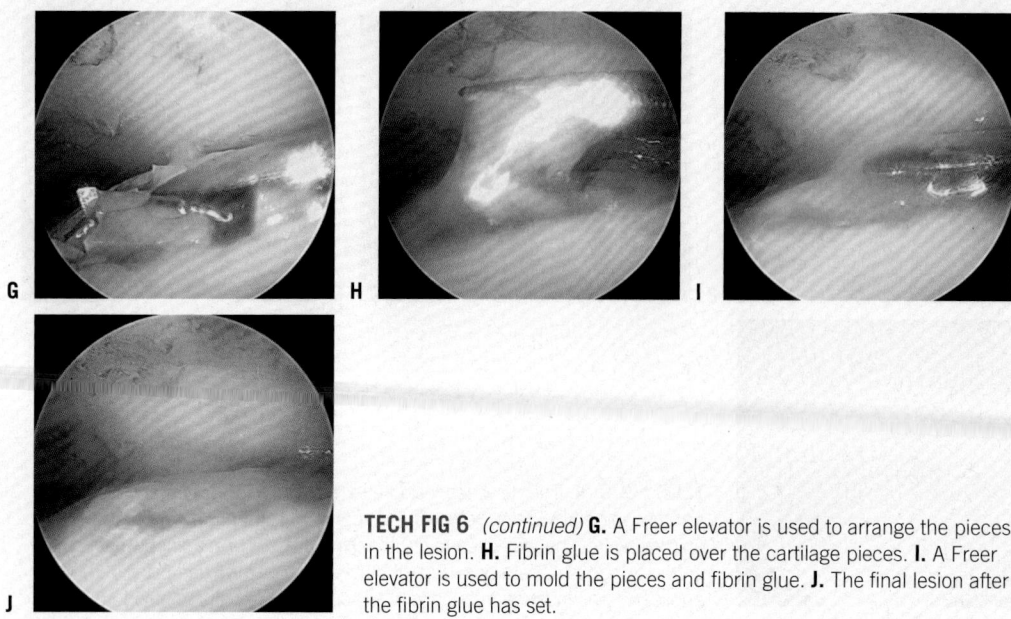

TECH FIG 6 *(continued)* **G.** A Freer elevator is used to arrange the pieces in the lesion. **H.** Fibrin glue is placed over the cartilage pieces. **I.** A Freer elevator is used to mold the pieces and fibrin glue. **J.** The final lesion after the fibrin glue has set.

TECHNIQUES

Pearls and Pitfalls

- PJCAT is indicated for focal osteochondral lesions and not for diffuse degenerative arthritis.

- If the osteochondral lesion is associated with a subchondral cyst, the cyst should be curetted and bone grafted prior to performing the PJCAT.

- Whether through an arthrotomy or arthroscopically, the PJCAT should be performed with the ankle joint as dry as possible before performing PJCAT.

- In PJCAT, the transplanted cartilage particles should fill the defect to the level of the native cartilage rim; stacking the particles so that they are proud may lead to shear of the transplanted cells.

- An excessive amount of fibrin glue is unnecessary. Glue that extends beyond the defect may adhere or impinge with ankle motion, creating tension on the glue covering in the defect, thereby potentially dislodging the cartilage particles.

POSTOPERATIVE CARE

- The patient is kept in the splint, non–weight bearing for 10 to 14 days. Sutures are removed at that point, and the patient is placed in a removable boot. The patient remains non–weight bearing. Gentle ROM exercises are started. ROM exercises are avoided in anterior lesions.
- At the 6-week postoperative time period, the patient may start progression to full weight bearing over the next 6 weeks.
- The boot can be removed at 12 weeks and a lace-up ankle brace can be worn.
  - Full ROM is allowed provided there is no contraindication based on concomitant performed procedures.
  - Physical therapy, strengthening exercises, stationary bicycle, and water activities may be initiated.
- Impact activities are not started until 6 months.

OUTCOMES

- Coetzee et al[6] presented a retrospective case series of 23 patients (24 ankles) treated with PJCAT at a mean follow-up of 16.2 months.
- The mean lesion surface size was 125 mm^2 (range, 50 to 300 mm^2) with a mean depth of 7 mm (range, 3 to 20 mm). All lesions had at least one dimension greater than or equal to 10 mm.
- The lesions were accessed via an open approach in 12 cases, an arthroscopic approach in 3 cases, and through an extended portal open approach in 9 cases. Bone grafting was performed on lesions deeper than 5 mm.
- Postoperative outcome scores were similar to published reports on patients who were treated with bone marrow stimulation, autologous chondrocyte implantation, and matrix-induced autologous chondrocyte implantation.

- Dekker and colleagues[7] retrospectively reviewed 15 patients who underwent PJCAT.
  - Unfortunately, the failure rate was 40%. Failure was defined as no improvement or worsening in symptoms or the need for an additional cartilage procedure.
  - Preoperative MRI lesion volume, intraoperative OLT area, and male sex were predictive of failure.
- A systematic review including 10 studies comprising 132 patients was recently performed.[2] However, strong conclusions about this technique could not be made. The review did show that improvement in functional outcomes was generally exhibited by these patients.

COMPLICATIONS

- An intraoperative complication specific to this technique is premature dislodging the graft material from the lesion. This is especially important for the arthroscopic technique, and the authors caution about using the arthroscopic technique in inexperienced hands. Currently, there are no known differences in outcomes between the open and arthroscopic techniques.
- Postoperative complications include inadequate take/fill of the OLT and graft material hypertrophy. Symptomatic inadequate take/fill should be assessed at the time of a second-look procedure. The lesion should be assessed for revision PJCAT versus another treatment procedure based on the progression of the OLT. Graft hypertrophy can be managed with arthroscopic débridement.

REFERENCES

1. Adams SB Jr, Yao JQ, Schon LC. Particulated juvenile articular cartilage allograft transplantation for osteochondral lesions of the talus. Tech Foot Ankle Surg 2011;10(2):92–98.
2. Aldawsari K, Alrabai HM, Sayed A, et al. Role of particulated juvenile cartilage allograft transplantation in osteochondral lesions of the talus: a systematic review [published online ahead of print February 26, 2020]. Foot Ankle Surg. doi:10.1016/j.fas.2020.02.011.
3. Anderson IF, Crichton KJ, Grattan-Smith T, et al. Osteochondral fractures of the dome of the talus. J Bone Joint Surg Am 1989;71(8): 1143–1152.
4. Bauer RS, Ochsner PE. Nosology of osteochondrosis dissecans of the trochlea of the talus [in German]. Z Orthop Ihre Grenzgeb 1987;125(2):194–200.
5. Campbell CJ, Ranawat CS. Osteochondritis dissecans: the question of etiology. J Trauma 1966;6(2):201–221.
6. Coetzee JC, Giza E, Schon LC, et al. Treatment of osteochondral lesions of the talus with particulated juvenile cartilage. Foot Ankle Int 2013;34(9):1205–1211.
7. Dekker TJ, Steele JR, Federer AE, et al. Efficacy of particulated juvenile cartilage allograft transplantation for osteochondral lesions of the talus. Foot Ankle Int 2017;39(3):278–283.
8. Elias I, Zoga AC, Morrison WB, et al. Osteochondral lesions of the talus: localization and morphologic data from 424 patients using a novel anatomical grid scheme. Foot Ankle Int 2007;28(2): 154–161.
9. Kappis M. Weitere beitrage zur traumatisch-mechanischen entstehung der "spontanen" knorpelablosungen (sogen osteohondrisit dessecans). Dtsch Z Chir 1922;171:13–20.
10. Lee KB, Bai LB, Park JG, et al. A comparison of arthroscopic and MRI findings in staging of osteochondral lesions of the talus. Knee Surg Sports Traumatol Arthrosc 2008;16(11):1047–1051.
11. McCullough CJ, Venugopal V. Osteochondritis dissecans of the talus: the natural history. Clin Orthop Relat Res 1979;(144):264–268.
12. McGahan PJ, Pinney SJ. Current concept review: osteochondral lesions of the talus. Foot Ankle Int 2010;31(1):90–101.
13. Peters PG, Parks BG, Schon LC. Anterior distal tibia plafondplasty for exposure of the talar dome. Foot Ankle Int 2012;33(3): 231–235.
14. Pettine KA, Morrey BF. Osteochondral fractures of the talus. A long-term follow-up. J Bone Joint Surg Br 1987;69(1):89–92.
15. Stroud CC, Marks RM. Imaging of osteochondral lesions of the talus. Foot Ankle Clin 2000;5(1):119–133.
16. Tol JL, Struijs PA, Bossuyt PM, et al. Treatment strategies in osteochondral defects of the talar dome: a systematic review. Foot Ankle Int 2000;21(2):119–126.

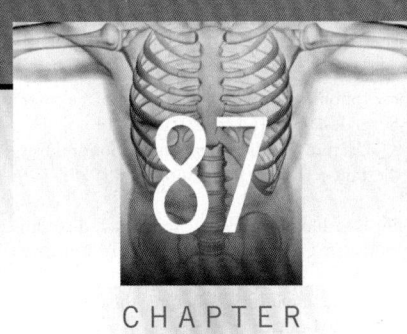

87

CHAPTER

Osteochondral Transfer for Osteochondral Lesions of the Talus

Mark E. Easley and Justin Orr

DEFINITION

- Medium-sized osteochondral defects of the talar dome
  - May approach the talar shoulder (transition of superior dome cartilage to the medial or lateral talar cartilage)
  - Often associated with subchondral cysts
- Osteochondral defect is reconstructed with a cylindrical osteochondral graft. To provide stability to this graft, the osteochondral defect in the native talus must be *contained* (have circumferential cartilage and subchondral bone).

ANATOMY

- Sixty percent of the talus' surface area is covered by articular cartilage.
- The talus is contained within the ankle mortise.
  - Superior talar dome articulates with the tibial plafond.
  - Medial dome articulates with the medial malleolus.
  - Lateral dome articulates with the lateral malleolus.
- Talar blood supply
  - Posterior tibial artery
    - Artery of the tarsal canal
    - Deltoid ligament branch
  - Peroneal artery
    - Artery of the tarsal sinus
  - Dorsalis pedis artery

PATHOGENESIS

- The pathogenesis for osteochondral lesions of the talus (OLTs) is not fully understood.
- Theories include the following:
  - Trauma
  - Idiopathic focal avascular necrosis

NATURAL HISTORY

- In general, OLTs do not progress to diffuse ankle arthritis.
- However, large volume OLTs may lead to subchondral collapse of a substantial portion of the talus and thus create deformity, higher contact stresses, and a greater concern for eventual ankle arthritis if left untreated.

PATIENT HISTORY AND PHYSICAL FINDINGS

- Patients may or may not report a history of trauma.
- Ankle pain, typically on the anterior aspect of the ankle, is a common complaint.
  - Pain is usually experienced on the side of the ankle that corresponds with the OLT, but it may be poorly localized to the site of the OLT. In fact, sometimes, medial OLTs produce lateral ankle pain and vice versa.
  - Pain is rarely sharp, unless a fragment of the OLT should act as an impinging loose body in the joint.
  - Typically, the pain is a deep ache, with and after activity, and is usually relieved with rest.
- Antalgic gait
- May be associated with malalignment or ankle instability
- Typically, tenderness on side of ankle that corresponds with OLT but not always
- Rarely crepitance or mechanical symptoms
- With chronic OLT, some degree of ankle stiffness is anticipated.

IMAGING AND OTHER DIAGNOSTIC STUDIES

- Plain radiographs
  - Obtain weight bearing, three views of the ankle
  - Small OLTs may be missed.
  - Large OLTs are usually identified on plain radiographs (FIG 1).
  - Often limited in characterizing OLT because the two-dimensional study cannot define the three-dimensional OLT
  - Particularly useful in assessing lower leg, ankle, or foot malalignment that needs to be considered in the management of OLTs
  - May detect incidental OLTs (patient has a radiograph for a different problem and an OLT is incidentally identified on plain radiographs)
- Magnetic resonance imaging (MRI)
  - Excellent screening tool when OLT or other foot–ankle pathology is suspected
  - Will identify incidental OLT but defines other potential soft tissue pathology
  - Demonstrates associated marrow edema that may lead to overestimation of the OLT's size
- Computed tomography (CT) (FIG 2)
  - Ideal for characterizing OLT, particularly large volume defects
  - Defines OLT size without distraction of associated marrow edema
  - Defines the character of the OLT and extent of its involvement in the talar dome
- Diagnostic injection
  - Intra-articular
  - An anesthetic versus anesthetic plus corticosteroid
  - May have some therapeutic effect, even for several months
  - If the source of pain is the OLT, then intra-articular injection should relieve symptoms from OLT. If the pain is not relieved, then other diagnoses should be considered.

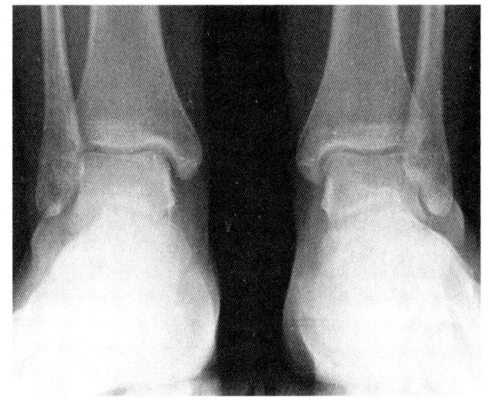
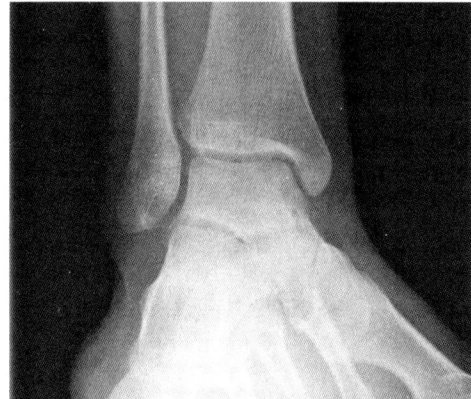
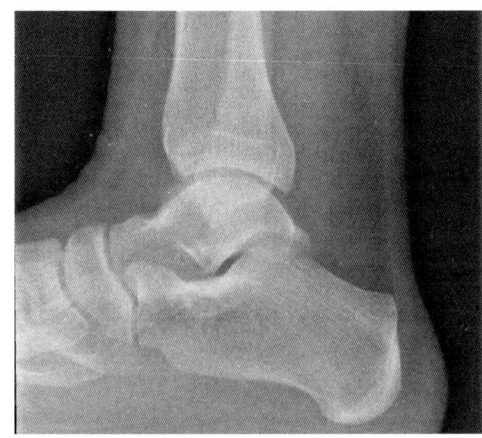

FIG 1 Radiographs. **A.** AP radiograph of the ankle suggests symmetric alignment and a medial talar dome defect. **B.** Mortise view also suggests medial OLT. **C.** Lateral view shows anatomic alignment, with OLT less obvious.

DIFFERENTIAL DIAGNOSIS

- Loose body in ankle joint
- Ankle impingement (anterior or posterior)
- Chronic ankle instability (medial, lateral, or syndesmotic)
- Ankle synovitis or adjacent tendinopathy
- Early ankle degenerative change

NONOPERATIVE MANAGEMENT

- Activity modification
- Bracing
- Physical therapy if associated ankle instability
- Nonsteroidal anti-inflammatories or COX-2 inhibitors
- Corticosteroid injection
- Viscosupplementation

SURGICAL MANAGEMENT

Preoperative Planning

- Indications for this surgery include the following:
  - Medium-sized OLTs not amenable to other joint-sparing procedures. If associated with a large subchondral cyst,

then arthroscopic débridement and microfracture may not be effective, and some surgeons recommend osteochondral transfer as a primary procedure.
  - Failed arthroscopic (débridement and microfracture) management
- Potential sites for graft harvest
  - Patient's ipsilateral knee (superolateral femoral condyle, intracondylar notch)
  - Allograft talus
- Ipsilateral knee versus talar allograft
  - Knee is autograft; however, knee cartilage is thicker than ankle cartilage and may have different biomechanical properties.
  - Allograft talus offers nearly the same cartilage thickness and harvest from the exact location of the native talus defect; however, it is not the patient's own tissue.
- The surgeon should check for associated pathology that may need to be addressed at the time of allograft talar reconstruction:
  - Osteophyte removal
  - Ligament reconstruction
  - Corrective osteotomies (calcaneal, supramalleolar)

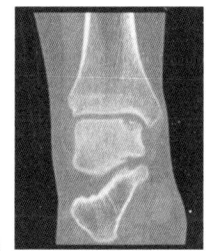
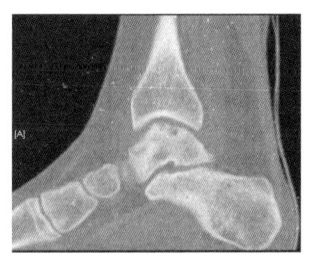
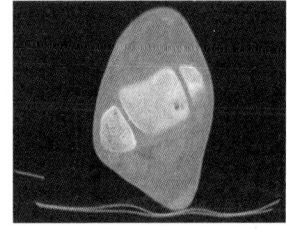

FIG 2 CT. **A.** Coronal view with medial OLT that approaches talar shoulder but appears contained. **B.** Sagittal view demonstrating rather medial OLT. **C.** Axial view with posteromedial OLT.

- Patient education
  - This is a complex procedure.
  - The patient must understand that the intent is to transfer cartilage and bone from one location to another and expect it to incorporate into the native talus.
  - If allograft is used, there is a negligible but real risk of disease transmission and possible graft rejection by the host.
  - There is no guarantee that the procedure will work, and a revision procedure may be required, such as structural allograft reconstruction or potentially ankle arthrodesis.

Positioning

- The patient is positioned supine (**FIG 3**).
- For a lateral OLT, a bolster under the ipsilateral hip typically affords better access to the lateral talar dome.
- We routinely use a thigh tourniquet.

Approach

- The surgeon must determine the optimal surgical approach:
  - Medial talar dome (usually centromedial or posteromedial) typically warrants a medial malleolar osteotomy.

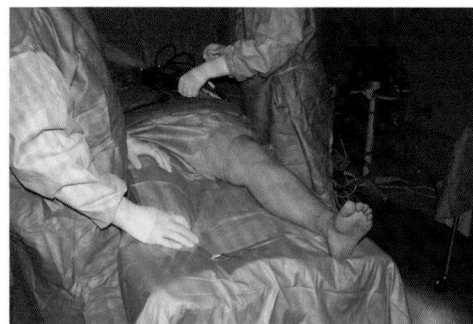

FIG 3 Positioning is supine, with easy access to the medial ankle but without too much external rotation, which would make access to the lateral knee cumbersome.

- Lateral talar dome (often centrolateral) typically necessitates ligament releases (anterior talofibular and calcaneofibular) with or without lateral malleolar osteotomy.
- The key is that exposure must allow perpendicular access to the OLT; otherwise, the dedicated instrumentation for the osteochondral transfer cannot be used.

TECHNIQUES

MEDIAL APPROACH FOR A MEDIAL OSTEOCHONDRAL LESION OF THE TALUS

- Make a longitudinal incision centered over the medial malleolus (**TECH FIG 1A**).
- Anterior ankle arthrotomy
  - Identify the joint line (**TECH FIG 1B**).
  - Visualize the anterior talus and possibly anterior OLT (**TECH FIG 1C**).
- Open the flexor retinaculum (**TECH FIG 1D**).
  - Identify and protect the posterior tibial tendon (PTT) (**TECH FIG 1E**).

- Predrill the intended screw holes for fixation of the osteotomy.
  - Two parallel drill holes in the same orientation are typically used for open reduction and internal fixation of a medial malleolar fracture (**TECH FIG 1F**).
  - Consider tapping the screw holes as well (traditional malleolar screws are not self-tapping) (**TECH FIG 1G**).
- Trajectory of the oblique osteotomy
  - Should target tibial plafond at lateral extent of OLT
  - Allows perpendicular access to the OLT with the dedicated instrumentation

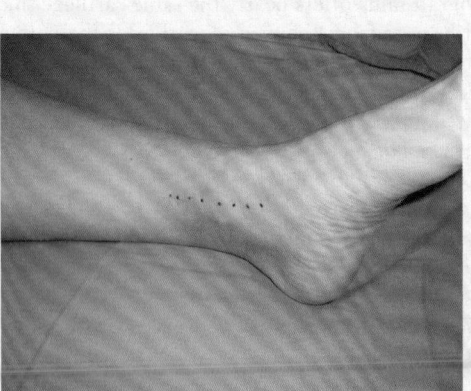
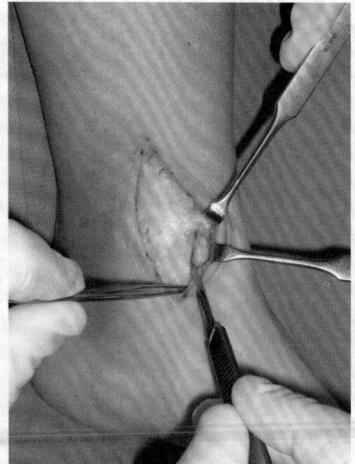
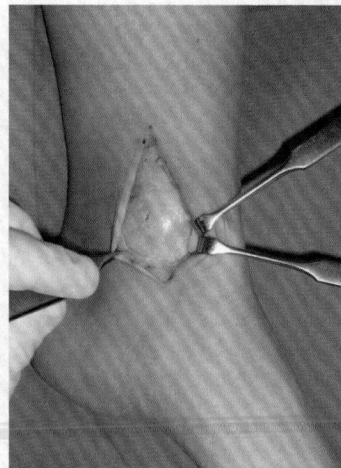

TECH FIG 1 **A.** Medial approach is similar to that for open reduction and internal fixation for a medial malleolar fracture. **B,C.** Anterior ankle arthrotomy. **B.** Locating joint and performing the medial capsulotomy. **C.** Medial talar dome visible through the arthrotomy with capsule retracted. This defines the anterior margin for the osteotomy. Rarely, the OLT may be accessed via arthrotomy alone, but this is more common for lateral lesions. *(continued)*

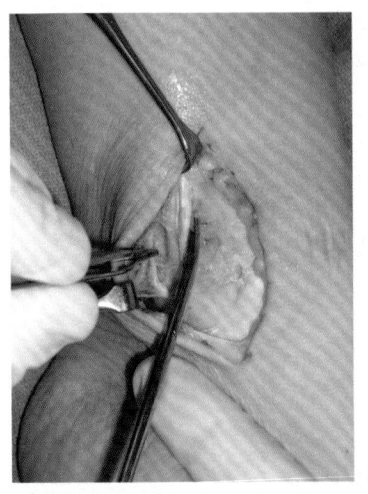
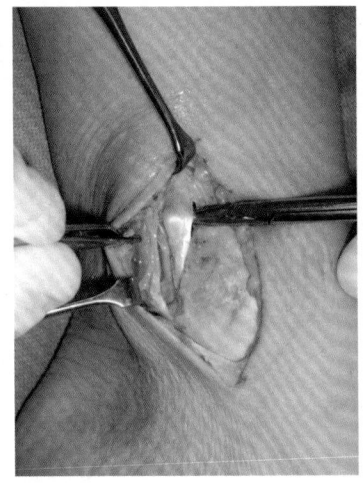
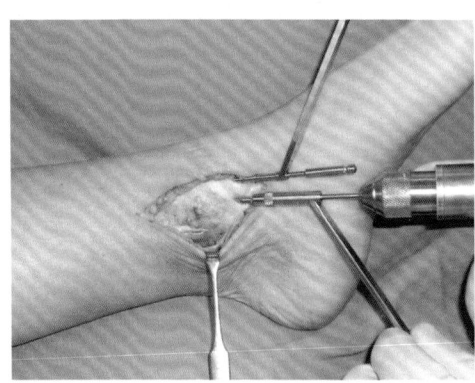

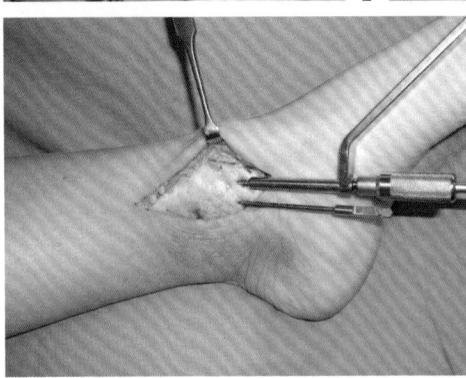

TECH FIG 1 *(continued)* **D,E.** Defining posterior tibia for the osteotomy. **D.** Opening the flexor retinaculum. **E.** Identifying the PTT (to be protected during the osteotomy). **F,G.** Predrilling the medial malleolus. **F.** Drill bit directed as it would be for medial malleolar screws for open reduction and internal fixation of a medial malleolar fracture. **G.** Tap used for screws that are not self-tapping.

- We routinely use a Kirschner wire to determine the trajectory for the osteotomy.
  - Place the wire slightly proximal and lateral to the planned osteotomy so as not to interfere with the saw blade and chisel **(TECH FIG 2A)**.
  - Confirm desired Kirschner wire trajectory with fluoroscopy.
- Mark the osteotomy.
  - Across the periosteum and with minimal periosteal stripping **(TECH FIG 2B)**
  - Perpendicular to the tibial shaft axis
- Protect the soft tissues.
  - Tibialis anterior retracted
  - PTT retracted. Do not mistake the flexor digitorum longus for the PTT (PTT rests in a groove directly on the posterior aspect of tibia).

- Performing the osteotomy
  - Microsagittal saw **(TECH FIG 2C)**
    - To the subchondral bone
    - Use cool saline irrigation to limit risk of heat necrosis of the bone.
- Chisel **(TECH FIG 2D)**
  - Complete the osteotomy with a chisel.
- Periodically check the progress of the osteotomy fluoroscopically to confirm trajectory and to avoid injury to the talar dome.
- Reflect medial malleolus on the deltoid ligament **(TECH FIG 2E)**.
  - The PTT sheath must be released from the malleolus to allow full reflection of the malleolus.

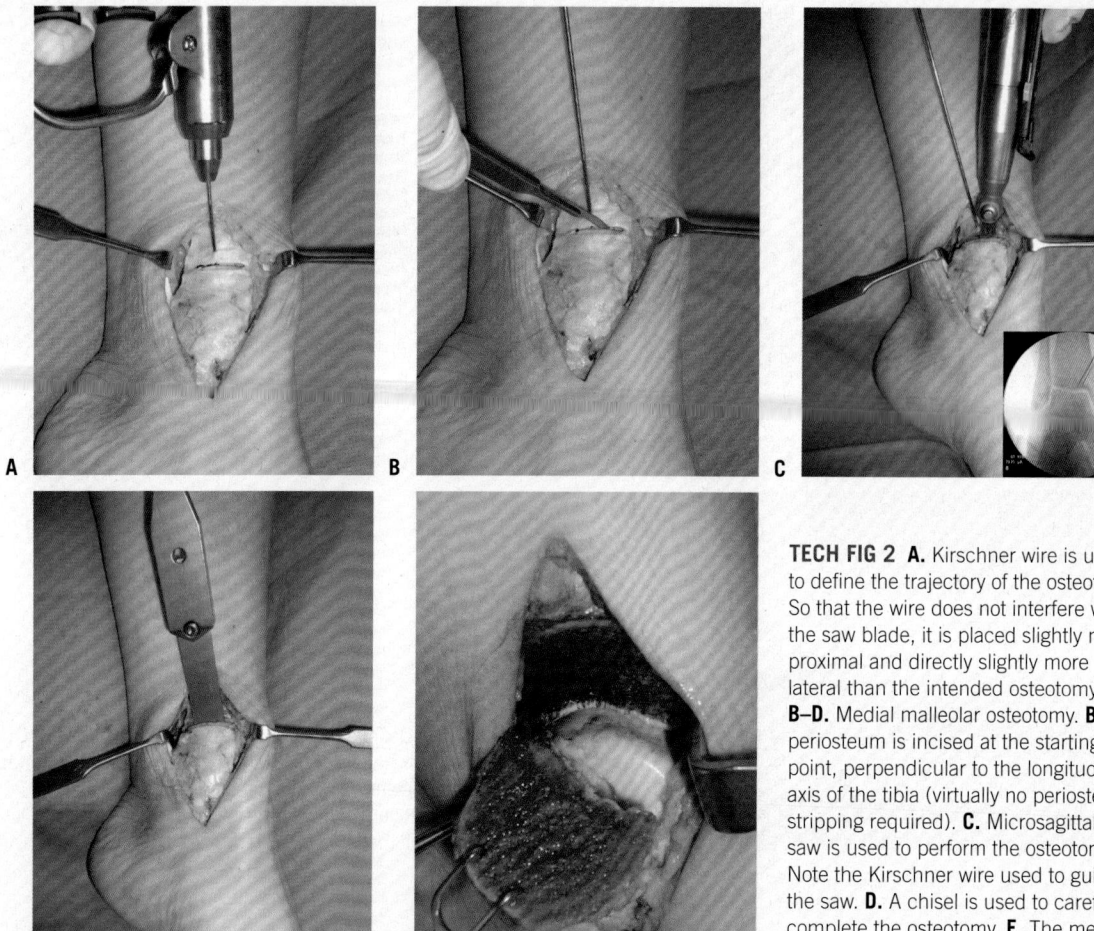

TECH FIG 2 A. Kirschner wire is used to define the trajectory of the osteotomy. So that the wire does not interfere with the saw blade, it is placed slightly more proximal and directly slightly more lateral than the intended osteotomy. **B–D.** Medial malleolar osteotomy. **B.** The periosteum is incised at the starting point, perpendicular to the longitudinal axis of the tibia (virtually no periosteal stripping required). **C.** Microsagittal saw is used to perform the osteotomy. Note the Kirschner wire used to guide the saw. **D.** A chisel is used to carefully complete the osteotomy. **E.** The medial malleolus is reflected, exposing the OLT.

LATERAL APPROACH FOR A LATERAL OSTEOCHONDRAL LESION OF THE TALUS

- Ideal for lateral OLT associated with lateral ankle instability
- Lateral ligaments may be released even without ligament instability.
- Make a longitudinal incision over the distal lateral fibula and curve it slightly anteriorly at the distal margin.
  - Protect the sural nerve and lateral branch of the superficial peroneal nerve.
- Identify the inferior extensor retinaculum and mobilize it to be used as augmentation to lateral ligament repair at the conclusion of the cartilage procedure.
- Identify the peroneal tendons and protect them throughout the procedure.
- Release the joint capsule, with anterior talofibular and calcaneofibular ligaments, from the distal fibula.
- In many patients, plantarflexion and inversion allows sufficient anterior subluxation of the talus to perform osteochondral transfer with the dedicated instruments perpendicular to the osteochondral defect.

- If the exposure is not sufficient with soft tissue release alone, a fibular osteotomy may be performed to gain access to the more posteriorly situated lateral OLT.
- Fibular osteotomy
  - We routinely perform an oblique fibular osteotomy, similar to the pattern of a Weber B ankle fracture.
  - When performed with the ligament release described earlier, exposure is markedly enhanced.
  - Before performing the osteotomy, we place a small fragment plate on the lateral fibula that spans the proposed osteotomy and predrill the holes.
  - With the peroneal tendons and superficial peroneal nerve protected, perform the osteotomy obliquely using a microsagittal saw.
    - Cool saline irrigation to limit bone heat necrosis
    - Avoid injuring intact articular cartilage on talus.
- Syndesmotic ligaments remain intact

OSTEOCHONDRAL TRANSFER

- Single-stage operation
- Donor options
  - Autograft from ipsilateral knee
    - Arthrotomy versus arthroscopy
    - Superolateral femoral condyle versus intracondylar notch
    - Moderate amount of donor graft available
  - Autograft from ipsilateral talus
    - Limited donor graft available
  - Allograft talus
    - Fresh allograft ideal
    - Ideally same side as the native talus to replace the deficient cartilage with cartilage from the exact same location
    - Maximum donor graft available
    - Advantage over knee or talar autograft if the OLT proves not to be contained
- Recipient site preparation
  - Débride the OLT sharply to stabilize circumferential rim of articular cartilage **(TECH FIG 3A)**.
  - Be sure that the defect is contained.
    - Bony rim circumferentially
    - Interference fit will be compromised if medial talar dome at the defect lacks integrity.
    - If not, then a structural allograft reconstruction should be considered.
  - Assess defect size and orientation with the sizing guide and with reference to preoperative CT scan **(TECH FIG 3B)**. Larger defects may warrant two or even three grafts.
  - Recipient site chisel
    - Assistant will need to position foot in maximal inversion or eversion for medial and lateral OLTs, respectively **(TECH FIG 4A)**.
    - Select appropriate chisel size.
    - Orient chisel perpendicular to defect **(TECH FIG 4B)**.
  - We routinely advance the chisel 11 to 12 mm into the talus **(TECH FIG 4C)**.
    - Maintain proper chisel orientation to the desired depth.
    - Do not attempt to change orientation of the chisel once the chisel has been advanced into the subchondral bone.

- Once at the desired depth, twist the chisel forcefully 90 degrees and then 90 degrees again **(TECH FIG 4D)**.
- Gently toggle the chisel to free the diseased cartilage from the surrounding healthy cartilage.
- Extract the diseased osteochondral cylinder **(TECH FIG 4E)**.
- If the subchondral bone is sclerotic, a reamer of corresponding size from an anterior cruciate ligament set may be used to create the recipient site.
  - Use cool saline irrigation to limit the risk of heat necrosis to surrounding native talus.
  - Predrill the guide pin to ensure that the reamer maintains position and proper orientation.
- Donor site preparation and graft harvest (superolateral femoral condyle)
  - Superolateral arthrotomy
    - Knee extended
    - Longitudinal approach immediately lateral to patella **(TECH FIG 5A,B)**, about 5 cm long
    - Avoid injuring cartilage.
  - Choose optimal site for graft harvest **(TECH FIG 5C)**.
    - Use the same sizing guide as you did for the recipient site to determine the proper trajectory for the harvesting chisel and to determine the ideal location for graft harvest.
  - If multiple grafts are needed, be sure to leave an adequate bridge between harvest sites.
    - Avoid fracturing one harvest site into another, thereby creating a large defect.
  - Select the corresponding donor chisel.
    - This chisel is 1 mm larger in diameter than the recipient chisel. This allows for interference fit of the graft into the recipient site.
    - The chisel must be perpendicular to the harvest site **(TECH FIG 5D)**.
    - Be sure not to contact the cartilage surface with the chisel until proper position has been obtained. The chisel is sharp and will cut into the cartilage, even with light pressure.

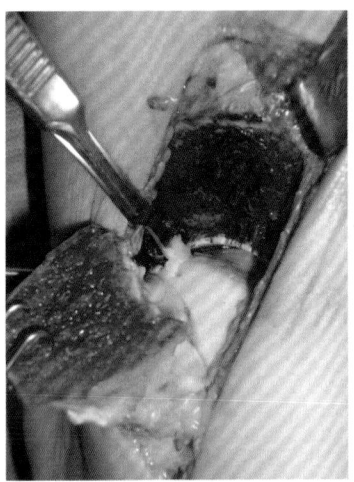 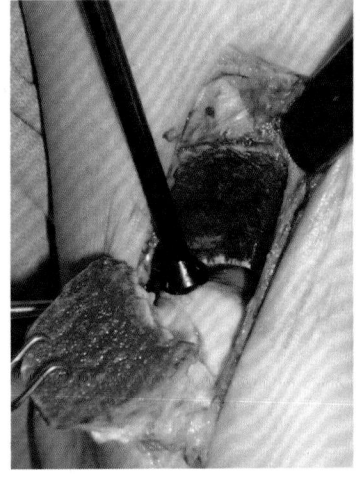

A   **B**

TECH FIG 3 A. The surgeon probes and débrides the OLT to define its superficial dimensions. **B.** The defect is sized to determine optimal recipient chisel size.

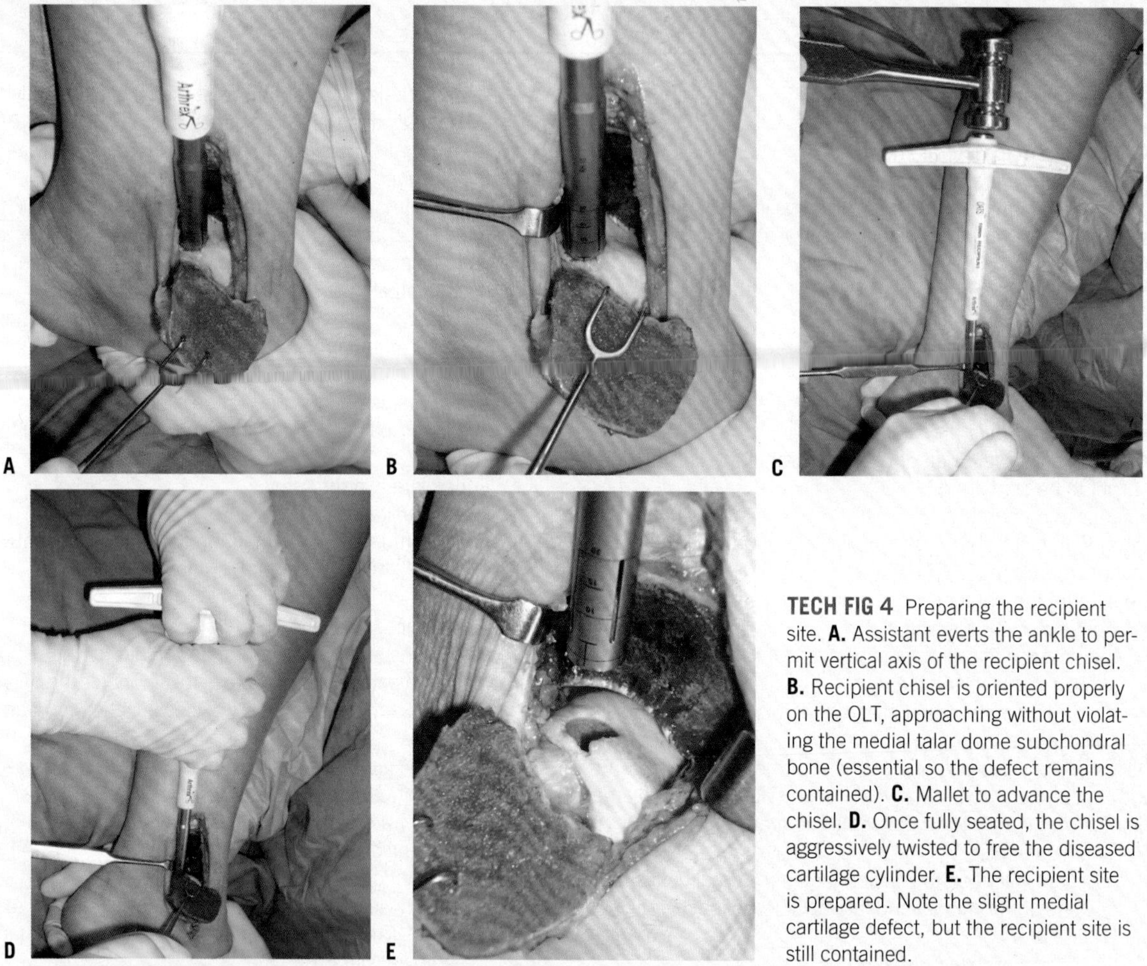

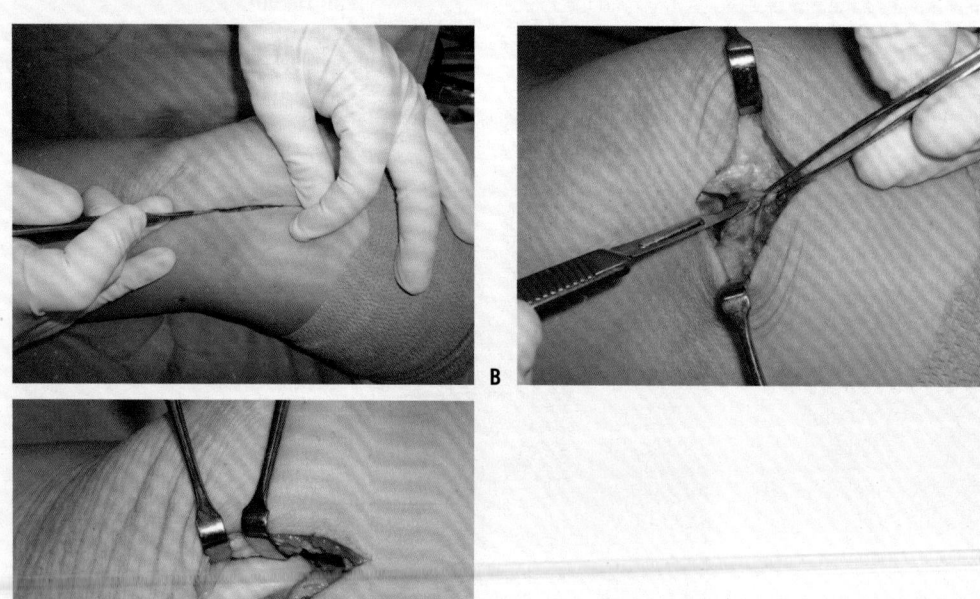

TECH FIG 4 Preparing the recipient site. **A.** Assistant everts the ankle to permit vertical axis of the recipient chisel. **B.** Recipient chisel is oriented properly on the OLT, approaching without violating the medial talar dome subchondral bone (essential so the defect remains contained). **C.** Mallet to advance the chisel. **D.** Once fully seated, the chisel is aggressively twisted to free the diseased cartilage cylinder. **E.** The recipient site is prepared. Note the slight medial cartilage defect, but the recipient site is still contained.

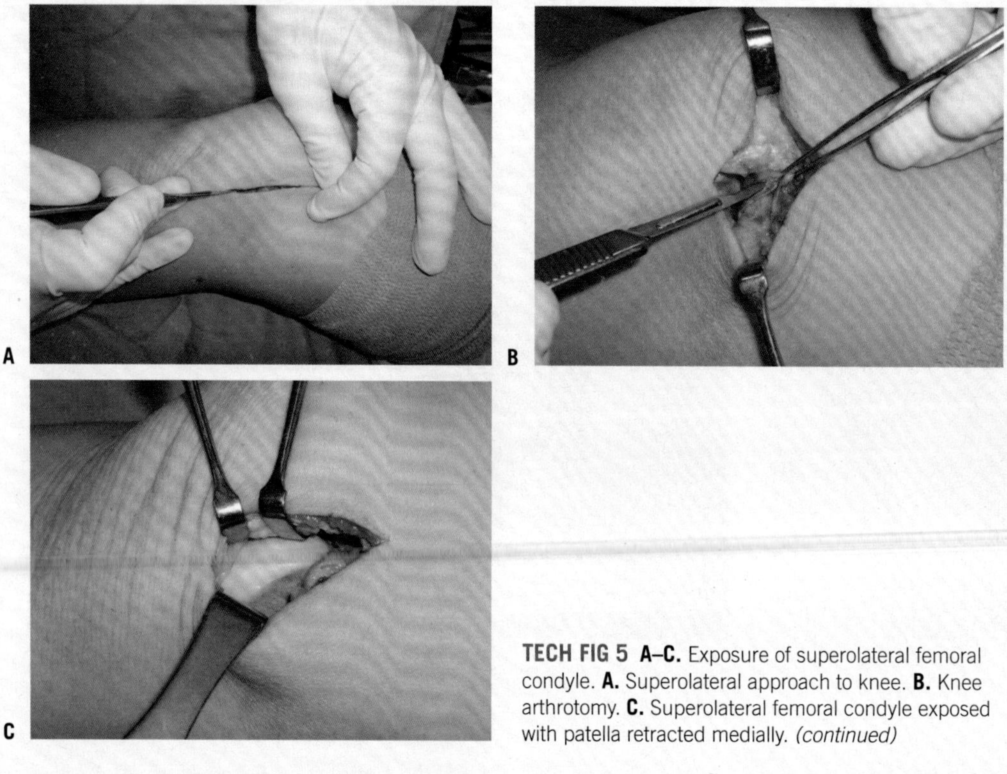

TECH FIG 5 A–C. Exposure of superolateral femoral condyle. **A.** Superolateral approach to knee. **B.** Knee arthrotomy. **C.** Superolateral femoral condyle exposed with patella retracted medially. *(continued)*

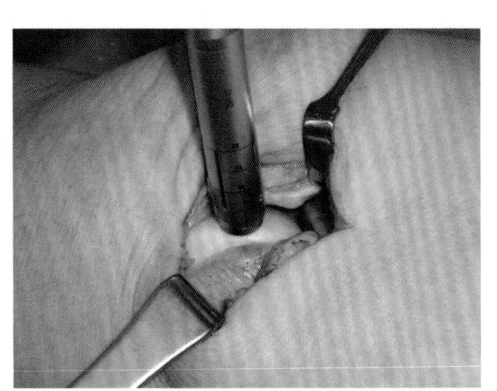
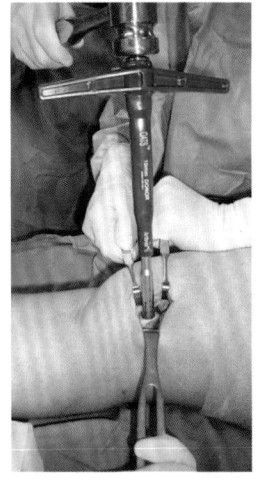
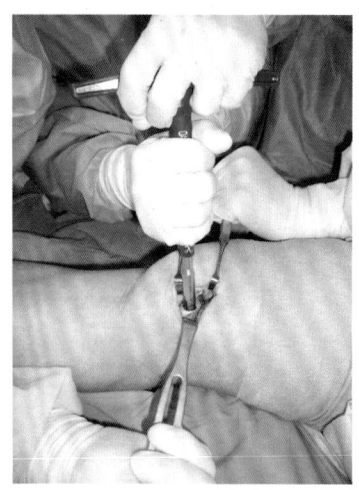

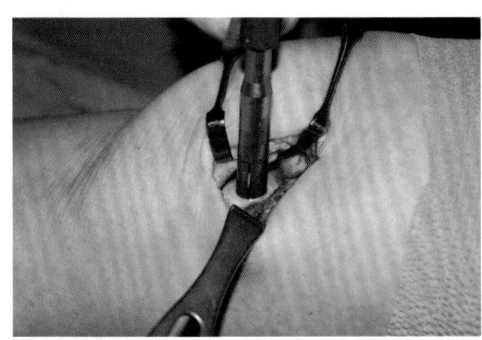
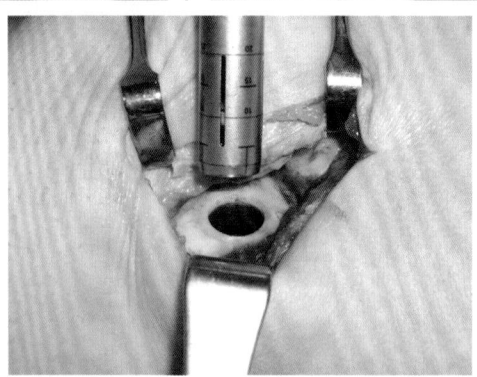

TECH FIG 5 *(continued)* **D–H.** Harvesting donor graft. **D.** Donor chisel oriented to allow optimal graft harvest. **E.** Harvesting chisel impacted without changing trajectory once chisel introduced. **F.** Once chisel is fully seated, it is aggressively twisted to free the cylindrical graft. **G.** Chisel is carefully withdrawn (fenestrations within chisel confirm that the graft is advancing with the chisel). **H.** Graft extracted and harvest site evident.

- Impact the chisel to a depth of 10 mm **(TECH FIG 5E)**.
  - Do not change the orientation of the chisel once it has been advanced into the subchondral bone.
- Once desired depth has been achieved
  - Rotate the chisel 90 degrees and then 90 degrees again **(TECH FIG 5F)**.
  - Toggle the chisel lightly to release the graft.
- Extract the graft from the knee.
  - A fenestration in the chisel allows for visualization of the graft to ensure it is free and advancing from the harvest site with the chisel **(TECH FIG 5G,H)**.
- The graft does not leave the chisel until it is secured in the recipient site.
- Graft transfer to the recipient site
  - Properly orient the donor chisel over the recipient site, maintaining contact with the chisel directly over the defect **(TECH FIG 6A,B)**.

- Advance the graft into the recipient site by advancing the tamp in the donor chisel **(TECH FIG 6C)**. Fenestrations in the chisel permit visualization of the graft being advanced.
- Remove the chisel when the graft is nearly fully seated **(TECH FIG 6D,E)**.
- The goal is to place the graft flush with the surrounding native articular cartilage.
- A corresponding tamp or sizing guide may then be used to carefully achieve the final position of the graft **(TECH FIG 6F,G)**.
- We routinely harvest a 10-mm osteochondral cylinder but prepare an 11- to 12-mm recipient site. Although countersinking the graft is a risk, the interference fit typically limits this from occurring. In our opinion, it is safer than creating a recipient site that is too shallow, thus potentially leading to forceful tamping of the graft that may lead to shearing of the graft cartilage from its osseous cylinder.

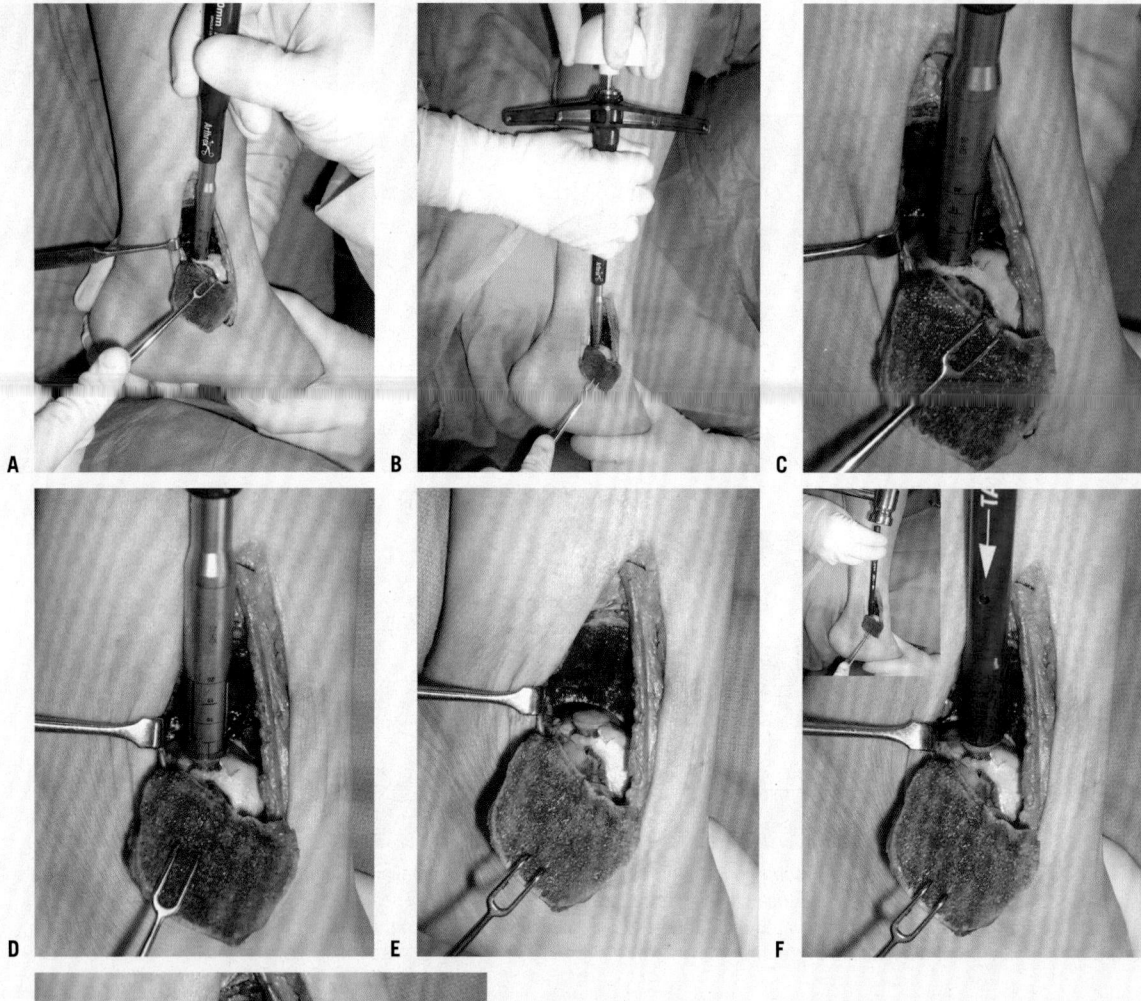

TECH FIG 6 Transfer of graft to recipient site. **A.** Donor chisel with graft oriented with recipient site. **B.** Tamp within chisel is advanced to transfer the graft into the recipient site. **C.** Fenestrations in chisel confirm that graft is advancing. **D.** Chisel typically releases graft before it is fully seated (in our hands, preferred so we can control the final graft position). **E.** Graft sitting slightly proud relative to the adjacent native cartilage. **F.** Dedicated smooth tamp used to perform final seating of graft. *Inset* shows that the tamp is tapped lightly to advance graft in a graduated manner. **G.** Graft seated flush with surrounding native cartilage. (Note medial articular defect not fully resurfaced, but majority of OLT is resurfaced with stable graft.)

OSTEOCHONDRAL TRANSFER INCORPORATING A SMALL PORTION OF MEDIAL OR LATERAL TALAR DOME CARTILAGE

- This technique is used when the OLT involves some of the cartilage on the medial or lateral sides of the talar dome while still being contained.
- Recipient site
  - The recipient site chisel approaches the talar shoulder but is not advanced beyond the subchondral border of the medial or lateral talus.
  - This will extract the dorsal shoulder of the talus, leaving the medial or lateral talar subchondral bone and cartilage intact (still contained).
- Donor site
  - As for the recipient site and chisel, the donor chisel approaches the superolateral femoral condyle's shoulder but is not advanced beyond its border.

- The dorsal shoulder of the graft will be included in the harvest without violating the lateral femoral condyle's subchondral bone on its lateral margin.
- Transfer
  - Medial OLT
    - The chisel will need to be rotated 180 degrees to fill the articular cartilage defect that extends over the shoulder from the dorsal talar dome.
    - Mark the donor chisel during graft harvest to avoid malrotation of the graft in the recipient site.
  - For a lateral OLT, this rotation is not necessary when transferring from the ipsilateral knee.

CLOSURE

- Medial closure
  - Reduction of the medial osteotomy after cartilage reconstruction
  - Temporarily place a drill bit in one of the predrilled holes to orient the reduction.
  - Confirm reduction by visualizing the anterior and posterior aspects of the osteotomy at the joint line.
  - We routinely use two partially threaded small fragment cancellous screws to fix the osteotomy under compression **(TECH FIG 7A,B)**.
    - If fixation is suboptimal, two fully threaded cortical screws may be used to engage the opposite cortex. It may be necessary to use longer cortical screws from a pelvic set to reach the opposite cortex.

- A buttress plate placed at the superior aspect of the osteotomy provides an antiglide effect **(TECH FIG 7C)**.
- Confirm fluoroscopically that the osteotomy is anatomically reduced at the plafond.
  - A minimal gap will be present at the osteotomy site despite anatomic reduction due to the thickness of the saw blade.
  - Reapproximate the flexor retinaculum with the PTT in its anatomic position **(TECH FIG 7D)**.
  - Close the anterior arthrotomy **(TECH FIG 7E)**.
  - The periosteum over the osteotomy may be reapproximated but must be coordinated with the antiglide plate.
- Lateral closure

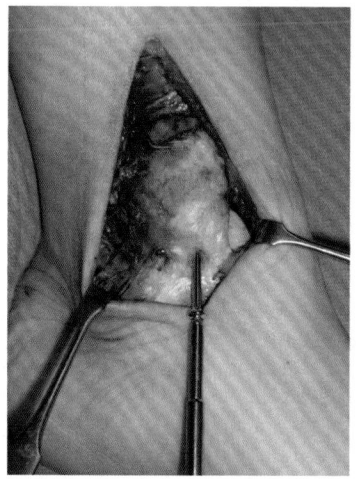 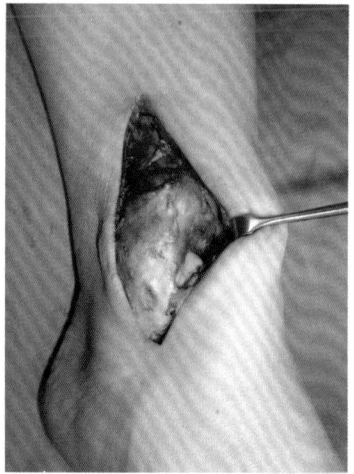 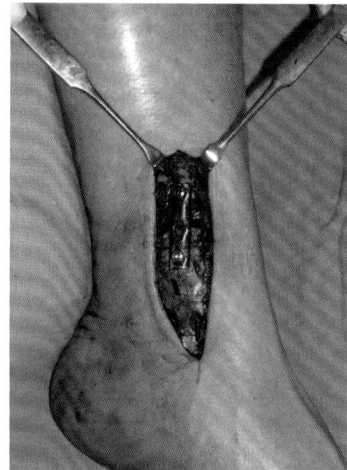

A B C

TECH FIG 7 Reducing medial malleolar osteotomy. **A.** Reduced osteotomy is secured with two malleolar screws placed in the predrilled holes. **B.** View through arthrotomy confirms reduction of anterior tibial plafond. **C.** Medial buttress plate. *(continued)*

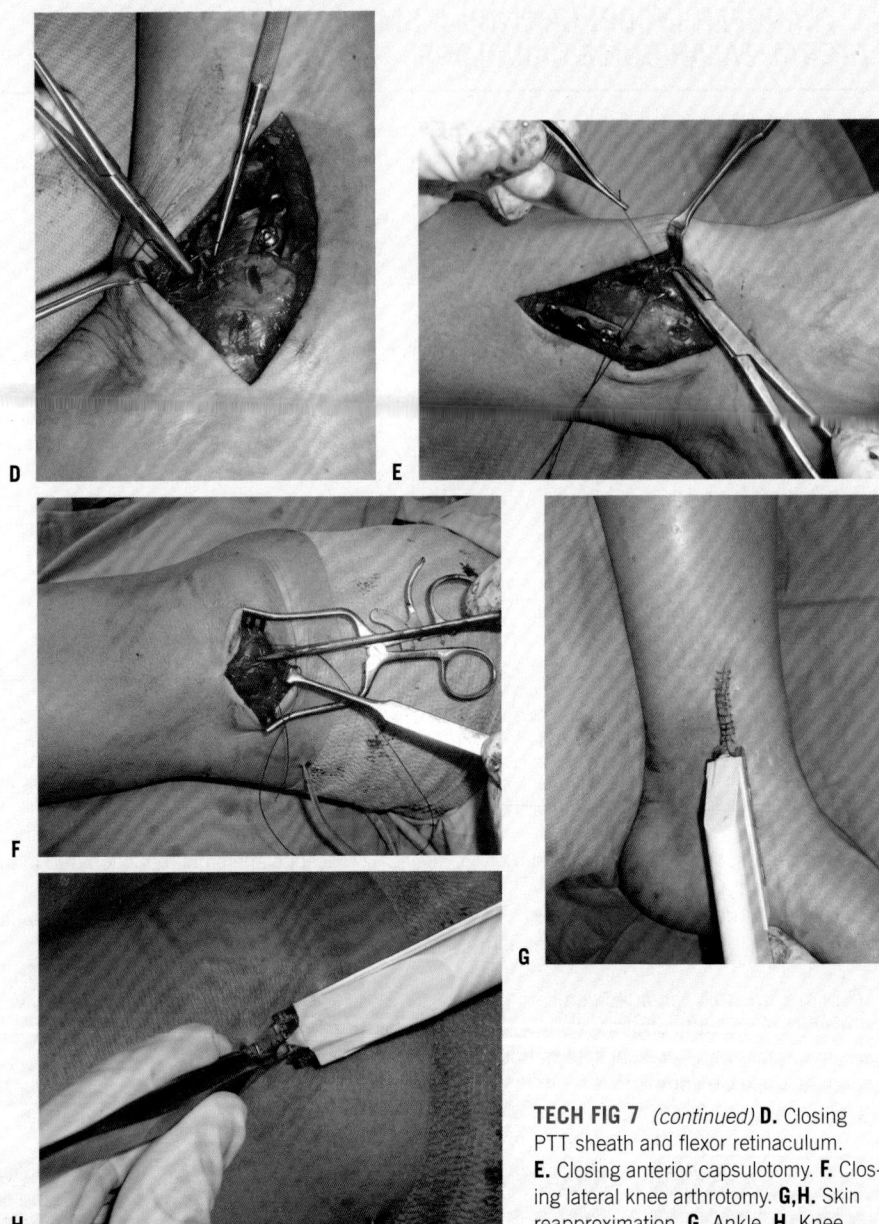

TECH FIG 7 *(continued)* **D.** Closing PTT sheath and flexor retinaculum. **E.** Closing anterior capsulotomy. **F.** Closing lateral knee arthrotomy. **G,H.** Skin reapproximation. **G.** Ankle. **H.** Knee.

- Fibular osteotomy reduction, ligament repair, and closure after cartilage procedure
  - Fibular osteotomy is reduced, plate is positioned, and screws are placed in predrilled holes. A small gap at the osteotomy site may be visible on fluoroscopic confirmation despite anatomic clinical reduction; this is secondary to saw blade thickness.
  - A modified Brostrom ligament repair serves to reattach the anterior talofibular and calcaneofibular ligaments and augment with the inferior extensor retinaculum. We routinely use suture anchors to reattach the ligaments to the fibula. We use a modified Brostrom ligament reattachment after osteochondral transfer for lateral OLTs.
- Close the superolateral capsule of the knee **(TECH FIG 7F)**.
- Close the subcutaneous layer and skin after tourniquet release and meticulous hemostasis for both the knee and ankle **(TECH FIG 7G,H)**.
- We use a drain, unless the wounds have minor residual bleeding.

Pearls and Pitfalls

Perpendicular Access	• The dedicated chisel must be oriented perpendicular to the articular cartilage. Thus, the exposure (osteotomy) must be adequate to accommodate the perpendicular position of the chisel.
Do not reorient the chisel once it has been advanced into the subchondral bone.	• Carefully obtain the proper orientation of the chisel before advancing it. If orientation is changed during impaction, you may not be able to extract an intact osteochondral graft.
Graft Height and Recipient Site Depth	• The graft must not be longer than the recipient site. Impaction may lead to shear of the graft's articular cartilage from its osseous cylinder.
Using Multiple Grafts	• Do not allow one graft harvest site to fracture into an adjacent harvest site. However, grafts may be overlapped (intersecting circles) to fill the recipient site optimally.
Malleolar Osteotomy	• The medial malleolar osteotomy must have perfect congruency at the tibial plafond when reduced.

POSTOPERATIVE CARE

- We routinely observe these patients overnight for pain control.
- Follow-up is done in about 10 to 14 days.
- Provided the wound and osteotomy (if one was performed) are stable, the patient is transferred into a touchdown weight-bearing cam boot. If not, a touchdown weight-bearing short-leg cast is continued until the wound and osteotomy are stable.
- Intermittent minimal, gentle ankle range of motion (ROM) is encouraged, three or four times a day. If financially feasible, we arrange for an ankle continuous passive motion device.
- Touchdown weight bearing is maintained for 8 to 10 weeks, with progressively increasing ankle ROM exercise.
- We routinely obtain simulated weight-bearing radiographs at 6 weeks and 10 weeks, and again at 14 to 16 weeks, depending on the progression of healing. If there was a concern

about fixation of the graft or osteotomy, then radiographs are also obtained at the first postoperative visit (FIG 4).

- Knee cartilage has a different thickness than ankle cartilage; therefore, an appropriately placed osteochondral graft from the knee may appear recessed on the postoperative radiograph (FIG 5).

OUTCOMES

- Good to excellent results with osteochondral autografting at short to intermediate follow-up can be obtained in 90% to 94% of patients.
  - Excellent functional outcomes
  - Improvement in ROM
  - Improved pain scores
- Best results for smaller defects (those that can be managed with a single graft)

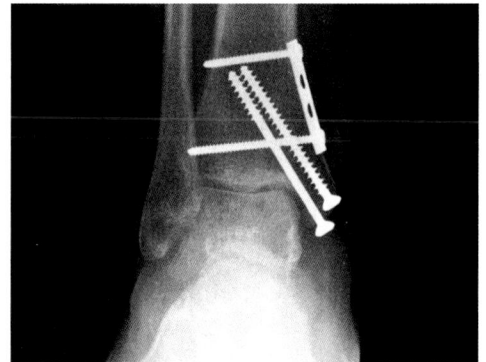
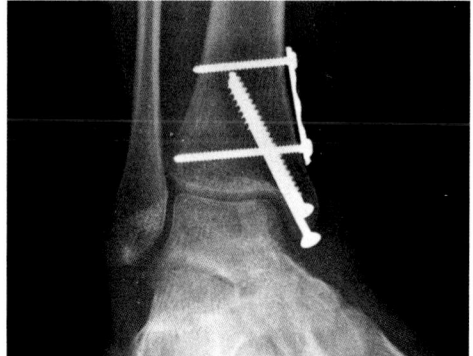
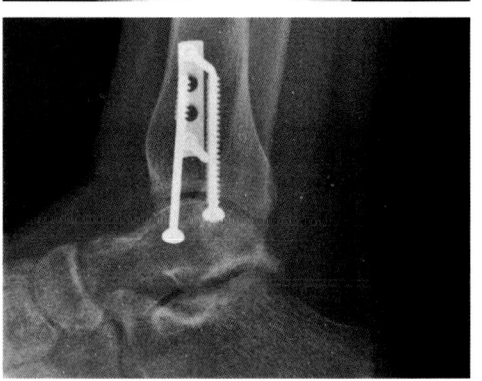

FIG 4 Postoperative radiographs. **A,B.** AP and mortise views showing anatomic reduction of medial malleolar osteotomy. **C.** Sagittal view.

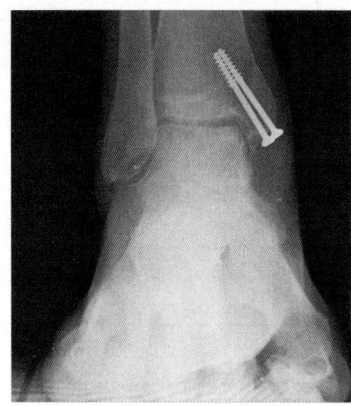

FIG. 5. Different patient undergoing osteochondral transfer. Knee cartilage is thicker than ankle cartilage; thus, despite having anatomic congruency of the graft and adjacent native cartilage, the graft may appear countersunk.

- Good to excellent results for OLTs associated with subchondral cysts
- Donor site morbidity was found to be minimal except in a single study, which found poor knee functional scores in 36%.
- No reported complications from malleolar osteotomy
- Results are not worse for osteochondral transfer performed as a secondary procedure after failed arthroscopic treatment compared to osteochondral transfer as a primary procedure. Additionally, there may be no benefit of osteochondral autograft transplantation over chondroplasty or microfracture in the management of primary lesions without subchondral cysts, as demonstrated in a recent randomized prospective trial comparing the three procedures.

COMPLICATIONS

- Infection
- Wound complication
- Failure of graft incorporation
- Graft failure and potential risk of developing degenerative change
- Articular cartilage delamination or fissuring of the graft

- Malleolar osteotomy nonunion
- Persistent pain despite radiographic suggestion of graft incorporation
- Disease transmission with allograft, but with the current screening practices of tissue banks, this risk is negligible
- Donor site morbidity at the knee

SUGGESTED READINGS

Al-Shaikh RA, Chou LB, Mann JA, et al. Autologous osteochondral grafting for talar cartilage defects. Foot Ankle Int 2002;23:381–389.
Baltzer AW, Arnold JP. Bone-cartilage transplantation from the ipsilateral knee for chondral lesions of the talus. Arthroscopy 2005;21:159–166.
Easley ME, Scranton PE Jr. Osteochondral autologous transfer system. Foot Ankle Clin 2003;8:275–290.
Garras DN, Santangelo JA, Wang DW, et al. A quantitative comparison of surgical approaches for posterolateral osteochondral lesions of the talus. Foot Ankle Int 2008;29:415–420.
Gobbi A, Francisco RA, Lubowitz JH, et al. Osteochondral lesions of the talus: randomized controlled trial comparing chondroplasty, microfracture, and osteochondral autograft transplantation. [Erratum appears in Arthroscopy 2008;24(2):A16]. Arthroscopy 2006;22(1):1085–1092.
Hangody L, Fules P. Autologous osteochondral mosaicplasty for the treatment of full-thickness defects of weight-bearing joints: ten years of experimental and clinical experience. J Bone Joint Surg Am 2003;85A(suppl 2):25–32.
Hangody L, Kish G, Modis L, et al. Mosaicplasty for the treatment of osteochondritis dissecans of the talus: two to seven year results in 36 patients. Foot Ankle Int 2001;22:552–558.
Imhoff AB, Paul J, Ottinger B, et al. Osteochondral transplantation of the talus: long-term clinical and magnetic resonance imaging evaluation. Am J Sports Med 2011;39(7):1487–1493.
Orr JD, Heida KA. Osteochondral autograft transfer system procedure for posterior osteochondral lesions of the talus through prone midline Achilles tendon-splitting approach. J Surg Orthop Adv 2017;26(1):58–64.
Sammarco GJ, Makwana NK. Treatment of talar osteochondral lesions using local osteochondral graft. Foot Ankle Int 2002;23:693–698.
Scranton PE Jr, Frey CC, Feder KS. Outcome of osteochondral autograft transplantation for type-V cystic osteochondral lesions of the talus. J Bone Joint Surg Br 2006;88:614–619.
Tochigi Y, Amendola A, Muir D, et al. Surgical approach for centrolateral talar osteochondral lesions with an anterolateral osteotomy. Foot Ankle Int 2002;23:1038–1039.

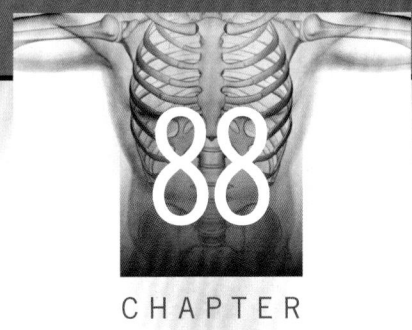

88

CHAPTER

Anterior Tibial Osteotomy for Osteochondral Lesions of the Talus

G. James Sammarco and V. James Sammarco

DEFINITION

- Osteochondral lesion of the talus (OLT) may cause significant pain and mechanical symptoms in the involved ankle.
- The talar articular surface is enclosed within the osseous structures of the ankle mortise.
- Sammarco and Makwana[3] described treatment of OLT through a "trap door" osteotomy with an autogenous talar autograft obtained from a non–weight-bearing portion of the talus.
- Surgical reconstruction of OLT may require osteotomy of the tibia or fibula for adequate exposure. Traditionally, osteotomy of the malleoli (medial and lateral) has been described in order to obtain access for cartilage grafting of these lesions. Malleolar osteotomies are unstable and typically require an extended period of non–weight bearing for adequate osseous healing. Nonunion of malleolar osteotomies may occur and may require further surgery.
- The anterior trap door osteotomy was developed as a stable alternative to malleolar osteotomies. This osteotomy is intrinsically stable and can be fixed with absorbable pins, facilitating postoperative imaging.

INDICATIONS

- The anterior trap door osteotomy is indicated for exposure during surgical treatment of OLT. Typically, this type of exposure is necessary for cartilage grafting procedures such as osteochondral allograft or autograft reconstruction of a defect.
- The osteotomy can be used for lesion of the anterior two-thirds of the talar dome. The osteotomy can be placed medially, centrally, or laterally, depending on the location of the talus which requires exposure.

SURGICAL MANAGEMENT

Patient Positioning

- The patient is positioned supine under appropriate anesthesia, with thigh tourniquet control. The patient is placed on a bean-bag patient positioner to facilitate positioning of the extremity. The patient can be rolled laterally toward the operative extremity to facilitate exposure of medial lesions or alternately can be rolled medially for central and lateral lesions. The leg, ankle, and foot are prepared and draped from below the knee distally.

Approach

- For a medial lesion, a 7-cm anteromedial longitudinal incision is made over the ankle joint parallel to the medial talar facet. Dissection is carried medial to the tibialis anterior tendon, taking care to identify and protect the saphenous vein and nerve.[3]
- Central lesions use a midline incision centered over the ankle mortise. The superficial peroneal nerve is identified in the subcutaneous tissue over the anterior ankle and the extensor retinaculum is divided. The interval between the tibialis anterior and extensor hallucis longus (EHL) tendons is used, identifying the deep peroneal nerve and anterior tibial artery, which must be protected and retracted laterally with the EHL tendon.[2]
- An anterolateral osteotomy can be used for OLT in the lateral talar dome.[1] An incision is made centered over the tibiofibular joint and dissection carried out through the extensor retinaculum. The superficial peroneal nerve will be directly in the field and must be identified and protected. Dissection over the anterior tibia is done, and the anteroinferior tibiofibular ligament must be incised in its midportion to remove the tibial trapdoor fragment. This should be sutured for repair during closure.
  - The soft tissue is dissected to the ankle joint and a capsulotomy performed.
  - Enough capsule is stripped from the tibia to expose the medial half of the joint.
  - A synovectomy is performed if needed.

TIBIAL OSTEOTOMY USING THE TRAP DOOR

Opening the Tibial Trap Door

- Elevate the periosteum proximally along the distal tibial metaphysis to the upper limit of the wound.
  - Make a 1-cm mark on the medial tibial plafond beginning at the angle of Hardy (**TECH FIG 1A**).
  - Make a second mark 3 cm above the joint line.
- Predrill the fixation for the osteotomy prior to its completion. This helps decrease the likelihood of creating an articular step-off when the trap door is replaced. Drill two transverse parallel holes across the tibial metaphysis beneath the cortex where the tibial trap door is to be removed. Absorbable pins will be inserted into these predrilled holes when the trap door is replaced after the graft has been inserted in the talar dome.
- Make two vertical parallel saw cuts with a micro-oscillating saw using a 10 × 20 mm long blade. The osteotomy needs to be of adequate depth that vertical exposure of the lesion can be achieved drilling of the defect and placement of the graft. A depth of 2 cm at the joint surface is usually adequate (**TECH FIG 1B**).
  - Taper these cuts proximally and upward to the anterior tibial metaphysis 3 cm above the joint.
  - To protect the talar articular surface, insert a Freer elevator between the tibia and talus.

- Make a third horizontal saw cut connecting the sagittal cuts at their upper limit.
  - Angle the saw inferiorly and 22 degrees posteriorly from the anterior metaphysis toward the joint surface.
- Use a thin, sharp 10-mm osteotome or chisel to mobilize the trap door. Remove the trap door and place it aside (**TECH FIG 1C**).

Coring Out the Lesion

- Plantarflex the ankle to deliver the osteochondral lesion into view (**TECH FIG 2**).
- Probe the lesion to determine its exact location.
- Select the appropriate-size coring instrument: 6, 8, or 10 mm.
- Place the coring instrument at right angles to the talar dome and extract the lesion.
- Save the osteochondral plug by placing it in a normal saline–soaked sponge to backfill the donor site.

Harvesting and Inserting the Graft

- Expose the medial facet of the talar body using a mini-Hohmann retractor with the ankle in plantarflexion.
- Position the harvesting instrument on the medial facet 4 mm beneath the talar dome.

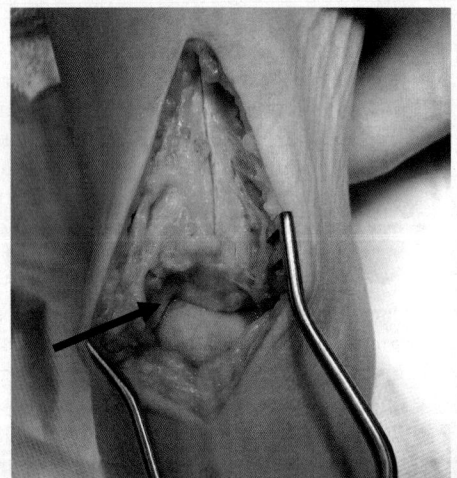

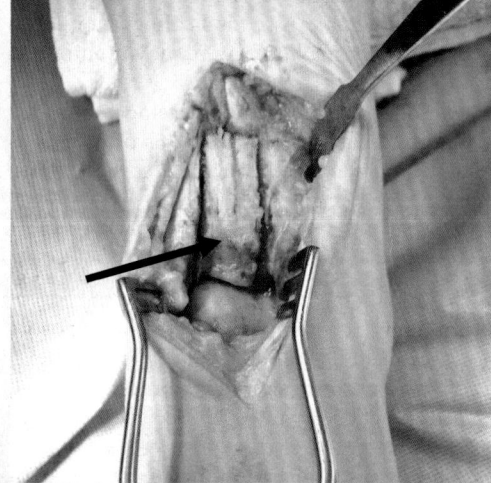

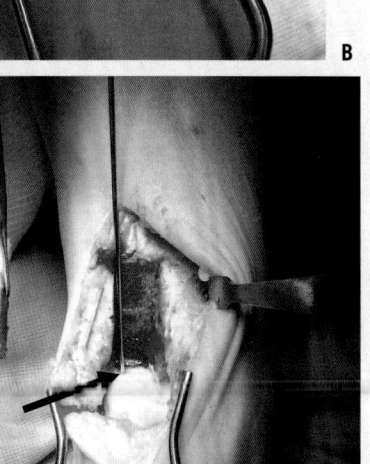

TECH FIG 1 A. A 7-cm anteromedial incision exposing the medial half of the ankle joint, showing the angle of Hardy (*arrow*) **B.** Saw cuts are made 1 cm wide, 3 cm high, and 2 cm deep (not seen), creating a trap door (*arrow*). **C.** The trap door is removed and set aside to be replaced after the graft is inserted. A probe has been inserted into the lesion (*arrow*).

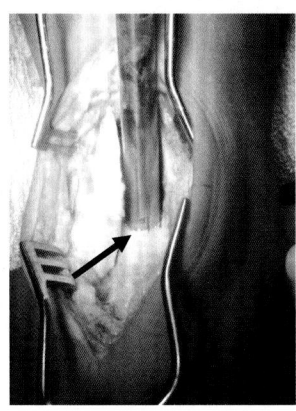

TECH FIG 2 The ankle is plantarflexed to expose the lesion, and a premeasured 8-mm coring device is used to remove the lesion (*arrow*).

- Harvest the graft in such a way that when inserted into the recipient site, the slightly elevated inferior margin of the graft from the medial facet will be oriented toward the medial border of the talar dome, approximating the shape of the normal talar weight-bearing surface (**TECH FIG 3A**).

- Débride the talar recipient site and tap the osteochondral graft into place with the inferior medial facet portion oriented toward the medial border of the talus (**TECH FIG 3B**).

Completion

- The donor site can be backfilled with the plug obtained from the weight bearing articular surface including the deficient chondral lesion. Minimal axial loading occurs in this facet with weight bearing, which makes area more tolerant to chondromalacia.
- The donor site can be augmented with cancellous bone taken from the distal tibia or demineralized allograft bone if needed.
- Insert the tibial bone block back into its bed and insert bioabsorbable pins (Orthosorb [Biomet, Warsaw, IN]) into the predrilled holes to secure the bone block in place (**TECH FIG 4**).
- The extensor retinaculum must be repaired meticulously to prevent bowstringing of the tendons. Approximate the deep tissues with 3-0 absorbable suture and close the skin with 3-0 monofilament nylon.
- Apply a compression dressing and posterior splint.

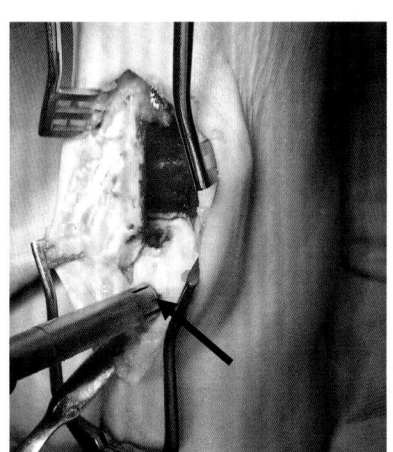

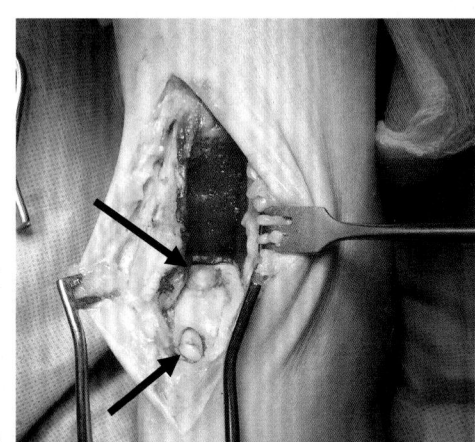

TECH FIG 3 A. The osteochondral graft is harvested from the anterior portion of the medial facet 4 mm below the articular surface of the talar dome and at least 10 mm away from the recipient site (*arrow*). **B.** The osteochondral graft has been inserted into the recipient site (*upper arrow*) and the bony material removed, including attached remaining cartilage from the defect that has been inserted into the donor site (*lower arrow*).

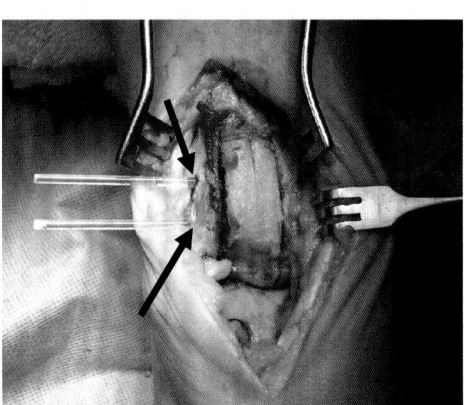

TECH FIG 4 The trap door is replaced and secured with bioabsorbable pins (*arrows*) placed into predrilled holes.

ADDITIONAL TECHNIQUE

- The lateral and central exposures are done in a similar manner to best expose the associated talar defect. The lateral osteotomy can use the incisura fibularis as a part of the exposure as an alternative to the lateral sagittal saw cut. In this instance, repair of the anterior–inferior tibiofibular ligament must be performed at the end of the procedure.

- The technique describes harvesting the donor osteochondral graft from a non–weight-bearing articular portion of the ipsilateral talar body. The trap door osteotomy is useful for treatment of osteochondral lesions where full open access is required for a weight-bearing articular surface lesion. Implantation of osteochondral grafts harvested from other sites or fresh osteochondral allografts can be implanted with this technique if indicated.

TECHNIQUES

Pearls and Pitfalls

- This technique avoids the need for a medial malleolar osteotomy. It provides excellent visualization of and access to the lesion through a single incision. Harvesting the donor graft from the ankle avoids creating an articular defect in an asymptomatic knee.
- The procedure is best suited for lesions up to 10 mm in diameter and up to 10 mm deep located in the anterior two-thirds of the medial or lateral talar dome margins.
- The graft can be harvested from the medial or lateral facet of the talus because these surfaces bear minimal weight. No complications have been noted in the medial or lateral gutters due to donor site morbidity.
- Saw kerf can cause articular step-off of the osteotomy if the trap door is compressed in place when the tibial osteotomy fragment is replaced. Predrilling the transverse fixation pins avoids this. If gapping occurs at the trapdoor osteotomy site, this can be backfilled with an injectable demineralized bone graft.
- The surgeon should avoid making the vertical saw cuts more than 3 cm deep at the joint surface or 4 cm in height because this increases the risk of a medial malleolar stress fracture.
- In harvesting the osteochondral graft, the surgeon should avoid taking the graft too near the talar surface or too near the recipient site in order to avoid a stress fracture of the talar dome.
- The most common complaint is pain at the anteromedial joint line with activity which can persist up to a year following the procedure.

POSTOPERATIVE CARE

- The compression dressing and posterior splint are changed at the first follow-up visit within the first week following surgery.
- Sutures are removed at 2 weeks, and a non–weight-bearing short-leg cast is used for 1 month.
- A range-of-motion boot is then prescribed allowing 50% weight bearing for 2 weeks with active and passive range of motion initiated.
- After 6 weeks, full weight bearing is allowed in the boot walker, and the boot is discontinued after 8 weeks.

REFERENCES

1. Garras DN, Santangelo JA, Wang DW, et al. A quantitative comparison of surgical approaches for posterolateral osteochondral lesions of the talus. Foot Ankle Int 2008;29(4):415–420.
2. Kreuz PC, Lahm A, Haag M, et al. Tibial wedge osteotomy for osteochondral transplantation in talar lesions. Int J Sports Med 2008;29(7):584–589.
3. Sammarco GJ, Makwana NK. Treatment of talar osteochondral lesions using local osteochondral graft. Foot Ankle Int 2002;23(8):693–698.

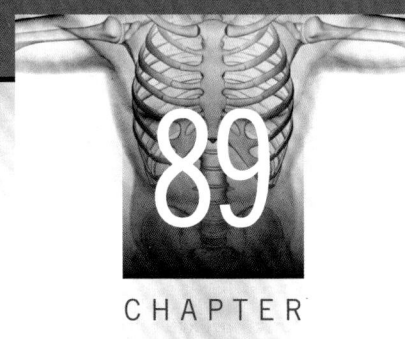

89
CHAPTER

Osteochondral Lesions of the Talus:
Structural Allograft

Samuel B. Adams, James A. Nunley II, and Mark E. Easley

DEFINITION

- Large osteochondral defects of the talar dome, typically involving the talar shoulder (transition of superior dome cartilage to the medial or lateral talar cartilage) and also often associated with large-volume subchondral cysts

ANATOMY

- Sixty percent of the talus's surface area is covered by articular cartilage.
- The talus is contained within the ankle mortise.
  - Superior talar dome articulates with the tibial plafond.
  - Medial dome articulates with the medial malleolus.
  - Lateral dome articulates with the lateral malleolus.
- Talar blood supply
  - Posterior tibial artery
    - Artery of the tarsal canal
    - Deltoid ligament branch
- Peroneal artery
  - Artery of the tarsal sinus
- Dorsalis pedis artery

PATHOGENESIS

- The pathogenesis for osteochondral lesions of the talus (OLTs) is not fully understood.
- Theories include the following:
  - Trauma
  - Idiopathic focal avascular necrosis

NATURAL HISTORY

- In general, OLTs do not progress to diffuse ankle arthritis.
- However, large-volume OLTs may lead to subchondral collapse of a substantial portion of the talus and thus create deformity, higher contact stresses, and a greater concern for eventual ankle arthritis if left untreated.

PATIENT HISTORY AND PHYSICAL FINDINGS

- Patients may or may not report a history of trauma.
- Ankle pain, typically on the anterior aspect of the ankle, is a common complaint.
  - Pain is usually experienced on the side of the ankle that corresponds with the OLT, but it may be poorly localized to the site of the OLT. In fact, sometimes, medial OLTs produce lateral ankle pain and vice versa.
  - Pain is rarely sharp, unless a fragment of the OLT should act as an impinging loose body in the joint.

- It is typically a deep ache, with and after activity, and is usually relieved with rest.
- Antalgic gait
- May be associated with malalignment or ankle instability
- Typically, tenderness on side of ankle that corresponds with OLT, but not always
- Rarely, crepitance or mechanical symptoms
- With chronic OLT, some degree of ankle stiffness is anticipated.

IMAGING AND OTHER DIAGNOSTIC STUDIES

- Plain radiographs
  - Small OLTs may be missed.
  - Large OLTs are usually identified on plain radiographs, three views of the ankle, weight bearing.
  - Radiographs are often limited in characterizing OLTs because the two-dimensional study cannot define the three-dimensional OLT.
  - Particularly useful in assessing lower leg, ankle, or foot malalignment, which needs to be considered in the management of OLTs
  - May detect incidental OLTs (Patient has radiograph for a different problem, and an OLT is incidentally identified on plain radiographs.)
- Magnetic resonance imaging
  - Excellent screening tool when OLT or other foot–ankle pathology is suspected
  - Will identify incidental OLT but defines other potential soft tissue pathology
  - Demonstrates associated marrow edema that may lead to overestimation of the OLT's size
- Computed tomography (CT)
  - Ideal for characterizing OLTs, particularly large-volume defects
  - Defines OLT size without distraction of associated marrow edema
  - Defines the character of the OLT and extent of its involvement in the talar dome
- Diagnostic injection
  - Intra-articular
  - An anesthetic versus anesthetic plus corticosteroid
  - May have some therapeutic effect, even for several months
  - If the source of pain is the OLT, then intra-articular injection should relieve symptoms from OLT (and any intra-articular pathology). If the pain is not relieved, then extra-articular diagnoses should be considered.

DIFFERENTIAL DIAGNOSIS

- Loose body in ankle joint
- Ankle impingement (anterior or posterior)
- Chronic ankle instability (lateral or syndesmosis)
- Ankle synovitis or adjacent tendinopathy
- Early ankle degenerative change

NONOPERATIVE MANAGEMENT

- Activity modification
- Bracing
- Physical therapy if associated ankle instability
- Nonsteroidal anti-inflammatories or COX-2 inhibitors
- Corticosteroid injection
- Viscosupplementation

SURGICAL MANAGEMENT

Preoperative Planning

- Indications for this surgery include the following:
  - Large-volume OLTs not amenable to other joint-sparing procedures
  - Failed arthroscopic surgery (débridement and microfracture)
  - Failed open procedures (cylindrical osteochondral transfer)
- Large-volume OLTs typically are not amenable to autologous osteochondral transfer (talus or knee).
- We favor reconstruction of the large talar defect with an allograft talus. Although we prefer fresh allograft tissue, we have on occasion used fresh frozen tissue.
- Scheduling of this procedure with fresh allograft tissue is similar to organ transplantation but with a wider window for implantation after procurement.
  - Multiple tissue banks have the ability to obtain fresh allograft tali.
  - Once a donor talus is identified, the tissue bank performs appropriate screening.
  - If the talus is deemed safe for implantation and represents a match based on radiographic size, on average 14 to 21 days of reasonable chondrocyte viability remain for the talar allograft to be used.
- Although fresh structural talar allograft reconstruction for large-volume OLTs has gained a foothold as an accepted treatment among reconstructive foot and ankle surgeons, not all third-party payers cover this procedure. We do not seek an allograft talus for our patients from the tissue banks until our patient has secured insurance coverage for the procedure.
- In seeking an allograft talus that is suited for the patient, the surgeon must:
  - Be sure that the talus is the correct side (right or left).
  - Provide the tissue bank with the optimal size of talar graft. Tissue banks use different methods for talar sizing.
    - Plain radiographic dimensions (If the defect in the diseased talus is particularly large, making measurements difficult, radiographs of the healthy, contralateral talus may be needed.)
    - CT scan measurements (may be more accurate, with measurements possible in three dimensions)

- The surgeon should check for associated pathology that may need to be addressed at the time of allograft talar reconstruction:
  - Osteophyte removal
  - Ligament reconstruction
  - Corrective osteotomies
    - Calcaneal
    - Supramalleolar
- The surgeon determines the optimal surgical approach.
  - In our hands, this depends on the amount of talus that will be reconstructed.
  - A portion of the medial talar dome (usually posteromedial) typically warrants a medial malleolar osteotomy.
  - A portion of the lateral talar dome (often centrolateral) typically necessitates ligament releases (anterior talofibular and calcaneofibular) with or without lateral malleolar osteotomy.
  - Involvement of the majority of the medial or lateral talar dome, particularly if involving its respective talar shoulder, usually can be performed through an anterior approach without osteotomy by replacing one-third to one-half of the talar dome.
- Patient education
  - This is a complex procedure.
  - The patient must understand that the intent is to implant allograft tissue.
  - There is a negligible, but real, risk of disease transmission and possible graft rejection by the host.
  - There is no guarantee that the procedure will work, and a revision procedure may be required, such as arthrodesis, which will eliminate joint motion.

Positioning

- Before anesthesia and moving the patient into the operating room, the surgeon should inspect the allograft to be sure it is the correct side (right or left) and for cartilage defects that may be present directly at the site that the graft is to be harvested.
- The patient is positioned supine.
- For a lateral OLT, a bolster under the ipsilateral hip typically affords better access to the lateral talar dome.
- We routinely use a thigh tourniquet.

Approach

- As noted earlier, the approach depends on the size and location of the OLT.
- For medial OLTs amenable to reconstruction of only a portion of the medial talar dome: direct medial approach, similar to that for open reduction and internal fixation (ORIF) of a medial malleolar fracture, with a medial malleolar osteotomy
- For lateral OLTs amenable to reconstruction of only a portion of the lateral talar dome: lateral approach, combining typical approaches for ORIF of a fibular fracture and the extensile exposure for a modified Brostrom procedure
- For large-medial or lateral OLTs, involving the majority of the medial or lateral talar shoulder: anterior approach, similar to that for ankle arthrodesis or total ankle arthroplasty; typically, no malleolar osteotomy is required.

STRUCTURAL ALLOGRAFT RECONSTRUCTION OF CONTAINED MEDIAL OSTEOCHONDRAL LESIONS OF THE TALUS

Approach and Oblique Medial Malleolar Osteotomy

- Make a curvilinear incision over the medial malleolus, similar to that for ORIF of a medial malleolar fracture.
- Protect the saphenous vein and accompanying saphenous nerves.
- Anterior ankle arthrotomy (**TECH FIG 1A**)
  - Defines anterior joint margin for safe performance of medial malleolar osteotomy
  - Allows partial visualization of the OLT and allows confirmation that there is no diffuse articular cartilage degeneration
- Open the posterior tibial tendon sheath–flexor retinaculum, directly on the posterior margin of the tibia and medial malleolus (**TECH FIG 1B**). Protect the posterior tibial tendon: It rests in a groove immediately posterior to the tibia and is at great risk with a medial malleolar osteotomy.

- Predrill the medial malleolus across the proposed osteotomy site (**TECH FIG 1C**).
  - We routinely use two small fragment malleolar screws and predrill with the corresponding drill.
  - Obtain fluoroscopic confirmation that the drill bits are in the proper trajectory.
  - Consider passing a tap as well.
- Place a Kirschner wire obliquely to define the trajectory of the medial malleolar osteotomy (see **TECH FIG 1C**).
  - Place it slightly proximal to the desired osteotomy, so it can function as a guide but not interfere with the saw (**TECH FIG 1D**).
  - Confirm the optimal Kirschner wire trajectory with intraoperative fluoroscopy.
  - Ideally, the Kirschner wire will extend to the lateral margin of the OLT but with large-volume OLTs that may be too much

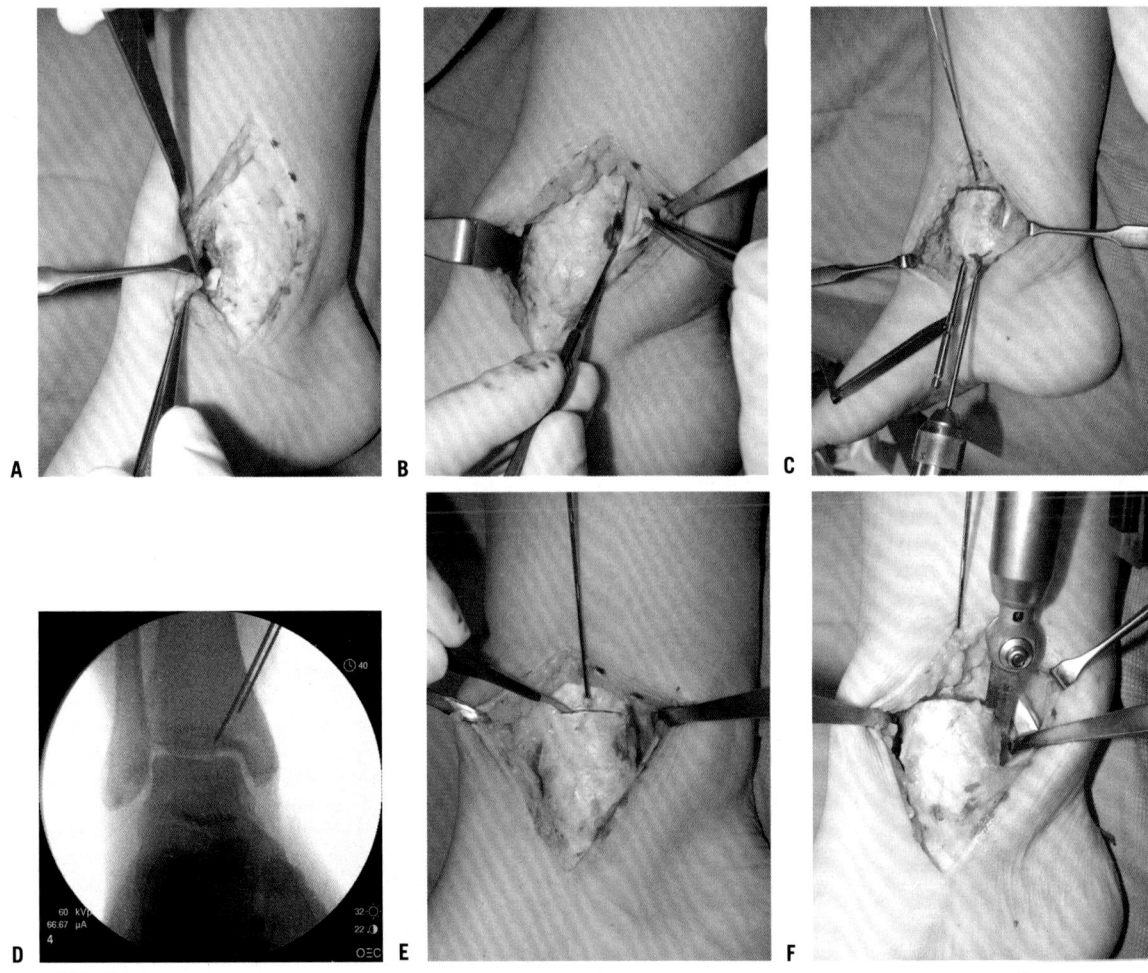

TECH FIG 1 A. Medial incision and anterior ankle arthrotomy. **B.** Opening of the posterior tibial tendon sheath. **C.** Predrilling of medial malleolus. Kirschner wire for trajectory of medial malleolar osteotomy has already been inserted and its position confirmed with fluoroscopy. **D.** Fluoroscopic image demonstrating Kirschner wire being used as a guide to direct the saw. **E.** The periosteum is scored perpendicular to the tibial shaft, at the level of the osteotomy. *(continued)*

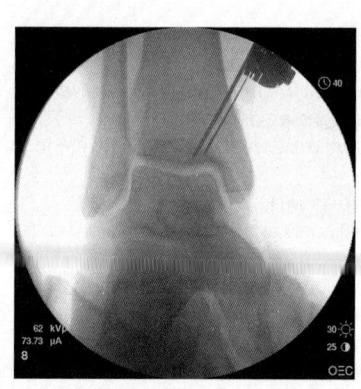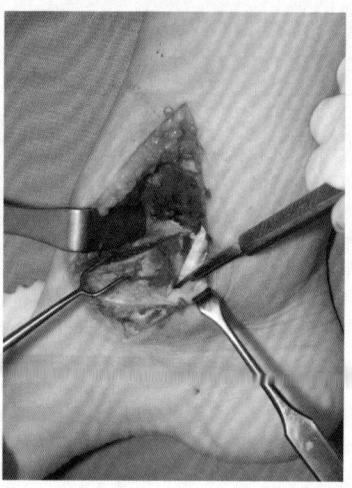

TECH FIG 1 *(continued)* **F.** Medial malleolar osteotomy. Care must be taken to protect the posterior tibial tendon. **G.** Fluoroscopic image showing near-complete bone cut. **H.** Release of posterior tibial tendon sheath from distal medial malleolus to allow mobilization.

and unnecessary. However, in our experience, making the osteotomy only to the axilla of the tibial plafond where it meets the medial malleolus will not allow adequate access to perform ideal recipient site preparation.

- Determine a plane for the osteotomy in the anteroposterior (AP) plane that is perpendicular to the longitudinal axis of the tibia. We find it helpful to score the osteotomy in the periosteum from anterior to posterior to determine this level **(TECH FIG 1E)**.
- Periosteal stripping is unnecessary; it may be limited to the osteotomy site.
- With a microsagittal saw oriented correctly in both planes, the osteotomy is initiated **(TECH FIG 1F)**.
  - Use cool saline to limit the risk of heat necrosis to the bone.
  - Obtain intraoperative fluoroscopy shortly after initiating the osteotomy; leave the saw blade in place to confirm proper trajectory. If incorrect, a subtle adjustment is still possible **(TECH FIG 1G)**.
- Continue the osteotomy with the saw to the subchondral bone and then complete the osteotomy with a chisel.
  - A fluoroscopic spot view allows the surgeon to confirm that the osteotomy is appropriate and is not violating the talar cartilage.
  - There may be some irregularity to the osteotomy at the posterior margin; this is typical as the osteotomy is mobilized. It may

be advantageous, as it allows for an interference fit during reduction of the osteotomy and perhaps greater stability.
- Reflect the medial malleolus.
  - The posterior tibial tendon sheath must be released to the distal aspect of the posterior medial malleolus to allow the malleolus to reflect adequately and to gain optimal exposure of the medial talar dome **(TECH FIG 1H)**. Protect the deltoid ligament fibers.

Preparing the Recipient Site

- Define the extent of the OLT **(TECH FIG 2A,B)**.
  - Clinical inspection
  - Review of CT scan
- If the talar defect appears amenable to structural allograft reconstruction, have the donor talus placed on the back table and protected in a saline-soaked sponge.
- Excise the diseased portion of the talus **(TECH FIG 2C–F)**.
  - Reciprocating and microsagittal saw (Use cool saline to limit risk of heat necrosis.)
  - May need a small curette and rasp as well
- Define the dimensions of the recipient site. Use a caliper and a ruler and double-check the measurements.

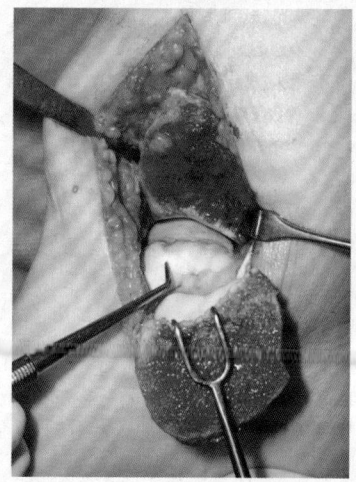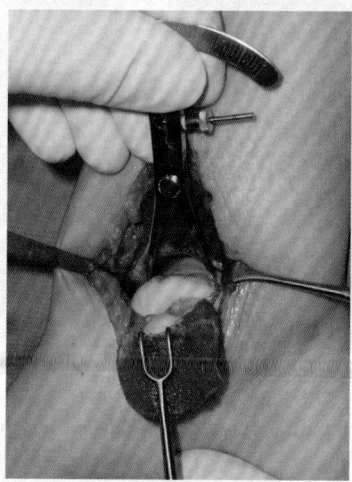

TECH FIG 2 A,B. Identifying the extent of the talar shoulder lesion. *(continued)*

TECHNIQUES

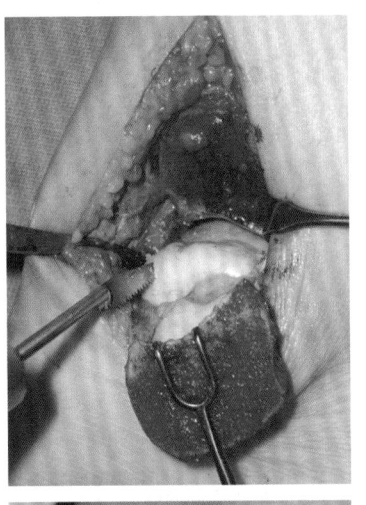
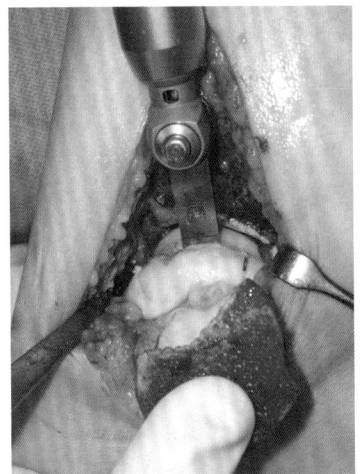
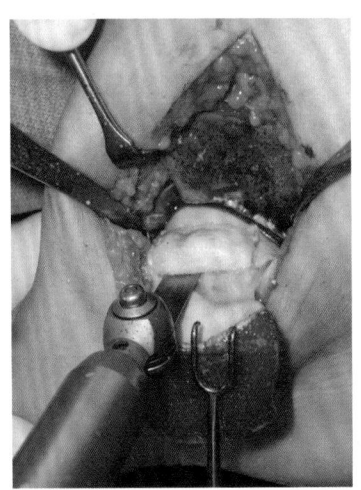

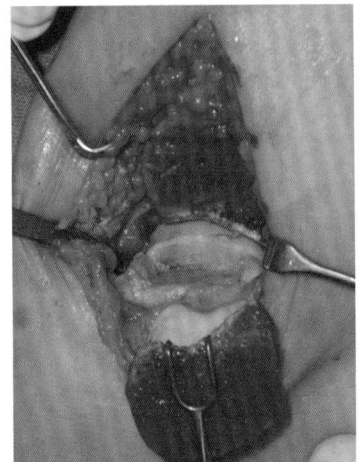

TECH FIG 2 *(continued)* **C–E.** Excision of the talar shoulder lesion using the microsagittal and oscillating saws. **F.** Talar shoulder lesion removed.

Harvesting Graft from Donor Talus

- Handle the allograft talus with bone forceps.
- Properly orient the talus (compare to native talus) to ensure that the cuts will be congruent and in the same plane as those for the recipient site.
- Carefully mark the dimensions for graft harvest on the allograft (**TECH FIG 3A**).
  - Same location on the allograft talus as the recipient site on the native talus

- If you err, err to have the graft slightly too large. Be sure to account for saw blade thickness.
- "Measure twice and cut once."
  - You have only one opportunity, so be sure the measurements and orientation of the saw blade for each cut are optimal.
- The allograft can be stabilized with two large pointed reduction clamps (**TECH FIG 3B**).

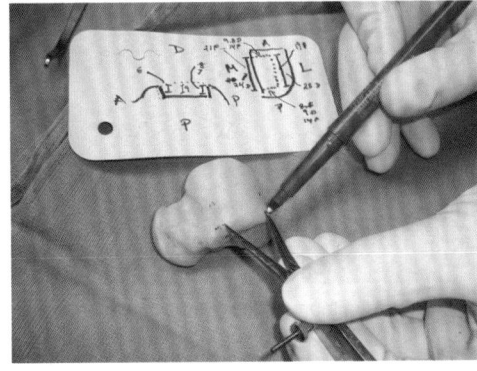
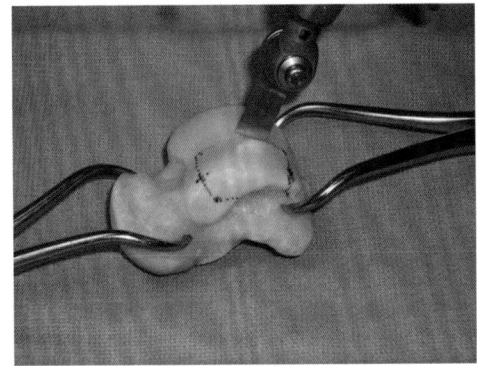

TECH FIG 3 A. The dimensions of the recipient site are carefully recorded and transferred to the allograft. **B.** Two pointed reduction clamps are used to stabilize the allograft during preparation. *(continued)*

TECHNIQUES

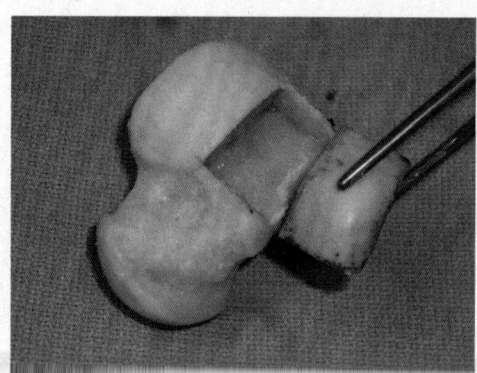

TECH FIG 3 *(continued)* **C.** Donor allograft with newly prepared graft removed.

- Extract the graft from the donor talus (**TECH FIG 3C**).
- Reduce the immunogenic load from the graft by washing the graft's cancellous surfaces with saline.

Implanting and Securing the Graft into the Recipient Site

- Only once have we had a graft match perfectly on the first attempt. The graft and recipient site will almost always need to be tailored slightly to allow optimal graft fit.
- It is unlikely that a perfect clinical and fluoroscopic match will be achieved. Attempt to achieve the best clinical match of the graft's articular surface with the surrounding native cartilage (**TECH FIG 4A**).
- If the clinical match is appropriate, then the fluoroscopic match is not important.
  - There is a lot of variability in cartilage thickness and talar architecture in the human talus.
  - It is difficult to get four surfaces to congruently match.
- Graft fixation
  - Ideally, the graft will have some interference fit.
  - We routinely secure the graft with one or two small-diameter solid screws (1.5 or 2.0 mm in diameter). One is typically

placed from dorsal to plantar and the other from medial to lateral (if the depth of the graft will allow) (**TECH FIG 4B,C**).
- Place the screws in lag fashion.
- Countersink the screw heads below the articular surface (**TECH FIG 4D,E**).
- Using fluoroscopy, confirm that the graft and hardware are in optimal position (**TECH FIG 4F–H**).
  - The graft will not look perfect fluoroscopically, but as long as the clinical appearance is acceptable, the outcome has a good chance to be favorable.
  - The hardware may appear slightly proud fluoroscopically despite being countersunk. The talar dome is not a flat plane, and therefore, the screw may seem to be protruding. Moreover, the articular cartilage is rather thick compared to such a low-profile screw head.

Medial Malleolar Osteotomy Reduction and Closure

- Irrigate the joint.
- Reduce the medial malleolus. Confirm the reduction through the anteromedial arthrotomy and posteriorly behind the posterior tibial tendon.
- Place the two screws in the predrilled holes and tighten the screws.
- Although not essential for healing, we favor placing an antiglide plate over the proximal aspect of the osteotomy.
- Using fluoroscopy, confirm reduction of the graft and medial malleolus (see **TECH FIG 4**).
  - Anticipate some incongruencies of the graft–native talus bony interfaces. It is difficult to achieve perfectly congruent apposition.
  - There will be a slight gap at the medial malleolar osteotomy site despite anatomic reduction of the medial malleolus. This is due to the thickness of the saw blade. However, it is not acceptable to see a step-off at the osteotomy site where it enters the tibial plafond; this must be anatomic.
  - The slight gaps at the graft and medial malleolus do not typically impair healing and should obliterate with eventual remodeling.

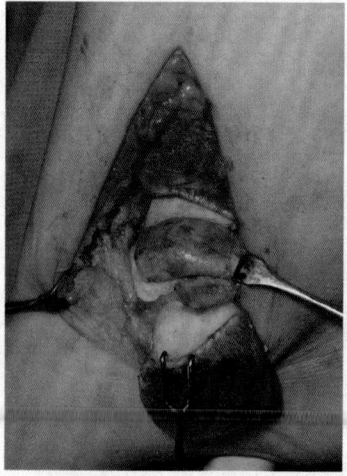
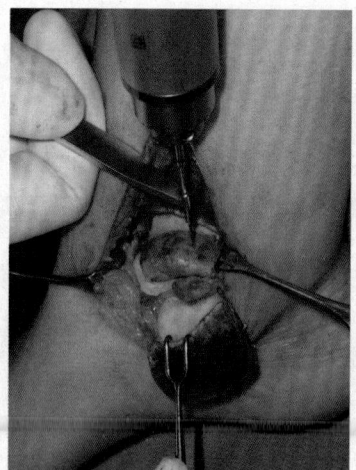
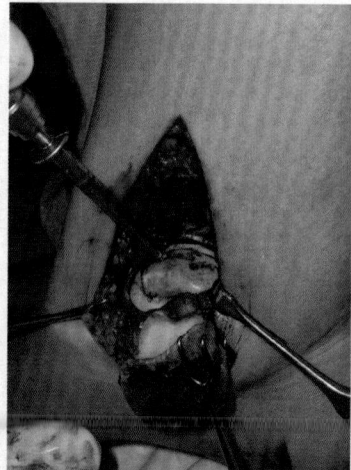

TECH FIG 4 A–C. Fitting and securing the graft to the native talus. **A.** After contouring the graft (some minor discoloration from debris while manipulating graft on back table; it is easily washed away). **B.** Drill hole perpendicular to graft. **C.** Securing graft with two countersunk screws. *(continued)*

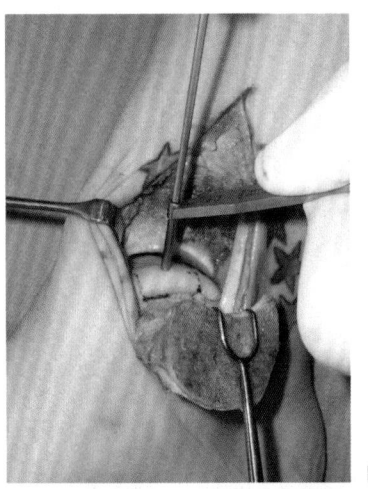
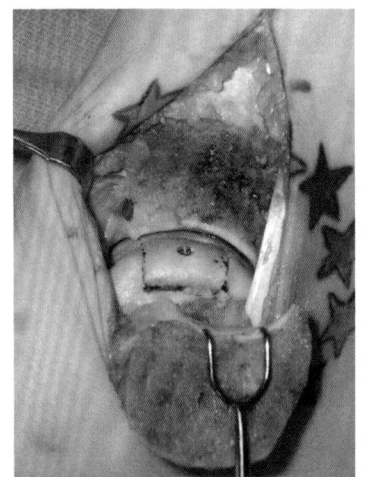
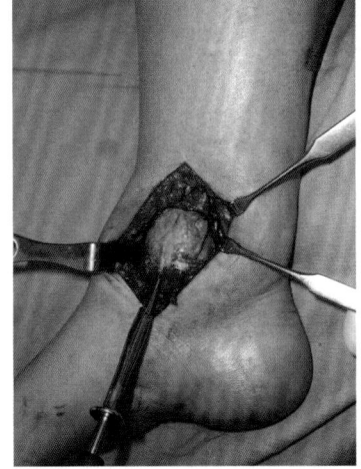
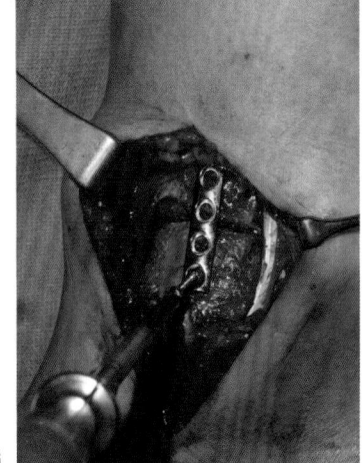
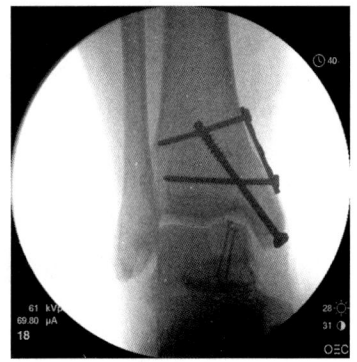

TECH FIG 4 *(continued)* **D,E.** A different patient with similar graft, excellent interference fit, and secured with a single screw. **D.** Screw is inserted in lag fashion. **E.** Screw head is countersunk. **F–H.** Reduction of the medial malleolar osteotomy. **F.** Screw fixation through the predrilled holes. **G.** Antiglide plate. **H.** Final fluoroscopic evaluation of graft and reduction of medial malleolar osteotomy. Despite optimal clinical fit of the graft, rarely does the fluoroscopic appearance suggest anatomic graft match to the native talus, typically due to differing cartilage thicknesses between the donor and the host. Although the screws may appear prominent, two-dimensional fluoroscopy is deceiving because the screws are countersunk below the articular surface of the graft, and the talar dome is curved.

- Closure
  - Posterior tibial tendon sheath and flexor retinaculum
  - Anterior arthrotomy
  - Subcutaneous layer

- Skin to a tensionless closure
- We routinely use a drain.
- Dressings, padding, and a posterior sugar-tong splint with the ankle in neutral position

HEMITALUS RECONSTRUCTION OF MEDIAL OSTEOCHONDRAL LESION OF THE TALUS

Preoperative Evaluation

- Patient is a 40-year-old man with chronic ankle pain failing prior arthroscopic débridement and microfracture, feels he is overloading lateral border of foot.

- Preoperative weight-bearing radiographs suggest large medial OLT and varus malalignment with some varus talar tilt **(TECH FIG 5A,B)**.
- CT demonstrates large-volume medial OLT **(TECH FIG 5C–E)**.

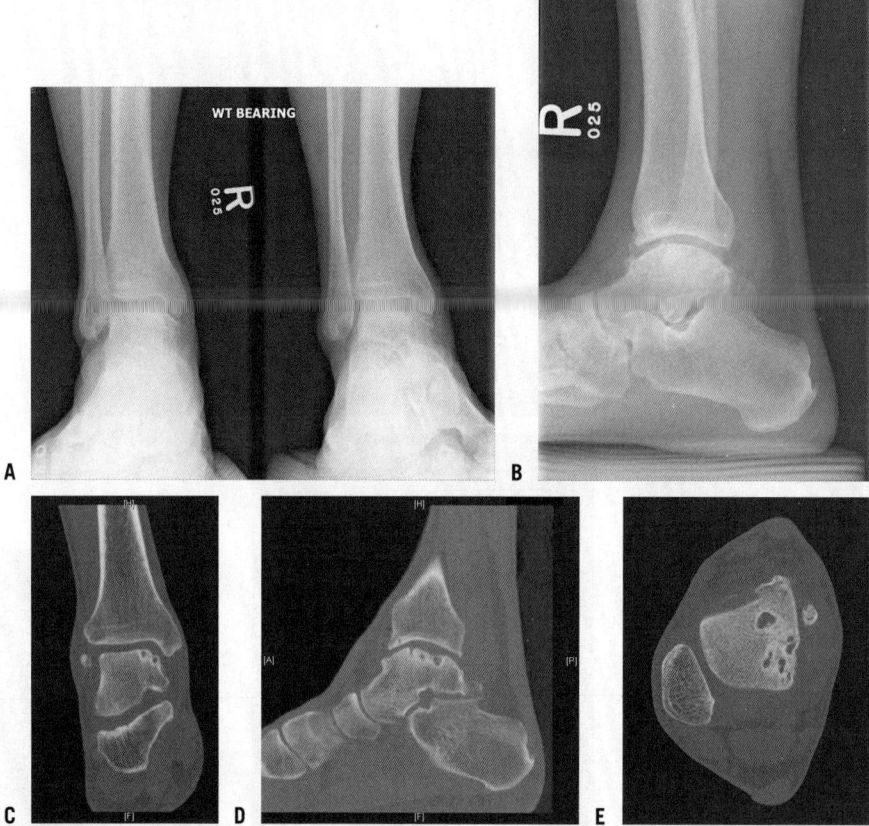

TECH FIG 5 A,B. Preoperative radiographs. **A.** AP and mortise ankle views suggest large medial talar dome OLT and varus alignment. **B.** Lateral radiograph. **C–E.** Preoperative CT of large-volume OLT. **C.** Coronal view. **D.** Sagittal view. **E.** Axial view.

- Before proceeding to the operating room, confirm that the allograft talus is the one intended for this patient, is available, and has not expired.

Approach

- Anterior approach (**TECH FIG 6**)
  - Similar to anterior approach for ankle arthrodesis and total ankle arthroplasty
  - Protect the superficial peroneal nerve.
  - Divide the extensor retinaculum over the extensor hallucis longus tendon.
  - Protect the deep neurovascular bundle.
  - Anterior capsulotomy, unlike ankle arthrodesis and total ankle arthroplasty, must protect ankle cartilage.
  - Expose OLT with plantarflexion. Assess mediolateral dimensions and attempt to assess AP dimensions.
- If the talus appears appropriate for an allograft talus, ask to have the donor talus opened and soaked in a warm saline-soaked sponge on the back table. At this point, though, this only expedites the procedure; it is not as though the talus may be returned.

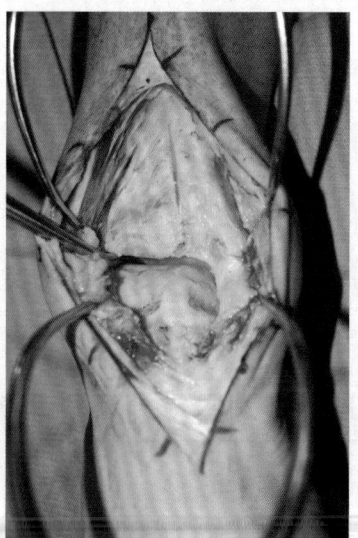

TECH FIG 6 Anterior approach, similar to that performed for total ankle arthroplasty. Because the entire medial one-third to one-half of the talar dome will be restructured, a medial malleolar osteotomy is typically not necessary.

Preparing the Recipient Site

- Joint distraction, preferably with an extra-articular distraction device
- Determine dimensions of diseased talus:
  - Clinical assessment
  - Review and correlate with CT.
- Determine exact lateral sagittal border of OLT.
- Make a vertical (sagittal) cut in the talus 1 mm lateral to the lateral extent of the OLT. The depth of this cut should be conservative until the exact superior to inferior dimensions of the OLT can be mapped out on the talus **(TECH FIG 7A)**.
- Horizontal (axial) resection in the talus **(TECH FIG 7B)**
  - To maintain the proper axis, we routinely use a Kirschner wire placed from anterior to posterior, with its trajectory and depth confirmed on intraoperative fluoroscopy, to avoid misdirection of the axial resection.

- We use a thin oscillating saw for this cut and also with cold saline irrigation to cool the blade in an attempt to avoid heat necrosis to the bone.
- Protect the medial malleolar cartilage. Consider using a malleable ribbon retractor in the medial gutter.
- Extract the resected bone **(TECH FIG 7C,D)**.
- Revisit the vertical and horizontal resections with the saw, a rasp, or both. If there is residual OLT in either or both of the prepared surfaces, then consider curetting these and bone grafting or resecting more native talus **(TECH FIG 7E)**.
- Fluoroscopic evaluation sometimes affords a useful appreciation of the recipient site.
- Determining the exact dimensions of the recipient site:
  - Calipers **(TECH FIG 7F)**
  - Ruler **(TECH FIG 7G)**
  - We routinely sketch the dimensions on a drawing of the recipient site on a surgical glove envelope or a sterile label on the back table.

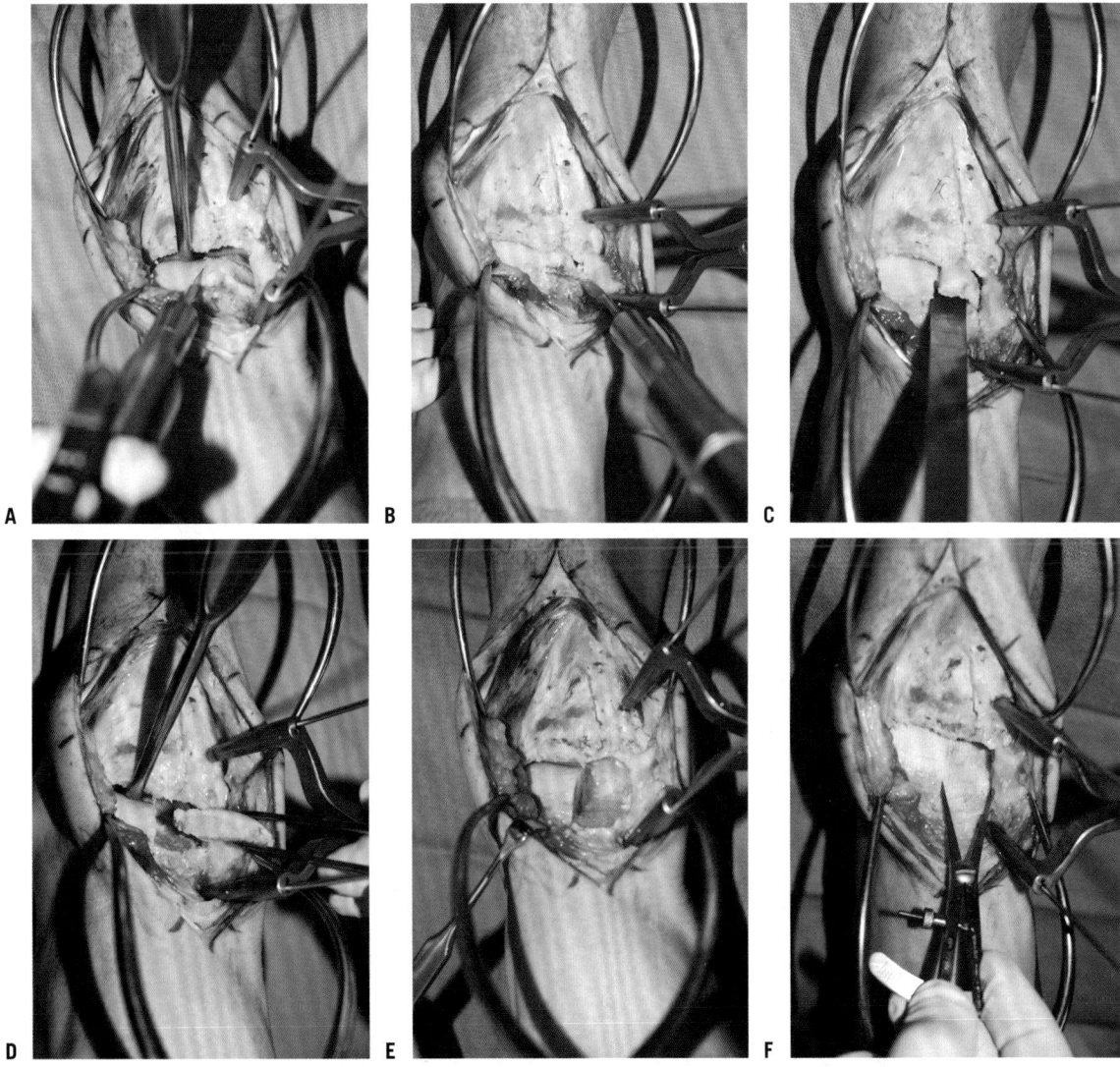

TECH FIG 7 A–D. Preparing the recipient site. **A.** Sagittal cut with reciprocating saw. **B.** Axial cut also with reciprocating saw. **C.** Elevating diseased portion of talus with osteotome. **D.** Extracting diseased portion. **E.** Further extraction of diseased cartilage until healthy-appearing cancellous surface is apparent. • **F,G.** Measuring dimensions of recipient site. **F.** Caliper. *(continued)*

TECHNIQUES

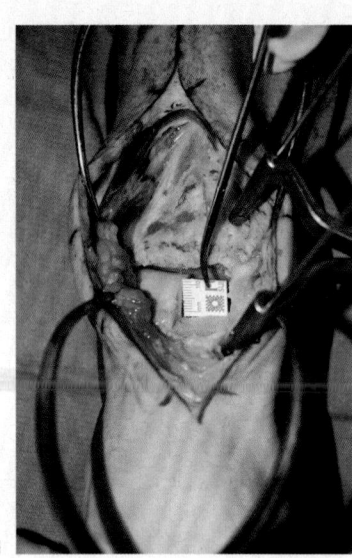

G

TECH FIG 7 *(continued)* **G.** Modified ruler.

Harvesting Graft from the Donor Talus

- Secure the allograft that has been placed on the back table with a bone-holding forceps.
- Mark the dimensions of the recipient site talus on the donor talus. One challenge is to orient the talus properly to ensure that the two cuts will be in the optimal planes to congruently match the recipient site.
- Double-check the measurements.
  - You have only one chance to harvest this graft.
  - Measure twice and cut once.
- Make the cuts to harvest the talus **(TECH FIG 8)**.
  - Attempt to match the recipient site dimensions exactly, taking into account the thickness of the saw blade.

- If you have to err, then err on the side of harvesting a graft that is too large. Fine-tuning the graft is sometimes difficult, but it is still possible to downsize it or increase the size of the recipient site; it is not possible to augment the graft or reduce the size of the recipient site once the graft has been harvested.
- We routinely wash the graft's cancellous surfaces with saline in an attempt to decrease the immunogenic load before implantation. However, we have no evidence to support this practice and perform this purely on an empiric basis.

Implanting and Securing Graft into Recipient Site

- Place the graft in the recipient site **(TECH FIG 9A,B)**.
- We have never had a perfect match on the first attempt at seating the graft in the recipient site.
- Tailoring the graft to match the recipient site is often challenging.
  - In our hands, this requires a slight deepening of the recipient site and a slight thinning of the graft.
  - Making the corresponding sagittal and axial talar cuts congruently is the most important step in achieving an optimal fit of the graft.
- Only once have we achieved a perfect graft match clinically and fluoroscopically.
  - The human talus is quite variable and regardless of the match, some inconsistencies will be present.
  - Although the clinical appearance may suggest a near-perfect match, we routinely see slight incongruencies in the sagittal and axial preparations and what appears to be a slight mismatch to the native subchondral bone.
  - In our experience, however, these are not clinically relevant and some degree of remodeling during graft incorporation is anticipated.
- Fixation of the graft to the native talus **(TECH FIG 9C–G)**
  - We routinely use two solid small-diameter screws (1.5 or 2.0 mm) placed in lag fashion to secure the graft to the native talus.

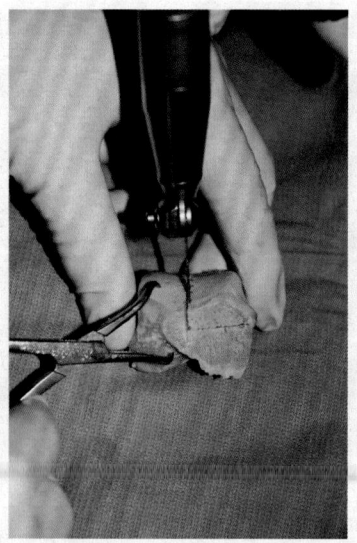

A   **B**

TECH FIG 8 Harvesting graft from donor talus. **A.** Sagittal cut with oscillating saw. **B.** After completion of axial cut.

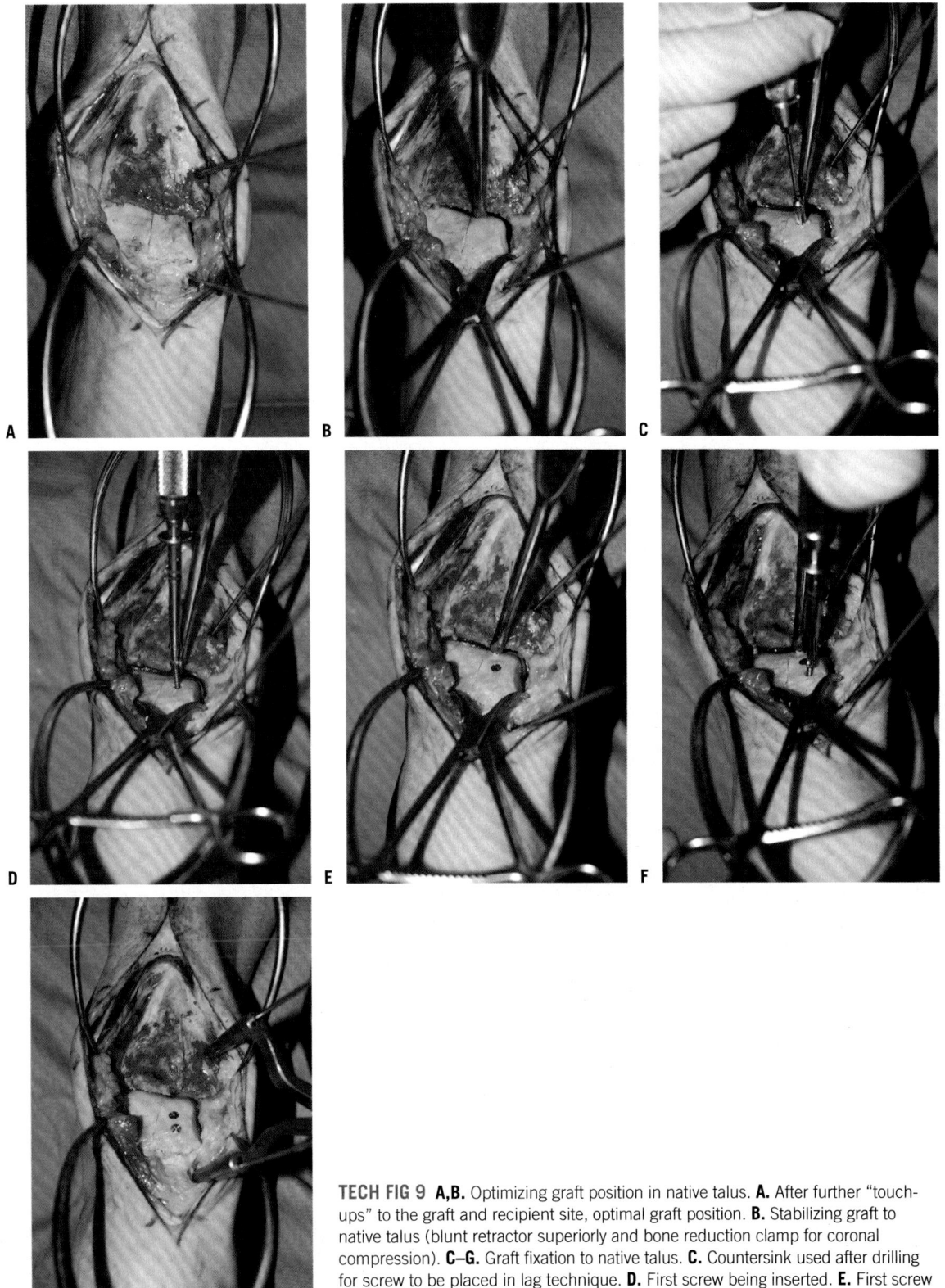

TECH FIG 9 A,B. Optimizing graft position in native talus. **A.** After further "touch-ups" to the graft and recipient site, optimal graft position. **B.** Stabilizing graft to native talus (blunt retractor superiorly and bone reduction clamp for coronal compression). **C–G.** Graft fixation to native talus. **C.** Countersink used after drilling for screw to be placed in lag technique. **D.** First screw being inserted. **E.** First screw with compression and countersunk. **F.** Second screw being inserted. **G.** Both screws countersunk.

- These are placed anteriorly and countersunk below the articular surface, typically anterior to the tibial plafond with the ankle in neutral position.
- Although we would prefer to avoid violating the cartilage surface, to date, we are not aware of any compromised outcome related to the articular defect created by placing the screws.
- Because the talus is contained within the ankle mortise, in our experience, posterior screw fixation is unnecessary.
- We routinely assess graft position after screw placement fluoroscopically. Because the articular cartilage is not visible and the physiologic talar dome is not in a single plane, the countersunk screws may appear proud fluoroscopically.

Axial Realignment

- Based on the preoperative plan and intraoperative reassessment, consider correction of axial malalignment. This improves the weight-bearing axis of the lower extremity and potentially unloads and protects the graft (eccentric load on the talus may have contributed to development of OLT). The preoperative plan dictates the amount of desired correction. As a rule, 1 mm of medial opening equals 1 degree of correction.
- Through the same incision, perform supramalleolar osteotomy for varus malalignment.
  - Medial opening wedge **(TECH FIG 10)**
    - Greenstick principle: Leave lateral cortical hinge if possible.
    - With or without fibular osteotomy, depending on degree of deformity

- Minimal periosteal stripping
  - Attempt to limit to osteotomy site.
- Protect soft tissues.
- Judicious osteotomy
- Consider a slightly oblique trajectory to increase surface area.
- Careful medial opening
  - Protect lateral hinge.
  - If hinge is weak, maintain proper contact, control rotation of two fragments, and consider using two plates in two planes for fixation.
  - We routinely bone graft the opening wedge osteotomy site. However, this is not recommended by all who perform these osteotomies.

Closure

- Perform thorough irrigation.
- Close the capsule.
- Release the tourniquet.
- Reapproximate the extensor retinaculum while protecting the deep neurovascular bundle, extensor tendons, and the superficial peroneal nerve.
- We routinely use a drain for 24 hours.
- Perform subcutaneous closure and tensionless skin reapproximation.
- Dressings, adequate padding, and posterior sugar-tong splint with the ankle in neutral or even a slightly dorsiflexed position

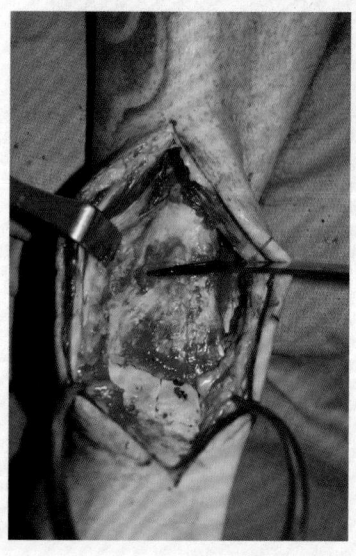 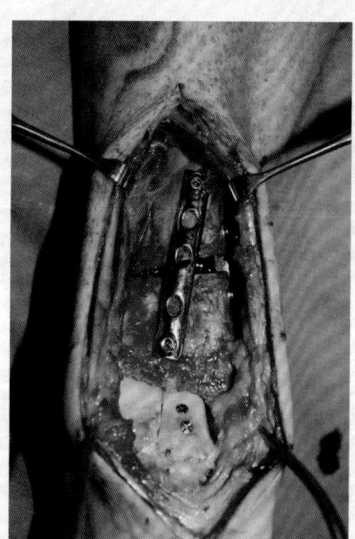

TECH FIG 10 Realignment medial opening supramalleolar osteotomy. **A.** Osteotomy being carefully opened with an osteotome while preserving the lateral cortical hinge. **B.** Plate fixation.

TECHNIQUES

Pearls and Pitfalls

Procuring a Talar Allograft	• Be sure it is the correct side (right or left). Be sure the tissue bank leaves the cartilage on the talus (we have had tali delivered from tissue banks that routinely remove the cartilage from the allograft talus).
Harvesting the Graft from the Donor Talus	• Measure twice and cut once. You have only one opportunity to harvest the graft. Use a caliper and a ruler and double-check the measurements.
Orienting the Donor Talus during Graft Harvest	• Take care to orient the donor talus properly, as it should rest in the ankle mortise (compare to the native talus). The sagittal and axial cuts must be congruent for the graft to have an optimal match.

Reducing the Immunogenic Load of the Graft	• Wash the graft's cancellous surfaces with saline before implantation.
Graft Position Relative to the Native Talus	• Rarely, if ever, is the graft a perfect clinical and fluoroscopic match; there is too much variability in the human talus. Anticipate some remodeling, provided the graft congruency is satisfactory to allow graft incorporation.
Screw Fixation	• Countersink the screws below the articular surface.
Malleolar Osteotomy	• Predrill the position for the screws to fix the malleolus at the conclusion of the surgery. Take into account the thickness of the saw blade; a perfect reduction clinically will demonstrate a slight gap due to bone loss from the saw blade. In our experience, the malleolus heals despite this narrow gap.

POSTOPERATIVE CARE

- We routinely observe these patients overnight for pain control.
- Follow-up is done in about 10 to 14 days.
- Provided the wound and osteotomy (if one was performed) are stable, the patient is transferred into a touchdown weight-bearing CAM boot. If not, a touchdown weight-bearing short-leg cast is continued until the wound and osteotomy are stable.
- Intermittent minimal, gentle ankle range of motion (ROM) encouraged, three or four times a day. If financially feasible, we arrange for an ankle continuous passive motion device.
- Touchdown weight bearing is maintained for 10 to 12 weeks, with progressively increasing ankle ROM exercise.
- We routinely obtain simulated weight-bearing radiographs at 6 and 10 weeks and again at 14 to 16 weeks, depending on the progression of healing. If there was a concern about fixation of the graft or osteotomy, then radiographs are also obtained at the first postoperative visit (**FIGS 1** to **3**).

OUTCOMES

- Gross et al[3] reported on nine patients who underwent fresh osteochondral allograft transplantation. At a mean follow-up of 11 years, six grafts remained in situ. The three failed allografts demonstrated radiographic and intraoperative evidence of fragmentation or resorption, and these patients went on to ankle fusion. Standardized outcomes measures for comparison were not used in that study.
- Raikin[4] recently reported on 15 patients who underwent bulk fresh osteochondral allografting for large-volume cystic lesions of the talus. The mean volume of the cystic lesions was 6059 mm³. At a mean follow-up of 4.5 years, the mean American Orthopaedic Foot & Ankle Society (AOFAS) ankle–hindfoot score was 83 points. Only two grafts failed and went on to have an ankle arthrodesis. Some form of graft collapse, graft resorption, or joint space narrowing was seen in all patients.
- A retrospective review by Adams et al[2] showed significant improvement in pain and the Lower Extremity Functional Scale at a mean follow-up of 48 months in eight patients who underwent osteochondral allograft transplantation of the talus. The mean postoperative AOFAS ankle–hindfoot score was 84 points. Three grafts were found to have graft–host lucencies in one plane on plain radiography. These patients were doing well and no further imaging was obtained. One patient continued to be symptomatic and was thought to have a nonunion of the graft due to circumferential lucency. Second-look arthroscopy demonstrated partial graft cartilage delamination but a stable graft. The patient did not wish to have any further treatment.

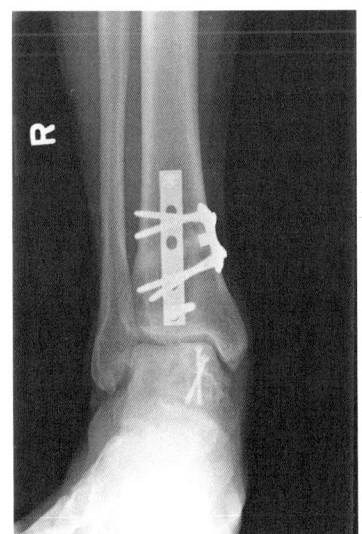 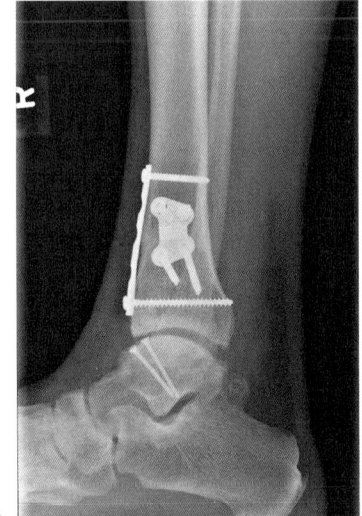 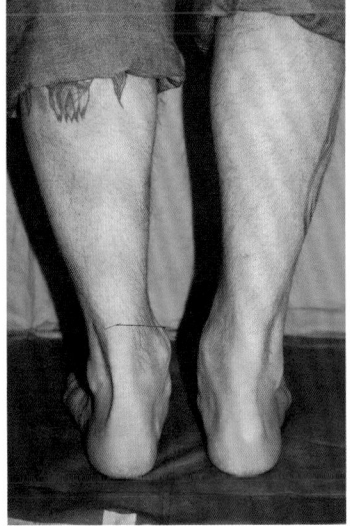

FIG 1 Two-and-a-half-year follow-up. **A.** AP radiograph. **B.** Lateral radiograph. **C.** Clinical correlation.

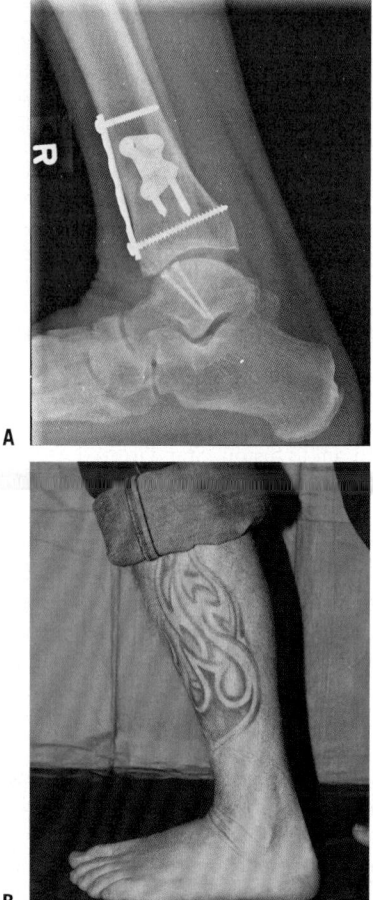

FIG 2 Dorsiflexion. **A.** Radiograph (although the joint appears to narrow anteriorly, this phenomenon has not changed in 2 years, and the patient experiences no pain or impingement). **B.** Clinical appearance.

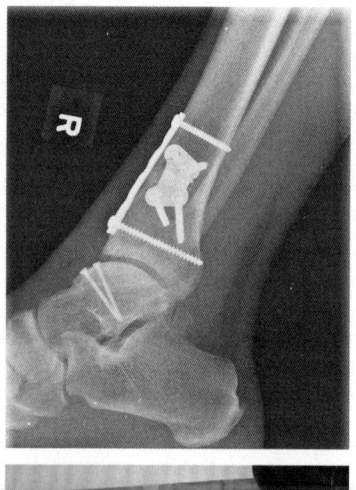

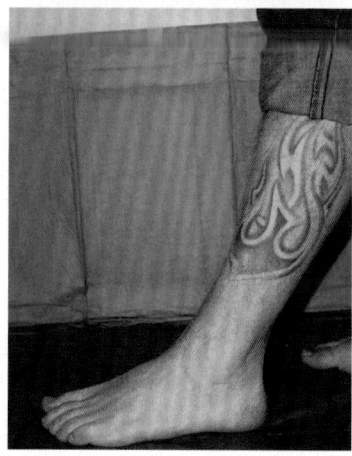

FIG 3 Plantarflexion. **A.** Radiograph. **B.** Clinical correlation.

- A follow-up prospective study by the same group included 14 patients with a mean follow-up of 55 months.[1] These patients demonstrated significant improvement in pain, AOFAS scale, short form-36 (SF-36), and short musculoskeletal function assessment (SMFA) scores at most recent follow-up.

COMPLICATIONS

- Hardware migration. Our most common reason for reoperation is removal of prominent screw from the graft.
- Infection
- Wound complications
  - Particularly for anterior approach (as is performed for total ankle replacement)
  - Deep retraction only, avoiding direct tension on wound margins, reduces this risk.
- Failure of graft incorporation
- With large structural grafts, graft failure, and development of degenerative change
- Articular cartilage delamination or fissuring of the graft
- Malleolar osteotomy nonunion
- Persistent pain despite radiographic suggestion of graft incorporation
- Disease transmission, although with the current screening practices of tissue banks, this risk is negligible

REFERENCES

1. Adams SB, Dekker TJ, Schiff AP, et al. Prospective evaluation of structural allograft transplantation for osteochondral lesions of the talar shoulder. Foot Ankle Int 2018;39(1):28–34.
2. Adams SB Jr, Viens NA, Easley ME, et al. Midterm results of osteochondral lesions of the talar shoulder treated with fresh osteochondral allograft transplantation. J Bone Joint Surg Am 2011;93(7):648–654. doi:10.2106/JBJS.J.00141.
3. Gross AE, Agnidis Z, Hutchison CR. Osteochondral defects of the talus treated with fresh osteochondral allograft transplantation. Foot Ankle Int 2001;22:385–391.
4. Raikin SM. Fresh osteochondral allografts for large-volume cystic osteochondral defects of the talus. J Bone Joint Surg Am 2009;91(12):2818–2826.

SUGGESTED READINGS

Adams SB, Viens NA, Easley ME, et al. Structural allograft transplantation for osteochondral lesions of the talus. JBJS Essent Surg Tech 2012;2(1):e4.
Gross CE, Adams SB, Easley ME, et al. Role of fresh osteochondral allografts for large talar osteochondral lesions. J Am Acad Orthop Surg 2016;27(1):e9–e17.

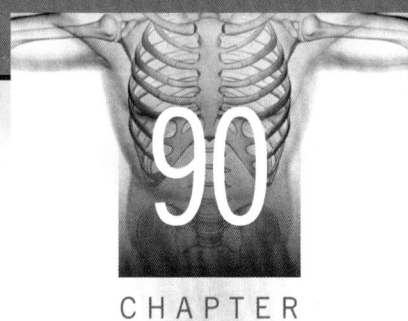

90

CHAPTER

Autologous Chondrocyte Transplantation

Markus Walther

DEFINITION

- There are several reasons for cartilaginous defects of the ankle:
  - Traumatic injury
  - Osteochondritis dissecans (OCD)
  - Degenerative changes
- The necessity to treat a cartilage defect of the ankle depends on the clinical presentation. Osteochondral lesions of the talus (OLTs) are often found incidentally on screening magnetic resonance imaging (MRI) obtained for reasons other than suspected intra-articular pathology.[50]
- Autologous chondrocyte transplantation, also known as *autologous chondrocyte implantation* (ACI), is one of several surgical treatment options for symptomatic cartilage defects. In my opinion, ACI is best suited for patients between 18 and 50 years of age.
- ACI is indicated for management of symptomatic OLTs failing to respond to débridement, drilling, or microfracture.[1,9,39]
- Primary ACI can be considered in lesions larger than 2 cm^2 or in osteochondral lesions associated with expansive subchondral cysts (stage V lesion).[66]
- Advantages of ACI include the following:
  - ACI provides a stable cartilage rim that can be maintained at the site of the OLT.
  - Large defects can be readily addressed with this technique.[19]
  - The periosteal flap can be harvested from the adjacent medial tibia.
  - With carefully executed suture technique or with matrix-induced chondrocytes, shoulder lesions can be managed.
- Disadvantages of the ACI for the talar dome are as follows:
  - ACI has U.S. Food and Drug Administration (FDA) approval only for the knee. ACI at the talus as well as matrix-induced autologous chondrocyte implantation (MACI) is considered investigational (as of January 2015).
  - The cost from industry for chondrocyte culture is considerable.
  - The procedure requires two stages to allow time for chondrocyte culture.
- Reports of the traditional technique that requires a periosteal flap under which the transplanted chondrocytes are positioned suggested limitations of the technique for the talus.[63] Many OLTs involve, at least in part, the talar shoulder, an anatomic region poorly suited for anatomic coverage with a periosteal flap. Recently introduced MACI may afford advantages because it does not require coverage of

the defect with a periosteal flap. Histologic investigations have shown that MACI may offer an improved alternative to traditional treatments for cartilage injury by regenerating hyaline-like cartilage.[66]

- Informed consent and patient education are imperative for ACI. ACI for the ankle lacks FDA approval. However, for larger OLTs, OLTs failing to respond to prior surgical management, or OLT with subchondral cysts, ACI provides patients and their surgeons with a potentially successful treatment avenue that did not exist before ACI. Early favorable outcomes with ACI applied to difficult OLTs justify the extra effort; education; and communication among physicians, patients, and third-party payers who may be required to proceed with ACI in the ankle.
- In Europe, harvesting cells for culturing is considered part of a drug-producing process. Therefore, special permission must be sought from the local health care administration. Standard operating procedures for harvesting and transportation of the cartilage cells are mandatory for the accreditation process.
- Latest developments focus on one-step, membrane-based, scaffold-enhanced cartilage repair. Mesenchymal progenitor cells migrate toward and adhere to the porous layer of the matrix, which is implanted analogue to the technique described in the following text in a one-step surgery. Whereas in Europe, different membranes are approved for use in the talus, the FDA approval is still in progress.[13,25,27,50,61,64]

ANATOMY

- A slight majority of OLTs are on the medial shoulder of the talus.[18,55]
  - Sixty-two percent of lesions are located at the medial talar shoulder; many of these are thought to be a result of OCD rather than posttraumatic.
  - Thirty-four percent of the lesions are located at the lateral talar shoulder; most are thought to be of traumatic origin.
  - Central OLTs are rare (<5%).
  - In the anteroposterior (AP) direction, the midtalar dome (equator) is much more frequently involved (80%) than the anterior (6%) or posterior (14%) thirds of the talar dome.
- Classification of osteochondral lesions is based on arthroscopic findings.[30]
  - Grade I: intact lesions
  - Grade II: lesions showing signs of early separation

- Grade III: partially detached lesions
- Grade IV: craters with loose bodies
- ACI is performed for symptomatic grade II-plus lesions (full-thickness cartilage defects).

PATHOGENESIS

- Traumatic cartilage injuries are caused by short, intensive, greater-than-physiologic strain on the joint resulting in partial detachment of the talar dome cartilage. The depth of these lesions varies from superficial chondral abrasions to full-thickness osteochondral defects.[44,60]
- OCD is a condition most frequently found in adolescents or young adults. Although the cause remains poorly defined, theories include the following:
  - Chronic overload
  - Local disturbance of blood supply to the subchondral bone associated with the affected cartilage[34]
- Degenerative cartilage defects (degenerative osteoarthritis) develop from wear and tear of the cartilage surface as part of the aging process. An individual's risk of developing primary osteoarthritis most likely depends on a genetically determined quality of the cartilage. Ankle instability and other conditions that impart eccentric or nonphysiologic loads to the cartilage may accelerate the process of degeneration. In exceptional cases, when such a degenerative process is limited to a focal portion of the talar dome, ACI may be considered for degenerative cartilage defects, provided the underlying cause leading to focal degeneration (ie, malalignment or chronic instability) is corrected.

NATURAL HISTORY

- The natural history of a focal cartilage injury has not been linked to diffuse ankle arthritis.
  - Posttraumatic arthritis, which differs from an OLT, develops from diffuse injury to the cartilage surface that results in cartilage fibrillation and eventual eburnation. ACI is contraindicated for diffuse ankle arthritis.
  - Injury to a focal portion of the talar dome spans the spectrum from a bone bruise to a detached focal osteochondral fragment. Although an osteochondral fragment may be created at the time of injury, the focal talar dome pathology probably evolves. Many OLTs are probably asymptomatic; we know this from numerous OLTs that are found incidentally on imaging studies of the ankle obtained for reasons other than suspected intra-articular pathology. However, with persistent eccentric stresses, greater-than-physiologic loads, inadequate local blood supply, or inadequate healing time, a stable OLT may progress to an unstable one.
  - The difficulty is also in the symptomatology. Although some apparently unstable lesions may be asymptomatic, other OLTs that are clearly stable result in considerable symptoms directly related to the OLT.[40]

PATIENT HISTORY AND PHYSICAL FINDINGS

- Although many patients report a specific ankle injury to account for the OLT, many do not present until months after ankle injury.[14] A symptomatic OLT is in the differential diagnosis for an ankle sprain that does not heal. However, many patients with symptomatic OLTs do not recall a specific traumatic event leading to the OLT.[53]

- In our practice, most patients presenting with symptomatic OLTs are between 20 and 50 years of age.[61]
- Men are more commonly affected than women (ratio 1.6:1).[53]
- Patients typically describe an ache in the ankle with activity or with the first steps after a period of rest. Occasionally, sharp ankle pain is noted with weight bearing. In our experience, mechanical symptoms of locking or catching are noted only with a completely detached osteochondral fragment. Paradoxically, OLTs may produce symptoms on the opposite side of the joint from the location of the cartilage defect.
- Our preferred physical examination methods are listed here. Occasionally, symptoms may not be elicited on clinical examination.
  - Locking or catching: found when something interrupts the normal movement of the joint. However, it says nothing about the cause of this condition (eg, scar, joint body, osteochondral fragment, and synovitis).
  - Inversion test (calcaneofibular ligament [CFL]): strongly dependent on the cooperation of the patient. If positive, it is highly specific for a ruptured CFL.
  - Medial stability: strongly dependent on the cooperation of the patient. If positive, it is highly specific for a ruptured deltoid ligament.
  - Anterior drawer test (anterior talofibular ligament [ATFL]): strongly dependent on the cooperation of the patient. If positive, it is highly specific for a ruptured ATFL.
  - The medial and lateral corner of the talar dome should be palpated with the ankle maximally flexed to identify anterior or central OLTs; posteromedial palpation immediately posterior to the posterior tibial tendon (PTT) with the ankle maximally dorsiflexed may reproduce symptoms for posteromedial OLTs. Although anterolateral OLTs are relatively easy to palpate, posteromedial lesions are difficult to access adequately on physical examination.
- We find it useful to compare the symptomatic ankle to the uninvolved contralateral ankle.
  - The medial and lateral corner of the talar dome should be palpated with the ankle maximally flexed to identify anterior or central OLTs; posteromedial palpation immediately posterior to the PTT with the ankle maximally dorsiflexed may reproduce symptoms for posteromedial OLTs. Although anterolateral OLTs are relatively easy to palpate, posteromedial lesions are difficult to access adequately on physical examination.
  - We typically dorsiflex and plantarflex the ankles with axial pressure while simultaneously applying eversion and inversion stresses to reproduce symptoms at the talar defect.
  - Despite appropriate provocative maneuvers, our experience has been that posterior OLTs rarely exhibit obvious clinical findings.
- Associated injuries and other considerations in the differential diagnosis of chronic ankle pain should be evaluated, particularly because OLTs may be incidental findings. These include the following:
  - Ankle instability: positive anterior drawer test and inversion testing
  - Chondromatosis of the ankle: Recurrent locking of the joint and persistent effusions are typical physical findings.

- Intra-articular scarring with load-dependent pain, mostly at the anterolateral aspect of the ankle joint
- Inflammatory arthropathy: Although effusion and deep joint pain with weight bearing are commonly present, pain at rest and persistent joint warmth are also common features of inflammatory disease.
- Pigmented villonodular synovitis (PVNS): Organized nodules of synovitis can mimic loose bodies with locking and effusion. Synovial swelling is not typical for osteochondral defects. MRI with contrast typically confirms the diagnosis of PVNS.
- Hindfoot malalignment with local osteoarthritis: Edge loading of the talus can cause symptomatic local cartilage lesions. Typically, those defects include the tibial cartilage as well as the talus, which can be visualized with MRI.

IMAGING AND OTHER DIAGNOSTIC STUDIES

- Plain radiographs of the ankle joint, including AP, mortise, and lateral views, are obtained to rule out late-stage degenerative arthritis.
- MRI with contrast is highly sensitive and specific in diagnosing osteochondral lesions as well as associated injuries.[32,47]
- Osteochondral lesions were first classified by Berndt and Harty[8] based on plain radiographs:
  - Stage I: compression lesion; no visible fragment
  - Stage II: beginning avulsion of a chip
  - Stage III: chip, completely detached but in place
  - Stage IV: displaced chip
- Plain films typically offer limited information on the size and extent of the lesion and may even miss the OLT. MRI, computed tomography (CT), and arthroscopic evaluation provide greater detail of OLTs than plain radiographs.
- DiPaolo classification of osteochondral lesions based on MRI[15]
  - Stage I: thickening of articular cartilage and low-signal changes
  - Stage II: articular cartilage breached, low-signal rim behind fragment indicating fibrous attachment
  - Stage III: articular cartilage breached, high-signal changes behind fragment indicating synovial fluid between fragment and underlying subchondral bone **(FIG 1)**
  - Stage IV: loose body
- Based on the greater detail of pathologic anatomy, Hepple et al[32] revised the classification and included a stage V (subchondral cyst formation).
  - Stage I: articular cartilage damage only
  - Stage IIa: cartilage injury with underlying fracture and surrounding bony edema
  - Stage IIb: stage IIa without surrounding bony edema
  - Stage III: detached but undisplaced fragment
  - Stage IV: detached and displaced fragment
  - Stage V: subchondral cyst formation
- The Ferkel and Sgaglione CT classification is used for preoperative planning purposes and to learn the size of the subchondral defect.[21]
  - Stage I: cystic lesion of the talar dome with an intact roof
  - Stage IIa: cystic lesion with communication to the talar dome surface
  - Stage IIb: open articular surface lesion with an overlying, nondisplaced fragment

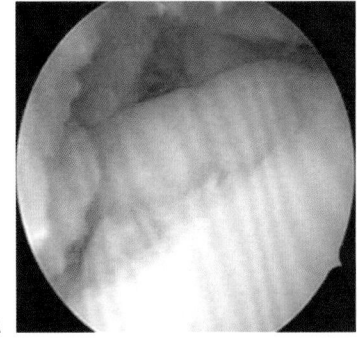

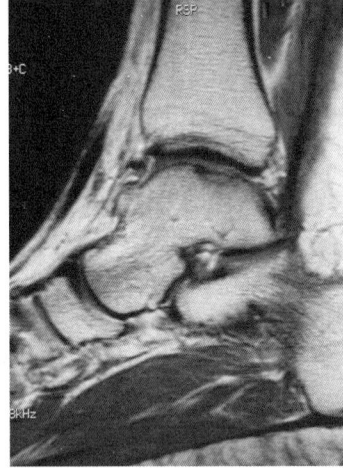

FIG 1 A. Arthroscopic view of a full-thickness osteochondral defect at the talar dome. **B.** Corresponding MRI.

- Stage III: nondisplaced lesion with lucency
- Stage IV: displaced osteochondral fragment

DIFFERENTIAL DIAGNOSIS

- Syndesmosis injury
- Intra-articular scarring
- Subluxation or tear of peroneal tendons
- Fracture or disruption of the os trigonum
- Malleolar avulsion fracture
- Interosseous ligament injury
- Anterior process fracture of the calcaneus
- Lateral shoulder fracture of the calcaneus
- Chondromatosis
- Inflammatory joint disease
- PVNS
- Degenerative arthritis

NONOPERATIVE MANAGEMENT

- In young patients with open physes, OCD can be managed conservatively with a high rate of complete remission **(FIG 2)**.[7,62]
- Acute osteochondral lesions may be treated conservatively. Acute lesions (stages I and II) require 3 weeks of immobilization. Stages III and IV lesions should be treated with a walker and partial weight bearing of 20 kg for 6 weeks.[53] However, unstable osteochondral lesions, particularly those with detached fragments, should be managed operatively.

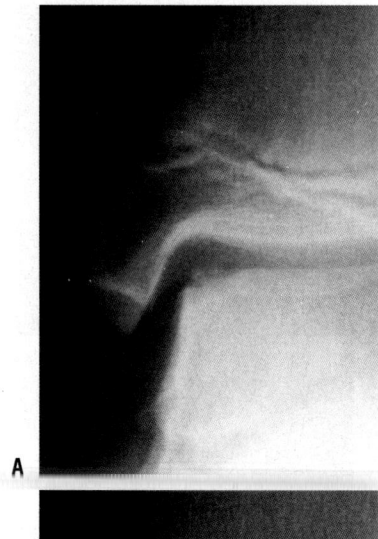

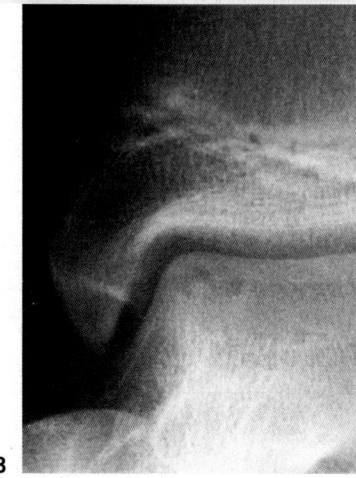

FIG 2 A. OCD in a child with open physis. **B.** Six months later, the lesion is healed with conservative treatment.

- Incidentally discovered OLTs and OCD cases in adults are generally treated expectantly with regular follow-up.[17,40]
- The literature suggests that chronic OLTs, even larger lesions, may be treated nonoperatively as well.[55] Nonoperative treatment comprises nonsteroidal anti-inflammatory agents, ankle bracing, physiotherapy, corticosteroid injection, viscosupplementation, and platelet-rich plasma. Currently, no conservative treatment of OLTs allows resurfacing or healing of the cartilage defect.

SURGICAL MANAGEMENT

- Microfracture
  - Arthroscopic débridement and microfracture generally represent the initial surgical management for the vast majority of OLTs, with satisfactory results in 65% to 90% of patients (see Chaps. FA-80 and 81).[6,33,52]
  - The biomechanical properties of fibrocartilage are different from those of hyaline cartilage; the fibrocartilage does not function in concert with the surrounding physiologic hyaline cartilage. The literature suggests that microfracture is successful in a majority of relatively small OLTs (up to 2 cm²).[6,26]
- Autologous osteochondral transfer (osteochondral autograft transplantations [OATS] or mosaicplasty) and ACI are typically secondary surgical procedures when arthroscopic débridement, microfracture, and drilling fail.[31]

- Due to inferior outcome of microfracture in OLTs larger than 2 cm², ACI can be considered as primary surgery in large defects.[12]
- Autologous osteochondral cylinder transplantation (OATS or mosaicplasty)[31,54]
  - In the OATS or mosaicplasty technique, osteochondral cylinders or plugs are harvested either from a low load-bearing area of the knee or from the medial or lateral facet of the talus.[51] These plugs are transplanted into the defect area, which has been prepared to the appropriate size.
  - This procedure fills large portions of the defect surface with high-quality hyaline cartilage.[31]
  - The results of this technique are satisfactory, but donor site morbidity occurs in up to 50% of cases.[49,56]
  - To limit these harvesting symptoms, osteochondral cylinder transplantation can be successfully applied for cartilage defects of up to only about 3 cm². Matching defects on the talar shoulder are difficult with this technique, despite technique modifications described by Hangody.[31] Moreover, the characteristics of talar cartilage differ from those of cartilage from the knee.[11]
- Allograft osteochondral cylinder transplantation[29]
  - If available, osteochondral cylinders can be taken from a fresh or fresh frozen cadaver talus.
  - Immunologic reactions have posed little problem to date.[42]
- Recent studies reported an increased risk of necrotic changes of the osteochondral transplant and cyst formation in the long-term follow-up. Autograft was inferior in the direct comparison to allograft.[57,58]

Preoperative Planning

- All imaging studies are reviewed, with MRI providing detail of the cartilage defect and CT providing detail of subchondral bone involvement.[2,16,53]
- Pure cartilage defects or shallow osteochondral defects can be managed with the conventional ACI procedure; deeper osteochondral defects require a "sandwich technique."
- The sandwich technique involves two layers of periosteum. The defect is prepared and bone grafted to recreate the subchondral bone architecture. On this, the first layer of periosteum is placed cambium layer up. Then, the defect can be treated in the conventional manner: The second layer of periosteum is placed cambium side down. The cultured cartilage cells are injected between these two layers. Alternatively, the cartilage defect may be bone grafted in a first stage, with a conventional ACI procedure being performed in a second stage. This is feasible in the knee but more challenging in the ankle, which may require ligament release or osteotomy for adequate exposure, procedures that should not be performed more than once if not necessary.
- Matrix-based chondrocytes that do not require a periosteal flap can be placed directly on a bone graft, which makes the management of stage V lesions less demanding. Matrix-based chondrocytes can be glued into the defect, which often allows to address the lesion without medial malleolar osteotomy.[65]
- Ankle malalignment and instability should be identified and corrected in conjunction with ACI if possible.

Positioning

- Harvesting chondrocytes: standard arthroscopy of the ankle or the knee

- Giannini et al[24] have demonstrated that the detached OLT fragment at the time of index arthroscopy may be an acceptable source of chondrocytes in ACI. Another possible source is the anterior aspect of the talus.[5]
- Transplantation of chondrocytes: Depending on the location of the defect, the patient is positioned supine with a slightly internally or externally rotated leg. If iliac crest graft is to be obtained, the pelvis needs to be prepared and draped as well and the ipsilateral pelvis supported with a bump. Alternatively, bone graft may be harvested from the calcaneus, distal tibia, or proximal tibia, all locations within the surgical field typically prepared for ACI.[20,22,48] A vacuum mattress can be helpful to adjust the patient's position during the procedure (**FIG 3**).

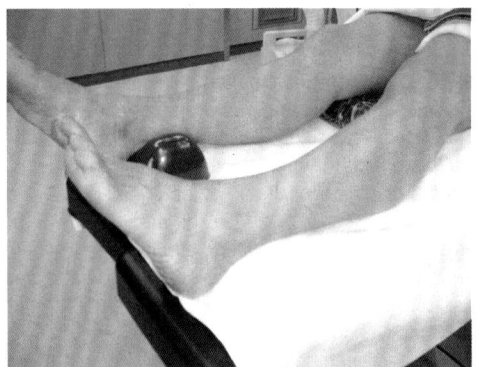

FIG 3 Standard positioning in a supine position.

T E C H N I Q U E S

APPROACH

- Harvesting chondrocytes: Medial and lateral anterior portals and a posterolateral portal give an adequate overview of the joint and allow the harvesting of chondrocytes.
- Transplantation: Depending on the location of the OLT, a medial approach between the medial malleolus and the PTT, a medial transmalleolar approach with osteotomy, or a lateral approach (with or without osteotomy) can be considered. ACI demands adequate exposure to properly suture a periosteal patch circumferentially around the OLT.[23] Except for OLTs at the anterior or posterior margins of the talar dome, ACI cannot be performed properly without medial malleolar osteotomy for extensive medial OLTs and ATFL–CFL release, lateral malleolar osteotomy, or both for extensive lateral OLTs.
- A major advantage compared to mosaicplasty or OATS is that a perpendicular access is not required. Muir et al[41] demonstrated that the majority of the talar dome can be accessed without osteotomy but acknowledged that osteotomies are required to adequately expose extensive OLTs.

MEDIAL OSTEOCHONDRAL LESIONS OF THE TALUS

- Occasionally, the ACI procedure can be performed for medial OLTs with an anteromedial or posteromedial arthrotomy.[41] In our experience, these are exceptional cases, often requiring extreme intraoperative ankle plantarflexion and dorsiflexion for anteromedial and posteromedial lesions, respectively. An intact deltoid ligament permits little if any translation of the talus relative to the tibia. Access to an anterior defect can be enhanced with a groove created in the anteromedial tibia but leaves a permanent defect in the anterior weight-bearing surface of the plafond. We appreciate that extreme dorsiflexion allows visualization of some posteromedial OLTs; however, we caution against extreme dorsiflexion that tensions the posteromedial neurovascular bundle in combination with the simultaneous required retraction of the neurovascular bundle to allow proper access to the lesion. One author suggested that a medial malleolar window can be created, obviating the need for osteotomy,[45] but we have no experience with this approach.

Oblique Medial Malleolar Osteotomy

- A longitudinal incision is centered over the medial malleolus, similar to that performed for open reduction and internal fixation of medial malleolar fractures.
- An anterior arthrotomy serves to identify the junction between the medial malleolar and tibial plafond articular surfaces and may allow visualization of the anterior aspect of the OLT.

- Posteriorly, the flexor retinaculum is opened, and the PTT is identified directly on the posterior tibia. The PTT rests in a groove in the posterior aspect of the medial tibia in its own sheath; the flexor digitorum longus tendon lies directly posterior to the PTT and should not be mistaken for the PTT.
- With the PTT properly retracted, the posteromedial neurovascular bundle will also be protected.
- The medial malleolar osteotomy requires minimal periosteal stripping; in fact, we advise leaving as much of the periosteum as possible on the medial malleolar fragment to maintain blood supply for healing.
- To optimize reduction of the medial malleolar osteotomy after the cartilage repair procedure, we recommend predrilling the medial malleolus. Two parallel drill holes are placed extra-articularly perpendicular across the desired osteotomy, in the same orientation as screws placed for conventional open reduction and internal fixation for medial malleolar fractures. The proper course for these drill holes is confirmed fluoroscopically, both in the AP and lateral planes.
- Under fluoroscopic guidance, a Kirschner wire pin is introduced obliquely to dictate the desired plane of the osteotomy. Typically, we introduce this guide pin slightly more proximal and medial than the intended course of the osteotomy to allow access for the saw blade, chisel, or both without having to remove the pin that guides our osteotomy.

- The osteotomy can be planned more conservatively as in mosaicplasty because a perpendicular access to the OLT is not needed. As a rule, we plan to have the osteotomy enter the tibial plafond at the medial extent of the OLT.
- With the plan for the osteotomy determined, the periosteum is divided transversely, again leaving the majority of the periosteum intact. With cold saline or sterile water irrigation to reduce the risk of osseous heat necrosis, a microsagittal saw is used to perform the oblique osteotomy to the level of the tibial plafond subchondral bone.
- The joint is penetrated with an osteotome or a chisel. Intermittent fluoroscopic guidance is recommended to confirm proper saw blade or chisel orientation and that the talar dome is not injured during the final stages of the osteotomy.
- The medial malleolus is then reflected, suspended by the deltoid ligament.
- Even with careful technique, the osteotomy rarely separates in a uniform plane. Particularly posteriorly, a slight irregularity is observed. This is of little concern, however, as these irregularities will provide greater stability when the osteotomy is reduced.

- To fully displace the medial malleolar fragment, the PTT sheath must be released from the medial malleolus.
- At the conclusion of the cartilage-resurfacing procedure, the medial malleolus is reduced and secured with two malleolar screws placed in the predrilled tracks with compression.
- To limit a vertical shear effect, an antiglide screw or plate may be placed at the proximal aspect of the osteotomy. Alternatively, a third screw can be carefully placed from medial to lateral eccentrically across the osteotomy in addition to the two predrilled compression screws.
- Anatomic reduction is confirmed clinically by visualizing the anterior and posterior aspects of the osteotomy and fluoroscopically in the AP and oblique planes. Fluoroscopy in all three routine views of the ankle confirms proper extra-articular position of the screws.
- Due to the thickness of the saw blade, a slight, incomplete gap may be visualized at the osteotomy site in select cases; despite this immediate postoperative finding, our anecdotal experience has been that the oblique medial malleolar osteotomy heals in its anatomic position with few complications.

LATERAL OSTEOCHONDRAL LESIONS OF THE TALUS

- ATFL and CFL release: Some lateral OLTs are associated with lateral ankle instability.[35] This combination of pathology is well suited to surgical management because a modified Broström procedure is required to stabilize the ankle. If a lateral OLT is identified without lateral ankle instability, lateral ligament release to allow access to the OLT is readily repaired with a modified Broström technique, particularly because the lateral ankle ligaments are not attenuated.[53]
- The fibula is exposed through a longitudinal incision. If ligament release is inadequate, the extensile longitudinal incision facilitates the addition of a lateral malleolar osteotomy. Moreover, if associated pathology involves the peroneal tendons, the extensile longitudinal approach is necessary.
- With the sural nerve protected posteriorly and inferiorly and the lateral branch of the superficial peroneal nerve protected anteriorly, the inferior flexor retinaculum is identified and isolated.
- Deep to the retinaculum and at the distal and posterior margin of the fibula, the peroneal tendons are identified and protected throughout the procedure.
- The ATFL and CFL lie within the lateral ankle capsular complex. Leaving a 1-mm cuff of capsule on the distal fibula, the capsule and the ATFL and CFL are released. The ankle is plantarflexed and inverted; the talus is subluxated anteriorly out of the ankle mortise to expose the OLT.
- After the cartilage resurfacing, the talus is reduced in the ankle mortise and a modified Broström procedure is performed. This can be done with suture anchors in the distal fibula, placed to secure the ATFL and CFL components of the lateral ankle capsule in particular or with transosseous sutures.
- During tensioning of the ligament repair, the talus is maintained posteriorly (avoiding anterior translation), with the ankle in a neutral sagittal plane position and the hindfoot in slight eversion. As described by Gould,[28] the inferior extensor retinaculum is advanced to the distal fibula to lend greater stability to the repair.

Lateral Malleolar Osteotomy

- Several different patterns for lateral malleolar osteotomies exist; surprisingly, few have been described in detail. We typically employ an oblique fibular osteotomy, similar to the pattern created by a simple Weber B ankle fracture. The approach is as described for the ligament release earlier. As for a medial malleolar osteotomy, periosteal stripping is kept to a minimum, predrilling is preferred, and cold saline or sterile water irrigation is applied to the osteotomy site to limit osseous heat necrosis.
- Before performing the osteotomy, we position a small fragment plate in the desired position and predrill the holes. With the soft tissues protected, in particular the superficial peroneal nerve and the peroneal tendons, the oblique osteotomy is created from anterior to posterior using a microsagittal saw. The syndesmotic ligaments are not disrupted. Release of the ATFL and CFL in combination with the fibular osteotomy can be considered to improve exposure of larger posterolateral OLTs with medial extension.
- At the conclusion of the cartilage repair procedure, the fibula is reduced and secured with the predrilled lateral fibular plate. Reduction is confirmed with intraoperative fluoroscopy. Before placing the plate, a lag screw may be placed across the osteotomy, but we do not routinely do so.
- As for the medial malleolar osteotomy, the thickness of the saw blade may lead to a slight, incomplete gap at the fibular osteotomy site in select cases. Again, despite this immediate postoperative finding, our anecdotal experience has been that the oblique medial malleolar osteotomy heals in its anatomic position with few complications.

CENTRAL DEFECTS

- As observed in the cadaver model of Muir et al,[41] perpendicular access to the central talar dome is not possible via medial and lateral osteotomies. Tochigi et al[59] described a Chaput lateral tibial osteotomy, similar to a Tillaux fracture, to allow greater medial exposure to extensive lateral OLTs; however, Muir et al[41] noted that this osteotomy still fails to allow access to the central talar dome.

- The trapdoor osteotomy described by Sammarco and Makwana,[51] in which an anterior osteochondral wedge is removed from the distal tibia, may permit access to select antero-central OLTs. Although attractive, the osteotomy must be carefully planned to accommodate the instrumentation at the ideal location for sufficient access, as coronal plane translation of the talus is not possible. Moreover, access to relatively rare posterocentral lesions is still not possible despite this novel approach.

HARVESTING OF CHONDROCYTES

- Complete diagnostic arthroscopy and identify all pathology.
- Using a curette, harvest two or three full-thickness articular grafts that include the superficial layer of subchondral bone (**TECH FIG 1**). The grafts are transferred to a sterile container and transported to the laboratory. Using a patented procedure, the articular cartilage matrix is enzymatically disrupted to isolate the chondrocytes. Culturing of chondrocytes requires about 2 to 6 weeks, depending on the company and the preferred culturing process.
- Ensure that the cells are sent to the company immediately, the "cool chain" is sustained, and the required documents are included in the box.

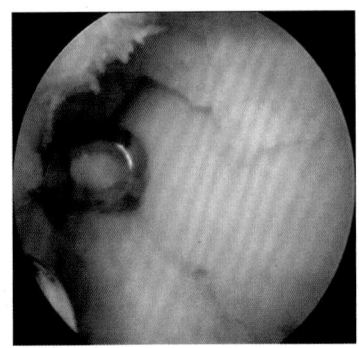 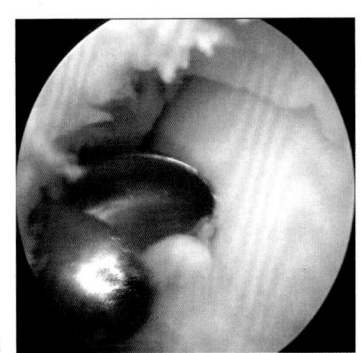

TECH FIG 1 A. Harvesting cartilage with a curette from the ventral aspect of the talus. **B.** Grasping the small piece of cartilage for culturing.

AUTOLOGOUS CHONDROCYTE TRANSPLANTATION

- To avoid compromising chondrocyte viability, use a tourniquet to maintain a bloodless field.
- We typically use a thigh tourniquet; although a calf tourniquet is possible, compression of the lower leg musculature may restrict exposure and manipulation of the ankle, thereby compromising exposure.
- Expose the transplantation site. Despite adequate exposure with appropriate osteotomies or ligament releases, performing the second ACI stage for the ankle, in particular suturing the periosteal flap, may prove tedious. Matrix-based transplants, where the chondrocytes for transplantation are already grown in a collagen matrix, provide a significant advantage. These membranes can be fixed with fibrous glue; sutures are optional. For the knee, both techniques have proven to have similar clinical outcomes.[3] At the talus, there is still a lack of scientific

evidence, but our extended anecdotal experience has shown similar results in both techniques.
- Débride all unstable cartilage with a curette to create a healthy, stable cartilage rim. The subchondral bone in the defect should be intact.
- If a shallow bony defect exists, remove the sclerotic bone. Despite tourniquet use, some bleeding may be encountered; it should be controlled with an epinephrine sponge or a minimal amount of fibrin glue.
- In the event of a deeper defect, use the sandwich technique described earlier to recreate subchondral support for the transplanted chondrocytes. Any bony cyst has to be filled with autologous bone graft, preferably from the iliac crest or the proximal tibia.[22]

- Impact the graft to provide a smooth surface for the transplantation site.
- Measure the defect and create a template using a small piece of paper (from a sterile glove pack) or aluminum foil (from a suture pack).

Technique with Periosteal Flap

- By exposing the distal tibia just proximal to the ankle, identify an appropriate area for periosteal flap harvest; exposure is to the level of the periosteum without violating it.
- Place the template on the periosteum and mark an outline 1 to 2 mm greater than the template on the periosteum. The periosteal harvest should be slightly larger than the template, as periosteum tends to recoil or shrink slightly after harvest.
- Perform sharp dissection to bone on the marked periosteum circumferentially. With a sharp periosteal elevator, elevate the periosteum, with its cambium layer, directly off the underlying tibia without creating defects in the periosteal graft. We routinely place a mark on the superficial layer of periosteum before detaching the periosteal flap from the tibia to be certain we can identify the cambium layer at the time of transfer to the talus.
- Carefully separate overlying fibrous tissue or fat from the periosteal graft.
- After ensuring that the OLT is bloodless, transfer the periosteal flap to the OLT, with the cambium layer facing the defect.
- Suture it using interrupted 6-0 Vicryl to the surrounding articular cartilage, with sutures spaced at intervals of about 3 mm. To optimize tensioning, the corners can be anchored first. Place the knots on the articular cartilage rather than the periosteal flap. The final suture is omitted at this point, with the residual defect being at the area of easiest access for chondrocyte transplantation.
- Apply fibrin glue around the periphery of the periosteal flap's junction with the healthy articular cartilage, particularly between the sutures.
- Using a flexible angiocatheter, inject sterile saline into the residual opening to confirm a watertight seal; any leakage of saline should emanate only from the residual opening. Add sutures, fibrin glue, or both as needed.

- The chondrocytes are delivered in a vial that is sterile internally but not externally. The vial can be placed on a separate back table while the surgeon maintains sterile technique while resuspending and extracting the chondrocytes from the vial into a sterile angiocatheter.
- Through the residual opening under the periosteal flap, introduce the angiocatheter into the defect. The chondrocytes are evenly distributed with the surgeon gently injecting the suspension.
- Remove the angiocatheter and seal the residual aperture with a final suture and more fibrin glue.
- After the fibrin glue has cured, ankle range of motion confirms that the periosteal flap is stable.
- Stabilize the ankle joint with repair of the ligaments or osteotomy, depending on the particular approach.
- ACI has not been perfected for shoulder lesions of the talus. However, as for the femoral trochlea, a carefully executed suture pattern can allow the periosteum to be draped over a shoulder lesion to recreate, at least to some degree, the physiologic contour of the talus. With the periosteum first tensioned at the shoulder and secondarily on the dorsal and mediolateral aspects of the talus, ACI can be effective for select talar shoulder OLTs.

Technique with Matrix-Induced Autologous Chondrocytes Implantation

- The technique with matrix-induced chondrocytes requires no further preparation after the size of the defect is measured. The matrix is stable and can be fixed directly to the OLT.
- Take care when removing the transplant from the transport container. In particular, avoid squeezing the transplant (**TECH FIG 2A,B**).
- Cut the transplant according to the size of the defect. Some companies provide special punches for this step. The size of the transplant should meet exactly the size of the defect. Preparing the transplant 2 mm larger, as recommended for the periosteal flap, can lead to overlaying edges and a lack of stability.

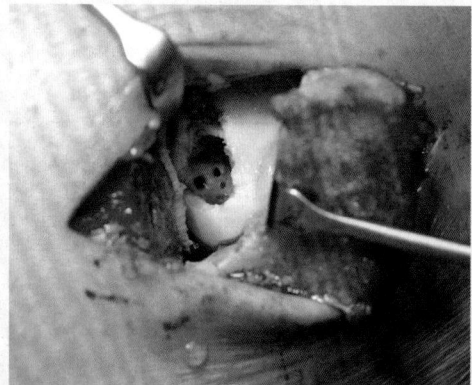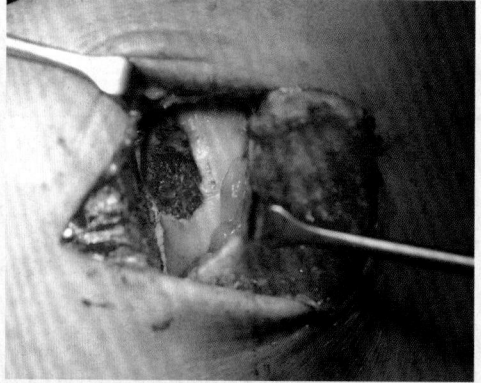

TECH FIG 2 A. Traumatic osteochondral lesion at the medial talar dome after removing the unstable cartilage and the subchondral cyst. The sclerotic wall of the cyst shows several drill holes. **B.** Defect filled with autologous bone graft. *(continued)*

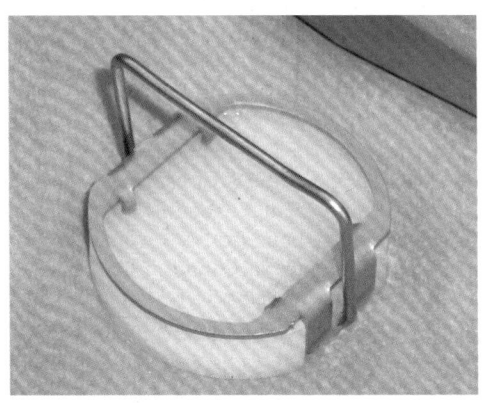
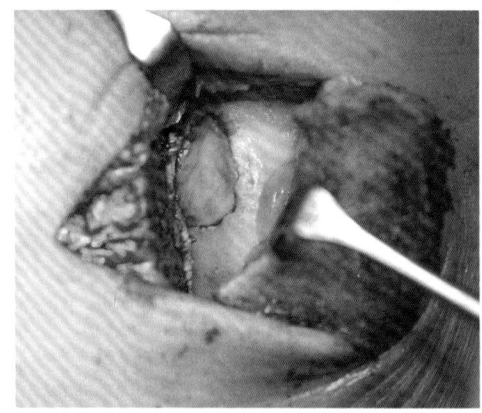

C   D

TECH FIG 2 *(continued)* **C.** Container with the matrix-induced chondrocytes, ready for transplantation. **D.** Matrix-induced chondrocytes transplanted into the defect and fixed with fibrin glue.

- Place the transplant into the defect. A first fixation happens due to adhesion forces. The edge can then be stabilized with 6-0 sutures and fibrin glue **(TECH FIG 2C,D)**.
- Check the transplant for stability by carefully moving the ankle joint into dorsiflexion and plantarflexion. We recommend that postoperative mobilization be limited so that the transplant is always covered at least partially by the tibial plafond to prevent shear forces. The optimal postoperative range of motion can be checked in this step.
- Insert one intra-articular tube before closing the wound. Stabilize the ankle joint with repair of the ligaments or osteotomy, depending on the particular approach.

TECHNIQUES

Pearls and Pitfalls

Indications and Planning	• Address associated pathology. • Generalized osteoarthritis or inflammatory arthritis is a contraindication. • Absence of clinical instability • Intact cartilage at the corresponding tibial side • The extent of cartilaginous detachment is often underestimated on MRI, whereas the bony reaction tends to be overestimated. • OLTs with subchondral cysts respond poorly to drilling or microfracturing. In these cases, ACI or MACI can be considered as a primary procedure. • ACI and MACI are *not* indicated in the face of diffuse ankle arthritis; these procedures are intended for focal defects only.
Harvesting	• Take extreme care when harvesting the chondrocytes from the ankle or ipsilateral knee joint. • If not completely destroyed, the detached cartilage can be harvested. • Ensure that the cool chain for transport is appropriate.
Cultivation	• This service is provided by several companies. They provide the medium for harvesting the chondrocytes and, in some cases, special tools for harvesting and transplantation.
Transplantation	• Be careful to prepare the transplant large enough. • Adequate exposure is mandatory for ACI or MACI. This often requires a malleolar osteotomy. • Intraoperative radiographs should be taken before performing an osteotomy and after the osteosynthesis. The osteotomy should be adequate to gain sufficient access to the OLT. • Do not squeeze the transplant (MACI). • Be sure that the periosteal flap is watertight before injecting the chondrocytes (ACI).
Rehabilitation	• Follow the rehabilitation plan; it takes time for the graft to gain its final stability and strength. • "Too much, too fast" is the most common reason for failures

POSTOPERATIVE CARE

- After covering the wounds with sterile dressings, the ankle joint is stabilized with a dorsal splint.
- Immediately postoperatively, the patient should have 48 hours of bed rest. The ankle should not be moved and is fixed with a brace to avoid bleeding.
- Forty-eight hours postoperatively, drainage tubes are removed, and the joint is mobilized with continuous passive motion. Limitations can occur in large defects or extended ligament repair.
- During the first 6 weeks postoperatively, the patients are allowed partial weight bearing (10 kg) and mobilization without weight bearing including accompanying physiotherapy (similar to the postoperative scheme in complex ankle fractures with open reduction and internal fixation).
- After 6 weeks, a gradual increase in joint loading is allowed (20 to 30 kg every 2 weeks) up to full body weight.
- After 12 weeks, full weight bearing in activities of daily life is allowed, including cycling with moderate resistance and swimming.
- After 6 months, increased athletic activities (eg, jogging and skating) can be considered. However, there is little experience in bringing patients with an ACI or MACI back to professional sports. In our anecdotal experience, we have seen most patients able to return to recreational sports.
- It is unclear whether patients can return to contact sports and sports that place high physical demands on the ankle joint. So far, there are no data available.

OUTCOMES

- Within the last years, there is increasing evidence that ACI improves pain and ankle function in OLTs. The majority of papers reports American Orthopaedic Foot & Ankle Society (AOFAS) scores between 85 and 90 points in a follow-up longer than 1 year.
- Brittberg et al[9] reported the results of their first 14 consecutive patients managed with ACI for the ankle. At an average follow-up of 45 months, 12 were considered improved, with 11 having good to excellent outcomes.
- Baums et al[5] found an improvement in the AOFAS ankle score from 43.5 to 88.4 in a prospective study of 12 patients.
- Giannini et al[23] reported an average AOFAS hindfoot–ankle score improvement from 26 points to 91 points at a mean follow-up of 26 months. Histologic analysis of biopsies obtained at 12 months suggested hyaline cartilage in all eight specimens.
- In another series, Giannini et al[24] demonstrated no statistically significant difference in 16 patients undergoing ACI with chondrocytes cultured from the detached OLT fragment compared to 7 patients undergoing ACI with chondrocytes harvested from the patient's ipsilateral knee. In both groups, the average AOFAS hindfoot–ankle score improved from 54 points to about 89 or 90 points. Histologic appearance, expression of specific cartilage markers, cell viability, cell proliferation in culture, and redifferentiation were favorable, and the morphologic and molecular characters of the cultured chondrocytes from the detached fragment were similar to those of physiologic hyaline cartilage.[23]
- The first studies with a follow-up from 5 to 10 years report an AOFAS score of 78 to 90 points.[36,37,46]

- The size of the lesion and patient's age seem to be the most relevant influential factors for the outcome.[38]
- By culturing the chondrocytes from the detached chondral fragment, donor site morbidity can be avoided.[24] However, by taking small chips of cartilage from an unloaded area of the knee, the risk of donor site problems should be significantly lower, as reported for harvesting osteochondral grafts from the ipsilateral knee joint.[49]
- MRI imaging after ACI can be challenging, edema can be found more than 12 months after implantation, especially in extended bone grafts. Incomplete integration of bone graft, nonintact subchondral lamina, high signal intensity, and extended edema were found to correlate with worse clinical functional outcomes.[10]
- Improvement of results can continue for several years.[4,46]

COMPLICATIONS

- In rare cases, the harvested chondrocytes are not suitable for culture. Typical causes are dead cells or contamination. In this case, the physician is informed by the laboratory that cultures the cartilage cells. One possibility is to do another arthroscopy to get cartilage cells; however, other treatment options like OATS or allograft can be considered.
- Delayed union in the malleolar osteotomy: Provided progression toward healing, even if very gradual, is observed on serial radiographs, our experience has been that the osteotomies eventually heal without complications. However, prompt revision open reduction and internal fixation with bone grafting is warranted if progression toward healing is not noted to limit the risk of displacement of the osteotomy.
- Failure of the transplanted tissue includes detachment, delamination, or ossification. Especially in the periosteal flap technique, ossification is a common cause of failure.[43] Ossification in the MACI technique has not yet been reported.
- Resorption of the subchondral bone graft in stage V lesions treated using the sandwich technique can lead to a graft failure.
- Hypertrophy: Fibrous tissue may form at the graft–host articular junction or within the ankle, causing impingement, and can be effectively débrided to relieve symptoms. ACI in particular is subject to fibrillation or hypertrophy, and arthroscopic débridement, in select cases, is essential to remove mechanical symptoms and avoid delamination of the graft.[9]
- The source of pain from an OLT remains ill defined, and the success of cartilage resurfacing procedures is certainly not 100%. Therefore, even without any obvious complication, pain may persist.
- If the clinical outcome is not satisfactory and follow-up imaging studies suggest graft compromise, ankle arthroscopy is warranted. Although failure of graft incorporation or delamination of the resurfaced articular segment is perhaps irreversible, not all persistent symptoms are necessarily due to such phenomena. Second-look arthroscopy may demonstrate that the cartilage resurfacing procedure was successful but was inadequate to resurface what proved to be a larger area of diseased talus than originally identified.
- In ACI for which the cartilage cells are harvested from the knee, there is a risk of persistent knee symptoms. The reported prevalence of persistent knee symptoms ranges from

less than 10%[23,31,54] to 50%.[49] It is important to educate patients about this risk preoperatively. Because Giannini et al[24] has demonstrated no statistically significant difference between chondrocytes cultured from the detached OLT fragment versus chondrocytes harvested from the patient's ipsilateral knee, we always harvest chondrocytes from the ankle joint to minimize the risk of donor site problems.[5] Based on our extended anecdotal experience doing so, we have seen no disadvantage with this concept.

- General surgical complications such as deep venous thrombosis, wound healing problems, or infection are also possible.

REFERENCES

1. Al-Shaikh RA, Chou LB, Mann JA, et al. Autologous osteochondral grafting for talar cartilage defects. Foot Ankle Int 2002;23: 381–389.
2. Barnes CJ, Ferkel RD. Arthroscopic debridement and drilling of osteochondral lesions of the talus. Foot Ankle Clin 2003;8:243–257.
3. Bartlett W, Skinner JA, Gooding CR, et al. Autologous chondrocyte implantation versus matrix-induced autologous chondrocyte implantation for osteochondral defects of the knee: a prospective, randomised study. J Bone Joint Surg Br 2005;87(5):640–645.
4. Battaglia M, Vannini F, Buda R, et al. Arthroscopic autologous chondrocyte implantation in osteochondral lesions of the talus: mid-term T2-mapping MRI evaluation. Knee Surg Sports Traumatol Arthrosc 2011;19:1376–1384.
5. Baums MH, Heidrich G, Schultz W, et al. Autologous chondrocyte transplantation for treating cartilage defects of the talus. J Bone Joint Surg Am 2006;88(2):303–308.
6. Becher C, Thermann H. Results of microfracture in the treatment of articular cartilage defects of the talus. Foot Ankle Int 2005;26: 583–589.
7. Benthien RA, Sullivan RJ, Aronow MS. Adolescent osteochondral lesion of the talus. Ankle arthroscopy in pediatric patients. Foot Ankle Clin 2002;7:651–667.
8. Berndt AL, Harty M. Transchondral fractures (osteochondritis dissecans) of the talus. J Bone Joint Surg Am 1959;41-A:988–1020.
9. Brittberg M, Peterson L, Sjögren-Jansson E, et al. Articular cartilage engineering with autologous chondrocyte transplantation. A review of recent developments. J Bone Joint Surg Am 2003;85-A(suppl 3): 109–115.
10. Caumo F, Russo A, Faccioli N, et al. Autologous chondrocyte implantation: prospective MRI evaluation with clinical correlation. Radiol Med 2007;112:722–731.
11. Cole AA, Margulis A, Kuettner KE. Distinguishing ankle and knee articular cartilage. Foot Ankle Clin 2003;8:305–316.
12. Cuttica DJ, Smith WB, Hyer CF, et al. Osteochondral lesions of the talus: predictors of clinical outcome. Foot Ankle Int 2011;32: 1045–1051.
13. Dickhut A, Dexheimer V, Martin K, et al. Chondrogenesis of human mesenchymal stem cells by local transforming growth factor-beta delivery in a biphasic resorbable carrier. Tissue Eng Part A 2010;16:453–464.
14. DiGiovanni BF, Fraga CJ, Cohen BE, et al. Associated injuries found in chronic lateral ankle instability. Foot Ankle Int 2000;21:809–815.
15. Dipaola JD, Nelson DW, Colville MR. Characterizing osteochondral lesions by magnetic resonance imaging. Arthroscopy 1991;7: 101–104.
16. Easley ME, Scranton PE Jr. Osteochondral autologous transfer system. Foot Ankle Clin 2003;8:275–290.
17. Elias I, Jung JW, Raikin SM, et al. Osteochondral lesions of the talus: change in MRI findings over time in talar lesions without operative intervention and implications for staging systems. Foot Ankle Int 2006;27:157–166.
18. Elias I, Zoga AC, Morrison WB, et al. Osteochondral lesions of the talus: localization and morphologic data from 424 patients using a novel anatomical grid scheme. Foot Ankle Int 2007;28:154–161.
19. Erickson B, Fillingham Y, Hellman M, et al. Surgical management of large talar osteochondral defects using autologous chondrocyte implantation. Foot Ankle Surg 2018;24(2):131–136.
20. Feeney S, Rees S, Tagoe M. Tricortical calcaneal bone graft and management of the donor site. J Foot Ankle Surg 2007;46:80–85.
21. Ferkel RD, Sgaglione NA. Arthroscopic treatment of osteochondral lesions of the talus: long-term results. Orthop Trans 1993;17:1011.
22. Geideman W, Early JS, Brodsky J. Clinical results of harvesting autogenous cancellous graft from the ipsilateral proximal tibia for use in foot and ankle surgery. Foot Ankle Int 2004;25:451–455.
23. Giannini S, Buda R, Grigolo B, et al. Autologous chondrocyte transplantation in osteochondral lesions of the ankle joint. Foot Ankle Int 2001;22:513–517.
24. Giannini S, Buda R, Grigolo B, et al. The detached osteochondral fragment as a source of cells for autologous chondrocyte implantation (ACI) in the ankle joint. Osteoarthritis Cartilage 2005;13: 601–607.
25. Giannini S, Buda R, Vannini F, et al. One-step bone marrow-derived cell transplantation in talar osteochondral lesions. Clin Orthop Relat Res 2009;467:3307–3320.
26. Giannini S, Vannini F. Operative treatment of osteochondral lesions of the talar dome: current concepts review. Foot Ankle Int 2004;25:168–175.
27. Gottschalk O, Altenberger S, Baumbach S, et al. Functional medium-term results after autologous matrix-induced chondrogenesis for osteochondral lesions of the talus: a 5-year prospective cohort study. J Foot Ankle Surg 2017;56(5):930–936.
28. Gould N. Repair of lateral ligament of ankle. Foot Ankle 1987;8: 55–58.
29. Gross AE, Agnidis Z, Hutchison CR. Osteochondral defects of the talus treated with fresh osteochondral allograft transplantation. Foot Ankle Int 2001;22:385–391.
30. Guhl JF. Arthroscopic treatment of osteochondritis dissecans. Clin Orthop Relat Res 1982;(167):65–74.
31. Hangody L. The mosaicplasty technique for osteochondral lesions of the talus. Foot Ankle Clin 2003;8:259–273.
32. Hepple S, Winson IG, Glew D. Osteochondral lesions of the talus: a revised classification. Foot Ankle Int 1999;20:789–793.
33. Kelbérine F, Frank A. Arthroscopic treatment of osteochondral lesions of the talar dome: a retrospective study of 48 cases. Arthroscopy 1999;15:77–84.
34. Koch S, Kampen WU, Laprell H. Cartilage and bone morphology in osteochondritis dissecans. Knee Surg Sports Traumatol Arthrosc 1997;5:42–45.
35. Komenda GA, Ferkel RD. Arthroscopic findings associated with the unstable ankle. Foot Ankle Int 1999;20:708–713.
36. Kreulen C, Giza E, Walton J, et al. Seven-year follow-up of matrix-induced autologous implantation in talus articular defects. Foot Ankle Spec 2018;11(2):133–137.
37. Kwak SK, Kern BS, Ferkel RD, et al. Autologous chondrocyte implantation of the ankle: 2- to 10-year results. Am J Sports Med 2014;42(9):2156–2164.
38. Lee KT, Lee YK, Young KW, et al. Factors influencing result of autologous chondrocyte implantation in osteochondral lesion of the talus using second look arthroscopy. Scand J Med Sci Sports 2012;22(4):510–515.
39. Mandelbaum BR, Gerhardt MB, Peterson L. Autologous chondrocyte implantation of the talus. Arthroscopy 2003;19(suppl 1):129–137.
40. McCullough CJ, Venugopal V. Osteochondritis dissecans of the talus: the natural history. Clin Orthop Relat Res 1979;(144):264–268.
41. Muir D, Saltzman CL, Tochigi Y, et al. Talar dome access for osteochondral lesions. Am J Sports Med 2006;34:1457–1463.
42. Myerson MS, Neufeld SK, Uribe J. Fresh-frozen structural allografts in the foot and ankle. J Bone Joint Surg Am 2005;87(1):113–120.
43. Nehrer S, Spector M, Minas T. Histologic analysis of tissue after failed cartilage repair procedures. Clin Orthop Relat Res 1999;(365): 149–162.
44. Outerbridge RE. The etiology of chondromalacia patellae. J Bone Joint Surg Br 1961;43-B:752–757.
45. Oznur A. Medial malleolar window approach for osteochondral lesions of the talus. Foot Ankle Int 2001;22:841–842.

46. Pagliazzi G, Vannini F, Battaglia M, et al. Autologous chondrocyte implantation for talar osteochondral lesions: comparison between 5-year follow-up magnetic resonance imaging findings and 7-year follow-up clinical results. J Foot Ankle Surg 2018;57(2):221–225.

47. Radke S, Vispo-Seara J, Walther M, et al. Osteochondral lesions of the talus—indications for MRI with a contrast agent [in German]. Z Orthop Ihre Grenzgeb 2004;142:618–624.

48. Raikin SM, Brislin K. Local bone graft harvested from the distal tibia or calcaneus for surgery of the foot and ankle. Foot Ankle Int 2005;26:449–453.

49. Reddy S, Pedowitz DI, Parekh SG, et al. The morbidity associated with osteochondral harvest from asymptomatic knees for the treatment of osteochondral lesions of the talus. Am J Sports Med 2007;35: 80–85.

50. Rothrauff BB, Murawski CD, Angthong C, et al. Scaffold-based therapies: proceedings of the International Consensus Meeting on Cartilage Repair of the Ankle. Foot Ankle Int 2018;39(suppl 1):41S–47S.

51. Sammarco GJ, Makwana NK. Treatment of talar osteochondral lesions using local osteochondral graft. Foot Ankle Int 2002;23: 693–698.

52. Schuman L, Struijs PA, van Dijk CN. Arthroscopic treatment for osteochondral defects of the talus. Results at follow-up at 2 to 11 years. J Bone Joint Surg Br 2002;84(3):364–368.

53. Scranton PE. Osteochondral lesions of the talus. In: Nunley JA, Pfeffer GB, Sanders RW, et al, eds. Advanced Reconstruction Foot and Ankle. Rosemont, IL: American Academy of Orthopaedic Surgeons, 2004:261–266.

54. Scranton PE Jr, Frey CC, Feder KS. Outcome of osteochondral autograft transplantation for type-V cystic osteochondral lesions of the talus. J Bone Joint Surg Br 2006;88(5):614–619.

55. Shea MP, Manoli A II. Osteochondral lesions of the talar dome. Foot Ankle 1993;14:48–55.

56. Shearer C, Loomer R, Clement D. Nonoperatively managed stage 5 osteochondral talar lesions. Foot Ankle Int 2002;23:651–654.

57. Shimozono Y, Hurley ET, Nguyen JT, et al. Allograft compared with autograft in osteochondral transplantation for the treatment of osteochondral lesions of the talus. J Bone Joint Surg Am 2018;100(21): 1838–1844.

58. Shimozono Y, Yasui Y, Hurley ET, et al. Concentrated bone marrow aspirate may decrease postoperative cyst occurrence rate in autologous osteochondral transplantation for osteochondral lesions of the talus. Arthroscopy 2019;35(1):99–105.

59. Tochigi Y, Amendola A, Muir D, et al. Surgical approach for centrolateral talar osteochondral lesions with an anterolateral osteotomy. Foot Ankle Int 2002;23:1038–1039.

60. Toth AP, Easley ME. Ankle chondral injuries and repair. Foot Ankle Clin 2000;5:799–840.

61. Walther M, Martin K. Scaffold based reconstruction of focal full thickness talar cartilage defects. Clin Res Foot Ankle 2013;1:115.

62. Wester JU, Jensen IE, Rasmussen F, et al. Osteochondral lesions of the talar dome in children. A 24 (7–36) year follow-up of 13 cases. Acta Orthop Scand 1994;65:110–112.

63. Whittaker JP, Smith G, Makwana N, et al. Early results of autologous chondrocyte implantation in the talus. J Bone Joint Surg Br 2005;87(2):179–183.

64. Wiewiorski M, Leumann A, Buettner O, et al. Autologous matrix-induced chondrogenesis aided reconstruction of a large focal osteochondral lesion of the talus. Arch Orthop Trauma Surg 2011;131:293–296.

65. Young KW, Deland JT, Lee KT, et al. Medial approaches to osteochondral lesion of the talus without medial malleolar osteotomy. Knee Surg Sports Traumatol Arthrosc 2010;18:634–637.

66. Zheng MH, Willers C, Kirilak L, et al. Matrix-induced autologous chondrocyte implantation (MACI): biological and histological assessment. Tissue Eng 2007;13:737–746.

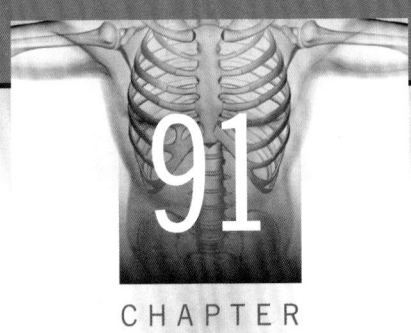

Arthroscopic Brostrom Lateral Ankle Ligament Repair

Jorge I. Acevedo, Peter Mangone, and Rishin J. Kadakia

DEFINITION

- Ankle sprains are one of the most common musculoskeletal injuries seen in emergency rooms and outpatient clinics.
- Around 85% of all ankle sprains are inversion injuries resulting in damage to the lateral ankle ligament complex.[4,11]
- Lateral ligament injury can lead to chronic pain and instability in approximately 20% to 40% of patients who sustain an ankle sprain.[5,6,8]

ANATOMY

- The lateral ankle ligament complex consists of the anterior talofibular ligament (ATFL), calcaneofibular ligament (CFL), and the posterior talofibular ligament (PTFL).
- The ATFL is the weakest component of the lateral ligament complex and thus is most frequently injured.[1,7]
- The ATFL originates approximately 10 to 14 mm superior and anterior from the tip of the fibula and attaches to the lateral talar neck.[9]
- The CFL originates approximately 5 to 9 mm superior and anterior from the tip of the fibula and travels deep to the peroneal tendons to attach to the lateral calcaneal wall.[9]
- The PTFL is the strongest ligament and travels from the posterior aspect of the distal fibula to the talar body; it is rarely torn in lateral ligament injuries.
- The intermediate branch of the superficial peroneal nerve (SPN) is found an average distance of 32 mm from the center of the ATFL origin, and this nerve travels anteriorly.[8]

PATHOGENESIS

- Lateral ligament injuries are typically the result of an inversion force to the plantarflexed ankle.
- The ATFL is most frequently injured as it is under the most tension in plantarflexion, and the CFL is the second most commonly injury ligament. Furthermore, the ATFL is the weakest of the three ligaments.
- Patients with generalized ligamentous laxity or hindfoot or ankle varus deformity may be predisposed to lateral ligament injuries.

NATURAL HISTORY

- Most ankle sprains recover with appropriate conservative care. Patients routinely present with acute-onset swelling and pain with weight bearing after an injury. The swelling and pain frequently subside over the course of a week.
- Physical therapy and supportive ankle braces can be used once the patient recovers from the immediate injury,

and these conservative modalities often lead to complete resolution of symptoms over the course of several weeks.
- Some patients develop chronic and debilitating lateral ankle pain and/or ankle instability that does not respond to conservative care.

PATIENT HISTORY AND PHYSICAL FINDINGS

- Patients with chronic lateral ankle instability typically have a history of multiple inversion ankle injuries.
- In addition to lateral ankle pain, patients will endorse instability, imbalance, and sensations that their ankle gives out on them.
- The anterior drawer test specifically tests the integrity of the ATFL and should be performed on both limbs to have a normal comparison.
  - This physical exam maneuver is performed with the knee bent to 90 degrees and the ankle plantarflexed. The tibia must be stabilized, and the talus is then drawn anteriorly. The displacement is quantified and can be compared to the contralateral ankle. The endpoint should also be appreciated.
- A complete physical examination of the lower extremity is necessary with particular attention to certain aspects.
  - Standing alignment of the ankle and hindfoot must be assessed as patients with varus deformity may be at an increased risk of lateral ankle instability and deformity may need to be addressed at the time of the repair.
  - Ankle and subtalar joint range of motion must be examined and compared to the contralateral extremity to examine for any soft tissue impingement or mechanical blocks.
  - Peroneal tendons must be evaluated as peroneal pathology can present with or be confused for lateral ligament injuries.
  - Chronic ankle instability and multiple sprains can lead to intra-articular pathology such as osteochondral lesions or loose bodies, which can present as joint line pain or mechanical pain.

IMAGING AND OTHER DIAGNOSTIC STUDIES

- Imaging studies begin with standard anteroposterior, lateral, and mortise views of the ankle.
  - Although these radiographs are routinely normal, they must be obtained especially in patients with tenderness to rule out a fracture (eg, lateral malleolus, lateral talar process).
- Magnetic resonance imaging without contrast is routinely obtained to evaluate the lateral ankle ligaments and can

provide useful information on other possible etiologies of lateral ankle pain such as an osteochondral lesion of the talus (OLT) or peroneal tendon tears.

- Computed tomography (CT) scans are rarely used except in cases where a fracture is suspected but not adequately visualized on imaging. CT can also help appreciate any periarticular cysts or OLTs.
- Stress radiographs can also be used to diagnose instability. Anterior drawer examination and talar tilt can be obtained using fluoroscopy but is often not tolerated acutely by the patient.

DIFFERENTIAL DIAGNOSIS

- OLT
- Peroneal tendon tear or subluxation
- Syndesmotic injury
- Lateral process talus fracture
- Fifth metatarsal base fracture
- Ankle impingement
- Lateral malleolus fracture

NONOPERATIVE MANAGEMENT

- Nonoperative management should be the first line treatment for all patients presenting with an ankle sprain or chronic instability.
- A consistent course of physical therapy with emphasis on proprioception and strengthening of the dynamic stabilizing muscles surrounding the ankle can completely alleviate symptoms in many cases.
- Ankle-stabilizing orthosis braces can provide a sense of stability for patients especially in situations where patients experience pain and instability only with certain activities.

SURGICAL MANAGEMENT

- Surgical treatment is warranted in cases of chronic lateral ligament instability that has failed the appropriate conservative treatment modalities.

Preoperative Planning

- All appropriate clinical data and imaging studies must be reviewed to ensure that the correct indications are present and that other pathology is not present that needs to be addressed at the time of surgery as well.
- Patients must be extensively counseled on the risks of the surgery and the postoperative protocol.

Positioning

- The procedure can be performed using either general or regional anesthesia depending on surgeon preference and certain patient characteristics.
- The patient is placed in the supine position with a bump under the ipsilateral hip.
- A distraction apparatus can be attached but is based on surgeon preference. It is important to note that distraction must be removed prior to tying down the repair.
- A thigh high tourniquet is placed, and the leg is prepped and draped per operating room protocol.

Approach

- Standard anteromedial and anterolateral portals are used for this procedure and a small ancillary incision to pass and tie sutures.
- Anatomic "safe zone" for suture passing **(FIG 1)**
  - To limit damage to surrounding nerves/tendons, the authors recommend mapping out the safe zone for percutaneous suture passing based on surrounding anatomy.
  - The anterior distal border of the distal fibula, the superior border of the peroneal tendons, and the path of the intermediate branch of the SPN are drawn. The "safe zone" for suture passing is 1.5 cm distal to the anterior border of the fibula within the zone in order to capture the inferior extensor retinaculum (IER) in the repair.[1-3]

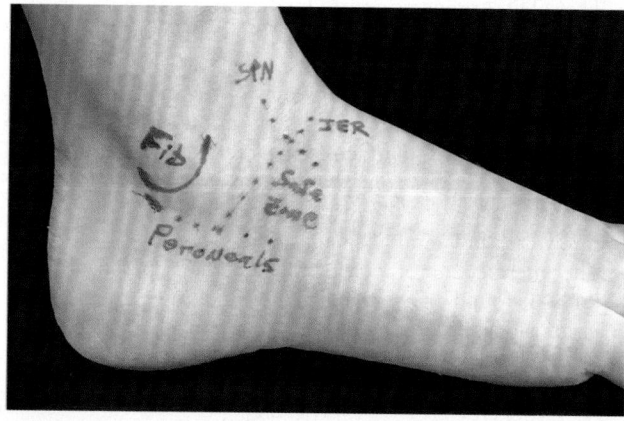

FIG 1 Anatomic "safe zone". The anatomic safe zone depicts the areas for passing suture. *SPN*, superficial peroneal nerve; *IER*, inferior extensor retinaculum; *Fib*, fibula.

DIAGNOSTIC ARTHROSCOPY

- A diagnostic arthroscopic evaluation of the ankle joint is first performed using the standard anteromedial and anterolateral portals.
- At this time, any other intra-articular pathology (anterior impingement, OLT, etc.) can be addressed.
- It is imperative to perform a thorough débridement of the lateral gutter to ensure adequate visualization of the fibula for anchor placement and to remove any soft tissue that may cause impingement, which can commonly be seen in patients with chronic lateral ankle instability.
- The anterior border of the fibula is carefully denuded with an arthroscopic shaver in preparation for anchor placement.

PLACEMENT OF FIRST ANCHOR

- The arthroscope is kept in the anteromedial portal, and the drill for the first suture anchor is passed through the anterolateral portal.
- The site for insertion is approximately 1 cm superior and anterior to the distal tip of the fibula and angled slightly cephalad **(TECH FIG 1A)**.
- After drilling, the anchor is placed into the fibula through the anterolateral portal, and the sutures will be exiting through this portal **(TECH FIG 1B)**.
- The sutures from this anchor are then passed individually using a sharp suture passer from inside the joint out through the skin **(TECH FIG 1C)**.
- It is imperative to pass the sutures through the safe zone described earlier and at least 1.5 cm distal to the tip of the fibula to capture the IER as part of the repair.
- The first suture is passed just superior to the peroneal tendons, and the second suture is passed 1 cm dorsal and anterior to the first suture.

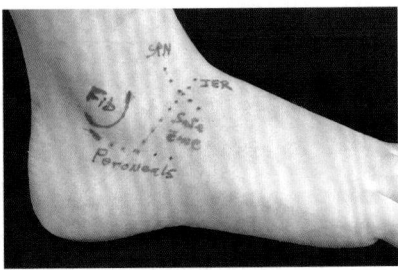

A

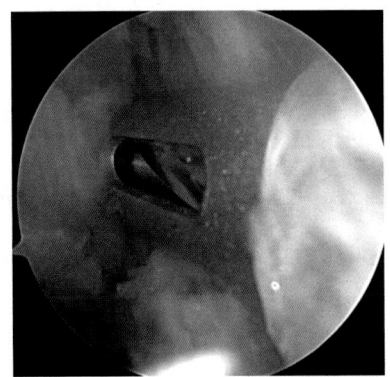

B

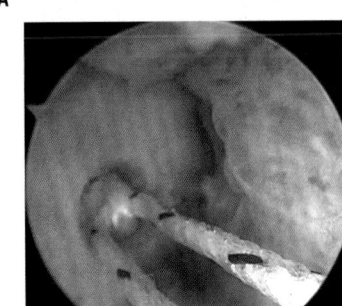

C

TECH FIG 1 A. Site for first anchor is 1 cm superior and anterior to the distal tip of the fibula. **B.** First anchor placement. **C.** The suture passer is placed intra-articular and passed through the skin in the safe zone. The first suture is passed just superior to the peroneal tendons.

PLACEMENT OF SECOND ANCHOR

- The arthroscope is kept in the anteromedial portal, and the drill is again inserted through the anterolateral portal for second anchor placement.
- The second anchor is inserted approximately 1 cm above the first anchor along the anterior border of the fibula. It is important to ensure that this anchor is placed below the superior border of the talar dome.
- The sutures are then passed in a similar fashion as earlier through the skin in the marked safe zone.
- The first suture limb is passed 1 cm anterior to the second suture from the first anchor along the arc of the IER **(TECH FIG 2)**.
- The second suture limb is passed 1 cm anterior and dorsal to the second suture.

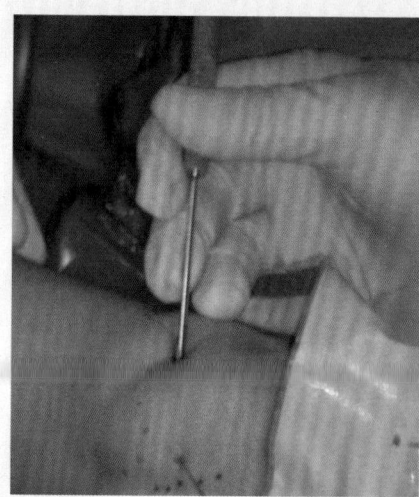

TECH FIG 2 The first suture limb has been passed through the safe zone. The second limb is being passed anterior to the first limb along the arc of the IER.

SUTURE TYING TO REPAIR THE LATERAL LIGAMENT COMPLEX

- A 3- to 4-mm skin incision is made between the two sets of sutures from the two anchors **(TECH FIG 3)**.
  - The sutures are all then passed through this skin incision subcutaneously with the assistance of a small probe.
  - Care is taken to keep the sutures from each anchor separate for tying purposes.
- The incision can be made larger, and blunt dissection is used if there is concern for nerve entrapment when passing the sutures.
- Prior to tying the sutures, it is important to remember to remove any distraction, and the ankle is held in eversion and neutral dorsiflexion while tying.
- The imbrication can be visualized with the arthroscope either during suture tying or after it is completed.

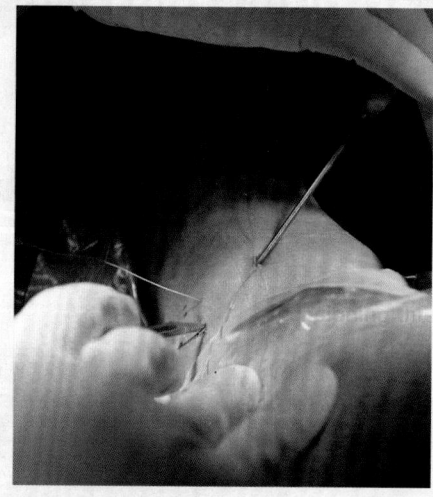

TECH FIG 3 Subcutaneous incision for suture passing.

CONFIRMATION OF STABILITY AND CLOSURE

- The ankle is then tested for stability using the anterior drawer test. It is compared to the stability preoperatively; thus, it is important to perform this exam at the start of the case.
- If the arthroscopic repair is not sufficient, the procedure can very easily be converted to an open procedure, and direct inspection/revision of the repair can be performed.
- Any augmentation of repair (internal brace, etc.) can be performed at this time.

- Arthroscopic equipment is removed once satisfactory repair is achieved, and the wounds are irrigated with normal saline.
- Arthroscopic portals and incisions for suture tying are closed with 3-0 nylon.
- Sterile dressings are applied, the tourniquet is released, and a well-padded posterior slab splint is applied.

Pearls and Pitfalls

Portal Placement	• Mark the "safe zone" and the intermediate branch of the SPN to avoid injury to these structures.
Anchor Placement	• Ensure the anchor is centered in the mediolateral plane prior to placing the anchor. • Fluoroscopy can be used to ensure appropriate anchor placement and angulation if there is a concern.
Suture Tying	• Release distraction prior to tying the sutures to ensure appropriate repair and tension on the repair. • When tying, avoid puckering of the skin by dissecting off subcutaneous tissue under the incision.

POSTOPERATIVE CARE

• Patients are placed into a splint postoperatively and kept non–weight bearing for approximately 10 to 14 days. The patient then returns to clinic for a wound check and suture removal.

• The patient is transitioned into a CAM boot at the first appointment and allowed to begin partial weight bearing (50%). Weight bearing is progressed gradually over the course of several weeks. Weight bearing may start at a later date depending on any other concomitant procedures performed.

• Gentle range of motion is started with only plantarflexion and dorsiflexion exercises. Any inversion or eversion is avoided until approximately 6 to 8 weeks postoperatively.

• Physical therapy is initiated at approximately 6 to 8 weeks postoperatively, and gentle inversion/eversion is started at this time in addition to gait training and strengthening.

• The patient begins to transition out of the boot into regular shoes at around 6 to 8 weeks as physical therapy begins. A lace-up brace is recommended for up to 3 months postoperatively, but many patients wear the brace for up to a year postoperatively.

OUTCOMES

• There are a few variations in technique with regard to arthroscopic lateral ligament repair. The technique described in this text uses two standard arthroscopy portals and a small incision for knot tying.[1-3] Other variations included arthroscopy-assisted techniques with larger incisions and all-inside techniques using accessory portals.

• There are several studies reporting good outcomes with the specific technique described in this chapter.

• Acevedo et al[3] first published on this technique in 2011 on a cohort of 24 patients and reported a 96% satisfaction rate at around 1 year of follow-up.

• Nery et al[10] reported on 26 patients with chronic ankle instability who underwent arthroscopic lateral ligament repair with a similar technique described in this study. With a mean follow-up of 27 months, they demonstrated a mean American Orthopaedic Foot & Ankle Society score of 90, an improvement of 32 points.

• Acevedo et al[1] reported on a cohort of 73 patients who underwent arthroscopic lateral ligament repair, the largest sample size to date. With a mean follow-up of 28 months, the patients demonstrate improvement in Karlsson-Peterson scores from 28.3 to 90.2. Only one patient reported recurrent instability, and only four patients were dissatisfied.

COMPLICATIONS

• Injury to surrounding structures during portal placement
  • Intermediate branch of SPN
  • Sural nerve
  • Peroneal tendons
• Infection
• Wound dehiscence
• Skin irritation from suture materials/anchors
• Recurrent instability

REFERENCES

1. Acevedo JI, Mangone PG. Ankle instability and arthroscopic lateral ligament repair. Foot Ankle Clin 2015;20(1):59–69.
2. Acevedo JI, Mangone PG. Arthroscopic Brostrom technique. Foot Ankle Int 2015;36(4):465–473.
3. Acevedo JI, Mangone PG. Arthroscopic lateral ankle ligament reconstruction. Tech Foot Ankle Surg 2011;10(3):111–116.
4. Ferran NA, Maffuli N. Epidemiology of sprains of the lateral ankle ligament complex. Foot Ankle Clin 2006;11(3):659–662.
5. Freeman MA, Dean MR, Hanham IW. The etiology and prevention of functional instability of the foot. J Bone Joint Surg Br 1965;47(4):678–685.
6. Gribble PA, Bleakley CM, Caulfield BM, et al. 2016 consensus statement of the International Ankle Consortium: prevalence, impact and long-term consequences of lateral ankle sprains. Br J Sports Med 2016;50(24):1493–1495.
7. Hossain M, Thomas R. Ankle instability: presentation and management. Orthopaed Trauma 2015;29(2):145–151.
8. Jorge JT, Gomes TM, Oliva XM. An anatomical study about the arthroscopic repair of the lateral ligament of the ankle. Foot Ankle Surg 2018;24(2):143–148.
9. Matsui K, Takao M, Tochigi Y, et al. Anatomy of anterior talofibular ligament and calcaneofibular ligament for minimally invasive surgery: a systematic review. Knee Surg Sports Traumatol Arthrosc 2017;25(6):1892–1902.
10. Nery C, Fonseca L, Raduan F, et al. Prospective study of the "inside-out" arthroscopic ankle ligament technique: preliminary result. Foot Ankle Surg 2018;24(4):320–325.
11. Shakked RJ, Karnovsky S, Drakos MC. Operative treatment of lateral ligament instability. Curr Rev Musculoskeletal Med 2017;10(1):113–121.

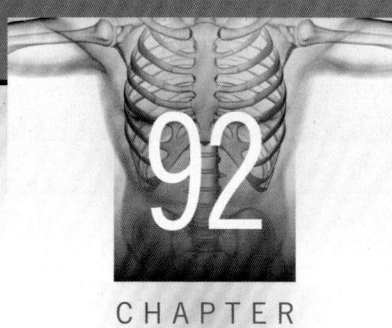

Modified Brostrom and Brostrom-Evans Procedures

Paul J. Hecht, Justin S. Cummins, Dean C. Taylor, and Mark E. Easley

DEFINITION

- Lateral ankle injuries are among the most common musculoskeletal injuries in the athletic population.
- Rates as high as 7 per 1000 person-years have been reported in the general population.
- From 10% to 20% of sprains progress to some kind of chronic symptoms.
- Determining whether the patient's instability is functional (ie, subjective giving way) or mechanical (ie, motion beyond the normal physiologic limits) is important for formulating treatment recommendations.

ANATOMY

- The lateral ankle ligament complex consists of the anterior talofibular ligament (ATFL), calcaneofibular ligament (CFL), and posterior talofibular ligament.
- The ATFL originates from the anterior aspect of the distal fibula and inserts on the lateral aspect of the talar neck. It is often ill defined and, in the chronically sprained ankle, may be manifest as a capsular expansion.
- The ATFL limits anterior translation of the talus with the ankle in neutral and becomes the primary restraint to inversion when the ankle is plantarflexed.
- The CFL originates from the distal tip of the fibula and inserts on the lateral wall of the calcaneus (FIG 1).
  - The CFL measures 4 to 6 mm in diameter and 13 mm in length and is directed posteriorly 10 to 45 degrees from the tip of the fibula.
  - The CFL functions to resist inversion with the ankle in neutral.

- The anterior margin of the talus is wider than the posterior margin, which makes the ankle more susceptible to inversion injuries while in plantarflexion.
- The peroneal tendons provide dynamic stability to the ankle joint.

PATHOGENESIS

- An inversion force with the ankle in plantarflexion is the most common mechanism of injury.
- The ATFL typically is the first ligament injured, followed by the CFL.
- Ligament ruptures are most commonly midsubstance tears or avulsions off of the talus.

NATURAL HISTORY

- Despite a relatively high incidence of lateral ankle injuries, most patients do well with nonoperative management.
- Patients are at increased risk for recurrent lateral ankle sprains after sustaining the initial injury and failing to rehabilitate completely.
- Chronic lateral instability may lead to progressive loss of function and osteoarthritic changes of the ankle.

PATIENT HISTORY AND PHYSICAL FINDINGS

- Patients with chronic ankle instability frequently present with pain as well as complaints of multiple sprains caused by minor provocation.
- Duration of symptoms, the type of incidents that cause sprains, the need for functional bracing, and previous treatments are important for determining treatment recommendations.

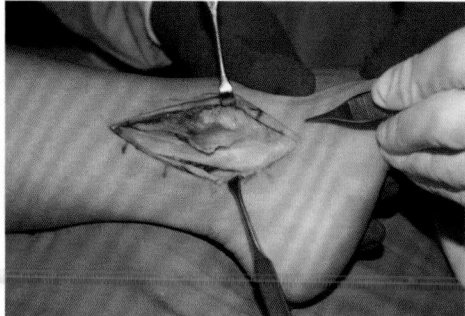
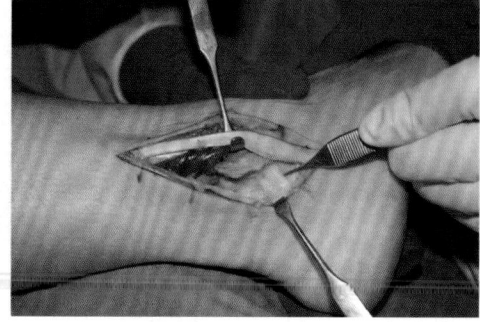

A   B

FIG 1 The CFL is directly deep to the peroneal tendons as demonstrated by this surgery to repair peroneal tendon dislocation. **A.** Peroneal tendons in their anatomic location. **B.** CFL identified when peroneal tendons are retracted.

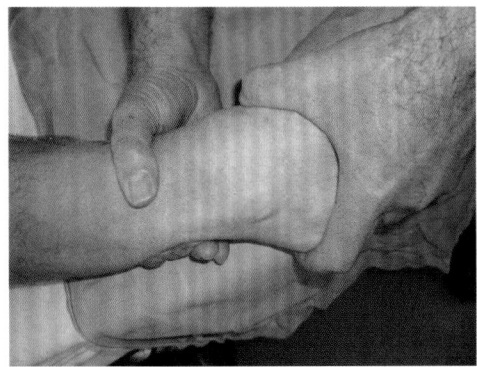

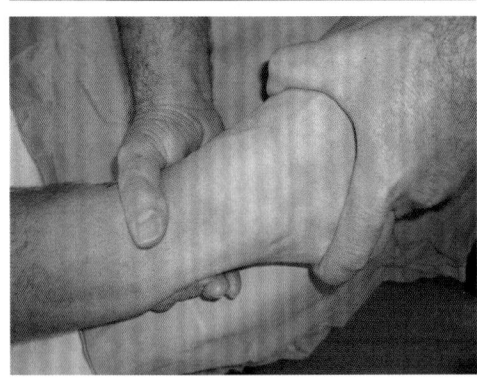

FIG 2 Anterior drawer test. **A.** Ankle reduced. **B.** Anterior subluxation.

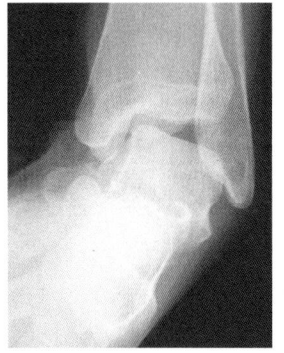
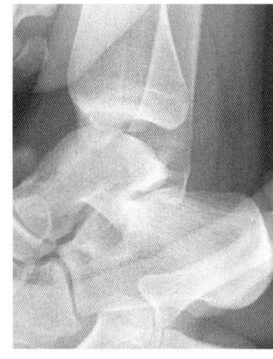

FIG 3 Radiographic stress tests. **A.** Positive talar tilt test. **B.** Positive anterior drawer test.

- If pain is present between episodes of instability, other lesions about the ankle should also be considered.
- An anterior drawer test with a bony end point that is distinctly different from that of the contralateral ankle is considered markedly positive.
- Physical examination techniques include the following:
  - Palpation. Palpate the ATFL, CFL, syndesmosis, medial and lateral malleoli, peroneal tendons, base of the fifth metatarsal, and anterior process of the calcaneus.
  - Anterior drawer test (**FIG 2**). The ankle is held in plantarflexion, and the talus is translated forward relative to the tibia. With intact medial structures, the displacement is rotatory. Translation of 5 mm more than the contralateral ankle or absolute translation of 9 to 10 mm is a positive test and suggests an incompetent ATFL. Grading ATFL injuries: I, stretching; II, partial tearing; III, complete rupture; most useful in the acute setting to determine which structures are injured.
  - Talar tilt. The heel is inverted with the ankle in neutral. Range of motion is compared to the contralateral ankle. Increased inversion is suggestive of a CFL injury.
  - Alignment. Assess the standing alignment of the hindfoot. Varus hindfoot alignment predisposes the ankle to inversion injury.

IMAGING AND OTHER DIAGNOSTIC STUDIES

- Standard radiographs should include standing anteroposterior, lateral, and mortise views to evaluate for anterior tibial marginal osteophytes, talar exostoses, osteochondral lesions of the talus, or intra-articular loose bodies.
- Talar tilt can be assessed with inversion stress mortise views of the ankle (**FIG 3A**).
  - Comparison views of the contralateral ankle should also be obtained.

- A talar tilt angle greater than 10 degrees, or 5 degrees greater than the contralateral ankle, is considered pathologic laxity.
- Anterior translation stress radiographs can be obtained by performing the anterior drawer test and shooting a lateral radiograph (**FIG 3B**).
  - Comparison stress views of the contralateral ankle should also be obtained.
  - Anterior translation 5 mm greater than the contralateral ankle, or an absolute value of greater than 9 mm, is suggestive of instability.
- Stress radiographs may be helpful, but physical examination remains the gold standard for evaluation of instability.
- Magnetic resonance imaging can be useful to evaluate the ligamentous injury as well as peroneal tendon pathology and suspected osteochondral injuries.

DIFFERENTIAL DIAGNOSIS

- Lateral process talar fracture
- Anterior process calcaneus fracture
- Base of the fifth metatarsal fracture
- Tarsal coalition
- Osteochondral lesion of the talus or tibia
- Subtalar instability
- Syndesmosis injury
- Neurapraxia of the superficial peroneal or sural nerve
- Peroneal tendon tear
- Peroneal instability
- Sinus tarsi syndrome
- Anterolateral ankle soft tissue impingement

NONOPERATIVE MANAGEMENT

- Physical therapy should be the initial treatment for patients with chronic instability.
  - Proprioceptive training and peroneal tendon strengthening are the most important features.
  - The duration of therapy varies based on strength deficiencies and the intensity of the program.
- External stabilization of the ankle with taping or bracing can be effective.
  - Taping provides tibiotalar stability but quickly deteriorates with activity.
  - Reusable braces provide similar stability but do not lose effectiveness with activity.
- Orthotic devices and shoe wear modification can also be used when foot or ankle malalignment contributes to the instability.

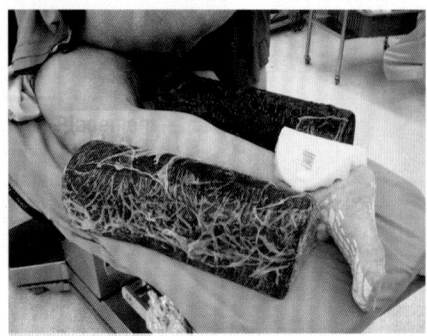
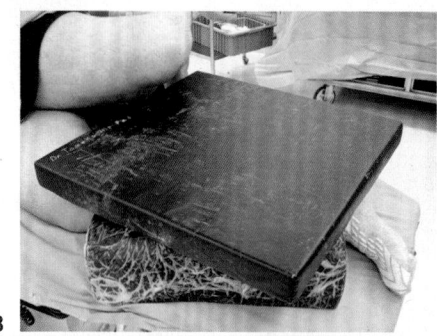
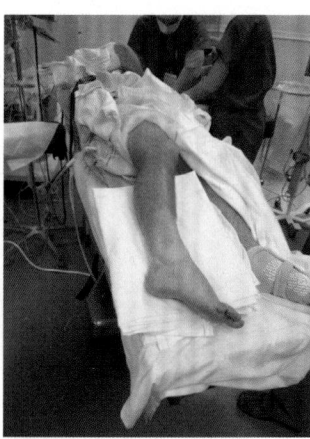

FIG 4 With the patient in the lateral decubitus position, the nonoperated extremity should be well padded. **A.** Nonoperated leg in a gel pad. **B.** With the nonoperated leg protected, a platform may be used to facilitate positioning of the operated leg. **C.** Alternatively, positioning in the lateral decubitus position, using a stack of folded sheets to serve as a rest for the operated leg.

SURGICAL MANAGEMENT

- If the patient fails 3 to 6 months of conservative treatment and has persistent signs and symptoms of functional and mechanical instability, he or she becomes a candidate for the modified Brostrom procedure or the modified Brostrom-Evans procedure, which is a combination of the modified Brostrom procedure and the Evans procedure, in which the anterior 50% of the peroneus brevis (PR) is tenodesed to the fibula.
- Indications for the Brostrom-Evans procedure
  - Athlete or patient in whom greater restraint against inversion is desired, such as football lineman who does not need as much hindfoot flexibility as a running back
  - Anatomic repair planned but greater than anticipated instability, particularly with inversion stress, and an intraoperative determination that more restraint to inversion is needed than can be afforded by the modified Brostrom procedure alone.
  - Lateral ankle instability in a patient with preexisting longitudinal split tear of the PR

Preoperative Planning

- The history must be considered. A relative contraindication for this anatomic repair is generalized ligamentous laxity as might be encountered in Ehlers-Danlos syndrome.
- Carefully review the physical examination. If a varus heel exists, a Dwyer-type calcaneal osteotomy should be considered.

- If an osteochondral lesion is present, the ligamentous reconstruction should be done in conjunction with arthroscopic or open treatment of the osteochondral defect.

Positioning

- The patient is placed in the lateral decubitus position with appropriate padding at bony prominences to avoid damage to subcutaneous structures **(FIG 4A,B)**.
- An operative platform is created using bolsters or blankets.
- A "bump" made of four or five towels is used either proximal to the ankle to create a varus or inverted position for better exposure or distal to the ankle to create a valgus or everted position to approximate the edges of the repair **(FIG 4C)**.

Approach

- Two commonly used approaches
  - J incision **(FIG 5A)**
    - The incision is made from the distal tip of the fibula along its anterior margin proximally to the level of the ankle mortise.
    - Does not afford optimal access to the peroneal tendons
  - Curvilinear extensile exposure **(FIG 5B)**
    - Curvilinear incision over posterior tip of fibular, extending to sinus tarsi area
    - Affords comprehensive exposure to anterior ankle, ATFL, CFL, and peroneal tendons

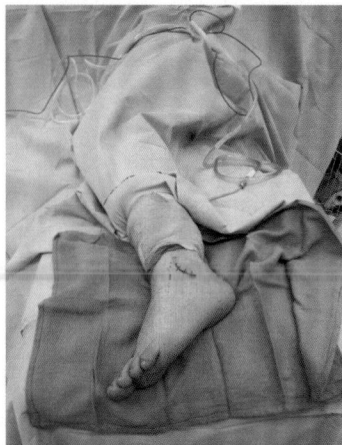
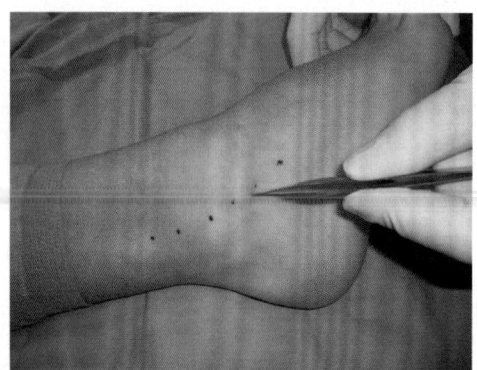

FIG 5 A. A traditional J approach on the anterior distal fibula. **B.** An extensile curvilinear exposure to the lateral ankle. This approach facilitates access to the peroneal tendons, should there be associated peroneal tendon pathology.

MODIFIED BROSTROM ANATOMIC LATERAL ANKLE LIGAMENT REPAIR WITH SUTURE ANCHORS

- Perioperative antibiotics are given.
- The patient is positioned as described, a thigh tourniquet is placed, and a standard orthopaedic prep and drape is carried out. The tourniquet is inflated.
- The incision is made as described under Approach in the Surgical Management section **(TECH FIG 1A)**.
- With the bump placed proximal to the ankle, a dissection is carried out to isolate the inferior extensor retinaculum.
- The joint capsule is then incised in line with the skin incision and just distal to the leading edge of the fibula. The ATFL may or may not be visible as a capsular expansion.
- The CFL is inspected. This inspection, along with the preoperative evaluation, is used to decide whether or not a repair of this ligament is needed.
- The joint is inspected for chondral injury.
- A subperiosteal dissection is carried out at the anterior and lateral aspect of the fibula, raising a flap 3 to 6 mm wide.
- Using curettes and rongeurs, a trough is made in the anterior and lateral aspect of the fibula at its leading edge, about 3 mm deep and 3 mm wide.
- If no CFL repair is needed, a single corkscrew anchor double-armed with no. 2 FiberWire suture (Arthrex, Inc., Naples, FL)

is inserted centrally in the trough. If a CFL repair is performed, a second anchor with no. 2 FiberWire suture is used **(TECH FIG 1B)**.
- The joint is thoroughly irrigated, and the actual repair begins. Move the bump, so it sits under the lateral border of the foot, placing the subtalar and ankle joints into an everted position before repairing the CFL if necessary.
- The capsular ligament and ATFL repair is now performed by bringing the sutures from deep to superficial in a horizontal mattress pattern. The "ligament" is shortened by creating the trough at the fibula. If further shortening is needed, the capsule may be trimmed from the distal cut edge.
- A second reinforcing layer of repair is created by suturing the inferior extensor retinaculum to the periosteal flap with absorbable 2-0 figure-8 sutures.
- The skin is closed in layers with 3-0 absorbable suture in the subcutaneous layers and staples or subcuticular suture used in the skin.
- Dressings are applied, and a short-leg non–weight-bearing splint is applied.

Case Example (Courtesy of Mark E. Easley)

- Confirm ankle instability with examination under anesthesia.
- A curvilinear incision is made over posterior tip of the fibula and extending to the sinus tarsi **(TECH FIG 2)**.
  - Protect sural nerve posteriorly and superficial peroneal nerve anteriorly.
- Prepare the inferior extensor retinaculum.
  - Identify and mobilize the inferior extensor retinaculum **(TECH FIG 3A,B)**.
  - Relatively thin superficial structure
- Identify, inspect, and protect the peroneal tendons **(TECH FIG 3C,D)**.
- Anterior arthrotomy
  - Detach the capsule, including the ATFL and CFL **(TECH FIG 4A,B)**.
  - Protect the peroneal tendons **(TECH FIG 4C)**.
  - Excise the anterior inferior tibiofibular ligament (Bassett ligament) **(TECH FIG 4D)**.
    - Usually present in patients after ankle sprain
    - Potential for anterolateral soft tissue ankle impingement
- Inspect the lateral talar dome for cartilage defect.

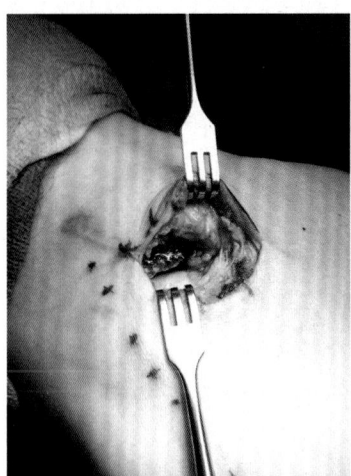

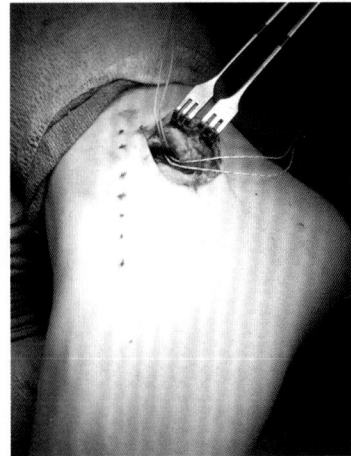

TECH FIG 1 A. Traditional approach to perform the modified Brostrom repair. **B.** Suture anchors placed in the distal fibula.

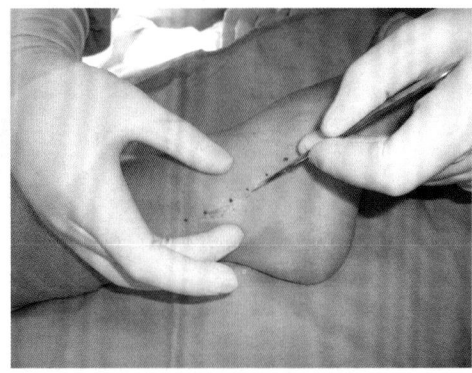

TECH FIG 2 Curvilinear extensile exposure to the lateral ankle ligaments.

TECHNIQUES

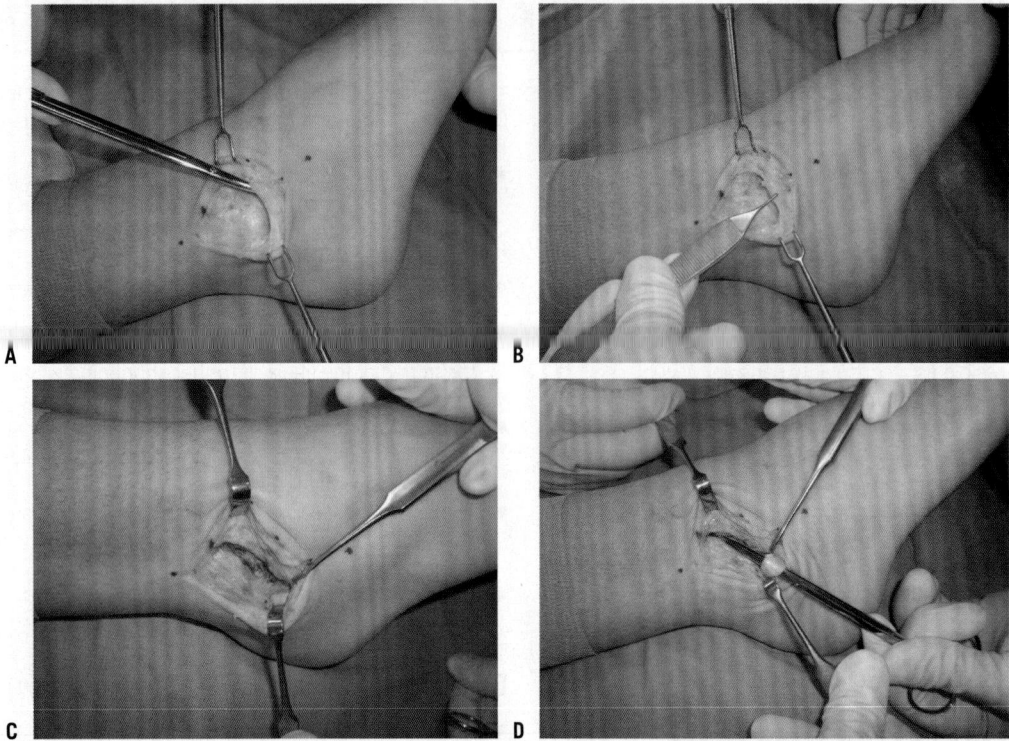

TECH FIG 3 A,B. Mobilize the inferior extensor retinaculum to be used to augment the repair (Gould modification of the Brostrom procedure). **A.** Identify the inferior extensor retinaculum. **B.** Demonstrate that the retinaculum can be advanced. **C,D.** Identify, inspect, and protect the peroneal tendons. **C.** Identify the tendons. **D.** Inspect the tendons.

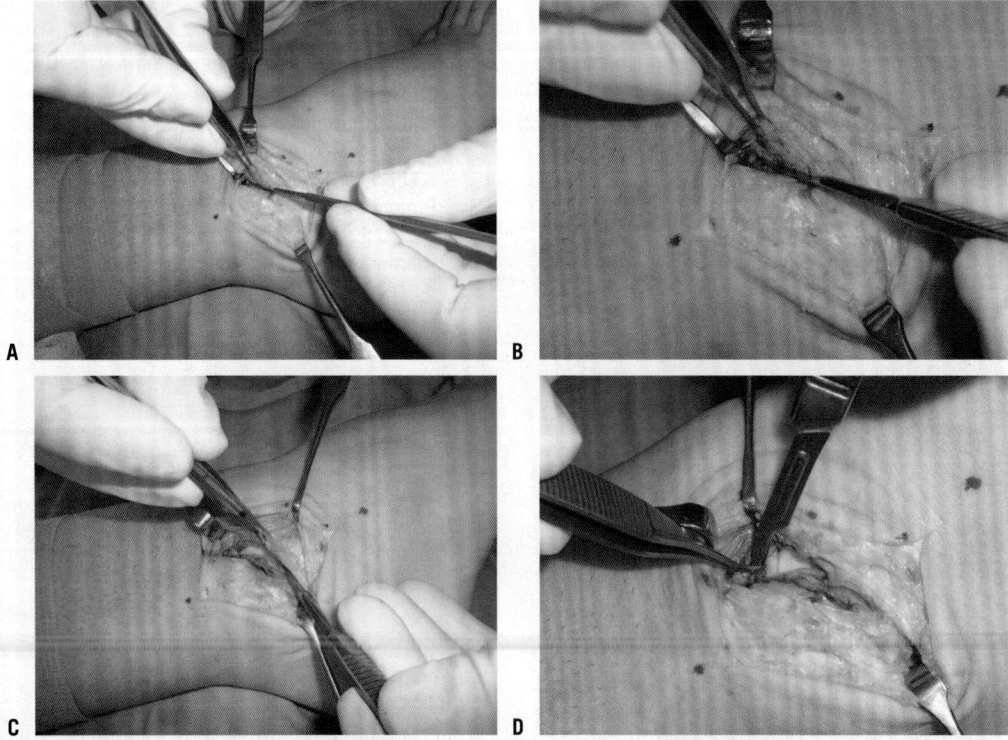

TECH FIG 4 Anterior arthrotomy. **A–C.** The anterolateral capsule is elevated from the distal fibula. **D.** With the anterolateral tibiotalar joint exposed, the talar articular cartilage may be inspected, and the hypertrophied anterior inferior tibiofibular ligament (Bassett ligament) may be excised. (Following multiple ankle sprains, anterolateral soft tissue ankle impingement frequently develops.)

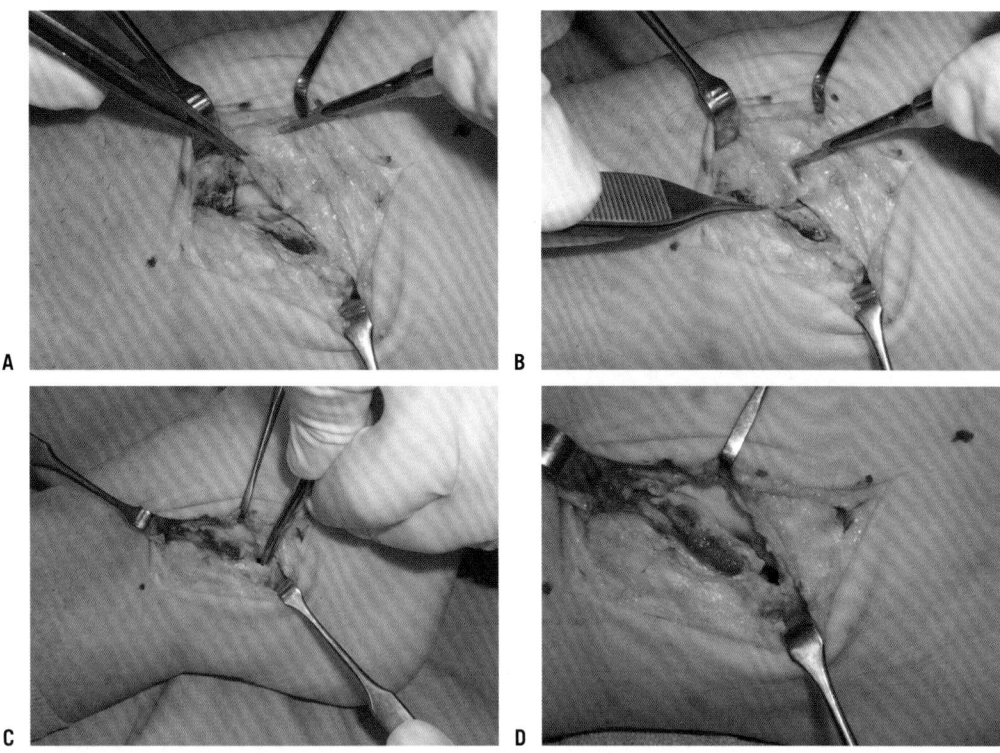

TECH FIG 5 Identify the ATFL and CFL within the lateral capsule; these structures represent condensations within the lateral capsule. **A,B.** ATFL and its anatomic location on the fibula identified. **C,D.** CFL identified and its competency tested with ankle/hindfoot inversion.

- Identify the ATFL and CFL **(TECH FIG 5)**; these are condensations within the capsular sleeve.
- Develop a distal fibular periosteal flap **(TECH FIG 6A,B)** to use as an additional reinforcement of the repair.
- Prepare anterior distal fibula for reattachment of capsule and ligaments.
  - Create a trough using a rongeur **(TECH FIG 6C)**.
  - Predrill anatomic footprints for ATFL and CFL suture anchor placement **(TECH FIG 6D,E)**.
- Place suture anchors **(TECH FIG 7A,B)**.
  - Orient them so that they do not
    - Interfere with one another
    - Violate the joint
    - Violate the posterior cortex of the fibula and irritate the PR

- Test the stability of the suture anchors **(TECH FIG 7C)**.
  - Lift the limb by the anchors; if the anchors are going to fail, we want them to do so now, so the problem can be rectified.
- Pass the respective sutures through the CFL, the adjacent capsule, and the ATFL **(TECH FIG 7D–F)**.
- Test the sutures to ensure that they indeed advance the appropriate portion of the capsule to the desired location on the distal fibula **(TECH FIG 7G)**.
- Position the ankle properly for securing the sutures **(TECH FIG 8A)**.
  - Reduce the talus within the ankle mortise.
  - Avoid anterior translation of the talus within the mortise.
  - Dorsiflex the ankle to neutral.
  - Maintain slight hindfoot valgus.

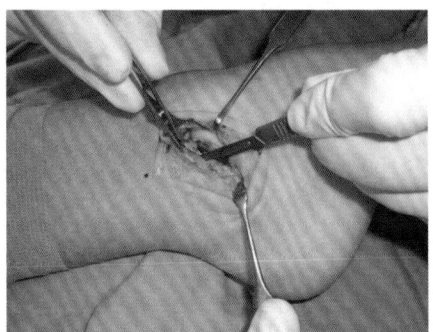
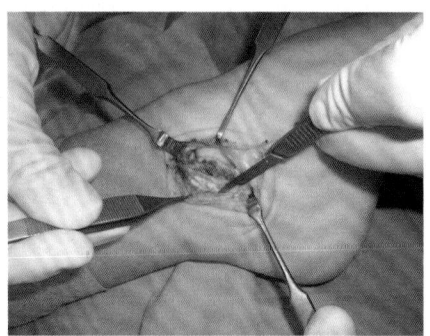

TECH FIG 6 Distal fibular periosteal flap. This flap may be developed to create another layer for repair. **A,B.** Mobilizing distal fibular flap. *(continued)*

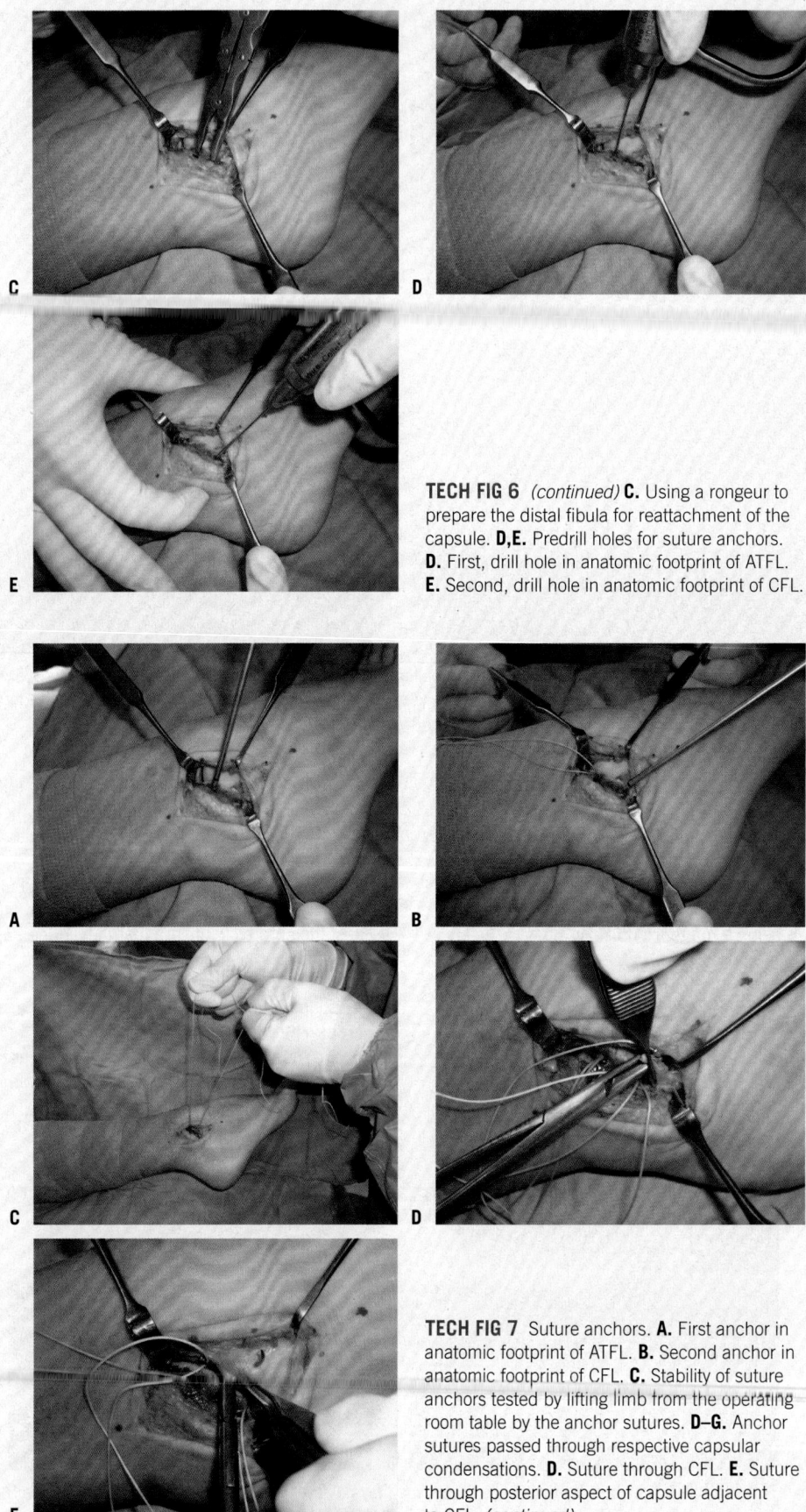

TECH FIG 6 *(continued)* **C.** Using a rongeur to prepare the distal fibula for reattachment of the capsule. **D,E.** Predrill holes for suture anchors. **D.** First, drill hole in anatomic footprint of ATFL. **E.** Second, drill hole in anatomic footprint of CFL.

TECH FIG 7 Suture anchors. **A.** First anchor in anatomic footprint of ATFL. **B.** Second anchor in anatomic footprint of CFL. **C.** Stability of suture anchors tested by lifting limb from the operating room table by the anchor sutures. **D–G.** Anchor sutures passed through respective capsular condensations. **D.** Suture through CFL. **E.** Suture through posterior aspect of capsule adjacent to CFL. *(continued)*

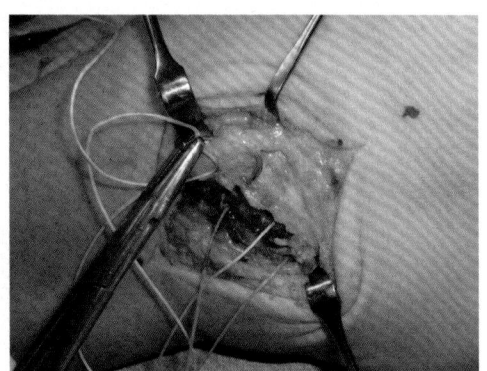
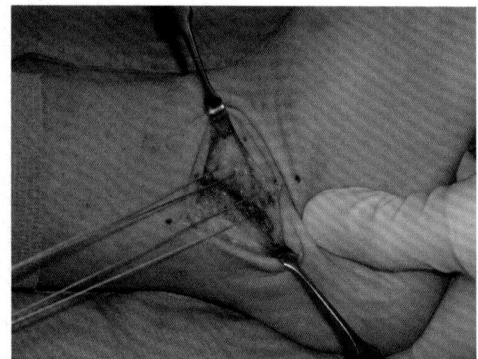

TECH FIG 7 *(continued)* **F,G.** Suture through ATFL.

- Tie the sutures (**TECH FIG 8B–D**).
- Check the stability of the repair after the anchor sutures have been tied (**TECH FIG 8E**).
- Pass the anchor sutures through the distal fibular periosteal flap (**TECH FIG 9A–C**).
  - This reinforces the repair.
  - Place additional sutures from the periosteum to the capsule that has been advanced to the distal fibula (**TECH FIG 9D,E**).
  - Augment the repair further with the inferior extensor retinaculum.

- Protect the peroneal tendons because they are in close proximity to the inferior extensor retinaculum (**TECH FIG 10A**).
- Advancing the inferior retinaculum to the distal fibula over the capsular advancement is the (Nathaniel) Gould modification of the Brostrom lateral ankle ligament reconstruction (**TECH FIG 10B–D**).
- If possible, advance the inferior retinaculum so that the tissue covers the sometimes prominent permanent anchor suture knots. Final check of the anterior drawer and talar tilt tests to ensure that ankle stability has been reestablished (**TECH FIG 11A**).
- Closure (**TECH FIG 11B**)

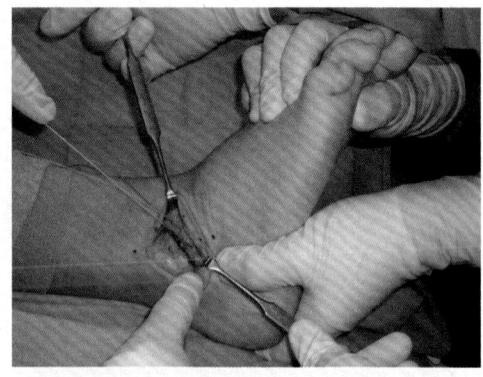
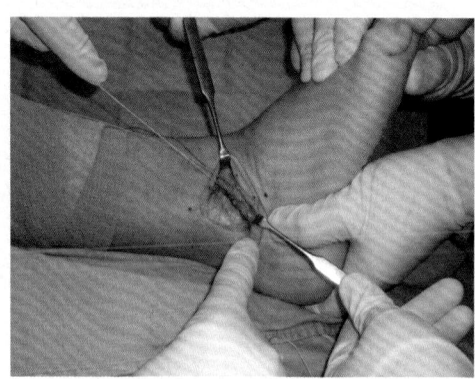
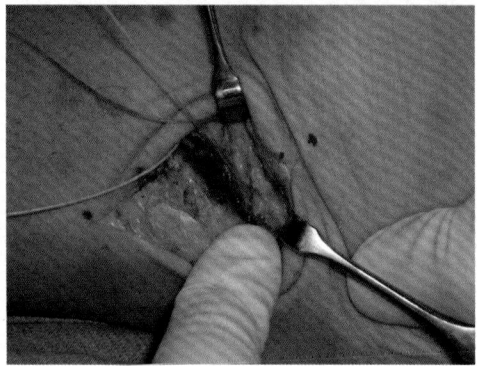

TECH FIG 8 A. Reduce the talus within the ankle mortise before reattaching the ligaments and capsule. The ankle is held in dorsiflexion, with a posterior force maintaining the talus within the ankle mortise. Although covered, a bump has been placed under the distal tibia to allow the heel to translate posteriorly without interfering with the operating table. The heel is maintained in slight valgus. **B–D.** Secure the sutures while ankle is maintained in optimal position. **B.** Protect the peroneal tendons. **C.** Secure the CFL and more posterior capsule. *(continued)*

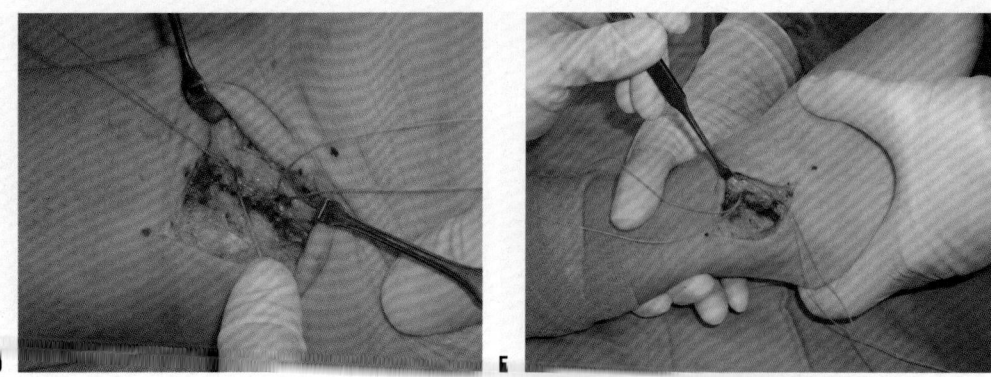

TECH FIG 8 *(continued)* **D.** Secure the ATFL. **E.** Recheck the anterior drawer test to determine if the primary sutures are securely maintaining ankle stability.

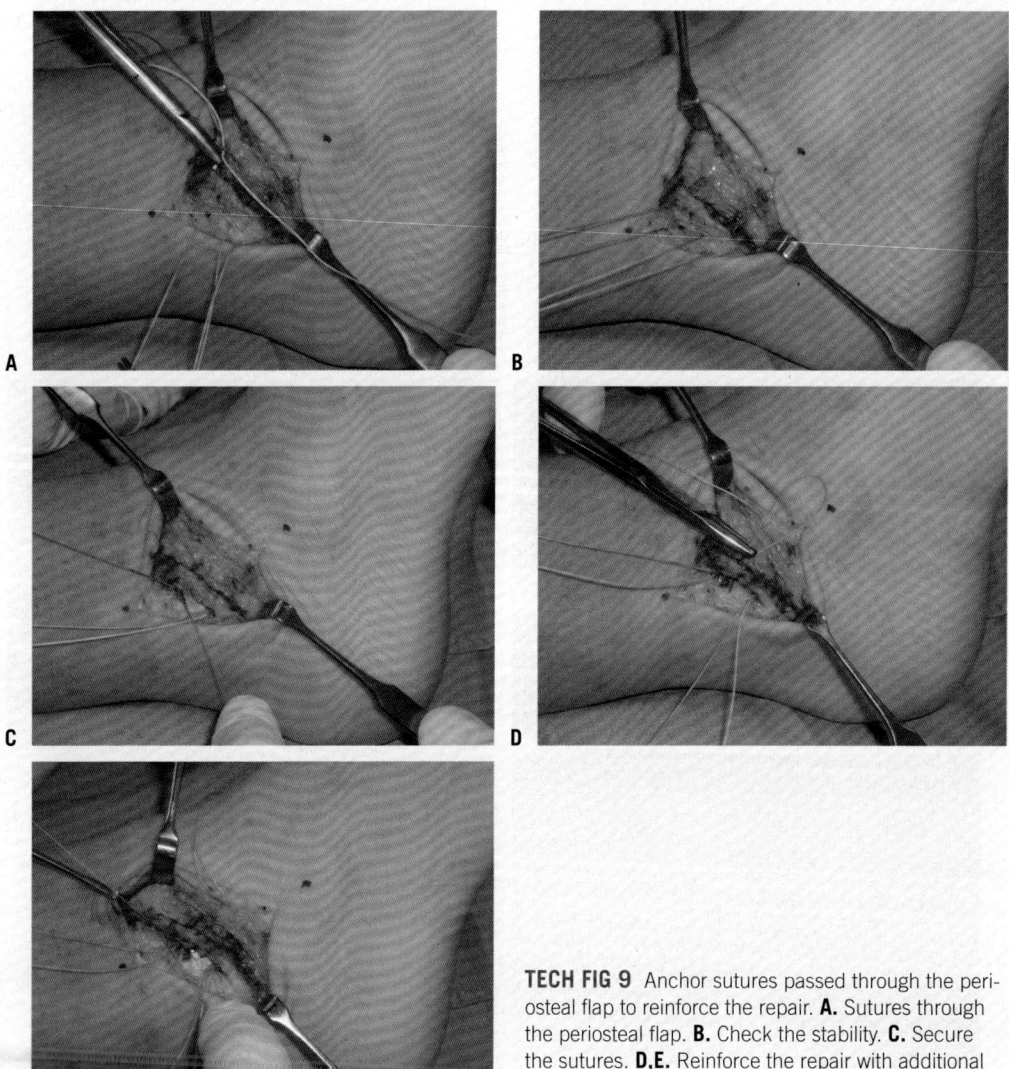

TECH FIG 9 Anchor sutures passed through the periosteal flap to reinforce the repair. **A.** Sutures through the periosteal flap. **B.** Check the stability. **C.** Secure the sutures. **D,E.** Reinforce the repair with additional sutures. **D.** Pass sutures from the capsule through the periosteal flap. **E.** Secure these sutures.

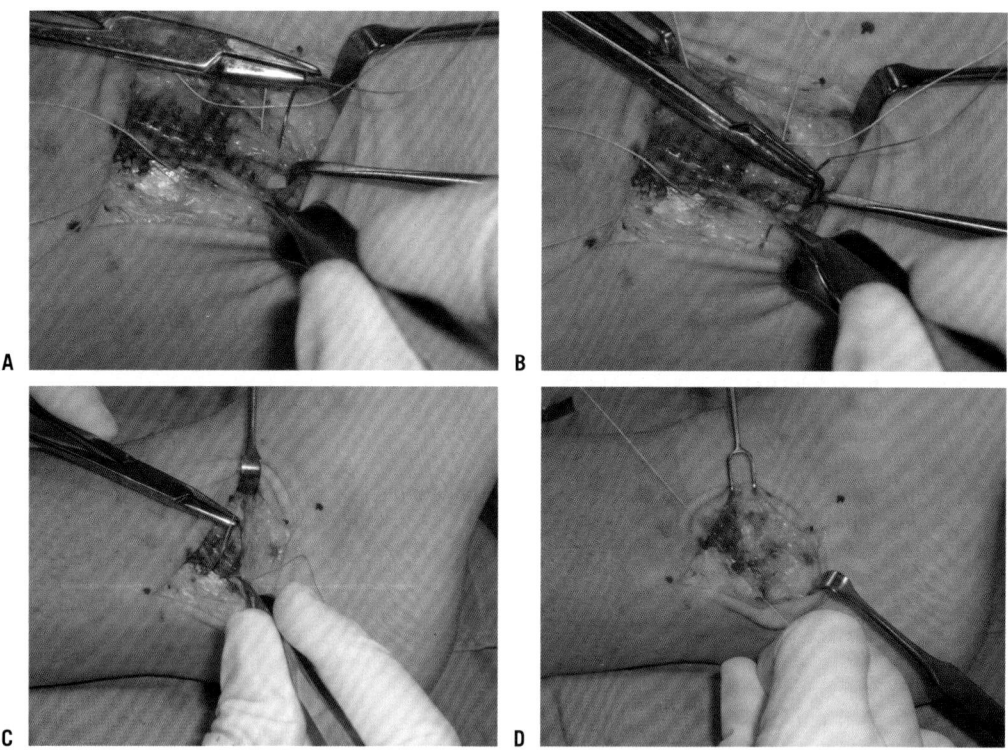

TECH FIG 10 Gould modification of the Brostrom procedure. **A.** Protect peroneal tendons. **B.** More posterior advancement of the inferior extensor retinaculum. **C.** Anterior advancement. **D.** Attempt to cover the permanent anchor sutures with the retinaculum.

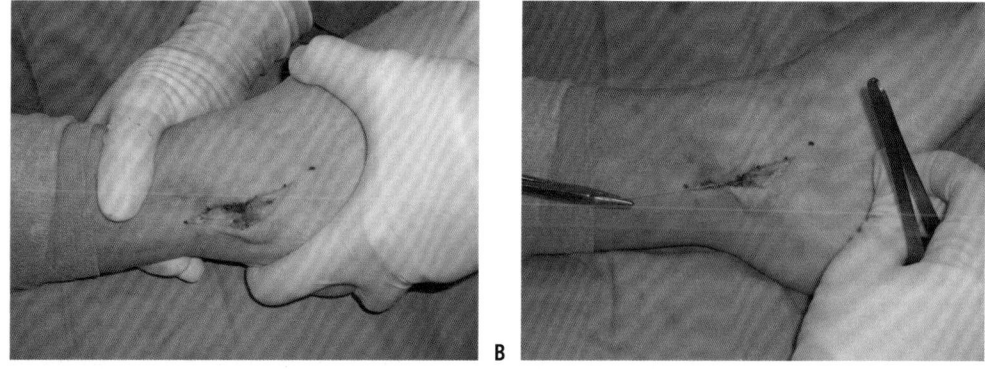

TECH FIG 11 A. Final check of anterior drawer and talar tilt tests to be sure repair is satisfactory. **B.** Closure.

MODIFIED BROSTROM-EVANS PROCEDURE

- Same positioning and approach as for a modified Brostrom procedure
- The ATFL and CFL are released with the capsular sleeve from the fibula, the same way as for the modified Brostrom procedure **(TECH FIG 12A)**.
- Preparing the PR tendon
  - The PR is isolated distal and proximal to the superior peroneal retinaculum (SPR) that is left intact.

- The PR is split longitudinally, and the anterior 50% is released proximally **(TECH FIG 12B)**.
  - While keeping the SPR intact, the PR is split using a suture that is passed beneath the SPR that is used to separate the PR into anterior and posterior limbs, acting as a "saw" to divide the tendon along its longitudinal fibers.
  - After being released proximally, the anterior limb of the PR is passed beneath the SPR distally.

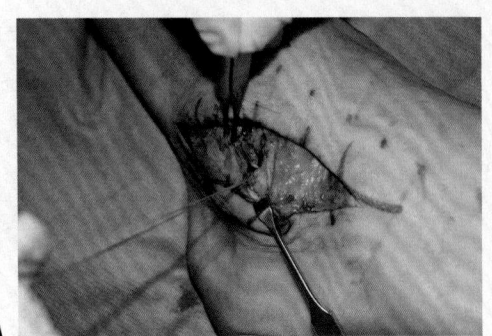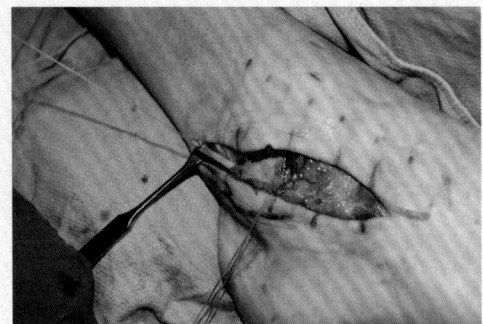

TECH FIG 12 A. Prepare the lateral ankle ligament complex as is done for the isolated modified Broström procedure. **B.** Isolate the anterior 50% of the PR tendon.

- Passing the anterior limb of the PR through the fibula
  - Drill an oblique tunnel in the distal fibula **(TECH FIG 13A)**.
  - Pass the anterior 50% of the PR through the tunnel from distal to proximal **(TECH FIG 13B)**.
  - Complete the modified Broström procedure **(TECH FIG 13C,D)**.
    - The ankle is held in neutral position.
    - The talus is maintained in the ankle mortise.
  - Slight valgus is maintained in the hindfoot.

- Augment the modified Broström with the Evans modification.
  - The anterior slip of the PR is secured to the fibular periosteum, both at the anterior and posterior aspects of the tunnel.
    - Avoid excessive valgus or excessive tensioning, as overtightening could occur; the goal is to have a restraint to inversion, not a complete lack of inversion.
    - Typically, the anterior slip of the PR can be sewn over the fibula after being passed through the tunnel to further augment the repair **(TECH FIG 13E,F)**.
- Check ankle stability with anterior drawer test and particularly inversion stress test **(TECH FIG 13G,H)**.

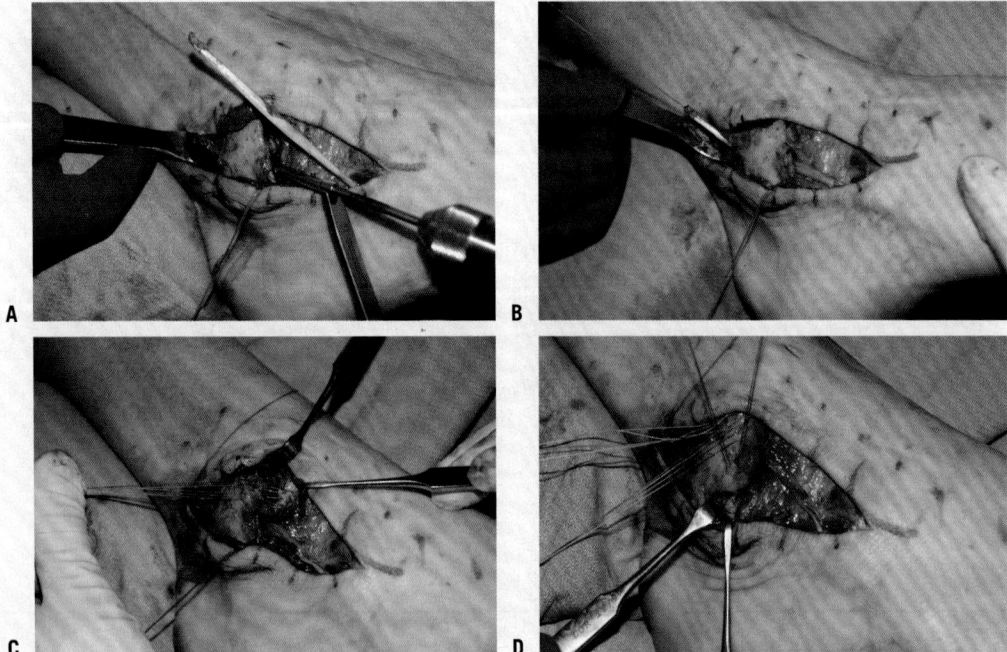

TECH FIG 13 A. Transect the anterior 50% of the tendon proximally and pass this half of the PR tendon beneath the intact superficial peroneal retinaculum. Drill a fibular tunnel from distal to proximal. **B.** Pass the anterior slip of the PR through the tunnel from distal to proximal. **C,D.** Complete the modified Broström procedure. *(continued)*

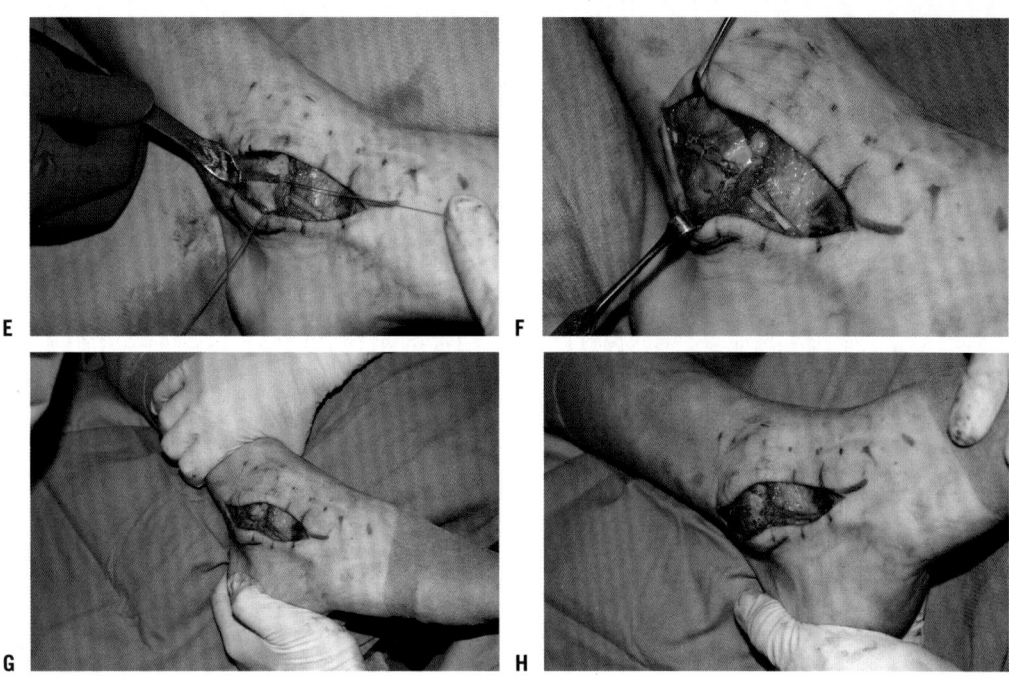

TECH FIG 13 *(continued)* **E,F.** After passing through the fibular tunnel, the anterior slip of the PR may be folded distally over the fibula to augment the repair. Check the ankle stability: anterior drawer (**G**) and inversion stress tests (**H**).

TECHNIQUES

Pearls and Pitfalls

Incision	• When making the traditional J incision, be sure it is positioned over the distal fibula and not the lateral process of the talus. Palpate the landmarks carefully.
Use a bump/bolster.	• Position is everything. A bolster under the ipsilateral hip ensures that the leg is maintained in the optimal position, thereby maintaining adequate exposure to the lateral ankle. A bolster under the operated ankle is also useful and improves access to the lateral ankle.
Ankle Position when Securing the Sutures	• Reduce the talus within the ankle mortise. Dorsiflex the ankle, push the talus posteriorly within the mortise, and maintain slight hindfoot valgus. It is useful to use a bump under the distal tibia so that the foot can be pushed posteriorly.
Protect the superficial peroneal nerve.	• The superficial peroneus nerve crosses the anterior aspect of the surgical approach for the classic J incision and potentially for the extensile exposure as well. Be careful not to injure the nerve.

POSTOPERATIVE CARE

- The patient is to remain non–weight bearing until seen in the clinic for the first cast change in 10 to 14 days.
- At this first postoperative visit, the splint is removed and wound evaluated. If no problems are seen, the skin closure is removed, and the patient is placed in a short-leg weight-bearing cast for the subsequent 4 to 5 weeks. Consider early mobilization with an ankle brace. Recent work has demonstrated that this leads to an earlier return to sport and work with fewer patients experiencing less satisfactory function.
- At the next visit, the cast is removed, and a physical therapy program is initiated for range-of-motion, proprioceptive training, and progressive resistive exercises.
- Gradual return to sport is possible at 12 to 16 weeks following surgery.

COMPLICATIONS

- Minimal; avoid injury to the superficial peroneal and sural nerves.
- Infection
- Wound dehiscence

- Failure of repair
- Peroneal weakness (Postoperative physical therapy program is important.)
- If the talus was not reduced within the ankle mortise when the sutures were secured, then the repair may prove inadequate.
- With an anatomic repair, overtightening is unlikely.

SUGGESTED READINGS

Black HM, Brand RL, Eichelberger MR. An improved technique for the evaluation of ligamentous injury in severe ankle sprains. Am J Sports Med 1978;6:276–282.

Broström L. Sprained ankles. VI. Surgical treatment of "chronic" ligament ruptures. Acta Chir Scand 1966;132:551–565.

Burks RT, Morgan J. Anatomy of the lateral ankle ligaments. Am J Sports Med 1994;22:72–77.

Cho BK, Kim YM, Kim DS, et al. Outcomes of the modified Brostrom procedure using suture anchors for chronic lateral ankle instability—a prospective randomized comparison between single and double suture anchors. J Foot Ankle Surg 2013;52(1):9–15.

Colville MR. Surgical treatment of the unstable ankle. J Am Acad Orthop Surg 1998;6:368–377.

Colville MR, Marder RA, Boyle JJ, et al. Strain measurement in lateral ankle ligaments. Am J Sports Med 1990;18:196–200.

Colville MR, Marder RA, Zarins B. Reconstruction of the lateral ankle ligaments. A biomechanical analysis. Am J Sports Med 1992;20:594–600.

de Vries JS, Krips R, Sierevelt IN, et al. Interventions for treating chronic ankle instability. Cochrane Database Syst Rev 2006;(4):CD004124.

Hølmer P, Søndergaard L, Konradsen L, et al. Epidemiology of sprains in the lateral ankle and foot. Foot Ankle Int 1994;15:72–74.

Hsu AR, Ardoin GT, Davis WH, et al. Intermediate and long-term outcomes of the modified Brostrom-Evans procedure for lateral ankle ligament reconstruction. Foot Ankle Spec 2016;9(2):131–139.

Huang B, Kim YT, Kim JU, et al. Modified Broström procedure for chronic ankle instability with generalized joint hypermobility. Am J Sports Med 2016;44(4):1011–1106.

Johnson EE, Markolf KL. The contribution of the anterior talofibular ligament to ankle laxity. J Bone Joint Surg Am 1983;65(1):81–88.

Peters JW, Trevino SG, Renstrom PA. Chronic lateral ankle instability. Foot Ankle 1991;12:182–191.

Porter DA, Kamman KA. Chronic lateral ankle instability: open surgical management. Foot Ankle Clin 2018;23(4):539–554.

Yu HY, Choi MS, Kim MS, et al. Gender differences in outcome after modified Broström procedure for chronic lateral ankle instability. Foot Ankle Int 2016;37(1):64–69.

Xu HX, Lee KB. Modified Broström procedure for chronic lateral ankle instability in patients with generalized joint laxity. Am J Sports Med 2016;44(12):3152–3157.

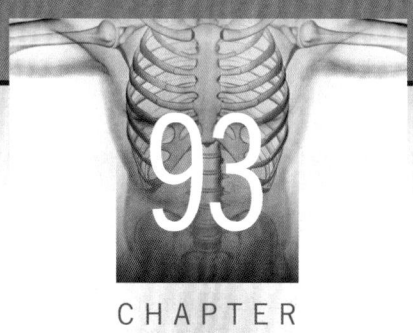

93

CHAPTER

Surgical Repair of Lateral Ankle Instability

Gregory C. Berlet, B. Collier Watson, Christopher F. Hyer, Travis M. Langan, and Jared M. Maker

DEFINITION

- Ankle sprains are the most common athletic-associated injury: They represent up to 40% of all sports-related injuries. The incidence of this inversion type of ankle sprain is around 10,000 people per day.[12]
- Literature has cited that about 50% of patients with ankle sprains have some long-term sequelae of their injury. Many of these people develop ankle instability.[10,12]
- Ankle instability can be divided into two categories, functional and mechanical.
  - Functional instability refers to the subjective feeling of the ankle giving way during activity.
  - Mechanical instability is the term used when patients show excessive ankle motion, beyond the normal physiologic barriers.

ANATOMY

- The lateral ankle is supported by both dynamic and static structures **(FIG 1)**.
- Static structures include the bony architecture of the joints and the ligaments. This bony configuration contributes about 30% of the stability, whereas the remaining 70% of stability comes from the soft tissues.

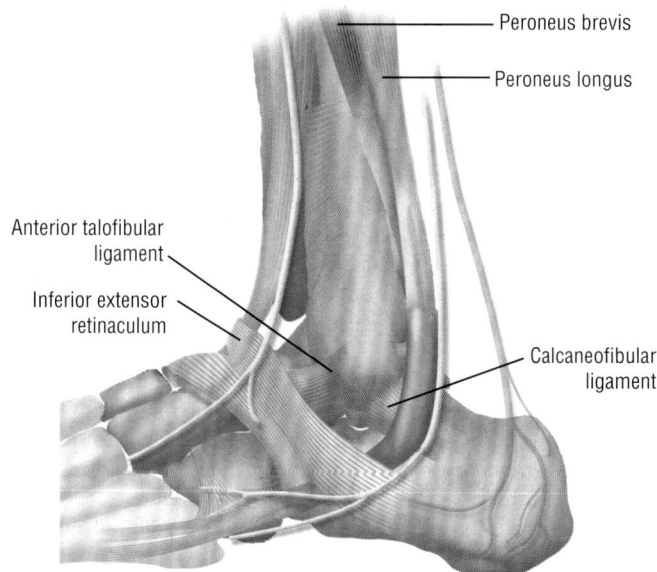

Peroneus brevis

Peroneus longus

Anterior talofibular ligament

Inferior extensor retinaculum

Calcaneofibular ligament

FIG 1 The relative positions of the sural nerve, the lateral branch of the superficial peroneal nerve, and the inferior extensor retinaculum.

- The dynamic structures that aid in the stability of the ankle include the peroneus longus and peroneus brevis tendons. These tendons run posterior to the fibula in the peroneal groove. They are kept in this groove by the superior peroneal retinaculum.
- Once the tendons pass the distal tip of the fibula, they alter their course and run along the lateral border of the calcaneus, under the inferior peroneal retinaculum, with the peroneus brevis inserting on the base of the fifth metatarsal and the peroneus longus making another turn at the cuboid tunnel and inserting on the plantar first metatarsal base and medial cuneiform.
- These two tendons act as the primary evertors of the ankle and participate in plantarflexion of the ankle. As a result of their course and function, they work in a dynamic fashion to provide stability to the ankle and subtalar joints.
- In addition to the bony configuration of the joint, the static restraints for the lateral aspect of the ankle include the anterior talofibular ligament (ATFL), the calcaneofibular ligament (CFL), and the posterior talofibular ligament (PTFL).
- The ATFL is the most frequently injured ligament and the weakest of the three ligaments. It is flat and broad and originates from the anterior border of the lateral malleolus and continues anteromedially to insert on the talar body, anterior to the articular surface.
- The CFL originates just inferior to the ATFL at the tip of the lateral malleolus and runs deep to the peroneal tendons and in a posterior, inferior, and medial direction to insert on the posterior aspect of the lateral calcaneus.
- The PTFL is the strongest of this lateral ankle complex and is rarely injured. It originates from the posterior aspect of the distal fibula, deep to the peroneals, and inserts on the posterolateral tubercle of the talus, laterally to the flexor hallucis longus groove.
- With the ankle plantarflexed, the ATFL is taut and becomes vertical, acting as a collateral ligament. In dorsiflexion, the same is true for the CFL.
- The ATFL has been shown to be the primary restraint to inversion in the ankle.

PATHOGENESIS

- Injury to the lateral ligamentous complex of the ankle is common. These inversion ankle injuries often result in attenuation or rupture to one or more of these ligaments.
- With the loss of these static restraints, the ankle becomes mechanically unstable, moving past the normal physiologic restraints for the ankle joint **(FIG 2)**.
- Ankle sprains are classified from grade I to grade III **(TABLE 1)**.[1]

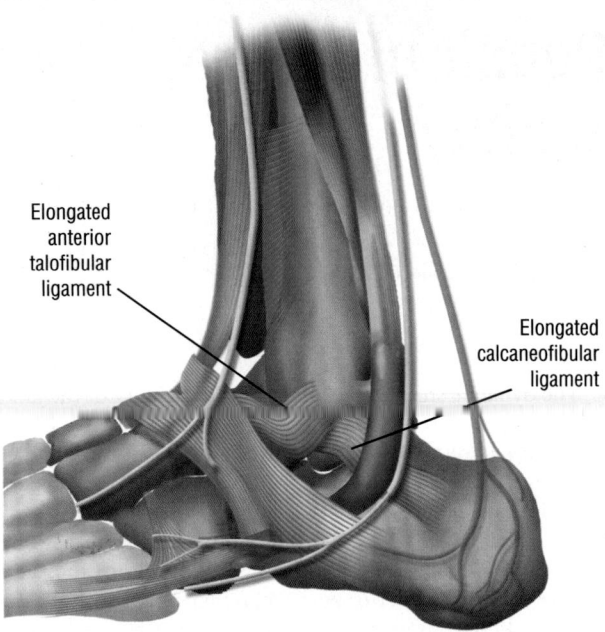

Elongated
anterior
talofibular
ligament

Elongated
calcaneofibular
ligament

FIG 2 Position of the elongated ATFL and CFL.

NATURAL HISTORY

- Once injury to the lateral stabilizers of the ankle has occurred, the patient should undergo immobilization followed by progressive rehabilitation.
- If this approach fails, it is usually related to peroneal weakness, proprioceptive defects, subtalar instability, and mechanical or functional instability.
- Chronic ankle instability can lead to repetitive inversion injuries, with the potential for fracture, osteochondral lesions of the talus, peroneal tendon injury and dislocation, and significant posttraumatic arthritis.

PATIENT HISTORY AND PHYSICAL FINDINGS

- Patients with chronic lateral ankle instability will describe an inversion injury in the past. As a result, they will report that they have problems with consistent repetitive ankle sprains and a feeling of looseness in the ankle with or without pain.
- The physician should inquire whether the patient is experiencing pain between intervals of repetitive injury. This would point toward the possibility of a secondary problem from instability (ie, osteochondritis dissecans, impingement lesion, synovitis).

TABLE 1 Grading Ankle Sprains	
Ankle Sprain Grade	**Pathology**
Grade I	• Stretching or attenuation of ATFL • Stretching or attenuation of CFL
Grade II	• Partial/complete tear of ATFL • Intact CFL
Grade III	• Complete tear of ATFL and CFL

ATFL, anterior talofibular ligament; CFL, calcaneofibular ligament.

- The examination for chronic lateral ankle instability includes evaluation of the joint above (knee) and below (subtalar). Assessment should include overall alignment, range of motion, point of maximal tenderness, anterior drawer testing, evaluation of the peroneal tendons for pathology, ankle proprioception, and evaluation for associated injuries.
- Alignment should be evaluated for both the overall lower limb and the hindfoot. Patients with hindfoot varus alignment are predisposed to ankle inversion injuries and instability. The alignment is assessed in both the seated and standing positions. The flexibility of the hindfoot should be checked.
- Patients whose malalignment cannot be corrected with orthoses should have the alignment addressed at the time of operative ligament repair.
- Tibiotalar as well as subtalar joint motion should be evaluated. Ankle motion has been described as ranging from 13 to 33 degrees of dorsiflexion and 23 to 56 degrees of plantarflexion.
  - The variability is dependent on the operator and the mode of measurement.
  - Accepted values for functional range of motion are 10 degrees of dorsiflexion and 25 degrees of plantarflexion.
  - Range-of-motion testing can always be compared to the uninjured side for comparison.
  - Subtalar motion occurs about an oblique axis running from the medial side of the talar neck to the posterolateral wall of the calcaneus. Total motion for inversion and eversion is an arc of 20 degrees, but this is extremely difficult to assess accurately. The predominance of this motion is inversion.
- The anterior drawer test is designed to test the competency of the ATFL.
  - The test is performed with the patient seated and the knee flexed to 90 degrees. The tibia is stabilized with one hand while the ankle rests in relaxed plantarflexion. The contralateral hand is used to draw the talus anteriorly.
  - If the medial restraints are intact, then the movement has a rotatory component. Increased talar displacement when compared to the contralateral limb indicates a positive test. In addition, excessive motion alone can signify incompetency of the ATFL. There may also be a dimple or "pucker" noted in the area anterior to the distal fibula as a vacuum is created when the talus slides out of the mortise (see Part 8 Foot and Ankle Exam Table at the end of the book).
  - Most sources cite an absolute value of 10 mm for a positive test. A firm end point should also be noted when testing for ATFL competency.
  - Stress radiographs can also be performed to evaluate the ATFL. The talus will sublux anteriorly in a positive test.
- The talar tilt test is designed to test the competency of the CFL.
  - The test is again performed with the patient seated and the knee flexed to 90 degrees. While the tibia is stabilized with one hand, the other had is used to place a strait inversion/varus stress on the calcaneus. This will stress the stability of the ankle and subtalar joint.
  - Generally, greater than 15 degrees of talar tilt indicates a positive test of an incompetent CFL.
  - Stress radiographs can be performed to evaluate the CFL. The talus will tilt abnormally in the ankle joint indicating a positive test.

- Proper examination of the ankle for chronic instability includes the evaluation of the peroneal tendons. These tendons can easily be injured at the time of the varus stress that injures the ligaments as well as with the recurrent instability that follows.
  - Evaluation for swelling in the retrofibular space is performed.
  - Simple palpation of the tendons (for tenderness) and strength testing are mandatory.
  - Peroneal weakness warrants a search for peroneal pathology.
  - The peroneal compression test can be helpful as well. The patient should be examined in a dynamic way to elicit peroneal subluxation or dislocation if it is present.
- Proprioception testing is an essential part of evaluating chronic ankle instability. Defects in proprioception following ankle sprains are well documented in the literature.
  - The modified Romberg test or stabilimetry is the best way to assess proprioception. A modified Romberg test is performed by having the patient stand first on the uninjured limb, with eyes open and then closed; this is then repeated on the injured side.
  - The difference in balance is related to the proprioception pathways of each limb.
  - The limitation of this test is that, to be accurate, there should be a full range of motion of the ankle and the subtalar joint and no pain with full weight bearing.
  - The advantage of the Romberg test is that it requires no special equipment.
  - Stabilimetry measures postural equilibrium and correlates with functional instability, but data generated on total sway in the vertical and horizontal planes require a force plate and computer analysis.
- Finally, the examiner must rule out other possibilities on the differential diagnosis and determine whether there is more than one source of pathology.
  - Point tenderness in the area of the fifth metatarsal base, the anterior calcaneal process, and the lateral talar process could represent fracture.
  - Full evaluation of the ankle joint for loose bodies, osteochondritis dissecans lesions, and impingement lesions should be performed.

IMAGING AND OTHER DIAGNOSTIC STUDIES

- The use of imaging in the patient with the symptoms of ankle instability should begin with three plain radiographic views of the ankle.
  - These films should be evaluated for fractures of the fifth metatarsal, lateral talar process and anterior process of the calcaneus, as well as fractures to the malleoli.
  - In addition, the examiner should be looking for exostoses of the tibia and talus, osteochondral lesions of the talus, and tarsal coalitions.
- Stress radiography can be used to evaluate anterior talar translation and talar tilt. A standardized apparatus improves reliability and consistency in this measure. The use of the contralateral limb as a control can be included when using this measure for a surgical indication.
- Further studies to evaluate the lateral aspect of the ankle include the use of magnetic resonance imaging (MRI). MRI can delineate peroneal tendon pathology as well as provide needed information about osteochondral lesions of the talus **(FIG 3)**.

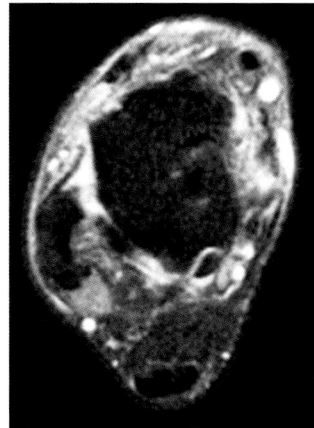

FIG 3 MRI with torn ATFL.

DIFFERENTIAL DIAGNOSIS

- Bone
  - Anterior process of calcaneus fracture
  - Lateral posterior talar process fracture
  - Lateral malleolus fracture
  - Base of fifth metatarsal fracture
  - Tibiotalar bony impingement
  - Tarsal coalition
- Cartilage
  - Osteochondral lesions of talus or tibia
  - Subtalar cartilage flap tear
- Ligamentous
  - Functional lateral ankle instability
  - Mechanical lateral ankle instability
  - Subtalar instability
  - Syndesmosis injury
- Neural
  - Neurapraxia of the superficial peroneal nerve
  - Neurapraxia of the sural nerve, reflex sympathetic dystrophy
- Tendons
  - Peroneus brevis tendon tear
  - Peroneus longus tendon tear
  - Painful os peroneum syndrome
  - Peroneal subluxation or dislocation
- Soft tissue
  - Anterolateral ankle impingement lesion
  - Sinus tarsi syndrome

NONOPERATIVE MANAGEMENT

- Nonsurgical treatment of lateral ankle instability focuses on functional rehabilitation through immobilization, restricted activity, and physical therapy.
- Physical therapy should focus on proprioception and peroneal tendon strengthening.
- In addition, braces and shoe wear modification can be used. The use of a lateral heel wedge, a flared sole, and a reinforced counter can provide increased stability.
- External stabilization of the ankle joint with taping or wrap dressings can provide some stabilization. Studies have shown superior initial resistance to inversion with taping, but taping has been shown to lose 50% of this initial effectiveness after 10 minutes of exercise.[14]

- As a result, the use of over-the-counter reusable braces such as an ankle stabilization orthosis is recommended for non-operative stabilization of the ankle joint. A University of California Berkeley orthosis, an ankle–foot orthosis (AFO), or a hinged AFO may also be used to help patients avoid surgery.
- In more sedentary patients, these modalities may provide adequate treatment, but for most athletes, they are unacceptable for long-term care.

SURGICAL MANAGEMENT

- Surgery for chronic ankle instability is indicated following a trial of failed nonoperative management.
- Patients with persistent, symptomatic mechanical instability will benefit from ligament reconstruction. This is often the case for athletes as well as patients who cannot tolerate bracing on a long-term basis.
- In high-level athletes, surgeons may consider early repair of acute grade III injuries. This allows for earlier return to sport in this patient population.[16]
- Relative contraindications for surgery include pain with no instability, peripheral vascular disease, peripheral neuropathy, and inability to comply with postoperative restrictions.
- Many procedures have been described for the management of ankle instability. They can be subdivided into anatomic and nonanatomic reconstruction techniques.
- The authors' choice for lateral ankle ligament reconstruction is influenced and based on the patient's body habitus, activity pattern, and physical demands.
- In healthy patients with normal body mass index (BMI) and alignment, primary anatomic repair is recommended. Primary repair is also used in patients with the need for full ankle range of motion, such as dancers.[16]
- In patients who are obese, are at risk for repetitive external varus stresses, have malalignment, have connective tissue disorders (Ehlers-Danlos), or are undergoing revision surgery, a nonanatomic reconstruction such as the Chrisman-Snook or Watson-Jones is preferred.
- In patients with attenuated tissue, the advent of bioengineered tissue has allowed us to augment the anatomic repair.

- Arthroscopy of the ankle is indicated for patients who have osteochondral lesions of the talus, tibial and talar exostoses, and anterior impingement lesions. The authors have had excellent results in treating chronic lateral ankle instability with arthroscopic techniques.

Preoperative Planning

- Preoperative planning in the case of chronic ankle instability is based on the cause of the instability.
- Patients should be thoroughly evaluated for the possibility of a tarsal coalition.
- Hindfoot alignment should be addressed. Patients with a varus hindfoot are predisposed to suffer inversion injuries and the possibility of a Dwyer calcaneal osteotomy in addition to the ligament repair should be considered.
- The presence of intra-articular pathology should also be addressed. Patients with clear pathology should have this addressed at the time of surgery.
- Peroneal tendon injuries often accompany ankle instability and should be evaluated and treated at this setting.

Positioning

- Positioning patients for lateral ankle ligament repair and reconstruction should be based on the chosen procedure.
- For anatomic ligament repair, we prefer to place the patient in the lateral decubitus position. This allows direct access to the lateral aspect of the ankle and the ability to address peroneal pathology and perform a calcaneal osteotomy if necessary.
- Patients who are undergoing arthroscopy can be placed in the supine position. If the surgeon then chooses open ligament repair techniques, a bump can be placed under the ipsilateral hip after the arthroscopic portion of the surgery is complete. The patient may also be placed in the lateral position. For the arthroscopic portion, we prefer the lateral position with the hip externally rotated of the operative limb. The operative limb is placed into a well leg holder, and the ankle is placed into a distractor once the limb is prepped **(FIG 4)**. Following the arthroscopic portion of the procedure, the leg is taken out of the distractor and leg

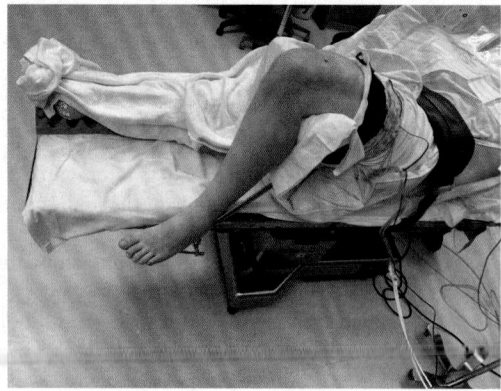
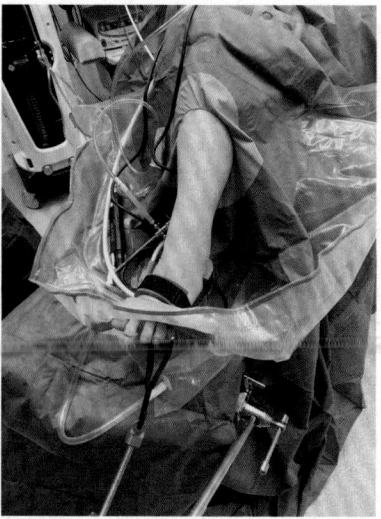

FIG 4 A. Patient in a lateral position with leg externally rotated in the well leg holder. **B.** Extremity draped and in the ankle distractor.

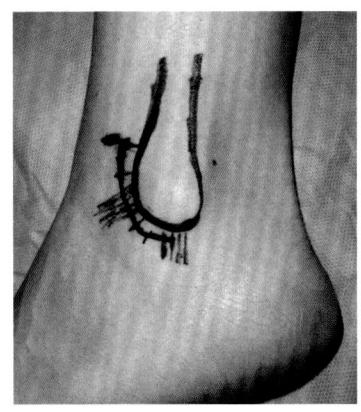
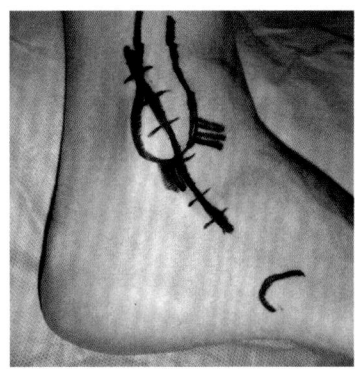

FIG 5 **A.** Anterior J incision. **B.** Posterior curvilinear incision.

holder and placed into a true lateral position while maintaining a sterile field.

Approach

- The incision for the Brostrom-Gould procedure was originally described as a J-shaped incision, just anterior to the fibula **(FIG 5A)**. This allows easy exposure to the anterolateral capsule and ATFL and CFL.
- An alternative to the J incision is a posterior curvilinear incision that allows the surgeon to repair the peroneal tendons and repair the lateral ligament complex **(FIG 5B)**. We prefer this curvilinear incision.

MODIFIED BROSTROM ANATOMIC LATERAL LIGAMENT RECONSTRUCTION

- In 1966, Brostrom reported a series of 60 patients on whom he performed a direct lateral repair of the lateral ligaments of the ankle.[8] The ligaments of the ATFL and the CFL were found to be disrupted but present, and the torn ends were shortened and repaired directly by midsubstance suturing.
- In 1980, Gould[6] modified this procedure by advancing the lateral aspect of the inferior extensor retinaculum to the fibula, reinforcing the repair of the ATFL.
- In addition to reinforcement, the modification limits subtalar instability and provides a checkrein to inversion.
- In this technique, the patient is placed in the lateral decubitus position. All bony prominences are padded, and an axillary roll is placed to protect the upper extremity. A well-padded thigh tourniquet is placed.
- The choice of an anterior incision or a posterior incision is surgeon preference.
- The curvilinear incision **(see FIG 5B)** extends from 4 to 5 cm proximal to the tip of the fibula and follows the course of the peroneal tendons.
- Distally, carry the incision toward the base of the fifth metatarsal.
- Take care to avoid the superficial peroneal and the sural nerves.
- Take dissection down to the level of the fibular periosteum.
- Mobilize the flaps anteriorly and posteriorly.
- Identify the anterolateral capsule, the peroneal tendons, and the inferior extensor retinaculum.
- The peroneal sheath can be opened proximally and distally, allowing preservation of the superior peroneal retinaculum. Peroneal tendon pathology can then be addressed.
- Make the anterior J-shaped incision along the anterior and distal aspects of the fibula. The incision begins at the level of the ankle joint and stops at the peroneal tendons.

- Carry dissection down to the anterolateral joint capsule, just anterior to the fibula. Take care to avoid any branch of the superficial peroneal nerve.
- In the distal aspect of either incision, identify the inferior extensor retinaculum and mobilize it for later Gould modification. A tag suture can be placed to help retract this tissue during the anatomic repair.
- Identify the lateral gutter of the ankle joint and divide the capsule. Leave a cuff of tissue on the fibula to allow for advancement and imbrication of this tissue.
- Carry the arthrotomy from the level of the tibiotalar joint to the peroneal tendons **(TECH FIG 1A)**. Care to protect these tendons during this part of the procedure is paramount.
- This arthrotomy will divide both the ATFL and the CFL in their midsubstance. At this time, the surgeon can evaluate the tibiotalar joint.
- Resect scar tissue; up to 5 mm of tissue can be excised.
- Imbricate the ligaments in a pants-over-vest fashion with 0 Vicryl stitches **(TECH FIG 1B–D)**.
- Place the sutures but do not tie them until the ankle is held in dorsiflexion and eversion. Be sure to prevent anterior subluxation of the talus at this time.
- After the repair, take the ankle through a range of motion to ensure that the sutures hold.
- Once repair of the arthrotomy has been performed, advance the extensor retinaculum and secure it to the periosteum of the fibula, covering the ligament and capsular repair.
- Perform irrigation and then subcutaneous and skin closure.
- Apply a dressing and splint, placing the ankle in a slightly everted position.

T E C H N I Q U E S

TECHNIQUES

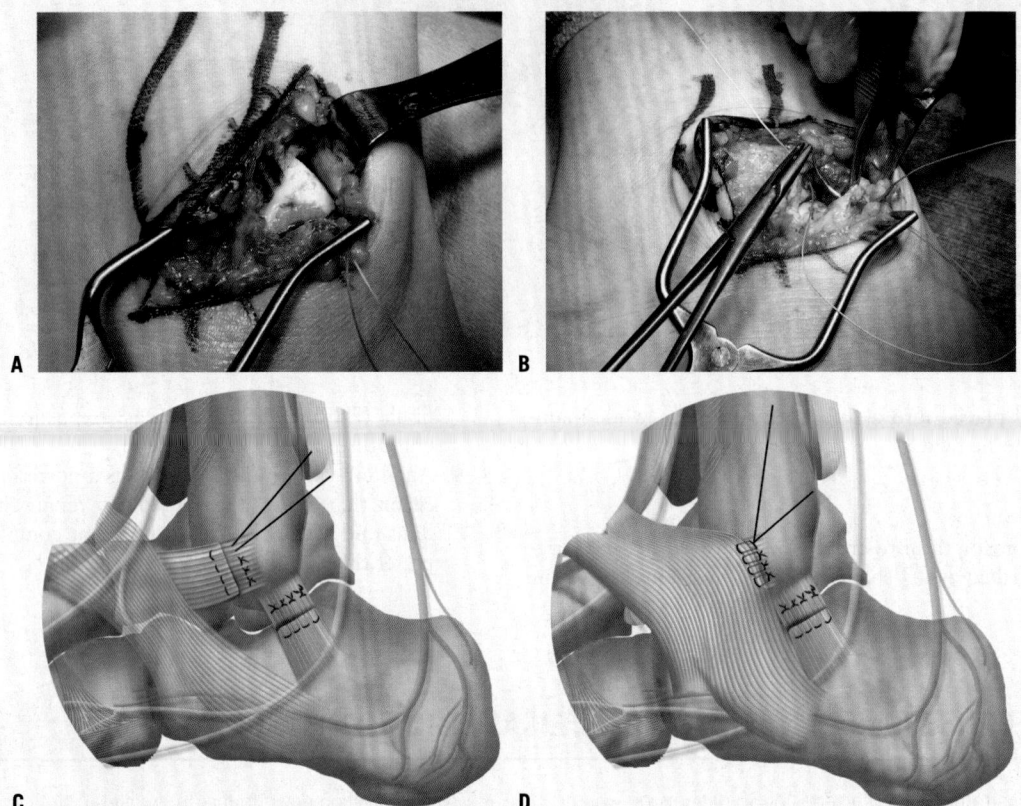

TECH FIG 1 A. Arthrotomy. **B.** Suturing ATFL with pants-over-vest stitch. **C.** After suturing the CFL and ATFL, the ankle is ready for inferior extensor retinaculum translocation. **D.** Suturing of the inferior extensor retinaculum to the anterior aspect of the fibula.

MODIFIED BROSTROM ANATOMIC LATERAL LIGAMENT RECONSTRUCTION WITH BIOENGINEERED TISSUE AUGMENTATION

- In patients who have suffered from chronic lateral ankle instability with repeated inversion injuries, often, the tissue at the time of surgery is attenuated and of poor quality. In the past, this might have caused failure of the anatomic repair or caused the surgeon to consider using an autologous tendon augmentation. If the native tissue is damaged beyond anatomic repair, there are now many different ways to augment the repair including suture anchors, interference screws, fiber tape/suture, and allograft/autograft tendon materials.
- With the growing orthobiologics market, we have found that these bioengineered tissue augments can provide the surgeon with another option in the case of poor tissue quality, without the morbidity of autogenous tendon harvest.
- The approach is the same as for the standard modified Brostrom repair.
- After performing the exposure and arthrotomy, select the preferred tissue graft and prepare it as recommended by the manufacturer.
- One type of repair is performed using FiberTape (**TECH FIG 2**). This technique has been shown to allow for complete recovery and can allow for a quicker return to sport/activity.[4,17]

- There is concern for overtightening as this material does not allow for any plasticity. Surgeon should be diligent when selecting the appropriate tension for the repair when using this technique.

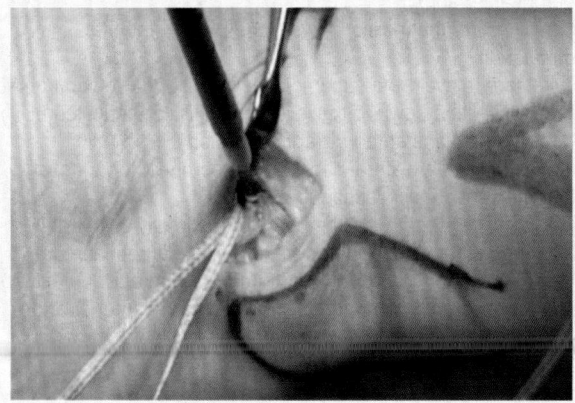

TECH FIG 2 Internal brace anchored from the fibula into the talus.

TECHNIQUES

- **TECH FIG 3A** shows a bioengineered graft that has excellent strength while allowing for more anatomic plasticity.[13] We feel this allows for the proper tension of the lateral ligaments without overtightening.
- Following the anatomic Brostrom ligament repair, the graft can be oversewn over the native ligaments to augment and strengthen the repair. The inferior extensor retinaculum is then advanced over the repair for the Gould modification.
- The graft may also be used to augment the repair by weaving it through the ligament tissues **(TECH FIG 3B)**. As seen, the graft is anchored distally into the talus with a suture anchor

(this can also be anchored into the fibula depending on the quality of tissues needing the augmentation). The graft is then placed through the robust tissue off the distal fibula. The standard pants-over-vest repair is performed, and the graft is tensioned appropriately. The graft is then secured back onto itself with the remaining nonabsorbable suture from the anchor **(TECH FIG 3C,D)**. The inferior extensor retinaculum is then advanced over the repair for the Gould modification.

- A nonanatomic repair can also be performed with the bioengineered tissue graft. This can be done in place of an allograft offering the same advantages previously discussed. This graft

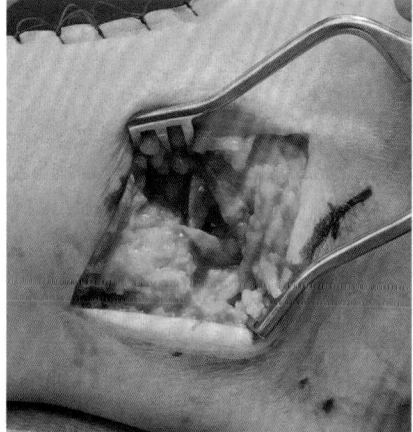

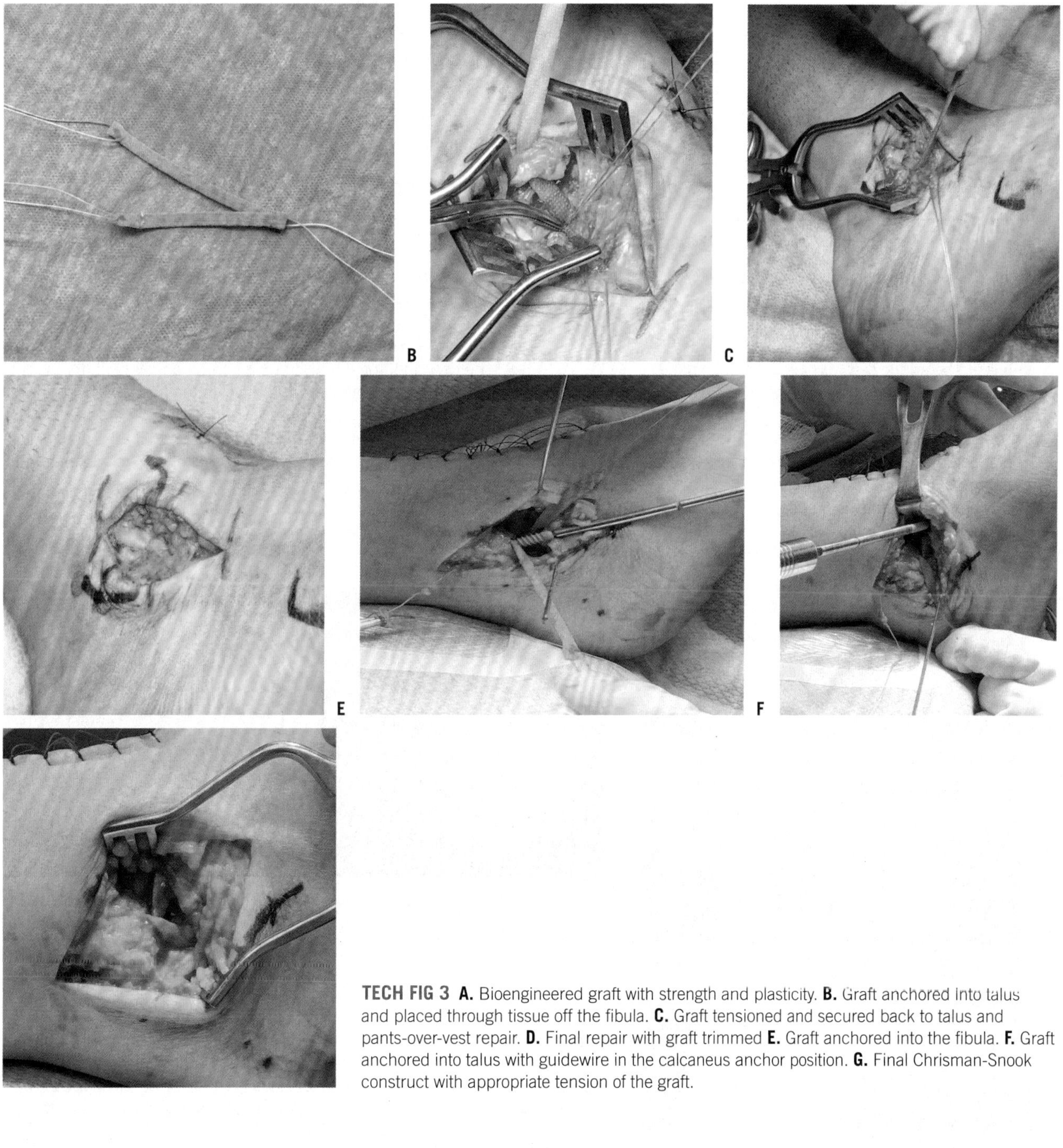

TECH FIG 3 A. Bioengineered graft with strength and plasticity. **B.** Graft anchored into talus and placed through tissue off the fibula. **C.** Graft tensioned and secured back to talus and pants-over-vest repair. **D.** Final repair with graft trimmed **E.** Graft anchored into the fibula. **F.** Graft anchored into talus with guidewire in the calcaneus anchor position. **G.** Final Chrisman-Snook construct with appropriate tension of the graft.

is less bulky than allograft and allows for proper tension while maintaining a degree of flexibility as to not overtighten the repair.

- A Chrisman-Snook style repair is shown in **TECH FIG 3E–G**. The graft is first anchored into the fibula 50% between the origin of the ATFL and CFL. Pilot holes are placed into the lateral talus at the insertion of the ATFL and the lateral calcaneus at the insertion of the CFL. The graft is fed into the insertion drill holes, the foot is everted to the appropriate tension, and the graft is secured with interference screws. Again, this graft allows for proper tension without overtightening. The same can be done utilizing a Watson-Jones technique (**TECH FIG 4**).

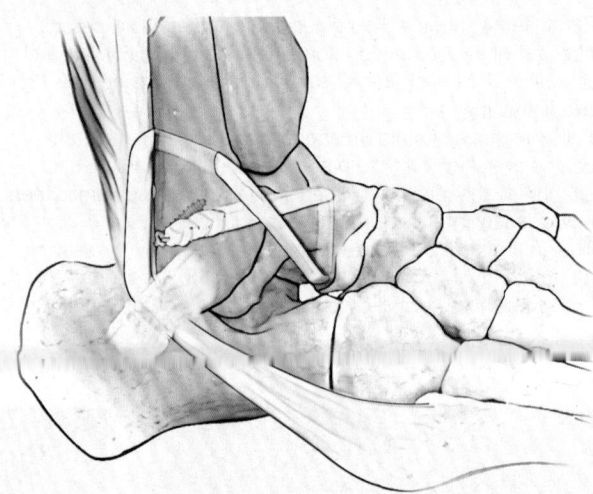

TECH FIG 4 Watson-Jones nonanatomic ligament repair.

ALL-INSIDE ARTHROSCOPIC ANATOMIC REPAIR FOR LATERAL ANKLE INSTABILITY

- Recently, an all-inside arthroscopic technique for anatomic repair of lateral ankle instability has been developed.[5,11,15]
  - Many times, there is intra-articular pathology associated with chronic lateral ankle instability, and the all-inside arthroscopic technique allows the advantage of both pathologies to be addressed with the same technique.
- The patient is placed supine on the operating table.
- A well-padded thigh tourniquet is placed on the upper thigh of the operative leg.
- The affected extremity is placed on a well leg holder located behind the knee.
- The operative extremity is prepped and draped in the usual manner.

- The peroneal tendons, peroneus tertius, superficial peroneal nerve as well as tibialis anterior tendon are marked out. The safe zone is between the superficial peroneal nerve and peroneal tendons.
- A noninvasive ankle distractor is used during the procedure.
- The described procedure requires three portals, with the accessory portal made anterior and distal to the fibula between the exit marks for the suture wire (**TECH FIG 5A**).
- A standard arthroscopic examination is performed, noting for any intra-articular pathology (osteochondral lesions, bone, and soft tissue impingement) and treated accordingly.

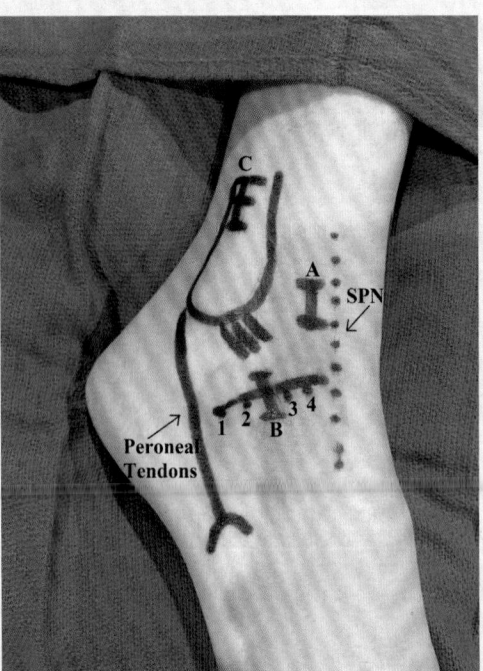

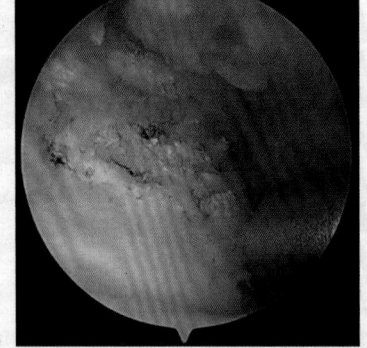

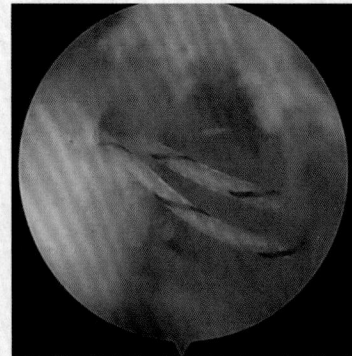

TECH FIG 5 A. Standard anterolateral portal (*A*), accessory anterolateral portal (*B*), and proximal incision for additional suture anchor (*C*). Exit points for each strand of suture wire through the inferior extensor retinaculum (*1–4*). *SPN*, Superficial Peroneal Nerve. **B.** Ablator used to clear tissue off anterior fibula. **C.** Anchors placed into anterior fibula and delivered through the skin.

- The anterior fibula is débrided with a shaver followed by an ablator for remaining soft tissue attachment through the anterolateral portal **(TECH FIG 5B)**.
- The drill guide is introduced through the anterolateral portal and positioned central and approximately 1 cm superior to the distal tip of the fibula.[5]
  - The drill guide is directed from anterior to posterior on the distal fibula parallel to the plane of the lateral gutter.
- Drilling is performed, and the guide is left in place.
- The anchor is seated into position through the guide. The guide is removed, and the sutures are delivered through the anterolateral portal **(TECH FIG 5C)**.
- A Micro SutureLasso (Arthrex, Inc., Naples, FL) is then used to capture the remaining ATFL, ankle capsule, and inferior extensor retinaculum.[5]
  - First pass is positioned approximately 1.5 to 2 cm anterior and inferior to the distal anterior fibula, exiting the anterior lateral portal.
    - The nitinol wire is then advanced capturing the first strand and pulling to exit the skin.
  - This is then repeated for the second strand with the second strand exiting the skin anterior and superior to the first strand.
- The same technique is used for placement of the second bone anchor (see **TECH FIG 5C**). The first strand of the second bone anchor is placed 1 cm anterior to the last strand of the previous placed anchor.
- A small accessory portal is made between the two sets of sutures with care to only incise the skin.[5]
  - A probe is used to gather the sutures and pull through the accessory portal.
- The extremity is removed from the distractor. The foot is then everted and slightly dorsiflexed, and suture knots are then placed for each anchor and tensioned appropriately.
- At this point, the strands are not cut, and a separate small incision approximately 3 cm proximal to the distal fibula is made (see **TECH FIG 5A**).[5]
  - Once the fibula is visualized, a drill hole is made for a bioabsorbable suture anchor.
  - A soft tissue tunnel is then made with a hemostat connecting the fibular incision to the accessory portal incision. The strands are then captured with the hemostat and advanced proximally exiting the fibular incision.
  - The strands are secured into the fibula using the bioabsorbable anchor tensioned appropriately, creating a double row construct with three suture anchors.
- Following the repair, the portals are closed with a standard portal stitch and a posterior plaster splint applied with the ankle in neutral position.

TECHNIQUES

Pearls and Pitfalls

Negative Anterior Drawer Test with History Consistent with Instability	• Be aware of the restraint of anterior tibial osteophytes. They can cause an abnormally negative drawer test despite a clinical picture of instability.
Failed Primary Brostrom Procedure	• Be sure to evaluate hindfoot anatomy. If there is a cavovarus foot structure, combine cavus correctional osteotomies or procedures in order to protect your ligament repair. Also, consider augmenting the repair as described.
Patient Activity Level	• Larger patients (>115 kg) and high-demand patients (football players) may require augmentation to the simple Brostrom-Gould procedure.
Anterolateral Ankle Joint Pain, No Chronic Instability Pattern, History of Previous Ankle Sprain	• An ankle impingement lesion can act as a primary pain generator. Consider performing an ankle arthroscopy along with the ligament repair.
Global Pain in Lateral Ankle Region	• Look carefully for secondary pathology. Recurrent instability can result in osteochondritis dissecans of the talus, subluxing or dislocating peroneal tendons, subtalar instability, and other intra-articular lesions of the ankle.

POSTOPERATIVE CARE

- Postoperatively, the patient course is divided into 3-week increments.
  - The first 4 weeks is non–weight bearing, and the second 4 weeks is weight bearing to tolerance in a boot.
- At the 8-week mark, the patient is weaned into an ankle stirrup brace and placed into a physical therapy program to begin range of motion, strengthening, and proprioceptive training.
- Patients are then progressed as tolerated until physical therapy goals are met.

- Patients are allowed to discontinue the brace for daily activities but are asked to brace in situations at risk for 1 year after reconstruction.

OUTCOMES

- The clinical and functional outcome from anatomic repair for chronic lateral ankle instability is good.[2] For older than 50 years, the modified Brostrom-Gould procedure has held up with good outcomes.[9] The open anatomic repair can be performed quickly and efficiently with consistent effective results.

- Recently, performing the lateral ligament repair through a minimally invasive arthroscopic approach has become popular. The results of the arthroscopic procedure have been promising and have comparable outcomes to the traditional open procedure.[7] Surgeons should be mindful of the at-risk nerve structures when performing the arthroscopic procedure.

- The advent and popularization of suture tape and soft tissue anchors has allowed for advances in lateral ligament repair. These techniques show good outcomes and earlier return to sport when used in an active population.[4,17] The authors caution surgeons to set the proper tension when using these techniques in order to prevent overtightening.

- A prospective outcome comparison study of the Chrisman-Snook and modified Brostrom procedure by Hennrikus et al[8] demonstrated that both operations provided good or excellent stability in more than 80% of patients, but the Brostrom procedure resulted in higher Sefton scores and a statistically significant decrease in complications when compared to the Chrisman-Snook. For this reason, the authors reserve nonanatomic reconstructions for those patients with revision surgery; high BMI; moderate to severe deformity; and those who have poor tissues, which do not allow for a robust anatomic repair.

- We now advocate bioengineered tissue that allows for a more anatomic tissue response for nonallograft repair.[13] The authors have had good results when using bioengineered tissue for nonanatomic repair of the lateral ligaments.

COMPLICATIONS

- The most common complications after repair of the lateral ligament complex are nerve related. The incidence of nerve complaints after surgery is reported around 10%.[3] We caution surgeons when performing the arthroscopic procedure to be mindful of the at-risk nerve structures.

- In addition to nerve complications, wound complications and infection, stiffness, and deep venous thrombosis have been reported. These complications are, of course, present with all surgeries and should be covered with patients when discussing possible complications of the procedure.

- The possibility of recurrent instability is also a possible complication of surgery. This is most often a result of inadequate rehabilitation but can also result if the patient is not appropriately evaluated for hindfoot varus or connective tissue disease.

REFERENCES

1. Balduini FC, Tetzlaff J. Historical perspectives on injuries of the ligaments of the ankle. Clin Sports Med 1982;1(1):3–12.
2. Berlet GC, Anderson RB, Davis WH. Chronic lateral ankle instability. Foot Ankle Clin 1999;4:713–728.
3. Brown AJ, Shimozono Y, Hurley ET, et al. Arthroscopic versus open repair of lateral ankle ligament for chronic lateral ankle instability: a meta-analysis. Knee Surg Sports Traumatol Arthrosc 2020;28(5):1611–1618.
4. Coetzee JC, Ellington JK, Ronan JA, et al. Functional results of open Broström ankle ligament repair augmented with a suture tape. Foot Ankle Int 2018;39(3):304–310.
5. Cottom JM, Baker JS, Richardson PE. The "all-inside" arthroscopic Broström procedure with additional suture anchor augmentation: a prospective study of 45 consecutive patients. J Foot Ankle Surg 2016;55(6):1223–1228.
6. Gould KG, Engel PC. Modification of mouse testicular lactate dehydrogenase by pyridoxal 5′-phosphate. Biochem J 1980;191(2):365–371.
7. Guelfi M, Zamperetti M, Pantalone A, et al. Open and arthroscopic lateral ligament repair for treatment of chronic ankle instability: a systematic review. Foot Ankle Surg 2018;24(1):11–18.
8. Hennrikus WL, Mapes RC, Lyons PM, et al. Outcomes of the Chrisman-Snook and modified-Broström procedures for chronic lateral ankle instability. A prospective, randomized comparison. Am J Sports Med 1996;24:400–404.
9. Hsu AR, Ardoin GT, Davis WH, et al. Intermediate and long-term outcomes of the modified Brostrom-Evans procedure for lateral ankle ligament reconstruction. Foot Ankle Spec 2016;9(2):131–139.
10. Kemler E, Thijs KM, Badenbroek I, et al. Long-term prognosis of acute lateral ankle ligamentous sprains: high incidence of recurrences and residual symptoms. Family Pract 2016;33(6):596–600.
11. Lopes R, Andrieu M, Cordier G, et al. Arthroscopic treatment of chronic ankle instability: prospective study of outcomes in 286 patients. Orthop Traumatol Surg Res 2018;104(8 suppl):S199–S205.
12. McCriskin BJ, Cameron KL, Orr JD, et al. Management and prevention of acute and chronic lateral ankle instability in athletic patient populations. World J Orthop 2015;6(2):161–171.
13. Shoaib A, Mishra V. Surgical repair of symptomatic chronic Achilles tendon rupture using synthetic graft augmentation. Foot Ankle Surg 2017;23(3):179–182.
14. van den Bekerom MPJ, van Kimmenade R, Sierevelt IN, et al. Randomized comparison of tape versus semi-rigid and versus lace-up ankle support in the treatment of acute lateral ankle ligament injury. Knee Surg Sports Traumatol Arthrosc 2016;24(4):978–984.
15. Vega J, Golanó P, Pellegrino A, et al. All-inside arthroscopic lateral collateral ligament repair for ankle instability with a knotless suture anchor technique. Foot Ankle Int 2013;34:1701–1709.
16. White WJ, McCollum GA, Calder JD. Return to sport following acute lateral ligament repair of the ankle in professional athletes. Knee Surg Sports Traumatol Arthrosc 2016;24(4):1124–1129.
17. Yoo JS, Yang EA. Clinical results of an arthroscopic modified Brostrom operation with and without an internal brace. J Orthop Traumatol 2016;17(4):353–360.

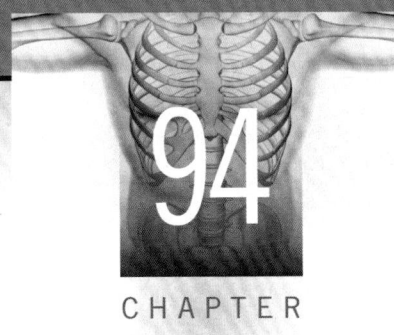

94

CHAPTER

Hamstring Autografting/ Augmentation for Lateral Ankle Instability

Anna-Kathrin Leucht, Alastair Younger, Heather Barske, and Mark Glazebrook

DEFINITION

- Lateral ligament instability occurs in some patients after an inversion injury of the ankle.[37] Although an inversion injury is common, only a few patients have ongoing ankle instability severe enough to require surgery. Persistent instability may occur in 20% to 30% of patients.[5,10,16,19,33,46,51,53,54,56,60]
- Hindfoot varus, hyperlaxity, coalitions as well as anatomic variations of tibiotalar axis, talar dome radius, and a posterior position of the lateral malleolus are considered as predisposing factors for ankle sprains.[4,9,20,50,52,58,64]
- Lateral ligament disruption may occur in combination with osteochondral defects, peroneal tendon tears, syndesmotic injuries, loose bodies, anterior lateral joint impingement, or a tight heel cord.[31,48,62] Any of these concomitant pathologies needs to be sought during the clinical examination and treated if it represents a significant component of the ongoing symptoms.
- Medial ankle instability may occur in combination with lateral ankle instability.[25] In these cases, the medial ligament instability may need to be addressed at the same time.

ANATOMY

- The lateral collateral ligaments include the anterior talofibular ligament (ATFL), the calcaneofibular ligament (CFL), and the posterior talofibular ligament (PTFL).[13,40] These are condensations within the lateral capsule.
- The ATFL arises from the inferior anterior portion of the distal fibula and inserts onto the lateral side of the talar neck (**FIG 1**).

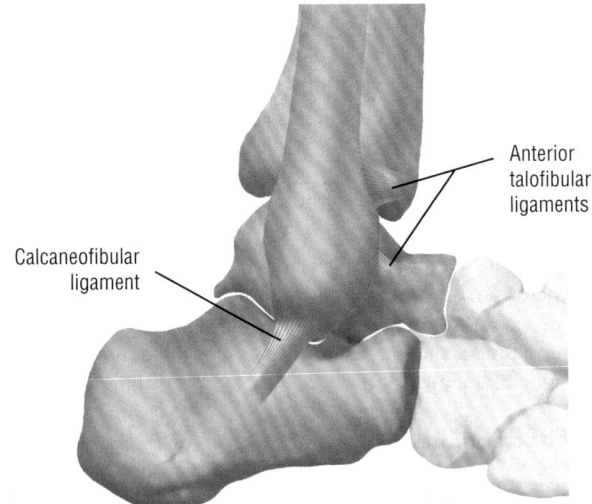

Anterior talofibular ligaments

Calcaneofibular ligament

FIG 1 Anatomy of the CFL and ATFL.

- The CFL runs from the anterior tip of the fibula to the lateral wall of the calcaneus. The ligament passes superficial to the lateral margin of the posterior facet of the subtalar joint and courses deep to the peroneal tendons to insert via a broad base onto the lateral side of the calcaneus.
- The PTFL runs from the inside of the posterior tip of the fibula to the lateral tuberculum of the posterior process of the talus.

PATHOGENESIS

- Lateral ankle instability occurs after an inversion injury to the lateral ligament complex. The injury typically occurs in plantarflexion. An isolated ATFL ruptures occur in approximately 65% of cases, a combined ATFL and CFL rupture in 20%, and a total rupture of the lateral ligaments in 10% to 15%.[10,27] Although traditional concepts indicate this combination, we feel that isolated calcaneofibular injury can also exist.
- A cavus (high arched) foot may predispose the ankle to recurrent instability.
- Osteochondral defects of the talus and peroneal tendon tears are known associated pathologies.[2,25]

NATURAL HISTORY

- Most ankle sprains resolve without the need for surgery.[21,41,60] However, a recurrently unstable ankle treated with appropriate physical therapy protocols may benefit from lateral ankle ligament repair or reconstructions.
- Left untreated, persistent lateral ankle instability may result in fixed varus tilt to the talus within the ankle mortise and eventual ankle arthritis.[57] Most patients present because of the disability associated with the recurrent sprains.
- Physiotherapy and bracing will improve symptoms in some patients with recurrent instability.
- There does not appear to be a role for immediate surgery on ruptures of the lateral ligaments.[18,29,33,47,49]

PATIENT HISTORY AND PHYSICAL FINDINGS

- Patients should remove their socks and shoes before the history is taken, so they can directly point to where the symptoms occur. Patients should be asked about pain and its relationship to activity and instability. Pointing to the foot or ankle with one finger will help focus the patient on the area of maximum discomfort and focuses the examination.
- Ankle instability may be difficult for the patient to convey; it may be more subtle than recurrent inversion injuries. Patients should be asked if the ankle gives way; if possible,

the position of the foot during the instability episode and circumstances (running, cutting left, cutting right, etc.) should be determined.

- The impact of the instability on sports and work should be determined.

- On physical examination, the patient should be examined standing and walking. He or she should be asked to heel walk and toe walk. The examiner should look for a cavus alignment to the foot. A "peek-a-boo" heel sign may assist in the diagnosis.

- Using the Coleman block: If heel varus corrects, the hindfoot is considered flexible; if heel varus does not correct, the cavus deformity is secondary to a forefoot varus and correction of forefoot will correct the hindfoot through the mobile midfoot. A severe cavus deformity that is rigid may require a valgenous osteotomy in addition to forefoot correction.

- The area of maximum discomfort and instability should be elicited. Examination of the ankle and hindfoot through a range of motion independent of one another is performed to determine the joint of maximum discomfort.

- Peroneal tendon pathology may accompany lateral ankle instability. A resisted contraction of ankle eversion should be performed and the tendons palpated for pain and fullness (suggestive of tenosynovitis). Rupture may also be present. The peroneal tendons, which are flexors, are best isolated with the ankle in plantarflexion and testing eversion against resistance. Peroneal tendon weakness accompanies most peroneal pathology due to pain; marked weakness may signify a peroneal tendon tear. In our experience, the combination of chronic ankle instability, varus hindfoot, and marked peroneal tendon weakness should raise the suspicion for a peroneal tendon tear. Occasionally, an equinus contracture may be associated with lateral ankle instability. A Silfverskiöld test (ankle dorsiflexion with the knee flexed contrasted with ankle dorsiflexion with the knee extended) allows the examiner to determine whether the contracture is isolated to the gastrocnemius or involves both the gastrocnemius and soleus components of the Achilles complex.

- The ATFL resists anterior translation and medial rotation of the talus on the tibia. A direct anterior draw (pulling the talus anteriorly without plantarflexion and internal rotation) may fail to elicit instability in an unstable ankle as an intact deltoid ligament medially will prevent translation. Instead, the examiner should hold the tibia posteriorly with the left hand while translating the calcaneus anteriorly and internally rotating the foot at the same time. Side-to-side comparison to the contralateral, physiologically stable ankle assists in identifying ankle instability.

- An inversion stress test determines the integrity of the CFL.

- An injury to the syndesmosis (ie, "high ankle sprain") may be elicited with a squeeze test and by rotating and translating the talus in the ankle mortise in dorsiflexion. A syndesmotic injury must be distinguished from lateral ankle instability because treatment is different.

- We also routinely examine the medial ankle for deltoid instability because medial and lateral instability may coexist.

IMAGING AND OTHER DIAGNOSTIC STUDIES

- We usually obtain weight-bearing anteroposterior and lateral ankle radiographs and a mortise view. Osteochondral defects, anterior osteophytes, and tibiotalar arthritis associated with

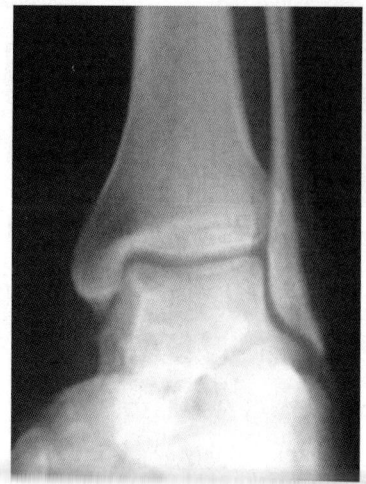

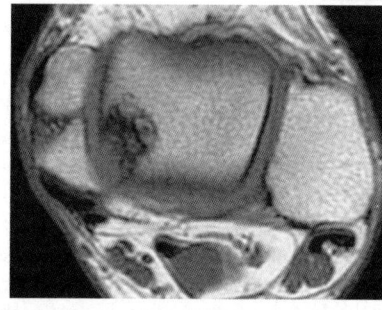

FIG 2 A. Radiologic finding of osteochondral lesion of talar dome. **B.** MRI finding of osteochondral lesion of posteromedial talar dome.

recurrent instability are generally visualized on standard radiographs of the ankle (**FIG 2A**).

- On occasion, we add a calcaneal axial view, Saltzman view, or tibial views if we need additional information on limb alignment. Recurrent ankle instability may be secondary to tarsal coalition; if the hindfoot is stiff on clinical examination, then calcaneal axial view and standard foot radiographs may identify the coalition. Computed tomography (CT) provides greater detail of osteochondral defects, osteophytes, arthritis, and tarsal coalition and should be obtained if these associated findings are suggested on plain radiographs.

- A magnetic resonance imaging (MRI), particularly a magnetic resonance arthrogram, can detect an ATFL or a CFL tear with a high accuracy.[12,61] Associated chondral and osteochondral defects (**FIG 2B**) as well as soft tissue impingement or peroneal tendon lesions may also be visualized by an MRI examination.

- Selective, diagnostic local anesthetic blocks of the ankle, subtalar, or talonavicular joints may be required to determine localized joint pain.

- When the diagnosis of ankle instability is suspected but remains in question, an inversion stress test done under fluoroscopy, compared to the physiologically stable contralateral ankle, may be useful. Bone scans can assist in determining associated pathology.

DIFFERENTIAL DIAGNOSIS

- Loose body in ankle
- Osteochondral defect
- Syndesmotic instability

- Peroneal tendinopathy or rupture
- Peroneal retinaculum tear
- Medial ankle instability
- Cavus foot
- Tarsal coalition

NONOPERATIVE MANAGEMENT

- Nonoperative treatment includes initial bracing and early functional rehabilitation.[17,18] Patients with recurrent ankle instability may develop peroneal tendon weakness and loss of proprioception.[32,36] Physiotherapy via proprioceptive training and strengthening can resolve the ankle instability. Bracing may help a patient to recover from a sprain and prevent future sprains by strengthening the dynamic, stabilizing peroneal tendons.
- Nonoperative treatment is less effective if ankle instability is associated with fixed hindfoot varus. Flexible hindfoot varus may be compensated for with a lateral wedge orthotic. If hindfoot varus is driven by a plantarflexed first ray (as determined by the Coleman block test), the orthotic should be "welled out" under the first metatarsal head, permitting further progression of the hindfoot into physiologic valgus.

SURGICAL MANAGEMENT

- The indication for surgical management of lateral ligament instability is chronic symptoms despite appropriate nonoperative management, including physiotherapy and bracing.[42]
- Surgical management of lateral ankle ligament instability includes repair (anatomic tightening of the lateral ankle ligaments) and reconstruction (reconstitution of the lateral ankle ligaments using more than the local physiologic tissue in the lateral ankle ligamentous complex).
- Lateral ankle ligament reconstruction may be anatomic or nonanatomic.[13] Anatomic reconstruction implies that the ligaments are rebuilt in the physiologically occurring orientation. Nonanatomic reconstruction suggests that lateral ankle support is reconstituted with tissue (typically tendon transfer to substitute for ligament deficiency) that does not follow a physiologic orientation of the ATFL and CFL.
- The literature on this topic favors anatomic over nonanatomic reconstruction (eg, Watson-Jones or Evans procedure) due to the higher incidence of early degenerative changes following nonanatomic reconstruction.[11,23,42,44,63]
- We recommend repairing the lateral ankle ligaments analog the classic Brostrom procedure whenever possible. A transfer of the inferior extensor retinaculum (Gould modification) can be added. If the ligaments are not repairable or require an augmentation, however, we perform an anatomic reconstruction of the ATFL and CFL.
  - Graft options for reconstruction include autograft (peroneus brevis, plantaris, gracilis) or allograft tendon.

Preoperative Planning

- Plain radiographs, and if further detail is needed other imaging studies of the ankle, must be evaluated for associated conditions, such as malalignment, osteochondral defects, tendon pathology, and arthritis. Adjuvant procedures must be planned so that they may be safely performed in concert with ligament reconstruction.

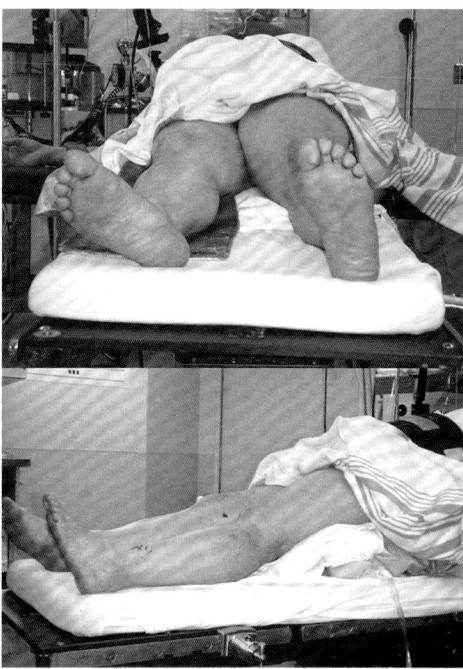

FIG 3 Patients positioned using beanbag to allow good exposure to the lateral aspect of the ankle.

- We recommend performing stress testing with the patient under anesthesia. In our opinion, the gold standard tests to determine lateral collateral ligament integrity are open anterior drawer and inversion stress tests on the table.

Positioning

- Apply a wide thigh tourniquet. Prepare and drape the leg to just above the knee. Perform anterior drawer and inversion stress tests on the table to confirm the diagnosis.
- We routinely use a beanbag or large bump under the ipsilateral hip to rotate the operated extremity and allow full access to the lateral ankle (**FIG 3**).
- A full lateral position is avoided, as it limits access to the proximal medial tibia, making harvest of the gracilis tendon autograft more challenging.
- Use regional anesthetic blocks if possible to ensure appropriate postoperative pain relief.

Approach

- We recommend an extensile approach (ie, a longitudinal curvilinear approach) in lieu of the traditional J-shaped incision popularized by Brostrom[10]. The extensile approach affords access to not only the lateral ankle ligaments but also the distal tibia, peroneal tendons, sinus tarsi, and lateral calcaneus for adjuvant procedures that may be warranted.
- We prefer a gracilis autograft tendon, anchored via drill holes, for the anatomic lateral ankle reconstruction and aim to obtain immediate stable fixation, biologic ingrowth to bone in time, and an anatomic reconstruction. The technique is a modification of the plantaris reconstruction described by Anderson[1] (**FIG 4A**).
- If intra-articular pathology has been preoperatively identified or is suspected, we routinely address this with ankle arthroscopy before lateral ankle reconstruction (**FIG 4B**).

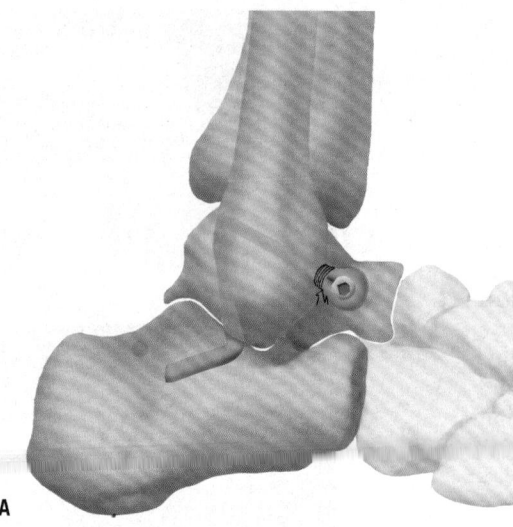

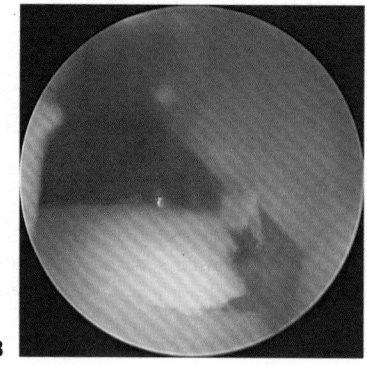

FIG 4 A. Free gracilis lateral ligament reconstruction. **B.** Osteochondral defect of the talus found on arthroscopy before ligament reconstruction.

T E C H N I Q U E S

GRACILIS RECONSTRUCTION THROUGH DRILL HOLES

Exposure

- Start the extensile longitudinal lateral incision on the distal fibula, continue it over the lateral malleolus, and curve it anteriorly toward the sinus tarsi **(TECH FIG 1A)**.
- Expose the superior extensor retinaculum anterior to the fibula while protecting the deep branch of the peroneal nerve, which has variable anatomy. Strip the extensor retinaculum off the fibula so that the extensor compartment is exposed. Carry the dissection distally toward the ankle joint to the junction between the tibia, talus, and fibula. Open the joint at this level. This dissection will ensure that no ligaments are damaged during the exposure **(TECH FIG 1B)**.
- Remove anterior osteophytes using an osteotome.

Stress Testing

- Perform an open anterior drawer and inversion stress tests **(TECH FIG 2)** to assess the integrity of the lateral collateral ligaments as a final check before proceeding with reconstruction. We will perform a repair if the ligaments are clearly torn off bone, if they are not obviously scarred or thickened, if there is enough length to bridge the gap, or if they have been avulsed with a bone fragment.[7]
- If the ligaments are not considered repairable, reconstruction is warranted. We favor an autograft gracilis reconstruction and, therefore, optimal patient positioning and preparation and draping of the operated extremity are important.

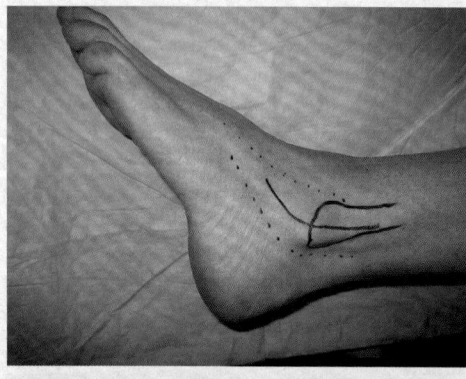

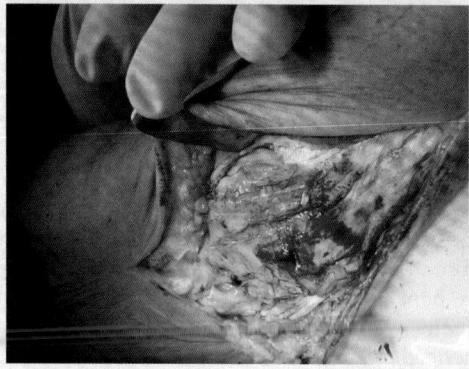

TECH FIG 1 A. Lateral incision (*solid line*) with course of sural and superficial peroneal nerves marked (*dotted lines*). **B.** Lateral dissection anterior to the fibula, sparing the ATFL.

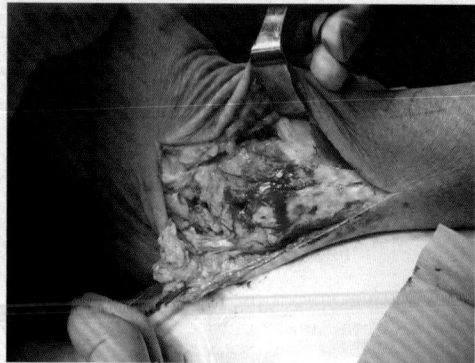

TECH FIG 2 Open anterior drawer test. Talus is anterior and internally rotated relative to fibula, indicating a positive test and insufficiency of the ATFL.

Tendon Harvest and Drill Hole Creation

- Perform a standard gracilis tendon harvest with an incision over the medial aspect of the tibial tubercle at the pes anserinus insertion. Carry dissection down through the sartorius fascia and onto the gracilis tendon. Isolate the gracilis with the knee flexed and use a tendon stripper to release it from its muscle proximally. Reef the tendon using a baseball whipstitch.
- Divide the tendon at its insertion into bone and measure it. Select a drill bit matching the size of the tendon (typically a 3.5-, 4.5-, or 6-mm drill bit).
  - Alternatively, a tendon-anchoring interference screw system may be used, size matched to the harvested tendon's diameter.
- Expose the fibula first by removing part of the peroneal fascia so that the peroneal tendons and the posterior fibula are exposed **(TECH FIG 3A)**. We typically examine the peroneal tendons at this time to rule out or treat associated peroneal tendon pathology.
  - If needed, the peroneal retinaculum is incised with a step cut to allow complete exposure of the peroneal tendons for débridement or repair.[31]

- Incise the collateral ligaments and expose the insertions of the CFL and ATFL. Dissect to the origin of both ligaments on the calcaneus and talus. Both areas are dissected clear onto bone **(TECH FIG 3B)**. Use a curette to clear the area of the junction of the body and neck of the talus.
- Make a medial incision at the anterior border of the Achilles tendon and carry the dissection down to the bone and tendon at this level **(TECH FIG 3C)**.
- Drill through the calcaneus from medial to lateral, adjacent to the Achilles tendon, with the appropriately sized drill bit (depending on harvest tendon diameter), exiting laterally at the origin of the CFL **(TECH FIG 3D)**. A cannulated drill or a combined aiming device can be used to target this drill to the calcaneofibular footprint on the calcaneus.
- Make a fibular drill hole starting at the insertion of the CFL and exiting the posterior fibula. Make another fibular drill hole starting at the insertion of the talofibular ligament and exiting in the posterior fibula about 1 cm above the exit point of the previous fibular drill hole **(TECH FIG 3E)**.
- Then, make a 2.5-mm drill hole in the center of the junction between the talar body and neck **(TECH FIG 3F)**. Measure its depth. A fully threaded cancellous small fragment screw with a small and large fragment washer is readied on the back table.

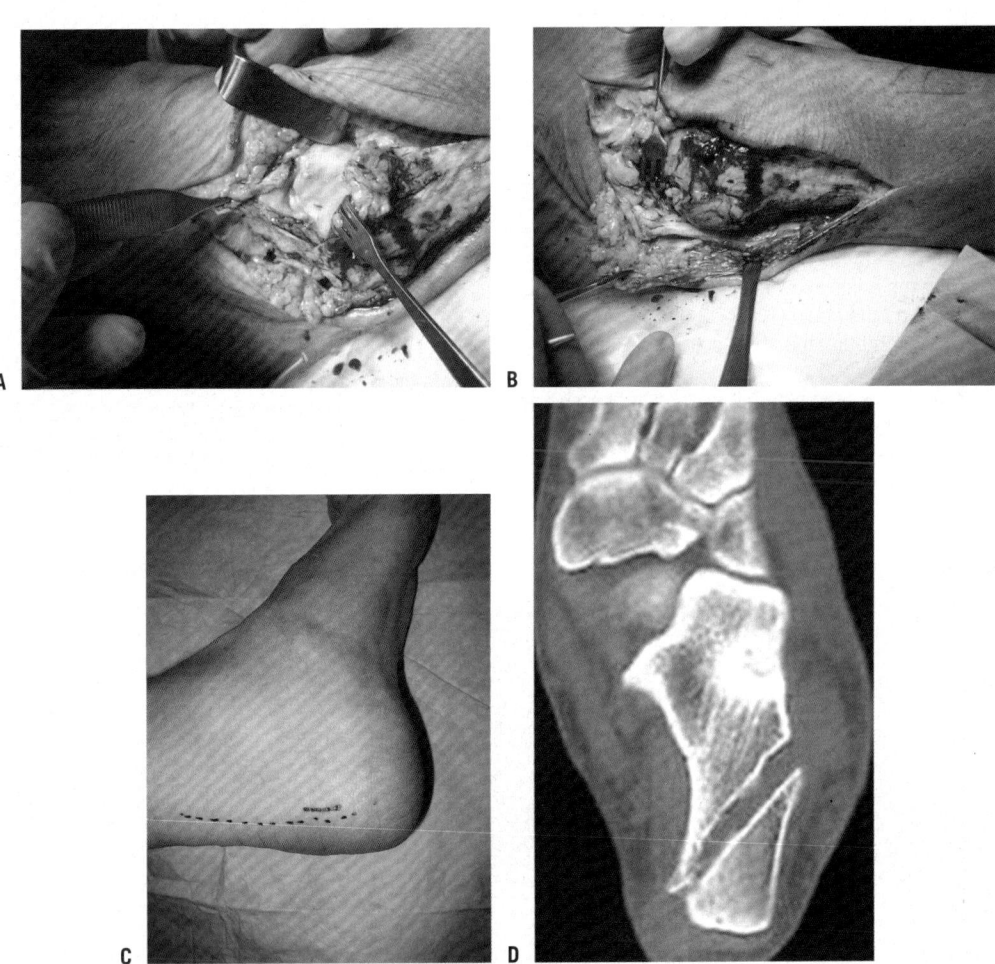

TECH FIG 3 A. Dissection of the talus with exposure of the insertion of the ATFL. **B.** Dissection posterior to the fibula to expose the peroneal tendons. **C.** Location of medial incision. **D.** Postoperative CT demonstrating drill path through calcaneus. *(continued)*

TECHNIQUES

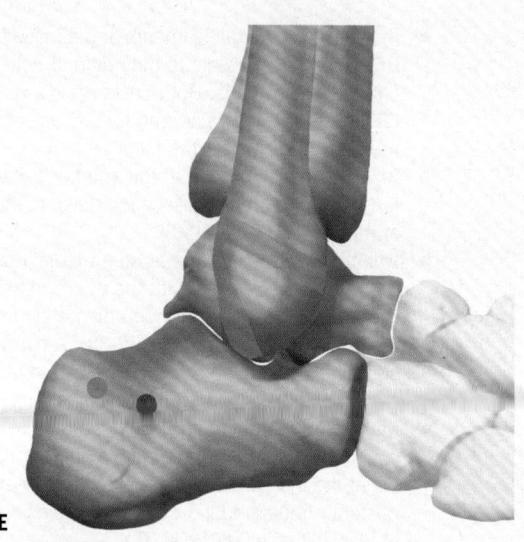

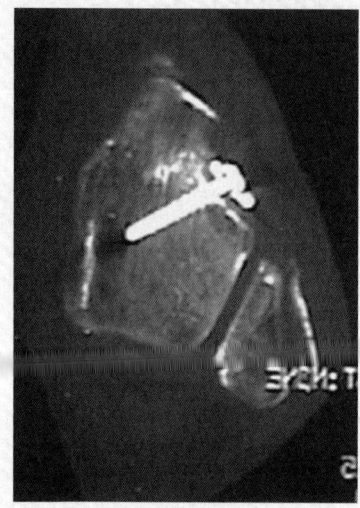

TECH FIG 3 *(continued)* **E.** Drill paths through calcaneus and fibula. **F.** Postoperative CT scan demonstrating orientation of screw in talus.

Passing and Securing the Graft

- With a no. 2 braided nonabsorbable polyester suture, suture the tendon onto the edge of the Achilles medially, using a Kessler stitch on the nonbraided end of the gracilis tendon. Leave 1 cm of loop between the Achilles and the end of the gracilis to prevent buildup of suture and ligament medially, which may cause irritation. Place the knot in the middle of this segment.
- Use a tendon passer to pass the tendon graft through the calcaneal tunnel to the lateral calcaneus.
- Cycle the tendon a few times to make it tight.
- Pass the tendon through to the posterior aspect of the fibula and pull it tight with the ankle in eversion. Suture the tendon to any remaining tissue on the fibula **(TECH FIG 4A)**.
- Bring the tendon back through the fibula so that it exits anteriorly at the second drill hole.
- Cycle the tendon in tension and suture it to the cuff of tissue on the fibula at the insertion of the talofibular ligament.
- Start the selected small fragment screw with the large and small washer into the 2.5-mm hole in the talar neck.

- Place the split tendon end over the washer (right side) and under the washer (left side) and secure it around the washer in a clockwise direction. Hold the foot in dorsiflexion and eversion.
- Hold the tendon tight around the washer and screw and tighten the screw home. The tendon will tighten as the screw is placed home **(TECH FIG 4B)**. Although interference screw systems are effective, we method using standard screws and a simple ligament washer is cost-effective and consistently affords immediate ankle stability.
- Suture the free end of the tendon back onto the tendon segment between the fibula and washer.
- Suture the remainder of the tendon back onto the lateral side of the fibula and trim the residual tendon end.
- To confirm stability and proper ligament tension of the reconstruction, place the ankle through repeat open anterior drawer and inversion stress tests. Close the wounds using nylon or staples. Use of a drain is at the surgeon's discretion.

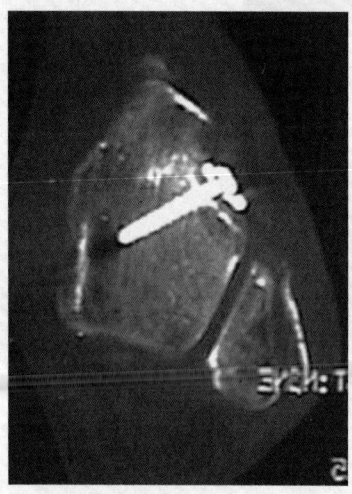

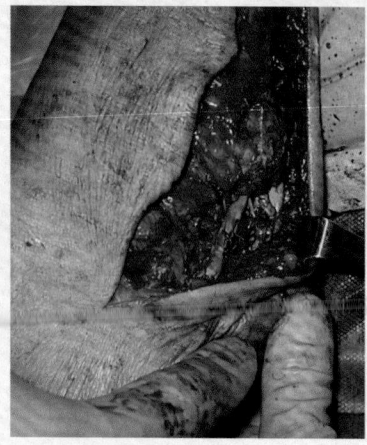

TECH FIG 4 A. Gracilis graft passed from calcaneus to fibula. **B.** Gracilis graft tensioned from fibula to talus.

COUGHLIN DRILL HOLES IN BONE

- An alternative technique is to use drill holes through the bone made on the lateral side only.[15] This is a variation of the Emslie technique **(TECH FIG 5)**.
- Use a similar exposure, with no medial incision.
- Make two drill holes on the lateral wall of the calcaneus on each side of the origin of the CFL.
- Pass the tendon through the drill holes and suture it back onto itself.
- Make a single drill hole on the tip of the fibula, joining the insertion of both lateral collateral ligaments.
- Make two drill holes on each side of the insertion of the talofibular ligament.
- Pass the tendon through the fibula and through the drill holes on the talus and tension it and suture it back onto itself.
- We consider this variation more challenging than our described technique, specifically in passing the tendon through bone without fracturing the bone bridges. Moreover, we find it more difficult to ensure anatomic location of the ligaments and optimal tendon tensioning. In our opinion, prolonged postoperative immobilization may be required, depending on the strength of the bone bridges.

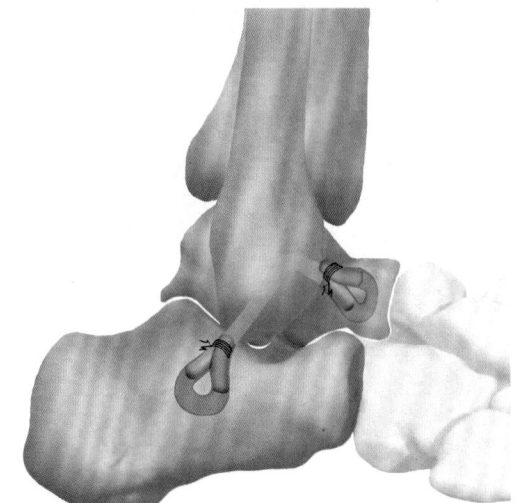

TECH FIG 5 Coughlin drill holes in bone technique.

BIO-TENODESIS SCREW TECHNIQUE

- With this technique, a similar exposure and tendon harvest are used **(TECH FIG 6)**. No medial exposure is required.
- Make a drill hole on the lateral side of the calcaneus at the CFL origin. Place the tendon over the tip of a tenodesis screw and secure it to the lateral wall of the calcaneus.
- Pass the tendon through two fibular tunnels at the anatomic locations of the CFL and talofibular ligament, exiting over a posterior fibular bone bridge as described in our technique.
- Make a second drill hole on the lateral side of the talus at the junction of the body and neck to accommodate the tendon and a second Bio-Tenodesis screw.
- Our concerns with this alternative are as follows:
  - Quality of fixation via interference screw in the relatively weak cancellous bone of the calcaneus
  - The relatively large talar drill hole, which may serve as a stress riser and cause of talar neck fracture

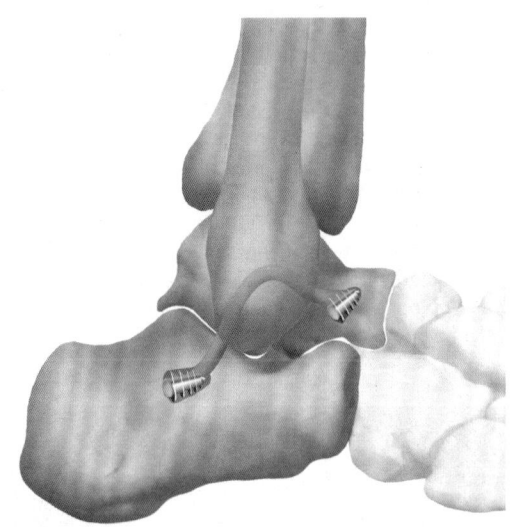

TECH FIG 6 Bio-Tenodesis screw fixation technique.

MYERSON MINIMAL INCISION TECHNIQUE

- This technique **(TECH FIG 7)** is similar to the Coughlin technique but is performed through two small incisions.
- Make one incision over the calcaneal drill holes and a second over the region of the talar drill holes. Carry dissection down to bone. Make two connecting drill holes in each location. Tunnel a drill bit and guide subcutaneously to drill the pathway through the fibula.
- Harvest the graft and route it in the same fashion as in the Coughlin technique described earlier.
- Although this is a reasonable alternative, as for the Coughlin technique, we have difficulty passing and tensioning the tendon using this technique.

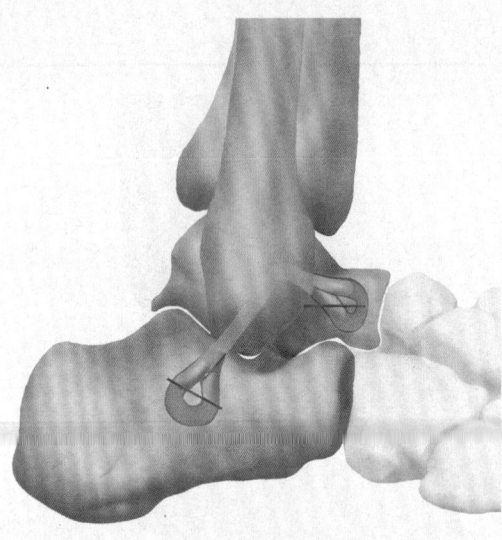

TECH FIG 7 Myerson minimally invasive technique. *Red lines* indicate skin incisions.

PERCUTANEOUS ANKLE RECONSTRUCTION OF LATERAL LIGAMENTS M GLAZEBROOK ET AL[22] (FILM)

- Positioning/exposure
  - A lateral or semilateral position with support under the leg is suggested.
  - The bony landmarks of origin and insertion of the ATFL and CFL are marked on the skin under fluoroscopy or palpation. The landmark for the origin of AFTL and CFL on the fibula is the fibular obscure tubercle (FOT). The landmark for the talar insertion of the ATFL is the talar obscure tubercle (TOT) at the anterolateral border of the talar body. The landmark for the insertion of the CFL is the tuberculum ligamenti calcaneofibularis (TLC) **(TECH FIG 8)**.[39,40]
- Constructing the anatomic y-graft
  - An autograft from the ipsilateral knee (eg, gracilis tendon) or an appropriate allograft at least 135 mm length and ~5 mm diameter are used.

- The anatomic "Y" configuration is prepared by doubling the graft to a looped stem (15 mm) for the talar, fibula, and calcaneal end.
- The loops are used for anchorage in the bone; the free 15-mm and 30-mm parts represent the reconstruction of the ATFL and CFL, respectively **(TECH FIG 9)**.
- Constructing of bone tunnels and insertion of passing threads
  - Three skin incisions are made for the construction of the fibular, talar, and calcaneal bone tunnel.

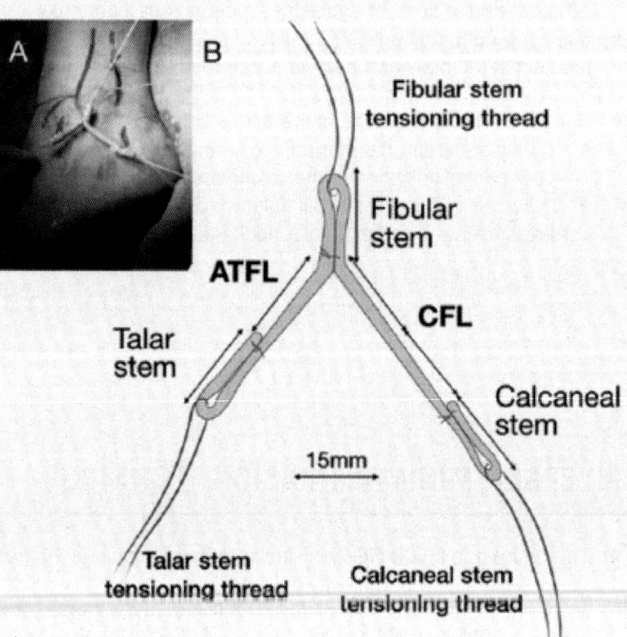

TECH FIG 9 Preparing the y-graft. **A.** Skin incisions. **B.** Graft preparation and position. *ATFL*, anterior talofibular ligament; *CFL*, calcaneofibular ligament.

TECH FIG 8 Bony landmarks of origin and insertion of the ATFL and CFL.

- A guidewire is inserted at the FOT and directed 30 degrees to the long axis of the fibula through the far cortex and the skin. The position is controlled under fluoroscopy in two planes.
- A bone tunnel diameter of 6 mm with a length of 20 mm is created with a cannulated drill.
- The talar guidewire is inserted at the TOT and directed slightly posterior and proximal to a point proximal to the medial malleolus. Again, a 6- × 20-mm bone tunnel is created.
- The calcaneal is pin inserted at the TLC and directed to the inferior, medial, and posterior areas of the calcaneus. The bone tunnel is drilled with the same diameter but a depth of 30 mm.
- A passing thread doubled into a loop is passed through each bone tunnel, the loop facing toward the insertion/origin sides of the ligaments. The loose ends are clamped with a Mosquito forceps.
- Delivery of each loop of the graft (TECH FIG 10)
  - A tension thread is passed through each looped stem of the y-graft.
  - The fibular stem is delivered first in an inside-out technique using the passing threads.
  - Next, the talar and calcaneal stems are inserted.
- Fixation of y-graft
  - With the ankle in neutral position, the y-graft is balanced and tensioned using the tension threads.
  - An interference screw guide pin is inserted into the fibular tunnel first, and a 6- × 15-mm interference screw is used to fix the fibular stem of the y-graft. The talar stem and the calcaneal stem are fixed likewise in their corresponding bone tunnel.
  - The tension threads are removed, and the incision sides are closed with nylon sutures.
  - Sterile wound dressings and a below-knee cast are applied.

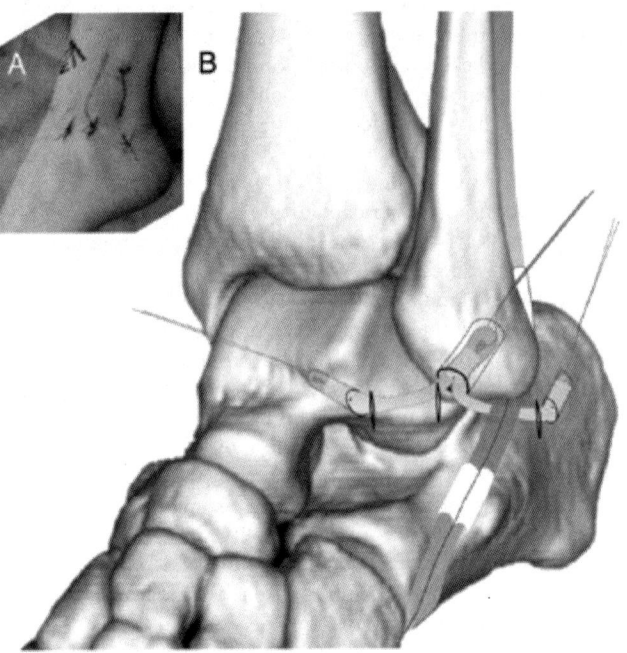

TECH FIG 10 Final position of graft. **A.** Skin incisions. **B.** Graft preparation and position.

TECHNIQUES

Pearls and Pitfalls

Exposure	• Ensure that the exposure goes through the anterior compartment and down into the ankle. This will avoid damage to the ligaments before the open anterior drawer test.
Positioning	• Use a beanbag to ensure that the ankle is internally rotated to allow access to the lateral side of the ankle. Different patients have different amounts of internal rotation, and this needs to be accommodated. However, avoid a full lateral position if you plan a gracilis tendon harvest.
Drill Holes	• Drill the calcaneal hole from medial to lateral. The vector guide can be used to ensure correct positioning of the exit hole and the CFL footprint on the lateral calcaneus.
Drill Hole Size	• The drill hole should closely match the size of the graft to ensure osseous integration. The drills and taps from the anterior cruciate ligament set can be used. The drill hole should be large enough to pass the tendon.
Graft Preparation	• The graft should be prepared with a whipstitch to ensure that it passes easily through the bone tunnels.
Graft Tensioning	• Avoid anterior translation of the talus within the ankle mortise when the tendon reconstruction is tensioned. In particular, place a bump under the distal tibia and avoid placing a bump under the heel, which tends to translate the foot and talus anteriorly. Also, after each pass of the tendon through a tunnel, cycle the ankle with the tendon under tension to gain optimal final tension.

POSTOPERATIVE CARE

- With our preferred technique, patients are placed in a walker boot at the time of surgery.
- At 1 week, they are allowed to bear weight as tolerated.
- The sutures are removed at 2 weeks. Ankle range of motion, supervised by physiotherapy, is initiated at this time.
- Patients are kept in the walker boot until 10 weeks after surgery during weight bearing. Gait training is started 8 weeks after surgery.
- Proprioception and single toe raises are started 12 weeks out.
- Patients may return to sports after 4 months.

OUTCOMES

- There are few retrospective reviews of anatomic reconstructions using various autografts. Despite the paucity of literature, all studies have reported good results, with 88% to 100% of patients reporting good outcomes.[1,14,16,55]
- Few studies have specifically looked at the outcome of a gracilis ligament reconstruction. A review of 29 ankles in 28 patients by Coughlin et al[16] reported a successful outcome in terms of American Orthopaedic Foot & Ankle Society and Karlsson scores in all patients; postoperative follow-up averaged 23 months
- A recent systematic review compares anatomic to nonanatomic stabilization techniques and concludes that anatomic repair and anatomic reconstruction provide a better functional outcome.[63] In addition, there are sufficient studies with poor outcomes in the current literature to recommend against nonanatomic reconstruction of the lateral ankle ligaments.[3,6,24,26,28,30,34,35,43,45,59]
- A systematic review comparing different minimal invasive approaches for chronic ankle instability showed that there is need for studies with a higher level of evidence on minimally invasive surgery (MIS) approach for chronic ankle instability to support the use of MIS.[38]
- There is a paucity of studies with higher level of evidence comparing allograft and autograft for anatomic lateral ligament reconstruction; therefore, no difference can be determined.[8]

COMPLICATIONS

- Wound healing
- Recurrent instability
- Nerve injury
- Loss of range of motion

REFERENCES

1. Anderson ME. Reconstruction of the lateral ligaments of the ankle using the plantaris tendon. J Bone Joint Surg Am 1985;67(6):930–934.
2. Becker HP, Rosenbaum D. Chronic recurrent ligament instability on the lateral ankle [in German]. Orthopade 1999;28(6):483–492.
3. Becker HP, Rosenbaum D, Zeithammer G, et al. Gait pattern analysis after ankle ligament reconstruction (modified Evans procedure). Foot Ankle Int 1994;15(9):477–482.
4. Bonnel F, Toullec E, Mabit C, et al. Chronic ankle instability: biomechanics and pathomechanics of ligaments injury and associated lesions. Orthop Traumatol Surg Res 2010;96(4):424–432.
5. Bosien WR, Staples OS, Russell SW. Residual disability following acute ankle sprains. J Bone Joint Surg Am 1955;37-A(6):1237–1243.
6. Boszotta H, Sauer G. Chronic fibular ligament insufficiency at the upper ankle joint. Late results after modified Watson-Jones plastic surgery. Unfallchirurg 1989;92(1):11–16.
7. Boyer DS, Younger AS. Anatomic reconstruction of the lateral ligament complex of the ankle using a gracilis autograft. Foot Ankle Clin 2006;11(3):585–595.
8. Brambilla L, Bianchi A, Malerba F, et al. Lateral ankle ligament anatomic reconstruction for chronic ankle instability: allograft or autograft? A systematic review. Foot Ankle Surg 2020;26(1):85–93.
9. Brennan SA, Kiernan C, Maleki F, et al. Talonavicular synostosis with lateral ankle instability—a case report and review of the literature. Foot Ankle Surg 2012;18(3):e34–e36.
10. Broström L. Sprained ankles. V. Treatment and prognosis in recent ligament ruptures. Acta Chir Scand 1966;132(5):537–550.
11. Cao Y, Hong Y, Xu Y, et al. Surgical management of chronic lateral ankle instability: a meta-analysis. J Orthop Surg Res 2018;13(1):159.
12. Chandnani VP, Harper MT, Ficke JR, et al. Chronic ankle instability: evaluation with MR arthrography, MR imaging, and stress radiography. Radiology 1994;192(1):189–194.
13. Colville MR. Surgical treatment of the unstable ankle. J Am Acad Orthop Surg 1998;6(6):368–377.
14. Colville MR, Grondel RJ. Anatomic reconstruction of the lateral ankle ligaments using a split peroneus brevis tendon graft. Am J Sports Med 1995;23(2):210–213.
15. Coughlin MJ, Matt V, Schenck RC Jr. Augmented lateral ankle reconstruction using a free gracilis graft. Orthopedics 2002;25(1):31–35.
16. Coughlin MJ, Schenck RC Jr, Grebing BR, et al. Comprehensive reconstruction of the lateral ankle for chronic instability using a free gracilis graft. Foot Ankle Int 2004;25(4):231–241.
17. de Vries JS, Krips R, Sierevelt IN, et al. Interventions for treating chronic ankle instability. Cochrane Database Syst Rev 2011;(8):CD004124.
18. Doherty C, Bleakley C, Delahunt E, et al. Treatment and prevention of acute and recurrent ankle sprain: an overview of systematic reviews with meta-analysis. Br J Sports Med 2017;51(2):113–125.
19. Freeman MA. Instability of the foot after injuries to the lateral ligament of the ankle. J Bone Joint Surg Br 1965;47(4):669–677.
20. Frigg A, Magerkurth O, Valderrabano V, et al. The effect of osseous ankle configuration on chronic ankle instability. Br J Sports Med 2007;41(7):420–424.
21. Gerber JP, Williams GN, Scoville CR, et al. Persistent disability associated with ankle sprains: a prospective examination of an athletic population. Foot Ankle Int 1998;19(10):653–660.
22. Glazebrook M, Stone J, Matsui K, et al. Percutaneous ankle reconstruction of lateral ligaments (Perc-Anti RoLL). Foot Ankle Int 2016;37(6):659–664.
23. Guillo S, Bauer T, Lee JW, et al. Consensus in chronic ankle instability: aetiology, assessment, surgical indications and place for arthroscopy. Orthop Traumatol Surg Res 2013;99(8 suppl):S411–S419.
24. Hedeboe J, Johannsen A. Recurrent instability of the ankle joint. Surgical repair by the Watson-Jones method. Acta Orthop Scand 1979;50(3):337–340.
25. Hintermann B, Boss A, Schäfer D. Arthroscopic findings in patients with chronic ankle instability. Am J Sports Med 2002;30(3):402–409.
26. Horstman JK, Kantor GS, Samuelson KM. Investigation of lateral ankle ligament reconstruction. Foot Ankle 1981;1(6):338–342.
27. Hunt KJ, Pereira H, Kelley J, et al. The role of calcaneofibular ligament injury in ankle instability: implications for surgical management. Am J Sports Med 2019;47(2):431–437.
28. Juliano PJ, Jordan JD, Lippert FG, et al. Persistent postoperative pain after the Chrisman-Snook ankle reconstruction. Am J Orthop (Belle Mead NJ) 2000;29(6):449–452.
29. Kaikkonen A, Kannus P, Järvinen M. Surgery versus functional treatment in ankle ligament tears. A prospective study. Clin Orthop Relat Res 1996;(326):194–202.
30. Karlsson J, Bergsten T, Lansinger O, et al. Lateral instability of the ankle treated by the Evans procedure. A long-term clinical and radiological follow-up. J Bone Joint Surg Br 1988;70(3):476–480.
31. Karlsson J, Brandsson S, Kälebo P, et al. Surgical treatment of concomitant chronic ankle instability and longitudinal rupture of the peroneus brevis tendon. Scand J Med Sci Sports 1998;8(1):42–49.
32. Karlsson J, Wiger P. Longitudinal split of the peroneus brevis tendon and lateral ankle instability: treatment of concomitant lesions. J Athl Train 2002;37(4):463–466.
33. Kerkhoffs GM, Handoll HH, de Bie R, et al. Surgical versus conservative treatment for acute injuries of the lateral ligament complex of the ankle in adults. Cochrane Database Syst Rev 2007;(2):CD000380.
34. Krips R, Brandsson S, Swensson C, et al. Anatomical reconstruction and Evans tenodesis of the lateral ligaments of the ankle. Clinical and radiological findings after follow-up for 15 to 30 years. J Bone Joint Surg Br 2002;84(2):232–236.
35. Labs K, Perka C, Lang T. Clinical and gait-analytical results of the modified Evans tenodesis in chronic fibulotalar ligament instability. Knee Surg Sports Traumatol Arthrosc 2001;9(2):116–122.
36. Larsen E, Lund PM. Peroneal muscle function in chronically unstable ankles. A prospective preoperative and postoperative electromyographic study. Clin Orthop Relat Res 1991;(272):219–226.
37. Mack RP. Ankle injuries in athletics. Clin Sports Med 1982;1(1):71–84.

38. Matsui K, Burgesson B, Takao M, et al. Minimally invasive surgical treatment for chronic ankle instability: a systematic review. Knee Surg Sports Traumatol Arthrosc 2016;24(4):1040–1048.

39. Matsui K, Oliva XM, Takao M, et al. Bony landmarks available for minimally invasive lateral ankle stabilization surgery: a cadaveric anatomical study. Knee Surg Sports Traumatol Arthrosc 2017;25(6): 1916–1924.

40. Matsui K, Takao M, Tochigi Y, et al. Anatomy of anterior talofibular ligament and calcaneofibular ligament for minimally invasive surgery: a systematic review. Knee Surg Sports Traumatol Arthrosc 2017;25(6):1892–1902.

41. Medina McKeon JM, Bush HM, Reed A, et al. Return-to-play probabilities following new versus recurrent ankle sprains in high school athletes. J Sci Med Sport 2014;17(1):23–28.

42. Michels F, Pereira H, Calder J, et al. Searching for consensus in the approach to patients with chronic lateral ankle instability: ask the expert. Knee Surg Sports Traumatol Arthrosc 2018;26(7):2095–2102.

43. Nimon GA, Dobson PJ, Angel KR, et al. A long-term review of a modified Evans procedure. J Bone Joint Surg Br 2001;83(1):14–18.

44. Noailles T, Lopes R, Padiolleau G, et al. Non-anatomical or direct anatomical repair of chronic lateral instability of the ankle: a systematic review of the literature after at least 10 years of follow-up. Foot Ankle Surg 2018;24(2):80–85.

45. Orava S, Jaroma H, Weitz H, et al. Radiographic instability of the ankle joint after Evans' repair. Acta Orthop Scand 1983;54(5):734–738.

46. Pijnenburg AC, Bogaard K, Krips R, et al. Operative and functional treatment of rupture of the lateral ligament of the ankle. A randomised, prospective trial. J Bone Joint Surg Br 2003;85(4):525–530.

47. Pijnenburg AC, Van Dijk CN, Bossuyt PM, et al. Treatment of ruptures of the lateral ankle ligaments: a meta-analysis. J Bone Joint Surg Am 2000;82(6):761–773.

48. Rubin A, Sallis R. Evaluation and diagnosis of ankle injuries. Am Fam Physician 1996;54(5):1609–1618.

49. Safran MR, Zachazewski JE, Benedetti RS, et al. Lateral ankle sprains: a comprehensive review part 2: treatment and rehabilitation with an emphasis on the athlete. Med Sci Sports Exerc 1999;31(7 suppl): S438–S447.

50. Sammarco GJ, Burstein AH, Frankel VH. Biomechanics of the ankle: a kinematic study. Orthop Clin North Am 1973;4(1):75–96.

51. Sammarco VJ. Complications of lateral ankle ligament reconstruction. Clin Orthop Relat Res 2001;(391):123–132.

52. Scranton PE Jr, McDermott JE, Rogers JV. The relationship between chronic ankle instability and variations in mortise anatomy and impingement spurs. Foot Ankle Int 2000;21(8):657–664.

53. Smith RW, Reischl SF. Treatment of ankle sprains in young athletes. Am J Sports Med 1986;14(6):465–471.

54. Staples OS. Result study of ruptures of lateral ligaments of the ankle. Clin Orthop Relat Res 1972;85:50–58.

55. Sugimoto K, Takakura Y, Kumai T, et al. Reconstruction of the lateral ankle ligaments with bone-patellar tendon graft in patients with chronic ankle instability: a preliminary report. Am J Sports Med 2002;30(3):340–346.

56. Takao M, Miyamoto W, Matsui K, et al. Functional treatment after surgical repair for acute lateral ligament disruption of the ankle in athletes. Am J Sports Med 2012;40(2):447–451.

57. Valderrabano V, Hintermann B, Horisberger M, et al. Ligamentous posttraumatic ankle osteoarthritis. Am J Sports Med 2006;34(4):612–620.

58. Van Bergeyk AB, Younger A, Carson B. CT analysis of hindfoot alignment in chronic lateral ankle instability. Foot Ankle Int 2002;23(1): 37–42.

59. van der Rijt AJ, Evans GA. The long-term results of Watson-Jones tenodesis. J Bone Joint Surg Br 1984;66(3):371–375.

60. van Rijn RM, van Os AG, Bernsen RM, et al. What is the clinical course of acute ankle sprains? A systematic literature review. Am J Med 2008;121(4):324–331.e6.

61. Verhaven EF, Shahabpour M, Handelberg FW, et al. The accuracy of three-dimensional magnetic resonance imaging in the diagnosis of ruptures of the lateral ligaments of the ankle. Am J Sports Med 1991;19(6):583–587.

62. Vertullo C. Unresolved lateral ankle pain. It's not always 'just a sprain.' Aust Fam Physician 2002;31(3):247–253.

63. Vuurberg G, Pereira H, Blankevoort L, et al. Anatomic stabilization techniques provide superior results in terms of functional outcome in patients suffering from chronic ankle instability compared to non-anatomic techniques. Knee Surg Sports Traumatol Arthrosc 2018;26(7):2183–2195.

64. Wikstrom EA, Hubbard TJ. Talar positional fault in persons with chronic ankle instability. Arch Phys Med Rehabil 2010;91(8):1267–1271.

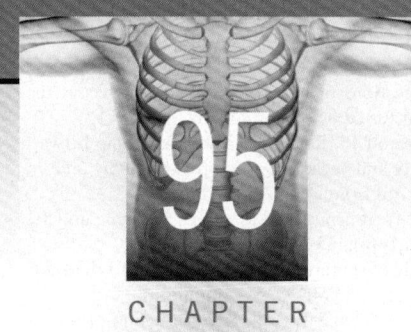

95

CHAPTER

Lateral Ankle Ligament Reconstruction Using Allograft and Interference Screw Fixation

Taggart T. Gauvain, William C. McGarvey, and Thomas O. Clanton

DEFINITION

- Lateral ankle sprains are the most common injury in sports, accounting for 15% or more of all athletic injuries in some parts of the world. These injuries result in compromise or complete disruption of the lateral ankle and, often subtalar, ligamentous complexes.[13,16]
- Ankle sprains range in severity from mild stretching to complete disruption of the ligamentous structures. Often, the injuries of moderate or medium severity are the most difficult to accurately diagnose and, therefore, manage properly.
- Eighty percent of acute ankle sprains respond well to a course of nonoperative therapy. Treatments include standard rest, ice, compression, and elevation (RICE) methods; a period of functional bracing or boot immobilization; and functional rehabilitation program focused on strengthening, balance, and proprioception.
- Thirty percent to 40% of patients will have persistent problems related to pain and swelling for up to 6 months after the injury, and 10% to 20% will have difficulties with recurrent sprains, leading to chronic ankle instability.[11]
- Chronic ankle instability can be debilitating and can result in chronic pain, repeat injuries during basic activity, inability to participate in sport activity, and arthritic changes in the ankle joint due to abnormal joint mechanics.

ANATOMY

- The lateral ankle ligamentous complex is made up of three distinct ligaments: the anterior talofibular ligament (ATFL), the calcaneofibular ligament (CFL), and the posterior talofibular ligament (PTFL). Other structures contributing to overall lateral ankle stability are the inferior extensor retinaculum and subtalar ligamentous complex.[2]
- The ATFL, which blends with the anterolateral joint capsule, is 15 to 20 mm long, 6 to 8 mm wide, and 2 mm thick. There are usually two distinct bands of the ATFL.[2]
- The ATFL originates from the anterior and distal fibula to insert on the lateral process of the talus, forming an angle of about 75 degrees to the floor.[2]
- The CFL is 20 to 30 mm long, 4 to 8 mm wide, and 3 to 5 mm thick. It originates from the posteromedial portion of the distal fibula tip to travel within the peroneal tendon sheath, under the tendons, and attaches to the lateral wall of the calcaneus. The orientation is 10 to 45 degrees posterior to the longitudinal axis of the fibula. The angle formed between the ATFL and CFL is 100 to 105 degrees.[2]

- The PTFL is the largest of the lateral ankle ligaments, at 30 mm in length, 5 mm in width, and 1 to 4 mm in thickness. It has a broad insertion on nearly the entire posterior lip of the talus.[2]
- The ATFL has the lowest load to failure of the three ligaments. Conversely, it has a much higher capacity to withstand strain than the CFL or PTFL, thereby allowing the greatest deformation before failure of all three structures.[17,2]
- The ATFL is taut with the ankle in plantarflexion, whereas the CFL is relatively loose. The reverse is true for the dorsiflexed ankle. The strength of the CFL and the stability afforded by the bony mortise at the malleoli in a neutral or dorsiflexed ankle make maximal plantarflexion the position of vulnerability for lateral ankle ligament injuries.[1,3,2]
- The subtalar joint is stabilized by the lateral talocalcaneal ligament, cervical ligament, interosseous talocalcaneal ligament, and the CFL. The stability of the subtalar joint does provide some measure of stability to the lateral ankle.[2]
- The lateral ankle is also stabilized by the peroneal tendons during dynamic activity. The peroneal tendons can, at times, be injured when the lateral ligaments are disrupted, and this additional pathology is vital to identify and treat as well.[2]

PATHOGENESIS

- Ankle instability is thought to be either acquired, as a result of repetitive trauma, or inherited due to ligamentous laxity, biomechanical abnormality (eg, heel varus, cavus foot position), or a combination of both.
- The ATFL is most commonly injured, accounting for about 75% of injuries to the ligaments of the ankle, followed by the CFL, which accounts for about 20% to 25% of these injuries. Injury to the ligaments occurs when they are either stretched, partially torn, or completely torn, either by avulsion from bone, or, more commonly, from midsubstance tearing.
- Neuromuscular deficits also result from these inversion injuries, leading to slower firing of the peroneal muscles in response to inversion stress, decreased responsiveness in the peroneal nerve branches, weakness, and restricted dorsiflexion range of motion due to inadequate muscle forces.
- Repetitive injury can result in accumulated scarring leading to anterolateral mechanical impingement or even sinus tarsi involvement.[7,15]
- Subtalar ligaments also may be injured, although usually to a lesser extent.

NATURAL HISTORY

- Even though most ankle sprains and instability receive some form of treatment, there is little consistency in treatment regimens.
- In one long-term study, one-third of patients treated functionally for ankle sprains had continued complaints of pain, swelling, or instability in the form of recurrent sprains.[11]
- Nearly 75% had some level of impairment on return to sporting activity, with almost 20% incurring repeated sprains and 4% with pain at rest or severe disability.
- Dysfunction after an acute sprain will persist for 6 months in 40% of injured athletes.[6]
- It has been suggested that long-term lateral ankle instability and repeated traumatic events to the ankle can lead to advanced stages of degenerative disease; however, the published literature has not proven this to be a direct relationship.
- It is presumed that continued ankle injuries as a result of lateral ankle instability can, and often will, lead to osteochondral injuries, abnormal joint mechanics, and neuromuscular dysfunction, predisposing the individual to risk of more severe injury to the extremity or disabling degenerative arthritis of the ankle and, possibly, the subtalar joints.

PATIENT HISTORY AND PHYSICAL EXAMINATION

- Patients experiencing acute ankle sprains often describe a painful tearing or pop after sustaining an inversion type injury. Longer standing instabilities will cause complaints of lack of confidence in the joint under high demands or frequent giving way. Pain, bruising, and swelling often are common complaints with acute injury but less so in cases of chronic instability.
- Findings on examination in the acute situation are reliably present and include anterolateral ankle pain, swelling, ecchymosis, and pain on passive plantarflexion or inversion. In the patient with a chronically unstable ankle, the examination focuses more on the anterior drawer and talar tilt tests. A grossly unstable drawer test can reveal a "suction sign" on the lateral ankle as the talus is allowed to displace anteriorly from the ankle mortise. The drawer test should be done in 20 degrees of plantarflexion to place maximal stress on the ATFL.
- Assessment for structural abnormalities also is important. Heel position should be examined in every patient, by looking at the patient from behind while he or she is standing, to determine the possible presence of varus malalignment.
- Neuromuscular function is another important part of the examination. Peroneal muscle group function, specifically, is critical. Strength and stability of the peroneals should be assessed by resistive muscle grading against plantarflexion and eversion. Provocative maneuvers such as the plantarflexion eversion stress test also should be performed to ensure that the peroneal tendons do not subluxate from the retrofibular groove.
- Sensory nerves should always be inspected to ensure no neurapraxia has taken place as a result of the traction from the injury.
- Syndesmotic integrity should be tested with palpation, the "squeeze" test, and dorsiflexion–external rotation provocative manipulations.

IMAGING AND OTHER DIAGNOSTIC TESTING

- According to the Ottawa Ankle Rules,[12] nearly 100% sensitivity is approached if the following criteria are used in the acute setting:
  - Tenderness at the posteroanterior edge or tip of the medial or lateral malleolus
  - Inability to bear weight (four steps) right after the injury or in the emergency room
  - Pain at the base of the fifth metatarsal
- If radiographs are required, anteroposterior (AP), lateral, and mortise views, preferably weight bearing, should be performed, looking for avulsion fractures of the tip of either malleolus or, less frequently, the lateral calcaneus. One also should inspect for osteochondral fractures, joint malposition, and other fractures that may mimic lateral ankle sprains.
- Stress views can be obtained in either the AP (talar tilt) or lateral (anterior drawer) position. Performing the study while stressing the ankle can give meaningful information regarding the stability of the joint. More than 15 degrees of varus tilt and 5 mm of anterior translation are reasonably considered abnormal.
- Magnetic resonance imaging (MRI) is valuable for determining the extent of the ligamentous injury, quality of ligamentous tissue, and the presence or absence of scar tissue and additional injury. Attenuation, wavy fibers, or disruption in the face of fluid accumulation suggests recent injury, whereas thickening or intrasubstance signal change gives rise to suspicion for a more remote injury. Infrequently, an absence of ligament tissue is noted, reflecting repeated injuries leading to degeneration of the complex.

DIFFERENTIAL DIAGNOSIS

- Acute
  - Lateral malleolar fracture
  - Fifth metatarsal fracture
  - Lateral talar process or "snowboarder's" fracture
  - Peroneal tendon dislocation
  - Osteochondral defect
  - Superficial peroneal neurapraxia
- Chronic
  - Peroneal instability
  - Peroneal split tears
  - Subtalar instability
  - Osteochondral defect
  - Tibiotalar or subtalar arthritis

NONOPERATIVE MANAGEMENT

- Nonoperative management is imperative for treatment of both acute and chronic instabilities. Most patients will respond to conservative management, and these efforts should be exhausted prior to surgical intervention.
- Acute swelling and pain, whether from a new injury or recent repeat injury, are best managed with RICE. Immobilization in a CAM boot should be considered for anyone demonstrating a positive drawer or talar tilt after an acute injury. Lower profile bracing is often used more frequently in the chronic setting.
- Once the acute symptoms have subsided, functional strapping, taping, or bracing should be instituted along with an

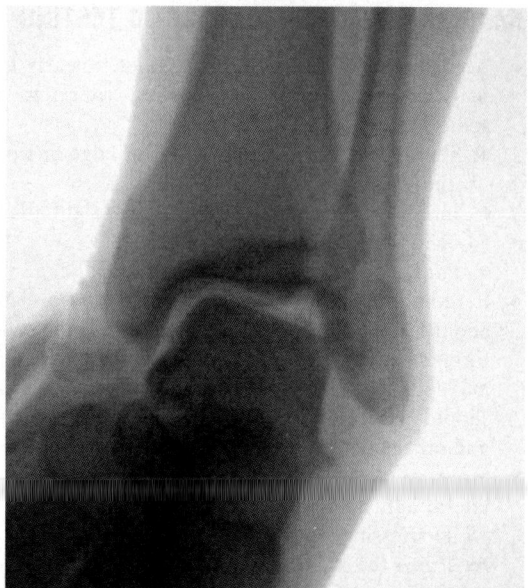 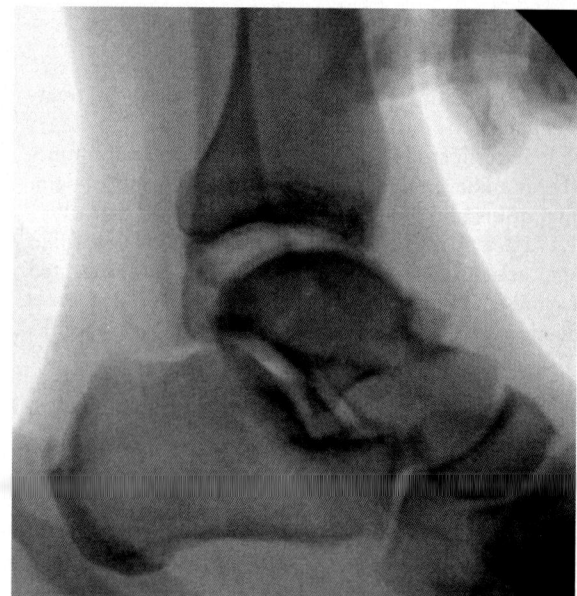

FIG 1 A. Plain radiograph x-ray demonstrating unstable tilt test. **B.** Plain radiograph x-ray demonstrating unstable anterior drawer test.

exercise regimen emphasizing peroneal strengthening, proprioceptive training, and Achilles tendon stretching.

- In the patient with a chronically unstable ankle, shoe wear modifications can be added as the individual returns to sports or activities. Orthoses with lateral heel and sole wedges or flare on the lateral sole of the shoe can promote a valgus moment and help avoid injury in the vulnerable patient. Reducing heel height and stiffening the sole of the shoe also can be helpful.
- Prophylactic brace wear or taping has been shown to have some benefit in prevention of injury. It also has a positive effect on reduction in severity of sprains if reinjury occurs while these measures are in effect.

SURGICAL MANAGEMENT

- Surgery rarely is indicated for an initial acute injury.
  - Acute injuries failing appropriate conservative care, in our opinion, are best treated with an anatomic repair and reinforcement using a modified Brostrom procedure.
- Chronic instability failing appropriate conservative measures may be improved with surgical intervention.
  - In a previously unoperated patient with MRI evidence of tissue remnants, an anatomic repair (modified Brostrom procedure) is very effective.
  - In patients who have repeated injuries and are left without evidence of ATFL or CFL remnant by MRI, or in patients who have previously undergone an attempt at surgical correction, reconstruction with free tendon graft is our preferred method.[4,5,8,14,18]

Preoperative Planning

- All imaging studies, including MRI, are reviewed, and any adjunctive pathology that may need to be addressed at the time of surgery, such as fragments of bone, osteochondral lesions, or peroneal tendon pathology, is noted.

- The joint (and the contralateral joint) is examined under anesthesia to determine the true nature of instability and also to gauge the effect of the repair **(FIG 1)**.
- Graft choice also is an important preoperative consideration. An autogenous hamstring graft can be chosen and harvested in similar fashion to that of anterior cruciate ligament graft harvests.[4,5,8,14,18] Alternatively, should the patient be averse to violating his or her own knee, an allograft gracilis tendon has been shown to be a very suitable alternative. Advantages include reduced pain, no donor site morbidity, and low incidence of inflammatory response or infection transmission.
- The presence of a varus heel may necessitate the addition of a laterally based closing wedge calcaneal osteotomy.

Positioning

- The patient is placed in the lateral position, typically with the torso supported by a beanbag positioner and the operative leg supported on foam board. Alternatively, the procedure can be performed in the supine position with a hip roll on the operative side to allow better access to the posterolateral ankle.
- Arthroscopic examination can be performed to identify any unseen intra-articular pathology.[10] The leg can be externally rotated while in the lateral position and placed in an ankle distractor to accommodate arthroscopic examination.

Approach

- One of two approaches may be chosen, depending on the degree of pathology that is to be addressed.
  - To perform the reconstruction and address peroneal pathology or anterior osteophytes, a 4- to 6-cm extensile lateral malleolar incision is used. The incision is centered along the fibula and then gently curves anteriorly after the tip of the fibula **(FIG 2A)**. The approach will require

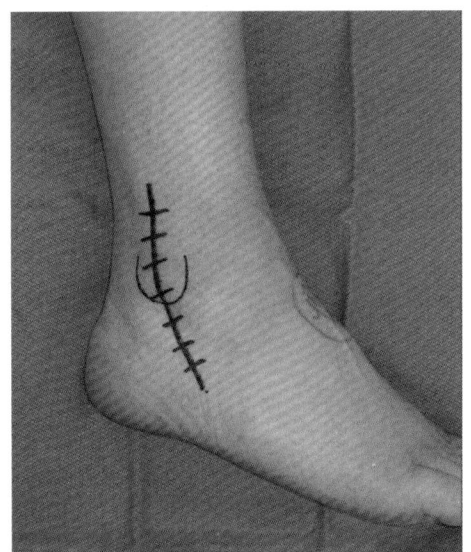
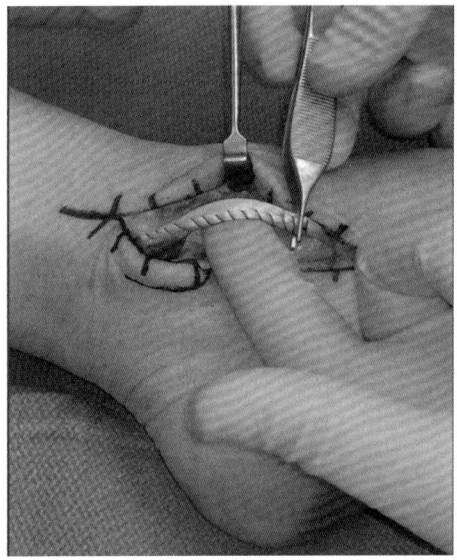

FIG 2 A. Surgical approach paralleling the posterior border of the fibula is marked on the skin. **B.** After approach is made, any peroneal tendon pathology can be easily addressed.

you to take down the peroneal retinacular tissue, which should be tagged and later repaired fully. Peroneal pathology can be easily addressed at this time **(FIG 2B)**.

- For ankle ligament reconstruction alone, an anterior curvilinear incision bordering the distal inferior tip of the fibula can be combined with small vertical incisions of approximately 2 cm each, posterior to the fibula, to

accept the graft passage. An additional incision on the lateral calcaneal wall is used to pass and secure the calcaneofibular limb of the graft.

- An oblique incision over the calcaneus usually can be added to either approach without great concern for increased wound morbidity if a calcaneal osteotomy is necessary to promote a valgus hindfoot.

TALAR TUNNEL PLACEMENT

- The lateral ankle is exposed by one of two incisions, as previously described.
- The origin sites of both ATFL and CFL are identified on the distal fibula.

- Dissection proceeds to expose the insertion of the ATFL on the lateral talus just at the corner of the lateral process as it blends from the body to the neck **(TECH FIG 1A,B)**.
- A 15- to 20-mm deep tunnel is drilled across the talus at this point with a 4.5- to 6-mm drill to accept the first limb of the tendon graft **(TECH FIG 1C,D)**.

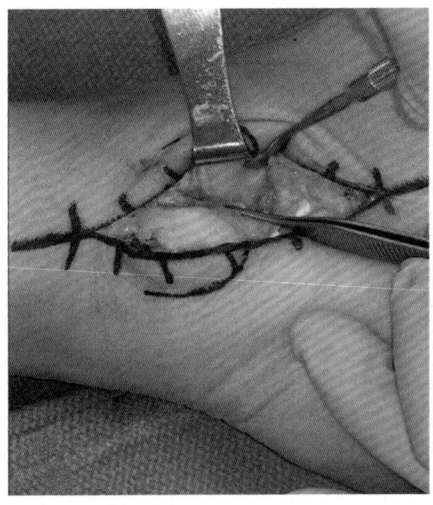
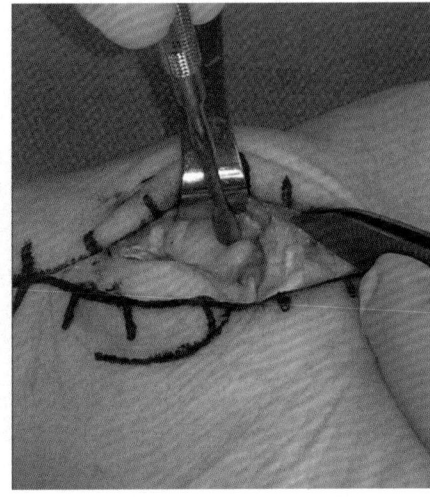

TECH FIG 1 A. Forceps mark the origin of the ATFL on the fibula, and the elevator marks the insertion on the talus lateral process. **B.** The talar tunnel is placed on the anterior border of the lateral process just off the leading edge of cartilage at the insertion of the ATFL. The tip of the elevator marks this position. *(continued)*

TECHNIQUES

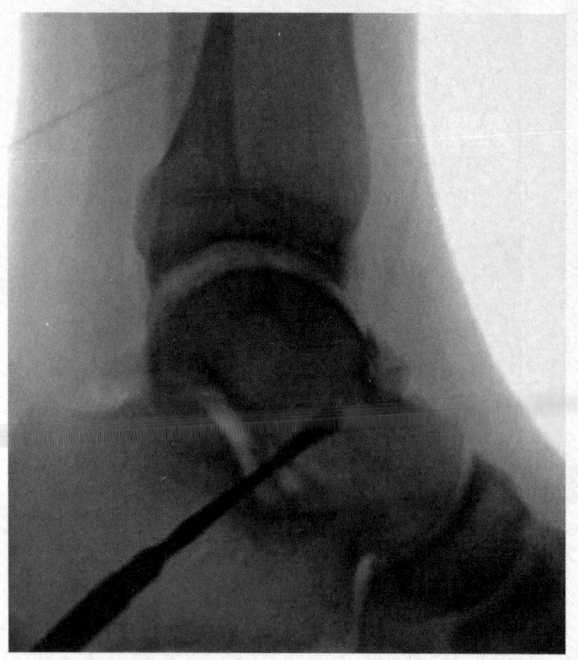
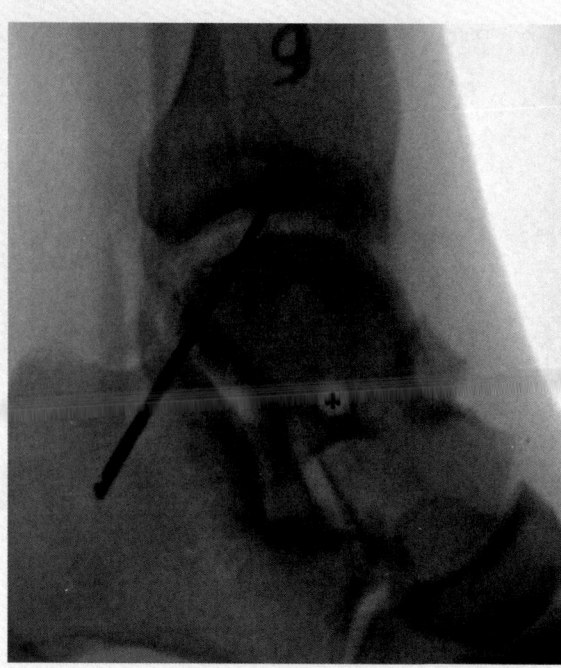

TECH FIG 1 *(continued)* **C.** The tunnel site is identified on lateral x-ray by the tip of elevator. **D.** Guide pin is drilled across the talus, and the tunnel is reamed over this pin. This is a unicortical tunnel *(asterisk)* and should not breach the medial talar wall or the joint surfaces above and below the horizontal tunnel position.

FIBULAR TUNNEL PLACEMENT

- The fibula is exposed, and two guide pins are placed in the fibula at the insertions of the ATFL and the CFL. The pins exit the posterior fibula cortex leaving a bony bridge between the two tunnels that are to be made next with the reamer. A 4.5- to 6-mm wide tunnel is then drilled over the guide pins to create two independent tunnels separated by 3 to 4 mm at the exit on the posterior fibula cortex **(TECH FIG 2A,B)**. This allows for graft passage over a cortical bridge and, in addition, the graft can be sutured to periosteum to prevent sliding **(TECH FIG 2C,D)**.

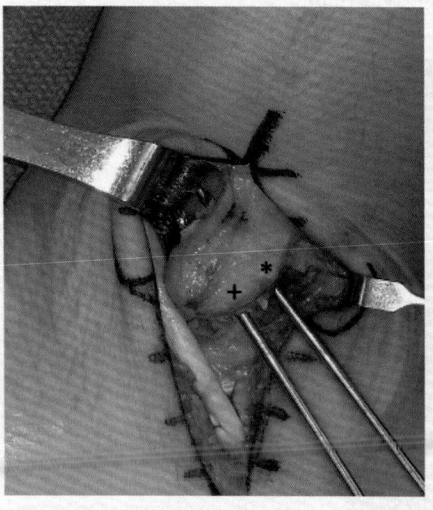
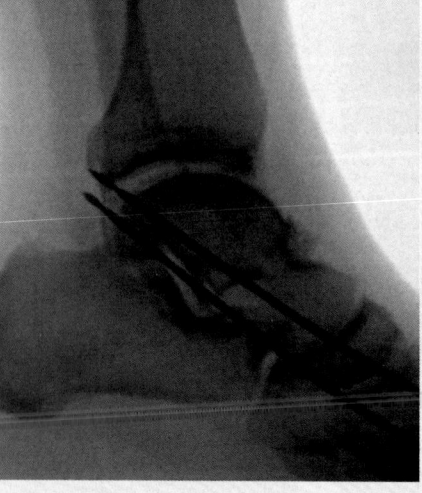

TECH FIG 2 A. The origin of the ATFL *(asterisk)* is used as the entry point for the first fibular tunnel. The guide pin is inserted, aiming superior and posterior at 45 to 60 degrees to allow for another more inferior tunnel for the CFL limb of the graft (+). **B.** The lateral x-ray shows the guide pin trajectory and illustrates the bony bridge that is to be left between the exit points of the two pins. *(continued)*

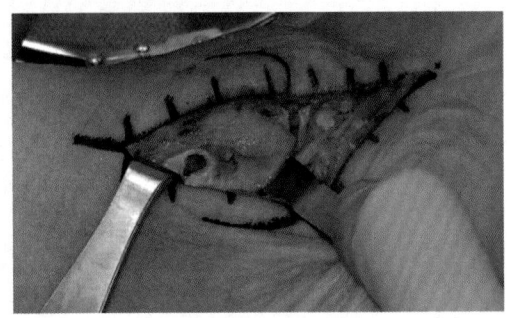 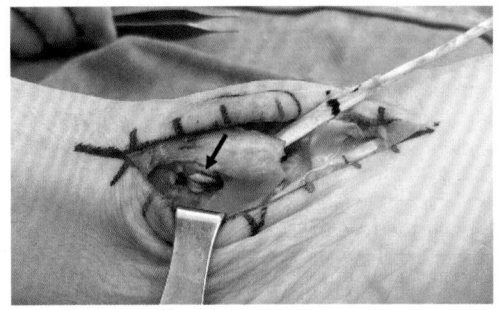

TECH FIG 2 *(continued)* **C.** Shown is the posterior surface of the fibula. A bony bridge is preserved between fibular tunnels after reaming of the tunnels is completed. **D.** After later graft passage, you can see how the bony bridge prevents subsidence of the graft between the two tunnels (*arrow*).

CALCANEAL TUNNEL PLACEMENT

- A guide pin is then placed at the CFL insertion on the calcaneus tuberosity. It is drilled bicortically in a posterior medial direction and its leading end is captured on the medial heel with a hemostat. A tunnel 4.5 to 6 mm wide is then drilled unicortically over the guide pin to a depth of 25 to 30 mm through the lateral calcaneal wall at the level of the CFL insertion **(TECH FIG 3)**. Be sure to leave the guide pin in to use later to shuttle the passing suture from the CFL limb of the graft.

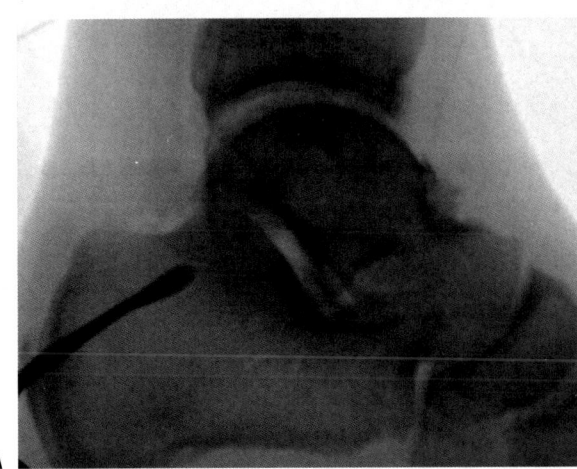

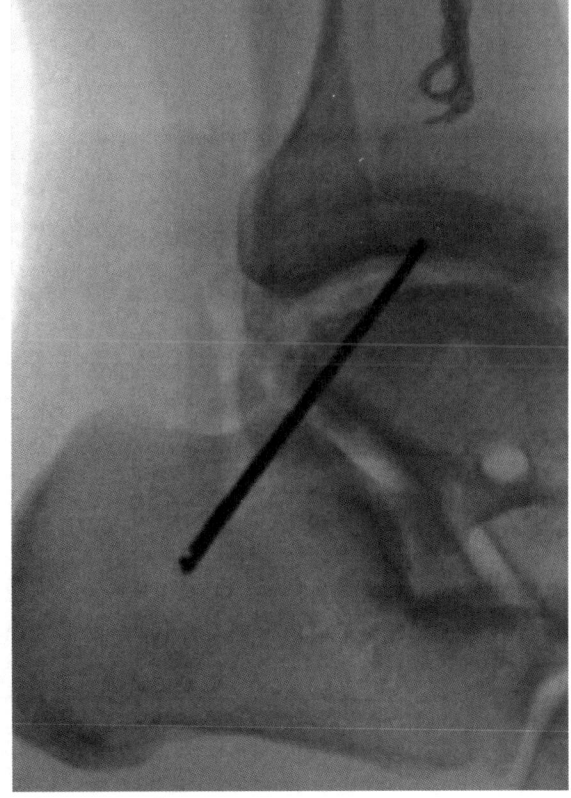

TECH FIG 3 A. The calcaneal tunnel is placed just inferior to the insertion point of the CFL as marked by the instrument on this lateral x-ray. **B.** The guide pin for the calcaneal tunnel is placed with the peroneal muscle group swept posteriorly and travels posteromedially to exit the medial heel.

GRAFT PASSAGE

- The sutured tendon is inserted first into the talar tunnel and fixed with an interference screw. If you are augmenting your ATFL limb with a suture tape, it is inserted into the talus with the graft (**TECH FIG 4A–C**).
- The graft and the suture tape, if used, are then passed through the fibular tunnel from the ATFL insertion, through the more proximal posterior exit tunnel. The foot is held neutral and slightly everted, with a slight posterior drawer force to insure proper mortise reduction as the graft and suture tape are appropriately tensioned. The first interference screw is then placed into the ATFL tunnel to secure the graft and the suture tape (**TECH FIG 4D**).
- Only the graft is then woven back through the more inferior fibular hole and out the CFL origin. The suture tape can be cut at the exit point of the proximal tunnel. This weaving pattern gives the most anatomic origin and insertion points (**TECH FIG 4E**).

- The remainder of the graft is then appropriately trimmed to leave 20 mm of graft that will be secured within the CFL tunnel. The new cut end is sutured and these passing sutures are taken through the CFL tunnel and out the medial heel using the guide pin (**TECH FIG 4F**). Be sure the CFL passes deep to the peroneal tendons.
- The CFL limb of the graft is appropriately tensioned with the foot in dorsiflexion, and a second interference screw is placed in the calcaneus (**TECH FIG 4G**).
- Range of motion and stability are assessed. If tension does not feel appropriate, the calcaneal screw can be removed, the graft retensioned, and the screw replaced.
- The tendon can receive a few sutures at the fibular tunnels to maintain tension of the individual limbs representing ATFL and CFL.
- Peroneal retinacular tissue must be fully repaired to prevent peroneal tendon subluxation and instability.

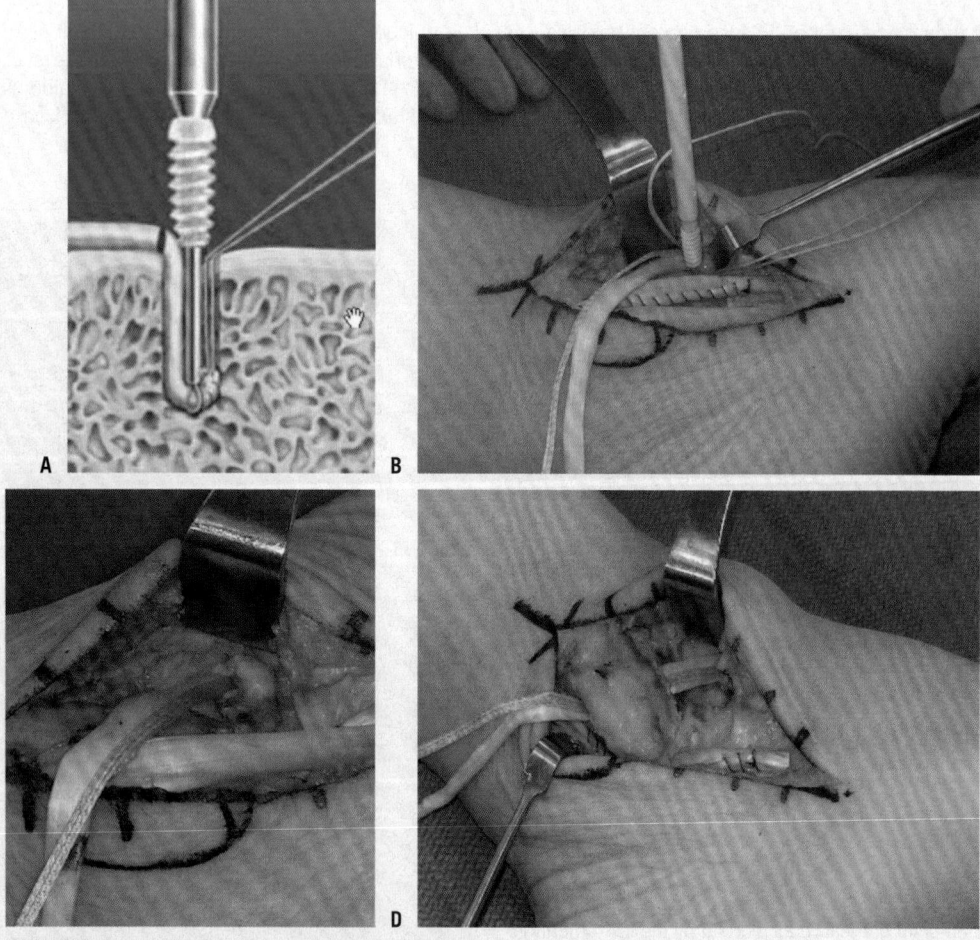

TECH FIG 4 A. Schematic of interference fit tenodesis screw. **B.** Allograft tendon is mounted for insertion into the tibia tunnel with the first interference screw. Shown here are both the tendon graft and the suture tape augmentation being placed into the tunnel and secured with an interference screw. **C.** After screw insertion, the suture tape should be superficial to the graft and remain untwisted so it lays flat with the tendon. **D.** The graft and suture tape are passed through the ATFL tunnel and fixated at the appropriate tension with an interference screw. The ankle is held in neutral dorsiflexion and slight eversion while tensioning and securing the graft in the first tunnel. (continued)

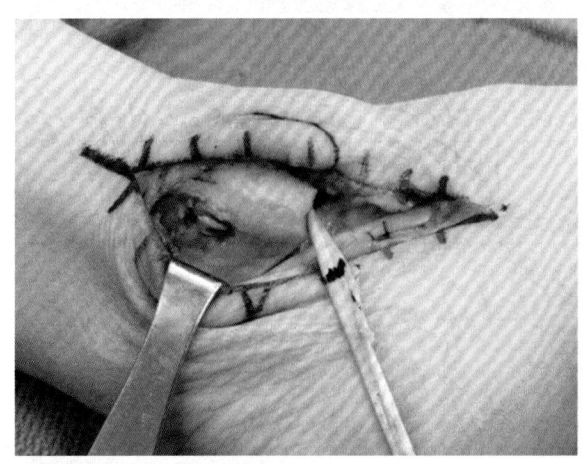

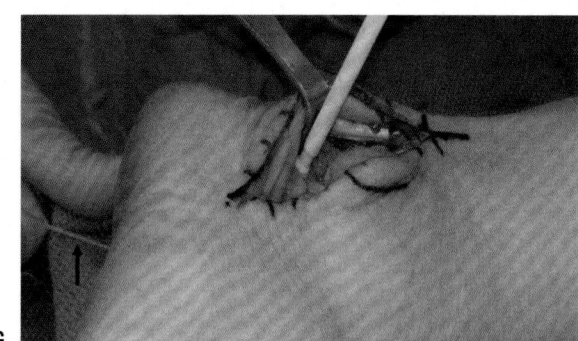

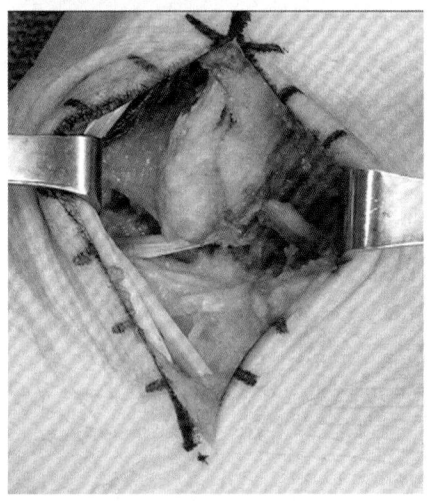

TECH FIG 4 *(continued)* **E.** The graft is then passed back through the CFL tunnel to exit the distal fibula as shown. The suture tape is not passed through, and it is cut off at the exit of the ATFL tunnel. **F.** The CFL limb is then measured to ensure 20 mm of graft with be within the calcaneal tunnel. The graft is drawn into the tunnel with the guide pin and passing sutures. The passing sutures are brought out through the medial heel and will be used to tension the CFL. **G.** The graft is tensioned by pulling the suture exiting the medial heel *(arrow)*. The interference screw is then placed. Note the CFL graft is deep to the peroneal tendons.

WOUND CLOSURE

- Layered closure is performed, usually with a subcutaneous layer of 2-0 Vicryl or 3-0 Monocryl followed by skin sutures with 3-0 nylon.

CALCANEAL OSTEOTOMY

- If heel varus is present, a laterally based closing wedge calcaneal osteotomy may be performed.
- An oblique incision is carried out directly over the area of the planned osteotomy (usually about 2 cm posterior to any other concurrent incision).
- Periosteum is raised in each direction.

- A 1 to 1.5 cm width is marked on the lateral wall of the calcaneal tuberosity, verifying that the osteotomy will not breach the bone tunnel.
- Saw cuts are made convergently to meet just before violating medial cortex.
- The wedge is removed and the osteotomy closed.
- Fixation can be achieved through either a large axially directed screws or staples.

Pearls and Pitfalls

Graft Handling	• Great care must be taken in harvesting autograft so as to get enough length on the native gracilis. • If allograft is used, it must be ordered properly, with enough length to span the distance of the tendon weave (25 cm is plenty). • Once the allograft is thawed, it should be bathed in antibiotic solution until ready for use.
Tunnel Placement	• Avoid tunnel break out. • Make two separate tunnels on the posterior fibula divided by a cortical bridge between them. This will help resist the chance of graft migration on cancellous bone within the V-shaped tunnel.
Heel Alignment	• Persistent heel varus can destroy a perfectly performed ligament reconstruction if not addressed. • If necessary, do a calcaneal osteotomy.
Tensioning the Graft	• Hold the foot in the desired neutral position (to about 5 degrees of eversion), pull the graft taut, and fix it in this position. Ensure mobility and stability at this time. Retensioning can be done now with interference screw fixation, but it will not be possible to compensate for this later. • Do not overshorten the graft. This will leave the repair too tight or require another harvest.

POSTOPERATIVE CARE

- A well-padded and molded trilaminar splint in a neutral ankle position is maintained for 10 to 14 days postoperatively.
- Once wounds are healed satisfactorily, the patient may begin protected weight bearing in a boot until 6 weeks postoperatively.
- Physical therapy is begun at postoperative week 2 with active range of motion/passive range of motion within tolerances, edema control, and gentle strengthening.
- Rehabilitation is increased after postoperative week 6 with stretching, proprioceptive training, and peroneal strengthening.
- Boot is weaned after postoperative week 8, and patient is transitioned to a brace.
- Brace is discontinued after postoperative week 12.
- Athletic activity usually is withheld for 4 to 6 months, and all physical therapy goals have been reached.

OUTCOMES

- Anatomic reconstruction for failed acute and chronic instability patterns continues to be our preferred method of lateral ankle ligament reconstruction. This has been shown in the literature to be extremely successful for return to function and reduction or elimination of symptoms in appropriately selected patients.
- When a patient has lost reliable lateral soft tissue structures by virtue of repetitive injury or previous failed procedures, an anatomic free graft lateral ligament reconstruction provides a very good alternative.
- Reconstruction using this method reconstitutes the ATFL and CFL, thus providing restoration of both ankle and subtalar stability.
- Anatomic reconstruction coupled with the preservation of native peroneal tendon function provides an optimum environment for return to function.
- Paterson et al[14] showed 81% complete or substantial symptom resolution in 26 patients at 2-year follow-up by performing reconstruction of the ATFL alone. No significant differences were noted between operated and contralateral ankles with respect to range of motion or uniaxial balancing.
- Coughlin et al[4,5] reported on 2-year follow-up in 28 patients. All patients were rated to have good or excellent

outcomes with objective improvement in talar tilt measurements (13 degrees preoperatively vs. 3 degrees postoperatively) and anterior drawer testing (on average, 10 mm preoperatively vs. 5 mm postoperatively).
- Addition of tenodesis or interference screw fixation adds the advantage of being able to promote range of motion earlier with less concern for graft loosening.[9,18]

COMPLICATIONS

- Nerve injury
- Wound problems
- Infection
- Joint stiffness
- Deep venous thrombosis
- Subjective under- or overtightening

REFERENCES

1. Ardèvol J, Bolíbar I, Belda V, et al. Treatment of complete rupture of the lateral ligaments of the ankle: a randomized clinical trial comparing cast immobilization with functional treatment. Knee Surg Sports Traumatol Arthrosc 2002;10:371–377.
2. Clanton TO, Campbell KJ, Wilson KJ, et al. Qualitative and quantitative anatomic investigation of the lateral ligaments for surgical reconstruction procedures. J Bone Joint Surg Am 2014;96(12):e98.
3. Colville MR, Grondel RJ. Anatomic reconstruction of the lateral ankle ligaments using a split peroneus brevis tendon graft. Am J Sports Med 1995;23:210–213.
4. Coughlin MJ, Matt V, Schenck RC Jr. Augmented lateral ankle reconstruction using a free gracilis graft. Orthopedics 2002;25: 31–35.
5. Coughlin MJ, Schenck RC Jr, Grebing BR, et al. Comprehensive reconstruction of the lateral ankle for chronic instability using a free gracilis graft. Foot Ankle Int 2004;25:231–241.
6. Gerber JP, Williams GN, Scoville CR, et al. Persistent disability with ankle sprains: a prospective examination of an athletic population. Foot Ankle Int 1998;19:653–660.
7. Hertel J. Functional instability following lateral ankle sprain. Sports Med 2000;29:361–371.
8. Jeys LM, Harris NJ. Ankle stabilization with hamstring autograft: a new technique using interference screws. Foot Ankle Int 2003;24: 677–679.
9. Jeys LM, Korrosis S, Stewart T, et al. Bone anchors or interference screws? A biomechanical evaluation for autograft ankle stabilization. Am J Sports Med 2004;32:1651–1659.

10. Komenda GA, Ferkel RD. Arthroscopic findings associated with the unstable ankle. Foot Ankle Int 1999;20:708–713.
11. Konradsen L, Bech L, Ehrenbjerg M, et al. Seven years follow-up after ankle inversion trauma. Scand J Med Sci Sports 2002;12:129–135.
12. Lynch SA. Assessment of the injured ankle in the athlete. J Athl Train 2002;37:406–412.
13. Maehlum S, Daljord OA. Acute sports injuries in Oslo: a one year study. Br J Sports Med 1984;18:181–185.
14. Paterson R, Cohen B, Taylor D, et al. Reconstruction of the lateral ligaments of the ankle using semi-tendinosis graft. Foot Ankle Int 2000;21:413–419.
15. Richie DH Jr. Functional instability of the ankle and the role of neuromuscular control: a comprehensive review. J Foot Ankle Surg 2001;40:240–251.
16. Sandelin J. Acute Sports Injuries: A Clinical and Epidemiological Study [dissertation]. Helsinki, Finland: University of Helsinki, 1988.
17. Siegler S, Block J, Schneck CD. The mechanical characteristics of the collateral ligaments of the human ankle joint. Foot Ankle 1988;8:234–242.
18. Takao M, Oae K, Uchio Y, et al. Anatomical reconstruction of the lateral ligaments of the ankle with a gracilis autograft: a new technique using an interference fit anchoring system. Am J Sports Med 2005;33:814–823.

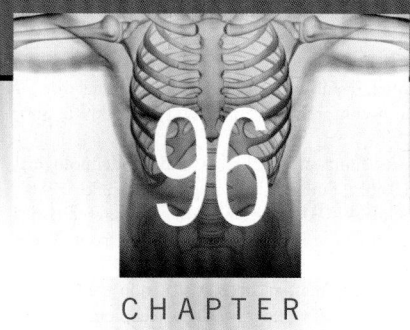

96
CHAPTER

Management of Chronic Lateral Ankle Instability with an Autologous Plantaris Longus Graft

Markus Walther

DEFINITION

- Acute lateral ligament injuries of the ankle are treated conservatively with good results in most cases. However, several factors may lead to chronic ankle instability with recurring ankle sprains:
  - Inadequate primary treatment
  - Incomplete healing of the ligaments
  - Repetitive trauma with deteriorated tissue quality
- Patients with chronic ankle instability can be divided into two groups:
  - Patients with sufficient tissue quality to perform a local repair
  - Patients with inadequate tissue quality for a local repair
- A Broström procedure for lateral ankle reconstruction is possible as long as there is sufficient tissue (see Chaps. FA-92 and 93).
- In patients with insufficient local tissue, an augmentation is needed to rebuild or reinforce the lateral ligaments. There are different options of tendon grafts, each with certain advantages and disadvantages:
  - Tenodesis
  - Semitendinosus tendon or gracilis tendon (see Chap. FA-94)
  - Plantaris longus tendon
  - Allograft (see Chap. FA-95)
- Another surgical option is the augmentation of the ligaments with fibular periosteal flap.[2,21]

ANATOMY

- Laterally, the ankle is stabilized by the anterior talofibular ligament (ATFL), posterior talofibular ligament (PTFL), and the calcaneofibular ligament (CFL) **(FIG 1)**.[7]
- Additional stability is provided by the bony structures. Especially in dorsal extension, the talus is locked between the medial and lateral malleolus.

PATHOGENESIS

- Torn lateral ligaments are the result of an ankle sprain. Depending on the severity of the sprain, one to three of the lateral ligaments are injured. A rupture of the ATFL is involved in most cases.
- Anatomic classification
  - Grade I: ATFL sprain
  - Grade II: ATFL and CFL sprain
  - Grade III: ATFL, CFL, and PTFL sprain
- American Medical Association standard nomenclature system by severity
  - Grade I: ligament stretched
  - Grade II: ligament partially torn
  - Grade III: ligament completely torn
- Grading by clinical presentation symptoms
  - Mild sprain: minimal functional loss, no limp, minimal or no swelling, point tenderness, pain with reproduction of mechanism of injury

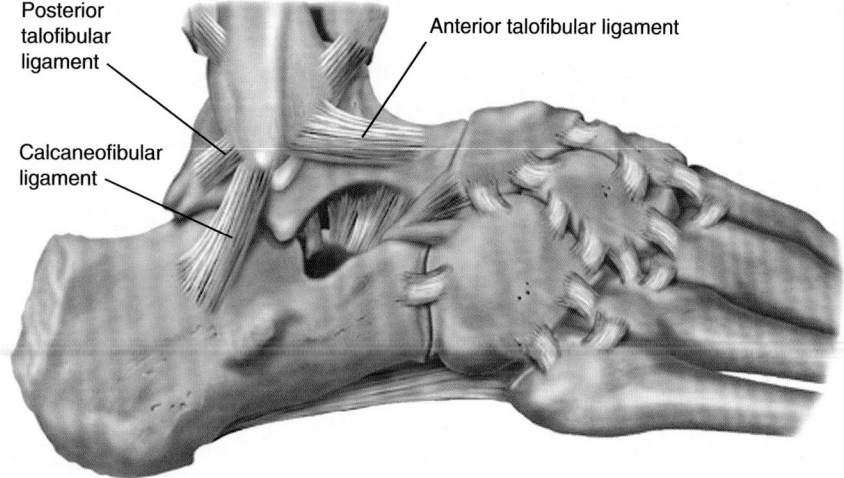

Posterior talofibular ligament

Anterior talofibular ligament

Calcaneofibular ligament

FIG 1 Anatomy of the lateral ankle showing the three ligaments: ATFL, PTFL, and the CFL.

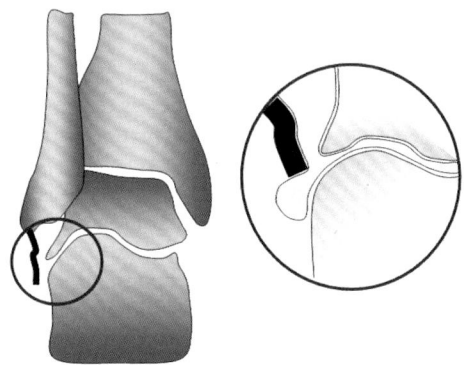

FIG 2 Synovial fluid between the two ends of torn ligaments can prevent the injury from healing.

- Moderate sprain: moderate functional loss, unable to toe rise or hop on injured ankle, limp when walking, localized swelling, point tenderness
- Severe sprain: diffuse tenderness and swelling, crutches preferred by patient for ambulation
- With each ankle sprain, proprioception of the ankle joint is compromised.
  - The risk for another ankle sprain increases after each injury. In an uninjured person, an ankle sprain will occur in 1:1,000,000 steps. This risk increases to 1:1000 steps after a severe ankle sprain.[14]
- Chronic ankle instability is the combination of insufficient active and ligament stabilization mechanisms.
- There is some evidence that special anatomic variations increase the risk of developing chronic ankle instability after an injury.[17]
- The healing of the ligaments can be compromised by synovial fluid between ligament and bone **(FIG 2)**.

NATURAL HISTORY

- Chronic instability is a risk factor for degenerative arthritis of the ankle joint. Valderrabano et al[25] have shown an increased prevalence of arthritis in patients with chronic ankle instability.
- Recurrent ankle sprains are likely in the future, but this is strongly dependent on lifestyle and sports activities.[26]

PATIENT HISTORY AND PHYSICAL FINDINGS

- The patient history includes sustained injuries, frequency of ankle sprains, and causes of pain as well as restrictions in daily living and sports.
- The degree of disability experienced by the patient depends on the degree of instability and the physical demands.
- A varus malalignment of the hindfoot increases the load on the lateral ligaments and the peroneal tendons. If a varus deformity of the hindfoot is present, there is a significant risk of failure of an isolated soft tissue ligament reconstruction. Simultaneous hindfoot alignment surgery has to be discussed with such patients (see Chap. FA-58).[15]

- Many tests for ankle instability are strongly dependent on patient cooperation. If positive, however, they can be highly specific.
  - The examiner should check the range of motion of the ankle joint with a stretched and a bent knee to rule out a shortening of the gastrocnemius or soleus muscle (or both). Restricted dorsiflexion with a stretched knee joint that is not found with a flexed knee is specific for a shortening of the gastrocnemius muscle (Silfverskiöld test).
  - The inversion test is used to assess for a ruptured CFL.
  - Medial ankle stability is checked in a plantarflexed position of the ankle to avoid a locking of the talus in the joint, which can mimic ligamentous stability. If positive, it is highly specific for a ruptured deltoid ligament. In the loaded situation, patients with deltoid instability may impress with a hindfoot valgus which can be compensated standing tiptoe by the intact posterior tibial tendon.
  - Insufficiency of the fibulocalcaneus ligament often affects the stability of the subtalar joint. The stability is checked in dorsiflexion of the ankle to lock the talus in the upper ankle joint. If positive, it is highly specific for a ruptured CFL in combination with subtalar instability.[18]
  - Effusion can be palpated ventrally, but smaller amounts of fluid are difficult to detect.
  - The ankle drawer test strains the ATFL and is highly specific for rupture of this ligament.

IMAGING AND OTHER DIAGNOSTIC STUDIES

- Plain radiographs should be obtained to evaluate potential bony pathology.
- Stress radiographs: The anteroposterior view shows the lateral opening of the joint. An anterior talar shift can be seen on the lateral stress view **(FIG 3)**.
- In patients with clinical signs of hindfoot varus, a hindfoot alignment view is recommended as well as loaded x-rays of the foot and ankle.[6]
- Magnetic resonance imaging (MRI) gives valuable information on the lateral ligaments and other pathology. In chronic instability scarring, effusion and synovitis was often found.

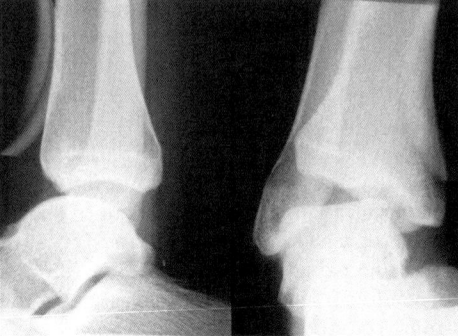

FIG 3 Stress radiographs of a patient with a chronic high-grade instability of the ankle joint.

However, it is impossible to judge functional stability in an MRI. Frequent additional pathologies visible on MRI are tears of the peroneal tendons, osteochondral lesions, and bone edema.

- Ultrasound of the lateral ligaments while performing the stress tests can visualize the displacement of the talus against the fibula. Effusion can also be detected by ultrasound. Ultrasound is always diagnosed in relation the other healthy ankle.[22]

DIFFERENTIAL DIAGNOSIS

- Articular injury (chondral or osteochondral fractures)
- Nerve injuries (sural, superficial peroneal, posterior tibial)
- Tendon injury (peroneal tendon tear or dislocation, tibialis posterior)
- Other ligamentous injuries (syndesmosis, subtalar, bifurcate, calcaneocuboid)
- Impingement (anterior osteophyte, anteroinferior tibiofibular ligament, scars)
- Unrelated pathology, masked by routine sprain (undetected rheumatoid condition, diabetic neuroarthropathy, tumor)
- Lateral ankle instability with hindfoot varus deformity[15,24]

NONOPERATIVE MANAGEMENT

- The goals of nonoperative treatment are improving proprioception and strength. This can be achieved by physiotherapy and exercises.
- Shoe modifications include a lateral wedge or a flare.
- Means of external fixation are orthoses, braces, or taping. However, those methods are limited.
  - Tape loses 30% of its stability after 200 steps. Skin problems are reported in up to 28%.
  - Within the group of orthoses, semirigid, warped types provide the highest degree of stability.[3]
- For many patients with symptomatic instability or pain, nonsurgical measures are not acceptable as a long-term solution. Usually, these patients require a lateral ligament repair.

SURGICAL MANAGEMENT

- In patients with no previous surgery and good tissue quality, the Broström procedure is a good option, reinserting the original ligaments in place.[5] Especially with modern anchor techniques, this procedure has regained a great deal of popularity. Broström[4] showed in his work that even after a longer period of chronic instability, a reconstruction of the original ligaments is possible, providing sufficient stability and function of the ankle joint.
- Due to improvements in suture anchor techniques, the possibilities of local, anatomic repair either open or arthroscopically have broadened over the last years.[9]
- However, some patients with a history of recurrent inversion trauma do not have adequate tissue quality to perform a Broström procedure.[8,13,20]
- Insufficient local tissue can be augmented or replaced by a tendon graft or a periosteal flap.

- There are different options of tendon grafts, each with certain advantages and disadvantages.
  - Tenodesis: The major disadvantage of tenodesis procedures (eg, Evans or Watson-Jones) is that they often end up in persistent pain[19,20] in combination with an increasing lack of stability over time.[16,23]
  - Autologous or homologous semitendinosus tendon or gracilis tendon can be used as graft. Although, in general, tolerated well, there is some risk of donor-site morbidity after harvesting those tendons.[1] If a homologous graft is used, there is a small risk of infection.
  - A local tendon that can easily be harvested with a minimum of donor-site morbidity is the plantaris longus tendon.[10]

Preoperative Planning

- In about 9% of the patients, no plantaris longus tendon can be found or it is not long enough for transplantation. A strategy has to be discussed with the patient as to how to proceed in this case. An option is to change to a technique using another transplant (eg, the gracilis or semitendinosus tendon) or to use a periosteal flap.
- Examinations performed under anesthesia include range of motion of the ankle joint and the ankle stress tests to confirm the previous results, without an active stabilization of the ankle joint by the patient.
- Additional intra-articular pathology is a common finding. In most cases, it is advisable to do an arthroscopy of the ankle joint before the ligament reconstruction.[11]

Positioning

- The patient is positioned supine with a sand sack under the injured side.
- The procedure is performed with a tourniquet (**FIG 4**).

Approach

- The plantaris longus tendon is harvested using a medial cut between the soleus and gastrocnemius muscle (**FIG 5A**).
- The procedure is performed with a standard lateral approach, straight, from the fibula directed to the base of the fifth metatarsal (**FIG 5B**).

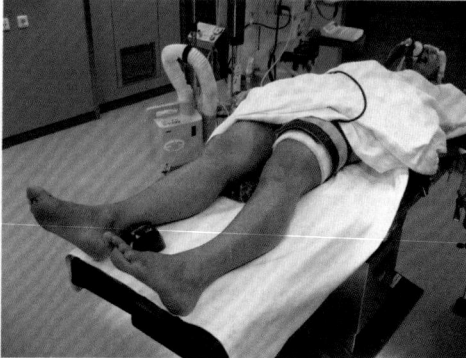

FIG 4 The patient is positioned supine with a sand sack under the injured side.

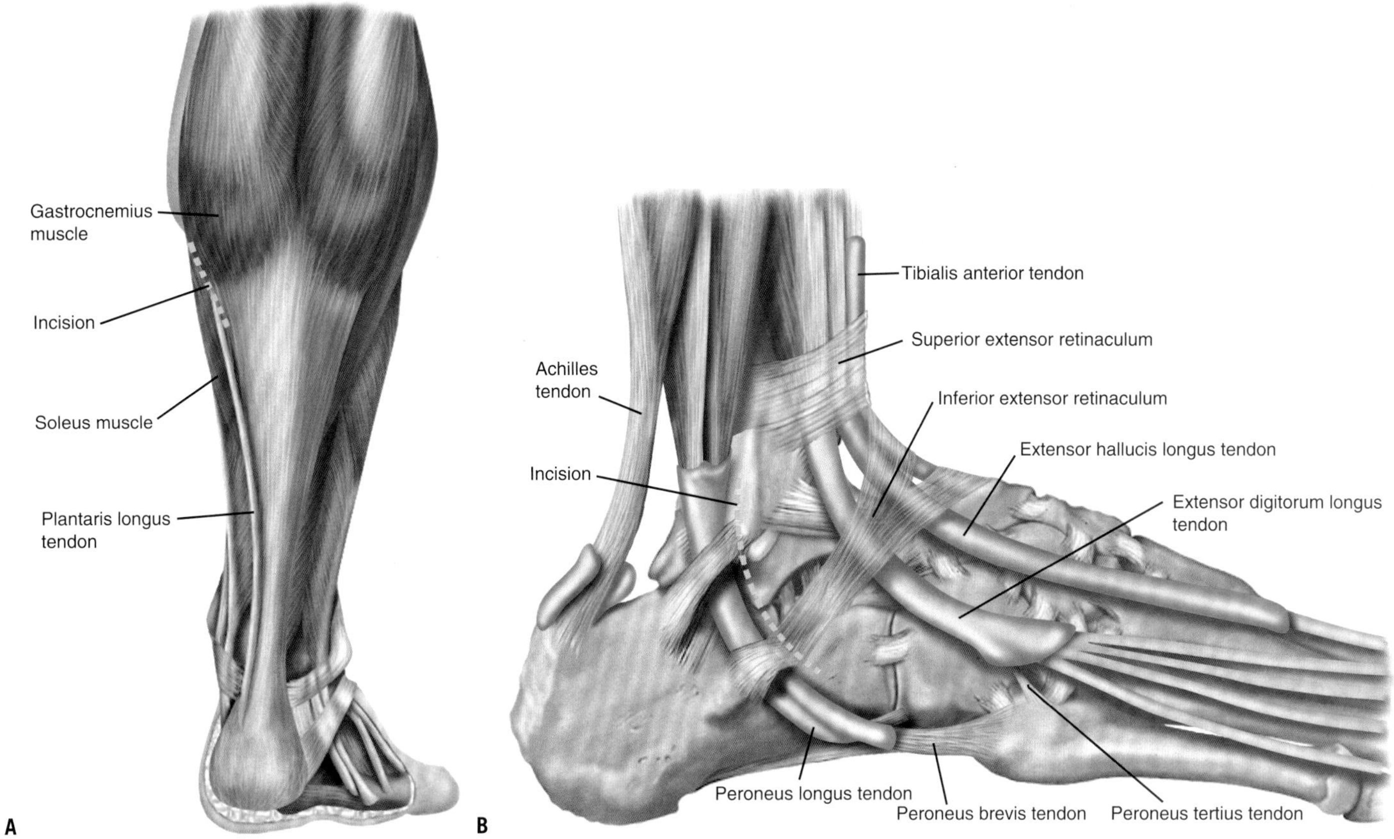

Gastrocnemius
muscle

Incision

Soleus muscle

Plantaris longus
tendon

Tibialis anterior tendon

Superior extensor retinaculum

Achilles
tendon

Incision

Inferior extensor retinaculum

Extensor hallucis longus tendon

Extensor digitorum longus
tendon

Peroneus longus tendon

Peroneus brevis tendon   Peroneus tertius tendon

A   **B**

FIG 5 A. Medial approach to harvest the plantaris longus tendon. **B.** Lateral approach with a 6- to 8-cm cut from the fibula toward the base of the fifth metatarsal.

HARVESTING OF PLANTARIS LONGUS

- Make a 3-cm cut at the medial aspect of the calf where the muscle has its highest volume **(TECH FIG 1)**.
- When the muscular fascia is split, the soleus and the gastrocnemius can be bluntly separated.
- The tendon structure found medially between the two muscles is the plantaris longus tendon, which can easily be harvested with a tendon stripper. The plantaris longus tendon often is much easier to identify at this location than at the medial aspect of the calcaneus.

- If it is not possible to mobilize the plantaris longus tendon distally with the tendon stripper, the tendon can be cut through a small longitudinal incision (about 1 cm).
- Free the tendon from any muscular or fatty tissue.
- Reinforce one end of the tendon with a 0 nonabsorbable suture.
- Store the tendon in a moist compress.

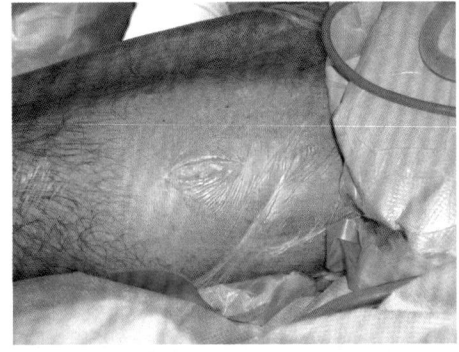
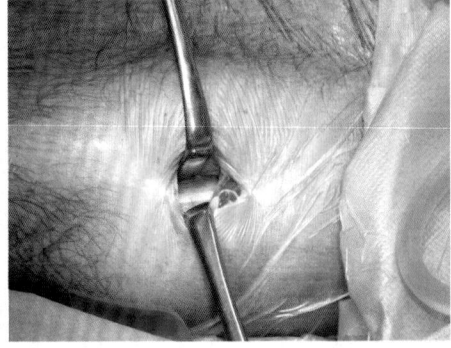

A   **B**

TECH FIG 1 Harvesting of the plantaris longus tendon. **A.** Medial incision between the soleus and gastrocnemius muscle. The fascia is directly under the fatty tissue. **B.** After a longitudinal incision of the fascia, the plantaris longus tendon is found right between the soleus and gastrocnemius muscle. *(continued)*

T E C H N I Q U E S

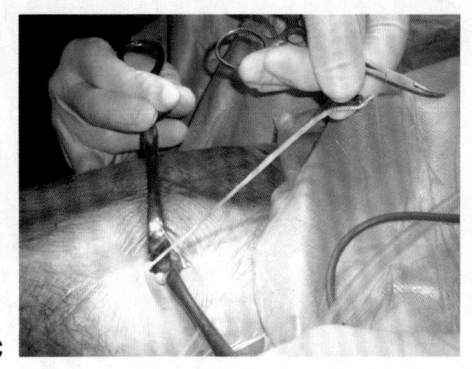
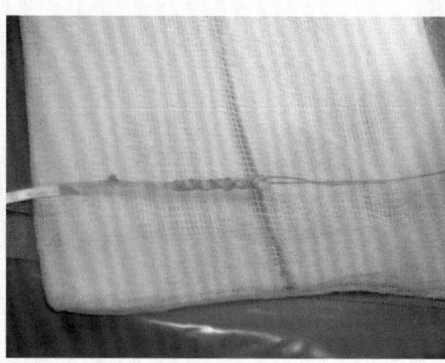

TECH FIG 1 *(continued)* **C.** The tendon is mobilized with a tendon stripper. **D.** The end of the plantaris longus is reinforced with a 0 non-absorbable suture and stored in a moist compress.

ANATOMIC RECONSTRUCTION OF THE LATERAL LIGAMENTS WITH THE PLANTARIS LONGUS TENDON

- Expose the lateral ligaments and the distal fibula via a lateral approach.
- The tissue of the sinus tarsi can be reamed, especially if there is any evidence of inflammation.
- Inspect the quality of ligaments and local tissue.
- Drill two holes at the ventral aspect of the fibula with a diameter of 3.2 mm and a distance of 7 and 13 mm from the tip of the fibula **(TECH FIG 2)**.
- Drill a third hole on the lateral side.
- With a small Weber forceps, connect the ventral holes and flatten the sharp edges surrounding them.
- Drill another two holes at the lateral aspect of the neck of the talus with a diameter of 3.2 mm and a distance of about 8 mm. The holes are located just at the border of the cartilage. In quite a few cases, remnants of the original ligaments can be found at this location.

- Again, create a canal with the Weber forceps.
- Retract the peroneal tendons and have the assistant position the hindfoot in maximum pronation. Drill two holes and connect them, 13 mm from the joint line of the subtalar joint, similar to the technique mentioned before.
- The plantaris longus transplant (which is armed with 0 nonabsorbable sutures) can be pulled through the holes with a sharp needle.
- When bringing the transplant under tension, the foot should be in a neutral position.
- Connect both ends of the transplant with 0 nonabsorbable sutures.
- If there are parts of the transplant left, they can be used to augment the reconstructed ligaments and held in place with side-to-side sutures.

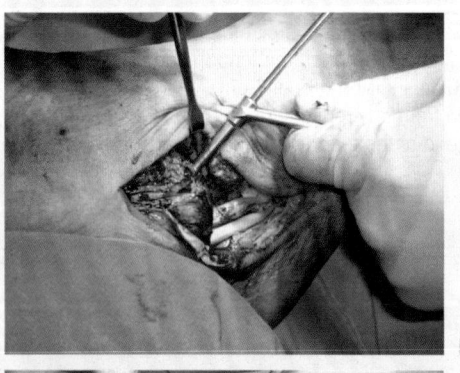
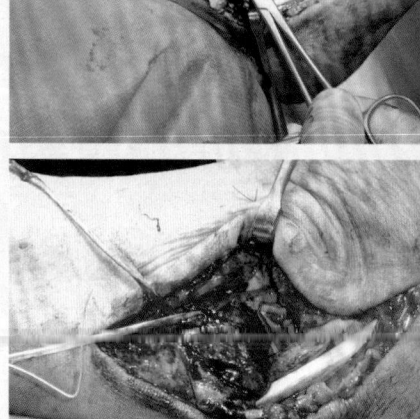
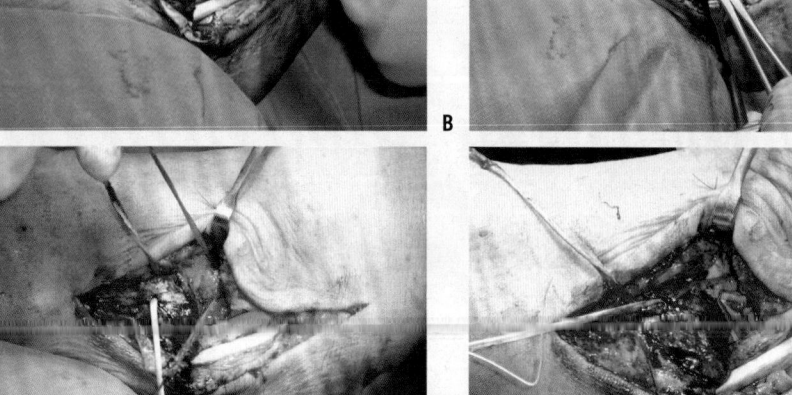

TECH FIG 2 Anatomic reconstruction with the plantaris longus tendon. **A.** Drilling a hole at the anatomic insertion of the ATFL. **B.** Creating a canal between the drill holes with a Weber forceps. **C.** Routing the tendon through the drill holes. **D.** Any spare tissue of the tendon can be used for a further reinforcement. *(continued)*

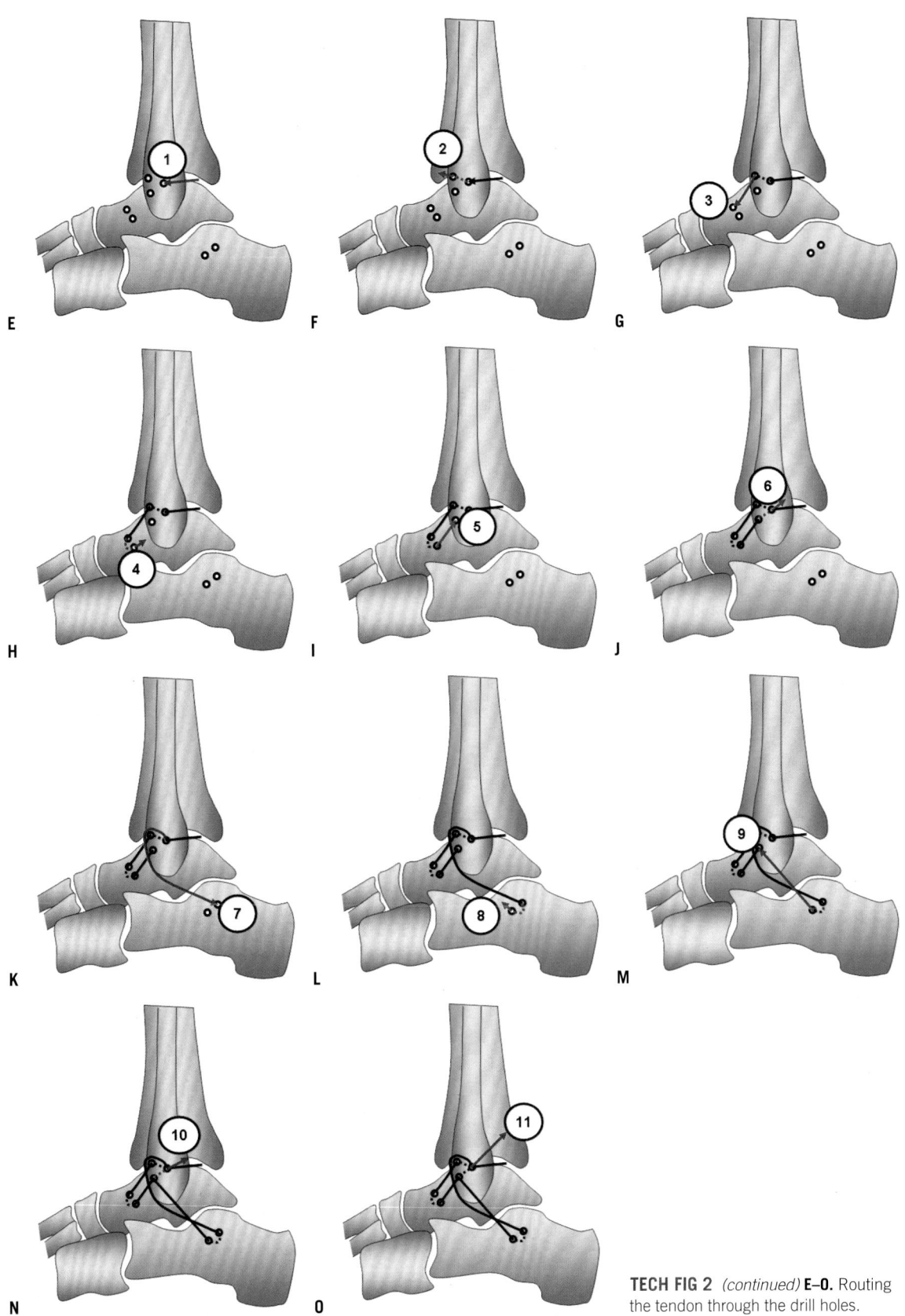

TECH FIG 2 *(continued)* **E–O.** Routing the tendon through the drill holes.

Pearls and Pitfalls

Indications	• A complete history and physical examination should be performed.
	• Care must be taken to address associated pathology.
	• Graft augmentation is always indicated when the local tissue is insufficient.
	• A preexisting hindfoot varus causes an increased load to the lateral ligaments. Simultaneous hindfoot realignment surgery has to be considered in those cases.
Graft Management	• A strategy has to be discussed with the patient if the plantaris longus tendon cannot be identified or is not suitable for transplantation.
	• Extreme care should be taken when harvesting and preparing grafts.
	• Graft should be secured at all times and handled carefully.
Fixation Problems	• If the tendon does not go through the holes, try again to smooth the edges with a Weber forceps.
	• If the plantaris longus tendon is too short for the whole routing, use a single layer, where the local tissue is best. An additional periosteal flap can be used to further augment the reconstruction site.
	• Fracture of the bony bridge between the drill holes can be managed with suture anchors or with a transosseous suture of the graft.

POSTOPERATIVE CARE

• All patients are kept in a walking boot or walking cast for 2 weeks, and weight bearing is limited to 10 kg. After 2 weeks, they get a rigid ankle brace for another 4 weeks with full weight bearing in normal shoes. The ankle brace should be used day and night. In addition, physiotherapy with active stabilization is started in the third week. Cycling is normally possible after 4 to 6 weeks and running after 8 to 10 weeks. The patient should avoid contact sports, including soccer, for 3 to 5 months.

OUTCOMES

• Hintermann and Renggli[12] published a series on this technique and found 78% excellent, 18% good, and 4% satisfying results in the American Orthopaedic Foot & Ankle Society hindfoot score. Those good results match our experience.

• Especially active patients benefit from anatomic repair of the ligaments, leading to a more physiologic mobility of the ankle and subtalar joint than tenodesis.[20]

COMPLICATIONS

• Intraoperative graft mishandling
• Graft failure or rupture
• Fracture of the fibula
• Deep venous thrombosis
• Infection
• Loss of motion

REFERENCES

1. Adachi N, Ochi M, Uchio Y, et al. Harvesting hamstring tendons for ACL reconstruction influences postoperative hamstring muscle performance. Arch Orthop Trauma Surg 2003;123(9):460–465.
2. Benazzo F, Zanon G, Marullo M, et al. Lateral ankle instability in high-demand athletes: reconstruction with fibular periosteal flap. Int Orthop 2013;37(9):1839–1844.
3. Reynnon B. The use of taping and bracing in treatment of ankle injury. In: Chan KM, Karlson J, eds. ISAKOS-FIMS World Consensus Conference on Ankle Instability. Stockholm, Sweden: International Federation of Sports Medicine, 2005:38–39.
4. Broström L. Sprained ankles. V. Treatment and prognosis in recent ligament ruptures. Acta Chir Scand 1966;132(5):537–550.
5. Broström L. Sprained ankles. VI. Surgical treatment of "chronic" ligament ruptures. Acta Chir Scand 1966;132(5):551–565.
6. Büber N, Zanetti M, Frigg A, et al. Assessment of hindfoot alignment using MRI and standing hindfoot alignment radiographs (Saltzman view). Skeletal Radiol 2018;47(1):19–24.
7. Burks RT, Morgan J. Anatomy of the lateral ankle ligaments. Am J Sports Med 1994;22(1):72–77.
8. Colville MR, Marder RA, Zarins B. Reconstruction of the lateral ankle ligaments. A biomechanical analysis. Am J Sports Med 1992;20(5):594–600.
9. Giza E, Shin EC, Wong SE, et al. Arthroscopic suture anchor repair of the lateral ligament ankle complex: a cadaveric study. Am J Sports Med 2013;41:2567–2572.
10. Hintermann B. Anatomische Rekonstruktion des Außenbandkomplexes am Sprunggelenk. Operat Orthop Traumatol 1998;10:210–218.
11. Hintermann B, Boss A, Schäfer D. Arthroscopic findings in patients with chronic ankle instability. Am J Sports Med 2002;30(3):402–409.
12. Hintermann B, Renggli P. Anatomic reconstruction of the lateral ligaments of the ankle using a plantaris tendon graft in the treatment of chronic ankle joint instability [in German]. Orthopade 1999;28(9):778–784.
13. Karlsson J, Bergsten T, Lansinger O, et al. Surgical treatment of chronic lateral instability of the ankle joint. A new procedure. Am J Sports Med 1989;17(2):268–273.
14. Konradsen L, Olesen S, Hansen HM. Ankle sensorimotor control and eversion strength after acute ankle inversion injuries. Am J Sports Med 1998;26(1):72–77.
15. Krause F, Seidel A. Malalignment and lateral ankle instability: causes of failure from the varus tibia to the cavovarus foot. Foot Ankle Clin 2018;23(4):593–603.
16. Krips R, van Dijk CN, Halasi PT, et al. Long-term outcome of anatomical reconstruction versus tenodesis for the treatment of chronic anterolateral instability of the ankle joint: a multicenter study. Foot Ankle Int 2001;22:415–421.
17. Mei-Dan O, Kahn G, Zeev A, et al. The medial longitudinal arch as a possible risk factor for ankle sprains: a prospective study in 83 female infantry recruits. Foot Ankle Int 2005;26(2):180–183.
18. Ringleb SI, Dhakal A, Anderson CD, et al. Effects of lateral ligament sectioning on the stability of the ankle and subtalar joint. J Orthop Res 2011;29(10):1459–1464.
19. Rosenbaum D, Becker HP, Sterk J, et al. Long-term results of the modified Evans repair for chronic ankle instability. Orthopedics 1996;19(5):451–455.

20. Rosenbaum D, Becker HP, Wilke HJ, et al. Tenodeses destroy the kinematic coupling of the ankle joint complex. A three-dimensional in vitro analysis of joint movement. J Bone Joint Surg Br 1998;80(1):162–168.

21. Rudert M, Wülker N, Wirth CJ. Reconstruction of the lateral ligaments of the ankle using a regional periosteal flap. J Bone Joint Surg Br 1997;79(3):446–451.

22. Salat P, Le V, Veljkovic A, et al. Imaging in foot and ankle instability. Foot Ankle Clin 2018;23(4):499.e28–522.e28.

23. Snook GA, Chrisman OD, Wilson TC. Long-term results of the Chrisman-Snook operation for reconstruction of the lateral ligaments of the ankle. J Bone Joint Surg Am 1985;67(1):1–7.

24. Strauss JE, Forsberg JA, Lippert FG III. Chronic lateral ankle instability and associated conditions: a rationale for treatment. Foot Ankle Int 2007;28(10):1041–1044.

25. Valderrabano V, Hintermann B, Horisberger M, et al. Ligamentous posttraumatic ankle osteoarthritis. Am J Sports Med 2006;34(4):612–620.

26. Walther M, Kriegelstein S, Altenberger S, et al. Lateral ligament injuries of the ankle joint [in German]. Unfallchirurg 2013;116:776–780.

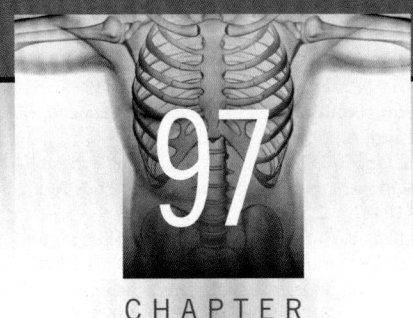

97

CHAPTER

Deltoid Ligament Reconstruction

Eric M. Bluman and Richard J. de Asla

DEFINITION

- Deltoid ligament deficiency is present when both the deep and superficial components of the medial collateral ligament complex of the ankle are ruptured or are insufficient.
- Deltoid ligament deficiency may result from degenerative (eg, late-stage adult acquired flatfoot deformity [AAFD]), postoperative,[6–8] or traumatic or athletic[4] causes.

ANATOMY

- The deltoid ligament complex is a multiunit structure that provides support and restraint for the tibiotalar joint, subtalar joint, spring ligament, and talonavicular joint.
- There is wide agreement that the deltoid ligament complex is made up of both deep and superficial components.
- The deep portion of the complex originates from the intercollicular groove and posterior colliculus of the medial malleolus and inserts on the medial face of the talar body near the center of rotation of the tibiotalar joint. These short and stout fibers are intra-articular but extrasynovial. It is made up of anterior and posterior fascicles.
- There has not been agreement over the superficial components of the complex. In one of the more detailed anatomic studies, Pankovich and Shivaram[5] described the superficial layer as being made up of the tibionavicular, tibiocalcaneal, and tibiotalar ligaments. These fibers represent a triangular array originating on the distal medial malleolus and extending in a fan shape to their respective insertions. The relative contribution of these components to both ankle and foot biomechanics is still a topic of investigation.

PATHOGENESIS

- The most common cause of deltoid ligament disruption is supination–external rotation (SER) ankle fractures. The most severe form of these fractures has either a medial malleolus fracture or a deltoid ligament rupture, in conjunction with a lateral malleolus fracture. The variant with an intact medial malleolus and disrupted medial collateral ligaments is termed *SER IV-deltoid*. This latter form is the most common form of deltoid ligament disruption.
- It has been very well established that deltoid reconstruction is not indicated for disruptions that occur in conjunction with ankle fractures. Reduction and fixation of the fracture component with reestablishment of the mortise morphology leads to healing of the deltoid ligament in the vast majority of those with these combined injuries.[9]

- A smaller proportion of patients with deltoid ligament insufficiency will have developed this as a component of stage IV AAFD.[2]
- Deltoid ligament insufficiency without concomitant ankle fractures resulting from the acute injury has been described but will not be discussed here. This chapter concentrates on deltoid ligament insufficiency arising from degenerative causes.

NATURAL HISTORY

- As the posterior tibial tendon becomes deficient, the ability to bring the hindfoot into varus actively is lost.
- As the mechanical axis of the leg is shifted medially (relative to the foot) and the hindfoot deformity becomes more severe and eventually stiff, tension is progressively increased on the soft tissues of the medial ankle. The medial collateral ligament complex becomes unable to resist the loads placed on it, with eventual insufficiency and lengthening.[7,8]
- Progression to stage IV AAFD occurs when the deltoid ligament becomes incompetent and the valgus force from the preexisting hindfoot deformity causes the talus to tilt within the mortise.

PATIENT HISTORY AND PHYSICAL FINDINGS

- Aspects of the history and physical examination of stage IV AAFD will be similar to those found in the earlier stages of this AAFD.
- There will be hindfoot valgus.
- Because of the chronic nature of posterior tibial tendon involvement, strength will be greatly diminished and likely absent because of rupture. The patient will neither be able to resist hindfoot eversion nor actively bring the forefoot across midline.
- Because of the decreased working length of the triceps surae resulting from chronic hindfoot valgus, there will be contracture of these muscles. A fixed hindfoot deformity may give a falsely optimistic impression of tibiotalar dorsiflexion. Reestablishment of ankle and hindfoot alignment without an appropriate lengthening of the heel cord will create or exacerbate an equinus deformity.
- There may be significant forefoot supination.
- Lateral pain may represent sinus tarsi or subfibular impingement, lateral ankle joint arthritis, or, in severe cases, distal fibular stress fracture.
- Pain in the sinus tarsi is frequently unrecognized or underappreciated before palpation by the clinician.
- Callosity and pain below the talar head may be present if substantial dorsolateral peritalar subluxation has caused a prominence in the medial plantar midfoot.

- It is essential to determine whether the tibiotalar valgus deformity that is a hallmark of stage IV AAFD is rigid or reducible. This is further explained under Surgical Management.
- Clinical determination of the presence of valgus tibiotalar deformity is greatly enhanced with radiologic examination.
- The integrity of the lateral collateral ligament complex needs to be determined. A severe valgus deformity may lead to erosion and incompetence of these structures.
- The surgeon must also evaluate for the presence of ipsilateral knee valgus. If this is significant, consideration should be given to correcting the proximal deformity before the foot and ankle surgery. Correction of the leg-ankle-foot axis without attention to knee deformity may not adequately relieve valgus stress through the reconstructed lower limb and result in recurrence of deformity.
- Methods for examining the deltoid ligament include the following:
  - Palpating the area inferior to the medial malleolus. Tenderness may represent incipient or recent deltoid rupture and may only be present early in stage IV disease.
  - Joint line palpation. The presence of valgus tilt indicates insufficiency of the deltoid ligament.
  - Weight-bearing anteroposterior (AP) ankle radiographs. Valgus tilt greater than 4 degrees indicates deltoid ligament insufficiency.

IMAGING AND OTHER DIAGNOSTIC STUDIES

- The preferred radiologic views include the three-view weight-bearing series. The AP standing view will provide the most information. Patients with deltoid ligament insufficiency will demonstrate tibiotalar valgus tilting **(FIG 1)**.
- Cross-sectional imaging is required only when plans are made for performing reconstruction using native peroneus longus tendon (discussed later). In this case, magnetic resonance imaging (MRI) is used to confirm the integrity of the peroneus brevis before the longus is harvested.
- Selective intra-articular blocks often help the clinician localize the exact source of pain.

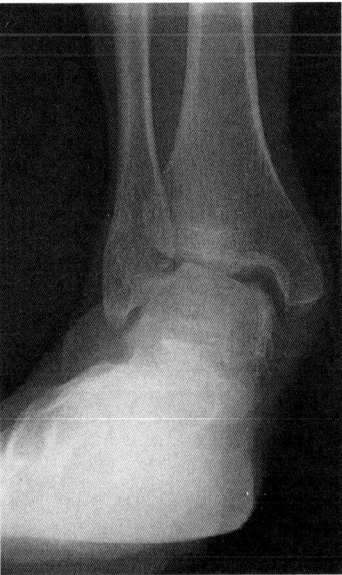

FIG 1 Standing AP weight-bearing radiograph of the ankle demonstrating valgus tibiotalar tilt resulting from insufficiency of the deltoid complex.

DIFFERENTIAL DIAGNOSIS

- Stage II or III AAFD
- Medial malleolus fracture nonunion
- Tibiotalar arthritis (with eccentric lateral joint erosion)
- Osteonecrosis of the talus with lateral collapse
- Distal tibial supramalleolar valgus malalignment (resulting from distal tibiofibular fracture or pilon fracture)
- Valgus malunion of pronation–abduction-type ankle fracture with lateral plafond impaction or comminution

NONOPERATIVE MANAGEMENT

- In contrast to acute deltoid deficiency presenting in conjunction with an ankle fracture, we believe that nonoperative care has a very limited place in patients with chronic deltoid ligament insufficiency resulting from degenerative causes (eg, stage IV AAFD). All but patients with medical comorbidities contraindicating surgery should undergo surgical reconstruction.
- Conservative therapy may also be needed to relieve pain and temporize deformity while related orthopaedic conditions are corrected.
- Should conservative therapy be chosen, custom-molded rigid orthotics that extend to the calf, such as the Arizona brace, provide the best chances of preventing progression of the disease.
- Although halting the progression of the disease may be possible with conservative therapy, the deformities of stage IV cannot be corrected with bracing alone.

SURGICAL MANAGEMENT

- Healing of a chronically insufficient deltoid ligament to a functional structure does not occur in AAFD. Reefing and other surgical techniques attempting to incorporate this diseased tissue into the repair do not produce reliable results. Allograft or autograft reconstructions of the deltoid ligament give the best chances for success.
- Once a diagnosis of stage IV AAFD is made, an operative plan to correct all components of the deformity is needed.
- Evaluation of the ability to passively correct the tibiotalar deformity is central to whether the deltoid ligament may be reconstructed for salvage of the ankle joint.
- Tibiotalar valgus deformity that can be corrected passively may benefit from deltoid reconstruction in conjunction with bony and tendon work. Rigid tibiotalar deformity of stage IV AAFD should be reconstructed with tibiotalocalcaneal or pantalar fusion.
- It is essential to correct all components of the foot deformity along with deltoid reconstruction so that the forces that resulted in the native deltoid ligament insufficiency are neutralized and do not cause failure of the reconstructed ligament.
- If lateral collateral ligament insufficiency is found on examination, the surgical plan should include reconstruction of these structures.

Preoperative Planning

- Imaging studies are reviewed.
- Examination under anesthesia (EUA) should be accomplished before positioning the patient. Intraoperative fluoroscopy may be very useful during the EUA.

- It is also important to reevaluate the lateral collateral ligaments during the EUA.
- All foot reconstructive procedures needed to restore plantigrade alignment should be done at the same surgical setting if possible. These procedures should be done immediately before deltoid ligament reconstruction.

Positioning

- The patient should be positioned supine on the operating table.
- Retrograde application of an Esmarch bandage followed by inflation of an upper thigh tourniquet may be used to create a relatively bloodless field.
- Access to the medial ankle may be improved by placing a soft support under the contralateral hip.
- The surgeon should ensure that the lower extremity is prepared and draped to a level above the knee so that limb–foot alignment may be evaluated intraoperatively.

Approach

- The approach for the minimally invasive deltoid ligament reconstruction (MIDLR) requires a longitudinal incision from the tip of the medial malleolus to just inferior to the prominence of the sustentaculum tali. This incision may need to be carried through incompetent fibers of the superficial deltoid ligament (**FIG 2**).

- The approach for the peroneal grafting method uses a straight longitudinal incision over the peroneal tendons to harvest the peroneus longus tendon and then a medial incision through which the tendon is brought before threading it through and securing it to the tibia. The patient should be initially positioned with a bump under the ipsilateral hip, which may be removed when increased access to the medial ankle is required.

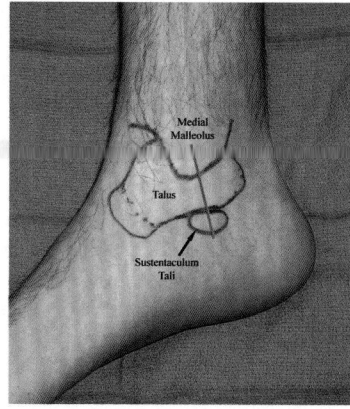

FIG 2 Approach for the minimally invasive deltoid ligament reconstruction technique marked out on the medial ankle. The locations of the medial malleolus, talus, and sustentaculum tali are indicated.

MINIMALLY INVASIVE DELTOID LIGAMENT RECONSTRUCTION

TECHNIQUES

- This technique[1,2] reconstructs components of both the superficial and deep layers of the deltoid ligament without sacrificing any host tissue for graft.

Forked Allograft Preparation

- Cadaveric allograft from the posterior tibial tendon or the peroneal tendon provides a graft of good size. Larger grafts (eg, Achilles tendon) may be used but should be cut to appropriate thickness. Do not use grafts smaller than the posterior tibial tendon or peroneals.
- The graft should be about 20 cm in length and 6 to 7 mm in diameter. Split one end longitudinally, leaving about 5 cm of the opposite end unsplit.
- Place Krackow stitches of no. 0 nonabsorbable woven suture in all three limbs of the tendon (**TECH FIG 1**).
- After preparation, wrap the graft in moistened gauze and set it aside.

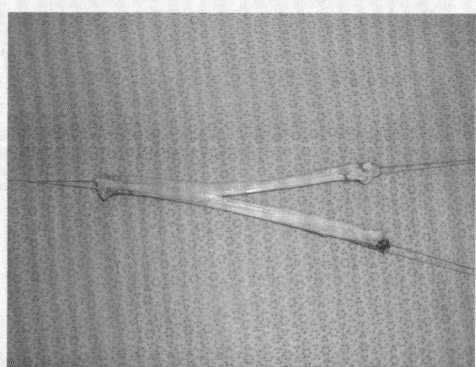

TECH FIG 1 Preparation of forked graft. An allograft tendon about 20 cm long and 7 mm in diameter is chosen and split longitudinally for about two-thirds of its length. Final appearance of the forked graft, showing Krackow sutures placed in all three ends of its limbs.

Tibial Limb Placement

- Above the medial malleolus, in the midcoronal plane, choose a level about 1 cm above the plafond at which the tibial limb of the graft will be anchored. This is approximated well by the level of the distal tibial physeal scar. Intraoperative fluoroscopy is very helpful in locating a proper site. The saphenous vein and nerve should be anterior to the entry site chosen.

- At the level of insertion, make a 1-cm longitudinal incision down to medial tibial cortex. Advance a guidewire from medial to lateral parallel to the plafond (**TECH FIG 2**). Make a 6.0-mm blind tunnel over the guidewire for a distance of 25 mm. Remove the guidewire.
- Secure the tibial limb (unsplit end) of the forked graft in the blind tibial tunnel using a 6.25-mm soft tissue interference screw (**TECH FIG 3**). Use manual testing to ensure that the graft is adequately anchored in the tunnel.

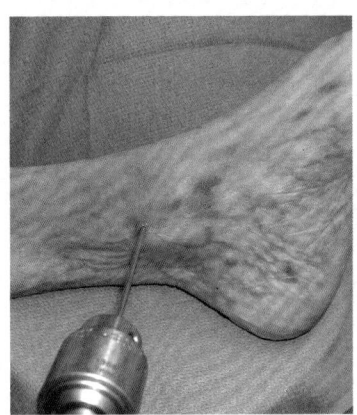
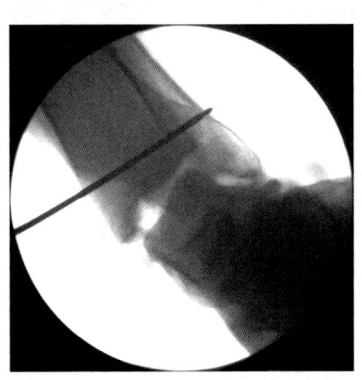
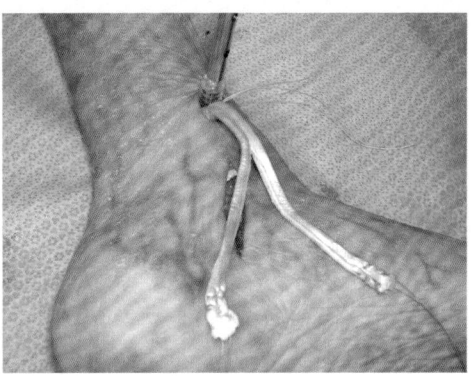

TECH FIG 2 Insertion of tibial limb. **A.** Starting point for tibial guidewire placement should be at the level of the distal tibial physeal scar. **B.** Tibial guidewire placement as shown by AP view with fluoroscopy. **C.** Securing the tibial limb of the graft with a soft tissue interference screw.

Talar Limb Placement

- The path of the tunnel through the talus starts at the medial center of tibiotalar rotation. This is most easily approximated by drilling the insertion point for the native deep deltoid ligament. The lateral exit of the tunnel is located at the lateral junction of the talar dome and neck. This lateral exit point is located by palpation. If this junction cannot be palpated, a small incision may need to be made to locate the lateral neck–body junction.

Advance a guidewire for a cannulated 5.0-mm drill along this axis. Confirm the position of the guidewire with AP and lateral fluoroscopic views.

- Drill a 5.0-mm tunnel over the guidewire. Pass one end of the sutured tendon through the tunnel from medial to lateral using a suture passer. Place appropriate tension on the graft and place a 5.0-mm soft tissue interference screw in the medial aspect of the tunnel to secure the graft. Advance the interference screw so that it is countersunk 1 to 2 mm into the tunnel.

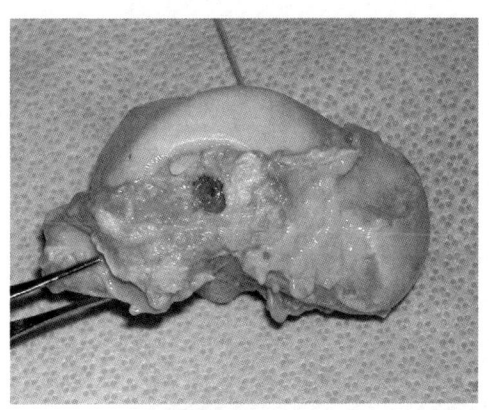
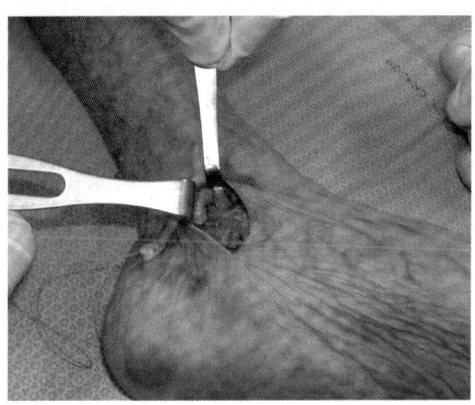
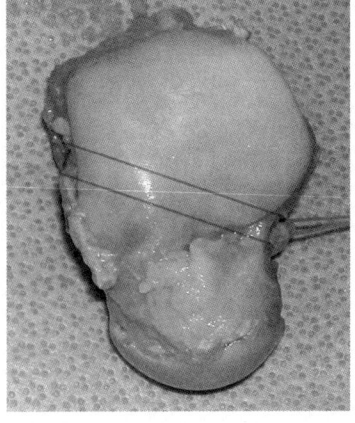

TECH FIG 3 Talar limb placement. **A.** Starting point for the talar tunnel is approximated by the footprint of the deep deltoid ligament insertion on the medial face of the talus. Shown is the medial talar surface of a cadaveric dissection specimen. A soft tissue interference screw has been placed in the medial portion of the talar tunnel. The talar head is oriented to the right in this image. **B.** Path of the talar tunnel as seen from a dorsoplantar view of a cadaveric talus. The talar head is toward the bottom and the medial talus is at the left side of the image. The lines represent the path of the tunnel through the talus. **C.** Medial aspect of ankle after talar limb has been inserted, tensioned, and secured.

Calcaneal Limb Placement

- Using palpation, locate the medial border of the sustentaculum tali. Once it is found, carefully dissect the posterior tibial tendon sheath away from the bone and retract it inferiorly. Insert the guidewire to the cannulated drill along an axis from the mid-portion of the sustentaculum tali to a point about 1 cm superior to the peroneal tubercle on the lateral side of the calcaneus (**TECH FIG 4A**). Placing the guidewire in this location allows for centralization in the sustentaculum and minimizes the chances of breaching the subtalar joint. Check the position of the guidewire using fluoroscopy.
- Create a 5.0-mm tunnel over this guidewire.

- Pass the free end of the remaining limb of the tendon graft through the sustentacular tunnel and out the skin overlying the lateral calcaneus. A small slit may need to be made to allow the graft to be pulled fully through. Perform tensioning and tibiotalar joint position manually and check it under fluoroscopy.
- When appropriate tension is achieved, insert a 5.0-mm interference screw from medial to lateral into the sustentacular tunnel.
- The appearance of the final construct in situ is illustrated in **TECH FIG 4B**. An illustration of the position of the graft after insertion and fixation is shown in **TECH FIG 4C**.
- Close the wounds in a layered fashion.

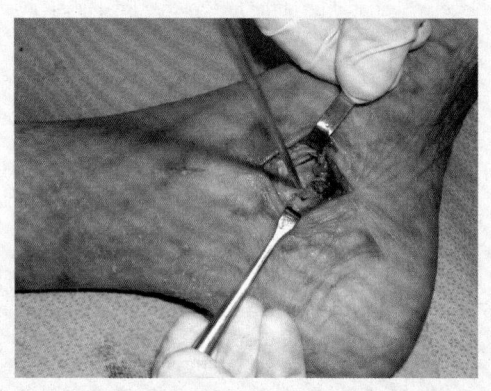 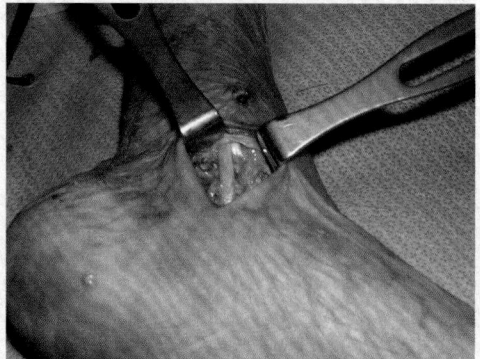

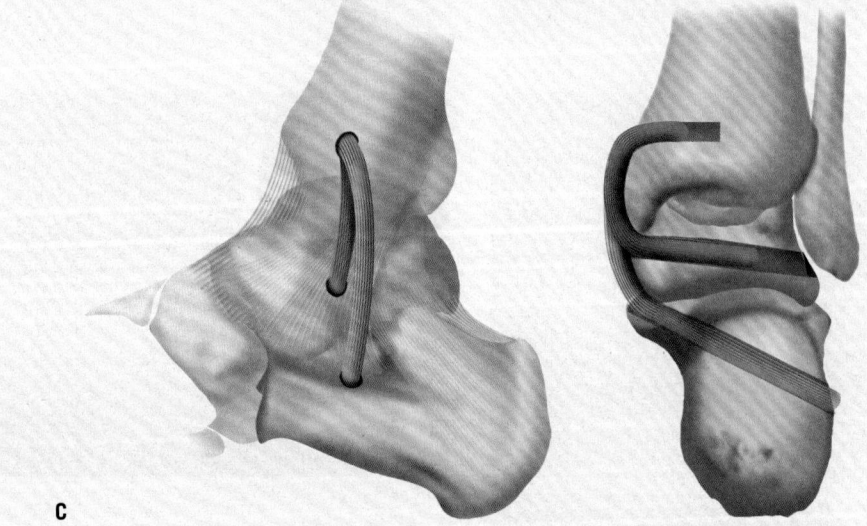

TECH FIG 4 Calcaneal limb placement. **A.** Starting point for the calcaneal limb with guidewire advanced so as to avoid the subtalar joint and exit out the lateral calcaneal cortex. **B.** Completed minimally invasive deltoid ligament reconstruction in situ from the medial aspect. **C.** Completed minimally invasive deltoid ligament reconstruction from the medial aspect and from a posteroanterior view.

PERONEUS LONGUS GRAFT TENDON HARVESTING

- Harvest the peroneus longus tendon through a lateral incision that extends from the fourth metatarsal base to about midway up the calf.[3]
- Tenodese the proximal stump of the transected peroneus longus tendon to the peroneus brevis.
- After securing a Krackow locking suture to the free end of the peroneus longus tendon, wrap it in a piece of moist gauze.

Talar Tunnel Construction

- Make a medial incision centered over the medial malleolus, extending distally over the fibers of the superficial deltoid.
- Divide the fibers of the attenuated deltoid ligament, exposing the medial aspect of the talus.
- Pass an intraosseous guidewire from the lateral talar neck–body junction to the estimated center of rotation on the medial aspect of the talus inferior to the tip of the medial malleolus.
- Verify guidewire position fluoroscopically and clinically by dorsiflexing and plantarflexing the ankle to determine if the center of rotation has been localized.
- Create a tunnel using a cannulated reamer about 4 to 5 mm in diameter.

Tibial Tunnel Construction

- Create a second bony tunnel from the tip of the medial malleolus to a point in the lateral distal tibia. The exit point is about 5 to 6 cm proximal to the tibial plafond and anterior to the fibula. We recommend saving the shavings from the reamer to be used later as bone graft.

Graft Passage and Fixation

- Pass the tendon through the tibial tunnel from distal medial to proximal lateral.

- Tension the tendon first at the medial talar tunnel and then at the lateral tibial exit site, with correction of valgus talar tilt.
- Secure the tendon to the lateral tibia under maximal tension with a soft tissue washer or staple. Pack bone graft obtained from reaming in the bony tunnels. A schematic of the final construct is depicted in **TECH FIG 5**.
- Close the wounds.

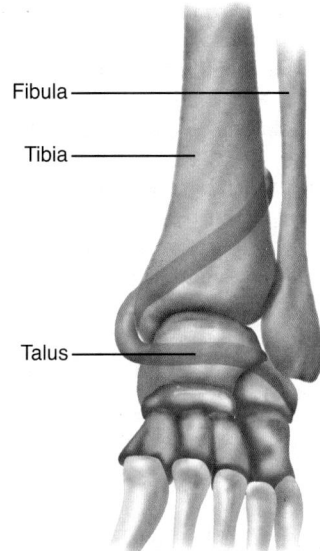

TECH FIG 5 Peroneus longus autograft construct. Completed peroneus longus autograft has been passed through the talar tunnel, into the medial malleolus, and out the lateral tibia, where it is fixed to the lateral cortex.

T E C H N I Q U E S

Pearls and Pitfalls

Need for Concomitant Procedures	• Deltoid reconstruction as described here is intended to reconstitute a functional restraint to valgus tibiotalar tilting. • Be sure to correct any malalignment or deformity that will tend to produce valgus angulation at the tibiotalar joint at the same time that the deltoid reconstruction is done. • Failure to do this may result in the correction being inadequate or may even lead to outright failure of the graft.
Fixation Problems: Graft Pullout	• Ensure that the tendon ends are reinforced with Krackow sutures to allow for secure passage of the tendons and to prevent interference screw laceration of the graft.
Tunnel Placement	• Make sure the talar tunnel starts medially at the insertion of the deep deltoid ligament. Substantial deviation of the starting point of the talar tunnel from this location will result in increased shearing forces across the tendon. • The superficial (calcaneal) limb of the graft must be centered within the sustentaculum. Eccentric placement may result in the medial facet of the subtalar joint or the inferior cortex of the sustentaculum being breached. Breaching the medial facet could lead to subtalar arthritis. Breaching the inferior sustentacular cortex could result in flexor hallucis longus paratenonitis or abrasion.
Nerve Injury	• Make small incisions over the exit of the talar and calcaneal limbs to prevent damage to branches of the superficial peroneal and sural nerves.
Indications	• These techniques are designed to aid in the surgical correction of stage IV AAFD. Other treatment methods may need to be used for either acute deltoid injuries or deltoid insufficiency associated with disease processes other than AAFD.

POSTOPERATIVE CARE

- In the immediate period after tibiotalar joint–sparing reconstruction of stage IV posterior tibial tendon rupture, a plaster splint is applied in neutral position. Physiotherapy starts after the incisions have healed, usually about 2 weeks postoperatively. Therapy consists of passive and active mobilization of the ankle joint as well as intrinsic muscle exercises. Weight bearing is started progressively but is not full until 12 weeks postoperatively. Gait training is instituted as needed after weight bearing is commenced.

OUTCOMES

- There are no long-term results for these methods because both were recently developed. Studies on outcomes are made difficult by the small number of patients who present with stage IV AAFD. Ongoing studies are evaluating the ability to maintain the correction and stability obtained with these methods.
- Two-year clinical results for the forked graft method are just becoming available at the time of the writing of this chapter. Initial short-term results are promising, with maintenance of tibiotalar joint motion and stability in those who have undergone the procedure.
- Short-term follow-up data are available for the peroneus longus graft method. In the five patients evaluated after undergoing this procedure, four had tibiotalar valgus correction to 4 degrees or less that was maintained 2 years after the procedure.

COMPLICATIONS

- Breaching tibiotalar joint with misplaced tibial or talar tunnel
- Breaching subtalar joint with misplaced calcaneal tunnel (forked graft method)
- Damage to superficial peroneal nerve
- Damage to deep peroneal nerve (peroneal graft method)
- Damage to the sural nerve on calcaneal limb pull-through (forked graft method)
- Infection
- Graft failure or rupture

REFERENCES

1. Bluman EM, Khazen G, Haraguchi N, et al. Minimally invasive deltoid ligament reconstruction: a biomechanical and anatomic analysis. Presented at American Orthopaedic Foot and Ankle Society 21st Annual Summer Meeting, Boston, MA, 2005.
2. Bluman E, Myerson M. Stage IV posterior tibial tendon rupture. Foot Ankle Clin 2007;12:341–362.
3. Deland JT, de Asla RJ, Segal A. Reconstruction of the chronically failed deltoid ligament: a new technique. Foot Ankle Int 2004;25:795–799.
4. Hintermann B, Valderrabano V, Boss A, et al. Medial ankle instability: an exploratory, prospective study of fifty-two cases. Am J Sports Med 2004;32:183–190.
5. Pankovich AM, Shivaram MS. Anatomical basis of variability in injuries of the medial malleolus and the deltoid ligament. I. Anatomical studies. Acta Orthop Scand 1979;50:217–223.
6. Pell RF IV, Myerson MS, Schon LC. Clinical outcome after primary triple arthrodesis. J Bone Joint Surg Am 2000;82(1):47–57.
7. Resnick RB, Jahss MH, Choueka J, et al. Deltoid ligament forces after tibialis posterior tendon rupture: effects of triple arthrodesis and calcaneal displacement osteotomies. Foot Ankle Int 1995;16:14–20.
8. Song SJ, Lee S, O'Malley MJ, et al. Deltoid ligament strain after correction of acquired flatfoot deformity by triple arthrodesis. Foot Ankle Int 2000;21:573–577.
9. Zeegers AV, van der Werken C. Rupture of the deltoid ligament in ankle fractures: should it be repaired? Injury 1989;20:39–41.

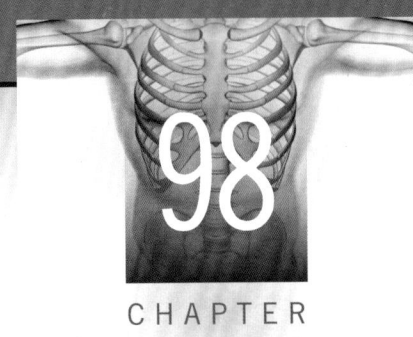

98

CHAPTER

Medial Ankle/Deltoid Ligament Reconstruction

Beat Hintermann and Roxa Ruiz

DEFINITION

- Pronation and exorotation/abduction injuries of the ankle joint complex may result in a partial or complete disruption of the superficial anterior bundles of the deltoid ligament.
- Medial ankle instability may be also the result of peritalar instability with progressive collapsed valgus foot deformity
- Chronic medial ankle instability may cause a secondary posterior tibial dysfunction over time, as the tendon may become elongated, ruptured, or both.
- Conversely, medial ankle instability may also result from a posterior tibial dysfunction with chronic overload of the deltoid ligaments and consecutive step-by-step disruption.
- Medial ankle instability must be suspected if the patient complains of "giving way," especially medially, when walking on even ground, downhill, or downstairs. Further signs can be pain at the anteromedial aspect of the ankle, and sometimes pain on the lateral ankle, especially during dorsiflexion of the foot.

ANATOMY

- The deltoid ligament is a multibanded complex with superficial and deep components.
- It may be wise to differentiate the superficial and deep portions of the deltoid complex with respect to the joints they are spanning. The superficial ligaments cross two (the ankle and the subtalar joints) and the deep ligaments cross one joint (only the ankle joint), although differentiation is not always absolutely clear.[14]
- The three superficial and more anterior bands are the tibionavicular, tibiospring, and tibiocalcaneal ligaments; the three deep bands are the anterior, superficial, and posterior tibiotalar ligaments **(FIG 1).**[1]

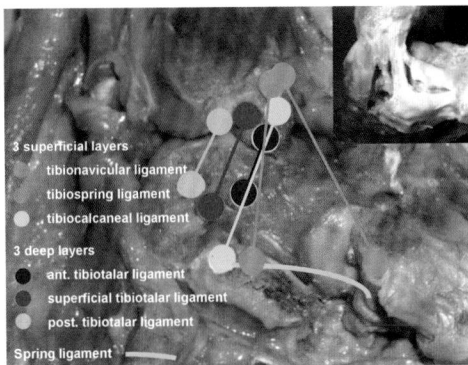

FIG 1 Anatomic situs of the medial ankle. The superficial and deep deltoid consists of three distinct bundles each.

- As the tibioligamentous portion of the superficial deltoid has a broad insertion on the "spring ligament," this ligament complex may interplay with the deltoid ligament in the stabilization of the medial ankle joint and thus is not functionally separated from it (see **FIG 1**).[5]

PATHOGENESIS

- Acute injuries to the medial ankle ligaments can occur during running downstairs, landing on an uneven surface, and dancing while the body is simultaneously rotated in the opposite direction. A key feature is whether the patient has sustained a pronation (eversion) trauma—for instance, an outward rotation of the foot during simultaneous inward rotation of the tibia.
- Complete deltoid ligament ruptures are sometimes seen in association with lateral malleolar fractures or in specific bimalleolar fractures.[4]
- Chronic deltoid ligament insufficiency can be seen in a number of conditions, including progressive collapsed valgus deformity of the foot, posterior tibial tendon disorder, traumatic and sports-related deltoid disruptions, as well as valgus talar tilting in patients with previous triple arthrodesis or total ankle arthroplasty.

NATURAL HISTORY

- There is evidence that the medial ankle ligaments are more often injured than generally believed.[6-9]
- Several structures contribute to the stabilization of the medial ankle, and in the case of injury, they are not involved in a uniform way. Medial ankle instability is thus not a single entity, and this has important consequences on the treatment strategy.
- The findings of an exploratory, prospective study on 51 patients (53 ankles) has supported our belief that medial ankle instability without posterior tibial tendon dysfunction does exist as an entity.[10] It is, however, not clear yet whether, or to what extent, such a medial ankle instability may cause a secondary posterior tibial dysfunction over time, as the tendon may become elongated, ruptured, or both.
- What is clear from the literature is that a coexisting pronation deformity and progressive collapse of medial arch of the foot will lead to further deterioration over time, as the medial ankle ligaments are chronically overstretched.

PATIENT HISTORY AND PHYSICAL FINDINGS

- The diagnosis of medial ankle instability is made on the basis of the patient's history and the results of physical examination, including special maneuvers, and plain radiographs.

- As mentioned earlier, medial instability is suspected if the patient complains of "giving way," especially medially, when walking on even ground, downhill, or downstairs. Further signs can be pain at the anteromedial aspect of the ankle, and sometimes pain on the lateral ankle, especially during dorsiflexion of the foot.
- A history of chronic instability, manifested by recurrent injuries with pain, tenderness, and sometimes bruising over the medial and lateral ligaments, is considered to indicate combined medial and lateral instability that is thought to result in rotational instability of the talus in the ankle mortise.
- Acute injuries may present with tenderness and hematoma at the medial side of the ankle.
- Physical examination methods for chronic medial ankle instability should include:
  - Standing test. Inspect for malalignment, deformity, asymmetry, and swelling. Asymmetric planus and pronation deformity of the affected foot may indicate medial ankle instability: distinct, moderate, important.
  - Palpation of anteromedial ankle. Pain in the medial gutter is typically provoked by palpation of the anterior border of the medial malleolus. It is the result of underlying synovitis due to chronic shifting of the talus within the ankle mortise.
  - Anterior drawer test is a highly sensitive test for medial ankle instability.
- A complete examination of the hindfoot should also include evaluating associated injuries and ruling out other possible causes. These include, among others:
  - Fractures of the medial malleolus: After an acute injury, radiographic analysis must be performed routinely to exclude a fracture of the medial malleolus (eg, bony avulsion of the deltoid ligament) or fibula fracture with or without syndesmotic disruption.

- Loss of posterior tibial function after partial or complete rupture: The patient cannot correct the deformity while standing or cannot create supination power to the foot.
- Talonavicular coalition: The subtalar joint is not mobile, so there is no varization of the heel while going into the tiptoe position.
- Neurologic disorder: There is partial or complete palsy of one or more muscles due to deficient neurologic control.

IMAGING AND OTHER DIAGNOSTIC STUDIES

- Acute injury: Plain radiographs, including anteroposterior (AP) and lateral views, should be obtained to rule out bony avulsion fractures or associated injuries.
- Chronic injury: Plain weight-bearing radiographs, including AP views of the foot and ankle (**FIG 2**), a lateral view of the foot and a hindfoot alignment view,[17] should be obtained to rule out old bony avulsion fractures, secondary deformities of the foot (eg, valgus malalignment of the heel, dislocation at the talonavicular joint), and tibiotalar alignment (eg, medial gapping of the joint due to incompetence of the deltoid ligament).
- Stress radiographs may be helpful to identify incompetence of the deltoid ligament in the treatment of acute ankle fractures,[18] but they are not helpful in chronic conditions.[5,10]
- A computed tomography (CT) scan may be obtained to detect a talocalcaneal coalition or bony fragmentation that involves the articular surfaces. A weight-bearing CT may be beneficial to recognize the specific position of talus within the ankle mortise and a potential incongruency in the subtalar joint, as given by an accompanying peritalar instability (**FIG 3**).
- Magnetic resonance (MR) imaging may show an injury to the deltoid ligament (**FIG 4**), particularly in acute conditions,[11,13] and it may also reveal pathologic conditions of the posterior tibial tendon.

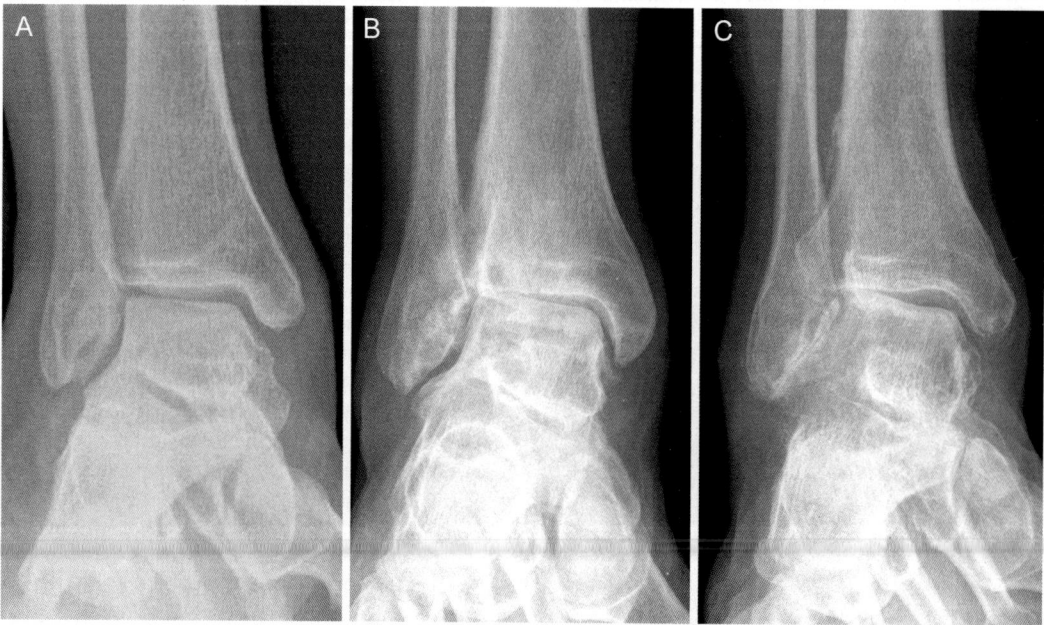

FIG 2 Incompetence of the deltoid ligament. **A.** Distinct instability: AP weight-bearing radiograph shows a gapping of less than 5 degrees of the medial tibiotalar joint. **B.** Moderate instability: AP weight-bearing radiograph shows a gapping of 5 to 11 degrees of the medial tibiotalar joint. **C.** Severe instability: AP weight-bearing radiograph shows a gapping of more than 11 degrees of the medial tibiotalar joint.

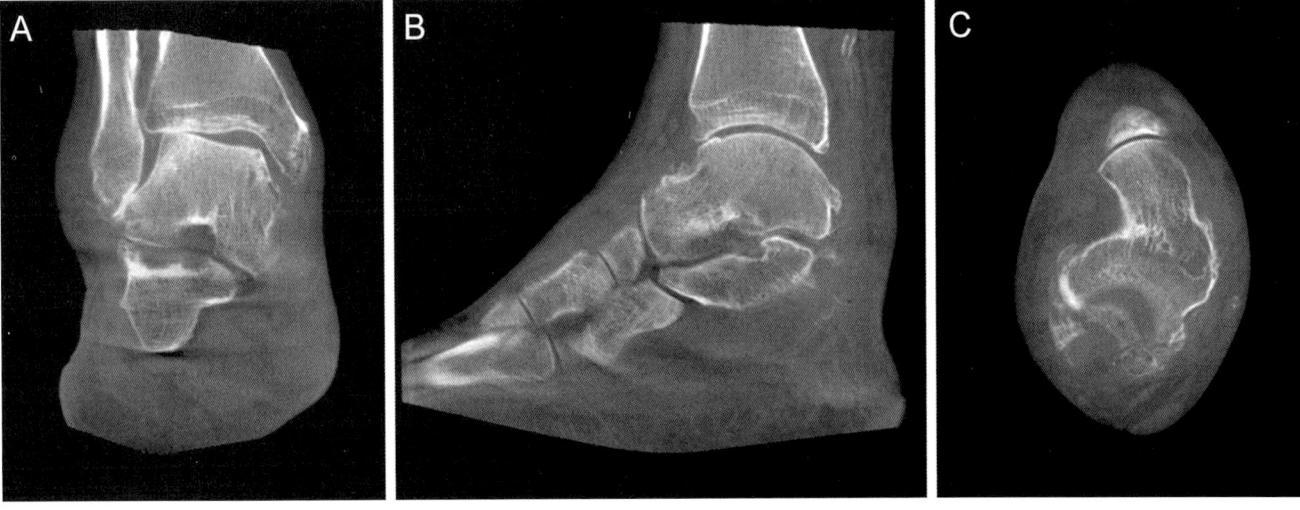

FIG 3 Weight-bearing CT in a patient with severe instability showing the peritalar instability with subsequent sinus tarsi and subfibular impingement (same patient as in **FIG 2C**). **A.** AP coronal plane. **B.** Sagittal plane. **C.** AP horizontal plane.

DIFFERENTIAL DIAGNOSIS

- Bony avulsion fracture of the medial malleolus (with or without fracture of the fibula or syndesmotic disruption)
- Fixed flatfoot deformity (eg, acquired flatfoot deformity in adults after posterior tibial dysfunction)
- Osteochondral injury
- Talocalcaneal coalition

NONOPERATIVE MANAGEMENT

- Although nonoperative management is controversial, patients with less instability, particularly those who have less of a "giving-way" feeling and those who are less involved with high-level pronation sports activities, may be treated nonoperatively.

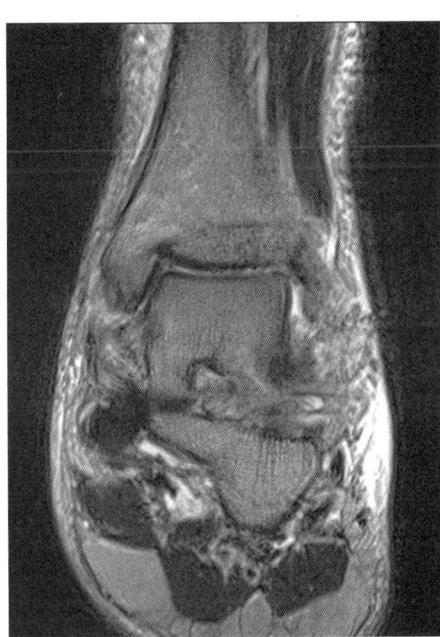

FIG 4 Proximal avulsion of the deltoid ligament. AP MR imaging reveals a complete avulsion of the deltoid ligament to the medial malleolus.

- Nonoperative treatment consists of three components:
  - Medial foot arch supports
  - Physiotherapy for strengthening the invertor muscles
  - A neuromuscular rehabilitation program

SURGICAL MANAGEMENT

Preoperative Planning

- All imaging studies are reviewed.
- Plain films should be reviewed for fractures, cartilage lesions, hindfoot and midfoot malalignment, and the presence of any hardware (from previous procedures) or foreign bodies.
- Associated fractures, cartilage lesions, foot malalignment, and tendon disruption should be addressed concurrently.
- Examination under anesthesia should be performed to compare with the contralateral ankle.

Positioning

- The patient is in a supine position with the feet at the edge of the table.
- A commercially available knee holder is used to support the distal femur and to place the foot into a hanging position **(FIG 5)**.
- This allows the surgeon to move the foot freely while arthroscopy is done before open reconstruction.
- After the arthroscopy, the knee holder is removed, leaving the foot on the table.

Approach

- An anteromedial approach is used for ankle arthroscopy.[7]
- A gently curved incision of 3 to 5 cm is made, starting 1 cm cranially of the tip of the medial malleolus and running toward the medial aspect of the navicular bone.
- If there is additional instability of the lateral ankle ligaments, as found on the clinical examination and confirmed by arthroscopy, a lateral approach to the ankle is also performed to explore the anterior talofibular and calcaneofibular ligaments.

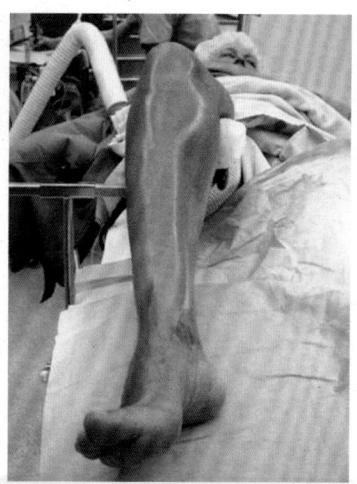

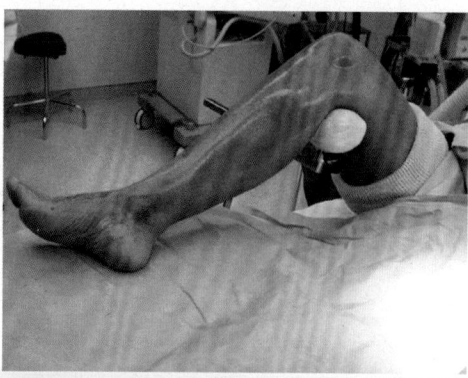

FIG 5 Positioning for arthroscopy and medial ligament reconstruction. A knee holder is used to support the distal femur so that the foot is hanging on the table. **A.** View from the bottom of the table. **B.** Medial view.

TECHNIQUES

ANKLE ARTHROSCOPY

- Arthroscopy is done to visualize the internal structures and to assess medial and lateral ankle stability.[7]
- After visual evaluation of the ligaments, test lateral and medial ligament stability by applying gentle varus, valgus, and anterior pull stress to the ankle joint under arthroscopic control.
- Ligament lesions are graded as distended if the ligament is thinned or elongated and as ruptured if continuity is lost.[10] Most ligament tears are located on the proximal insertion this is best seen by a completely free insertion area of the ligament on the malleoli **(TECH FIG 1)**.
- As the foot is everted and pronated, the deltoid ligament is considered incompetent when it is tensioned, but obviously, no strong medial buttress is created with this maneuver **(TECH FIG 2)**. An excessive lifting away of the talus from the medial malleolus by pulling the foot anteriorly is also considered an indicator of stretching of this ligament.

- Lateral instability is considered to be present when talar tilting occurs by supination stress of the foot.
- As evaluated for both the medial and lateral side, the ankle joint is graded as stable when there is some translocation of the talus but not enough to open the tibiotalar joint by more than 2 mm (as measured by the 2-mm hook) and not enough to introduce the 5-mm arthroscope into the tibiotalar space; as moderately unstable when the talus moves to some extent out of the ankle mortise, allowing introduction of the 5-mm arthroscope into the tibiotalar space but not enough to open the tibiotalar joint by more than 5 mm; and as severely unstable when the talus moves easily out of the ankle mortise, typically allowing free insight into the posterior aspect of the ankle joint without significant pulling stress on the heel.[10]

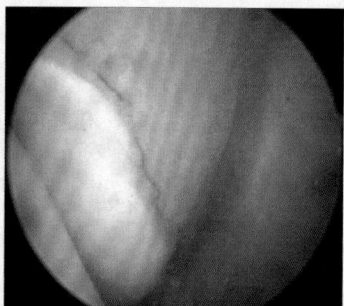

TECH FIG 1 Avulsion of the anterior superficial layers from the medial malleolus. Arthroscopy typically reveals a completely free insertion area of the ligament on the medial malleolus.

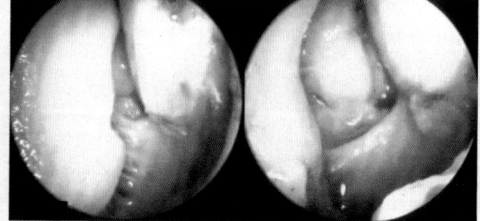

TECH FIG 2 Incompetent deltoid ligament. **A.** As the foot is everted and pronated, the deltoid ligament is considered incompetent when it is tensioned, but obviously, no strong medial buttress is created with this maneuver. **B.** An excessive lifting away of the talus from the medial malleolus by pulling the foot anteriorly is also considered an indicator of stretching of this ligament.

MEDIAL ANKLE LIGAMENT RECONSTRUCTION

Complete Acute Rupture

- Because the rupture is mostly situated at the proximal end of the deltoid ligament **(TECH FIG 3)**, reattachment to the medial malleolus is achieved by interosseous sutures; a bony anchor can also be used for refixation to the bone.[8]

Chronic Rupture of the Superficial Deltoid Ligament

- Classification of these injuries is shown in **TABLE 1**.[8,10]

Type I Lesion

- Expose the anterior border of the medial malleolus by making a short longitudinal incision between the tibionavicular and tibio-spring ligaments, where there is usually a small fibrous septum without adherent connective fibers between the two ligaments **(TECH FIG 4A)**.

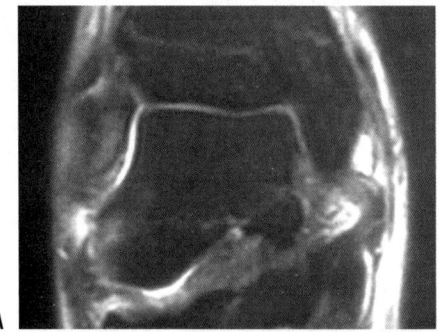

A

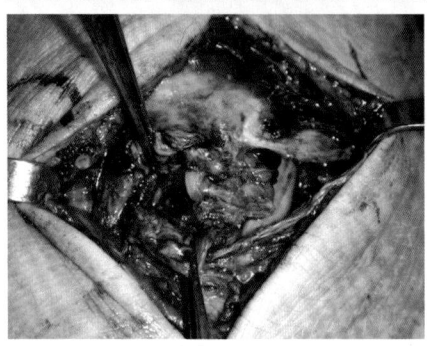

B

TECH FIG 3 Acute deltoid rupture. This 28-year-old soccer player sustained a valgus trauma, causing an acute "giving way" of the foot. **A.** MR imaging reveals complete disruption of the ligament close to its proximal insertion to the medial malleolus. **B.** Surgical exploration confirms complete disruption of the deltoid ligament, although the posterior tibial tendon remained intact.

TABLE 1 Classification of Chronic Superficial Lesions of Deltoid Ligament		
Lesion	**Location of Tear**	
Type I lesion	Proximal tear/avulsion of the deltoid ligament	
Type II lesion	Intermediate tear of the deltoid ligament	
Type III lesion	Distal tear/avulsion of the deltoid and the spring ligaments	

TECHNIQUES

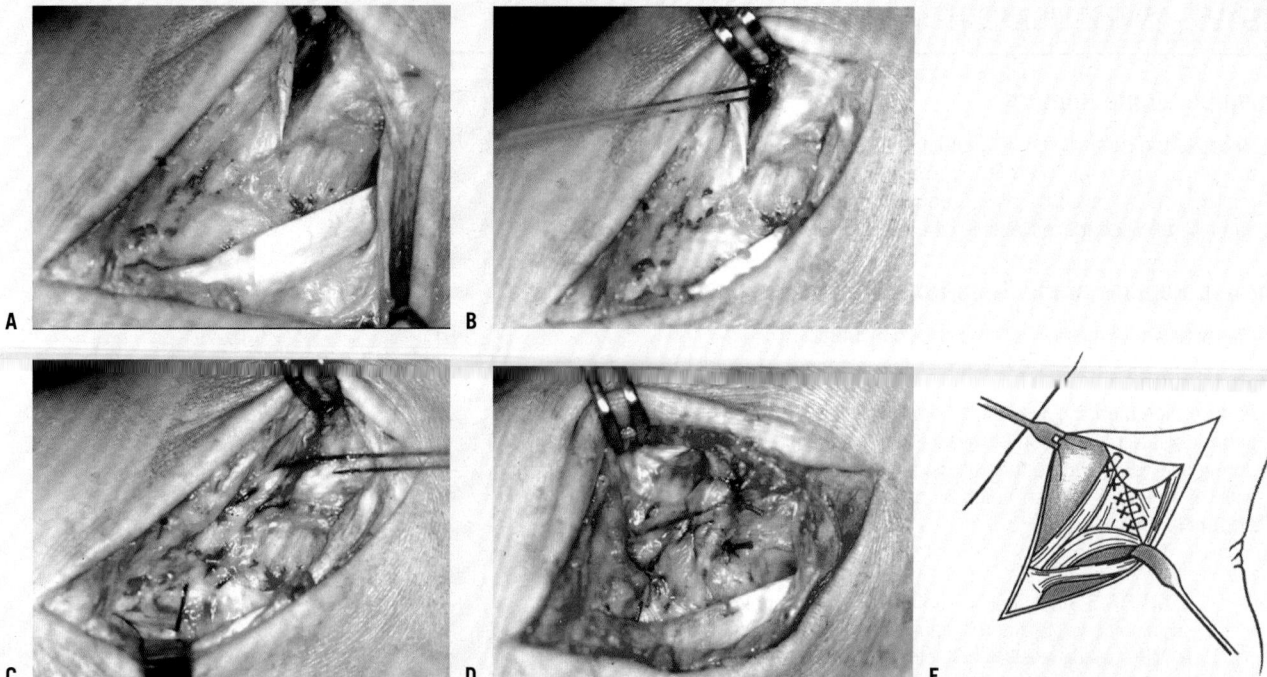

TECH FIG 4 Chronic rupture of the superficial deltoid ligament (type I lesion). **A.** The rupture is located between the tibionavicular and tibiospring ligaments, where a small fibrous septum without adherent connective fibers between the two ligaments is usually present. **B.** After roughening the medial aspect of the medial malleolus, an anchor (FASTak) is placed 6 mm above the tip of the malleolus. **C.** It serves for refixation of the tibionavicular and tibiospring ligaments to the medial malleolus and to shorten both ligaments. **D.** Final reconstruction after some additional no. 0 resorbable sutures. **E.** Principle of reconstruction.

- After roughening the medial aspect of the medial malleolus, place an anchor (FASTak [Arthrex, Inc., Naples, Florida]) 6 mm above the tip of the malleolus (**TECH FIG 4B**); this serves for refixation of the tibionavicular and tibiospring ligaments to the medial malleolus and to shorten both the tibionavicular and tibiospring ligaments (**TECH FIG 4C–E**).
- Use additional no. 0 resorbable sutures to refix the tibionavicular and tibiospring ligaments.

Type II Lesion
- Divide the scarred insufficient ligament (**TECH FIG 5A**) into two flaps: The deep flap remains reattached distally; the superficial flap remains reattached to the medial malleolus.
- Place two anchors (FASTak) 6 mm above the tip of the malleolus (**TECH FIG 5B**) and place one anchor (FASTak) at the superior edge of the navicular tuberosity (**TECH FIG 5C**).

Two anchors serve for refixation of the deep flap to the medial malleolus (**TECH FIG 5D**) and the superficial flap to the navicular tuberosity (**TECH FIG 5E**), thereby creating a strong and well-tightened ligament reconstruction (**TECH FIG 5F**). The second superior anchor on the medial malleolus serves for reattachment of the tibionavicular ligament (**TECH FIG 5G**).
- Use additional no. 0 resorbable sutures to further stabilize the reconstructed tibionavicular and tibiospring ligaments (**TECH FIG 5H,I**).

Type III Lesion
- If necessary, débride the tear (**TECH FIG 6A**).
- Place two nonresorbable sutures in the spring ligament (**TECH FIG 6B**).
- If the tibionavicular ligament is completely detached from its insertion, place an anchor (FASTak) at the superior edge of the navicular tuberosity.

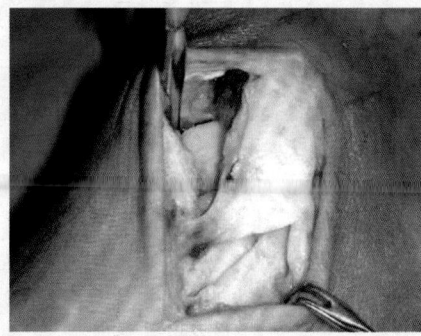

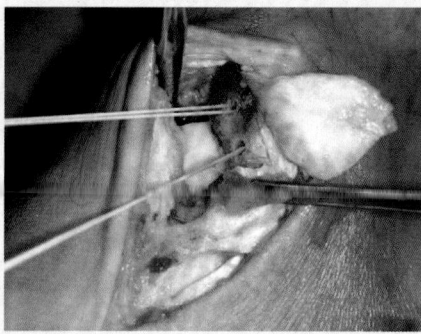

TECH FIG 5 Chronic rupture of the superficial deltoid ligament (type II lesion). **A.** The superficial deltoid ligament is scarred and incompetent. **B.** Two anchors (FASTak) are placed 6 and 9 mm above the tip of the medial malleolus. *(continued)*

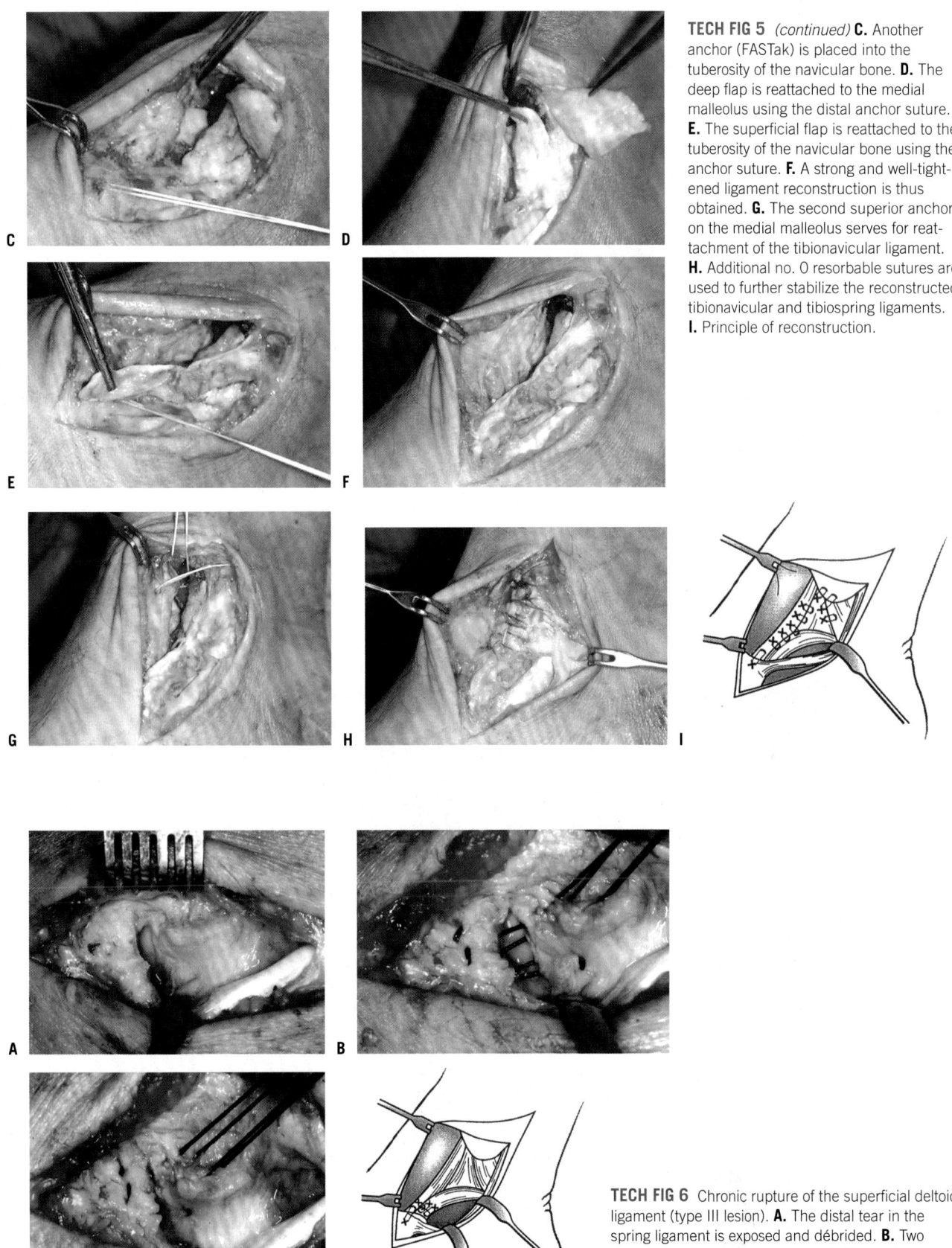

TECH FIG 5 *(continued)* **C.** Another anchor (FASTak) is placed into the tuberosity of the navicular bone. **D.** The deep flap is reattached to the medial malleolus using the distal anchor suture. **E.** The superficial flap is reattached to the tuberosity of the navicular bone using the anchor suture. **F.** A strong and well-tightened ligament reconstruction is thus obtained. **G.** The second superior anchor on the medial malleolus serves for reattachment of the tibionavicular ligament. **H.** Additional no. 0 resorbable sutures are used to further stabilize the reconstructed tibionavicular and tibiospring ligaments. **I.** Principle of reconstruction.

TECH FIG 6 Chronic rupture of the superficial deltoid ligament (type III lesion). **A.** The distal tear in the spring ligament is exposed and débrided. **B.** Two nonresorbable sutures are placed in the spring ligament. **C.** The sutures are tightened. **D.** Principle of reconstruction.

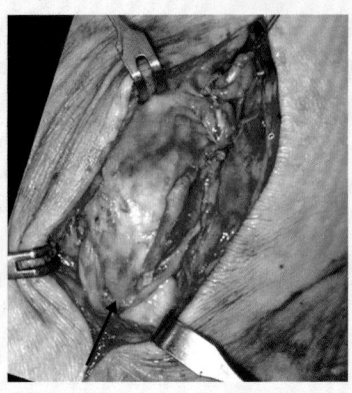

TECH FIG 7 Chronic rupture of the deep deltoid ligament. After the posterior tibial tendon has been split into two bundles, both bundles are inserted into a drill hole at the tip of the medial malleolus (*arrow*). One bundle is conducted through the anterior tunnel at the anterior aspect of the medial malleolus, and the other bundle is conducted through the posterior tunnel at the posterior aspect of the medial malleolus.

- After tightening the sutures **(TECH FIG 6C,D)**, use additional no. 0 resorbable sutures to further stabilize the reconstructed tibionavicular and spring ligaments.

Chronic Rupture of the Deep Deltoid Ligament

- Because this condition usually includes an extended tear of the superficial anterior bundles of the deltoid ligament, any reconstructive surgery should attempt to address the whole deltoid ligament.
- The posterior tibial tendon can be used as a graft for augmentation of the reconstructed deltoid ligament by passing it through a drill hole from the tip of the medial malleolus to the medial aspect of the distal tibia **(TECH FIG 7)**.

- However, this technique was found to be disappointing as it does not sufficiently reinforce the deep tibiotalar ligaments. Most recently, the use of a bone–tendon–bone transplant has been proposed for reconstruction of the deltoid ligament **(TECH FIG 8)**.[2] In this in vitro study, two limbs were created on a distal transplant: one was fixed to the medial aspect of the talus and the other to the sustentaculum tali. The proximal end was fixed to the distal tibia, the medial malleolus, or the lateral tibia. Less than 2.0 degrees of angulation was found while applying valgus stress of 5 daN for all fixation methods. However, the authors advised against fixation of the proximal limb to the medial malleolus. Other techniques with the use of an allograft have been also proposed, but they need to proof their efficiency over time.[3]

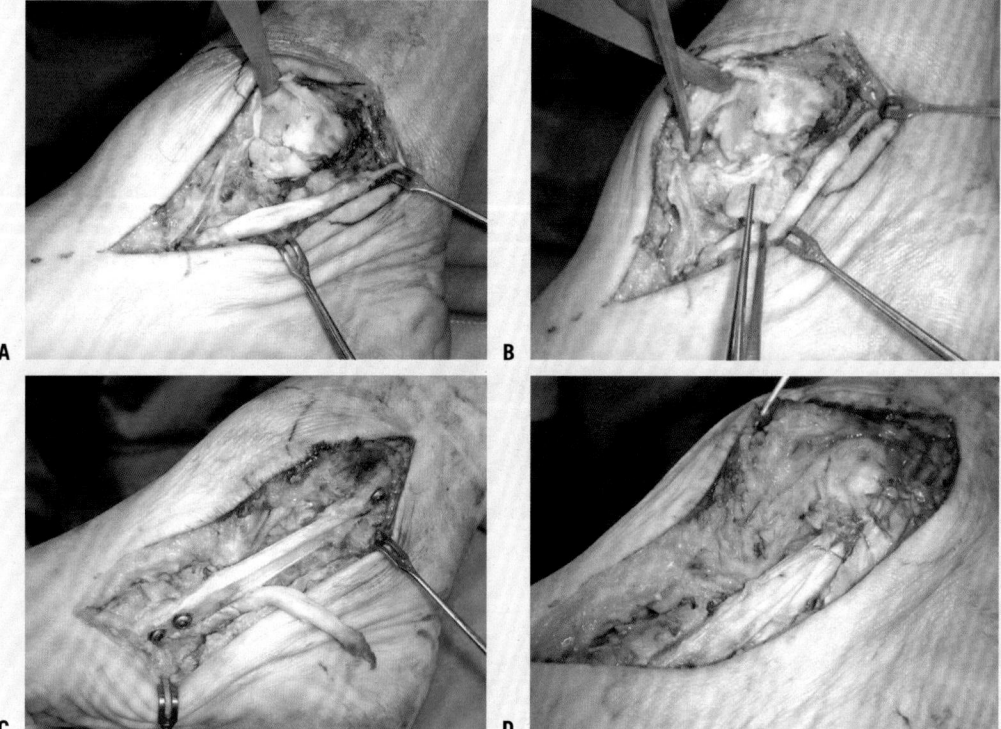

TECH FIG 8 Chronic rupture of the deep deltoid ligament. **A.** Exposure of the posterior tibial tendon reveals a tear. **B.** Exposure of the deltoid ligament reveals an extended disruption and incompetence of the superficial and deep layers. **C.** A bone–tendon–bone transplant is fixed by screws distally into the navicular bone and, after tightening, proximally to the posterior aspect of the medial malleolus. **D.** Multiple nonabsorbable and absorbable sutures are used for further reconstruction of the ligament.

LATERAL ANKLE LIGAMENT RECONSTRUCTION

- About 75% of patients with chronic medial ankle instability were found to have an associated avulsion of the anterior talofibular ligament that resulted in a complex rotational instability of the talus within the ankle mortise.[10]
- If the condition of the anterior talofibular ligament and the calcaneofibular ligament allows an adequate primary repair, these ligaments can be reconstructed by shortening and reinsertion (**TECH FIG 9**).
- When no substantial ligamentous material is present, augmentation with a free plantaris tendon graft is performed (**TECH FIG 10**).[16]

Posterior Tibial Débridement and Reconstruction

- Inspect the posterior tibial tendon meticulously during surgery, especially in the case of a type II or type III lesion of the anterior deltoid ligament.
- If there is degeneration of the tendon, débride the tendon.
- If there is elongation of the tendon, consider shortening the tendon.
- If there is an accessory bone (os tibiale externum), consider reattaching the bone with the tendon insertion; the posterior tibial tendon can also be tightened if the bone is reattached more distally to the navicular bone (**TECH FIG 11**).[12]
- A transfer of the flexor digitorum tendon might be considered in the case of a diseased or ruptured tendon, but this is seldom the case.

Lateral Lengthening Calcaneal Osteotomy

- This procedure is considered in the case of a preexisting valgus and pronation deformity of the foot (eg, when a valgus and pronation deformity is also present on the contralateral, asymptomatic foot) or in the case of a severe attenuation or defect of the tibionavicular, tibiospring, or spring ligaments.
- A calcaneal osteotomy is performed along and parallel to the posterior facet of the subtalar joint, from lateral to medial, preserving the medial cortex intact (**TECH FIG 12A–D**).[9]
- As the osteotomy is widened usually by 6 to 8 mm, the pronation deformity of the foot disappears (**TECH FIG 12E**).
- Fashion a tricortical graft from the iliac crest to the length required or an allograft and place it into the osteotomy site (**TECH FIG 12F–H**). Also, the use of a metallic wedge may be considered.

Double Arthrodesis

- This procedure is considered when the medial ankle instability is so excessive that a valgus tilt of the talus within the mortise of more than 12 degrees is seen on a standard AP view of the ankle while the foot is loaded.[15]
- Be sure to fully correct the whole deformity (eg, valgus malalignment of the heel, and the peritalar dislocation of talus).
- Expose the talonavicular joint from medially through the same incision (**TECH FIG 13A,B**).

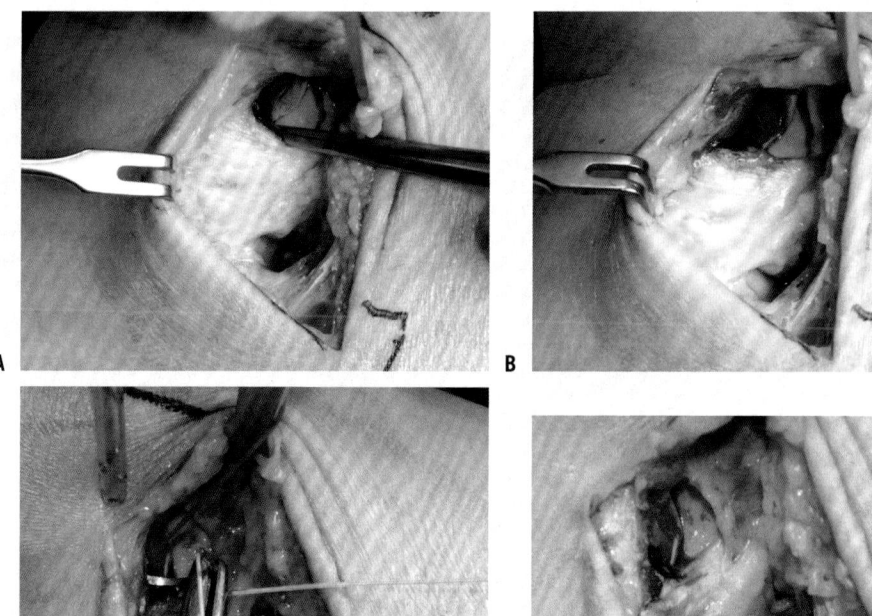

TECH FIG 9 Primary anatomic repair of lateral ankle ligaments. **A.** Exposure of lateral ligaments and arthrotomy of the ankle and subtalar joints that are débrided. The scarred anterior portion of the lateral ligaments is widely disconnected from the anterior border of the fibula. **B.** The anterior border of the fibula is roughened. **C.** An anchor or transosseous sutures are used to reattach the avulsed lateral ligaments (eg, the anterior tibiofibular and calcaneofibular ligaments at their common insertion 8 to 10 mm above the tip of lateral malleolus). **D.** A strong and well-tightened ligament reconstruction is thus obtained.

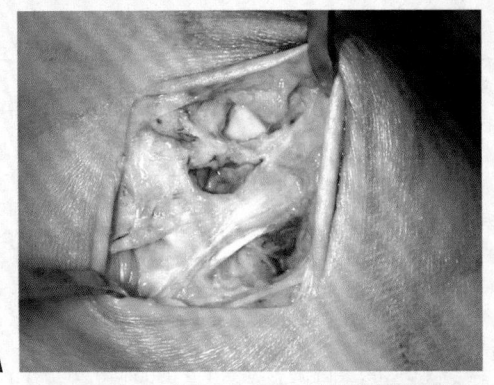
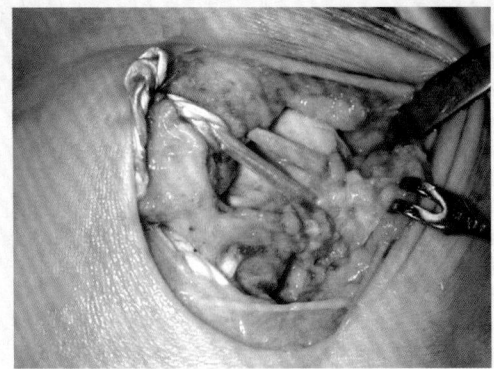
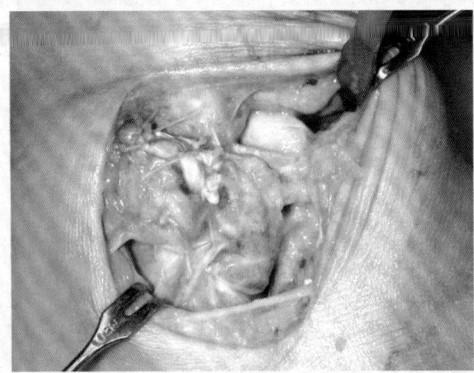

TECH FIG 10 Reconstruction of the lateral ankle ligaments with a free plantaris tendon graft. **A.** The remaining scarred ligaments do not allow primary repair of lateral ankle ligaments. **B.** A free plantaris tendon graft is used for reconstruction of the anterior talofibular and the calcaneofibular ligaments. **C.** A strong and well-tightened ligament reconstruction is thus obtained.

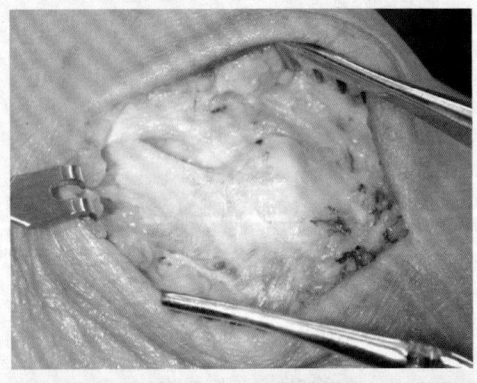
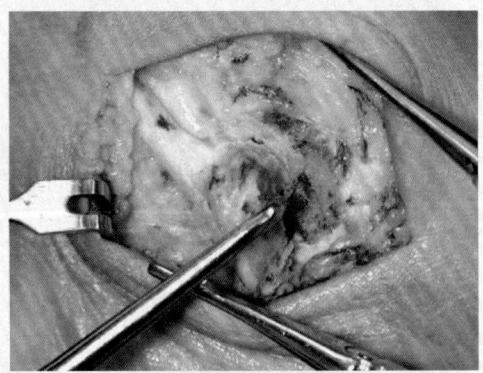
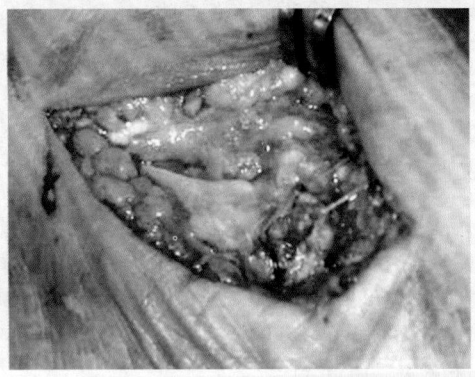

TECH FIG 11 Unstable os tibiale externum. **A.** An unstable accessory bone (os tibiale externum) is found to weaken the pull of posterior tibial tendon. **B.** The accessory bone is mobilized, and 3 to 5 mm of bone is removed on both sides of the pseudarthrosis. **C.** This allows for reattachment of the accessory bone more distally to the navicular bone, using screws and nonabsorbable sutures

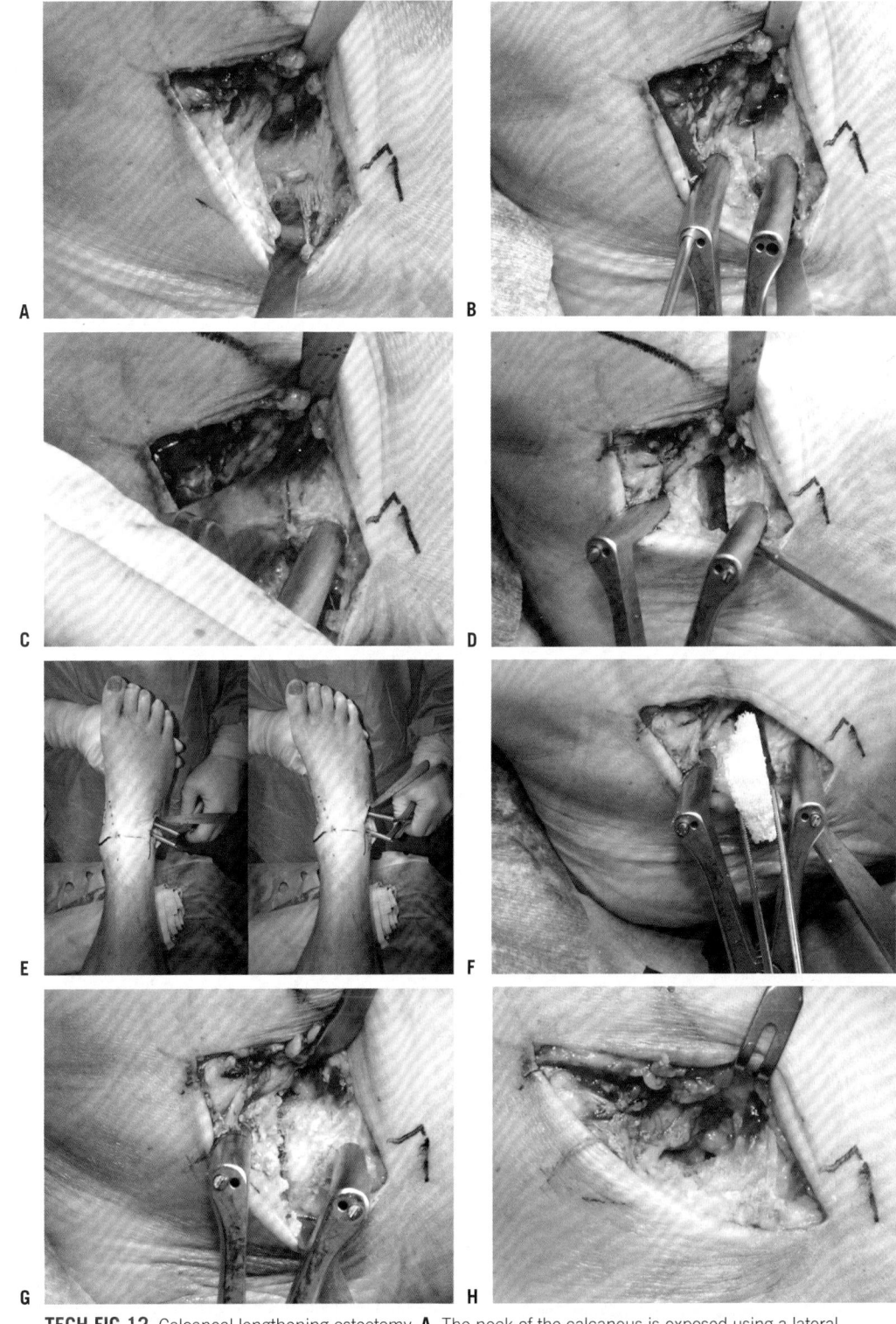

TECH FIG 12 Calcaneal lengthening osteotomy. **A.** The neck of the calcaneus is exposed using a lateral incision. **B.** The osteotomy is marked by a chisel to be directed through the sinus tarsi along the anterior border of the posterior facet of the subtalar joint. Two Kirschner wires for the Hintermann retractor are inserted. **C.** Osteotomy is performed using a saw. **D.** The osteotomy is opened using the retractor. **E.** As the osteotomy is widened, the pronation deformity of the foot disappears. **F.** A tricortical graft from the iliac crest or an allograft is fashioned to the length required and placed into the osteotomy site. **G.** The border of the inserted graft is smoothed. **H.** A regular bony contour on the bottom of the sinus tarsi is thus obtained.

- Use a distraction spreader (Hintermann spreader) to open the joint; this allows for cartilage removal and débridement **(TECH FIG 13C,D)**.
- Expose the subtalar joint from medially through the same incision.
- Use the distraction spreader to open the joint; this allows for cartilage removal and débridement **(TECH FIG 13E–G)**.
- Correct the deformity first by reducing the former talonavicular joint, making sure to correct the frontal plane position of the navicular (eg, to achieve full correction of any forefoot supination deformity) **(TECH FIG 13H–L)**.
- Stable fixation is achieved by triple screw fixation at the talonavicular and double screw fixation at the subtalar joint **(TECH FIG 13M–O)**.

Wound Closure

- Close the wounds in layers.
- Close the subcutaneous tissue and skin in standard fashion.

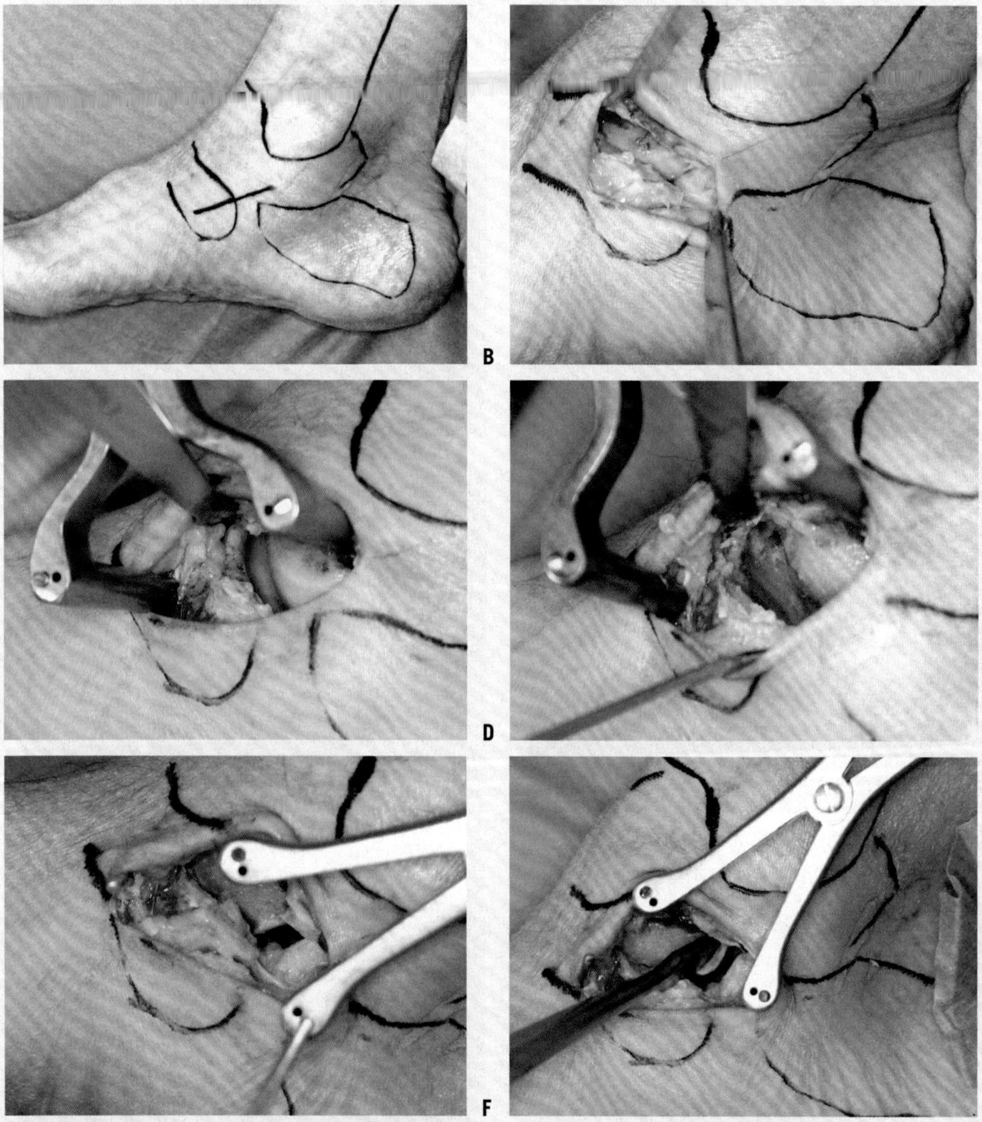

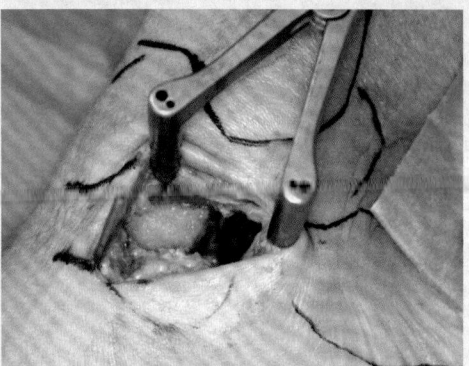

TECH FIG 13 Double arthrodesis. **A.** Skin incision just above the posterior tibial tendon; the surgeon should stop proximally at a perpendicular line through the medial malleolus (eg, so as not to damage the deep bundles of the deltoid ligament). **B.** Incision of skin and dissection of the medial ankle ligaments by sharp incision along the spring ligament. **C.** The talonavicular joint is exposed first. The Hintermann retractor serves to expose the joint. **D.** Cartilage is removed, and the joint is cleaned to subchondral bone. **E.** A third Kirschner wire is inserted into the sustentaculum tali of the calcaneus. This allows the surgeon to open the subtalar joint using the Hintermann distractor. **F.** The cartilage is removed. **G.** Final inspection shows complete débridement of the subtalar joint, including the sinus tarsi. *(continued)*

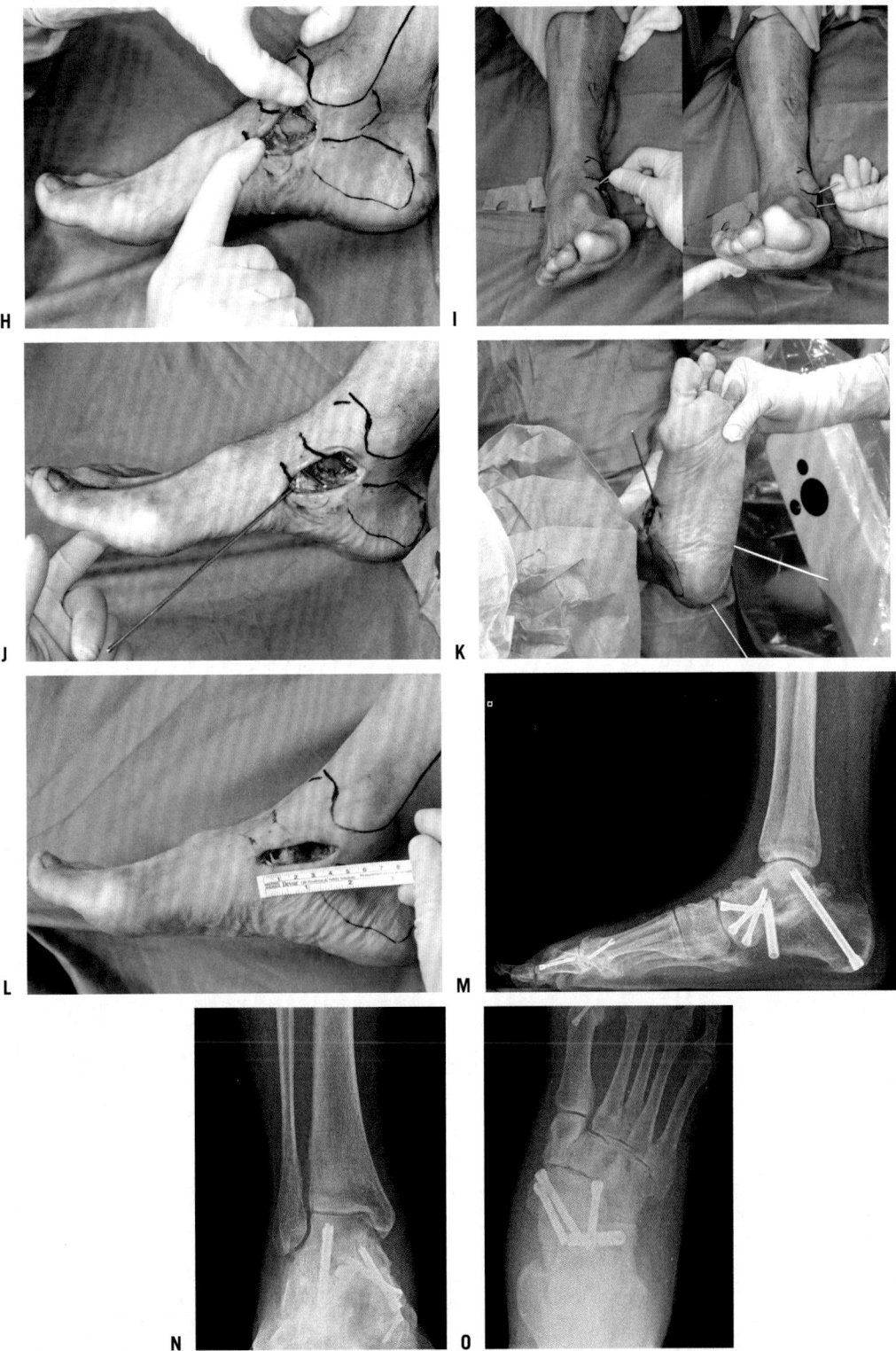

TECH FIG 13 *(continued)* **H.** The Kirschner wires in the navicular and talar bones are kept in place and serve to reduce the talonavicular joint properly. **I.** Frontal view showing the frontal realignment at the talonavicular joint using both Kirschner wires as joysticks. **J.** A first guiding Kirschner wire is inserted through the tuberosity of the navicular into the talus. Two further guidewires will be used to properly stabilize the talonavicular joint in the frontal plane. **K.** After inserting two additional guidewires from the bottom through the subtalar joint, fluoroscopy is used to insert the cannulated screws (QWIX, Newdeal/Integra, Princeton, NJ). **L.** The deltoid ligament is reattached to the spring ligament using nonabsorbable sutures. The foot looks properly positioned at the end of surgery. Note the short incision that is used for this procedure. At 2 months, weight-bearing radiographs are obtained. **M.** Lateral view. **N.** AP view of the ankle. **O.** AP view of the foot.

Pearls and Pitfalls

Diagnosis	• Medial ankle instability is a clinical diagnosis; therefore, a complete and careful patient history and physical examination should be performed.
Indication	• Care must be taken to address associated pathologies.
Suture Techniques	• Transosseous sutures or anchor sutures should be used for proper fixation of the ligaments to the bone. • Slowly resorbable or nonresorbable suture material should be used for fixation to bone.
Ligament Reconstruction	• Nonanatomic reconstruction of ligaments is responsible for most failures. • Careful exploration of the injured or incompetent ligament should be done routinely.
Additional Procedures	• Careful assessment of the foot while weight bearing is mandatory to identify associated malalignment and deformity problems. • Reconstruction of the medial ankle ligaments will fail if such associated problems are neglected or inappropriately addressed.

POSTOPERATIVE CARE

- The foot is protected by a plaster cast or a walking booth for 6 weeks, and full weight bearing is allowed as soon as pain-free loading is possible. In the case of double arthrodesis, initial plaster immobilization for 8 weeks is recommended.
- The rehabilitation program starts after cast removal. It includes passive and active mobilization of the ankle joint, training of the muscular strength, and protection with a walker or stabilizing shoe when walking.
- A walker or stabilizing shoe can be used for 4 to 6 weeks after cast removal, depending on regained muscular balance of the hindfoot.
- We recommend continued use for walks on uneven ground, for high-risk sports activities, and for professional work outside.

OUTCOMES

- With an appropriate surgical technique, success rates for ligament reconstruction of the medial ankle are on the order of 85% to 90% in terms of return to former sports and professional activities.[10]
- As associated malalignment has been addressed more aggressively in the last years, the success rate has further increased.
- The most troubling problem remains a chronic incompetence of the deep deltoid ligament, which results in valgus tilt of the talus while loading the foot. Despite the use of tendon augmentation, most attempts at isolated ligament reconstruction have failed; a main treatment step is probably a double arthrodesis in getting a stable and well-aligned hindfoot. An alternative may be a tibiocalcaneal arthrodesis.

COMPLICATIONS

- Deficient stability because of inappropriate ligament reconstruction
- Recurrent instability because valgus deformity was not addressed
- Suture granuloma at the anterior margin of the medial malleolus when using nonresorbable sutures and placing the suture knot onto a bony surface
- Deep venous thrombosis
- Infection

- Scarring in the anteromedial ankle causing soft tissue impingement

REFERENCES

1. Boss AP, Hintermann B. Anatomical study of the medial ankle ligament complex. Foot Ankle Int 2002;23:547–553.
2. Buman EM, Khazen G, Haraguchi N, et al. Minimally invasive deltoid ligament reconstruction: a comparison of three techniques. Paper presented at: Proceedings of the 36th Annual Winter Meeting, Specialty Day, AOFAS; March 25, 2006; Chicago, IL.
3. Deland JT, de Asla RJ, Segal A. Reconstruction of the chronically failed deltoid ligament: a new technique. Foot Ankle Int 2004;25:795–799.
4. Gougoulias N, Sakellariou A. When is a simple fracture of the lateral malleolus not so simple? How to assess stability, which ones to fix and the role of the deltoid ligament. Bone Joint J 2017;99-B(7):851–855.
5. Harper MC. Deltoid ligament: an anatomical evaluation of function. Foot Ankle 1987;8:19–22.
6. Hintermann B. Medial ankle instability. Foot Ankle Clin 2003;8: 723–738.
7. Hintermann B, Boss A, Schäfer D. Arthroscopic findings in patients with chronic ankle instability. Am J Sports Med 2002;30:402–409.
8. Hintermann B, Knupp M, Pagenstert GI. Deltoid ligament injuries: diagnosis and management. Foot Ankle Clin 2006;11:625–637.
9. Hintermann B, Valderrabano V. Lateral column lengthening by calcaneal osteotomy. Techn Foot Ankle Surg 2003;2:84–90.
10. Hintermann B, Valderrabano V, Boss AP, et al. Medial ankle instability: an exploratory, prospective study of fifty-two cases. Am J Sports Med 2004;32:183–190.
11. Jeong MS, Choi YS, Kim Y, et al. Deltoid ligament in acute ankle injury: MR imaging analysis. Skeletal Radiol 2014;43(5):655–663.
12. Knupp M, Hintermann B. Reconstruction in posttraumatic combined avulsion of an accessory navicular and the posterior tibial tendon. Techn Foot Ankle Surg 2005;4:113–118.
13. Lee S, Lin J, Hamid KS, et al. Deltoid ligament rupture in ankle fracture: diagnosis and management. J Am Acad Orthop Surg 2019;27(14):e648–e658.
14. Milner CE, Soames RW. The medial collateral ligaments of the human ankle joint: anatomical variations. Foot Ankle Int 1998;19:289–292.
15. Nelson DR, Younger A. Acute posttraumatic planovalgus foot deformity involving hindfoot ligamentous pathology. Foot Ankle Clin 2003;8:521–537.
16. Pagenstert GI, Hintermann B, Knupp M. Operative management of chronic ankle instability: plantaris graft. Foot Ankle Clin 2006;11:567–583.
17. Saltzman CL, El Khoury GY. The hindfoot alignment view. Foot Ankle Int 1995;16:572–576.
18. Tornetta P III. Competence of the deltoid ligament in bimalleolar ankle fractures after medial malleolar fixation. J Bone Joint Surg Am 2000;82:843–848.

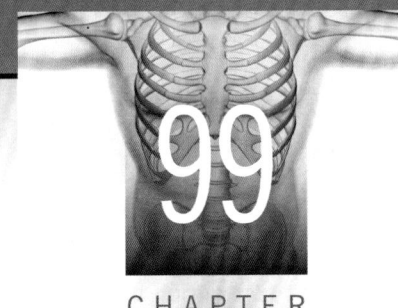

99

CHAPTER

Open Achilles Tendon Repair

Sameh A. Labib and Rishin J. Kadakia

DEFINITION

- The Achilles tendon is the strongest tendon in the body and is the primary plantarflexor of the ankle joint.[25]
- Sudden stretch of the tendon tissue can result in complete or partial rupture, with an estimated incidence of 8 to 18 per 100,000 persons.[1,4]
- With complete rupture, the ruptured ends of the tendon may pull apart, leading to a significant plantar flexion weakness and to the creation of a gap that is palpated clinically.
- A common source of confusion is that patients may continue to have active ankle plantar flexion due to the action of other flexors of the ankle.
- As a result, the diagnosis is initially missed in an estimated 20% to 25% of cases.[7]

ANATOMY

- Three calf muscles—the medial and lateral gastrocnemius, and soleus—converge together to form the "triceps surae" or the Achilles tendon (FIG 1).

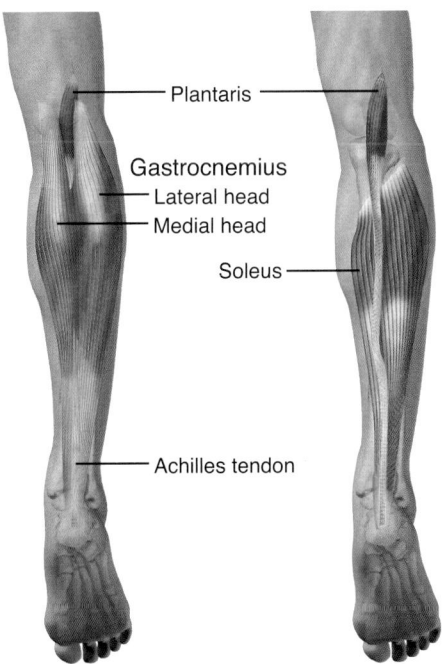

- Plantaris
- Gastrocnemius
  - Lateral head
  - Medial head
- Soleus
- Achilles tendon

FIG 1 The triceps surae (Achilles tendon) is formed by the convergence of the medial and lateral gastrocnemius, and soleus muscles.

- The plantaris muscle originates from the lateral femoral condyle and passes obliquely between the gastrocnemius and soleus to reside medial to the Achilles tendon and inserts into it or the calcaneus. In an anatomic study, the plantaris muscle was absent in 7.3% of specimens.[25]
- The Achilles tendon courses distally, rotates 90 degrees internally, the soleus contribution being medial to that of the gastrocnemius, and inserts into the middle third of the flat surface of the posterior calcaneal tuberosity.[14]
- The middle section of the tendon, 2 to 6 cm proximal to its insertion site, is a hypovascular zone.
  - This zone is the narrowest in cross-section and corresponds to the most common site of tendon pathology, including paratenonitis, tendinosis, and tendon rupture.[14]
- The tendon is surrounded by a paratenon that has a single layer of cells with variable structure, not a true tenosynovium.
- A recent study utilizing ultrasound to evaluate anatomic properties of the Achilles tendon found that nearly all tendon parameters (length, width, thickness, and cross-sectional area) correlated positively with certain patient characteristics such as height, weight, and foot size.[24]
  - Males also had significantly higher values for all tendon parameters, but this could be influenced by height and weight.
  - Only the cross-sectional area of the tendon was positively associated with increased activity level.
- Webb et al[27] documented the highly variable position of the sural nerve in relation to the Achilles tendon.
  - As measured from the calcaneal insertion, the sural nerve crossed the tendon from medial to lateral at a mean distance of 9.8 cm and then coursed distally to lie a mean of 18.8 mm laterally (FIG 2).

PATHOGENESIS

- Achilles ruptures are usually caused by noncontact injuries. Common injury mechanisms leading to Achilles rupture are forceful push-off with an extended knee, sudden unexpected ankle dorsiflexion, or violent dorsiflexion of a plantarflexed foot.[19]
- Achilles rupture can occur high, near the muscle–tendon juncture (9%), at the tendon midportion (72%), or at the calcaneal insertion (19%).[7]
- Concomitant injuries such as ankle ligament sprains or ankle or tarsal fractures should be ruled out.

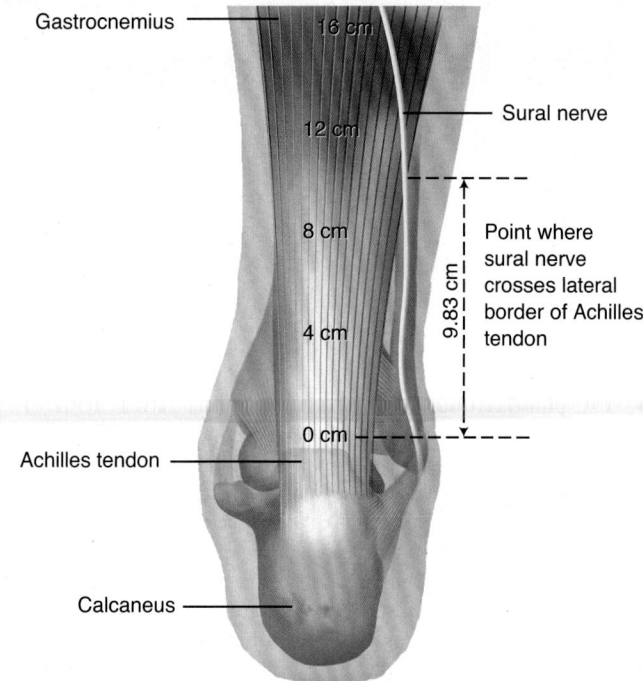

Gastrocnemius — 16 cm

Sural nerve

12 cm

8 cm

Point where
sural nerve
crosses lateral
border of Achilles
tendon

4 cm

9.83 cm

Achilles tendon —

0 cm

Calcaneus —

FIG 2 Position of the sural nerve in relation to the Achilles tendon. (Adapted with permission from Webb J, Moorjani N, Radford M. Anatomy of the sural nerve and its relation to the Achilles tendon. Foot Ankle Int 2000;21[6]:475–477. Copyright © 2000 SAGE Publications.)

NATURAL HISTORY

- Most Achilles ruptures do not have any antecedent symptoms.
  - A study of histologic scores comparing ruptured tendons with unruptured tendons, however, showed that there were significant histopathologic changes in the ruptured group that were not present in the older, asymptomatic, and unruptured group. Therefore, tendinosis may play a role, but the extent of this role remains unknown.[20]
- Achilles rupture is more common in men. Studies have shown a male-to-female ratio of up to 12:1.
- From an epidemiologic standpoint, middle-aged men with white-collar professions and recreational athletic activity constitute most of the patients.
  - Other predisposing factors are leg muscle imbalance, training errors, foot pronation, and use of corticosteroids and fluoroquinolones.[19]
- In a longitudinal observational study, there was a contralateral Achilles rupture in 6% of patients who had a previously repaired Achilles rupture with a median delay of 3.1 years.[1]

PATIENT HISTORY AND PHYSICAL FINDINGS

- Most ruptures occur during athletic activity. Patients usually describe a sudden painful snap or shooting pain followed by sudden weakness to foot push off.
- Athletes will be unable to bear weight and will report distal leg swelling and stiffness.
- Examination for ruptured Achilles tendon can include the following:
  - Palpable gap test. A gap present indicates complete Achilles rupture with separation of the ruptured ends. It is more reliable when done early after rupture. It is 73% sensitive.[19]

- Calf squeeze test (Thompson test). With patient prone, squeeze the calf and observe foot movement. Compare with the contralateral side. It is 96% sensitive.[19]
- Prone knee flexion/Matles test. With patient prone, patient actively flexes knee. Observe foot position and compare with other. It is 88% sensitive.[19]
- Active plantar flexion. This is poorly sensitive and unreliable because powerful plantar flexion may still be possible due to the action of other ankle plantarflexors.
- Contralateral ankle resting angle. With the patient prone, the knee of the uninjured limb is flexed to 90 degrees, and the patient is asked to relax the ankle and the foot. The angle formed between the long axis of the leg and the foot is measured. Originally described by Carmont et al,[6] this angle can be estimated visually or precisely measured using a goniometer with one arm centered along the fibular shaft and the other arm aligned with the fifth metatarsal. A study examining the ankle resting angle among health controls found that while there is variation between patients, there is no significant difference between limbs in a single patient. The study found a mean resting angle to be approximately 45 degrees.[24] Thus, this angle can be used to intraoperatively when tensioning the surgical repair and determining appropriate length.

IMAGING AND OTHER DIAGNOSTIC STUDIES

- Anteroposterior, lateral, and mortise view plain radiographs of the ankle should be obtained to rule out concomitant fractures or calcific changes of the Achilles tendon.
  - On a lateral view, the examiner should look for a disruption of the normal triangular fat pad seen anterior to the Achilles tendon (Kager triangle; **FIG 3A**).
- Ultrasonography can provide a dynamic study of the tendon structure and accurately measure gapping of the ruptured tendon ends.
  - The quality of ultrasound images is highly dependent on the equipment and operator (**FIG 3B**).
- Magnetic resonance imaging (MRI) is highly sensitive and specific in diagnosing Achilles tendon rupture.
  - It provides valuable information about tendon degeneration or other associated injuries (**FIG 3C**).
  - MRI was found to be superior to ultrasound in diagnostic specificity of chronic Achilles tendinopathy.[2]

DIFFERENTIAL DIAGNOSIS

- Rupture of the medial gastrocnemius
- Plantaris tendon rupture
- Baker cyst rupture
- Acute deep venous thrombosis
- Leg or calf contusion
- Tibia distal shaft fracture
- Posterior ankle impingement or symptomatic os trigonum

NONOPERATIVE MANAGEMENT

- Traditionally, nonoperative treatment usually entailed casting the foot in plantar flexion to allow apposition of the tendon ends, followed by casting the foot in neutral. Treatment continues for 12 weeks.
  - In a recent retrospective review, early recognition and initiation of nonoperative management within 48 hours of injury resulted in a successful functional outcome that was comparable to surgical repairs.[28]

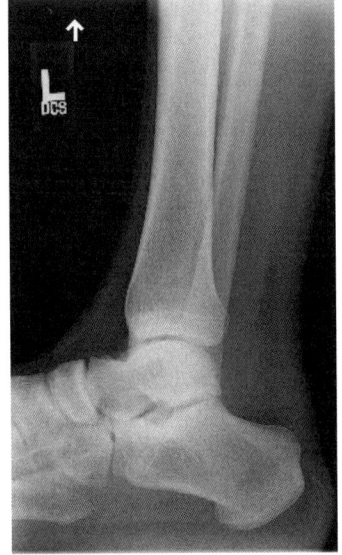
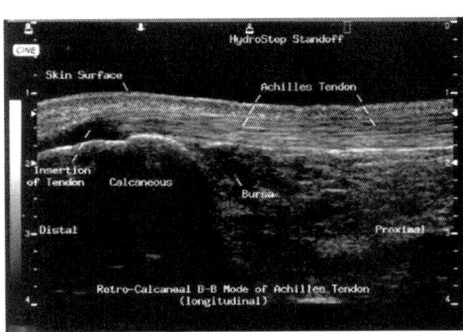
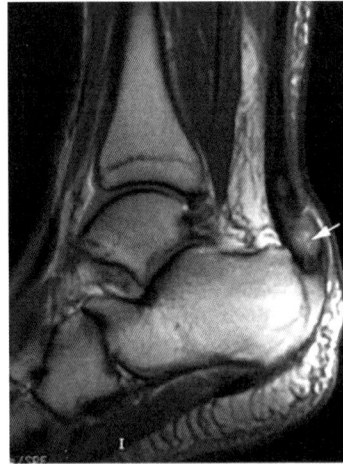

FIG 3 A. Ankle radiograph showing a disrupted Kager triangle. **B.** Normal Achilles ultrasound image. **C.** Ankle MRI (T1-weighted image) showing a distal Achilles tendon rupture (*white arrow*).

- Several level 1 studies have showed comparable results of patient reported outcomes between operative repair and nonoperative treatment with an accelerated rehabilitation protocol.[22,29,30] There is ongoing debate as to whether rerupture rates are higher with nonoperative treatment. Although several studies suggest that rerupture rates are significantly higher with nonoperative treatment,[8,21,29] some argue that rerupture rates are similar when early motion and functional rehabilitation is employed.[26] Functional rehabilitation can have promising results when initiated early, but it requires patient compliance and close monitoring.[9] Regardless, operative treatment has been shown to have several advantages with regard to strength and function. Surgical repair provides an improvement in plantar flexion isokinetic strength as documented with Biodex testing,[30] isokinetic dynamometer,[18] and jump and hop testing.[22] Furthermore, literature demonstrates that patients managed operatively return to work sooner than those who undergo nonoperative treatment.[8,26]
- Based on the aforementioned information, it is still our practice to offer young, active individuals surgical repair with full disclosure of the possible use of nonoperative treatment.
- In our hands, nonoperative treatment is often reserved for elderly; sedentary patients; and also for patients with diabetes, tobacco use, and steroid use who are at high risk for surgical wound healing.[5]

SURGICAL MANAGEMENT

- Operative repair and early mobilization is considered the treatment of choice for younger patients with active lifestyles. In most patients, it is established that operative repair results in a favorable functional outcome, and there is literature to suggest lower rerupture rates with operative management.[8,21,29]
- Numerous surgical techniques have been described, including open repair, percutaneous repair, limited open repair, and open repair with augmentation.
    - In a comprehensive review of the recent literature, Wong et al[31] concluded that in terms of outcome and

the complication rate, the best results could be achieved with open repair and early mobilization.

Preoperative Planning

- Plain radiographs are reviewed, and any displaced fractures are treated at the same surgical sitting.
- MRIs are reviewed to evaluate the quality of tendon tissue and the level of rupture and to measure the tendon gap if present.
- Severe tendon degeneration or a large gap may require a larger incision or tendon lengthening or augmentation; the surgeon should take this into account during preoperative patient counseling.

Positioning

- Achilles tendon repair is performed with the patient prone (**FIG 4**). We prefer to use a Wilson frame and commercially available foam headrest.
- A thigh tourniquet is used for intraoperative hemostasis. A leg tourniquet is not recommended because it may tether the calf muscles and prevent intraoperative tendon apposition.

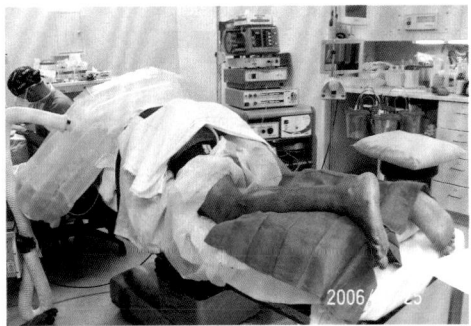

FIG 4 Patient is in prone position with both legs prepared and draped for surgery.

- Some surgeons prefer to drape both legs for intraoperative comparison and accurate restoration of the resting tendon length. The operated leg should be clearly marked.

Approach

- Open Achilles repair is usually performed through a longitudinal medial, midline, or lateral incision.
- Primary end-to-end repair is done with heavy nonabsorbable suture.
- Modified Bunnell, Kessler, Krackow, and triple-bundle techniques have been described.[7]
  - In a biomechanical study, Jaakkola et al[10] showed that the triple-bundle technique **(FIG 5)** provided the strongest suture repair. They credited its superior strength to the use of multiple strands and to tying the knots away from the repair site. However, the authors expressed concern over the large amount of suture material used and its possible negative effect on the vascularity of the tendon.
- At our institution, we have designed a modification of the Krackow technique in which the free ends of one suture are passed peripherally to encircle the transverse limb of the opposite suture **(FIG 6)**.
- We likened this scheme to wrapping a gift box and named it the *gift box technique.*
- We have performed biomechanical pullout studies on 13 Achilles cadaveric pairs comparing the gift box technique to the standard Krackow suture and documented more than a twofold increase in suture pullout strength.[17]
- A retrospective review of a cohort of 44 patients who underwent repair using the gift box technique demonstrated good patient satisfaction and patient reported outcomes. The mean American Orthopaedic Foot & Ankle Society ankle–hindfoot score was 93.2 ± 6.8%, and the Foot Function Index score was 7.0 ± 10.5. There were no reruptures, wound complications, or infections observed in this cohort.[16]
- We believe that the modification is simple to perform, minimizes suture material use, and preserves the vasculature of the healing tendon.

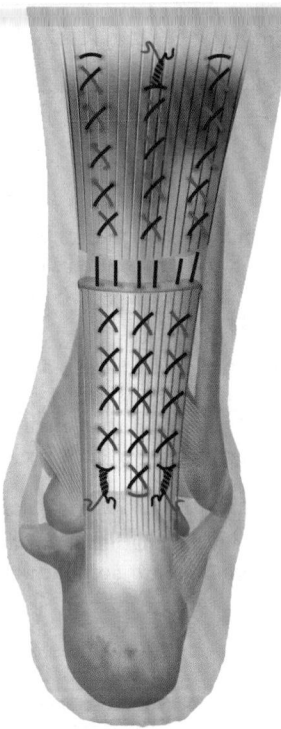

FIG 5 Triple-bundle technique of Achilles repair.

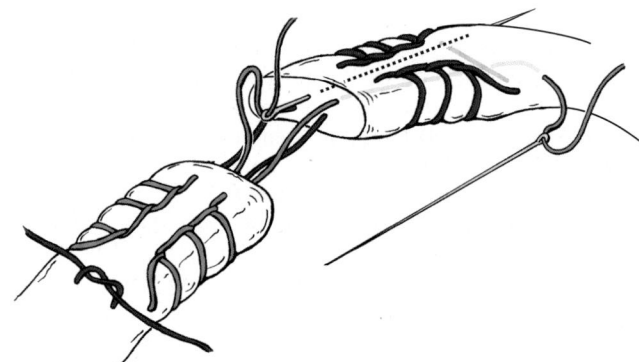

FIG 6 Our modification of Krackow suture or the gift box technique. (Copyright Sam Labib, MD.)

EXPOSURE

- A 7 cm-longitudinal incision over the medial border of the tendon provides excellent exposure and access to the plantaris tendon and avoids the sural nerve **(TECH FIG 1)**.
  - Mobilize the thick skin and subcutaneous layer laterally and take great care to preserve the paratenon.
  - Protect the sural nerve and lesser saphenous vein as they course lateral to the paratenon.
  - Enter the paratenon through a midline incision (away from the skin incision).
  - Limit dissection at the tendon–paratenon plane, especially anterior to the tendon, to preserve the vascular supply of the tendon.

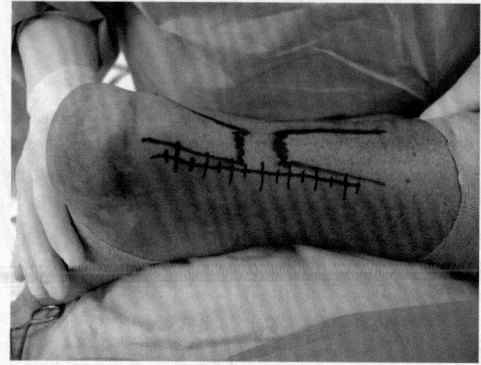

TECH FIG 1 Medial longitudinal incision centered over the rupture site.

TECHNIQUES

MODIFIED KRACKOW SUTURE (GIFT BOX) TECHNIQUE

- Débride the ends of the ruptured tendon in a limited manner.
- Two 2-mm width tape sutures (FiberTape, Arthrex, Inc., Naples, FL) are used. In the past, we used no. 2 fortified polyester sutures (FiberTape, Arthrex, Inc., Naples, FL) with good clinical results. There is biomechanical data to suggest improved pullout strength with tape suture in tendon repairs, and we now use tape suture.[23]
  - Four-loop Krackow locking sutures[13] are passed on the medial side and four on the lateral side, avoiding the middle third of the tendon width.
  - Unlike the classic Krackow suture, we pass our transverse limb in the middle of the tendon as we transition from one side to the other **(TECH FIG 2A)**.
- Use straight Keith needles to pass the free suture ends across the rupture site into the opposite end of the tendon.
  - Sutures should emerge one superficial and one deep to the transverse limb of the opposite Krackow suture **(TECH FIG 2B)**.
  - Thus, four-suture strands are passed across the rupture site.
- Tie the surgical knots away from the rupture site—in other words, proximal and distal to the Krackow suture.
  - Excellent apposition is usually achieved as the knots push on the transverse limbs of opposing sutures, and the desired tendon length is recreated **(TECH FIG 2C,D)**.
- The repair is tensioned to match the ankle resting angle of the contralateral limb, which must be clinically evaluated either preoperatively or can be evaluated intraoperatively if both limbs are included in the surgical field.
- Use epitendinous running 2-0 FiberWire (Arthrex, Inc., Naples, FL) to oversew the tendon ends together.
- Meticulously repair the paratenon with 3-0 braided polyglycolic absorbable suture (Vicryl, Ethicon, Inc., Somerville, NJ) **(TECH FIG 2E)**.
  - This can be facilitated by placing the ankle in maximum plantar flexion to relax the tendon tissue.
  - We believe that midline placement of the paratenon incision facilitates its repair and minimizes the chance of skin tethering to the repaired tendon.
- Perform subcuticular skin closure with 4-0 monofilament absorbable suture (Monocryl, Ethicon, Inc., Somerville, NJ).

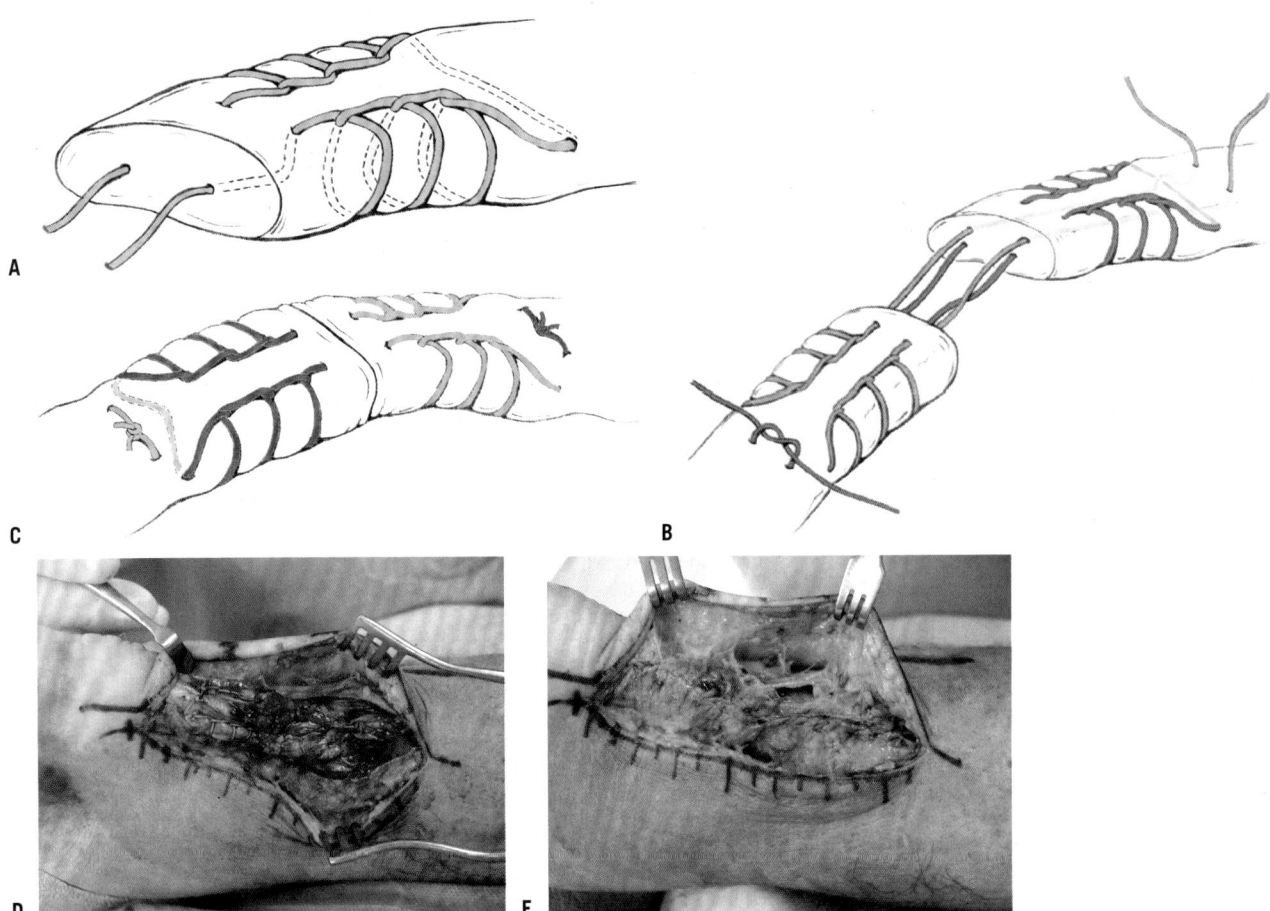

TECH FIG 2 A. The transverse limb of the gift box suture is passed through tendon midsubstance. **B.** One suture limb from the opposite limb passes superficial to the transverse limb, whereas the other passes deep to it as depicted by the blue sutures above. **C.** The gift box suture completed and tied. Note the tension created on the transverse limb of the suture, which helps tendon apposition. **D.** Completed gift box suture. **E.** Photo after closure of the Achilles paratenon. **(A–C:** Copyright Sam Labib, MD.)

TRIPLE-BUNDLE SUTURE TECHNIQUE

- Jaakkola et al[10] popularized an open repair of the Achilles tendon using no. 1 nonabsorbable polyester suture (Ethibond, Ethicon, Inc., Somerville, NJ).
- Three rows of sutures are placed, creating six strands of suture that are tied away from the rupture site.
- The technique provides the strongest suture repair available to date but is technically difficult to perform, requires a large amount of suture material, and may lead to vascular compromise of the tendon during healing.[10]

- A recently published study examining a cohort of patients who underwent repair with a triple-bundle technique found that similar complications rates as other open repair techniques and good functional and patient reported outcomes.[3] Thus, this method of repair is a valid and can have good results for those who have experience with this technique.

PRIMARY REPAIR WITH AUGMENTATION

- Multiple authors have advocated primary augmentation of Achilles repair, with some preferring plantaris tendon, flexor tendon **(TECH FIG 3)**, or artificial tendon implants.[19]
- A study by Jessing and Hansen,[11] however, found no evidence that such augmentation was superior to a nonaugmented end-to-end repair.

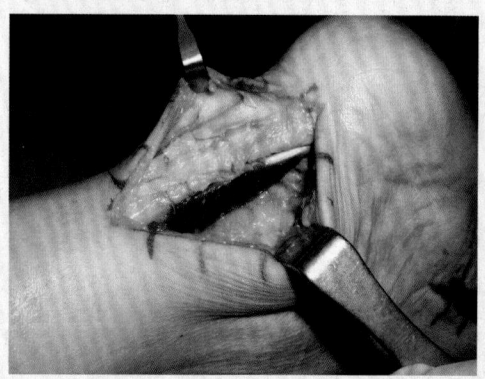

TECH FIG 3 Flexor hallucis longus tendon used to augment Achilles tendon repair.

TECHNIQUES

Pearls and Pitfalls

Clinical Evaluation	• Diagnosis of complete rupture can be missed due to other active ankle flexors. • Ultrasonography or MRI may be needed to verify the diagnosis. • Care is taken to evaluate concomitant bony or tendon injury.
Nonoperative Treatment	• Should be initiated early, with cast application in plantar flexion preferably within 48 hours of injury • Tendon gapping should be looked for and corrected. • Strongly considered for patients with poor skin or vascular compromise. Poorly controlled diabetes and tobacco or steroid use are relative contraindications for surgical treatment.
Approach	• Midline incisions may result in a painful scar. • A lateral incision places the sural nerve at an added risk of injury. • Poor tissue handling may result in wound slough or dehiscence.
Tendon Tension	• Aggressive trimming of tendon ends may result in significant shortening and undue tension on the repair. • Use the contralateral limb as your guide to appropriate restoration of resting tendon length.
Suture Technique	• Avoid strangulating locking suture techniques, which may compromise tendon healing and promote scar formation. • Paratenon preservation and repair is mandatory for tendon repair and healing.

POSTOPERATIVE CARE

- Early functional mobilization was shown to yield improved tendon healing.[12]
- A posterior splint holding the site in mild plantar flexion is used for 14 days. Labib et al[15] showed no significant difference in tension when the repaired tendon was positioned in 30, 20, and 10 degrees of plantar flexion.
- Wound inspection is done, a non–weight-bearing cast boot is applied with heel lifts, and daily active range of motion is started.
- The patient is kept non–weight bearing for the first 3 weeks and then is transitioned to partial weight bearing in a boot with two heel lifts until 8 weeks postoperatively. The patient then transitions to full weight bearing at 8 weeks postoperatively and gradually is weaned out of the boot.
- The patient is kept non–weight bearing for a total of 6 weeks, but recent evidence suggests that weight bearing can be started before 6 weeks with no added risk of rerupture or gap formation.[12]
- The patient is allowed gradual return to full weight bearing over an additional 6 weeks.
- At 3 months, full weight bearing is permitted, with low-impact activities.
- At 6 months, full activities are permitted as tolerated.

OUTCOMES

- Several studies have identified favorable outcomes following open operative repair and early functional mobilization of Achilles tendon ruptures. Despite ongoing debate as to rerupture rates with nonoperative treatment, operative management consistently leads to low rerupture rates estimated to be around 3.6%.[29]
- Patients who undergo operative treatment have greater strength and resulting functional outcomes. A recent meta-analysis found that three different studies have determined that patients who undergo open surgical repair return to work and activity earlier.[8,26]
- Wong et al[31] conducted an extensive literature review and concluded that the best results regarding outcome and complication rate could be achieved with open repair and early mobilization.
- Although functional rehabilitation and early range-of-motion protocols have decreased rerupture rates and improved outcomes in nonoperative management, most authors agree that surgical repair in the healthy active individual leads to better functional and patient reported outcomes, but these advantages should be weighed against the possible risks of wound dehiscence or infection.

COMPLICATIONS

- Delayed or missed diagnosis
- Intraoperative devitalization of tendon, leading to wound infection
- Failure to preserve and repair the paratenon, leading to scarring and skin tethering
- Sural nerve injury and neuroma formation
- Wound dehiscence
- Tendon rerupture
- Loss of ankle motion
- Calf weakness

REFERENCES

1. Årøen A, Helgø D, Granlund OG, et al. Contralateral tendon rupture risk is increased in individuals with a previous Achilles tendon rupture. Scand J Med Sci Sports 2004;14(1):30–33.
2. Aström M, Gentz CF, Nilsson P, et al. Imaging in chronic Achilles tendinopathy: a comparison of ultrasonography, magnetic resonance imaging and surgical findings in 27 histologically verified cases. Skeletal Radiol 1996;25:615–620.
3. Bevoni R, Angelini A, D'Apote G, et al. Long term results of acute Achilles repair with triple-bundle technique and early rehabilitation protocol. Injury 2014;45(8):1268–1274.
4. Bhandari M, Guyatt GH, Siddiqui F, et al. Treatment of acute Achilles tendon ruptures: a systematic overview and metaanalysis. Clin Orthop Relat Res 2002;(400):190–200.
5. Bruggeman NB, Turner NS, Dahm DL, et al. Wound complications after open Achilles tendon repair: an analysis of risk factors. Clin Orthop Relat Res 2004;(427):63–66.
6. Carmont MR, Silbernagel KG, Mathy A, et al. Reliability of Achilles tendon resting angle and calf circumference measurement techniques. Foot Ankle Surg 2013;19:245–249.
7. Coughlin MJ, Mann RA, eds. Athletic injuries to the soft tissues of the foot and ankle. In: Surgery of the Foot and Ankle, ed 7. St. Louis: Mosby, 1999:835–850.
8. Erickson BJ, Mascarenhas R, Saltzman BM, et al. Is operative treatment of Achilles tendon ruptures superior to nonoperative treatment? A systematic review of overlapping meta-analyses. Orthop J Sports Med 2015;3(4):2325967115579188.
9. Glazebrook M, Rubinger D. Functional rehabilitation for nonsurgical treatment of acute Achilles tendon rupture. Foot Ankle Clin 2019;24(3):387–398.
10. Jaakkola JI, Hutton WC, Beskin JL, et al. Achilles tendon rupture repair: biomechanical comparison of the triple bundle technique versus the Krackow locking loop technique. Foot Ankle Int 2000;21:14–17.
11. Jessing P, Hansen E. Surgical treatment of 102 tendo Achillis ruptures—suture or tenontoplasty? Acta Chir Scand 1975;141:370–377.
12. Kangas J, Pajala A, Ohtonen P, et al. Achilles tendon elongation after rupture repair: a randomized comparison of 2 postoperative regimens. Am J Sports Med 2007;35:59–64.
13. Krackow KA, Thomas SC, Jones LC. A new stitch for ligament-tendon fixation. Brief note. J Bone Joint Surg Am 1986;68(5):764–766.
14. Labib SA, Gould JS. Achilles tendonitis. Orthopedic Board Review Hyperguide. Available at: http://www.ortho.hyperguide.com/Sports Medicine. Accessed July 12, 2019.
15. Labib SA, Hage WD, Sutton K, et al. The effect of ankle position on the static tension in the Achilles tendon before and after operative repair: a biomechanical cadaver study. Foot Ankle Int 2007;28:478–481.
16. Labib SA, Hoffler CE II, Shah JN, et al. The gift box open Achilles tendon repair method: a retrospective clinical series. J Foot Ankle Surg 2016;55(1):39–44.
17. Labib SA, Rolf R, Dacus R, et al. The "giftbox" repair of the Achilles tendon: a modification of the Krackow technique. Foot Ankle Int 2009;30:410–414.
18. Lantto I, Heikkinen J, Flinkkila T, et al. A prospective randomized trial comparing surgical and nonsurgical treatments of acute Achilles tendon ruptures. Am J Sports Med 2016;44(9): 2406–2414.
19. Maffulli N. The clinical diagnosis of subcutaneous tear of the Achilles tendon. A prospective study in 174 patients. Am J Sports Med 1998;26(2):266–270.
20. Maffulli N, Barrass V, Ewen SW. Light microscopic histology of Achilles tendon ruptures. A comparison with unruptured tendons. Am J Sports Med 2000;28:857–863.
21. Ochen Y, Beks RB, van Heijl M, et al. Operative treatment versus nonoperative treatment of Achilles tendon ruptures: systematic review and meta-analysis. BMJ 2019;364:k5120.
22. Olsson N, Silbernagel KG, Eriksson BI, et al. Stable surgical repair with accelerated rehabilitation versus nonsurgical treatment for acute Achilles tendon ruptures: a randomized controlled study. Am J Sports Med 2013;41(12):2867–2876.
23. Ono Y, Joly DA, Thornton GM, et al. Mechanical and imaging evaluation of the effect of sutures on tendons: tape sutures are

protective to suture pulling through tendon. J Shoulder Elbow Surg 2018;27(9):1705–1710.

24. Patel NN, Labib SA. The Achilles tendon in healthy subjects: an anthropometric and ultrasound mapping study. J Foot Ankle Surg 2018;57(2):285–288.

25. Sarrafian SK. Anatomy of the Foot and Ankle: Descriptive, Topographic, Functional, ed 2. Philadelphia: JB Lippincott, 1993.

26. Soroceanu A, Sidhwa F, Aarabi S, et al. Surgical versus nonsurgical treatment of acute Achilles tendon rupture: a meta-analysis of randomized trials. J Bone Joint Surg Am 2012;94(23):2136–2143.

27. Webb J, Moorjani N, Radford M. Anatomy of the sural nerve and its relation to the Achilles tendon. Foot Ankle Int 2000;21:475–477.

28. Weber M, Niemann M, Lanz R, et al. Nonoperative treatment of acute rupture of the Achilles tendon: results of a new protocol and comparison with operative treatment. Am J Sports Med 2003;31:685–691.

29. Wilkins R, Bisson LJ. Operative versus nonoperative management of acute Achilles tendon ruptures: a quantitative systematic review of randomized controlled trials. Am J Sports Med 2012;40(9):2154–2160.

30. Willits K, Amendola A, Bryant D, et al. Operative versus nonoperative treatment of acute Achilles tendon ruptures: a multicenter randomized trial using accelerated functional rehabilitation. J Bone Joint Surg Am 2010;92(17):2767–2775.

31. Wong J, Barrass V, Maffulli N. Quantitative review of operative and nonoperative management of Achilles tendon ruptures. Am J Sports Med 2002;30:565–575.

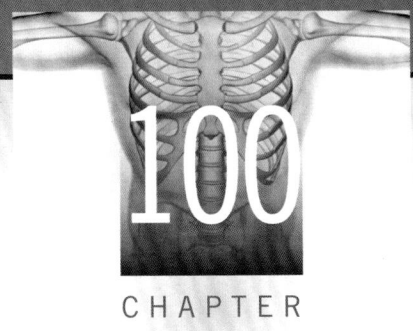

100
CHAPTER

Mini-Open Achilles Tendon Repair:
Perspective 1

Mathieu Assal, Marc Merian-Genast, and Mark E. Easley

DEFINITION

- Achilles tendon ruptures usually occur 3 to 4 cm above the calcaneal tuberosity.
- Although most injuries are "complete" ruptures, "partial" injuries have been described.

ANATOMY

- The Achilles tendon is about 9 cm long and 0.9 cm in diameter.
- The proximal part is composed of the gastrocnemius and soleus tendons.
- The distal portion inserts onto the posterior aspect of the tuberosity of the calcaneus.
- The Achilles tendon is surrounded by the paratenon, a delicate envelope that contributes to tendon vascularization.
- There is an area of poor vascularity located between 2.5 and 5 cm above the calcaneal tuberosity.

PATHOGENESIS

- Rupture of the Achilles tendon is a common injury among high-level athletes, recreational sports enthusiasts, or even sedentary individuals.
- Rupture of the Achilles tendon usually occurs during forceful dorsiflexion of the ankle.
- Patients often describe hearing or feeling a "pop" in the back of their ankle.
- Intratendinous degeneration can be found histologically.
- Association with cortisone and fluoroquinolone use has been demonstrated.
- This is typically a lesion of middle age, with peak incidence during the third and fourth decades.

NATURAL HISTORY

- There is a great deal of controversy concerning the treatment of an acute rupture of the Achilles tendon.
- Conservative treatment is found to have a higher rate of tendon rerupture and loss of strength because the tendon heals in an elongated position.
- The major factor motivating surgeons to use a nonoperative approach appears to be avoiding the wound complications that occur with an operative repair.
- An increasing number of reports in the literature have tended to favor operative treatment of an acute rupture of the Achilles tendon.

- The exact type of operative procedure and the postoperative regimen remain controversial. Mini-invasive techniques are associated with a lower complication rate.
- If soft tissue complications are avoided, excellent functional results and full return to previous activity can be expected.

PHYSICAL FINDINGS

- Physical examination reveals moderate swelling about the posterior aspect of the ankle.
- Patients are usually able to walk, although with moderate pain.
- With the patient prone, spontaneous excess dorsiflexion of the involved ankle is noted.
- In most cases, a tender defect ("soft spot") can be palpated in the Achilles tendon between 2.5 and 5 cm proximal to its insertion into the calcaneal tuberosity.
- The Thompson squeeze test is positive.
- Patients have difficulty walking on their toes or rising up on their heels.

IMAGING AND DIAGNOSTIC STUDIES

- History and physical examination are sufficient to confirm the diagnosis.
- Because these injuries occur in a traumatic setting, plain radiographs of the ankle are strongly advised.
- There have been many reports of associated ankle fractures (medial malleolus).
- Calcaneal (tuberosity) avulsion will appear on the lateral view.
- Ultrasound and magnetic resonance imaging are not required for the diagnosis of Achilles tendon rupture but may be of value when the diagnosis is questionable.

DIFFERENTIAL DIAGNOSIS

- Ankle sprain
- Ankle fracture
- Tennis leg (gastrocnemius tear)
- Acute paratenonitis
- Calcaneal (tuberosity) avulsion
- Plantaris tendon rupture

NONOPERATIVE MANAGEMENT

- Nonoperative treatment of acute Achilles tendon ruptures involves prolonged immobilization.

- Prolonged immobilization is associated with musculoskeletal changes (atrophy), increased time necessary for rehabilitation, and delayed return to work and preinjury activities.
- In randomized studies, the rerupture rate has been found to be much higher in the nonoperative group.
- However, nonoperative treatment avoids surgical complications.
- Nonoperative treatment should be considered in elderly patients with limited functional expectations, patients with significant tobacco or alcohol addictions, patients receiving chronic cortisone treatment, patients with vascular disease, and patients with severe comorbidities such as renal failure.

Indications and Contraindications

- The indication for this technique is an acute (<3 weeks) Achilles tendon rupture, occurring 2 to 7 cm above the tuberosity of the calcaneus.
  - Over 90% of ruptures of the Achilles tendon occur in the area 2 to 8 cm above the calcaneal tuberosity.
  - We believe that ruptures occurring more than 8 cm above the tuberosity (muscular ruptures) can be treated nonoperatively and ruptures occurring less than 2 cm from the tuberosity necessitate fixation directly to bone.
- Contraindications include chronic rupture greater than 3 weeks in duration, previous local surgery, steroid use, open ruptures and lacerations greater than 6 hours in duration, complex open ruptures with soft tissue defects, and ruptures not occurring between 2 and 8 cm above the tuberosity of the calcaneus.

SURGICAL MANAGEMENT

Preoperative Planning

- Plain films should be reviewed for fracture, avulsion, and calcific tendinopathy.
- All imaging studies are reviewed.
- An examination under anesthesia should be performed before positioning the patient to reconfirm the side of injury.

Positioning

- The patient is placed prone on the operating table.
- A tourniquet is applied around the upper thigh.

- Both legs are included in preparation and draping to compare Achilles tendon tension and spontaneous plantarflexion intraoperatively.
- Plastic draping is not used (the technique involves percutaneous steps).
- Patients receive antibiotic prophylaxis.

Instrumentation

- The Achillon (Integra LifeScience, Plainsboro, NJ) was designed by Matthieu Assal and is made of either a rigid polymer or a stainless steel (**FIG 1**).
- It is designed to guide the passage of the sutures.
- It is composed of a pair of internal branches connected to a pair of external branches, with each branch having a line of apertures at the same level to allow easy and accurate passage of the sutures through all four branches.
- The two internal branches are at an 8-degree angle to each other, following the V-shaped anatomic form of the tendon.
- A micrometric screw allows for varying the opening of the branches according to tendon morphology.
- A straight needle loaded with a suture is passed through the device, soft tissues, and tendon. A cap for the needle facilitates applying pressure to the end of the needle.

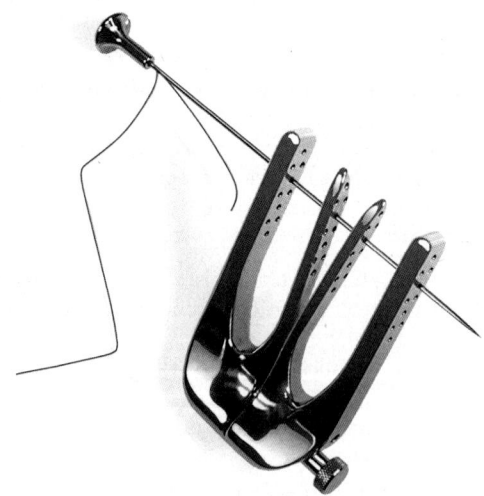

FIG 1 The Achillon instrument, with a straight needle and suture passed through one of the levels of holes.

OPEN REPAIR ILLUSTRATED

Exposure

- Palpate the site of injury, represented by the gap or soft spot (**TECH FIG 1A**).
- The incision is paratendinous and medial (**TECH FIG 1B**), beginning at the soft spot and extending about 2.0 cm proximally.
- Gently retract the skin and subcutaneous tissue with hooks and identify the paratenon (**TECH FIG 1C**).
- Carefully open the sheath and tag each edge with a stay suture (**TECH FIG 1D**).
- Identify both stumps of the ruptured tendon (**TECH FIG 1E**) and carefully note the exact site of rupture.

Introducing the Achillon

- Introduce the Achillon in the closed position under the paratenon in a proximal direction, holding the tendon stump with a small clamp under the instrument (**TECH FIG 2A**).
- The tendon stump is located between the two internal branches (**TECH FIG 2B**).
- As the instrument is introduced, progressively widen it, holding the tendon stump firmly with the clamp.
- Confirm the position of the guide by external palpation; you should feel the tendon between the central (internal) branches of the instrument.

TECHNIQUES

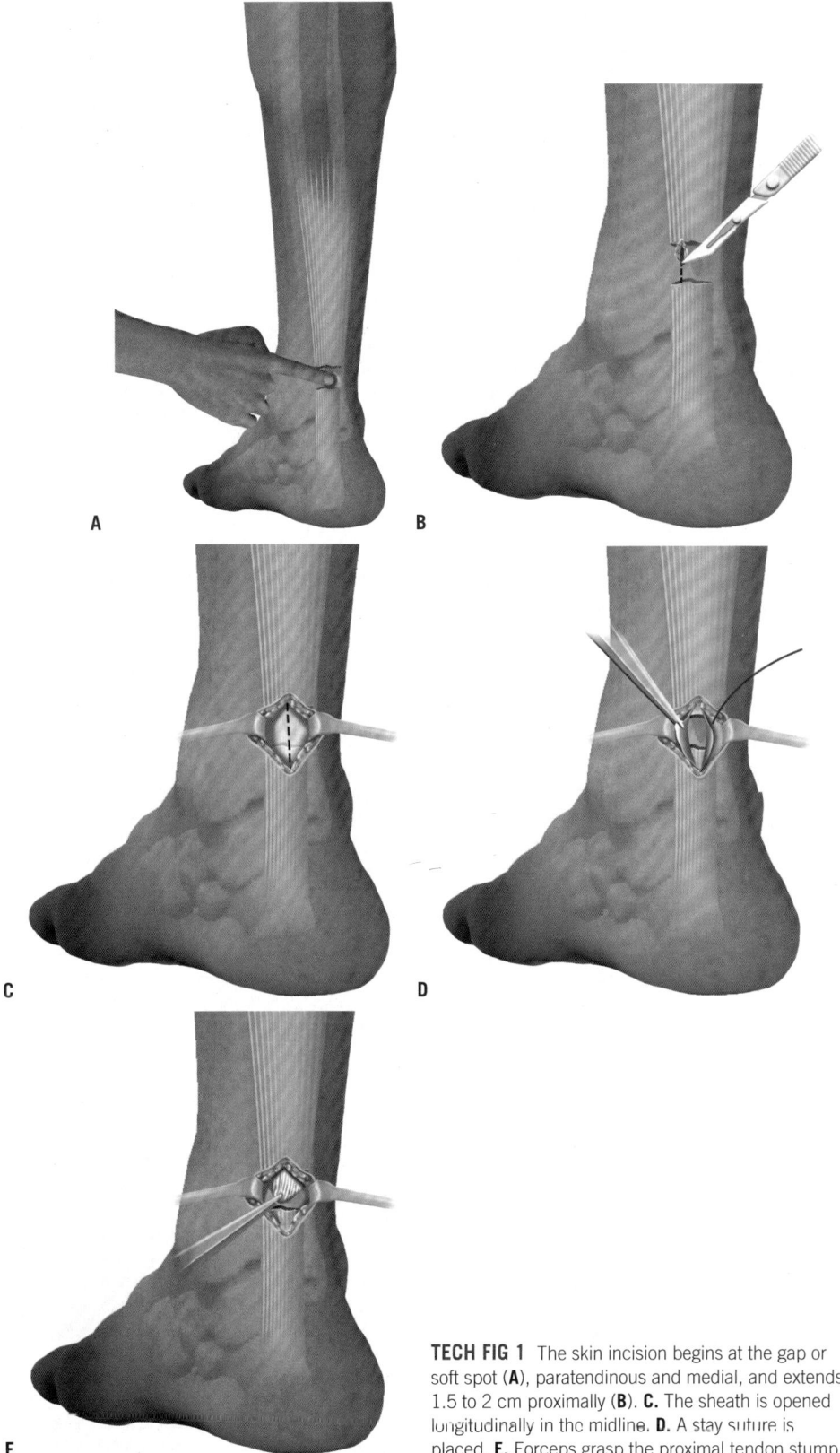

TECH FIG 1 The skin incision begins at the gap or soft spot (**A**), paratendinous and medial, and extends 1.5 to 2 cm proximally (**B**). **C.** The sheath is opened longitudinally in the midline. **D.** A stay suture is placed. **E.** Forceps grasp the proximal tendon stump.

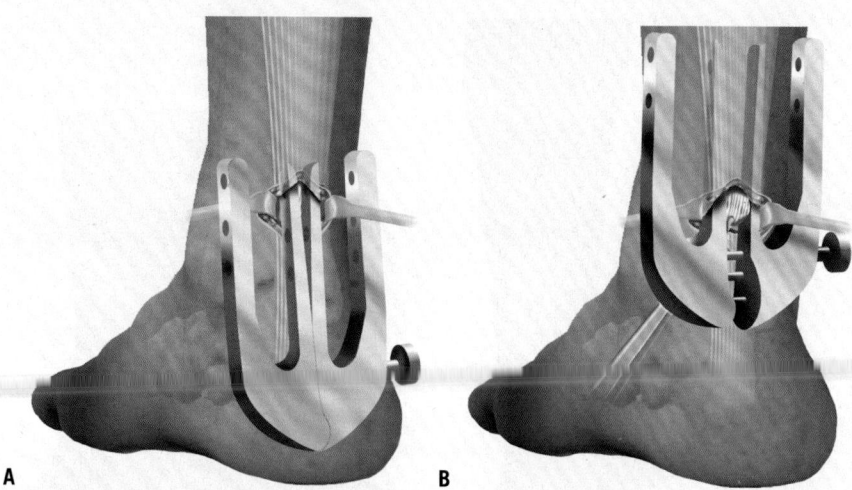

TECH FIG 2 A,B. Introduction of the instrument proximally under the paratenon.

Suturing

- Pass three sutures from lateral to medial, usually beginning with the most proximal hole of the instrument (**TECH FIG 3A,B**).
- Hold the end of each suture with a small clamp to keep them separate from each other.
- Slowly withdraw the instrument while progressively closing the branches (**TECH FIG 3C**).
- This maneuver results in the sutures sliding from an extracutaneous position to a peritendinous position, and thus, the tendon itself is the only tissue held by the sutures (**TECH FIG 3D**).
- Apply traction to the three suture pairs to ensure they are firmly anchored in the tendon and individually clamp them to prevent any confusion.
- Perform the same sequence on the distal stump: Introduce the instrument under the tendon sheath and push it until it touches the calcaneus (**TECH FIG 3E**).

- All the sutures are now organized for tightening (**TECH FIG 3F**), which is carried out with corresponding pairs, and the tendon reduction is under direct visual control (**TECH FIG 3G**).
- If it is difficult to ascertain tendon length and reduction because the ends are too frayed, compare the tendon tension to the opposite leg.

Closure

- Close the tendon sheath and then the skin with intradermal sutures (**TECH FIG 4**).
- No drain is used.
- Apply a splint holding the ankle in 30 degrees of flexion before moving or waking up the patient.

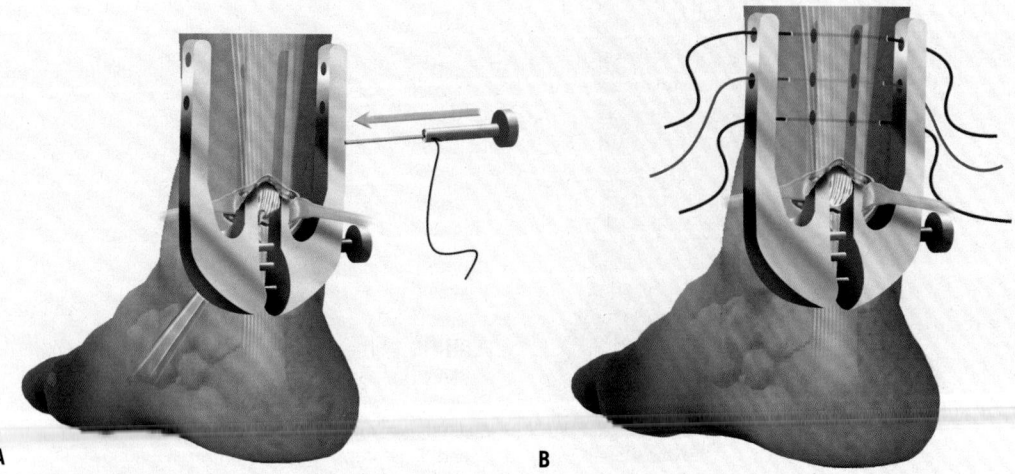

TECH FIG 3 A. The first needle is introduced. **B.** All three sutures in the proximal tendon. *(continued)*

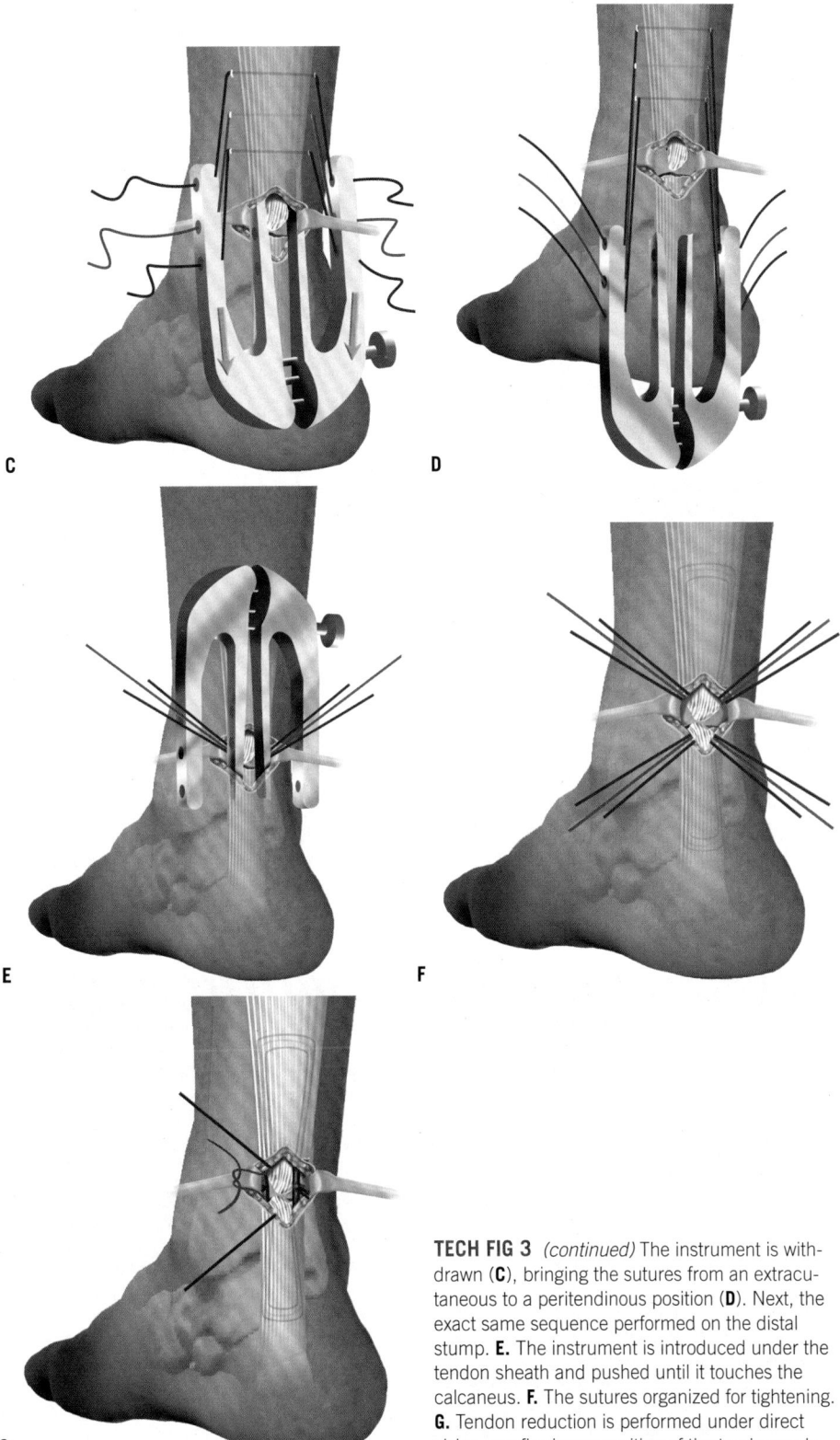

C

D

E

F

G

TECH FIG 3 *(continued)* The instrument is withdrawn (**C**), bringing the sutures from an extracutaneous to a peritendinous position (**D**). Next, the exact same sequence performed on the distal stump. **E.** The instrument is introduced under the tendon sheath and pushed until it touches the calcaneus. **F.** The sutures organized for tightening. **G.** Tendon reduction is performed under direct vision, confirming apposition of the tendon ends.

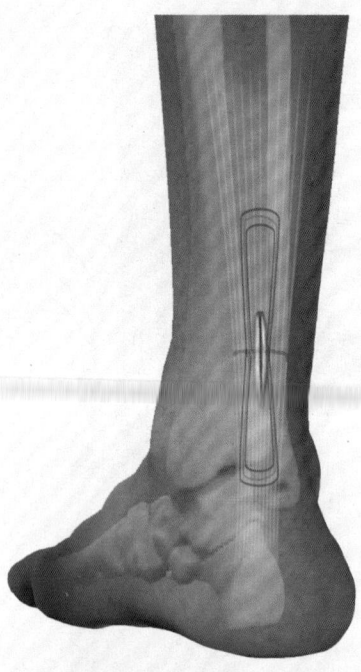

TECH FIG 4 Closure of the skin with intradermal sutures.

OPEN REPAIR IN INTRAOPERATIVE PHOTOGRAPHS

Approach and Identification of Ruptured Tendon Ends

- Mini-open incision **(TECH FIG 5A)**
  - Make a longitudinal skin incision about 2 cm long at the level of the rupture.
    - The incision is longitudinal in the event the procedure has to be converted to a full open procedure.

- Divide the paratenon to gain control of the ruptured tendon ends **(TECH FIG 5B)**.
  - The plantaris tendon may occasionally be intact despite complete Achilles tendon rupture **(TECH FIG 5C)**.
  - Tag the two tendon ends with suture **(TECH FIG 5D,E)**.

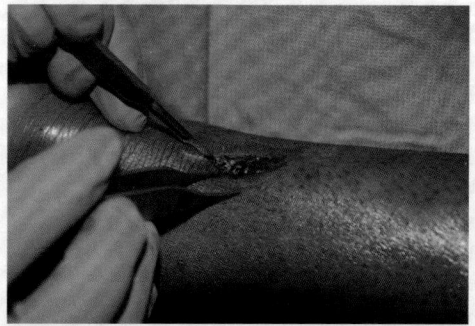

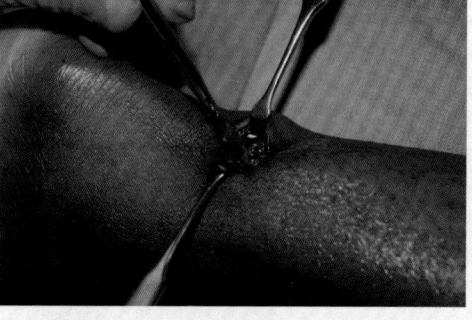

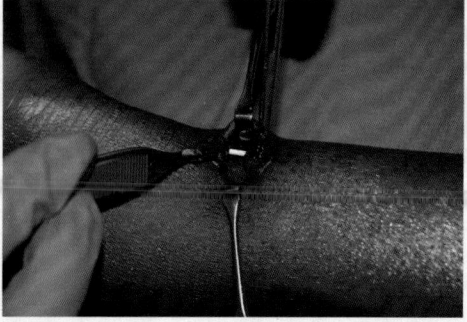

TECH FIG 5 A. Mini open longitudinal incision directly over tendon rupture. **B.** Paratenon is divided to gain access to tendon ends. **C.** The plantaris tendon may remain intact despite complete Achilles tendon rupture. *(continued)*

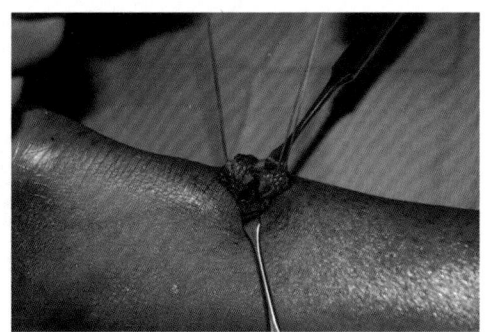
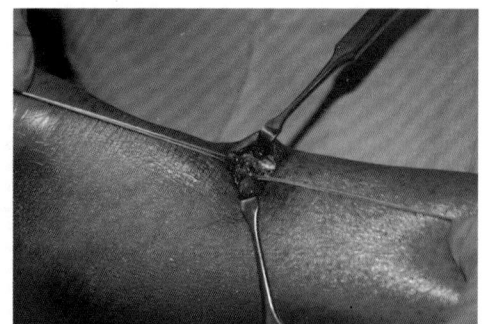

TECH FIG 5 *(continued)* **D.** Tag sutures are placed on the mobilized tendon ends. **E.** Tension is applied to tag sutures, approximating the tendon ends.

Placing Permanent Sutures in Proximal Aspect of the Ruptured Tendon

- Using the proximal tag sutures, apply tension to the proximal tendon stump.
- Place retractors within the paratenon to define the interval between the tendon and the paratenon.
- Advance the Achillon device within the paratenon on the medial and lateral aspects of the tensioned proximal tendon **(TECH FIG 6A,B)**.
- Typically, the tendon is palpable between the arms of the Achillon device.
- In succession from closest to farthest from the rupture, pass three sutures through the tensioned proximal tendon **(TECH FIG 6C–F)**.

- By retracting the Achillon device distally back into the wound, secure the sutures in the tendon, within the paratenon, and exiting within the wound **(TECH FIG 6G,H)**.
- Tension must be placed on the sutures before proceeding to the next step to ensure the sutures are properly anchored in the proximal tendon **(TECH FIG 6I)**.
- If the sutures pull out, repeat the three aforementioned steps, with careful palpation to be sure that the tendon is indeed between the arms of the Achillon device.

Placing Permanent Sutures in Distal Aspect of the Ruptured Tendon

- This is essentially the mirror image of placing sutures in the proximal tendon.

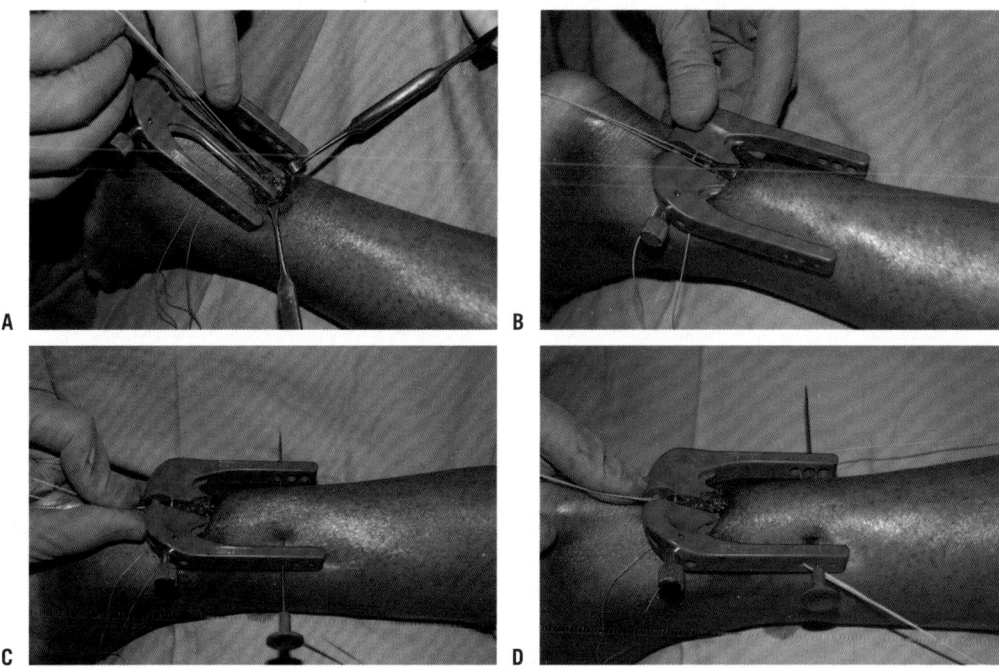

TECH FIG 6 A. The Achillon device is advanced within the paratenon. **B.** Longitudinal tension placed on the tag suture while advancing the Achillon device facilitates optimal positioning of the tendon between the two arms of the Achillon device. **C.** The suture closest to the rupture is inserted first. Tension is maintained on the tag suture. **D.** The second suture is passed through the tendon. *(continued)*

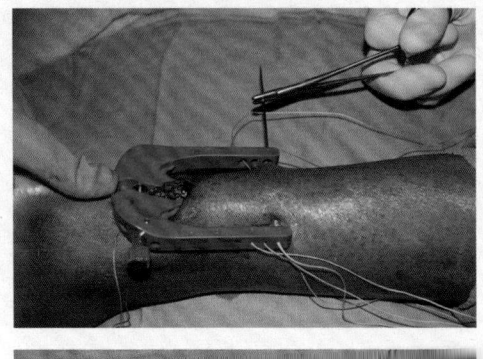

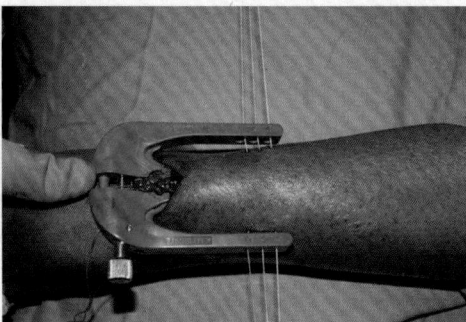

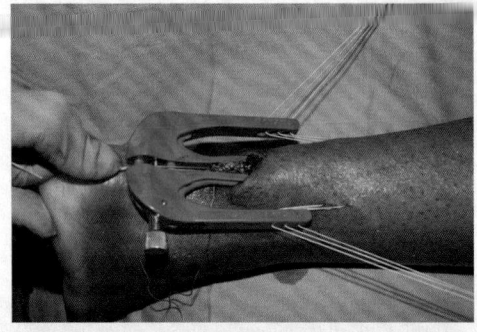

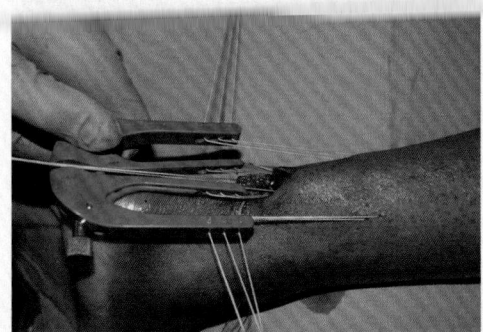

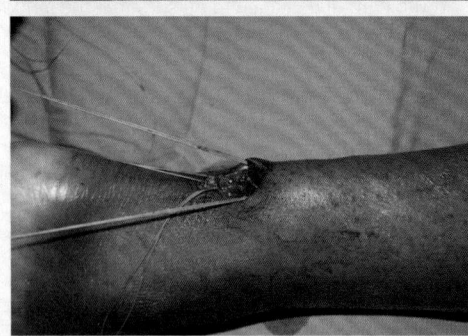

TECH FIG 6 *(continued)* **E.** The third suture is passed. Tension is still maintained on the tag suture, and the tendon is centered between the two arms of the Achillon device that are within the paratenon. **F.** All three sutures are passed through the proximal tendon and organized. **G,H.** By retracting the device from the wound, the three sets of sutures remain in the tendon, are within the paratenon, and exit at the wound.
I. Longitudinal traction is placed on the sutures to ensure that they are secured within the proximal tendon.

- With distal ruptures, the Achillon device must be advanced as close to the Achilles insertion on the calcaneus as possible to optimize the sutures' purchase in tendon.
- Advance the Achillon device's inner arms on either side of the Achilles tendon, within the paratenon **(TECH FIG 7A)**.
  - Palpate to be sure that the tendon is indeed between the two arms of the Achillon device.
- Place the three sutures (similar to those in the proximal tendon), from closest to farthest from the rupture, into the distal tendon, with tension applied to the tag sutures **(TECH FIG 7B–E)**.
- Retract the Achillon device from the wound, thereby bringing the three sutures within the paratenon and into the wound, ready for repairing the rupture **(TECH FIG 7F)**.
- To ensure that the purchase of the sutures in the distal tendon is satisfactory, apply forceful tension to the sutures.
  - Tension should plantarflex the ankle **(TECH FIG 7G)**.
  - Should the sutures pull out, repeat the steps described earlier so that acceptable purchase of the sutures in the distal tendon is achieved. In our opinion, palpation of the tendon between the arms of the Achillon device is helpful.

Tendon Repair

- Approximate the two tendon ends by tensioning the sutures **(TECH FIG 8A)**.

- The sutures must be carefully organized so that corresponding sutures are secured to one another.
- Passive plantarflexion of the ankle with a bump placed under the dorsum of the foot or maintained by an assistant takes tension off the tendon during repair.
- Secure the two sets of sutures closest to the rupture to one another first.
  - With tension maintained on one side, secure the other side with a surgeon's knot **(TECH FIG 8B)**.
  - Then secure the other side, applying tension first to remove residual slack in the suture **(TECH FIG 8C)**.
- Repeat the suture technique described for the initial set of sutures for the other sets **(TECH FIG 8D)**.
  - Secure the intermediate set of sutures to one another, followed by the sets farthest from the rupture.
  - If the sutures more distant from the rupture are overtensioned during the repair, then the tension gained with the previously secured sutures is forfeited. Therefore, overtensioning of each successive set of sutures is unnecessary.
- With the opposite, uninjured extremity prepared into the operative field, the resting tension of the repair may be compared to what is deemed physiologic **(TECH FIG 8E)**.
  - Setting the resting tension of the repair slightly greater than that of the contralateral extremity is acceptable and, in our opinion, preferred.
  - Avoid undertensioning of the repair.

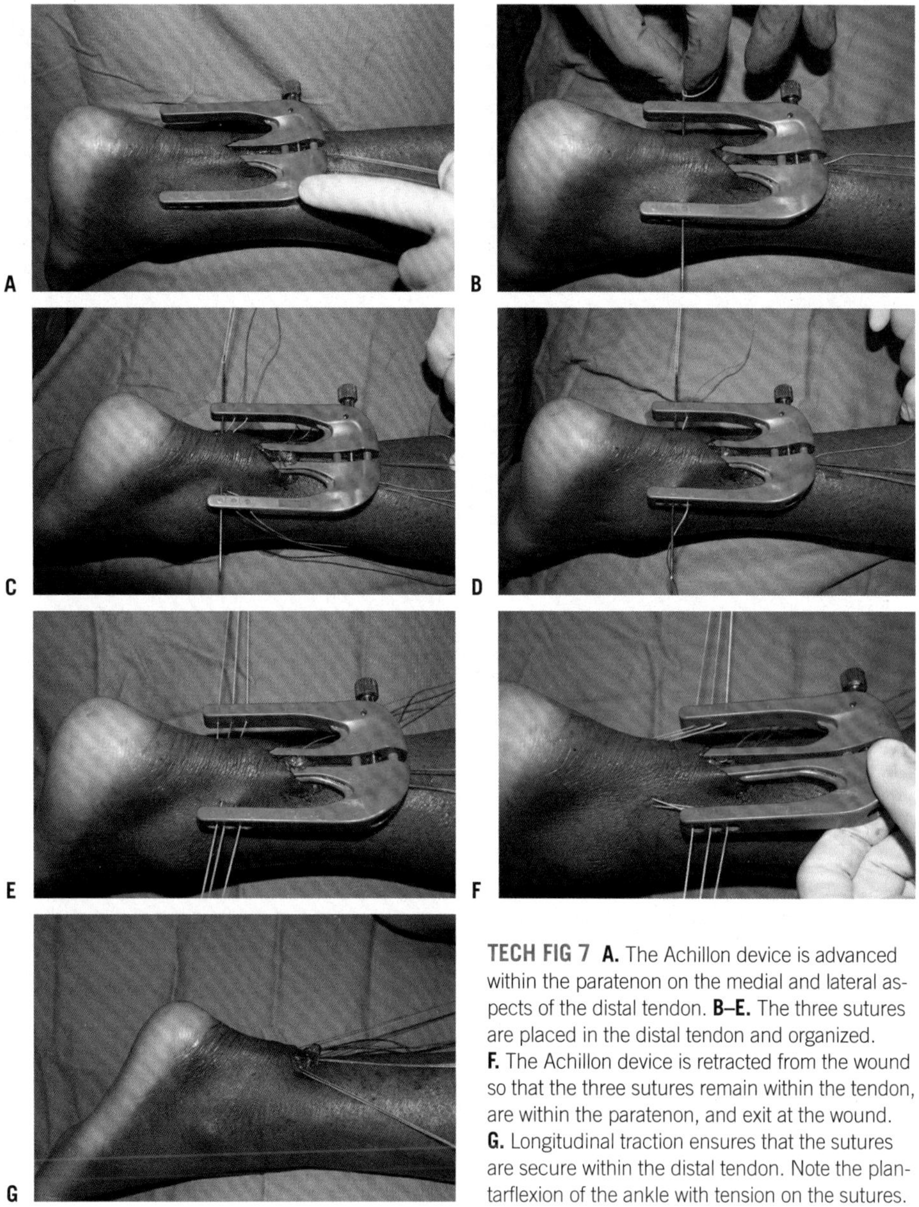

TECH FIG 7 A. The Achillon device is advanced within the paratenon on the medial and lateral aspects of the distal tendon. **B–E.** The three sutures are placed in the distal tendon and organized. **F.** The Achillon device is retracted from the wound so that the three sutures remain within the tendon, are within the paratenon, and exit at the wound. **G.** Longitudinal traction ensures that the sutures are secure within the distal tendon. Note the plantarflexion of the ankle with tension on the sutures.

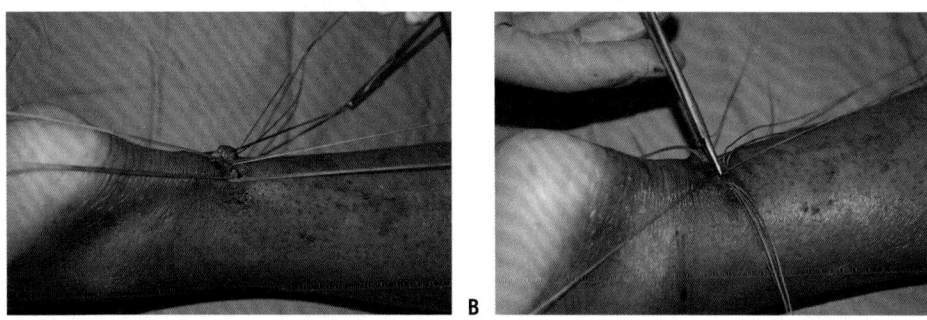

TECH FIG 8 A. The ruptured tendon ends are approximated by tensioning both sets of sutures. **B.** One side of the corresponding sutures closest to the rupture is tied. Tension should be maintained on the other side of this set of sutures. *(continued)*

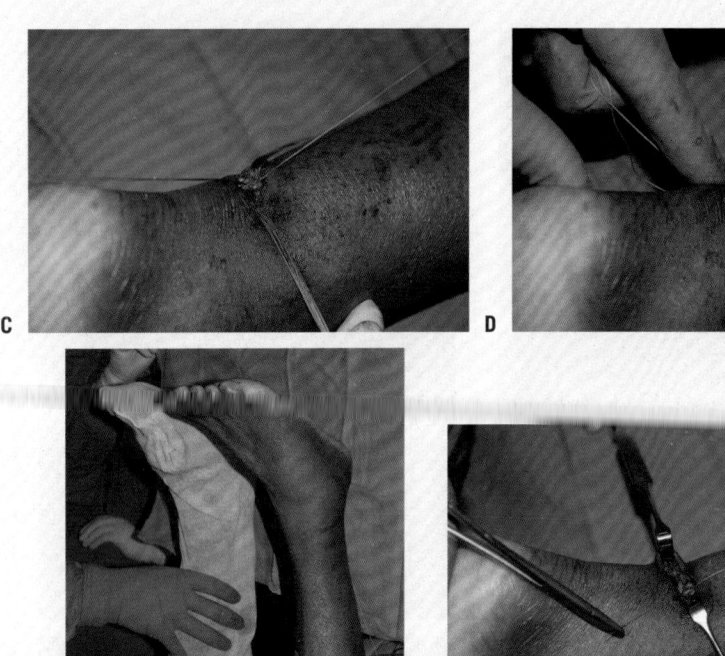

TECH FIG 8 *(continued)* **C.** After removing slack in the suture, the other side of this first set of sutures is tied. **D.** The second and third set of sutures are secured. Overtensioning of each successive set of sutures should be avoided because this will cause the previous set to lose its tension. **E.** The resting tension of the repair should match that of the other uninjured extremity. Preferably, the tension should be slightly greater in the repair. **F.** The repair is reinforced with a single running or multiple interrupted sutures directly at the rupture.

- As for flexor tendon repairs for the hand, we recommend reinforcing the repair with additional sutures directly at the rupture **(TECH FIG 8F)**.
  - In our opinion, this is important because the mini-open technique described earlier only serves the function of an internal splint. When the repair site is directly palpated after repair with only the three sets of sutures, invariably, there is mostly suture at the repair site and relatively little collagen.
  - We routinely perform this reinforcement with a running, absorbable suture.
  - This not only reinforces the tendon repair but also tends to bring more tendon collagen directly to the repair site.

- Place the running or alternatively multiple interrupted sutures circumferentially at the repair site.
- A similar system for mini-open Achilles tendon repair allows one of the three sutures to be locked in either tendon end. This may afford a stronger repair and improved suture anchoring in the each tendon end **(TECH FIG 9)**.

Closure

- Repair the paratenon and fascial layer over the tendon to a "water-tight" closure **(TECH FIG 10A)**.
- Reapproximate the subcutaneous layer and skin to a tensionless closure **(TECH FIG 10B,C)**.

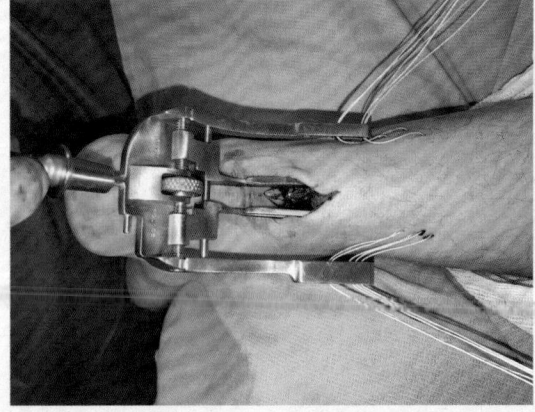
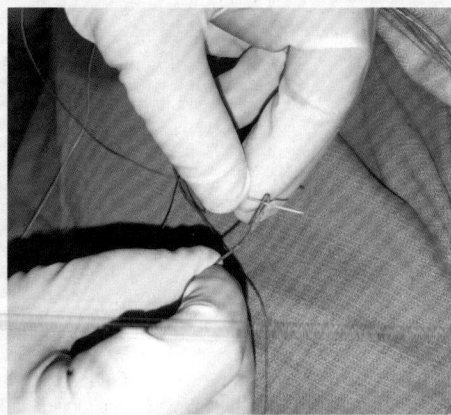

TECH FIG 9 Different patient using a similar mini-open repair system that locks one of the sutures on each side of the repair. **A.** Device being retracted after proximal sutures passed. **B.** One of the proximal sutures locked. *(continued)*

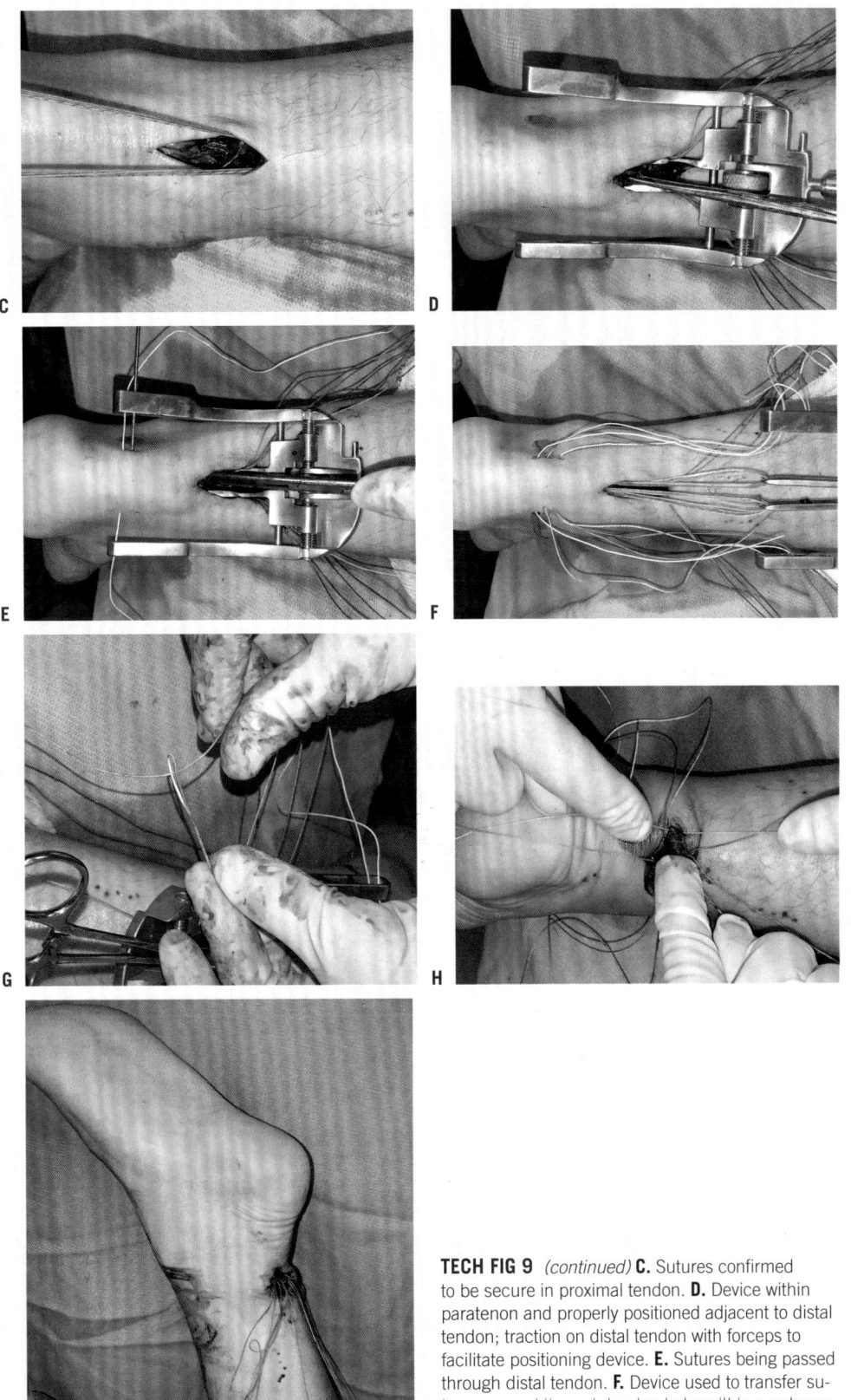

TECH FIG 9 *(continued)* **C.** Sutures confirmed to be secure in proximal tendon. **D.** Device within paratenon and properly positioned adjacent to distal tendon; traction on distal tendon with forceps to facilitate positioning device. **E.** Sutures being passed through distal tendon. **F.** Device used to transfer sutures passed through tendon to be within paratenon. **G.** One of the distal sutures being locked. **H.** With ankle held in plantarflexion, three corresponding sutures being tied to repair proximal and distal tendon stumps. **I.** Proper resting tension confirmed for the repair.

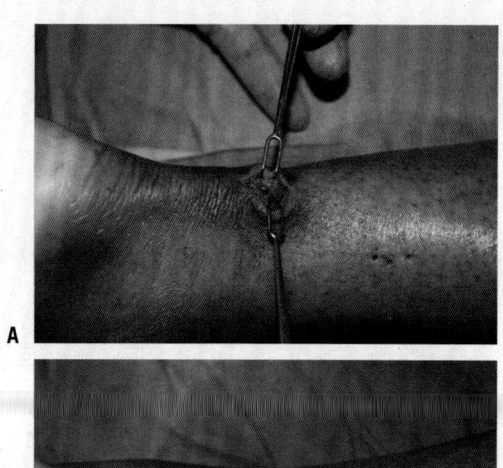

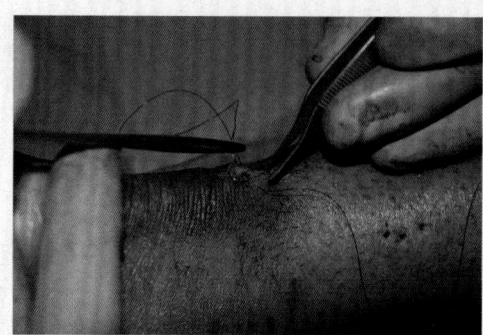

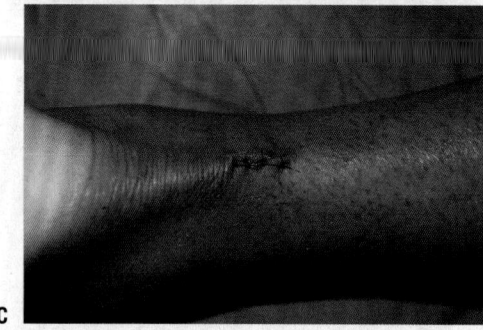

TECH FIG 10 A. The paratenon and fascial layer are reapproximated. **B,C.** The subcutaneous layer and skin are reapproximated to a tensionless closure.

TECHNIQUES

Pearls and Pitfalls

Ensure that the tendon is between the arms of the Achillon device.	• Palpate the tendon between the Achillon device arms during suture insertion.
Gain maximum purchase of the sutures in the tendon.	• Use tag sutures in the ruptured tendon ends to apply tension while advancing the Achillon device and while passing sutures through the tendon.
Organize the sutures.	• Use three different colors for the sutures on either side of the repair to facilitate coordinating corresponding sutures for the repair.
Ensure that the sutures are indeed secured in the tendon ends before repair.	• Apply tension to the sutures after they have been passed through the tendon and have been organized within the paratenon; if they should pull out, then they will need to be passed again.
Optimal Tensioning of the Repair	• In our experience, setting the tension slightly greater than the opposite extremity's physiologic resting tension is appropriate and leads to an optimal outcome.
Assess the rupture pattern.	• Although mini-open, the tendon ends may be assessed through the limited approach. Occasionally, shear patterns of the rupture are not amenable to this technique and a more traditional open technique is warranted. We, therefore, recommend that the mini-open technique be performed through a short longitudinal incision that can easily be extended if necessary.

POSTOPERATIVE CARE

- Low-molecular-weight heparin (subcutaneous administration) is used to prevent deep vein thrombosis for 3 weeks postoperatively.
- Our early functional rehabilitation program, carefully supervised by the physical therapist, is divided into four stages.
- For the first 2 weeks, patients are allowed partial weight bearing (30 to 45 lb) and maintained in the splint full-time.
- Then, gentle ankle range of motion (flexion and extension) is begun as well as thigh muscle exercises and the use of a stationary bicycle.
- The goal is to reach a neutral ankle position by the end of the third week.
- After 3 weeks, full weight bearing is allowed with continuous use of the protective splint.
- At the end of 8 weeks, the splint is discontinued, and weight bearing is allowed without any external support.
- A more intensive program of ankle range of motion, stretching, and isometric and proprioceptive exercises is instituted.
- Jogging is allowed at 3 months and more demanding sports at 5 months.

OUTCOMES

- This limited open procedure with use of the Achillon instrument provides the advantage of an open repair but avoids the soft tissue problems associated with open repair.
- We published a prospective multicenter study in 2002 including 82 patients. Results showed no wound healing problems and no infections. No patient noted a sensory disturbance in the sural nerve distribution. All patients returned to their previous professional or sporting activities. The mean American Orthopaedic Foot & Ankle Society score was 96 points (range, 85 to 100 points).
- Complications occurred in three patients. Two of them were noncompliant and removed the orthosis within the first 3 weeks postoperatively, thus disrupting the repair by a new injury. One patient fell 12 weeks after the surgery and sustained a rerupture. All three new injuries were repaired with an open surgical procedure.
- Isokinetic results: The concentric peak torque was performed with the ankle in plantarflexion at 30 and 60 degrees per second of angular velocity, after correction for dominance. There was no significant difference between the injured and uninvolved sides **(TABLE 1)**. Endurance testing at 120 degrees per second also revealed no difference between sides.
- Three recent reports describe similar excellent results using the exact surgical technique and Achillon instrument, thus providing further confirmation of its important role in the repair of acute Achilles tendon ruptures.

TABLE 1 Concentric Peak Torque Measured with Isokinetic Dynamometry in 50 Patients

Angular Velocity (degrees/s)	Mean Torque (Nm ± SD)	
	Injured Side	Unaffected Side
30	111.4 ± 19	118.9 ± 30
60	95.4 ± 19	101.3 ± 25

SD, standard deviation.

COMPLICATIONS

- Disruption of the repair related to the patient's noncompliance with the rehabilitation protocol (before the third month postoperatively)
- Rerupture of the healed Achilles tendon (after the third month postoperatively)
- Sural nerve injury
- Infection
- Deep venous thrombosis

SUGGESTED READINGS

Anathallee MY, Liu B, Budgen A, et al. Is Achillon repair safe and reliable in delayed presentation Achilles tendon rupture? A five-year follow-up. Foot Ankle Surg 2018;24(4):296–299.

Assal M, Jung M, Stern R, et al. Limited open repair of Achilles tendon ruptures: a technique with a new instrument and findings of a prospective multicenter study. J Bone Joint Surg Am 2002;84-A(2): 161–170.

Assal M, Stern R, Peter R. Fracture of the ankle associated with rupture of the Achilles tendon: case report and review of the literature. J Ortho Trauma 2002;16:358–361.

Bradley JP, Tibone JE. Percutaneous and open surgical repairs of Achilles tendon ruptures: a comparative study. Am J Sports Med 1990;18: 188–195.

Calder JD, Saxby TS. Independent evaluation of a recently described Achilles tendon repair technique. Foot Ankle Int 2006;27:93–96.

Cetti R, Christensen SE, Ejsted R, et al. Operative versus nonoperative treatment of Achilles tendon rupture: a prospective randomized study and review of the literature. Am J Sports Med 1993;21:791–799.

Clanton TO, Haytmanek, CT, Williams BT, et al. A biomechanical comparison of an open repair and 3 minimally invasive percutaneous Achilles tendon repair techniques during a simulated, progressive rehabilitation protocol. Am J Sports Med 2015;43(8):1957–1964.

Cretnik A, Kosanovic M, Smrkolj V. Percutaneous versus open repair of the ruptured Achilles tendon: a comparative study. Am J Sports Med 2005;33:1369–1379.

DiStefano VJ, Nixon JE. Achilles tendon rupture: pathogenesis, diagnosis, and treatment by a modified pullout wire technique. J Trauma 1972;12:671–677.

Haji A, Sahai A, Symes A, et al. Percutaneous versus open tendo Achillis repair. Foot Ankle Int 2004;25:215–218.

Kakiuchi M. A combined open and percutaneous technique for repair of tendo Achillis. Comparison with open repair. J Bone Joint Surg Br 1995;77:60–63.

Leppilahti J, Orava S. Total Achilles tendon rupture. A review. Sports Med 1998;25:79–100.

Ma GW, Griffith TG. Percutaneous repair of acute closed ruptured Achilles tendon: a new technique. Clin Orthop Relat Res 1977;(128): 247–255.

Maffulli N. Rupture of the Achilles tendon. J Bone Joint Surg Am 1999;81:1019–1036.

Mandelbaum BR, Myerson MS, Forster R. Achilles tendon ruptures. A new method of repair, early range of motion, and functional rehabilitation. Am J Sports Med 1995;23:392–395.

McCullough KA, Shaw CM, Anderson RB. Mini-open repair of Achilles rupture in the National Football League. J Surg Orthop Adv 2014;23(4):179–183.

Orr JD, McCriskin B, Dutton JR. Achillon mini-open Achilles tendon repair: early outcomes and return to duty in U.S. military service members. J Surg Orthop Adv 2013;22(1):23–29.

Rippstein P, Easley M. "Mini-open" repair for acute Achilles tendon ruptures. Tech Foot Ankle Surg 2006;5:3–8.

Soldatis JJ, Goodfellow DB, Wilber JH. End-to-end operative repair of Achilles tendon rupture. Am J Sports Med 1997;25:90–95.

Tasatan E, Emre TY, Demircioglu DT, et al. Long-term results of mini-open repair technique in the treatment of acute Achilles tendon rupture: a prospective study. J Foot Ankle Surg 2016;55(5): 971–975.

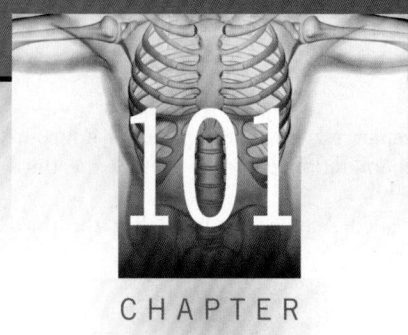

101
CHAPTER

Mini-Open Achilles Tendon Repair:
Perspective 2

Emilio Wagner and Cristian Ortiz

DEFINITION

- Spontaneous Achilles tendon rupture are defined as a partial or complete loss of continuity of the distal tendinous portions of the gastrocnemius and soleus muscles with the consequent loss in physiologic equinus of the ankle.

ANATOMY

- The gastrocnemius muscle merges with the soleus muscle to form the Achilles tendon, which inserts onto the calcaneus.
  - The gastrocnemius muscle is the most superficial muscle and is responsible of plantarflexion of the ankle and propelling the body forward. The soleus muscle is a postural muscle, with no action on the knee joint (it inserts only on the tibia), and also acts as a peripheral vascular pump.
  - The Achilles tendon is approximately 15 cm long, flattened at both its proximal and distal end but rounded in the middle portion. On its anterior surface receives muscular fibers from the soleus up to its insertion.[6]
- The Achilles tendon is enclosed by a paratenon, which is a thin gliding membrane, continuous proximally with fascia overlying muscles and distally continuous with the periosteum of the calcaneus. This structure is the most important regarding blood supply to the middle portion of the tendon. Most blood vessels arise from the anterior aspect of the paratenon, which is also the area where neovascularization occurs in tendinopathic patients. A relatively avascular area of the tendon is described near its insertion. Regarding vascular density, the middle portion of the tendon possesses the lesser density compared to its proximal or distal parts.[6]

PATHOGENESIS

- The Achilles tendon transmits all the tension generated by the gastrocnemius–soleus complex to the calcaneus. The tendon is elastic and has the capability of deforming and recovering its original length if the strain does not exceed 4%. If the strain is between 4% and 8%, the tendon fibers start to become damaged. At a strain level of approximately 8%, the Achilles tendon may rupture.[5]
- The exact reason why the Achilles tendon ruptures is not known, but there are two main theories: one a degenerative theory and one a mechanical theory. In the mechanical

theory, the tendon just suffers strain that exceeds its limit with subsequent failure of the collagen fibrils. In the degenerative theory, a chronic degeneration of the tendon leads to rupture without the need of applying excessive loads.

- Degenerative tendinopathy is present in most histologic samples from spontaneous tendon ruptures.[8] It can be assumed that degenerated tendons will have less tensile strength and rupture under physiologic forces. It has been shown that ruptured tendons have more advanced intratendinous changes than tendinopathic tendons. Degenerative changes are described as hypoxic, mucoid, tendolipomatous, and calcific changes. These changes are found just in 31% of control tendons.[5]
- The origin of tendinopathy is the subject of debate, but the overload theory is the most accepted one, where repeated loading of a musculotendinous unit may result in weakening of the structure and, in some cases, a failure of tendon tissue. If the overload persists and the tendon is unable to heal and/or respond to load over time, this weakening may increase and compromise a higher percentage of the total tissue.[8] The failed healing response of the tendon may relate to numerous factors, such as genetics, age, and gender, among others.
- Other reasons for Achilles tendon ruptures relate to drug-related effects. Corticosteroids (local and systemic) have been described as risk factors for tendon ruptures. Fluoroquinolone antibiotic use is also a risk factor for Achilles tendon ruptures. Inflammatory conditions, collagen abnormalities, infectious diseases, and hyperlipidemia have also been associated with tendon ruptures.

NATURAL HISTORY

- When left untreated, Achilles ruptures are named *chronic ruptures*, and they cause great difficulty with ankle plantarflexion. Besides atrophy of the muscle belly, the tendon sheath becomes thickened and adherent to the tendon ends. There is a scar tissue bridging the defect, but this tissue is of poor quality, not as strong as the intact tendon, and may elongate with time.[4]
- Chronic ruptures of the Achilles tendon are mainly surgically treated, and conservative measures such as ankle–foot orthoses are only used in low-demand individuals or if the surgery is contraindicated.

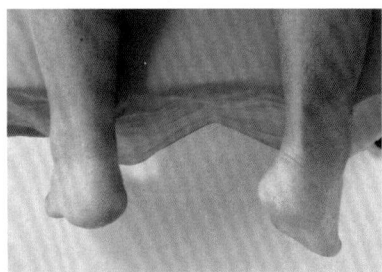

FIG 1 Patient positioned prone at the end of the table. Observe normal physiologic equinus position of the ankle at the left of the picture compared to the nonphysiologic dorsiflexed position of the ankle at the right side, representing a complete Achilles tendon rupture.

PATIENT HISTORY AND PHYSICAL FINDINGS

- Almost all the time, patients present with a typical history of feeling suddenly a "pop" in the calf, often believing that they were hit by someone or somebody. After that, they feel pain and weakness to bear weight. Achilles tendon ruptures can be missed in up to 25% of patients.[5] The diagnosis is clinical, and physical examination is paramount.
- The identification of loss of physiologic equinus of the ankle will ascertain the diagnosis of a complete Achilles tendon rupture.
  - This can be evaluated by the knee flexion test, where the patient is prone holding the knee flexed and the foot falls into neutral or dorsiflexion position.
  - This same test can be performed prone but with the knee extended, and the relative equinus of the ankle can be compared between the healthy and injured side. Any difference in the plantarflexion resting position of the ankle will indicate a loss of continuity of the Achilles tendon (**FIG 1**). A gap can be palpated in the rupture site, but this maneuver can be painful.
  - The Thompson test can also be performed, where squeezing of the calf should produce ankle plantarflexion. The test is positive when there is no or limited plantarflexion of the ankle, indicating an Achilles tendon rupture.

IMAGING AND OTHER DIAGNOSTIC STUDIES

- Generally speaking, no diagnostic studies are needed to complete the diagnosis of Achilles tendon ruptures.
- Ultrasonography and magnetic resonance imaging (MRI) have been used as an adjunct to assure clinical diagnosis, but they should be used to evaluate other diagnoses, which may individually change the approach.
  - Tendinopathy can be evaluated by MRI, which may have a role for follow-up studies.
  - Ultrasonography may have a role when long-standing ruptures are being evaluated, as it will show if there still is hematoma left at the rupture site. If not, this may hinder a minimally invasive approach and incline the surgeon to perform an open repair. Also, ultrasound will detect the presence of deep vein thrombosis, which may delay the operative intervention.
- Sometimes, imaging studies could be misleading when they show partial continuity of the tendon. In these cases, clinical diagnosis based on loss of physiologic equinus confirms the diagnosis.

DIFFERENTIAL DIAGNOSIS

- Plantaris rupture, leg contusion, muscle strain, leg fracture, posterior tibialis tendon rupture, deep venous thrombosis, etc.

NONOPERATIVE MANAGEMENT

- Classically, nonoperative treatment has not been the treatment of choice because of the high rerupture rate associated to this treatment.
- In the past few years, more information has become available which suggests that functional rehabilitation associated with early weight bearing can deliver rerupture rates similar between operative and nonoperative treatments.[9]
- In the article by Glazebrook,[9] 10 studies comparing operative versus nonoperative treatment for Achilles tendon ruptures were chosen to be analyzed regarding rerupture rates, complications, and time to return to work, among other factors. No difference was found between both groups except in the time to return to work, which was faster in the operative group.
- Regarding functional outcomes, only four studies were available for comparison, and it is still a matter of controversy because most experts feel that only surgery can yield a better functional outcome.
- Relative to conservative treatment, it should consider functional rehabilitation as stated earlier, which stands for fast weight bearing and protected motion.

SURGICAL MANAGEMENT

- The best candidates for a minimally invasive approach are patients with acute Achilles tendon rupture less than 10 days from the injury due to the presence of hematoma at the rupture site, which supposedly keeps growth factors present, and the absence of scar tissue, which will hinder a correct healing afterward.
- Minimally invasive options should be known to orthopaedic surgeons, as there is evidence showing decreased postoperative complications and increased likelihood of a good to excellent subjective outcome compared to open surgery.[2]
- Patients should be physiologically active, independent of age, who desire the best probability of returning back to work and sporting activities as close as possible to preoperative levels.
- Main contraindications should consider general surgical contraindications, as serious medical comorbidities, local infection, and very low physical demand patients or nonambulatory patients.
- The technique presented here corresponds to a modification of the Dresden surgical technique presented and developed by Amlang et al[1] in 2005. The unique characteristics of the Dresden technique rely on suturing through an interval between the superficial fascia of the leg and the paratenon and accessing through a mini-open incision away from the rupture site, thereby avoiding the disturbance of the rupture hematoma and growth factors present at the site, hopefully obtaining a better repair tissue. Further modifications of the technique are being studied and include different ways of suturing the repair proximally and reattaching distally the tendon to the calcaneus through suture anchors, variations already included in other techniques.[7]

Preoperative Planning

- The level of injury should be evaluated preoperatively, clinically, and/or through ultrasound.
- A sensory evaluation should be performed right before surgery and also to ascertain if there is any preoperative sural damage in order to report it to the patient.

Positioning

- Under regional anesthesia, the patient is placed in prone position with both legs in the operative field.
- We regularly leave both legs on top of a bolster and sufficiently distal on the operating table to have both feet hanging free from the edge of the table in order to evaluate the physiologic equinus.
- No tourniquet is used.

EXPOSURE

- A 2.5-cm paramedial longitudinal incision is made 3 cm above the proximal end of the ruptured Achilles tendon.
- It is vital to determine in the operating room, by palpation, the location of proximal stump of the tendon. In this way, we are sure we will be on top of healthy paratenon and tendon **(TECH FIG 1A)**.

- The superficial fascia is identified with the thin free thin subcutaneous fat **(TECH FIG 1B)**.
- The superficial fascia is incised, but the paratenon is not opened and the interval between the fascia and the paratenon is developed.
  - We regularly use a rounded tip instrument to free up the superficial fascia from the paratenon **(TECH FIG 1C)**.

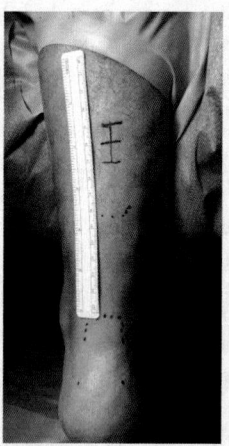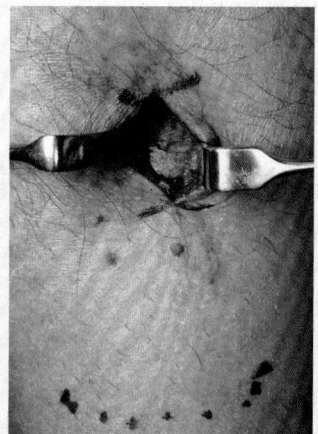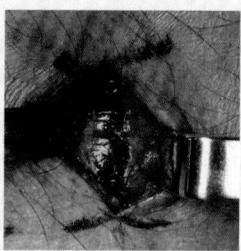

TECH FIG 1 A. The skin incision is 3 cm proximal to the most proximal aspect of the gap identified by palpation. The incision measures 2.5 cm long and is slightly medial to avoid damaging the sural nerve. **B.** After skin and subcutaneous dissection, the superficial fascia of the leg is identified, as a fibrous whitish layer. Care is to be taken to isolate it from subcutaneous tissue and eventually the sural nerve. **C.** The superficial fascia is opened longitudinally with a knife and then with scissors, showing the deeply situated Achilles paratenon, as a red structure. With a rounded tip instrument as a mosquito clamp or suture scissors, the fascia is gently separated from the underlying paratenon in the area surrounding the incision and distally toward the calcaneus.

PASSING THE SUTURES

- Through this developed interval, the suture passers are introduced distally until the calcaneus is reached, one on each side of the tendon **(TECH FIG 2A,B)**.
- The suture passers are used to pass three 2-0 polyblend sutures through the distal end of the Achilles tendon, each spaced 1 cm proximal to the previous one, using straight-eyed needles.
- The slot in the tip of each instrument measures 3 cm in length and therefore can hold the three needles with their sutures at one time, which aids in the aiming and positioning of each consecutive needle.

- To check that the needles went through the needle passers, these instruments can be twisted slightly and corresponding bending effect on the needles observed **(TECH FIG 2C)**.
- The instruments are then retrieved proximally through the skin incision, one at a time, taking care that the sutures are being secure on one side while being pulled by the contralateral instrument **(TECH FIG 2D)**.
- The grip of the three sutures is tested by pulling them hard and being able to obtain plantarflexion at the ankle joint **(TECH FIG 2E,F)**.

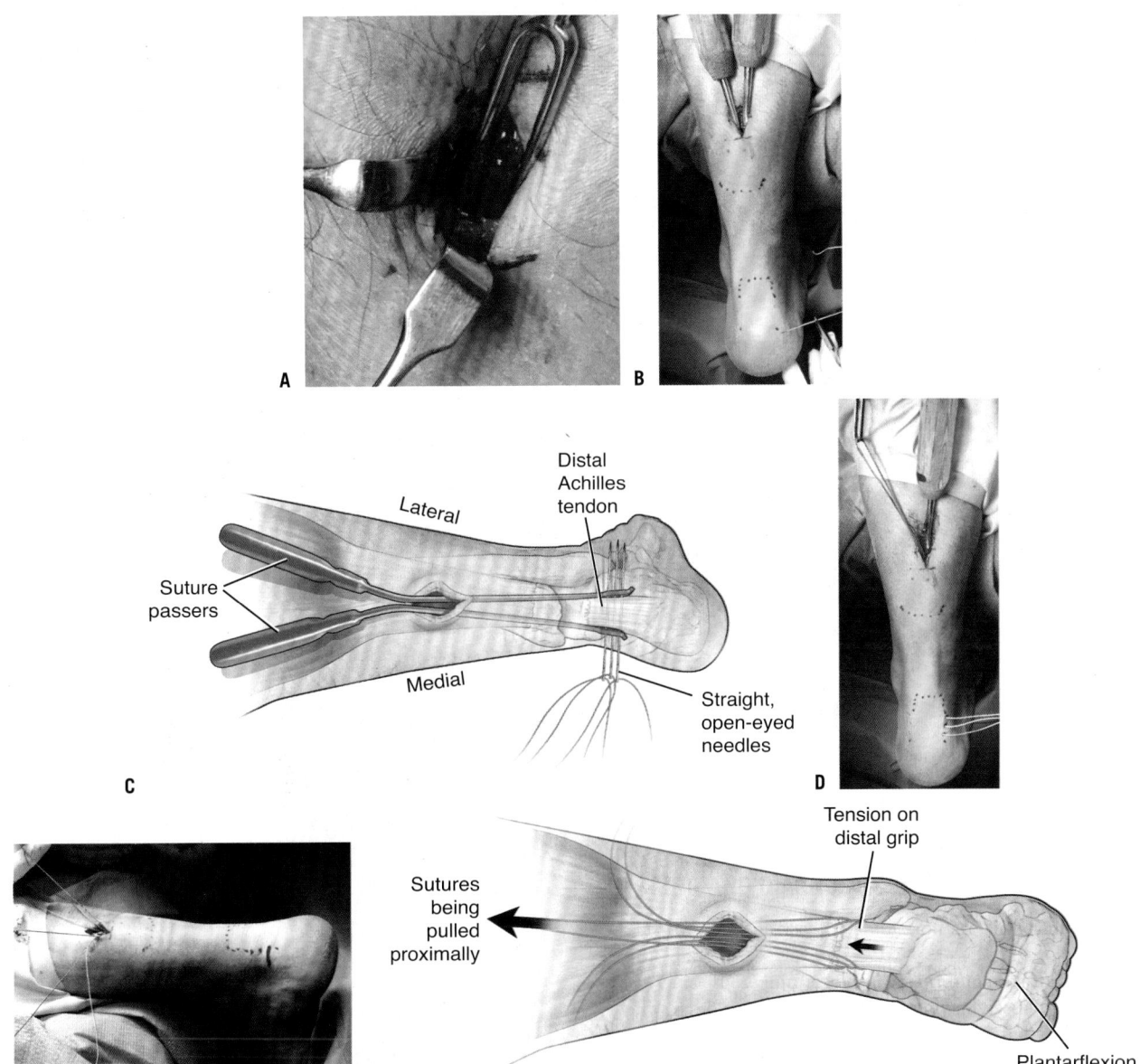

TECH FIG 2 A. One of the suture passers is introduced through the interval between the superficial fascia and the paratenon, being helped by a soft tissue retractor. The suture passer should be introduced gently and superficially, trying to avoid damaging the paratenon and aiming toward either the dorsomedial or dorsolateral aspects of the distal Achilles tendon. **B.** After getting as near as possible to the calcaneal Achilles tendon insertion, the second suture passer is introduced in the same way and both are held as distal as possible in symmetric positions. Twisting the instruments will allow to appreciate the orientation of the distal aspect of the instrument with its hollow slot, which will be the aiming point of the straight needles to be used in the next step. **C.** Three straight, open-eyed needles, each with an independent 2-0 polyblend suture, are passed from one side of the ankle, through the Achilles tendon and through both suture passers and out through the skin on the opposite side. Care has to be taken to ensure correct aiming of the needles through the suture passers. This can be achieved by twisting each suture passer and observing the corresponding twist of the needles. Pulling or pushing the suture passer will correspondingly bend the needles, which is another method to ensure correct positioning of the sutures. After this is done, the needles are passed through and disengaged from the sutures. **D.** One of the suture passers is retrieved from the proximal incision, pulling all three sutures with it, taking care to hold the opposite suture ends with one hand. Then, the second suture passer is retrieved in the same way, finally retrieving all three sutures through the proximal incision. **E.** Correct identification of the sutures is performed, matching one end on one side of the repair with its opposite. In this way, all three sutures are identified and kept apart correspondingly. It is of no importance which suture is the most distal one or the most proximal one. **F.** Each of the sutures is tested, pulling each pair of limbs proximally in order to test the distal grip on the tendon. It is vital to perform this test, as this will tension the distal grip and assure the suture was passed through a healthy portion of the tendon. On the picture, plantarflexion is achieved by pulling on one pair of limbs of a suture, and this test is repeated for each of the three sutures.

TECHNIQUES

TYING THE SUTURES AND COMPLETION

- The sutures are driven through the proximal stump with an open-eyed tapered needle, one at a time, in a crisscross fashion, grabbing the paratenon and tendon underneath as one layer, suturing them consecutively, and assuring that at least 5 degrees of additional plantarflexion is achieved compared to the normal physiologic equinus **(TECH FIG 3A–C)**.
- One of the threads of the polyblend suture is used with an eyed needle to drive and hide underneath the paratenon the bulk of the knots.

- The superficial fascia is closed with interrupted 3-0 Vicryl sutures, so as to cover the knots with the fascia. Subcutaneous layer and skin are closed afterward **(TECH FIG 3D)**.
- A CAM walker is applied keeping the ankle in 30 degrees of equinus, which corresponds to 3 cm of surgical towels. An alternative is a hinged CAM walker boot, which is our preference now.

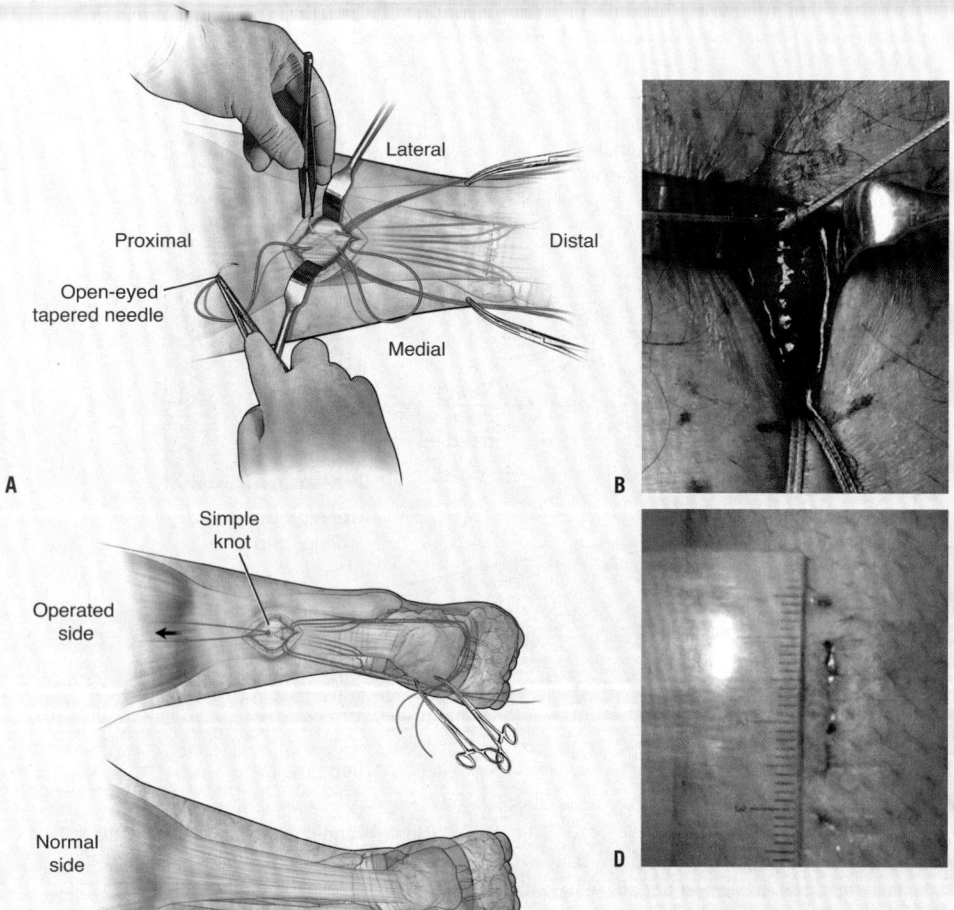

TECH FIG 3 A. With an open-eyed tapered needle, one limb of each suture is passed in a crisscross fashion from distal–medial to proximal–lateral (or the opposite depending on the suture position relative to the tendon) and the opposite is done with the other limb of the suture. **B.** A double surgeon knot is done and tied over the paratenon and slid distally until the knot reaches the distalmost aspect of the incision, helping gently the ankle to achieve plantarflexion. **C.** After the first knot is initially tied, a correct physiologic equinus position of the ankle has to be achieved, adjusting the tension as needed in order to achieve 5 degrees in excess of plantarflexion. Five additional simple knots are added after each initial double knot. All three sutures are tied the same way assuring that not more equinus is produced, as this may create too much tension in one of the sutures. Attention is placed on trying to hide each knot by pulling one limb of the knot with an open-eyed needle under the paratenon. **D.** The superficial fascia is closed with interrupted 4-0 Vicryl sutures, and the skin is closed with intradermal 4-0 Monocryl.

Pearls and Pitfalls

Sutures Passed Distally Did Not Grab the Distal Stump	• Make sure the straight needles really go through the suture passers. A twisting motion of the instrument will bend the needle and confirm the correct position. Pulling and pushing the suture passers should deform consequently the needle, also as a confirmation of the correct needle position.
Sutures Slipped Proximally When Testing the Distal Grip	• Probably due to a too superficial or deep pass of the sutures. When piercing the distal end of the tendon, make sure to palpate the tendon and have a feel of how superficial it is.
Irregular Tension of One of the Sutures	• The first suture sets the equinus position of the ankle. The second suture should be sutured in order to obtain tension but not increase equinus. It should be tied until it deforms slightly the visible paratenon.

POSTOPERATIVE CARE

- The ankle is protected in equinus position in a removable boot, allowing weight bearing as tolerated for 2 weeks.
- At the second week, dorsiflexion active motion is allowed to obtain as close to 90 degrees of dorsiflexion, basically to avoid stiffness and scar adherence.
- Stitches are removed at 2 weeks postoperatively.
- Patients are stimulated to bear weight as tolerated and get rid of crutches as soon as the second week postoperatively.
- Generally, full weight bearing is achieved at the end of the third week, and physiotherapy is started.
- The boot is removed at the end of the sixth week. Impact sports are allowed after 12 weeks from surgery.
- Return to sports is achieved at 5 months postoperatively.

OUTCOMES

- We reported on 100 consecutive patients with acute Achilles ruptures, operated with the minimally invasive technique described, with a mean follow-up of 42.1 months.[3]
  - The mean time to return to work was 56.0 days, and the mean time to return to sports was 18.9 weeks.
  - The mean American Orthopaedic Foot & Ankle Society score was 97.7; 98% of patients were satisfied.
  - The isokinetic evaluation showed good recovery of the involved muscles.
- It is worth to mention that instruments are reusable and in this way less costly than the most commonly used devices for percutaneous Achilles tendon ruptures.
- These results and the lack of complications compare favorably with other published series.

COMPLICATIONS

- No complications regarding soft tissues and sural nerve damage were reported nor was there any need to remove sutures.
- Two reruptures and five cases of deep venous thrombosis were observed.

REFERENCES

1. Amlang MH, Christiani P, Heinz P, et al. Percutaneous technique for Achilles tendon repair with the Dresden instruments [in German]. Unfallchirurg 2005;108(7):529–536.
2. Grassi A, Amendola A, Samuelsson K, et al. Minimally invasive versus open repair for acute Achilles tendon rupture: meta-analysis showing reduced complications, with similar outcomes, after minimally invasive surgery. J Bone Joint Surg Am 2018;100:1969–1981.
3. Keller A, Ortiz C, Wagner E, et al. Mini-open tenorrhaphy of acute Achilles tendon ruptures: medium-term follow-up of 100 cases. Am J Sports Med 2014;42(3):731–736.
4. Maffulli N, Ajis A. Management of chronic ruptures of the Achilles tendon. J Bone Joint Surg Am 2008;90(6):1348–1360.
5. Movin T, Ryberg A, McBride DJ, et al. Acute rupture of the Achilles tendon. Foot Ankle Clin 2005;10:331–356.
6. O'Brien M. The anatomy of the Achilles tendon. Foot Ankle Clin 2005;10(2):225–238.
7. Patel M, Kadakia A. Minimally invasive treatments of acute Achilles tendon ruptures. Foot Ankle Clin 2019;24(3):399–424.
8. Rees JD, Maffulli N, Cook J. Management of tendinopathy. Am J Sports Med 2009;37(9):1855–1867.
9. Soroceanu A, Sidhwa F, Aarabi S, et al. Surgical versus nonsurgical treatment of acute Achilles tendon rupture: a meta-analysis of randomized trials. J Bone Joint Surg Am 2012;94(23):2136–2143.

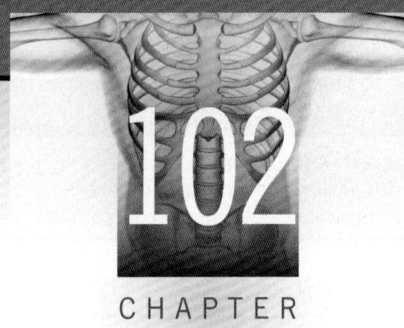

CHAPTER 102

Percutaneous Achilles Tendon Repair: Perspective 1

Karen M. Sutton, Sandra L. Tomak, Kristin C. Caolo, and Mark C. Drakos

DEFINITION

- Achilles tendon ruptures typically occur about 2 to 6 cm proximal to the tendon's insertion site on the calcaneus.
- This injury is relatively common among both high-performance athletes and the recreational athlete, particularly the "weekend warrior."
- Ruptures occur most often in men between 30 and 50 years of age; Achilles tendon ruptures have a large male predominance with a male-to-female ratio ranging from 5.5:1 to 30:1.[18,51]
- Percutaneous Achilles tendon repair is a minimally invasive procedure that can be used instead of the open Achilles tendon repair and involves a small incision and the use of a metal jig to pass locking and nonlocking sutures.

ANATOMY

- Tendinous portions of the gastrocnemius and soleus muscles coalesce to form the Achilles tendon (**FIG 1**).

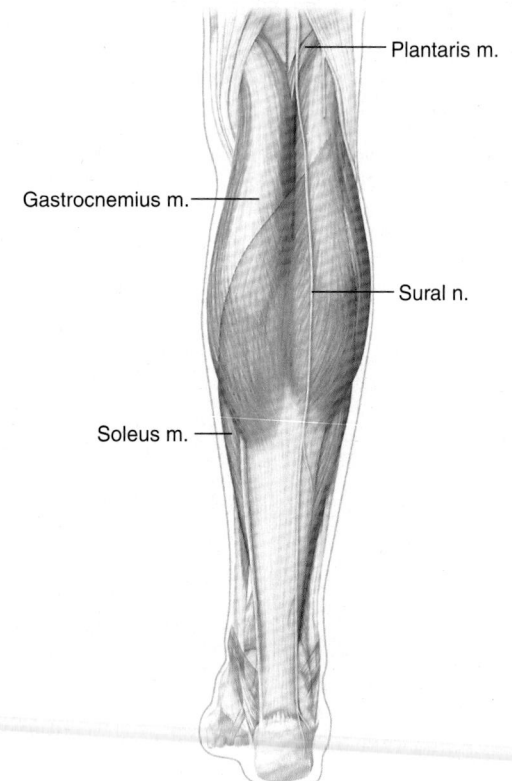

FIG 1 Merging of the gastrocnemius and soleus muscles to form the Achilles tendon.

Plantaris m.

Gastrocnemius m.

Sural n.

Soleus m.

- The plantaris muscle is a distinct entity medial to the Achilles tendon but is absent in 10% to 20% of limbs and is often ruptured with the Achilles.[45]
- The Achilles tendon originates as a band proximally on the posterior surface of its muscle, and the gastrocnemius tendon emerges from the distal margin of the muscle bellies.
- The length of the tendon formed from the gastrocnemius and soleus range from 11 to 26 cm and 3 to 11 cm, respectively.
- Viewed from proximal to distal, the Achilles tendon progressively becomes thinner in its anteroposterior dimensions, particularly from 4 cm proximal to the calcaneus to its insertion on the calcaneus, it also rotates through 90 degrees as it descends.[13,40]
- The Achilles is a viscoelastic tissue.[48] Ninety-five percent of the tendon collagen is type I collagen; a small percentage is elastic. Seventy percent of the dry weight of the tendon is collagen.[39,44]
- The blood supply to the Achilles tendon arises from the musculotendinous junction, the osseous insertion, and multiple mesotenal vessels.
- The tendon is most poorly vascularized at its midportion, receiving its blood supply from the paratenon.[44] The mesotenal vessels decrease in number 2 to 6 cm proximal to the osseous insertion.[47] The lack of vascular perfusion makes the tendon susceptible to injury and reduced healing.[10] Injuries at this location in the tendon almost always heal, but the midportion of the tendon is a common site for Achilles tendinosis.[34,38]
- The Achilles tendon receives much of its nutrition from the tenosynovial fluid that bathes the tendon and is contained within the paratenon.

PATHOGENESIS

- Ruptures occur most commonly during athletic activities, especially during eccentric exercises such as coming out of a backpedal.
- The most common sports for sports-related Achilles tears are basketball as the most common, followed by soccer, tennis and racquet sports, football, baseball, and volleyball.[7,53] The injury mechanisms and activities causing Achilles tendon ruptures change with age groups as well.[33]
- Ruptures are most common in "weekend warrior" recreational athletes who are active intermittently.
- Hyperpronation is associated with Achilles tendon injuries.[43]
- Inconsistent training, including sudden increases in training intensity; excessive training, training on hard surfaces; and running on sloping, hard, or slippery roads, have been implicated in Achilles tendon problems.[43]

- Mechanisms of injury, leading to eccentric loads on the Achilles tendon, include pushing off with the weight-bearing forefoot while extending the knee, unexpected dorsiflexion of the ankle, or violent dorsiflexion of a plantarflexed foot.[2]
- With normal aging, the Achilles tendon decreases in cell density, collagen fibril diameter and density, and fiber waviness. These changes may make the aging athlete more susceptible to injury.[47]
- Spontaneous rupture of the Achilles tendon has been associated with corticosteroid injections,[31] inflammatory or autoimmune conditions,[17,36] collagen abnormalities,[15] infectious diseases,[3] neurologic conditions,[36] kidney transplant recipients,[28] long-term dialysis,[28] and fluoroquinolone use.[42]

PATIENT HISTORY AND PHYSICAL FINDINGS

- The patient reports sudden pain in the affected leg.
- Some patients recall an audible pop or snap.
- With Achilles tendon ruptures, patients occasionally experience a sensation as though they were "kicked," "hit," or "shot" in the injured calf.
- Patients can often still bear weight and flex their ankle after an Achilles tendon rupture. They can ambulate but are unable to push-off; their ankle passively dorsiflexes.
- Physical examination should include the following:
  - Palpation of gap: Palpate along the posterior aspect of the lower leg, and a gap may be felt along the course of the tendon.
    - Positive: appreciable gap
  - Thompson test: With the patient prone and with feet off of the table, squeeze the proximal portion of the calf.
    - Positive: no plantarflexion of the ankle
    - False-positive results may be obtained with an intact plantaris tendon.
  - Knee flexion test: With the patient in prone position, actively flex both knees to 90 degrees.
    - Positive: asymmetric resting tension of both ankles; the affected foot may even fall into neutral or dorsiflexion.

IMAGING AND OTHER DIAGNOSTIC STUDIES

- Plain radiographs
  - In a lateral radiograph, the fat-filled triangular space (ie, Kager triangle) anterior to the Achilles tendon and between the posterior aspect of the tibia and the superior aspect of the calcaneus loses its regular configuration.
  - Preoperative lateral radiographs can be analyzed to detect the presence of bony avulsion fragments from an insertional tear as well as a posterior calcaneal tuberosity fracture or midsubstance calcium deposits, which would indicate tendinopathy in the tendon.[29]
- Magnetic resonance imaging (MRI) **(FIG 2)**
  - T1- and T2-weighted images in the axial and sagittal planes should be used to evaluate Achilles tendon ruptures.
    - T1 weighted: A complete rupture of the Achilles tendon is identified as a disruption of the signal within the tendon.
    - T2 weighted: A complete rupture is demonstrated as a generalized increase in signal intensity, and the edema and hemorrhage at the site of the rupture are seen as an area of high signal intensity.[30]
  - Helpful in surgical planning for insertion and avulsion tears

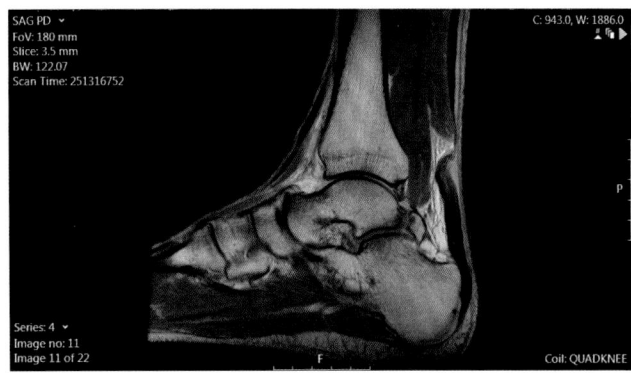

FIG 2 T1-weighted MRI scan showing complete Achilles tendon rupture 8.1 cm away from its calcaneal insertion near the myotendinous junction.

  - Can be used for chronic ruptures, tendinopathy, proximal tears of musculotendinous junction
  - MRI can be used to find extensive tendon degeneration that has implications for optimal surgical treatment.[4]
  - Physical exam diagnosis takes precedence over MRI diagnosis as MRI only has a sensitivity of 90.9% for the interpretation of a complete tear when measured against intraoperative observation, whereas the sensitivity of a physical exam (including positive Thompson test, palpable defect, and decreased resting ankle tension) is 100% for interpreting a complete tear.[19]
- Ultrasound
  - Useful because it can be performed in the office setting
  - Rupture seen as an acoustic vacuum with thick irregular edges
  - May also be used for postoperative evaluation to assess the structure of the tendon and integrity of repair[35]
  - Nonoperatively treated Achilles tendons have a different sonographic appearance than operatively treated tendons.[24]
  - Ultrasound can differentiate full-thickness Achilles tears from partial-thickness tears or tendinosis with 92% accuracy.[22]

DIFFERENTIAL DIAGNOSIS

- Typically, acute rupture of the Achilles tendon does not have a large differential diagnosis.
- Because four other muscles plantarflex the ankle, Achilles tendon ruptures may be initially mistaken for ankle sprains; although increasingly less common, it has been reported that up to 20% of Achilles tendon ruptures may be missed by the first doctor to examine the patient.[29] Since the advent of urgent care centers, patients require urgent follow-up with an orthopaedic surgeon or musculoskeletal specialist.

NONOPERATIVE MANAGEMENT

- Weeks 0 to 2: Immediately after injury, patients are placed in a posterior slab/splint and are non–weight bearing with crutches.
- Weeks 2 to 4: Patients are placed in an Aircast walking boot with a 2-cm heel lift; they are to follow protected weight bearing with crutches. Patients can actively plantarflex and dorsiflex to neutral and invert and evert below neutral. At physical therapy, they can undergo modalities to control swelling and incision mobilization as well as do hip and knee exercises

with no ankle involvement such as leg lifts from sitting, prone, or side-lying position. Patients can do non–weight-bearing fitness and cardiovascular exercises such as bicycling with one leg or deep-water running as well as hydrotherapy.

- Weeks 4 to 6: Patients are weight bearing as tolerated and can follow the protocol from weeks 2 to 4.
- Weeks 6 to 8: Remove the heel lift from the boot; patients are weight bearing as tolerated. They can do slow dorsiflexion stretching; graduated resistance exercises (open and closed kinetic chain as well as functional activities); proprioceptive and gait retraining; modalities such as ice, heat, and ultrasound as indicated; and incision mobilization. Patients can also do fitness and cardiovascular exercises to include weight bearing as tolerated such as bicycling, elliptical machine, walking and/or running on a treadmill, using the StairMaster, as well as doing hydrotherapy.
- Weeks 8 to 12: Patients can begin to wean off of the boot; they can return to using crutches or a cane as necessary and gradually wean off of it. Continue to progress range of motion, strength, and proprioception.
- >Week 12: Continue to progress range of motion, strength, and proprioception. Retrain strength, power, and endurance. Increase dynamic weight-bearing exercise and include plyometric training and sport specific retraining.[53]
- Considered for elderly or sedentary patients, poor surgical candidates (vascular compromise and/or poor skin quality), patients favoring nonoperative treatment, or patients who are diabetic[46] or are smokers[1]
- In studies comparing rerupture rates in patients with operative or nonoperative management, rerupture rates have been steadily decreasing in patients undergoing nonoperative treatment **(TABLE 1)**.
  - Hufner et al[27] examined the cases of 168 patients with less than 10 mm of gap with the foot in neutral position and complete apposition of the tendon stumps in 20 degrees of plantarflexion as observed on ultrasound. They found a rerupture rate of 6.4% with 92 patients (73.5%) reporting good or better results at 5.5 years postinjury.[27]
  - Kotnis et al[32] examined the use of ultrasound in patients with a 5-mm gap or more in their Achilles tendon with foot in equinus who were treated either operatively or nonoperatively. Operative treatment had a rerupture rate

of 1.5%; nonoperative treatment had a rerupture rate of 3.4% (not statistically significant). There were also no statistically significant differences between groups in complications such as chronic pain, numbness, wound infection, or deep venous thrombosis.[32]
- Willits et al[53] conducted a randomized study in which patients diagnosed with Achilles tendon rupture were assigned to operative or nonoperative treatment paired with accelerated functional rehabilitation. Rerupture occurred in two patients in the operative group (2.7%) and in three patients in the nonoperative group (4.2%).[53]
- Barfod et al[5] compared immediate weight-bearing and non–weight-bearing protocols in nonoperative Achilles tendon ruptures.
  - Patients in the intervention group were weight bearing immediately, whereas the control group was weight bearing after 6 weeks.
  - The weight-bearing group was found to have better health-related quality of life at 12 months.
  - The mean Achilles Tendon Total Rupture Score (ATRS) at 12 months and the total heel-rise work performed by the injured limb relative to the uninjured limb had no significant differences between groups.
  - There were three reruptures in the weight-bearing group and two reruptures in the control group.
  - Immediate weight bearing can be a recommended option in nonoperative Achilles tendon rupture recovery.

SURGICAL MANAGEMENT

- In our hands, percutaneous repair can be used for acute tears, a minimal tendon gap, and compliant patients.
- The procedure should occur ideally 7 to 14 days postinjury.[16]
- Advantages of percutaneous repair are as follows:
  - Low risk of wound complications
  - Preservation of blood supply for tendon healing
  - Performed as outpatient procedure
  - Uses neuraxial block as anesthetic
  - Maintenance of tendon length
  - Earlier return to function when compared to closed treatment
  - Improved cost-effectiveness over open repair[8]

TABLE 1 Summary of Nonoperative Repair Studies

Study	Evidence Level	N	Age[a]	Male[b] (%)	Most Common Activity (%)	Sport Injury (%)	Injury to Surgery (days)	Follow-up (years)	Return to Baseline (%)	Complication (%)	Rerupture (%)	Sural Nerve Injury (%)	ATRS	AOFAS AHS
Willits et al[53]	I	72	41.1 (8)	81.9	Racket sport (33.3)	—	—	—	—	8.3	4.2	—	—	—
Kotnis et al[32]	II	58	43.9	70.4	—	77.6	—	—	—	6.9	3.4	0	—	—
Hufner et al[27]	III	168	39.8	84	—	—	—	5	73.5	18.4	6.4	0	—	—

ATRS, Achilles Tendon Total Rupture Score; AOFAS, American Orthopaedic Foot and Ankle Society; AHS, Ankle-Hindfoot Scale.
[a]Mean (standard deviation).
[b]Percentage male may apply to the whole study sample and not those patients only receiving nonoperative repair.

- Smaller mean scar length (2.9 vs. 9.5 cm)[23]
- Faster return to sport and athletic activities[37]
- Disadvantages include the following:
  - Potential sural nerve injury
  - Limited patient population
  - Need for compliance postoperatively
- Percutaneous repair is contraindicated in chronic tears, tendon gap, noncompliant patients, and high-level athletes (relative).

Positioning

- Prone position with feet hanging off of the table with a small bump under the anterior aspect of the ankle to adjust the amount of ankle plantarflexion during the operation[25]
- Thigh tourniquet is placed while the patient is supine before flipping the patient prone.
- Injured foot is placed in about 25 degrees of plantarflexion.
- The repair is performed under neuraxial block.

INCISION AND SETUP

- Measure and mark a 2.5-cm incision over the defect in the center of the tendon **(TECH FIG 1)**.
- A 15-blade knife is used to incise the skin and subcutaneous tissues.
- A 2.5-cm incision is made through the paratenon followed by evacuation of a hematoma and confirmation of the location of the tendon tear.
- An Allis clamp is inserted into the tendon sheath and grabs the proximal stump to pull it approximately 1 cm through the wound; if the rupture site has frayed ends, the proximal tendon may need to be grabbed greater than 1 cm.

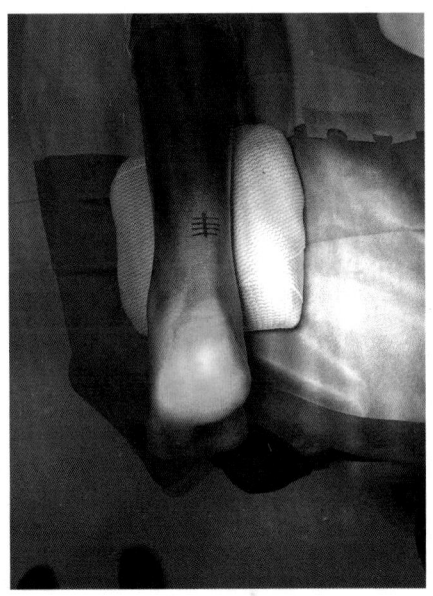

TECH FIG 1 Patient is in prone position with feet hanging off of the table and a small bump placed under the anterior aspect of the ankle. A 2.5-cm incision is made medial to the midline. Dissection is completed through layers of skin and subcutaneous tissue. Blunt dissection is carried out to the level of the peritenon, which is incised sharply in line with its fibers. This is followed by mobilization of the tendon ends.

PARS JIG INSERTION AND SUTURE PASSING (TECH FIG 2)

- Test the percutaneous Achilles repair system (PARS) jig to make sure the prongs open and close smoothly as well as test that the needles pass freely through the jig.
- The PARS jig is inserted through the wound with the prongs in the narrowest opening possible.
- The jig is slid proximally along the tendon with the prongs gradually opening, the jig is then slid back and forth a few times to ensure placement within the paratenon sheath and around the tendon. There will be minimal resistance during insertion once in the correct location. The proximal tendon can be palpated through the skin to check for the centering of the tendon in the jig.
- The jig needs to be stabilized in a central position, making sure that it does not rotate medially or laterally. This will help to prevent sutures from missing the tendon causing iatrogenic injury to the medial neurovascular bundle or sural nerve.

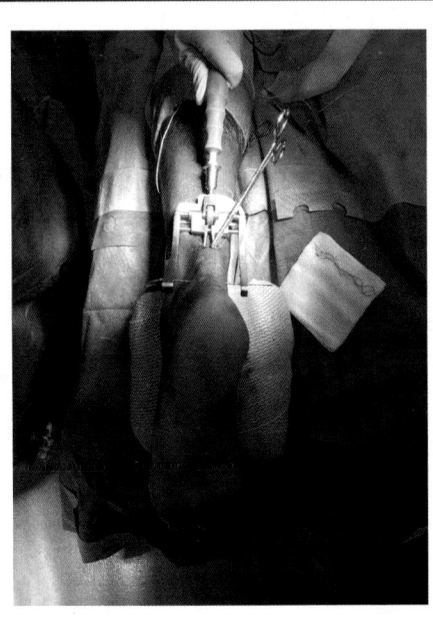

TECH FIG 2 A PARS jig is inserted into the incision starting in the narrowest position. The tendon is then tagged percutaneously with locking and nonlocking sutures.

SUTURING

- Insert needles 1 and 2 without sutures into the jig and through the tendon to maintain two points of fixation between the tendon and jig.
- Use no. 2 FiberWire (Arthrex, Inc., Naples, FL) sutures in multiple colors (blue, white, green stripe, black stripe).
- The first suture (blue) is put through the first hole with the assistance of the needle suture passer, making sure the length is even on both sides. The first suture is then passed through the third hole following an oblique orientation before passing the second suture (white).

- The third and fourth sutures (green stripe) have a loop at one end and a tail on the other; they are passed through a crossing pattern in a slightly oblique direction.
- The fifth suture (black stripe) is passed directly across the tendon like the first suture.
- The sixth and seventh holes in the jig are reserved for heavy laborers, morbidly obese patients, or elite athletes. They can pass additional looped sutures, creating an additional locking suture near the rupture site.

JIG REMOVAL AND LOCKING SUTURE CREATION (TECH FIG 3)

- To remove the jig, first remove the Allis clamp and then apply gentle, even tension distally while also closing the prongs.
- Confirm that sutures are pulled through the wound by the jig. Remove any frayed tendon fragments using pickups.
- Gently pull on both sides of all five sutures to ensure fixation and proximal tendon control.
- If any sutures pull out of the tendon, the tendon was not centered in the jig, and all sutures must be removed, and the jig must be reinserted.
- Place the following sutures spread apart on the medial and lateral sides from proximal to distal in order of blue, white, looped green stripe, tail green stripe, and black stripe.
- Loop the white suture twice distally around the two green stripe sutures and then back through the looped end of the green stripe suture. To create a locking suture, pull the green stripe tail from each side through the tendon onto the opposite side.
- After the suture passing is complete, there should be two nonlocking sutures (blue and black stripe) and one locking suture (white) through the tendon. To confirm that the sutures are securely fixed within the proximal tendon, pull on each pair of suture ends to remove the remaining slack.
- The distal jig is inserted, and sutures are passed following the same steps for the proximal jig insertion.

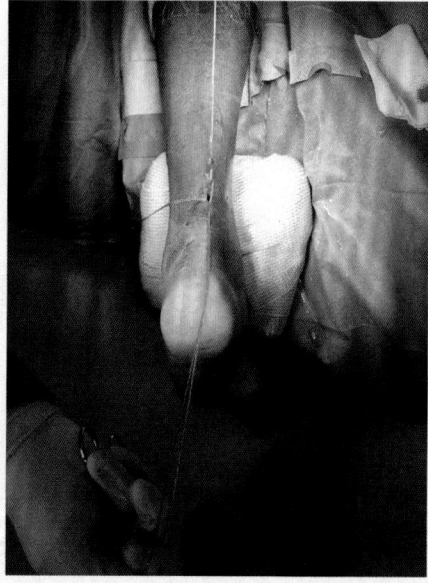

TECH FIG 3 After removal of the PARS jig, sutured ends of the tendon are tied together.

ACHILLES TENSIONING AND CLOSING (TECH FIG 4)

- Place the ankle in maximum plantarflexion to obtain a secure end-to-end repair during suture tying. Tie the sutures starting with those farthest from the rupture site and finish with those closest to the rupture site.
- The first nonlocking suture that is tied is a stay stitch and will slide. The locking suture will not slide.
  - Pull all remaining slack within the suture and secure them with five to six surgeon's knots.
  - After irrigation, check suture knots with a small hemostat to ensure they will not cause skin irritation.

- Following completion of the suture tying, the ankle should remain in plantarflexion with improved resting tension and have a negative Thompson test.
- The paratenon should be closed with 2-0 Vicryl, and subcutaneous tissue should be closed with 3-0 Monocryl. Skin is closed with 3-0 Nylon sutures followed by placement of a non–weight-bearing splint with the ankle in resting plantar flexion.[25]

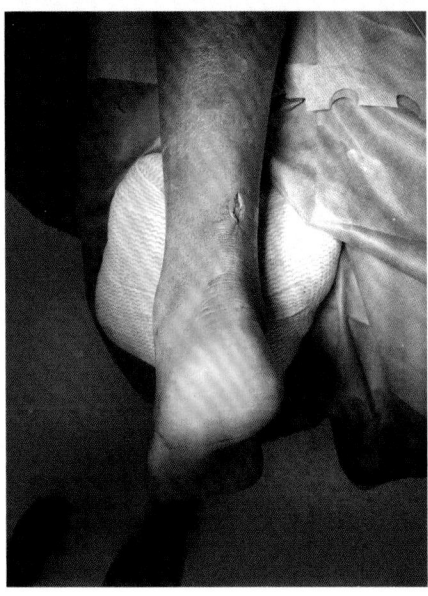

TECH FIG 4 After suturing of the tendon is completed, the paratenon is sutured closed followed by subcutaneous tissue closure. Following closure of the skin, patient is placed into a non–weight-bearing splint in plantarflexion for 2 weeks postoperatively.

TECHNIQUES

Pearls and Pitfalls

- Physical exam (including positive Thompson test, palpable defect, and decreased resting ankle tension) is the most accurate way to diagnose a complete tear.[19]
- PARS jig allows for smaller incisions and minimal soft-tissue disruption leading to fewer wound complications.
- Know sural nerve location as, often, it is not visualized during the operation.
- Avoid use in patients with chronic tears, tendon gap, and noncompliant patients.
- Complications can include rerupture, sural nerve injury, palpable suture knot, and deep venous thrombosis.[5]

POSTOPERATIVE CARE

- Weeks 1 to 2: Patients are kept in a plantar flexion non–weight-bearing splint.
- Weeks 3 to 6: Patients are weight bearing as tolerated in a boot with a heel lift.
- Weeks 7 to 12: Patients are weight bearing as tolerated in a boot without a heel lift.
- Months 6 to 9: Patients can progress return to sport, with the understanding that they will not be at full capacity until a year.
- Patel et al[41] described allowing patients to immediately bear weight on a percutaneous Achilles tendon repair.
  - Postoperatively, patients were placed in a plantigrade short-leg cast and allowed immediate weight bearing.
  - At week 2, patients were in a plantigrade walking boot and encouraged to ambulate to tolerance and start Thera-Band exercises.
  - At week 6, physical therapy is started with range of motion and strengthening.
  - The average American Orthopaedic Foot and Ankle Society (AOFAS) scale was 96 (range, 81 to 100) points. Ninety percent of patients were able to return to desired level of activity.
- De la Fuente et al[14] found that 20 patients who had undergone aggressive therapy using early progressive controlled mobilization had higher ATRS, lower verbal pain scores, an earlier return to work, and higher tendon strength.

OUTCOMES

- Retrospective review of 10 consecutive patients with acute Achilles tendon ruptures[49]:
  - No reruptures
  - No major complications
  - One sural nerve injury
  - Mean return to full activity at 6.1 months
  - AOFAS ankle hindfoot rating: average score, 94
  - Mean difference of 1.58 cm in calf circumference, with the involved leg having the smaller circumference
  - Mean plantarflexion peak torque of the uninvolved leg and the involved leg of 67.8 and 52.8 ft-lb, respectively (at a speed of 30 degrees per second)
- Comparative studies of percutaneous versus open Achilles tendon repair **(TABLES 2** and **3)**
  - Haji et al[21] reported mean operative times of 28.5 and 25.9 minutes (statistically significant) and rerupture rates of 2.6% versus 5.7% (not statistically significant), respectively, for percutaneous versus open repair.
  - Cretnik et al[12] noted significant increased tendon thickness and increased loss of dorsiflexion in the openly treated patients.
    - Out of 132 percutaneously repaired tendons, 1 patient (0.7%) sustained a complete rerupture, and 4 patients (3%) sustained a partial rupture, compared with 3 (2.8%) and 0 patients, respectively, in the open repair group.

TABLE 2 Summary of Percutaneous Achilles Repair System (PARS) Studies

Study	Evidence Level	N	Age[a]	Male[b] (%)	Most Common Activity (%)	Sport Injury (%)	Injury to Surgery (days)[a]	Follow-up (weeks)[a]	Return to Baseline (%)	Complication (%)	Rerupture (%)	Sural Nerve Injury (%)	ATRS[a]	AOFAS AHS
Hsu et al[26]	III	101	40 (10)	86.5	Basketball (39)	—	6 (3)	34 (24)	98	5	0	0	—	—
Chiu et al[11]	IV	19	38.7	94.7	Judo (31.6)	100	5.8	96	95	16	0	—	—	92
Maffuli et al[38]	IV	27	73.4 (8.7)	76.3	Golf (25.9)	68.6	2	196	50	60	7	11	69.4 (14)	—
Carmont et al[9]	IV	73	45.5 (11.6)	82.2	Football (22)	85	6 (3.7)	—	—	13.7	1.4	5.5	89 (18)[c]	—
Bisaccia et al[6]	II	20	53	71.4	—	—	—	—	—	0	0	0	87.67 (2.3)	—
Ververidis et al[50]	I	670	36.9	—	—	—	—	—	—	11.3	2.1	3.3	89	96.1
Wagnon and Akayi[52]	II	22	43	85.7	Football (37)	58	—	160	40	4.6	4.6	0	—	—
Haji et al[21]	III	38	41.4	71.3	—	48.3	—	—	—	26.3	2.6	10.5	—	—
Cretnik et al[12]	II	132	40.3	93.9	Soccer (41)	78	2.1	3, 6, 8, 12	—	9.7	3.7	4.5	—	96.3

ATRS, Achilles Tendon Total Rupture Score; AOFAS, American Orthopaedic Foot and Ankle Society; AHS, Ankle-Hindfoot Scale.
[a]Mean (standard deviation).
[b]Percentage male may apply to the whole study sample and not those patients only receiving PARS.
[c]At 1-year postoperation.

TABLE 3 Summary of Open Repair Studies

Study	Evidence Level	N	Age[a]	Male[b] (%)	Most Common Activity (%)	Sport Injury (%)	Injury to Surgery (days)[a]	Follow-up (weeks)[a]	Return to Baseline (%)	Complication (%)	Rerupture (%)	Sural Nerve Injury (%)	ATRS[a]	AOFAS AHS
Hsu et al[26]	III	169	41 (10)	86.5	Basketball (47)	—	10 (6)	37 (56)	82	10.6	0	3	—	—
Bisaccia et al[6]	II	36	53	71.4	—	—	—	—	—	0	0	—	85.2 (1.93)	—
Wagnon and Akayi[52]	II	35	43	85.7	Football (47)	—	—	160	40	14.3	5.7	0	—	—
Haji et al[21]	III	70	42.3	71.3	—	58	—	—	—	15.7	5.7	1.4	—	—
Cretnik et al[12]	II	105	37.6	94.3	Soccer (51)	48.3	1.4	3, 6, 8, 12	—	21.3	2.8	2.8	—	—
Willits et al[53]	I	72	39.7 (11)	81.9	Racket sport (33.3)	65	—	—	—	18.1	2.8	—	—	96.1

ATRS, Achilles Tendon Total Rupture Score; AOFAS, American Orthopaedic Foot and Ankle Society; AHS, Ankle-Hindfoot Scale.
[a]Mean (standard deviation).
[b]Percentage male may apply to the whole study sample and not those patients only receiving open repair surgery.

- Sural nerve injury occurred in 6 patients (4.5%) in the percutaneous repair group and 3 patients (2.8%) in the open repair group.
  - Hsu et al[26] found an overall complication rate of 8.5% with no reruptures, with 88% of patients returning to baseline activities.
    - Percutaneous repairs were associated with a 5.0% complication rate, and open repairs were associated with a 10.6% complication rate (not statistically significant).
    - Percutaneous repairs had a 98% return to baseline physical activities, compared to the open repair, which had 82% of patients return to baseline activities.
  - Chiu et al[11] found that 18 out of 19 patients (95%) who had percutaneous Achilles repairs returned to baseline sporting activity.
- Wagnon and Akayi[52] compared the Webb-Bannister percutaneous technique to open repair.
  - The open repair group had an 8.6% incidence of wound complications (no wound dehiscence occurred in the percutaneous repair group).
  - Two patients out of 35 experienced rerupture after open repair; 1 patient (out of 22) experienced a rerupture after percutaneous repair.
  - Patients returned to work a mean of 4 months after open repair and 3.75 months after the Webb-Banister percutaneous repair.
  - No sural nerve complications occurred.
- Ververidis et al[50] reviewed 13 studies with 670 patients in total to evaluate percutaneous repairs in an athletic population:
  - There was a rerupture rate of 2.1%, and the rate of deep venous thrombosis was 0.6%.
  - Patients returned to previous level of athletic activity in 78% to 84% of cases; 91.4% of patients returned to some level of sporting activity.
- Maffulli et al[38] evaluated percutaneous repairs in a population of patients older than 65 years:
  - Only 50% of the athletic involved population returned to preinjury levels of activity.
  - They found an 11% incidence of superficial infection, 11% sural nerve injury, and 7% deep vein thrombosis.
- Bisaccia et al[6] reviewed 56 patients who underwent either open suture Achilles tendon repairs or percutaneous ultrasound-assisted repairs and found that ultrasound-assisted tenorrhaphy is a reliable treatment with good clinical outcomes including an average ATRS of 87.67 and a McComis score of 56.25.
- Carmont et al[9] evaluated 73 patient outcomes using ATRS at 3, 6, 9, 12 months postoperatively and found that ATRS improved over time, with a marked improvement in function occurring between 3 and 6 months postoperatively.
- Grassi et al[20] performed a meta-analysis of eight studies and 182 total patients and found that patients who had undergone minimally invasive surgery were more likely to report good or excellent subjective results.

COMPLICATIONS

- Sural nerve injury
- Palpable suture knot, which may necessitate excision
- Rerupture
- Deep venous thrombosis[5]

REFERENCES

1. Ağladıoğlu K, Akkaya N, Güngör HR, et al. Effects of cigarette smoking on elastographic strain ratio measurements of patellar and Achilles tendons. J Ultrasound Med 2016;35(11):2431–2438.
2. Arner O, Lindholm A. Subcutaneous rupture of the Achilles tendon; a study of 92 cases. Acta Chir Scand Suppl 1959;116(suppl 239):1–51.
3. Arner O, Lindholm A, Orell S. Histologic changes in subcutaneous rupture of the Achilles tendon; a study of 74 cases. Acta Chir Scand 1959;116:484–490.
4. Bäcker HC, Wong TT, Vosseller JT. MRI assessment of degeneration of the tendon in Achilles tendon ruptures. Foot Ankle Int 2019;40:895–899.
5. Barfod KW, Bencke J, Lauridsen HB, et al. Nonoperative dynamic treatment of acute Achilles tendon rupture: the influence of early weight-bearing on clinical outcome: a blinded, randomized controlled trial. J Bone Joint Surg Am 2014;96(18):1497–1503.
6. Bisaccia M, Rinonapoli G, Meccariello L, et al. Validity and reliability of mini-invasive surgery assisted by ultrasound in Achilles tendon rupture. Acta Inform Med 2019;27(1):40–44.
7. Caldwell JE, Lightsey HM, Trofa DP, et al. Seasonal variation of Achilles tendon injury. J Am Acad Orthop Surg Glob Res Rev 2018;2(8):e043.
8. Carmont M, Heaver C, Pradhan A, et al. Surgical repair of the ruptured Achilles tendon: the cost-effectiveness of open versus percutaneous repair. Knee Surg Sports Traumatol Arthrosc 2013;21:1361–1368.
9. Carmont MR, Silbernagel KG, Edge A, et al. Functional outcome of percutaneous Achilles repair: improvements in Achilles Tendon Total Rupture Score during the first year. Orthop J Sports Med 2013;1(1):2325967113494584.
10. Chen TM, Rozen WM, Pan W, et al. The arterial anatomy of the Achilles tendon: anatomical study and clinical implications. Clin Anat 2009;22(3):377–385.
11. Chiu C, Yeh W, Tsai M, et al. Endoscopy-assisted percutaneous repair of acute Achilles tendon tears. Foot Ankle Int 2013;34(8):1168–1176.
12. Cretnik A, Kosanovic M, Smrkolj V. Percutaneous versus open repair of the ruptured Achilles tendon: a comparative study. Am J Sports Med 2005;33:1369–1379.
13. Cummins E, Anson B. The structure of the calcaneal tendon (of Achilles) in relation to orthopedic surgery, with additional observations on the plantaris muscle. Surg Gynecol Obstet 1946;83:107–116.
14. De la Fuente C, Peña y Lillo R, Carreño G, et al. Prospective randomized clinical trial of aggressive rehabilitation after acute Achilles tendon ruptures repaired with Dresden technique. Foot 2016;26:15–22.
15. Dent CM, Graham GP. Osteogenesis imperfecta and Achilles tendon rupture. Injury 1991;22:239–240.
16. DeVries JG, Scharer BM, Summerhays BJ. Acute Achilles rupture percutaneous repair: approach, materials, techniques. Clin Podiatr Med Surg 2017;34(2):251–262.
17. Dodds WN, Burry HC. The relationship between Achilles tendon rupture and serum uric acid level. Injury 1984;16:94–95.
18. Egger AC, Berkowitz MJ. Achilles tendon injuries. Curr Rev Musculoskelet Med 2017;10(1):72–80.
19. Garras DN, Raikin SM, Bhat SB, et al. MRI is unnecessary for diagnosing acute Achilles tendon ruptures: clinical diagnostic criteria. Clin Orthop Relat Res 2012;470(8):2268–2273.
20. Grassi A, Amendola A, Samuelsson K, et al. Minimally invasive versus open repair for acute Achilles tendon rupture: meta-analysis showing reduced complications, with similar outcomes, after minimally invasive surgery. J Bone Joint Surg Am 2018;100(22):1969–1981.
21. Haji A, Sahai A, Symes A, et al. Percutaneous versus open tendo Achillis repair. Foot Ankle Int 2004;25:215–218.
22. Hartgerink P, Fessell DP, Jacobson JA, et al. Full- versus partial-thickness Achilles tendon tears: sonographic accuracy and characterization in 26 cases with surgical correlation. Radiology 2001;220(2):406–412.
23. Henriquez H, Munoz R, Carcuro G, et al. Is percutaneous repair better than open repair in acute Achilles tendon rupture? Clin Orthop Relat Res 2012;470(4):998–1003.
24. Hollenberg GM, Adams MJ, Weinberg EP. Sonographic appearance of nonoperatively treated Achilles tendon ruptures. Skeletal Radiol 2000;29(5):259–264.

25. Hsu AR, Anderson RB. Mini-open Achilles tendon rupture repair. Tech Foot Ankle Surg 2017;16(2):55–61.
26. Hsu AR, Jones CP, Cohen BE, et al. Clinical outcomes and complications of percutaneous Achilles repair system versus open technique for acute Achilles tendon ruptures. Foot Ankle Int 2015;36(11):1279–1286.
27. Hufner TM, Brandes DB, Thermann H, et al. Long-term results after functional nonoperative treatment of Achilles tendon rupture. Foot Ankle Int 2006;27(3):167–171.
28. Humbyrd CJ, Bae S, Kucirka LM, et al. Incidence, risk factors, and treatment of Achilles tendon rupture in patients with end-stage renal disease. Foot Ankle Int 2018;39(7):821–828.
29. Inglis AE, Scott WN, Sculco TP, et al. Ruptures of the tendo Achillis. An objective assessment of surgical and non-surgical treatment. J Bone Joint Surg Am 1976;58:990–993.
30. Kabbani YM, Mayer DP. Magnetic resonance imaging of tendon pathology about the foot and ankle. Part I. Achilles tendon. J Am Podiatr Med Assoc 1993;83:418–420.
31. Kennedy JC, Willis RB. The effects of local steroid injections on tendons: a biomechanical and microscopic correlative study. Am J Sports Med 1976;4:11–21.
32. Kotnis R, David S, Handley R, et al. Dynamic ultrasound as a selection tool for reducing Achilles tendon reruptures. Am J Sports Med 2006;34(9):1395–1400.
33. Lemme NJ, Li NY, DeFroda SF, et al. Epidemiology of Achilles tendon ruptures in the United States: athletic and nonathletic injuries from 2012 to 2016. Orthop J Sports Med 2018;6(11):2325967118808238.
34. Lopez RGL, Jung H-G. Achilles tendinosis: treatment options. Clin Orthop Surg 2015;7(1):1–7.
35. Maffulli N. Rupture of the Achilles tendon. J Bone Joint Surg Am 1999;81:1019–1036.
36. Maffulli N, Irwin AS, Kenward MG, et al. Achilles tendon rupture and sciatica: a possible correlation. Br J Sports Med 1998;32:174–177.
37. Maffulli N, Longo UG, Maffulli GD, et al. Achilles tendon ruptures in elite athletes. Foot Ankle Int 2011;32(1):9–15.
38. Maffulli N, Longo UG, Ronga M, et al. Favorable outcome of percutaneous repair of Achilles tendon ruptures in the elderly. Clin Orthop Relat Res 2010;468(4):1039–1046.
39. O'Brien M. Functional anatomy and physiology of tendons. Clin Sports Med 1992;11:505–520.
40. O'Brien M. The anatomy of the Achilles tendon. Foot Ankle Clin 2005;10(2):225–238.
41. Patel VC, Lozano-Calderon S, McWilliam J. Immediate weight bearing after modified percutaneous Achilles tendon repair. Foot Ankle Int 2012;33:1093–1097.
42. Royer RJ, Pierfitte C, Netter P. Features of tendon disorders with fluoroquinolones. Therapie 1994;49:75–76.
43. Saltzman CL, Tearse DS. Achilles tendon injuries. J Am Acad Orthop Surg 1998;6:316–325.
44. Schmidt-Rohlfing B, Graf J, Schneider U, et al. The blood supply of the Achilles tendon. Int Orthop 1992;16:29–31.
45. Spina AA. The plantaris muscle: anatomy, injury, imaging, and treatment. J Can Chiropr Assoc 2007;51(3):158–165.
46. Spoendlin J, Meier C, Jick SS, et al. Achilles or biceps tendon rupture in women and men with type 2 diabetes: a population-based case-control study. J Diabetes Complications 2016;30(5):903–909.
47. Strocchi R, De Pasquale V, Guizzardi S, et al. Human Achilles tendon: morphological and morphometric variations as a function of age. Foot Ankle 1991;12:100–104.
48. Suydam SM, Soulas EM, Elliott DM, et al. Viscoelastic properties of healthy Achilles tendon are independent of isometric plantar flexion strength and cross-sectional area. J Orthop Res 2015;33(6):926–931.
49. Tomak SL, Fleming LL. Achilles tendon rupture: an alternative treatment. Am J Orthop 2004;33:9–12.
50. Ververidis AN, Kalifis KG, Touzopoulos P, et al. Percutaneous repair of the Achilles tendon rupture in athletic population. J Orthop 2015;13(1):57–61.
51. Vosseller JT, Ellis SJ, Levine DS, et al. Achilles tendon rupture in women. Foot Ankle Int 2013;34(1):49–53.
52. Wagnon R, Akayi M. The Webb-Bannister percutaneous technique for acute Achilles' tendon ruptures: a functional and MRI assessment. J Foot Ankle Surg 2005;44:437–444.
53. Willits K, Amendola A, Bryant D, et al. Operative versus nonoperative treatment of acute Achilles tendon ruptures: a multicenter randomized trial using accelerated functional rehabilitation. J Bone Joint Surg Am 2010;92(17):2767–2775.

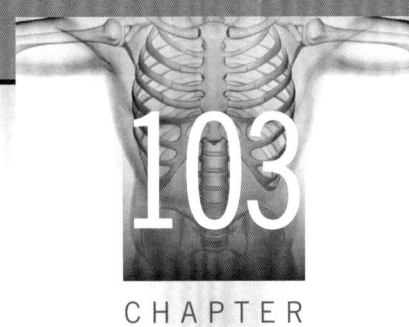

103 CHAPTER

Minimally Invasive Achilles Tendon Repair: Perspective 2

Alessio Giai Via, Francesco Oliva, and Nicola Maffulli

DEFINITION

- Acute Achilles tendon ruptures are more common in recreational middle-aged athletes, between 30 and 50 years, and in active patients involving in running and jumping activities, such as soccer, basketball, and tennis. However, 25% of ruptures occur in older sedentary patients.[22]
- The incidence ranges from 6 to 18 per 100,000 people per year, and it has been increasing during the past few decades.[1]
- More than 20% of acute Achilles tendon ruptures are misdiagnosed, leading to chronic ruptures, which are defined as an untreated Achilles tendon rupture presenting more than 4 weeks from the initial injury.[22]

ANATOMY

- The Achilles tendon is the thickest and strongest tendon of the human body. It is about 15 cm long.[25]
- The Achilles tendon arises near the middle of the calf, from the gastrocnemius and soleus muscles, in the superficial compartment of the calf, and extends distally to insert into the posterior surface of the calcaneus. It may have also a small contribution from the plantaris. Through the Achilles tendon, the gastrocnemius and soleus muscles are the main plantar flexors of the ankle.
- The Achilles tendon is subjected to the highest loads in the body, with tensile loads up to 10 times body weight during running, jumping, hopping, and skipping. It can receive a load stress 3.9 times body weight during walking and 7.7 times body weight when running.[9]

PATHOGENESIS

- The pathogenesis of Achilles tendon ruptures is multifactorial and includes both intrinsic and extrinsic factors, although their precise role still remains unclear. Usually, Achilles tendon ruptures do not occur in a healthy tendon, and histologic signs of tendinopathy are always present at the time of the injury.[8]
- Achilles tendon ruptures usually occur between 2 and 6 cm proximally to the insertion of the tendon into the calcaneus. The tendon is at the greatest risk when it is obliquely loaded, the muscle is contracting maximally, and the tendon length is short. The most common mechanism of injury is pushing off with the weight-bearing forefoot while extending the knee. Sudden unexpected dorsiflexion of the ankle or violent dorsiflexion of a plantar flexed foot may also result in a rupture.[15]

- Corticosteroids, rheumatoid arthritis, and renal transplantation have been associated with Achilles tendon ruptures.[2]
- The use of fluoroquinolones is a well-recognized risk factor for Achilles tendinopathy and ruptures.[3]
- There is a higher risk of tendon injuries in patients affected by diabetes mellitus, hypothyroidism, and obesity.[21]

NATURAL HISTORY

- Although Achilles tendon ruptures mostly occur in previously asymptomatic tendons as a consequence of trauma, it is the end result of a single eccentric contraction on a histologically abnormal tendon. It is the end-stage of profound asymptomatic histochemical changes in the Achilles tendon.[24]
- A delay in treatment results in the formation of a gap between the ruptured tendon ends, which may fill with fibrous nonfunctional scar. Patients may find walking and ascending stairs difficult and standing on tiptoes on the affected limb impossible.
- The clinical diagnosis of a chronic Achilles tendon rupture may be more difficult because the fibrous scar may fill the gap, which becomes less discernible at palpation. Furthermore, active plantarflexion of the foot is usually preserved because of the action of tibialis posterior, the peroneal tendons, and the long toe flexors tendons. Ultrasound and magnetic resonance imaging are useful for diagnosis of chronic Achilles tendon tears, but clinical examination (calf squeeze test and knee flexion test) reigns prince.[17]

PATIENT HISTORY AND PHYSICAL FINDINGS

- Patients usually report a sensation of having been hit on the posterior aspect of the ankle and an audible snap. They also refer acute pain and inability to weight bearing.
- In acute Achilles tendon ruptures, a gap in the Achilles tendon is usually palpable. In delayed presentations, edema may fill this gap, which can be more difficult to appreciate at palpation.
- Many clinical tests have been described. The most popular is the calf squeeze test, which was first described by Simmonds in 1957,[23] but it is often credited to Thompson. The patient is prone with the ankles clear of the table, and the examiner squeezes the middle part of the calf. When the tendon is uninjured, squeezing of the calf results in plantarflexion of the foot, which is not observable in case of the tendon's tear. The affected leg should be always compared with the contralateral side.
- The knee flexion test (Matles test) is performed with the patient prone and the knees flexed at 90 degrees. The foot

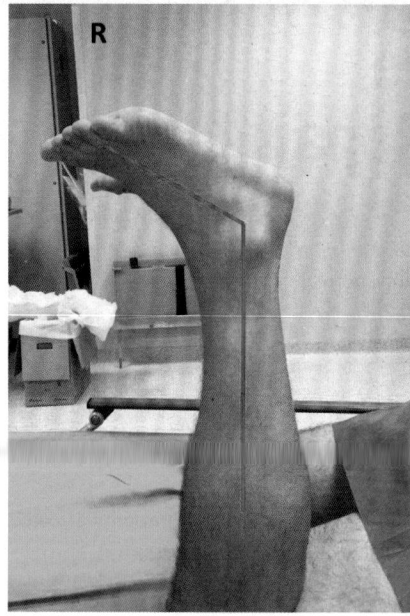
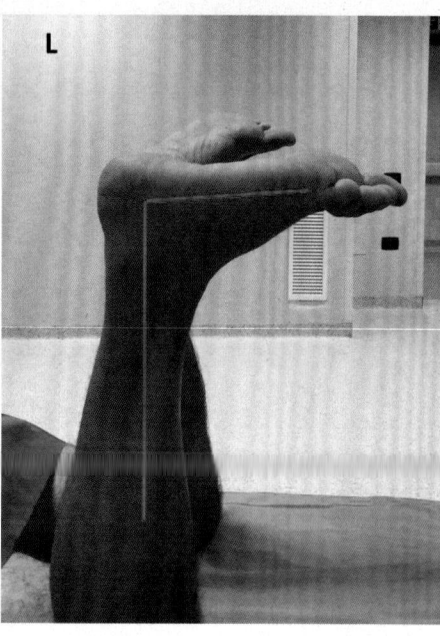

FIG 1 The knee flexion test (or Matles test): The patient is prone with both knees at 90 degrees of flexion. The foot of the injured side falls into neutral or slight dorsiflexion position.

of the uninjured side will be in slight plantarflexion from the tension exerted by the Achilles tendon in continuity. The foot of the affected side falls into neutral or slight dorsiflexed position **(FIG 1)**.[18]

- Other tests are the Copeland and O'Brien tests. The single leg rise is usually difficult to perform in case of acute ruptures. [22]
- Active plantarflexion of the foot is usually preserved given the action of the tibialis posterior, peroneal tendons, and the long toe flexors.
- If two or more of these tests are positive, the diagnosis of an Achilles tendon tear is highly probable.[16] According to recent guidelines, the presence of a palpable gap, positive calf squeeze test, and flexion knee test are the most useful clinical signs to diagnose the Achilles tendon tear.[22]

IMAGING AND OTHER DIAGNOSTIC STUDIES

- The diagnosis of acute Achilles tendon rupture is usually clinical. Accurate history taking and clinical examination allow to make a correct diagnosis.
- Plain radiographs of the ankle and the foot are usually prescribed to identify possible associate injuries as fractures. Lateral view of the ankle may reveal an irregular configuration of the fat-filled triangular space anterior to the Achilles tendon and between the posterior aspect of the tibia and the superior aspect of the calcaneus.
- There is not enough evidence to recommend the routine use of ultrasound and magnetic resonance imaging to confirm the diagnosis of acute Achilles tendon rupture.[11] On the other hand, they are very useful tools in patients in whom a chronic rupture is suspected.

DIFFERENTIAL DIAGNOSIS

- Ankle sprain, fractures
- Achilles tendinopathy
- Chronic Achilles tendon tear

NONOPERATIVE MANAGEMENT

- With acceptable functional results and lower complication rates than operative treatment, nonoperative treatment of acute Achilles tendon ruptures is indicated for patients with increased surgical risk factors and lower functional demands. Functional treatment is superior to immobilization for conservative treatment of Achilles tendon ruptures, and the most recent protocols are based on early weight bearing and mobilization.[22]
- Better functional outcomes and higher return to sports have been reported after surgical repair compared to conservative treatment. However, the complication rate, including impaired wound healing, postoperative infections, and sural nerve injuries, is higher in patients treated surgically. Patients managed nonoperatively did not significantly differ from the ones undergoing surgery in the amount of time to return to work.[7,14]
- Higher rerupture rate has been reported after conservative treatment compared to surgical repair, although a recent systematic review reported the difference in rerupture rate is small and possibly not clinically relevant. However, conservative management may result in tendon lengthening, thus altering function, and different studies have shown that patients take longer to return to sport and have less confidence in their Achilles tendon.[1,20]

SURGICAL MANAGEMENT

- Minimally invasive repair consists in a little skin incision to suture the tendon stumps. It was originally described as a compromise between open surgery and conservative management. Recent studies report good to excellent results regarding functional outcomes, return to sports, and rerupture rate, similar to open procedures. On the other hand, the advantages of minimally invasive procedures are that the procedure is less expensive and less time demanding, with a lower risk of local complications.[6,13]

- The use of absorbable sutures and early weight bearing reduce the risk of complications. However, iatrogenic neurologic complications, such as sural nerve injury, may be more frequent after minimally invasive procedures if performed by inexperienced surgeons.[22]

Preoperative Planning

- Once the diagnosis is made, an assessment of general health and comorbidities should be performed. The preoperative functional status should be noted.
- The skin quality and neurovascular status of the affected limb should be examined. The status of the sural nerve should be documented.
- We recommend deep venous thrombosis prophylaxis after surgery.
- The procedure can be performed under locoregional anesthesia or a local anesthetic, with a mixture of 20 mL of 1% lignocaine hydrochloride and 10 mL of 0.5% bupivacaine hydrochloride injected medially and laterally around the Achilles tendon starting from an area 10 cm proximal to the calcaneal insertion of the tendon.
- The surgical approaches can be planned with a surgical marker **(FIG 2)**.

Positioning

- The patient is placed prone, and a pillow is placed beneath the anterior aspect of the ankles to allow the feet to hang free.
- The operating table is angled down 20 degrees cranially to reduce venous pooling in the feet and ankles.
- The affected leg is prepared in the usual sterile fashion. We do not use a tourniquet.
- Local anesthetic injection is used. Instill a mixture of 20 mL of 2% lignocaine hydrochloride and 10 mL of 0.25%

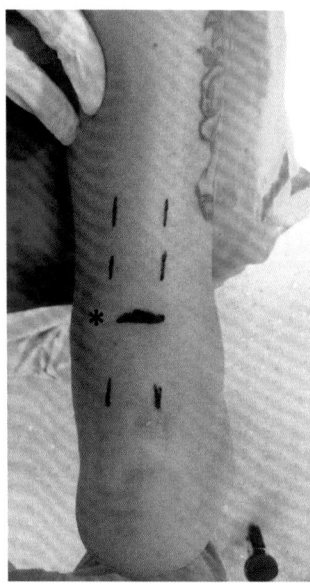

FIG 2 The skin incisions are planned with a surgical marker before surgery. The palpable tendon defect is palpated and marked (*asterisk*). Six longitudinal stab incisions are marked, four proximal and two distal to the palpable defect.

bupivacaine hydrochloride into an area 8 to 10 cm around the ruptured Achilles tendon.

Approach

- Previous approaches such as those described by Ma and Griffith[13] using three medial and three lateral stab incisions carry a relatively high incidence of sural nerve entrapment.
- We describe in the following text the surgical technique we described and employ.[4]

MINIMALLY INVASIVE REPAIR OF ACUTE ACHILLES TENDON RUPTURE

- A 10 to 15 mm transverse incision is made over the tendon defect to expose the tendon stumps. If necessary, the tendon stumps can be débrided through such incision.
- Four longitudinal stab incisions are made about 6 cm proximal to the palpable defect, two lateral and two medial to the tendon. Two further longitudinal incisions on either side of the tendon are made just proximal to the insertion of the Achilles tendon on the calcaneus.
- If necessary, forceps are used to gently mobilize the tendon from beneath the subcutaneous tissues. We normally do not use them.
- We use two no. 2 double loop Vicryl sutures. In this way, each throw of the needle carries four suture strands, and a total of eight core sutures are therefore present within the substance of the operated tendon.
- The first suture is passed from the transverse incision, with a distal to proximal direction, through the bulk of the tendon, and the needle is withdrawn from the first lateral longitudinal incision **(TECH FIG 1)**.

- The suture is passed from the same longitudinal incision, with a diagonal direction, and it is withdrawn from the most proximal medial longitudinal incision **(TECH FIG 2)** and then transversely between the two proximal stab incisions through the bulk of the tendon from medial to lateral.
- The procedure is repeated with a proximal to distal direction, resulting in an X configuration of the suture. The needle is introduced from the proximal lateral stub incision to medial longitudinal incision and finally it pass from this stub incision, and it is withdrawn from the transverse incision over the tendon defect **(TECH FIG 3)**. In this way, a Bunnell type of configuration of suture is achieved.
- The suture is then tested for strength and security by pulling the ends of the Vicryl suture distally through the transverse incision **(TECH FIG 4)**.
- The procedure is repeated for the distal Achilles tendon stump. A new double loop no. 2 Vicryl suture is passed from the transverse incision to the distal medial longitudinal incision, then between the two distal stabs incisions through the tendon,

TECHNIQUES

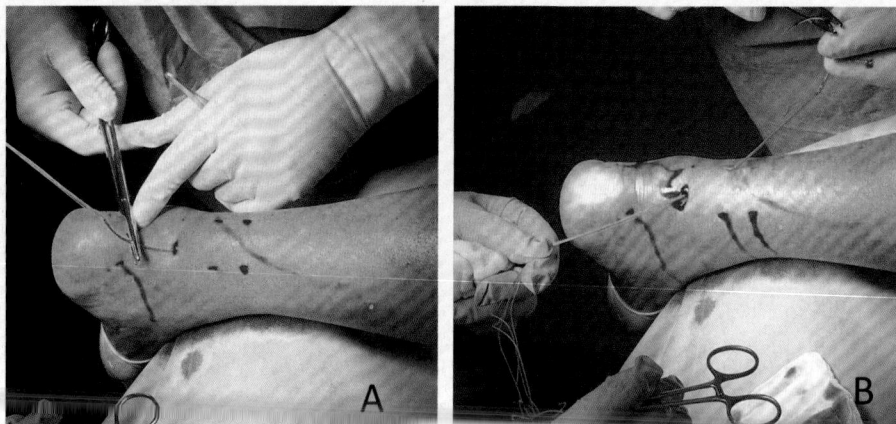

TECH FIG 1 A. A 10 to 15 mm transverse incision is made over the tendon defect, four longitudinal stab incisions are made proximal and two distal to the palpable defect. **B.** The suture is passed from the transverse incision, and the needle is withdrawn from the first lateral longitudinal incision.

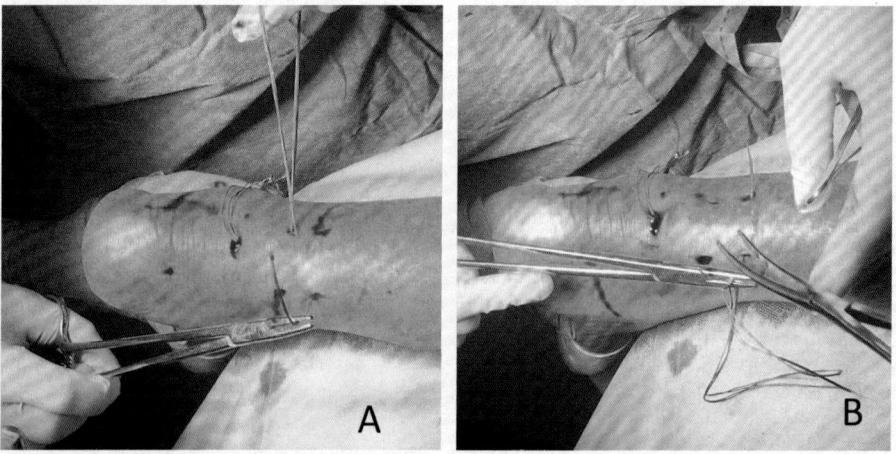

TECH FIG 2 A. The suture is passed from the first longitudinal lateral stub incision, with a diagonal direction, to the proximal medial longitudinal incision. **B.** Then the needle is passed transversely between the two proximal stab incisions through the bulk of the tendon.

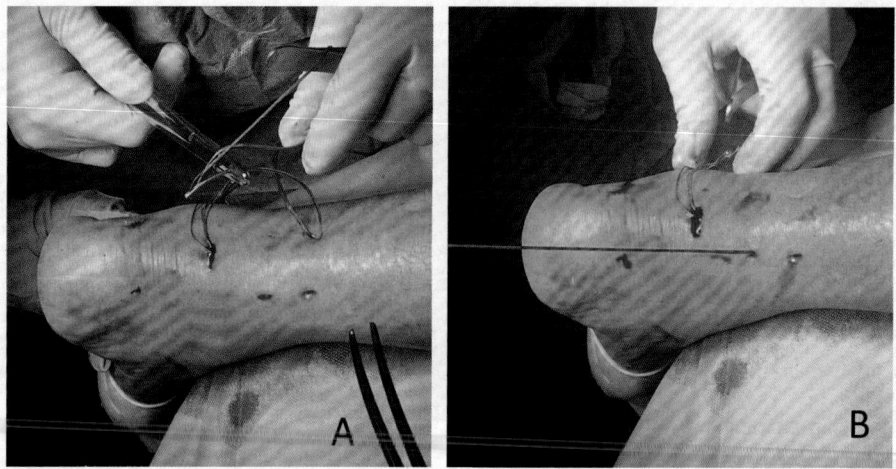

TECH FIG 3 A,B. The needle is passed from proximal lateral stub incision to medial longitudinal incision, resulting in an X configuration of the suture.

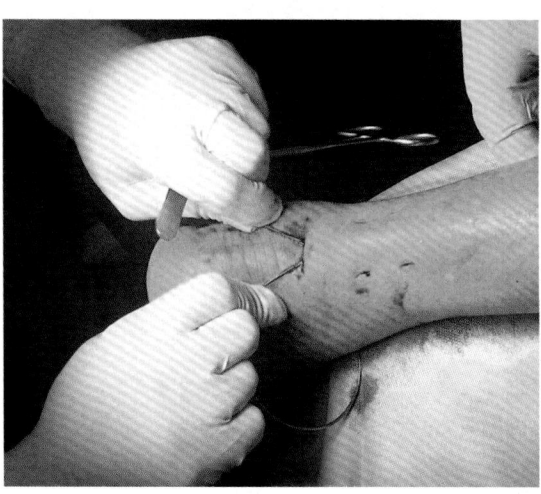

TECH FIG 4 The suture finally came out from the transverse incision over the tendon defect and it is tested for security.

and finally back from the transverse incision in a half Kessler fashion **(TECH FIG 5)**. The suture is then tested for security by pulling both ends of the Vicryl suture proximally through the transverse incision. The ankle should plantar flex freely.

- The ankle is held in full plantarflexion by an assistant, and in turn, the opposing ends of the Vicryl suture are tied together with a double knot **(TECH FIGS 6 and 7)**. The knots are buries in the substance of the tendon through the transverse incision.

- After the repair, we control if the physiologic plantarflexion of the ankle is restored, and the Thompson test is performed **(TECH FIG 8)**.

- A subcuticular Biosyn suture 3.0 (Tyco Healthcare, Norwalk, CT) is used to close the transverse incision, and Steri-Strips (3M Health Care, St Paul, MN) are applied to the stab incisions. Finally, a Mepore dressing (Mölnlycke Health Care, Gothenburg, Sweden) is applied, and an anterior cast slab with the ankle in full plantarflexion is applied.

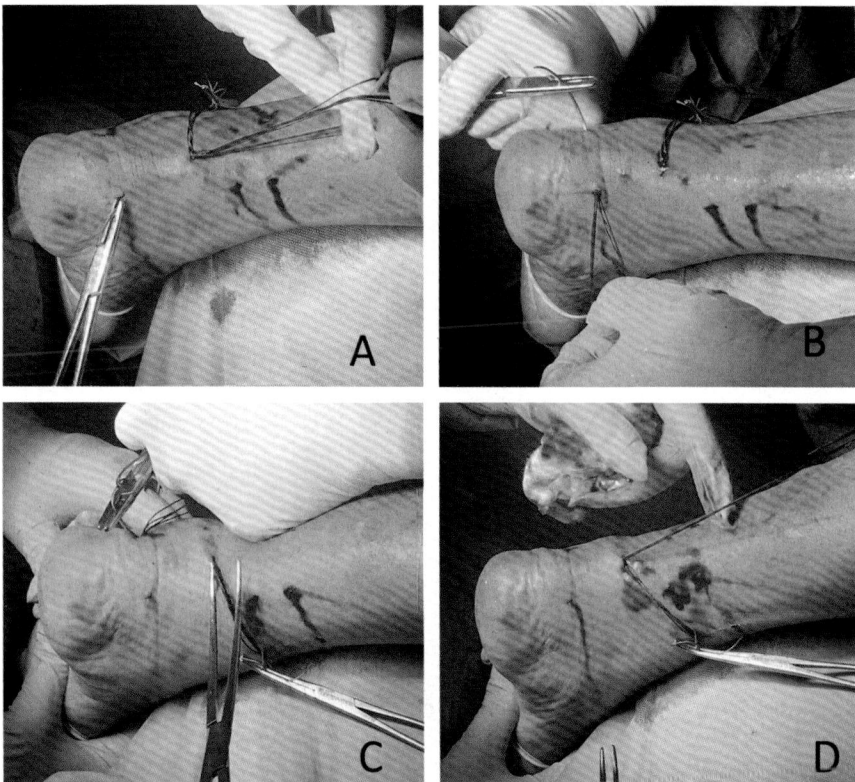

TECH FIG 5 The same procedure is repeated for the distal tendon stump. The needle is passed from the transverse incision to the distal medial longitudinal incision (**A**), then transversely between the two distal stabs incisions through the tendon (**B**), and finally the suture is passed back coming out from the transverse incision (**C,D**).

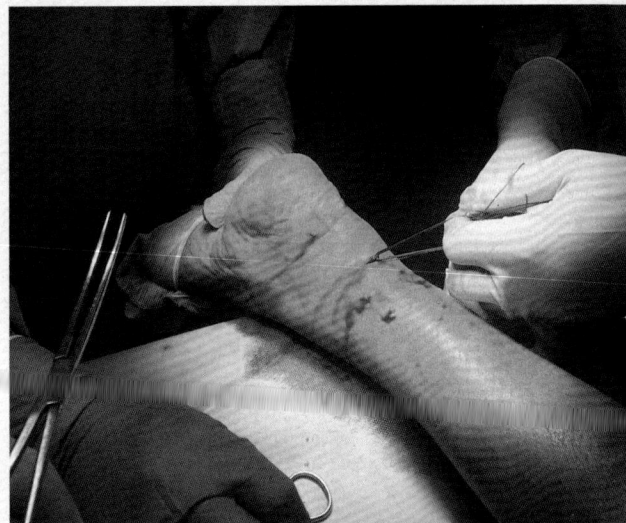

TECH FIG 6 After testing the suture for security, the ankle is held in full plantarflexion, and the suture is performed by knotting together the opposing ends of the Vicryl wire.

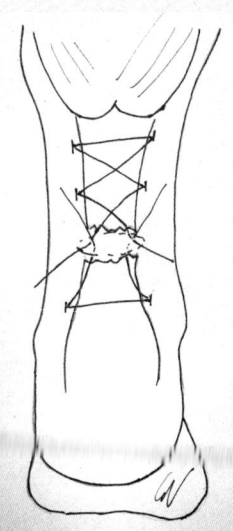

TECH FIG 7 Schematic representation of the minimally invasive suture technique described.

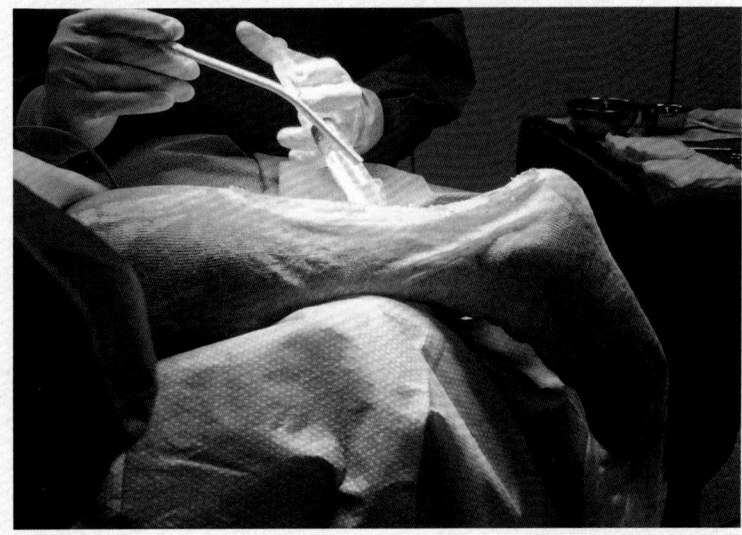

TECH FIG 8 The physiologic plantarflexion of the ankle is restored after the minimally invasive repair. The Thompson test is repeated.

TECHNIQUES

POSTOPERATIVE CARE

- The patient is discharged on the same day of the operation, after having ensured that the neurovascular status of the limb is normal, and that a physiotherapist has ensured that the patient is safe and comfortable in the cast slab.
- The anterior slab is retained for 2 weeks, and the patient is allowed to bear weight on the tiptoes as tolerated.
- At 2 weeks, the patient is reviewed as outpatient, and the wounds are inspected. A walker boot is prescribed with the foot in full plantarflexion for a further 4 weeks. The patients is advised to walk with two crutches and partial weight bearing initially, increasing to weight bearing as able by 2 weeks. Gentle active mobilization of the subtalar joint with the help of physiotherapist is indicated, avoiding

dorsiflexion of the ankle. Stretching and massage are not allowed.
- After 8 weeks, the boot is removed. Physiotherapy for full recovery of ankle motion is indicated. The patient continues isometric strengthening exercises, and light weight-bearing exercise can be started. Patients are normally fully weight bearing by this time.
- At 12 weeks postoperatively, patients are assessed as to whether they are able to undertake more vigorous physiotherapy.
- Eccentric exercises are indicated after 3 months from surgery.
- Patients are then followed up at 3-month intervals and discharged 12 months after the operation, once they are able to perform at least five toe raises unaided on the operated leg and after they returned to their work or sport.

OUTCOMES

- Recent guidelines are unable to recommend for or against minimally invasive surgery for patients with acute Achilles tendon rupture because few high-level studies comparing the two procedures are published in literature. However, retrospective comparative study reported similar functional outcomes, return to sport activities, and rerupture rate between the two procedures.[5,10,14]
- Lim et al,[12] in a randomized controlled trial, advocated percutaneous repair over open surgical techniques after finding no significant differences in functional results, lower infection rate with the percutaneous repair, and subjectively better cosmetic appearance.
- Systematic reviews of literature and meta-analyses comparing open versus minimally invasive and percutaneous repair reported no significant differences in respect to the incidence of rerupture, tissue adhesion, deep infection, and deep vein thrombosis. However, minimally invasive techniques significantly reduced the risk of superficial wound infection, reduced the operatory time, and improved patient satisfaction.[6,19,26]
- The incidence of sural nerve injuries is higher after minimally invasive and percutaneous repair.[26]
- Optimal outcomes and functional recovery have been reported up to 85% of patients treated with minimally invasive repair.[22]
- The use of absorbable suture and early postoperative weight bearing reduce the risk of complications.[22]

COMPLICATIONS

- Early complications include sural nerve damage and hematoma.
- Middle term (<6 weeks) complications: superficial and deep wound infections
- Late complication (>6 weeks): rerupture, deep infections

REFERENCES

1. Baumfeld D, Baumfeld T, Spiezia F, et al. Isokinetic functional outcomes of open versus percutaneous repair following Achilles tendon tears. Foot Ankle Surg 2019;25:503–506.
2. Beason DP, Abboud JA, Kuntz AF, et al. Cumulative effects of hypercholesterolemia on tendon biomechanics in a mouse model. J Orthop Res 2011;29:380–383.
3. Bisaccia DR, Aicale R, Tarantino D, et al. Biological and chemical changes in fluoroquinolone-associated tendinopathies: a systematic review. Br Med Bull 2019;130:39–49.
4. Carmont MR, Maffulli N. Modified percutaneous repair of ruptured Achilles tendon. Knee Surg Sports Traumatol Arthrosc 2008;16:199–203.
5. Chan AP, Chan YY, Fong DT, et al. Clinical and biomechanical outcome of minimal invasive and open repair of the Achilles tendon. Sports Med Arthrosc Rehabil Ther Technol 2011;3:32.
6. Del Buono A, Volpin A, Maffulli N. Minimally invasive versus open surgery for acute Achilles tendon rupture: a systematic review. Br Med Bull 2014;109:45–54.
7. Ebinesan AD, Sarai BS, Walley GD, et al. Conservative, open or percutaneous repair for acute rupture of the Achilles tendon. Disabil Rehabil 2008;30:1721–1725.
8. Giai Via A, Papa G, Oliva F, et al. Tendinopathy. Curr Phys Med Rehabil Rep 2016;4:50–55.
9. Giddings VL, Beaupré GS, Whalen RT, et al. Calcaneal loading during walking and running. Med Sci Sports Exerc 2000;32:627–634.
10. Guillo S, Del Buono A, Dias M, et al. Percutaneous repair of acute ruptures of the tendo Achillis. Surgeon 2013;11:14–19.
11. Kou J. AAOS clinical practice guideline: acute Achilles tendon rupture. J Am Acad Orthop Surg 2010;18:511–513.
12. Lim J, Dalal R, Waseem M. Percutaneous vs. open repair of the ruptured Achilles tendon—a prospective randomized controlled study. Foot Ankle Int 2001;22:559–568.
13. Ma GW, Griffith TG. Percutaneous repair of acute closed ruptured Achilles tendon: a new technique. Clin Orthop Relat Res 1977;(128): 247–255.
14. Maffulli G, Del Buono A, Richards P, et al. Conservative, minimally invasive and open surgical repair for management of acute ruptures of the Achilles tendon: a clinical and functional retrospective study. Muscles Ligaments Tendons J 2017;7:46–52.
15. Maffulli N. Rupture of the Achilles tendon. J Bone Joint Surg Am 1999;81:1019–1036.
16. Maffulli N. The clinical diagnosis of subcutaneous tear of the Achilles tendon. A prospective study in 174 patients. Am J Sports Med 1998;26:266–270.
17. Maffulli N, Giai Via A, Oliva F. Chronic Achilles tendon rupture. Open Orthop J 2017;11:3–12.
18. Matles AL. Rupture of the tendo Achilles: another diagnostic sign. Bull Hosp Joint Dis 1975;36:48–51.
19. McMahon SE, Smith TO, Hing CB. A meta-analysis of randomised controlled trials comparing conventional to minimally invasive approaches for repair of an Achilles tendon rupture. Foot Ankle Surg 2011;17:211–217.
20. Ochen Y, Beks RB, van Heijl M, et al. Operative treatment versus nonoperative treatment of Achilles tendon ruptures: systematic review and meta-analysis. BMJ 2019;364:k5120.
21. Oliva F, Berardi AC, Misiti S, et al. Thyroid hormones and tendon: current views and future perspectives. Concise review. Muscles Ligaments Tendons J 2013;3:201–203.
22. Oliva F, Ruggiero C, Giai Via A, et al. I.S.Mu.L.T. Achilles tendon ruptures guidelines. Muscle Ligaments Tendon J 2018;8:310–363.
23. Simmonds FA. The diagnosis of the ruptured Achilles tendon. Practitioner 1957;179:56–58.
24. Tallon C, Maffulli N, Ewen SW. Ruptured Achilles tendons are significantly more degenerated than tendinopathic tendons. Med Sci Sports Exerc 2001;33:1983–1990.
25. Williams PL. Gray's Anatomy, ed 38. Edinburgh: Churchill Livingstone, 1995.
26. Yang B, Liu Y, Kan S, et al. Outcomes and complications of percutaneous versus open repair of acute Achilles tendon rupture: a meta-analysis. Int J Surg 2017;40:178–186.

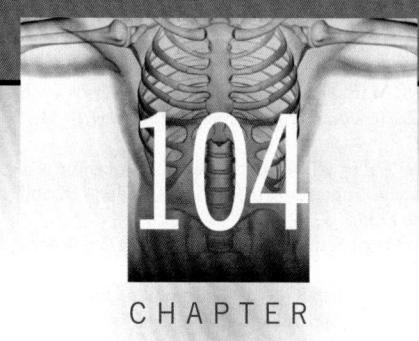

104 CHAPTER

Retrocalcaneal Bursoscopy (Endoscopic Removal of Bone, Bursa, and Paratenon)

Fred W. Ortmann

DEFINITION AND INTRODUCTION

- Patrick Haglund in 1928 described an enlarged posterior border of the os calcis.[1]
- This anatomy (Haglund deformity) becomes very important when external shoeing/heel counter and repeated hyperdorsiflexion causes contact between the Achilles tendon, the posterior vertical surface of the calcaneus, and the interposed retrocalcaneal bursa.
  - As a result, Haglund syndrome is commonly characterized by inflammation within the retrocalcaneal or Achilles tendon bursa and often secondarily presents as insertional Achilles tendinopathy.
- The posterior heel pain and swelling associated with Haglund syndrome is the result of mechanical irritation by the calcaneal prominence on the surrounding soft tissues and the anterior paratenon of the Achilles tendon.
- After conservative/nonoperative measures have failed and imaging does not show significance, Achilles tendinopathy, Haglund deformity, and retrocalcaneal bursitis can be treated surgically using an endoscopic technique. General indications are pain, limp, alteration of workstyle or lifestyle, and, lastly, significant night pain.
  - The endoscopic technique is an outpatient treatment that is associated with low morbidity and high outpatient satisfaction. There is a short recovery time and a short time to gain prior activity level.
  - Appropriate visualization of the Achilles tendon and its paratenon and removal of the calcaneal prominence and retrocalcaneal bursa can be effectively accomplished using an endoscopic technique.

PATHOGENESIS

- The retrocalcaneal space has been described as a disc space bursa covering the posterior superior angle of the calcaneus.[3] The bursa walls may become diseased and hypertrophied with repeated hindfoot movement. Increased pressure can occur and become chronic with secondary calcaneal bone edema and paratenon reactive fibrosis at the insertion.
- Achilles tendinopathy is a degenerative process within the tendon substance causing microtears, which can progress to macrotears, edema, and reactive fibrosis with scar formation. These changes can cause secondary mechanical irritation of the surrounding tissues and can even stimulate an inflammatory process.[9]

PATIENT HISTORY AND PHYSICAL FINDINGS

- Clinical evaluation may be difficult between retrocalcaneal bursitis and Achilles tendinopathy, although the two often coexist.
- Pathology within the retrocalcaneal space is detected on clinical examination with point tenderness along the anteromedial and anterolateral aspects of the Achilles tendon and an associated prominence of the calcaneus.
- Palpation of the affected hindfoot often reveals tenderness at the distal portion of the Achilles tendon proximal to its insertion on the calcaneus. The pain can be reproduced with passive or active dorsiflexion. The retrocalcaneal bursa and the more directly posterior Achilles tendon bursa can become confluent and "wrap around."

IMAGING AND OTHER DIAGNOSTIC STUDIES

- Imaging can assist with documenting the presence or absence of tendinopathy (FIG 1A).
- It can be difficult to distinguish whether symptoms are caused by retrocalcaneal bursitis or insertional Achilles tendinosis or tendinitis. These two conditions often coexist.
- Magnetic resonance imaging (MRI) should be used preoperatively to better demonstrate or differentiate coexistence of these diagnoses (FIG 1B–D).
- Normal-appearing and diseased tendons can usually be distinguished endoscopically.
- Ultrasound can help rule out a distal Achilles noninsertional tendinopathy or tendinitis.
- Limited bone scan can help with differential diagnosis with its sensitivity (FIG 1E).

NONOPERATIVE MANAGEMENT

- Nonoperative measures for the treatment of posterior heel pain include the use of nonsteroidal anti-inflammatory medication, shoe wear modification (such as using backless shoes and avoiding irregular counters), physical therapy for icing or other modalities, stretching exercises, pressure-release inserts, and hands-on friction massage.
- Local injections can be given in the retrocalcaneal space for diagnostic purposes. The concomitant use of local anesthesia and corticosteroids can further weaken the substance of the Achilles tendon and risk weakness and further micro- or macrorupture of the tendon.[5]

We would like to respectfully acknowledge the contributions made by Dr. Angus M. McBryde to the second edition of this chapter.

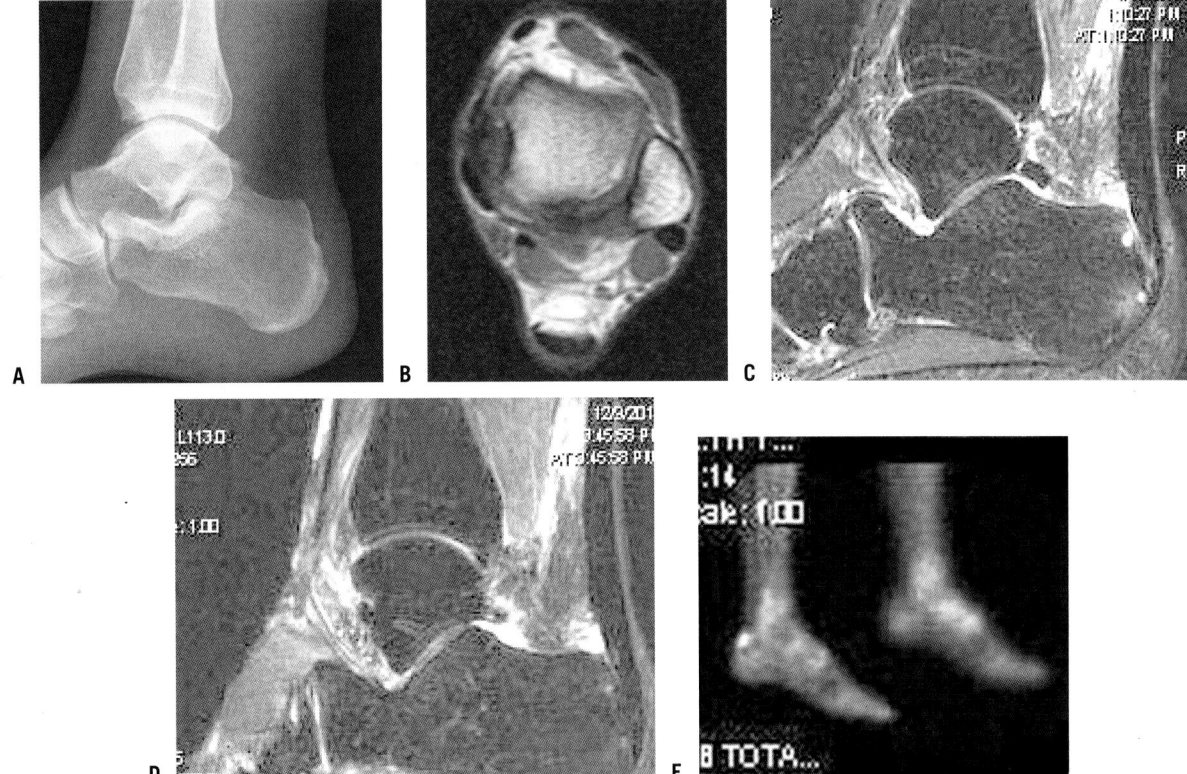

FIG 1 A. Preoperative lateral foot film showing Haglund exostosis. **B.** MRI showing retrocalcaneal bursa involvement and insertional tendinopathy. **C.** Sagittal view; the Achilles tendon insertional involvement, the distinctive and extensive calcaneal response (including cystic change), and a clinical treatment nonresponse makes an open approach preferable. **D.** Sagittal view; the intact Achilles, the lesser reactive calcaneal signal, and a more modest functional disability, although recalcitrant to a nonoperative approach makes endoscopy preferred. Axial views are necessary to quantitate any tendinopathy component. **E.** Triple-phase bone scan, particularly the delayed phase, can help rule out adjacent problems and further target/quantitate the calcaneal or bursal involvement. (**A,B:** Reprinted with permission from Ortmann FW, McBryde AM. Endoscopic bony and soft-tissue decompression of the retrocalcaneal space for the treatment of Haglund deformity and retrocalcaneal bursitis. Foot Ankle Int 2007;28[2]:149–153. Copyright © 2007 SAGE Publications.)

SURGICAL MANAGEMENT

- The goal of treatment for Haglund deformity and associated inflammation and tendinopathy is to remove the calcaneal prominence and to decompress the inflamed surrounding soft tissues.
- Open surgical correction is an alternative for patients who have failed to respond to nonoperative measures and if there is an estimated tendinopathy with ~25% involvement on axial Achilles serial images. In that case, augmentation (authors' preference) or alternate open Achilles tendon surgery is advisable.
  - Open procedures generally include the following:
    - Resection of the calcaneal prominence (Haglund deformity) proximal to the Achilles tendon insertion
    - Retrocalcaneal bursa removal
- Rarely, a dorsal closing wedge osteotomy can rotate the posterior calcaneus to a lesser prominent position.
- Achilles tenolysis and partial resection of the diseased portion of the tendon may be necessary, often with augmentation by the flexor hallucis longus or flexor digitorum.
- Complete Achilles removal at its insertion with multianchor reinsertion is occasionally necessary.
- Complications associated with these procedures can include hematomas, tendon or skin breakdown, nonunion, Achilles tendon avulsion, tenderness around the operative scar, cosmetic problems, altered sensation around the heel, and stiffness.[1,7,12,14,15] Rehabilitation following open surgery can be prolonged.
- The endoscopic technique of decompressing the retrocalcaneal space but with an "intact" Achilles tendon insertion was developed to reduce morbidity and decrease the functional time to recovery for patients with retrocalcaneal bursitis.[11,16,17]
  - The endoscopic technique has been shown to have fewer complications and a better cosmetic appearance than an open procedure.[8]
- Here, authors describe retrocalcaneal bursoscopy using our method of endoscopic bony and soft tissue decompression of the retrocalcaneal space and the results from our patient series.[13] Hindfoot endoscopy is being increasingly used for numerous problems.

Positioning

- The operation is performed with the patient in the supine position and under either general or regional anesthesia. Monitored anesthesia care is occasionally used. The foot should be adjusted on the table until in a neutral position.
  - A high thigh tourniquet is inflated to 300 mm Hg after Esmarch ischemia. A sequential compression device is used on the contralateral leg, ankle, or foot.

- The heel is positioned at the leading edge of the operating table. This enables the surgeon to place the foot against his or her body while using both hands to operate the arthroscopic instruments.
- The leg rests on a firm padded 12-inch long and 4-inch wide diameter cylindrical (bump) that allows the surgeon ample room to use both hands and to control ankle dorsiflexion and plantarflexion.
- Alternatively, the prone position can be used.[2]
- Both positions allow the patient's foot to be controlled against the chest of the surgeon, who can then have both hands free for use of arthroscopic instruments.

PORTAL PLACEMENT AND EXPOSURE

- Make a lateral portal with a vertical incision at the level of the superior aspect of the calcaneus (**TECH FIG 1A**).
- The incisions are slightly anterior to the Achilles tendon and posterior to the sural nerve. It is important to bluntly dissect and spread the soft tissues when making the lateral portal to minimize the risk of injury to the sural nerve.
- Establish the second portal similarly just anterior to the Achilles tendon, using the light of the arthroscope or a hemostat as a guide (**TECH FIG 1B**).
- Enter the retrocalcaneal space with a blunt trocar to develop a working space.
- Place a 4.0-mm arthroscope into the retrocalcaneal space.

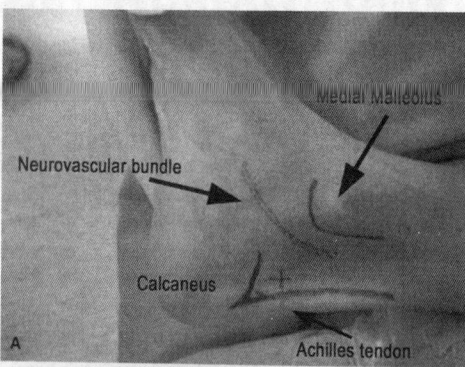

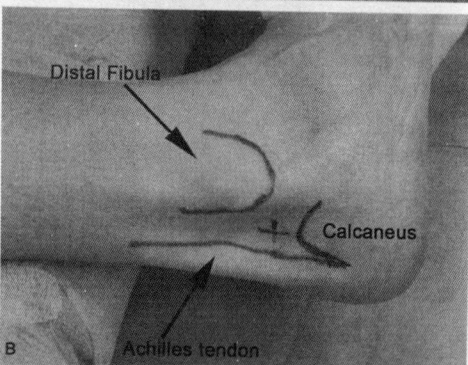

TECH FIG 1 Establishing landmarks and planning portal placement medially (**A**) and laterally (**B**).

RESECTION AND DECOMPRESSION

- Introduce a 3.5-mm arthroscopic shaver (for larger hindfeet, a 4.5-mm arthroscope can be used) through the portal and remove the bursal tissue. This expanded working space creates visualization and access to the posterior calcaneus and the Achilles tendon attachment.
- Depending on the quality of the bone, use either the arthroscopic shaver and/or a 4-mm arthroscopic burr to resect the posterosuperior calcaneal prominence (**TECH FIG 2**).
- Keep the hooded portions of the instruments toward the anterior direction. A short sleeve can be helpful. Switching portals promotes symmetry of bone removal.
- Take special care to stop the rotating or oscillating shaver or burr usage when the instrumentation enters or exits the portal.
- Carry out the resection both medially and laterally into the sulcus of the calcaneal tendon (retrocalcaneal bursa) space and distally stopping at the attachment of the Achilles tendon.

Old chronic scarring can make the Achilles attachment hard to identify; requiring mini C-arm check.
- Visually confirm adequate exposure and resection of the osseous prominence until there are no areas of Achilles tendon impingement.
  - Protocol dictates the use of the mini C-arm (Mini 6600 series [GE OEC Medical Systems, Salt Lake City, UT] or a similar unit) pre- and post-bony resection to determine bony removal, confirm adequate resection, and to document completion.
- Damaged or diseased Achilles tendon can be selectively exposed and with a nerve hook or probe identified. Small lesions and ossification can be removed with mixed use of the burr and/or rongeur.
- Limited bone or tendinopathy can be removed with the arthroscopic shaver.

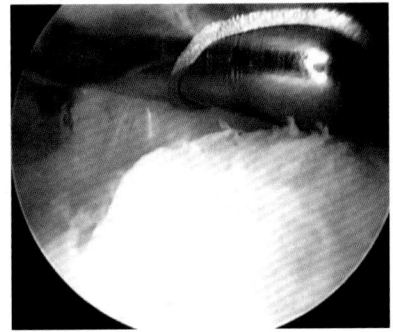 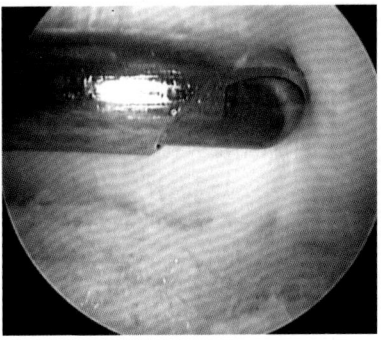

A   B

TECH FIG 2 A,B. An arthroscopic shaver is used to resect the posterior superior calcaneal prominence. A 4-mm arthroscopic burr is also used. (Reprinted with permission from Ortmann FW, McBryde AM. Endoscopic bony and soft-tissue decompression of the retrocalcaneal space for the treatment of Haglund deformity and retrocalcaneal bursitis. Foot Ankle Int 2007;28[2]:149–153, with permission. Copyright © 2007 SAGE Publications.)

- An 18-gauge needle can be inserted several times into the tendon to promote blood ingress and collagen scar where there is hemosiderin deposit, myxoid, or degenerative change or frank tear.
  - The rationale for this is to initiate a vascular response within the tendons for healing; it is performed with or without débridement. Platelet-rich plasma is not used.

- Insert an image-guided arthroscopic probe into the retrocalcaneal space to confirm continuing effective attachment of the Achilles tendon. Clinical pre- and postoperative palpation of the tendon is also important.

COMPLETION AND WOUND CLOSURE

- Hyperplantar and dorsiflex the foot with the anterior chest and abdomen to verify any last areas of impingement. Also, medial and lateral oblique hindfoot views are taken to make sure medial and lateral corners are clear of bone.
- Irrigate and suction the retrocalcaneal space to remove any loose bone/tissue.

- Close the portal sites with two 4-0 or 5-0 nylon horizontal mattress skin sutures.
- Inject local anesthetic (0.5% Marcaine without epinephrine) into the portal sites.
- Apply a compression dressing and splint the foot into slight 5-degree equinus with the posterior splint and sugar-tong (trilaminar splint).

TECHNIQUES

Pearls and Pitfalls

- Set up with heels directly at the end of operating room table so can manage position of ankle/foot in dorsiflexion and plantarflexion with chest/abdomen.
- Develop operative field from posteromedial to posterolateral corner so panoramic view of Achilles tuberosity attachment in its entirety.
- MRI is necessary preoperatively to document insertional tendinopathy. If more than 25% of the cross-sectional area of the tendon is involved, open repair may be necessary (authors' opinion).
- Do not use an "extremity" MRI, as most are ~8 inches diameter and cannot be positioned with the ankle in a neutral "90 degrees." Tendon distortion and crimp occur and prevent adequate interpretation.
- Experience enables removal of paratenon and further removal/débridement of small ruptures and/or ossification in selected cases and situations. The so-called "tug lesion" or exostosis present in many insertions can be partially or completely removed in many cases, that is, stress fracture at its base and bony bulk symptoms posteriorly.[10]
- Postoperative routine are as follows:
  - Non–weight bearing for 2–3 weeks
  - Walker boot with partial weight bearing for 2–3 weeks
  - Maximize posterior tibial and peroneal strength as soon as possible.
  - Variation of rehab is necessary with condition of the tendon, premature sport-specific loading, and patient factors such as weight and compliance.

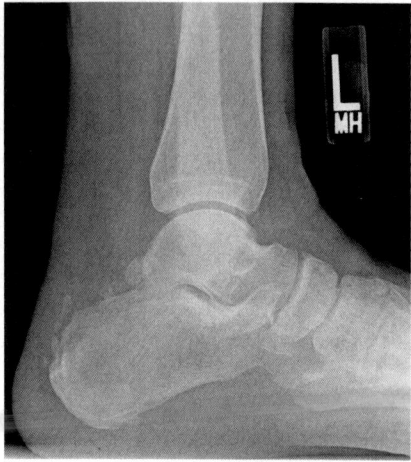

FIG 2 A typical postoperative lateral at 4 months postoperative.

POSTOPERATIVE CARE

- The average time until full weight bearing in a walker boot is 4 weeks.
- Patients wear shoes with a heel counter and return to normal daily function in 6 to 8 weeks.
- All athletes returned to their previous level of activity in an average of 12 weeks.
- Patients may need a longer period of cast/boot immobilization after débridement of the Achilles tendon or significant Achilles tendinopathy. Generally, an open procedure would be used in this event.
- There are frequently small islands of calcification or ossification at the endoscopic site on postoperative lateral films of the hindfoot. They are of no consequence **(FIG 2)**.

OUTCOMES

- In our study of endoscopic bony and soft tissue decompression of the retrocalcaneal space for the treatment of Haglund deformity and retrocalcaneal bursitis,[13] 32 heels in 30 consecutive patients underwent endoscopic decompression. The timing for surgery after diagnosis of retrocalcaneal

bursitis averaged 20 months. All patients had failed to respond to nonoperative measures, and none had undergone previous surgery.

- Indications for operative intervention included failed nonoperative measures, history, and physical examinations consistent with retrocalcaneal bursitis and Haglund deformity causing mechanical impingement or Achilles tendinopathy.
- Patients were prospectively followed from 1997 to 2003, with a mean follow-up of 35 months (range, 3 to 62 months).
- Thirty heels completed subjective and objective measures using the American Orthopaedic Foot & Ankle Society ankle–hindfoot scale.[6]
  - Twenty-six patients had excellent results and three had good results. There was one poor outcome and one major complication. An excellent result was defined as pain-free activity with complete return to activity, and a poor result was defined as having persistent symptoms and inability to return to activity.
  - The cohort was stratified into "daily athletic activity" and "athletic" groups, and the groups were compared. No statistical differences in outcome between the two groups existed.
  - All patients reported satisfaction with the cosmetic appearance of their portal sites.
  - These results compared with those published by van Dijk et al[18]: Their 20 patients resumed participating in sports at an average of 12 weeks.

COMPLICATIONS

- One major complication occurred among the 30 heels: A patient sustained a proximal Achilles tendon rupture (of an unprotected tendon) 19 days after having undergone endoscopic decompression while ambulating without a prescribed protected walker boot.[13]
- There were no intraoperative or skin or soft tissue complications (ie, wound dehiscence and postoperative infection).
- No patients reported a painful scar or neuroma-type symptoms.
- Stress fracture can result if there is "irregular" bony removal coupled with early leg-based activity **(FIG 3)**.

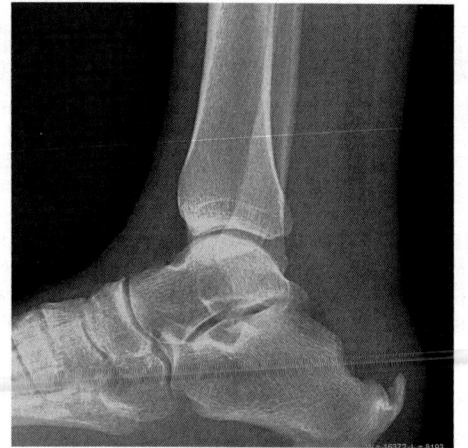
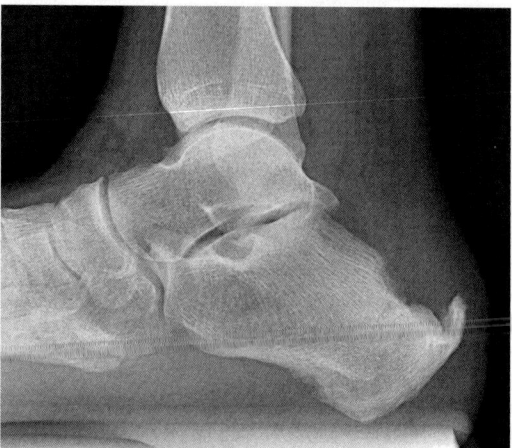

FIG 3 **A.** An irregular and an operatively slightly deep tuberosity bone removal endoscopically. **B.** At 7 weeks, a radiographic lucency accompanied increased pain, limp, and tenderness with calcaneal medial/lateral compression pain compatible with stress fracture. *(continued)*

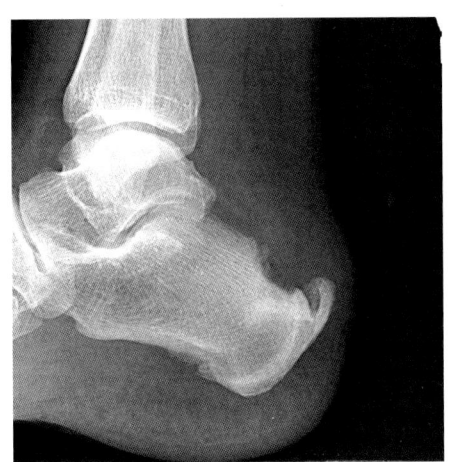
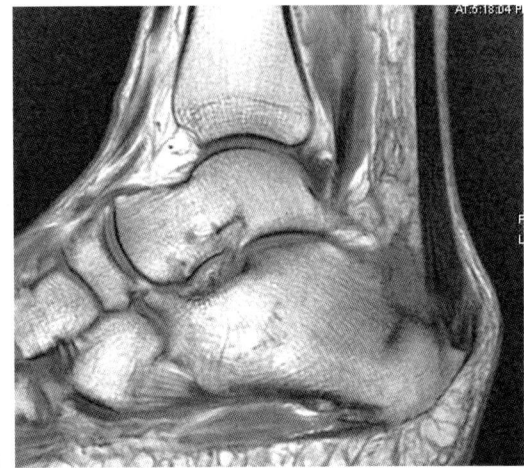

FIG 3 *(continued)* **C.** At 9 weeks, clear condensation of bone further confirms stress fracture. **D.** Sagittal T1 optional MRI shows unequivocal stress fracture of bone.

REFERENCES

1. Angermann P. Chronic retrocalcaneal bursitis treated by resection of the calcaneus. Foot Ankle 1990;10:285–287.
2. Bohu Y, Lefèvre N, Bauer T, et al. Surgical treatment of Achilles tendinopathies in athletes. Multicenter retrospective series of open surgery and endoscopic techniques. Orthop Traumatol Surg Res 2009;95(8)(suppl 1):S72–S77.
3. Frey C, Rosenburg Z, Shereff MJ, et al. The retrocalcaneal bursa: anatomy and bursography. Foot Ankle 1992;13:203–207.
4. Haglund P. Beitrag zur Klinik der Achillessehne. Zeitschr Orthop Chir 1928;49:49–58.
5. Kennedy JC, Willis RB. The effects of local steroid injections on tendons: a biomechanical and microscopic correlative study. Am J Sports Med 1976;4:11–21.
6. Kitaoka HB, Alexander IJ, Adelaar RS, et al. Clinical rating systems for the ankle-hindfoot, midfoot, hallux, and lesser toes. Foot Ankle Int 1994;15:349–353.
7. Leach RE, Dilorio E, Harney RA. Pathologic hindfoot conditions in the athlete. Clin Orthop Relat Res 1983;(177):116–121.
8. Leitze Z, Sella EJ, Aversa JM. Endoscopic decompression of the retrocalcaneal space. J Bone Joint Surg Am 2003;85(8):1488–1496.
9. Lohrer H, Nauck T. Retrocalcaneal bursitis but not Achilles tendinopathy is characterized by increased pressure in the retrocalcaneal bursa. Clin Biomech (Bristol, Avon) 2014;29(3):283–288.
10. Lohrer H, Nauck T, Dorn NV, et al. Comparison of endoscopic and open resection for Haglund tuberosity in a cadaver study. Foot Ankle Int 2006;27(6):445–450.
11. Lui TH, Lo CY, Sui YC. Minimally invasive and endoscopic treatment of Haglund syndrome. Foot Ankle Clin 2019;24(3):515–531.
12. Miller AE, Vogel TA. Haglund's deformity and the Keck and Kelly osteotomy: a retrospective analysis. J Foot Surg 1989;28:23–29.
13. Ortmann FW, McBryde AM. Endoscopic bony and soft-tissue decompression of the retrocalcaneal space for the treatment of Haglund deformity and retrocalcaneal bursitis. Foot Ankle Int 2007;28:149–153.
14. Pauker M, Katz K, Yosipovitch Z. Calcaneal ostectomy for Haglund disease. J Foot Surg 1992;31:588–589.
15. Scheider W, Niehus W, Knahr K. Haglund's syndrome: disappointing results following surgery—a clinical and radiographic analysis. Foot Ankle Int 2000;21:26–30.
16. Syed TA, Perera A. A proposed staging classification for minimally invasive management of Haglund's syndrome with percutaneous and endoscopic surgery. Foot Ankle Clin 2016;221(3):641–664.
17. van Dijk CN, Scholten PE, Krips R. A 2-portal endoscopic approach for diagnosis and treatment of posterior ankle pathology. Arthroscopy 2000;16:871–876.
18. van Dijk CN, van Dijk GE, Scholten PE, et al. Endoscopic calcaneoplasty. Am J Sports Med 2001;29:185–189.

Insertional Achilles Tendinopathy

Mark E. Easley and Matthew J. DeOrio

DEFINITION

- Insertional Achilles tendinopathy is posterior heel pain at the insertion of the Achilles tendon.
- The clinical diagnosis is acute and chronic pathology of the Achilles tendon insertion and its surrounding tissues.

ANATOMY

- The Achilles tendon, the condensation of the gastrocnemius and soleus tendons, inserts on the posterior calcaneal tuberosity.
- The insertion is not only posterior but also on the medial and lateral aspects of the calcaneus.
- A dorsal posterior calcaneal prominence is most obvious on a lateral radiograph. The Achilles tendon inserts distal to this, directly posterior on the calcaneus.
- Between the distal Achilles tendon and the dorsal posterior calcaneal prominence, immediately proximal to the Achilles insertion, is the retrocalcaneal bursa.
- A pre-Achilles bursa is superficial to the distal Achilles tendon.

PATHOGENESIS

- Although not fully understood, repetitive microtrauma to the Achilles tendon insertion is thought to be the cause.
- Most likely, some initial injury occurs, followed by multiple minor reinjuries that lead to chronic symptoms.
- In the acute phase, the process may have some inflammatory characteristics; however, the chronic process is degenerative, with a relative paucity of inflammatory tissue.
- Without histologic confirmation, the diagnosis of Achilles tendinitis or tendinosis cannot be made; therefore, the pathologic process at the Achilles tendon insertion is viewed as "tendinopathy" without tissue confirmation.

PATIENT HISTORY AND PHYSICAL FINDINGS

- The patient may recall an inciting event but typically reports chronic activity-related aching or even sharp pain at the posterior heel.
- In addition, the patient notes a progressively enlarging prominence on the posterior heel.
- This ache is usually accompanied by exquisite tenderness directly posteriorly on the calcaneus, at the Achilles tendon insertion, with manual pressure, on contact from the shoe's heel counter, or when the posterior heel is rested on a hard surface.

- Putting the Achilles tendon on stretch aggravates the symptoms, such as when the patient walks uphill.
- Physical examination reveals the following:
  - A prominence is evident on the posterior heel at the Achilles tendon insertion (FIG 1).
  - Tenderness is felt directly on the posterior calcaneal prominence.
  - No tenderness is found in the Achilles tendon proximal to its insertion on the calcaneus.
  - Thompson test is negative.

IMAGING AND OTHER DIAGNOSTIC STUDIES

- A lateral weight-bearing radiograph of the foot often demonstrates irregularities and calcifications at the Achilles tendon insertion on the posterior calcaneus (FIG 2A).
- Although unnecessary to make the diagnosis, magnetic resonance imaging (MRI) defines the extent of tendon involvement at the insertion and the presence of retrocalcaneal and perhaps even pre-Achilles bursitis (FIG 2B).

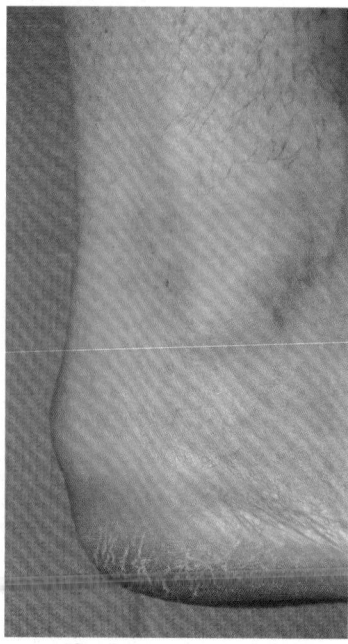

FIG 1 Example of posterior calcaneal prominence characteristic of insertional Achilles tendinopathy.

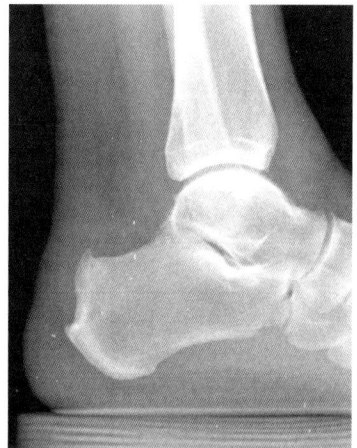 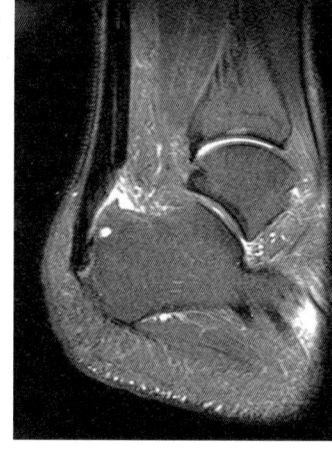

FIG 2 A. Lateral foot radiograph demonstrating the posterior calcaneal prominence and calcification within the Achilles tendon insertion. **B.** T2-weighted sagittal MRI of patient with insertional Achilles tendinopathy. Signal change in the distal tendon and retrocalcaneal bursitis can be seen.

DIFFERENTIAL DIAGNOSIS

- Pre-Achilles bursitis
- Retrocalcaneal bursitis
- Calcaneal stress fracture
- Haglund deformity (prominent dorsal posterior calcaneal tuberosity impinging on the Achilles tendon)
- Calcaneal stress fracture
- Posterior ankle impingement
- Plantar fasciitis
- Noninsertional Achilles tendinopathy

NONOPERATIVE MANAGEMENT

- Activity modification (avoidance of activities that place the Achilles tendon on stretch)
- Nonsteroidal anti-inflammatory agents
- Heel lift or a shoe with a heel to unload the Achilles tendon
- Open-backed shoe or a shoe with a soft heel counter
- Physical therapy
  - Focus on eccentric strengthening exercises
  - In our experience, the common practice of aggressive Achilles stretching must be avoided as it will aggravate the symptoms.
  - Modalities: ultrasound, iontophoresis
- Extracorporeal shockwave therapy may have some benefit but is largely unproven.
- Corticosteroid injection may lead to Achilles rupture and is contraindicated unless the process is isolated to retrocalcaneal bursitis, in which case, a judicious injection of only the retrocalcaneal bursa can be performed.

SURGICAL MANAGEMENT

- The primary surgical indication is nonoperative management.
- Up to 50% of insertional Achilles tendinopathy can be successfully managed without surgery, even when there is a large posterior calcaneal prominence.
- Insertional Achilles tendinopathy with central calcific tendinosis may be less amenable to nonoperative management.

Preoperative Planning

- Preoperative medical clearance
- Even in healthy patients, the thin skin on the posterior heel is at risk. Carefully inspect skin to be sure that the patient is a reasonable candidate for a posterior approach to the Achilles tendon insertion.
- With extensive Achilles tendon degeneration (confirmed with preoperative MRI), an augmentation of the insertion may be warranted. Therefore, preoperative planning should include the anticipation that the flexor hallucis longus (FHL) tendon may need to be harvested and transferred to the posterior calcaneus. The FHL tendon lies immediately deep to the deep compartment fascia that is anterior to the Achilles tendon and can readily be harvested through the same approach.
  - As a rough estimate, we perform an FHL augmentation in less than 10% of cases but routinely have our preferred anchoring system available should the transfer be warranted.
  - We educate all of our patients undergoing surgical management for insertional Achilles tendinopathy that, based on our intraoperative findings, an FHL tendon transfer may be necessary.
- The recovery following surgical management for insertional Achilles tendinopathy is prolonged and may take a full year before the patient returns to full activity. We educate our patients that the recovery is not rapid.

Positioning

- The patient is placed prone on the operating table.
- We routinely inflate the thigh tourniquet with the patient supine on the stretcher and then flip the patient to the prone position on the operating room table. This facilitates proper tourniquet position and avoids stressing the patient's lumbar spine, which may be stressed when placing the tourniquet with the patient in the prone position.
- The chest and pelvis are well padded.
- The brachial plexuses and ulnar nerves at the elbows are protected and relaxed.
- The genitalia are protected.

EXPOSURE AND REFLECTION OF THE ACHILLES TENDON INSERTION

Approach

- A central approach is undertaken, directly over Achilles tendon and posterior calcaneus (**TECH FIG 1A**).
- The scalpel is moved through skin and into central portion of distal Achilles tendon. Deep incision is continued distally, directly to bone.
  - The goal is to avoid unnecessary delamination of the soft tissues and to elevate full-thickness flaps.
- We then elevate medial and lateral slips of Achilles tendon from the calcaneus (**TECH FIG 1B,C**).
  - More than half of the Achilles tendon insertion can be elevated without compromising the integrity of the insertion. One study suggests that up to 75% can be released.

- We elevate the Achilles tendon until all the diseased portion of tendon can be excised.
- Another study suggests that the entire insertion of the Achilles tendon should be routinely elevated and excised to ensure that all diseased tissue is removed. Reattachment is facilitated by a proximal Achilles tendon lengthening that also serves to unload the Achilles tendon.
- We do not routinely elevate the entire Achilles tendon, but should one or both of the Achilles tendon slips become detached, we have uniformly been able to reattach the tendon to the calcaneus with a successful outcome.

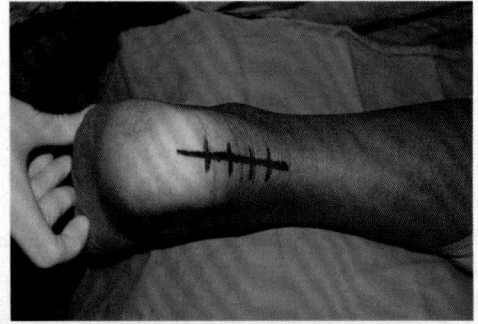
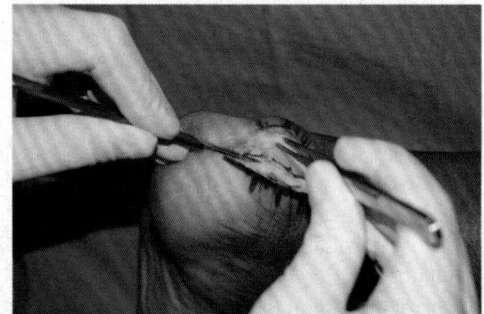
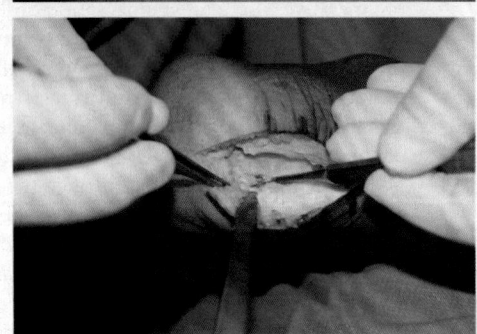

TECH FIG 1 A. Central posterior approach. The foot is hanging from the end of the bed. After a full-thickness incision is made through the diseased portion of the tendon, lateral (**B**) and medial (**C**) tendon slips are developed.

DÉBRIDEMENT OF THE DISEASED PORTION OF ACHILLES TENDON

- The diseased portion of tendon is gradually pared from the Achilles insertion, until only healthy fibers remain (**TECH FIG 2A–C**).
  - Healthy Achilles fibers have an organized, longitudinal pattern.
  - Degenerated Achilles tendon substance is unorganized and may be likened to crab meat (**TECH FIG 2D,E**).
- Calcific tendinosis may be present, and all calcifications within the residual Achilles tendon must be excised (**TECH FIG 2F**).

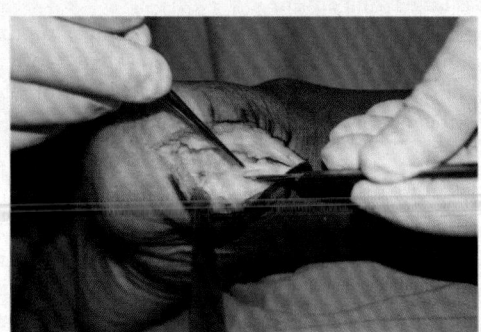

TECH FIG 2 Débriding the diseased portion of the tendon. **A.** Medial tendon slip débridements. *(continued)*

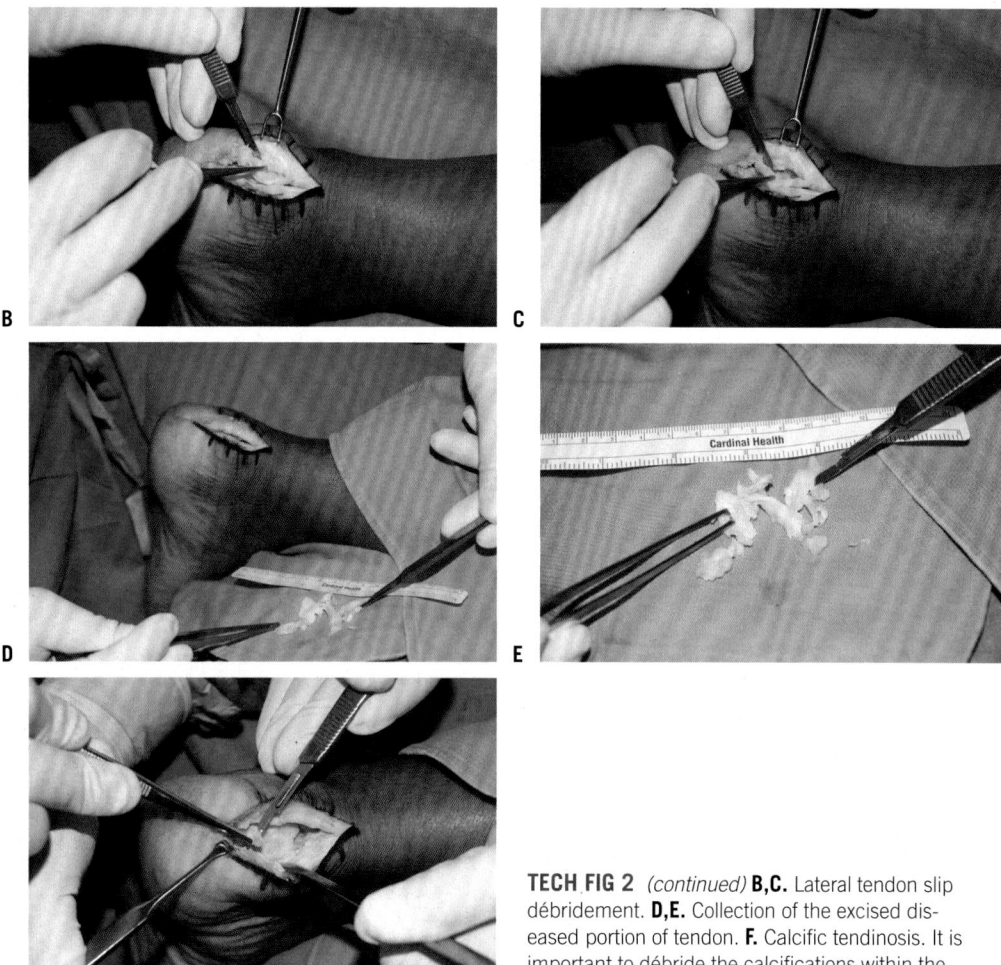

TECH FIG 2 *(continued)* **B,C.** Lateral tendon slip débridement. **D,E.** Collection of the excised diseased portion of tendon. **F.** Calcific tendinosis. It is important to débride the calcifications within the residual tendon.

CALCANEAL EXOSTECTOMY

- Retractors are used to protect the medial and lateral Achilles tendon slips.
- We routinely use a microsagittal saw to perform the exostectomy.
- We first define the exit point on the dorsal calcaneus in order to avoid the tendency to take unnecessary calcaneal bone **(TECH FIG 3A)**.
  - If necessary, a single fluoroscopy spot image may be used to define the trajectory of the saw blade.
  - As a general rule, it is steeper (more vertical) than anticipated **(TECH FIG 3B)**.
- The bony prominence is mobilized with a chisel and removed with a rongeur **(TECH FIG 3C,D)**.
- Commonly, the exostectomy must be "touched up" to remove all of the prominence **(TECH FIG 3E)**.
- With the Achilles tendon slips still protected, the medial and lateral chamfers are removed **(TECH FIG 3F,G)**.
  - This helps narrow the heel and reduce the bulk of the residual calcaneal, medial, and lateral prominences that may lead to persistent pressure and impingement experienced by the patient.

- Although these chamfers are near the medial and lateral insertion points of the Achilles tendon, typically, they can be excised without compromising the residual tendon attachment.

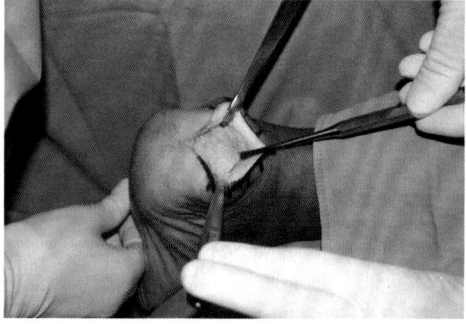

TECH FIG 3 Calcaneal exostectomy. **A.** Planning the trajectory for the saw blade. *(continued)*

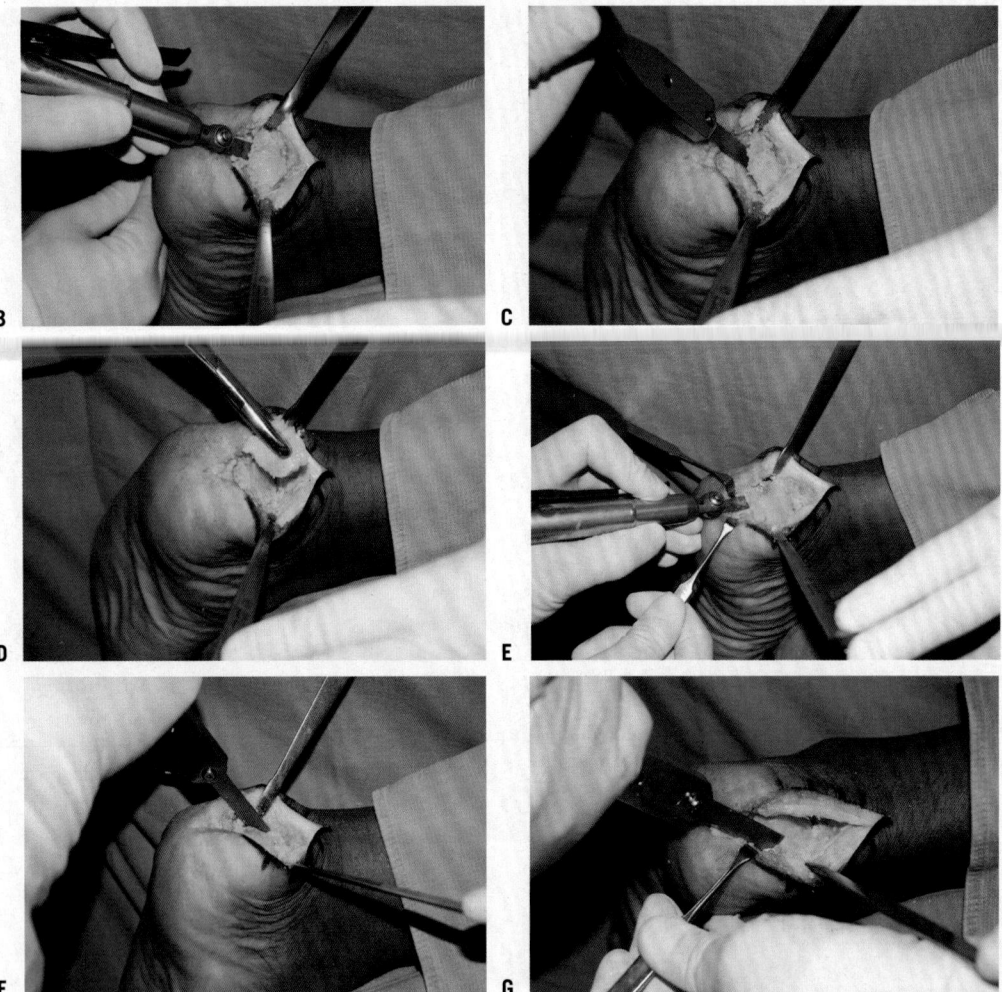

TECH FIG 3 *(continued)* **B.** A microsagittal saw is used to perform the exostectomy. **C.** A chisel is used to mobilize the excised fragment. **D.** A rongeur is used to remove the resected bone. **E.** Touch up to ensure an appropriate amount of bone was removed, and an adequate "healing" cancellous surface is exposed. Chamfer preparation to decompress the lateral **(F)** and medial **(G)** dimensions of the prominent calcaneus.

REATTACHMENT OF RESIDUAL HEALTHY ACHILLES TENDON

Primary Sutures

- With only healthy Achilles tendon fibers remaining and the calcaneus decompressed posteriorly, medially, and laterally, the Achilles tendon should be reattached to the calcaneus.
- Although one study suggested that up to 75% of the tendon attachment can be released without compromising the integrity of the insertion, we routinely reattach the elevated portion of tendon to the exposed cancellous calcaneal surface.
- In our opinion, reattachment not only strengthens the repair but also facilitates direct tendon healing to the calcaneus.
- We routinely use two or three suture anchors:
  - One anchor for each tendon slip
  - Occasionally, an additional anchor to augment the reattachment of both tendon slips
- The anchors are positioned relatively symmetrically on the exposed cancellous surface, in a position that will allow for each

respective tendon slip to be reapproximated to the calcaneus in a balanced fashion **(TECH FIG 4A,B)**.
- The anchors must be strong enough to lift the foot from the bed **(TECH FIG 4C–E)**. If they should fail, we would prefer for them to fail now, so we can rectify the problem.

Balancing and Securing the Sutures

- The anchor sutures are then passed in through their respective tendon slip also in a balanced manner to ensure that the tendon slips have near-equal tension once the sutures are secured **(TECH FIG 5A–C)**.
- We routinely check the anticipated tension by pushing the tendon slip to bone while tensioning the sutures after they have been passed through the tendon.
- If the tension does not appear to be equal in the two slips, we readjust the position of the sutures.

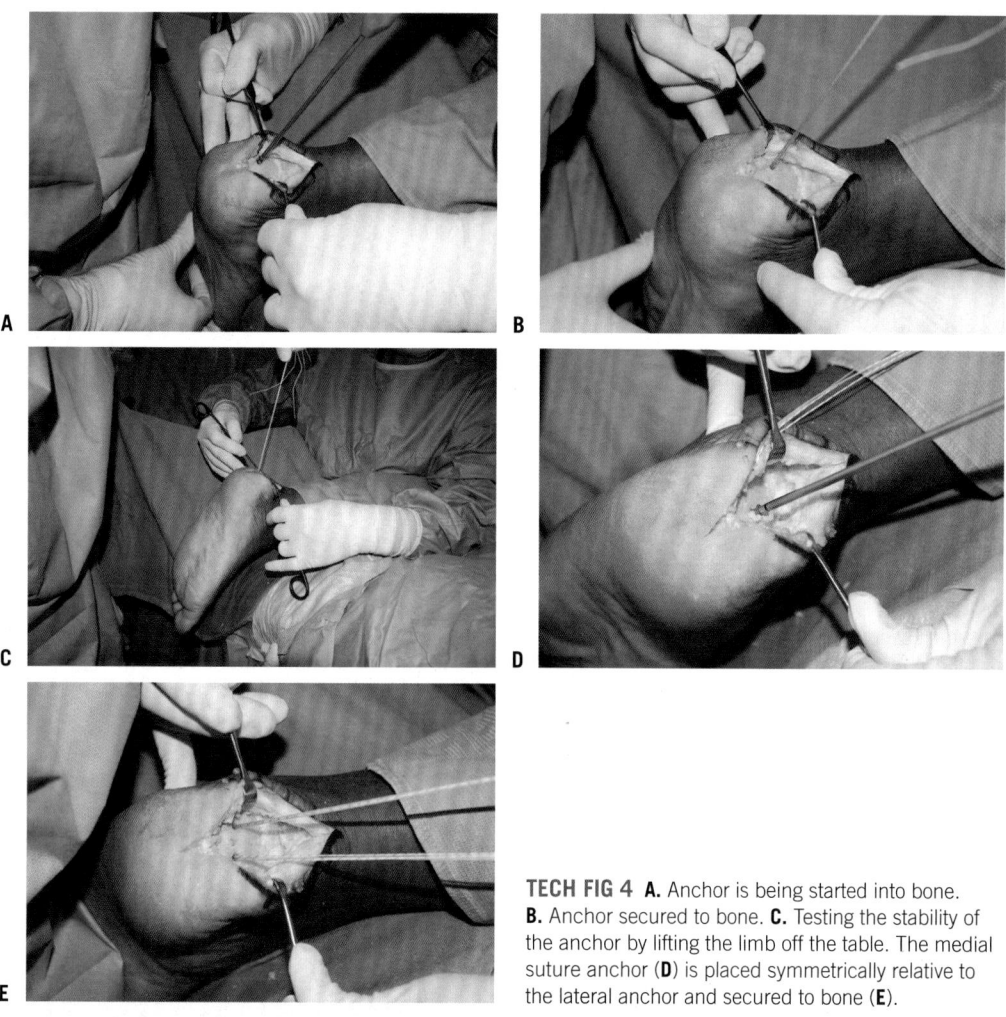

TECH FIG 4 A. Anchor is being started into bone. **B.** Anchor secured to bone. **C.** Testing the stability of the anchor by lifting the limb off the table. The medial suture anchor (**D**) is placed symmetrically relative to the lateral anchor and secured to bone (**E**).

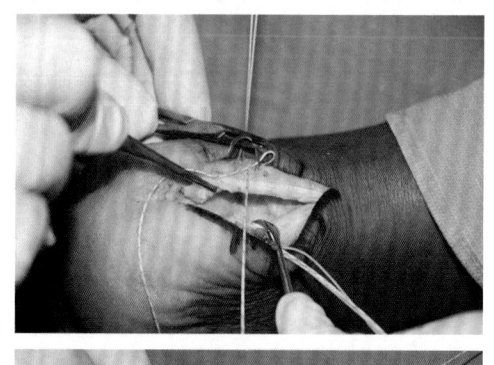
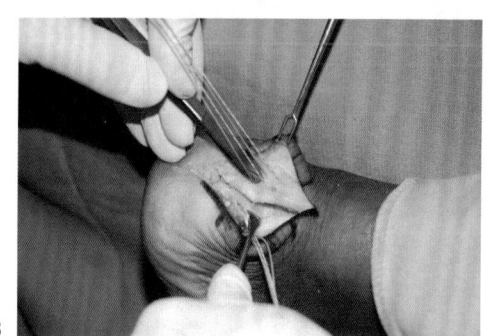
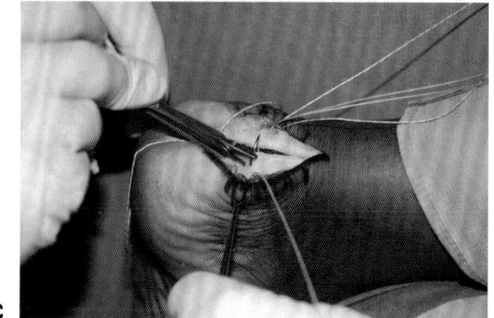

TECH FIG 5 A. The suture is passed through the tendon. **B.** Confirming the optimal balance of the tendon slip on the anchor. **C.** Passing the sutures through the second tendon slip. *(continued)*

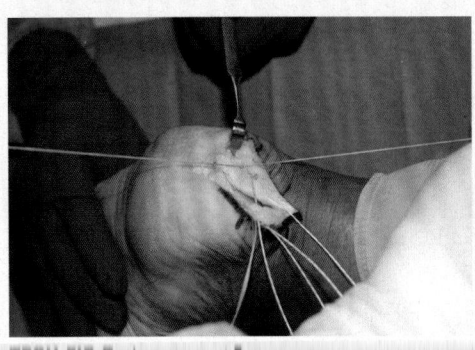
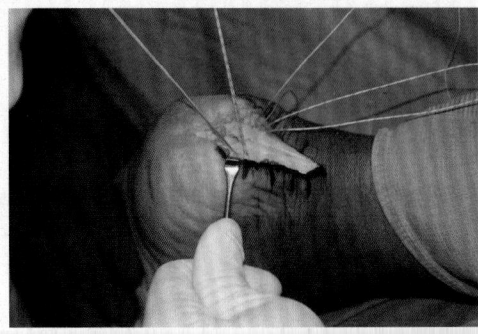

TECH FIG 5 *(continued)* **D.** Lateral tendon slip fully approximated to bone. Note that the ankle is held in plantarflexion to facilitate tendon approximation. **E.** Medial tendon slip being attached.

- The sutures must not only be tensioned appropriately in the longitudinal plane but must also be balanced well in the medial to lateral plane so that the two tendon slips may also be reapproximated side to side and reconfigure the physiologic Achilles attachment.
- The sutures are then secured **(TECH FIG 5D,E)**. Have the assistant hold the ankle in plantarflexion so that the tendon slips fully contact the calcaneus.

Additional Sutures

- We have a low threshold to place a third suture anchor to further stabilize both Achilles slips distally on the calcaneus **(TECH FIG 6A–C)**.

- Finally, the most distal Achilles fibers are reapproximated to the fascial tissue immediately distal to the calcaneus **(TECH FIG 6D,E)**.
  - Avoid trapping fat in this portion of the repair, as it may lead to fat necrosis.
- The two Achilles slips are then reapproximated to one another with an absorbable suture **(TECH FIG 6F)**.
- Gently test dorsiflexion. The ankle should typically still reach neutral without compromising the repair. If it does not, however, it is not a problem.
  - Patients rarely, if ever, develop equinus contracture.
  - Once the Achilles tendon insertion is again healthy and asymptomatic, it has been our experience that the gastrocnemius and soleus muscles accommodate.

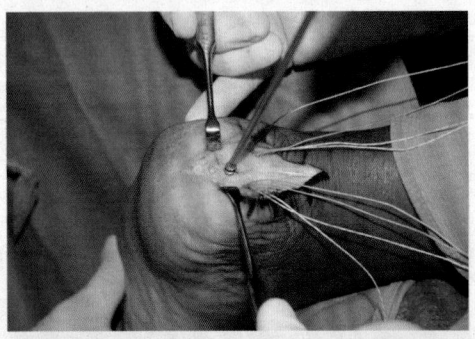
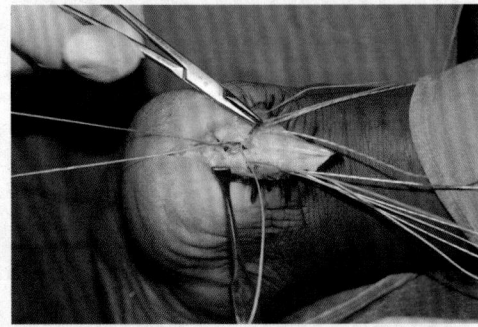
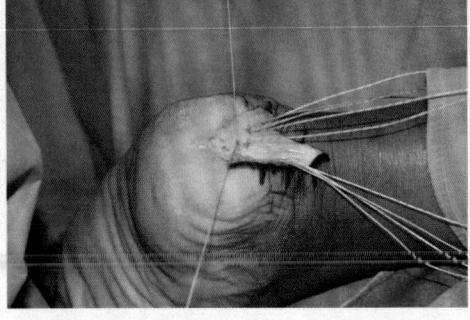

TECH FIG 6 A. A third anchor is being placed centrally and distal to the other anchors. **B.** Securing these sutures to both tendon slips. **C.** Tightening these sutures to bring distal tendon slips to bone. *(continued)*

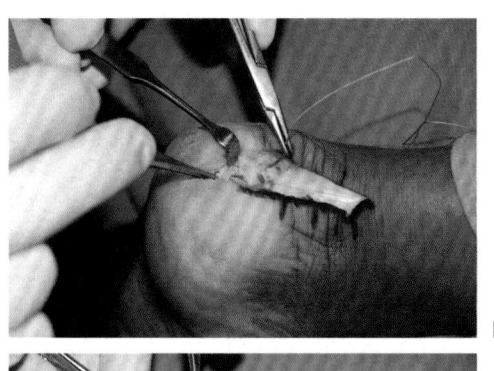

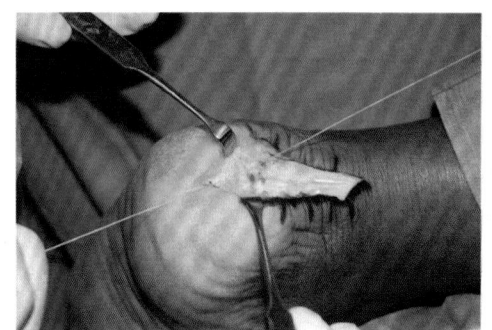

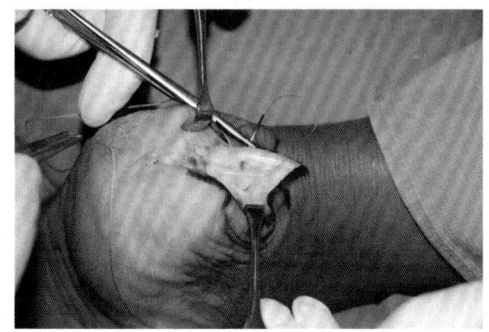

TECH FIG 6 *(continued)* **D–F.** Reapproximating the tendon slips to the distal fascia. **D.** Passing suture. **E.** Fully closing the gap between the distal tendon and the fascia. **F.** Reapproximating two tendon slips proximal to the reattachment.

CLOSURE

- Close the paratenon **(TECH FIG 7A)**.
- Reapproximate the subcutaneous tissues **(TECH FIG 7B)**.
- Perform a tensionless closure. We routinely use staples in the proximal wound but favor suture in the

distal wound, where the skin does not evert as readily **(TECH FIG 7C)**.

- Sterile dressings, abundant padding, and a posterior splint with the ankle in its resting tension complete the closure.

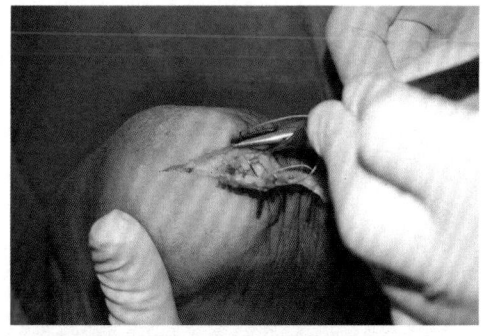

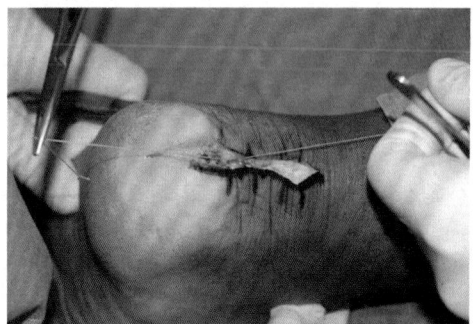

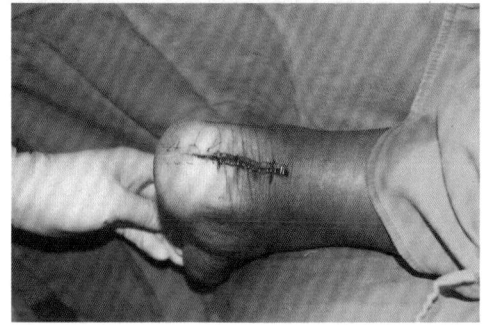

TECH FIG 7 Closure. **A.** Paratenon. **B.** Subcutaneous tissue. **C.** Skin. (Sutures are used distally to ensure that skin margins did not invert.)

FLEXOR HALLUCIS TENDON AUGMENTATION

- Only rare patients present with a combination of insertional and noninsertional Achilles tendinopathy.
- Extensive débridement of diseased tendon is required (TECH FIG 8A,B).
- After fasciotomy of the deep compartment, the FHL tendon is identified, the tibial nerve is protected, and the FHL is harvested from its medial fibro-osseous tunnel with the ankle and hallux interphalangeal joint in maximum plantarflexion (TECH FIG 8C).
- With this local (short) harvest of the FHL, in contrast to a long harvest from the plantar foot via a separate incision,

the tendon length is ample for augmentation of the Achilles reattachment (TECH FIG 8D).
- The FHL tendon is anchored via an interference screw in the central calcaneus, within the exposed cancellous surface created after exostectomy (TECH FIG 8E).
  - A suture goes through the plantar calcaneus to allow optimal tensioning of the FHL tendon (TECH FIG 8F).
- Suture anchors for reattachment of the Achilles slips are balanced on either side of the FHL anchor point (TECH FIG 8G).

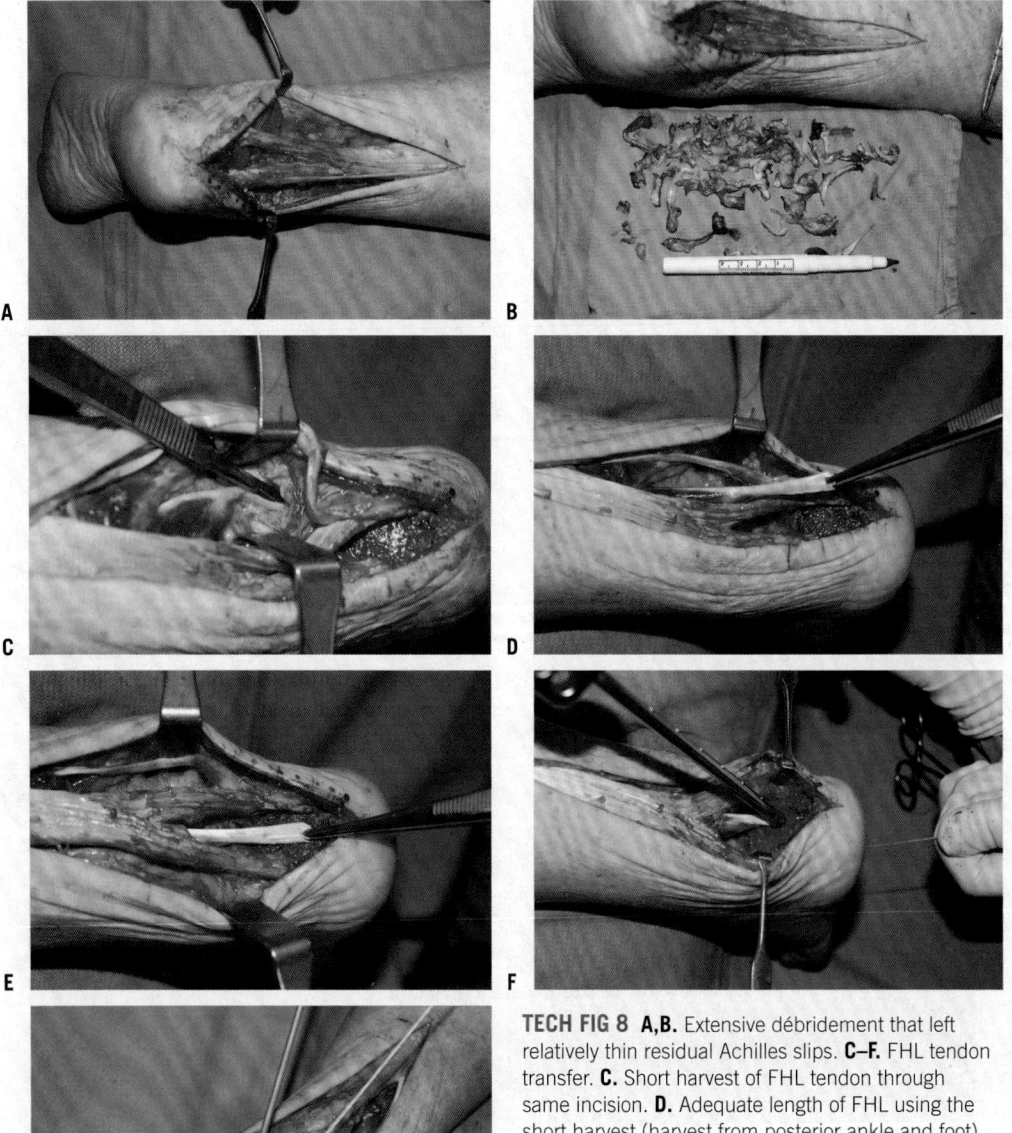

TECH FIG 8 **A,B.** Extensive débridement that left relatively thin residual Achilles slips. **C–F.** FHL tendon transfer. **C.** Short harvest of FHL tendon through same incision. **D.** Adequate length of FHL using the short harvest (harvest from posterior ankle and foot). **E.** Determining the optimal position to anchor the FHL (ideally, as posterior as possible to maximize mechanical advantage). **F.** Interference screw fixation of FHL. (Note the suture through plantar foot to appropriately tension the FHL.) **G.** Suture anchors are placed symmetrically for reattachment of Achilles slips, without interfering with the FHL anchor point.

Pearls and Pitfalls

Calcific Tendinosis	• Be sure not only to débride the unhealthy tendon fibers but also to remove all calcifications within the tendon.
Reattachment of the Healthy Achilles Tendon to the Calcaneus	• The two Achilles tendon slips should be reattached in a balanced manner on the exposed cancellous surface of the calcaneus. • Before tying the sutures of the suture anchors, check that the tension appears nearly equal for the two tendon slips.
Paratenon	• As for repair of acute Achilles tendon ruptures, be sure to close the paratenon over the tendon.
Flexor Hallucis Longus Tendon Augmentation	• This is an intraoperative decision and, in our experience, rarely necessary. If augmentation is needed, perform an FHL harvest through the same incision via a deep compartment fasciotomy. Be sure to identify and protect the tibial nerve that will be immediately adjacent to the FHL tendon. Transfer the tendon as far posteriorly on the exposed cancellous surface of the calcaneus as possible for the greatest mechanical advantage.

POSTOPERATIVE CARE

• Weeks 0 to 2: posterior splint with the ankle in resting tension of plantarflexion
• At 2 weeks: Return to clinic for suture removal and casting.
• Weeks 2 to 5: short-leg, plantarflexed (5 to 10 degrees) weight-bearing cast, with weight bearing permitted but use of an assistive device encouraged
• At 5 weeks: Return to clinic for cast removal and transfer to a cam boot.
• Weeks 5 to 8: cam walker boot with a 5- to 10-degree heel lift; initiate a physical therapy program, with a gradual progression to careful resistance exercises.
• Weeks 8 to 12: progression to a regular shoe with a heel lift or an open-back shoe with a slight heel, physical therapy with a progressive eccentric strengthening exercises
• Between 3 and 6 months: Return to full activities, home program for physical therapy.
• It may take a full year before patients "can forget about this Achilles tendon."
• Maintain independent basic physical therapy exercises for a lifetime.

OUTCOMES

• Most patients undergoing surgical management of insertional Achilles tendinopathy have good to excellent results, albeit without returning to full activity for 6 to 12 months.
• However, most studies note that there are patients that do not return to full activity and although they are improved, they are not pain-free.
• Johnson et al reported a mean improvement in the American Orthopaedic Foot and Ankle Society ankle outcomes score from 53 to 89 points for 22 patients at 34 months' average follow-up.
• McGarvey et al noted an 82% satisfaction rate in 22 patients at mean follow-up of 33 months. Thirteen of 22 patients were pain-free, and an equal number could return to full activities.

COMPLICATIONS

• Wound dehiscence
• Infection
• Avulsion of Achilles tendon from anchors on calcaneus
• Persistent pain despite apparent successful procedure
• Suture reaction or irritation

SUGGESTED READINGS

Barg A, Ludwig T. Surgical strategies for the treatment of insertional Achilles tendinopathy. Foot Ankle Clin 2019;24(3):533–559.

Calder JD, Saxby TS. Surgical treatment of insertional Achilles tendinosis. Foot Ankle Int 2003;24:119–121.

Chimenti RL, Cychosz CC, Hall MM, et al. Current concepts review update: insertional Achilles tendinopathy. Foot Ankle Int 2017;38(10):1160–1169.

Den Hartog BD. Insertional Achilles tendinosis: pathogenesis and treatment. Foot Ankle Clin 2009;14:639–650.

DeOrio MJ, Easley ME. Surgical strategies: insertional Achilles tendinopathy. Foot Ankle Int 2008;29:542–550.

Dilger CP, Chimenti RL. Nonsurgical treatment options for insertional Achilles tendinopathy. Foot Ankle Clin 2019;24(3):505–513.

Furia JP. High-energy extracorporeal shock wave therapy as a treatment for insertional Achilles tendinopathy. Am J Sports Med 2006;34:733–740.

Johnson KW, Zalavras C, Thordarson DB. Surgical management of insertional calcific Achilles tendinosis with a central tendon splitting approach. Foot Ankle Int 2006;27:245–250.

Knobloch K, Kraemer R, Lichtenberg A, et al. Achilles tendon and paratendon microcirculation in midportion and insertional tendinopathy in athletes. Am J Sports Med 2006;34:92–97.

Kolodziej P, Glisson RR, Nunley JA. Risk of avulsion of the Achilles tendon after partial excision for treatment of insertional tendonitis and Haglund's deformity: a biomechanical study. Foot Ankle Int 1999;20:433–437.

Maffulli N, Testa V, Capasso G, et al. Calcific insertional Achilles tendinopathy: reattachment with bone anchors. Am J Sports Med 2004;32:174–182.

McGarvey WC, Palumbo RC, Baxter DE, et al. Insertional Achilles tendinosis: surgical treatment through a central tendon splitting approach. Foot Ankle Int 2002;23:19–25.

Nicholson CW, Berlet GC, Lee TH. Prediction of the success of nonoperative treatment of insertional Achilles tendinosis based on MRI. Foot Ankle Int 2007;28:472–477.

Nunley JA, Ruskin G, Horst F. Long-term clinical outcomes following the central incision technique for insertional Achilles tendinopathy. Foot Ankle Int 2011;32(9):850–855.

Rompe JD, Furia J, Maffulli N. Eccentric loading compared with shock wave treatment for chronic insertional Achilles tendinopathy. A randomized, controlled trial. J Bone Joint Surg Am 2008;90(1):52–61.

Shakked RJ, Raikin SM. Insertional tendinopathy of the Achilles: debridement, primary repair, and when to augment. Foot Ankle Clin 2017;22(4):761–780.

Wagner E, Gould J, Bilen E, et al. Change in plantarflexion strength after complete detachment and reconstruction of the Achilles tendon. Foot Ankle Int 2004;25:800–804.

Wagner E, Gould JS, Kneidel M, et al. Technique and results of Achilles tendon detachment and reconstruction for insertional Achilles tendinosis. Foot Ankle Int 2006;27:677–684.

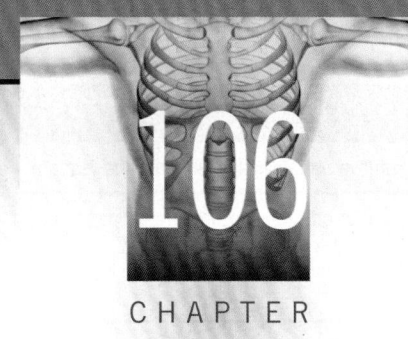

106

CHAPTER

Flexor Hallucis Longus Tendon Augmentation for the Treatment of Insertional Achilles Tendinosis

Taggart T. Gauvain, William C. McGarvey, and Thomas O. Clanton

DEFINITION

- Insertional Achilles tendinosis can be defined as a degenerative condition involving the insertion of the Achilles tendon and represents 10% to 20% of all Achilles pathology.[2] It is traditionally referred to as *insertional Achilles tendinitis*, but this is a misnomer and does not reflect the more chronic, degenerative process as it is known to be.[5,8–10,16] It is a painful, inflammatory condition that occurs at the insertion of the *tendo Achilles* (TA) on the posterior aspect of the calcaneal tuberosity. Often, there is associated calcification of the tendon fibers in the local area and in advanced cases can involve the formation of large enthesophytes.
  - Most commonly seen as an overuse injury in athletes; for example, runners and "push-off" athletes such as basketball and volleyball players.
  - Also seen in sedentary patients as a chronic and painful degenerative process

ANATOMY

- The Achilles tendon is the largest tendon in the body and is the confluence of three tendons—the medial and lateral gastrocnemius muscles and the soleus muscle, all contribute to the Achilles tendon.
- It is viscoelastic and strong, elongating up to 15% under loads and bearing up to 10 times body weight in single-legged stance during running.[5,10]
- The Achilles insertion is a broad expanse that envelops the entire posterior tuberosity of the calcaneus and sends Sharpey fibers to the medial, lateral, and plantar borders of the bone.[1]
- Immediately anterior to the Achilles are the retrocalcaneal bursa and a variably sized posterolateral prominence of the calcaneus known as the *Haglund deformity*.
- Further anterior lies the deep posterior compartment with its fascial covering. The flexor hallucis longus (FHL) and the posteromedial neurovascular bundle (tibial nerve, posterior tibial artery, and veins) are contained in this compartment in close proximity.
- The FHL originates laterally and central from the midfibula and interosseous membrane. It travels obliquely and distally in a medial direction to enter its fibro-osseous tunnel posteromedial to the talus. It then passes under the sustentaculum tali, passing the flexor digitorum longus at the master knot of Henry as it heads toward its insertion on the plantar surface of the hallux.

PATHOGENESIS

- Repetitive stress and microtearing can lead to a combination of inflammatory and degenerative changes.
- Degeneration and tendinosis occur as the already compromised vascularity is further reduced by age and injury.[9,10]
  - Microscopic and macroscopic changes occur, leading to scarring and slow regeneration or repair.
  - Tenocytes are reduced in quality and quantity, contributing to poor repair potential.
- Inflammatory changes are manifested as paratenonitis involving the investing layer surrounding the Achilles. The paratenon begins to thicken and adhere to the tendon itself reducing tendon gliding causing further pain and discomfort.
- Additionally, the continuum of injury and inadequate repair capacity create a cycle of collagen and calcium deposition in an effort to stabilize the tendinous enthesis. Enthesophytes can develop resulting in local irritation of the poor-quality tissues resulting in pain and further thickening of the insertion of the Achilles tendon.

NATURAL HISTORY

- Untreated insertional disease leads to chronic pain, discomfort, and difficulty with activity and shoe wear.
- Pain and swelling locally are common and can increase over time leading to disability.
- A vicious cycle occurs in which further injury induces more attempts at repair and scar formation, leading to more irritation of local tissues, decreased vascularity, and further microscopic injury.
- Range of motion (ROM) is reduced, leading to increased susceptibility to Achilles injury with any activity that places the tendon under strain.
- Calcific debris is generated as a reactive tissue response to injury and intratendinous hematoma formation. This compromises the viscoelasticity and, therefore, the integrity of the tendon, making it more apt to tear, either partially or completely.[4,16]
- A painful, less pliable, less resilient Achilles tendon is the end product. Insertional avulsion or rupture may occur, presenting a difficult treatment dilemma.

PATIENT HISTORY AND PHYSICAL FINDINGS

- Patients consistently complain of pain in the heel at the bone–tendon interface posteriorly.
- On occasion and with advanced disease, there may be some pain found along the tendon proper.

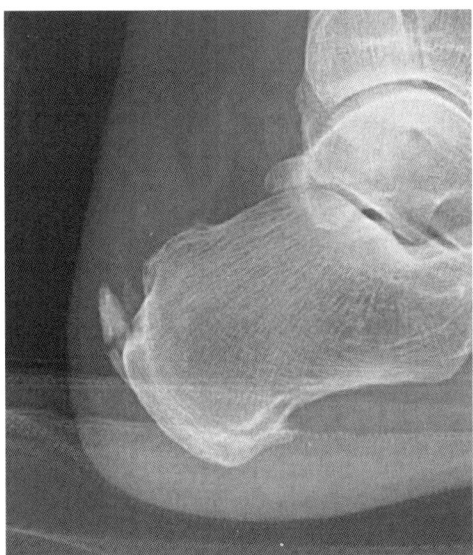

FIG 1 Lateral radiograph of the calcaneus showing a large enthesophyte and calcification of the Achilles insertion.

- Pain may be worse after activity but gradually becomes more pervasive.
- Examination demonstrates tenderness directly posteriorly on the heel or, often, posterolaterally.
- In advanced cases, thickening, nodularity, or hardening of the tendon can be palpated.
- Dorsiflexion of the ankle may be reduced compared to the contralateral leg.
- Methods for examining the Achilles tendon and its insertion include the following:
  - Direct palpation
    - The posterior heel and TA are inspected for visual or palpable swelling, tenderness, nodularity,

or gapping, all of which are suggestive of diseased tendon.
- Thompson test
  - With the patient prone, squeeze the calf at the gastrocnemius–soleus junction to elicit plantar flexion of the foot. Compare with the contralateral side. A positive test is identified when the excursion of the injured side is far less than its uninjured counterpart. A positive test is evidence for complete rupture.

IMAGING AND OTHER DIAGNOSTIC STUDIES

Radiographs

- Radiographs are not required for diagnosis, but they are helpful in determining the presence of calcific debris, which is a poor prognostic sign (**FIG 1**).[16]
- Plain lateral and axial radiographic views of the calcaneus are usually sufficient.

Ultrasonography

- Ultrasonography is a relatively inexpensive and accurate way to determine tendon quality, integrity, and function.
- It has the advantage of being used dynamically to watch active tendon excursion, if so desired. It may also be used to follow the course of healing.
- It is a highly user-dependent tool.

Magnetic Resonance Imaging

- Magnetic resonance imaging (MRI) probably is the most comprehensive study available for investigation and evaluation of a damaged Achilles tendon (**FIG 2**).
- This study gives the most accurate information regarding degree of TA involvement, quality of the surrounding tissue,

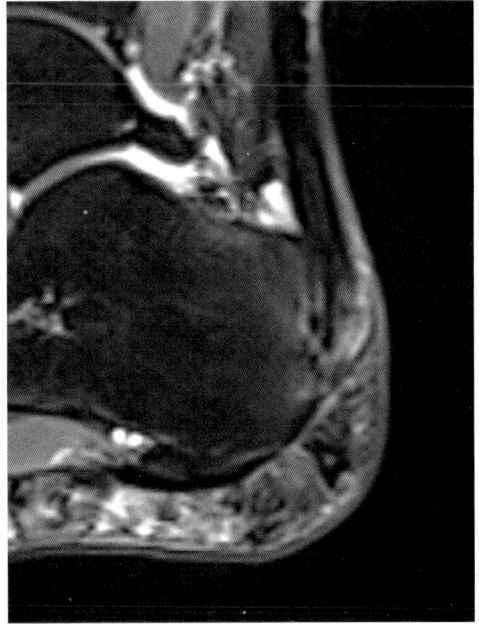
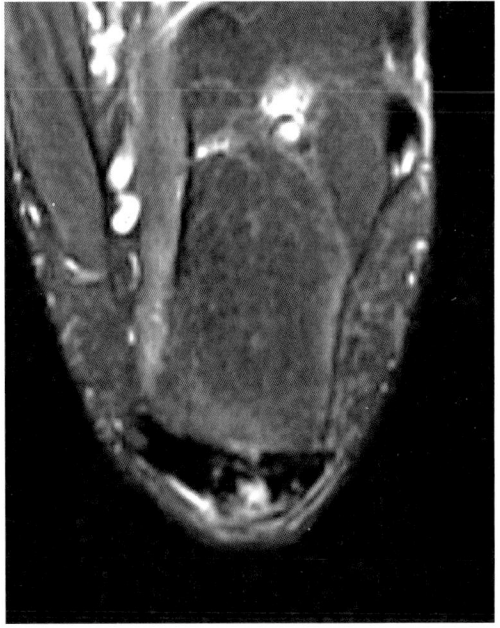

FIG 2 A. This sagittal T2 weighted MRI scan demonstrates increased signal in the Achilles tendon insertion. **B.** This axial T2 weighted MRI scan of the Achilles insertion shows extensive degenerative changes.

presence or absence of rupture, and other concomitant pathology.

DIFFERENTIAL DIAGNOSIS

- Retrocalcaneal bursitis
- Haglund syndrome
- Inflammatory arthritides
- Seronegative spondyloarthropathies
- Gout
- Familial hyperlipidemia
- Sarcoidosis
- Diffuse idiopathic skeletal hyperostosis
- Pharmacologically induced pathology
  - Chronic corticosteroid use

NONOPERATIVE MANAGEMENT

- Nonoperative treatment is successful in 85% to 90% of patients with this process.[5,9]
- Success rates decline in the face of greater age at time of presentation, long-standing symptoms, and evidence of calcific tendinosis.[9]
- Initial phases of treatment include nonsteroidal anti-inflammatory drug use, heel lifts, eccentric stretching, and shoe modification to widen and soften the heel counter.
- More advanced situations may call for formal orthoses to correct any biomechanical abnormality, night splinting to apply continual stretch to the TA, and therapy modalities such as ice, extracorporeal shockwave therapy, and iontophoresis.
- Severe cases may require immobilization in a cast or boot, followed by gradual reintroduction to cross-training before return to regular sports activities.
- There is no role for steroid injections into the insertion of the TA and can potentially cause tendon rupture.

SURGICAL MANAGEMENT

- Surgical decision making should reflect failed conservative efforts and continued symptoms with functional impairments.
- Younger, more athletic patients often respond to simple débridement of damaged TA, which usually accounts for less than 50% of the total tendon. A midline tendon splitting approach to this débridement is our preferred procedure for these patients.
- FHL tendon transfer should be considered if severe Achilles tendon disease is present, the patient is older than 50 years old, the patient has a high body mass index, or greater than 50% of the native Achilles tendon is débrided during surgery.[6,12]

Preoperative Planning

- Structural integrity becomes questionable with involvement of more than 50% of the tendon, so augmentation is thus considered. The extent of tissue disease may become evident on preoperative testing or, alternatively, on intraoperative evaluation.
- Ideally, the surgeon will already have a good idea before beginning the procedure as to whether an augmentation is necessary.
- This is readily apparent on lateral ankle imaging. MRI can also identify the extent of pathology but is not required.
- One must be ready to perform the FHL transfer if it is found to be necessary intraoperatively.

Positioning

- The patient is placed in the prone position with the foot hanging just off the end of the table.
- Both feet may be prepped into the surgical field, up to the level of the knee. Alternatively, only the operative limb is prepped in; however, this limits your ability to compare resting tone during the procedure.

Approach

- A 6-cm incision is made directly in the posterior midline of the heel. Incision starts 2 to 3 cm above the insertion of the Achilles tendon on the calcaneus and ends just distal to the glabrous–nonglabrous skin junction (FIG 3).
- The entire insertion of the TA is exposed.

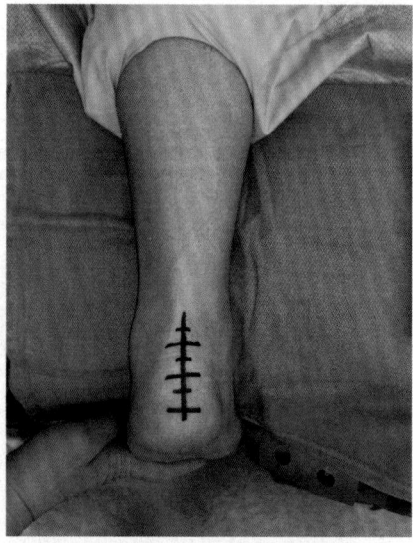

FIG 3 A 6-cm midline posterior incision is used for this procedure to provide enough exposure for the FHL transfer.

CHAPTER 106 • Flexor Hallucis Longus Tendon Augmentation for the Treatment of Insertional Achilles Tendinosis   **5791**

T E C H N I Q U E S

RETROCALCANEAL DÉBRIDEMENT

- Full-thickness dissection down to the level of the paratenon which is then incised vertically along the tendon in the midline.
- Tendon and its insertion are split in the midline with the scalpel for the full length of the skin incision. The insertion is then subperiosteally dissected off of the calcaneus tuberosity leaving the far medial and far lateral insertional fibers intact.
- The tendon is now sharply débrided of all degenerative tissue and calcifications.
- Deep to the tendon layer is the retrocalcaneal bursa. There is fatty tissue and small veins present in this area. This tissue should be removed with the assistance of electrocautery as it is fairly vascular tissue. You are safe in the midline and superficial to the deep posterior compartment fascial layer.
- Any posterior spur on the calcaneus, including the Haglund deformity, can now be removed with osteotome or oscillating saw. An aggressive decompression of this area is desired.
- The calcaneus can then be shaped with a power rasp to round and smooth the medial and lateral edges as well as the convexity of the posterior calcaneus.
- Inspect the remaining Achilles tendon. Transfer of the FHL should be considered if 50% or more of the native tendon has been débrided during the procedure.

FLEXOR HALLUCIS LONGUS HARVEST

- Deep to the retrocalcaneal bursa space, the fascia of the deep posterior compartment will be identified. The retrocalcaneal fat must be removed to reveal the fascia (**TECH FIG 1**).
  - Open the fascia in the midline vertically using blunt-tipped Metzenbaum scissors with the tips pointed laterally to avoid injury to the neurovascular bundle medially.
- The FHL muscle belly will be easily identified with its tendon as it runs from lateral to medial and inters its fibro-osseous tunnel.
  - Pull on the FHL tendon to be sure the great toe flexes to confirm you have the correct tendon.
- The tibial nerve and posterior tibial artery and veins are located medial to the tendon of the FHL, just outside the fibro-osseous tunnel.
- Maximally plantarflex the foot and great toe to allow maximal excursion of the tendon back into the posterior ankle area. Pull then tendon with the blade side of a Senn retractor laterally (**TECH FIG 2**).

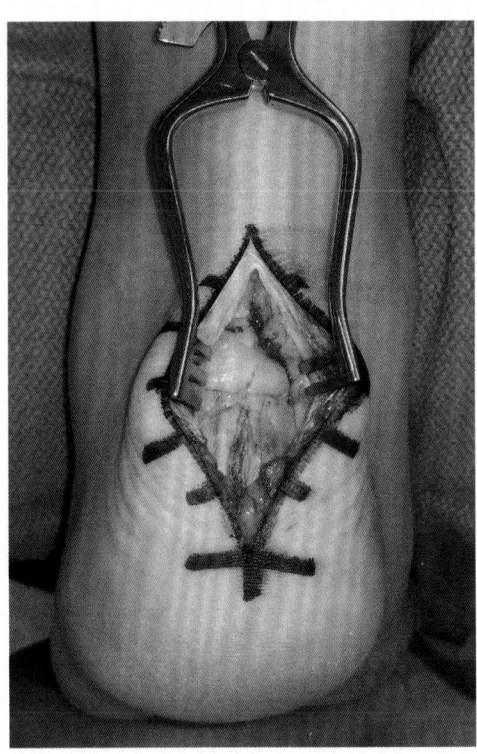

TECH FIG 1 Retrocalcaneal fat (*yellow*) must be removed to reveal the fascia of the deep posterior compartment.

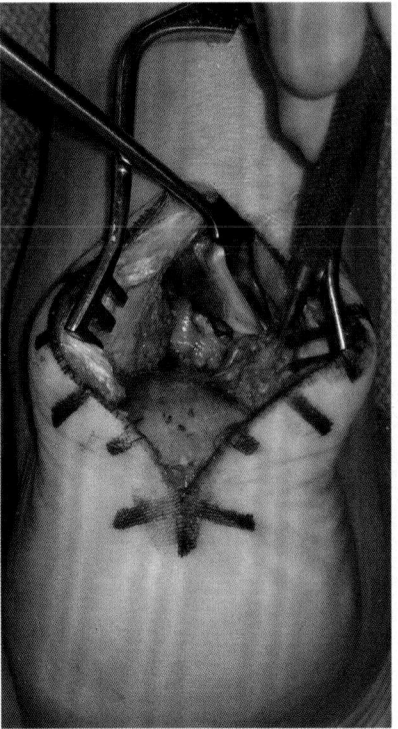

TECH FIG 2 FHL is retracted laterally, and the tendon can be seen diving into its fibro-osseous tunnel. Visualizing the red muscle belly attached to the tendon helps to ensure you have selected the tendon and not the tibial nerve.

- Using a no. 15 blade scalpel, transect the tendon as distally as possible within the fibro-osseous tunnel. Cut the tendon from medial to lateral, so the blade of the knife is always facing away from the neurovascular bundle.
- Then tendon end then can be secured with a whipstitch using a 2-0 braided, nonabsorbable looped suture (**TECH FIG 3**).
    - Size the tendon using a tendon sizer.

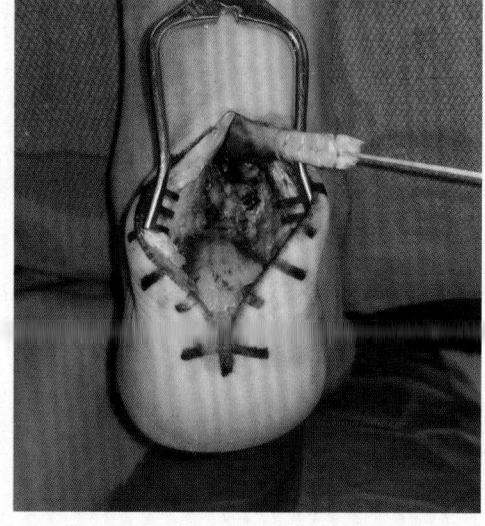

TECH FIG 3 Secure the tendon with 2-0 nonabsorbable suture which will be used to pass the FHL tendon into the prepared bone tunnel in the next step.

ATTACHING THE GRAFT

- Plan for your anchor placement in the heel. The tunnel for the FHL transfer should be located in the midline, approximately 1 cm deep to the Achilles tendon insertion (**TECH FIG 4**).
- Pass the guide pin through the calcaneus and out the bottom of the foot.

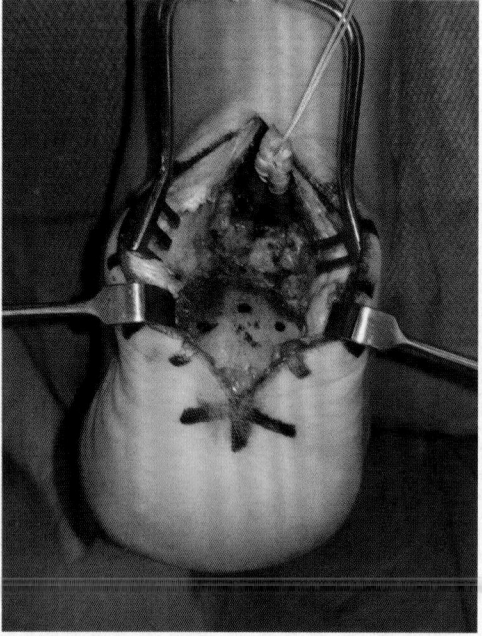

TECH FIG 4 The *center dot* marks the position for the FHL transfer. The marks (*dots*) on either side represent the position of the suture anchors for the Achilles repair.

- Ream the bone tunnel over the wire. The bone tunnel should be sized appropriately to accommodate the size of the tendon and the interference screw.
    - Example: For a 5-mm tendon, ream a 5.5-mm bone tunnel and place a 5.5-mm interference screw for a tight but accommodative fit.
    - Do not ream through the plantar cortex. The depth of the tunnel only needs to accommodate the length of the interference screw plus a few millimeters. If the tendon is too long, it can be trimmed back to 20 to 25 mm as that is all that is needed in the tunnel.
- The sutures on the FHL are brought through the tunnel and out the bottom of the foot using the guide pin.
    - Use the pin driver on oscillating mode to pull the guide pin through without spinning up the FHL sutures.
- Pull the tendon into the tunnel and tension it appropriately to recreate the normal resting tone as compared to the contralateral side. Average resting tone is 15 to 20 degrees of plantarflexion. Also, the far medial and lateral insertional fibers of the Achilles tendon that were left intact can serve as a tensioning guide.
    - Grasp the sutures at the plantar skin interface with a hemostat to hold the desired tension (**TECH FIG 5**).
    - Interference screw is placed into the bone tunnel to secure tendon transfer (**TECH FIG 6**).
- Additional bone tunnels can now be made for the repair of the Achilles tendon.
- Repair insertion of Achilles tendon using suture and bone anchors in a double suture row construct per standard technique.
- FHL muscle belly and tendon can then be sewn to the deep side of the Achilles tendon as its remaining tissue is repaired at the midline split with 2-0 absorbable suture.
    - This helps promote vascularity and improves integrity of the healing tendon to help restore power and push-off.

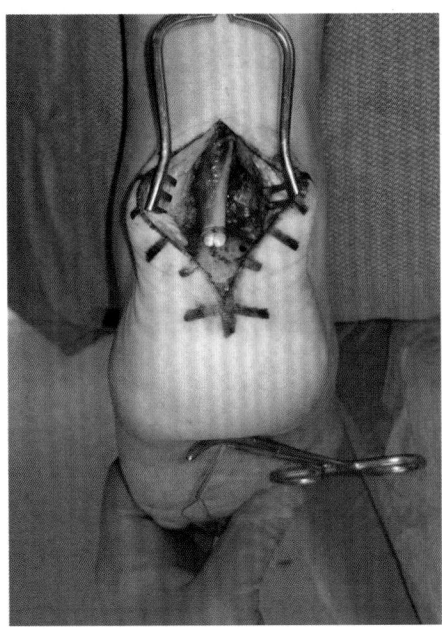

TECH FIG 5 Note the FHL is held in the bone tunnel by the hemostat. Set the tension of the FHL to match the resting tone of the native Achilles.

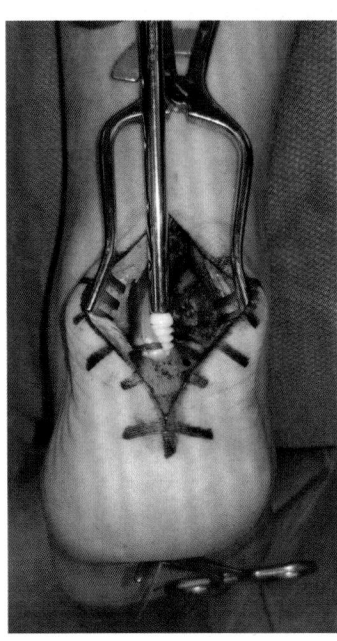

TECH FIG 6 The interference screw fixating the FHL should be placed behind the tendon as shown. This will help keep the FHL closer to the Achilles as the suture tenodesis is completed between the two.

WOUND CLOSURE

- Repair paratenon with 3-0 absorbable monofilament.
- A 3-0 absorbable monofilament is also used to close the subcutaneous tissue layer.

- Skin closure is completed with interrupted, horizontal mattress 3-0 nylon sutures.
  - A 0.25-inch Steri-Strips can be placed in between sutures to decrease tension across the wound.

TECHNIQUES

Pearls and Pitfalls

Decision to Augment	• All studies must be evaluated thoroughly, and the tendon inspected carefully at the time of surgery to ensure TA insertional integrity. Any question regarding stability of the insertion should prompt consideration for augmentation.
Incision	• Full-thickness flaps are essential for reliable healing. Avoid undermining the skin. Perform the débridement through the tendon. • A midline incision appears to better preserve angiosomal blood supply than either medial or lateral incisions. • Place retractors only within the tendon. Do not place static retractors on the skin as this can cause local necrosis.
FHL Harvest	• The muscle belly is easy to identify, but the tendon and tibial nerve are similar in appearance, consistency, and location as they course into the foot. • Follow the FHL from muscle to tendon and stay within the fibro-osseous tunnel under the sustentaculum. • Transect the tendon from medial to lateral up against the medial calcaneal wall.
Insertional Débridement	• Be aggressive in removal of injured TA tissue and inflamed bursa. • Be generous in resecting the calcaneal process and decompressing the heel.
Bone Tunnel	• Do not wallow out the tunnel while drilling. The calcaneus is predominantly cancellous, and this is easy to do.
Tensioning	• Leaving some of the TA insertion attached medially and laterally can demonstrate the patient's natural resting tension to help with this step.

POSTOPERATIVE CARE

- Immediately postoperatively, the foot is splinted in 20 to 30 degrees of plantar flexion for 2 weeks until clinical follow-up.
- At 2 weeks, the sutures are removed if wound is doing well, and the foot is placed into a walking boot with a 2-inch lift to maintain a plantarflexed position. Physical therapy is initiated to allow edema control, gentle ROM below neutral dorsiflexion, and weight bearing in the boot is allowed.
- At 4 weeks postoperative, the patient begins to wean the lift by removing 1 inch per week. Once the lift is gone, the patient will spend 1-week plantigrade in the boot before the boot can be removed for walking at approximately 7 weeks postoperative. Weaning process can be slowed dependent on patient's response.
- Avoid excessive dorsiflexion until 12 weeks postoperative.
- Physical therapy is used from weeks 2 to 16 with progression of strengthening and activity as the patient recovers.

OUTCOMES

- Treatment of insertional Achilles tendinosis is generally successful in younger patients but more unpredictable as the extent of disease or age of patient increases.[9]
- Several studies have shown substantial healing times after tendon débridement alone and poor predictability of recovery when intratendinous calcific debris is present.[16]
- The success of the procedure depends on how thoroughly débridement of involved tissue is performed; however, beyond 50% tendon compromise, the stability of the insertion comes into question.
- Augmentation with the FHL tendon has been shown to be technically reproducible and statistically successful.[7,13,15,17]
  - In one series, 20 patients undergoing the procedure for chronic Achilles tendon insufficiency revealed no postoperative reruptures, tendinopathy recurrences, or wound complications.[17]
  - Despite presumed and reported differences in calf circumference and push-off strength, these differences seem well tolerated and acceptable to patients when compared to the substantial amount of pain relief and restoration of function they receive.[17]
- The technique, as described, modifies classic descriptions in several ways:
  - Deviation from the classic two-incision technique,[7,13,15] thus reducing morbidity of additional surgical site.
  - Maintains more native FHL bulk and function by preserving distal vincular tendon attachments at the master knot of Henry.[14] Theoretically, this will reduce the push-off strength morbidity associated with this procedure.
  - Decision regarding augmentation can be made after débridement of the Achilles tendon is complete, thus basing it on perceived insertional integrity. The FHL harvest is done through the same incision, so there is no increased incisional morbidity if the transfer is thought to be indicated.

- Less tendon is needed because tendon transfer fixation is equal to or better than the side-to-side single-looped method because of interference screw fixation of the tendon directly to the bone.[3,11]

COMPLICATIONS

- Wound complications
- Inadequate tendon débridement
- Inadequate bone resection and decompression of the posterior tuberosity
- Tibial nerve injury
- Fracture through bone tunnel
- Over- or under tensioning the transfer

REFERENCES

1. Chao W, Deland JT, Bates JE, et al. Achilles tendon insertion: an in vitro anatomic study. Foot Ankle Int 1997;18:81–84.
2. Clain MR, Baxter DE. Achilles tendinitis. Foot Ankle 1992;13:482–487.
3. Cohn JM, Sabonghy EP, Godlewski CA, et al. Tendon fixation in flexor hallucis longus transfer: a biomedical study comparing a traditional technique versus bioabsorbable interference screw fixation. Tech Foot Ankle Surg 2005;4:4214–4221.
4. Fiamengo SA, Warren RF, Marshall JL, et al. Posterior heel pain associated with a calcaneal step and Achilles tendon calcification. Clin Orthop Relat Res 1982;167:203–211.
5. Gerken AP, McGarvey WC, Baxter DE. Insertional Achilles tendinitis. Foot Ankle Clin 1996;1:237–248.
6. Hunt KJ, Cohen BE, Davis WH, et al. Surgical treatment of insertional Achilles tendinopathy with or without flexor hallucis longus tendon transfer: a prospective, randomized study. Foot Ankle Int 2015;36:998–1005.
7. Kann JN, Myerson MS. Surgical management of chronic ruptures of the Achilles tendon. Foot Ankle Clin 1997;2:535–545.
8. Marks RM. Achilles tendinopathy, peritendinitis, pantendinitis, and insertional disorders. Foot Ankle Clin 1999;4:789–810.
9. McGarvey WC, Palumbo RC, Baxter DE, et al. Insertional Achilles tendinosis: surgical treatment through a central tendon splitting approach. Foot Ankle Int 2002;23:19–25.
10. Myerson MS, McGarvey WC. Disorders of the Achilles tendon insertion and Achilles tendinitis. Instr Course Lect 1999;48:211–218.
11. Sabonghy EP, Wood RM, Ambrose C, et al. Tendon transfer fixation: comparing a tendon to tendon technique vs. bioabsorbable interference-fit screw fixation. Foot Ankle Int 2003;24:260–262.
12. Schon LC, Shores JL, Faro FD. Flexor hallucis longus tendon transfer in treatment of Achilles tendinosis. J Bone Joint Surg Am 2013;95(1):54–60.
13. Wapner KL, Hect PJ. Repair of chronic Achilles tendon rupture with flexor hallucis longus tendon transfer. Oper Tech Orthop 1994;4:132–137.
14. Wapner KL, Hect PJ, Shea JR, et al. Anatomy of second muscular layer of the foot: consideration for tendon selection in transfer for Achilles and posterior tibial tendon reconstruction. Foot Ankle Int 1994;15:420–423.
15. Wapner KL, Pavlock GS, Hect PJ, et al. Repair of chronic Achilles tendon rupture with flexor hallucis longus tendon transfer. Foot Ankle 1993;14:443–449.
16. Watson AD, Anderson RB, Davis WH. Comparison of results of retrocalcaneal decompression for retrocalcaneal bursitis and insertional Achilles tendinosis with calcific spur. Foot Ankle Int 2000;21:638–642.
17. Wilcox DK, Bohay DR, Anderson JG. Treatment of chronic Achilles tendon disorders with flexor hallucis longus tendon. Foot Ankle Int 2000;21:1004–1010.

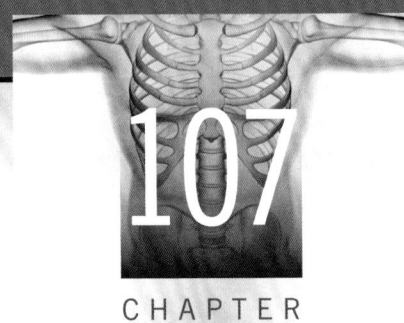

107

CHAPTER

Open Management of Achilles Tendinopathy

Rocco Aicale, Francesco Oliva, and Nicola Maffulli

DEFINITION

- "Tendinopathy" refers to a clinical condition characterized by pain, swelling, and functional limitations of tendons.[2] Traditionally, several terms have been used to describe it, such as *tendinitis*, *tendinosis*, and *paratenonitis*, but the demonstration of absence of overt inflammatory response prompted to use the term *tendinopathy* to describe these disorders.[15]
- Tendon damages can be acute or chronic and caused by intrinsic or extrinsic factors, alone or in combination.[1] Intrinsic factors directly affect the health and composition of the tendon, whereas extrinsic factors influence the tendon environment from the outside and can cause injuries and impair healing in both acute and chronic situations.[15]
- Achilles tendinopathy (AT) can be divided in insertional (at the calcaneus–Achilles tendon junction) and noninsertional (2 to 6 cm proximal to the insertion of the Achilles tendon into the calcaneus) according to the anatomic location of the pathology.[2]

ANATOMY

- The two heads of gastrocnemius (medial and lateral) arise from the condyles of the femur, with the fleshy part of the muscle extending to about the midcalf. As the muscle fibers descend, they insert into a broad aponeurosis, which gradually narrows down and receives the tendon of soleus on its deep surface to form the Achilles tendon.[14]
- The Achilles tendon is the thickest and strongest tendon in the body. About 15 cm long, it originates in the midcalf and extends distally to insert into the posterior surface of the calcaneum. Throughout its length, it receives muscle fibers from the soleus on its anterior surface.[1]

PATHOGENESIS AND NATURAL HISTORY

- AT may be a cause of disability in athletes because of continuous prolonged intense functional demands imposed on the Achilles tendon. This is common in runners and athletes participating in racquet sports, track and field, volleyball, and soccer.[12]
- In AT, there is a disordered proliferative angioblastic reaction with random blood vessels orientation. Inflammatory lesions and the presence of granulation tissue are uncommon; however, if present, they are associated with tendon ruptures.[11]
- The etiopathogenesis of AT remains unclear despite being currently considered multifactorial and the result of interaction between intrinsic and extrinsic factors.[18] Changes in training pattern, poor technique of exercise execution, previous injuries, and environmental factors are extrinsic factors that may predispose to AT.[18]
- Fluoroquinolones (such as ciprofloxacin) and corticosteroids have been implicated as risk factors in tendinopathy.[4] Imbalance of matrix metallo-proteases activity in response to repeated injury or mechanical strain may result in tendinopathy.[23] Metabolic diseases and genetic component seem to play a role.[21]
- The management of AT lacks evidence-based support, and tendinopathy sufferers are at risk for long-term morbidity with unpredictable clinical outcome.[20]
- Most patients respond to conservative measures, and the symptoms can be controlled, especially if the patients accept that a decreased level of activities may be necessary.[10]

PHYSICAL FINDINGS AND PATIENTS HISTORY

- AT is clinically characterized by pain and swelling in and around the tendon, commonly arising from overuse but evident in middle-aged overweight patients with no history of increased physical activity.[10]
- Pain is the main symptom of AT, but the underlying mechanism is not fully understood. It may originate from a combination of mechanical and biochemical causes[6] and occurs at the beginning and after the end of a training session, but with the pathologic process progressing, it occurs during the entire daily living activities.[21]
- Pain is typically located 2 to 6 cm above the calcaneum insertion of the tendon; pain on palpation is reliable and accurate for diagnosis.[10]
- The foot and the heel should be inspected for malalignment, deformity, obvious asymmetry in the size of the tendon, localized thickening, a Haglund heel, and any previous scars.[22]
- The Achilles tendon should be palpated for tenderness, heat, thickening, nodule, and crepitation,[27] and tendons excursion must be estimated to determine any tightness.[7]
- Other used and reliable clinical diagnostic tests for AT are palpation, the painful arc sign, and the Royal London Hospital test.[17]

IMAGING AND DIAGNOSTIC TOOLS

- Diagnostic imaging, such as plain radiography, ultrasonography (US) and magnetic resonance imaging (MRI), may be required to verify a clinical suspicion or to exclude other musculoskeletal disorders.[29]
- US, although operator-dependent, correlates well with histopathologic findings; only in case of unclear US, an additional MRI study should be performed.[24]

- MRI provide extensive information about internal tendon morphology and external anatomy; it is useful to evaluate chronic degeneration, with differentiate between paratendinopathy and tendinopathy of tendon main body.
- Areas of mucoid degeneration in the AT are shown at MRI as high–signal intensity zone on T1- and T2-weighted images. Furthermore, MRI is superior to US to detect incomplete tendon rupture,[10] which is, however, rare.

NONOPERATIVE MANAGEMENT

- Management is primarily conservative, and many patients show good outcomes. If conservative management fails, surgery is recommended.[26]
- Topical laser therapy, low-dose heparin, heel pads, and peritendinous steroid injection produced no difference in outcome when compared with no treatment.[19]
- The drugs proven to be effective in randomized controlled trials include administration of peritendinous injection of aprotinin, topical application of glyceryl trinitrate, and the use of US-guided sclerosing injections in the area of neovascularization.[20] However, when these substances have been used by independent researchers, the results have of them been disappointing.
- Eccentric loading and low-energy shock wave therapy show comparable results.[26]
- Only few available studies were able to produce promising results, for example, positive effectiveness was demonstrated in both randomized studies investigating polidocanol.[28]
- Interesting results for prolotherapy that shown potential improvement in pain and functionality, but no improvements in long-term results compared to typical physical therapy program have been reported.[30]

SURGICAL MANAGEMENT

- Conservative management fails in 24% to 45.5% of patients with AT within 6 months of presentation, and surgery is recommended.[13]
- The aim of surgery is excision of fibrotic adhesions, removing areas of failed healing response, making multiple longitudinal incisions in the tendon to detect intratendinous lesions and restore vascularization and stimulate the remaining viable cells to initiate cell-matrix response and healing.[5]

- Multiple longitudinal tenotomies induce neoangiogenesis in the Achilles tendon, with increased blood flow and, consequentially, improved nutrition and a more favorable environment for healing.[9]
- No prospective randomized studies comparing operative and conservative treatment of AT have been published, and the treatment efficacy is based on clinical experience and descriptive studies.
- If significant loss of tendon tissue occurs during the débridement, consideration could be given to a tendon augmentation or transfer. Gastrocnemius flap, plantaris weave, or the tendon of the flexor hallucis longus can be used for this purpose.
- In rabbit model, after longitudinal tenotomy and soleus pedicle grafting within the operated tendon, it has been shown that transplanted muscle. After the same time, graft tissue hypervascularization, probably, owing to the operation, was also observed, together with neoangiogenesis.[3]

Preoperative Planning and Positioning

- Preoperative imaging can guide surgeon in placement of the incision and to incise the tendon sharply in line with the diseased tendon fiber bundles.
- Under locoregional anesthesia, the patient is placed prone with the ankles clear of the operation table. Prone position allows excellent access to the affected area.
- Alternatively, the patient can be positioned supine with a sandbag under the opposite hip and the affected leg positioned in a figure-of-four position.
- A tourniquet is applied to the limb to be operated on. The limb is exsanguinated, and a tourniquet is inflated to 250 mm Hg.[15]

Approach

- An incision is made on the medial side of the tendon to avoid injury to the sural nerve and short saphenous vein.
- A midline straight posterior incision may also be more bothersome with the edge of the heel counter pressing directly on the incision.
- Maintaining thick skin flaps is vital to reduce the incidence of wound breakdown.

TECHNIQUES

- The paratenon and the Achilles tendon are exposed, and then the paratenon is incised **(TECH FIG 1)**.
- In patients with evidence of coexisting paratendinopathy, scarred and thickened tissue is generally excised.
- The Achilles tendon is incised sharply in line with the tendon fiber bundles, according to preoperative imaging studies **(TECH FIG 2)**.
- Tendinopathic tissue can be identified as it generally has lost its shiny appearance and frequently contains disorganized fiber bundles, which have more of a "crabmeat" appearance, then, this tissue is sharply excised **(TECH FIG 3)**.

- The remaining gap can be repaired using a side-to-side repair. We leave it unsutured **(TECH FIG 4)**.
- The subcutaneous tissues are sutured with absorbable material.
- The skin edges are juxtapproximated with Steri-Strips (3M Surgical Products, St. Paul, MN) before a routine compressive bandage. The limb is then immobilized in a below-knee synthetic weight-bearing cast with the foot plantigrade.
- If significant loss of tendon tissue occurs during the débridement, consideration could be given to a tendon augmentation or transfer.

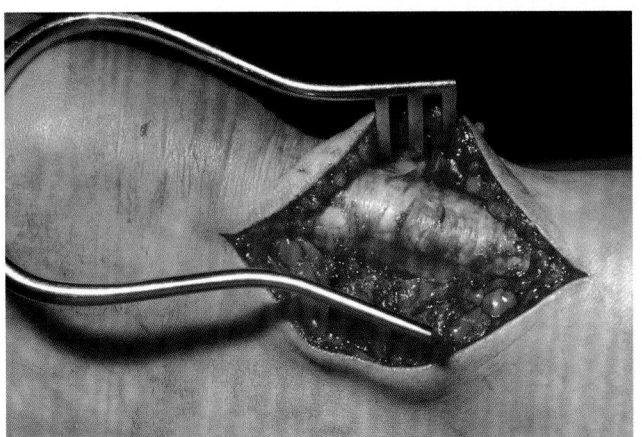

TECH FIG 1 Paratenon and the Achilles tendon exposed.

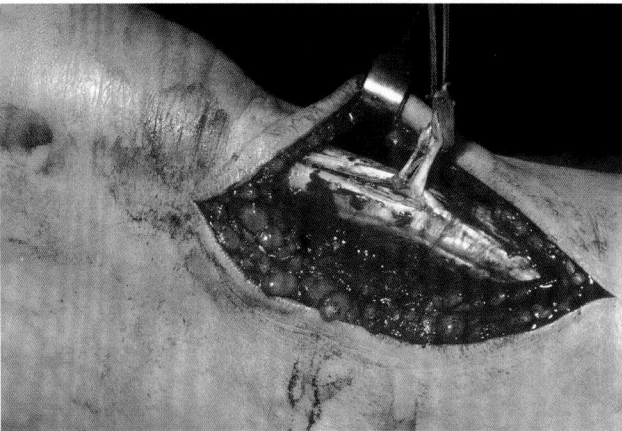

TECH FIG 3 The tendinopathic tissue is excised.

- A tendon turndown flap, a plantaris weave, has been described for this purpose.
- The plantaris tendon can be found on the medial edge of the Achilles tendon. It can be traced proximally as far as possible and detached as close as possible to the muscle tendon junction to gain as much length as possible.

- The plantaris tendon can be left attached distally to the calcaneus, looped and weaved through the proximal Achilles tendon, and sewn back onto the distal part to the tendon. Alternatively, the plantaris can be detached distally as well and used as a free graft.
- The tourniquet is deflated and the time recorded.

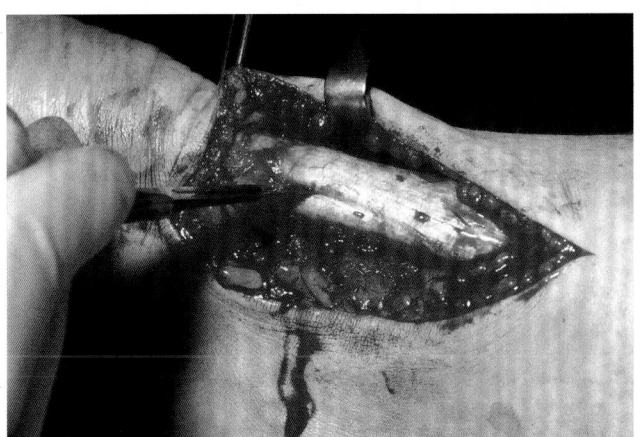

TECH FIG 2 Longitudinal tenotomy along the tendon fibers. Note that, as the tendon fibers rotate 90 degrees, the longitudinal tenotomy has to follow them.

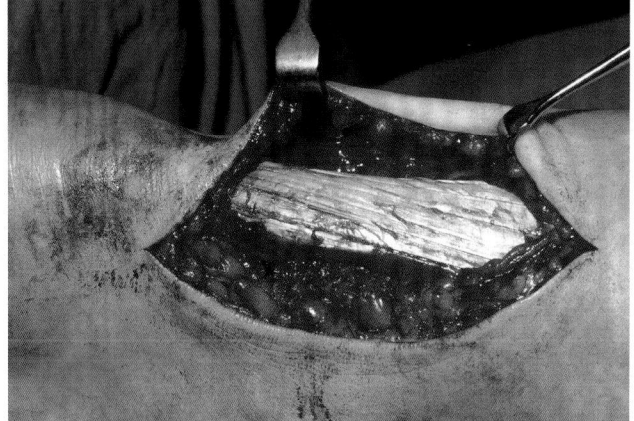

TECH FIG 4 Appearance at the end of the procedure.

TECHNIQUES

Pearls and Pitfalls

Diagnosis	• Diagnosis is usually made on a clinical basis, including a careful history and physical examination. • Ultrasound can identify hypoechoic areas, which have been shown at surgery to consist of degenerated tissue, and increased thickness of the tendon. • MRI studies should be performed only if the ultrasound scan remains unclear.
Positioning	• Prone position, with thigh tourniquet
Incision	• An incision placed medial and anterior to the medial border of the Achilles tendon reduces the likelihood of injury to the sural nerve and short saphenous vein.

POSTOPERATIVE CARE

- Initial splinting and crutch walking is generally used to allow pain and swelling to subside. In addition, the initial period of immobilization in the cast may promote skin healing to avoid wound complications.
- After 14 days, the cast is removed, and motion exercises are initiated. Patients are encouraged to start daily active and passive ankle range of motion exercises. Weight bearing is not limited according to the degree of débridement needed at surgery, and we encourage early weight bearing. Extensive débridements and tendon transfers may require protected weight bearing for 4 to 6 weeks postoperatively.
- After 6 to 8 weeks of mostly range of motion and light resistive exercises, initial tendon healing will have completed. More intensive strengthening exercises are started, gradually progressing to plyometrics and eventually running and jumping.[25,26]

OUTCOMES

- Surgical procedure is commonly successful, but patients should be informed of potential failure, risks of wound complications, and prolonged recovery time.[18]
- Rehabilitation is focused on early motion and avoidance of overloading the tendon in the initial healing phase.
- Two systematic review reports surgical success rates in over 70% of cases. This is not always observed in clinical practice: indeed, the articles that reported success rates higher than 70% had poorer methods scores.[8] This finding could be used as evidence that the discrepancy between published results and clinical outcomes may well be the result of poor research methodology.[16]

COMPLICATIONS

- Wound healing problems
- Infection
- Sural nerve injury
- Rupture of Achilles tendon
- Deep vein thrombosis

REFERENCES

1. Aicale R, Tarantino D, Maffulli N. Basic science of tendons. In: Bio-orthopaedics. Berlin, Germany: Springer-Verlag GmbH, 2017: 249–273.
2. Aicale R, Tarantino D, Maffulli N. Non-insertional Achilles tendinopathy: state of the art. In: Canata GL, d'Hooghe P, Hunt KJ, et al, eds. Sports Injuries of the Foot and Ankle: A Focus on Advanced Surgical Techniques. Berlin, Germany: Springer-Verlag GmbH, 2019:359–367.
3. Benazzo F, Stennardo G, Mosconi M, et al. Muscle transplant in the rabbit's Achilles tendon. Med Sci Sports Exerc 2001;33:696–701.
4. Bisaccia DR, Aicale R, Tarantino D, et al. Biological and chemical changes in fluoroquinolone-associated tendinopathies: a systematic review. Br Med Bull 2019;130(1):39–49.
5. Kannus P, Józsa L. Histopathological changes preceding spontaneous rupture of a tendon. A controlled study of 891 patients. J Bone Joint Surg Am 1991;73:1507–1525.
6. Khan KM, Maffulli N. Tendinopathy: an Achilles' heel for athletes and clinicians. Clin J Sport Med 1998;8:151–154.
7. Longo UG, Ronga M, Maffulli N. Achilles tendinopathy. Sports Med Arthrosc Rev 2009;17:112–126.
8. Longo UG, Ronga M, Maffulli N. Achilles tendinopathy. Sports Med Arthrosc Rev 2018;26:16–30.
9. Maffulli N. Re: Etiologic factors associated with symptomatic Achilles tendinopathy. Foot Ankle Int 2007;28:661.
10. Maffulli N, Aicale R. Update on non-insertional Achilles tendinopathy. Fu & Sprunggelenk 2019;17:248–256.
11. Maffulli N, Barrass V, Ewen SW. Light microscopic histology of Achilles tendon ruptures. A comparison with unruptured tendons. Am J Sports Med 2000;28:857–863.
12. Maffulli N, Binfield PM, King JB. Tendon problems in athletic individuals. J Bone Joint Surg Am 1998;80:142–144.
13. Maffulli N, Kader D. Tendinopathy of tendo Achillis. J Bone Joint Surg Br 2002;84:1–8.
14. Maffulli N, Kenward MG, Testa V, et al. Clinical diagnosis of Achilles tendinopathy with tendinosis. Clin J Sport Med 2003;13:11–15.
15. Maffulli N, Khan KM, Puddu G. Overuse tendon conditions: time to change a confusing terminology. Arthroscopy 1998;14:840–843.
16. Maffulli N, Longo UG, Kadakia A, et al. Achilles tendinopathy. Foot Ankle Surg 2020;26:240–249. doi:10.1016/j.fas.2019.03.009.
17. Maffulli N, Oliva F, Loppini M, et al. The Royal London Hospital test for the clinical diagnosis of patellar tendinopathy. Muscles Ligaments Tendons J 2017;7:315–322.
18. Maffulli N, Sharma P, Luscombe KL. Achilles tendinopathy: aetiology and management. J R Soc Med 2004;97:472–476.
19. Maffulli N, Testa V, Capasso G, et al. Similar histopathological picture in males with Achilles and patellar tendinopathy. Med Sci Sports Exerc 2004;36:1470–1475.
20. Maffulli N, Testa V, Capasso G, et al. Surgery for chronic Achilles tendinopathy yields worse results in nonathletic patients. Clin J Sport Med 2006;16:123–128.
21. Maffulli N, Via AG, Oliva F. Chronic Achilles tendon disorders: tendinopathy and chronic rupture. Clin Sports Med 2015;34:607–624.
22. Maffulli N, Wong J, Almekinders LC. Types and epidemiology of tendinopathy. Clin Sports Med 2003;22:675–692.
23. Magra M, Maffulli N. Nonsteroidal antiinflammatory drugs in tendinopathy: friend or foe. Clin J Sport Med 2006;16:1–3.
24. Neuhold A, Stiskal M, Kainberger F, et al. Degenerative Achilles tendon disease: assessment by magnetic resonance and ultrasonography. Eur J Radiol 1992;14:213–220.
25. Rompe JD, Nafe B, Furia JP, et al. Eccentric loading, shock-wave treatment, or a wait-and-see policy for tendinopathy of the main body of tendo Achillis: a randomized controlled trial. Am J Sports Med 2007;35:374–383.
26. Sayana MK, Maffulli N. Eccentric calf muscle training in non-athletic patients with Achilles tendinopathy. J Sci Med Sport 2007;10:52–58.
27. Teitz CC, Garrett WE Jr, Miniaci A, et al. Tendon problems in athletic individuals. Instr Course Lect 1997;46:569–582.
28. Willberg L, Sunding K, Ohberg L, et al. Sclerosing injections to treat midportion Achilles tendinosis: a randomised controlled study evaluating two different concentrations of polidocanol. Knee Surg Sports Traumatol Arthrosc 2008;16:859–864.
29. Williams JG. Achilles tendon lesions in sport. Sports Med 1986;3:114–135.
30. Yelland MJ, Sweeting KR, Lyftogt JA, et al. Prolotherapy injections and eccentric loading exercises for painful Achilles tendinosis: a randomised trial. Br J Sports Med 2011;45:421–428.

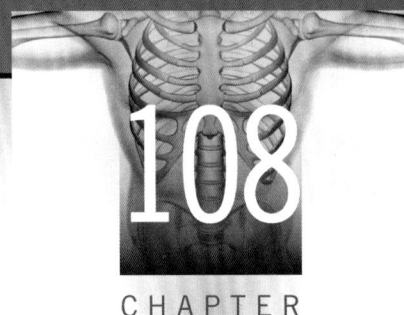

108

CHAPTER

Flexor Hallucis Longus Transfer for Achilles Tendinosis

Bryan D. Den Hartog

DEFINITION

- Insertional and midsubstance Achilles tendinosis is a painful degenerative process that arises due to mechanical and vascular factors and affects the paratenon and collagen fibers.
- It is most commonly seen in patients in their mid-40s and older.

ANATOMY

- The Achilles tendon, the largest tendon in the body, connects the gastrocsoleus complex to the calcaneus (FIG 1).
- It is covered by a paratenon without a definite tendon sheath.
- The blood supply of the tendon arises distally from calcaneal arterioles and proximally from intramuscular branches. There is a relatively hypovascular, or watershed, area 2 to 4 cm proximal to the tendon insertion.

PATHOGENESIS

- Mechanical and vascular factors contribute to the development of tendinosis. The process begins with mechanical pressure on the insertion of the Achilles tendon from internal factors, a Haglund deformity, or external factors, such as a firm heel counter. Retrocalcaneal bursitis develops initially without Achilles tendon involvement. Increasing prominence of the posterolateral calcaneal tuberosity or hindfoot malalignment (ie, varus heel) can cause tendon collagen fiber injury and further inflammation of the retrocalcaneal bursa.

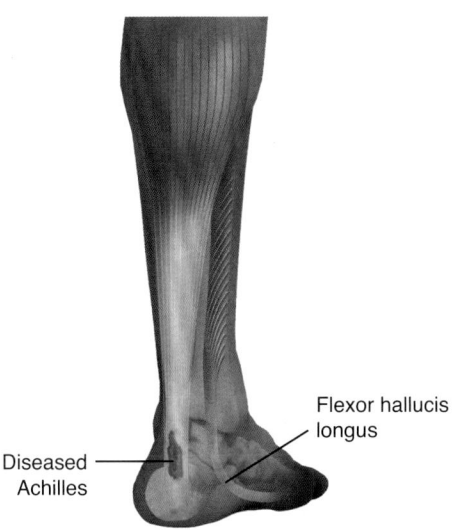

Flexor hallucis longus

Diseased Achilles

FIG 1 The Achilles tendon and its relationship to the FHL tendon.

- Progressive thickening of the retrocalcaneal bursa and peritendinous tissue increases mechanical pressure on the tendon, impeding blood flow, and hampering the normal repair process, leading to a thickened, degenerative tendon.
- With dysvascular changes associated with aging, the tendon becomes increasingly thick and painful. Radiographs at this point may show a spur or calcification at the Achilles insertion.

NATURAL HISTORY

- The natural history of the pathologic process most likely is a continuum that begins with retrocalcaneal bursitis and ends in chronic Achilles tendinosis.
- Patient activity becomes more restricted due to increased pain and weakness.
- Age-dependent changes in collagen quality and decreased vascularity contribute to the development of tendinosis.
- As the degenerative process becomes chronic, the tendon becomes mechanically deficient and more susceptible to rupture.
- Symptoms become unremitting as the disease progresses.

PATIENT HISTORY AND PHYSICAL FINDINGS

- Achilles tendinosis causes pain and swelling of the diseased segment of tendon.
- Pain increases with physical activity and with direct pressure on the affected tendon.
- Patients with seronegative arthropathies, spondyloarthropathies, hypercholesterolemia, sarcoidosis, and renal transplant have an increased incidence of Achilles tendinopathy.
- The patient should be assessed for hyperpronation or heel varus deformities, which can cause eccentric Achilles tendon loading. If either is present, an orthosis to keep the hindfoot in neutral may be necessary.
- Ankle dorsiflexion is measured with the knee flexed and extended to assess for gastrocnemius or Achilles tendon tightness. If excessive tightness is present, a gastrocnemius recession should be considered along with the flexor hallucis longus (FHL) transfer.
- With the patient prone on the examining table, the Achilles tendon is palpated to localize the area of thickening and tenderness (either insertional or noninsertional). Assess the size of the calcaneal tuberosity; if it is enlarged, excision of this prominence should be considered to reduce mechanical pressure on the diseased Achilles tendon.

IMAGING AND OTHER DIAGNOSTIC STUDIES

- Radiographs are useful in evaluating the extent of tendon calcification and presence of a Haglund deformity (FIG 2A).

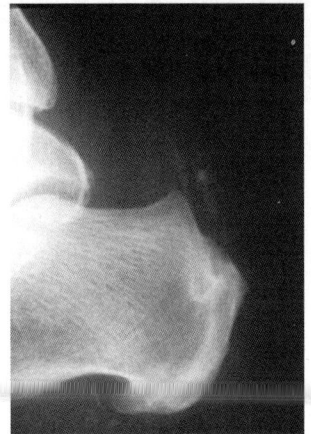 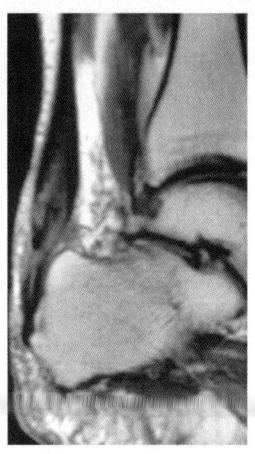 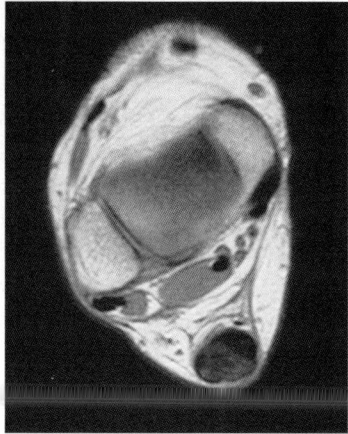

FIG 2 A. Lateral radiograph of the heel revealing a prominent calcaneal tuberosity and calcification of the Achilles insertion. **B.** This sagittal MRI scan demonstrates increased signal in the Achilles insertion. **C.** This axial MRI scan of the Achilles insertion reveals diseased fibers.

- Although magnetic resonance imaging (MRI) scanning is not essential for preoperative planning, it can be beneficial in estimating the amount of degenerative tendon to be excised (**FIG 2B,C**).

DIFFERENTIAL DIAGNOSIS

- Haglund deformity
- Os trigonum
- Retrocalcaneal bursitis
- Peritendinitis
- Seronegative spondyloarthropathy
- Insertional tendinopathy
- Achilles tendinosis

NONOPERATIVE MANAGEMENT

- Nonsurgical treatment of insertional or noninsertional Achilles tendinosis includes rest, immobilization, and rehabilitation.
- Immobilization can include casting, a cast brace, and a custom-molded ankle–foot orthosis.
- Structural abnormalities such as heel varus are addressed with wedges or orthotics, or both.
- Training regimens are modified to reduce stress on the affected tendon.
- Physical therapy for heavy load eccentric strengthening exercises has been found to be effective for Achilles tendinopathy and may be superior to conventional treatment regimens and comparable to open débridement of the tendon.

SURGICAL MANAGEMENT

- Surgery is performed only on those patients who have intractable pain and impaired function or those who have failed previous tendon débridement or Haglund resection alone.
  - Most people in this patient group have a chronic Achilles tendon deficiency and are sedentary, overweight, and have radiographic or MRI evidence of a thickened, calcific Achilles insertion.
- Most treatments that have been described focus on removing mechanical pressure from the diseased tendon (eg, excising the posterosuperior calcaneal tuberosity), débridement of the diseased tendon, or augmentation of the remaining, débrided tendon (ie, FHL, peroneus brevis, plantaris).
- The bulk of surgical treatment is discussed in the following sections and in the Techniques section.

Preoperative Planning

- The extent and location of diseased tendon must be identified. The area of tendon degeneration most often is the distal 2 to 4 cm. The degeneration also may be isolated at the midsubstance.
- The patient must understand preoperatively that the time to maximum improvement could be prolonged (average 8.2 months).
- If the surgeon wants to loop the transferred FHL through the calcaneus at the time of the transfer and more tendon length consequently will be needed, the FHL should be harvested from the midmost at Henry knot and pulled out the posterior incision.

Positioning

- The patient is placed prone on the operating table with a soft bump anterior to the ankle (**FIG 3**).

Approach

- Various incisions have been used to approach the diseased tendon.
  - Incisions that have been recommended include central splitting, medial and/or lateral longitudinal pretentious, or medial with a transverse L-shaped extension distally.
  - All of these incisions can be used successfully to expose and débride diseased tissue, but if augmentation of the Achilles tendon is anticipated, a medial incision will give the best access to the FHL.
- Whatever incision is selected, it should be done sharply through the subcutaneous tissue to the paratenon, taking care not to dissect horizontally, thus reducing the risk of vascular compromise of the soft tissues overlying the tendon.

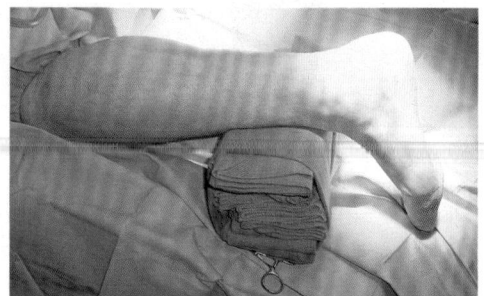

FIG 3 The patient is positioned prone on the operating table.

EXPOSURE AND TENDON PREPARATION

- A 10-cm posteromedial incision is made starting near the junction of the proximal and middle thirds of the Achilles tendon and stopping distally at the tendinous insertion into the calcaneal tuberosity.
- The incision is made sharply through the subcutaneous tissue to the paratenon, taking care not to dissect horizontally, thereby reducing the risk of vascular compromise of the soft tissue overlying the Achilles tendon.
- An L-shaped extension of the incision distally is performed if extensive débridement of the Achilles tendon is anticipated and better exposure of the lateral tendon insertion is needed **(TECH FIG 1A)**.
- The substance of the tendon is carefully inspected. Any amorphous (codfish-flesh appearing), calcified, or ossified tissue of

the tendon is excised, leaving only relatively healthy, normally striated tissue. Usually, more than 50% of the cross-section is removed.
- The degenerative, calcified area of tendon is best excised by removing a wedge-shaped piece of tissue from the insertion of the Achilles tendon **(TECH FIG 1B,C)**.
- In all cases, a partial calcaneal ostectomy is performed at the superoposterior aspect to decompress the Achilles tendon insertion **(TECH FIG 1D–F)**. This also improves exposure to the anterior aspect of the tendon, aiding in tendon inspection and débridement.
- With the degenerative tissue removed, the triangular fat pad anterior to the Achilles tendon is excised, exposing the deep posterior fascia **(TECH FIG 1G)**.

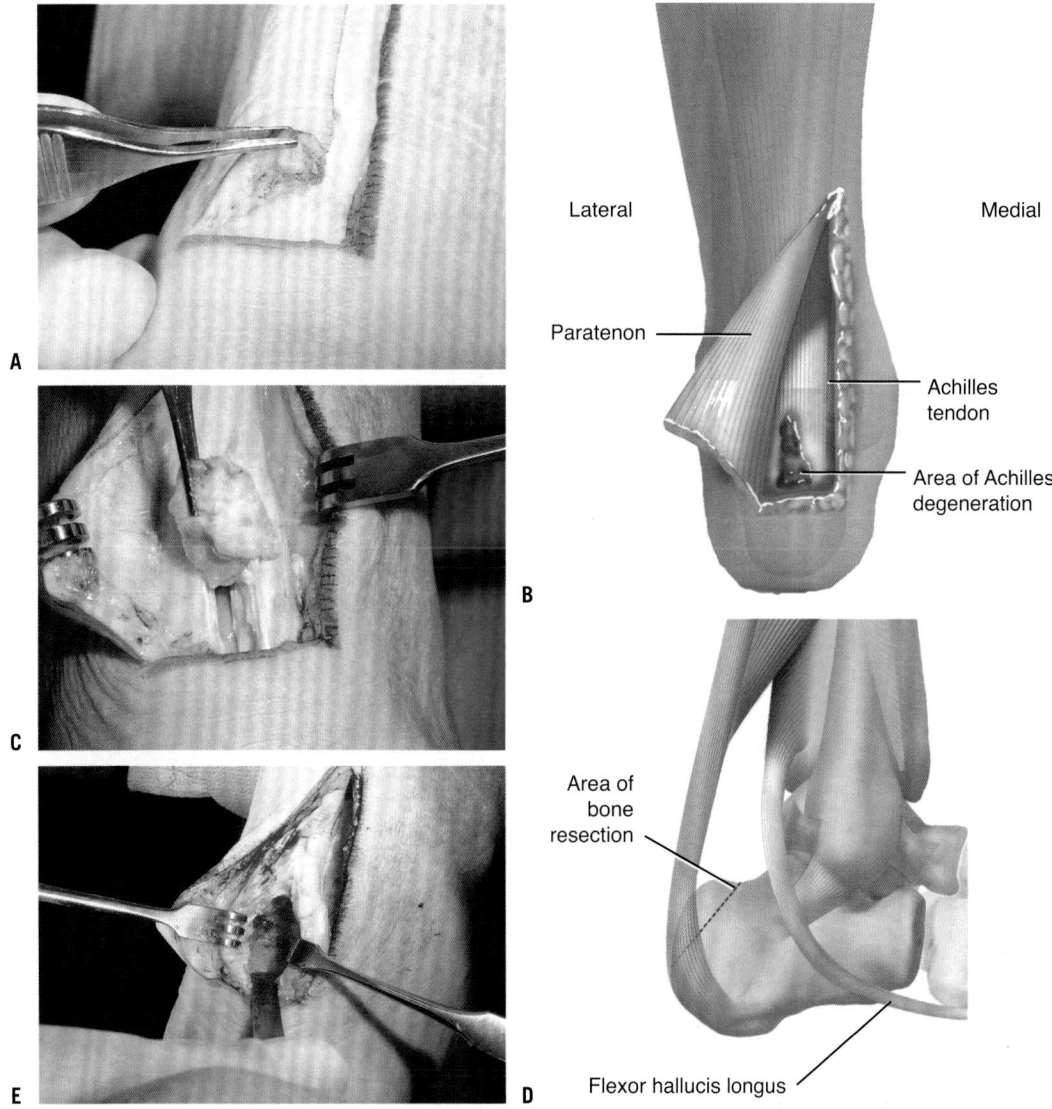

Lateral   Medial

Paratenon

Achilles tendon

Area of Achilles degeneration

Area of bone resection

Flexor hallucis longus

TECH FIG 1 A. Full-thickness, L-shaped incision to increase exposure of the diseased Achilles tendon. **B.** Typical location of diseased Achilles. **C.** Area of wedge resection of the Achilles insertion in preparation for repair. **D.** Area of bone resection. **E.** Partial ostectomy performed through the resected tendon. *(continued)*

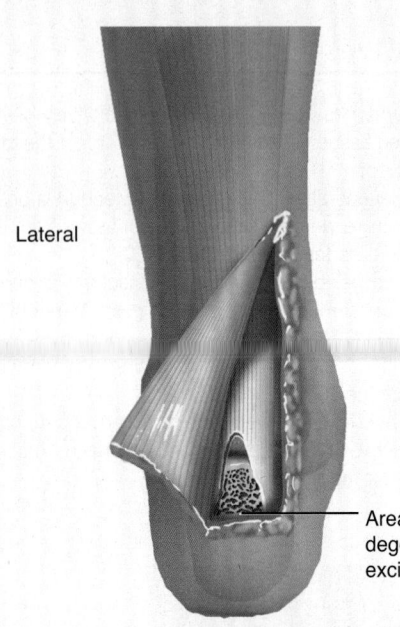

Lateral

Medial

Area of
degeneration
excised

F

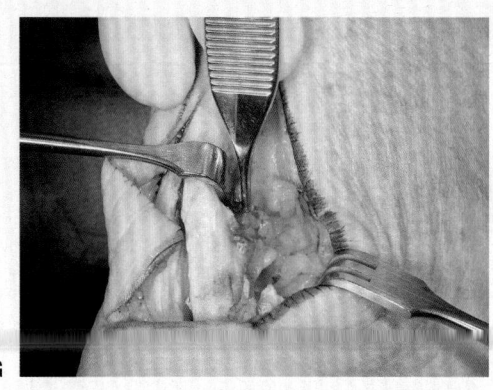

G

TECH FIG 1 *(continued)* **F.** Resected bone and decompressed tendon insertion. **G.** The triangular fat pad is excised, and the deep posterior fascia is exposed.

TENDON TRANSFER

- The fascia overlying the posterior compartment of the leg is incised longitudinally to the proximal extent of the FHL muscle body. The FHL tendon is identified (**TECH FIG 2A**). The flexor retinaculum is released along the medial aspect of the hindfoot to further expose the FHL.
- Gentle retraction of the neurovascular bundle with a blunt retractor allows safe visualization of the tendon distally (**TECH FIG 2B,C**).
  - The FHL is transected as far distal as possible with the ankle and hallux in maximum plantarflexion.
  - Transection of the tendon is done medial to lateral to avoid accidental injury to the neurovascular structures.

- The tendon is brought posteriorly and positioned at the calcaneus between the two limbs of the remaining débrided Achilles insertion (**TECH FIG 2D–F**).
  - If more length of the FHL is needed, the origin of the more distal muscle fibers of the FHL can be detached bluntly from the fibula and interosseous ligament to increase the excursion of the FHL.
  - Proper tensioning of the FHL transfer is determined by dorsiflexing the ankle to place the Achilles tendon at maximal stretch. With the FHL appropriately tensioned, any excess length of the tendon is removed to allow optimal pull of the transferred tendon to the calcaneus.

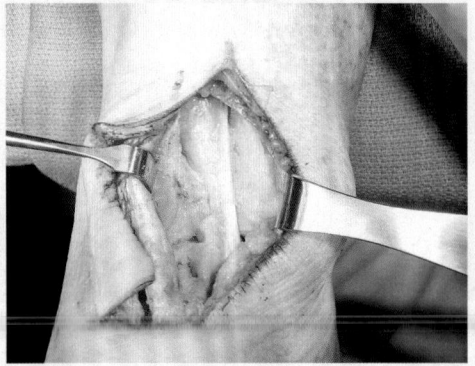

A

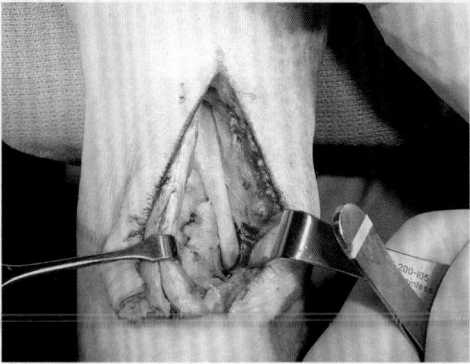

B

TECH FIG 2 A. The flexor hallucis longus (*FHL*) tendon is exposed after the deep fascia is split. **B.** The flexor retinaculum is split to expose the FHL distally. *(continued)*

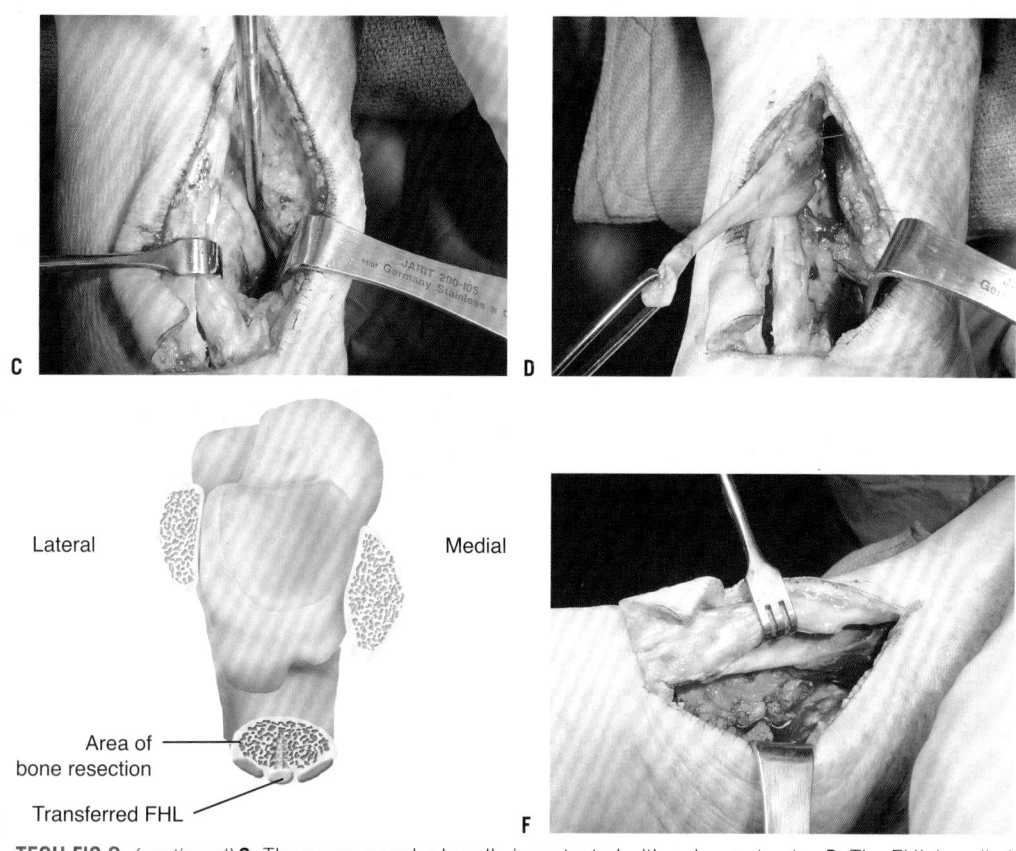

TECH FIG 2 *(continued)* **C.** The neurovascular bundle is protected with a deep retractor. **D.** The FHL is pulled posteriorly and checked for length. **E.** Drawing of FHL placement between the limbs of the remaining Achilles tendon. **F.** The FHL is tightly positioned against the Achilles tendon.

SECURING THE TENDON

- The transferred tendon is held with a two-strand suture anchor (**TECH FIG 3A**).
- The first strand of suture is used in modified Kessler fashion to secure the FHL to the calcaneus at the proper tension (**TECH FIG 3B**).

- The second strand is used as a whipstitch to add pullout strength (**TECH FIG 3C,D**).
- The FHL tendon is sutured to the Achilles tendon in side-to-side fashion with nonabsorbable braided suture (**TECH FIG 3E,F**).
- A careful, layered closure of the paratenon, subcutaneous tissue, and skin is performed.

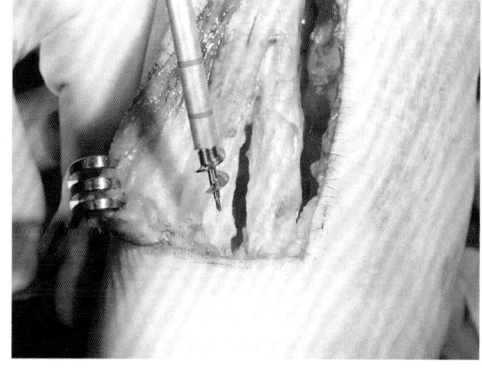

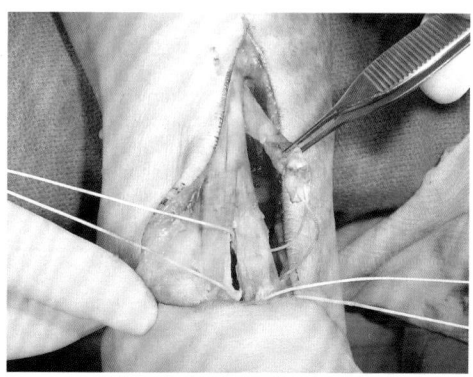

TECH FIG 3 A. Two-strand suture anchor. **B.** A positioning stitch is applied to the tendon, and appropriate FHL tension is determined. *(continued)*

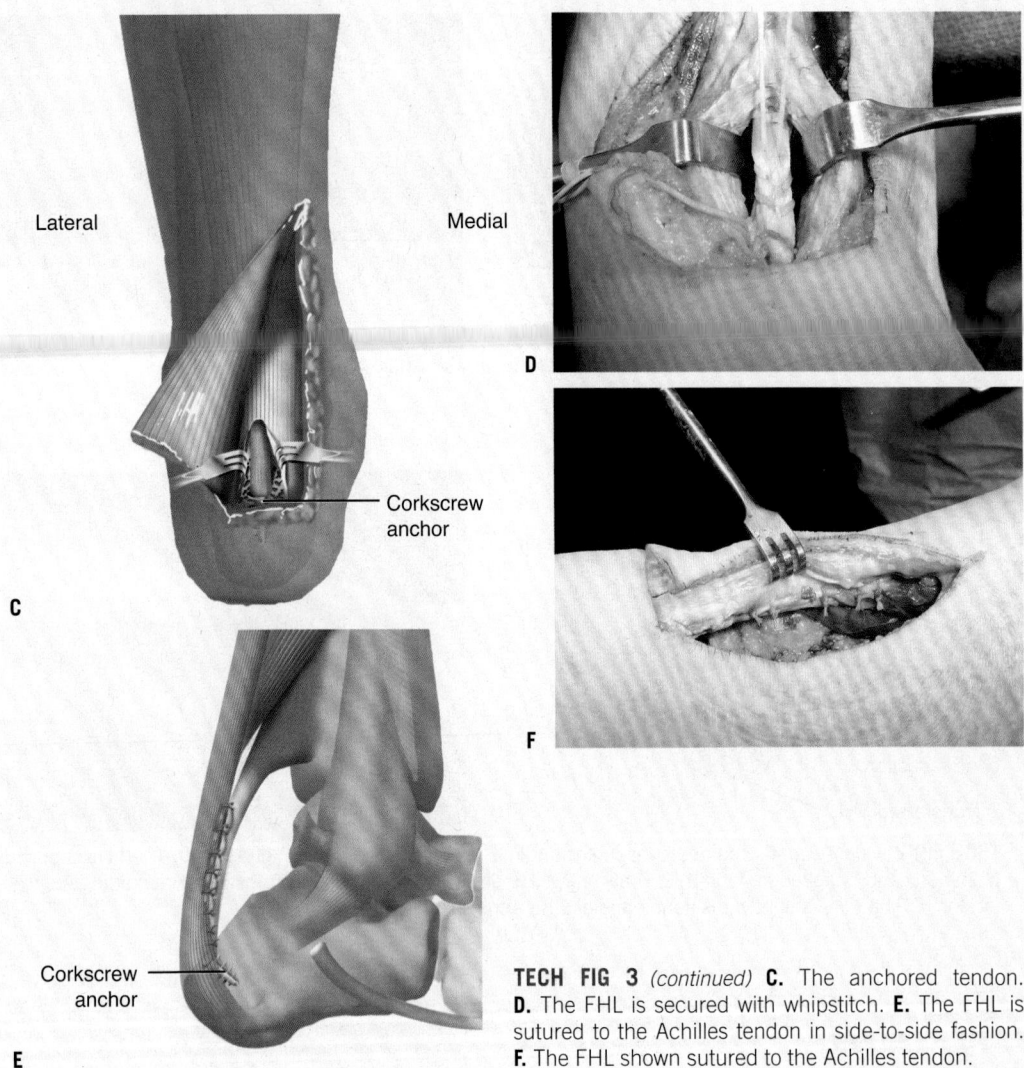

Lateral   Medial

Corkscrew
anchor

C

D

F

Corkscrew
anchor

E

TECH FIG 3 *(continued)* **C.** The anchored tendon.
D. The FHL is secured with whipstitch. **E.** The FHL is
sutured to the Achilles tendon in side-to-side fashion.
F. The FHL shown sutured to the Achilles tendon.

TECHNIQUES

Pearls and Pitfalls

Skin Incision	• Care must be taken to make a full-thickness incision from the skin to the paratenon without undermining the soft tissue layer to avoid skin slough.
Achilles Tendon Débridement	• Make sure to excise all diseased Achilles tendon to reduce the risk of persistent pain postoperatively.
FHL Harvest	• Protect the neurovascular bundle with a deep retractor through the medial incision while exposing the FHL for transfer to avoid injuring adjacent vital structures. • Cut the tendon with a no. 15 blade medial to lateral to avoid injury to the neurovascular bundle. • Maximally plantarflex the ankle and great toe and pull on the FHL before cutting the tendon to obtain adequate length of the transferred tendon.
FHL Transfer	• Dorsiflex the foot while placing the FHL transfer at maximal stretch to determine the proper insertion point and tensioning of the transferred tendon. • Make sure there is good apposition between the FHL and remaining Achilles tendon by excising all interposed fat and using nonabsorbable sutures to hold the repair.
Skin Closure	• Perform careful, separate layer closure, starting with the paratenon, to avoid excessive scarring.

POSTOPERATIVE CARE

- A compressive dressing with splints is applied in the operating room with the ankle in neutral position. The initial dressing is kept in place for 10 to 14 days. At that time, if the incision is well healed and the reconstruction was deemed stable at the time of operation, the patient is placed in a controlled ankle movement (CAM)–soled walker and weight bearing as tolerated is allowed.
- If more than 75% of the Achilles tendon has been débrided, a weight-bearing cast is applied for 4 weeks to provide extra support for the healing tendon.
- Range-of-motion and strengthening exercises are begun 6 to 8 weeks postoperatively if clinical improvement (decreased pain and swelling) is evident.
- The patient is weaned from the CAM-soled walker at 10 to 12 weeks as symptoms of pain and swelling allow.

OUTCOMES

- Hansen reported a proximal FHL transfer technique with good or excellent results. Emphasis was placed on thoroughly excising the diseased tendon.
- Wapner et al reported good to excellent pain relief and improved function in seven patients with Achilles débridement and FHL transfer harvested from the midfoot for tendinosis.
- Wilcox et al, using the American Orthopaedic Foot & Ankle Society (AOFAS) hindfoot score and the 36-Item Short Form Survey Health Survey, reported overall good results with FHL transfer in 20 patients with recalcitrant Achilles tendinosis but found that patient function may not improve.
- Den Hartog reported significant improvement in the postoperative AOFAS hindfoot scores in 29 patients who underwent FHL transfer for severe Achilles tendinosis.

COMPLICATIONS

- Rerupture of the augmented Achilles
- Wound necrosis secondary to undermining of soft tissues
- Infection
- Scarring secondary to inadequate repair of the paratenon
- Persistent pain and swelling

SUGGESTED READINGS

Carr AJ, Norris SH. The blood supply of the calcaneal tendon. J Bone Joint Surg Br 1989;71(1):100–101.

Cottom JM, Hyer CF, Berlet GC, et al. Flexor hallucis tendon transfer with an interference screw for chronic Achilles tendinosis: a report of 62 cases. Foot Ankle Spec 2008;1(5):280–287.

Coull R, Flavin R, Stephens MM. Flexor hallucis longus tendon transfer: evaluation of postoperative morbidity. Foot Ankle Int 2003;24:931–934.

Den Hartog BD. Flexor hallucis longus transfer for chronic Achilles tendonosis. Foot Ankle Int 2003;24:233–237.

Den Hartog BD. Use of proximal flexor hallucis longus transfer in severe calcific Achilles tendinosis. Tech Foot Ankle Surg 2002;1:145–150.

Elias I, Raikin SM, Besser MP, et al. Outcomes of chronic insertional Achilles tendinosis using FHL autograft through single incision. Foot Ankle Int 2009;30(3):197–204.

Hansen ST. Trauma to the heel cord. In: Jahss MH, ed. Disorders of the Foot and Ankle, ed 2. Philadelphia: WB Saunders, 1991:2357.

Mann RA, Holmes GB Jr, Seale KS, et al. Chronic rupture of the Achilles tendon: a new technique of repair. J Bone Joint Surg Am 1991;73(2):214–219.

McGarvey WC, Palumbo RC, Baxter DE, et al. Insertional Achilles tendinosis: surgical treatment through a central tendon splitting approach. Foot Ankle Int 2002;23:19–25.

Puddu G, Ippolito E, Postacchini F. A classification of Achilles tendon disease. Am J Sports Med 1976;4:145–150.

Rahm S, Spross C, Gerber F, et al. Operative treatment of chronic irreparable Achilles tendon ruptures with large flexor hallucis longus tendon transfers. Foot Ankle Int 2013;34(8):1100–1110.

Schepsis AA, Leach RE. Surgical management of Achilles tendinitis. Am J Sports Med 1987;15:308–315.

Turco VJ, Spinella AJ. Achilles tendon rupture—peroneus brevis transfer. Foot Ankle 1987;7:253–259.

Wapner KL, Pavlock GS, Hecht PJ, et al. Repair of chronic Achilles tendon rupture with flexor hallucis longus tendon transfer. Foot Ankle 1993;14:443–449.

Watson AD, Anderson RB, Davis WH. Comparison of results of retrocalcaneal decompression for retrocalcaneal bursitis and insertional Achilles tendinosis with calcific spur. Foot Ankle Int 2000;21:638–642.

Wilcox DK, Bohay DR, Anderson JG. Treatment of chronic Achilles tendon disorders with flexor hallucis longus transfer/augmentation. Foot Ankle Int 2000;21:1004–1010.

Will RE, Galey SM. Outcome of single incision flexor hallucis transfer for chronic Achilles tendinopathy. Foot Ankle Int 2009;30(4):315–317.

Young A, Redfern DJ. Simple method of local harvest and fixation of FHL in Achilles tendon reconstruction: technique tip. Foot Ankle Int 2008;29(11):1148–1150.

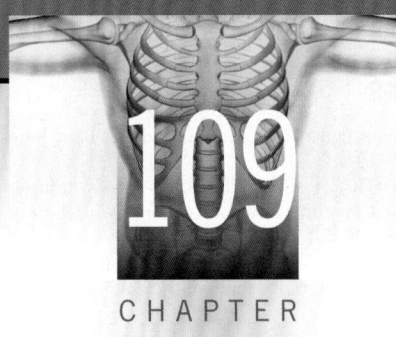

109

CHAPTER

Achilles Tendon Lengthening

Jeremy M. LaMothe and David S. Levine

DEFINITION

- A plantarflexion contracture is defined as the inability to passively dorsiflex the ankle ≥5 degrees past neutral, with a neutral hindfoot, and suggests contracture of the gastrocsoleus complex (FIG 1).
- Plantarflexion contracture may be secondary to contracture the gastrocnemius, soleus, or both components of the complex.
- Plantarflexion contractures are commonly associated with a variety of adult foot/ankle conditions.[6] Up to 65% patients presenting with foot and ankle pathology may have some degree of contracture of the gastrocsoleus complex.[2]

ANATOMY

- The superficial posterior compartment contains the gastrocnemius, soleus, and plantaris muscles.
- The gastrocnemius muscle has two heads (medial and lateral) and originates above the knee from the posterior distal femur, which makes the gastrocnemius a three-joint muscle.
- The soleus originates from the posterior aspect of the proximal fibula, interosseous membrane, and the posterior aspect of the middle one third of the tibia, which makes the soleus a two-joint muscle.
- The gastrocnemius tendon is longer than that of the soleus, and they blend together to form the Achilles tendon approximately 5 cm from the calcaneal tuberosity, which has a broad enthesis.
- As the Achilles tendon shifts from its origin to insertion, it spirals 90 degrees so that the medial border of the proximal tendon rests posterolaterally.
- The gastrocsoleus complex can be considered in three zones[4]: zone 1 is from the femoral origins of the gastrocnemius muscle to the distal extent of the bluntly separable interval between the gastrocnemius and soleus, which is usually at the level of the medial gastrocnemius muscle belly, zone 2 is from the distal aspect of the medial gastrocnemius muscle belly to the distal end of the soleus muscle, and zone 3 is the Achilles tendon from the distal end of the soleus muscle to the insertion on the calcaneus (FIG 2).

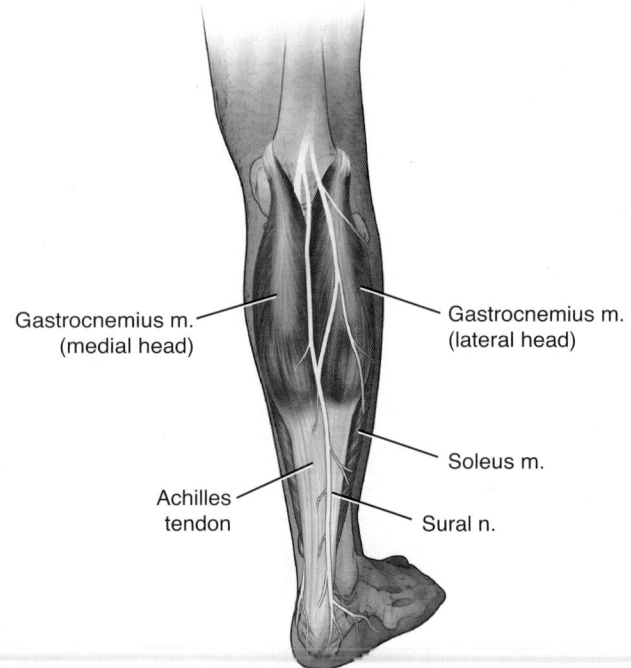

FIG 1 The gastrocsoleus complex, as viewed from a posterolateral angle, including the location of the sural nerve.

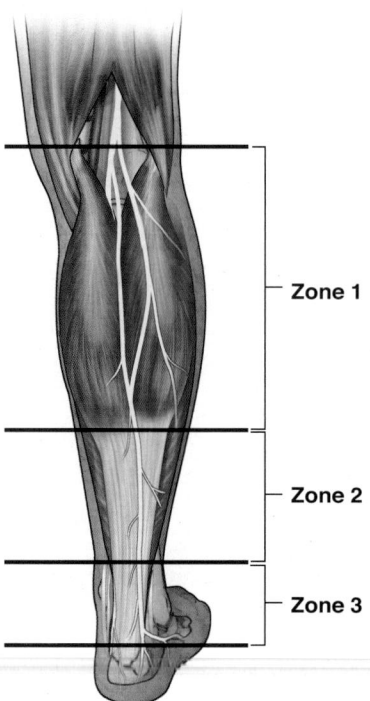

FIG 2 Three zones of gastrocsoleus lengthening.

- The gastrocnemius and soleus muscles can be differentially lengthened in zones 1 and 2 (ie, separate fascial releases can be performed for each of these muscles).

PATHOGENESIS

- The etiologies of gastrocsoleus contractures are broad and include metabolic/endocrine (eg, diabetes mellitus), posttraumatic, congenital, neurologic, and idiopathic origins. The natural history of the contracture is dependent on the etiology.
- Gastrocsoleus contractures have implications for coronal and sagittal plane pathologies.
- Sagittal plane pathologies include forefoot overloading and its sequelae including metatarsalgia, plantar plate pathology, or bunions.
- Coronal plane pathologies include flatfoot and hallux valgus deformities.
- Contracture may also be associated with midfoot pain/arthritis, planar fasciitis, or Achilles tendinopathy.
- In patients with peripheral vascular disease and/or neuropathy, contracture may predispose to Charcot midfoot breakdown or serious foot ulcerations; treatment may require a gastrocsoleus complex lengthening.

NATURAL HISTORY

- In general, conditions caused by a gastrocsoleus complex contracture will fail to completely resolve without some form of gastrocsoleus stretching/lengthening. This concept can be critical in diabetic forefoot and midfoot ulcers.

PATIENT HISTORY AND PHYSICAL FINDINGS

- The patient history should be used to determine if there is a specific etiology of the contracture (eg, posttraumatic, diabetes, cerebral palsy, stroke).
- Associated medical conditions should be ascertained on history (eg, diabetes, neuropathy).
- Physical examination should assess the overall lower extremity alignment, including hindfoot, midfoot, and forefoot alignment.
- Look for any signs of forefoot overloading, such as metatarsophalangeal joint tenderness, prominent metatarsal calluses, or ulcerations.
- Special attention should be paid to ankle range of motion with the knee extended and flexed, with the hindfoot held in a neutral/varus position as is described with the Silfverskiöld test, which may help distinguish an isolated gastrocnemius contracture from a tight gastrocsoleus complex (see Part 8 Foot and Ankle Exam Table at the end of the book). Holding the hindfoot in a neutral/varus position during the test is critical to lock the Chopart joint and minimize dorsiflexion through the hindfoot.

IMAGING AND OTHER DIAGNOSTIC STUDIES

- Standard radiographic workup should include a weight-bearing foot and ankle series. Weight bearing is critical to determine alignment.
- Radiographs should be assessed for foot alignment and any structural causes for decreased ankle dorsiflexion

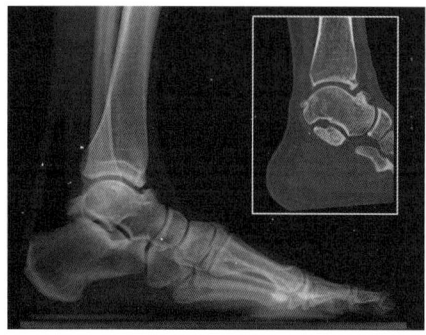

FIG 3 Lateral radiograph demonstrating an osseous etiology for a plantarflexion contracture. Note the large talar neck osteophytes.

(eg, talar neck/anterior tibial osteophytes, malunion, ankle arthritis; **FIG 3**)
- Targeted imaging should be performed for the symptoms the patient is experiencing (eg, magnetic resonance imaging for Achilles tendinopathy).

DIFFERENTIAL DIAGNOSIS

- Ankle arthritis
- Anterior ankle impingement (bony or soft tissue)
- Posttraumatic malunion of the tibia
- Syndesmotic malreduction
- Neglected foot drop
- Spasticity/neuromotor conditions

NONOPERATIVE MANAGEMENT

- Calf stretching is indicated in patients with a gastrocsoleus contracture and foot symptoms/pathology that can be attributed to or exacerbated by this contracture.
- Static calf stretching may provide small increases in ankle dorsiflexion.[7,13]
- Eccentric calf stretching exercises may be helpful in managing Achilles tendinopathy.[1]
- Night splints may be indicated in the treatment of plantar fasciitis, but the effectiveness of night splints in treating other conditions is unknown.

SURGICAL MANAGEMENT

- Failure of nonoperative management of the pathology associated with a tight gastrocsoleus complex is an indication for surgery.
- Lengthening of the gastrocsoleus complex can be a critical component of a more extensive surgical plan (eg, Achilles tendon lengthening in addition to a flatfoot reconstruction), or it may be the sole treatment (eg, gastrocnemius recession in patients with noninsertional Achilles tendinopathy, metatarsalgia, plantar fasciitis, diabetic foot ulcerations). Accordingly, surgical decision making is individualized for each patient.

Preoperative Planning

- The patient should be medically optimized for surgery; this is of particular importance in patients with diabetes mellitus.

- Deformities of the lower extremity should be examined, and joint ranges of motion should be measured.
- Preoperative performance of a Silfverskiöld test is of critical importance to determine if the plantarflexion contracture is secondary to an isolated gastrocnemius contracture, or a combined gastrocsoleus contracture.
- If gastrocsoleus lengthening is indicated as part of a larger surgical plan, it is controversial if the lengthening should be performed at the beginning or the end of the case and is left to the discretion of the treating surgeon.

Positioning

- Although positioning is determined by the specific surgical case, supine positioning is generally appropriate to perform most gastrocsoleus lengthenings. An assistant can elevate the leg to facilitate lengthenings such as the Hoke or Vulpius lengthening **(FIG 4)**.
- Prone positioning is preferred for an Achilles Z-lengthening, but it can also be done supine with the leg in a figure-of-four position if the lengthening is a component of a larger procedure requiring supine positioning.
- Occasionally, concomitant procedures may require repositioning.

Approach

- The particular surgical approach is determined by the lengthening that will be performed.
- More proximal lengthenings (eg, Baumann, or Strayer lengthenings) are more mechanically stable, are able to differentially lengthen the gastrocnemius and soleus, provide smaller corrections, and may require less postoperative protection than distal lengthenings **(TABLE 1)**.[4]
- More distal lengthenings (eg, Hoke or Z-lengthening) are less mechanically stable, lengthen the gastrocsoleus complex as a unit, and elicit larger corrections but may require more postoperative protection.[4]

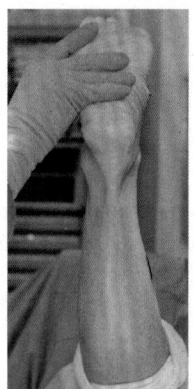

FIG 4 If the patient is in a supine position, elevation of the leg enables access to perform some two or three lengthenings.

- In general, the location of the sural nerve needs to be considered for each approach. The sural nerve has an inconsistent course and may be superficial to the deep fascia of the leg (42.5%), deep to the deep fascia of the leg (57.5%), or deep and adherent to the gastrocnemius tendon (12.5%).[12]
- Plantarflexion contracture secondary to isolated gastrocnemius contracture is typically treated with a more proximal lengthening such as a Baumann or Strayer procedure **(FIG 5)**.
- Plantarflexion contracture secondary to combined gastrocsoleus contracture is generally treated with a more distal procedure such as a Vulpius, Hoke, or Z-lengthening procedure.
- More complex plantarflexion contractures secondary to posttraumatic cases may require a Z-lengthening with posterior ankle/subtalar joint capsular releases and may require external fixation to facilitate a safe and gradual correction.

TABLE 1 Different Techniques for Gastrocsoleus Lengthenings and Their Relative Characteristics

Lengthening	Indication	Zone	Possibility for Differential Lengthening of the Gastrocnemius and Soleus	Capacity for Lengthening	Mechanical Stability	Postoperative Protection
Baumann	Gastrocnemius or gastrocsoleus contracture	Proximal 1	Yes	Smallest	Stable	WBAT
Strayer	Gastrocnemius or gastrocsoleus contracture	Distal 1	Yes		Stable	WBAT
Vulpius/Baker	Gastrocsoleus contracture	2	No		Stable	WBAT
Hoke	Gastrocsoleus contracture	3	No		Unstable	Protected
Z-lengthening	Gastrocsoleus contracture	3	No	Largest	Unstable	Protected

WBAT, weightbearing as tolerated.
Reprinted with permission from Firth GB, McMullan M, Chin T, et al. Lengthening of the gastrocnemius-soleus complex: an anatomical and biomechanical study in human cadavers. J Bone Joint Surg Am 2013;95-A(16):1489–1496.

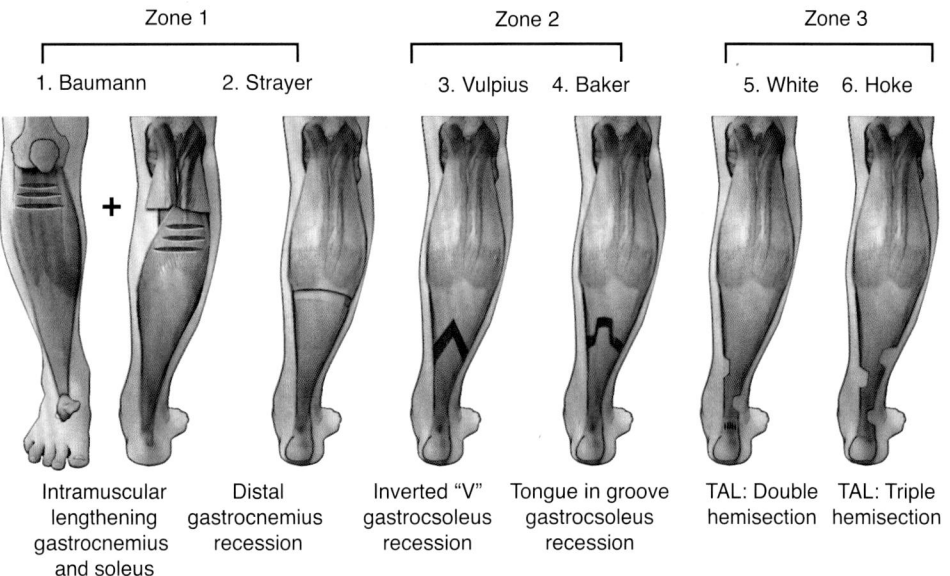

Zone 1
1. Baumann   2. Strayer

Zone 2
3. Vulpius   4. Baker

Zone 3
5. White   6. Hoke

Intramuscular lengthening gastrocnemius and soleus

Distal gastrocnemius recession

Inverted "V" gastrocsoleus recession

Tongue in groove gastrocsoleus recession

TAL: Double hemisection

TAL: Triple hemisection

FIG 5 Commonly used gastrocsoleus lengthenings and their position along the gastrocsoleus complex. *TAL*, tendo achilles lengthening.

BAUMANN LENGTHENING

- The patient is placed supine, and the surgeon stands on the contralateral side.
- A 5-cm incision is made two fingerbreadths posterior to the posteromedial tibial crest at junction of the proximal and middle third of the leg.
- Bluntly develop the plane to the superficial fascia of the leg (crural fascia) and retract the saphenous neurovascular bundle if encountered.
- Longitudinally incise the crural fascia at the interval between the gastrocnemius and soleus muscle bellies.

- Use finger dissection to bluntly develop the plane between the gastrocnemius and soleus from their palpable medial to lateral borders. It is critical to identify the lateralmost margin of the gastrocnemius muscle.
- Identify the plantaris tendon and transect it.
- Once the anterior gastrocnemius and posterior soleal fascial are identified, place the ankle in dorsiflexion and use a long handle knife to incise the anterior gastrocnemius fascia from medial to lateral. Take care not to incise the underlying muscle belly. Repeat the Silfverskiöld test. Up to three fascial incisions of the gastrocnemius can be performed, each <1.5 cm from each other **(TECH FIG 1)**.

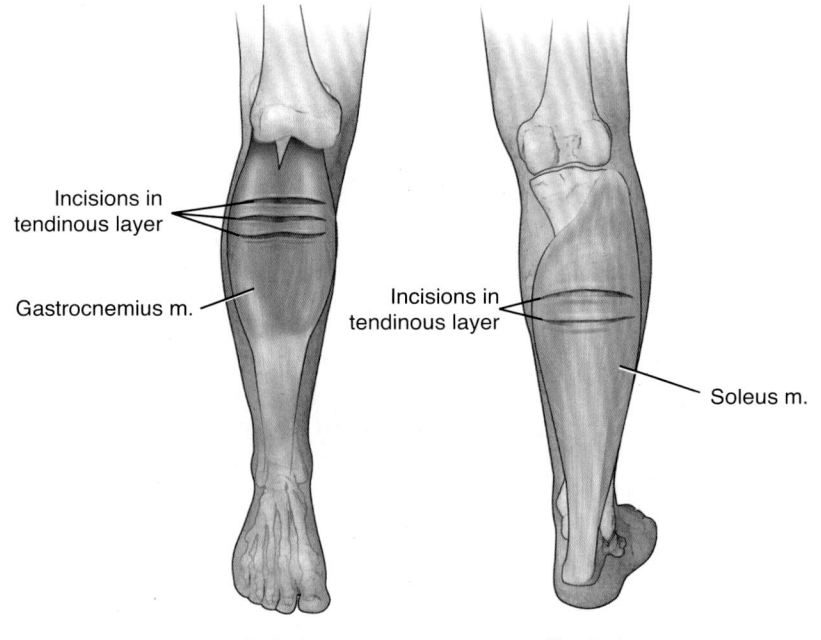

Incisions in tendinous layer

Gastrocnemius m.

Incisions in tendinous layer

Soleus m.

Anterior

Posterior

TECH FIG 1 View of the proximal gastrocsoleus interval for a Baumann recession, and recessions of the anterior gastrocnemius fascia, and posterior soleal fascia.

T E C H N I Q U E S

- If the ankle still requires more dorsiflexion, the surgeon can perform a posterior soleal recession distal to the gastrocnemius recessions. Place the soleal recession ~1.5 cm distal to the gastrocnemius recessions to avoid postoperative adhesions between the gastrocnemius and soleus.

- Close the crural fascia with an absorbable suture and close the skin.
- The Baumann procedure has the benefit of being relatively more cosmetic because the distal gastrocnemius confluence with soleus tendon is preserved.

STRAYER LENGTHENING

- The patient is placed in the supine position and the distal aspect of the medial gastrocnemius muscle belly is identified visually and by palpation. In legs with a larger subcutaneous fat layer, dorsiflexing and plantarflexing the ankle can assist in defining this landmark.
- An incision is made from this muscle belly extending 3 cm distally two fingerbreadths posterior to the posteromedial tibial crest (**TECH FIG 2**).
- Bluntly develop the plane of dissection to the superficial fascia of the leg (crural fascia) and retract the saphenous neurovascular bundle if encountered.
- Longitudinally incise the crural fascia over the visible gastrocnemius tendon where it meets the soleus muscle. This interval is visible through the crural fascia (**TECH FIG 3**).
- Use finger dissection to bluntly develop the plane between the gastrocnemius and soleus to the point where they converge distally (approximately 2 cm distal to the most distal aspect of the medial gastrocnemius muscle belly).
- It is critical to develop this plane from the medial border to the lateral border. A small blunt elevator can help palpate the lateral margin.
- Identify the plantaris tendon and transect (**TECH FIG 4**).
- Identify the distal extent of the medial gastrocnemius muscle, and identify the sural nerve posterior to the gastrocnemius myotendinous junction, being mindful of the variations in location of the sural nerve (**TECH FIG 5**). If the medial gastrocnemius muscle belly is not encountered on the posterior side of the presumed gastrocnemius fascia, repeat the dissection and ensure that the tissue plane being dissected is not the crural or soleal fascia.
- Dorsiflex the ankle and place the gastrocnemius tendon on tension. A vaginal speculum or large nasal speculum will function as an excellent retractor if placed on the anterior and posterior sides of the gastrocnemius tendon (**TECH FIG 6**).

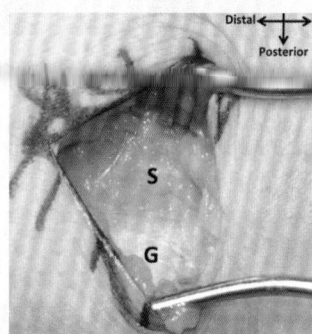
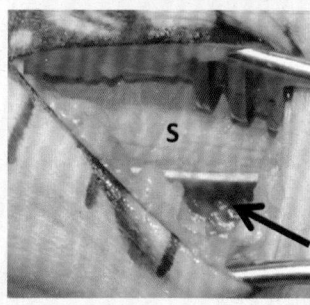

TECH FIG 3 A. Superficial dissection to the crural fascia at the medial gastrocnemius myotendinous junction demonstrating the visible interval between the underlying soleus (*S*) and gastrocnemius (*G*). **B.** Dissection through the crural fascia at the visible interval with proximal retraction of the mobile skin window demonstrating the soleus (*S*) and distal extent to the medial gastrocnemius muscle (*arrow*).

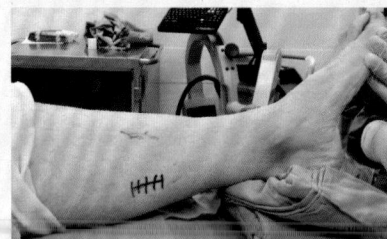

TECH FIG 2 Skin incision for a Strayer recession.

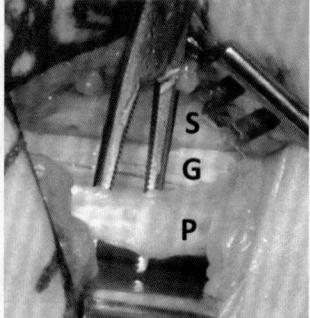

TECH FIG 4 The plantaris (*P*) is identified in the interval between the soleus (*S*) and gastrocnemius (*G*) and brought into the surgical field with a snap for easy transection.

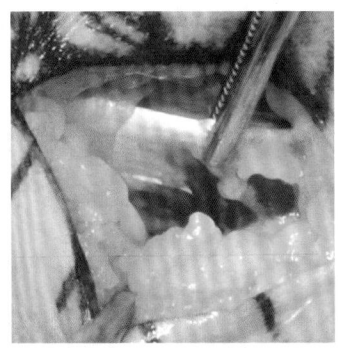

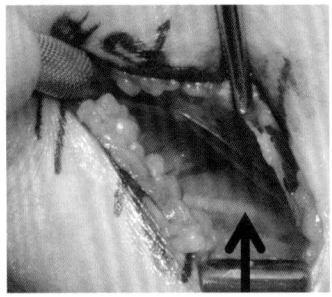

TECH FIG 5 A. The distal extent of the medial gastrocnemius muscle is identified and a Kocher clamp is used to retract the gastrocnemius tendon anteriorly to allow for inspection of the sural nerve, which may be adherent to the posterior gastrocnemius tendon in some cases. **B.** The sural nerve (*arrow*) is identified posterior to the gastrocnemius tendon on most cases and must be identified for safe gastrocnemius recession at this level.

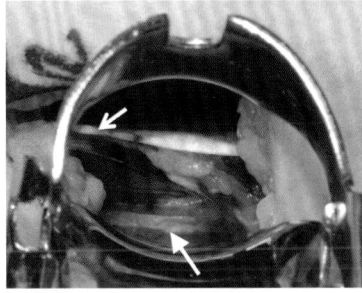

TECH FIG 6 A vaginal speculum can be used for safe anterior and posterior retraction of the gastrocnemius tendon at the level of the myotendinous junction (*open arrow*). The sural nerve can be identified (*closed arrow*) and retracted with the posterior tine of the speculum.

- If just proximal to the myotendinous junction, the medial belly of the gastrocnemius can be swept off of the distal aspect of the posterior gastrocnemius tendon with a blunt soft tissue elevator. Use a long-handle knife or scissors to incise the gastrocnemius tendon **(TECH FIG 7)**.
- Ensure there are no fibers of the tendon intact laterally.
- The Silfverskiöld test is repeated, and if there is still an equinus contracture, the underlying soleal fascial may be recessed as well.
- The gastrocnemius fascia does not need to be sutured to the soleal fascia and should be allowed to find its new resting position following the recession.
- The gastrocnemius–soleus recession occurs in an approximate 2:1 ratio.[4]
- The crural fascia is closed with an absorbable suture.

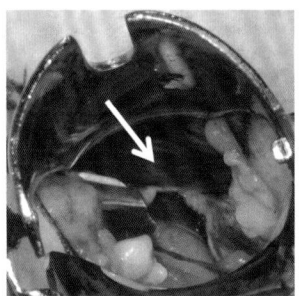

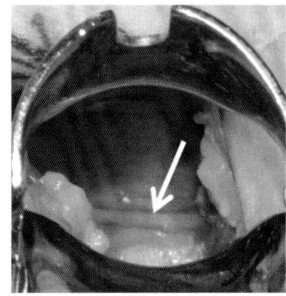

TECH FIG 7 A. The gastrocnemius tendon is sharply divided with a long-handle knife. Often, a secondary inspection will reveal that the lateralmost margin of the gastrocnemius tendon is still intact and a second pass with the knife is required to complete the recession. Using a long-handle clamp to deliver the lateral margin of the tendon into the surgical field may provide easier access to the lateral tendon. A finger should be used to palpate the tendon and verify that the recession is complete. **B.** Once the recession is complete, the sural nerve can be identified in the interval where the recession occurred.

VULPIUS AND BAKER LENGTHENINGS

- The Vulpius and Baker procedures lengthen at the same level (through the conjoined tendon of the gastrocnemius aponeurosis and soleus fascia) and only differ in the geometry of the cut (see **FIG 5**).
- If this is an isolated procedure, prone positioning allows for better visualization of the cut. However, if associated procedures are performed, these lengthenings can be performed with

an assistant elevating the leg and the surgeon positioned at the end of the bed (see **FIG 4**).
- A midline 2-cm incision is made at the junction between the distal and middle one-third of the leg.
- Carry the dissection bluntly down to the crural fascia and palpate the medial and lateral margins of the conjoint tendon with blunt soft tissue elevator **(TECH FIG 8)**.

- Incise the conjoint tendon from its medial to lateral margin and do not incise the deep soleus muscle belly. Vulpius's original description indicated that cuts could be made "horizontally, diagonally, or best of all, in the form of an upside down 'V'."[4] The Baker lengthening describes an upside down "U" cut, which forms a tongue and groove-shaped defect.
- Identify the deep median soleal raphe and incise this (TECH FIG 9).
- Close the crural fascia and skin.

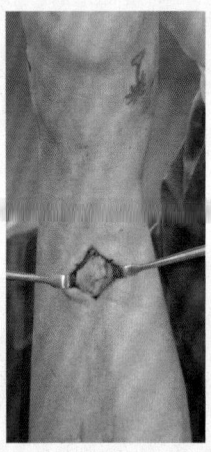

TECH FIG 8 The conjoint gastrocsoleus tendon, exposed for a Vulpius or Baker lengthening.

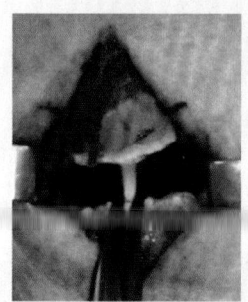 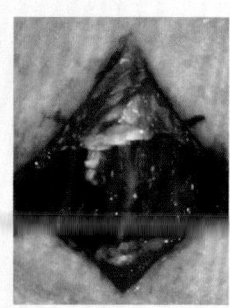

TECH FIG 9 Median soleal raphe exposed after recession of the overlying gastrocsoleus conjoint tendon before (**A**) and after (**B**) transection.

HOKE ACHILLES TRIPLE HEMISECTION LENGTHENING

- This procedure can be performed in the supine position with an assistant elevating the leg.
- The proximal and distal margins of the Achilles tendon are palpated with the ankle in dorsiflexion.
- Mark the proximal, middle, and distal central points of the Achilles tendon (ie, a total of three marks; TECH FIG 10).
- Place the ankle in dorsiflexion and make a longitudinal percutaneous stab incision in the distal most mark with a no. 15 or no. 11 blade. Place the blade in the tendon just to the anterior aspect of the tendon; it is critical not to plunge with the blade as there are vital structures nearby.
- Turn the blade 90 degrees medially and place a thumb on the medial border of the Achilles tendon adjacent to the blade. Complete the hemisection using the thumb to palpate when the blade completes the hemisection.
- Repeat the percutaneous hemisection, except for a lateral direction, at the middle mark.
- Repeat the percutaneous medial hemisection for the proximal mark.
- Some surgeons prefer to perform proximal–lateral/ middle–medial/distal–lateral hemisections in patients with valgus hindfeet to theoretically decrease the lateral/valgus moment arm of the Achilles tendon pull. If this is the case, extra precautions need to be taken to avoid damaging the sural nerve, especially at the proximal most incision.

- Place Steri-Strips type dressings on the percutaneous stab incisions.
- Care must be taken not to plunge the blade when performing the hemisections as there are critical structures nearby; the flexor hallucis longus and tibial nerve are less than 1 cm from the proximal cut if directed medially, and the sural nerve is less than 1 cm from the middle cut if directed laterally.[14]

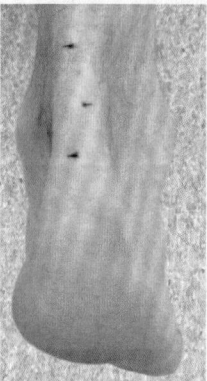

TECH FIG 10 Skin markings demonstrating appropriate placement of the percutaneous stab incisions for a Hoke lengthening.

Z-LENGTHENING

- This procedure is routinely performed in the prone position.
- The proximal and distal aspects of the Achilles tendon are identified, and a longitudinal incision is made either in the midline of the Achilles tendon, or on the medial border of the Achilles tendon, extending the length of the Achilles tendon.
- The paratenon is identified and incised sharply in line with the length of the incision. Raise the paratendon flaps as a medial and lateral soft tissue layer for later closure over the Achilles tendon.
- Perform a full-thickness incision of the Achilles tendon in the midline from its proximal to distal extent.
- At the proximal margin of the tendon-splitting incision, turn the knife 90 degrees and come out of the tendon medially (exiting laterally proximally puts the sural nerve at higher risk of inadvertent laceration).
- At the distal margin of the tendon-splitting incision, turn the knife 90 degrees to come out of the tendon laterally, once again being mindful of the nearby sural nerve.
- For more serious contractures, reflect the Z-lengthening and continue the dissection deep to the posterior ankle and subtalar joints. Perform capsular releases as necessary.
- Dorsiflex the ankle to the desired tension and suture the Achilles tendon back to itself with a heavy nonabsorbable suture. Take care to ensure that the knot pillars are not prominent **(TECH FIG 11)**.
- Close the skin and paratenon with an absorbable suture.

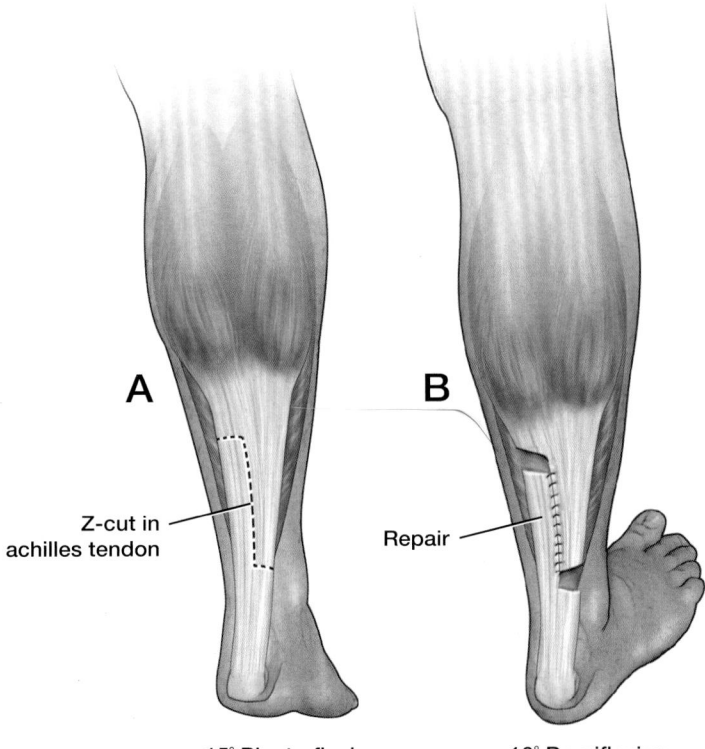

A — Z-cut in achilles tendon — 15° Plantarflexion

B — Repair — 10° Dorsiflexion

TECH FIG 11 Illustration of a Z-lengthening demonstrating the Z-cuts in the tendon before (**A**) and after (**B**) ankle dorsiflexion.

TECHNIQUES

Pearls and Pitfalls

Rule out other causes of decreased ankle range of motion.	• Bony impinging lesions and ankle arthritis are readily apparent on weight-bearing radiographs.
Determining if the contracture is isolated to the gastrocnemius or combined gastrocsoleus will help indicate the proper lengthening procedure.	• Preoperative and intraoperative Silfverskiöld testing, with the hindfoot held in a neutral/varus position, is an important physical examination maneuver.
It is important to obtain adequate ankle dorsiflexion intraoperatively.	• The Baumann and Strayer procedures can be supplemented with a release of the soleal fascia to improve ankle dorsiflexion.
Good visualization is key.	• A vaginal or nasal speculum and headlamp can be very helpful.
Avoid nerve injuries.	• Be mindful of the variable anatomy of the sural nerve; identifying it with the Strayer procedure may help decrease inadvertent injury.

POSTOPERATIVE CARE

- All patients should be examined at ~2 weeks for a wound check.
- When performed in conjunction with larger surgical reconstructions, the postoperative care is determined by the reconstruction.
- In the case of isolated gastrocsoleus lengthenings, all lengthenings described herein except Hoke and Z-lengthenings may be weight bearing as tolerated in a controlled ankle motion (CAM) boot for 2 weeks followed by a gradual transition out of the boot and range-of-motion protocol.
- The author's preferred method is to remove the CAM boot on postoperative day 4 and mobilize in a sneaker to allow for range of motion. The patient should sleep with the boot to help maintain the correction for 4 to 6 weeks.
- Hoke and Z-lengthenings should be maintained non–weight bearing in a boot for 2 to 4 weeks, followed by gradual progression of weight bearing to full weight bearing over 2 to 4 weeks. The patient should be maintained in a CAM boot for 6 to 8 weeks.

OUTCOMES

- Lengthening the gastrocsoleus complex increases passive ankle range of motion, and gains are maintained late in the postoperative period.[6]
- Lengthening may cause a slight weakness in the gastrocsoleus complex,[5,10] the long-term sequelae of which is unknown.[11]
- Forefoot plantar pressure decreases following lengthening[15]; this may be secondary to increased ankle range of motion or weakness in the gastrocsoleus complex.
- Clinical outcomes are dependent on the pathology being treated; however, results for a variety of pathologies including plantar fasciitis and metatarsalgia[8] are encouraging.
- Achilles tendon lengthening may significantly decrease the early and late risk of ulcer recurrence in patients with diabetes and neuropathic ulcers.[9]
- Isolated gastrocnemius recession has a high rate of success in treating chronic Achilles tendinopathy.[3,10]

COMPLICATIONS

- Complications may occur in up to 15% of cases[5,6] and may include sural nerve injury, poor cosmesis secondary to scar adhesions or proximal gastrocnemius muscle retraction, overlengthening and subsequent heel pain or calf weakness, complete Achilles tendon rupture (for distal lengthenings), or wound healing problems.

REFERENCES

1. Alfredson H, Cook J. A treatment algorithm for managing Achilles tendinopathy: new treatment options. Br J Sports Med 2007;41:211–216.
2. DiGiovanni CW, Kuo R, Tejwani N, et al. Isolated gastrocnemius tightness. J Bone Joint Surg Am 2002;84:962–970.
3. Duthon VB, Lübbeke A, Duc SR, et al. Noninsertional Achilles tendinopathy treated with gastrocnemius lengthening. Foot Ankle Int 2011;32:375–379.
4. Firth GB, McMullan M, Chin T, et al. Lengthening of the gastrocnemius-soleus complex: an anatomical and biomechanical study in human cadavers. J Bone Joint Surg Am 2013;95:1489–1496.
5. Gianakos A, Yasui Y, Murawski CD, et al. Effects of gastrocnemius recession on ankle motion, strength, and functional outcomes: a systematic review and national healthcare database analysis. Knee Surg Sports Traumatol Arthrosc 2016;24:1355–1364.
6. Holtmann JA, Südkamp NP, Schmal H, et al. Gastrocnemius recession leads to increased ankle motion and improved patient satisfaction after 2 years of follow-up. J Foot Ankle Surg 2017;56(3):589–593.
7. Medeiros DM, Martini TF. Chronic effect of different types of stretching on ankle dorsiflexion range of motion: systematic review and meta-analysis. Foot (Edinb) 2018;34:28–35.
8. Molund M, Paulsrud Ø, Ellingsen Husebye E, et al. Results after gastrocnemius recession in 73 patients. Foot Ankle Surg 2014;20(4):272–275.
9. Mueller MJ, Sinacore DR, Hastings MK, et al. Effect of Achilles tendon lengthening on neuropathic plantar ulcers. A randomized clinical trial. J Bone Joint Surg Am 2003;85:1436–1445.
10. Nawoczenski DA, Barske H, Tome J, et al. Isolated gastrocnemius recession for Achilles tendinopathy: strength and functional outcomes. J Bone Joint Surg Am 2015;97(2):99–105.
11. Nawoczenski DA, DiLiberto FE, Cantor MS, et al. Ankle power and endurance outcomes following isolated gastrocnemius recession for Achilles tendinopathy. Foot Ankle Int 2016;37(7):766–775.
12. Pinney SJ, Sangeorzan BJ, Hansen ST Jr. Surgical anatomy of the gastrocnemius recession (Strayer procedure). Foot Ankle Int 2004;25:247–250.
13. Radford JA, Burns J, Buchbinder R, et al. Does stretching increase ankle dorsiflexion range of motion? A systematic review. Br J Sports Med 2006;40:870–875; discussion 75.
14. Salamon ML, Pinney SJ, Van Bergeyk A, et al. Surgical anatomy and accuracy of percutaneous Achilles tendon lengthening. Foot Ankle Int 2006;27:411–413.
15. Vinagre G, Alfonso M, Cruz-Morande S, et al. Efficacy of pedobarographic analysis to evaluate proximal medial gastrocnemius recession in patients with gastrocnemius tightness and metatarsalgia. Int Orthop 2017;41(11):2281–2287.

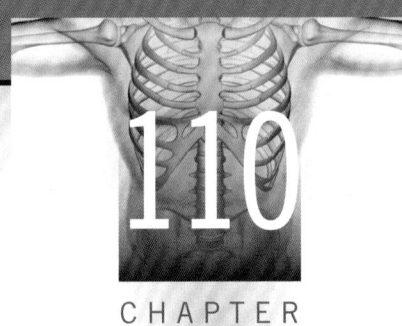

110
CHAPTER

Repair of Peroneal Tendon Tears

Christopher E. Gross, Selene G. Parekh, James A. Nunley II, and Mark E. Easley

DEFINITION

- Pathology of the peroneal tendons may be due to a singular traumatic episode or recurrent ankle sprains.
- In patients undergoing surgery for ankle instability, 25% have peroneal tendon tears; however, the true incidence is unknown.[4]
- Isolated tears of the peroneus brevis and longus are rare.
- When recognized early, direct repair is possible with good results.[2,3]
- Delays in diagnosis are common, as up to 40% of peroneal tendon disorders are missed at first evaluation.[5]

ANATOMY

- The peroneus brevis and longus are innervated by the superficial peroneal nerve and reside in the lateral compartment of the leg.
- The peroneal longus attaches to the base of the first metatarsal and medial cuneiform and is responsible for plantar flexion of the first ray and eversion. Its muscular antagonist is the tibialis anterior.
- The peroneal brevis attaches to the base of the fifth metatarsal and acts to evert and plantarflex the foot. Its muscular antagonist is the tibialis posterior. The brevis often has a low-lying muscle belly.
- At the level of the lateral malleolus, the peroneus brevis is directly posterior to the bone; the longus is posterior to the brevis.
- Both peroneal tendons are tethered at the level of the lateral malleolus in the fibular groove by the superior peroneal retinaculum, a 1- to 2-cm fibrous sling that extends from the tip of the lateral malleolus to the calcaneus. Disruption of this retinaculum can cause a subluxation of the tendons.
- The inferior peroneal retinaculum is continuous with the inferior extensor retinaculum anteriorly and passes obliquely down to insert onto the lateral surface of the calcaneus. At this level, the peroneal tubercle of the calcaneus is a bony ridge that separates the brevis and longus. Injury to the inferior retinaculum does not allow for tendon subluxation.

PATHOGENESIS

- The peroneal tendons may be injured acutely in an inversion ankle sprain (**FIG 1**) or in chronically unstable ankles.
- Contributing factors to tearing include tendon subluxation, superior retinacular stenosis,[1] a low-lying peroneal brevis muscle belly,[8] the presence of a peroneus quartus,[18] and tenosynovitis.
- The most common location for longitudinal peroneus brevis tendon tears is at the fibular groove,[13] whereas the most common location for a peroneus longus tear is at the peroneal tubercle, at the entry of the cuboid tunnel.

- At the fibula, both the peroneus longus and brevis have reduced vascularity.[14]

NATURAL HISTORY

- Peroneal tendon pathology can be commonly overlooked in a patient with chronic lateral ankle pain.
- Anatomic variants may predispose to peroneal tendon tears. For example, a shallow retromalleolar groove predisposes the peroneals to subluxation or dislocation.[16]
- Peroneal tendons that frequently subluxate or dislocate causes fraying at the tip of the fibula, as the tendons are constantly exposed to abnormal loads.
- Additionally, the fibrocartilage of the distal fibula may hypertrophy and cause splitting of the brevis tendon.

PATIENT HISTORY AND PHYSICAL FINDINGS

- Patients may present after a severe ankle sprain or chronic lateral ankle instability.
- Acute or chronic swelling and pain along the posterior border of the distal fibula is an important clinical indicator of peroneal pathology.
- Palpation along the course of the peroneal tendons is important in eliciting pain. Pain at the tip of the fibula is usually due to a tear of the peroneus brevis[11] as compared to the peroneus longus tear, which presents as pain close to the base at the fifth metatarsal or cuboid tunnel.
- Pain may be associated with active, resisted eversion and ankle dorsiflexion. The patient may also experience subluxation of the tendons with this maneuver.
- On eversion strength testing, patients can have considerable weakness and pain.

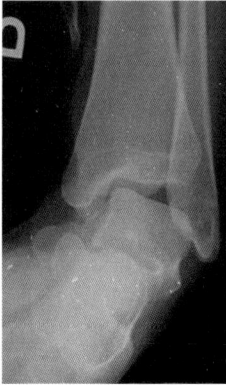

FIG 1 Radiograph of inversion stress test demonstrating left ankle instability.

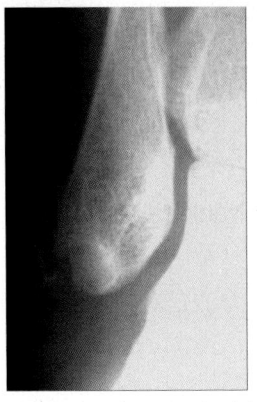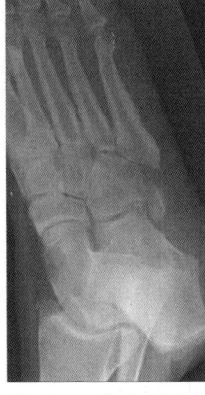

FIG 2 A. Fleck sign: Note avulsed bone fragment from distal lateral fibula. **B.** Oblique radiograph of right foot demonstrating irregular os peroneum. In some peroneus longus tears, the os peroneum will be separated into two distinct fragments.

- Alignment of the affected lower extremity must be assessed. A fixed hindfoot varus deformity may need to be corrected at the time of surgery.
  - The single heel rise is helpful to evaluate the normal inversion (varus) alignment of the hindfoot.
- The peroneal tunnel compression test is used to evaluate peroneus longus tears. One applies manual pressure along the peroneal tendon sheath in the retromalleolar groove with the knee flexed to 90 degrees and the foot in a resting plantarflexed position.[15] A peroneal longus tendon tear may be present if the first ray does not plantarflex.
- Circumduction of the foot may reveal subluxating or dislocating peroneal tendons.

IMAGING AND OTHER DIAGNOSTIC STUDIES

- Weight-bearing ankle and foot radiographs must be obtained.
  - Radiographs may show a "fleck sign" **(FIG 2A)** at the lateralmost border of the fibular tip. This represents an avulsion of the superior peroneal retinaculum and is pathognomonic.[6]
  - The os peroneum **(FIG 2B)**, if present, should be identified. Any fragmentation or displacement of this sesamoid may indicate peroneal longus disruption.

- Ultrasonography can identify peroneal tendon tears with 90% to 100% accuracy, 100% sensitivity, and 85% to 100% specificity.[9,12,17]
- Magnetic resonance imaging (MRI) is generally useful in confirming peroneal tendon pathology, demonstrating tears in the substance of the tendon and fluid in the sheaths. Associated pathology of the ankle can be identified as well **(FIGS 3 and 4)**.

DIFFERENTIAL DIAGNOSIS

- Stress fracture of fibula, cuboid, or fifth metatarsal
- Lateral ankle instability
- Acute fracture of os peroneum or lateral process of the talus
- Ankle or syndesmosis sprain
- Talar osteochondral lesions
- Sinus tarsi syndrome
- Calcaneocuboid syndrome
- Degenerative joint disease
- Accessory muscle/bone
- Hypertrophic peroneal tubercle
- Sural neuritis

NONOPERATIVE MANAGEMENT

- Functional rehabilitation includes range of motion for the ankle and hindfoot, concentric and eccentric muscle strengthening, endurance training with particular attention to the peroneal musculature, and proprioceptive exercises.
- Functional bracing or taping may be useful to help prevent recurrent injury during "at-risk" activities.
- A recent study[7] demonstrates that ultrasound-guided peroneal injections is safe and relatively effective in treating peroneal tendon tears or tendinopathy with only 25% of patients needing surgery after this intervention.

SURGICAL MANAGEMENT

Preoperative Planning

- All imaging studies must be reviewed so that the location of the lesion is identified. MRI is often useful in identifying the exact level of peroneal tendon pathology.
- Plain films must be reviewed for associated pathology, including degenerative changes, malalignment, and fractures. The ankle radiographs may reveal an avulsion of the superior peroneal retinaculum.

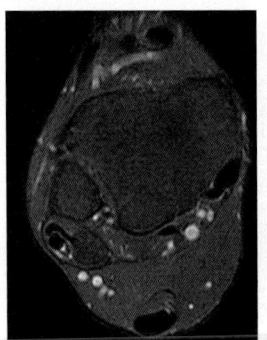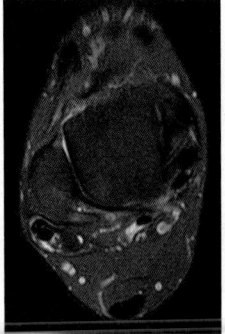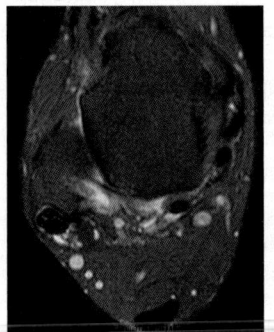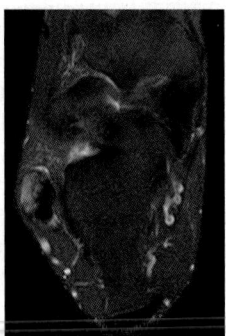

FIG 3 T2-weighted axial MRI scans demonstrating a peroneus brevis tear. **A.** Posterior to distal fibula, peroneus brevis, the more anterior tendon, appears intact. **B.** More distally, the peroneus brevis tendon demonstrates signal change. **C.** At the distal fibula, there is a greater signal change within the peroneus brevis tendon. **D.** Immediately distal to the tip of the fibula, more extensive signal change in peroneus brevis tendon, suggesting degenerative tear.

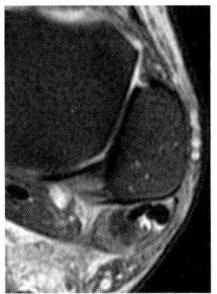 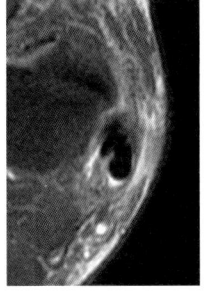 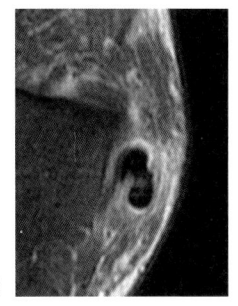 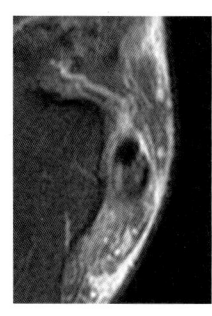

FIG 4 T2-weighted axial MRI scans demonstrating a peroneus longus tear. **A.** Posterior to distal fibula, peroneus longus, the more posterior tendon, appears intact. **B.** More distally, the peroneus longus tendon is thickened. **C.** More distally, adjacent to the talus, there is a signal change within the peroneus longus tendon. **D.** Even more distally, in the foot adjacent to the calcaneus, more extensive signal change in peroneus longus tendon, suggesting degenerative tear.

Positioning

- The patient is placed in a modified lateral or full lateral decubitus position.
- Saline bags or large blanket bumps are placed under the ipsilateral hip to achieve a lazy lateral position; a beanbag may be used to maintain a full lateral decubitus position.

- A well-padded thigh tourniquet is placed.
- The operative foot is elevated, with a bump made of blankets under the sterile field or with sterile towels within the sterile field.

PRELIMINARY STEPS

Exposure

- An 8- to 12-cm longitudinal incision is centered over the course of the peroneal tendons, beginning 1 cm posterior and proximal to the tip of the fibula.
- Depending on the preoperative plan, the incision may need to be extended to the base of the fifth metatarsal or just distal to the distal tip of the fibula.
- Care must be taken to identify and protect the saphenous vein and sural nerve in the distal aspect of the incision, which is subcutaneous and just posterior to the incision. A hemostat is often the best tool to achieve blunt dissection in this region.
  - The nerve, once identified, is tagged with a purple skin scribe or a vessel loop.
- The peroneal sheath is inspected for redundant tissue that may be suggestive of inflammation **(TECH FIG 1)**.
- The tendons are manipulated in order to elicit any subluxation.
- At this point, the superior retinaculum is incised.
- Usually, the peroneus longus tendon is encountered first.

Inspecting and Débriding the Peroneal Tendons

- The tendon is inspected both proximally and distally (in light of the preoperative MRI) in order to document any tearing or degeneration. Oftentimes, the inferior peroneal retinaculum must be incised to fully appreciate the longus.
- Once this tendon has been thoroughly inspected, a tenosynovectomy is performed sharply with a no. 15 blade scalpel.
- Degenerated or nonviable tendon is excised. Any low-lying peroneus muscle belly that may create impingement posterior to the fibula should also be excised.
- The peroneus brevis is then inspected, and any residual pathology is documented.

- After comprehensive tenosynovectomy and tendon débridement, repair is initiated.

Treatment Decision

- Once both tendons have had an extensive synovectomy and débridement, a treatment decision must be made. We conceptualize this similar to the algorithm proposed by Krause and Brodsky.[10]
- For tendons that have damage to less than 50% of their cross-sectional area, the tendon is considered salvageable.
- In tendons that have greater than 50% of their cross-sectional areas débrided due to degeneration, the stump is tenodesed to the other peroneal tendon (assuming it is viable).
- If both tendons have over 50% degeneration, another algorithm, based on Redfern and Myerson,[11] is used.
  - If the proximal muscle bellies are not mobile, then a tendon transfer is performed.
  - If there is some proximal muscle excursion
    - If the tissue bed is scarred: silicone rod–staged reconstruction
    - If the tissue bed is mobile: allograft or tendon transfer

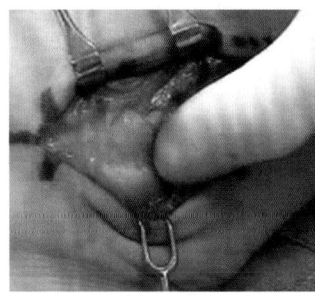

TECH FIG 1 Peroneal tendon sheath fullness suggests inflammation.

REPAIR OF A PERONEUS BREVIS TEAR IN ISOLATION

- MRI scan is typically accurate in identifying peroneal tendon tears and may be useful in determining the location of the tear (see **FIG 3**).
- If the damage is less than 50% of the cross-sectional area of the tendon
  - The area of the longitudinal split is inspected (**TECH FIG 2A,B**).
  - If present, a low-lying muscle belly that may impinge within the peroneal sheath should be excised (**TECH FIG 2C**).
  - The diseased/degenerated portion of the peroneus brevis tendon is excised (**TECH FIG 2D,E**).

- Using a 3-0 absorbable suture, the tendon is repaired in a tubularized fashion.
  - At one end of the longitudinal tear, a surgeon's knot is thrown (**TECH FIG 2F,G**).
  - In a whipstitch/running fashion or in an interrupted simple suturing technique, each end of the split is captured to reestablish a smooth tendon (**TECH FIG 2H**).
  - The superficial peroneal retinaculum is then repaired with a 0 absorbable suture (**TECH FIG 2I,J**).

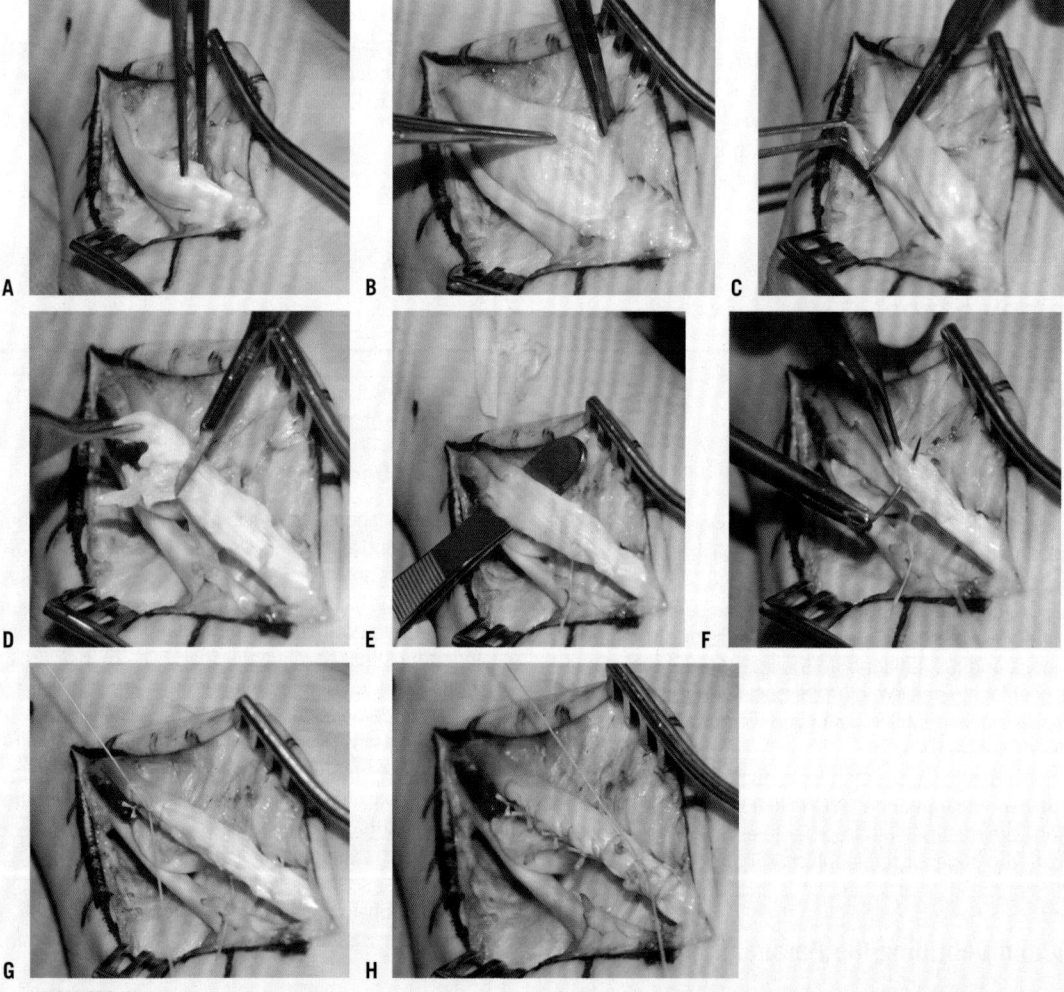

TECH FIG 2 A,B. Peroneus brevis tendon tear. **A.** Thickened tendon is consistent with MRI findings in **FIG 3D**. **B.** A longitudinal split tear creates a loss of contour of the tendon. **C.** Débridement of low-lying peroneus brevis muscle. The bulbous thickening of the peroneus brevis tendon is characteristic of chronic tendon tear/degeneration. **D.** Débridement of diseased portion of peroneus brevis tendon. **E.** Residual healthy fibers of débrided peroneus brevis tendon. **F–H.** Peroneus brevis tendon repair. **F.** Proximal anchoring suture. **G.** Repair via tubularization of the peroneus brevis tendon. **H.** Distal repair reinforced with a combination of interrupted and running sutures. *(continued)*

TECHNIQUES

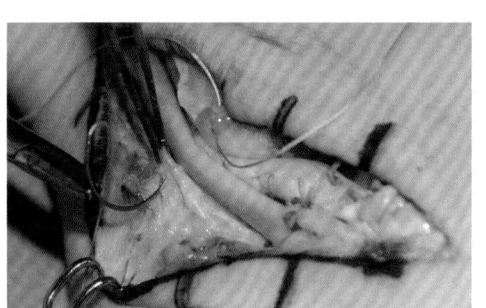
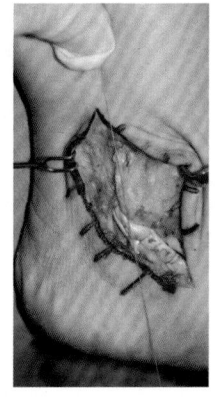

TECH FIG 2 *(continued)* **I,J.** Repair of the superficial peroneal retinaculum following peroneus brevis repair. **I.** Retinaculum being sewn after peroneal tendons reduced to their anatomic position. **J.** Imbrication of the superior peroneal retinaculum with tendons reduced posterior to fibula.

- If the damage is greater than 50% of the cross-sectional area of the tendon
  - The diseased tendon is excised with a scalpel.
  - The viable proximal and distal tendons are tenodesed to the peroneal longus tendon with a 2-0 absorbable suture where the stumps lie when the foot is in a neutral position. This should be done for at length of about 2 cm to improve strength of the repair.

- Usually, the proximal tenodesis is 3 to 4 cm proximal to the tip of the fibula and the distal tenodesis is 5 to 6 cm distal to the fibular tip.
- A (rare) rupture of the peroneal brevis from the base of the fifth metatarsal requires securing the tendon stump to its insertion.
  - Prepare a bleeding bone bed at the anatomic footprint of the base of the fifth metatarsal.
  - Use a 3.5-mm suture anchor to secure the stump to the bone.

REPAIR OF A PERONEUS LONGUS TEAR IN ISOLATION

- MRI scan is typically accurate in identifying peroneal tendon tears and may be useful in determining the location of the tear (see **FIG 4**).
- If the damage is less than 50% of the cross-sectional area of the tendon
  - The area of the longitudinal split is inspected **(TECH FIG 3A–C)**.
  - The diseased/degenerated portion of the peroneus brevis tendon is excised **(TECH FIG 3D,E)**.
  - Using a 3-0 absorbable suture, the tendon is repaired in a tubularized fashion **(TECH FIG 3F,G)**.
    - An imbricating suture pattern is used to create the tubularization **(TECH FIG 3H–J)**.
    - In a whipstitch/running fashion, each end of the split is captured to reestablish a smooth tendon **(TECH FIG 3K)**.
    - The superficial peroneal retinaculum is then repaired **(TECH FIG 3L,M)**.

- If the damage is over half of the cross-sectional area of the tendon, the tendon is tenodesed to the peroneal brevis tendon with a 2-0 absorbable suture where the residual tendon lies when the foot is in a neutral position.
- If the os peroneum is fractured and needs to be excised, then the dissection must be extended distally to visualize the tendon, diving below the cuboid. The abductor muscle must be retracted inferiorly.
  - If the tendon is disrupted transversely (after the os is removed), then the tendon ends are reapproximated and can be repaired end to end with a nonabsorbable suture.
  - If the tendon cannot be repaired end to end, then the tendon may be tenodesed to the peroneus brevis tendon.
  - If the tendon does not have excursion, then a tenodesis should not be performed because it may limit the function of the peroneus brevis tendon.

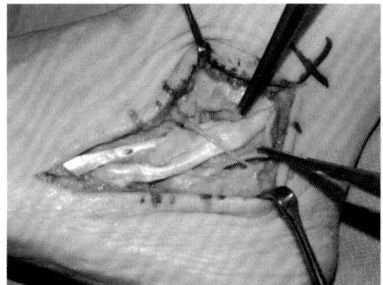
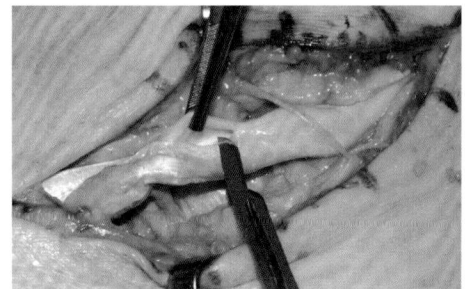

TECH FIG 3 A. Peroneus longus tendon degeneration identified, corresponding to MRI findings in **FIG 4C. B.** Tendon degeneration corresponding to MRI findings in **FIG 4D**. *(continued)*

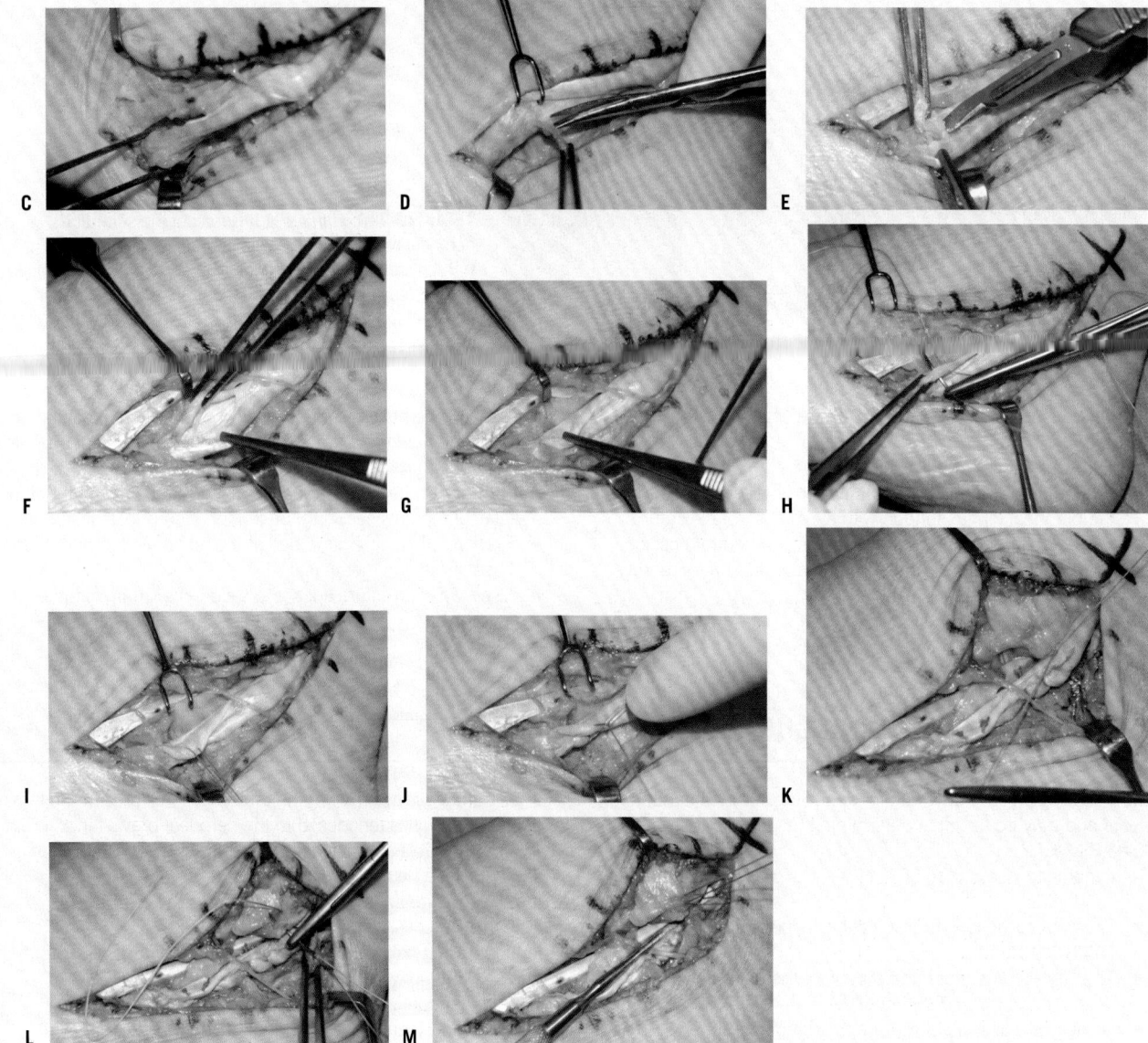

TECH FIG 3 *(continued)* **C.** Distal tendon degeneration at the os peroneum. **D,E.** Débridement of diseased portion of peroneus longus tendon. **D.** Tenosynovectomy and partial tendon excision. **E.** Excision of central tendon degeneration in more distal portion of tendon. **F.** Healthy tendon fibers after central portion of diseased tendon excised. **G.** Planned tubularization of residual healthy tendon. **H.** Suture pattern to create tubularization. **I.** Tendon overlapped to create tubularized repair. **J.** Tendon repair secured. **K.** More proximal interrupted suture to reinforce repair. **L,M.** Repair of the superficial peroneal retinaculum following peroneus longus repair. **L.** Retinaculum being sewn after peroneal tendons reduced to their anatomic position. **M.** Imbrication of the superior peroneal retinaculum with tendons reduced posterior to fibula.

REPAIR OF A PERONEUS BREVIS TEAR WITH FIBULAR GROOVE DEEPENING

- The peroneus brevis tendon may have a tear due to chronic subluxation around the distal fibula.
- The tear should be inspected **(TECH FIG 4A)**.
- Any structures that may cause impingement within the peroneal tendon sheath such as a low-lying peroneus brevis muscle belly or inflamed tenosynovium should be excised **(TECH FIG 4B)**.
- The diseased portion of tendon is excised **(TECH FIG 4C–E)**.
- The tendon is assessed for a persistent tendency to subluxate **(TECH FIG 4F)**.

- If subluxation persists, then a fibular groove deepening is performed **(TECH FIG 4G–I)**.
- The peroneus brevis tendon is repaired via tubularization using absorbable suture **(TECH FIG 4J)**.
- The peroneal tendons are reduced in their anatomic position, now without tendency to subluxate following fibular groove deepening **(TECH FIG 4K)**.
- The superior peroneal retinaculum is repaired **(TECH FIG 4L,M)**.

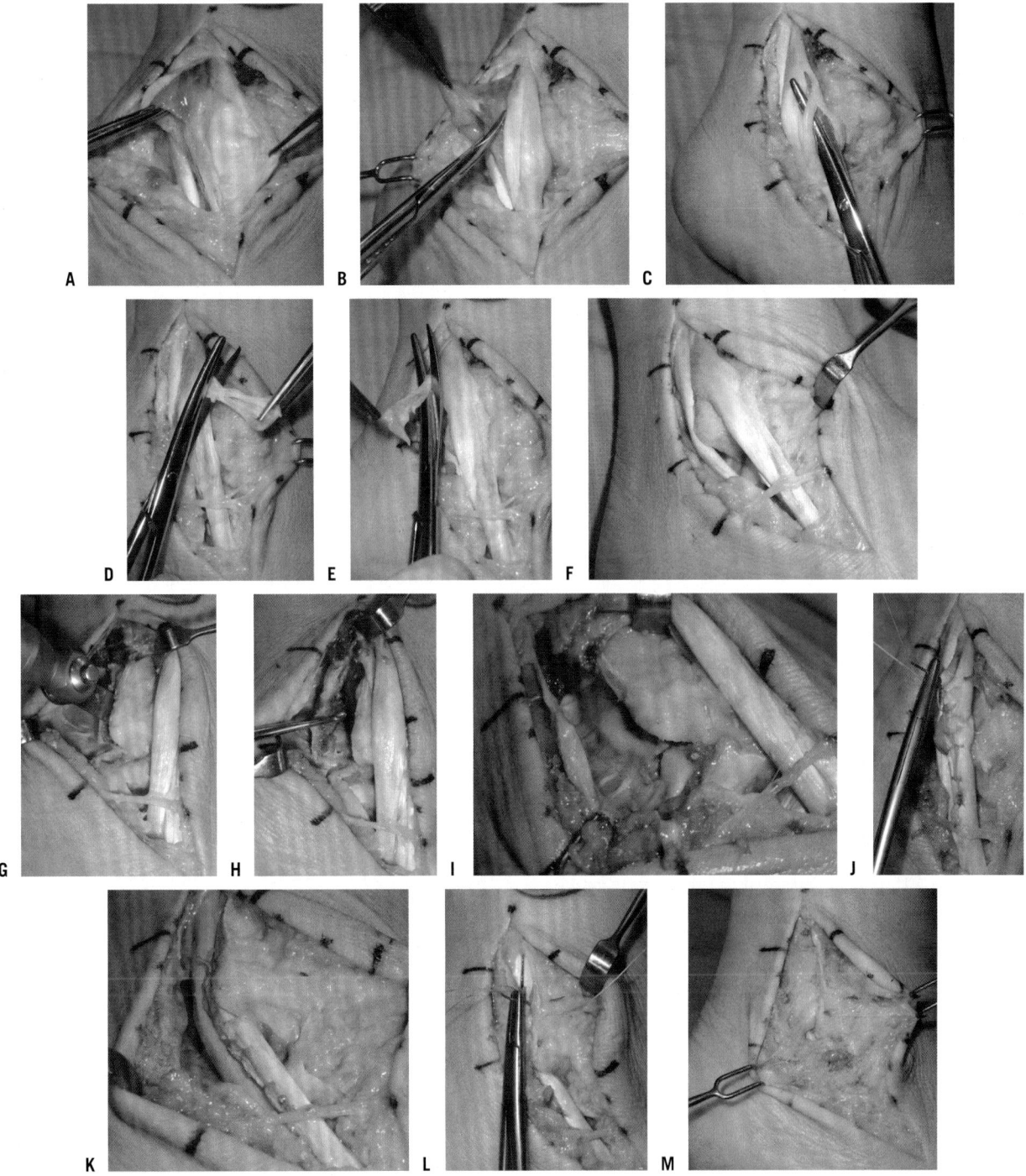

TECH FIG 4 **A.** Right peroneus brevis tear due to recurrent tendon subluxation at tip of fibula. **B.** Flexor tenosynovectomy. **C.** Identifying degenerative peroneus tendon tear. **D.** Débridement of degenerated portion of tendon anteriorly. **E.** Débridement of degenerated portion of tendon posteriorly. **F.** Despite débridement and tenosynovectomy, the peroneus brevis tendon continues to subluxate anterior to the fibula. **G.** Microsagittal saw creating "trapdoor" in posterior distal fibula. **H.** Trapdoor hinged open and distal fibula decancellated to create deeper fibular groove. **I.** With trapdoor reduced after decancellation, deeper fibular groove established. **J.** Peroneus brevis tendon repair via tubularization. **K.** Peroneal tendons now remain reduced even without superior peroneal retinacular repair. **L.** Superficial peroneal retinaculum being sewn after peroneal tendons reduced to their anatomic position. **M.** Imbrication of the superior peroneal retinaculum with tendons reduced posterior to fibula, with sutures passed through the bony ledge created by fibular groove deepening.

Pearls and Pitfalls

Indication	• Complete history and physical examination • Address associated malalignment and pathology such as ankle instability.
Incision	• Avoid injury to the sural nerve.
Débridement	• Perform adequate débridement of the peroneal tendons.
Tubularization	• The goal is to create a smooth tendon surface. One should try to bury the first and last knots of the suture.

POSTOPERATIVE CARE

- Patients are initially placed in a bulky Jones dressing for the first 2 weeks.
- Thereafter, they are allowed to bear weight as tolerated in a removable short-leg walking boot.
- They are instructed to remove the boot four times a day and perform active and passive range-of-motion exercises of the ankle and hindfoot in all planes of motion.
- Home strengthening exercises are begun at 8 weeks, and the patient is advanced to an ankle stirrup at 12 to 14 weeks based on his or her strength.
- All patients are enrolled in formal physical therapy for functional rehabilitation of the ankle starting at 8 weeks.

OUTCOMES

- Data on the 6.5-year follow-up of 18 patients has been published by Demetracopoulos et al.[3]
  - These patients had débridement and primary repairs (tubularization) of their peroneus longus and brevis tendons who had less than 50% débrided.
  - There were no reoperations or failures during this time interval.
  - There was a significant improvement in the postoperative visual analog scale and lower extremity functional scale scores.
  - Seventeen of 18 patients returned to full sporting activities without limitation.

COMPLICATIONS

- Wound complications
- Sural neuralgia or sural nerve injury
- Chronic pain
- Rerupture

REFERENCES

1. Burman M. Stenosing tendovaginitis of the foot and ankle; studies with special reference to the stenosing tendovaginitis of the peroneal tendons of the peroneal tubercle. AMA Arch Surg 1953;67(5):686–698.
2. Cox D, Paterson FW. Acute calcific tendinitis of peroneus longus. J Bone Joint Surg Br 1991;73(2):342.
3. Demetracopoulos CA, Vineyard JC, Kiesau CD, et al. Long-term results of debridement and primary repair of peroneal tendon tears. Foot Ankle Int 2014;35(3):252–257.
4. DiGiovanni BF, Fraga CJ, Cohen BE, et al. Associated injuries found in chronic lateral ankle instability. Foot Ankle Int 2000;21(10):809–815.
5. Dombek MF, Lamm BM, Saltrick K, et al. Peroneal tendon tears: a retrospective review. J Foot Ankle Surg 2003;42(5):250–258.
6. Eckert WR, Davis EA Jr. Acute rupture of the peroneal retinaculum. J Bone Joint Surg Am 1976;58(5):670–672.
7. Fram BR, Rogero R, Fuchs D, et al. Clinical outcomes and complications of peroneal tendon sheath ultrasound-guided corticosteroid injection. Foot Ankle Int 2019;40(8):888–894.
8. Geller J, Lin S, Cordas D, et al. Relationship of a low-lying muscle belly to tears of the peroneus brevis tendon. Am J Orthop (Belle Mead NJ) 2003;32(11):541–544.
9. Grant TH, Kelikian AS, Jereb SE, et al. Ultrasound diagnosis of peroneal tendon tears. A surgical correlation. J Bone Joint Surg Am 2005;87(8):1788–1794.
10. Krause JO, Brodsky JW. Peroneus brevis tendon tears: pathophysiology, surgical reconstruction, and clinical results. Foot Ankle Int 1998;19(5):271–279.
11. Redfern D, Myerson M. The management of concomitant tears of the peroneus longus and brevis tendons. Foot Ankle Int 2004;25(10):695–707.
12. Rockett MS, Waitches G, Sudakoff G, et al. Use of ultrasonography versus magnetic resonance imaging for tendon abnormalities around the ankle. Foot Ankle Int 1998;19(9):604–612.
13. Sammarco GJ, DiRaimondo CV. Chronic peroneus brevis tendon lesions. Foot Ankle 1989;9(4):163–170.
14. Sobel M, Geppert MJ, Hannafin JA, et al. Microvascular anatomy of the peroneal tendons. Foot Ankle 1992;13(8):469–472.
15. Sobel M, Geppert MJ, Olson EJ, et al. The dynamics of peroneus brevis tendon splits: a proposed mechanism, technique of diagnosis, and classification of injury. Foot Ankle 1992;13(7):413–422.
16. Title CI, Jung HG, Parks BG, et al. The peroneal groove deepening procedure: a biomechanical study of pressure reduction. Foot Ankle Int 2005;26(6):442–448.
17. Waitches GM, Rockett M, Brage M, et al. Ultrasonographic-surgical correlation of ankle tendon tears. J Ultrasound Med 1998;17(4):249–256.
18. Zammit J, Singh D. The peroneus quartus muscle. Anatomy and clinical relevance. J Bone Joint Surg Br 2003;85(8):1134–1137.

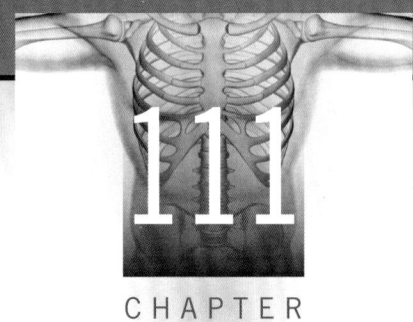

111
CHAPTER

Repair of Dislocating Peroneal Tendons:
Perspective 1

Kamil M. Amer and Sheldon Lin

DEFINITION

- Subluxation or dislocation of the peroneal tendon is a relatively uncommon injury, with the majority of the cases attributed to a traumatic event. Chronic subluxation has also been reported without any history of a specific event.
- Numerous surgical procedures have been described for the treatment of peroneal tendon subluxation, which may be classified into three categories: primary repair, soft tissue augmentation, and bony reconstruction.
- Primary repair of the superior peroneal retinaculum (SPR) is a commonly used surgical procedure. However, the effectiveness of primary repair depends on the quality of the retinaculum and its ability to contain the peroneal tendons. When the SPR tissue is deficient or insufficient, then other procedures are necessary.
- Soft tissue procedures other than primary repair involve the augmentation of tissue already present or the rerouting of tissue from other structures to recreate the SPR.
- Bony procedures attempt to recreate a more stable fibular sulcus by deepening the fibular groove or extending the fibular rim. In this chapter, we present a soft tissue augmentation procedure using a periosteal-based flap of the retrofibular sulcus.

ANATOMY

- Along the lateral aspect of the lower leg, there are two muscles in the lateral compartment, the peroneus longus (PL) and peroneus brevis (PB). These two muscles arise at the proximal fibula and become tendinous before crossing the ankle.
- The peroneal tendons are contained in a single sheath located posteriorly and immediately distal to the fibula. Roughly at the level of the peroneal tubercle on the lateral calcaneus, the tendons separate into separate sheaths. The PB muscle belly extends more distal than the PL, and it becomes tendinous about 1.5 cm before the tip of the fibula. The PB tendon lies directly posterior to the fibula and anteromedial to the PL tendon as the two tendons course behind the fibula.
- The peroneal tendon sheath comprises the SPR, the calcaneofibular ligament (CFL), and the fibular sulcus. Respectively, the fibular sulcus represents the anterior border, the SPR the lateral border, portions of the SPR and CFL the posterior border, and portions of the CFL and posterior talofibular ligament the medial border of the peroneal tendon sheath.[15]

- The PB inserts on the dorsal base of the fifth metatarsal, whereas the PL courses lateral to medial on the plantar aspect of the foot and inserts on the lateral sides of the base of the first metatarsal and medial cuneiform bones.
- The SPR is the primary restraint against subluxation of the peroneal tendons within the fibular groove. The SPR can have an extremely varied anatomy, with differences in width, thickness, and insertional patterns. Most commonly, the SPR inserts into both the Achilles tendon and the calcaneus.[3] There is no distinct insertion point of the SPR; instead, it blends into the periosteum of the fibula.
- The anatomy of the fibula is varied as well. About 50% of fibula have a bony ridge about 2 to 4 mm that augments the fibular sulcus.[2] A cadaveric study by Edwards[5] found that 82% of the time, a sulcus was present at the posterior edge of the distal fibula. The average sulcus dimension was 3 mm deep and 6 mm wide. He found that 11% of the cadavers had no groove and that 7% of the cadavers had a convex fibula. A fibrocartilaginous rim was deficient in 48% of all cadavers and was absent in 30%.

PATHOGENESIS

- According to Zoellner and Clancy,[23] in acute injury, the peroneal tendons tend to dislocate anteriorly over the lateral malleolus in people who have an anatomic predisposition. The fibular groove that serves as the pulley for the tendons can be shallow or convex, and the SPR may be absent or lax. A low-lying PB muscle belly can also cause subluxation (FIG 1). In a study of the effect of a low-lying PB muscle belly, Geller et al[8] measured the location of the musculotendinous junction (MTJ) in 30 cadaveric specimens with respect to the fibula tip and peroneal tubercle and also the width of the PB tendon. The PB MTJ was significantly more distal, and the tendons had a significantly greater diameter in torn (4 of 30) versus untorn (26 of 30) specimens (TABLE 1). The authors suggested that the location of the PB MTJ may have an influence on the development of degenerative tears.
- Recurrent dislocations are the result of an inciting acute traumatic episode of forceful ankle dorsiflexion with a simultaneous powerful contraction of the peroneal muscles that causes failure of the SPR. The dorsiflexion causes the SPR to tighten, thereby decreasing its diameter. This force is theorized to cause the retinaculum to be avulsed from its periosteal attachment. Eckert and Davis[4] stated that the SPR's attachment on the edge of the fibula does not adhere to a strong band of collagen but instead blends into the

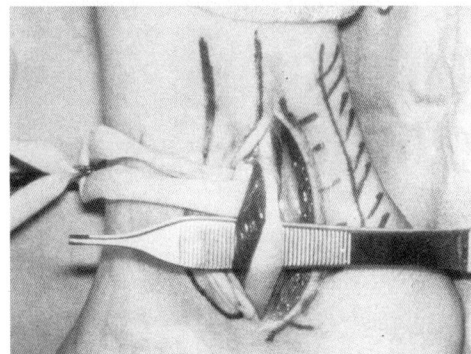

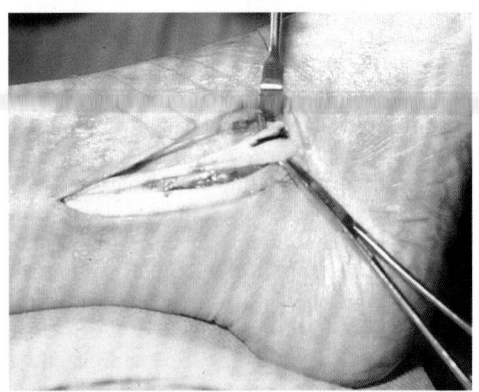

FIG 1 A,B. Anatomic dissection of a peroneus muscle belly that is too distal. Note the distance to the fibular tip.

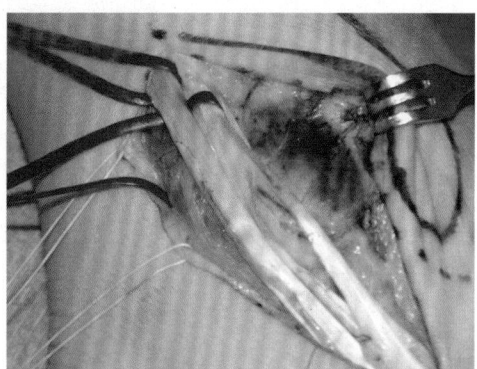

FIG 2 The split PB tendon, with the PL running more posterior.

periosteum of the lateral malleolus. They proposed that this weak insertion point is responsible for tendon dislocation secondary to avulsion of the fibular fibrocartilaginous lip and stripping of the SPR from the fibula.

- The prototypical mechanism is in skiers as they forcefully contract the peroneal muscles to grab the ski edge into the snow.
- Eckert and Davis[4] classified SPR injury into three different grades according to severity:
  - Grade 1 injury: separation of the retinaculum from the cartilaginous lip and the lateral malleolus
  - Grade 2 injury: The distal 1- to 2-cm dense fibrous lip is elevated along with the SPR.
  - Grade 3 injury: avulsion of a thin fragment of bone along with the collagenous lip attached to the deep surface of the SPR and deep fascia (Radiographically, this may be represented by a "fleck sign.")
  - In grade 1 injuries, the peroneal tendons are easily reducible and are unstable under tension only.
  - In grade 2 and 3 injuries, the peroneal tendons fail to remain reduced even without tension.
  - Normally, the peroneal tendons are contained within the fibular sulcus by the SPR.

NATURAL HISTORY

- Based on our experience, symptomatic recurrent subluxation does not resolve spontaneously.
- Often, peroneal tendon dislocation continues to be misdiagnosed as a chronic ankle sprain. As the tendons dislocate and relocate, direct tendon injury occurs due to repetitive trauma.
- Zone 1 tendon injuries occur at the fibular groove and usually involve the PB tendon. The action of the PB tendon snapping over the sharp ridge of the fibula leads to a longitudinal tear within the tendon substance **(FIG 2)**.
- Zone 2 injuries occur distal to the fibular tip, usually affecting the PL tendon. These injuries are caused by the PL coursing over the lateral wall of the calcaneus and turning 45 degrees at the cuboid facet. As the tears propagate, an inflammatory response may lead to tenosynovitis, tendinopathy, and potential tendon rupture. Peroneal tendon subluxation and dislocation is thought to accentuate the symptoms.

PATIENT HISTORY AND PHYSICAL FINDINGS

- The patient may not be able to recall a traumatic event preceding the usual complaints of lateral ankle swelling and pain posterior to the lateral malleolus. Most patients report that the pain radiates proximally. Patients complain of persistent lateral ankle pain and swelling with a sensation of snapping or popping and may note a "pop" laterally before the tendon gives way.
- On physical examination, the lateral ankle will be swollen and tender and may be ecchymotic in the acute setting. This can easily be confused with a lateral ankle sprain **(TABLE 2)**, but the location of the pain may be used to differentiate between the two. Tenderness posterior to the fibula is indicative of peroneal tendinopathy; in contrast, tenderness at the anterior distal fibula suggests an anterior talofibular ligament injury (ankle sprain). However, because the CFL is the floor of

TABLE 1 Low-Lying Muscle Belly of Peroneus Brevis and Its Relationship to Peroneus Brevis Tears			
Specimen Data	Average Distance to Fibula Tip (cm)	Average Distance of Peroneal Tuberosity (cm)	Average Width (cm)
No tear (n = 26)	1.62 ± 1.38	3.39 ± 1.3	1.19 ± 0.37
Tear (n = 4)	0.04 ± 1.51	2.13 ± 0.83	1.44 ± 0.39

TABLE 2 Clinical Differentiation of Ankle Subluxation from Ankle Sprain

Signs and Symptoms	Subluxation	Sprain
Tenderness	Proximal to tip of fibula	Distal to tip of fibula
Swelling	Posterolateral	Anteroinferior
History	Snapping	Giving way
Worse on uneven ground?	Possible	Probable
Worse on circumduction?	Yes	No
Worse on flexion–inversion?	No	Yes

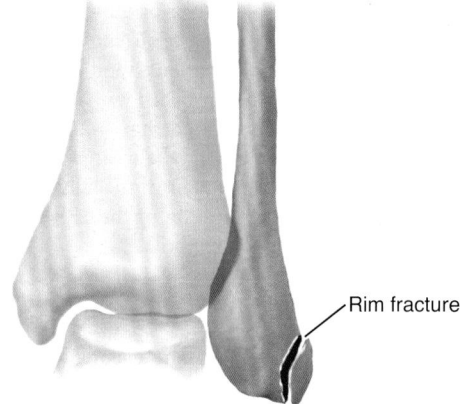

FIG 3 Fleck sign on a radiograph. The best view to see this on is the mortise view.

Rim fracture

the peroneal tendon sheath, there may still be some confusion with more severe ankle sprains. A negative anterior drawer test and pain experienced when the foot is stressed against resisted eversion are more indicative of an injury to the SPR.

- Peroneal tendon subluxation test: In the prone position, with the knee flexed to 90 degrees, ankle dorsiflexion and forced hindfoot eversion against resistance is performed. Apprehension and peroneal tendon subluxation or dislocation with this provocative maneuver typically confirms the diagnosis.[10]
- Acutely dislocated peroneal tendons are occasionally seen on physical examination, but more commonly, the tendons are reduced upon presentation and are dislocated only with the peroneal tendon subluxation test.
- Likewise, chronic peroneal tendon subluxation or dislocation may not present with the tendons frankly dislocated. Chronic subluxation and dislocation are generally best diagnosed by testing the ankle through a range of motion of inversion and plantarflexion to maximum eversion and dorsiflexion with resistance.
- Peroneal compression test: direct compression of the peroneal tendon sheath to identify peroneal tendon injury

IMAGING AND OTHER DIAGNOSTIC STUDIES

- Standard weight-bearing ankle radiographs (anteroposterior [AP], lateral, and mortise) define the bony ankle anatomy alignment. In cases of peroneal tendon subluxation, radiographs are usually negative. In a grade 3 injury, a "fleck" of bone can be seen off the posterior distal fibula and is considered pathognomonic of an SPR injury **(FIG 3)**.
- Magnetic resonance imaging (MRI) affords detail of the soft tissues. Injury to the SPR, the peroneal tendons, or other supporting tissues may be identified: Anomalous structures such as the peroneus quartus or a low-lying PB muscle belly may be suggested **(FIG 4)**. An MRI is useful for preoperative planning, as other pathology (PB tear, low-lying MJT, fibular sulcus) may also need to be surgically addressed concomitant with repair of the subluxation or dislocating peroneal tendons. We also use MRI to define the morphology of the fibular sulcus. Although MRI may identify dislocated or subluxated peroneal tendons, the tendons are often reduced while the patient is relaxed in the MRI scanner; however, occasionally, dislocated tendons may be identified on axial MRI views.
- Computed tomography scan is rarely indicated in preoperative planning of dislocated peroneal tendons.

DIFFERENTIAL DIAGNOSIS

- Injury to the lateral ligament complex
- Fracture of lateral malleolus, lateral process of the talus, anterior process of the calcaneus, or fracture at the base of the fifth metatarsal
- Osteochondral defect on the talar dome
- Peroneal tendon pathology

NONOPERATIVE MANAGEMENT

- Initial treatment of an acute injury consists of a well-molded, short-leg cast for 6 weeks.
- Successful outcomes of nonoperative management range from 14% in a study by Eckert and Davis[4] to up to 56% as reported by McLennan,[11] whereas other investigators have also reported variable outcomes in small case series.[6,12,14,19] At best, only half of all patients become better. Therefore, as part of initial injury counseling, it is necessary to inform the patient that an operation will still be necessary, in most instances, despite conservative treatment.

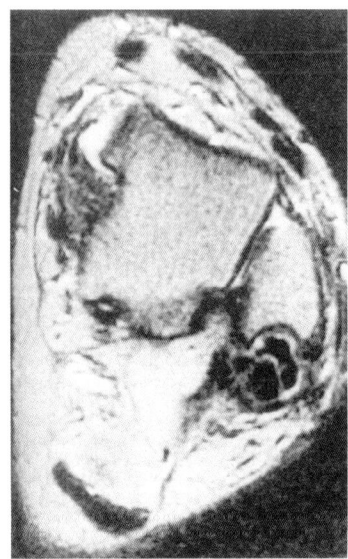

FIG 4 An MRI in the axial plane demonstrating the PB tendon splitting over the cartilage lip of the fibula.

- For patients with chronic subluxation, nonoperative treatment has not been shown to help; usually, pain and symptoms recur once the short-leg cast is removed. In addition, more athletic, higher demand patients tend to demand more reliable treatment and wish to proceed with operative repair.
- Recent studies have demonstrated that some acute grade I and possible grade III injuries maybe treated conservatively in a short-leg cast with foot in neutral to slight inversion for 6 weeks. This would allow healing of the SPR to adhere to the posterolateral aspect of the fibula.[16]

SURGICAL MANAGEMENT OF TENOSYNOVITIS

- The treatment of symptomatic peroneal tendinopathy and tears traditionally begins with nonsteroidal anti-inflammatory drugs, activity modification, physical therapy, and immobilization, with surgery typically reserved for those failing nonoperative treatment. Other treatment options recently studied include ultrasound-guided peroneal tendon sheath corticosteroid injections, which demonstrated increased pain relief.[7]
- Recent studies have also demonstrated that tendoscopy is a useful method for the diagnosis and treatment of many peroneal tendon pathologies including tears and tenosynovitis.[21]
  - The use of a diagnostic ultrasound-guided injection of a local anesthetic into the peroneal tendon sheath followed by surgical release of the peroneal tendon sheath and débridement of the calcaneal exostosis was shown to be effective in the diagnosis and treatment of stenosing peroneal tenosynovitis.[22]

SURGICAL MANAGEMENT OF PERONEAL SUBLUXATION AND DISLOCATION

- Illustrated here is a modified surgical technique for soft tissue augmentation representing an alternative procedure for the treatment of peroneal tendon subluxation. No absolute contraindications exist for the procedure, but relative contraindications include the following:
  - The presence of a previous fracture or surgery that alters the local morphology and tissue quality
  - An Eckert and Davis[4] grade 3 fracture, with a thin fragment of bone along the cartilaginous lip attached to the deep surface of the peroneal retinaculum; the anterior portion of the SPR is already compromised and would not make a good surgical candidate.

- Patients with collagen disorders (Marfan, Ehlers-Danlos), where the strength and integrity of the periosteal flap could be suspect

Preoperative Planning

- Routine ankle radiographs are essential to identify or rule out a rim fracture of the distal fibula, which occurs in 15% to 50% of all cases of peroneal subluxation.[1]
- Typically, the ankle radiographs appear normal. We routinely obtain an MRI to identify potential peroneal tendon tears, other soft tissue anomalies such as a peroneus quartus, or other causes of lateral ankle pain and instability that need to be addressed concomitant to SPR augmentation.[17]
- MRI axial cuts define the morphology of the fibular sulcus and are helpful in staging a bony procedure if necessary during the superior retinaculoplasty.
- When dealing with irreparable PB tendon tears, recent studies demonstrated that allograft reconstruction substantially restored distal tension of peroneal tendons when compared to tenodesis of the peroneal brevis to peroneal longus.[13]
- A recent study by Guelfi et al[9] demonstrated that there are two main subgroups of peroneal tendon injuries. These include chronic subluxations with SPR injury and those with intrasheath subluxation with SPR remaining intact. They used tendoscopic treatment for patients with intrasheath subluxation and demonstrated improved outcomes.[9]

Positioning

- Either general or regional anesthesia is acceptable for this procedure, and the surgeon's preference determines which anesthetic method to use.
- The patient is placed in an oblique lateral position using a beanbag or large support under the ipsilateral hip. Adequate rotation of the limb facilitates access to the posterior fibula.
- We routinely use a thigh tourniquet and carefully pad all bony prominences.
- An examination under anesthesia with provocative maneuvers such as the anterior drawer and rotary subluxation tests may identify associated instability and locking or popping of the unstable peroneal tendons.

Approach

- The standard lateral approach is used.
- Care should be taken not to injure the sural nerve.

TECHNIQUES

SUPERIOR PERONEAL RETINACULOPLASTY

- We use a standard lateral incision along the course of the peroneal tendons, taking care not to injure the sural nerve.
- Carry the incision down to the level of the peroneal tendon sheath (**TECH FIG 1A**).
- Inspect the SPR. Usually, it is attenuated and deficient, especially along its anterior border. The retinaculum often is lifted off its fibular attachment, thus allowing the peroneal tendons to subluxate.
- Make an incision in the peroneal sheath along the posterior border of the fibula.
- Retract the peroneal tendons anteriorly (**TECH FIG 1B**).

- Occasionally, a small tear may be noticed in the PB tendon, warranting débridement or repair.
- If a shallow or convex fibular groove is present, we typically perform a groove-deepening procedure.
- We routinely reinforce the SPR with a soft tissue periosteal flap elevated from the fibular groove from a posterior to anterior direction.
- Raise the periosteal flap, measuring about 1.0 × 3.0 cm, sharply, from posterior to anterior. After the flap is raised, a groove-deepening procedure may be performed when indicated.

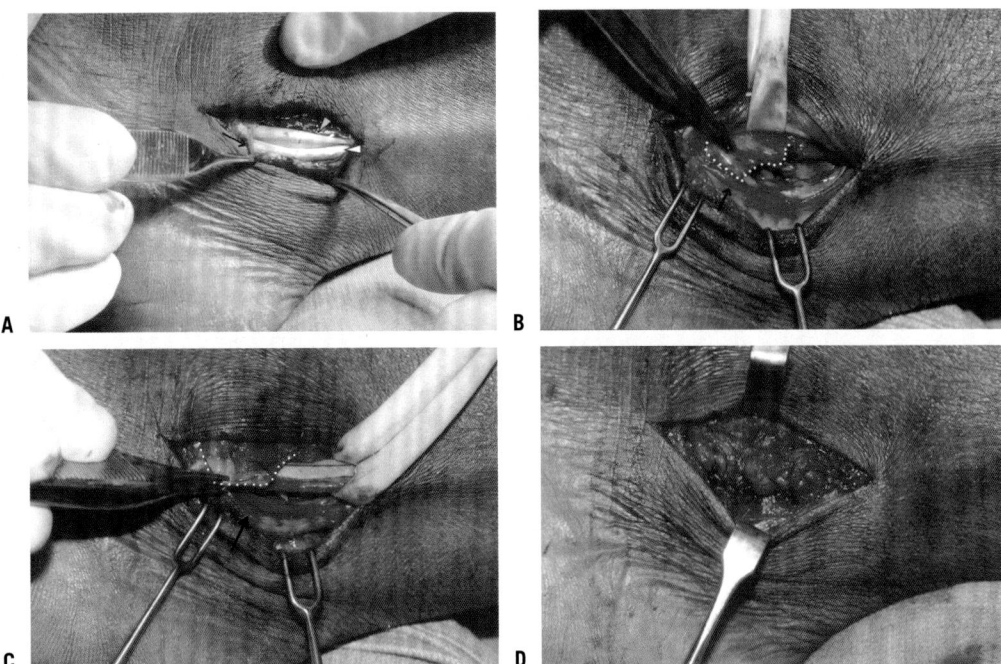

TECH FIG 1 **A.** Intraoperative photograph of a left ankle (lateral approach) shows the peroneal tendons sub-luxing anteriorly (brevis is the *gray arrowhead*, longus is the *white arrowhead*, SPR is the *black arrow*). **B.** The peroneal tendons have been retracted anteriorly by the Penrose drain. Elevation of an anterior-based periosteal flap (outlined by *white dots*) from the fibular groove has been completed. The *black arrow* shows the remnant of the SPR posteriorly. **C.** The tendons are relocated, after a groove-deepening procedure, into the recreated groove. The *white dots* outline the anteriorly based periosteal flap. It is then brought over to the posterior remnant of the SPR (*black arrow*). **D.** The flap is sutured to the remnant SPR with nonabsorbable sutures, completing the superior peroneal retinaculoplasty.

- Use a burr to deepen the groove 6 to 9 mm with all raw bony edges. The groove should extend from the fibular tip to 5 cm proximal. We use bone wax to smooth the groove.
- Reduce the peroneal tendons and use the periosteal flap to contain the tendons, with the visceral side of the periosteum facing the tendons (**TECH FIG 1C**).

- Suture the flap to the posterior remnant of the SPR with a series of 3-0 polybraided nonabsorbable sutures (**TECH FIG 1D**).
- Range the ankle to evaluate the soft tissue repair, being sure that the tendons are free to move within the reconstructed peroneal tendon sheath.
- Close the skin in usual fashion and place the leg into appropriate dressings and splints with compressive bandages.

DETAILED SURGICAL TECHNIQUE (COURTESY OF MARK E. EASLEY, MD, AND JAMES K. DEORIO, MD)

- Patient positioned in lateral decubitus position
- Regional anesthesia
- Thigh tourniquet
- Posterolateral approach
  - Immediately posterior to posterior margin of the distal fibula
  - Expose SPR.
  - Protect sural nerve.

- Release SPR 1 to 2 mm posterior from posterior fibular margin.
  - Peroneal tendons will be dislocated, so determining exactly where to release SPR will be distorted.
- Chronically dislocated tendon may be located in a "pocket" lateral to the distal fibula (**TECH FIG 2**).
- Inspect the tendons, particularly the more anterior PB, for a tear.
  - Peroneal tendon dislocations predispose the tendons to longitudinal split tears as the tendon repeatedly subluxates around the posterolateral fibula.

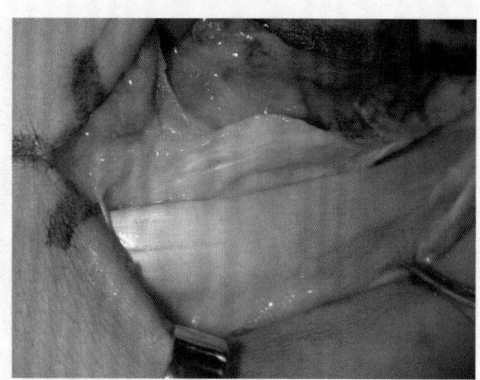 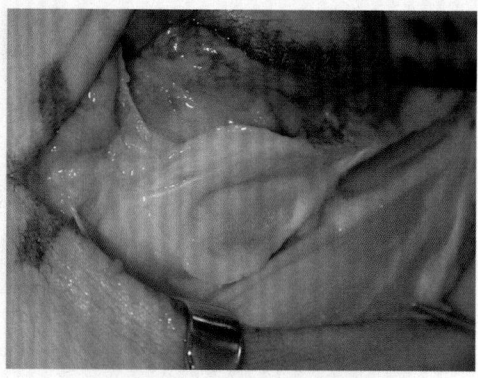

TECH FIG 2 Chronically dislocated peroneal tendons. **A.** Tendons in a pseudogroove on the lateral fibula. **B.** With peroneal tendons reduced, a "new gliding surface" and pocket of displaced SPR is evident.

TRADITIONAL GROOVE-DEEPENING PROCEDURE ("TRAPDOOR TECHNIQUE")

Creating the "Trapdoor" in the Posterior Distal Fibula

- Maintain the peroneal tendons dislocated anteriorly to protect them during the fibular groove deepening.
- Using a microsagittal saw, weaken the posterior cortex within the fibular groove (**TECH FIG 3A**).
- Although the fibula may be weakened only on the posterolateral margin, it is often necessary to weaken the "hinge" on the posteromedial margin as well (**TECH FIG 3B**).
- The fibular groove also needs to be weakened transversely, at the proximal margin of the trapdoor (**TECH FIG 3C**).
- Next, the trapdoor is completed at its distal margin, where the fibular groove rounds the distal fibula (**TECH FIG 3D**).
- Elevate the trapdoor and reflect it posteriorly on its hinge (**TECH FIG 3E,F**). If the hinge should be separated completely, it is not a problem.

Decancellating the Distal Fibula and Replacing the Trapdoor

- We typically use a high-speed burr to evacuate the cancellous bone from the distal fibula (**TECH FIG 4**), but a curette may also be used.

- Replace the trapdoor into the deepened fibular groove.
  - Impact the posterior fibular bone that was elevated but try to preserve the smooth surface so that the peroneal tendons have a smooth gliding surface with little risk of impingement or creation of adhesions (**TECH FIG 5A**).
  - The groove should be deep enough to keep the peroneal tendons reduced without manually restricting them (**TECH FIG 5B**). If it is not, then further decancellation may be necessary.

Repairing the Superior Peroneal Retinaculum

- With the tendons reduced, repair the SPR by advancing the intact leading edge of the SPR from its posterior position to the posterolateral rim of the distal fibula from which the SPR was displaced by the tendon dislocation and elevated for the surgical exposure (**TECH FIG 6A**).
- We routinely create drill holes in the distal posterolateral fibula to anchor the SPR (**TECH FIG 6B**).
- Be sure that the tendons glide well within the new fibular groove and are not stenosed by the repair (**TECH FIG 6C,D**).
- Standard closure

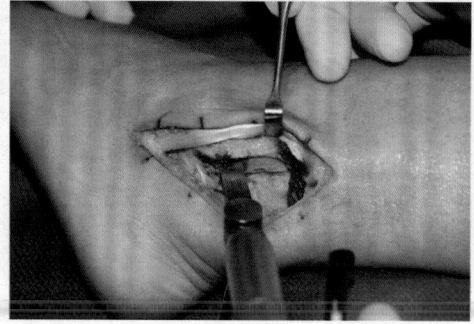 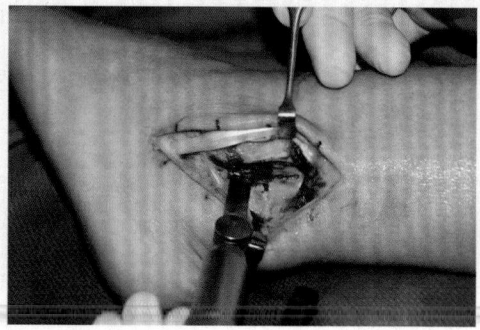

TECH FIG 3 A. Weakening the posterolateral aspect of the fibula to create the trapdoor. **B.** Weakening the hinge of the trapdoor. *(continued)*

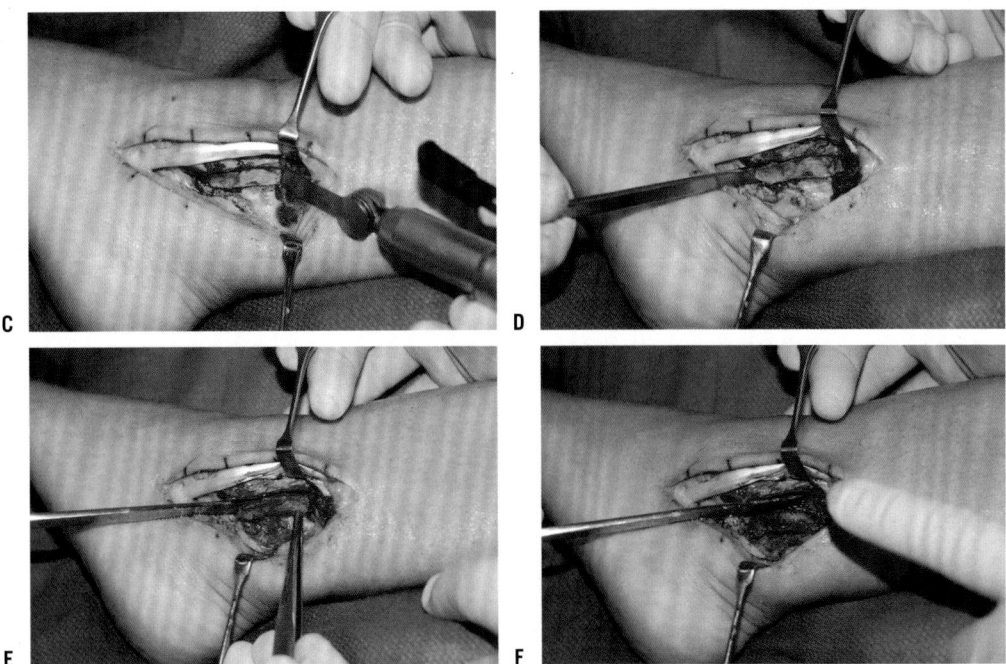

TECH FIG 3 *(continued)* **C.** Transverse osteotomy to ensure that the trapdoor can open. **D–F.** Elevating the trapdoor. **D.** Osteotome introduced into distal posterior fibula. **E.** Posterior fibula elevated at its posteromedial hinge. **F.** Trapdoor completely open.

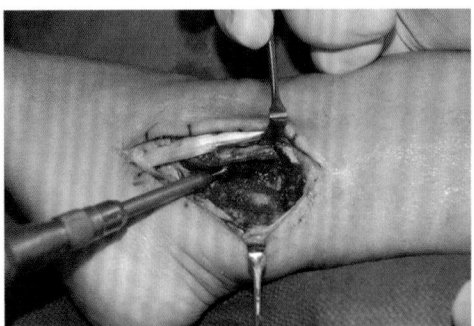

TECH FIG 4 High-speed burr is used to remove cancellous bone from distal fibula.

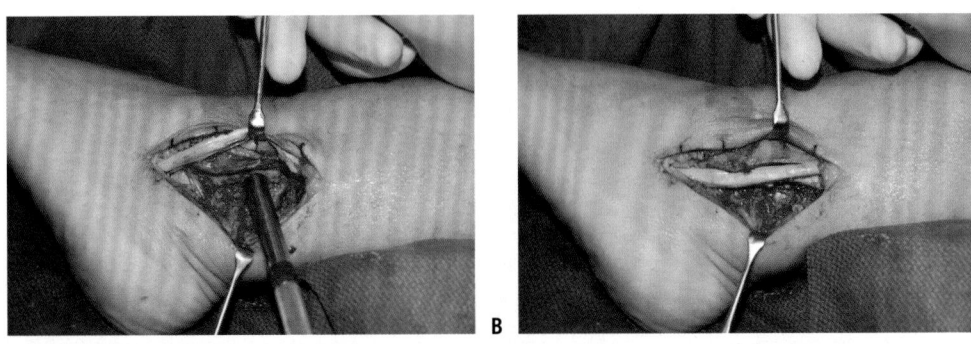

TECH FIG 5 **A.** Trapdoor reduced in deepened fibular groove, with impactor being used to recess the bone and deepen the groove maximally. **B.** Peroneal tendons remaining reduced, even without repair of the SPR.

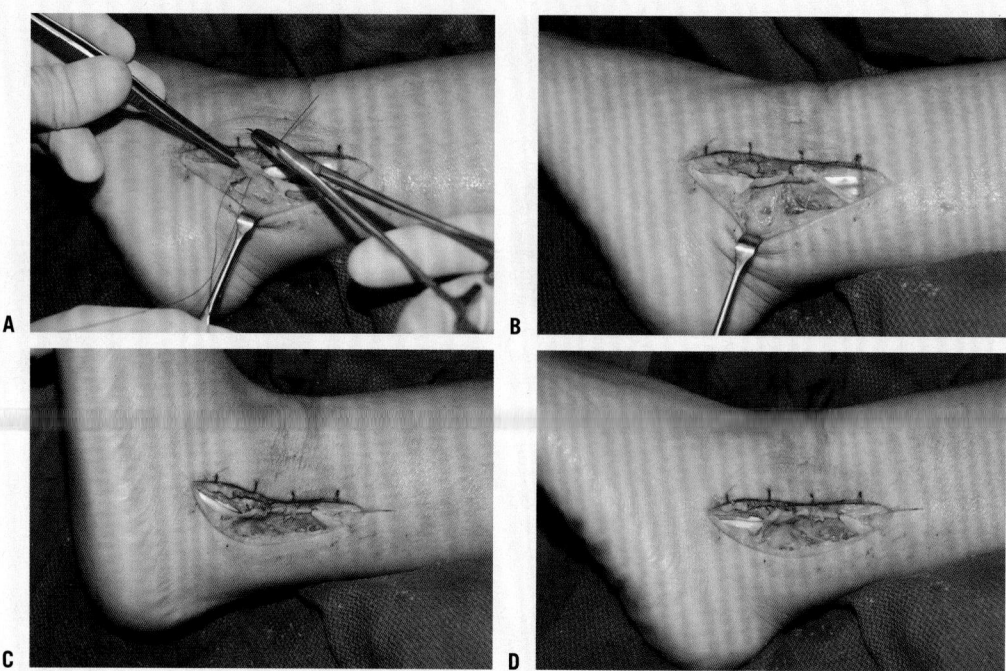

TECH FIG 6 A,B. SPR repair to posterior fibula. **A.** Sutures to the posterolateral fibula to advance the SPR. **B.** Drill holes used to anchor SPR to posterolateral fibula. **C,D.** Peroneal tendons gliding without being stenosed within new fibular groove. **C.** Dorsiflexion. **D.** Plantarflexion.

MODIFIED TECHNIQUE USING A LARGE-DIAMETER DRILL BIT
(AS DESCRIBED BY ROBERT B. ANDERSON, MD)

- Chronically dislocated peroneal tendons may create a new pocket and even gliding surface on the lateral fibula **(TECH FIG 7)**.
- Protect the dislocated tendons and adjacent soft tissues from the drill bit.
- From the distal fibular tip, introduce progressively larger diameter drill bits to weaken the distal fibula and ream away the distal fibular cancellous bone **(TECH FIG 8)**.
- Although simple impaction of the posterior fibula to deepen the groove is possible at this point, we prefer to first weaken the cortex with a microsagittal saw as described for the traditional fibular groove-deepening procedure **(TECH FIG 9A)**.

- To protect the smooth surface on the posterior fibula, a tamp can be placed longitudinally in the groove and impacted so as to avoid disruption of the smooth gliding surface for the peroneal tendons **(TECH FIG 9B)**.
- The peroneal tendons should remain reduced without manually restraining them **(TECH FIG 10A)**. If not, then deepen the groove further with a larger diameter drill bit and perform further impaction of the posterior fibular surface.
- Reattach the SPR to the posterolateral fibular margin via drill holes.
- Be sure the peroneal tendons glide well without restriction in the deeper fibular groove **(TECH FIG 10B)**.
- Standard closure

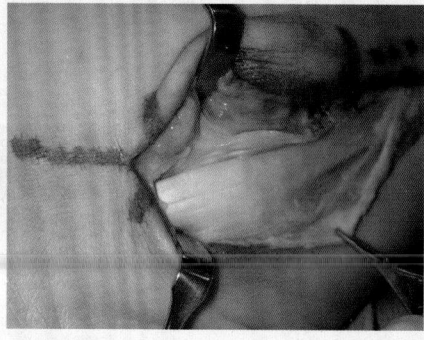 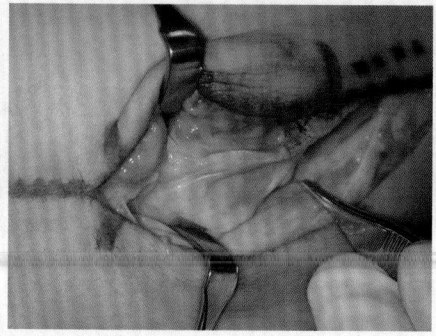

TECH FIG 7 Pseudogroove created on lateral fibula. **A.** Peroneal tendons lateral to fibula. **B.** With tendons reduced, the pseudogroove is visible, with the displaced and attenuated SPR.

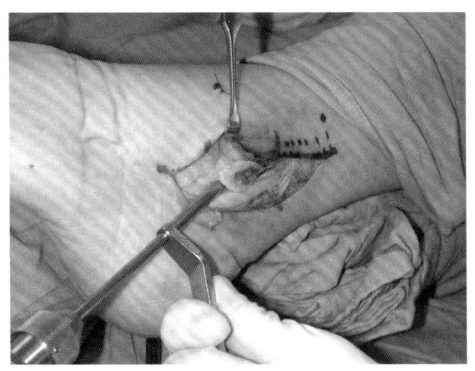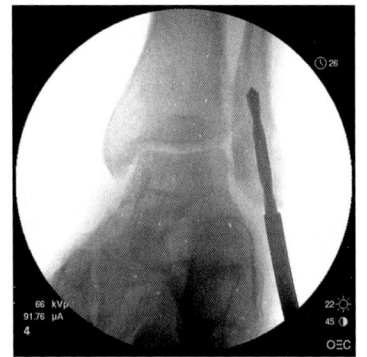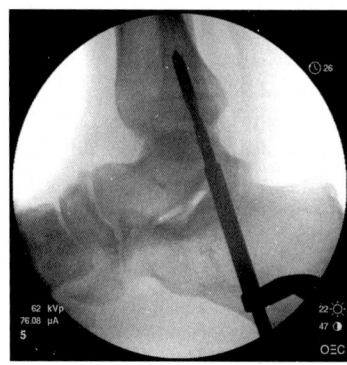

TECH FIG 8 A. Drill bit introduced to decancellate the distal fibula. **B,C.** Fluoroscopic confirmation of proper drill bit position in distal fibula. **B.** AP view. **C.** Lateral view.

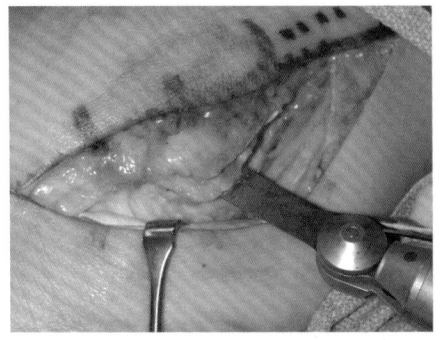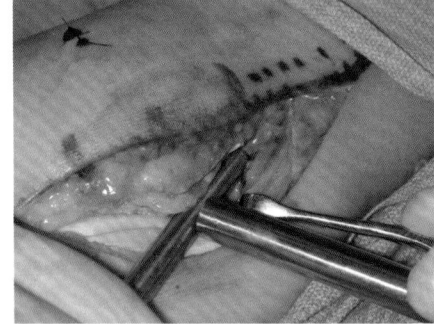

TECH FIG 9 Impaction of the posterior fibula to deepen the fibular groove. **A.** Weakening the posterolateral margin of the fibula to facilitate impaction. **B.** Use a tamp longitudinally to protect the gliding surface of the posterior fibula during its impaction.

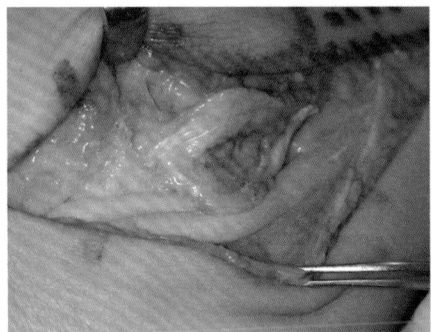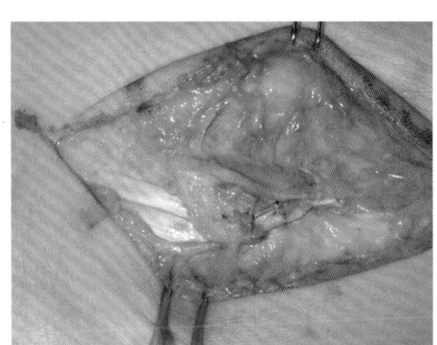

TECH FIG 10 A. Peroneal tendons remaining reduced in the deepened fibular groove, even without SPR repair. **B.** SPR repaired without stenosis of the peroneal tendons.

TECHNIQUES

Pearls and Pitfalls

Harvest of Periosteal Flap	• The peroneal tendons must be retracted anteriorly to allow visualization of the flap donor site to ensure sufficient harvest and to avoid damage to the peroneal tendons. • The flap should maintain its continuity, anteriorly, with the fibrocartilage ridge. Use of a no. 69 Beaver blade is critical for flap elevation. • The flap should be elevated before any groove-deepening procedure. If the groove is deepened before this, the periosteum will be destroyed.
Flap-to-Tendon Adhesions	• No issues with tendon-to-flap adhesions have been reported; nonetheless, early range of motion starting at 4 weeks minimizes any chance of adhesions developing.
Peroneal Tendon Tears	• Tears in the tendons need to be débrided and repaired or reconstructed. Successful peroneal tendon reduction with persistent symptoms secondary to peroneal tendon tears may lead to a poor outcome.
Avoid Overtightening of the Peroneal Tendon Sheath Reconstruction	• This will lead to stenosing flexor tenosynovitis. Overtightening is unnecessary; the tendons simply need to remain reduced.

POSTOPERATIVE CARE

- Postoperatively, the patient is immobilized in a short-leg cast and is kept non–weight bearing for a total of 6 weeks.
- After 4 weeks, the cast is removed and the patient is given a removable stiff-ankle rocker bottom boot and remains non–weight bearing for an additional 2 weeks while beginning physical therapy with ankle range-of-motion exercises.
- At the end of 6 weeks, the patient is progressed to weight bearing as tolerated in the brace, after which the patient is weaned from the stiff-ankle boot and is started with ankle strengthening with inversion and eversion exercises.

OUTCOMES

- A favorable outcome of the procedure depends not only on how well the surgical procedure is performed but also on the appropriate treatment of other associated conditions. Often, tendon injuries coexist with subluxation and dislocation and must be treated simultaneously. If tendon pathology such as a tear or degeneration is present and left untreated, pain may persist after surgery no matter how well the surgery was performed.
- In a preliminary study by Tan et al[20] conducted at two centers (University of Pennsylvania and University of Medicine and Dentistry of New Jersey), 10 patients with subluxation or dislocation of the peroneal tendons were treated with this technique. Nine of 10 patients had good to excellent results. One patient required a groove-deepening procedure.
- In a recent study by Steginsky et al,[18] 71 patients underwent primary repair of their peroneal brevis tendon and were available for follow-up at an average of 4.6 years. Of these patients, 59 (83.1%) reported a return to regular exercise and sports at final follow-up. There was significant improvement in functional outcomes and over 85% of patients were satisfied with their outcomes.[18]

COMPLICATIONS

- Peroneal tendon adhesions: Early range-of-motion exercises starting at 4 weeks can minimize this complication.
- Stenosing flexor tenosynovitis: Overtightening of the peroneal tendon sheath is unnecessary; the tendons simply need to remain reduced posterior to the fibula.
- Sural and superficial peroneal nerve injury

ACKNOWLEDGMENT

- The editor and coauthors of this chapter wish to acknowledge the contribution of Dr. Enyi Okereke. Dr. Okereke passed away while on a medical mission to Enugu, Nigeria.

REFERENCES

1. Church CC. Radiographic diagnosis of acute peroneal tendon dislocation. AJR Am J Roentgenol 1977;129(6):1065–1068.
2. Clanton TO, Porter DA. Primary care of foot and ankle injuries in the athlete. Clin Sports Med 1997;16(3):435–466.
3. Davis WH, Sobel M, Deland J, et al. The superior peroneal retinaculum: an anatomic study. Foot Ankle Int 1994;15(5):271–275.
4. Eckert WR, Davis EA Jr. Acute rupture of the peroneal retinaculum. J Bone Joint Surg Am 1976;58(5):670–672.
5. Edwards ME. The relations of the peroneal tendons to the fibula, calcaneus, and cuboideum. Am J Anat 1928;42(1):213–253.
6. Escalas F, Figueras JM, Merino JA. Dislocation of the peroneal tendons. Long-term results of surgical treatment. J Bone Joint Surg Am 1980;62(3):451–453.
7. Fram BR, Rogero R, Fuchs D, et al. Clinical outcomes and complications of peroneal tendon sheath ultrasound-guided corticosteroid injection. Foot Ankle Int 2019;40(8):888–894.
8. Geller J, Lin S, Cordas D, et al. Relationship of a low-lying muscle belly to tears of the peroneus brevis tendon. Am J Orthop (Belle Mead NJ) 2003;32(11):541–544.
9. Guelfi M, Vega J, Malagelada F, et al. Tendoscopic treatment of peroneal tendons intrasheath subluxation: a new subgroup with SPR injury. Foot Ankle Int 2018;39(5):542–550.
10. Magee DJ, ed. Lower leg, ankle, and foot. In: Orthopedic Physical Assessment Enhanced Edition, ed 4. St. Louis: Saunders Elsevier, 2005:765–845.
11. McLennan JG. Treatment of acute and chronic luxations of the peroneal tendons. Am J Sports Med 1980;8:432–436.
12. Oden RR. Tendon injuries about the ankle resulting from skiing. Clin Orthop Relat Res 1987;(216):63–69.
13. Pellegrini MJ, Glisson RR, Matsumoto T, et al. Effectiveness of allograft reconstruction vs tenodesis for irreparable peroneus brevis tears: a cadaveric model. Foot Ankle Int 2016;37(8):803–808.
14. Sarmiento A, Wolf M. Subluxation of peroneal tendons. Case treated by rerouting tendons under calcaneofibular ligament. J Bone Joint Surg Am 1975;57(1):115–116.
15. Sarrafian SK. Biomechanics of the subtalar joint complex. Clin Orthop Relat Res 1993;(290):17–26.
16. Selmani E, Gjata V, Gjika E. Current concepts review: peroneal tendon disorders. Foot Ankle Int 2006;27(3):221–228.
17. Sobel M, Bohne WH, Markisz JA. Cadaver correlation of peroneal tendon changes with magnetic resonance imaging. Foot Ankle 1991;11(6):384–388.
18. Steginsky B, Riley A, Lucas DE, et al. Patient-reported outcomes and return to activity after peroneus brevis repair. Foot Ankle Int 2016;37(2):178–185.
19. Stover CN, Bryan DR. Traumatic dislocation of the peroneal tendons. Am J Surg 1962;103:180–186.
20. Tan V, Lin SS, Okereke E. Superior peroneal retinaculoplasty: a surgical technique for peroneal subluxation. Clin Orthop Relat Res 2003;(410):320–325.
21. Urguden M, Gulten IA, Civan O, et al. Results of peroneal endoscopy with a technical modification. Foot Ankle Int 2019;40(3):356–363.
22. Watson GI, Karnovsky SC, Levine DS, et al. Surgical treatment for stenosing peroneal tenosynovitis. Foot Ankle Int 2019;40(3):282–286.
23. Zoellner G, Clancy W Jr. Recurrent dislocation of the peroneal tendon. J Bone Joint Surg Am 1979;61(2):292–294.

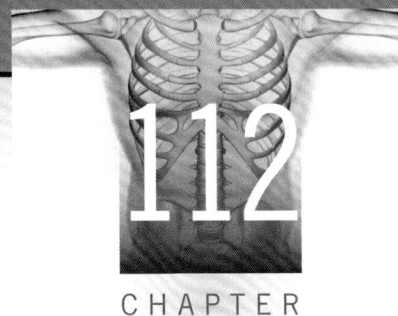

CHAPTER 112

Repair of Dislocating Peroneal Tendons:
Perspective 2

Florian Nickisch, Robert B. Anderson, and Miranda J. Rogers

DEFINITION

- Peroneal tendon subluxation or dislocation from the retrofibular groove is a rare cause of ankle pain and disability. The acute injury often remains unrecognized or is misdiagnosed as an ankle sprain.
- Untreated or misdiagnosed acute injury predisposes a patient to recurrent peroneal dislocation, potential peroneal tendon tear, or chronic dislocation.

ANATOMY

- The peroneus longus and brevis muscles are the two major structures within the lateral compartment of the leg, both arising from the proximal fibula (FIG 1A).
- Both structures become tendinous before crossing the ankle joint and remain in a common sheath. As they course distally, the tendon of the peroneus brevis lies against the posterior surface of the distal fibula, anterior, and medial to the tendon of the peroneus longus.
- Distal to the fibula, each tendon enters a distinct tendon sheath, separated by the peroneal tubercle.
- Posterior to the distal fibula, both tendons are stabilized in the retrofibular groove by the superior peroneal retinaculum (SPR) (FIG 1B).
- The posterior surface of the distal fibula is covered by a layer of fibrocartilage to allow smooth gliding of the peroneal tendons.

The depth and width of the retrofibular (peroneal) groove is variable. A definite groove is present in between 68% and 100%.[1,4,19] In the remaining cases, the posterior surface of the fibula is thought to be flat or convex,[9] although more recent studies have not found convexity to be a common variant.[1] A fibrocartilage rim on the lateral border of the fibula that adds an additional 2 to 4 mm to the depth of the sulcus is often present.

- The SPR, the primary restraint to peroneal instability, is composed of a band of the deep fascia that is continuous with the periosteum of the distal fibula but does not attach to the fibrocartilage rim or the posterolateral edge of the bone.[16] It is extremely variable in width and thickness, and five distinct insertional patterns have been described, the most common being a band to both the Achilles tendon and the calcaneus.[6]
- The fiber orientation of the SPR was thought to be parallel to those of the calcaneofibular ligament, and therefore, inversion injuries of the calcaneofibular ligament may also cause injury to the SPR.[10,14] More recent research found it to have fibers upward, backward, and medially, until it merged with deep transverse fascia of the leg.[1]

PATHOGENESIS

- Acute subluxation or dislocation of the peroneal tendons usually occurs while the foot is forcefully dorsiflexed with

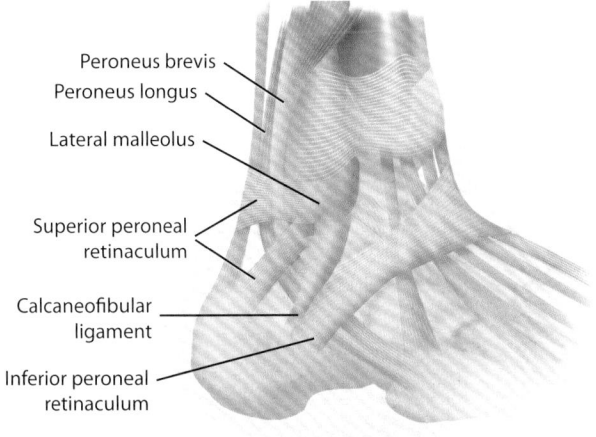

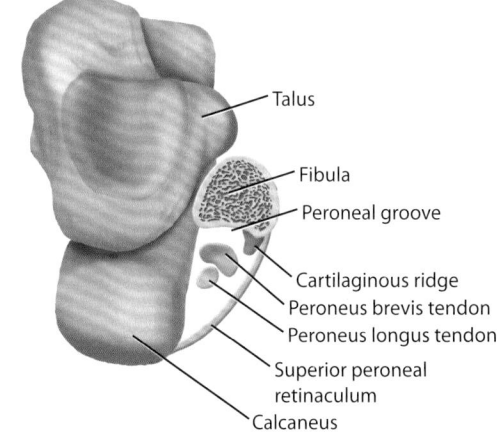

FIG 1 A. Lateral view of the ankle showing the peroneal tendons as well as the superior and inferior peroneal retinacula. Note the vertical orientation of a portion of the SPR that corresponds to the orientation of the calcaneofibular ligament. **B.** Superior view of the ankle region shows the relationship of the fibular groove, SPR, peroneal tendons, and cartilaginous ridge. (**A:** Reprinted with permission from Davis WH, Sobel M, Deland J, et al. The superior peroneal retinaculum: an anatomic study. Foot Ankle Int 1994;15[5]:273. Copyright © 1994 SAGE Publications. **B:** Reprinted from Coughlin MJ, Mann RA, eds. Surgery of the Foot and Ankle, ed 7. St. Louis: Mosby, 1999:819. Copyright © 1999 Elsevier. With permission.)

the peroneal muscles strongly contracted; it commonly occurs during a forward fall in Alpine skiing or in springboard diving.[13]

- Resisted plantarflexion and inversion while the peroneals contract may also cause subluxation or dislocation of the peroneal tendons, and in this case, it is commonly associated with lateral instability of the ankle.
- Peroneal dislocation may also occur as a sequela to severe calcaneal fractures with lateral displacement of the calcaneus.[8,12] Tendon displacement has been documented in 28% of calcaneal fractures and is more common with joint depression than tongue-type fractures.[24] Additionally, the risk of peroneal tendon dislocation increases if there is an associated fibula fracture accompanying a calcaneal fracture: 83% tendon dislocation with both and 30% with an isolated calcaneal fracture.[18]
- Peroneal dislocations can be classified into three grades per Eckert and Davis[8] depending on the pathoanatomy of the injury:
  - Grade I: SPR stripped from fibrous lip/lateral malleolus but still attached to periosteum on posterior fibula; peroneus longus dislocated anteriorly
  - Grade II: fibrous rim avulsed from posterolateral aspect of fibula along with SPR; peroneus longus dislocated anteriorly
  - Grade III: bony rim avulsion fracture attached to SPR with anterior dislocation of peroneus longus. Tendons can dislocate inside the fracture site.[27]
- An additional classification was added by Oden[17]:
  - Grade IV: SPR is elevated from posterior attachment and can be found lying deep to the tendons.
- There is also a category of intrasheath subluxation of peroneal tendons within the groove with an intact retinaculum that was diagnosed via dynamic ultrasound.[20]
- As a result of subluxation or dislocation, inherent injuries to the tendons can occur. Depending on the location of the tendon injury, they are divided into zones I, II, and III.[22]
  - Zone I injuries are defined as those involving the fibular groove and most often affect the peroneus brevis tendon. As the tendons sublux in the groove, the brevis is forced onto the sharp posterolateral bony ridge of the distal fibula, causing a longitudinal split in the tendon from the strain of a 45-degree course change as well as compression by the overlying longus tendon.
  - Zone II injuries are located between the tip of the fibula and the cuboid tunnel, as the peroneal tendon courses to the peroneal tubercle; often involves the peroneus longus
  - Zone III injuries are located in the cuboid tunnel and primarily involve the peroneus longus tendon and possibly a painful os peroneum.

NATURAL HISTORY

- Acute peroneal tendon dislocation often occurs after a traumatic injury. If diagnosed early, in acute peroneal dislocation, the tendons can be manually reduced and held in a reduced position for a 4- to 6-week period of immobilization. In this situation, functional rehabilitation leads to maintenance of tendon reduction and complete recovery in about 50% of cases.[2] It is important to note that the average duration of symptoms before diagnosis of acute tears is 7 to 48 months, which can complicate treatment.[22]

Additionally, there is a wide variety in treatment plans given the lack of established treatment algorithm and late presentation of patients.[3]

- Chronic dislocations and tears tend to be attritional and have an insidious onset. With delayed diagnosis and treatment, recurrent subluxation and chronic dislocation are common and may lead to degeneration and tearing of the peroneal tendons.[15]

PATIENT HISTORY AND PHYSICAL FINDINGS

- Most patients present well beyond the acute phase complaining of vague posterolateral ankle pain that radiates proximally with or without a popping sensation during activity.[21]
- There may be a history of forced dorsiflexion trauma associated with a pop on the lateral aspect of the ankle.
- Often, a history of an inversion–supination sprain and possible lateral ankle instability is reported.[14]
- On physical examination, peroneal tendinopathy is characterized as fullness along the tendons with diffuse tenderness. Localized tenderness over the posterior ridge of the fibula should raise suspicion for progression of the injury to a peroneal tendon split tear.
- Pain may be elicited with inversion stretch or active-resisted eversion.
- Tendon subluxation typically presents as snapping or popping and pain with eversion against resistance. The peroneal tunnel compression test consists of having the patient perform this motion while palpating the posterior border of the fibula. Circumduction of the ankle may demonstrate dislocation of the tendons with eversion and dorsiflexion and spontaneous relocation with plantarflexion and inversion (**FIG 2**).
- Chronic dislocation of the tendons is characterized by a palpable ridge over the lateral distal fibula often associated with chronic swelling.
- Eversion strength may be limited by pain. Significant weakness of active eversion without much pain should raise suspicion for a complete tear of the peroneal tendons.
- A complete examination of the ankle should also include evaluation of associated injuries, ruling out differential diagnoses. This includes (but is not limited to) the following:
  - Lateral ankle instability: history of frequent sprains, cavovarus foot, increased laxity with anterior drawer or inversion stress test compared to the contralateral side

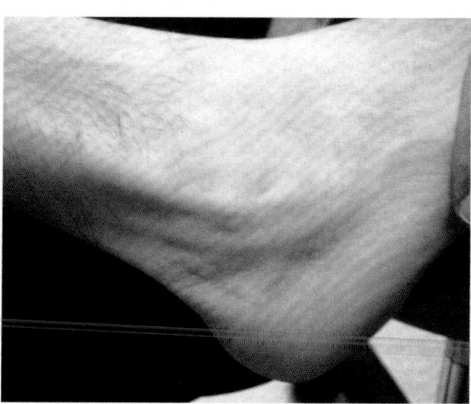

FIG 2 Dislocated peroneal tendons during resisted eversion.

- High ankle sprain (syndesmotic sprain): pain over anterior ankle syndesmosis, pain with provocative maneuvers (calf squeeze test, external rotation stress test)
- Painful os trigonum or posterior talar process fracture: pain with forced plantarflexion, pain with resisted plantarflexion of the great toe

IMAGING AND OTHER DIAGNOSTIC STUDIES

- Plain radiographs including anteroposterior (AP), mortise, and lateral views of the ankle should be obtained to rule out fracture or large osteochondral defects of the talus.
- Occasionally, a "fleck" sign, an avulsion fracture off the posterior distal fibula, can be seen on AP or mortise views. If present, this is considered pathognomonic for a grade III injury to the SPR with peroneal dislocation.[8] Peroneal tendons were found dislocated in 84.1% of cases in which a bony fleck was identified. As a diagnostic test, the presence of a fleck sign had a sensitivity of 0.31, specificity of 0.98, positive predictive value (PPV) of 0.84, negative predictive value (NPV) of 0.79, a positive likelihood ratio of 13.6, and a negative likelihood ratio of 0.70.[27]
  - As shown in **FIG 3A**, this may be difficult to see without the use of a "hot lamp."
- Stress views may be helpful to rule out lateral ankle instability.
- Computed tomography (CT) may be helpful in uncertain diagnosis to evaluate the anatomy of the fibular groove and detect small avulsion fractures, which may be difficult to see on plain films **(FIG 3B)**.[5,8] Axial CT scan images may also confirm peroneal tendon dislocation.

- Magnetic resonance imaging can identify injury to the SPR, subluxated or dislocated tendons, and intrasubstance degeneration and split tears of the tendons **(FIG 3C,D)**. Magnetic resonance imaging does have difficulty evaluating tears secondary to the magic angle effect—when signal intensity is seen because the tendon is oriented 55 degrees to the axis of the magnetic field.[3,4]
- Ultrasound, although operator dependent, allows a dynamic, real-time examination to evaluate subluxation during provocative maneuvers.

DIFFERENTIAL DIAGNOSIS

- Peroneal tendinopathy or tears
- Lateral ankle instability
  - Those with lateral ankle instability can also have peroneal tendon pathology, with tenosynovitis seen in 77%, SPR attenuation in 54%, and peroneus brevis tears in 25%.[3,7]
- High ankle sprain
- Osteochondral defect of the talus
- Painful os trigonum or posterior talar process fracture
- Retrocalcaneal bursitis

NONOPERATIVE MANAGEMENT

- Acute peroneal subluxation or dislocation can be treated nonoperatively if the peroneal tendons can be reduced and held in a reduced position.
- In this case, treatment consists of short-leg cast immobilization in slight plantarflexion and inversion for 4 to 6 weeks,

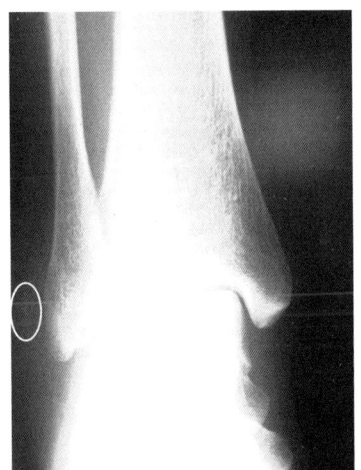
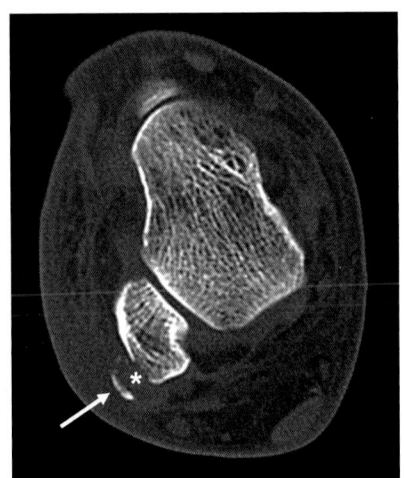
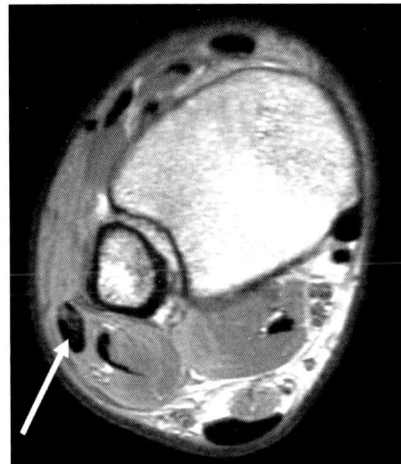
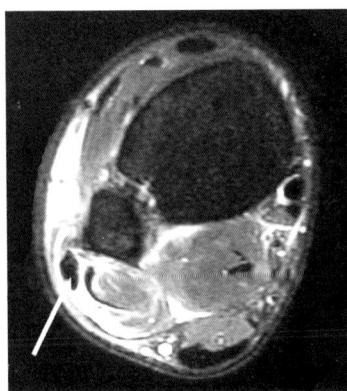

FIG 3 A. AP radiograph of the ankle under a hot lamp shows a lateral rim fracture off the distal fibula (fleck sign, *circle*). **B.** Axial CT scan shows a grade III injury with an avulsion fracture of the lateral edge of the distal fibula (fleck sign, *arrow*) and dislocated peroneal tendon (*asterisk*). **C,D.** T1- and T2-weighted axial magnetic resonance images, respectively, show dislocated peroneal tendons (*arrows*) with abundant tenosynovitis. Note the shallow retrofibular groove and the torn SPR.

followed by functional rehabilitation. U- or J-shaped foam or felt pads can be placed in the cast to apply pressure around the distal fibula and maintain the position of the peroneal tendons.

- In our opinion, there is no role for nonoperative treatment for symptomatic chronic peroneal dislocation or recurrent subluxation.

SURGICAL MANAGEMENT

- All irreducible peroneal tendon dislocations and those associated with a rim avulsion fibular fracture should be considered for acute surgical reduction and repair.
- Operative treatment is also indicated for all chronic injuries in patients with pain or functional limitations.
- Five basic categories of repair have been described[13]:
  - Anatomic reattachment of the retinaculum
  - Bone block procedures
  - Reinforcement of the SPR with local tissue transfers
  - Rerouting of the tendons behind the calcaneofibular ligament
  - Groove-deepening procedures
- The goal of groove-deepening procedures is to increase the height of the posterolateral fibular rim to prevent the peroneal tendons from subluxating.
- General contraindications to surgical intervention include peripheral vascular disease, skin breakdown or vasculitis, and patients who are "voluntary" subluxators. These are usually patients with generalized ligamentous laxity. Physical examination usually shows the peroneal tendons to subluxate to the lateral rim of the fibula on both ankles but not over it.
- The most commonly used procedures at this time include repair and/or reinforcement of the SPR +/− groove-deepening procedures. Bone-blocking procedures have the following report concerns: osteotomy complications, fracture, hardware failure, tendon irritation, nonunion, and recurrent subluxation. As for transposition of soft tissues, including rerouting tendons, there are limited reports with low sample size and a 19% complication rate documented by McGarvey and Clanton[14] as well as concerns for sural nerve injury and ankle ankylosis.[11]

Preoperative Planning

- We recommend reviewing all imaging studies preoperatively to plan for not only fibular groove deepening but also any procedures to address associated pathology. Plain films should be reviewed for fractures, loose bodies, ankle and foot alignment, and the presence of any hardware (from previous procedures).
- Associated fractures, osteochondral lesions, and lateral ankle instability should be addressed concurrently.

- We routinely perform an examination under anesthesia on the operating table before making an incision to assess the ankle and subtalar joint. The peroneal tendons may also be assessed under anesthesia, but without the patient being able to evert against resistance, this is of limited value.

Positioning

- The procedure is performed with the patient in the semilateral position.
- A beanbag is used to maintain the position of the body with a 10-lb sandbag underneath the ipsilateral hip.
  - This allows the physician to readily access the posterior fibula and obtain fluoroscopic AP and lateral views of the ankle without moving the C-arm from the standard AP position.
- Regional or general anesthesia can be used, and a thigh tourniquet is applied.

Approach

- The standard surgical approach is through a longitudinal, curvilinear incision on the posterior aspect of the fibula following the course of the peroneal tendons to roughly the level of the peroneal tubercle (**FIG 4**).
- This not only allows excellent visualization of the SPR, the peroneal tendons, and the posterior aspect of the distal fibula but also provides sufficient access to the lateral tibiotalar joint in cases where concomitant lateral ligament reconstruction is indicated.
- If lateral ankle instability and injury to the peroneal tendons distally have been ruled out preoperatively or with the examination under anesthesia, the approach can be limited to a longitudinal incision just posterior to the fibula.

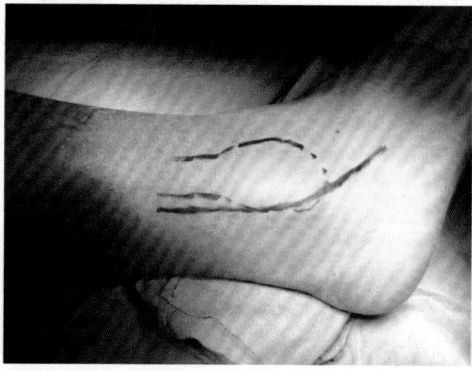

FIG 4 Utilitarian posterolateral approach for peroneal repair and indirect fibular groove deepening.

INDIRECT FIBULAR GROOVE DEEPENING

Exposure

- Make a curvilinear incision along the posterior aspect of the distal fibula. It extends toward the base of the fifth metatarsal but usually ends at the level of the peroneal tubercle.
- Develop full-thickness skin flaps to avoid skin necrosis.
  - Protect the sural nerve and branches of the superficial peroneal nerve.
- Incise the peroneal sheath distal to the fibula.
- If the SPR is still intact, incise it over the bone and then sharply elevate it off the fibula, leaving a cuff of tissue on the distal fibula. Retract the edges of the SPR posteriorly with two small hemostats to facilitate later repair.

Peroneal Preparation

- Inspect the peroneal tendons, excise inflamed tenosynovium, and débride and repair split tears in the tendons with buried nonabsorbable suture (**TECH FIG 1A,B**).
- Excise any low-lying peroneus brevis muscle from the tendon. Also excise a normal anatomic variant, the peroneus quartus, a supernumerary muscle of the lateral compartment of the leg, if present.
- These additional procedures tend to make room in the groove for the peroneal tendons (**TECH FIG 1C**).

Deepening the Groove

- Expose the distal fibular tip, avoiding injury to the calcaneofibular ligament.
- Place an intramedullary guide pin from distal to proximal inside the fibula, in line with the posterior cortex (**TECH FIG 2A**).

- Thin the posterior cortex by sequential reaming over the guide-wire (usually 7 to 8 mm) (**TECH FIG 2B,C**).[23]
  - We routinely use suitably sized reamers from the Bio-Tenodesis screw system (Arthrex, Inc., Naples, FL) or any anterior cruciate ligament instrument set.
  - Alternatively, consider using progressively larger drill bits from a standard trauma set or cannulated drills from a dedicated fifth metatarsal (Jones fracture) set (Wright Medical Group, Memphis, TN).
- Once the posterior cortex is sufficiently thinned, impact it into the void created by the reamers using an appropriately sized bone tamp (**TECH FIG 2D**). This preserves the physiologic gliding surface covering the groove, making it a smooth bed for tendon excursion.
  - If the bone is very hard and impaction cannot be performed easily, the posterolateral cortex of the fibula can be perforated with an osteotome or microsagittal saw to facilitate impaction of the posterior cortex (**TECH FIG 2E**).
- Also, tamp the very distal tip of the fibula inward to avoid a sharp edge that would otherwise impinge on the peroneal tendon as it courses into the foot.
- When done correctly, the entire peroneus brevis and at least 50% of the peroneus longus tendon should be covered by the fibular rim with the tendons in a resting position.

Superior Peroneal Retinaculum Repair

- After completing groove deepening, tendon débridement, and tendon repair, repair the SPR.
- Sharply elevate the remainder of the cuff on the fibula off bone, exposing the lateral cortex, which is then roughened to bleeding bone with a rasp or rongeur.

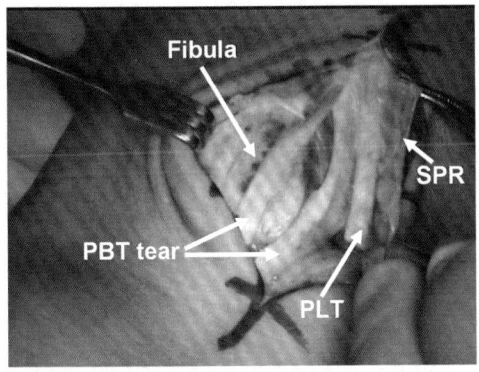

A

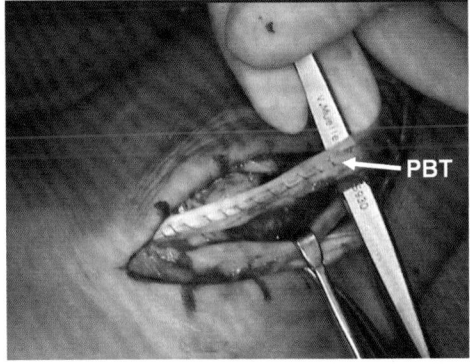

B

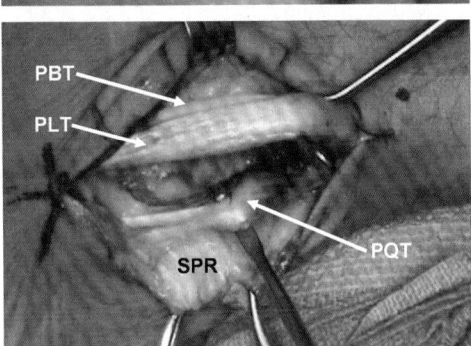

C

TECH FIG 1 **A.** The superior peroneal retinaculum (*SPR*) is incised longitudinally and retracted with two hemostats. A longitudinal split tear of the peroneus brevis tendon (*PBT*) is often identified in chronic dislocations. *PLT,* peroneus longus tendon. **B.** Split tears of the PBT are débrided or repaired. **C.** The low-lying peroneus brevis muscle and, if present, the peroneus quartus (*PQT*) are excised to create room for the peroneal tendons.

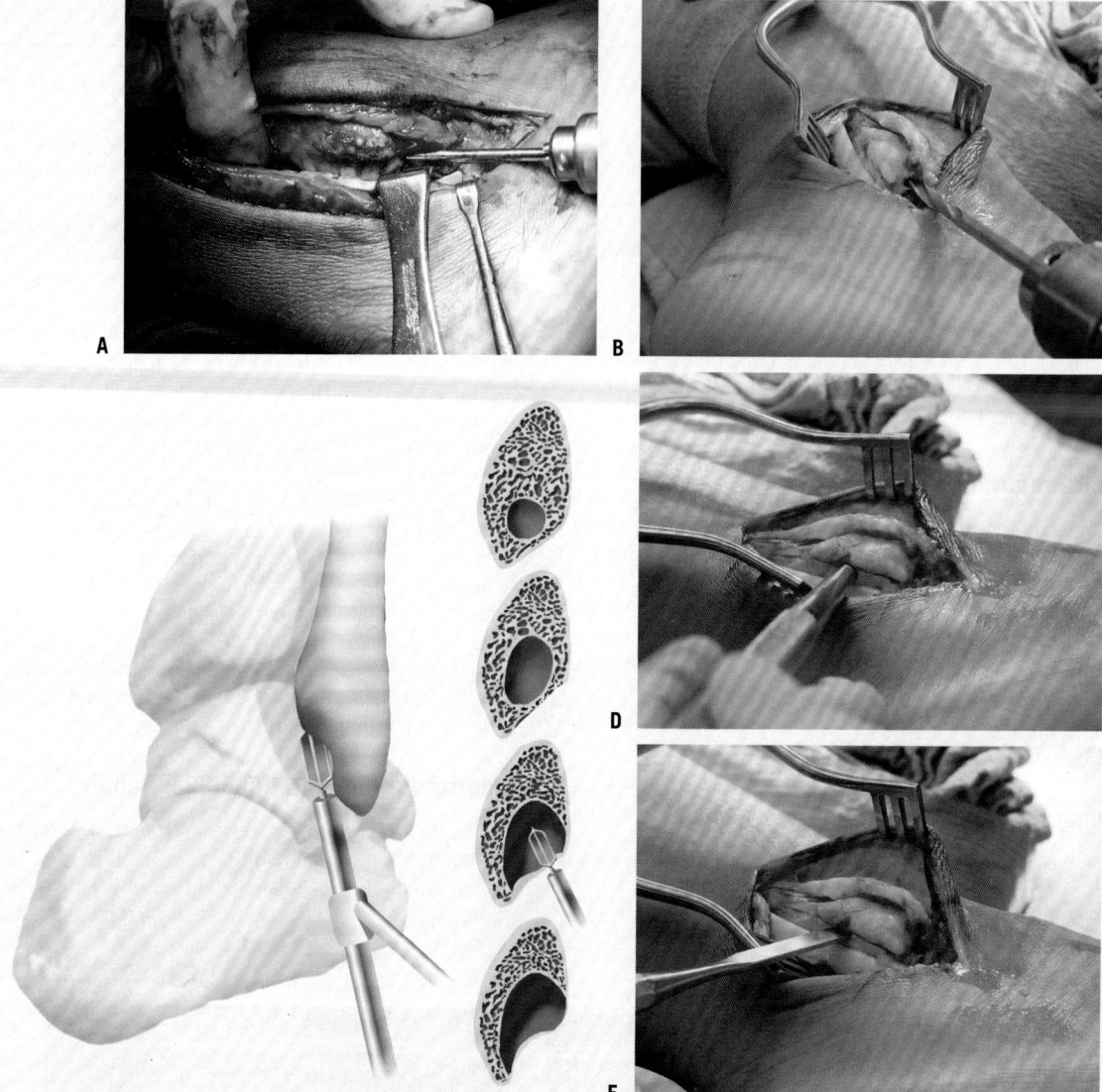

TECH FIG 2 A. An intramedullary guide pin is placed into the distal fibula parallel to the posterior cortex. **B.** The posterior cortex of the fibula is thinned by intramedullary reaming with cannulated reamers over the guide pin. **C.** Technique for indirect fibular groove deepening. **D.** The posterior cortex of the fibula is impacted into the void created by the reamers with an appropriate-sized tamp. **E.** To avoid fracture of the edge of the fibula during impaction, the posterolateral cortex is perforated with an osteotome (this is necessary only in very hard bone).

- Excise any redundant SPR tissue and advance the remaining SPR to the previously prepared cortical bed; secure it through either drill holes or suture anchors.
- Place three or four drill holes or suture anchors about 1 cm apart proximally from the tip of the fibula (**TECH FIG 3A**).
- Reattach the posterior flap of the SPR to the prepared bone with 2-0 suture in a "pants-over-vest" technique, making sure that the space between the bony surface of the lateral malleolus and the SPR is obliterated.

- Suture the anterior portion of the retinaculum over the repair with interrupted 2-0 suture (**TECH FIG 3B,C**).
- Test the stability of the repair by ranging the ankle through a full range of motion.
  - Verify free excursion of reduced tendons; the tendons should not be trapped by the repair.
  - Overtightening of the SPR repair is not necessary; the goal is to keep the peroneal tendons reduced posterior to the fibula.

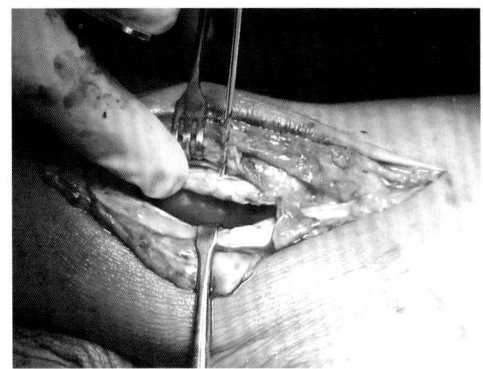

A

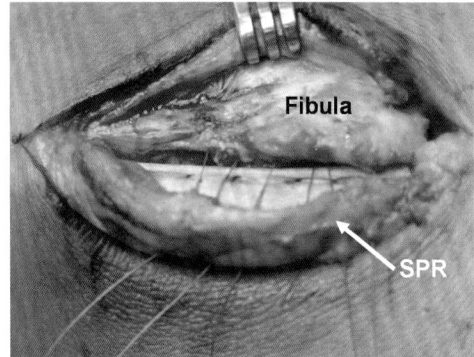

B

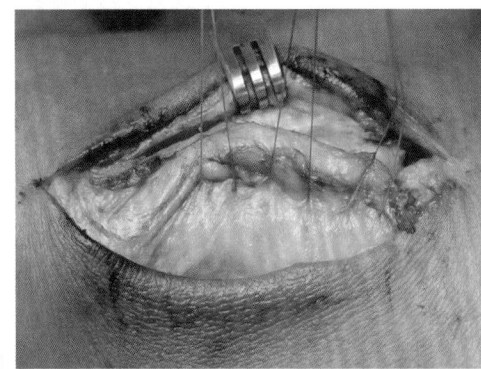

C

TECH FIG 3 After deepening of the retrofibular groove, the lateral cortex of the fibula is roughened with a rongeur or rasp and the superior peroneal retinaculum (*SPR*) is repaired. **A.** Six drill holes are created in the posterolateral edge of the fibula (alternatively, two or three suture anchors can be used). **B,C.** The SPR is then repaired to the distal fibula with 2-0 suture in a pants-over-vest fashion.

TECHNIQUES

Pearls and Pitfalls

Avoid surgery on voluntary dislocators.	• High risk of recurrence
Maintain the operated limb in a semilateral position (use a large bump under the ipsilateral hip or a beanbag).	• It is difficult to gain access to the posterior aspect of the fibula with the patient in a supine position.
Incise the SPR on the posterior margin of the fibula, not too far posteriorly.	• This allows excision of redundant tissue and a secure SPR repair to bone.
Create adequate room for the peroneal tendons.	• Excise all low-lying peroneus brevis muscle and the entire peroneus quartus if present.
Inspect both peroneal tendons for tears.	• Débride and repair as necessary.
Avoid fibular stress fracture.	• Reaming the fibula may not weaken the posterior fibula adequately, particularly in young, healthy patients with good bone quality. Weaken the posterior fibular cortex with an osteotome or microsagittal saw before impaction to control the fibular groove deepening.
Avoid creating stenosis of the peroneal tendons when repairing the SPR.	• Observe satisfactory tendon excursion with ankle and hindfoot range of motion after SPR repair.

POSTOPERATIVE CARE

• Immediately postoperatively, the leg and ankle are placed into a posterior and U-splint in neutral position, and the patient is kept non–weight bearing for 2 weeks.

• Sutures are removed at 2 weeks. A short-leg walking cast is applied, and the patient is allowed to bear weight as tolerated.

• At 6 weeks, the cast is removed and a cam walker boot is applied to avoid ankle inversion while allowing plantarflexion and dorsiflexion. Active range-of-motion exercises are initiated at that time.

• Peroneal strengthening is started at about 8 to 10 weeks after surgery.

- Full return to activities is expected between 4 and 6 months postoperatively.
- In elite athletes, given a stable reconstruction, we have been more aggressive with the rehabilitation to include biking and pool activities by 4 weeks.

OUTCOMES

- As many variations of fibular groove-deepening techniques have been described, all reported results in the literature are derived from small retrospective series. There are no published prospective randomized studies comparing different surgical techniques.
- In general, results of fibular groove-deepening techniques have been good as long as the underlying pathology is correctly addressed.[16]
- In our hands, indirect grooving has provided excellent overall results while minimizing the surgical dissection and morbidity.
- There is some outcome data after groove deepening that reveals a low recurrence rate (2% postoperative dislocation) and small number of patients who need revision surgery (7%). Majority of patients (84%) would undergo procedure again. There was some decreased strength identified after the procedure.[26]
- We recommend that fibular groove deepening should be performed with every SPR reconstruction for chronic peroneal dislocation.

COMPLICATIONS

- Infection
- Delayed wound healing
- Sural nerve injury
- Recurrent dislocation
- Loss of motion

REFERENCES

1. Athavale SA, Swathi, Vangara SV. Anatomy of the superior peroneal tunnel. J Bone Joint Surg Am 2011;93(6):564–571.
2. Brage ME, Hansen ST Jr. Traumatic subluxation/dislocation of the peroneal tendons. Foot Ankle 1992;13:423–431.
3. Brodsky JW, Zide JR, Kane JM. Acute peroneal injury. Foot Ankle Clin 2017;22(4):833–841.
4. Cerrato RA, Myerson MS. Peroneal tendon tears, surgical management and its complications. Foot Ankle Clin 2009;14(2):299–312.
5. Clanton TO, Porter DA. Primary care of foot and ankle injuries in the athlete. Clin Sports Med 1997;16:435–466.
6. Davis WH, Sobel M, Deland J, et al. The superior peroneal retinaculum: an anatomic study. Foot Ankle Int 1994;15:271–275.
7. DiGiovanni BF, Fraga CJ, Cohen BE, et al. Associated injuries found in chronic lateral ankle instability. Foot Ankle Int 2000;21(10):809–815.
8. Eckert WR, Davis EA Jr. Acute rupture of the peroneal retinaculum. J Bone Joint Surg Am 1976;58(5):670–672.
9. Edwards M. The relations of the peroneal tendons to the fibula, calcaneus, and cuboideum. Am J Anat 1927;42:213–252.
10. Geppert MJ, Sobel M, Bohne WH. Lateral ankle instability as a cause of superior peroneal retinacular laxity: an anatomic and biomechanical study of cadaveric feet. Foot Ankle 1993;14:330–334.
11. Hu M, Xiangyang X. Treatment of chronic subluxation of the peroneal tendons using a modified posteromedial peroneal tendon groove deepening technique. J Foot Ankle Surg 2018;57(5):884–889.
12. Karlsson J, Eriksson BI, Swärd L. Recurrent dislocation of the peroneal tendons. Scand J Med Sci Sports 1996;6:242–246.
13. Maffulli N, Ferran NA, Oliva F, et al. Recurrent subluxation of the peroneal tendons. Am J Sports Med 2006;34:986–992.
14. McGarvey W, Clanton T. Peroneal tendon dislocations. Foot Ankle Clin 1996;1:325–342.
15. McLennan JG. Treatment of acute and chronic luxations of the peroneal tendons. Am J Sports Med 1980;8:432–436.
16. Niemi WJ, Savidakis J Jr, DeJesus JM. Peroneal subluxation: a comprehensive review of the literature with case presentations. J Foot Ankle Surg 1997;36:141–145.
17. Oden RR. Tendon injuries about the ankle resulting from skiing. Clin Orthop Relat Res 1987;(216):63–69.
18. Ohashi K, Sanghvi T, El-Khoury GY, et al. Diagnostic accuracy of 3D color volume-rendered CT images for peroneal tendon dislocation in patients with acute calcaneal fractures. Acta Radiol 2015;56(2):190–195.
19. Ozbag D, Gumusalan Y, Uzel M, et al. Morphometrical features of the human malleolar groove. Foot Ankle Int 2008;29(1):77–81.
20. Raikin SM. Intrasheath subluxation of the peroneal tendons. Surgical technique. J Bone Joint Surg Am 2009;91(suppl 2, pt 1):146–155.
21. Sammarco GJ. Peroneal tendon injuries. Orthop Clin North Am 1994;25:135–145.
22. Saxena A, Ewen B. Peroneal subluxation: surgical results in 31 athletic patients. J Foot Ankle Surg 2010;49(3):238–241.
23. Shawen SB, Anderson RB. Indirect groove deepening in the management of chronic peroneal tendon dislocation. Tech Foot Ankle Surg 2004;3(2):118–125.
24. Toussaint RJ, Lin D, Ehrlichman LK, et al. Peroneal tendon displacement accompanying intra-articular calcaneal fractures. J Bone Joint Surg Am 2014;96(4):310–315.
25. van Dijk PA, Gianakos AL, Kerkhoffs GM, et al. Return to sports and clinical outcomes in patients treated for peroneal tendon dislocation: a systematic review. Knee Surg Sports Tramatol Arthrosc 2016;24(4):1155–1164.
26. Ward P, Anderson R, Ellington JK, et al. What is the rate of recurrence of peroneal groove deepening for subluxation/dislocation. Foot Ankle Orthop 2018;3.
27. Wong-Chung J, Tucker A, Lynch-Wong M, et al. The lateral malleolar bony fleck classified by size and pathoanatomy: the IOFAS classification. Foot Ankle Surg 2018;24(4):300–308.

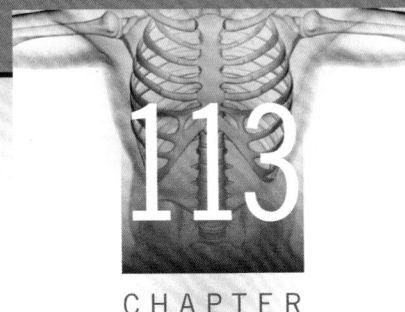

113

CHAPTER

Reconstruction of Tibialis Anterior Tendon Ruptures

James Santangelo and Mark E. Easley

DEFINITION

- Tibialis anterior rupture may present as an acute injury or as a chronic painless foot drop.[3]
- The diagnosis is often delayed.
- Recommended treatment is surgical for active patients and nonsurgical for low-demand patients. Surgical options include direct repair and reconstruction.

ANATOMY

- The tibialis anterior muscle originates from the lateral tibial condyle and interosseous membrane.
- Its insertion is the medial side of the medial cuneiform and the inferomedial base of the first metatarsal.
- The musculotendinous junction is at the junction of the middle and distal thirds of the tibia.
- The tendon courses within a synovial sheath from the musculotendinous junction to its insertion,[2] deep to the extensor retinaculum of the ankle and foot.
- Innervation is the deep peroneal nerve.
- The tibialis anterior muscle controls deceleration of the foot after heel strike and dorsiflexes the ankle.

PATHOGENESIS

- Younger individuals with healthy tibialis anterior tendons rarely suffer spontaneous rupture; instead, their mechanism of injury is laceration from penetrating trauma or distal tibia fracture.
- Spontaneous ruptures typically occur in older individuals with degenerative tendinopathy of the tibialis anterior tendon. Minor trauma may be associated with these ruptures, with a mechanism of plantarflexion–eversion. Ruptures typically occur within 3 cm of the tendon's insertion on the medial cuneiform.[1]

NATURAL HISTORY

- The natural history of tibialis anterior rupture is inferred from studies documenting the results of nonoperatively treated patients. These patients will ambulate with a slap foot gait and sometimes have difficulty negotiating uneven terrain. Most patients are functional; however, they may require a brace.
- Nonoperatively treated patients tend to be older and lower demand. The natural history for younger, more active patients may indicate less desirable results.
- Definite conclusions regarding the natural history of tibialis anterior ruptures are limited due to the low number of reported cases in the literature and lack of natural history studies.

PATIENT HISTORY AND PHYSICAL FINDINGS

- Physical examination methods include the following:
  - Examining for swelling. The examiner should palpate along the course of the tibialis anterior muscle–tendon. Swelling with discontinuity of the tendon indicates a tendon rupture. An anterior ankle mass may be the presenting complaint.
  - Gait disturbance. The examiner should observe the patient ambulating, looking for slap foot gait or foot drop. Chronic ruptures may present with minimal gait disturbance; the patient may have difficulty ambulating only when on uneven surfaces. Inability to heel walk indicates tibialis anterior dysfunction. The patient may need to hyperflex the hip and knee to clear the foot during the swing phase of gait because the ankle does not dorsiflex adequately.
  - Muscle strength is evaluated with manual motor testing. No contraction or weak ankle dorsiflexion suggests tibialis anterior dysfunction. Patients will substitute the toe extensors for the tibialis anterior during ankle dorsiflexion, exhibiting toe hyperextension when asked to dorsiflex the ankle.
- The examiner should note any heel cord tightness. Subacute and chronic injuries often present with heel cord contractures because the major antagonist to ankle plantarflexion is forfeited with tibialis anterior tendon rupture. As a rule, at least 10 degrees of ankle dorsiflexion must be present for a tibialis anterior repair or reconstruction, and thus, surgical management may require adding Achilles tendon or gastrocnemius lengthening.
- The examiner should completely assess the involved extremity to rule out other diagnoses. The most common errors in diagnosis are as follows:
  - Lumbar radiculopathy: presents with diminished sensation, positive straight-leg raise test
  - Peroneal nerve palsy: affects the toe extensors and peroneal musculature in addition to the tibialis anterior. Preservation of extensor hallucis longus (EHL) and toe extensor function will distinguish tibialis anterior rupture from peroneal nerve palsy.[1]

IMAGING AND OTHER DIAGNOSTIC STUDIES

- Imaging studies are generally not required in the evaluation of tibialis anterior tendon ruptures because the diagnosis is usually simple to make on clinical examination alone.

- Radiographs are nondiagnostic and rarely required in the evaluation of tibialis anterior tendon ruptures. Radiographs are, however, useful to assess associated injures (tibial fractures).
- Magnetic resonance imaging (MRI) may be useful in chronic cases where patients do not recall a history of trauma.[1] MRI demonstrates lack of continuity in the tibialis anterior and signal change in the tendon, particularly with preexisting tendinopathy. Because the tibialis anterior tendon courses from lateral to medial across the anterior ankle and retracts with rupture, occasionally, it is difficult to assess.
- If there is uncertainty in the diagnosis, electrodiagnostic studies may identify common peroneal palsy or lumbar radiculopathy.

DIFFERENTIAL DIAGNOSIS

- Peroneal nerve palsy
- Lumbar radiculopathy
- Rarely, a peripheral neuropathy may present as isolated tibialis anterior tendon dysfunction.

NONOPERATIVE MANAGEMENT

- Low-demand patients may be treated with an ankle–foot orthosis (AFO).

SURGICAL MANAGEMENT

- Direct repair of the tendon is occasionally possible, but delay in diagnosis may preclude direct repair due to muscle contracture.
- A sliding tibialis anterior tendon grafting technique has been described to gain tendon length to allow repair, and allograft tendon transfers have been proposed in the absence of tibialis anterior myofibrosis.

- Our preferred reconstruction for tendons that cannot be directly repaired is to augment the repair with the adjacent, native EHL tendon **(FIG 1)**.
- Indications for allograft tendon reconstruction[4]
  - Advanced tibialis anterior tendon degeneration
  - Tibialis anterior muscle excursion preserved
    - Minimal to no myofibrosis
    - Allograft reconstruction for a muscle that has no excursion, that is, is scarred, will result in a no more than a tenodesis without function.

Preoperative Planning

- Imaging studies are reviewed when available to appreciate the extent of preexisting tendinopathy and to potentially identify the approximate site of the rupture.
- The surgeon should prepare for Achilles tendon lengthening or gastrocnemius–soleus recession to achieve adequate (at least 10 degrees) dorsiflexion.

Positioning

- The patient is positioned supine. A bump may be placed under the ipsilateral hip, but this is typically not necessary because access is required only to the anteromedial ankle.

Approach

- An anterior approach is made directly over the course of the tibialis anterior tendon.
- As has been learned from total ankle arthroplasty and open reduction and internal fixation of tibial pilon fractures, careful soft tissue handling is essential.

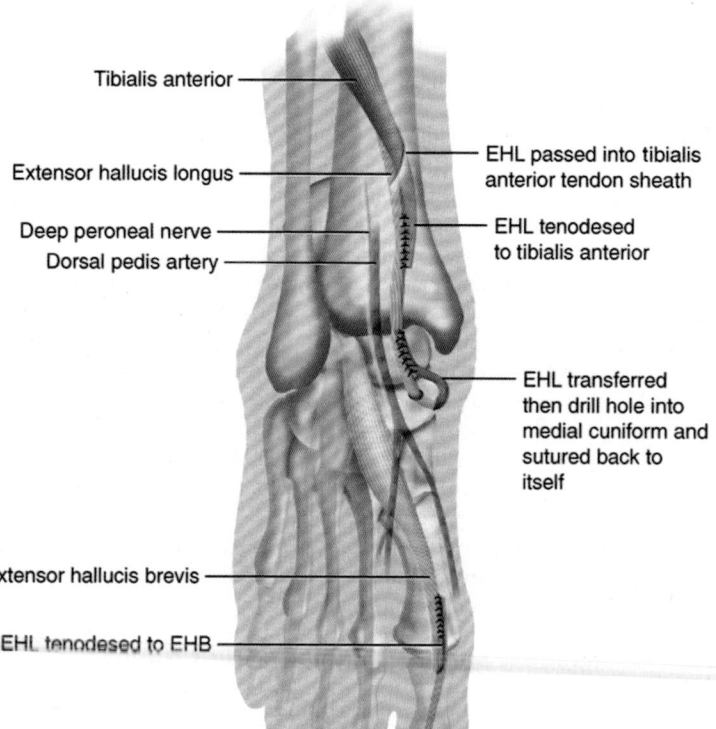

Tibialis anterior

Extensor hallucis longus

Deep peroneal nerve

Dorsal pedis artery

EHL passed into tibialis anterior tendon sheath

EHL tenodesed to tibialis anterior

EHL transferred then drill hole into medial cuniform and sutured back to itself

Extensor hallucis brevis

EHL tenodesed to EHB

FIG 1 EHL transfer to medial cuneiform. The proximal end of the tibialis anterior tendon is tenodesed to the EHL. Distally, the extensor hallucis brevis (*EHB*) is tenodesed to the EHL distal end to preserve hallux interphalangeal joint extension.

EXTENSOR HALLUCIS LONGUS TRANSFER TO MEDIAL CUNEIFORM

Exposure

- Perform gastrocnemius recession or Achilles tendon lengthening if indicated.
- Use an anterior approach with an incision over the course of the tibialis anterior tendon (**TECH FIG 1**).
- Divide the superior and inferior extensor retinaculum and tibialis anterior sheath.
- Isolate the remnant of the tibialis anterior tendon. Occasionally, direct repair is possible, rarely by advancing the residual tendon to bone but instead to the residual tendon stump on the medial cuneiform. If inadequate tendon is available or muscle excursion is poor, proceed with EHL transfer.

Extensor Hallucis Longus Transfer

- Expose the EHL tendon. Proximally, the EHL is in a separate sheath adjacent to the tibialis anterior.
- Through a separate 3- to 5-cm incision over the distal EHL immediately proximal to the first metatarsophalangeal joint, divide the EHL tendon distally. Leave enough distal stump to suture to the adjacent tendon of the extensor hallucis brevis. Place a whipstitch consisting of no. 2 nonabsorbable suture in the free end of the EHL.
- Pass the EHL under the skin bridge and through the tibialis anterior sheath proximally. The EHL will now occupy the previous sheath for the tibialis anterior (**TECH FIG 2**).

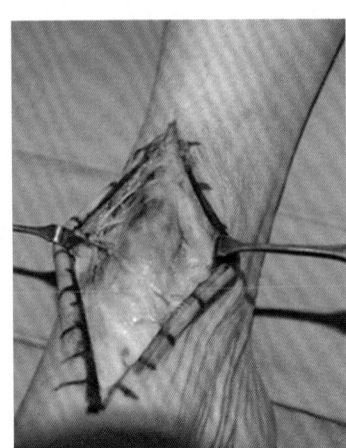

A

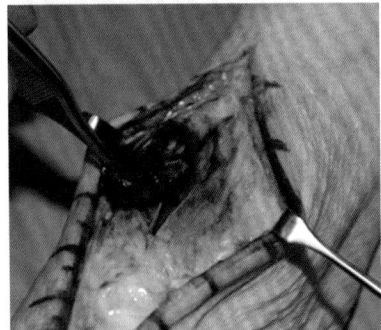

B

TECH FIG 1 A. Anterior approach over tibialis anterior. **B.** The tendon sheath is opened, exposing the torn retracted end of the tibialis anterior. The sheath is carefully preserved for later repair.

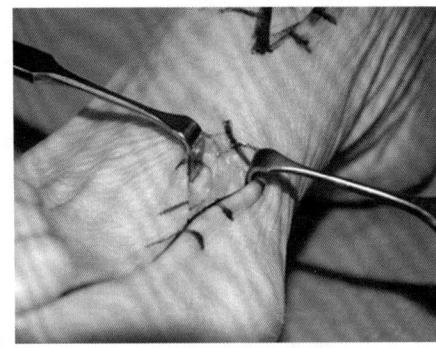

A

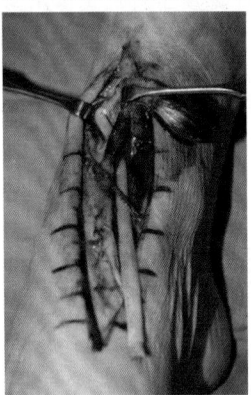

B

TECH FIG 2 A. The EHL tendon is harvested by dividing it at the level of the metatarsophalangeal joint. **B.** The EHL tendon sheath is entered proximally. The EHL tendon is passed into the tibialis anterior sheath and pulled distally.

- Drill a vertical hole in the medial cuneiform for attachment of the EHL. Sequentially drill using 2.5-, 3.5-, and 4.5-mm drill bits. Enlarge the hole with a curette as needed to allow graft passage. Leave enough periosteum to provide additional points of attachment for suturing the graft in place.

Fixation

- Secure the graft with the ankle in 10 degrees of dorsiflexion (**TECH FIG 3A–D**).

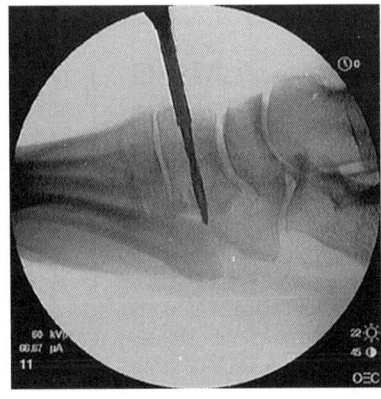

A

TECH FIG 3 A. A drill hole is placed from dorsal to plantar at the midpoint of the medial cuneiform. *(continued)*

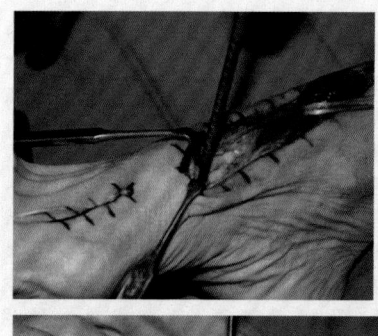
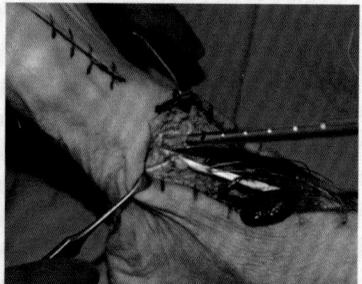
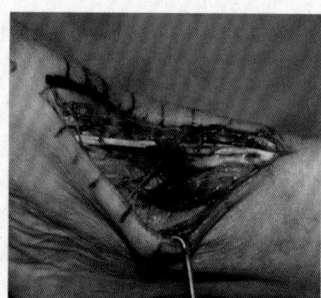

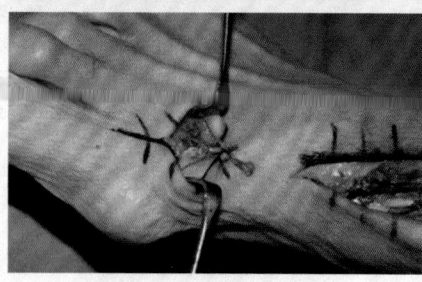

TECH FIG 3 *(continued)* **B.** The drill hole is sequentially enlarged. **C.** Fixation using a Bio-Tenodesis screw (Arthrex, Inc., Naples, FL). The graft is also looped around the medial cuneiform and sutured to itself and surrounding soft tissue. **D.** Proximally, the EHL is tenodesed to the tibialis anterior stump. **E.** The EHL stump is sutured to the extensor hallucis brevis.

- Pass the EHL graft from dorsal to plantar. Fixation may be accomplished with an interference screw or by looping the graft around the medial cuneiform and suturing it to surrounding periosteum and back on itself. The EHL tendon may be further anchored to the residual distal fibers of the torn tibialis anterior tendon.
- The transferred EHL tendon serves to bridge the gap created by the tibialis tendon rupture. However, the relative strength of the EHL muscle is far less than that of the tibialis anterior muscle. Therefore, in the absence of myofibrosis of the tibialis anterior, we recommend sewing the residual tibialis anterior tendon stump to the transferred EHL tendon under some tension.
- Attach the distal EHL stump to the extensor hallucis brevis, and we recommend dorsiflexing the hallux about 10 to 15 degrees to compensate for anticipated stretching of this tendon transfer postoperatively **(TECH FIG 3E)**.

Completion

- Close the tibialis anterior tendon sheath, superior extensor retinaculum, and wound in layers **(TECH FIG 4)**.
- Place a splint or bivalved cast with the ankle in 10 degrees of dorsiflexion. Avoid plantarflexion, as this places tension on the wound edges and tendon transfer.

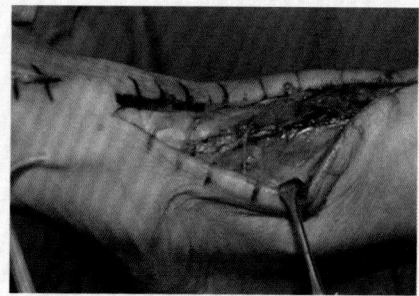

TECH FIG 4 The tibialis anterior sheath is closed.

ALLOGRAFT TENDON RECONSTRUCTION

Assess for Equinus Contracture

- Delay in diagnosis and treatment of a tibialis anterior tendon rupture may lead to an equinus contracture.
- Allograft tibialis anterior tendon reconstruction typically restores satisfactory dorsiflexion.
  - If no equinus contracture, then the Achilles tendon should not be lengthened.
  - However, it may not restore full physiologic function.
  - Cannot overcome an equinus contracture
- With an equinus contracture, consider judicious Achilles tendon lengthening or gastrocnemius–soleus recession.
  - If equinus indeed present, Achilles lengthening or gastrocnemius–soleus recession should be performed prior to allograft tibialis anterior tendon reconstruction.

- Although a utilitarian midline anterior approach to the ankle may be used, repair/reconstruction of distal tibialis anterior tendon avulsion is facilitated if the incision is directed medially toward the physiologic course of the tibialis anterior tendon.
  - This is important in allograft tendon reconstruction where exposure of the residual distal tendon and first cuneiform is important for securing the distal allograft.
- Create a longitudinal incision directly over the physiologic course of tibialis anterior tendon **(TECH FIG 5A)**.
- Protect the superficial peroneal nerve that courses superficial to the extensor retinaculum.
- Expose the extensor retinaculum **(TECH FIG 5B)**.

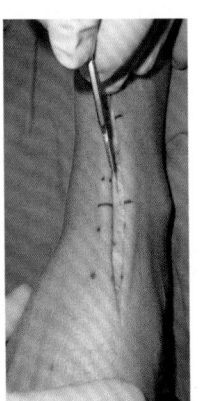 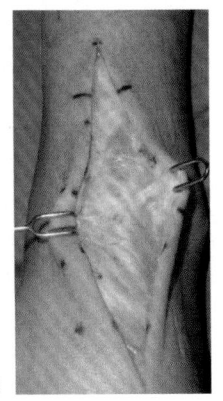 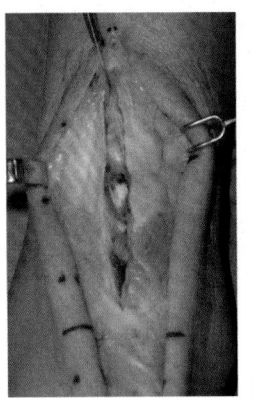 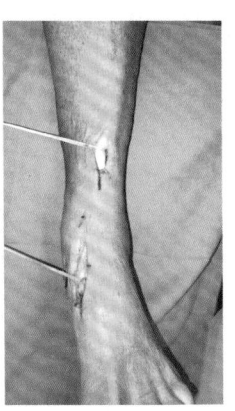

A   B   C   D

TECH FIG 5 A. Longitudinal incision directly over physiologic course of the tibialis anterior tendon. **B.** Expose the extensor retinaculum. **C.** Longitudinal incision in the extensor retinaculum to expose the tendon rupture. **D.** Leaving the central skin and retinaculum over the ankle intact allows for adequate exposure to anchor the allograft distally and to secure it to the native proximal tendon; this approach may lead to fewer wound complications and less chance for allograft tendon adhesion.

- Divide the extensor retinaculum.
  - The retinaculum may be divided directly over the ruptured tibialis tendon to expose the ruptured tibialis anterior tendon **(TECH FIG 5C)**.
- Alternatively, the tendon reconstruction may be performed through two separate approaches, one proximal and the other distal. This way, the central skin and retinaculum are left intact directly over the ankle, leading to less "bowstringing" of the reconstructed tendon into a repaired retinaculum. Although this limits visualization, it allows for adequate exposure to (1) excise the diseased tendon segment, (2) anchor the allograft tendon distally, and (3) secure the allograft to the native proximal tendon. Moreover, it may lead to less chance of allograft tendon adhesion **(TECH FIG 5D)**.

Assessing the Ruptured Tibialis Anterior Tendon

- Often, patients with tibialis anterior tendon ruptures do not present immediately after acute rupture.
- Proximal tendon
  - The proximal end of the tendon is typically retracted.
  - The example case demonstrates a subacute rupture with a bulbous proximal end of the tendon **(TECH FIG 6A,B)**.
  - To consider allograft reconstruction, the proximal tendon and muscle must have some excursion.
  - Place distally directed tension on the proximal tendon to assess excursion **(TECH FIG 6C)**.
  - Applying careful tension for several minutes typically restores some excursion.

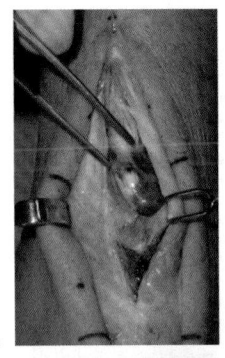 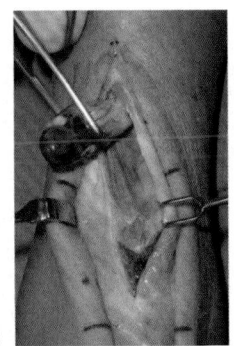 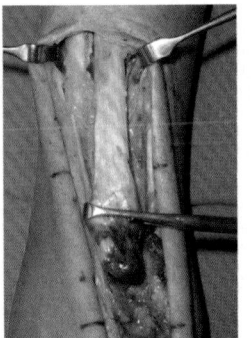 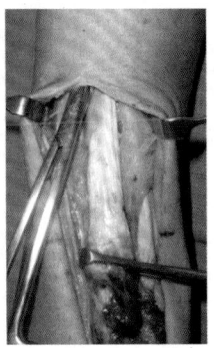 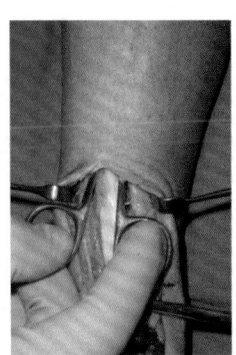

A   B   C   D   E

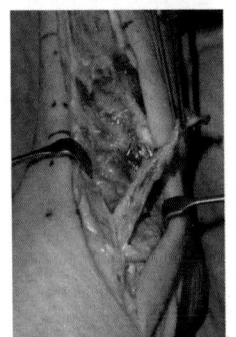 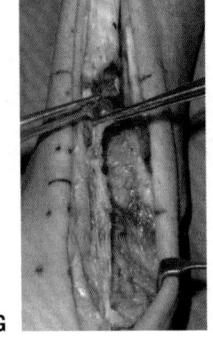

F   G

TECH FIG 6 A. Proximal tendon identified. **B.** Characteristic findings of a subacute rupture. **C.** The proximal tendon (and muscle) must have excursion for an allograft tendon reconstruction to restore dynamic ankle dorsiflexion. **D.** Release of proximal tendon adhesions. **E.** Adhesions released within the tibialis anterior tendon sheath deep to the proximal extensor retinaculum. **F.** Limited residual distal tendon is this patient with tibialis anterior tendon avulsion injury. **G.** After proximal tendon mobilization, the tendon ends can be approximated, but the poor quality of residual distal tendon is not conducive to direct repair.

- Lack of excursion does not necessarily indicate muscle fibrosis; limited excursion may be due to adhesions within the sheath from lack of motion.
- Release adhesions with blunt-tipped scissors advanced between the proximal tendon and its tendon sheath **(TECH FIG 6D,E)**.
- Distal tendon
  - The distal tendon, with its attachment to the base of the first metatarsal, is static without excursion.
  - In the example case, the tibialis tendon ruptured from its distal attachment.
    - Minimal residual tendon attachment remains **(TECH FIG 6F)**.
- Although the proximal and residual distal tendon ends may be approximated after proximal tendon and muscle mobilization, the lack of satisfactory distal tendon quality eliminates the option of direct repair **(TECH FIG 6G)**.

Reconstruction

- The allograft tibialis tendon should be pretensioned.
- Preserve the residual distal native tendon to be used in the distal allograft reconstruction.
- Assess the planned course of the allograft tendon **(TECH FIG 7A)**.
  - It should course to the plantar medial aspect of the first cuneiform.
- Place suture anchors in the medial aspect of the first cuneiform.
  - Consider fluoroscopic guidance to optimize anchor positioning **(TECH FIG 7B)**.
- Anchor the allograft tendon distally.
  - Suture anchors to the medial aspect of the first cuneiform **(TECH FIG 7C)**.
  - Suture the residual distal native tendon to the allograft tendon **(TECH FIG 7D)**.
    - A tendon weave may be considered.
    - In this example case, the residual native tendon was more conducive to a side-to-side repair.

- Confirm that the distal attachment is satisfactory.
  - By applying tension to the attached allograft tendon, ankle dorsiflexion should be possible **(TECH FIG 7E)**.

Proximal Allograft Tendon Attachment

- Support the ankle in neutral position **(TECH FIG 8A)**.
- Weave the allograft into the proximal native tendon.
- Carefully create the first longitudinal slit in the distal aspect of the native proximal tendon.
  - Create the slit sharply with a scalpel and avoid unnecessary injury to the tendon.
  - This initial slit should be no more than 1 cm in length affording optimal contact between tendons.
- Pass the proximal end of the allograft tendon through the distal proximal native tendon.
- Place proximally directed tension on the allograft.
- Place distally directed tension on the proximal native tension.
- Because the tendon reconstruction is intended to be dynamic and function physiologically, excessive overtensioning is typically not indicated.
  - However, because some stretch of the allograft and more proximal native tendon–muscle excursion is anticipated, slightly greater than physiologic tension should be considered.
- Secure the allograft to the native proximal tendon with nonabsorbable suture **(TECH FIG 8B)**.
- Weave the allograft tendon through the native tendon for a second time.
  - Perform the second longitudinal slit in the native tendon approximately 2 cm proximal from the first slit.
  - To avoid the two slits in the tendon becoming confluent, create the second slit at 90 degrees from the first.
  - The slit in the native tendon is performed sharply with a scalpel blade passed through the native tendon from the same direction intended for the allograft tendon to be passed.

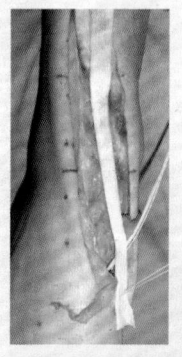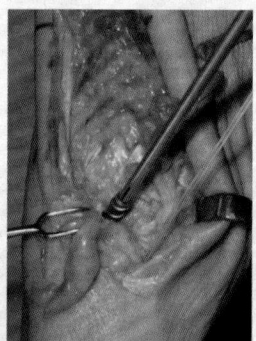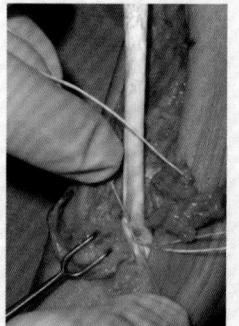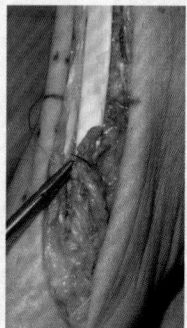
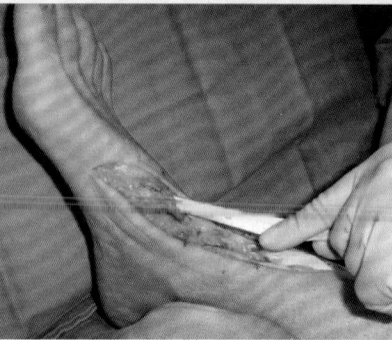

TECH FIG 7 A. Assessing course of allograft tendon with planned distal reattachment. **B.** Suture anchors placed in medial aspect of first cuneiform. **C.** Anchoring allograft to medial first cuneiform. **D.** Securing residual distal native tendon to anchored allograft tendon. **E.** Confirming satisfactory distal allograft tendon attachment.

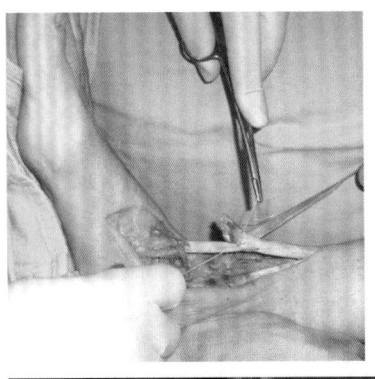
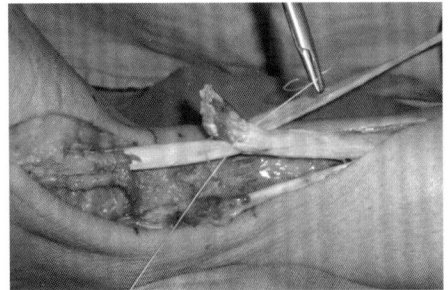
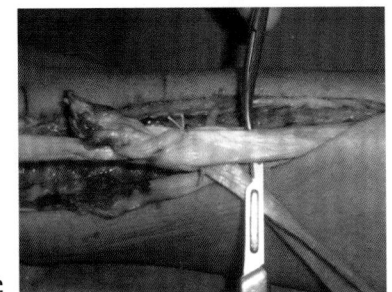
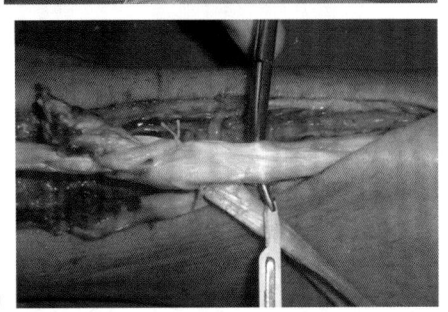
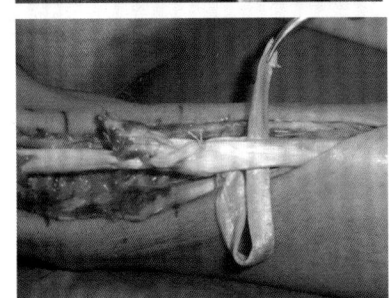

TECH FIG 8 Weaving allograft tendon to the proximal native tendon. **A.** Ankle held in neutral dorsiflexion. **B.** After first pass of allograft tendon through native tendon, tension applied to tendons and tendons secured with suture. **C.** Second weave created by passing scalpel blade through tendon at 90 degrees from initial weave in the direction intended for the allograft to be passed. **D.** Scalpel blade pushed back through slit in native tendon with a hemostat clamp. **E.** Allograft tendon pulled through the native tendon with the hemostat clamp.

- Once the tip of the scalpel blade has passed through the tendon, fasten a hemostat clamp to the scalpel's tip and push the scalpel blade back out of tendon so that the hemostat is safely passed through the same slit in the tendon without compromising the tendon (**TECH FIG 8C,D**).
- Pull the allograft tendon through the slit in the native tendon (**TECH FIG 8E**).
- Tension the two tendon ends and suture as described for the first weave earlier.
- A third weave and possibly a fourth weave are created to optimally secure the allograft to the native tendon.
  - Each slit is spaced at least 2 cm from the previous slit.
  - Each slit is created at 90 degrees from the previous slit.

Completion

- The excess allograft tendon is excised.
- Reinforce the distal and proximal allograft attachments to the native tendon with absorbable suture.
- Ensure that the tendon is intact and competent with ankle motion.

- Close the retinaculum over the reconstructed tendon (**TECH FIG 9A–D**).
  - Avoid a suture capturing the tendon reconstruction.
- Routine skin closure; consider using a drain.
- Consider temporary chemical weakening of the gastrocnemius muscle.
  - Although the tibialis anterior tendon reconstruction is healing and muscle function is restored, its antagonist, the gastrocnemius muscle, may be temporarily weakened with botulinum toxin injection (**TECH FIG 9E**).
  - Botulinum toxin injection to the gastrocnemius muscle for this purpose may be expensive and should be preauthorized prior to surgery (**TECH FIG 9F**).
  - Gastrocnemius weakness after botulinum toxin injection typically persists for 3 to 6 months, ideal for recovery of the tibialis anterior tendon reconstruction.
    - Because botulinum toxin has some potential side effects, the plan to inject botulinum toxin to the gastrocnemius muscle must be discussed with the patient as part of the informed consent process.
- Splint or cast with ankle in slight dorsiflexion.

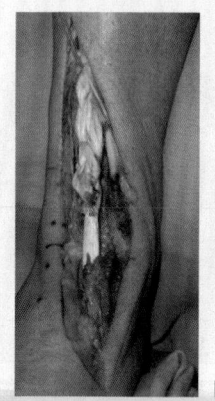 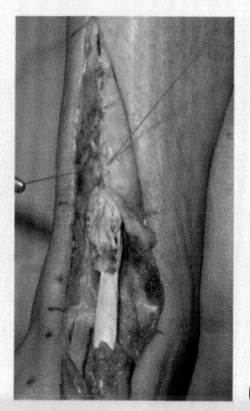 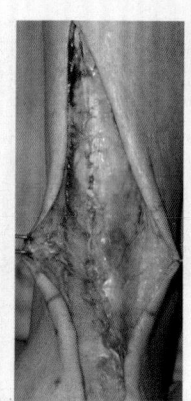

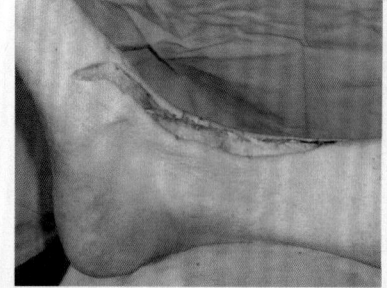 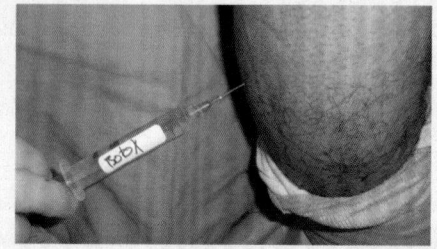 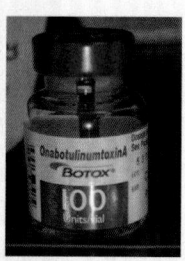

TECH FIG 9 Closing extensor retinaculum. **A.** After tendon reconstruction complete, begin closing extensor retinaculum proximally. **B.** Care to avoid trapping the tendon reconstruction in the retinacular closure. **C.** Important to completely close retinaculum over full length of tendon reconstruction. **D.** Note that tendon reconstruction well contained within retinaculum. **E,F.** Temporary chemical gastrocnemius weakening. **E.** Botulinum injection into gastrocnemius muscle (the antagonist to the tibialis anterior) may help protect the reconstruction during the 6 months of rehabilitation. **F.** Botulinum toxin is expensive and should be preapproved before surgery.

TECHNIQUES

Pearls and Pitfalls

Misdiagnosis	• Perform a complete history and physical examination to rule out conditions that may mimic tibialis anterior rupture.
Failure to Address Heel Cord Tightness	• Note ankle dorsiflexion as part of the preoperative evaluation and perform Achilles tendon lengthening or gastrocnemius recession as indicated.
Inadequate EHL Graft Length	• Expose and divide the distal end of the EHL at the metatarsophalangeal joint level.
Wound Breakdown	• Carefully close the tibialis anterior sheath, superior extensor retinaculum, and subcutaneous tissue before skin closure. Immobilization in at least 5 degrees of dorsiflexion is important to avoid tension on the wound edges.
Graft Failure	• Secure fixation with proper use of an interference screw and adequate graft length to suture back on itself and surrounding tissues. • Postoperative immobilization • Avoidance of early aggressive rehabilitation

POSTOPERATIVE CARE

- EHL transfer
  - A short-leg cast is worn for 6 weeks, followed by an AFO for an additional 6 weeks.
- Allograft tendon reconstruction
  - 2 to 3 weeks
    - Wound check and suture removal
    - Sturdy posterior splint with ankle in slight dorsiflexion

- 2 to 6 weeks
  - Reliable patient should perform intermittent gentle passive ankle range of motion.
    - Three or four times a day ankle removed from splint to perform passive ankle/hindfoot range of motion
    - No active ankle dorsiflexion unless physical therapist (PT) supervision available to perform active-assisted dorsiflexion
    - Touchdown weight bearing

■ Unreliable patient probably best casted in slight ankle dorsiflexion
- 6 to 10 weeks
  ■ Cam boot
  ■ Weight bearing as tolerated in cam boot
  ■ Physical therapy with active-assisted ankle dorsiflexion for first 2 weeks and gradually progressing to active dorsiflexion over second 2 weeks
- 10 to 14 weeks
  ■ Continue physical therapy and progress to active dorsiflexion.
  ■ Hinged AFO with a plantarflexion stop during day
  ■ Still use splint or boot with ankle in neutral position while sleeping.
- 14 to 24 weeks
  ■ Gradual return to activities of daily living without splint
  ■ Continue physical therapy to develop program to return to full activities by 6 months.

OUTCOMES

- Sammarco et al[7] presented a series of 18 patients with acute and chronic tibialis anterior tendon ruptures managed with direct repair or interpositional graft. There was significant improvement in the average hindfoot score. The authors concluded that surgical repair of a ruptured tibialis anterior tendon can be beneficial regardless of age, sex, medical comorbidities, or delay in diagnosis.
- Ouzounian and Anderson[6] reported on seven patients with tibialis anterior rupture treated with a variety of surgical reconstructive techniques. All patients had an increase in strength and function.
- Markarian et al[5] failed to show a significant difference between operative and nonoperatively treated groups. The lack

of statistical significance was possibly due to the bimodal age distribution in the study, with older, more sedentary patients receiving nonoperative treatment.
- The literature is scarce regarding the results and complications of surgical reconstruction of the tibialis anterior tendon due to the rarity of this injury.

COMPLICATIONS

- Intraoperative graft complications
- Neuroma
- Wound dehiscence
- Infection
- Graft failure

REFERENCES

1. Coughlin MJ. Disorders of tendons. In: Coughlin MJ, Mann RA, eds. Surgery of the Foot and Ankle, ed 7. St. Louis: Mosby, 1999:790–795.
2. Cracchiolo A. Anterior tibial tendon disorders. In: Nunley JA, Pfeffer GB, Sanders RW, et al, eds. Advanced Reconstruction Foot and Ankle. Rosemont, IL: American Academy of Orthopaedic Surgery, 2003: 173–177.
3. Harkin E, Pinzur M, Schiff A. Treatment of acute and chronic tibialis anterior tendon rupture and tendinopathy. Foot Ankle Clin 2017;22(4): 819–831.
4. Huh J, Boyette DM, Parekh SG, et al. Allograft reconstruction of chronic tibialis anterior tendon ruptures. Foot Ankle Int 2015;36(10): 1180–1189.
5. Markarian GG, Kelikian AS, Brage M, et al. Anterior tibialis tendon ruptures: an outcome analysis of operative vs. nonoperative treatment. Foot Ankle Int 1998;19:792–802.
6. Ouzounian TJ, Anderson R. Anterior tibial tendon rupture. Foot Ankle Int 1995;16:406–410.
7. Sammarco VJ, Sammarco GJ, Henning C, et al. Surgical repair of acute and chronic tibialis anterior tendon ruptures. J Bone Joint Surg Am 2009;91(2):325–332.

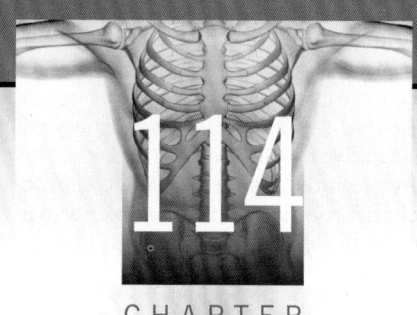

114

CHAPTER

Tendon Transfer for Foot Drop

Mark E. Easley and Aaron T. Scott

DEFINITION

- Pathology leading to a spectrum of motor function loss that includes loss of ankle dorsiflexion
  - Common peroneal nerve palsy, L5 radiculopathy, cerebrovascular accident
    - Loss of ankle dorsiflexion and hindfoot eversion
    - Retained posterior tibial tendon (PTT) function
  - Hereditary sensory motor neuropathy
    - A constellation of motor function deficits and associated deformity
    - Includes loss of dorsiflexion and hindfoot eversion
    - Retained PTT function
  - Flaccid paralysis
    - Global loss of motor function to the ankle and foot

ANATOMY

- Posterior tibialis
  - Muscle originates on the posterior tibia, interosseous membrane (IOM), and fibula.
  - Muscle and then tendon course in the deep posterior compartment.
  - Tendon travels directly posterior to the medial malleolus.
  - Tendon has numerous insertions on bones of plantar midfoot, spring ligament, and medial aspect of navicular.
- IOM and distal tibia–fibula syndesmosis
  - Thick fibrous bands between tibia and fibula
  - Distal tibia–fibula syndesmosis is narrow, with little space for tendon transfer even when a generous window is created in the distal IOM.
- Inferior extensor retinaculum
  - On the dorsum of the foot to prevent bowstringing of the extensor tendons as they transition across the anterior ankle to the dorsal foot
- Sciatic nerve
  - Comprises tibial and common peroneal nerves that separate immediately proximal to the popliteal fossa
  - Common peroneal nerve often affected in these neuropathies
  - Superficial peroneal nerve
    - Motor function to anterior and lateral compartment muscles
      - Dorsiflexion and eversion, respectively
    - Sensory distribution to dorsum of the foot
  - Deep peroneal nerve
    - Courses between tibialis anterior and extensor hallucis longus tendons proximal to the ankle

- Located directly on the dorsum of midfoot
  - Immediately deep to extensor hallucis brevis muscle belly
  - Motor function to intrinsic muscles of foot
  - Sensory distribution to first web space
- Tibial nerve function typically spared
- Tibial nerve must be intact to create a dynamic tendon transfer.
- If tibial nerve is not intact, then transfer can only be a tenodesis.
- Anterior ankle and dorsal midfoot neurovascular structures at risk
  - Superficial peroneal nerve (may be insensate as part of the neuropathy)
  - Deep neurovascular bundle
    - Anterior tibial artery
    - Deep peroneal nerve (may also be insensate as part of the neuropathy)
  - Peroneal artery branch
    - Situated directly on anterior distal IOM

PATHOGENESIS

- Loss of common peroneal nerve function
- Loss of ankle dorsiflexion and hindfoot eversion
- Loss of major antagonists
  - Eventual equinus contracture
    - Imbalance of hindfoot inverter (PTT) and everters (peroneus brevis and usually, but not always, peroneus longus)
  - Eventual hindfoot varus deformity
    - Imbalance of hindfoot inverters (PTT) and everter (peroneus longus)
- Flaccid paralysis
  - Tibial and common peroneal nerve palsies
  - No motor function distal to knee
  - Because both sets of major antagonists lost, typically no contractures

NATURAL HISTORY

- Foot drop may eventually recover.
  - Tendon transfers should not be considered until a chance for recovery has been ruled out.
- Common peroneal nerve palsy may lead to progressively worsening equinocavovarus foot deformity due to overpull of plantarflexors and inverters powered by intact tibial nerve and loss of dorsiflexors and everters powered by compromised common peroneal nerve.
- Flaccid paralysis remains relatively stable because both sets of antagonists are compromised.

PATIENT HISTORY AND PHYSICAL FINDINGS

- Gait abnormality
  - "Slap foot gait"
    - Inability to dorsiflex ankle and control tibialis anterior from heel strike to stance phase
  - Exaggerated hip and knee flexion
    - Inability to dorsiflex ankle or great toe from push-off through swing phase
    - Compensation to allow toes to clear during swing phase
  - Hindfoot inversion
    - Patient walks on lateral border of foot.
- Inability to dorsiflex ankle
  - May check by asking patient to walk on heels
  - Manual muscle testing with patient seated on examining table with knee flexed
- Lack of eversion
  - Varus hindfoot
  - Over time, may become a fixed inversion contracture
- In some disease processes (eg, Charcot-Marie-Tooth disease), toe dorsiflexion is spared, creating claw toe deformities.
  - Patient attempts to compensate for lack of ankle dorsiflexion with toe extensors, worsening claw toe deformities.
- Even when toe extensors are involved in the palsy, flexor tendons may become contracted.
  - Passive dorsiflexion of the ankle will reveal this.
- With equinocavovarus foot contracture, calluses may form under metatarsal heads, particularly the fifth.
- Sensation may be diminished on the dorsal and lateral aspects of the foot.

IMAGING AND OTHER DIAGNOSTIC STUDIES

- Imaging is typically unnecessary for patients with foot drop except in the following situations:
  - Consideration should be given to magnetic resonance imaging:
    - If there is concern for mass effect creating a compressive neuropathy: lumbar spine, common peroneal nerve at fibular head
    - To rule out tibialis anterior tendon rupture (should be evident on clinical examination alone)
- Consideration should be given to radiographs of foot or ankle:
  - To rule out stress fracture
  - To better define bony deformity (fixed deformity, associated ankle or foot arthritis; important because arthrodesis may need to be considered in lieu of or in combination with tendon transfer)
- Electrodiagnostic studies
  - Absence of recovery at 1 year and particularly at 18 months is highly suggestive that recovery of nerve function will not occur.
  - Nerve conduction studies and electromyography
  - Baseline and follow-up studies to determine if any recovery is evident
  - Important to determine if tendon transfer is warranted
  - Tendon transfer should not be performed if nerve function may recover.

- Absence of recovery at 1 year and particularly at 18 months is highly suggestive of no recovery.
- We recommend consultation with a neurologist to confirm interpretation of electrodiagnostic studies.
- Studies may also define function of PTT.
  - Important when considering dynamic PTT transfer versus PTT tenodesis
  - A tendon transfer of a healthy tendon immediately reduces its strength on manual muscle testing from 5/5 to 4/5, so if it is already compromised, then the tendon transfer will do little more than to create a tenodesis.
- Useful in determining if a more proximal compressive neuropathy exists

DIFFERENTIAL DIAGNOSIS

- Tibialis anterior tendon rupture
- Cerebrovascular accident
- Lumbar spine radiculopathy
- Hereditary sensorimotor neuropathy
- Leprosy
- Poliomyelitis
- Cerebral palsy (spastic)

NONOPERATIVE MANAGEMENT

- Bracing with an ankle–foot orthosis (AFO)
  - Requires a fixed AFO in flaccid paralysis
  - May be a flexible AFO with common peroneal palsy
    - Requires plantarflexion stop
  - Equinus contracture may need to be corrected to facilitate brace wear.
    - Achilles stretching
    - Botulinum toxin injection
    - Tendo Achilles lengthening (TAL)
  - Varus deformity
    - If flexible, may be corrected with bracing
    - If fixed, bracing is difficult.

SURGICAL MANAGEMENT

Preoperative Planning

- The surgeon must confirm that motor function will not recover before proceeding with tendon transfer.
  - Serial clinical examination
  - Serial electrodiagnostic studies (at least one compared to baseline)
- The surgeon must determine what motor function persists:
  - Tibial nerve
    - PTT (inversion)
    - Gastrocnemius–soleus (plantarflexion)
  - None (flaccid paralysis)
- The surgeon must evaluate for equinus contracture.
  - The surgeon should be prepared to perform TAL if necessary (see **TECH FIG 1A–D**).
- Flexible versus fixed deformities
  - Flexible deformity typically corrects with tendon transfer alone.
  - Fixed deformity
    - May require capsular release or even arthrodesis

- Toe contractures
  - Although claw toe deformity may not be evident with the ankle plantarflexed, once the deformity is corrected, toe contractures may become obvious.
    - Dorsiflexing the ankle will put the contracted flexor hallucis and digitorum on stretch, thereby revealing the toe contractures.
    - The surgeon should be prepared to address toe contractures as part of the procedure.
- Tendon transfer anchoring
  - We routinely use interference screws to anchor tendon transfers to bone.
  - Need to have an anchoring system available
  - Alternatively, anchoring to existing distal tendon or existing soft tissues in the foot may be possible.
- In our experience, anesthesia should maintain complete muscle relaxation and paralysis during the procedure; otherwise, the success of the tendon transfer may be compromised.
- At the conclusion of the procedure, we often perform botulinum toxin injections into the gastrocnemius–soleus complex to further protect the tendon transfer postoperatively.

Positioning

- Supine
- If the PTT will be transferred through the IOM or if a peroneal tendon will be used for correction of flaccid paralysis, we routinely place a bolster under the ipsilateral hip

to afford optimal lateral exposure. Once the lateral tendon is harvested or the PTT transferred through the IOM, the bolster may be removed.
- We routinely use a thigh tourniquet.

Approach

- Multiple relatively small incisions are needed; extensile exposures are unnecessary.
  - PTT harvest
    - Medial harvest over navicular
    - Posteromedial tibia at musculotendinous junction of PTT
  - PTT transfer through the IOM
    - Incision over distal IOM
    - Incision over dorsolateral foot
  - PTT transfer anterior to tibia
    - Incision over central midfoot
  - Bridle procedure
    - Same PTT harvest
    - PTT transfer through IOM with incision directly anterior over distal tibia; may be extended to dorsal foot. Alternatively, separate small incision over centrodorsal midfoot.
    - Lateral incisions: incision over musculotendinous junction of peroneus longus and another incision over lateral cuboid where peroneus longus courses around cuboid

ACHILLES LENGTHENING

- Indications
  - Not always necessary but typically required when foot drop occurs
    - Without active dorsiflexion, the gastrocnemius–soleus complex's antagonist is lost, often leading to an Achilles contracture.
    - Occasionally, patients maintain an active stretching program, thereby avoiding an Achilles contracture.
  - Weakening of the gastrocnemius–soleus complex may be beneficial because a transfer of a healthy muscle–tendon unit is subject to an automatic one-grade loss of power (5/5 manual muscle testing drops to 4/5 with transfer).
    - Occasionally, we use botulinum toxin in the gastrocnemius–soleus complex when performing a PTT transfer for foot drop.
- Technique
  - Determined by the Silfverskiöld test
    - Equinus contracture with the knee in extension and flexion (TECH FIG 1A)
    - Triple hemisection (Hoke procedure) because both the gastrocnemius and soleus are contracted (TECH FIG 1B–D)
    - Equinus contracture only with the knee in extension: gastrocnemius–soleus recession (Strayer procedure) because only the gastrocnemius is contracted

Posterior Tibial Tendon Transfer Anterior to the Tibia

- Advantages
  - PTT in direct line from its muscle through the IOM to the lateral cuneiform (our preferred site for tendon anchoring)
  - Anchor point slightly lateral of midline to promote dorsiflexion and eversion
- Disadvantage
  - PTT may be constricted and stenosed within narrow window created in distal IOM.

Posterior Tibial Tendon Harvest

- Make a 4-cm longitudinal incision over the medial navicular and PTT on the medial foot.
- Open the PTT sheath to expose the tendon.
- Release the PTT insertion on the medial navicular.
- Alternatively, use a chisel to elevate some medial navicular bone with the PTT release from the medial navicular (may allow for another centimeter of tendon for transfer) (TECH FIG 2A).
- Isolate the PTT attachment on the medial navicular and the tendon fibers that begin to course to the plantar midfoot (TECH FIG 2B).

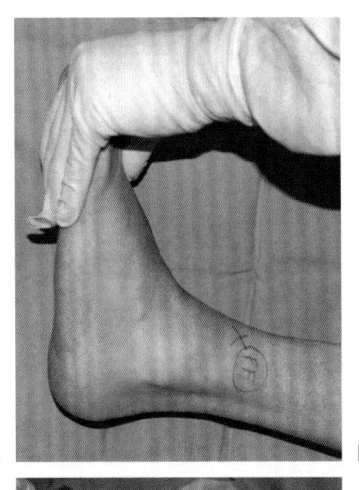
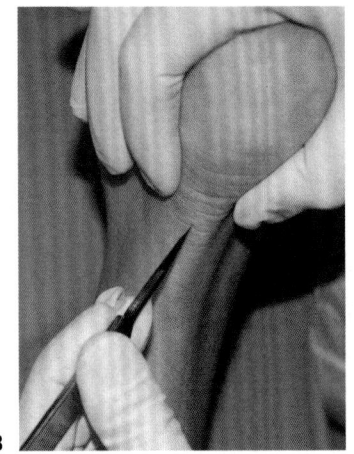
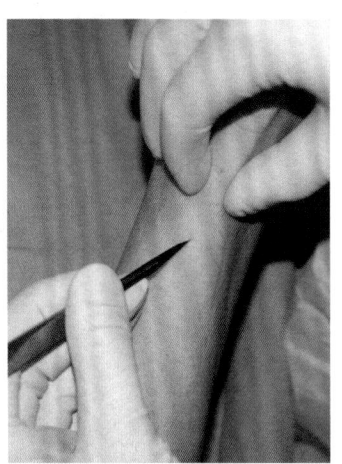

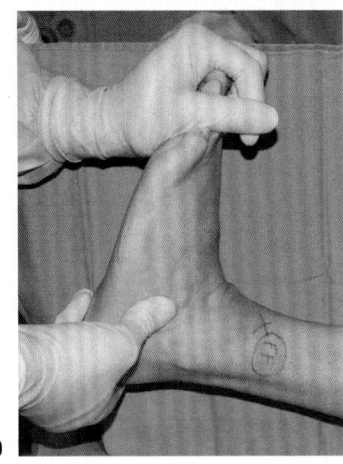

TECH FIG 1 TAL. **A.** Equinus with knee in flexion and extension suggests tight gastrocnemius and soleus. **B.** Initial Achilles hemisection. **C.** Second Achilles hemisection (opposite direction from first), to be followed by third and final hemisection in same direction as first. **D.** Dorsiflexion reestablished after Achilles lengthening.

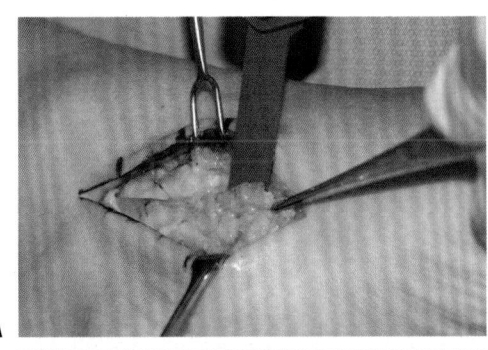
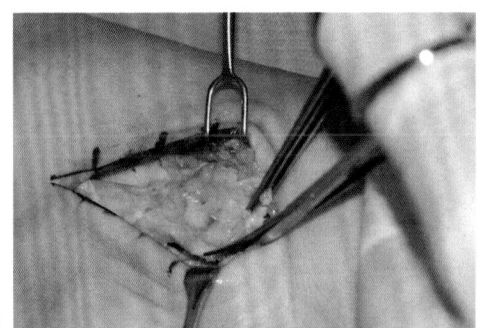

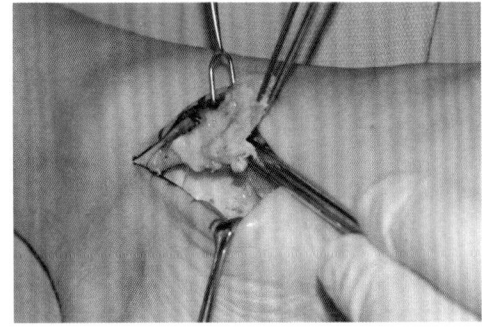

TECH FIG 2 PTT harvest. **A.** Elevating PTT with a sliver of medial navicular may allow longer tendon harvest. **B.** Isolating PTT. **C.** Distal PTT needs to be trimmed to allow it to pass into dorsal foot osseous tunnel. *(continued)*

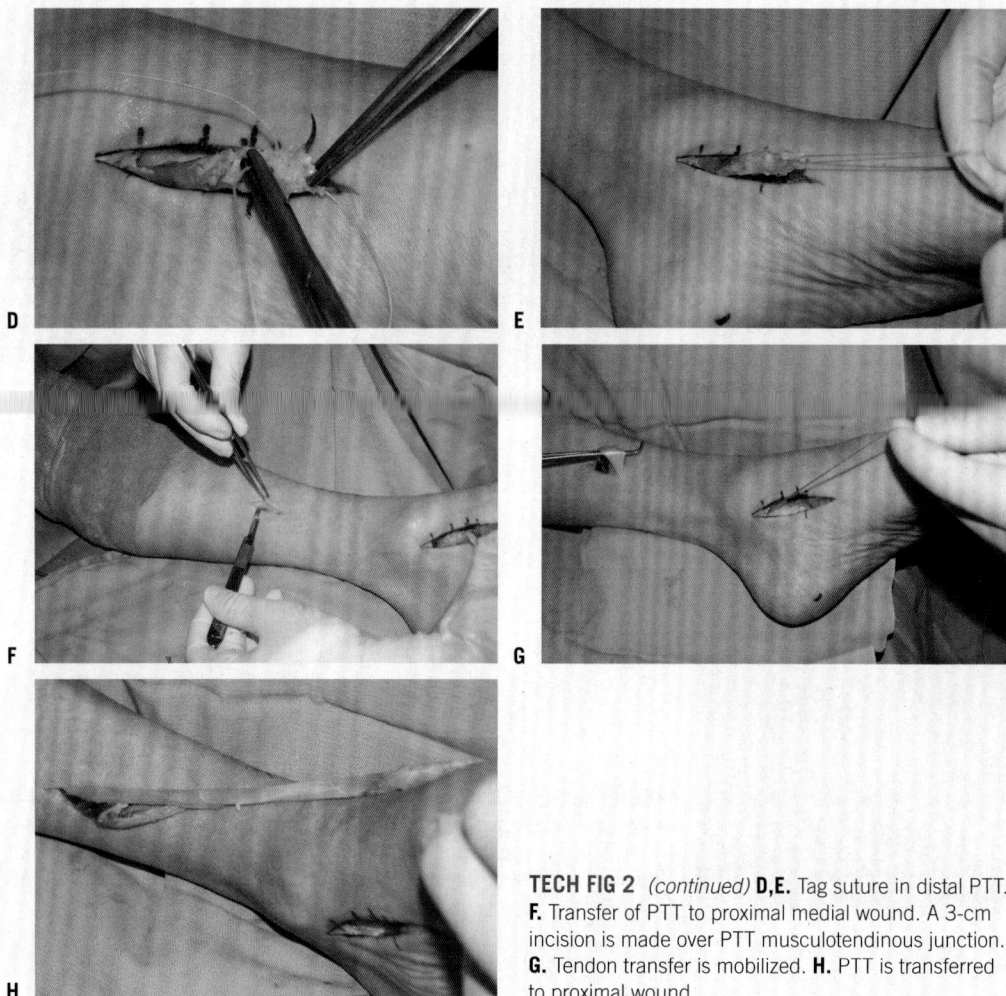

TECH FIG 2 *(continued)* **D,E.** Tag suture in distal PTT. **F.** Transfer of PTT to proximal medial wound. A 3-cm incision is made over PTT musculotendinous junction. **G.** Tendon transfer is mobilized. **H.** PTT is transferred to proximal wound.

- With the PTT fibers isolated, transect them to release the PTT distally.
  - Be sure to fully isolate the PTT fibers; the medial plantar nerve and the plantar medial complex of veins is in close proximity.
    - Accidentally transecting the nerve leads to loss of sensation in the plantar medial forefoot.
    - Violating the veins may make it difficult to achieve satisfactory hemostasis, as these veins may then retract under the foot.
- Thin the distal stump of the PTT to be transferred to facilitate its transfer into an osseous tunnel that will be created in the foot **(TECH FIG 2C)**.
- Place tag sutures in the distal PTT **(TECH FIG 2D,E)**.
- Make a more proximal medial incision at the PTT musculotendinous junction on the posterior tibia.
  - A 3-cm incision **(TECH FIG 2F)**
    - Flexor digitorum tendon is usually encountered first.
    - Deep to the flexor digitorum longus, directly on the posteromedial tibia, the PTT is identified.
    - Place a blunt retractor around the PTT through this more proximal wound to isolate it.

- Mobilize the distal PTT.
  - Alternate tension on the proximal tendon through the proximal wound and the distal tag sutures **(TECH FIG 2G)** and then apply tension proximally only.
  - This may not work.
  - The medial incision may need to be extended proximally to allow access to the posterior medial malleolus, a common location where the tendon may bind.
  - Once mobilized, the distal aspect of the PTT may be transferred to the proximal wound **(TECH FIG 2H)**.
  - Tendon will desiccate rapidly, so we keep it tucked in the proximal medial wound.

Posterior Tibial Tendon Transfer through the Interosseous Membrane

- Lateral incision on anterior aspect of distal fibula, at distal tibio-fibular syndesmosis
- Careful exposure of anterior IOM
  - Elevate the anterior compartment soft tissues
- A branch of the peroneal artery courses on the anterior IOM and is at risk.

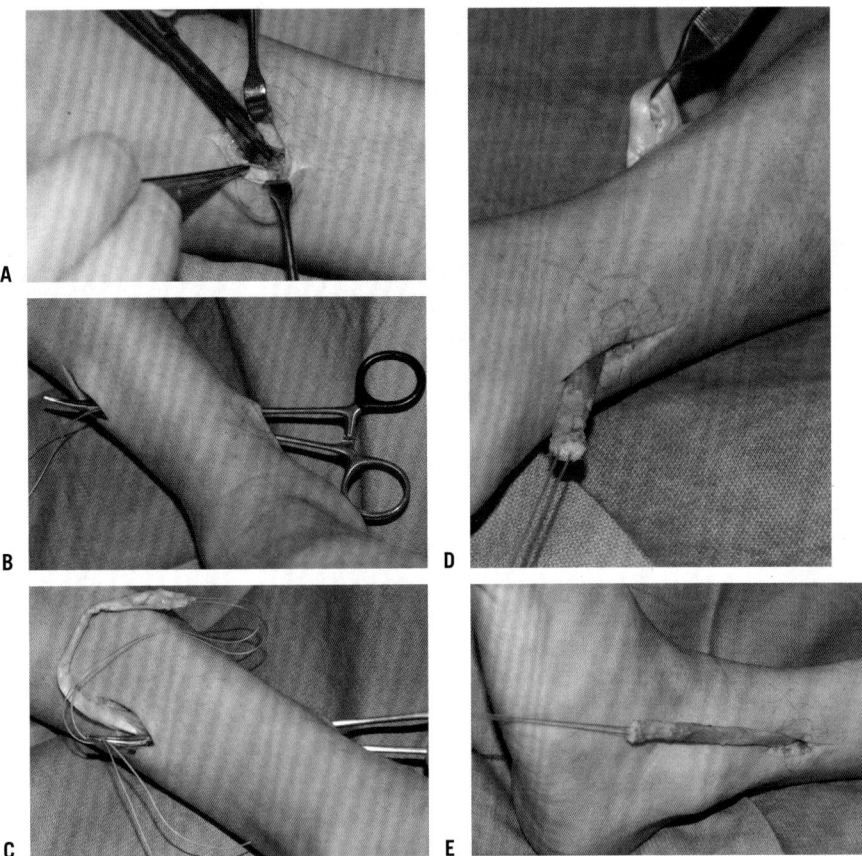

TECH FIG 3 PTT transfer through the IOM. **A.** A window is carefully created in the IOM (perspective with view of lateral distal leg [foot to the left and knee to the right]). **B.** A blunt clamp is passed through IOM, directly on posterior tibia. **C.** PTT tag sutures are grasped. **D.** PTT is transferred to anterolateral wound, with tendon immediately on posterior tibia. **E.** The surgeon must be sure tendon does not bind in IOM window.

- Create a generous window in the distal IOM **(TECH FIG 3A)**.
  - From tibia to fibula
  - About 3 to 4 cm long
- Pass a tonsil clamp through the IOM directly on the posterior aspect of the tibia to exit in the proximal medial wound **(TECH FIG 3B)**.
  - The posterior neurovascular structures (tibial nerve and posterior tibial artery) are at risk, so be sure the clamp is *directly* on the posterior tibia.
- Use the tonsil clamp to grasp the tag sutures of the PTT **(TECH FIG 3C)**.
- Pull the tag sutures and PTT from the medial wound to the lateral wound, keeping the tendon directly on the posterior aspect of the tibia **(TECH FIG 3D,E)**.
- Be sure that the window in the IOM does not impinge on the transferred tendon.
  - If there is stenosis, then further enlarge the window so that the tendon easily glides between the tibia and fibula.
- Keep the tendon end in the wound to limit desiccation.

Preparation of the Dorsal Foot Anchor Site

- Fluoroscopically identify the center of the lateral cuneiform.
  - Oblique foot views usually best define the lateral cuneiform **(TECH FIG 4A)**.
- Center a 3- to 4-cm longitudinal skin incision directly over the lateral cuneiform.

- Dissect to the lateral cuneiform.
  - Protect the superficial peroneal nerve and extensor tendons.
  - Deep neurovascular bundle is usually medial to this approach.
- Expose and define the cuneiform.
  - We routinely use small-gauge hypodermic needles or Kirschner wires to mark the joints surrounding the lateral cuneiform and fluoroscopically confirm that the lateral cuneiform is defined by these markers **(TECH FIG 4B)**.
  - Periosteum and capsular tissue are left intact.
- Create an osseous tunnel in the center of the lateral cuneiform.
  - We routinely predrill the center with a Kirschner wire and confirm the starting point and trajectory of the wire fluoroscopically.
  - Remove the wire and introduce sequentially larger drill bits to enlarge the tunnel **(TECH FIG 4C)**.
    - We use drill bits to a diameter of 4.5 mm.
    - With fluoroscopic confirmation, slight adjustments may be made with each successive drill bit to center the tunnel optimally in the cuneiform.
  - Introduce the reamer system for the interference screw system to enlarge the tunnel to the desired diameter **(TECH FIG 4D)**.
    - Typically, we enlarge the tunnel to 6.5 to 7.0 mm in the lateral cuneiform **(TECH FIG 4E)**.

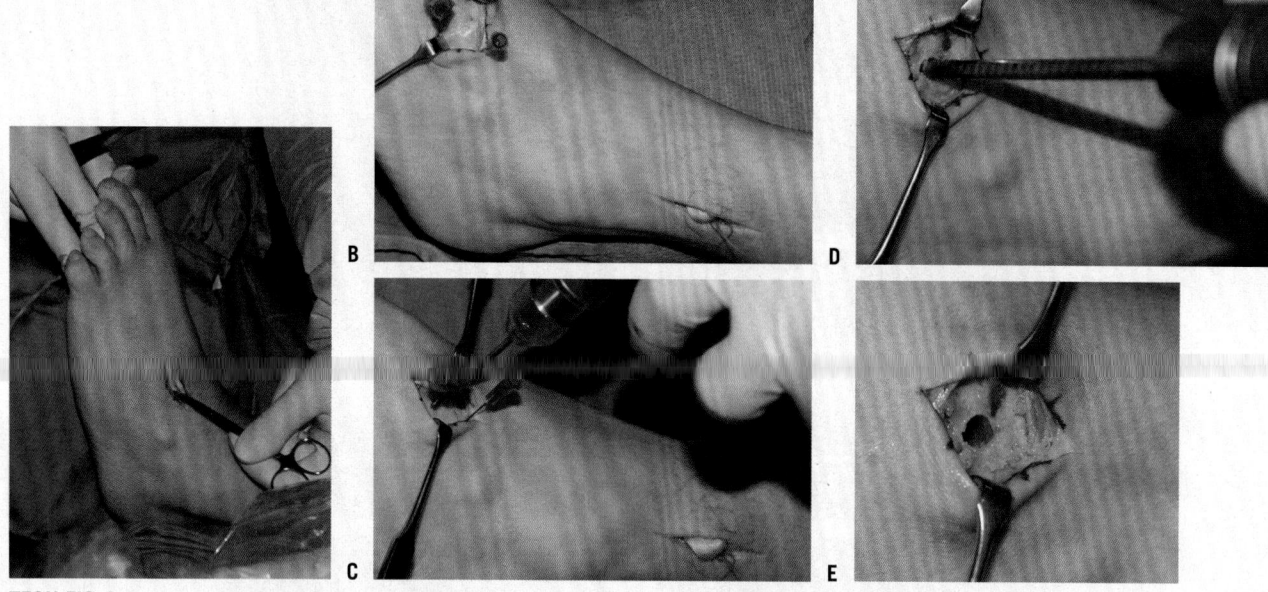

TECH FIG 4 Preparing dorsal foot osseous tunnel. **A.** Lateral cuneiform is identified fluoroscopically. **B.** Borders of lateral cuneiform are exposed and marked. **C.** Drill hole is created in lateral cuneiform, and proper position is confirmed fluoroscopically. **D.** Osseous tunnel is gradually enlarged, first with drill bits and then dedicated reamer system for interference screw. **E.** Prepared osseous tunnel in lateral cuneiform.

Posterior Tibial Tendon Transfer to Dorsum of Foot

- Transferring the PTT deep to the extensor retinaculum with the extensor tendons diminishes the power of the transfer (which is by definition already weakened by one grade with transfer).
- Create a subcutaneous soft tissue tunnel from the dorsal foot incision to the more proximal and lateral lower leg incision using a curved Kelly or tonsil clamp (**TECH FIG 5A**).
- Use the clamp to grasp the tag sutures and pull the tendon through the subcutaneous tunnel to the dorsal foot incision (**TECH FIG 5B**).
- Before anchoring the tendon in the osseous tunnel, pull the tendon via the tag sutures into the tunnel to be sure that the tunnel diameter is appropriate.
  - Pass a Beath pin or drill bit (has an eye to place suture) through the tunnel and the plantar skin (**TECH FIG 5C**).
    - Because of the midfoot arch and the drill hole centered in the lateral cuneiform foot, this pin or the drill bit will exit in the medial arch (**TECH FIG 5D**).
  - Dorsiflex the ankle.
- With the tag sutures secured, pull the pin or drill bit through the plantar skin, thereby pulling the distal tendon end into the tunnel (**TECH FIG 5E**).
    - If the tunnel does not accommodate the tendon, then the tendon and tag sutures must be withdrawn and the tunnel enlarged.
    - Because of the angle at which the tendon enters the tunnel, we often need to guide the tendon into the tunnel with a forceps.
  - Anchoring the tendon to bone
    - Some degree of stretching or accommodation is antici pated, so we routinely anchor the tendon with the ankle

maintained in 10 degrees of dorsiflexion and pull firmly on the plantar suture (**TECH FIG 5F,G**).
- A properly sized isolated interference screw is probably adequate.
- However, we typically augment the anchor point with several nonabsorbable sutures from the periosteum surrounding the tunnel to the tendon directly at the entrance to the tunnel.
- To further augment the anchor point, before advancing the tendon and tag suture into the tunnel, place one or two suture anchors within the tunnel (**TECH FIG 5H,I**). Then, advance the tendon into the tunnel and secure the tendon with the anchors (**TECH FIG 5J,K**). By tightening these sutures, the tendon may be pulled even further into the tunnel (**TECH FIG 5L**). An interference screw and periosteal sutures may still be used (**TECH FIG 5M–O**).
- Have the assistant maintain full ankle dorsiflexion and tension on the tag sutures on the plantar foot.
- We usually cut the tag sutures, so they retract beneath the skin.
- Rarely, we have used a well-padded button on the plantar foot to further augment the tendon's anchor point. We do not routinely do so because of the risk for plantar skin necrosis from the button despite adequate padding.
- In select patients, the dorsiflexed ankle will unmask claw toes due to flexor hallucis longus and flexor digitorum longus contractures. Consider flexor hallucis longus and flexor digitorum longus lengthenings, posterior to the ankle and tibia via the more proximal medial approach, or percutaneous tenotomies at the plantar toes.

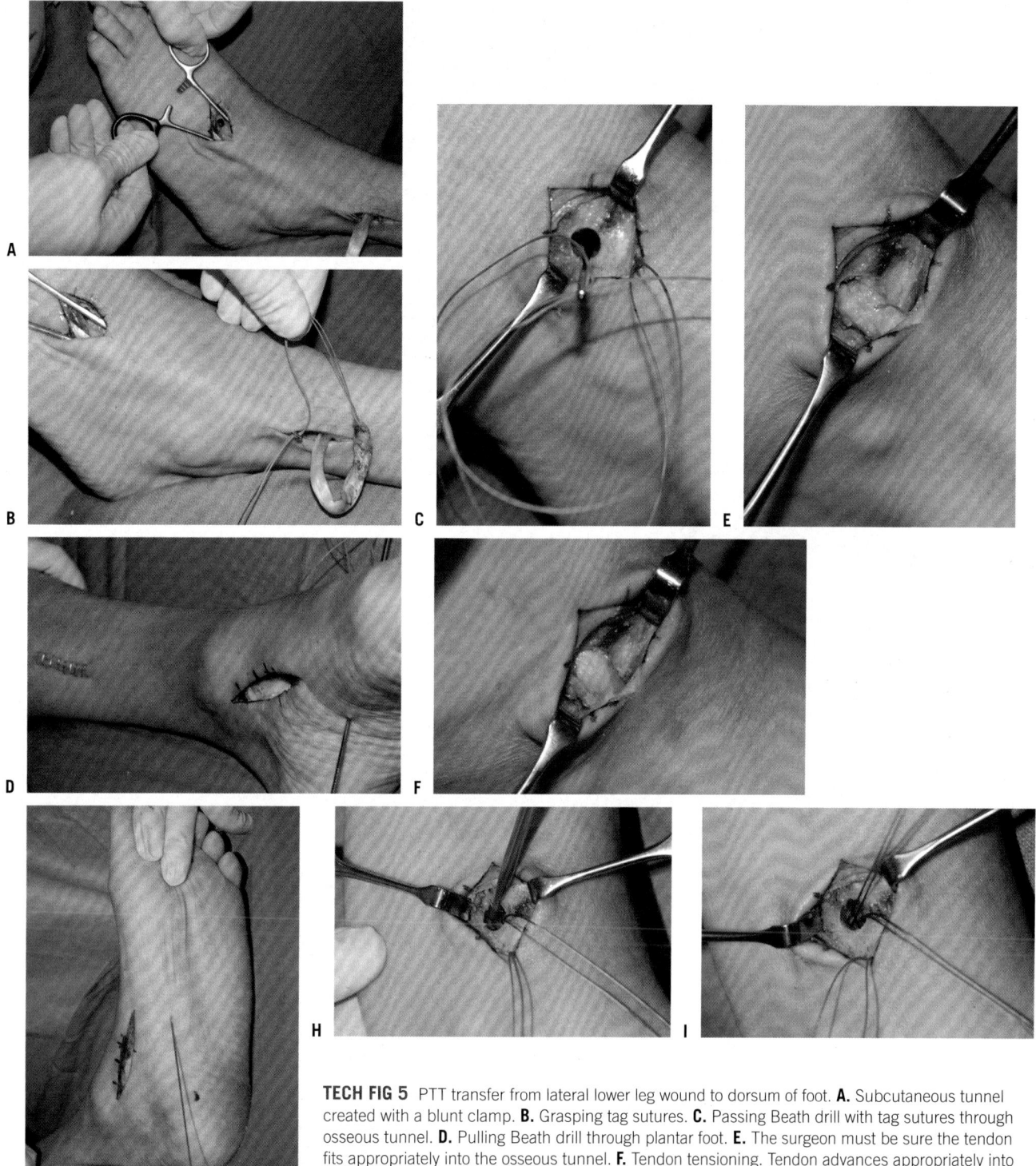

TECH FIG 5 PTT transfer from lateral lower leg wound to dorsum of foot. **A.** Subcutaneous tunnel created with a blunt clamp. **B.** Grasping tag sutures. **C.** Passing Beath drill with tag sutures through osseous tunnel. **D.** Pulling Beath drill through plantar foot. **E.** The surgeon must be sure the tendon fits appropriately into the osseous tunnel. **F.** Tendon tensioning. Tendon advances appropriately into osseous tunnel (note that ankle is held in dorsiflexion). **G.** Tension applied on plantar tag sutures. **H.** Augmenting anchoring. Suture anchor being placed within osseous tunnel. **I.** Two anchors secured in tunnel (note separate tag suture of PTT). *(continued)*

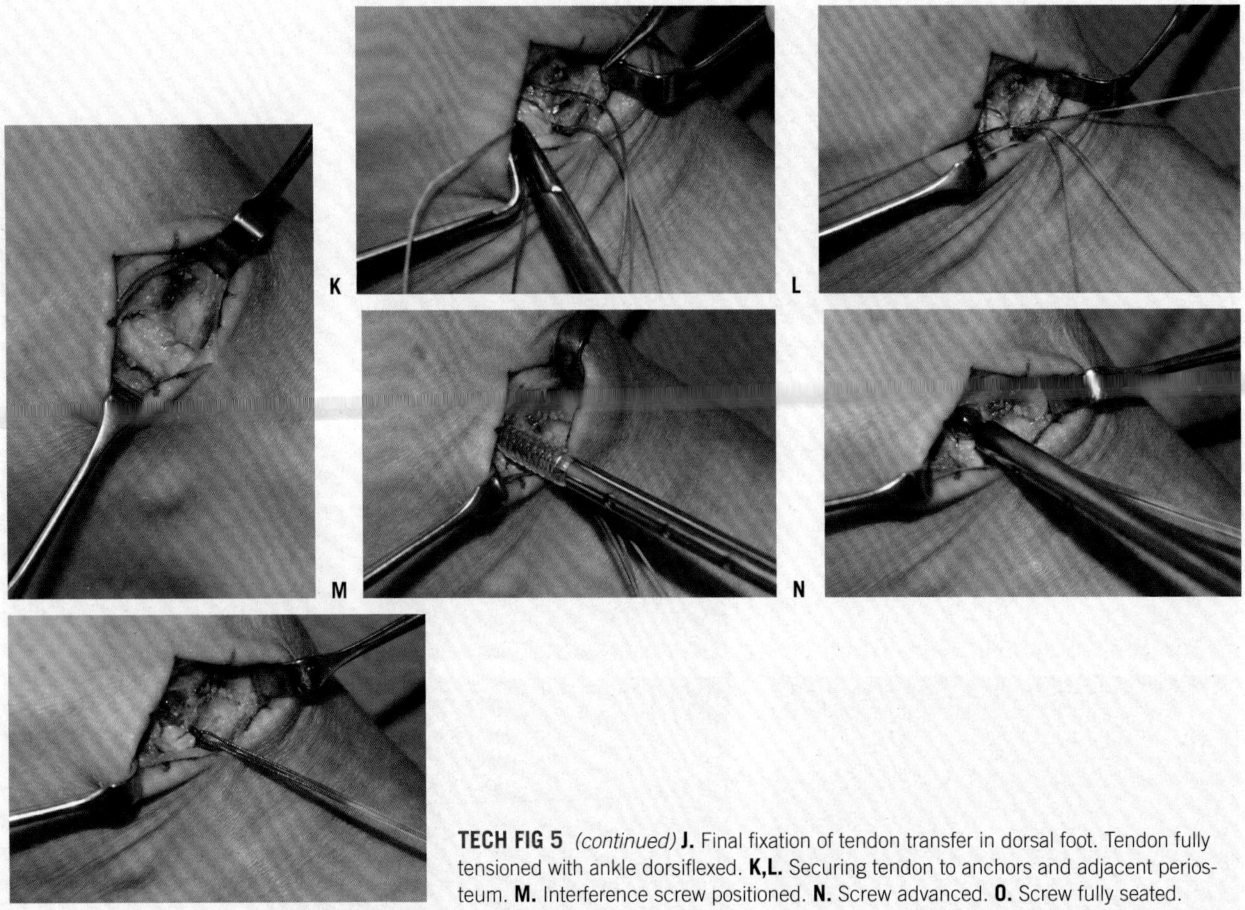

TECH FIG 5 *(continued)* **J.** Final fixation of tendon transfer in dorsal foot. Tendon fully tensioned with ankle dorsiflexed. **K,L.** Securing tendon to anchors and adjacent periosteum. **M.** Interference screw positioned. **N.** Screw advanced. **O.** Screw fully seated.

POSTERIOR TIBIAL TENDON TRANSFER ANTERIOR TO THE TIBIA

- Advantages
  - PTT has no opportunity to stenose in the IOM.
  - Glides smoothly around anteromedial tibia
  - Anchor point slightly lateral of midline to promote dorsiflexion and eversion
- Disadvantage
  - PTT is not in direct line from its origin to anchor point in the foot; it must travel around medial tibia.
  - Anchor point is in the middle (second) cuneiform.
    - Central location so it cannot provide an eversion moment
    - However, typically unimportant because with PTT transfer, the agonist–antagonist balance between PTT and peroneus brevis is again reestablished by being neutralized.

Achilles Lengthening

- Same as for PTT transfer through IOM described earlier **(TECH FIG 6)**

Posterior Tibial Tendon Harvest

- Same as for PTT transfer through IOM described earlier **(TECH FIG 7)**

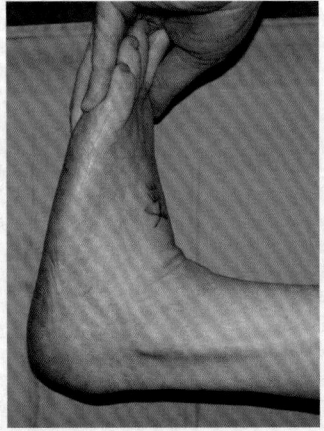

TECH FIG 6 Adequate dorsiflexion (essential for successful tendon transfer to reestablish dorsiflexion).

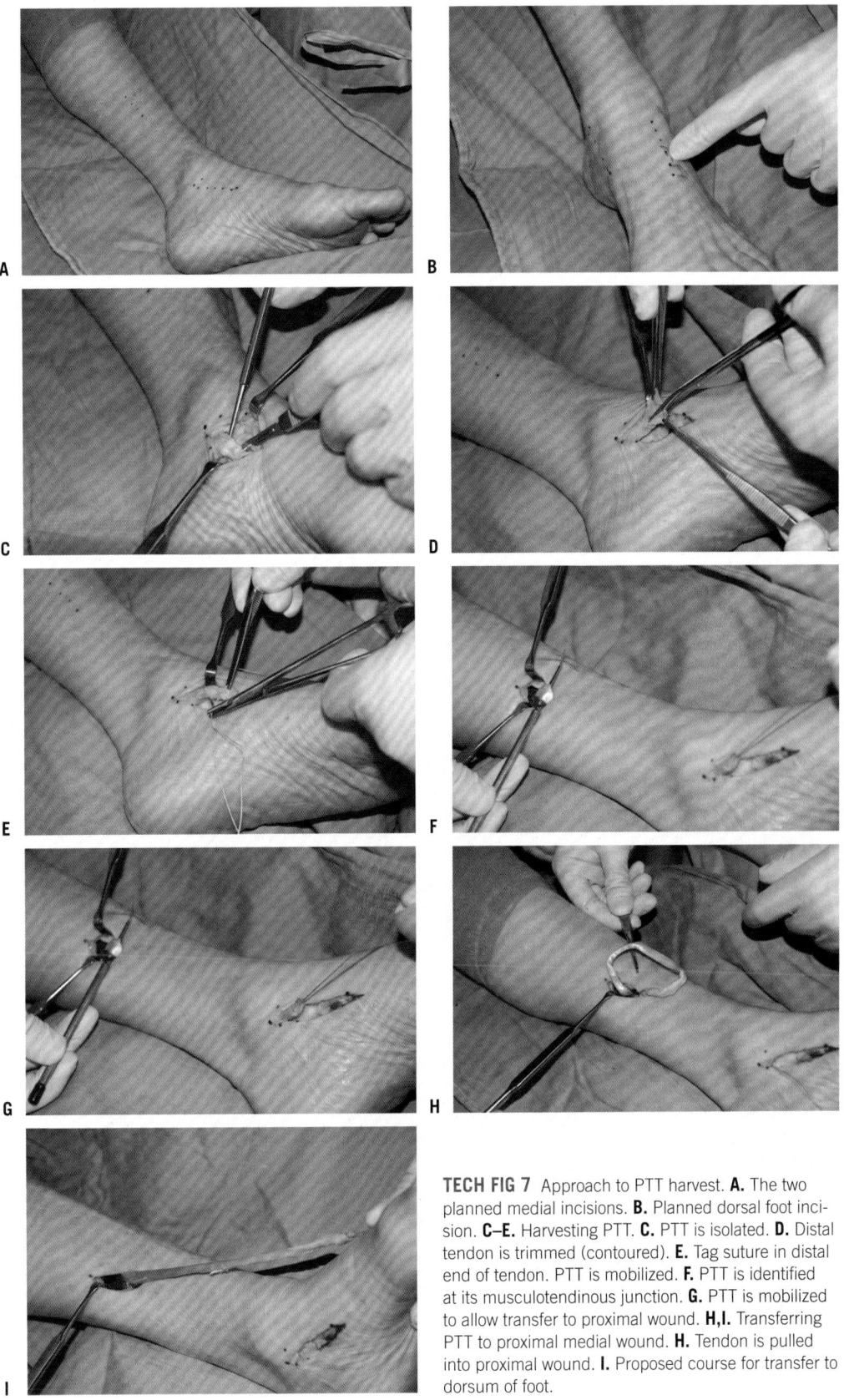

TECH FIG 7 Approach to PTT harvest. **A.** The two planned medial incisions. **B.** Planned dorsal foot incision. **C–E.** Harvesting PTT. **C.** PTT is isolated. **D.** Distal tendon is trimmed (contoured). **E.** Tag suture in distal end of tendon. PTT is mobilized. **F.** PTT is identified at its musculotendinous junction. **G.** PTT is mobilized to allow transfer to proximal wound. **H,I.** Transferring PTT to proximal medial wound. **H.** Tendon is pulled into proximal wound. **I.** Proposed course for transfer to dorsum of foot.

Preparation of the Dorsal Foot Anchor Site

- Similar to preparation of dorsal foot anchor site described earlier for PTT transfer through IOM
  - However, when transferring the PTT through the IOM, we typically anchor the tendon to the lateral (third) cuneiform.
  - In contrast, when we transfer the PTT anterior to the medial tibia, we typically anchor the tendon in the middle (second) cuneiform.
  - Middle cuneiform is smaller than the lateral cuneiform.
    - In our experience, greater risk of fracture with drill hole, tendon transfer, and interference screw
- Fluoroscopically identify the center of the middle cuneiform.
  - Anteroposterior and sometimes oblique foot views best define the middle cuneiform.
- Center a 3- to 4-cm longitudinal skin incision directly over the middle cuneiform.
- Dissect to the middle cuneiform.
  - Protect the superficial peroneal nerve and extensor tendons **(TECH FIG 8A)**.
  - Protect the deep neurovascular bundle, usually encountered in this approach; it is directly deep to the muscle of the extensor hallucis brevis.

- Expose and define the cuneiform.
  - We routinely use small-gauge hypodermic needles or Kirschner wires to mark the joints surrounding the medial cuneiform and fluoroscopically confirm that the medial cuneiform is defined by these markers **(TECH FIG 8B)**.
- Leave the periosteum and capsular tissue intact.
- Create an osseous tunnel in the center of the medial cuneiform.
  - We routinely predrill the center with a Kirschner wire and confirm the starting point and trajectory of the wire fluoroscopically.
  - Remove the wire and introduce sequentially larger drill bits to enlarge the tunnel **(TECH FIG 8C)**.
    - We use drill bits to a diameter of 4.5 mm.
    - With fluoroscopic confirmation, slight adjustments may be made with each successive drill bit to center the tunnel optimally in the cuneiform.
  - Use the reamer from the interference screw system to enlarge the tunnel to the desired diameter **(TECH FIG 8D)**.
- Typically, we enlarge the tunnel from 5.5 to 6.0 mm in the medial cuneiform.

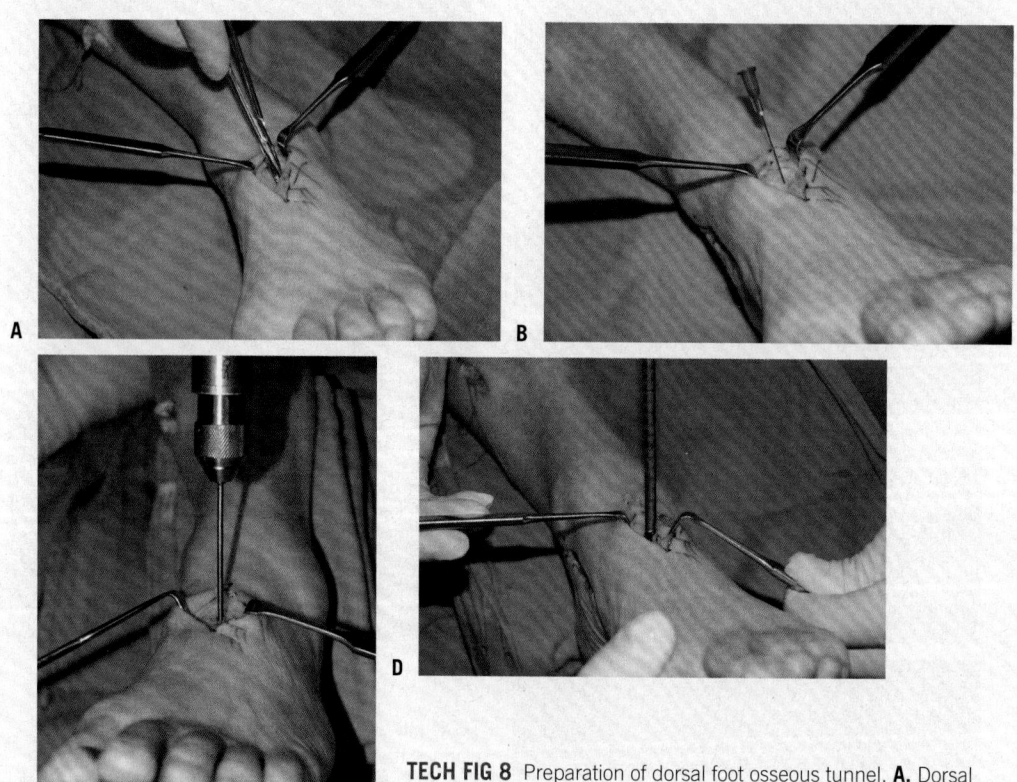

TECH FIG 8 Preparation of dorsal foot osseous tunnel. **A.** Dorsal incision over middle cuneiform. **B.** Middle cuneiform is identified and marked. **C.** Increasingly larger diameter drill bits. **D.** Increasingly larger reamers (judiciously because the middle cuneiform is not particularly large).

Posterior Tibial Tendon Transfer to Dorsum of Foot

- Transferring the PTT deep to the extensor retinaculum with the extensor tendons diminishes the power of the transfer (which is by definition already weakened by one grade with transfer).
- Create a subcutaneous soft tissue tunnel from the dorsal foot incision to the more proximal and medial lower leg incision using a curved Kelly or tonsil clamp **(TECH FIG 9A,B)**.
- Use the clamp to grasp the tag sutures and pull the tendon through the subcutaneous tunnel to the dorsal foot incision.
- Before anchoring the tendon in the osseous tunnel, pull the tendon via the tag sutures into the tunnel to be sure that the tunnel diameter is appropriate.
  - Pass a Beath pin or drill bit (has an eye to place suture) through the tunnel and the plantar skin **(TECH FIG 9C,D)**. Because of the midfoot arch, this pin or drill bit will exit in the medial arch **(TECH FIG 9E)**.
  - Dorsiflex the ankle.
  - With the tag sutures secured, pull the pin or drill bit through the plantar skin, thereby pulling the distal tendon end into the tunnel **(TECH FIG 9F)**.
    - If the tunnel does not accommodate the tendon, then the tendon and tag sutures must be withdrawn and the tunnel enlarged.
  - Because of the angle at which the tendon enters the tunnel, we often need to guide the tendon into the tunnel with a forceps.
- Anchoring the tendon to bone
  - Some degree of stretching or accommodation is anticipated in the posterior tibial muscle and tendon, so we routinely anchor the tendon with the ankle maintained in 10 degrees of dorsiflexion.
  - A properly sized isolated interference screw is probably adequate.
  - However, we typically augment the anchor point with several nonabsorbable sutures from the periosteum surrounding the tunnel to the tendon directly at the entrance to the tunnel.
  - To further augment the anchor point
    - Before advancing the tendon and tag suture into the tunnel, place one or two suture anchors within the tunnel **(TECH FIG 9G)**.
    - Then, advance the tendon into the tunnel and secure the tendon with the anchors. By tightening these sutures, the tendon may be pulled even further into the tunnel. An interference screw and periosteal sutures may still be used **(TECH FIG 9H)**.
- Have the assistant maintain full ankle dorsiflexion and tension on the tag sutures on the plantar foot.
- We usually cut the tag sutures, so they retract beneath the skin.
- Rarely, we have used a well-padded button on the plantar foot to further augment the tendon's anchor point **(TECH FIG 9I)**. We do not routinely do so because of the risk for plantar skin necrosis from the button despite adequate padding.

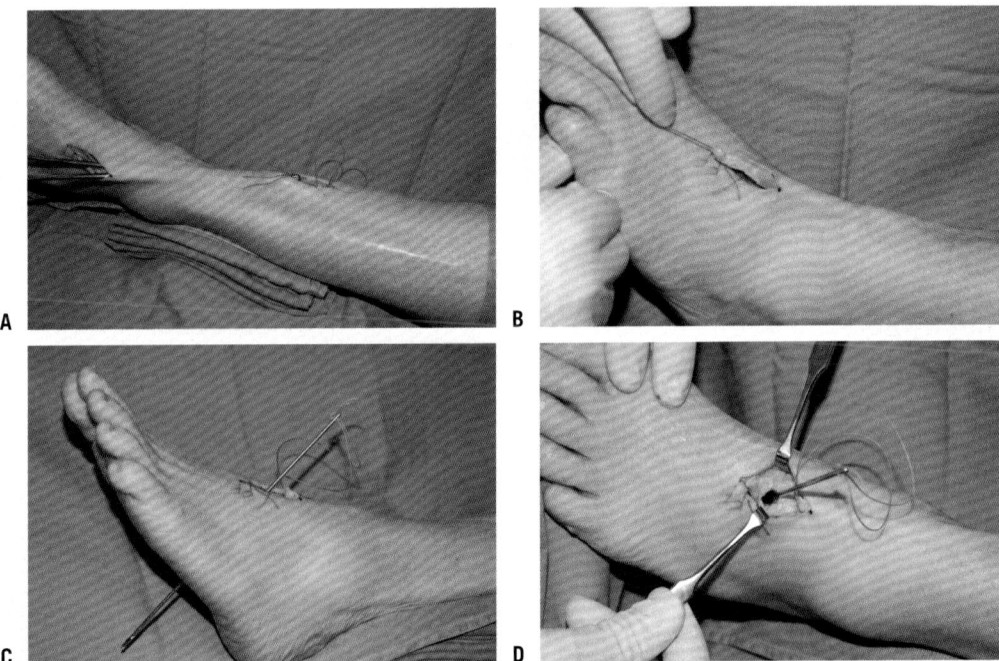

TECH FIG 9 Transfer of PTT to dorsum of foot. **A.** Subcutaneous tunnel for blunt clamp to grasp tag suture in PTT. **B.** PTT is transferred subcutaneously to dorsum of foot. **C–F.** Ensuring that PTT will pass through osseous tunnel in middle cuneiform. **C.** Beath drill through tunnel with tag suture from PTT secured. **D.** Entry point of Beath drill in dorsal tunnel. *(continued)*

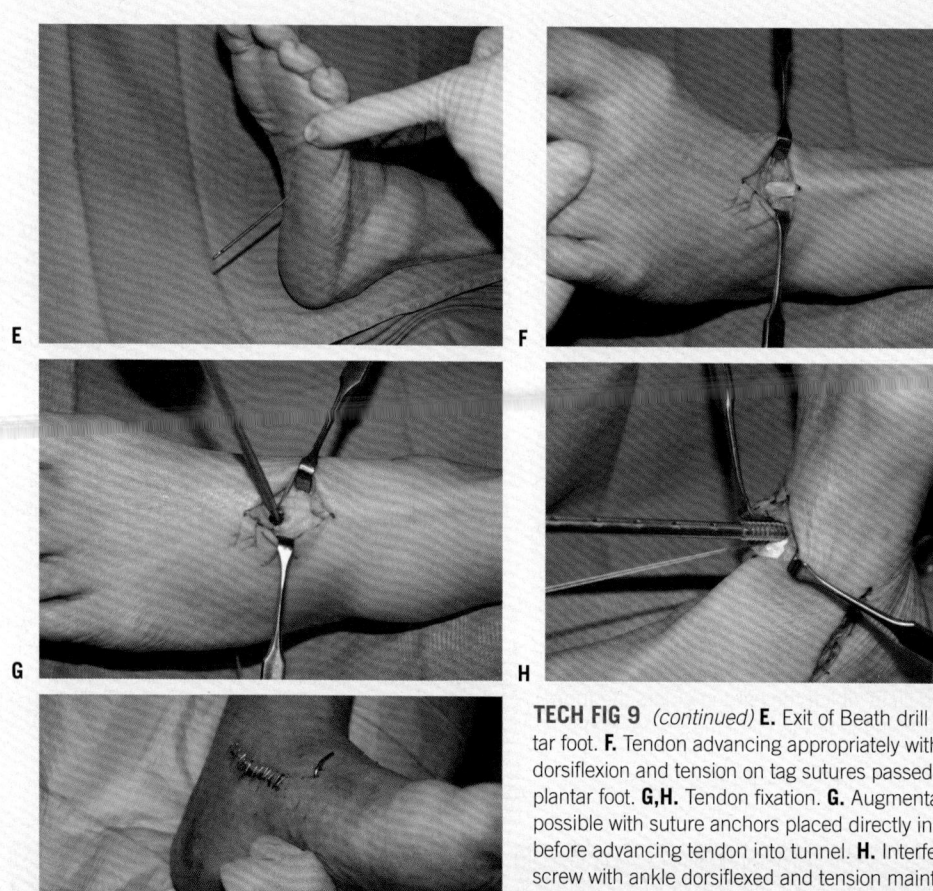

TECH FIG 9 *(continued)* **E.** Exit of Beath drill in plantar foot. **F.** Tendon advancing appropriately with ankle in dorsiflexion and tension on tag sutures passed through plantar foot. **G,H.** Tendon fixation. **G.** Augmentation possible with suture anchors placed directly in tunnel before advancing tendon into tunnel. **H.** Interference screw with ankle dorsiflexed and tension maintained on plantar tag suture. **I.** Suture button. In this case, middle cuneiform fractured with insertion of interference screw, and therefore, a suture button was used. Note also the use of two Kirschner wires in the medial foot to further stabilize fracture in cuneiform.

BRIDLE PROCEDURE

- Advantages
  - The "bridle" creates a balance to the foot and ankle.
  - Potentially can make the patient with flaccid paralysis brace-free
- Disadvantage
  - With flaccid paralysis, the tendon transfer is static, not dynamic.
  - Functions as a tenodesis
    - If procedure is successful, foot and ankle remain in neutral position at all times.

Achilles Lengthening

- Same as for PTT transfer through IOM described earlier

Posterior Tibial Tendon Harvest

- Same as for PTT transfer through IOM described earlier **(TECH FIG 10)**

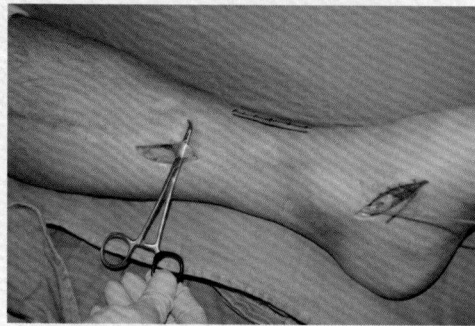

TECH FIG 10 Harvest of PTT for bridle procedure

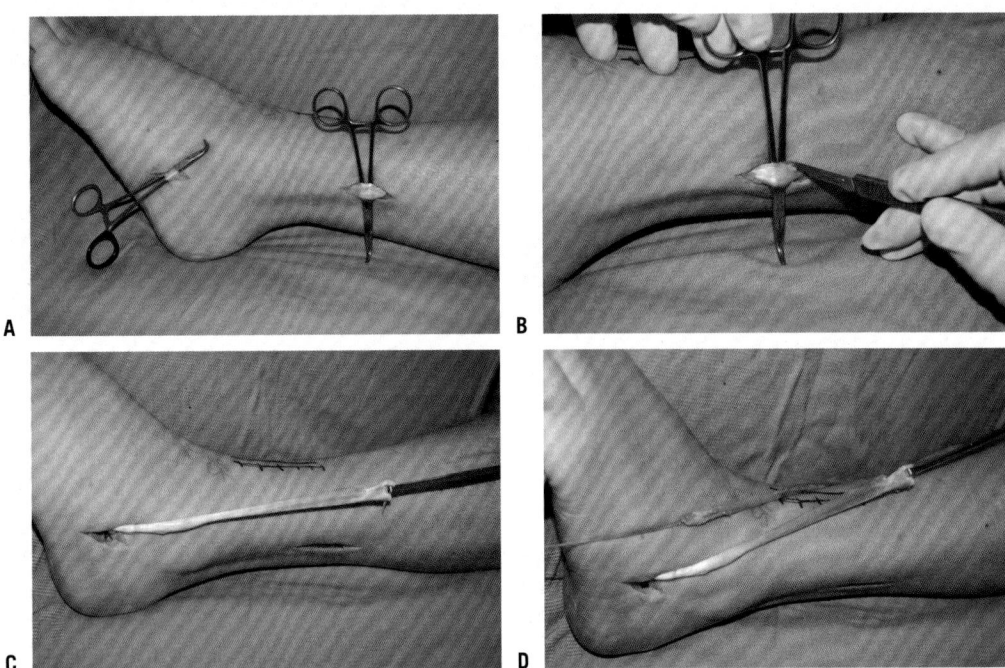

TECH FIG 11 A–C. Harvest of peroneus longus for bridle procedure. **A,B.** Two small incisions, the first at the musculotendinous junction of peroneus longus and the second where the tendon courses around the cuboid. **C.** Peroneus longus transferred to distal lateral incision. **D.** Anticipated course for peroneus longus in bridle procedure (note also approximate course of PTT transfer).

Harvest of the Peroneus Longus

- With an adequate skin bridge from the anterior ankle distal tibial incision, make a 2- to 3-cm incision immediately posterior to the fibula, about 8 cm proximal to the tip of the fibula at the level of the peroneus longus' musculotendinous junction **(TECH FIG 11A)**.
- Protect the superficial peroneal nerve. However, with common peroneal nerve palsy, an injury to this terminal sensory branch will probably be inconsequential.
- Sharply divide the peroneal retinaculum 2 to 3 cm longitudinally over the musculotendinous junction of the peroneus longus.
- Divide the peroneus longus tendon at its musculotendinous junction **(TECH FIG 11B)**.
- Place a tag suture in the transected distal end of the tendon.
- Make another 2- to 3-cm incision over the lateral cuboid (see **TECH FIG 11A**).
  - Protect the sural nerve.
  - Isolate the peroneus longus tendon and pull its released proximal portion through this lateral foot wound **(TECH FIG 11C,D)**.
- Tuck the peroneus longus tendon in the distal lateral foot wound to keep it from desiccating.
- The peroneus longus tendon will be passed to the anterior ankle wound (see in the following text).

Posterior Tibial Tendon Transfer through the Interosseous Membrane

- Make an incision over the lateral aspect of the distal anterior tibia.
- Carefully expose the anterior IOM **(TECH FIG 12A)**.

- Protect the superficial peroneal nerve.
  - Divide the extensor retinaculum over the tibialis anterior and extensor hallucis longus tendons.
  - Protect the deep neurovascular bundle **(TECH FIG 12B)**.
- Protect the peroneal artery branch that courses on the anterior IOM.
- Create a generous window in the distal IOM **(TECH FIG 12C)**.
  - From tibia to fibula
  - About 4 cm long
- Pass a curved Kelly or tonsil clamp through the IOM directly on the posterior aspect of the tibia to exit in the proximal medial wound **(TECH FIG 12D)**.
  - The posterior neurovascular structures (tibial nerve and posterior tibial artery) are at risk, so be sure the clamp is *directly* on the posterior tibia.
- Use the tonsil clamp to grasp the tag sutures of the PTT.
- Pull the tag sutures and PTT from the medial wound to the lateral wound, keeping the tendon directly on the posterior aspect of the tibia **(TECH FIG 12E)**.
- Be sure that the window in the IOM does not impinge on the transferred tendon. If there is stenosis, then further enlarge the window so that the tendon easily glides between the tibia and fibula.
- Keep the tendon end in the wound to limit desiccation.

Transfer of the Peroneus Longus

- Using a Kelly clamp, create a subcutaneous tunnel from the anterior distal tibial wound to the lateral foot wound **(TECH FIG 13A)**.
  - Spread this tissue carefully with the clamp to avoid any soft tissue impingement within the tunnel.
  - Grasp the tag suture in the peroneus longus and pull the tendon from the lateral foot wound to the anterior distal tibial wound **(TECH FIG 13B)**.

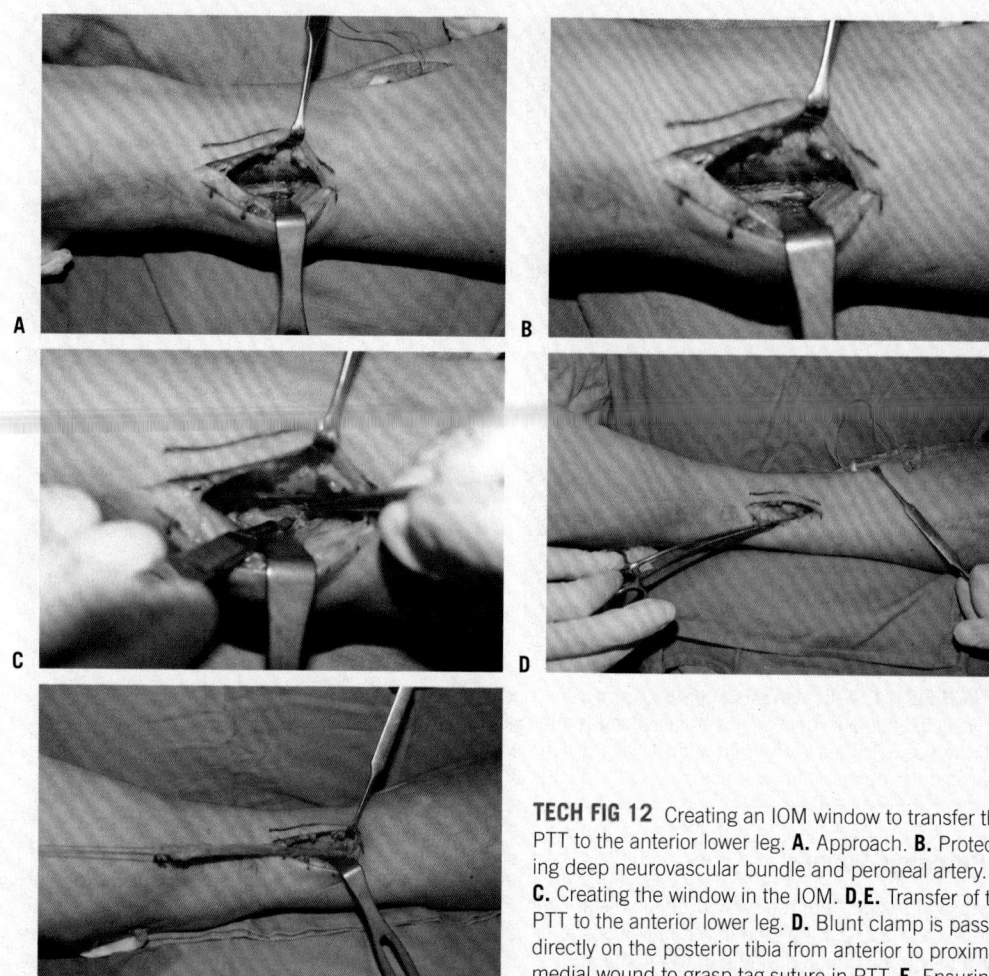

TECH FIG 12 Creating an IOM window to transfer the PTT to the anterior lower leg. **A.** Approach. **B.** Protecting deep neurovascular bundle and peroneal artery. **C.** Creating the window in the IOM. **D,E.** Transfer of the PTT to the anterior lower leg. **D.** Blunt clamp is passed directly on the posterior tibia from anterior to proximal medial wound to grasp tag suture in PTT. **E.** Ensuring that the tendon does not bind in the IOM window.

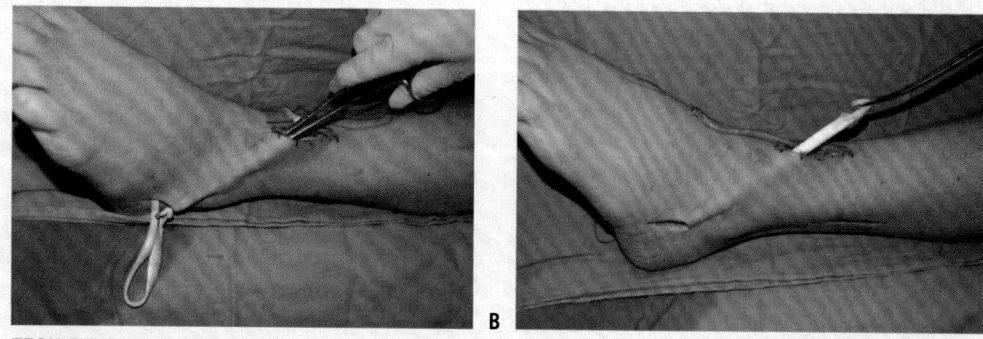

TECH FIG 13 Transferring peroneus longus tendon from distal lateral foot wound to anterior lower leg wound. **A.** Subcutaneous tunnel to grasp free end of peroneus longus. **B.** Tendon transferred.

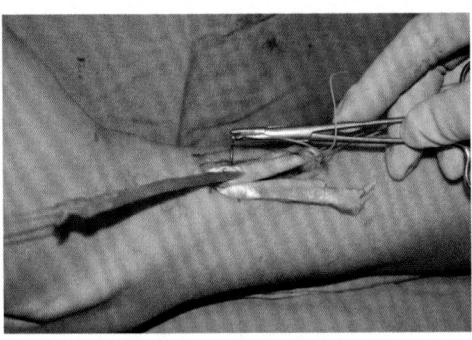

TECH FIG 14 PTT is transferred through the tibialis anterior. Note the pretensioning of the tibialis anterior to optimize tension in the bridle.

Transfer of Posterior Tibial Tendon through the Tibialis Anterior Tendon

- Make a stab incision in the tibialis anterior tendon with proximal tension placed on the tibialis anterior tendon while the ankle is held in dorsiflexion.
  - This will tension the distal extent of the tibialis anterior tendon before it is secured to the PTT.
  - Avoid simply creating an incision in the tibialis anterior tendon in situ; this will render the tension in the medial aspect of the bridle ineffective.
- Pass the PTT through this stab incision in the tibialis anterior **(TECH FIG 14)**.
- If a more secure fixation between the tibialis anterior and PTT is desired, then consider a Pulvertaft weave.
  - Although more weaving of the PTT through the tibialis anterior may afford greater fixation, it may in turn diminish the excursion of the PTT, thereby limiting the amount of distal PTT that will rest within the middle cuneiform's osseous tunnel.

Preparation of the Dorsum of the Foot and Anchoring the Posterior Tibial Tendon

- Similar to that described for PTT transfer anterior to the tibia (see earlier)
  - Transfer to the middle cuneiform
- A separate incision may be made (two limited incisions anteriorly) or the anterior distal tibial approach may be extended to the dorsum of the foot (single extensile anterior incision).
- Create an osseous tunnel in the middle cuneiform **(TECH FIG 15A)**.
- Create a subcutaneous soft tissue tunnel from the dorsal foot incision to the more proximal and anterior lower leg incision using a curved Kelly clamp.
- Use the clamp to grasp the tag sutures and pull the tendon through the subcutaneous tunnel to the dorsal foot incision **(TECH FIG 15B)**.
- Before anchoring the tendon in the osseous tunnel, pull the tendon via the tag sutures into the tunnel to be sure that the tunnel diameter is appropriate.
  - Pass a Beath pin or drill bit (has an eye to place suture) through the tunnel and the plantar skin **(TECH FIG 15C)**. Because of the midfoot arch, this pin or drill bit will exit in the medial arch **(TECH FIG 15D)**.
  - Dorsiflex the ankle.
  - With the tag sutures secured, pull the pin or drill bit through the plantar skin, thereby pulling the distal tendon end into the tunnel **(TECH FIG 15E)**.
- With the PTT properly tensioned in the second cuneiform's osseous tunnel, the PTT is anchored in a manner similar to that described earlier for the other techniques (interference screw with or without suture anchor in tunnel) **(TECH FIG 15F,G)**.

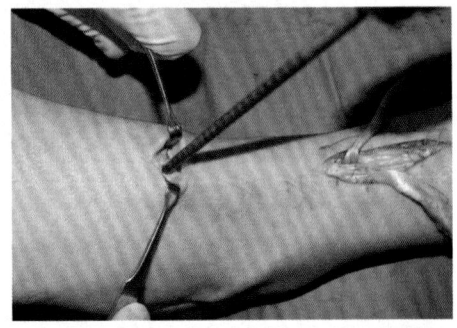

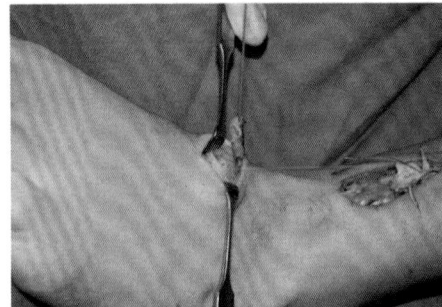

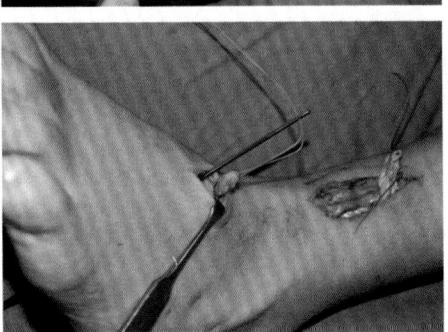

TECH FIG 15 A. Creating the osseous tunnel in middle cuneiform. **B–G.** Transferring PTT from anterior lower leg wound to dorsum of foot. **B.** Tendon passed through subcutaneous tunnel to dorsum of foot. **C.** Beath needle with tag sutures from PTT passed through osseous tunnel. *(continued)*

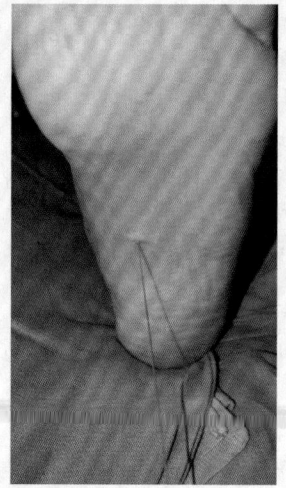 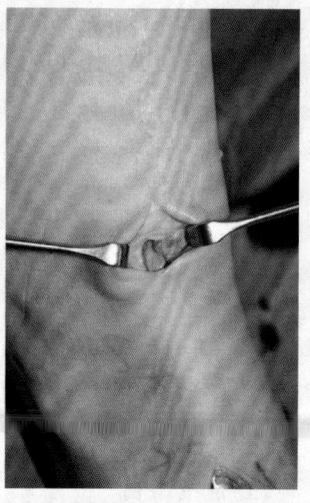 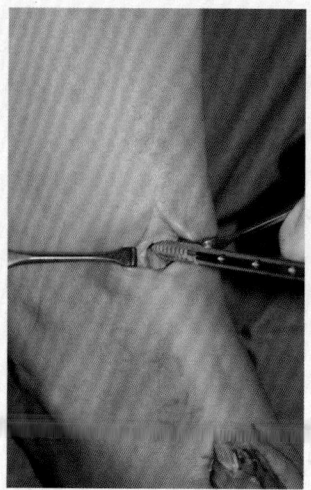 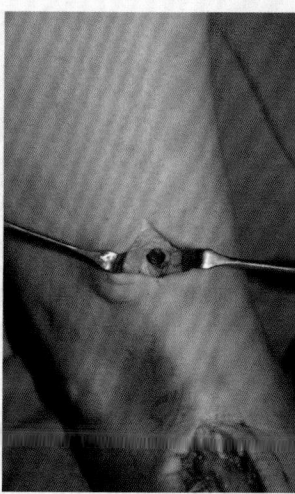

TECH FIG 15 *(continued)* **D.** Tension on tag sutures on plantar foot. **E.** Tendon passed into middle cuneiform osseous tunnel. **F.** Positioning interference screw. **G.** Interference screw fully seated with appropriate PTT tension achieved.

Securing and Tensioning Tibialis Anterior and Peroneus Longus to the Posterior Tibial Tendon

- Maintain the ankle in 10 degrees of dorsiflexion.
- Balance the foot with respect to varus or valgus; it should have a neutral to slight valgus heel.
- Tibialis anterior
  - Tension the tibialis anterior proximally and suture the tibialis anterior and PTT to one another at the point where the PTT passes through the tibialis anterior.
  - Reinforce this connection with several more side-to-side sutures between the two tendons, both proximal and distal to where the PTT passes through the tibialis anterior.
- Peroneus longus
  - Approximate the peroneus longus to the PTT where it passes anterior to the distal tibia and ankle, with maximum tension applied **(TECH FIG 16)**.
- Without support, the ankle should maintain dorsiflexed ankle and neutral hindfoot positions.

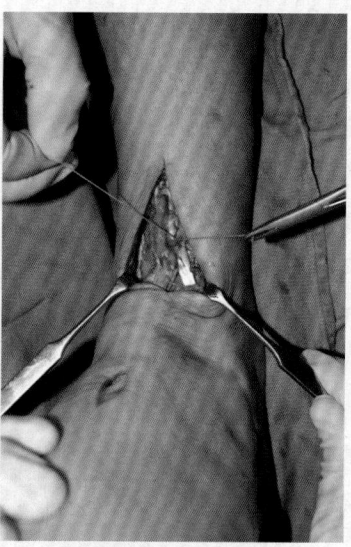

TECH FIG 16 With the foot balanced, tibialis anterior and peroneus longus are secured to PTT transfer to create the bridle.

TECHNIQUES

Pearls and Pitfalls

Tension of Tendon Transfer	• Overtension rather than undertension, as some "stretching out" of the transfer is anticipated
Achilles Lengthening	• The threshold to lengthen the gastrocnemius–soleus complex should be low. Obviously, with an Achilles contracture, lengthening is warranted. Transferring the PTT immediately reduces its power by one grade, so weakening the transfer's antagonist may be prudent. Overlengthening must be avoided.
Residual Muscle Function	• Be sure the PTT is fully functional; if not, the transfer will not be dynamic but instead simply a tenodesis. This is the objective in flaccid paralysis but not for a foot drop secondary to a common peroneal nerve palsy.

Route of PTT Transfer	• PTT transfer through the IOM may lead to stenosis. Provided there is no residual peroneal (eversion) function, then transferring the PTT anterior to the tibia may lead to an effective transfer without the risk of stenosis.
Bridle Procedure	• Balance the foot with proper tensioning of the tibialis anterior and peroneus longus components of the transfer.
Anchoring the Transfer	• With newer anchoring techniques, placing a suture button on the plantar foot secured to the tag suture is typically unnecessary.

POSTOPERATIVE CARE

- We routinely place a well-padded short-leg cast in the operating room to protect the transfer, with the ankle in maximum dorsiflexion.
- At first follow-up (2 to 3 weeks), we remove the cast while maintaining ankle dorsiflexion.
  - To protect the transfer, the ankle should not be allowed to plantarflex.
  - A new short-leg cast is applied, one that allows touchdown weight bearing.
- Follow-up at 5 to 6 weeks from surgery.
  - The short-leg cast is removed, again protecting dorsiflexion.
  - Wound inspection
    - Without allowing the ankle to plantarflex, the cast is removed.
  - Consideration may be given to creating a temporary AFO.
  - We typically place the patient in a short-leg walking cast at this point, with the ankle in near-maximum dorsiflexion. The patient is encouraged to walk.
- At 8 to 10 weeks
  - The patient can typically discontinue use of the cast.
  - AFO for ambulation is typically worn until 4 to 5 months after surgery. During the final month of brace wear, the surgeon can consider hinging the AFO and placing a plantarflexion stop at neutral.
  - A CAM boot is used for sleeping; it is typically worn until 4 to 5 months after surgery.
  - A physical therapy program is initiated to train the PTT to function as an ankle dorsiflexor.
- Return to brace-free full function is not recommended before 6 months.

OUTCOMES

- Select case series of PTT transfers for foot drop and bridle procedures suggest a satisfactory outcome in a majority of cases.

COMPLICATIONS

- Infection
- Wound dehiscence. The wound must be healed before initiating active dorsiflexion (usually not a problem because cast is maintained for at least 8 weeks).
- Failure of the tendon transfer anchoring point; less common with newer anchoring system
- Imbalance of bridle procedure: Tibialis anterior and peroneus longus must be properly tensioned intraoperatively.

SUGGESTED READINGS

Cho BK, Park KJ, Choi SM, et al. Functional outcomes following anterior transfer of the tibialis posterior tendon for foot drop secondary to peroneal nerve palsy. Foot Ankle Int 2017;38(6):627–633.

Dreher T, Wolf SI, Heitzmann D, et al. Tibialis posterior tendon transfer corrects the foot drop component of cavovarus foot deformity in Charcot-Marie-Tooth disease. J Bone Joint Surg Am 2014;96(6):456–462.

Elsner A, Barg A, Stufkens SA, et al. Lambrinudi arthrodesis with posterior tibialis transfer in adult drop-foot. Foot Ankle Int 2010;31:30–37.

Hove LM, Nilsen PT. Posterior tibial tendon transfer for drop-foot. 20 cases followed for 1-5 years. Acta Orthop Scand 1998;69:608–610.

Johnson JE, Paxton ES, Lippe J, et al. Outcomes of the bridle procedure for the treatment of foot drop. Foot Ankle Int 2015;36(11):1287–1296.

Mizel MS, Temple HT, Scranton PE Jr, et al. Role of the peroneal tendons in the production of the deformed foot with posterior tibial tendon deficiency. Foot Ankle Int 1999;20:285–289.

Molund M, Engebretsen L, Hvaal K, et al. Posterior tibial tendon transfer improves function for foot drop after knee dislocation. Clin Orthop Relat Res 2014;472(9):2637–2643.

Morita S, Muneta T, Yamamoto H, et al. Tendon transfer for equinovarus deformed foot caused by cerebrovascular disease. Clin Orthop Relat Res 1998;(350):166–173.

Rodriguez RP. The Bridle procedure in the treatment of paralysis of the foot. Foot Ankle 1992;13:63–69.

Schweitzer KM Jr, Jones CP. Tendon transfers for the drop foot. Foot Ankle Clin 2014;19(1):65–71.

Soares D. Tibialis posterior transfer for the correction of foot drop in leprosy. Long-term outcome. J Bone Joint Surg Br 1996;78(1):61–62.

Sundararaj GD. Tibialis posterior transfer (circumtibial route) for foot-drop deformity. Indian J Lepr 1984;56:555–562.

Wagner E, Wagner P, Zanolli D, et al. Biomechanical evaluation of circumtibial and transmembranous routes for posterior tibial tendon transfer for dropfoot. Foot Ankle Int 2018;39(7):843–849.

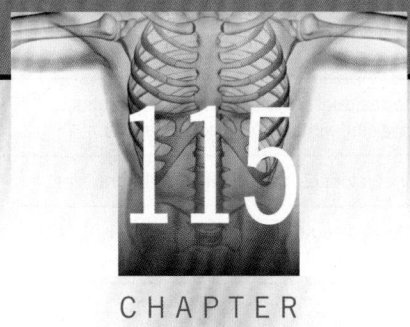

115
CHAPTER

Surgical Management of Proximal Fifth Metatarsal Fractures

Jeannie Huh and Mark E. Easley

DEFINITION

- The fifth metatarsal is the most frequently fractured metatarsal bone. Of these, proximal fractures are the most common.[10]
- Proximal fifth metatarsal fractures are traditionally classified into three types, based on the zone or location of the fracture (FIG 1):
  - Zone I: tuberosity avulsion fracture that may extend to the fifth metatarsal–cuboid articulation
  - Zone II: classic "Jones fracture" at the metaphyseal–diaphyseal junction that extends into, but not beyond, the fourth and fifth intermetatarsal articulation
  - Zone III: proximal diaphyseal stress fracture
- Identifying the correct zone is important because the healing characteristics and management differ for fractures occurring in each.

ANATOMY

- The fifth metatarsal consists of a head, diaphysis, metaphysis, and tuberosity.
- The tuberosity is the most proximal and plantar structure of the fifth metatarsal.
- Proximally, the fifth metatarsal has articulations with the cuboid and fourth metatarsal.
- There are four main soft tissue attachments to the proximal aspect of the fifth metatarsal:
  - The peroneus brevis tendon inserts on the dorsolateral tuberosity.
  - The peroneus tertius tendon attaches on the dorsal aspect of the metaphysis.

- The lateral band of the plantar fascia attaches to the plantar aspect of the fifth metatarsal base.
- Dorsal, plantar, and interosseus ligaments attach between the bases of the fourth and fifth metatarsals.
- Blood supply to the proximal fifth metatarsal is derived from two sources (FIG 2):
  - Metaphyseal vessels supply the tuberosity.
  - An intramedullary nutrient artery enters from the medial cortex at the proximal diaphysis and flows retrograde, terminating at the metaphyseal–diaphyseal junction.
  - The region at which these blood vessels converge corresponds to a relatively avascular watershed area, making it a tenuous area for healing.[15]
- The dorsolateral branch of the sural nerve usually lies approximately 2 to 3 mm proximal to the tuberosity and often courses at the incision site used for surgical fixation.[5]
- The peroneus longus courses lateral to and then plantar to the cuboid, immediately proximal to the fifth metatarsal base (FIG 3).

PATHOGENESIS

- Different mechanisms of injury have been associated with the different fracture zones:
  - Zone I (tuberosity) fractures result from forces exerted on the peroneus brevis tendon or the lateral band of the plantar fascia with foot inversion.
  - Zone II (Jones) fractures result from an indirect, large adduction force applied to the forefoot with the ankle in plantarflexion.
    - The ligaments at the base of the fourth and fifth metatarsals are resistant to displacement, resulting in fracture just distal to them, at the level of the fourth and fifth intermetatarsal joints.
  - Zone III (diaphyseal stress) fractures result from overuse or overload injuries.
    - These injuries may be acute or chronic.
- Underlying hindfoot varus alignment has been implicated in overloading the lateral foot and is considered a predisposing factor for proximal fifth metatarsal fractures as well as nonunion and refracture if not addressed at the time of surgical stabilization.[13]

NATURAL HISTORY

- Zone I (tuberosity) fractures nearly always heal with conservative management alone. Although patients can expect to return to their preinjury level of function, recovery may take 6 months or longer.[7]

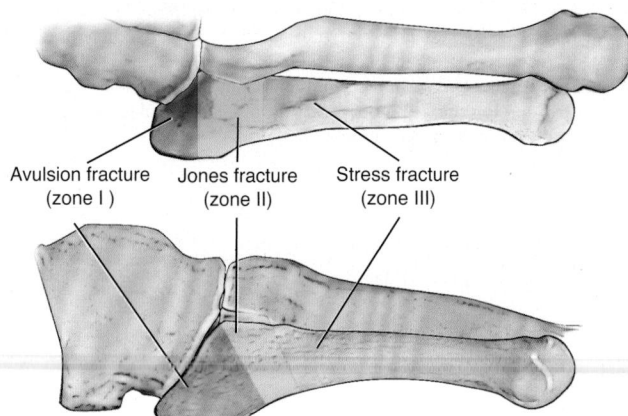

Avulsion fracture (zone I) Jones fracture (zone II) Stress fracture (zone III)

FIG 1 Three anatomic zones of the proximal fifth metatarsal with corresponding fracture types.

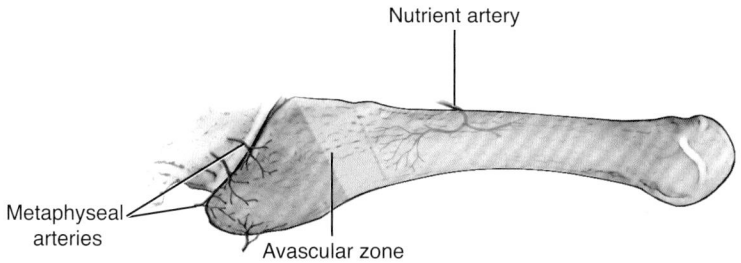

FIG 2 Vascular supply to the proximal fifth metatarsal. Note the watershed segment between the metaphyseal arteries and the intramedullary nutrient artery located at the metaphyseal–diaphyseal junction (zone II), where fractures are notoriously at high risk for delayed union and nonunion.

- Zone II (Jones) fractures are notorious for a high incidence of delayed union and nonunion (up to 28%)[2] when treated conservatively and are thought to be due to their tenuous location:
  - Relatively avascular watershed zone
  - The peroneus brevis and the lateral band of the plantar fascia cause continued motion at the fracture site despite immobilization.
- Zone III (diaphyseal stress) fractures are also notorious for their protracted healing time and risk of nonunion (shown to develop in up to 25% of nonoperatively treated cases).[3]

PATIENT HISTORY AND PHYSICAL FINDINGS

- History
  - Usually entails injury to the foot during sports activity, especially basketball or football
  - In the nonathlete, tripping off a curb with the foot inverted is a common mechanism.
  - In the setting of an overuse injury, the patient may describe prodromal symptoms.
  - The patient will complain of painful weight bearing and tenderness over the lateral border of the foot that is reproducible with direct palpation.
- Physical examination
  - Swelling and ecchymosis over the lateral border of the foot is often present.
  - Pain and/or weakness with eversion may be noted.
  - Evaluate for potential sources of lateral foot overload (ie, hindfoot varus), which can have implications on

healing after fixation of a proximal fifth metatarsal fracture, if not simultaneously addressed.
- Assess for signs of Lisfranc injury with direct palpation over the tarsometatarsal joint complex and presence of plantar ecchymosis.

IMAGING AND OTHER DIAGNOSTIC STUDIES

- Anteroposterior (AP), lateral, and oblique radiographs of the affected foot are sufficient to diagnose a proximal fifth metatarsal fracture **(FIG 4A–C)**.
- If there is suspicion for Lisfranc injury, weight-bearing radiographs of the affected foot should be obtained.
- Computed tomography (CT) scan is rarely indicated but may assist in differentiating between acute and chronic fractures and degree of union after treatment **(FIG 4D,E)**.

DIFFERENTIAL DIAGNOSIS

- Cuboid fracture
- Fifth metatarsal shaft fracture
- Lisfranc injury

NONOPERATIVE MANAGEMENT

- Conservative treatment is typically reserved for the following:
  - Zone I fractures
  - Patients of low-activity demand with a zone II or III fracture
  - Patients with medical comorbidities that preclude surgery

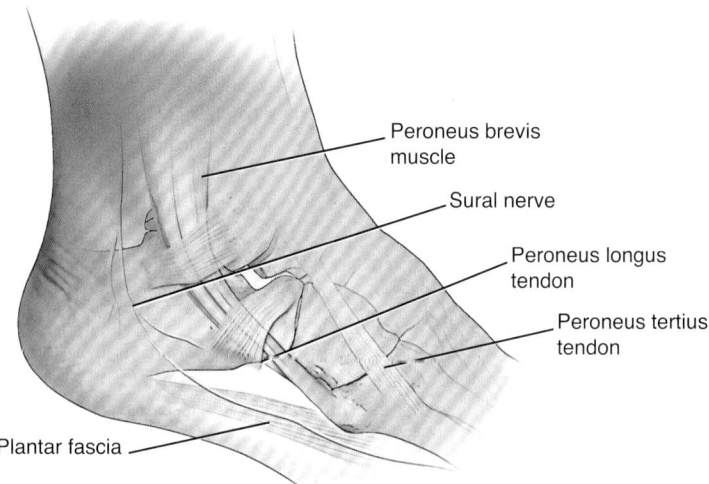

FIG 3 Structures at risk during surgical fixation of proximal fifth metatarsal fractures. Typically, the sural nerve and peroneus brevis tendon are retracted dorsally, whereas the peroneus longus tendon is retracted plantarward.

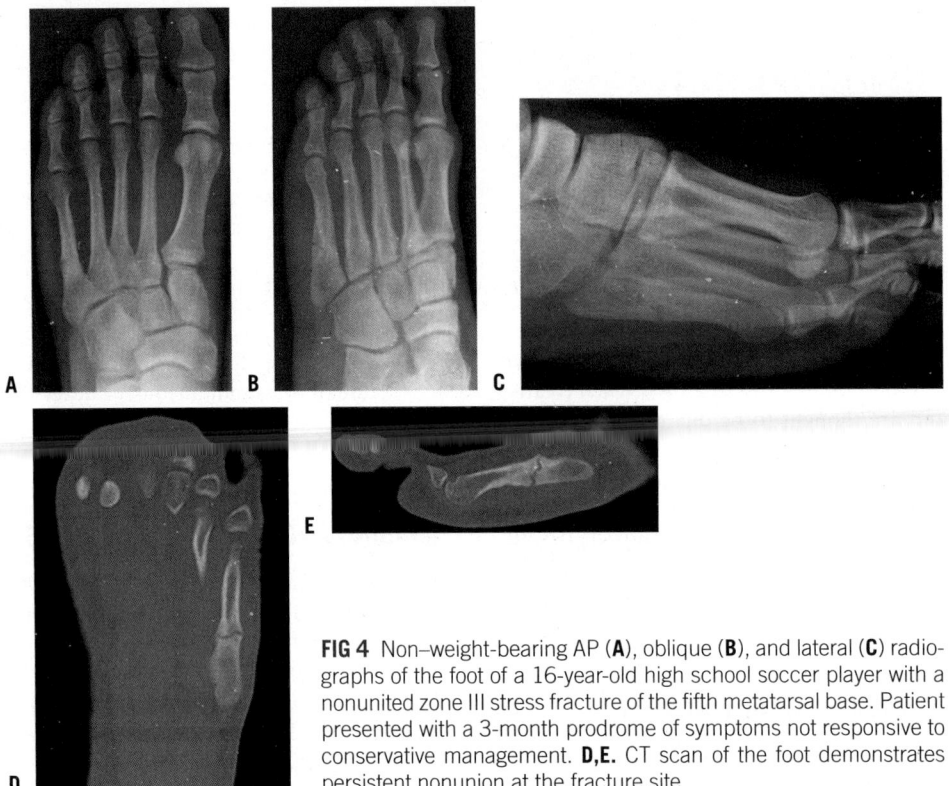

FIG 4 Non–weight-bearing AP (**A**), oblique (**B**), and lateral (**C**) radiographs of the foot of a 16-year-old high school soccer player with a nonunited zone III stress fracture of the fifth metatarsal base. Patient presented with a 3-month prodrome of symptoms not responsive to conservative management. **D,E.** CT scan of the foot demonstrates persistent nonunion at the fracture site.

- Zone I fracture: weight bearing as tolerated in a hard-soled shoe or boot (6 to 8 weeks)
- Zone II/III fractures: 6 weeks of cast immobilization and non–weight bearing, followed by an additional 6 weeks of boot immobilization with gradual advancement of weight bearing

SURGICAL MANAGEMENT

- The indications for surgical fixation of proximal fifth metatarsal fractures remain.
- Surgical treatment is indicated in the following:
  - Zone II or III fracture in athletes or individuals desiring a quicker return to activity[2,3,9]
  - Informed patients who prefer surgery to the risk of nonunion with nonsurgical treatment[2,3,9]
  - Zone III fractures with symptomatic delayed union/nonunion[3,4]
  - Zone I fractures with symptomatic delayed union/nonunion

Preoperative Planning

- Determine the appropriate type and method of fixation.
  - Percutaneous intramedullary screw fixation is the most widely used technique.
    - A variety of screw options exist, and each have their advantages and disadvantages (ie, solid vs. cannulated, stainless steel vs. titanium, fully threaded vs. partially threaded vs. variable pitch).
    - Although the biomechanical properties of various screws have been shown to vary, no single type of screw has clinically been shown to be superior.

- Recently, low-profile, precontoured proximal fifth metatarsal fracture plates have become popularized as an alternative fixation option. Lateral hook plates have tines or "hooks" at one end, which serve to engage the proximal fracture fragment and provide rotational control.[8] Tension-sided plantar plating[1,17] has gained interest, as it offers several potential advantages over intramedullary screw fixation, including biomechanical superiority due to improved resistance to both rotational and tensile forces,[6] better fixation of the proximal metaphyseal fragment, and an approach that allows direct assessment and access to the fracture site. Indications for plate fixation may include the following:
  - Comminuted zone II fractures (**FIG 5**)
  - Osteoporotic bone
  - Revision cases after failed intramedullary screw fixation
  - Cases in which intramedullary screw fixation is less than optimal (ie, loss of cortical integrity, canal diameter too small to accommodate a minimum 4.5-mm screw)
  - Symptomatic delayed union or nonunion of zone I fractures
- Determine if bone graft is desired.
  - We typically use bone graft harvested from the ipsilateral calcaneus in cases of comminution, osteoporotic bone, delayed, and nonunions.
- Determine if an underlying source of lateral foot overload (ie, hindfoot varus, chronic lateral ankle instability, etc.) is present and ensure that it is addressed, either surgically or conservatively (ie, orthotics, bracing), in conjunction with stabilization of the proximal fifth metatarsal fracture.

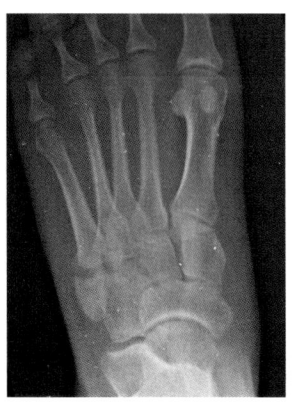 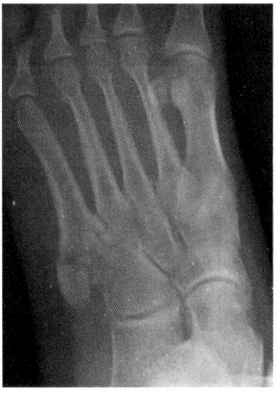 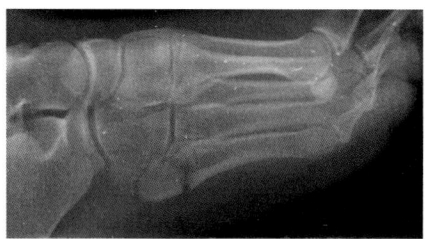

FIG 5 Non–weight-bearing AP (**A**), oblique (**B**), and lateral (**C**) radiographs of the foot of a 34-year-old female with a displaced and comminuted zone II fracture of the fifth metatarsal base.

Positioning

- The patient is placed supine with a bolster under the ipsilateral hip to internally rotate the leg, providing better access to the lateral foot.
- Place the surgical foot at the lateral edge of the operating table. This facilitates use of a mini-fluoroscopy unit that

will serve as a lateral extension of the table for portions of the case.

- A calf tourniquet is used to avoid bleeding that may obscure structures at risk in the surgical field. Ensure it is placed distal to the fibular head to avoid pressure on the common peroneal nerve.

PERCUTANEOUS INTRAMEDULLARY SCREW FIXATION

Incision and Dissection

- The surgical approach is similar to intramedullary fixation of a long bone.
- Make a 2-cm longitudinal incision, approximately 1 cm proximal to the base of the fifth metatarsal, in line with the longitudinal axis of the shaft. Avoid referencing solely off the tip of the tubercle, as this will put you more plantar than the actual axis of the shaft.
- Identify and protect the following three structures:
  - Dorsolateral branch of the sural nerve, which courses directly at the incision site
  - Peroneus brevis tendon, which inserts on the dorsolateral tuberosity
  - Peroneus longus tendon, which courses lateral to and then plantar to the cuboid, immediately proximal to the fifth metatarsal base

- Keep the sural nerve and peroneus brevis tendon protected by retracting them dorsally, whereas the peroneus longus is retracted plantarward.
- Throughout the duration of the case, a soft tissue guide should be used during pinning, drilling, and tapping to further protect the structures at risk.

Guide Pin Positioning and Drilling

- Place the guide pin at the "high and inside" starting position. This corresponds to the dorsal and medial aspects of the proximal end of the fifth metatarsal, which will optimally keep the pin within the longitudinal axis of the metatarsal **(TECH FIG 1A,B)**.

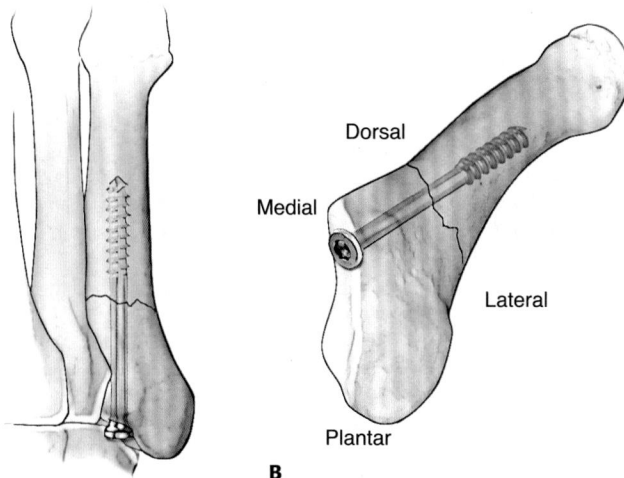

Dorsal

Medial

Lateral

Plantar

A   **B**

TECH FIG 1 The high and inside starting position and resultant screw position during intramedullary fixation of proximal fifth metatarsal fractures. The dorsal and medial starting position aligns the screw with the intramedullary canal. **A.** Coronal view of screw position relative to the fifth metatarsal. **B.** End-on view of the proximal fifth metatarsal with screw in place. *(continued)*

TECHNIQUES

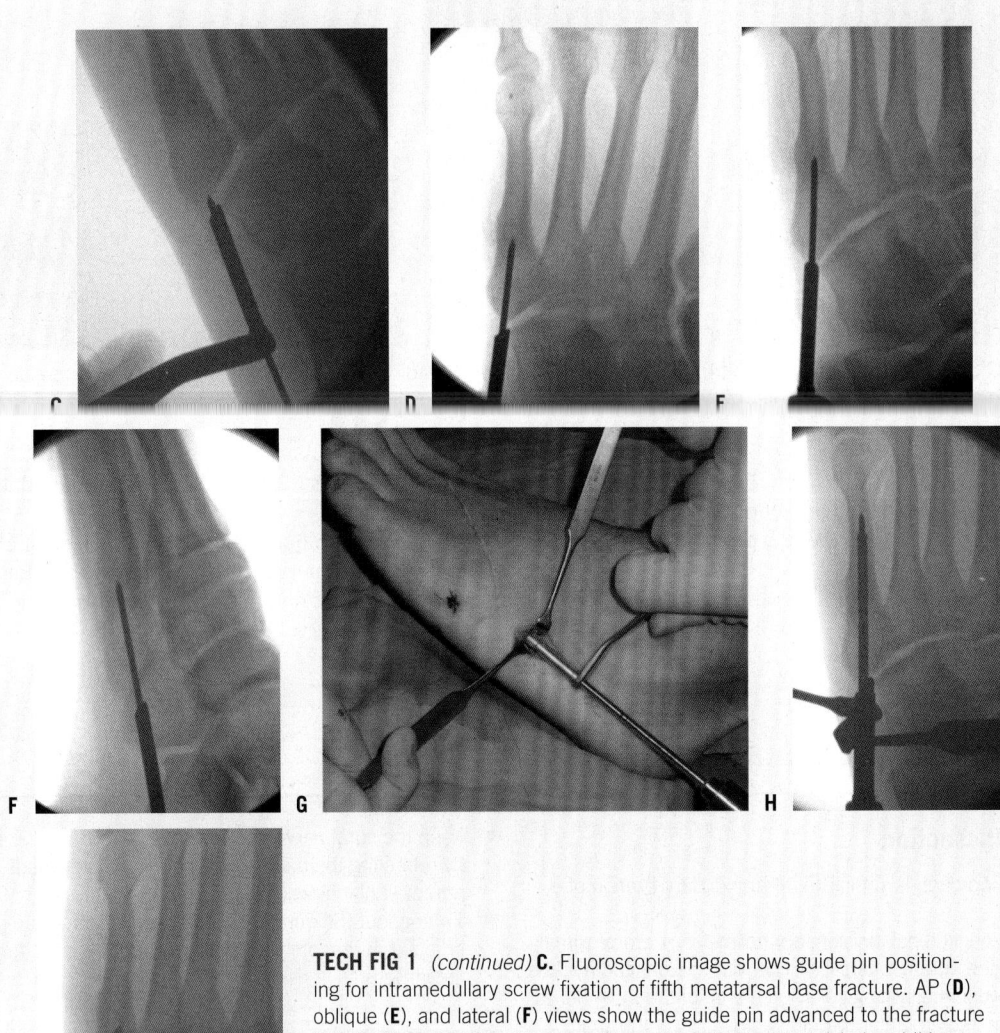

TECH FIG 1 *(continued)* **C.** Fluoroscopic image shows guide pin positioning for intramedullary screw fixation of fifth metatarsal base fracture. AP (**D**), oblique (**E**), and lateral (**F**) views show the guide pin advanced to the fracture site. **G.** Protective drill sleeve used to protect structures at risk, in addition to retraction of the peroneal tendons and sural nerve, when drilling for intramedullary screw fixation of a proximal fifth metatarsal fracture. **H.** Fluoroscopic image. Drilling is necessary only to the level that will allow the threads of the partially threaded screw to cross the fracture site. **I.** Fluoroscopic image shows drilling of sclerotic bone to promote fracture healing at the nonunion site.

- Confirm the starting position under fluoroscopy. It is important to use all three planes (AP, lateral, and oblique).
  - Start with the oblique plane, as this places the metatarsal in profile and is the easiest position in which to interpret the pin's position on fluoroscopy **(TECH FIG 1C)**.
  - Refrain from advancing the pin until its proper position has then been confirmed in the other two planes. It is difficult to make subtle adjustments with a guide pin once a hole has been created near the ideal starting position, as the pin will tend to fall back into the improperly placed hole.
- Once the optimal starting point is confirmed, aim the pin so that it is directed into the center of the fifth metatarsal intramedullary canal and partially advance **(TECH FIG 1D–F)**.
- Confirm that the trajectory of the guide pin is appropriate and then advance it across the fracture or nonunion site.
  - Because the fifth metatarsal is a curved bone and intramedullary fixation is performed with a straight screw, the guide

pin, drill, tap, and screw only need to be advanced so that all of the screw's threads are distal to the fracture/nonunion site. This typically only involves the proximal 50% of the metatarsal. If the final screw is too long, it may impinge on the distal medial cortex of the curved fifth metatarsal, thereby creating a lateral cortical gap at the fracture site and potentially promoting nonunion.
- If there is a concern that the guide pin will dislodge during drilling or tapping, then the guide pin may be advanced farther down the metatarsal, but there is no need to drill or tap that far.
- Use the cannulated drill (with drill sleeve) to overdrill the guide pin, just beyond the fracture site **(TECH FIG 1G,H)**.
- In the setting of nonunion, a small-diameter drill bit may be used to disrupt the sclerotic bone at the nonunion site to promote fracture healing **(TECH FIG 1I)**.

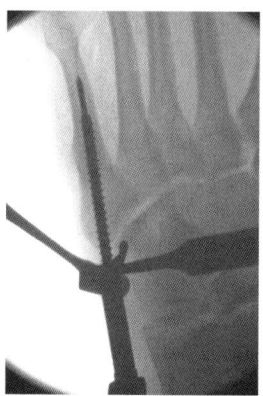

TECH FIG 2 Use of the tap in intramedullary screw fixation of a proximal fifth metatarsal fracture. Fluoroscopic image shows the tap engaged with the inner cortex of the metatarsal shaft. Note that the tap is advanced only far enough to allow the threads of the partially threaded screw to cross the fracture.

Use of the Tap

- The tap is introduced over the guide pin with its soft tissue sleeve **(TECH FIG 2)**.
- The tap serves two purposes:
  - Prepares the canal for the screw
  - Gauges the size of screw that will afford the best purchase in the distal fragment. This is performed using a set of graduated taps of increasing diameter.
- While advancing the tap with one hand, the surgeon holds the distal aspect of the metatarsal with the other hand to gauge and resist torque that is created.
- The tap only needs to be advanced far enough for all threads of the eventual screw to cross the fracture/nonunion site.
- The optimal screw diameter is determined by the tap size that creates a firm torque on the distal fragment with each turn of the tap.

Determining Screw Size

- Screw diameter
  - Optimal screw diameter is determined by the diameter of the tap that best engages the distal fragment.
  - A screw that is too large in diameter risks cortical compromise and stress shielding.
  - Although biomechanical data exist that suggest improved fracture fixation with a larger screw diameter, the clinical evidence to support this is weak.
  - In general, most advocate use a screw diameter of at least 4.5 mm in skeletally mature patients.[11,14]
- Screw length
  - Optimal screw length is that which will allow all screw threads to cross the fracture site, without contacting the distal medial cortex, as this may lead to gapping of the lateral cortex and potentially nonunion.
  - Screw length can be determined by any of the following three methods:
    - Use a cannulated depth gauge with the intramedullary guide pin tip at the desired position for the tip of the screw. Ensure the gauge is flush against bone.

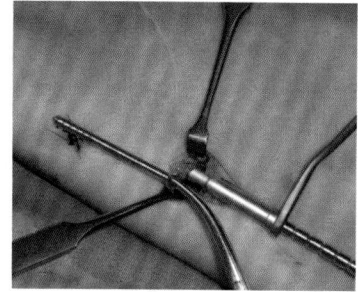

TECH FIG 3 Determining screw length for open reduction and internal fixation of a proximal fifth metatarsal fracture. Intraoperative photograph shows the surgeon holding the screw adjacent to the metatarsal for a fluoroscopic image. Although the surgeon must account for magnification error, this technique provides some guidance as to the length of screw needed for the threads to cross the fracture.

- Use two guide pins and measure the difference, with the intramedullary guide pin in the optimal position and the second placed to the level of the base of the fifth metatarsal.
- Hold the screw immediately adjacent to the fifth metatarsal base to determine if the threads will cross the fracture site (must account for a slight magnification effect) **(TECH FIG 3)**.

Screw Insertion

- With the ideal diameter and length determined, the screw is advanced into the prepared canal.
- As the screw engages the distal fragment, the surgeon must use the opposite hand to **(TECH FIG 4A)**:
  - Resist the torque that is created by the screw in the distal fragment so that the screw fully advances in the metatarsal without excessive rotation at the fracture site.
  - Apply an axial force on the distal fragment to provide compression and ensure that the screw fully advances without distraction at the fracture site.
- Final fluoroscopic images in all three planes are checked to confirm that the screw is fully seated with all threads beyond the fracture site and that the fracture is reduced and compressed **(TECH FIG 4B–D)**.

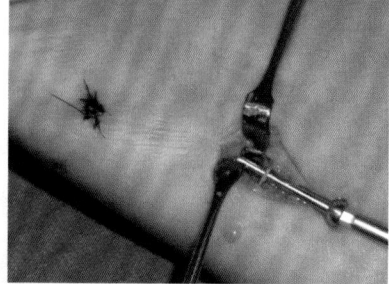

A

TECH FIG 4 Screw insertion in intramedullary screw fixation of a proximal fifth metatarsal fracture. **A.** Intraoperative photograph shows the surgeon holding the distal fragment with one hand while placing the screw with the other. This technique allows for axial compression and assessment of how well the screw is engaging the inner cortex of the distal fragment. *(continued)*

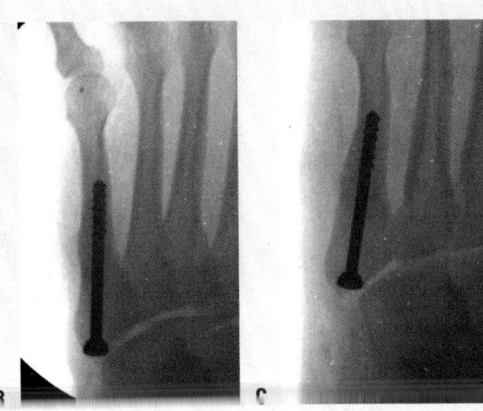
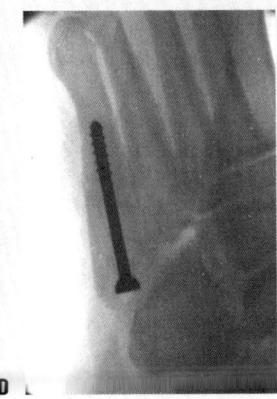

TECH FIG 4 *(continued)* Intraoperative AP (**B**), oblique (**C**), and lateral (**D**) fluoroscopic images confirm that the screw is in proper position, with all threads across the fracture site; the fracture is reduced; and there are no associated stress fractures.

OPEN REDUCTION AND INTERNAL FIXATION USING A LOW-PROFILE, PRECONTOURED PROXIMAL FIFTH METATARSAL FRACTURE PLATE

Incision and Dissection

- Make a 5-cm longitudinal incision directly along the lateral border of the fifth metatarsal, starting 1 cm proximal to the tuberosity, extending distally (**TECH FIG 5A**).
  - Identify and protect the dorsolateral branch of the sural nerve.
  - Identify and protect the peroneus brevis dorsally and peroneus longus plantarly.
  - Gently retract the sural nerve in the direction with the least resistance.
- Develop dorsal and plantar skin flaps along the length of the incision to expose the proximal metatarsal.
  - Avoid soft tissue and periosteal stripping, except for at the tip of the tuberosity, which will serve as an anchor point for the proximal tines of the plate (**TECH FIG 5B**).

Initial Reduction

- Sometimes, the fracture may be nondisplaced and obviate the need for formal reduction.
- If reduction is needed, remove 2 mm of periosteum and soft tissue only at the fracture site.
  - Gently débride and irrigate any interposed soft tissue and hematoma.
  - If desired, place bone graft into the fracture site at this time (**TECH FIG 6A**).
  - Use a pointed reduction forcep or Kirschner wire (K-wire) to obtain provisional reduction of the fracture.
- Seat the plate guide along the lateral border of the proximal metatarsal in the position where it best contours and lies flush against the bone. Secure the plate with its accompanying K-wires.
- Confirm satisfactory fracture reduction and guide position under fluoroscopy (**TECH FIG 6B–D**).
- Use the proximal guide holes to drill two holes through the outer cortex of the tuberosity with a 1.75-mm drill bit.

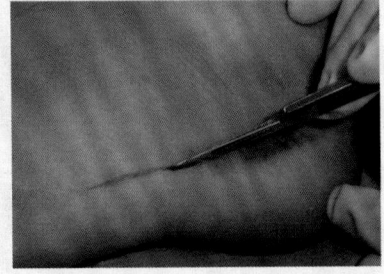
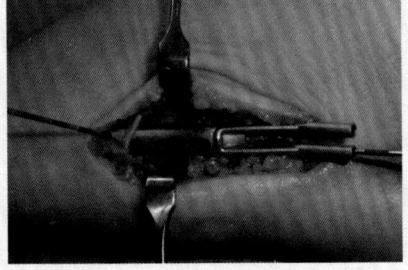

TECH FIG 5 A. Skin incision for plate fixation of proximal fifth metatarsal fracture. The longitudinal incision should center along the axis of the proximal metatarsal and extend approximately 1 cm proximal to the tubercle. **B.** The plate guide in proper position about the proximal metatarsal. Note a crossing branch of the sural nerve, which should be protected through the duration of the case. Also note that the fifth metatarsal soft tissue and periosteum has been preserved under the guide.

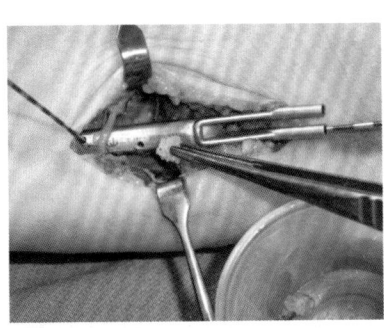
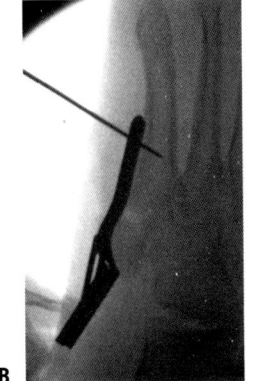
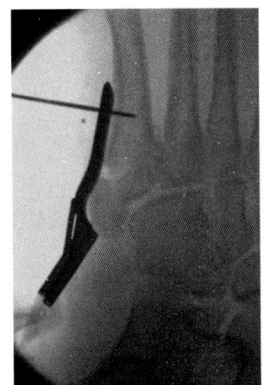
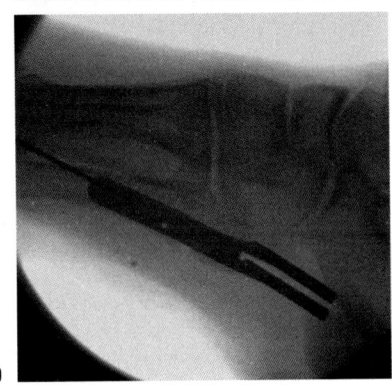

TECH FIG 6 A. If desired, bone graft may be placed into the fracture site at this time. Fluoroscopic AP (**B**), oblique (**C**), and lateral (**D**) images demonstrate the position of the guide, which is well contoured and flush to the native metatarsal cortex.

Applying the Plate

- Determine the appropriate length plate for the fracture.
- Remove the guide and engage the proximal tines or hooks of the plate into the drilled holes at the tuberosity (**TECH FIG 7A**).
- Use the mini-impactor to completely seat the tines into bone (**TECH FIG 7B**).

- The plate should lie centered and flush against the proximal metatarsal. Confirm appropriate plate position under fluoroscopy (**TECH FIG 7C,D**).
- Secure the distal end of the plate to the metatarsal shaft using the 1.75-mm drill bit in the oblong hole, followed by the appropriate sized 2.3-mm bicortical screw.
  - If compression at the fracture site is desired, drill eccentrically in the hole (away from the fracture) (**TECH FIG 7E**).
  - Leave the screw slightly untightened (**TECH FIG 7F**).

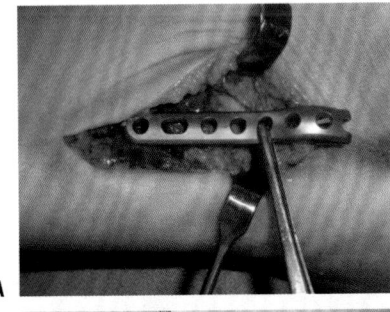
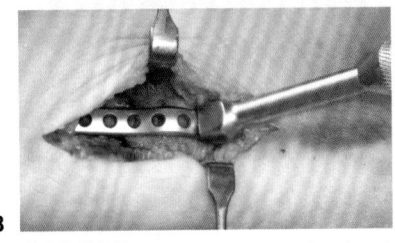
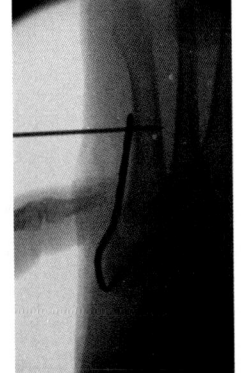
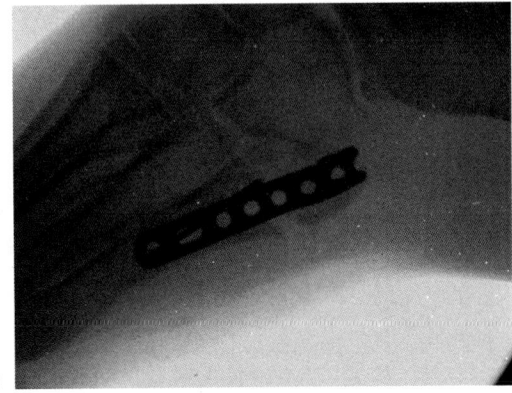

TECH FIG 7 Inserting and securing the plate. **A.** Intraoperative photograph shows the plate ready to be inserted. This is done by engaging the hooks into the previously drilled holes in the tubercle created with the guide. **B.** A tamp is used to seat the plate so that it is flush to bone. Intraoperative oblique (**C**) and lateral (**D**) fluoroscopic images confirm plate position. *(continued)*

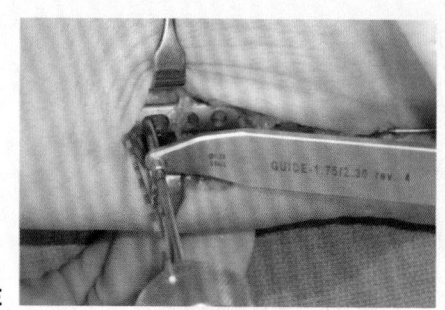
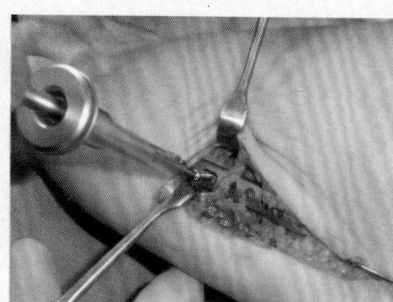

TECH FIG 7 *(continued)* **E.** Eccentric drilling of the oblong hole, furthest away from the fracture, to provide compression through the plate. **F.** The screw is engaged to the plate and bone but not fully tightened.

Compressing the Fracture

- If compression is not desired (ie, excessive comminution), this step may be skipped.
- Engage the screwdriver tip of the expander/compression tool into the head of the screw.
- Insert the opposite jaw of the tool into the adjacent distal hole in the plate.

- Gently squeeze the handle of the tool until the desired amount of compression is obtained **(TECH FIG 8A)**.
- Maintaining compression, completely tighten and seat the screw **(TECH FIG 8B)**.
- Evidence of compression is depicted by a more proximal position of the screw in the oblong hole **(TECH FIG 8C)**.

Final Fixation

- Place additional 2.3-mm screws in the distal and proximal fragments as needed.
  - Proximally, ensure the screws are directed appropriately to maintain intraosseous position.
- Obtain final fluoroscopic images in three planes to evaluate reduction and hardware position **(TECH FIG 9)**.

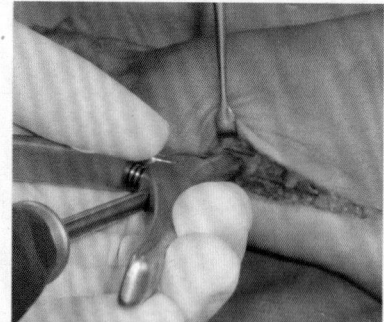
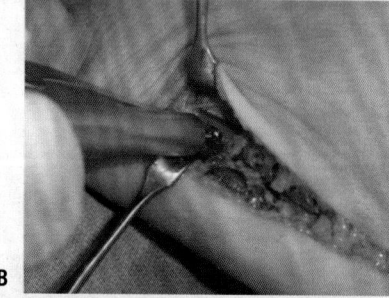
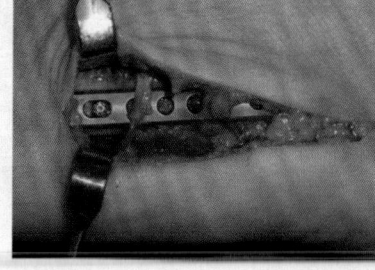

TECH FIG 8 Compression is applied (**A**), and the screw is completely tightened to the plate (**B**), maintaining the compression across the fracture site. **C.** The screw head is now closest to the fracture site in the oblong hole. Also note preservation of the crossing branch of the sural nerve as well as the periosteum over the metatarsal shaft.

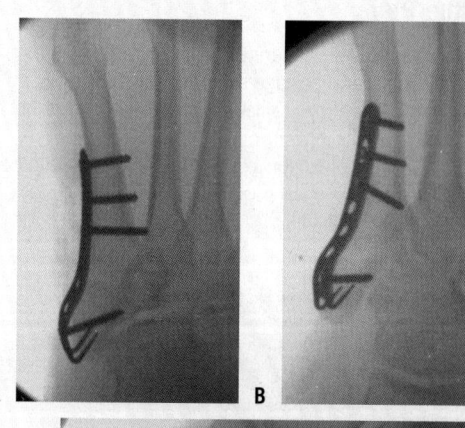
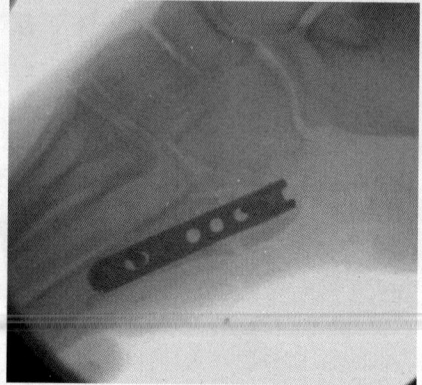

TECH FIG 9 AP (**A**), oblique (**B**), and lateral (**C**) fluoroscopic images confirm that the hardware is appropriately seated against bone and that the fracture is reduced.

OPEN REDUCTION AND INTERNAL FIXATION USING A TENSION-SIDED PLANTAR PLATE

Incision and Dissection

- Make a longitudinal incision along the lateral glabrous border of the fifth metatarsal, centered over the fracture site **(TECH FIG 10A)**.
  - Identify and protect the sural nerve.
  - Identify and gently retract the abductor digiti minimi inferiorly.
- Develop a plantar skin flap along the length of the incision to expose the proximal metatarsal and fracture site **(TECH FIG 10B)**.
- Avoid soft tissue and periosteal stripping, except for plantarly where the plate will lie.

Initial Reduction

- Sometimes, the fracture may be nondisplaced and obviate the need for formal reduction.
- If reduction is needed, remove 2 mm of periosteum and soft tissue only at the fracture site.
  - Gently débride and irrigate any interposed soft tissue and hematoma.
  - If desired, place bone graft into the fracture site. Cancellous autograft from the calcaneus is a common source. Bone marrow aspirate is another option.

- Use a pointed reduction forcep to obtain provisional reduction and compression of the fracture.

Applying the Plate

- Determine the appropriate-length plate and position for the fracture. Some plating systems have a trial or template that can be used **(TECH FIG 11)**.
- Seat a precontoured, low-profile plate along the plantar aspect of the proximal metatarsal, centered over the fracture site and flush against the bone. Secure the plate with its accompanying olive wires **(TECH FIG 12A,B)**.
- Confirm satisfactory fracture reduction and position under fluoroscopy **(TECH FIG 12C–E)**.
- Secure the proximal end of the plate to the metatarsal **(TECH FIG 13A)**, followed by the distal end **(TECH FIG 13B)**.
  - If compression at the fracture site is desired, drill eccentrically in the hole (away from the fracture).

Final Fixation

- Place additional screws in the distal and proximal fragments as needed. Ensure the screws are directed appropriately to maintain intraosseous position.
- Obtain final fluoroscopic images in three planes to evaluate reduction and hardware position **(TECH FIG 14)**.

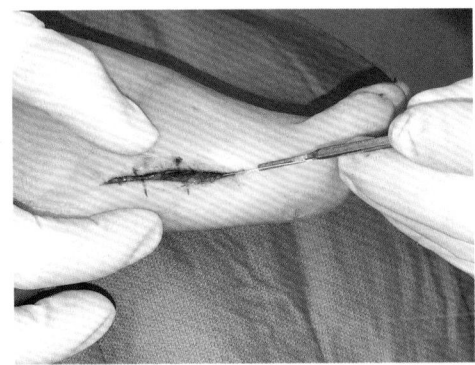
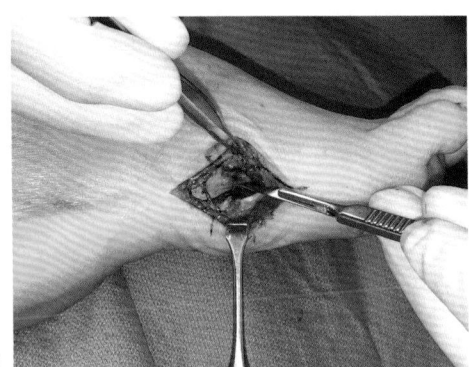

TECH FIG 10 A. Skin incision made along glabrous border of the foot for plantar plate fixation of proximal fifth metatarsal fracture. **B.** Fracture site exposed and plantar skin flap created along the length of the incision.

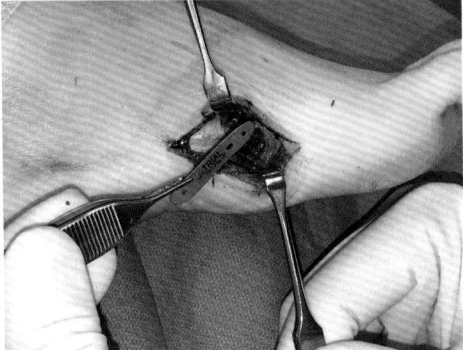

TECH FIG 11 A template may be used to determine the appropriate-length plate and position for the fracture.

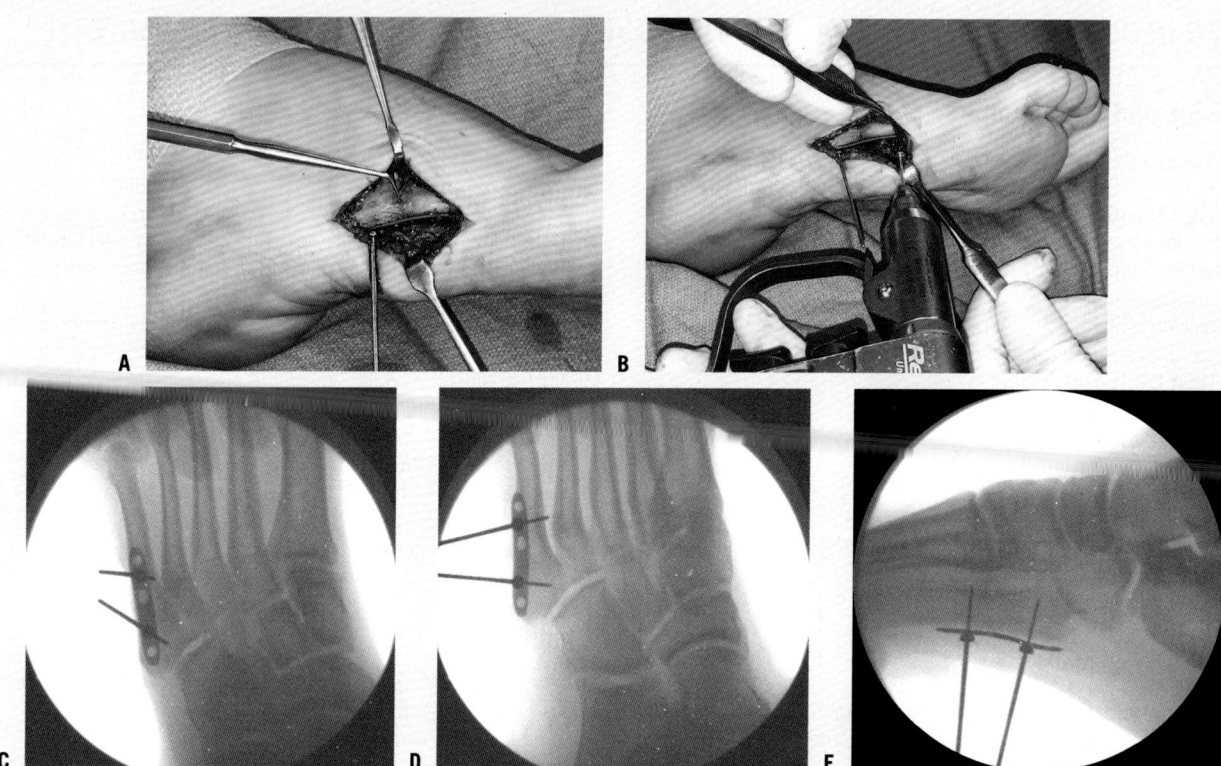

TECH FIG 12 A precontoured, low-profile plate is seated along the plantar aspect of the metatarsal, centered over the fracture site and secured with its accompanying olive wires proximally **(A)** and distally **(B)**. **C–E.** Satisfactory fracture reduction and hardware position confirmed under fluoroscopy.

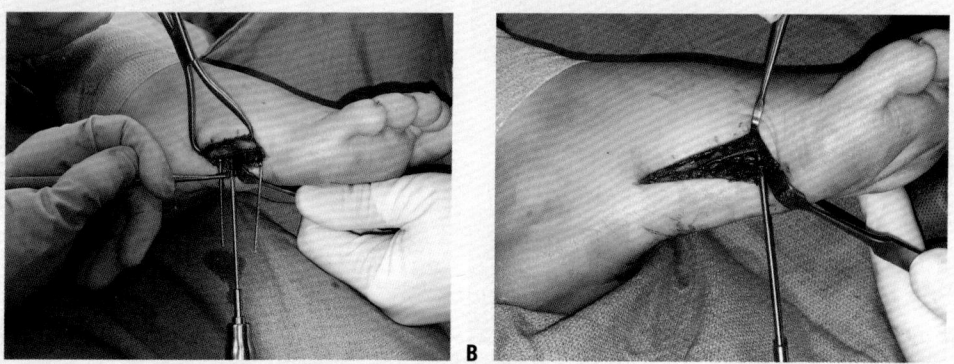

TECH FIG 13 The proximal end of the plate **(A)** is secured to the metatarsal, followed by the distal end **(B)**.

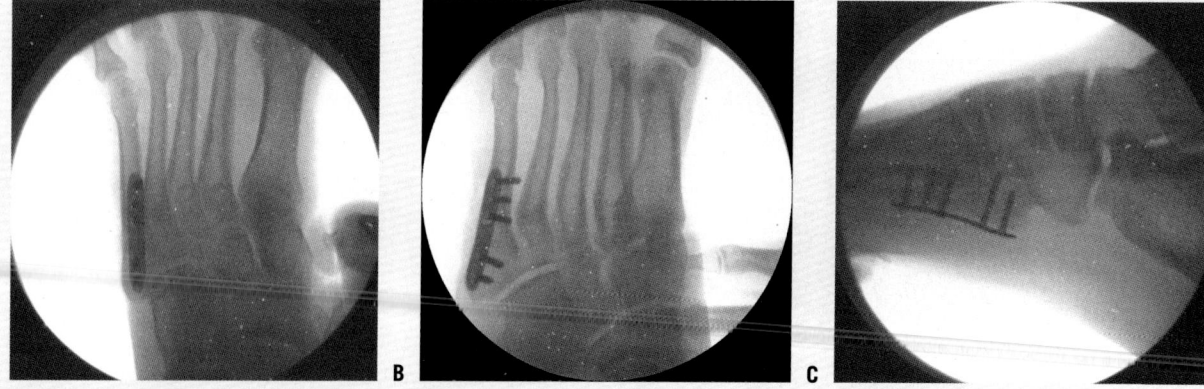

TECH FIG 14 AP **(A)**, oblique **(B)**, and lateral **(C)** fluoroscopic images confirm the plate is appropriately seated against bone, and the fracture is reduced.

Pearls and Pitfalls

Operating Room Setup	• Position the foot at the distal lateral border of the operating table so that it can be easily moved onto the adjacently positioned fluoroscopy unit when needed. • Use a bolster under the ipsilateral hip to internally rotate the foot and provide easy access to its lateral border.
Intramedullary Screw Fixation	
Avoid iatrogenic injury to the sural nerve and peroneal tendons.	• Use retractors and a drill guide or sleeve when drilling, tapping, and upon screw application.
Ideal Starting Position	• Use the high and inside starting position, dorsal and medial on the proximal end of the fifth metatarsal.
Ideal Screw Diameter	• Must allow adequate endosteal bite of the screw threads • Avoid too large a diameter, as this risks cortical compromise and stress shielding.
Ideal Screw Length	• Screw threads must cross the fracture site for compression to occur. • Avoid too long a screw, as this risks gapping at the fracture site as the screw attempts to straighten the native distal curve of the bone.
Plate Fixation	
Avoid excessive soft tissue stripping.	• If direct reduction is needed, only expose directly at the fracture site.
Avoid compression when there is significant fracture comminution.	• Instead, bridge the comminution and use the plate as a template for fracture reduction.
Prevent hardware irritation.	• Use precontoured plate or manually contour the plate with plate benders as needed to ensure it sits flush against bone its entire length.

POSTOPERATIVE CARE

- The patient is kept immobilized in a postoperative splint for the first 2 weeks after surgery to allow their incision to heal.
- They are then transitioned to a short-leg cast or CAM walker and kept protected weight bearing until 6 weeks postoperatively.
- Gradual progression of weight bearing in a CAM walker is instituted at 6 weeks postoperatively, followed by transition to regular shoes.

- Return to full activities and athletics is allowed once complete radiographic healing is observed and the patient is nontender at the fracture site (10 to 12 weeks postoperatively) (**FIGS 6** and **7**). Consider obtaining CT scan before returning high-level athletes to play (see **FIG 6**).[16]
- In the patient with preoperative flexible hindfoot varus, we recommend a custom rigid orthotic insert (lateral hindfoot wedge extended to a lateral forefoot post) to offload the fifth metatarsal base and potentially reduce the risk of refracture.[13]

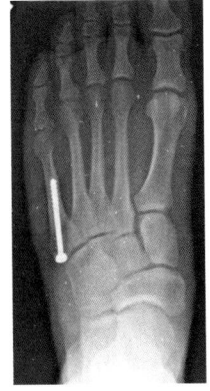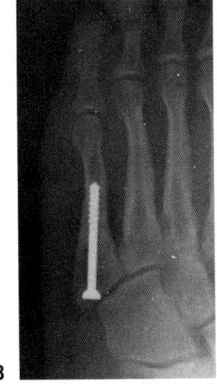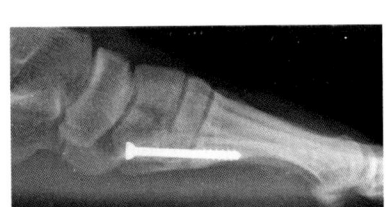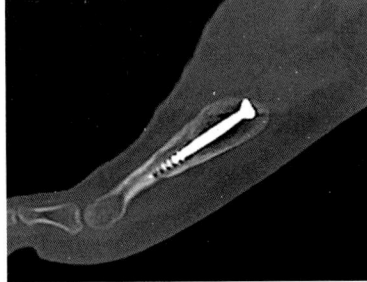

A   **B**   **C**   **D**

FIG 6 AP (**A**), oblique (**B**), and lateral (**C**) radiographs obtained at 3-month follow-up after intramedullary screw fixation of the zone III proximal fifth metatarsal stress fracture in the 16-year-old soccer player presented in this chapter. Bridging trabeculation at the fracture site was suggested on all three radiographs. **D.** CT scan at 4-month follow-up confirmed complete healing across the fracture site. The foot was nontender on clinical examination, and the patient was released to full return to athletics without complications.

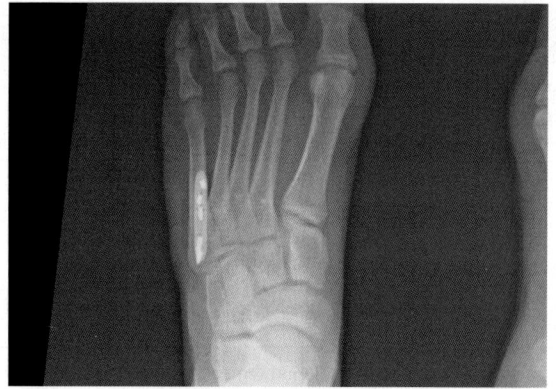
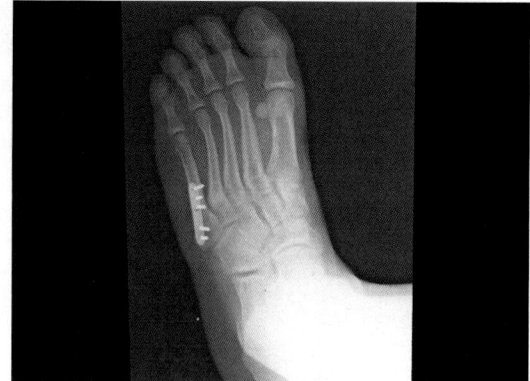
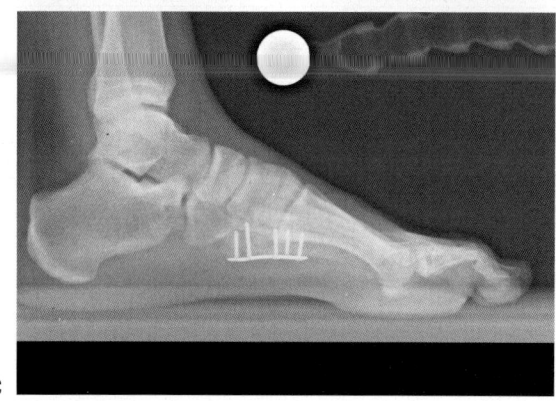

FIG 7 AP (**A**), oblique (**B**), and lateral (**C**) radiographs obtained at 3-month follow-up after open reduction and internal fixation with a plantar plate for a zone III proximal fifth metatarsal stress fracture, demonstrating bridging trabeculation at the fracture site in all three planes.

OUTCOMES

- Compared to nonoperative management, surgical management of proximal fifth metatarsal fractures has been shown to result in faster time to union and return to sports activities.[9]
- The overall healing rate with intramedullary screw fixation has been reported to be better than 90%.[4,9,12]
- Proximal fifth metatarsal plate
  - The literature on outcomes after plate fixation of proximal fifth metatarsal fractures is limited to level IV case series.
  - Lee et al[8] treated 19 patients with zone I (12) and zone II (7) proximal fifth metatarsal fractures with a locking compression distal ulna hook plate. Radiographic bony union occurred in all patients at an average of 7.4 weeks (range, 4 to 16). All patients returned to their regular sports activities and daily life at a mean of 11.2 weeks (range, 9 to 19).[8]
  - In 2018, Bernstein et al[1] reported the outcomes of plantar plating in eight elite athletes (four primary fractures, four refractures) with a minimum follow-up of 2 years. There were no incisional complications, delayed unions or nonunions, refractures, hardware loosening, or complaints of hardware prominence. Clinically asymptomatic radiographic union was observed in 100% of the athletes at 6.5 ± 1.1 weeks, and full release to activities was given at 12.3 ± 1.9 weeks. All athletes returned to sport at the same level of competition.
  - In 2020, Young et al[17] retrospectively evaluated 38 athletes who underwent plantar plating with a minimum follow-up of 1 year and found a mean time to radiographic union of 9.3 (range, 8 to 16) weeks. There were no nonunions or delayed unions; however, 4 refractures

developed (10.5%). All but 1 patient were able to return to their previous level of sporting activity at an average of 22 (range, 12 to 40) weeks.

COMPLICATIONS

- Intramedullary screw
  - Delayed union, nonunion, and refractures have been associated with use of screw diameters smaller than 4.5 mm, incomplete reaming of a sclerotic canal, and early return to vigorous activity.
  - Refracture can occur after healing and screw removal. As a result, some recommend the following[16]:
    - Leaving the screw in place until the end of the patient's athletic career
    - Considering functional bracing, shoe modification, or an orthosis with return to play
    - Using advanced imaging to help document complete healing before returning to play
  - Distal fracture at the tip of the screw (peri-implant fracture)
  - Prominent screw head
  - Sural neuralgia
  - Injury to the peroneus brevis or longus tendons
- Proximal fifth metatarsal plate
  - Refracture hardware irritation, requiring removal
  - Sural neuralgia
  - Delayed wound healing

REFERENCES

1. Bernstein DT, Mitchell RJ, McCulloch PC, et al. Treatment of proximal fifth metatarsal fractures and refractures with plantar plating in elite athletes. Foot Ankle Int 2018;39:1410–1415.

2. Clapper MF, O'Brien TJ, Lyons PM. Fractures of the fifth metatarsal. Analysis of a fracture registry. Clin Orthop Relat Res 1995;(315): 238–241.

3. Dameron TB Jr. Fractures of the proximal fifth metatarsal: selecting the best treatment option. J Am Acad Orthop Surg 1995;3:110–114.

4. DeLee JC, Evans JP, Julian J. Stress fracture of the fifth metatarsal. Am J Sports Med 1983;11:349–353.

5. Donley BG, McCollum MJ, Murphy GA, et al. Risk of sural nerve injury with intramedullary screw fixation of fifth metatarsal fractures: a cadaver study. Foot Ankle Int 1999;20:182–184.

6. Duplantier NL, Mitchell RJ, Zambrano S, et al. A biomechanical comparison of fifth metatarsal jones fracture fixation methods. Am J Sports Med 2018;46:1220–1227.

7. Egol K, Walsh M, Rosenblatt K, et al. Avulsion fractures of the fifth metatarsal base: a prospective outcome study. Foot Ankle Int 2007;28(5):581–583.

8. Lee SK, Park JS, Choy WS. Locking compression plate distal ulna hook plate as alternative fixation for fifth metatarsal base fracture. J Foot Ankle Surg 2014;53(5):522–528.

9. Mologne TS, Lundeen JM, Clapper MF, et al. Early screw fixation versus casting in the treatment of acute Jones fractures. Am J Sports Med 2005;33(7):970–975.

10. Petrisor BA, Ekrol I, Court-Brown C. The epidemiology of metatarsal fractures. Foot Ankle Int 2006;27:172–174.

11. Porter DA, Duncan M, Meyer SJ. Fifth metatarsal Jones fracture fixation with a 4.5-mm cannulated stainless steel screw in the competitive and recreational athlete: a clinical and radiographic evaluation. Am J Sports Med 2005;33(5):726–733.

12. Portland G, Kelikian A, Kodros S. Acute surgical management of Jones' fractures. Foot Ankle Int 2003;24:829–833.

13. Raikin SM, Slenker N, Ratigan B. The association of a varus hindfoot and fracture of the fifth metatarsal metaphyseal-diaphyseal junction: the Jones fracture. Am J Sports Med 2008;36:1367–1372.

14. Shah SN, Knoblich GO, Lindsey DP, et al. Intramedullary screw fixation of proximal fifth metatarsal fractures: a biomechanical study. Foot Ankle Int 2001;22:581–584.

15. Smith JW, Arnoczky SP, Hersh A. The intraosseous blood supply of the fifth metatarsal: implications for proximal fracture healing. Foot Ankle 1992;13:143–152.

16. Wright RW, Fischer DA, Shively RA, et al. Refracture of proximal fifth metatarsal (Jones) fracture after intramedullary screw fixation in athletes. Am J Sports Med 2000;28:732–736.

17. Young K, Kim JS, Lee HS, et al. Operative results of plantar plating for fifth metatarsal stress fracture. Foot Ankle Int 2020;41:419–427.

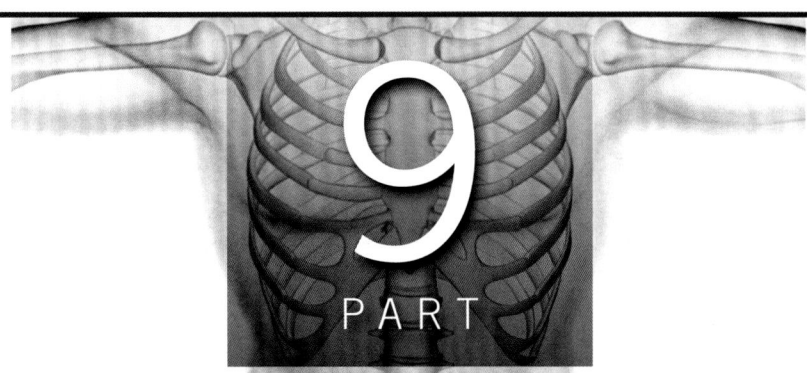

9

PART

Spine

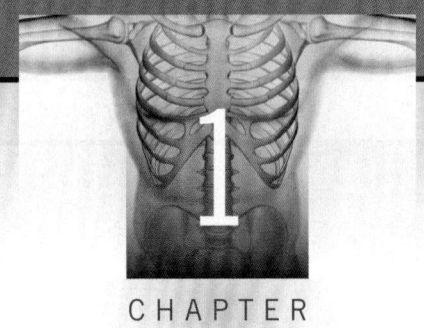

CHAPTER 1

Cervical
Anterior Cervical Discectomy and Fusion with and without Instrumentation

John M. Rhee, Claude Jarrett, and Sam W. Wiesel

DEFINITION

- Cervical spondylosis refers to degenerative conditions affecting the cervical spine, including disc degeneration, herniation, facet arthrosis, and osteophytic spur formation. Depending on the nature and location of the spondylotic changes, pathologic compression of neural structures in the cervical spine may occur.
- This chapter focuses on anterior cervical discectomy and fusion (ACDF) as a surgical treatment option for patients with cervical radiculopathy. Cervical myelopathy can also be treated with ACDF as long as the spinal cord compression occurs at the disc rather than the retroverteberal level.
- All techniques described in this chapter can apply to the decompression of the spinal cord in myelopathic patients as well as the nerve root in radiculopathic patients. However, for the purposes of organization, cervical myelopathy is discussed in the chapter on anterior cervical corpectomy.

ANATOMY

- The anterior longitudinal ligament is a wide band of ligaments stretching along the anterior surface of the vertebral

bodies. Its dense longitudinal fibers widen as they travel caudally and are intimately associated with the intervertebral discs as well as the vertebral endplates.
- The posterior longitudinal ligament (PLL) is a smooth and shiny group of dense ligaments that course along the posterior surface of the vertebral bodies within the spinal canal. The PLL tends to be thicker centrally and thins out laterally as it attaches to the uncinate regions. Bulging or ossification of the PLL (OPLL) can cause spinal cord compression.
- The intervertebral disc comprises the outer annulus fibrosus and the central gelatinous nucleus pulposus. Each disc is attached to the subchondral bone of the adjacent vertebral bodies. The outermost rim of the vertebral endplate is not attached to the disc, leaving a ring of exposed bone that may be more prone to forming arthritic spurs.
- The uncovertebral joints are critical bony landmarks for anterior cervical decompression (FIG 1). Spurs commonly arise from these articulations and cause impingement of the exiting roots as they enter the foramen.
- Depending on the cervical level, the vertebral artery may be as close as 5 mm away from the medial aspect of the uncinate process.

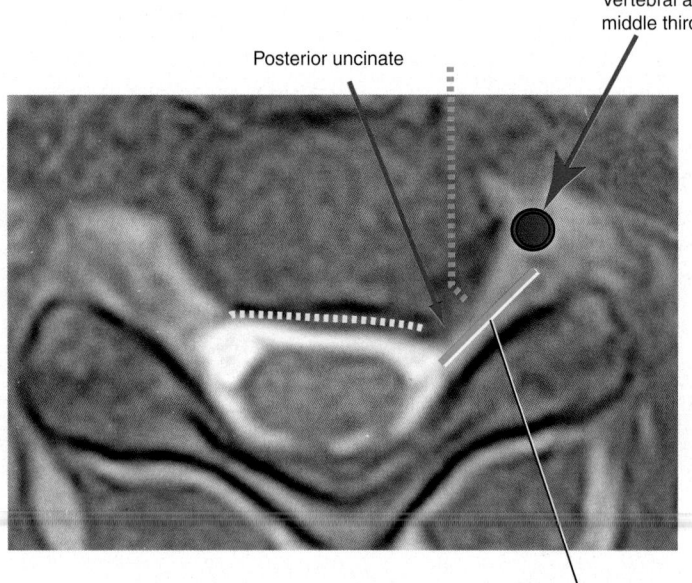

Posterior uncinate

Vertebral artery, middle third

Root exits ventrally at 45-degree angle

FIG 1 Anterior foraminotomy anatomy: important anatomic relationships to consider when performing anterior cervical spine surgery. The exiting nerve root enters the foramen at a 45-degree ventrolateral angle. The posterior aspect of the uncinate joint marks the entry zone of the neuroforamen, and it is where osteophytes commonly arise to impinge the exiting root. Thus, the uncus should be decompressed when performing foraminotomy. It is critical to hug the posterior aspect of the uncinate during foraminotomy to avoid injuring the exiting root, which lies immediately dorsal. The vertebral artery is less likely to be injured while working in the posterior disc space (eg, during decompression) because it is located at roughly the level of the middle third of the vertebra. The trajectory of discectomy should be bounded by the uncinates at all times, but it can widen posteriorly at the level of the nerve root to thoroughly decompress the root while avoiding vertebral artery injury (*dashed blue line*). The PLL (*dashed yellow line*) tends to be thicker and better defined centrally; it thins out laterally.

TABLE 1	Neurologic Examination of the Cervical Spine		
Root	Sensory	Motor	Reflex
C2	Sensation to posterior occiput		
C3	Sensation to neck		
C4	Sensation to upper shoulder, chest		
C5	Sensation along lateral arm	Motor to deltoid	Biceps reflex
C6	Sensation to lateral forearm and radial two digits	Motor to biceps, wrist extension, pronation	Brachioradialis reflex
C7	Sensation to middle finger	Motor to triceps and wrist flexion	Triceps reflex
C8	Sensation to medial forearm and ulnar two digits	Motor to finger flexors—grip	
T1	Sensation to medial arm	Motor to interossei	

- Each cervical spinal nerve is composed of dorsal and ventral roots. The ventral root lies dorsal to the uncovertebral joint, whereas the dorsal root is ventral to the superior articular facet.
  - It is important to keep in mind when performing uncovertebral osteophyte resection that the nerve root leaves the spinal cord at roughly a 45-degree angle ventrolaterally in the axial plane. Thus, care must be taken to hug the posterior surface of the uncinate to avoid injury to the exiting root.[4]

PATHOGENESIS

- Neural impingement occurs in two main locations: within the spinal canal, affecting the spinal cord, the nerve root, or both; or within the foramen, where the exiting root can be affected.
- Depending on whether the involved structure is the spinal cord or the nerve root, patients can present with symptoms of myelopathy, radiculopathy, or both.

NATURAL HISTORY

- The natural history of cervical radiculopathy is generally favorable with most patients having spontaneous resolution or considerable improvement of their symptoms over time.
- It is not common for radiculopathic patients to progress to myelopathy.[10,11]

HISTORY AND PHYSICAL FINDINGS

- Patients with radiculopathy typically present with radiating pain, paresthesia, or motor weakness (TABLE 1). However, the pattern of symptoms is not always dermatomal (FIG 2).[8]
- On examination, patients with radiculopathy may have motor, sensory, or reflex changes along the affected nerve root distribution. However, the neurologic examination findings may be normal.
- Patients may express exacerbation of radicular pain with particular head positions (ie, head positions that narrow the size of the neural foramen such as neck extension with rotation to the affected extremity).
  - This can be elicited by performing the Spurling test. The Spurling sign is very helpful in differentiating cervical radiculopathy from extraspinal causes, such as cubital or carpal tunnel syndromes, as reproduction of symptoms should occur only with a cervical source of compression.

IMAGING AND OTHER DIAGNOSTIC STUDIES

- Plain radiographs, although of limited value in evaluating neural compression, remain a commonly acquired initial study and can be used to evaluate overall alignment, spinal instability, or bony pathology, including spur formation.
- Magnetic resonance imaging (MRI) is the modality of choice for evaluating neural compression.
- Computed tomography (CT) myelography provides outstanding resolution of bony and neural anatomy, but it is less appealing as it requires an invasive procedure. It is typically recommended for patients with contraindications to

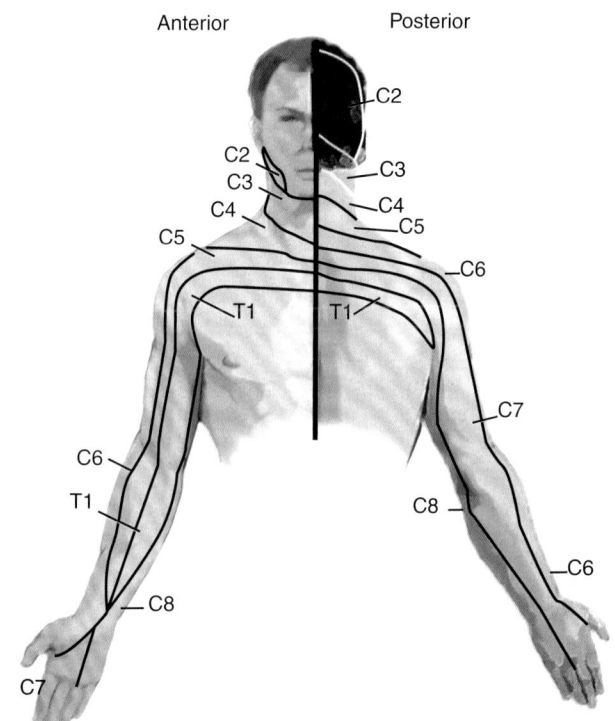

FIG 2 Dermatomes of the cervical nerve roots. Symptoms do not always follow the textbook distribution of dermatomes. In particular, radiculopathies involving various nerve roots, such as C5, C6, or C7, can all produce periscapular pain, not uncommonly in the absence of radiating pain down the arm. If in doubt as to the offending level, a selective nerve root block can be performed for diagnostic purposes.

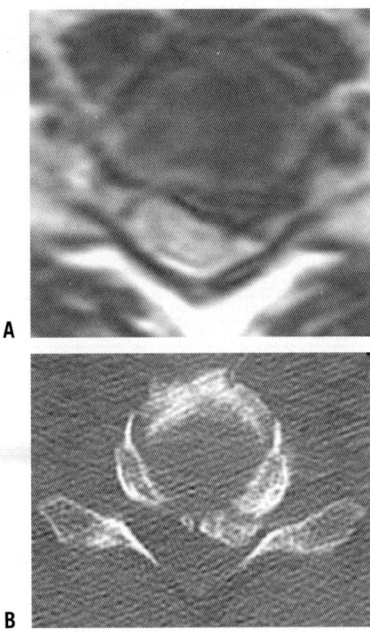

A

B

FIG 3 MRI and CT scans may provide complementary information in delineating bony versus soft tissue masses. **A.** On the axial MRI, the compressive lesion has the appearance of a soft disc. **B.** A CT scan through the same level, however, demonstrates the pathology to be an ossified disc. Similarly, CT scans can help differentiate disc herniations from OPLL.

MRI (eg, prosthetic heart valve, pacemaker) or when MRI fails to provide sufficient detail.

- If a high-quality MRI is available but questions remain regarding bony anatomy for the purposes of surgical planning, a noncontrast CT scan provides complementary information (eg, differentiating soft disc versus ossified disc or OPLL) **(FIG 3)**.

DIFFERENTIAL DIAGNOSIS

- Cervical radiculopathy
- Cervical myelopathy
- Brachial plexus injury
- Complex regional pain syndrome or reflex sympathetic dystrophy
- Thoracic outlet syndrome
- Inflammatory arthropathy
- Spinal cord tumor
- Angina
- Shoulder pathology
- Peripheral nerve compression (eg, carpal or cubital tunnel syndrome)
- Diabetic neuropathy
- Multiple sclerosis
- Syringomyelia
- Stroke
- Guillain-Barré syndrome
- Normal pressure hydrocephalus
- Spinal cord tumor

NONOPERATIVE MANAGEMENT

- Nonoperative management should be considered as the initial mode of treatment for most patients with radiculopathy.
- Nonsurgical treatment typically includes physical therapy, traction, pain medication, cervical collars, and epidural

injections. It is not clear if nonoperative modalities alter the natural history, but they can provide pain relief while the natural history runs its course.

SURGICAL MANAGEMENT

- Surgical intervention is indicated for radiculopathy in patients with persistent symptoms resistant to nonoperative care, progressive weakness, or instability.
- Common surgical approaches to radiculopathy include ACDF versus posterior laminoforaminotomy.[12]

Preoperative Planning

- The surgeon should evaluate imaging studies for anatomic variations, such as medial aberrancy of the vertebral artery.
- To perform a safe but complete and adequate neural decompression, high-quality illumination and magnification are essential.
  - An operating microscope provides illumination and visualization superior to that of loupes and headlights, but either method can be used.
  - Another advantage of the microscope is that the view obtained by the assistant is the same as that of the operating surgeon.
  - If the surgeon chooses to use the microscope, given the smaller field of view, it is imperative to continuously adjust the viewing angle such that a line of sight parallel to the disc space is achieved **(FIG 4)**. If this is not done, the surgeon may inadvertently stray away from the disc space, veer into

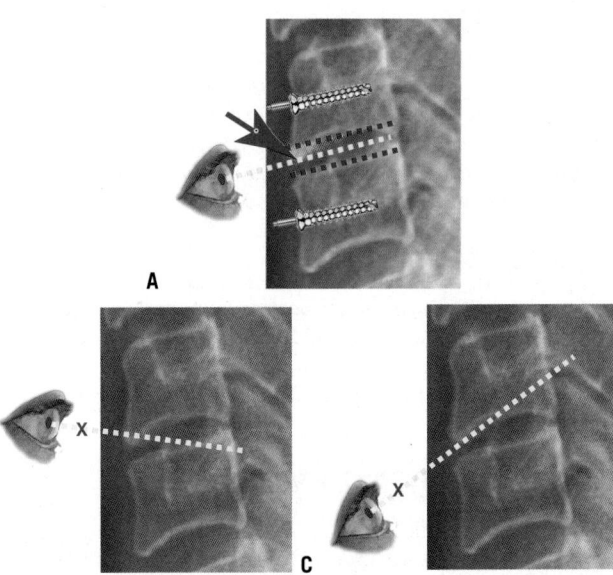

A

B   **C**

FIG 4 Line of sight. When using the microscope, it must be angled properly to provide a parallel view of the disc space to facilitate decompression and endplate preparation. **A.** Endplate preparation should proceed in a parallel fashion (*dotted red lines*) centered on the disc space to achieve a rectangular space for graft insertion. Parallel, wide preparation of the disc space also makes decompression easier to perform and ensures that the decompression is centered on the disc space. To achieve parallel surfaces, the inferior endplate of the cepahalad vertebra typically requires greater preparation because it is concave. In contrast, the superior endplate of the caudal vertebra is flatter and requires less preparation. Proper line of sight is facilitated by removing the anterior lip (*arrow, shaded yellow*) which allows for better visualization of, and access to, the posterior disc space. **B,C.** If the line of sight is not maintained, one may err into the vertebral bodies above and below rather than progressing toward the area at the disc level that requires decompression.

one vertebral body or the other, and not proceed to the back of the disc space where the decompression needs to occur.

Positioning

- The patient is positioned with a bump under the scapula and the occiput on a foam doughnut to prevent pressure necrosis.

- The amount of extension tolerated preoperatively without excessive pain or neurologic symptoms is recreated.

Approach

- A standard Smith-Robinson approach to the anterior cervical spine is used for most cases from C2 to T2.

ANTERIOR CERVICAL DISCECTOMY AND FUSION WITH INSTRUMENTATION

Initial Discectomy

- Once the disc is exposed, it is sharply incised with a no. 15 blade and removed with a combination of curettes and pituitary rongeurs.
- The disc and cartilaginous material should be removed until the PLL and both uncinate processes are visualized (**TECH FIG 1A**).
- An important maneuver to facilitate disc space visualization and neural decompression is to remove the anterior portion of the inferior endplate of the superior vertebral body (the anterior lip). Doing so provides a direct line of sight into the posterior disc space, which facilitates later foraminotomy and resection of the PLL, if necessary.
- This surface is almost always concave, with the anterior portion overhanging the disc space, thus preventing direct visualization of the posterior disc space.
- Removal can be done with either a Kerrison rongeur or a high-speed burr.
- Flattening this surface also facilitates optimal graft–endplate contact (**TECH FIG 1B,C**).
- Use of the burr to fashion the endplates, alternating with use of the curettes and pituitary rongeur to remove cartilage and disc material, is performed.

Use of Distraction: Pins, Tongs, and Spreaders

- Intervertebral body distraction pins can be placed to gently distract the disc space and improve visualization.
  - Generally, this is done after an initial superficial discectomy, which allows greater disc space mobilization with the pins.
- Because greater preparation of the inferior endplate of the superior vertebra is usually needed, the Caspar pin should be placed more cephalad in the cephalad vertebral body (**TECH FIG 2**).
- Overdistraction of the disc space is not desired. If the disc space is fused in an overdistracted position, postoperative neck pain may result. If there is a significant compressive lesion on the spinal cord, distraction should be avoided until the compression has been relieved to prevent stretching or tenting of the cord over that lesion.
- An additional benefit of the Caspar pins is that they help to retract the soft tissues in a cephalocaudal direction without the use of a secondary set of retractor blades.
- Alternatively, a small laminar spreader can be used in the contralateral disc space instead of Caspar pins to provide distraction.

Endplate Preparation

- The inferior endplate of the cephalad level is concave, whereas the superior endplate of the inferior level tends to be relatively flatter. Thus, to achieve intimate contact of bone graft with both

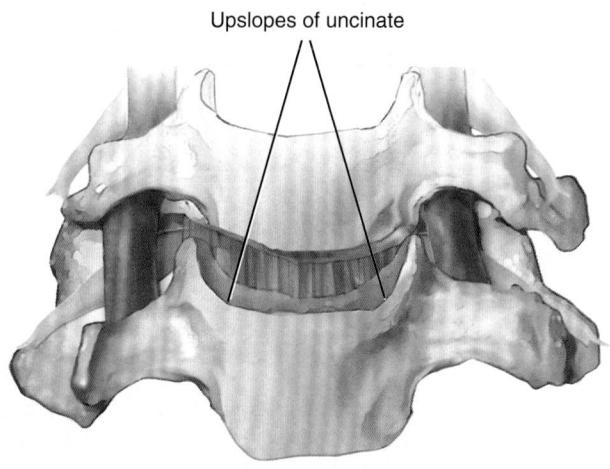

Upslopes of uncinate

A

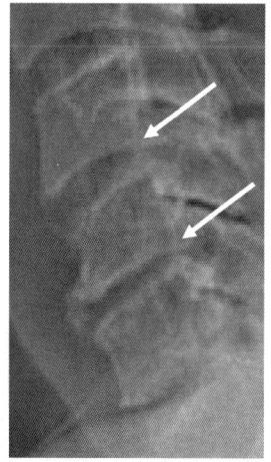

B

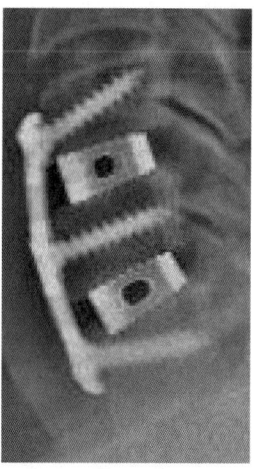

C

TECH FIG 1 A. The discectomy should be performed from uncus to uncus. The upslope of the uncinate is clearly defined with curettes and Kerrison rongeurs until these borders are unquestionably identified. Having a wide discectomy allows for placement of larger grafts or supplemental grafts in the uncinate regions. **B,C.** ACDF graft carpentry in a patient with two level cervical spondylotic myelopathy. Creating parallel disc spaces facilitates graft–host bone contact, securing an intimate fit as well as allowing for wide decompression of spurs arising from the posterior disc space (*white arrows* in figure B). Posterior spurs along the floor of the canal have been removed at each level, decompressing the spinal cord. The central portion of each endplate is maintained as much as possible to optimize structural integrity. Titanium interbody cages were used for structural grafting at both levels.

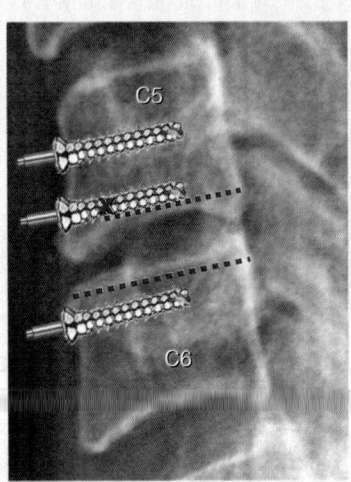

TECH FIG 2 Caspar pin placement. Because greater preparation of the inferior endplate on the cephalad vertebra is necessary, the surgeon should place the upper Caspar pin (C5) further away from the endplate (eg, in the midbody of C5 or more cephalad) while being cognizant of not entering the adjacent disc space above. The Caspar pins are placed in the midline to avoid compromising later screw fixation during plating. To achieve parallel distraction, the pins should be placed parallel to the disc space. If the tips (ie, the leading ends) converge, relative kyphosis of the disc space occurs with placement of the Caspar pin spreader and distraction; if the tips diverge, relative segmental lordosis occurs with placement of the Caspar pin spreader and distraction. It may be desirable at times to try to increase lordosis through this mechanism.

endplates, a rectangular space is created by parallel decortication of the endplates.

- This generally requires greater preparation of the inferior endplate of the cephalad level versus the superior endplate of the inferior level.
- It is important not to remove too much bone off the inferior endplate of the cephalad level, however, as doing so limits the bone available in the vertebra to accommodate a plate and screws. This is particularly the case in smaller patients who have smaller vertebrae.
- A high-speed burr is helpful in decorticating the endplates.
- The creation of a parallel rectangular space within the disc space allows insertion of a graft appropriately sized to match the larger height present at the center of the disc space.
- Both endplates should be thoroughly denuded of cartilage and decorticated to reveal bleeding bony surfaces to enhance the chance of successful fusion.[5]
- Alternating use of the high-speed burr, curettes, and the pituitary rongeur will allow the surgeon to reach the posterior disc space and the PLL.
- During ACDF, we are more aggressive with endplate preparation than during corpectomy because ACDF grafts tend to be more stable than corpectomy grafts.
  - If major endplate resection is performed during corpectomy, significant settling or pistoning of the graft may occur (see Chap. SP-7), which is less likely with ACDFs. Furthermore, in cases of extensive spondylosis, wide disc space preparation facilitates decompression along the floor of the canal in ACDF surgery.
  - When performing corpectomy, on the other hand, the additional room is not usually necessary because removing the vertebral body creates wide access for work at the disc level.

Anterior Foraminotomy

- The discectomy is performed to the level of the PLL, with complete removal of the posterior annulus. It is safer to leave the PLL intact during the initial foraminotomy or resection of posterior osteophytes when the burr is being used because it acts as a protective layer to the neural elements. Once the bony removal is complete, the PLL can then be resected.[2]
- The medial half of the posterior uncinate is thinned under direct visualization with a high-speed burr to unroof the entry zone of the foramen (**TECH FIG 3**).
  - The microscope is angled appropriately to visualize the uncinate.
- In general, it is easier to decompress the contralateral rather than the ipsilateral foramen, although decompression of both is certainly possible. Thus, in cases of unilateral radiculopathy, we prefer to approach the spine from the side opposite to the patient's symptoms.
- It is important not to force a large instrument into a severely narrowed foramen if it does not fit easily. Instead, the surgeon

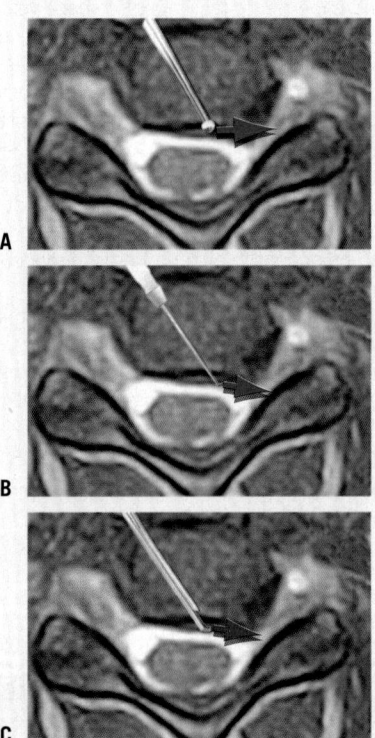

TECH FIG 3 Anterior foraminotomy. **A.** The burr is used to thin down bone in the lateral aspect of the canal (*arrow*) until only a thin shell is left. The PLL is left intact as a protective layer to the neural elements until burring is completed. **B.** A curette is used to outline the bony edges and ensure that they are thin enough for passage of a curette or Kerrison rongeur. The PLL does not necessarily need to be resected during foraminotomy if the pathology is due solely to uncinate bone spurs, although we routinely do so and do not consider the decompression complete until the lateral edge of the dura and the exiting root are clearly visualized and palpated to be free of compression. **C.** A 2-mm Kerrison is then used to remove bone spurs. It is critical to hug the posterior margin of the uncinate during this move to avoid injuring the root underneath, which exits the canal ventrolaterally at about 45-degree angle. Note also that the vertebral artery is typically at the level of the mid-disc space. Thus, it is important to stay posterior when removing osteophytes off of the uncus rather than straying anteriorly where the vertebral artery is at greater risk.

should use the burr to thin the uncus until the instrument can easily be passed into the foramen.

- Constant irrigation is performed to prevent thermal injury and to clear away bone debris.
- If visualization is adequate, continued thinning of the osteophyte can progress until only a thin shell of bone is left.
- A microcurette or 2-mm Kerrison is then used to resect the thinned osteophytes.
- Alternating between microcurettes or a Kerrison and the burr, the foramen can be gently and progressively carved out laterally.
  - The nerve root exits the spinal canal at roughly 45-degree angle ventrolaterally. Thus, it is imperative to avoid blindly placing a burr, curette, or Kerrison deep to the uncinate to avoid root injury. Instead, one should closely hug the uncinate while entering and decompressing the foramen (see **FIG 1**).
- Foraminotomy is complete when a micro nerve hook or curette can easily be passed into the foramen anterior to the exiting root without resistance.[6]

When and How to Resect the Posterior Longitudinal Ligament

- With soft disc herniations, a defect in the PLL is often present through which the nuclear material extrudes **(TECH FIG 4A,B)**.

- By delicately probing with a microcurette, the extruded fragment can be fished out from behind the PLL.
  - If necessary, the defect in the PLL should be enlarged with a 2-mm Kerrison until a satisfactory portal is available to remove the herniation and ensure that all loose disc fragments have been removed.
- It is debatable whether the PLL needs to be resected in every case. In general, we prefer to do so, especially in cases of disc extrusion, and do not consider the decompression complete until the dural sac or exiting nerve root (depending on which is compressed based on preoperative imaging) is inspected for the absence of any further compression.
  - If, however, the compressive lesion is an uncinate spur, with no evidence of subligamentous disc extrusion, satisfactory decompression can be achieved by removing the spurs without necessarily removing the PLL.
- If there is no rent in the PLL, one can be created by teasing a microcurette between the longitudinal fibers of the PLL until the curette is posterior to the PLL **(TECH FIG 4C,D)**.
- Once the plane is identified between the PLL and dura, the fibers of the PLL can be resected with a curette or Kerrison rongeur.
- Placing tension on the PLL with gentle distraction will facilitate its removal.

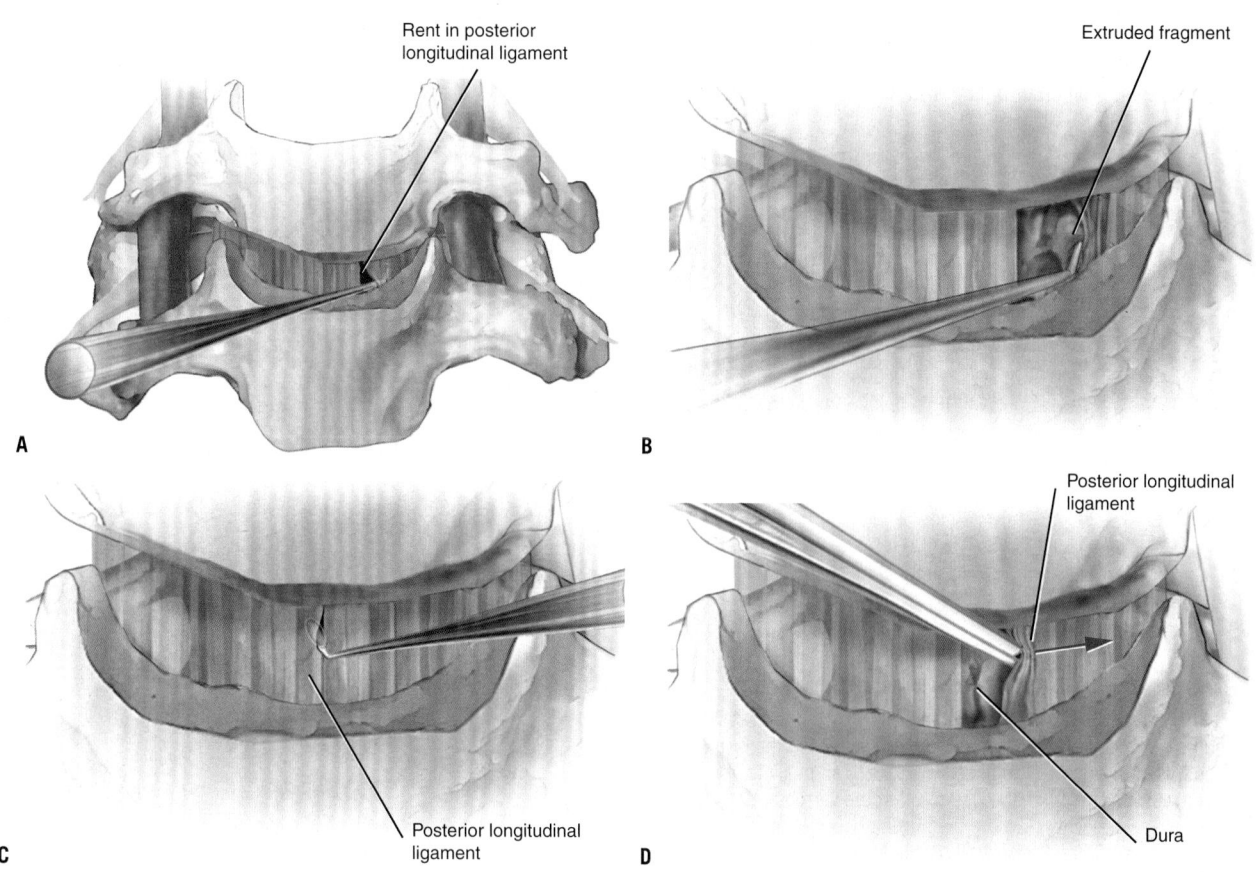

TECH FIG 4 A,B. Removing herniated nucleus pulposus. **A.** With extruded herniations, a rent in the longitudinal fibers of the PLL may be identified. A curette is then used to delineate the edges of the rent in the PLL. Once this is defined and the surgeon is certain of a plane between the PLL and underlying dura, a Kerrison is used to enlarge the edges of the rent. **B.** The rent has been enlarged to provide more room for finding the herniation. Curettes are then used to fish out the fragments and decompress the cord or root. **C,D.** Removing the PLL. **C.** If the PLL is intact, it can be removed by teasing in between the longitudinal fibers with a microcurette. Once a plane is established, a Kerrison can be used to remove the PLL. **D.** It is often easier to find this plane in the central portion of the PLL, where it is thicker, than laterally, where it is thinner and less defined.

TECHNIQUES

- We generally find it easier to define a plane in the PLL centrally, where it tends to be thicker, than laterally, where it is thinner and the plane with the dura is less distinct. Often, there are multiple layers of PLL, and usually in chronic cases, there is a membranous layer between the PLL and the dural sac that can be confused with dura itself. In general, if it does not look like dura, it probably is not.
- The portion of the PLL contralateral to the disc herniation or symptomatic foraminal stenosis does not routinely need to be removed.

Avoiding Vertebral Artery and Neural Injury

- Before surgery, the surgeon should always scrutinize the position of the vertebral arteries on the preoperative scans to rule out the presence of aberrancies in their course **(TECH FIG 5)**.
- Aberrations typically occur within the vertebral body. However, it is not uncommon for one vertebral artery to be closer to the uncinate on one side versus the other, which would mandate greater caution when approaching that side.[3]
- In the absence of vertebral artery aberrancy, laceration to the vertebral artery is most likely to occur from the surgeon's loss of orientation to the uncinates. The uncinates define the safe zone for the vertebral artery and the effective zone for the decompression.
  - It is imperative to define and maintain orientation with both uncinates at all times during anterior cervical surgery.
- The vertebral artery is typically in the anterior two-thirds of the disc space. When curetting disc material in this area, a

- vertebral artery laceration might occur if the curette strays lateral to the lateral border of the uncinate.
- If in doubt, a Penfield dissector can be used to identify the lateral border of the uncinate processes to avoid straying laterally and injuring the vertebral arteries, which are generally a few millimeters from the lateral edge of the uncinate **(TECH FIG 5C)**.

Graft Sizing and Placement

- Ultimate graft height can be estimated preoperatively from the preoperative lateral film. In many cases, a graft height of 2 to 3 mm more than that measured on the preoperative lateral film will be the optimal choice.
- Ideally, the anteroposterior depth of the graft should be a few millimeters less than that of the disc space, such that the graft can be countersunk 2 mm without entering the spinal canal.
- The final height of the graft can be determined after endplate preparation with sizers that accompany commercial grafts **(TECH FIG 6)**.
  - The trials should be lightly malleted into position under gentle Caspar pin distraction.
- A snug fit in the distracted position will ensure an excellent fit after removal of distraction pins.
- If the trial does not fit but the next smaller trial seems too loose, the surgeon should identify the area of impingement and lightly decorticate that area. Then, the trial is reinserted.
- For multilevel ACDF, we prefer to decompress and graft each segment before proceeding to the next level.
- One way to enhance fusion rates is to place as much bone into the interspace as possible. A wide decompression also provides greater room for bone graft.
  - Space lateral to the structural bone graft in the uncinate regions can be packed with bone or bone graft substitutes. If the space is wide enough, two grafts can be placed side by side to fill the entire space.

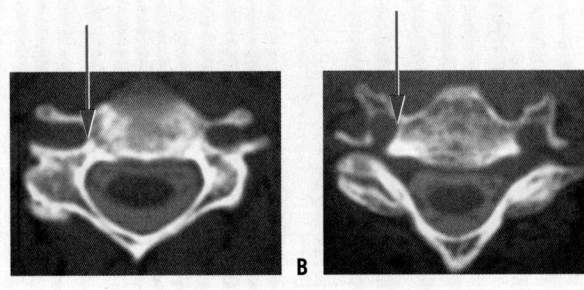

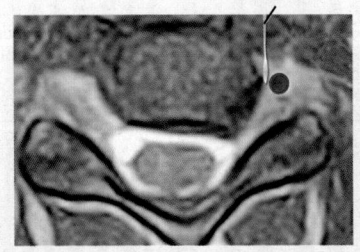

Dissector

TECH FIG 5 A,B. Vertebral artery anomalies. **A.** The right transverse foramen (*arrow*) courses somewhat more medially than the one on the left. This is a subtle but potentially important anomaly to observe preoperatively. **B.** The anomaly occurs within the vertebral body rather than at the disc space level where the right transverse foramen is now more normally positioned (*arrow*). **C.** Penfield lateral to the uncinate. In certain cases, especially if there is a deformity, the location of the lateral border of the uncinate (ie, the safe zone for the vertebral artery) may not be obvious after elevation of the longus colli. Placing a Penfield dissector no. 4 gently underneath the longus colli, retracting it laterally, and then hooking the dissector lateral to the uncinate will allow for safe orientation to the vertebral artery.

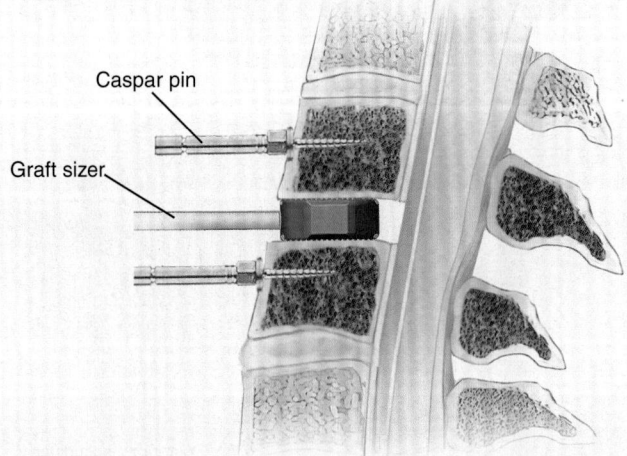

Caspar pin

Graft sizer

TECH FIG 6 Commercially available sizers are used to determine optimal graft size. A trial that fits snugly under gentle Caspar distraction will suffice. If autograft is used, the appropriate trial is used as a template for cutting the autograft bone. The surgeon should try to place a graft that fills the space as much as possible without overdistracting, which can cause posterior neck pain, or entering the spinal canal.

- We generally prefer to use commercially prepared cortical allografts for ACDF, except in patients with poor healing potential. Alternatively, autograft iliac crest bone can be used.

Determining Plate Length

- Plating is optional for one-level ACDF with autograft. If allograft or multilevel surgery is performed, plating is recommended.
- Once the graft has been placed, the size of the plate is then determined.
- Optimal plate length is one that allows for the screws to be immediately adjacent to the endplates **(TECH FIG 7)**.
  - This plate length allows for screws that angle away from the disc space, which in turn allows for screws that are longer than ones directed parallel to the disc space, yet are short enough to avoid entry into the supra- and infra-adjacent disc spaces.
  - This length also prevents impingement of the plate into the adjacent disc spaces.

Plating Techniques

- The plate should be contoured into lordosis to lie flush against the vertebral bodies.
  - It should also be centered coronally within the margins of the uncinate processes.
- Screws should also be angled medially to decrease the chance of lateral injury to nerve roots or vertebral arteries.

- The screw length can be estimated preoperatively by measuring the depth of the vertebral body on CT or MRI scans. Ideally, screws are as long as possible within the vertebral body to maximize fixation.
- Dynamic plates can be used if desired **(TECH FIG 8)**. They have the theoretical benefit of improving load sharing on the graft. There are several types of dynamic plates.
  - Variable screw systems allow for toggling within a fixed screw hole with settling of the construct. A potential downside is that the screw can loosen within bone as toggling occurs.
  - Slotted plates have holes that allow screws to translate longitudinally as the construct shortens. The screws are rigidly fixed to bone and do not toggle, but excessive translation may lead to adjacent-level plate impingement.
  - Telescoping plates use fixed screws in nonslotted holes, but the ends of the plate telescope with respect to each other as settling occurs. Postoperative adjacent-level plate impingement will not occur with this design if the plate is properly positioned at the time of surgery, as the distance from the end of the plate to the endplate does not change with construct shortening. However, these plates tend to be somewhat thicker.
- If dynamic plates are used, the surgeon must perform the plating procedure to accommodate the anticipated settling without overlapping uninvolved adjacent discs.[9] In general, we prefer rigid plating in most cases to avoid excessive construct settling. Variable plating has not been clearly demonstrated to improve outcomes or fusion rates.

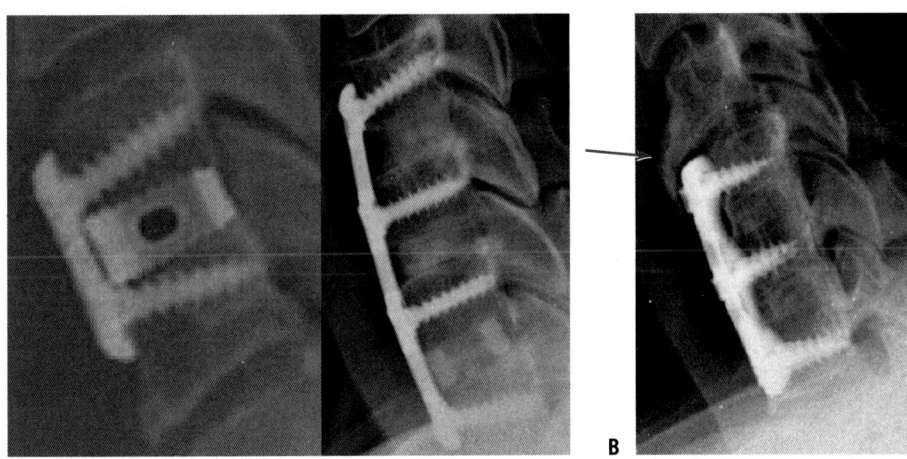

TECH FIG 7 Proper plate sizing. **A.** Two patients whom we treated with one (*left*) and three (*right*) level ACDF. The length of an optimally sized plate is such that the screw holes at the top and bottom of the construct are as close as possible to their respective endplates. Long screws provide stronger fixation. Screws should be angled away from the disc space to provide greater length and divergent fixation, which may better resist pullout. In the three-level patient (*right*), the distal segment has been grafted with two allografts rotated 90 degrees to the usual orientation in order to better fill the large disc space (as a result, note the different appearance of the grafts at this level vs. the proximal two levels). **B.** This patient was sent to us for adjacent segment disease after surgery elsewhere. The plate was placed too close to the adjacent disc, resulting in adjacent-level ossification disease (*arrow*). The cephalad screws are not immediately adjacent to the endplate but rather inserted at roughly the midpoint of the vertebral body. Similarly, the caudal screws begin in the midportion of the vertebral body. The plate is too long distally and comes close to the subjacent disc as well.

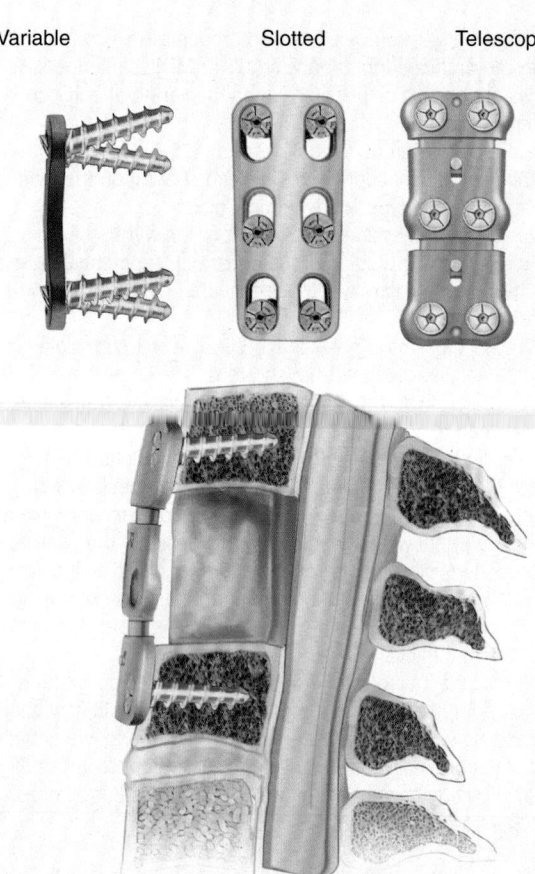

Variable   Slotted   Telescoping

TECH FIG 8 Dynamic plates generally fall into three categories: those with variable screws that fit into round holes that allow for toggling of the screws, those with slotted holes to allow for translation, and those in which the ends of the plate telescope are shortened. In contrast to the variable and slotted plates, with the telescoping plate design shown, the relationship between the ends of the plate and the adjacent disc spaces remains fixed as the plate dynamizes because the plate shortens internally. Thus, progressive adjacent-level disc impingement is less likely to occur with settling over time if it did not occur at the initial placement of the device.

ANTERIOR CERVICAL DISCECTOMY AND FUSION WITHOUT INSTRUMENTATION

Sam W. Wiesel

- ACDFs were traditionally performed without plating.
- Although plates may better preserve lordosis and achieve higher fusion rates in multilevel cases, avoiding plates may decrease operative time, decrease the amount of retraction on the soft tissue structures of the neck during surgery, and avoid plate-related complications such as screw backout or esophageal erosion.
- However, if one chooses not to use a plate, autograft should be used rather than allograft, and rigid postoperative immobilization in a cervical orthosis is mandatory.
- Up to three adjacent interbody cervical fusions can be safely performed without instrumentation.
  - The interspaces should be fused sequentially, meaning a decompression and fusion is completed at one interspace before the next is addressed.

Measuring the Space

- After appropriate decompression, the depth and height of the interspace are measured without distraction (**TECH FIG 9A,B**).

- A laminar spreader is then inserted to distract the interspace, and the height is again measured (**TECH FIG 9C,D**).
- Without distraction, the height is generally 6 mm; with distraction, it can be up to 12 mm.
- This distraction is important in shaping the tricortical graft. The height of the graft should be greater than the resting height but less than the distracting height so that the inherent compression of the vertebral bodies will hold the graft firmly in place.

Inserting the Graft

- After the appropriate size of cortical graft is obtained, it is inserted with the laminar spreader distracted (**TECH FIG 10A,B**).
- The graft should have at least a 2-mm offset anteriorly, and the posterior edge of the graft should be 4 mm anterior to the dura and PLL.
- After the distraction is released (**TECH FIG 10C,D**), the graft should be tested for stability by trying to dislodge it using a smooth right angle probe.
- Postoperatively, if the graft is stable, a simple soft collar should be used for 4 to 6 weeks.

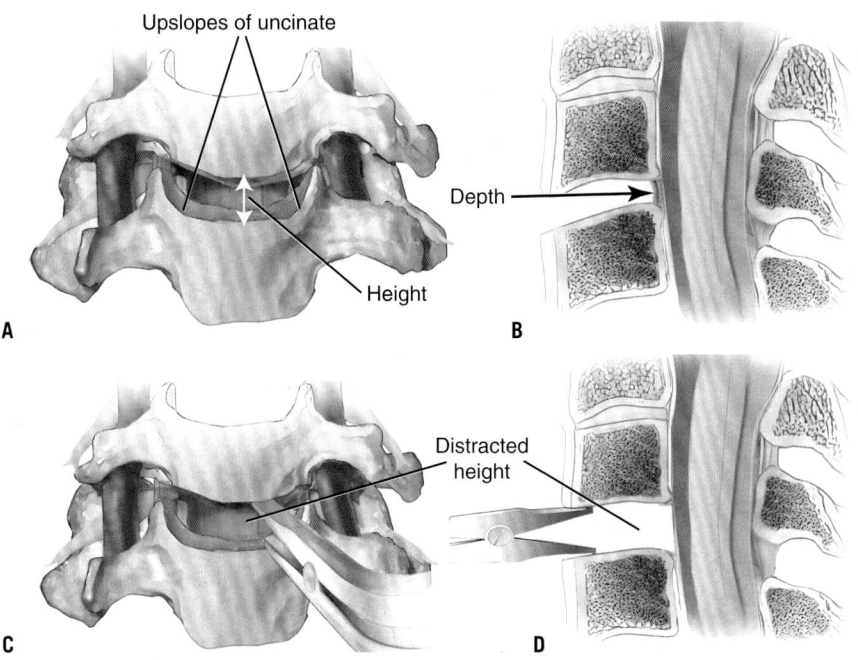

TECH FIG 9 Measuring the interspace without (**A,B**) and with (**C,D**) distraction.

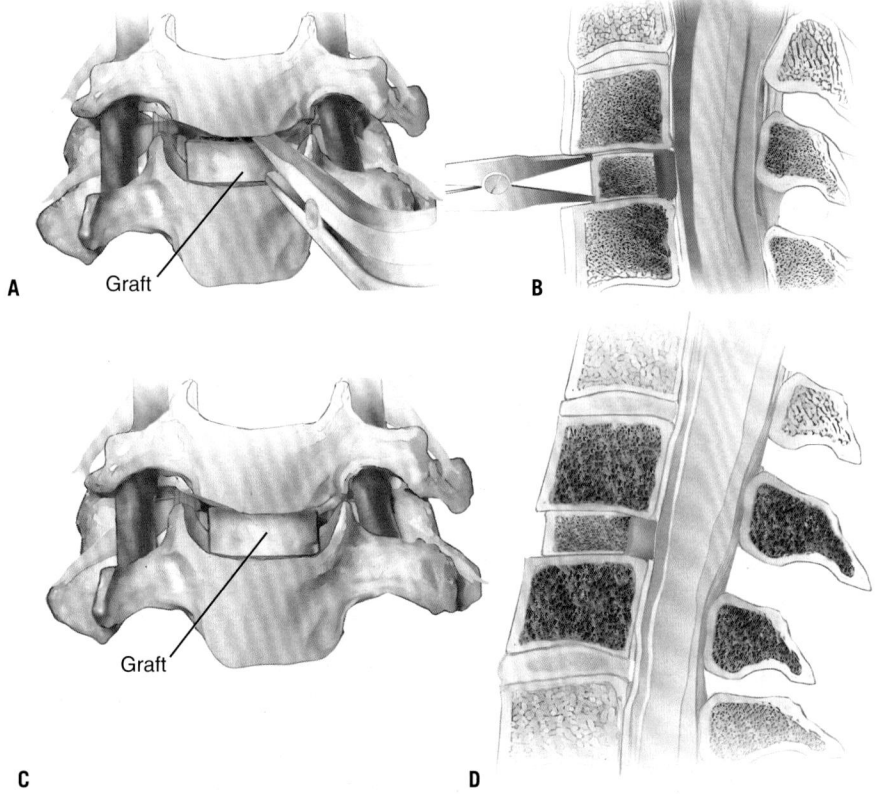

TECH FIG 10 The cortical graft in place with (**A,B**) and without (**C,D**) distraction. Without distraction, the graft is compressed by the natural elasticity of the cervical spine. There is about 2 to 6 mm of free space between the posterior surface of the graft and the spinal cord.

Pearls and Pitfalls

Discectomy	• Removing the anterior portion of the inferior endplate allows for better visualization of the posterior disc space, particularly in narrow spondylotic discs, and facilitates subsequent decompression.
Endplate Preparation	• The surgeon should create a rectangular space with parallel endplates. This will generally require greater preparation of the inferior endplate of the cephalad vertebrae. Excessive bone removal should be avoided to prevent excessive graft settling.
Foraminotomy	• The uncinate is the guide to the foramen. The surgeon should maintain orientation to it at all times. When entering the foramen to remove bone spurs, the curette or Kerrison should hug the posterior aspect of the uncinate to avoid the nerve root, which exits ventrally at a 45-degree angle. The uncinate should be thinned first with a burr so that a small instrument can be inserted into the foramen to complete the foraminotomy without injuring the underlying root.
Plate Fixation	• The surgeon should choose the shortest plate that will fit, such that the screw holes are immediately adjacent to the endplates, to avoid adjacent-level plate or screw impingement.
Multiple Fusions in ACDF without Instrumentation	• In cases of multiple fusions, each decompression and fusion must be completed before the next interspace is addressed. If all the interspaces to be fused are decompressed before the first graft is inserted, it will lead to unbalanced grafts, with one bone plug being significantly wider than the others because of the inherent elasticity of the vertebral bodies. In general, the vast majority of ACDFs are now plated, especially multilevel cases.

POSTOPERATIVE CARE

- The use of bracing after plated ACDF is debatable.
- We typically place the patient in a cervical collar for 6 weeks.
- A deep drain is placed in the retropharyngeal space to prevent hematoma formation. It is typically removed the morning after surgery unless its output is greater than 30 mL in the last 8 hours.
- The postoperative diet may be rapidly advanced as tolerated. Cold beverages and ice cream may help with dysphagia and reduce swelling in the immediate postoperative period.

OUTCOMES

- Over 90% of patients experience excellent relief of radicular symptoms with ACDF.
- Midline axial neck pain may improve if it is associated with radicular pain, but patients should be counseled that the primary goal of treatment is neural decompression and relief of radicular or myelopathic symptoms.
  - Similarly, unilateral neck pain can be a manifestation of radiculopathy and also generally improves.
  - However, isolated axial neck pain without radicular complaints does not predictably improve with surgery, and we recommend nonoperative treatment in most such patients.

COMPLICATIONS

- Complications potentially associated with ACDF include dysphagia, dysphonia, pseudarthrosis, implant failure, neurologic injury, esophageal injury, airway compromise from swelling or hematoma, and vertebral artery injury.[1]
- Some degree of dysphagia is almost universal immediately after surgery. The majority of patients with dysphagia have only mild symptoms, with clinical improvement within 3 weeks. Long-term significant dysphagia is not common (about 4%).
- The superior laryngeal nerve innervates the cricothyroid muscle, which adjusts the tension on the vocal folds and also provides supraglottic sensation. Superior laryngeal nerve palsies therefore may lead to difficulty with singing high notes as well as aspiration.

- The recurrent laryngeal nerve innervates the muscles responsible for abducting the vocal folds. Recurrent laryngeal nerve palsy most commonly presents as hoarseness. Bilateral injuries can lead to airway obstruction and require tracheostomy.
- Even with modern surgical techniques, nonunions still occur. However, many cervical nonunions are asymptomatic and do not require further treatment. Symptomatic nonunions can be addressed with revision ACDF or posterior laminoforaminotomy and fusion.
- It is often argued that fusion accelerates adjacent segment degeneration. Although biomechanical studies show increased disc pressures and mobility at discs adjacent to fusions, clinical series have not confirmed that adjacent segment degeneration is truly accelerated by fusion versus simply being a manifestation of the patient's propensity toward spondylosis. In fact, the available evidence suggests that about 3% of patients will have symptomatic adjacent segment disease regardless of whether the index operation was ACDF, anterior cervical discectomy without fusion, or posterior foraminotomy without fusion.[7]

REFERENCES

1. Bazaz R, Lee MJ, Yoo JU. Incidence of dysphagia after anterior cervical spine surgery: a prospective study. Spine (Phila Pa 1976) 2002;27:2453–2458.
2. Brigham CD, Tsahakis PJ. Anterior cervical foraminotomy and fusion. Surgical technique and results. Spine (Phila Pa 1976) 1995;20:766–770.
3. Curylo LJ, Mason HC, Bohlman HH, et al. Tortuous course of the vertebral artery and anterior cervical decompression: a cadaveric and clinical case study. Spine (Phila Pa 1976) 2000;25:2860–2864.
4. Ebraheim NA, Lu J, Haman SP, et al. Anatomic basis of the anterior surgery on the cervical spine: relationships between uncus-artery-root complex and vertebral artery injury. Surg Radiol Anat 1998;20:389–392.
5. Emery SE, Bolesta MJ, Banks MA, et al. Robinson anterior cervical fusion comparison of the standard and modified techniques. Spine (Phila Pa 1976) 1994;19:660–663.
6. Henderson CM, Hennessy RG, Shuey HM Jr, et al. Posterior-lateral foraminotomy as an exclusive operative technique for cervical radiculopathy: a review of 846 consecutively operated cases. Neurosurgery 1983;13:504–512.

7. Hilibrand AS, Carlson GD, Palumbo MA, et al. Radiculopathy and myelopathy at segments adjacent to the site of a previous anterior cervical arthrodesis. J Bone Joint Surg Am 1999;81(4):519–528.

8. McAnany SJ, Rhee JM, Baird EO, et al. Observed patterns of cervical radiculopathy: how often do they differ from a standard, "Netter diagram" distribution? Spine J 2019;19(7):1137–1142.

9. Park JB, Cho YS, Riew KD. Development of adjacent-level ossification in patients with an anterior cervical plate. J Bone Joint Surg Am 2005;87(3):558–563.

10. Radhakrishan K, Litchy WJ, O'Falon WM, et al. Epidemiology of cervical radiculopathy. A population-based study from Rochester, Minnesota, 1976 through 1990. Brain 1994;117:325–335.

11. Sampath P, Bendebba M, Davis JD, et al. Outcome in patients with cervical radiculopathy. Prospective, multicenter study with independent clinical review. Spine (Phila Pa 1976) 1999;24:591–597.

12. Smith GW, Robinson RA. The treatment of certain cervical-spine disorders by anterior removal of the intervertebral disc and interbody fusion. J Bone Joint Surg Am 1958;40-A(3):607–624.

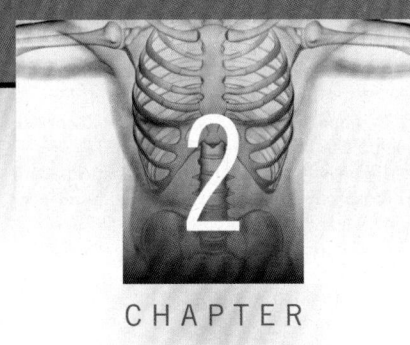

2

CHAPTER

Anterior Cervical Corpectomy and Fusion with Instrumentation

John M. Rhee and Claude Jarrett

DEFINITION

- Cervical myelopathy describes a constellation of signs and symptoms resulting from cervical spinal cord compression. Common symptoms include gait instability, clumsiness and loss of manual dexterity, and glove-like (rather than dermatomal) numbness of the hands.
- Because the presentation of myelopathy can be subtle, especially in its early manifestation, the diagnosis can be missed or wrongly attributed to "aging."
- Surgical decompression is the mainstay of treatment and can be accomplished anteriorly (ie, corpectomy, discectomy and fusion, or both), posteriorly (ie, laminectomy and fusion or laminoplasty), or through a combined anterior-posterior approach depending on the pattern of spinal cord compression.
- Anterior corpectomy and fusion are discussed in this chapter. Corpectomy is performed when retrovertebral compression of the spinal cord exists. If the compression is purely disc-based, corpectomy is not necessary, and an anterior cervical discectomy and fusion approach can be used instead.

PATHOGENESIS

- Spondylotic changes (eg, bone spurs, disc degeneration with annular bulging, disc herniations) are the most common causes of cervical cord compression.
- Ossification of the posterior longitudinal ligament (OPLL) is another not uncommon cause of cord compression. It may arise in discrete locations or be continuous (**FIG 1A,B**).[6]
- Kyphosis, whether primary or occurring after laminectomy, can also cause cord compression and myelopathy.
- Cervical myelopathy often arises in the setting of a congenitally narrowed cervical canal (**FIG 1C,D**). In these patients, the cord may have escaped compression during relative youth but not after the accumulation of a threshold amount of space-occupying spondylotic changes.
  - Although cervical spondylotic myelopathy tends to be a disorder seen in patients 50 years of age or older, depending on the degree of congenital stenosis and the magnitude of the accumulated spondylotic changes, it can be seen in patients who are much younger.

NATURAL HISTORY

- Patients with cervical myelopathy are generally thought to have a poor prognosis without surgical treatment, with a gradual stepwise progression of symptoms.[1]

HISTORY AND PHYSICAL FINDINGS

- Patients with cervical myelopathy present with a spectrum of upper and lower extremity complaints.
  - Upper extremity complaints include a generalized feeling of clumsiness of the arms and hands, "dropping things," inability to manipulate fine objects such as coins or buttons, trouble with handwriting, and diffuse (nondermatomal) numbness.
  - Lower extremity complaints include gait instability, a sense of imbalance when walking, and "bumping into walls" when walking. Family members may comment that the patient walks as if he or she is intoxicated.
- Patients with severe spinal cord compression may also complain of Lhermitte symptoms: electric shock-like sensations that radiate down the spine or into the extremities with certain offending positions of the neck (can occur with either flexion or extension).
- Many myelopathic patients deny any loss of motor strength. Similarly, bowel and bladder symptoms, if present, may arise in the later stages of disease. Despite advanced degrees of spondylosis, many myelopathic patients may have no neck pain.
- Symptomatic nerve root compression can coexist in patients with myelopathy and presents as a myeloradiculopathy.
- Physical examination should include the following:
  - Scapulohumeral reflex testing, which is positive with hyperactive elevation of the scapula or abduction of humerus upon tapping the spine of the scapula. This finding may be associated with high cervical cord compression from C1 to C3.
  - Jaw jerk reflex, which is positive with hyperactive jerking of the jaw upon tapping
  - Test for the Babinski sign, which is positive if the great toe extends while the remaining toes fan apart upon stroking the lateral sole of the foot and then curving across the metatarsal heads medially
  - Test for the Hoffman sign, which is positive with spastic flexion of the index finger and thumb upon flicking the distal phalanx of the middle finger
  - Inverted radial reflex test, which is positive if one observes flexion of fingers rather than a reflex contraction of the brachioradialis upon tapping the brachioradialis tendon. Positive result suggests cord and root compression at the C5–C6 level.
  - Test for finger escape sign, which is positive if the little finger (also possibly the ring finger) cannot be held in this position without falling into abduction and flexion for more than 30 seconds. This is suggestive of cervical myelopathy.

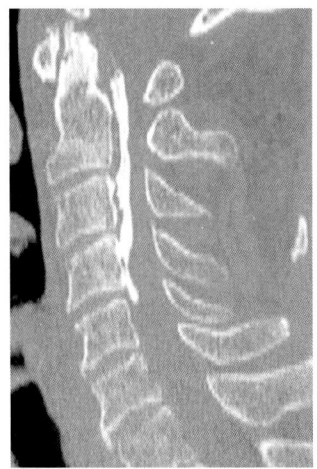

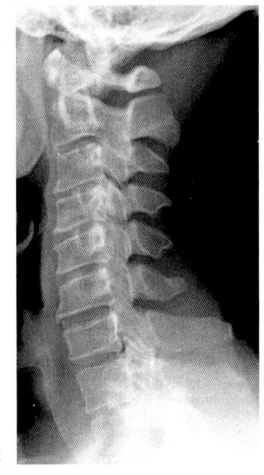

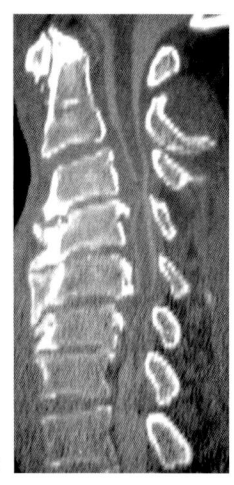

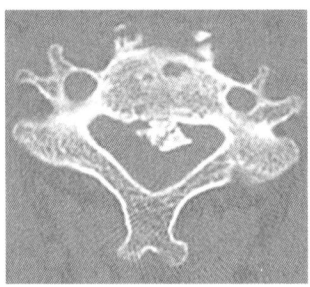

FIG 1 OPLL. **A.** Continuous OPLL causing severe spinal canal stenosis from C1 to C4. **B.** Axial CT scan in a different patient demonstrating a central stalk of OPLL. **C,D.** Congenital canal in different patients. *Congenital stenosis* is defined as a ratio of the canal to the vertebral body of 0.8 or less, and it can be measured on lateral radiographs (**C**) or advanced imaging such as CT-myelography (**D**). The CT-myelogram shows superimposed spondylotic changes that further narrow the canal dimensions and cause cord compression.

- Tandem gait test, which is positive if the patient demonstrates significant instability. A positive result confirms gait imbalance but in no way specifies the source of the imbalance as being the cervical spinal cord.
- It is important to note, however, that patients with cervical myelopathy may not necessarily have "classic" physical findings. One study[3] demonstrated that about 20% of patients with myelopathy do not display any obvious physical findings (eg, hyperreflexia, Hoffman sign). Thus, the absence of physical findings does not necessarily exclude the diagnosis of cervical myelopathy.

IMAGING AND OTHER DIAGNOSTIC STUDIES

- A lateral radiographic view can be helpful in showing the amount of congenital cervical stenosis as well as sagittal alignment.
- Lateral views are consistent with congenital stenosis when the ratio of the diameter of the canal to the diameter of the vertebral body is less than 0.8.
- Particularly if OPLL is suspected, computed tomography (CT) scans (with or without myelograms, depending on whether a high-quality magnetic resonance imaging [MRI] is available) are helpful in delineating bony versus soft tissue pathology.

DIFFERENTIAL DIAGNOSIS

- Of cervical myelopathy
  - Amyotrophic lateral sclerosis
  - Myopathies
  - Peripheral neuropathy
  - Syringomyelia
  - Multiple sclerosis
  - Diabetic neuropathy
  - Brachial plexopathy

NONOPERATIVE MANAGEMENT

- Surgery is generally the treatment of choice for symptomatic cervical myelopathy.
- Nonoperative treatment of cervical myelopathy is typically reserved for patients who cannot tolerate surgery.[4]
- Controversy exists regarding the management of patients with asymptomatic spinal cord compression. In those with severe asymptomatic compression, consideration should be given to prophylactic surgery, particularly if cord signal changes are present, to prevent spinal cord injury with trauma (eg, central cord syndrome) **(FIG 2)**.

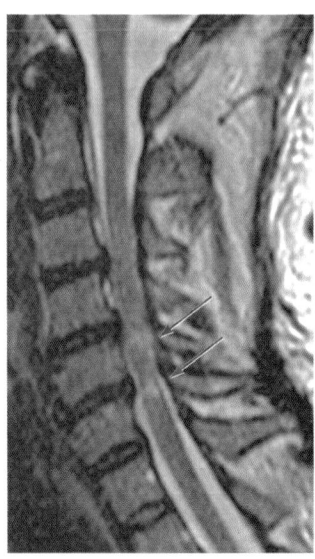

FIG 2 Sagittal T2-weighted MRI demonstrating spinal cord signal changes (*red arrows*).

SURGICAL MANAGEMENT

- The most common surgical options include anterior decompression and fusion (discectomy vs. corpectomy, depending on the absence or presence of retrovertebral cord compression, respectively), laminoplasty, and laminectomy with fusion.
- In general, anterior surgery is preferred when cord compression arises from three or fewer disc segments, as the incidence of fusion and graft complications increases substantially with greater number of segments fused. The presence of kyphosis or significant spondylotic neck pain also favors an anterior approach.
- Conversely, posterior approaches such as laminoplasty are favored when myelopathy arises from three or more motion segments and the cervical alignment is neutral or lordotic, particularly if the patient has minimal to no neck pain.
  - For posterior surgery to adequately decompress the cord, however, enough lordosis must be present to allow cord to drift back after removal of the posterior tethers (lamina, flavum).
- Combined anterior and posterior surgery should be considered in cases of significant kyphosis, whether primary or postlaminectomy.
- Multilevel corpectomy as a stand-alone operation is generally not recommended due to a relatively high propensity for frank construct failure or sagging into kyphosis. Plating does not reliably prevent such failures. Failures of stand-alone multilevel corpectomies are even more likely in patients with significant postlaminectomy kyphosis. In cases where multilevel corpectomy is needed, supplemental posterior fixation should be considered.

Preoperative Planning

- Preoperative CT and MRI scans should be scrutinized to analyze the course of the vertebral arteries and the width of the spinal canal requiring decompression.

- CT scans may provide additional information to MRI scans when it is unclear whether the compressive lesions are bony (OPLL, osteophytes) or soft disc material.

Positioning

- For anterior cervical corpectomy and fusion, patients are positioned as described in Chapter SP-01.
- However, greater caution is necessary in positioning the myelopathic versus radiculopathic patient. In particular, one must ensure that the patient is not excessively extended beyond the tolerance of the compressed cord. The amount of extension tolerated preoperatively should be assessed and not exceeded intraoperatively.
- Gardner-Wells tongs traction is optional when performing corpectomy, especially if a multilevel corpectomy is needed. In general, traction can be generated intraoperatively for one or even two-level corpectomies through Caspar pins without need for external tong traction.
- Significant distraction on the cervical spine should be avoided until after the cord has been decompressed to avoid stretching the cord over compressive pathology.

Approach

- The approach is similar to that for anterior cervical discectomy and fusion but generally needs to be more extensile to access multiple levels. (Please see Chap. SP-01 for further details.)
- The surgeon should ensure that wide exposure beyond the medial border of the uncinates is achieved, with appropriate elevation of the longus colli muscles bilaterally, to achieve a stable base for the self-retaining retractors as well as to provide orientation to the uncinates, which remain the critical landmarks for either corpectomy or discectomy surgery.

TECHNIQUES

EVALUATING THE LIMITS FOR THE CORPECTOMY

- The corpectomy is performed after the initial discectomies above and below the vertebra to be resected. The discectomies are performed from uncinate to uncinate as detailed in Chapter SP-11.
- The width of the corpectomy required to decompress the cord should be based on preoperative imaging studies **(TECH FIG 1)**.
  - Generally, sufficient decompression will occur if the width of the decompression spans from uncinate to uncinate.

- Wider decompressions beyond the medial border to the uncinates are typically performed at the disc level, where a combination of cord and root compression may occur, but are not necessary at the vertebral body level, where only the spinal cord is compressed.
- Staying within the uncinates will allow for thorough decompression while avoiding vertebral artery injury, unless a vertebral artery anomaly exists. Such anomalies are more likely to occur within the vertebral body rather than the disc spaces, and they should be recognized on preoperative imaging to avoid injury.

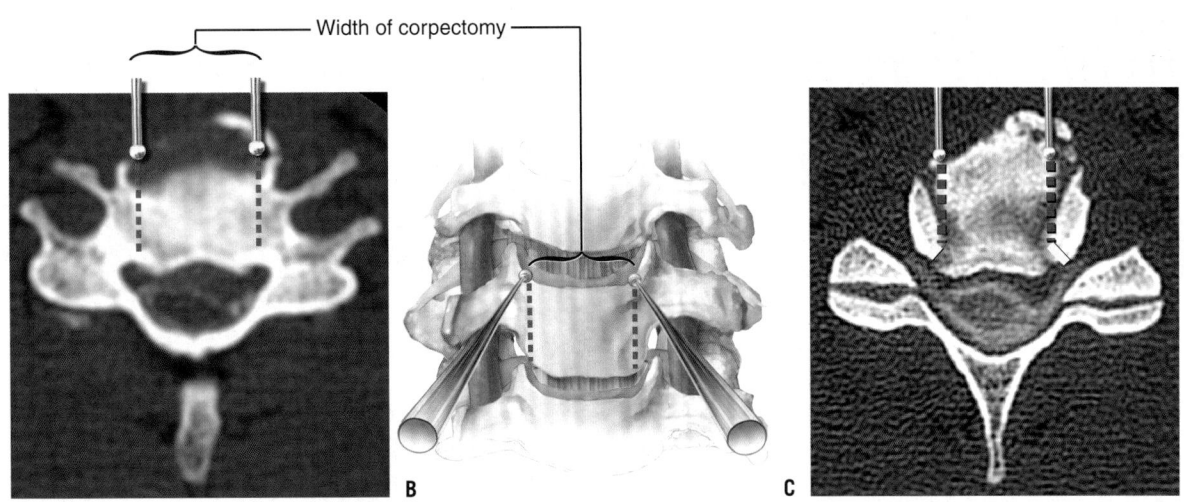

TECH FIG 1 Limits of corpectomy. **A.** The width of the corpectomy is based on that necessary to decompress the spinal cord and can be estimated on preoperative imaging. **B.** In general, a corpectomy spanning from the medial border of one uncinate to the other will be sufficient at the vertebral body level. **C.** At the level of the disc space, a wider decompression may be necessary for satisfactory root decompression (*yellow lines*).

CERVICAL CORPECTOMY

- The edges of the corpectomy are longitudinally delineated with a high-speed burr from uncinate to uncinate to define the safe limits of the decompression.
- Next, a Leksell rongeur can be used to quickly remove large fragments of vertebral body bone (**TECH FIG 2**). This bone should be saved for grafting.
- Once the cancellous bone is removed grossly, fine decompression then proceeds with a high-speed burr.
- Under direct visualization, a high-speed burr is used to remove bone until a thin shell of posterior cortex remains.
- Microcurettes and Kerrisons are then used to flake off the remaining bone.
- Attention should be paid to maintaining the width of the corpectomy as it proceeds posteriorly toward the canal, as the tendency is to cone the decompression narrowly as one proceeds posteriorly.
- Vertebral body bleeding often hinders visualization during bone removal.
  - The surgeon should take time to achieve hemostasis using bone wax (gently applied when the remaining vertebra is still thick) or powdered Gelfoam–thrombin (when the remnant vertebral body is very thin).
  - Significant dorsal pressure should be avoided during these maneuvers to avoid inadvertently plunging into the spinal canal.
- Epidural bleeding is best controlled with bipolar cautery as well as Gelfoam–thrombin.

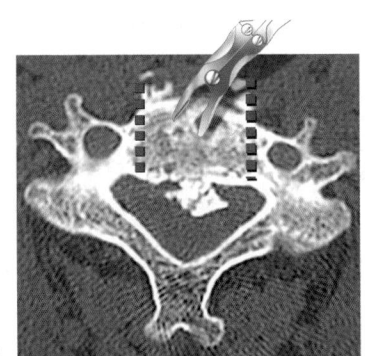
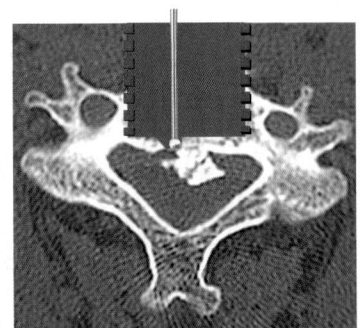
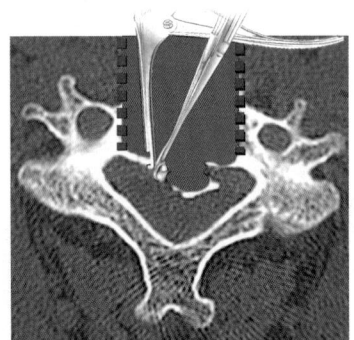

TECH FIG 2 Steps in bone removal. **A.** Leksell rongeur is used to remove large pieces of vertebral body bone after delineating the lateral edges of the corpectomy longitudinally along the medial border of the uncinates with a high-speed burr. **B.** After removing the bulk of the vertebra, a burr is used to sequentially remove bone in layers until only a thin remnant of bone remains. **C.** Finally, curettes and Kerrison rongeurs are used to remove the remaining bone. Adequate thinning of all bone to be removed allows the passage of smaller instruments that do not exert pressure on the spinal cord.

REMOVING THE POSTERIOR LONGITUDINAL LIGAMENT

- If cord compression arises strictly from bony osteophytes or congenital narrowing of the spinal canal, the posterior longitudinal ligament (PLL) does not necessarily need to be resected. In general, we favor removing the PLL to confirm adequate decompression.
- If, however, there is an extruded or sequestered herniated disc behind the vertebral body or if OPLL is the cause of compression, the PLL should be resected.
- When resecting the PLL, a small curette is used to probe in between longitudinal fibers of the PLL until it can be passed dorsal to it. Once a plane is created, larger curettes or 2- or 3-mm Kerrisons can be used to complete the resection of the PLL **(TECH FIG 3)**.
- If severe OPLL is present, the dura may be deficient or absent, and the surgeon should be prepared to perform a dural patch and possibly a subarachnoid lumbar drain.
  - The presence of severe OPLL may favor a posterior approach, all other factors being equal, to avoid complications related to dural deficiencies.
- In severe OPLL, instead of removing the entire OPLL, an alternative technique is to allow it to float anteriorly by releasing its tethers at nonossified portions, then allowing the ossified portion to float anteriorly along with the underlying adherent dura. However, one downside to this approach can be the potential for regrowth of the OPLL.[9]

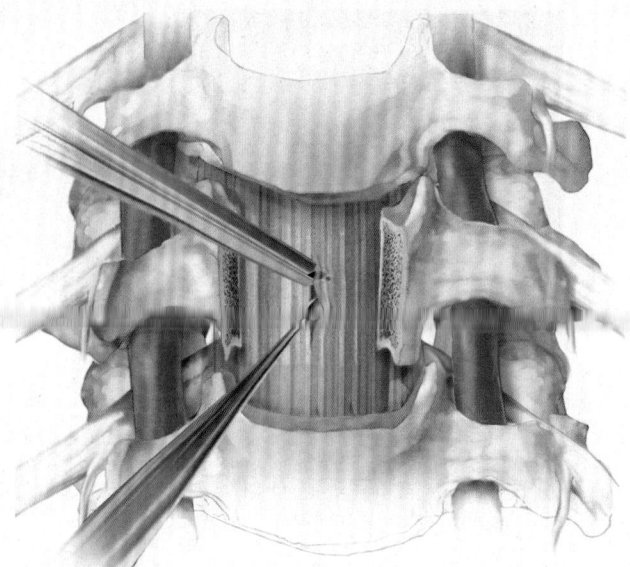

TECH FIG 3 A curette is used to tease apart the longitudinal fibers and create a plane dorsal to the PLL. Once this plane is identified, a curette or pituitary rongeur is used to elevate the PLL while a small Kerrison removes it. The surgeon must be careful never to exert compression on the cord by passing large instruments.

GRAFTING OPTIONS

- Autograft, allograft, or cages can be used.
- Autograft options include structural iliac crest or autologous fibula. Both are excellent graft materials but can be associated with significant donor site morbidity. Because of its shape, iliac crest is generally suitable for one- or sometimes two-segment corpectomy reconstruction. Fibula is favored for two-segment or more corpectomy reconstruction.[8]
- Because of donor site morbidity issues, allograft fibula or cages filled with local autograft remain popular choices for corpectomy reconstruction.
- Local corpectomy bone can be used to provide the biologic stimulus for healing, allowing the allograft to serve both structural and osteoconductive roles. Local bone is packed in and around the allograft **(TECH FIG 4)**.

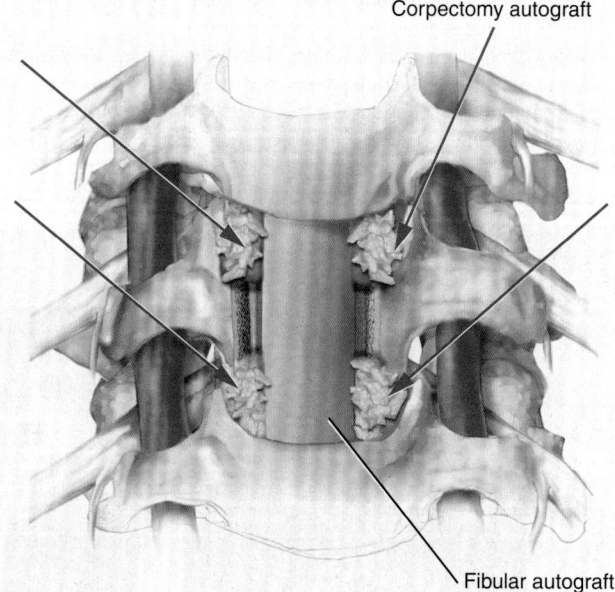

Corpectomy autograft

Fibular autograft

TECH FIG 4 Local morselized autograft (*arrows*) is packed around the strut graft and into the cleared-out uncinate regions. An additional benefit of wide discectomy is the ability to fuse the uncinate regions.

ENDPLATE PREPARATION

- The endplates above and below the corpectomy should be thoroughly decorticated and denuded of all cartilaginous material.
  - To prevent excessive subsidence, we prefer not to remove as much endplate when performing corpectomy reconstruction as is done when performing anterior cervical discectomy and fusion.
- Nevertheless, it is helpful to remove the anterior lip on the caudal surface of the cephalad vertebra to allow for better contact of the graft to the endplate. The anterior lip is flattened to be level with the central concavity of the endplate (**TECH FIG 5A**).
- The structural integrity of the endplate is maintained in the central third to allow a stable loading surface for the graft.

- Preserving the curvature on the posterior third of the endplate protects the graft from kicking posteriorly into the canal.
- If the posterior lip needs to be removed to decompress the cord, it can be done along the floor of the canal with a Kerrison after the corpectomy is completed.
- Kick out is most likely to occur at the caudal end of the construct where the compressive loads on the graft are translated into a shear force due to the relative lordosis of the caudal vertebra. To prevent kick out, the caudal endplate may be prepared parallel to the floor, such that the shear vector is minimized. The trade-off is that doing so will result in a greater likelihood of subsidence (**TECH FIG 5B,C**).

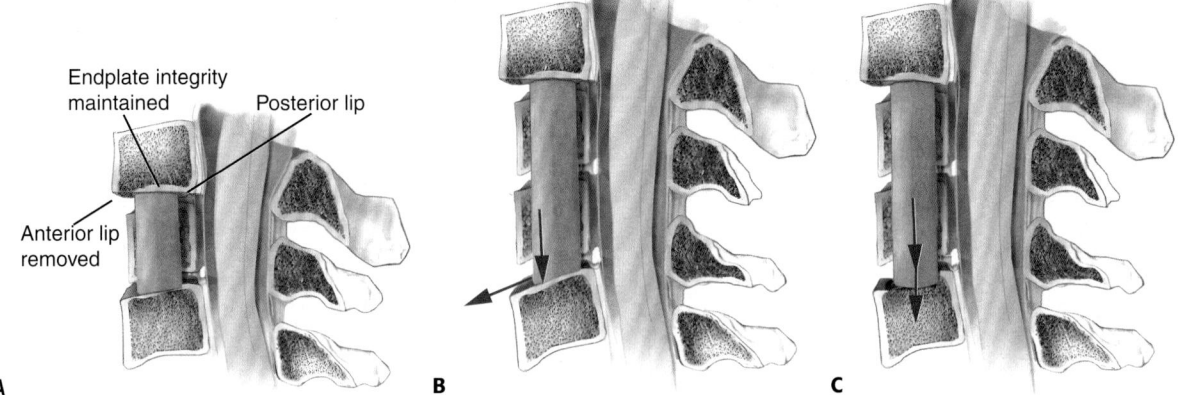

Endplate integrity maintained   Posterior lip

Anterior lip removed

A   **B**   **C**

TECH FIG 5 A. Carpentry of the inferior endplate of the cephalad level: preparing the inferior endplate of the cephalad segment (eg, the inferior endplate of C5 during a C6 corpectomy). Flattening the anterior lip and the anterior third of the endplate allows for proper insertion of a strut graft. They are flattened to be level with the central concavity of the endplate. The central third of the endplate is left as structurally sound as possible to resist excessive subsidence. The posterior third may be left intact to act as a barrier to posterior migration of the graft into the canal. The posterior lip, which is often a source of spondylotic compression, can be removed with a Kerrison after the corpectomy is completed to decompress the floor of the spinal canal. **B,C.** Carpentry of the superior endplate of the distal level. **B.** When performing corpectomy reconstructions in which the distal level is lordotic, if the superior endplate of that vertebra is not level with the ground, the graft may be more likely to kick out anteriorly as the compressive loads on the graft are converted into shear at the graft–endplate interface. **C.** One solution is to flatten the superior endplate of the caudal vertebra. The graft is now less likely to kick out, but the trade-off is that it may be more likely to piston.

GRAFT SIZING

- If a total corpectomy is performed, care is taken to find a graft that will fill most of the depth of the vertebral body but will still be small enough to stay well clear of the decompressed cord when recessed by 2 to 3 mm from the front of the vertebral body.
- A reasonable amount of distraction should be performed after the decompression. This can be done by the application of weights to cervical tongs or, in one- or some two-level situations, by Caspar pin distraction (the Caspar spreader is usually not long enough to span multilevel corpectomies).

- Care should be taken not to distract the spine until all compressive lesions on the cord have been removed to avoid tenting the cord over the compressive lesions.
- In general, the amount of distraction should result in overall vertebral column length that is slightly longer than it was preoperatively. Excessive distraction is more likely to result in subsequent graft pistoning and subsidence, as the spine naturally recoils to its initial state once the patient is upright.
- The wooden end of a cotton applicator can be whittled away until it just fits into the corpectomy. This can be used as a template for cutting the graft to appropriate length (**TECH FIG 6**).

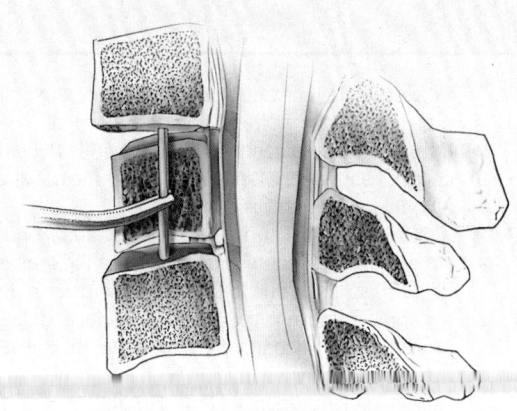

TECH FIG 6 After applying distraction, a wooden applicator (Q tip) serves as a useful device for measuring the length of the graft.

GRAFT INSERTION

- The graft is gently tamped into the distracted corpectomy site **(TECH FIG 7)**.
- Distraction is then released, and the stability of the graft is tested by gently pulling on the graft with a clamp.
- Because bony union is desired not only at the ends of the graft but also side to side between the shaft of the strut graft and the remaining vertebral bodies, intimate contact of graft to host is desirable in all regions. Any open spaces can be grafted with the local bone from the corpectomy.

- If autograft is scarce, it is best to save it for the ends of the allograft strut and fill the middle portion of the marrow cavity with a bone graft substitute.
- The uncinate regions at each disc level are a good surface for fusion and can be grafted with local bone. The residual disc spaces lateral to the medial border of the uncinates can be packed with local bone to facilitate fusion.

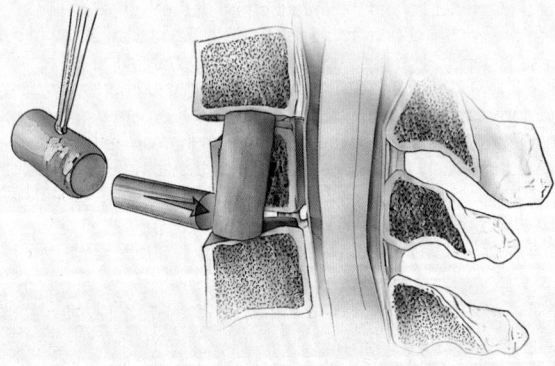

TECH FIG 7 The graft is inserted under either tong traction or Caspar pin distraction. The superior end of the graft is inserted first, and then the inferior end is gently tamped into position.

ANTERIOR CERVICAL PLATING

- Plating is performed as noted during anterior cervical discectomy and fusion.
- Stand-alone plated multilevel corpectomies (three or more disc levels) have been reported to be associated with high failure rates. Consideration should be given in such cases to supplemental posterior fixation.[7]

RESECTION OF SUPERIOR ARTICULAR FACET

- Once the inferior articular facet is resected, the superior articular facet underneath is resected out to the lateral border of the pedicles, completing the decompression **(TECH FIG 3)**.
- During the decompression, copious irrigation (20-mL syringe with a 2-inch long 18-gauge angiocatheter) must be used to prevent thermal damage to the surrounding tissues. It also aids in visualization.

- Typically, we recommend the use of a burr over Kerrison rongeurs because inserting instruments (such as Kerrison rongeur, which may have a relatively thick footplate) into the already stenotic canal and foramen can cause neurologic damage. However, once most of the roof of the foramen has been removed, it is usually safe to use a 1-mm Kerrison rongeur to clean up any overhanging bone.

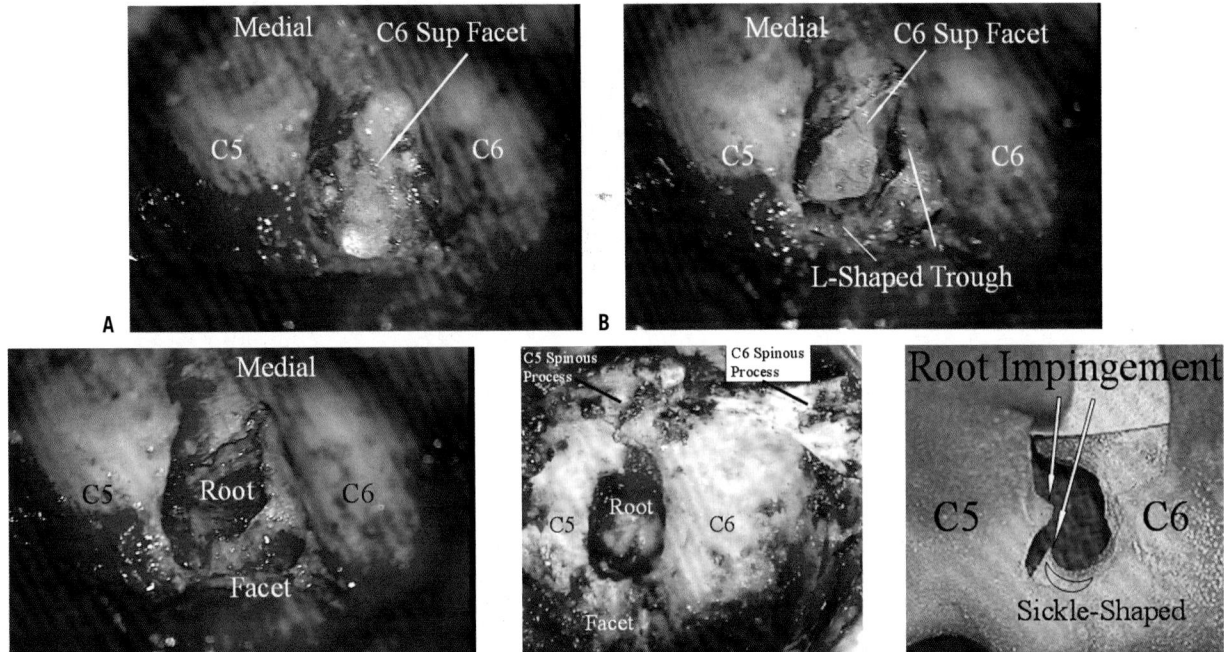

TECH FIG 3 A. An intraoperative image showing that once the inferior articular facet is resected, the superior articular facet underneath can be identified. **B.** The superior articular facet is resected out to the lateral border of the pedicles; this is best performed using an L-shaped resection, as shown in the intraoperative image, to ensure there is no iatrogenic impingement on the nerve root, which can occur if a keyhole or a C-shaped resection of the superior articular facet is performed (see **E**). **C.** An intraoperative image showing the complete resection of the superior articular facet. The remaining small ledge of bone can be removed using a small angled microcurette or 1-mm Kerrison rongeur. **D.** An intraoperative image showing the completed foraminotomy. **E.** Model of the cervical spine showing the C5–C6 interspace showing C- or sickle-shaped decompression, which can lead to iatrogenic impingement on the nerve root.

DISCECTOMY

- If the patient has an intraforaminal disc herniation, then the nerve root must be manipulated to expose the herniated disc fragment that is ventral to the nerve root.
- If there is little room for the root to migrate cranially, the cranial 2 to 3 mm of the caudal pedicle may have to be

burred down, and a microscopic right angle probe can then be placed into this space and rotated ventrally to the root to sweep any herniated disc fragment out from under the root, and micropituitary rongeurs can be used to remove the disc fragment.

CONFIRMATION OF ADEQUATE DECOMPRESSION

- After completing the decompression, a hemostatic agent such as Floseal or Surgiflo is used to control any bleeding surfaces.

- Once the foraminotomy is completed, the lateral walls of the cranial and caudal pedicles should be readily palpable, and there should be no bone overhanging the medial and superior aspect of the caudal pedicle (**TECH FIG 4**).

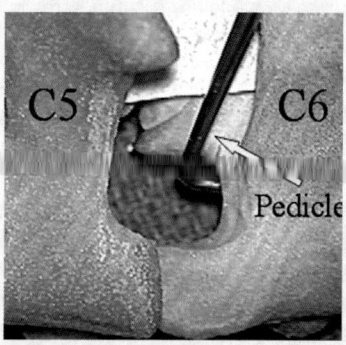
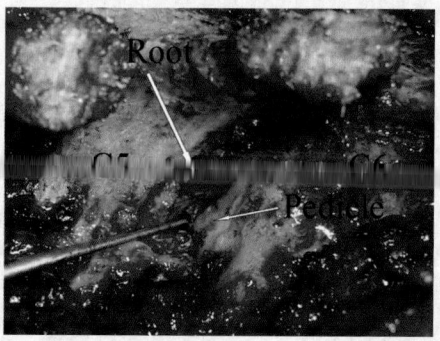

TECH FIG 4 A. Model showing completion of the foraminotomy with complete decompression of the foramen. The microprobe shows the medial pedicle border. **B.** An intraoperative image showing palpation of the medial pedicle border after completion of the foraminotomy.

WOUND CLOSURE

- The posterior wound is closed in multiple layers.
- If meticulous midline exposure was performed, the preserved interspinalis muscle is the first layer to be reapproximated. The amount of muscle incorporated into the suture is minimized because all such muscle will necrose.
- With a well-exposed spine, one can find a thin fascial layer enveloping the muscle that can be used to close the layers.

- The closure progresses from deep to superficial with the placement of a drain if needed. For unilateral foraminotomy, a drain is often not needed, but a drain can be necessary in a multilevel, bilateral operation.
- The drain prevents isolated pockets of hematoma, which can act as a nidus for infection.

TECHNIQUES

Pearls and Pitfalls

Positioning	• Bivector traction with the neck placed in flexion when the foraminotomy is being performed is crucial, as neck flexion unshingles the facets and exposes the underlying superior articular facet. • Reverse Trendelenburg position helps to decrease blood loss. • Good coordination and communication with the anesthesia providers during change of positioning of the head is critical.
Exposure	• Meticulous midline dissection through avascular raphe decreases blood loss and allows better closure. • Care must be taken not to detach the semispinalis cervicis from the spinous process of C2 if a C2–C3 foraminotomy is required. • Care must be taken to remain superficial to the facet capsules during dissection to preserve them, as they provide some protection against postoperative kyphosis.
Decompression	• Adequate decompression requires resection of the superior articular facet (the roof of the foramen) to the lateral margin of the pedicles. • About 50% (mediolateral) of the overlying inferior articular facet must be resected to expose the underlying superior articular facet. • Any overhang of the superior facet over the caudal pedicle can result in persistent nerve root compression.
Closure	• The posterior wound is closed in multiple layers to more closely reapproximate the normal anatomy.
Postoperative Course	• Postoperatively, patients do not have any range-of-motion restrictions nor are they required to wear a brace.

POSTOPERATIVE CARE

- Postoperative pain regimen includes patient-controlled analgesia and ketorolac (Toradol) for 36 to 48 hours in patients younger than age 65 years who have normal renal function and no history of congestive heart failure.
- Patients undergoing single level and unilateral procedures can often be discharged the same day from the recovery room. Patients undergoing bilateral or multilevel operations can remain in the hospital for 24 to 48 hours, depending on drain output and pain control. Patients are discharged on oral pain medication and are instructed to return to the clinic for routine follow-up at 6 weeks postoperatively.
- Although a soft collar is given for comfort, patients are encouraged to discontinue using the collar as soon as they can.
- There are no range-of-motion restrictions, and therapy with immediate motion can begin.
- Rapid return to normal activities and aerobic exercise is encouraged.

OUTCOMES

- Results of posterior cervical foraminotomy are encouraging, with good or excellent outcomes reported in about 90% to 95% of patients.

COMPLICATIONS

- Neurologic injury or worsening radiculopathy
- Infection
- Inadequate decompression or failure to relieve symptoms
- Instability and deformity secondary to overly aggressive decompression
- Air embolism if the procedure is done in a sitting position

SUGGESTED READINGS

Albert TJ, Murrell SE. Surgical management of cervical radiculopathy. J Am Acad Orthop Surg 1999;7:368–376.

Aldrich F. Posterolateral microdiscectomy for cervical monoradiculopathy caused by posterolateral soft cervical disc sequestration. J Neurosurg 1990;72:370–377.

Brodsky A. Management of radiculopathy secondary to acute cervical disc degeneration and spondylosis by the posterior approach. In: Kehr P, Weidner A, eds. The Cervical Spine. Philadelphia: J. B. Lippincott Co., 1983:395–402.

Emery SE. Cervical disc disease and cervical spondylosis. In: An HS, ed. Principles and Techniques in Spine Surgery. Philadelphia: Williams & Wilkins, 1998:401–412.

Epstein JA. The surgical management of cervical spinal stenosis, spondylosis, and myeloradiculopathy by means of the posterior approach. Spine (Phila Pa 1976) 1988;13:864–869.

Epstein NE. A review of laminoforaminotomy for the management of lateral and foraminal cervical disc herniations or spurs. Surg Neurol 2002;57:226–234.

Fager CA. Management of cervical disc lesions and spondylosis by posterior approaches. Clin Neurosurg 1977;24:488–507.

Fager CA. Posterior surgical tactics for the neurological syndromes of cervical disc and spondylotic lesions. Clin Neurosurg 1978;25:218–244.

Fager CA. Posterolateral approach to ruptured median and paramedian cervical disk. Surg Neurol 1983;20:443–452.

Grob D. Surgery in the degenerative cervical spine. Spine (Phila Pa 1976) 1998;23:2674–2683.

Henderson CM, Hennessy RG, Shuey HM Jr, et al. Posterior-lateral foraminotomy as an exclusive operative technique for cervical radiculopathy: a review of 846 consecutively operated cases. Neurosurgery 1983;13:504–512.

Herkowitz H, Kurz LT, Overholt DP. Surgical management of cervical soft disc herniation. A comparison between the anterior and posterior approach. Spine (Phila Pa 1976) 1990;15:1026–1030.

Levine MJ, Albert TJ, Smith MD. Cervical radiculopathy: diagnosis and nonoperative management. J Am Acad Orthop Surg 1996;4:305–316.

Ma DJ, Gilula LA, Riew KD. Complications of fluoroscopically guided extraforaminal cervical nerve blocks: an analysis of 1036 injections. J Bone Joint Surg Am 2005;87A:1025–1030.

Parker WD. Cervical laminoforaminotomy. J Neurosurg 2002;96(2 suppl):254.

Williams RW. Microcervical foraminotomy. A surgical alternative for intractable radicular pain. Spine (Phila Pa 1976) 1983;8:708–716.

Witzmann A, Hejazi N, Krasznai L. Posterior cervical foraminotomy: a follow-up study of 67 surgically treated patients with compressive radiculopathy. Neurosurg Rev 2000;23:213–217.

Woertgen C, Holzschuh M, Rothoerl RD, et al. Prognostic factors of posterior cervical disc surgery: a prospective, consecutive study of 54 patients. Neurosurgery 1997;40:724–729.

Zeidman SM, Ducker TB. Posterior cervical laminoforaminotomy for radiculopathy: review of 172 cases. Neurosurgery 1993;33:356–362.

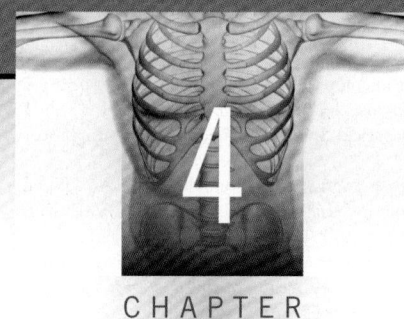

4

CHAPTER

Cervical Laminoplasty

Steven K. Leckie, James S. Kercher, and S. Tim Yoon

DEFINITION

- Cervical laminoplasty is a surgical technique first described in 1983 that is used to decompress the cervical spinal cord from a posterior approach.[3] The procedure is designed to open the spinal canal by reconstructing the cervical lamina without fusing across the motion segments of the spine. This procedure is typically performed over multiple levels, thus decompressing multiple compressed levels and preserving motion. It is distinctly different from a laminectomy in that the lamina is largely preserved and laminoplasty is thought to be much less likely to lead to cervical kyphosis.

- Cervical spondylosis is a degenerative condition, which can lead to multilevel spinal cord compression resulting in myelopathy. Congenital stenosis superimposed on spondylosis may predispose patients to myelopathy. Other conditions such as ossification of the posterior longitudinal ligament (OPLL), trauma, infection, and neoplasm can also result in myelopathy.

- The goal of laminoplasty is to alleviate compression of the spinal cord by decompressing the posterior aspect of the spinal canal and allowing the spinal cord to drift away from ventral compressive structures. A lordotic alignment of the cervical spine is helpful in the cord drift back.

ANATOMY

- The cervical spine is composed of seven vertebrae normally arranged in lordotic alignment. The occiput–C1 articulation is responsible for 50% of neck flexion and extension and the C1–C2 atlantoaxial articulation is responsible for 50% of total rotation. Lateral bending below the C2–C3 level is coupled with rotation due to the 45-degree inclination of the cervical facet joints.

- The subaxial vertebral segments of C3–C7 are similar to each other and distinct from C1 (atlas) and C2 (axis). The subaxial vertebrae articulate via zygapophyseal (facet) joints posteriorly and uncovertebral joints of Luschka laterally.

- Intervertebral discs are located between the vertebral bodies of C2–C7. The discs are composed of an inner nucleus pulposus and an outer annulus fibrosus.

- Anteriorly, the spinal canal is bounded by the vertebral bodies, the intervertebral discs, and the posterior longitudinal ligament. The pedicles form the lateral boundary of the spinal canal. Posteriorly, the ligamentum flavum runs from the anterior surface of the superior lamina to the anterior and posterior surface of the inferior lamina (**FIG 1**).

PATHOGENESIS

- Cervical spondylotic changes are the most common reason for cervical myelopathy.

- Spondylosis is characterized by intervertebral disc desiccation and height loss, which leads to annular bulging and osteophyte formation around the uncovertebral and facet joints. In the dorsal spinal canal, thickening or buckling of the ligamentum flavum further decreases canal and foraminal cross-sectional area.

- Spinal cord compression causes derangement at a cellular level, which leads to clinical deficits. In addition to static spinal cord compression, instability leads to motion that may aggravate myelopathy.

NATURAL HISTORY

- There is a lack of recent literature that documents the long-term natural history of cervical spondylotic myelopathy because modern practice is to perform a surgical decompression once significant myelopathy has been diagnosed. Early studies described a stepwise decline in neurologic function punctuated by stable periods, although some patients exhibited a continuous functional decline or no decline at all.

- The clinical course may be stable or worsen over a period of years. Sensory symptoms may be transient, but motor symptoms tend to persist and progress. Irreversible muscle atrophy can occur in long standing or severe myelopathy. Although surgical intervention may relieve symptoms and halt progression, neurologic deficits may be permanent.

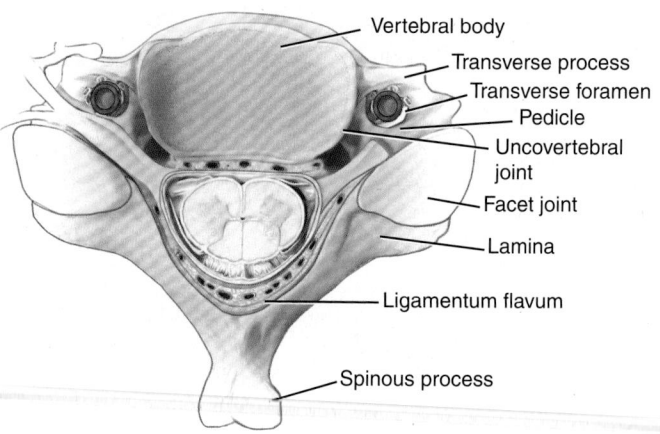

Vertebral body
Transverse process
Transverse foramen
Pedicle
Uncovertebral joint
Facet joint
Lamina
Ligamentum flavum
Spinous process

FIG 1 Anatomy of cervical vertebrae.

PATIENT HISTORY AND PHYSICAL FINDINGS

- The diagnosis of cervical myelopathy may be difficult secondary to the variability in clinical findings. Pain is frequently not a significant complaint in myelopathic patients unless it is associated with root compression or facet arthrosis. Patients may present with subtle findings or profound neurologic deficits.
- Patients can present with the insidious onset of gait disturbance, trouble with balance, and hand clumsiness. They may report numbness or other sensory disturbance in the upper extremities, difficulty with handwriting and fine motor control, or weakness of grasp. Weakness of the intrinsic muscles of the hand is often the first motor deficit. Advanced cases can present with motor weakness or bowel and bladder dysfunction.
- The physical examination should include an assessment of gait, which may be wide based, hesitant, stiff, or spastic. Inability to walk heel-to-toe is a sensitive physical finding. Patients may also display poor balance during toe raise.
- Sensory findings may be variable. Pain, temperature, vibratory, and light touch sensation may be decreased.
- Mixed upper and lower motor neuron findings may be present depending on the degree of cord compression, concomitant nerve root compression, or peripheral nerve dysfunction.
- The L'Hermitte sign is positive when extreme neck flexion or extension results in electrical sensation down the arms or body and is a sign of spinal cord compression. Pathologic reflexes include the scapulohumeral reflex (indicating compression above the C3 level) or inverted radial reflex (indicating compression at C5 or C6). Other findings include the Hoffman sign, clonus (more than three beats), Babinski sign, slow grip and release, unsteady Romberg (posterior column), and abnormal finger escape (T1 level).

IMAGING AND OTHER DIAGNOSTIC STUDIES

- Plain anteroposterior and lateral standing radiographs of the cervical spine are useful for initial evaluation of sagittal alignment and the extent of spondylotic changes (such as disc space narrowing, osteophytes, kyphosis, joint subluxation, and spinal canal stenosis; **FIG 2A**).
  - Flexion and extension views provide information about possible spinal instability.
- Typically, magnetic resonance imaging (MRI) is the imaging modality of choice for diagnosing spinal cord compression. It can visualize the spinal cord and canal dimensions without any ionizing radiation. The spinal cord parenchyma can be visualized to help evaluate the extent of spinal cord damage. MRI is also useful for visualization of compressive soft tissue such as ligamentum hypertrophy and disc herniation (**FIG 2B**). Because it is usually obtained supine, MRI is less reliable than standing x-ray for evaluation of sagittal alignment.
- Computed tomography (CT) is superior to MRI for defining bony anatomy and is useful for evaluating OPLL (**FIG 2C,D**). The addition of contrast dye myelogram combined with the CT (CT-myelogram) can improve the ability to assess spinal cord compression in the setting of previous hardware placement that would obscure an MRI with scatter artifact.

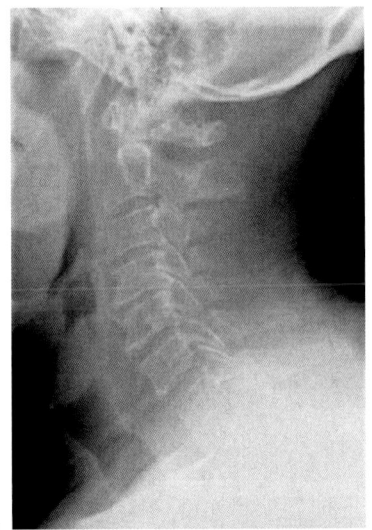

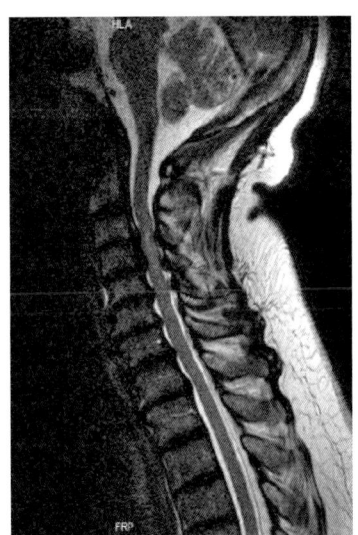

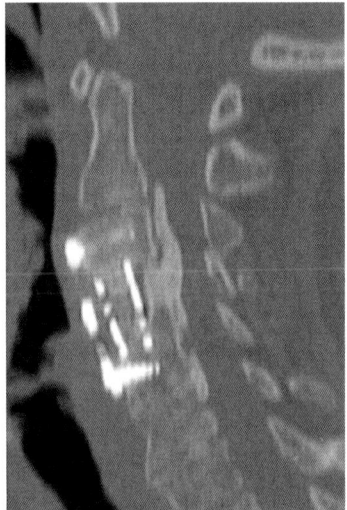

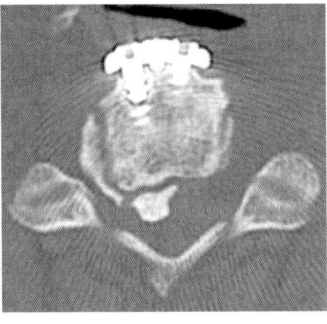

FIG 2 A. Preoperative lateral cervical spine radiograph demonstrating spondylotic changes: diffuse disc height loss and osteophyte formation. **B.** Sagittal T2-weighted MRI showing multilevel cervical disc protrusions and circumferential stenosis at C3–C4, C4–C5, and C5–C6, resulting in cord deformation. Cord signal changes can be seen at C3–C4 and C4–C5, indicative of cord damage. **C.** Sagittal CT reconstruction showing large ossified posterior longitudinal ligament extending from C2 to C6. There is evidence of failed anterior decompression by an outside facility. **D.** Axial CT image demonstrating a large ossified posterior longitudinal ligament.

DIFFERENTIAL DIAGNOSIS

- Stroke
- Peripheral compression neuropathy (ie, carpal tunnel syndrome, cubital tunnel)
- Parkinson disease
- Muscular dystrophy or dystonia
- Syringomyelia
- Tumor
- Vascular disease
- Autoimmune disorders
- Epidural abscess
- Nerve injury
- Drug intoxication
- Multiple sclerosis
- Amyotrophic lateral sclerosis
- Cerebellar dysfunction
- Idiopathic movement disorder
- Peripheral neuropathy (vitamin B_{12} deficiency)

SURGICAL MANAGEMENT

- Laminoplasty was specifically designed to decompress the spinal cord while avoiding the kyphotic deformities that had previously complicated laminectomy alone. Laminoplasty may be associated with fewer complications than laminectomy and fusion[2,8] and has lower implant costs. It may also have fewer complications than multilevel anterior corpectomy.[1]
- Laminoplasty creates effective posterior decompression of the subaxial cervical spine by allowing for dorsal cord expansion and drift while preserving motion.[5] Dome laminectomy of C2 can be added if needed.
- Theoretical advantages of laminoplasty over laminectomy and fusion include relative motion preservation, less soft tissue dissection, shorter operative time, diminished blood loss (in experienced hands), and less concern about smoking status and nonsteroidal anti-inflammatory drug use (which would increase the nonunion risk in fusion surgery).
- Laminoplasty can be performed via open door (lateral opening trough with a single hinge) or French door (midline opening trough with bilateral hinges) technique. Although the French door technique requires an additional hinge, it results in less epidural bleeding than the open door technique because the veins tend to be lateral. Both techniques are effective in treating myelopathy.[7]
- Indications
  - Spinal stenosis due to either cervical spondylosis, congenital stenosis, or OPLL that results in multilevel cord compression and cervical myelopathy[6]
- Contraindications
  - Kyphotic sagittal alignment of more than 10 to 14 degrees can lead to worsening of kyphosis and poor neurologic outcomes because the spinal cord is unable to drift back.
  - Significant segmental instability
- Relative contraindications
  - Previous posterior cervical surgery such as foraminotomies: Scar formation can produce adhesions that impede safe opening of the laminar arch.
  - Primary axial neck pain in the setting of myelopathy: Laminoplasty preserves motion, and hence the procedure is not designed to address pain generation from

facet arthrosis and disc degeneration. Fusion procedures may provide greater benefit to patients with significant complaints of axial neck pain.

Preoperative Planning

- Evaluation of the patient's active range of motion in flexion and extension assists with head positioning. Passive flexion and extension beyond the patient's natural range during positioning can lead to dangerous impingement or stretching of the tenuous cord and subsequent neurologic dysfunction.
- Careful examination of CT scans to determine the bony anatomy of the dorsal cortices is helpful, with special attention given to the lamina-to-lateral mass junction.
- French door laminoplasty may also be used in conjunction with fusion (in lieu of laminectomy) to increase the size of the fusion bed, although this makes instrumentation more challenging. A unilateral open door technique can also be used with fusion and lateral mass instrumentation if needed.

Positioning

- Intubation is performed with caution in the myelopathic patient, starting with advanced notification to anesthesia personnel. Care should be taken not to extend the neck more than the patient's comfortable range of motion before sedation. The use of fiberoptic assistance should be considered in high-risk cases.
- Application of a Mayfield head holder provides a stable platform during the procedure (**FIG 3A**).
- The patient is placed prone onto chest bolsters. The abdomen should be as free as possible to reduce venous bleeding and prevent ventilatory difficulty. Arms are padded and tucked at the patient's side (**FIG 3B**). Shoulders can be taped in gentle traction, although care must be taken to avoid stretching the brachial plexus.

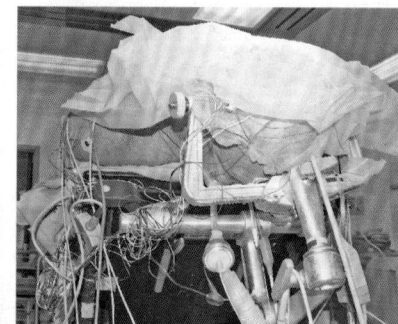
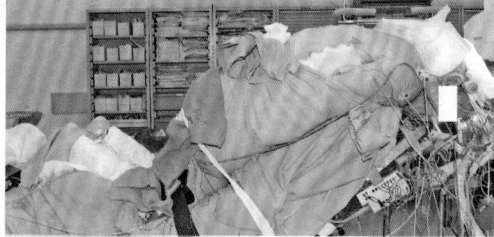

FIG 3 A. The patient's head is placed in a Mayfield head holder. **B.** The patient is placed prone onto chest bolsters with arms tucked at the sides. The head is placed in slight flexion. Spinal cord monitoring equipment is also seen.

- The head is positioned in slight cervical flexion, which tensions the skin on the posterior neck folds and decreases shingling of lamina.
- Intraoperative modification of neck flexion–extension is possible if needed by adjustment of the Mayfield tongs.
- The bed is placed in reverse Trendelenburg to decrease venous bleeding and allow for a more horizontal surgical field.

- Spinal cord monitoring is often performed in myelopathic patients. This helps to monitor neurologic problems related to positioning as well as with the laminoplasty procedure itself.
- Hair should be clipped to above the base of the occiput. The surgical field should be prepared from the nuchal line to roughly T4 to allow for possible wound extension.

INCISION AND DISSECTION

- In the typical situation where C3–C7 lamina need to be decompressed, a posterior midline approach to the spinous processes is made using a longitudinal incision extending from C2 to T1. In situations where fewer levels need decompression, avoiding exposure of C2 or C7 can reduce postoperative pain and instability.
- Electrocautery is used to divide the subcutaneous fat in the midline to reach the tips of the spinous processes.
- Once the tips of the spinous processes have been found, a meticulous subperiosteal dissection is performed to expose the lamina. Careful attention should be paid to stay in the midline avascular plane to reduce bleeding.
  - The dissection should extend laterally to fully expose the junction of the lateral mass and the lamina.
  - Exposure should not extend beyond the midportion of the lateral masses, unlike a traditional laminectomy and fusion exposure, which requires wider access.

- The extensor muscle attachment to the C2 spinous process is carefully preserved to prevent iatrogenic kyphosis. The inferior C2 laminar margin is usually broad and should be exposed to aid in visualization of the C2–C3 junction.
- The spinous processes can be amputated at their base. In certain situations, the spinous processes can be for strutting open the lamina or for local morselized bone grafting of the hinge side. Avoid placing bone graft in the interlaminar spaces or across facet joints.
  - Removing the spinous processes significantly improves exposure and reduces asymmetric posterior displacement of paraspinal musculature (**TECH FIG 1A**).
- The interlaminar ligamentum flavum between levels C2–C3 and C7–T1 (or the top and bottom interspaces) is removed. First, a rongeur is used to create a small opening in the interlaminar ligament flavum. Then, a combination of curettes and Kerrison rongeurs is used to divide the remainder of the interlaminar ligamentum flavum (**TECH FIG 1B**).

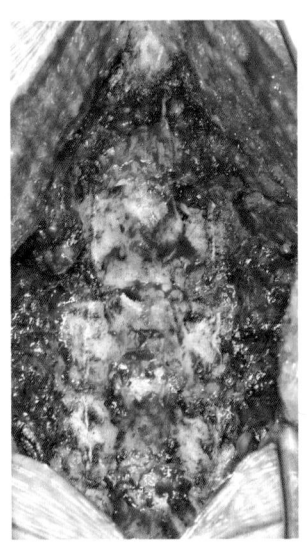 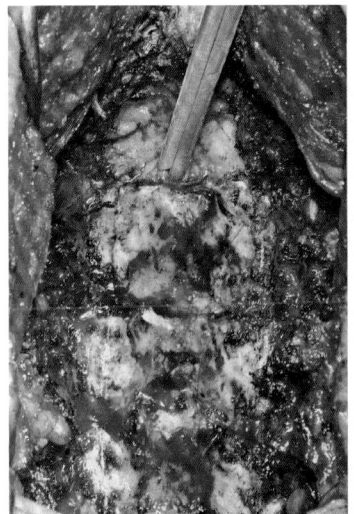

TECH FIG 1 A. Lamina exposure after subperiosteal dissection and spinous process removal. The dissection should extend laterally to expose the junction of the lateral mass and lamina. Attempts should be made to minimize disruption of the facet capsule. This will decrease long-term postoperative neck pain. Planned lines for opening and hinge trough creation have been marked using electrocautery and marking pen. **B.** A Kerrison rongeur is used to divide the interlaminar ligamentum flavum.

TROUGH PREPARATION

Open-Side Trough

- The open side should be on the side with the more severe foraminal stenosis.
- A 4.0-mm round or oval low-aggression high-speed burr is used to form the trough.
- The trough location is at the junction of the lamina and lateral mass.

- For the opening side, bony layers should be removed in sequence: the outer cortex, then the cancellous middle layer, followed by most of the ventral cortex (**TECH FIG 2A**).
- If the trough gets deeper than the diameter of the 4.0-mm burr without reaching the ventral cortex, the trough may be too lateral and heading toward the vertebral artery and should be redirected medially.

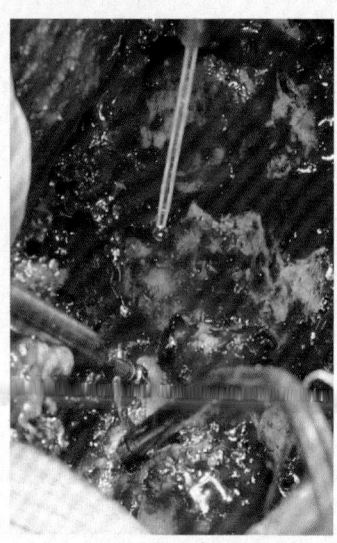
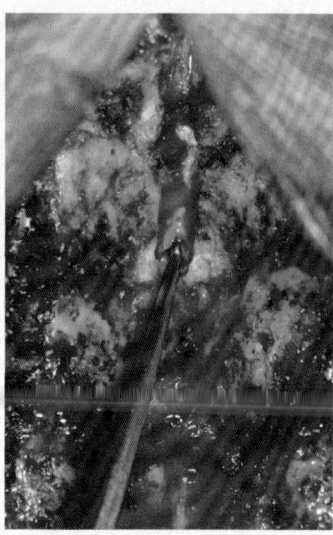

TECH FIG 2 A. Creation of the opening trough requires sequential removal of bony layers with a burr (open door technique depicted). **B.** After the initial burring, completion of the trough can be performed using a microcurette, a 2.0-mm Kerrison rongeur, or a diamond burr (French door technique depicted).

- Once the ventral laminar bone is thinned sufficiently, complete the trough with a microcurette, a 2.0-mm Kerrison rongeur, or a diamond burr to reduce the chance of durotomy from burring directly onto the dura **(TECH FIG 2B)**.
- Care should be used at this time to avoid the epidural veins, which can create significant bleeding. Thrombin-soaked powdered Gelfoam and bipolar electrocautery can be used to control bleeding epidural veins.

French Door (Midline Splitting)

- The French door technique involves creation of a midline opening trough and two lateral hinge troughs **(TECH FIG 3A)**.
- The midline of the posterior arch can be split by a variety of methods. One method is to remove the spinous process and use a 4.0-mm low-aggression burr to create a complete midline trough **(TECH FIG 3B)**.

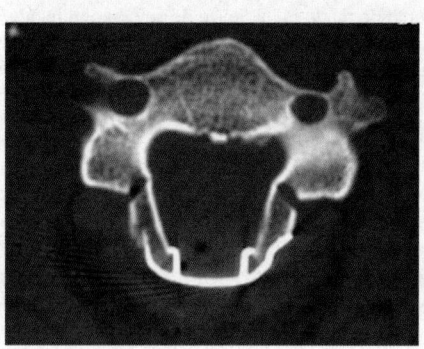
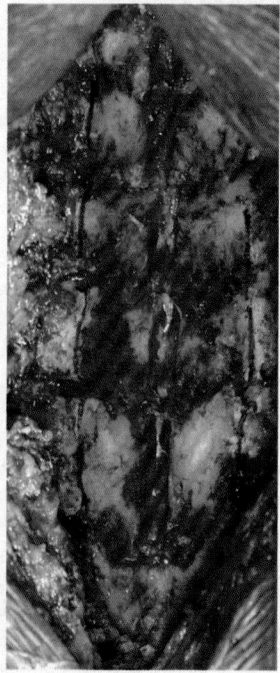

TECH FIG 3 A. Axial CT of a French door laminoplasty showing a large bilateral surface area available for bone grafting. **B.** The French door technique uses a midline opening trough. In this image, the midline trough has been created. Planned lines for the hinge troughs are shown on either side.

Hinge-Side Trough

- The hinge side should be prepared after the opening trough has been created so that greenstick fracture of the hinge can be carefully assessed for pliability.
- Preparing the hinge trough entails removal of the dorsal cortex, cancellous layer, and some of the ventral cortex **(TECH FIG 4)**. Often, areas of thicker cortical bone preventing hinge closure are found at the most caudal and cephalad edges of each lamina.
- Stiffness of the hinge should be tested periodically during preparation. The goal is to create a pliable yet firm hinge that yields to moderate opening force without breaking the inner cortex.
- Hinge troughs used for the French door technique are prepared in the same anatomic location as troughs created for the open door technique. Similar to the open door technique, ventral laminar cortex should be preserved to create stable hinges.

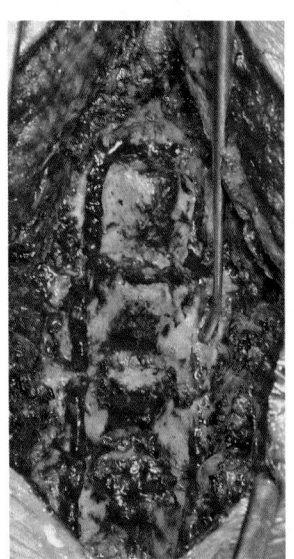

TECH FIG 4 Opening and hinge troughs for the open door technique. Preserved ventral cortex for the hinge trough is seen at the tip of the Penfield dissector.

OPENING THE LAMINOPLASTY

- Proceeding from caudal to cranial, a nerve hook or curved curette is used to elevate the lamina away from the spinal cord. A Kerrison rongeur can be used to divide ligamentous attachments, and bipolar forceps are used for cauterization of epidural veins.
- The laminae are then opened sequentially. This can be done with the assistance of a curved microcurette to raise the opening side and gently bend open each lamina hinge. Care

should be taken to identify and lyse any epidural adhesions **(TECH FIG 5A)**. Do not allow the newly opened door to fall violently back onto dorsal spinal cord.
- Starting from C3 and proceeding to C7 allows for blood to flow away from the working area and reduces the overhang of the inferior edge of the superior lamina due to lamina shingling.
- Completion of opening lamina is carried out carefully with small curettes **(TECH FIG 5B)**.

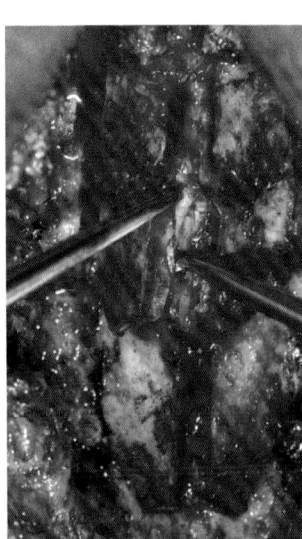

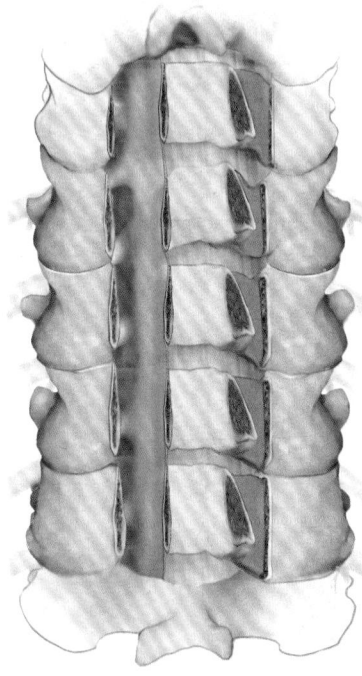

TECH FIG 5 A. Completing the opening for the French door technique. With the assistance of a curved microcurette, the lamina is gently bent back on its hinge. Care should be taken to identify and lyse epidural adhesions. **B.** Completion of open door laminoplasty.

A B

TECHNIQUES

POSTERIOR ARCH RECONSTRUCTION

- The laminoplasty door is held open using a variety of techniques.
- Plate reconstruction has become popular because of the immediate mechanical security that plates provide **(TECH FIG 6A,B)**. However, eventual mechanical stability relies on hinge-side bony healing to permanently hold the posterior arch open.
- Bone struts can also be used; this was the most frequently used method for many years. Autogenous grafts fashioned from the spinous processes of C6 and C7 can be used as well as rib allograft or machined cortical grafts **(TECH FIG 6C)**.
- Reconstruction with bone has the advantage of allowing for full bony reconstruction of the lamina arch, as the bone struts usually fully incorporate. Furthermore, bone can be easier and

faster to place than plates and screws, but bone provides less initial mechanical stability to the arch and may (rarely) dislodge before healing of the hinge.
- Hybrid reconstruction with alternating plate and bone graft can also be used **(TECH FIG 6D)**.
- With the French door technique, midline plates can be applied. Other materials have been used to keep the door open, including autograft, allograft, or hydroxyapatite **(TECH FIG 6E,F)**.
- Alternatively, the door can be held open with sutures that go from the lamina to the lateral mass or facet capsules. Suture anchors have also been used.

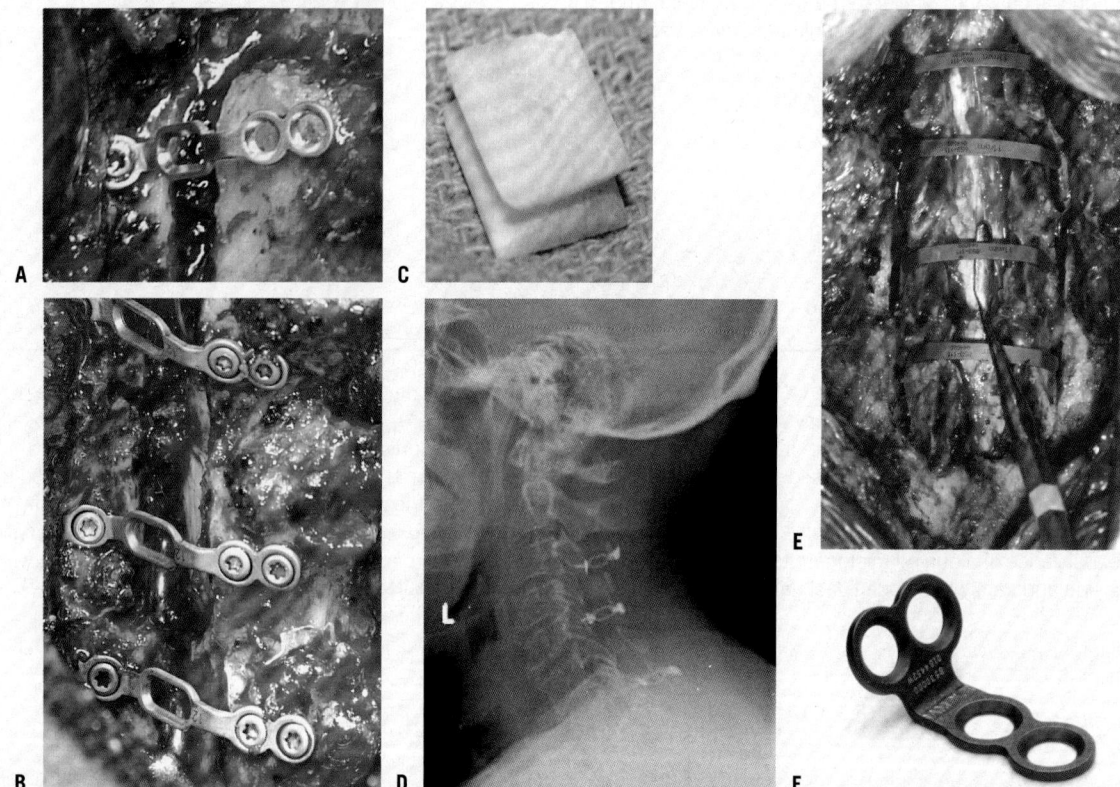

TECH FIG 6 A,B. Open door plates. **A.** First, a 6-mm lateral mass screw is placed. **B.** Then the lamina is opened and held in place with 4-mm screws. **C.** Machined cortical allograft. Grooves allow for better stability when interpositioned between lamina and lateral mass. **D.** Postoperative lateral radiograph after laminoplasty performed with alternating plate and graft technique. **E.** French door posterior arch reconstruction using midline plates. Adequate space must be maintained between the plate and cord to allow for expansion. **F.** A salvage plate can fix the lamina to the lateral mass in the event that the hinge is disrupted.

WOUND CLOSURE

- A deep drain is placed, followed by a layered fascial and subcutaneous closure.
- Skin is closed using a subcuticular stitch.

Pearls and Pitfalls

Physical Examination	• The Hoffman reflex can indicate spinal cord compression but can be positive in normal individuals.
Patient Position	• Slight cervical flexion facilitates exposure and closure by eliminating redundant posterior skin folds and decreases overlap of lamina (laminar shingling) for improved identification of adjacent levels.
Opening Side	• If foraminotomies are planned, then the opening side should be made over the ipsilateral side of nerve root compression. If asymmetric compression is present, it may be beneficial to open the more affected side. • While creating the opening hinge, a color change in the cortex can be appreciated. As the deep (ventral) cortex is thinned, yellow areas (which correspond to ligamentum flavum) and blue areas (which correspond to veins or dura) can be seen through the bone. Care should be taken at this point, as the ventral bone is now very thin.
Hinge-Side Trough	• The surgeon should avoid removing excessive bone on the hinge side, which would create a floppy hinge. • The surgeon should always recheck that the opening side is complete if there is any difficulty elevating the lamina, instead of focusing solely on thinning the hinge side. • If the hinge is completely incompetent, then it can be reconstructed with a salvage plate that fixates on the hinge side (see **TECH FIG 6F**).
Epidural Vein Ligation	• The epidural veins should be ligated as far dorsal as possible. This decreases bleeding by avoiding the ventral longitudinal veins.

POSTOPERATIVE CARE

- A soft collar can be worn for comfort for 2 to 4 weeks after surgery.
- When plate fixation has been used, immediate gentle active neck motion should be permitted to prevent stiffness.
- Drain output is monitored and drains and removed when output is low enough, typically at 48 hours after surgery.

OUTCOMES

- Cervical laminoplasty is a valuable treatment option for myelopathic patients with multilevel stenosis. It provides cord decompression while preserving some motion. With proper patient selection, this procedure provides excellent neurologic outcomes with few complications.
- When compared to laminectomy with fusion, outcomes regarding neurologic improvement are similar. However, laminectomy with fusion has more frequent fusion-related complications such as nonunion, instrumentation failure, persistent pain from bone graft harvest site, subjacent degeneration requiring reoperation, and a higher deep infection rate.[2]
- When compared to corpectomy in patients without kyphotic alignment, outcomes regarding neurologic improvement are similar. However, laminoplasty patients have fewer complications and require less pain medication.[8]

COMPLICATIONS

- Segmental nerve root palsy: This is most commonly a motor deficit affecting the C5 root that occurs a day or two after surgery and typically improves over the course of months.[4]
- Axial neck pain has been reported at a high rate. However, the pain is typically mild and often described as stiffness.
- Loss of cervical motion: Up to 50% loss of range of motion has been reported with some laminoplasty techniques.
- Dural tears are infrequent but can be handled with either direct repair or glue with or without the addition of a lumbar diverting cerebrospinal fluid drain.
- Hardware failure leading to laminar door closure has been reported.
- Infection and epidural hematoma can occur; however, the rates are very low.

REFERENCES

1. Edwards CC II, Heller JG, Murakami H. Corpectomy versus laminoplasty for multilevel cervical myelopathy: an independent matched-cohort analysis. Spine 2002;27(11):1168–1175.
2. Heller JG, Edwards CC II, Murakami H, et al. Laminoplasty versus laminectomy and fusion for multilevel cervical myelopathy: an independent matched cohort analysis. Spine 2001;26(12):1330–1336.
3. Hirabayashi K, Watanabe K, Wakano K, et al. Expansive open-door laminoplasty for cervical spinal stenotic myelopathy. Spine 1983;8(7):693–699.
4. Imagama S, Matsuyama Y, Yukawa Y, et al. C5 palsy after cervical laminoplasty: a multicentre study. J Bone Joint Surg Br 2010;92(3):393–400.
5. Machino M, Yukawa Y, Hida T, et al. Cervical alignment and range of motion after laminoplasty: radiographical data from more than 500 cases with cervical spondylotic myelopathy and a review of the literature. Spine 2012;37(20):E1243–E1250.
6. Matsumoto M, Chiba K, Toyama Y. Surgical treatment of ossification of the posterior longitudinal ligament and its outcomes: posterior surgery by laminoplasty. Spine 2012;37(5):E303–E308.
7. Okada M, Minamide A, Endo T, et al. A prospective randomized study of clinical outcomes in patients with cervical compressive myelopathy treated with open-door or French-door laminoplasty. Spine 2009;34(11):1119–1126.
8. Yoon T, Hashimoto R, Raich A, et al. Outcomes following laminoplasty compared with laminectomy and fusion in patients with cervical myelopathy: a systematic review. Spine 2013;38(22 suppl 1):S183–S194.

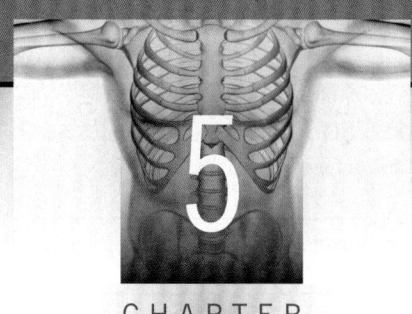

5

CHAPTER

Posterior Cervical Fusion with Instrumentation

Shalin Patel and Raj Rao

SURGICAL MANAGEMENT

- Operative intervention in the posterior subaxial cervical spine is frequently carried out for decompression or stabilization.
  - Fusion and instrumentation of the posterior cervical spine may be required for unstable fractures or after extensive decompressive procedures.
  - Instrumentation reduces the need for postoperative immobilization and orthosis wear, augments fusion success, and allows better maintenance of sagittal alignment of the cervical spine and prevents kyphotic deformity of the spine.

Interspinous Wiring

- Interspinous wiring can be an alternative to lateral mass or pedicle screw fixation in stabilization of the posterior cervical spine.
  - Although it resists flexion reasonably well, it is generally not as strong in resisting extension, axial load, rotation, and lateral bending.
- The most commonly used implants are 18- or 20-gauge stainless steel wire or 1- to 1.2-mm titanium braided cable.
- In modern spine surgery, wiring techniques are generally limited to cases in which biomechanically superior techniques such as lateral mass fixation cannot be used, a somewhat less invasive midline-only exposure is desired, or the additional rigidity of lateral mass fixation is not necessary (eg, for posterior repair of relatively stable pseudarthroses or to provide a tension band effect as an adjunct to anterior instrumentation).
- Techniques of wiring include simple interspinous wiring (eg, Rogers), Bohlman triple wiring (can be used also for occipitocervical fixation), and oblique wiring.
  - As a result of the direction of its stabilizing forces, oblique wiring may counter rotational instability better than simple interspinous wiring.

Lateral Mass Screw Fixation

- The lateral mass of the subaxial cervical vertebra is a quadrangular column of bone formed by the complex of the superior and inferior articular processes and the intervening bone.
- Lateral mass screws are the most commonly used and widely evaluated implants for posterior fixation of the subaxial cervical spine.

- Lateral mass screws are versatile in that they can be used when the spinous processes and laminae are unavailable as fixation points (eg, from trauma, tumors, or surgical resection for decompression).
- Lateral mass screw fixation techniques provide superior flexion and torsional stiffness compared to posterior wiring.[5]
  - The improved strength of fixation allows instrumentation to be limited to the levels of fusion. When wiring techniques are used, the construct occasionally needs to be extended proximally or distally to obtain additional points of fixation.
  - A lower incidence of postoperative kyphosis is achieved with lateral mass screws versus wiring techniques.[5]
  - Lateral mass screws are easier to insert and have a low incidence of complications when compared to cervical pedicle screws.
- The Magerl technique of lateral mass screw fixation has been shown to have superior pullout strength and higher load to failure when compared to screws inserted with the Roy-Camille technique.[22] This may be related to the longer screw length generally possible with the Magerl technique.
  - Anatomic variations in screw lengths occur at each subaxial level, with either technique; from C3 to C6, the Magerl technique can safely afford a screw length of 14 mm as compared to the Roy-Camille technique, which can afford a screw length of 12 mm. At C7, the reported screw lengths are 2 mm shorter for the Roy-Camille technique and 3 to 4 mm shorter for the Magerl technique. Screw lengths are greater in males compared to females at all levels. Assessment of lateral masses on preoperative computed tomography (CT) scans is recommended to ascertain screw lengths while using either technique.[5]
- Pullout strength is significantly greater with a bicortical screw than with a unicortical purchase.
  - Because bicortical purchase engenders potential risk to nerve roots and the vertebral artery, unicortical purchase is used in most cases. A cadaveric study by Seybold et al[21] found a 5.8% incidence of direct artery injury and 17.4% of direct nerve root injury with bicortical screws compared to unicortical screws.

Pedicle Screw Fixation of the Cervical Spine

- Pedicle screw fixation allows simultaneous stabilization of all three columns of the cervical spine and has been reported to be biomechanically superior to lateral mass fixation.[18]

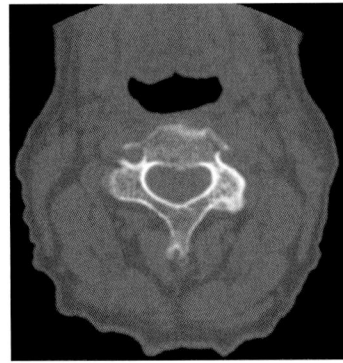

FIG 1 Axial CT image of a subaxial cervical vertebra depicting variability in the pedicle diameter at the same level.

TABLE 1 Cervical Pedicle Outer Width	
Pedicle	Width (mm)
C2	6.9 ± 1.6
C3	5.3 ± 0.8
C4	5.4 ± 0.8
C5	5.7 ± 0.8
C6	5.9 ± 0.9
C7	6.7 ± 1.0

- Biomechanical testing shows cervical pedicle screws have improved strength with constant uniplanar toggle in the sagittal plane. This fatigue testing shows lower levels of bone implant loosening compared to lateral mass fixation.[21]
- Although cervical pedicle screws are commonly used in Asian countries, they are not as popular in United States. The risk of neurovascular injury from broaching the walls of the small cervical pedicles from C3 to C6 and variability in pedicle size sometimes even at the same level (**FIG 1**) makes this procedure technically difficult and restricts its widespread use.[10]
- Pedicle screws are most commonly used at C2 and C7 where the pedicles are largest in the cervical spine and the risk of neurovascular injury is lower.
- At C7, most patients do not generally have a vertebral artery in the foramen transversarium, making pedicle screw fixation safer at this level.
  - At C2, the vertebral artery is generally lateral to the insertion site and trajectory of the pedicle, making pedicle screw fixation feasible.
  - From C3 to C6, the proximity of the vertebral artery and the small diameter of the pedicles make pedicle screw fixation challenging and not feasible for routine use.
  - Whenever pedicle screw fixation in the cervical spine is contemplated, careful scrutiny of preoperative CT and magnetic resonance imaging scans is essential to measure the dimensions and angulation of the pedicles and rule out congenital anomalies.
- The cervical pedicle is generally taller than it is wide, with the mean height of all cervical pedicles around 7 mm (range 6 to 11 mm).[23]
  - The width of the pedicle is the critical dimension for feasibility of pedicle screw placement.
  - Pedicle outer diameters less than 4 mm generally preclude pedicle screw insertion.[10]
  - Multiple morphologic studies have found that the mean cervical pedicle outer width varies from 4 to 7 mm, with significant variation in the width at different levels (**TABLE 1**).[10]
  - The pedicles of C2 and C7 are, however, generally large enough to accommodate either 3.5- or 4-mm screws.

- The length of the pedicles from C3 to C6 ranges from 12 to 18 mm.[10] Screw lengths are generally slightly longer to obtain purchase within the vertebral body.
- The axial angle of the pedicle (medial angle to the sagittal plane) is the least at C2 (25 to 30 degrees)[9] and increases to a mean of 44 degrees (25 to 55 degrees) at C3. From C3 to C7, it gradually reduces to a mean of 37 degrees (33 to 55 degrees).[11]
- Preoperative CT-based navigation[4] and, more recently, the use of intraoperative three-dimensional imaging-based navigation[9] have been reported to reduce the cervical pedicle screw malpositioning and, consequently, the risk of neurovascular complication.

C2 Translaminar Screw Fixation

- Wright[25] first introduced translaminar screw fixation in 2004 as a method for instrumentation of the axis using a cross trajectory technique.
- This technique is particularly useful in cases of a high-riding or aberrant vertebral artery, thus preventing safe instrumentation of C2 via a pedicle or pars screw.
- Up to 20% of patients have a vertebral artery anomaly that precludes placement of C2 pars/pedicle screw.[25]
- Evaluation of preoperative CT scan is critical to determine appropriateness of the axis for translaminar screw placement.
- The C2 translaminar screw requires intact posterior element of C2 and a laminar width that can accommodate a minimum of a 3.5-mm diameter screw.
- Average screw length for C2 translaminar screw is between 25 and 35 mm.
- C2 translaminar screw technique allows for instrumentation of the axis under direct visualization and is thus a very safe and effective method of fixation.
- The C2 translaminar screw can be a useful salvage procedure in cases of a failed C2 pedicle screw.
- Rod fixation of either the C1 or C3 lateral mass to the screw head of the contralateral C2 laminar screw allows increased rotational stability of the construct.[25]
- One notable disadvantage of this technique involves increased difficulty with connecting the rod to the subaxial screw heads within a multilevel construct due to the medially positioned tulip head of the C2 translaminar screw.

POSTERIOR CERVICAL FUSION

- Although it is tempting to focus on instrumentation techniques, performing a meticulous fusion technique is just as important, if not more so, to the success of surgery.
- In virtually all cases, posterior fusion is supplemented by some form of instrumentation.
- To maximize the surface area for fusion, all posterior bony surfaces that do not need to be resected for the decompression should be left intact for fusion.
- Following exposure, all soft tissues, including the interspinous ligaments and muscles, facet joint capsules, and paraspinal soft tissue, are meticulously resected so that the posterior cortical surfaces are exposed.
- In patients who require a laminectomy, the lateral masses and facet joints form the fusion bed.
- Facet joint cartilage is removed with a curette or 3-mm burr within the facet joint. It is easier to decorticate the facet joints if done before the insertion of lateral mass screws.
- The posterior cortical surfaces of the lateral masses, laminae, and spinous processes are decorticated with a 3-mm burr to expose bleeding subcortical bone **(TECH FIG 1)**.
- Bone graft obtained from the iliac crest or local bone from laminectomy is morselized into small cancellous and cortico-cancellous chips and onlaid over the bleeding bone.
- Cancellous chips of bone are inserted directly into the facet joint.

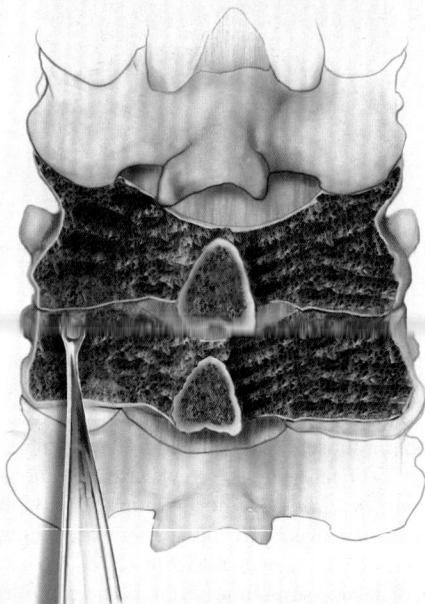

TECH FIG 1 Decortication of the laminae and facet joints at the levels selected for fusion. Only iliac crest bone graft is placed over the decorticated areas.

INTERSPINOUS WIRING

Simple Interspinous Wiring

- The spinous processes and laminae at the level to be instrumented should be confirmed to be intact and instrumentable on preoperative imaging studies.
  - Closed or operative reduction of spinal fracture-dislocations should be carried out before instrumentation if possible.
  - In some cases of flexion–distraction injury, sequential tightening of the wires can be done to reduce the spine.

- Two- to 3-mm drill holes are made through the cortex at the junction of the spinous process and laminae bilaterally at the levels to be included in the fusion.
- Attention should be paid to the ventral location of the dural sac, and the drill should be directed coronally to minimize the risk of inadvertent spinal cord injury **(TECH FIG 2A)**.
- The drill holes should be positioned at the proximal aspect of the cephalad spinous process and the distal aspect of the caudal spinous process to provide the widest margin of safety against the wire cutting through the spinous process.

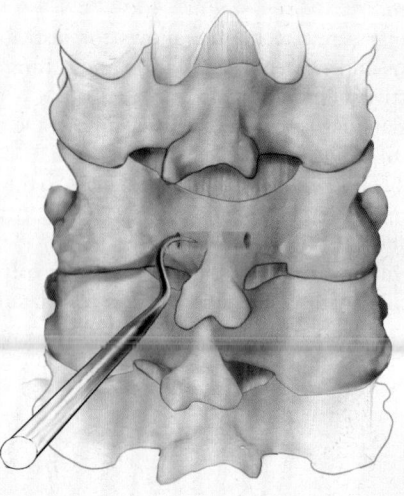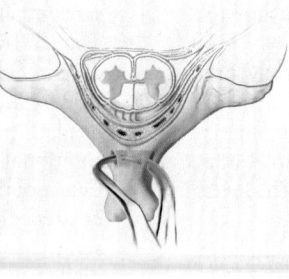

TECH FIG 2 Simple interspinous wiring. **A.** Safe position of the drill hole for passage of spinous process wire is dorsal to the spinal laminar line. *(continued)*

A

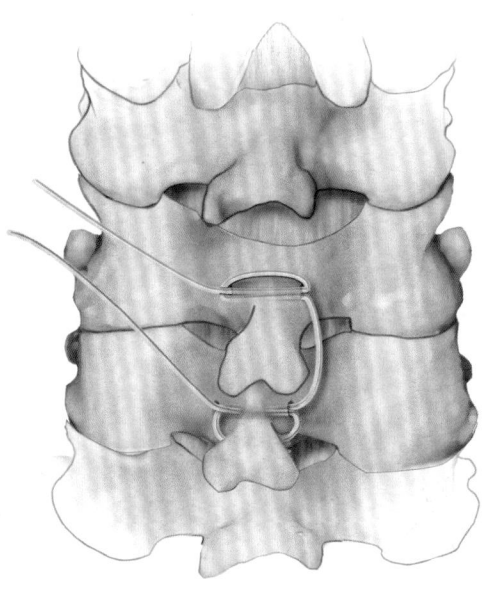
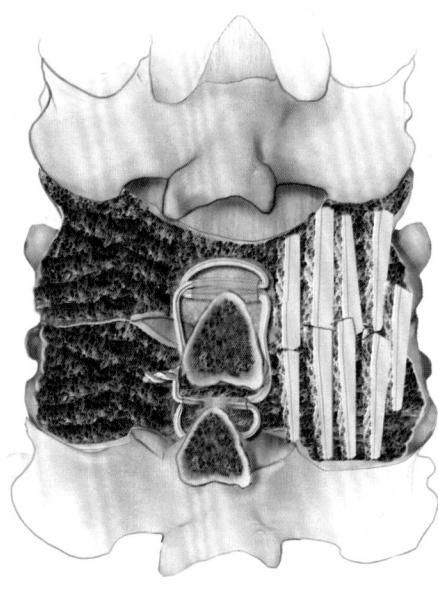

B   C

TECH FIG 2 *(continued)* **B.** The wire or cable selected is passed through and around the base of the cranial and caudal spinous processes at the levels selected for fusion so that both ends of the wire are on the same side of the spine. **C.** Ends of wire are twisted together after releasing any cervical traction.

- The tips of a towel clip or a tenaculum clamp are placed in the cortical holes on either side of the base of the spinous process.
  - A gentle side-to-side rocking movement is used to create a continuous tract in the cancellous bone at the base of the spinous process.
- The wire or cable selected for use is passed through and around the base of the cranial spinous process **(TECH FIG 2B)**.
  - One end of this wire is similarly passed through and around the base of the caudal spinous process so that both the ends of the wire end up on the same side of the spine.
  - The free ends of the wire are tightened **(TECH FIG 2C)**.
  - Cancellous bone graft is placed bilaterally on the decorticated laminae and spinous processes and within the facet joint at the fusion levels.
- Modification of the technique can include a plate of cortico-cancellous bone graft harvested from the iliac crest and placed under the wire or cable bilaterally prior to tightening.

Triple Wire Technique

- The wire or cable selected is passed through and around the spinous processes at the cephalad and caudal ends of the fusion levels, as with routine interspinous wiring.
- A pair of corticocancellous plates of bone graft including the full thickness of the cancellous bone of the iliac crest but excluding the inner cortical table is harvested from the posterior iliac crest.
  - The length of the bone block should be adequate to span the fusion construct and wide enough to cover the decorticated laminae within the fusion levels.
- Two- to 3-mm drill holes are created in the proximal and distal portions of the harvested bone grafts.
  - Two additional 22-gauge wires are passed through the holes in the proximal and distal spinous processes.

- These wires are then passed on either side through the holes made in the bone graft.
- The wires are tightened over the grafts on both sides to hold the bone graft rigidly against the decorticated lamina and spinous process **(TECH FIG 3)**.

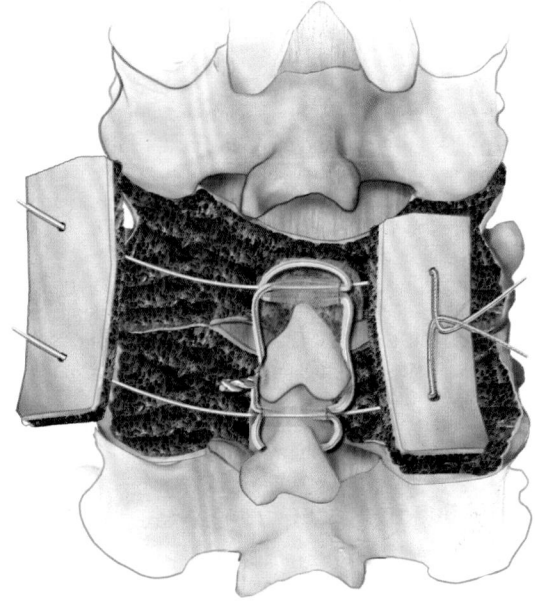

TECH FIG 3 Triple wiring technique. After simple interspinous wiring, additional wires are passed through the cranial and caudal spinous processes at the levels selected for fusion. These wires are used to firmly hold corticocancellous plates of bone graft against the decorticated laminae at the fusion levels.

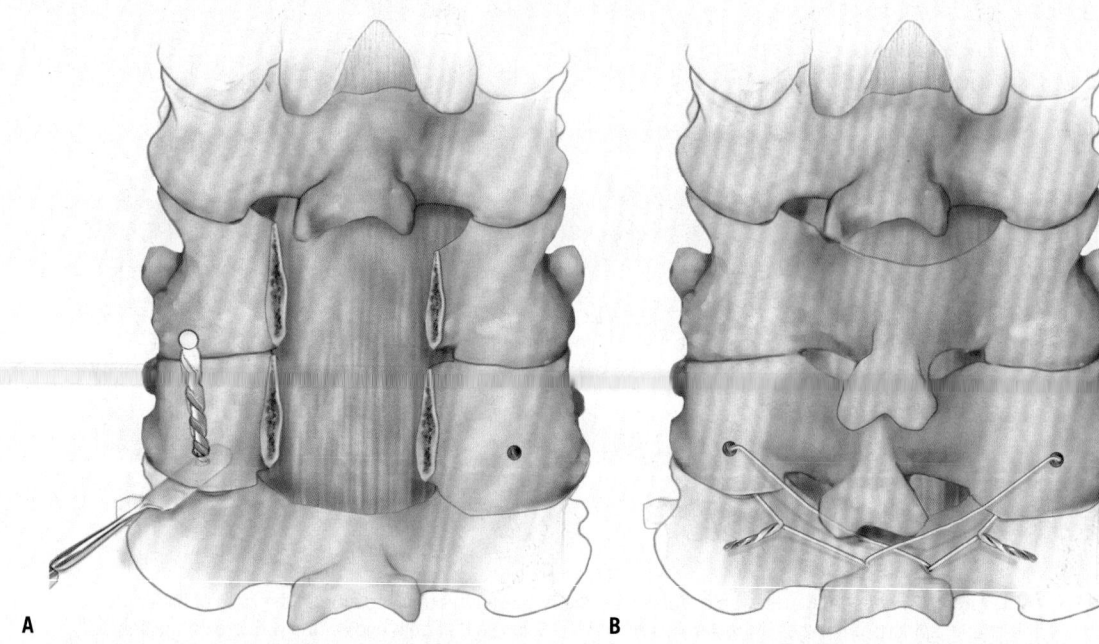

TECH FIG 4 Facet wiring techniques. **A.** A channel is drilled in the sagittal plane through the midportion of the inferior articular process, exiting through the articular surface into the joint. A periosteal elevator held within the joint space prevents overpenetration by the drill and can be used to guide the wire out through the joint space. **B.** Facet wires may be obliquely looped around the spinous process when the lamina is deficient at a level.

Oblique Wiring

- A periosteal elevator is carefully inserted into the facet joint to slightly distract and clearly identify the plane of the facet joint.
- A 2-mm drill bit is used to make a channel in the sagittal plane through the midportion of the inferior articular process, exiting through the articular surface into the joint.
  - The periosteal elevator within the joint confirms penetration by the drill and prevents overpenetration by the drill **(TECH FIG 4A)**.
- A 20-gauge wire or cable is passed through this drill hole and is guided distally through and out of the facet joint using a periosteal elevator in a "shoehorn" fashion.
  - One end of the wire is then passed either around or through a hole in the intact spinous process of the vertebra one or two levels caudal to the level of injury.
  - This procedure is done bilaterally, and the free ends of the ipsilateral wires are twisted together to the appropriate tension **(TECH FIG 4B)**. The absence of laminae or spinous processes is often a reason to consider oblique wiring over interspinous wiring.
- Supplemental midline interspinous or triple wiring is frequently added when the bony anatomy permits.

Multilevel Buttress Facet Wiring

- Posterior stabilization after multilevel laminectomy can also be obtained by posterolateral facet fusion with multilevel facet wiring.
- Oblique facet wires are passed bilaterally through the inferior articular processes at all facet joints included in the fusion.
  - Two wires are passed through a hole in the spinous process of the most caudal vertebra.

- Rib grafts, iliac crest strut grafts, or metal rods have all been used for stabilization with the multilevel facet wires **(TECH FIG 5)**.[6,12]
- The bone graft is placed over the decorticated lateral masses and in between the free ends of the wires, and the wires are twisted together at each level to the appropriate tension.

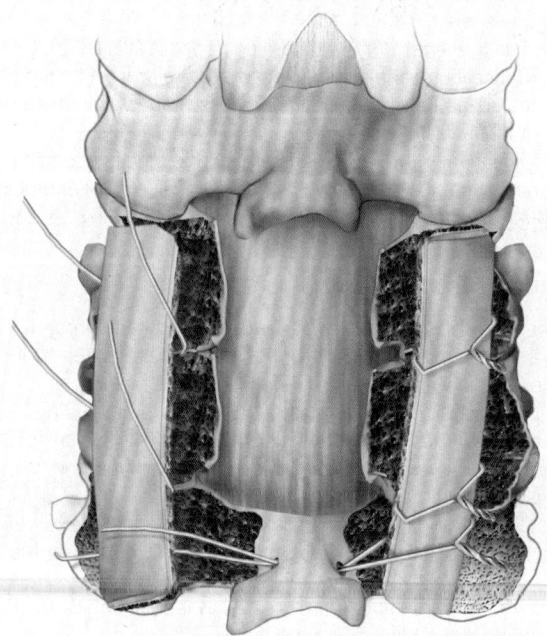

TECH FIG 5 Facet wires may be tightened over rib grafts bilaterally in cases of multilevel laminectomy.

Postoperative Immobilization

- Rigid external bracing is recommended in all posterior cervical wiring procedures until solid bony fusion is obtained. Six to 12 weeks of halo vest or rigid cervicothoracic bracing should be used after interspinous or oblique wiring, depending on the stability of the construct and the number of levels included in the fusion.
- Radiographs should show a continuous fusion mass and absence of mobility in flexion and extension before immobilization is discontinued.

LATERAL MASS SCREW FIXATION

- The quadrilateral posterior surface of the lateral mass is clearly exposed.
  - A ridge between the lamina and lateral mass helps identify the medial border. This distinction is less prominent at C7.
  - The lateral edge of the lateral mass can be easily palpated.
  - The joint lines above and below delineate the superior and inferior borders.
- The center of the quadrilateral posterior surface of the lateral mass is identified.
- Several techniques have been described for lateral mass screw insertion. The goal is to avoid damage to the vertebral artery and the nerve root in the foramen and avoid violating the facet joint while inserting a lateral mass screw of adequate length.
- Roy-Camille et al[19] proposed an entry point for the lateral mass screw at the center of the posterior surface of the lateral mass.
  - The screw is directed perpendicular to the posterior surface of the lateral mass, angled laterally 10 degrees to the sagittal plane.
  - This trajectory aims to exit lateral to the vertebral artery and inferior to the exiting nerve root **(TECH FIG 6A–C)**.

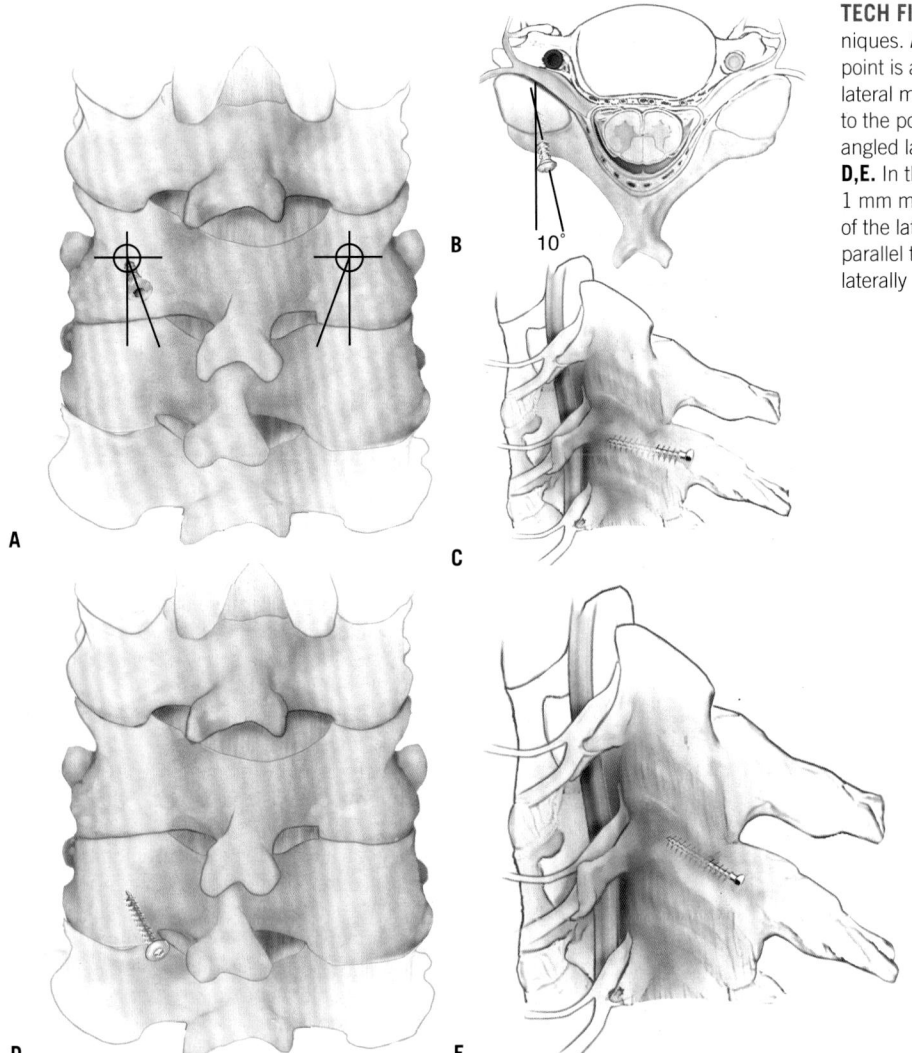

TECH FIG 6 Lateral mass screw insertion techniques. **A–C.** In the Roy-Camille method, the entry point is at the center of the posterior surface of the lateral mass, with the screw directed perpendicular to the posterior surface of the lateral mass and angled laterally 10 degrees to the sagittal plane. **D,E.** In the Magerl technique, the entry point is 1 mm medial to the center of the posterior surface of the lateral mass, and the screw is directed parallel to the plane of the facet joint and angled laterally 25 degrees to the sagittal plane.

- Magerl proposed an entry point 1 mm medial to the center of the posterior surface of the lateral mass.
  - The screw is directed parallel to the plane of the facet joint with 25 degrees of lateral angulation in the axial plane.
  - Magerl recommended inserting a needle into the facet joint to determine the plane of the joint.
  - Lateral plane fluoroscopy can help accurately determine the direction of the screw in the sagittal plane, aiming to keep the screw parallel to and between the articular surfaces of the lateral mass.
  - This trajectory aims to exit lateral to the vertebral artery and superior to the exiting nerve root (**TECH FIG 6D,E**).
- A modification of the Magerl technique by An et al[3] uses a similar starting point but recommends angling the screw 30 degrees laterally in the axial plane and 15 degrees cranially in the sagittal plane.
  - This trajectory again aims to exit laterally to the vertebral artery and superiorly to the exiting nerve root at the junction of the transverse process and the lateral mass.
- Enlarged and bulbous tips of the spinous processes can be rongeured if they interfere with appropriate angulation of the instruments.
- When the lateral masses are sclerotic, a high-speed 2-mm burr is used to penetrate the outer cortex of the lateral mass at the entry point before a drill is used. This will also prevent the drill tip slipping on the surface of the lateral mass.
- A tap is used prior to screw insertion in sclerotic bone.
- Most current instrumentation systems use a rod to connect the screws after they have been precisely positioned and inserted into the lateral mass.
  - Lining up the screw heads for subsequent rod fixation is easier if the most proximal and distal screws are inserted initially followed by the screws in between.
  - Polyaxial screw heads compensate for minor variations in insertion or anatomy.
  - The rods can be contoured in multiple planes and allow for application of compressive, distractive, and rotatory forces for correction of deformity.
  - A rod–screw construct can easily be extended to the occipital and thoracic region.
- Bicortical screws provide better pullout strengths as compared to unicortical screws; however, they can cause nerve root irritation or damage if too long. Bicortical screws should be considered in certain cases:
  - Patients with rheumatoid arthritis or metastatic bone tumors in whom bone quality may be suboptimal
  - Longer fixation constructs extending to the occipital or thoracic regions to reduce the chances of implant pullout

PEDICLE SCREW FIXATION OF THE CERVICAL SPINE

Insertion of Pedicle Screws from C3 to C7

- Preoperative radiographs and CT images should be reviewed to assess pedicle dimensions and orientation and to confirm the feasibility of obtaining intraoperative radiographs; this is especially important in patients with short, stocky necks.
- Inserting pedicle screws before decompression allows better identification of morphologic landmarks and reduces the risk of inadvertent injury to an exposed spinal cord during the insertion process.
- Anatomic studies provide broad guidelines on locations of the pedicle entry point at each subaxial cervical level.[10]
- The most commonly used technique relies on identification of topographic landmarks combined with fluoroscopy.[1]
- The entry point to the pedicle is 1 to 2 mm inferior to the caudal edge of the inferior articular process and 2 to 3 mm lateral to the midline of the lateral mass or 2 to 3 mm medial to the lateral edge of the lateral mass.
  - Occasionally, degenerative changes at the joint obscure true landmarks.
- The dorsal cortex of the lateral mass is penetrated using a high-speed burr.
  - The cancellous bone of the pedicle in many cases can be visualized in this pilot hole.
- A blunt, fine pedicle probe is advanced through this cancellous bone to find the medially angled pedicle (**TECH FIG 7A**).
- Fluoroscopy is used to guide the trajectory in the sagittal plane.
  - In general, the screws should be parallel to the superior endplate of the vertebral body from C5 to C7 and angled slightly rostral to the endplate from C2 to C4.
- Some authors recommend that a keyhole laminoforaminotomy be performed after locating the entry point.[4]
  - The superior and medial walls of the pedicle are directly palpated through this foraminotomy with a right-angled nerve hook to direct the trajectory of the pedicle probe (**TECH FIG 7B**).
- The pilot hole is tapped before inserting the screw.
  - Size 3.5- or 4-mm screws are generally used based on preoperative imaging of pedicle dimensions.
  - Small pedicle diameters may require a 2.7-mm screw.[20]
- The length of the screw ranges from 18 to 26 mm, depending on the length of the pedicle as determined on preoperative CT scans.
  - The screw should be inserted to a depth no longer than two-thirds of the anteroposterior width of the vertebral body, as confirmed on the lateral fluoroscopy image.
  - Because the C7 pedicle is longer, a screw up to 30 mm can usually be inserted at this level.
- Computer-assisted image guidance systems have been used for pedicle screw insertion in the cervical spine.
  - Preoperative CT data are used by the computer-assisted system to prepare a three-dimensional model of the vertebra.
  - Alternatively, intraoperative CT of the cervical spine is obtained following exposure. This data is transferred to the navigation system.
  - After registration of surface landmarks during surgery, a registered probe or drill bit can be used to locate the pedicle screw entry point and trajectory and guide a fine drill bit through the pedicle into the vertebral body.

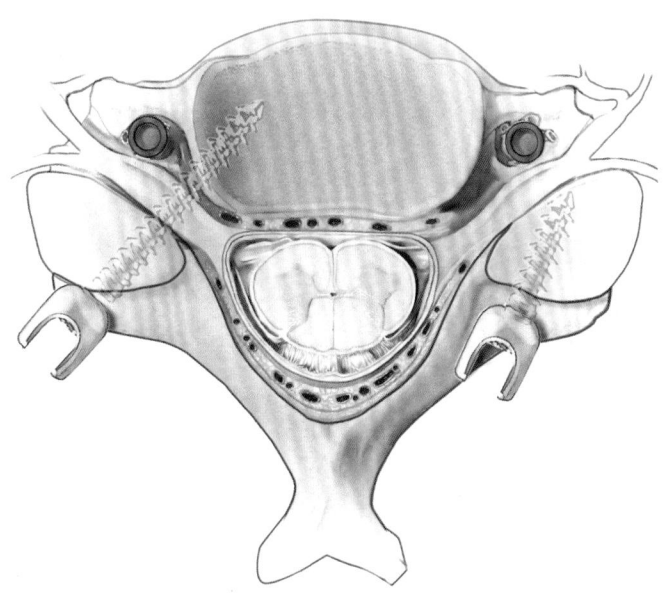

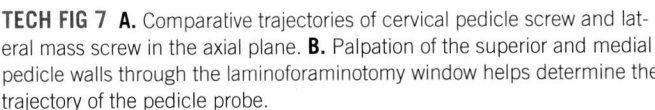

A

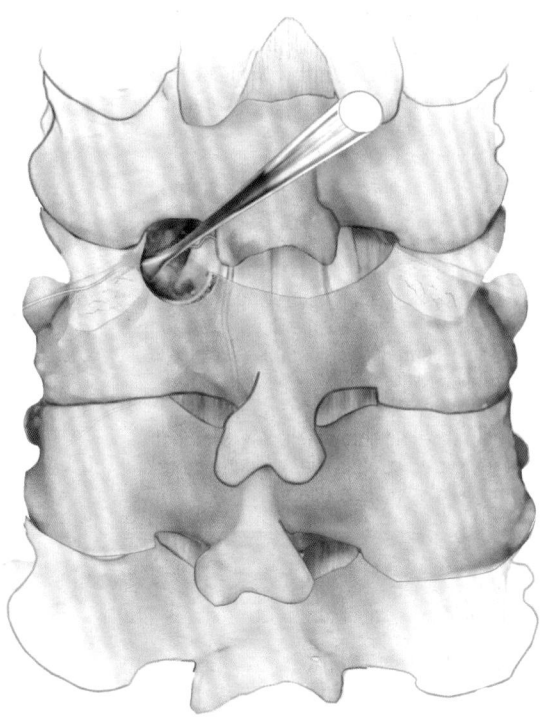

B

TECH FIG 7 A. Comparative trajectories of cervical pedicle screw and lateral mass screw in the axial plane. **B.** Palpation of the superior and medial pedicle walls through the laminoforaminotomy window helps determine the trajectory of the pedicle probe.

C2 Pedicle Screw Insertion

- The entry point for the C2 pedicle is located on the superior medial quadrant of the posterior aspect of the lateral mass of C2, 3 mm lateral to the medial edge of the isthmus, and in line with or slightly distal to the superior margin of the C2 lamina.
- The entry point and trajectory for subsequent drilling are confirmed by palpating the medial and superior margins of the C2 pedicle with a Penfield probe to determine medial angulation and with fluoroscopy to determine sagittal angulation.
  - The cortex is penetrated with a 3-mm burr.
  - The underlying cancellous bone is probed with a fine curette or pedicle probe to locate the pedicle channel. A 2.7-mm drill bit can also be used under fluoroscopy control to cannulate the pedicle.
  - The drill is generally angled 15 to 25 degrees medially and 20 to 30 degrees cranially.
  - The integrity of the drilled hole is verified with a blunt probe and tapped, and a 3.5- to 4.0-mm screw is inserted.
- Twenty- to 22-mm screw lengths are generally used. C2 pedicle screws longer than 24 mm are likely to penetrate the anterior surface of the vertebral body and may provide superior fixation in some situations. The pullout strength of C2 pedicle screw is reported to be twice that of C2 pars screw.[4]
- The varying screw entry points and trajectories in the cervical spine occasionally create challenges in contouring the connecting rods. Using a polyaxial screw head provides some tolerance in placement of the rod connecting C2 to subaxial levels.

C2 Pars Screw Insertion

- The entry point for a C2 pars screw is located on the lateral mass of C2, 3 mm cranial and 3 mm lateral to medial edge of the inferior articular facet of C2.

- After a pilot hole is drilled at this location, a 2.7-mm drill bit is used to cannulate the pars under fluoroscopy control. The drill is angled 10 to 15 degrees medially. A Penfield dissector can be used to feel the medial edge of the C2 pars, which can help with directing the drill. Fluoroscopy is used to assist with sagittal trajectory, which is generally around 25 degrees cranially directed, more caudally oriented than a C1–C2 transarticular screw.
- The C2 pars screw is shorter than the C2 pedicle and can measure up to 16 mm.

C2 Translaminar Screw Insertion

- The axial CT slice of C2 should be evaluated, and the width and length of the lamina should be measured to determine appropriateness for screw placement.
- It is imperative that the entire lamina of C2 be thoroughly exposed from the lateral edge of the lateral mass on each side.
- The junction of the base of the bifid spinous process and the dorsal lamina should be identified as the starting point for the contralateral translaminar screw. One can identify this starting point by appreciating the rostral margin of the C2 lamina.
- Using a 3-mm high-speed burr, a small pilot hole should be made to breach the cortex in the midpoint of the cranial/caudal plane of the spinal laminar junction.
- A cervical gearshift or a hand drill is advanced in a collinear trajectory to the contralateral lamina to develop an interosseous tract within cancellous channel of the lamina.
- The use of a hand drill or cervical gearshift allows for greater control and tactile feel, thus reducing the chance of cortical wall penetration.

- Penetration of the ventral lamina can result in a dural laceration. This can be prevented through slow, controlled, and steady advancement of the cervical gearshift in a colinear trajectory to the lamina. The gearshift should advance with minimal resistance along the angle of the exposed contralateral laminar surface.[25]
- A ball-tip probe is then used to confirm the entire path is interosseous. Particular care should be taken to ensure that there is no ventral breach of the cortex.
- Once the pathway is confirmed to be completely interosseous, it can be tapped and screw placed **(TECH FIG 8)**.
- Bilateral screw placement is preferred to allow for more rigid fixation of the axis, thus allowing for more rotational stabilization.
- With bilateral screw placement, care must be taken such that the traversing screw trajectories do not intersect. To prevent this, starting points are placed eccentrically on either side of the bifid spinous process.

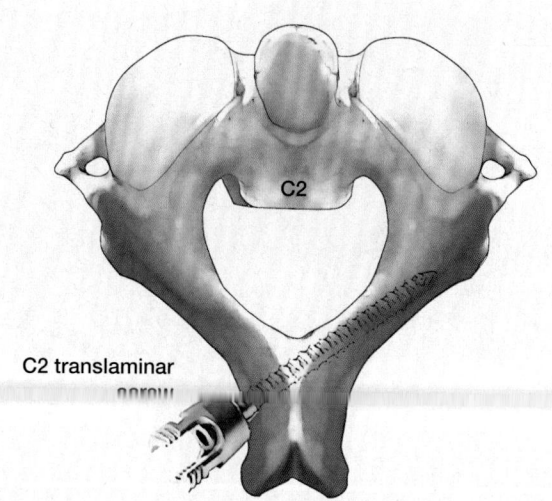

TECH FIG 8 C2 translaminar screw. Axial view with screw in C2 lamina.

TECHNIQUES

Pearls and Pitfalls

Posterior Cervical Infusion	• The surgeon should ensure meticulous decortication of the laminae and spinous processes within the fusion levels. • Facet joint cartilage should be resected at fused levels.
Posterior Cervical Instrumentation	• Insert lateral mass or pedicle screws before neural decompression. This allows better identification of morphologic landmarks and offers a degree of protection against inadvertent injury to the spinal cord.
Posterior Wiring Techniques	• Drill holes should be positioned at the proximal aspect of the cephalad spinous process and the distal aspect of the caudad spinous process to allow greater purchase of the wires in bone. • Wires should be positioned dorsal to the spinolaminar line.
Lateral Mass Fixation	• Preoperative templating allows selection of appropriate screw length to minimize the risk of spinal nerve injury. • Linking the screws to the rod is easier if the most proximal and distal screws are inserted initially followed by the screws in between.
Pedicle Screw Fixation	• Pedicle screw dimensions and orientation should be identified on preoperative imaging studies. • Osteophytes can distort bony margins and should be resected to allow identification of morphologic landmarks for screw insertion. • A burr is used to expose cancellous bone at the pedicle screw insertion point. A blunt, fine pedicle probe is advanced through this cancellous bone to find the medially angled pedicle. • The screw should be inserted to a depth no greater than two-thirds of the anteroposterior width of the vertebral body.
C2 Translaminar Screw	• Preoperative axial CT of C2 must be evaluated and the diameter of the C2 lamina assessed. • This technique is a useful fixation method for patients with a high-riding vertebral artery. • Care should be taken prevent ventral breach of the lamina. • Screw lengths generally range from 25 to 35 mm in length with a minimum diameter of 3.5 mm.

OUTCOMES

- Posterior wiring techniques
  - Long-term successful fusion rates of 94% to 96% have been reported with interspinous wiring techniques when used for trauma, degenerative conditions, and tumors of the cervical spine.[5]
  - Weiland and McAfee[24] reported a fusion rate of 100% when a triple wire technique was used for subaxial posterior cervical fusion in 60 patients. Two of the 60 patients required halo vest immobilization, whereas the rest fused with a two-poster orthosis.
  - Fusion rates with interspinous wiring have been found to be comparable to those obtained from lateral mass plating.[14]
- Lateral mass screw fixation
  - Ebraheim et al[6] retrospectively reviewed the radiographic and clinical outcomes in 36 patients treated with lateral mass plate–screw fixation for traumatic instability, postlaminectomy instability, or metastatic disease. Fusion occurred at an average of 3 months in all patients. One patient demonstrated postoperative neurologic deterioration, but this is resolved with subsequent decompression.
  - Fehlings et al[7] reported successful arthrodesis in 39 (93%) of 42 patients treated with lateral mass plate–screw fixation for cervical instability at a mean follow-up of 46 months. Revision of posterior plating was required in 2 patients for a screw pullout. Another patient required supplementary anterior plating for progressive postoperative kyphosis.
  - Katonis et al[12] reported on insertion of 1662 lateral mass screws in 225 patients. The fusion rate in their group was 97.4% at the mean follow-up of 18 months. Intraoperatively, 27 (1.6%) screws were associated with lateral mass fracture without any neurovascular deficits. Screw removal was required in 3 (1.3%) patients for radiculopathy due to bicortical screws causing nerve root irritation. Screw pullout as a late complication developed in 3 (1.3%) patients within 14 weeks of surgery. The total reoperation rate was 6.2% (14 cases) for nerve injury, hematoma formation, pseudarthrosis, and screw pullout.
  - A systematic review by Coe et al[5] showed that rod and/or screw pullout occurred in 13 out of 5404 screws placed in 818 patients over eight separate studies. Additionally, the overall rate of nerve injury in this systematic review occurred in only 1% of 1041 patients. No cases of vertebral artery injury were identified in 758 patients. The authors conclude that the lateral mass screw fixation is both safe and highly effective.
- Cervical pedicle screws
  - Screw loosening or pullout has not been an issue with cervical pedicle screw use.
  - Abumi et al[2] used pedicle screw–rod fixation after correction of cervical kyphosis in 30 patients and reported excellent correction and no adverse mechanical or neurovascular sequelae related to the pedicle screws.
  - Yukawa et al[27] reported on cervical pedicle screw fixation in 100 patients with unstable cervical injuries.

A total of 419 pedicle screws were inserted. They reported a 4% incidence of pedicle perforation (more than 50% of the screw diameter outside the pedicle). Instrumentation failure associated with loss of correction was found in 2 patients, whereas an additional 3 patients had a loss of correction of more than 10 degrees on follow-up. Local vertebral alignment around the injured segment measured 6 degrees of kyphosis preoperatively and 6.7 degrees of lordosis postoperatively. Successful bony fusion was achieved in all patients other than 3 patients who died shortly after surgery.
  - Kotil et al[15] reported on placement of 210 cervical pedicle screws via freehand technique for fixation of C3 to C7. Patients were followed for 35.7 months on average. In 205 of 210 pedicles (97.6%), the screws were in the correct position as confirmed by postoperative CT scan. Two pedicle screws (0.9%) violated the vertebral foramen. Postoperative angiography demonstrated normal blood flow. The fusion rate in their cohort was 100%.
- C2 translaminar screws
  - The largest single-surgeon series to date indicates that the 7-year outcomes of C2 translaminar screw fixation have been favorable with a 97.6% fusion rate.[9]
  - Meyer et al[16] reviewed 27 patients treated with C2 translaminar screws fixation for upper cervical spine instability. The author reported no intraoperative complication and reported a fusion rated of 92.9% with no hardware failures at follow-up.
  - Gorek et al[8] reported on an in vitro biomechanical study that there was no statistically significant difference between C2 intralaminar and pedicle screw constructs in cadaver models who had undergone odontoidectomy and subsequent C1–C2 fusion.

COMPLICATIONS

Wiring

- The most common complications reported with interspinous wiring are loss of reduction and recurrence of the deformity. Loss of reduction is more common when posterior wiring is done across a level with fractured posterior elements by bypassing that level.
- Osteoporosis or excessive tensioning of the wires can result in intraoperative or postoperative fracture of a spinous process.
- Wire breakage can occur with use of a single-strand wire. Use of multistrand cable reduces the risk of wire breakage.[4]
- Inadvertent passage of spinous process wire through the spinal canal can lead to spinal cord injury. Appropriate placement of drill holes at the spinolaminar line and avoiding a ventrally placed tract between the holes on either side should avoid this complication.

Lateral Mass Screw Fixation

- In a cadaveric comparison of different screw placement techniques, Xu et al[26] found that violation of either the dorsal or ventral nerve root was least likely using the modification of the Magerl technique described by An et al.[3]

- Clinical studies with lateral mass screw insertion have reported a 6% incidence of nerve root injury[15] and a 6% incidence of screw malposition.[13]
  - Three percent of the patients required screw removal for radiculopathy.[13]
  - Screw loosening is reported to occur with an incidence ranging from 2% to 6%.[11,13,15]
  - In addition to direct contact of the nerve root by the screw, radiculopathy can also occur from foraminal stenosis as the lateral mass gets pulled up to the rod during final tightening of the construct.
  - Precise screw length and placement and appropriate contouring of the rod should minimize the incidence of this problem.
- Preoperative planning with evaluation of CT scan can minimize risk of intragenic nerve root injury by allowing for determination of appropriate screw length. The risk of vertebral artery injury and foramen transversarium violation is increased when the divergent angle of the screw in the axial plane are smaller.
- Incidence of foramen transversarium penetration is low with Magerl technique and reported in literature as low as 0.876%. Additionally, violation of the adjacent facet joint was determined to be 1.433%, with the most common joint violation occurring with the C3 lateral mass screw.[27]

Cervical Pedicle Screws

- The medial pedicle wall is the thickest, making medial perforation and spinal cord injury less likely.
  - The lateral pedicular wall is thin, increasing the risk of lateral perforation during pedicular screw insertion.
  - There is little to no space between the superior border of the pedicle and the superior nerve root, whereas there is a mean gap of 1.4 to 1.6 mm between the inferior border of the pedicle and the inferior nerve root.[4]
  - Thus, cortical perforations of the pedicle walls by the pedicular screws are more likely to damage the vertebral artery or superior nerve roots.
- Abumi et al[1] reported a 6.7% (45 out of 669 pedicle screws) incidence of cortical perforation by the screw in 180 consecutive patients.
  - Three of the 180 patients developed screw-associated neurovascular complications, with 2 patients developed radiculopathy that resolved with nonoperative management.
  - One patient developed vertebral artery injury without neurologic sequelae.
- Kast et al[11] reported lateral cortical perforation with more than 25% narrowing of the vertebral artery foramen in 4 of 94 pedicular screws implanted in 26 patients.
  - No vascular or neurologic sequelae occurred with these breaches.
  - Three screws encroached on the intervertebral foramen; one of these screws was revised for a sensory radiculopathy.
- Nakashima et al[17] reported data from a multicenter study on complications of pedicle screw fixation in 84 patients. A total of 390 cervical pedicle screws were inserted. The incidence of pedicle screw misplacement was 19.5%, with 16 (4.1%) of these screws showing more than 50% of the screw diameter outside the pedicle. Complications directly attributable to screw insertion were observed in 5 patients,

with nerve root injury in 3 and vertebral artery injury in 2 patients.

- Yukawa et al[27] reported on insertion of 620 cervical pedicle screws in 144 cervical trauma patients. The incidence of pedicle breach (<50% of the screw diameter outside the pedicle) was 9.2%, whereas the incidence of pedicle perforation (>50% of pedicle diameter outside the pedicle) was 3.9%. There was 1 patient in whom a pedicle probe penetrated the vertebral artery without further complications and 1 patient with transient radiculopathy.
- Kotani et al[14] reported an improvement in the incidence of pedicle perforation when an image-guided system was used.
- Ishikawa et al[9] reported on use of intraoperative CT-assisted navigation system for cervical pedicle screw insertion. Of the 108 pedicle screws inserted, 88.9% were completely contained inside the pedicle with no perforation, 8.3% perforated the pedicle with less than 50% of the screw diameter exposed, and 2.8% perforated the pedicle with more than 50% of the screw diameter exposed. There were no instances of complete pedicle perforation with 100% of the screw diameter outside the pedicle.
- Uehara et al[23] reported on 129 consecutive patients who underwent cervical C2–C7 pedicle screw placement using CT navigation. The combined rate of pedicle perforation was determined to be 20% (116 out of 579). There were, however, no clinically significant complications such as vertebral artery injury, spinal cord injury, or nerve root injury caused by the pedicle breech.

C2 Translaminar Screws

- Ventral laminar breach is the greatest concern of C2 translaminar screw fixation. A ventral breach can result in dural laceration and lead to persistent cerebrospinal fluid leakage and cutaneous fistula.
- The medial location of the C2 translaminar screw heads prevents decortication and maximal placement of bone graft dorsally, thus potentially contributing to less fusion potential.
- No major vascular or neurologic injuries have been reported with C2 translaminar screw placement in the literature.

REFERENCES

1. Abumi K, Shono Y, Ito M, et al. Complications of pedicle screw fixation in reconstructive surgery of the cervical spine. Spine (Phila Pa 1976) 2000;25(8):962–969.
2. Abumi K, Shono Y, Taneichi H, et al. Correction of cervical kyphosis using pedicle screw fixation systems. Spine (Phila Pa 1976) 1999;24(22):2389–2396.
3. An HS, Gordin R, Renner K. Anatomic considerations for plate-screw fixation of the cervical spine. Spine (Phila Pa 1976) 1991;16(10 suppl):S548–S551.
4. Bransford R. Posterior fixation of the upper cervical spine: contemporary techniques. J Am Acad Orthop 2011;19(2):63–71.
5. Coe D, Vaccaro R, Dailey T, et al. Lateral mass screw fixation in the cervical spine: a systematic literature review. J Bone Joint Surg 2013;95(23):2136–2143.
6. Ebraheim NA, Klausner T, Xu R, et al. Safe lateral-mass screw lengths in the Roy-Camille and Magerl techniques: an anatomic study. Spine (Phila Pa 1976) 1998;23(16):1739–1742.
7. Fehlings MG, Cooper PR, Errico TJ. Posterior plates in the management of cervical instability: long-term results in 44 patients. J Neurosurg 1994;81(3):341–349.

8. Gorek J, Acaroglu E, Berven S, et al. Constructs incorporating intralaminar C2 screws provide rigid stability for atlantoaxial fixation. Spine (Phila Pa 1976) 2005;30(13):1513–1518.

9. Ishikawa Y, Kanemura T, Yoshida G, et al. Intraoperative, full-rotation, three-dimensional image (O-arm)-based navigation system for cervical pedicle screw insertion. J Neurosurg Spine 2011;15(5):472–478.

10. Johnston T, Karaikovic E, Lautenschlager E, et al. Cervical pedicle screws vs. lateral mass screws: uniplanar fatigue analysis and residual pullout strengths. Spine J 2006;6(6):667–672.

11. Kast E, Mohr K, Richter HP, et al. Complications of transpedicular screw fixation in the cervical spine. Eur Spine J 2006;15(3):327–334.

12. Katonis P, Papadakis SA, Galanakos S, et al. Lateral mass screw complications: analysis of 1662 screws. J Spinal Disord Tech 2011;24(7):415–420.

13. Kim H-S, Suk K-S, Moon S-H, et al. Safety evaluation of freehand lateral mass screw fixation in the subaxial cervical spine: evaluation of 1256 screws. Spine (Phila Pa 1976) 2015;40(1):2–5.

14. Kotani Y, Abumi K, Ito M, et al. Improved accuracy of computer-assisted cervical pedicle screw insertion. J Neurosurg 2003;99(3 suppl):257–263.

15. Kotil K, Akçetin M, Savas Y. Neurovascular complications of cervical pedicle screw fixation. J Clin Neurosci 2012;19(4):546–551.

16. Meyer D, Meyer F, Kretschmer T, et al. Translaminar screws of the axis—an alternative technique for rigid screw fixation in upper cervical spine instability. Neurosurg Rev 2012;35(2):255–261.

17. Nakashima H, Yukawa Y, Imagama S, et al. Complications of cervical pedicle screw fixation for nontraumatic lesions: a multicenter study of 84 patients. J Neurosurg Spine 2012;16(3):238–247.

18. Ra I-H, Min W-K. Radiographic and clinical assessment of a freehand lateral mass screw fixation technique: is it always safe in subaxial cervical spine? Spine J 2014;14(9):2224–2230.

19. Roy-Camille R, Sallient G, Mazel C. Internal fixation of the unstable cervical spine by posterior osteosynthesis with plates and screws. In: The Cervical Spine Research Society Editorial Committee, ed. The Cervical Spine, ed 2. Philadelphia: JB Lippincott, 1989:390–404.

20. Savage J, Limthongkul W, Park H, et al. A comparison of biomechanical stability and pullout strength between an intralaminar screw and pedicle screw construct for a C1-C2 instability model. Spine J 2010;10(9):S19.

21. Seybold E, Baker J, Criscitiello A, et al. Characteristics of unicortical and bicortical lateral mass screws in the cervical spine. Spine (Phila Pa 1976) 1999;24(22):2397–2403.

22. Stemper BD, Marawar SV, Yoganandan N, et al. Quantitative anatomy of subaxial cervical lateral mass: an analysis of safe screw lengths for Roy-Camille and Magerl techniques. Spine (Phila Pa 1976) 2008;33(8):893–897.

23. Uehara M, Takahashi J, Ikegami S, et al. Screw perforation features in 129 consecutive patients performed computer-guided cervical pedicle screw insertion. Eur Spine J 2014;23(10):2189–2195.

24. Weiland DJ, McAfee PC. Posterior cervical fusion with triple-wire strut graft technique: one hundred consecutive patients. J Spinal Disord 1991;4(1):15–21.

25. Wright NM. Posterior C2 fixation using bilateral, crossing C2 laminar screws: case series and technical note. J Spinal Disord Tech 2004;17(2):158–162.

26. Xu R, Haman SP, Ebraheim NA, et al. The anatomic relation of lateral mass screws to the spinal nerves: a comparison of the Magerl, Anderson, and An techniques. Spine (Phila Pa 1976) 1999;24(19):2057–2061.

27. Yukawa Y, Kato F, Ito K, et al. Placement and complications of cervical pedicle screws in 144 cervical trauma patients using pedicle axis view techniques by fluoroscope. Eur Spine J 2009;18(9):1293–1299.

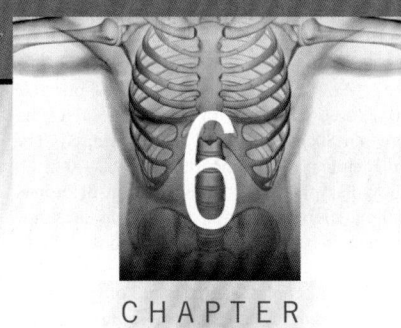

CHAPTER

6

Occipitocervical and C1–C2 Fusion with Instrumentation

S. Babak Kalantar, John M. Rhee, and John G. Heller

DEFINITION

- The terms *occipitocervical* and *atlantoaxial instability* encompasses a number of varied conditions that include disruption of the normal function of the O–C1 and C1–C2 joints, resulting in either pain, spinal cord dysfunction, or the threat thereof.
- Instability can result from trauma, including fractures of the articular masses and occipital condyles, rupture of the transverse ligament, odontoid fracture, or Jefferson fracture. Nontraumatic causes include inflammatory arthropathy (most commonly rheumatoid arthritis), osteoarthritis, congenital anomalies, rotatory subluxation, tumor, and infection.
- Several methods have been described for stabilizing the atlantoaxial complex, as well as the occipitocervical junction, including wiring techniques, transarticular screw fixation, plate and screw fixation, and screw and rod fixation.
- We describe a group of techniques for occipitocervical plating; transarticular screw fixation; articular mass screw and rod construct to achieve atlantoaxial arthrodesis with C2 pars, pedicle, and translaminar screw fixation; and C1–C2 wiring techniques.

ANATOMY

- The base of the skull is composed of the external occipital protuberance (EOP), the occipital condyles (which articulate with the C1 lateral masses), and foramen magnum. Landmarks noted on posterior dissection are the posterior edge of the foramen magnum, the superior nuchal line, the inferior nuchal line, and the EOP (**FIG 1**).
- The nuchal lines serve as attachments to the paired neck muscles. The trapezius attaches to the superior line, and the rectus capitis attaches to the inferior line.
- The nuchal ligament attaches to the external protuberance.
- The thickness of the bone in the suboccipital region varies depending on location. In the midline, the internal occipital crest has a mean thickness of 8.3 mm at the level of the inferior nuchal line, increasing to a mean of 13.8 mm at the EOP. The lateral bone is thinner, ranging from a mean of 3.7 mm at the level of the inferior nuchal line and increasing to a mean of 8.3 mm at the level of the superior nuchal line.[24]
- The first cervical vertebra, or the atlas (C1), is unlike any other in that it lacks a vertebral body and spinous process. It consists of an anterior and posterior arch connected by two articular masses, forming a ring that pivots about the odontoid process of C2 (**FIG 2A**).
- On each side of the cranial surface of the C1 posterior arch, there is a groove for the vertebral artery, the first cervical nerve, and their associated venous complex (**FIG 2B**). In a small subset of the population, this groove is covered by an arch of bone, the ponticulus posticus. The resulting foramen is identified as the *arcuate foramen*.[25]

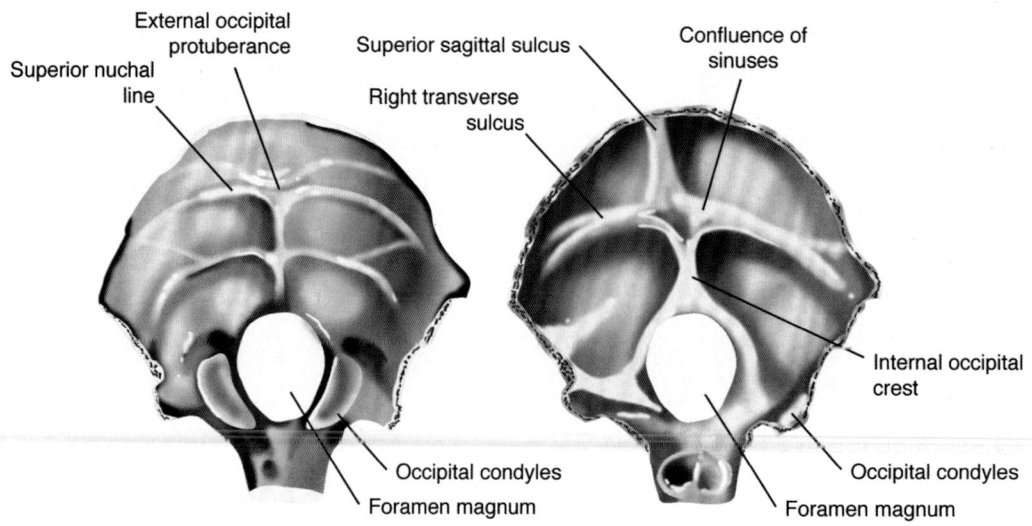

FIG 1 Anatomic landmarks and features of the occiput.

Transverse ligament
of axis

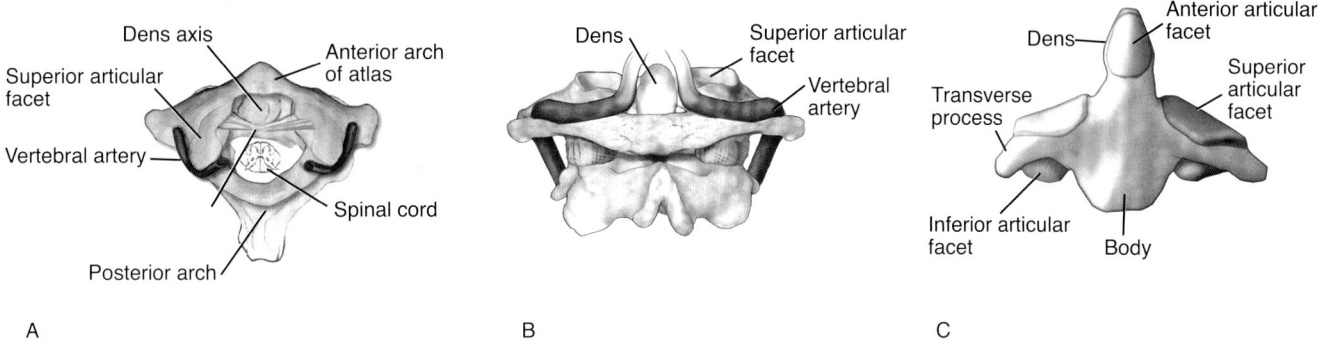

A

B

C

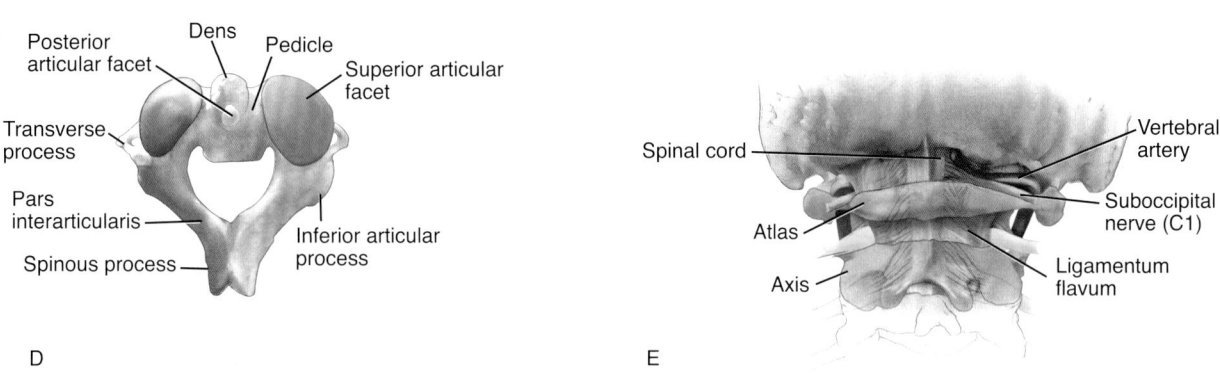

D

E

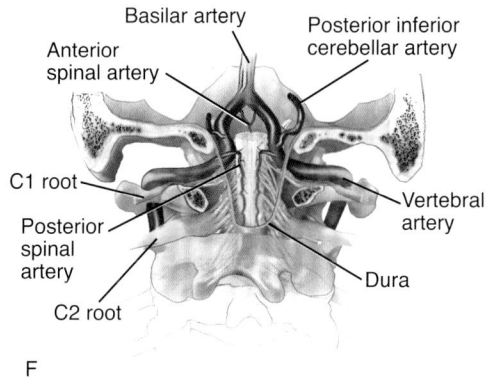

F

FIG 2 A. The atlas consists of an anterior and posterior arch connected by two articular masses. **B.** Posteroanterior view of first and second cervical vertebrae. Anterior (**C**) and superior (**D**) views of the axis, demonstrating the odontoid process projecting upward from the vertebral body. The pedicle connects the lamina and the vertebral body, projecting superomedially. The pars interarticularis lies between the superior and inferior articular processes. **E.** The vertebral artery ascends through the foramina transversaria from C6 to C3. It takes a turn laterally through C2 underneath the pars interarticularis. Once it traverses the transverse foramen at C1, it turns medially and lies on the superior surface of the C1 ring. **F.** After passing medially on the superior surface of the C1 ring, the vertebral artery passes through the foramen magnum and merges with its counterpart to form the basilar artery.

- The articular masses of C1 give rise to the superior and inferior articular facets, which are broad and articulate with the occipital condyles superiorly and the axis inferiorly. A synovial joint also is located between the anterior arch of C1 and the odontoid process of the axis.

- The axis (C2) has thicker laminae and a larger bifid spinous process than the subaxial cervical vertebra. It is characterized further by an odontoid process that projects upward from the vertebral body. Lateral to the odontoid process, or dens, are the sloping superior articular surfaces, which articulate with the inferior articular facets of C1, forming the atlantoaxial joint. The C2 pedicle can be identified in

a zone between the lamina and vertebral body, projecting superomedially (**FIG 2C,D**).

- O–C1 articulation: The kidney-shaped lateral masses of the atlas articulate cranially with the kidney-shaped occipital condyles. The joint allows for 15 to 20 degrees flexion and extension with 5 to 10 degrees of lateral bending.[26] Stability depends on the associated ligaments, the tectorial membrane, and the longitudinal bands of the cruciate ligaments.

- C1–C2 articulation: The C1–C2 complex includes three articulations—two laterally composed of the inferior C1 and superior C2 articular facets, and one anteriorly between the dens and the posterior aspect of the anterior C1 arch.

- The C1–C2 articulation allows up to 47 degrees of rotation to either side, which is approximately 50% of the lateral rotation of the entire cervical spine.[27] Panjabi and associates[23] showed that in the healthy spine, C1–C2 flexion is 11.5 degrees, extension is 10.9 degrees, lateral bending is 6.7 degrees, and axial rotation to each side is 38.9 degrees.

- The vertebral artery, which is the first branch of the subclavian artery medial to the anterior scalene muscle, ascends behind the common carotid artery. It then ascends through the foramina transversaria from C6 to C1. After traversing through the foramina transversaria at C1, the artery takes a sharp turn medially and posteriorly to course behind the C1 articular mass along the groove in the posterior arch of C1. It then passes through the posterior atlanto-occipital membrane before ascending through the foramen magnum, as it merges with its counterpart to form the basilar artery **(FIG 2E,F)**.

- The C1 nerve root, or the suboccipital nerve, exits cranial to the posterior arch of C1 and innervates muscles of the suboccipital triangle. The C2 nerve root, or greater occipital nerve, exits between the posterior arches of C1 and C2, posterior to the superior C1–C2 articulation. It does not exit through a true foramen like the remaining subaxial cervical nerve roots. It traverses inferior to the obliquus capitis inferiorly to ascend through the semispinalis capitis to lie superficial to the rectus capitis. Injury to the greater occipital nerve can lead to dysesthesia of the posterior scalp and can be troublesome to patients.

PATHOGENESIS

- Stability of the O–C1 articulation relies on the ligamentous support and anatomic contour of the occipital condyles on the lateral masses of C1. Occipital condyle fractures may be stable or represent the osseous component of an occipitocervical dissociation (OCD). OCD involves disruption of the ligamentous restraints and/or osseous structures resulting in an injury with high mortality rate.[1]

- Stability of the C1–C2 articulation relies heavily on its ligaments, including the transverse, alar, and apical ligaments, and the facet capsules. Trauma may disrupt these ligamentous restraints. Also, with the advanced degeneration found in arthritic conditions, these ligamentous structures may become incompetent.

- Up to 3 mm of anterior translation of C1 on C2, as measured by the anterior atlantodental interval (AADI) on a lateral cervical radiograph, is normal. An atlantodental interval of 3.5 to 5 mm in an adult indicates potential damage to the transverse ligament, whereas an interval greater than 5 mm indicates probable injury to the transverse ligament and accessory ligaments **(FIG 3A)**.

- In cases of trauma, an atlantodental interval greater than 3.5 mm probably is an indication for further evaluation and most likely requires C1–C2 arthrodesis.

- In patients with inflammatory arthropathy, including rheumatoid arthritis, a canal diameter identified as posterior atlantodental interval (PADI) smaller than 14 mm is associated with a worse outcome and is an indication for

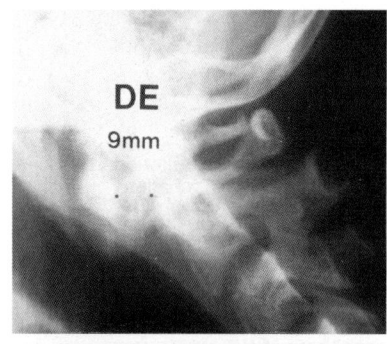

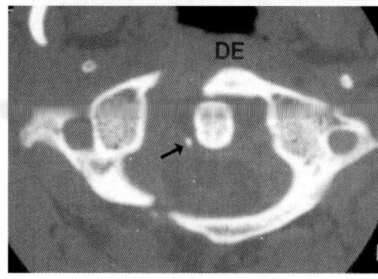

FIG 3 A. An AADI greater than 5 mm indicates likely injury to the transverse ligament and, in the setting of trauma, necessitates operative stabilization. **B.** An avulsion (*arrow*) of the transverse ligament from the ring of C1 indicates instability and may require arthrodesis of C1–C2.

decompression and fusion.[2] The exact AADI measurement is not as relevant in these patients as with trauma patients.

- Fractures that involve the osseous structures of C1 and C2 also may result in atlantoaxial instability and require arthrodesis **(FIG 3B)**.

NATURAL HISTORY

- In the event of trauma to the occipital condyles, careful evaluation with computed tomography (CT) and possibly magnetic resonance imaging (MRI) is indicated to rule out an OCD. In the setting of an OCD, patient mortality can be high, and operative management is recommended. Any translation or distraction at that level is an indication for intervention. Traction is contraindicated. Immediate immobilization followed by occipitocervical fusion is indicated.

- In the event of C1–C2 trauma, ligamentous instability, fractures, or a combination of the two may require surgical treatment. Atlantoaxial instability due to rupture of the transverse ligament represents a threat to the cervical spinal cord with a low likelihood of successful healing. Thus, C1–C2 fusion is indicated.

- Transverse ligament disruption in association with a Jefferson fracture may represent an exception to this rule, in that, successful nonoperative fracture treatment (halo vest) can lead to a "stable" C1–C2 segment on flexion–extension radiographs.

- Fractures of the odontoid process may represent a primary indication for C1–C2 fusion if nonoperative means (eg, halo vest immobilization) cannot obtain or maintain an appropriate reduction, if primary odontoid screw fixation is contraindicated, or if a patient elects surgery to avoid the use of a halo. Displaced odontoid fractures have an

MAGERL METHOD OF C1–C2 TRANSARTICULAR SCREW FIXATION[16]

- Sagittal and axial CT images are scrutinized preoperatively. The isthmus of the C2 pars must measure at least 4.5 mm in height and width to accommodate a transarticular screw.[18] An abnormally large or malpositioned vertebral artery might lead to increased risk of harm to this important structure.
- C1–C2 reduction and the ability to obtain a true lateral view of C1–C2 with a fluoroscope are confirmed.
- A midline incision is made from the occiput far enough caudally to allow a steep enough angulation of the drill and other instruments.
- Posterior C1 and C2 exposure is carried out laterally to visualize the superior and medial surfaces of the C2 pars. Care also should be taken to avoid disturbing the C2–C3 facet capsule.
- The starting point for the transarticular screw is at the posterior cortex of the C2 inferior articular process, 2 mm cephalad and 2 to 3 mm lateral to the medial border of the C2–C3 facet joint. The appropriate location is confirmed by a combination of lateral fluoroscopic images and observing the location of the point relative to the medial border of the C2 pars.
- The starting point is confirmed with a direct lateral C-arm image and marked with a 2-mm burr to provide a secure starting point for the tip of the drill bit. Caudal–cranial angulation is determined via lateral C-arm fluoroscopic guidance. The sagittal plane orientation is confirmed visually with reference to the superior and medial surfaces of the C2 pars. A Penfield no. 4 dissector can be placed on the dorsal surface of the C2 pars to serve as a guide on the lateral fluoroscopy view.
- The Kirschner wire (K-wire) is directed superiorly along the C2 pars while aiming toward the anterior arch of C1, as seen on the lateral fluoroscopic images, with slight medial angulation of 0 to 10 degrees **(TECH FIG 3A,B)**. Advance the drill or wire slowly with frequent fluoroscopic visualization.
- We recommend leaving the drill bit or K-wire in place on the initial side to transfix the C1–C2 joint and then proceeding to the opposite side. The screw on the second side is inserted before returning to the initial side to remove the drill bit and then tap and insert the second screw. This avoids any problems with loss of reduction **(TECH FIG 3C–F)**.
- Bone grafting is performed with autologous iliac crest. After careful decortication of the posterior arches, a modified Gallie technique is employed using either heavy suture or braided titanium cable to secure the graft in place (as described under Gallie Method of Sublaminar Wiring and Grafting section) (see **TECH FIG 10**).
- The extensors at C2 are repaired with drill holes placed through the spinous process.

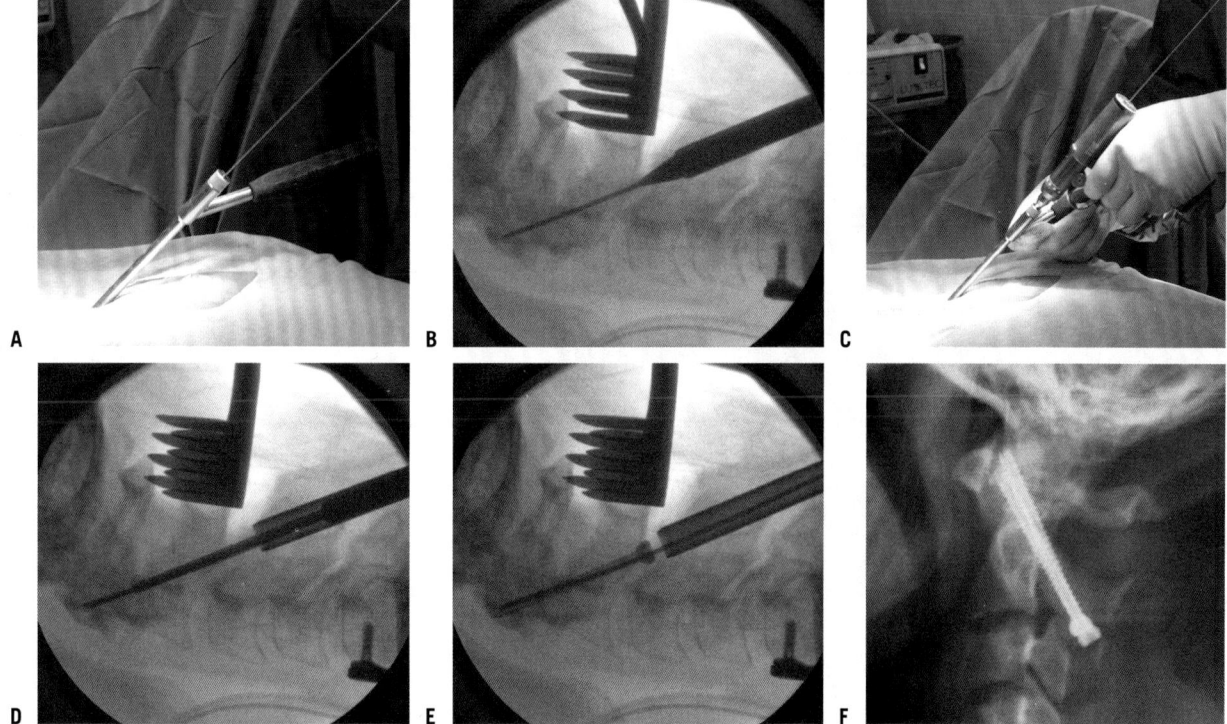

TECH FIG 3 A,B. The guidewire is placed superiorly through the pars, aiming toward the anterior arch of C1 on lateral fluoroscopic images. With the first guidewire in place, a second guidewire is placed on the other side. The K-wire is overdrilled with a drill bit **(C,D)** and tapped, and the screw is placed on the second side **(E)** before the same is done on the first side. **F.** Postoperative radiograph of transarticular screw fixation in a patient who sustained a C1–C2 fracture-dislocation.

GOEL-HARMS METHOD OF C1 ARTICULAR MASS FIXATION[10]

- The ponticulus posticus is a common anomaly that can easily be mistaken for a broad posterior arch of the atlas, and the lateral radiograph must be reviewed to check for the presence of an arcuate foramen to avoid injuring the vertebral artery.[29]
- The starting point for the C1 screw is in the middle of the junction of the C1 posterior arch and the midpoint of the posterior inferior part of the C1 lateral mass. The entry point is marked with a 2-mm high-speed burr **(TECH FIG 4)**.
- The C2 nerve root is retracted in a caudal direction for proper screw placement. At times, ligation of the C2 root will be required due to either altered local anatomy or excessive bleeding from the associated venous plexus. If the root is divided, some patients may experience troubling neuralgia and numbness postoperatively.
- The initial drill hole is made in a straight or slightly convergent trajectory in the axial plane and parallel to the plane of the C1 posterior arch in the sagittal plane, with the tip of the drill aimed toward the anterior arch of C1 **(TECH FIG 5A)**.
- The hole is tapped and measured, and a 3.5-mm partially threaded polyaxial screw of appropriate length is placed allowing the polyaxial portion of the screw to lie above the arch of C1. The partially threaded screw helps minimize any irritation to the greater occipital (C2) nerve.
- Care should be taken when dissecting around the C1–C2 articulation to avoid excessive bleeding from the epidural venous

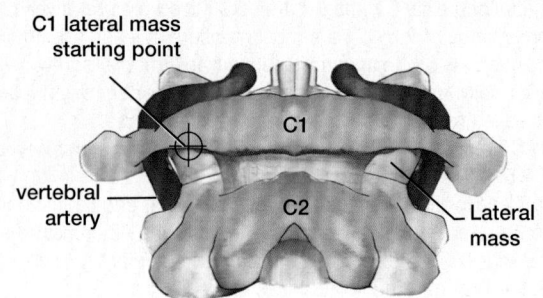

TECH FIG 4 C1 lateral mass starting point.

plexus in this area. Hemostasis can be achieved using bipolar electrocautery, powdered Gelfoam with thrombin, and cotton pledgets.
- The center of the lateral mass of C1 is the ideal exit point of the C1 lateral mass screw, and the proximity of the internal carotid artery (ICA) places it in danger when placing a bicortical screw. The ICA can vary in location from side to side and may be within 1 mm of the ideal exit point of a bicortical transarticular screw or a C1 lateral mass screw.[7]
- Medial angulation of the screw in the lateral mass of C1 may increase the margin of safety for the ICA, but care should be taken to avoid penetrating the occipitocervical joint by aiming caudally.

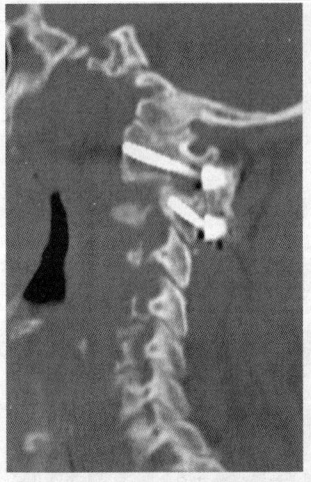
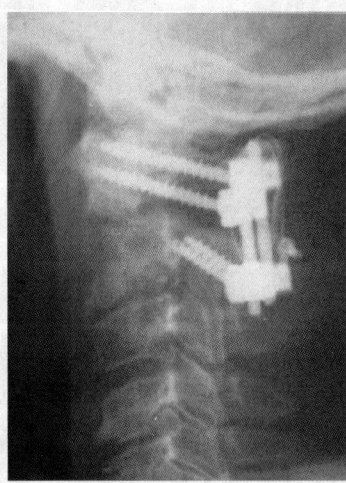

TECH FIG 5 Postoperative CT scan (**A**) and lateral radiograph (**B**) of a patient with a displaced, kyphotic, chronic C2 fracture who underwent C1–C2 posterior fusion using C1 articular mass screws and C2 pars screws.

C2 PEDICLE/PARS SCREW PLACEMENT

- The starting point of the C2 pedicle is in the midline of the C2–C3 facet joint, 3 to 5 mm cranial to the C2–C3 articulation. The trajectory is 25 degrees of medial convergence and is aimed 25 degrees cephalad while keeping in mind that individual anatomy will vary **(TECH FIG 6A)**.

- The starting point of the C2 pars screw is 2 mm superior and lateral to the inferior C2–C3 articulation. It is placed in a craniocaudal trajectory similar to the transarticular screw but does not need to be aimed as much cephalad. It is aimed 20 to 25 degrees medial **(TECH FIG 6B)**.

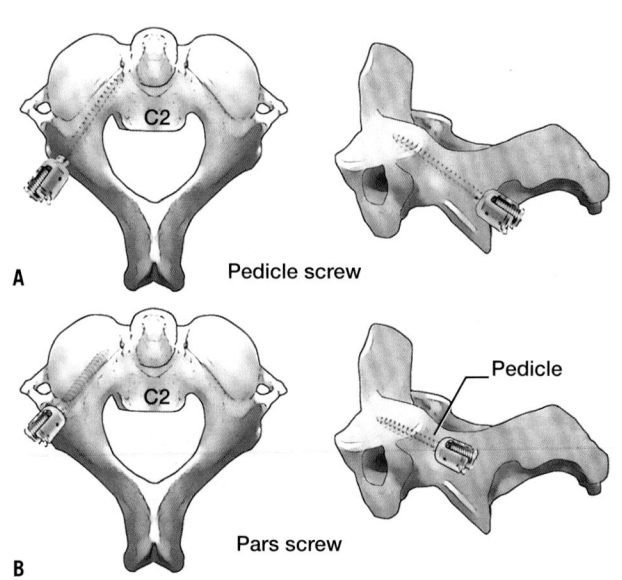

A   Pedicle screw

B   Pars screw

TECH FIG 6 Screw trajectory and correct identification of the pedicle (**A**) and pars (**B**) of the C2 or axis.

- A no. 4 Penfield dissector is used to feel the medial border of the C2 pars interarticularis, and the superior and medial aspects of the isthmus are palpated during the drilling process.
- The drilled hole is then palpated with a blunt ball-tipped probe. The hole is tapped, and a 3.5- or 4.0-mm polyaxial screw is inserted.
- C2 pars screw length is typically 16 to 22 mm, depending on the anatomy of the vertebral artery and thickness of the pars. Preoperative CT will aid in estimating length.
- The polyaxial screw heads are connected with two rods. If necessary, a reduction of the C1–C2 articulation is performed before fixation with the rods.
- The posterior elements of C1 and C2 are decorticated, and a corticocancellous H graft is secured using a modified Gallie technique (**TECH FIG 5B**).
- The extensors at C2 are repaired using drill holes through the spinous process.

C2 TRANSLAMINAR SCREW PLACEMENT[21]

- A high-speed burr with a 2-mm tip is used to open a small cortical hole at the junction of the C2 spinous process and lamina starting on the right side. This is done in the cranial half of the C2 lamina.
- A hand drill is used to drill the contralateral or left lamina with the drill aligned along the angle of that lamina. This is done to a depth of 25 to 30 mm. Care must be taken to allow the trajectory to be slightly less than the downslope of the lamina so that any cortical breakthrough would occur dorsally and not ventrally toward the spinal canal.
- A small ball probe is used to evaluate the drilled hole for any cortical breaches.
- Typically, a 4.0- × 30-mm screw is placed with the head of the screw at the junction of the spinous process and lamina on the right. A smaller diameter screw may be needed

depending on the height of the lamina in order to accommodate two screws.
- Using the high-speed burr, a small cortical hole is made at the junction of the spinous process and lamina on the left in the caudal half of the lamina. Using a similar technique as described earlier, a 4.0- × 30-mm screw is placed in the right lamina with the screw head at the junction of the spinous process and lamina on the left (**TECH FIG 7A–C**).
- C1 lateral mass screws and/or subaxial screws are placed as described.
- The posterior elements of C1 and C2 are decorticated, and a corticocancellous H graft is secured using a modified Gallie technique (see **TECH FIG 10**).
- If possible, the extensors at C2 are repaired using drill holes through the spinous process.

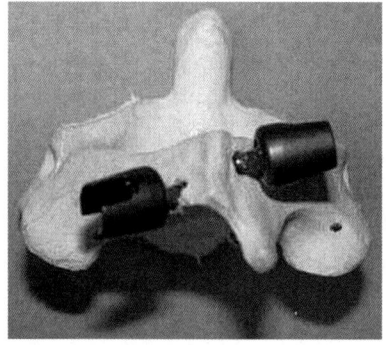
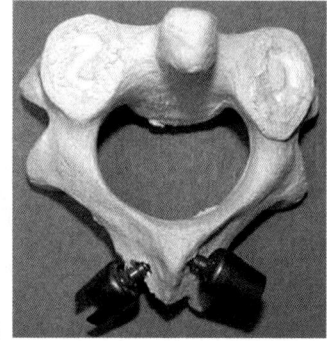
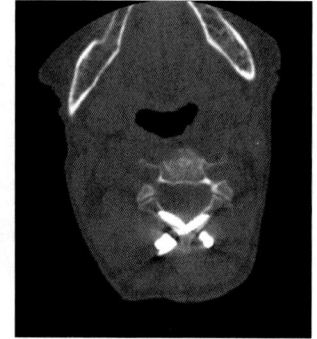

A   **B**   **C**

TECH FIG 7 Saw bones model demonstrating coronal (**A**) and axial (**B**) appearance of the translaminar screw technique. **C.** Axial CT image of translaminar fixation.

BROOKS METHOD OF WIRE FIXATION

- Brooks wiring is the most reliable of the traditional wire fixation methods. It does not provide as much stability as the newer screw options. Thus, it requires more significant postoperative immobilization, often a halo vest, for optimal likelihood of fusion.[3] It also requires passing sublaminar wires at C2, which can be technically demanding with some risk of spinal cord injury.
- Midline posterior subperiosteal exposure of C1 and C2 laminae is carried out with careful attention to dissect from midline laterally at C1 to prevent injury to the vertebral artery. The occipital nerves emerge through the interlaminar space between C1 and C2.
- The ligamentum flavum between C1 and the occiput and also between C1 and C2 is sharply divided. A Woodson instrument is used to confirm that there are no dural adhesions in the sublaminar space.
- Although Brooks originally described the use of two doubled 20-gauge stainless steel wires passed under each side of the arch of C1 followed by C2 in a cephalad to caudal direction, we routinely use pairs of braided titanium cables rather than stainless steel wire, but it is crucial to ensure that there is sufficient subarachnoid space to safely pass wires or cables beneath the laminae without injuring the spinal cord.

- After the cables are passed with a loop at the end, two full-thickness rectangular bone grafts measuring approximately 1.25 × 3.5 cm are taken from the iliac crest. The sides of each graft are beveled to fit in the interval between the C1 and C2 laminae and placed on each side.
- The bone grafts are then held in place by securing the cables (**TECH FIG 8**).

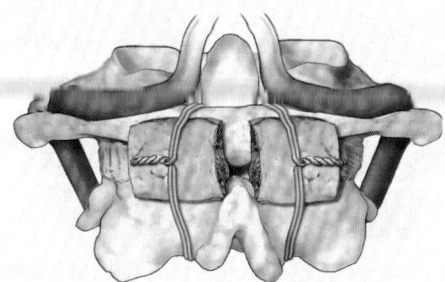

TECH FIG 8 Brooks wiring technique.

GALLIE METHOD OF SUBLAMINAR WIRING AND GRAFTING

- The Gallie method is less stable than the Brooks method and is relatively contraindicated in the presence of any posterior C1–C2 instability.[9] Biomechanically, this method provides less stability in rotation with only comparable stability in anteroposterior translation.[12] It also requires significant postoperative immobilization.
- Dissection similar to that of the Brooks method is performed.
- A sublaminar wire or braided titanium cable is passed under the arch of C1 and looped around the spinous process of C2. We use a suture for this technique when the Gallie graft is employed in conjunction with Magerl transarticular fixation

because the Gallie configuration is relied on for maintenance of graft position, not for mechanical stability (**TECH FIG 9**).
- A corticocancellous bone graft from the iliac crest (**TECH FIG 10A**) is taken and placed with the cancellous side facing down on the posterior elements after the cortical bone has been burred to reveal a nice bleeding cancellous bed (**TECH FIG 10B**). The small grooves are placed on the superior and inferior edges of the graft to hold the cables in place.
- The cable is tightened or the suture is tied, and the graft is secured (**TECH FIG 10C**).

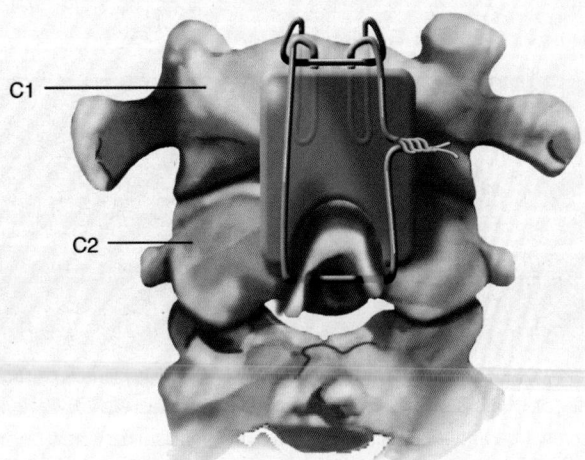

C1

C2

TECH FIG 9 Gallie wiring technique.

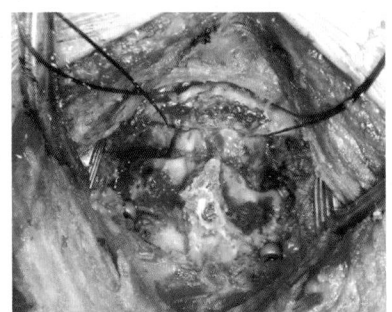
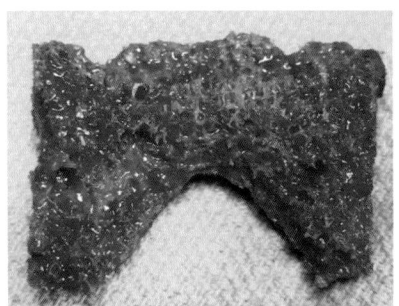
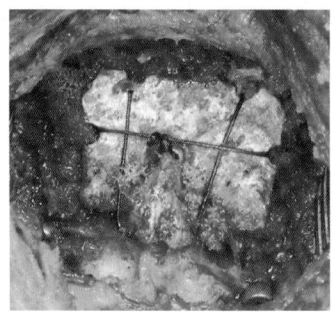

A   **B**   **C**

TECH FIG 10 A. The posterior arches of C1 and C2 are decorticated. **B.** A corticocancellous graft is taken from the iliac crest. This is fashioned into an H shape, and the cancellous side is placed facing down on the decorticated posterior elements of C1–C2. **C.** A modified Gallie technique is used to secure the graft in place.

TECHNIQUES

Pearls and Pitfalls

Bone Grafting	• A Gallie H graft is fashioned from the iliac crest and contoured to fit over the posterior arches of C1 and C2, with its cancellous surface applied directly opposing the decorticated surfaces of C1 and C2.
Frameless Stereotactic Navigation	• This method registers only one vertebra, and the relation of C1 and C2 obtained on the CT scan may differ from that resulting after positioning on the operating table, resulting in aberrant screw placement and possible injury to the vertebral artery, whereas intraoperative fluoroscopy yields real-time information. Caution should be used in interpreting the information presented on the "virtual" images during surgery.
Injury to the Vertebral Artery	• Careful preoperative planning will guide selection of the appropriate procedure to reduce the risk of injury. In the event of injury to a vertebral artery during a Magerl procedure, a short screw may be placed to contain the bleeding. If this occurs while drilling or tapping the first side, it is unwise to attempt a C1–C2 screw on the contralateral side. An alternative fixation technique, which does not place the contralateral artery at risk, should be employed, such as a Brooks or Gallie procedure.
Venous Bleeding Near the C1 Lateral Mass	• Gentle tamponade of the venous sinuses, along with application of hemostatic agents, is recommended. Once the surgical instruments are removed along with the pressure from the retractors, the bleeding is usually controlled with ease. Avoid indiscriminate use of cautery. If necessary, ligate the C2 root proximal to the dorsal root ganglion to gain access to the veins and stop the bleeding.
Supplemental Wire/Cable Fixation	• Supplemental wiring in conjunction with screw fixation methods at C1 and C2 provides no significant mechanical advantage. It does add technical difficulty, risk, and cost. However, a suture configuration of a similar nature will hold the graft surfaces in proper apposition to the decorticated host bone, possibly improving the fusion rates.
C1–C2 Facet Fusion	• Originally described as a component of the Magerl procedure, direct exposure, decortication, and grafting of the posterior aspect of the C1–C2 facets is not routinely necessary. It may be indicated for revision procedures, patients with incompetent posterior C1 arches, certain fracture patterns, or for high-risk hosts.

POSTOPERATIVE CARE

- Whereas patients undergoing the Brooks or Gallie procedure obtain a maximal fusion rate with postoperative halo vest immobilization, the modern screw fixation methods yield fusion rates in excess of 90% with only cervical collars worn for 6 to 12 weeks.
- The type of collar used and duration of wear should be in accordance with surgeon judgment about host bone, security of fixation, anticipated patient compliance, and so forth.

OUTCOMES

- Jeanneret and Magerl[16] achieved solid fusion in 13 of 13 patients stabilized with the transarticular screw technique.
- McGuire and Harkey[20] showed solid fusion in 8 of 8 patients using a transfacet screw technique.
- Fielding and associates[8] achieved fusion in 45 of 46 patients with fractures using the Gallie technique.
- Brooks and Jenkins[3] used a C1–C2 sublaminar wiring technique to achieve fusion in 14 of 15 patients.
- Harms and Melcher[14] reported fusion in all 37 patients with C1 lateral mass and C2 pedicle minipolyaxial screw and rod construct.

COMPLICATIONS

- Vertebral artery and ICA injuries
- Infection
- Malpositioned screw
- Nonunion
- C2 neuralgia
- C1–C2 hyperextension with Brooks or Gallie procedure if the C1 and C2 arches are compressed together

REFERENCES

1. Ben-Galim PJ, Sibai TA, Hipp JA, et al. Internal decapitation: survival after head to neck dissociation injuries. Spine (Phila Pa 1976) 2008;33(16):1744–1749.
2. Boden SD, Dodge LD, Bohlman HH, et al. Rheumatoid arthritis of the cervical spine. A long term analysis with predictors of paralysis and recovery. J Bone Joint Surg Am 1993;75:1282–1297.
3. Brooks AL, Jenkins EW. Atlanto-axial arthrodesis by the wedge compression method. J Bone Joint Surg Am 1978;60(3):279–284.
4. Brown T, Reitman CA, Nguyen L, et al. Intervertebral motion after incremental damage to the posterior structures of the cervical spine. Spine (Phila Pa 1976) 2005;30(17):E503–E508.
5. Chaudhary A, Drew B, Orr RD, et al. Management of type II odontoid fractures in the geriatric population: outcome of treatment in a rigid cervical orthosis. J Spinal Disord Tech 2010;23(5):317–320.
6. Cothren CC, Moore EE, Ray CE Jr, et al. Cervical spine fracture patterns mandating screening to rule out blunt cerebrovascular injury. Surgery 2007;141(1):76–82.
7. Currier BL, Todd LT, Maus TP, et al. Anatomic relationship of the internal carotid artery to the C1 vertebra: a case report of the cervical reconstruction for chordoma and pilot study to assess the risk of screw fixation of the atlas. Spine (Phila Pa 1976) 2003;28(22):E461–E467.
8. Fielding JW, Hawkins RJ, Ratzan SA. Spine fusion for atlanto-axial instability. J Bone Joint Surg Am 1976;58(3):400–407.
9. Gallie W. Fractures and dislocations of the cervical spine. Am J Surg 1939;46:495–499.
10. Goel A, Laheri V. Plate and screw fixation for atlanto-axial subluxation. Acta Neurochir (Wien) 1994;129(1–2):47–53.
11. Gorek J, Acaroglu E, Berven S, et al. Constructs incorporating intralaminar C2 screws provide rigid stability for atlantoaxial fixation. Spine (Phila Pa 1976) 2005;30(13):1513–1518.
12. Grob D, Crisco JJ III, Panjabi MM, et al. Biomechanical evaluation of four different posterior atlantoaxial fixation techniques. Spine (Phila Pa 1976) 1992;17(5):480–490.
13. Haher TR, Yeung AW, Caruso SA, et al. Occipital screw pullout strength. A biomechanical investigation of occipital morphology. Spine (Phila Pa 1976) 1999;24(1):5–9.
14. Harms J, Melcher RP. Posterior C1–C2 fusion with polyaxial screw and rod fixation. Spine (Phila Pa 1976) 2001;26(22):2467–2471.
15. Hwang H, Hipp JA, Ben-Galim P, et al. Threshold cervical range-of-motion necessary to detect abnormal intervertebral motion in cervical spine radiographs. Spine (Phila Pa 1976) 2008;33(8):E261–E267.
16. Jeanneret B, Magerl F. Primary posterior fusion of C1/2 in odontoid fractures: indications, techniques, and results of transarticular screw fixation. J Spinal Disord 1992;5(4):464–475.
17. Madawi AA, Casey AT, Solanki GA, et al. Radiological and anatomic evaluation of the atlantoaxial transarticular screw fixation technique. J Neurosurg 1997;86(6):961–968.
18. Mandel IM, Kambach BJ, Petersilge CA, et al. Morphologic considerations of C2 isthmus dimensions for the placement of transarticular screws. Spine (Phila Pa 1976) 2000;25(12):1542–1547.
19. McCulloch PT, France J, Jones DL, et al. Helical computed tomography alone compared with plain radiographs with adjunct computed tomography to evaluate the cervical spine after high-energy trauma. J Bone Joint Surg Am 2005;87(11):2388–2394.
20. McGuire RA Jr, Harkey HL. Modification of technique and results of atlantoaxial transfacet stabilization. Orthopedics 1995;18(10):1029–1032.
21. Menendez JA, Wright NM. Techniques of posterior C1-C2 stabilization. Neurosurgery 2007;60(1 suppl 1):S103–S111.
22. Muchow RD, Resnick DK, Abdel MP, et al. Magnetic resonance imaging (MRI) in the clearance of the cervical spine in blunt trauma: a meta-analysis. J Trauma 2008;64(1):179–189.
23. Panjabi M, Dvorak J, Duranceau J, et al. Three-dimensional movements of the upper cervical spine. Spine (Phila Pa 1976) 1988;13(7):726–730.
24. Roberts DA, Doherty BJ, Heggeness MH. Quantitative anatomy of the occiput and the biomechanics of occipital screw fixation. Spine (Phila Pa 1976) 1998;23(10):1100–1108.
25. Stubbs D. The arcuate foramen. Variability in distribution related to race and sex. Spine (Phila Pa 1976) 1992;17(12):1502–1504.
26. Wang JC, Mummaneni PV, Haid RW Jr. Fixation options in the occipitocervical junction. In: Mummaneni PV, Lenke LG, Haid RW Jr, eds. Spinal Deformity: A Guide to Surgical Planning and Management. St. Louis: Quality Medical Publishing, 2008:223–2400.
27. White A III, Panjabi M. The clinical biomechanics of the occipitoatlantoaxial complex. Orthop Clin North Am 1978;9(4):867–878.
28. Wright NM. Posterior C2 fixation using bilateral, crossing C2 laminar screws: case series and technical note. J Spinal Disord Tech 2004;17(2):158–162.
29. Young JP, Young PH, Ackermann MJ, et al. The ponticulus posticus: implications for screw insertion into the first cervical lateral mass. J Bone Joint Surg Am 2005;87(11):2495–2498.

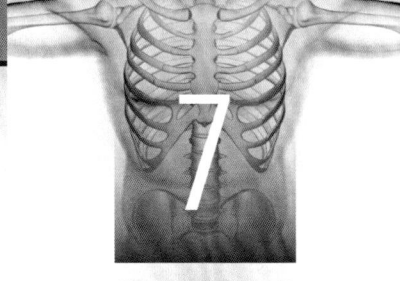

7

CHAPTER

Cervical Disc Replacement

Michael A. Finn, Arianne J. Boylan, and Gregory Kuzmik

ANATOMY

- Familiarity with the anterior cervical anatomy is a necessity, particularly in regard to muscular, fascial, vascular, aerodigestive, nervous, and bony structures (**FIG 1**).
- Approach level can be estimated by overlying anatomy:
  - C3: hyoid bone
  - C4–C5: thyroid cartilage
  - C6: cricoid cartilage, carotid tubercle
- Muscular anatomy
  - The only muscle transected in the approach is the platysma, which lies superficially, just under the subcutaneous fat layer.
  - The sternocleidomastoid extends from the mastoid inferomedially to the sternomanubrial articulation and provides a lateral border for the exposure.
  - The omohyoid traverses the approach to the anterior cervical spine at approximately the C6 level and may be retracted or resected.
  - The longus colli muscles lie on the anterolateral surface of the cervical spine and are more widely spaced in the caudal direction than the cephalad. The position of the longus muscles is helpful in identifying the midline of the vertebral bodies.
- Fascial planes
  - Superficial cervical fascia—lies just deep to the dermis and surrounds the platysma
  - Deep cervical fascia
    - Superficial layer: Also called the *investing layer*, this forms a collar around the neck and contains the sternocleidomastoid, among other structures, and blends with the lateral aspect of the carotid sheath.

- Middle layer: Muscular part surrounds the strap muscles and great vessels, whereas the visceral part (also known as *pretracheal fascia*) encloses the anteromedial structures of the neck (aerodigestive tract and thyroid gland). It blends laterally with the carotid sheath.
  - Deep layer: The prevertebral part closely surrounds the vertebral column and prevertebral muscles. The alar part lies between the prevertebral and pretracheal fascia and defines the posterior border of the retropharyngeal space.
- Vascular structures
  - The anterior and external jugular veins take variable courses superficial to the sternocleidomastoid and deep to the platysma.
  - The carotid artery and internal jugular vein are contained in the carotid sheath and help define the lateral margin of the deep exposure.
  - The vertebral arteries enter the transverse foramen at the C6 level in most (~90%) of cases. The vertebral artery lies around 1.5 mm laterally to the uncovertebral joints in the middle cervical spine, although this is somewhat variable. The course of the vertebral artery takes is more medial, closer to the uncinate processes more rostrally.[26]
- Neural structures
  - The recurrent laryngeal nerve ascends from the thoracic cavity in the tracheoesophageal groove to innervate all the intrinsic muscles of larynx with the exception of the cricothyroid.
  - The right recurrent laryngeal nerve arises in anterior to the subclavian artery and takes a more anterior course in the neck than does the left nerve, which arises more distally near the arch of the aorta.
  - Superiorly, the superficial laryngeal nerve crosses lateral to medial at the level of the hyoid to pierce the thyrohyoid membrane, at the level of the C3–C4 interspace and provides innervation to the cricothyroid muscle as well as sensory innervation to the posterior pharynx.[21,31]
  - The spinal radicular nerve exits the spinal canal through the neural foramen at approximately 45-degree angle to the cord in the axial plane.
- Bony and ligamentous structures
  - The anterior longitudinal ligament (ALL) overlies the anterior aspect of the vertebral column and closely adheres to the intervertebral disc and endplate.
    - The disc underlies the ALL and is composed of a tough outer annulus fibrosus surrounding a soft gelatinous core, the nucleus pulposus.
    - The annular fibers are attached to the subchondral bone of the adjacent vertebral bodies.

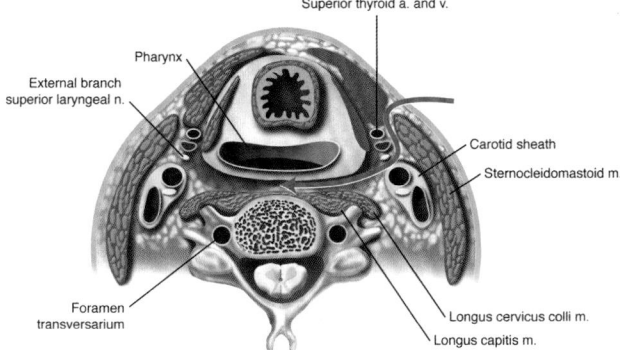

FIG 1 Cross-sectional view of the cervical spine with avenue of Smith-Robinson approach drawn.

Superior thyroid a. and v.

Pharynx

External branch superior laryngeal n.

Carotid sheath

Sternocleidomastoid m.

Foramen transversarium

Longus cervicus colli m.

Longus capitis m.

- The posterior longitudinal ligament (PLL) runs down the posterior aspect of the vertebral column and is more robust centrally.
- The uncovertebral joints, or uncinate joints, are situated laterally in the intervertebral space and serve as a landmark for anterior cervical decompressions.
  - Foraminal stenosis is often caused by hypertrophic degeneration of the uncinate joints.

PATHOGENESIS

- Arthritic degeneration can affect any mobile joint in the spine.
  - Facet joint: neck pain (not treated with arthroplasty)
  - Uncovertebral joints: foraminal stenosis causing radiculopathy
  - Disc space
    - Osteophytic degeneration can cause central stenosis and myelopathy or radiculopathy.
    - Herniated disc fragments can be associated with significant inflammatory response and profound acute symptoms of radiculopathy or myelopathy.[24]
- Risk factors for arthritic degeneration[10,35]
  - Genetic predisposition
  - Age
  - Tobacco use
  - Activity/occupation (heavy manual labor)
  - Obesity (body mass index >30)

NATURAL HISTORY

- The natural history of cervical radiculopathy is most often benign, with about 70% of patients having spontaneous improvement.[11,15,29]
  - Symptoms can recur or take on a waxing and waning course.
  - Between 6% and 35% matriculate to surgical intervention.
- The natural history of myelopathy is controversial and appears to most often have a course of episodic or steady decline while improving with conservative treatment in only a minority of patients.[17]

HISTORY AND PHYSICAL FINDINGS

- Radiculopathy
  - Patients often present with dermatomal pain, sensory changes (numbness, paresthesias), and weakness (TABLE 1).
  - May have dull ache in neck, shoulder, and scapula

- Often worse with extension; lateral rotation and bending toward symptomatic side; or when straining, sneezing, or coughing
- Neurologic examination may be normal or reveal segmental weakness and reflex deficit.
- Myelopathy
  - Over 50% of patients may present without significant painful complaints.[4]
  - Often presents as insidious decline of upper and lower extremity motor function
    - Clumsiness of hands
    - Gait instability
    - Sensory dysfunction
  - Physical examination can reveal the following:
    - Weakness, often greatest in hands
    - Muscle wasting, often greatest in hands
    - Spasticity
    - Hyperreflexia with pathologic reflexes (Hoffman sign, Babinski sign)

IMAGING AND OTHER DIAGNOSTIC STUDIES

- Plain x-rays may demonstrate arthritic changes such as disc space narrowing, subchondral sclerosis, osteophyte formation, and foraminal stenosis (with oblique views) as well as overall alignment of neck and evidence of instability.
- Computed tomography (CT) clearly delineates bony changes and may demonstrate bony foraminal compression. CT may be useful in evaluating for suspected ossification of the PLL when considering arthroplasty. CT myelography is useful in evaluating for the presence of neural compression in patients who are unable to undergo magnetic resonance imaging (MRI) and in those who have been previously instrumented.
- MRI is the imaging modality of choice for the evaluation of cervical radiculopathy or myelopathy and is sensitive in detecting disc herniations, osteophytes, spinal cord signal abnormalities, and central and foraminal stenosis.
- Other modalities, including electrodiagnostic studies (electromyography) and injections, may be used to clarify a diagnosis in difficult cases.

DIFFERENTIAL DIAGNOSIS

- Cervical radiculopathy
- Cervical myelopathy
- Tumor (cranial or spinal)
- Stroke
- Motor neuron disease

TABLE 1 Cervical Radicular Function			
Root	Motor Function	Sensory Distribution	Reflex
C3	Diaphragm	Upper neck	
C4	Diaphragm	Neck, upper shoulder, and chest	
C5	Shoulder abduction (deltoid), elbow flexion (biceps), external rotation of arm (supraspinatus/infraspinatus; diaphragm)	Shoulder, lateral arm to anterior forearm	Biceps, brachioradialis
C6	Wrist extension, elbow flexion, forearm supination	Anterior arm and forearm to thumb and index finger	Biceps, brachioradialis
C7	Elbow extension, wrist flexors, finger extensors	Lateral arm, dorsal forearm to middle three fingers	Triceps
C8	Intrinsic, thumb extension, wrist ulnar deviation	Back of arm to little and index fingers	Pronator

- Multiple sclerosis
- Syringomyelia
- Brachial plexopathy
  - Parsonage-Turner syndrome
  - Thoracic outlet syndrome
  - Radiation plexopathy
- Peripheral nerve entrapment
- Musculoskeletal
  - Shoulder disease (eg, rotator cuff)
  - Myofascial pain syndrome
  - Infection
  - Tumor
  - Tendinitis
  - Inflammatory arthropathy
- Cardiac ischemia
- Chest pathology
- Reflex sympathetic dystrophy

NONOPERATIVE MANAGEMENT

- Nonoperative treatment should be attempted in most patients with radiculopathy.
  - Physical therapy or placement of a cervical collar have both been shown to be efficacious in acute (<1 month duration) symptoms and nonefficacious in cases of long-standing (>3 months) radiculopathy.[15,25]
  - Medications
    - Anti-inflammatory medications
    - "Nerve medications"—gabapentin, amitriptyline, pregabalin
    - Narcotics—limited role
  - Injections—epidural steroid injection and selective nerve root block can be therapeutic and predictive of surgical outcome.[33]
- Cervical myelopathy can be treated conservatively with a collar in patients unable or unwilling to undergo surgical decompression.[14]

SURGICAL MANAGEMENT

- Surgical intervention is indicated in cases of radiculopathy resistant to conservative care and in cases of progressive weakness.
- Surgical intervention is indicated for cervical myelopathy in the presence of a compressive spinal cord lesion.

Indications

- Treatment of symptomatic degenerative disease of the cervical spine, including disc degeneration, herniation, and osteophyte formation causing radiculopathy or myelopathy
- Symptoms resistant to conservative care for over 6 weeks or progressive neurologic deficit
- Treatment of degeneration or disc disease in cervical levels C2–C3 and C6–C7
- The Mobi-C cervical disc was U.S. Food and Drug Administration (FDA)-approved in 2013 for two-level cervical arthroplasty.
- Cervical disc replacement remains controversial for the treatment of adjacent level disease.

Contraindications

- Significant sagittal plane deformity (angulation >20 degrees)
- Instability (>3.5 mm of motion in flexion/extension or spondylolisthesis)

- Severe disc space collapse with limited range of motion (<2 degrees of motion)
- Significant facet arthrosis
- Ossification of the PLL
- Treatment of fractures, infections, and tumors
- Osteoporosis

Preoperative Planning

- Films should be thoroughly examined for anomalous anatomy, such as an aberrant vertebral artery course, and for other possible causes of the patient's symptoms. The depth and height of the disc space can be measured to estimate the size of the potential implant.
- Preoperative measurements should always be confirmed intraoperatively as endplate preparation will alter dimensions.

Positioning

- The patient is positioned supine with a small bump under the shoulders and the head in a doughnut in slight extension. A radiolucent table is used to allow for anteroposterior (AP) and lateral fluoroscopy.
- The shoulders may need to be retracted inferiorly with tape to allow visualization of more caudal levels in large patients. Overly aggressive retraction should be avoided to reduce risk of brachial plexus injury.

Approach

- A standard Smith-Robinson approach is used to access the anterior cervical spine.
- On initial exposure, the level of interest is confirmed radiographically, and the midline of immediately adjacent cephalad and caudad levels are marked with Bovie electrocautery prior to elevation of the longus muscles (FIG 2).
  - Using a marking pen over the cauterized bone can help to more clearly delineate and preserve midline markings.
- After the midline is clearly marked, the medial border of the longus colli muscle is incised with the Bovie electrocautery,

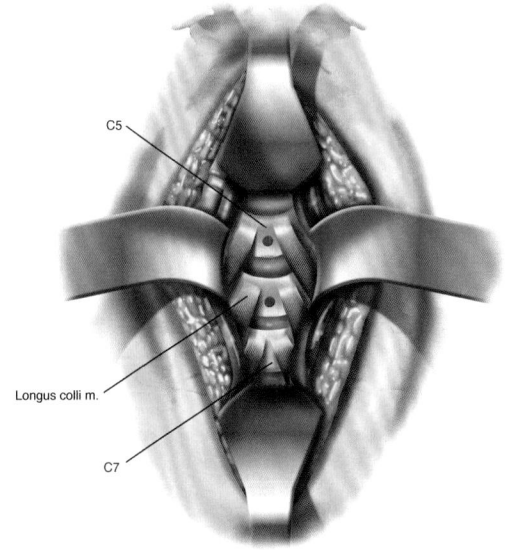

FIG 2 Exposure of the anterior cervical spine. The longus colli are used to identify the midline, which is then marked with Bovie electrocautery and a marking pen.

and a longus flap is elevated. The longus should be elevated over approximately half the height of the adjacent vertebral body with care taken to preserve the annular attachments of the adjacent level. A self-retaining retractor is placed underneath the flap.

- Care should also be taken not to transect or perform extensive dissection of the ventral surface of the longus colli, which risks damage to the sympathetic chain and a resultant Horner syndrome. A self-retaining retractor is placed underneath the elevated muscle flap.

DISCECTOMY

- The disc space is incised with a no. 15 blade scalpel, and a partial discectomy is performed with pituitary rongeurs.
- A 3-0 curette is then used to separate the attachment of the annular fibers to vertebral endplate at the lateral margins of the disc space.
  - The separation with the curette proceeds from lateral to medial and superficial to deep, allowing for the lateral aspect of the disc to be removed en bloc.
  - This technique allows for rapid identification and exposure of the uncovertebral joints and thus the lateral margins of the exposure.
- The disc is removed posteriorly to the PLL.

Use of Distraction: Pins, Tongs, Spreaders

- Distraction posts may be placed before or after the discectomy, although placing posts after the discectomy allows better definition of the vertebral endplates and an improved understanding of their trajectory.
- Although we place distraction posts in a mildly divergent trajectory when performing fusion, to reestablish cervical lordosis, we place them parallel in arthroplasty so as not to introduce hyperlordosis and for better fitment of the implant. The ProDisc system comes with unique distraction posts, which should be placed parallel to the adjacent endplate as outlined in the following text.
- The superior post should be placed high in the vertebral body so as not to interfere with endplate preparation, as the anteroinferior margin of the superior vertebral body often

has an overhang, which must be milled flush with the rest of the endplate to accommodate the implant.

- Distraction about the endplate should be employed only to aid in visualization for neural decompression. Overdistraction during implant sizing and placement may lead the placement of an oversized implant, which will have suboptimal mobility.

Endplate Preparation

- The cartilaginous endplates are removed with care taken to preserve the integrity of the bony endplate as this will provide the structure to prevent subsidence. The cartilaginous endplates can often be removed with curettes. Alternatively, the high-speed drill can be used.
- The inferior endplate of the superior level is most often concave, with an inferiorly protruding lip at the anteroinferior aspect. A high-speed drill is used to mill this flush with the posterior aspect of the endplate to create a broad, flat surface for implant apposition.
- The superior endplate of the inferior level requires less preparation to create a flat surface. It is often slightly concave in the coronal plane, and the high-speed drill is used to mill down the proud lateral aspects and create a flat surface to accommodate the implant.
- The final endplate preparation should be performed without distraction across the disc space to ensure flush and parallel endplates in the neutral position. A rasp can be used after burring to remove any small irregularities.

FORAMINOTOMY AND OSTEOPHYTECTOMY

- An aggressive foraminotomy is needed with arthroplasty as motion will be preserved and incomplete decompression will result in recurrent symptoms. Furthermore, foraminal expansion by means of distraction is not used in arthroplasty as an oversized implant will result in reduced motion due to increased ligamentous tension.
- The PLL is left intact for the initial foraminotomy to protect the underlying neural elements.
- The high-speed burr is used to perform the majority of the foraminotomy. We use the burr with a horizontal back and forth motion to remove posteriorly protruding osteophytes off the uncinate process. The burr can also be used in circular motion at the foraminal opening to enlarge the foramen. The burr should be operated under continuous motion and

with frequent irrigation to prevent thermal injury to the underlying nerve root.

- Final osteophytectomy can be accomplished with a small upgoing curette used in a rotational motion. The cutting edge of the curette can be angled in to bone for safe removal with minimal intrusion into the foraminal space.
- A small (2-mm) Kerrison rongeur can also be used to expand the foraminotomy. Care should be taken to angle the butt of the instrument directly against the thecal sac to minimize chances of injuring the underlying exiting nerve.
- Small instruments should be used when enlarging to foraminal opening to avoid traumatic damage to the exiting nerve.

- Adequate foraminal decompression is confirmed by placing a nerve hook out the neural foramen without resistance.
- The high-speed burr can also be used to remove posteriorly protruding osteophytes. The burr should be angled to attack the junction of the osteophyte and normal vertebral body, to reduce the chances of drilling out the endplate, and to more efficiently disconnect and remove the osteophyte. Final osteophytectomy can be accomplished with an upward angle curette used in a twisting motion.
- Resection of posterior osteophytes can be confirmed by placing a nerve hook or upgoing curette posterior to the vertebral bodies and taking a fluoroscopic image. The instrument should lie flush with the posterior aspect of the vertebral body **(TECH FIG 1)**.
- Anterior osteophytes should also be removed, either with rongeurs or a high-speed burr, to ensure flush fitment of devices with anterior flanges (eg, Prestige ST).

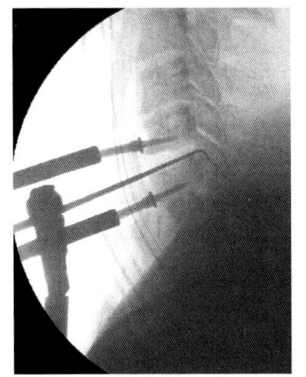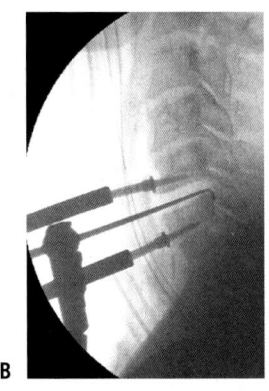

TECH FIG 1 A. Fluoroscopic image demonstrating residual posterior osteophyte underlying nerve hook. **B.** Image after osteophyte has been removed, showing flush apposition of the nerve hook to the posterior vertebral body.

POSTERIOR LONGITUDINAL LIGAMENT RESECTION

- The question of whether to resect the PLL in all cases of cervical arthroplasty is controversial.
  - PLL resection results in increased segmental motion without instability, which may aid the goal of arthroplasty.[30]
  - PLL resection may further aid in the adequate posterior positioning of the implant, especially in cases of significant arthritic degeneration, and may aid in restoration of a physiologic instantaneous axis of rotation.
  - PLL resection should be performed in all cases of posterior disc extrusion in which a fragment may be situated dorsal to the ligament.
- The first step in resecting the PLL is the creation (or identification) of a rent in the ligament, allowing access to the epidural space. A rent may be present in cases of posteriorly herniated fragments, whereas one can otherwise be created with an upgoing curette.
  - The curette can be used in a rotational cephalocaudal fashion to slip between the fibers of the PLL and enter the epidural space.
- Once the rent is identified or created, it can be expanded with an upgoing curette.
- A small (2-mm) Kerrison can then be used to resect the ligament. Using the Kerrison at the intersection of the ligament and vertebral body ensures efficient resection.
  - Care must be taken to minimize dorsal pressure on herniated fragment behind the PLL with the butt end of the Kerrison rongeurs.
  - Care is also taken when resecting the ligament laterally to avoid grasping the exiting nerve root with the Kerrison rongeur.

PRESTIGE IMPLANT

Sizing

- Indicated for the treatment of radiculopathy or myelopathy at one or two cervical disc spaces in adults
- The footprint size of the Prestige ST implant **(TECH FIG 2)** can be estimated preoperatively by measuring endplate depth and width on the preoperative MRI or CT.
- As large a footprint as possible should be chosen.
- The height of the device can more accurately be determined intraoperatively, as the height of the disc space, and thus that of the appropriate implant, will be altered by the endplate preparation.
- After the decompression is complete, a trial spacer is used to confirm implant size.
- The spacer should slide smoothly into the disc space without distraction applied.

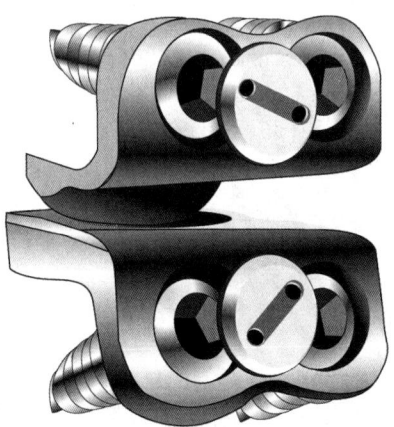

TECH FIG 2 The Prestige ST implant.

- If distraction is needed to place the trial, a smaller trial should be placed or the endplates should be further milled.
- Care is taken to ensure midline placement of the trial, as marked previously.
- Final position is confirmed with biplanar fluoroscopy with AP views used to confirm midline position.

Placement

- Anterior osteophytes are removed with rongeurs or the high-speed burr to ensure that the implant sits flush with anterior vertebral body.
- The profile trial, which is angled to slide into the prepared disc space, is then used to confirm adequate anterior osteophyte resection and flush fitment of the implant **(TECH FIG 3A)**.

- Following preparation, the appropriate-size implant is loaded into the loading block and inserted into the disc space.
  - The implant is directional, with a slight cranial inclination, and should slide easily into the disc space, although gentle tamping with a mallet is sometimes needed.
- Prospective screw tracts are then created using the drill placed through a guide in line with the holes in the insertion device. The 13-mm drill guide is typically used **(TECH FIG 3B,C)**.
- The drill guide is removed, and the screws are then partially placed through the inserter. All four screws are then sequentially tightened, and the inserter is removed.
- Locking screws are placed over the screw heads to prevent back out.
- Final position of the implant is confirmed with AP and lateral fluoroscopy. Motion can be confirmed by manipulating the patient's head through the drapes.

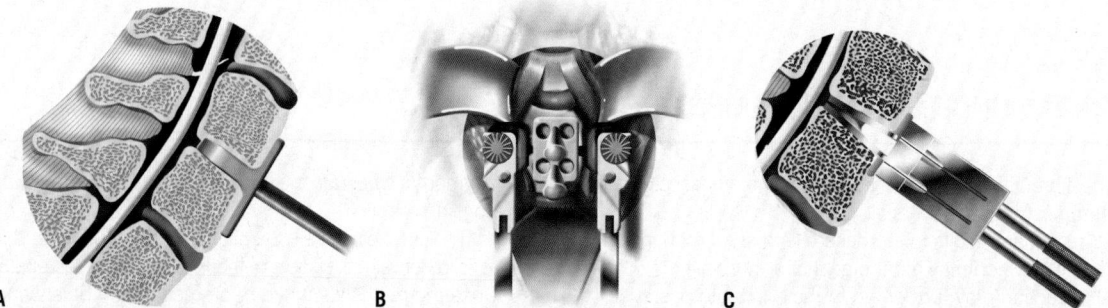

TECH FIG 3 A. The profile trial spacer is used to confirm adequate milling of anterior osteophytes. Anterior (**B**) and lateral (**C**) views of the implant inserted into the disc space, mounted on the inserter with incorporated drill guide.

PRODISC-C

Sizing and Distraction

- ProDisc-C is indicated for the treatment of radiculopathy or myelopathy at one cervical disc space due to herniated disc, spondylosis, or loss of disc height.
- The size of the implant **(TECH FIG 4A)** can be estimated on preoperative imaging studies.
- On initial exposure, the midline is marked using the fluoroscopy. A lasting mark is made by using the Bovie to burn down the bone and then using a marking pen over this mark.
- The distraction screws are placed in the distal one-third of the adjacent vertebral bodies.

- An initial perforation of the anterior cortex is created, and the screws are placed parallel to the adjacent endplates. The screws are placed under fluoroscopic guidance as deeply as possible.
  - It is important to place the screws distally enough to allow for the implant keels to be placed between them **(TECH FIG 4B)**.
- The retainer is then placed over the screws, and a partial discectomy is performed.
- The vertebral distractor is placed in the disc space, and the distraction is applied across the operated level. The distraction is maintained in a parallel fashion with the retainer, and the distractor is removed.

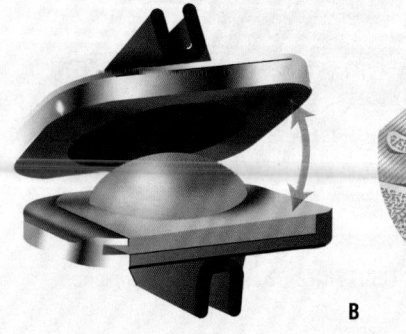
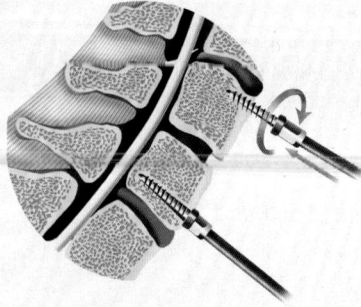

TECH FIG 4 A. The ProDisc-C implant. **B.** The distraction posts are placed parallel to the adjacent endplates.

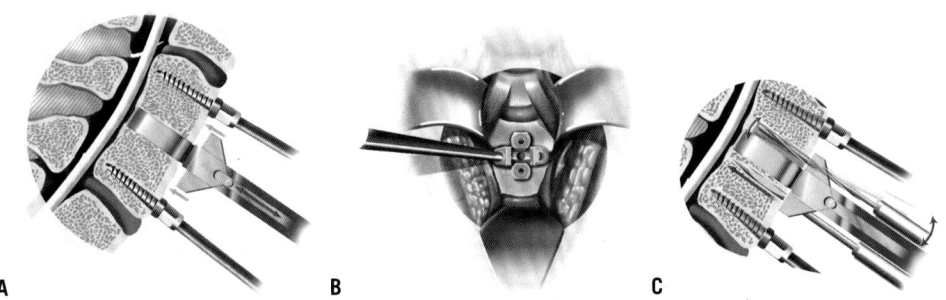

TECH FIG 5 A. The trial is placed to be flushed with the posterior vertebral body line. The stops can be adjusted for optimal depth positioning. Anterior (**B**) and lateral (**C**) depictions of the milling guide placed over the trial. The guide sets the limits of bone removal to accommodate the implant keel.

Trial Fitting

- The discectomy and decompression are completed.
- Trial implants are then placed into the disc space. The implant with the largest possible footprint is chosen. The trial should be inserted flush with the posterior aspect of the vertebral body in the midline.
- Distraction is released, and the trial handle is removed to leave the trial in the disc space. Care is taken not to over distract the interspace, which may compromise implant motion.
- A 5-mm implant is most commonly selected. AP and lateral fluoroscopy images are then taken to confirm adequate position (**TECH FIG 5A**).
- The milling guide is next placed over the shaft of the trial implant and secured with a locking nut. A retention pin is placed through the superior hole of the guide.
- A power drill is used to create the inferior hole under fluoroscopic guidance. The drill is sunk to the level of the stop and then rotated to the limits of the stop in a cephalad and caudal angulation. The drill is removed, a retention pin is placed in its spot, and the process is repeated at the cephalad level (**TECH FIG 5B,C**).
- The box chisel is then placed over the shaft of the trial and advanced into the vertebral bodies with a mallet under fluoroscopic visualization. Prior to impaction, it is confirmed that the trial stop is seated securely against the anterior face of the vertebral bodies.
- The box-cutting chisel is next used over the implant. Prior to removal of the box-cutting chisel, a small amount of distraction is reintroduced around the operated level through the distraction pins.

- Excess bone is removed from the keel tracts with the keel cut cleaner. Symmetric depth of the superior and inferior keel cuts is also confirmed—the posterior edge of both keels should be identical when measured from the posterior vertebral body wall.
- A position gauge can be used to confirm adequacy of the final bone work to accept the implant.

Placement

- The implant is prepared in the implant inserter with the appropriately sized spacer and keels with care taken to maintain the superior and inferior directionality of the keels.
- The implant is then advanced into the prepared disc space under fluoroscopic control.
- The inserter, retainer, and retainer screws are then removed, and final implant position is confirmed with AP and lateral fluoroscopy (**TECH FIG 6**).

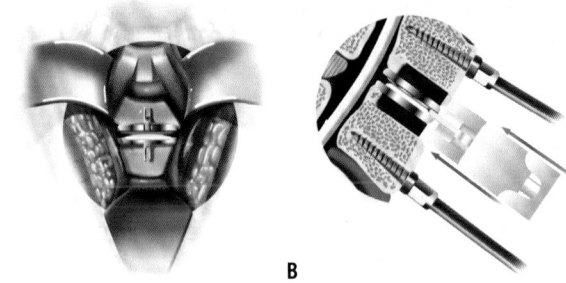

TECH FIG 6 A. The implant is tamped into the defect under fluoroscopic guidance with care taken to ensure that it is fully seated posteriorly. **B.** Anterior view of the final implant.

BRYAN CERVICAL DISC

Selection Criteria

- There are strict criteria for a Bryan cervical disc prosthesis (**TECH FIG 7A**).
  - Patients are not eligible if they exhibit hypermobility, instability, degenerative disease, facet joint pathology, or severe osteoporosis.

- The prosthesis is most appropriate for single-level radiculopathy or myelopathy from a herniated disc or uncovertebral osteophyte at C4–C5 or C5–C6, although C3–C4 and C6–C7 may be appropriate based on patient anatomy.[34]
- The implant size and sagittal slope are determined based on preoperative imaging (**TECH FIG 7B,C**).[34]

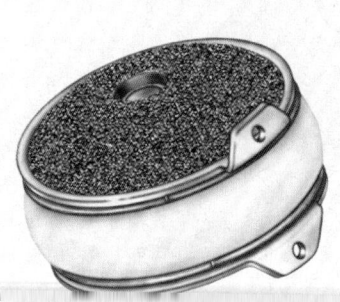
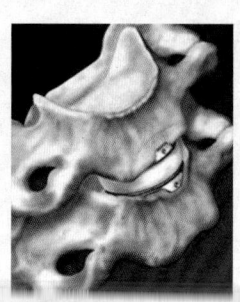
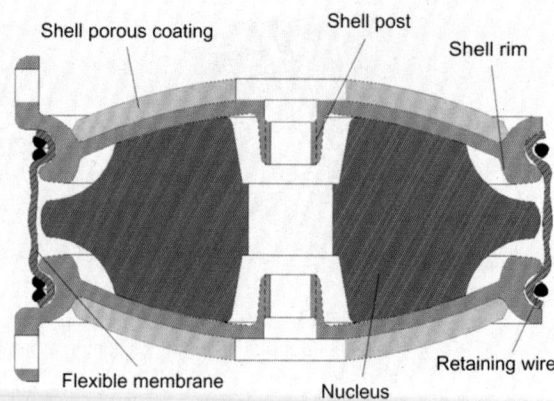

Shell porous coating
Shell post
Shell rim
Flexible membrane
Nucleus
Retaining wire

TECH FIG 7 A. The Bryan disc implant is made of two porous convex shells over a central access port. There are two anterior stops that will sit on the vertebral endplate. **B.** The Bryan disc in situ. **C.** Cross-section of the Bryan disc prosthetic. The void is around the center post between the endplates and the nucleus. The nucleus is convex at the center and concave at the border.

Exposure and Decompression

- The patient is placed supine with the neck in a neutral position, which can be achieved by placing a rolled towel under the neck (**TECH FIG 8A**).[34]
- The initial exposure and discectomy is carried out using the usual Smith-Robinson approach.
- A 0.5-mm sagittal cam distractor is then used to measure the disc space height and segment mobility.
  - At this point, if there is hypermobility, the case may be converted to a standard anterior cervical fusion.
- The gravitational referencing system is then constructed, and the extensions are attached to the operating table side rails.
  - The retractor frame is centered a few centimeters above the wound in parallel with the spine. This will be used to determine the intraoperative sagittal angle of the disc space (**TECH FIG 8B**).
- The center of the disc is defined using the milling jig, which sits between the uncovertebral joints and finds the center.
  - A sagittal wedge is placed into the disc space under fluoroscopic guidance (**TECH FIG 8C**).
- The milling fixture is set to the sagittal slope measurement and screwed into the vertebral body above and below the disc space.
  - The milling technique, drilling along the y-axis, creates concave surfaces to exactly match the convex porous-coated Bryan disc endplates.

- The lateral dimension for the implant is then verified with fluoroscopy (**TECH FIG 8D,E**).
- Final decompression of the neural foramen and canal can then be completed while preserving the uncovertebral joints.

Sizing and Placement

- The correct size of the Bryan disc is determined by preoperative review of imaging and intraoperative measurements using a milling depth gauge.
- The trial prosthesis size burring block ring is attached to the frame and inserted to the level of the PLL using fluoroscopic guidance.
- The anchor screws are left in place as the burr and assembly is removed.
- The Bryan disc is then filled with sterile saline and attached to the introducer via the superior and inferior projections of the Bryan disc (**TECH FIG 9A**).
- An intervertebral distractor is inserted, and the disc is hammered into position under lateral fluoroscopy. Correct positioning is confirmed with AP imaging and ensures a low profile in the intervertebral space (**TECH FIG 9B**).
- The anchor screws are removed, and the wound is closed in the standard fashion.[34]

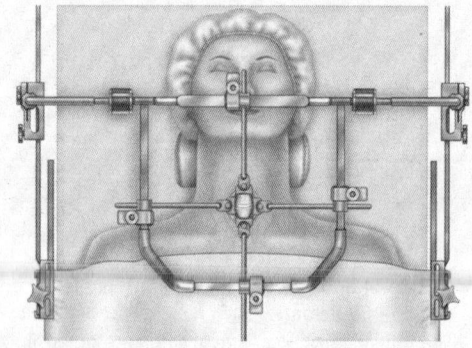
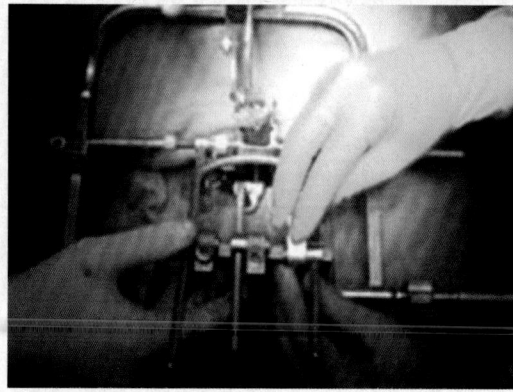

TECH FIG 8 A. Positioning for the Bryan disc. **B.** The Bryan frame in its final position. A towel has been rolled behind the neck to support physiologic cervical lordosis. *(continued)*

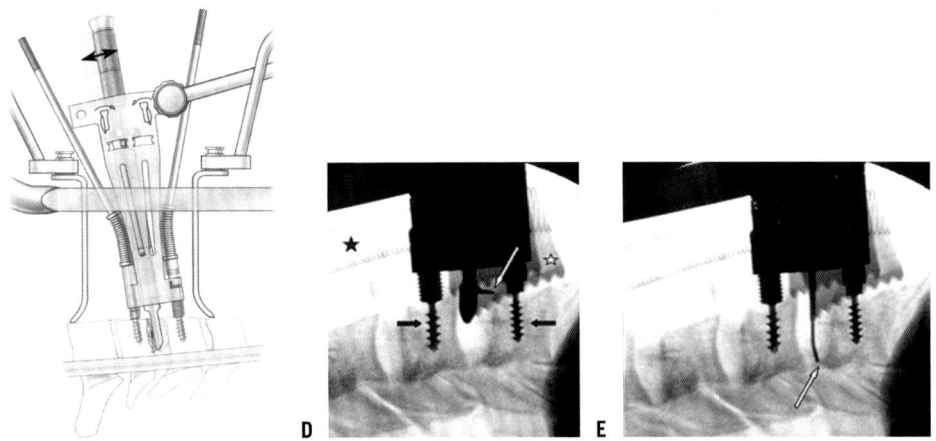

TECH FIG 8 *(continued)* **C.** The milling disc moves along the x-axis to prepare the vertebral recess. There is a hook in the slit of this apparatus, which prevents damage to the thecal sac. **D.** Intraoperative lateral fluoroscopy showing milling depth gauge at the anterior edge of the vertebra (*white arrow*), anchor screws (*black arrows*), retractor blades (*white asterisk*), and endotracheal anesthesia tube (*black asterisk*). **E.** Intraoperative lateral fluoroscopy showing burring depth gauge at the posterior vertebral edge and the remainders of the PLL (*white arrow*). (**D,E:** Reprinted with permission from Wenger M, Markwalder TM. Bryan total disc arthroplasty: a replacement disc for cervical disc disease. Med Devices [Auckl] 2010;3:11–24. Copyright © 2010 Dove Medical Press Ltd.)

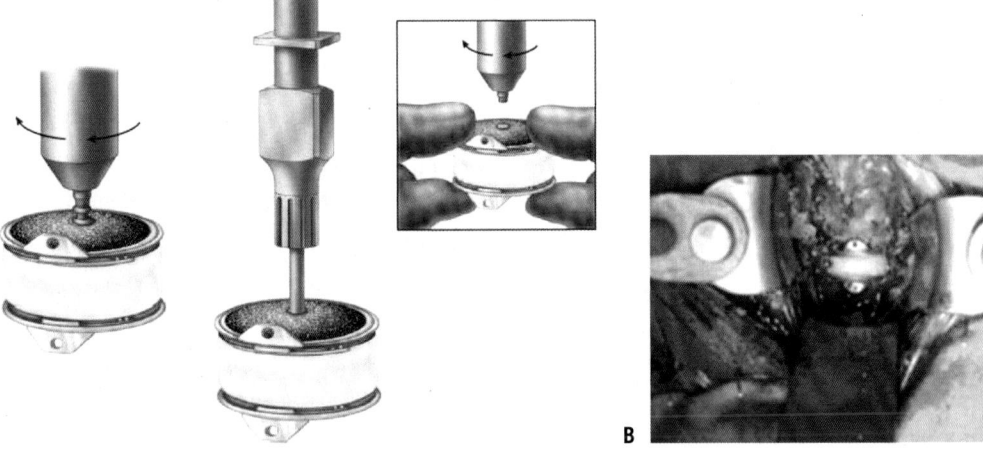

TECH FIG 9 A. Before implantation the Bryan disc is filled with saline. **B.** In situ Bryan disc with low profile in the intervertebral space at the end of the procedure. (**A:** Reprinted from Sasso R, Martin L Jr. The Bryan artificial disc. In: Yue JJ, Bertagnoli R, McAfee PC, et al, eds. Motion Preservation Surgery of the Spine: Advanced Techniques and Controversies. Philadelphia: Saunders, 2008:196. Copyright © 2008 Elsevier.)

MOBI-C DISC

Selection

- The Mobi-C disc **(TECH FIG 10A)** is approved for one- and two-level cervical arthroplasty from C3 to C7 for degenerative disease or herniated nucleus pulposus with radiculopathy or myelopathy.
  - Patients with severe osteoporosis, malignancy, prior cervical spine surgery, obesity, or heavy tobacco use are not candidates for this procedure.[3]

- Preoperative measurements on CT and MRI are used to estimate the size of the implant(s) **(TECH FIG 10B)**.

Exposure and Distraction

- The patient is positioned with a neutral neck in anatomic lordosis. A towel can be placed under the patient's head or neck to achieve this position. Halter traction may be used for positioning.

TECHNIQUES

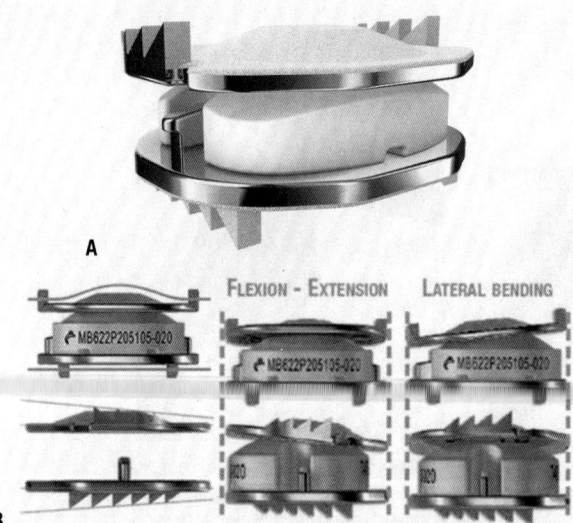

TECH FIG 10 A. The Mobi-C disc endplates are made of components of cobalt–chromium alloy coated with plasma-sprayed titanium and hydroxyapatite coating. The insert nucleus is polyethylene. The goal is to restore height while maintaining rotation of the segment. **B.** Range of motion in flexion–extension and lateral bending for the Mobi-C disc. (**A:** Courtesy of Zimmer Biomet. **B:** Reprinted with permission from Kim SH, Shin HC, Shin DA, et al. Early clinical experience with the Mobi-C disc prosthesis. Yonsei Med J 2007;48[3]:457–464. Copyright © 2007 The Yonsei University College of Medicine.)

- A standard Smith-Robinson anterior exposure is performed at the most diseased level first to obtain restoration of disc height as well as lordosis and sagittal balance.[16]
- The Caspar retractor fixation pins are then inserted 5 mm from the superior and inferior vertebral body endplates **(TECH FIG 11)**.
- Resection of the PLL is at the discretion of the surgeon.
- Osteophytes are removed, and the uncovertebral joint identified bilaterally to ensure bilateral decompression of the foramen.[16]
- Minimal endplate milling is advised for this procedure.

Sizing and Placement

- The width gauge is used to estimate the size of the implant. The implants are 15, 17, and 19 mm.

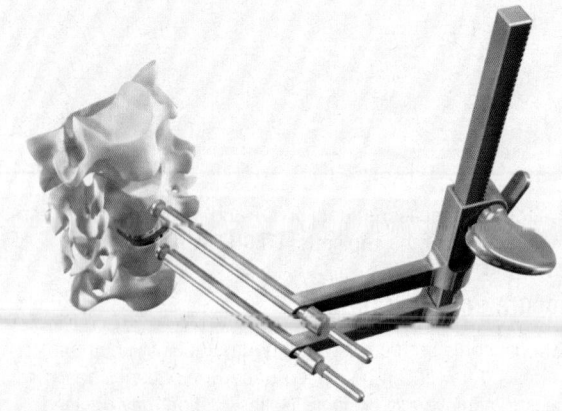

TECH FIG 11 Caspar pin distraction. (Courtesy of Zimmer Biomet.)

- The depth of the disc space can be measured by a hook placed behind the posterior edge of the vertebral endplate. There are 13- or 15-mm depth implants **(TECH FIG 12A)**.
- The available implant heights are 5, 6, and 7 mm. One should start with the shortest trial, and the implant should not exceed the height of healthy adjacent discs.
- A trial implant is tamped into place using a self-retracting inserter under fluoroscopic guidance within 1 mm of the posterior vertebral body wall **(TECH FIG 12B)**.
- The self-retracting inserter has a stop, which is set to 0 to 5 mm by the surgeon.
- An implant holder is used to place the Mobi-C disc in alignment with the disc space and to keep contact with the anterior wall of the vertebral body as the implant is hammered into place under fluoroscopy.
  - The groove in the inserter should be at the midline of the disc space **(TECH FIG 12C)**.
- At this point, the universal implant inserter and disposable implant holder are released **(TECH FIG 12D)**.
- The Caspar pins are compressed to seat the teeth of the implant into the vertebral bodies. The position of the implant is confirmed using AP and lateral fluoroscopy **(TECH FIG 12E)**.
- This technique is repeated for desired adjacent levels **(TECH FIG 12F)**.
- Closure is undertaken in the standard fashion.[6,16]

M6-C Disc

- The M6-C implant is approved for reconstruction of the disc following single-level discectomy in skeletally mature patients with intractable degenerative cervical radiculopathy with or without spinal cord compression at one level from C3 to C7 **(TECH FIG 13A,B)**.
- The patient's head and neck are placed in a neutral position, and fluoroscopy is used to ensure that there is no flexion, extension, or rotation of the cervical spine. The neck is supported with a soft roll, and tape is used to secure the head and prevent unwanted movement.
- A standard anterior cervical approach is used to expose the treatment levels. Care is taken to preserve the longus coli muscles to maintain a reference for the midline.
- Using fluoroscopic guidance, cervical retainer pins are placed into the vertebral bodies above and below the index disc space. Each pin should be inserted in the midline and parallel to the endplate.
- A total, symmetric discectomy is performed. Anterior and posterior osteophytes are removed using drills and rongeurs.
- The endplates are prepared by removing the cartilaginous endplate with curettes. Care is taken not to remove or damage the cortical endplate bone.
- An intervertebral paddle distractor is used to mobilize the treatment level and restore disc height **(TECH FIG 13C,D)**. The cervical retainer is then used to maintain the desired disc height.
- A footplate template is then used to determine the correct implant size. The template should fit within the medial boundaries of the uncovertebral joints and be within 1 to 2 mm of the posterior vertebral border.
- A trial spacer is then inserted into the disc space under fluoroscopic guidance, ensuring that the midline marking guide on the trial aligns with the anatomic midline **(TECH FIG 13E,F)**. The center alignment port on the trial is used to align the C-arm in place with the disc space **(TECH FIG 13G,H)**. With the trial in position, evaluate the disc space height, facet joints, and

spinous processes compared to adjacent levels to ensure there is no overdistraction.

- A fin cutter chisel is then tapped into the disc space under fluoroscopic guidance with care to maintain midline alignment in order to create tracks in the vertebral bodies for the final implant **(TECH FIG 13I)**. The tracks will determine the final position of the implant, and care must be taken to not advance the chisel too far posteriorly.

- The appropriately sized implant is then loaded on to the inserter. The center keel of the implant is then aligned with the center track from the chisel, and the inserter handle is oriented in line with the disc space. The implant is then tapped into the disc space under fluoroscopic guidance. The inserter is then removed, and final position of the implant is confirmed with lateral and AP fluoroscopy images.

- The incision is then closed in standard fashion.[12]

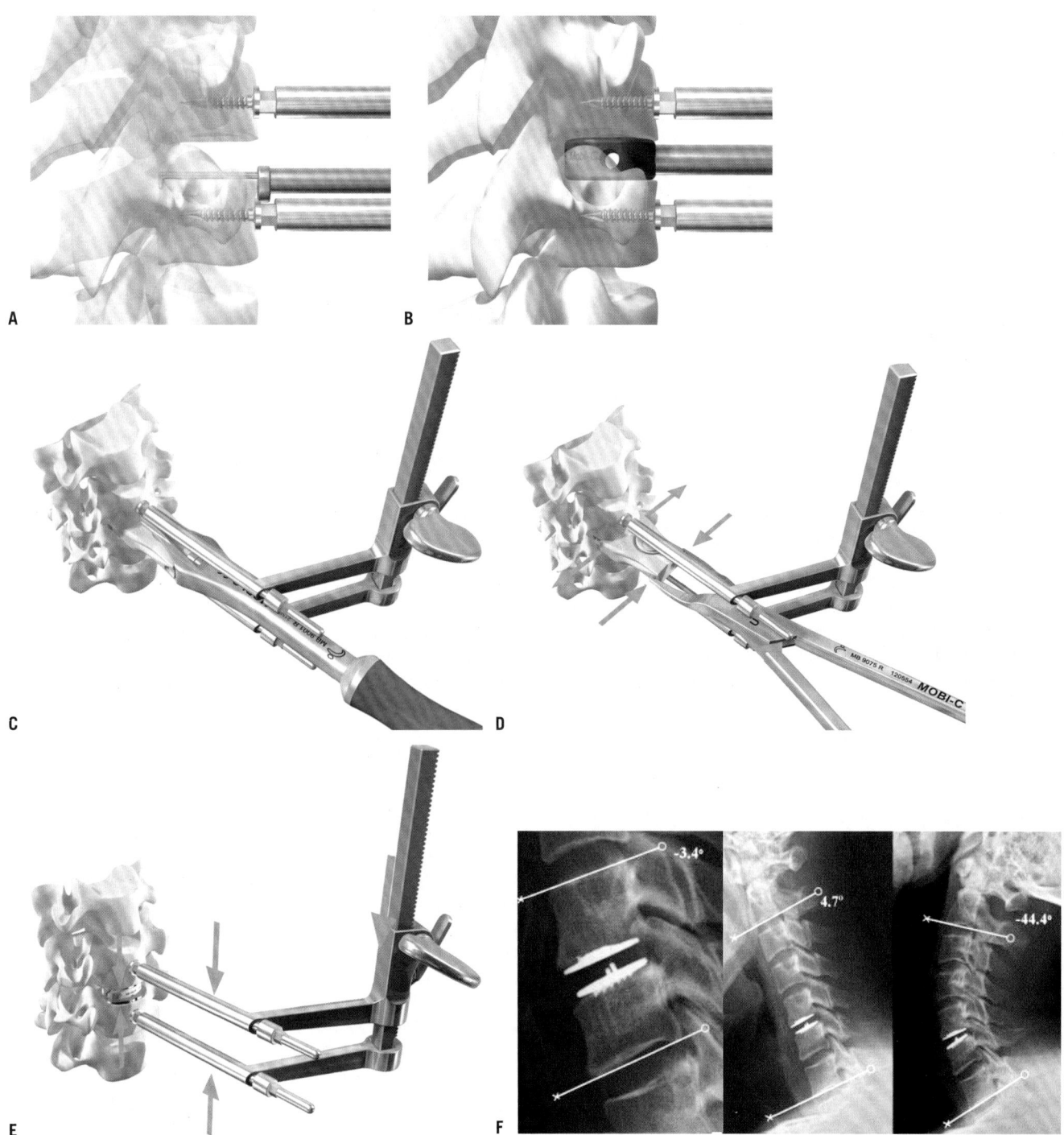

TECH FIG 12 A. Measurement of trial depth. **B.** Insertion of trial Mobi-C implant. **C.** Insertion of Mobi-C disc using universal inserter. **D.** Removal of universal inserter. **E.** Removal of Caspar distractors. **F.** Radiographic range of motion for Mobi-C implant. (**A–E:** Courtesy of Zimmer Biomet. **F:** Reprinted with permission from Kim SH, Shin HC, Shin DA, et al. Early clinical experience with the Mobi-C disc prosthesis. Yonsei Med J 2007;48[3]:457–464. Copyright © 2007 The Yonsei University College of Medicine.)

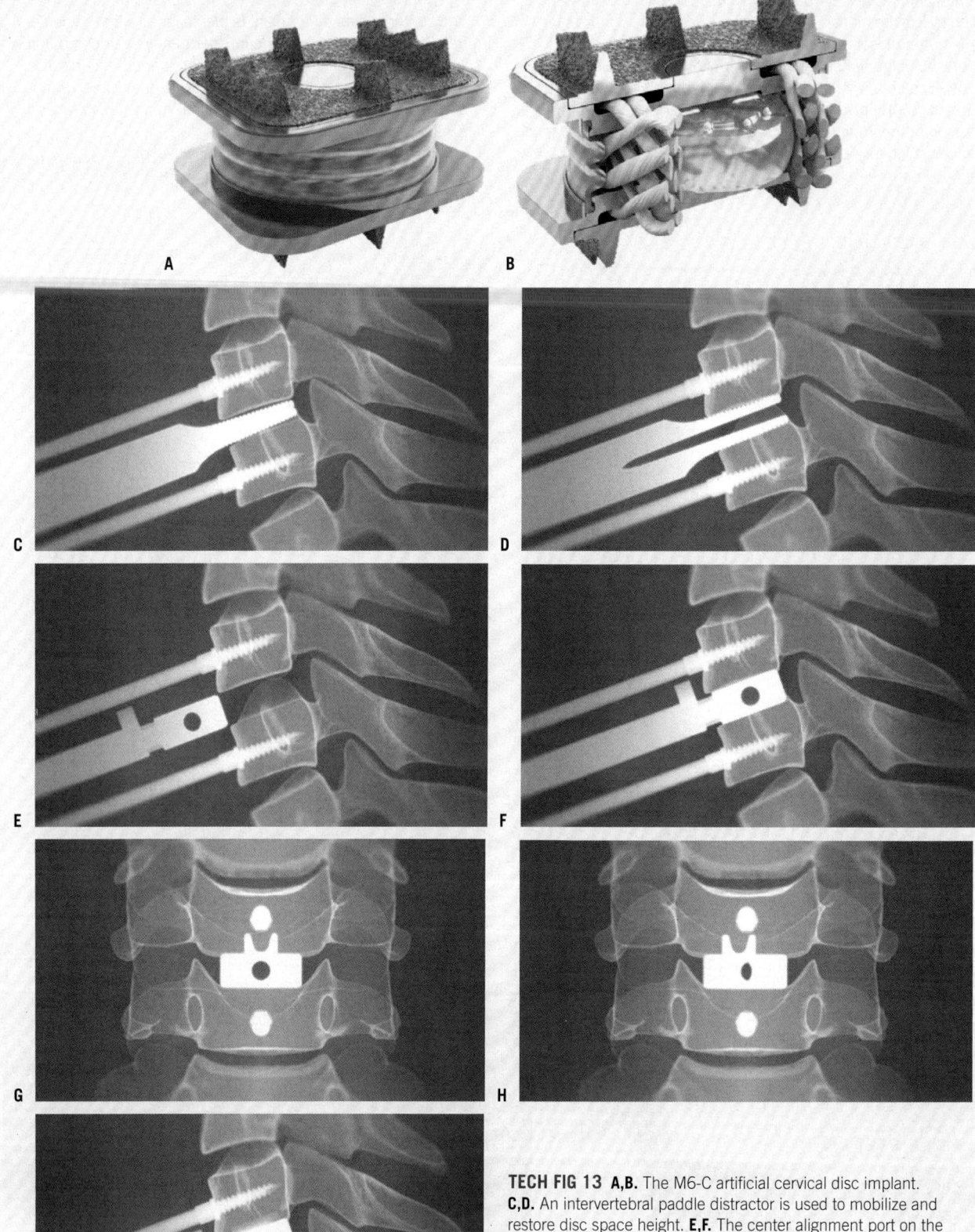

TECH FIG 13 A,B. The M6-C artificial cervical disc implant.
C,D. An intervertebral paddle distractor is used to mobilize and restore disc space height. **E,F.** The center alignment port on the trial is used to align the C-arm in place with the disc space. The C-arm is aligned when the center alignment port appears as a perfect circle on AP fluoroscopic image, as shown in **G**; **H** is misaligned. **I.** A fin cutter chisel is tapped into the disc space to create tracks for the final implant position. (Images of the M6-C artificial cervical disc and instrumentation are provided courtesy of Orthofix Medical, Inc.)

POSTOPERATIVE CARE

- Bracing is not typically used postoperatively.
- A drain may be placed depending on surgeon preference.
- Most patients are admitted for a single hospital day, although some surgeons perform single and two-level arthroplasty on an outpatient basis.
- Diet is advanced as tolerated. Dysphagia, when experienced, is usually transient and may mandate a slower advance of diet.
- Nonsteroidal anti-inflammatory drugs (NSAIDs) may be given postoperatively and may have a role in decreasing the incidence of heterotopic ossification.
- Activity is restricted with no heavy lifting or high-impact activity for 6 weeks. After 6 weeks, patients are encouraged to slowly resume their activity to preoperative levels.

OUTCOMES

- Pain and disability: Randomized trials of the five devices described in this chapter demonstrate significant improvements or trends toward improvements in Neck Disability Index (NDI), arm pain, neck pain, SF-36, visual analog scale (VAS) neck pain score, and VAS arm pain score postoperatively.[10,12,20]
  - Seven-year data from trials of the Mobi-C device showed significant improvement from baseline NDI scores, VAS neck and arm pain scores, and SF-12 MCS/PCS scores.[28]
  - There are trends toward improved return to work following arthroplasty compared to fusion, although these outcomes are not conclusive.[22]
- Perioperative complications: Studies have shown that cervical arthroplasty is associated with decreased operative time, decreased length of stay, and increased likelihood of discharge to home over rehab compared to anterior cervical discectomy and fusion (ACDF).[36]
  - A meta-analysis of randomized controlled trials of the eight FDA-approved disc arthroplasty devices showed no statistical differences compared to ACDF in dysphagia/dysphonia, hardware-related complications, heterotopic ossification, death, and overall neurologic adverse events.[1]
- Adjacent level disease: Although adjacent segment disease is noted after arthroplasty, there appears to be a lower rate of symptomatic patients requiring reoperation. Long-term follow-up is needed.[37]
  - A randomized clinical trial showed that at 7 years of follow-up, the Bryan and Prestige discs had significantly lower rates of symptomatic adjacent level disease requiring surgery compared to ACDF. Ten-year data from the Bryan disc likewise showed lower rates of symptomatic adjacent level disease requiring surgery, although this did not reach statistical significance.[7] Seven-year data from the Mobi-C disc likewise showed there was a lower rate of adjacent level secondary surgery in arthroplasty patients versus ACDF patients.[28]
  - Pooled meta-analysis results of several randomized trials of approved devices corroborate the finding that rates of symptomatic adjacent segment disease are significantly lower in arthroplasty versus fusion,[18] resulting in lower rates of reoperation for adjacent segment disease at this time.[3]
- Range of motion: In biomechanical models, cervical arthroplasty has been demonstrated to maintain segmental and global spinal range of motion similar to the native spine. This flexibility may reduce the physical demands on adjacent segments, which may lessen or slow the development of arthritic disease.[6]
  - Adjacent level cervical range of motion has been shown to be maintained up to 2 years postoperatively among patients who underwent arthroplasty.
  - However, imaging has demonstrated a potential trend toward reduced range of motion and worsening alignment in arthroplasty constructs after 2 years. Of note, no clinical symptoms were reported by these patients.
  - Studies have yet to show definitively whether cervical arthroplasty will have similar or reduced risk of aseptic loosening of hardware in comparison to large joint arthroplasty.[16]
- Postoperative kyphosis: Some groups have reported worsening cervical kyphosis after arthroplasty. However, it has been shown that cervical lordosis and sagittal balance can be restored by selecting appropriate patients, avoiding over-milling the endplates, and choosing appropriate insertion angles and depth.[2,32,39]
- Multilevel constructs: Compared with multilevel ACDF, two-level disc arthroplasty has superior outcomes in neurologic deterioration, adverse neurologic events, neck and arm VAS scores, device failure requiring subsequent operation, and maintenance of range of motion at superior and inferior adjacent levels up to the 7-year[13,40] and 10-year[7] time points.
  - A hybrid technique using fusion and arthroplasty at alternate levels for multilevel disease has been described with good results. This has been shown to reduce adjacent-level hypermobility and increasing moment loads **(FIG 3)**.[19,23]

COMPLICATIONS

- Approach-related complications
  - Dysphagia is a frequent complication and often is self-limited. The incidence and severity of dysphagia may be lower after arthroplasty compared with fusion, potentially as a result of the lower profile of the constructs or the decreased need for esophageal retraction.[20]

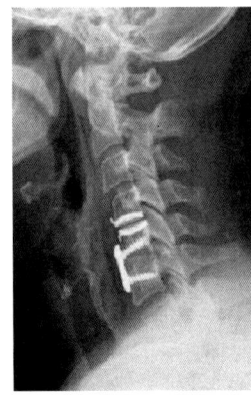

FIG 3 Hybrid arthroplasty/fusion construct. (Reprinted with permission from Laratta JL, Shillingford JN, Saifi C, et al. Cervical disc arthroplasty: a comprehensive review of single-level, multilevel, and hybrid procedures. Global Spine J 2018;8[1]:78–83. Copyright © 2018 SAGE Publications.)

- Nerve palsies—recurrent laryngeal nerve, superior laryngeal nerve
- Nerve root injury
- Spinal cord injury
- Cerebrospinal fluid leak
- Hematoma
  - Prevertebral
  - Epidural
- Esophageal injury
- Device-related complications
  - Device failure: Loosening or migration is rare but has been reported more frequently in the perioperative period in devices not secured with screw fixation.[8]
  - Arthrosis of the facet at the operated level and heterotopic ossification have been reported to occur in up to 20% and 50% of patients, respectively, but neither have been shown to have a correlation with clinical outcome.[38]
    - The incidence of same-level facet arthrosis may be influenced by suboptimal positioning of the implant.
    - The incidence of heterotopic ossification may be reduced by thoroughly irrigating the wound to eliminate bone dust, coagulating exposed bone with electrocautery, and administering NSAIDs in the perioperative period.
  - Segmental kyphosis is likely attributable to improper endplate preparation and device insertion.[27] Arthroplasty is not likely to correct preoperative segmental kyphosis and should be avoided in such cases.
  - Risk of subsidence is increased with osteoporosis and minimized by placing as large an endplate footprint as possible.
  - Continued neurologic deficit can be caused by the maintenance of motion in the setting of inadequate decompression.
    - Persistent radiculopathy may be treatable with a posterior foraminotomy.
    - Persistent myelopathy or pain may require fusion.
  - Sagittal split fracture of the vertebral body is rare and may be predisposed by osteoporosis and the use of a keeled device.[5]
  - Studies have shown that implants with metal-on-metal components may have similar complication rates to large joint arthroplasty.[9]

REFERENCES

1. Anderson PA, Nassr A, Currier BL, et al. Evaluation of adverse events in total disc replacement: a meta-analysis of FDA summary of safety and effectiveness data. Global Spine J 2017;7(1 suppl):76S–83S.
2. Anderson PA, Sasso RC, Riew KD. Comparison of adverse events between the Bryan artificial cervical disc and anterior cervical arthrodesis. Spine (Phila Pa 1976) 2008;33(12):1305–1312.
3. Chang KE, Pham MH, Hsieh PC. Adjacent segment disease requiring reoperation in cervical total disc arthroplasty: a literature review and update. J Clin Neurosci 2017;37:20–24.
4. Crandall PH, Batzdorf U. Cervical spondylotic myelopathy. J Neurosurg 1966;25(1):57–66.
5. Datta JC, Janssen ME, Beckman R, et al. Sagittal split fractures in multilevel cervical arthroplasty using a keeled prosthesis. J Spinal Disord Tech 2007;20(1):89–92.
6. Davis RJ, Kim KD, Hisey MS, et al. Cervical total disc replacement with the Mobi-C cervical artificial disc compared with anterior discectomy and fusion for treatment of 2-level symptomatic degenerative disc disease: a prospective, randomized, controlled multicenter clinical trial; clinical article. J Neurosurg Spine 2013;19(5):532–545.
7. Ghobrial GM, Lavelle WF, Florman JE, et al. Symptomatic adjacent level disease requiring surgery: analysis of 10-year results from a prospective, randomized, clinical trial comparing cervical disc arthroplasty to anterior cervical fusion. Neurosurgery 2019;84(2):347–354.
8. Goffin J, Van Calenbergh F, van Loon J, et al. Intermediate follow-up after treatment of degenerative disc disease with the Bryan cervical disc prosthesis: single-level and bi-level. Spine (Phila Pa 1976) 2003;28(24):2673–2678.
9. Golish SR, Anderson PA. Bearing surfaces for total disc arthroplasty: metal-on-metal versus metal-on-polyethylene and other biomaterials. Spine J 2012;12:693–701.
10. Hassett G, Hart DJ, Manek NJ, et al. Risk factors for progression of lumbar spine disc degeneration: the Chingford study. Arthritis Rheum 2003;48(11):3112–3117.
11. Heckmann JG, Lang CJ, Zöbelein I, et al. Herniated cervical intervertebral discs with radiculopathy: an outcome study of conservatively or surgically treated patients. J Spinal Disord 1999;12(5):396–401.
12. Hui N, Phan K, Kerferd J, et al. Comparison of M6-C and Mobi-C cervical total disc replacement for cervical degenerative disc disease in adults. J Spine Surg 2019;5(4):393–403.
13. Jackson R, Johnson DE. Neurological outcomes of two-level total disk replacement versus anterior discectomy and fusion: 7-year results from a prospective, randomized, multicenter trial. Neurosurgery 2016;63(1):164.
14. Kadanka Z, Mares M, Bednařík J, et al. Predictive factors for spondylotic cervical myelopathy treated conservatively or surgically. Eur J Neurol 2005;12(1):55–63.
15. Kuijper B, Tans JT, Beelen A, et al. Cervical collar or physiotherapy versus wait and see policy for recent onset cervical radiculopathy: randomized trial. BMJ 2009;339:b3883.
16. LDR. Mobi-C® cervical disc. Surgical technique: two-level. Zimmer Biomet. Available at: http://us.ldr.com/Portals/1/PDF/2LST.pdf. Accessed October, 2020.
17. Lees F, Turner JW. Natural history and prognosis of cervical spondylosis. Br Med J 1963;2(5373):1607–1610.
18. Luo J, Wang H, Peng J, et al. Rate of adjacent segment degeneration of cervical disc arthroplasty versus fusion meta-analysis of randomized controlled trials. World Neurosurg 2018;113:225–231.
19. Martin S, Ghanayem AJ, Tzermiadianos MN, et al. Kinematics of cervical total disc replacement adjacent to a two-level, straight versus lordotic fusion. Spine (Phila Pa 1976) 2011;36:1359–1366.
20. McAfee PC, Cappuccino A, Cunningham BW, et al. Lower incidence of dysphagia with cervical arthroplasty compared with ACDF in a prospective randomized clinical trial. J Spinal Disord Tech 2010;23(1):1–8.
21. Melamed H, Harris MB, Awasthi D. Anatomic considerations of superior laryngeal nerve during anterior cervical spine procedures. Spine (Phila Pa 1976) 2002;27(4):E83–E86.
22. Mummaneni PV, Amin BY, Wu JC, et al. Cervical artificial disc replacement versus fusion in the cervical spine: a systematic review comparing long-term follow-up results from two FDA trials. Evid Based Spine Care J 2012;3(suppl 1):59–66.
23. Murrey D, Janssen ME, Delamarter RB, et al. Results of the prospective, randomized, controlled multicenter Food and Drug Administration investigational device exemption study of the ProDisc-C total disc replacement versus anterior discectomy and fusion for the treatment of 1-level symptomatic cervical disc disease. Spine J 2009;9(4):275–286.
24. Olmarker K, Blomquist J, Stromberg J, et al. Inflammatogenic properties of nucleus pulposus. Spine (Phila Pa 1976) 1995;20(6):665–669.
25. Pain in the neck and arm: a multicentre trial of the effects of physiotherapy, arranged by the British Association of Physical Medicine. Br Med J 1966;1(5482):253–258.
26. Pait TG, Killefer JA, Arnautovic KI. Surgical anatomy of the anterior cervical spine: the disc space, vertebral artery, and associated bony structures. Neurosurgery 1996;39(4):769–776.
27. Pickett GE, Sekhon LH, Sears WR, et al. Complications with cervical arthroplasty. J Neurosurg Spine 2006;4(2):98–105.

28. Radcliff K, Davis RJ, Hisey MS, et al. Long-term evaluation of cervical disc arthroplasty with the Mobi-C© cervical disc: a randomized, prospective, multicenter clinical trial with seven-year follow-up. Int J Spine Surg 2017;11:31.

29. Radhakrishnan K, Litchy WJ, O'Fallon WM, et al. Epidemiology of cervical radiculopathy. A population-based study from Rochester, Minnesota, 1976 through 1990. Brain 1994;117(pt 2):325–335.

30. Roberto RF, McDonald T, Curtiss S, et al. Kinematics of progressive circumferential ligament resection (decompression) in conjunction with cervical disc arthroplasty in a spondylotic spine model. Spine (Phila Pa 1976) 2010;35(18):1676–1683.

31. Sant'Ambrogio G, Sant'Ambrogio FB. Role of laryngeal afferents in cough. Pulm Pharmacol 1996;9(5–6):309–314.

32. Sasso RC, Anderson PA, Riew KD, et al. Results of cervical arthroplasty compared with anterior discectomy and fusion: four-year clinical outcomes in a prospective, randomized controlled trial. Orthopedics 2011;34:889.

33. Sasso RC, Macadaeg K, Nordmann D, et al. Selective nerve root injections can predict surgical outcome for lumbar and cervical radiculopathy: comparison to magnetic resonance imaging. J Spinal Disord Tech 2005;18(6):471–478.

34. Sekhon L. Cervical artificial disc replacement using the Bryan. SpineUniverse. Available at: https://www.spineuniverse.com/treatments /emerging/artificial-discs/cervical-artificial-disc-replacement-using -bryan. Accessed October, 2020.

35. Shiri R, Karppinen J, Leino-Arjas P, et al. Cardiovascular and lifestyle risk factors in lumbar radicular pain or clinically defined sciatica: a systematic review. Eur Spine J 2007;16(12):2043–2054.

36. Upadhyayula PS, Yue JK, Curtis EI, et al. A matched cohort comparison of cervical disc arthroplasty versus anterior cervical discectomy and fusion: evaluating perioperative outcomes. J Clin Neurosci 2017;43:235–239.

37. Wang QL, Tu ZM, Hu P, et al. Long-term results comparing cervical disc arthroplasty to anterior cervical discectomy and fusion: a systematic review and meta-analysis of randomized controlled trials. Orthop Surg 2020;12(1):16–30.

38. Yi S, Kim KN, Yang MS, et al. Difference in occurrence of heterotopic ossification according to prosthesis type in the cervical artificial disc replacement. Spine (Phila Pa 1976) 2010;35(16):1556–1561.

39. Yi S, Shin HC, Kim KN, et al. Modified techniques to prevent sagittal imbalance after cervical arthroplasty. Spine (Phila Pa 1976) 2007;32: 1986–1991.

40. Zou S, Gao J, Xu B, et al. Anterior cervical discectomy and fusion (ACDF) versus cervical disc arthroplasty (CDA) for two contiguous levels cervical disc degenerative disease: a meta-analysis of randomized controlled trials. Eur Spine J 2017;26(4):985–997.

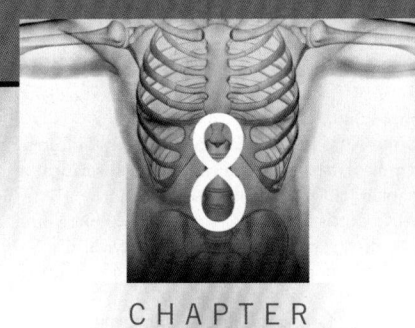

8

Cervical Osteotomies for Kyphosis

Michael P. Kelly and K. Daniel Riew

DEFINITION

- The precise definition of cervical kyphosis is not clearly described. Normal alignment from C2 to C7 in the sagittal plane is approximately 20 degrees of lordosis.

ANATOMY

- With normal alignment, the load-bearing axis of the cervical spine lies in the posterior third of the vertebral bodies.
- The foramen transversarium of C7 generally contains only veins; however, vertebral artery anomalies do exist and careful examination of the preoperative magnetic resonance imaging (MRI) is necessary.[4]
- As the C7 foramen transversarium is usually "empty," this level is the most amenable to a pedicle subtraction osteotomy (PSO).

PATHOGENESIS

- There are many etiologies of cervical kyphosis, including degenerative disease, trauma (acute and chronic onset), tumor, infection, inflammatory arthropathies, and iatrogenic causes.
- Ankylosing spondylitis is the most common inflammatory cause.
  - Caused by contraction and ossification of the ligaments of the spine
  - Associated with the human leukocyte antigen B27 haplotype in 80% to 90% of patients.
- Iatrogenic causes include postlaminectomy kyphosis, pseudarthrosis, and postradiation syndromes.

NATURAL HISTORY

- As there are many etiologies of cervical kyphosis, the natural history is quite variable.
  - In patients with fixed deformities, such as ankylosing spondylitis, the deformity may progress due to stress fracture or an unrecognized fracture, often indicated by an acute increase in the magnitude of the deformity or the level of pain.
  - As the axis of loading moves anterior to the vertebral body, the tendency is for progression of the deformity.
  - With more deformity, the spinal cord may become draped over the vertebral bodies, and the patient may become myelopathic, quadriparetic, or quadriplegic.

PATIENT HISTORY AND PHYSICAL FINDINGS

- The chief complaint of the patient should be elicited. The patient may present with swallowing and/or breathing difficulties.

Forward gaze is often affected. Patients may also note low back pain, as they hyperextend the lumbar spine to maintain a horizontal gaze.
- The patient should be asked to stand with hips and knees extended, allowing for an accurate assessment of the deformity and sagittal balance.
- Any sudden change in deformity or pain should be considered a fracture until proven otherwise.
- An accurate history of previous cervical procedures is needed, as this is essential for preoperative planning.
- The patient should be asked to lay supine to assess the rigidity of the deformity.
- The gait should be observed for evidence of myelopathy. Other affected joints should be assessed to determine the need for treatment prior to addressing the cervical deformity; for example, hip flexion contractures.
- The exam should include a full neurologic examination to check for evidence of myelopathy or spinal cord dysfunction.
- All patients should undergo a full medical evaluation, as respiratory and gastrointestinal dysfunctions are not uncommon in this population. In severe cases of respiratory compromise, a preoperative tracheostomy may be advisable.

IMAGING AND OTHER DIAGNOSTIC STUDIES

- Radiographic evaluation should begin with anteroposterior (AP), lateral, and flexion/extension radiographs of the cervical spine (FIG 1A–F).
  - This allows for assessment of both the degree and flexibility of the deformity.
- Standing AP and lateral radiographs of the entire spine, with the hips and knees in maximal extension, are obtained to assess global coronal and sagittal balance.
  - Full-spine radiographs inform levels of instrumentation, as stopping at the apex of a cervicothoracic deformity is not advised given the risk of distal junctional kyphosis.
  - Similarly, a C7 PSO is often not appropriate in cases of cervicothoracic deformity, increasing the risk of the procedure while reducing overall correction. A T2 or T3 three-column osteotomy is preferred, both for safety and correction.
- A computed tomography (CT) scan with 1-mm cuts and sagittal, coronal, and three-dimensional reconstructions are obtained. This allows for assessment of the fusion mass and helps provide landmark guidance for instrumentation (FIG 1G).
- If one is deciding between posterior column osteotomies (PCO, Ames type 2, eg, Smith-Petersen type) and a PSO (Ames type 6), then careful evaluation of the disc spaces

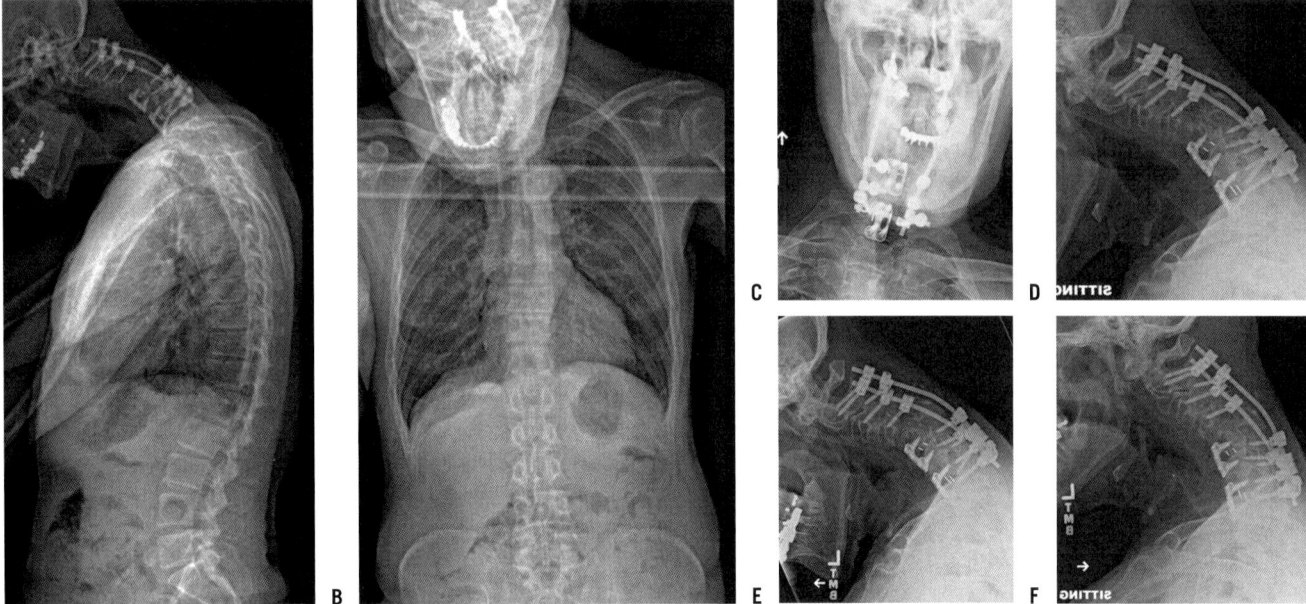

FIG 1 A,B. Standing AP and lateral radiographs, respectively, of a 69-year-old man who presented with fixed coronal and sagittal plane deformities after multiple prior anterior and posterior procedures. The fixed deformity was confirmed by AP (**C**), lateral (**D**), flexion (**E**), and extension (**F**) radiographs. **G.** Midsagittal CT scan shows a fixed cervical kyphosis at C4–C6.

is necessary. If there is a circumferential fusion, a PSO is required.

- An MRI is obtained to visualize the neural elements. If the patient cannot tolerate a closed MRI (sometimes precluded by the deformity), then an open MRI or CT myelogram may be obtained.

DIFFERENTIAL DIAGNOSIS

- Degenerative disease
- Inflammatory arthropathy
  - Ankylosing spondylitis
  - Rheumatoid arthritis
- Posttraumatic kyphosis
  - Acute
  - Chronic
- Infection
- Tumor: includes intradural pathologies
- Iatrogenic
  - Postlaminectomy
  - Pseudarthrosis
  - Postradiation

NONOPERATIVE MANAGEMENT

- Nonoperative management of symptomatic cervical kyphosis is limited, as the patient has minimal compensatory mechanisms to maintain horizontal gaze.

- Pain may be controlled with anti-inflammatory and narcotic medications.
- Bracing of flexible deformities is not ideal, as any improvement in symptoms will only occur when the brace is worn. Bracing of fixed deformities is not possible.
  - Chronic brace use runs the risk of pressure ulcer formation.

SURGICAL MANAGEMENT

- Surgical management is necessary when the patient is suffering from respiratory compromise, has difficulty eating, or has significant difficulty maintaining horizontal gaze.
- In many cases, correction of cervical kyphosis is an elective procedure that is performed when the patient can no longer tolerate the symptoms, most of which are not life-threatening.

Preoperative Planning

- All joints should be evaluated prior to a cervical osteotomy because hip and knee flexion contractures may require intervention prior to addressing the cervical spine.
- Patients may present with concomitant, fixed thoracolumbar (TL) kyphosis, and a corrective osteotomy of the TL spine may be necessary. In this case, the TL procedure should be performed first, as horizontal gaze may correct with the TL osteotomy.[9] If the cervical osteotomy is performed first, a subsequent TL osteotomy may leave the patient in a position with the head fixed in excessive extension.

- The chin–brow angle should be measured.
  - We measure this angle of deformity with a midsagittal CT scan image. This allows for more accurate planning in severe deformities.
  - The goal of correction should be to create a chin–brow angle of approximately 10 degrees.
    - With the head in slight flexion, the patient is able to see both feet and straight ahead.
- We aim to align the posterior vertebral line of C2 with the anterior vertebral line of C7.
- Although aesthetically pleasing to the layman, a neutral chin–brow angle is not well tolerated by the patients, as they cannot see directly in front of their body.[9]
  - For smaller deformities, with only a posterior fusion, we may perform single or multiple PCOs. For larger deformities (>50 degrees) or circumferential fusion, we will perform a PSO.
    - Anterior osteotomies or a corpectomy, combined with a posterior approach, may offer impressive corrections, avoiding the increased risks associated with three-column osteotomies.
    - Also, combined anterior/posterior approaches may be more appropriate for segmental kyphosis above C7.

Positioning

- Gardner-Wells tongs are used to secure the head, and 15 lb of traction is applied.
  - Bivector traction is applied through the frame. One vector pulls axially and is used to position the head until the osteotomy closure. At the time of closure, an extension moment is applied by switching the weight to the second rope, which facilitates closure and holds the head in the appropriate position until the head is fixed in place (**FIG 2**).
  - Although many prefer a Mayfield head holder, this complicates a Stagnara wake-up test, should one be required. We have had excellent results with the freedom of Gardner-Wells tongs.

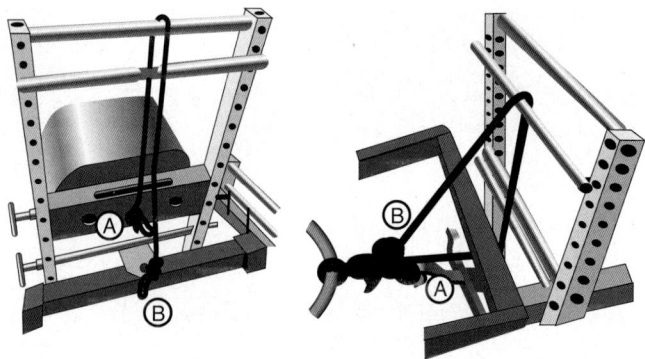

FIG 2 Bivector traction is achieved through two traction ropes. Rope *A* pulls longitudinally. Rope *B* is placed over the "H-bar" and pulls with an extension moment.

- We position the patient prone on a Jackson frame with a chest bolster, anterior iliac crest pads, and a leg sling. In the case of severe deformity, the chest bolster may be built up with pillows to allow appropriate positioning of the surgical field.
  - Although historically performed in a seated position, we prefer the prone position, as upper cervical implant placement is easier.[7]
- The arms are wrapped with blankets at the patient's side, and the elbows and wrists are padded.
- Gentle traction is applied to the shoulders with tape.
- The patient is placed in a maximal reverse Trendelenburg position. This brings the operative site into the surgeon's field of view and allows for pooling of blood in the lower extremities.

Approach

- A standard midline approach is used. We minimize blood loss by staying within the midline raphe down to the spinous processes.
- The lateral masses are exposed in their entirety but not more laterally in an effort to minimize bleeding from the venous plexus.

TECHNIQUES

POSTERIOR COLUMN OSTEOTOMY (AMES TYPE 2)

Osteotomy

- This technique relies on open disc spaces or a prior anterior release/osteotomy.
- The inferior facet of the cranial vertebra is removed using a matchstick burr. A chevron shape is created to maximize bony apposition after osteotomy closure and provide some increased stability.
  - The ligamentum flavum is excised with Kerrison rongeurs or curettes. If ossified, it is removed with a high-speed burr.
- Ensure that the exiting nerve root passes freely by resecting the superior articular process of the caudal vertebral to the level of the pedicle (akin to a foraminotomy), without the creation of iatrogenic foraminal stenosis.
  - The entire superior facet at the pedicle and medial to it should be removed as any residual fragment increases the risk of stenosis.

Osteotomy Closure

- After the osteotomies and implant placement, the surgeon takes a firm hold of the Gardner-Wells tongs and the traction weight is shifted to the extension rope. The surgeon lifts the head, thereby extending the neck, and the osteotomies is closed.
  - Stainless steel cables around spinous processes can assist with posterior column shortening and osteotomy closure. This can be done across multiple levels to maximize total correction.
- The rods are placed in the screw heads and fixed in place.
- Intraoperative radiographs are obtained to check implant position and to check the correction of the deformity.
- The wound is closed as described later.

PEDICLE SUBTRACTION OSTEOTOMY (AMES TYPE 6)

Placement of Instrumentation

- Similar to the PCO. At C2, pedicle screws are placed if the anatomy allows. Laminar screws may also be used, although rod placement may require lateralizing connectors. A combination of laminar screws and pedicle screws may be used as well. We often extend to skull if the occipitocervical junction is already fused, as this affords excellent implant purchase.
- From C3 to C5, lateral mass screws are placed. Attention is paid to place the screws in line with one another, as this facilitates placement of the final rod.
  - It is infrequent that subaxial pedicle screws are used above C7. Although recent reports may encourage their use, the added risk of this seems to be without added benefit in our experience, as lateral mass screw failure is uncommon provided implants are placed at C2 or higher.
- Lateral mass screws are placed at C6 if T1 is not instrumented.
  - This is because the tulip heads will be closely approximated, although will be out of plane complicating rod placement after osteotomy closure.
- Pedicle screws are placed from T1 to T3 or T4, with T1 omitted if C6 is instrumented. The instrumentation is placed distally to T3 or T4 to ensure six to eight points of distal fixation (TECH FIG 1).

C7 Laminectomy

- A laminectomy of C7 is performed using a high-speed burr. The lamina is removed in one piece and reserved for use as local bone graft (TECH FIG 2A).
- The laminae of C6 and T1 are undercut to provide additional room for the neural elements following closure of the osteotomy.
  - The C6 laminectomy should be performed to the caudal extent of the C6 pedicle. After closure, additional midline resection may be required.
  - The T1 laminectomy should be performed to the cranial extent of the T1 pedicle.
- The ligamentum flavum is excised with Kerrison rongeurs and/or curettes. If ossified, a burr is used.
  - All ligamentum flavum must be resected, through the ventral capsule attachments, to reduce the risk of iatrogenic stenosis after closure.

- The lateral masses of C7 are removed in piecemeal fashion, with a Leksell rongeur and a high-speed burr. A chevron-shaped cut is made so that there is rotational stability after closing the osteotomy (TECH FIG 2B).
- The inferior facets of C6 and superior facets of T1 are excised. The inferior borders of the C6 pedicles and superior borders of the T1 pedicles must be visualized. This allows adequate room for the C7 and C8 nerve roots following osteotomy closure.

Decancellation

- Cotton patties and Penfield retractors are place around the C7 pedicle to protect the C7 and C8 nerve roots. Resection of the C7 pedicle begins by passing the high-speed burr down the pedicle.
  - Care must be taken to preserve the walls of the pedicle.
  - Decancellation can be done with sequential taps, increasing by 0.5 mm with each pass.
  - Box-cutter osteotomes can be used as well, although one must be careful with manipulation of the C7 and C8 roots as they can be intolerant of manipulation.

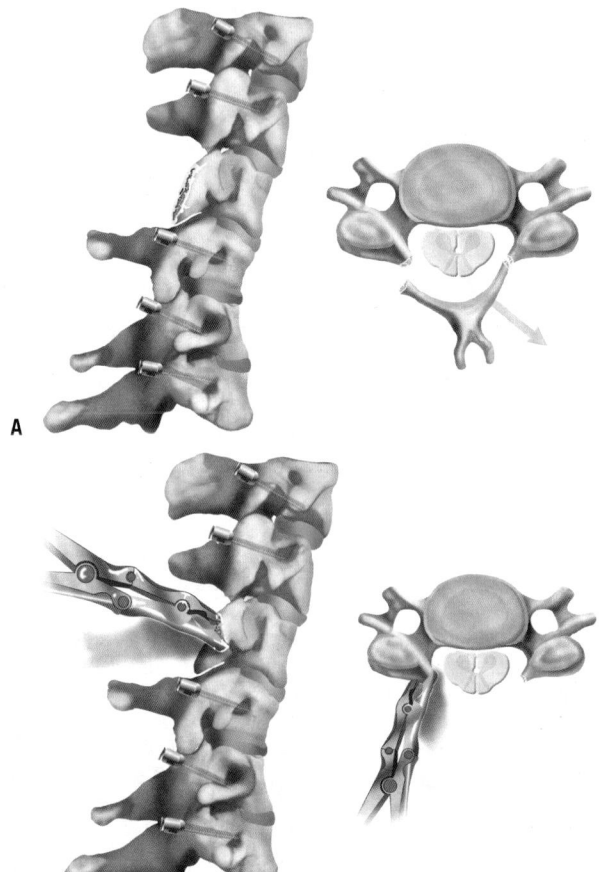

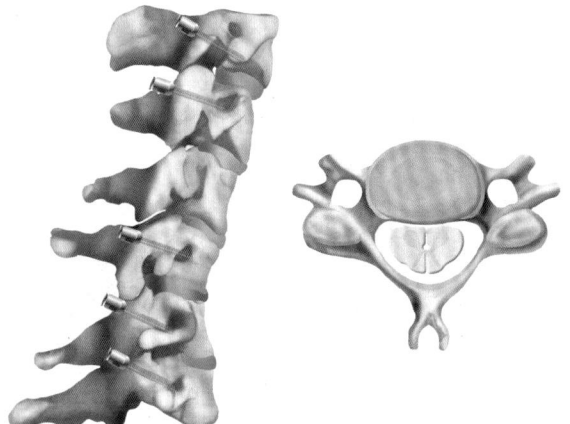

TECH FIG 1 Instrumentation has been placed.

TECH FIG 2 A. The laminectomy is performed en bloc and the bone is saved for use as bone graft. B. The lateral masses are removed with the Leksell rongeur, and the superior facets of T1 and inferior facets of C6 are removed.

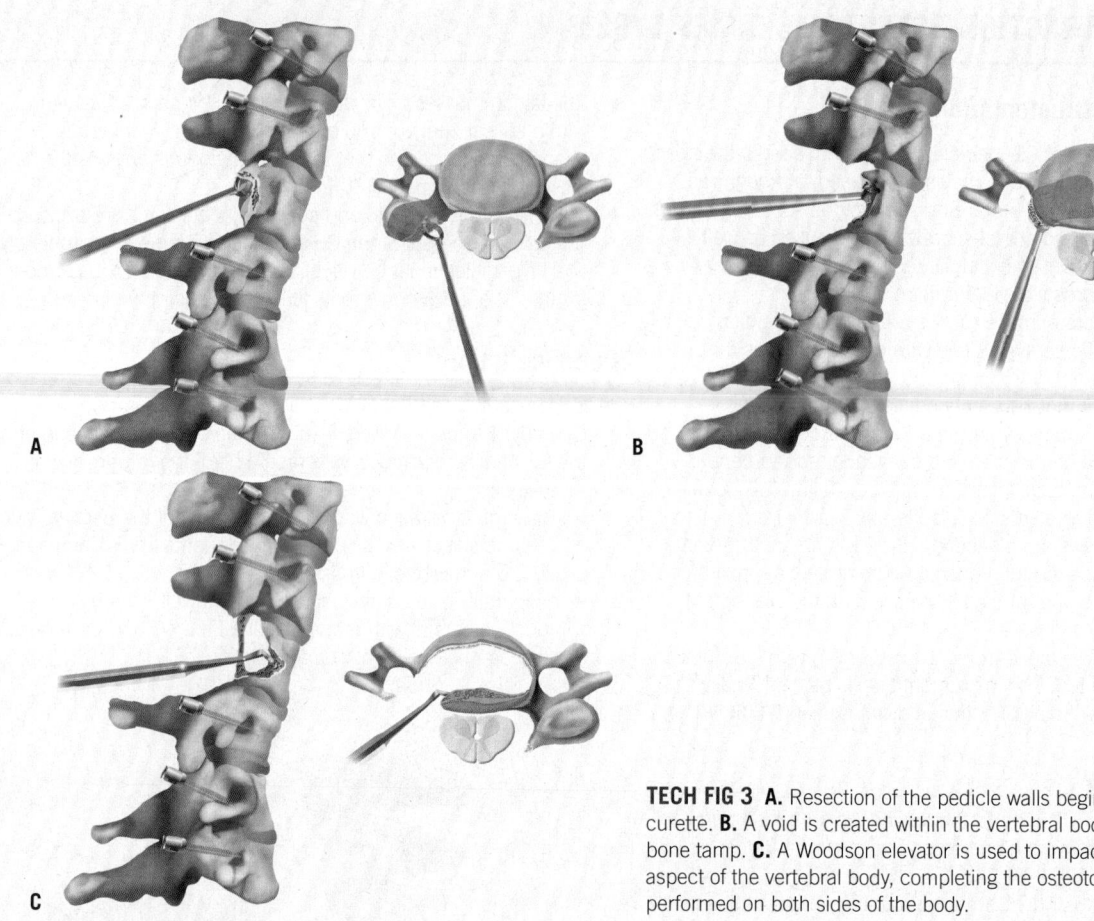

TECH FIG 3 A. Resection of the pedicle walls begins with a curette. **B.** A void is created within the vertebral body with a small bone tamp. **C.** A Woodson elevator is used to impact the posterior aspect of the vertebral body, completing the osteotomy. This is performed on both sides of the body.

- The pedicle walls are then removed, piecemeal, with pituitary rongeurs and reverse angle curettes **(TECH FIG 3A)**.
  - The pedicle walls must be removed entirely to prevent nerve root impingement following closure of the osteotomy.
- A void is created in the posterosuperior portion of the vertebral body, with reverse angle curettes or small bone tamps **(TECH FIG 3B)**.
- Decancellation is completed with curettes and pituitary rongeurs, with the cancellous bone removed and preserved for local graft or pushed anteriorly within the vertebral body **(TECH FIG 3C)**.
- A rod must be placed on the side of the resection prior to beginning the other side. This will prevent subluxation with the potential for neurologic monitoring changes or neurologic deficits.
- The same procedure is performed at the contralateral pedicle. Decancellation should continue until the void communicates from side to side.
  - An "egg shell" of C7 should now remain.
- With a Woodson elevator or elevator down-pushing curette, the posterior wall of the vertebral body is impacted, completing the osteotomy of C7. This should not require much force. If it does, then more decancellation of the body is necessary **(TECH FIG 3D)**.

Osteotomy Closure

- Prebent rods, or articulating rods (our preference), are placed in the distal screw heads **(TECH FIG 4A)**.
- The surgeon now holds the Gardner-Wells tongs and the weight is switched to the extension moment rope. The neck is gently extended by the surgeon to the desired position **(TECH FIG 4B)**.
- If enough bone has been removed from C7, this action should take little force.
- The rods are fixed in place into the proximal tulip heads.
- The C7 and C8 nerve roots are checked with a Woodson elevator; ensure that there is no impingement.
- The electrophysiologist checks the neuromonitoring signals to ensure there have been no changes during closure of the osteotomy.
  - If there are changes, we relax the closure and perform a rehearsed Stagnara wake-up test.
- Radiographs are checked to assess implant position, deformity correction, and the integrity of the anterior column.
  - In some cases, the anterior column may open. This usually happens when corrections greater than 40 degrees are attempted. In these cases, we will perform a staged anterior approach, with allograft into the void and an anterior cervical plate. We also do this in osteoporotic patients with poor fixation. If we instrumented to the skull and the screws have excellent purchase, this is not necessary.

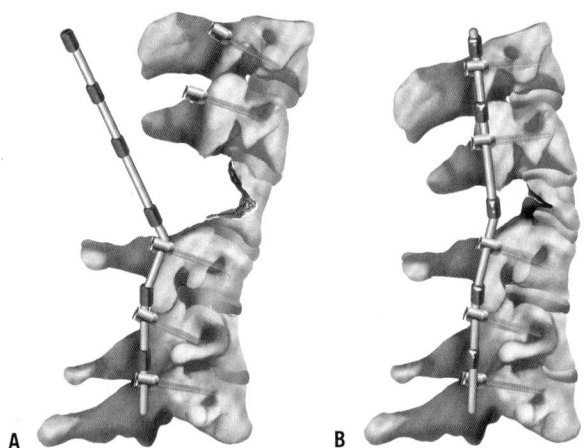

TECH FIG 4 A. An articulating or contoured rod is then placed. **B.** The head is extended, and the osteotomy site is closed.

Bone Grafting

- The laminae, spinous processes, and lateral masses/transverse processes of C6 and T1 are decorticated with a high-speed burr.
  - Irrigation is used to minimize thermal necrosis.
- The C7 lamina, which had been preserved, is split in the sagittal plane. The two pieces are then placed along the decorticated

spinous processes of C6 and T1 and then cabled or sutured in place.
- The remainder of the local bone graft is packed around the closed osteotomy site.

Wound Closure

- Meticulous attention is paid to wound closure to minimize dead space and to ensure a good cosmetic appearance.
- We close the paraspinals in multiple layers, minimizing the amount of muscle within each suture bite.
- Prior to closure of the fascial layer, 500 to 1000 mg of vancomycin are placed in the wound.
- Redundant skin is inevitable, but, with an accurate closure, the wound will smooth as it heals.
  - In the case of excessive redundancy, we will excise ellipses of full-thickness skin from the proximal and distal aspects of the wound.
  - Changing the traction rope to the "straight ahead" rope after implants are tightened assists with closure of the redundant tissue.
- Drains are placed deep and superficial to the fascia.
  - These drains are removed when over 8 hours output is less than 30 mL, usually on postoperative day 1.
- Hemostasis is verified after the closure of each layer.
  - Pressure is applied for 30 seconds after the closure of each layer.

TECHNIQUES

Pearls and Pitfalls

Preoperative Planning	• The preoperative physical examination should evaluate other joints that may be affected by the disease process and require intervention before the cervical spine. • TL kyphosis, if severe enough to warrant surgery, should be corrected before the cervical spine. • Careful examination of the vertebral artery using preoperative imaging will minimize the risk of injury **(FIG 3)**. • A detailed pulmonary history and examination is necessary, as some extreme cases may require a preoperative tracheostomy. • The medical comorbidity burden of cervical deformity patients must be scrutinized, as these are complex surgeries with risks of major complication. • The goal of correction should be to 10–20 degrees of flexion, allowing the patient to see directly in front of their body. • Use Gardner-Wells tongs and bivector traction to help with intraoperative positioning of the head. • Position the patient prone, in maximal reverse Trendelenburg. This brings the operative site into the field of view and minimizes blood loss through pooling in the lower extremities.

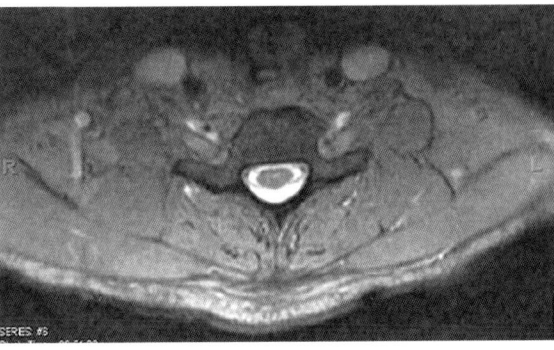

FIG 3 Axial T2-weighted MRI of a 34-year-old man with a fixed cervical deformity, showing intraforaminal vertebral artery at C7. For this reason, multiple Smith-Petersen osteotomy were performed.

Implant Placement	• Laminar screws may be placed at C2 if the anatomy is not amenable to pars screws. Laminar screws may also be placed as an adjunct to pars screws in cases of poor bone stock. • Place the implants in a straight line so that contouring of the rods is minimized.
Osteotomy	• Remove the C7 lamina in one piece and reserve for use as local bone graft. • The inferior articular facet of C6 and superior articular facet of T1 must be removed entirely to reduce the risk of C7 or C8 nerve root impingement. • Protect the nerve roots with cotton patties and Penfield retractors. • Impaction of the posterior wall should proceed with minimal force. If significant force is required, then remove more bone from the body itself.
Wound Closure	• Close the wound in many layers, with meticulous attention to tissue apposition. • Achieve hemostasis with compression and pharmacologic means (thrombin, Gelfoam, etc.) after closure of each layer. • Application of vancomycin to the wound may reduce infection rates. • Place drains deep and superficial to the fascia. This will minimize dead space. • In cases of extreme tissue redundancy, ellipses may be excised from the proximal and distal aspects of the wound. • A plastic surgery consultation may be appropriate in the most extreme cases (redundant skin, previous surgery, etc.).
Postoperative Care	• Immobilize the patient in a hard collar for 6–12 weeks. • Mobilize the patient on postoperative day 1.

POSTOPERATIVE CARE

- Most patients can be extubated without difficulty immediately following the procedure.
- All patients are immobilized in a hard collar for 6 to 12 weeks.
- All patients are out of bed and walking on postoperative day 1.
- Patients are generally discharged to home on postoperative day 1 or 2.

OUTCOMES

- With proper planning, horizontal gaze is reliably restored **(FIG 4)**.[1,2,5-7,10]
- Belanger et al[1] reported improved neck pain scores in 88% (21 out of 24) of ankylosing spondylitis patients.
  - Subjective dysphagia was improved in 95% (18 out of 19).
- Subjective satisfaction scores are often good to excellent.[7,10]

COMPLICATIONS

- Neurologic injury, including paralysis, has been reported with extension osteotomies, with an overall rate of approximately 23%.[3]
  - The most commonly affected nerve root is C8, with transient palsies more common than permanent injury.[10]
- In cases of osteoporosis and osteopenia, implant failure and pseudarthrosis are concerns.
  - Pseudarthrosis rates with modern implants have been reported from 0% to 13%.[1,5,6,10]
- The vertebral artery is at risk; however, performing the osteotomy at C7 and careful planning may minimize the risk. Make sure that there is no anomalous vertebral artery in the foramen transversarium of C7.
- As with any posterior procedure, wound infection and wound dehiscence are potential risks. A plastic surgery consultation is appropriate for the most extreme wounds.

- One-year mortality rates for cervical deformity patients has been reported as high as 9%. This underscores the complex nature of these patients and procedures, necessitating an experienced surgeon and complete, informed decision-making process.[8]

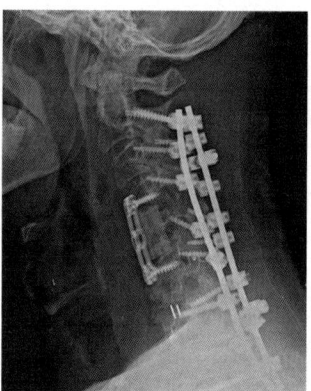

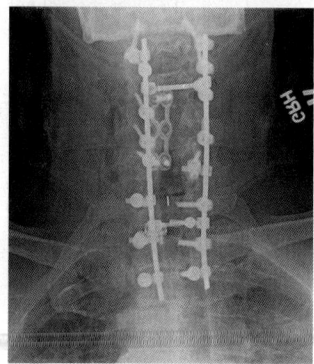

FIG 4 Postoperative radiographs of the patient in **FIG 1**. He underwent posterior osteotomies (C4–C5, C5–C6) and removal of instrumentation, anterior C5 corpectomy and C7–T1 anterior cervical discectomy and fusion, and posterior instrumentation C2–T3.

REFERENCES

1. Belanger TA, Milam RA, Roh JS, et al. Cervicothoracic extension osteotomy for chin-on-chest deformity in ankylosing spondylitis. J Bone Joint Surg Am 2005;87(8):1732–1738.
2. El Saghir H, Boehm H. Surgical options in the treatment of the spinal disorders in ankylosing spondylitis. Clin Exp Rheumatol 2002;20(suppl 28):S101–S105.
3. Etame AB, Than KD, Wang AC, et al. Surgical management of symptomatic cervical or cervicothoracic kyphosis due to ankylosing spondylitis. Spine (Phila Pa 1976) 2008;33(16):E559–E564.
4. Hong JT, Park DK, Lee MJ, et al. Anatomical variations of the vertebral artery segment in the lower cervical spine: analysis by three-dimensional computed tomography angiography. Spine (Phila PA 1976) 2008;33(22):2422–2426.
5. Langeloo DD, Journee HL, Pavlov PW, et al. Cervical osteotomy in ankylosing spondylitis: evaluation of new developments. Eur Spine J 2006;15(4):493–500.
6. McMaster MJ. Osteotomy of the cervical spine in ankylosing spondylitis. J Bone Joint Surg Br 1997;79(2):197–203.
7. Simmons ED, DiStefano RJ, Zheng Y, et al. Thirty-six years experience of cervical extension osteotomy in ankylosing spondylitis: techniques and outcomes. Spine (Phila Pa 1976) 2006;31(26):3006–3012.
8. Smith JS, Shaffrey CI, Kim HJ, et al. Prospective multicenter assessment of all-cause mortality following surgery for adult cervical deformity. Neurosurgery 2018;83(6):1277–1285.
9. Suk KS, Kim KT, Lee SH, et al. Significance of chin-brow vertical angle in correction of kyphotic deformity of ankylosing spondylitis patients. Spine (Phila Pa 1976) 2003;28(17):2001–2005.
10. Tokala DP, Lam KS, Freeman BJ, et al. C7 decancellisation closing wedge osteotomy for the correction of fixed cervico-thoracic kyphosis. Eur Spine J 2007;16(9):1471–1478.

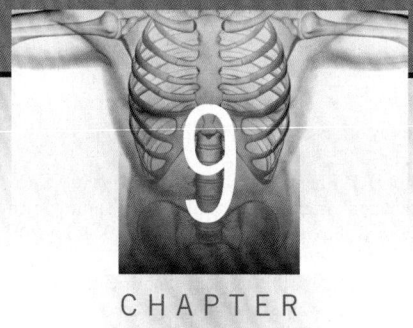

9
CHAPTER

Reduction Techniques for Cervical Fractures and Dislocations

Adam M. Pearson, Keith W. Lyons, and Alexander R. Vaccaro

BACKGROUND

- Cervical spine fractures are seen in approximately 5% of trauma patients being evaluated at level I trauma centers.
- Dislocations and displaced fractures require reduction and frequently surgical stabilization.
- This chapter focuses on the cervical fractures that often require reduction and the closed and open techniques used to manage them.

GENERAL PRINCIPLES OF CLOSED REDUCTION

Traction

- Application of longitudinal traction assists in the reduction of cervical spine fractures through ligamentotaxis and the ability to apply rotational moments to the cervical spine.
- Traction can be performed urgently in the emergency room.
- Successful reduction requires an understanding of the biomechanics of both injury and reduction.
- Traction is contraindicated in extension distraction injuries and type IIA hangman's fractures (see section Traumatic Spondylolisthesis).
- Placement of a towel roll between the scapulae can help to raise the head off the bed and allow for better control of the flexion or extension moment.
- Low weight (10 lb) should initially be placed in order to ensure that there is no craniocervical instability or unsuspected distraction.

- Weight is generally added in 10-lb increments with lateral radiographs obtained every 10 to 15 minutes after adding weight in order to allow for the viscoelastic tissues to creep and for the muscles to fatigue. Serial neurologic examinations should also be performed and documented with each addition of weight.
- If not successful, open reduction in the operating room is generally indicated.

Gardner-Wells Tongs

- Imaging of the skull (plain films or computed tomography [CT] scan) should be obtained prior to pin placement to ensure there are no skull fractures.
- Pin placement is extremely important. The pins should generally be placed 1 cm above the pinna, in line with the external auditory meatus and below the equator of the skull (**FIG 1**). Placement more anteriorly results in an extension moment, whereas placement more posteriorly results in a flexion moment (sometimes desirable for facet dislocations).
- The pin sites should be prepped with Betadine. Because these pins are temporary, the hair does not need to be shaved. Lidocaine is injected subcutaneously and subperiosteally at the planned pin sites.
- Pins should be tightened until the indicator protrudes at least 1 mm, which corresponds to 30 lb of compression at the pin site. Undertightened pins can disengage and cause scalp lacerations. Do not overtighten pins, as penetration of the inner table of the skull can occur.

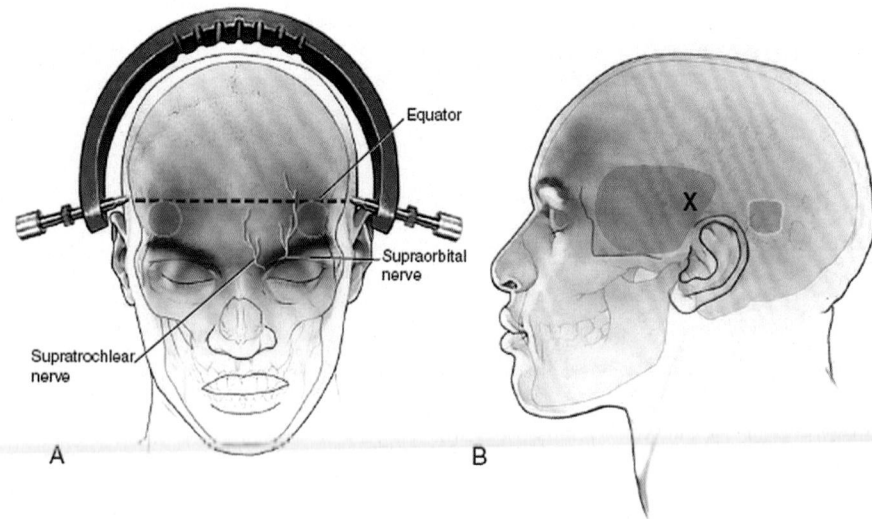

A

B

FIG 1 A,B. Gardner-Wells tongs are to be placed with pins approximately 1 cm above the pinna in line with the external auditory meatus, below the equator of the skull ("X" in Figure B). Anterior halo pins are placed over the lateral third of the eyebrow in order to avoid the supraorbital and supratrochlear nerves, whereas posterior pin sites are posterior to the pinna, below the equator of the skull.

- Gardner-Wells tongs are temporary devices used for reduction. Use of halo ring traction should be considered if a halo is to be used for definitive management, although the amount of weight that can be applied to a halo ring is also less than what can be added to stainless steel Gardner-Wells tongs. We generally prefer to perform a reduction using Gardner-Wells tongs and then convert to a halo if surgery is going to be delayed, and the patient needs to be stabilized in the interim.

Halo Vest Application

- Most halo vest systems are now magnetic resonance imaging (MRI) compatible.
- Proper application of the ring is essential to prevent nerve injury, skin problems, and provide a method of immobilization with long-term durability.
- At least two providers familiar with halo application are required.
- The first step is to size the vest and the ring using the manufacturer's instructions. The vest should extend down to the level of the xiphoid and be snug but allow access to the skin. The ring should fit as close to the skull as possible without contacting the skin at any point.
- The patient can be logrolled to place the posterior portion of the vest.
- One person then holds the halo ring in place, ensuring that it does not contact the ears or the head, is symmetrically and appropriately aligned, and is below the equator of the skull.
- Another person then plans the pin placement (see **FIG 1**). The two anterior pins are generally placed 1 cm cranial to the lateral third of the orbital rim to avoid the supraorbital and supratrochlear nerves. The pins can be placed into the eyebrow in patients concerned about scar cosmesis. The posterior pins are generally placed 1 cm above the helix of the ear, posterior to the external auditory meatus, and below the equator of the skull.
- If the halo is going to remain in place for an extended period, the posterior pin sites should be shaved prior to starting the procedure. The pin sites should be prepped with Betadine, and lidocaine should be injected subcutaneously and subperiosteally.
- While one person holds the ring in place (various devices such as suction cups and blunt pins can be used to assist with this), the other person screws the pins in until they all just contact the skin. Opposing pins should then be tightened simultaneously, going back and forth between the two pairs. The pins should be tightened to 8-inch lb using either a torque-limiting breakaway applicator or a torque wrench.
- The halo ring can then be attached to traction using the appropriate metal bail or to the uprights of the halo vest. The head should be positioned appropriately, and radiographs should be obtained to determine if the alignment is appropriate.
- Pins should be retightened to 8-inch lb in 24 to 48 hours.
- Loose pins can be retightened once and should then be replaced through another hole if they loosen again.
- Meticulous pin site care is required, although pin site infection can still occur. If infection is present but the pin is still tight, it can be treated with local care and oral antibiotics. If the pin loosens in the presence of infection, it should be replaced.

Bivector Traction

- Bivector traction allows for simultaneous control of longitudinal traction and a flexion moment using a specially designed traction apparatus on a RotoRest bed **(FIG 2)**.

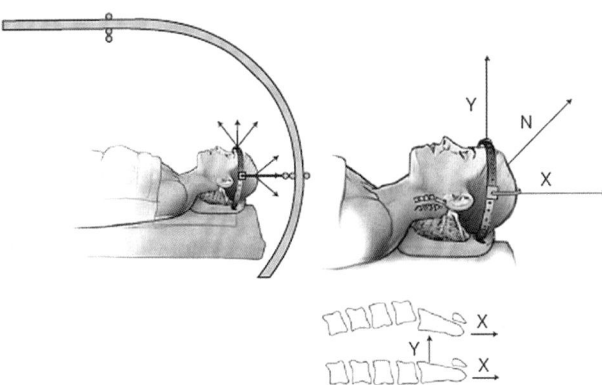

FIG 2 Bivector traction with Gardner-Wells tongs. Two cables are used in order to adjust anterior and superior traction individually in order to affect a reduction.

- The patient is positioned on a RotoRest bed with the head pad removed and shoulder roll in place to allow for freedom of motion of the head in the sagittal plane.
- Longitudinal traction is applied to the ring using an S-clip and anterior traction is applied via a cord attached to both of the pins. The two forces should initially be at 90 degrees to each other and can then be fine-tuned as needed.
- Application of weight to the anterior pulley allows flexion to be "dialed-in" without having to change the position of the longitudinal traction, which can be difficult when heavy weight has been applied.
- Bivector traction is indicated for most cervical spine reductions as it allows for more precise control of the traction vector than a single-vector traction setup.

ODONTOID FRACTURES

DEFINITION

- Fracture through the odontoid process that can be located from the tip of the dens to its base.
- Odontoid fractures are very common, accounting for almost 20% of all cervical fractures.

ANATOMY

- Two ossification centers fuse in utero, separating the dens ossification center from the primary ossification center of the C2 vertebral body. These two ossification centers are separated by the dentocentral synchondrosis, which fuses by age 7 years. Another secondary ossification center, the ossiculum terminale, forms at the tip of the dens around age 9 years and fuses by age 13 years.
- There is a rich vascular supply around the dens originating from the vertebral arteries and ascending pharyngeal artery. Although it was thought that type II dens fractures were predisposed to nonunion due to the presence of a watershed area at the base of the dens, this has been shown to be untrue.[8]
- The transverse atlantal ligament runs posterior to dens and connects to the posterior aspect of the anterior C1 ring bilaterally, preventing anterior translation of C1 on C2. The alar ligaments run from the tip of the dens to the skull base and restrict axial rotation. The weak apical ligament connects the tip of the dens to the occiput **(FIG 3)**.

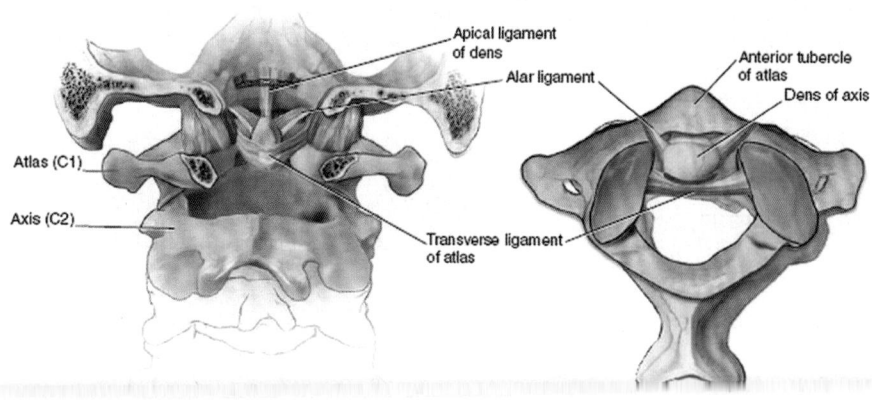

FIG 3 Ligamentous anatomy of the upper cervical spine.

- The C2 nerve root exits posterior to the C1–C2 joint in contrast to nerve roots below this level, which exit anterior to the facet joints. This puts the C2 nerve root at risk during posterior C1–C2 fusions.
- Fifty percent of axial rotation of the cervical spine occurs at C1–C2.
- A fracture of the dens results in atlantoaxial instability.

CLASSIFICATION

- Anderson and D'Alonzo[2] **(FIG 4)**
- Type I fractures are avulsions of the apical portion of dens and generally represents a stable fracture with a high union rate. Occipital cervical dissociation should be suspected and ruled out.
- Type II fractures involve the base of the odontoid and do not extend into the C2 body. These are generally considered unstable and are associated with a nonunion rate of at least 32% with nonoperative treatment.[5]

- Type III fractures extend into the vertebral body of C2. These are relatively stable fractures that have a union rate of 85% to 90% with nonoperative treatment.[11]

PATIENT PRESENTATION

- The majority of patients present neurologically intact.
- Delayed presentation is common, and patients frequently present with neck pain and may have varying degrees of myelopathy.

IMAGING

- Plain films including an open mouth view of the odontoid should be obtained.
- CT scan with thin cuts and sagittal and coronal reformations is the study of choice to detect and characterize odontoid fractures.

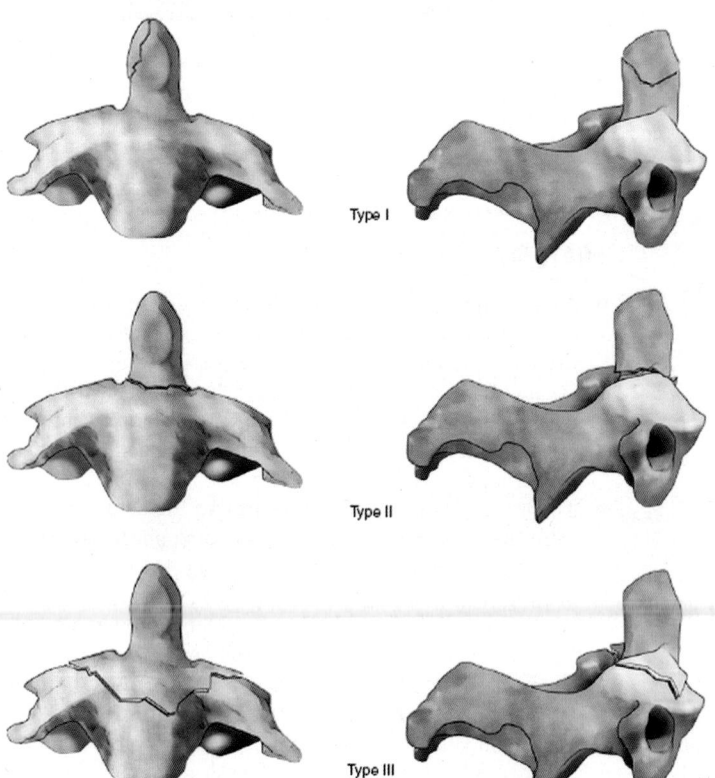

FIG 4 Anderson and D'Alonzo classification of odontoid fractures. Type I involves the apex, type II involves the base of the dens, and type III enters the body of C2.

- MRI is indicated in patients with neurologic deficit and can be useful to assess the ligaments of the upper cervical spine.

CLOSED REDUCTION AND TREATMENT

- Gardner-Wells tongs are applied and bivector traction is used to reduce displaced odontoid fractures. If definitive treatment in a halo vest is planned, reduction can be performed with a halo ring. Although single-vector traction can be used for the reduction of odontoid fractures, bivector traction allows for more precise control of the traction vector.
- In posteriorly displaced fractures, there is a risk of respiratory compromise during the reduction maneuver that typically requires flexion of the neck. This is most likely due to compression of the airways by the retropharyngeal hematoma, although others have suggested that it is due to the displaced odontoid compressing the respiratory pathways that run in the anterolateral portion of the upper spinal cord.[20] As such, nasotracheal intubation of these patients prior to reduction is recommended.

- A relatively low amount of weight is generally required (20 to 30 lb), and serial plain x-rays or fluoroscopy should be used with bivector traction to fine-tune the reduction.
- Type I and III fractures rarely need reduction and can be managed with a halo vest or cervical collar. It has been recommended that type II fractures, particularly in elderly patients who cannot tolerate a halo vest, should be treated surgically.[15]

SURGICAL TREATMENT

- Indicated for elderly patients with type II fractures and for failure to hold reduction or nonunion in younger patients
- Options include odontoid screw, transarticular C1–C2 fusion, and Harms posterior C1–C2 fusion **(FIG 5)**. Posterior C1–C2 wiring is an older technique that also had acceptable results, although a lower fusion rate than transarticular

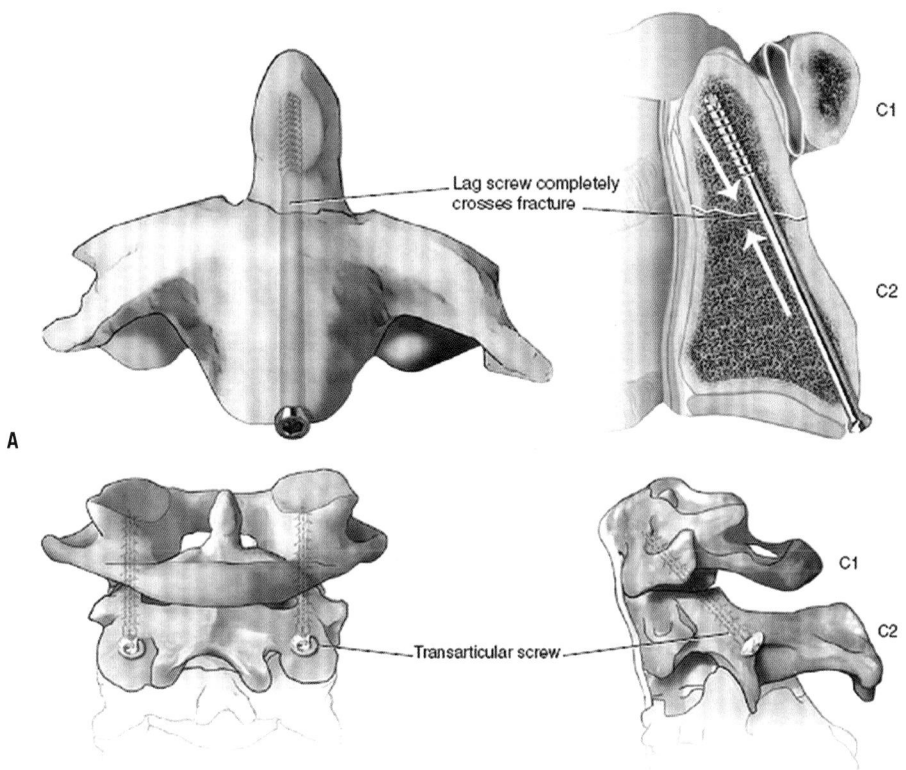

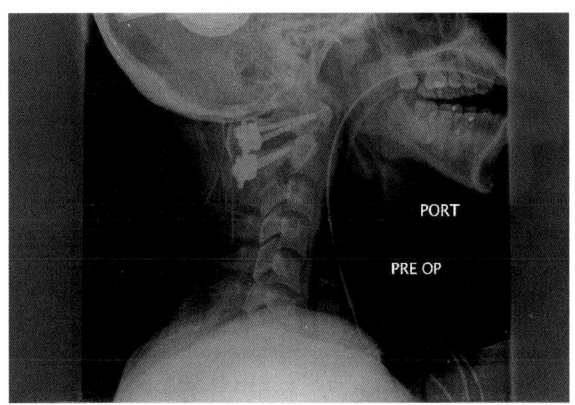

FIG 5 Fixation techniques for odontoid fractures. **A.** Anterior lag screw. **B.** Transarticular fusion. **C.** Harms fusion.

fixation. Anterior screw fixation allows for some preservation of C1–C2 rotation, although it is associated with a higher rate of technical problems and nonunions compared to posterior C1–C2 fusion.[30]

OUTCOMES

- In type II fractures, union rates are approximately 51% with collar treatment, 65% with halo vest orthosis, 82% with odontoid screw fixation, and 93% with posterior C1–C2 fusion.[9]
- In type III fractures, collar immobilization results in a union rate of approximately 92% compared to 95% with halo vest orthosis.[9]

COMPLICATIONS

- In patients older than 70 years old, inpatient mortality can be as high as 35%.[5]
- In patients older than 65 years old treated with a halo vest orthosis, mortality can be as high as 42%, primarily due to pneumonia and cardiac arrest.[24]
- Operative treatment of dens fractures in the elderly is also associated with high mortality rates of 40% with anterior screw fixation and 22% for posterior C1–C2 fusion.[6,18]
- Anterior screw fixation can result in nonunion and screw cut out, particularly in elderly, osteoporotic bone.
- Posterior screw placement at C1 and C2 can result in vascular injury to the vertebral or internal carotid arteries.[10]

Pearls and Pitfalls

Bivector Traction	• Can be extremely helpful in the reduction of displaced odontoid fractures
Posteriorly Displaced Fractures	• Should be intubated prior to closed reduction
Elderly Patients with a Halo Vest	• Treatment is associated with high morbidity and mortality in elderly patients, so operative treatment is often favored. • We prefer a posterior Harms C1–C2 fusion in these patients.

TRAUMATIC SPONDYLOLISTHESIS OF THE AXIS ("HANGMAN'S FRACTURE")

DEFINITION

- Fracture through the C2 pars interarticularis. A similar lesion is seen in judicial hangings, although the mechanisms and outcomes are obviously quite different.

ANATOMY

- C2 is a unique vertebra in that it serves as the transition from the upper cervical spine to the lower cervical spine.
- The superior articular processes (SAPs) are anterolateral to the spinal canal, biconcave, articulate with the inferior articular processes (IAPs) of C1, and allow for rotation around the dens. The IAPs are posterolateral to the spinal canal and articulate with the SAPs of C3. The pars connects the superior and IAPs of C2 and is an area of frequent injury due to its relative weakness **(FIG 6)**.
- The vertebral artery runs through the C2 foramen on the lateral aspect of the C1–C2 joint.
- The spinal canal is quite capacious at C2, explaining the low rate of neurologic injuries with fractures at this level.

PATHOGENESIS AND CLASSIFICATION

- The most commonly used classification is Levine and Edward's[17] modification of Effendi's classification system **(FIG 7)**.
- Type I fractures are nondisplaced (<3 mm) and nonangulated vertical fractures just posterior to the vertebral body that are parallel and symmetric to each other. These typically result from hyperextension and axial loading. The

discal and ligamentous structures are generally intact, and these represent stable fractures.
- Type IA, or atypical, fractures are nondisplaced (<3 mm) and nonangulated vertical fractures that are asymmetric (ie, the fracture lines are located at slightly different locations in the neural arch and are not parallel). These typically result from hyperextension and lateral bending. These generally represent stable fractures. Starr and Eismont[23] also described two displaced "atypical" hangman's fractures that were associated with neurologic deficit due to the spinal cord becoming impaled on the posterior fragment at the fracture site.
- Type II fractures are displaced (>3 mm), angulated fractures that tend to be vertically oriented just posterior to the vertebral body. The pars fractures occur with initial hyperextension, which is then followed by flexion that disrupts the disc, elevates the anterior longitudinal ligament (ALL) off of C3, and often fractures the anterosuperior corner of C3.
- Type IIA fractures are angulated (often >15 degrees), minimally translated fractures that are oriented obliquely, running from anteroinferior to posterosuperior through the pars. The mechanism of injury is distraction-flexion, resulting in the pars failing in tension. The disc fails from posterior to anterior, and the ALL is usually intact. It is important to recognize this variant because traction will exacerbate the deformity rather than reduce it.
- Type III fractures are typically type I fractures through the pars combined with a bilateral C2–C3 facet dislocation. The mechanism leading to type III fractures is unclear, but it has been hypothesized that a distraction-flexion injury resulting in facet dislocation occurs initially followed by an extension force that fractures the pars. Due to the discontinuity between the vertebral body and the dislocated facets, closed reduction generally fails, and this injury requires operative treatment.

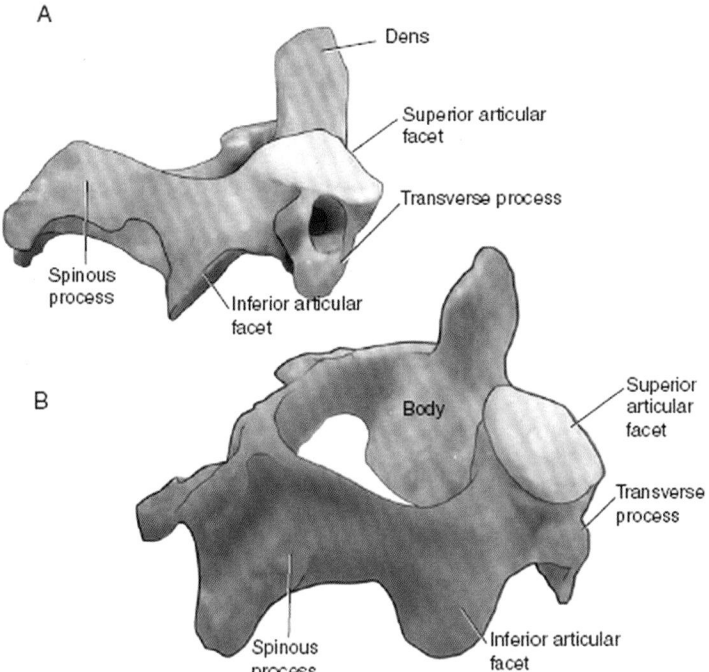

FIG 6 A,B. C2 bony anatomy.

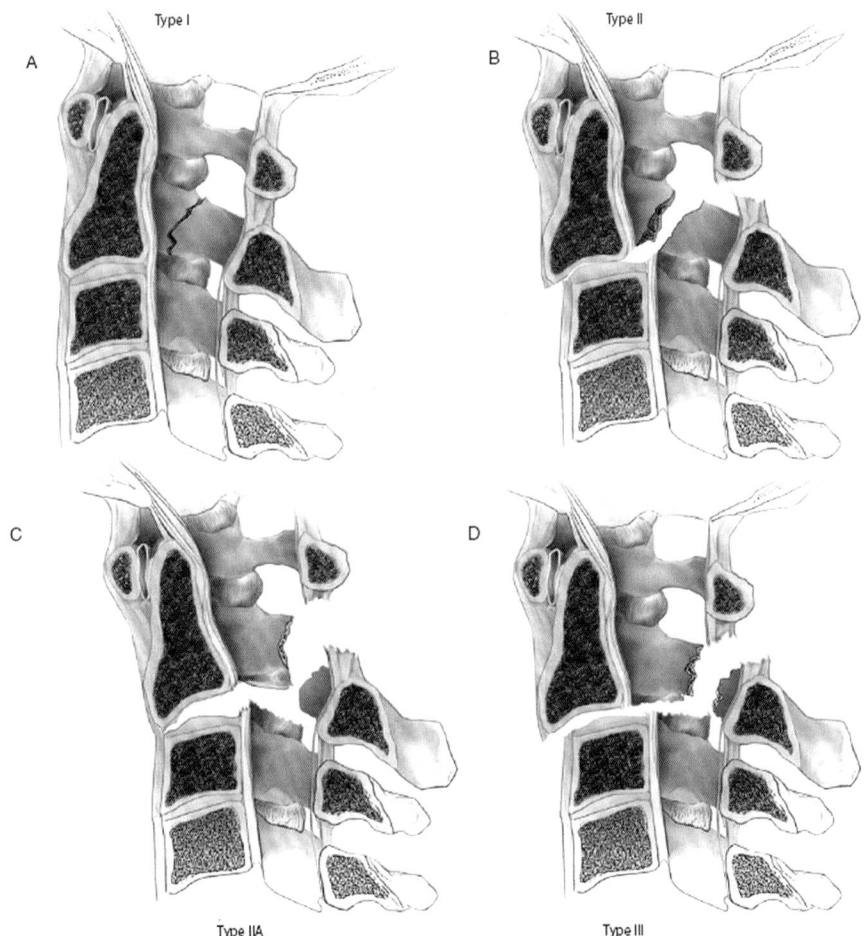

FIG 7 A–D. Levine and Edward's classification of traumatic spondylolisthesis of the axis (hangman's fracture). Type I fractures are minimally displaced (<3 mm). Type II fractures are displaced (>3 mm), angulated fractures. Type IIA fractures are angulated but minimally translated, usually with an intact ALL. Type III fractures have an accompanying bilateral facet dislocation.

PATIENT HISTORY AND PHYSICAL FINDINGS

- The most common mechanism of injury is motor vehicle accident.
- Neurologic injury is uncommon due to the large diameter of the spinal canal at this level. The majority of patients with neurologic injuries have type III fractures, although neurologic injury can also be seen in atypical type IA fractures due to asymmetric canal narrowing.
- Concomitant fractures elsewhere in the spine are common, so the remainder of the spine needs to be assessed with physical examination and imaging.

IMAGING

- Cross-table lateral radiographs generally demonstrate the fracture lines through the pars and the traumatic spondylolisthesis if present. The exception is the type IA fracture, in which the fracture lines are in different planes and are not always seen on the x-ray.
- Type II fractures can reduce when the patient is supine, so upright x-rays should be obtained in patients with type I fractures. Some authors have even suggested physician supervised flexion–extension radiographs in neurologically intact patients with apparent type I fractures to ensure that it does not actually represent a type II fracture.[16]
- CT scan of the cervical spine should be obtained to better characterize the fracture and rule out other cervical spine fractures. Imaging of the thoracic and lumbar spine should also be obtained to rule out noncontiguous fractures.
- MRI is indicated in patients with neurologic deficits or type III fractures, which must be evaluated for a disc herniation in association with the facet dislocation.

NONOPERATIVE MANAGEMENT

- Type I and type IA fractures can be treated with a cervical collar for 3 months. Upright x-rays are obtained to make sure the fracture is not actually a type II fracture.
- Type II fractures often are reduced by closed reduction. Because the mechanism causing displacement of these fractures is flexion and compression, reduction requires extension and traction.
- This is generally best performed using halo ring traction, as it allows for conversion to a halo vest orthosis.

- To obtain reduction, a towel roll is generally placed at approximately C6 to extend the spine, and traction is applied. Reduction is generally obtained with 25 to 40 lb.
- Following reduction, a halo vest orthosis is applied, and upright x-rays are obtained to ensure that reduction can be maintained with the halo vest.
- In patients with more than 5 mm of anterior translation or 11 degrees of angulation, reduction is difficult to maintain in the halo vest.[28] These patients can be treated with prolonged skeletal traction (up to 6 weeks) followed by halo vest immobilization after the fracture becomes stable or with surgery. Many physicians forgo prolonged traction due to patient discomfort and cost and will accept fracture displacement while immobilized in a halo orthosis.
- Type IIA fractures result from flexion-distraction, so traction is *absolutely contraindicated* and will increase the deformity. These fractures are characterized by angulation without translation and oblique fracture lines.
- Type IIA fractures should be reduced with gentle hyperextension and axial compression. An acceptable reduction is less than 10 degrees of angulation. Prior to reduction, a halo ring should be placed and then attached to the halo vest with the neck in mild extension and compression in order to maintain the reduction. The halo vest is generally maintained for 3 months. Failure to obtain or maintain an acceptable reduction is an indication for surgery.
- Type III fractures cannot be managed with closed treatment.

SURGICAL MANAGEMENT

Indications

- For type II and type IIA fractures in which an acceptable reduction cannot be maintained with a halo vest, surgery is indicated. Open reduction and osteosynthesis with placement of C2 pedicle screws across the fracture site is the surgical treatment of choice.
- A C2–C3 anterior cervical decompression and fusion (ACDF) is another option for fractures that lose reduction or go onto nonunion.
- Type III fractures require open reduction and fixation of the facet dislocation and subsequent positioning of the head in an extended position if needed to reduce the spondylolisthesis.

C2 OSTEOSYNTHESIS

- A posterior approach is used, with Mayfield tongs or a halo ring attached to the operating table to hold the head in a reduced position.
- The posterior elements of C2 are completely exposed, and the isthmus of C2 is palpated to help guide screw placement. Care is taken to protect the C2 nerve root.
- Lag screws are placed across the fracture site using fluoroscopy guidance, if desired (**TECH FIG 1**).

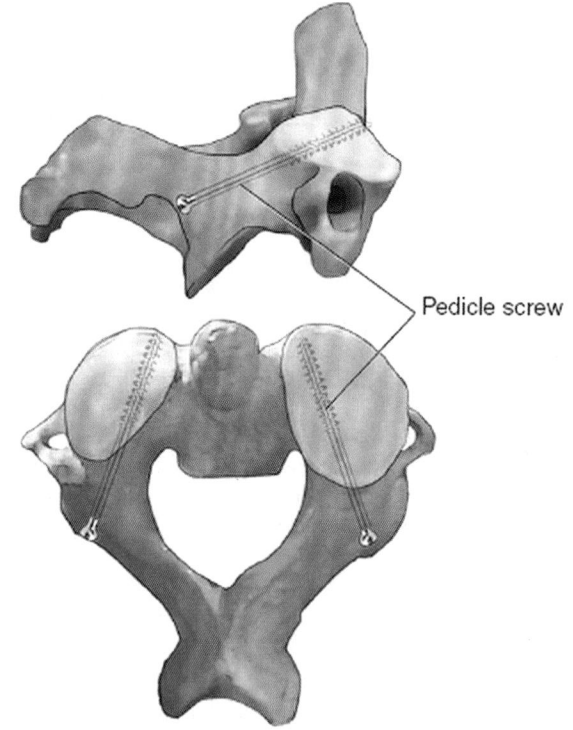

Pedicle screw

TECH FIG 1 C2 osteosynthesis using pedicle screws placed across the pars fractures in traumatic spondylolisthesis of the axis (hangman's fracture).

C2 pedicle screws for osteosynthesis

OPEN REDUCTION INTERNAL FIXATION OF FACET DISLOCATION

- The head is positioned in Mayfield tongs, and the posterior elements of C2 and C3 are completely exposed.
- Towel clips or tenaculums are then used to reduce the dislocated facets, and any remaining spondylolisthesis is reduced by positioning the head in extension.
- Following reduction, C2 pedicle screws are placed across the fracture site using a lag technique to promote osteosynthesis of the pars fractures.

- Lateral mass screws are then placed at C3 and connected to the C2 pedicle screws using rods.
- The remaining cartilage in the C2–C3 facet joint is removed using a burr and bone graft applied in order to obtain a C2–C3 fusion (**TECH FIG 2**).
- Alternatively, the pars fracture may be treated nonoperatively with halo immobilization.

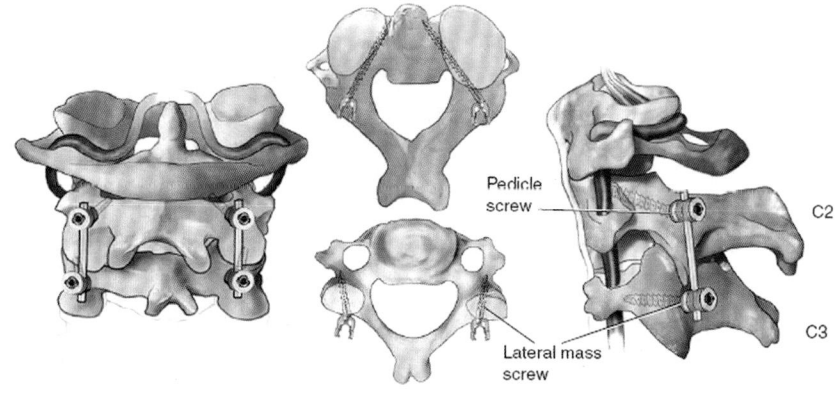

Pedicle screw

Lateral mass screw

C2

C3

C2-C3 fusion with C2 pedicle screws and C3 lateral mass screws

TECH FIG 2 C2–C3 posterior fusion for type III traumatic spondylolisthesis of the axis (hangman's fracture) using C2 pedicle screws across the pars fractures and lateral mass fixation at C3 following open reduction of the facet dislocation.

Pearls and Pitfalls

Type I and IA Fractures	• Stable and should not be overtreated • A collar is sufficient.
Type IIA Fracture	• Must be identified and traction is *absolutely contraindicated* in these patients as it will increase the deformity • These patients should undergo closed reduction with gentle extension and axial compression.
Type III Fracture	• The only absolute indication for surgery

OUTCOMES

- The union rate for type I and IA fractures approaches 100%.[16]
- Some patients can develop C2–C3 facet arthritis due to cartilage damage that occurs with hyperextension at the time of injury.
- Patients with type II fractures usually develop anterior ankylosis at C2–C3 due to the injury to the disc and elevation of the ALL. If this fails to occur, nonunion can occur, although the rate of this is unknown.
- Patients with type III fractures typically have worse outcomes if they suffered a neurologic injury. No long-term outcome data on this group are available, likely due to the very low incidence of this injury.

COMPLICATIONS

- Nonunion is rare and can be treated with C2 pedicle screw osteosynthesis or a C2–C3 ACDF.
- Injury to the spinal cord or vertebral artery can occur with improper C2 pedicle screw placement. Characterization of the course of the vertebral artery is necessary prior to performing this procedure.

SUBAXIAL FACET DISLOCATIONS AND FRACTURES

DEFINITION

- Facet dislocations occur when the IAP of the cranial vertebra dislocates anterior to the SAP of the caudal vertebra.
- This occurs with a distraction-flexion mechanism.
- Distraction-flexion injuries can present as subluxations with gapping of the facet joint, "perched" facets with the IAP resting on the SAP or "jumped" facets where the IAP has dislocated anterior to the SAP.
- These injuries can be unilateral or bilateral.
- Facet fractures involve a combination of flexion-distraction or hyperextension with lateral bending or rotation. They often represent part of the spectrum of injuries from these mechanisms that can also lead to subluxations or dislocations.
- The superior facet is involved 80% of the time. These injuries may represent rotational instability.[22]

ANATOMY

- The cervical spine can be viewed as having an anterior column (ALL, vertebral body, disc, posterior longitudinal ligament [PLL]) and a posterior column (pedicle, lateral masses, facet joints, facet capsules, ligamentum flavum, inter- and supraspinous ligaments) that provide stability.

- The facet joints in the subaxial cervical spine are oriented in the coronal plane and inclined approximately 45 degrees horizontally (**FIG 8**). This orientation allows for axial rotation, lateral bending, and flexion–extension, with coupled lateral bending and axial rotation.
- The cervical nerve roots exit directly laterally and exit above the pedicle of the vertebra for which they are named (ie, C7 nerve root exits above the C7 pedicle), posterior to the vertebral artery.
- The vertebral artery runs through the foramina transversarium from C2 through C6 but generally not through the foramen at C7. It is located anteriorly to the medial aspect of the lateral masses.

PATHOGENESIS AND CLASSIFICATION

- A popular classification for subaxial cervical spine injuries was published by Allen et al[1] in 1982.
- Facet dislocations are classified in the distractive flexion (DF) phylogeny (**FIG 9**).

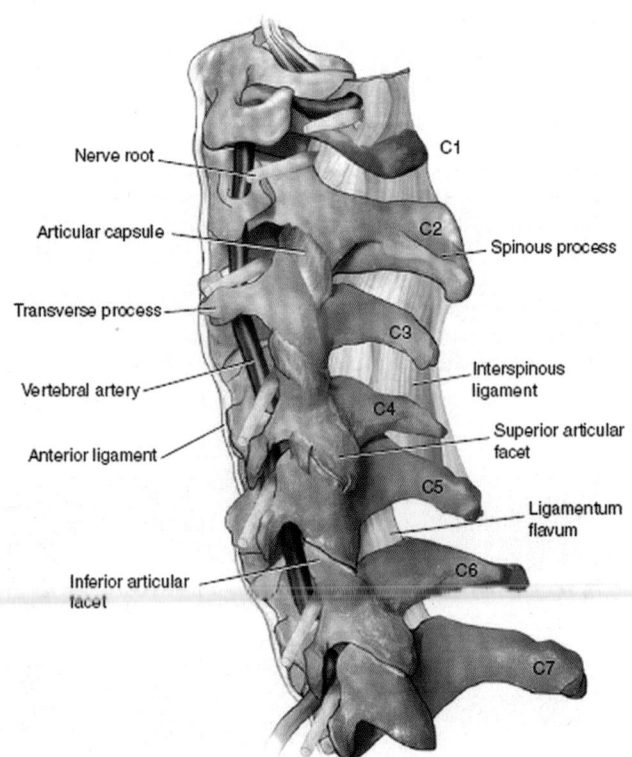

Nerve root

Articular capsule

Transverse process

Vertebral artery

Anterior ligament

Inferior articular facet

C1
C2 — Spinous process
C3
Interspinous ligament
C4
Superior articular facet
C5
Ligamentum flavum
C6
C7

FIG 8 Osteoligamentous anatomy of the cervical spine.

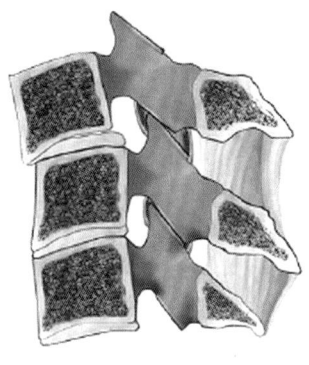

DF-1

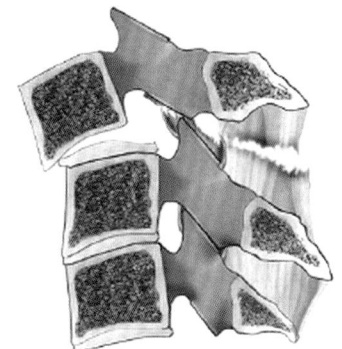

DF-2

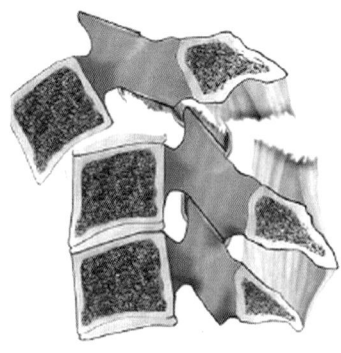

DF-3

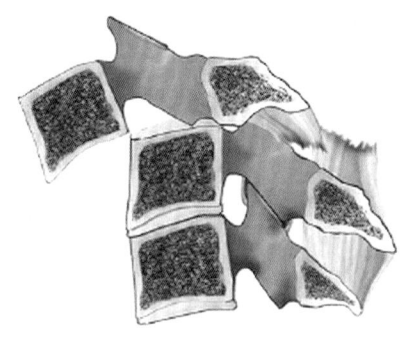

DF-4

Distractive flexion phylogeny

FIG 9 Allen and Ferguson's DF phylogeny. DF stage 1 (*DF-1*) injuries involve subluxation of the facet joints. DF stage 2 (*DF-2*) is a unilateral dislocation. DF stage 3 (*DF-3*) is a bilateral dislocation. DF stage 4 (*DF-4*) is 100% anterior translation of the vertebra.

- The subaxial cervical spine injury classification system would classify this injury as a translational cervical injury with facet dislocation, with disruption of the discoligamentous complex with or without a neurologic deficit.
- The majority of facet dislocations are due to shallow diving injuries or motor vehicle accidents in which the head is axially loaded anterior to the midsagittal plane, resulting in flexion and posterior distraction.
- A biomechanical model demonstrated that the posterior ligamentous structures fail first, allowing for flexion and separation of the facet joints. As anterior column soft tissue structures fail, including the PLL and posterior anulus, anterior translation and facet dislocation can then occur.[19]
- In Allen's DF phylogeny, DF stage 1 (DF-1) injuries include facet subluxation without dislocation, DF-2 injuries are unilateral facet dislocations with approximately 25% anterior translation of the cranial vertebra on the caudal vertebra, DF-3 injuries are bilateral facet dislocations with approximately 50% anterior translation, and DF-4 injuries represent 100% anterior translation (ie, the "floating vertebra").

PATIENT HISTORY, PHYSICAL FINDINGS, AND INITIAL MANAGEMENT

- There is a high rate of spinal cord injury (SCI) associated with facet dislocations: at least 25% with unilateral dislocations and over 50% with bilateral dislocations.[29]
- Patients should undergo full trauma resuscitation with immobilization of the cervical spine in the field.

- The use of methylprednisolone in SCI patients is controversial. The National Acute Spinal Cord Injury Study 2 and 3 trials concluded that SCI patients presenting within 8 hours of injury should receive methylprednisolone (30 mg/kg bolus followed by 5.4 mg/kg/hour infusion for 24 hours if presentation is within 3 hours of injury and for 48 hours if presentation is between 3 and 8 hours after injury).[3,4] However, these recommendations are based on minimal neurologic improvements found only in subgroup analyses, and many centers have abandoned the use of steroids in SCI.[13]
- An attempt should be made to maintain mean arterial pressure above 85 mm Hg for the first 5 to 7 days following SCI in order to maintain perfusion of the injured cord.[7]

IMAGING

- Standard radiographic evaluation of a suspected cervical spine injury includes anteroposterior, lateral, and open mouth views. In order to be sufficient, both the occipitocervical and the cervicothoracic junctions should be visualized.
- Most trauma centers now obtain CT scans of the cervical spine in all trauma patients as they are much more sensitive in diagnosing subtle cervical spine fractures and fractures at the occipitocervical and cervicothoracic junctions.
- MRI is indicated in all patients with facet dislocations to assess the status of the spinal cord, ligamentous structures, and the intervertebral disc. The timing of MRI relative to reduction is controversial. Many physicians experienced in the management of cervical dislocations advocate an immediate closed skeletal reduction in the absence of MRI only in an awake, alert,

oriented, and cooperative patient in order to closely follow the patient's neurologic status during the process of reduction.[27]

- There is almost absolute consensus that patients with a complete SCI should also undergo immediate closed reduction prior to MRI because the potential downside neurologically is small compared to the potential benefit of immediate neurologic decompression. Obtunded patients should undergo MRI prior to closed reduction because they are unable to cooperate with serial neurologic examinations.
- All patients need an MRI prior to surgical treatment to assess the need for an anterior discectomy.
- Imaging of the entire spine should be performed due to the high rate of noncontiguous injuries.
- Patients with facet dislocations are at high risk for vertebral artery injury. Numerous studies have demonstrated that these patients, along with other high-risk subsets (fractures in ankylosed spines, multilevel fractures, atlanto-occipital injuries, fractures extending into the transverse foramen, etc.) should be evaluated with CT-angiography.[14,25]

NONOPERATIVE MANAGEMENT

- All patients with facet dislocations need to undergo reduction in order to decrease the pressure on the spinal cord as soon as possible. The timing of MRI relative to closed reduction is discussed earlier.
- Most facet dislocations occur in the lower cervical spine, and large amounts of weight can be required (up to 140 lb) to obtain a closed reduction. As such, stainless steel Gardner-Wells tongs should be used.
- An initial flexion moment should be applied along with axial traction in order to unlock the facet joints. This may be accomplished with bivector traction, although positioning the tongs posterior to the external auditory meatus will also produce a flexion moment.
- Once the facets are perched, the physician can then gently extend the patient's neck in order to obtain a reduction.

This is done by using the treating physician's thumbs to control the traction pins while the other fingers are used to provide an anterior counterforce to the posterior aspect of the lower cervical spine. A towel roll between the scapulae and removal of the foam pad beneath the patient's head on the RotoRest bed can allow for unencumbered extension (**FIG 10**).

- During the reduction maneuver, an assistant can decrease the amount of traction. If reduction is successful (it is often-times accompanied by a palpable clunk), the patient can be left with 10 lb of traction in extension to control the head and maintain reduction.
- Reduction should be confirmed radiographically, and the patient's neurologic status should be documented. A decline in neurologic function with reduction suggests possible cord compression by herniated disc material.
- An MRI should be obtained prior to going to the operating room in order to assess for the possibility of a herniated disc impinging on the cord. If present in a neurologically intact or incomplete patient, an anterior discectomy is indicated.
- If operative treatment is delayed, application of a halo vest orthosis should be considered to maintain the reduction.
- For unilateral facet dislocations, a reduction maneuver is often required. Following the application of traction, the physician must axially rotate the head away from the side of the dislocation while flexion is applied in order to unlock the facet. Once imaging suggests the facet is perched, a reduction maneuver can be performed in which the neck is extended and axially rotated toward the side of the dislocation.
- The majority of isolated unilateral facet fractures can be managed nonoperatively. This includes those without neurologic deficits, ones that are nondisplaced, and with fractures that involve less than 40% of the absolute height of the intact lateral mass or that are less than 1 cm in absolute height. Fractures that involve greater than 40% of the intact lateral mass or are less than 1 cm in height are at high risk for failure of nonoperative treatment.[22]

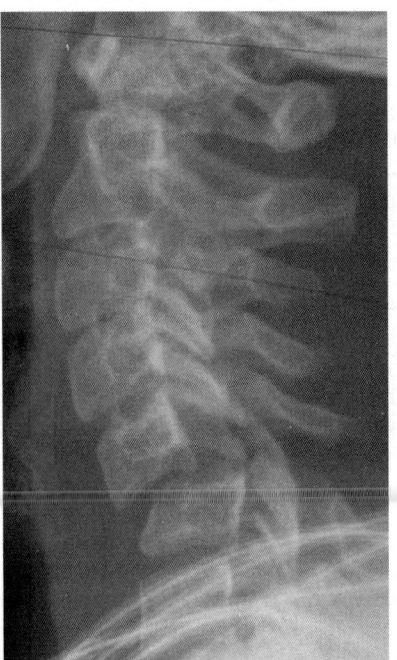 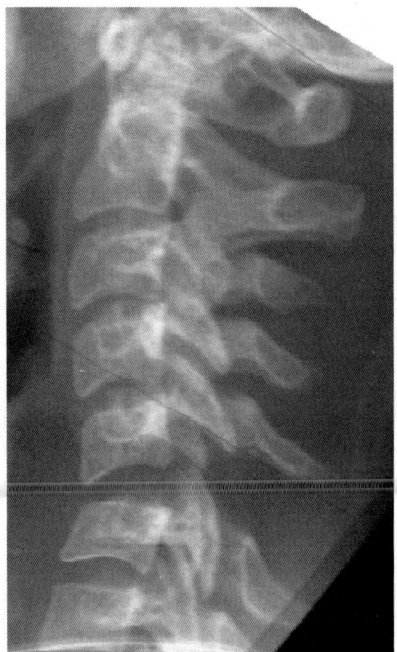 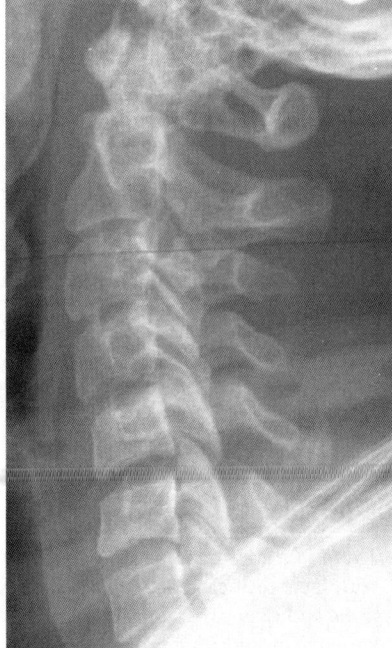

A   B   C

FIG 10 Reduction of C5–C6 bilateral facet dislocation. **A.** Injury film showing dislocated facets. **B.** Axial traction with slight flexion has been applied, and the facets are perched. **C.** Extension was applied at this point, resulting in reduction.

SURGICAL TREATMENT

- Facet dislocations represent unstable injuries, and surgical intervention should be strongly considered. A variety of situations can be encountered that necessitate different approaches to treatment **(FIG 11)**.
- If the dislocation is irreducible, the patient should be taken to the operating room for an open reduction and stabilization. An MRI should be obtained prior to going to the operating room in order to assess for a disc herniation and the need for an anterior discectomy prior to reduction.
- For anesthesia, awake fiberoptic intubation avoids excessive cervical extension and allows for a neurologic examination after intubation. Neurophysiologic baselines are recorded after the administration of general anesthesia as well as after prone positioning and shoulder taping.

We generally obtain prepositioning baselines in all patients, and it is required in neurologically intact patients or those with incomplete SCIs.
- Neurophysiologic spinal cord monitoring during open reduction is extremely helpful. If a change in neurologic status is detected, the reduction maneuver can readily be reversed, potentially avoiding permanent neurologic injury.
- Multimodality monitoring is preferred, including motor evoked potentials, somatosensory evoked potentials, and spontaneous electromyogram recordings.
- Large unilateral facet fractures (>1 cm in height, >40% of the absolute height of the intact lateral mass) can represent unstable injuries, these injuries may benefit from operative fixation. Recent studies have demonstrated that operative treatment provides more successful outcomes in terms of failure of treatment to maintain reduction.[12,22]

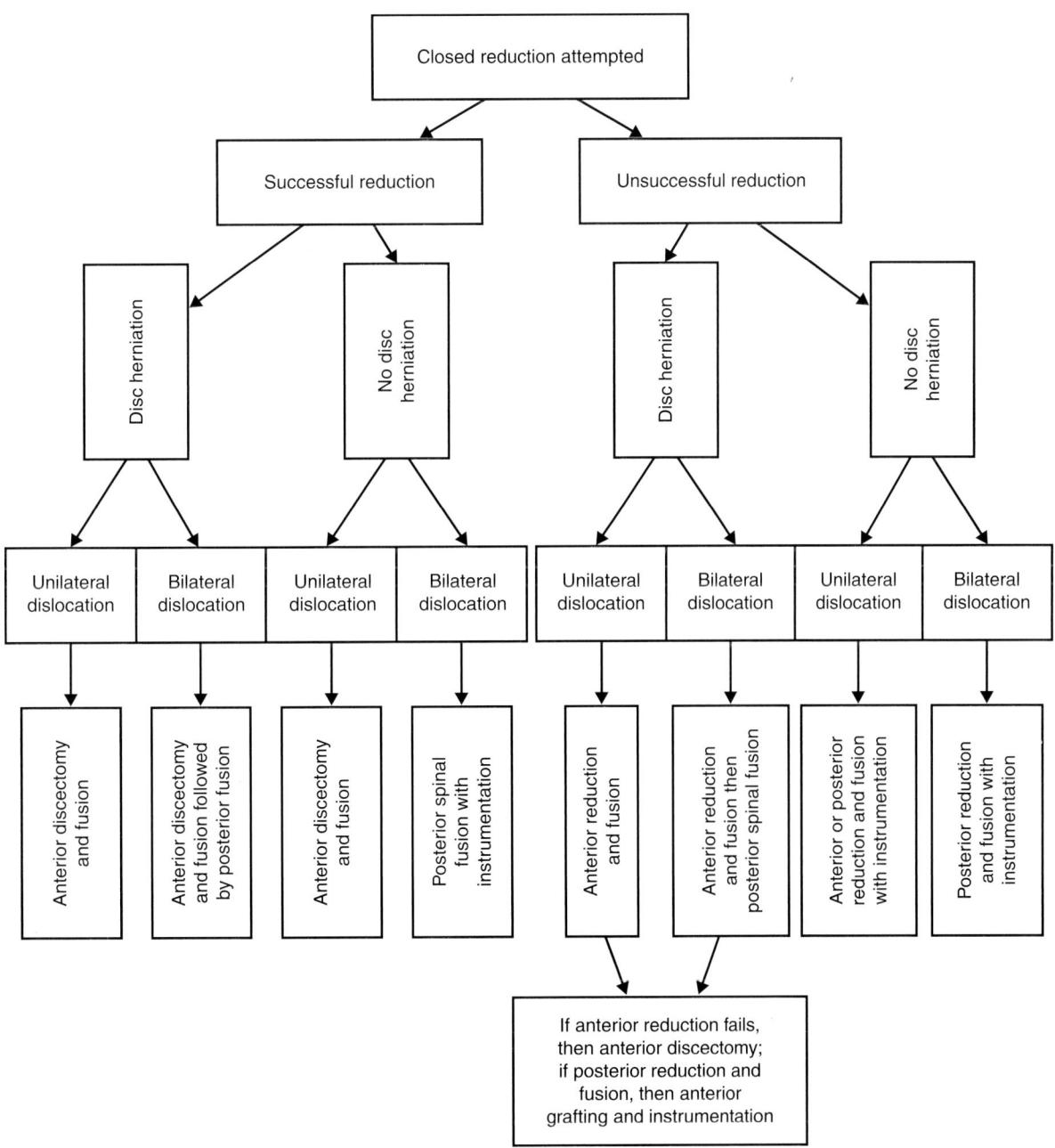

FIG 11 Algorithm for treatment of facet dislocations.

POSTERIOR OPEN REDUCTION

- If the dislocation is irreducible with closed methods and there is no significant disc herniation, a posterior open reduction is favored because it allows direct access to the dislocated facet joints (**TECH FIGS 3** and **4**).
- For prone positioning, the patient can remain in their halo ring or Mayfield tongs can be applied. The patient can then be rotated into the prone position on a Stryker frame or Jackson table. Traction can be applied during the rotation maneuver in order to increase stability.
- After prone positioning and establishment of neurophysiology baseline recordings, a standard subperiosteal dissection of the posterior cervical spine is performed.
- Care should be taken to avoid violating the facet capsules and interspinous ligaments of levels not involved in the intended fusion.
- The dislocated level can often be detected by a step-off between the spinous processes and the presence of hematoma and posterior ligamentous injury.
- Once the dislocation is identified clinically and/or radiographically, the lateral masses are exposed completely.
- The dislocation can be reduced by grasping the involved cephalad and caudal spinous process with a tenaculum or towel clip at the spinolaminar junction.
- The neurophysiologist should be warned of the possibility of an acute signal change. If any significant neurophysiologic changes are detected, the procedure should be halted.
- Axial caudal traction is applied to the caudal tenaculum. A gentle distraction and kyphotic moment is applied to the cephalad tenaculum to disengage the dislocated IAP.
- A rotational force may also be required for unilateral facet dislocations. The maneuver is applied until the IAP(s) of the cephalad vertebra is freed from the SAP(s) of the caudal vertebra.
- After disengaging the IAP(s), reduction can be obtained by applying cranial traction to the cranial vertebra until the IAP(s) clear the SAP. Caudal traction is then performed to reduce the IAP(s) posterior to the SAP(s).
- If this maneuver fails to achieve reduction, a Penfield or nerve hook along with the traction maneuvers can be used to lever the dislocated IAP over the SAP. Care must be taken to avoid fracturing the articular processes.
- The cranial edge of the SAP can also be trimmed using the burr in order to eliminate a barrier to reduction, although the surgeon should avoid overresection of the SAP as this decreases stability.
- Following reduction, lateral mass or pedicle screws are then placed in the standard fashion at the level of the dislocation. A one-level fusion can be performed if there is no soft tissue injury at the adjacent levels and the lateral masses are intact and allow for good screw purchase. If these criteria are not met, additional levels must be included in the fusion.
- Many surgeons use local bone and bone graft extender for the fusion, although autograft harvested from the iliac crest is widely used.
- To achieve anatomic alignment, compression can be applied across the lateral mass screws.

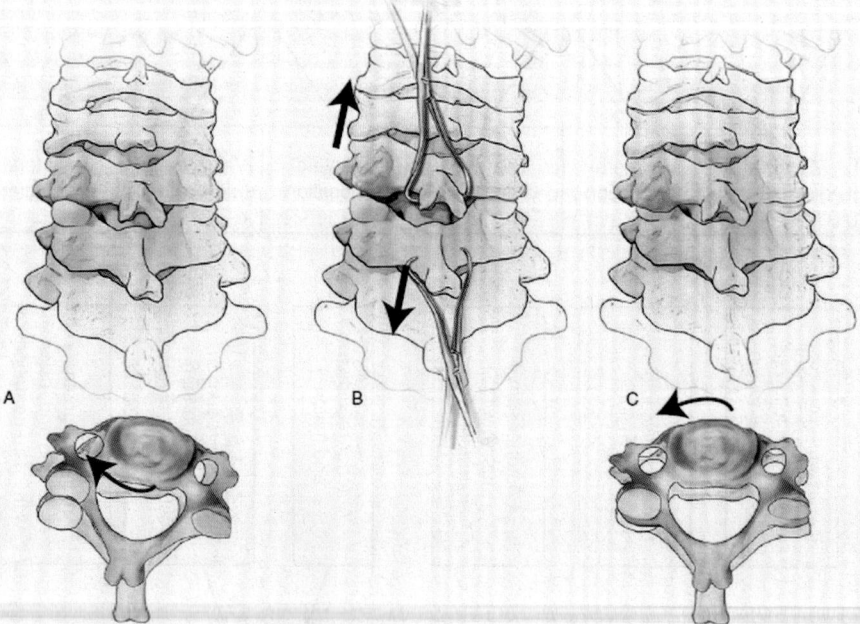

TECH FIG 3 A–C. Posterior open reduction technique for unilateral facet dislocation. Tenaculums can be used to apply rotational and flexion moments to unlock the facet followed by axial traction and reduction.

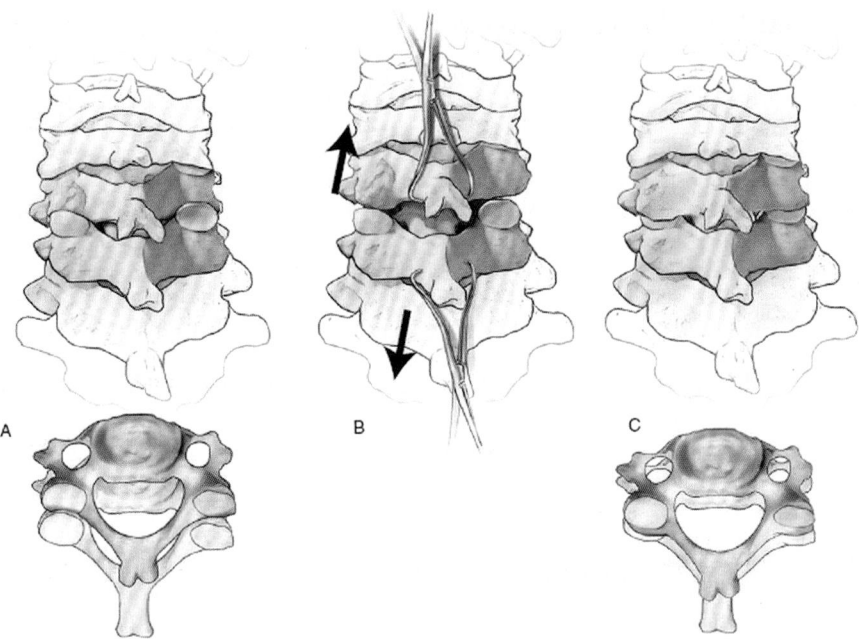

TECH FIG 4 A–C. Posterior open reduction technique for bilateral facet dislocation. Tenaculums can be used to unlock the facet joints with axial traction and slight flexion followed by extension to affect the reduction.

ANTERIOR OPEN REDUCTION

- Although posterior open reduction is generally preferred for unreducible facet dislocations, if a disc herniation is present, an initial anterior approach is required. If the dislocation can be reduced through an anterior approach following discectomy, a posterior procedure may be avoided.
- The patient is positioned supine with a shoulder roll and the head supported in slight extension on a gel roll.
- Plain x-ray or fluoroscopy is essential to monitor the reduction maneuver.
- A standard ACDF approach is used.
- Once adequate exposure had been obtained, a discectomy is performed along with resection of the PLL. A complete, aggressive discectomy prior to reduction is of paramount importance to reduce the risk of neurologic injury.
- Vertebral body pins (Caspar or equivalent devices) are placed into the vertebral bodies, diverging from each other approximately 10 to 20 degrees in order to produce a bending moment.
- Gently manipulating the pins into parallel orientation in the distraction device creates a flexion moment to unlock the facets. Subsequent distraction often results in perching of the facets.
- The cranial vertebral body is then translated dorsally with leverage through an interbody distractor or Cobb in order to obtain reduction. This can be done with simple manual manipulation of the distraction pins or by placing a Cobb under the inferior endplate of the dislocated vertebra and applying a gentle superoposterior force once the facets are perched. Clearly, care

must be taken to avoid overly aggressive reduction maneuvers or plunging into the spinal canal with the Cobb.
- In the case of a unilateral dislocation, the distraction pins should be applied with a divergent angle in the axial plane to accentuate the rotational deformity as traction is applied in order to unlock the facets. For example, if the right C5–C6 facet joint is dislocated, the C5 pin would be placed rotated toward the right (in the opposite direction that the C5 vertebra is rotated) such that a rotational moment will be applied that will help to unlock the dislocation after traction is applied. Once the facet is perched, manual pressure or a Cobb can be used to affect reduction.
- Following radiographic confirmation of reduction, an interbody structural bone graft and anterior plate are placed. In general, we prefer to use allograft in the traumatic setting to prevent creating a wound at the iliac crest harvest site that could be at higher risk for infection in the trauma population.
  - Autograft could be considered in patients at high risk for nonunion (ie, smokers).
- We use traditional fixed plates rather than dynamic plates when treating trauma patients because we are usually fixing a single level, and there is no evidence that dynamic plates improve fusion rates in single-level cases. In addition, if an anterior-only construct is performed, a dynamic plate could allow for collapse into kyphosis due to injury to the posterior ligamentous complex that accompanies these injuries.

TECHNIQUES

STABILIZATION FOLLOWING REDUCTION

- If a successful closed reduction is performed, the surgeon must determine what approach to use for stabilization (ie, anterior, posterior, or circumferential).
- Posterior fixation has been shown to be biomechanically superior to ACDF[26]; however, clinical results of ACDF have been shown to be equivalent to posterior fusion even for bilateral facet dislocations.[21] Posterior surgery is generally associated with more surgical morbidity and postoperative pain due to the stripping of the paraspinal muscles off the posterior elements.
- Circumferential fusion is certainly the strongest construct and is preferred for bilateral facet dislocations by some authors.

Additionally, it can avoid the need for multiple-level fusion, which is sometimes necessary if a posterior-only approach is used.

- If an anterior approach is necessary to remove herniated disc material, an ACDF is probably sufficient. Posterior fixation can also be added to improve the strength of the construct.
- If a posterior approach is needed to obtain reduction, posterior fixation alone is typically sufficient. An ACDF can also be performed to strengthen the construct.
- In cases where closed reduction is successful and there is no disc herniation, the approach is left to the surgeon's discretion.

TECHNIQUES

Pearls and Pitfalls

Closed Reduction	• Should be performed urgently, and prereduction MRI is not necessary in awake, alert, cooperative patients who can comply with a neurologic examination
Closed Reduction of Lower Cervical Spine Facet Dislocations	• Can sometimes require high amounts of weight (up to 140 lb), but efforts should be made to obtain a rapid closed reduction in order to decrease pressure on the cord and simplify surgical treatment
Preoperative MRI	• Always required to determine if a disc herniation is present
Open Reduction	• Much easier to perform via a posterior approach, although reduction with an anterior approach is technically feasible and often performed

OUTCOMES

- The neurologic status of the patient is the main determinant of outcome.
- Union rates following operative stabilization of facet dislocations are over 90%.[21]

COMPLICATIONS

- Neurologic deterioration during closed reduction or surgery is a feared complication. This risk can be minimized with frequent neurologic examinations in an awake, alert, cooperative patient during closed reduction and neurologic monitoring during surgery.
- Vertebral artery injuries occur occasionally. However, the majority are asymptomatic and treatment is controversial. For patients who are symptomatic, anticoagulation is an option, but the risks and benefits of anticoagulation in the presence of a spine injury must be weighed.
- Cervical SCI patients are at risk for many complications including deep venous thrombosis, decubitus ulcers, contractures, osteoporosis, and respiratory failure (particularly with higher SCI). Coordination of care with an SCI rehabilitation team is essential to avoid these and other complications.

REFERENCES

1. Allen BJ, Ferguson R, Lehman T, et al. A mechanistic classification of closed, indirect fractures and dislocations of the lower cervical spine. Spine (Phila Pa 1976) 1982;7(1):1–27.
2. Anderson L, D'Alonzo R. Fractures of the odontoid process of the axis. J Bone Joint Surg Am 1974;56(8):1663–1674.
3. Bracken M, Shepard M, Collins W, et al. A randomized, controlled trial of methylprednisolone or naloxone in the treatment of acute spinal-cord injury. Results of the Second National Acute Spinal Cord Injury Study. N Engl J Med 1990;322(20):1405–1411.
4. Bracken M, Shepard M, Holford T, et al. Administration of methylprednisolone for 24 or 48 hours or tirilazad mesylate for 48 hours in the treatment of acute spinal cord injury. Results of the Third National Acute Spinal Cord Injury Randomized Controlled Trial. National Acute Spinal Cord Injury Study. JAMA 1997;277(20):1597–1604.
5. Clark C, White AA III. Fractures of the dens. A multicenter study. J Bone Joint Surg Am 1985;67(9):1340–1348.
6. Frangen T, Zilkens C, Muhr G, et al. Odontoid fractures in the elderly: dorsal C1/C2 fusion is superior to halo-vest immobilization. J Trauma 2007;63(1):83–89.
7. Hadley MN, Walters BC, Grabb PA, et al. Blood pressure management after acute spinal cord injury. Neurosurgery 2002;50(3 suppl):S58–S62.
8. Haffajee M. A contribution by the ascending pharyngeal artery to the arterial supply of the odontoid process of the axis vertebra. Clin Anat 1997;10(1):14–18.

9. Hsu W, Anderson P. Odontoid fractures: update on management. J Am Acad Orthop Surg 2010;18(7):383–394.

10. Inamasu J, Guiot B. Vascular injury and complication in neurosurgical spine surgery. Acta Neurochir (Wien) 2006;148(4):375–387.

11. Julien T, Frankel B, Traynelis V, et al. Evidence-based analysis of odontoid fracture management. Neurosurg Focus 2000;8(6):e1.

12. Kepler CK, Vaccaro AR, Chen E, et al. Treatment of isolated cervical facet fractures: a systematic review. J Neurosurg Spine 2016;24(2): 347–354.

13. Kwon B, Vaccaro A, Grauer J, et al. Subaxial cervical spine trauma. J Am Acad Orthop Surg 2006;14(2):78–89.

14. Lebl DR, Bono CM, Velmahos G, et al. Vertebral artery injury associated with blunt cervical spine trauma: a multivariate regression analysis. Spine (Phila Pa 1976) 2013;38(16):1352–1361.

15. Lennarson P, Mostafavi H, Traynelis V, et al. Management of type II dens fractures: a case-control study. Spine (Phila Pa 1976) 2000;25(10):1234–1237.

16. Levine A, Dacre A. Traumatic spondylolisthesis of the axis. In: Clack CR, Benzel EC, eds. The Cervical Spine, ed 4. Philadelphia: Lippincott Williams & Wilkins, 2005:629–650.

17. Levine A, Edwards C. The management of traumatic spondylolisthesis of the axis. J Bone Joint Surg Am 1985;67(2):217–226.

18. Müller E, Wick M, Russe O, et al. Management of odontoid fractures in the elderly. Eur Spine J 1999;8(5):360–365.

19. Panjabi M, Simpson A, Ivancic P, et al. Cervical facet joint kinematics during bilateral facet dislocation. Eur Spine J 2007;16(10):1680–1688.

20. Przybylski G, Harrop J, Vaccaro A. Closed management of displaced type II odontoid fractures: more frequent respiratory compromise with posteriorly displaced fractures. Neurosurg Focus 2000;8(6):e5.

21. Razack N, Green B, Levi A. The management of traumatic cervical bilateral facet fracture-dislocations with unicortical anterior plates. J Spinal Disord 2000;13(5):374–381.

22. Spector LR, Kim DH, Affonso J, et al. Use of computed tomography to predict failure of nonoperative treatment of unilateral facet fractures of the cervical spine. Spine (Phila Pa 1976) 2006;31(24):2827–2835.

23. Starr J, Eismont F. Atypical hangman's fractures. Spine (Phila Pa 1976) 1993;18(14):1954–1957.

24. Tashjian R, Majercik S, Biffl W, et al. Halo-vest immobilization increases early morbidity and mortality in elderly odontoid fractures. J Trauma 2006;60(1):199–203.

25. Tobert DG, Le HV, Blucher JA, et al. The clinical implications of adding CT angiography in the evaluation of cervical spine fractures: a propensity-matched analysis. J Bone Joint Surg Am 2018;100:1490–1495.

26. Ulrich C, Woersdoerfer O, Kalff R, et al. Biomechanics of fixation systems to the cervical spine. Spine (Phila Pa 1976) 1991;16(3 suppl): S4–S9.

27. Vaccaro A, Falatyn S, Flanders A, et al. Magnetic resonance evaluation of the intervertebral disc, spinal ligaments, and spinal cord before and after closed traction reduction of cervical spine dislocations. Spine (Phila Pa 1976) 1999;24(12):1210–1217.

28. Vaccaro A, Madigan L, Baurle W, et al. Early halo immobilization of displaced traumatic spondylolisthesis of the axis. Spine (Phila Pa 1976) 2002;27(20):2229–2233.

29. Vives MJ, Garfin SR. Flexion injuries. In: Clark CR, ed. The Cervical Spine, ed 4. Philadelphia: Lippincott-Raven, 2005:660–670.

30. White A, Hashimoto R, Norvell D, et al. Morbidity and mortality related to odontoid fracture surgery in the elderly population. Spine (Phila Pa 1976) 2010;35(suppl 9):S146–S157.

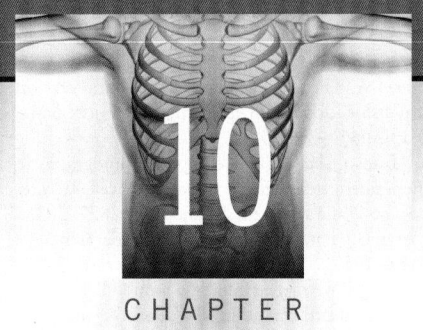

10

Minimally Invasive Posterior Cervical Laminoforaminotomy

Laura A. Snyder, S. Harrison Farber, Andrew Platt, Ernest J. Wright, and Richard G. Fessler

DEFINITION

- Cervical radiculopathy is a neurologic condition characterized by dysfunction of a cervical spinal nerve, the roots of the nerve, or both.
- It usually presents with unilateral pain that radiates from the neck to the arm and/or the hand.
- Patients may experience a combination of sensory loss, loss of motor function, and reflex changes in the affected nerve root distribution.
- This chapter focuses on minimally invasive posterior cervical laminoforaminotomy as a surgical treatment option for patients with cervical radiculopathy.

ANATOMY

- The external occipital protuberance (EOP) can be palpated in the midline of the skull. The superior nuchal line is the thickened ridge that extends laterally from the EOP (**FIG 1A**).
- The superficial fascia is located beneath the skin and subcutaneous fat of the posterior cervical spine (**FIG 1B**).
- Deep to the superficial fascia, structures are anatomically compartmentalized by an organized deep fascia and several interfascial planes (**FIG 2**).
- There are three principal fascial layers: a superficial, middle, and deep layer.
  - One layer is attached to the EOP, the superior nuchal line, the ligamentum nuchae, and the spinous processes of the cervical vertebrae; it divides to surround the trapezius.
  - The deep layer of the deep cervical fascia is attached to the ligamentum nuchae in the midline.
- The most superficial muscle on the posterior aspect of the neck is the trapezius, which arises from the EOP and the medial part of the superior nuchal line of the occipital bone, the spinous processes of C7–T1 through T12, the supraspinal ligament, and the ligamentum nuchae (**FIG 3**).
- The next muscle is the splenius capitis and arises from the ligamentum nuchae and spinous processes of C7 through T3 and inserts on the lateral portion of the superior nuchal line (see **FIG 1B**).
- The erector spinae lie deep in the cervical region and include the iliocostalis cervicis, the longissimus cervicis, the splenius cervicis, and the splenius capitis.
- The deep layer of the deep cervical musculature includes the semispinalis cervicis and the semispinalis capitis (see **FIG 1B**).
- The spinous process projects posteriorly from the junction of the laminae.

- The lateral mass forms at the junction of the lamina and pedicle and gives rise to the superior and inferior articular processes or facets (**FIG 4**).
- The superior facet at each level faces upward and posteriorly; the inferior facet faces downward and anteriorly.
- A superior facet articulates with the corresponding inferior facet of the vertebral body cephalad to form the osseous elements of the zygapophyseal joints.
- A vertebral notch is located on the superior and inferior aspect of each pedicle, such that adjacent notches contribute to the intervertebral foramen, through which the spinal nerve exits the spinal canal.
- The foramen is bound superiorly and inferiorly by the pedicle; posteriorly by the facets; and anteriorly by the intervertebral discs, uncovertebral joints, and vertebral bodies (**FIG 5**).
- The vertical diameter of the foramen is approximately 9 mm, the horizontal diameter is 4 mm, and the length ranges from 4 to 6 mm.
- Foramina exit at an angle of 45 degrees from the midsagittal plane.
- The spinal cord is cylindrical and slightly flattened in the anteroposterior (AP) direction and thus usually has a larger transverse than AP diameter.
- The spinal cord enlarges from C3 to C6 where it usually attains a maximal transverse diameter of 13 to 14 mm (**FIG 6**).
- In the lower cervical spine, the anterior and posterior root entry zones are located approximately one disc level higher than the corresponding intervertebral foramen through which will pass the nerve root formed from its rootlets.
- The rootlets pass obliquely laterally and caudally within the canal, entering the root sleeve where the sensory and motor roots are separated by the interradicular septum, a lateral extension of the dura mater.
- Each dorsal root presents an oval enlargement, the spinal ganglion, as it approaches or enters the intervertebral foramen.
- Just distal to this ganglion, the dorsal and ventral roots combine to form a spinal nerve.
- The cervical nerve root occupies one-third of the foraminal space in a normal spine, usually the inferior aspect, with the superior aspect being filled with fat and associated veins.
- The ventral (motor) roots emerge from the dura mater more caudally than the dorsal (sensory) roots, and the ventral roots course along the caudal border of the dorsal roots within the intervertebral foramina.
- Thus, compression of the ventral roots, dorsal roots, or both depends on the anatomic structures around the nerve roots, such as a prolapsed disc (ventral root compression) or osteophytes from the facet joint (dorsal root compression).

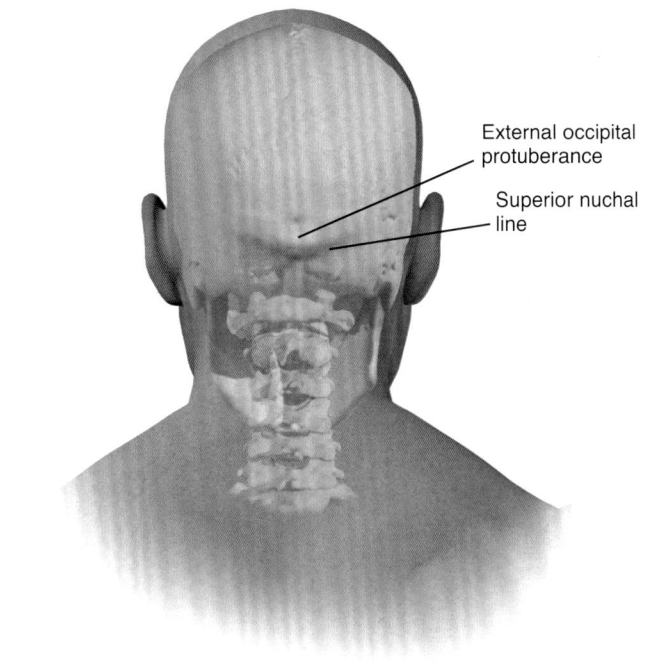

External occipital
protuberance

Superior nuchal
line

A

Internal jugular vein and
the carotid artery

Scalenus anterior

Scalenus medius

Levator scapula

Trapezius

Semispinalis
colli

Semispinalis
capitis

Splenia capita

B

FIG 1 A. Superficial anatomic landmarks of the posterior cervical spine. **B.** Cross-sectional anatomy of the posterior cervical spine: superficial fascial layer (*blue*) and the muscles underneath.

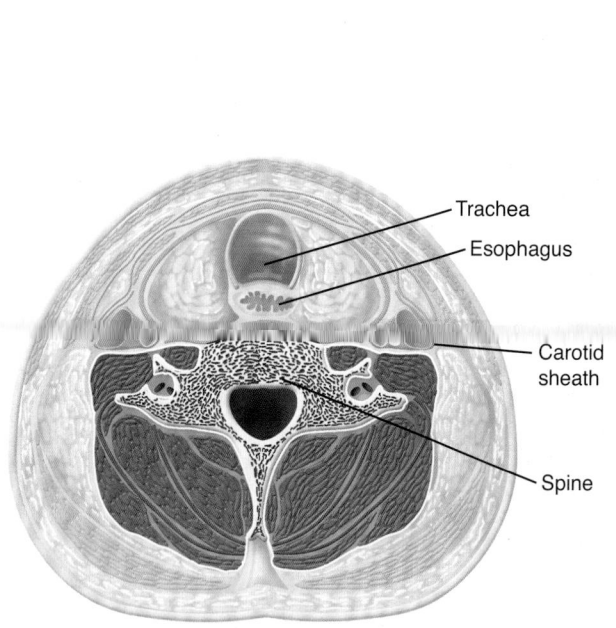

FIG 2 Cross-sectional anatomy of the posterior cervical spine: deep fascial layer (*blue*) and the muscles underneath.

Trachea

Esophagus

Carotid sheath

Spine

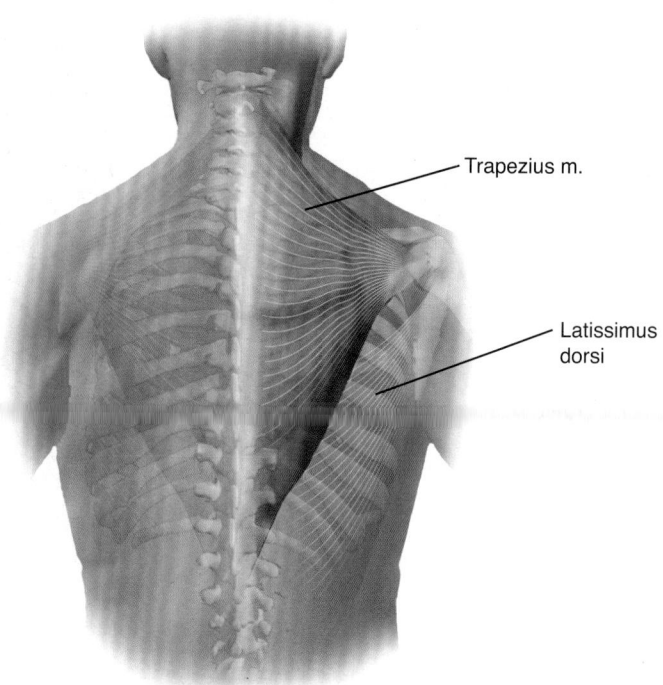

FIG 3 Trapezius muscle anatomy and its insertion points.

Trapezius m.

Latissimus dorsi

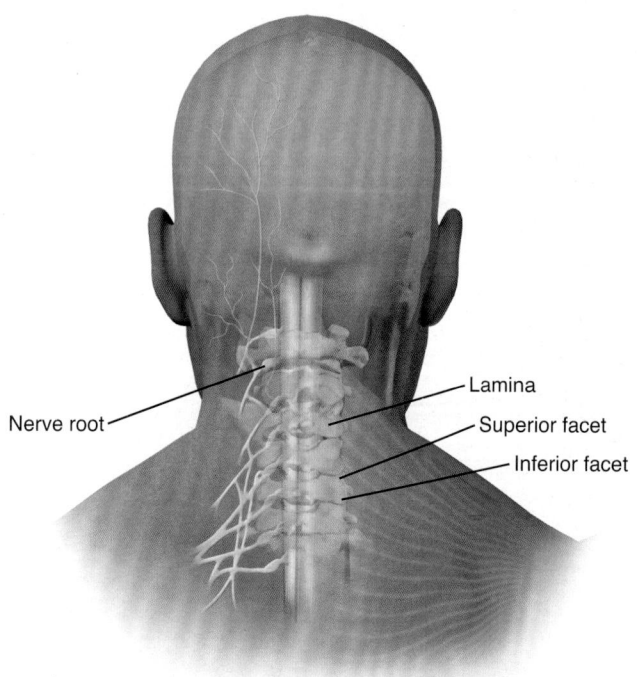

FIG 4 Bone anatomy of the posterior cervical spine demonstrating the relationships of the superior and inferior facets, the lamina, and the exiting nerve roots.

Nerve root

Lamina

Superior facet

Inferior facet

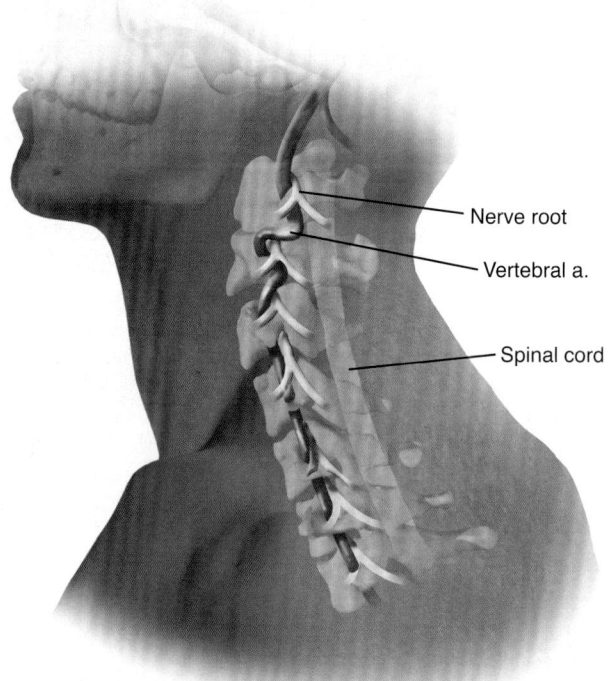

FIG 5 Lateral view of cervical spine depicting the exiting nerve roots and vertebral artery within the region of the neural foramen.

Nerve root

Vertebral a.

Spinal cord

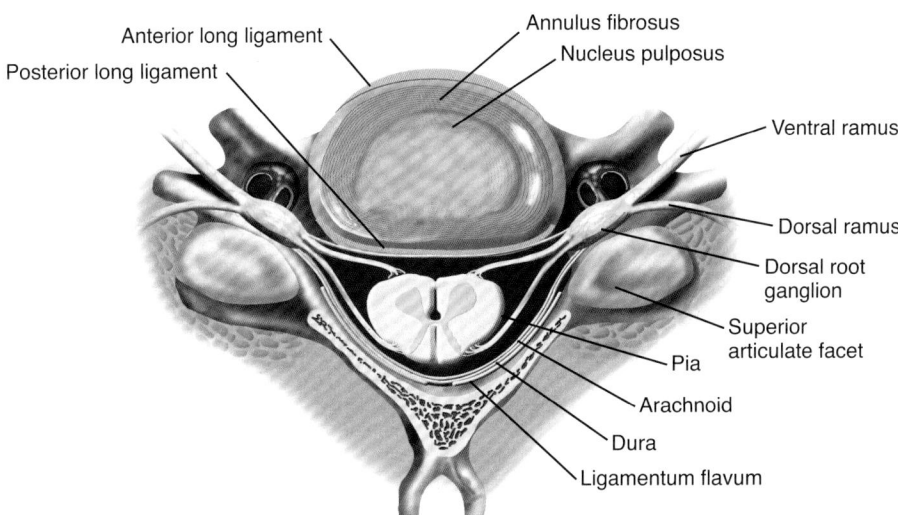

FIG 6 Cross-sectional anatomy of the cervical spine.

- The most likely site of compression of the radicular nerve is at the entrance zone of the intervertebral foramen because the medial entrance zone of the foramen is smaller in diameter than the lateral exit zone, whereas the nerve roots are widest at their takeoff from the central thecal sac and become more narrow laterally.
- Nerves C2–C7 exit above the correspondingly numbered vertebrae.
- The C8 nerve root exits the intervertebral foramen formed between C7 and T1.
- The dorsal root ganglion is usually located between the vertebral artery and the superior articular process.
- In the sagittal plane, cervical nerve roots C3–C8 in the intervertebral foramina lie midway between the posterior midpoints of the lateral masses situated an average of 5.5 mm above or below each lateral mass point.
- Thus, cervical nerve roots enter their intervertebral foramina and leave the spinal canal at the level of the disc and above the pedicle of the same numbered level, except for C8, which exits above the T1 pedicle.
- The vertebral artery enters the transverse foramen of C6 and ascends through the transverse foramen to the level of the atlas.
- In this region, it lies just in front of (ventral) to the ventral rami of cervical nerves C2–C6 and is surrounded by a venous plexus and sympathetic nerve fibers.
- The transverse interforaminal distance and thus the transverse distance between vertebral arteries at the same cervical level increase slightly from C3 to C6.

PATHOGENESIS

- The most common cause of cervical radiculopathy is foraminal compression of the spinal nerve.
- Contributing factors include disc herniations and bulges, decreased disc height, degenerative changes of the uncovertebral joints anteriorly, and the zygapophyseal joints posteriorly **(FIG 7A–D)**.

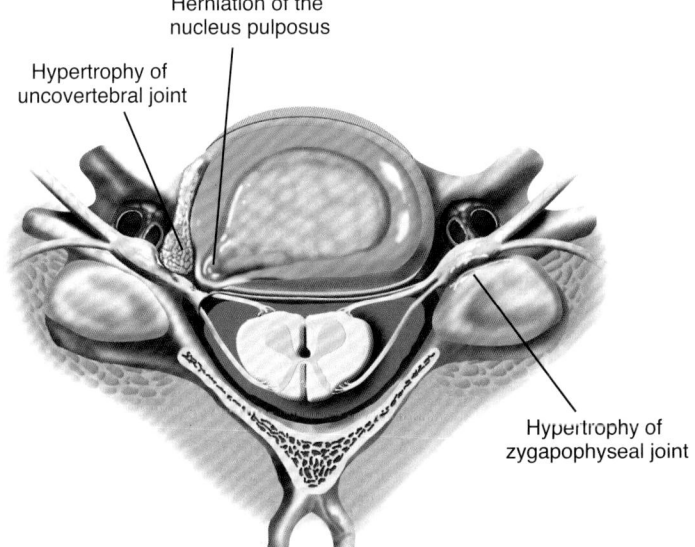

FIG 7 A. Cross-sectional anatomy of the cervical spine depicting several pathologic states: hypertrophy of the uncovertebral joints, hypertrophy of zygapophyseal joints, and herniation of the nucleus pulposus. *(continued)*

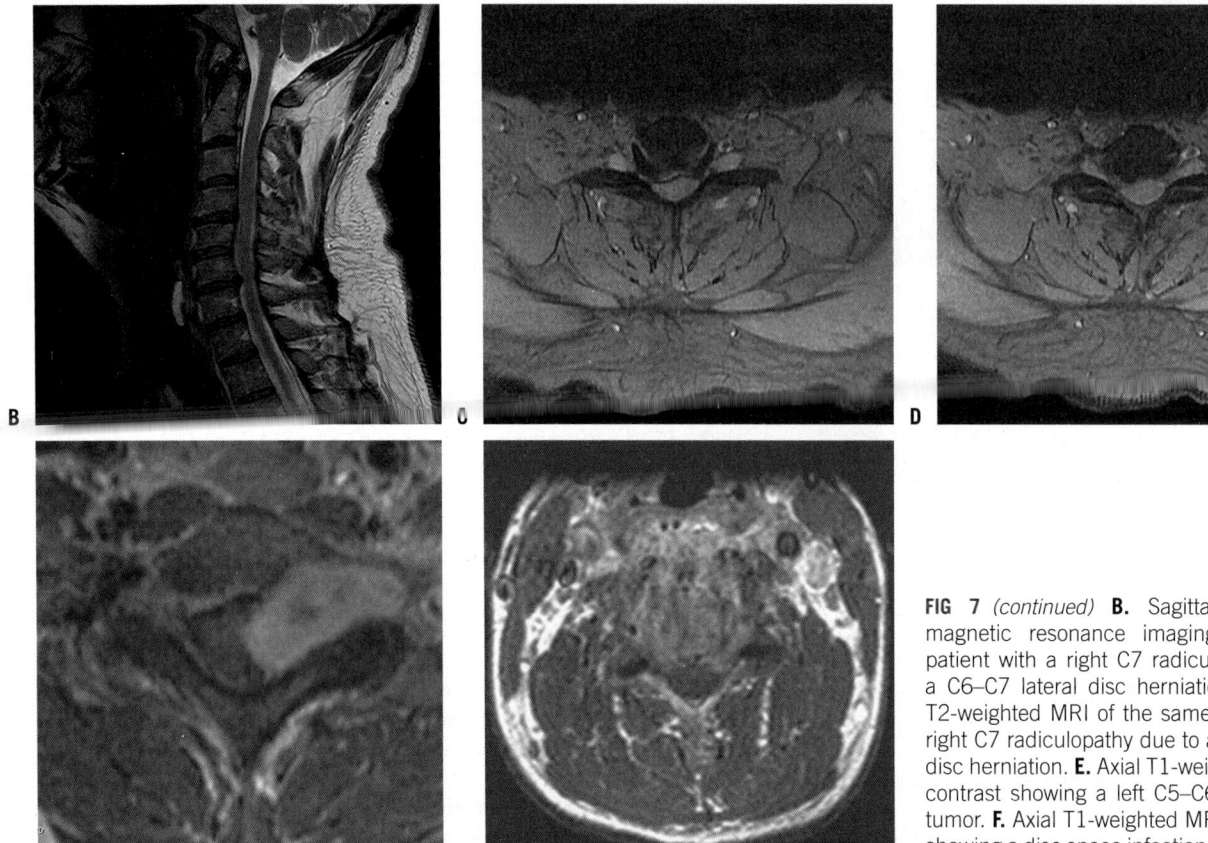

FIG 7 (continued) **B.** Sagittal T2-weighted magnetic resonance imaging (MRI) of a patient with a right C7 radiculopathy due to a C6–C7 lateral disc herniation. **C,D.** Axial T2-weighted MRI of the same patient with a right C7 radiculopathy due to a C6–C7 lateral disc herniation. **E.** Axial T1-weighted MRI with contrast showing a left C5–C6 nerve sheath tumor. **F.** Axial T1-weighted MRI with contrast showing a disc space infection with left foraminal epidural abscess.

- Other rare causes include tumors and spinal infections **(FIG 7E,F).**
- Normal disc itself does not contain nociceptive nerve fibers and is insensitive to pain.
- When the nucleus pulposus ruptures through the annulus fibrosus, there is little or no localized pain until nociceptive fibers of the sinuvertebral nerves in the lateral posterior ligament and the dura of the nerve root sleeves are stimulated.
- This stimulation generates localized back and neck pain.
- In cases of cervical spondylosis, vertebral bodies subside and lose height, and the ligamentum flavum and facet joint capsule tend to fold, which further decreases foraminal dimensions.
- Some have postulated that nerve root compression by itself does not always lead to pain and note that the dorsal root ganglion must also be compressed before pain is felt.[11]
  - Mechanical distortion of the nerve root leads to a cascade of events in the microenvironment of the nerve.
- Hypoxia of the nerve root and dorsal ganglion can aggravate the effect of compression.
- Evidence indicates that inflammatory mediators—including matrix metalloproteinases, prostaglandin E, interleukin-6, substance P, and nitric oxide—are released by herniated cervical intervertebral discs.
  - These observations underlie the reason that anti-inflammatory agents often suffice to treat the radicular pain.

NATURAL HISTORY

- Cervical radiculopathy occurs annually in 85 out of 100,000 people.
- It is estimated that 75% to 90% of patients with acute cervical radiculopathy due to disc herniation will improve without surgery.
- In a 1994 population-based study from Rochester, Minnesota, 26% of patients with cervical radiculopathy underwent surgery within 3 months of the diagnosis (typically for the combination of radicular pain, sensory loss, and muscle weakness), whereas the remainder were treated medically.
  - Recurrence, defined as the reappearance of symptoms of radiculopathy after a symptom-free interval of at least 6 months, occurred in 32% of patients during a median follow-up of 4.9 years. At the last follow-up, 90% of the nonoperated patients had normal findings or were only mildly incapacitated owing to cervical radiculopathy.

PATIENT HISTORY AND PHYSICAL FINDINGS

- Patients with cervical radiculopathy exhibit the hallmark symptoms of unilateral neck and/or arm pain, sensory disturbances, and possibly motor deficits **(TABLE 1).**
- Central to the patient's history are descriptors that include location, onset, duration, severity, associated symptoms, and triggers.

TABLE 1   Distribution of Cervical Disc Herniations and Anatomic Correlates

Level	Percentage of Cervical Disc Herniations	Compressed Root	Muscles Affected	Sensory Region	Reflex
C4–C5	2%–5%	C5	Deltoid	Shoulder	Deltoid and pectoralis
C5–C6	15%–20%	C6	Forearm flexion	Upper arm, thumb, radial forearm	Biceps and brachioradialis
C6–C7	65%–70%	C7	Triceps and forearm extenders	2nd and 3rd fingers	Triceps
C7–T1	10%	C8	Hand intrinsics	4th and 5th fingers	Finger jerk

- Pain is most prominent in acute cervical radiculopathy, and it may be described as sharp, electric, achy, or burning.
- Pain can be located in the neck, shoulder, arm, or chest, depending on the nerve root involved.
- Classically, a patient with an acute radiculopathy presents with pain radiating in a myotomal distribution.
- Sensory symptoms, predominantly paresthesias and numbness, are more common than motor loss and diminished reflexes.
- The clinician should keep in mind that the sensory symptoms frequently do not follow classic dermatomal patterns, as there is normal anatomic variation from individual to individual **(FIG 8)**.
- For patients with acute cervical radiculopathy, arm pain is present in nearly 100%, sensory deficits in 85%, neck pain in 79%, reflex deficits in 71%, motor deficits in 68%, scapular pain in 52%, anterior chest pain in 17%, headaches in 9%, anterior chest and arm pain in 5%, and left-sided chest and arm pain in 1%.
- Radicular pain is often accentuated by maneuvers that stretch the involved nerve root, such as coughing, sneezing, Valsalva, and certain cervical movements and positions.

- The Spurling test is performed by maximally extending and rotating the neck toward the involved side **(FIG 9)**.
- When positive, this test is particularly useful in differentiating cervical radiculopathy from other etiologies of upper extremity pain, such as peripheral nerve entrapment disorders, because the maneuver stresses only the structures within the cervical spine.
- It is important to note that the physical examination can be normal in patients with cervical radiculopathy.
- The presence of "red flags" in the patient's history (including fever, chills, unexplained weight loss, unremitting night pain, previous cancer, immunosuppression, or intravenous drug use) should alert clinicians to the possibility of more serious disease such as tumor or infection.

IMAGING AND OTHER DIAGNOSTIC STUDIES

Plain Films

- Plain films offer the advantage of showing the spinal column in a weight-bearing state.

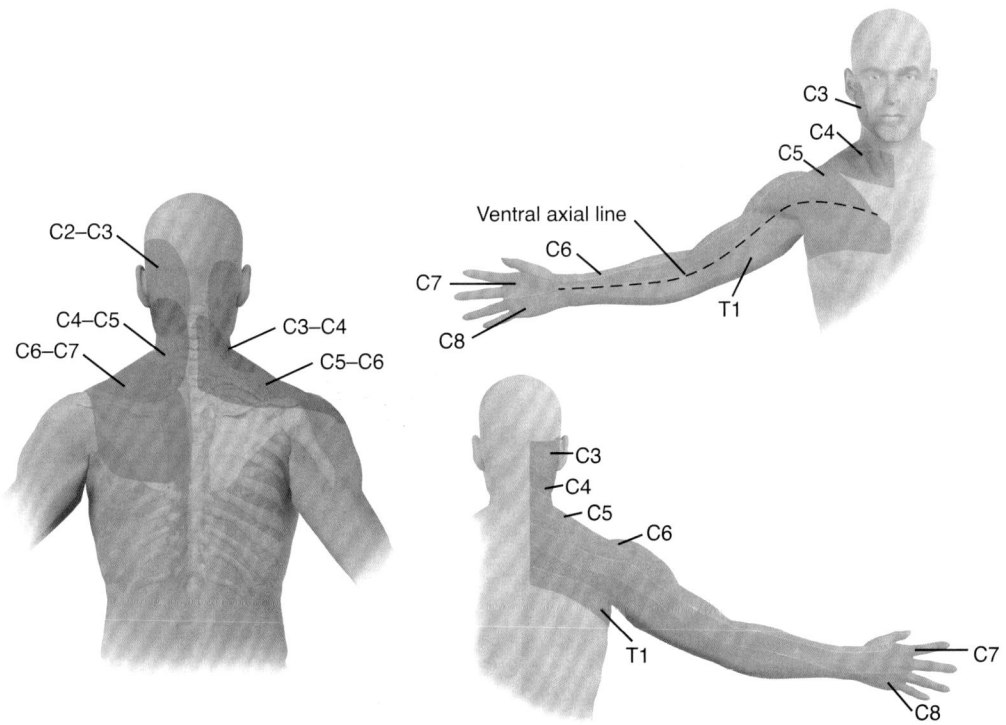

FIG 8 Cervical dermatomes and sites of sensory symptoms.

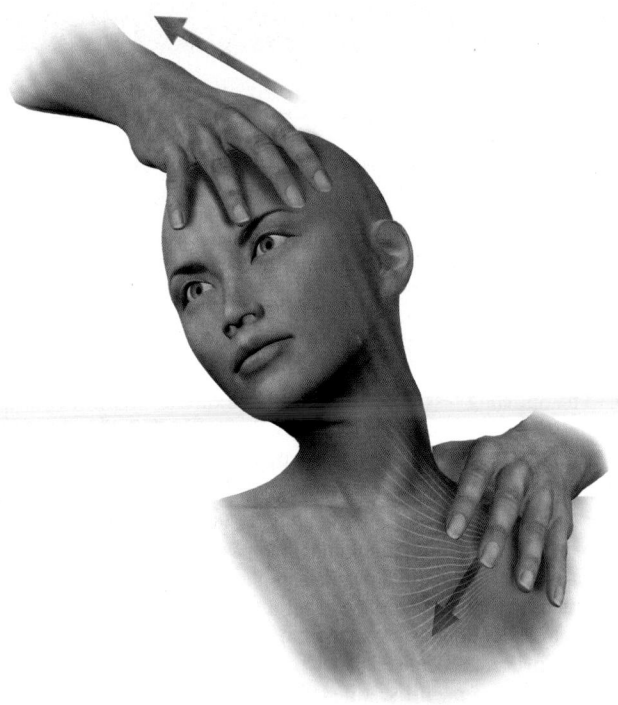

FIG 9 Spurling maneuver.

- Degenerative changes on plain radiographs become more prevalent as individuals age.
  - However, it has been shown that degenerative changes are present in both symptomatic and asymptomatic individuals.
- Radiographs are inexpensive, readily available, and provide information regarding sagittal balance, congenital abnormalities, fractures, deformity, and instability.
- Flexion–extension lateral cervical spine radiographs can reveal instability that may be the cause of intermittent or positional symptoms.
- Standing scoliosis films allow the surgeon to assess the overall global alignment of the spine.

Myelography

- Changes in the contrast-filled spinal canal can serve as an indirect measure of neural compression.
- The major disadvantage of plain myelography is its invasive nature.
- Accuracy rates for cervical myelography in the diagnosis of clinical nerve root compression range between 67% and 92% when compared with intraoperative findings.
- Myelography is associated with few false-positive results, a 15% false-negative rate, and an overall accuracy rate of 85% in a study of 53 patients who had surgical confirmation of the cervical spine pathology.
- See the Exam Table for Spine at the back of the book for methods for examining the cervical spine for nerve root syndromes.

Computed Tomography

- Computed tomography (CT) allows for the direct visualization of pathology causing compression of neural structures.
- CT also has a high-spatial resolution and is especially helpful in visualizing the foraminal region.

- Another important advantage of CT is that it can distinguish neural compression caused by soft tissue from compression related to bony structures such as facet hypertrophy.
- The main disadvantage of CT is the partial volume averaging effect and streak artifacts.
  - These can cause distortion of images, particularly at the lower cervical levels, or in individuals with wide shoulders.
- The reported accuracy of CT of the cervical spine ranges from 72% to 91%.
- By combining myelography with CT, the diagnostic accuracy approaches 96%.
- CT angiography may be considered to evaluate for an anomalous course of the vertebral artery.

Magnetic Resonance Imaging

- Magnetic resonance imaging (MRI) can detect neural structures directly and noninvasively.
- The accurate assessment of disc herniations and spinal stenosis is due to the intrinsic contrast and good spatial resolution.
- MRI correctly predicts 88% of the lesions as opposed to 81% for CT myelography, 57% for plain myelography, and 50% for CT.
- Disc herniations are commonly observed on MRI of asymptomatic individuals.
- Disc herniations may be observed in 10% of asymptomatic people younger than 40 years of age and 5% of those older than 40 years of age.
- Degenerative disc disease may be observed in 25% of asymptomatic people younger than 40 years of age and 60% of those older than 40 years of age.
- Therefore, the imaging findings should be carefully correlated with the neurologic examination.

Electrodiagnostic Studies

- Electrodiagnostic studies identify physiologic abnormalities of the nerve root and rule out other neurologic causes of the patient's symptoms.
- However, in patients with well-defined radiculopathy and good imaging correlation, the pain and added expense of electrodiagnostic studies are usually not justified.
- The electrodiagnostic study has two parts: the nerve conduction velocity (NCV) and the needle electrode examination (electromyography [EMG]).
- The NCV study is performed to exclude peripheral nerve pathology.
- The EMG is performed by analyzing multiple muscles within the same myotome and in adjacent myotomes.
- The presence of fibrillation potentials and positive sharp waves at rest is indicative of denervation, but these changes may not occur until 3 weeks after the onset of neural injury.
- Abnormalities are noted in the paraspinal musculature before they become apparent in the appendicular muscles.
- The EMG may be normal in the presence of mild radiculopathy or a predominantly sensory radiculopathy and is less likely to be positive in patients with no demonstrable weakness.
- NCV studies and EMG have been shown to be useful in diagnosing nerve root dysfunction and distinguishing cervical radiculopathy from other lesions that are unclear on physical examination.
- These studies also correlate well with findings on myelography and surgery.

DIFFERENTIAL DIAGNOSIS

- Carpal tunnel syndrome
- Cubital tunnel syndrome
- Anterior interosseous syndrome
- Posterior interosseous syndrome
- Suprascapular nerve entrapment
- Infection (discitis, osteomyelitis, epidural abscess)
- Primary bone neoplasm
- Nerve sheath tumor
- Metastatic disease (epidural and/or bony element)
- Inflammatory arthropathy
- Cervical facet syndrome
- Peripheral brachial plexus nerve tumor
- Acute brachial neuritis (Parsonage-Turner syndrome)
- Cervical sprain/strain injuries
- Disorders of rotator cuff and shoulder
- Thoracic outlet syndrome
- Herpes zoster
- Pancoast tumor
- Sympathetically mediated syndromes
- Myocardial infarction/angina

NONOPERATIVE MANAGEMENT

- Activity modification
  - Patients should be educated regarding the cause of their pain and basic activity modifications that may improve it.
  - Simple activity modifications to keep the head and neck in a midline and unflexed position may minimize stress on the cervical spine and thereby relieve pain and reduce root compression.
  - The effectiveness of these measures, however, is unproven.[21] Cervical orthoses (or collars) sometimes are recommended for this same purpose but should be used for less than 1 to 2 weeks, given the counterproductive effects of prolonged immobilization.
  - Patients are generally advised to avoid lifting objects greater than 5 to 10 lb during an acute stage of cervical radiculopathy.
- Physical therapy
  - Core strengthening of neck musculature
  - Arm and hand exercises
  - Cervical traction
- Medications
  - Nonsteroidal anti-inflammatory drugs (NSAIDs) and acetaminophen generally are the medications recommended most frequently early in the course of radiculopathy.
  - NSAIDs are believed to reduce the inflammatory response that may underlie the pain in these conditions. These agents have the potential for renal and gastric toxicity.
  - Toxicity risks are important to remember in high-risk patients (eg, the elderly or those treated with anticoagulants).
    - Coadministration of gastric protective agents, such as proton pump inhibitors, may be needed.
  - Steroids often are used in the acute period of radiculopathy as a pulse treatment.
  - Many regimens are described, but generally, an initial oral dose (approximately 1 mg/kg of ideal body weight daily) is followed by a tapered reduction over 2 to 3 weeks.
    - Steroids are associated with adverse effects, such as impaired glycemic control, worsening hypertension, and gastritis, but short-term use generally results in few long-term complications.
- Epidural injections
  - Few randomized clinical trials are available and those available generally do not provide assessment with validated outcome measures.
  - Multiple studies suggest that epidural injections may be beneficial, with decreased pain reported in up to 60% of patients.
    - These procedures may have significant complications, although the current use of fluoroscopic guidance may minimize the risk.

SURGICAL MANAGEMENT

- The primary indication for a posterior cervical foraminotomy is unilateral cervical radiculopathy that can be correlated to radiographic findings of a lateral herniated cervical disc or cervical foraminal stenosis.
- Open posterior cervical foraminotomy was historically the treatment for foraminal stenosis.
- Advances in the anterior approach to cervical disease made the anterior cervical discectomy and fusion (ACDF) the preferred method for spine surgeons.
- The anterior cervical approach is allowed for decreased muscle injury, decreased postoperative pain, and decreased length of stay as compared to the classic open posterior foraminotomy.[3,8,23]
- Many studies have shown that posterior cervical foraminotomy is still a highly effective treatment option.[4,7,8,17]
- Posterior cervical laminoforaminotomy has been shown to provide symptomatic relief in 92% to 97% of these patients.[8]
- Other indications for cervical foraminotomy include multilevel foraminal narrowing without central stenosis, persistent radicular symptoms after ACDF, and patients with relative contraindications for anterior cervical surgery (infection, prior radiation, multiple anterior surgeries).
- However, the posterior open procedure has several major drawbacks. These include the need for extensive subperiosteal stripping of the paraspinal musculature. This approach-related morbidity leads to significant postoperative pains and muscle spasms. This pain and dysfunction can be debilitating in 18% to 60% of patients.[6,10,21]
- Compared with an ACDF, several key advantages to the posterior approach include the direct visualization of the lateral cervical spinal cord and exiting cervical nerve root. The nerve root can be followed out into the neuroforamen, and the source of compression can be directly visualized and addressed. The posterior approach also avoids complications related to anterior cervical approaches such as esophageal injury, dysphagia, or recurrent laryngeal nerve palsy.[20]
- The other significant advantage of the posterior approach is the preservation of motion segments in the cervical spine. This approach does not destabilize the facet joints. This is especially important in young patients and athletes. In the elderly population, by avoiding a fusion, the risk of accelerated degenerative changes at the levels above and below the pathologic segment (adjacent level disease) can be avoided as well.[6,26]
- The posterior cervical minimally invasive laminoforaminotomy and discectomy are minimally invasive approaches that were developed to exploit the advantages of a posterior

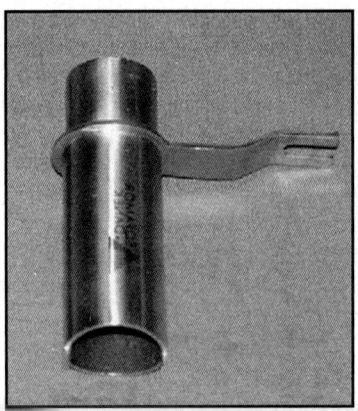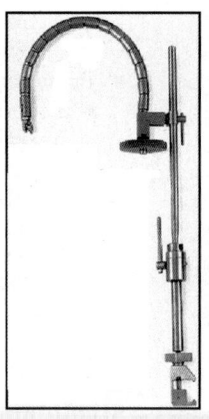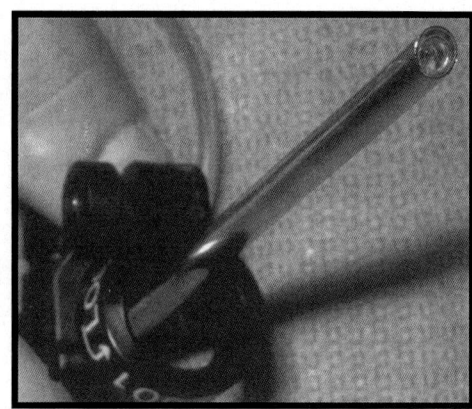

FIG 10 The METRx system of endoscopic retractors, camera, and instruments for our microendoscopic foraminotomy procedures.

cervical decompression while minimizing the approach-related morbidity. This procedure can be performed with the use of a microscope or a microendoscope.

- Advantages of the minimally invasive posterior approach compared to the open approach include decreases in operative time, blood loss, hospital length of stay, and postoperative pain.[1,5,16,24]
- The major contraindication for posterior cervical minimally invasive laminoforaminotomy and discectomy is the presence of a large central herniated disc causing symptoms of radiculopathy.
- Using a posterior approach, the cervical cord cannot be retracted to adequately address a central pathology. The anterior approach is favored when there is clinical evidence of myelopathy in the setting of a central pathology.
- Other major contraindications include cervical segmental instability or a kyphotic cervical deformity. Other relative contraindications include patients with primary symptom of axial neck pain and patients with foraminal stenosis due to ventral osteophytes.[2]

Preoperative Planning

- A complete history and physical examination identifies patients with probable cervical pathology.
- Acute onset of symptoms, report of pain or paresthesias in a dermatomal distribution, and weakness are good historical clues that nerve root compression may exist.
- If this history is corroborated on examination by findings of weakness, decreased sensation, presence of the Spurling sign, or diminished reflexes in a specific nerve root distribution, there is high clinical suspicion of root compression.
- It is paramount to exclude the presence of myelopathy (hyperreflexia, ataxia, presence of upper motor signs), which would suggest spinal stenosis and not root pathology.
- Plain cervical spine radiographs with flexion and extension views are essential for beginning the evaluation process.
- Oblique views are sometimes helpful in correlating foraminal stenosis with clinical symptoms.
- These radiography studies reveal areas of foraminal stenosis, significant osteophytes, and the presence of spinal instability.
- A cervical spine MRI is next used to look for any disc herniations or foraminal stenosis and to exclude the presence of central stenosis.

- In patients with previous cervical surgery in whom hardware was implanted or in patients whose clinical history and examination findings do not correlate with MRI findings, a CT myelogram of the cervical spine is warranted.
- MRI is notorious for inadequately showing the degree of compression from osteophytes—these can be clearly seen on CT myelograms.
- The senior author employs the METRx system (Medtronic, Dublin, Ireland) of endoscopic retractors, camera, and instruments for the microendoscopic foraminotomy procedure (**FIG 10**).

Positioning

- The patient is placed under general endotracheal anesthesia in the standard fashion. Throughout the procedure, somatosensory evoked potentials and myotomal EMG monitoring are used to monitor the spinal cord. An arterial line and a precordial Doppler may be used as well.
- The patient's head is secured in the three-point Mayfield head clamp.
- The patient is positioned in a semisitting position with the head slightly flexed. All extremities are carefully padded, and the neck is once again examined to ensure adequate venous drainage (**FIG 11A**).
  - This position significantly reduces the blood loss and allows for better visualization of the affected stenosis and disc pathology.
  - The semisitting position is contraindicated in patients with a patent foramen ovale.
- Alternatively, the patient may be placed in the prone position, and a microscope instead of a microendoscope can be used. The head may be secured with the Mayfield clamp or with Gardner-Wells tongs. Patients can be placed in reverse Trendelenburg position to decrease venous bleeding. If the patient is well taped to the bed, the bed can be turned to improve visualization.
- The organization of the microendoscopic operating room is as follows:
  - The anesthesiologist is located to the left of the operating table; the scrub table, fluoroscopic monitor, and video cart are on the right side (**FIG 11B**).
  - The fluoroscopy unit is brought in from the right side as well.

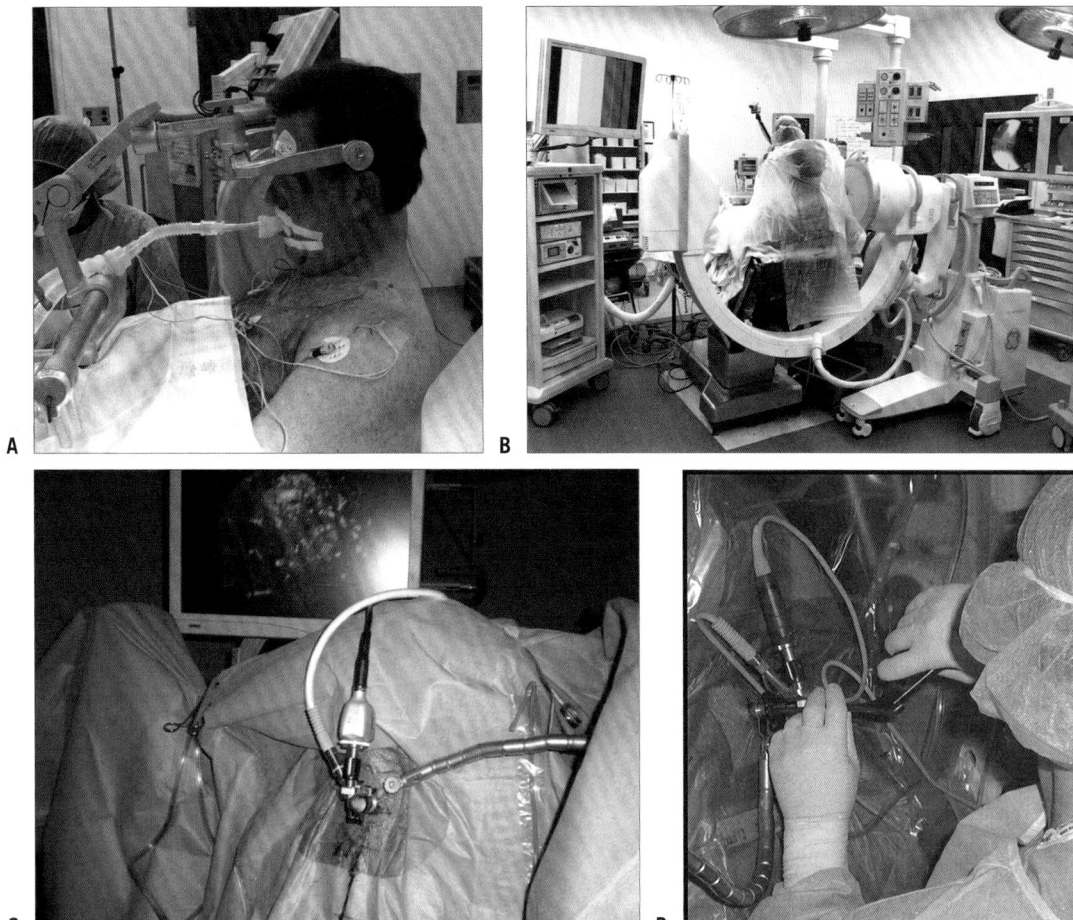

FIG 11 A. Intraoperative picture of the patient in the Mayfield three-point fixation device and the sitting position. **B.** Intraoperative picture of the operating room setup. **C.** Intraoperative picture showing the operative field with the sterile drape over the C-arm and the surgeon's operating screen in view. **D.** Example of this operative arrangement with a close-up view of the endoscopic apparatus in place, as it would appear during the procedure.

- The C-arm is brought either over or under the patient's head, according to the surgeon's preference.
- Suction canisters and a Bovie unit are generally located at the patient's feet.
- The Midas drill is placed on a sterile Mayo stand on the left side behind the patient.
- We use a standard blue sterile drape, similar to the one used for routine hip surgery, to create our surgical field **(FIG 11C,D)**.
- A single dose of antibiotics (either cefazolin or vancomycin) is routinely given before skin incision.
- Intravenous steroids are not routinely administered.
- A central venous line is usually not required because of the quick nature of the procedure.
- A Foley catheter is generally not needed.
- A C-arm fluoroscopic image is taken to identify the correct operative level.

Approach

- Traditionally, the posterior cervical laminoforaminotomy is performed via a midline incision in the region of interest.
- This approach, typically referred to as an *open technique*, requires an incision long enough such that the exposure can be carried laterally to the facet complex.
- The paraspinal muscles are then stripped from the spinous process, which requires violation of their ligamentous attachments to the midline. The muscular attachments are also stripped from their position on the bony elements of the facet capsule, spinous process, and lamina.
- To achieve this amount of muscular retraction, it is necessary to mobilize muscles above and below the targeted region **(FIG 12)**.

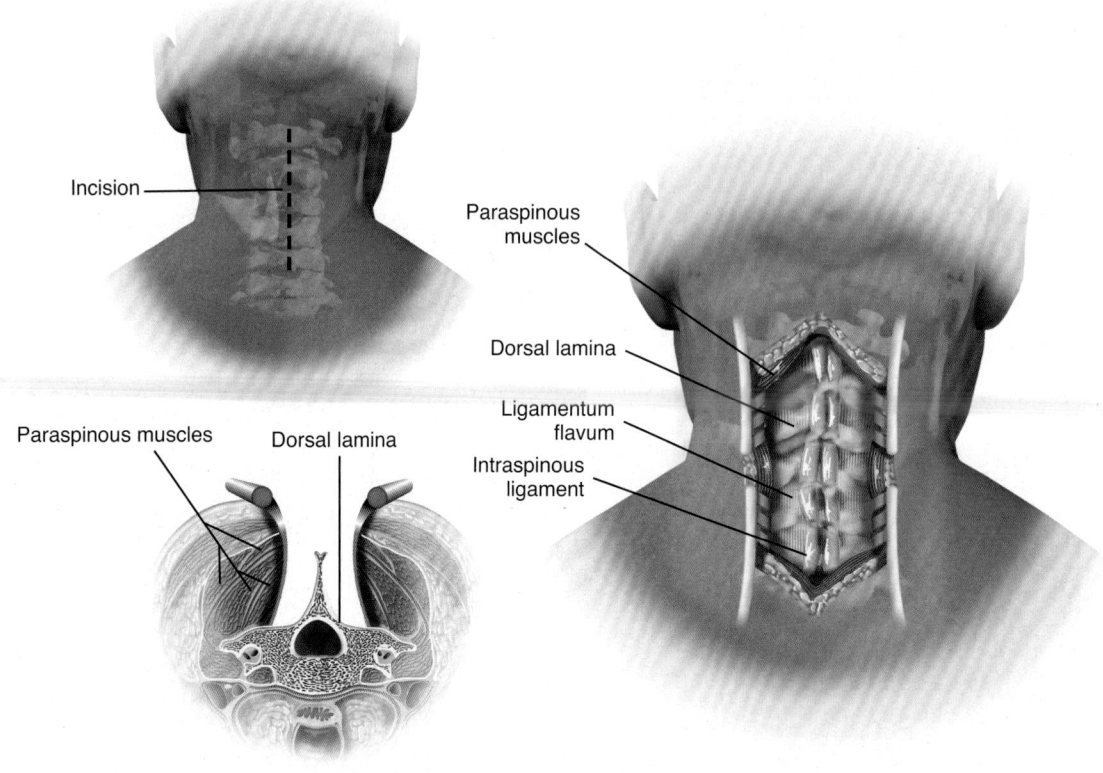

FIG 12 Sample picture of traditional "open" posterior approach to the cervical spine.

MINIMALLY INVASIVE CERVICAL LAMINOFORAMINOTOMY

Localization and Exposure

- An 18-mm longitudinal incision is made at the appropriate level, 1.5 cm off the midline (incisions 0.5 to 2 cm off the midline also have been described).
- The muscle is spread, and the fascia is incised under direct vision to the length of the incision.
- After the fascia is opened, a pair of Metzenbaum scissors is used to carefully dissect down to the facet.

- The smallest dilator is introduced slowly in a perpendicular trajectory with no medial angulation.
- Fluoroscopy is used to visualize the dilator docking onto the inferomedial edge of the rostral lateral mass of the appropriate level **(TECH FIG 1A)**. The tubular muscle dilators are placed in a sequential fashion to the width of the retractor and endoscopic system that is used **(TECH FIG 1B,C)**. A final dilator size of 13 to 16 mm is used, depending on surgeon comfort.
- Radiography is used to ensure that the tubular retractor is docked at the C6–C7 interspace **(TECH FIG 1D,E)**.

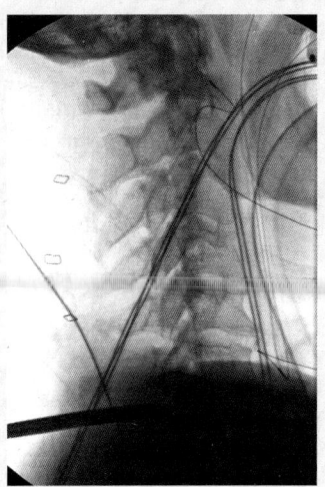
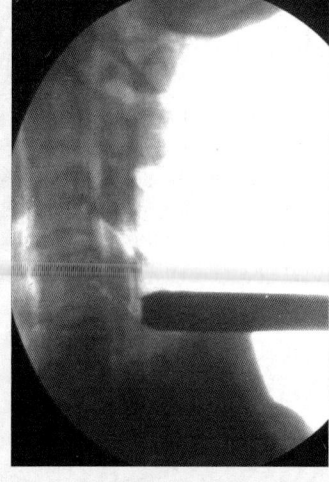

TECH FIG 1 A. First dilator in position at C6–C7. **B.** Intraoperative x-ray of the final tube docked on the facet complex. *(continued)*

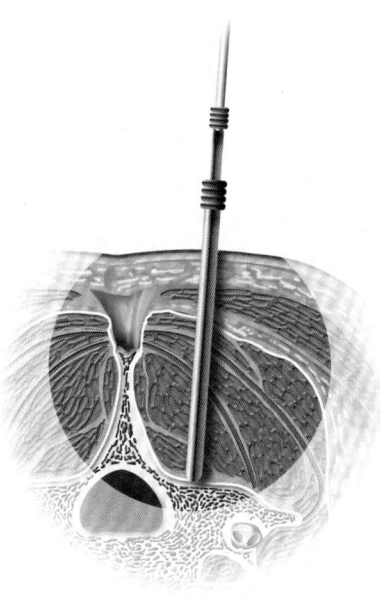

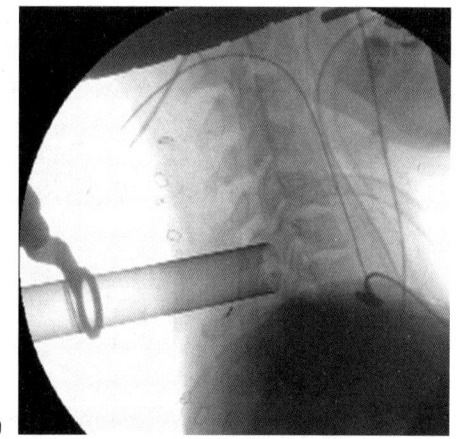

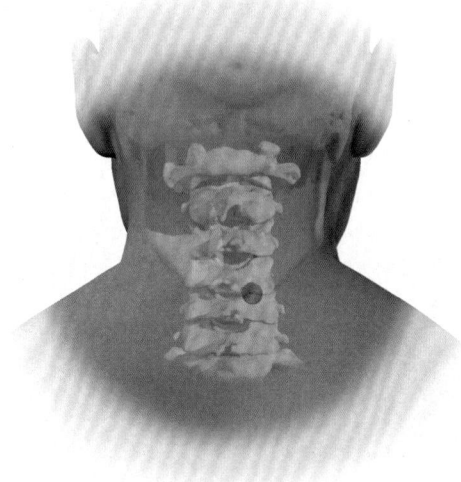

TECH FIG 1 *(continued)* **C.** Drawing of the final tube docked on the facet complex. **D.** Intraoperative x-ray of the tube secured at the C6–C7 level. **E.** Schematic drawing of the area on the facet used to dock the dilators and working channel.

- A 25-degree angled endoscope can be then affixed to the retractor system, or the surgeon can use a microscope to visualize further dissection.

Initial Dissection

- Monopolar cautery and pituitary rongeurs are used to identify the lateral mass and lamina.
- It is best to begin this dissection laterally where the bone is clearly felt. The dissection can then be continued medially to expose the laminofacet junction, with attention paid to not slip into the interlaminar space at this point.
- The possibility exists that there is a large interlaminar space medially, and care must be used to remain over bony landmarks during this dissection.
- Care should be taken to avoid dissection lateral to the facet to preserve the joint capsule.

- For a minimally invasive cervical laminoforaminotomy procedure, it is important to visualize the medial one-third of the rostral and caudal lateral mass and lateral one-third of the rostral and caudal lamina of interest **(TECH FIG 2A)**.
- A small-angled curette is used to detach the ligamentum flavum from the undersurface of the inferior edge of the rostral lamina **(TECH FIG 2B)**.
- Proper placement of the curettes can be confirmed under fluoroscopy to double-check that it is indeed under the lamina of the correct level. Good dissection of the underlying flavum and dura from the bone defines the relevant anatomy and helps to prevent incidental dural tears.
- Bleeding from epidural veins and the edge of the flavum is controlled via a long-tipped endoscopic bipolar cautery. For bleeding underneath the edge of the lamina, angled bipolar forceps with a 45-degree angle are often useful.

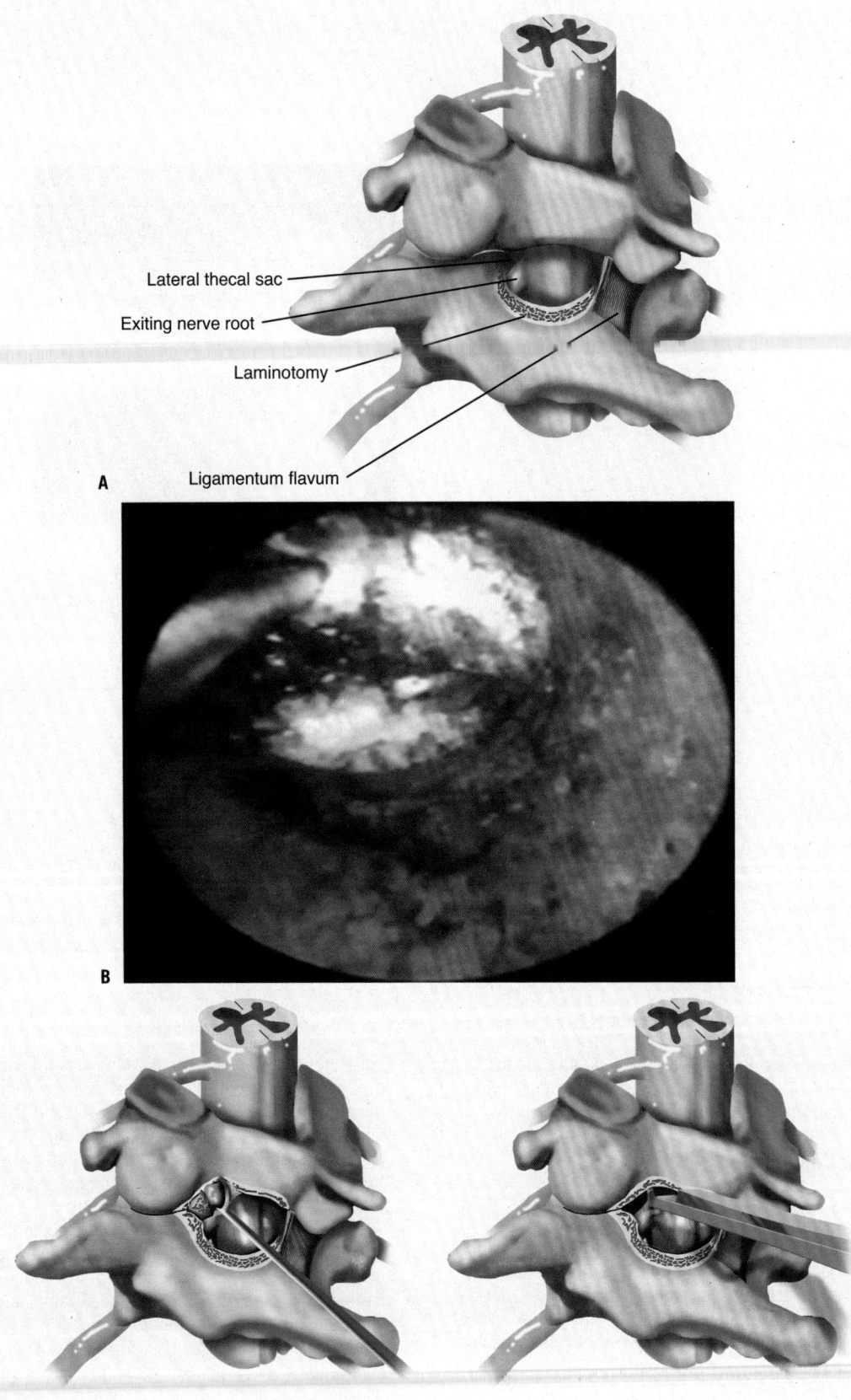

Lateral thecal sac

Exiting nerve root

Laminotomy

Ligamentum flavum

A

B

C

TECH FIG 2 A. Illustration of the area of desired bone resection with the exiting nerve root and lateral thecal sac in view. **B.** Frequent dissection of the soft tissue off the bone with an angled curette facilitates safe use of the Kerrison rongeur. **C.** After the rongeur work.

Bone Decompression

- A 1-mm or 2-mm Kerrison rongeur is then used to create a small laminotomy to visualize the lateral border of the cervical dura and the proximal exiting cervical nerve root.
- The Kerrison is used to begin the medial facetectomy over the exiting cervical root **(TECH FIG 3A)**.
- Periosteal and bone bleeding is addressed with bone wax and cautery.
- Often, the lamina can be oriented in quite a vertical fashion, making it difficult to bite it with a Kerrison punch.
- In such instances, it is best to use a drill to simultaneously thin and flatten the lamina down.
- Frequent dissection of the soft tissue off the bone with an angled curette facilitates safe use of the Kerrison rongeur.
- The drill with a fine cutting bit is often useful to finish the medial facetectomy and guarantee an adequate foraminal decompression **(TECH FIG 3B)**.
- We prefer a drill bit with a safety shield on one side to prevent inadvertent injury to the thecal sac **(TECH FIG 3C)**.
- Preferably no more than 50% of the facet joint should be removed to prevent destabilization at the level.

Nerve Root Exposure

- After the bony decompression of the dorsal cervical foramen is complete, bipolar coagulation is used to dissect the venous plexus that surrounds the nerve root.
- The nerve root can then be mobilized in a superior or inferior direction to visualize and palpate the ventral foramen and to identify the osteophytes or cervical disc fragments.
- To increase exposure to this ventral space without over distraction of the nerve root, the superomedial quadrant of the caudal pedicle can be drilled.
- Disc fragments can be teased out with the use of a nerve hook and micropituitary rongeur **(TECH FIG 4A)**. Osteophyte fragments can be manipulated and fractured through the use of angled curettes or tamped down with down-angled curettes.
- The foramen should be inspected one final time to assure no ventral or dorsal compression of the exiting nerve root **(TECH FIG 4B–D)**.
- After hemostasis is achieved and the wound is irrigated with antibiotic irrigation, the tubular retractor is removed, the wound is closed in layers, and Dermabond (Ethicon, Inc., Somerville, NJ) is applied over the incision.

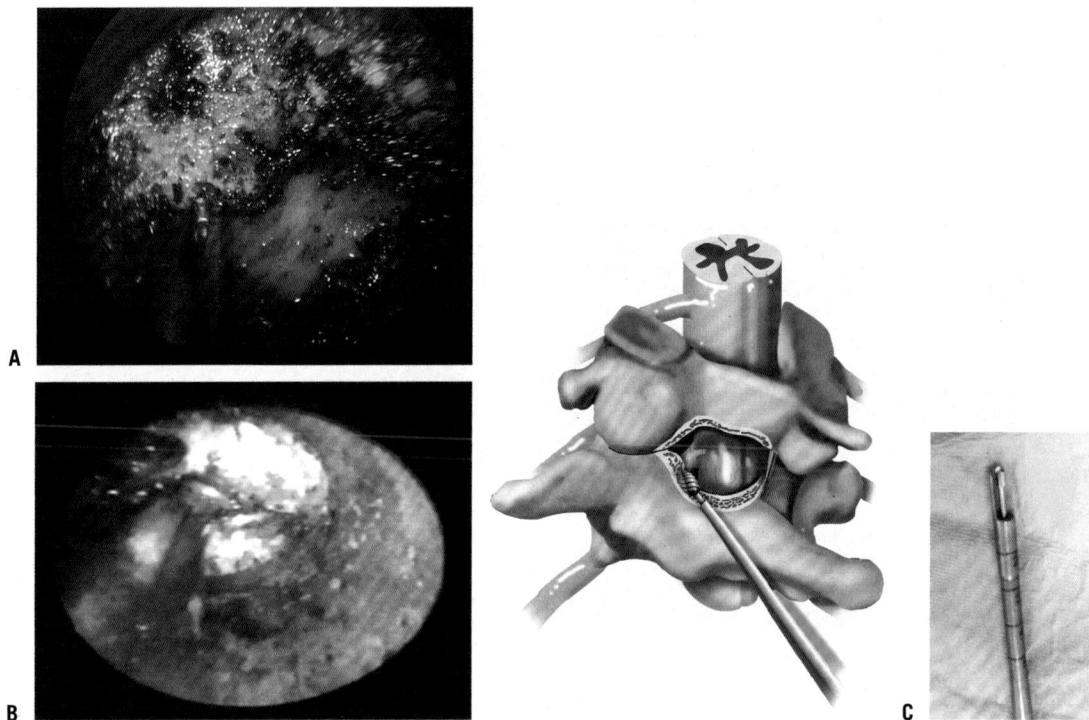

TECH FIG 3 A. Kerrison punch with joint synovium in view. **B.** A drill with a long endoscopic bit (eg, AM-8 bit with Midas Rex or TAC bit with MedNext drill) can be used to further thin the medial facet and lateral mass. **C.** Drill bit with safety shield.

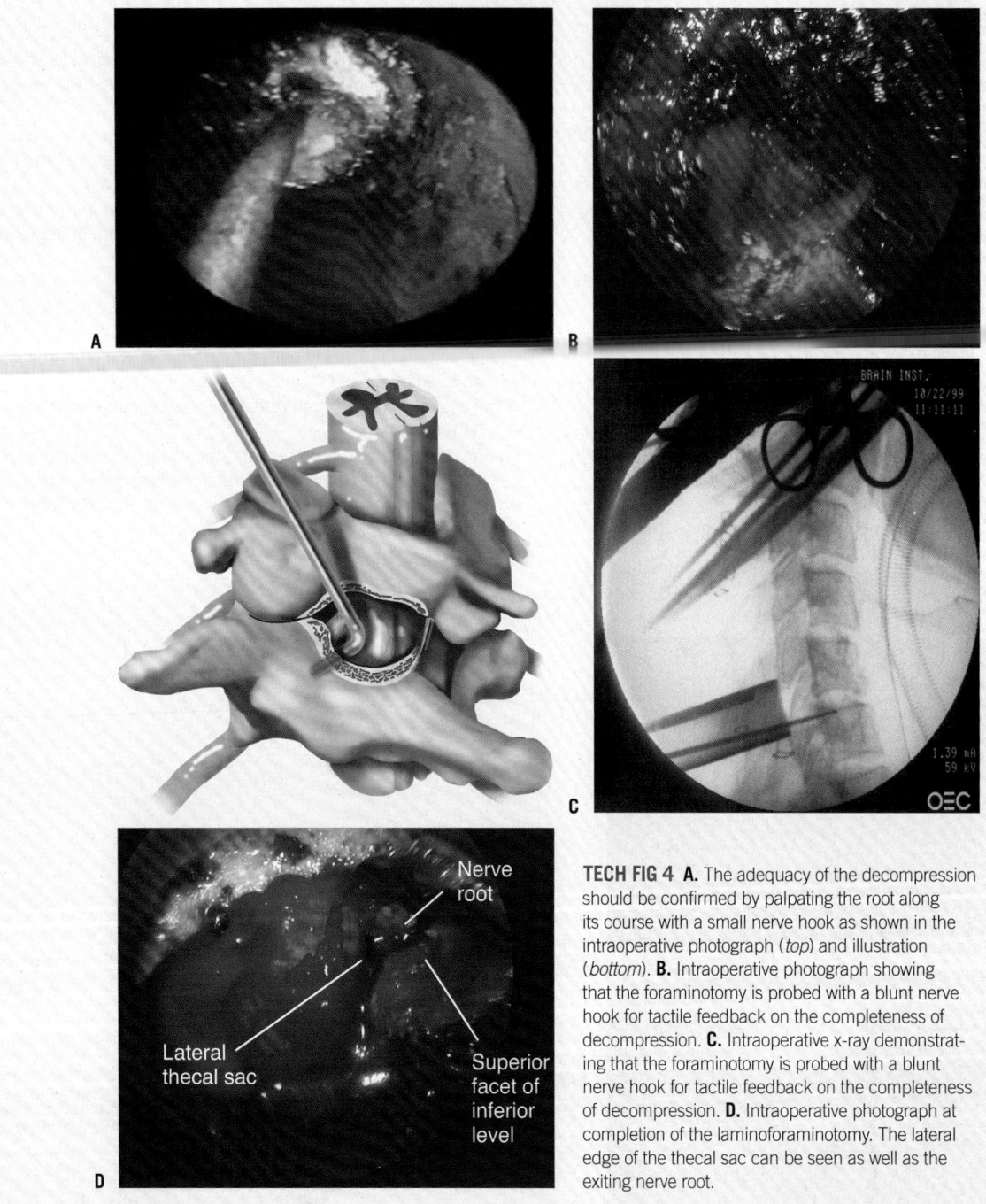

TECH FIG 4 A. The adequacy of the decompression should be confirmed by palpating the root along its course with a small nerve hook as shown in the intraoperative photograph (*top*) and illustration (*bottom*). **B.** Intraoperative photograph showing that the foraminotomy is probed with a blunt nerve hook for tactile feedback on the completeness of decompression. **C.** Intraoperative x-ray demonstrating that the foraminotomy is probed with a blunt nerve hook for tactile feedback on the completeness of decompression. **D.** Intraoperative photograph at completion of the laminoforaminotomy. The lateral edge of the thecal sac can be seen as well as the exiting nerve root.

TECHNIQUES

Pearls and Pitfalls

Positioning	• Care should be directed to ensuring that the cervical spine and neck musculature are not kinked or held in an unfavorable position. The neck, chin, and chest must be allowed to remain loose and free of compression. Precordial Doppler monitoring can be used to detect air emboli within the atrium.
Localization	• The incision should be 1.5 cm from the midline to ensure that the surgical exposure is not too medial. The incision length and the tubular retractor width should be the same to ensure adequate stability of the final tube.

Incision and Tube Dilation	• A mini-open approach is used to avoid the need for Kirschner wire insertion, and potential spinal cord injury, in the cervical spine. The first dilator is docked directly on the bony lamina. As sequential dilators are placed, care is taken to not apply too much pressure, which could result in an inadvertent plunge through the interlaminar space.
Surgical Approach	• After the initial induction of anesthesia, we have refrained from the use of neuromuscular paralytics to allow for improved feedback from the nerve root during the operation. It is best to begin this dissection laterally where the bone is clearly felt. The dissection can then be continued medially to expose the laminofacet junction with attention paid to not slip into the interlaminar space at this point.
Bone Exposure	• Good dissection of the underlying flavum and dura from the bone defines the relevant anatomy and helps to prevent incidental dural tears. For bleeding underneath the edge of the lamina, angled bipolar forceps with a 45-degree angle are often useful.
Foraminotomy	• Often, the lamina can be oriented in quite a vertical fashion, making it difficult to bite it with a Kerrison punch. In such instances, it is best to use a drill to simultaneously thin and flatten the lamina down. Frequent dissection of the soft tissue off the bone with an angled curette facilitates safe use of the Kerrison rongeur. The adequacy of the decompression should be confirmed by palpating the root along its course with a small nerve hook.

POSTOPERATIVE CARE

- Most of our patients can be safely discharged home the same day of surgery.
- Patients are counseled to expect neck/muscle and incisional pain for the first week or two after surgery.
- They are given prescriptions for a narcotic pain medication and a muscle relaxant; we typically prescribe hydrocodone/acetaminophen and methocarbamol.
- Patients are also placed on a bowel regimen consisting of daily stool softeners to avoid constipation from the narcotic medication.
- They are encouraged to walk as tolerated and discouraged from lifting more than 10 lb.
- Most patients can return to light work duties by 4 weeks.
- All patients begin a short course of physical therapy 4 to 6 weeks after surgery to improve neck strength and mobility.
- Most patients return to work, are able to drive, and have discontinued narcotic pain medication by 6 to 8 weeks following surgery.

OUTCOMES

- Good to excellent outcomes are reported in up to 97% of patients with neuroforaminal stenosis or lateral disc herniations following laminoforaminotomy performed for radiculopathy.[8,9,13,15,22]
- Poor prognostic factors include long-term preoperative complaints and long-standing preoperative neurologic deficits.[25]
- Posterior cervical microendoscopic foraminotomy and discectomy have been demonstrated to be safe and effective procedures with improvement in patients' neck disability index and visual analog scale for both the neck and arm after 1-year and 2-year follow-up.[18]
- Additionally, patients appear to exhibit continued good long-term outcomes in which 86% of patients were still doing well 15 years later (**FIG 13**).[25]

COMPLICATIONS

- Potential complications following a minimally invasive cervical decompression include injury to the cervical spinal cord

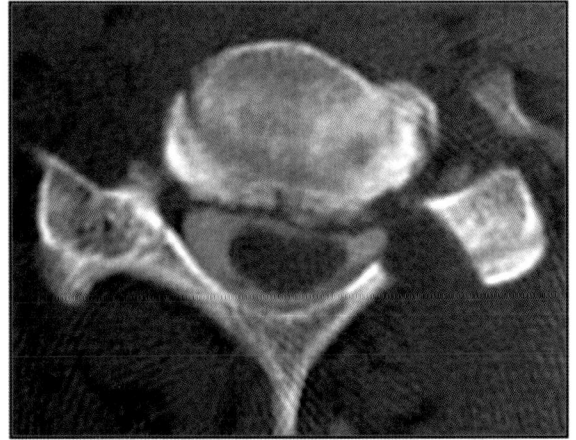
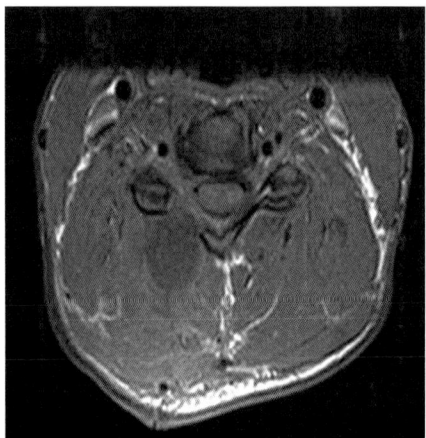

FIG 13 A. Postoperative computed tomography demonstrating the typical foraminotomy defect that is obtained after a microendoscopic foraminotomy with good preservation of the lateral mass integrity. **B.** Postoperative magnetic resonance imaging.

or nerves, cerebrospinal fluid leak, and infections. The incidence of complications following this procedure is low.[15,19]

- The treatment of an unintended durotomy include direct repair of a visible tear or placement of muscle, fat, or Gelfoam (Pfizer, New York, NY) over the tear and the application of a dural sealant such as DuraSeal (Integra LifeSciences, Plainsboro Township, NJ).
- The limited volume of dead space created with the minimally invasive approach has led to a decreased incidence of postoperative pseudomeningocele. Adequate layered closure should also minimize the risk of pseudomeningocele.
- The potential exists for injury to the cervical cord or the cervical nerve root. Careful dilation technique can minimize this risk of injury to the spinal cord. The cervical fascia should be opened under direct visualization, and the first dilator tube placed directly perpendicular to the spine without any medial angulation.
- To minimize injury to the cervical nerve root, adequate bony decompression must be achieved prior to manipulation of the nerve root.
- Venous bleeding from the plexus surrounding the cervical nerve root must be carefully monitored and controlled with bipolar coagulation and Gelfoam packing. The use of the semisitting position helps decrease the amount of this venous blood loss. The potential exists for a symptomatic air embolus in this semisitting position, although this has not been observed in the authors' series to date. Other series have reported rates of air embolism to be 0% to 2.3%.[1,12,14,26] The use of a precordial Doppler can help in identifying an air embolus, and the appropriate treatment can be performed.
- The vertebral artery runs immediately anterior to the cervical nerve root. When manipulating the cervical nerve root and osteophytes that may exist in this space, the surgeon should carefully monitor for an increase in venous bleeding. Because the vertebral artery is surrounded by a rich venous plexus, this venous bleeding is a good indicator of the proximity to the artery itself.
- Cervical instability following surgery can be avoided by preserving at least 50% of the facet complex during the bony decompression. When drilling the superomedial quadrant of the pedicle, careful attention must be paid to drill only the volume necessary to allow a nerve hook access behind the cervical nerve root.

ACKNOWLEDGMENT

- The authors thank the staff of Neuroscience Publications at Barrow Neurological Institute for assistance with manuscript preparation.

REFERENCES

1. Adamson TE. Microendoscopic posterior cervical laminoforaminotomy for unilateral radiculopathy: results of a new technique in 100 cases. J Neurosurg 2001;95:51–57.
2. Baaj AA, Mummaneni PV, Uribe JS, et al. Handbook of Spine Surgery, ed 2. New York: Thieme Medical Publishers, 2016.
3. Bailey RW, Badgley CE. Stabilization of the cervical spine by anterior fusion. J Bone Joint Surg Am 1960;42-A:565–594.
4. Bohlman HH, Emery SE, Goodfellow DB, et al. Robinson anterior cervical discectomy and arthrodesis for cervical radiculopathy. Long-term follow-up of one hundred and twenty-two patients. J Bone Joint Surg Am 1993;75:1298–1307.
5. Coric D, Adamson T. Minimally invasive cervical microendoscopic laminoforaminotomy. Neurosurg Focus 2008;25:E2.
6. Fessler RG, Khoo LT. Minimally invasive cervical microendoscopic foraminotomy: an initial clinical experience. Neurosurgery 2002;51:S37–S45.
7. Grieve JP, Kitchen ND, Moore AJ, et al. Results of posterior cervical foraminotomy for treatment of cervical spondylitic radiculopathy. Br J Neurosurg 2000;14:40–43.
8. Henderson CM, Hennessy RG, Shuey HM Jr, et al. Posterior-lateral foraminotomy as an exclusive operative technique for cervical radiculopathy: a review of 846 consecutively operated cases. Neurosurgery 1983;13:504–512.
9. Holly LT, Moftakhar P, Khoo LT, et al. Minimally invasive 2-level posterior cervical foraminotomy: preliminary clinical results. J Spinal Disord Tech 2007;20:20–24.
10. Hosono N, Yonenobu K, Ono K. Neck and shoulder pain after laminoplasty. A noticeable complication. Spine (Phila Pa 1976) 1996;21:1969–1973.
11. Howe JF, Loeser JD, Calvin WH. Mechanosensitivity of dorsal root ganglia and chronically injured axons: a physiological basis for the radicular pain of nerve root compression. Pain 1977;3:25–41.
12. Jadik S, Wissing H, Friedrich K, et al. A standardized protocol for the prevention of clinically relevant venous air embolism during neurosurgical interventions in the semisitting position. Neurosurgery 2009;64:533–539.
13. Jagannathan J, Sherman JH, Szabo T, et al. The posterior cervical foraminotomy in the treatment of cervical disc/osteophyte disease: a single-surgeon experience with a minimum of 5 years' clinical and radiographic follow-up. J Neurosurg Spine 2009;10:347–356.
14. Jödicke A, Daentzer D, Kästner S, et al. Risk factors for outcome and complications of dorsal foraminotomy in cervical disc herniation. Surg Neurol 2003;60:124–130.
15. Khoo LT, Perez-Cruet MJ, Fessler RG. Posterior cervical microendoscopic foraminotomy. In: Khoo LT, Perez-Cruet MJ, Fessler RG, eds. Outpatient Spinal Surgery. St. Louis: Quality Medical Publishing, 2006:71–93.
16. Kim KT, Kim YB. Comparison between open procedure and tubular retractor assisted procedure for cervical radiculopathy: results of a randomized controlled study. J Korean Med Sci 2009;24:649–653.
17. Klein GR, Vaccaro AR, Albert TJ. Health outcome assessment before and after anterior cervical discectomy and fusion for radiculopathy: a prospective analysis. Spine (Phila Pa 1976) 2000;25:801–803.
18. Lawton CD, Smith ZA, Lam SK, et al. Clinical outcomes of microendoscopic foraminotomy and decompression in the cervical spine. World Neurosurg 2014;81:422–427.
19. O'Toole JE, Eichholz KM, Fessler RG. Surgical site infection rates after minimally invasive spinal surgery. J Neurosurg Spine 2009;11:471–476.
20. Perez-Cruet MJ, Fessler RG, Wang MY. An Anatomic Approach to Minimally Invasive Spine Surgery, ed 2. New York: Thieme Medical Publishers, 2018.
21. Ratliff JK, Cooper PR. Cervical laminoplasty: a critical review. J Neurosurg 2003;98:230–238.
22. Ruetten S, Komp M, Merk H, et al. Full-endoscopic cervical posterior foraminotomy for the operation of lateral disc herniations using 5.9-mm endoscopes: a prospective, randomized, controlled study. Spine (Phila Pa 1976) 2008;33:940–948.
23. Smith GW, Robinson RA. The treatment of certain cervical-spine disorders by anterior removal of the intervertebral disc and interbody fusion. J Bone Joint Surg Am 1958;40-A:607–624.
24. Winder MJ, Thomas KC. Minimally invasive versus open approach for cervical laminoforaminotomy. Can J Neurol Sci 2011;38:262–267.
25. Woertgen C, Holzschuh M, Rothoerl RD, et al. Prognostic factors of posterior cervical disc surgery: a prospective, consecutive study of 54 patients. Neurosurgery 1997;40:724–729.
26. Zeidman SM, Ducker TB. Posterior cervical laminoforaminotomy for radiculopathy: review of 172 cases. Neurosurgery 1993;33:356–362.

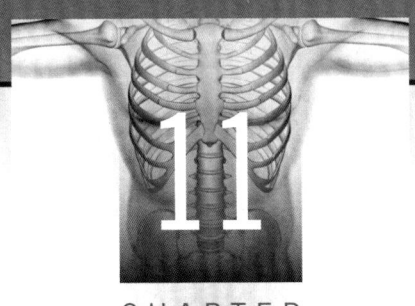

11
CHAPTER

Thoracolumbar
Lumbar Discectomy

Bradley K. Weiner and Rachel Bratescu

DEFINITION

- Clinically, significant lumbar disc herniations are characterized by a focal distortion of the normal anatomic configuration of discal material resulting in compression *and* subsequent dysfunction of the lumbar nerve roots.

ANATOMY

- The functional components of the intervertebral disc are the annulus fibrosus (fibrous concentric rings, type I collagen) enclosing the central nucleus pulposus (gelatinous, type II collagen, proteoglycans) and the vertebral endplates (hyaline cartilage).
- The anatomic unit of the lumbar spine is the vertebral body with its attached posterior elements and the disc below (**FIG 1A**).
- The nerve roots travel within the common dural sac (the cauda equina) and then exit at each level. They are numbered according to the pedicle beneath, which they pass.
- The spinal canal is divided into zones from medial to lateral: central canal, subarticular zone, foraminal zone, and extraforaminal (far lateral) zone (**FIG 1B**).
- Disc herniations are best classified based on the following ways:
  - Based on the integrity of the annulus fibrosus and whether there is a connection of herniated discal material with the disc space (**FIG 2**)

- Based on the anatomic location of the herniated material relative to the disc space, the canal, and the compressed nerve root using the nomenclature mentioned earlier (**FIG 3**).
- Accurate anatomic classification of disc herniations facilitates preoperative planning and can minimize the risk of surgical complications such as missed pathology and iatrogenic nerve root injury.
- The importance of a complete knowledge of spinal anatomy and understanding of the particular patient's pathoanatomy cannot be overstated.

PATHOGENESIS

- In the normal disc, the nucleus pulposus imbibes and releases water to balance mechanical loads. The annulus fibrosus converts these loads to hoop stresses, thereby containing the nuclear material. The endplates allow diffusion of nutrition into, and waste products out of, the nucleus.
  - Together, they allow for the three basic spinal segmental functions: mobility, stability, and protection of the nearby neurologic structures.
- With early or intermediate disc degeneration (natural aging with or without minor repetitive trauma), the endplates fail to allow adequate diffusion, the nucleus fails to replace degraded proteoglycans, and annular support weakens (failure of cross-linking, development of clefts). Biomechanical dysfunction occurs, with possible herniation of nuclear material.

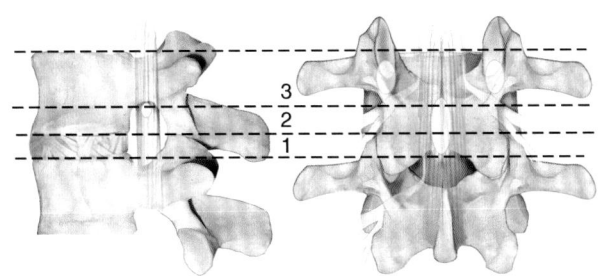

A

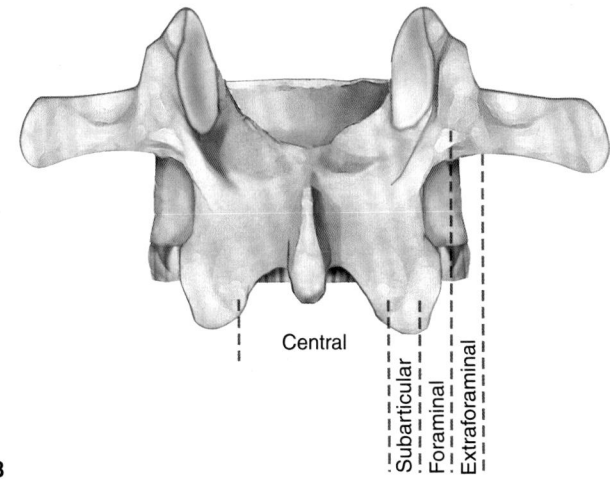

Central

Subarticular
Foraminal
Extraforaminal

B

FIG 1 A. Anatomic unit. The first floor is the disc level, the second floor is the foraminal level, and the third floor is the pedicle level. **B.** Regions of the canal.

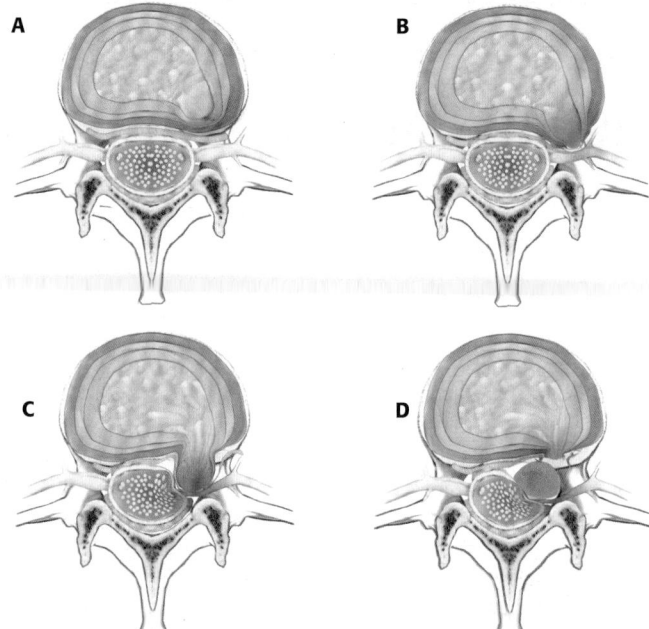

FIG 2 Classification of disc herniations based on relation to outer annulus: protrusion (**A**), subannular extrusion (**B**), transannular extrusion (**C**), and sequestration (**D**).

- Many disc herniations do not cause pain or neurologic symptoms. A combination of herniation, nerve root compression, and an inflammatory interface is required for nerve root dysfunction and associated radiculopathy and sciatica.

NATURAL HISTORY

- Many studies have shown that with time and nonoperative treatment, over 90% of patients with a first-time lumbar disc herniation will get better without surgery. Accordingly, to propose surgery requires clear indications.
  - Absolute indications
    - Bladder or bowel involvement secondary to a massive disc herniation and cauda equina syndrome: immediate surgical intervention
    - Progressive (ie, worsening) neurologic deficit: the earlier, the better prognostically
  - Relative indications
    - Failure of conservative measures greater than 6 weeks to 3 months

- Multiply recurrent sciatica
- Significant neurologic deficit
- In each case, the properly informed patient must clearly understand the current best evidence: Most patients get better quickly with nonoperative care. For those with significant symptoms that are not better within 6 weeks, short-term and long-term (8 years) outcomes are better in patients treated with discectomy as compared with continued nonoperative care.

HISTORY AND PHYSICAL FINDINGS

- The most common complaint is pain with or without associated paresthesias or weakness in a specific monoradicular anatomic distribution.

IMAGING AND OTHER DIAGNOSTIC STUDIES

- Magnetic resonance imaging (MRI) is the imaging study of choice for the diagnosis and anatomic classification of lumbar disc herniations. It is highly sensitive and specific and provides, along with the clinical picture, adequate information for detailed preoperative planning.
- Computed tomography myelography is invasive and less specific than MRI but provides excellent sensitivity when MRI is unavailable or contraindicated.
- Plain radiographs may show disc space narrowing, early formation of osteophytes, or a "sciatic scoliosis." Although providing no direct evidence of a herniated disc, they may be helpful to rule out unexpected destructive pathology (eg, infection, tumor, fracture) in patients who have failed to respond to nonoperative intervention or those with red flags. They also allow excellent delineation of bony anomalies that may prove vital to preoperative planning and intraoperative localization, such as transitional lumbosacral articulations or spina bifida occulta.

DIFFERENTIAL DIAGNOSIS

- Intraspinal, extrinsic compression, or irritation at the level of the nerve root: spinal stenosis, osteomyelitis or discitis, neoplasm, epidural fibrosis (scar)
- Intraspinal, extrinsic compression, or irritation proximal to the nerve root: conus and cauda lesions such as neurofibroma or ependymoma
- Intraspinal, intrinsic nerve root dysfunction: neuropathy (diabetic, idiopathic, alcoholic, iatrogenic [chemotherapy]), herpes zoster, arachnoiditis, nerve root tumor

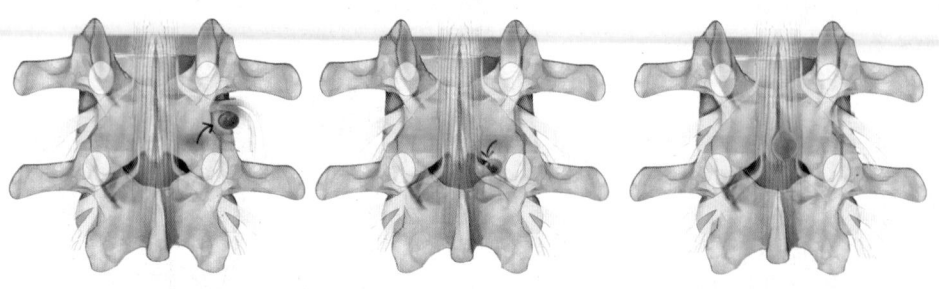

FIG 3 The patterns of disc migration can be characterized relative to the structures of the anatomic unit (eg, at the disc level or at the pedicle level). The area of root compression can be described relative to the nerve root anatomy (eg, at the shoulder of the traversing root, in the axilla of the exiting root).

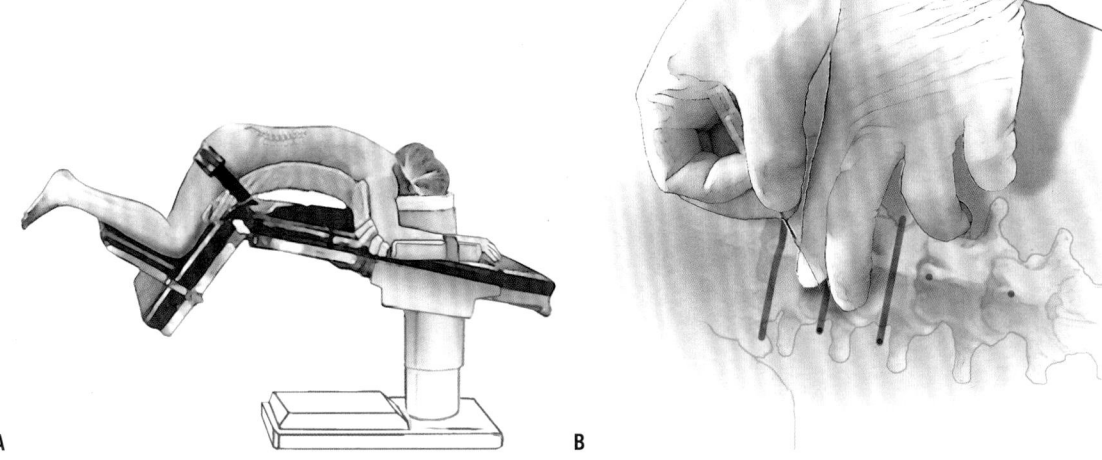

FIG 4 A. The kneeling position obtained with the Andrews, Wilson, or Jackson frames. **B.** The marking needle.

- Extraspinal sources distal to the nerve root: pelvic or more distal neoplasms with associated sciatic or femoral nerve compression, sacroiliac disease (eg, infection, osteoarthritis), osteoarthritis of the hip, peripheral vascular disease

NONOPERATIVE MANAGEMENT

- The evidence base is still a bit unclear, but the following are commonly recommended.
  - Rest: bed rest (no more than 2 or 3 days), activity or job modification, weight loss
  - Medication: analgesics (very short term for severe pain only), nonsteroidal anti-inflammatories, tapered doses of oral steroids
  - Exercise: physical therapy (McKenzie program)
  - Injections: epidural or selective root blocks (may provide some temporary relief while the natural history takes over)—no impact on long-term outcomes
  - Time: 6 weeks to 3 months (unless absolute indications for surgery exist as noted earlier)

SURGICAL MANAGEMENT

- The evidence base is clear: Open discectomy and microdiscectomy are the operative techniques with the best-documented short-term and long-term outcomes and are the gold standards of surgery for lumbar disc herniations.

Preoperative Planning

- This is *vital* and should aim to answer three questions:
  - What nerve root is involved (answered by history and physical examination)?
  - Where is the herniated material relative to the disc space, the canal, and the nerve root (answered by MRI)?
  - What approach will afford the best visualization and access to the herniated material while minimizing injury to tissues not directly involved in the pathologic process?

Positioning

- A "kneeling" position is generally used, with the patient stabilized on an Andrews frame, a Wilson frame, or the Jackson table (**FIG 4A**).
  - Some hip and knee flexion will decrease lumbar lordosis and facilitate an approach through the interlaminar window.
  - The abdomen must be free to decrease intra-abdominal pressure and venous backflow through the plexus of Batson into the spinal canal.
- Shoulders should be abducted less than 90 degrees and with some flexion. The neck should be neutral or gently flexed.
- Eyes must be protected and elbows, knees, and feet well padded.
- A needle is passed between and lateral to the spinous processes at the involved level, and C-arm imaging is used to confirm that the proper level will be approached (**FIG 4B**). The needle is removed, and the level is marked and labeled on the skin.
- The involved side will be determined preoperatively by patient complaint and location of herniation on MRI but should also be marked on the patient's skin at this point.

Approach

- The interlaminar window approach is used in about 90% of lumbar disc herniations requiring surgery. It is appropriate for herniations within the central canal or subarticular zones from L1 to S1 and for herniations within the foramen at L5–S1.
- The intertransverse window approach is used in about 10% of lumbar disc herniations requiring surgery. It is appropriate for herniations within the foraminal and extraforaminal zones from L1 to L5.
- For each step in the procedure, incision, excision, and retraction of tissues should be minimized. The goal is to *get the job done completely and safely with minimal trauma to tissues not directly involved in the pathologic process.*

INCISION AND DISSECTION

- The skin incision is made directly midline posteriorly and extends from the top of the cephalad spinous process to the bottom of the caudal spinous process, about 1.5 inches for single-level pathology.

- The subcutaneous tissues are then gently and bluntly mobilized and retracted to allow visualization of the dorsolumbar fascia.
- From here, one of two windows of approach will be undertaken based on the location of the disc herniation: the interlaminar window or the intertransverse window.

INTERLAMINAR WINDOW

- The dorsolumbar fascia is incised just off the midline in a gentle curvilinear fashion on the involved side at a length to match the skin incision.
- A Cobb elevator is used to gently elevate the muscle (multifidus) from the spinous processes to the midportion of the facet joint laterally.
  - The degree of muscle elevation should be limited to what is necessary to allow adequate laminar exposure for laminotomy.

- A retractor is then placed. We prefer a retractor with a medial hook for the interspinous ligament and a blade for gentle lateral muscular retraction (**TECH FIG 1A**).
- An intraoperative C-arm image is then obtained to confirm the level. Alternatively, a lateral radiograph can be taken.
- A cylindrical retractor, placed transmuscularly using a sequential dilation technique, is a reasonable alternative as long as great care is taken to expose the correct portion of the interlaminar window (there is a tendency to be "pushed" too far laterally resulting in failure of the pars).

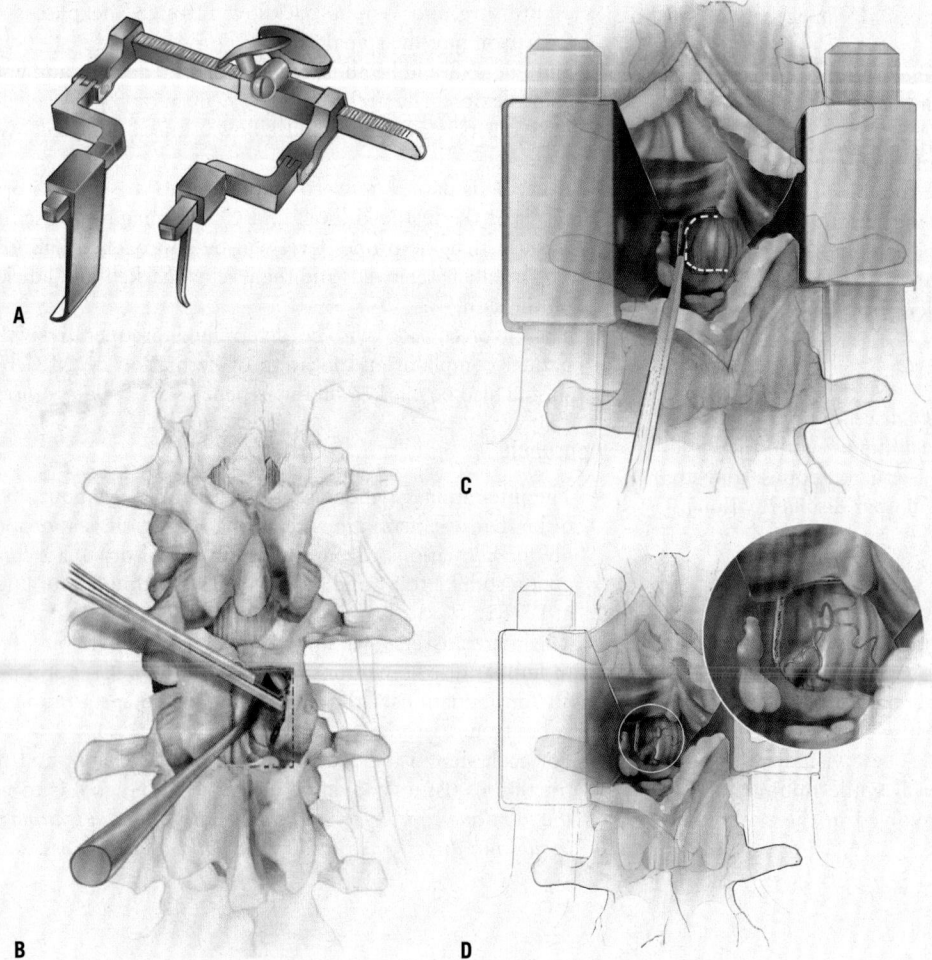

TECH FIG 1 A. Muscle retractor. **B.** Laminotomy. **C.** Laminotomy and the ligamentum. Bony excision used for the typical disc herniation in the canal or subarticular zones. It may need to be extended cephalad for herniations extending upward into the second story or may need to include the upper portion of the caudal lamina for herniations extending downward into the third story of the level below. The ligamentum is either freed from its insertions on the undersurface of the lamina above and the undersurface of the facet capsule laterally using a sharp curette, creating a flap, or is incised and split as depicted. **D.** Identifying the lateral edge of the root. The traversing root is readily identified by vessels that travel along its lateral edge longitudinally, rise up onto its shoulder, and form a plexus in its axilla. Further caudally, the root is closely associated with the medial border of the pedicle.

T
E
C
H
N
I
Q
U
E
S

- At this point, illumination and magnification are gained by the use of the operative microscope (our preference) or a headlamp and loupes.
  - Outcomes are similar for the two when used properly, and the surgeon should decide on his or her preference based on experience and comfort level.
- A laminotomy on the undersurface of the cephalad lamina and minimal medial facetectomy is then performed using a Kerrison rongeur **(TECH FIG 1B)**.
  - The degree of laminotomy and facetectomy should be enough to allow full visualization of the underlying nerve root at the area of compression and to allow access for excision of herniated disc material—no more and no less.
    - For small disc herniations in the canal or subarticular zones (the "typical disc herniation"), minimal bony excision is required at lower lumbar levels.
    - For larger disc herniations and those extending cephalad into the second story, a larger laminotomy or even hemilaminectomy may be required. The key in these situations is to preserve at least 5 mm of the lateral pars interarticularis and at least 50% of the medial facet.
- Laminotomy of the upper surface of the caudal lamina is generally not needed unless the herniated material has migrated caudally to the third story of the level below adjacent to the pedicle.
- The ligamentum flavum is then addressed. One of two techniques is used: the Rick Delamarter and John McCulloch flap or the Rob Fraser split **(TECH FIG 1C)**.
  - The former preserves the ligamentum flavum as a complete barrier to minimize scar formation from posterior, whereas the latter offers a little less coverage but preserves the ligament's biomechanical integrity.
- The lateral edge of the traversing nerve root is then identified.
  - This is readily identified by consistent lateral veins and the root's association with the pedicle **(TECH FIG 1D)**.
  - These veins can then be gently mobilized to allow exposure of the underlying annulus.
  - Occasionally, anomalous roots lateral to the traversing root may be present. Again, safety is ensured by identifying the veins directly overlying the annulus and using these to provide a window to access.

Herniation Exposure

- For herniations within the canal or subarticular zones and in the first or second story (85% of encountered discs), the traversing nerve root is gently mobilized medially, allowing exposure of the herniated disc.
  - If the root is immobile, the surgeon should excise more bone within the subarticular region (medial facetectomy) to afford visualization and palpation of the medial border of the pedicle associated with the traversing root.
  - Access to the disc cephalad to this will be within a safe zone lateral to the traversing root and within the axilla of the exiting root.
  - Once larger fragments are teased out, the traversing root will become mobile, allowing greater access.
  - Retraction should be minimal at upper levels (L1–L3 due to presence of the conus) and limited to about 40%, that is,

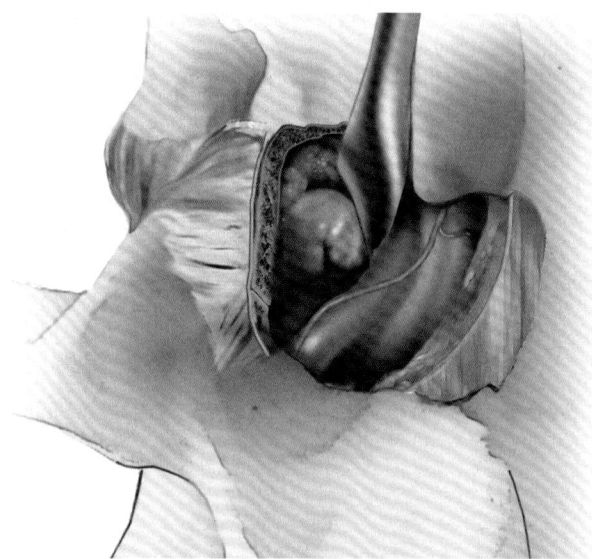

TECH FIG 2 Root retraction is minimal and intermittent.

to less than half the width of the unilateral hemilaminotomy below this **(TECH FIG 2)**.
- Retraction should be relaxed during periods in which no active work is undertaken in or near the disc space: The nerve is rested while the pituitary rongeur is being cleaned and gently re-retract when it returns. This will minimize trauma to the root.
- Hemostasis is then obtained by gently tucking small pieces of Gelfoam or thrombin cephalad and caudally to the exposed disc space. These are to be removed at the end of the case.
  - If bipolar cautery is used, it should be done with caution to avoid root injury.
- Herniations extending caudally to the third story of the level below (uncommon, 5%) are most often within the "axilla" of the traversing root. Retraction of the root is not used; rather, the herniation (usually sequestered) is gently teased out from the axilla.

Discectomy

- Once visualized, any free disc material is removed with a pituitary rongeur. A ball-tipped probe is used to tease out any additional free fragments hiding further out in the subarticular zone or under the common dural sac or root.
- The disc space is then entered (this will be the first step in "contained" herniations) by annulotomy. A long-handled no. 15 blade facing away from the traversing root is used, preferably with a longitudinal orientation.
- Within the disc space, any loose fragments are removed with the pituitary rongeur **(TECH FIG 3)**, and the disc space is irrigated.
  - More aggressive excision ("complete discectomy") may slightly decrease the risk of recurrence but at the price of increased back pain and a potential for accelerating the degenerative process.

- Depth of work should be limited to avoid anterior perforation and potential vascular injury. The surgeon should respect the anterior portion of the annulus and avoid perforating it with an instrument.
- Discectomy is complete when no additional loose fragments can be removed from the disc space and free mobility of the nerve root is confirmed.
- The root retractor is then removed, along with the pieces of Gelfoam.
- The wound is thoroughly irrigated. This "washing," coupled with removing the root retractor, is usually adequate to stop any epidural bleeding.
  - If it persists, temporarily placing Gelfoam again is almost always adequate.
- Unless there is still a bit of oozing, drains are generally not indicated, and the wound is closed in three layers (fascia, subcutaneous tissue, and skin [absorbable, subcuticular]).

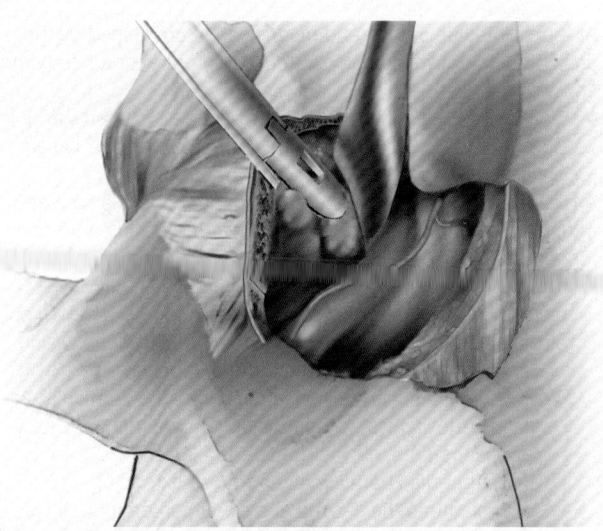

TECH FIG 3 Discectomy. After annulotomy, the pituitary rongeur is used to remove the herniation and loose fragments within the disc space.

INTERTRANSVERSE WINDOW

- The dorsolumbar fascia is incised 1.5 fingerbreadths off the midline longitudinally **(TECH FIG 4A)**.
- The plane between the multifidus medially and the longissimus laterally is freed by finger dissection, allowing palpation of the facet joint.
- A retractor is placed within this plane **(TECH FIG 4B)** and an intraoperative C-arm image is obtained to confirm the level.
- The tip of the superior articular process and the lateral pars interarticularis are exposed with electrocautery and partially resected **(TECH FIG 4C,D)**.
- The intertransverse membrane is gently retracted laterally using a ball-tipped probe.

- Gentle blunt dissection is used to identify the exiting nerve root and the underlying herniated material. Gentle technique, patience, and really good lighting and magnification are required here (again, we prefer the operative microscope but outcomes are similar regardless). There is plenty of adipose tissue and a venous plexus surrounding the dorsal root ganglion of the root that must be identified before introducing the pituitary rongeur.
- A ball-tipped probe and pituitary rongeur are used to gently tease out the loose fragment, with minimal to no retraction applied to the root. This can be traced back into the disc space, as necessary, and any loose fragments are removed.
- The wound is irrigated, hemostasis is obtained, and closure is performed, as described earlier.

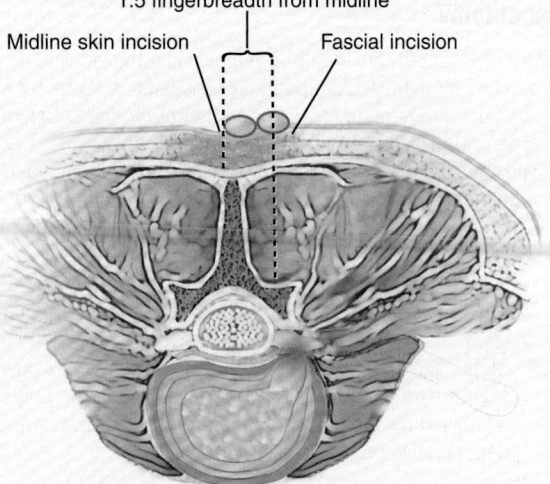

1.5 fingerbreadth from midline

Midline skin incision   Fascial incision

A

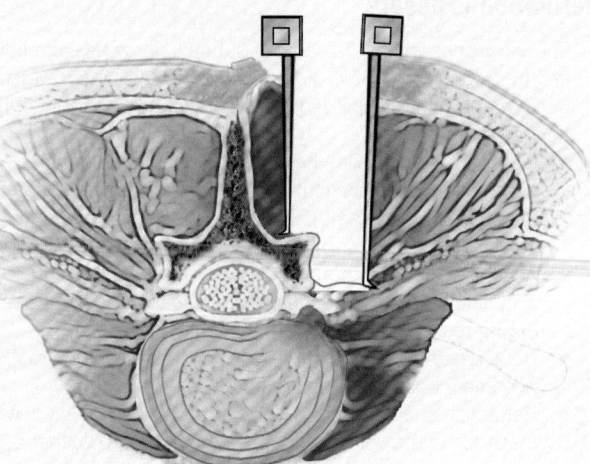

B

TECH FIG 4 A. The fascial incision is made 1.5 fingerbreadths from the midline. **B.** Retraction. *(continued)*

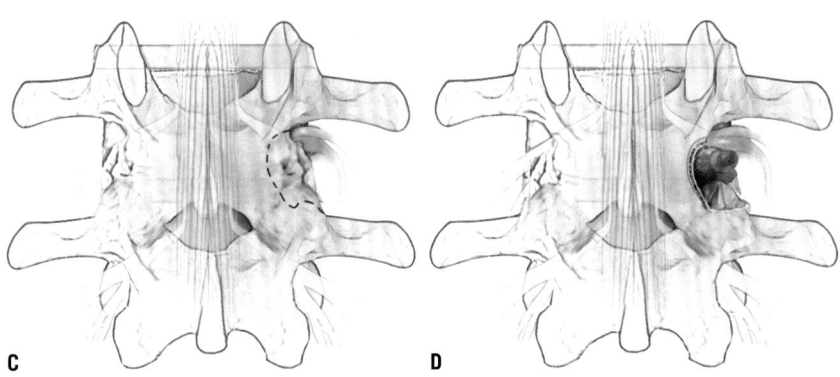

C   D

TECH FIG 4 *(continued)* **C.** The *dashed lines* represent the area of bony excision during discectomy. **D.** The intertransverse membrane is then gently mobilized laterally, allowing exposure and excision of the herniated disc.

TECHNIQUES

Pearls and Pitfalls

Wrong-level exposure, exploration, or surgery is always a risk. The level is marked preoperatively and intraoperatively, as noted earlier.	• The surgeon should beware of obese patients with a significant lumbar lordosis. It is very common to expose the wrong level despite proper localization of the skin incision. Thus, the correct level must be ensured radiographically before entering the spinal canal. • The surgeon should also beware of patients with "transitional" lumbar vertebrae (sacralization or lumbarization). Here, it is often best to correlate the level on intraoperative images with the preoperative MRI, which will clearly show the disc herniation as well as the immobile, uninvolved transitional levels (narrow disc space with maintained bright signal intensity on T2 with or without poorly developed facet joints).
Certain differences exist between revision discectomy via the interlaminar window and primary surgery.	• In revision surgery, the laminotomy and facetectomy should be extended cephalad and laterally to allow exposure of "normal" dura (above and lateral to areas of epidural fibrosis [scar]). • Identification of the traversing root may be difficult (scar, loss of characteristic veins), but it will still *always* be associated with its pedicle. The medial border of the pedicle is readily identified, and tissues medial to it (scar, root) are gently mobilized to identify the fragment and disc space. • If the root is completely immobile, further medial facetectomy will be required, and the disc space should be entered in line with the subjacent pedicle to ensure being lateral to the traversing root and medial to the exiting root.
Revision discectomy via the intertransverse window for foraminal or extraforaminal disc herniations is not recommended, as the planes will be distorted and safe surgery is difficult.	• Using the interlaminar window instead, with resection of the inferior articular process of the cephalad vertebra with or without arthrodesis, is safer and affords excellent visualization.
Anomalous neural anatomy can be best identified preoperatively on MRI.	• The surgeon should beware of large, perfectly round soft tissue masses within the foramen on parasagittal imaging or in the canal on axial imaging. If it does not look like the other roots (mimicking a large round disc herniation) but has their signal intensity, it is likely an anomalous or conjoined root.

POSTOPERATIVE CARE

• After surgery, patients may be fitted with a light lumbar corset if desired and are encouraged to walk once anesthesia has worn off and pain permits. About 85% are discharged as outpatients. Fifteen percent who are older (less mobile) or have nausea and vomiting require an overnight stay and 23-hour observation.

• Once home, patients engage in a program of progressive walking, stretching, and corset use for comfort. For those progressing slowly, physical therapy may be introduced.

Heavy lifting and excessive bending and twisting should be avoided in the first few weeks.

• If all is well, they may drive in about a week and return to light work once they feel up to it. Heavy labor should be avoided for 6 to 12 weeks to ensure proper soft tissue healing (skin, muscle, annulotomy). Long-term activities are not restricted.

OUTCOMES

• There is an 85% likelihood of an excellent or good outcome 8 years postoperatively.

- Patients with significant medical or social comorbidities (eg, diabetes, heavy smoking), worker's compensation or litigation, and psychological problems (depression) are less likely to do well. The same is true for patients who receive no care for more than 6 months before presentation.
- Anatomically, patients with larger disc herniations (sac compression one-third or more) and those at higher levels (L2–L3 or L3–L4) have a better prognosis. Those with a retrolisthesis at L5–S1 do not do as well.
- Truly informed consent is mandatory.

COMPLICATIONS

- Surgeon dependent: wrong level, wrong side, missed pathology, iatrogenic instability, "battered root syndrome," dural tear, hemorrhage, positioning (eg, eyes, ulnar nerve)
- Operative environment or patient dependent: wound infection, disc space infection, urinary retention, thrombophlebitis, or pulmonary embolism

SUGGESTED READINGS

Atlas SJ, Deyo RA, Keller RB, et al. The Maine Lumbar Spine Study, part II. 1-year outcomes of surgical and non-surgical management of sciatica. Spine 1996;21:1777–1786.

Boden SD, Davis DO, Dina TS, et al. Abnormal magnetic-resonance scans of the lumbar spine in asymptomatic subjects. A prospective investigation. J Bone Joint Surg Am 1990;72(3):403–408.

Lurie J, Weinstein J, Lurie JD, et al. Surgical versus nonoperative treatment for lumbar disc herniation: eight-year results for the spine patient outcomes research trial. Spine 2014;39:3–16.

McCulloch JA. Microdiscectomy. In: Frymoyer JW, ed. The Adult Spine: Principles and Practice. New York: Raven Press, 1991:1765–1783.

McCulloch JA, Weiner BK. Microsurgery in the lumbar intertransverse interval. Instr Course Lect 2002;51:233–241.

Spangfort EV. The lumbar disc herniation. A computer-aided analysis of 2,504 operations. Acta Orthop Scand 1972;142:1–95.

Weber H. Lumbar disc herniation. A controlled prospective study with ten years of observations. Spine 1983;8(2):131–140.

Weiner BK, Dabbah M. Lateral lumbar disc herniations treated with a paraspinal approach: an independent assessment of longer-term outcomes. J Spinal Disord Tech 2005;18(6):519–521.

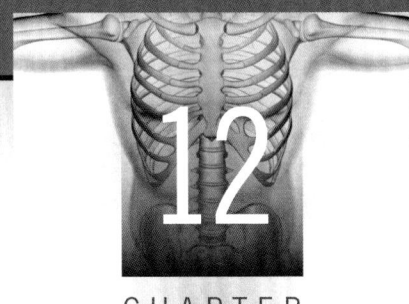

12

CHAPTER

Lumbar Decompression

Bradley K. Weiner and Rachel Bratescu

DEFINITION

- Degenerative changes that are part of the aging process may lead to compression of neurologic tissues within the spinal canal or subarticular zones (with or without the foraminal zone) of the lumbar spine.
- This *spinal canal stenosis* may lead to neurogenic claudication or a monoradiculopathy.

ANATOMY

- The functional vertebral unit is depicted in **FIG 1**. More details are given in the anatomy section of Chapter SP-11.
- Spinal canal stenosis is best classified based on vertical extent of compression, regions of the canal involved, and severity of the involvement.
- Accurate anatomic classification facilitates preoperative planning and can minimize the risk of surgical complications such as missed pathology and iatrogenic root injury.

PATHOGENESIS

- Degenerative changes can affect the disc, the soft tissues, and the facet joints of the spinal unit.
- Annular bulging of the disc, ligamentum flavum hypertrophy and infolding, and osteophyte formation on the facet joints can contribute to neurologic compression. Occasionally, epidural lipomatosis also contributes to spinal stenosis.
- Stenosis/compression progresses slowly and gradually affects the blood supply (arterial inflow and venous outflow) of traversing nerve roots and the free flow of cerebrospinal fluid within the common dural sac. When increased demands are placed, as in walking, the nutritional needs of the nerve roots cannot be met and noxious by-products of metabolism cannot be removed, resulting in neurophysiologic malfunction characterized clinically by paresthetic and cramping symptoms in the legs.
- As in lumbar disc herniations, many patients with spinal stenosis are asymptomatic, suggesting that other factors

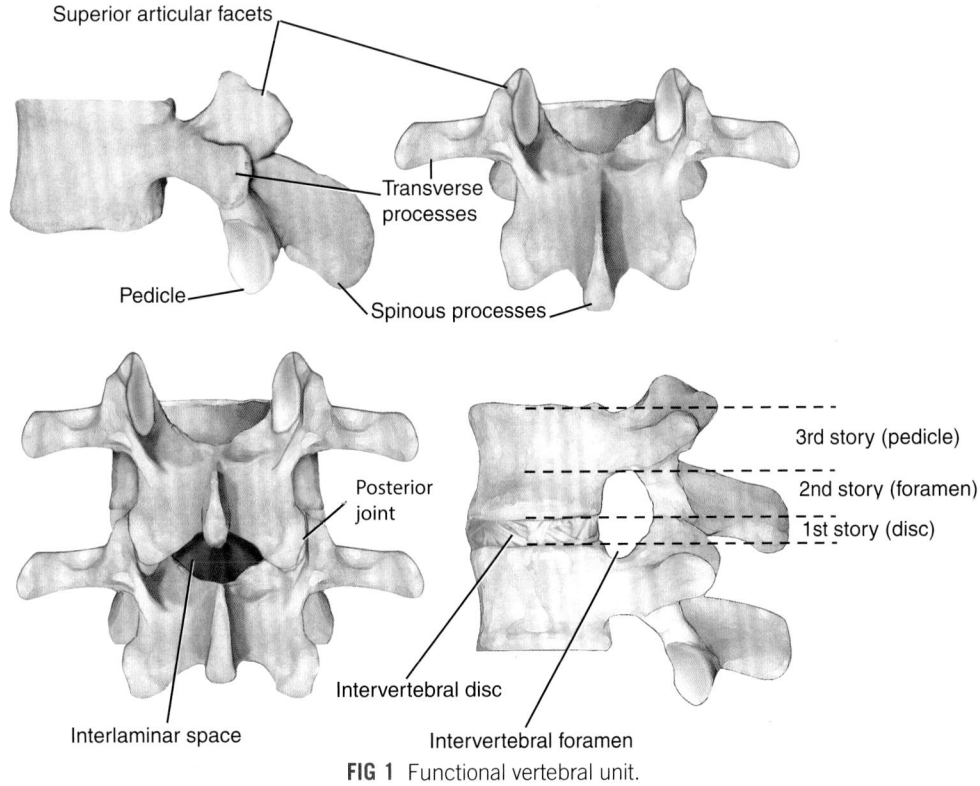

FIG 1 Functional vertebral unit.

intrinsic to nerve root function and adaptability are equally important (eg, smoking, vascular disease, diabetes).

NATURAL HISTORY

- Patients with mild to moderate symptoms and mild to moderate neurologic compression may respond to conservative care. Unless the compression increases, symptoms generally remain stable, with minimal resolution and minimal worsening.
- The more severe the symptoms and the more severe the neurologic compression, the more likely symptoms will progress, the less likely they will respond to conservative measures, and the more likely patients will seek surgical intervention.

HISTORY AND PHYSICAL FINDINGS

- Symptomatic patients with spinal canal stenosis generally present with neurogenic claudication (70%), monoradiculopathy (15%), or a combination of the two. Note that a small group of patients within the claudication group will present primary with low back pain that has uniquely claudicant characteristics.
- Foraminal stenosis (10% to 15% of cases) is best diagnosed clinically by a severe monoradiculopathy of an exiting nerve root and radiographically on parasagittal magnetic resonance imaging (MRI) or computed tomography (CT) sagittal reconstruction (**FIG 2**).

IMAGING

- As described in Chapter SP-11, MRI is the imaging study of choice for the diagnosis and anatomic classification of spinal canal stenosis.
- CT myelography is invasive and can better resolve the bony component of stenosis compared to MRI. Myelograms taken in flexion–extension may demonstrate a dynamic component to the stenosis. CT myelograms may be particularly useful in patients who have had prior surgery (where MRI may be difficult to interpret due to scarring) and in those with associated spinal deformity (eg, scoliosis).
- Plain radiographs are useful in demonstrating instability in the coronal (lateral listhesis) or sagittal (spondylolisthesis) planes that may need to be addressed with fusion in addition to decompression. Upright anteroposterior, lateral, and flexion–extension views can be obtained.

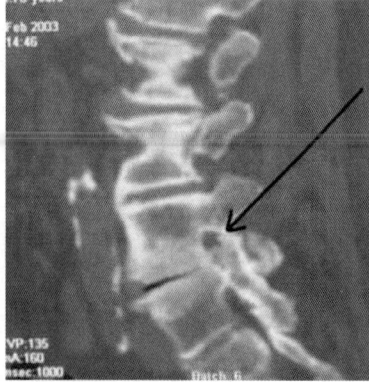

FIG 2 Classic foraminal stenosis due to osteophyte formation on the tip of the superior articular facet demonstrated on CT sagittal reconstruction.

DIFFERENTIAL DIAGNOSIS

- Vascular claudication, bilateral hip osteoarthritis, peripheral neuropathy, and "pump problems" such as congestive heart failure or coronary artery disease resulting in poor peripheral vascular flow

NONOPERATIVE MANAGEMENT

- Patients with mild claudicant symptoms *or* a monoradiculopathy may respond to physical therapy, nonsteroidal anti-inflammatories, and epidural or root sleeve steroid injections. Although some patients may relapse into symptoms, many in this group are content to repeat these efforts or to live with their symptoms.
- Patients with significant claudication or radiculopathies generally do not respond to nonoperative measures, or they respond only temporarily. Most will elect to undergo operative decompression. Similar to disc herniations, absolute surgical indications include a cauda equina syndrome and progressive neurologic deficits.

SURGICAL MANAGEMENT

- The evidence base is clear: Decompressive laminectomy or laminotomy is the operative technique with the best-documented long-term outcomes and is the gold standard of surgery for spinal canal stenosis. In those patients having failed basic conservative measures, the long-term outcomes of decompression are superior to continued nonoperative measures.

Preoperative Planning

- Planning is *vital* and should aim to answer several questions:
  - What is the patient's clinical syndrome?
  - What levels are involved?
  - Is the involvement "intersegmental"?
  - Are the foramina involved?
  - Is there associated pathology: disc herniation, synovial cyst, or degenerative spondylolisthesis or lateral listhesis?
- The answers to these questions will direct the surgical approach, with the goal being complete and safe decompression of compressed neurologic tissue while minimizing damage to tissues not directly involved in the pathologic process.

Positioning

- Prone positioning on a well-padded frame is used (generally the Andrew, Wilson, or Jackson; see **FIG 4A** in Chap. SP-11). The hips and knees are gently flexed to decrease lumbar lordosis and to facilitate the interlaminar approach. The abdomen is free to decrease intra-abdominal pressure and venous backflow into the canal.
- Shoulders should be gently flexed and abducted to less than 90 degrees; eyes, elbows, knees, and feet need to be well padded.
- A needle is passed between and lateral to the spinous processes at the involved level or levels and C-arm imaging used to confirm the level. The needle is removed and the level or levels are marked and labeled on the skin (see **FIG 4B** in Chap. SP-11).

Approach

- After initial dissection, one of two windows will be undertaken based on the location of stenosis: the interlaminar window or the intertransverse window.

- The traditional interlaminar approach for laminotomy or laminectomy is used in about 90% of cases of spinal canal stenosis requiring operative intervention.
  - It is used to decompress soft and bony tissues that compress the neurologic structures within the central canal and subarticular zones throughout the lumbar spine.
- Two less invasive approaches may also be used and have outcomes similar to those seen with the more traditional approach: microdecompression via a unilateral approach and microdecompression via spinous process osteotomies.
  - Both techniques afford bilateral decompression of spinal canal stenosis via a unilateral approach.

INCISION

- The skin incision is made directly midline posteriorly and extends from the top of the most cephalad involved spinous process to the bottom of the most caudally involved spinous process (about 1.5 inches for single-level pathology).
- The subcutaneous tissues are gently mobilized and retracted to allow visualization of the dorsolumbar fascia.

Traditional Interlaminar Window for Decompression

- The dorsolumbar fascia is incised in the midline along the length of the skin incision, allowing exposure of spinous processes at each level.
- A Cobb elevator is then used to gently elevate the muscles (multifidus) from the spinous processes and laminae to the midportion of the facet joints bilaterally.
- A retractor is then placed and an intraoperative fluoroscopic image obtained to confirm the levels.
- At this point, illumination or magnification, based on surgeon preference and experience, is gained by the use of the operative microscope or headlamp and loupes.
- A midline laminotomy is performed on the undersurface of the cephalad lamina to above the level of the insertion of the ligamentum flavum.
  - The insertion point is invariably in line with the most cephalad portion of the facet joint.
- This laminotomy is then continued into the subarticular zone laterally (medial facetectomy) and then to include the superior surface of the caudal lamina (**TECH FIG 1**).
- This bony work allows for exposure and excision of soft and hard tissues compressing the common dural sac and nerve roots and should be enough to get the job done safely and completely while avoiding iatrogenic injury.
  - The surgeon should aim to limit the medial facetectomies to less than 50% bilaterally and to preserve at least 5 mm of the lateral pars intra-articularis.
- In cases with concomitant congenital stenosis (involvement in the anatomic "third story" [see Chap. SP-11]; about 15% of cases), complete midline laminectomy may be needed because the lamina itself is part of the pathologic compressive process.
- In the absence of congenital stenosis or deformity, a decompressive procedure that spans the distance from the top to the bottom of the facet joint will adequately decompress the central portion of the canal in most cases. This is because in most cases, central stenosis occurs where the disc, ligamentum flavum, and facets converge to impinge on neural structures.
- Soft and hard compressive tissue are then excised, allowing for decompression of the common dural sac and nerve roots.
  - This includes the ligamentum flavum in its entirety (in the midline decompression of the central canal, its insertion on the undersurface of the capsule, a trumpeted decompression within the subarticular zone via medial facetectomy) and undercutting of the tip of the superior articular process and osteophytes from the facet joints.

- Generally, no retraction of the underlying dura and roots is needed because most pathology is visible and accessible posteriorly.
- Concomitant pathology will also need to be addressed if present.
  - Unstable degenerative spondylolisthesis should be treated by spinal fusion with or without instrumentation. There is controversy regarding the need for fusion if the spondylolisthesis is mild and/or stable.
  - Synovial cysts will need to be completely excised and the pseudocapsule gently peeled from the dura.
  - Disc herniation should be addressed as described in Chapter SP-11.
- The process is repeated at each clinically involved level. Generally, a residual laminar bridge is maintained at each level for routine decompression for degenerative stenosis. Cases of congenital stenosis require midline laminectomy given the compression within the "third story."
- The wound is then irrigated and hemostasis obtained. The use of a drain is optional, depending on the degree of oozing. The wound is then closed in three layers (fascia, subcutaneous tissue, and skin in running subcuticular fashion).

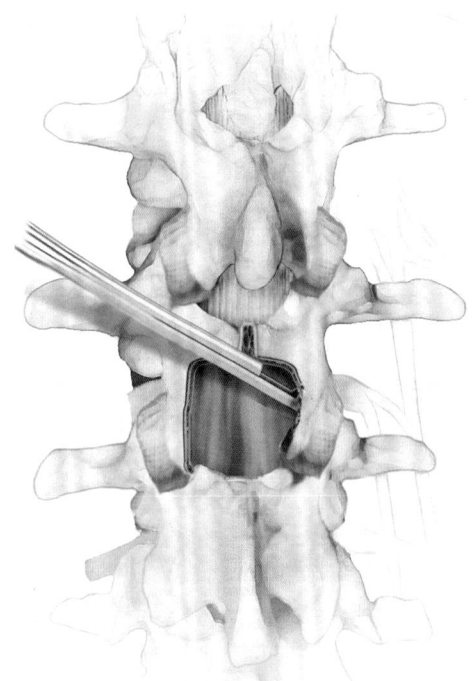

TECH FIG 1 Laminotomy or laminectomy is performed to allow access to the ligamentum flavum, which is excised in its entirety in a trumpeted fashion throughout the segment. Medial facetectomy is included to address any bony stenosis in the subarticular zones.

TECHNIQUES

MICRODECOMPRESSION VIA THE INTERLAMINAR WINDOW

Unilateral Approach

- Microdecompression via a unilateral approach may be used for patients with a predominant monoradiculopathy with or without neurogenic claudication and degenerative stenosis with minimal to no spondylolisthesis.
  - In other words, it is a good option in any case that may be adequately decompressed via laminotomy.
- A unilateral approach and decompression similar to that described earlier is undertaken on the ipsilateral side.
- The contralateral side is decompressed via excision of the inferior half of the spinous process and laminar junction (this is a key step to afford adequate contralateral decompression), allowing exposure and excision (by working underneath the interspinous ligament) of the contralateral ligamentum flavum via progressive angulation of the microscope, progressive resection of the contralateral laminae (covering the entire area where the ligamentum inserts), and ligamentum resection in its entirety **(TECH FIG 2)**.
- This operation is technically demanding but affords a recovery similar to that seen with unilateral microdiscectomy.

Spinous Process Osteotomy Approach

- Microdecompression via spinous process osteotomies may be used as a less invasive alternative for surgeons more comfortable with the traditional approach.
  - It affords the visualization of traditional midline approaches while preserving the spinous process and interspinous and supraspinous ligaments.
- A unilateral approach is used similar to typical discectomy.
- The spinous processes are then osteotomized just posterior to their junction with the laminae.
- When the retractor is placed, the typical bilateral interlaminar window is exposed and decompression, as described earlier, is undertaken **(TECH FIG 3)**.
- Once the retractor is removed, the spinous processes fall back into place and generally heal back to the residual laminar ring.

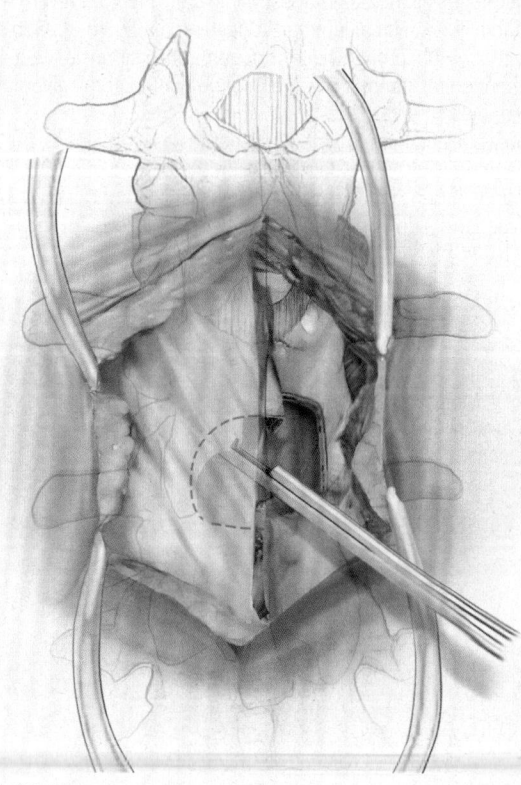

TECH FIG 2 Microdecompression. A unilateral approach is used and a unilateral decompression is performed. The contralateral side is decompressed by angulating under the interspinous ligament in a trumpeted fashion.

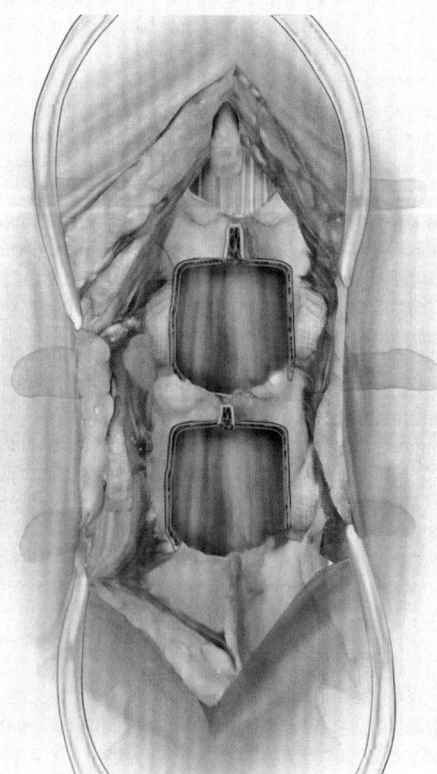

TECH FIG 3 Spinous process osteotomies. A unilateral approach is used and the spinous processes are osteotomized near their base. The spines are then retracted, allowing exposure of the "usual" interlaminar window. After decompression, the spines fall back into place and generally heal to the residual laminar bridge.

FORAMINAL DECOMPRESSION VIA THE INTERTRANSVERSE WINDOW

- Foraminal stenosis may be present with or without associated stenosis within the central canal and subarticular zone (addressed separately as previously). With the exception of L5–S1, where it is accessible via an interlaminar window, it is best addressed via the intertransverse window.
- Adequate decompression of foraminal stenosis via an interlaminar approach requires resection of the lateral pars and results in potential instability at the level. The intertransverse window is a less morbid and easier approach to the foraminal zone and requires minimal resection of the lateral pars.
- The multifidus is taken medially and the longissimus is taken laterally by finger dissection, allowing placement of a retractor in this intermuscular–nervous plane.

- The tips of the superior articular process and the lateral pars interarticularis are exposed with electrocautery.
- Staying within the capsule of the facet joint to protect the underlying exiting root, the surgeon excises the tip of the superior articular process entirely, affording a bony decompression of the foramen (**TECH FIG 4**). Concomitant soft tissue stenosis (ligamentum flavum insertion in the subarticular zone or lateral disc herniation) can then be easily addressed if present.
- Irrigation, hemostasis, and closure are performed as described earlier.

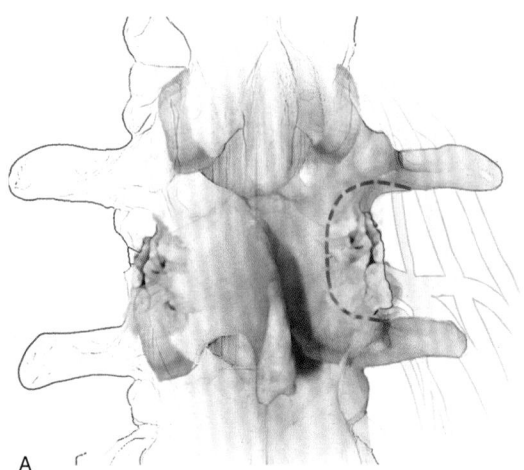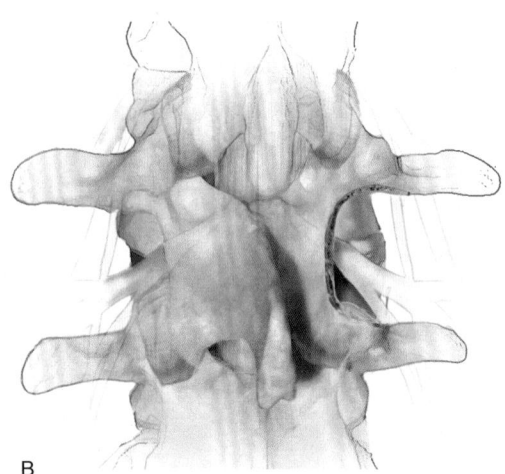

A   B

TECH FIG 4 Foraminal decompression. Excision of the tip of the superior articular process and part of the pars interarticularis via a paraspinal approach (**A**) affords decompression of the exiting root in the foramen (**B**).

TECHNIQUES

Pearls and Pitfalls

Wrong-level exposure, exploration, and surgery are always a concern.	• The recommendations in Chapter SP-11 discuss how to limit these possibilities.
Revision decompression is difficult due to significant midline scar formation.	• The goals should be to find residual lamina and to excise this cephalad and laterally, allowing exposure of previously undistributed dura and roots. The decompression can then be carried caudally and medially using this normal dura as a guide.

POSTOPERATIVE CARE

- After surgery, patients are fitted with a light lumbar corset and are encouraged to walk once anesthesia has worn off and pain permits. About 90% will be ready for discharge as outpatients or 23-hour observation patients. The others (older patients and those with comorbidities) are discharged once they are medically stable and can mobilize adequately.

- Once home, patients engage in a program of progressive walking, stretching, and corset use for comfort. For those progressing slowly, physical therapy may be introduced.
- If all is well, they may drive in about a week and return to light work once they feel up to it. Heavy labor should be avoided for 6 to 12 weeks to ensure proper soft tissue healing. Long-term activities are not restricted.

OUTCOMES

- In most patients, there is an 80% likelihood of an excellent or good outcome, short and long term, after surgery. Reoperation rates are about 15%.
- Patients with significant medical comorbidities (eg, diabetes, heavy smoking, peripheral vessel disease, coronary artery disease) are less likely to do well. There is some evidence that those patients with significant claudication who undergo epidural injections prior to surgery have worse surgical outcomes. Those with primarily leg pain appear to do better.
- Truly informed consent is recommended, as these procedures are not benign in this population.

COMPLICATIONS

- Dependent on the surgeon: wrong level, wrong side, missed pathology, iatrogenic instability, root injury, dural tear, hemorrhage, positioning (eg, eyes, ulnar nerve)
- Dependent on the operative environment and patient: wound infection, urinary retention, thrombophlebitis, or pulmonary embolism

SUGGESTED READINGS

Johnsson KE, Rosén I, Udén A. The natural course of lumbar spinal stenosis. Clin Orthop Relat Res 1992;(279):82–86.

Katz JN, Lipson SJ, Chang LC, et al. Seven- to 10-year outcome of decompressive surgery for degenerative lumbar spinal stenosis. Spine (Phila Pa 1976) 1996;21:92–98.

Lurie JD, Tosteson TD, Tosteson A, et al. Long term outcomes of lumbar spinal stenosis: eight-year results of the Spine Patient Outcomes Research Trial (SPORT). Spine (Phila Pa 1976) 2015;40: 63–76.

Weiner BK, Fraser RD, Peterson M. Spinous process osteotomies to facilitate lumbar decompressive surgery. Spine (Phila Pa 1976) 1999; 24:62–66.

Weiner BK, Walker M, Brower RS, et al. Microdecompression for lumbar spinal canal stenosis. Spine (Phila Pa 1976) 1999;24: 2268–2272.

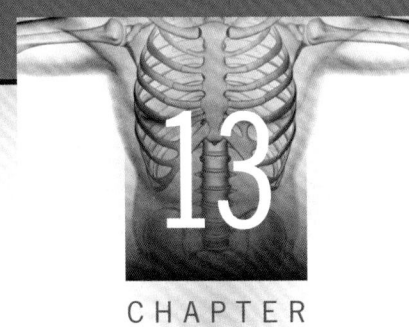

13

CHAPTER

Posterolateral Thoracolumbar Fusion with Instrumentation

James M. Parrish, Joon S. Yoo, Nathaniel W. Jenkins, Sreeharsha V. Nandyala, Alejandro Marquez-Lara, Junyoung Ahn, and Kern Singh

ANATOMY

- Pedicle morphology is detailed in **TABLE 1**.

IMAGING AND OTHER DIAGNOSTIC STUDIES

- Standing posteroanterior and lateral radiographs should be obtained whenever feasible.
- Additional flexion–extension views may provide insight into subtle instabilities (**FIG 1**).
- Full-length posteroanterior and lateral radiographs are obtained in cases of spinal deformity to assess for global balance (coronal or sagittal).
- Lateral bending views can help determine the flexibility of the curvature and levels for fusion.
- Axial computed tomography (CT) images can provide invaluable clinical information about pedicle morphology, particularly in the setting of deformity.

SURGICAL MANAGEMENT

Indications

- Degenerative
  - Spondylolisthesis
  - Iatrogenic instability
  - Discogenic back pain
  - Pseudarthroses
- Adult deformity
  - Curve progression
  - Neurologic deficit
  - Back pain refractory to nonoperative care
  - Pulmonary compromise secondary to deformity
  - Coronal or sagittal imbalance
- Pediatric deformity
  - Progressive scoliosis greater than 50 degrees
  - Kyphosis greater than 75 degrees

TABLE 1 Pedicle Morphology				
Region	**Thoracic**	**Lumbar**	**Sacral**	**General Points**
Size	Width increases cephalad and caudal to T5. T5 is the smallest pedicle (mean 4.5 mm).	Width decreases moving cephalad.	S1 pedicle is the widest of all pedicles (mean 18 mm).	Narrowest in mediolateral dimension
Horizontal angulation	Medial angulation increases gradually to 30 degrees at T1. T12 is angled laterally; T11 is neutral.	Medial angulation increases to 30 degrees at L5. Angulation is 10 degrees medial at L1.		Angulation is medial at all levels except T12.
Vertical angulation	Angulation increases gradually to T2 and then slightly decreases. There is a large increase in superior angulation between L1 (2 degrees) and T12 (10 degrees).	L5 is angled slightly inferior. L3 and L4 are neutral. L1 and L2 are angled slightly superior.		
Length	Pedicles become shorter cephalad and caudal to T8. Longest pedicle is at T8 (45 mm).	Average length is 50 mm throughout the lumbar spine.		There is a high standard deviation in the length of T12 pedicle.

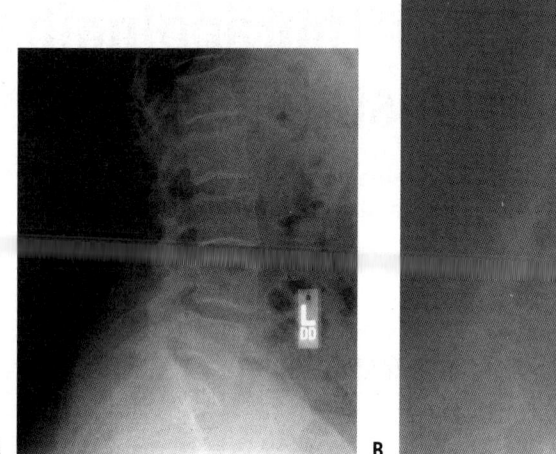
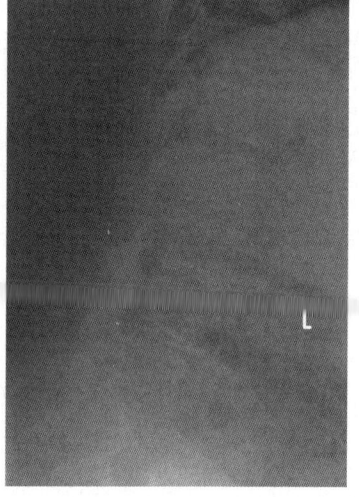
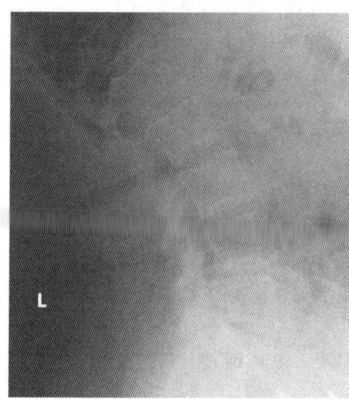

FIG 1 A–C. Flexion and extension lumbar lateral spine radiographs can show evidence of spondylolisthesis as seen here at the L4–L5 level.

- Curve progression, in spite of bracing, in a skeletally immature individual
- Isthmic spondylolisthesis more than 50%

Preoperative Planning

- Pedicle anatomy can be best assessed on CT **(FIG 2)**.
- A general assessment of whether a pedicle is instrumentable can be obtained by examining its size on an anteroposterior radiograph of the pedicle.
- Pedicle diameter/length and starting points can be determined from the axial image.

Positioning

- Patients should be placed in the prone position on a radiolucent table **(FIG 3)**.
- Care is taken to ensure that the neck is in a neutral position to avoid hyperextension.
- The arms are abducted at 90 degrees or less to minimize the likelihood of rotator cuff impingement. The arms are allowed to hang down in a forward-flexed position at approximately 10 degrees. The axilla should be clear from any padding to prevent an inadvertent brachial plexus palsy.

- Elbow pads are placed along the medial epicondyle in order to protect the ulnar nerve.
- The chest pad is placed just proximal to the level of the xiphoid process and distal to the axilla. In women, extra care is taken to reposition the breasts and ensure that the nipples are pressure free.
- The iliac pads are placed two fingerbreadths distal to the anterior superior iliac spine, allowing the abdomen to hang free, thus reducing any unnecessary epidural bleeding.
- Proper placement of the chest and iliac pads allows for optimal restoration of sagittal alignment via gravity.

Approach

- Two approaches are used: the midline approach and the paraspinal approach.
- The midline approach is used for most spinal procedures because it enables direct access to the spinal canal.
- The paraspinal approach, also known as the *Wiltse approach*, was initially described for spondylolisthesis but is also used for far lateral discectomies and minimally invasive muscle-sparing techniques (eg, minimally invasive pedicle screw instrumentation or transforaminal lumbar interbody fusion).
- Specific screw entry points are detailed in **TABLE 2**.

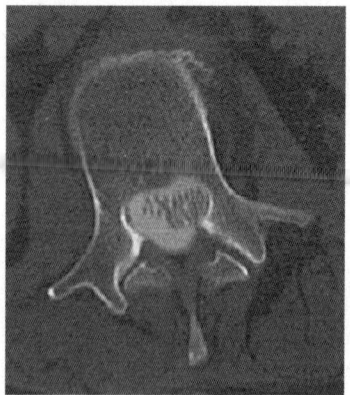
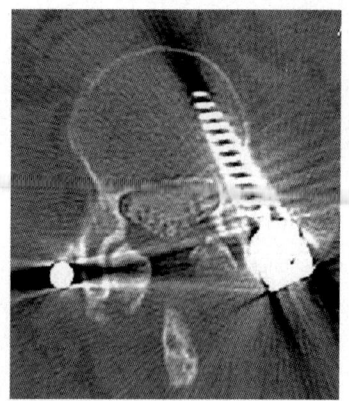

FIG 2 A,B. Pedicle anatomy for screw placement can be assessed with CT scan.

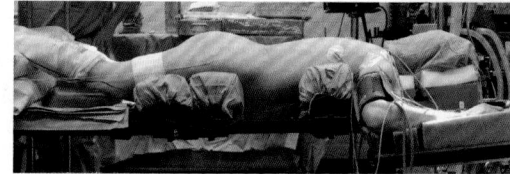

FIG 3 The patient is positioned prone on the Jackson frame.

TABLE 2 Pedicle Screw Starting Points

Region	Starting Point
Proximal thoracic (T1–T3)	Junction of the midpoint of the transverse process and the lateral pars
Midthoracic (T4–T9)	Junction of the proximal transverse process and the lateral third of the superior articular process
Distal thoracic (T10–T12)	Junction of the midpoint of the transverse process and the lateral pars
Lumbar	Junction of the midpoint of the transverse process and 2 mm lateral to the pars
Sacral	At the inferolateral aspect of the L5–S1 facet joint

THORACOLUMBAR PEDICLE SCREW PLACEMENT

Pedicle Start Point

- Once the bony anatomy of the dorsal elements is meticulously exposed, the proper position of the pedicle entry point is defined. Anatomic landmarks include the lateral edge of the facet joint, the pars interarticularis, and the transverse processes **(TECH FIG 1A)**.
- The actual pedicle starting point may vary substantially from the commonly quoted "norms" in many patients. General guidelines follow. Preoperative imaging studies (such as CT scan, or even the relationship between the pedicle and the lateral aspect of the pars on an anteroposterior radiograph) can elucidate anatomic variations in a given patient or level.
- In both the lower (T10–T12) and upper (T1–T3) thoracic spine, the entry point is at the intersection of the bisected transverse process and the lateral edge of the pars interarticularis.
  - In the midthoracic region (T5–T9), the starting point is more medial and cephalad. In this figure, it is at the junction of the superior margin of the transverse process and the lateral third of the superior articular process **(TECH FIG 1B)**.

- In the lumbar spine, the point of entry is at the midpoint of the transverse process and 2 mm lateral to the pars interarticularis.
- The sacral entry point is at the inferolateral aspect of the L5–S1 facet joint.
- Using a 4-mm high-speed burr, the posterior cortex is breached to a depth of approximately 5 mm **(TECH FIG 1C)**.
- Alternatively, fluoroscopic imaging may be used with the bull's-eye technique to ascertain the correct starting point, particularly when patient anatomy is complex **(TECH FIG 1D)**.

Cannulating the Pedicle

- A 3.2-mm hand drill is positioned into the starting hole and advanced along the axis of the pedicle **(TECH FIG 2A,B)**. The drill is advanced under fluoroscopic guidance into the vertebral body to a depth of 35 to 40 mm in the lumbosacral spine, 25 to 30 mm in the lower and upper thoracic spine, and 30 to 35 mm in the midthoracic spine.
  - Measurements of pedicle length can be made on axial CT or magnetic resonance imaging scans and used to guide screw length.

TECH FIG 1 A. Posterior anatomy of the lumbar spine. **B.** Starting points for pedicle screws in the thoracic spine. **C.** The posterior cortex is breached with a 4-mm burr. **D.** The "bull's-eye" technique with fluoroscopy can be used to correctly identify the starting point.

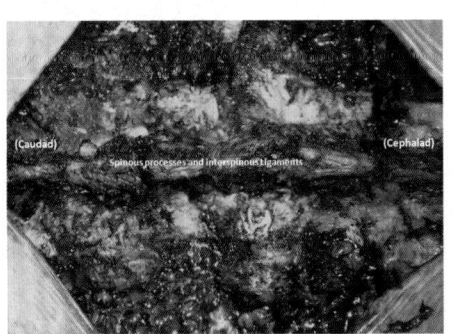

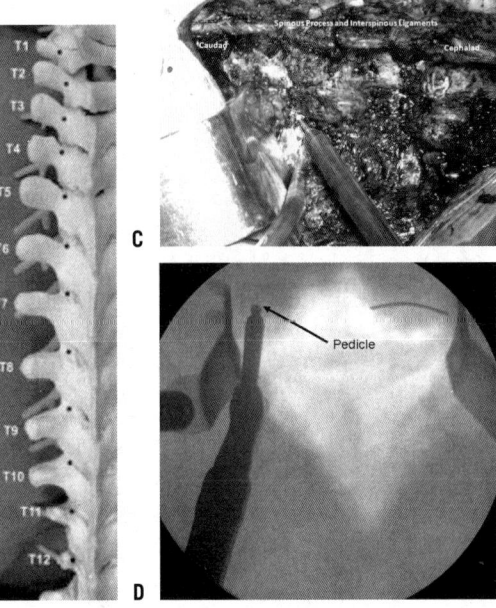

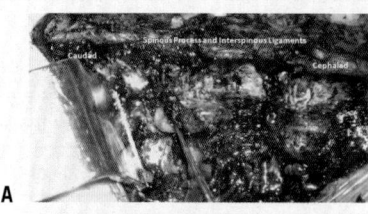

TECH FIG 2 A. The hand drill is advanced into the pedicle. **B.** Path for the tricortical sacral pedicle screw. **C.** L5–S1 instrumentation with tricortical sacral fixation.

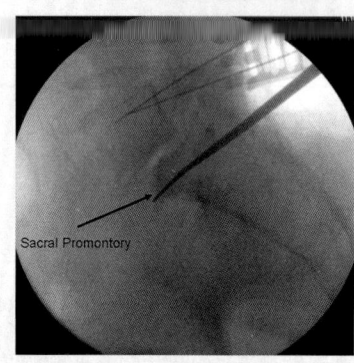

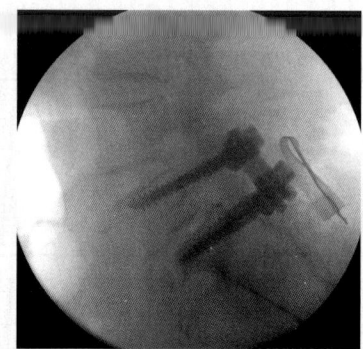

- The advantage of using a hand drill is that cortical violations are minimized. When resistance is met (cortex), the drill is unable to advance, and, as a result, the angle is adjusted.
- Alternatively, a "gearshift" type of device can be used to sound the pedicle. The gearshift should be gently rotated or wiggled as it is advanced. This technique enables the instrument to find the proper path within cancellous bone as opposed to being pushed forcefully through a cortical wall. The process is analogous to feeding a guidewire into a vein during central line placement: The concept is to provide guidance, not force, to the instrument as it navigates a path within the cortical margins of the bone.
- For the S1 pedicle, the drill is guided 25 degrees medially and 10 degrees inferiorly toward the sacral promontory. A lateral fluoroscopic image is used to identify the sacral promontory **(TECH FIG 2C)**.
  - Ideally, the screw tip should achieve tricortical purchase (engaging the anterior and posterior cortex and superior endplate of S1) (see **TECH FIG 2C**).
- Next, a flexible, ball-tipped probe is advanced down the pedicle tract. Bone should be encountered at the base of the tract as well as along all four walls of the pedicle. Medial and lateral

cortical breaching is most common as the pedicle is narrowest in this plane.
- A medial pedicle breach is most likely to occur at a depth between 15 and 20 mm ventral to the transverse process, which is the depth at which the spinal canal is reached in most levels.
- If a proper start site is chosen, lateral breaches are more likely to occur at a depth of 20 mm or greater due to failure to medialize and follow the proper trajectory as the pedicle transitions into the vertebral body. However, if the start site is too lateral, a lateral breach may occur more superficially.

Pedicle Screw Sizing

- With the ball-tipped probe advanced along the length of the pedicle tract, the surgeon measures the tract depth with a hemostat and a ruler **(TECH FIG 3A)**.
- In general, pedicles are tapped 1 mm smaller than the diameter of the screw to be used to optimize screw purchase. If the pedicle is sclerotic, "line-to-line" tapping should be performed. If the patient is osteoporotic, tapping is not needed.
- After tapping, the ball-tipped probe is again advanced through the pedicle tract to ensure that the pedicle cortices and anterior vertebral body are intact.

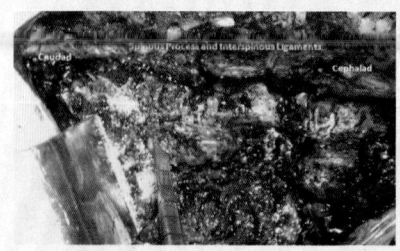

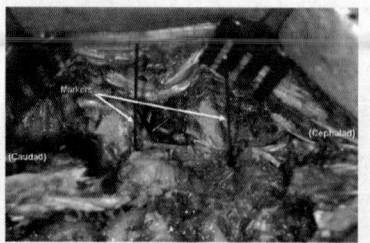

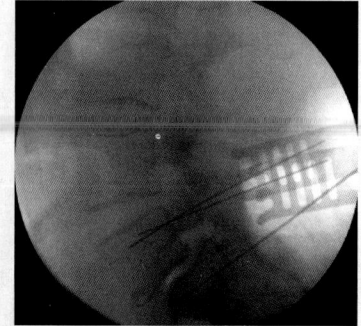

TECH FIG 3 A. A gearshift is inserted in a twisting motion to cannulate the pedicle. The starting point is the mammillary process found at the junction of the transverse process and the superior articular facet. **B,C.** Pedicle marker positions are confirmed with fluoroscopy.

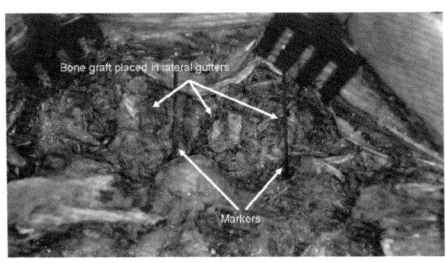

TECH FIG 4 After decortication, bone graft is placed over the decorticated areas.

- A Kirschner wire is then positioned into the pedicle while the remaining pedicle tracts are cannulated.
- Proper placement of all Kirschner wires is confirmed via fluoroscopy. At this point, fusion bed preparation may occur **(TECH FIG 3B,C)**.

Fusion Bed Preparation

- The wound is extensively irrigated before decortication to preserve the local bone graft generated with high-speed burring.
- Using a high-speed burr, the transverse process, the pars interarticularis, and the lateral wall of the facet joint of each level to be fused are decorticated.

- Bone graft is placed over the decorticated areas. The fusion bed can be created with any combination of autogenous iliac crest bone graft, autogenous local bone graft (from the spinous processes and lamina), allograft, demineralized bone matrix, or bone morphogenic protein **(TECH FIG 4)**.
  - Decorticating and bone grafting the intertransverse, lateral pars, and lateral facet regions are performed before placing the screws to optimally prepare the fusion bed without the instrumentation getting in the way.
- Once the bone graft has been positioned, the Kirschner wires function as identifying landmarks for pedicle screw cannulation. Care is taken to advance the screw slowly in the same angulation noted with the Kirschner wire in place.

PELVIC FIXATION

- Sacropelvic fixation can be used in the setting of long deformity reconstructions and tumors and in traumatic settings involving the lower lumbosacral spine.
- Modern pelvic fixation is most simply accomplished via modular iliac screw placement.
- After dissection of the posterior superior iliac spine, a starting point is identified 1.5 cm distal to the tubercle.
- A burr or rongeur is used to a recessed defect, such that the iliac screw head will lie recessed within the posterior superior iliac spine.

- A gearshift is then inserted into the starting point and advanced between the inner and outer tables of the pelvis, with the medial point of the probe scraping along the medial wall.
  - The trajectory should generally aim toward the hip joint.
  - The cortex of the medial wall is thicker than the lateral, making lateral violations more likely than medial violations.
- A ball-tipped probe is used to assess the inner and outer tables.
- Depth is measured and the screw is inserted. The screw is typically 7.5 to 8.5 mm in diameter and roughly 60 to 80 mm long **(TECH FIG 5)**.

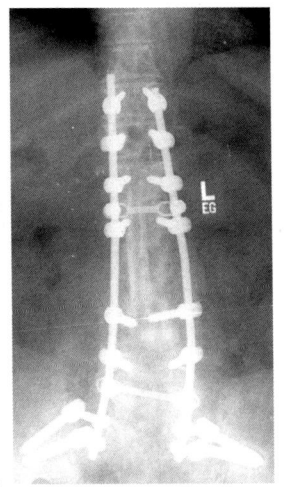
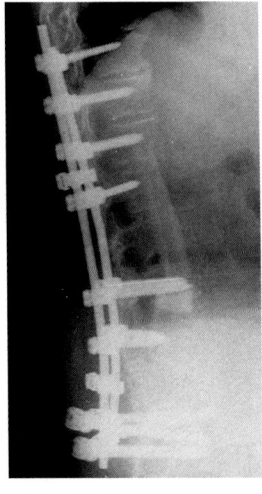

TECH FIG 5 A,B. Fusion to pelvis with iliac screws.

CROSS-CONNECTORS

- Cross-connectors can significantly increase the rotational and bending stiffness of a multilevel construct.

- One, two, or three cross-links can be used, depending on the length of the construct. If multiple cross-connectors are used, they should be separated as far apart as possible from each other to maximize construct rigidity.

HOOK INSERTION

- Hooks can be placed about the pedicle, transverse process, or lamina.
- Fixation is increased with a claw configuration.
- A claw figuration is made of two hooks directed toward each other, separated by one or two levels. Claws are primarily used at the ends of a construct (**TECH FIG 6A**).
- Pedicle hooks provide the strongest fixation of all hook constructs. The pedicle hook is placed between the lamina of the superior vertebra and the superior articular process of the inferior vertebra in a cephalad orientation (**TECH FIG 6B**). The U-shaped tip fits around the pedicle and allows for increased stability.
  - The inferior facet of the vertebra can be removed with an osteotome. It is beneficial to resect enough of the facet so that the lateral edge of the spinal canal is identified so it can be avoided during implant placement. The cartilage of the superior facet is removed with a curette. A pedicle hook developer is positioned in the facet to develop the plane before placing the hook itself (**TECH FIG 6C**).

- Laminar hooks can be placed on the superior (downgoing) or inferior (upgoing) laminae (**TECH FIG 6D**). They should be used with caution, as a portion of the implant is placed within the spinal canal. Generally, placing two laminar hooks into the canal at the same level (eg, two downgoing hooks or two upgoing hooks on the same lamina) should be avoided to minimize implant volume in the canal.
  - The ligamentum flavum is dissected off the lamina, and the laminar surface receiving the hook is prepared with a Kerrison rongeur to ensure that the hook will be flushed against the bone.
- Transverse process hooks can be used when sublaminar or pedicle hooks are not possible (**TECH FIG 6E**). They can be oriented either cephalad or (more commonly) caudad. A transverse process hook developer helps create a plane for the implant. Although weaker than sublaminar or pedicle hooks, they avoid violation of the spinal canal.

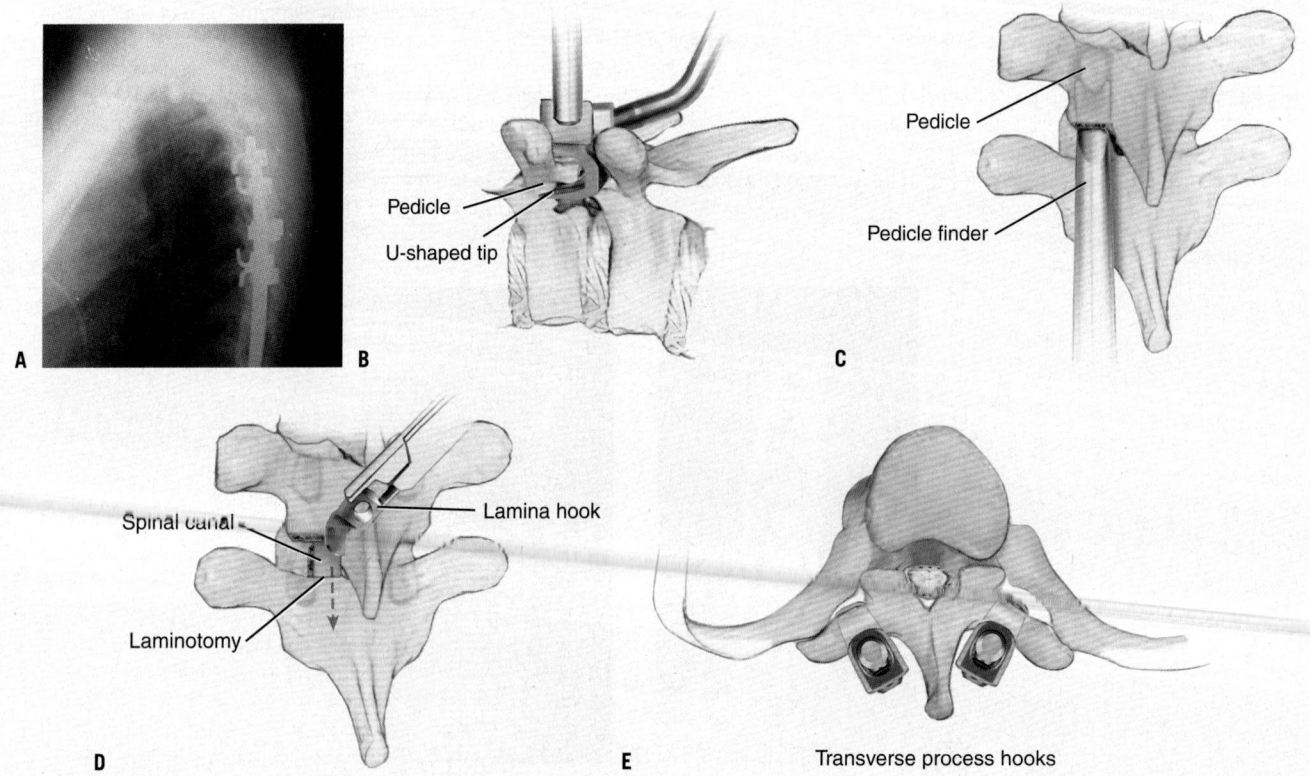

TECH FIG 6 A. Thoracic hooks oriented in the claw configuration. **B.** Placement of a thoracic pedicle hook. **C.** A pedicle hook developer developing a plane for the pedicle hook. **D.** Placement of an upgoing laminar hook. **E.** Upgoing and downgoing transverse process hooks.

Pearls and Pitfalls

- Careful assessment of preoperative imaging (CT) allows for more accurate pedicle screw placement.

- Fluoroscopy can be used to identify proper pedicle starting points when patient anatomy is distorted.

- Breaching the medial or inferior pedicle cortex endangers the exiting nerve root. Medial pedicle breaches are typically identified at a depth of 15–20 mm.

- Too medial of a starting point for pedicle screw entry may injure the supra-adjacent facet joint.

POSTOPERATIVE CARE

- With secure multilevel pedicle screw fixation, it is likely not necessary to brace patients postoperatively, although that decision should be individualized based on the patient's pathology.

COMPLICATIONS

- Infection
  - The incidence of infection for posterior spine surgery increases with the addition of an instrumented fusion.
  - A 1% infection rate has been noted for discectomies; a 6% infection rate for discectomies and fusion.
  - Although there is a wide range reported for instrumented posterior fusions, the overall infection rate appears to be around 5% to 6%.
- Pseudarthrosis (nonunion rates, particularly crossing the lumbosacral junction)
  - The incidence of nonunion after posterior lateral inter-transverse fusion ranges from 3% to 25%.
  - Smoking has been demonstrated to be a risk factor for nonunion.
  - A wide range of fusion rates across the lumbosacral junction have been reported (22% to 89%).
  - A 92.5% fusion rate is reported across the L5–S1 junction when using iliac screws.
- Neurologic and vascular injury
  - Although there is potential for severe vascular injury with pedicle screws in the thoracolumbar spine, vascular complications are rare, outside of a few reports.
- The risk of nerve root irritation has been reported to be very low (0.2%) from pedicle screw instrumentation.

SUGGESTED READINGS

Ali RM, Boacjie-Adjei O, Rawlins BA. Functional and radiographic outcomes after surgery for adult scoliosis using third-generation instrumentation techniques. Spine (Phila Pa 1976) 2003;28: 1163–1169.

Andrés-Cano P, Cerván A, Rodríguez-Solera M, et al. Surgical infection after posterolateral lumbar spine arthrodesis: CT analysis of spinal fusion. Orthop Surg 2018;10:89–97.

Bernard TN Jr, Seibert CE. Pedicle diameter determined by computed tomography. Its relevance to pedicle screw fixation in the lumbar spine. Spine (Phila Pa 1976) 1992;17:S160–S163.

Bernhardt M, Swartz DE, Clothiaux PL, et al. Posterolateral lumbar and lumbosacral fusion with and without pedicle screw internal fixation. Clin Orthop Relat Res 1992;(284):109–115.

Bridwell KH, Lewis SJ, Edwards C, et al. Complications and outcomes of pedicle subtraction osteotomies for fixed sagittal imbalance. Spine (Phila Pa 1976) 2003;28:2093–2101.

Brown CW, Orme TJ, Richardson HD. The rate of pseudarthrosis (surgical nonunion) in patients who are smokers and patients who are nonsmokers: a comparison study. Spine (Phila Pa 1976) 1986;11: 942–943.

Brox JI, Sørensen R, Friis A, et al. Randomized clinical trial of lumbar instrumented fusion and cognitive intervention and exercises in patients with chronic low back pain and disc degeneration. Spine (Phila Pa 1976) 2003;28:1913–1921.

Fischgrund JS, Mackay M, Herkowitz HN, et al. 1997 Volvo award winner in clinical studies. Degenerative lumbar spondylolisthesis with spinal stenosis: a prospective, randomized study comparing decompressive laminectomy and arthrodesis with and without spinal instrumentation. Spine (Phila Pa 1976) 1997;22:2807–2812.

Fritzell P, Hägg O, Wessberg P, et al. Chronic low back pain and fusion: a comparison of three surgical techniques: a prospective multicenter randomized study from the Swedish Lumbar Spine Study group. Spine (Phila Pa 1976) 2002;27:1131–1141.

Gibby JT, Swenson SA, Cvetko S, et al. Head-mounted display augmented reality to guide pedicle screw placement utilizing computed tomography. Int J Comput Assist Radiol Surg 2019;14:525–535.

Horowitch A, Peek RD, Thomas JC Jr, et al. The Wiltse pedicle screw fixation system. Early clinical results. Spine (Phila Pa 1976) 1989;14: 461–467.

Horwitz NH, Curtin JA. Prophylactic antibiotics and wound infections following laminectomy lumbar disc herniation. J Neurosurg 1997;86:975–980.

Kato S, Fok KL, Lee JW, et al. Dynamic fluctuation of truncal shift parameters during quiet standing in healthy young individuals. Spine (Phila Pa 1976) 2018;43:E746–E751.

Keller A, Brox JI, Gunderson R, et al. Trunk muscle strength, cross-sectional area, and density in patients with chronic low back pain randomized to lumbar fusion or cognitive intervention and exercises. Spine (Phila Pa 1976) 2004;29:3–8.

Kornblum MB, Fischgrund JS, Herkowitz HN, et al. Degenerative lumbar spondylolisthesis with spinal stenosis: a prospective long-term study comparing fusion and pseudarthrosis. Spine (Phila Pa 1976) 2004;29:726–733.

Lenke LG, Fehlings MG, Shaffrey CI, et al. Neurologic outcomes of complex adult spinal deformity surgery: results of the prospective, multicenter Scoli-RISK-1 study. Spine (Phila Pa 1976) 2016;41:204–212.

Leufvén C, Nordwall A. Management of chronic disabling low back pain with 360 degrees fusion. Results from pain provocation test and concurrent posterior lumbar interbody fusion, posterolateral fusion, and pedicle screw instrumentation in patients with chronic disabling low back pain. Spine (Phila Pa 1976) 1999;24:2042–2045.

Lonstein JE, Denis F, Perra JH, et al. Complications associated with pedicle screws. J Bone Joint Surg Am 1999;81(11):519–528.

Lu T, Lu Y. Comparison of biomechanical performance among posterolateral fusion and transforaminal, extreme, and oblique lumbar interbody fusion: a finite element analysis. World Neurosurg 2019;129:e890–e899.

Lynn G, Mukherjee DP, Kruse RN, et al. Mechanical stability of thoracolumbar pedicle screw fixation. The effect of crosslinks. Spine (Phila Pa 1976) 1997;22:1568–1572.

Matsunaga S, Sakou T, Morizono Y, et al. Natural history of degenerative spondylolisthesis. Pathogenesis and natural course of the slippage. Spine (Phila Pa 1976) 1990;15:1204–1210.

Molinari RW, Bridwell KH, Lenke LG, et al. Complications in the surgical treatment of pediatric high-grade, isthmic dysplastic spondylolisthesis. A comparison of three surgical approaches. Spine (Phila Pa 1976) 1999;24:1701–1711.

Moore KR, Pinto MR, Butler LM. Degenerative disc disease treated with combined anterior and posterior arthrodesis and posterior instrumentation. Spine (Phila Pa 1976) 2002;27:1680–1686.

Parker LM, Murrell SE, Boden SD, et al. The outcome of posterolateral fusion in highly selected patients with discogenic low back pain. Spine (Phila Pa 1976) 1996;21:1909–1916.

Rechtine GR, Sutterlin CE, Wood GW, et al. The efficacy of pedicle screw/plate fixation on lumbar/lumbosacral autogenous bone graft fusion in adult patients with degenerative spondylolisthesis. J Spinal Disord 1996;9:382–391.

Sato H, Kikuchi S. The natural history of radiographic instability of the lumbar spine. Spine (Phila Pa 1976) 1993;18:2075–2079.

Sciubba DM, Yurter A, Smith JS, et al. A comprehensive review of complication rates after surgery for adult deformity: a reference for informed consent. Spine Deform 2016;4:575–594.

Steinmann JC, Herkowitz HN. Pseudarthrosis of the spine. Clin Orthop Relat Res 1992;(284):80–90.

Suk SI, Kim WJ, Lee SM, et al. Thoracic pedicle screw placement in deformity: are they really safe? Spine (Phila Pa 1976) 2001;26:2049–2057.

Urquhart JC, Alnaghmoosh N, Gurr KR, et al. Posterolateral versus posterior interbody fusion in lumbar degenerative spondylolisthesis. Clin Spine Surg 2018;31:E446–E452.

Weinstein SL, Dolan LA, Spratt KF, et al. Health and function of patients with untreated idiopathic scoliosis: a 50-year natural history study. JAMA 2003;289:559–567.

Weinstein SL, Ponseti IV. Curve progression in idiopathic scoliosis. J Bone Joint Surg Am 1983;65(4):447–455.

Zindrick MR, Wiltse LL, Doornik A, et al. Analysis of the morphometric characteristics of the thoracic and lumbar pedicles. Spine (Phila Pa 1976) 1987;12:160–166.

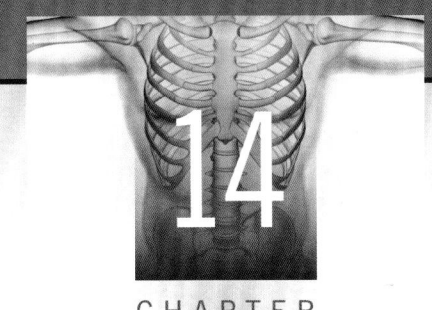

14
CHAPTER

Transforaminal and Posterior Lumbar Interbody Fusion

Christopher M. Mikhail and Saad B. Chaudhary

DEFINITION

- Several arthrodesis techniques are available to address the various pathologic processes in the lumbar spine.
- The standard lumbar arthrodesis techniques include the following:
  - Anterior lumbar interbody fusion (ALIF)
  - Posterior spinal fusion (PSF), which includes two subtypes
    - Posterior interlaminar and facet fusion
    - Posterior lateral intertransverse fusion
  - Combined anterior and posterior fusion (AP fusion or 360-degree fusion)
  - Posterior lumbar interbody fusion (PLIF) and its variant, the transforaminal lumbar interbody fusion (TLIF)
- The PLIF procedure uses a posterior approach to the spine that involves radical discectomy and endplate preparation combined with an interbody fusion using a structural graft or cage with or without supplemental posterior instrumentation.
- The TLIF procedure is similar to PLIF with the modification that the interbody region is accessed unilaterally via a more lateral approach in conjunction with pedicle screw instrumentation.
- PLIF and TLIF are versatile techniques that offer several advantages over the other fusion methods.[4]
  - They allow for pathology in all three columns of the spine to be addressed and for a circumferential fusion to be achieved through a single posterior approach.
  - They directly address the disc as a potential pain generator in patients with discogenic pain syndromes.
  - They have demonstrated a high rate of fusion that approximates the arthrodesis rate achieved with a more extensive combined AP fusion procedure.
  - They allow for direct decompression of the spinal canal if necessary.
  - They facilitate correction of spinal deformities, including asymmetric disc space collapse, spondylolisthesis, and mild kyphosis.
- PLIF and TLIF procedures also avoid some of the drawbacks inherent to ALIF procedures, such as the following:
  - Vascular injury, higher rates of thromboembolic disease, and retrograde ejaculation in males[8]
- PLIF and TLIF have a few disadvantages associated with a standard posterior approach and proximity to neural structures:
  - Potential nerve root injury from dissection, preparation, and instrumentation of the disc space through a posterior approach

- The TLIF implant, unlike an ALIF cage, is often smaller or expandable, which may lead to higher incidence of subsidence.[12,20]
- Longer operative time and higher transfusion rate compared to ALIF[8]

ANATOMY

- The standard posterior approach to the lumbar spine is used for posterior interbody fusion techniques.
- Applied surgical anatomy considerations for TLIF and PLIF are nearly identical, with both techniques using a midline incision and standard posterior exposure.
- Both PLIF and TLIF techniques require interbody access via a posterior annulotomy.
- The major difference is that the PLIF procedure uses a bilateral and more medial approach to access the interbody region, whereas the TLIF technique involves a unilateral approach with complete removal of one facet joint to allow more lateral access to the disc space (FIG 1).
  - As a result, the exiting root is at a greater risk when performing a TLIF, whereas the traversing root and thecal sac are at greater risk with a PLIF.
- A masterful understanding of the triangular working window to the annulus and the local neurologic anatomy is critical in order to safely execute the TLIF or PLIF procedure.
- The triangular working window consists of the following:
  - The traversing nerve root and thecal sac form the medial border of the triangle.
  - The exiting nerve root from the proximal vertebral level forms the lateral border (eg, L4 for an L4–L5 TLIF or PLIF).
  - The superior aspect of the pedicle of the distal vertebra forms the base of the triangle.
- A confluence of epidural veins traveling longitudinally and transversely drapes the floor of the spinal canal and neuroforamen.
- With careful exposure, a triangular working window measuring up to 1.5 cm wide and of slightly greater height can be created.
- A noncollapsed disc space of an adult lumbar spine averages between 12 and 14 mm in height, with an AP diameter of about 35 mm.[6]

PATHOGENESIS

- The PLIF and TLIF techniques are most commonly used when addressing the degenerative pathologies of the lumbar spine. The pathophysiologic discussion of the degenerative cascade is beyond the scope of this chapter and is touched on elsewhere in this book.

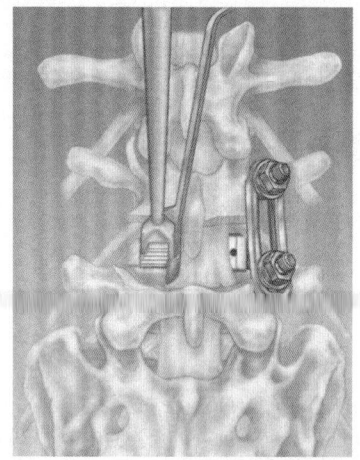

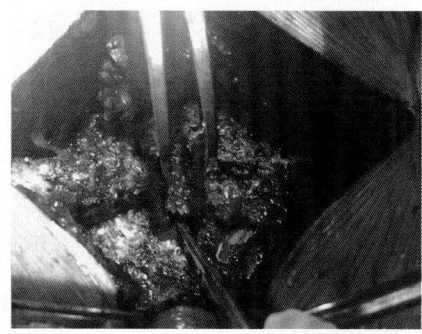

FIG 1 **A.** PLIF technique, demonstrating the bilateral approach to the interbody region with complete facetectomies. Medial retraction of the neurologic elements is necessary to facilitate access to the disc space. **B.** TLIF technique, demonstrating the more lateral approach to the disc space with unilateral facetectomy. With the TLIF technique, medial retraction of the neurologic elements is frequently not needed. (**A:** Reproduced with permission of Medtronic, Inc.)

- Common pathologies include the following:
  - Spondylolisthesis
  - Adult deformity
  - Recurrent disc herniation
  - Degenerative disc disease/discogenic back pain
- The PLIF and TLIF procedures allow for fusion of the anterior column of the spine in the interbody region, which offers several biologic and biomechanical advantages over PSFs:
  - The anterior column of the spine is known to support 80% of the body's compressive load; consequently, intervertebral structural grafts are subjected to compressive loading, which facilitates arthrodesis.
  - Because interbody structural grafts are load sharing, they significantly reduce the cantilever bending forces applied to posterior spinal implants, thus protecting them from failure.
  - The interbody space has been shown to provide an optimal milieu for promoting arthrodesis for several reasons:
    - A large surface area of highly vascular cancellous bone is available.
    - The disc space represents a relatively shorter gap to span when compared to intertransverse fusion.
    - The outer annulus serves as a barrier that reduces fibrous tissue ingrowth into the fusion mass during healing of an interbody arthrodesis.

INDICATIONS

- Discogenic pain syndromes due to internal disc disruption or degeneration as well as postdiscectomy chronic low back pain are well suited to PLIF or TLIF for several reasons[13,16]:
  - These procedures directly address the disc as the pain generator and have been shown to have superior clinical outcomes in treating discogenic pain compared to isolated PSFs, which do not remove and fuse the painful disc.
  - They allow for restoration of intervertebral height and some correction of local kyphosis without putting undue stress on the posterior implants.
  - They permit decompression of the exiting and traversing nerve roots indirectly by restoring foraminal height and directly via open laminectomy and foraminotomy. Because of this, PLIF and TLIF are ideally suited to patients with discogenic pain syndromes occurring in conjunction with radicular symptoms caused by herniated disc pathology or stenosis (**FIG 2**).
- Low-grade (grade 1 or 2) degenerative or isthmic spondylolisthesis can also be treated successfully with PLIF and TLIF procedures as an alternative to performing a combined AP fusion.[13]
  - In addition to direct and indirect decompression of neural elements, PLIF and TLIF raises the arthrodesis rate over stand-alone posterior fusion.

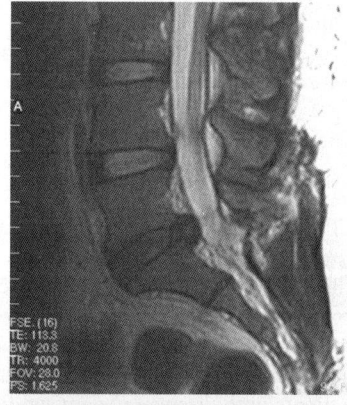

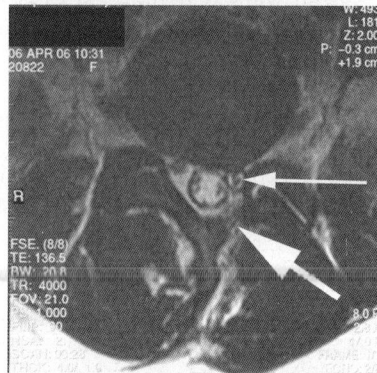

FIG 2 **A.** T2-weighted sagittal MRI demonstrating L5–S1 disc degeneration with a recurrent disc herniation in this patient who had undergone a previous L5–S1 discectomy. **B.** T2-weighted axial image of the same patient. Note the dorsal displacement of the traversing left S1 nerve root (*thin arrow*) by the disc and the previous left-sided laminotomy defect (*thick arrow*).

- When clinically indicated and with proper instrumentation, PLIF and TLIF allow for reduction of the spondylolisthesis and slip angle, with restoration of lordosis. In experienced hands and in conjunction with a wide decompression and intraoperative neurologic monitoring, some higher grade (grade >2) spondylolistheses can also be successfully reduced and stabilized with the PLIF and TLIF procedures.
- PLIF and TLIF procedures can be a useful adjunct to adult deformity surgeries such as degenerative scoliosis and spondylolisthesis and offer several advantages:
  - They can be used to provide anterior column support at the caudal end of fusion constructs and the lumbosacral junction without requiring an additional anterior approach to the spine.
  - They improve the arthrodesis rate, which can be helpful when an interlaminar fusion is not possible because a midline decompression was necessary to address spinal stenosis.
  - They allow for some additional deformity correction by releasing asymmetrically collapsed disc spaces and providing interbody structural support.
- PLIF and TLIF can also help raise the fusion rate in clinically challenging situations posing a high risk for nonunion, such as:
  - Patients unwilling or unable to quit smoking
  - Patients with diabetes mellitus or on systemic corticosteroids
  - Patients on chemotherapy or with an irradiated fusion bed
  - Revision spinal fusion procedures in which the posterolateral fusion bed is fibrotic and hypovascular

CONTRAINDICATIONS

- PLIF should not usually be attempted at the level of the conus medullaris (typically L1–L2) or above, and great caution must be taken using the TLIF procedure at the level of the cord or conus.
- Severe osteoporosis is a relative contraindication to these procedures as disc space preparation can result in major endplate violations with subsequent implant subsidence.
- Anomalous neural anatomy such as a conjoined nerve root can make the performance of a PLIF or TLIF procedure impossible.
  - Even in some cases of "normal" nerve root anatomy, local variations in takeoff angles of the exiting and traversing roots can place the roots at risk during interbody approaches. Caution should be exercised in such cases and interbody fusion abandoned if not felt to be safe.
- Severe focal kyphosis is poorly addressed with a PLIF or TLIF procedure and is usually better treated with an anterior procedure that allows for release of the anterior longitudinal ligament and annulus fibrosus.
- Irreducible higher grade (grade >2) spondylolistheses are not well treated with the PLIF and TLIF procedures as the surface area of the opposing vertebral endplates is minimized.
- Severe epidural fibrosis and an active infectious process can result in dural tears, neurologic injury, and possible meningitis.

NONOPERATIVE MANAGEMENT

- Before considering PLIF and TLIF surgeries, standard nonoperative management options for the pathologic conditions being addressed should typically be exhausted.

- Nonsurgical treatment usually involves a combination of analgesic medications, physical therapy, and activity and lifestyle modification. When applicable, interventional pain management techniques such as trigger point injections, facet blocks, or epidural steroid injections should be considered.
- Surgical intervention is usually reserved for patients who remain symptomatic despite several months of nonoperative treatment and whose symptoms are severe enough to justify the risks associated with operative care.

SURGICAL MANAGEMENT

- As mentioned earlier, PLIF and TLIF procedures are capable of addressing a wide variety of pathologic conditions and, in specific situations, offer several compelling advantages.
- Given their versatility, the well-trained spinal surgeon needs to be aware of the indications for these procedures and must be capable of executing them properly.
- Although the usefulness of the PLIF and TLIF procedures is clear, one must remain mindful that these procedures are technically demanding and should be undertaken only after careful training and preoperative planning and with meticulous surgical technique.

Preoperative Planning

- Preoperative imaging studies should be reviewed to determine the appropriate size and trajectories necessary for pedicle screw insertion as well as the AP diameter of the disc space.
- Disc space height as well as adjacent disc height and overall lumbar alignment should be measured to help determine optimal interbody implant size.
- An assessment should be made whether direct or indirect neurologic decompression will be necessary.
- When using the TLIF technique, the interbody approach should be performed on the patient's symptomatic side if he or she has radicular complaints or from the side of maximal neurologic compression if the lower extremity symptoms are of equal severity.
- Although sometimes difficult to assess, the patient's magnetic resonance imaging (MRI) needs to be studied carefully to identify anomalous neural anatomy such as a conjoined nerve root.
  - If a conjoined nerve root is suspected, the TLIF should be performed from the opposite side, and the patient should be counseled preoperatively that the interbody portion of the procedure may not be possible because the contralateral side may demonstrate intraoperative nerve root anomalies as well.
  - For the PLIF procedure, the presence of a conjoined nerve root usually necessitates a unilateral PLIF. If identified preoperatively, conversion to a TLIF should be strongly considered.
- Deformity at the level of the planned fusion needs to be assessed so that intraoperative measures can be taken to provide for correction.

Positioning

- The patient should be positioned prone on an operating room table that allows for fluoroscopic imaging, such as a Jackson spine table (**FIG 3**).

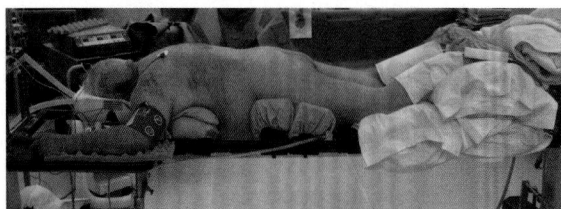

FIG 3 Prone positioning with the abdomen free of compression, lower extremity compression devices in place, knees flexed, and all bony prominences padded. All tubes and wires are secured so that the area under the patient is free of obstruction, which facilitates later use of the fluoroscopy unit.

- The abdomen should be free to decompress the vena cava. This maneuver has been found to reduce epidural venous engorgement and bleeding.
- A Foley catheter and lower extremity sequential compression devices should be used routinely.
- Pillows should be used to keep the knees slightly flexed to minimize tension on the lumbar nerve roots.
- Intraoperative physiologic monitoring with somatosensory evoked potentials and "free running" electromyographic monitoring should be considered. Physiologic monitoring will also allow for the option of pedicle screw stimulation testing to help detect any inadvertent pedicle wall breaches.

Approach

- The standard posterior approach to the lumbar spine is used, including exposure out to the tips of the transverse processes so that an adequate intertransverse fusion can be performed.
  - Some surgeons choose to perform a more limited dissection and do not perform the posterolateral portion of the fusion, hoping that by preserving the blood supply and muscular attachments in the intertransverse region, there will be reduced erector muscle dysfunction and fibrosis with improved outcomes.
  - Minimally invasive TLIF options have been developed and are described in Chapter SP-19.
- For the standard TLIF procedure, the spinous processes and interspinous ligaments can usually be left intact. Preserving these structures minimizes epidural scarring and provides a larger surface area for the posterior fusion.
  - If decompression of the contralateral side of the spinal canal is required, the TLIF procedure can be modified to include a central laminectomy.
- Two exposure options exist for the PLIF procedure, each of which is discussed in more detail later in the chapter:
  - Extensive resection, including wide laminectomy with bilateral facetectomies
  - Limited resection using bilateral laminotomies and medial facetectomies

TRANSFORAMINAL LUMBAR INTERBODY FUSION

TECHNIQUES

Pedicle Screw Insertion

- After exposure, pedicle entry points are identified at the junction of the transverse process with the superior articular process of each vertebra.
- A high-speed burr or awl is then used to access each pedicle, followed by use of a pedicle probe and tap to create a proper path for the screws.
- Polyaxial pedicle screws are then placed bilaterally in the standard fashion.
- Fluoroscopy or image guidance systems and electromyographic responses can be used to aid in proper screw positioning.
- Medial breach may be effectively ruled out by direct palpation of the medial wall in the setting of a wide laminectomy.
- The transverse processes should be decorticated using a high-speed burr or curette before screw insertion. This facilitates the posterior arthrodesis, as access to the transverse processes becomes somewhat limited once the pedicle screws are in place.

Disc Space Distraction

- After screw placement, the next step is to provide posterior distraction to open the posterior portion of the disc space.
  - Lumbar disc spaces are normally lordotic, which can make insertion of an appropriate-sized interbody cage through the narrow posterior portion of the disc space difficult.
  - With distraction, the disc space alignment can be neutralized, thereby facilitating access to the interbody region with minimal bony resection.
- Several methods of achieving interbody distraction exist, and these can be combined as needed to achieve the

desired alignment. The choice of distraction technique is largely based on surgeon preference, as all three methods have been found to be effective.
- Distraction option 1: use of rods and screws
  - Rods can be loaded bilaterally into the pedicle screws, followed by provisional placement of the system's locking nuts. However, unilateral rod insertion on the contralateral side alone is preferred for unencumbered disc space approach and preparation.
  - Distraction is then carried out using the rod(s) and a standard distractor (**TECH FIG 1A–C**).
  - To allow for the distraction, the rods need to be slightly longer than will ultimately be necessary.
  - If bilateral rod placement is considered, the polyaxial screw heads should be angled as laterally as possible to maximize the volume of space medial to the rods. This maneuver facilitates later access to the disc space without requiring rod removal.
  - Alternatively, several systems have pedicle screw distractor instruments that provide distraction off the screws obviating rod insertion.
    - Lateral fluoroscopy should be used to judge the amount of distraction obtained at the posterior margin of the disc space.
    - Once adequate alignment is obtained, the system's locking nuts are tightened to maintain the distraction.
    - Care should be taken not to excessively distract off the screws in osteoporotic patients as this could lead to screw loosening or cutout.
- Distraction option 2: spinous process distraction
  - Distraction can also be achieved by using a lamina spreader placed between the spinous processes (**TECH FIG 1D**).

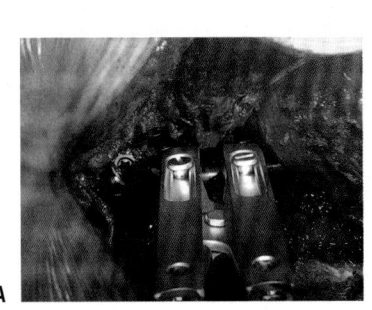
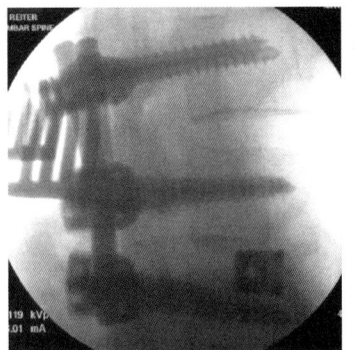
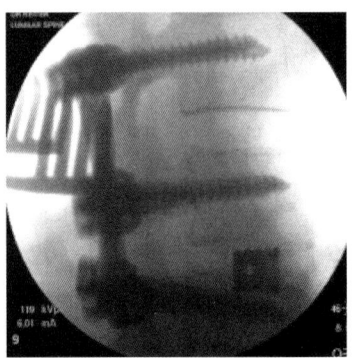
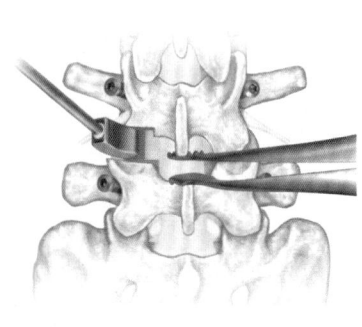
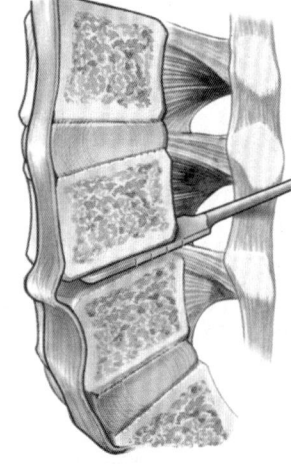

TECH FIG 1 Interbody distraction techniques. **A.** A distractor is placed over the rod between the pedicle screws. **B.** A two-level TLIF procedure. The upper level disc space remains slightly lordotic before distraction using the rods and screws. **C.** Distraction has neutralized the upper disc space, which facilitates access for endplate preparation and graft insertion. **D.** Lamina spreader placed between the spinous processes. **E.** A dilator or shaver is placed into the disc space.(**E:** Courtesy of Aesculap.)

- Distracting off the spinous process can reduce the risk of screw loosening that might occur with excessive distraction on the pedicle screws.
  - This technique should also be done with great care in osteoporotic patients as to avoid fracture of the spinous process and possible dural injury with the distraction device.
- Distraction option 3: interbody dilators
  - Another option available to facilitate interbody distraction is to use interbody dilators, which are placed into the disc space and rotated to restore disc space height (**TECH FIG 1E**).
- This technique minimizes stress applied to the posterior implants and provides the most powerful method of vertebral body distraction.
- Use of interbody distractors, however, is not possible until access to the disc space has been achieved, which may be challenging in a collapsed disc space.
- Another limitation of this method is that it requires a bilateral disc approach to maximize disc preparation and insertion. It is not possible to work within the disc space with an interbody dilator in place on the ipsilateral side.

Complete Unilateral Facetectomy

- The inferior articular process of the cephalad vertebra should be exposed and removed using an osteotome or rongeurs (**TECH FIG 2A**).
- The superior articular process of the caudal vertebra is then dissected free of the ligamentum flavum with curettes and removed using Kerrison rongeurs. To maximize access to the disc space, the entire superior articular process down to the cephalad aspect

of the pedicle should be removed so that the top of the pedicle can be easily seen and palpated (**TECH FIG 2B**).
- The lateral aspect of the hemilamina and the caudal portion of the pars interarticularis are resected using Kerrison rongeurs to provide access to the neural foramen and posterolateral annulus.
- Kambin's triangular working zone between the exiting and traversing nerve roots and the superior aspect of the pedicle should be identified (**TECH FIG 2C**).
  - The exiting nerve root is present just below the pedicle of the cephalad vertebra.
    - The exiting nerve can be identified visually or palpated but should not be deliberately manipulated as the sensitive dorsal root ganglion is in this region.
    - Although it is critical to identify the location of the exiting nerve root, care should be taken not to unnecessarily dissect the nerve out of its sleeve of fatty tissue; in some cases, the nerve will be located and palpated but never fully visualized.
  - The traversing nerve root and the lateral aspect of the thecal sac will be present in the medial portion of the triangle. Nerve root retractors can be used to mobilize the neurologic elements medially to provide additional access to the posterolateral annulus (**TECH FIG 2D**).
  - As in all lumbar spinal surgical procedures, if trouble is encountered locating a nerve root, the surgeon should find or palpate the associated pedicle and look along the medial and inferior pedicle wall.
- With the neurologic elements accounted for, the posterolateral annulus can be accessed through the previously described

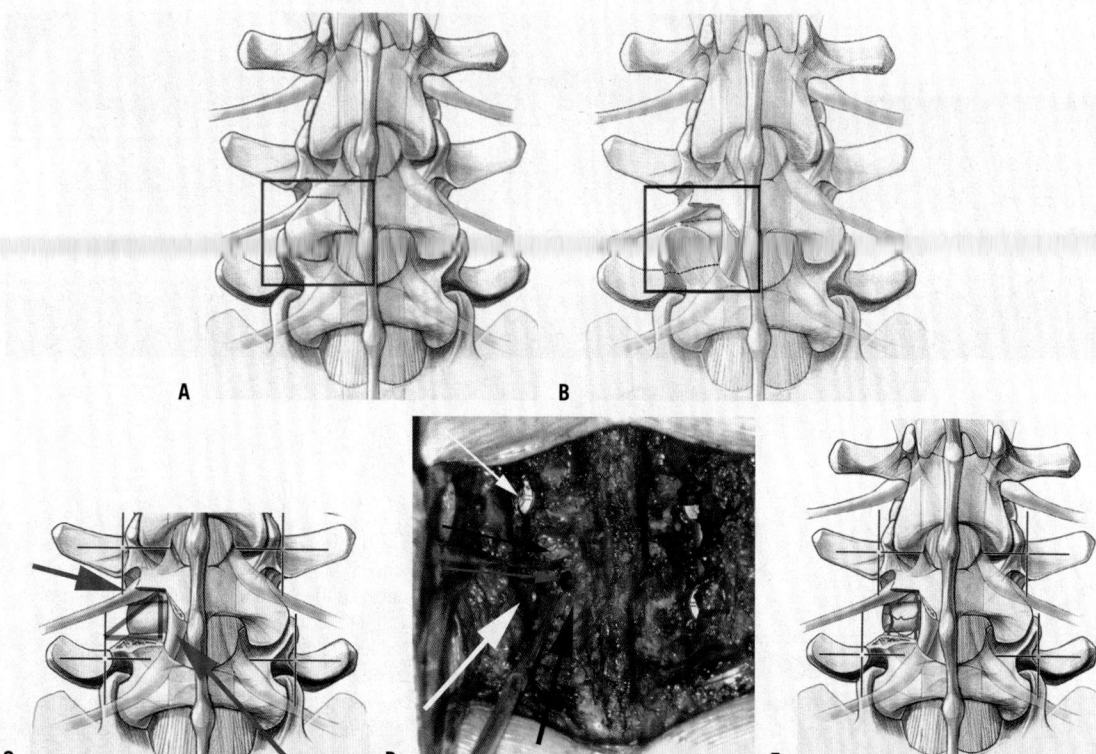

TECH FIG 2 A. Removal of inferior articular process. **B.** Removal of superior articular process. **C.** Exposure after unilateral facetectomy, with the triangular working zone outlined in gray. The exiting nerve root (*red arrow*) forms the lateral border, and the traversing nerve root and thecal sac (*blue arrow*) form the medial border of the working zone. **D.** Intraoperative picture following facetectomy and discectomy. Pedicle screws at L4 and L5 are marked by the *small* and *large white arrows*, respectively. The exiting L4 nerve root (*small black arrow*) and the traversing L5 nerve root (*large black arrow*) are both being gently retracted, with the annular window into the interbody region (*blue arrow*) seen between them. **E.** Posterolateral annulus with overlying epidural veins. To avoid inadvertent injury while obtaining hemostasis, one must constantly be aware of the location of the neurologic elements when working in the epidural space.

triangular working zone by carefully coagulating and dividing the obstructing epidural veins using bipolar cautery **(TECH FIG 2E)**.

- Significant bleeding can be encountered at this stage, and the use of cottonoids in conjunction with hemostatic agents such as Gelfoam (Pfizer, New York, NY), Floseal (Baxter, Deerfield, IL), or Surgiflo (Ethicon, Inc., Somerville, NJ) can be helpful.
- The use of perioperative intravenous tranexamic acid can also be considered in patients with no contraindications.
- If the surgeon is not careful, the exiting or traversing nerve roots can be damaged while dealing with the bleeding arising from the epidural venous plexus. Working methodically while remaining constantly aware of the location of these neural structures is critical.

Disc Space Preparation

- A nerve root retractor is used to mobilize the thecal sac and traversing nerve root medially to improve exposure of the posterolateral annulus. An advantage of the TLIF procedure is that minimal neural retraction is necessary to access the interbody region. Depending on the local nerve root anatomy, however, retraction of the traversing root may be necessary even with a TLIF.

- A scalpel is then used to incise a rectangular region of the annulus lateral to the traversing nerve root to create a window into the disc space **(TECH FIG 3A)**.
- It is extremely important to have proper instruments available to facilitate the critical step of disc space preparation. These instruments are frequently provided by the vendor of the graft or implants to be used in the interbody region and should include the following **(TECH FIG 3B)**:
  - Interbody paddle scrapers to dilate and prepare the endplates
  - Offset curettes to facilitate access to the contralateral side of the disc space
  - Rasps, ring curettes, and reverse curettes to assist in endplate preparation
  - Osteotomes or box chisels to improve access to the interbody region when the disc space is narrowed posteriorly
  - Long, straight and up-biting pituitary rongeurs for débridement of the interbody region
- After creation of the annular window, typically shavers or dilators of increasing size are serially introduced into the disc space and rotated **(TECH FIG 3C,D)**.
  - Lateral fluoroscopy can be helpful in determining the proper depth of penetration into the disc space. The anterior and anterolateral annulus should be palpated by the instrument and never violated or catastrophic vascular injury could occur.

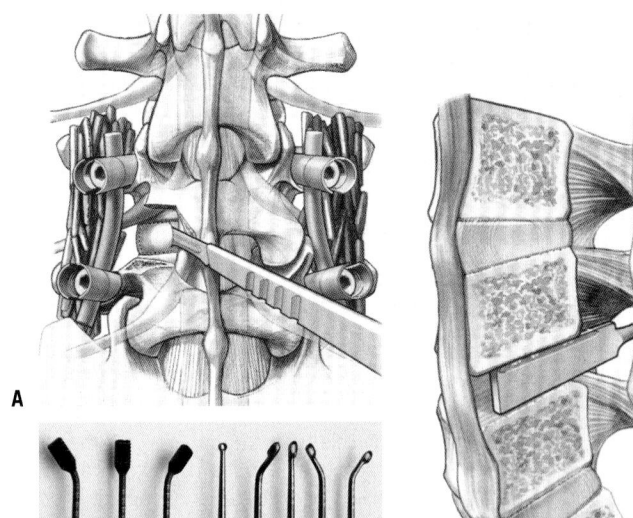

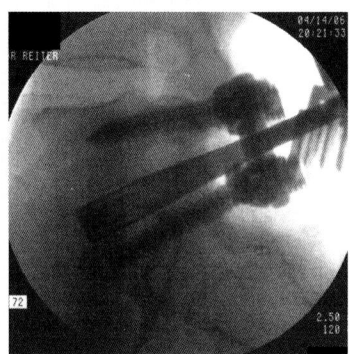

TECH FIG 3 A. With the TLIF's lateral approach, annular incision is frequently possible without neurologic retraction. **B.** Disc space preparation instruments (from left to right): left offset, straight, and right offset rasps; ring curette; reverse curette; straight, left, and right offset curettes. Other instruments not shown may include dilators, shavers, osteotomes, and straight and angled pituitary rongeurs. **C.** Schematic of a shaver introduced into a disc space. Rotation of the shaver should remove endplate cartilage to facilitate arthrodesis. **D.** Lateral fluoroscopic image of a shaver within the disc space at L5–S1. To avoid violation of the endplates, care must be taken when working in the interbody region to maintain a parallel trajectory to the disc space. (**A,C:** Courtesy of Aesculap. **B:** Courtesy of Zimmer Biomet.)

- Instruments used within the disc space are typically marked so that they are not overinserted to avoid potentially catastrophic violation of the anterior annulus. It is helpful to preoperatively estimate disc space length (posterior to anterior) on MRI or computed tomography (CT) scan to have an idea of how far the instruments can be inserted.
- After dilation and shaving, a combination of curettes and rongeurs is used to perform a thorough discectomy and endplate preparation down to bleeding bone.
  - Care should be taken not to violate the endplates in regions expected to load share with the interbody implant as this can make implant placement difficult and lead to settling of the structural graft.
  - Several TLIF techniques do call for perforation of the endplates to expose cancellous bleeding bone in non–load-sharing interbody regions using osteotomes for the anterior portion of the disc space or curettes and awls for other areas.
  - Because of the concave nature of the endplates, it is sometimes necessary to use osteotomes or box chisels to remove a rim of bone from the posterior aspect of the vertebral bodies to improve access to the disc space and allow for placement of a properly sized graft. The surgeon should remember that aggressive removal of the posterior lip may lead to a greater risk of implant backout with root compression.
- To minimize the risk of neurologic injury and postoperative dysesthetic pain, several recommendations should be followed during the disc space preparation and graft insertion:
  - Retraction on the neurologic elements should be minimized, and it should be released intermittently throughout the procedure.
  - The thecal sac should never be retracted across the midline of the spinal canal.

- Particularly in revision cases, the neurologic elements should be carefully mobilized off the floor of the canal and disc space before retraction.
- Implants should be selected that can be inserted without excessive neural retraction.
  - This can be an issue with use of threaded cylindrical cages because the height and width of the device must be equal; consequently, a cage of the appropriate height might be too wide to be safely inserted.

Graft Placement

- A variety of interbody grafting techniques have been described for use in the TLIF procedure:
  - Placement of two vertical fibular allografts or vertical titanium mesh cages posteriorly in the disc space with cancellous graft packed anteriorly
  - Use of an oblique threaded cylindrical cage or machined cortical allograft bone dowel
  - Use of an obliquely placed polyetheretherketone (PEEK) cage or bullet-shaped cortical allograft
  - Placement of a curved titanium cage, PEEK cage, or machined cortical allograft anteriorly and as centrally as possible within the disc space, with cancellous graft placed behind the device
- Although it has been shown that anterior and midline cage placement is biomechanically superior to posterior and lateral cage placement, studies comparing the clinical efficacy of these various techniques do not exist.[2]
- When choosing an interbody graft and grafting technique, surgeons should consider several factors:
  - Ability to insert the device without requiring excessive neurologic retraction
  - Volume of cancellous graft that can be packed within and around the cage or allograft

- The effect of the graft's position and shape on the ability to restore lordosis with later compression of the posterior instrumentation[9]
- The remainder of this section describes the technique in which a single-curved titanium or PEEK cage or allograft is placed anteriorly and centrally within the disc space.
- After endplate preparation, graft trials should be used to determine the proper size for the interbody spacer. Fluoroscopic imaging should be used to confirm proper sizing of the trial.
- The anterior and lateral aspects of the disc space should then be tightly packed with morselized graft material.
  - Several options are available for use as morselized graft material, including autogenous iliac crest bone graft, local bone graft from the removed facet and lamina, allograft corticocancellous bone, allograft demineralized bone matrix, ceramic bone graft extenders, and bone-inducing substances such as bone morphogenetic protein (BMP).
  - Although the use of recombinant human bone morphogenetic protein #2, has shown tremendous success in the area of radiographic fusion without any donor site morbidity, there have been recent concerns about BMP-related complications, including radiculitis, osteolysis, and heterotopic ossification.[1] In the absence of high-level data suggesting optimal dosing of BMP in the TLIF/PLIF technique, it is the authors' recommendation to use this product with high clinical restraint for this procedure.
  - The choice of graft should depend on surgeon experience, host factors that may affect fusion, patient preference, cost, and availability.
- Graft impactors should be used to maximize the amount of bone that can be placed into the interbody space. For the technique using a central and anteriorly placed cage, the anterior 25% of the disc space should be filled initially with tightly packed morselized graft material.

- Before inserting the actual cage or graft, the trial should be reinserted to confirm that the morselized graft has not blocked the pathway for insertion of the structural graft.
- The implant should then be inserted into the interbody space and placed anteriorly and as centrally as possible.
  - Implant position should be confirmed with AP and lateral fluoroscopy during insertion.
  - Straight and offset impactors can be used to facilitate proper cage positioning.
- Additional morselized graft material should then be packed into the posterior aspect of the disc space behind the implant.

Compression and Posterolateral Grafting

- With the implant in place, distraction is released from the spinous processes or pedicle screws. Compression is then applied to the pedicle screw construct, and the locking nuts are finally tightened.
- Compression both loads the anterior implant and restores lordosis to the spine.
- The contralateral spinous processes, lamina, facet joint, and transverse processes should then be decorticated (ideally, the transverse processes were decorticated at the time of screw insertion).
- Morselized graft can then be placed into the contralateral interlaminar, facet, and intertransverse regions **(TECH FIG 4)**.
  - The interspinous ligament, if preserved, will serve to prevent graft migration into the exposed portion of the spinal canal and foramen.
  - Some surgeons may also wish to place graft on the ipsilateral side in the intertransverse region, but care must be taken to avoid allowing graft to enter the spinal canal or compress the exiting nerve root.
- Final AP and lateral fluoroscopic images should be obtained.

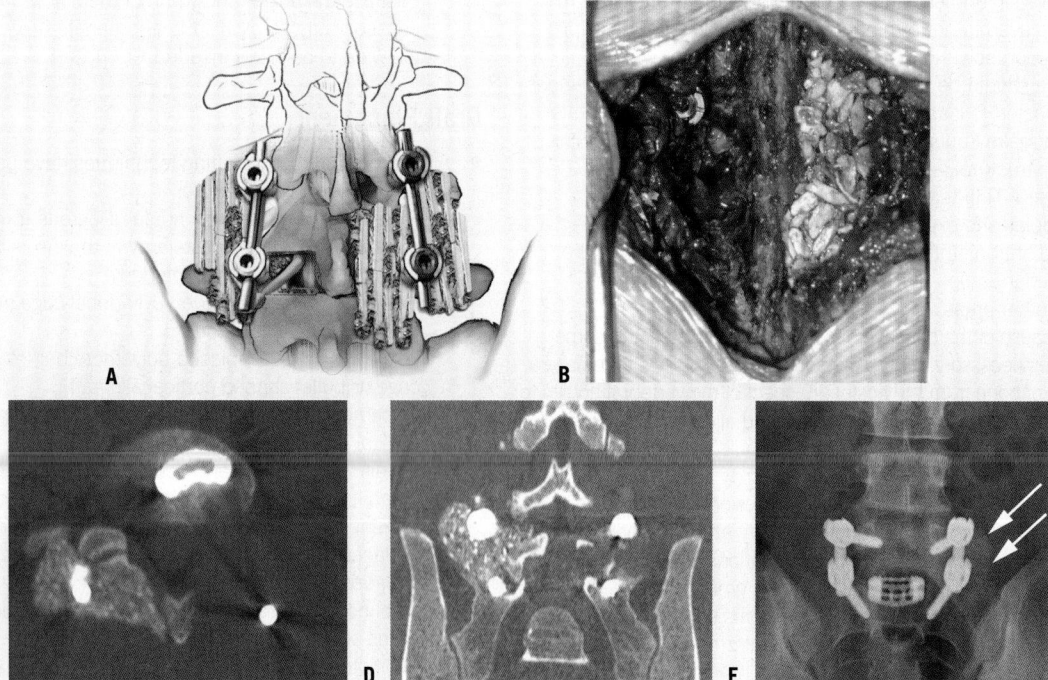

TECH FIG 4 A. Schematic demonstrating posterolateral and interlaminar bone grafting. **B.** Intraoperative photograph with unilateral posterior morselized graft in place on right. Axial (**C**) and coronal (**D**) CT images demonstrating posterolateral and interlaminar graft in place. **E.** Postoperative radiograph demonstrating a solid unilateral arthrodesis (*white arrows*) in the posterolateral region. Assessing fusion status in the posterolateral region is sometimes easier than assessing fusion within the interbody space.

Closure

- Before closure, final hemostasis should be obtained, and the neurologic elements are inspected to ensure that no graft material has fallen into the spinal canal.

- A Valsalva maneuver can also be performed to confirm the integrity of the dural sac.
- A standard layered closure over a drain is then carried out.

POSTERIOR LUMBAR INTERBODY FUSION

- Most of the technique for PLIF is similar to that described earlier for TLIF, except that a bilateral and more medial approach to the interbody space is used.
- This section describes the PLIF procedure by highlighting the differences between the TLIF and PLIF techniques.
- As noted in the exposure section, two PLIF exposure options are available (**TECH FIG 5**):
  - Extensive resection, including wide laminectomy with bilateral complete facetectomies
  - Limited resection using bilateral laminotomies and medial facetectomies
- The decision to use the wide laminectomy with total facetectomies is affected by several considerations:
  - It provides maximal exposure and minimizes the amount of neural retraction necessary to place the interbody grafts or implants. This is essentially a bilateral TLIF.
  - It should be strongly considered when fusing levels with a smaller interpedicular distance such as in patients of short stature and in the upper lumbar spine.
  - It results in iatrogenic instability and therefore must be supplemented with pedicle screw instrumentation. Even with pedicle screws, a bilateral PLIF represents a more unstable situation. In patients with poor bone quality, the pedicle screws can loosen and lead to instability of the construct, with possible cage migration.
  - It eliminates the ability to fuse the facet joints posteriorly and reduces the host bone contact area available for the posterolateral fusion.

- Limited resection using bilateral laminotomies and medial facetectomies
  - Preserves the segment's biomechanical stability by preserving the spinous processes, the interspinous ligaments, and, most importantly, the lateral half of the facet joints and associated pars interarticularis
  - Must be employed for cases in which posterior instrumentation is not being used
  - May be difficult in patients with a tall disc space as there may not be enough room for passage of the larger interbody graft required without more extensive resection of the facets
  - Should only be attempted by surgeons very familiar with the PLIF procedure as additional neural retraction is necessary, with a consequent higher risk of neurologic injury
- After the exposure, pedicle screws are inserted, and disc space distraction is applied as described for the TLIF procedure.
  - The PLIF procedure can be performed without pedicle screws if one uses the limited resection technique during exposure and care is taken not to destabilize the segment.

Laminotomy and Partial Facetectomy

- If the partial resection technique is being used, a laminotomy is performed by using curettes to detach the ligamentum flavum from each of the adjacent lamina as well as the superior articular process of the caudal vertebra.
- Kerrison rongeurs are then used to remove lateral portions of the adjacent lamina and the medial half of the superior and inferior articular processes.
- This process should be repeated bilaterally and should result in working windows for approaching the disc space on each side of spinal canal.
  - When using the limited resection technique, care should be taken to preserve the spinous process, interspinous ligaments, lateral pars, and lateral half of the facet joints.
- As in the TLIF procedure, the exiting and traversing nerve roots need to be identified and appropriate caution used to avoid traumatizing these sensitive neurologic structures during the procedure. To minimize root injury, one should remove enough lateral bone to be able to access the disc space without major retraction of the traversing root.
- The wide laminectomy and bilateral facetectomy technique simply involves enlarging the earlier approach.
  - Resection of the spinous process and interspinous ligaments medially will improve the ability to retract the thecal sac toward the midline.
  - For a maximally sized working window, total facetectomies can be performed to allow for more lateral access to the disc space (see **TECH FIG 2E**).

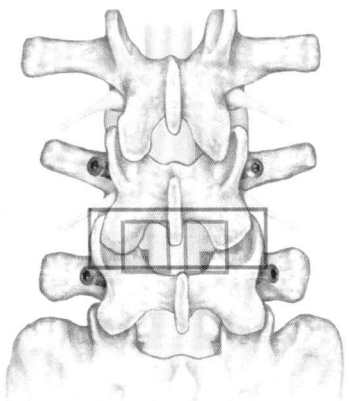

TECH FIG 5 Bony resections necessary for each of the two PLIF exposures. Wide laminectomy and complete facetectomies are demonstrated by the *gray rectangle*. Laminotomy and partial facetectomies are shown by the *red rectangles*.

- After exposure, the posterolateral annulus can be accessed through the previously described triangular zone cephalad to the pedicle of the inferior vertebra, medial to the exiting nerve root, and lateral to the traversing nerve root and thecal sac (see **TECH FIG 2C**).
- Epidural veins are carefully coagulated and divided in the same way as described for the TLIF procedure.

Disc Space Preparation

- Disc space preparation is performed in an identical fashion as described earlier for the TLIF procedure, except that bilateral annular windows are created somewhat more medially than for a TLIF.
- The thecal sac and traversing nerve root are mobilized medially, and a combination of shavers, curettes, and rongeurs is used to perform a thorough discectomy down to exposed endplate.
- In noninstrumented PLIF procedures, achieving adequate interbody graft contact area is critical to reduce the risk of graft subsidence.
  - Closkey et al[3] demonstrated that in patients of average bone density and size, interbody graft contact area should exceed 6.2 cm^2 or an area roughly 2.5 × 2.5 cm.
  - Instrumentation reduces the risk of subsidence but has not been shown to improve the clinical outcome when compared to properly performed noninstrumented PLIF procedures.[19]

Graft Placement

- The PLIF procedure requires the placement of structural interbody grafts inserted from each side of the spinal canal (**TECH FIG 6**).

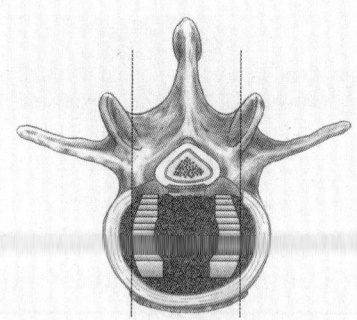

TECH FIG 6 Bilateral PLIF grafts surrounded by cancellous bone. (Reproduced with permission of Medtronic, Inc.)

- As in the TLIF, many graft options exist, including structural autograft or allograft bone as well as threaded or rectangular titanium or PEEK implants.
- Herkowitz and Simeone[6] and Lee et al[11] have cautioned that most commercially available implants typically do not meet the surface area requirements for noninstrumented PLIF and should be used only when supplemented with pedicle screws.
- Regions of the interbody space not filled with structural graft should be packed as tightly as possible with morselized graft material.
- Fluoroscopy can be used to ensure appropriate midline and anterior interbody implant position.

Compression, Posterolateral Grafting, and Closure

- Compression (when pedicle screw instrumentation has been used), posterolateral grafting, and closure are all accomplished in a fashion similar to that described for the TLIF procedure.

TECHNIQUES

Pearls and Pitfalls

Indications	• As in all lumbar fusion surgeries, clinical success will depend largely on proper patient selection. • Spondylolisthesis, degenerative scoliosis, high risk for pseudarthrosis, and selective refractory cases of degenerative disc disease • Fusions performed primarily for discogenic back pain have a limited success rate, and realistic expectations will enhance patient satisfaction with the procedure. • Revision procedures with extensive epidural scarring are technically challenging and benefit from a more lateral approach to the disc space to minimize retraction of neurologic elements typically surrounded by fibrous tissue.
Interbody Access and Preparation	• Distraction techniques are used to neutralize the alignment of the adjacent endplates as much as technically feasible. • Concave endplates may require use of an osteotome or box chisel to facilitate access to the disc space and allow for placement of a properly sized graft. • An array of interbody preparation instruments, including offset curettes, must be available to facilitate comprehensive removal of endplate cartilage and disc material. • Because achieving an interbody fusion is critical to the success of the procedure, adequate time and effort must be spent in disc space preparation. The surgeon must not rush in interbody preparation. • To avoid serious endplate violation, care must be taken to maintain a parallel trajectory to the disc space when working with instruments in the interbody region.

Neurologic Injury	• Identifying the location of the exiting nerve root is a vital step in the procedure and should occur before incising the annulus.
	• Insufficient laminectomy can result in poor visualization and excessive neural retraction with inadvertent neurologic injury.
	• Exiting nerve roots with a more acute angle of takeoff from the thecal sac can result in a smaller triangular working zone and should be gently retracted laterally.
	• Medial retraction of the thecal sac and traversing nerve root should be minimized and must never cross the midline.
	• Neurologic retraction should be released frequently to allow for reperfusion of these sensitive structures.
	• Free-running electromyographic monitoring can provide live feedback and help reduce the risk of neurologic injury from overzealous neurologic retraction.
	• Great care must be taken to account for the dura and neurologic elements every time that an instrument or graft is inserted into the disc space.
	• Should significant difficulties arise such as obstructing anomalous neural anatomy, major epidural bleeding, or a complex dural tear, one must be willing to abandon the interbody portion of the fusion rather than risk causing a catastrophic injury.
Epidural Bleeding	• Epidural bleeding can be troublesome in the posterior annular region, and use of hemostatic agents such as Gelfoam, Floseal, or Surgiflo should be strongly considered.
	• Great care must be taken to identify the neurologic structures when using bipolar cautery.
	• Should a dural tear occur, it should be repaired as soon as technically possible, as reduced intrathecal pressure will produce engorgement of the epidural veins with significantly more bleeding.
Graft Placement	• Bony resection must allow sufficient access to the interbody region to allow placement of an adequately sized graft.
	• Graft type should be chosen carefully in situations where access to the disc is limited or a tall disc space exists.
	• Due to their narrower widths, rectangular grafts or cages can be inserted more easily into a tall disc space than cylindrical grafts (fallen out of favor), which require a larger transverse exposure.
	• Fluoroscopy and offset impactors should be used during graft insertion to facilitate optimal final implant position.

POSTOPERATIVE CARE

- The patient is typically mobilized out of bed the day after surgery.
- Postoperative bracing is typically not required for the TLIF or instrumented PLIF procedures but can be used according to surgeon preference.
- Most physicians prefer to use a thoracolumbosacral orthosis during the postoperative period for noninstrumented PLIF procedures.
- Serial radiographs are used to assess for fusion.

OUTCOMES

- Fusion rates for the PLIF and TLIF procedures are similar, with studies finding rates of obtaining a solid arthrodesis varying between 89% and 100%. Several studies have reported fusion rates above 95%.[10,14,15]
- Although clinical success rates vary between studies, most series report similar outcomes with PLIF and TLIF as for anterior interbody and combined AP fusion procedures.
- Most of the studies on PLIF and TLIF using visual analog scale and Oswestry Disability Index scores as outcome measures demonstrate an overall patient satisfaction rate of about 80% with the procedure.[5,10,11,18]
- Longer term studies indicate that the results of PLIF and TLIF procedures tend to be durable once a solid arthrodesis has been achieved.

COMPLICATIONS

- Neurologic injury is an uncommon complication of PLIF and TLIF and has been reported to occur in between 0% and 4% of patients. Many of these injuries represent a neurapraxia due to excessive nerve root retraction and resolve spontaneously.[17,21]

- Dural tears are a more common complication and have historically been reported to occur in 0.5% to 18% of PLIF and TLIF procedures.
  - The dural tear rate appears to be significantly lower with the TLIF procedure compared to the PLIF, likely related to the fact that less neural retraction is necessary when using the TLIF's more lateral approach to the disc space.[7]
  - More recent studies demonstrate a trend toward much lower rates of dural tears in both PLIF and TLIF procedures, with a reported incidence in the range of 1% to 5%.
- Implant migration or failure is a rare complication in the TLIF procedure but has been reported to occur in up to 2.4% of cases in which a noninstrumented PLIF is performed. Properly sizing the interbody implants and fully packing the disc space with graft material can help reduce the risk of this complication.
- Other complications of posterior lumbar fusions that are not specific to the PLIF and TLIF procedure include wound infection, excessive bleeding, pedicle screw malposition, and epidural hematoma.

REFERENCES

1. Carragee EJ, Hurwitz EL, Weiner BK. A critical review of recombinant human bone morphogenetic protein-2 trials in spinal surgery: emerging safety concerns and lessons learned. Spine J 2011;11(6):471–491.
2. Castellvi AD, Thampi SK, Cook DJ, et al. Effect of TLIF cage placement on in vivo kinematics. Int J Spine Surg 2015;9:38.
3. Closkey RF, Parsons JR, Lee CK, et al. Mechanics of interbody spinal fusion. Analysis of critical bone graft area. Spine (Phila Pa 1976) 1993;18(8):1011–1015.
4. Enker P, Steffee AD. Interbody fusion and instrumentation. Clin Orthop Relat Res 1994(300):90–101.
5. Hackenberg L, Halm H, Bullmann V, et al. Transforaminal lumbar interbody fusion: a safe technique with satisfactory three to five year results. Eur Spine J 2005;14(6):551–558.

6. Herkowitz HN, Simeone FA. Rothman-Simeone: the Spine, ed 5. Philadelphia: Elsevier, 2006.

7. Humphreys SC, Hodges SD, Patwardhan AG, et al. Comparison of posterior and transforaminal approaches to lumbar interbody fusion. Spine (Phila Pa 1976) 2001;26(5):567–571.

8. Katz AD, Mancini N, Karukonda T, et al. Approach-based comparative and predictor analysis of 30-day readmission, reoperation, and morbidity in patients undergoing lumbar interbody fusion using the ACS-NSQIP dataset. Spine (Phila Pa 1976) 2019;44(6):432–441.

9. Kwon BK, Berta S, Daffner SD, et al. Radiographic analysis of transforaminal lumbar interbody fusion for the treatment of adult isthmic spondylolisthesis. J Spinal Disord Tech 2003;16(5):469–476.

10. Lauber S, Schulte TL, Liljenqvist U, et al. Clinical and radiologic 2-4-year results of transforaminal lumbar interbody fusion in degenerative and isthmic spondylolisthesis grades 1 and 2. Spine (Phila Pa 1976) 2006;31(15):1693–1698.

11. Lee CK, Vessa P, Lee JK. Chronic disabling low back pain syndrome caused by internal disc derangements. The results of disc excision and posterior lumbar interbody fusion. Spine (Phila Pa 1976) 1995;20(3):356–361.

12. Lee N, Kim KN, Yi S, et al. Comparison of outcomes of anterior, posterior, and transforaminal lumbar interbody fusion surgery at a single lumbar level with degenerative spinal disease. World Neurosurg 2017;101:216–226.

13. Lin PM. Posterior lumbar interbody fusion (PLIF): past, present, and future. Clin Neurosurg 2000;47:470–482

14. McAfee PC, DeVine JG, Chaput CD, et al. The indications for interbody fusion cages in the treatment of spondylolisthesis: analysis of 120 cases. Spine (Phila Pa 1976) 2005;30(6 suppl):S60–S65.

15. Miura Y, Imagama S, Yoda M, et al. Is local bone viable as a source of bone graft in posterior lumbar interbody fusion? Spine (Phila Pa 1976) 2003;28(20):2386–2389.

16. Moskowitz A. Transforaminal lumbar interbody fusion. Orthop Clin North Am 2002;33(2):359–366.

17. Okuda S, Miyauchi A, Oda T, et al. Surgical complications of posterior lumbar interbody fusion with total facetectomy in 251 patients. J Neurosurg Spine 2006;4(4):304–309.

18. Potter BK, Freedman BA, Verwiebe EG, et al. Transforaminal lumbar interbody fusion: clinical and radiographic results and complications in 100 consecutive patients. J Spinal Disord Tech 2005;18(4):337–346.

19. Prolo LM, Oklund SA, Zawadzki N, et al. Uninstrumented posterior lumbar interbody fusion: have technological advances in stabilizing the lumbar spine truly improved outcomes? World Neurosurg 2018;115:490–502.

20. Teng I, Han J, Phan K, et al. A meta-analysis comparing ALIF, PLIF, TLIF and LLIF. J Clin Neurosci 2017;44:11–17.

21. Villavicencio AT, Burneikiene S, Bulsara KR, et al. Perioperative complications in transforaminal lumbar interbody fusion versus anterior-posterior reconstruction for lumbar disc degeneration and instability. J Spinal Disord Tech 2006;19(2):92–97.

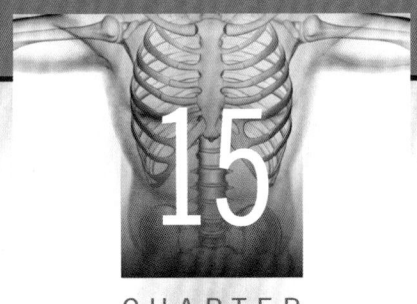

CHAPTER 15

Iliac Crest Bone Graft Harvesting

Joon S. Yoo, Nathaniel W. Jenkins, James M. Parrish, Sreeharsha V. Nandyala, Alejandro Marquez-Lara, Junyoung Ahn, and Kern Singh

DEFINITION

- The use of autogenous bone graft is considered by most spine surgeons to be the gold standard for achieving arthrodesis in the spine.
- Autogenous bone graft can be used at any spinal level, anterior or posterior.
- The posterior iliac crest is the most frequently harvested site for nonstructural, cancellous bone graft used in lumbar interbody fusions.
- Tricortical, structural bone grafts for cervical interbody fusions are typically harvested from the anterior ilium.

ANATOMY

- Anterior ilium
  - The anterior ilium has a concave anterosuperior surface.
  - The anterior iliac crest is thickest at the iliac tubercle, which is 2 to 3 cm posterior to the anterior superior iliac spine (ASIS) **(FIG 1A)**.

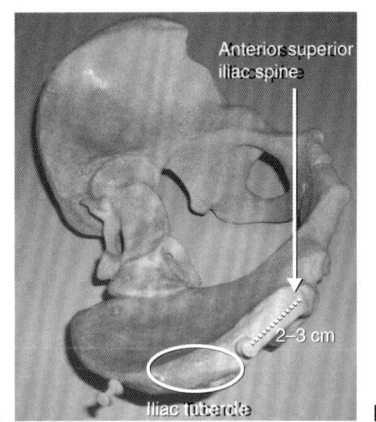

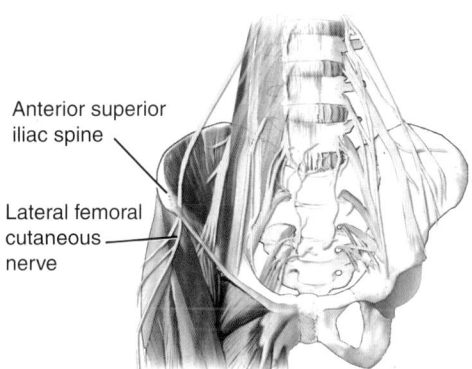

FIG 1 A. Ideal anterior iliac crest bone graft is obtained 2 to 3 cm posterior to the ASIS. **B.** The lateral femoral cutaneous nerve generally traverses medial to the ASIS. **C.** The superior cluneal nerves cross the posterior iliac crest 8 cm anterior to the PSIS. **D.** The superior gluteal artery exits from the greater sciatic foramen.

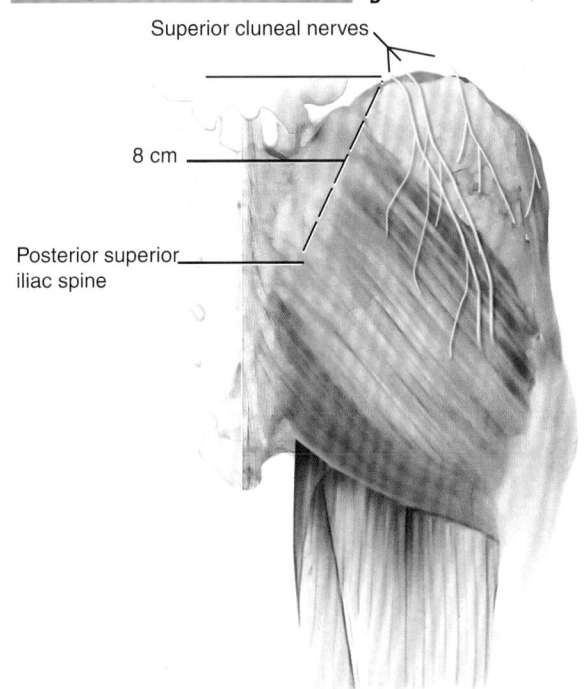

C

D

- The lateral femoral cutaneous nerve typically courses medially to the ASIS; however, it can infrequently cross laterally to the ASIS and be at risk for injury (**FIG 1B**).
- Posterior ilium
  - The thickness of the posterior iliac crest ranges from 14 to 17 mm.
  - The superior cluneal nerve passes over the iliac crest 7 to 8 cm laterally to the posterior superior iliac spine (PSIS) and is at risk for injury with a lateral incision (**FIG 1C**).

- The superior gluteal artery exits the pelvis from the greater sciatic notch and can be injured if bone harvesting approaches the sciatic notch (**FIG 1D**).

SURGICAL MANAGEMENT

Positioning

- A bump of towels or a rolled blanket beneath the ipsilateral ischial tuberosity can facilitate access to the anterior iliac crest.

SURGICAL APPROACH

Anterior Iliac Crest

- A skin incision is made parallelly to the iliac crest and is centered over the iliac tubercle.
- The incision is carried down to the fascia overlying the iliac crest. Subperiosteal dissection is then performed to expose the iliac wing. Care is taken to preserve the fascia so that it can be repaired, minimizing postoperative pain from the graft site (**TECH FIG 1**).
  - The tensor fasciae latae, gluteus medius, and gluteus minimus muscles originate from the lateral aspect of the ilium. These muscles are innervated by the superior gluteal nerve.
  - The abdominal muscles are also attached to the iliac crest and are segmentally innervated; therefore, the incision over the crest is internervous and safe.

Posterior Iliac Crest

- The posterior superior iliac crest is often palpable underneath the skin dimple in the superomedial aspect of the gluteal region.
  - A vertical incision over the PSIS is made to minimize injury to the cluneal nerves.
  - An oblique or curvilinear incision can be made over the posterior iliac crest. The cluneal nerves cross the iliac crest 7 to 12 cm anterolateral to the PSIS; therefore, the incision should be made medially to this cutaneous innervation.
- The subcutaneous tissue is divided to the level of the iliac crest.
- Using a Bovie electrocautery, the iliac crest is incised.
- The muscles are elevated subperiosteally from the posterolateral surface of the ilium.
  - The gluteus maximus, medius, and minimus muscles originate from the lateral surface of the ilium. The superior gluteal nerve innervates the gluteus medius and minimus muscles, and the inferior gluteal nerve innervates the gluteus maximus muscle.
  - The paraspinal musculature is innervated segmentally.

Posterior Iliac Crest: Midline Skin Incision

- A midline spine incision may be extended distally and the posterior iliac crest approached laterally under the skin and subcutaneous fat. This can help avoid a second skin incision.
- The fascia overlying the PSIS is incised on the medial surface where it is more robust. This facilitates fascial closure upon completion of the bone graft harvesting.
- The PSIS is exposed on its outer surface with the aid of an electrocautery via subperiosteal dissection.

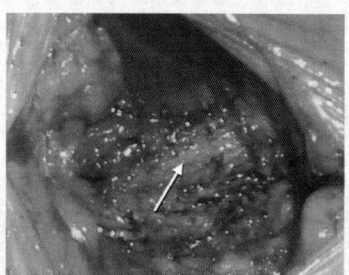

TECH FIG 1 The anterior iliac crest (*arrow*).

ANTERIOR TRICORTICAL ILIAC CREST BONE GRAFT

- After exposure of the anterior iliac crest, an oscillating saw can be used to make parallel cuts through the inner and outer table (**TECH FIG 2A**).

- Curved osteotomes can be used to make longitudinal cuts in the inner and outer tables to complete the tricortical bone graft harvesting (**TECH FIG 2B,C**).

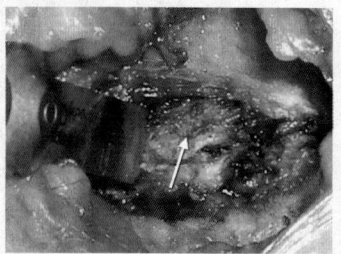
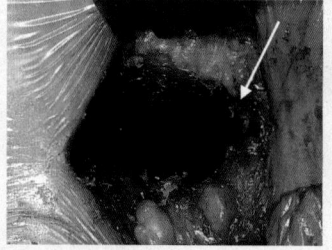
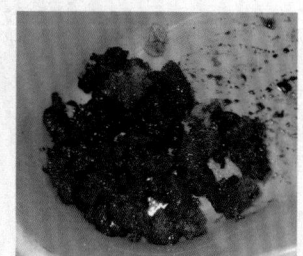

TECH FIG 2 A. An oscillating saw is used to make two parallel cuts in the anterior iliac crest (*arrow*). **B.** The void left by anterior iliac crest harvest (*arrow*). **C.** Resected tricortical anterior iliac crest bone graft.

POSTERIOR ILIAC CREST BONE GRAFT

Corticocancellous Strips

- After exposure of the posterior iliac crest, adequate visualization can be obtained with the use of a Taylor retractor.
- Caution should be taken to avoid penetrating the sciatic notch and potentially injuring the superior gluteal artery.
- The removal of bone in the vicinity of the sciatic notch can weaken the thick bone that forms the notch, resulting in pelvic instability.
  - It is important to stay cephalad to the sciatic notch and remove bone only from the false pelvis. The false or greater pelvis is the portion of pelvis that lies cephalad to the pelvic brim, which defines the inner diameter of the pelvis.
  - For a landmark, an imaginary line dropped anteriorly from the PSIS with the patient in the prone position can be used as the caudal limit of bone removal (TECH FIG 3A).

- Using a straight osteotome, multiple corticocancellous vertical strips can be cut from the iliac crest edge. A curved osteotome can be used to complete the cuts distally (TECH FIG 3B,C).
- After removal of the corticocancellous strips, gouges or curettes can be used to harvest additional cancellous bone (TECH FIG 3D).

Uncapping the Posterior Superior Iliac Spine

- With a rongeur, an osteotome, or both, the cap of the PSIS can be removed, allowing for harvesting of the cancellous bone between the two tables (TECH FIG 4A).
- Using a curette or gouge, the cancellous graft is then harvested through this window (TECH FIG 4B).

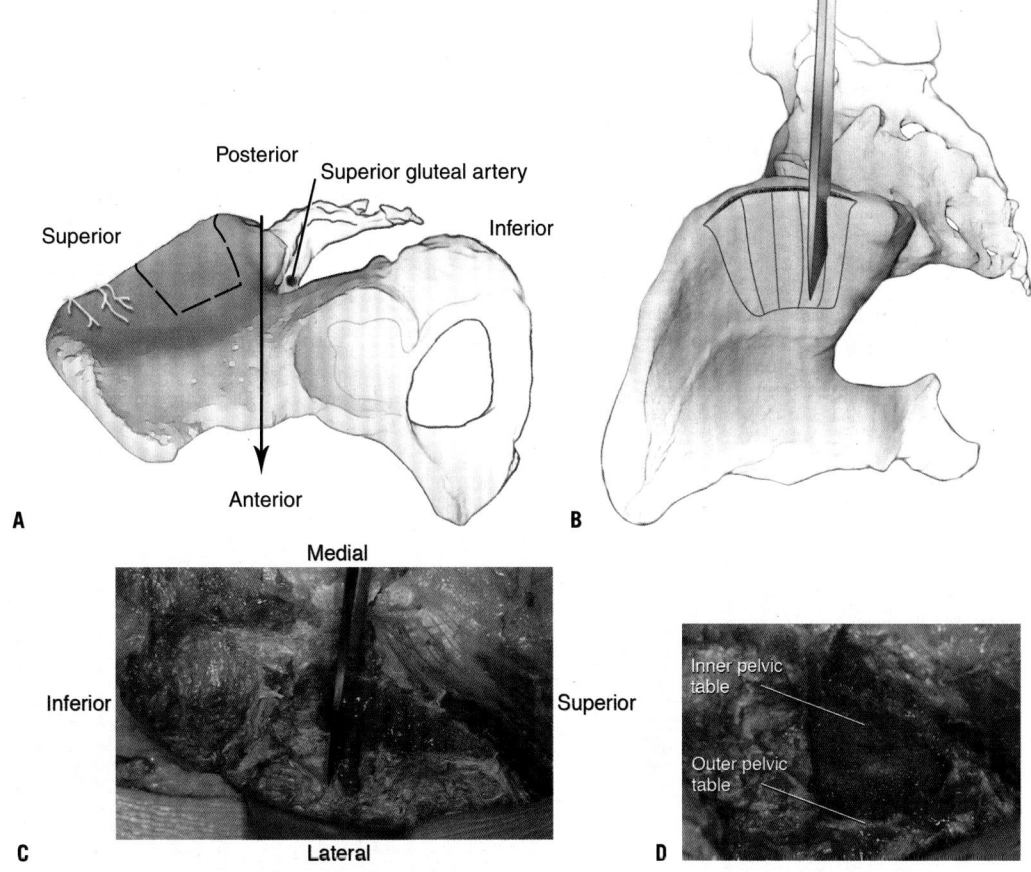

TECH FIG 3 **A.** Line directed anteriorly from the PSIS marks the caudal safe zone for bone grafting to avoid injury to the contents of the sciatic notch. **B,C.** Using osteotomes, several corticocancellous strips can be created from the posterior iliac crest. **D.** The void left after posterior bone graft harvesting.

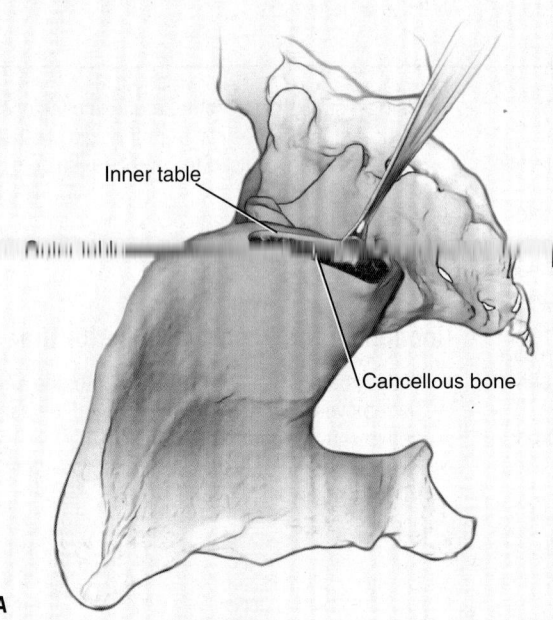

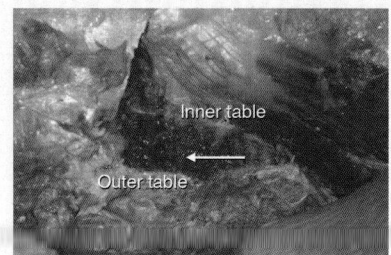

TECH FIG 4 A. The cap of the PSIS can be removed to expose cancellous bone. **B.** After removal of the cap of the PSIS, cancellous bone is exposed for harvesting (*arrow*).

ILIAC CREST GRAFT SITE RECONSTRUCTION

- Several graft site techniques have been described to improve cosmesis and function as well as to potentially reduce the onset of chronic dysesthesia.
- Malleable bone cement contoured to the void can be used, particularly when structural bone graft has been harvested **(TECH FIG 5A).**

- Crushed allograft bone chips can also be packed into the ilium between the inner and outer table, allowing for bone reconstitution.
- After filling the defect with allograft or demineralized bone matrix, malleable polymerized lactide sheets can be contoured to the defect to allow for reconstitution of the external iliac anatomy **(TECH FIG 5B).**

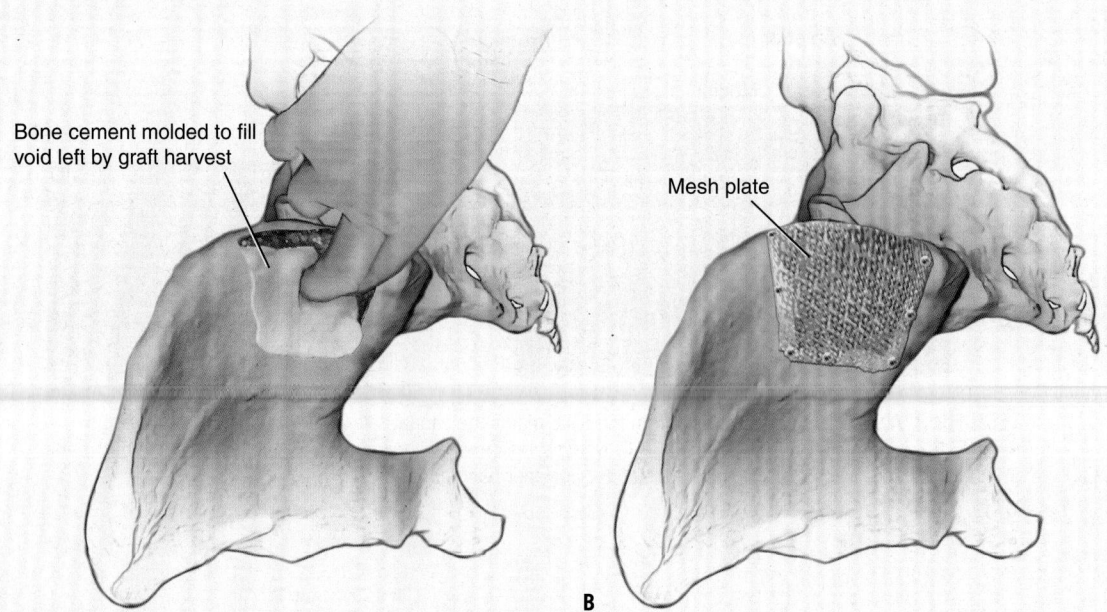

TECH FIG 5 A. After bone graft harvest, cement can be molded to fit the void left from the harvest. **B.** A mesh sheet can be used to traverse the bone graft void to restore the crest.

Pearls and Pitfalls

Posterior Iliac Crest Exposure	• Preservation of the outer table spares the nociceptors located in the posterior periosteum. Preserving the most distal portion of the iliac crest may allow for placement of iliac screws adjacent to the harvest site.
Lateral Femoral Cutaneous Nerve	• The lateral femoral cutaneous nerve passes 2–3 cm medial to the ASIS. Avoiding this area can minimize the risk of injury and meralgia paresthetica.
Superior Cluneal Nerves	• The superior cluneal nerves cross the posterior cortex 8 cm lateral to the posterior iliac spine. Injury to these nerves can cause numbness to the posterior buttocks and occasionally painful neuromas. Vertical incisions are preferred.
Superior Gluteal Artery	• Special care should be taken when working near the sciatic notch. The superior gluteal artery exits the sciatic notch and can be injured if graft is taken too close to the notch. If injured, this vessel may retract into the pelvis and cause significant hemorrhage.

COMPLICATIONS

- Donor site pain is common after bone graft harvesting.
  - However, most symptoms resolve within 3 months.
  - Chronic donor site pain that persists beyond 3 months can be debilitating.
- Anteriorly, nerves at risk for injury include the lateral femoral cutaneous, ilioinguinal, and iliohypogastric nerves.
  - Injury to the lateral femoral cutaneous nerve may give rise to meralgia paresthetica, or paresthesia, along the lateral aspect of the thigh.
  - The ilioinguinal nerve may be injured when the abdominal wall is retracted medially from the anterior iliac crest. The nerve may be compressed beneath the retractor on the inner part of the wall of the ilium. Ilioinguinal neurologic injury is characterized by pain radiating from the iliac toward the inguinal and genital areas.
- Posteriorly, nerves at risk for injury include the cluneal, superior gluteal, and sciatic nerves.
  - The sciatic nerve may be injured when the dissection is extended down to the sciatic notch. A surgical instrument such as an osteotome may be passed deep to the sciatic notch to cause this injury. The bony rim of the notch should be palpated before the dissection is carried to this area.
  - Injury to the cluneal nerve gives rise to numbness to the buttocks or, more rarely, painful cluneal neuromas.
- Injury to the superior gluteal artery is rare but may occur with bone graft harvesting too close to the sciatic notch or via inappropriate placement of retractors or elevators.
  - If cut, the superior gluteal artery may retract into the pelvis.
  - If the superior gluteal vessel is lacerated, it can be compressed locally and exposed for ligation or clipping. A finger may be used to apply direct pressure to the vessel against the bone.
  - If the bleeding vessel is still not accessible, the area should be packed and then accessed anteriorly via a retroperitoneal or transperitoneal approach.
  - Arterial occlusion by embolization or by use of a Fogarty catheter is another option.
- The deep circumflex iliac artery, the iliolumbar artery, or the fourth lumbar artery may cause troublesome bleeding when working on the inner table of the ilium.
- A hernia through the iliac bone graft donor site may occur after the removal of a full-thickness bone graft from that site. Symptoms may appear as an iliac swelling, sometimes associated with pain or symptoms of bowel obstruction. Strangulated hernia and volvulus are very rare occurrences.

- Fracture
  - Removal of a large quantity of bone graft from the posterior ilium may disrupt the mechanical keystone effect of the sacroiliac joint and the posterior sacroiliac ligament, causing instability.
  - The ensuing instability transfers the stress forces to the pelvic ring, causing fractures of the superior and inferior pubic rami.
  - Patients with such instability may develop symptoms indistinguishable from other spinal disorders. History of clicking or thudding, as well as pain in the thigh and gluteal region, may be characteristic.
  - Anteriorly, bone resection less than 3 cm from the ASIS may result in an avulsion fracture of the ASIS from the attached muscle groups (sartorius or tensor fascia lata).
- The incidence of infection of the bone graft site ranges from 1% to 5%.
- Careful subperiosteal dissection can limit hematoma formation. Hemostasis after bone graft harvesting with clotting agents (Gelfoam) should be used to limit hematoma formation.
- The harvesting of tricortical grafts, particularly in thin patients, can result in a cosmetic deformity. Careful closure of fascial attachments should be performed to minimize soft tissue defects.

SUGGESTED READINGS

Armaghani SJ, Even JL, Zern EK, et al. The evaluation of donor site pain after harvest of tricortical anterior iliac crest bone graft for spinal surgery: a prospective study. Spine (Phila Pa 1976) 2016;41(4):E191–E196.

Haws BE, Khechen B, Narain AS, et al. Iliac crest bone graft for minimally invasive transforaminal lumbar interbody fusion: a prospective analysis of inpatient pain, narcotics consumption, and costs. Spine (Phila Pa 1976) 2018;43(18):1307–1312.

Lehr AM, Oner FC, Hoebink EA, et al. Patients cannot reliably distinguish the iliac crest bone graft donor site from the contralateral side after lumbar spine fusion: a patient-blinded randomized controlled trial. Spine (Phila Pa 1976) 2019;44(8):527–533.

Lopez GD, Hijji FY, Narain AS, et al. Iliac crest bone graft: a minimally invasive harvesting technique. Clin Spine Surg 2017;30(10):439–441.

Merritt AL, Spinnicke A, Pettigrew K, et al. Gluteal-sparing approach for posterior iliac crest bone graft: description of a new technique and assessment of morbidity in ninety-two patients after spinal fusion. Spine (Phila Pa 1976) 2010;35(14):1396–1400.

Sheha ED, Meredith DS, Shifflett GD, et al. Postoperative pain following posterior iliac crest bone graft harvesting in spine surgery: a prospective, randomized trial. Spine J 2018;18(6):986–992.

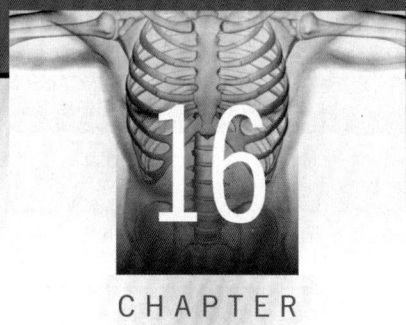

Anterior Lumbar Interbody Fusion, Disc Replacement, and Corpectomy

James W. Klunk, Brad W. Moatz, and P. Justin Tortolani

DEFINITION

- Lumbar disc degeneration is an age-related process heralded by a loss of disc height and gradual changes to the biochemical structure and biomechanical behavior of the intervertebral disc.
- Disc degeneration is not painful in most individuals, but in some patients, the degenerative changes do become painful and lead to the clinical entity known as *degenerative disc disease* (DDD). It is unclear why disc degeneration is painful in some but not in most.
- The etiology of DDD is multifactorial, including genetic and environmental determinants.
- *Discogenic pain* is the term used to describe pain due to a degenerative disc.

ANATOMY

- The intervertebral disc is composed of the outer annulus fibrosus and the inner nucleus pulposus (FIG 1A).
- The vertebral endplate is composed of cancellous bone in the center and strong, dense, cortical bone along the periphery.

- Magnetic resonance imaging (MRI) provides information about the extent of hydration within the disc nucleus. The degenerated disc nucleus will have low signal characteristics (appear dark) on T2-weighted MRI images (FIG 1B).
  - Dark discs on MRI do not necessarily correlate with symptomatic low back pain.[2]
- Lumbar vertebral bodies are ovoid shaped with a rounded circumference on axial cross-section, except for L5, which is more triangular with a slightly wider base posteriorly bordering the central canal and flattened sides leading to an anterior apex. Care should be taken with transbody screw placement at this level.

PATHOGENESIS

- Various mechanisms have been proposed to explain disc degeneration with age:
  - Reduced nutrition and waste transport
  - Decreased concentration of viable cells
  - Loss of matrix proteins, proteoglycans, and water
  - Degradative enzyme activity
  - Fatigue failure of the matrix

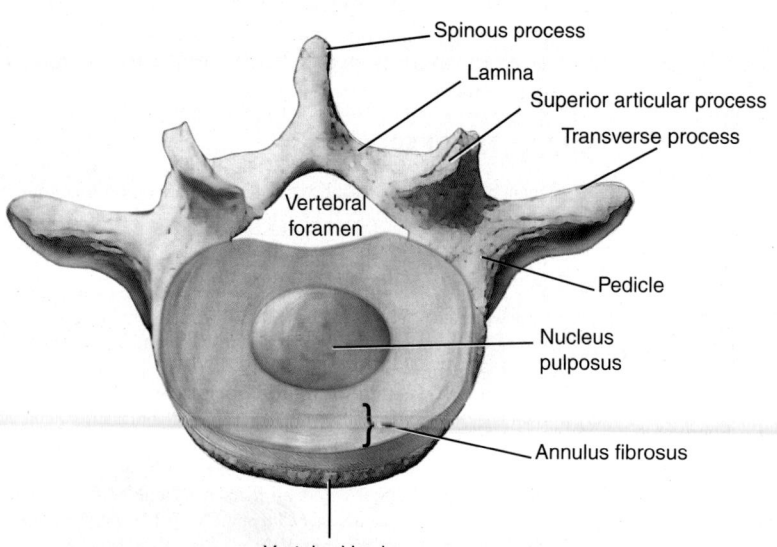

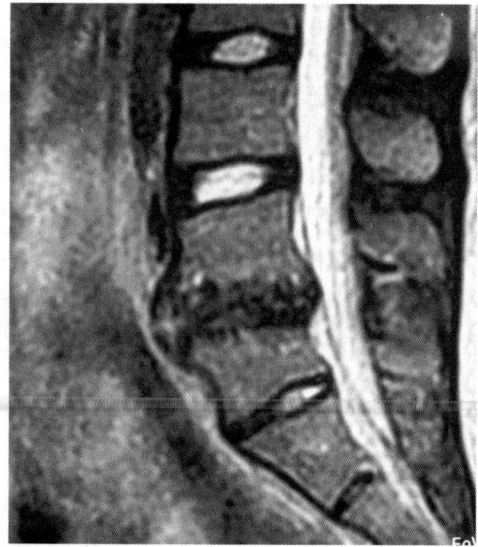

Spinous process
Lamina
Superior articular process
Transverse process
Vertebral foramen
Pedicle
Nucleus pulposus
Annulus fibrosus
Vertebral body

A

B

FIG 1 **A.** The intervertebral disc is composed of the outer annulus fibrosus (radial orientation of collagen fibers) and the inner nucleus pulposus (relatively higher water content and proteoglycans). The cancellous center of the lumbar vertebral body is surrounded by a peripheral rim of relatively strong cortical bone. **B.** T2-weighted sagittal MRI showing DDD at the L4–L5 disc space. The nucleus pulposus is low signal intensity (dark) compared to the adjacent discs, which are high signal intensity (bright) due to relatively higher water concentration. The vertebral body endplates are irregular, with anterior vertebral osteophytes.

- Herniated nucleus pulposus
- Subclinical, indolent disc space infection
- Alterations to the vertebral endplate microenvironment such as venous pooling and reduced oxygen tension are additional factors.
  - Nicotine has known detrimental effects on the intervertebral disc, perhaps via these mechanisms.
- Several factors have been implicated in the generation of discogenic pain: altered disc structure and function, release of inflammatory cytokines, and nerve ingrowth into degenerated discs, which under normal conditions are only minimally innervated in the outermost portion of the annulus.

NATURAL HISTORY

- Radiographic findings of disc degeneration typically appear around age 30 years.
- Posttraumatic disc herniations, vertebral endplate injuries, and genetic factors may predispose patients to earlier presentation.
- As structural changes occur within the intervertebral disc, associated changes in the vertebral body endplate become apparent:
  - Anterior, lateral, or posterior osteophyte formation
  - Schmorl nodes and cystic cavities along the endplate can be visualized.
  - Endplate sclerosis
- The degenerative changes at the level of the disc, bony endplate, and ultimately the posterior facet joint complex restrict motion at the affected level or levels. At this stage, patients will typically complain more of back stiffness and soreness rather than pain. Neurogenic claudication due to narrowing of the spinal canal and spinal stenosis typically becomes more limiting than complaints of back pain.
- The final stage in the natural history of disc degeneration is autofusion.
- Patients should be counseled that disc degeneration itself is an inevitable process of aging and that any back pain experienced could, but may not necessarily, be associated with the disc degeneration.
- The overwhelming majority of patients have only occasional episodes of low back pain. Long-term disability resulting from DDD is rare.

PATIENT HISTORY AND PHYSICAL FINDINGS

- No pathognomonic history or physical examination findings exist for the diagnosis of lumbar DDD.
- Discogenic back pain is typically worst in situations in which an axial load is applied to the lumbar spine, as in prolonged sitting or standing with a forward-bent posture (ie, washing dishes, vacuuming, shaving, or brushing teeth).
- Conversely, positions such as side lying (ie, the fetal position) or floating erect in water place the least amount of strain across the intervertebral disc and should therefore provide some pain relief.
- Leg pain (in the absence of neural compression), if present, is nonradicular and "referred" in that it does not follow lumbar dermatomes into the lower leg and is not typically associated with loss of motor power, reflex changes, numbness, or tingling.
- Patients will occasionally describe a discrete traumatic disc injury in which they first experienced back pain. Imaging

studies that depict an old endplate fracture above or below a degenerative disc help corroborate this history.
- Loss of truncal musculature fitness from abdominal wall hernias, obesity, and prior abdominal wall surgery (ie, rectus muscle transfer procedures) may worsen discogenic back pain.
- Other causes of back pain should be sought in the history, physical examination, and imaging studies, including muscular strain, spondylolysis or spondylolisthesis, herniated nucleus pulposus, compression fracture, pseudarthrosis, tumor, and discitis.
- Patients with isolated DDD by definition should have a normal neurologic examination.

IMAGING AND OTHER DIAGNOSTIC STUDIES

- Standing plain radiographs
  - Lateral radiographs allow for measurement of the intervertebral disc height and allow comparison to other lumbar intervertebral discs (**FIG 2A**).
  - Anteroposterior (AP) radiographs allow for determination of asymmetric, coronal plain disc degeneration, which may be a precursor to lumbar degenerative scoliosis.
  - Flexion–extension radiographs may be helpful in diagnosing an occult spondylolisthesis or spondylolysis.
- MRI provides excellent visualization of the discs, the degree to which they have degenerated, and the relationship of the discs to the adjacent endplate and surrounding neurologic structures (**FIG 2B**).
  - "Modic changes" characterize the endplate on MRI:
    - Type 0: no changes
    - Type 1: dark on T1 and bright on T2 (represent marrow edema and inflammation)
    - Type 2: bright on T1 and isointense/bright on T2 (represent conversion from normal red into yellow marrow)
    - Type 3: dark on T1 and T2 (subchondral sclerosis)
  - Modic changes do not always follow DDD but are rare in healthy individuals. They may represent a shifting biomechanical stress distribution across the endplate.[14]
- Provocative discography attempts to reproduce the patient's typical back pain by pressurizing the disc with normal saline. The patient needs to be awake to provide subjective feedback as to the quality and intensity of the pain. Architectural changes to the disc are inferred by contrast administered with the saline.
  - Studies have shown that provocative discography leads to accelerated disc degeneration.[5]
- Computed tomography (CT) discography provides more detailed information about the disc morphology after contrast administration (**FIG 2C**).
- Normal laboratory tests, including complete blood count, erythrocyte sedimentation rate, and C-reactive protein, can help rule out a disc space infection; severe disc degeneration can sometimes mimic infection radiologically.

DIFFERENTIAL DIAGNOSIS

- DDD
- Discitis
- Pyogenic vertebral osteomyelitis

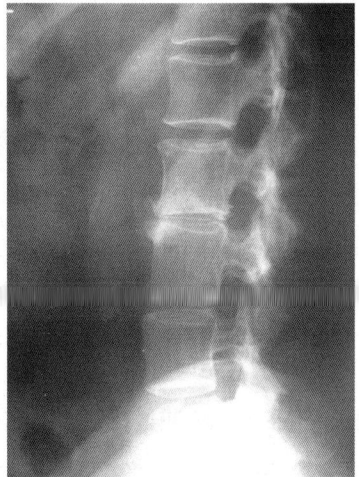 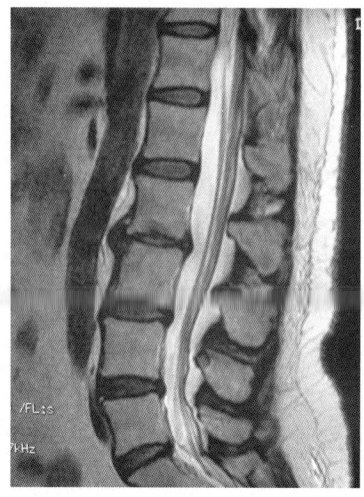 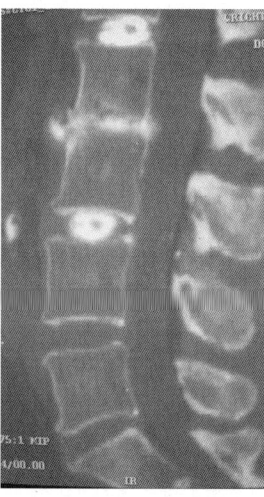

FIG 2 A. Lateral radiograph showing DDD at the L2–L3 level. **B.** Sagittal T2-weighted MRI of the same patient with low signal intensity in the nucleus of the L2–L3 disc. Anterior and posterior disc bulges are present. **C.** Sagittal CT discogram of the same patient showing dramatic loss of integrity of the L2–L3 nucleus and annulus with leakage of contrast anteriorly. The patient's pain was concordant at the L2–L3 disc level. The L1–L2 and L3–L4 discs served as negative controls with regard to both disc architecture and pain.

NONOPERATIVE MANAGEMENT

- DDD is analogous to hip and knee osteoarthritis in that the intervening cartilage (in the case of the disc: collagen, water, and proteoglycans) fails under compressive loads.
- Weight reduction and activity modification (avoidance of exacerbating activities) may be effective first-line treatments.
- Nonsteroidal anti-inflammatory medications
- Acupuncture or massage therapy
- Physical therapy with aquatic or dry land exercises
- Gentle pelvic traction
- Methylprednisolone (Solu Medrol) taper
- Epidural injections
- Narcotic medications for severe episodes of pain

SURGICAL MANAGEMENT

- Indications
  - Discogenic back pain refractory to nonoperative management
  - Discitis with pyogenic vertebral osteomyelitis refractory to nonoperative management
  - Spinal deformity requiring radical discectomy
  - Revision cases for pseudarthrosis
- A thorough and complete discectomy improves the effectiveness of anterior interbody fusion by creating a wide surface area of exposed bone.
- Interbody reconstruction and fusion can be accomplished by a variety of methods, including structural autogenous bone graft (iliac crest or fibula), structural allograft (ie, femoral or humeral ring, femoral head, machined bone dowel), or synthetic device (titanium, polyetheretherketone [PEEK], carbon fiber, composite) packed with cancellous bone or collagen sponges impregnated with bone morphogenetic protein 2 (BMP-2).
- Lumbar total disc replacement (LTDR) was initially adopted in Europe for preservation of segmental motion and avoidance of adjacent-level disc disease; however, prospective randomized investigational device exemption trials in

the United States failed to reveal superiority of LTDR when compared to anterior fusion. This information plus the rare but catastrophic complications associated with LTDR migrations have precluded widespread use in the United States.
- Regardless of the method used, prerequisites are that the interbody spacer be strong enough to resist intervertebral compressive loads and provide an appropriate biologic environment for healing.

Preoperative Planning

- Plain radiographs, MRI, or CT scans should be carefully evaluated for undiagnosed spondylolysis or spondylolisthesis, which may alter the surgical plan.
- Templates can be used with plain radiographs or MRI scans to gauge the size of the final implant to be used.
  - Oversized implants can lead to undesired stretch on neurologic structures and reduced motion of lumbar disc replacements.
  - Screw trajectories in stand-alone anterior lumbar interbody fusion (ALIF) devices must be templated to avoid violation of the central canal or neuroforamina.
- The level of the confluence of the common iliac veins into the inferior vena cava and the bifurcation of the aorta can be located on the axial MRI scans.
- At L5–S1, the pubic symphysis occasionally precludes appropriate visualization and instrumentation of the disc space in patients with a deep-seated L5–S1 relative to the pelvis. Evaluation of the lateral radiograph with the pubis on the film is critical to visualize the trajectory into the disc space and avoid this miscalculation.

Positioning

- See Chapter SP-35.
- The patient is placed over an inflatable pillow over a 1-inch thick foam pad, which is placed on the mattress of the operating table. The pillow allows for modulation of lordosis throughout the procedure and the foam pad props the pa-

tient up, allowing the arms to be tucked posteriorly out of the plane of the spine during imaging.

- Positioning over the break in the table allows for increased lordosis if needed.
- The use of fluoroscopic C-arm imaging is crucial for appropriate patient and implant positioning. It is helpful to verify that adequate fluoroscopic imaging of operative landmarks can be achieved after the patient is positioned but before the incision is made.

Approach

- See Chapter SP-35 on Anterior Lumbar Approach.
- Anterior retroperitoneal approaches will typically allow access to the lumbar discs from L2 to L3 to the sacrum.
- The renal vessels limit more proximal extension of the exposure.
- Lateral exposures to the lumbar spine are required for access to the L2 vertebra and above.

ANTERIOR LUMBAR RADICAL DISCECTOMY

Exposure

- Identify the intervertebral disc and mark the midline with a spinal needle or screw placed into the vertebral body (we prefer not to place a needle into the disc space because this may create unwanted disc injury) **(TECH FIG 1A)**.
- Use AP and lateral fluoroscopic imaging to check the midline. The midline marker also serves to verify the spinal level.
- At L5–S1, retract the left common iliac artery and vein to the patient's left and the right common iliac artery and vein to the right. At levels above L5–S1, the aorta and inferior vena cava must be mobilized to the patient's right.
- The great vessels can be held in their retracted position using handheld Hohmann retractors, custom-designed pins, or Kirschner wires, all of which can be advanced directly into the vertebral bodies (virtually eliminating the risk of vessel migration into the field of interest) **(TECH FIG 1B)**.
  - Alternatively, stainless steel vein retractors or radiolucent retractors can be fixed to the arms of an abdominal retractor system (Omni) or floating, Endo ring–type retractor system. These blade retractors have the disadvantage of allowing vessel migration into the field by sliding under the retractor blades as motion occurs during the procedure. The advantage of the radiolucent retractors is that better visualization of the operative field is possible with fluoroscopy. In addition, blade-type retractors can be easily manipulated during the procedure without having to reinsert into the vertebral body.
- Attempt to retract the vessels as far lateral as you can to allow for the widest possible view of the intervertebral disc.

Poor visualization at this stage will compromise the quality of the discectomy and any ensuing interbody device placement.

Removing the Disc

- Using a no. 10 blade on a long handle, incise the intervertebral disc starting laterally along the superior endplate and move toward midline. Always move away from the vessels to avoid an accidental lateral plunge into the great vessels. The blade should be inserted between the cartilage endplate and bone if possible, and we use both hands on the knife shank for optimal control and coordination **(TECH FIG 2A,B)**.
- A large, sharp Cobb elevator is then used to release as much of the cartilaginous endplate as possible from the superior and inferior endplates. By angling the Cobb blade toward the bone and pronating and supinating the hand, almost the entire disc (annulus and nucleus) can be removed, as if peeling an orange in one large piece **(TECH FIG 2C)**.
- Long-handled no. 2 and no. 3 Cobb curettes are used to remove the remaining disc, taking the dissection all the way to the posterior longitudinal ligament **(TECH FIG 2D)**. Systematic removal of endplate cartilage enhances thorough removal. Thus, start anteriorly on the superior endplate and move posteriorly. Then, start anteriorly on the inferior endplate and move posteriorly.
  - The curette will function much more effectively if it is used as a cutting instrument rather than a scraper. For this reason, we prefer that curettes be sharp, nonangled, and used with a pronating–supinating motion with the edge of the curette between the cartilage endplate and the endplate bone.

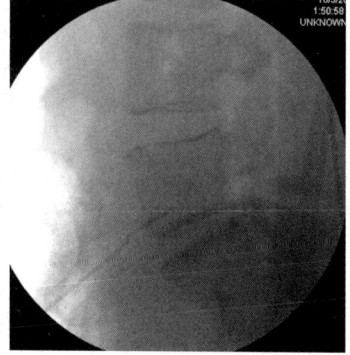
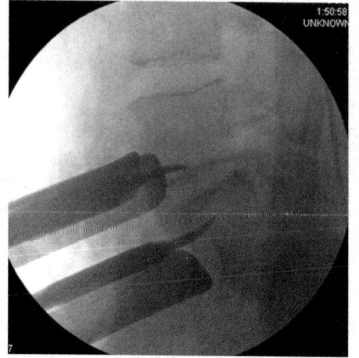

TECH FIG 1 **A.** Lateral radiograph showing the spinal needle inserted into the L4 vertebral body above the L4–L5 disc to be removed. **B.** Lateral radiograph showing sharp Hohmann retractors placed into the L4 vertebral body above and L5 vertebral body below. Blade-type retractors can be left in place lateral to the Hohmann retractors for additional visibility, as shown.

T E C H N I Q U E S

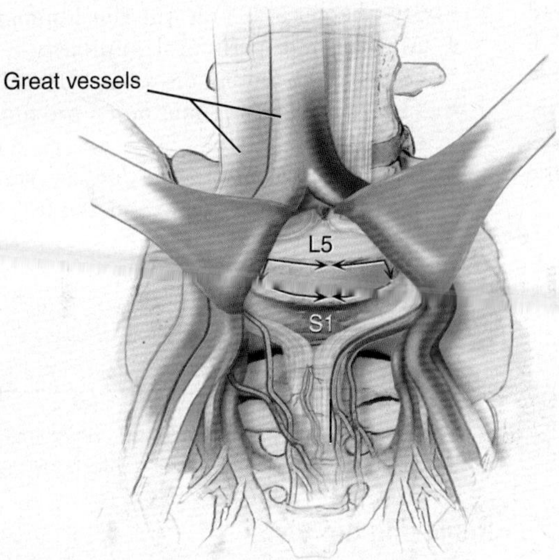

Great vessels

L5

S1

A

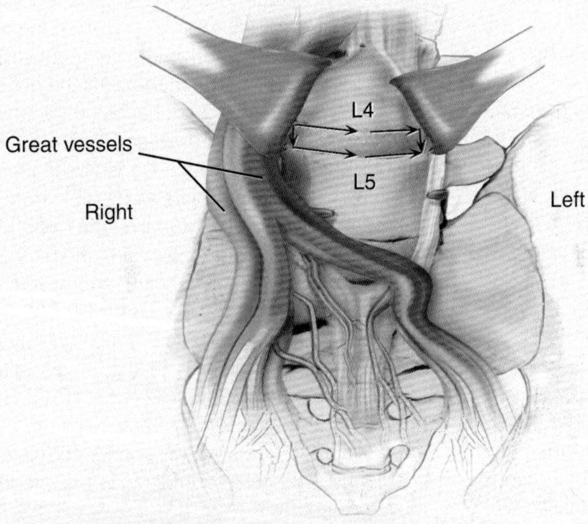

Great vessels

Right

L4

L5

Left

B

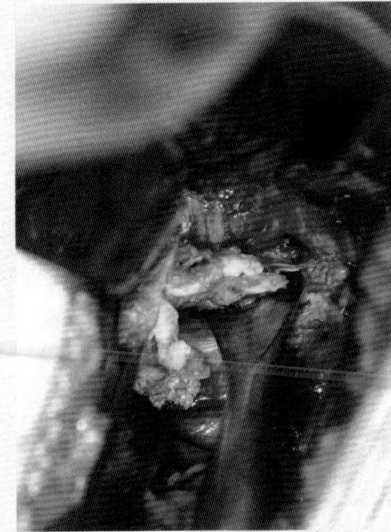

C

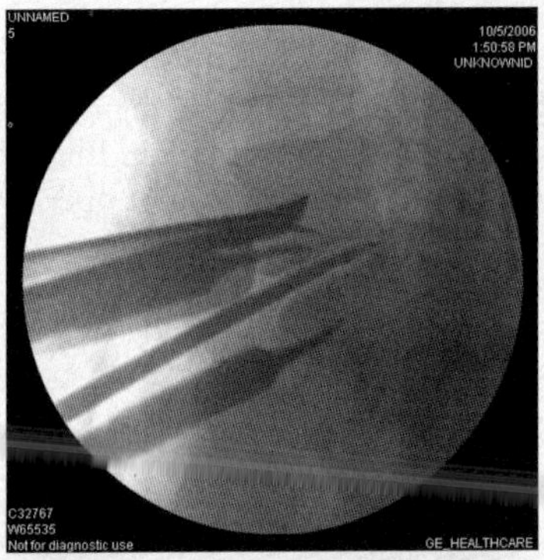

D

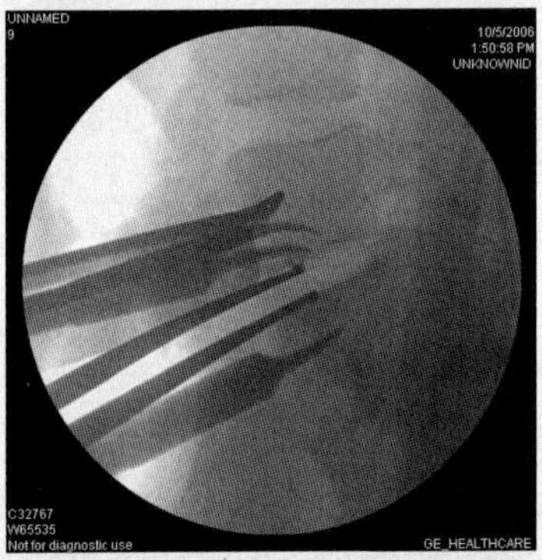

E

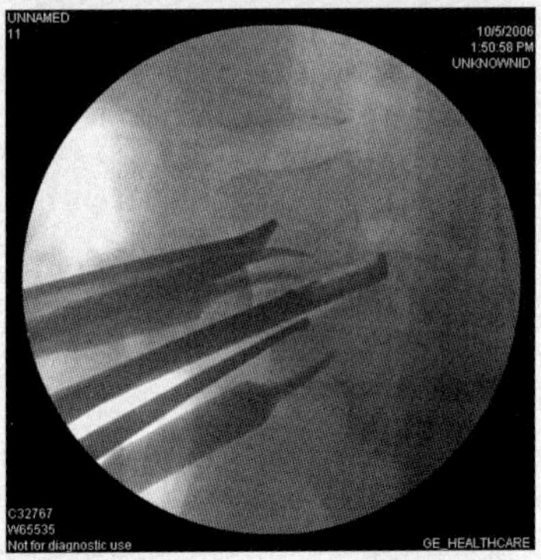

F

TECH FIG 2 A,B. Direction of movement of the surgical blade. At L5–S1, the surgical field is within the bifurcation of the great vessels, so the surgical knife should always be directed toward the midline and inferiorly—away from vascular structures. At L4–L5 and above, the vascular structures are retracted to the patient's right, and therefore, movements with the knife blade are directed to the patient's left and inferiorly. **C.** A large Cobb is used between the disc cartilage and the vertebral body to remove as much as possible in one large piece. **D.** Lateral radiograph showing a no. 2 Cobb curette used to remove the cartilaginous disc endplate. **E.** Lateral radiograph demonstrating a lamina spreader creating distraction within the disc space. The distractor enhances visualization of the posterior portion of the disc space. Care should be taken to make sure that the distractor is seated anteriorly and laterally on strong endplate bone to avoid damage to the central cancellous region. **F.** Lateral radiograph showing the use of a 4-mm long Kerrison rongeur to decompress the neural foramen.

- The posterior longitudinal ligament is not routinely removed, but the posterolateral corners of the disc space must be thoroughly débrided of disc material for several reasons:
  - Periphery of the endplate is the strongest bone and therefore provides the most stable support of an interbody device.
  - Disc material that is left over can be pushed posteriorly into the epidural space, causing an iatrogenic disc herniation during implant insertion.
  - If anterior decompression of the neural foramen is one of the goals of surgery, visualization and removal of a herniated disc or disc–osteophyte complex will not be possible without proper visualization in this region.
- The lateral extent of the discectomy is determined by the width of the device to be inserted, but care must be taken to maintain the width of the discectomy posteriorly as the natural tendency is to remove less disc laterally in the posterior portion of the disc space.
- A lamina spreader can be gently distracted in the anterolateral interbody region to gain enhanced visibility of the posterior disc space **(TECH FIG 2E)**.
- Removal of a posterior or foraminal disc herniation can be accomplished by passing an angled Kerrison rongeur posteriorly and into the neural foramen. Identification of the ventral aspect of the dura enhances the safety of this maneuver **(TECH FIG 2F)**.
- Epidural bleeding can be brisk during posterior disc removal, but thrombin-soaked Gelfoam gauze and removal of intervertebral distraction can be used to control it.

ANTERIOR LUMBAR INTERBODY FUSION

Threaded Devices

- Once the discectomy has been completed, disc space distractors are inserted to gauge the size of the final implant **(TECH FIG 3A)**. Appropriate distractor size can be gauged by comparing the operative level with a normal disc above or below. In addition, the interface between the distractor and the bony endplate should be less than 1 mm. This ensures good interference fit of the final device.
- For threaded devices such as the lumbar tapered (LT) cage, a cannulated guide channel is inserted over the disc distractors. This working channel serves to prevent inadvert migration of the great vessels into the disc space.
- Endplate reamers are then inserted to appropriate depth as determined by lateral fluoroscopic imaging **(TECH FIG 3B)**. Care should be taken to aim the reamer for the midportion of the disc space posteriorly on lateral fluoroscopy rather than through one endplate or the other.
  - Asymmetric reaming will result in excessive removal of one endplate compared to another and the final implant will be more likely to fail in subsidence. Because the reamer tends to follow the path of least resistance, an exceptionally sclerotic endplate will predispose one to asymmetric reaming by this mechanism.
  - Alternatively, an "exact-fit" approach may be selected in which the endplate is left intact. However, proper sizing of the implant may be difficult, and the intact endplate does not provide an optimal vascular environment for fusion.
- Final threaded implants are then screwed into the appropriate depth and orientation **(TECH FIG 3C,D)**. The first cage (in a dual-cage system) is inserted in the same trajectory as the reamers, and lateral fluoroscopic imaging during cage placement ensures that the cage is not placed too anteriorly or posteriorly. The cage should not be inserted beyond the depth of the reamer or else the threads will strip and the cage will lose a large percentage of its fixation strength.
  - Saving the C-arm image of the final reamer depth allows the surgeon to reference this image when inserting the cage.
- The second cage is inserted using the first cage as a reference for trajectory and depth. Final images should be true AP and lateral projections showing the cage devices to be in good position.

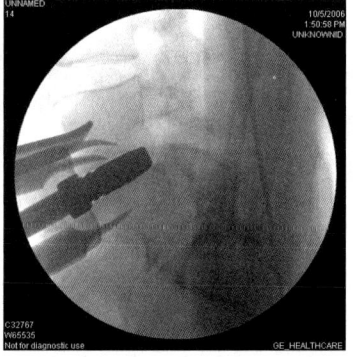 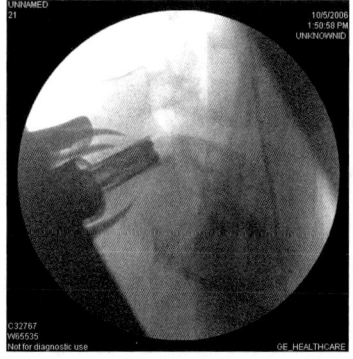 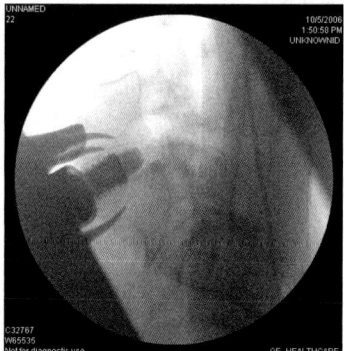

A   B   C

TECH FIG 3 A. Lateral radiograph showing a radiopaque disc distractor within the intervertebral disc. The distractor approximates the height of the disc space above (L3–L4), and there is at most 1 mm of space between the intervertebral endplate and the distractor. **B.** Lateral radiograph showing reaming of the intervertebral channel for the anterior interbody device. Because the vertebral body is shallower in the AP plane away from the midline, reaming should stop shy of the posterior vertebral body line, as shown. **C.** Lateral radiograph showing threaded cage entry into the disc space. The cage is directed parallel to the vertebral endplates. *(continued)*

TECHNIQUES

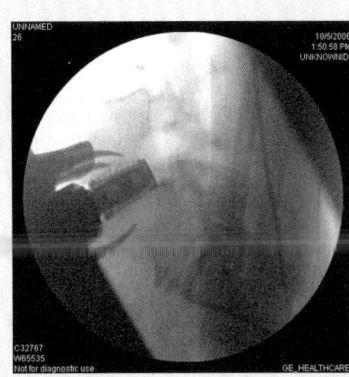 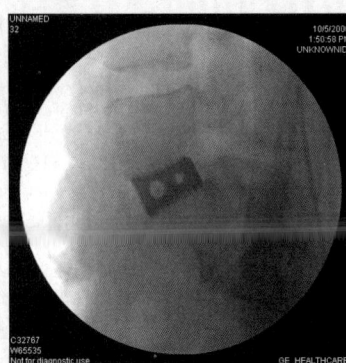 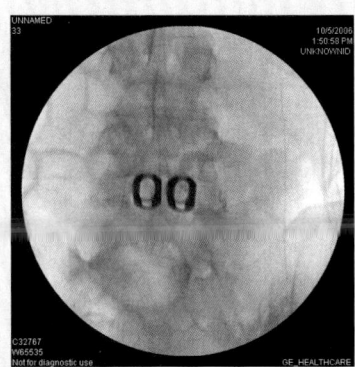

TECH FIG 3 *(continued)* **D.** Final cage placement should not extend beyond the depth of the reamer. **E.** Lateral radiograph showing final cage placement. The overlapping pedicles confirm true lateral positioning. **F.** AP radiograph showing parallel positioning of paired cages.

Overlapping pedicles on the lateral image will appear sharp, confirming true lateral positioning **(TECH FIG 3E,F)**.
- Cages should be positioned within the footprint of the endplate as near to the periphery as possible to dissipate compressive force over a wider area. Cages placed anteriorly may have a biomechanical advantage through increased compressive loading.[6]

Nonthreaded, Stand-Alone Anterior Lumbar Interbody Fusion Devices

- A subtotal discectomy, whereby the lateral most aspects of the annulus are preserved, is advised to provide increased stability via the remaining annulus. A trial implant can serve as a guide for optimal disc resection.
- The interspace can be distracted, and then the entire cartilage endplate region covered by the trial implant is removed on both vertebral bodies.
- Typically, a single interbody cage that spans the disc space is selected, with graft material packed on both sides within the implant. This is positioned in the center of the interspace using product-specific instruments **(TECH FIG 4A)**.

- Locking screws are directed cephalad and caudad either through the cage device or through a metal faceplate that attaches to the cage **(TECH FIG 4B)**. Knowledge of product-specific screw trajectories and starting points is paramount as they may be either symmetric about the midline or translated left or right to allow safe passage of the drill between the iliac vessels.

Adjunct Treatments

- Autograft material or a BMP-2–impregnated collagen sponge may be used to fill the graft. BMP-2 has been approved by the U.S. Food and Drug Administration (FDA) for single-level ALIF in the titanium LT interbody devices (Medtronic Sofamor Danek, Memphis, TN).[4]
- Concomitant posterior fusion increases construct stiffness and is indicated in the setting of instability. Transpedicular fixation theoretically reduces the force transmitted through the ALIF cage and provides immediate stability. Facet screw fixation provides less stability but reduces stiffness to permit more force anteriorly. Scant evidence exists to differentiate these options based on outcomes.[8]

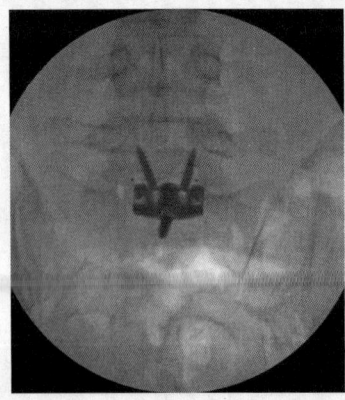 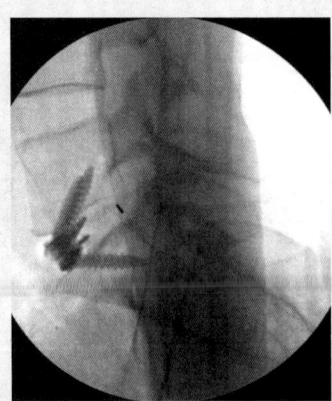

TECH FIG 4 AP (**A**) and lateral (**B**) fluoroscopic images showing midline positioning and screw trajectories of stand-alone ALIF device.

LUMBAR TOTAL DISC REPLACEMENT

- Under fluoroscopic guidance, determine the midline on a true AP image of the vertebral body above or below the disc (**TECH FIG 5A**). A bone screw may be inserted as a reference.
- Sizing guides are trialed to fill the entire footprint of the endplate (**TECH FIG 5B**). Height and lordosis are then set using trial

wedges (**TECH FIG 5C–E**) and should match the resected gap and preoperative templating.
- An implant-specific chisel is then directed straight posteriorly through the bodies to cut a groove for the keel or teeth that align the implant and prevent rotation (**TECH FIG 5F**) and the final implant inserted (**TECH FIG 5G–I**).

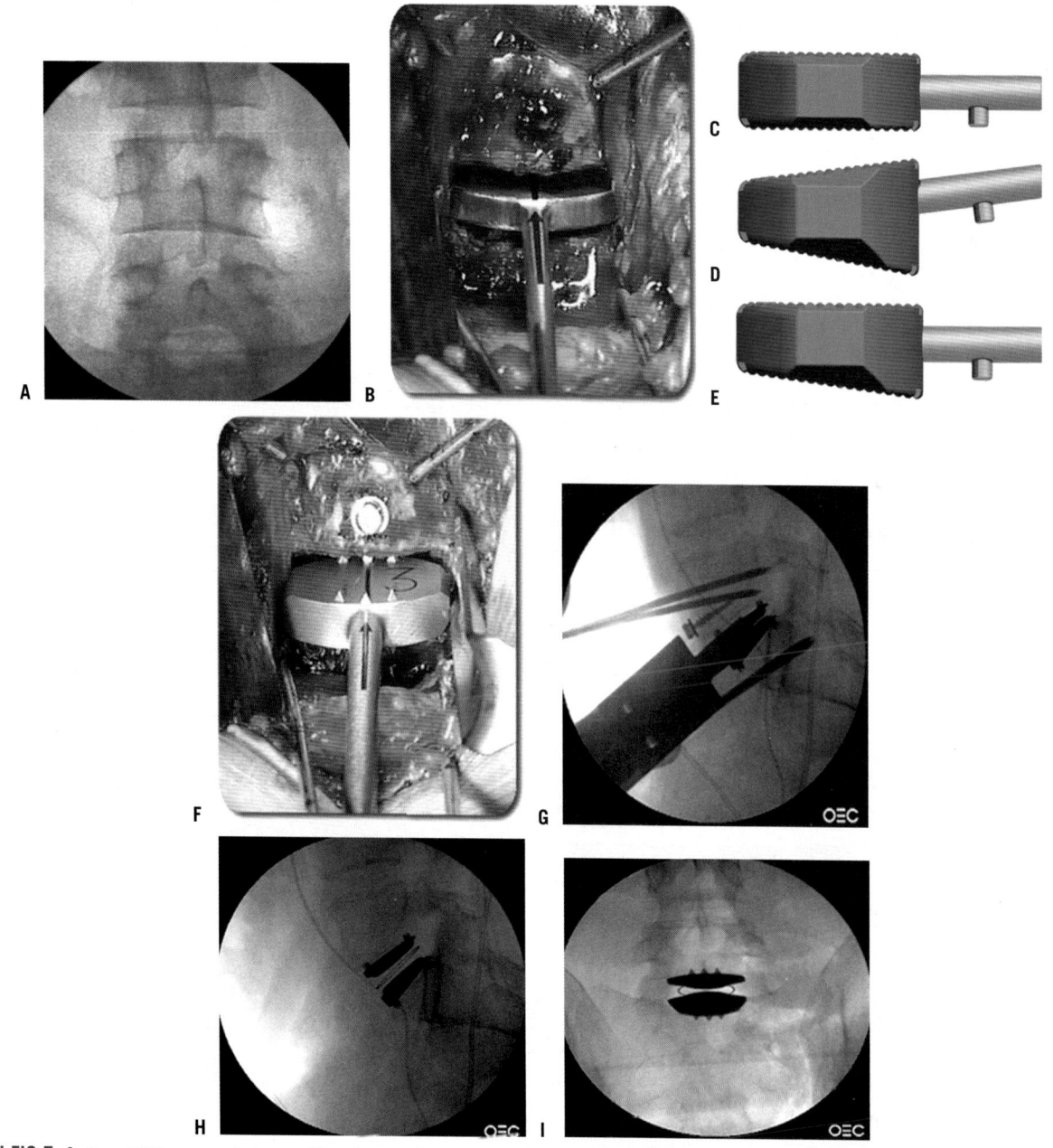

TECH FIG 5 A. True AP fluoroscopic image. The distance between the midpoint of the vertebra and the pedicles should be the same. The cortical margins of the pedicles themselves should be the same size (ensuring the spine is not rotated). Finally, the spinous processes should bisect the vertebra. The spinous processes are the least reliable landmark as they can be malformed, especially at L5 and S1. **B.** A sizing guide, or "lollipop," demonstrates how well the endplate will be covered by the final implant. The largest size that allows good peripheral endplate coverage in both the sagittal and coronal planes is desired. **C–E.** Using radiolucent trial wedges of varying height and lordosis allows the final device to be individualized to the patient's anatomy. **F.** Introduction of the channel cutter into the disc space. **G.** Lateral fluoroscopic image showing implant insertion. The insertion instruments are still connected, which allows for fine adjustment to the final positioning. **H,I.** Lateral and AP fluoroscopic images of the final TDR placement with all of the instruments removed. The final implant should be in the center of the vertebral body on the AP image and in the center (sagittal midline) or just posterior to the center of the vertebral body on the lateral image. (**B–E:** Courtesy of DePuy Spine, Raynham, MA.)

ANTERIOR LUMBAR CORPECTOMY

Vertebra Removal

- The indications for anterior corpectomy in the lumbar spine are lumbar burst fracture, catastrophic failure of lumbar disc replacement or interbody device (ie, vertebral fracture), lumbar vertebral osteomyelitis, correction of kyphosis, and vertebral body malignancy.
  - In cases of corpectomy for vascular tumors, preoperative embolization should be performed **(TECH FIG 6A)**.
  - In cases of corpectomy, radical discectomies are performed above and below the vertebral body to be removed (see discectomy technique discussed earlier).
  - This enables the surgeon to become oriented to the midline and also to judge the depth and width of the corpectomy to be performed.
  - The discectomy space also allows the surgeon to use a large rongeur efficiently to remove the vertebral body **(TECH FIG 6B)**.
- Retractors should be placed above and below the entire vertebra to be removed, so there is an unobstructed view for the surgeon and the assistants. The vertebral body bleeds more rapidly than the endplates, so the assistants need to be able to visualize the operative field to suction effectively.
- A Leksell rongeur can be used to remove all of the vertebral body back to the level of the posterior cortex. If this needs to be removed, angled curettes are used to develop the plane behind the vertebra, starting at the disc space. Kerrison punches or angled curettes are then used to lift the posterior cortex off the ventral dura.
  - Healthy vertebral body bone should be saved for interbody fusion.

Filling the Interbody Space

- Once the corpectomy is completed, bone graft or an interbody device is contoured to fit into the defect. The wooden end of a cotton-tipped applicator can be cut to the length of the defect and can then be used as a size gauge for the final interbody device. This is particularly useful when cutting and contouring a bone graft because calipers and rulers do not always fit easily into the central portion of the corpectomy defect to give an accurate height measurement.
- Check the height of the corpectomy defect with the wooden applicator throughout its entire depth from anterior to posterior. Keep in mind that the shape of the corpectomy site may be lordotic, and thus, the bone graft or implant needs to be fashioned appropriately.
- Autogenous tricortical iliac crest and autogenous fibula have the greatest healing potential but are also associated with significant harvest site morbidity.
- Metal cages generally are the easiest to fashion to fit the corpectomy space and can be packed with morselized corpectomy bone **(TECH FIG 7A)**. The disadvantages are their expense and relatively reduced surface area at the endplate for fusion compared to bone.

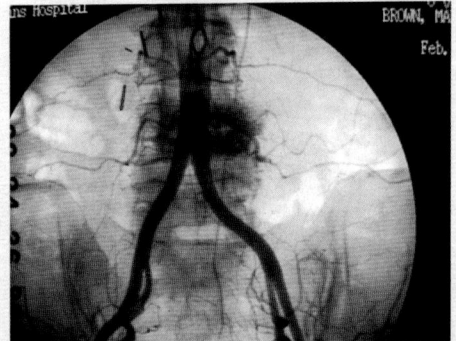

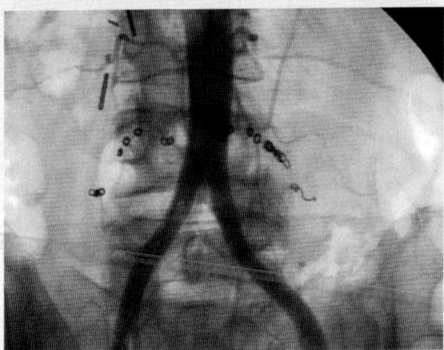

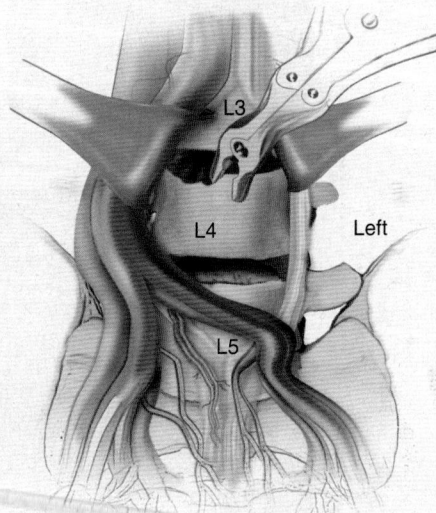

TECH FIG 6 A. Preembolization angiogram depicting the aortic bifurcation in a 65-year-old patient with metastatic renal cell carcinoma to the L4 vertebra. Note the degree of vascularity of the L4 vertebral body. **B.** Postembolization angiogram depicting a striking reduction in contrast entering the L4 vertebral body. Small embolization coils are seen in the vascular network surrounding the vertebral body. **C.** Anterior discectomy enables the surgeon to use a large rongeur to gain access to the edge of the vertebra and thereby remove the vertebral body bone.

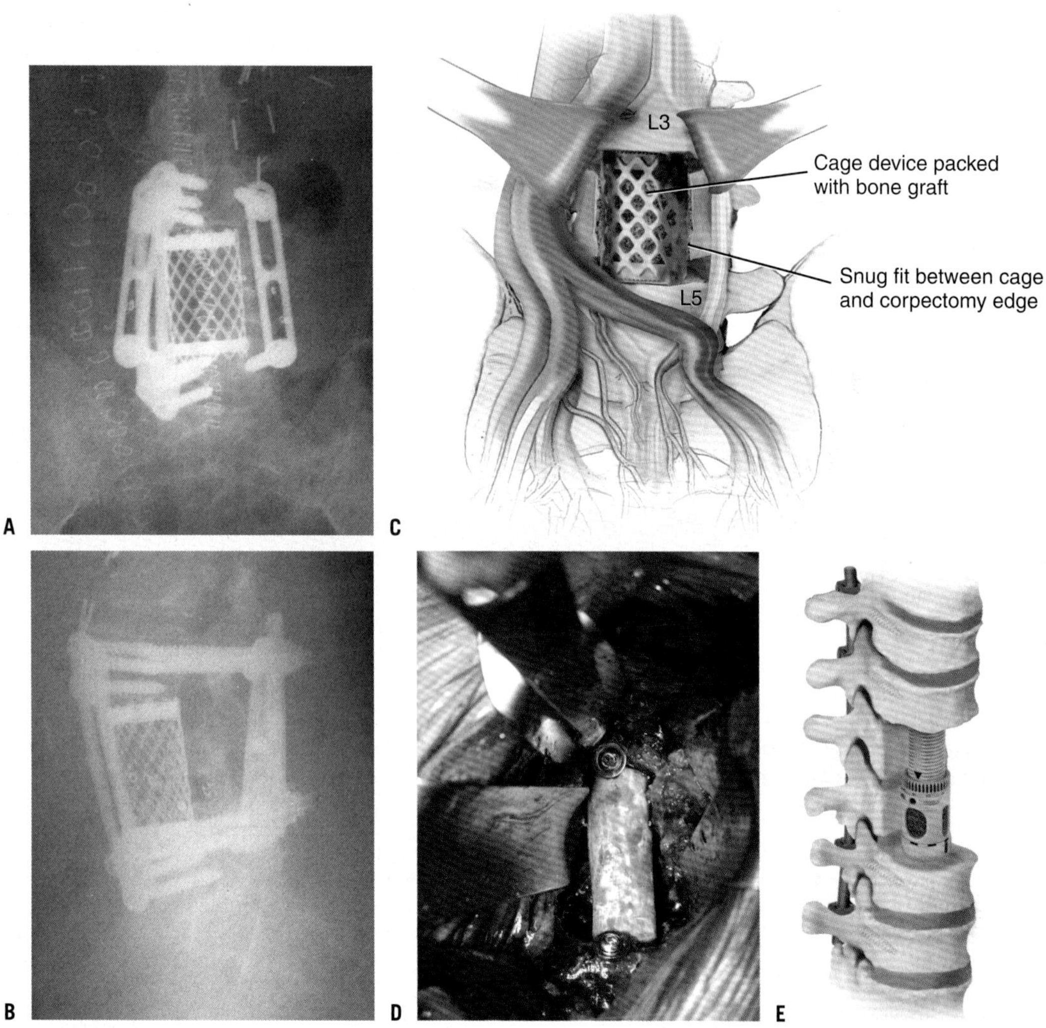

TECHNIQUES

Cage device packed
with bone graft

Snug fit between cage
and corpectomy edge

L3

L5

A

B

C

D

E

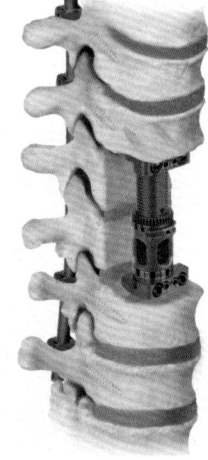

F

TECH FIG 7 A,B. AP and lateral postoperative radiographs of a patient in whom posterior element resection followed by fusion and instrumentation with pedicle screws was performed as a first stage followed by complete anterior corpectomy and reconstruction with a cylindrical titanium mesh cage packed with autogenous bone graft. An anterior side plate was applied as the lateral vertebral body wall was completely removed. **C.** The corpectomy strut device should fit snugly against the cut edge of the vertebral body to promote side-to-side fusion from host bone to strut graft. **D.** Intraoperative image of anterior allograft reconstruction after corpectomy, irrigation, and débridement of the L3 vertebra in a 62-year-old man with L3 vertebral body destruction from pyogenic vertebral osteomyelitis. A 4.5-mm cortical screws with washers are used to prevent allograft kickout. **E,F.** PEEK polymer and titanium expandable cages should fill the interspace snugly and are useful for precise reconstruction of the defect space. (**E,F:** Fortify®. Courtesy of Globus Medical, Inc., Audubon, PA.)

- The width of the corpectomy should be kept as narrow as possible without compromising decompression or removal of pathologic bone **(TECH FIG 7B)**.
  - Allows bone ingrowth from the corpectomized vertebral body into the interbody bone graft
  - Enhances the stability of the interbody strut
- A bone screw with a washer can be used above and below large defects as an "anti-kickout" buttress for allografts **(TECH FIG 7C)**.
- Allograft strut grafts such as femoral head, humerus, or fibular shafts can be cut using an oscillating saw to fit snugly into the interbody space **(TECH FIG 7D)**. The advantages of allograft are it can be packed with morselized autogenous bone, it has a similar modulus of elasticity to host vertebral bone, and it will become osseointegrated over time.

- Expandable corpectomy devices have been developed to facilitate anterior column reconstruction following single- or multilevel corpectomy. These devices are inserted and expanded until there is good interference fit at the endplates **(TECH FIG 7E)**.
  - Their use in single-level cases also permits more accurate height restoration and simplifies the carpentry because the height of the device can be expanded to fill virtually any defect.
  - One potential disadvantage of the expandable corpectomy devices is the reduction in bone graft volume and bone graft apposition to the vertebral endplate. Concomitant posterior fusion is advocated given the large amount of resection and potential instability.

TECHNIQUES

Pearls and Pitfalls

Use of a pulse oximeter on the left great toe provides real-time feedback to the surgeon about perfusion to the distal extremity during great vessel retraction.	• There should be a low threshold for prophylactic inferior vena cava filter placement in patients with venous injuries requiring repair, as pulmonary embolism, although rare, carries potentially catastrophic consequences.
Perforation of the cancellous vertebral body endplates with Cobb curettes or the lamina spreader increases the likelihood of implant subsidence.	• Early (<2 weeks) implant malpositions or migrations can be easily revised as the anterior tissue planes are still preserved.
Epidural bleeding can be effectively controlled quickly with thrombin-soaked Gelfoam gauze and release of any disc space distractors.	• Overdistraction of the disc space with a lumbar disc replacement implant will result in compromised motion and may be associated with new postoperative leg pain related to stretch injury to the lumbosacral nerve trunks.
Marking the location of the dorsalis pedis and posterior tibial pulses with a marking pen facilitates reassessment of pulses in the postoperative setting when lower extremity swelling is more prevalent.	

POSTOPERATIVE CARE

- As soon as the patient emerges from anesthesia, a complete neurologic examination and brief history should be performed. Specifically, patients should be asked if they have any new leg pain. If present, CT myelography or plain CT scans should be obtained to ensure that no bone, disc material, or portion of an implanted device is impinging on the lumbar nerve roots.
- Nasogastric tubes for the first 12 to 24 hours help to minimize abdominal wall distention and postoperative ileus.
- Patients are encouraged to walk on postoperative day 1.
- Lumbar corsets or abdominal binders are prescribed at the discretion of the surgeon and may reduce the tension on the abdominal incision in the early postoperative period.
- Return to heavy manual labor is restricted in patients undergoing anterior interbody fusion until the fusion is solid. Fine-cut CT scans are useful in documenting solid fusion if there is doubt on AP, lateral, or flexion–extension radiographs **(FIG 3)**. Manual labor should be restricted in patients undergoing disc replacement until the bone–prosthesis interface is judged to be stable.

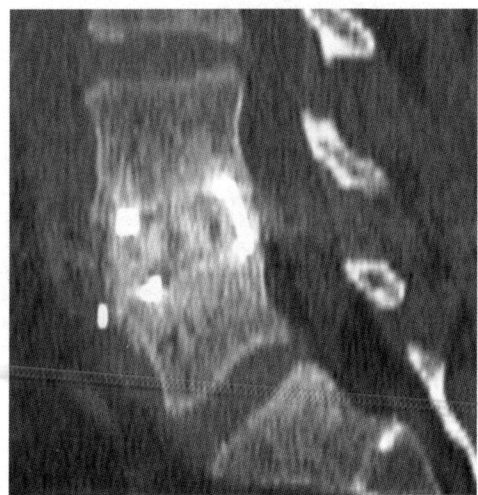

FIG 3 Sagittal fine-cut CT image depicting trabecular bone bridging across the disc space 3 months after anterior interbody fusion with a threaded titanium cage packed with collagen sponges impregnated with BMP-2.

OUTCOMES

- Level IV evidence reported by Tropiano et al[18] showed significant improvements in back pain, radiculopathy, and disability at mean of 8.7 years after insertion of the ProDisc lumbar disc replacement.
  - However, a Cochrane review of seven randomized controlled trials of LTDR versus fusion failed to demonstrate a clinically significant difference in outcomes and called into question selection and reporting bias in studies supporting LTDR.[9]
- ALIF with titanium cages and iliac crest bone graft has been shown to yield significantly greater fusion rates (97%) versus allograft dowels packed with iliac crest bone graft (48%).[15]
- Stand-alone ALIF devices (those without posterior fusion or instrumentation) demonstrated a fusion rate of 88% overall, 94% with an anterior plate, and 94% with rhBMP-2 versus 84% without.[10]
- BMP-2 is FDA approved for use in LT interbody devices for single-level ALIF. Improved fusion rates and clinical outcomes were reported in patients who had ALIF cages packed with BMP-2–impregnated collagen sponges compared to patients in whom the cages were packed with iliac crest bone graft.[4]
  - Subsequent investigation has called into question the safety and efficacy of BMP-2. A longitudinal study[6] of 472 patients and an independent review of industry data[16] both demonstrated an increased rate of retrograde ejaculation (7% vs. 1%) with nearly equivalent functional outcomes in groups treated with ALIF and BMP-2 as opposed to autograft. They also noted a small, but clinically insignificant, increased cancer risk associated with the use of BMP-2.
  - A review of a cohort of 146,278 Medicare patients undergoing lumbar fusion surgery revealed no difference in new cancer diagnosis rates between those who received BMP-2 and those who had not (15% vs. 17% of patients with a new cancer diagnosis, respectively).[7] The relationship between BMP-2 and carcinogenesis is uncertain at this point.
- Clinical outcomes and flexion–extension range of motion correlate with surgical technical accuracy of lumbar disc replacement.[11]
- The addition of posterolateral fusion with or without instrumentation (360-degree fusion) may be efficacious in carefully selected individuals; however, identification of the most appropriate patients and the outcomes of this approach have not been clearly established in the literature.[13]

COMPLICATIONS

- Most complications associated with anterior lumbar discectomy, interbody fusion, disc replacement, and corpectomy are approach related (see Chap. SP-35).[1,3,12,18]
- The most common complications of ALIF are pseudarthrosis and device failures such as migration or breakage.
- The complications of lumbar disc replacement depend on the exact type of device being inserted but generally can be categorized as follows[17,19]:
  - Device failures: metal endplate breakage, core dislodgement or fracture, polyethylene degradation
  - Bone implant failures: subsidence, vertebral body fracture, implant migration or dislocation
  - Iatrogenic deformity: kyphosis, scoliosis
  - Host response: osteolysis, heterotopic ossification
  - Infection
- Revision approaches to the anterior lumbar spine carry six times the risk of major bleeding or thromboembolic complications.[12] Preoperative intravenous filter insertion, ureteral stenting, and percutaneous venous access wires are critical to reduce these risks.

REFERENCES

1. Bertagnoli R, Zigler J, Karg A, et al. Complications and strategies for revision surgery in total disc replacement. Orthop Clin North Am 2005;36:389–395.
2. Boden SD, Davis DO, Dina TS, et al. Abnormal magnetic-resonance scans of the lumbar spine in asymptomatic subjects. A prospective investigation. J Bone Joint Surg Am 1990;72(3):403–408.
3. Brau SA, Delamarter RB, Schiffman ML, et al. Vascular injury during anterior lumbar surgery. Spine J 2004;4:409–412.
4. Burkus JK, Heim SE, Gornet MF, et al. Is INFUSE bone graft superior to autograft bone? An integrated analysis of clinical trials using the LT-CAGE lumbar tapered fusion device. J Spinal Disord Tech 2003;16:113–122.
5. Carragee EJ, Don AS, Hurwitz EL, et al. 2009 ISSLS prize winner: does discography cause accelerated progression of degeneration changes in the lumbar disc: a ten-year matched cohort study. Spine (Phila Pa 1976) 2009;34(21):2338–2345.
6. Comer GC, Smith MW, Hurwitz EL, et al. Retrograde ejaculation after anterior lumbar interbody fusion with and without bone morphogenetic protein-2 augmentation: a 10-year cohort controlled study. Spine J 2012;12(10):881–890.
7. Cooper GS, Kou TD. Risk of cancer after lumbar fusion surgery with recombinant human bone morphogenic protein-2 (rh-BMP-2). Spine (Phila Pa 1976) 2013;38(21):1862–1868.
8. Hueng DY, Chung TT, Chuang WH, et al. Biomechanical effects of cage positions and facet fixation on initial stability of the anterior lumbar interbody fusion motion segment. Spine (Phila Pa 1976) 2014;39(13):E770–E776.
9. Jacobs W, Van der Gaag NA, Tuschel A, et al. Total disc replacement for chronic back pain in the presence of disc degeneration. Cochrane Database Syst Rev 2012;(9):CD008326.
10. Manzur M, Virk S, Jivanelli B, et al. The rate of fusion for stand-alone anterior lumbar interbody fusion: a systematic review. Spine J 2019;19(7):1294–1301.
11. McAfee PC, Cunningham BW, Holtsapple G, et al. A prospective, randomized, multicenter Food and Drug Administration investigational device exemption study of lumbar total disc replacement with the CHARITE artificial disc versus lumbar fusion: part II: evaluation of radiographic outcomes and correlation of surgical technique accuracy with clinical outcomes. Spine (Phila Pa 1976) 2005;30:1576–1583.
12. McAfee PC, Geisler FH, Saiedy SS, et al. Revisability of the CHARITE Artificial Disc Replacement: analysis of 688 patients enrolled in the U.S. IDE study of the CHARITE Artificial Disc. Spine (Phila Pa 1976) 2006;31:1217–1226.
13. Mummaneni PV, Dhall SS, Eck JC, et al. Guideline update for the performance of fusion procedures for degenerative disease of the lumbar spine. Part 11: interbody techniques for lumbar fusion. J Neurosurg Spine 2014;21(1):67–74.
14. Rahme R, Moussa R. The modic vertebral endplate and marrow changes: pathologic significance and relation to low back pain and segmental instability of the lumbar spine. AJNR Am J Neuroradiol 2008;29(5):838–842.
15. Sasso RC, Kitchel SH, Dawson EG. A prospective, randomized controlled clinical trial of anterior lumbar interbody fusion using a titanium cylindrical threaded fusion device. Spine (Phila Pa 1976) 2004;29(2):113–122.
16. Simmonds MC, Brown JV, Heits MK, et al. Safety and effectiveness of recombinant human bone morphogenetic protein-2 for spinal fusion: a meta-analysis of individual-participant data. Ann Intern Med 2013;158(12):877–889.
17. Tortolani PJ, McAfee PC, Saiedy S. Failures of lumbar disc replacement. Semin Spine Surg 2006;18:78–86.
18. Tropiano P, Huang RC, Girardi FP, et al. Lumbar total disc replacement. Seven to eleven year follow-up. J Bone Joint Surg Am 2005;87(3):490–496.
19. van Ooij A, Oner FC, Verbout AJ. Complications of artificial disc replacement: a report of 27 patients with the SB Charité disc. J Spinal Disord Tech 2003;16(4):369–383.

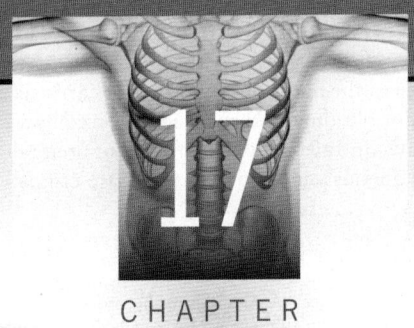

17

CHAPTER

Anterior Thoracic Corpectomy

Sheeraz A. Qureshi, Samuel C. Overley, Morgan N. Chen, and Andrew C. Hecht

DEFINITION

- Anterior thoracic approaches provide a means of decompression, stabilization, and fusion for a variety of spinal pathologies, such as deformity, trauma, infection, tumors, and disc herniations.

ANATOMY

- The thoracic vertebral bodies are heart-shaped in the axial plane.
  - The thoracic pedicles are oval and are larger superoinferiorly than mediolaterally.
  - The T4 pedicle is the smallest in width with a mean[10] of just 4.4 mm.
  - The progression of width starts with the largest at T12, decreasing to T4, and increasing again from T3 to T1.
  - The average height is 8 to 15 mm, and the average width is 3 to 10 mm.
- The medial cortex is the thickest; however, there is no epidural space between the medial cortical edge and the dura.[19]
- The facet joints are situated more anteriorly and articulate superiorly and inferiorly with a rib. As the transition from the thoracic to lumbar spine occurs, the thoracic vertebrae begin to resemble the lumbar vertebrae and the facets change from a coronal orientation to one that is more sagittal.

PATHOGENESIS

Intervertebral Disc Herniation

- Thoracic disc herniations are uncommon, making up only 1% of all operable intervertebral disc herniations.[16]
- Seventy-five percent of thoracic disc herniations occur between T8 and L1, with T11–T12 being most common. They are classified as central, centrolateral, lateral, or paramedian.
  - Most herniations occur central or centrolateral and are often calcified.
- Bimodal distribution with traumatic etiology (discussed in the following text) is common in acute herniated nucleus pulposus in the young and degenerative herniated nucleus pulposus in the elderly.[16]
- The spinal canal in the thoracic spine is relatively small.
  - Neurologic consequences occur from direct anterior compression of the spinal cord from a herniated disc. There can be posterior displacement of the cord and local vascular insufficiency.

Infection

- The mechanism of spinal infections is controversial. Proposed routes of infection include hematogenous spread from other infected foci, local extension from nearby infections, and direct inoculation.
  - The two proposed routes of hematogenous spread are venous and arterial.
  - Advocates of venous hematogenous spread argue that organisms are carried to the spine via the plexus of Batson, similar to the mechanism of tumor metastasis.[2]
  - Proponents of arterial hematogenous spread note that the metaphyseal bone near the anterior longitudinal ligament is an area where infections typically begin. This region has an end-arteriole network that is susceptible to bacterial seeding.[22]

Tumor

- Most spine tumors are of metastatic origin. The spinal column is the most frequent site of skeletal metastasis.[21]
- Malignant cells are carried to the spine through the valveless, extradural venous plexus of Batson.[2,8] A recent anatomic model suggests that malignant cells can also metastasize through the segmental arteries.[23]

Trauma

- The articulation of the vertebral column, ribs, and sternum makes the thoracic spine relatively stable.[1]
- High-energy injuries are frequently required to produce injury to the thoracic spine.
- Forces associated with injury are axial compression, flexion, lateral compression, flexion–rotation, shear, flexion–distraction, and extension.
- Traumatic herniations are most common at T11–T12 secondary to true costovertebral joint and transition to more sagittally oriented facets, both allowing for increased flexion–extension moments.

NATURAL HISTORY

Intervertebral Disc Herniation

- Surgical indications are similar to lumbar/cervical: myelopathy, intractable radicular pain that has not improved with conservative measures, and progressive neurologic deterioration.
- Wood et al[24] described 20 patients with asymptomatic thoracic disc protrusions followed by magnetic resonance imaging (MRI). All patients remained asymptomatic at

an average of 26 months, and most disc herniations were smaller or unchanged on repeat MRI.

- It is unknown how often asymptomatic thoracic herniations become symptomatic.
- Brown et al[3] reported on 55 patients with 72 thoracic disc herniations. Fifty-four were treated initially with conservative therapy, and 15 eventually required surgery. Nine of 11 patients with lower extremity complaints went on to have surgery. Two patients had myelopathy and were treated surgically. All 55 patients ultimately returned to their previous level of activity.
  - Patients with lower extremity symptoms and myelopathy are likely to require surgical intervention.

Infection

- Vertebral osteomyelitis is rare and accounts for 2% to 4% of all cases of osteomyelitis.
- *Staphylococcus aureus* is the most common organism, accounting for almost 50% of pyogenic infections.[5]
- The incidence is rising as a result of a growing immunocompromised and elderly patient population, increased intravenous drug abuse, and an increase in invasive diagnostic and therapeutic procedures.
- Before medical and surgical treatment, spinal osteomyelitis carried a mortality rate of greater than 70%.[12] The advent of antibiotics and anterior spinal débridement techniques has reduced mortality to less than 15%.[6,15]
- Carragee[6] reported on 72 patients treated nonoperatively with antibiotics. Over 33% of them required surgical débridement. Results were related to patient age and immune status.

Tumor

- Over 90% of spinal tumors are metastatic lesions with a distant primary source.
- Primary tumors from the breast, prostate, lung, kidney, and thyroid are most likely to metastasize to the vertebral column.[21]
- Tumors that affect the anterior elements of the spine can be benign or malignant.
- Benign primary tumors that have a predilection for the anterior elements include giant cell tumors and hemangiomas. Malignant tumors that commonly affect the anterior elements include osteosarcomas, chondrosarcomas, myelomas, and lymphomas.[18]
- Improved diagnostics have allowed for more accurate diagnosis and improved staging.[11]
- Chemotherapy and radiotherapy have improved survival and local control.[17]
- Treatment goals include preservation of neural function, spinal stability, margin-free tumor resection, and correction of deformity.

Trauma

- Fractures of the thoracolumbar spine are the most common spinal injuries.
- The thoracic spine configuration of vertebrae, sternum, and rib cage confers an inherent stability.[1]
- Injuries to this region require significant force, and unstable injuries are usually a result of high-energy injuries such as motor vehicle accidents, falls from heights, and crush injuries.
- Patients can have associated injuries such as pneumothoraces, pulmonary contusions, and vascular injuries.

- Although most thoracic injuries do not involve neurologic deficit, complete neurologic deficits are more common with thoracic spine injuries due to the small neural canal, the tenuous blood supply, and the high energy needed to cause injury.[4]

PATIENT HISTORY AND PHYSICAL FINDINGS

- Neurologic status is examined.
  - Manual motor testing of the lower extremities may detect a mass effect on the corticospinal tract.
  - Pinprick and light touch sensory examination may help to localize the cord level of injury based on dermatome.
  - Babinski reflex and clonus are upper motor neuron signs, indicating a potential thoracic cord compression.
  - Reflex examination of the patellar and Achilles tendons: Hyperactivity is an upper motor neuron sign.

IMAGING AND OTHER DIAGNOSTIC STUDIES

- It is often useful to obtain an MRI and a computed tomography (CT) myelogram preoperatively. MRI is the key radiologic study to confirm the diagnosis and localize pathology. Plain CT scans are helpful in delineating bony anatomy. As with all spinal imaging, it is imperative to correlate imaging with physical examination findings.
- A plain CT scan should be obtained in concert with MRI on every patient with a destructive bony process, such as tumor or infection, to preoperatively assess the degree of bony loss and determine the optimal strategy for reconstruction.
- CT myelography may be needed if MRI scans cannot be obtained or if quality of the MRI is suboptimal due to patient movement, metal artifact from prior implants, or other factors.
  - CT can detail ossification of the posterior longitudinal ligament (PLL) or ligamentum flavum.
  - CT myelography can also clarify whether cord compression is primarily anterior secondary to a disc fragment or circumferential due to stenosis.

DIFFERENTIAL DIAGNOSIS

- Spinal tumors
- Infections
- Transverse myelitis
- Ankylosing spondylitis
- Fractures
- Intercostal neuralgia
- Herpes zoster
- Cervical and lumbar herniated discs
- Disorders of thoracic and abdominal viscera
- Amyotrophic lateral sclerosis
- Multiple sclerosis
- Arteriovenous malformations

NONOPERATIVE MANAGEMENT

Intervertebral Disc Herniation

- In the absence of myelopathy, most patients can be treated conservatively.
- A conservative treatment plan should include nonsteroidal anti-inflammatories, activity modification, and physical therapy focusing on trunk stabilization.[3]
- Other options include selective intercostal nerve blocks and pharmacotherapy such as narcotics, tricyclic antidepressants, serotonin reuptake inhibitors, and certain antiepileptics.

Infection

- Carragee[6] showed that white blood cells is normal in over half of patients with vertebral osteomyelitis, whereas erythrocyte sedimentation rate was elevated in all with normal immune status.
- Vertebral infections should be treated nonoperatively with culture-specific antibiotics and spinal immobilization.
- Open or CT-guided biopsy can aid in targeting appropriate antibiotic treatment.
- Treatment frequently involves 6 weeks of parenteral antibiotics followed by a course of oral antibiotics.
- An infectious disease consultant can help guide the antibiotic regimen.
- External immobilization with an orthosis can help stabilize the spine, decrease pain, and prevent deformity.
- Bracing is particularly important in patients with greater than 50% destruction of the vertebral body because they are at greater risk for deformity.[7]
- Response to treatment can be followed clinically with erythrocyte sedimentation rate.

Tumor

- A multidisciplinary approach including a neuroradiologist, pathologist, oncologist, and spine surgeon is used to treat spinal tumors.
- A CT-guided biopsy can help establish a diagnosis in 76% to 93% of lesions.[11,21]
- Metastatic lesions that do not compromise spinal stability and without rapid neurologic progression can be managed nonoperatively.[21]
- Nonoperative treatment can include radiation, chemotherapy, embolization, and bracing.
- Most primary spinal tumors require operative treatment.

Trauma

- Most thoracic and thoracolumbar spine injuries can be effectively treated nonoperatively.
- Conservative treatment can include recumbency, bracing, and pain management for patients without neurologic deterioration and with a structurally stable injury.[13,20]
- Decubitus ulcers, thromboembolism, urinary tract infections, and late pain are complications reported with nonoperative treatment.[14]

SURGICAL MANAGEMENT

- Indications for discectomy
  - Presence of myelopathy on presentation
  - Progressive neurologic symptoms, primarily weakness or paralysis
  - Radicular pain refractory to conservative therapy
  - Deformity correction
- Indications for corpectomy
  - Fractures with anterior spinal cord compression
  - Metastatic or primary thoracic tumors
  - Osteomyelitis
  - Sequestered disc herniations that have migrated behind the vertebral body
  - Ossification of the PLL
- Indications for bone grafting and cage or allograft placement
  - Infection
    - Although somewhat counterintuitive, anterior spinal infections can be successfully managed with allograft, cage, or instrumentation reconstruction if a thorough débridement of infected tissues is performed and postoperative antibiotics are administered.
  - Tumor
  - Trauma
  - Degenerative disease
  - Deformity correction (scoliosis, kyphosis)
- Indications for polymethylmethacrylate (PMMA) use
  - Anterior column reconstruction of tumors in patients with a life expectancy of less than 1 year
  - Patients in whom the use of radiation or chemotherapy is anticipated
- Indications for plate fixation
  - Anterior and middle column instability
  - Revision of failed posterior fusion
  - Pseudarthrosis
- Indications for use of solid rod instrumentation
  - Patient younger than 30 years of age
  - Thoracic and thoracolumbar curves of less than 65 degrees (Cobb angle)
  - Thoracic or lumbar compensatory curves that correct to less than 20 degrees with side bending
  - Hypokyphosis (<20 degrees from T5 to T12)

TECHNIQUES

THORACIC DISCECTOMY

- After elevating the articular ligaments of the costotransverse and costovertebral articulations, the remaining rib head is excised (**TECH FIG 1**).
- The superior edge of the pedicle of the caudal vertebra is resected with a rongeur to expose the dural tube.
- To find the disc herniation, the surgeon follows the superior edge of the pedicle to the vertebral body and disc space.
- The disc herniation is removed using small-angled curettes and pituitary rongeurs.
- Discectomy can be facilitated by removing a small portion (1 to 2 cm) of the adjacent vertebral bodies. If the disc is extremely calcified or has migrated behind the vertebral body, it is helpful to perform hemicorpectomies of the adjacent vertebral bodies.

- The portion of the disc that lies away from the ventral aspect of the spinal cord should be removed first. Once a cavity is created by removing this initial disc and bone, the rest of the disc can be removed into this cavity, ensuring that all forceful maneuvers are directed anteriorly away from the thecal sac.
- We prefer to keep the PLL intact whenever possible, as its removal often results in substantial epidural bleeding. We will pass an elevator or nerve hook through a rent in the PLL if one is present to ensure adequate decompression from pedicle to pedicle. If the PLL needs to be removed, we use bipolar cautery to cauterize the PLL and then carefully remove it with either a Kerrison or a combination of pituitary rongeur and curette.

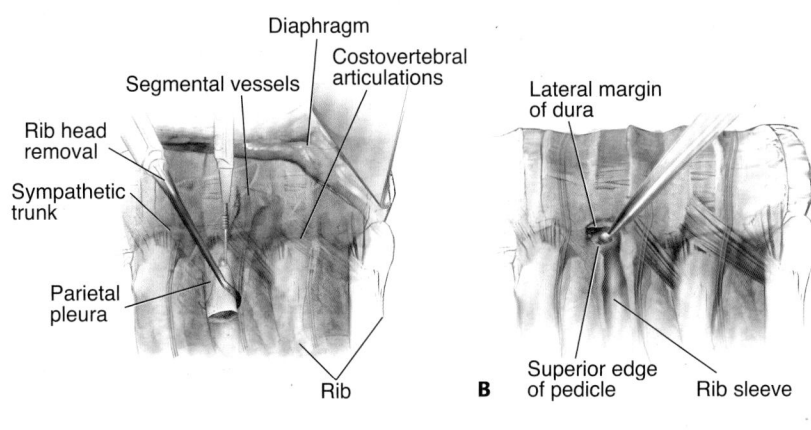

TECH FIG 1 A,B. The rib head can be removed with a high-speed burr once the costotransverse and costovertebral articulations are excised.

MINIMALLY INVASIVE THORACIC DISCECTOMY

- The patient is positioned prone on radiolucent Jackson-type table.
- C-arm anteroposterior localization of desired level with attention to cephalocaudal orientation for flat-appearing endplates
- A 2- to 3-cm vertical incision is made through skin and fascia lateral to midline, just lateral to facet so that an obliquely oriented working tube may dock with medial third over the lateral facet complex overlying desired disc space (**TECH FIG 2**).
- Blunt dissection may be carried out manually with a finger down to the facet complex or the surgeon may begin initial blunt dissection with progressive tubular dilators such as the METRx port system docking in the desired position described earlier.

- Confirmation of appropriate position of the dilator tubes is obtained with anteroposterior (medial third of tube over lateral facet) and lateral radiographs (disc space at center of tube with flat endplate appearance).
- Lock tube to secure table-mounted flexible arm and bring in microscope.
- Insulated unipolar and bipolar cautery along with pituitary and Kerrison are used to dissect remaining overlying tissue until facet complex/transverse process junction is encountered.
- Using the high-speed burr, remove the cranial portion of the transverse process and lateral aspects of the facet joint until the ligamentum flavum is encountered.

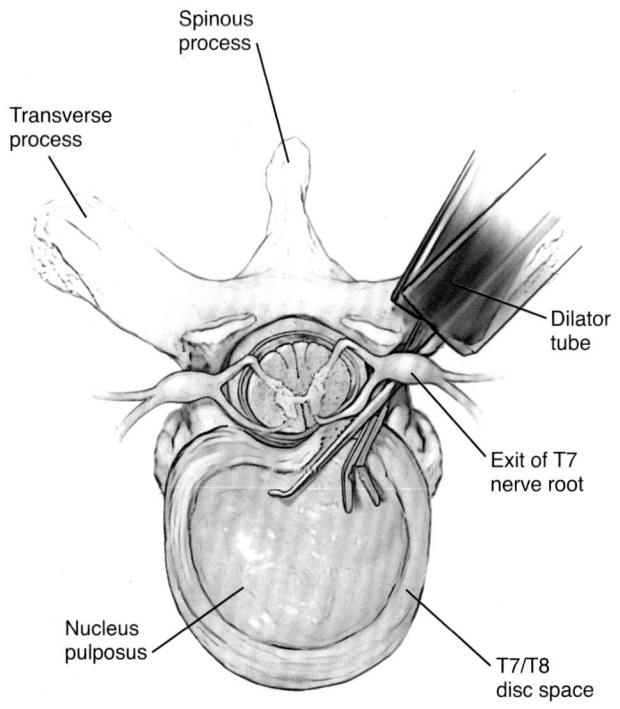

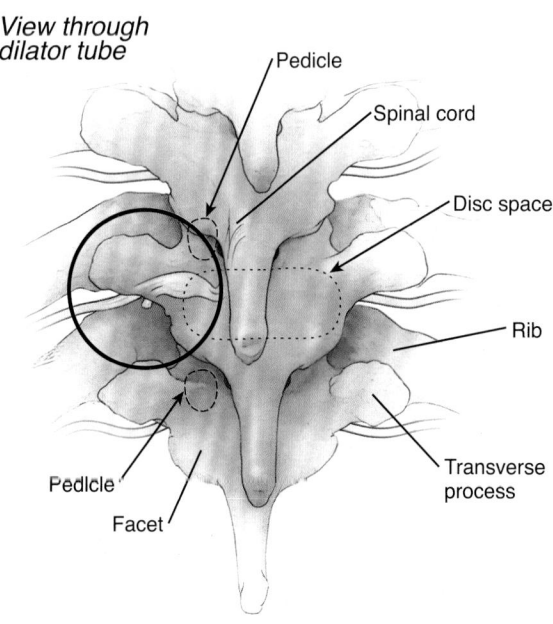

TECH FIG 2 A. Posterolateral approach to the thoracic disc space. **B.** The obliquity of the dilator tube allows for bilateral decompression without spinal cord manipulation.

- Carefully remove the ligamentum flavum from the underlying nerve root and lateral edged of the spinal cord. The herniated disc should now be visible and may be removed under direct visualization without any retraction of the spinal cord.
- The obliquity of the approach provides almost a lateral view of the disc space interface, allowing for bilateral decompression through a single annulotomy.

- Using a no. 11 blade with nerve root retractors protecting the cord medially and the exiting nerve root inferolaterally, a cruciate or box annulotomy is made.
- The desired amount of degenerative nucleus pulposus is removed; the disc space is pressure-irrigated through the annulotomy and after hemostasis is achieved, the tube is removed.[9]

THORACIC OR THORACOLUMBAR CORPECTOMY

- The posterior aspect of the vertebral body is identified.
  - Discectomy is performed above and below the level of the corpectomy.
  - The lateral annulus is incised using a no. 10 blade to the anterior midline.
  - An elevator is then used to separate the disc from the endplates.
  - Discectomy is completed using curettes and rongeurs.
- Attention is turned to the vertebrectomy. Using a 4-mm burr, the surgeon removes most of the bone from the vertebral body.
  - Corpectomy is completed by removing the remaining bone with a rongeur (**TECH FIG 3**).
  - Depending on the nature of the pathology, the PLL may need to be removed for the purposes of decompression.
- For retropulsed fracture fragments, the fragments are first thinned using a high-speed, 4-mm, ball-tipped burr.
- Then a thin, sharp curette is used to peel the fragments away from the dura and into the created trough.
  - It is important to work quickly but carefully at this point as there can be a significant amount of epidural bleeding.
- The posterior cortical fragments are removed from the contralateral (deep) side of the canal first so that the bulging dura will not obscure the rest of the fragments.
- Decompression is adequate when the dura can be seen bulging into the corpectomy trough and the spinal canal has been decompressed throughout its complete width.

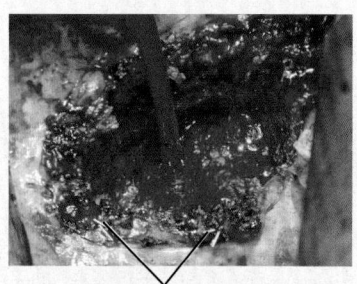

Ligated segmental vessels

TECH FIG 3 Corpectomy site.

Plating

- A flat surface is prepared for the plate by removing lateral endplate prominences and rib heads with a high-speed burr.
- Using an awl insertion guide, a posterior bicortical thoracic bolt is placed at the cephalad and caudad fixation levels.
- The trajectory should be parallel to the endplate and angled slightly anteriorly to avoid penetrating the canal (**TECH FIG 4A**).

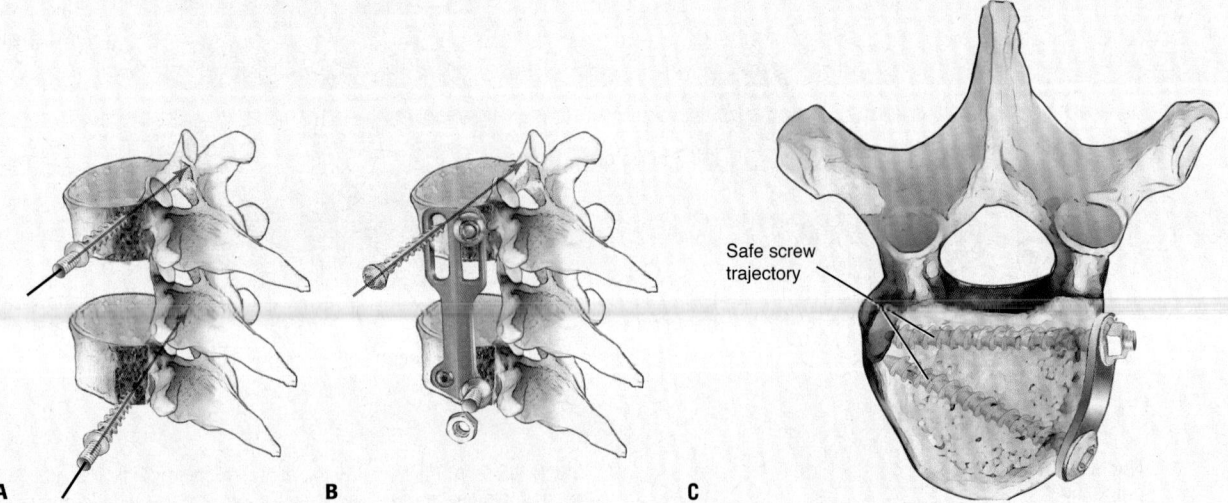

Safe screw trajectory

A   **B**   **C**

TECH FIG 4 Application of plate and screws. **A.** Osteophytes are removed, and a trajectory is planned parallel to the endplate and angled slightly anteriorly to avoid penetration of the canal. **B.** Nuts secure the posterior bolts, and screws are applied anteriorly. **C.** It is important for the screws to be a safe distance from the dural covering of the spinal cord.

- If sagittal correction or interbody graft placement is needed, distraction is performed on the endplates using a lamina spreader.
- A correct length plate is applied over the bolts without extending into the adjacent disc spaces **(TECH FIG 4B,C)**. Nuts are applied loosely to secure the plate to the posterior bolts.

- Using a drill or awl, correct length anterior screws are placed angling slightly posteriorly.
  - In general, bicortical screws are preferred because the cancellous bone of the vertebral body provides relatively weak purchase, especially in patients with tumors or infections.

SCREW–ROD INSTRUMENTATION

- Use of an anterior screw–rod construct allows for correction of coronal plane deformity through fusion of fewer spinal motion segments compared with posterior instrumentation.
- The entry position for the anterior vertebral screws is determined based on the location of the vertebral foramen, as this identifies posterior body cortex.

- The surgeon inserts the most cephalad and caudal screws first in the midlateral vertebral body at the same distance from the posterior cortex **(TECH FIG 5)**.
- The screw tips should engage the far cortex of each vertebra and should be directed toward the posterolateral corner of the vertebra.
- The rest of the screws are placed in similar fashion.
- The rods are inserted as directed by the particular system, and alignment is corrected before tightening.

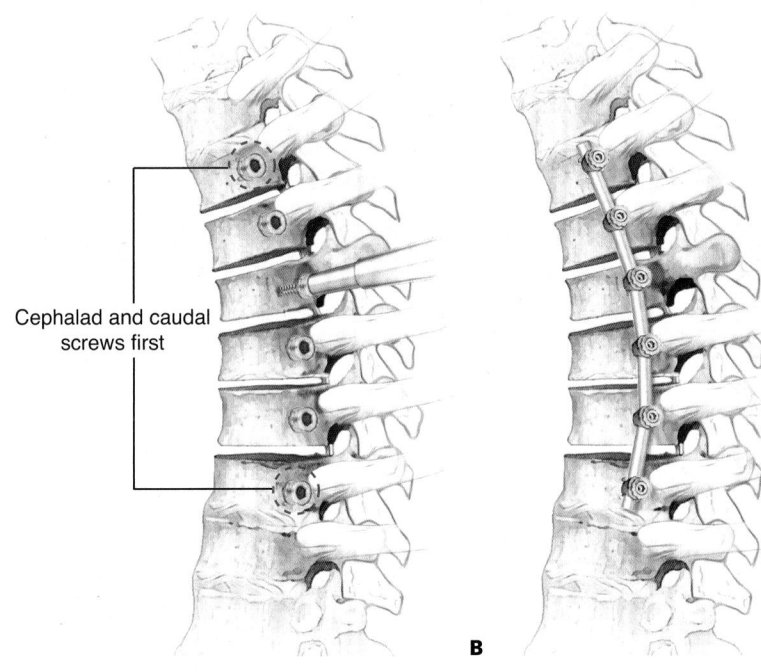

Cephalad and caudal screws first

A   **B**

TECH FIG 5 Application of screw–rod instrumentation.

BONE GRAFTING AND CAGES

- It is of utmost importance to prepare an adequate fusion bed.
- A thorough decortication is performed.
- Although placement of the graft on preserved bleeding subchondral endplates is preserved, creating a slot or peg hole in the adjacent vertebral bodies can help to prevent graft extrusion.
- Before graft placement, kyphotic deformity can be corrected by distracting adjacent vertebrae.
  - Extreme care must be taken to avoid injury to the adjacent endplates during distraction, especially in patients with osteoporosis or other states with compromised bone quality (tumors, infections).

- After the graft has been anchored, compression locks the graft in position.
- If tricortical iliac crest bone is used, we prefer to have the cortical smooth surface face the spinal canal.
- Single-level corpectomy defects can be supported with tricortical iliac crest grafts, whereas larger defects are better stabilized with autogenous fibular strut grafts or shaft allografts.
  - Depending on the size of the patient, humeral shafts often provide the best fit in the thoracic spine.

- For cage placement, the ends of the cage can be trimmed to create the necessary cage configuration **(TECH FIG 6A)**.
  - Alternatively, stackable cages (eg, those made of polyetheretherketone) can be measured to fit the space.
- The packed cage is implanted between the distracted adjacent endplates **(TECH FIG 6B)**.
- The cage is stabilized when the distraction is released.
- Bone graft should be packed in and around the cage.

Polymethylmethacrylate

- PMMA may be used in patients with spinal tumors who have poor life expectancy or who are unlikely to heal anterior bone grafts due to poor bone quality or healing potential.
- It provides immediate spinal stability and is strongest in compression.
- The PMMA can be reinforced and anchored with Steinmann pins drilled into the adjacent vertebral bodies.
- Bends in the Steinmann pins can prevent pin migration.
- To increase interdigitation of the cement, multiple drill holes are placed in the adjacent vertebral bodies.

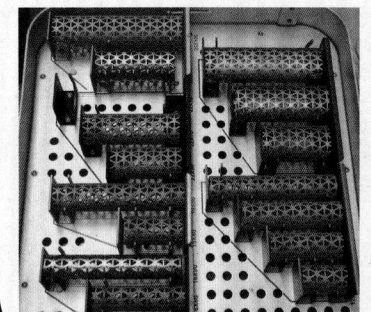 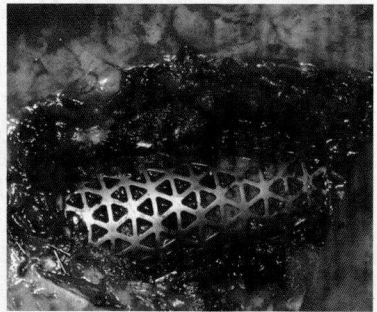

TECH FIG 6 A. Titanium mesh cages. **B.** Cage placement.

TECHNIQUES

Pearls and Pitfalls

Thoracic Corpectomy	• By keeping the PLL intact until the end of procedure, epidural bleeding can be minimized.
Choice of Graft	• Patients with short life expectancies and those who will need adjuvant chemotherapy or radiation should be reconstructed with PMMA to provide the maximal short-term stability.
Graft Sizing	• It is important not to undersize the graft, as it is more prone to migration.
Thoracic Discectomy	• When removing herniated disc fragments, the surgeon should always direct the angled curettes away from the dura.

POSTOPERATIVE CARE

- Chest tubes remain until output is less than 150 mL over 24 hours.

COMPLICATIONS

- The exiting nerve root can be injured while removing the pedicle.
- Vascular injury
- Intercostal neuralgia
- Atelectasis
- Neurologic injury
- Wrong-level surgery
- Significant bleeding can be encountered when entering the epidural space.

REFERENCES

1. Andriacchi TP, Schultz A, Belytschko T, et al. A model for studies of mechanical interactions between the human spine and rib cage. J Biomech 1974;7:497–507.
2. Batson OV. The role of the vertebral veins in metastatic processes. Ann Intern Med 1942;16:38–45.
3. Brown CW, Deffer PA Jr, Akmakjian J, et al. The natural history of thoracic disc herniation. Spine 1992;17(6 suppl):S97–S102.
4. Burke DC, Murray DD. The management of thoracic and thoracolumbar injuries of the spine with neurological involvement. J Bone Joint Surg Br 1976;58:72–78.
5. Butler JS, Shelly MJ, Timlin M, et al. Nontuberculous pyogenic spinal infection in adults: a 12-year experience from a tertiary referral center. Spine 2006;31:2695–2700.
6. Carragee EJ. Pyogenic vertebral osteomyelitis. J Bone Joint Surg Am 1997;79(6):874–880.
7. Frederickson B, Yuan H, Olans R. Management and outcomes of pyogenic vertebral osteomyelitis. Clin Orthop Relat Res 1978;(131):160–167.
8. Harada M, Shimizu A, Nakamura Y, et al. Role of the vertebral venous system in metastatic spread of cancer cells to the bone. Adv Exp Med Biol 1992;324:83–92.
9. Khoo LT, Smith ZA, Asgarzadie F, et al. Minimally invasive extracavitary approach for thoracic discectomy and interbody fusion: 1-year clinical and radiographic outcomes in 13 patients compared with a cohort of traditional anterior transthoracic approaches. J Neurosurg Spine 2011;14(2):250–260.

10. Kretzer RM, Chaput C, Sciubba D, et al. A computed tomography-based morphometric study of thoracic pedicle anatomy in a random United States trauma population. J Neurosurg Spine 2011;14(2): 235–243.

11. Lis E, Bilsky MH, Pisinski L, et al. Percutaneous CT-guided biopsy of osseous lesion of the spine in patients with known or suspected malignancy. AJNR Am J Neuroradiol 2004;25:1583–1588.

12. Makins GH, Abbott FC. On acute primary osteomyelitis of the vertebrae. Ann Surg 1896;23:510–539.

13. Mumford J, Weinstein JN, Spratt KF, et al. Thoracolumbar burst fractures. The clinical efficacy and outcome of nonoperative management. Spine 1993;18:955–970.

14. Rechtine GR II, Cahill D, Chrin AM. Treatment of thoracolumbar trauma: comparison of complications of operative versus nonoperative treatment. J Spinal Disord 1999;12:406–409.

15. Rezai AR, Woo HH, Errico TJ, et al. Contemporary management of spinal osteomyelitis. Neurosurgery 1999;44:1018–1025.

16. Sekhar LN, Jannetta PJ. Thoracic disc herniation: operative approaches and results. Neurosurgery 1983;12(3):303–305.

17. Simmons ED, Zheng Y. Vertebral tumors: surgical versus nonsurgical treatment. Clin Orthop Relat Res 2006;443:233–247.

18. Simon MA, Springfield D. Surgery of Bone and Soft-Tissue Tumors. Philadelphia: Lippincott-Raven, 1998.

19. Vaccaro AR, Rizzolo SJ, Allardyce TJ, et al. Placement of pedicle screws in the thoracic spine. Part I: morphometric analysis of the thoracic vertebrae. J Bone Joint Surg Am 1995;77(8):1193–1199.

20. Weinstein JN, Collalto P, Lehmann TR. Long-term follow-up of nonoperatively treated thoracolumbar spine fractures. J Orthop Trauma 1987;1:152–159.

21. White AH, Kwon B, Lindskog D, et al. Metastatic disease of the spine. J Am Acad Orthop Surg 2006;14:587–598.

22. Wiley AM, Trueta J. The vascular anatomy of the spine and its relationship to pyogenic vertebral osteomyelitis. J Bone Joint Surg Br 1959;41-B:796–809.

23. Willis TA. Nutrient arteries of the vertebral bodies. J Bone Joint Surg Am 1949;31(3):538–540.

24. Wood KB, Garvey TA, Gundry C, et al. Magnetic resonance imaging of the thoracic spine. Evaluation of asymptomatic individuals. J Bone Joint Surg Am 1995;77(11):1631–1638.

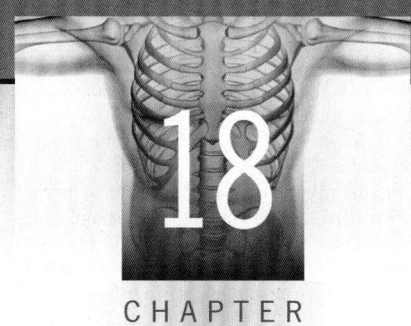
Lateral Approaches to Interbody Fusion

Keith W. Michael and S. Tim Yoon

DEFINITION

- Lateral approach to interbody fusion
- Many different names including lateral lumbar interbody fusion, extreme lateral interbody fusion, direct lateral interbody fusion, or oblique lumbar interbody fusion. It is often called the *transpsoas* or *antepsoas approach* because in the lumbar spine, it requires traversing or passing anterior to the psoas muscle. The lateral approach can be used to access thoracic spine as well.
- The transpsoas technique relies on a combination of neuromonitoring and direct visualization to safely navigate through the lateral lumbosacral neurologic plexus. The antepsoas approach uses the interval between the aorta and the psoas to access the spine ventral to the lumbar plexus.

ANATOMY

- After the superficial dissection, the lateral abdominal wall muscles are split to approach the lumbar spine. This leads directly into the retroperitoneal space.
- The psoas muscle flanks the lateral lumbar spine and is covered by a thin, slippery fascia.

- Within the psoas muscles traverse the lumbosacral plexus, genitofemoral nerve, and lateral cutaneous nerve (**FIG 1**).[1,7]
- Moro et al[5] identified and counted the location of the lumbar plexus and genitofemoral nerve relative to each disc space in 12 cadavers. Although there are general trends for each disc level in an anterior to posterior distribution, each individual has significant variability that can be different from the "typical" situation.[5]
- As one progresses distally in the lumbar spine, the lumbosacral plexus covers more of the ventrolateral aspect of the lumbar spine.
- The lateral iliac crests are typically slightly below or at the level of the L4–L5 disc space. However, there is variability between patients, and at times, high iliac crest (or deep seated L4–L5 disc space) may prevent parallel access to the L4–L5 disc space from a direct lateral approach (**FIG 2**). Angled tools may enable access when this situation arises.
- When approaching the upper lumbar levels, the ribs may interfere with direct lateral approach to the spine. This may require choosing an incision that is not perfectly lateral to the disc space or excising a rib to improve access (see **FIG 2**).

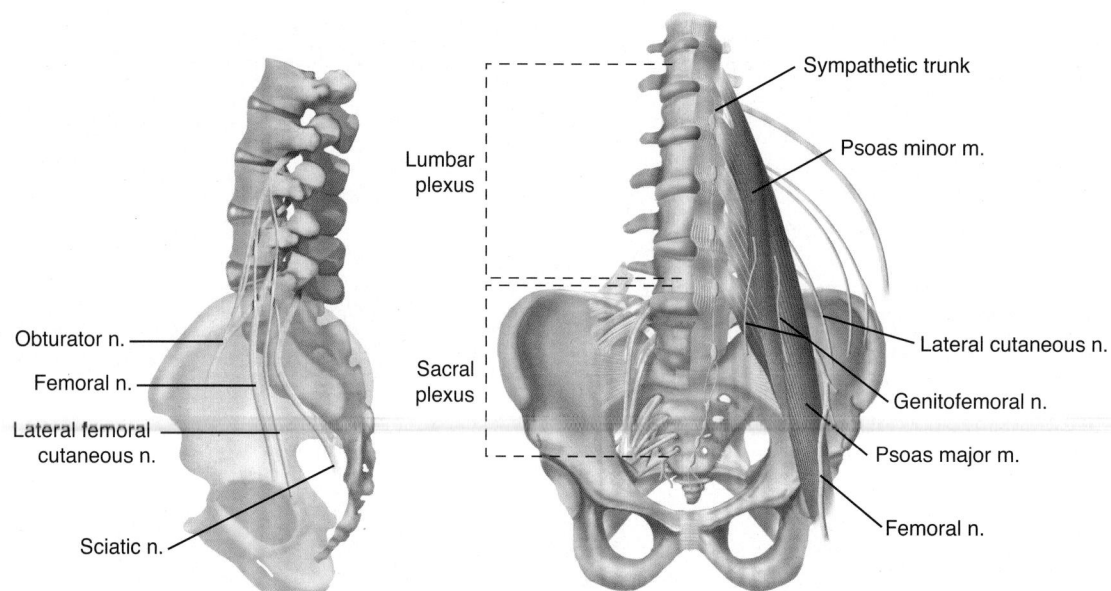

FIG 1 The lumbar plexus exits the foramen traveling through the psoas muscle while moving more ventral as it progresses caudally.

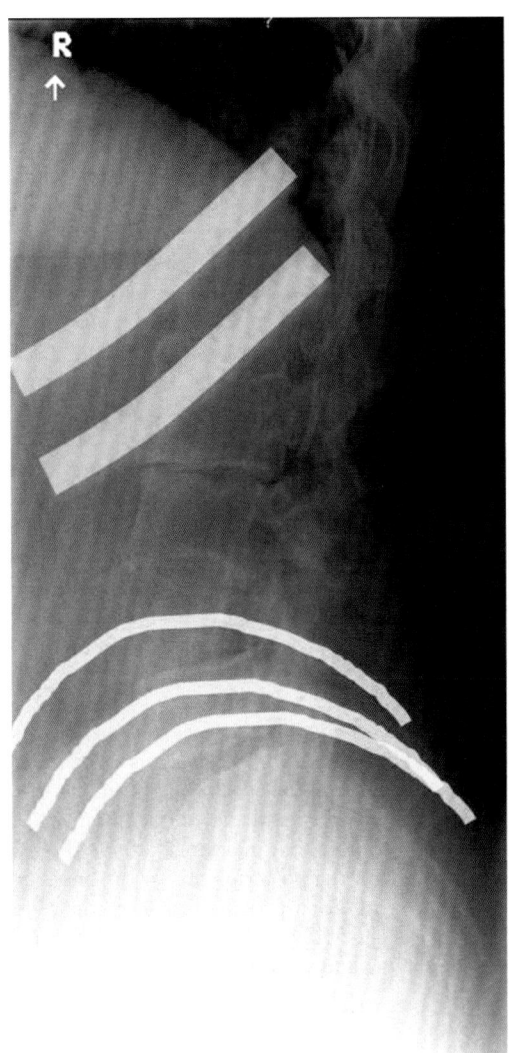

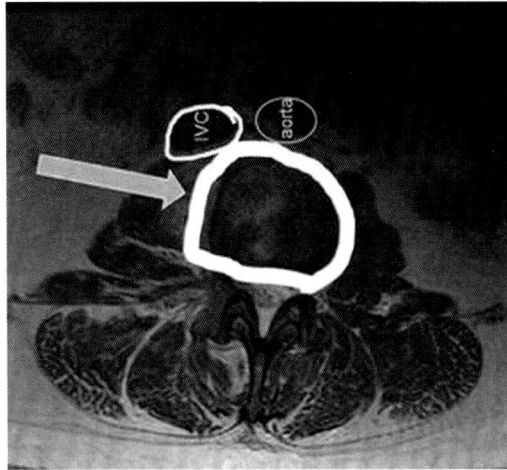

FIG 3 Axial imaging allows preoperative planning of the working window (*red arrow*) to access the disc space (*white oval*), including evaluating the proximity of the aorta and inferior vena cava (*IVC*).

- Discitis after failure of medical management
- Other situations when interbody fusion is necessary

Preoperative Planning

- AP and lateral radiographs allow assessment of accessibility of each disc level relative to the iliac crest and ribs.
- Determine side of approach. Typically, the disc is approached from the convex side (ie, the more open side of the disc) to facilitate intradiscal work. However, in scoliosis cases, when the approach to the L4–L5 level (the convex side) dictates the side of the approach, this may place the other levels on the concave side. Surgeons often perform the surgery on the same side (convex at L4–L5 and concave at the other lumbar levels) and work around the inconvenience of working in the concavity (**FIG 4**). In flexible curves, bending the patient can alleviate this problem significantly. Rarely, some surgeons may choose to flip the patient to work on the convex side for the rest of the curve.
- Establish a neuromonitoring plan. Typically, electromyography (EMG) monitoring is performed if the approach is transpsoas. This can consist of both free-running EMG as well as stimulated proximity sensing. EMGs help to monitor the motor branches of the lumbosacral plexus; however, sensory nerves cannot be monitored. The genitofemoral and lateral cutaneous nerves cannot be monitored. Approaches anterior to the psoas may not require neuromonitoring because this is within safe corridor ventral to the lumbar plexus.
- Ensure the anesthetic plan is compatible with the neuromonitoring plan. The patient must have muscle twitches during the surgery to allow for EMG monitoring. If no monitoring is performed, then the patient can be paralyzed chemically to facilitate the exposure.

Positioning

- Positioning on the operative table is extremely important in lateral interbody fusion.
- Typically, the procedure is performed on a regular operative bed with the capacity to break or flex in the middle. Usually, the table's orientation is reversed such that the base is attached to the feet, allowing the C-arm to pass freely underneath the thoracolumbar spine.

FIG 2 Lateral lumbar radiographs superimpose the ribs (*thick yellow lines*) and iliac crest (*think yellow lines*) over the disc spaces to determine which levels are accessible with a lateral approach.

- Anteroposterior (AP) and lateral lumbar radiographs are useful to assess the rib and iliac crest position relative to the level that needs to be approached.
- Aorta, inferior vena cava, and common iliac vessels run on the ventral surface of the anterior longitudinal ligament (ALL). Axial imaging allows preoperative localization of these structures to understand the safe zone for each patient (**FIG 3**).

SURGICAL MANAGEMENT

Indications

- Spondylolisthesis low grade
  - Isthmic
  - Degenerative
- Deformity
  - Scoliosis
  - Kyphosis
  - Flat back
  - In combination with pedicle subtraction osteotomy (PSO)
- Foraminal stenosis with vacuum disc and instability
- Adjacent segment disease with instability

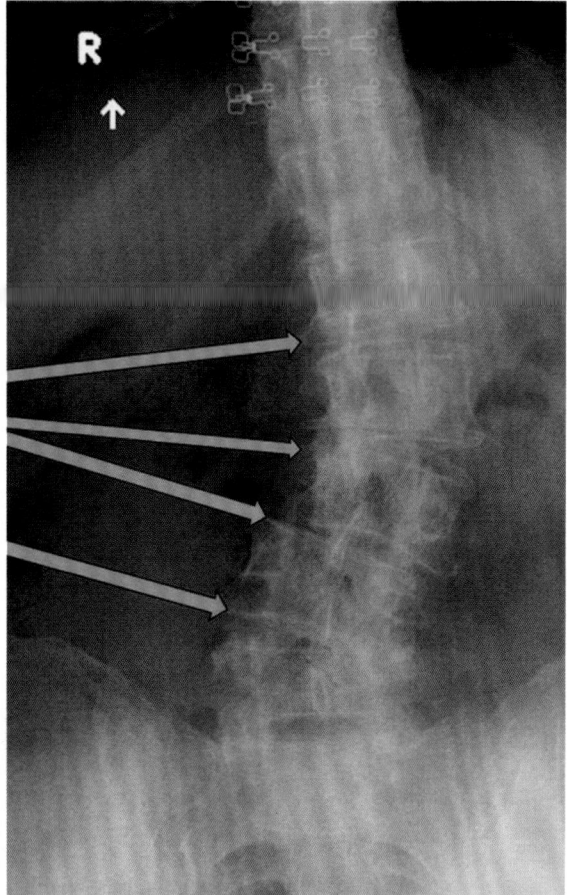

FIG 4 AP lumbar radiographs help determine the best approach side in preoperative planning. Approach angles are indicated by the *blue arrows*. The approach side is often determined by the orientation of the L4–L5 disc or by the convexity of the curve. Bending films can be used to determine the flexibility of the curve, which is often reproduced by flexing the operating room table.

- The patient is positioned in a true lateral position as close to vertical as possible. This can be fine-tuned under fluoroscopy by tilting the bed. Select the appropriate position, front versus back, on the table to facilitate any additional fixation, that is placing the patient posterior on the table to prevent interference on the down side if posterior screws are placed while the patient is in the lateral position (single position surgery).

- The iliac crest should be positioned approximately 4 inches cephalad to the center of the break in the table. This allows the flexion of the table to open the disc space while still giving enough room for the C-arm to pass underneath the table to provide a perfect lateral of the L4–L5 disc space **(FIG 5A)**.
- Hips are flexed approximately 30 degrees to take tension off the iliopsoas. Knees are flexed approximately 30 degrees to compensate for the hip flexion and to keep the feet in a good position on the bed.
- Once positioned and prior to flexing the table, the patient is taped to the table. First, tape the patient horizontally at the hip (just inferior to the iliac crests) and at the chest (just below the axilla). Next, a crossing pattern of tape holds the legs in position because the table will be tilted throughout the case **(FIG 5B)**.
- After taping, it may be necessary to flex the table. Flexing typically requires reverse Trendelenburg at the base while flexing the long end of the table. The goal is to have the involved disc space perpendicular to the floor. Feel the tension of the abdominal oblique muscles on the convex side to determine when sufficient flexion has been achieved and then use reverse Trendelenburg to make the lumbar spine parallel with the floor. Another round of taping of the hip area may be necessary.
- Flexing the table may not be necessary for more oblique or anterior approaches. The approach is designed to work ventral to the iliac crest. It is still helpful to tilt the bed to align the disc space perpendicular to the floor.
- It is important to note that in a direct lateral approach, the surgeon will be on the posterior side of the patient. For an oblique approach, the surgeon will stand on the ventral side of the patient. This will influence how the fluoroscopy machine and mayo stand will be arranged.

Approach

- The approach technique in the lumbar spine can be divided into the one-incision or two-incision technique, direct lateral techniques, or an oblique approach.
- With the one-incision technique, a single incision is created directly lateral to the disc space in a position that is as parallel as possible to the two endplates of the disc **(FIG 6A)**.
- With the two-incision technique, an initial incision is made posterior to the direct lateral position. Then, a second incision is made directly lateral to the spine in a manner similar to the one-incision technique.

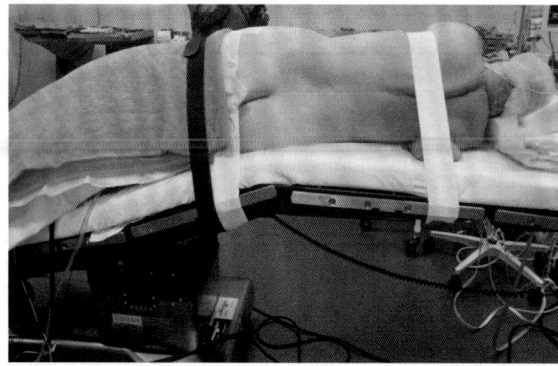
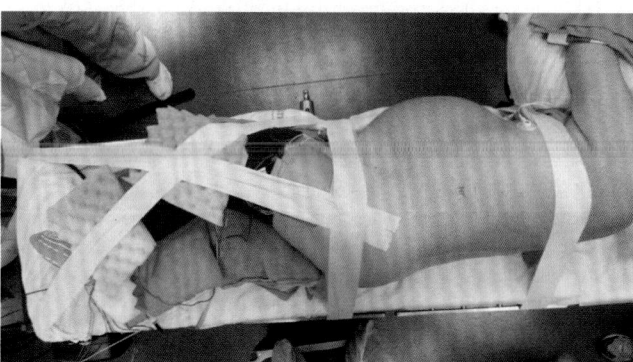

FIG 5 A. The iliac crest is positioned approximately 4 inches cephalad of the break in the table. This allows the disc space to be opened by flexing the table while allowing the C-arm to pass freely underneath the table. **B.** Horizontal tape straps are placed at the hip and the chest followed by a crossing pattern of tape on the lower extremities to secure them while the table is tilted during surgery.

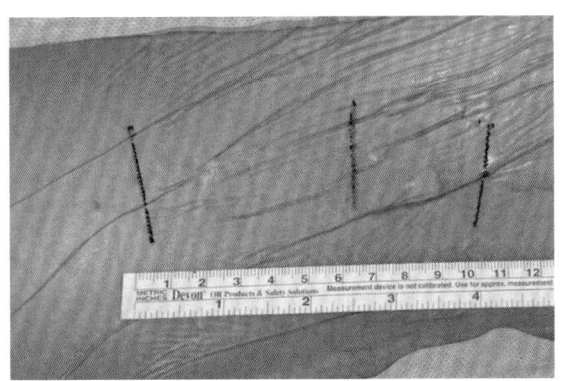

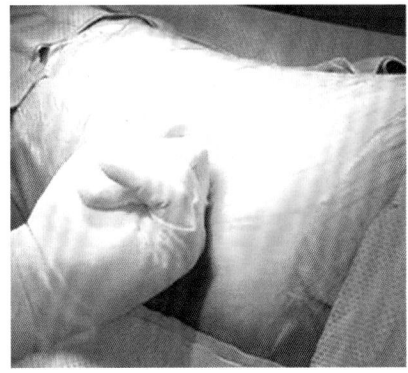

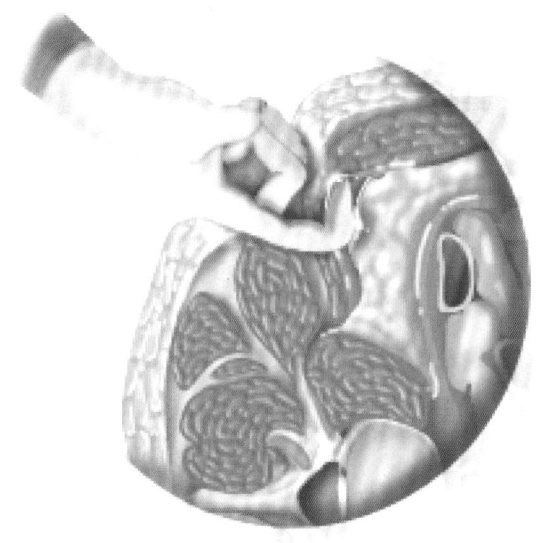

FIG 6 **A.** Three incisions are planned, each parallel to the respective disc space. This is the one-incision technique as the posterior incision is omitted. **B,C.** The posterior incision allows finger localization of the disc space and direct finger-guided delivery of instruments to the lateral disc space.

- The addition of the posterior incision allows finger localization of the retroperitoneal space prior to incising the lateral abdominal musculature and facilitates finger-guided (through the posterior incision) placement of the instruments to the lateral disc space (**FIG 6B,C**).
- The single-incision technique can also be used safely, but extra care must be taken to identify the retroperitoneal space, and a larger incision may be necessary to allow a finger to be placed through the direct lateral incision as opposed to through the posterior incision.

- With the oblique approach, an incision is made 4 to 6 cm ventral to the midvertebral body point, in line with the disc space. It may be possible to combine two levels in one ventral incision.
- If multiple levels are involved, a single longitudinal incision or multiple, small transverse incisions paralleling each of the involved disc spaces can be used. Multiple well-localized, transverse incisions at each disc space have the advantage of ensuring one is able to work directly aligned over each disc space without undue soft tissue tension.[6]

LOCALIZING THE INCISION[2,6]

- The C-arm should be turned parallel to the floor (ie, beam is horizontal). Adjustments are made to the table to obtain a perfect AP view of the disc space. The body, pedicles, and spinous processes are used as guides.
- Once the true AP is obtained (ie, beam is horizontal in orientation), arc the C-arm 90 degrees into the lateral position. Then, adjust the bed angle to get a parallel view of the endplates. Although these steps, to align the disc space to the vertical and horizontal planes, are not absolutely necessary, it can be very helpful for the surgeon to maintain orientation and help the surgeon stay within the safe zone throughout the case.

- Using a guidewire or other radiopaque instrument, mark the anterior and posterior border of the involved disc on the skin while the C-arm captures a true lateral of the disc space. Mark the incision such that it exactly parallels the orientation of the disc, which may change at each level based on the changes in lordosis or kyphosis (**TECH FIG 1**).
- In the oblique approach, the incision is typically longitudinal and can be planned as shown in **FIG 5** by looking at the approach angle and is centered in line with disc space approximately 4 to 6 cm ventral to the middle of the disc.

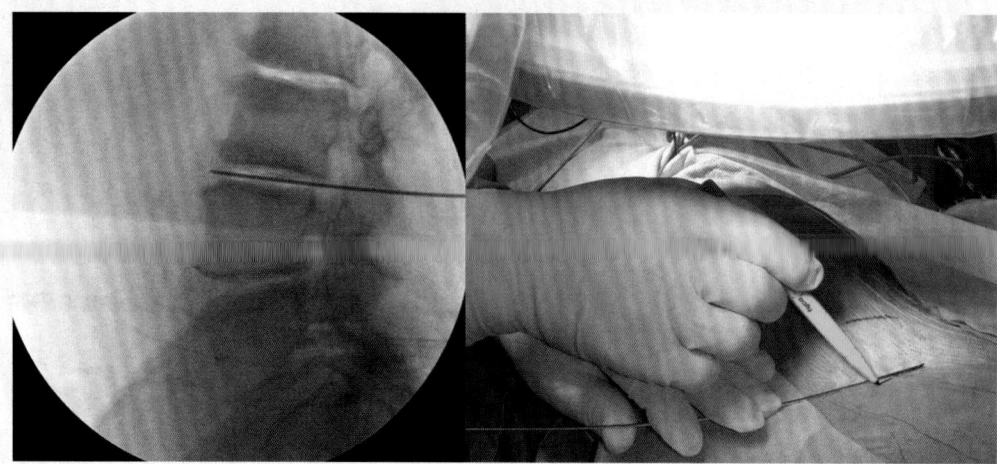

TECH FIG 1 The guidewire is used to localize the incision parallel to the disc space using fluoroscopy at each surgical level.

APPROACH AND DISSECTION

Single-Incision Technique

- After incising the skin sharply, dissect through the subcutaneous tissue to the fascia overlying the external oblique muscle.
- Dissect through the external oblique, internal oblique, and transversus muscles and fascia to enter the retroperitoneum. Sharp, blunt, or electrocautery dissection can be performed through the external layers of the abdominal muscles, but careful, blunt dissection is recommended beyond that to minimize chances of damage to the peritoneum. Minimizing disruption to the muscle and innervation of the abdominal wall may reduce the risk of pseudohernia.
- Characteristic features of the retroperitoneum include the presence of retroperitoneal fat causing a very slippery feel to the tissues and the ability to feel striations in the psoas musculature. In many situations, it is possible to directly palpate the disc and vertebral body undulations (**TECH FIG 2**).

Two-Incision Technique

- A longitudinal 4-cm incision is made approximately 5 to 8 cm posterior to the planned transverse incision overlying the disc space.
- Dissection is carried through the fascia and abdominal muscles into the retroperitoneal space, which is confirmed by feel.
- Approach is made through the skin and subcutaneous tissue down to the level of the fascia through the standard transverse incision.
- A finger is passed into the retroperitoneal space via the posterior incision and used to push up underneath the muscle and fascia in line with the transverse incision. Monopolar electrocautery can then be used to safely divide the abdominal muscles and fascia to enter the retroperitoneal space.

Oblique Technique

- A longitudinal incision is made 4 to 6 cm ventral to the midpoint of the disc. External oblique fascia is divided in line with its fibers. External, internal, and transverse musculature is divided in line with the fibers. Transversalis fascia is divided and the retroperitoneal fat is identified.
- Once in the retroperitoneal space, the peritoneum is mobilized off the lateral wall and then gently swept down and ventral with a finger.
- The ventral border of the psoas is mobilized with Penfield, endoscopic Kittner, or cobb. Once the psoas is fully mobilized, the guidewire entry point can be selected.

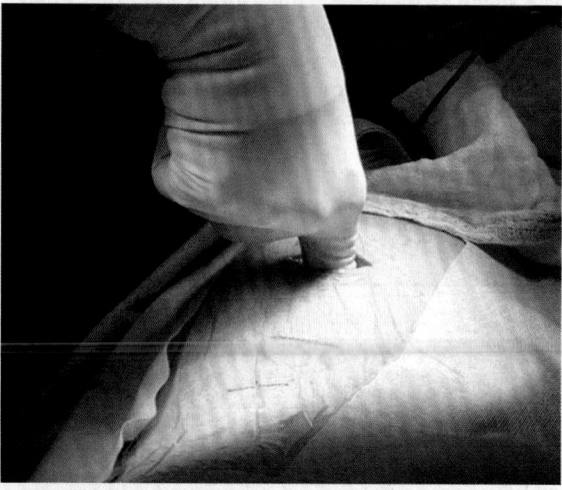

TECH FIG 2 Gentle finger sweeps allow localization of the retroperitoneal space, psoas, and lateral disc space.

PLACING THE GUIDEWIRE

- After ensuring the approach is retroperitoneal, a small dilator is then placed through the psoas onto the disc space. Neuromonitoring during this step will alert the surgeon to proximity of motor nerves and redirection of the dilator may be necessary. Once the dilator is docked on the lateral aspect of the disc and neuromonitoring is safe, then the guidewire is placed into the disc space.
- If the incision was localized correctly, the guidewire will be oriented perfectly vertical and centered in the incision in order to fall at the center of the disc.
- Care should be taken to pass the initial dilator to the lateral aspect of the disc by shuttling it with a finger (either through the same incision or the second posterior incision). This will prevent inadvertent bowel injury.
- The ideal position for the guidewire varies from level to level. Although it is more convenient to place the guidewire slightly posterior to midpoint, because of the lumbar plexus, it is advisable to start at the midpoint or slightly anterior at L4–L5 or any level at which neuromonitoring warning is present at the more posterior position. The orientation of the guidewire should be in line with the fluoroscopy beam, resulting in a single superimposed circle (TECH FIG 3).

Oblique Approach

- In this approach, the guidewire is placed under direct visualization. Once in the retroperitoneal space, the ventral portion of the psoas is visualized and mobilized. The guidewire will be placed here under direction visualization but should be confirmed with a lateral fluoroscopy.

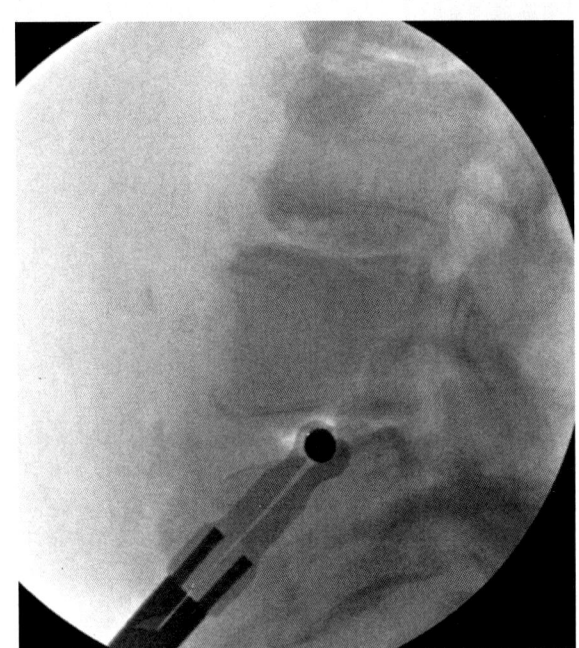

TECH FIG 3 Under fluoroscopy, the guidewire is positioned on the lateral disc space just posterior to the midpoint of the disc parallel with the fluoroscopy beam.

EXPOSURE

- Once the guidewire is in position, a series of larger soft tissue dilators are used to bluntly spread the soft tissue and psoas muscle. Each dilator connects to the EMG neuromonitoring system to help localize the motor nerves of the lumbosacral plexus.
- Starting with the smallest dilator, slide it over the guidewire. Rotate the dilator clockwise and counterclockwise with gentle pressure to advance to the lateral aspect of the disc. Attach the neuromonitoring system during dilation to determine if it is safe to proceed. Ensure the EMG electrode is oriented posteriorly, typically marked by a line on the dilator probe, as this is where the lumbosacral plexus and exiting nerve roots are most likely to be encountered.
- Repeat this step until the largest dilator is passed to the lateral disc space and reveals safe monitoring parameters.
- Many surgeons prefer the "dock shallow" approach where the dilators are placed on the psoas muscle instead of through the muscle. Once the retractor is placed on the psoas, the dissection can occur under direct visualization. This reduces the risk of neurologic injury, especially to sensory nerves that are not detected by EMG neuromonitoring.

DOCKING AND OPENING THE RETRACTOR

- Attach the retractor arm to the mount affixed to the anterior side of the bed for a lateral approach or the posterior side of the bed for an oblique approach.
- Connecting the neuromonitoring clip to the retractor will allow for neuromonitoring during the placement of the retractor.
- Connect the retractor arm to the retractor (TECH FIG 4).

TECHNIQUES

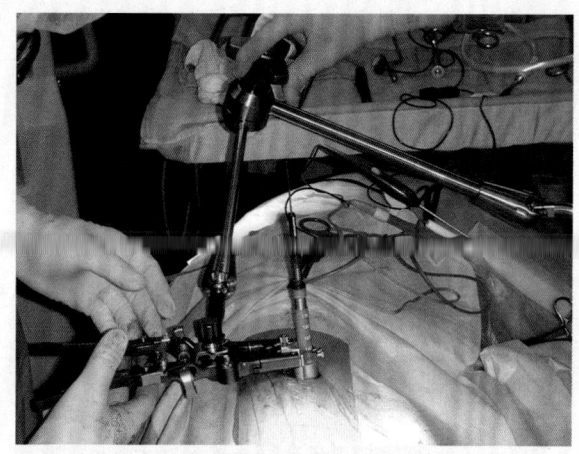

TECH FIG 4 Once the dilator is in place, the blades are oriented so as to open in line with the disc space prior to locking the position with the holding arm.

- Depending on the system and where you attach the retractor arm, the blades will open anteriorly or posteriorly. Typically in the lumbar spine, it is often more favorable to dock posteriorly and open the blades anteriorly.[5]
- Open the blades anteriorly, cephalad, and caudad. Affix the light sources. At this time, using a combination of direct visual inspection and the neuromonitoring probe tip, explore the remaining soft tissue over the lateral disc space. When "shallow docking," dissection through the psoas may be necessary. Remember, the neuromonitoring system will not detect sensory nerves. It is important to check for nervous structures before proceeding with the discectomy or using bipolar electrocautery.
- Once the wound bed is confirmed to be free of nervous structures, the posterior blade can be affixed with the docking blade into the disc space. This should be done under direct vision to avoid entry to adjacent nervous structures. An optional anterior retractor can be placed over the ALL to help retract anterior soft tissues and provide a reference to prevent disruption of the ALL during discectomy.

DISCECTOMY

- With the lateral annulus exposed, perform a rectangular annulotomy and remove the nucleus pulposus with a pituitary rongeur.
- Pass a Cobb elevator along the cartilaginous surface of the superior and inferior endplate, with special care not to violate the bony endplate. Use AP fluoroscopy to ensure the Cobb takes down the annulus at both the superior and inferior endplate on the far lateral side (**TECH FIG 5**). This step allows the disc space to open and allows the cage to pass to the far lateral cortex. Depending on the level, orientation, and shape of the disc endplate, an angled or straight Cobb may be preferred.
- Using a combination of curettes and pull shavers, perform a complete discectomy. Rotary shavers can facilitate discectomy; however, judicious use is encouraged as they can result in a high incidence of endplate violation.
- Kerrison rongeur is used to débride any overlying annulus or osteophyte at the opening of the discectomy to improve visualization.

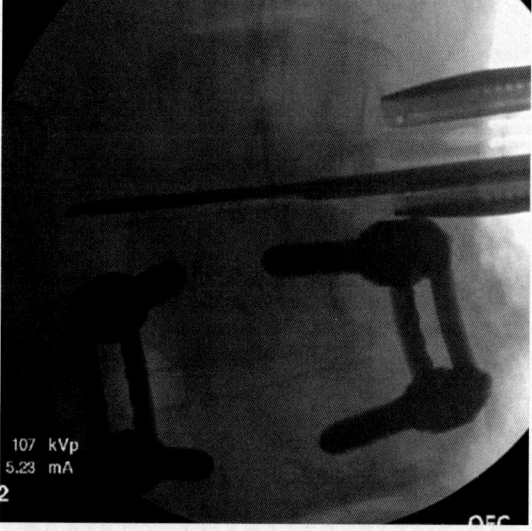

TECH FIG 5 AP fluoroscopy image is used to monitor the position of the Cobb as the far annulus is released.

TRIALING AND SIZING

- Once a complete discectomy is performed, size the interbody cage using the sizing trials. In addition to choosing the appropriate height, select the depth and width.
- When trialing cages, it is important to obtain both AP and lateral fluoroscopy views to ensure the cage is well positioned in all planes.
- Placing a cage that extends to both lateral rims of the endplates improves coronal plane correction and reduces the potential for

cage collapse through the endplate. This can be confirmed on AP fluoroscopy images (**TECH FIG 6A**).
- AP cage size depends on the anatomic situation. Larger cages are biomechanically superior, but the bigger footprint requires more dissection and hence more chance of encountering neurologic structures (**TECH FIG 6B**).

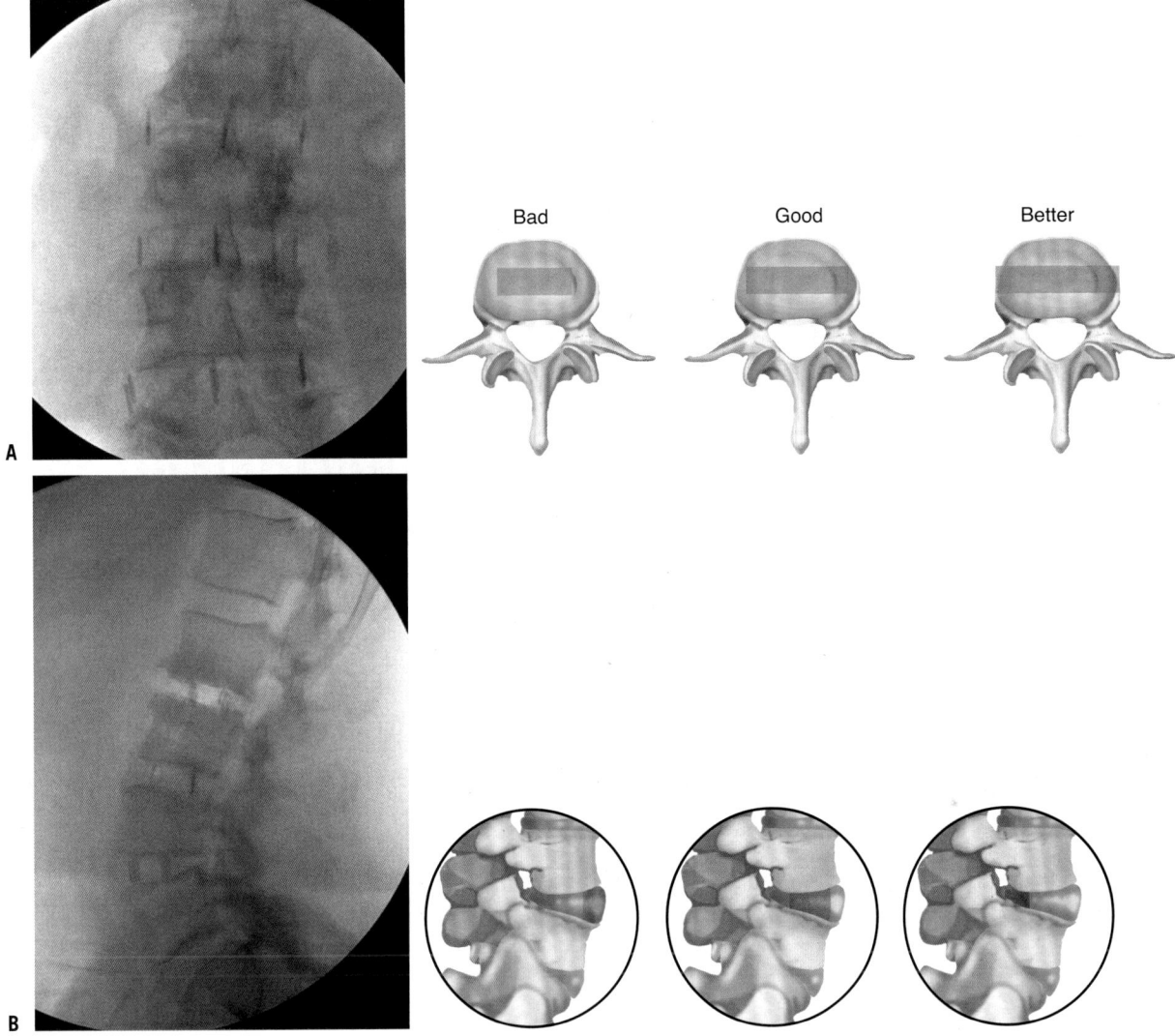

TECH FIG 6 A. AP fluoroscopy is used to confirm that the cage covers both lateral cortices to reduce the chance of collapse. **B.** Increased AP width provides increased contact surface area to prevent collapse without compromising fusion surface area. The cage should be centered in the AP direction. Red areas indicate potential location of cage.

ANTERIOR LONGITUDINAL LIGAMENT RELEASE

- Intentional ALL release can be performed to achieve additional lordosis in cases of sagittal imbalance. This procedure is called the *anterior column realignment* or *ACR* by some surgeons.
- The ALL release can be done as part of an anterior and posterior case when a moderate degree of correction is required, or it can be done as part of a posterior (osteotomy), anterior, then posterior (compression and fixation) case when even more correction is required.
- This requires careful dissection anterior to the ALL and a retractor to protect the aorta and vena cava. Typically, the lateral annulus on both sides is released, the disc space cleaned out, and then trials inserted.

- Once reasonable tension is obtained with the initial trials, the ALL is resected under direct vision.
- Then, taller cages or hyperlordotic cages are trialed and inserted. Restraint should be observed to avoid placing an overly lordotic or tall cage that merely leads to anterior placement of the cage.
- Screw fixation of the cage is typically required when the ALL is released to prevent migration.
- Hyperlordotic cages of 20 or 30 degrees with vertebral body tabs that allow screw fixation are available that facilitate this procedure.

GRAFT PREPARATION AND DELIVERY

- Most available cages are made of polyetheretherketone or titanium. The cage should be filled with bone graft material. This can be held in place with circumferential sutures during delivery or by using a graft slider.
- The graft can be delivered by impacting it into place; however, there is a risk for endplate violation. The graft slider can

safely deliver the graft while reducing the chance for endplate violation (**TECH FIG 7**).
- Graft delivery should be checked on AP fluoroscopy to ensure the radiographic markers in the graft extend to or slightly beyond the lateral body cortex.

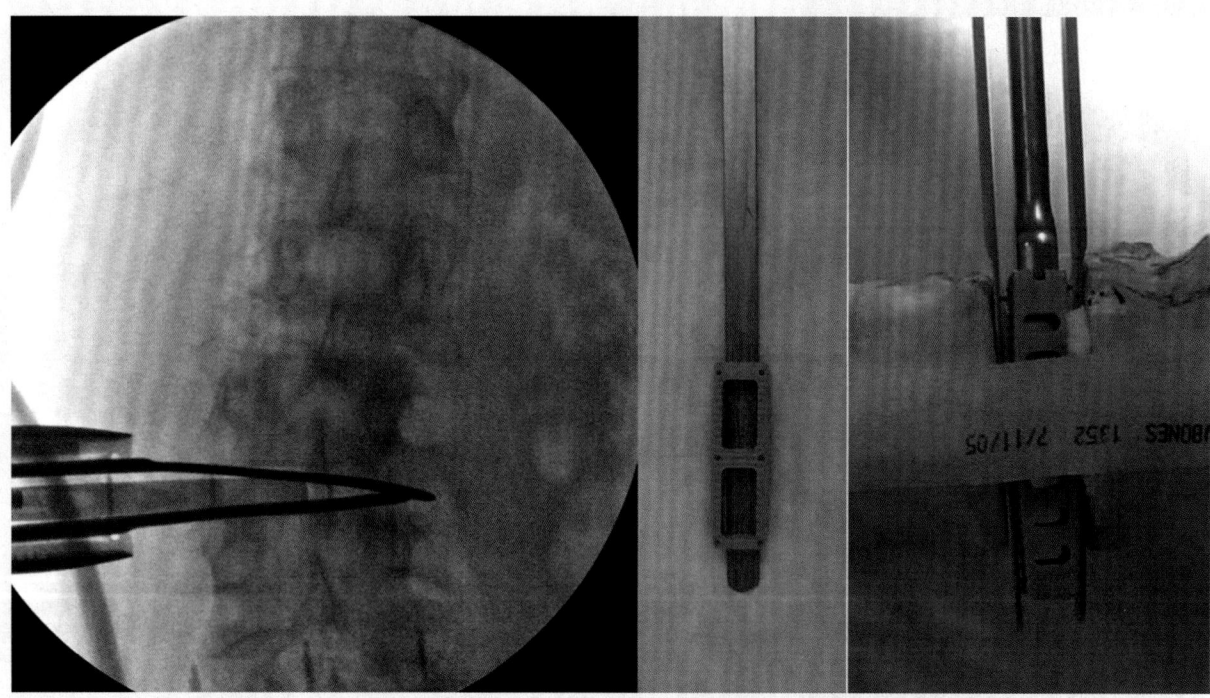

TECH FIG 7 The graft slider delivers the graft while preventing endplate violation.

CLOSURE

- Confirm graft location with final AP and lateral fluoroscopic images.
- Obtain hemostasis prior to retractor removal. Partially collapse the retractor and gently remove while inspecting for bleeding along the walls.

- Layered closure is then performed, including the external abdominal fascia.
- If the thoracic cavity was entered, a chest tube may be indicated.

ADDITIONAL FIXATION

- When posterior instrumentation is planned, additional anterior fixation is not required.
- Percutaneous pedicle screws, either unilateral or bilateral, are commonly used to augment the lateral interbody graft. This can be performed while in the lateral position or after moving the patient to the prone position.

- If the ALL is disrupted intraoperatively, there is a marked increase in the risk of graft dislodgement. In this case, additional anterior fixation may be indicated.
- In some instances, vertebral body screw fixation with rod, plate, or through the cage itself can be performed to improve biomechanics. However, this typically requires more dissection of the psoas and increases morbidity.

Pearls and Pitfalls

Maintain Vertical Orientation	• Rotating and tilting the bed rather than the C-arm to fine-tune images improves the surgeon's sense of orientation. This method keeps the retractor vertical. This is more important in multilevel cases and with cases that have rotational malalignment. • Working vertically within the confines of the retractor will prevent excessive anterior dissection that may threaten the ALL or posterior dissection that may encroach on the posterior longitudinal ligament and dura. • It will also help place the graft perfectly lateral.
Cage Size	• Cages that have undersized footprints increase the risk of collapse, especially in osteoporotic patients. • Passing the Cobb elevator through the far side of the annulus, on both the superior and inferior endplate, will allow placement of a cage that spans the entire width of the body lateral rim to lateral rim.
Endplate Violation	• Passing the Cobb elevator too aggressively across the endplate can cause a disruption. • The rotatory shavers commonly violate the endplate if they are used too aggressively. • Delivery of a large cage that is not perfectly parallel with the disc space risks endplate violation. This can be avoided with use of the graft slider.
Preservation of the ALL	• The ALL serves as an anterior tension band that allows the cage to distract the foramina and the posterior structures, enabling indirect decompression. • Furthermore, ALL incompetence dramatically increases the risk of graft dislodgement, especially if the plan includes prone lordotic positioning that may open up the disc space further. • If the ALL disruption is recognized intraoperatively, it is prudent to fix the graft either with direct screw fixation or anterior compression plating to minimize the risk of graft dislodgement. • Understanding where the anterior blade of the retractor is docked relative to the ALL, localizing the ALL, and protecting it with additional retractors may reduce the risk of disruption.
ALL Release	• Can be used in cases of sagittal imbalance to achieve additional lordosis • Use with PSO to achieve additional correction **(FIG 7)**. • Must protect adjacent vascular structures • Screw fixation of cage is often required to prevent migration once the ALL is released.

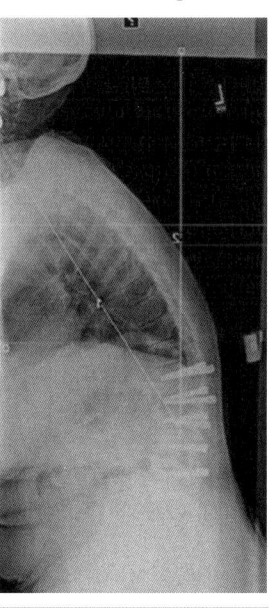 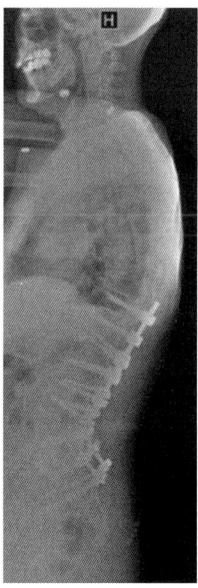

FIG 7 Preoperative (**A**) and postoperative (**B**) lateral radiographs demonstrate the correction in sagittal balance achieved with an L4 PSO and T12–L1 lateral interbody cage with ALL release.

POSTOPERATIVE CARE

• No additional postoperative protocols or restrictions are required after lateral interbody fusion than is standard for posterolateral or anterior fusion.
• With both anterior and posterior column support (assuming posterior augmentation is performed), postoperative bracing is typically not necessary.
• Generally, because of the minimally invasive retroperitoneal approach, patients typically mobilize quickly and with less pain than open posterolateral fusions.[10]

OUTCOMES

• Less intraoperative blood loss compared with open posterior fusion[4]
• No significant difference in outcomes or complication profile in obese patients[9]
• Early and midterm outcome data for the treatment of adult degenerative scoliosis suggests less morbidity, blood loss, and overall complication rate compared with open posterior fusion historical cohorts.[2,8]

COMPLICATIONS[3,4,9,11]

- Psoas palsy
- Lumbosacral plexus injury
- Quadriceps palsy
- Meralgia paresthetica (lateral femoral cutaneous nerve)
- Genitofemoral nerve injury
- Implant subsidence
- Broken cage
- Cage displacement
- Endplate violation
- ALL disruption
- Vascular injury
- Hernia/pseudohernia
- Bowel injury

REFERENCES

1. Benglis DM, Vanni S, Levi AD. An anatomical study of the lumbosacral plexus as related to the minimally invasive transpsoas approach to the lumbar spine. J Neurosurg Spine 2009;10(2):139–144.
2. Dakwar E, Cardona RF, Smith DA, et al. Early outcomes and safety of the minimally invasive, lateral retroperitoneal transpsoas approach for adult degenerative scoliosis. Neurosurg Focus 2010; 28(3):E8.
3. Galan TV, Mohan V, Klineberg EO, et al. Case report: incisional hernia as a complication of extreme lateral interbody fusion. Spine J 2012; 12(4):e1–e6.
4. Knight RQ, Schwaegler P, Hanscom D, et al. Direct lateral lumbar interbody fusion for degenerative conditions: early complication profile. J Spinal Disord Tech 2009;22(1):34–37.
5. Moro T, Kikuchi S, Konno S, et al. An anatomic study of the lumbar plexus with respect to retroperitoneal endoscopic surgery. Spine (Phila Pa 1976) 2003;28(5):423–428.
6. Ozgur BM, Aryan HE, Pimenta L, et al. Extreme Lateral Interbody Fusion (XLIF): a novel surgical technique for anterior lumbar interbody fusion. Spine J 2006;6(1):105–110.
7. Park DK, Lee MJ, Lin EL, et al. The relationship of intrapsoas nerves during a transpsoas approach to the lumbar spine: anatomic study. J Spinal Disord Tech 2010;23(4):223–228.
8. Phillips FM, Isaacs RE, Rodgers WB, et al. Adult degenerative scoliosis treated with XLIF: clinical and radiographical results of a prospective multicenter study with 24-month follow-up. Spine (Phila Pa 1976) 2013;38(21):1853–1861.
9. Rodgers WB, Cox CS, Gerber EJ. Early complications of extreme lateral interbody fusion in the obese. J Spinal Disord Tech 2010;23(6):393–397.
10. Rodgers WB, Cox CS, Gerber EJ. Experience and early results with a minimally invasive technique for anterior column support through eXtreme Lateral Interbody Fusion (XLIF). Musculoskelet Rev 2007;1:28–32.
11. Tonetti J, Vouaillat H, Kwon BK, et al. Femoral nerve palsy following mini-open extraperitoneal lumbar approach: report of three cases and cadaveric mechanical study. J Spinal Disord Tech 2006;19(2):135–141.

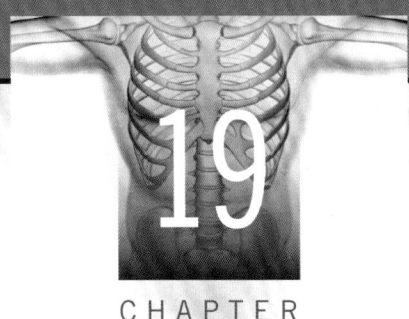

Minimally Invasive Transforaminal Interbody Fusion

Choll W. Kim

DEFINITION

- Minimally invasive transforaminal interbody fusion (MIS TLIF) is a modification of the Wiltse exposure for decompression and interbody fusion of the motion segment using specialized retractor and instrumentation systems and fluoroscopic guidance to minimize the surgical corridor.
- Standard TLIF is a well-established technique for decompression and fusion of a vertebral motion segment, which uses a midline exposure to perform a unilateral facetectomy and exposure of Kambin triangle to access the disc space for interbody fusion.
- TLIF, in comparison to standard posterolateral fusion, allows for improved fusion rates, indirect decompression via restoration of intervertebral disc height, and anterior column support without the need for an anterior retroperitoneal/transperitoneal exposure. The increased risk of neurologic injury to the exiting and traversing nerve roots with TLIF must be weighed against these advantages.
- MIS TLIF, in comparison to standard open TLIF, is performed through small paramedian incisions and is typically coupled with minimally invasive posterior instrumentation. Typically, formal posterolateral fusion is not done, consequently, MIS TLIF relies heavily on the interbody fusion for avoidance of pseudarthrosis and successful outcomes.
- MIS TLIF has been shown to have less blood loss, earlier postoperative recovery, decreased opioid use, and decreased rates of infection in comparison to standard surgery. MIS TLIF may potentially have improved long-term outcomes as a result of the preservation of important musculotendinous attachments and the maintenance of integrity of the dorsolumbar fascia.
- MIS TLIF is much more reliant on fluoroscopic imaging in comparison to standard TLIF, thus there is increased radiation exposure to the surgeon, staff, and patient. The amount of radiation exposure lessens with surgeon experience. Navigation with fluoroscopic or computed tomography (CT) imaging may allow for decreased radiation exposure to the surgeon and staff.

ANATOMY

Paraspinal Muscles

- The lumbar multifidus muscle is a key stabilizer of the lumbar spine.
  - Largest and most medial of the deep lumbar paraspinal musculature

- Originates from the spinous process and inserts on the superior articular process of the vertebra one to two levels caudally **(FIG 1)**
- Designed for short, powerful movements with maximum force generated during lumbar flexion to optimize its ability to stabilize the lumbar spine motion segments during movement
- Detachment of the multifidus tendon with traditional midline laminectomy compromises multifidus function.
- A paramedian approach, in contrast, preserves the multifidus tendon attachments.

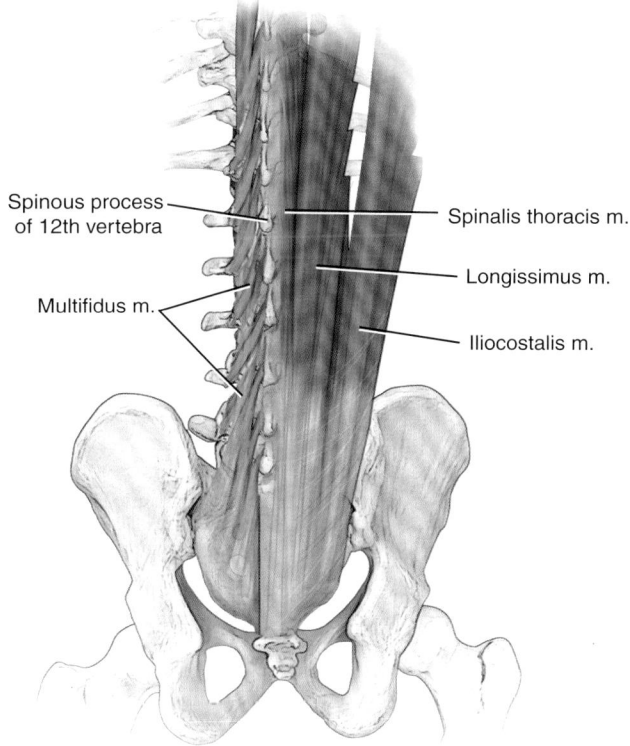

Spinous process of 12th vertebra —
Spinalis thoracis m. —
Longissimus m. —
Multifidus m. —
Iliocostalis m. —

FIG 1 The multifidi are the deepest and most medial of the lumbar paraspinal musculature. They originate from the spinous process and insert on the superior articular process of the vertebra one to two levels caudally. They are unique among the lumbar paraspinal muscles in that they generate a significant amount of force despite their limited excursion. These characteristics suggest that they play a key role in motion segment stability.

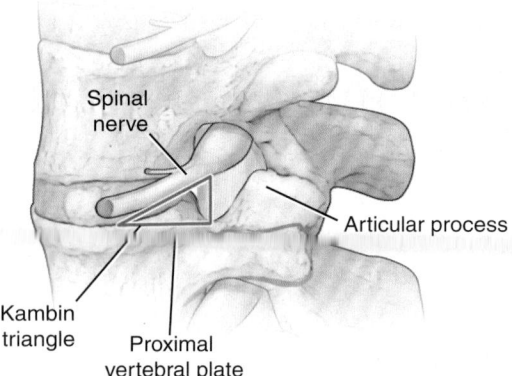

FIG 2 Kambin triangle is a safe corridor to the disc space bounded medially by the traversing nerve root, superiorly by the exiting nerve root, and inferiorly by the pedicle.

Surgical Target Site

- Kambin triangle is an anatomic safe corridor to the intervertebral disc space bounded medially by the dural tube/traversing nerve root, laterally by the exiting nerve root, and caudally by the pedicle (**FIG 2**).
- Exposure of Kambin triangle is accomplished by facetectomy. In the technique we described, a total facetectomy is performed. The inferior articular process is removed; however, the pars is maintained (to protect the dorsal root ganglion on cage insertion). The superior articular process is removed up to the cranial aspect of the pedicle.
- The exiting nerve root hugs the medial and inferior border of its associated pedicle. The sensitive dorsal root ganglion typically lies inferior to the pedicle.

Radiographic Anatomy

- Percutaneous pedicle screw placement requires understanding the topographic anatomy of the posterior elements as well as the radiographic projection of the pedicle on various radiographic views.
- The anatomic starting point for pedicle screw placement is typically at the intersection of a horizontal line that bisects the transverse process and a vertical line at or just lateral to the lateral aspect of the pars. The upslope of the facet–transverse process junction is a palpable anatomic landmark.
  - The more lateral the starting point, the more medial angulation is needed. This can be problematic in a patient with a narrow pelvis as the posterior iliac crests can limit the ability to medialize pedicle screw tracts.
  - The more medial the starting point, the greater the risk of facet violation.
- The radiographic starting point for pedicle screw placement is typically at the lateral aspect of the radiographic pedicle. At the low lumbar spine, because of medial pedicle angulation, an anatomic starting point may be preferred that may not necessarily coincide with the lateral aspect of the radiographic pedicle.
- The radiographic pedicle correlates with the anatomic isthmus of the pedicle for hourglass-shaped pedicles. In the lower lumbar spine, where the pedicles are more cylindrical (ie, without an isthmus) and medially angulated, the anatomic correlate of the radiographic pedicle is less clear.

- Pedicles in the upper lumbar spine have a more sagittal orientation and angulate progressively medial as one moves caudal. At L5 and S1, the pedicles typically project well more than 20 degrees medial.

PATIENT HISTORY AND PHYSICAL FINDINGS

- The earlier postoperative recovery associated with MIS TLIF is advantageous in elderly patients.
- Patients with severe osteoporosis are not ideal candidates for MIS TLIF because of the difficulty in avoiding endplate violation and subsequent graft subsidence.
- MIS TLIF is challenging in obese patients because of the difficulty in obtaining good radiographic imaging and the difficulty in manipulating instruments through a long working corridor. The advantages in terms of postoperative recovery, however, are most apparent in obese patients as the difference in the extent of soft tissue dissection between MIS and standard techniques is greatest.
- MIS TLIF can be a useful in patients with previous midline surgery as dissection through scar tissue can be avoided. However, scar tissue from intracanal epidural bleeding at levels adjacent to previous surgery can complicate the exposure of Kambin triangle.

IMAGING AND OTHER DIAGNOSTIC STUDIES

- Pedicles should be evaluated radiographically prior to surgery to ensure that pedicle screw placement is feasible. If not, alternative means of fixation should be considered.
- A narrow pelvis (decreased distance between the posterior iliac crests) can make medial angulation of lower lumbar pedicle screws challenging. A more medial starting point with a straightforward pedicle screw trajectory or alternative means of fixation may need to be considered in these situations.
- CT and magnetic resonance imaging axial sections can be used to identify pedicle screw starting points and to approximate screw diameters and lengths.
- Nerve root anomalies can be identified on preoperative imaging and, if unilateral, should prompt consideration for MIS TLIF exposure on the contralateral side. Alternative techniques that do not require nerve root retraction can also be considered (eg, standard posterolateral fusion without interbody reconstruction, anterior fusion through an anterior, or lateral retroperitoneal exposure with posterior MIS fusion and instrumentation).
- TLIF, in general, should be pursued with care at the level of the cord or conus medullaris as the risk of significant neurologic injury is increased.

SURGICAL MANAGEMENT

- Indications
  - One- or two-level lumbar pathology in the presence of the following:
    - Spinal stenosis with instability (eg, degenerative or isthmic spondylolisthesis)
    - Symptomatic degenerative disc disease
- Relative contraindications
  - High-grade spondylolisthesis (Meyerding grade 3 or 4)
  - Severe osteoporosis
  - Nerve root anomalies

- There are multiple methods of performing an MIS TLIF. The different techniques are similar with respect to the decompression and discectomy but can differ with respect to the method used for distraction of the disc space, the fusion technique used to supplement the interbody fusion, and the instrumentation used for stabilization of the motion segment.
  - The technique we described involves subtotal discectomy using interbody spacer trials to sequentially distract the disc space and contralateral facet fusion with bilateral pedicle screw placement.
  - Posterior interlaminar, contralateral facet, or posterolateral bone grafting can be performed to supplement the interbody fusion.
  - Alternative means of posterior instrumentation/stabilization include unilateral pedicle screw placement, unilateral pedicle screw placement with a contralateral facet screw, unilateral pedicle screw placement with a spinous process plate, and isolated spinous process plate fixation.

Preoperative Planning

- Patients should be evaluated for the following:
  - Osteoporosis
  - Potential issues with bone healing (eg, nicotine, diabetes mellitus, steroids, chemotherapy, previous pseudarthrosis)
  - Previous surgery and the potential for epidural scarring
  - Obesity and retractor blade depth requirements
  - Need for contralateral decompression
- Imaging should be evaluated for the following:
  - Mobility of the motion segment
  - Extent and nature of canal stenosis
    - Determines cranial/caudal extent of decompression
    - Need for osteophyte removal at the contralateral recess

- Nerve root anomalies—best seen on T1-weighted axial imaging
- Pedicle orientation, diameters, and pedicle deformities

Positioning

- Patients are positioned prone on a radiolucent spine table. We prefer to position our patients using a Wilson frame attachment for the Jackson table to aid exposure of the interlaminar window and distraction of the motion segment. With release of the disc space and careful attention to the radiographic alignment, inadvertent kyphosis can be avoided.
- Upper limbs are carefully positioned to avoid iatrogenic injury (eg, brachial plexus palsy, ulnar nerve compression, rotator cuff tendinitis).
- Flexion of the knees reduces root tension for the lower lumbar levels.
- Room setup (**FIG 3**)
  - C-arm from opposite side of TLIF
    - This is a key point. With the C-arm coming in from the opposite side of the exposure, the C-arm base can be locked, and the boom can be "wagged" in and out of the field. This allows for frequent imaging and decreases the need for the surgeon to step out of the surgical field. This is especially critical in the initial phases of the learning curve where inadequate imaging often leads to technical complications.
- Table mount on opposite side of TLIF at level of hip

Imaging

- Consistent terms for intraoperative fluoroscopic imaging improves communication with the radiology technician and increases operating room (OR) time efficiency. We use the following:
  - Push in/out: brings the image intensifier closer or farther from the patient

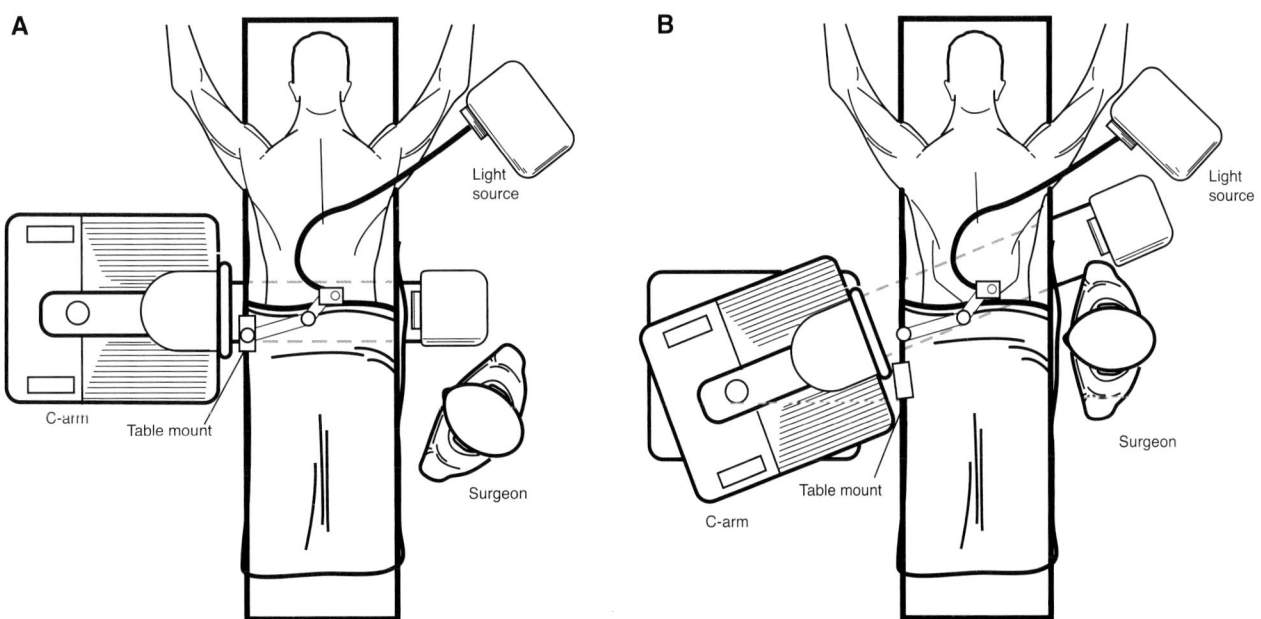

FIG 3 Room setup. **A.** The C-arm should come from the side opposite the surgeon. **B.** This allows the C-arm to be easily moved to the side ("wagged") allowing the surgeon access to the surgical exposure. The C-arm can be brought back into position to expedite frequent imaging.

- Tilt north/south: allows for Ferguson and anti-Ferguson views
- Rainbow over/under: uses the arc of the C-arm to obtain oblique views of the spine, as in a Scotty dog view of the pedicles
- Roll north/south: translates entire base of C-arm cephalad or caudad

- Wag north/south: angles the field generator out and out of the field without moving the base of the C-arm
- Properly aligned anteroposterior (AP) and lateral images are crucial for the MIS TLIF technique. The best method for identifying the "perfect" image is to sequentially image from "imperfect" to "perfect" back to "imperfect."

PLANNING OF INCISION SITES

- True AP positioning
  - The C-arm should start in a direct upright position ("90–90").
  - The table should be rotated ("airplane") until a perfectly AP image of the index level is obtained. The C-arm should then be "tilted" until level endplates are obtained. The C-arm should not be "rainbowed." This ensures that the index level is truly AP relatively to the floor, thereby ensuring that the under-the-table lateral image is also a true lateral.
  - A properly aligned AP image of the vertebral body should show the superior endplate as a single, dense line. The pedicles should be symmetric and located just below the superior endplate. The spinous process should be in the midline (although this can be misleading in the presence unusual the spinous process anatomy, as in scoliosis or trauma) **(TECH FIG 1A)**.

- A horizontal line on the back marking the disc space can be used to guide the orientation of the C-arm for a properly aligned lateral image.
- A properly aligned lateral image should show the superior endplate as a single, dense line. The pedicles should be superimposed.
- For discs with significant angulation to a vertical plumb line (eg, L5–S1), the patient can be placed into reverse Trendelenburg to ease access to the disc.
- Planning incisions
  - Mark the centerline on a properly aligned AP image **(TECH FIG 1B)**.
  - Mark two parallel paramedian lines approximately 4 cm lateral to the center line **(TECH FIG 1C)**.
  - Using lateral imaging, mark the point in line with the disc space on the paramedian skin markings **(TECH FIG 1D,E)**.
  - This point will be the center of a 3-cm incision.

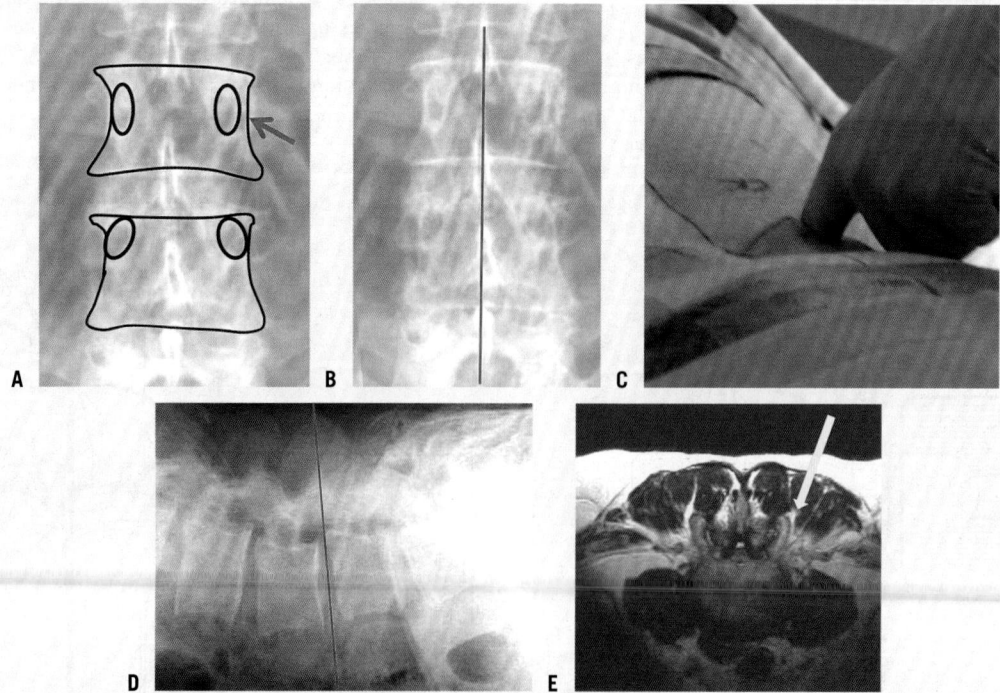

TECH FIG 1 A. A "perfect" AP image of the vertebra should have the spinous process in the midline; the pedicles should be symmetric and just inferior to the superior endplate; and the superior endplate should be a single, dense line. The inferior vertebra (L4) in this image is a "perfect" AP image. The superior vertebra (L3) in this image is rotated; note the asymmetric pedicles *(red arrow)*. **B.** After a perfect AP image is obtained of the surgical levels, the midline is marked. Parallel lines 4 cm lateral to the midline are also marked. Paramedian incisions (2.5 cm long) will be made on these paramedian lines **(C)**, with the midpoint of these incisions at a point in line with the disc space on lateral imaging **(D)**. After the skin is incised, the paraspinal fascia is incised in line with the skin incision. **E.** Finger dissection then proceeds between the multifidus and longissimus muscles to the lateral aspect of the facet joint *(yellow arrow)*.

EXPOSURE OF THE TARGET SITE

- The skin incision is made with a no. 11 blade followed by a fascial incision in line with skin incision. Finger dissection proceeds along the interval between the multifidus and longissimus to the lateral aspect of the facet joint.
- The multifidus tendinous attachments at the target facet joint are released with a Cobb elevator using C-arm for localization. Because the facet joints at the lower lumbar levels are in close proximity due to the lordotic alignment of the lower lumbar spine, it is easy to inadvertently release the tendons from the wrong facet joint. This leads to increased bleeding and increased muscle creep and can be avoided by careful fluoroscopic localization prior to tendon release.

- Release of the tendinous attachments at the facet joint allows the serial dilator tubes to "surround" the facet joint **(TECH FIG 2)**. Twisting the dilators as they are placed aids in the release of the tendinous attachments.
- Blade lengths are measured at the lateral aspect of the dilator tube, and the retractor with appropriately sized blades is placed over the dilators. Rotating the retractor back and forth as they are placed over the dilating tubes can be helpful, like the twisting motion used when pulling a tight ring off one's finger.
- The retractor blades should be positioned so that they are in line with the disc space and are directed medially toward the facet joint and base of the spinous process.

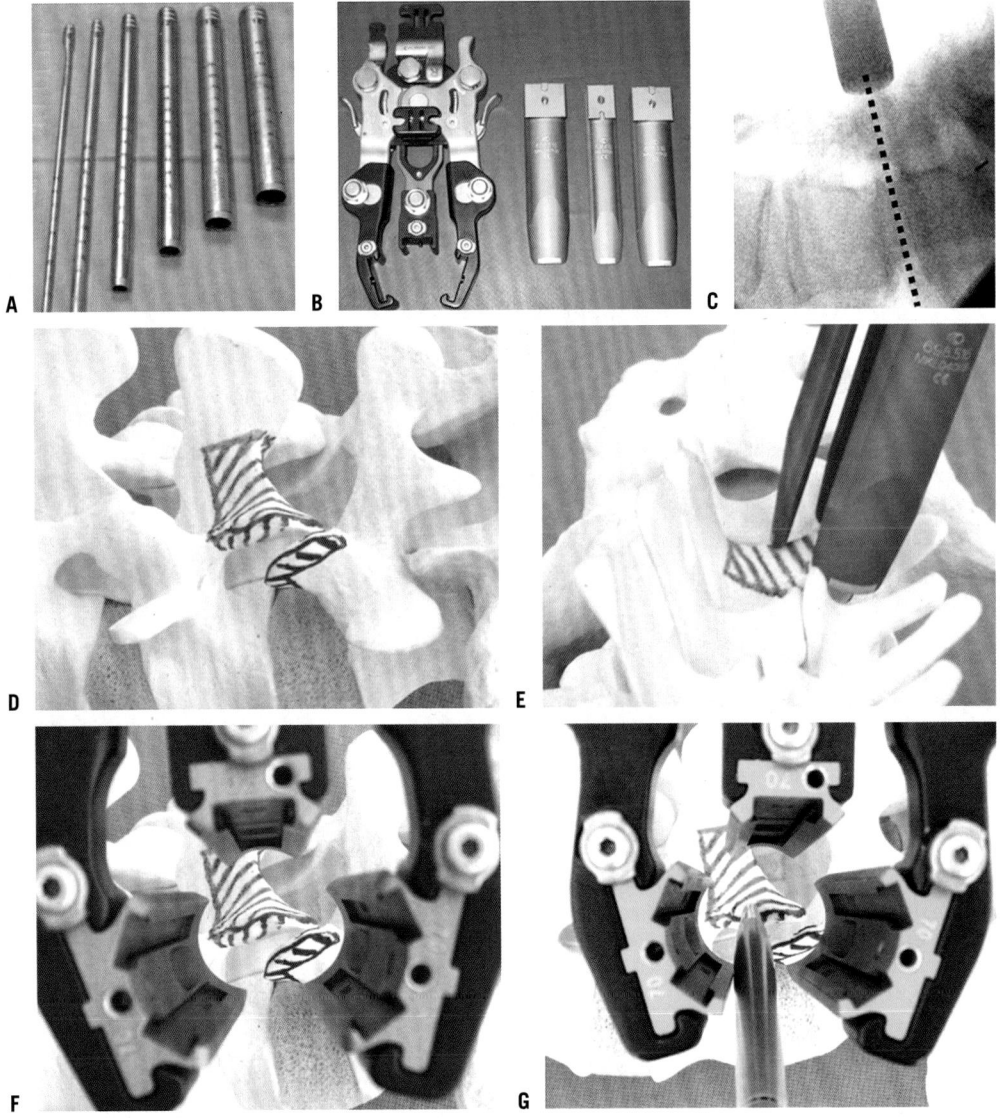

TECH FIG 2 A. After the multifidus tendinous attachments are released from the facet joint, dilators are used to expand the surgical corridor and encircle the facet joint. The expandable tubular retractor (**B**) is inserted over the last dilator and should be medially angulated and positioned in line with the disc space (**C**) *(broken line)*. **D,E.** The key anatomic landmarks are the base of the spinous process medially and the facet joint line laterally. The amount of retractor blade distraction should be optimized to visualize these landmarks. Opening the retractor more than necessary will lead to significant muscle creep. **F,G.** We prefer retractor systems with gaps between the blades (as opposed to closed tubes), as they allow angulation of instruments to be angulated out of the visual field.

TECHNIQUES

- Key landmarks
  - Medially: base of spinous process
  - Laterally: facet joint line
- Minimizing retractor opening decreases amount of muscle creep.

- We prefer retractors with gaps between the retractor blades, which allows for angulation of instrumentation (see **TECH FIG 2G**).

FACETECTOMY AND CONTRALATERAL DECOMPRESSION

- Paraspinal muscle fibers within the surgical field are gently cauterized to expose the base of the spinous process and the facet joint.
- The facet joint line is identified (**TECH FIG 3A,B**).
- The cranial limit of bony resection is sufficient to allow the residual pars to be in line with the inferior endplate of the cranial vertebra (**TECH FIG 3C**).
- The ligamentum flavum is maintained for protection of the dural tube during removal of the inferior articular process.

- Ligamentum flavum is released with a curved curette and resected with Kerrison rongeurs to expose the dural tube (**TECH FIG 3D**).
- The contralateral ligamentum flavum and joint capsule are resected to achieve contralateral decompression. Additional bone at the base of the spinous process can be removed if more access is needed to the contralateral side. The angulation of the retractor is the key to obtaining a surgical corridor that allows access to the contralateral lateral recess (**TECH FIG 3E,F**). Alternatively, contralateral exposure can be used to decompress the contralateral lateral recess.

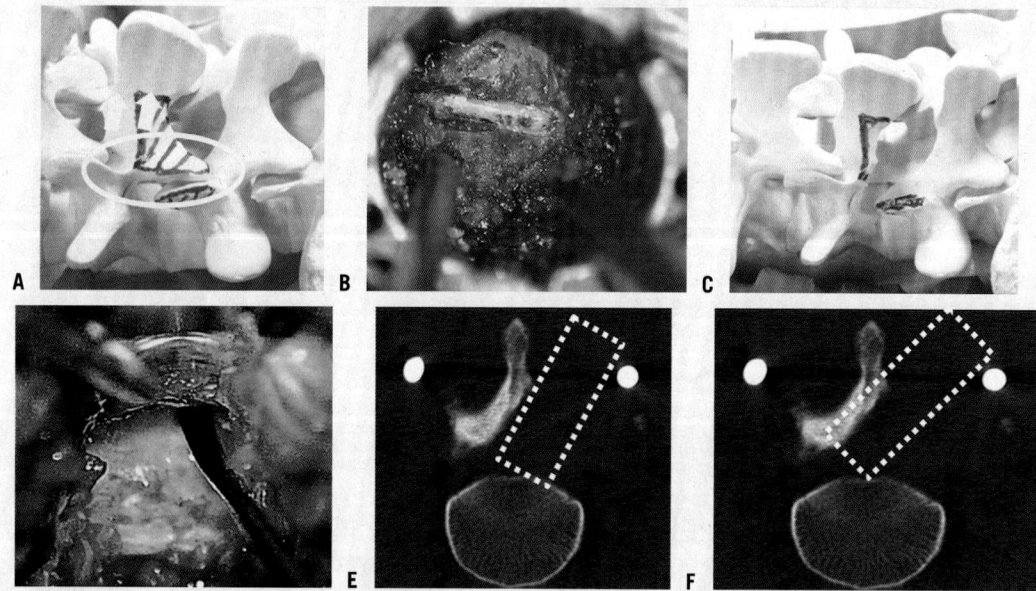

TECH FIG 3 A. The facet joint line is a key anatomic landmark demarcating the lateral extent of exposure *(yellow circle)* and the rise of the spinous process is the medial margin of the surgical exposure *(yellow arrows)*. **B.** The burr is used to remove bone from the inferolateral edge of the inferior articular process to the base of the spinous process. **C,D.** A thorough contralateral decompression can be performed via a unilateral exposure with appropriate angulation of the retractor. **E,F.** The retractor is angulated, and bone is resected from the base of the spinous process to allow adequate visualization of the contralateral lateral recess for decompression. (**E**) Broken rectangle shows the surgical corridor used for the interbody reconstruction). (**F**) Broken rectangle shows the surgical corridor used for the contralateral decompression.

EXPOSURE OF KAMBIN TRIANGLE, DISCECTOMY, AND ENDPLATE PREPARATION

- The retractor blades are maintained in line with the disc space but are redirected laterally toward Kambin triangle (**TECH FIG 4A**).
- The superior articular process is removed up to the cranial aspect of the caudad pedicle. Care must be taken to remove bone cranial to the pedicle within the corridor used for interbody cage

placement. Residual bone (typically at the lateral aspect of the superior articular process cranial to the pedicle) will cause the larger size cages to migrate medially into the traversing nerve root. When all bone cranial to the pedicle has been removed, retraction of the dural tube is not typically necessary for safe cage insertion.

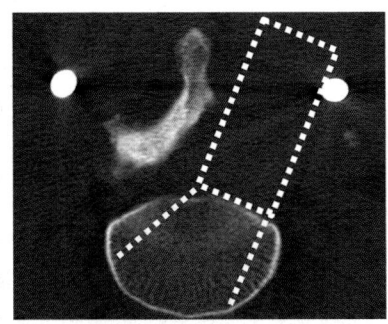
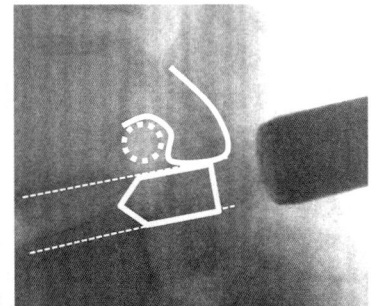
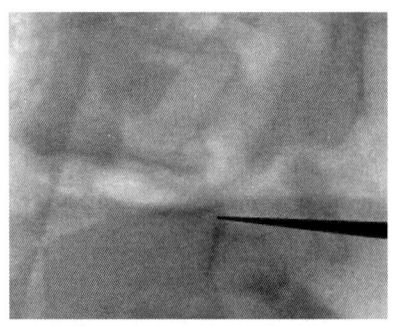
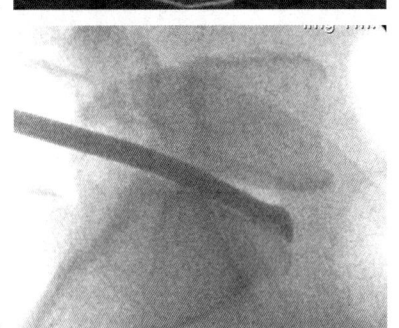

TECH FIG 4 A. After completion of the facetectomy and contralateral decompression, the retractor is repositioned to redirect the surgical corridor for the discectomy and interbody preparation. Broken rectangle shows the orientation for the surgical corridor during interbody preparation. The broken yellow lines show the access within the disc space when a full complement of disc preparation instruments are used. **B.** The inferior articular process and pars are resected, leaving a residual amount of pars sufficient to protect the dorsal root ganglion. The exiting nerve root position is shown by the broken white circle. The interbody spacer is represented by the yellow diagram. **C.** Bone cranial to the pedicle (superior articular process) is completely resected, and if necessary, an osteotome is used to remove overhanging osteophytes from the caudad endplate. **D.** Intraoperative imaging is used to confirm that a thorough discectomy and endplate preparation is accomplished, especially anteriorly.

- The pars interarticularis is preserved to protect the exiting nerve root during cage insertion (**TECH FIG 4B**).
- The dural tube should be released from the posterior vertebral body to allow the traversing nerve root to move out of the way of the spacers/cage. This is especially important in revision settings when the dural tube is commonly adherent to the posterior vertebral bodies as a result of previous epidural bleeding and scarring and thus at increased risk for injury.
- The disc within Kambin triangle is exposed.
- Epidural veins are cauterized with bipolar electrocautery. The location of the traversing and exiting nerve roots should be assessed at all times to prevent inadvertent neural injury.
- A horizontal slit annulotomy is made with a no. 15 blade scalpel and is subsequently opened with a rotary shaver.
- Posterior disc osteophytes are removed with rongeurs/osteotomes. Removal of the posterior lips can ease access to the disc space (**TECH FIG 4C**). We typically maintain the posterosuperior lip to decrease the chance for impingement of the exiting nerve root by the cage and the chance for cage migration posteriorly.
- Subtotal discectomy and endplate preparation are accomplished using a combination of straight and angled curettes and rasps.
  - Smooth rotating paddle sizers and spacer trials can be used to dilate and release disc space. We avoid use of the rotary shaver, especially in osteoporotic bone, because of the risk of endplate violation.
  - Fluoroscopic guidance can be used to ensure thorough discectomy. The most commonly missed portions of the disc are the ipsilateral lateral disc, the contralateral posterior disc, and the anterior disc (**TECH FIG 4D**).
  - Concave endplates can make discectomy challenging unless posterior osteophytes/lips are removed and/or the curettes are appropriately bent to accommodate the concavity.
  - Thorough release of the disc space and restoration of disc height aid in reduction of spondylolisthesis.

CAGE SELECTION AND INSERTION

- Solid trial spacers are sequentially inserted to dilate the annulotomy window. Expandable trials are used to determine optimum cage height. Undersizing the cage can increase the stress on posterior instrumentation, risking failure. Oversizing the cage risks endplate compromise and subsequent graft subsidence.
- Options for cage selection include oblique and banana-shaped cages.
  - Oblique cages are easier to insert but can have suboptimal purchase in the presence of concave endplates if the implant is not appropriately contoured.
  - Banana-shaped cages are more difficult to insert but are more biomechanically sound when placed at the anterior margin of the disc space, which also make them less likely to migrate posteriorly.
- Bulleted cages (a modification for ease of insertion) should be used with caution as violation of the anterior annulus is possible with aggressive insertion.
- Expandable cages allow for cage insertion at a contracted height, decreasing the risk of nerve root irritation during insertion. Once inside the disc space and safely past the exiting nerve root, it can be expanded until optimal fit and elevation is appreciated (**TECH FIG 5**).
- Bone graft is packed anteriorly within the disc space. A combination of local autograft bone together with bone graft extender is used to fill the disc space.

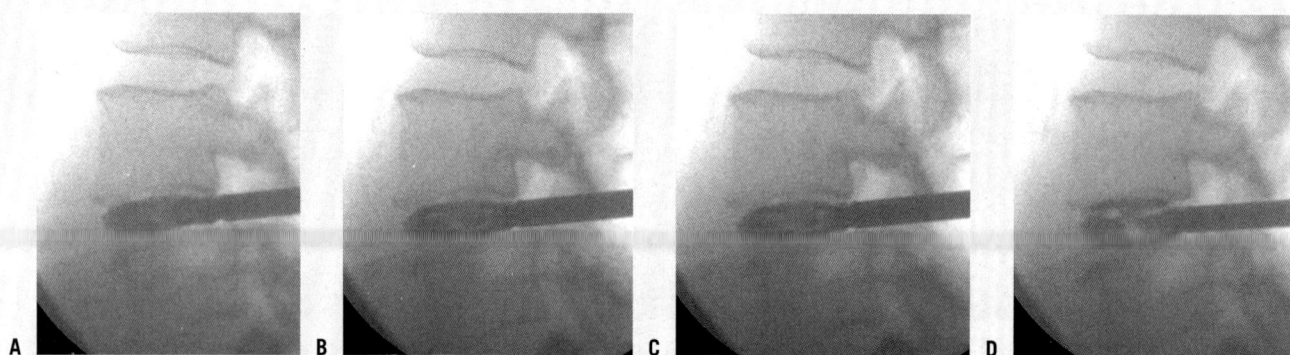

TECH FIG 5 A. Expandable cages are inserted at a contracted height to allow safe entry into the disc space with less chance for impingement of the traversing and exiting nerve roots. **B–D.** The cage is then expanded in the interbody space to restore disc height and obtain interbody cage purchase.

- The cage is inserted with care taken to avoid impingement of both the traversing and exiting nerve root. The residual pars protects the exiting nerve root during cage insertion (see **TECH FIG 4C**).
- If endplate violation occurs and the cage settles into an endplate defect, there is a risk for graft subsidence. In this situation, the cage can be "pushed" to the contralateral side of the disc space using the trial spacers, and a second cage can be inserted into the location of the endplate defect to prevent migration of the initial cage back into the defect.
  - Alternatively, cage insertion can be performed through a fresh approach through the contralateral side.
- The annulotomy window is sealed with fibrin sealant.

PEDICLE SCREW TRACT CANNULATION

- Bilateral pedicle screw placement is the most stable construct. A unilateral construct may be acceptable in a young patient with normal bone density and excellent pedicle screw purchase.
- Properly aligned AP images are obtained at the target vertebrae. This is the most crucial step for safe percutaneous pedicle screw placement. We prefer to cannulate all pedicles under AP imaging before moving to lateral imaging (**TECH FIG 6**).
- A Jamshidi needle is docked at the appropriate starting point via a combination of radiographic localization and anatomic palpation with the tip of the Jamshidi needle. As the Jamshidi needle is "walked" along the bone, the surgeon should appreciate the rise of the superior articular process as the needle moves from lateral to medial along the transverse process. The anatomic starting point identified through palpation should match the radiographic starting point on imaging. If not, ensure that true AP imaging has been obtained.
- The needle is gently tapped to seat the needle tip into the bone. A line is drawn on the needle shaft 20 mm above the skin. This represents the length of the pedicle, from the starting point to the base of the pedicle.
- The needle is aligned parallel to the endplate and held in the appropriate amount of mediolateral angulation for the level being performed. The needle is advanced toward the medial border of pedicle using gentle taps with the mallet. The tip should be just medial to the medial border of the pedicle when the 20-mm mark reaches the skin. On lateral imaging, the tip should be just past the posterior vertebral line.
- Oblique imaging (bull's-eye view, Scotty dog view) can be used to check for medial and lateral breaches.
  - Starting with the AP view, the C-arm is "rainbowed" to line the beam up with the pedicle axis.
  - The needle should be advanced down the center of the radiographic pedicle, keeping the needle shaft in line with the C-arm beam.
- Guidewires are placed after ensuring that there is an adequate fascial incision to accommodate placement of the pedicle screw (muscle/fascia can become entrapped underneath the head of the pedicle screw). Guidewires are inserted past the tip of the Jamshidi needle into "crunchy" cancellous bone. If the bone is too hard to manually insert the guidewire, a needle driver clamped to the guidewire 5 mm above the top of the Jamshidi needle can be gently tapped with a mallet. The position of the guidewires on AP, lateral, and oblique imaging is confirmed prior to tapping and screw insertion.

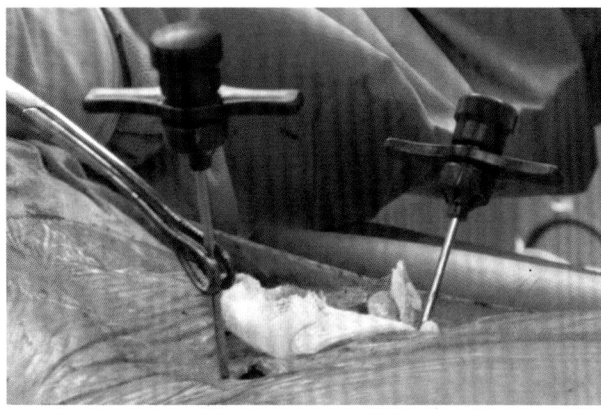

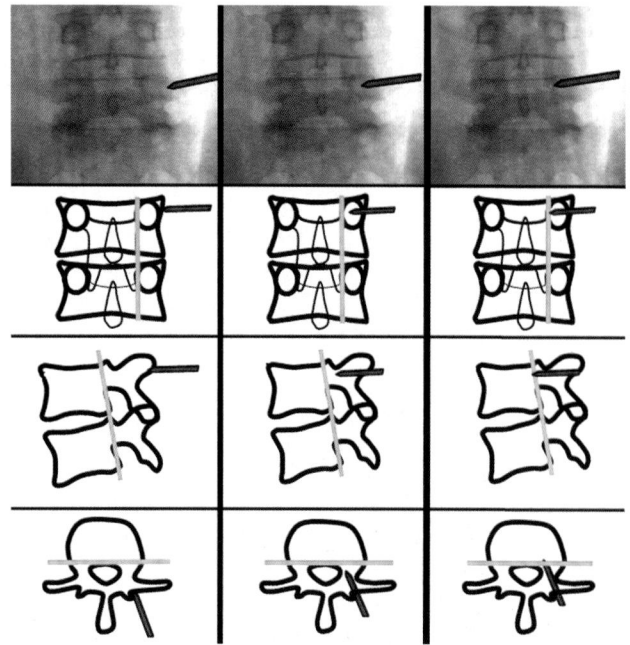

TECH FIG 6 A. Jamshidi needles are docked on the optimum pedicle starting points and their positions checked on AP image. **B.** Traversing the pedicle with a Jamshidi needle radiographically requires an understanding of the anatomic correlates to radiographic imaging findings. Once the Jamshidi needle has approached the medial pedicle wall on anteroposterior imaging, it should be just ventral to the posterior vertebral body wall on lateral imaging. The solid blue line represents the intersection between the posterior vertebral body line and medial border of the pedicle.

PEDICLE SCREW INSERTION

- The pedicle is tapped over the guidewire. We typically undertap by 1 mm. Tapping should be done under fluoroscopic imaging to prevent potentially catastrophic advancement of the guidewire **(TECH FIG 7)**.
- The guidewire or tap can be tested for pedicle breach with triggered electromyography.
  - Electrodiagnostic evidence of pedicle breach (threshold <10 mA) should prompt careful radiographic assessment of the pedicle screw tract with AP and oblique imaging. Redirecting the guidewire or aborting screw placement should be considered if there is concern for pedicle breach.
- Screws are placed over the guidewire, again, under fluoroscopic imaging to prevent inadvertent guidewire advancement. The guidewire can be removed once the screw tip is past the posterior vertebral body wall.
- Insert screws deep to avoid prominent hardware. The radiographic projection of the transverse process can aid in proper placement with regard to depth. If two levels are being performed and segmental fixation is desired, care must be taken to properly align screw heights to achieve a smooth contour for rod seating.

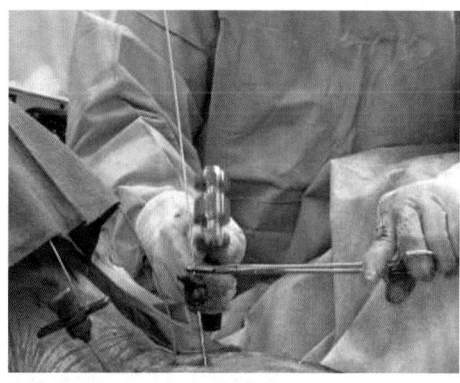

TECH FIG 7 Uncontrolled advancement of the guidewire risks catastrophic vascular or visceral injury. **A.** Grasping the guidewire with a needle driver 5 to 10 mm above the Jamshidi needle followed by gentle tapping of the needle driver allows for controlled insertion of the guidewire. *(continued)*

TECHNIQUES

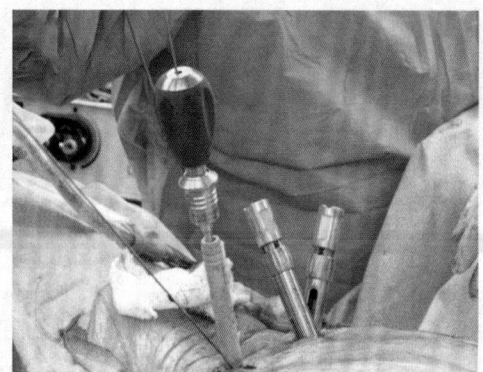

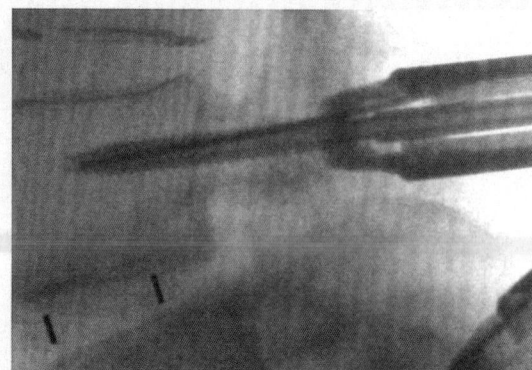

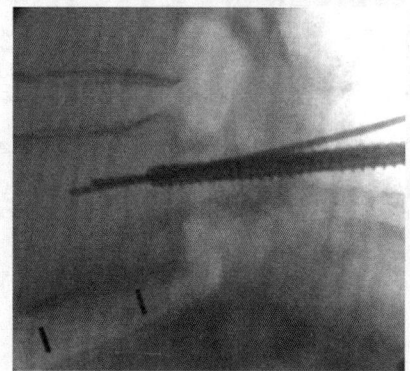

TECH FIG 7 *(continued)* **B–D.** The pedicles are tapped with cannulated taps, neuromonitoring is checked, and then screws are inserted. This should be done under lateral imaging to monitor for inadvertent advancement of the guidewire. Guidewires should be removed once the screw tip is 5 mm past the posterior vertebral body wall to minimize the chances of the guidewire binding within the screw cannula and inadvertently advancing. Screws should be inserted deep to avoid prominent hardware; the radiographic transverse process can be a useful guide. For multilevel fusions with segmental instrumentation, screws should be inserted to a depth where the polyaxial motion of the screw head is maintained to ease rod insertion and capture.

ROD PASSAGE

- The rod length is determined with MIS calipers.
- If necessary, the rod should be contoured after attachment to its holder to prevent issues with the attachment mechanism.
- The rods are passed under the fascia and through the rod sleeves under lateral fluoroscopic imaging **(TECH FIG 8)**.

Entrapment of fascia underneath the screw heads/rod must be avoided as this can result in severe postoperative pain.
- Confirm rods are seated within the sleeves, visually or with a tester.

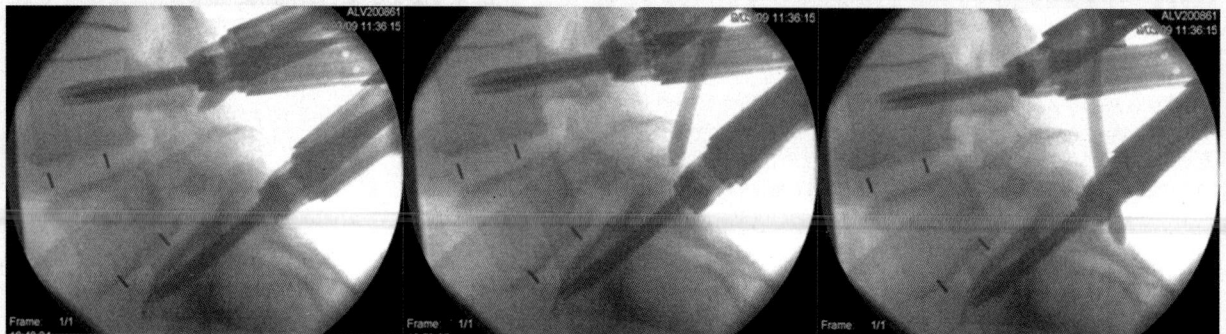

TECH FIG 8 Appropriate-length rods are contoured and then introduced into the screw sleeves, reduced into the screw heads, and captured with set screws.

ROD REDUCTION

- A rod reducer can be used to reduce the rod to the screw heads. If this is difficult, ensure that polyaxial motion of the screw heads is present.
- Screw caps are placed, and compression or distraction can then be performed as needed.
- The rod sleeves are removed, and a final check for entrapment of the muscle/fascia is done prior to closure.

- If reduction of a spondylolisthesis is desired, the rods can be fixed into the caudal vertebrae, and the pedicle screws from the cranial vertebra can be reduced to the rod. This technique is dependent on good screw purchase to prevent pullout **(TECH FIG 9)**.

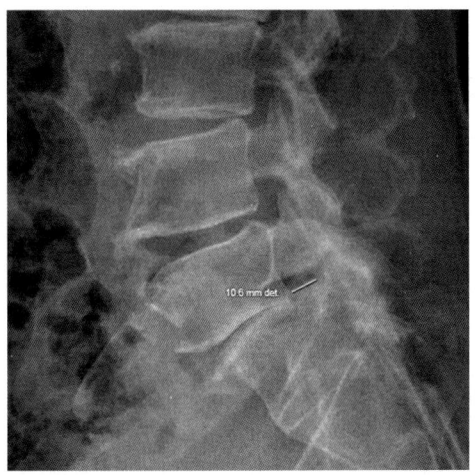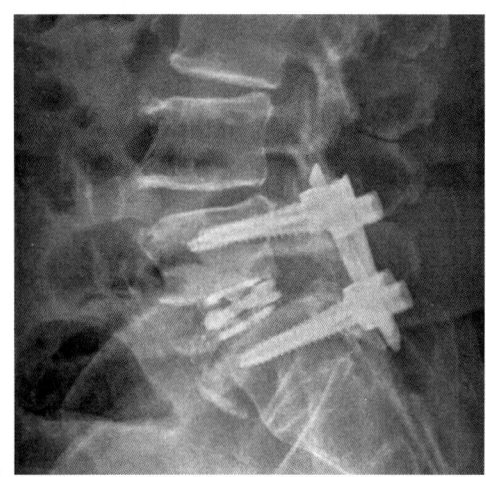

A   B

TECH FIG 9 Reduction of spondylolisthesis (**A**) using rod reduction technique after thorough discectomy and minimally invasive interbody cage placement (**B**).

CLOSURE

- The surgical sites are compressed for 2 to 3 minutes to tamponade muscle bleeding.
- The epidural space is checked. We typically do not find it necessary to use a subfascial drain.
- Muscle fascia is closed with 0 Vicryl on a tapered needle.

- The surgical sites are compressed again for 2 to 3 minutes.
- The dermis is closed with 2-0 Vicryl on a tapered needle.
- A topical skin adhesive (eg, Dermabond) is used to seal the skin.

INCIDENTAL DUROTOMY

- The patient can be placed into Trendelenburg to minimize leakage.
- A suture repair is performed, if possible.
- For small durotomies (<5 mm), we have found a layered patch to be effective. A collagen matrix patch (eg, DuraGen) is sealed with fibrin glue (eg, Tisseel). This is repeated with progressively larger collagen matrix patches. We typically use three layers

(ie, patch, fibrin glue, second patch, fibrin glue, third patch, fibrin glue).
- Cerebrospinal fluid leakage is rarely a problem because of the minimal dead space.
- Patients are placed supine with the head of bed flat postoperatively for 6 to 12 hours.

Pearls and Pitfalls

Patient Selection	• As with all spinal surgery, proper patient selection is the key to successful outcomes. Osteoporotic patients, obese patients, and patients with isthmic spondylolisthesis are challenging and should be avoided during the initial learning curve for this minimally invasive technique.
C-arm Placement	• The C-arm should be placed on the opposite side of the TLIF exposure to allow for frequent image capture.
Retractor Positioning for Contralateral Decompression	• The angulation of the retractor is the key to obtaining adequate exposure to perform a contralateral decompression. Removal of the base of the spinous process can aid in obtaining adequate visualization.
Preservation of Pars	• Preserving the pars protects the exiting nerve root and helps avoid nerve irritation/injury during cage insertion.
Removal of Bone Superolateral to Pedicle	• Ensuring removal of anterior longitudinal ligament bone superolateral to the caudad pedicle clears the corridor for cage placement and prevents medial migration of the cage into the traversing root during insertion.
Removal of Posterior Lip	• Lessens the risk of endplate disruption from discectomy instrumentation and eases graft sizing and placement
Endplate Violation	• Avoid aggressive use of discectomy instruments, especially in osteoporotic patients. If an endplate defect occurs, placement of a second cage may be helpful to avoid graft subsidence. Alternatively, a fresh, contralateral approach can be used.
Pedicle Cannulation	• Properly aligned AP and lateral imaging is crucial to safe pedicle screw placement. Serial imaging going from "imperfect" to "perfect" back to "imperfect," improves identification of "perfect" imaging. Oblique imaging is useful for medially angulated pedicles.
Inadvertent Guidewire Advancement	• Images should be taken frequently during tapping and screw placement.
Muscle/Fascia Entrapment	• Finger palpation around the rod and screws heads easily identifies muscle/fascia that get entrapped under the rod. These should be released prior to wound closure.

POSTOPERATIVE CARE

- Perioperative antibiotic prophylaxis.
- Patients are mobilized early (ie, day of surgery)
- Antispasmodic medications are a useful addition to the postoperative pain control regimen.
- Oral steroids can be used for postoperative radiculitis. This should be a diagnosis of exclusion; new or unexpected postoperative neurologic symptoms or signs should be investigated with imaging.

OUTCOMES

- The literature supports earlier postoperative recovery, less blood loss, less opioid use, and decreased rates of infection in comparison to standard TLIF. Fusion rates are comparable to open posterior interbody fusion techniques.

COMPLICATIONS

- Infection
  - The risk of infection with MIS TLIF appears to be decreased in comparison to standard techniques.
- Bleeding
  - Bleeding is rarely enough to require transfusion.
  - Epidural bleeding can lead to epidural hematoma. Risk of epidural hematoma is minimized with meticulous technique and careful use of bipolar electrocautery and flowable hemostatic agents.
- Nerve injury
  - Releasing the dural tube from the posterior vertebral body minimizes the risk of injury to the traversing nerve root during cage insertion, which is especially important in revision cases.
  - Maintaining the pars protects the exiting nerve root during cage insertion.
  - The procedure may need to be aborted or done on the contralateral side if conjoined or anomalous nerve root anatomy is identified.
  - New or unexpected postoperative neurologic deficit should be worked up expeditiously. Reexploration to evacuate epidural hematoma and ensure there is no neural entrapment should be considered in the perioperative period as necessary.
- Cerebrospinal fluid leakage
  - Suture repair is usually not necessary. Most durotomies tend to be small and can be sealed with layered collagen matrix patch and fibrin sealant.

- Hardware issues
  - Graft subsidence can occur with endplate violation and lead to pedicle screw failure. Care must be taken to avoid endplate violation, especially with elderly osteoporotic patients.
  - Pedicle screw breach is possible. Medial breaches may occur more frequently in comparison to standard techniques because of the ease of medial angulation through the paramedian exposure. Accurate, reliable radiographic imaging is crucial. Neuromonitoring is a useful adjunct.
- Adjacent segment degeneration
  - May be minimized in comparison to standard techniques as a result of the preservation of adjacent segment musculotendinous attachments. Compromise of the cranial facet during screw placement must be avoided.

SUGGESTED READINGS

Goldstein CL, Macwan K, Sundararajan K, et al. Perioperative outcomes and adverse events of minimally invasive versus open posterior lumbar fusion: meta-analysis and systematic review. J Neurosurg Spine 2016;24:416–427.

Hockley A, Ge D, Vazquez-Montes D, et al. Minimally invasive versus open transforaminal lumbar interbody fusion surgery: an analysis of opioids, nonopioid analgesics, and perioperative characteristics. Global Spine J 2019;9(6):624–629.

Kim CW, Garfin SR, Fessler RG. Rationale of minimally invasive spine surgery. In: Herkowitz HN, Garfin SR, Eismont FJ, et al, eds. Rothman-Simeone The Spine, ed 6. Philadelphia: Elsevier Saunders, 2011:998–1006.

McGirt MJ, Parker SL, Lerner J, et al. Comparative analysis of perioperative surgical site infection after minimally invasive versus open posterior/transforaminal lumbar interbody fusion: analysis of hospital billing and discharge data from 5170 patients. J Neurosurg Spine 2011;14(6):771–778.

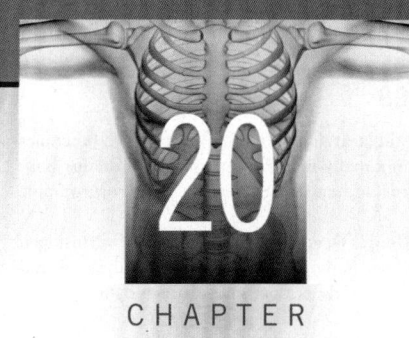

CHAPTER 20

Minimally Invasive Lumbar Microdiscectomy and Laminectomy

Michael Chang, Jose A. Canseco, Christopher K. Kepler, and David Greg Anderson

DEFINITION

- Lumbar microdiscectomy is the most common spinal operation.[2,10,15]
- Lumbar spinal stenosis is the most common indication for spinal surgery in elderly patients.[10]
- The pathology of lumbar spinal stenosis is a combination of degenerative changes involving the disc space, facet joints, and ligamentum flavum, which ultimately leads to compression of the neural elements and, in some cases, neurogenic symptoms.[14]
- Studies have shown favorable outcomes from surgery for patients with herniated disc disease and lumbar stenosis, especially after a failed course of nonoperative management.[2,3,10,15,23]
- Minimally invasive (as opposed to traditional open) lumbar decompression has been shown to decrease trauma to myoligamentous structures surrounding the spine, lessen perioperative morbidity, and quicken patient recovery.[1,8,12,14,17,24,26]
- This chapter reviews the technique of performing minimally invasive lumbar decompression for herniated disc disease and lumbar stenosis via microendoscopy.

HISTORY AND PHYSICAL FINDINGS

- Although the exact clinical presentation varies from person to person, most patients with herniated disc disease and lumbar stenosis present with pain radiating into the lower extremities, or sciatica.
- The classic presentation of herniated disc disease involves pain radiating into a single extremity, usually along a dermatomal distribution between L4 and S1. There are often associated neurologic findings, including changes in strength, sensation, and reflexes.
- The classic presentation of lumbar stenosis is neurogenic claudication, which involves crampy pain radiating into one or both extremities when standing and walking. The pain commonly progresses from proximal to distal and is improved or relieved by spinal flexion (ie, leaning forward or sitting down). This pain ameliorating behavior is usually termed the *shopping cart sign*, as this is the activity that is most commonly described by patients to provide symptom relief.
  - This is in contrast to vascular claudication, which is relieved by standing still. Significant neurologic deficits in lumbar stenosis are uncommon; however, those with herniated disc disease will commonly show changes in reflexes, motor, and sensory functioning. Acute loss of bowel or bladder control in the setting of significant compression of the cauda equina is a surgical emergency.
- Nonsurgical measures that may be considered for both herniated disc disease and lumbar stenosis include nonsteroidal anti-inflammatory drugs, epidural steroids, and physical therapy.[5]

SURGICAL MANAGEMENT

Preoperative Planning

- Surgical intervention may be considered for patients with severe, ongoing symptoms of leg pain that are unresponsive to nonsurgical therapy.[13]
- Patients who are elderly, obese, and/or medically frail may particularly benefit from the minimally invasive nature of microendoscopic lumbar decompression.[26]
- It is important to demonstrate anatomic compression of lumbar nerve roots in a distribution that correlates to the clinical symptoms. This is usually done with either magnetic resonance imaging or computed tomography myelography.[13]

Positioning

- The procedure is typically done under general anesthesia, although epidural or spinal anesthesia may be used according to surgeon's preference.
- Prior to surgery, prophylactic antibiotics and lower extremity compression stockings are administered.
- The patient is positioned prone on a spinal frame, which allows fluoroscopic imaging of the spine (FIG 1).
- Care should be taken to ensure no compression of the abdominal region.
- Care should be taken to ensure accessibility for fluoroscopic imaging.
- A standard sterile preparation and drape of the lumbar region is performed.

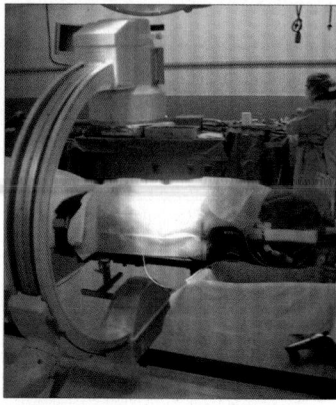

FIG 1 Positioning of the patient in the prone position on a radiolucent operative table.

UNILATERAL MICROENDOSCOPIC DECOMPRESSION

Incision

- Palpable landmarks, including posterior superior iliac spine, intercrestal line, and spinous processes, are demarcated and used to determine the approximate level for the skin incision.
- A spinal needle is introduced lateral to the midline in the proposed location of the surgical incision and directed to avoid penetration of the spinal canal (minimizing inadvertent penetration of the dura) **(TECH FIG 1)**.
- The C-arm is used to obtain a lateral projection of the spine and spinal needle so the location and trajectory of the needle can be used to plan the incision.
- A skin incision equal in length to the diameter of the tubular retractor is made through the skin and underlying fascia. The incision is placed lateral to the spinous process.

Placement of the Tubular Retractor

- In cases of herniated disc disease, the incision is made on the side of the herniation.
- In cases of lumbar stenosis, the incision is positioned on the side that will give the best access to both sides of the spinal canal or will allow decompression of the region of symptomatic stenosis without sacrificing excessive facet joint or overthinning the pars interarticularis region.
- For ipsilateral decompression, the skin incision is generally positioned about 1.5 to 2 cm from the midline.
- For bilateral decompression, the skin incision is generally positioned 3 to 4 cm lateral to the midline to allow angulation of the tubular retractor across the midline to reach the contralateral side of the spinal canal.
- A small Cobb elevator is used to elevate the periosteum at the site of the operative exposure **(TECH FIG 2A)**. We prefer to use this rather than dilation over a Kirschner wire (K-wire), which has the risk of penetrating the dura and is less effective in creating the working space adjacent to the lamina.

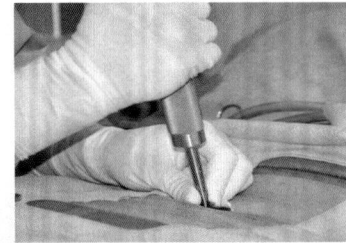

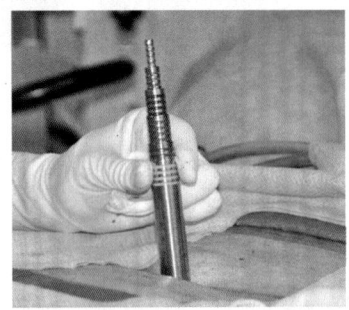

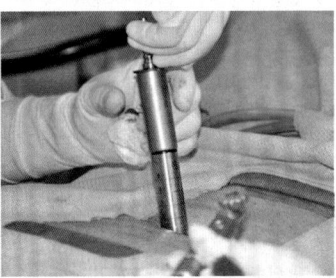

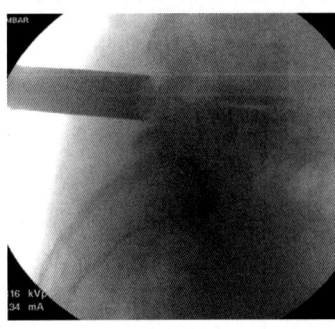

TECH FIG 2 A. Use of a Cobb elevator to perform subperiosteal dissection. **B.** Serial dilators are placed to allow placement of the tubular retractor. **C.** Placement of the tubular retractor. **D.** Lateral fluoroscopic image to confirm appropriate level and position of the tubular retractor.

- Dilators are placed through the incision to expand the operative portal **(TECH FIG 2B)**.
- A tubular retractor of appropriate length is selected and placed over the dilators to the level of the spine **(TECH FIG 2C)**.
- The diameter of the tubular retractor used depends on the nature of the planned surgical procedure. As a general rule, a 14- to 18-mm diameter tubular retractor is used for a

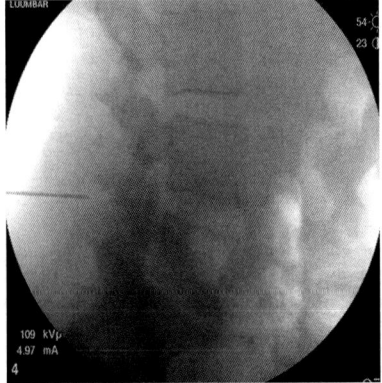

TECH FIG 1 Spinal needle is used to demarcate the proposed location for the surgical incision.

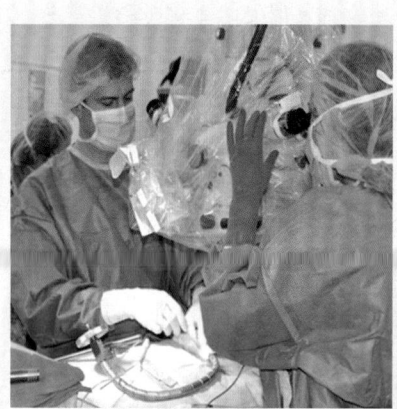
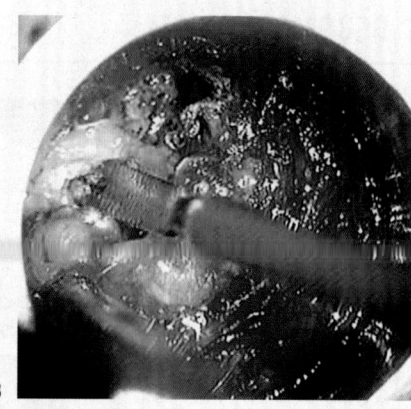

TECH FIG 3 A. Positioning of the microscope to visualize the tissue at the base of the tubular retractor. **B.** Use of the electrocautery to clear soft tissue and expose the bony anatomy.

microdiscectomy procedure, whereas an 18- to 20-mm tubular retractor is used for spinal stenosis cases.

- The tubular retractor is secured to the table-mounted retractor holder, and the position of the retractor is verified with lateral fluoroscopy **(TECH FIG 2D)**.
- If necessary, the position of the tubular retractor is adjusted to allow optimal access to the spinal pathology.
- Use of a sharp K-wire prior to sequential dilation is avoided as an incidental dural puncture can occur.
- An appropriate length of the tubular retractor should reach from the skin edge to the spine to minimize soft tissue creep at the base of the retractor.

Visualization through the Tubular Retractor

- An operative microscope is focused on the tissue at the base of the tubular retractor **(TECH FIG 3A)**.
- The residual soft tissue at the base of the tubular retractor should be resected with electrocautery to allow good visualization of the bony elements **(TECH FIG 3B)**.
- Care should be taken to avoid injury to the facet joint capsule during soft tissue clearance.

Ipsilateral Decompression

- Before the decompression begins, the inferior edge of the lamina, underlying ligamentum flavum, and medial portion of the facet joint should be identified.
- It is helpful to palpate the lateral edge of the pars interarticularis to avoid excessive resection of bone, which could result in an iatrogenic pars fracture.
- The ligamentum flavum is released from the undersurface of the lamina using a curved curette.
- The medial lamina is removed using a Kerrison rongeur.
- The ligamentum flavum is traversed with a straight curette by dividing the ligamentum in line with its fibers.
- The ligamentum flavum is resected with a Kerrison rongeur as necessary to visualize and remove the spinal pathology.
- The pedicle is identified by palpation within the spinal canal and used as a landmark for identification of the spinal pathology.
- The ventral surface of the spinal canal and intervertebral discs can be visualized by gentle retraction of the dura.
- Any sequestered disc material is removed by "sweeping" the free disc fragments into the laminotomy site using a ball-tipped probe.

- Extruded disc material is generally removed by breaking the thin, inflammatory membrane over the herniation with a Penfield no. 4 instrument and working through the existing annular tear.
- The use of large annular incisions is discouraged, as they may predispose to recurrent disc herniation.
- If lateral recess stenosis is present, the medial portion of the superior articular process is trimmed using a curved-tip Kerrison rongeur.
- Ipsilateral foraminal stenosis can also be addressed by using a curved-tip Kerrison rongeur to trim the superior tip of the superior articular process.
- After an adequate decompression of the neural elements has been achieved and confirmed with palpation using a ball-tipped probe, hemostasis of the wound should be achieved prior to closure.
- Avoid overthinning the inferior articular process or pars interarticularis, which may fracture, leading to instability or persistent pain.
- If the high-speed burr (drill) is to be used to thin the bone prior to resection, leave the ligamentum flavum intact during drilling to protect the dura **(TECH FIG 4)**. We prefer to use a 3-mm round burr rather than a matchstick style of burr, as it is felt to be more controllable, especially when "end cutting."
- Palpate between the dura and the overlying bone to ensure that an adequate plane exists prior to resection of the bone, as this will lessen the risk of an iatrogenic dural laceration.
- Neovascularization around the nerve root can easily be appreciated while working under the microscope and is a good clinical sign of a symptomatic lesion.

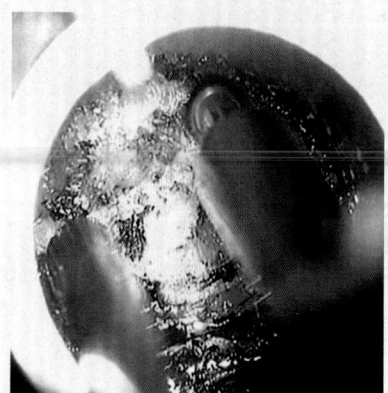

TECH FIG 4 Use of a high-speed burr/drill to thin the lamina.

BILATERAL DECOMPRESSION THROUGH A UNILATERAL TUBULAR APPROACH

- When stenotic changes affect both sides of the spinal canal and cause bilateral neurogenic symptoms, a bilateral decompression of the neural elements should be performed (**TECH FIG 5A**).
- The side of the incision is generally chosen to allow optimal access to the pathology, remembering that foraminal stenosis is often easiest to decompress on the contralateral side.
- The incision is localized in a fashion similar to the unilateral decompression but is placed 3 to 4 cm lateral to the midline to allow the tubular retractor to be angulated to reach the contralateral side of the spinal canal.
- After docking the tubular retractor on the lamina and confirming the localization of the tubular retractor with fluoroscopy, an ipsilateral bony laminotomy is performed, leaving the ligamentum in place.
- The tubular retractor is then angled toward the contralateral side of the spinal canal and the operating table is tilted to provide the most direct microscopic visualization of the contralateral side.
- Drilling is carried out to provide access to the contralateral side of the spinal canal by removal of the base of the spinous process and the undersurface of the contralateral lamina.
- As the drilling proceeds, the surgeon will notice the cancellous bone of the inferior articular process.

- The drilling should continue until the facet joint is thin enough that it can be trimmed (medial facetectomy) with a Kerrison rongeur.
- Throughout drilling, the ligamentum flavum should be preserved to protect the underlying dura.
- On the contralateral side, the ligamentum flavum is released ventral to the facet joint, and the thickness of the residual facet joint can be palpated and assessed.
- After the facet joint is sufficiently thinned and drilling is completed, a curette is used to release the bony attachments of the ligamentum flavum, which is then removed.
- The contralateral pedicle is identified by palpation.
- The exiting and traversing nerve roots are identified.
- Bone and ligament decompression is achieved as needed to decompress the neural structures (**TECH FIG 5B**).
- After completion of the contralateral decompression, the tubular retractor is wanded back to the ipsilateral side. Decompression of the ipsilateral side is achieved in a similar manner as described.
- Meticulous hemostasis is performed, followed by tube withdrawal and wound closure.

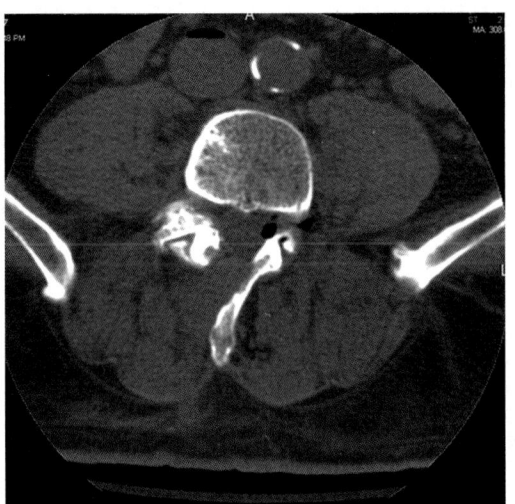

Midline

Dural sac

Foot   Head

Nerve root

Right side

A   B

TECH FIG 5 **A.** Bilateral decompression of the spinal canal is accomplished by drilling away the base of the spinous process and traversing to the contralateral side of the spinal canal. The contralateral facet is trimmed as needed to decompress the spinal canal. The tube is then redirected, and the ipsilateral side of the spinal canal is decompressed until the dura is free of any compression. **B.** Adequate decompression is achieved when no further compression of the dura is present.

WOUND CLOSURE

- Deep tissue (thoracolumbar fascia, if possible) is closed with interrupted suture followed by closure of the subcutaneous tissue and skin.

- The subcutaneous incision is infiltrated with a long-acting local anesthetic agent, and a surgical dressing is placed.

Pearls and Pitfalls

- Localize the incision fluoroscopically.
- Use a small Cobb elevator to separate the soft tissues from the lamina prior to inserting the tubular retractor.
- Use a surgical microscope for optimal visualization of the surgical field.
- Palpate the plane of the nerve root prior to bone removal to reduce the odds of a dural tear.
- Keep the ligamentum flavum intact during use of the surgical drill to reduce the risk of dural injury.
- Ensure adequate decompression of the neural elements of direct palpation and visualization.
- Ensure meticulous hemostasis at the conclusion of the procedure.

POSTOPERATIVE CARE

- Routine postanesthesia recovery is performed.
- The patient is then mobilized for ambulation and activities of daily living.
- Discharge is generally performed on the day of surgery. A 30-minute-per-day walking program is recommended.
- Pain management is achieved with either a mild oral narcotic or an over-the-counter medication, such as ibuprofen or acetaminophen, depending on the patient's individual pain control requirements.
- An office visit and wound check is performed 10 to 14 days after surgery.
- Early outpatient physical therapy to assist in rehabilitation is often recommended.

OUTCOMES

- Studies have reported improved outcomes with lumbar decompression when compared to nonoperative modalities with respect to mobility, endurance, and pain control.[2,3,7,10,22]
- The benefits of minimally invasive versus traditional open approaches in the degenerative lumbar spine, in relation to symptom relief and quality of life, are largely equivocal.[8,23,25]
- However, microendoscopic lumbar decompression has the advantage of reduced intraoperative blood loss, limited soft tissue dissection, and preserved posterior stability. All of which correlates with shorter hospital stays.[4,8,11,18,19,20,24,26]

COMPLICATIONS

- As with all surgical procedures, complications occur with minimally invasive spinal decompression procedures.
- The incidence of problems can be minimized with careful technique and experience with these procedures. Microendoscopic lumbar surgery, more so than other approaches, exhibits a steep learning curve. One study demonstrated an 18% incidence of neurologic complications for the first third of cases and then a marked decrease to 6.3% for the last two-thirds.[8,13,26]
- The incidence of dural tear for minimally invasive spine surgery varies and according to the largest studies likely hovers around 5.3% to 9.4%.[13,21]
- When using a tubular retractor, very little soft tissue dead space is created, and thus, even with small dural tears, the incidence of pseudomeningocele or dural cutaneous fistula is very low even if formal dural suture repair is not used.[25]
- Small dural tears (<1 cm) with no nerve rootlet extrusion may be successfully treated with a small pledget of Gelfoam followed by dural sealant.[21,23,25]
- Larger tears or those with exposed nerve roots should undergo a formal dural repair with suture in a watertight fashion.[25]
- Suture repair should be accomplished working through the tubular retractor using a micropituitary instrument as a needle holder and using double-armed 6-0 Gore-Tex suture. An arthroscopic knot pusher is used to tie knots during the repair.[6,9]
- Infection rates from tubular decompression surgery are very low. In the rare event of a wound infection, treatment with débridement and appropriate antibiotic therapy should be employed.[16]

CONCLUSION

- Minimally invasive surgery for lumbar spinal stenosis and/or intervertebral disc herniation is an effective procedure with many advantages compared with traditional open lumbar decompression.

REFERENCES

1. Asgarzadie F, Khoo LT. Minimally invasive operative management for lumbar spinal stenosis: overview of early and long-term outcomes. Orthop Clin North Am 2007;38(3):387–399.
2. Atlas SJ, Keller RB, Robson D, et al. Surgical and nonsurgical management of lumbar spinal stenosis: four-year outcomes from the Maine Lumbar Spine Study. Spine (Phila Pa 1976) 2000;25(5):556–562.
3. Atlas SJ, Keller RB, Wu Y, et al. Long-term outcomes of surgical and nonsurgical management of lumbar spinal stenosis: 8 to 10 year results from the Maine Lumbar Spine Study. Spine (Phila Pa 1976) 2005;30(8):936–943.
4. Benz RJ, Garfin SR. Current techniques of decompression of the lumbar spine. Clin Orthop Relat Res 2001;(384):75–81.
5. Birkmeyer N, Weinstein J, Tosteson A, et al. Design of the Spine Patient Outcomes Research Trial (SPORT). Spine (Phila Pa 1976) 2002;27(12):1361–1372.
6. Chou D, Wang V, Khan A. Primary dural repair during minimally invasive microdiscectomy using standard operating room instruments. Neurosurgery 2009;64(5 suppl 2):356–358.
7. Cummins J, Lurie J, Tosteson T, et al. Descriptive epidemiology and prior healthcare utilization of patients in the Spine Patient Outcomes Research Trial's (SPORT) three observational cohorts: disc herniation, spinal stenosis, and degenerative spondylolisthesis. Spine (Phila Pa 1976) 2006;31(7):806–814.
8. Garg B, Nagraja U, Jayaswal A. Microendoscopic versus open discectomy for lumbar disc herniation: a prospective randomised study. J Orthop Surg (Hong Kong) 2011;19(1):30–34.
9. Ghobrial G, Maulucci C, Viereck M, et al. Suture choice in lumbar dural closure contributes to variation in leak pressures: experimental model. Clin Spine Surg 2017;30(6):272–275.
10. Gibson J, Waddell G. Surgery for degenerative lumbar spondylosis: updated Cochrane review. Spine (Phila Pa 1976) 2005;30(20):2312–2320.
11. Guiot BH, Khoo LT, Fessler RG. A minimally invasive technique for decompression of the lumbar spine. Spine (Phila Pa 1976) 2002;27(4):432–438.
12. Ikuta K, Tono O, Oga M. Clinical outcome of microendoscopic posterior decompression for spinal stenosis associated with degenerative spondylolisthesis—minimum 2-year outcome of 37 patients. Minim Invasive Neurosurg 2008;51(5):267–271.

13. Ikuta K, Tono O, Tanaka T, et al. Surgical complications of microendoscopic procedures for lumbar spinal stenosis. Minim Invasive Neurosurg 2007;50(3):145–149.
14. Khoo LT, Fessler RG. Microendoscopic decompressive laminotomy for the treatment of lumbar stenosis. Neurosurgery 2002;51(suppl 5):S146–S154.
15. Lurie J, Tosteson T, Tosteson A, et al. Surgical versus nonoperative treatment for lumbar disc herniation: eight-year results for the Spine Patient Outcomes Research Trial. Spine (Phila Pa 1976) 2014;39(1):3–16.
16. Ogihara S, Yamazaki T, Inanami H, et al. Risk factors for surgical site infection after lumbar laminectomy and/or discectomy for degenerative diseases in adults: a prospective multicenter surveillance study with registry of 4027 cases. PLoS One 2018;13(10):e0205539.
17. Palmer S, Turner R, Palmer R. Bilateral decompression of lumbar spinal stenosis involving a unilateral approach with microscope and tubular retractor system. J Neurosurg 2002;97(2 suppl):213–217.
18. Park P, Foley KT. Minimally invasive transforaminal lumbar interbody fusion with reduction of spondylolisthesis: technique and outcomes after a minimum of 2 years' follow-up. Neurosurg Focus 2008;25(2):E16.
19. Podichetty VK, Spear J, Isaacs RE, et al. Complications associated with minimally invasive decompression for lumbar spinal stenosis. J Spinal Disord Tech 2006;19(3):161–166.
20. Rosen DS, O'Toole JE, Eichholz KM, et al. Minimally invasive lumbar spinal decompression in the elderly: outcomes of 50 patients aged 75 years and older. Neurosurgery 2007;60(3):503–509.
21. Ruban D, O'Toole J. Management of incidental durotomy in minimally invasive spine surgery. Neurosurg Focus 2011;31(4):E15.
22. Shriver M, Xie J, Tye E, et al. Lumbar microdiscectomy complication rates: a systematic review and meta-analysis. Neurosurg Focus 2015;39(4):E6.
23. Turner JA, Ersek M, Herron L, et al. Surgery for lumbar spinal stenosis. Attempted meta-analysis of the literature. Spine (Phila Pa 1976) 1992;17(1):1–8.
24. Wang Y, Liang Z, Wu J, et al. Comparative clinical effectiveness of tubular microdiscectomy and conventional microdiscectomy for lumbar disc herniation. Spine (Phila Pa 1976) 2019;44(14):1025–1033.
25. Wolff S, Kheirredine W, Riouallon G. Surgical dural tears: prevalence and updated management protocol based on 1359 lumbar vertebra interventions. Orthop Traumatol Surg Res 2012;98(8):879–886.
26. Wong A, Smith Z, Lall R, et al. The microendoscopic decompression of lumbar stenosis: a review of the current literature and clinical results. Minim Invasive Surg 2012:2012:325095.

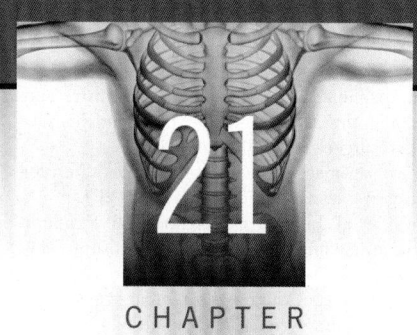

21
CHAPTER

Percutaneous Pedicle Screw Fixation and Fusion for Trauma

Jacob J. Bruckner, David J. Love, Jael E. Camacho, and Steven C. Ludwig

DEFINITION

- The advancement of minimally invasive techniques in spinal surgery, specifically percutaneous pedicle screw fixation, has reduced approach-related morbidity.
- Minimally invasive techniques have been shown to be advantageous in patients with spine tumors and deformities and have become increasingly applicable for managing complex spinal trauma, including thoracolumbar trauma.
- Allows internal bracing of unstable fractures while maintaining sagittal alignment
- The goals of treatment of traumatic spine fracture remain the same whether an open or percutaneous approach is used: Stabilize the spine to facilitate rehabilitation; enhance neurologic recovery; and prevent neurologic deterioration, delayed pain, and postoperative deformity.

ANATOMY

- Traditional open posterior surgical approaches can result in extensive soft tissue damage, muscle denervation, and ischemia, with subsequent paraspinal muscular atrophy and decreased strength.
- In addition, open approaches can lead to increased blood loss, protracted postoperative pain, and higher infection rates.
- In contrast, minimally invasive procedures involve less extensive and thus less disruptive dissection. Important relevant anatomy and anatomic landmarks are discussed in following text.

PATHOGENESIS

- The most common mechanisms of traumatic injury to the thoracolumbar spine are both simple and high-energy falls, motor vehicle collisions, sports injuries, and violence.
- When traumatic injury results in spinal cord injury, the loss of neurologic function is attributed to both a primary and a secondary injury process.
- The primary injury is sustained when the spinal cord and spinal column absorb energy from the trauma, with resultant spinal deformation and persistent postinjury compression.
- A cascade of secondary effects ensues, including vascular changes, cell membrane lipid peroxidation, free radical formation, electrolyte shifts, neurotransmitter accumulation, and inflammation. This cascade results in expansion of the initial area of injury in a craniocaudal fashion, leading to further gray matter loss and white matter degeneration.

IMAGING AND OTHER DIAGNOSTIC STUDIES

- Preoperative advanced imaging is a critical tool for understanding the patient's pathoanatomy and preoperative planning.
- Commonly, computed tomography (CT) and magnetic resonance imaging (MRI) scans are obtained to assess bony and spinal cord injury, respectively.
- Additionally, MRI can be used to assess the competency of the posterior ligamentous structures, which can assist in determining the overall stability of the injury.
- Using preoperative images as a guide, the fluoroscope can then be precisely rotated in the axial plane to the degree of medial angulation seen on axial view CT or MRI scans at the respective level.

NONOPERATIVE MANAGEMENT

- Thoracolumbar trauma has historically been managed with conservative treatment in the form of traction, casting, and bed rest.
- However, nonoperative treatment can be complicated by the morbidity of prolonged immobilization, namely pneumonia, deep vein thrombosis, and decubitus ulcers.
- Nonoperative management can take several forms but typically is achieved with thoracolumbar orthosis for 8 to 12 weeks with frequent follow-up and radiographic imaging to ensure healing.

SURGICAL MANAGEMENT

- Indications for minimally invasive percutaneous pedicle screw fixation are dependent on fracture type, patient characteristics, and surgeon preference. Single-level thoracolumbar burst fractures have better outcomes when done through minimally invasive spine surgery (MISS).[5]
- Relative indications include unstable thoracolumbar burst fractures, stable burst fractures that have failed nonoperative management, flexion/extension injuries, and unstable pelvic fractures that require lumbopelvic fixation.
- Multiple variables are important when considering surgical intervention, including fracture morphology, neurologic involvement, and the status of the posterior ligamentous complex.
- Some patients may not be amenable to percutaneous fixation, due to obesity, osteopenia, and rotational deformities that can make fluoroscopic targeting difficult.
- Other contraindications may include multilevel vertebral fractures, pedicle fractures, adjacent body fractures, and severe neural deficits requiring canal decompression, although further data is required.[9]

- The Thoracolumbar Injury Classification and Severity Score can be used to help guide the surgeon's decision-making process for operative versus nonoperative fracture management.
- MISS provides several benefits over traditional open surgery, such as decreased surgical time, decreased blood loss, reduction in postoperative surgical site infections, reduced rates of returning to the operating room, avoiding muscle damage secondary to muscle denervation and ischemia, and improved ability to weight-bear immediately without restriction. This leads to reduced length of stay and improved postoperative mobility.[3,13]
- Recent evidence suggests additional benefits of MISS may include decreased incidence of pneumonia, decreased length of stay in the intensive care unit, shorter number of ventilator-dependent days, and decreased hospital charges.[1,2,8]
- The application of these principles in the setting of spine trauma offers the patient earlier mobilization and rehabilitation.

Preoperative Planning

- Before the surgical procedure, a thorough understanding of the patient's surgical anatomy is essential. Due to the nature of MISS, traditional visual and tactile landmarks for pedicular fixation are not present. Thus, without optimal preoperative fluoroscopic visualization, the surgeon must keep in mind the potential risk for screw malposition.
- Corrective maneuvers for fracture reduction need to be planned. Fracture reduction can be accomplished with a mini-open technique at the fracture level **(FIG 1A)**, through patient positioning, or with more standardized compression-distraction forces through the pedicular implants.
- Achieving biologic fusion is challenging in multilevel traumatic cases, and the benefit of doing so is not entirely clear. If necessary, the fusion procedure can be performed in a staged fashion through a standardized midline approach when the patient is physiologically stable ("damage control").

- Alternatively, in cases in which anterior reconstruction or decompression is indicated, fusion can be achieved anteriorly with stabilization performed in a minimally invasive fashion posteriorly using percutaneous pedicle screws.
- Other options for achieving fusion include the use of a posterior cannula through a midline posterior approach to the facet joint. **FIG 1B** shows a hybrid approach to facet fusion, combining percutaneous fixation and a mini-open technique.

Positioning

- The operative setup and positioning for minimally invasive spine procedures are the same as for conventional open posterior procedures.
- The patient is positioned prone on a radiolucent table.
- Ensure that the eyes are well protected, the cervical spine is in a neutral position, the arms are positioned in 90 degrees of abduction and 90 degrees of elbow flexion, the bony prominences are well padded, and vital structures and distal extremities are protected from incidental injury during the operation. Additionally, the abdomen must be free of compression to improve venous return.

Approach

- Percutaneous pedicle instrumentation can be performed by one of four methods: true anteroposterior (AP) targeting, Magerl (or owl's eye) technique, image-guided navigation, and biplanar fluoroscopy.
- The first two methods are the authors' preferred techniques for the following reasons:
  - By using only a true AP view, the setup is more time efficient.
  - Sterility is better maintained when not alternating between AP and lateral views.
  - Two surgeons can operate simultaneously on both sides, thereby reducing procedure time and radiation exposure.

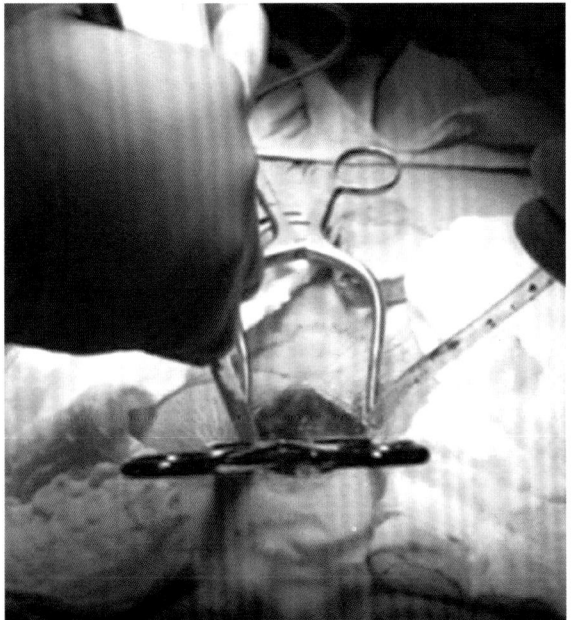
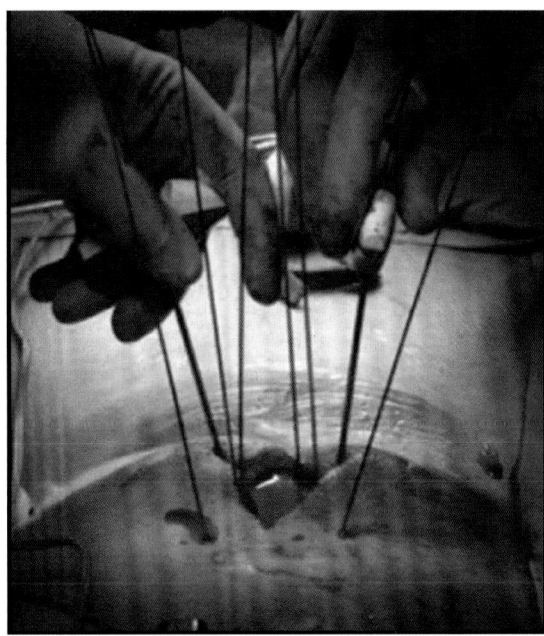

A   B

FIG 1 A. The mini-open technique is used to achieve biologic fusion in addition to percutaneous pedicle screw placement. **B.** Patient with spine trauma being treated with a minimally invasive technique.

FLUOROSCOPIC IMAGING

- When performing MISS, fluoroscopic imaging is essential. The vertebral bodies that require treatment need to be able to be viewed in the AP and lateral views radiographically.
- Following positioning and prior to incision, the surgeon should obtain a true AP view radiograph. A true AP radiograph is when the center of the x-ray beam is parallel to the superior endplate of the vertebra. This creates a single superior endplate shadow, as the anterior and posterior margins of the vertebra are superimposed.

- The spinous processes should be equal distances from the pedicles.
- The pedicle shadows should be just inferior to the superior endplate shadow (TECH FIG 1).
- Upper thoracic imaging may be difficult due to kyphosis. Mayfield head holders may assist in imaging of the upper thoracic spine.

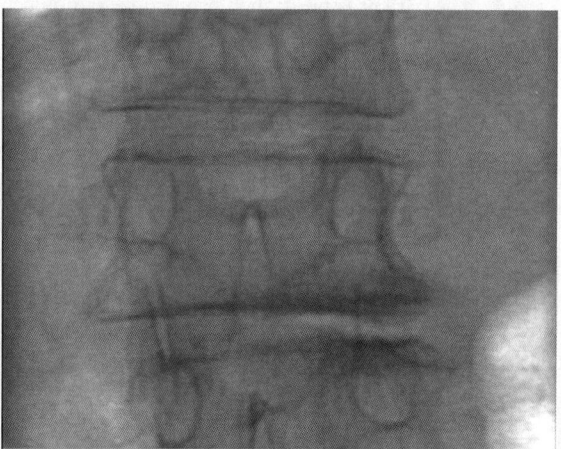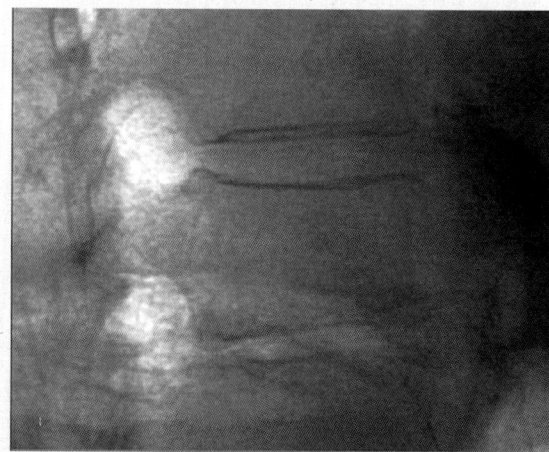

TECH FIG 1 True AP (**A**) and lateral (**B**) view fluoroscopic images obtained before commencing percutaneous needle placement.

PEDICLE STARTING POINTS

- After a true AP fluoroscopy view is obtained, the surgeon defines the starting points on the patient's skin by placing a Kirschner wire (K-wire) longitudinally over the lateral border of the pedicles on either side of the spine, using a skin marker to mark the lateral border.

- A second line is marked through the center of the pedicle, intersecting the first two longitudinal lines.
- Next, skin incisions are marked 1 cm lateral to the intersection of the skin marks. This accounts for the divergent trajectory of the pedicles and helps to better align the skin and fascial incisions with the bony target (TECH FIG 2).

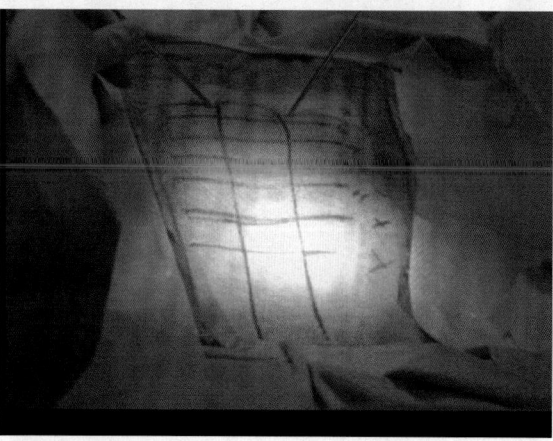

TECH FIG 2 Preoperative skin markings show the minimally invasive screw starting points.

TRUE ANTEROPOSTERIOR VIEW METHOD

- Contraindications: radiographic visualization cannot be obtained (eg, osteopenia, morbid obesity, severely deformed anatomy).
- The skin and fascia are incised, and the muscular tissues are dissected bluntly until the transverse process is palpated. Fascial incisions should be slightly larger than the screw head.
- Jamshidi needles are inserted into the incisions and are docked at the correct starting point for each pedicle: at the intersection of the lateral border of the upgoing facet, the midline of the transverse process, and the upslope of the pars interarticularis.
- A true AP view image is obtained to verify this location, and the needle tip should overlie the midlateral wall of the pedicle (the 3 o'clock position for the patient's right pedicle and the 9 o'clock position for the patient's left pedicle).
- The craniocaudal direction of the needle can be simultaneously verified on fluoroscopy. Once the proper position of the Jamshidi needle is confirmed, it is tapped with a mallet to penetrate a few millimeters into the cortex.
- At that time, the needle shaft can be realigned to be parallel to the superior vertebral endplate.

- The shaft of the Jamshidi needle is then marked 2 cm above the skin to track the depth of penetration into the pedicle. The depth is confirmed by checking the preoperative imaging studies and measuring the length of the pedicle at each level.
- With the needle shaft parallel to the endplate on the true AP view and with 10 to 12 degrees of lateral to medial angulation, the needle is tapped to the depth of the mark on the shaft.
- The tip of the needle should be at the base of the pedicle, anterior to the posterior wall of the vertebral body **(TECH FIG 3)**. A blunt-tipped guidewire is driven through the needle into the cancellous bone and advanced 10 to 15 mm past the tip of the needle.
- Placement is confirmed with lateral fluoroscopy, with the tip of the guidewire just ventral to the pedicle vertebral body junction.
- The needle is removed as the guidewire is held in position, the pedicle is tapped, and a cannulated pedicle screw is inserted. A true lateral view radiograph can be used to confirm the appropriate depth of the screw.
- All the aforementioned steps are performed at each vertebral level to be instrumented.

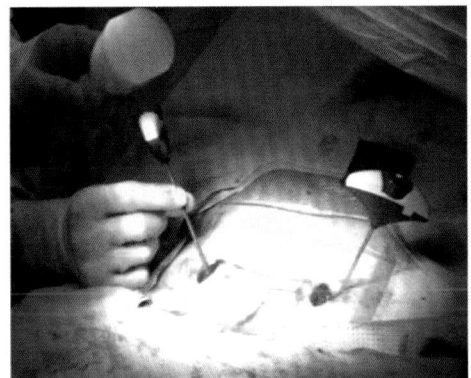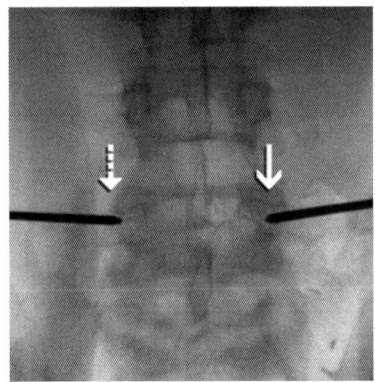

TECH FIG 3 A. The Jamshidi needle being advanced into the pedicle. **B.** AP view fluoroscopic image confirms appropriate placement of the Jamshidi needles within the pedicles.

MAGERL, OR OWL'S EYE, TECHNIQUE

- This method involves a fluoroscopic view along the axis of the pedicle. To obtain the owl's eye (or en face) view, the x-ray beam is positioned directly in line with the pedicle axis.
- First, a true AP view of the vertebra of interest is obtained. The C-arm is then rotated until the x-ray beam is parallel to the pedicle (typically 10 to 30 degrees oblique to the true AP view) **(TECH FIG 4)**.
- Once a proper view has been obtained, the skin incision should be made directly over the pedicle.
- Placement of the Jamshidi needle, K-wire exchange, and pedicle cannulation or screw placement should then be performed in the same manner as with other techniques.

- Intermittent lateral view fluoroscopic images or preoperative images can aid in determining the depth of instrument positioning.
- Obtaining an en face view of the S1 pedicle is achieved in a slightly different manner. Because the pedicle is not cylindrical at the S1 level, only the medial wall is visible on its projection.
- The surgeon must first align the C-arm in the sagittal plane such that the superior sacral endplate appears as a single line. The C-arm is then rotated axially to obtain the maximum resolution of the medial pedicle wall.
- As with the lumbar spine, determination of the medial angulation of the pedicle can be aided with preoperative axial view CT or MRI scans.

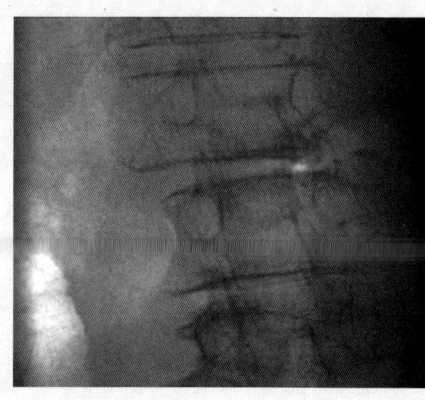

TECH FIG 4 Fluoroscopic image shows the Magerl technique of screw insertion.

IMAGE-GUIDED NAVIGATION[4]

- Ideal reference frame placement is dependent on goals of surgery and anatomy. Common locations are the left ilium inferior to posterior superior iliac spine for short-segment instrumentation or a midline percutaneous incision over a proximal spinous process. The workstation and detector camera were placed at the foot of the bed and head of the bed, respectively.
- Pay careful attention to line of sight issues in order to maximize workflow.
- Using an O arm, three-dimensional CT images are obtained.
- Paramedian lateral based skin incisions are planned with navigating probe as well as planning the pedicle screw trajectories. This ensures accurate incision placement and length.
- Navigated dilator is inserted through the paraspinal muscle interval and docked at ideal pedicle screw starting point.
- Serial dilators are inserted.

- Using a lateral to medial trajectory, a Jamshidi needle is used to enter the center of the bony pedicle canal with the assistance of the axial, coronal, and sagittal guidance.
- Guidewires are inserted through the Jamshidi to maintain trajectory.
- Navigated tap is used to assess the bony pedicle tract and to determine the proper size and length of the screw.
- Rods are then inserted.
- Care should be taken to avoid excessive forces on the operated spine, as they can lead to misplaced instrumentation and inaccuracies from minor spinal displacement.
- Recommend withdrawing guidewires several centimeters after screw is placed in proximal pedicle, reducing the risk of inadvertently advancing guidewires into the abdominal cavity.

ROD PLACEMENT

- A few basic principles allow the successful and efficient percutaneous placement of rods. Screw positioning is of critical importance, with special attention paid to align the screw heads in the coronal and sagittal planes.
- Screw depth is determined by advancing the screws to a position at which they meet slight resistance against the lateral border of the facet joint.
- The tops of the screw extensions and cannulae should demonstrate a smooth transition between levels and symmetric angulation.
- The tops of the screw extensions can be used to assess rod contouring in the appropriate coronal and sagittal planes.
- A precontoured rod should be inserted in a cranial to caudal manner because of the protective, shingling effect of the thoracic and lumbar lamina.
  - To maximize sensory feedback, a two-handed technique should be used (**TECH FIG 5**). The surgeon's dominant hand is placed on the rod holder, and the nondominant hand remains free to manipulate the screw heads.

- An example of the workflow for rod insertion during a multilevel procedure is as follows:
  - First, rod length is measured and the rod is contoured before passage.
  - While pushing the rod, the surgeon can rotate each screw head to allow passage. To confirm successful placement, the surgeon can attempt to rotate the screw heads.
  - If rotation of the screw head is possible, the rod passage must be reattempted.
  - Alternatively, the surgeon can use another instrument, such as a screwdriver, for tactile feedback as the rod passes through each screw head.
- AP and lateral views should be obtained prior to removal of screw extenders.
- Several factors can inhibit rod placement: uneven screw head height, poor rod contouring, interposed muscle and fascia, and bony obstruction.
- If problems encountered during rod placement, screw height or rod contouring can be adjusted.

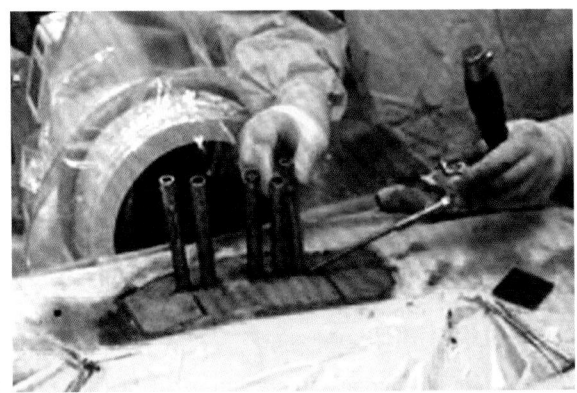

A

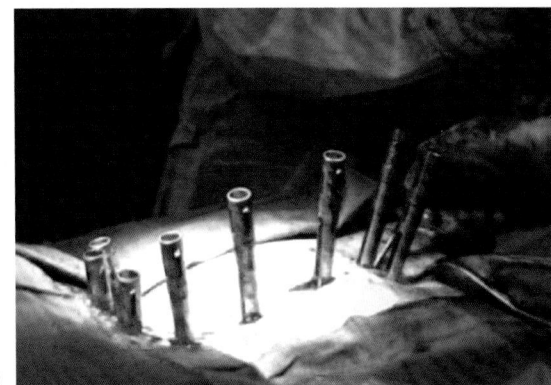

B

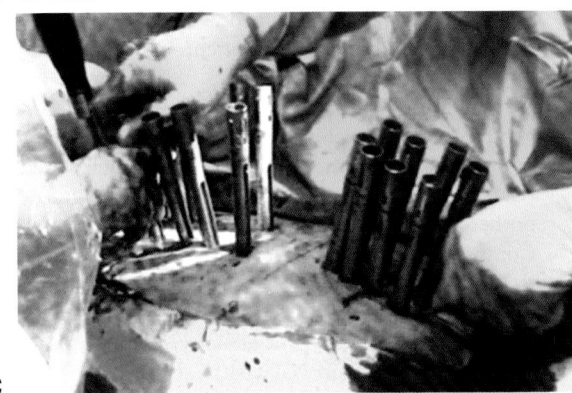

C

TECH FIG 5 A–C. Three different angles and stages of rod placement and passage and technique.

TECHNIQUES

Pearls and Pitfalls

- The owl's eye method can provide an excellent view of the pedicle, but certain disadvantages are associated with the technique.
  - This technique precludes working simultaneously on either side of the patient, requiring realignment of the C-arm twice per level. This increases radiation exposure to the patient and the surgical team.
  - This technique is associated with a higher rate of medial pedicle wall violation, likely secondary to the more medial starting position of the pedicle screws. Because the spinal canal is not well visualized with the en face projection, a medial violation might not be recognized. Therefore, it is critical that pedicle cannulation is started in a lateral position at the junction of the transverse process and facet.
- When longer or curved rods are needed, insertion and positioning of these rods can be challenging.
- Precise and careful positioning of the pedicle screws is essential and should not be overlooked. It is important to remain deep to the fascia and to use the rod's bend to steer the tip and facilitate the passage.
- The development of more advanced implant systems has made multilevel procedures easier to perform.
- Determining proper rod length for multilevel constructs can also be challenging. Although most implant manufacturers have equipment to aid in this process, multiple inspections should be performed using lateral view fluoroscopy to confirm that the rod length is correct.
- Percutaneous pedicle fixation of the upper thoracic spine is more difficult and deserves special consideration because of the inherent magnitude of upper thoracic kyphosis. Poor radiographic visualization is a contraindication to MISS.
- To aid in fluoroscopic imaging, placing the patient's head into a skeletal pin headrest and simultaneously flexing the cervical spine and translating the spine anteriorly may facilitate the process.
  - Positioning the head in this fashion also enables the rod and the rod holder to be manipulated through the upper screw extensions without maneuvering around the patient's head.
- Percutaneously placed multilevel constructs that cross the thoracolumbar junction can also present a challenge.
  - Although the lordotic portion of the rod might pass easily across the thoracic kyphosis, passage of the rod from the upper thoracic region toward the lumbosacral junction generally becomes more difficult as the kyphotic portion of the rod is passed across the thoracic apex.
- Manipulation of the kyphotic portion of the rod into a more coronal plane or a frank lordotic position usually assists the passage of the rod across the thoracic spine. Rod inserters that allow in situ rotation of the rod can help to overcome these challenges.

POSTOPERATIVE CARE

- Standard postoperative care should be delivered to all patients after percutaneous pedicle fixation, including pain control, deep vein thrombosis prophylaxis, and progressive physical therapy.

OUTCOMES

- The literature evaluating the results of MISS with percutaneous pedicle fixation continues to evolve. Several studies have examined the rates of postoperative surgical infection associated with minimally invasive techniques.
- Sun et al[11] performed a meta-analysis and showed that percutaneous approach was superior to open approach in Cobb correction loss; however, open approach was superior in postoperative Cobb angle and vertebral body angle (VBA) correction.
- O'Toole et al[7] reported three surgical site infections among 1338 minimally invasive spinal procedures in 1274 patients with a mean age of 55.5 years. The surgical site infection rate was 0.10% for simple decompressive procedures, 0.74% for fusion and/or fixation procedures, and 0.22% overall. The authors compared their rate with the 2% to 6% reported rates in large clinical series of open spinal procedures and concluded that minimally invasive techniques might reduce postoperative wound infections by nearly 10-fold.
- Wang et al[12] compared 20 patients with type A thoracolumbar fractures treated with traditional open pedicle screw fixation, with 17 patients treated with percutaneous pedicle screw techniques. The authors found that the percutaneously treated cohort had significantly smaller incisions, less estimated blood loss, shorter intraoperative time, decreased lengths of stay, and less postoperative pain.
- Poelstra et al[10] conducted a retrospective review of 10 patients managed with damage control orthopaedics and minimally invasive techniques for unstable thoracolumbar fractures associated with life-threatening injuries.
  - Nonoperative brace treatment was not possible because of fracture type, associated injuries, or body habitus (>300 lb), and all patients were too hemodynamically unstable to undergo open spinal stabilization.
  - Patients were followed for a minimum of 1 year. Postoperative CT scans confirmed that a total of 82 screws in 10 patients were placed without pedicle breaches. Blood loss was an average of 177 mL, and the average length of surgery from time of incision to transfer of the patient to the intensive care unit was 95 minutes.
  - All patients underwent minimally invasive spinal stabilization within 48 hours after injury, all patients survived their trauma, and no revision surgery was performed.
  - The authors concluded that damage control spinal stabilization via a minimally invasive technique is appropriate for patients who have suffered multisystem trauma and complex unstable spinal injuries. However, further studies are needed to assess whether immediate patient survival and eventual functional outcomes are truly improved with an MISS damage control approach.
  - In a patient with multiple traumatic injuries, minimally invasive spinal fixation might play an important role in allowing early stabilization of thoracolumbar spinal fractures and could consequently minimize the morbidities associated with delayed fixation.

- McHenry et al[6] retrospectively reviewed risk factors of respiratory failure in 1032 patients at a level 1 trauma center after operative stabilization of thoracolumbar spinal fractures.
- They found the following five independent risk factors for respiratory failure: age older than 35 years, Injury Severity Score greater than 25 points, Glasgow Coma Scale score below 12 points, blunt chest injury, and surgical stabilization performed more than 2 days after admission.
- They concluded that early operative stabilization of thoracolumbar fractures—the only risk factor that can be controlled by the physician—might decrease the risk of respiratory failure in multiply injured patients.

COMPLICATIONS

- As with any surgical intervention, the benefits of operative stabilization must be weighed against the risks of surgery, especially in a critically ill patient suffering from multiple systemic traumatic injuries.
- Although the risk of blood loss is less compared with conventional open techniques, care should be coordinated among the entire medical team to optimize preoperative risks in cases of hemodynamic instability, coagulopathy, hypothermia, or elevated serum lactate levels.
- Compared with open surgical techniques, postoperative infection rates associated with minimally invasive techniques are substantially reduced. In addition, it has been shown that operative times were shorter, hospital stays were shorter, and there were improved visual analog scale (VAS) functional outcomes with percutaneous approaches to surgery.
- There is no difference in screw malpositioning between open and percutaneous procedures. Studies have also shown that there is no difference between postoperative Cobb angle, postoperative body angle, and postoperative anterior body height.[9]

CONCLUSIONS

- Percutaneous pedicle screw fixation provides a means of internal bracing in fractures while preserving the innervation, blood supply, and musculature of the back.
- The benefits of MISS are reduction of blood loss, shorter operative times, shorter hospital stays, and, importantly, reduction in infection rates.
- When a surgeon is deciding whether to use minimally invasive techniques for traumatic thoracolumbar disorders, he or she needs to establish the proper indications for the procedure, offer the procedure for those cases in which it is superior to performing a conventional open procedure, establish revision strategies if the technique is not effective, and minimize complications.

REFERENCES

1. Cengiz SL, Kalkan E, Bayir A, et al. Timing of thoracolumber spine stabilization in trauma patients; impact on neurological outcome and clinical course. A real prospective (rct) randomized controlled study. Arch Orthop Trauma Surg 2008;128(9):959–966.
2. Croce MA, Bee TK, Pritchard E, et al. Does optimal timing for spine fracture fixation exist? Ann Surg 2001;233(6):851–858.
3. Kerwin AJ, Frykberg ER, Schinco MA, et al. The effect of early surgical treatment of traumatic spine injuries on patient mortality. J Trauma 2007;63(6):1308–1313.
4. Kim TT, Johnson JP, Pashman R, et al. Minimally invasive spinal surgery with intraoperative image-guided navigation. Biomed Res Int 2016;2016:5716235.

5. Kumar A, Aujla R, Lee C. The management of thoracolumbar burst fractures: a prospective study between conservative management, traditional open spinal surgery and minimally interventional spinal surgery. Springerplus 2015;4:204.

6. McHenry TP, Mirza SK, Wang J, et al. Risk factors for respiratory failure following operative stabilization of thoracic and lumbar spine fractures. J Bone Joint Surg Am 2006;88(5):997–1005.

7. O'Toole JE, Eichholz KM, Fessler RG. Surgical site infection rates after minimally invasive spinal surgery. J Neurosurg Spine 2009;11(4): 471–476.

8. Pakzad H, Roffey DM, Knight H, et al. Delay in operative stabilization of spine fractures in multitrauma patients without neurologic injuries: effects on outcomes. Can J Surg 2011;54(4):270–276.

9. Phan K, Rao PJ, Mobbs RJ. Percutaneous versus open pedicle screw fixation for treatment of thoracolumbar fractures: systematic review and meta-analysis of comparative studies. Clin Neurol Neurosurg 2015;135:85–92.

10. Poelstra KA, Gelb D, Kane B, et al. The feasibility of damage control spinal stabilization (MISS) in the acute setting for complex 1 thoracolumbar fractures. Paper presented at: 23rd Meeting of the North American Spine Society; October 14–18, 2008; Toronto, Canada.

11. Sun XY, Zhang XN, Hai Y. Percutaneous versus traditional and paraspinal posterior open approaches for treatment of thoracolumbar fractures without neurologic deficit: a meta-analysis. Eur Spine J 2017;26(5):1418–1431.

12. Wang HW, Li CQ, Zhou Y, et al. Percutaneous pedicle screw fixation through the pedicle of fractured vertebra in the treatment of type A thoracolumbar fractures using Sextant system: an analysis of 38 cases. China J Traumatol 2010;13(3):137–145.

13. Williams SK, Quinnan SM. Percutaneous lumbopelvic fixation for reduction and stabilization of sacral fractures with spinopelvic dissociation patterns. J Orthop Trauma 2016;30(9): e318–e324.

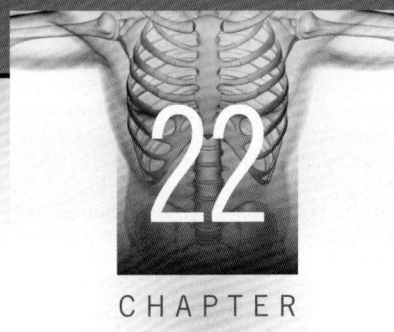

Costotransversectomy for Canal Decompression and Anterior Column Reconstruction via a Posterior Approach

Yu-Po Lee, Saifal-Deen Farhan, and Steven R. Garfin

DEFINITION

Posterolateral (Costotransversectomy) Approach to the Thoracic Spine

- The costotransversectomy uses a posterolateral approach to the thoracic spine. This approach provides access to the posterior spine (**FIG 1A**), the lateral spinal canal (**FIG 1B**), and also to the anterolateral portion of the vertebral body (**FIG 1C**).
- The costotransversectomy approach was first described by Menard in 1894 for drainage of tuberculous abscesses in patients with Pott paraplegia.[1] Various modifications of this procedure have been developed for removal of anterior thoracic disc herniation, traumatic lesions, and metastatic tumors of the spine.[1,4] Other indications now include biopsy and removal of neoplastic tissue(s), resection of fractured bone fragments, spinal cord decompression, and to facilitate various spinal fusions (**FIG 2A–D**).[2–5,7]
- In comparison to the formal anterior thoracotomy, the costotransversectomy approach allows extrapleural access to the thoracic spine. Because the pleural cavity is not violated, this reduces the risk of pulmonary complications.[6,8] Additionally, whereas anterior thoracotomy provides limited access in the regions of the upper thoracic spine and the levels near the diaphragm, the costotransversectomy approach can expose any level of the entire thoracic spine.
- Limitations of the costotransversectomy approach center around its poor visualization of the ventral canal. This makes addressing midline pathology such as broad-based calcified discs or central herniation more difficult via the costotransversectomy approach. Furthermore, a transthoracic approach may be advantageous in situations of multilevel involvement in order to avoid operative blood loss and thoracic cage instability from rib resection.

ANATOMY

- The thoracic vertebrae are chiefly distinguished from the adjacent cervical and lumbar spinal regions by the presence of complex osteoligamentous articulations with the ribs.[9,10]
- Two major articulations account for the costovertebral joint.
  - Ventrally, each thoracic rib articulates with the adjacent vertebral body and rostral intervertebral disc by the anterior costovertebral ligament, also known as the *radiate ligament*. Dorsolaterally, the costotransverse ligaments support the costal articulation with the transverse process.
    - The superior costotransverse ligament extends from the inferior edge of the transverse process to the superior margin of the caudally adjacent vertebrae.
    - The medial costotransverse ligament, also known as the *capsular ligament*, attaches the posterior neck of the rib with the anterior margin of the transverse process.
    - Finally, the lateral costotransverse ligament attaches the transverse process to the posterior costal tubercle.

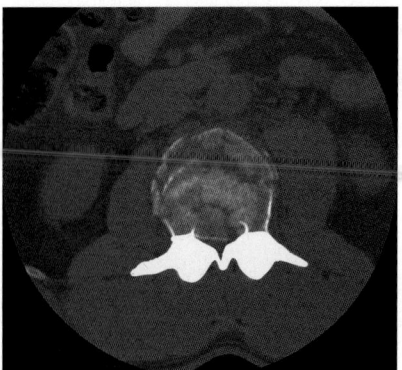
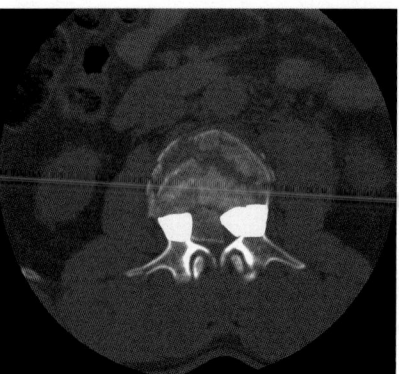
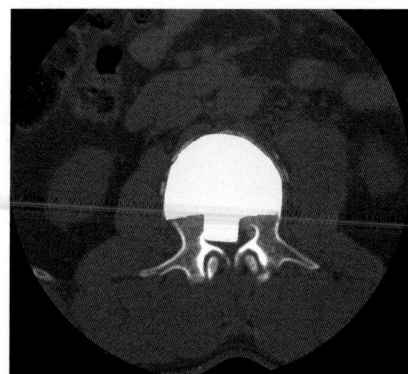

FIG 1 The costotransversectomy approach allows access to the posterior spine (highlighted in *white*) (**A**), the lateral spinal canal (highlighted in *white*) (**B**), and also to the anterolateral portion of the vertebral body (highlighted in *white*) (**C**).

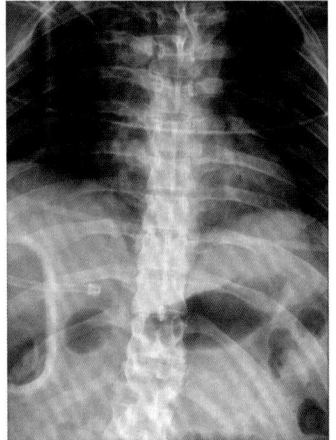 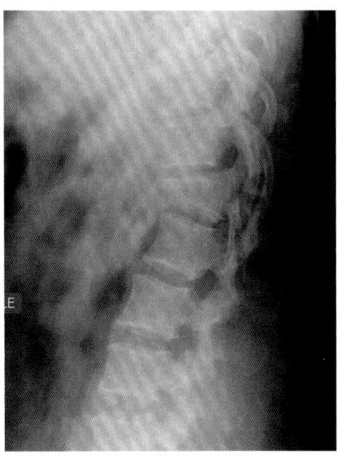 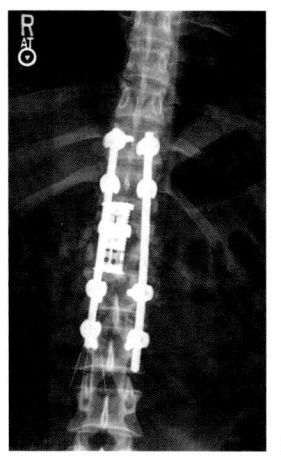 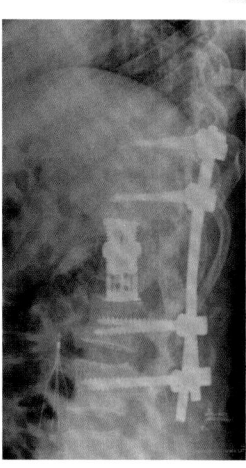

FIG 2 A. AP view of T12 fracture dislocation. **B.** Lateral view of T12 fracture dislocation. The decision was made to perform a costotransversectomy to avoid taking down the diaphragm. **C.** Postoperative AP view of T12 corpectomy and posterior T10–L2 spinal fusion. **D.** Lateral view of T12 corpectomy and reconstruction with lateral expandable cage.

- The osseous variability along the length of the spine adds to the complex three-dimensional anatomy of the region, making thoracic spine surgery a technical process requiring a thorough understanding and proper preoperative planning.
- There are 12 thoracic vertebrae, each with slight variations in measurable dimensions. Specifically, variations exist between vertebral body diameter, facet positioning, pedicle dimensions, and transverse process and spinous process dimensions.[9,10]
- Pedicle widths gradually decrease from T1 to T4 and increase from T4 to T12. Pedicle width is approximately 4.5 mm at T4, whereas pedicle width at T12 is approximately 7.8 mm. Pedicle height and length tend to increase from T1 to T12. Medial orientation and transverse pedicle angle tend to decrease from T1 to T12.[9,10]

NATURAL HISTORY

- The natural history of the disease depends on the underlying pathology.

PATIENT HISTORY AND PHYSICAL FINDINGS

- A thorough history and physical examination is the basis of complete preoperative planning. The history should include medical and surgical history, social history addressing functional disability and socioeconomic issues, and history of pain or neurologic symptoms.
- The physical examination should consist of observation of deformity and gait, palpation for tenderness or masses, range of motion of the spine and joints, assessment of intact neurologic function with a sensory/motor examination, and rectal examination.

IMAGING AND OTHER DIAGNOSTIC STUDIES

- As previously mentioned, safe preoperative planning relies on understanding the complex three-dimensional anatomy of the costovertebral articulations, vertebrae dimensions, and locations of the neurovascular bundles.
- Proper imaging including radiographs and/or advanced imaging modalities is essential to preoperative planning.
- Magnetic resonance imaging (MRI) is the imaging modality of choice for most pathologies to characterize the soft tissue

of the involved region, especially cases involving spinal cord compression.
- Computed tomography (CT) myelography may offer comparable visualization of the neural elements and is especially beneficial in cases where spinal instrumentation has been used previously.
- For bony anatomy, CT is the preferred modality. Sagittal reconstruction and three-dimensional CT imaging may be useful supplements to axial sequences.
- Frequently, both MRI and CT imaging are obtained for preoperative planning, to characterize both the regional soft tissue and bony anatomy, respectively.

DIFFERENTIAL DIAGNOSIS

- Indications for costotransversectomy include:
  - Anterolateral spinal decompression of infection/abscess
  - Vertebral body biopsy or partial resection (neoplastic, traumatic)
  - Anterior intraspinal tumor
  - Removal of paracentral herniated disc
  - Congenital kyphosis or kyphoscoliosis
  - Sympathectomy
  - Various fusions, including limited anterior spinal fusion
  - Rib pain

NONOPERATIVE MANAGEMENT

- The decision to treat a patient operatively or nonoperatively is dependent on the underlying disease. With some tumors, radiation may be the first line of treatment. With most thoracic disc herniations and other degenerative diseases, nonoperative treatment is often tried prior to consideration for surgery unless there is neurologic deterioration.
- Nonoperative treatment is dependent on the underlying disease.

SURGICAL MANAGEMENT

- In thoracic disc resection, the costotransversectomy approach should be performed on the affected side. This is usually the side with greater deficit on neurologic examination, which should correlate with imaging studies obtained preoperatively.

- In cases of central herniations without lateralizing deficits or root pain, the right-sided approach has been favored to avoid injury to the artery of Adamkiewicz, which usually originates from the left intercostal arteries from T8 to L2.
- The side of approach for other pathologies depends on the location of the lesion.

Preoperative Planning

- A thorough history and physical examination is essential. In cases where a tumor or infection is suspected, the history may provide clues as to the origin of the tumor or infection.
- Appropriate laboratory values should be obtained. These include a basic metabolic panel, complete blood count, prothrombin time, and partial thromboplastin time. In cases where tumors or infections are suspected, an erythrocyte sedimentation rate and C-reactive protein are also recommended. In cases where infections are suspected, blood cultures may be helpful in identifying an organism.
- Arranging for appropriate blood products is recommended. In the case of tumors and infections, there can be considerable blood loss and hemostasis may be difficult to achieve. In addition to packed red blood cells, fresh frozen plasma and platelets may also need to be called for ahead of time.

- Appropriate imaging, including radiographs, MRI, and CT, are essential.
- If time permits, a biopsy is recommended in the cases where tumors are suspected and a primary is not known. Embolization of tumors that have a propensity to bleed (renal cell carcinoma, hemangioma, hemangiosarcoma) is recommended.
- Discussion with anesthesia regarding maintaining mean arterial pressure above 80 mm Hg to ensure adequate perfusion to the spinal cord

Positioning

- Various positioning techniques are available depending on the surgeon's preference. It is the authors' preference to use a prone position on the operating table. Longitudinal chest rolls with the arms tucked in on a radiolucent table is our preferred method to maintain stability during the corpectomy and allow access for fluoroscopy.
- After desired positioning is achieved, the patient should be draped wide enough to allow adequate exposure of the ribs laterally. Additionally, the posterior iliac crests are commonly prepped and draped in the field on both sides in the event bone graft is necessary.

INCISION AND EXPOSURE

- The spinous process of the level desired should be palpated and confirmed using a lateral radiograph. Be aware that the thoracic spinous processes are relatively long and thin and tend to overlap adjacent levels. The incision should span over 2 to 3 levels above and below the level where the costotransversectomy is going to be performed.
- Depending on the level of the lesion and extent of exposure required, various incisions may be used. Incisions vary from a straight midline incision, a midline incision with a "T" over the rib to be resected, a paramedian incision made midway between the spinous process and medial scapular border for proximal lesions above T7, or a curvilinear incision. It is the authors' preference to use a midline incision that can be extended as needed to allow adequate exposure to resect the ribs. The importance of draping widely is emphasized here again.
- Following skin incision through the subcutaneous fat, the trapezius is cut in a longitudinal direction in line with the incision to expose underlying muscles (**TECH FIG 1A**). Depending on the region of thoracic spine, the rhomboid muscles, latissimus dorsi, and thoracodorsal fascia are divided next to access the paraspinal muscles.
- The paraspinal muscles are elevated off of the spinous processes and laminae to gain access to the spine. A subperiosteal dissection will minimize blood loss. The muscles are then elevated off of the transverse processes and ribs to expose the costotransverse articulation (**TECH FIG 1B**).
- Pedicle screw fixation may be performed at this point if a fusion is planned, and a rod can be placed on the side opposite from the costotransversectomy. This will provide stability during the corpectomy.

- The anterior surface of the rib can then be elevated subperiosteally with caution not to disrupt the neurovascular bundle nestled under the inferior aspect of the rib (**TECH FIG 1C**). Take care not to enter the pleural cavity.
  - In cases where the pleural cavity is violated, the pleura may be repaired with 6-0 or 4-0 Prolene in running locked fashion. To ensure adequate closure of the pleural cavity, immerse the wound in saline and perform a Valsalva maneuver. If bubbles persist, a chest tube can be placed at the end of the procedure.
- The rib is cut approximately 6 to 10 cm from the costovertebral articulation (**TECH FIG 1D**). The transected rib can be elevated and the pleura swept away from the undersurface of the rib. Any remaining muscle attachments to the rib should be cleared to visualize the costotransverse ligament, which can be removed. With careful reflection of the pleura from the anterolateral surface of the vertebral body, the costovertebral joint can be disarticulated by dissecting the anterior costovertebral ligament to free the rib.
- Once disarticulation of the rib is complete, the transverse process can be removed to visualize the disc space.
- The intercostal artery and nerve should be ligated or retracted to avoid significant bleeding during rib resection.
- If a corpectomy is planned, a laminectomy can be useful to improve visualization and resection of the vertebral body. A laminectomy can be performed to visualize the spinal cord in standard fashion.
- To gain access to the discs above and below the vertebra and to avoid retraction on the spinal cord, the nerve roots above and below the pedicle may need to be tied off and transected. We generally use 2-0 silk ties (**TECH FIG 1E**). This is generally well tolerated without significant side effects.

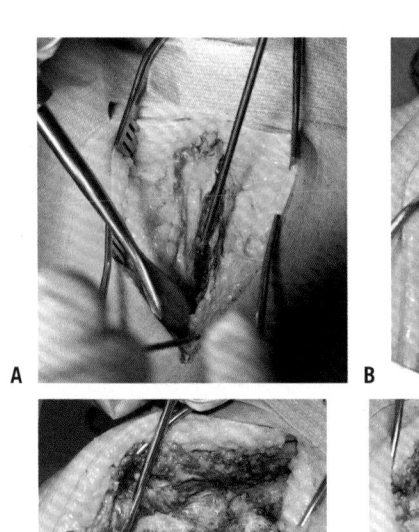
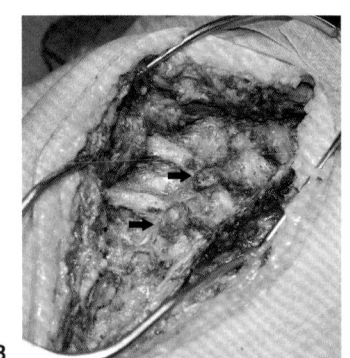
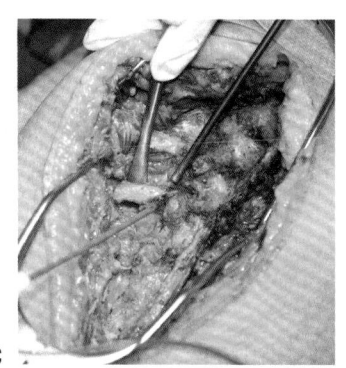
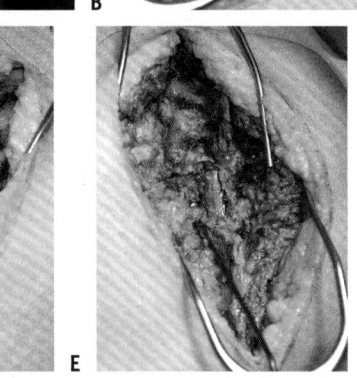

TECH FIG 1 A. We prefer a standard midline approach. Following skin incision through the subcutaneous fat, the trapezius is cut in a longitudinal direction in line with the incision to expose underlying muscles. **B.** The muscles are then elevated off of the transverse processes and ribs to expose the costotransverse articulation (*black arrows*). **C.** The anterior surface of the rib can then be elevated subperiosteally with caution not to disrupt the neurovascular bundle nestled under the inferior aspect of the rib. **D.** The rib is cut approximately 6 to 10 cm from the costovertebral articulation. The transected rib can be elevated and the pleura swept away from the undersurface of the rib. **E.** To gain access to the discs above and below the vertebra and to avoid retraction on the spinal cord, the nerve roots above and below the pedicle may need to be tied off and transected. Figure of the nerve root passing underneath the pedicle.

CORPECTOMY

- Using a high speed burr, the center of the pedicle can be burred down into the vertebral body.
- Then, the lateral portion of the pedicle may be removed with a rongeur and the medial portion may be removed by pushing the pedicle wall laterally to avoid injury to the spinal cord.
- In cases of infection, purulent drainage should be encountered at this point and the cavity should be irrigated and débrided. In tumor cases, lytic or solid tumor masses may be encountered. With lytic lesions, the tumor may be débrided from the cavity and hemostasis obtained. With solid tumors, it might be possible to resect the tumor en bloc. These specimens may be sent to pathology for the appropriate tests.
  - Use of thrombin and Gelfoam and other hemostatic agents may be necessary, and preparation of these materials is recommended prior to entering the cavity.
  - Tranexamic acid can be used to decrease blood loss as well. But be aware of potential deep venous thrombosis, pulmonary embolus, and myocardial infarction as potential risks.
  - Use of a cell saver can be considered but in cases of tumor or infection, the use of an autogenous blood recovery system is not recommended.
- Next, a Penfield no. 1 may be used to elevate the periosteum off of the vertebral body and separate the pleura away from the vertebra if more exposure is needed **(TECH FIG 2A)**. To avoid injury to the segmental vessels, try to get the Penfield no. 1 under the periosteum and elevate the soft tissues subperiosteally from the lateral and anterior portions of the vertebral body.
  - If the segmental vessels are injured, clamp the vessels to obtain hemostasis. Then, tie them with 2-0 silk ties or vessel clips.

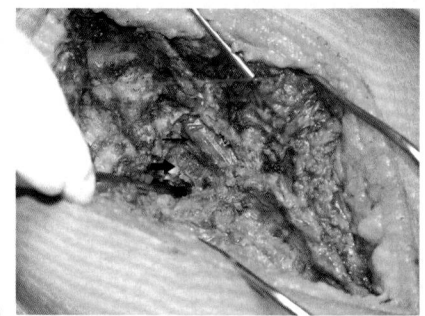
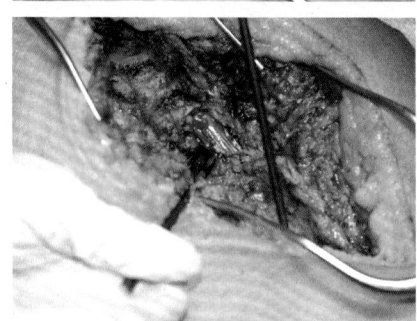

TECH FIG 2 A. Elevate the periosteum off of the vertebral body with a Penfield no. 1 or periosteal elevator and separate the pleura away from the vertebra if more exposure is needed. The *thin arrow* is pointing at the dura. The *larger arrow* is pointing at the pedicle. **B.** Figure of the cavity created from resection of bone from the costotransversectomy approach.

TECHNIQUES

- Then, the vertebra may be removed posterolaterally with curettes and pituitary rongeurs **(TECH FIG 2B)**. Be careful not to retract the spinal cord as this could lead to neurologic injury. With tumors or infections, there is often a cavity. Clean this cavity out using curettes and pituitaries.
- Once the tumor or pus has been excavated from this cavity, the lateral wall of the vertebral body may be removed with a rongeur. If you need more exposure, knock the posterior wall of the vertebral body into the cavity that you have created with a downward facing curette and remove the pieces with a pituitary. This reduces the risk of spinal cord injury.
  - Always be cognizant of the integrity of the anterior wall of the vertebral body because the aorta and vena cava are just anterior to the anterior wall of the vertebral body. If the anterior wall has been destroyed by tumor or infection, elevate the periosteum off of the anterior wall of the vertebral body or define the anterior border of the vertebra prior to performing the corpectomy to reduce the risk of vessel injury.
  - If further exposure is necessary, removal of another rib may provide better visualization and access.
- Once the tumor, pus, and granulation tissue have been adequately resected, remove enough of the vertebral body to allow space for a strut or cage.

DISCECTOMY AND APPLICATION OR INTERBODY CAGE

- Remove the disc at each end of the cavity to expose the endplates of the vertebrae above and below.
- Tying and ligating the exiting nerve roots will improve visualization of the discs and facilitate the discectomy. Make a box annulotomy with a no. 15 scalpel blade and remove the disc above and below the corpectomy site. Start with a pituitary and remove as much of the disc as you can.
- Use curettes to thoroughly remove the cartilaginous endplates. Remove the endplate in a posterolateral direction to avoid sending any material into the ventral portion of the spinal cord. Angled curettes and scrapers can be useful here to avoid injury to the spinal cord. Scrape the endplates in a mediolateral direction versus anteroposterior (AP) direction to avoid injury to the vessels anteriorly or the spinal cord posteriorly.

CAGE PLACEMENT

- Place an allograft strut or cage posterolaterally to sit securely on the endplates. Our preference is to use an expandable cage. An expandable cage can be helpful in these cases to avoid retraction on the spinal cord and potential neurologic injury because it is smaller than standard cages or allograft struts when it is initially inserted.
- The resected ribs provide an excellent source of graft material. If necessary, iliac crest may be obtained for additional graft. Demineralized bone matrix or other extenders may be necessary to obtain a fusion.
- Calipers and trials are used to get the exact size of the cage. Evaluation of radiographs of the disc and vertebral body above and below the corpectomy site should give a rough estimation of the size of the cage.
- Fill the expandable cage with the harvested graft. Insert the cage in a posterolateral direction to avoid injury to the spinal cord.
- Expand the cage to secure the cage in place and get AP and lateral fluoroscopic views to check for good positioning of the cage. Leave the handle on the cage when taking the radiographs in case the cage must be repositioned. Expand the cage to obtain a good interference fit. You should be able to pull on the cage with a Kocher clamp without it moving.
- Decorticate and pack the remaining graft in the posterolateral gutters and place the ipsilateral rod.
- After the appropriate procedure is completed, closure is performed in routine fashion.
- Use of a drain is recommended especially in the case of tumors or infections to continue evacuation of infected material or tumor cells. Closure with unbraided, nonabsorbable suture is recommended to decrease the risk of infection or wound dehiscence.

Pearls and Pitfalls

Imaging	• For any lesion requiring costotransversectomy, proper intraoperative imaging is helpful. Use of a radiolucent table will facilitate images. Tucking the arms in will also facilitate fluoroscopy.
Exposure	• Inadequate rib resection may create a more posterior directed approach than anticipated, which restrains the view of more anterior structures. This could lead to improper exposure of the lesion necessitating spinal cord manipulation, which should always be avoided. This can be avoided by an adequately lateral rib resection to establish a proper posterolateral approach. • Tying off the nerve roots will also allow easier access to the vertebral body and endplates.
Pleural Injury	• In the case of pleural disruption, repair should proceed immediately. Flooding the operative field with irrigation while searching for air leakage during ventilation can check for undiscovered pleural leaks. A chest tube can be placed at the end of the case if need be.
Corpectomy	• The key to doing an adequate corpectomy is visualization and access. To gain adequate access, tie off the nerve roots and resect the rib as far lateral as necessary to view as much of the vertebra as you need.
Discectomy	• Obtaining adequate exposure will facilitate the discectomy. Angled instruments will also help. During the discectomy, move the curettes and rasps in a mediolateral direction to avoid injury to the ventral spinal cord.
Hemostasis	• Hemostasis should be maintained throughout surgery. Take time to obtain good vascular access and to ensure adequate blood products are available. • When dealing with tumors, embolization of vascular tumors may decrease blood loss.

POSTOPERATIVE CARE

• Management of the patient after spinal surgery of any region depends greatly on the pathology, level of surgery, and general health of the patient. It is the authors' normal practice to drain cavities created by costotransversectomy using bulb suction drainage.

• Pain management: Proper pain management is necessary to alleviate pain during respiratory movements, decreasing incidence of atelectasis or other respiratory problems.

• Prophylaxis: Pulsatile compression stockings may be continued postoperatively.

• Positioning in bed: During the first 12 postoperative hours, the patient is allowed to lie supine, as pressure on the wound discourages hematoma development. The patient is rolled every 2 hours to prevent wound maceration and pressure ulcers. Dressings are changed at 48 hours and daily thereafter as needed. Sutures are removed after 14 to 17 days, and the wound is not soaked during this time. In patients who have had radiation to the area, the sutures are left longer to allow the wound to heal completely.

• Ambulation: Patients are encouraged to ambulate on postoperative day 1. Those with residual neurologic deficits can be mobilized to chair with assistance when possible; otherwise, repositioning with log rolling every 2 hours to prevent skin breakdown is necessary. Patients with neurologic deficits begin physical rehabilitation 48 hours after surgery, with both passive and active exercises performed in bed.

• Bracing: Bracing is not usually required. However, if fixation is a concern, thoracolumbar orthosis with or without thigh extension may be instituted until radiographs suggest adequate osseous support.

OUTCOMES

• The outcomes for surgical procedures involving costotransversectomy vary depending on the type of pathology, preoperative extent of the lesion, and anatomic location.

• Chandra et al[2] described the results of 46 patients who underwent an extracavitary approach to treat traumatic fractures, tuberculosis, and tumors. Thirty-five of 46 patients (76%) demonstrated improvement in the performance status. The major complications included pneumonitis (3), pneumothorax (3) and neurologic deterioration (3; improved in 2), deep venous thrombosis (2), and recurrent hemoptysis (1). No implant failures were noted. There were two mortalities: one because of myocardial infarction and another because of respiratory complications.

• In another study, Kapoor et al[5] studied the results of 33 patients who had large thoracic disc herniations. A total of 23 patients underwent thoracotomy, 9 costotransversectomy, and 2 transpedicular approaches for excision of thoracic discs. The outcome was favorable in the majority (84.4%) of patients. However, significant approach-related complications were noted in patients undergoing thoracotomies.

• Similar results were noted in a study by Sciubba et al.[11] The authors reviewed seven cases where a costotransversectomy was used in conjunction with an expandable cage to correct thoracolumbar kyphosis resulting from spinal tumors, osteomyelitis, or fractures. A costotransversectomy was chosen in these cases because a transthoracic approach was deemed too risky due to medical comorbidities. The authors noted a 53% kyphosis correction. None of the patients had a decline in neurologic function, and pain management consisted of minimal use of oral narcotics.

• Lastly, the costotransversectomy approach for tumor resection has also been studied. In a study by Elsamadicy et al,[3] the authors compared the results of costotransversectomy versus transpedicular approach to treat metastatic tumors causing impinging on the thoracic spine. A total of five (45.5%) complications occurred in the costotransversectomy group and seven (58.3%) in the transpedicular group. An improvement in American Spinal Injury Association Impairment Scale grades was observed in three (27.3%) patients in the costotransversectomy group and one (8.3%) in transpedicular group. No patient worsened in the costotransversectomy group, whereas one (8.3%) patient in transpedicular group worsened. The median survival was 12.2 months in the costotransversectomy group and 19.0 months in the transpedicular group.

- Hence, the costotransversectomy approach can be a very useful method to treat pathologies of the thoracic spine. As noted in the studies cited earlier, there are many risks associated with this procedure and a thorough discussion with the patient regarding the risks and benefits of the surgery is recommended prior to surgery. However, it can have very good results when used for the right indications. It seems to have maximum benefit when a transthoracic approach is deemed too risky or morbid for the patient to tolerate.

COMPLICATIONS

- Possible complications following costotrasversectomy are those typical of spine surgery. The immediate proximity of osseous structures with neurovascular and visceral anatomy establishes a technical challenge with several possible complications to be aware of. But overall, complications tend to be uncommonly observed.
- Intraoperatively, care should be taken to avoid pleural compromise. This complication is more common when the pleura is thickened in cases involving neoplasm, infection, or previous surgery. If necessary, a chest tube can be placed at the end of surgery.
- Historically, blood loss has been recognized as a concern for posterolateral approaches, but with recent attention to hemostasis, blood loss can be well controlled. Special attention to penetrating arteries is required during dissection and removal of portions of the pedicle and anterior aspect of the vertebral body.
- The intercostal artery and nerve should be ligated or retracted to avoid significant bleeding during rib resection. Similarly, injury to the intercostal nerve should be avoided to prevent intercostal neuralgia.
- Other nervous injuries, including nerve root injuries or dural tears, are possible. Dural tears should be closed intraoperatively to prevent cerebrospinal fluid leakage.

- Postoperatively, infectious complications such as pneumonia and urinary tract infection have been noted. Patients who undergo costotransversectomy usually suffer multiple comorbidities, which further complicates postoperative course. Postoperative atelectasis may result secondary to pain and immobility. Wound infections are not common but can be treated with appropriate irrigation and débridement and intravenous antibiotics.

REFERENCES

1. Alderstone OD, Benzel EC. History: Menard's costotransversectomy. In: Benzel EC, ed. Spine Surgery: Techniques, Complications, Avoidance, and Management, ed 2. Philadelphia: Elsevier, 2005:8.
2. Chandra SP, Ramdurg SR, Kurwale N, et al. Extended costotransversectomy to achieve circumferential fusion for pathologies causing thoracic instability. Spine J 2014;14(9):2094–2101.
3. Elsamadicy AA, Adogwa O, Sergesketter A, et al. Posterolateral thoracic decompression with anterior column cage reconstruction versus decompression alone for spinal metastases with cord compression: analysis of perioperative complications and outcomes. J Spine Surg 2017;3(4):609–619.
4. Herkowitz HN, Garfin SR, Eismont FJ, et al, eds. Rothman-Simeone The Spine, ed 5. Philadelphia: Elsevier, 2006:308–319.
5. Kapoor S, Amarouche M, Al-Obeidi F, et al. Giant thoracic discs: treatment, outcome, and follow-up of 33 patients in a single centre. Eur Spine J 2018;27(7):1555–1566.
6. Kerezoudis P, Rajjoub KR, Goncalves S, et al. Anterior versus posterior approaches for thoracic disc herniation: association with postoperative complications. Clin Neurol Neurosurg 2018;167:17–23.
7. Lau D, Song Y, Guan Z, et al. Perioperative characteristics, complications, and outcomes of single-level versus multilevel thoracic corpectomies via modified costotransversectomy approach. Spine (Phila Pa 1976) 2013;38(6):523–530.
8. Lubelski D, Abdullah KG, Steinmetz MP, et al. Lateral extracavitary, costotransversectomy, and transthoracic thoracotomy approaches to the thoracic spine: review of techniques and complications. J Spinal Disord Tech 2013;26(4):222–232.
9. Lubelski D, Steinmetz M. Lateral extracavitary approach. In: Steinmetz MP, Benzel EC, eds. Benzel's Spine Surgery: Techniques, Complication Avoidance, and Management, ed 4. Philadelphia: Elsevier, 2017:424–428.
10. Martinez-del-Campo E, Soriano-Baron H, Theodore N. Extraspinal anatomy and surgical approaches to the thoracic spine. In: Steinmetz MP, ed. Benzel's Spine Surgery: Techniques, Complication Avoidance, and Management, ed 4. Philadelphia: Elsevier, 2017:397–405.
11. Sciubba DM, Gallia GL, McGirt MJ, et al. Thoracic kyphotic deformity reduction with a distractible titanium cage via an entirely posterior approach. Neurosurgery 2007;60(4 suppl 2):223–230.

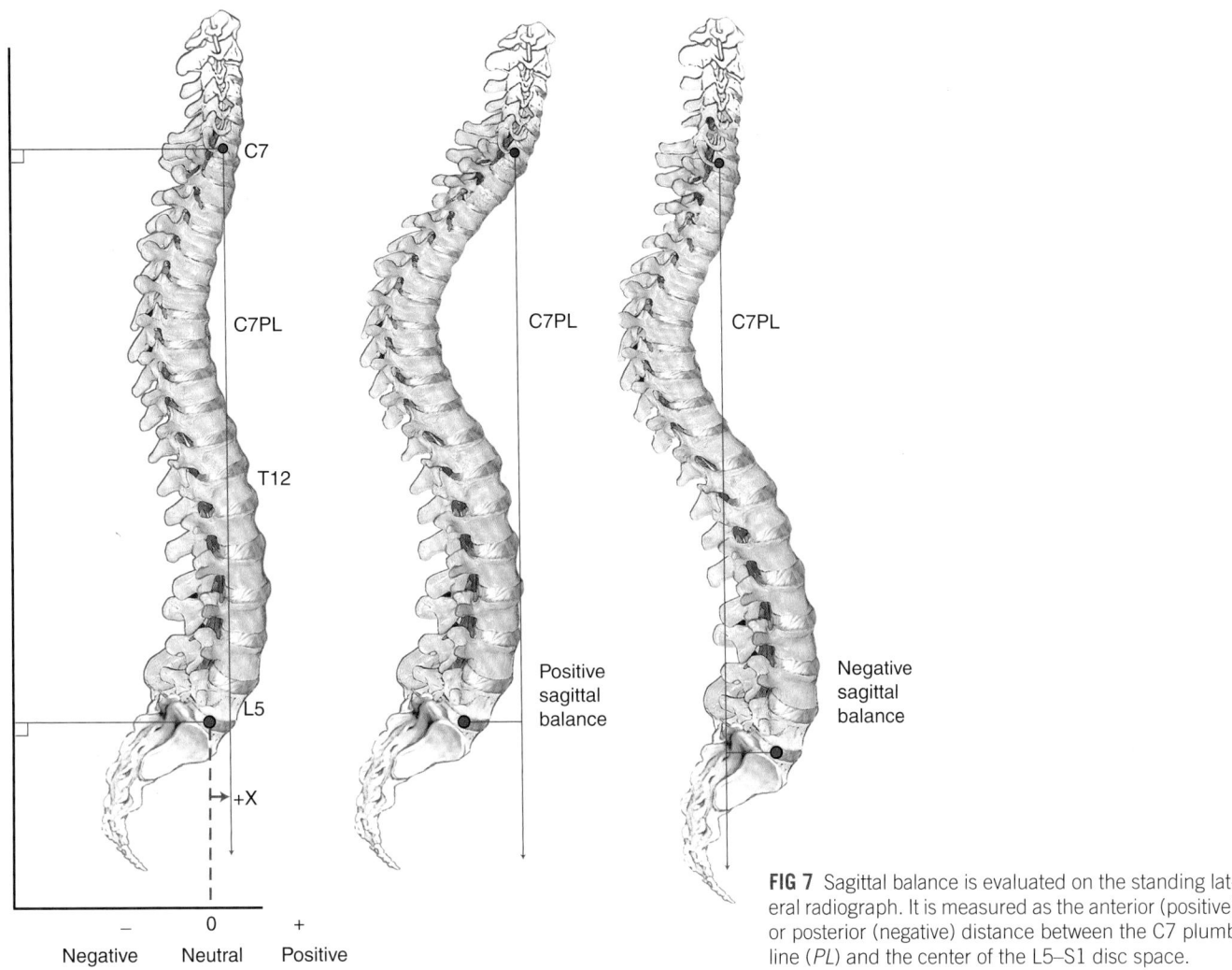

C7

C7PL

T12

L5

+X

−　　0　　+

Negative　Neutral　Positive

C7PL

Positive sagittal balance

C7PL

Negative sagittal balance

FIG 7 Sagittal balance is evaluated on the standing lateral radiograph. It is measured as the anterior (positive) or posterior (negative) distance between the C7 plumb line (*PL*) and the center of the L5–S1 disc space.

correction), and assess local bone quality (osteoporosis, sclerosis, osteophyte density); all of which is used for preoperative planning.

- Plain radiographs and CT images can be used to assess the degree of bone loss and tailor the reconstructive techniques to the bone quality of the patient.
- Three-dimensional reconstruction provides intricate details of the deformity when major osteotomy or vertebral column resection (VCR) is contemplated.
- CT scan data may also be used for preoperative planning of screw trajectories on various robotic-assisted planning softwares. Intraoperative robotic/stereotactic assistance for screw placement is becoming common for these extensive surgeries.

Magnetic Resonance Imaging

- MRI is used to assess neurologic compression **(FIG 11)** as well as the status of the disc, ligamentum flavum, and other soft tissues.
- Thoracic spine MRI should be evaluated when thoracic instrumentation is contemplated.
- CT as well as the MRI images should be carefully assessed to determine location of major vessels, level of aortic bifurcation.

Dual-Energy X-Ray Absorptiometry

- Dual-energy x-ray absorptiometry is often performed for patients with identified risk factors:
  - History of fracture as an adult or fracture in a first-degree relative
  - White race
  - Advanced age
  - Smoking
  - Low body weight
  - Female gender
  - Dementia
  - Poor health or general fragility

Provocative Tests

- Discography, although not 100% accurate, can be useful to assess for painful segments and evaluate the competence of the disc annulus, particularly in the lower lumbar spine.
- Facet blocks have been employed to determine levels that should be included, or need not be included, in the fusion. This may be particularly relevant at the lumbosacral junction.

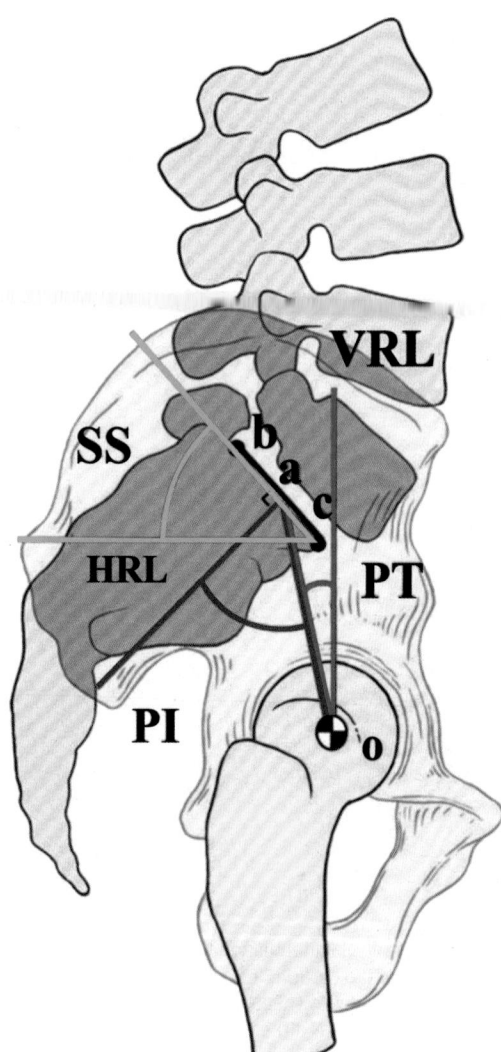

FIG 8 Diagrammatic representation showing spinopelvic parameters. Pelvic incidence (*PI*) is the angle between a line perpendicular to the midpoint of the sacral endplate (*b*) and the line from this point to the midpoint of femoral heads. PI is constant for each person and does not change with age. Sacral slope (*SS*) is the angle formed by the sacral endplate with the horizontal reference line (*HRL*). Pelvic tilt (*PT*) is the angle formed by the line joining midpoint of sacral endplate and center of femoral heads with vertical reference line (*VRL*). PT is a measure of pelvic retroversion. PT increases and SS decreases with increasing pelvic retroversion. (Image reproduced with permission from O'Brien MF, et al. Radiographic Measurement Manual: Memphis, TN: Medtronic Sofamor Danek, 2004.)

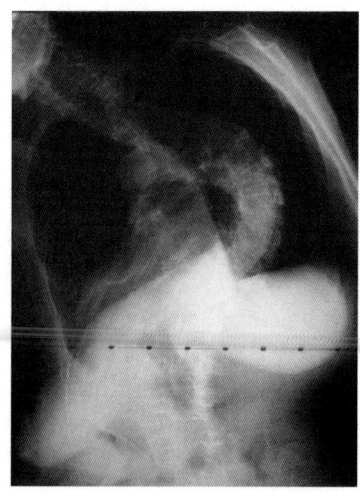
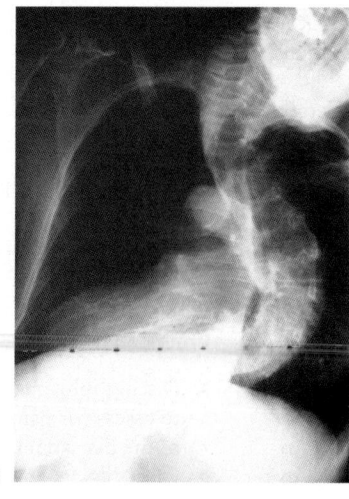

FIG 9 A,B. Bending radiographs aid in determining the flexibility of the spinal curves and are also used to determine the structural or nonstructural nature of the curves. This patient has a relatively rigid deformity.

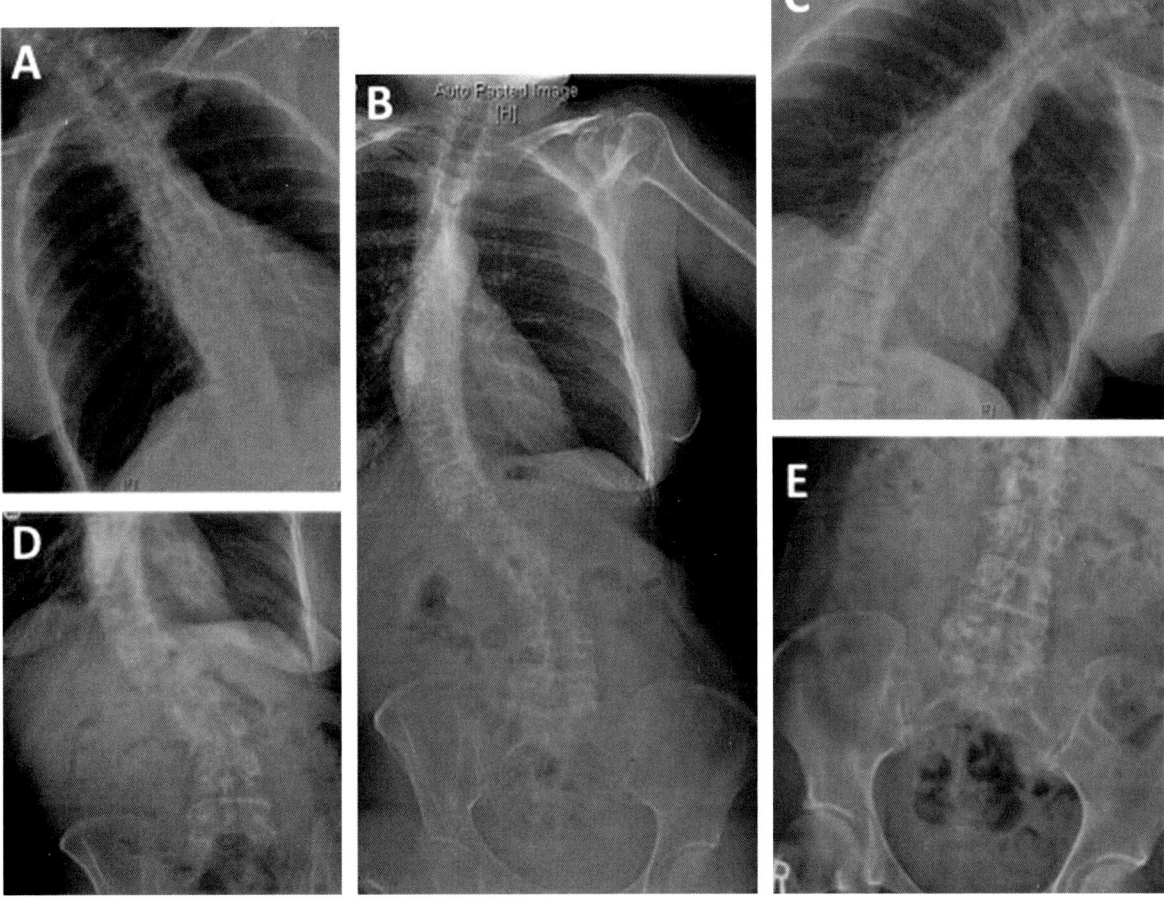

FIG 10 Regional bending (**A,C–E**) and full-length standing (**B**) radiographs characterize this as a flexible deformity. **A,C.** The thoracic bending films demonstrate near-complete correction of the thoracic curve. **D,E.** The lumbar bending films also demonstrate near-complete correction of the lumbar curve.

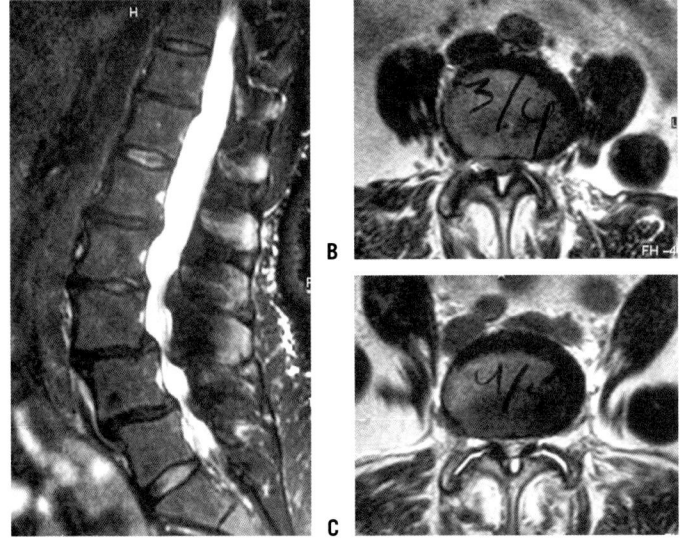

FIG 11 A–C. MRI is particularly useful in evaluating patients with neurologic symptoms such as claudication. It is used to assess neurologic compression as well as the status of the disc, ligamentum flavum, and other soft tissues.

MANAGEMENT OF ADULT SCOLIOTIC DEFORMITY

- Adult deformity patients can be categorized by their clinical presentation.[15]
  - One group, predominantly defined by lumbar stenosis and neurogenic claudication with degenerative deformity, has surgical management typically achieved by posterior lumbar procedures.
  - A second group, categorized by progressive deformity, with or without back pain, is more frequently treated with combination anterior and posterior procedures that may involve the thoracic spine to achieve surgical goals.
- Although the surgical principles and techniques used to address these different categories are similar, important variations exist.

Nonoperative Management

- A physical therapy regimen may be tried, focusing on the following:
  - Stretching and core-strengthening exercises
  - Postural training
  - Gait training
  - Resolution of hip and knee flexion contractures
  - General conditioning
- Nonsteroidal anti-inflammatory medications may be used if safely tolerated.

Surgical Management

- The treatment of adult scoliosis is complex because of the global nature of the spinal deformity and the multiple causes of this disorder.
- Efficiency, safety, and effectiveness in meeting surgical goals are each optimized by a well-designed procedure that is tailored for individual patient.
- Surgical treatment is considered for patients who are refractory to prolonged multimodal conservative management, when there is documented progression of the curvature, deterioration of sagittal and coronal balance with or without presence of back and or leg pain.

Preoperative Planning

- Preoperative planning is instrumental to a successful treatment algorithm; avoiding both short- and long-term complications is paramount.
- The patient with adult scoliosis may carry a myriad of comorbidities that may increase the risk of a spinal operation or even contraindicate it. A complete preoperative assessment of those considering surgical treatment provides the opportunity to minimize risks by optimizing health status.
- Modifiable conditions that affect surgical risk include the following:
  - Tobacco smoking
  - History of asthma or chronic obstructive pulmonary disease
  - Coronary or cerebrovascular disease
  - Diabetes
  - Nutritional deficiency
  - Osteoporosis
  - Depression
  - Current significant life stressors

- Collaboration with consulting medical specialists who are trained in perioperative management is an important technique to optimize outcomes for patients with adult scoliosis.
- Anesthesia colleagues familiar with this surgical course may also reduce risks.
- Certain medical considerations directly affect the selection of surgical techniques for a patient with adult scoliosis.
  - Assessment of bone quality plays a critical role in the design of the operation.
  - Osteoporosis is the rule, not the exception.[18] Although bisphosphonate medications may be helpful (and common) in treating osteoporosis, they inhibit osteoclastic bone resorption, which may have a negative impact on fusion biology.

Surgical Planning
Goals

- The surgical procedure is planned according to the individual patient and the main complaints of the patient. Overall, the surgery is designed to adequately decompress the neurologic elements and to restore the sagittal and coronal balance of the patient.
- The surgical treatment is centered mainly at restoration of the coronal and sagittal profile of the patient as well as the spinopelvic alignment. Correction of coronal curve magnitude is considered secondary.

Importance of Spinal Balance

- Optimal sagittal spinopelvic alignment is considered as a major determinant of overall health-related quality of life and pain in patients with adult spinal deformity.[11,12,27]
- Important determinants of the spinal balance are as follows:
  - Positive sagittal balance (>50 mm)—most reliable determinant of disability in this group of patients
  - Coronal imbalance (>40 mm)
  - PI-LL mismatch ≥9 degrees: PI helps in understanding magnitude of lumbar lordosis that is needed to restore the sagittal balance of the patient.
  - PT less than 22 degrees—determinant of the pelvic retroversion. Pelvic retroversion serves as compensatory mechanism in patients and can mask their sagittal imbalance.

Classification

- The Scoliosis Research Society (SRS)-Schwab classification[31] provides a well-validated classification system, which helps in surgical decision making for treatment of this complex clinical problem.
- The classification system incorporates important outcome predictors in decision making along with the coronal and sagittal characteristics of the deformity.
- The classification system (**FIG 12**) consists of four coronal curve types and three sagittal modifiers.

Surgical Treatment Options

- Magnitude of the surgical intervention is decided based on patient's symptoms, age, overall health, bone quality, and expectations. Preoperative optimization of the health

Coronal Curve Types	Sagittal Modifiers
	PI minus LL
Thoracic (T)	0: <10°
- lumbar curve <30°	+: moderate 10–20°
	++: marked >20°
Thoracolumbar/Lumbar (L)	
- thoracic curve <30°	**Global Alignment**
	0: SVA <4 cm
Double Curve (D)	+: SVA 4–9.5 cm
- T and TL/L curves >30°	++: SVA >9.5 cm
No Major Coronal	**Pelvic Tilt**
Deformity (N)	0: PT <20°
- all coronal curves <30°	+: PT 20–30°
	++: PT >30°

FIG 12 SRS-Schwab classification for adult spinal deformity. The adult spinal deformity curves are classified into coronal curve types based on the location of the major curve. The curves are classified into thoracic (*T*), thoracolumbar (*TL*)/lumbar (*L*), double curve (*D*), and no major coronal deformity (*N*) type. Sagittal modifiers are used to evaluate spinopelvic and global alignment of the patient. *PI*, pelvic incidence; *LL*, lumbar lordosis; *SVA*, sagittal vertical axis; *PT*, pelvic tilt. (Reprinted with permission from Schwab F, Ungar B, Blondel B, et al. Scoliosis Research Society—Schwab adult spinal deformity classification: a validation study. Spine [Phila Pa 1976] 2012;37[12]:1077–1082.)

and the bone quality is of utmost importance. The surgical treatment options are as follows:

Decompression Alone

- Decompression alone can be considered as the treatment of choice for carefully selected patients.
- Ideally, suited for patients with relatively smaller curves, good sagittal and coronal balance, presence of collapsed discs and bridging osteophytes, predominantly radicular or claudicatory symptoms with minimal axial back pain, and in absence of significant listhesis or instability.
- Decompression is also considered for patients who are not suitable for extensive surgical procedures.
- Higher incidence of revision surgery[13] and postoperative instability[32] has been reported in patients undergoing decompression only surgery in presence of deformity.

Decompression with Posterior Instrumented Fusion

- Decompression with instrumented fusion is the treatment of choice for majority of the symptomatic patients with adult degenerative scoliosis.
- Special consideration should be given while deciding the extent of fusion (short segment vs. long segment), caudal extent of fusion (L5 vs. S1 vs. pelvis), rostral extent of fusion (upper lumbar/lower thoracic/upper thoracic).
- Following basic principles of deformity correction can help in decision making.
  - Proximal instrumented vertebra should be a neutral and a stable vertebra.
  - In presence of thoracic hyperkyphosis—fusion is extended to upper thoracic spine (T2–T4)
  - Stopping at physiologic apex of the thoracic kyphosis (T5–T6) should be avoided.

- In presence of thoracic hypokyphosis, we believe that T9–T10 is ideal for upper extent of the fusion.
- Fusion to the sacrum versus pelvis:
  - Extension of the fusion to the sacrum and pelvis for the adult scoliosis patient is an important and controversial subject. There is no consensus as to the best strategy for all clinical scenarios, but certain guidelines and lessons have been developed.
  - There is a relatively high rate of pseudarthrosis (and other complications) after L5–S1 fusion.[8] For these reasons, in part, avoiding fusion to the sacrum whenever possible has been advocated.
  - Certain scenarios do require lumbosacral fusion:
    - *Symptomatic L5–S1 spondylolisthesis*
    - *Other instability*
    - *Oblique takeoff with over 15 degrees of scoliosis at the L5–S1 segment often requires reduction and fusion for adequate correction of deformity.*
    - *For correction of lumbar hypolordosis to achieve proper sagittal balance*
- The risk of pseudarthrosis at the lumbosacral junction can be limited by the following:
  - Employing combined approaches to perform a meticulous 360-degree fusion at the L5–S1 segment
  - Bone morphogenetic protein (BMP) may be applied within an interbody device at L5–S1 to increase the chances of solid arthrodesis.
  - Extending the fusion construct to the ilium, using iliac screws, S2 alar screws, sacroiliac screws, or other distal fixation methods
- To summarize, posterior approach forms the mainstay of deformity correction. The posterior surgical techniques offer versatility, familiarity with the approach. The approach also provides flexibility of including transforaminal interbody fusion techniques (usually carried out at L4–L5 and L5–S1 to restore the lordosis) and can also be expanded to include various forms of osteotomies.

Combined Anterior and Posterior Approach

- Anterior surgical approaches provide a unique advantage for deformity surgery.
- Anterior approaches allow better discectomy, ability to insert bigger spacers with greater footprint and better correction of lordosis, restoration of the disc height.
- Anterior surgery can be performed using traditional anterior lumbar interbody fusion (ALIF), transpsoas lateral lumbar interbody fusion (LLIF) or an oblique lumbar interbody fusion (OLIF). Each of these techniques has several advantages and disadvantages which are described later in this chapter.
- Anterior thoracolumbar release procedures are rarely performed for adult deformity surgery.

Osteotomies

- Osteotomies involve resection of part of the vertebral body or complete resection of the vertebrae (VCR).
- Selection of the osteotomy procedure is based on rigidity of the deformity, magnitude of coronal and sagittal balance, magnitude of the coronal Cobb angle, number of segments the correction needs to be achieved.
- Osteotomies involve excision from a simple facetectomy to a three-column resection of the vertebra.

- Smith-Petersen osteotomy (SPO), which involves resection of posterior elements (bilateral facets, inferior lamina, the spinous process, and the ligaments) followed by closure of the osteotomy. The osteotomy allows extension through an intact mobile disc space. This increases segmental lordosis by 5 to 10 degrees. SPO is performed at multiple segments mainly to address moderate sagittal imbalance (sagittal vertical axis [SVA] <10 cm) or to increase flexibility of the curve.
- Pedicle subtractions osteotomy (PSO) is reserved for sharp angular deformities deformities in previously fused spine, and when there is severe sagittal imbalance (SVA > 10 cm) PSO is performed by removing all posterior elements, bilateral pedicles, and a wedge of the vertebral body. PSO improves the segmental lordosis by approximately 30 degrees. An asymmetrical PSO may be used for coronal correction.
- VCR entails total resection of the entire vertebral body with the disc above and below. It is reserved severe focal deformities in the coronal and sagittal plane.

Complications

- Surgical treatment of adult spinal deformity is associated with high rate of complications.[1,25,28,30]
- The complications may include spinal fluid leak, infection, pseudarthrosis, hardware failure, neurologic deficit, proximal junctional failure/fracture.
- Patient may also develop medical/systemic complications like deep vein thrombosis, pulmonary embolism, myocardial infarction, urinary tract infection, pneumonia, stroke.
- The risk of complications is higher in patients undergoing revision surgeries, combined approaches and needing complex osteotomies.[25]
- The overall complication rate with these surgeries has been reported to be 13.4%.[25]
- The complication rate is found to increase with increasing age and has been reported to be as high as 71% in patients between 65- and 85-year age group.[30]

PEDICLE SCREW SELECTION AND PLACEMENT

- Screw pullout strength is improved when high insertional torque is achieved with the following:
  - Undertapping (or not tapping) the screw path
  - Tapered screws. These are limited by the absolute restriction that they cannot be reversed or backed out; such an action would remove the screw's contact with the bone.
  - Larger diameter screws. Increased cortical contact may increase insertional torque but may increase the risk of pedicle fracture as well.

- Longer screws: Bicortical purchase can increase screw pullout strength but may pose the possibility of injury to abdominal or vascular structures.
- Loss of proximal fixation in the thoracic spine can be reduced by placing thoracic pedicle screws with alternating "anatomic" and "straight ahead" trajectories; this increases fixation by changing the mode of potential failure from straight "pull out" to a required "plow out" mode. This principle has been effective with long bone fracture treatment, using fixed-angle divergent or convergent fixation in metaphyseal bone (TECH FIG 1).

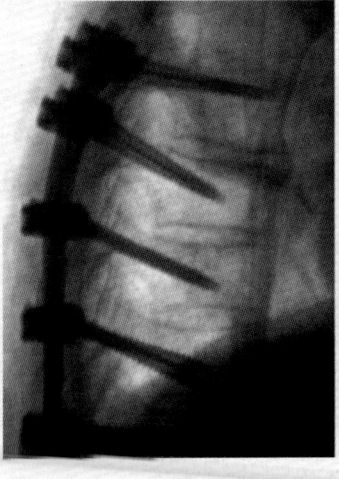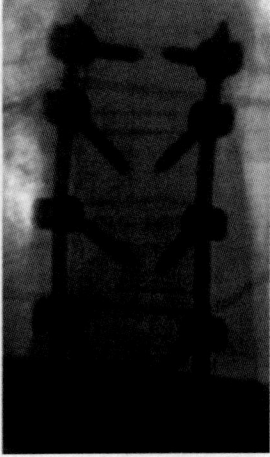

TECH FIG 1 These radiographs depict both the straight ahead trajectory (uppermost and lowermost vertebrae on these images) and the anatomic trajectory (central three vertebrae on these images) for thoracic pedicle screws. Alternating trajectories at adjacent segments may help improve fixation.

FIXATION STRATEGIES FOR OSTEOPOROTIC BONE

- Pedicle screw fixation is less effective in osteoporotic bone.[5]
  - Trabecular bone is predominantly affected by osteoporosis.
  - Because pedicle screws have cortical contact limited to the pedicle isthmus, a "windshield wiper" mode of failure may lead to screw loosening.

- Fixation strategies for osteoporotic bone include the following[4]:
  - Taking advantage of the relatively stronger cortical bone
  - Augmenting the fixation of a pedicle screw within the existing trabecular bone

TECHNIQUES

- Extending the fixation, that is, to the pelvis, in order to "protect" the fixation in the sacrum, to prevent sacral fracture
- Bone implant interface complications in the osteoporotic spine can be reduced by various methods.
  - Sublaminar wires, laminar hooks, and pediculolaminar fixation take advantage of the cortical bone composition of the posterior spinal lamina.
  - Fixation of pedicle screws within osteoporotic trabecular bone may be improved by polymethylmethacrylate (PMMA) cement augmentation.[26]

- Fluoroscopy is used to visualize the placement of 2 to 3 mL of PMMA per pedicle to ensure that cement does not migrate to the neural elements.
- Calcium sulfate paste may also be used; this has the theoretical advantage of becoming replaced by bone over time.
- Modified pedicle screws may also be used, including conical screws, hydroxyapatite-coated screws, and expandable screws.

FUSION AND BONE GRAFTING

- Establishment of a solid fusion is critical.
- The pseudarthrosis rate in one large series of adult deformity patients after long fusion procedures was 24%. Statistically significant risk factors for pseudarthrosis in that study included
  - Thoracolumbar kyphosis
  - Hip osteoarthritis
  - Use of a thoracoabdominal (vs. paramedian) approach
  - Positive sagittal balance greater than 5 cm
  - Age older than 55 years
  - Incomplete sacropelvic fixation
- These risk factors emphasize the importance of surgically establishing the proper mechanical environment, including overall sagittal balance and appropriate fixation.

Bone Graft Selection

- Appropriate graft selection may reduce pseudarthrosis risk.
- Bone grafts and alternatives may serve multiple roles in the surgical treatment of adult scoliosis; fusion–promotion and deformity–correction techniques both may influence graft selection.
  - An anterior interbody graft may need to be structural to correct a deformity.
  - If a structural graft is used anteriorly first, it is with the anticipation that further deformity correction at that segment will be limited by posterior manipulation.
  - Anterior structural interbody grafts can be instrumental in preventing a kyphosis when the convexity of a deformity is compressed in a reduction maneuver.
  - Structural grafts can be placed with a bias toward the concavity in order to assist in the deformity correction.
  - Structural interbody grafts serve a critical role in supplementing the stability of a reconstruction, particularly at the caudal end of a construct, at the lumbosacral junction.
- Morselized grafts may allow for deformity correction by subsequent posterior manipulation.
- Our typical strategy is as follows:
  - Use structural grafts at the caudal end of the construct (two to four levels).
  - Overzealous posterior manipulation can cause loosening or displacement of an anterior structural graft.

- Use morselized graft rostrally.
  - Subsequent deformity correction during the posterior procedure will be limited mainly to those levels with morselized (or no) anterior graft.

Interbody Graft Materials

- Graft selection is guided by the following:
  - The goal of fusion success
  - The potential use of structural roles for the graft
  - The risk of potential complications and other shortcomings
  - Costs
- Interbody grafts may be composed of the following:
  - Bone (autograft or allograft)
  - Metal
  - Carbon fiber
  - Polyetheretherketone (PEEK)
  - Other synthetic materials
- To reduce the risk of graft subsidence, a graft with a modulus of elasticity similar to that of the native bone can be employed.
  - Iliac crest autograft may be the best modulus match but is associated with well-established harvest-related morbidity.
  - In osteoporosis, we have used allograft harvested from the iliac crest of a donor, which offers the following:
    - A relatively high proportion of trabecular to cortical bone compared to a long bone allograft and an appropriate modulus match
    - More rapid biologic incorporation of trabecular grafts
  - Carbon fiber and PEEK interbody cages offer a lower (and more closely matched) modulus compared to metal cages; we typically avoid metal cages in the reconstruction of osteoporotic spinal deformities.
- Autograft remains the gold standard material for establishing a solid arthrodesis but has shortcomings:
  - Morbidity of iliac crest autograft harvest
    - Chronic donor site pain
    - Postoperative hematoma, infection
    - Nerve or vessel injury
  - Iliac graft harvest may be undesirable when iliac instrumentation is planned.
  - Autograft may be insufficient for an extensive thoracolumbar fusion.
  - Autograft alternatives include allograft products, synthetics, and BMP.

Bone Morphogenetic Protein

- The fusion efficacy of bone morphogenetic protein 2 (BMP-2) has been demonstrated in patients with adult spinal deformity.
  - Seventy adult patients underwent scoliosis fusion with anterior or posterior BMP-2 application, with either local bone graft only (posterior) or no bone graft (anterior), obviating rib, iliac crest, or other autograft harvest morbidity.
  - Fusion rates were satisfactory, with 96% anterior fusion success and 93% posterior fusion success.[19]
- The use of BMP-2 in spine surgery has been popularly criticized, however. Independent meta-analyses organized through the Yale Open Data Access project have reported decreased efficacy and increased risk, as compared to what was reported in prior industry supported trials.[10,29]
- Attention to certain surgical techniques may reduce the risk of complications and may also improve efficacy.
- The risks associated with the use of BMP in the cervical spine include
  - Complications related to soft tissue swelling
  - Inappropriate bone formation
  - Accelerated graft resorption
- In the lumbar spine, there also have been reports of undesirable effects, including
  - Inappropriate bone formation around neural elements[20]
  - Postoperative radiculitis
  - Retrograde ejaculation
  - Accelerated resorption of interbody grafts, increasing the risk of pseudarthrosis, has also been reported in a study of single-level uninstrumented ALIF.[24]
- Structural allograft with appropriate doses of BMP at the lower two to four levels in adult thoracolumbar fusions can, however, be used with minimal risks of complications.
- Example: BMP-augmented transforaminal lumbar interbody fusion (TLIF)
  - Care is taken to reduce the risk of inappropriate bone formation.
  - These steps may help ensure maintenance of the BMP and limit the BMP from affecting adjacent tissues:
    - Irrigate before the placement of the BMP packed cage, not afterward.
    - Pack the BMP sponge entirely within the cage, avoiding "overstuffing."
    - Place additional sponge only anterior to the cage.

TRANSFORAMINAL LUMBAR INTERBODY FUSION FOR DEFORMITY CORRECTION AND RECONSTRUCTION

- TLIF may achieve these goals with a posterior-only approach.
- To assist in correction of the deformity, the cage may be biased to the concavity of the scoliosis to address the coronal plane.
- After facetectomy and posterior compression, lordosis can be restored.
  - In general, a posterior interbody technique (posterior or thoracic lumbar interbody fusion) is less effective than an anterior interbody approach for restoring lordosis.
  - The use of an operating table that produces extension of the lumbar spine (Jackson) to maximize positional lordosis is critical.
- The decision of the levels to include in the treatment of a degenerative lumbar deformity may be determined by a variety of influences.
  - It can be useful to preoperatively determine which segments contribute to a patient's pain.
  - The apex of the deformity is included (typically L3 or L4).
  - Levels that are severely degenerated may also be included, particularly if they exhibit lateral or rotary listhesis.

TRANSPSOAS LATERAL LUMBAR INTERBODY FUSION FOR DEFORMITY CORRECTION AND INTERBODY FUSION

- LLIF is an alternative to anterior and posterior interbody fusion, with excellent applications to deformity.[21]
  - The lateral approach provides excellent access for discectomy and interbody fusion **(TECH FIG 2)**.
- It also accommodates excellent deformity correction via
  - The placement of large interbody devices, which span the apophyseal ring and marginal vertebral cortex
  - Complete resection of the lateral annulus and lateral osteophytes, without disruption of the anterior and posterior longitudinal ligaments
- In many cases, it can also provide indirect decompression of the neural elements by restoring segmental height and alignment.[14,22]
- LLIF has been found to be generally safe and effective in comparison to ALIF and TLIF, but it has been frequently associated with adverse anterior thigh symptoms, particularly when operating at L4–L5.[3,6]
- Surgical techniques proposed to limit the risk of adverse anterior thigh symptoms include the following:
  - Direct visualization of the transpsoas approach (via single incision)
  - Direct dissection through psoas (to limit crush or other trauma to muscle and nerve plexus)
  - Accessing the disc through a portal just anterior to midbody; this may limit the risk of encountering a nerve (typically found posterior) and may also limit the pressure on the nerve between the retractor and the transverse processes (TP).

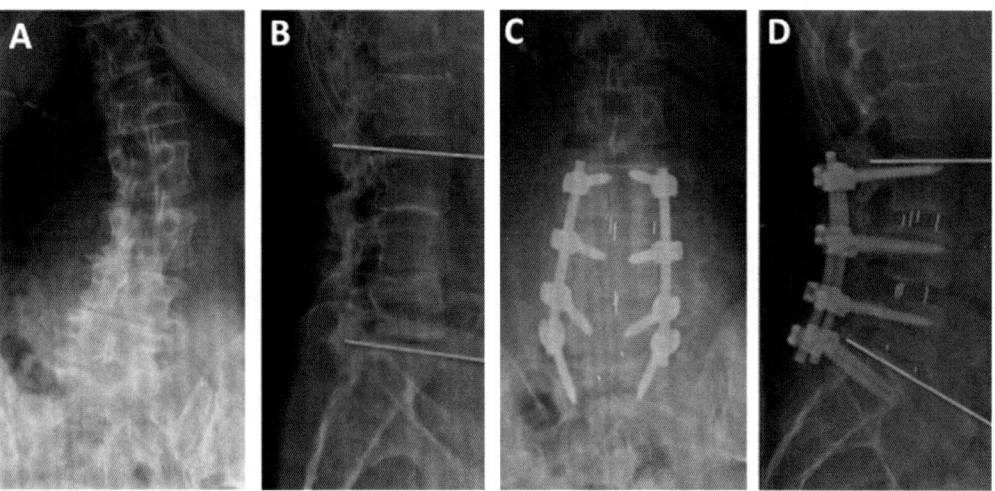

TECH FIG 2 These standing radiographs depict the coronal and sagittal correction associated with interbody reconstruction from a lateral (L3–L4 and L4–L5) and posterior (L5–S1) approach. Note that little to no deformity correction was required from the posterior instrumentation. The coronal correction (**A–C**) and the sagittal correction (**B–D**) were achieved with interbody surgery alone. Panel **A** depicts that the preoperative apical vertebrae is L2, and the central sacral line bisects T11. By maximizing the interbody correction at the focal segments, however, this patient required a relatively short-segment fusion from L3 to S1.

- Performing discectomy and fusion expeditiously; this may limit the nerve injuries related to prolonged compression between the retractor and the TP.
- Avoiding or limiting opening the retractor to limit the degree of compression on the nerves that lie between the retractor and the TP.
- Using intraoperative neuromonitoring (IONM) that includes motor-evoked potentials (MEP), almost all nerve injuries have gone undetected by the traditionally used mode of IONM (electromyography) because the most typical mode of nerve injury (prolonged compression) does not generate a nerve depolarization. MEP however can be used to detect nerve dysfunction related to this slow and progressive mode of injury. We have found this to be very useful in our practice.
- Other LLIF surgical techniques that have been helpful when treating spinal deformity in our practice include the following:
  - Being aware of the effect of the deformity on the location of the retroperitoneal structures (vessels, psoas, lumbosacral plexus) in relation to the planned approach
  - Determine the side of the approach (left vs. right) by the coronal plane deformity; L4–L5 typically can only be approached from the convexity due to the relationship with the iliac crest. Other levels may be best approached from the concavity, however, so that multiple levels can be accessed through a single small lateral incision (**TECH FIG 3**).
  - Ensuring that the patient is positioned with the operative vertebrae orthogonal to the walls and floor of the room will ensure that a path straight down is also straight across the disc. This may reduce the risk of inadvertently traversing posteriorly (into spinal canal and contralateral foramen) or anteriorly (into vessels).
  - Positioning the interbody device anteriorly to favor lordosis while positioning the device posteriorly bias to favor restoration of the foramen height and improve the degree of indirect neurologic decompression

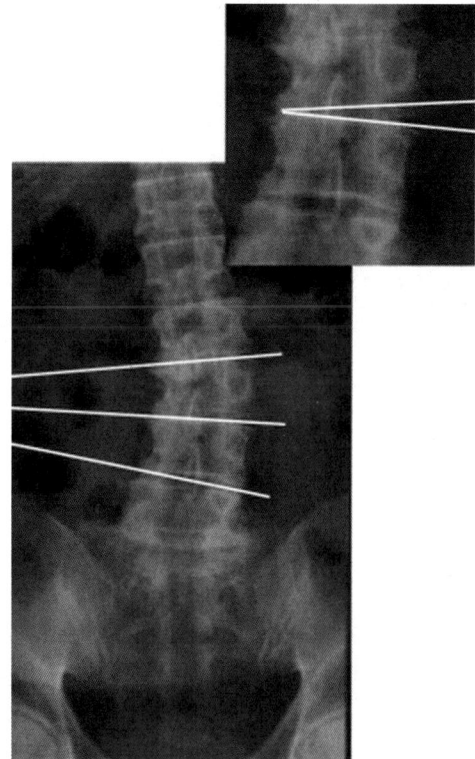

TECH FIG 3 Approaching from the concavity of the lumbar curve (in this case, from patient's right side) may allow multiple levels to be approached from a small single-skin incision. Also, L4–L5 can typically be approached only from the concavity of lumbar curves because the iliac crest typically would prevent the approach from the other side. In this case, L4–L5 is best approached from the patient's right side. In treating single-level, coronal-deformed segments, however, it may be easier to enter the interbody space from the convexity because interbody access is less frequently prevented by osteophytes and because it may be easier to perform the discectomy from the "open" side of the disc.

TECHNIQUES

OBLIQUE LATERAL INTERBODY FUSION

- OLIF uses the corridor between the anterior border of the psoas muscle and the great vessels. This corridor has been shown to increase with mild posterior retraction of the psoas.[7]
- The oblique approach uses the corridor with for levels L2–L5. For L5–S1 the approach uses the corridor caudal to the bifurcation.
- The advantages of the oblique approach are as follows:
  - Allows complete resection of the intervertebral disc, lateral annulus, and osteophytes
  - Large interbody spacers can be placed, which allows correction of the deformity. The spacers are supported by stronger apophyseal bone of the vertebrae.
  - The oblique approach avoids dissection through the psoas and significantly decreases the risk of femoral nerve injury especially at L4–L5 disc space where the risk of injury is higher in transpsoas approach.[3,6]
  - The oblique lateral technique allows anterior interbody fusion from L2 to S1 in single position, thus eliminating the limitations of ALIF and LLIF techniques.

- Pertinent technical details are as follows:
- Patient is positioned right decubitus position (left-side up) **(TECH FIG 4A)** in such a way that the discs are orthogonal for lateral access similar to the LLIF technique. Ensuring that the patient is positioned with the operative vertebrae orthogonal to the walls and floor of the room will ensure that a path straight down is also straight across the disc. This may reduce the risk of inadvertently traversing posteriorly (into spinal canal and contralateral foramen) or anteriorly (into vessels).
- Fluoroscopic images are used to carry out surface markings delineating the disc levels. Incisions are accordingly marked **(TECH FIG 4B)**.
- Initial dissection through the oblique muscles and transversalis to gain access to the retroperitoneum to reach the corridor between the great vessels and the psoas **(TECH FIG 4C)**.

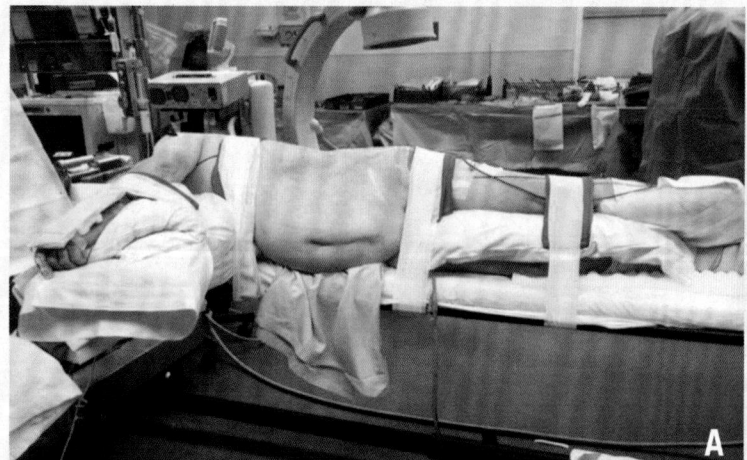
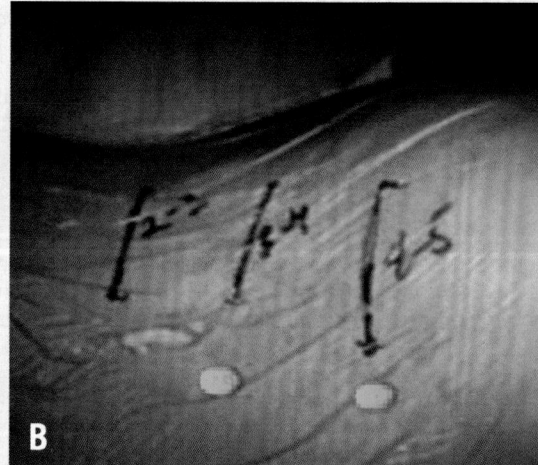

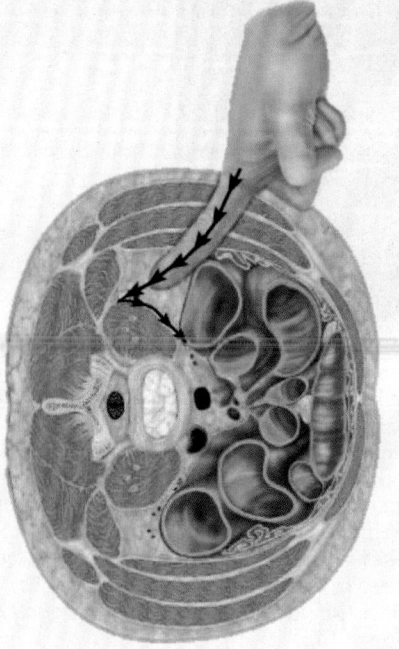
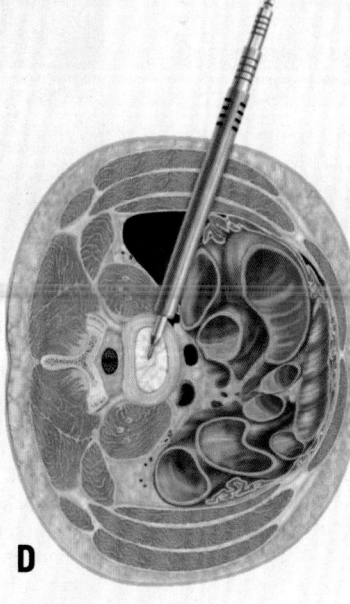

TECH FIG 4 Diagrammatic representation of OLIF. **A.** Patient is positioned in lateral decubitus position. **B.** Fluoroscopic images are used to carry out surface markings delineating the disc levels. Incisions are accordingly marked. *Green circles* describe the incision. **C.** Initial dissection is carried out through abdominal musculature directing obliquely toward the psoas muscle and the TP *(arrows)*. **D.** Sequential dilators are then used, and final retractor is placed. *(continued)*

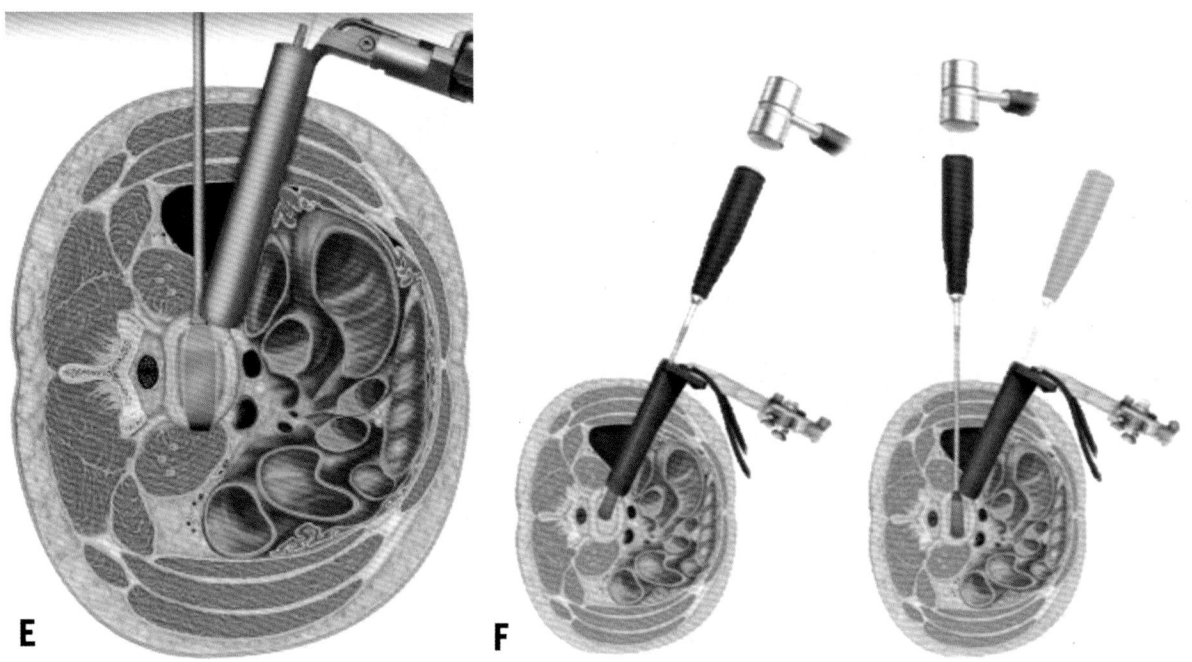

TECH FIG 4 *(continued)* **E.** Disc material is excised, and endplates are prepared. **F.** Orthogonal maneuver for spacer placement.

- Preoperative planning from axial images is of utmost to study relationship of the vessels with psoas, the width of the corridor at the level of L4–L5, level of bifurcation, mobility of the psoas, and left common iliac vein and artery (shape of the vein on the axial cuts [flattened vs. presence of fat underneath the vein and psoas]).
- For L5–S1, the left common iliac vessels are retracted laterally
- Retractors are placed and attached to the table mount **(TECH FIG 4D,E)**.
- An annulotomy is performed in the anterior one-third to one-half of the disc space, a thorough efficient discectomy is carried out, and endplates are prepared carefully.

- Contralateral annulotomy is carried out with the help of a Cobb elevator under C-arm image intensifier.
- An appropriately sized trial and spacer is inserted in the disc space. Insertion of spacer is carried out with a careful orthogonal maneuver **(TECH FIG 4F)**.
- Positioning the interbody device anteriorly to favor lordosis while positioning the device posteriorly bias to favor restoration of the foramen height and improve the degree of indirect neurologic decompression.
- OLIF can be effectively used in degenerative **(TECH FIG 5A–C)** (L4–L5 degenerative spondylolisthesis) and isthmic spondylolisthesis **(TECH FIG 5D–F)** (L5–S1 isthmic spondylolisthesis) from L2 to S1 in a single lateral position.

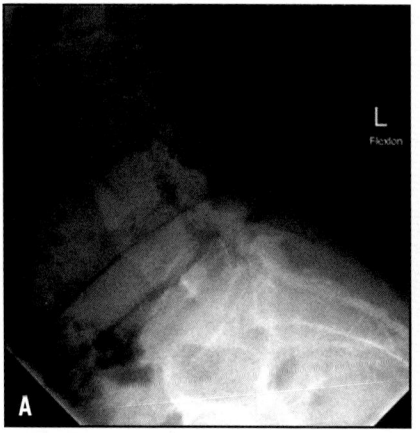
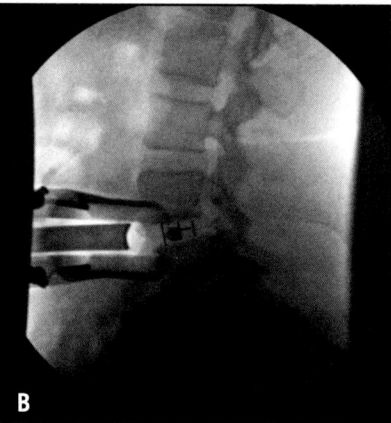
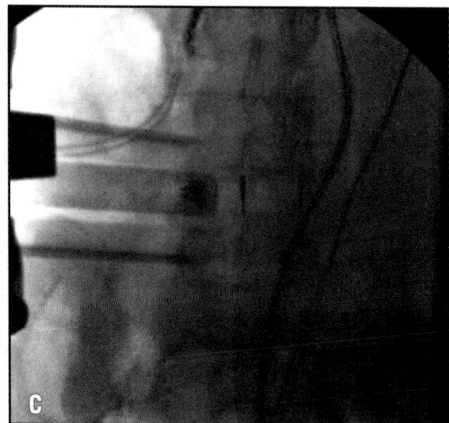

TECH FIG 5 A–C. OLIF used in treatment of L4–L5 degenerative spondylolisthesis. **A.** Lateral flexion view of lumbar spine showing instability and spondylolisthesis. **B,C.** Intraoperative fluoroscopic lateral and AP images showing optimal placement of the spacer in the disc space with reduction of the spondylolisthesis. *(continued)*

TECHNIQUES

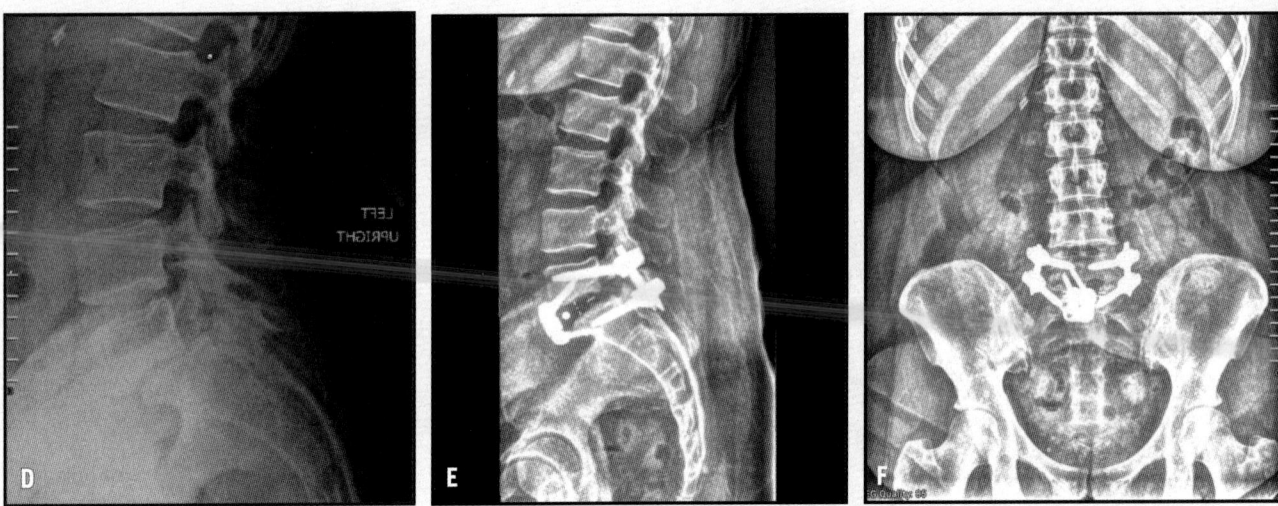

TECH FIG 5 *(continued)* **D–F.** OLIF at the level of L5–S1 for treatment of lytic spondylolisthesis. **D.** Preoperative lateral radiograph showing grade 1 lytic spondylolisthesis at L5–S1. Final postoperative lateral (**E**) and AP (**F**) radiographs showing placement of the spacer, anterior lumbar plate instrumentation, and posterior pedicle screw fixation.

SELECTION OF FUSION LEVEL

- There is no general consensus as to where a lumbar construct should terminate cranially, but it should be at least at a stable-end vertebra (ie, the cranial-end level of the fusion construct should be bisected by the center sacral line on a lateral radiograph).
- If the goal is to treat neurogenic claudication, relieve stenosis, and prevent future progression, a short-segment construct (often L2–L5) is sufficient if adequate lordosis is attained, and the cranial and caudal vertebrae are well balanced.
- In many scenarios, however, such as when the Cobb angle is from L1 to L5, it is necessary to continue the fusion cranially past the thoracolumbar junction.
- When this is the case, one should take care not to end the fusion at the thoracolumbar junction or at the apex of the thoracic kyphosis.
- Extending the fusion to the thoracolumbar junction provides fixation into the more stable rib-bearing vertebrae and is more likely to terminate within the sagittal plumb line, reducing the risk of instrumentation failure or junctional kyphosis.
- A frequent decision-making dilemma is where to end the caudal end of the fusion reconstruction.
- Accepted indications to fuse to the sacrum include the following[2]:
  - Spondylolisthesis or previous laminectomy at L5–S1 (**TECH FIG 6A**)
  - Stenosis requiring decompression at L5–S1
  - Severe degeneration
  - An oblique takeoff (above 15 degrees) of L5 (see **TECH FIG 6A**)

- Fusions to the sacrum in adults with lumbar scoliosis have been found to
  - Require more additional surgery than those to L5
  - Have more postoperative complications
- On the other hand, fusions to L5 have been associated with the following:
  - A 61% rate of adjacent segment disease
  - An associated shift in sagittal balance
- When fusion to the sacrum is performed, iliac fixation should be considered, particularly if the fusion includes more than three levels (**TECH FIG 6C,D**).
- Augmentation of the lumbosacral reconstruction with interbody fusion at L5–S1
  - Improves biomechanical stability[23]
  - Reduces the risk of lumbosacral pseudarthrosis[17]
- A structural graft at L5–S1 can
  - Recreate lordosis, partially restoring sagittal balance
  - Diminish stenosis by restoring intervertebral height
- Hip and knee flexion contractures can be common in this group, with patients accustomed to ambulating with flexed posture.
  - A flexion contracture at the hip limits the patient's ability to extend the sagittal plumb line posterior to the hips.
  - It may be necessary to address the patient's hip pathologies before planning any surgical correction of a spinal deformity.

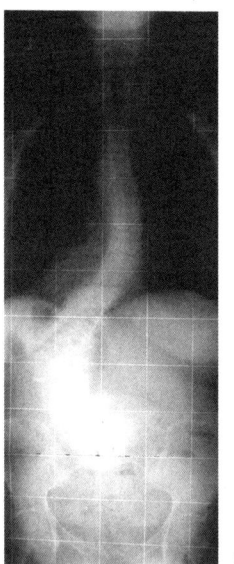
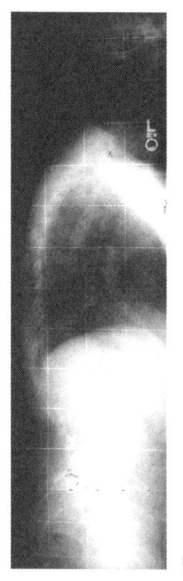
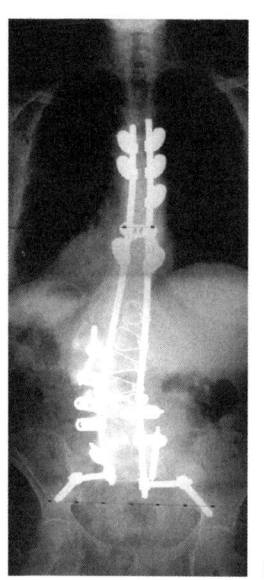
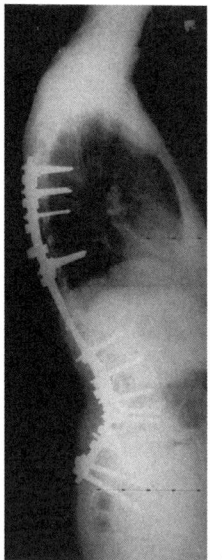

A   B   C   D

TECH FIG 6 These standing radiographs were performed on 36-inch cassettes before and after scoliosis fusion from T4 to the ileum. **A,B.** Iliac fixation was motivated, in part, by the obliquity at the lumbosacral junction. Concerns related to this patient's osteoporosis led the surgeons to use a combination of fixation techniques, including pedicle screw fixation and sublaminar wiring, to take advantage of the relatively well-preserved cortical bone. There is restoration of coronal (**C**) and sagittal (**D**) balance.

THORACIC AND LUMBAR (DOUBLE CURVE) SCOLIOSIS

- Patients with double major adult scoliosis may present with axial skeletal pain.
- Complaints of progressive deformity may be manifested as follows:
  - Changes in balance
  - Gait abnormalities
  - Alterations in cosmesis
- The surgical treatment of double-curve scoliosis often combines anterior and posterior procedures (**TECH FIG 7**).
  - Long deformities that are relatively inflexible may require anterior releases to accomplish effective reduction and fusion with posterior surgery.
- In part, because of the typical degeneration in adult patients, fusions into the caudal lumbar spine are more frequently required.
  - Bending films determine whether the lumbar flexibility is adequate for the scoliosis to "bend out" (see **FIGS 6** and **7**).
  - Curve stiffness is related to both patient age and curve magnitude.

- Flexibility decreases by 10% with every 10-degree increase in coronal deformity beyond 40 degrees.
- Flexibility decreases by 5% to 10% with each decade of life.
- The correction of a double-curve deformity can be accomplished with a variety of methods. The primary goal of achieving a proper sagittal balance must be emphasized. Reduction of the coronal and rotational deformities follows in priority, with the goal of establishing coronal balance and reduction of rib asymmetry for enhanced cosmesis and patient satisfaction, if possible.
- Analogous to the design of the operation for adult lumbar deformities, the decision of whether to extend the fusion to the sacrum may be difficult.
- Lumbosacral fusion is recommended when
  - Decompression of L5–S1 stenosis is required
  - There is a fixed obliquity over 15 degrees at L5–S1 (see **TECH FIG 6B**)

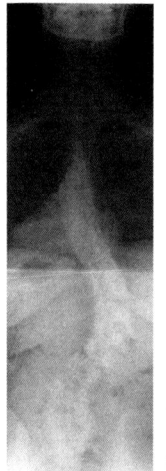
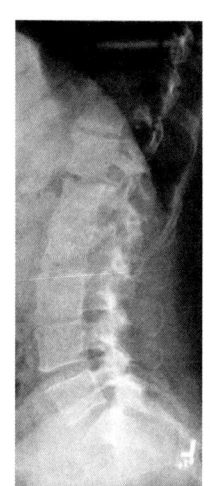
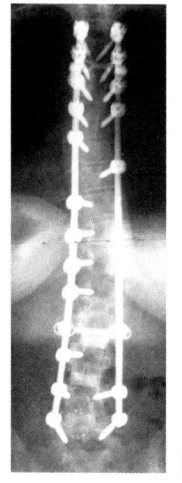
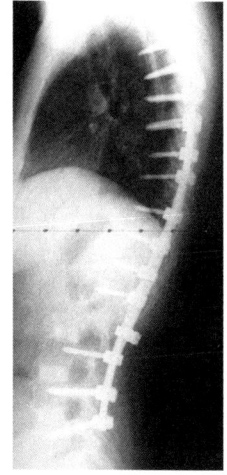

A   B   C   D

TECH FIG 7 A–D. This long thoracolumbar scoliosis was treated with a fusion from the upper thoracic spine to L5. To reduce the risk of pseudarthrosis at the caudal end of the construct and to assist in the recreation of lordosis, structural interbody grafts were placed in the three most caudal disc spaces of the fusion, with morselized graft above, after release of the anterior interbody soft tissues were performed. Subsequently, a posterior fusion was performed with pedicle screw instrumentation.

- Long fusions to the sacrum increase the risk of pseudarthrosis and reoperation. These may be minimized by anterior augmentation and iliac fixation, as previously discussed (see **TECH FIG 7**).
- The cranial end of the fusion should include the thoracic curve and should not stop caudal to any structural aspect of it.
- All fixed deformities and subluxations should be included in the fusion.
- Rod cross-links increase the stiffness of long constructs and are recommended (see **TECH FIG 7C**). They should be avoided at the thoracolumbar junction, however, where they may increase the risk of pseudarthrosis.[15]

- Vertebral derotation
  - Curve stiffness may limit the surgeon's ability to reduce the rotational deformity in the adult population.
  - For relatively flexible rotational deformities, rotational reduction can be achieved with effective improvement in trunk symmetry, which can significantly improve patient satisfaction (**TECH FIG 8**).
  - Additional release maneuvers may be necessary in stiff curves, including thoracoplasty, concave rib osteotomies, and aggressive facetectomies.

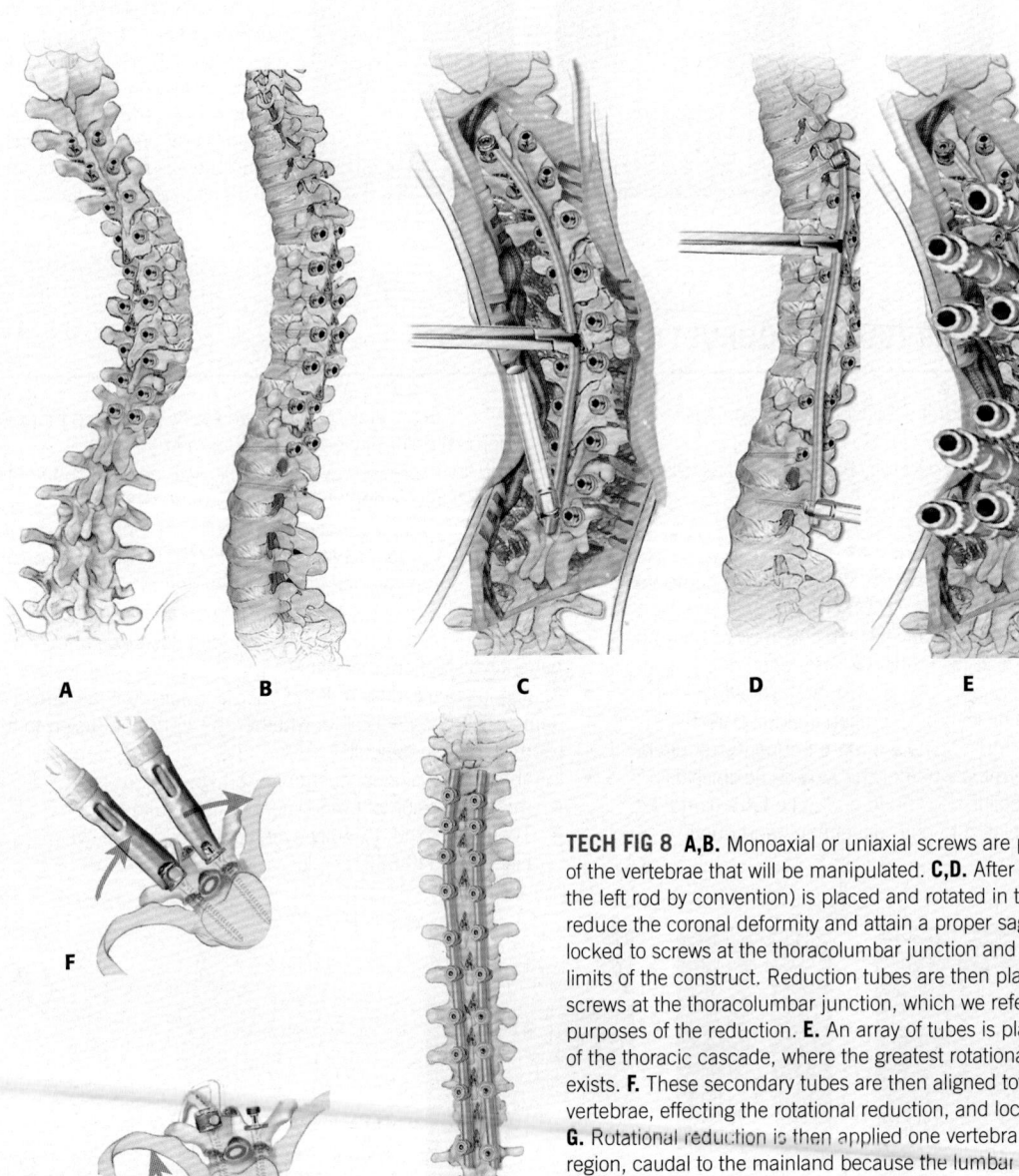

TECH FIG 8 A,B. Monoaxial or uniaxial screws are placed into the pedicles of the vertebrae that will be manipulated. **C,D.** After one prebent rod (usually the left rod by convention) is placed and rotated in the usual manner to reduce the coronal deformity and attain a proper sagittal relationship, it is locked to screws at the thoracolumbar junction and at the cranial and caudal limits of the construct. Reduction tubes are then placed onto the fixed screws at the thoracolumbar junction, which we refer to as the *mainland* for purposes of the reduction. **E.** An array of tubes is placed onto the screws of the thoracic cascade, where the greatest rotational deformity typically exists. **F.** These secondary tubes are then aligned toward the mainland vertebrae, effecting the rotational reduction, and locked to the rods (*arrows*). **G.** Rotational reduction is then applied one vertebra at a time in the lumbar region, caudal to the mainland because the lumbar lordosis often limits the application of more than one set of reduction tubes concurrently (*arrows*). **H.** The prebent contralateral rod is then placed and locked to screws at the thoracolumbar junction as well.

Pearls and Pitfalls

Reduction of Complications Associated with Bone Morphogenetic Protein	• The surgeon should minimize the dose of BMP specific to each application.
	• The surgeon should minimize diffusion of the protein from the site of desired action.
	  • Meticulous hemostasis should be achieved before BMP implantation; a postoperative hematoma may provide an avenue for the spread of the protein.
	  • Wound irrigation should be performed before BMP implantation, not afterward.
	  • The BMP should be contained within a rigid structure to limit compression of the implant to prevent pressure-induced diffusion.
	  • A barrier should be created between the protein implant and sensitive tissues. Thrombin glue has been used to seal the epidural space from the BMP.
	  • Hemostatic sponges and suction drains may permit protein to migrate to adjacent tissues and should not be placed adjacent to the protein implant.

Prevention of Adjacent Segment Disease	• The preoperative status (or health) of the segment or disc is the greatest predictor for the development of adjacent segment disease.
	• For the population with adult scoliosis, where some identifiable degenerative disease is nearly ubiquitous, this is particularly relevant.
	  • The surgeon should not end a fusion adjacent to a severely degenerated disc.
	  • The surgeon should not end a fusion adjacent to a segment with fixed obliquity or subluxation.
	  • The surgeon should preserve the supra-adjacent facet.
	  • The surgeon should preserve the intraspinous and the supraspinous ligaments.
	  • The surgeon should not violate the cranial disc space or facet joint with pedicle screws.

POSTOPERATIVE CARE

• If a brace is used, it must be custom-molded postoperatively after surgical deformity correction is accomplished.

• Application of a preoperatively molded brace is counterproductive and should be avoided.

• Postoperative physical therapy regimen should focus on the following:

　• Range-of-motion and flexibility improvement, often in response to chronic hip and knee loss of motion or contractures

　• Gait training, to include balance rehabilitation

　• General conditioning

REFERENCES

1. Baron EM, Albert TJ. Medical complications of surgical treatment of adult spinal deformity and how to avoid them. Spine (Phila Pa 1976) 2006;31(19 suppl):S106–S118.
2. Bridwell KH. Selection of instrumentation and fusion levels for scoliosis: where to start and where to stop. Invited submission from the Joint Section Meeting on Disorders of the Spine and Peripheral Nerves, March 2004. J Neurosurg Spine 2004;1(1):1–8.
3. Cahill KS, Martinez JL, Wang MY, et al. Motor nerve injuries following the minimally invasive lateral transpsoas approach. J Neurosurg Spine 2012;17(3):227–231.
4. Coe JD, Warden KE, Herzig MA, et al. Influence of bone mineral density on the fixation of thoracolumbar implants. A comparative study of transpedicular screws, laminar hooks, and spinous process wires. Spine (Phila Pa 1976) 1990;15(9):902–907.
5. Cook SD, Salkeld SL, Stanley T, et al. Biomechanical study of pedicle screw fixation in severely osteoporotic bone. Spine J 2004;4(4):402–408.
6. Cummock MD, Vanni S, Levi AD, et al. An analysis of postoperative thigh symptoms after minimally invasive transpsoas lumbar interbody fusion. J Neurosurg Spine 2011;15(1):11–18.
7. Davis TT, Hynes RA, Fung DA, et al. Retroperitoneal oblique corridor to the L2–S1 intervertebral discs in the lateral position: an anatomic study. J Neurosurg Spine 2014;21(5):785–793.
8. Eck KR, Bridwell KH, Ungacta FF, et al. Complications and results of long adult deformity fusions down to l4, l5, and the sacrum. Spine (Phila Pa 1976) 2001;26(9):E182–E192.
9. Faraj SS, Holewijn RM, van Hooff ML, et al. De novo degenerative lumbar scoliosis: a systematic review of prognostic factors for curve progression. Eur Spine J 2016;25(8):2347–2358.
10. Fu R, Selph S, McDonagh M, et al. Effectiveness and harms of recombinant human bone morphogenetic protein-2 in spine fusion: a systematic review and meta-analysis. Ann Intern Med 2013;158(12):890–902.
11. Glassman SD, Berven S, Bridwell K, et al. Correlation of radiographic parameters and clinical symptoms in adult scoliosis. Spine (Phila Pa 1976) 2005;30(6):682–688.
12. Glassman SD, Bridwell K, Dimar JR, et al. The impact of positive sagittal balance in adult spinal deformity. Spine (Phila Pa 1976) 2005;30(18):2024–2029.
13. Kelleher MO, Timlin M, Persaud O, et al. Success and failure of minimally invasive decompression for focal lumbar spinal stenosis in patients with and without deformity. Spine (Phila Pa 1976) 2010;35(19):E981–E987.
14. Kepler CK, Sharma AK, Huang RC, et al. Indirect foraminal decompression after lateral transpsoas interbody fusion. J Neurosurg Spine 2012;16(4):329–333.
15. Kim YJ, Bridwell KH, Lenke LG, et al. Pseudarthrosis in long adult spinal deformity instrumentation and fusion to the sacrum: prevalence and risk factor analysis of 144 cases. Spine (Phila Pa 1976) 2006;31(20):2329–2336.
16. Kobayashi T, Atsuta Y, Takemitsu M, et al. A prospective study of de novo scoliosis in a community based cohort. Spine (Phila Pa 1976) 2006;31(2):178–182.
17. Kuklo TR, Bridwell KH, Lewis SJ, et al. Minimum 2-year analysis of sacropelvic fixation and L5-S1 fusion using S1 and iliac screws. Spine (Phila Pa 1976) 2001;26(18):1976–1983.
18. Lin JT, Lane JM. Osteoporosis: a review. Clin Orthop Relat Res 2004;(425):126–134.
19. Luhmann SJ, Bridwell KH, Cheng I, et al. Use of bone morphogenetic protein-2 for adult spinal deformity. Spine (Phila Pa 1976) 2005;30(17 suppl):S110–S117.
20. McKay B, Sandhu HS. Use of recombinant human bone morphogenetic protein-2 in spinal fusion applications. Spine (Phila Pa 1976) 2002;27(16 suppl 1):S66–S85.
21. Metkar U, McGuire KJ, White AP. Indirect decompression and interbody fusion for treatment of isthmic and degenerative lumbar spondylolisthesis by minimally invasive trans-psoas approach. Orthop J Harv Med Sch 2011;13.
22. Oliveira L, Marchi L, Coutinho E, et al. A radiographic assessment of the ability of the extreme lateral interbody fusion procedure to

indirectly decompress the neural elements. Spine (Phila Pa 1976) 2010;35(26 suppl):S331–S337.

23. Polly DW Jr, Klemme WR, Cunningham BW, et al. The biomechanical significance of anterior column support in a simulated single-level spinal fusion. J Spinal Disord 2000;13(1):58–62.

24. Pradhan BB, Bae HW, Kropf MA. Graft resorption with rhBMP-2 in anterior cervical discectomy and fusion: a radiographic characterization of the effect of rhBMP-2 on structural allografts. Spine J 2005;5:181S–189S.

25. Sansur CA, Smith JS, Coe JD, et al. Scoliosis Research Society morbidity and mortality of adult scoliosis surgery. Spine (Phila Pa 1976) 2011;36(9):E593–E597.

26. Sarzier JO, Evans AJ, Cahill DW. Increased pedicle screw pullout strength with vertebroplasty augmentation in osteoporotic spines. J Neurosurg 2002;96(3 suppl):309–312.

27. Schwab FJ, Blondel B, Bess S, et al. Radiographical spinopelvic parameters and disability in the setting of adult spinal deformity: a prospective multicenter analysis. Spine (Phila Pa 1976) 2013;38(13):E803–E812.

28. Silva FE, Lenke LG. Adult degenerative scoliosis: evaluation and management. Neurosurg Focus 2010;28(3):E1.

29. Simmonds MC, Brown JV, Heirs MK, et al. Safety and effectiveness of recombinant human bone morphogenetic protein-2 for spinal fusion: a meta-analysis of individual-participant data. Ann Intern Med 2013;158(12):877–889.

30. Smith JS, Shaffrey CI, Glassman SD, et al. Risk-benefit assessment of surgery for adult scoliosis: an analysis based on patient age. Spine (Phila Pa 1976) 2011;36(10):817–824.

31. Terran J, Schwab F, Shaffrey CI, et al. The SRS-Schwab adult spinal deformity classification: assessment and clinical correlations based on a prospective operative and nonoperative cohort. Neurosurgery 2013;73(4):559–568.

32. Transfeldt EE, Topp R, Mehbod AA, et al. Surgical outcomes of decompression, decompression with limited fusion, and decompression with full curve fusion for degenerative scoliosis with radiculopathy. Spine (Phila Pa 1976) 2010;35(20):1872–1875.

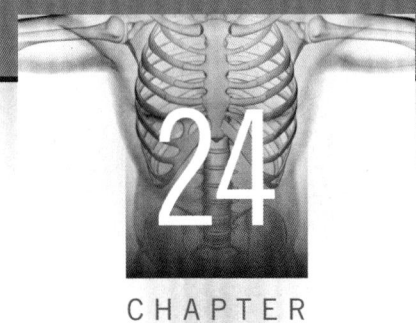

24

CHAPTER

Posterior Column Osteotomy and Pedicle Subtraction Osteotomy

Michael P. Kelly, Lukas P. Zebala, and Keith H. Bridwell

DEFINITION

- A posterior column osteotomy (PCO) is a chevron resection of the posterior elements that shorten the posterior column and lengthen the anterior column upon closure (**FIG 1A**). The chevron osteotomy is called a *Smith-Petersen osteotomy* (SPO) if performed through a prior fusion or a *Ponté osteotomy* if done through a nonfused spinal segment. These are Schwab type 2 osteotomies.[6]
- Pedicle subtraction osteotomy (PSO) is a posterior-based osteotomy that requires resection of the posterior elements, pedicles, and decancellation of the vertebral body in a V-shaped fashion through the transpedicular corridor (**FIG 1B**). The osteotomy hinges on the anterior column with closure of the middle and posterior columns creating a large cancellous bone footprint for fusion. These are Schwab type 3 and 4 osteotomies.

ANATOMY

- A thorough understanding of spinal anatomy including spinal cord, nerve root, and vertebral segments is needed to safely perform these procedures. For a PCO, understanding the relationship of the interspinous ligaments, ligamentum flavum, facet joints, nerve roots, and spinal cord is important to resect enough posterior elements to allow osteotomy closure without posterior impingement. In a PSO, it is important to understand these same relationships, but in addition, the relationship of the exiting and traversing nerve roots to the corresponding pedicle is necessary to allow safe osteotomy closure.
- PCO involves creating a chevron trough in the posterior elements by resecting the posterior elements through the facet joints and pars intra-articularis and posterior ligaments (supraspinous, intraspinous, and ligamentum flavum). A mobile disc space allows for closure of the middle and posterior columns and spontaneous opening of the anterior column.
- A PSO requires a wide laminectomy from the pedicle above to pedicle below the osteotomy level, resection of the bilateral pedicles at the PSO level, and vertebral body decancellation to the anterior vertebral body in a wedge shape.

PATHOGENESIS

- Sagittal imbalance may be classified into two types.
  - Type I sagittal imbalance is when there is a region of the spine that is fused in a hypolordotic or kyphotic position, but overall, sagittal balance is satisfactory (sagittal C7 plumb falling through the L5–S1 disc space or slightly behind it on a standing long cassette lateral radiograph) as the patient is able to compensate through nonfused segments.

- A type II imbalance is one in which the patient cannot compensate due to adjacent level degeneration resulting in a positive sagittal imbalance (patient leans forward in the sagittal plane).
- Type I patients often maintain their balance by hyperextending through mobile lumbar segments below the kyphotic segment. In type II imbalance, vertebral segments above or below the kyphotic area are substantially degenerated or fused, and therein, the spine is unable to hyperextend and maintain balance (**FIG 2**).
- Kyphosis can be smooth and span several segments, such as in Scheuermann kyphosis (**FIG 3**), or sharp and angular, over one or two segments, such as in congenital or posttraumatic kyphosis.

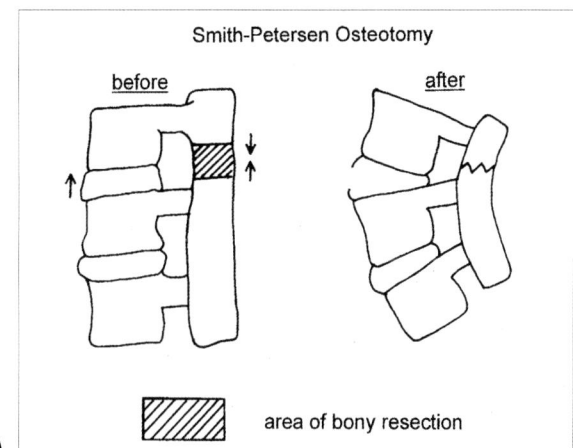

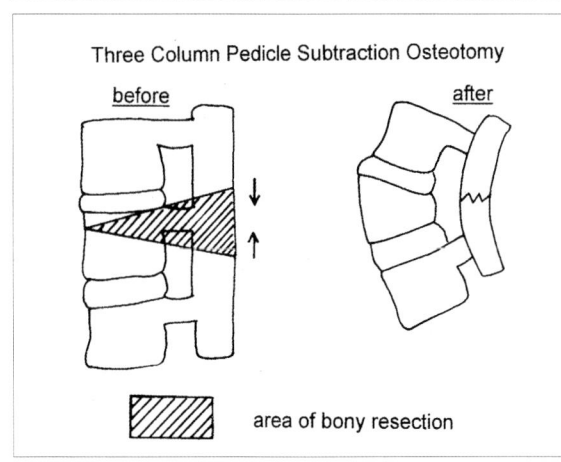

FIG 1 A. Area of bone resection for an SPO. **B.** Area of bone resection for a PSO.

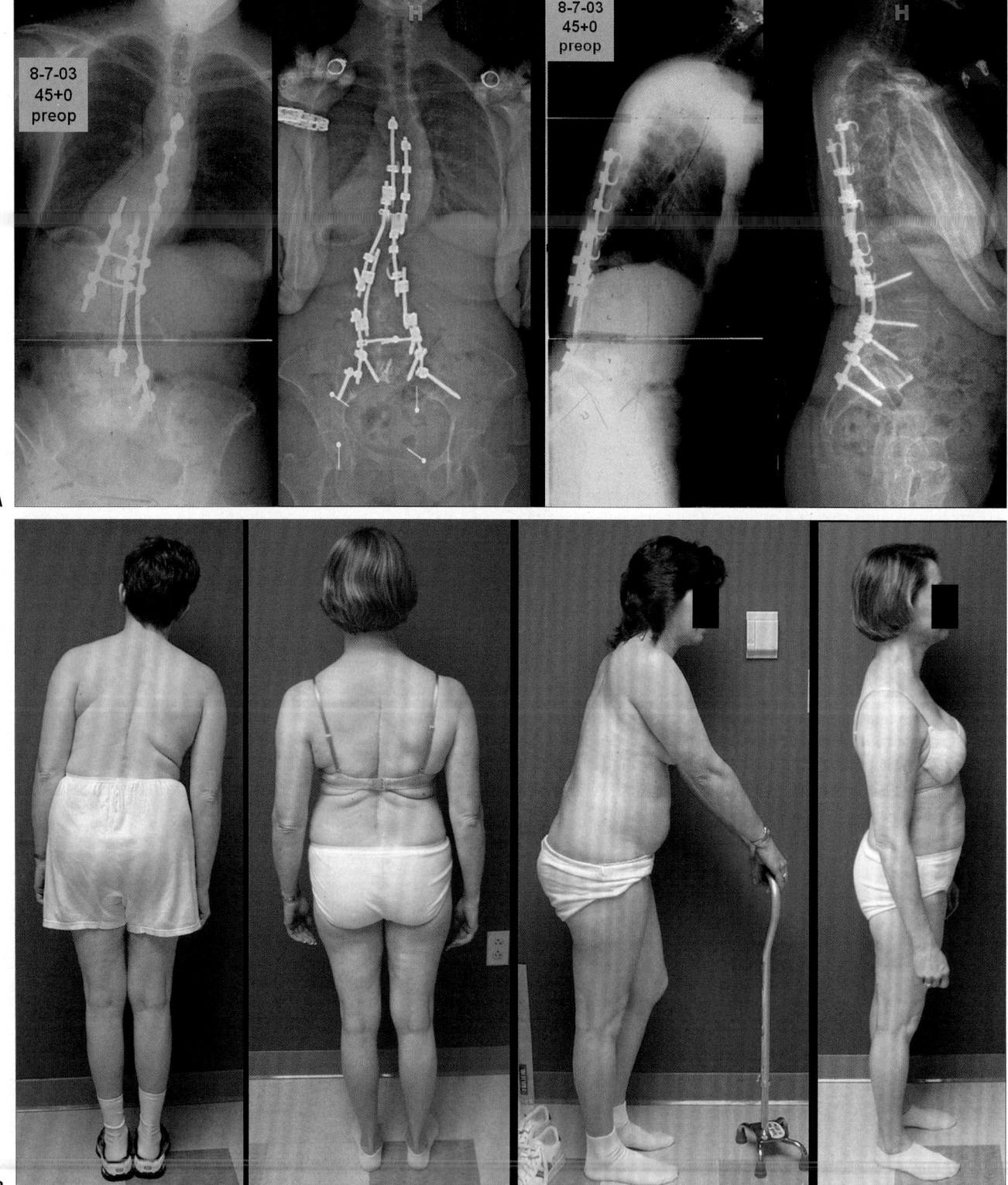

FIG 2 A,B. Patient (45-year-old woman) with eight prior spinal fusions presenting with fixed sagittal and coronal imbalances. An asymmetric L2 PSO was performed for spinal realignment. At 6-year follow-up, a solid fusion was achieved with improvement in radiographic and clinical appearance.

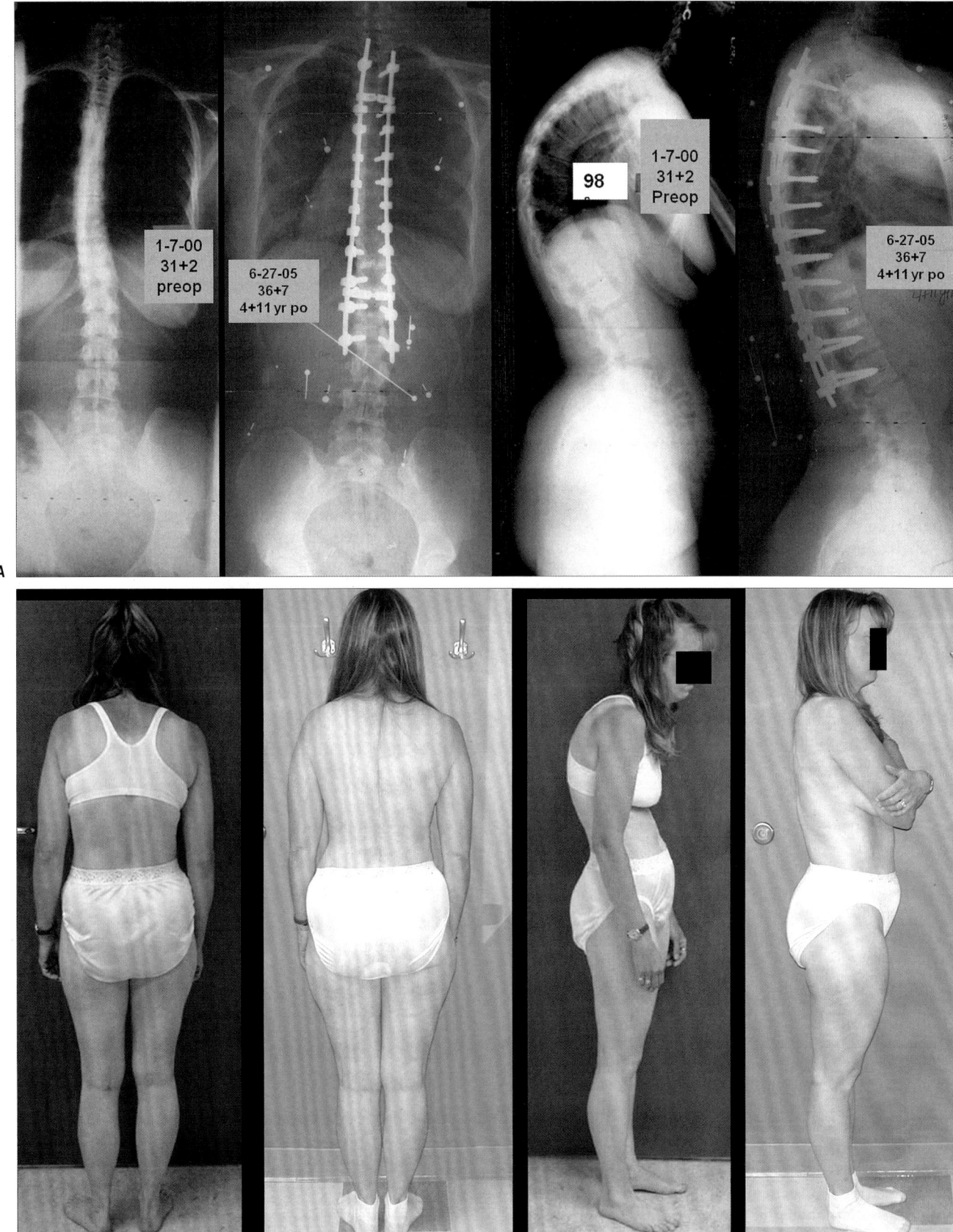

FIG 3 A,B. Patient (31-year-old woman) with three prior posterior spinal fusions at outside institution for treatment of Scheuermann kyphosis presented with worsened thoracic kyphosis, multiple pseudarthrosis, and sagittal imbalance. A revision T3–L2 posterior spinal fusion with SPOs T5–T12 and anterior spinal fusion was performed for spinal realignment. At 5-year follow-up, a solid AP fusion was achieved with improvement in radiographic and clinical appearance.

- These osteotomies are most often used for the correction of sagittal imbalance or kyphosis. PCOs are most often used to correct sagittal imbalance between 5 and 10 cm or smooth gradual kyphosis, whereas a PSO is used to treat sagittal imbalance greater than 10 cm or sharp, angular kyphosis within the lumbar spine. An asymmetric PSO can be done for a deformity that has both a coronal imbalance and sagittal imbalance together. A vertebral column resection can be used to treat sharp, angular kyphosis within the thoracic or thoracolumbar spine.

NATURAL HISTORY

- The natural history of the diseases/conditions leading to sagittal imbalance and kyphosis is variable, and a complete workup is necessary before recommending an osteotomy as a corrective operation.
- Deformities that progress become rigid and, uncompensated, may present with intolerable pain, decreased ability to perform activities of daily living, or myelopathy and nerve root impingement.

PATIENT HISTORY AND PHYSICAL FINDINGS

- The thorough history should include an understanding of the patient's main reason(s) for seeking treatment, for example, progressive deformity, pain, loss of function, and neurologic deterioration.
- The history should include a careful assessment of current pain medication usage as preoperative narcotic usage may complicate the perioperative care. Additionally, any medications that may confer a risk of increased bleeding (eg, acetylsalicylic acid) should be noted, and the patient is cautioned to stop them prior to surgery.
- Patients should be questioned on their use of nicotine-containing products, particularly cigarettes, as the risk of perioperative complications and pseudarthrosis is increased in these patients and is a relative contraindication to these procedures.
- Those patients with diabetes mellitus must have well-controlled blood glucose levels before and after surgery, as uncontrolled blood glucose levels are associated with increased risk of perioperative infection. Our target hemoglobin A1c for elective spine surgery is 7.5%.
- A patient's nutritional status should be assessed and optimized prior to surgery. In addition, a bone density test should be performed to assess for osteoporosis, and appropriate treatment of these deficiencies or referral for their treatment should be initiated.
- Patients with respiratory disease may require consultation with a pulmonologist or assessment of lung function by pulmonary function tests. Cardiac history should be assessed with the assistance of a cardiologist. Often, coordination with the patient's primary care physician is necessary to get the patient ready for these surgeries.
- The overall coronal and sagittal plane balance should be observed with the patient standing upright.
- The deformity should be assessed for its flexibility by placing the patient prone and supine on the examination table. Several minutes of supine positioning will allow one to assess the flexibility of a kyphotic deformity.
- A detailed neurologic examination assessing sensation, strength, reflexes, and pathologic reflexes is necessary.

A complete neurologic examination should assess for signs of myelopathy (gait disturbance such as a wide-based gait, imbalance) or nerve root palsies (foot drop). In addition, assessment of hip and knee contractures is required as these conditions may make osteotomy correction and postoperative recovery more difficult.

IMAGING AND OTHER DIAGNOSTIC STUDIES

- Radiographic assessment includes a series of standing full-length 36-inch radiographs in the anteroposterior (AP) and lateral planes and full-length supine or prone radiographs to assess spontaneous deformity correction.
- Hyperextension radiographs (bolster placed at apex of kyphosis) and hyperflexion radiographs (bolster at apex of lordosis) help assess sagittal plane rigidity.
- For sagittal plane deformity, comparison of standing AP and lateral radiographs to prone and/or supine fulcrum hyperextension long-cassette radiographs will help assess deformity flexibility.
- Computed tomography (CT) scan is often obtained to assess prior fusion masses, bone quality, relevant bone anatomy at proposed osteotomy site, and bone anomalies (small pedicles) that may preclude safe fixation point placement. A CT myelogram may help assess areas of stenosis.
  - CT scans will also show vacuum discs. These can be exploited for sagittal plane correction with a PCO at the level of the degeneration.
- Magnetic resonance imaging is often obtained to evaluate the spinal cord and nerve roots in addition to assessing for neural axis anomalies.
- If PCOs are planned, assessment for mobile disc spaces or vacuum discs is paramount as they are a requirement for this osteotomy.

DIFFERENTIAL DIAGNOSIS

- Smooth global kyphosis (Scheuermann kyphosis)
- Sharp angular kyphosis (posttraumatic)
- Sagittal imbalance (types I and II) (flat back syndrome, postlaminectomy kyphosis)

NONOPERATIVE MANAGEMENT

- Patients with static deformities and only mild pain or physical impairment should be managed with a trial of nonoperative therapy.
- This includes a directed physical therapy program to include cardiovascular conditioning, postural training, and abdominal strengthening.
- For those patients with moderate to severe pain, a referral to a pain specialist, most notably for those patients with complaints of pain not consistent with their presenting pathology or other signs of nonorganic causes of pain.
- Epidural and transforaminal steroid injections offer a less invasive, potentially diagnostic, and/or therapeutic intervention for patients with nerve root compression.

SURGICAL MANAGEMENT

- PCO is often used to treat semirigid, smooth, gradual kyphotic deformities or positive sagittal imbalance of 5 to 10 cm.
- Usually, multiple PCOs are performed through the apex of the deformity.

- It is important to perform a wide facetectomy as posterior compression closes down the neural foramina and may cause nerve root impingement. In general, the degree of kyphotic correction with a single SPO is 10 degrees per level or 1 degree per millimeter of bone resected.
  - Removal of all ligamentum flavum is necessary to avoid central stenosis after closure.
- A PSO is most often performed for sharp angular kyphosis, gradual kyphosis that lacks mobile disc spaces, or positive sagittal imbalance greater than 10 cm. In general, the degree of kyphotic correction with a lumbar PSO is approximately 30 to 40 degrees.

Preoperative Planning

- A multidisciplinary team approach is often necessary in the treatment of patients with complex deformity that requires multilevel PCOs or a PSO.
- Preoperative assessment of the patient's cardiovascular, pulmonary, nutritional, hematologic, and metabolic systems is required to maximize the patient's preoperative reserve.
  - PCOs can be performed within any region of the spine, most often in the thoracic or lumbar spine.
  - PSOs are most often performed in the lumbar spine. They are also performed at the cervicothoracic junction for sagittal plane deformities. The smaller vertebral bodies here limit shortening and angular correction, however.

Positioning

- An Orthopedic Systems, Inc., Jackson frame with six pads or an articulating frame is our preferred operative table when performing corrective deformity surgery. The pads are strategically placed to allow the abdomen to rest free, reducing intra-abdominal pressure and intraoperative bleeding. In addition, the axilla should be free to help reduce the risk of brachial plexus injury.
- We prefer to place a halo or Gardner-Wells tongs with 5 to 15 lb of traction that allows for rigid positioning of the skull and allows the face and eyes to remain free during surgery.
  - We will often use a halo for positioning for semirigid kyphotic deformities as the halo pushes the upper spine dorsally.
- Arms are placed in a 90/90 position on padded arm boards with no pressure on the axillae and elbow padding to decrease the risk of brachial plexopathy or ulnar nerve neuropathy.
- The hips are gently extended, and the knees are slightly flexed. For PSO correction, the hips can be extended further to help close down the osteotomy.
- Spinal cord monitoring leads are placed to monitor the sensory and motor function of the lower extremities.

Approach

- The standard posterior subperiosteal approach is used from the transverse processes of the most superior instrumented level to the most distal vertebra or ilium that are to be fused.
- The approach can be done in stages, lumbar followed by thoracic or vice versa, to help reduce blood loss if adequate surgical help is not available. In conjunction with the anesthesiologist, hypotensive anesthesia is used to help reduce blood loss.
- In addition, the use of antifibrinolytic medications can assist in helping reduce blood loss during these procedures. In general, we use tranexamic acid with a 30 mg/kg loading bolus and 10 mg/kg/hour infusion until wound closure.

POSTERIOR COLUMN OSTEOTOMY

- Identify the pedicles at all levels where PCOs are planned by placing pedicle screws.
  - Alternatively, PCOs can be done prior to placement of pedicle screws. For large deformities or abnormal pedicle anatomy, performing a PCO first can help identify the medial and superior borders of the pedicle to assist in locating of the starting point for pedicle screw placement.
- Remove the interspinous ligaments down to level of ligament flavum and identify the median raphe. Ensure adequate space between ligament flavum and dura with a Woodson elevator and use Kerrison punches to resect a V of bone that starts centrally and works out laterally through the facet joints and pars (see **FIG 1A**).

- Closure of the osteotomy is through a combination of compression and cantilever forces **(TECH FIG 1)**.
  - In treatment of a smooth gradual kyphosis, bilateral rods are contoured to the desired sagittal plane profile and secured into the cephalad pedicles.
  - Gradual cantilever (downward) force is applied, and the rods are sequentially captured within the caudally located pedicle screws.
  - Once the rod is captured within the pedicle screws, sequential compression through the pedicle screws toward the deformity apex can be added to close down the PCOs.
  - Compressive forces reduce spinal kyphosis.

TECHNIQUES

TECHNIQUES

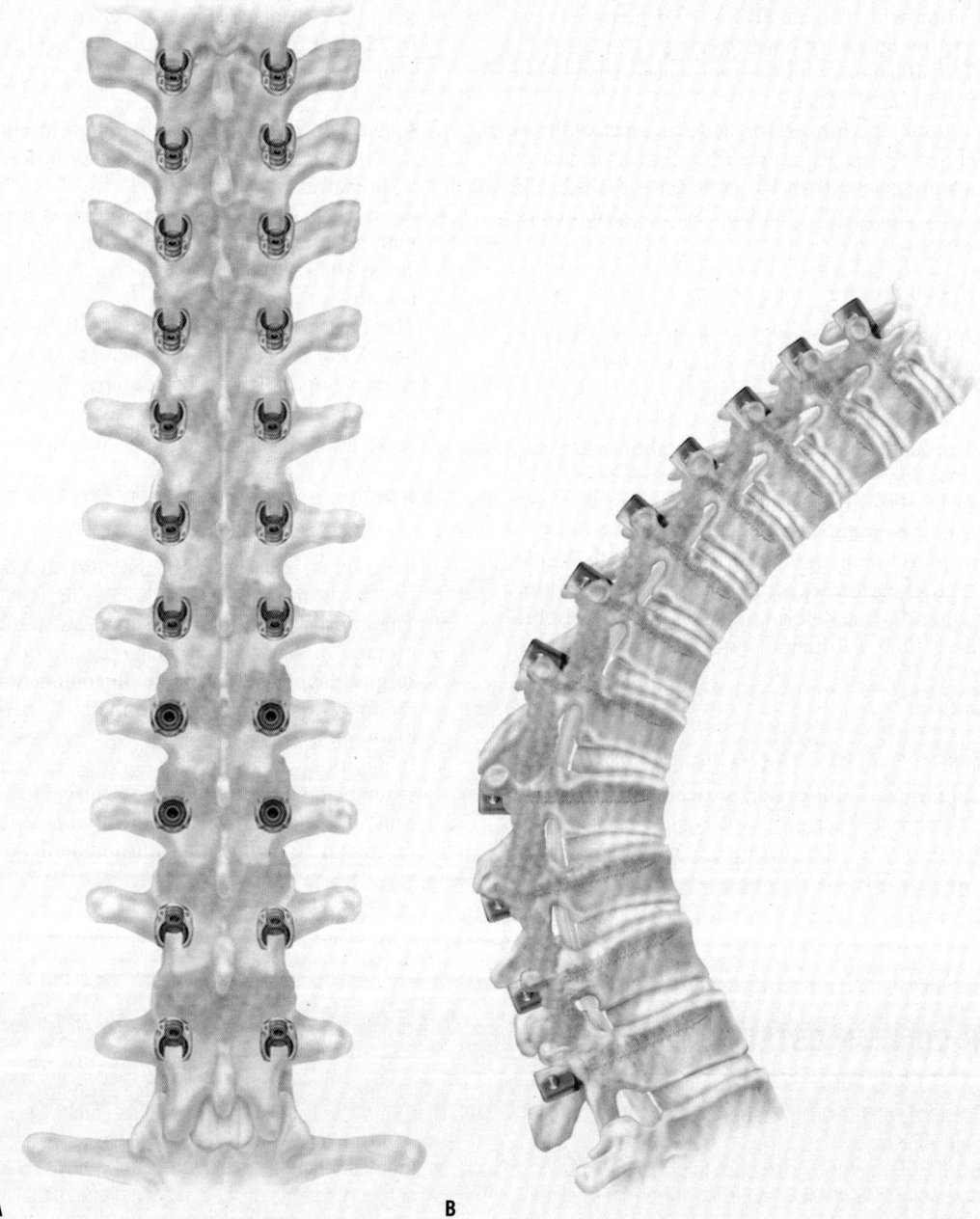

A   B

TECH FIG 1 A,B. Gradual, smooth thoracic kyphosis with multilevel pedicle screw placement. *(continued)*

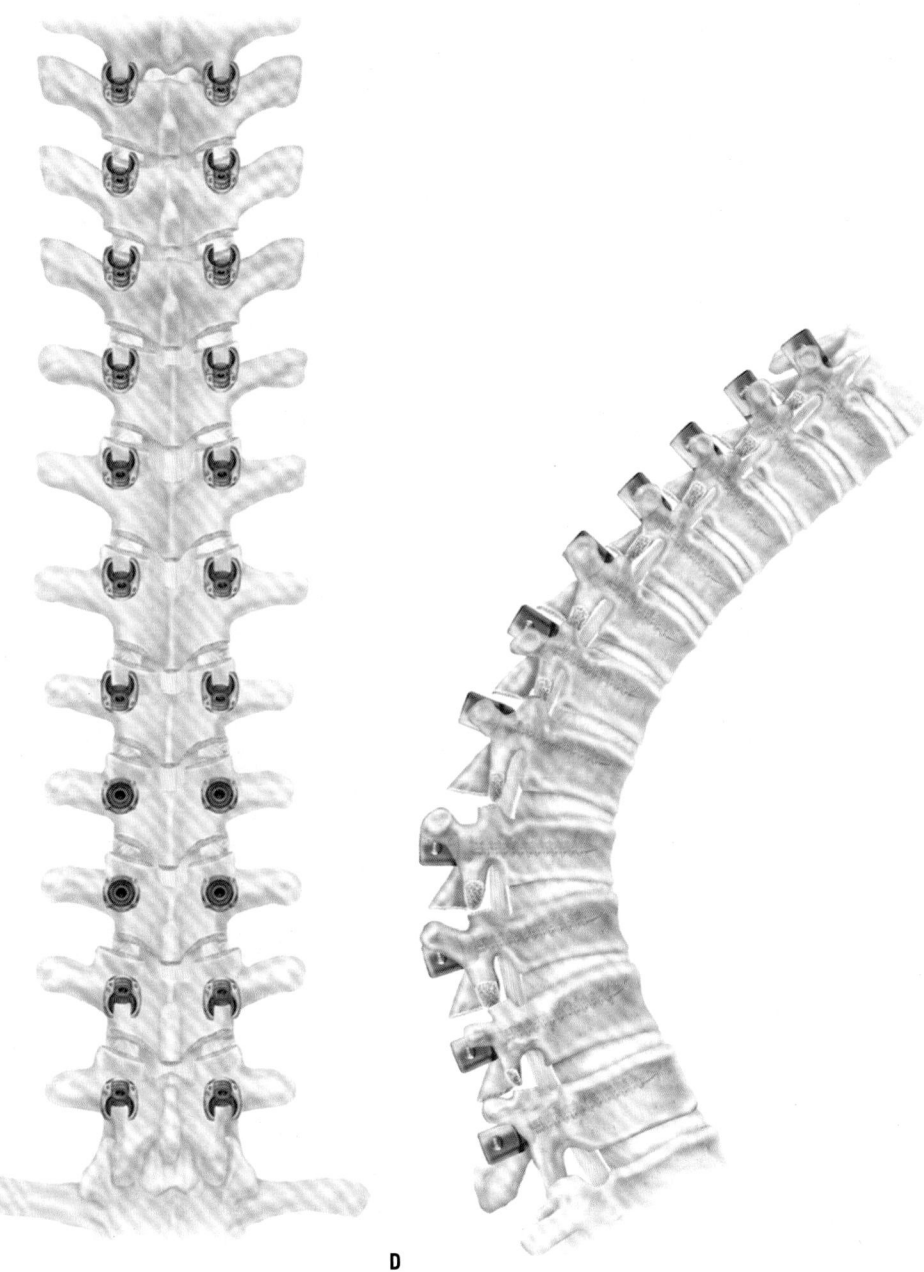

C

D

TECH FIG 1 *(continued)* **C,D.** Multiple thoracic SPOs performed through the apex of the smooth kyphosis; an ideal situation for sagittal correction with multiple SPOs. *(continued)*

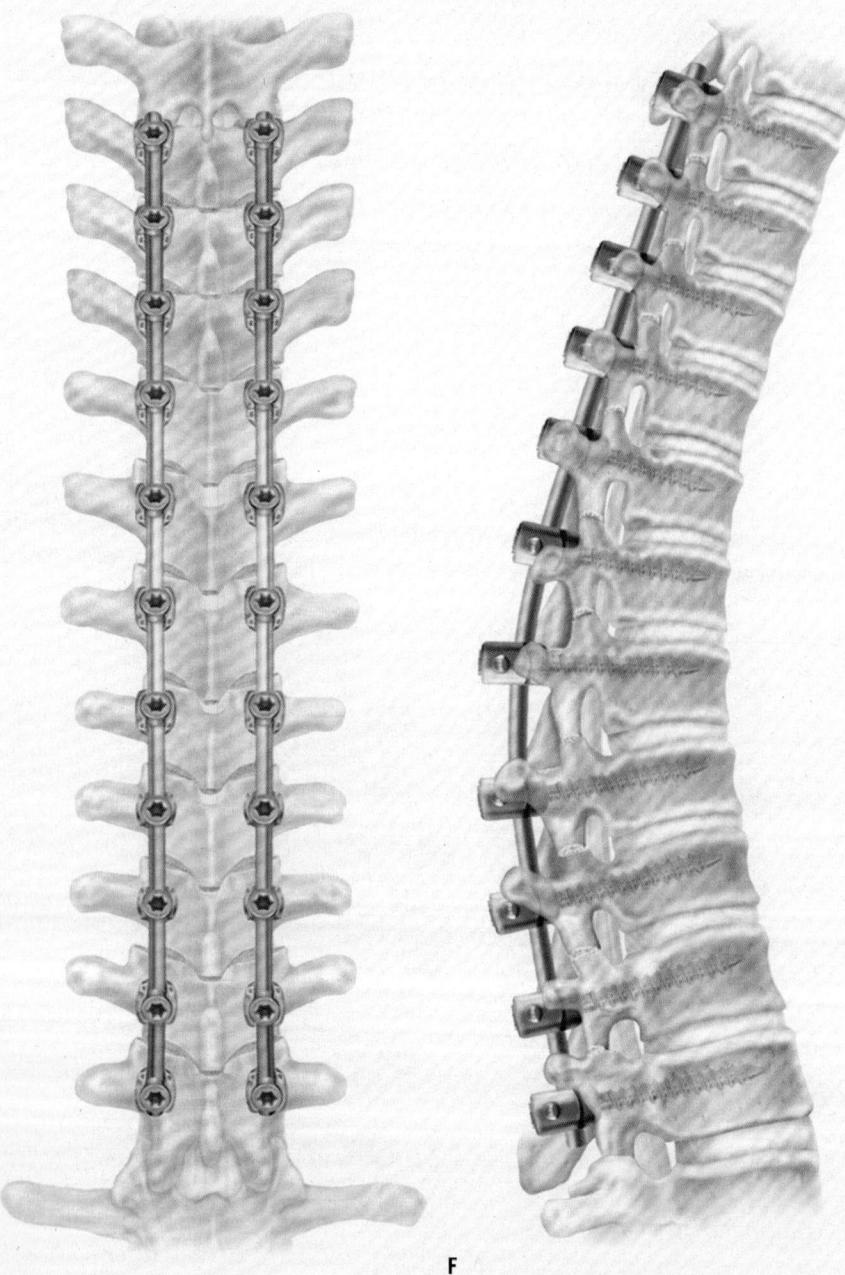

E   F

TECH FIG 1 *(continued)* **E,F.** Cantilever and compression forces through bilateral rods allow for gradual, controlled correction of the smooth kyphosis by closing down of the SPOs.

PEDICLE SUBTRACTION OSTEOTOMY

- Resect all the posterior elements around the pedicles with a combination of Leksell rongeurs, high-speed burr, and Kerrison ▢ches.
  - ▢rr can outline the bone to be removed, and then ▢ is completed with an osteotome. This may speed ▢ ▢articularly in cases of large fusion masses.

- The pedicles are surrounded medially, laterally, superiorly, and inferiorly **(TECH FIG 2A)**.
- A partial laminectomy and pars resection of the level above the PSO is performed to the level of the caudal pedicle. A partial laminectomy and superior facetectomy is performed at the caudal level. This allows visualization of the two exiting roots and the traversing root.

- In cases of revision laminectomies, all of the scar must be removed from the dura. If this is not done, it may buckle and case a neurologic deficit after osteotomy closure.
  - Penfield no. 1, no. 15 blade, and fine Metzenbaum scissors are all useful when dissecting scar from the dura.
- At L5, we resect the entire transverse process. Above L5, the transverse process is detached at the lateral pedicle and the psoas attachments are preserved. This offers another area for posterolateral fusion (**TECH FIG 2B**).
  - When performing L5 PSO, we resect the top of the sacral ala and trace the L5 root into the pelvis.
- Subperiosteal dissection is performed along the lateral pedicle and vertebral body wall to reach the front of the spine.
  - We then pack this with cotton or place a "spoon" retractor to retract lateral structures.

- A box osteotome resects the pedicle after a temporary rod is placed on the contralateral side.
  - Two cuts are frequently needed. We begin with the superior cut along the top of the pedicle. The second cut removes the inferior portion of the pedicle. This large pedicle fragment is removed with vertebral body.
  - Working within the void, we remove the remainder of the vertebral body as planned to allow for the appropriate correction.
  - One must be careful to preserve the anterior cortex. It must not collapse with closure, or else one will lose angular correction.
  - A rod is placed on the side of the resection, and the same procedure performed on the other side.
- Thin the posterior vertebral body wall with a curette until it is wafer thin. Greenstick the posterior vertebral cortex with a Woodson elevator or reverse-angled curette (**TECH FIG 2C**).

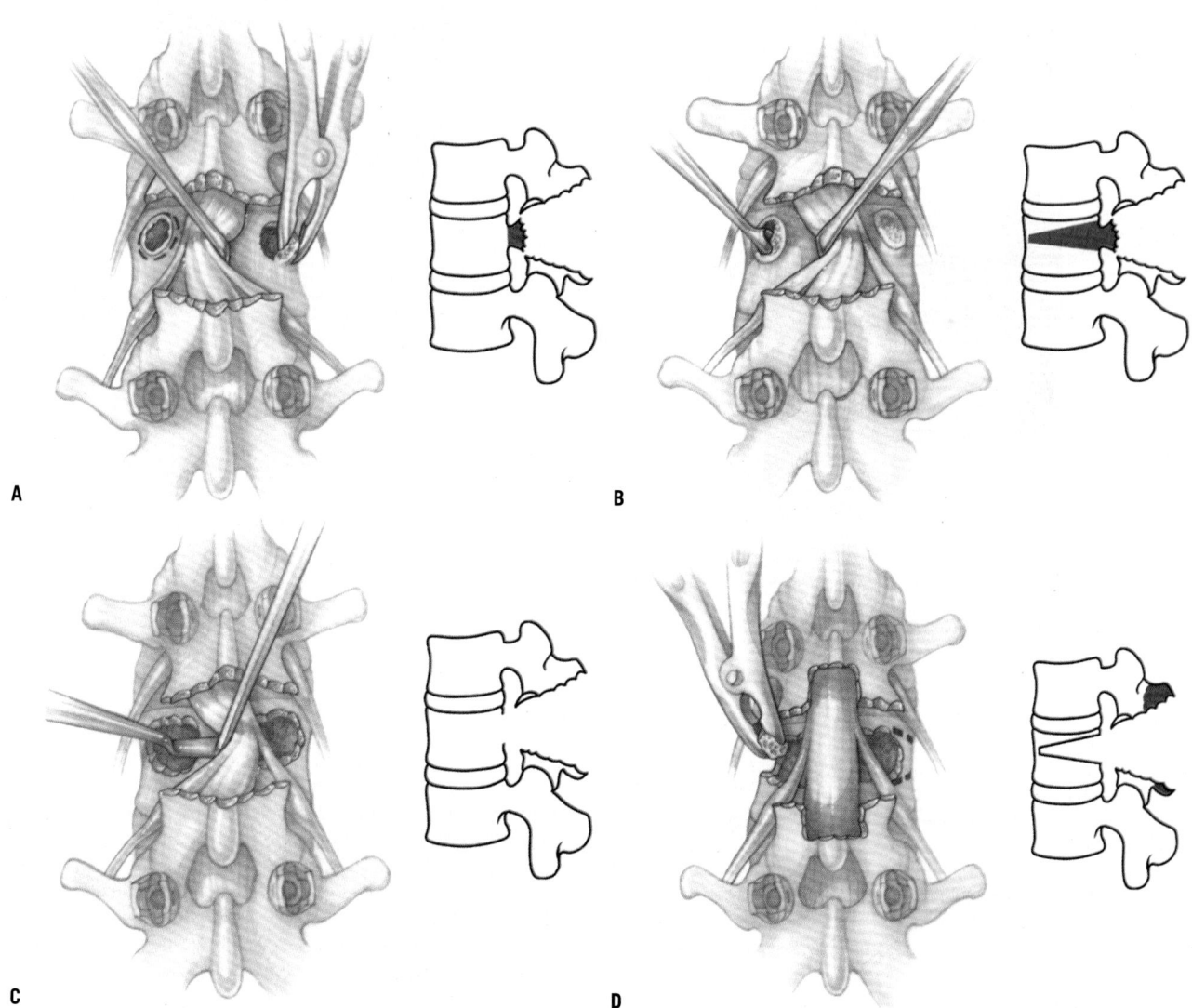

A   **B**

C   **D**

TECH FIG 2 A. All posterior elements around the pedicles are resected. **B.** The pedicles and vertebral bodies are decancellated. **C.** The posterior vertebral cortex is greensticked with a Woodson elevator or reverse-angled curette. **D.** The lateral vertebral cortex is resected with Leksell bilaterally. *(continued)*

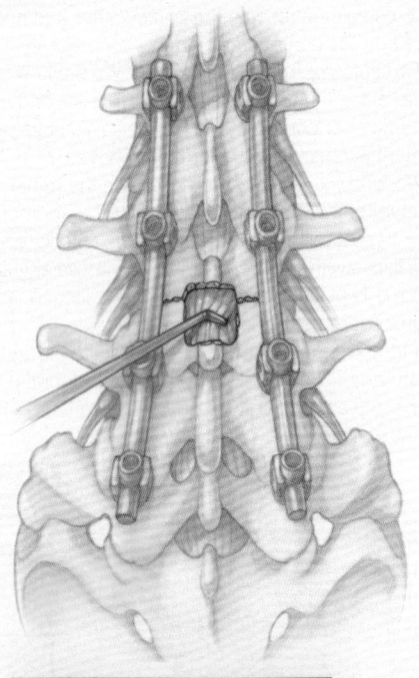

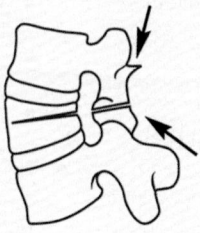

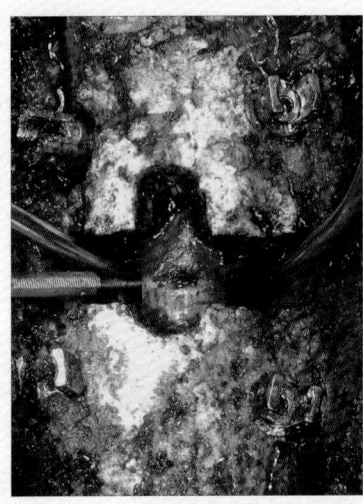

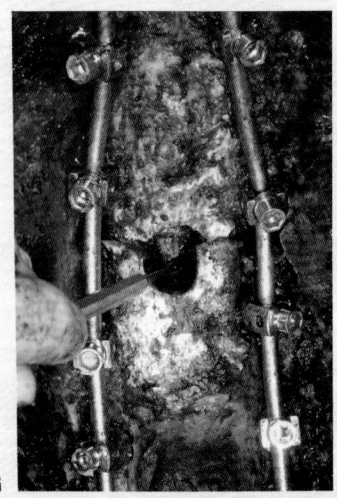

TECH FIG 2 *(continued)* **E.** The osteotomy is closed (*arrows*) with compression, cantilever, and extension of the chest and lower extremities. **F,G.** Intraoperative photographs showing the surgeon assessing for adequate decompression posteriorly at the PSO site prior to and after PSO closure to help prevent iatrogenic impingement of neural elements with PSO closure.

- Resect the lateral vertebral cortex with a Leksell rongeur bilaterally **(TECH FIG 2D)**.
- To close the osteotomy, apply gentle downward pressure on the two segments along with compression through the pedicle screws and rods to approximate the two osteotomy edges **(TECH FIG 2E)**.
  - If using an articulating bed, the bed is bent to close the osteotomy. Rods should be engaged in the tulip heads to minimize the risk of subluxation.
  - Cantilevering through the rods can also assist in osteotomy closure.
  - Sometimes, placing more pillows/pads underneath the patient's hips and legs can extend the pelvis/hips and help with osteotomy closure.
  - ___ third rod technique can also be used. This relies on estab- ___ midline fixation points, often through a prior fusion ___ ove and below the PSO site. A rod within these ___ s can then be used to use sequential compres- ___ g the osteotomy to closure.

- Inspect the osteotomy site to make sure that there is adequate decompression without dorsal impingement of the thecal sac or nerve roots after the osteotomy is closed **(TECH FIG 2F,G)**.
  - One must check the dural buckling to ensure that it is not fixed. We will palpate with a Woodson to ensure the folds are "mobile" and not fixed. If fixed, then an expansive duraplasty may be advisable.
- An asymmetric PSO requires resection of more bone on the convex side of the deformity when creating the wedge resection so that during closure, the convex side is closed more than the concave side, allowing rebalancing of the patient in the coronal plane and sagittal plane.
  - Not only is the posterior column resection bigger on the convexity, but the middle and anterior columns have to be resected more generously on the convexity as well.
  - This involves turning the corner on the vertebral body and what amounts to resecting two-thirds of the convexity of the vertebral body both laterally and anteriorly, which otherwise would not be necessary with a standard PSO.

Pearls and Pitfalls

PCO	• Fixation points can be placed before or after the osteotomies are performed. • For large deformities or abnormal pedicle anatomy, performing a PCO first, prior to pedicle screw placement, can help in identifying the medial and superior borders of the pedicle to assist in locating the starting point. • Undercut the lamina as much as possible to remove all ligamentum flavum. • If possible, limit the amount of forces placed on the pedicle screws and apply forces more through the posterior elements.
PSO	• Resect a symmetric wedge of bone within the vertebral body to minimize the potential for coronal decompensation with osteotomy closure. • Ensure that the ventral dura is free from the posterior vertebral cortex and that the posterior vertebral cortex is adequately thin to allow for controlled implosion of the bone into the osteotomy site. • Attempting to greenstick the posterior vertebral cortex that is too thick may require too much force and increases the risk of a ventral dural tear. • Remember, as the osteotomy is closed, the contour in the rods will have to change. As more closure is achieved, more lordosis is needed in the rods. • If possible, limit the amount of forces placed on the pedicle screws and apply forces more through the posterior elements. • With pedicle subtraction procedures, there is some risk of dural buckling and the posterior elements impinging on the dura. Our preference is to enlarge the field centrally to observe dural buckling and to "feel" the dorsal canal with nerve hooks/Woodson elevators. Watch carefully for vertebral subluxation at the osteotomy site. • Neuromonitoring is followed for up to 1 hour after final osteotomy compression. A formal wake-up test is often done after the osteotomy closure, as neuromonitoring is at times unable to detect nerve root injury. A formal wake-up test is performed prior to leaving the operating room.

POSTOPERATIVE CARE

• Patients are mobilized on postoperative day 1.
• Drains are retained until recorded output is less than 30 mL per 8-hour shift.
• Diet is advanced slowly, with the return of bowel sounds.
• Deep vein thrombosis prophylaxis is provided with sequential compressive devices and thromboembolic deterrent hose.
• Avoid flexion and axial loading of the spine for at least 4 months postoperatively.
• No cast or brace is necessary.

OUTCOMES

• Studies have shown improvement (20% to 30%) in Scoliosis Research Society and Oswestry Disability Index scores in most patients at 2- and 5-year follow-up.[1-3]
• Three PCOs accomplish approximately what is accomplished with one pedicle subtraction procedure. The blood loss is greater with a pedicle subtraction procedure.[1,5]
• In general, one should try to reserve PSO for cases of fixed deformities.

COMPLICATIONS

• Substantial complications associated with PSOs include neurologic deficit, substantial blood loss, and adding on to the sagittal deformity if the entire thoracic and lumbar spine is not fused.[2]
• The neurologic risk with performing a pedicle subtraction procedure in the lumbar spine exceeds the risk associated with three SPOs. The complications associated with the procedure in older patients are more substantial.[4]
• A review of 108 PSOs revealed an intraoperative and postoperative neurologic deficit rate of 11.1%, with 2.8% of deficits being permanent.[4]
• Multiple SPOs can accomplish substantial correction of major fixed sagittal imbalance. However, there is a risk of pitching the patient to the concavity because of the fact that the osteotomies are often performed through areas of residual scoliosis and the SPO shortens the concavity/posterior elements and lengthens the convexity/anterior disc spaces.[1]

REFERENCES

1. Booth KC, Bridwell KH, Lenke LG, et al. Complications and predictive factors for the successful treatment of flatback deformity (fixed sagittal imbalance). Spine 1999;24(16):1712–1720.
2. Bridwell KH, Lewis S, Edwards C, et al. Complications and outcomes of pedicle subtraction osteotomies for fixed sagittal imbalance. Spine 2003;28(18):2093–2101.
3. Bridwell KH, Lewis SJ, Rinella A, et al. Pedicle subtraction osteotomy for the treatment of fixed sagittal imbalance. Surgical technique. J Bone Joint Surg Am 2004;86A(suppl 1):44–50.
4. Buchowski JM, Bridwell KH, Lenke LG, et al. Neurological complications of lumbar pedicle subtraction osteotomy: a 10-year assessment. Spine 2007;32(20):2245–2252.
5. Cho K, Bridwell KH, Lenke LG, et al. Comparison of Smith-Petersen versus pedicle subtraction osteotomy for the correction of fixed sagittal imbalance. Spine 2005;30(18):2030–2037.
6. Schwab F, Blondel B, Chay E, et al. The comprehensive anatomical spinal osteotomy classification. Neurosurgery 2014;74(1):112–120.

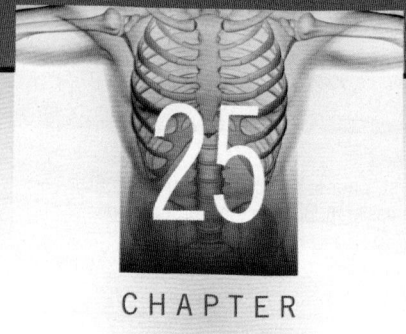

CHAPTER 25

Vertebral Column Resection for Severe Rigid Spinal Deformity through an All Posterior Approach

Michael P. Kelly, Lukas P. Zebala, and Lawrence G. Lenke

DEFINITION

- Posterior vertebral column resection (VCR) entails the removal of the anterior, middle, and posterior columns of the vertebra(e) through a posterior-alone approach.
- VCR is often performed at the apex of a deformity for severe, rigid scoliotic, and kyphotic spinal deformities.

ANATOMY

- A thorough understanding of the anatomy of the vertebral segment and spinal cord is needed to safely perform this procedure. This includes understanding the peculiarities of rotated vertebral segments in severe scoliotic deformities. The morphologic and iatrogenic changes of the posterior elements must be appreciated, as must the course of the spinal cord and nerve roots.

PATHOGENESIS

- The origins of these deformities are multiple and varied, including congenital, idiopathic, neoplastic, traumatic, and iatrogenic causes.

NATURAL HISTORY

- The natural history of the diseases leading to severe scoliotic, kyphotic, or combined deformities are variable.
- Those who do progress to severe, rigid deformities may present with intolerable deformity, severe pain, decreased ability to perform activities of daily living, myelopathy/spinal cord compression, and pulmonary dysfunction.
- Those patients with fixed deformities who are asymptomatic (ie, a well-balanced patient without complaint) may be managed nonoperatively. However, one must obtain careful follow-up to assess for possible deformity progression over time.

PATIENT HISTORY AND PHYSICAL FINDINGS

- The overall coronal and sagittal plane balance should be observed with the patient standing upright.
- deformity should be assessed for any flexibility by placing patient prone and supine on the examination table. utes of supine positioning will allow one to assess of a kyphotic deformity. Often, we will have ine on the examining table, turn the lights to 20 minutes for repeat evaluation.

- The history should include a careful assessment of current pain medication usage as preoperative narcotic usage may complicate the perioperative care. Additionally, any medications that may confer a risk of increased bleeding (eg, aspirin) should be noted and the patient cautioned to stop them prior to surgery.
- The use of nicotine-containing products, particularly cigarettes, is a relative contraindication to this procedure as the risk of pseudarthrosis is increased as well as perioperative complications.
- Those patients with diabetes mellitus must have well-controlled blood glucose levels before surgery as uncontrolled blood glucose levels are associated with increased risk of perioperative infection. Our goal is hemoglobin A1c <7.5%.
- A patient's nutritional status should be assessed and optimized prior to surgery. In addition, a bone density test should be performed to diagnose presence of osteoporosis and initiate preoperative treatment of any deficiencies. Our preference is 3 months of preoperative anabolic therapy (eg, teriparatide) followed by a minimum of 3 months postoperative anabolic therapy.
- The patient's gait should be assessed for evidence of myelopathy (eg, wide-based, shuffling gait). In our experience, myelopathy substantially increases the neurologic risk of surgery.
- A detailed neurologic examination must be performed and documented, including examination for pathologic reflexes such as asymmetric abdominal reflexes, Babinski response, and sustained clonus. Pathologic reflexes must alert the surgeon to possible intraspinal pathologies (eg, Chiari II, syrinx, tethered cord) that may need attention prior to the deformity correction.
- Preoperative examinations by a primary care physician, a cardiologist (including stress testing as indicated), and an anesthesiologist is mandatory to mitigate any risks of perioperative morbidity and mortality.
- A review of systems should include a review of the respiratory system and any history of respiratory compromise or distress. Preoperative pulmonary function tests should be obtained in all patients with a deformity severe enough to be considered for a VCR procedure.

IMAGING AND OTHER DIAGNOSTIC STUDIES

- A radiographic spinal deformity series is obtained, which includes standing anteroposterior (AP) and lateral long-cassette radiographs, left- and right-side bending, full AP, and lateral supine or prone images (FIG 1).

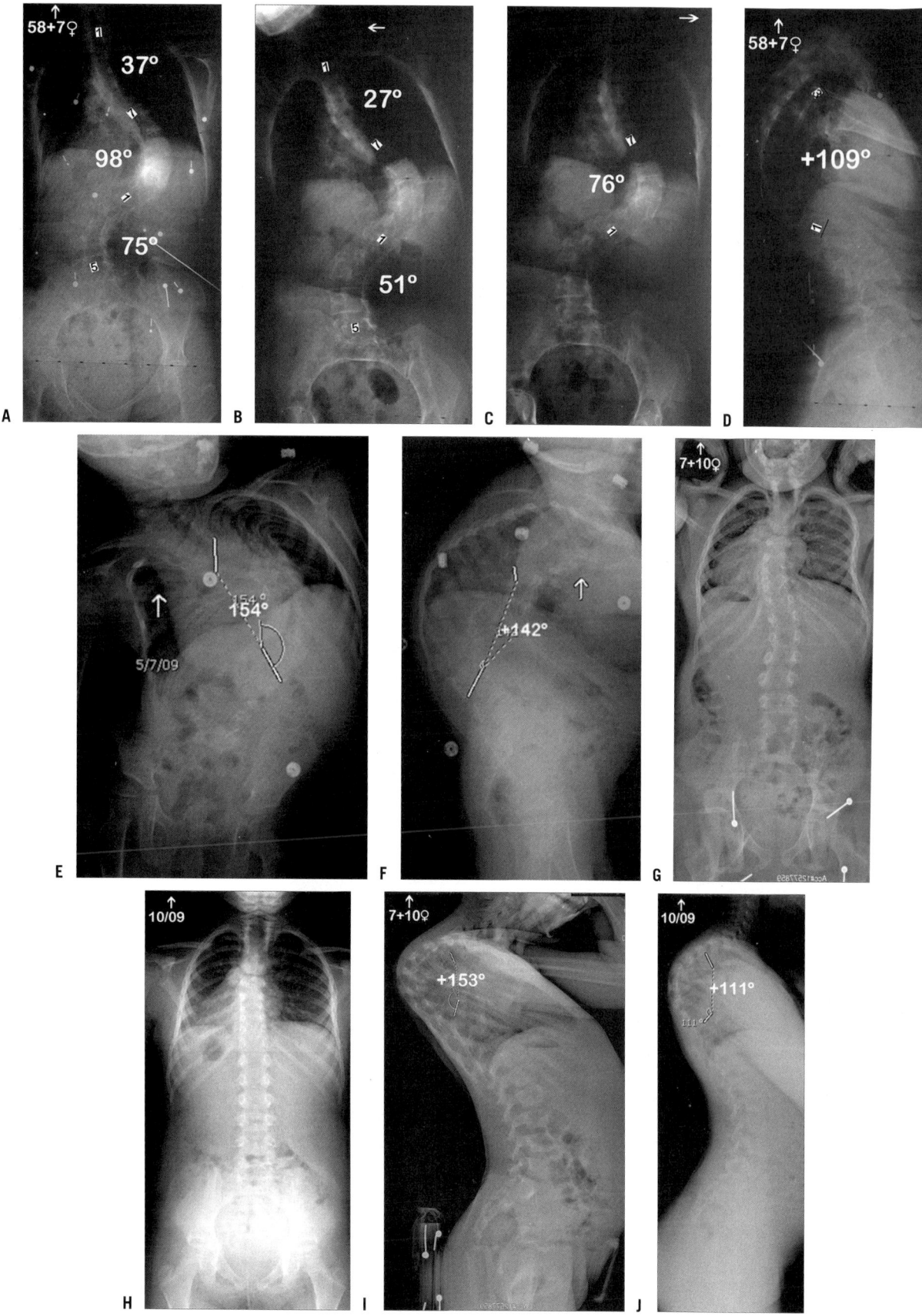

FIG 1 A–D. Case 1. Fifty-eight-year-old woman with adult idiopathic thoracic kyphoscoliosis. **E,F.** Case 2. Six-year-old boy with severe congenital kyphoscoliosis. **G–J.** Case 3. Seven-year-old girl with a severe 153-degree postlaminectomy kyphosis with myelopathy. She was placed in preoperative halo-gravity traction.

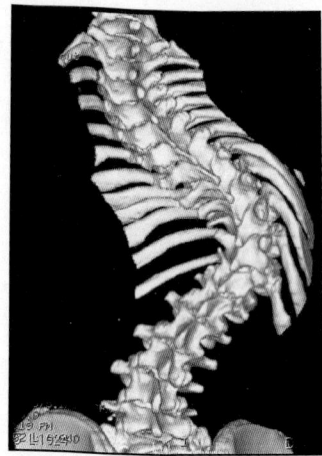
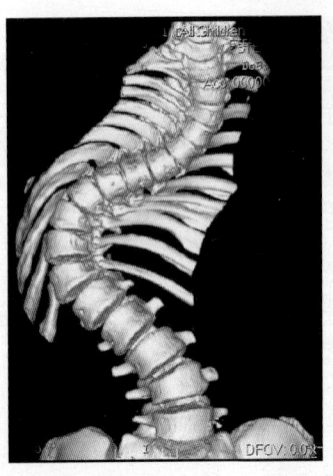
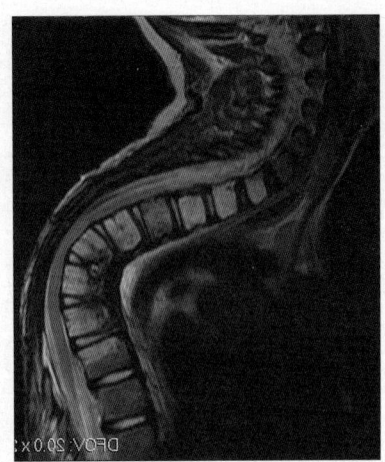
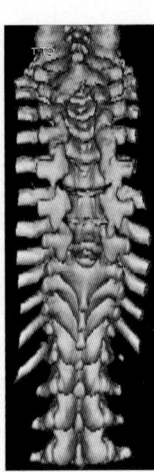

FIG 2 A,B. Posterior and anterior 3-D CT scans, respectively, of a patient with severe idiopathic scoliosis. **C.** Case 3. Preoperative sagittal MRI scan shows postlaminectomy kyphosis with draping of the spinal cord. **D.** Case 3. Preoperative 3-D CT scan shows the laminectomy defect.

- Flexibility radiographs include push-prone and axial traction x-rays and help assess coronal plane rigidity.
- Hyperextension radiographs (bolster placed at apex of kyphosis) and hyperflexion radiographs (bolster at apex of lordosis) help assess sagittal plane rigidity.
- A three-dimensional (3-D) computed tomography (CT) scan is obtained to evaluate the entire anterior and posterior spinal column. This aids in the identification of important vertebral landmarks **(FIG 2)**.
- Skull to sacrum magnetic resonance imaging (MRI) is necessary to evaluate the entire neural axis (eg, Chiari malformation, syringomyelia, tethered spinal cord) **(FIG 3)**.

DIFFERENTIAL DIAGNOSIS

- Severe scoliosis
- Global kyphosis
- Angular kyphosis
- Kyphoscoliosis
- Fixed coronal and sagittal imbalance syndrome (eg, status post-Harrington rod instrumentation)

NONOPERATIVE MANAGEMENT

- Patients with static deformities and only mild pain or physical impairment should be managed with a trial of nonoperative therapy.

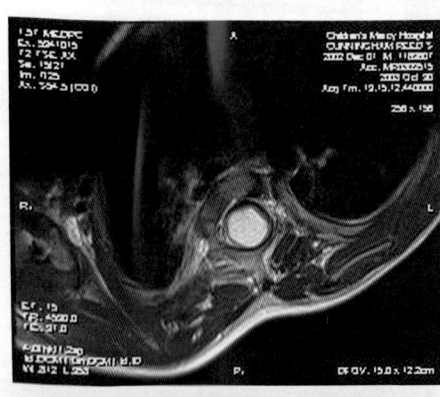
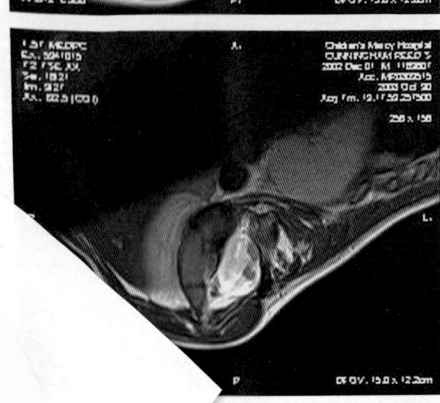
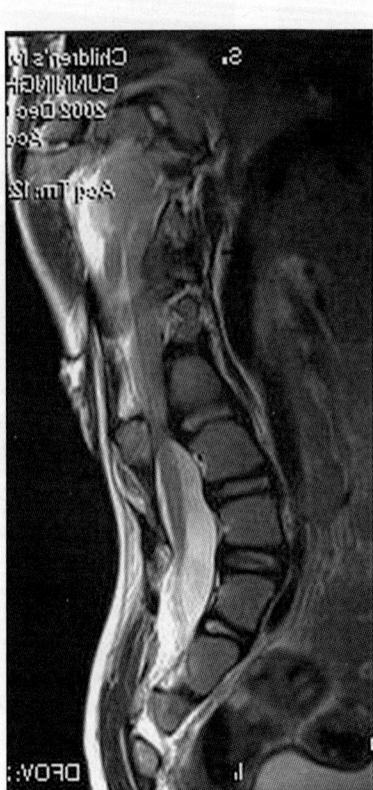

FIG 3 A–C. Case 2. Patient's total spine MRI demonstrated a syringomyelia, diplomyelia, and a tethered spinal cord.

- This includes a directed physical therapy program, to include cardiovascular conditioning, postural training, and abdominal strengthening.
- For those patients with moderate to severe pain, a referral to a pain specialist, most notably for those patients with complaints of pain not consistent with their presenting pathology or other signs of nonorganic causes of pain
- As with nerve root compression, epidural and transforaminal steroid injections offer a less invasive, potentially diagnostic, and/or therapeutic intervention.

SURGICAL MANAGEMENT

- Classically, rigid deformities were treated with staged anterior and posterior procedures to resect and reconstruct the spine through the rigid segment.[2,3,5] The posterior VCR allows a similar correction of deformity, with the benefits of shorter total operative time and lower total blood loss.[8]
- Location of the deformity often determines whether a VCR (thoracic) or pedicle subtraction osteotomy (lumbar) will assist in correction of sagittal imbalance. For less severe and flexible deformity with mobile disc spaces, multilevel Ponté/Smith-Petersen osteotomies may be adequate for deformity correction.[1]
  - Flexibility films will help determine whether a three-column osteotomy is needed versus posterior column osteotomies alone. Posterior column osteotomies may correct up to 10 degrees of kyphosis per level of depending on their location. For large, angular deformities, a three-column osteotomy allows for greater correction in the coronal and sagittal planes.
  - We perform VCR in place of anterior and posterior procedures, electing to perform the correction through one single approach.
  - The VCR is almost invariably performed at the apex of the deformity.

Preoperative Planning

- A multidisciplinary team approach is often necessary in the treatment of patients with complex deformity that requires a VCR.
- Preoperative assessment of the patient's cardiovascular, pulmonary, nutritional, hematologic, and metabolic systems is required to maximize the patient's preoperative reserve.
- Careful examination of the preoperative CT scan should alert the surgeon to areas of bony deficiency in the posterior elements to prevent incidental durotomies (see **FIG 2C,D**).
- In many cases of thoracic kyphosis, preoperative halo-gravity traction improves alignment before surgery. This usually requires open disc spaces and stiff, although not fixed, deformities. In some instances, however, slow deformation of the fusion mass is possible. Our goal traction weight is one-third body weight. In our experience, most correction occurs by 6 weeks.
  - Prolonged halo-gravity traction is particularly useful when other systems (eg, nutritional) need optimization.

Positioning

- The patient is positioned prone on an Orthopedic Systems, Inc., Jackson frame with six pads, which are placed strategically to allow the abdomen to rest free, reducing intra-abdominal pressure and intraoperative bleeding.
- We prefer to place a halo or Gardner-Wells tongs with 5 to 15 lb of traction that allows for rigid positioning of the skull with the face free.
  - A halo is useful in cases of stiff cervicothoracic deformities (eg, proximal junctional kyphosis) when positioning can provide some correction.
- The arms are placed in a 90–90 position with care to position the axillae free and elbows well padded to decrease the risk of brachial plexopathy or ulnar nerve neuropathy.
- Pressure areas are carefully padded as the length of the procedure increases the risk of position-related complications (eg, skin macerations, plexopathies).
- The hips are gently extended and the knees slightly flexed with the use of multiple pillows.
  - In cases of severe lumbar kyphosis, a sling may be needed to allow for positioning. After the VCR, the boards may be placed, putting the hips in extension and correcting the kyphosis.
- Spinal cord monitoring leads are placed to monitor the sensory and motor function of the lower extremities.
  - In some cases (eg, myelopathy), transcranial motor-evoked potentials (tcMEP) may not be available. This is the "unmonitorable" patient. In these situations, we perform Stagnara wake-up test at the following intervals. Although it may seem onerous, the neurologic risks in "unmonitorable" patients are high, and all efforts must be made to minimize these risks.
    1. After prone positioning
    2. After exposure
    3. After facetectomies and osteotomies
    4. After closure of the VCR
    5. 1 hour after closure of the VCR
    6. After turning the patient supine to the hospital bed, prior to extubation

Approach

- The standard posterior, subperiosteal approach is used.

TECHNIQUES

EXPOSURE

- A subperiosteal approach is undertaken from the transverse processes of the most superior instrumented level to the most distal vertebra or ilium to be instrumented/fused **(TECH FIG 1)**.
- Thoracoplasties may be necessary at apical vertebrae to obtain adequate exposure of the transverse processes at the apex of a severe scoliosis or kyphoscoliosis deformity.
- Intraoperative radiographs or fluoroscopy should always be used to confirm vertebral levels.

- An efficient, meticulous exposure is necessary to minimize blood loss.
  - Tranexamic acid is used throughout the case to reduce blood loss. Pediatric cases are dosed with a 50 mg/kg loading bolus followed by 10 mg/kg/hour infusion. Adult cases are dosed at 30 mg/kg bolus followed by 10 mg/kg/hr infusion.

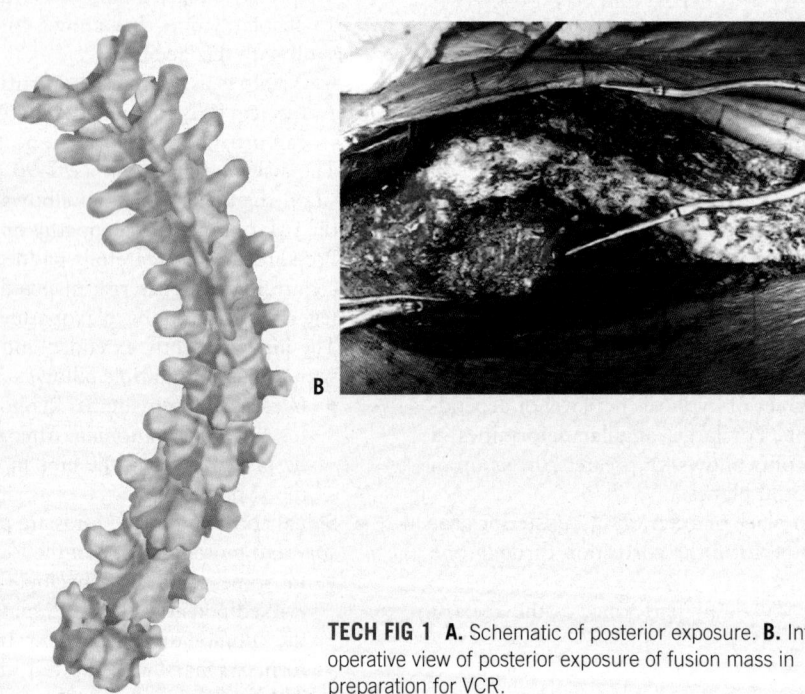

TECH FIG 1 **A.** Schematic of posterior exposure. **B.** Intraoperative view of posterior exposure of fusion mass in preparation for VCR.

FACET OSTEOTOMIES

- Inferior facetectomies are performed at every level where motion exists, resecting approximately 3 to 4 mm of the inferior facet joint.
- Ponté or Smith-Petersen osteotomies are performed around the apex of the deformity, usually from the upper end vertebra to one level below the lower end vertebra. The ligamentum flavum and facet joints are excised.
  - These osteotomies allow for more harmonious correction of the deformity as well as offering access to the medial

pedicle to aid in screw placement at the concavity of the deformity.
- In those patients with severe apical kyphosis, we will place pedicle screws prior to any osteotomies. A temporary rod is placed prior to any osteotomy to prevent sagging of the vertebral column, which can put the spinal cord at risk of neurologic impairment.

SCREW PLACEMENT

...lified anatomic freehand technique with a ...w trajectory to increase pedicle pullout ...ment of preoperative imaging allows for

assessment of pedicle screw diameter and length at each vertebra **(TECH FIG 2)**.
- Pedicle screw placement is performed in a sequential fashion from distal to proximal.

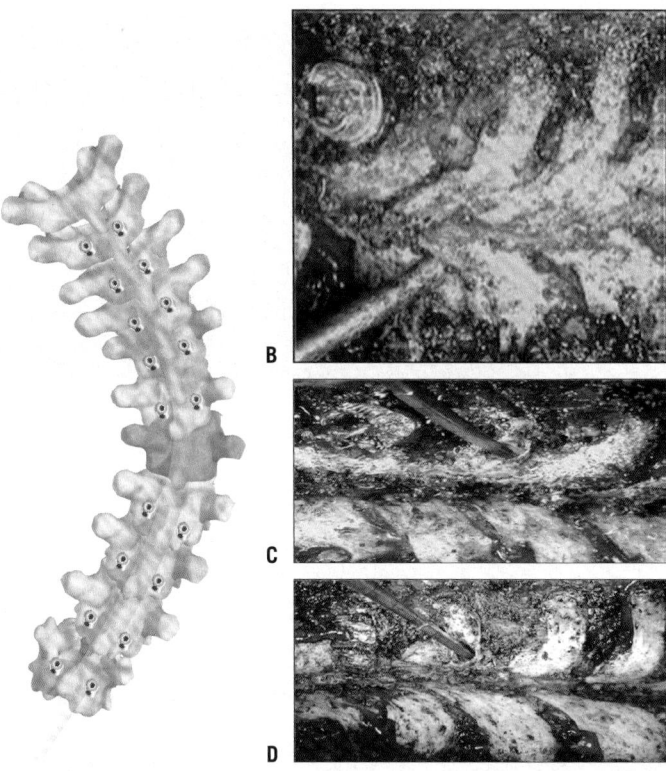

A

B

C

D

TECH FIG 2 A. Pedicle screws placed segmentally except at shaded apical level where resection is planned. **B–D.** Freehand pedicle screw placement.

- Placement of segmental apical screws is important to ensure rigid stabilization of the VCR site.
- Intraoperative use of fluoroscopy, CT scan, or navigation may be used in assisting the placement of screws, especially through areas of prior fusion with distorted anatomy.

- Multiaxial screws (or multiaxial reduction screws) are most commonly used.
  - Reduction screws are used when cantilever bending is needed for reduction of the rod and deformity. This is often at the distal end of a construct and in areas of hyperlordosis, where rod reduction may be difficult.

VERTEBRAL COLUMN RESECTION

Costotransversectomy and Laminectomy

- A stabilizing rod is placed, capturing three segments above and three below. In some deformities, a "construct to construct" closure is planned. In these cases, rods connect the segments above and below the level of resection. These two "constructs" are then connected via dominoes, thereby spanning the level of resection.
- In the thoracic spine, bilateral costotransversectomies are performed at the level of resection (**TECH FIG 3A**).
  - Five to 6 cm of medial rib is resected prior to the laminectomy to minimize the risk of canal intrusion.
  - After subperiosteal dissection, the medial rib fragment is removed, ideally with the rib head attached. Often, however, the rib head remains attached at the vertebral body and can be removed later during the corpectomy. Dissection of the costovertebral joint with a Cobb elevator is helpful.
- The ribs are kept intact, not morselized, and are used as structural grafts to bridge the laminectomy site after osteotomy closure. Next, a wide laminectomy is performed extending from the cranial vertebral pedicles of the level(s) of resection to the caudal vertebra pedicles (**TECH FIG 3B,C**).

- A thorough central decompression is necessary to prevent dorsal dural compression with osteotomy closure. Exiting nerve roots are isolated by removing the facet joints and pedicles bilaterally.
- The nerve roots at the level of the osteotomy are temporarily clamped with a bulldog-type vascular clamp for 5 to 10 minutes, and attention is turned to any spinal cord, monitoring data changes.
  - In the thoracic spine, we prefer to ligate the nerve roots medial to the dorsal root ganglion.
    - If spinal cord monitoring data remains stable, then the nerve root is ligated with two 2-0 silk sutures.
    - In our experience, two or three contiguous, unilateral thoracic roots can be sacrificed without neurologic deficits, except for occasional chest wall numbness.
    - In general, we ligate the root on the convexity facilitating placement of an anterior structural support. The concave root is spared.
  - In the lumbar spine, the nerve roots are preserved. Sacrifice of the L1 nerve root is generally safe. There are data to support the safety of L2 sacrifice, although we attempt to preserve this root.[4]

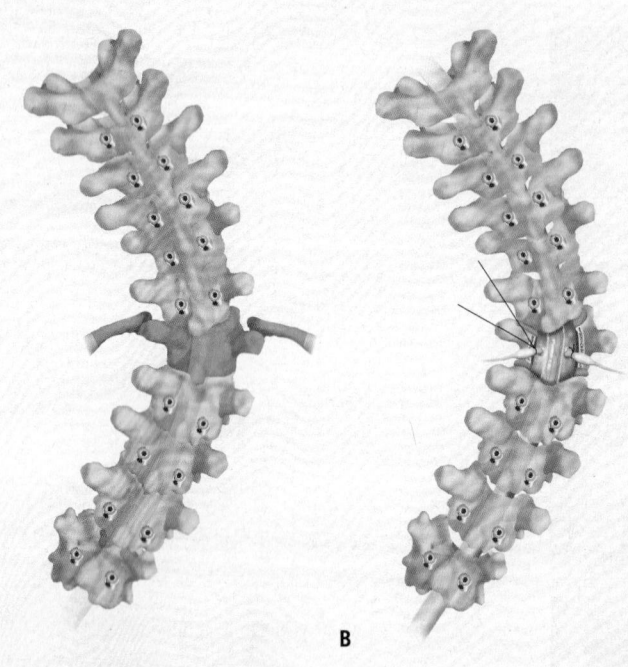

A   B

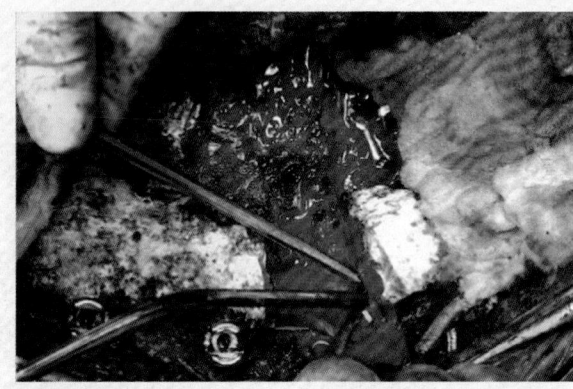

C

TECH FIG 3 A. Shaded area on ribs adjoining to vertebra to be resected via bilateral costotransversectomy. **B.** Laminectomy and nerve root ligation. **C.** Laminectomy and undercutting of ventral aspect of fusion mass.

Stabilizing Rod Placement

- In preparation for the vertebral body resection, a unilateral stabilizing rod is placed with pedicle screws two or three levels above and below the level of resection **(TECH FIG 4)**.
  - For extreme angular kyphotic or kyphoscoliotic deformities, bilateral rods are used to prevent subluxation of the vertebral column.
  - If a "construct to construct" correction is planned, we will place rods the length of the deformity above and below, connecting these "constructs" through a third rod and dominoes.

〒G 4 Stabilizing rod placement.

Vertebral Body Removal and Discectomy

- The cancellous bone of the vertebral body is accessed via a lateral pedicle body window. Subperiosteal dissection on the lateral vertebral body is done with a combination of blunt dissection tools and electrocautery. The paraspinal structures are carefully peeled away until access to the anterior vertebral body is gained. Special retractors or cotton patties may help protect these structures during the corpectomy **(TECH FIG 5A)**.
  - The cancellous bone is then curetted and saved for use as local bone graft.
  - Resecting the concave pedicle poses a challenge, as it is very cortical.
    - In a pure scoliosis deformity, the dural sac and cord rest on the medial pedicle, with no ventral body due to rotation.
  - We prefer to use a matchstick burr to remove this cortical bone in these situations.
    - In these deformities, most of the vertebral body will be removed from the convexity.
    - The concave pedicle is removed first as blood may obscure the field if the convexity is removed first. This also allows the cord to drift medially, away from the majority of the resection.
    - A Penfield retractor should be placed on medial dura during concave resection. One must not retract the dura in these cases, as the neural elements may be stretched to the maximum tolerable state.
  - The entire vertebral body is removed. The anterior longitudinal ligament is sectioned at some point to allow for anterior column lengthening, which allows for maximum correction in all planes **(TECH FIG 5B,C)**.
- Discectomies are performed at the levels above and below the vertebral body resection **(TECH FIG 5D,E)**.
  - Care must be taken to preserve the endplates for cage placement.

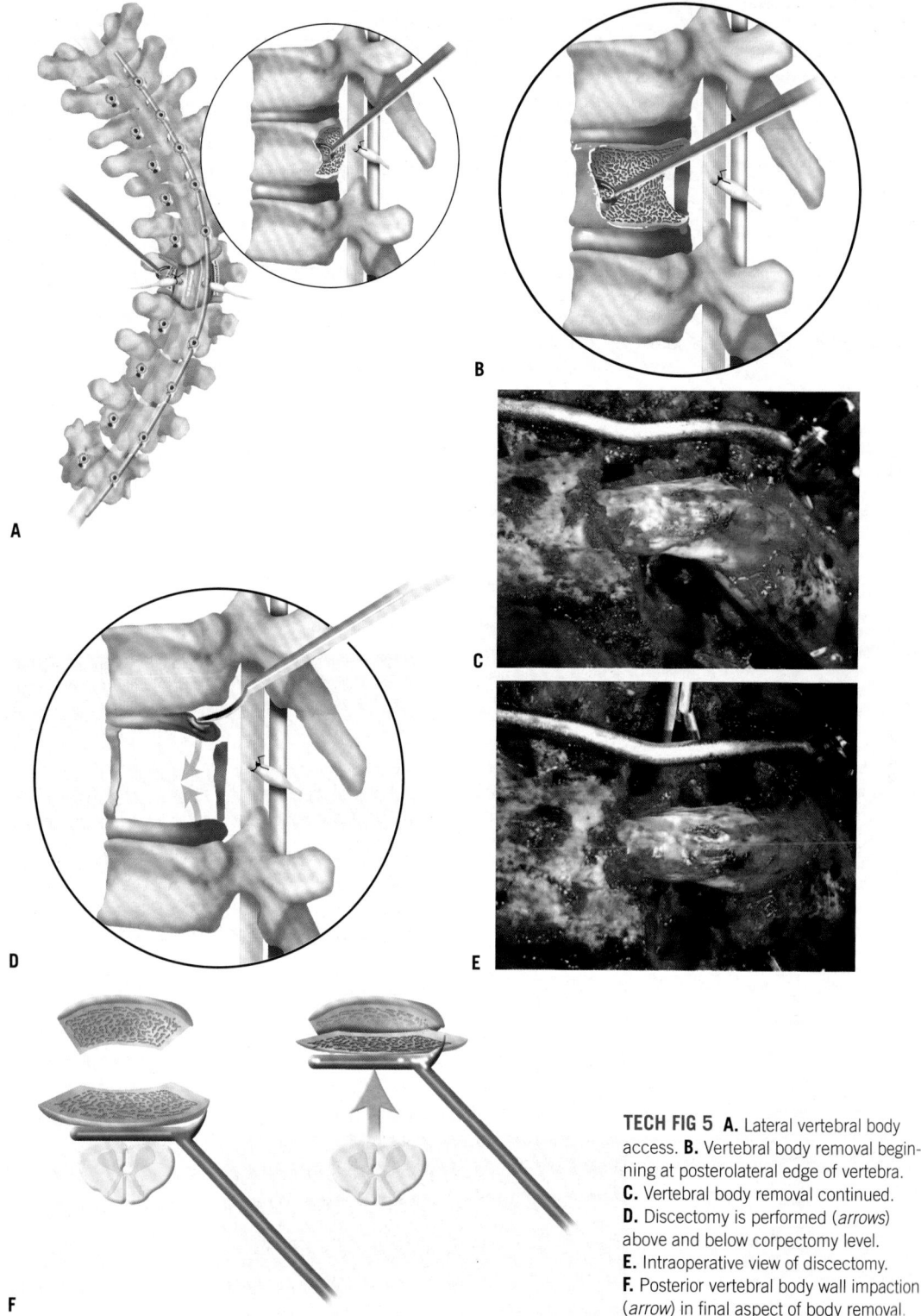

TECH FIG 5 A. Lateral vertebral body access. **B.** Vertebral body removal beginning at posterolateral edge of vertebra. **C.** Vertebral body removal continued. **D.** Discectomy is performed (*arrows*) above and below corpectomy level. **E.** Intraoperative view of discectomy. **F.** Posterior vertebral body wall impaction (*arrow*) in final aspect of body removal.

- The last section of the vertebral body, which is removed by impaction, is the posterior vertebral body wall or ventral spinal canal (**TECH FIG 5F**).
- The dural sac must be freed from the posterior longitudinal ligament.

- The posterior body wall is removed with reverse-angled curettes, Woodson elevators, or a specialized posterior wall resector (pedicle subtraction osteotomy tool set; Medtronic Spinal and Biologics, Memphis, TN).
- Care must be taken to remove any posterior osteophytes to prevent cord impingement during the correction.

CLOSURE OF RESECTION SITE

- Closure of the resected area is now performed with compression **(TECH FIG 6A)**. Compression of the convexity allows for shortening of the spinal column. Sequential compression on the convexity and distraction of the concavity, performed in an alternating fashion, allows for safe reduction of the deformity through a shortening procedure. Distraction is not an initial technique as this may put traction on the spinal cord and cause a neurologic deficit.
  - Compression, followed by in situ bending to lengthen the anterior column, is useful. Shortening should always precede any lengthening action, and these should be performed in multiple sequences to shorten the posterior column,

lengthen the anterior column, and keep the middle column static or shortened. The spinal cord must not be stretched.
- In cases with large degrees of kyphosis, a structural cage is placed anteriorly. This prevents overshortening and acts as a hinge for greater correction of the kyphotic deformity **(TECH FIG 6B,C)**.
  - To choose the cage height, close the osteotomy approximately 50%. Ensure that no excessive dural buckling has occurred and that neurologic monitoring data are unchanged. After using trial sizers, place a cage that fits approximately endplate to endplate and compress around the cage.

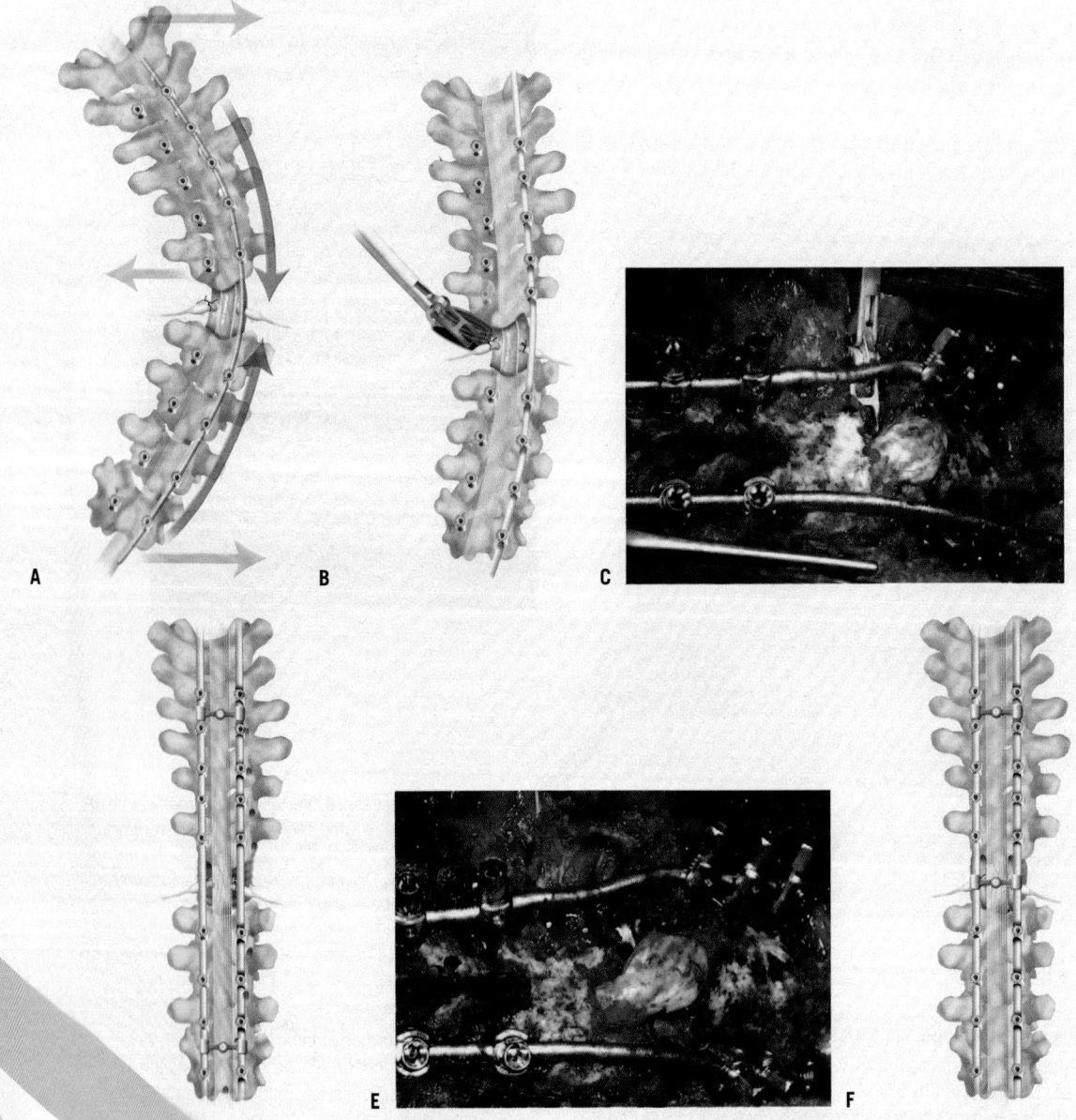

posterior shortening (via compression of the convexity [*arrows*]) is always the initial corrective maneuver. **B,C.** Cage erformed before final closure. **D,E.** Final correction with both rods placed. **F.** Rib grafts placed over laminectomy defect.

- The spinal cord can tolerate 2.5 to 3 cm of shortening before buckling affects blood flow. Thus, the posterior column can be shortened more than 3 cm without issue, although constant attention to the amount of dural buckling and tcMEP data is necessary.
- In cases with good pedicle fixation, compression is applied through the screws.
- In cases with less rigid pedicle fixation, a "construct to construct" closure is performed, with dominoes at the level of the resection.
  - Care must be taken to watch for subluxation or dural sac impingement during closure.
- After the closure is performed, a contralateral rod is placed. The temporary stabilization rod is removed, and a final rod is placed **(TECH FIG 6D,E)**.

- In situ contouring of the rods is performed, again with care taken to watch for subluxation at the resection or dural sac impingement.
- Intraoperative radiographs are obtained to check alignment.
- Decortication of dorsal laminae and transverse processes is performed with a matchstick burr.
- The laminectomy defect at the site of resection is covered with the resected rib sections (from the previously performed costo-transversectomy) **(TECH FIG 6F)**.
  - The ribs are split longitudinally, and placed, cancellous side down, from the lamina above to the lamina below.
  - The ribs may be secured with sutures or a cross-link, if space allows.
  - A final circumferential check of the dura is performed to ensure no dural sac impingement.

WOUND CLOSURE

- Deep drains are placed, and the fascial layer closed using 0 Vicryl (Ethicon, Inc., Somerville, NJ). A suprafascial drain is placed and the subcutaneous layer closed using 2-0 Vicryl suture. The skin is closed using absorbable 3-0 Vicryl suture.
- Vancomycin is placed in the wound in all cases without allergies to vancomycin.

- A rehearsed wake-up test is performed prior to extubation. Deleting an intraoperative wake-up test is performed.
- Final radiographs are obtained to confirm implant position and overall alignment.

TECHNIQUES

Pearls and Pitfalls

Preoperative Planning	• A multispecialty approach to preoperative surgical clearance should include cardiac, pulmonary, hematologic, and bone mineral density workups. • Use of neuromonitoring of motor and sensory pathways is mandatory. • Stagnara wake-up tests must be rehearsed, and all participants (patient included) ready to use these if necessary.
VCR	• Prior to starting VCR, mean arterial pressure should be kept at 80 mm Hg to help with spinal cord perfusion, hemoglobin should be close to 30%, and room should be warmed. • Subperiosteal dissection of lateral vertebral body wall with careful attention to save segmental vessels will minimize blood loss. • Temporary rod placement prior to decompression to prevent subluxation • Wide laminectomy from superior to inferior level pedicles with complete facetectomies • Identification of bilateral nerve roots. In the thoracic spine, often, only one nerve root needs to be sacrificed. Tieing off nerve root should be done medial to dorsal root ganglion. • Resection of vertebral body should be accomplished as much as possible from one side to minimize the number or exchanges necessary of the temporary rods. • The spinal cord should be free from the posterior longitudinal ligament/dorsal vertebral body prior to removal of the posterior vertebral body wall. • Osteotomy closure should be done slowly with constant neuromonitoring. • Limit spinal cord shortening to 2.5 cm. The dorsal column may be shortened 3–4 cm. • Use of an anterior intervertebral cage will limit amount of spine shortening and should be placed after initial round of osteotomy closure.
After Resection Complete	• Neuromonitoring is followed for up to 1 hour after final osteotomy compression, and a formal neurologic examination is performed prior to leaving the operating room. • Rib autograft should be used as a bridge over osteotomy site to protect neural elements. • Deep and superficial drains may reduce postoperative hematoma/seroma formation.

POSTOPERATIVE CARE

- Patients are often sent to the intensive care unit for close monitoring (for 24 to 48 hours as needed) and then transitioned to the hospital ward.
- Patients are mobilized on postoperative day 1.
- Drains are retained until recorded output is less than 30 mL per 8-hour shift.
- Diet is advanced slowly with the return of bowel sounds.
- Deep vein thrombosis prophylaxis is provided with sequential compressive devices and thromboembolic deterrent hose.

OUTCOMES

- **FIGS 4** and **5** show postoperative results in two of the patients in **FIG 1**.
- One of the authors (LGL) has performed over 107 consecutive posterior VCRs:
  - 63 pediatric and 44 adult
  - 47 primary and 60 revision

- 99 in the spinal cord region and 8 in the lumbar spine
- 73 were one level, 28 were two levels, and 6 were three levels
- Diagnoses: severe scoliosis (29), global kyphosis (16), angular kyphosis (25), kyphoscoliosis (37)
- Average correction: severe scoliosis (69%), global kyphosis (54%), angular kyphosis (63%), kyphoscoliosis (56%)
- Mean estimated blood loss: 1300 mL; mean operative time: 9 hours, 37 minutes

COMPLICATIONS

- Twelve spinal cord monitoring changes: all reversed with intraoperative measures to restore spinal cord blood flow (increased mean arterial pressure, wider decompression, larger interbody cage, reduced subluxation); no neurologic deficits upon wake up
- Two neurologic deficits: Spinal cord monitoring is not available on either because of preexisting severe myelopathic disease. Both awoke paraplegic with intact sensation. Both have improved and are able to walk.

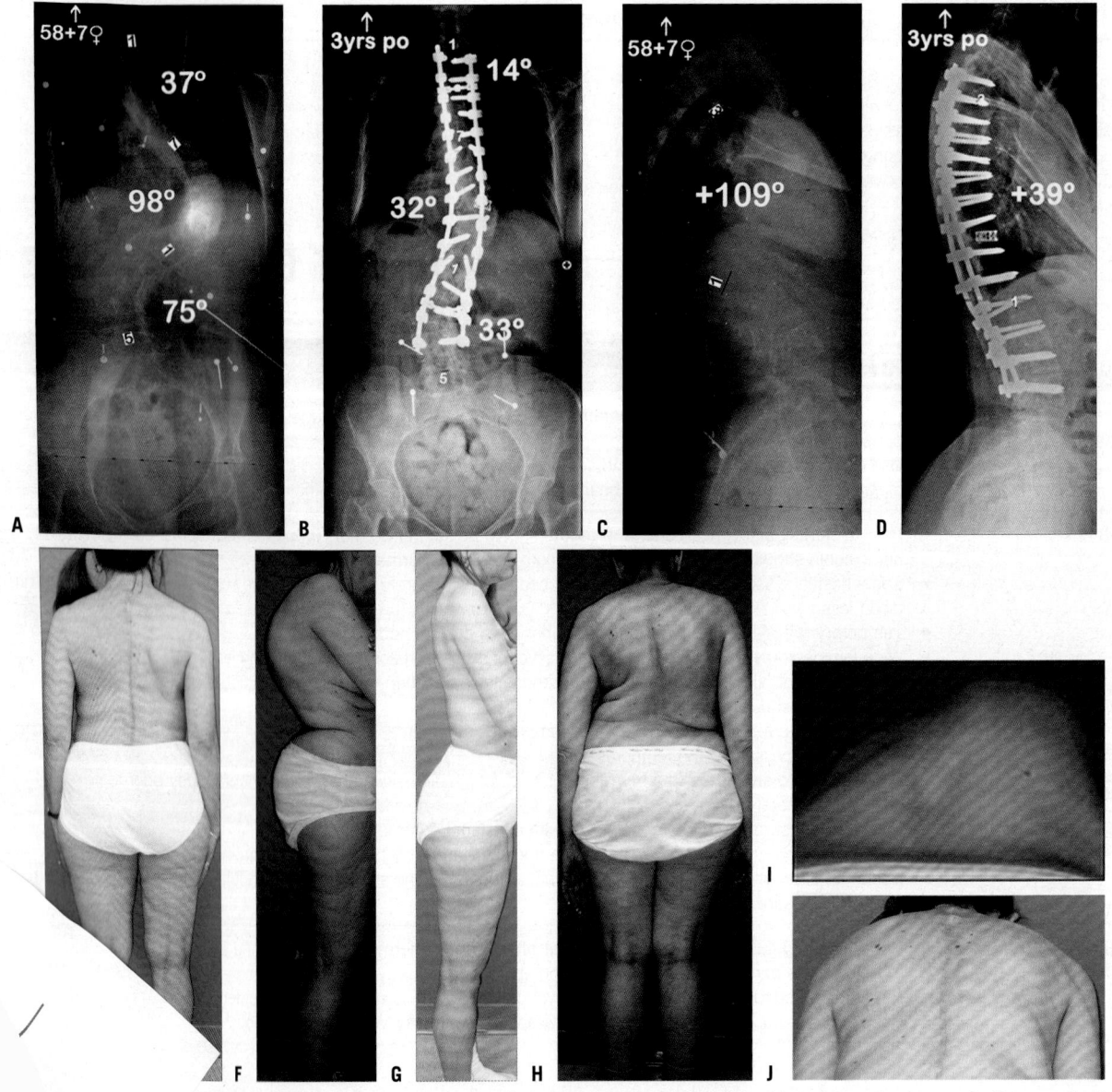

FIG 1. Patient underwent a posterior spinal fusion T2–L4 with a T10 VCR with radiographs demonstrating excellent ... 3 years postoperatively. **E–J.** Preoperative and postoperative clinical photos.

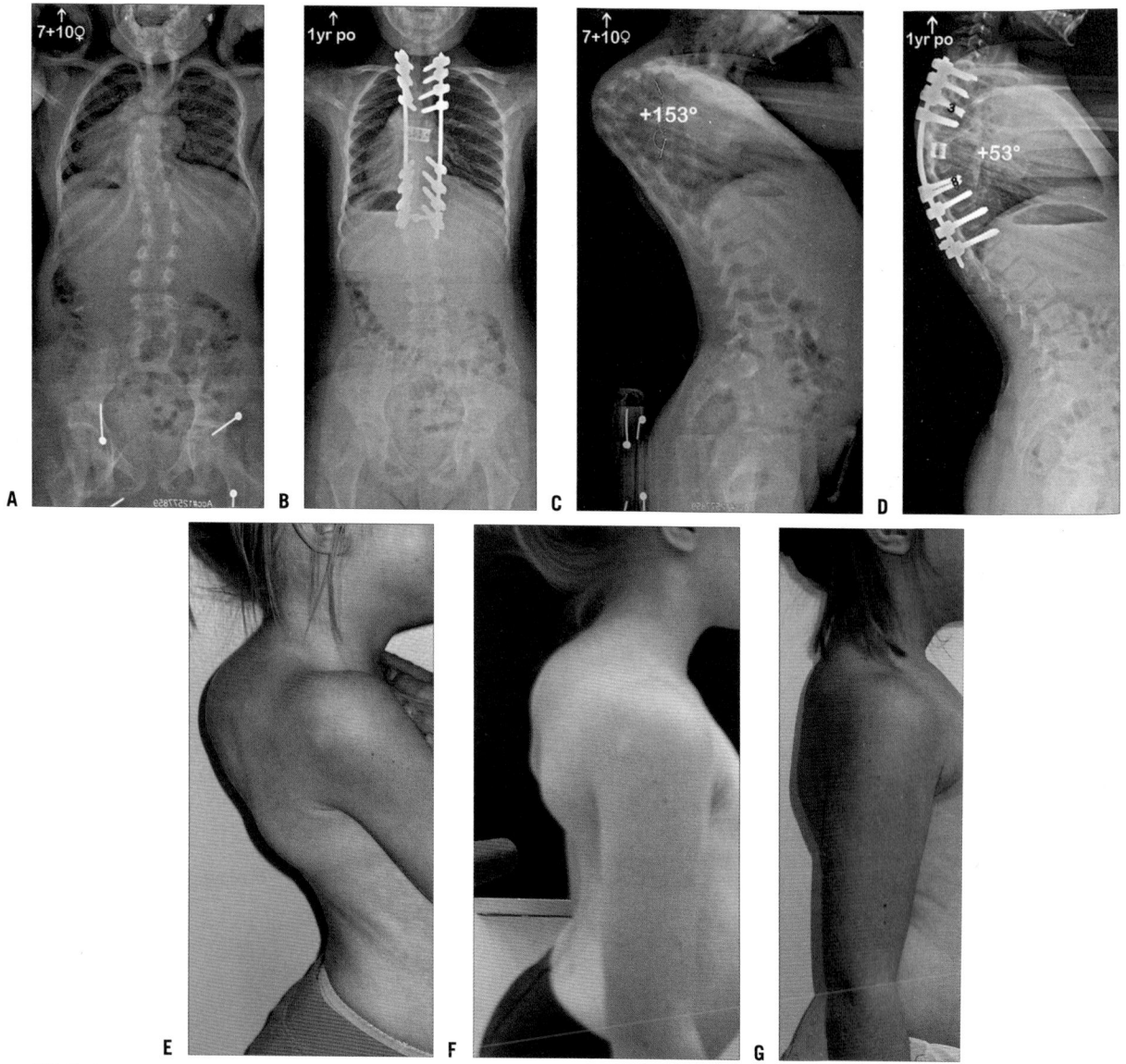

FIG 5 A–D. Case 3. Patient underwent a two-level posterior VCR and posterior spinal fusion T1–T11 with complete relief of her myelopathy. **E–G.** Preoperative, traction, and 1-year postoperative clinical photos, respectively.

- The Scoli-Risk-1 study provided excellent data regarding the risk of new neurologic deficits and outcomes after complex spinal deformity surgeries.[7] New neurologic deficits occurred in approximately 20% of patients. At 2 years after surgery, half of these patients had returned to baseline or improved, with a 10% rate of permanent new neurologic deficits.

REFERENCES

1. Cho KJ, Bridwell KH, Lenke LG, et al. Comparison of Smith-Petersen versus pedicle subtraction osteotomy for the correction of fixed sagittal imbalance. Spine (Phila Pa 1976) 2005;30(18):2030–2038.
2. Dick J, Boachie-Adjei O, Wilson M. One-stage versus two-stage anterior and posterior spinal reconstruction in adults. Comparison of outcomes including nutritional status, complications rates, hospital costs, and other factors. Spine (Phila Pa 1976) 1992;17(8 suppl): S310–S316.
3. Johnson JR, Holt RT. Combined use of anterior and posterior surgery for adult scoliosis. Orthop Clin North Am 1988;19(2):361–370.
4. Kato S, Murakami H, Demura S, et al. Motor and sensory impairments of the lower extremities after L2 nerve root transection during total en bloc spondylectomy. Spine (Phila Pa 1976) 2019;44(16):1129–1136.
5. Leatherman KD, Dickson RA. Two-stage corrective surgery for congenital deformities of the spine. J Bone Joint Surg Br 1979;61-B(3): 324–328.
6. Lehman RA Jr, Polly DW Jr, Kuklo TR, et al. Straight-forward versus anatomic trajectory technique of thoracic pedicle screw fixation: a biomechanical analysis. Spine (Phila Pa 1976) 2003;28(18): 2058–2065.
7. Lenke LG, Shaffrey CI, Carreon LY, et al. Lower extremity motor function following complex adult spinal deformity surgery: two-year follow-up in the Scoli-RISK-1 prospective, multicenter, international study. J Bone Joint Surg Am 2018;100(8):656–665.
8. Lenke LG, Sides BA, Koester LA, et al. Vertebral column resection for the treatment of severe spinal deformity. Clin Orthop Relat Res 2010;468(3):687–699.

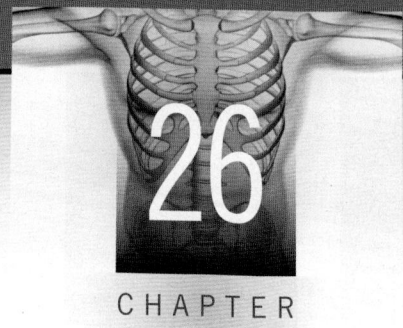

26
CHAPTER

Smith-Petersen Osteotomy for the Management of Sagittal Plane Spinal Deformity

Selvon St. Clair

DEFINITION

- A number of osteotomy techniques have been described to treat severe or rigid sagittal plane spinal deformity.
- These include multilevel anterior interbody radical discectomy and release, posterior pedicle subtraction osteotomy (PSO), vertebral column resection, and Smith-Petersen osteotomy (SPO).
- This chapter reviews the SPO (also known as *chevron* or *Ponté osteotomy*), a mainstay in the treatment of sagittal deformity since it was first described in 1945 by Smith-Petersen and associates.[16]

ANATOMY

- The SPO is indicated for correction of a fixed or partially fixed sagittal plane spinal deformity, including hyperkyphosis typified by Scheuermann kyphosis (FIG 1).

- Although commonly used in the thoracic spine, it has also been used in the lumbar region to correct flat back syndrome or loss of normal lordosis.

PATHOGENESIS

- The various causes of flat back syndrome include Harrington distraction instrumentation,[5,11,12] anterior column degeneration, chronic vertebral compression fractures, adjacent segment degeneration, and iatrogenic causes with pseudarthrosis resulting in loss of sagittal plane correction.[1,4]
- Additionally, the concepts behind SPO have been applied at the cervicothoracic junction for kyphosis such as in ankylosing spondylitis.
- Regardless of the etiology, the clinical presentation of patients with sagittal plane spinal deformity is quite similar.

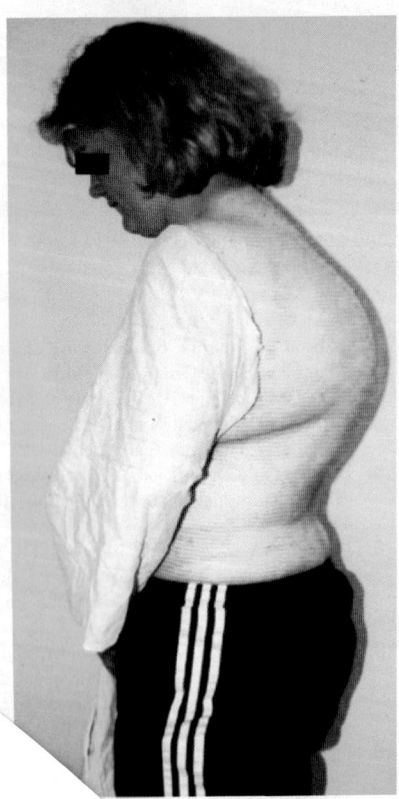
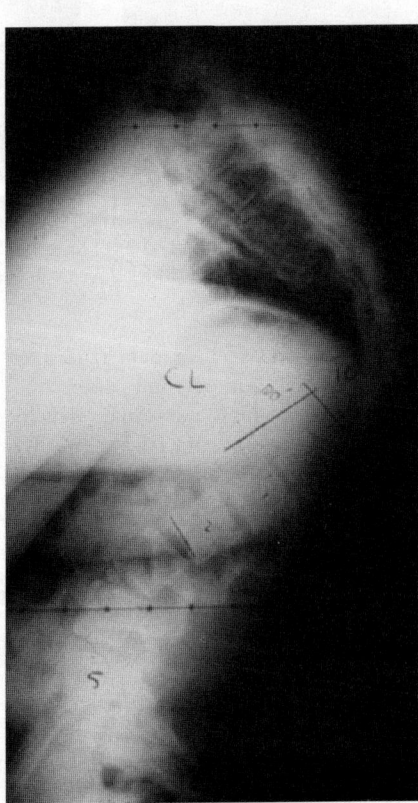

Preoperative clinical photograph (**A**) and lateral radiograph (**B**) of 100-degree Scheuermann kyphosis.

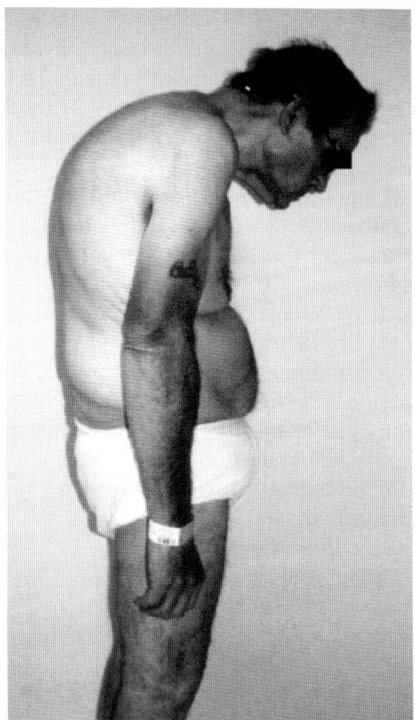

FIG 2 Clinical photograph of a patient with sagittal plane deformity.

PATIENT HISTORY AND PHYSICAL FINDINGS

- Patients usually complain of back pain due to muscle fatigue but can also present with the inability to stand erect without compensating by bending their knees, stumbling while walking, and a feeling of leaning forward **(FIG 2)**.[10]

IMAGING AND OTHER DIAGNOSTIC STUDIES

- The flexibility of the deformity should be evaluated by both physical examination and preoperative planning radiographic evaluation.
- Radiographically, sagittal spinal deformity is evaluated with anteroposterior, posteroanterior, and lateral full-length radiographs with the knees extended and the hands resting on the clavicles **(FIG 3A,B)**.[9]
- The bolster supine hyperextension lateral radiograph or the push prone radiograph is also helpful to assess the rigidity of the deformity **(FIG 3C)**. Further detailed analysis of coronal plane and segmental anatomy can be determined by computed tomography scan.
- Sagittal imbalance is usually determined by the vertical plumb line technique[9,10,13] as assessed on 36-inch plain film.
- Neutral sagittal balance: Vertical plumb line falls at the center of dens or middle of C7 vertebral body aligned with the posterosuperior aspect of the S1 endplate on standing upright films.
- Positive sagittal balance: Vertical plumb line falls anterior to posterosuperior aspect of S1 by a minimum of 2 to 3 cm.
- Types of sagittal imbalance include the following:
  - Compensated abnormalities with neutral sagittal balance
  - Uncompensated abnormalities with positive sagittal balance that can be rigid or fixed
- Attention must also be placed on the femurs and on pelvic parameters in evaluating global balance and in preoperative planning.[14]

SURGICAL MANAGEMENT

- Standard SPO essentially involves complete resection of the facet complex bilaterally as well as any overlapping lamina and spinous process.
- The posterior column bone resection must extend from pedicle to pedicle in a cephalocaudal direction. Facetectomies

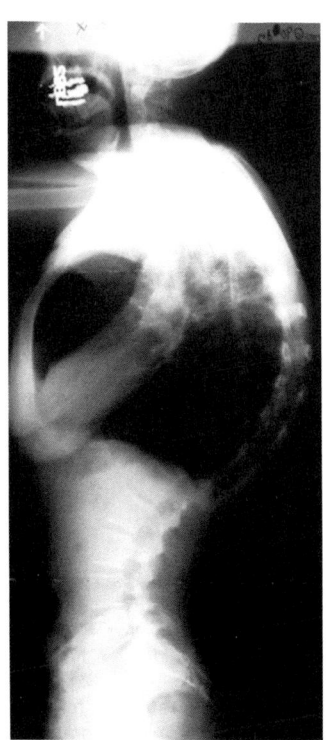

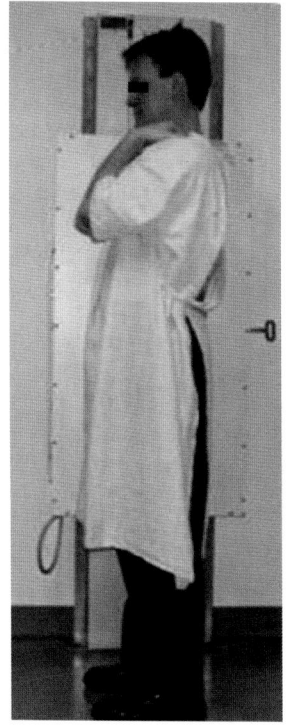

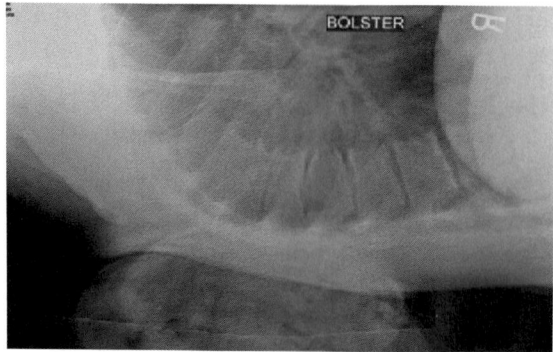

FIG 3 A. A 36-inch film with arms straight out obs[...] view of C7–T4 area. **B.** Demonstration of correct pos[...] 36-inch film to allow view of upper thoracic spine a[...] fect balance. **C.** Supine bolster lateral x-ray.

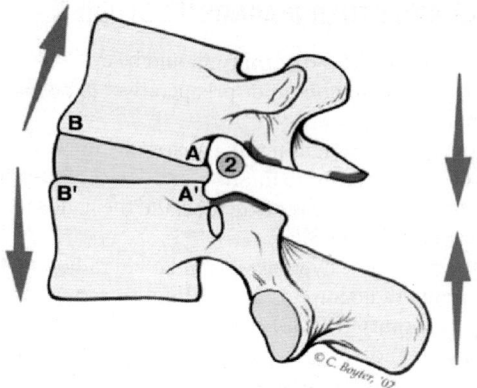

FIG 4 Schematic illustration of the bony resection required for and the angular correction that is obtainable with SPO.

allow for shortening of the posterior column and a component of subsequent lengthening of the anterior column with middle column as fulcrum (**FIG 4**).

- If done in the thoracic spine, the rib head and costovertebral articulation will also act with the middle column as the fulcrum for extension.
- The end objective is increased lordosis by shortening the posterior column to restore the sagittal balance such that the head is centered over the sacrum.[13]
- Modification of the SPO involves placement of an interbody graft or spacer in the disc space after complete discectomy and interbody arthrodesis. This method permits a greater degree of lordosis without compromising neural foraminal height and can be used to address coronal plane deformity by placing the interbody spacer asymmetrically in the disc space.[13]
- It must be recognized that the degree of correction is governed by the flexibility of the anterior column and the effective preoperative disc height.
- Ankylosis or bridging anterior osteophytes may significantly block the correction (**FIG 5**). In cases of rigid deformity, true anterior column osteoclasis helps to achieve a correction of up to 40 to 50 degrees, as may be seen with ankylosing spondylitis.[15]
- Although it is commonly estimated that 1 mm of posterior bone resection results in approximately 1 degree of sagittal correction, this may vary depending on the flexibility through the disc. If a radical anterior release is performed before extension osteotomy, the combined anterior distraction and posterior shortening can increase the segmental correction by a factor of 2.5.[14]

- Indications[2,3,13]
  - Type I smooth thoracic and/or lumbar kyphosis
  - Type I sharp, angular kyphosis in the thoracic spine
  - Type II smooth kyphotic deformity of thoracic and/or lumbar spine when associated with minor (6 to 8 cm) positive sagittal balance
  - Type II smooth kyphotic deformity of thoracic spine when associated with major sagittal imbalance (>12 cm)
  - In scoliosis, for three-dimensional deformity correction
- Contraindications
  - Sharp, fixed angular type II deformity that cannot be corrected by SPO[2,3,13]
  - Anterior fixation, a collapsed or immobile disc space, or an anterior bridging osteophyte at the level of a planned SPO (an open mobile disc space is prerequisite)
  - Posterior wound infection
  - Anterior or lateral bridging osteophytes or congenital bars that cannot be released
- Relative contraindications
  - Calcification of the great vessels
  - Ossification of the dura
  - Inability to achieve appropriate segmental control with fixation

Preoperative Planning

- The more caudal the level considered for an SPO, the greater the effect will be on overall alignment.
- More mobile and taller interbody disc spaces allow for greater correction than severely degenerated, less mobile disc spaces.
- Due to the potential for natural long-term postoperative degeneration of adjacent disc levels that may have a kyphogenic effect, overestimating the required correction by a few degrees is preferred.
- Disperse SPO over multiple levels.
- Avoid SPO adjacent to the lowest instrumented vertebra or upper instrumented vertebra to minimize the risk of end vertebrae fixation pullout.

Equipment

- Posterior-based segmental instrumentation system
- Open frame that will allow the kyphosis to reduce radiolucent operating table
- Neurologic intraoperative monitoring is highly recommended.
  - Transcranial motor evoked potential: essential in kyphosis correction
  - Somatosensory evoked potentials: essential in kyphosis correction

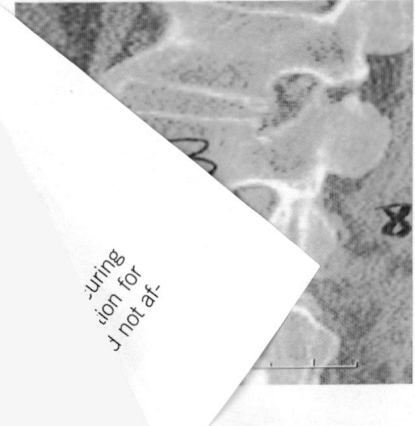

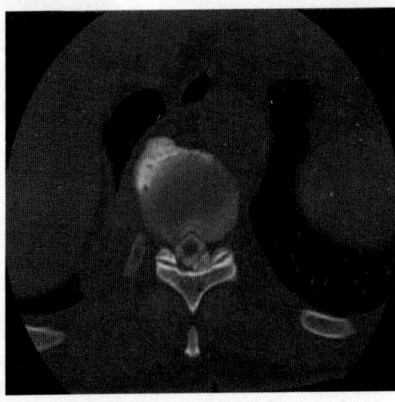

FIG 5 A. Patient with ankylosing spondylitis with only one disc that might move with SPO. **B.** Patient with ossification of the ligamentum flavum, which if not resected, might prevent SPO closure and neurologic compromise.

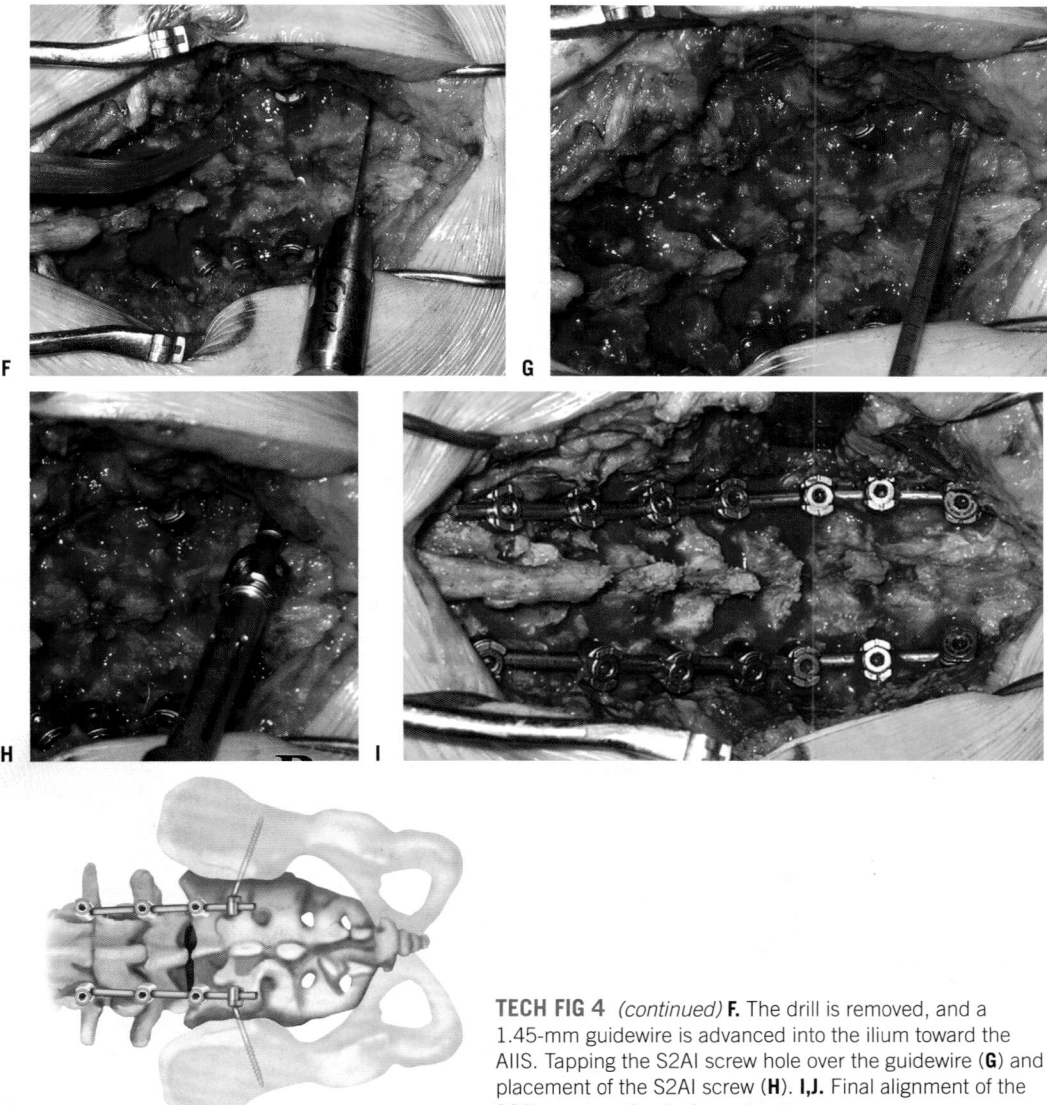

TECH FIG 4 *(continued)* **F.** The drill is removed, and a 1.45-mm guidewire is advanced into the ilium toward the AIIS. Tapping the S2AI screw hole over the guidewire (**G**) and placement of the S2AI screw (**H**). **I,J.** Final alignment of the S2AI screw and spinal construct.

- When using a freehand technique, the trajectory can be confirmed by placing two fingers over the tip of the greater trochanter and aiming toward that point.
- A 2.5-mm drill bit (extended length) is used to drill through the sacral ala, across the SI joint, this distance is roughly 30 to 45 mm in most patients (**TECH FIG 4E**).
- At this point, the 2.5-mm drill bit may be replaced with a larger 3.2-mm drill bit in order to reduce the risk of breakage in harder bone. The drill is then advanced for a total depth of approximately 90 to 100 mm. The drill should continue to be directed toward the AIIS. A hard bony end point should always be insured to avoid breaching the lateral cortex (most common error) or the medial cortex (less common).
- The drill is then removed. A depth gauge is inserted into the path created by the drill in order to determine the length of the screw.
- Next, a 1.45-mm guidewire is placed into the prepared path, again a hard bottom should be confirmed (**TECH FIG 4F**).

- Intraoperative fluoroscopy can be helpful especially in patients with difficult anatomy and early in the surgeon's learning curve.
- Placing the S2AI free hand and using robotic guidance have also been shown to be safe and equally accurate.[20]
- The prepared screw path is then manually tapped over the guidewire using a cannulated tap (**TECH FIG 4G**), and an appropriate length cannulated screw is placed over the guidewire (**TECH FIG 4H**).
  - Screw sizes of 8 to 10 mm in diameter and at minimum 80 to 100 mm long
  - A partially threaded screw with a larger shaft and non-threaded proximal portion is preferred, this minimizes screws breakage and avoids the threads from being located across the SI joint.
- Because the screws are in line with the rest of the spinal construct, no additional cross-connectors are required to connect to the longitudinal rod (**TECH FIG 4I,J**).

PERCUTANEOUS S2AI TECHNIQUE

- Because the S2AI screw falls in line with the more cephalad spinal construct, the S2AI technique allows for the sacropelvic fixation to placed percutaneously, using a minimally invasive approach.[13,17]
- The percutaneous sacropelvic fixation is frequently combined with a minimally invasive percutaneous instrumentation of the lumbar spine.
- The approach to the sacrum is a 3-cm midline incision at a level midway between the S1 and S2 dorsal foramen.
- The starting point, located in line with the lateral edge of the S1 foramen and midway between the S1 and S2 dorsal foramina (see **TECH FIG 4B**), is identified using standard AP and pelvic inlet fluoroscopic views.
- A Jamshidi needle is directed toward the AIIS and advanced 30 to 40 mm into the sacral ala and across the SI joint by about 10 mm. The ideal S2AI trajectory is the same as in the open procedure and averages 40 degrees of lateral angulation and 20 to 30 degrees caudally, the trajectories varies with pelvic obliquity and pelvic tilt (see **TECH FIG 4C,D**).
  - A teardrop view is then obtained to verify the needle trajectory (**TECH FIG 5A**).
    - The teardrop view is a fluoroscopic view obtained by angling the C-arm roughly 30 degrees lateral and 30 degrees caudal, which creates an overlap of the AIIS and the PSIS and the image of a teardrop.

- The needle position is adjusted to be coaxial with the teardrop and then advanced 30 to 40 mm into the ilium and toward the AIIS, until the adequate length is reached.
- Next, a guidewire is passed through the Jamshidi needle and advanced and additional 20 to 30 mm past the tip of the needle.
- The Jamshidi needle is removed, and the guidewire is left in place (**TECH FIG 5B**).
- Positioning and angulation of the wire can be confirmed with fluoroscopic views as needed.
- Screw lengths are then measured by marking the depth of the guidewire. Screw sizes of 8 to 10 mm by 80 to 100 mm should be used in the adults and pediatric patients.
- The prepared path is manually tapped over the guidewire using a cannulated tap (**TECH FIG 5C**), and an appropriate length screw is placed (**TECH FIG 5D**).
- Because the screws are in line with the rest of the spinal construct, no additional cross-connectors are required.
- In cases in which a percutaneous lumbar spinal procedure has also been performed, the S2AI screw can be attached to the main spinal construct by threading a rod percutaneously from proximal to distal and maneuvering the rod and screws tulips to align.
- The final trajectory and placement of the screw is identical to that of the open S2AI technique.

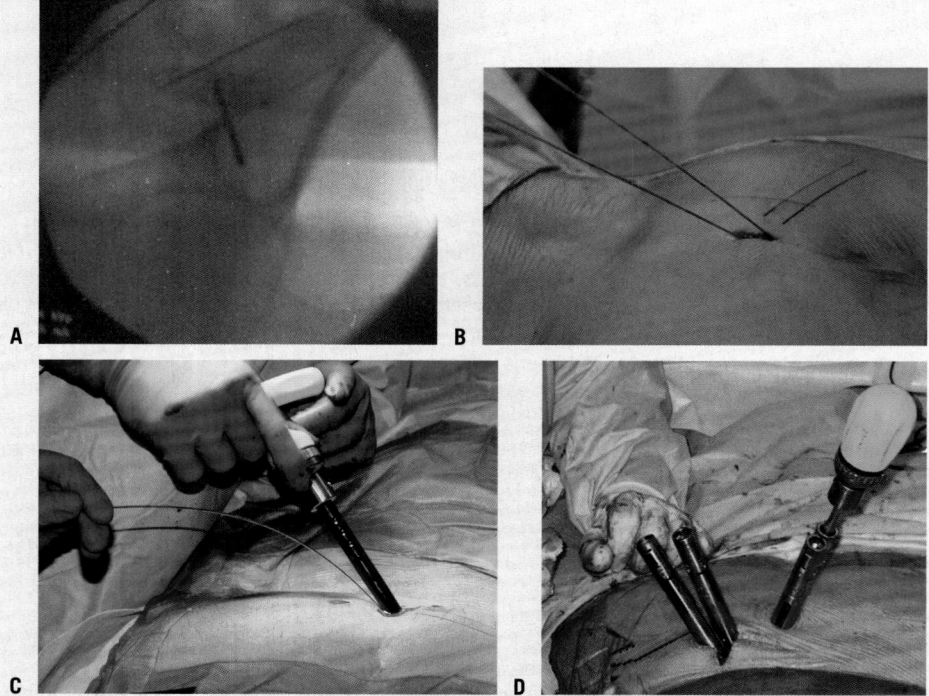

TECH FIG 5 A. Representative fluoroscopic teardrop view is obtained by rolling the C-arm approximately 30 degrees lateral and 30 degrees caudal, which creates an overlap of the AIIS and PSIS and the image of a teardrop. **B.** Percutaneous guidewire placement. **C.** A cannulated handheld tap is used to tap the screw hole over the guidewire. **D.** The screw is placed with a handheld driver (*green handle*). In cases in which a minimally invasive lumbar spine procedure has also been done, the rod can be attached to the main spinal construct by passing it underneath the skin with the assistance of special tubes attached to the screws tulips. (**A,D:** From Martin CT, Witham T, Kebaish KM. Sacropelvic fixation: two case reports of a new percutaneous technique. Spine [Phila Pa 1976] 2011;36[9]:e618–e621.)

Pearls and Pitfalls

Indications	• Long spinal fusions to the sacrum are the most common indication for sacropelvic fixation.
Teardrop Fluoroscopic View	• The teardrop is created by the overlap of the AIIS and PSIS and represents a bony canal through which the pelvic fixation can be safely placed.
Damage to Surrounding Soft Tissues	• Structures in the sciatic notch can be at risk. • Minimized by verifying that the screw pathway has a bony end point with a blunt probe prior to screw placement • Use of C-arm to verify the trajectory; the teardrop view is the most helpful.
Implant Prominence	• Common reason for revision • Minimized by creating a notch prior to placement of the iliac screw by burying the screw beyond the PSIS or by using the S2AI technique, which the screw tulip to be at least 15 mm less superficial than the iliac screw
Instrumentation Loosening	• Minimized by using the largest diameter screw that the anatomy allows • Addition of an anterior fusion increases construct stability. • Using the S2AI technique, which is associated with less incidence of implant loosening • Using a partially threaded screws with a large diameter shank
Authors' Preferred Technique	• At our institution, the S2AI technique has been adopted as the procedure of choice for sacropelvic fixation in both adult and pediatric patients.

POSTOPERATIVE CARE

- The patient should be awoken in the operating room, and a detailed neurologic examination should be conducted immediately following surgery. If a neurologic deficit is detected, appropriate imaging and surgical intervention may be necessary.
- The postoperative diet and patient pain control can be managed as per routine postoperative care.
- No additional external immobilization such as an orthotic is necessary.
- The patient should be placed in a regular hospital bed, and early ambulation should be encouraged.
- Physical therapy should be started as soon as feasible following the surgical procedure.
- After discharge, follow-up at regular intervals is important, including appropriate radiographs as indicated depending on the procedure performed.

OUTCOMES

- Excellent fusion rates have been achieved with all three techniques.[2,8,11,22]
- Implant prominence and pain is a common reason for instrumentation removal in both the iliac screw and the Galveston techniques. However, less than 2% of patients with S2AI screws require implant removal after 2 years, as compared to up to 22% of patients with iliac screws.[7]
- The screw in the S2AI technique breaches the synovial cartilage of the SI joint in approximately 60% of cases. However, a recent study showed no adverse effects on the SI joint at 2 years follow-up.[22]
- Multiple investigators have found that the S2AI screw provide superior stability and is biomechanically strong anchor for long-segment constructs.[21]

COMPLICATIONS

- Modern techniques for sacropelvic fixation have helped to minimize the incidence of complications. However, serious complications still can and do occur. A brief discussion of these complications and ways to minimize them is presented here.
- In the young pediatric patients, the S2AI technique was not associated with growth disturbance even though the implant crossed the SI joint.[5]
- A recent meta-analysis reviewed multiple showing that the S2AI screws with their lower profile have made a significant impact in reducing complications associated with conventional iliac screws.[9]
- Instrumentation misplacement and injuries to adjacent structures
  - The structures in the greater sciatic foramen and those overlying the anterior surface of the sacrum are at risk during placement of the instrumentation.[10]
  - However, injury to these structures is very uncommon,[10] and the risk can be minimized by using a blunt probe to ensure a proper bony end point prior to screw placement.
  - Fluoroscopic imaging can also be useful, particularly in patients with difficult anatomy.
  - Freehand placement of the S2AI screws has been shown to be safe and reliable.[21]
  - Both methods, free hand and robotic guidance, are safe and equally accurate.[20]
- Implant prominence
  - Implant prominence following traditional iliac screws can lead to significant pain and discomfort and is the most common reason for revision of this procedure.[10]
  - The risk of this complication is highest in thin patients and is only seen in patients who had the iliac screw and Galveston techniques.[10]
  - The risks can be minimized by creating a notch prior to placement of the iliac screw, by burying the screw beyond the PSIS, by choosing a medial starting point for the iliac screw, or by using the S2AI technique, which on average allows for 15-mm deeper placement of the screw head as compared to the iliac screw technique.[4]
- Implant loosening
  - Loosening is a second common reason for implant removal, but it may remain asymptomatic if fusion can be achieved prior to its onset.[10]

- Loosening is caused by repeated micromotion of the implants and is visible radiographically as a radiolucency around the screw or rod.
- In the Galveston L-rod technique, loosening of the short arm of the L-rod is particularly common, and this complication is called the *windshield wiper effect*.[3,8]
- In some patients treated with the Galveston technique, the windshield wiper effect may lead to pain and the need for implant removal.[3,8]
- With the S2AI and iliac screw techniques, choosing the largest diameter screw possible (usually 8 to 10 mm in adults) can help to delay implant loosening and maximize the chances of a successful fusion.
- Wound problems and infection
  - Few studies have reported definitive infection rates associated with sacropelvic fixation.
  - Furthermore, the infection rate associated with sacropelvic fixation alone is difficult to ascertain because these techniques are often combined with fusions of the mobile spine above, which requires additional incisions and soft tissue dissection.
  - Infection rates associated with the Galveston L-rod have been reported to range from 3% to 10%.[8,16]
  - In a study of 81 patients treated with iliac screw fixation, the infection rate was reported as 4%.[11]
  - A study of 27 patients treated with the S2AI technique showed an infection rate of 0%.[22]
  - Significantly less dissection is required for the S2AI technique, which may account for the lower infection rates reported with that procedure.
- Nonunion and instrumentation failure
  - If bony fusion does not occur, the instrumentation is destined to fail, often through implant failure or breakage.
  - Augmentation of sacropelvic fixation with an anterior interbody lumbar fusion at L4–L5 and L5–S1 can optimize fusion stability and increase the chances of a successful fusion.

REFERENCES

1. Allen BL Jr, Ferguson RL. The Galveston technique for L rod instrumentation of the scoliotic spine. Spine (Phila Pa 1976) 1982;7(3):276–284.
2. Allen BL Jr, Ferguson RL. The Galveston technique of pelvic fixation with L-rod instrumentation of the spine. Spine (Phila Pa 1976) 1984;9(4):388–394.
3. Broom MJ, Banta JV, Renshaw TS. Spinal fusion augmented by Luque-rod segmental instrumentation for neuromuscular scoliosis. J Bone Joint Surg Am 1989;71:32–44.
4. Chang TL, Sponseller PD, Kebaish KM, et al. Low profile pelvic fixation: anatomic parameters for sacral alar-iliac fixation versus traditional iliac fixation. Spine (Phila Pa 1976) 2009;34(5):436–440.
5. Cottrill E, Margalit A, Brucker C, et al. Comparison of sacral-alar-iliac and iliac-only methods of pelvic fixation in early-onset scoliosis at 5.8 years' mean follow-up. Spine Deform 2019;7(2):364–370.
6. Cunningham BW, Lewis SJ, Long J, et al. Biomechanical evaluation of lumbosacral reconstruction techniques for spondylolisthesis: an in vitro porcine model. Spine (Phila Pa 1976) 2002;27:2321–2327.
7. Emami A, Deviren V, Berven S, et al. Outcome and complications of long fusions to the sacrum in adult spine deformity: Luque-Galveston, combined iliac and sacral screws, and sacral fixation. Spine (Phila Pa 1976) 2002;27(7):776–786.
8. Gau YL, Lonstein JE, Winter RB, et al. Luque-Galveston procedure for correction and stabilization of neuromuscular scoliosis and pelvic obliquity: a review of 68 patients. J Spinal Disord 1991;4(4):399–410.
9. Hasan MY, Liu G, Wong HK, et al. Postoperative complications of S2AI versus iliac screw in spinopelvic fixation: a meta-analysis and recent trends review. Spine J 2020;20(6):964–972.
10. Kebaish KM. Sacropelvic fixation: techniques and complications. Spine (Phila Pa 1976) 2010;35(25):2245–2251.
11. Kuklo TR, Bridwell KH, Lewis SJ, et al. Minimum 2-year analysis of sacropelvic fixation and L5–S1 fusion using S1 and iliac screws. Spine (Phila Pa 1976) 2001;26(18):1976–1983.
12. Lehman RA Jr, Kuklo TR, Belmont PJ Jr, et al. Advantage of pedicle screw fixation directed into the apex of the sacral promontory over bicortical fixation: a biomechanical analysis. Spine (Phila Pa 1976) 2002;27(8):806–811.
13. Martin CT, Witham TF, Kebaish KM. Sacropelvic fixation: two case reports of a new percutaneous technique. Spine (Phila Pa 1976) 2011;36(9):E618–E621.
14. Mirkovic S, Abitbol JJ, Steinman J, et al. Anatomic consideration for sacral screw placement. Spine (Phila Pa 1976) 1991;16(6 suppl):S289–S294.
15. Moshirfar A, Rand FF, Sponseller PD, et al. Pelvic fixation in spine surgery. Historical overview, indications, biomechanical relevance, and current techniques. J Bone Joint Surg Am 2005;87(suppl 2):89–106.
16. Nectoux E, Giacomelli MC, Karger C, et al. Complications of the Luque-Galveston scoliosis correction technique in paediatric cerebral palsy. Orthop Traumatol Surg Res 2010;96(4):354–361.
17. O'Brien JR, Matteini L, Yu WD, et al. Feasibility of minimally invasive sacropelvic fixation: percutaneous S2 alar iliac fixation. Spine (Phila Pa 1976) 2010;35(4):460–464.
18. O'Brien JR, Yu WD, Bhatnagar R, et al. An anatomic study of the S2 iliac technique for lumbopelvic screw placement. Spine (Phila Pa 1976) 2009;34(12):E439–E442.
19. O'Brien MF. Sacropelvic fixation in spinal deformity. In: Dewlad RL, ed. Spinal Deformities: The Text. New York: Thieme, 2003:601–614.
20. Shillingford JN, Laratta JL, Park PJ, et al. Human versus robot: a propensity-matched analysis of the accuracy of free hand versus robotic guidance for placement of S2 alar-iliac (S2AI) screws. Spine (Phila Pa 1976) 2018;43(21):E1297–E1304.
21. Shillingford JN, Laratta JL, Tan LA, et al. The free-hand technique for S2-alar-iliac screw placement: a safe and effective method for sacropelvic fixation in adult spinal deformity. J Bone Joint Surg Am 2018;100(4):334–342.
22. Sponseller PD, Zimmerman RM, Ko PS, et al. Low profile pelvic fixation with the sacral alar iliac technique in the pediatric population improves results at two-year minimum follow-up. Spine (Phila Pa 1976) 2010;35(20):1887–1892.
23. Wiggins GC, Ondra SL, Shaffrey CI. Management of iatrogenic flatback syndrome. Neurosurg Focus 2003;15(3):E8.

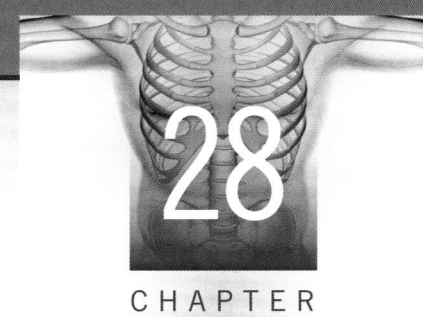

28

CHAPTER

Complications
Management of Intraoperative Cerebrospinal Fluid Leaks

Christopher G. Kalhorn and Kevin M. McGrail

BACKGROUND

- Management of intraoperative durotomies and the postoperative management of cerebrospinal fluid (CSF) leaks can pose serious problems in spinal surgery.
- This chapter discusses risk factors that can predispose patients to the occurrence of an intraoperative durotomy.
- We review the surgical instruments, biologic agents, and drainage catheters that are of assistance with repair of durotomies.
- A discussion then occurs with respect to the particular challenges at varying locations within the spinal axis when it is approached either anteriorly or posteriorly.

AVOIDANCE OF DUROTOMY

- Careful study of preoperative imaging studies may yield valuable information with respect to potential pitfalls during exposure of the spine.
- Look out for postoperative changes from previous laminectomies or laminotomies.
- Spina bifida occulta is reported in up to 10% to 15% of normal healthy adults and is a potential site for durotomy during exposure.
- Incomplete ossification of the C1 laminar arch should be kept in mind during any posterior approach to the high cervical spine or craniocervical junction.
- The L5–S1 interspace is a widened interspace and is a frequent area for incidental durotomy during exposure of the lumbar spine.
- Ossification of the posterior longitudinal ligament, especially in the cervical and thoracic spine can often be recognized on preoperative imaging studies and carries a high risk of intraoperative CSF leak.

PRINCIPLES OF REPAIR

- Often, these durotomies occur in the midline and can be repaired primarily with simple interrupted or running sutures. A 4-0 or 5-0 monofilament suture such as Prolene (Ethicon, Inc., Somerville, NJ) or nylon are appropriate.
- We prefer a repair with a small tapered needle such as an RB-1 in a simple running fashion.
- A good needle driver such as Castro-Viejo can be helpful to repair a tear in the lateral recess.

GENERAL PRINCIPLES AND PATIENT SAFETY

- When an intraoperative durotomy has occurred, care should be taken to avoid any injury to the underlying neural elements.

- Surgical cautery (Bovie) use should be limited when in proximity to neural elements.
- Minimize the use of high-speed cutting drill bits near the spinal canal. A diamond drill bit is a much safer instrument especially in less experienced hands.
- The use of appropriate-sized suction tips is recommended once a durotomy has occurred. The smallest suction tip that can be used to keep the surgical field clear should be employed.
  - Suction tips that allow for regulation of the strength of the suction at the handpiece are extremely useful.
  - Suction tips that have their apertures on the side and not on the tip (Grossman suction tips) are also very useful in these situations.
  - Suction lines that are soft and flexible allow for rapid "clamping off" when a durotomy has occurred. This can prevent a suction tip from inadvertently sucking up nerve roots.
- Make sure that you have a capable and experienced assistant. Sometimes, what you really need is an extra pair of experienced hands to maximize your exposure so that you can work on primary repair of the dural defect.
- Once a durotomy has taken place, protect the neural elements with a soft Cottonoid (Codman, Warsaw, IN).
- Focus is then directed toward minimizing and further extension of the durotomy and attaining sufficient bone exposure to allow for primary dural repair when possible.
- Whenever possible, achieve a watertight primary dural repair and reinforce with dural sealant when indicated.
- Decompression of the lumbar cistern through the release of spinal fluid can also alleviate the extramural forces on the epidural venous plexus. This can result in large amounts of bleeding, which can normally be controlled with bipolar cautery or thrombin-soaked Gelfoam (Baxter Healthcare Corp., Hayward, CA).

PRODUCTS

Dural Substitutes

- There are a number of commercially available dural substitute materials, most of which are derivatives of bovine collagen.
- They are available as suturable or onlay dural grafts.
- Bovine pericardium is also commercially available as a suturable dural graft. There are case reports of aseptic or chemical meningitis associated with bovine pericardial grafts.
- Autologous grafting materials include pericranium, fascia lata, and autologous muscle grafts that can be used as a plug to prevent a leak.

Dural Sealants

- There are a number of commercially available dural sealants, most of which are derivatives of fibrin glue.
- Thin layers of these sealants can be applied with aerosolizers to reinforce a dural repair.
- Some of these products have been reported to swell postoperatively. For this reason, a minimum of product should be used to reinforce the repair and avoid postoperative compression of the neural elements.

DUROTOMIES DURING POSTERIOR LUMBAR SURGERY

- Lumbar dural tears may occur during exposure of the lumbar spine, during the course of decompression of the neural elements, or during the placement of spinal hardware.
- If possible, avoid a leak in the first place. This can be done by avoiding sharp bone edges along the margins of a decompressive laminectomy.
- Make good use of your assistant. In the lumbar spine, have your assistant use a blunt nerve hook or a no. 4 Penfield to gently displace the dura away from the bone edge while you are doing your decompression.
- Most midline durotomies lend themselves to primary dural repair.
- Durotomies, which occur in the lateral recess or overlying the exiting nerve root sheath, are more difficult to repair.
- When a CSF leak occurs in the lateral recess, first obtain wider bone exposure. A primary dural repair should then be attempted.

- Large dural defects that cannot be repaired primarily should be grafted (eg, with bovine pericardial graft or dural substitute). These grafts should be sewn in place in a watertight manner when possible.
- For dural tears that cannot be repaired primarily or patched, consider an onlay dural substitute graft reinforced with a dural sealant.
- When CSF leaks occur over the nerve root sheath, these are often difficult to repair primarily and can be treated successfully with dural sealant or fibrin glue.
- Occasionally, one can face a fairly small lumbar durotomy through which multiple rootlets of the cauda equina can herniate. In this situation, it may be necessary to enlarge the durotomy and even to drain some spinal fluid to allow for safe reduction of the rootlets back into the spinal canal followed by primary repair of the dura.

DUROTOMIES DURING REVISION LUMBAR SURGERY

- Patients with a history of CSF leak with previous surgery should be counseled preoperatively that they are likely at a higher risk of recurrent CSF leak.
- During exposure of the spine, sharp curettes can be used to define normal facet and bone anatomy.

- The use of a diamond drill around the margins of a previous laminectomy may help prevent a leak.
- When scar is densely adherent to the underlying dura, it may be prudent to leave areas of adherent scar attached to avoid a CSF leak.

DUROTOMIES DURING POSTERIOR THORACIC SURGERY

- Many of the same principles as outlined in repair of CSF leaks during posterior lumbar surgery apply in the posterior thoracic spine.
- If a leak occurs over a thoracic nerve root sheath, the root itself can be ligated and sacrificed to prevent further leakage of CSF.

- With CSF leak in the setting of posterior lumbar or thoracic surgery, we will often recommend a period of flat bed rest for the first 48 hours to allow for short-term healing of the repair.
- After 48 hours, we will mobilize the patients ad lib.

DUROTOMIES DURING POSTERIOR CERVICAL SURGERY

- Durotomies during posterior spinal surgery normally are midline or paramedian in location and lend themselves to primary dural repair.
- This can be supplemented with dural sealant.

TECHNIQUES

DUROTOMIES DURING ANTERIOR CERVICAL SPINAL APPROACHES

- CSF leaks are not as common in anterior cervical approaches as they are in lumbar spinal procedures.
- Most leaks that we have observed during anterior cervical discectomy and fusion (ACDF) have been in association with the use of high-powered drills.
- These leaks normally occur at the site of the takeoff of the cervical root sheath. In this location, the dura takes a slight superior course as the nerve root exits the foramen, making the dura more likely to be injured in this location.

- Durotomies during ACDF can be extremely difficult to repair primarily.
- Most of these durotomies can be treated with an onlay dural substitute and a widely fitting bone graft that occupies the width of the discectomy defect.
- Consideration should be given to the placement of a lumbar subarachnoid drain.

DUROTOMIES DURING ANTERIOR THORACIC SPINAL APPROACHES

- Durotomies that occur during anterior thoracic approaches are of concern because of the large potential space of leak and frequent requirements for postoperative chest tubes.
- Attempt should be made to repair the dura primarily if possible.
- Often, these leaks can only be repaired with onlay dural substitute and dural sealant together.
- Attention should be given to the postoperative chest tube output.
- If there is a question about whether chest tube fluid represents normal pleural fluid or CSF, a sample of fluid can

be collected and sent for beta-2 transferrin testing, which is positive in CSF.
- With a persistent CSF leak occurring in the setting of a chest tube with CSF coming out of the chest tube, we recommend taking the chest tube off of negative pressure suction when feasible and continuing the lumbar drain until the chest tube can be removed.
- Our experience has been that recurrent CSF leaks in the chest are unusual.

PLACEMENT OF LUMBAR SUBARACHNOID DRAINS

- We will most often place a lumbar drain in cases of recurrent CSF leak after primary repair or in cases that are deemed to be high risk for postoperative CSF leak.
- Lumbar subarachnoid drains can either be placed surgically at the time of a lumbar decompressive laminectomy or separately through a 14-gauge Tuohy needle.
- The purpose of a lumbar drain is to divert spinal fluid and alleviate pressure to allow for the repaired area of CSF leak to heal.

- Care should be taken at the time of lumbar catheter placement; do not attempt to reposition the drain catheter while the spinal needle is in place. This can result in inadvertent shearing of the catheter.
- Lumbar drains are connected to a sterile drainage system.
- Most common site of insertion is from L2 to L5.

TECHNIQUES

POSTOPERATIVE MANAGEMENT

- Lumbar drains
  - Careful postoperative orders must be given regarding the management of lumbar drains.
  - Drainage systems are most commonly placed at the level of the patient's spine, and the height of the drainage collection device is adjusted to maintain a CSF output of approximately 80 mL of spinal fluid per 8-hour shift.
  - Patients are frequently maintained on intravenous antibiotics while the spinal drain is in place. We use prophylactic Ancef until the drain is removed.

- The drain is normally left open for 3 to 7 days to allow time for healing of the durotomy.
- The lumbar drainage system is clamped, and the patient is observed for signs or recurrent CSF leak.
- If there is no further evidence of CSF leak after the drain has been clamped for 24 hours, the lumbar subarachnoid drain is removed.
- Overdrainage of CSF through a lumbar drain can result in tearing of cranial bridging veins and acute subdural hematoma formation.
- The risk of infection with prolonged indwelling drains can be minimized with good sterile technique. Drains can

also be tunneled, which also helps to minimize infection risk. It has been our practice to maintain our patients on intravenous antibiotics while the drain is in place, and we make an effort not to extend CSF diversion through a lumbar drain beyond 7 days.

- Wound drains (wound Hemovac)
  - We will place wound drains in the setting of a repaired CSF leak to help prevent the postoperative occurrence of an epidural hematoma.
  - Epidural hematoma is of concern due to a loss of turgor pressure within the thecal sac and decompression of the lumbar epidural venous plexus.
  - These drains can later be removed or taken off of suction if the drain outputs are high or the patient develops a spinal headache.

COMPLICATIONS

- Clinical signs of CSF leak
  - Low-pressure (spinal) headaches will be present when the patient is in the upright position and will resolve or improve when the patient is recumbent.
  - New-onset cranial nerve palsies (abducens nerve palsy)
    - As the sixth cranial nerve has the longest intracranial course, this is presumably due to traction on the sixth nerve with excessive CSF drainage.
  - Nausea and vomiting
- For cases of recurrent CSF cutaneous fistulas or recurrent symptomatic CSF leaks that have not resolved with CSF diversion, often, the only option is reexploration and attempted repair of the leak if it can be located.

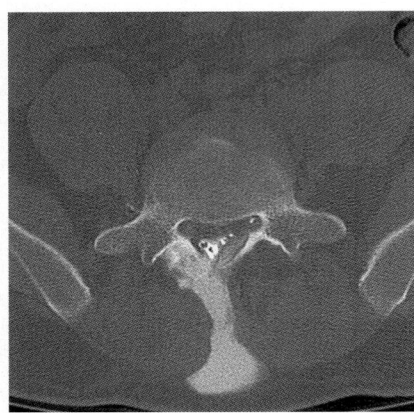

FIG 1 Axial computed tomography myelogram demonstrating dye extravasation into a pseudomeningocele cavity consistent with CSF leak.

- Pseudomeningocele should be divided according to small or asymptomatic collections and larger, symptomatic, or cosmetically disfiguring collections.
  - Small, asymptomatic collections can be observed.
  - Large, symptomatic collections will usually require reexploration and repair with possible CSF diversion through a lumbar subarachnoid drain.
  - Patients who have symptomatic pseudomeningocele may complain of pain or swelling at the surgical site or symptoms of low CSF pressure. These symptoms include persistent positional headache, nausea, vomiting, or occasionally photophobia. These symptoms are exacerbated in the upright position **(FIG 1)**.

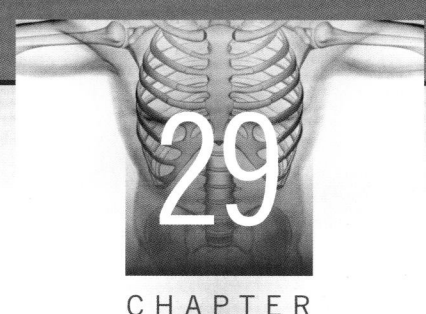

29
CHAPTER

Revision Lumbar Surgery

Shyam A. Patel, Alan H. Daniels, Kevin J. DiSilvestro, and Jeffrey A. Rihn

DEFINITION

- *Revision lumbar surgery* is a catch-all term, which can include any repeat surgical intervention in a patient after primary lumbar surgery. Reasons may include persistent pain and radiculopathy, infection, trauma, tumor, and both degenerative and nondegenerative deformity.
- The term *failed back syndrome* has been used to describe patients that experience poor clinical outcomes following lumbar surgery; however, this term usually refers specifically to degenerative causes often involving the intervertebral disc.[7]

ANATOMY

- During revision lumbar surgery, spinal anatomy can be distorted. Normal bony landmarks may or may not be present, especially in the presence of fusion masses. Dense fibrous scar can cause adherence of natural anatomic planes, which is particularly concerning when there is dural involvement. In these circumstances, unintended durotomy can occur if dissection is not carried out with caution.
- Preoperative preparation is critical with these cases. Weight-bearing films to visualize and localize the relevant anatomy can be of tremendous aid, especially when identifying hardware and intact bony elements as reference for the correct operative level. Computed tomography (CT) can also be of use if the bony anatomy is particularly complex.
- When exposing during revision lumbar surgery, it is important to identify regions of normal anatomy before proceeding to expose previously operated-on areas. Once the lateral wall of the bony canal is identified, one can use it as a reference to identify neural elements. Residual bone lateral to the spinal canal (eg, the facet joints or bony fusion mass) and implanted instrumentation can also serve as valuable and reliable landmarks.
- If hardware is in place, dissection is best started laterally by identifying the facets or hardware. From here, the surgeon can work medially to remove scar and identify dura, if necessary.

PATHOGENESIS

- Up to 15% of those who have an operation for degenerative lumbar disease will require a revision for a number of reasons.[3,6]
- The pathogenesis is dependent on the specific need for revision, which may or may not be related to the primary surgery.
- Reasons may include persistent pain and radiculopathy, infection, trauma, tumor, and both degenerative and nondegenerative deformity.

NATURAL HISTORY

- The natural history of recurrent pathology following primary surgery is not completely understood but is likely similar to that of the original condition. In other words, the natural history of a recurrent disc herniation, for example, is likely similar to that of the original herniation: spontaneous resolution of symptoms in many cases.
- Hence, conservative treatment can be tried before surgical intervention. Of course, in situations where this concerns for infection or progressive neurologic instability, prompt surgical intervention should not be delayed.

PATIENT HISTORY AND PHYSICAL FINDINGS

- A complete and thorough history and physical exam is important, especially if the primary surgery was performed by a different surgeon and outside records are limited or acquisition of them is difficult.
  - In particular, it is important to establish a surgical timeline. Note the onset and characteristics of the initial symptoms, the pathology at the time of presentation, and surgery performed.
  - It is helpful to review preoperative clinical notes and operative reports. These should be obtained whenever possible. The operative note should be scrutinized for comments about potential intraoperative adverse events such as durotomy.
  - A detailed description of all subsequent spinal surgical interventions and the presence or absence of symptom-free periods should be documented.
  - All medications, especially narcotic analgesics, anticoagulants, and anything that may increase risk of infectious or prevent wound healing must be recorded.
  - As with nonrevision patients, it is useful to categorize the patient's new chief complaint into one of three groups: leg pain predominant, back pain predominant, or equal parts leg and back pain.
    - Predominant leg pain suggests a neurogenic cause.
      - The quality and pattern of the patient's leg pain can provide significant information about the nature of the pain.
      - Leg pain that is described as *burning*, for example, suggests neuropathic pain, which is generally unresponsive to further surgical intervention.
      - Similarly, leg pain that is present constantly and is unchanged by activity generally suggests the presence of underlying changes in the nerve that are unlikely to be significantly changed by

additional surgery. Such nonmechanical pain is not typical of neurogenic pain that is amenable to surgery, which is generally mechanical in nature.

- In patients with leg pain, careful examination of the lower extremity joints and pulses is important to rule out nonspinal causes. This is particularly important in older patients in whom spinal disease frequently coexists with other degenerative conditions such as peripheral vascular disease and joint arthritis.
- Predominant back pain suggests the pain is likely not due to a neurogenic causes and the etiology is typically much more difficult to identify.

- From the original records or postoperative timeline, one must determine whether or not the patient's original diagnosis and treatment were appropriate.
  - Three broad questions need to be determined and asked:
    - Was the original diagnosis correct?
    - Was the specific surgical treatment appropriate?
    - Was the surgical treatment performed adequately?
- The duration of symptom relief following the initial surgery and timing of symptoms presentation can narrow down the list of possible causes.
  - If the patient had no symptom relief following surgery, either the surgeon did not identify/address all of the pathology (eg, lateral recess stenosis, foraminal stenosis, or disc herniation) or an inappropriate surgical procedure was performed.
    - Other factors to consider if there is no improvement after surgery include whether it was a work-related injury, particularly if associated with a pending compensation claim.
      □ The likelihood of secondary gain is a potentially significant factor in these patients.
      □ The surgeon must also be cognizant of psychosocial issues before planning a revision operation. This includes depression and narcotic addiction.
      □ The presence of these psychosocial factors (worker's compensation, depression, anxiety, litigation, etc.) can have a significant negative impact on patient outcome after lumbar surgery.[8]
      □ When in doubt about potential significance of such psychosocial factors, a psychological evaluation should be obtained.
    - The presence of Waddell signs should also be documented, if present. One of the more significant Waddell signs is overreaction to pain. Other signs include superficial skin tenderness, regional disturbances, distraction phenomena, and simulation.
      □ The presence of three or more Waddell signs indicates that the patient's pain is likely nonorganic and portends a poor prognosis, particularly with further surgery.[9]
    - Distraction testing includes the "flip test" in which a patient demonstrates a positive straight-leg raise test in the supine position but not in the seated position (FIG 1). A straight-leg raise test in a patient who is exhibiting pain behavior will be easily achieved to 90 degrees, whereas a patient with pain from a true radiculopathy will "flip" back on their hands when attempting a sitting straight-leg raise in order to relieve tension in the sciatic nerve.

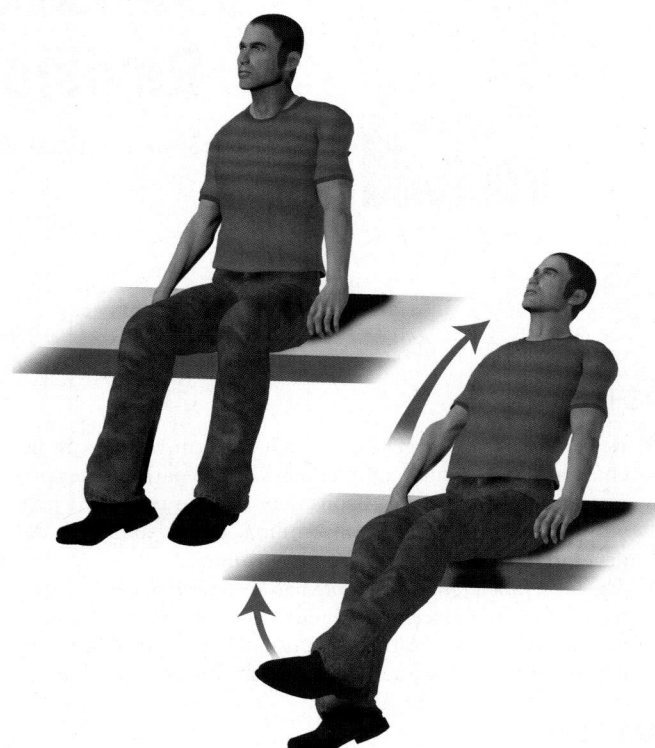

FIG 1 Flip test. Patient should flip back on hands if straight-leg raise test is truly positive.

- With simulation, anticipatory behavior can be elicited through simulated movement. For example, the patient will report back pain through maneuvers that do not typically move the back such as mild trunk rotation through hip rotation (TABLE 1).

TABLE 1 Vascular versus Neurogenic Claudication		
Examination	**Vascular**	**Neurogenic**
Walking distance	Fixed	Variable
Palliative factors	Standing	Sitting/bending
Provocative factors	Walking	Walking/standing
Walking uphill	Painful	Painless
Bicycle test	Positive (painful)	Negative (painless)
Pulses	Absent	Present
Skin	Loss of hair/shiny	Normal
Back pain	Occasionally	Commonly
Back motion	Normal	Limited
Pain character	Cramping/distal to proximal	Numbness/aching/proximal to distal
Atrophy	Uncommon	Occasionally

- Transient relief of symptoms (<6 months) suggests the development of scar tissue, infection, or disc reherniation.
  - Some element of scarring occurs after all surgeries. The presence of peridural fibrosis following decompressive spinal surgery does not necessarily implicate it as a cause of the patient's symptoms. However, patients undergoing lumbar revision surgery tend to have poor outcomes when significant fibrosis is present.[4]
  - The risk of developing a recurrent lumbar disc herniation after discectomy is approximately 5% to 18%.[1,2]
- If the patient experienced a long duration of relief of his or her symptoms (typically longer than 6 to 12 months), this suggests the development of new pathology at either the same level or at a new (often adjacent) level. This may include postoperative instability (eg, spondylolisthesis, scoliosis, kyphosis, and flat back deformity), pseudoarthrosis, or adjacent level disease.
  - Pseudarthrosis in the setting of spinal fusion surgery refers to the radiologic failure of new bone to form across the intended joint space.

IMAGING STUDIES

- Ideally, all of the patient's preoperative and immediate postoperative imaging should be available for review. From this, the surgeon can ensure that pathology was initially present and addressed adequately in terms of the correct level and extent of decompression/stabilization.
- All patients being evaluated for revision lumbar surgery should have a current standing anteroposterior (AP) and lateral plain x-ray of their lumbar spine.
  - This should also include a coned-down spot lateral view of the lumbosacral level, especially in patients with prior surgery at L5–S1. This provides valuable information about sagittal and coronal alignment, hardware position and integrity, and bony anatomy.
  - Standing AP and lateral 3-foot films including the external auditory meatus and femoral heads should be performed in nearly all cases of revision fusion and are mandatory in all cases of spinal deformity. Spinopelvic parameters should also be measured, and surgical planning should be completed with consideration of age-appropriate alignment correction.
  - If iatrogenic injury to the pars interarticularis is suspected, oblique views of the lumbar spine can be useful, although CT scan is more sensitive for detecting pars fracture.
- Flexion–extension lateral views of the lumbar spine can be used to evaluate for segmental instability.
- Most patients who have persistent back pain or leg pain after lumbar surgery will have a magnetic resonance imaging (MRI) of their lumbar spine.
  - In patients with a suspected recurrence of a disc herniation, depending on the acuteness of the reherniation, it is important to distinguish between recurrence and scar, as the former is more responsive to surgery. A precontrast and postcontrast (gadolinium) MRI is helpful to distinguish scar from recurrent disc herniation. Disc material is avascular and will not enhance after gadolinium administration, whereas scar will.

- There are times when an MRI may be of little clinical value or cannot be obtained and a combined myelogram/CT scan study may be necessary.
  - For example, in patients with older stainless steel implants, MRI is generally not useful because significant metal artifact will obscure detail.
  - Although distortion with titanium implants is less of an issue, it can occur on occasion. For both instances, a myelogram/CT scan can be used to identify neural compression.
  - Patients who have an implantable pacemaker or internal defibrillator or who are claustrophobic may not be candidates for MRI and should have a myelogram/CT scan to visualize compressive pathology.
- CT without myelography using coronal and sagittal reconstructions is useful to evaluate hardware placement (especially pedicle screws) and to evaluate an interbody fusion for evidence of pseudarthrosis. Vacuum discs indicate pseudarthrosis and highlight areas for possible deformity correction via anterior realignment.

DIFFERENTIAL DIAGNOSIS

- Incorrect diagnosis
  - Pathology not present at time of original surgery
  - Pathology present but not symptomatic
- Pathology originally present but not adequately addressed
  - Wrong-level surgery
  - Inadequate surgery (pathology incompletely addressed)
- New pathology
  - At same level as prior surgery
    - Recurrent herniated nucleus pulposus
    - Recurrent stenosis
    - Arachnoiditis
    - Epidural scar tissue
    - Iatrogenic instability or deformity
      - Iatrogenic flat back
      - Pars destabilization and resulting spondylolisthesis
    - Hardware failure
      - Hardware breakage or loosening
      - Hardware misplacement
  - At different level
    - Adjacent segment
      - Herniated nucleus pulposus
      - Spondylolisthesis
      - Stenosis
      - Fracture
    - Trauma
    - Other pathology (eg, tumor)
- Complications
  - Infection
    - Discitis
    - Osteomyelitis
    - Superficial or deep wound infection
    - Infection associated with hardware
    - Pseudoarthrosis
    - Durotomy
- Other
  - Noncompressive pathology
    - Nonspinal pathology (eg, neuropathy, hip pathology)

- Psychosocial issues (including chronic pain behavior, opioid dependence, depression, worker's compensation, or litigation)
- Sacroiliac disease or extraspinal joint disease
- Peripheral nerve syndromes

NONOPERATIVE MANAGEMENT

- It is reasonable to try a course of conservative management, similar to that used for the index condition, for recurrent disc herniation or stenosis.
  - Many patients will improve with physical therapy, non-steroidal anti-inflammatory drugs, injection therapy, or other pain management treatments.
- Injections with a local analgesic and steroid may provide relief in patients with sacroiliac disease or other extraspinal joint disease, such as hip arthritis.
  - Spinal epidural injections are unpredictable in the setting of failed back surgery, although they may have a role.
  - Transforaminal injections may be useful as a diagnostic aid in localizing radicular pain to a particular nerve root.
- Patients with multilevel degenerative disease and primary back pain refractory to other treatments may benefit from a multidisciplinary chronic pain management program. These programs typically include pain management specialists, physical therapists, physiatrists, and psychiatrists/psychologists who focus on a physical and cognitive approach to chronic back pain treatment.
- Spinal cord stimulation is an option in patients with persistent and refractory back or leg pain in whom no identifiable cause for the pain can be identified.

SURGICAL MANAGEMENT

Preoperative Planning

- Carefully consider the initial indication for surgery. Operating on the wrong patient or for the wrong indication is a recipe for failure.

- Again, evaluation of the patient's symptoms, physical examination, and radiographic findings will help the surgeon tailor the operative plan most appropriately.
  - It is imperative that the surgeon performs a careful history and physical examination and that imaging findings are correlated with clinical findings.
  - Patients who have predominant back pain and a prior failed fusion surgery may have a pseudarthrosis or another hardware-related problem that might explain the pain.
  - Patients with leg pain as their primary complaint may have neural compression from stenosis or disc herniation.

Positioning

- It is generally important that the patient's abdomen be free of compression to minimize epidural bleeding. There are many options to accomplish this, and the authors prefer a Jackson table (Mizuho OSI, Union City, CA).
  - This table allows the abdomen to hang freely, thereby reducing intra-abdominal pressure and minimizing epidural bleeding. It also facilitates lumbar lordosis (FIG 2A).
- The kneeling position can also be used for simple revision decompressions and discectomies (FIG 2B). It is not advised for multilevel revision fusions as it produces pressure on the knees and may result in iatrogenic flat back.
- Gardner-Wells tongs are recommended for lengthy procedures in order to avoid pressure on the globe and to reduce the likelihood of pressure or abrasions on the patient's face.
- Elevate the head of the bed to reduce facial edema and reduce intraocular pressure.
- Padding of all bony prominences is advised to prevent compressive neuropathies. This included the ulnar nerve at the elbow and the lateral femoral cutaneous nerve at the anterior superior iliac spine.

Approach

- In general, when possible, try to avoid operating through a prior anterior or lateral exposure for revision unless

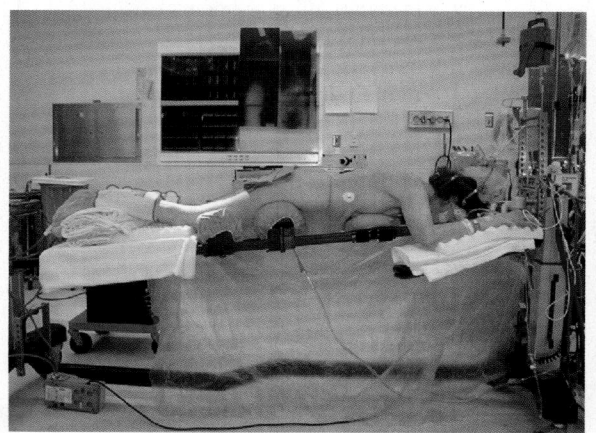 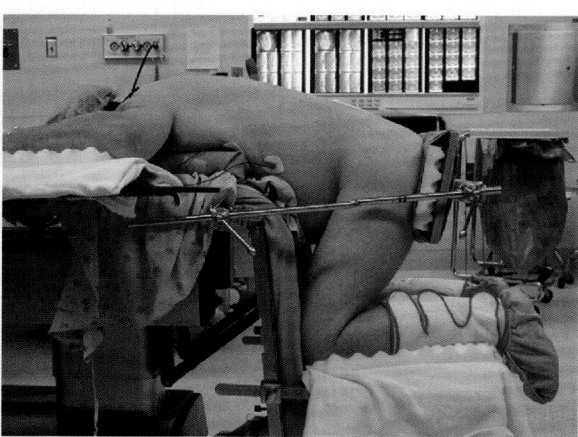

FIG 2 A. The Jackson table allows the patient's abdomen to hang freely below the surgical field, minimizing epidural bleeding and enhancing lumbar lordosis. This position is preferred for lumbar fusion cases to preserve lumbar lordosis during instrumentation. **B.** The abdomen is also allowed to hang freely in the kneeling position. This position is advantageous for revision discectomies or decompressions not requiring instrumentation and fusion, as this position flattens the lumbar spine, distracting the posterior elements and facilitating approach to the disc.

absolutely necessary. The scar tissue from these procedures can make the revision approach difficult and dangerous.

- If an anterior approach is absolutely required, the approach can be made from the opposite side.

- Posterior
  - The posterior approach is popular and most familiar to spine surgeons. Most pathology in patients having had prior surgery can be addressed with this approach. The posterior approach gives the surgeon easy access to the pedicles when instrumentation is needed, permits exposure of the entire lumbar and thoracolumbar spine if needed, and provides adequate access to the intervertebral discs.
  - Bleeding during revision lumbar surgery is typically greater than that of primary surgeries. To some extent, the presence of avascular scar tissue reduces the amount of bleeding (although at times, scar tissue can be considerably vascular). Furthermore, the amount of dissection is generally considerable. To a large extent, the amount of bleeding is directly related to the length of the incision and the length (duration) of the surgery. In many, if not most, posterior revision cases, both are considerable.
    - Careful hemostasis is necessary. This can be facilitated by the use of electrocautery such as the Aquamantys (Medtronic, Portsmouth, NH), which is a hemostatic device that uses a combination of radiofrequency and saline to reduce blood loss.
    - Additional blood conservation can be achieved by the use of cell salvage in which intraoperative blood loss is given back to the patient.
    - Preoperative and intraoperative antifibrinolytic agents such as tranexamic acid and Amicar are also effective at decreasing blood loss.

- Anterior or lateral
  - Anterior or lateral procedures can be used to augment a posterior procedure in order to increase fusion rates. They can also be useful to treat a pseudarthrosis following a posterior fusion by providing direct access to the disc through an unoperated tissue plane. In addition, these approaches enable a more thorough removal of disc material and facilitate placement of a large graft to increase the likelihood of achieving fusion. This avoids the potential difficulty of trying to achieve a posterior fusion in the presence of a previously operated and scarred posterior fusion site.
  - Anterior lumbar interbody fusion (ALIF) is also a useful technique for spinal realignment in cases of positive sagittal balance even in the presence of posterior instrumentation by overpowering the existing construct.
  - The anterior or lateral approach may also be used in unusual situations such as to address an anteriorly extruded intervertebral graft or cage.
  - A major disadvantage of lateral and anterior approaches is that they generally provide a more limited exposure to the lumbar spine. Hence, they are often reserved for focal revision lumbar surgery when the initial approach was posterior. Additionally, particularly for an anterior approach, one might also require an approach surgeon for the exposure.
- Minimally invasive techniques
  - Minimally invasive techniques are an option for select patients.
  - This may include obese patients with a recurrent disc herniation or a new herniation at a different level.
  - It is generally not advisable to perform a minimally invasive surgery in a patient requiring extensive reconstruction and instrumentation for deformity or pseudarthrosis, although exceptions do exist and are often related to surgeon comfort and experience with such techniques.

POSTERIOR APPROACH: LAMINECTOMY AND DISCECTOMY

Positioning

- After induction of anesthesia and intubation, the patient is positioned with the abdomen hanging freely, either prone on a Jackson table or on another frame that eliminates abdominal compression such as a Wilson frame or a four-poster frame.
  - A Wilson frame offers the advantage of reducing lumbar lordosis and distracting the posterior elements, thereby facilitating the approach to the intervertebral discs.
  - Alternatively, the patient may be placed in the kneeling position.
  - For lengthy cases, it is recommended that the patient be placed on a Jackson table with the head placed in Gardner-Wells tongs with 10 to 15 lb of traction. It is imperative that all extremities and bony prominences are carefully padded.

Exposure

- The preoperative films should be studied to provide optimal exposure.
  - Generally, the surgeon will be going through the same incision as the previous surgery.
  - However, the normal bony landmarks may be significantly distorted or absent. In cases in which the posterior bony

elements have been completely removed, the surgeon may choose to lengthen the incision proximally or distally to include adjacent normal bony landmarks as a reference.
  - It is generally safer to proceed from normal anatomy to abnormal (previously operated) levels.
- The incision is deepened, identifying any remnants of normal anatomy that may be present such as the spinous processes, laminae, and facet joints. Care must be taken to avoid injury to the dura, which may be unprotected if a prior laminectomy has been performed.
- In many revision surgeries, there will be significant scar tissue present, which may be firm and adherent to surrounding structures (including the dura).
- In general, dissection should be carried out laterally along the bony wall of the canal rather than diffusely in the midline because the area of interest is the nerve root. Separation of the lateral edge of the dural sac and nerve root is facilitated by the use of either a no. 1 Penfield or a small curette.
  - Care must be taken not to carry the dissection too far laterally so as to avoid inadvertent injury to the pars. Some surgeons prefer to identify the lateral extent of the pars in order to visualize it, thereby minimizing the risk of injury to it.

- The nerve should be followed along its entire course, including the lateral recess and neural foramen, if necessary.

Decompression

- As with nonrevision surgery, the key to proper orientation is identifying the pedicle because the nerve passes beneath it.

This is more important in revisions because other landmarks are often absent.

- At the end of the decompression, the nerve should be relatively easily retractable medially, and a probe should be able to be passed dorsally and ventrally to the nerve root. The pedicles can be palpated with a Woodson.

POSTERIOR APPROACH: FUSION AND INSTRUMENTATION

Positioning

- The patient is positioned prone on a Jackson table. Pressure points are padded, and care is taken to ensure that the chest pad is not compressing breast tissue in female patients.
- Standard Jackson table attachments (iliac and thigh pads) are used to allow maximum natural lumbar lordosis and allow the abdomen to hang freely.

Exposure

- Regions of normal anatomy, such as preexisting spinous processes that were not removed during the initial surgery, are an excellent starting point for dissection. The amount, if any, of any such remaining bone varies depending on the type and extent of the previous surgery.
- Because implanted hardware provides an excellent known landmark for exposure, it is generally useful to initially identify and expose laterally placed hardware.
- After the dissection is carried through the deep fascial layer, the dissection should be skived (angled) laterally

toward the hardware rather than plunging deeply toward the unprotected dura.
- This will bring the dissection down to the rods and screw heads.
- Once the screw heads are exposed, the facets are easily identified (TECH FIG 1).
- Care should be taken to avoid inadvertent injury to facet joints proximal and distal to the existing fusion unless they are to be included in an extension of the fusion. Once the hardware is visualized, the lateral edge of the bony canal is easily identified. From here, dissection can be carried out medially.
- Attention is first turned to separating the scar and pseudomembrane from the lateral bony canal. There is generally little to be gained by trying to remove scar from the midline dura and such attempts may lead to inadvertent durotomy.

Screw and Rod Replacement

- Once the hardware is exposed, the next step is to remove the screws and rods. Corresponding screw widths and lengths should be recorded at each level.

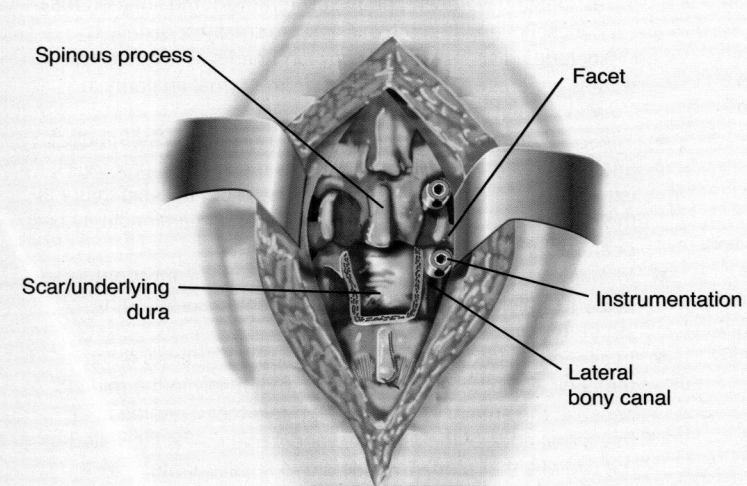

Spinous process

Facet

Scar/underlying dura

Instrumentation

Lateral bony canal

TECH FIG 1 When performing revision exposure, the safest strategy is to proceed from normal anatomy above or below and from lateral to medial, identifying the edges of the prior laminectomy from known to unknown.

- The preexisting posterior fusion mass is then exposed, noting any evidence of pseudarthrosis.
  - Fibrous tissue within the pseudarthrosis is removed using curettes in order to preserve the intact fusion mass as much as possible.
- Preexisting holes that contained the pedicle screws are probed to check integrity and length of the hole measured.
  - When possible, it is recommended that a slightly longer and wider diameter screw be used for the revision hardware.
  - If larger diameter screws are not available, additional augmentation may be provided by the application of polymethylmethacrylate bone cement, especially in osteoporotic patients.
- If broken screws are encountered, several solutions are possible.
  - If the broken screw is in the middle of a construct, that level can usually be skipped, and a cross-connector can be added to provide additional stability.
  - If the broken screw is at the terminal end of a construct, the instrumentation may be extended at a level below or above the involved level, if feasible.
  - If it is thought that instrumentation at the level of the broken screw is necessary, the screw can be removed using a removal kit or by removing additional bone to expose the broken screw. The latter may necessitate additional augmentation with cement (**TECH FIG 2**).
- Fusion mass may be augmented by the use of autologous iliac crest bone graft, by local bone from laminectomy if available, by graft extenders such as demineralized bone matrix, or by the off-label use of bone morphogenetic protein (BMP).

Transforaminal Lumbar Interbody Fusion

- Pseudarthrosis after a posterolateral instrumented fusion is often most optimally treated by the addition of an interbody fusion through nonoperated and therefore unscarred tissue. This provides a healthy focus for fusion.
- When a posterior approach is being used, this is most efficiently achieved through a transforaminal lumbar interbody fusion (TLIF).
  - A TLIF may not be advisable or possible in the presence of significant scar from prior surgery. But if scarring is minimal,

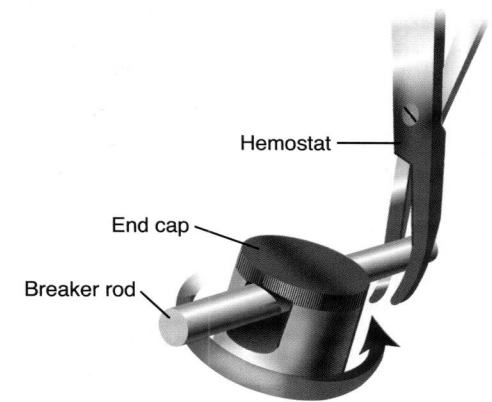

Hemostat

End cap

Breaker rod

TECH FIG 2 Salvage technique for saw removal.

a TLIF provides a safe and effective way to achieve additional anterior column support to facilitate fusion.
- This is achieved by a unilateral (or if desired, bilateral) facetectomy with a pedicle-to-pedicle exposure, thereby unroofing the neural foramen entirely and allowing the root and thecal sac to be gently retracted medially.
- The intervertebral disc is then sharply incised with a scalpel, and the disc is removed piecemeal using curettes and pituitary rongeurs.
- The cartilaginous endplates are then removed by using a special set of dilators and scrapers.
- Once cartilage has been removed from the bony endplates, spacers are used to estimate proper graft size. An interbody graft or synthetic cage (usually a polyetheretherketone or PEEK) is then filled with autologous bone, allograft bone, and/or a collagen sponge soaked in BMP used in an off-label manner and placed in the disc space.
- Placement is verified using x-ray, and the interbody graft or cage is locked into place by compressing across the previously placed pedicle screws and rods.

ANTERIOR APPROACH

- ALIF, when feasible, provides excellent exposure to the intervertebral disc and allows the surgeon maximal access to the disc space. It is a good adjunct to a posterior fusion, especially in the presence of a pseudarthrosis after posterolateral instrumented fusion.
- The ALIF allows access to disc spaces that may be difficult to access posteriorly because of scar. It also allows for the placement of larger grafts that cannot be inserted through a TLIF approach; this maximizes endplate contact with the graft

and increases the chances of fusion and decreases the risk of subsidence.[5]
- A standard anterior retroperitoneal approach to the lumbar spine is used.
- Revision anterior procedures in patients with previous anterior lumbar surgery can be difficult and dangerous due to significant scarring. The risk of vascular injury is significant, and exposure by an experienced vascular surgeon is recommended.

ANTEROLATERAL RETROPERITONEAL APPROACH

- This approach is beneficial to address interbody pathology that is not otherwise accessible from a purely anterior or posterior approach.
- The patient is placed on a standard operating room table in a right lateral decubitus position. The hip is positioned behind the table break so as to create separation between the ribcage and the iliac crest.
- This position can treat pathology from L3 to L5. If L2 exposure is needed, it will likely be necessary to resect the 12th rib.
- In certain circumstances, it may be advantageous to approach from the right side, but in general, avoidance of the inferior vena cava and the liver via the right lateral decubitus position is favorable.
- The patient is secured to the table with tape. The left arm is suspended in an arm sling and padded and secured to the sling with tape.
- Fluoroscopy is used to demarcate the level of pathology. This general area is marked on the skin to plan the incision.
- A curvilinear incision is planned beginning in front and superior to the iliac crest, curving under the 12th rib and following this rib to the insertion on the spine.

- Once the incision is made, the subcutaneous tissue is retracted, and the first muscle that is visible will be the latissimus dorsi. This muscle is sharply divided and retracted.
- The next layer will be the posterior inferior serratus muscle and the internal and external oblique muscles. These muscles are also divided sharply by using Bovie cautery. Care must be taken not to violate the peritoneum directly below these muscles.
- The peritoneal layer is retracted anteriorly while the ureter and the kidney are retracted to the right, bringing into view the quadratus lumborum. The 12th rib is also identified and may be resected if higher approaches are to be attempted. The neurovascular bundle should be preserved; if this is not possible, it can be tied off and divided.
- The retroperitoneal tissue overlying the lumbar spine is bluntly dissected and brought anteriorly.
  - Care is taken to preserve the ilioinguinal and iliohypogastric nerves that will run between the quadratus lumborum and the psoas muscle.
- Once this is performed, the lateral surfaces of the lumbar vertebrae are brought into view.

TECHNIQUES

Pearls and Pitfalls

Diagnostic Pitfalls	• Account for proper pathology. • Double check surgical indications. • Take into account other pathology (vascular, joints, etc.). • Back pain versus radiculopathy recurrence: Back pain is much less amenable to reoperation than radiculopathy.
Surgical Planning Pitfalls	• Obtain proper imaging studies. Pre- and postgadolinium MRI should be performed on patients evaluated for recurrent disc pathology or stenosis. If there is a question of global imbalance or deformity, obtain standing 3-foot x-rays. • Select correct procedure. • Examine all old medical records. • Ensure proper operating room tools are available (eg, a universal driver set for removing hardware). • Prepare the iliac crest in every patient for possible use.
Surgical Technique Pitfalls	• Properly position the patient. Elevate the head of the bed and ensure the abdomen hangs free in the prone position to minimize epidural bleeding. Use a head holder with pins if prolonged surgery is planned. • Address neural compression. • Pay attention to overall alignment. Standing x-rays can help the surgeon evaluate this. • Start at known and work toward the unknown. • No central scar tissue removal, stay lateral where there is bone present, and work toward the midline. • Ensure adequate lateral recess decompression.

POSTOPERATIVE CARE

- Standard postoperative care of spine surgery patients is indicated in most patients undergoing revision surgery.
- Pain control can be a significant issue in patients undergoing revision lumbar surgery. These patients often have substantial preoperative narcotic requirements making postoperative pain control difficult.
  - When possible, the use of an epidural pain catheter can be considered. This may not always be possible if there is significant epidural scar tissue present, making the passage of the catheter difficult.

- Another option for pain control is patient-controlled analgesia, in which the patient controls, within certain predetermined limits, the amount of narcotic analgesic delivered.
- If the surgery was lengthy (6 hours or more) and required significant amounts of blood products and fluids, it may be advantageous to leave the patient intubated overnight and admitted to an intensive care unit.
  - Reasons for prolonged postoperative intubation are often related to the amount of facial and airway swelling present. The use of the Jackson table with Gardner-Wells

tongs and head of bed elevation can reduce facial and airway edema, making it more likely that the patient can be extubated in the operating room.
- Multilevel revision surgery or extensive front–back procedures can usually require an admission to intensive care.
- Standard neurologic checks in the immediate postoperative period are performed to assess for neural recovery or new deficits.
- Upright x-rays are obtained in patients with hardware placement. These are usually performed within a few days of surgery or as soon as the patient is able to comfortably stand for the x-rays. These must be assessed for early junctional failure prior to discharge.

OUTCOMES

- Patient outcomes depend largely on the initial patient diagnosis. There is a wide variety of pathology that a patient can present with after lumbar surgery, and the surgeon must carefully assess all of the information at hand to make the most informed decision.
- The patient with recurrent leg pain or leg pain in a different distribution than before the initial surgery has a good chance of benefitting from a second operation.[9] Recurrent leg pain in the same distribution as preoperative suggests reherniation of the same disc, whereas new leg pain may represent a different disc herniation.
- The patient with predominant axial back pain (and normal sagittal and coronal alignment), however, will most likely not benefit from another operation. In these patients, it is very difficult for the surgeon to pinpoint the source of the back pain.

COMPLICATIONS

- Neural injury is one of the most feared complications of revision surgery. To a large extent, the magnitude of this risk is dictated by the distortion of the normal anatomy and by the presence of scar tissue. Careful adherence to the principles outlined in this chapter will help reduce this risk.
- Durotomy is a relatively common occurrence in revision lumbar surgery as the dura is often adherent to and obscured by the overlying scar and pseudomembrane.
  - When a durotomy is encountered, it should be repaired immediately, if possible. Failure to repair a durotomy promptly can result in the loss of thecal sac turgor and the tamponade effect that a turgid sac produces on the epidural veins. This can result in more blood loss and more difficulty with repair of the durotomy.
  - If the overlying scar is thick enough, it may be included in the suture line. If not, work to expose the free edges of the dura and close primarily.

- A patch of muscle or fascia may be sewn under the suture line to attempt to tightly appose the defect. An absorbable hemostatic agent such as Surgicel (Ethicon, Menlo Park, CA) and/or fibrin glue may be used to cover the suture line as well.
- Infection is always possible after revision surgery. It should be treated in the standard manner that all spine postoperative infections are treated: antibiotics and surgical débridement and washout if the wound is frankly purulent and draining.
  - With an initial infection following an instrumented fusion, it is generally recommended that the instrumentation be kept in place if it is providing stability. This requires a period of parenteral antibiotics often followed by a prolonged period of oral antibiotics, with some infectious disease consultants recommending that oral antibiotics be continued indefinitely as long as the hardware is present. In general, the initial surgical débridement is accompanied by wound closure.
  - If a subsequent episode of infection occurs, use of vacuum dressing may be required with delayed wound closure.
- Pseudarthrosis may occur following an initial surgery or revision surgery. Smokers have a higher risk of pseudarthrosis than nonsmokers. Consequently, patients should be counseled to stop smoking preoperatively and refrain from smoking postoperatively.

REFERENCES

1. Ambrossi GL, McGirt MJ, Sciubba DM, et al. Recurrent lumbar disc herniation after single-level lumbar discectomy: incidence and health care cost analysis. Neurosurgery 2009;65(3):574–578.
2. Cinotti G, Roysam GS, Eisenstein SM, et al. Ipsilateral recurrent lumbar disc herniation. A prospective, controlled study. J Bone Joint Surg Br 1998;80(5):825–832.
3. Diwan AD, Parvartaneni H, Cammisa F. Failed degenerative lumbar spine surgery. Orthop Clin North Am 2003;34(2):309–324.
4. Jönsson B, Strömqvist B. Repeat decompression of lumbar nerve roots. A prospective two-year evaluation. J Bone Joint Surg Br 1993;75(6):894–897.
5. Lee S-H, Kang B-U, Jeon SH, et al. Revision surgery of the lumbar spine: anterior lumbar interbody fusion followed by percutaneous pedicle screw fixation. J Neurosurg Spine 2006;5(3):228–233.
6. Malter AD, McNeney B, Loeser JD, et al. 5-year reoperation rates after different types of lumbar spine surgery. Spine (Phila Pa 1976) 1998;23(7):814–820.
7. Onesti ST. Failed back syndrome. Neurologist 2004;10:259–264.
8. Trief PM, Grant W, Fredrickson B. A prospective study of psychological predictors of lumbar surgery outcome. Spine (Phila Pa 1976) 2000;25(20):2616–2621.
9. Waddell G, Kummel EG, Lotto WN, et al. Failed lumbar disc surgery and repeat surgery following industrial injuries. J Bone Joint Surg Am 1979;61(2):201–207.

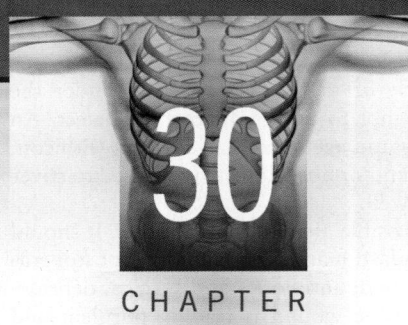

30

CHAPTER

Revision Cervical Surgery

Yoshihiro Katsuura and Todd J. Albert

DEFINITION

- Cervical spine surgery is used to treat a number of common spinal pathologies including the following:
  - Cervical spinal stenosis
  - Deformity
  - Disc herniation
  - Myelopathy
  - Trauma
  - Pathologic conditions such as neoplasia, infection, and metabolic and inflammatory disease
- Revision cervical surgery may be required to treat the complications of prior operations, progression of the primary cervical pathology, or unexpected sequelae of life events such as trauma or malignancy. The more common complications and conditions are covered in this chapter.
  - Pseudarthrosis is a failure of bone fusion at the site of attempted arthrodesis (ie, a "false joint" or nonunion). The diagnosis is typically made anywhere from 6 months to 2 years following the index surgery. Pseudarthrosis may occur following anterior or posterior cervical procedures.
  - Adjacent segment degeneration (ASD) occurs when there are spondylotic changes at unfused levels proximal or distal to prior cervical fusion. Some controversy exists whether the degeneration occurs secondary to compensation from a prior arthrodesis or as a result of natural progression in an individual already prone to degenerative disc disease.
  - Postlaminectomy kyphosis (PLK) is a deformity of the cervical spine that develops as a result of resection or damage to the posterior tension band composed of the spinous process, lamina, supraspinous and interspinous ligaments, and muscle.
  - Hardware/construct failure: Plates, screws, and rods may loosen or break if bone healing at the fusion site fails or is prolonged. Structural grafts used to support of the spine may collapse or subside as a result of poor bone quality or surgical technique. Moreover, modern disc arthroplasty devices may also fail and require revision.
  - Same segment disease/residual compression is persistent or recurrent pain that is present at the level of previous decompression. Same segment disease results from failed stabilization or inadequate decompression at the site of the initial cervical procedure.
  - Pathologic conditions may be the inciting event for the index surgical procedure or may occur after and result in

the need for revision surgery. Tumor, infection, trauma, and inflammatory conditions such as rheumatoid arthritis and ankylosis spondylitis may lead to instability, deformity, or neurocompression after an index cervical procedure.

ANATOMY

- Vertebrae
  - The cervical spine consists of seven specialized vertebrae.
    - C1 is ringed shaped with two large lateral masses and is unique in that it has no vertebral body.
    - C2 has a caudal projection at the vertebral body known as the *dens* or *odontoid process*, which articulates with C1.
    - C3–C6 are all composed of a vertebral body, which is connected to two lateral masses via small pedicles. Each lateral vertebral body is flanked by two uncinate processes cranially.
    - C7 is a transitional vertebrae more closely resembles a thoracic vertebrae with larger pedicles and thinner lateral masses than the cranial cervical vertebrae.
  - Transverse foramina are present bilaterally for the passage of the vertebral artery.
  - The vertebral artery generally enters the cervical spine at C6 in 95% of cases. Occasionally, it will enter at C7 or C5. The artery may also enter the spine at different levels on either side of the cervical spine in the same patient. Magnetic resonance imaging (MRI) should be obtained prior to surgical intervention to ascertain the site of vertebral artery entry and any anomalies present along its excursion (FIG 1).
  - The spinous processes of C6–C2 are bifid. The C7 spinous process is not bifid and is more prominent than the others and thus referred to as *vertebra prominens*.
- Discs
  - An intervertebral disc is present between each of the cervical vertebrae from C2 through T1.
  - The occiput to C1 and the C1–C2 articulation do not have intervertebral discs and articulate through true synovial joints.
  - Each disc consists of an outer annulus fibrosus and inner nucleus pulposus. However, cervical discs differ from lumbar discs as they lack a continuous annular fibrosis.
  - A cartilaginous endplate exits between the annulus fibrosus/nucleus pulposus complex and the vertebral body. The removal of this cartilaginous endplate is crucial to a successful interbody arthrodesis.

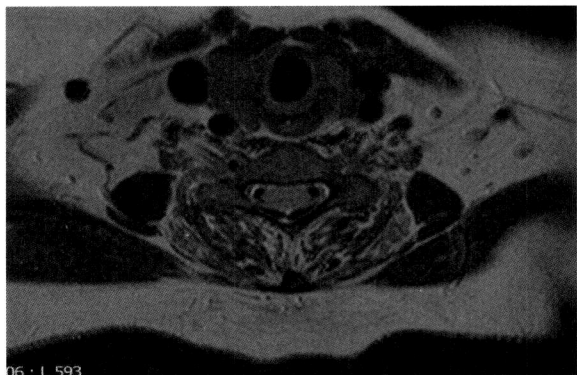 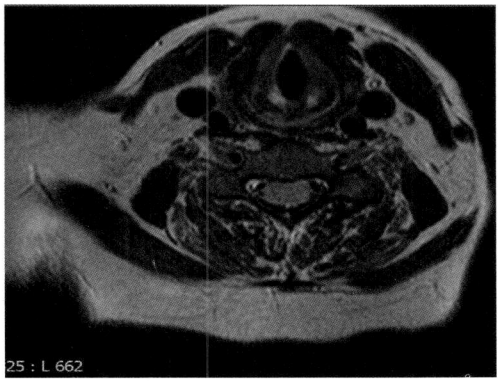

FIG 1 A. Axial T2-weighted image through the C6 vertebral body. Note in this patient that the vertebral artery is anomalous, and only the right-sided artery enters the spine at this level. **B.** Axial T2-weighted image through the C5 vertebral body in the same patient as **FIG 1A**. At this level, both right and left vertebral arteries have entered the cervical spine.

- Ligaments
  - A supraspinous ligament runs dorsally over the top of the spinous processes.
  - An interspinous ligament is present between spinous processes at each level.
  - The anterior longitudinal ligament runs along the front of the spine adherent to the ventral aspect of the vertebral body.
  - The posterior longitudinal ligament (PLL) runs along the dorsal aspect of the vertebral body and intervertebral discs. It forms a barrier between the discs and the dura/spinal cord.
- There is a large range of what can be considered normal lordosis of the cervical spine (4.89 to 14.4 degrees).[25,59]
- Unlike the lumbar spine, the weight-bearing axis of the cervical spine passes through the posterior neural arch and articular processes).[34,38]
- Loss of the posterior tension band, particularly the insertion of the semispinalis cervicis muscle after resection of the lamina and spinous processes may lead to kyphosis and an anterior shift in the weight-bearing axis.

PATHOGENESIS

- Pseudarthrosis
  - Pseudarthrosis occurs when bone fails to fuse at the site of attempted arthrodesis. Multiple factors may play a role in the formation of pseudarthrosis. It has been reported to occur at a rate of 2.9% to 44% in cervical surgery.
  - Risk factors include the following[60]:
    - Excessive motion at arthrodesis site cause by use of interbody alone without plate[12]
    - Use of allograft rather than autograft[43]
    - Multilevel fusions[4,10]
    - Metabolic abnormalities
    - Smoking[15]
    - Infection
    - Patient factors: chronic steroid use, malnutrition, obesity, osteoporosis
    - Specific radiographic parameters: excessive motion (>12 degrees segmental motion) and higher preoperative T1 slope[6]
    - Specific segments: typically, the most caudal segment of the construct (especially the C6–C7 level)[38]

- Excessive motion at the surgical site following an anterior cervical discectomy and fusion is associated with increased rates of pseudarthrosis. Use of anterior cervical plating has been shown in multiple studies to decrease the rate of pseudarthrosis.[7,54]
- Interestingly, uncinate resection for complete foraminotomy has been shown to not affect the pseudoarthrosis rates.[24,37]
- ASD
  - As previously noted, some controversy exists whether the degeneration of adjacent segments occurs as a result of prior arthrodesis, which may place increased demands on a level above or below a fusion, or whether the degeneration is a result of natural progression in an individual already prone to degenerative disc disease.
  - Eck et al[9] measured cadaveric disc pressures at C4–C5 and C6–C7 before and after simulated fusion at C5–C6 and found a 73% increase in cranial and 45% in caudal disc pressures during flexion.
  - In vitro studies have failed to show changes in segmental motion adjacent to a fused cervical level.[36,37,39] However, alteration in the sagittal configuration of the cervical spine has been associated with ASD.
  - Moreover, a plate to disc distance <5 mm has been implanted in increased ossification of the adjacent disc.
- Deformity (PLK)
  - Causes of PLK include the following:
    - Damage to the posterior restraints of the cervical spine (neural bony arch, the supraspinous and interspinous ligaments or the extensor musculature) increases the risk of PLK particularly in those with preexisting kyphotic alignment. Resection of greater than 50% of the facet has also been shown to lead to instability.[32]
    - Younger patients (<30 years) are typically more at risk for this complication than older patients.
    - The risks of PLK as summarized by Lonstein[28] are as follows:
      - Age younger than 30 years
      - Aggressive facetectomy
      - Removal of more than four laminae
      - Preoperative deformity
      - Removal of C2 posterior elements (major semispinalis insertion)
      - Paraspinal muscle weakness
      - Anterior instability following fracture

- Kyphosis causes the weight-bearing axis of the spine to shift anteriorly resulting in extensor musculature fatigue and progression of the deformity.[1]
- The load from the skull, typically born mostly by the posterior elements, is then transferred to the anterior vertebral bodies and discs which in animal models has been shown to accelerate endplate chondrocyte apoptosis.[20] Thus, kyphosis can result in decreasing disc height and endplate degeneration with increased deformity.
- As a kyphotic deformity worsens, the spinal cord may lengthen, impairing microcirculation, and result in worsening myelopathy.
- Nowinski et al[32] studied the effects of progressive facetectomy and recommend posterior fusion when over 25% of the facets are sacrificed for decompression.
- Of note, the term *postlaminectomy kyphosis* must be differentiated from *dropped head syndrome*, where a neuromuscular disease (myasthenia gravis, amyotrophic lateral sclerosis, or multiple systems atrophy) results in weakness of the cervical paraspinal extensor musculature.[45]
- Hardware/construct failure[29,30]
  - Hardware-related complications following ACDF have been characterized in 22% to 36% of cases.[23]
  - Screw breakage or loosening is often the result of a nonunion or pseudarthrosis.
  - Infection, osteoporosis, tumor, and trauma can also lead to hardware failure or graft subsidence after cervical fusion with or without instrumentation.
  - The use of multilevel interbody fusion versus corpectomies with strut grafting has been shown to decrease the risk of graft extrusion.
  - Dynamic plates have also been shown to have lower rates of hardware failure compared to static plates in ACDF surgery.
- Same segment disease/residual compression
  - Same segment disease results from failed stabilization or inadequate initial surgical decompression
  - Truumees and McLain[55] outline four general causes for residual compression after cervical surgery:
    - Failure to perform a complete decompression at the injured/involved level
    - Failure to decompress adjacent involved levels
    - Migration of graft or fixation materials into the canal or foramen
    - Wrong-level surgery (initial surgery performed at a level that was not responsible for the patient's symptoms)
    - Moreover, residual neck pain is common in patients incorrectly treated with motion preserving procedures such as laminoplasty, cervical foraminotomy, and disc arthroplasty.
- Pathologic conditions
  - The pathogenesis of tumor, infection, and inflammatory conditions such as rheumatoid arthritis and ankylosis spondylitis is beyond the scope of the current text. Failure of the cervical spine as it relates to these conditions is a progressive deterioration of the structural integrity of the bones or erosion of the ligamentous support of the spine. Loss of these structures leads to instability, deformity, or compression of the neural elements.

NATURAL HISTORY

- Pseudarthrosis
  - The most common cause of pain or radiculopathy after ACDF is pseudarthrosis.[46,56]
  - The diagnosis of cervical pseudoarthrosis is made difficult by the high rate of patients who are asymptomatic and the lack of a diagnostic test with high sensitivity and specificity.[26]
  - Lowery et al[30] defined pseudarthrosis as follows:
    - Continued or worsening axial/mechanical pain 6 months after the initial procedure
    - Complete radiolucency at the host–graft interface
    - Vertebral body motion greater than 2 mm on flexion and extension films
  - Phillips et al[38] followed a large series of patients with radiographic pseudarthrosis:
    - Sixty-seven percent developed symptoms.
    - A younger age was associated with a pseudoarthrosis becoming symptomatic.
    - Sixteen patients remained asymptomatic for 5.1 years.
    - Twenty-eight percent of symptomatic patients were pain free for 2 years before trauma caused development of symptoms.
    - Eighty-two percent of patients developed pseudarthrosis at the most caudal level after multilevel fusion.
    - Revision surgery led to good or excellent results in all cases (anterior or posterior).
  - In a later study, Lee et al[24] studied the fate of pseudoarthroses detected at 1 year and found that by 2 years, 70% had gone onto fusion independently. However, 40% of three level fusions persisted at 3 years.[24] Thus, the authors suggested that a definitive diagnosis of pseudoarthrosis could not be made until 2 years; however, revision surgery could be considered for those with refractory neck pain or multilevel ACDF patients.
  - Posterior fusion with lateral mass screws leads to high rate of fusion from 100% to 98.6%.
- ASD
  - Radiographic ASD occurs at a rate of 25% at an average of 2.9 years.[2]
  - Symptomatic ASD occurs at a rate of 2.9% per year, with 25% of patients developing ASD within 10 years.[14]
  - Patients with degenerative changes at C5–C6 or C6–C7 at time of initial procedure are at greatest risk for development of ASD.
- Deformity (PLK)
  - Lonstein[28] described PLK as a focal, dramatic angulation of the cervical spine after posterior decompression.
  - Patients with PLK generally have a pain-free period following the index surgical procedure followed by the development of persistent pain with decompensation of the head.
  - As the deformity worsens, myelopathic symptoms may increase as well as symptomatic muscle spasm and neck pain.
  - Patients will have increasing difficulty holding the head upright and maintaining horizontal gaze.
- Hardware/construct failure
  - When failure occurs, the risk of injury to the tracheoesophageal structures is generally low.[29]

- Immediate removal of failed hardware is typically unnecessary and should only be considered if there is evidence of dysphagia or risk to the spinal cord or nerve roots.
- Careful and long-term follow-up in patient with loose or broken hardware assures that it does not progress.
- Same segment disease/residual compression
  - Posterior osteophytes may be a significant source of residual compression and have limited remodeling potential after ACDF.[51,55,58]
  - Kozak et al[21] has advocated PLL resection to achieve a more complete decompression and decrease the likelihood of residual symptoms.
  - Decompression of the neural elements may be needed at the time of surgery for cervical trauma to decrease the potential for the later development of stenosis.[41]
  - Neck pain resulting from motion preservation operations as noted earlier may best be treated with fusion surgery.
- Pathologic conditions: tumor, infection, and inflammatory arthropathies
  - The natural history of the pathologic condition affecting the postsurgical cervical spine is highly dependent on the individual entity.
  - In general, nonoperative treatment is rarely indicated for fractures and hardware complications in the face of trauma, infection, or tumor. Such conditions should be dealt with promptly with appropriate stabilization procedures.
  - Infection of the cervical spine typically begins as a spondylodiscitis causing destruction of the intervertebral disc, which can then spread to the vertebral bodies causing collapse and kyphosis.
  - Metastatic lesions of the cervical spine typically start in the vertebral body and cause progressive destruction and instability.
  - Inflammatory arthropathies may cause progressive deformity despite previous surgery leading to kyphosis, atlantoaxial subluxation, cranial settling, and subaxial subluxation.

PATIENT HISTORY AND PHYSICAL FINDINGS

- Symptomatic patients with prior cervical surgery typically present with single or multiple complaints of axial neck pain, radiculopathy, myelopathy, or progressive deformity. A general neurologic history should be performed in addition to specifics regarding the prior surgery.
- The evaluation must include a complete review of all prior cervical procedures, pain-free periods, and trauma.[3,55]
- It is helpful to know whether the current symptoms are similar or different from the symptoms experienced before the initial surgery. Moreover, understanding the timing of the symptoms is important: Did the original symptoms resolve after their first surgery? If so, for how long?
- Ask about any complications following surgery.
- If possible, obtain preoperative imaging and medical records to fully understand the nature and indication for the primary surgery.
  - It is also helpful to examine the surgical report to learn the type of instrumentation used if any for planning a revision.

- Physical examination
  - A general examination including posture and range of motion (ROM) of the head and neck should be performed. If the head is dropped in kyphosis, the examiner should determine if the deformity flexible or rigid by having the patient lay supine.
  - A complete motor and sensory examination is essential for correct diagnosis of the offending cervical level.
  - Evaluate the reflexes including the biceps (C5), brachioradialis (C6), and triceps (C7). Note that normal reflexes diminish with age, and an elderly patient with normal reflexes may in fact be hyperreflexic.
  - Evaluate for signs of myelopathy; include Hoffman sign, dysdiadochokinesia, inverted radial reflex, and the ulnar escape test. In the lower extremities, signs of myelopathy include clonus, an upgoing Babinski reflex, or a wide-based gait.
  - Finally, rule out other potential causes of upper extremity dysfunction, including thoracic outlet syndrome, shoulder impingement/rotator cuff pathology, and/or peripheral nerve compression (cubital tunnel, radial tunnel, carpal tunnel syndromes).
  - Neck and shoulder pathology commonly overlap. A patient with failed cervical surgery and persistent neck pain should have a careful examination of the shoulder to rule out referred pain.[18]

IMAGING AND OTHER DIAGNOSTIC STUDIES

- Plain radiographs, including anteroposterior, lateral, flexion, and extension views of the cervical spine should be obtained as part of the initial evaluation.
  - Evaluation of plain radiographs allows for comparison with prior studies to determine if there is deformity, hardware failure, graft subsidence, or spondylosis.
  - In the case of deformity or PLK, there are several radiographic parameters which should be measured.
    - Cervical lordosis: measured as the Cobb angle between the inferior endplate of C2 and C7. Normal value is 12.2 degrees.[17]
    - C2–C7 sagittal vertical axis (SVA): distance from a C2 plumb line to the posterior superior corner of C7. Normal value is 21.3 mm.
    - Chin–brow vertical angle: measured by taking the angle between a line connecting the chin and the brow and a vertical line from the brow. This is a measure of horizontal gaze. This is typically measured from full body EOS® x-rays. Normal value is 1.7 degrees.
  - Flexion/extension view allows for evaluation of motion at a level suspected of pseudarthrosis or ASD.
  - For detecting pseudoarthrosis, Song et al[48] popularized the interspinous method where the lateral dynamic x-rays viewed at 150% magnification are examined for ≥1 mm interspinous motion with ≥4 mm superior (nonfused segment) to confirm adequate effort. This method has a sensitivity and specificity of 86% and 96%, respectively.
  - In the case of spinal deformity, flexion/extension views provide information with respect to the reducibility of the cervical deformity to return to normal lordosis.

- Oblique views of the cervical spine allow evaluation of the neural foramina, uncovertebral joint spurring, facet joints, and fusion mass.
- Computed tomography (CT) scans
  - CT scans provide the best overall evaluation of the bony architecture of the cervical spine.
  - CT is the modality of choice for the evaluation of a fusion mass and to rule out pseudarthrosis.
  - Riew et al[40] in a comparison of four measurement techniques (including interspinous motion) showed that the presence of extra graft bridging bone on CT (any bridging bone outside the graft or cage without a transverse lucent line crossing the peripheral margin of the operated disc space) was the most sensitive and specific way of detecting a pseudarthrosis.
  - In the case of PLK, the CT scan should be scrutinized for areas of fusion and ankylosis, which may necessitate an osteotomy type procedure.
  - Myelography of the cervical spine can be used in cases where an MRI scan is contraindicated. It is also useful in revision cervical surgery as instrumentation often obscures MRI imaging.
- MRI
  - MRI is the modality of choice for evaluation of the soft tissues and neural elements and is sensitive to detect edema and any pathologic changes.
  - In cases of revision surgery, intravenous contrast medium is used to distinguish between scar tissue, which enhances with gadolinium, and recurrent disc herniation, which does not enhance as it lacks a blood supply.
  - MRI may be contraindicated in patients with pacemakers, spinal cord stimulators, and some cardiac stents.
- Others modalities: nerve conduction studies/electromyography (EMG), bone scans, and pain blocks
  - Nerve conduction studies and EMG can be used to rule out peripheral nerve compression in cases where a peripheral cause is suspected. EMG can also assist with determination of the offending cervical level in cases where physical examination findings are unclear.
  - Nuclear tests such as bone scans and single-photon emission computed tomography (SPECT) scan can assist in the diagnosis of pseudarthrosis. Both show increased uptake at the site of stress fracture or pseudarthrosis. The SPECT scan provides a better spatial representation of the cervical spine.
  - Selective nerve root blocks can provide therapeutic relief of pain symptoms and are often incorporated into the nonoperative management for recurrent cervical pain and radiculopathy. In addition, selective root blocks can provide diagnostic data in cases with complex pain or sensory distributions.
  - All patients scheduled to undergo a revision anterior procedure should have a referral for fiberoptic laryngoscopy to evaluate the status of the vocal chords. Recurrent laryngeal nerve palsy may be asymptomatic and should be identified to prevent a contralateral palsy, which could result in airway obstruction. As many as 17% to 22% of revision, patients referred for laryngoscopy may be diagnosed with a unilateral vocal ford paralysis.[8,35]

- Laboratory workups including blood counts, chemistries, and inflammatory markers such as erythrocyte sedimentation rate and C-reactive protein should be obtained prior to revision surgery to rule out infection as a potential cause of pain or dysfunction.
  - In the case of pseudoarthrosis, it may be helpful to order specific laboratory tests which may indicate an abnormality in bone metabolism:
    - 25-Hydroxy vitamin D
    - Low urinary calcium
    - Thyroid-stimulating hormone
    - Parathyroid hormone
    - Recently, a low preoperative measurement of urinary-N-telopeptide (a bone turnover marker) has been shown to be a potential predictor of nonunion.[49]
- Physical examination (see Part 9 Spine Exam Table at the end of the book for details)
  - Spurling test
  - Lhermitte phenomenon
  - Hoffman reflex
  - Inverted radial reflex
  - Finger escape sign (ulnar escape sign)
  - Impingement sign
  - Hawkins modified impingement sign
  - Adson test

DIFFERENTIAL DIAGNOSIS

- Discogenic, myofasciocutaneous, and cervical facet joint pain
- ASD
- Deformity (PLK)
- Hardware/construct failure
- Pseudarthrosis
- Recurrent pain from inadequate decompression during initial surgical procedure
- Peripheral neuropathies and pain syndromes that may mimic cervical pathology
  - Thoracic outlet syndrome
  - Parsonage-Turner syndrome
  - Carpal tunnel syndrome
  - Cubital tunnel syndrome
  - Radial tunnel syndrome
  - Wartenberg syndrome
  - Ulnar tunnel syndrome
  - Shoulder impingement/rotator cuff disease

NONOPERATIVE MANAGEMENT

- Surgical outcomes for revision cervical surgery are less predictable than for primary procedures. Every effort should be made to relieve the patient's symptoms with nonoperative measures prior to consideration of revision surgery. Nonetheless, surgery should be considered in cases of progressive neurologic deficit or gait impairment, persistent disabling pain (3 months), and progressive deformity with significant axial or radicular pain.[55]
- Nonoperative modalities
  - Nonsteroidal anti-inflammatory drugs (NSAIDs)
  - Isometric cervical strengthening/physical therapy
  - Selective cervical root injections
  - Epidural steroid injections
  - Pain management clinic
  - Psychological evaluation

SURGICAL MANAGEMENT

- A thorough understanding of the cause of the patient's symptoms is essential for appropriate surgical planning and management.
- Surgical intervention should be considered in patients who have failed a trial of nonoperative intervention and who meet the indication for surgery as described earlier.
- The goals of surgical intervention are the following[42]:
  - Stabilization of unstable segments
  - Decompression of the spinal cord or nerve roots in cases of myelopathy or radiculopathy
  - Correction of spinal deformity: This can be accomplished through an anterior, posterior, or combined approach and must be tailored for each case.
- Pseudarthrosis
  - In cases of symptomatic pseudarthrosis, the goal is to achieve fusion of the failed segment. This can be accomplished through an anterior or posterior approach.
  - Posterior fusion is an excellent alternative to a second anterior attempt at stabilization. Posterior stabilization reinforces the anterior instrumentation and increased the chances for eventual fusion while avoiding the risks of an additional anterior procedure.[11,27]
    - However, the posterior approach is generally unable to correct kyphosis as effectively or correct hardware which may have migrated anteriorly.[54]
  - Posterior revision for pseudarthrosis is generally very successful has a 94% to 100% fusion rate.[22]
  - Anterior revision for pseudarthrosis has less blood loss and shorter hospital stays compared to the posterior approach. However, need for a second revision is 44% in some series.[5]
  - Although some authors support the use of the anterior approach, in Phillips' series, only 86% of anterior revisions went on to union, whereas 100% of posterior revisions went on to union.[7,38,61]
  - Moreover, most recent literature supports the use of the posterior approach. Kuhns et al[22] published a 100% fusion rate with the posterior approach for anterior pseudoarthrosis. In a pooled analysis of fusion results between anterior and posterior approaches, McAnany et al[31] showed the posterior approach demonstrated a significantly greater fusion rate.
- ASD, residual compression **(FIG 2)**
  - ASD is managed with ACDF at the adjacent level.
  - Management of residual compression or recurrent disc herniation is determined by the site of neurologic compromise. A revision ACDF or corpectomy may be required for significant anterior compression. A posterior keyhole foraminotomy can be made to decompress a soft disc herniation.
  - For extension of an anterior fusion to an adjacent level, previous hardware must be removed to allow for extension of the instrumentation. Knowledge of the hardware manufacturer and required tools for removal are essential. Recently, stand-alone interbody devices have been introduced on the market that allow instrumentation at an adjacent level without removal of previous hardware.
  - In the case of a solid fusion mass, the previous ACDF plate may be removed and replaced with a smaller plate spanning the newly symptomatic level. However, fractures of the unprotected fusion mass have been reported.[44]

- Hardware/construct failure
  - Surgical intervention is indicated in hardware failure patients with neurologic compression or soft tissue compromise, instability, or progressive deformity.
  - The approach is determined by the location of the hardware failure (anterior failure is approached anteriorly and vice versa).
  - Hardware failure is often associated with significant inflammatory reaction and care should be taken as this can obscure the surgical approach.
  - In general, revision instrumentation can be replaced at the site of previous failure. If significant instability is present, a combined anterior/posterior stabilization should be considered.
- Revision cervical disc replacement (CDR)
  - Artificial disc replacements were developed to reduce the rate of adjacent segment disease compared to the ACDF procedure. Currently, there are multiple implant designs on the market.
  - Although multiple studies have shown a lower revision rate with this procedure compared to ACDF, significant heterotopic ossification (42%) and complete ankylosis (18%) at the level of surgery have been described. However, this tends to be clinically inconsequential.[52]
  - Due to their recent widespread use, there has been relatively little written regarding the complications and strategies of revising these implants.
  - Causes for revision include improper patient selection, incomplete decompression with persistent radiculopathy or myelopathy, infection, malposition of the implant (in kyphosis or off center), improper sizing, mechanical failure of the implant from bearing surface wear, subsidence from fracture or osteolysis, and metallosis.[47]
  - Revision strategies will be dependent on the design of the implant, but in general, there are three main categories: reoperation (foraminotomy/laminectomy/posterior fusion), revision (modification of original implant), and removal with replacement.
  - Skovrlj et al[47] summarized the mean rate of reoperation, revision, and removal at 2.3 years as 1%, 0.2%, and 0.2%, respectively.
  - Reoperation with foraminotomy is indicated for recurrent foraminal disc herniation or foraminal stenosis.
  - Revision is indicated when there is device malfunction or malalignment noticed in the immediate postoperative period.
  - General indications for removal and fusion include gross malposition (extrusion, subsidence, or retropulsion) infection, or mechanical failure of the device. In these cases, a corpectomy may be required depending on the amount of bone loss.
  - A posterior fusion alone may be used to produce a fusion across a symptomatic implant which does not require anterior retrieval.
  - Onken et al[33] reported on the revision of 16 third-generation-type disc protheses due to an industry call back. In this series, six patients were converted to ACDF, where 10 patients received an alternative prosthesis. They reported an 18% complication rate including a malposition of a replanted prosthesis, a C6 hyperesthesia, and a

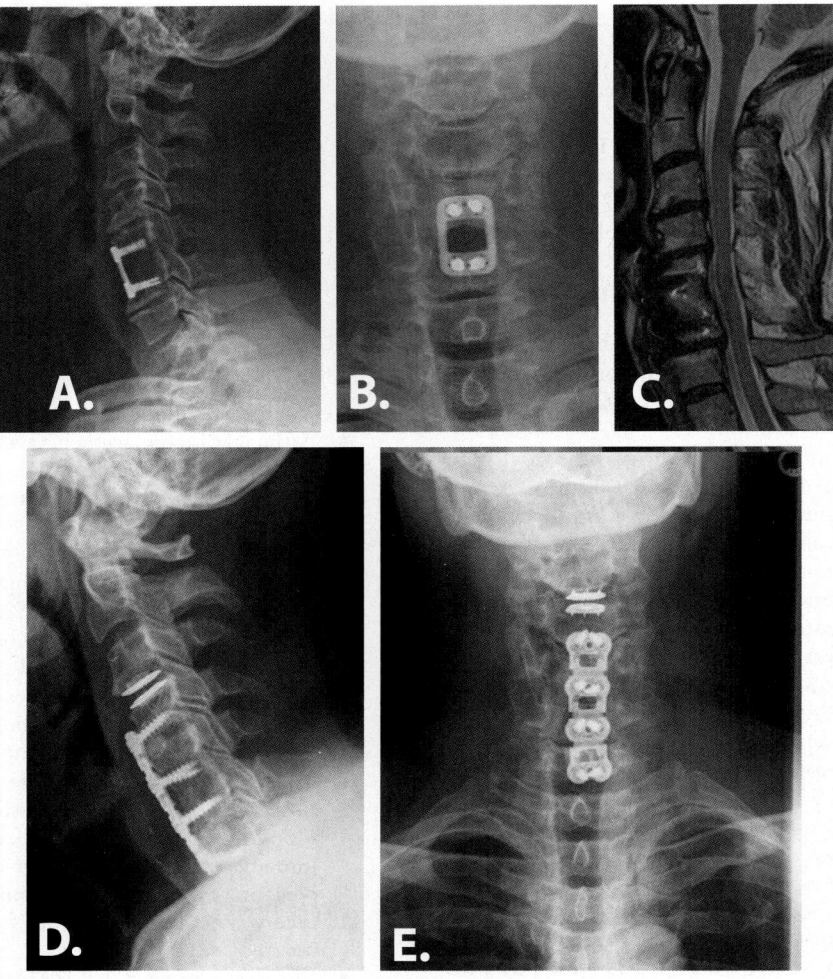

FIG 2 X-rays (**A,B**) and sagittal T2-weighted MRI (**C**) of a 61-year-old male who is 20 years status post a C5–C6 ACDF showing ASD and stenosis above and below the construct. Images (**D,E**) show revision ACDF from C4–C7 with a C3–C4 CDR. The choice was made for a hybrid construct to decrease the fusion surfaces and hopefully prevent future ASD.

recurrent laryngeal nerve palsy. Histologic analysis was performed on four devices, which showed fibrocartilage formation in early removals (<24 months) and vascular-rich granulation tissue in late removal (60 months). There was no metallic debris or inflammatory infiltrate noted.

- Kyphosis
  - There are no absolute guidelines for treatment of kyphosis; however, surgery is indicated in cases of deformity combined with neurologic deficit, severe mechanical pain, or a functional deficit such as dysphagia or horizontal gaze loss.[50]
  - The goals of surgical correction of kyphosis are to decompress stenotic areas and realign the spine such that horizontal gaze is possible.
  - The radiographic alignment goals are as follows: C2–C7 SVA <40 mm, chin–brow vertical angle between −10 degrees and +20 degrees, and T1 slope minus C2–C7 lordosis <15 degrees.[53]
  - The surgical principles of cervical deformity correction are to shorten the posterior column, lengthening the anterior column, and use the PLL as a hinge to facilitate correction.

- Three general approaches are used to address kyphosis:
  - Anterior approach is indicated to addresses ventral compressive pathology or focal cervical kyphosis caused by a compromised anterior column through corpectomy and strut grafting or multilevel ACDF.[42] An anterior approach may be used in isolation to correct deformity so long as the facet joints are not fused. Anterior approaches allow lengthening of the anterior column through placement of interbody devices or strut grafts to a greater degree than posterior osteotomies to shorten the posterior column. For this reason, an anterior procedure with or without a posterior approach has become the preferred method of deformity correction.[60]
  - Posterior approach: This approach uses lateral mass instrumentation with or without posterior osteotomies of the cervical spine to correct the deformity. Posterior strategies are typically indicated for flexible deformities if adequate fixation (six fixation points) can be achieved above and below the apex of the deformity in nonosteoporotic bone. However, posterior fixation may be limited by poor bone stock following previous laminectomy.

- Anterior/posterior combined approach: This approach is useful for cases with focal deformity requiring longer fusions over four segments. This approach is typically indicated in cases where there is fusion of the anterior and posterior elements with ventral compressive pathology which must be treated. The combined approach allows for powerful correction of the sagittal plane deformity with the cost of the added risk of a second procedure. Of note, in some patients with significant deformity with posterior arthrosis or fusions, a three-stage procedure may be required. The first stage performed is a posterior osteotomy of autofusion or levels of arthrosis with placement of instrumentation. The second stage is performed anteriorly with corpectomy and strut grafting or multilevel ACDF. The final stage is performed to secure the posterior fixation.
- Posterior osteotomies for correction of kyphosis
  - Posterior osteotomies are indicated in cases of rigid kyphosis which do not require anterior column lengthening.
  - Smith-Petersen osteotomy (SPO): This is an osteotomy through the posterior elements only. The lateral masses between two pedicles are resected at the levels of kyphosis, allowing extension of the spine. SPOs can be performed at any level between C3 and C7.
  - Pedicle subtraction osteotomy (PSO): This is a three-column osteotomy involving resection of the posterior elements, pedicles, and a wedge-shaped resection of the vertebral body. A PSO allows for approximately 30 degrees of cervical extension. As the osteotomy passes through all three columns, acceptable levels for PSO are limited to C7 and T1. The vertebral artery passing through the foramen transversarium at C1–C6 makes PSO at these levels impossible. As such, cervical PSOs are generally used for correction of focal kyphosis at the cervicothoracic junction.

Preoperative Planning

- In most cases, an approach through a previously unexploited plane is the safest.
- If the initial procedure was performed through a right-sided approach, then revision may be performed through a left-sided approach.
- In cases of anterior surgery, consultation with an otolaryngologist for inspection of the vocal cords confirms that no injury has occurred to the recurrent laryngeal nerve. If vocal fold mobility is abnormal, the approach should be performed through the abnormal side to prevent injury to the healthy fold.

Positioning

- Neuromonitoring should typically be employed in most cases with the potential for spinal cord manipulation.
- This also allows for the detection of positioning related neurocompromise in the prone and supine positions for almost all procedures.
- Supine positioning: anterior cervical procedures **(FIG 3A)**
  - Patient is supine on a flat Jackson table or standard operating room (OR) table.
  - A bump or towel role is placed between the scapulae to generate cervical extension.
  - In the case of rigid cervical kyphosis, the head may float in midair and a stack of sheets should be placed underneath with a foam doughnut to support the head.
  - Gardner-Wells tongs may be placed for inline traction using 2 to 9 lb of weight.
  - Tape is used to draw the shoulders down allowing for visualization of the cervicothoracic junction. Care must be taken not to place too much pressure on the shoulders as this may result in a brachial plexus injury.
  - Arms are tucked at the sides with foam around the wrists and elbows to prevent neurapraxia.
  - Padding is placed behind the knees and heels.

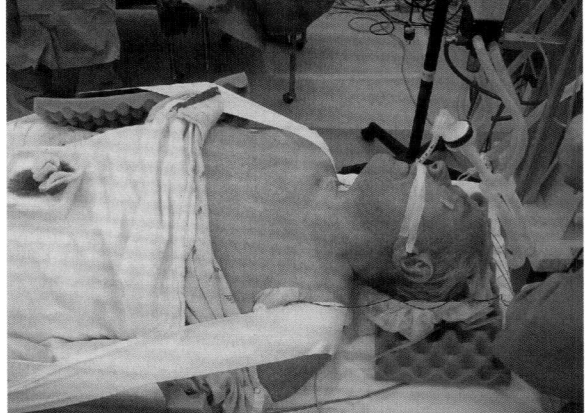 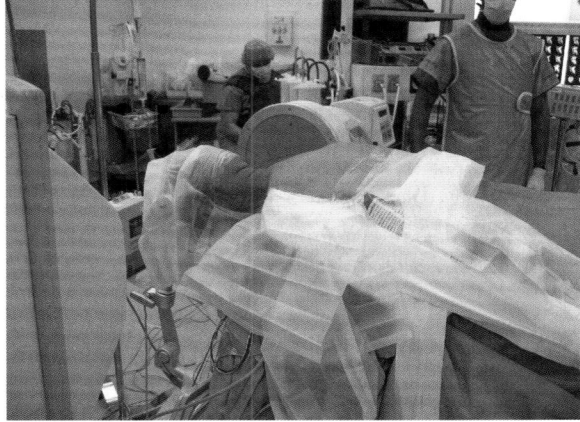

A **B**

FIG 3 A. Patient in the supine position with a bolster between the scapulae, the head slightly extended. The shoulders are taped caudally to allow for visualization of the lower cervical levels. Ask the anesthesiologist to place the tube in the side of the mouth opposite the side anticipated for the approach. **B.** Patient in the prone position using the Mayfield headrest. The patient may also be placed in a prone view or soft face holder during the procedure. The arms are padded and tucked to the sides. The shoulders are taped caudally to allow for visualization of the lower cervical levels. For upper cervical surgery, the hairline must be trimmed prior to predraping.

- If using a standard OR table, the headrest can be extended to allow further lordosis. Flexion of headrest after placement of interbody grafts provides some compression prior to anterior plating.
- Baseline neuromonitoring parameters should be established prior to draping.
- Prone positioning: posterior cervical approaches **(FIG 3B)**
  - If a Mayfield head holder is to be used, this is placed with the patient in the supine position prior to flipping to the prone position.
  - During placement of the Mayfield tongs, the adjustment arm should be in the forward position directly over the patient's nose. This allows the surgeon to confirm the tongs will not impinge on the nose during intraoperative adjustment of the tongs.
  - Alternatively, bivector traction may be used with a Jackson table. In this strategy, two separate ropes—one for extension and another for flexion—are attached and may be used in different parts of the procedure to correct the deformity.
  - Neuromonitoring is attached prior to prone positioning.
  - The patient is gently turned to the prone position with the torso on bolsters or a four-point frame.
  - If Mayfield tongs are used, attachment to the operating frame is the first priority following the flip.
  - All bony prominences are padded to prevent neurapraxia.
  - Elbows and hands are padded and the arms tucked to the sides.
  - Tape is used to draw the shoulders down, allowing for visualization of the cervicothoracic junction.
  - Fluoroscopy is used to confirm cervical alignment.
  - Baseline neuromonitoring parameters should be established prior to draping.
- Deep vein thrombosis prophylaxis with thromboembolic deterrent hose and sequential compression devices should be initiated. A warming blanket should be placed prior to draping.

Approach

- Revision anterior approach
  - Superficial landmarks are used to determine the level of the incision. These landmarks are the following:
    - Hard palate: arch of the atlas
    - Lower border of the mandible: C2–C3
    - Hyoid bone: C3
    - Thyroid cartilage: C4–C5
    - Cricoid cartilage: C6
    - Carotid tubercle: C6
  - A transverse incision is made at the level of pathology.
  - If an ipsilateral vocal cord palsy is detected, the previous incision is used to avoid damage to the intact recurrent laryngeal nerve.
  - For more extensile exposures, a longitudinal "carotid" type incision is made just medial to the sternocleidomastoid (SCM) muscle. However, these incisions have a less desirable cosmetic result.
  - The platysma is split in line with the incision.

- An interval is then developed between the SCM and carotid sheath laterally and the strap muscles with the tracheoesophageal structures medially.
- As there may be scarring in the area obscuring vital structures, careful blunt dissection is used as much as possible.
- The omohyoid muscle if present may be incised to provide increased exposure.
- The prevertebral fascia, a loose connective tissue layer, will be encountered over the anterior longitudinal ligament. The fascia is incised and stripped from the spine, exposing the anterior longitudinal ligament and longus colli muscles.
- At higher cervical levels (C3–C4), the superior thyroid artery may be encountered crossing the surgical interval. However, if ligation is necessary for exposure, it should be carefully isolated from the superior laryngeal nerve, which often travels in its proximity.
- The tracheoesophageal bundle should be carefully released the entire length of the exposure to protect the esophagus and decrease retraction pressure.
- The level of pathology is marked with a spinal needle or disc marker and an x-ray obtained to confirm the correct level of pathology.
- Tips for finding the correct level include palpation of the carotid tubercle and careful evaluation of preoperative x-ray for anterior osteophytes and their relation to the level of interest.
- Once the level is confirmed, the longus colli muscles are elevated bilaterally, and soft tissue retractors are placed below the muscle belly to expose the anterior body and uncinate processes.
- Posterior approach
  - The bony prominences of the posterior spine are palpated. C2 has a prominent spinous process as does C7 and T1.
  - A longitudinal incision is made in line with the spinous processes at the levels of pathology.
  - Electrocautery is used to maintain hemostasis throughout the case.
  - The nuchal ligament is followed and divided as it courses down to the spinous processes. The paraspinal muscles in the cervical region often cross midline. The nuchal ligament appears as a lightly colored pale streak that follows the course of the paraspinal muscles. Following this streak will avoid cutting through muscle fibers and will ultimately lead to the spinous process.
  - X-rays are obtained with marker on spinous process to confirm correct-level surgery.
  - The deep layer of muscle is stripped from the spinous process and lamina close to the bone with the aid of electrocautery.
  - Subperiosteal dissection is carried to the lateral border of the lateral masses; however, one should be mindful not to go beyond the lateral mass where a venous plexus exits. Moreover, dissection lateral to the facet joint may destroy the medial branch of the dorsal cervical rami, which will result in denervation of the paraspinal musculature.
  - Soft tissue retractors are placed for optimal visualization.

ANTERIOR REVISION FUSION FOR PSEUDARTHROSIS OR RECURRENT STENOSIS

- After an anterior approach, the previous anterior instrumentation is removed from the spine carefully protecting the esophagus. There may often be a fibrotic rind covering the plate or hardware, which can be exploited to help release the tracheoesophageal bundle.
- Distraction pins are placed in the levels above and below the pseudarthrosis.
- In cases requiring added lordosis, the distraction pins should be placed in a convergent manner to allow the generation of lordosis with distraction.
- Alternatively, the plate may be exploited as a lever arm with the use of a lamina spreader to help pry open the disc space. Additionally, a cervical Cobb may be used to aid the development of the plane.
- Once the segment has been mobilized, the residual graft and fibrous tissue are removed with a curette or pituitary rongeur.
- In cases of severe collapse, the pseudarthrosis may literally be bone on bone. In these instances, a high-speed burr is used to follow the "scar" or cleft left by the pseudarthrosis. This can be less than 1 mm wide.
- Periodically, stop and check the scar to confirm you are still in the correct plane. Opening and closing the distraction pins while looking at the pseudarthrosis will show micromotion in the plane of the nonunion.
- As the posterior cortex is thinned, a small forward-angled curette or micro-Kerrison can be used to remove the posterior cortex.
- In cases of radiculopathy, the removal of the posterior cortex can be carried out laterally toward the foramen until a nerve hook can be passed without impingement.
- In primary anterior surgery, resection of the PLL has been advocated for complete decompression. However, this should not be attempted in cases of previous PLL resection as there will be no true plane between the scarred PLL and the dura, increasing the risk of dural tear. If previous operative notes suggest the PLL was undisturbed, it can be resected at the time of revision.
- Following decompression, the interbody space is shaped to accommodate a graft. The graft can be tricortical autograft or cortical cancellous allograft.
- The graft is fashioned using a clamp and high-speed burr **(TECH FIG 1)**.
- Following graft preparation, the block is inserted into the interbody space.
- Anterior plating is recommended in all cases of pseudarthrosis unless a standalone device is used.
- X-rays are obtained to confirm appropriate placement of the graft and anterior plate.
- The incision is closed over a drain.
- Cervical collar is placed for immobilization.

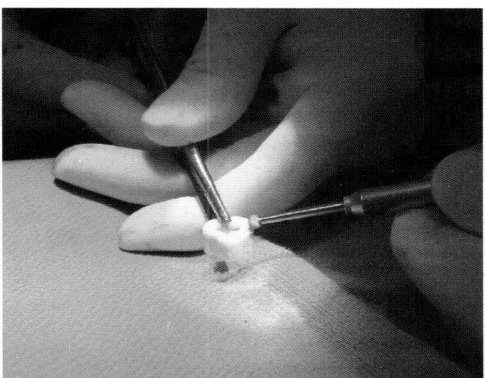

TECH FIG 1 Graft preparation.

POSTERIOR SPINAL FUSION FOR ANTERIOR PSEUDARTHROSIS

- Posterior exposure is performed at the levels of anterior pseudarthrosis.
- If radiculopathy is present, a laminoforaminotomy is performed. This technique is described in later text.
- Several methods of posterior instrumentation exist. At our institution, posterior fixation with lateral mass screws and rods is most frequently performed.
- A 2-mm high-speed burr is used to make a starting hole 1 mm medial to the center point on the lateral mass.
- A 2.4-mm drill bit is used to create a pilot hole for the 3.5-mm lateral mass screw.
- The direction of the drill hole is 15 degrees cephalad and 30 degrees lateral.
- Drilling begins with a 12-mm depth sleeve and can be increased by 2-mm increments.
- After drilling, a depth gauge is used to confirm appropriate screw length.
- The hole is tapped with a slightly undersized tap.
- The screw is inserted in the same trajectory as the drill and tap.
- These steps are repeated until all lateral mass screws are placed.
- The lateral masses and lamina are then decorticated using the burr.
- Appropriate length rods are contoured and then inserted into the heads of the screws bilaterally. Set screws are placed and tightened to appropriate torque.
- Bone graft is then placed over the decorticated lateral masses.
- Closure of the wound in layers.
- Cervical collar is placed for immobilization (typically for longer segmental reconstruction).

ANTERIOR TREATMENT OF POSTLAMINECTOMY KYPHOSIS

- After anterior exposure, scar may be found over the apex of the deformity. Resection of the scar will allow for increased exposure and mobility of the spine.
- Flexible deformity correction can be achieved by several methods including the use of a laminal spreader in the disc space or convergent distraction pin insertion to generate lordosis as described earlier.
- At each level of deformity, the intervertebral discs are excised using a pituitary rongeur, curettes, and a micro-Kerrison when needed. The discectomy should be carried down to the level of the PLL.
- Care should be taken to completely remove the cartilaginous endplate to prevent pseudarthrosis.
- In cases of associated radiculopathy, the foramen is decompressed. A nerve hook passed laterally into the foramen confirms the decompression is adequate.
- If multiple interbody grafts are to be used, trial spacers are inserted into the interbody spaces, and appropriate grafts are selected for each level.
- The lordotic grafts are preferred to help deformity correction.
- If strut grafting is desired or required for adequate decompression, a corpectomy is performed.
- First, a trough is created 16 mm wide in the vertebral body. The majority of bone in this trough may then be removed efficiently with a rongeur.
- As the posterior cortex is approached, a high-speed burr is used to thin the bone.
- A small angled curette or micro-Kerrison can be introduced below the posterior cortex and used to carefully perform the final resection.
- The superior and inferior vertebral endplates are prepared with the high-speed burr, creating decorticated bleeding cancellous beds with posterior lips to prevent displacement of the graft into the spinal canal.
- A cortical strut is then fashioned from allograft fibula.
- Twenty pounds of traction is placed on the skull with an extension moment to allow for insertion of the lordotic graft.
- The graft is inserted and tapped into place with extreme caution to avoid injury to the spinal cord or nerves. The weight is then removed, which loads the graft.
- Anterior cervical plating is recommended in all cases. In multilevel ACDF, there are several sites for screw fixation. For strut grafting, screws are placed above and below the strut. Screws should not be placed through the graft as risk of graft fracture is substantial. If concerned about graft displacement, a nonabsorbable suture can be used to tie the graft to the plate.
- To generate more lordosis, the anterior plate may be contoured to increase its lordotic shape. Next, screws are placed at the apex of the deformity rather than at the ends of the plate. This allows the mechanical drawing of the spine to the plate with progressive tightening of the screws. Once correction is achieved, the distal screws are placed.

ANTERIOR TREATMENT OF RIGID POSTLAMINECTOMY KYPHOSIS

- In cases of rigid cervical deformity, a complete osteotomy of the anterior column may be performed according to the technique described by Kim et al.[19]
- Prior to performing this procedure, the surgeon must have a complete understanding of the course of the vertebral arteries by carefully studying the preoperative MRI or CT angiogram.
- Exposure is performed as described earlier and distractions pins are placed above and below the kyphotic segment.
- Bony resection is performed perpendicular to the disc space/fusion mass with a high-speed matchstick burr. Resection may be asymmetric to correct any coronal deformity.
- Lateral bony resection of the uncinates is usually necessary. To perform this, the lateral edge of the uncinates is exposed, and a Penfield 4 is used to protect the vertebral artery, whereas a burr is used to thin the uncinate at its base. Following this, a microcurette is used to break the wafer of bone medially.
- The deformity correction may now be achieved using a combination of removing sheets from under the head, placing gentle pressure on the forehead while expanding the distraction pins to achieve desired correction.
- A graft and plate are placed as described earlier.

POSTERIOR APPROACHES FOR FLEXIBLE OR RIGID POSTLAMINECTOMY KYPHOSIS

- Prior to the procedure, the Mayfield head holder is positioned on the patient.
- Alternatively, a bivector traction setup may be used as described earlier.
- After prone positioning, the Mayfield is secured with the neck in flexion.
- Following lateral mass instrumentation as outlined earlier, the flexible deformity may be reduced into lordosis by propositioning the head in extension using the Mayfield. In this position, the lordotic rods are placed and secured to the lateral mass screws.

- If rigid kyphosis is present, an osteotomy technique such as the SPOs or PSOs may be required. These must be performed prior to lateral mass fixation.
- SPOs are performed by resecting the superior and inferior articulating facets as well as all posterior elements of the cervical spine.
- PSOs are indicated in rigid kyphotic deformities typically for conditions where the posterior elements are fused such as in an iatrogenic deformity or ankylosing spondylitis. PSOs are performed at either the C7 or T1 level to avoid the vertebral artery. The resection includes removal of the posterior elements of the vertebrae including the pedicle and decancellation of the vertebral body to allow for collapse. A complete description is provided by Wollowick et al.[57]
- If the osteotomy renders the posterior bone inadequate for isolated posterior fixation, anterior fusion may become necessary.
- If adequate bone stock is present after osteotomy, then posterior instrumentation with lateral mass screws and fusion is performed as outlined previously.

Combined Anterior Posterior for Postlaminectomy Kyphosis

- Unless significant posterior fusions or arthrosis are present, the combined approach begins with anterior discectomy or corpectomy as outlined under the discussion of isolated anterior treatment of cervical kyphosis.
- Once the anterior instrumentation is complete, the patient is turned to the prone position for lateral mass fixation with or without an osteotomy.
- In general, short anterior procedures of three levels or less do not require posterior stabilization. In cases of four or more levels of reconstruction, posterior instrumentation should be considered.
- Posterior fixation should also be considered in patients with poor bone stock or risks for pseudarthrosis.
- Posterior instrumentation is discussed in detail in the previous section.
- Following combined anterior posterior fusion and instrumentation, the patient should be immobilized in a cervical collar for a minimum of 6 weeks.

Revision for Adjacent Segment Degeneration (Revision Anterior Cervical Discectomy and Fusion)

- Revision surgery for ASD is similar in many ways to primary ACDF.
- A major difference is the need for approach from a previously unexploited plane. Ear, nose, and throat consultation should be obtained, and if vocal cords function normally, the anterior spine is approached from the side opposite that is used during the primary procedure.
- A second difference is the potential need for hardware removal at the site of previous fusion. Every effort should be made to identify the hardware prior to revision surgery.
- With these two exceptions, anterior treatment for ASD is ACDF as outlined under treatment of cervical disc herniation.

Laminoforaminotomy

- Posterior laminoforaminotomy is useful for treatment of nerve root compression in cases of adjacent level degeneration or recurrent disc herniation at the site of previous anterior fusion.[11]
- A unilateral posterior approach at the level of nerve compression is performed, and the lamina and lateral mass are identified.
- A curved curette is used to create a plane between the medial aspect of the facet and the ligamentum flavum.
- A burr is used to thin the lateral lamina and medial facet.
- The anterior facet capsule and additional bone are resected to visualize the exiting nerve root. (Care should be taken to avoid excessive resection of the facet; >50% of this may cause iatrogenic instability to the cervical spine.)
- The ligamentum is resected, and the laminotomy is widened to expose the junction of the thecal sac and nerve root.
- The foramen is probed with a Woodson or nerve hook to confirm decompression; if disc herniation is found, the PLL is incised, and the disc fragment is removed.
- The spine is closed in layers.
- Soft cervical collar is provided for comfort.

Removal of Cervical Disc Replacement

- Removal of an arthroplasty implant depends on its specific design features and manufacturer guidelines on removal should be studied prior to surgery.
- It is recommended to approach the device through the original incision.
- After identification of the implanted level using fluoroscopy, the disc removal procedure should be performed under Caspar pin distraction.
- The original anterior longitudinal defect is typically filled with scar and or ectopic bone, which is carefully removed using a high-speed burr or curette.
- It is preferable to remove the device piecemeal by its individual components, starting with the removal of the polyethylene insert using an inlay separator.
- The metal endplates may be removed with a Cobb in the case of nonkeeled implants or forked osteotomes in the case of keeled implants.

Pearls and Pitfalls

Patient Selection	• Appropriate patient selection is the single most important step to reducing the number of patients requiring revision cervical surgery.
Implants	• Identify all previously placed implants prior to revision surgery. Have specific removal equipment available at the time of cervical revision surgery.
Nonoperative Management	• Nonoperative interventions including NSAIDs, physical therapy, and epidural injections should be attempted prior to surgical intervention.
Imaging	• Correlate patient symptoms with positive imaging findings to optimize patient outcomes.

POSTOPERATIVE CARE

- Immediate postoperative care after revision cervical surgery involves immobilization of the spine for 2 to 12 weeks, depending on the number of levels addressed during the surgery and the likelihood of instability or nonunion.
- Short fixation over one to two segments is immobilized in a cervical collar for 2 weeks. At that time, the patient is allowed to gradually return to activities of daily living. Formal physical therapy evaluation for ROM and strengthening of the cervical spine is typically reserved until fusion mass is seen on plain radiographs.
- Patients with longer fusion and those at risk for poor wound healing and pseudarthrosis are treated in a rigid cervical collar for a minimum of 6 weeks. Formal therapy is started once the fusion is visualized on plain x-rays.
- Physical therapy following revision cervical surgery involves isometric strengthening and ROM prior to returning to unlimited activity.

OUTCOMES

- Overall, revision surgery has less favorable outcomes when compared with primary surgical procedures.
- Outcomes for revision for pseudarthrosis vary with the approach used for revision. Anterior revision surgery is associated with a 57% fusion rate. Several studies reported fusion rates of 94% following posterior revision for pseudarthrosis.
- Zdeblick et al[61] and Coric et al[7] reported 100% fusion rates with anterior revision of interbody pseudarthrosis. Both autograft and anterior plating were advocated to increase fusion rates.
- The rate of arthrodesis following surgery for ASD is lower in patients treated with interbody grafting (63%) versus those treated with corpectomy and strut grafting (100%). No statistical significance was found in the clinical outcomes between those treated with interbody fusion and corpectomy with strut grafting.[16]

COMPLICATIONS

- The risk of complications after revision cervical surgery is significantly higher than the risk associated with primary surgery. The overall risk of complication is reported at 27%.[13]
- For each approach, the risk of complication associated with the primary surgery remains with the addition of risks associated with revision circumstances.
- Anterior complications include the following:
  - Esophageal injury: a life-threatening injury; one-third recognized at time of surgery. Early recognition associated with 15% mortality; late recognition associated with 30% mortality.
  - Vocal cord paralysis: 15% of cases[13]
  - Dysphagia: 10% of cases
  - Neurologic injury/monoradiculopathy: 7% of cases
  - Durotomy
  - Graft site complication
- Posterior complications include the following:
  - Neurologic injury
  - Durotomy
  - Significant wound complications/infection occurs at a rate of 1.2%.

ACKNOWLEDGMENT

- The authors wish to express gratitude to the author of this chapter in the previous edition, Dr. Casey C. Bachison for providing the strong foundation to build on.

REFERENCES

1. Albert TJ, Vacarro A. Postlaminectomy kyphosis. Spine (Phila Pa 1976) 1998;23(24):2738–2745.
2. Baba H, Furusawa N, Imura S, et al. Late radiographic findings after anterior cervical fusion for spondylotic myeloradiculopathy. Spine (Phila Pa 1976) 1993;18(15):2167–2173.
3. Boden SD, Bohlman H. The Failed Spine. Philadelphia: Lippincott Williams & Wilkins, 2003.
4. Bolesta MJ, Rechtine G III, Chrin AM, Three- and four-level anterior cervical discectomy and fusion with plate fixation: a prospective study. Spine (Phila Pa 1976) 2000;25(16):2040–2044.
5. Carreon L, Glassman SD, Campbell MJ. Treatment of anterior cervical pseudoarthrosis: posterior fusion versus anterior revision. Spine J 2006;6(2):154–156.
6. Choi SH, Cho JH, Hwang CJ, et al. Preoperative radiographic parameters to predict a higher pseudarthrosis rate after anterior cervical discectomy and fusion. Spine (Phila Pa 1976) 2017;42(23):1772–1778.
7. Coric D, Branch CL Jr, Jenkins JD. Revision of anterior cervical pseudoarthrosis with anterior allograft fusion and plating. J Neurosurg 1997;86(6):969–974.
8. Curry AL, Young WF. Preoperative laryngoscopic examination in patients undergoing repeat anterior cervical discectomy and fusion. Int J Spine Surg 2013;7:e81–e83.
9. Eck JC, Humphreys SC, Lim TH, et al. Biomechanical study on the effect of cervical spine fusion on adjacent-level intradiscal pressure and segmental motion. Spine (Phila Pa 1976) 2002;27(22):2431–2434.
10. Emery SE, Fisher RS, Bohlman HH. Three-level anterior cervical discectomy and fusion: radiographic and clinical results. Spine (Phila Pa 1976) 1997;22(22):2622–2624.
11. Farey ID, McAfee PC, Davis RF, et al. Pseudarthrosis of the cervical spine after anterior arthrodesis. Treatment by posterior nerve-root decompression, stabilization, and arthrodesis. J Bone Joint Surg Am 1990;72(8):1171–1177.
12. Fraser JF, Hartl R. Anterior approaches to fusion of the cervical spine: a metaanalysis of fusion rates. J Neurosurg Spine 2007;6(4):298–303.

13. Gok B, Sciubba DM, McLoughlin GS, et al. Revision surgery for cervical spondylotic myelopathy: surgical results and outcome. Neurosurgery 2008;63(2):292–298.

14. Hilibrand AS, Carlson GD, Palumbo MA, et al. Radiculopathy and myelopathy at segments adjacent to the site of a previous anterior cervical arthrodesis. J Bone Joint Surg Am 1999;81(4):519–528.

15. Hilibrand AS, Fye MA, Emery SE, et al. Impact of smoking on the outcome of anterior cervical arthrodesis with interbody or strut-grafting. J Bone Joint Surg Am 2001;83(5):668–673.

16. Hilibrand AS, Yoo JU, Carlson GD, et al. The success of anterior cervical arthrodesis adjacent to a previous fusion. Spine (Phila Pa 1976) 1997;22(14):1574–1579.

17. Iyer S, Lenke LG, Nemani VM, et al. Variations in occipitocervical and cervicothoracic alignment parameters based on age: a prospective study of asymptomatic volunteers using full-body radiographs. Spine (Phila Pa 1976) 2016;41(23):1837–1844.

18. Katsuura Y, Bruce J, Taylor S, et al. Overlapping, masquerading, and causative cervical spine and shoulder pathology: a systematic review. Global Spine J 2020;10(2):195–208.

19. Kim HJ, Piyaskulkaew C, Riew DK. Anterior cervical osteotomy for fixed cervical deformities. Spine (Phila Pa 1976) 2014;39(21):1751–1757.

20. Kong D, Zheng T, Fang J, et al. Apoptosis of endplate chondrocytes in post-laminectomy cervical kyphotic deformity. Eur Spine J 2013;22(7):1576–1582.

21. Kozak JA, Hanson GW, Rose JR, et al. Anterior discectomy, microscopic decompression, and fusion: a treatment for cervical spondylotic radiculopathy. J Spinal Disord 1989;2(1):43–46.

22. Kuhns CA, Geck MJ, Wang JC, et al. An outcomes analysis of the treatment of cervical pseudarthrosis with posterior fusion. Spine (Phila Pa 1976) 2005;30(21):2424–2429.

23. Lawrence J, White A, Hilibrand A. Same segment disease after cervical spine surgery. Spine J 2007;7(5):55S.

24. Lee DH, Cho JH, Hwang CJ, et al. What is the fate of pseudarthrosis detected 1 year after anterior cervical discectomy and fusion? Spine (Phila Pa 1976) 2017;43(1):E23–E28.

25. Le Huec JC, Demezon, Aunoble S. Sagittal parameters of global cervical balance using EOS imaging: normative calues from a prospective cohort of asymptomaytic volunteers. Eur Spine J 2015;24(1):63–71.

26. Leven D, Cho S. Pseudarthrosis of the cervical spine: risk factors, diagnosis and management. Asian Spine J 2016;10(4):776–786.

27. Lindsey RW, Newhouse KE, Leach J, et al. Nonunion following two-level anterior cervical discectomy and fusion. Clin Orthop Relat Res 1987;(223):155–163.

28. Lonstein JE. Post-laminectomy kyphosis. Clin Orthop Relat Res 1977;(128):93–100.

29. Lowery GL, McDonough RF. The significance of hardware failure in anterior cervical plate fixation. Patients with 2- to 7-year follow-up. Spine (Phila Pa 1976) 1998;23(2):181–187.

30. Lowery GL, Swank ML, McDonough RF. Surgical revision for failed anterior cervical fusions. Articular pillar plating or anterior revision? Spine (Phila Pa 1976) 1995;20(22):2436–2441.

31. McAnany SJ, Baird EO, Overley SC, et al. A meta-analysis of the clinical and fusion results following treatment of symptomatic cervical pseudarthrosis. Global Spine J 2015;5(2):148–155.

32. Nowinski GP, Visarius H, Nolte LP, et al. A biomechanical comparison of cervical laminaplasty and cervical laminectomy with progressive facetectomy. Spine (Phila Pa 1976) 1993;18(14):1995–2004.

33. Onken J, Reinke A, Radke J, et al. Revision surgery for cervical artificial disc: surgical technique and clinical results. Clin Neurol Neurosurg 2017;152:39–44.

34. Pal GP, Sherk HH. The vertical stability of the cervical spine. Spine (Phila Pa 1976) 1988;13(5):447–449.

35. Paniello RC, Martin-Bredahl KJ, Henkener LJ, et al. Preoperative laryngeal nerve screening for revision anterior cervical spine procedures. Ann Otol Rhinol Laryngol 2008;117(8):594–597.

36. Park JB, Cho YS, Riew KD. Development of adjacent-level ossification in patients with an anterior cervical plate. J Bone Joint Surg Am 2005;87-A:558–563.

37. Park MS, Kelly MP, Lee DH, et al. Sagittal alignment as a predictor of clinical adjacent segment pathology requiring surgery after anterior cervical arthrodesis. Spine J 2014;14(7):1228–1234.

38. Phillips FM, Carlson G, Emery SE, et al. Anterior cervical pseudarthrosis. Natural history and treatment. Spine (Phila Pa 1976) 1997;22(14):1585–1589.

39. Reitman CA, Hipp JA, Nguyen L, et al. Changes in segmental intervertebral motion adjacent to cervical arthrodesis: a prospective study. Spine (Phila Pa 1976) 2004;29(11):E221–E226.

40. Riew KD, Yang JJ, Chang DG, et al. What is the most accurate radiographic criterion to determine anterior cervical fusion? Spine J 2019;19(3):469–475.

41. Robertson PA, Ryan MD. Neurological deterioration after reduction of cervical subluxation. Mechanical compression by disc tissue. J Bone Joint Surg Br 1992;74(2):224–227.

42. Robinson RA, Walker AE, Ferlic DC, et al. The results of anterior interbody fusion of the cervical spine. J Bone Joint Surg 1962;44(8):1569–1587.

43. Samartzis D, Shen FH, Matthews DK, et al. Comparison of allograft to autograft in multilevel anterior cervical discectomy and fusion with rigid plate fixation. Spine J 2003;3(6):451–459.

44. Sellin JN, Burks SS, Levi AD. Fracture of fusion mass following anterior cervical plate removal: case report. J Clin Neurosci 2018;47:128–131.

45. Sharan AD, Kaye D, Charles Malveaux WM, et al. Dropped head syndrome: etiology and management. J Am Acad Orthop Surg 2012;20(12):766–774.

46. Simmons EH, Bhalla SK. Anterior cervical discectomy and fusion. A clinical and biomechanical study with eight-year follow-up. J Bone Joint Surg Br 1969;51(2):225–237.

47. Skovrlj B, Lee DH, Caridi JM, et al. Reoperations following cervical disc replacement. Asian Spine J 2015;9(3):471–482.

48. Song KS, Piyaskulkaew C, Chuntarapas T, et al. Dynamic radiographic criteria for detecting pseudarthrosis following anterior cervical arthrodesis. J Bone Joint Surg Am 2014;96(7):557–563.

49. Steinhaus ME, Hill PS, Yang J, et al. Urinary N-telopeptide can predict pseudarthrosis after anterior cervical decompression and fusion: a prospective study. Spine (Phila Pa 1976) 2019;44(11):770–776.

50. Steinmetz MP, Stewart TJ, Kager CD, et al. Cervical deformity correction. Neurosurgery 2007;60(1 suppl 1):S90–S97.

51. Stevens JM, Clifton AG, Whitear P. Appearances of posterior osteophytes after sound anterior interbody fusion in the cervical spine: a high-definition computed myelographic study. Neuroradiology 1993;35(3):227–228.

52. Suchomel P, Jurák L, Benes V III, et al. Clinical results and development of heterotopic ossification in total cervical disc replacement during a 4-year follow-up. Eur Spine J 2010;19(2):307–315.

53. Tan LA, Riew D, Traynelis VC. Cervical spine deformity—part 1: biomechanics, radiographic parameters, and classification. Neurosurgery 2017;81(2):197–203.

54. Tribus CB, Corteen DP, Zdeblick TA. The efficacy of anterior cervical plating in the management of symptomatic pseudoarthrosis of the cervical spine. Spine (Phila Pa 1976) 1999;24(9):860–864.

55. Truumees E, McLain R. Failed and revision cervical spine surgery. In: Chapman MW, ed. Chapman's Orthopaedic Surgery, ed 3. Philadelphia: Lippincott Williams & Wilkins, 2001:3846–3860.

56. Whitecloud TS III, Seago RA. Cervical discogenic syndrome. Results of operative intervention in patients with positive discography. Spine (Phila Pa 1976) 1987;12(4):313–316.

57. Wollowick AL, Kelly MP, Riew KD. Pedicle subtraction osteotomy in the cervical spine. Spine (Phila Pa 1976) 2012;37(5):E342–E348.

58. Wu W, Thuomas KA, Hedlund R, et al. Degenerative changes following anterior cervical discectomy and fusion evaluated by fast spin-echo MR imaging. Acta Radiol 1996;37(5):614–617.

59. Zdeblick TA, Abitbol JJ, Kunz DN, et al. Cervical stability after sequential capsule resection. Spine (Phila Pa 1976) 1993;18(14):2005–2008.

60. Zdeblick TA, Ducker TB. The use of freeze-dried allograft bone for anterior cervical fusions. Spine (Phila Pa 1976) 1991;16(7):726–729.

61. Zdeblick TA, Hughes SS, Riew KD, et al. Failed anterior cervical discectomy and arthrodesis. Analysis and treatment of thirty-five patients. J Bone Joint Surg Am 1997;79(4):523–532.

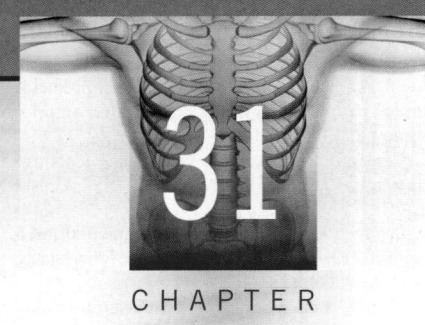

31
CHAPTER

Intradural Surgery
Surgical Excision of Intradural Spinal Tumors

Geoffrey Stricsek, Gerald E. Rodts, Jr., and Daniel Refai

PATHOGENESIS

- The main categories of intradural tumors are intradural extramedullary and intradural intramedullary. Some tumors will exhibit characteristics of both intramedullary and extramedullary or exophytic growth.
- Intradural tumors of the spine are less common than primary or metastatic tumors of the bone or epidural space. Their surgical removal requires delicate technique and maximal avoidance of injury to the spinal cord and nerve roots.
- The most common types of tumor found in the intradural extramedullary space are benign: meningioma, schwannoma, and neurofibroma. Intradural tumors are rarely the result of metastatic spread of malignant cells.
- Teratoma is a rare intradural tumor that often is both intramedullary and extramedullary.
- The most common intramedullary tumors are spinal cord ependymoma, hemangioblastoma, lipoma, astrocytoma, and glioblastoma. They are rarely exophytic except for ependymomas that occur at the conus medullaris.
- Nerve sheath tumors (schwannoma, neurofibroma) usually present with radicular symptoms; myelopathic symptoms develop once the tumor has enlarged to the point where it is causing compression of the spinal cord.
- In the lumbar spine (below the conus medullaris), intradural extramedullary tumors commonly cause radicular symptoms (pain, paresthesias, weakness); low back pain can develop and rapidly progress to an excruciating level when the tumors grow to occupy the majority of the spinal canal.
- Intradural intramedullary tumors can cause axial or radicular pain, but the most common presentation is myelopathy. The progression is typically very slow over many months, unless the pathology is a malignant glioblastoma of the spinal cord. A careful preoperative evaluation must eliminate other pathology of the spinal cord parenchyma such as sarcoidosis, transverse myelitis, multiple sclerosis, etc.

PATIENT HISTORY AND PHYSICAL FINDINGS

- Presenting symptoms of both intramedullary and extramedullary spinal cord tumors include axial or appendicular/radicular pain. The pain is usually persistent when either active or at rest.
- Myelopathic symptoms present as numbness, tingling (paresthesias), gait instability, small motor/hand incoordination (cervical), increasing urinary voiding frequency, difficulty voiding, and general motor weakness.

- Upper motor neuron signs such as hyperreflexia, Hoffman sign, spreading of reflexes, myoclonus, and Babinski signs are typical.

IMAGING AND OTHER DIAGNOSTIC STUDIES

- Magnetic resonance imaging (MRI) is the imaging technology of choice for intramedullary and extramedullary spinal cord tumors. Contrast enhancement is necessary.
  - Intramedullary tumors have fairly characteristic appearances on MRI.
    - Astrocytomas will demonstrate variable contrast enhancement and almost never have a solid, homogenous area of enhancement.
    - Ependymomas consistently have a homogenously enhancing mass within the parenchyma of the spinal cord (FIG 1A), often with cystic component.
    - T1-weighted images will show low intensity within the tumor mass that enhances brightly on contrast administration.
    - Often, T2-weighted images will demonstrate surrounding edema within the spinal cord.
    - Hemangioblastomas typically have a cystic area of low-signal intensity on T1-weighted images with a smaller contrast-enhancing nodule on the inside wall of the cyst.
    - Intramedullary lipomas will be nonenhancing and exhibit the typical high signal on T1- and T2-weighted images, as seen in bodily adipose tissue.
  - Extramedullary tumors such as meningiomas will usually enhance positively with contrast in a very homogenous pattern, and often, a "tail" of enhancement will be seen in the location of attachment to the dura (FIG 1B,C).
  - Schwannomas and neurofibromas can have homogeneous or heterogeneous enhancement patterns. Some schwannomas will exhibit little to no enhancement, but this is less common.
  - Advanced imaging of the entire neuraxis should be obtained to evaluate for other tumor foci.
- For patients who cannot undergo an MRI (eg, those with pacemakers, defibrillators, spinal cord stimulators), computed tomography (CT) myelography can be used and can delineate an area of spinal cord swelling or even myelographic block that would indicate the location of intramedullary tumors. Extramedullary tumors are usually well outlined by CT myelography.

T E C H N I Q U E S

- Electromyography: free running of lower extremities and evoked with pedicle screw fixation (optional)
- D-wave monitoring

Patient Positioning

- The patient is placed in the prone position with the hips flexed initially.
- For lumbar deformities, the hips can be extended in the case during correction to help close the osteotomy.

Approach

- Posterior extension osteotomies are done at the apex of the deformity. The procedure's objective is to shorten the posterior column by closing down the disc space posteriorly pivoting on the posterior longitudinal ligament and to thereby extend the anterior column (see **FIG 5**).[16]
- The rule of thumb is for every 1 mm of posterior bone resection, 1 degree of correction can be expected.[8]

SMITH-PETERSEN OSTEOTOMY

- Obtain meticulously clean, wide exposure of spinous process, lamina, pars, facets, out to the tips of transverse process (TP), as well as the lateral border of any old fusion. Strive for meticulous hemostasis; use bipolar cautery respecting bilateral segmental perfusion dynamics. Avoid Gelfoam, or if needed, it should be removed before osteotomy closure (**TECH FIG 1**).
- Remove overlapping spinous processes to cleanly delineate ligamentum flavum and its midline raphe.
- Remove inferior facets bilaterally at the desired spinal level, exiting inferior to the base of the TP.
- Undertake ligamentum flavum resection from pedicle to pedicle to avoid any mass effect from redundant ligament dorsally on the neural structures once the SPO is closed down.
- Perform bilateral superior articular facet resection, which ends flush to the top of the TP.
- Smooth out cut edges to avoid any obstruction to closure or possible iatrogenic injury to dura or nerves.
- If there is no coronal deformity to be corrected, the osteotomy should be symmetric.
- To address a coronal deformity, an asymmetric SPO can be used with the wider osteotomy on the side of convexity.[13]

- Removal of laminar bone should be adequate and account for possible desired contact between the superior and inferior lamina after closure that may aid fusion. Typically, the osteotomy width is between 6 and 10 mm cephalocaudally.
- The gap created by the osteotomy is compressed, hinging on the posterior aspect of the disc space, causing posterior column shortening and anterior column extension.
- The compression is held in place with posterior spinal instrumentation (**TECH FIG 2**).
- If multiple SPOs are planned, dorsal compression should be performed in a way that redistributes forces over the largest area possible, using either the cantilever reduction technique (**TECH FIG 3A**) or the apical compression technique (**TECH FIG 3B**). If using the cantilever method, manipulate two rods simultaneously to distribute corrective loads and carefully monitor stress on the end vertebrae fixation.
- The lamina and the spinous process of the upper and lower vertebra are decorticated in preparation for arthrodesis.

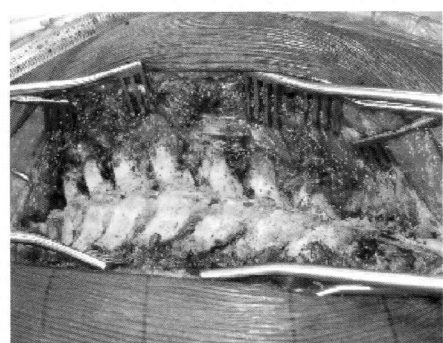
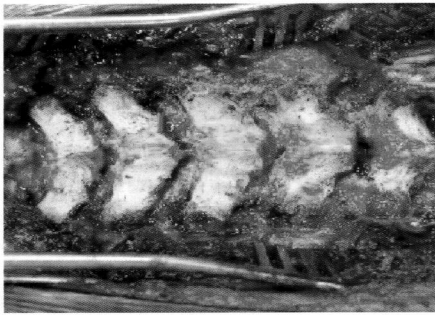

TECH FIG 1 Intraoperative photographs before (**A**) and after (**B**) SPO.

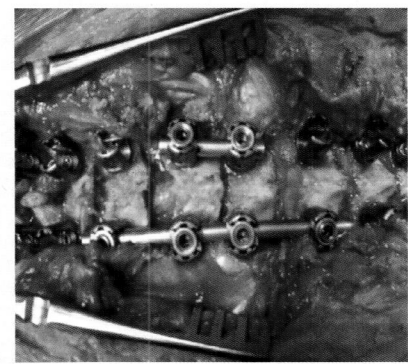
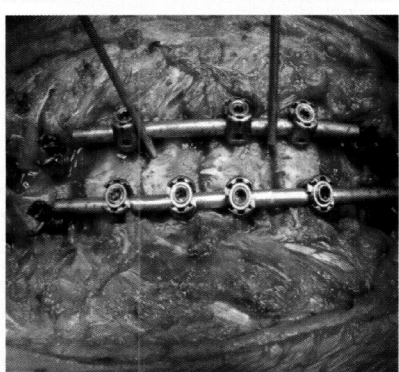

TECH FIG 2 A,B. Sequential temporary apical rod technique for segmental reduction.

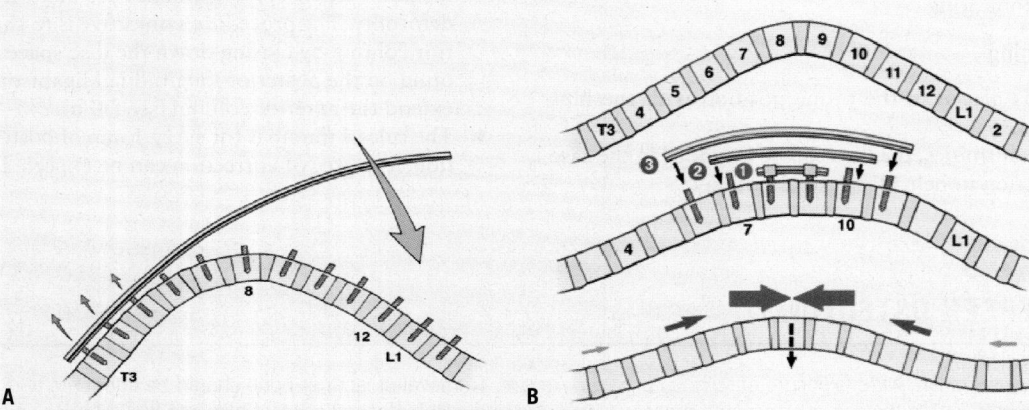

TECH FIG 3 A. Cantilever reduction technique. **B.** Apical-based sequential temporary apical rod technique.

TECHNIQUES

Pearls and Pitfalls

- Attention to cardiovascular parameters can assist with limiting blood loss.
  - In adults, mild hypotension during exposure can help reduce blood loss; however, during osteotomy and manipulation, the pressure should be elevated; mean arterial pressures over 80 mm Hg are ideal.
  - In the pediatric population, mean arterial pressures are maintained between 50 and 60 mm Hg during the approach with an increase from 70 to 80 mm Hg before deformity correction.[6]
  - Avoid bone wax where it can inhibit fusion.

- Carefully plan for soft tissue coverage. Initial exposure should meticulously preserve full-thickness flaps especially at the deformity apex. Flaps may be necessary to get tensionless closure in revision cases. Low-profile instrumentation or monoaxial screws may need to be considered in kyphosis with severe gibbus deformity and thin tissue cover.

- Beware of ossification of the ligamentum flavum, which can best be seen on preoperative scans (see **FIG 5B**). These areas are frequently stenotic and adhered to dura dorsally. Ligamentum flavum must be fully resected before any closure is attempted.

- During the SPO, the pedicles should remain undisturbed. One must be especially careful with osteotomes, which may propagate a crack into the pedicle if dull or not well directed. Invasion of pedicles may weaken critical fixation points requiring an alternate approach to adequately allow for closure of the osteotomy.

- Avoid the use of large Kerrisons; size 2 or 3 mm is recommended, particularly when working on the concavity of deformity with associated scoliosis.

- Look out in rare cases with dorsal displacement of spinal cord or roots, which may have frequent adhesions that need to be resected.

- End segments are most likely to pullout, so optimization of screw length and diameter is critical.

- In higher degree thoracic kyphotic patients, cranial traction may be helpful. In severe lumbar deformity, extending the table during correction may facilitate osteotomy closure, but beware of pressure on the thighs and tibiae or the patient shifting under the drapes.

- Before closing any osteotomy, the neural foramina should be probed gently to ensure they are patent. It is common to discover a small superior tip of a resected superior facet retained in the foramen (especially in thoracic spine) or a remaining spike of either facet base.

- In cases where osteotomy fails to close down, check for residual lateral facet bone or bridging osteophytes or anterior column obstruction. You may need to do more SPOs or convert to PSO if the anterior column will not release.

- During closure, anteriorly directed manual pressure near the apex can help provide additional corrective force. Any time instruments are used for pushing down on the apex to assist reduction, be certain that the canal is safe and there is no risk if an instrument inadvertently slips.

- In the lumbar spine where lordosis increases during closure, the dura may buckle slightly. If this is seen, create additional central opening by resecting and beveling the midline lamina to provide extra space.

- Ensure TP decortication laterally and, in the midline, use careful decortication technique mindful of fixation points and any exposed neural elements. Carefully pack generous bone around all osteotomy points avoiding any material into the canal.

- Cross-table postreduction lateral imaging should be done to ensure that adequate correction has been obtained.

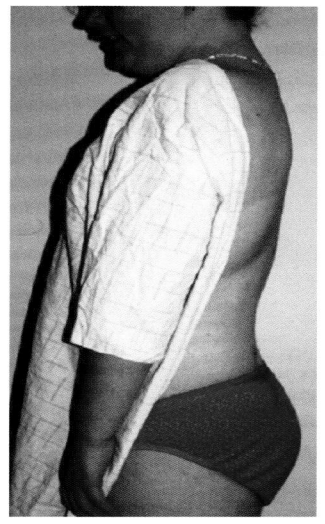 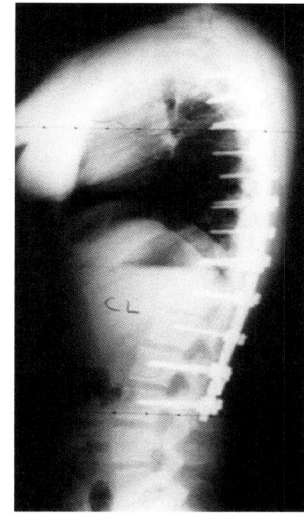

FIG 6 Clinical photograph (**A**) and lateral radiograph (**B**) after SPO correction of 100-degree Scheuermann kyphosis.

OUTCOMES

- A good result is pictured in **FIG 6**.

COMPLICATIONS

Intraoperative

- Subluxation
- Dorsal root compression
- Spinal cord traumatic injury
- Dural buckling
- Cerebrospinal fluid leak
- Great vessel injury
- Pedicle fracture

Postoperative

- New neurologic deficits secondary to intraoperative spinal cord or nerve root injury
- Radiculopathy from neural foraminal compression (rare unless there is baseline foraminal stenosis)[12]
- Superior mesenteric artery syndrome, intestinal obstruction,[7,8] and prolonged ileus
- Epidural or intraspinal hematoma
- Deep venous thrombosis and pulmonary embolism
- Pseudarthrosis is another reported complication.
- Adjacent segment disease/junctional kyphosis

ACKNOWLEDGMENTS

- The author would like to acknowledge the assistance of Dr. William C. Horton III in proofreading the original draft of the chapter.

REFERENCES

1. Berven SH, Deviren V, Smith JA, et al. Management of fixed sagittal plane deformity: results of the transpedicular wedge resection osteotomy. Spine 2001;26(18):2036–2043.
2. Booth KC, Bridwell KH, Lenke LG, et al. Complications and predictive factors for the successful treatment of flat back deformity (fixed sagittal imbalance). Spine 1999;24(16):1712–1720.
3. Bridwell KH. Decision making regarding Smith-Petersen vs. pedicle subtraction osteotomy vs. vertebral column resection for spinal deformity. Spine 2006;31(19 suppl):S171–S178.
4. Bridwell KH, Lenke LG, Lewis SJ. Treatment of spinal stenosis and fixed sagittal imbalance. Clin Orthop Relat Res 2001;(384): 35–44.
5. Casey MP, Asher MA, Jacobs RR, et al. The effect of Harrington rod contouring on lumbar lordosis. Spine 1987;12(8):750–753.
6. Diab MG, Franzone JM, Vitale MG. The role of posterior spinal osteotomies in pediatric spinal deformity surgery: indications and operative technique. J Pediatr Orthop 2011;31(1 suppl): S88–S98.
7. Dorward IG, Lenke LG. Osteotomies in the posterior-only treatment of complex adult spinal deformity: a comparative review. Neurosurg Focus 2010;28(3):E4.
8. Gill JB, Levin A, Burd T, et al. Corrective osteotomies in spine surgery. J Bone Joint Surg Am 2008;90(11):2509–2520.
9. Horton WC, Brown CW, Bridwell KH, et al. Is there an optimal patient stance for obtaining a lateral 36″ radiograph? A critical comparison of three techniques. Spine 2005;30(4):427–433.
10. Joseph SA Jr, Moreno AP, Brandoff J, et al. Sagittal plane deformity in the adult patient. J Am Acad Orthop Surg 2009;17(6): 378–388.
11. LaGrone MO. Loss of lumbar lordosis. A complication of spinal fusion for scoliosis. Orthop Clin North Am 1988;19(2): 383–393.
12. LaGrone MO, Bradford DS, Moe JH, et al. Treatment of symptomatic flatback after spinal fusion. J Bone Joint Surg Am 1988;70(4): 569–580.
13. La Marca F, Brumblay H. Smith-Petersen osteotomy in thoracolumbar deformity surgery. Neurosurgery 2008;63(3 suppl):163–170.
14. Lee MJ, Wiater B, Bransford RJ, et al. Lordosis restoration after Smith-Petersen osteotomies and interbody strut placement: a radiographic study in cadavers. Spine 2010;35(25):E1487–E1491.
15. Simmons EH. Kyphotic deformity of the spine in ankylosing spondylitis. Clin Orthop Relat Res 1977;(128):65–77.
16. Smith-Petersen MN, Larson CB, Aufranc OE. Osteotomy of the spine for correction of flexion deformity in rheumatoid arthritis. J Bone Joint Surg Am 1945;27:1–11.

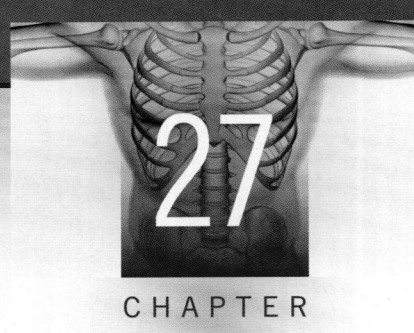

CHAPTER

Sacropelvic Fixation Techniques

Floreana A. Kebaish and Khaled M. Kebaish

DEFINITION

- *Sacropelvic fixation* is a term used to describe instrumentation that spans the sacrum and the iliac bone.
- The most common indication in adult patients is a long spinal fusion to the sacrum. Other indications include high-grade spondylolisthesis, sagittal or coronal malalignment requiring corrective osteotomy, and reconstruction following resection of neoplasms. The most common indication in the pediatric population is long fusion in neuromuscular deformities.
- The purpose is to provide secure and reliable foundation at the base of the spinal column that resist the strong flexion moments and cantilever forces present at the lumbosacral junction.
- Multiple techniques are used, including the Galveston rod, the traditional iliac screws, and the S2 alar iliac (S2AI) technique.

ANATOMY

- A clear understanding of the anatomy of the sacrum and pelvis is crucial to the safe and accurate placement of sacral and pelvic instrumentation. Familiarity with the anatomy of the sacrum, ilium, and sacroiliac (SI) joint is of particular importance.

The Sacrum

- The sacrum lies at the junction between the mobile and fixed portions of the spine and functions as a keystone that unites the two iliac bones and transfer the weight from the torso to the pelvis and subsequently to hip joints and lower extremities.
- Embryologically, the sacrum is formed by five sacral vertebrae that are fused together, and the transverse processes merge into the expanded lateral sacral ala.
- The majority of the bone in the sacrum has a cancellous osseous structure. The trabecular density is greatest in the pedicle and body of the sacral vertebrae and least in the sacral ala. Therefore, S1 sacral pedicle screws are best directed toward the midline.[15]
- The first sacral segment does not contain a true pedicle but rather a confluence of cancellous bone between the sacral body and the ala. Compared to pedicles in the mobile spine, this area is capacious. The S1 pedicle has a mean length of 46.9 ± 3.3 mm in women and 49.7 ± 3.7 mm in men and is angled roughly 40 degrees from the midline (**FIG 1**).

- Numerous critical structures—including the internal iliac artery and vein, middle sacral artery and vein, sympathetic chain, lumbosacral trunk, and sigmoid colon—lie directly on the sacrum at some point and could potentially be injured by the instrumentation used in sacropelvic fusions (**FIG 2**).[14]

The Ilium

- The ilium is the most superior of the three bones that make up the os coxa.
- In adolescents, the ilium is connected to the pubis and the ischium through the triradiate cartilage. Fusion of this cartilage completes between 13 and 16 years of age in most patients.
- In a relatively thin patient, the posterior superior iliac spine (PSIS) is marked by an overlying dimple in the skin. A transverse line drawn between these two dimples crosses the sacrum at the level of S2.
- The structures of the greater sciatic foramen are at risk for damage during instrumentation of the pelvis.[10]

The Sacroiliac Joint

- The SI joint is an L-shaped synovial joint that connects the sacral ala to the iliac bone with an irregularly contoured surface that interlocks in order to resist movement. The joint functions to transfer axial load from the torso onto the hemipelvises.
- The joint is stabilized by the anterior SI ligament, interosseous SI ligament, and the posterior SI ligament (**FIG 3**).

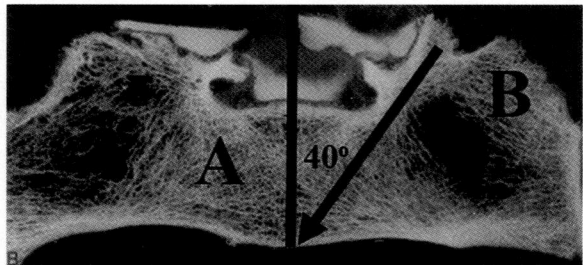

FIG 1 Cross-section of sacrum. The bone density is greatest in the pedicle and body of the vertebrae (*A*) and lowest in the ala (*B*). *Arrow* marks the location of S1 pedicle.

- Furthermore, the density of bone in the sacrum is generally suboptimal, and obtaining adequate fixation can be a challenge in some patients.
- The lumbosacral pivot point **(FIG 4)** is defined as the middle of the osteoligamentous column at the junction between L5 and S1.
  - The farther that the sacropelvic anchor progresses anterior to this point, the more stable the construct. Furthermore, instrumentation that crosses the SI joint without extending anterior to this pivot point is not effective.
- O'Brien[19] introduced the concept of three zones of sacropelvic fixation **(FIG 5)**. Fixation in zone 3 has the highest biomechanical strength as it allows for the placement of the instrumentation farthest anterior to the pivot point.

IMAGING

- Standing full length lateral and posteroanterior plain radiographs should be obtained on all patients with a spinal deformity, to evaluate overall alignment of the spine.
- Due to the complex and variable anatomy of the sacrum, computed tomography imaging may be helpful for planning of screw placement in patients with complex anatomy but is not always necessary as a routine preoperative workup.
- Identification of anatomic abnormalities such as dural ectasia and Tarlov cyst that might alter the necessary surgical approach should be completed prior to the surgical procedure.
- A prior iliac crest autograft harvest may interfere with placement of iliac screws but is unlikely to impact the placement of S2AI screws.

SURGICAL MANAGEMENT

Indications

- Long spinal fusions to the sacrum
  - The most common indication for sacropelvic fixation is a long spinal fusion to the sacrum.[10] The definition of a long spinal fusion is controversial. Most investigators

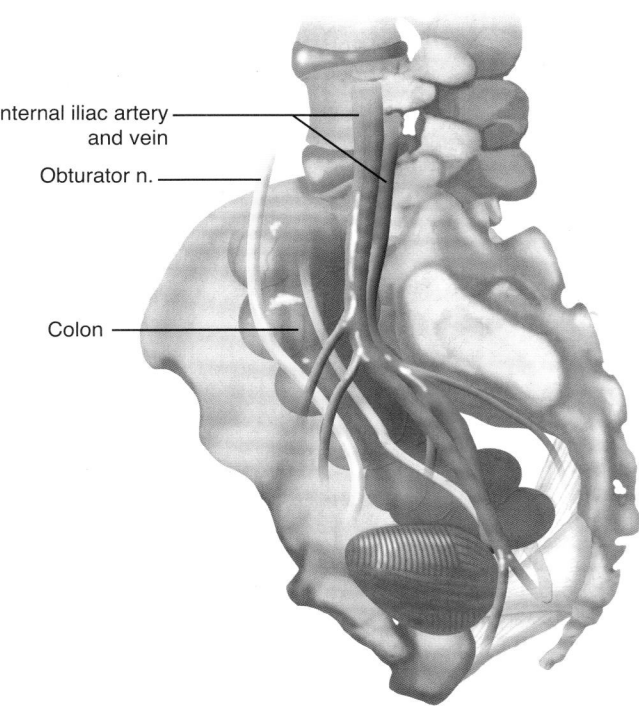

FIG 2 Important anatomic structures overlying the sacrum.

BIOMECHANICS

- Fusions across the lumbosacral junction are a particular challenge for spine surgeons and it has a relatively high incidence of pseudarthrosis.[10]
- Substantial biomechanical forces are concentrated at the lumbosacral junction. Multiple instrumented spine segments above the sacrum act as a long lever arm that transmits flexion, extension, and torsional forces from the spine above. These forces cause motion at the lumbosacral junction that may increase the risk of pseudarthrosis.

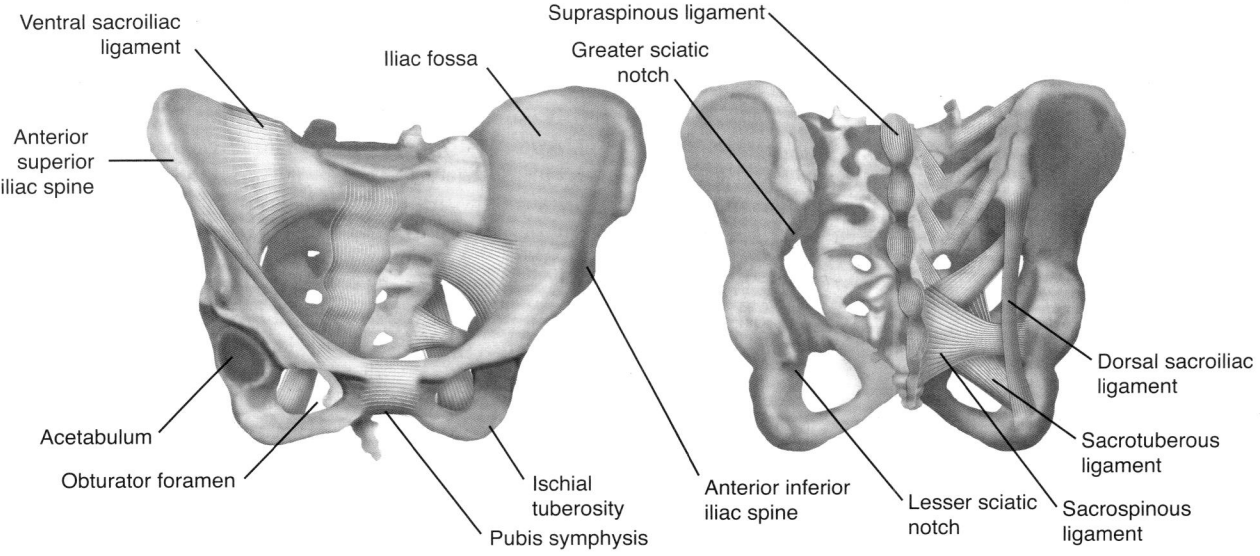

FIG 3 Ligamentous support and bony anatomy of the pelvis.

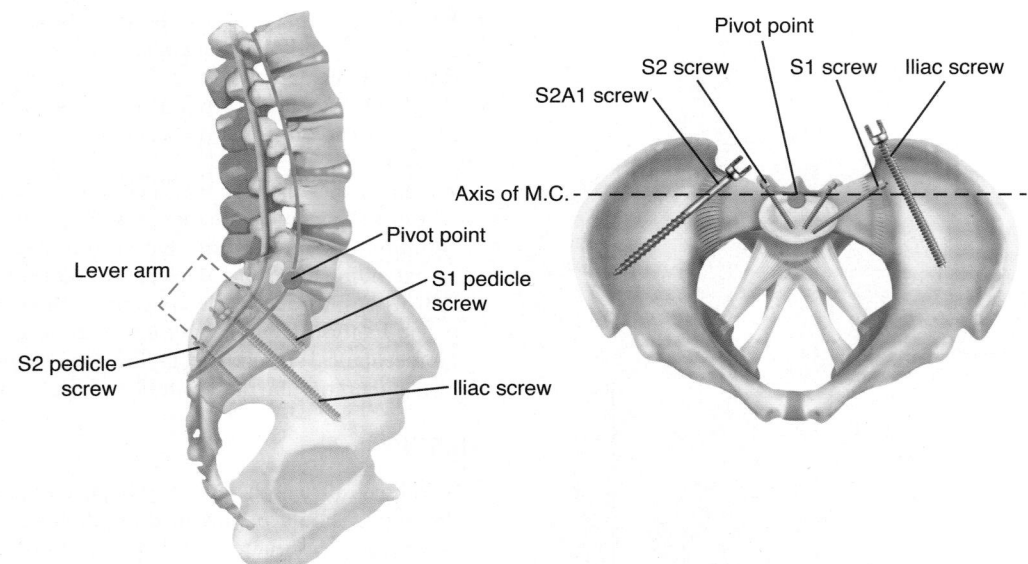

FIG 4 Lumbosacral pivot point. Lateral (**A**) and axial (**B**) views of the pivot point.

currently agree that fusions that cross the thoracolumbar junction and progress to the sacrum should be augmented with pelvic anchors. However, we believe that pelvic anchors should also be considered in fusions that extend above L2 and progress to the sacrum.
- Conditions that commonly require a long spinal fusion include degenerative lumbar scoliosis, flat back deformities, and fixed sagittal malalignment. In children, common indications include neuromuscular spinal deformities, structural lumbosacral scoliotic curves, and congenital scoliosis.[15]
- High-grade spondylolisthesis
  - Correction of high-grade spondylolisthesis, grade III or higher, places excessive force on the S1 pedicle screws.[6]
  - Extending the instrumentation into the ilium serves as an adjunct to the S1 pedicle screws and may reduce the incidence of pseudarthrosis and distal implant failure.[22]
- Sagittal malalignment requiring corrective osteotomy
  - Flat back syndrome refers to the loss of lumbar lordosis following a posterior spinal fusion.[23] Patients present with pain, loss of sagittal balance, and caudal disc degeneration.

- Correction of this often rigid deformity frequently requires osteotomies and a long fusion to the sacrum.[23] These fusions should be supplemented with pelvic instrumentation to decrease the risk of S1 failure and pseudarthrosis.
- Correction of pelvic obliquity
  - Pelvic obliquity is common in young patients with neuromuscular deformities.
  - Correction of the coronal malalignment at the lower lumbar spine frequently requires pelvic fixation.[8]
- Other indications
  - Less common indications include sacrectomy performed for sacral tumors, sacral fracture, and severe osteoporosis in patients requiring lumbosacral fusion.[15]
  - Although many techniques exist for sacropelvic fixation, only two are currently used,[10] and we focus only on those: the traditional iliac screw (iliac bolts) technique[11] and the S2AI technique.[4,18] We also briefly discuss the Galveston L-rod technique[2] because of its historical importance as the precursor of the two modern techniques, which are discussed in more details.

Preoperative Planning

- Planning the extent and type of procedure to be performed requires a thorough understanding of the anatomy of the patient's deformity.
- Patients with significant pelvic obliquity may have significant differences between the two sides of the pelvis, and the trajectory of the anchors may need to be modified accordingly.
- Patients with significant osteoporosis may require larger size screws, up to 10 mm, in order to obtain adequate purchase.
- Patients who have had bone harvested from the iliac crest may not be candidates for iliac bolts, and the S2AI technique should be used instead.
- Patients with deficient iliac bone—for example, patients with sacropelvic resection for tumor—may require additional points of fixation on the contralateral side.
- A C-arm should be available for intraoperative imaging if necessary, especially in patients with more complex pelvic bones anatomy.

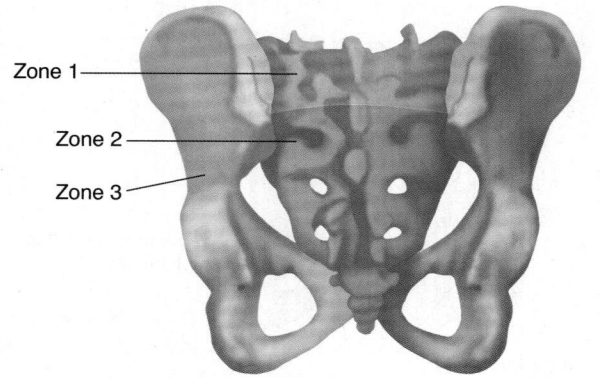

FIG 5 Zones of pelvic fixation. Biomechanical strength increases as you progress from zone 1 to zone 3. Furthermore, zone 3 allows placement of the instrumentation the farthest anterior to the pivot point.

Positioning

- The patient is positioned prone on a radiolucent frame, per routine for posterior spinal procedures.
- A transverse pad should run across the chest at the level of the shoulders. Two-side pads support each iliac crest at the level of the anterior superior iliac spine (ASIS). The abdomen should be free to expand without touching the table to ensure that the abdominal and pelvic blood vessels are not under compression, which helps minimize blood loss. This positioning method also helps ensure adequate lumbar lordosis is achieved when arthrodesis is performed.
- The caudal drapes should be applied distal to the PSIS, leaving that area and the iliac crests accessible during the procedure.

Approach

- The approach depends on the technique used and specific points for each technique are discussed in the following text.
- In general, the approach for the open procedures is an extension of the midline incision, centered over the spinous processes, and with some modification distally based on the technique.
- The goal should be to effectively expose the entire area of the spine that is going to be instrumented.
- The exposure should extend caudally enough to expose the dorsal S1 sacral foramen.
- The iliac screw and Galveston techniques require additional soft tissue dissection laterally over the iliac crest in order to expose the starting point on the PSIS.

SACRAL TRICORTICAL PEDICLE SCREWS

- The iliac screw and S2AI methods for sacropelvic fixation begin with placement of sacral (S1) screws, which should be completed prior to placement of the pelvic fixation.
- Sacral pedicle screws can be placed through either two or three (through the sacral promontory) cortices. Tricortical screws have been shown to have twice the insertional torque of bicortical screws, and this is the preferred technique.[12]
- An awl is used to breach the dorsal cortex of the sacrum at the starting point 1 cm proximal and immediately lateral to the S1 sacral foramen (TECH FIG 1A).
- A slightly curved large pedicle finder (gearshift type) is used to sound the cancellous bone. The path should be directed 30 to 40 degrees anteromedially and 15 degrees cephalad toward the anterior tip of the sacral promontory (TECH FIG 1B).

- The direction toward the anterior tip of the promontory can be estimated from preoperative plain radiographs and confirmed intraoperatively with lateral radiograph or by fluoroscopy prior to placement of the screw (TECH FIG 1C).
- The pilot hole is tapped using a tap size 1 mm less than the screw to be inserted, typically a 6-mm tap is used, and a 7-mm screw is placed (TECH FIG 1D).
- All five boundaries of the screw hole are sounded using a ballpoint probe to verify that the bony cortex has not been breached.
- Screw length is then measured using a depth gauge. Screws are typically placed with a bicortical purchase.
- The screws are then placed under direct visualization.

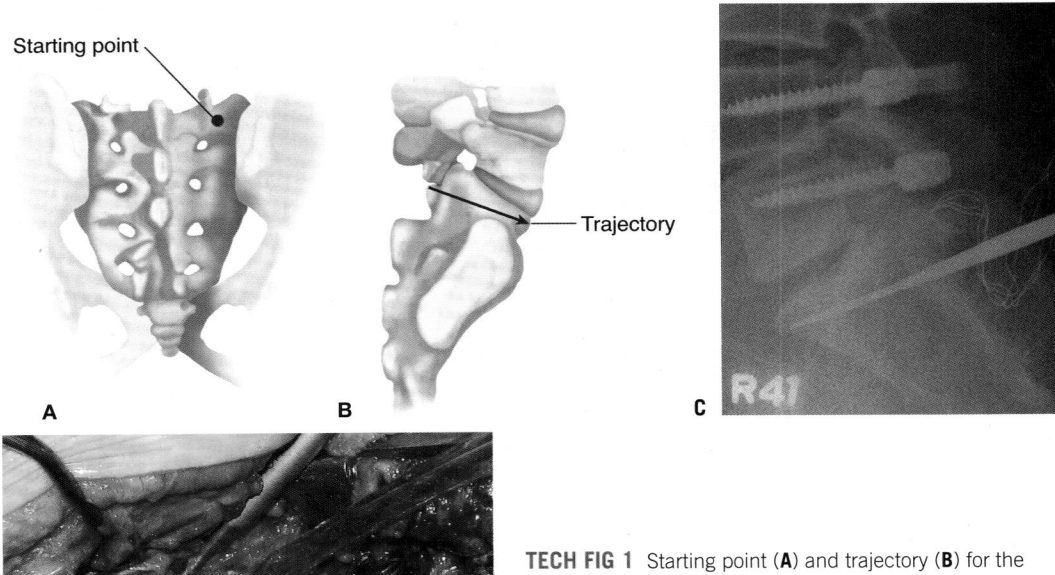

TECH FIG 1 Starting point (**A**) and trajectory (**B**) for the tricortical S1 screws. **C.** Intraoperative lateral radiograph showing the trajectory of the pedicle finder, which is 30 to 40 degrees anteromedially and 15 degrees cephalad toward the anterior tip of the sacral promontory. **D.** Placement of the S1 tricortical screw. The pilot hole is tapped using a tap size 1 mm less than the screw to be inserted, the depth is measured using a ballpoint depth gauge, and an appropriate length screw is placed along the path obtaining a bicortical purchase.

TECHNIQUES

THE GALVESTON L-ROD TECHNIQUE

- Placement of the Galveston rods proceeds after a standard midline exposure to the facet joint. Here, we focus only on those steps necessary for placement of pelvic fixation. Specific steps necessary for placement of the sublaminar wires or pedicle screws or for correction of the deformity in scoliotic or myelodysplastic spines are beyond the scope of this chapter but can be found elsewhere.[1]
- After placement of sublaminar wires or pedicle screws at the spinal segments that are to be instrumented, exposure of the ilium is begun by palpating the PSIS and then dissecting off the subcutaneous tissue from the lumbosacral fascia starting in the midline and proceeding out bilaterally toward the PSIS using Cobb elevators and electrocautery.
- The gluteal musculature should be subperiosteally dissected away from the outer cortex of the ilium until the greater sciatic notch is accessible with a finger.
- A longitudinal or oblique incision is made in the fascia overlying the PSIS.

- A 3/16-inch stainless steel pelvic pin is then driven into the ilium toward the anterior inferior iliac spine (AIIS) to a depth of 6 to 9 cm. The starting point is just posterior to the SI joint at the level of the PSIS. Placement of a finger into the sciatic notch can help guide the pin toward the AIIS.[2]
- The pin is left in place in order to facilitate correct bending of the L-rod, which is a 3/16-inch diameter stainless steel rod.
- The first bend in the L-rod creates the short end, which will be placed into the table of the ilium and can be approximated by placing the short end of the rod parallel to the pelvic pin in the table of the ilium. The second bend turns the long end of the rod cephalad (TECH FIG 2A).
- Next, the pelvic pin is removed, and the short end of the L-rod is driven in-between the two tables of the ilium.
- The long end of the L-rod is then attached to the mobile spine by using the previously placed sublaminar wires (TECH FIG 2B,C).
- Alternatively, some surgeons choose to attach the Galveston rod to the heads of pedicle screws.

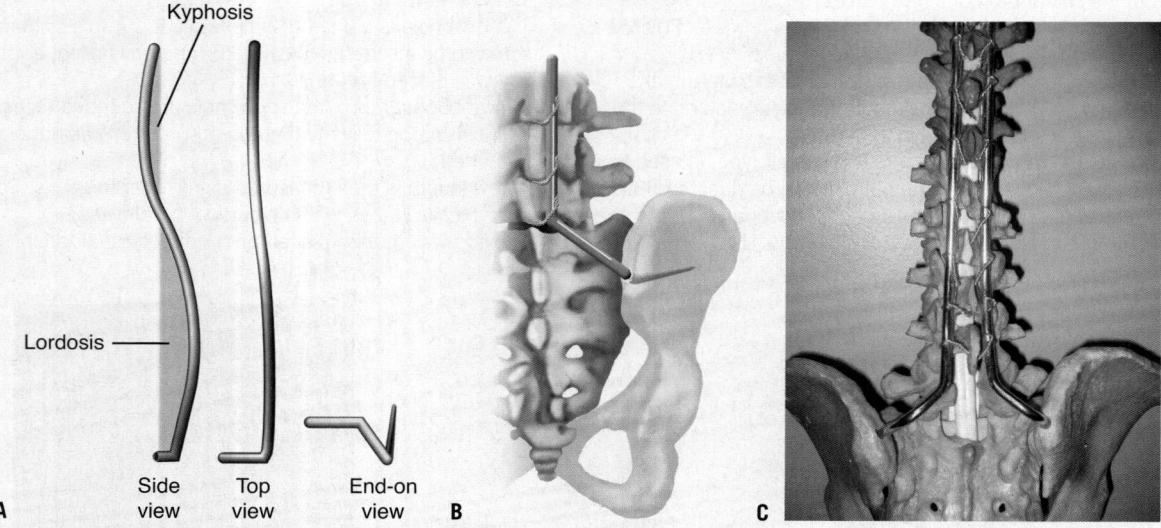

Kyphosis

Lordosis

| Side view | Top view | End-on view |

A   **B**   **C**

TECH FIG 2 A. Appropriate shaping of the L-rod. **B,C.** Line diagram and model, respectively, showing proper placement of the Galveston rod into the table of the ilium.

THE ILIAC SCREW (ILIAC BOLTS) TECHNIQUE

- We recommend that the iliac screw be placed only after other points of fixation, including the S1 screws, have already been completed.
- The PSIS is palpated, and the subcutaneous tissue is dissected off the lumbosacral fascia bilaterally toward the PSIS using Cobb elevators and Bovie electrocautery (TECH FIG 3A).
- A longitudinal or oblique incision is made in the fascia overlying the PSIS.
- The incision is extended both caudally and cephalad along the ilium with respect to the PSIS.

- A rongeur or burr is used to breach the cortex overlying the PSIS, approximately 1 cm from the distal ilium. The amount of bone resected depends on the bulkiness of the implant, and the goal should be to minimize implant prominence.[11]
- With a pedicle seeker or curette, the path into the ilium down toward the AIIS is then developed (TECH FIG 3B).
- The path averages 25 degrees lateral to midsagittal plane and 30 to 35 degrees caudal to the transverse plane toward the ASIS (TECH FIG 3C). Fluoroscopy can be used to confirm the path. Alternatively, placement of a finger into the sciatic

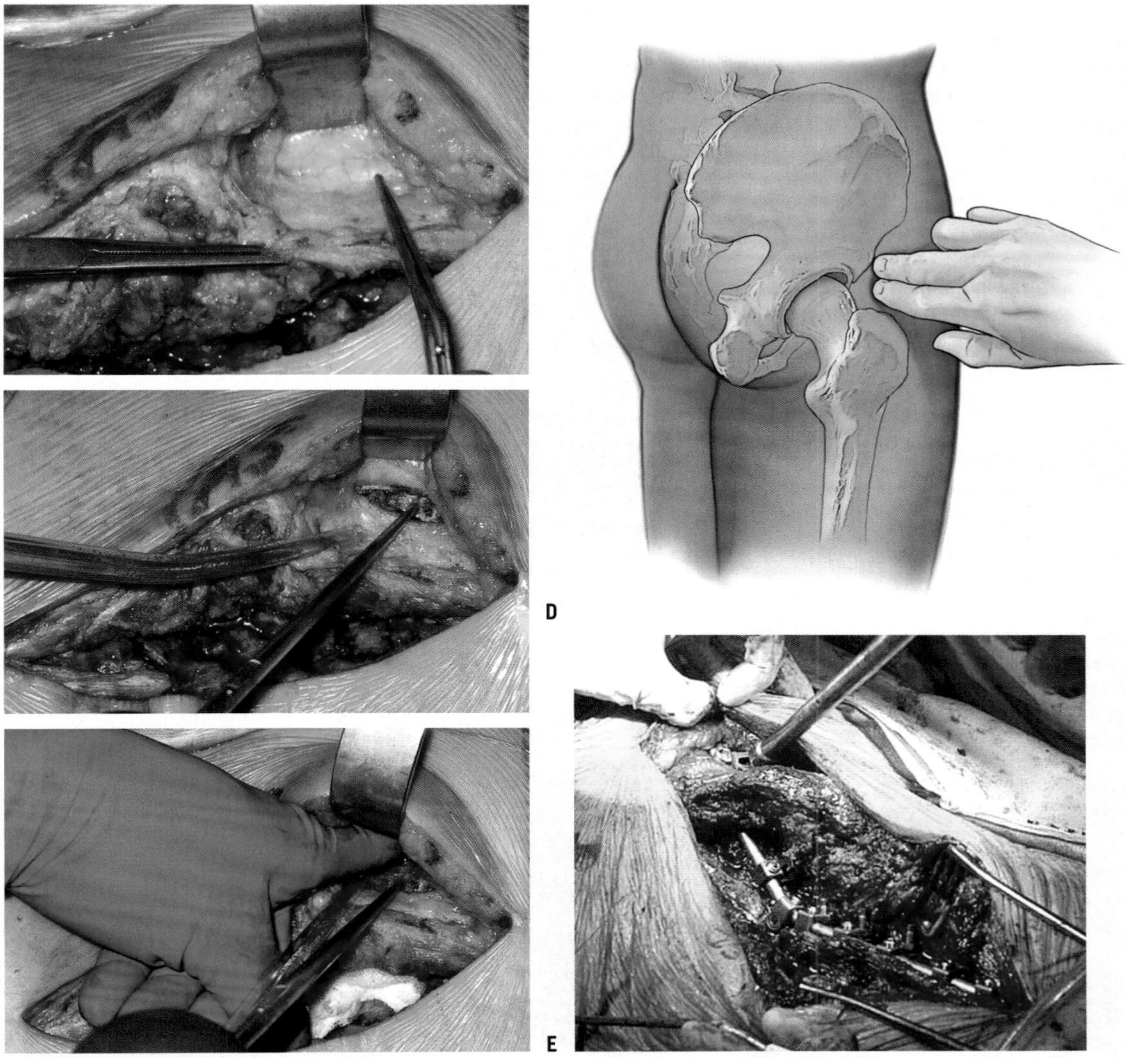

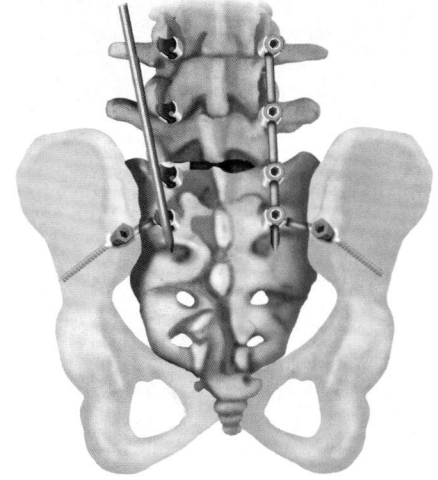

TECH FIG 3 A. Extension of the midline incision out to the PSIS for placement of the iliac screws. The paraspinal muscles are held out of the field with a clamp, and the PSIS is marked by the forceps. An oblique incision is made in the fascia overlying the PSIS. **B.** Subsequently, the pedicle seeker is driven into the table of the ilium, angled toward the ASIS. **C.** Placement of a finger into the greater sciatic notch can help guide the pedicle seeker. **D.** Line diagram of trajectory. **E,F.** The iliac screw is attached to the main spinal construct by using a modular connector system, which is tunneled anterior to the paraspinous muscles. (**B,C,E:** Reprinted with permission from Moshirfar A, Rand FF, Sponseller PD, et al. Pelvic fixation in spine surgery. Historical overview, indications, biomechanical relevance, and current techniques. J Bone Joint Surg Am 2005;87[suppl 2]:89–106. Copyright © 2005 by The Journal of Bone and Joint Surgery, Incorporated.)

TECHNIQUES

notch provides an anatomic landmark that can help guide the path (**TECH FIG 3D**).[15]

- The path is palpated with a ballpoint probe to verify that neither the medial nor lateral iliac crest cortex has been breached.
- Screw lengths are then measured by marking the depth on the ballpoint probe. Common screw sizes are 8 to 10 mm in diameter and 70 to 90 mm in length.
- The screw path is tapped using a handheld tap, and an appropriate length screw based on the measurement is inserted.
- Finally, the screw must then be attached to the longitudinal rods connecting the remaining proximal screws of the main construct by using a modular connectors. The connectors are tunneled anterior to the paraspinal muscles (**TECH FIG 3E,F**).
- Radiographs or C-arm fluoroscopic images may be taken to confirm placement. The trajectory and starting point of the screw should be assessed.
  - For the iliac screw, the starting point should be over the PSIS and directed toward the AIIS, proximal to the sciatic notch.
  - For the S2AI screw, the starting point is midway between S1 and S2 sacral foramina and directed toward the AIIS, using an anteroposterior (AP) view will ensure the cephalad/caudal position; a teardrop view will ensure no breach to the medial or lateral cortices of the ilium.

OPEN S2 ALAR ILIAC TECHNIQUE (AUTHORS' PREFERRED TECHNIQUE)

- When placing the iliac screws using the S2AI technique, inserting the proximal screws, especially the S1 pedicle screw first, helps in guiding the surgeon in accurately planning the lateral/medial starting point for the S2AI screws so as to end with straight in-line anchors at the lumbosacral junction facilitating rod contouring.
- The position of the S1 and S2 dorsal foramina are identified using a Woodson elevator (**TECH FIG 4A**).

- An awl is used to breach the dorsal cortex over the starting point, located in line with the lateral edge of the S1 dorsal foramen and midway between S1 and S2 dorsal foramina (**TECH FIG 4B**).
- In most patients, the S2AI trajectory averages 40 degrees of lateral angulation to the posterior surface of the sacrum and 20 to 30 degrees of caudal angulation in the sagittal planes directed toward the AIIS (**TECH FIG 4C,D**).

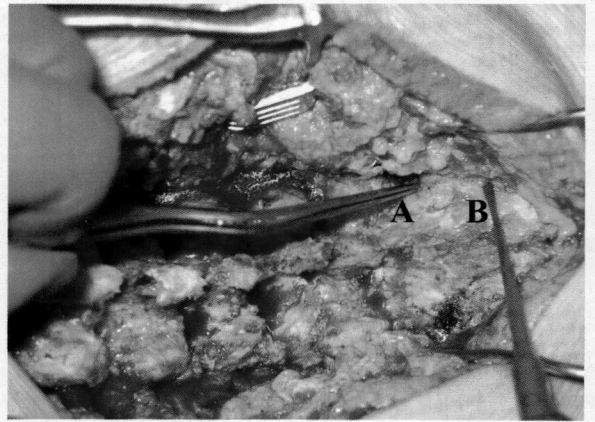

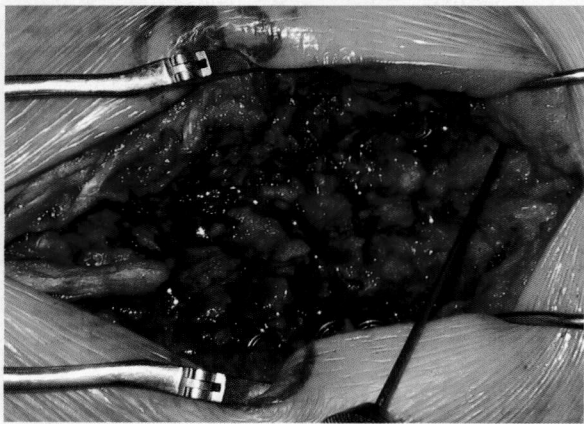

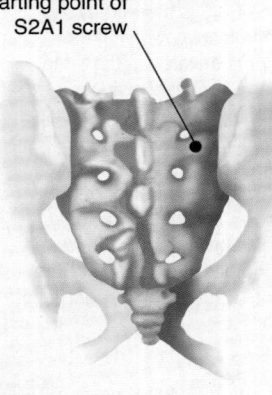

Starting point of S2A1 screw

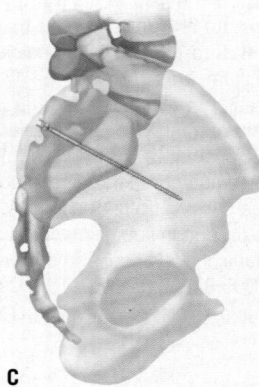

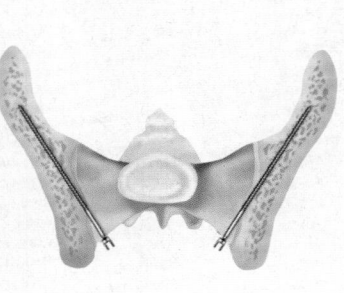

TECH FIG 4 **A.** Standard midline exposure. Probes mark the location of the S1 and S2 dorsal sacral foramina at points *A* and *B*, respectively. **B.** Starting point for the S2AI screw. **C,D.** Sagittal and coronal views, respectively, of the final trajectory of the S2AI screw. **E.** A drill is used to go across the SI joint. *(continued)*

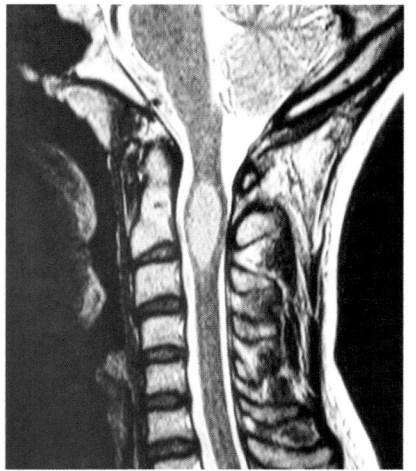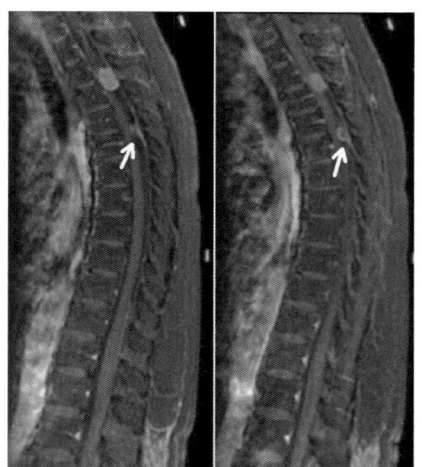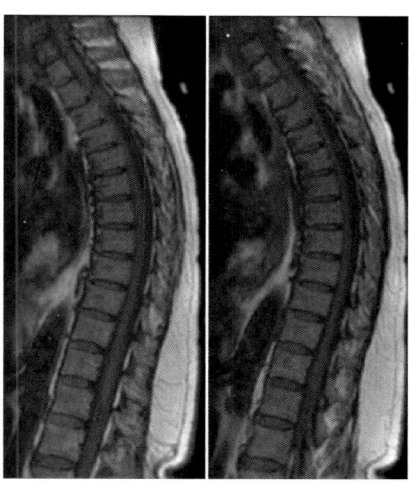

FIG 1 A. Ependymoma on contrast-enhanced MRI. **B,C.** T1-weighted MRIs with and without contrast, respectively. Intradural extramedullary meningioma enhanced with contrast. Note dural tail sign (*arrows* in **B**).

NONOPERATIVE MANAGEMENT

- Asymptomatic patients with minimal or no upper motor neuron signs can be watched closely with serial neurologic and MRI examination.
- Patients with lumbar intradural tumors that are asymptomatic can similarly be watched carefully, but one needs to make sure that even subtle signs of lower motor neuron bladder dysfunction are in fact not present.

SURGICAL MANAGEMENT

Intradural Extramedullary Tumors

- The indications to proceed with surgical resection of intradural tumors of the spine include severe, progressive axial, or radicular pain; progressive weakness due to nerve root compression or involvement; myelopathic symptoms of an upper motor neuron bladder, spastic gait disturbance, incoordination of the upper extremities, generalized weakness, and sensory loss or disturbance; and/or progressive enlargement of an asymptomatic lesion.

Preoperative Planning

- Surgery for intradural extramedullary tumors is usually done via a posterior approach. The amount of bone removal (laminectomy vs. transpedicular vs. costotransversectomy) is dependent on tumor location within the spinal canal and should be planned with the goal of maximizing tumor visualization while minimizing spinal cord manipulation.
- Preoperative intravenous antibiotics with good central nervous system penetration such as Nafcillin or Ancef are administered within 1 hour of the skin incision. Consider steroid administration as well.
- Strongly consider the use of neuromonitoring (somatosensory evoked potentials, motor evoked potentials, D-wave) to optimize extent of resection while minimizing risk of permanent neurologic deficit.
- The need for fusion should also be considered in patients undergoing resection of intradural tumors. Patients who require removal of a joint or pedicle to access ventral pathology, surgery spanning junctional levels, or multilevel laminectomy

(three or more) in the cervical spine may be at increased risk for kyphotic deformity in the absence of stabilization.

Positioning

- Patients with tumors located between the skull base and the upper thoracic spine (approximately T4–T5) are positioned on chest rolls on a regular operating room table with the head in the table-mounted, three-pin head holder or using an open Jackson frame with C-Flex attachment.
- A slightly flexed position is used for most cervical tumors.
- If posterior fusion with instrumentation is planned, a more neutral sagittal position is preferred.
- Mid- and lower thoracic as well as lumbar tumors can be positioned using an open Jackson frame.
- Consider placement of arterial line and urethral catheter.

Intradural Intramedullary Spinal Cord Tumors

Preoperative Planning

- The most common tumor types encountered within the parenchyma of the spinal cord are ependymoma, astrocytoma, hemangioblastoma, and lipoma.
- The presenting symptoms of intramedullary tumors are less radicular and mostly myelopathic.
- Deep axial or radicular pain is uncommon. Numbness, spasticity, disturbance of bladder function, and quadriparesis are most commonly the presenting symptoms.
- Needle biopsy is not recommended due to the risk of spinal cord injury and hemorrhage. Therefore, open biopsy and resection are the standard practice for primary intramedullary tumors.
- Patients should be counseled extensively regarding the much higher risk and expectation of new postoperative deficits compared with extramedullary tumors.
- Almost all patients will experience some degree of new or increased sensory or motor disturbance as a result of removal of an intramedullary spinal cord tumor.
- In the early postoperative state, it is difficult to ascertain what new deficits will be transient and which changes may be permanent. Most patients, however, experience improvement of new neurologic findings over time. Some patients

will have new permanent deficits, and in some patients, there will be progressive neurologic deficits as seen in patients with a malignant, incompletely resected astrocytoma of the spinal cord. Often, these tumors respond poorly to radiation therapy and chemotherapy.

Positioning

- Positioning is essentially identical to that performed for extramedullary tumors; bone removal for intramedullary tumor removal can usually be limited to laminectomy.
- The dural opening is usually made in the midline regardless of the eccentricity of the tumor within the spinal cord.

- Although the techniques of internal debulking and tumor capsule dissection are fairly consistent with all solid extramedullary tumors, the strategies of resection for intramedullary tumors vary with tumor type.
- MRI characteristics of the tumor preoperatively usually allow the surgeon to anticipate whether there is going to be a demarcation between tumor capsule and spinal cord tissue (as with ependymoma), or whether there is going to be a diffuse blending of tumor tissue with the spinal cord tissue at the periphery of the tumor (astrocytoma, lipoma), or whether there is a large cystic area containing a smaller mural nodule of tumor (hemangioblastoma).

MICROSURGICAL RESECTION OF INTRADURAL EXTRAMEDULLARY TUMORS

TECHNIQUES

Incision and Exposure

- After the skin preparation, a midline incision is made and a subperiosteal exposure of the spine is accomplished.
- The dural opening for most intradural extramedullary tumors will usually need to include a lamina above and below the pathology, so the number of laminae to be removed is usually clear from the sagittal and axial MRI or CT myelogram images. Some surgeons may use intraoperative ultrasound to confirm tumor location prior to dural opening.
- The dural opening is usually midline, but the opening can be paramedian in patients with tumors eccentric to one side.
- Large schwannomas and neurofibromas will often be visible on exposure as a dura-covered mass extending out and expanding the neural foramen. In these cases, the dural opening is often lateral, with a T-shape extension of the midline opening.
- As with all tumors located in or extending out laterally to the neural foramina in the cervical spine, the location of the vertebral artery must be clearly known from preoperative imaging studies. This artery is most commonly displaced anteriorly and can remain patent.
- In such cases, the vertebral artery can almost always be spared following resection.
- For tumors in which the vertebral artery is encased within the mass of the tumor, consideration can be given to preoperative endovascular test occlusion and subsequent obliteration via coiling/embolization.

Resection

- Once the dura is opened, the microscope is brought into the field.
- For extramedullary tumors such as schwannoma, neurofibroma, and meningioma, the essential techniques of tumor removal consist of internal debulking of the tumor, delicate dissection of the tumor capsule from the pial surface of the spinal cord, and meticulous sparing and protection of surrounding nerve rootlets.
- An ultrasonic aspirator is most useful for internal debulking of these tumors.
- The surgeon must be careful to avoid going through the capsule of the tumor.
- It is helpful to pause from resection every few minutes and three-dimensionally reassess the extent of tumor mass remaining by careful palpation and manipulation of the tumor capsule and remaining tumor mass using microinstruments.
- All three of these tumor types typically allow for successful peeling of the final capsule off of the pial surface of the spinal cord.

- In cases in which the tumor capsule is very adherent to the pial surface or to the surface of posterior or ventral nerve rootlets, the surgeon may elect to leave behind that material and coagulate it with bipolar cautery.
- With large, ventral dural-based (meningioma) or nerve root sleeve tumors, it is usually necessary to cut the denticulate ligaments at the equator of the spinal cord. This should be done at several levels so that manipulation of tumor does not result in excessive torquing of the spinal cord tissue in a small area.
- Microscopic monofilament suture (eg, 6-0, 8-0 Prolene [Ethicon, Inc., Somerville, NJ]) can be placed through the base of the denticulate ligaments to provide a means of gently rotating the spinal cord.
- If rotation is necessary to gain access to large ventral tumors, then the denticulate ligament should be released over several levels (not just in the vicinity of the tumor).
- Blood pressure should be maintained at normal levels and, if used, motor evoked and somatosensory evoked potentials can be checked at regular intervals during and following tumor resection.
- Changes in neuromonitoring during rotation of the spinal cord can allow the surgeon to release the traction to help prevent injury.
- In removal of a meningioma, the surgeon should assess the location of the dural attachment and decide whether dural resection and patching is possible or whether coagulation (alone) of the area is best.
- Ideally, resection of the area of dura from which the tumor arose provides the best protection against recurrence. Local fascia or lyophilized bovine pericardium or synthetic materials can be used for sewing in a patch.
- With final removal of a schwannoma, all nerve fibers that are not the source of the tumor are carefully dissected off the capsule and preserved. Those that clearly enter the bulk of the tumor are cut and removed with the tumor.
- Prior to final closure, meticulous inspection for bleeding is performed. One should limit the amount of bipolar coagulation of pial blood vessels. Often, holding a thrombin-soaked collagen sponge with gentle pressure over a small bleeding venule or arteriole is sufficient to stop microscopic hemorrhage.
- The dural is then closed with a running (locking or unlocked) monofilament or braided nylon or Prolene suture. Interrupted dural closure is also acceptable. Fibrin glue or other synthetic glue products are often used to reinforce the suture closure.
- The adjuvant use of external lumbar cerebrospinal fluid draining is up to the judgment of the surgeon and may be helpful particularly in cases where weeping of cerebrospinal fluid is seen despite a good suture closure of the dura.

MICROSCOPIC RESECTION OF INTRAMEDULLARY TUMORS

Incision and Exposure

- One important decision involves where to enter the spinal cord. For tumors that come to the pial surface, it is obviously safest to enter there.
- Many tumors, however, have normal spinal cord tissue between the tumor and the pial surface. They may be eccentric to one side.
- For centrally located tumors, a midline myelotomy should be considered (**TECH FIG 1**).
- For eccentric tumors that do not come to the surface, the dorsal root entry zone should be considered.
- Ultrasound can be helpful in assessing the location and outline of the tumor. The pia is coagulated using microbipolars at low settings, and a no. 11 blade scalpel or microscissors are used to open the pial layer.
- Microinstruments are then used to gently tease open the tissue from inside out, working up and down along the extent of the tumor and respecting the cephalocaudal orientation of the long tracts.

Resection

- With an ependymoma, the tumor capsule will be a distinctly different color (gray-red) than the surrounding white spinal cord parenchyma (**TECH FIG 2A**).
- When a portion of the tumor capsule has been exposed, the capsule is coagulated and incised with a no. 11 blade scalpel.
- The ultrasonic aspirator and hand instruments such as cupped forceps or micropituitary rongeur are used to internally debulk the tumor tissue.
- A portion should be sent for frozen section analysis.
- The important step in internal debulking of an ependymoma is making sure that one does not penetrate the capsule because there is often normal tissue ventral and lateral to the capsule (**TECH FIG 2B**).
- With this tumor type, there is almost always a ventrally located artery supplying the tumor that one will encounter and need to coagulate as the final, ventral portions of the capsule are resected (**TECH FIG 2C**).
- Small Cottonoid patties (Codman, Warsaw, IN) are very useful in "claiming territory," as the capsule becomes soft and floppy. Multiple Cottonoids placed between the capsule and the tumor tissue serve as further protection against instrument damage. Gross total removal of an ependymoma is often feasible.
- With a spinal cord astrocytoma, the demarcation between tumor tissue and spinal cord parenchyma is often difficult to identify.

- The goals of surgery are different from an ependymoma removal where gross total resection can be achieved.
- With an astrocytoma, the surgeon must carefully judge the appearance of the tumor tissue under the microscope. Clearly, abnormal tissue that is more yellow or gray can usually be safely removed without devastating consequences.
- Once the demarcation is no longer clear, one should consider avoiding further tumor removal, as it can lead to permanent neurologic deficit.
- In cases where the frozen section results show a high-grade (malignant) astrocytoma or glioblastoma, then the prognosis is very poor and the risk of creating devastating neurologic loss may not be of value to the patient.
- Spinal cord lipomas are usually solid, bright yellow tissue, and easily distinguished from normal spinal cord parenchyma.
- In rare cases, the tumor mass may be discovered to be in liquid, oily form rather than solid tissue. These tumors usually are visible on the pial surface and can even be exophytic, but ventrally and laterally, the fatty tissue can blend in with the normal parenchyma. Thus, gross total resections may not be

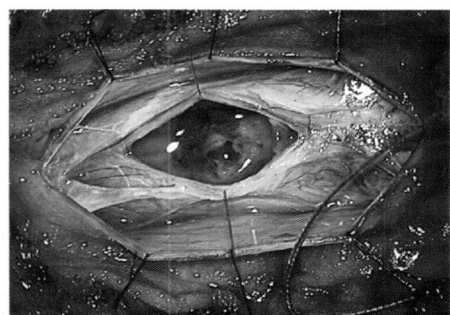

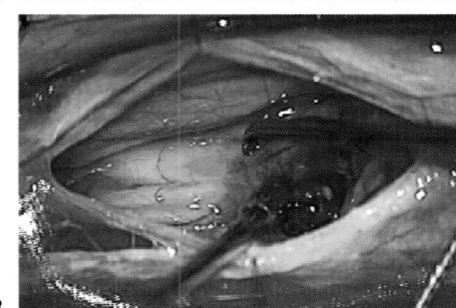

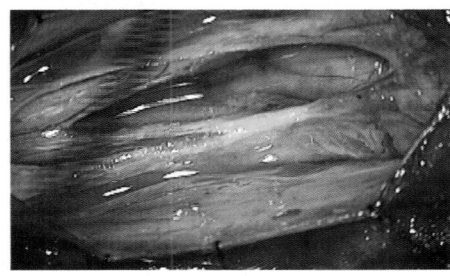

TECH FIG 2 A. Myelotomy complete, exposing tumor mass within parenchyma of the spinal cord. Small pia–arachnoid sutures can be seen superiorly and inferiorly holding open myelotomy. **B.** Final portions of tumor being removed with normal spinal cord tissue at base of cavity within spinal cord. **C.** Tumor removed, pial sutures released.

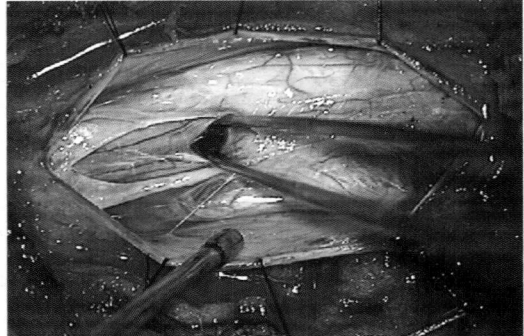

TECH FIG 1 Initial dissection of the arachnoid, preparing for midline myelotomy. Note dural tack-up sutures.

possible without the increased risk of neurologic injury. Often, a small rim of lipomatous tissue is left behind.

- With cystic hemangioblastomas, the surrounding spinal cord tissue does not necessarily have to be opened along the entire extent of the cystic cavity.
- Attention is paid to where the mural nodule of tumor is located.
- The myelotomy should be performed closest to the level where the nodule is located, and often, only a portion of the cystic

cavity is exposed that allows adequate visualization of the tumor.

- Vessels identified under magnification that are feeding and draining the tumor are coagulated and cut, and the tumor can often be dissected off of the wall of the cystic cavity.
- The fluid of the cavity typically drains out spontaneously after working and irrigating during tumor removal. Meticulous hemostasis (as always) is confirmed prior to dural closure.

TECHNIQUES

Pearls and Pitfalls

- The essence of surgery for removal of intradural extramedullary tumors is internal debulking of the tumor and careful dissection of tumor capsule from the pial surface of the spinal cord.
- In removing intradural intramedullary tumors of the spinal cord, preoperative knowledge of the anatomic characteristics such as the presence of a cyst, the sharpness of demarcation on imaging of the tumor, the presence of a mural nodule, etc, all help guide the surgeon in deciding the location of the initial myelotomy and the approach to the tumor.
- With ventral intradural extramedullary tumors, multiple levels of release of the denticulate ligaments are helpful to rotate the spinal cord and increase tumor visualization.
- When dissecting or manipulating normal or tumor tissue, use fine, slow movements to minimize tissue trauma.
- Always dissect during the initial myelotomy with the idea of the cephalocaudal orientation of the long tracts.
- Avoid using coagulation on normal pial vessels (gently apply Gelfoam sponge [Baxter Healthcare Corp., Hayward, CA] and micro-Cottonoid and, most bleeding will stop in tiny vessels).
- Frequently zoom out and take in the larger picture of how far along the tumor resection has progressed.
- The "backside" or "side walls" of the tumor or tumor capsule will come up faster than you think; avoid breaching that final layer of tumor tissue and injuring normal tissue on the blind side of the tumor.

POSTOPERATIVE CARE

- Intensive care unit observation of immediate postoperative patients is recommended following resection of an intradural intramedullary or extramedullary spinal cord tumor so that blood pressure can be monitored, and frequent neurologic examinations can be performed to identify those rare patients with a complication such as a postoperative epidural or intramedullary hemorrhage.
- The use of corticosteroids is at the discretion of the surgeon.
- External cerebrospinal fluid diversion via a lumbar intrathecal drain may be used.
  - Patients with cervical or upper thoracic tumors can be nursed in a partially upright or sitting position, as this will decrease the cerebrospinal fluid pressure in the area of the dural closure.
  - Lower thoracic (and lumbar) tumor patients are often kept at flat bed rest, although no guidelines exist for this issue, and the decision is at the discretion of the surgeon.
  - Progressive mobilization and ambulation can begin very soon after surgery or a period of bed rest.

COMPLICATIONS

- The most concerning complication is quadriplegia, and this may occur even when very delicate handling of spinal cord and tumor tissue has been performed. This complication can sometimes not be avoided, but short amplitude; delicate movements of the microinstruments; maintenance of

normal blood pressure and oxygenation; and preservation of normal arteries, arterioles, veins, and venules are of great importance.

- Postoperative intramedullary hemorrhage is rare and meticulous confirmation of hemostasis while under the microscope is essential; risk is higher with incompletely resected tumors.
- Cerebrospinal fluid leak is a more common complication. Attention to watertight closure suturing technique is important, and many surgeons use various forms of fibrin glue or synthetic materials to help seal the suture closure.
- In patients with thin or easily torn dura and/or leaking of cerebrospinal fluid through the suture holes, postoperative external cerebrospinal fluid drainage via a lumbar intrathecal catheter can be helpful. Three to 5 days of drainage in those patients is commonly practiced.

SUGGESTED READINGS

Angevine PD, Kellner C, Hague RM, et al. Surgical management of ventral intradural spinal lesions. J Neurosurg Spine 2011;15(1):28–37.

Boström A, von Lehe M, Hartmann W, et al. Surgery for spinal cord ependymomas: outcome and prognostic factors. Neurosurgery 2011; 68(2):302–308.

Kucia EJ, Bambakidis NC, Chang SW, et al. Surgical technique and outcomes in the treatment of spinal cord ependymomas, part 1: intramedullary ependymomas. Neurosurgery 2011;68(1 suppl):57–63.

Kucia EJ, Maughan PH, Kakarla UK, et al. Surgical technique and outcomes in the treatment of spinal cord ependymomas: part II: myxopapillary ependymoma. Neurosurgery 2011;68(1 suppl):90–94.

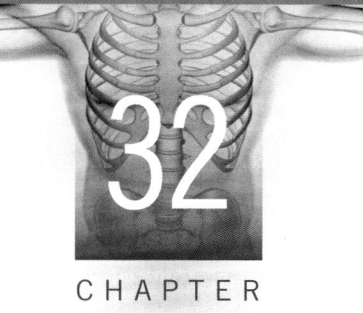

32

CHAPTER

Approaches
Anterior Cervical Approaches

John Heflin and John M. Rhee

GENERAL CONSIDERATIONS

Anterior Approach (Smith-Robinson)

- The approach chosen depends on a number of factors, including the spinal segments that must be exposed, the nature of the procedure to be performed, and the patient's body habitus.
- In general, the Smith-Robinson approach allows access from C2 down to T1 in most patients. However, local variations in patient morphology may either limit or increase the extent of available exposure.
- Ease of access to the C2–C3 disc depends on the location of the mandible and can be assessed on the preoperative lateral radiograph.
- Nasal intubation is preferable when approaching this level as it allows the mandible to be maximally closed, away from the line of sight of the disc.
  - Depending on the location of the mandible with respect to C3–C4, nasal intubation may be preferable in certain instances of C3–C4 access as well.
- For pathology at C7–T1 or distal, careful scrutiny of the disc space with respect to the sternal notch on lateral radiographs will help to assess whether a sternal-splitting approach may be necessary.
  - In some patients with long necks, access to T2 or even T3 may be possible with a standard Smith-Robinson approach.
  - In those with short or stocky necks, even getting to C7 may be a challenge (**FIG 1**).

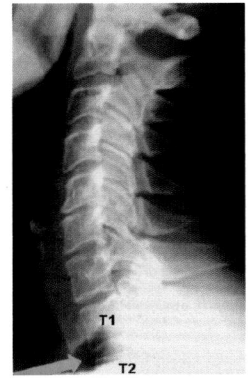
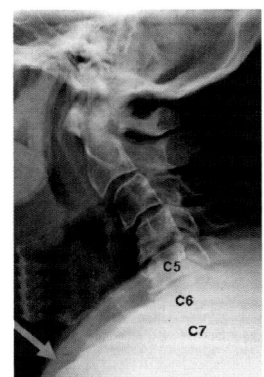

FIG 1 Long versus short necks. **A.** In patients with long necks, anterior exposure through a standard Smith-Robinson approach readily provides far distal access (eg, down to T1–T2 disc space [*arrow*]). **B.** In those with short necks, however, even getting to C6–C7 may be difficult if the sternum blocks the necessary trajectory to the disc space (*arrow*), although it can almost always be done.

- Imaging studies should be evaluated for anatomic variations such as medial aberrancy of the vertebral artery.
- Considerable debate exists whether the "sidedness" of approach affects the rate of postoperative recurrent laryngeal nerve palsy. The literature is not conclusive but suggests higher rates with right-sided approaches.
  - If a patient has had prior neck surgery and it is desirable to approach the spine from the opposite side to avoid scar, a preoperative indirect laryngoscopy should be performed by ear, nose, and throat consultation to rule out a recurrent laryngeal nerve palsy.
  - If one exists, the spine must be approached from the side of the injury to avoid the possibility of bilateral vocal cord palsy. If one does not exist, the spine can be approached from either side.

Lateral Retropharyngeal Approach (Whitesides)

- This approach can be used for anterior access to the upper cervical spine but not the basiocciput.
- It is often used for high cervical bony lesions, including tumors or infections for which a posterior approach is not possible, unstable fractures or dislocations with deficient or incompetent posterior elements, or posterior nonunions (particularly for fusions of C1–C2).
- It is also useful for access to high cervical ventral or ventrolateral intradural lesions such as neurofibromas or meningiomas.
- It allows unilateral access from C1 to C3. Access to the far contralateral side requires a second approach.
- Potential complications include injury to the spinal accessory nerve and the vertebral artery. The jugular vein also lies within the operative field and can be a site of significant bleeding if inadvertently injured.
- Significant retropharyngeal swelling has occurred and can result in prolongation of intubation if the patient's airway becomes obstructed.

Anterior Approach to the Cervicothoracic Junction (Transmanubrial–Transclavicular Approach)

- There are several different approaches for exposing the cervicothoracic junction, including the transmanubrial–transclavicular and the sternal-splitting (median sternotomy) approaches.
  - The sternal-splitting (median sternotomy) approach may be useful in providing improved distal access to the upper thoracic spine.

- Deep dissection is essentially the same for the two approaches.
  - Cranial to caudal dissection is recommended to avoid injury to the major crossing vessels distally (eg, the left brachiocephalic vein).
- With a left-sided approach, the thoracic duct is at greater risk. It passes into the left venous angle between the subclavian artery and the common carotid artery.
- With a right-sided approach, the recurrent laryngeal nerve is at greater risk because of its greater variability versus the left side where the nerve is more constant in its location in the tracheoesophageal groove.

POSITIONING

Anterior Approach (Smith-Robinson)

- The patient is positioned supine with the neck slightly extended.
- The amount of extension tolerated by the patient without developing neurologic symptoms should be assessed preoperatively and not exceeded during positioning **(FIG 2)**.
- A bump (eg, rolled sheets) under the shoulders facilitates gentle extension of the spine.

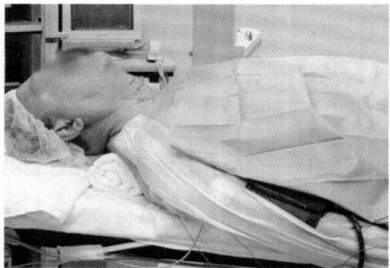

FIG 2 Positioning. Especially in patients with myelopathy, the amount of preoperative extension tolerated without worsening of neurologic symptoms should be assessed and never exceeded during positioning. A rolled sheet is placed under the scapulae to help gently extend the neck.

- A halter or Gardner-Wells tongs is optional but not routinely necessary for anterior cervical discectomy and fusion surgery.
- A foam doughnut is placed behind the occiput to prevent pressure necrosis.
- The head is placed in neutral rotation. Doing so provides landmarks (the nose and the sternal notch) that are in line with the longitudinal axis of the spine for orientation during decompression and instrumentation.
- Depending on the relationship of the mandible to the upper cervical spine, proximal approaches to C2–C3 may be easier if the head is gently rotated away from the side of the approach.
  - The amount of rotation should be kept in mind to prevent disorientation during surgery.
- The shoulders are gently taped down to facilitate intraoperative radiographic visualization.
  - Excessive force should be avoided when taping down the shoulders to avoid brachial plexus injuries.
- Spinal cord monitoring (eg, somatosensory evoked potentials and motor evoked potentials) can be used to help prevent positioning-related nerve injuries, but it is not completely sensitive in detecting injury.

Lateral Retropharyngeal Approach (Whitesides)

- The patient is placed supine with the head turned away from the side from which the approach will be performed unless the patient is constrained in a halo for instability.
  - If this is the case, the exposure will be more challenging but still possible.
- Nasotracheal intubation opposite the side of the approach is desirable as it allows the jaw to be fully closed, offering the least inhibited exposure.
- The pinna (earlobe) can be retracted forward and sewn anteriorly to allow better access to the styloid process and posterior ear area.
- The entire cervical region and lower face is prepared and draped.

ANTERIOR APPROACH (SMITH-ROBINSON)

Incision and Superficial Dissection

- A transverse incision placed in a skin crease is more cosmetic and suffices for accessing three or more disc levels in most instances.
  - A longitudinal incision, although less cosmetic, allows for a more extensile approach (C2–thoracic spine) and may be considered when three or more discs require access or if the patient has a very thick, muscular neck.
- The incision is made using palpable anterior structures as a guide (ie, C3 hyoid bone, C4–C5 thyroid cartilage, C6 carotid tubercle, C7 cricoid cartilage) **(TECH FIG 1A)**.
  - The preoperative lateral radiograph can also be used to determine roughly where to make the incision to allow optimal access to the desired disc(s).
  - The surgeon should try to make the incision such that it will be in line with the "line of sight" of the intended disc space **(TECH FIG 1B)**.

- Transverse incisions may extend from the anterior two-thirds of the sternocleidomastoid (SCM) to the midline.
- Longer incisions and greater tissue mobilization facilitate multilevel procedures and will heal with a nearly imperceptible scar if placed within a natural skin crease.
- Vertical incisions, if used, are placed along the medial border of the SCM.
- The incision is continued through the subcutaneous fat to the platysma **(TECH FIG 1C)**.
  - After dividing the platysma, blunt dissection with scissors undermines the edges of the platysma.
  - This allows for greater mobilization of the soft tissues, which is helpful in accessing multiple disc levels and getting enough exposure to place plates and screws.
- Superficial veins crossing the field of dissection may need to be ligated to facilitate exposure **(TECH FIG 1D)**.

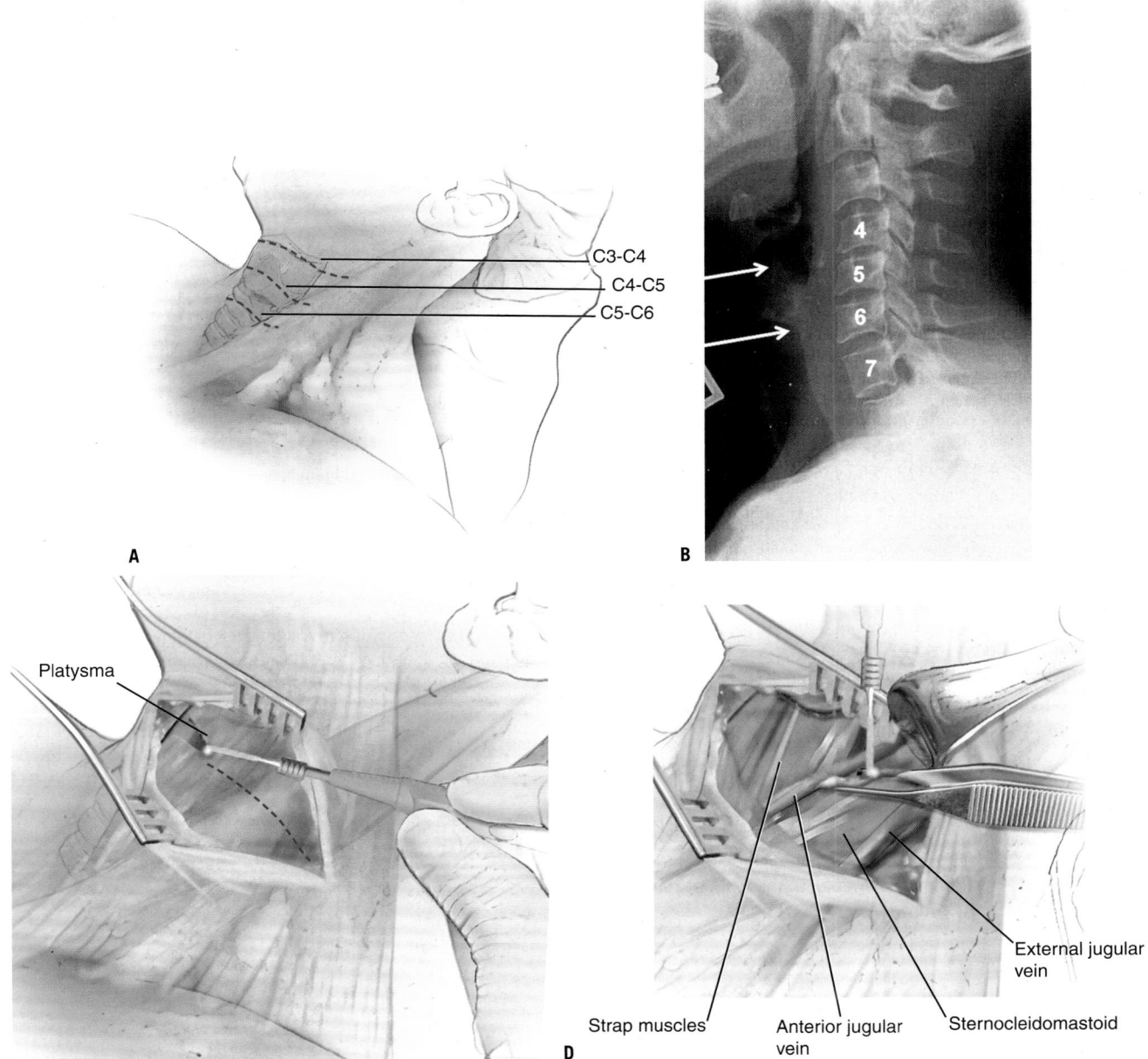

TECH FIG 1 Incision. **A.** The location of the incision is determined by palpating for known landmarks. Generally, these landmarks overlie specific vertebrae or disc spaces such as the hyoid bone (C3), thyroid cartilage (C4–C5), cricoid cartilage (C7), and carotid tubercle (C6). **B.** Alternatively, by looking at the preoperative lateral radiograph, one can estimate the optimal location for the skin incision. (*Top arrow* indicates the C4–C5 approach; *bottom arrow*, the C5–C7 approach.) **C.** The incision is continued through the subcutaneous fat to the platysma. Platysma is then divided. **D.** The surgeon should avoid injuring crossing structures when possible. Superficial veins crossing the field of dissection may need to be ligated to facilitate exposure, however.

Deep Dissection

- The anterior border of the SCM is identified.
- Blunt dissection is then carried through the deep cervical fascia directly medial to the SCM.
- The SCM is retracted laterally to allow palpation and identification of the carotid artery **(TECH FIG 2A)**.
  - The carotid artery should be visualized and will form the lateral border of the approach; the esophagus will define the medial border of the approach.

- Once the carotid is identified, a plane through the pretracheal fascia lying between the carotid sheath and the medial structures (thyroid gland, trachea, and esophagus) is created **(TECH FIG 2B)**.
  - Finger dissection in this plane is useful in allowing extensile exposure.

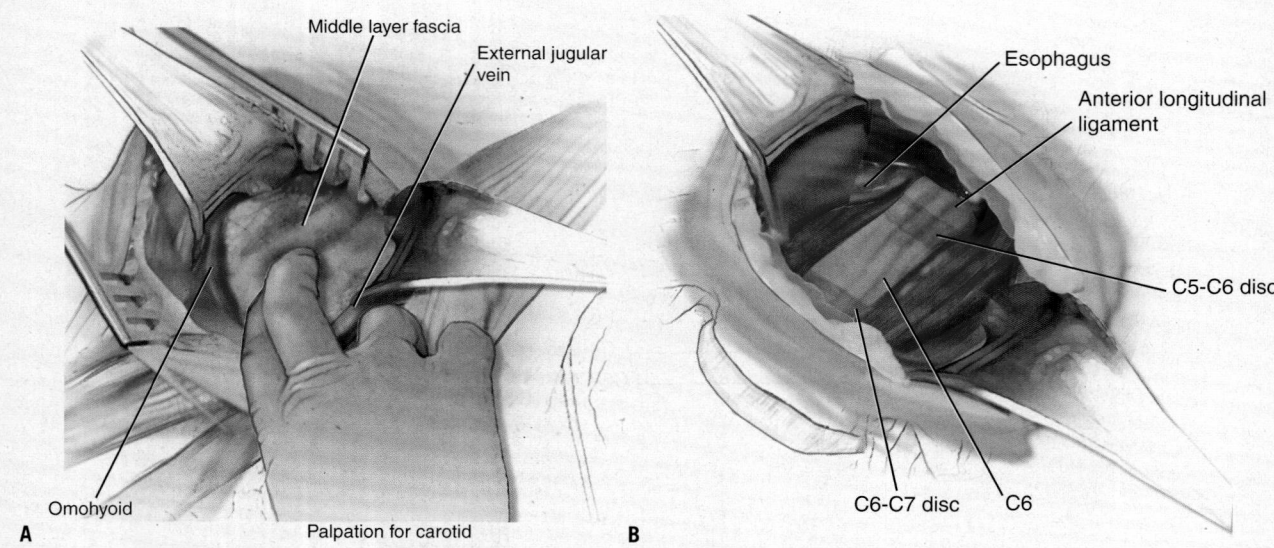

TECH FIG 2 A. The SCM is retracted laterally using blunt retractors. This will allow palpation and identification of the carotid artery. **B.** After the carotid artery is identified, a plane is created between the carotid sheath and the medial structures (thyroid gland, trachea, and esophagus). Blunt dissection techniques are most effective in developing this plane.

Extending the Exposure

- If surgery involves one level, minimal mobilization may be necessary. If the surgery involves multiple levels or the skin incision is not collinear with the desired disc space, greater mobilization is helpful.
- In general, crossing structures should be preserved, if possible, to avoid potential injury to neural structures (eg, laryngeal nerves). Blunt dissection with scissors, Kittners, or fingers works best.
  - The superior thyroid vessels typically overlie C3–C4, and the inferior thyroid vessels generally overlie C6–C7.
- The omohyoid is encountered crossing distal lateral to cephalomedial in the interval medial to the SCM at roughly the C6 level. It can be divided with electrocautery or left intact.
- Dividing the omohyoid will allow for a more extensile cephalocaudal exposure and less tension on the wound for easier placement of plates and screws in multilevel or very distal constructs.

Elevation of Longus Colli and Identification of Levels

- Using bipolar electrocautery, subperiosteal elevation of the longus colli should be done to the level of the uncinate processes bilaterally and at least from the midportion of the vertebral body above to the midportion of the body below the level for which discectomy is planned (**TECH FIG 3A**).
- Time and care spent on carefully elevating the longus colli facilitates proper, stable placement of self-retaining retractors, which in turn facilitates decompression and accurate placement of hardware.

- Retractor blades are then placed beneath the elevated longus colli (**TECH FIG 3B**).
  - Careful placement of retractors will help avoid injury to the esophagus and sympathetic chain (which runs along the ventral surface of the longus colli).
- The plane of dissection for the Smith-Robinson approach is shown in a cross-sectional view at the C5 level in **TECH FIG 3C**.
- Location of the appropriate level should be ensured by intraoperative radiographs before disruption of the disc.

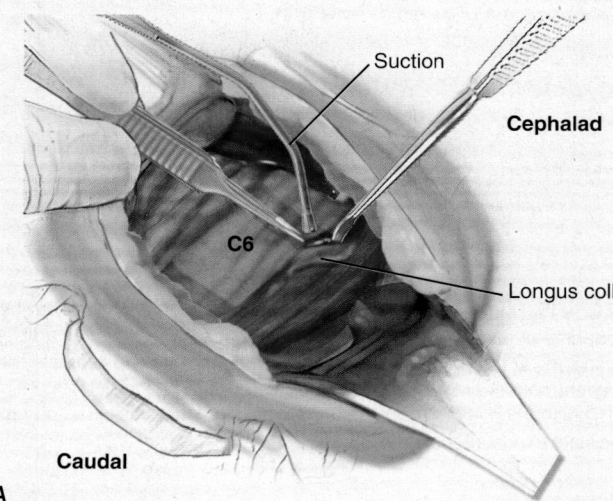

TECH FIG 3 A. Bipolar electrocautery is used to elevate the longus colli in a subperiosteal fashion to the level of the uncinate processes bilaterally. *(continued)*

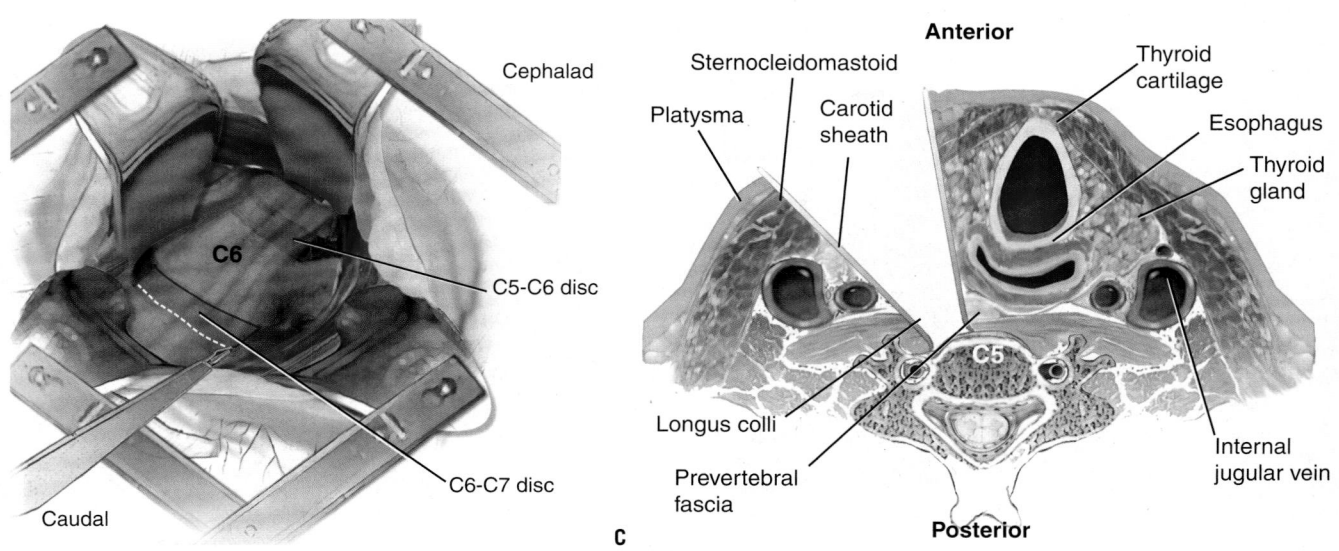

B **C**

TECH FIG 3 *(continued)* **B.** Self-retaining retractors can be placed beneath the elevated longus colli to allow an unimpeded view of the anterior spine. Care should be taken to avoid injuring the esophagus and sympathetic chain during placement of the retractors. The use of cephalad/caudal retractors is optimal but not necessary in most cases. **C.** A cross-sectional view through the neck at C5 demonstrating the plane of dissection.

LATERAL RETROPHARYNGEAL APPROACH (WHITESIDES)

Incision and Superficial Dissection

- A transverse incision is extended from the mastoid tip, posterior to the ear, and is carried along the inferior border of the mandible, preferably in a natural skin crease.
- The incision is then directed caudally along the anterior border of the SCM **(TECH FIG 4A)**.

- This incision can be extended as needed according to the amount of distal cervical spine exposure required. It can be carried as far as the sternal notch.
- The incision is then carried through the subcutaneous tissues and platysma muscle using electrocautery.
- Dissection is carried out using blunt dissection techniques in the subplatysmal plane, allowing the creation of superior–anterior and inferior–posterior musculocutaneous flaps **(TECH FIG 4B)**.

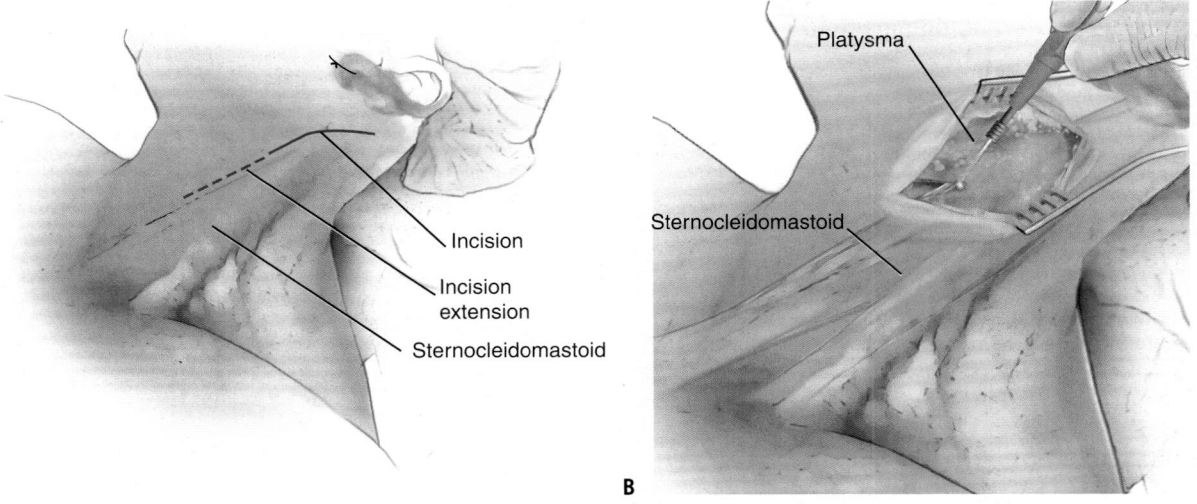

A **B**

TECH FIG 4 A. A transverse incision is extended from the mastoid tip and is carried along the inferior border of the mandible, turning caudally and continuing along the anterior border of the SCM muscle. **B.** The incision is carried through the subcutaneous tissues and platysma muscle using electrocautery in line with the incision. Subplatysmal flaps are developed with blunt dissection techniques to allow adequate mobilization of tissue. *(continued)*

TECHNIQUES

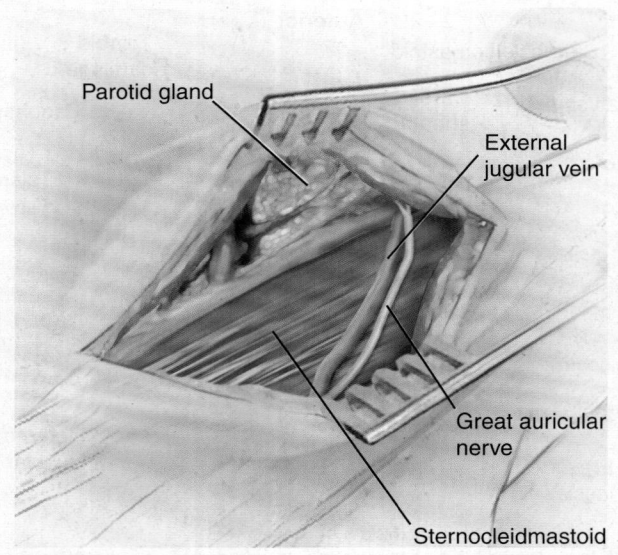

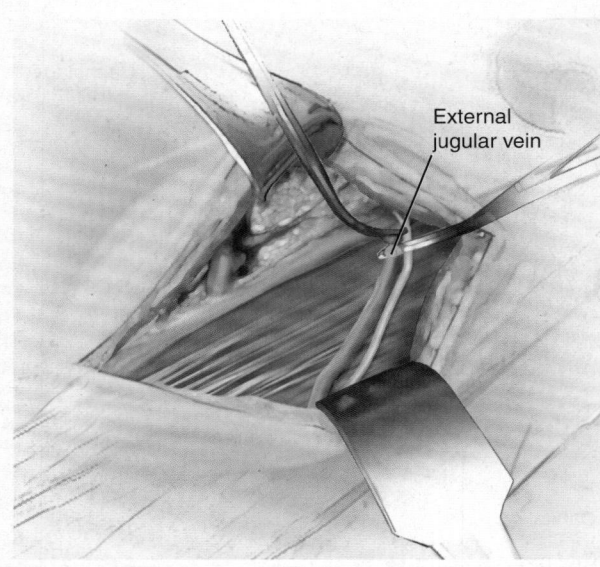

TECH FIG 4 *(continued)* **C.** The greater auricular nerve is identified and mobilized from the subcutaneous tissues to allow adequate retraction. It is sometimes necessary to sacrifice the greater auricular nerve. This will result in a small area of insensate skin but otherwise has no functional significance. **D.** The external jugular vein and collaterals are mobilized or ligated as needed. The SCM is mobilized anteriorly with the carotid sheath. For additional exposure, the SCM can be taken down from the mastoid prominence by sectioning through the tendinous insertion.

- The superior–anterior flap is elevated to the inferior border of the parotid gland.
- The greater auricular nerve is identified and dissected out of the subcutaneous tissue both caudally and cephalad to allow adequate retraction (**TECH FIG 4C**).
- It is occasionally necessary to sacrifice the greater auricular nerve; this will leave the patient with a small insensate patch of skin but no long-term functional deficit.
- The external jugular vein is identified and then mobilized or ligated as needed (**TECH FIG 4D**).
- The SCM is mobilized and retracted medially and anteriorly with the carotid sheath.

Mobilization of Sternocleidomastoid

- Depending on the amount of exposure required, the SCM may be detached partially or entirely from its tendinous insertion at the mastoid prominence.
  - Be sure to leave enough tissue cuff to allow reapproximation of the muscle on closure.
- Take care to identify and protect the spinal accessory nerve, which enters the SCM about 3 cm distal to the tip of the mastoid process.
  - For limited exposure, the spinal accessory nerve can be retracted anteromedially with the SCM (**TECH FIG 5**).
  - For more extensive exposure, it can be dissected off the jugular foramen in a cephalad direction and retracted posterolaterally while the SCM is everted.

Deep Dissection

- Lymph nodes found in the field of dissection and around the spinal accessory nerve can be excised.
- The lateral process of C1 is now easily palpable about 1 cm distal to the mastoid process.
- The interval between the jugular vein and the longus capitis muscles is then created, allowing access to the retropharyngeal space.

- The retropharyngeal space can be opened further with blunt dissection techniques employing scissors, Kittners, or fingers.
- A sharp elevator or bipolar electrocautery can then be used to elevate the longus capitis and longus colli muscles from the transverse processes and lateral masses of C1 and C2 (**TECH FIG 6A**).
- Retraction is best accomplished by bending a malleable retractor so that it can be used as a lever against the contralateral transverse process, thus elevating the soft tissues anteriorly and medially (**TECH FIG 6B**).

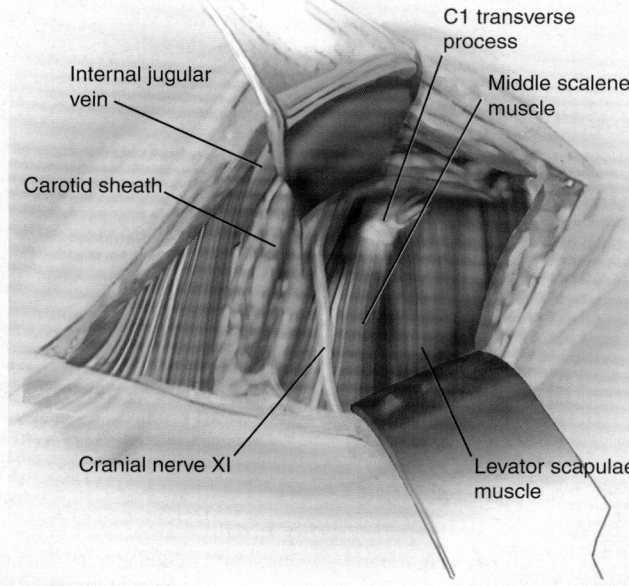

TECH FIG 5 The spinal accessory nerve is identified as it enters the SCM about 3 cm distal to the tip of the mastoid process and retracted anteriorly with the SCM. The lateral process of C1 will lie essentially in the middle of the field of dissection, about 1 cm distal to the mastoid process.

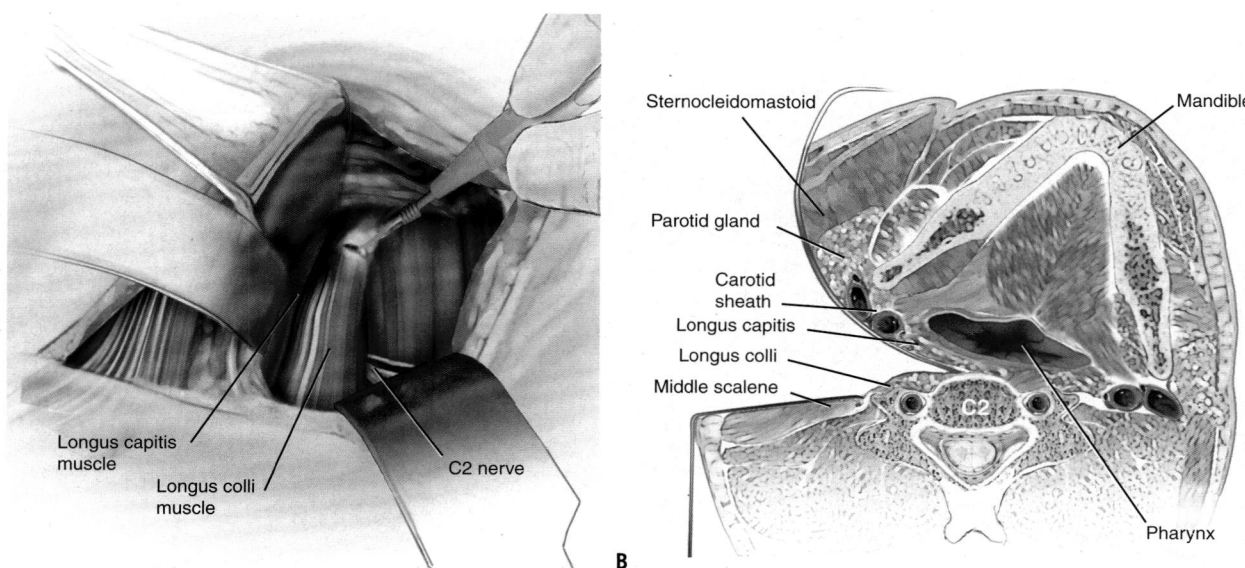

TECH FIG 6 A. Bipolar electrocautery can be used to elevate the longus capitis and longus colli muscles subperiosteally from the transverse processes and lateral masses of C1 and C2. **B.** Plane of dissection for the retropharyngeal approach. For deep retraction, a malleable retractor can be used as a lever against the contralateral transverse process, allowing elevation of the soft tissues anteriorly and medially.

ANTERIOR APPROACH TO THE CERVICOTHORACIC JUNCTION (TRANSMANUBRIAL–TRANSCLAVICULAR APPROACH)

Incision and Superficial Dissection

- A standard Smith-Robinson approach is taken, with the incision extended distally over the manubrium (**TECH FIG 7A**).
- The sternal and clavicular heads of the SCM are released at the tendinous attachments and retracted proximally and laterally. Be sure to leave enough tissue cuff to allow reapproximation of the muscle on closure.
- Likewise, the sternohyoid and sternothyroid are sectioned and retracted proximally and medially (**TECH FIG 7B**).
  - The omohyoid is also generally sectioned for better exposure. It does not need to be repaired.

Mobilization of Clavicle

- The medial third of the clavicle and the left side of the manubrium are then cleared of any remaining soft tissue.
- The clavicle is then divided (typically with a Gigli saw) at the junction of the medial and middle thirds (**TECH FIG 8A**).
  - Care must be taken to avoid injuring the left subclavian vein, which is normally closely apposed to the undersurface of the clavicle.
- At this point, the medial third of the clavicle can be disarticulated from the manubrium (**TECH FIG 8B**).
  - If more exposure is needed, the left side of the manubrium can be removed in a piecemeal fashion by a rongeur.
  - Alternatively, the medial third of the clavicle and a section of the manubrium can be removed together by careful sectioning. This will allow plate or wire reconstruction of the clavicle and manubrium if desired.

- If the manubrium and medial third of the clavicle are removed in this manner, the sternal head of the SCM can be left in continuity with the manubrium and reflected en bloc (**TECH FIG 8C**).

Deep Dissection

- The inferior thyroid vein and artery are often encountered with deeper dissection and may need to be ligated for better exposure.
- Careful blunt dissection proceeds in the same interval as for the standard Smith-Robinson approach (ie, between the carotid sheath laterally and the trachea and esophagus medially).
  - The recurrent laryngeal nerve is almost always found between the esophagus and trachea on the left side of the neck within this plane.
- Blunt retractors are then placed, and the carotid sheath, left brachiocephalic artery, and innominate vein are retracted inferolaterally (**TECH FIG 9A**).
- Likewise, a blunt retractor is used to retract the trachea, esophagus, left recurrent laryngeal nerve, and right brachiocephalic vessels inferolaterally to the patient's right.
- The prevertebral fascia is then identified and incised to expose the vertebral bodies. Once adequately dissected, the surgeon can visualize and access as far distally as T3 or T4.
- **TECH FIG 9B** represents a cross-sectional view at the cervicothoracic junction demonstrating the plane of dissection for the transmanubrial–transclavicular approach.
- At the completion of the procedure, the clavicle is replaced and plated.

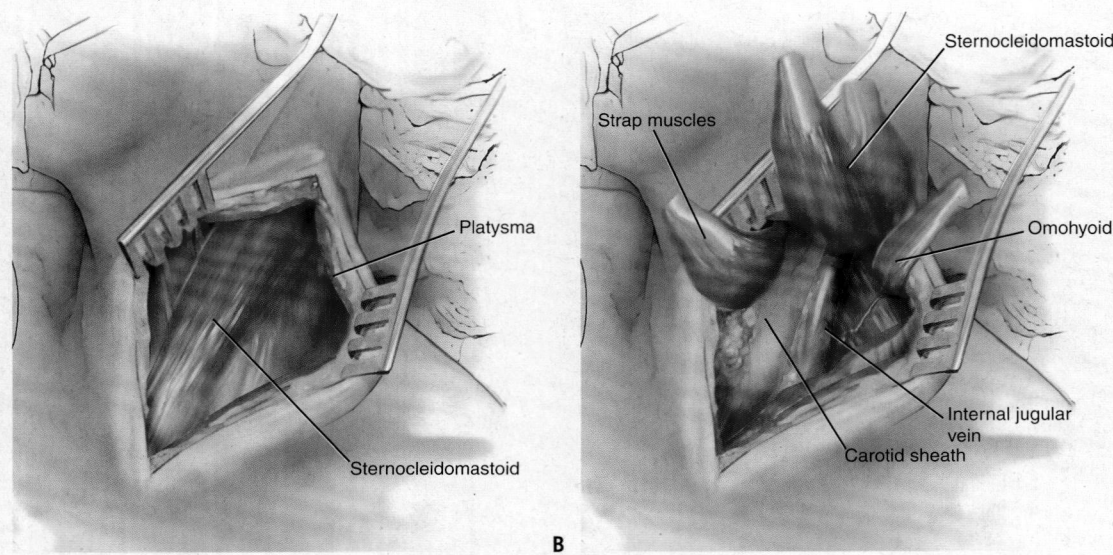

A **B**

TECH FIG 7 A. The incision for a low Smith-Robinson approach can be extended along the anterior border of the SCM to the midsagittal plane at roughly the sternal notch and then extended vertically to just beyond the manubrial–sternal junction. **B.** The sternal and clavicular heads of the SCM are released and reflected laterally, whereas the sternohyoid and sternothyroid muscles are sectioned and reflected medially. The omohyoid is usually released during the exposure. It does not need to be repaired.

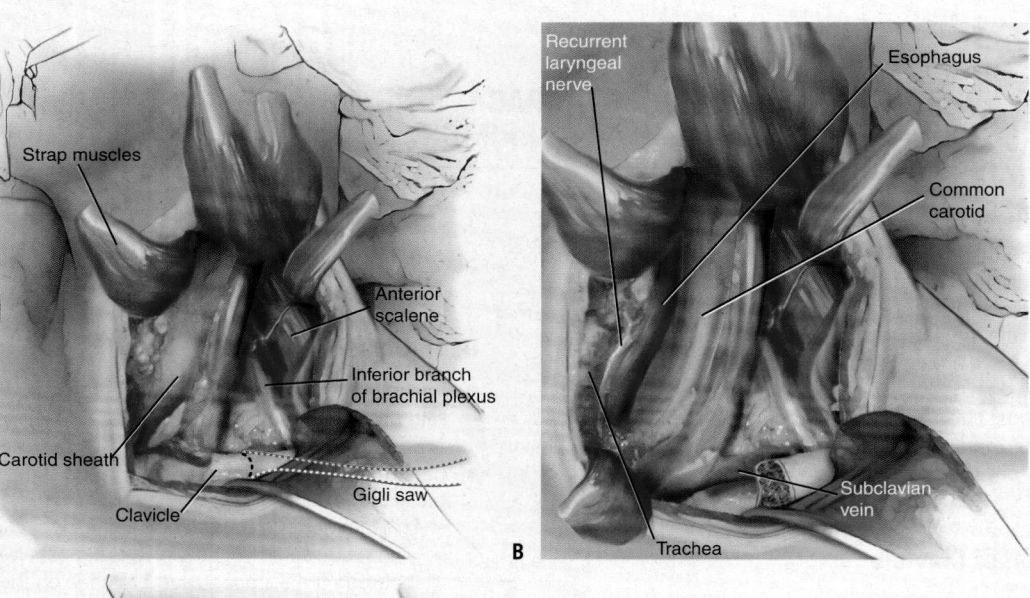

A **B**

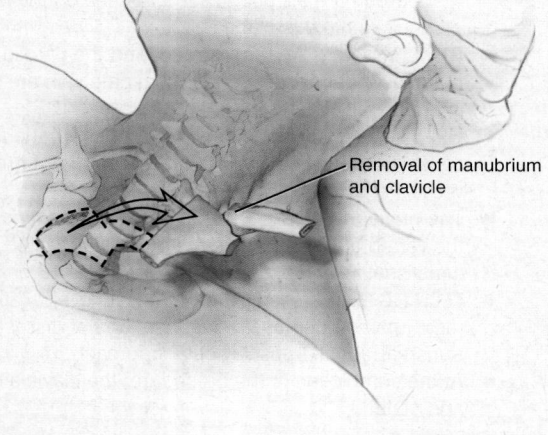

C

TECH FIG 8 A. The clavicle is divided at the junction of the medial and middle thirds, taking care to avoid injuring the left subclavian vein, which is normally closely apposed to the undersurface of the clavicle. **B.** The medial third of the clavicle can be disarticulated from the manubrium at the manubrioclavicular joint. This will generally provide adequate exposure to the C7–T1 level. **C.** For additional exposure, the left side of the manubrium can be removed piecemeal using a rongeur. A second option involves careful sectioning of the manubrium, which will allow lateral reflection of both the manubrium and medial third of the clavicle without disarticulation of the manubrioclavicular joint.

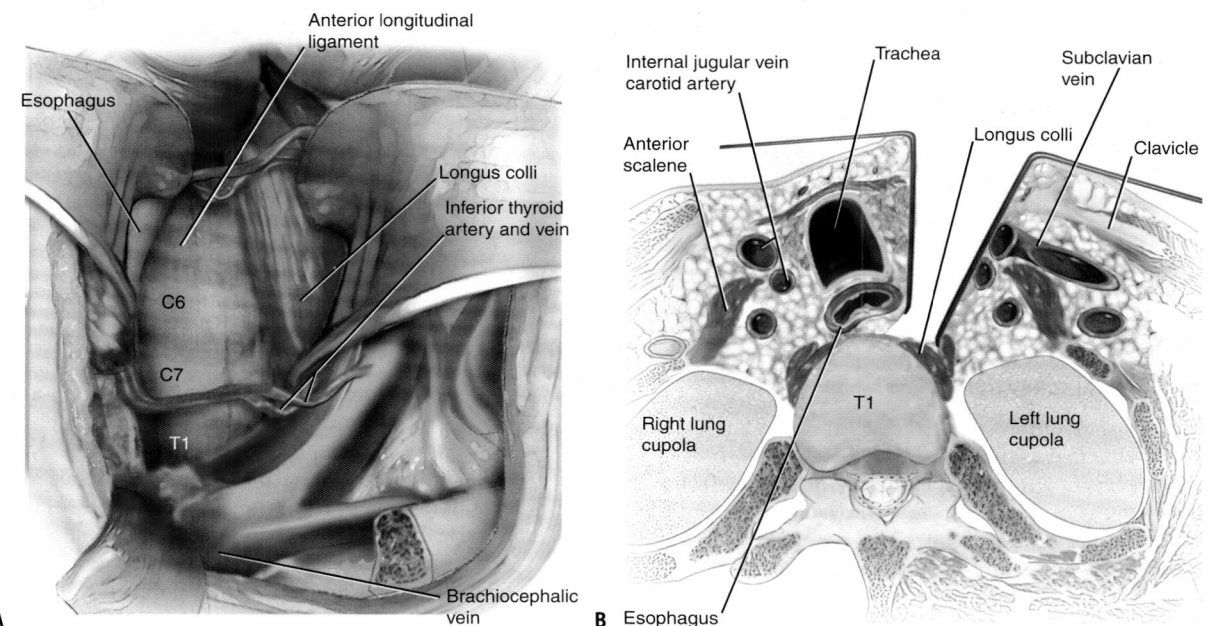

TECH FIG 9 A. Blunt retractors are used to carefully retract the carotid sheath, left brachiocephalic artery, and innominate vein inferolaterally, whereas the trachea, esophagus, left recurrent laryngeal nerve, and right brachiocephalic vessels are retracted inferomedially. **B.** Cross-sectional view through the cervicothoracic junction demonstrating the plane of dissection for the transmanubrial–transclavicular approach.

TECHNIQUES

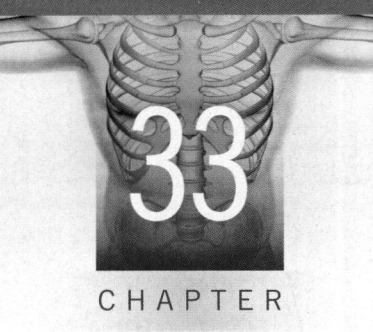

CHAPTER 33

Posterior Cervical Approach

Raj Rao, Satyajit V. Marawar, and George S. Ibrahim

ANATOMY

Posterior Cervical Musculature

- The muscles covering the posterior aspect of the cervical spine are arranged in three layers (**FIG 1**).
- Superficial layer: The trapezius muscle originates from the superior nuchal line of the occiput, the ligamentum nuchae, and the spinous processes of the upper thoracic spine. It inserts into the spine of the scapula and the acromion.
- Intermediate layer: The splenius capitis arises from the lower half of the ligamentum nuchae and upper six thoracic vertebrae, inserting onto the mastoid process and the lateral half of the superficial nuchal line under the sternocleidomastoid.
- The deep layer consists of the semispinalis capitis, the semispinalis cervicis, the multifidus, and the rotators, arranged from superficial to deep layers, respectively.
  - The semispinalis capitis arises from the transverse processes of the upper six thoracic vertebrae and the articular processes of the midcervical vertebrae and inserts

onto the occiput between the superior and inferior nuchal lines.
  - The semispinalis cervicis arises from the transverse processes of the upper six thoracic vertebrae and inserts onto the spinous processes of C2–C5.
  - The multifidus muscle lies deep to the semispinalis cervicis. It originates from the articular processes of the lower cervical vertebrae and inserts onto the spinous processes of the upper cervical vertebrae.
  - The rotators lie deep to the multifidus. They originate from the transverse process of one vertebra and ascend obliquely to insert on the spinous process of the vertebra one or two levels cranial to their origin.

Suboccipital Musculature

- The rectus capitis posterior minor originates from the posterior tubercle of the atlas and inserts onto the medial half of the inferior nuchal line.

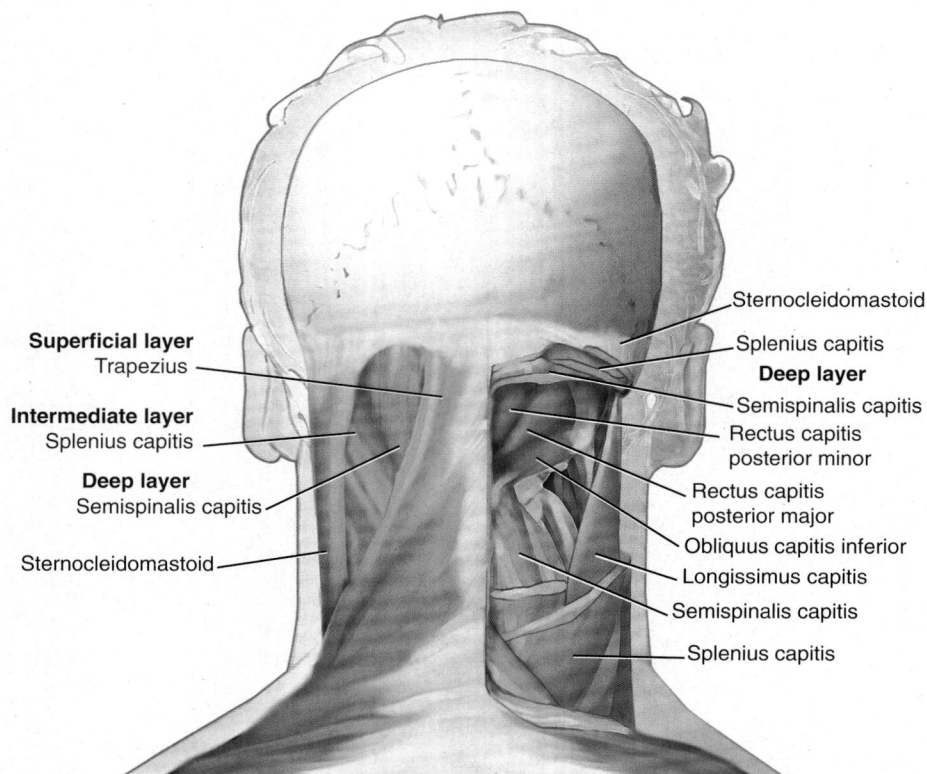

Superficial layer
Trapezius

Intermediate layer
Splenius capitis

Deep layer
Semispinalis capitis

Sternocleidomastoid

Sternocleidomastoid
Splenius capitis
Deep layer
Semispinalis capitis
Rectus capitis posterior minor
Rectus capitis posterior major
Obliquus capitis inferior
Longissimus capitis
Semispinalis capitis
Splenius capitis

FIG 1 Superficial, intermediate, and deep layers of the posterior cervical musculature are shown on the *left*. The suboccipital muscles lie deep to these muscles and are shown on the *right*.

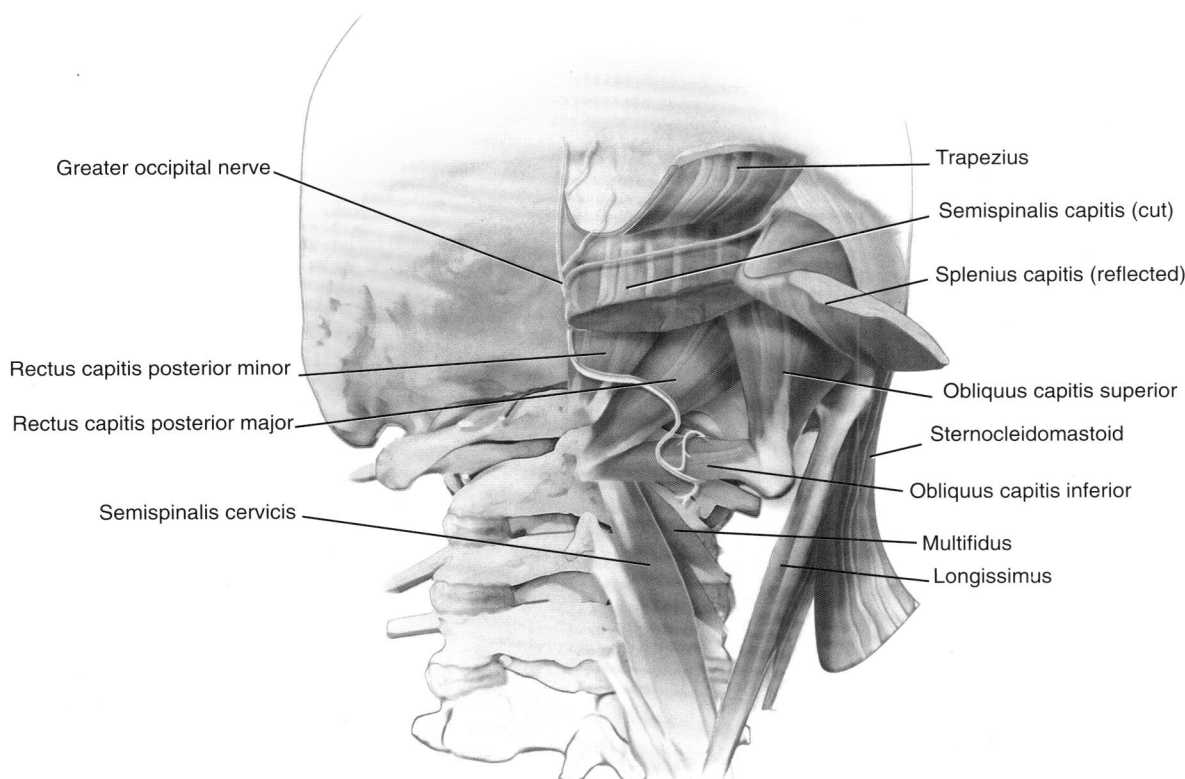

FIG 2 Anatomy of the suboccipital triangle. The suboccipital triangle lies between the rectus capitis posterior major, the obliquus superior, and the obliquus inferior. The greater occipital nerve is seen crossing the suboccipital triangle along its medial angle. The posterior arch of the atlas with the vertebral artery is seen in the floor of the suboccipital triangle.

- The rectus capitis posterior major originates from the spinous process of the axis and inserts onto the lateral half of the inferior nuchal line.
- The obliquus capitis superior originates from the transverse process of the atlas and inserts onto the occiput laterally between the superior and inferior nuchal lines.
- The obliquus capitis inferior muscle originates from the spinous process of the axis and inserts onto the transverse process of the atlas.
- The suboccipital triangle lies between the rectus capitis posterior major and the superior and the inferior obliques.
  - The greater occipital nerve is the medial branch of the posterior division of the second cervical nerve at the medial angle of the suboccipital triangle. It runs cephalad between the semispinalis capitis and the obliquus inferior toward the occiput where it pierces the semispinalis capitis and the trapezius. It is responsible for cutaneous innervation of the back of the scalp (**FIG 2**).

Osteoligamentous Anatomy

- The external occipital protuberance or inion is an easily palpable bony landmark in the midportion of the occiput. The superior nuchal line extends as a bony ridge on either side of this prominence. A small ridge or crest, called the *median nuchal line*, descends in the medial plane from the external occipital protuberance to the foramen magnum. The inferior nuchal line runs parallel to the superior nuchal line, midway between the inion and foramen magnum (**FIG 3**).

- The atlas does not have a spinous process but has a posterior tubercle marking the center of the posterior arch.
- The spinous process of the axis is tall, bifid, and broadest in the cervical spine.
- A broad sheet of thick fibrous tissue called the *posterior atlanto-occipital membrane* extends from the posterior border of the foramen magnum to the superior border of the posterior arch of the atlas.
- The posterior atlantoaxial membrane is a broad, thin membrane extending from the inferior border of the posterior arch of the atlas to the superior border of the lamina of the axis.
- The tectorial membrane is the cranial extension of the posterior longitudinal ligament, running posterior to the transverse ligament to attach onto the anterior border of the foramen magnum.
- The anterior atlantoaxial ligament is the continuation of the anterior longitudinal ligament, extending from the inferior border of the anterior arch of the atlas to the front of the body of the axis (**FIG 4**).
- The supraspinous ligament is absent in the cervical spine. Ligamentum nuchae is a midline avascular fibroelastic structure that is composed of dorsal and ventral components. The dorsal component is a median raphe that extends from the spinous process of C7 to the occipital protuberance, whereas the ventral component is a fascial septum that extends anteriorly from the dorsal component to merge with the interspinous ligament. The interspinous ligament in the cervical spine is thin and less developed.

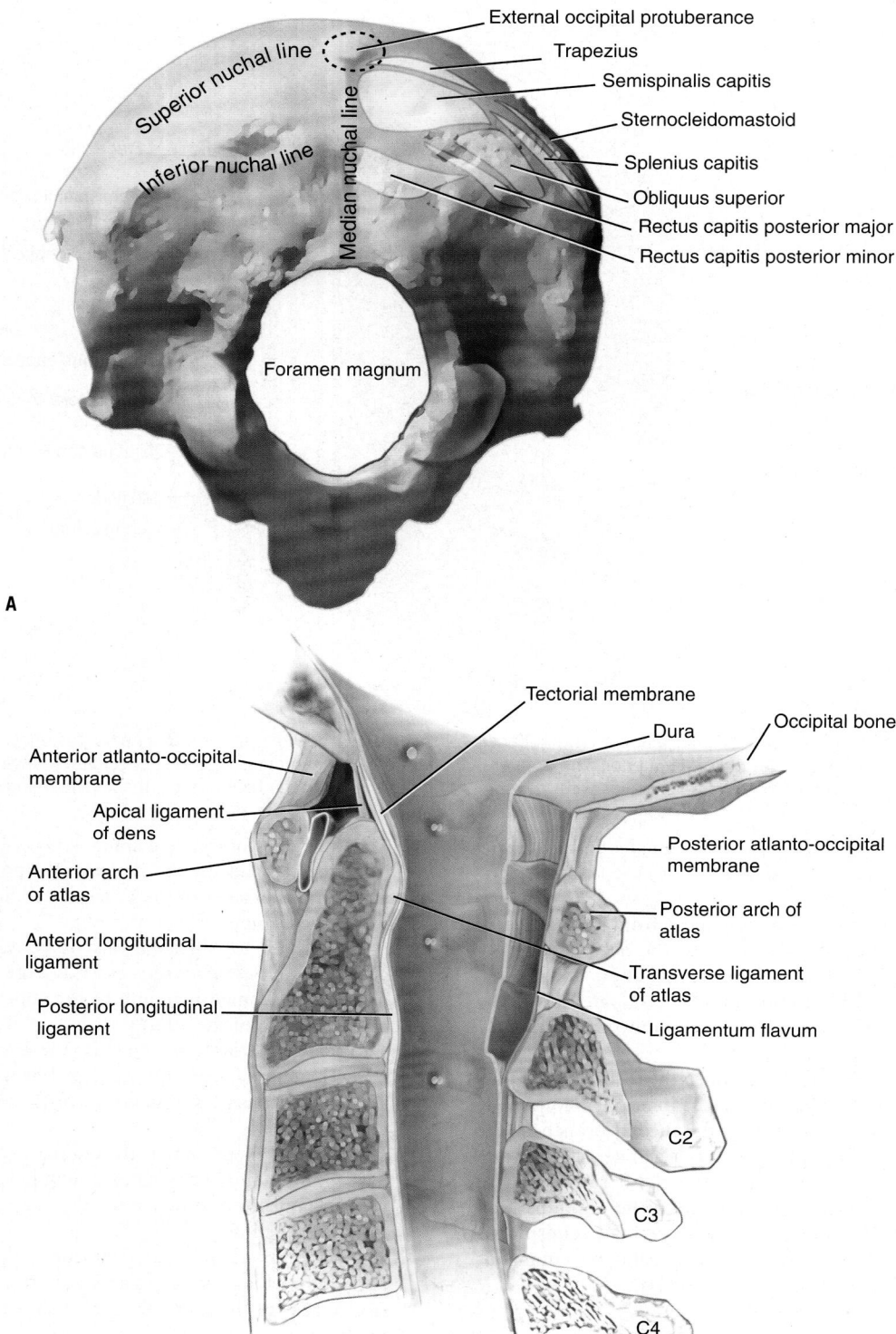

A

B

FIG 3 **A.** Bony anatomy of the occiput with muscular insertions. Superior, inferior, and median nuchal lines are the prominent bony ridges on the posterior occipital surface. The major posterior cervical muscles and muscles of the suboccipital triangle insert on these bony ridges and on the posterior occipital surface between these ridges. **B.** Sagittal cross-section showing the ligamentous architecture of the proximal cervical spine. Anterior and posterior atlanto-occipital as well as atlantoaxial ligaments and the ligaments stabilizing the odontoid process are depicted: the apical ligament of the dens and the transverse ligament of the atlas.

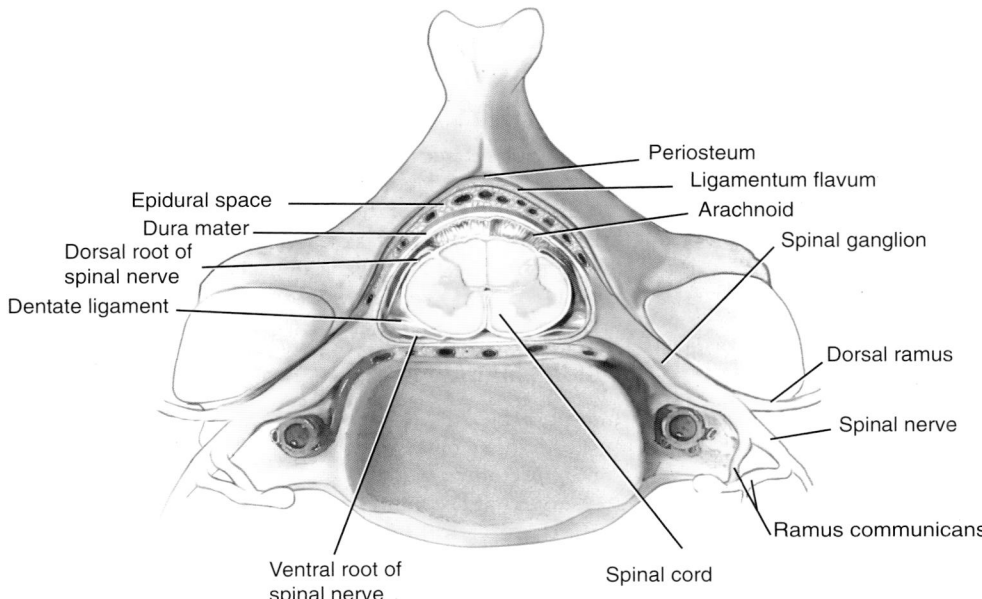

FIG 4 Axial section showing nerve root anatomy. The spinal rootlets join to form the ventral and the dorsal roots of the spinal nerve. The dorsal root ganglion is seen as the enlargement of the dorsal root lying between the facet joint and the vertebral artery. The roots merge outside the intervertebral foramen to form the spinal nerve.

- The ligamentum flavum extends from the superior margin of the inferior lamina to anterior surface of the superior lamina. Laterally, it extends to the articular processes. Infolding of the ligamentum flavum with loss of intervertebral disc height due to degenerative changes can contribute to spinal stenosis.
- The pars interarticularis or isthmus of C2 is the waist of the posterior arch of C2, connecting the superior and inferior articular processes. The medial margin of the pars interarticularis along the superior border of the C2 lamina is a guide to the medial margin of the C2 pedicle.
- The C1–C2 facet joint is oriented largely in the axial plane, whereas the C2–C3 and remaining subaxial cervical facet joints are oriented 45 degrees to the coronal plane of the spine.
- The spinous processes from C3 to C6 are small and bifid. The C7 spinous process tends to be straight and long and terminates in a single tubercle. It is usually the longest of the cervical spinous processes.
- The laminae in the cervical spine do not override as much as in the thoracic spine. There is a risk of inadvertent penetration of instruments in the spinal canal through the wide interlaminar windows during surgical exposure.
- The lateral mass of the cervical spine refers to the lateral column of each vertebra that includes the superior and inferior articular processes and the transverse foramen on either side.
  - It offers a secure fixation anchor for screw insertion from C3 to C6, particularly when the spinous process and lamina are fractured or removed.
  - A faint longitudinal groove marks the separation between the laminae and lateral masses.
  - The exiting nerve root and posterior portion of the transverse process lie anterior to the lateral mass.
  - The anteroposterior depth of the lateral mass reduces gradually from C3 (about 8.9 mm) to C7 (about 6.4 mm).[3]
  - The lateral mass of C7 is elongated superoinferiorly but is thinner in the anteroposterior plane than the other cervical vertebrae.

- The pedicles of the cervical vertebrae are smaller than those in the lumbar spine. Imaging studies should be obtained in all patients prior to screw fixation to verify pedicle morphology and rule out congenital anomalies. Pedicle dimensions generally allow for screw fixation at C2 and C7.
- The intervertebral foramen in the cervical spine is bound anteriorly by the uncinate process, the intervertebral disc, and the inferior portion of the superior vertebral body; superiorly and inferiorly by the pedicles; and posteriorly by the facet joint and the superior articular facet of the inferior vertebra.

Nerve Root Anatomy

- The dorsal and ventral nerve roots formed from the respective rootlets enter a common sleeve of the arachnoid and dura mater.
- The nerve root runs 45 degrees anterolaterally and 10 degrees inferiorly to enter the intervertebral foramen by passing over the top of the corresponding pedicle.
- The dorsal nerve root lies anterior to the superior articular process, positioned at the tip of the superior articular facet medially, and then coursing inferiorly to lie on top of the pedicle laterally.
- The ventral root lies anteroinferiorly adjacent to the uncovertebral joint.
- The cervical nerve roots occupy the lower third of the intervertebral foramen, whereas the upper two-thirds of the foramen is filled with fat.
- In the lateral part of the intervertebral foramen, the dorsal nerve root is enlarged to form the dorsal root ganglion, which lies between the vertebral artery and a groove on the anterolateral aspect of the superior articular process (see **FIG 4**).
- The dorsal and the ventral nerve roots join distal to the dorsal root ganglion outside the intervertebral foramen to form the spinal nerve.

Vertebral Artery

- The vertebral artery is a branch of the first part of the sub-clavian artery, lying anterior to the transverse process of the seventh cervical vertebra at its origin.
- The vertebral artery courses medially and posteriorly through the subaxial cervical spine within the transverse foramina of the sixth through the first cervical vertebrae.
  - It is at risk for injury where it lies unprotected between the transverse foramina and during anterior procedures lateral to the disc space, particularly at the upper cervical levels (**FIG 5**).
  - Anatomic variations in the course of the vertebral artery are not infrequent. Following its origin off of the sub-clavian artery, the vertebral artery typically enters the C6 transverse foramen. Bruneau et al[1] reported entry into the C3, C4, C5, or C7 transverse foramina in 0.2%, 1.0%, 5.0%, and 0.8% of patients, respectively.
    - A 2% incidence of tortuosity of the vertebral artery has been reported, leading to a potentially dangerous medial course of the vessel within the vertebral body.[1,2]
- More cephalad, after emerging from the transverse foramen of C2, the artery lies lateral to the C1–C2 facet joint before it enters the transverse foramen of the atlas.
- The artery exits the transverse foramen of the atlas and continues posteromedially in a groove on the superior surface of the posterior arch of the atlas.
- It enters the foramen magnum by piercing the atlanto-occipital membrane about 10 mm from the midline.[1]
- In approaches to the posterior cervical spine, the vertebral artery is at risk for injury during exposure of the posterior arch of the atlas and in the transverse foramina of C1 and C2 during screw insertion for occipitocervical or atlantoaxial fusion procedures.
  - To protect the vertebral artery during these procedures, dissection should be limited to within 12 mm of the midline on the posterior aspect of C1 and within 8 mm of the midline on the superior surface of the posterior arch of the atlas.[1] Further lateral dissection can be performed on the inferior surface of the C1 arch versus the superior surface because the vertebral artery runs on the superior surface of the C1 arch.
- The width of the lateral mass of the atlas averages 11.6 ± 1.4 mm. The height of the portion of the lateral mass of the atlas inferior to its posterior arch averages 4.1 ± 0.7 mm.[2] The lateral mass of C1 thus can generally safely accommodate a 3.5-mm screw below its attachment to the posterior arch.

SURGICAL MANAGEMENT

- Indications
  - Posterior spinal cord decompression via laminoplasty or laminectomy
  - Nerve root decompression via foraminotomy
  - Occipitocervical or atlantoaxial decompression, fusion, and instrumentation
  - Posterior cervical fusion
  - Cervical pedicle or lateral mass instrumentation

Positioning

- The patient's cervical spine should be ranged in flexion and extension in the preoperative area to determine a safe range that does not produce symptoms. Movements of the neck during intubation should be minimized, particularly in myelopathic patients.
- Awake intubation and positioning should be considered in myelopathic patients with markedly reduced canal dimensions. Use of fiberoptic imaging also allows neutral positioning of the neck during intubation. Careful monitoring of mean arterial pressure using an arterial line is recommended in patients with severe cervical stenosis.

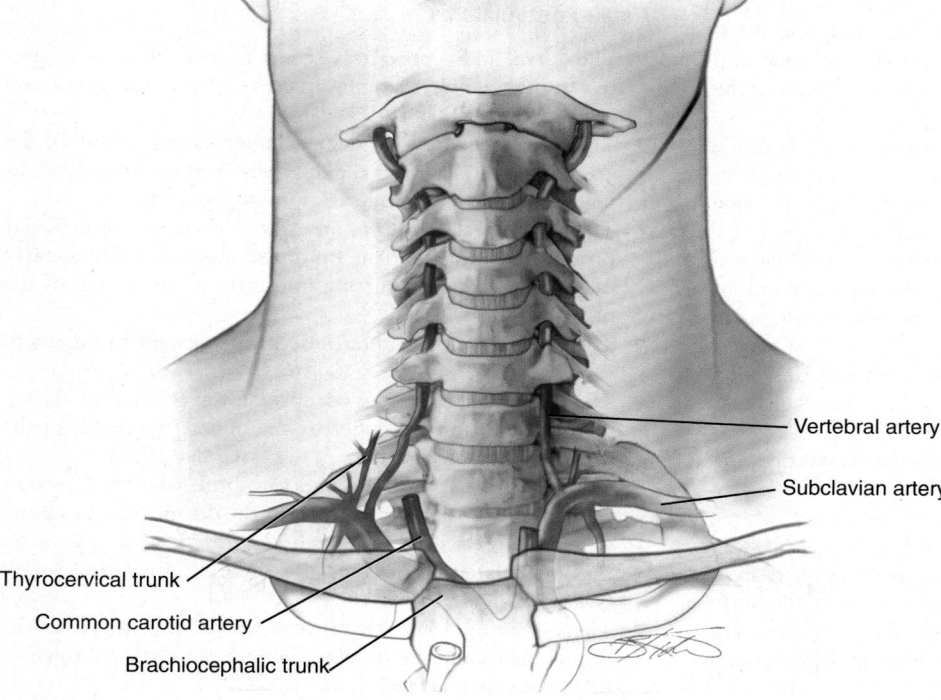

Vertebral artery

Subclavian artery

Thyrocervical trunk

Common carotid artery

Brachiocephalic trunk

FIG 5 Origin and course of the vertebral artery. The vertebral artery branches out from the first part of the subclavian artery. It passes through the transverse foramina of the upper six cervical vertebrae and has a significantly tortuous course in the proximal cervical spine.

- Spinal cord monitoring is initiated prior to positioning when required or in severely myelopathic patients.
- In patients undergoing occipitocervical and atlantoaxial procedures, the chin should be tucked to facilitate exposure of the occipitocervical region. For subaxial procedures, slight flexion of the neck reduces overlap of the laminae and facet joints, making deep dissection easier and facilitating decompression of the central and lateral canal. The neck should be brought back into neutral position for fusion or instrumentation procedures.
- Hyperextended or hyperflexed positions under anesthesia, particularly when held for prolonged periods of time, may contribute to spinal cord injury.
- We recommend use of the Mayfield three-point clamp to hold the cranium during posterior occipitocervical and posterior cervical surgery. The clamp is secured to the operating table with an adaptor.
- We infrequently use intraoperative tong traction because we believe the amount of traction transmitted to the operative site is variable.
- The patient is positioned prone on a frame of surgeon's choice. Adequate padding of the chest, axillae, hips, and knees is ensured. The shoulders are pulled down and taped to the distal end of the bed when necessary to facilitate intraoperative radiographic visualization (FIG 6). Excessive traction on the shoulders should be avoided to minimize the risk of brachial plexus injury or aggravation of underlying shoulder pathology. Upper limbs are held snug to the side of the patient's torso using bed sheets or tape.
- Slight reverse Trendelenburg position reduces epidural venous congestion and intraoperative bleeding and may provide mild traction effect on the cervical spine. We avoid the

sitting position to minimize the risk of intraoperative air embolism.
- Bony prominences and peripheral nerves in the upper and lower extremities should be well padded to protect against intraoperative decubiti or neurapraxia.
- Allowing the abdomen to hang freely facilitates venous return to the heart, maintains cardiac output, and decreases the required peak inspiratory pressure.
- Radiographs are obtained after positioning to verify cervical alignment. Placement of a radiopaque marker before obtaining these radiographs facilitates planning of the incision.

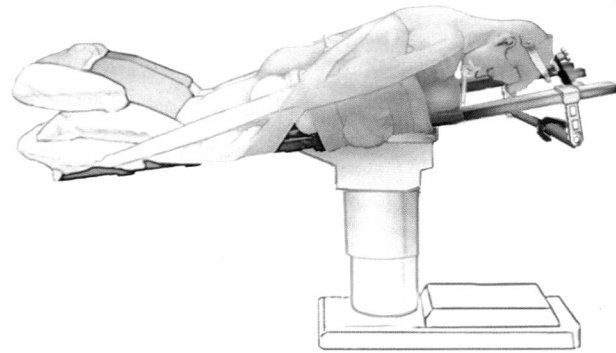

FIG 6 Positioning of the patient for posterior cervical surgery. In the prone position, the patient's head is stabilized with a Mayfield three-point clamp while traction is applied through the shoulders by taping them down. The patient is in the reverse Trendelenburg position with the abdomen allowed to hang free.

POSTERIOR APPROACH TO SUBAXIAL SPINE

- A midline skin incision is used for most surgical procedures to the subaxial spine. Palpation of the prominent spinous processes of C2 and C7 beneath the skin or the use of intraoperative radiographs can help restrict the incision to the area that requires exposure.
- The incision is deepened through the relatively avascular median raphe, which appears as a "white line" in the midline.
- Electrocautery is then used to incise the ligamentum nuchae.
  - Troublesome bleeding from the paraspinal muscles can be minimized by staying within the avascular median raphe.
  - Intermittent palpation of the spinous processes helps the surgeon stay oriented to the midline. The posterior cervical paraspinal musculature generally originates laterally and caudally, passing obliquely cephalad.
  - Reduction of intraoperative bleeding is facilitated at each segment by dissecting caudal to cephalad in a subperiosteal fashion.

- There is usually a venous plexus deep to the fascia around the cervicothoracic junction. Coagulating these blood vessels before dissection of the paraspinal muscles in this area can help reduce bleeding.
- For laminoplasty or multilevel laminectomy, the interspinous tissues are cauterized to minimize bleeding and then stripped off the spinous processes.
  - Deep retractors are inserted beneath the fascial layers directly on bone. Deep dissection is carried further laterally along the laminae.
- Localization of level is facilitated by identifying the large C2 and C7 spinous processes and the bifid spinous processes from C2 to C6.
- An intraoperative lateral radiograph should be obtained to confirm the operative levels.
- If facet fusion is not planned, the dissection should stop at the medial third of the facet joint, and the facet joint capsule should be preserved.
  - If facet fusion or instrumentation is required, the dissection is extended to the lateral border of the lateral mass.

TECHNIQUES

POSTERIOR APPROACH TO OCCIPITOCERVICAL REGION

- The external occipital protuberance and the prominent bifid C2 spinous process can be palpated in most patients beneath the skin. A midline skin incision is made extending from just above the occipital protuberance to the cervical level required.
- The incision on the scalp is deepened down to bone, and the occiput is exposed in subperiosteal fashion from the inion down to the foramen magnum.
  - The attachment of the trapezius can be elevated from the nuchal crest to allow lateral dissection.
  - The dissection is carried laterally for a distance of 2.5 cm on either side of the median occipital crest. Excessive lateral dissection or retraction can injure the greater occipital nerve.
- The incision is extended caudally through the ligamentum nuchae in the midline. Staying in the midline reduces blood loss.
  - Self-retaining retractors are applied at both ends of the incision.
- The large bifid spinous process of C2 is easily identified. It is exposed subperiosteally by dissecting the attachments of the rectus capitis posterior major and obliquus capitis inferior muscles from these structures.
  - The greater occipital nerve exits posteriorly along the inferior border of the obliquus capitis inferior muscle and can be preserved by limiting the dissection to the subperiosteal plane over the lamina of C2.
  - Muscular attachments to the distal and lateral aspect of C2 spinous process, specifically, that of semispinalis cervicis, should be preserved to maintain subaxial stability postoperatively.

- The C1 ring lies deep in the space between the occiput and C2. The posterior arch of C1 has no muscular attachments.
- Soft tissue from the posterior arch of C1 is dissected subperiosteally, taking care to stay within 12 mm of the midline on the posterior aspect of the posterior ring of C1 and within 8 mm of the midline on the superior aspect of the posterior ring of C1 to avoid vertebral artery injury (**TECH FIG 1**).[4]

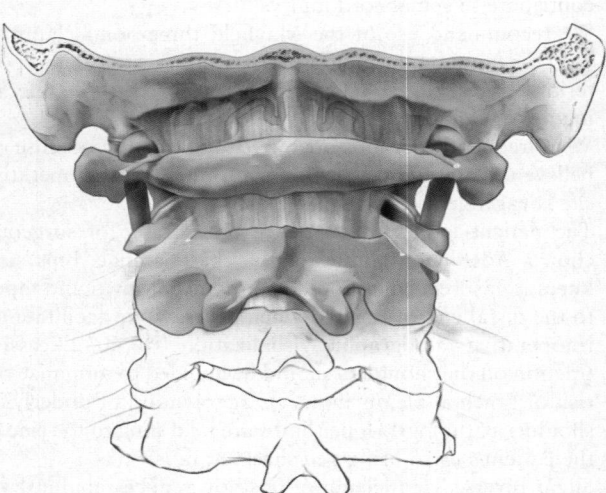

TECH FIG 1 The vertebral artery emerges from the transverse foramen of the atlas and courses medially in the groove on the superior surface of the posterior arch of the atlas. At the medial end of the groove, it turns anteriorly and pierces the atlanto-occipital membrane about 10 mm from the midline.

EXPOSURE OF C1–C2 FACET JOINT

- Exposure of the C1–C2 facet joint is required for insertion of the C1 lateral mass screw and fusion of the facet joint.
- The spinous process and lamina of C2, as well as the posterior arch of C1, are exposed with careful subperiosteal dissection.
- After self-retaining retractors are positioned appropriately, the lamina of C2 is exposed laterally as it continues to the pars. The medial border of the pars of C2 is identified. Dissection is continued cranially over the posterior aspect of the pars until the C2 nerve root is identified. A venous plexus around the nerve root can lead to significant bleeding. Bipolar coagulation, thrombin-soaked Gelfoam, and Cottonoids should be used to control bleeding. Following adequate hemostasis, C2 nerve root

is retracted caudally to expose the C1–C2 articulation. Alternatively, the nerve can be sacrificed for better exposure of the joint.[5] Medial and lateral dissection with a Freer elevator will expose the entire width of this facet joint.
- Exposure of the C1 lateral mass can be obtained by following the caudal edge of the posterior arch laterally. Once lateral to the medial border of the pars of C2, careful ventral dissection with a Penfield or a Freer elevator will expose the lateral mass of C1. During insertion of C1 lateral mass screws, C2 nerve root will need to be retracted distally.[6]
- Dissection lateral to the C1–C2 facet joint should be avoided to protect the vertebral artery.

MUSCLE-SPARING APPROACHES

- To reduce postoperative symptoms of pain, excessive stiffness, and muscle atrophy, the deep extensor muscles can be spread apart rather than detached, preserving their insertions onto the spinous processes.

Lower Cervical Spine

- Localization of the correct levels is performed as described earlier.
- Following a midline skin incision, the deep cervical fascia is divided laterally to allow better visualization of the intermuscular planes.
- The intermuscular triangle between the interspinalis muscle medially and the upper and lower semispinalis muscles at the level is exploited to access the lateral bony canal (**TECH FIG 2**).
- A plane is developed between the semispinalis cervicis muscles in line with their fibers.
- For exposure of the midline interlaminar space, exposure is through the interval between the right and left interspinalis muscles as they run longitudinally along the spinous process.
  - By separating the interspinalis muscles on both sides, the spinous process and lamina can be segmentally accessed from C2–C3 to C6–C7.
  - The spinous process can be divided longitudinally in the midline with a high-speed burr or surgical wire, maintaining the attachments of the semispinalis and multifidus on each side.[7]

Upper Cervical Spine

- Dissecting the intermuscular plane between the semispinalis cervicis and the obliquus capitis inferior can expose the intervertebral joints of C1–C2 and C2–C3 as well as the lamina and pedicle of C2.
- A plane can also be developed between the rectus capitis posterior major and the obliquus capitis inferior, and the lateral aspect of the posterior arch of the atlas and axis are then exposed.[8]

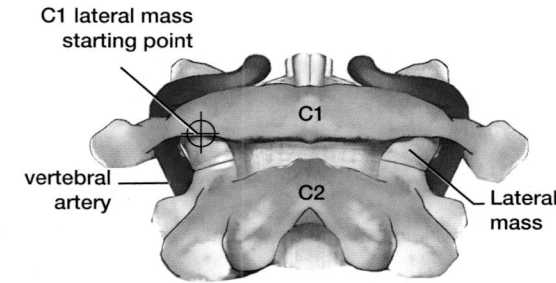

TECH FIG 2 In the muscle-sparing approach, the semispinalis muscles are separated to access the lateral bony canal.

MINIMALLY INVASIVE APPROACH TO THE CERVICAL SPINE

- Minimally invasive techniques are aimed at preservation of soft tissue structures of the posterior cervical spine to maintain strength of the neck and stability after surgery and reduce postoperative morbidity.
- For obese patients, adequate visualization can be obtained with minimally invasive approaches using tubular retractor systems.[9]
- Tubular retractor placement follows sequential dilators inserted through limited incisions on either side of the midline to access the foramen and underlying disc space.

- After docking the tubular retractor on the target region of the posterior bony canal, the lateral mass and lamina are denuded of overlying soft tissue using electrocautery and sharp instruments to complete exposure.[10]
- For bilateral decompression, a midline skin incision is made with subcutaneous dissection mobilizing laterally as necessary. Alternatively, small incisions can be made on either side of the midline.

TECHNIQUES

Pearls and Pitfalls

Posterior Vertebral	• Unstable or fractured fragments should be stabilized with a clamp during dissection to avoid arch fragments inadvertent contusion of the spinal cord.
Stenotic Canal	• Excessive manipulation of the posterior elements in a patient with a stenotic canal should be avoided as it may inadvertently result in spinal cord injury.
Excessive Bleeding	• Venous bleeding from epidural veins can occasionally be profuse. The patient should be positioned in reverse Trendelenburg position to decrease the blood loss. Hemostatic agents and bipolar cautery are used to control bleeding from these veins.
Vertebral Artery	• The vertebral artery is endangered at lower cervical levels (C3–C6) if the transverse processes at these levels are destroyed by tumor or infection or if the dissection is markedly lateral.
Spina Bifida	• Cervical spina bifida is a rare condition that can lead to cord damage during dissection if not recognized.

REFERENCES

1. Bruneau M, Cornelius JF, Marneffe V, et al. Anatomical variations of the V2 segment of the vertebral artery. Neurosurgery 2006;59 (1 suppl 1):20–24.
2. Curylo LJ, Mason HC, Bohlman HH, et al. Tortuous course of the vertebral artery and anterior cervical decompression: a cadaveric and clinical case study. Spine 2000;25(22):2860–2864.
3. Ebraheim NA, An HS, Xu R, et al. The quantitative anatomy of the cervical nerve root groove and the intervertebral foramen. Spine (Phila Pa 1976) 1996;21(14):1619–1623.
4. Ebraheim NA, Xu R, Ahmad M, et al. The quantitative anatomy of the vertebral artery groove of the atlas and its relation to the posterior atlantoaxial approach. Spine (Phila Pa 1976) 1998;23(3):320–323.
5. Gala VC, O'Toole JE, Voyadzis JM, et al. Posterior minimally invasive approaches for the cervical spine. Orthop Clin North Am 2007;38(3):339–349.
6. Hong X, Dong Y, Yunbing C, et al. Posterior screw placement on the lateral mass of atlas: an anatomic study. Spine (Phila Pa 1976) 2004;29(5):500–503.
7. Joseffer SS, Post N, Cooper P, et al. Minimally invasive atlantoaxial fixation with a polyaxial screw-rod construct: technical case report. Neurosurgery 2006;58(4 suppl 2):ONS–E375.
8. Santiago P, Fessler R. Minimally invasive surgery for the management of cervical spondylosis. Neurosurgery 2007;60(1 suppl 1): S160–S165.
9. Shiraishi T, Kato M, Yato Y, et al. New techniques for exposure of posterior cervical spine through intermuscular planes and their surgical application. Spine (Phila Pa 1976) 2012;37(5): E286–E296.
10. Xu Y, Xiong W, Han S II, et al. Posterior bilateral intermuscular approach for upper cervical spine injuries. World Neurosurg 2017;104:869–875.

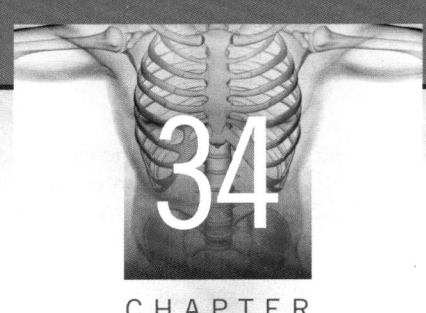

34

CHAPTER

Anterior Thoracic Approach

Christopher M. Mikhail, James E. Dowdell, Sheeraz A. Qureshi, and Andrew C. Hecht

DEFINITION

- The anterior approach can be used to access the thoracic spine for decompression, deformity correction, and stabilization.
- This approach allows for access to treat conditions such as intervertebral disc herniation, infection, tumor, and trauma.[1]

ANATOMY

- The thoracic spinal cord may have a tenuous blood supply, particularly in patients with congenital anomalies and kyphosis.
- The midthoracic cord represents a watershed zone for vascularity. The artery of Adamkiewicz supplies the thoracic cord but can have a variable origin. Its origin is usually (80%) from the left side at the T10 level but can vary from T5 to L5.[2]
- Because of the thoracic spine's tenuous blood supply and the potential for anterior spinal artery compression caused by thoracic disc herniations, indirect approaches were developed, obviating the need for wide laminectomy and direct visualization of the cord. The goal of these techniques, including the posterolateral transpedicular and transthoracic anterior approaches, is to minimize direct cord manipulation via retraction and prevent subsequent microcontusion and cord ischemia.

SURGICAL MANAGEMENT

Preoperative Planning

- Location of pathology is a key element to choosing the optimal approach to the thoracic spine.
  - In terms of disc pathology, evidence has shown that more centrally located disc herniations are better treated with an anterior approach, whereas a posterolateral approach is better suited for lateral or foraminal disc herniations.
- Radiographs of the thoracic spine and chest should be obtained to determine the level of surgery and help in "rib counting."
  - It is often helpful to obtain lumbar radiographs also to determine the number of lumbar segments below the most distal thoracic rib. Knowing this information preoperatively helps in counting "up" from the sacrum intraoperatively if needed.
  - In the absence of obvious bony pathology such as fractures, infections, or tumors, it is very easy to inadvertently localize the wrong level in the thoracic spine. The surgeon should be sure to have a strategy for intraoperative-level identification based on careful scrutiny of radiographs and magnetic resonance imaging (MRI) or computed tomography (CT) scans before surgery, understanding that the quality of intraoperative fluoroscopy may not be optimal.

- When obtaining an MRI to better understand the nature of the pathology in relation to the thoracic spinal cord, the surgeon should ask for a topogram to be performed so that there is no question as to the level or levels of involvement.
  - On CT or MRI scans, the surgeon should pay close attention to the position of the aorta and inferior vena cava, especially on the axial cuts, as this may affect the side from which the spine is approached, especially if a corpectomy will be performed.
- Anesthesia considerations include the use of an oral gastric tube and double-lumen endotracheal tube, which allows for collapse of the ipsilateral lung.
  - If the surgical site is T10 or caudal, selective deflation of the ipsilateral lung is usually not necessary. Additionally, a left-sided approach may prove more advantageous at the thoracolumbar junction, as the elevated right hemidiaphragm may prevent adequate exposure.
  - If the surgical site is proximal to T10, selective deflation is helpful in keeping the lung out of the field, but it may lead to more postoperative issues with atelectasis.
- We routinely use neurologic monitoring when performing thoracic operations.

Positioning

- The patient should be in the lateral decubitus position with the arms in prayer position.
- The thorax vertex should be positioned over the break of the bed, all pressure points should be padded, pillows should be placed between legs and arms, and an axillary roll should be used to prevent compression of the axillary vessels (FIG 1).

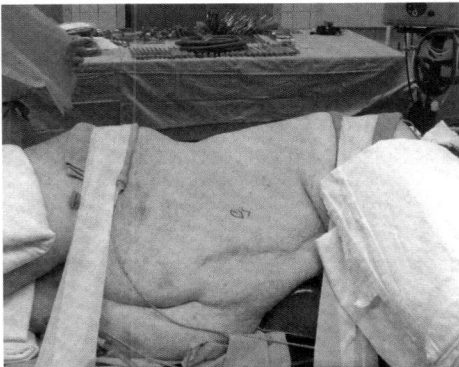

FIG 1 Patient placed in the lateral decubitus position. It is important to ensure that all bony prominences are well padded.

- The operating surgeon typically stands behind the patient during the exposure. However, it may be helpful to stand in front of the patient when performing the decompression, as the line of sight into the spinal canal is better from that vantage point.

Approach (Right versus Left)

- Considerations for thoracic approaches include the following:
  - Approach from the side of herniation in cases of posterolateral or lateral herniation.
  - Look at the axial CT or MRI scans to determine the location of the heart and great vessels. In most thoracic cases, these structures are either on the left or central.

Thus, all other factors being equal, a right-sided approach is favored in most cases.
- In the distal thoracic spine (eg, T10–T12), the elevated right hemidiaphragm and liver may be in the way of a right-sided approach. As retracting the liver is more difficult than the kidney or spleen, a left-sided approach may be favorable.
- Considerations for thoracolumbar approaches include the following:
  - The left-sided approach is generally favored, as it is easier to mobilize the great arteries (aorta, iliacs) from their left central position to the right rather than mobilizing the more friable great veins (which lie further to the right).

T E C H N I Q U E S

ANTERIOR THORACIC APPROACH FROM T1 TO T4

- For upper thoracic exposures, a right-sided approach is preferred to avoid the heart and great vessels.
- The surgeon makes a curved skin incision below the tip of the scapula (**TECH FIG 1A**).
- This incision is carried down to the latissimus dorsi muscle and then the latissimus is incised, leaving a cuff of the muscle on the scapula for later closure (**TECH FIG 1B**).
- A large retractor (ie, Richardson retractor) can then be held by the assistant while the surgeon incises the periosteum over the appropriate rib and then resects the rib as far anteriorly and posteriorly as possible (**TECH FIG 1C**).

- At this point, the chest is entered through the rib bed and a Finochietto or Omni retractor can be placed, with one of the blades holding the scapula up and out of the way.
  - Now, the lung can be deflated and retracted anteriorly and inferiorly (**TECH FIG 1D**).
- The pleura overlying the spine is now sharply incised. Placing suture into the edges of the pleura makes subsequent closure easier.
- Segmental vessels are identified and ligated as needed, and the vertebral bodies (the "valleys") and disc spaces (the "hills") are identified.

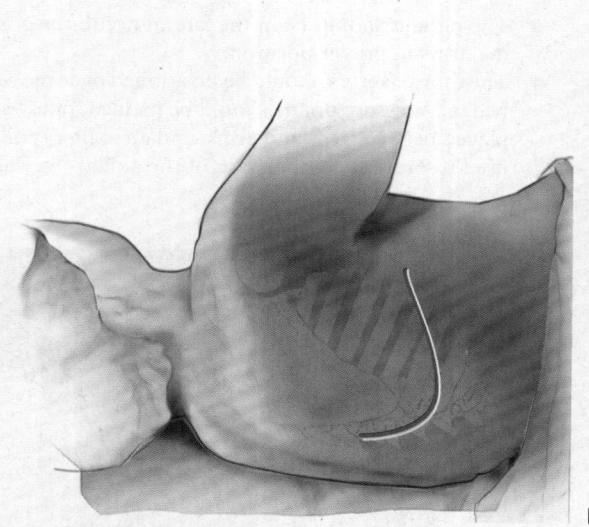
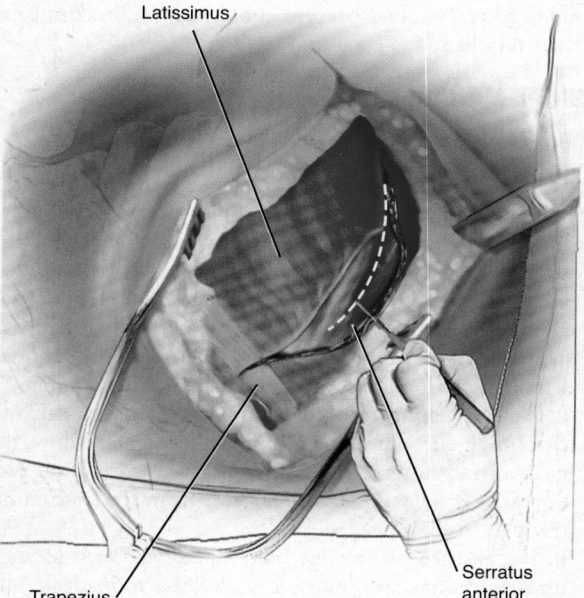

TECH FIG 1 Anterior thoracic approach from T1 to T4. **A.** A curved incision should be made just under the tip of the scapula. **B.** The incision is carried down to the latissimus dorsi. A cuff of muscle is left attached to the scapula for repair upon closure. *(continued)*

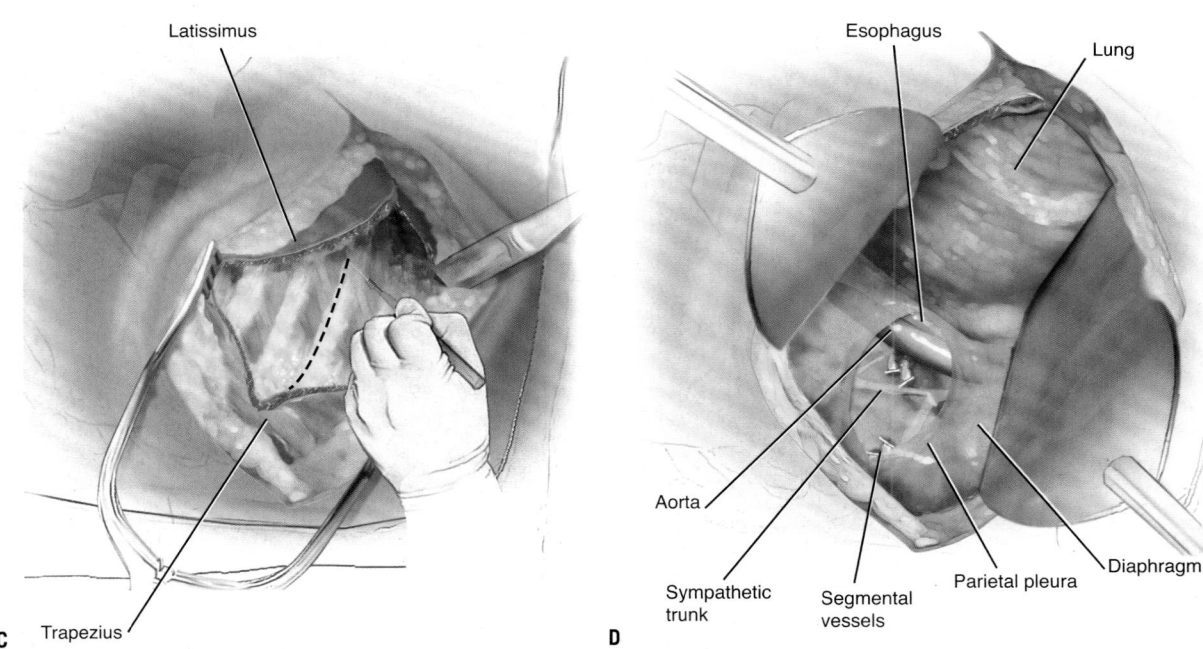

TECH FIG 1 *(continued)* **C.** The surgeon incises the periosteum over the rib. **D.** The deflated lung is retracted anteriorly and inferiorly while protecting the esophagus and great vessels.

ANTERIOR THORACIC APPROACH FROM T5 TO T12

- The surgeon should plan the incision directly over the desired rib (ie, 10th rib for T9–T10 disc). A curvilinear skin incision is made along the path of the rib from the anterior border of the latissimus dorsi to the costochondral junction anteriorly **(TECH FIG 2A)**.
  - Due to the downslope of the ribs, it is generally preferable to make an incision that is more proximal rather than distal. If the incision is too distal, the ribs may impede access to the more proximal segment, necessitating a second thoracotomy. In contrast, it is easier to access levels that are distal to the rib that is resected. Thus, if in doubt as to the exact rib to be resected, the incision should be made more proximal. ·
- Skin and subcutaneous fat are incised to expose the trapezius and latissimus dorsi.
- The trapezius and latissimus dorsi are divided in line with the incision using electrocautery. The rhomboids may need to be split to gain more exposure cephalad.
- Once the correct rib is identified, the surgeon divides the periosteum over the upper border of the rib to avoid injury to the intercostal nerve and vessels **(TECH FIG 2B)**.
- The rib is stripped subperiosteally anteriorly to the costochondral angle and as far posteriorly as possible **(TECH FIG 2C)**.
- The rib is removed with a rib cutter and passed off the field. The rib is cut at the midaxillary line anteriorly and as far posteriorly as possible. The rib can be used as a strut graft or autologous bone graft.
- The periosteal rib sleeve and parietal pleura are incised to enter the thorax. A rib spreader is placed to hold the ribs apart **(TECH FIG 2D)**.
- The ipsilateral lung is deflated and retracted medially to expose the parietal pleura overlying the spine.
- The parietal pleura overlying the spine is incised and retracted medially. Stitches can be placed in the parietal pleura to make

closure easier. The underlying segmental vessels are visualized **(TECH FIG 2E)**.
- The segmental arteries arising from the aorta can run in ascending, recurrent, horizontal, or descending direction depending on the level of involvement.
- The surgeon carefully ligates as few segmental vessels as possible to gain adequate exposure to the spine. Ligating more segmental vessels than necessary places the spinal cord at increased risk for ischemia because the thoracic spinal cord has a tenuous blood supply **(TECH FIG 2F)**.
  - In cases of suspected vascular anomalies, such as congenital kyphosis, the surgeon should consider temporary occlusion of the segmental vessels and check evoked potentials before vessel ligation. If a patient has had a prior spine exposure on one side, the surgeon should be wary of ligating the contralateral segmental vessels. Instead, the surgery should be performed through the previously exposed side, or a preoperative angiogram should be obtained to identify the important arterial feeders to the spinal cord.
- The intrathoracic vertebral bodies and intervertebral discs are now exposed. To gain access to the posterior intervertebral disc, the rib head may need to be removed.
- The costotransverse and costovertebral articulations are removed to excise the rib head **(TECH FIG 2G)**.
- The soft tissues overlying the transverse process, pedicle, and vertebral body are removed.
- The superior edge of the pedicle is identified and followed back to the intervertebral space.
- The superior edge of pedicle is burred to expose the posterior intervertebral disc and lateral margin of the dura **(TECH FIG 2H)**.

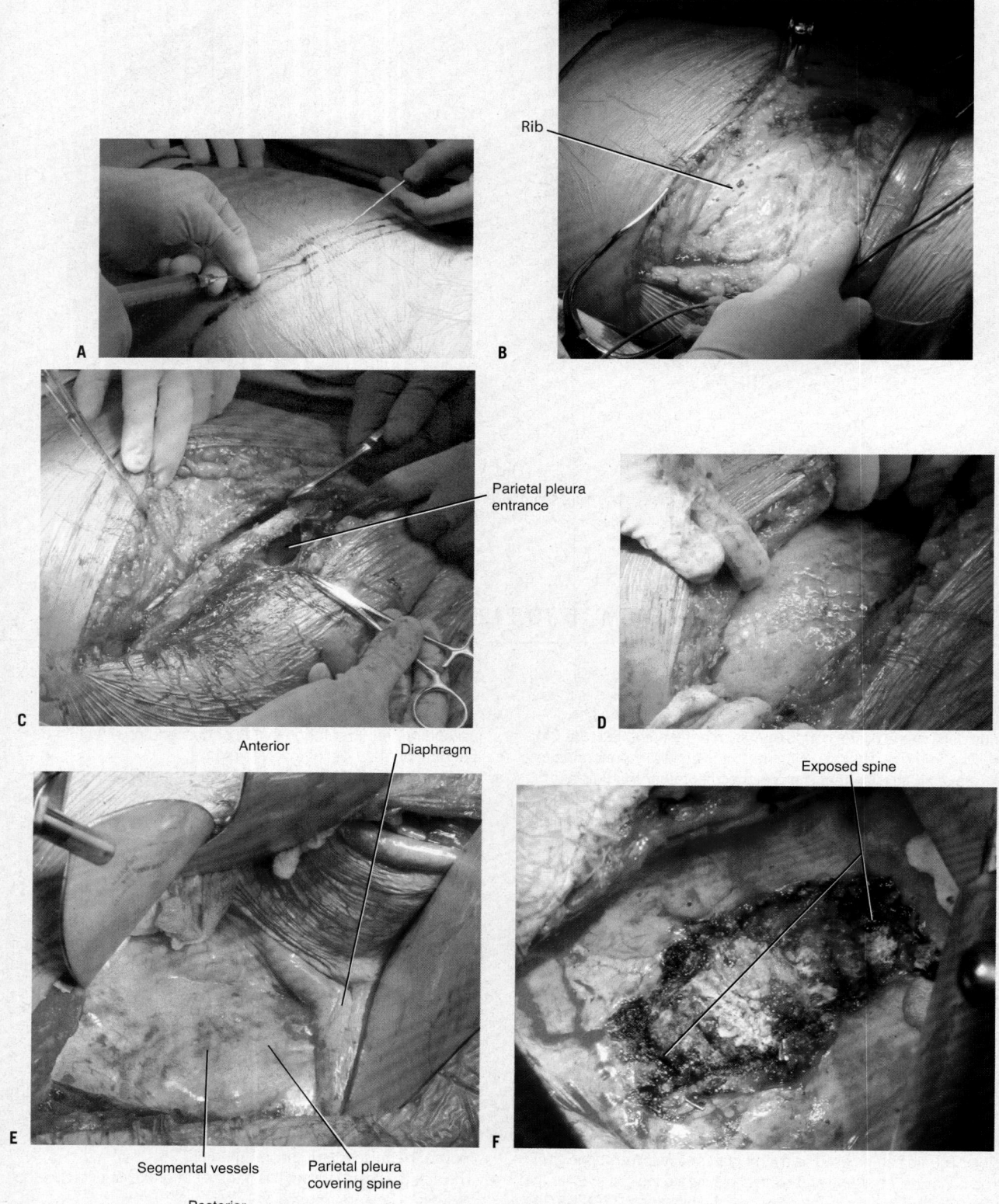

TECH FIG 2 Anterior thoracic approach from T5 to T12. (In these images, the patient's head is to the upper left and the patient's back is toward the surgeon.) **A.** The incision is planned directly over the rib. Injecting the subcutaneous tissues with a combination of anesthetic and epinephrine aids in hemostasis. **B.** The skin and subcutaneous tissues have been divided, exposing the desired rib. **C.** Subperiosteal exposure of the rib before excision. Note the thin parietal pleura beneath the rib bed. **D.** After excision of the rib the parietal pleura is entered, exposing the ipsilateral lung. **E.** The parietal pleura and the underlying segmental vessels. **F.** The vertebral bodies and intervertebral discs are exposed after segmental arteries are ligated, and the overlying soft tissues are removed. *(continued)*

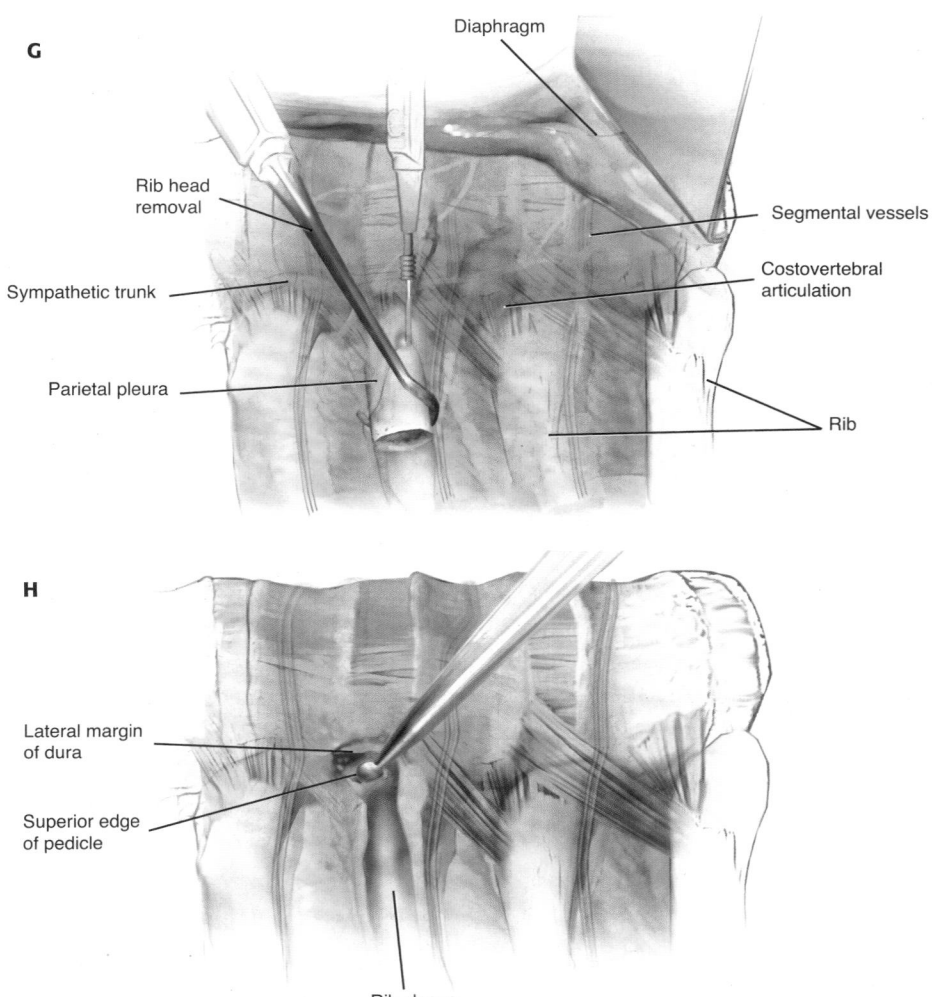

G

Diaphragm

Rib head removal

Segmental vessels

Costovertebral articulation

Sympathetic trunk

Parietal pleura

Rib

H

Lateral margin of dura

Superior edge of pedicle

Rib sleeve

TECH FIG 2 *(continued)* Once the costotransverse and costovertebral articulations are excised (**G**), the rib head can be removed with a high-speed burr (**H**).

MINI TRANSTHORACIC ANTERIOR APPROACH

Exposure

- Patient is positioned in the lateral decubitus position.
- Fluoroscopic evaluation is used to identify desired levels to gain access to, and the level of these vertebral bodies are marked with a skin pen directly over their position on a lateral projection.
- A skin incision is made parallel to the ribs medially extending 5 to 10 cm laterally.
- Using a pair of curved scissors, bluntly split the latissimus dorsi and serratus anteriorly in line with their fibers until you encounter the underlying rib.
- Using the rib spreading, create a space between the two ribs.
  - The rib need only be resected if exposure is not adequate with the rib spreader

- Deflate the lung and sharply split the visceral pleura and retract it medially to expose the desired vertebra and confirm with fluoroscopy.
- Bring the microscope into the field and identify the costovertebral junction.
- Using a high-speed burr, resect the rib head, superolateral portion of the caudal vertebral body, and the inferolateral portion of the cranial vertebra, and the superior portion of the pedicle below the desired disc, exposing the longitudinal ligament, which is incised to provide clear visualization of the intervertebral disc (**TECH FIG 3**).

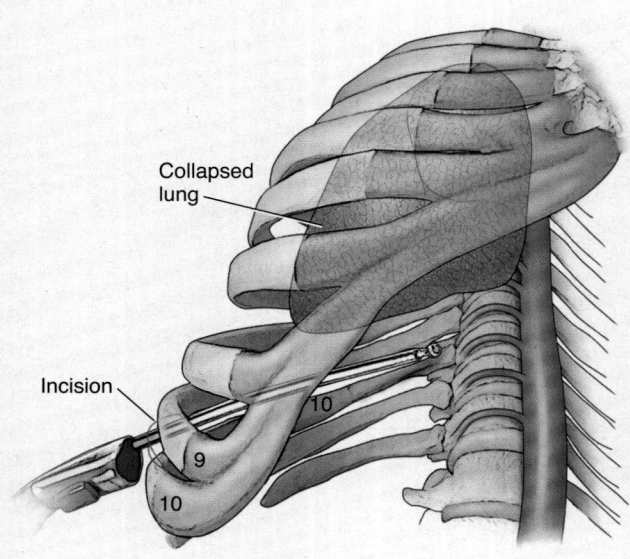

Collapsed lung

Incision

10

9

10

TECH FIG 3 In the mini transthoracic approach, a 5- to 10-cm incision is made just cranial to the 10th rib through the parietal and visceral pleura, bypassing the inflated lung. This approach provides access to the T9–T10 disc space to allow for a variety of procedures, including corpectomy and plating, interbody fusion, and discectomy.

VIDEO-ASSISTED THORASCOPIC SURGERY ANTERIOR THORACIC APPROACH

Exposure

- Patient is positioned in the lateral decubitus position.
- Fluoroscopic evaluation is used to identify desired levels to gain access to, and the levels of these vertebral bodies are marked with a skin pen directly over their position on a lateral projection.
- A 10-cm skin incision is made parallel to the centered just anterior to the midaxillary line.
- Split the latissimus dorsi and serratus anteriorly in line with their fibers until you encounter the underlying rib.
- The lung is deflated by the anesthesia team.
- Sharply split the intercostal muscles and visceral pleura to enter the pleural cavity. Using the rib spreading, create a space between the two ribs.
  - The rib need only be resected if exposure is not adequate with the rib spreader.
- Introduce the thoracoscope and retract the deflated lung medially to expose the anterior thoracic spinal column.
- A 5-mm camera port is then placed at a useable intercostal space at the anterior axillary line under video-assisted visualization.
- Once thoracoscope is in position, a working 15-tmm port along the midaxillary line is placed.
  - The level of placement for the working port is determined with fluoroscopic guidance of desired level.
  - Once adequate visualization and access is obtained, exposure is carried out with use of bipolar and harmonic cautery ensuring adequate ligation of the segmental vessels lying over the vertebral bodies.
  - Using a high-speed burr, resect the rib head, superolateral portion of the caudal vertebral body, and the inferolateral portion of the cranial vertebra, and the superior portion of the pedicle below the desired disc, exposing the longitudinal

ligament, which is incised to provide clear visualization of the intervertebral disc (TECH FIG 3).
- This approach may be also be used for anterior correction of scoliosis deformity.

Detaching the Diaphragm

- Exposure of T12–L1 may require detaching the diaphragm.
  - The diaphragm inserts and originates from the xiphoid and the inferior six ribs.
  - The lateral arcuate ligament arises from the transverse process of L1.
  - The crura extend more distally on the right.
  - The diaphragm is innervated centrally by the phrenic nerves.
- The surgeon starts at the costal angle and incises the costodiaphragmatic reflection until extraperitoneal fat is visualized.
- The diaphragm is divided off the anterior chest wall (TECH FIG 4). The surgeon should leave a 1- to 2-cm cuff of diaphragm on the anterior chest wall to allow for diaphragm repair at closure. To avoid diaphragm denervation, the diaphragm should be incised only at its periphery. The diaphragm is split up to the lateral arcuate ligament.
- The medial and lateral crura are detached, exposing the underlying peritoneum.
- The peritoneum is swept medially until the retroperitoneal space is visualized.
- The surgeon bluntly dissects and sweeps the fascia of Gerota medially to expose the spine and the overlying parietal pleura.
- The aorta and vena cava are identified.
- The surgeon can elevate the psoas muscle if needed.
- The parietal pleura is incised to expose the spine.

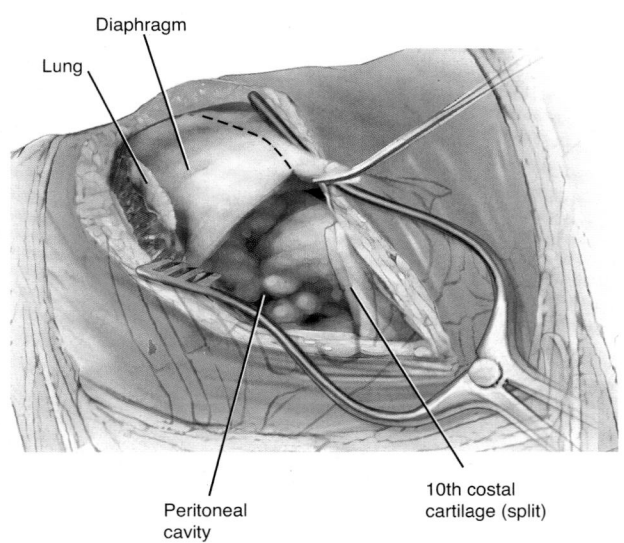

TECH FIG 4 The diaphragm is incised circumferentially 2 cm from its peripheral attachment to the chest wall. Marker stitches should be placed for resuturing upon closure.

THORACOABDOMINAL RETROPERITONEAL LUMBAR SPINE APPROACH FROM T10 TO L3

- The patient is positioned in the lateral decubitus position with the right side down. The approach should be made from the left side to avoid the liver and inferior vena cava.
- The crura of the diaphragm are detached as described earlier.
- An oblique incision is made from the quadratus lumborum to the lateral border of the rectus abdominis **(TECH FIG 5)**.
  - This approach can be extended to L5 in most patients and even to S1 in those with low-riding iliac crests.
- The subcutaneous tissue is incised, and the fascia of the external oblique is divided.
- The external and internal obliques, transverse abdominis, and transversalis fascia are incised.

- The peritoneum is exposed and bluntly reflected anteriorly.
- The ureter is identified and reflected anteriorly with retroperitoneal fat.
- The vertebral bodies, psoas, and great vessels are identified.
- The genitofemoral nerve lies on anterior psoas muscle, and excessive traction should be avoided.
- The segmental vessels that lie over the middle of the vertebral bodies are identified and ligated.
- The psoas is bluntly dissected off the vertebrae and retracted laterally.
- The vertebral body, pedicle, and neuroforamen can be visualized.

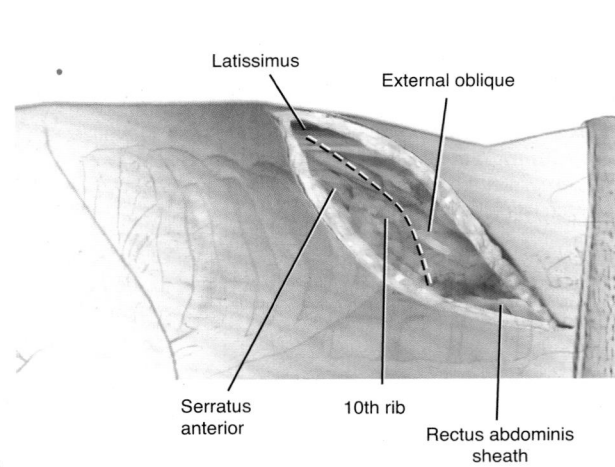

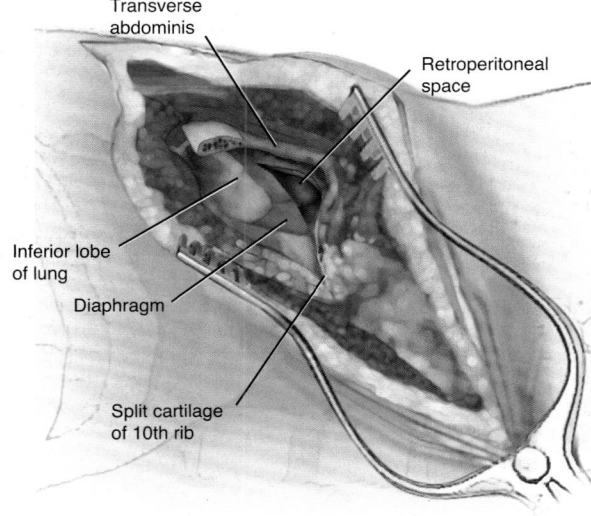

TECH FIG 5 Thoracoabdominal approach. **A.** A curvilinear incision is made over the 10th rib, and the muscle layers are identified. **B.** The retroperitoneal space is entered through the costal cartilage after removing the 10th rib. *(continued)*

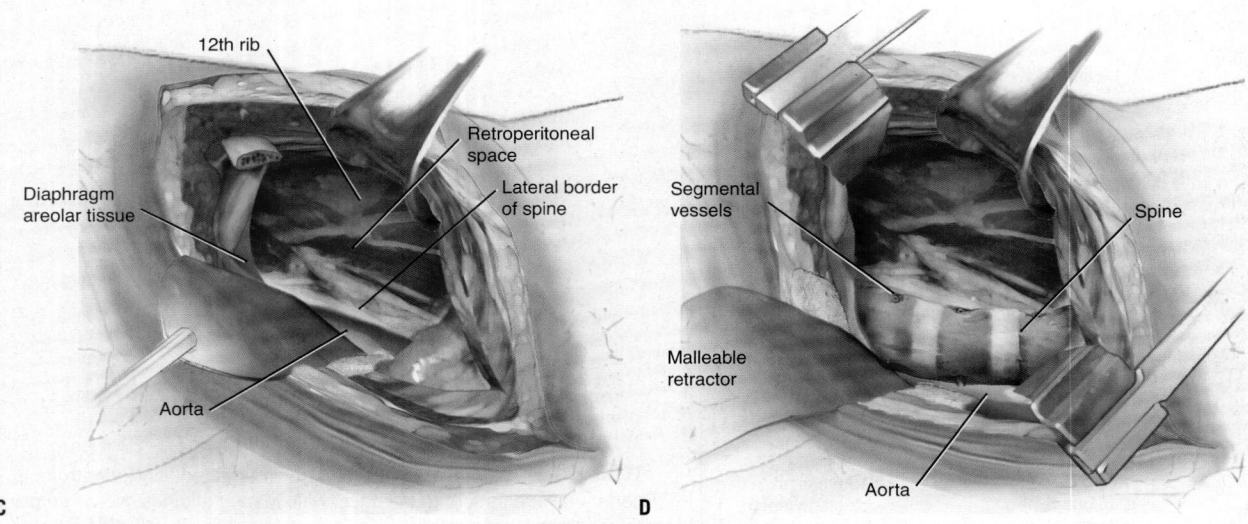

TECH FIG 5 *(continued)* **C.** The light areolar tissue that signifies the retroperitoneal space is identified, and the peritoneum is mobilized from the undersurface of the diaphragm and abdominal wall as well as the aorta. **D.** Exposure of the spine is done after ligation of segmental vessels.

TECHNIQUES

Pearls and Pitfalls

Neurologic Compromise	• The surgeon should consider preoperative angiography before left-sided approaches between T8 and T12 to identify the artery of Adamkiewicz and prevent spinal cord infarction. • The surgeon should consider temporarily clamping the segmental arteries before ligation and assessing for changes in evoked potentials to avoid vascular catastrophe because blood supply to the spinal cord is tenuous in the thoracic region, especially in the "critical zone" from T4 to T9.
Avoiding Wrong-Level Surgery	• The surgeon should place a hand under the scapula and count rib spaces. The first rib is often difficult to feel, but the second rib space is the largest. • Preoperative anteroposterior and lateral chest radiographs can aid in rib counting, especially in kyphotic patients. • Consider intraoperative navigation for further confirmation of correct levels
Exposure	• Using a double-lumen endotracheal tube will allow deflation of the ipsilateral lung and improve exposure. • Detaching the psoas muscle off the transverse processes can improve exposure of the intervertebral disc space and neuroforamen. The transverse processes can also be removed to further increase exposure. • Flexing the patient's hips can decrease tension on the psoas and improve visualization of the lumbar spine. • More ribs may need to be excised to gain better exposure, especially in older patients, in whom the ribs may not be as compliant to the rib spreader. • From T2 to T5, it may help to detach the serratus anterior muscle from the anterior chest wall and reflect it cephalad to gain better exposure. The surgeon should avoid cutting the long thoracic nerve at this level. • If scapular manipulation is needed to gain better exposure, the rhomboids, trapezius, and dorsal scapular muscles can be divided, allowing the scapula to be mobilized laterally.
Visceral Injury	• When approaching from the right side, the surgeon should dissect the soft tissues away from the spine as close as possible to the bone with a blunt gauze or finger to prevent injury to the cisterna chyli and thoracic duct.

POSTOPERATIVE CARE

- Chest tubes are left in place until output is less than 150 mL over 24 hours.

COMPLICATIONS

- The exiting nerve root can be injured while removing the pedicle.
  - Care should be taken to tie the nerve root off proximal to the dorsal root ganglion.
- Vascular injury
- Intercostal neuralgia
- Atelectasis
- Neurologic injury
- Wrong-level surgery
- Significant bleeding can be encountered when entering the epidural space.
- Visceral injury

REFERENCES

1. Arts MP, Bartels RHMA. Anterior or posterior approach of thoracic disc herniation? A comparative cohort of mini-transthoracic versus transpedicular discectomies. Spine J 2014;14(8):1654–1662.
2. Grace RR, Mattox KL. Anterior spinal artery syndrome following abdominal aortic aneurysmectomy. Case report and review of the literature. Arch Surg 1977;112:813–815.

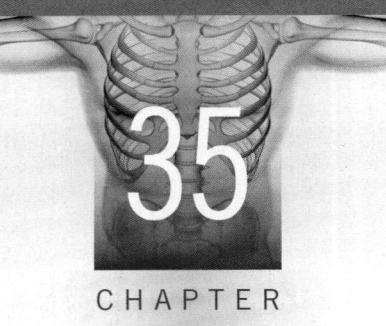

CHAPTER

35

Anterior Lumbar Approach

James W. Klunk, Brad W. Moatz, and P. Justin Tortolani

DEFINITION

- The anterior lumbar approach provides excellent access to the lumbar spine extending from the L2–L3 disc to the first segment of the sacrum (S1).

ANATOMY

- The anterior abdominal wall has a layered configuration that changes depending on whether the approach is proximal or distal to the arcuate line.
- Above the arcuate line, the layers in order are skin, subcutaneous fat (containing fascia of Camper and Scarpa), anterior rectus sheath (aponeurosis of the external and internal oblique muscles), rectus muscle, posterior rectus sheath (aponeurosis of the internal oblique and transversus abdominis muscles), transversalis fascia, and peritoneum (FIG 1).
- Below the arcuate line, the posterior rectus sheath is not present, and thus the rectus muscle lies directly on the transversalis fascia.
- For retroperitoneal exposures, the approach goes through the abdominal wall to the layer of the transversalis fascia and then progresses laterally until this fascia ends, exposing the retroperitoneal fat.
- For transperitoneal exposures, the transversalis fascia is divided in the midline, as is the peritoneum, and the exposure proceeds directly posterior to the level of the sacral prominence.

- The abdominal contents are retracted to expose the great vessels overlying the anterior lumbar spine.
- Key vascular structures with relationship to the spine are shown in FIG 2.
- Vascular
  - The abdominal aorta and the bifurcation into the left and right common iliac arteries lie anterior to the venous system, and the left iliac artery is typically encountered first (L4–L5). In most people, the bifurcation occurs at L4–L5.
    - Preoperative scrutiny of magnetic resonance imaging (MRI) or computed tomography (CT) scans can help identify the location of the bifurcation, which can be important in planning.
  - The left renal artery and vein (L2) restrict exposure proximal to L2.
  - The inferior vena cava (IVC) lies posteriorly and to the right of the aorta, whereas the superior hypogastric plexus lies to the left of the IVC. Because of its deep, right-sided position, mobilization of the IVC from right to left (although less injurious to the sympathetic chain) risks side wall rupture. By contrast, mobilization from left to right places tension on the side wall of the left iliac vein and appropriate precautions must be taken.[4]
  - The L5–S1 disc occupies a position between the bifurcation of the aorta and the IVC in most patients, so mobilization of the large vessels is rarely required for access.

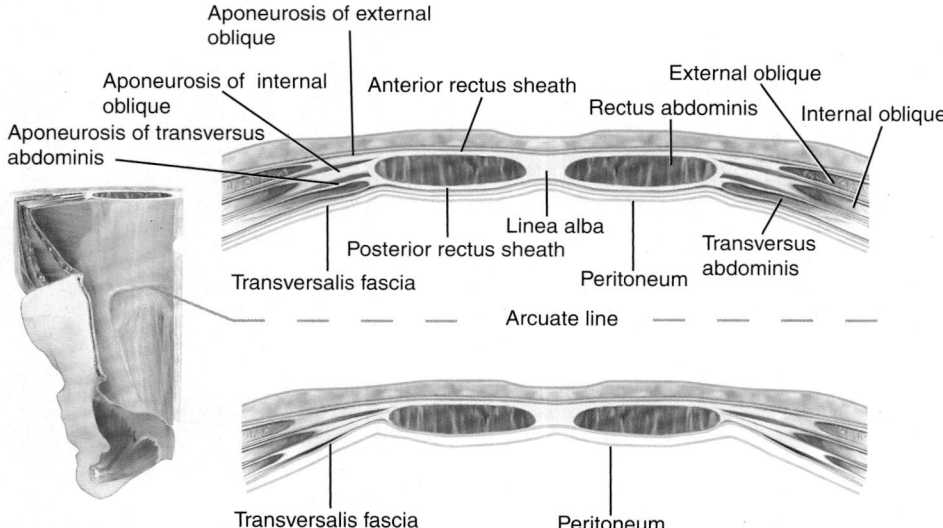

Aponeurosis of external oblique
Aponeurosis of internal oblique
Aponeurosis of transversus abdominis
Anterior rectus sheath
External oblique
Rectus abdominis
Internal oblique
Transversalis fascia
Posterior rectus sheath
Linea alba
Peritoneum
Transversus abdominis
Arcuate line
Transversalis fascia
Peritoneum

FIG 1 Above (proximal to) the arcuate line, the posterior rectus sheath is present and contains fibers from the internal oblique and transversus abdominis aponeuroses. Below (distal to) the arcuate line, the posterior rectus sheath is no longer present. Exposures to the L4–L5 disc space generally require identification and incision of the posterior rectus sheath.

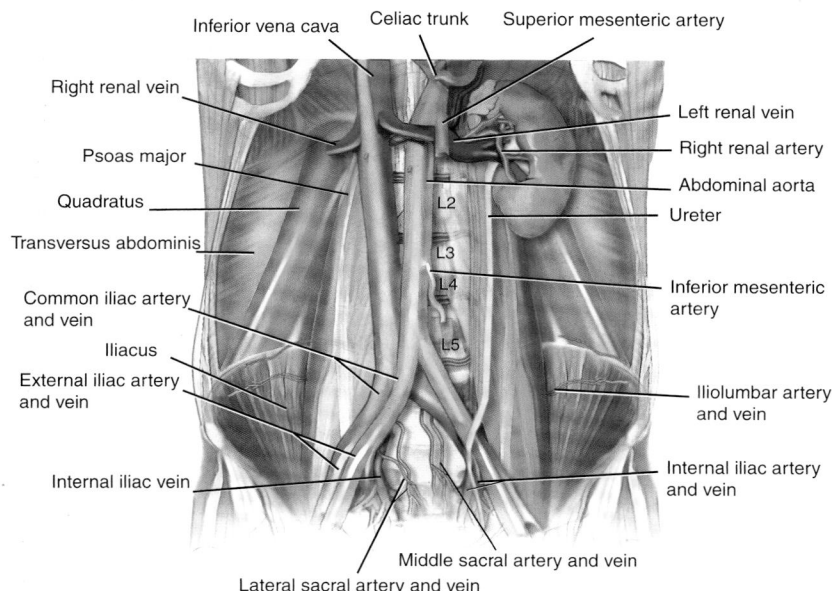

Inferior vena cava   Celiac trunk   Superior mesenteric artery

Right renal vein

Psoas major

Quadratus

Transversus abdominis

Common iliac artery
and vein

Iliacus

External iliac artery
and vein

Internal iliac vein

Left renal vein

Right renal artery

Abdominal aorta

Ureter

Inferior mesenteric
artery

Iliolumbar artery
and vein

Internal iliac artery
and vein

Middle sacral artery and vein

Lateral sacral artery and vein

L2
L3
L4
L5

FIG 2 Vascular and anatomy of the retroperitoneal space.

The middle sacral artery and vein generally branch off of the left common iliac artery and vein and should be ligated or cauterized if small.

- Exposures above L5–S1, however, require mobilization of the great vessels to the right. To do this, the iliolumbar vein, which branches off the left common iliac, must be identified and ligated (see Techniques section).
- Genitourinary
  - Left kidney: rarely visualized, surrounded by perinephric fat (L1–L2)
  - Left ureter: easily retracted anteriorly with peritoneal contents and can be identified by stimulated peristalsis or intraoperative administration of intravenous indigo carmine
- Muscular
  - Psoas (paraspinal, L1–L5)
- Neurologic
  - Sympathetic chain (paraspinal, anterior and medial to psoas)
  - Presacral plexus (directly over sacrum)
  - Lumbosacral plexus (posteromedial to and within psoas muscle)
  - Genitofemoral nerve (lies on anterior aspect of psoas)
- Lymphatic
  - Paraspinal lymphatics and lymph nodes
  - Lymphatic drainage will appear as a milky white fluid, which is rarely of clinical consequence.

PATIENT HISTORY AND PHYSICAL FINDINGS

- Previous abdominal surgery (eg, hysterectomy, hernia repair) can create challenges during this exposure. The presence of midline abdominal mesh, cellulitis or abscess, and a colostomy are relative contraindications to the anterior approach.
- Previous exposure of the anterior lumbar spine, particularly if it involved mobilization of the great veins, makes revision approaches much more risky due to the greater likelihood of vascular injury.

- Obesity (body mass index above 40 kg/m²) is a relative contraindication to anterior exposure of the lumbar spine due to the depth of the operative field.

IMAGING AND OTHER DIAGNOSTIC STUDIES

- Plain radiographs are used to assess the degree of aortic calcification and lumbopelvic deformity.
- Preoperative axial MRI or CT allows for estimation of the level of the bifurcation of the aorta and IVC (**FIG 3**).
- Routine angiography, CT angiography, or magnetic resonance angiography is not necessary unless there is a concern for aberrant anatomy (eg, history of situs inversus).
- Preoperative arteriograms, venograms, and prophylactic IVC filters should be considered before any revision approaches to the anterior lumbar spine. Preoperative ureteral stents can also help prevent ureteral injury during revision exposure.

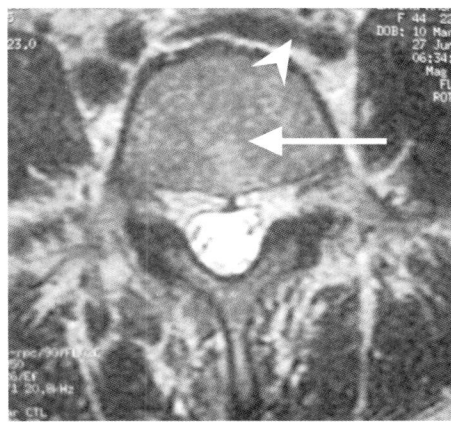

FIG 3 T2-weighted axial MRI image demonstrates the bifurcation of the IVC (*arrowhead*). In this case, the bifurcation occurs at the level of the L5 vertebra rather than the L4–L5 disc space. This configuration may make access easier at the L4–L5 disc but harder at the L5–S1 disc, as the left iliac vein may obliquely cross over it (*arrow*).

SURGICAL MANAGEMENT

- Indications for the anterior lumbar approach are as follows:
  - Anterior discectomy for interbody fusion, total disc replacement, disc débridement in cases of discitis and vertebral osteomyelitis, and radical discectomy for deformity correction
  - Anterior corpectomy for tumor resection, radical deformity correction, and vertebral body osteomyelitis
- Contraindications are relative and include the following:
  - Prior anterior approach or other abdominal surgery, fascial mesh, colostomy, pelvic radiation, low bifurcating aorta or vena cava for L5–S1 approaches, untreated paraspinal infection, obesity (body mass index >40 kg/m²), and severe atherosclerosis or aneurysms preventing vascular mobilization

Preoperative Planning

- When exposure of the L5–S1 disc is required, the direct anterior lumbar approach should be used in most cases, as the ilium blocks satisfactory access from a lateral approach.
- The direct anterior approach is less morbid than the lateral approach to the lumbar spine because the latter involves greater division of the abdominal wall musculature.[5]
- For these reasons, we prefer the direct anterior approach (vs. the lateral approach) even in cases of multilevel disc exposures (eg, lumbar scoliosis correction) unless the L1–L2 disc or L2 vertebra requires exposure or if anterior instrumentation in the form of screw–rod constructs is needed. Anterior plates can be used from a direct anterior approach at L5–S1 and, in some cases, L4–L5, depending on the vascular anatomy.
- However, greater mobilization of the great vessels at the level of the bifurcation is needed from a direct anterior versus lateral approach. Thus, a lateral approach may provide better exposure if mobilization of the great vessels is anticipated to be difficult.

Positioning

- The patient is positioned supine over an inflatable pillow **(FIG 4A)**. Inflation of the pillow allows extension of the spine during discectomy and graft placement, if needed. Slight Trendelenburg may aid to retract an obstructive pannus.
- The operating room table should allow for free passage of the fluoroscopic C-arm **(FIG 4B)**.
- Care should be taken to ensure that the pelvis is level so that true anteroposterior and lateral fluoroscopic images can be easily obtained.
- The patient's arms can be tucked to the side, placed into a "cross" position, or crossed over the chest but must not restrict appropriate fluoroscopic imaging **(FIG 4C)**.
- A pulse oximeter may be placed on the patient's first toe of the left foot in order to provide an early warning for left iliac artery thrombosis or excessive retraction. This is especially important with surgery involving the L4–L5 level.

Approach

- Various skin incisions can be used.
  - The Pfannenstiel can be used for L5–S1 exposures but is less extensile if additional proximal exposure is necessary.
  - The direct midline and paramedian incisions are useful for multilevel exposures as they are easily extended proximally or distally **(FIG 5A–D)**.

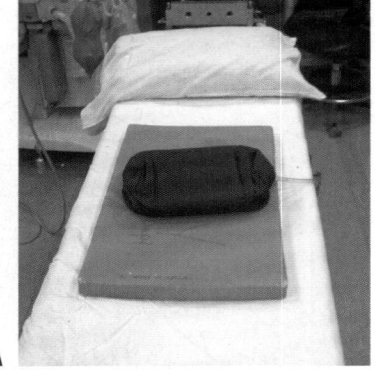
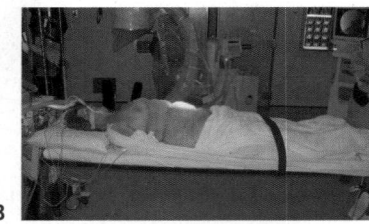
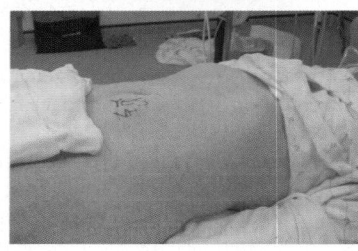

FIG 4 A. An inflatable pillow can be modulated during the case to allow increased or decreased lordosis. The pillow is placed over a thick foam pad (blue), which allows the patient's arms to be tucked along the side and thus out of the lateral fluoroscopic image beam. **B.** The operating room table is radiolucent and open underneath, allowing the fluoroscopic C-arm (in the distance) to pass under the table. **C.** The patient's arms are tucked to the side with a draw sheet after padding the elbows.

- Palpation of the sacral promontory allows more accurate placement of the skin incision **(FIG 5E)**. Alternatively, a lateral C-arm view can be taken to mark the location of the incision, keeping in mind that the trajectory needed to access the disc, especially at L5–S1, may require that the incision be placed where the path of this trajectory meets the skin rather than directly over the disc space itself.
- Retroperitoneal versus transperitoneal
  - The transperitoneal approach carries a higher risk of retrograde ejaculation due to the theoretically greater likelihood of injury to the presacral sympathetic nerve fibers.
  - This approach is useful, however, in revision approaches to L5–S1 in which the retroperitoneal exposure was used at the index procedure.
  - Transperitoneal approaches likely increase the risk of adhesion formation and possible small bowel obstruction. In addition, small or large bowel perforation and postoperative ileus are relatively more likely when the peritoneum is entered. Finally, extra time and care are required to retract the small intestines; this generally requires more retractors and large sponges to prevent interference during the remainder of the procedure.
- Right versus left retroperitoneal

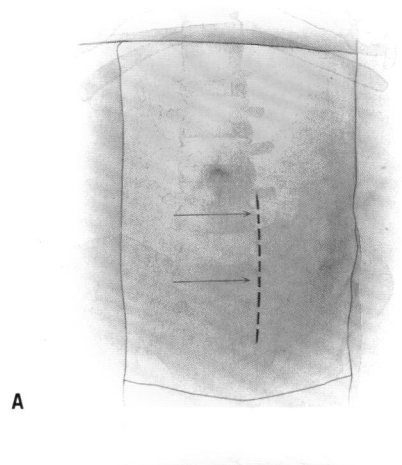

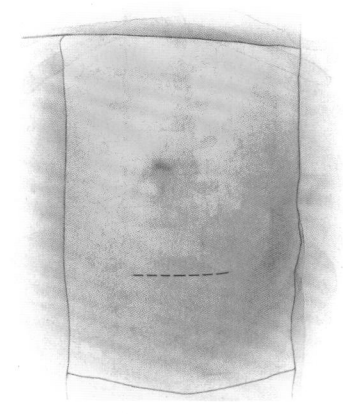

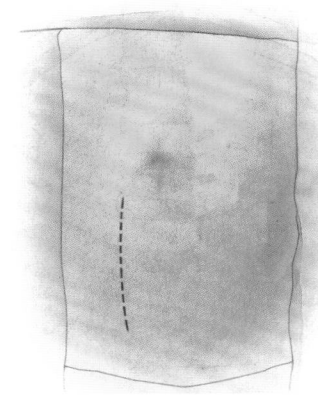

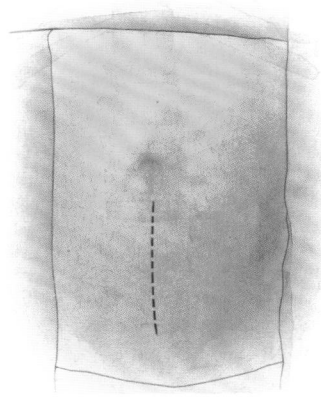

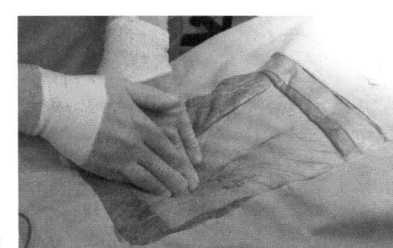

FIG 5 A. A left vertical paramedian incision allows excellent exposure of the anterior rectus sheath and not only facilitates closure but also provides easy access to the left retroperitoneal space. The *arrows* indicate the expected spinal levels (L4–L5, *upper arrow*; L5–S1, *lower arrow*). Other skin incision options are Pfannenstiel (**B**), right paramedian (**C**), and midline (**D**). **E.** Palpating the sacral promontory allows the surgeon to tailor the skin incision to the appropriate spinal level.

- With certain failures of lumbar disc replacement, revision exposures of the lumbar spine are necessary. To preserve the left retroperitoneal exposure for a potential revision exposure, some surgeons advocate performing a right-sided retroperitoneal incision at the index surgery.
  - Because optimal placement of a lumbar disc correlates with improved functional outcomes for the patient, we advocate performing the exposure that provides the ideal set of circumstances for accurate device placement at the outset.[7]
- Because the right common iliac artery and vein lie more vertical, crossing the L5–S1 disc space, whereas the left common iliac artery and vein traverse the disc diagonally, access to L5–S1 is easier and provides a more expansive exposure when performed from the left retroperitoneal approach.

ANTERIOR EXPOSURE OF LUMBAR SPINE (LEFT PARAMEDIAN INCISION AND RETROPERITONEAL APPROACH)

Dissection

- Once the skin is incised, the subcutaneous fat is divided in line with the skin incision to the level of the anterior rectus sheath.
- The anterior rectus sheath is identified and stripped clean of all fat to assist in identification of the fascial edges at the time of wound closure **(TECH FIG 1A)**.
- The anterior rectus sheath is incised in line with the skin incision—centered over the disc of interest—and then retracted laterally, exposing the underlying rectus abdominis muscle **(TECH FIG 1B)**.
- The rectus abdominis is then retracted laterally, exposing the underlying transversalis fascia **(TECH FIG 1C)**. The inferior epigastric vessels are noted here and should be preserved.
- With the rectus abdominis retracted, the transversalis fascia is followed laterally to its insertion on the abdominal wall. A sponge on a stick can be used to gently strip the transversalis fascia off this insertion **(TECH FIG 1D)**.
- Handheld retractors are then used to sweep the peritoneum and left ureter to the midline and beyond to the patient's right. Inadvertent tears in the peritoneum should be repaired with absorbable suture as encountered.
- Lateral dissection will reveal the spermatic cord (males) or round ligament (females may be divided for exposure).

TECHNIQUES

TECHNIQUES

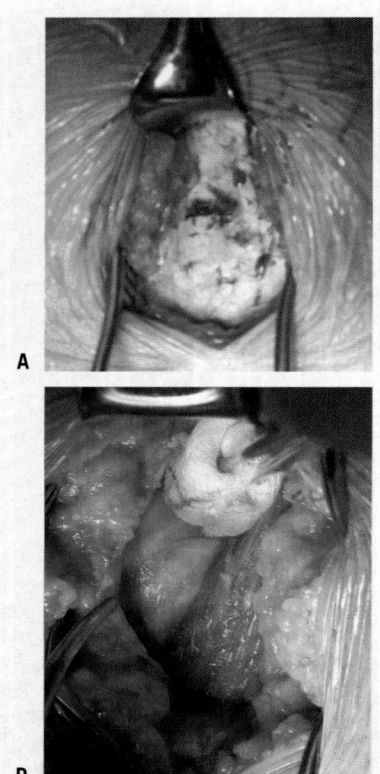
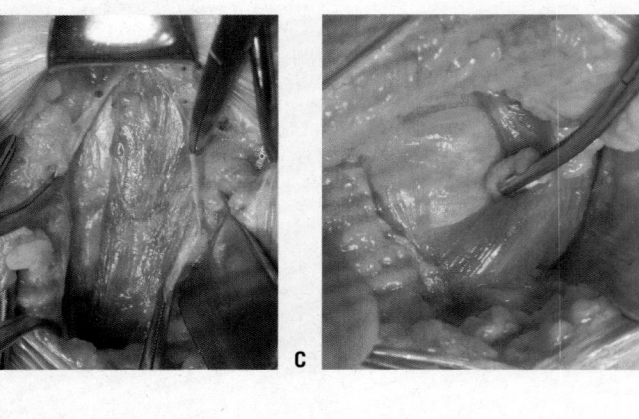

TECH FIG 1 **A.** The anterior rectus sheath can be clearly visualized. A small Richardson retractor has been placed at the top of the incision and a cerebellar retractor has been placed inferiorly. The *blue arrow* marks the center of the planned vertical fascial incision. **B.** The vertical fibers of the rectus abdominis muscle are visualized as the anterior rectus sheath is held to the patient's left with two Kocher clamps. **C.** The rectus abdominis muscle is retracted laterally with a Kittner, exposing the underlying transversalis fascia. **D.** A sponge on a stick is used to bluntly dissect the transversalis fascia off the undersurface of the rectus.

Further Exposure

- If exposure of L4–L5 is required, the arcuate line is identified and a small, 1-inch incision is created to allow more freedom in mobilization of the peritoneum (**TECH FIG 2A,B**).
- For exposure of the L4–L5 disc or above, the lateral border of the left common iliac artery and vein are first identified using

blunt dissection. These vessels are then retracted toward the midline to expose the iliolumbar veins coursing posteriorly (**TECH FIG 2C**).

- There is often more than one iliolumbar vein (up to 25% of patients),[8] and retracting the common iliac too forcefully can result in avulsion and significant bleeding that can be

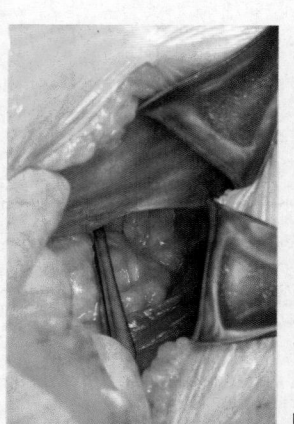
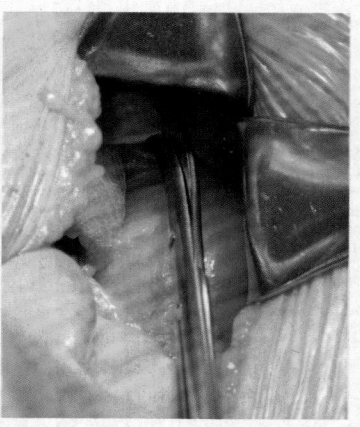
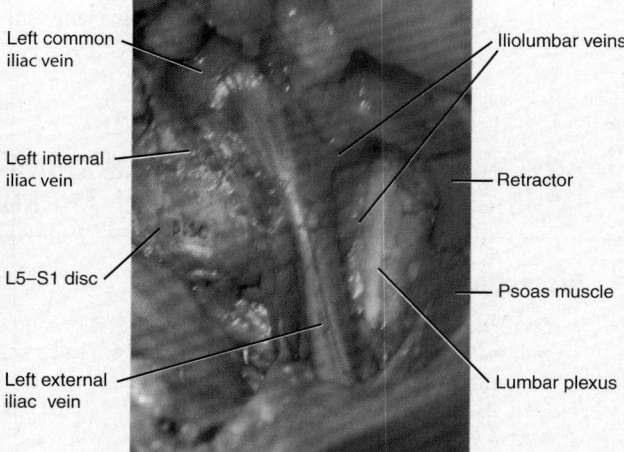

TECH FIG 2 **A.** For exposures at L4–L5, the posterior rectus sheath (arcuate line) is identified and the peritoneum is retracted away. **B.** Once the arcuate line is identified, it can be cut vertically; this enables the surgeon to safely retract the abdominal contents to the patient's right. **C.** In this cadaveric dissection, the iliolumbar veins can be visualized branching off the left common iliac vein, coursing posteriorly and laterally. By retracting the vein toward the midline and the psoas muscle laterally, the vein takes on a more transverse orientation and is easier to ligate. One of the lumbar nerve roots can be seen directly lateral to the iliolumbar vein. Excessive retraction pressure can injure these nerve roots. The arterial system has been removed.

difficult to control, especially if the wound is deep or the distal end of the vein retracts behind the psoas after avulsion.
- At L5–S1, blunt dissection with a Kittner exposes the disc space and defines the vascular anatomy. Palpation of the sacral promontory helps guide the blunt dissection.

Retractor Placement

- Although a vascular surgeon or assistant retracts the great vessels with handheld retractors, sharp, narrow Hohmann retractors are placed directly into the vertebrae.
  - Alternatively, blunt radiolucent retractors can be used. These retractors can be held by hand, can be fixed with transfixion pins, or can be clipped to an external frame (Omni) or ring (Endo Ring) for the remainder of the procedure.
- The optimal configuration of retractors for L5–S1 and L4–L5 exposures is depicted in **TECH FIG 3A,B**.
  - At L5–S1, placing a malleable retractor against the sacrum keeps the peritoneal contents and bladder out of the operative field and also provides a safety barrier to inadvertent movements of surgical instruments.

- For L5–S1 exposures, we prefer to use a sharp Hohmann retractor, which penetrates the bone on the (patient's) left side of the inferior vertebral body of L5. This ensures that the left common iliac vein will not slip under the retractor. Because this retractor is embedded in bone, there is no retraction on the lumbar nerve plexus.
- For L4–L5 exposures, because there are no vascular structures to retract on the (patient's) left side, a handheld retractor can be used to gently retract the psoas muscle. With a handheld retractor, it is critical that the blade does not extend too deep along the lateral edge of the vertebra, where it can impinge on the lumbar plexus. Surgical assistants need to pay attention to the force and location of their retraction effort.
- At L5–S1, retractors are positioned to retract the right and left common iliac artery and veins lateral to the superior margin of the disc.
- Before incising the disc, lateral fluoroscopic imaging should confirm the operative level and ensure that the retractors have not pierced the endplate **(TECH FIG 3C)**.
- For exposures at L4–L5 and above, mobilization of the aorta and IVC to the patient's right maybe difficult due to direct

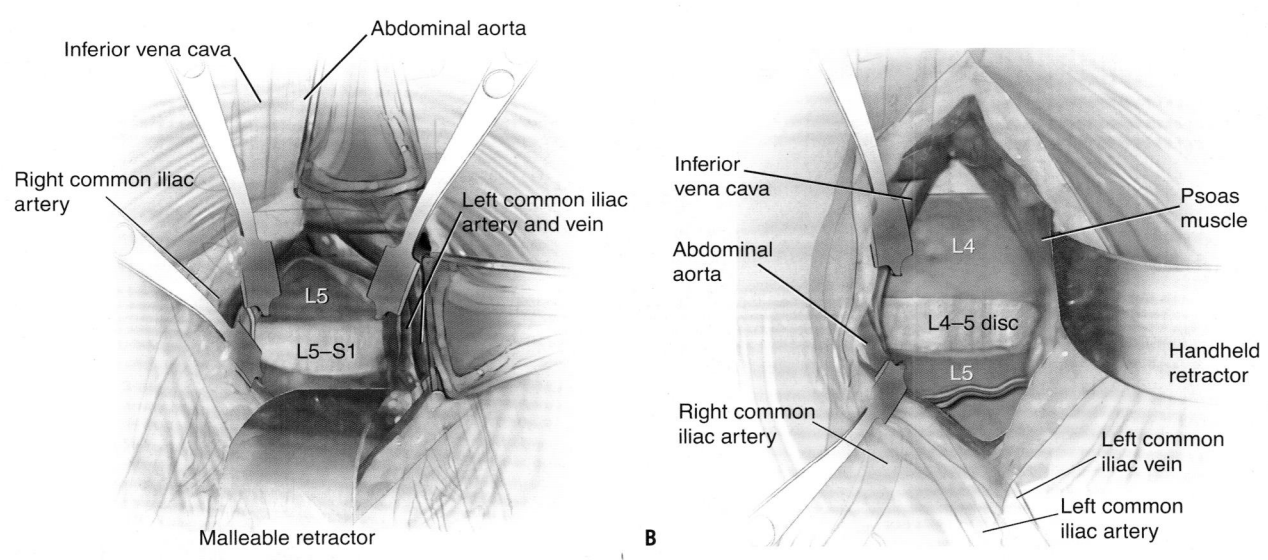

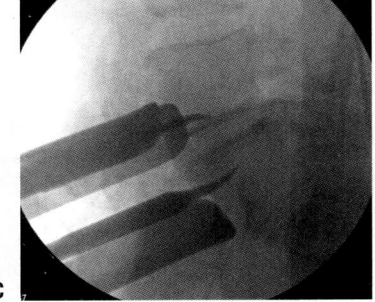

TECH FIG 3 A. Optimal configuration of retractors for exposure of the L5–S1 disc. **B.** Optimal configuration of retractors for exposure of the L4–L5 disc. Thin Hohmann retractors with sharp tips can be used to pierce the vertebral body and keep the great vessels out of the operative field. Handheld radiolucent blade retractors can also be used to retract the great vessels. Some retractors are cannulated, allowing them to be fixed with a transfixion pin into the vertebral body. **C.** The lateral fluoroscopic image confirms that the teeth of the Hohmann retractors are not in the disc space and that they are surrounding the disc of interest.

adhesions of the vessels to the anterior longitudinal ligament. Furthermore, anterior osteophytes may project into the great vessels making mobilization across the midline more risky.

- In these circumstances, we recommend retraction to the midline but not further **(TECH FIG 4A)**. Handheld retractors can hold the vessels in this position.

- Subsequent disc removal and interbody device placement can occur via an oblique trajectory into the disc, corresponding to the 12 o'clock to 3 o'clock position of the disc in the axial plane **(TECH FIG 4B)**.
- Interbody device placement can be made via a handle that attaches to the anterolateral position of the device **(TECH FIG 4C)**.

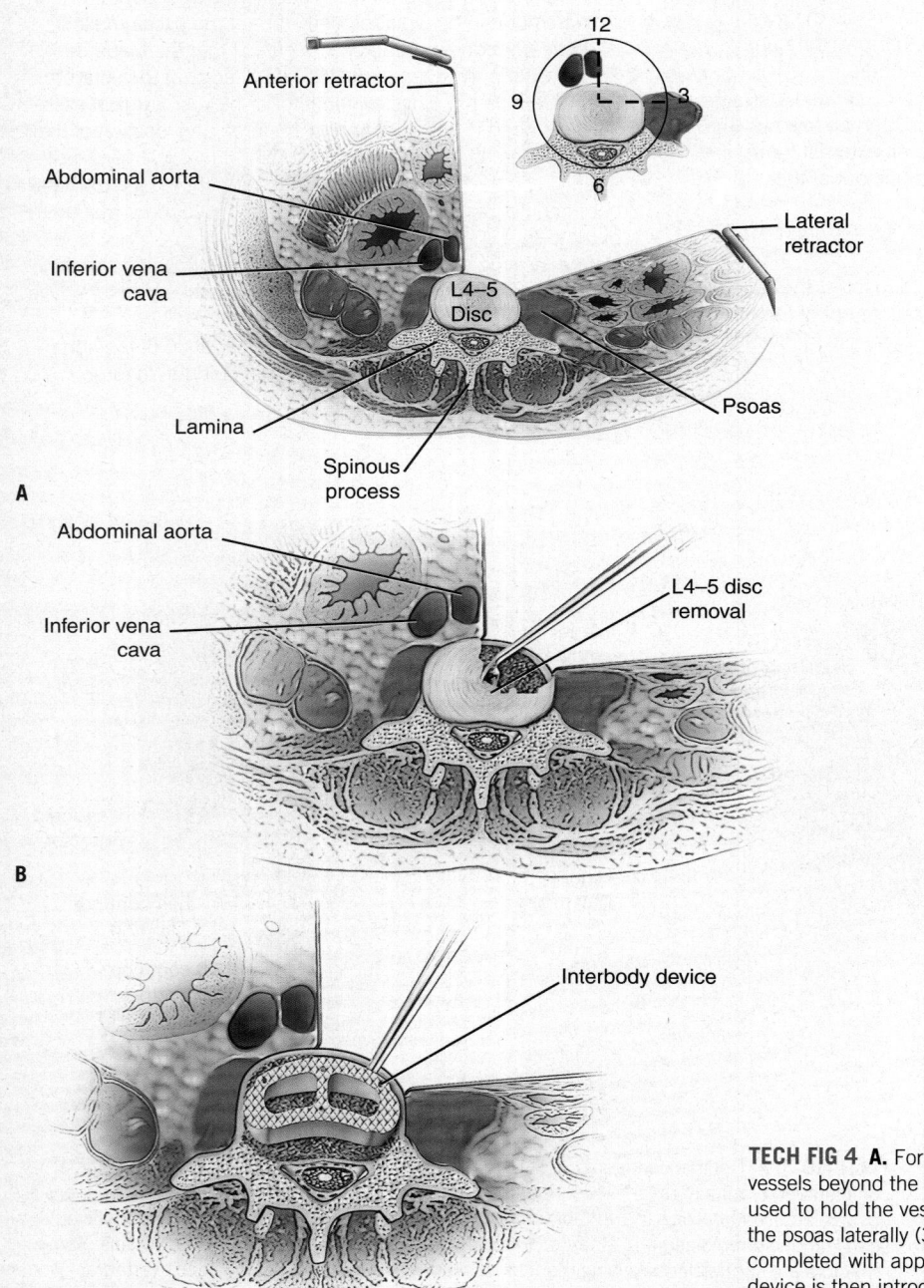

TECH FIG 4 A. For exposure at L4–L5, if retraction of the great vessels beyond the midline seems too risky, retractors can be used to hold the vessels to the midline (12 o'clock position) and the psoas laterally (3 o'clock position). **B.** Discectomy can be completed with appropriately angled curettes. **C.** The interbody device is then introduced through an anterolateral attachment handle.

Pearls and Pitfalls

- Cleaning the prerectus sheath of fat aids in finding this fascial edge at the end of the case.
- Use of bipolar and blunt dissection theoretically reduces the risk of presacral plexus injury and retrograde ejaculation.
- If the sympathetic chain is injured in the approach, the ipsilateral leg will feel warmer postoperatively; this is not to be confused with a cold contralateral leg.
- When ligating the iliolumbar veins, the surgeon should tie or clip each side of the vein twice to prevent loss of ligature.

POSTOPERATIVE CARE

- The patient is given 24 hours of antibiotics for wound infection prophylaxis.
- A perioperative nasogastric tube is used to reduce the incidence of postoperative ileus.
- The patient is mobilized on postoperative day 1 with a lumbar corset.
- Incentive spirometry is used.
- Skin staples are removed on postoperative day 10 or 14.
- Stool softeners and laxatives are used as needed to avoid fecal impaction.

OUTCOMES

- The prevalence of major vein lacerations was 1.4%, and the prevalence of left iliac artery thrombosis was 0.45% in a series of 1315 consecutive retroperitoneal exposures.[1,2]
- Ureteral and nerve injuries (lumbosacral nerve root or sympathetics) occur less frequently than major vascular injuries.[6]
- Mortality after anterior lumbar exposures is less than 1%.[6]
- Anterior approaches to the spine likely result in reduced patient satisfaction in terms of self-image and appearance.[3]
- The possibility of retrograde ejaculation should be discussed preoperatively with all male patients, as the prevalence ranges from 1% to 7%.[3,9] To preclude the need to harvest sperm from the bladder in affected men, donation before surgery is a viable option.

COMPLICATIONS

- Retrograde ejaculation
- Ureteral injury
- Abdominal or umbilical hernia
- Wound infection and dehiscence
- Bowel injury
- Bladder injury
- Lumbosacral plexus injury
- Deep venous thrombosis and pulmonary embolism
- Major vessel injury and massive blood loss
- Reflex sympathetic dystrophy

REFERENCES

1. Brau SA. Mini-open approach to the spine for anterior lumbar interbody fusion: description of the procedure, results, and complications. Spine J 2002;2(3):216–223.
2. Brau SA, Delamarter RB, Schiffman ML, et al. Vascular injury during anterior lumbar surgery. Spine J 2004;4(4):409–412.
3. Comer GC. Retrograde ejaculation after anterior lumbar interbody fusion with and without bone morphogenetic protein-2 augmentation: a 10-year cohort controlled study. Spine J 2012;12(10):881–890.
4. Edgard-Rosa G, Geneste G, Nègre G, et al. Midline anterior approach from the right side to the lumbar spine for interbody fusion and total disc replacement: a new mobilization technique of the vena cava. Spine (Phila Pa 1976) 2012;37(9):E562–E569.
5. Horton WC, Bridwell KH, Glassman SD, et al. The morbidity of anterior exposure for spinal deformity in adults: an analysis of patient-based outcomes and complications in 112 consecutive cases. In: Proceedings from the Scoliosis Research Society Annual Meeting; October 27–30, 2005; Miami FL.
6. Ikard RW. Methods and complications of anterior exposure of the thoracic and lumbar spine. Arch Surg 2006;141(10):1025–1034.
7. McAfee PC, Cunningham BW, Holtsapple G, et al. A prospective, randomized, multicenter Food and Drug Administration investigational device exemption study of lumbar total disc replacement with the CHARITE artificial disc versus lumbar fusion: part II: evaluation of radiographic outcomes and correlation of surgical technique accuracy with clinical outcomes. Spine (Phila Pa 1976) 2005;30:1576–1583.
8. Nalbandian MM, Hoashi JS, Errico TJ. Variations in the iliolumbar vein during the anterior approach for spinal procedures. Spine (Phila Pa 1976) 2013;38(8):E4445–E4450.
9. Sasso RC, Burkus KJ, LeHuec JC. Retrograde ejaculation after anterior lumbar interbody fusion: transperitoneal versus retroperitoneal exposure. Spine (Phila Pa 1976) 2003;28(10):1023–1026.

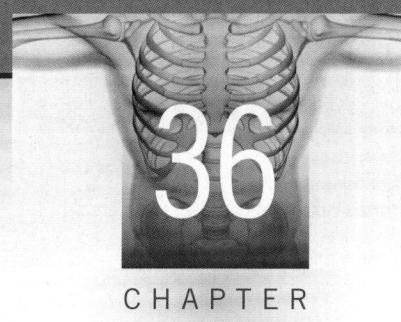

36
CHAPTER

Posterior Thoracic and Lumbar Approaches

Nathaniel W. Jenkins, James M. Parrish, Joon S. Yoo, Sreeharsha V. Nandyala, Alejandro Marquez-Lara, Junyoung Ahn, and Kern Singh

ANATOMY

- Superficial landmarks enable gross determination of the anatomic level. Proximally, C7 and T1 are the largest spinous processes and may serve as palpable anatomic landmarks. Distally, the intercristal line approximates the L4–L5 interspace.
- There are three layers of the posterior spinal musculature (**FIG 1; TABLE 1**):
  - Superficial layer: trapezius, latissimus dorsi, rhomboid major and minor, and the levator scapulae
  - Intermediate layer: superior and inferior serratus posterior and the levatores costarum
  - Deep layer: erector spinae, transversospinalis, interspinalis, and the intertransversarii
- The superficial and intermediate layers receive their nervous supply from peripheral nerves, which are not encountered through the posterior approach (**FIG 2**). The deep layer receives its nervous supply segmentally from the posterior dorsal rami. There is significant redundancy in deep layer innervation.
  - The midline approach is a true internervous plane. Nerve injury is more likely to occur with excessive lateral dissection.
- The vascular supply to the deep layer originates from segmental branches of the aorta. These vessels enter the operative field at the level of the intertransverse ligament and can be a source of significant bleeding.
- The facet joint capsules have a shiny white appearance and the individual fibers can be seen inserting onto the lateral edge of the laminar trough. Unless that segment is being fused, care should be taken to avoid violating the capsular fibers.
- The ligamentum flavum has a yellowish appearance with the fibers running in a cephalocaudal direction. The cephalad end of the ligament has a broad insertion from the base of the spinous process to between 50% and 70% of the anterior surface of the lamina. The caudal end of the ligament inserts from the superior edge of the lamina to between 2 and 6 mm of the anterior surface of the lamina.[6]

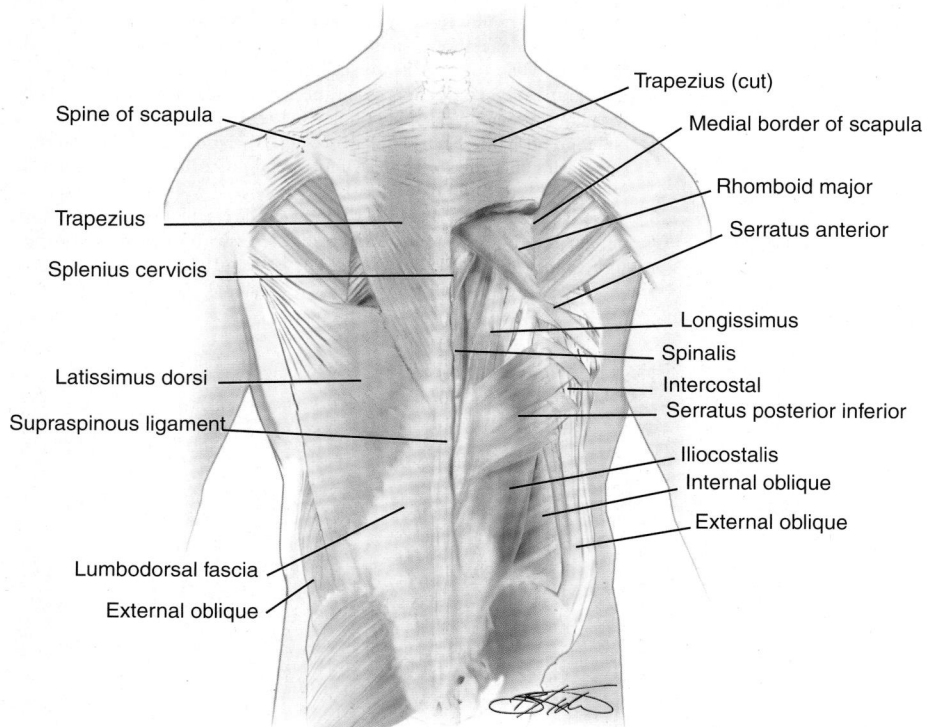

FIG 1 The superficial, intermediate, and deep musculature of the back.

TABLE 1 Musculature of the Back

Muscle	Origin	Insertion	Innervation	Blood Supply
Superficial Layer				
Trapezius	Medial third of superior nuchal line of occiput, external occipital protuberance, and ligamentum nuchae; spinous processes of C7–T12	Lateral third of clavicle, acromion, spine of scapula	Motor supply from spinal accessory nerve, sensory fibers from C3 to C4	Transverse cervical artery
Latissimus dorsi	Spinous processes of T7—sacrum, medial third of iliac crest, ribs 9–12, inferior angle of scapula	Floor of bicipital groove	Thoracodorsal nerve (C7, C8)	Thoracodorsal artery
Levator scapulae	Transverse processes of C1–C4	Medial border of scapula	Dorsal scapular nerve (C5), with branches of C3–C4 innervating upper part of muscle	Dorsal scapular artery
Rhomboid major	Spinous processes of T2–T5	Medial border of scapula	Dorsal scapular nerve (C5)	Dorsal scapular artery
Rhomboid minor	Caudal end of ligamentum nuchae, spinous processes of C7–T1	Medial border of scapula	Dorsal scapular nerve (C5)	Dorsal scapular artery
Intermediate Layer				
Serratus posterior superior	Spinous processes of C7–T3	Ribs 1–4	Intercostal nerves	Posterior intercostals arteries of T1–T4
Serratus posterior inferior	Thoracolumbar fascia, spinous processes of T11–L2	Ribs 9–12	Intercostal nerves	Posterior intercostal arteries, subcostal artery, and L1–L2 lumbar arteries
Levatores costarum	Tip of transverse process of C7–T11 vertebrae	Rib below level of origin	Posterior rami of thoracic spinal nerves	Dorsal intercostal arteries
Deep Layer				
Erector spinae (vertically oriented and superficial)				
Iliocostalis	Iliac crest, sacrum, transverse and spinous processes of vertebrae, and supraspinal ligament	Ribs, transverse and spinous processes of vertebrae, posterior aspect of skull	Segmental innervation by dorsal primary rami of spinal nerves C1–S5	Segmental supply by deep cervical arteries, posterior intercostal arteries, subcostal artery, and lumbar arteries
Longissimus				
Spinalis				
Transversospinalis (obliquely oriented and intermediate)				
Semispinalis	Transverse processes T1–T12	Spinous processes of C2–T5	Dorsal rami of spinal nerves	Segmental arteries from aorta
Multifidus	Articular processes of cervical vertebrae, transverse processes of thoracic vertebrae, mammillary processes of lumbar vertebrae, posterior superior iliac spine	Spinous processes of C2–L5	Dorsal rami of spinal nerves	Segmental branches from aorta
Rotatores	Transverse processes	Base of spinous processes above; Long skip one level; short attach at level above	Dorsal rami of spinal nerves	Segmental branches from aorta
Deepest muscle				
Interspinales	Spinous processes	Spinous processes one level above	Dorsal rami of spinal nerves	Segmental branches from aorta
Intertransversarii	Anterior and posterior transverse processes of cervical vertebrae, transverse and mammillary processes of lumbar vertebrae	Anterior and posterior processes of cervical vertebrae one level above, transverse and accessory processes of lumber vertebrae one level above	Dorsal rami of spinal nerves	Segmental branches from aorta

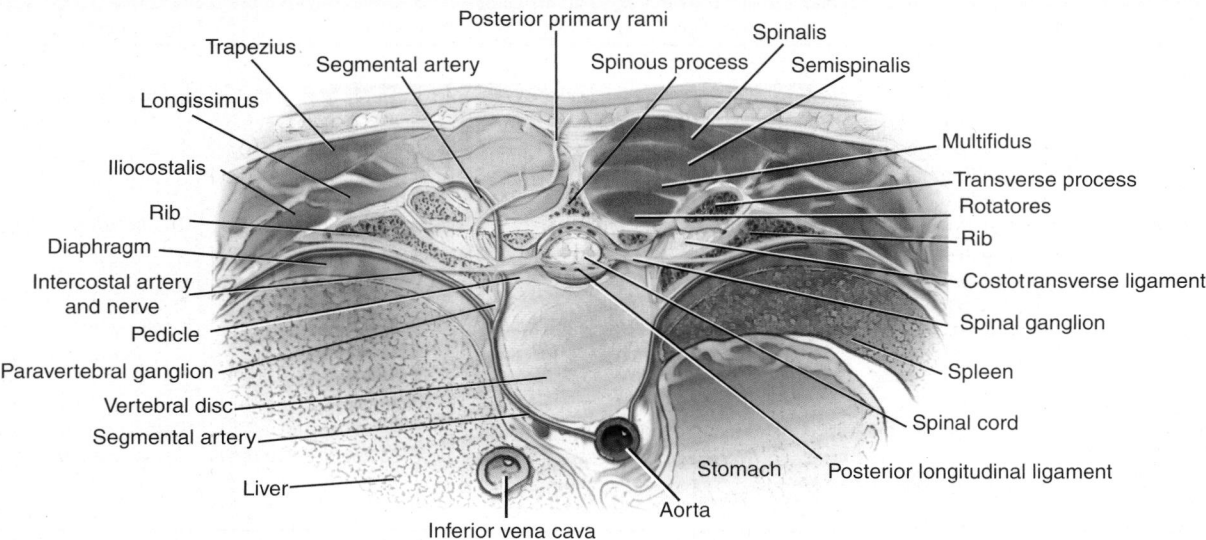

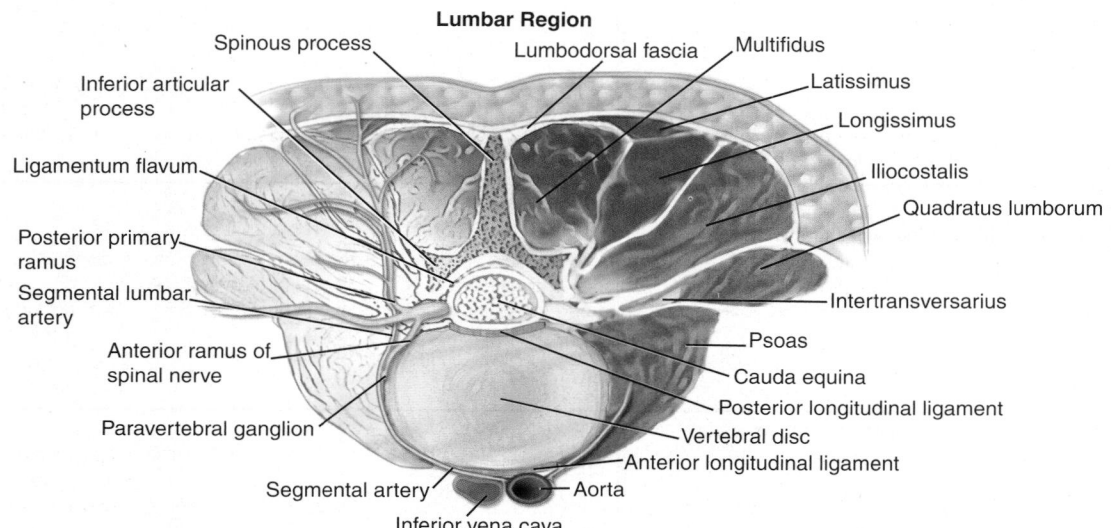

FIG 2 Cross-sectional anatomy of the thoracic and lumbar spine.

- Particularly at the L5–S1 level, the interspace may be widened or the posterior bony anatomy only partly formed. Caution should be taken when exposing this level as inadvertent plunging into the canal may occur.
- Laterally, the intertransverse membrane overlies the iliopsoas and protects the underlying neural structures.
- In children, the spinous process apophysis has not fused. During dissection, the apophysis is split down to the bone and then elevated with the paraspinal musculature.

SURGICAL MANAGEMENT

Positioning

- Patients should be placed in the prone position on a radiolucent table (**FIG 3A**).
- Vigilance is recommended to ensure the neck is in a neutral position with no hyperextension.
- The arms are abducted at 90 degrees or less to minimize the likelihood of rotator cuff impingement. The arms are

allowed to slightly hang down in a forward-flexed position about 10 degrees. The axilla should be clear from any padding to prevent brachial plexus palsy.
- Elbow pads are placed along the medial epicondyle to protect the ulnar nerve.
- Pads are placed at the chest and iliac crests.
- The chest pad is placed just proximal to the level of the xiphoid process and distal to the axilla. In women, care is taken to tuck the breasts and ensure that the nipples are pressure-free.
- The iliac pads are placed two fingerbreadths distal to the anterior superior iliac spine, permitting the abdomen to hang freely and reducing the potential for unnecessary epidural bleeding.
- Proper placement of the chest and iliac pads allows for restoration of normal sagittal alignment via gravity.
- Alternatively, for lumbar decompressive procedures alone, the knees are positioned in a sling, thereby allowing the hips to flex and eliminating lumbar lordosis and widening the laminar interspaces (**FIG 3B**). This position improves access

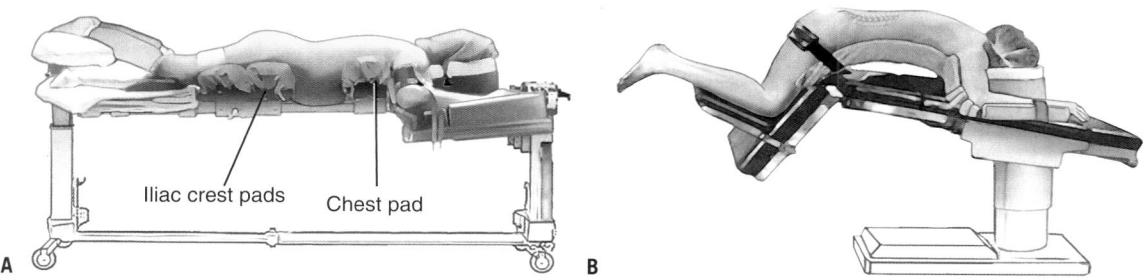

FIG 3 A. Prone position on a radiolucent table. The abdomen is not compressed. **B.** The knee-chest position is obtained using a Wilson frame.

to the lumbar spinal canal but should be avoided when instrumenting as lumbar lordosis is decreased.

Approach

- Two approaches are used: midline and paraspinal.
- The midline approach is used for most spinal procedures as it facilitates direct access to the spinal canal.

- The paraspinal approach, also known as the *Wiltse approach*, was initially described for spondylolisthesis but is now used for far lateral discectomies and minimally invasive muscle-sparing techniques.
  - There is increased interest in the paraspinal approach, particularly in conjunction with transforaminal lumbar interbody fusion procedures.[3]

MIDLINE POSTERIOR APPROACH

Incision and Dissection

- Anatomic landmarks are identified to appropriately center the skin incision **(TECH FIG 1A)**.
- A midline incision is made over the spinous processes down to the level of the fascia.
- A Cobb elevator is used to create 2-mm full-thickness skin flaps with subcutaneous fat. This allows for better visualization of the fascia during closure **(TECH FIG 1B,C)**.

- The location of the spinous processes is again verified, and electrocautery is used to reflect the fascia from the tips of the spinous processes.
- Electrocautery is used to subperiosteally elevate the paraspinal musculature laterally to the trough of the lamina. The surgeon should avoid going beyond this point to ensure protection of the insertion of the facet joint capsule.
- A sponge and Cobb are then used to gently dissect the paraspinal musculature off the facet joint capsule.

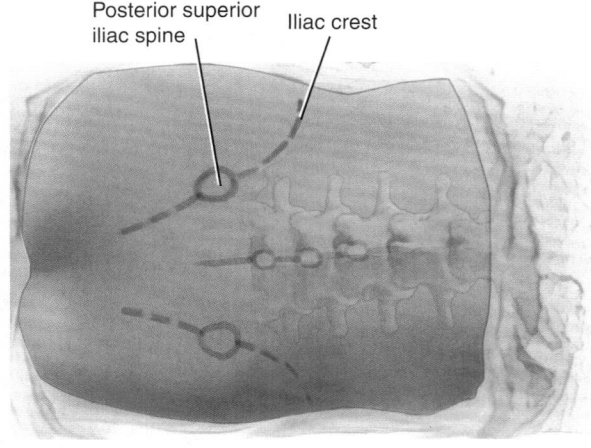

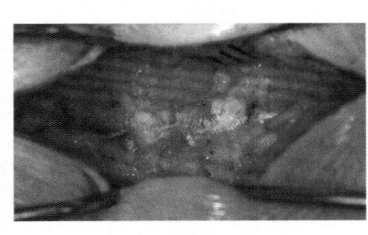

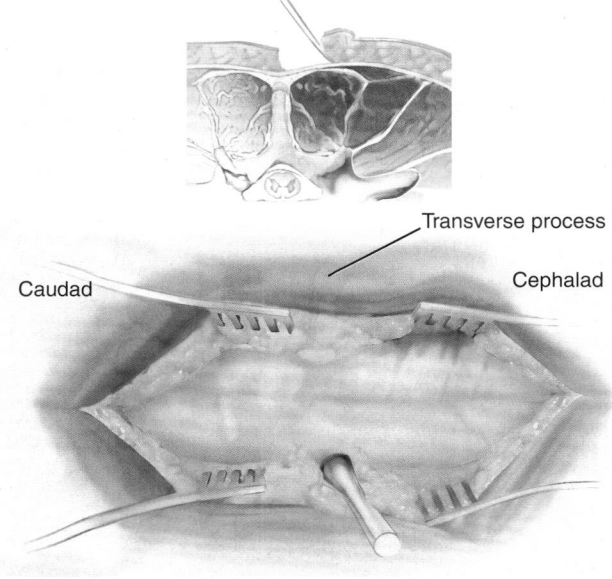

TECH FIG 1 A. Anatomic landmarks. **B,C.** The fascia is exposed with full-thickness skin flaps.

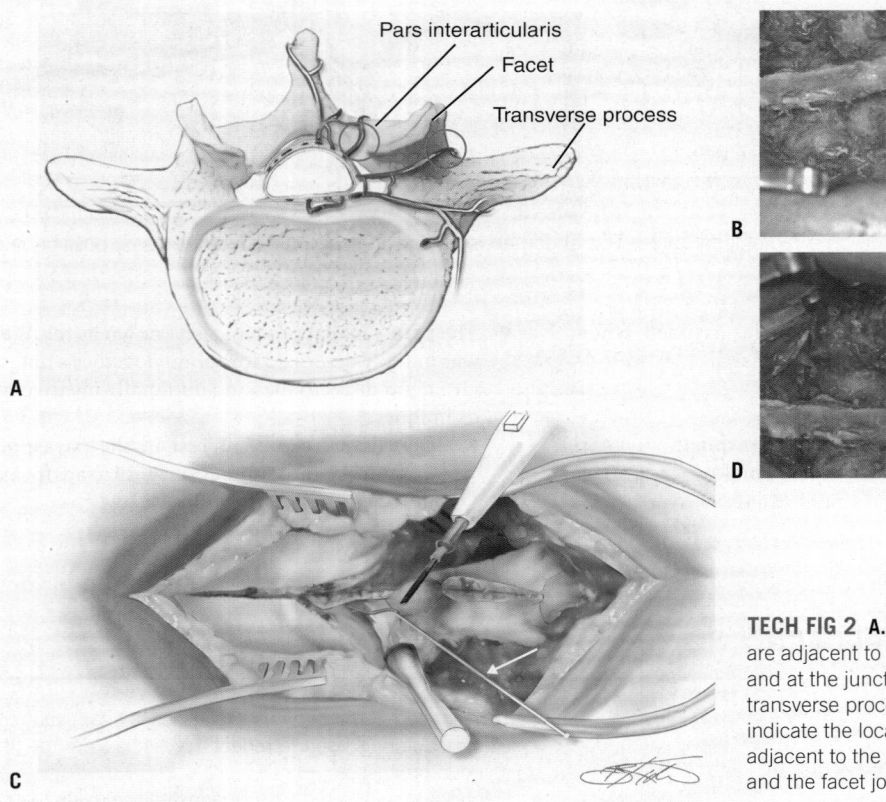

Pars interarticularis

Facet

Transverse process

A

B

D

C

TECH FIG 2 A. Venous bleeding sites are adjacent to the pars interarticularis and at the junction of the facet and the transverse process. **B,C.** Probes (*arrows*) indicate the location of venous bleeders adjacent to the pars interarticularis (**B,C**) and the facet joint (**D**).

Cautery

- Two venous bleeders are encountered that require electrocautery (**TECH FIG 2A**).
  - The first is located adjacent to the pars interarticularis (**TECH FIG 2B,C**).
  - The second is located just lateral to the facet joint (**TECH FIG 2D**).
- Electrocautery is used to elevate the paraspinal musculature off the transverse processes. Care should be taken to stay on the transverse process and to not violate the intertransverse membrane.

- Bipolar cautery should be used at the intertransverse ligament to avoid damage to the spinal nerves.

Paraspinal Resection

- In muscular patients or those with a larger body habitus, it is often necessary to excise a portion of the paraspinal muscles overlying the transverse processes that are to be fused.
- The muscle is resected beginning underneath the fascia and extending toward the lateral edge of the transverse processes. This creates a pocket over the transverse processes that serve as a bone graft cavity (**TECH FIG 3**).

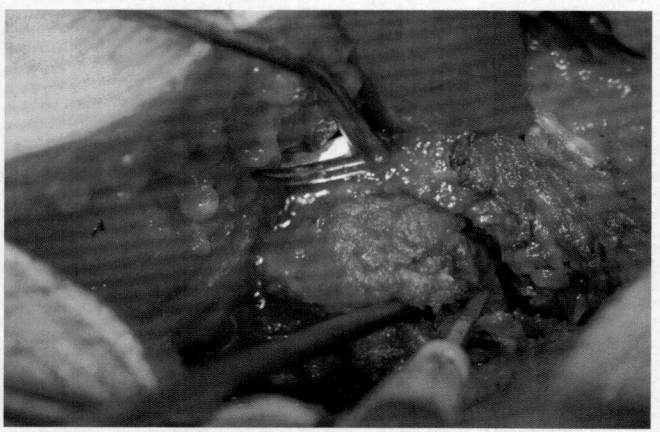

A

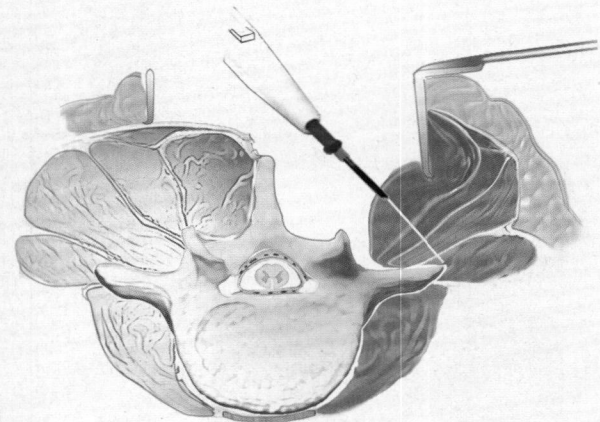

B

TECH FIG 3 A,B. Electrocautery is used to excavate a muscular pocket for the fusion mass. *(continued)*

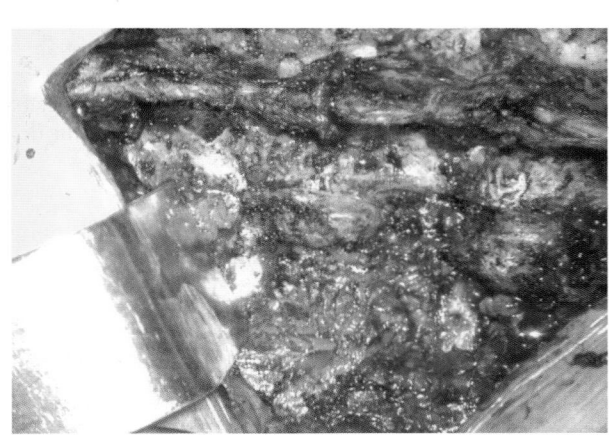

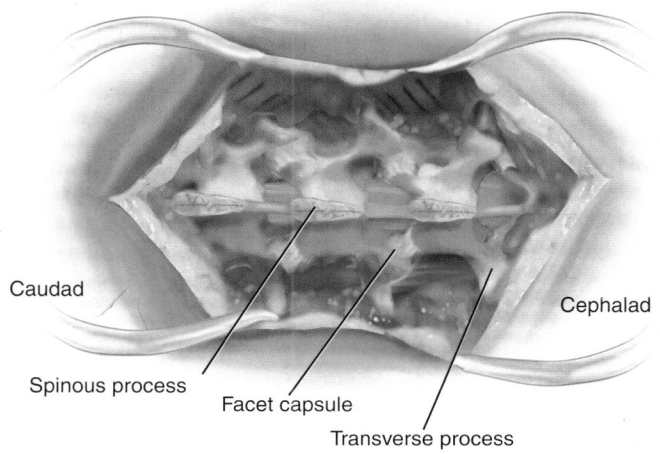

C

D

TECH FIG 3 *(continued)* **C,D.** Complete posterior exposure.

PARASPINAL APPROACH

- The approach is typically performed two fingerbreadths lateral to the spinous process.[7]
- After the fascia is exposed, the paraspinal muscles are palpated, and the interval between the multifidus medially and longissimus laterally is identified.
- A sharp incision through the fascia is made at this interval **(TECH FIG 4)**.
- The interval is defined with blunt dissection down to the lateral edge of the facet joint and transverse process junction.

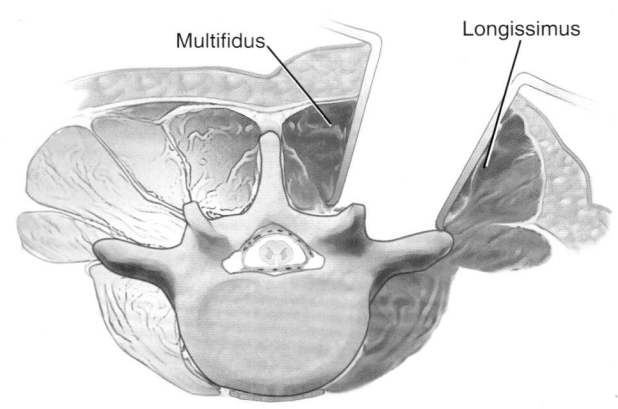

TECH FIG 4 Cross-section of spine showing Wiltse interval.

TECHNIQUES

Pearls and Pitfalls

Pars Interarticularis Bleeder	• Lateral to the pars; can be prophylactically identified and cauterized
Lateral Facet Bleeder	• A ball-tipped probe can be placed along the undersurface of the lateral edge of the superior articular process where the facet bleeder originates. Electrocautery can then be used to coagulate this vessel, which hinders intertransverse exposures.
Facet Capsule Preservation	• A sponge can be placed over the facet. Muscle stripping is then performed with a Cobb elevator as the sponge protects the capsular fibers from being disrupted and accidentally incised.
Widened Lower Lumbar Interspace	• An anteroposterior radiograph should be evaluated preoperatively to assess for spina bifida occulta and widened interlaminar windows. Extra caution should be employed when working in these areas to avoid inadvertent injury to the thecal sac.

TABLE 2 Complications Associated with the Posterior Approach

Complications	Occurrence
Major	
Wound infection	1%–10%
Pneumonia	5%
Renal failure	5%
Myocardial infarction	3%
Respiratory distress	2%
Neurologic deficit	2%
Congestive heart failure	2%
Cerebrovascular accident	1%
Minor	
Urinary tract infections	34%
Anemia requiring transfusion	27%
Confusion	27%
Ileus	22%
Arrhythmia	7%
Transient hypoxia	7%
Wound seroma	5%
Leg dysesthesia	2%

From Carreon LY, Puno RM, Dimar JR II, et al. Perioperative complications of posterior lumbar decompression and arthrodesis in older adults. J Bone Joint Surg Am 2003;85(11):2089–2092; Olsen MA, Mayfield J, Lauryssen C, et al. Risk factors for surgical site infection in spinal surgery. J Neurosurg 2003; 98(2 suppl):149–155.

COMPLICATIONS

- Major and minor complication rates of up to 80% have been reported in some series **(TABLE 2)**.[2]
- Risk factors for complications include patient age, length of surgery, levels exposed, blood loss, low serum albumin, low preoperative serum calcium, and postoperative urinary incontinence. Diabetes and other medical comorbidities have not been shown to be independent risk factors for the development of postoperative complications.[1,2,4,5,8]

REFERENCES

1. Benz RJ, Ibrahim ZG, Afshar P, et al. Predicting complications in elderly patients undergoing lumbar decompression. Clin Orthop Relat Res 2001;(384):116–121.
2. Carreon LY, Puno RM, Dimar JR II, et al. Perioperative complications of posterior lumbar decompression and arthrodesis in older adults. J Bone Joint Surg Am 2003;85(11):2089–2092.
3. Fujibayashi S, Neo M, Takemoto M, et al. Paraspinal-approach transforaminal lumbar interbody fusion for the treatment of lumbar foraminal stenosis. J Neurosurg Spine 2010;13:500–508.
4. Liu J-M, Deng H-L, Chen X-Y, et al. Risk factors for surgical site infection after posterior lumbar spinal surgery. Spine 2018;43:732–737.
5. Olsen MA, Mayfield J, Lauryssen C, et al. Risk factors for surgical site infection in spinal surgery. J Neurosurg 2003;98(2 suppl):149–155.
6. Olszewski AD, Yaszemski MJ, White AA III, et al. The anatomy of the human lumbar ligamentum flavum. New observations and their surgical importance. Spine (Phila Pa 1976) 1996;21(20):2307–2312.
7. Vialle R, Wicart P, Drain O, et al. The Wiltse paraspinal approach to the lumbar spine revisited: an anatomic study. Clin Orthop Relat Res 2006;445:175–780.
8. Wang MY, Widi G, Levi AD. The safety profile of lumbar spinal surgery in elderly patients 85 years and older. Neurosurg Focus 2015;39:E3.

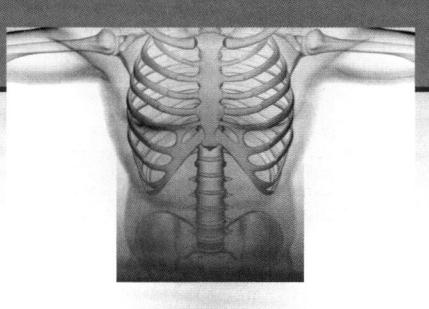

Exam Table for Foot and Ankle

Examination	Technique	Illustration	Grading and Significance
Achilles tendon rupture: active plantarflexion test	With the patient supine, active plantarflexion power is tested.		Positive: weak plantarflexion power graded 1–5 Poorly sensitive and unreliable, as powerful plantarflexion may still be possible due to the action of other ankle plantarflexors
Achilles tendon rupture: knee flexion test	While prone, the patient actively flexes the knee. The examiner observes foot position and compares it with the other side.		Positive: Foot falls into neutral or dorsiflexion. Negative: Foot maintains plantarflexion posture. Less reliable test; may be difficult to perform due to acute pain; 88% sensitive
Achilles tendon rupture: palpable gap test	Gentle palpation of the tendon reveals a defect at the rupture site.		Gap present or absent. Gap present indicates complete Achilles rupture with separation of the ruptured ends. More reliable when done early after rupture; 73% sensitive.
Achilles tendon rupture: Thompson or Simmonds test	With the patient in prone position, the examiner squeezed the calf at the gastrocsoleus muscle level. Limited ankle plantarflexion occurs (as compared to the unaffected side).		Positive test if ruptured, demonstrating limited ankle plantarflexion. Not as reliable in chronic ruptures as it is in acute ruptures due to formation of "pseudo tendon" scar between ruptured ends.
Ankle instability: anterior drawer test	The patient sits on the edge of the examination table with the legs dangling and the feet in a few degrees of plantarflexion. The examiner places one hand on the anterior aspect of the tibia and grasps the calcaneus with the palm of the other hand. The examiner then pulls the calcaneus anteriorly while pushing the tibia posteriorly. This tests the anterior talofibular ligament. To test the calcaneofibular ligament, the same maneuver is performed with the ankle in a dorsiflexed position.		Typically, anterior drawer is increased when the foot is externally rotated (vs. internally rotated); this is a highly sensitive test for medial ankle instability. The examiner should look for a difference of 3–5 mm in the relationship between the lateral talus and the anterior aspect of the fibula. On side-to-side comparison, the unstable side will have a greater degree of translation; indicates an insufficient anterior talofibular ligament

(continued)

1

Examination	Technique	Illustration	Grading and Significance
Ankle instability: suction sign test	Anterior drawer test as described for the anterior drawer test in the preceding exam technique		As the heel is delivered from the back of the ankle in an unstable ankle, a dimpling will occur in the region just anterior and inferior to the tip of the fibula as a vacuum is created by the talus sliding out from the mortise.
Digital purchase: paper pull-out test	A thin strip of paper is placed under the affected toe pulp. The examiner attempts to pull the paper strip out, while the patient attempts to resist with toe pressure against the ground.		The test is considered positive when there is no toe purchase present; it is considered reduced when the purchase is present but not powerful enough to resist the paper strip to being pulled out and is considered negative when the toe is able to prevent the paper strip to being pulled out.
Distal tarsal tunnel test	The examiner palpates for medial hindfoot tenderness (plus or minus swelling) at the "soft spot"—the distal edge of the abductor hallucis muscle about 5 cm anterior to the posterior of the heel at the intersection of the plantar and medial skin.		Tenderness corresponds with the course of the lateral plantar nerve and its first branch and is associated with nerve entrapment or neuritis.
Equinus contracture	The hindfoot is held in neutral position, and the midfoot is aligned by internal rotation of the navicular. Then, the forefoot is placed into pronation, and the medial ray is held firm. Then, the examiner manipulates the foot into dorsiflexion with the knee extended as well as with the knee flexed.		With knee extended: isolated gastrocnemius contracture when unable to achieve neutral dorsiflexion. Gastrocsoleus contracture is present when the examiner cannot get the ankle to neutral with the knee flexed; may need to perform a gastrocnemius recession or Achilles lengthening procedure concomitantly when there is 5 degrees of equinus in the ankle

Examination	Technique	Illustration	Grading and Significance
Equinus contracture: Silfverskiöld test	With the patient sitting, the ankle is maximally dorsiflexed with the knee extended and the foot held in a neutral position. The knee is then flexed and the ankle dorsiflexed again.		Positive: when the foot is held in equinus correcting to above neutral with the knee flexed; indicates a tight Achilles tendon within the gastrocnemius muscle. The deformity may aggravate an unstable ankle.
First metatarsophalangeal (MTP) joint grind test	The examiner grinds the MTP joint with an axially directed force.		Pain at MTP joint associated with osteochondral lesion or severe degeneration. Usually not symptomatic in mild cases. If this test causes severe pain, one may consider imaging studies. Not normally painful unless an osteochondral defect is present or degeneration is advanced. If painful, then arthrodesis is indicated.
First MTP joint hypertension test to distinguish hallux rigidus from sesamoid pathology	The big toe is hyperextended.		The examiner must discern between rising pain at the plantar (sesamoid) or dorsal (hallux rigidus) aspect of the MTP joint; high specificity with appropriate history but otherwise not specific
First tarsometatarsal hypermobility test (perspective 1)	The examiner grasps the lesser metatarsal heads with one hand and passively plantarflexes and dorsiflexes the first metatarsal with the other hand.		Hypermobility has been defined as an elevation of 5–8 mm above the level of the second metatarsal, but the diagnosis of hypermobility is often more subjective. Hypermobility at the tarsometatarsal joint creates a valgus moment at the MTP joint that may contribute to failure of distal hallux valgus correction.

(continued)

Examination	Technique	Illustration	Grading and Significance
First tarsometatarsal joint excursion (perspective 2)	One hand is placed with the thumb and index finger located plantar and dorsal to the first metatarsal head and the opposite thumb and index finger placed plantar and dorsal to the second metatarsal hand. The first ray is then dorsiflexed and plantarflexed to end range of motion (ROM) and the intervals between the thumb and index finger of both hands are noted and measured.		The normal first ray excursion is 10 mm (5 mm of dorsiflexion and 5 mm of plantarflexion). Hypermobility can be defined as total excursion >15 mm. Hypermobility of the first ray is significant when contemplating a surgical procedure for the hallux valgus deformity. If hypermobility is present, a first tarsometatarsal joint fusion may be more appropriate.
Fixed forefoot varus	The calcaneus is held in a neutral position (out of valgus), and any fixed elevation of the first ray relative to the fifth is noted.		The severity of deformity is noted in degrees. Fixed forefoot varus must be accounted for in any treatment algorithm and is usually the first component of the deformity to become rigid.
Flexor hallucis longus tenosynovitis	The pain is produced with active–passive motion of the hallux while a thumb palpates the tendon for tenderness and crepitus.		The presence of flexor hallucis longus tenosynovitis should be documented and treated accordingly.
Forced dorsiflexion of the first MTP joint	The examiner gradually increases dorsiflexion of the first MTP joint.		Pain is associated with impingement of the base of the proximal phalanx and metatarsal head. The amount of dorsiflexion obtained is measured as well. Maximum extension is characteristically limited, and pain is sometimes present. Also, the osteophytic ridge can be best palpated in the dorsolateral portion of the joint. Pain associated with stretching of the extensor hallucis longus, capsule, and inflamed synovium; often occurs earlier in the disease process. Maximal flexion is sometimes limited, but pain is best brought out. Tenderness is commonly identified in the dorsolateral aspect of the joint.

Examination	Technique	Illustration	Grading and Significance
Lesser MTP joint push-up test	With the patient seated and knee flexed, the examiner dorsiflexes the ankle to neutral by applying pressure under the metatarsal heads. The correction of the toe deformity with this maneuver is noted.		If the deformity is flexible, with the push-up test, the MTP joint will flex to its normal position. If not, it will remain extended defining a fixed deformity. Semiflexible deformities are those that correct partially with the push-up test. A flexible deformity is amenable to soft tissue procedures, including tendon transfers. Fixed deformities will need extensive procedures, including osteotomies. This test is also useful in the operating room to assess residual MTP joint contracture after the hammertoe has been corrected at the proximal interphalangeal joint. Residual MTP joint contracture necessitates additional surgical correction at the MTP joint, such as extensor tendon lengthening, capsular release, or collateral ligament release.
Lesser MTP joint stability test	The metatarsal bone and the proximal phalanx are stabilized, and stress is placed in a dorsoplantar direction, attempting to subluxate the joint.		Stage 0: no laxity to dorsal translation; stage 1: The base of the proximal phalanx can be subluxated with the dorsal stress; stage 2: The proximal phalangeal base can be dislocated and relocated; stage 3: The base of the proximal phalanx is fixed in a dislocated position. For the initial stages (0, 1, and 2), a tendon transfer associated with a dorsal MTP soft tissue release will stabilize the deformity. For fixed MTP dislocations, a bone-shortening procedure should be added to the soft tissue procedures.
Lesser toe manipulation test	Gentle manual straightening of the toe to assess the ability of the toe to correct to neutral		If the toe completely corrects to neutral, it is considered a flexible deformity. If the toe does not completely correct, it is considered a fixed deformity. A flexible deformity can be addressed with a soft tissue procedure such as a flexor-to-extensor tendon transfer. A fixed deformity will require bone resection for surgical correction.
MTP joint vertical Lachman test	The examiner stabilizes the hallux metatarsal with the thumb and index finger of one hand while attempting to translate the proximal phalanx in a dorsal–plantar direction with the thumb and index finger of the other hand.		A positive test is any laxity greater than the contralateral side.

(continued)

Examination	Technique	Illustration	Grading and Significance
Mulder test for Morton neuroma	With the patient prone and the knee flexed 90 degrees, the examiner deeply palpates the plantar aspect web space with the index finger. Maintaining this pressure, the examiner gently squeezes the forefoot.		Palpable "click" and reproduction of symptoms help confirm the diagnosis.
Percussion test for neuralgia	Percussion over the dorsomedial hallucal nerve or terminal hallucal branch of the deep peroneal nerve in the first web space.		Hypesthesias or radiating symptoms can occur in the terminal nerve branches because of compression from synovitis or dorsal osteophytes. Most clinicians simply note a positive or negative percussion test. Large dorsal osteophytes may compress the dorsal medial or lateral digital nerve.
Posterior ankle impingement: Maquirriain	In the seated position (90 degrees hip flexion, 90 degrees knee flexion, neutral ankle position), the subject is asked to slide both feet forward while maintaining full contact on the floor. Limited ankle plantarflexion or posterior ankle pain will be evidenced by the inability to maintain forefoot contact.		Positive: asymmetric motion due to posterior ankle pain or limited ankle plantarflexion Negative: symmetric motion Examiner should try to reproduce typical painful motion of posterior ankle impingement syndrome in closed position. It also allows the examiner to estimate the passive ROM limitation.
Posterior ankle impingement: passive forced plantarflexion test (perspective 1)	With the patient in prone position with both feet out of the table, the physician performs a forced plantarflexion maneuver. Limitation of ROM can also be estimated.		Discomfort; posterior ankle pain. Normal ankle ROM is 18 degrees dorsiflexion and 48 degrees plantarflexion. Examiner should try to reproduce typical painful motion of posterior ankle impingement syndrome. It also allows the examiner to estimate the passive ROM limitation.
Posterior ankle impingement: passive forced plantarflexion test (perspective 2)	The ankle is passively flexed while the subtalar joint is held in neutral position. The opposite thumb and index finger are used to palpate the retromalleolar regions for any crepitus.		Sharp pain or crepitus is produced at full plantarflexion with a positive test.

Examination	Technique	Illustration	Grading and Significance
Tibiotalar joint line palpation	Digital palpation of medial joint line with simultaneous application of valgus force.		Valgus tilt present or absent. Presence of valgus tilt indicates insufficiency of deltoid ligament.
Toe palpation	The examiner palpates the distal and proximal interphalangeal joints and the MTP joint for points of maximal tenderness.		The proximal interphalangeal joint should be the area of maximal tenderness, but the tip of the toe may be painful as well.
Windlass mechanism test	The examiner palpates the affected versus unaffected plantar fascia while recreating the windlass mechanism (by combining passive ankle dorsiflexion and 1–5 MTP joint dorsiflexion).		Less firm or tense plantar fascia compared to the opposite side indicates chronic attenuation or incompetence of the plantar fascia.

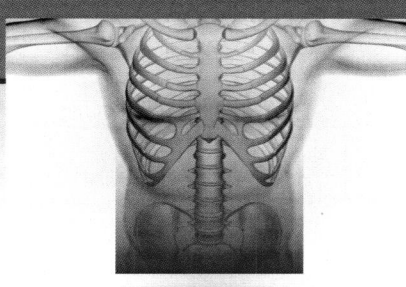

Exam Table for Spine

Examination	Technique	Illustration	Grading and Significance
Adams forward bend test	The examiner observes lumbar, thoracolumbar, and/or scapular hump with patient standing and then forward-flexed at the hips.		Mild, moderate, or severe. Rotational deformity may be a significant component of the patient's concern related to cosmesis. A scoliometer can be used to measure the degree of tilt from side to side.
Altered sensation evaluation	Sensation can be assessed by light touch, pin prick, pain, and temperature sensation.		Normal, decreased, or increased; can aid in diagnosis of nerve root or spinal cord level
Babinski reflex test	The outside of the plantar aspect of the foot is stimulated, beginning at the heel and going forward to the base of the great toe. The Babinski sign is manifest by the upturning of the big toe and by fanning of the other toes.		A positive Babinski sign is an upper motor neuron sign and may indicate the presence of cervical or thoracic myelopathy.
Clavicle (shoulder) asymmetry	The examiner observes and palpates the vertical relationship of the right and left acromion with the patient standing.	Negative (–) CHRL / Positive (+) CRL / ● Clavicle angle	Vertical discrepancy is measured in centimeters. Shoulder asymmetry may occur with certain patterns of scoliosis.
Coronal balance	Posterior observation of the patient standing. The examiner drops a plumb line from the occiput and measures deviation at the sacrum.		Leftward or rightward shift in centimeters. Centered posture is biomechanically and cosmetically desirable.

(continued)

1

Examination	Technique	Illustration	Grading and Significance
Hip flexion contractures	One hip is maximally flexed with the pelvis stabilized in order to evaluate a flexion contracture on the opposite side.		Measured in degrees. Longstanding sagittal plane deformities, as well as neurogenic claudication, may result in hip and knee flexion contractures.
Pelvic obliquity	The examiner observes and palpates the vertical relationship of the right and left iliac crests.		Vertical difference between posterosuperior iliac spines in centimeters. Pelvic obliquity may be a primary or compensatory mechanism with spinal deformity.
CERVICAL SPINE			
Adson test	Examiner stands behind the patient; radial pulse is palpated with the arm relaxed at the side. The arm is then abducted, extended, and externally rotated. Have patient take a deep breath and turn head to the side being tested. Evaluate pulse again.		Diminution or absence of the radial pulse. A positive Adson test indicates compression of the subclavian artery by a cervical rib or tight scalene muscle. This test is used to rule out thoracic outlet syndrome.
Finger escape sign (ulnar escape sign)	Performed with eyes closed, fingers adducted. Observe hands while patient is asked to maintain adducted finger position.		Abduction of the small finger indicates intrinsic muscle weakness associated with cervical myelopathy.

Examination	Technique	Illustration	Grading and Significance
CERVICAL SPINE			
Hawkins modified impingement sign	Forward flexion of the humerus with internal rotation		This test rotates the greater tuberosity under the coracoacromial ligament, and a painful response at anterolateral corner of the acromion is indicative of impingement syndrome.
Hoffman reflex	Elicited by taking the middle finger and flipping the distal phalanx		Pincer response between thumb and forefinger has a correlation with cervical spondylotic myelopathy. May be a normal variant. Comparison with contralateral side showing asymmetry may be a better indicator of myelopathy.
Impingement sign	With patient seated and examiner's hand on scapula to prevent rotation, the affected arm is forward flexed causing greater tuberosity to contact the acromion.		Pain at the anterolateral acromion indicates a positive result.
Inverted radial reflex	This reflex is demonstrated by tapping the brachioradialis tendon.		A diminished normal reflex is noted along with a reflex contraction of the finger flexors. Abnormal reflex denotes peripheral compression of the C6 nerve root. Compression at C6 allows pathologic upper motor neuron response.
Lhermitte phenomenon	Flexion and/or extension in sagittal plane. The test is generally positive at the extremes of flexion and/or extension.		Positive test causes shock-like sensation running down the spine. Pain in extension suggests spondylotic myelopathy, whereas symptoms in flexion are more suggestive of posttraumatic or iatrogenic kyphosis.
Spurling test	Ipsilateral axial rotation, extension, axial compression		Reproduces radicular symptoms when compressive pathology is present. Dermatomal distribution of pain should correlate with level of pathology.

(continued)

Examination	Technique	Illustration	Grading and Significance
CERVICAL SPINE NERVE ROOT SYNDROMES			
Biceps, wrist extension	Patient flexes elbow and extends wrist against examiner's resistance; sensation lateral forearm and radial two digits		Muscle strength graded 0–5. Deficits reveal abnormal function of C6 nerve root.
Deltoid	Patient abducts arm against examiner's resistance; sensation tested in deltoid region and along lateral arm		Muscle strength graded 0–5. Deficits reveal abnormal function of C5 nerve root.
Finger abduction	Sensation to medial arm; motor to interossei		Muscle strength graded 0–5. Deficits reveal abnormal function of T1 nerve root.
Handgrip	Sensation to medial forearm and ulnar two digits; motor to finger flexors—grip		Muscle strength graded 0–5. Deficits reveal abnormal function of C8 nerve root.

Examination	Technique	Illustration	Grading and Significance
CERVICAL SPINE NERVE ROOT SYNDROMES			
Triceps and wrist flexion	Patient extends elbow and flexes wrist; sensation to middle finger		Muscle strength graded 0–5. Deficits reveal abnormal function of C7 nerve root.

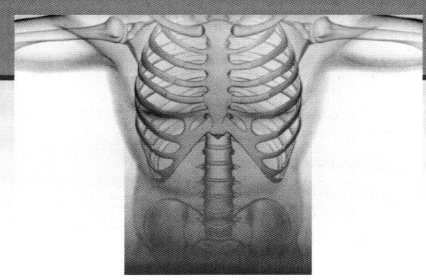

Index

Page numbers followed by *f* and *t* indicate figures and tables, respectively.

pull-through button technique for, 2969–70, 2969–70*f*
surgical approach in, 2968
surgical management of, 2967–73
suture anchors for, 2970
Jobe technique, modified, in ulnar collateral ligament reconstruction, 4556–58, 4556–58*f*
Joint reactive force (JRF), hip, 1112, 1113*f*
Jones fractures, 5868–81
anatomy and, 1093–94, 1093*f*, 5868
definition of, 1093, 5868, 5868*f*
differential diagnosis of, 1095, 5869
imaging and diagnostic studies of, 1094*f*, 1095, 5869, 5871*f*
natural history of, 1094, 5869
nonoperative management of, 1095, 5870
ORIF of, 1093–1102, 5870–80
complications of, 1101, 5880
low-profile, precontoured plate for, 5874–76, 5874–76*f*
outcomes of, 1101, 5880
patient positioning for, 1096, 1096*f*, 5871
percutaneous intramedullary screw fixation in, 1096–99, 1096–99*f*, 5871–73, 5871–74*f*
percutaneous intramedullary screw fixation with local bone graft in, 1099
plate fixation and calcaneal bone grafting for nonunion in, 1099–1100, 1100*f*
postoperative care in, 1101, 5879, 5879–80*f*
preoperative planning for, 5870–71, 5871*f*
tension-sided plantar plate for, 5877, 5877–78*f*
pathogenesis of, 1094, 5868
patient history and physical findings of, 1094–95, 5869
pearls and pitfalls in, 1101, 5879
surgical management of, 1095–96, 5870–71
treatment goals in, 1095–96
Jones procedure
for cavovarus foot, 5275, 5279, 5279*f*, 5285–86, 5285*f*, 5286*f*
modified, for equinocavovarus foot, 5294, 5294*f*, 5298–99*f*, 5298–5300
modified, for pediatric cavus foot, 2503, 2503*f*
JRA. *See* Juvenile rheumatoid arthritis
Judet approach, 4142
JuggerKnot anchor, 622, 623*f*
JuggerStitch, 363
Junctura tendinum, for extensor tendon centralization, 3571
Jungbluth clamp, in symphysis ORIF, 655, 655*f*
Juvenile rheumatoid arthritis (JRA), 4678
Juvenile scoliosis, 2181

K

K-wire fixation. *See also specific injuries and procedures*
acetabular, in triple innominate osteotomy, 2389, 2390*f*
capitellar, 4578

carpometacarpal, 3056*f*, 3058*f*, 3801–4, 3801*f*
clubfoot, 2539, 2539*f*
digital, in replantation, 3958–59, 3958–59*f*
distal femoral, in derotational osteotomy, 1884–86, 1884–86*f*
distal femoral physeal, 1742–44, 1743*f*, 1744*f*
distal humerus, 1655–56, 1656*f*, 1665, 1665*f*
distal humerus, in arthroplasty, 4589, 4589*f*
distal interphalangeal joint of hand, 2968, 2969*f*, 3746, 3748–49, 3748–49*f*
distal radioulnar, 3337, 3337*f*
distal radius, 3247–56, 3303, 3304
distal tibia, 1771, 1771*f*
epiphyseal, in modified Dunn procedure, 2452, 2452*f*
femoral neck, 706, 706*f*
first metatarsophalangeal joint, 4974, 4974*f*
lateral condyle of humerus, 1594, 1594–95*f*
lunate, 3159, 3159*f*
lunotriquetral ligament, 3446
medial cuneiform, 5146, 5146*f*
medial epicondyle, 1599, 1601, 1601*f*
metacarpophalangeal, 3076–77, 3078*f*, 3746, 3753–55, 3755*f*
metatarsal, 4750, 4751*f*, 4894–95, 4894–95*f*
pediatric radial neck, 1644
perilunate, 3242, 3243–44, 3243*f*, 3447, 3448*f*
phalangeal, 2977–78, 2979, 2979–81*f*, 2986, 2986*f*
phalangeal condylar, 2994, 2994*f*, 2996–98, 2997–98*f*
proximal humeral, pediatric, 1677
proximal interphalangeal joint of foot, 5039, 5041–42
proximal interphalangeal joint of hand, 3003, 3006–12, 3006–12*f*, 3025, 3025–26*f*, 3746, 3750
proximal phalanx, 4894–95, 4894–95*f*
proximal ulnar, 4632–33, 4632–34*f*
radial head and neck, 4613–14, 4614*f*
scapholunate ligament, 3189–91, 3190*f*, 3446, 3447*f*, 3453–54
thumb metacarpal, 3807
tibial tuberosity, 1761, 1762*f*
for vertical talus, 2553, 2555
wrist, 3822–23, 3823*f*
K-wire joystick technique, 3113, 3114*f*
Kambin triangle, 6072, 6072*f*, 6076–77, 6077*f*
Kapandji technique, for percutaneous pinning, 3251, 3251*f*, 3304
Kaplan approach, to elbow, 4154, 4578
Kaposi sarcoma of hand, 4088–89
Kaposiform hemangioendothelioma, 4084
Kasabach-Merritt syndrome, 4084
Kaufman technique, for radial head and neck fractures, 1642, 1643*f*
Kellgren-Lawrence classification, 5452
Kidner procedure, 5230
Kidner procedure, modified, 5230, 5231, 5231–32*f*, 5242

Kienböck disease, 3167–84
anatomy and, 3167, 3167*f*, 3178–79, 3178*f*, 3179*f*
capitate shortening osteotomy for, 3171, 3178, 3179, 3181–82, 3182*f*
classification of lunate vascularity/viability in, 3179, 3180*f*
core decompression for, 3175, 3175*f*, 3176
definition of, 3167, 3178
differential diagnosis of, 3170
imaging and diagnostic studies of, 3139, 3168–70, 3169*f*, 3179*f*, 3180*f*
natural history of, 3168
nonoperative management of, 3170
pathogenesis of, 3167–68, 3816, 3847
patient history and physical findings of, 3168
proximal row carpectomy for, 3171, 3816–20
radial osteotomy for, 3167–77, 3179
closing wedge, 3171, 3174, 3174*f*
complications of, 3176
dome, 3171
outcomes of, 3176
patient positioning for, 3171
pearls and pitfalls in, 3175
postoperative care in, 3175
preoperative planning for, 3171
shortening, 3170–74, 3172–74*f*, 3175
volar approach in, 3171, 3172*f*
radiographic classification of, 3168–70, 3169*f*
scaphocapitate arthrodesis for, 3179
scaphocapitate pinning for, 3179
surgical management of, 3140–41, 3170–71, 3179–80
total wrist arthroplasty in, 3847, 3847*f*
vascularized bone grafting for, 3171, 3178–84
approach in, 3180
complications of, 3184
elevation of dorsal capsular flap in, 3180–81, 3180–81*f*
graft placement in, 3182, 3183*f*
indications for, 3179, 3179*f*
lunate unloading procedure with, 3178, 3179, 3181–82, 3182*f*
medial femoral trochlea flap for, 3139–40, 3140*f*, 3147, 3147*f*
outcomes of, 3183–84
patient positioning for, 3180
pearls and pitfalls in, 3183
postoperative care in, 3183, 3183*f*
preoperative planning for, 3180
wrist arthrodesis for, 3171
wrist denervation for, 3171
Kiloh-Nevin syndrome, 3617
Kirschner wire. *See* K-wire fixation
"Kissing lesion," 1836, 1837
Klippel-Trenaunay syndrome, 4085, 4086
Knee. *See also specific disorders, injuries, and procedures*
anatomy of, 325–26, 325*f*, 856
articular cartilage of, 401, 401*f*, 420
chondral defects of, 390–400. *See also* Osteochondritis dissecans of knee
allograft cartilage transplantation for, 420–27, 1838–39, 1839*f*
anatomy and, 390, 401, 401*f*, 420

Quadratus femoris nerve compression, 297
Quadriceps. *See also specific disorders, injuries, and procedures*
   anatomy of, 607, 1439, 2891–93
   distal femoral fracture and, 813
   elevation, in SUPERhip procedure, 1907, 1907f
   release, in anterior flap hemipelvectomy, 2806, 2806f
   tumors of
      imaging and staging studies of, 2893–94, 2893f
      surgical management of, 2894. *See also* Quadriceps resection
Quadriceps biopsy, 2894, 2894f
Quadriceps recession, percutaneous, 1930, 1930f
Quadriceps resection, 2891–99
   anatomy and, 2891–92f, 2891–93
   background on, 2891
   biceps femoris transfer in, 2892f, 2896
   completion of, 2896, 2898f
   complications of, 2898–99
   exposure in, 2895, 2895–96f
   imaging and staging studies for, 2893–94, 2893f
   incision in, 2894, 2894f
   indications for, 2898
   outcomes of, 2898
   patient positioning for, 2894, 2894f
   pearls and pitfalls in, 2898
   postoperative care and rehabilitation in, 2898
   sartorius transfer in, 2892f
   semitendinosus transfer in, 2892f
   tumor resection in, 2896, 2897f
Quadriceps snip, 1531, 1532, 1532f, 1535–36, 1557, 1557f
Quadriceps tendinitis, 606–7
Quadriceps tendon graft
   for ACL reconstruction, 454, 456, 457f, 467, 472–73, 473f, 475, 475f, 529
   for ACL reconstruction, pediatric, 1810
   for multiligament-injured knee, 529
   for PCL reconstruction, 491, 491f, 529
Quadriceps tendon repair, 540–41
   acute, 540
   approach in, 540
   of chronic tears, 540
   outcomes of, 541
   patient positioning for, 540
   pearls and pitfalls in, 541
   postoperative care in, 541
   preoperative planning for, 540
Quadriceps tendon ruptures, 535, 539–41
   anatomy and, 539
   imaging and diagnostic studies of, 539–40
   nonoperative management of, 540
   pathogenesis of, 539
   patient history and physical findings of, 539
   surgical management of, 540–41. *See also* Quadriceps tendon repair
   total knee arthroplasty and, 1537, 1543–44
Quadriceps tenotomy, mini-open, 1931, 1931f
Quadriceps turndown
   in knee arthroplasty, 1531, 1533, 1533f, 1535–36
   in MPFL reconstruction, 1790, 1790f, 1794

Quadricepsplasty, V-Y, 1531, 1533, 1534f, 1535–36
Quadriplegia, functional, in spina bifida, 2210, 2210f

R
RAA. *See* Radial articular angle
Radial artery
   anatomy of, 3109, 4006–7, 4008, 4008f, 4135
   distal humeral resection and, 2706–7, 2707f
   hand flaps for finger coverage and, 3996, 3996f
   thumb CMC arthroscopy and, 3402, 3402f
Radial articular angle (RAA), 2140, 2140f, 2141
Radial bursa, anatomy of, 3938, 3938f
Radial collateral ligament, of elbow, anatomy of, 184, 4694
Radial collateral ligament, of thumb
   anatomy of, 3080
   injuries of
      definition of, 3080
      differential diagnosis of, 3082
      imaging and diagnostic studies of, 3081, 3082f
      natural history of, 3081
      nonoperative management of, 3082
      pathogenesis of, 3080, 3081f
      patient history and physical findings of, 3081
      surgical management of, 3082
   repair and reconstruction of, 3080–92
      acute repair, 3085–86, 3086f
      complications of, 3092
      outcomes of, 3092
      pearls and pitfalls in, 3092
      postoperative care in, 3092
      reconstruction using tendon graft, 3090–91, 3090–91f
Radial diaphyseal fractures, 3376–84
   anatomy and, 3376, 3376f, 3377f, 3378f
   imaging and diagnostic studies of, 3378
   malunion or nonunion of, 3385–94
      anatomy and, 3385–86, 3385f
      anterior (volar) approach to, 3389, 3390f
      complications of, 3393–94
      corrective osteotomy for, 3388–94
      definition of, 3385
      differential diagnosis of, 3387
      imaging and diagnostic studies of, 3387, 3387f
      natural history of, 3386
      nonoperative management of, 3387
      outcomes of, 3393
      pathogenesis of, 3386
      patient history and physical findings of, 3386–87, 3386f
      pearls and pitfalls in, 3393
      posterior (dorsal) approach to, 3389, 3390, 3390f
      postoperative care in, 3393, 3393f
      preoperative planning for, 3388–89, 3388–89f
      reduction, plating, and bone grafting in, 3391–92, 3391–92f
      surgical management of, 3388–89

nonoperative management of, 3378–79
ORIF of, 3378–82, 3384
   anterior (volar) approach in, 3379, 3380–81f, 3380–82
   approaches in, 3379
   complications of, 3384
   intraoperative imaging in, 3379
   outcomes of, 3384
   patient positioning for, 3379
   pearls and pitfalls in, 3384
   posterior (dorsal) approach in, 3379, 3382, 3382–83f
   postoperative care in, 3384
   preoperative planning for, 3379
pathogenesis of, 3377–78
patient history and physical findings of, 3378
surgical management of, 3378–79
Radial duplication, 2096. *See also* Polydactyly
Radial dysplasia
   anatomy and, 2131–32
   classification of, 2131, 2131t
   definition of, 2131
   imaging and diagnostic studies of, 2131t, 2132, 2132f
   natural history of, 2132
   nonoperative management of, 2132
   pathogenesis of, 2132
   patient history and physical findings of, 2132, 2132f
   surgical management of, 2132–36
      approach in, 2134
      centralization in, 2133, 2133f
      complications of, 2136
      options for, 2133, 2133f
      outcomes of, 2136, 2136f
      patient positioning for, 2134
      pearls and pitfalls in, 2136
      postoperative care in, 2136
      preoperative planning for, 2133–34
      radialization in, 2133, 2133f
      release of radial deviation of wrist in, 2135, 2135f
      skeletal augmentation in, 2133, 2133f
      skeletal realignment in, 2133, 2133f
      soft tissue reorganization in, 2133, 2133f
      volar bilobed flap in, 2133, 2134–36, 2134–36f
Radial (radial artery) forearm flaps
   for distal upper extremity injuries, 4006–13
      advantages and disadvantages of, 4008
      anatomy and, 4006–7, 4008, 4008f
      approach for, 4009
      complications of, 4013
      outcomes of, 4013
      pearls and pitfalls of, 4012
      postoperative care of, 4012
      selection of, 4008
   for oncology, 2614–15, 2619, 2619f, 4108
   reverse fascia-only, 4010, 4010–11f
   reverse fasciocutaneous, 4009, 4010f
   for upper extremity burn injuries, 4078
Radial head
   anatomy of, 1626–27, 1638, 4132–33, 4133f, 4606, 4606–7f, 4617, 4617f
   congenital dislocation of, Monteggia fracture-dislocation *vs.*, 1631, 1631f